CONTENTS

Circulation

JULY 1985 *Volume 72/Number 1*

FEATURES

Perspectives

1 Programmed electrical stimulation of the heart in patients with life-threatening ventricular arrhythmias: What is the significance of induced arrhythmias and what is the correct stimulation protocol?
Hein J. J. Wellens, Pedro Brugada, and William G. Stevenson

8 Some reflections on arteriosclerosis: past, present, and future. Presidential Address
Antonio M. Gotto, Jr.

Editorial

18 Human tissue-type plasminogen activator: from the laboratory to the bedside
D. Collen

Preludes and Progress

21 Cardiology in 1885
W. Bruce Fye

CLINICAL INVESTIGATION

PATHOPHYSIOLOGY AND NATURAL HISTORY

27 Fibrin formation and platelet aggregation in patients with severe coronary artery disease: relationship with the degree of myocardial ischemia
A. Gallino, A. Haeberli, H. R. Baur, and P. W. Straub

31 Risk factors for the development of prosthetic valve endocarditis
Stephen B. Calderwood, Lois A. Swinski, Christine M. Waternaux, Adolf W. Karchmer, and Mortimer J. Buckley

Hypertension

38 Participation of endogenous catecholamines in the regulation of left ventricular mass in progeny of hypertensive parents
Bruno Trimarco, Bruno Ricciardelli, Nicola De Luca, Antonio De Simone, Alberto Cuocolo, Maria D. Galva, Giovanni B. Picotti, and Mario Condorelli

47 Transient enhancement of sympathetic nervous system activity by long-term restriction of sodium intake
Massimo Volpe, Franco B. Müller, and Bruno Trimarco

53 Is hypertension more benign when associated with obesity?
Elizabeth Barrett-Connor and Kay-Tee Khaw

Congestive Heart Failure

61 Characteristics of vascular hydraulic load in patients with heart failure
Warren K. Laskey, William G. Kussmaul, Jack L. Martin, Joseph P. Kleaveland, John W. Hirshfeld, Jr., and Sanjeev Shroff

72 Effect of the sympathetic nervous system on limb circulation and metabolism during exercise in patients with heart failure
John R. Wilson, Nancy Ferraro, and David H. Wiener

DIAGNOSTIC METHODS

82 Transluminal, subselective measurement of coronary artery blood flow velocity and vasodilator reserve in man
Robert F. Wilson, Donald E. Laughlin, Peter H. Ackell, William M. Chilian, Myrl D. Holida, Craig J. Hartley, Mark L. Armstrong, Melvin L. Marcus, and Carl W. White

93 The ratio of plasma high-density lipoprotein cholesterol to total and low-density lipoprotein cholesterol: age-related changes and race and sex differences in selected North American populations. The Lipid Research Clinics Program Prevalence Study
Manfred S. Green, Gerardo Heiss, Basil M. Rifkind, Gerald Cooper, O. Dale Williams, and H. A. Tyroler

105 Quantitative analysis of the high-frequency components of the signal-averaged QRS complex in patients with acute myocardial infarction: a prospective study
Joseph A. Gomes, Rahul Mehra, Philip Barreca, Nabil El-Sherif, Robert Hariman, and Ronald Holtzman

Circulation

AN OFFICIAL JOURNAL OF THE American Heart Association

Editorial correspondence — Burton E. Sobel, M.D., Editor, Washington University School of Medicine, 660 South Euclid Ave., Box 8055, St. Louis, Missouri 63110.

Business correspondence — regarding advertising, subscriptions, change of address, etc. — American Heart Association, 7320 Greenville Ave., Dallas, Texas 75231.

Circulation (USPS 113720) is published twelve times a year at the Publications Office, American Heart Association, Dallas, Texas 75231.

Subscription rates — annually (subscriptions accepted at any time), $56 United States, $72 elsewhere, postage included. Single copies, postpaid $7.00 U.S., $9.00 elsewhere; single copies of supplements at additional cost. Interns, residents, medical students — special rate of $28 annually in the U.S., $36 Canada and Mexico. (Letter stating post held required.) Airmail rates available upon request. All orders for Europe must go through Bailliere Tindall 1st Anne's Road, Eastbourne, East Sussex BN21 3UN ENGLAND. All orders for Japan must go through Nankodo Co., Ltd., 42-6 Hongo-3 Chome, Bunkyo-Ku, Tokyo, JAPAN. Remittances for subscriptions should be made by check, draft, post office or express money order payable to the American Heart Association. Second class postage paid at Dallas, Texas, and additional mailing offices. POSTMASTER: Send address changes to Circulation, American Heart Association, 7320 Greenville Ave., Dallas, Texas 75231. The Publishing Director should be advised of change of address 30 days before date of issue with both the subscriber's old and new address given.

Therapy and Prevention

112 Lysis of left ventricular thrombi with urokinase
Peter Kremer, Rainer Fiebig, Volkmar Tilsner, Walter Bleifeld, and Detlef Mathey

Surgery

119 Left ventricular systolic and diastolic function in coronary artery disease: effects of revascularization on exercise-induced ischemia
John D. Carroll, Otto M. Hess, Heinz O. Hirzel, Marko Turina, and Hans Peter Krayenbuehl

130 Results of triple valve replacement in 91 patients: perioperative mortality and long-term follow-up
Bernard J. Gersh, Hartzell V. Schaff, Pierce J. Vatterott, Gordon K. Danielson, Thomas A. Orszulak, Jeffrey M. Piehler, Francisco J. Puga, James R. Pluth, and Dwight C. McGoon

138 Improved graft patency in patients treated with platelet-inhibiting therapy after coronary bypass surgery
B. Greg Brown, Ramon A. Cukingnan, Timothy DeRouen, Lacy V. Goede, Maylene Wong, Henry J. Fee, Jack A. Roth, and Joseph S. Carey

Arrhythmia

147 Periodic procainamide for paroxysmal tachycardia
D. Woodrow Benson, Jr., Ann Dunnigan, Thomas P. Green, David G. Benditt, and Shanda P. Schneider

153 Comparative efficacy of transvenous cardioversion and pacing in patients with sustained ventricular tachycardia: a prospective, randomized, crossover study
Sanjeev Saksena, Prathap Chandran, Yogesh Shah, Roberto Boccadamo, Demetris Pantopoulos, and Stephen T. Rothbart

161 Atrial fibrillation in patients with Wolff-Parkinson-White syndrome: incidence after surgical ablation of the accessory pathway
A. D. Sharma, G. J. Klein, G. M. Guiraudon, and S. Milstein

170 Efficacy and safety of transcatheter ablation of posteroseptal accessory pathways
Fred Morady, Melvin M. Scheinman, Stuart A. Winston, Lorenzo A. DiCarlo, Jr., Jessie C. Davis, Jerry C. Griffin, Michael Ruder, Joseph A. Abbott, and Michael Eldar

LABORATORY INVESTIGATION

178 A comparison of the thrombolytic and hemorrhagic effects of tissue-type plasminogen activator and streptokinase in rabbits
Giancarlo Agnelli, Michael R. Buchanan, Francoise Fernandez, Bernard Boneu, Joanne Van Ryn, Jack Hirsh, and Désiré Collen

Tissue Characterization

183 The dependence of myocardial ultrasonic integrated backscatter on contractile performance
Samuel A. Wickline, Lewis J. Thomas III, James G. Miller, Burton E. Sobel, and Julio E. Perez

193 Ultrasonic tissue characterization: detection of acute myocardial ischemia in dogs
Ingela Schnittger, August Vieli, Joseph E. Heiserman, Bruce A. Director, Margaret E. Billingham, Stephen G. Ellis, Robert S. Kernoff, Toshihiko Takamoto, and Richard L. Popp

Arrhythmia

200 Day-to-day variations in inducibility of ventricular tachyarrhythmias during the late postmyocardial infarction phase in conscious dogs
Stuart M. Cobbe, Ellen Hoffmann, Andreas Ritzenhoff, Johannes Brachmann, Wolfgang Kübler, and Jochen Senges

205 An enzyme histochemical study of human sinus node, coronary sinus, and mitral valve muscle
Claude Théry, Ivan Krivosic, Philippe Asseman, and A. E. F. Hugo Meijer

214 The effects of premature stimulation of the His bundle on epicardial activation and body surface late potentials in dogs susceptible to sustained ventricular tachyarrhythmias
Joseph F. Spear, David A. Richards, George J. Blake, Michael B. Simson, and E. Neil Moore

Coronary Blood Flow

225 Collateral conductance changes during a brief coronary occlusion in awake dogs
Susan Brazzamano, John M. Fedor, Judith C. Rembert, and Joseph C. Greenfield, Jr.

233 Effect of the combination of diltiazem and atenolol on exercise-induced regional myocardial ischemia in conscious dogs
Masunori Matsuzaki, Brian Guth, Tsukasa Tajimi, W. Scott Kemper, and John Ross, Jr.

News from the AHA

Begins on ad page . . . 13

Calendar of Meetings Ad page . . . 28

Instructions to Authors

Ad page 7

Circulation

An Official Journal of the American Heart Association

AUTHOR/SUBJECT INDEX TO

VOLUME 72

JULY-DECEMBER 1985

*

Cardiovascular Medicine:
Opportunities for Enhanced University-Industry Collaboration
Part II, Volume 72, Number 2, August 1985
Supplement I

*

Cardiovascular Surgery 1984
Part II, Volume 72, Number 3, September 1985
Supplement II

*

Cardiovascular Metabolic Imaging:
Physiologic and Biochemical Dynamics In Vivo
Part II, Volume 72, Number 5, November 1985
Supplement IV

*

Surgery in the Treatment of Coronary Artery Disease
Part II, Volume 72, Number 6, December 1985
Supplement V

AMERICAN HEART ASSOCIATION, INC.

CONTENTS

Circulation

AUGUST 1985 *Volume 72/Number 2*

FEATURES

Perspectives

245 Dopamine receptors: applictions in clinical cardiology
Leon I. Goldberg and Sol I. Rajfer

249 Atrial flutter: a synthesis of concepts
John P. Boineau

Editorial

258 Cardiology at a precipice
Robert A. O'Rourke

Preludes and Progress

262 The delayed diagnosis of myocardial infarction: it took half a century!
W. Bruce Fye

CLINICAL INVESTIGATION

PATHOPHYSIOLOGY AND NATURAL HISTORY

272 Local changes in myosin types in diseased human atrial myocardium: a quantitative immunofluorescence study
Patrice Bouvagnet, Jocelyne Léger, Claude A. Dechesne, Georges Dureau, Monique Anoal, and Jean J. Léger

280 Left ventricular aneurysm and the prediction of left ventricular enlargement studied by two-dimensional echocardiography: quantitative assessment of aneurysm size in relation to clinical course
Masayuki Matsumoto, Fumiko Watanabe, Akira Goto, Yutaka Hamano, Kiyoshi Yasui, Takazo Minamino, Hiroshi Abe, and Takenobu Kamada

287 Factors that modify the flow response to intracoronary injections
Håkan Emanuelsson, Stig Holmberg, Kjell Selin, and Jan Wallin

292 Coronary anatomy and left ventricular function in the first 12 hours of acute myocardial infarction: the Western Washington Randomized Intracoronary Streptokinase Trial
Michael L. Stadius, Charles Maynard, James K. Fritz, Kathryn Davis, James L. Ritchie, Florence Sheehan, and J. Ward Kennedy

Cardiomyopathy

302 Mildly dilated congestive cardiomyopathy
Andre Keren, Margaret E. Billingham, Dominique Weintraub, Edward B. Stinson, and Richard L. Popp

310 Diastolic abnormalities in patients with hypertrophic cardiomyopathy: relation to magnitude of left ventricular hypertrophy
Paolo Spirito, Barry J. Maron, Francesco Chiarella, Paolo Bellotti, Roberto Tramarin, Massimo Pozzoli, and Carlo Vecchio

DIAGNOSTIC METHODS

Nuclear Cardiology

317 Validation of attenuation-corrected equilibrium radionuclide angiographic determinations of right ventricular volume: comparison with cast-validated biplane cineventriculography
Louis J. Dell'Italia, Mark R. Starling, Richard A. Walsh, Frederick R. Badke, John C. Lasher, and Ralph Blumhardt

327 Quantification of myocardial infarction: a comparison of single photon–emission computed tomography with pyrophosphate to serial plasma MB–creatine kinase measurements
Donald E. Jansen, James R. Corbett, Christopher L. Wolfe, Samuel E. Lewis, Gregory Gabliani, Neil Filipchuk, Gregory Redish, Robert W. Parkey, L. Maximilian Buja, Allan S. Jaffe, Robert Rude, Burton E. Sobel, and James T. Willerson

for Everyone

In Hypertension*... When You Need to Conserve K+

For patients concerned about the cost of therapy **'DYAZIDE'** is more economical than beta blockers.

Potassium-Sparing

DYAZIDE®

25 mg Hydrochlorothiazide/**50 mg** Triamterene/SKF

The unique red and white Dyazide® capsule: Your assurance of SK&F quality.

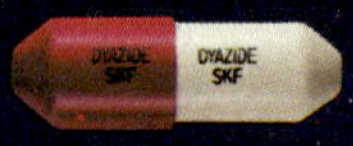

a product of
SK&F CO.
Carolina, P.R. 00630

Serum K+ and BUN should be checked periodically (see Warnings and Precautions).

hepatic function. They can precipitate coma in patients with severe liver disease. Observe regularly for possible blood dyscrasias, liver damage, other idiosyncratic reactions. Blood dyscrasias have been reported in patients receiving triamterene, and leukopenia, thrombocytopenia, agranulocytosis, and aplastic and hemolytic anemia have been reported with thiazides. Thiazides may cause manifestation of latent diabetes mellitus. The effects of oral anticoagulants may be decreased when used concurrently with hydrochlorothiazide; dosage adjustments may be necessary. Clinically insignificant reductions in arterial responsiveness to norepinephrine have been reported. Thiazides have also been shown to increase the paralyzing effect of nondepolarizing muscle relaxants such as tubocurarine. Triamterene is a weak folic acid antagonist. Do periodic blood studies in cirrhotics with splenomegaly. Antihypertensive effects may be enhanced in post-sympathectomy patients. Use cautiously in surgical patients. Triamterene has been found in renal stones in association with the other usual calculus components. Therefore, 'Dyazide' should be used with caution in patients with histories of stone formation. A few occurrences of acute renal failure have been reported in patients on 'Dyazide' when treated with indomethacin. Therefore, caution is advised in administering nonsteroidal anti-inflammatory agents with 'Dyazide'. The following may occur: transient elevated BUN or creatinine or both, hyperglycemia and glycosuria (diabetic insulin requirements may be altered), hyperuricemia and gout, digitalis intoxication (in hypokalemia), decreasing alkali reserve with possible metabolic acidosis. 'Dyazide' interferes with fluorescent measurement of quinidine. Hypokalemia is uncommon with 'Dyazide', but should it develop, corrective measures should be taken such as potassium supplementation or increased dietary intake of potassium-rich foods. Corrective measures should be instituted cautiously and serum potassium levels determined. Discontinue corrective measures and 'Dyazide' should laboratory values reveal elevated serum potassium. Chloride deficit may occur as well as dilutional hyponatremia. Concurrent use with chlorpropamide may increase the risk of severe hyponatremia. Serum PBI levels may decrease without signs of thyroid disturbance. Calcium excretion is decreased by thiazides. 'Dyazide' should be withdrawn before conducting tests for parathyroid function.

Thiazides may add to or potentiate the action of other antihypertensive drugs.

Diuretics reduce renal clearance of lithium and increase the risk of lithium toxicity.

Adverse Reactions: Muscle cramps, weakness, dizziness, headache, dry mouth; anaphylaxis, rash, urticaria, photosensitivity, purpura, other dermatological conditions; nausea and vomiting, diarrhea, constipation, other gastrointestinal disturbances; postural hypotension (may be aggravated by alcohol, barbiturates, or narcotics). Necrotizing vasculitis, paresthesias, icterus, pancreatitis, xanthopsia and respiratory distress including pneumonitis and pulmonary edema, transient blurred vision, sialadenitis, and vertigo have occurred with thiazides alone. Triamterene has been found in renal stones in association with other usual calculus components. Rare incidents of acute interstitial nephritis have been reported. Impotence has been reported in a few patients on 'Dyazide', although a causal relationship has not been established.

Supplied: 'Dyazide' is supplied as a red and white capsule, in bottles of 1000 capsules; Single Unit Packages (unit-dose) of 100 (intended for institutional use only); in Patient-Pak™ unit-of-use bottles of 100.

BRS-DZ:L39

Therapy and Prevention

334 The effects of coronary angioplasty and reperfusion on distribution of myocardial flow
D. W. Wahr, T. A. Ports, E. H. Botvinick, M. Dae, N. Schechtmann, J. Huberty, R. S. Hattner, J. W. O'Connell, and K. Turley

Pharmacology

344 Frequency-dependent effects of verapamil on atrioventricular nodal conduction in man
Kenneth A. Ellenbogen, Lawrence A. German, William G. O'Callaghan, Paul G. Colavita, Anne C. Marchese, Marcel R. Gilbert, and Harold C. Strauss

353 Improvement in regional wall motion and left ventricular relaxation after administration of diltiazem in patients with coronary artery disease
Harold Dash, Gary L. Copenhaver, and Susan Ensminger

364 Systemic and regional effects of captopril and milrinone administered alone and concomitantly in patients with heart failure
Thierry H. LeJemtel, Carol S. Maskin, Donna Mancini, Lawrence Sinoway, Harry Feld, and Brian Chadwick

LABORATORY INVESTIGATION

370 Dispersion of ventricular repolarization and arrhythmia: study of two consecutive ventricular complexes
Chien-Suu Kuo, Hirotsugu Atarashi, C. Pratap Reddy, and Borys Surawicz

377 A Doppler–two-dimensional echocardiographic method for quantitation of mitral regurgitation
Kathryn J. Ascah, William J. Stewart, Leng Jiang, J. Luis Guerrero, John B. Newell, Linda D. Gillam, and Arthur E. Weyman

Pharmacology

384 Coronary thrombolysis in dogs with intravenously administered human pro-urokinase
D. Collen, D. Stump, F. van de Werf, I. Jang, M. Nobuhara, and H. R. Lijnen

389 The effect of cyclooxygenase inhibition on vasomotion of proximal coronary arteries with endothelial damage
Gary E. Lane and Alfred A. Bove

397 Cyclic blood flow variations induced by platelet-activating factor in stenosed canine coronary arteries despite inhibition of thromboxane synthetase, serotonin receptors, and α-adrenergic receptors
P. Apprill, J. J. Schmitz, W. B. Campbell, G. Tilton, J. Ashton, S. Raheja, L. M. Buja, and J. T. Willerson

406 Survival after an experimental myocardial infarction: beneficial effects of long-term therapy with captopril
Mark A. Pfeffer, Janice M. Pfeffer, Cynthia Steinberg, and Peter Finn

Ventricular Function

413 Effects of propranolol and diltiazem alone and in combination on the recovery of left ventricular segmental function after temporary coronary occlusion and long-term reperfusion in conscious dogs
Larry R. Bush, L. Maximilian Buja, Gregory Tilton, Mark Wathen, Phillip Apprill, Juliet Ashton, and James T. Willerson

431 Immediate functional recovery and avoidance of reperfusion injury with surgical revascularization of short-term coronary occlusion
J. Vinten-Johansen, T. Arthur Edgerton, Harold R. Howe, Pamela A. Gayheart, Stephen A. Mills, George Howard, and Robert A. Cordell

440 Accuracy of volume measurement by conductance catheter in isolated, ejecting canine hearts
Daniel Burkhoff, Enno van der Velde, David Kass, Jan Baan, W. Lowell Maughan, and Kiichi Sagawa

News from the AHA

Begins on ad page . . . 8

Calendar of Meetings Ad page . . . 36

Instructions to Authors

Information regarding manuscripts suitable for publication in *Circulation* including format, review, and submission requirements, appears in the first issue of each volume (January and July).

Editorial correspondence — Burton E. Sobel, M.D., Editor, Washington University School of Medicine, 660 South Euclid Avenue, Box 8055, St. Louis, Missouri 63110.

Circulation

AN OFFICIAL JOURNAL OF THE American Heart Association

Editorial correspondence — Burton E. Sobel, M.D., Editor, Washington University School of Medicine, 660 South Euclid Ave., Box 8055, St. Louis, Missouri 63110.

Business correspondence — regarding subscriptions, change of address, single copies, missing issues, author reprint orders, etc. — American Heart Association, 7320 Greenville Ave., Dallas, Texas 75231.

Advertising — Pharmaceutical Media, Inc., 130 Madison Ave., New York, NY 10016. Advertising space is given only to copy approved by a special committee of the American Heart Association. Forms close first day of month preceding date of issue. Advertising rates and page sizes on application.

Circulation (USPS 113720) is published twelve times a year at the Publications Office, American Heart Association, Dallas, Texas 75231.

Subscription rates — annually (subscriptions accepted at any time), $56 United States, $72 elsewhere, postage included. Single copies, postpaid $7.00 U.S., $9.00 elsewhere; single copies of supplements at additional cost. Interns, residents, medical students — special rate of $28 annually in the U.S., $36 Canada and Mexico. (Letter stating post held required.) Airmail rates available upon request. All orders for Europe must go through Bailliere Tindall 1 St. Anne's Road, Eastbourne, East Sussex BN21 3UN ENGLAND. All orders for Japan must go through Nankodo Co., Ltd., 42-6 Hongo-3 Chome, Bunkyo-Ku, Tokyo, JAPAN. Remittances for subscriptions should be made by check, draft, post office or express money order payable to the American Heart Association. Second class postage paid at Dallas, Texas, and additional mailing offices. POSTMASTER: Send address changes to Circulation, American Heart Association, 7320 Greenville Ave., Dallas, Texas 75231. The Publishing Director should be advised of change of address 30 days before date of issue with both the subscriber's old and new address given.

CONTENTS

Circulation

SEPTEMBER 1985 Volume 72/Number 3

FEATURES

Editorial

449 Some unexpected lessons from large multicenter randomized clinical trials
Shahbudin H. Rahimtoola

Perspectives

456 Atherosclerosis, calcium, and calcium antagonists
Philip D. Henry

460 The radiographic assessment of coronary blood flow parameters
Robert A. Vogel

CLINICAL INVESTIGATION

PATHOPHYSIOLOGY AND NATURAL HISTORY

466 Effects of β-adrenoceptor–blocking drugs in patients with Raynaud's phenomenon
Jay D. Coffman and Helen M. Rasmussen

471 Abnormal distribution of pulmonary blood flow after the Glenn shunt or Fontan procedure: risk of development of arteriovenous fistulae
Alain Cloutier, Judith M. Ash, Jeffrey F. Smallhorn, William G. Williams, George A. Trusler, Richard D. Rowe, and Marlene Rabinovitch

Electrophysiology

480 The effects of overdrive pacing and lidocaine on atrioventricular junctional rhythm in man: the role of abnormal automaticity
József Tenczer, László Littmann, Miklós Rohla, and Tamás Fenyvesi

487 Programmed ventricular stimulation in survivors of acute myocardial infarction
Denis Roy, Etienne Marchand, Pierre Théroux, David D. Waters, Guy B. Pelletier, and Martial G. Bourassa

495 Change in ventricular cavity size: differential effects on QRS and T wave amplitude
Ted Feldman, Rory W. Childers, Kenneth M. Borow, Roberto M. Lang, and Alex Neumann

Ventricular Function

502 Are right and left ventricular ejection fractions equal? Ejection fractions in normal subjects and in patients with first acute myocardial infarction
Jens Marving, Poul F. Høilund-Carlsen, Bent Chræmmer-Jørgensen, and Niels Gadsbøll

515 Altered left ventricular mechanics in patients with valvular aortic stenosis and coarctation of the aorta: effects on systolic performance and late outcome
Kenneth M. Borow, Steven D. Colan, and Alexander Neumann

DIAGNOSTIC METHODS

523 A new approach to noninvasive evaluation of aortic regurgitant fraction by two-dimensional Doppler echocardiography
Akira Kitabatake, Hiroshi Ito, Michitoshi Inoue, Jun Tanouchi, Ken Ishihara, Toshio Morita, Kenshi Fujii, Yutaka Yoshida, Tohru Masuyama, Hideo Yoshima, Masatsugu Hori, and Takenobu Kamada

Circulation

AN OFFICIAL JOURNAL OF THE American Heart Association

Editorial correspondence — Burton E. Sobel, M.D., Editor, Washington University School of Medicine, 660 South Euclid Ave., Box 8055, St. Louis, Missouri 63110.

Business correspondence — regarding subscriptions, change of address, single copies, missing issues, author reprint orders, etc. — American Heart Association, 7320 Greenville Ave., Dallas, Texas 75231.

Advertising — Pharmaceutical Media, Inc., 130 Madison Ave., New York, NY 10016. Advertising space is given only to copy approved by a special committee of the American Heart Association. Forms close first day of month preceding date of issue. Advertising rates and page sizes on application.

Circulation (USPS 113720) is published twelve times a year at the Publications Office, American Heart Association, Dallas, Texas 75231.

Subscription rates — annually (subscriptions accepted at any time), $56 United States, $72 elsewhere, postage included. Single copies, postpaid $7.00 U.S., $9.00 elsewhere; single copies of supplements at additional cost. Interns, residents, medical students — special rate of $28 annually in the U.S., $36 Canada and Mexico. (Letter stating post held required.) Airmail rates available upon request. All orders for Europe must go through Bailliere Tindall 1 St. Anne's Road, Eastbourne, East Sussex BN21 3UN ENGLAND. All orders for Japan must go through Nankodo Co., Ltd., 42-6 Hongo-3 Chome, Bunkyo-Ku, Tokyo, JAPAN. Remittances for subscriptions should be made by check, draft, post office or express money order payable to the American Heart Association. Second class postage paid at Dallas, Texas, and additional mailing offices. POSTMASTER: Send address changes to Circulation, American Heart Association, 7320 Greenville Ave., Dallas, Texas 75231. The Publishing Director should be advised of change of address 30 days before date of issue with both the subscriber's old and new address given.

Therapy and Prevention

530 Influence of intimal dissection on restenosis after successful coronary angioplasty
Pierre P. Leimgruber, Gary S. Roubin, H. Vernon Anderson, Clayton E. Bredlau, Hall B. Whitworth, John S. Douglas, Jr., Spencer B. King III, and Andreas R. Gruentzig

Pharmacology

536 Improvement in symptoms and exercise tolerance by metoprolol in patients with dilated cardiomyopathy: a double-blind, randomized, placebo-controlled trial
Richard S. Engelmeier, John B. O'Connell, Ronald Walsh, Nancy Rad, Patrick J. Scanlon, and Rolf M. Gunnar

547 The interaction of verapamil and norverapamil with β-adrenergic receptors
Ross D. Feldman, Glen D. Park, and Chein-Yu Cynthia Lai

555 Electrophysiologic and antiarrhythmic effects of sotalol in patients with life-threatening ventricular tachyarrhythmias
Koonlawee Nademanee, Gregory Feld, JoAnn Hendrickson, Pramil N. Singh, and Bramah N. Singh

LABORATORY INVESTIGATION

565 Metabolic rate of radioiodinated heptadecanoic acid in the normal canine heart
Frans C. Visser, Machiel J. van Eenige, Gerrit Westera, Wim Den Hollander, Caspar M. B. Duwel, Ernst E. van der Wall, Guido A. K. Heidendal, and Jan P. Roos

572 Angle dependence of ultrasonic backscatter in arterial tissues: a study in vitro
Eugenio Picano, Luigi Landini, Alessandro Distante, Marco Salvadori, Fabio Lattanzi, Michele Masini, and Antonio L'Abbate

577 The accuracy of Doppler ultrasound measurement of pressure gradients across irregular, dual, and tunnellike obstructions to blood flow
Paul Teirstein, Paul G. Yock, and Richard L. Popp

Electrophysiology

585 Effects of unilateral stellate ganglion stimulation and ablation on electrophysiologic changes induced by acute myocardial ischemia in dogs
Michiel J. Janse, Peter J. Schwartz, Francien Wilms-Schopman, Ron J. G. Peters, and Dirk Durrer

596 Electrophysiologic and anatomic basis for fractionated electrograms recorded from healed myocardial infarcts
Phyllis I. Gardner, Philip C. Ursell, John J. Fenoglio, Jr., and Andrew L. Wit

612 Catheter-mediated electrical ablation of the posterior septum via the coronary sinus: electrophysiologic and histologic observations in dogs
Fernando Coltorti, Gust H. Bardy, Dennis Reichenbach, H. Leon Greene, Robert Thomas, Donald G. Breazeale, Clif Alferness, and Tom D. Ivey

Myocardial Infarction

623 Interruption of sympathetic and vagal-mediated afferent responses by transmural myocardial infarction
Michael J. Barber, Thomas M. Mueller, Becky G. Davies, Robert M. Gill, and Douglas P. Zipes

632 Left ventricular ejection fraction after acute coronary occlusion in conscious dogs: relation to the extent and site of myocardial infarction
Ricky M. Schneider, Alan Chu, Makoto Akaishi, William S. Weintraub, Kenneth G. Morris, and Frederick R. Cobb

639 Patterns of myoglobin release after reperfusion of injured myocardium
Avery K. Ellis, Thomas Little, A. R. Zaki Masud, and Francis J. Klocke

Ventricular Function

648 The superiority of maximum fiber elastance over maximum stress-volume ratio as an index of contractile state
Thomas Wisenbaugh, George Yu, and Joyce Evans

654 Effect of heart rate on the canine end-systolic pressure-volume relationship
W. Lowell Maughan, Kenji Sunagawa, Daniel Burkhoff, Willard L. Graves, Jr., William C. Hunter, and Kiichi Sagawa

660 A potential method of correcting intracavitary left ventricular filling pressures for the effects of positive end-expiratory airway pressure
Roy V. Ditchey, JoAnn Lindenfeld, E. Wayne Grogan, and Gary O. Zerbe

668 Diminished stroke volume during inspiration: a reverse thoracic pump
Craig O. Olsen, George S. Tyson, George W. Maier, James W. Davis, and J. Scott Rankin

546 Retraction

554 Erratum

News from the AHA

Begins on ad page . . . 8

Calendar of Meetings Ad page . . . 11

Instructions to Authors

Information regarding manuscripts suitable for publication in *Circulation* including format, review, and submission requirements, appears in the first issue of each volume (January and July).

Editorial correspondence — Burton E. Sobel, M.D., Editor, Washington University School of Medicine, 660 South Euclid Avenue, Box 8055, St. Louis, Missouri 63110.

CONTENTS

Circulation

OCTOBER 1985 *Volume 72/Number 4*

FEATURES

Perspectives

681 Sudden unexpected death in patients with congestive heart failure: a second frontier
Milton Packer

686 Cholesterol and cardiovascular disease: no longer whether, but rather when, in whom, and how?
Robert I. Levy

Editorial

692 Comprehensive health care and noncardiovascular mortality: an unlikely explanation of the findings from the Hypertension Detection and Follow-up Program
Siegfried Heyden, Kenneth Schneider, and George J. Fodor

SYMPOSIUM

Platelets and Vascular Occlusion

698 Inhibition of platelet function in thrombosis
Aaron J. Marcus, Lenore B. Safier, Harris L. Ullman, M. Johan Broekman, Naziba Islam, Thomas D. Oglesby, Robert R. Gorman, and Jean W. Ward

702 A review of possible roles of the platelet 12-lipoxygenase
Alan R. Brash

708 Evidence for 15-HETE synthesis by human umbilical vein endothelial cells
Robert R. Gorman, Thomas D. Oglesby, Gordon L. Bundy, and Nancy K. Hopkins

713 A role for PAF-acether (platelet-activating factor) in platelet-dependent vascular diseases?
J. Benveniste and M. Chignard

718 Production of platelet-activating factor by human vascular endothelial cells: evidence for a requirement for specific agonists and modulation by prostacyclin
Guy A. Zimmerman, Thomas M. McIntyre, and Stephen M. Prescott

728 Platelets, endothelium, and vasospasm
P. M. Vanhoutte and D. S. Houston

735 Locally acting growth factors for vascular smooth muscle cells: endogenous synthesis and release from platelets
Daniel F. Bowen-Pope, Russell Ross, and Ronald A. Seifert

741 Adenosine diphosphate as a mediator of platelet aggregation in vivo: an editorial view
G. V. R. Born

CLINICAL INVESTIGATION

PATHOPHYSIOLOGY AND NATURAL HISTORY

747 The effects of sublingually administered nitroglycerin on forearm vascular resistance in patients with heart failure and in normal subjects
Tsutomu Imaizumi, Akira Takeshita, Toshiaki Ashihara, and Motoomi Nakamura

753 Death and other time-related events after valve replacement
Eugene H. Blackstone and John W. Kirklin

768 Noninvasively diagnosed peripheral arterial disease as a predictor of mortality: results from a prospective study
Michael H. Criqui, Steven S. Coughlin, and Arnost Fronek

Myocardial Infarction

774 Prognostic significance and natural history of left ventricular thrombi in patients with acute anterior myocardial infarction: a two-dimensional echocardiographic study
Paolo Spirito, Paolo Bellotti, Francesco Chiarella, Stefano Domenicucci, Angela Sementa, and Carlo Vecchio

781 Non–Q wave perioperative myocardial infarction: assessment of the incidence and severity of regional dysfunction with quantitative two-dimensional echocardiography
Thomas Force, Andrew J. Kemper, Peter Bloomfield, Donald E. Tow, Shukri F. Khuri, Miguel Josa, and Alfred F. Parisi

for Everyone

In Hypertension*...
When You Need
to Conserve K+

For patients concerned about the cost of therapy **'DYAZIDE'** is more economical than beta blockers.

Potassium-Sparing

DYAZIDE®

25 mg Hydrochlorothiazide/**50 mg** Triamterene/SKF

The unique red and white Dyazide® capsule: Your assurance of SK&F quality.

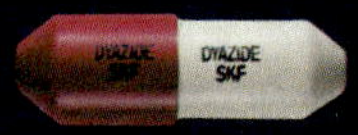

a product of
SK&F CO.
Carolina, P.R. 00630

Serum K+ and BUN should be checked periodically (see Warnings and Precautions).

hepatic function. They can precipitate coma in patients with severe liver disease. Observe regularly for possible blood dyscrasias, liver damage, other idiosyncratic reactions. Blood dyscrasias have been reported in patients receiving triamterene, and leukopenia, thrombocytopenia, agranulocytosis, and aplastic and hemolytic anemia have been reported with thiazides. Thiazides may cause manifestation of latent diabetes mellitus. The effects of oral anticoagulants may be decreased when used concurrently with hydrochlorothiazide; dosage adjustments may be necessary. Clinically insignificant reductions in arterial responsiveness to norepinephrine have been reported. Thiazides have also been shown to increase the paralyzing effect of nondepolarizing muscle relaxants such as tubocurarine. Triamterene is a weak folic acid antagonist. Do periodic blood studies in cirrhotics with splenomegaly. Antihypertensive effects may be enhanced in post-sympathectomy patients. Use cautiously in surgical patients. Triamterene has been found in renal stones in association with the other usual calculus components. Therefore, 'Dyazide' should be used with caution in patients with histories of stone formation. A few occurrences of acute renal failure have been reported in patients on 'Dyazide' when treated with indomethacin. Therefore, caution is advised in administering nonsteroidal anti-inflammatory agents with 'Dyazide'. The following may occur: transient elevated BUN or creatinine or both, hyperglycemia and glycosuria (diabetic insulin requirements may be altered), hyperuricemia and gout, digitalis intoxication (in hypokalemia), decreasing alkali reserve with possible metabolic acidosis. 'Dyazide' interferes with fluorescent measurement of quinidine. Hypokalemia is uncommon with 'Dyazide', but should it develop, corrective measures should be taken such as potassium supplementation or increased dietary intake of potassium-rich foods. Corrective measures should be instituted cautiously and serum potassium levels determined. Discontinue corrective measures and 'Dyazide' should laboratory values reveal elevated serum potassium. Chloride deficit may occur as well as dilutional hyponatremia. Concurrent use with chlorpropamide may increase the risk of severe hyponatremia. Serum PBI levels may decrease without signs of thyroid disturbance. Calcium excretion is decreased by thiazides. 'Dyazide' should be withdrawn before conducting tests for parathyroid function.

Thiazides may add to or potentiate the action of other antihypertensive drugs.

Diuretics reduce renal clearance of lithium and increase the risk of lithium toxicity.

Adverse Reactions: Muscle cramps, weakness, dizziness, headache, dry mouth; anaphylaxis, rash, urticaria, photosensitivity, purpura, other dermatological conditions; nausea and vomiting, diarrhea, constipation, other gastrointestinal disturbances; postural hypotension (may be aggravated by alcohol, barbiturates, or narcotics). Necrotizing vasculitis, paresthesias, icterus, pancreatitis, xanthopsia and respiratory distress including pneumonitis and pulmonary edema, transient blurred vision, sialadenitis, and vertigo have occurred with thiazides alone. Triamterene has been found in renal stones in association with other usual calculus components. Rare incidents of acute interstitial nephritis have been reported. Impotence has been reported in a few patients on 'Dyazide', although a causal relationship has not been established.

Supplied: 'Dyazide' is supplied as a red and white capsule, in bottles of 1000 capsules; Single Unit Packages (unit-dose) of 100 (intended for institutional use only); in Patient-Pak™ unit-of-use bottles of 100.

BRS-DZ:L39

790 Subendocardial infarction in retrospect: pathologic, cardiographic, and ancillary features
Harold D. Levine

DIAGNOSTIC METHODS

801 Detection of local abnormalities in ventricular activation sequence by body surface isochrone mapping in patients with previous myocardial infarction
Kozue Ikeda, Isao Kubota, Akira Igarashi, Michiyasu Yamaki, Kai Tsuiki, and Shoji Yasui

Echocardiography

810 Noninvasive estimation of valve area in patients with aortic stenosis by Doppler ultrasound and two-dimensional echocardiography
Terje Skjaerpe, Lars Hegrenaes, and Liv Hatle

819 Assessment and follow-up of patients with aortic regurgitation by an updated Doppler echocardiographic measurement of the regurgitant fraction in the aortic arch
Thierry Touche, Richard Prasquier, Alain Nitenberg, Dominique de Zuttere, and René Gourgon

825 Fetal atrioventricular valve insufficiency associated with nonimmune hydrops: a two-dimensional echocardiographic and Doppler ultrasound study
Norman H. Silverman, Charles S. Kleinman, Abraham M. Rudolph, Joshua A. Copel, Ellen M. Weinstein, Marlene A. Enderlein, and Mitchell Golbus

THERAPY AND PREVENTION

Surgery

833 Comparative long-term effects of coronary artery bypass graft surgery and percutaneous transluminal coronary angioplasty on regional coronary flow reserve
Eric R. Bates, Fred M. Aueron, Victor Legrand, Michael T. LeFree, John Mancini, John M. Hodgson, and Robert A. Vogel

840 Senning repair for transposition of the great arteries in the first week of life
G. Paul Matherne, Jerry D. Razook, Webb M. Thompson, Jr., Mary M. Lane, Cynthia K. Murray, and Ronald C. Elkins

Pharmacology

846 Comparative systemic and renal effects of dopamine and angiotensin-converting enzyme inhibition with enalaprilat in patients with heart failure
Carol S. Maskin, Steven Ocken, Brian Chadwick, and Thierry H. LeJemtel

853 Verapamil-induced improvement in left ventricular diastolic filling and increased exercise tolerance in patients with hypertrophic cardiomyopathy: short- and long-term effects
Robert O. Bonow, Vasken Dilsizian, Douglas R. Rosing, Barry J. Maron, Stephen L. Bacharach, and Michael V. Green

865 Importance of internal controls, statistical methods, and side effects in short-term trials of vasodilators: a study of hydralazine kinetics in patients with aortic regurgitation
Charles R. McKay, Michele Nanna, David T. Kawanishi, Uri Elkayam, P. Anthony N. Chandraratna, Joyce N. Weiss, and Shahbudin H. Rahimtoola

873 Use of an ultra short–acting β-blocker in patients with acute myocardial ischemia
James M. Kirshenbaum, Robert A. Kloner, Elliott M. Antman, and Eugene Braunwald

LABORATORY INVESTIGATION

881 Exercise thallium-201 scintigraphy in dogs: effects of long-term coronary occlusion and collateral development on early and late scintigraphic images
Michael V. Cohen and Richard M. Steingart

Pharmacology

892 Effects of synthetic atrial natriuretic peptide on renal function and renin release in acute experimental heart failure
Terry A. Scriven and John C. Burnett, Jr.

898 Frequency-dependent effects of amitriptyline on ventricular conduction and cardiac rhythm in dogs
Stanley Nattel

Myocardial Protection

907 Delayed effects of early infarct-limiting therapies on healing after myocardial infarction
Bodh I. Jugdutt

915 Enhancement of recovery of myocardial function by oxygen free–radical scavengers after reversible regional ischemia
Mary Lee Myers, Roberto Bolli, Raymond F. Lekich, Craig J. Hartley, and Robert Roberts

Electrophysiology

922 Effect of serial brief ischemic episodes on extracellular K^+, pH, and activation in the pig
William F. Fleet, Timothy A. Johnson, Chris A. Graebner, and Leonard S. Gettes

933 Autonomic control of ventricular tachycardia: sympathetic neural influence on spontaneous tachycardia 24 hours after coronary occlusion
James B. Martins

746 Tribute

809 Erratum

News from the AHA

Begins on ad page . . . 14

Calendar of Meetings Ad page . . . 24

Instructions to Authors

Information regarding manuscripts suitable for publication in *Circulation* including format, review, and submission requirements, appears in the first issue of each volume (January and July).

Editorial correspondence — Burton E. Sobel, M.D., Editor, Washington University School of Medicine, 660 South Euclid Avenue, Box 8055, St. Louis, Missouri 63110.

CONTENTS

Circulation

NOVEMBER 1985 *Volume 72/Number 5*

FEATURES

Perspectives

943 Atherogenic lipoproteins and coronary artery disease: concepts derived from recent advances in cellular and molecular biology
Robert W. Mahley

949 A consideration of antiarrhythmic therapy
Douglas P. Zipes

CLINICAL INVESTIGATION

PATHOPHYSIOLOGY AND NATURAL HISTORY

957 Increased lung vasoreactivity in children from Leadville, Colorado, after recovery from high-altitude pulmonary edema
James W. Fasules, James W. Wiggins, and Robert R. Wolfe

963 Complex ventricular arrhythmias in patients with Q wave and non–Q wave myocardial infarction
Alan S. Maisel, Neil Scott, Elizabeth Gilpin, Staffan Ahnve, Martin Le Winter, Hartmut Henning, Daniel Collins, and John Ross, Jr.

971 The relationship of white cell count, platelet count, and hematocrit to cigarette smoking in adolescents: the Oslo Youth Study
G. S. Tell, R. H. Grimm, Jr., O. D. Vellar, and L. Theodorsen

Exercise

975 Isometric exercise in patients with chronic advanced heart failure: hemodynamic and neurohumoral evaluation
Uri Elkayam, Arie Roth, Laura Weber, Willa Hsueh, Michele Nanna, Lindalee Freidenberger, P. Anthony N. Chandraratna, and Shahbudin H. Rahimtoola

982 The nature of opioid involvement in the hemodynamic respiratory and humoral responses to exercise
J. Staessen, R. Fiocchi, R. Bouillon, R. Fagard, P. Lijnen, E. Moerman, A. De Schaepdryver, and A. Amery

Ventricular Performance

991 Effects of reduced left ventricular mass on chamber architecture, load, and function: a study of anorexia nervosa
Martin G. St. John Sutton, Ted Plappert, Lon Crosby, Pamela Douglas, James Mullen, and Nathaniel Reichek

1001 Effects of sublingual nifedipine on hemodynamics and systolic and diastolic function in patients with hypertrophic cardiomyopathy
Sandro Betocchi, Richard O. Cannon III, Rita M. Watson, Robert O. Bonow, Harold G. Ostrow, Stephen E. Epstein, and Douglas R. Rosing

1008 Global and regional right ventricular function in normal infants and infants with transposition of the great arteries after Senning operation
Eckardt Trowitzsch, Steven D. Colan, and Stephen P. Sanders

DIAGNOSTIC METHODS

1015 Intraoperative detection of myocardial ischemia in high-risk patients: electrocardiography versus two-dimensional transesophageal echocardiography
John S. Smith, Michael K. Cahalan, David J. Benefiel, Benjamin F. Byrd, Francis W. Lurz, William A. Shapiro, Michael F. Roizen, Alain Bouchard, and Nelson B. Schiller

1022 Transcutaneous oxygen recovery and toe pulse reappearance time in the assessment of peripheral vascular disease
Harry B. Kram, Rodney A. White, Joseph Tabrisky, Paul L. Appel, Arthur W. Fleming, and William C. Shoemaker

1028 Computer detection of atrioventricular dissociation from surface electrocardiograms during wide QRS complex tachycardias
Janet Slocum, Ernest Byrom, Lynn McCarthy, Alan Sahakian, and Steven Swiryn

THERAPY AND PREVENTION

1037 Maintenance of exercise stroke volume during ventricular versus atrial synchronous pacing: role of contractility
Kalman Ausubel, Richard M. Steingart, Mona Shimshi, Peter Klementowicz, and Seymour Furman

1044 In-hospital morbidity and mortality in patients undergoing elective coronary angioplasty
Clayton E. Bredlau, Gary S. Roubin, Pierre P. Leimgruber, John S. Douglas, Jr., Spencer B. King III, and Andreas Gruentzig

Circulation

AN OFFICIAL JOURNAL OF THE **American Heart Association**

Editorial correspondence — Burton E. Sobel, M.D., Editor, Washington University School of Medicine, 660 South Euclid Ave., Box 8055, St. Louis, Missouri 63110.

Business correspondence — regarding subscriptions, change of address, single copies, missing issues, author reprint orders, etc. — American Heart Association, 7320 Greenville Ave., Dallas, Texas 75231.

Advertising — Pharmaceutical Media, Inc., 130 Madison Ave., New York, NY 10016. Advertising space is given only to copy approved by a special committee of the American Heart Association. Forms close first day of month preceding date of issue. Advertising rates and page sizes on application.

Circulation (USPS 113720) is published twelve times a year at the Publications Office, American Heart Association, Dallas, Texas 75231.

Subscription rates — annually (subscriptions accepted at any time), $56 United States, $72 elsewhere, postage included. Single copies, postpaid $7.00 U.S., $9.00 elsewhere; single copies of supplements at additional cost. Interns, residents, medical students — special rate of $28 annually in the U.S., $36 Canada and Mexico. (Letter stating post held required.) Airmail rates available upon request. All orders for Europe must go through Bailliere Tindall 1 St. Anne's Road, Eastbourne, East Sussex BN21 3UN ENGLAND. All orders for Japan must go through Nankodo Co., Ltd., 42-6 Hongo-3 Chome, Bunkyo-Ku, Tokyo, JAPAN. Remittances for subscriptions should be made by check, draft, post office or express money order payable to the American Heart Association. Second class postage paid at Dallas, Texas, and additional mailing offices. POSTMASTER: Send address changes to Circulation, American Heart Association, 7320 Greenville Ave., Dallas, Texas 75231. The Publishing Director should be advised of change of address 30 days before date of issue with both the subscriber's old and new address given.

Pharmacology

1053 The effects of the rate of intravenous infusion of streptokinase and the duration of symptoms on the time interval to reperfusion in patients with acute myocardial infarction
Allan S. Lew, Pierre Laramee, Bojan Cercek, Lois Rodriguez, Prediman K. Shah, and William Ganz

1059 Warfarin versus dipyridamole-aspirin and pentoxifylline-aspirin for the prevention of prosthetic heart valve thromboembolism: a prospective randomized clinical trial
C. K. Mok, John Boey, Rebecca Wang, T. K. Chan, K. L. Cheung, P. K. Lee, Joseph Chow, Ronald P. Ng, and T. F. Tse

1064 Amiodarone and its desethyl metabolite: tissue distribution and morphologic changes during long-term therapy
P. C. Adams, D. W. Holt, G. C. A. Storey, A. R. Morley, J. Callaghan, and R. W. F. Campbell

LABORATORY INVESTIGATION

1076 Effects of intravascular volume state on the value of pulsus paradoxus and right ventricular diastolic collapse in predicting cardiac tamponade
Terrence L. Cogswell, Gregory A. Bernath, L. Samuel Wann, Raymond G. Hoffman, Harold L. Brooks, and H. Sidney Klopfenstein

1081 Comparison of pathologic and angiographic findings in a porcine preparation of coronary atherosclerosis
Bonnie H. Weiner, Ira S. Ockene, John Jarmolych, Katherine E. Fritz, and Assaad S. Daoud

1087 Uptake of hematoporphyrin derivative by valvular vegetations in experimental infective endocarditis
Artur M. Spokojny, Nigel Sinclair, Stuart Schnitt, Sven Paulin, and J. Richard Spears

1092 Cesium chloride–induced long QT syndrome: demonstration of afterdepolarizations and triggered activity in vivo
Joseph H. Levine, Joseph F. Spear, Thomas Guarnieri, Myron L. Weisfeldt, Cees D. J. de Langen, Lewis C. Becker, and E. Neil Moore

Ischemia

1104 Effects of right ventricular ischemia on left ventricular geometry and the end-diastolic pressure-volume relationship in the dog
Yoichi Goto, Jin Yamamato, Muneyasu Saito, Kazuo Haze, Tetsuya Sumiyoshi, Kenichi Fukami, Katsuhiko Hiramori

1115 Contrast echocardiographic estimation of regional myocardial blood flow after acute coronary occlusion
Andrew J. Kemper, Thomas Force, Robert Kloner, Michele Gilfoil, Lorri Perkins, Sharon Hale, Kevin Alker, and Alfred F. Parisi

1125 Mechanisms of improving regional and global ventricular function by preload alterations during acute ischemia in the canine left ventricle
Wilbur Y. W. Lew and Ernesto Ban-Hayashi

NEWS FROM THE AHA

Begins on ad page . . . 11

Calendar of Meetings ad page . . . 24

Special Report page . . . 1135A

INSTRUCTIONS TO AUTHORS

Information regarding manuscripts suitable for publication in *Circulation* including format, review, and submission requirements, appears in the first issue of each volume (January and July).

Editorial correspondence — Burton E. Sobel, M.D., Editor, Washington University School of Medicine, 660 South Euclid Avenue, Box 8055, St. Louis, Missouri 63110.

CONTENTS

Circulation

DECEMBER 1985 *Volume 72/Number 6*

FEATURES

Editorials

1135 Physicians confront the nuclear peril
Bernard Lown

1144 Percutaneous transluminal coronary angioplasty: a surgeon's view
Nicholas T. Kouchoukos

Perspectives

1148 Has 'obstruction' hindered our understanding of hypertrophic cardiomyopathy?
John Michael Criley and Robert J. Siegel

1155 The virtual disappearance of rheumatic fever in the United States: lessons in the rise and fall of disease. T. Duckett Jones Memorial Lecture
Leon Gordis

SYMPOSIUM

Platelets and Vascular Occlusion

1164 The human pharmacology of platelet inhibition: pharmacokinetics relevant to drug action
Anders Kirstein Pedersen and Garret A. FitzGerald

1177 Clinical pharmacology of platelet cyclooxygenase inhibition
Carlo Patrono, Giovanni Ciabattoni, Paola Patrignani, Francesco Pugliese, Paola Filabozzi, Francesca Catella, Giovanni Davi, and Laura Forni

1185 Pharmacology of platelet inhibition in humans: implications of the salicylate-aspirin interaction
Giovanni de Gaetano, Chiara Cerletti, Elisabetta Dejana, and Roberto Latini

1194 The biochemical pharmacology of thromboxane synthase inhibition in man
Garret A. FitzGerald, Irene A. G. Reilly, and Anders K. Pedersen

1202 Thromboxane A_2 and prostaglandin endoperoxide receptors in platelets and vascular smooth muscle
David L. Saussy, Jr., Dale E. Mais, Daniel R. Knapp, and Perry V. Halushka

1208 AH23848: a thromboxane receptor–blocking drug that can clarify the pathophysiologic role of thromboxane A_2
R. T. Brittain, L. Boutal, M. C. Carter, R. A. Coleman, E. W. Collington, H. P. Geisow, P. Hallett, E. J. Hornby, P. P. A. Humphrey, D. Jack, I. Kennedy, P. Lumley, P. J. McCabe, I. F. Skidmore, M. Thomas, and C. J. Wallis

1219 Platelet actions of stable carbocyclic analogues of prostacyclin
Brendan J. R. Whittle and Salvador Moncada

CLINICAL INVESTIGATION

PATHOPHYSIOLOGY AND NATURAL HISTORY

1226 Effect of β-adrenergic blockers on the peripheral circulation in patients with peripheral vascular disease
William R. Hiatt, Sandra Stoll, and Alan S. Nies

1232 Significance of cardiac defects in the developing fetus: a study of spontaneous abortuses
Philip C. Ursell, Julianne M. Byrne, and Barbara A. Strobino

1237 Effect of isotonic exercise training on left ventricular volume during upright exercise
Michael H. Crawford, Michael A. Petru, and Charles Rabinowitz

1244 Survival and functional results after valve replacement for aortic regurgitation from 1976 to 1983: impact of preoperative left ventricular function
Robert O. Bonow, Anthony L. Picone, Charles L. McIntosh, Michael Jones, Douglas R. Rosing, Barry J. Maron, Edward Lakatos, Richard E. Clark, and Stephen E. Epstein

1257 Regional wave travel and reflections along the human aorta: a study with six simultaneous micromanometric pressures
Ricky D. Latham, Nico Westerhof, Pieter Sipkema, Bernard J. Rubal, Peter Reuderink, and Joseph P. Murgo

Congestive Heart Failure

1270 The pressure-flow response of the pulmonary circulation in patients with heart failure and pulmonary vascular disease
Joseph S. Janicki, Karl T. Weber, Mariell J. Likoff, and Alfred P. Fishman

1279 Right ventricular function in an operating room model of mechanical left ventricular assistance and its effects in patients with depressed left ventricular function
David J. Farrar, Peter G. Compton, James J. Hershon, and J. Donald Hill

Electrophysiology

1286 Intermittent failure of local conduction during ventricular tachycardia
John M. Miller, Joseph A. Vassallo, W. Clark Hargrove, and Mark E. Josephson

1293 Further observations on transient entrainment: importance of pacing site and properties of the components of the reentry circuit
Ken Okumura, Richard W. Henthorn, Andrew E. Epstein, Vance J. Plumb, and Albert L. Waldo

Diagnostic Methods

1308 Abnormal signal-averaged electrocardiograms in patients with nonischemic congestive cardiomyopathy: relationship to sustained ventricular tachyarrhythmias
David S. Poll, Francis E. Marchlinski, Rita A. Falcone, Mark E. Josephson, and Michael B. Simson

Therapy and Prevention

1314 Coronary angioplasty of multiple vessels: short-term outcome and long-term results
Michael J. Cowley, George W. Vetrovec, Germano DiSciascio, Stephen A. Lewis, Paul D. Hirsh, and Timothy C. Wolfgang

Myocardial Infarction

1321 The hypotensive effect of intravenous streptokinase in patients with acute myocardial infarction
Allan S. Lew, Pierre Laramee, Bojan Cercek, Prediman K. Shah, and William Ganz

1327 Comparative effects of volume loading, dobutamine, and nitroprusside in patients with predominant right ventricular infarction
Louis J. Dell'Italia, Mark R. Starling, Ralph Blumhardt, John C. Lasher, and Robert A. O'Rourke

1336 Systemic and transcardiac platelet activity in acute myocardial infarction in man: resistance to prostacyclin
Hiltrud S. Mueller, Parinam S. Rao, Mark A. Greenberg, Peter M. Buttrick, Ira I. Sussman, Howard A. Levite, Richard M. Grose, Vicente Perez-Davila, Janet E. Strain, and Theodore H. Spaet

LABORATORY INVESTIGATION

1346 Prevention of coronary thrombosis with subthrombolytic doses of tissue-type plasminogen activator
Keith A. A. Fox, Alice K. Robison, Robert M. Knabb, Thomas L. Rosamond, Burton E. Sobel, and Steven R. Bergmann

1355 Determination of left ventricular mass in dogs with rapid-acquisition cardiac computed tomographic scanning
Andrew J. Feiring, John A. Rumberger, Steven J. Reiter, David J. Skorton, Steven M. Collins, Martin J. Lipton, Charles B. Higgins, Steven Ell, and Melvin L. Marcus

1365 Treatment of canine permeability pulmonary edema: short-term effects of dobutamine, furosemide, and hydralazine
William D. Molloy, K. Y. Lee, Linda Girling, and Richard M. Prewitt

Electrophysiology

1372 Correlation between refractory periods and activation-recovery intervals from electrograms: effects of rate and adrenergic interventions
C. Kay Millar, Fany A. Kralios, and Robert L. Lux

1380 Kinetics of electrophysiologic changes during oral loading of amiodarone and after withdrawal of amiodarone in the unsedated dog
Ishik C. Tuna, Anchen Qi, Charles Gornick, R. Morton Bolman III, and David G. Benditt

1386 In Appreciation

1390 Index to Volume 72

News from the AHA

Begins on ad page . . . 13

Calendar of Meetings ad page . . . 20

Instructions to Authors

Information regarding manuscripts suitable for publication in *Circulation* including format, review, and submission requirements, appears in the first issue of each volume (January and July).

Editorial correspondence — Burton E. Sobel, M.D., Editor, Washington University School of Medicine, 660 South Euclid Avenue, Box 8055, St. Louis, Missouri 63110.

Circulation

AN OFFICIAL JOURNAL OF THE American Heart Association

Editorial correspondence — Burton E. Sobel, M.D., Editor, Washington University School of Medicine, 660 South Euclid Ave., Box 8055, St. Louis, Missouri 63110.

Business correspondence — regarding subscriptions, change of address, single copies, missing issues, author reprint orders, etc. — American Heart Association, 7320 Greenville Ave., Dallas, Texas 75231.

Advertising — Pharmaceutical Media, Inc., 130 Madison Ave., New York, NY 10016. Advertising space is given only to copy approved by a special committee of the American Heart Association. Forms close first day of month preceding date of issue. Advertising rates and page sizes on application.

Circulation (USPS 113720) is published twelve times a year at the Publications Office, American Heart Association, Dallas, Texas 75231.

Subscription rates — annually (subscriptions accepted at any time), $56 United States, $72 elsewhere, postage included. Single copies, postpaid $7.00 U.S., $9.00 elsewhere; single copies of supplements at additional cost. Interns, residents, medical students — special rate of $28 annually in the U.S., $36 Canada and Mexico. (Letter stating post held required.) Airmail rates available upon request. All orders for Europe must go through Bailliere Tindall 1 St. Anne's Road, Eastbourne, East Sussex BN21 3UN ENGLAND. All orders for Japan must go through Nankodo Co., Ltd., 42-6 Hongo-3 Chome, Bunkyo-Ku, Tokyo, JAPAN. Remittances for subscriptions should be made by check, draft, post office or express money order payable to the American Heart Association. Second class postage paid at Dallas, Texas, and additional mailing offices. POSTMASTER: Send address changes to Circulation, American Heart Association, 7320 Greenville Ave., Dallas, Texas 75231. The Publishing Director should be advised of change of address 30 days before date of issue with both the subscriber's old and new address given.

Circulation
VOL 72 NO 1
JULY 1985
An Official Journal of the American Heart Association, Inc.®

FEATURES

Programmed electrical stimulation of the heart in patients with life-threatening ventricular arrhythmias: What is the significance of induced arrhythmias and what is the correct stimulation protocol?

HEIN J. J. WELLENS, M.D., PEDRO BRUGADA, M.D., AND WILLIAM G. STEVENSON, M.D.*

FOLLOWING ITS INTRODUCTION into the practice of cardiology in 1972,[1] programmed electrical stimulation (PES) of the heart has developed from a technique used for diagnostic purposes into one used for clinical management of patients with life-threatening ventricular arrhythmias.

During the same years we have seen a gradual change from relatively simple pacing protocols using one or two premature stimuli during ventricular stimulation to "aggressive" protocols using up to four premature stimuli, many basic pacing rates, and different sites of ventricular stimulation.

During PES some factors can, but many cannot, be controlled by the investigator. Among those that are controllable are (1) stimulus (strength, duration, type of current, number and rate of basic stimuli, number and interval of premature stimuli), (2) stimulation site, (3) mode of stimulation (unipolar or bipolar), and (4) interelectrode distance. Some factors that are not controllable are (1) type of spontaneous tachycardia, (2) etiology of spontaneous tachycardia, (3) resting heart rate, (4) autonomic state, (5) electrophysiologic properties of the arrhythmia substrate, (6) autonomic response to pacing or the administration of drugs, and (7) hemodynamic and ischemic consequences of pacing and drug administration. In our opinion a discussion on the value of PES in the study and treatment of life-threatening ventricular arrhythmias and the importance of the stimulation protocol should include three aspects: (1) What is the significance of different ventricular arrhythmias induced during PES and how do these arrhythmias relate to the "aggressiveness" of the protocol? (2) What then is the most effective, safest, and least time-consuming protocol in relation to the clinical problem? (3) What implications do these considerations have for the use of PES in selecting antiarrhythmic treatment?

From the Department of Cardiology, Annadal Hospital, University of Limburg, Maastricht, The Netherlands.
Address for correspondence: Hein J.J. Wellens, M.D., Department of Cardiology, Annadal Hospital, University of Limburg, Maastricht, The Netherlands.
*Current address: UCLA Center for the Health Sciences, Division of Cardiology, Los Angeles.

The significance of different ventricular arrhythmias induced during PES and their relationship to the aggressiveness of the PES protocol

Our definitions of the different ventricular arrhythmias that can be induced during PES are as follows: Sustained arrhythmias are those greater than 30 sec in duration or requiring an intervention for termination. Spontaneously occurring arrhythmias must require an intervention for termination to be considered sustained. Nonsustained arrhythmias are those 6 beats to 29 sec in duration. Spontaneous nonsustained ventricular tachycardia is considered to be that of 3 or more beats in duration. Monomorphic ventricular tachycardia is a ventricular rhythm faster than 100 beats/min with a regular rate and consistent beat-to-beat morphology. Polymorphic ventricular tachycardia is a ventricular tachycardia characterized by frequent changes in QRS morphology and/or axis, which must occur at least every 1 to 2 sec or every 6 beats. Ventricular fibrillation is a ventricular rhythm characterized by totally disorganized activity and no discernible QRS complexes on the surface electrocardiogram. It is important to realize that these definitions vary in the different institutions performing PES. An induced arrhythmia is considered to be clinical when it is similar to the one occurring spontaneously.

Sustained monomorphic ventricular tachycardia. The observation that sustained monomorphic ventricular tachycardia could almost never be induced during PES in patients without a cardiac abnormality[2] and could be induced in up to 95% of patients with spontaneous episodes of sustained monomorphic ventricular tachycardia[3-5] led to the belief that the initiation of sustained monomorphic ventricular tachycardia during PES was a highly significant finding.

In patients with recurrent sustained monomorphic ventricular tachycardia the chance of reproducing the same arrhythmia in the catheterization laboratory is very high. With the use of one right ventricular stimulation site (the right ventricular apex) and two premature stimuli and at least two basic pacing rates, the incidence varies from 70% to 90% in patients with ventricular tachycardia occurring late (more than 5 weeks) after myocardial infarction.[5, 6]

Adding a third extrastimulus to the pacing protocol increases the rate of induction of the clinically documented arrhythmia by 12% to 24%.[3-5] Stimulation in the right ventricular outflow tract in addition to that from the usual site (the apex of the right ventricle) and pacing in the left ventricle have been described to lead to a further increase in rate of induction of ventricular tachycardia.[4, 7] The use of isoproterenol will facilitate the induction of ventricular tachycardia in those patients in whom the arrhythmia is related to exercise or emotions.

Recently we reported that a stimulation protocol using a single right ventricular stimulation site (the apex), three basic pacing rates, and a maximum of three extrastimuli induced the clinically documented arrhythmia in 93% of patients with recurrent sustained monomorphic ventricular tachycardia after myocardial infarction. Such a protocol can be performed in less than 1 hr. Increasing the stimulus strength of the premature beat to 20 mA or changing the stimulation site from the right ventricular apex to the outflow tract did not result in a higher incidence of induction of tachycardia than did the previously described protocol.[8]

The ability to induce the clinically occurring sustained monomorphic ventricular tachycardia depends on the cause of the arrhythmia. The arrhythmia can be initiated in close to 100% of patients with an old myocardial infarction, 75% to 90% of patients with idiopathic ventricular tachycardia, and 50% to 60% of patients with cardiomyopathy or prolapse of the mitral valve.[9]

Induction of sustained monomorphic ventricular tachycardia has been accepted as indicative of the presence of an arrhythmia substrate or pathway. The demonstration of such a situation in the survivor of myocardial infarction has been suggested as an independent marker of increased risk of sudden (arrhythmic) cardiac death.[10]

The problem is, however, that in our experience, using the protocol mentioned,[8] the initiation of sustained monomorphic ventricular tachycardia is nearly as common in patients resuscitated from sudden death as in patients after myocardial infarction who never suffered from life-threatening ventricular arrhythmias (60% vs 45%).[11] When only two ventricular premature depolarizations were used the rates of induction of sustained monomorphic ventricular tachycardia were 45% and 22%, respectively. Typically, and in contrast to the patient with clinically documented sustained monomorphic ventricular tachycardia, in these two groups of patients the monomorphic ventricular tachycardia is usually fast, poorly tolerated, and frequently deteriorates into ventricular fibrillation. While the work of the group of Richards et al.[10] indicates that induction of this arrhythmia carries a poor prognosis in the infarct survivor, this could not be confirmed by other groups, including our own.[11] This suggests to us that the induction of monomorphic sustained ventricular tachycardia in the arrhythmia-free survivor of infarct could be a nonspecific finding. Therefore, although initiation of such an arrhythmia in patients who have survived an episode of sudden death might reflect what happened clinically, since most survivors of sudden death have extensive coronary artery disease and 40% have had a previous myocardial infarction, one has to consider the possibility of a nonspecific event. The question of whether an event is specific or not cannot usually be answered because multiple-lead documentation of the arrhythmic event at the time of an episode of sudden death is usually not available and therefore comparison with the arrhythmia induced by PES is impossible.

Monomorphic nonsustained ventricular tachycardia. It is extremely uncommon to induce nonsustained monomorphic ventricular tachycardia in patients without structural heart disease and who have had no documented ventricular arrhythmias.[5] Ten years ago we found that the clinical arrhythmia could be induced by pacing in only 8% of patients with documented nonsustained monomorphic ventricular tachycardia but no heart disease.[9] Recently Buxton et al.[12] found a higher induction rate in patients with documented monomorphic nonsustained ventricular tachycardia and coronary artery disease than in patients with idiopathic ventricular tachycardia (83% vs 30%). Use of isoproterenol increased the rate of induction in the group with idiopathic ventricular tachycardia.

Our group found that shortly after myocardial infarction nonsustained monomorphic ventricular tachycardia could be initiated in 20% of patients,[11] regardless of the clinical occurrence of this arrhythmia. The arrhythmia could be induced in 14% of patients with one or two extrastimuli. These observations suggest that one should question the use of induction of a nonsustained ventricular tachycardia (from 3 beats to more than 10 sec) as an end point for assessing antiarrhythmic therapy or identification of risk for subsequent development of ventricular arrhythmias.[13] We conclude that the significance of induction of nonsustained monomorphic ventricular tachycardia is presently unknown.

Polymorphic ventricular tachycardia. Polymorphic ventricular tachycardia is the most frequent ventricular arrhythmia initiated by PES in patients without spontaneous sustained arrhythmias or structural heart disease and the incidence of this arrhythmia increases with the number of extrastimuli used in the stimulation protocol.[3, 14] This suggests that polymorphic ventricular tachycardia is a "non-specific response to aggressive stimulation protocols."[14]

Sustained polymorphic ventricular tachycardia is induced more frequently in patients resuscitated from sudden death than in those presenting with sustained ventricular tachycardia without cardiac arrest, suggesting that it may be a precursor of ventricular fibrillation. The initiation of nonsustained polymorphic ventricular tachycardia has also been interpreted to be indicative of a greater risk of ventricular fibrillation and sudden death.

We recently compared the incidence of inducible polymorphic ventricular tachycardia in 32 patients without structural heart disease who were evaluated for suspected supraventricular arrhythmias with that in 36 patients who had spontaneous sustained ventricular tachycardia or ventricular fibrillation more than 10 days after myocardial infarction.[15] We found no difference between the normal subjects and the patients with previous myocardial infarction with respect to the incidence of greater than 5 beats of polymorphic ventricular tachycardia when ventricular pacing protocols up to the step including three extrastimuli delivered at a cycle length of 600 msec were used. The cumulative risk of inducing this arrhythmia with up to two extrastimuli during sinus rhythm and ventricular pacing at cycle lengths of 600, 500, and 430 msec was 38% in the normal subjects and 51% in the myocardial infarction group ($p = NS$).

We therefore conclude that the initiation of polymorphic ventricular tachycardia per se during PES is a nonspecific finding. Its incidence increases with the use of more aggressive stimulation protocols. Polymorphic ventricular tachycardia can, however, initiate a sustained monomorphic ventricular tachycardia and therefore be the initiating mechanism of a clinically significant arrhythmia. In a consecutive series of 26 patients with clinically documented sustained monomorphic ventricular tachycardia we found that during PES polymorphic ventricular tachycardia preceded the monomorphic type in 19%.[15]

Ventricular fibrillation. Ventricular fibrillation can be induced during PES in patients with normal hearts, those with abnormal hearts without documentation of ventricular arrhythmias, those with abnormal hearts and documented ventricular arrhythmias, and in patients resuscitated from sudden death.[5, 13] The number of premature ventricular stimuli required to induce ventricular fibrillation in the normal heart is usually higher than that required in the abnormal heart.[5] In view of the overlap between the two groups, however, induction of ventricular fibrillation should in our opinion be considered an aspecific finding. The incidence of ventricular fibrillation induction increases with use of more aggressive stimulation protocols.

In patients with coronary heart disease we found no differences in the incidence of induction of ventricular fibrillation in patients with 3-week-old myocardial infarctions without spontaneous ventricular arrhythmias, patients with 3-week-old myocardial infarctions and documented nonsustained monomorphic ventricular tachycardia, patients suffering from clinically documented sustained monomorphic ventricular tachycardia after myocardial infarction, and patients with coronary heart disease resuscitated from sudden death.[11] These findings stress again the nonspecificity of induction of ventricular fibrillation.

What is the proper stimulation protocol?

PES is used in different categories of patients with proven or suspected ventricular arrhythmias. Since different protocols are used in different institutions and no unanimity of opinion exists as to the correct one to use to facilitate comparison, we favor presentation of the results of PES in the way shown in figure 1, which is similar to a survival analysis curve. A display of results in the way shown in this figure can be used to (1) analyze the sensitivity of different programmed stimulation protocols, (2) compare modes of induction

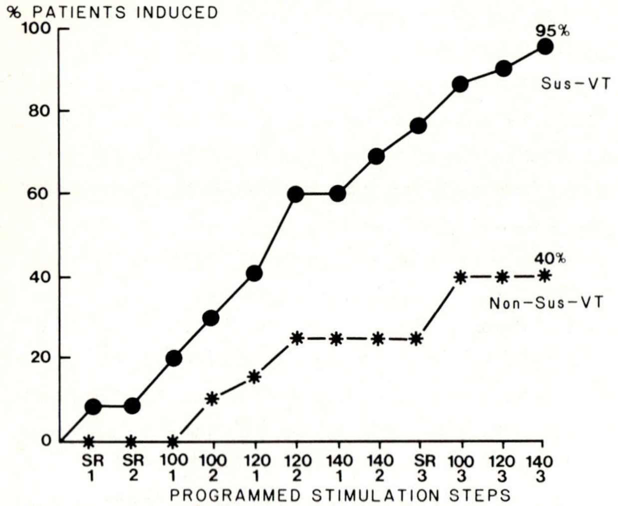

FIGURE 1. Visual display of the results of programmed ventricular stimulation of 100 patients. Fifty patients had documented sustained monomorphic ventricular tachycardia (sus-VT) and 50 patients had documented nonsustained VT (non-sus-VT) after myocardial infarction. A standardized programmed ventricular stimulation protocol with 12 different consecutive steps was used in all of these patients. The curves illustrate the cumulative percentage of patients at each step in whom a sustained monomorphic ventricular tachycardia was induced. The steps are shown on the horizontal axis in the order they were performed. (SR 1 = one extrastimulus during sinus rhythm; SR 2 = two extrastimuli during sinus rhythm; 100,1 = one extrastimulus during pacing at 100/min; etc.) All stimulation was done in the right ventricular apex. Display of results of PES in this way, which is similar to a survival analysis curve allows: (1) immediate recognition of the total percentage of patients in whom sustained monomorphic ventricular tachycardia was induced (95% and 40% in the figure), (2) recognition of stimulation steps that were ineffective (for instance, pacing with 140/min and one extrastimulus in both groups of patients) (3) log-rank test recognition of programmed stimulation steps that contributed significant differences in the results of the stimulation protocol between the two groups (for example, pacing at 120/min with two extrastimuli). (4) determination of the relative efficacy or lack thereof of the program by studying the area under the curve and comparing it with the total area, and (5) determination of the mean number of extrastimuli and stimulation steps required to induce a sustained ventricular tachycardia that can be calculated and compared between the two groups.

in different patient populations when the same protocol is used (as illustrated in figure 1), (3) refine programmed stimulation protocols in relation to type and cause of ventricular tachycardia, (4) assess significance of induced arrhythmias in relation to mode of induction, and (5) assess changes in inducibility pattern before and after drug treatment.

The patient with a documented sustained monomorphic ventricular tachycardia. In accordance with the findings with regard to monomorphic ventricular tachycardia that we discussed above, we believe that to reproduce the arrhythmia in patients with documented sustained monomorphic ventricular tachycardia, right ventricular apical stimulation using one site, three basic pacing rates, and a maximum of three extrastimuli is usually sufficient. Stimulation from another right ventricular site or the left ventricle is indicated only in the rare patient in whom this stimulation protocol does not result in initiation of the clinical arrhythmia and in whom endocavitary mapping is essential for subsequent surgical treatment.

The patient resuscitated from sudden death. Holter recordings have shown that most episodes of sudden death are the result of ventricular fibrillation. In patients in whom no acute ischemia is the underlying mechanism ventricular tachycardia frequently precedes fibrillation. Unfortunately, in these patients multiple-lead electrocardiographic documentation of QRS configuration of this ventricular tachycardia is not available. Therefore, determination of the end point of the stimulation study becomes difficult. Initiation of a monomorphic sustained ventricular tachycardia, which is frequently observed during PES in the patient resuscitated outside hospital, indicates that the substrate for sustained ventricular reentry is present.[13] In a recent study we found that in 60% of patients resuscitated from sudden death more than 3 weeks after a myocardial infarction a monomorphic ventricular tachycardia could be initiated.[15] Typically, and in contrast to the patient coming to the hospital with sustained monomorphic ventricular tachycardia, the arrhythmia in the patients we studied was fast and frequently required cardioversion because of hemodynamic compromise or deterioration into ventricular fibrillation. As already discussed, with the use of the same PES protocol the same arrhythmia can be induced in 45% of patients who have survived acute myocardial infarction but have never had an episode of a life-threatening ventricular arrhythmia.

In 20% to 40% of patients resuscitated outside the hospital no life-threatening ventricular arrhythmias can be induced by PES. In these patients other causes for their fatal arrhythmias, such as ischemia, electrolyte abnormalities, the administration of antiarrhythmic drugs, have to be identified and, when possible, corrected. This allows effective long-term management.

We conclude that in patients resuscitated from sudden death a rapid ventricular tachycardia resulting in severe hemodynamic changes or deteriorating into ventricular fibrillation can frequently be initiated with the pacing protocol described above for patients with documented sustained monomorphic ventricular tachycardia. The hemodynamic consequences of the arrhythmia initiated by this method usually do not allow endocardial mapping, so that PES is not helpful in localizing the site of origin of the arrhythmia under these conditions. Initiation of ventricular fibrillation by PES is in itself a nonspecific finding.

The patient with short-lasting ventricular tachycardia. The purpose of PES is to induce the clinically occurring arrhythmia. This requires electrocardiographic registration of the arrhythmia in several simultaneously recorded leads both before and during PES to document their similarity. Proving similarity of polymorphic ventricular tachycardias presents a formidable problem. Also, as discussed above, initiation of a nonsustained polymorphic ventricular tachycardia during PES is common, even in normal hearts. We do not believe, therefore, that PES is useful in patients with polymorphic ventricular tachycardia.

Initiation of clinically documented nonsustained monomorphic ventricular tachycardia seems to be more common in patients with coronary heart disease than in those without structural cardiac abnormalities. Therefore, PES is of dubious or no value in patients with nonstained polymorphic ventricular tachycardia and of questionable (cause-related) value in those with the nonsustained monomorphic type.

The patient with syncope. Syncope of cardiovascular origin can be related to bradycardia or tachycardia. In view of the previously discussed observations during PES in patients without documented ventricular arrhythmias, we believe that initiation of nonsustained polymorphic ventricular tachycardia or ventricular fibrillation is of no diagnostic value. Only when sustained ventricular tachycardia is induced can a causal relation to syncope be surmized and antiarrhythmic therapy instituted. The PES protocol should, in patients being evaluated because of syncope, not only consist of the steps mentioned above for patients with monomorphic ventricular tachycardia, but should also include steps to exclude the possibility of disease of the sinus node and the atrioventricular conduction system.

Identification of the patient at high risk of sudden death after myocardial infarction

It has been suggested that results of PES studies are independent markers in the recognition of infarct survivors at risk of dying suddenly.[10] The induction of ventricular tachycardia of 10 sec or more was found to be related to an important increase in arrhythmic death in the first year after myocardial infarction. However, there is no unanimous opinion about the value of PES in identifying those at high risk of sudden death after myocardial infarction.

Marchlinski et al.,[16] using up to two extrastimuli, induced sustained monomorphic ventricular tachycardia 2 to 8 weeks after myocardial infarction in 13% of 40 patients, none of whom subsequently died suddenly or developed sustained ventricular tachycardia over a mean follow-up of 18 months. Using up to three extrastimuli, we have found that a sustained monomorphic ventricular tachycardia could be induced in 45% of patients with previous myocardial infarction who had had no spontaneous episodes of sustained ventricular tachycardia.[11] None of these patients died during a mean follow-up of 6 months.

Since the risk of sudden death after hospital discharge in the first year after myocardial infarction was found to be less than 10% in two recent multicenter studies, the initiation of a sustained monomorphic ventricular tachycardia must be of limited prognostic significance in many patients who are not suffering from spontaneous occurrences of this arrhythmia before undergoing PES.

The value of PES in the selection of antiarrhythmic therapy. The possibility of reproducible initiation and termination of clinical arrhythmias in patients with recurrent sustained ventricular tachycardia by PES led to the use of this technique for rational selection of antiarrhythmic drug therapy. If one drug does not prevent initiation of ventricular tachycardia during PES, the effect of the next drug is studied. The protocol followed during serial drug testing in these patients is shown in figure 2. When such an approach is used patients with true- and false-negative test results after taking the drug are not identified. The value of this method, however, is supported by reports indicating that identification and use of a drug that prevents induction of ventricular tachycardia results in a much better prognosis than if no such drug can be found. Unfortunately, a drug that prevents induction of ventricular tachycardia can be identified in only 25% of patients with documented life-threatening ventricular arrhythmias, and this percentage will be even lower when aggressive stimulation protocols or left ventricular stimulation is used. Also, with newer antiarrhythmic agents like amiodarone and propafenone the drug may be clinically effective, but fail to prevent induction of ventricular tachycardia during PES. This finding led to the acceptance of other indicators during PES pointing to a beneficial effect of a drug such as slowing in rate of the induced tachycardia, change from sustained to nonsustained tachycardia, or the need for a more aggressive PES protocol to initiate the arrhythmia.

We believe that the predictive value of PES in the patient with documented sustained monomorphic ventricular tachycardia can be summed up as follows:

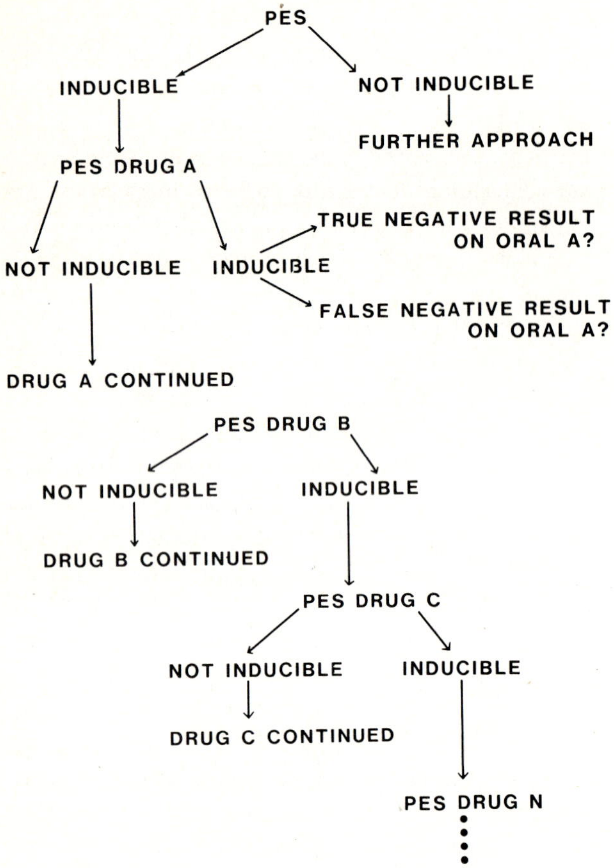

FIGURE 2. Currently used protocol for serial testing of drugs.

Excellent: prevention of induction of tachycardia during PES
Satisfactory: induced tachycardia has slower rate or is self-terminating
Questionable: more "aggressive" PES protocol required to initiate tachycardia
Unknown: no changes in induction of tachycardia

Taking into consideration our discussion of the significance of ventricular arrhythmias induced by PES, it seems clear that it is not acceptable to base therapeutic decisions on the effect of antiarrhythmic drugs on an induced arrhythmic response such as polymorphic ventricular tachycardia or ventricular fibrillation.

To find answers to the questions raised, especially in regard to the newer antiarrhythmic drugs, we favor the approach shown in figure 3. This will not only allow us to obtain information on the effectiveness of a drug for the prevention of the tachycardia initiating premature depolarization, but also will give us an idea about the true value of PES in the selection of antiarrhythmic therapy.

Conclusions

PES is being used increasingly in the management of patients with proven or suspected ventricular arrhythmias. In our opinion, however, only the induction of clinically documented sustained monomorphic ventricular tachycardia has convincingly been demonstrated to be a significant finding during PES, so that only in patients with this disorder can the value of PES for selecting antiarrhythmic therapy be tested.

Although one is tempted to accept the induction of sustained monomorphic ventricular tachycardia as an important finding in the patient with syncope, cardiac arrest, or myocardial infarction, our observations indicate that in diseased hearts such an arrhythmia may be induced but may never become clinically manifest. Further study is required to inform us about the significance of induction of sustained monomorphic ventricular tachycardia in the patient without documented arrhythmias of this type. As pointed out, no convincing evidence has been presented that the induction of nonsustained ventricular tachycardia, polymorphic ventricular tachycardia, or ventricular fibrillation is a reliable indicator of risk of arrhythmic death or a dependable method for evaluating efficacy of therapy with antiarrhythmic agents. We cannot exclude the possibility that refinements in characterization of the ventricular arrhythmias induced may lead to different conclusions.

The stimulation protocol used should be able to demonstrate the presence or absence of the substrate for sustained monomorphic ventricular tachycardia. A single right ventricular stimulation site, three basic pacing rates, and up to three extrastimuli can generally

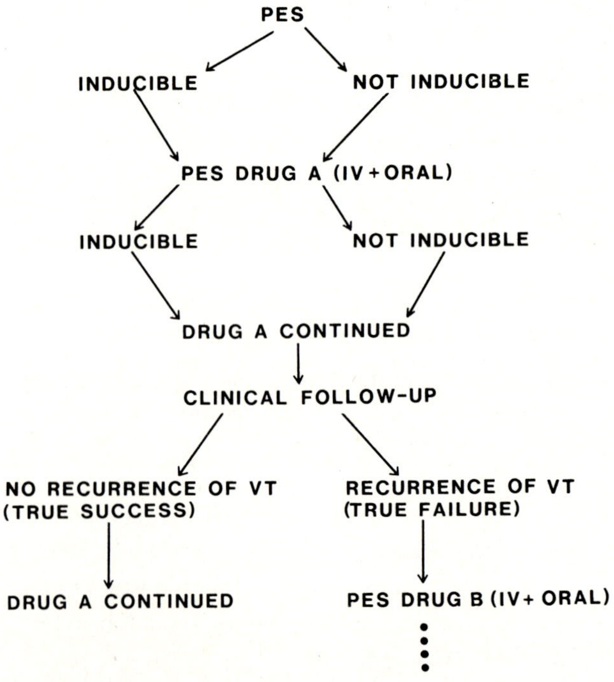

FIGURE 3. Suggested approach to testing the validity of use of PES of the heart in selecting drug treatment (so-called parallel testing).

be considered adequate. More study is needed, however, to reduce the steps necessary for the stimulation procedure. A reduction in time period of the investigation will have obvious financial benefits and will make PES more comfortable and possibly safer for patient and investigator.

Prevention of induction of ventricular tachycardia after drug administration is a useful therapeutic finding. Persistence of the arrhythmia after antiarrhythmic therapy, however, does not rule out clinical effectiveness of the drug.

References

1. Wellens HJJ, Schuilenburg RM, Durrer D: Electrical stimulation of the heart in patients with ventricular tachycardia. Circulation **46:** 216, 1972
2. Vandepol CJ, Farshidi A, Spielman SR, Greenspan AM, Horowitz LN, Josephson ME: Incidence and significance of induced ventricular tachycardia. Am J Cardiol **45:** 725, 1980
3. Buxton AE, Waxman HL, Marchlinski FE, Untereker WJ, Waspe LE, Josephson ME: Role of triple extrastimuli during electrophysiologic study of patients with documented sustained ventricular tachyarrhythmias. Circulation **69:** 532, 1984
4. Morady F, DiCarlo L, Winston S, Davis JC, Scheinman MM: A prospective comparison of triple extrastimuli and left ventricular stimulation in studies of ventricular tachycardia induction. Circulation **70:** 52, 1984
5. Brugada P, Green M, Abdollah H, Wellens HJJ: Significance of ventricular arrhythmias initiated by programmed ventricular stimulation: The importance of the type of ventricular arrhythmia induced and the number of premature stimuli required. Circulation **69:** 87, 1984
6. Josephson ME, Marchlinski FE, Buxton AE, Waxman HL, Doherty JU, Kienzle MG, Falcone R: Electrophysiologic basis for sustained ventricular tachycardia. *In* Josephson ME, Wellens HJJ, editors: Tachycardia, mechanisms, diagnosis, treatment. Philadelphia, 1984, Lea and Febiger, p 305
7. Wellens HJJ, Düren DR, Lie KI: Observations on mechanisms of ventricular tachycardia in man. Circulation **54:** 237, 1976
8. Brugada P, Wellens HJJ: A comparison in the same patient of 2 programmed ventricular stimulation protocols to induce ventricular tachycardia. Am J Cardiol **55:** 380, 1985
9. Wellens HJJ: Value and limitations of programmed electrical stimulation of the heart in the study and treatment of tachycardias. Circulation **57:** 845, 1978
10. Richards DA, Cody DV, Dennis AR, Russell PA, Young AA, Uther JB: Ventricular electrical instability: a predictor of death after myocardial infarction. Am J Cardiol **51:** 75, 1983
11. Brugada P, Waldecker B, Wellens HJJ: Characteristics of induced ventricular arrhythmias in four subgroups of patients with myocardial infarction. Circulation **70**(suppl II): II-29, 1984
12. Buxton AE, Marchlinski FE, Doherty JU, Cassidy DM, Vassalle JA, Flores BT, Josephson ME: Repetitive, monomorphic ventricular tachycardia: Clinical and electrophysiologic characteristics in patients with and patients without organic heart disease. Am J Cardiol **54:** 997, 1984
13. Ruskin JN, DiMarco JP, Garan H: Out-of-hospital cardiac arrest: Electrophysiologic observation and selection of long-term antiarrhythmic therapy. N Engl J Med **303:** 607, 1980
14. Brugada P, Abdollah H, Heddle W, Wellens HJJ: Results of a ventricular stimulation protocol using a maximum of four premature stimuli in patients without documented or suspected ventricular arrhythmias. Am J Cardiol **52:** 1214, 1983
15. Stevenson WG, Brugada P, Waldecker B, Zehender M, Wellens HJJ: Significance of polymorphic ventricular arrhythmias induced by programmed ventricular stimulation. Am J Cardiol (in press)
16. Marchlinski FE, Buxton AE, Waxman HL, Josephson ME: Identifying patients at risk of sudden death after myocardial infarction: value of response to programmed stimulation, degree of ventricular ectopic activity and severity of left ventricular dysfunction. Am J Cardiol **52:** 1190, 1983

Some reflections on arteriosclerosis: past, present, and future

Presidential Address

ANTONIO M. GOTTO, JR., M.D., D.PHIL.

THE EMPHASIS of the annual meeting of the American Heart Association and of the Presidential Address is usually on the most recent advances in cardiovascular disease and what these imply for the present and future. Instead, I would like to first present a historical perspective, and to attempt to give a panoramic view of arteriosclerosis as a circulatory disease — past, present, and future. I have selected certain individuals, their writings, their lectures, and their discoveries to serve as roadmarks in the long history of this disease. I am indebted to a number of medical writers and medical historians in the preparation of this review, but I would like to acknowledge in particular the books *The History of Coronary Heart Disease* by J. O. Leibowitz of the Hebrew University of Jerusalem, and *The History of the Heart and Circulation* by Fredrick A. Willius and Thomas J. Dry from the University of Minnesota.

I would like to begin with two physicians of antiquity because of the importance of their discoveries and because of their long-lasting influence on those studying the circulatory system. The first is an Egyptian physician named Erasistratus, who lived around 300 B.C. He was able to carry out an extensive study of organs of the body and described three pathways: veins, arteries, and nerves. His description of the heart and the heart valves is a very accurate one. However, Erasistratus believed that arteries contained a substance called pneuma that was replaced each time a person breathed. Pneuma may be taken to be synonomous with air or spirit, or soul. Erasistratus believed that veins carried blood to nourish the tissues and that the arteries contained pneuma only during life. When an artery was cut, blood rushed in as the pneuma escaped.[1]

I would like to shift in time to 120 A.D. and to the city of Pergamos in Asia minor where there lived a man named Claudius Galen who had more influence on medicine than any other individual for the next 1500 years (figure 1). It is astonishing today to think of the impact that Galen had on medicine. With knowledge gained from dissecting apes and other animals that were killed by the Roman gladiators, Galen demonstrated that the heart is made up of muscle and he described the presence and movement of blood in the arteries. He made many important contributions to medicine, but several of his erroneous views were documented as truth by the Church and accepted as dogma for 1500 years. It was not until the Renaissance that anyone dared challenge his authority. Galen believed that the liver, rather than the heart, was the central organ of the circulation (figure 2). He viewed blood in arteries as ebbing and flowing with the heart's pulsation. While his view of the circulation was erroneous, Galen was correct in suggesting that blood moved from one side of the heart to the other. He was faced with the problem of describing how blood passed from the right to the left side of the heart. He proposed the hypothesis that the interventricular septum contained small pores that allowed the blood to pass from the right side to the left where it entered the arteries to pass out to the tissues.[2, 3] Humility was not one of Galen's attributes. He once said that if anyone desired to become famous, one had only to accept what he had accepted.

Medical knowledge quickly declined between the time of Galen and that of the Renaissance. The Renaissance rekindled man's desire for discovery and exploration. Not only were there courageous explorers who sailed the oceans, there also came a new breed of scientists and physicians interested in studying the mysteries of life. The spirit of medical inquiry was recaptured.

During the Renaissance, Leonardo da Vinci, who lived from 1452 to 1519, illustrated the close relationship between art and medicine (figure 3). He prepared approximately 750 anatomical drawings, about 600 of

From the Department of Medicine, Baylor College of Medicine, The Methodist Hospital, Houston.

This *Perspective* summarizes Dr. Gotto's Presidential Address to the annual meeting of the American Heart Association, Nov. 12, 1984, Miami Beach.

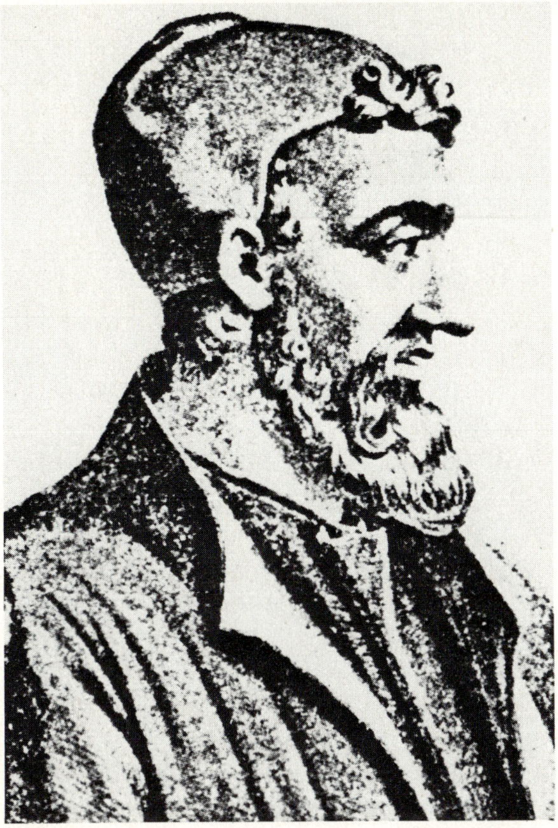

FIGURE 1. Claudius Galen. (Reprinted, with permission, from Willius and Dry.[3])

which remain today at Windsor Castle. Leonardo had problems drawing the coronary vessels since "they are surrounded by waxy fat." This was possibly why some early anatomists had failed to observe the coronary arteries. Leonardo demonstrated the origin of the coronary vessels, and his drawings indicate changes with aging. In his drawing *The Anatomy of the Old Man*, the vessels appear as tortuous. Leonardo wrote, "vessels in the elderly, through the thickenings of the tunics, restrict the transit of the blood," and "the artery and the vein in the aged which extend between the spleen and the liver, acquires so thick a covering that it contracts the passage of blood. . . ." This is one of the earliest descriptions of the changes of arteriosclerosis. In the *Anatomy of the Old Man* Leonardo describes, "debility through lack of blood and deficiency of the artery which nourishes the heart and the other lower members." This reference apparently refers to a diminished blood flow through the aorta.[2] Leonardo's illustrations of the coronary arteries are exquisite and very precise, and these, along with his descriptions, added much to the limited knowledge of the age.

Another great collection of medical illustrations is found in the book called *De Humani Corporis Fabrica Libri Septem*, published in 1555 by Andreas Vesalius (figure 4). Andreas, born in 1514, went to Paris when he was 18 years old to study anatomy (figure 5). At this time, the study of anatomy was greatly hampered by a 14th century edict of Pope Boniface VII that prohibited the dismemberment of corpses. Vesalius obtained his medical degree in Paris in 1537 and subsequently carried out his studies at the University of Padua, where he became a professor and discovered more than 200 errors of Galen. His lectures at Padua might be described as mob scenes. There was hysterical shouting and cheering as he was violently attacked by pro-Galenic forces. Vesalius wrote of one of his patients whom he called "the most noble and learned Dominus de Imersel," a member of the court of Charles V. Vesalius described a "sad feeling and pain in the heart of poor Imersel," explaining that, "in the left ventricle of his heart we found almost two pounds of glandulous flesh, whereby the heart distended like a belly around this flesh." This man "was, before his death, in a persistant melancholic and wakeful state, his pulse being really astonishingly unequal and changeable, manifestly demonstrating the contraction of the artery."[2] Vesalius made the inference that this "sad feeling and pain" was related to heart disease, an idea that

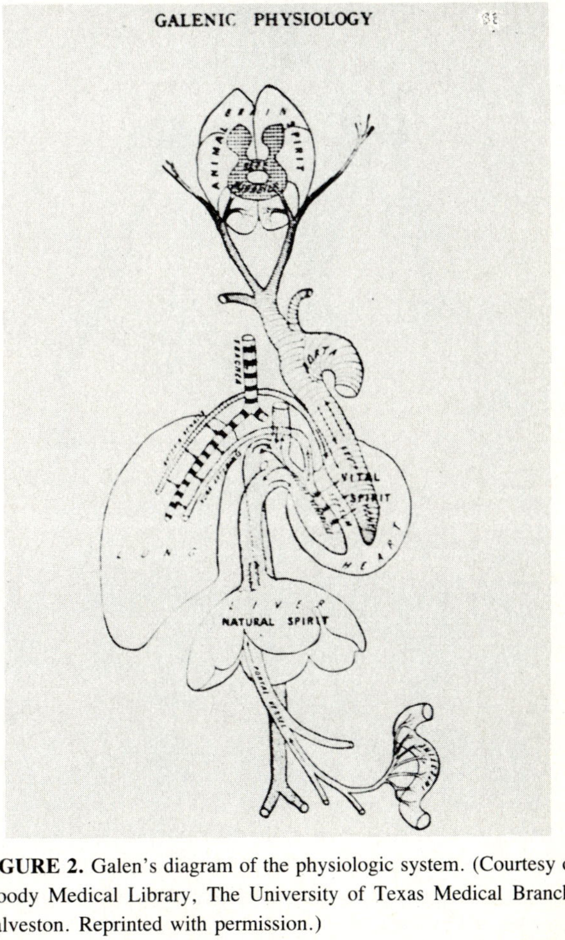

FIGURE 2. Galen's diagram of the physiologic system. (Courtesy of Moody Medical Library, The University of Texas Medical Branch, Galveston. Reprinted with permission.)

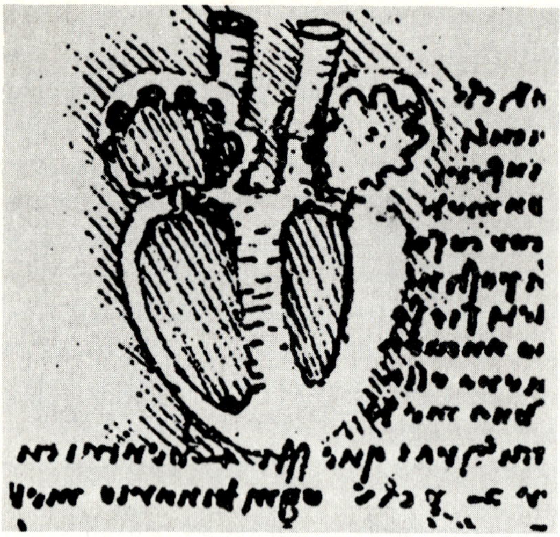

FIGURE 3. Leonardo da Vinci's drawing of the heart. (Reprinted, with permission, from Willius and Dry.[3])

was not to be accepted until more than 200 years later.

William Harvey is credited, and rightly so, with the discovery of the circulation, described in his book *De Motu Cordis*, or *The Motion of the Heart*, published in

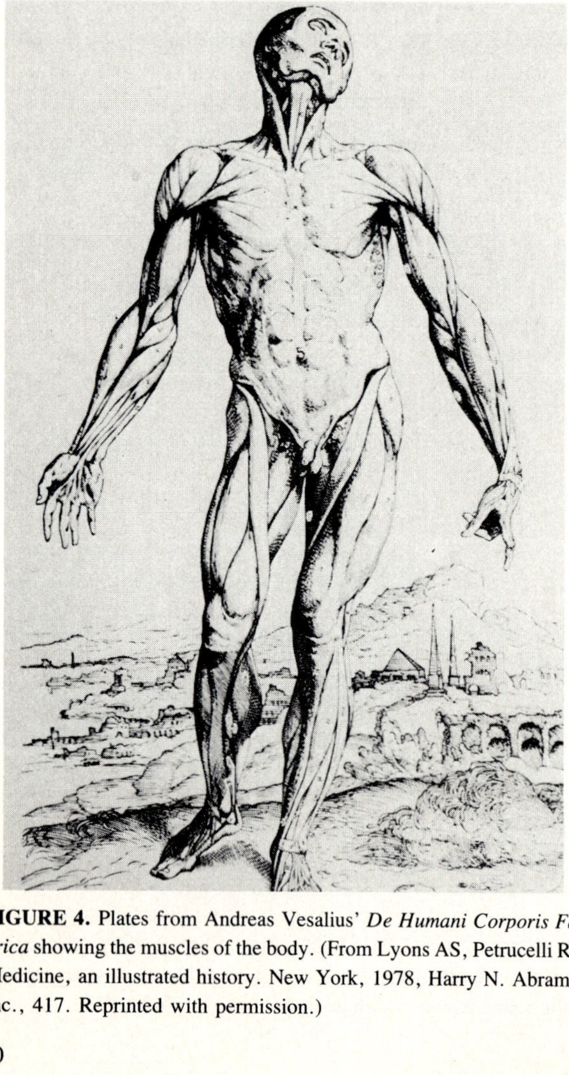

FIGURE 4. Plates from Andreas Vesalius' *De Humani Corporis Fabrica* showing the muscles of the body. (From Lyons AS, Petrucelli RJ: Medicine, an illustrated history. New York, 1978, Harry N. Abrams, Inc., 417. Reprinted with permission.)

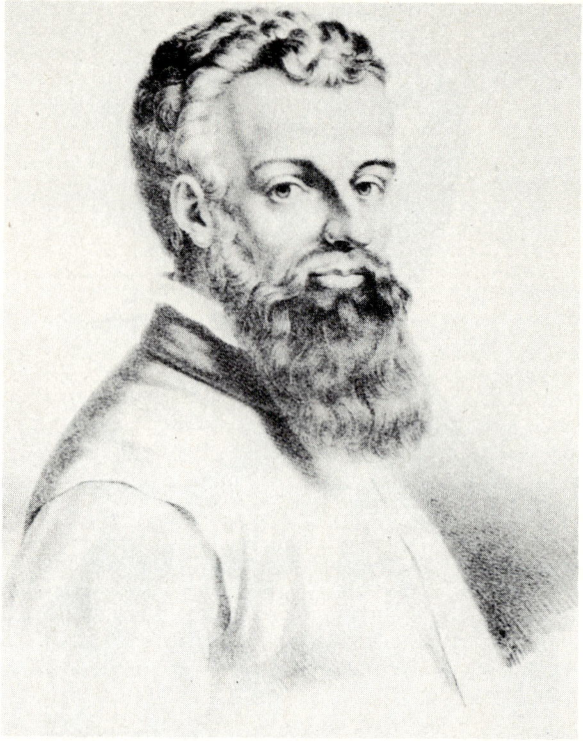

FIGURE 5. Andreas Vesalius. (Courtesy of Moody Medical Library, The University of Texas Medical Branch, Galveston. Reprinted with permission.)

1828 (figure 6). It is important to realize, though, that as much a landmark as was Harvey's discovery, it was not made in isolation. Great breakthroughs in medical knowledge are almost always dependent upon other discoveries and the intellectual climate of the time. Harvey benefited from the great advances in knowledge about the human body that occurred during the Renaissance and that were centered in Northern Italy. The intellectual lineage of Harvey's predecessors was as follows: Andreas Vesalius was a professor of anatomy at Padua, and was the teacher of Columbo, who in turn was the teacher both of Fabricus and of Andreas Cesalpino. Fabricus was also a professor of anatomy in Padua; he discovered the valves in the veins, and was the teacher of William Harvey.[3]

Andrea Cesalpino of Arezzo lived from approximately 1525 to 1603 and accurately described the circulation in several of his writings, one of which was published in 1571, and which actually used the words "blood circulation" (figure 7). Most of his scientific observations, unfortunately, were buried in long philosophical and religious treatises, one of which was devoted to the subject of demons. In about 1592, Cesalpino was called to Rome to serve as physician to the Pope. He also became Professor of Medicine at the University of Rome during this period. Cesalpino's description of the circulation was not nearly as clear

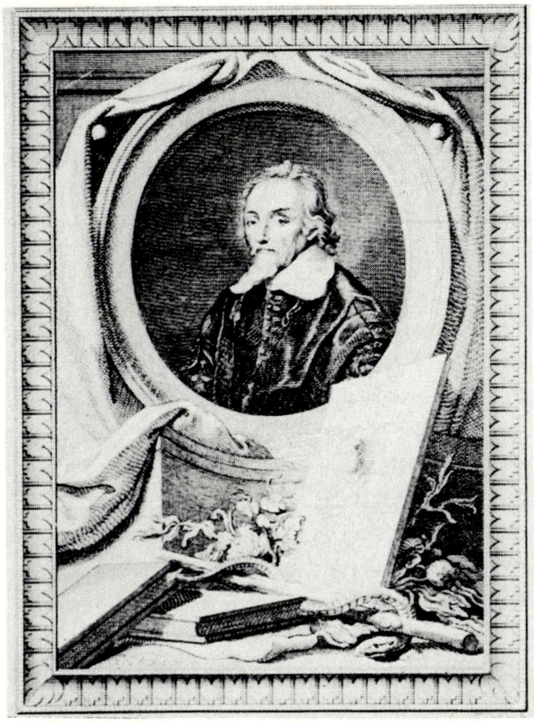

FIGURE 6. William Harvey. (Courtesy of Moody Medical Library, The University of Texas Medical Branch, Galveston. Reprinted with permission.)

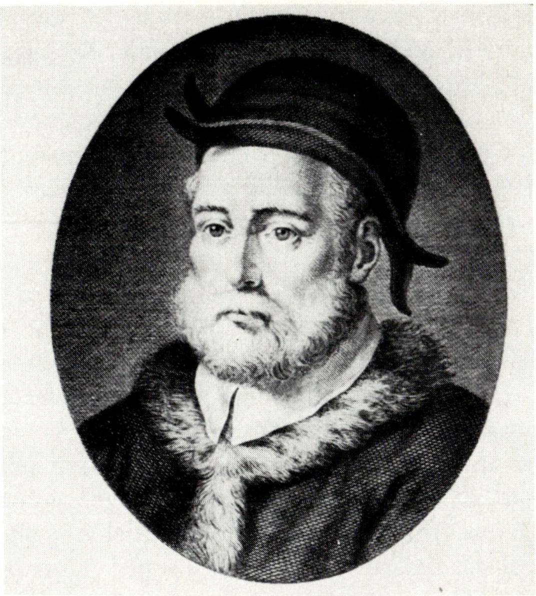

FIGURE 7. Andrea Cesalpino. (Courtesy of Moody Medical Library, The University of Texas Medical Branch, Galveston. Reprinted with permission.)

and precise as Harvey's, nor did it have the experimental evidence produced by Harvey to support its claims. Harvey closely observed the pumping action of the heart. His major achievement was in establishing the concept that the circulation was a closed system, and he was the first to establish the principal features of the circulation on a quantitative basis.[4, 5]

It was more than 200 years later that William Heberden described angina pectoris as a manifestation of heart disease (figure 8). Heberden, who lived from 1710 to 1801, read his article, "Some Account of a Disorder of the Breast" at the College of Physicians in 1768, and published it in 1772. Heberden was greatly admired and respected in his time for his high standards of scholarship and for his integrity. He stated that he made his observations in "the chambers of the sick"; he was not affiliated with a hospital. His interpretations were very conservative and today he would be considered slow to publish. While there certainly were inferences about angina pectoris by earlier writers, including Harvey, Heberden did not appear to have knowledge of these. He described heart pain on exertion as follows, "they who are afflicted with it, are seized while they are walking (especially if it be uphill, and soon after eating) with a painful and most disagreeable sensation in the breast, which seems as if it would extinguish life if it were to increase or to continue; but the moment they stand still, all this uneasiness vanishes." This is a typical description of angina with effort.[2]

On November 17, 1772, Heberden wrote a paper on

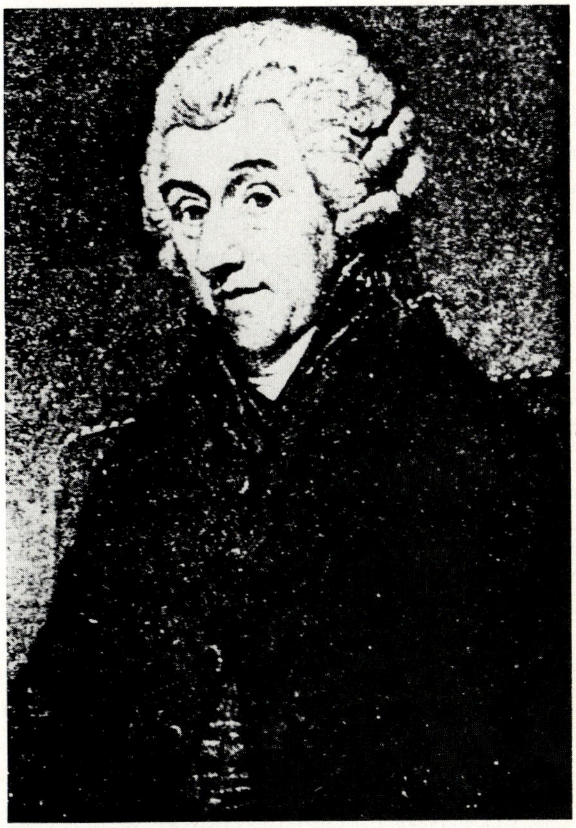

FIGURE 8. William Heberden. (Reprinted, with permission, from Willius and Dry.[3])

an individual he called "Doctor Anonymous" and published it 13 years later in 1785. Doctor Anonymous was a 52-year-old physician-patient who had a tendency toward obesity. He first experienced symptoms at age 47 when he had chest pain radiating down the left arm upon walking. "I attributed it to an obstruction in the circulation, sensations which to me seemed to indicate a sudden death." He described these symptoms in a letter to Heberden. After he died, Doctor Anonymous' serum was described as "thick like cream"; this possibly was the earliest description of hyperlipidemia. The doctor died suddenly after suffering an attack of angina pectoris. Heberden described the higher incidence of angina pectoris in men versus women, and he singled out angina pectoris from other types of heart conditions. His great contribution was in his emphasis of clinical description, rather than anatomical findings.[2]

Another interesting case involves the examination performed by the famous surgical pathologist John Hunter in 1775. Upon dissection of the coronary arteries Hunter found "(they) were transformed into one piece of bone . . . the blood had not in the least coagulated." The patient described here was a 63-year-old man who had complaints 3 or 4 years before his death. Hunter wrote, "In a sudden and violent transport of anger, he fell down and expired immediately." This description illustrates the importance of emotion, stress, and anger in precipitating coronary death.[2] Hunter himself suffered from angina pectoris and reportedly died suddenly after a violent argument with a hospital colleague.[3]

The Quaker physician, John Fothergill (1712–1780) gave interesting advice concerning the prevention of coronary disease and arteriosclerosis. On the first appearance of symptoms, he advised the patient to adopt a plan of restricted food, which "might greatly retard the progress of the disorder, and to restrain excesses of passion and anxiety, which perhaps contribute more to the increase of this disease than a combination of all other causes." Thus, Fothergill forecast the role of diet and psychosocial factors in the etiology of coronary heart disease.[2]

While Heberden related angina pectoris to disease of the heart, it remained for Edward Jenner (1749–1832), the discoverer of the smallpox vaccine, to make the essential link between angina pectoris and disease of the coronary arteries. Jenner wrote a letter to Heberden in 1778 about a patient who had died of the angina pectoris. He described the coronary artery of a deceased doctor as being ossified and like a "fleshy tube" that did not appear to have any connection with the coat of the artery, and that may have represented a recanalized thrombus. He added that "the heart . . . was loaded with fat and the vessels were concealed in that substance."[2]

With these observations of ossification or calcification of the coronary arteries and of a blood clot within an artery, we are getting closer to a more precise description of the pathogenesis of angina pectoris and myocardial infarction. The first clear description of arteriosclerosis was presented by the Italian surgeon and anatomist Antonio Scarpa, who lived from 1752 to 1832 (figure 9). In his book, *Sull Aneurisma, Riflession: ed Osservazioni Anatomico-chirurgiche* (figure 10) he described the cause of aneurysm as "slow, morbid ulcerated, steatomatous, fungus, squamous degeneration of the internal coat of the artery." He further wrote, "these diseases, which sometimes soften the substance of the heart and dispose it to ulceration and rupture, are likewise common in the arteries."[2] Here is a description of a fatty, ulcerated lesion, and a statement that the disorganization of the internal coat is responsible for the development of arteriosclerosis. Both the concepts of fatty infiltration and of intimal involvement are present in Scarpa's description. Scarpa predicted correctly that the process causing

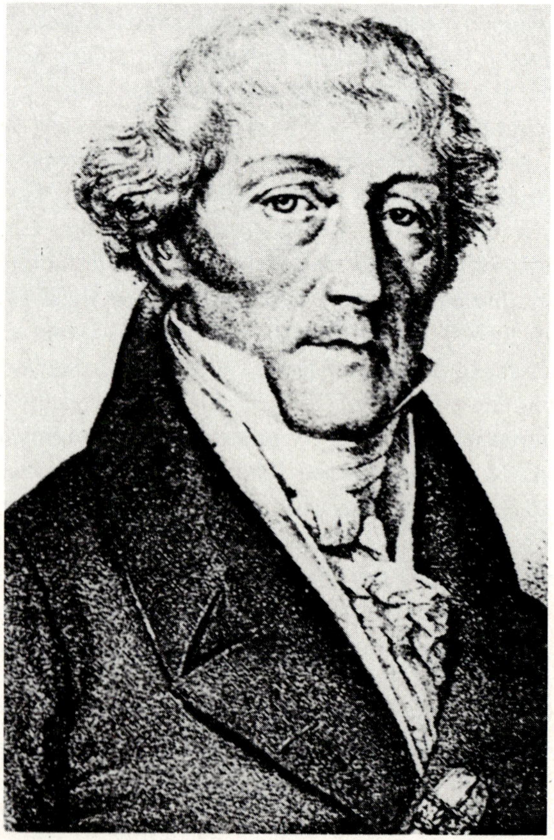

FIGURE 9. Antonio Scarpa. (Reprinted, with permission, from Willius and Dry.[3])

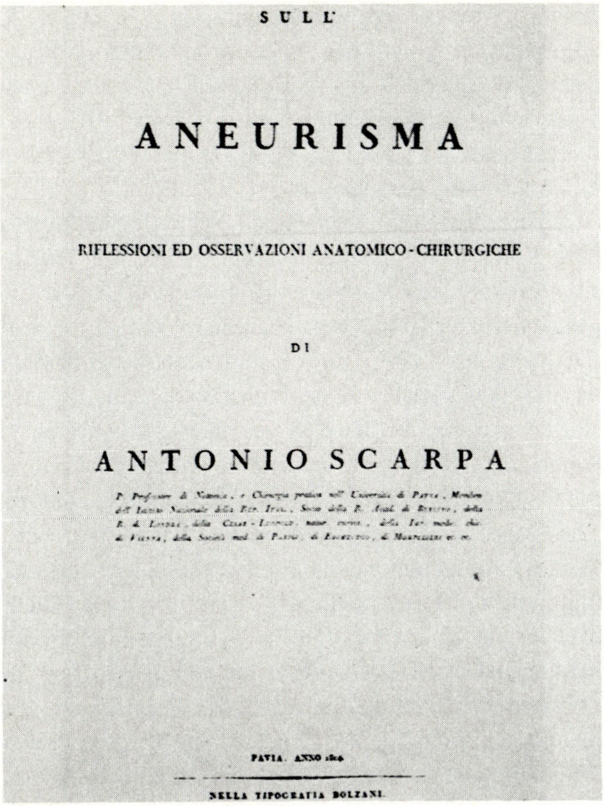
SULL'

ANEURISMA

RIFLESSIONI ED OSSERVAZIONI ANATOMICO-CHIRURGICHE

DI

ANTONIO SCARPA

PAVIA. ANNO [illegible]

NELLA TIPOGRAFIA BOLZANI

FIGURE 10. Title page from *Sull Aneurisma, Riflession: ed Osservazioni Anatomico-chirurgiche* by Antonio Scarpa. (Reprinted, with permission, from Leibowitz.[2])

arteriosclerosis is a long-term one, and that it has unknown causes.

The term "arteriosclerosis" was coined in 1833 by Jean-Frederick Lobstein, a pathologist working in Strassburg. He wrote two treatises in which he used the term and he refers to it as a thickening and a hardening of the arteries. "Atheroma" is derived from the Greek word meaning "groats" or "porridge," and was revived in 1755 by Albrecht von Haller of Bern.[2] Monckeburg, in 1903, stressed that calcification of the media was a pathologic entity separate and distinct from intimal arteriosclerosis.[6] The term "atherosclerosis," referring to the type of arteriosclerosis affecting the intimal coat of the artery, was coined in 1904 by Marchand, a pathologist from Leipzig.[2]

Rudolph Virchow (1821–1902), who authored over 1000 papers, was interested in both thrombosis and arteriosclerosis. Virchow adopted the word "thrombosis," which actually dates back to Galen, who described a vascular obstruction due to thrombosis. Virchow noted three conditions necessary for thrombosis to occur: (1) an increase in the coagulability of the blood, (2) an increased sluggishness in blood flow, and (3) development of a lesion in the coats of blood vessels. Virchow thought that the atheroma represented a chronic inflammation of the intima, and believed intimal damage to be a very early step in the development of an atheroma. He believed that cholesterol accumulation occurred late in the sequence of events, and he observed gelatinous swelling of the intima preceding the formation of an atherosclerotic plaque.[2]

Baron Karl von Rokitansky was one of the leading pathologists of his day. His *Manual of Pathological Anatomy*, published in the 1840s, ran counter to Virchow's view that inflammation was an important factor in the etiology of atherosclerosis. Instead, Rokitansky proposed that atherosclerosis developed in the intima because of the formation of many small blood clots that were eventually converted into scar tissue. Rokitansky's view was that "the deposit is an endogenous product derived from the blood, and for the most part from fibrin."[2]

The establishment of coronary thrombosis as a diagnosable clinical entity had to await the 20th century. We usually credit James Herrick with the first description in the article, "Clinical Features of Sudden Obstruction of the Coronary Arteries," published in the *Journal of the American Medical Association* in 1912. This report clearly related obstruction of the coronary arteries to chest pain and, in some instances, sudden death. Herrick described a sudden coronary blockage and emphasized the clinical recognition of coronary obstruction during a patient's life. Herrick said "the publication arroused no interest. It fell like a dud. Recognizing the radical nature of the view I held, I doggedly kept at the subject, doing what I called 'missionary work' . . . I hammered away at the topic. When in 1918, I showed lantern slides and electrocardiograms of coronary obstruction, physicians in America and later Europe woke up to the diagnosis, which was later to become a household word translated by the layman into 'heart attack.' "[2]

While Herrick generously credited earlier workers' contributions, he was unaware that two Russian clinicians from Kiev had published a similar description of the diagnosis of coronary artery thrombosis in 1910. W. P. Obrastzow and N. D. Straschesko described three cases in great detail. In two of these cases, diagnosis was made while the patient was still living. The two Russian doctors emphasized the role of physical exertion and emotional stress as precipitating events. They used the term thrombosis, while Herrick used the term coronary obstruction.[2]

The earliest descriptions of experimental arteriosclerosis are also attributable to Russian scientists. In 1908, A. I. Ignatovski demonstrated the relationship between diet and atherosclerosis by feeding milk and egg yolks to rabbits to induce severe atherosclerosis.[6] N. W. Stuckey, in 1912, found that while a diet high in egg yolk and brain caused arterial lesions, one containing sunflower seed and fish oil did not. N. Anichkov and S. Chalatov performed a classical experiment of cholesterol feeding in 1913 by adding pure cholesterol to a rabbit's diet to produce atherosclerosis. A very interesting summary of their work and of the research, carried out at the Anichkov school of pathology in Leningrad, was published in 1958 by A. L. Myasnikov.[2]

The 20th century brought many important contributions to the study of arteriosclerosis. These include the discovery of lipoproteins by Macheboef, the important discoveries concerning diet and atherosclerosis, the elaboration of the role of the endothelial injury hypothesis, the role of platelets, and the proliferative nature of plaque development.[7] Also important was the discovery of the relationship of risk factors, including plasma lipoproteins, hypertension, cigarette smoking, and diabetes, to the development and progression of coronary artery disease.

The study of atherosclerotic lesions continues to be an integral part of coronary heart disease research.[7, 8] Atherosclerotic lesions have been subdivided into fatty streaks, fibrous plaques, and complicated lesions. The proliferation of smooth muscle cells within the intima, the accumulation of cholesterol and cholesteryl esters, and the elaboration of connective tissue are accepted pathologic hallmarks of atherosclerosis. Injury to the endothelial cells may be provoked by hypercholesterolemia, hypertension, cigarette smoking, and diabetes. In hypercholesterolemic primates, blood monocytes can be seen adhering to the surface of endothelial cells. These cells may migrate into the intima, accumulate intracellular cholesterol, and become macrophages.[9, 10] Fatty streaks, which were described by Stary[11, 12] in the first decade of life, consist of mainly fat-filled macrophages and smooth muscle cells within the intima. If the endothelial lining becomes damaged, platelets from the blood adhere to the subendothelial matrix. A growth factor, originally discovered in platelets and called the platelet-derived growth factor (PDGF), may be released from platelets and from damaged endothelial cells, from macrophages, and possibly by altered smooth muscle cells under certain conditions. This growth factor stimulates the growth and proliferation of smooth muscle cells. This entire atherosclerotic process may represent an exaggerated form of wound healing. Thromboxane A_2 released from platelets is toxic to the arterial wall, while prostacyclin or PGI_2, produced by the endothelial cell, is protective. An angiogenesis growth factor, present in many tissues of the body, can stimulate endothelial cell growth, and could lead to capillary proliferation, manifested by an increase in the vasa vasorum, in the region of an atherosclerotic plaque.

Where do we go from here? What do we have to look forward to; what are the future directions of arteriosclerosis research in the 80s and the 90s? The first plenary session of this year's annual meeting dealt with the question — where do we stand with the cholesterol or LDL (low-density lipoprotein) hypothesis? Several studies reported in the past year have shown that the lowering of cholesterol by diet or drugs will decrease the rate of progression of an atherosclerotic plaque. The Coronary Primary Prevention Trial[13, 14] has provided the most conclusive evidence to date that lowering cholesterol and LDL will decrease coronary heart disease risk, defined as the sum of nonfatal and/or fatal myocardial infarctions. What we now need is a more effective and convenient way of lowering LDL and plasma cholesterol. The development of more potent drugs and the perfection of noninvasive methods for measuring the progression of arteriosclerosis should make it possible to test various treatment modalities more quickly and with fewer subjects.

There should be safe and effective ways of lowering LDL cholesterol by 50% or more by the end of this decade. One approach to reducing LDL is by stimulating the activity of the hepatic receptors that bind the lipoprotein and remove it from the circulation, an approach that is derived from the work of Brown and Goldstein. Figure 11 shows the inverse relationship between the relative number of LDL receptors in the liver and the concentration of plasma LDL. The Coronary Primary Prevention Trial used cholestyramine, which increases the activity of hepatic LDL receptors.

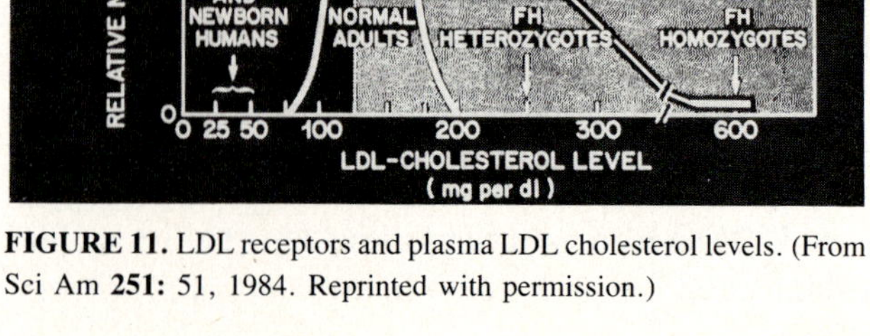

FIGURE 11. LDL receptors and plasma LDL cholesterol levels. (From Sci Am **251:** 51, 1984. Reprinted with permission.)

The combination of a bile acid sequestrant with a safe and effective inhibitor of hydroxymethylglutaryl coenzyme A reductase is one possible approach. Another potential approach is to devise ways of manipulating the activity of macrophage lipoprotein receptors. We do not know yet whether lipoprotein uptake by these receptors is harmful or protective to the arterial wall, but this question should be answerable.

Two other questions that demand answers are: Is it beneficial to raise high-density lipoprotein (HDL), and what are the long-term affects of doing so? Drugs that increase the activity of hepatic lipase, for example, might enhance cholesterol removal by the liver, decreasing the plasma level of HDL. Undoubtedly, if raising HDL concentrations does turn out to be beneficial, the pharmaceutical industry will devise new ways of accomplishing this. At the present time, the methods available include physical exercise, estrogen therapy, alcohol in moderate amounts, and drugs such as nicotinic acid and gemfibrozil. The use of estrogen would be restricted to postmenopausal females while moderate alcohol consumption has been shown to raise HDL in sedentary males, but not in exercising males or premenopausal females. In addition, alcohol has been found to raise the level of HDL_3, while the HDL_2 subfraction is thought to be associated with a decreased coronary risk. Because of the toxic effects of alcohol and the social hazards associated with its use, I cannot justify recommending alcohol consumption to the general public to prevent coronary disease, as popular as this approach might be with many of our patients.

More than likely, substances will be discovered that protect the arterial wall without exerting their primary effect on plasma lipids and lipoproteins. We do not yet know the precise cause of atherosclerosis. Once we do, we will be in a much stronger position to devise rational methods of treatment and prevention. Potential ways of protecting the arterial wall may be through reducing intracellular calcium overload with the use of slow-channel calcium blockers or other calcium antagonists. Other strategies are the development of agents that interfere with endogenous promoters of atherosclerosis such as PDGF or other growth factors, or through the manipulation of the metabolites of the arachidonic acid pathway. Specific vasodilator action is an appealing approach that might take advantage of the reactivity of blood vessel wall. The coronary arteries have a considerable ability to dilate. The blood flow of the coronary artery system might be increased severalfold, producing a potentially enormous coronary artery reserve, if we had the drugs to produce a specific coronary dilation.

In the next 20 years we will probably see less open heart surgery, more percutaneous transluminal coronary angioplasty, and more selective angioplasty with a multivessel approach. More heart transplants and heart-lung transplants will be done. Completely implantable heart support devices should be developed over the next two decades. Pacemakers will be programmed to intervene in potentially fatal arrhythmias. We should be able to diagnose arteriosclerosis much earlier in life with an array of diagnostic procedures ranging from B mode ultrasound to nuclear magnetic resonance, positron-emission tomographic scanning, and the use of fiber optics to look inside vessels.

Laser sources will be tested for their ability to remove atherosclerotic blockage at selected sites as an interoperative procedure. The percutaneous application of laser therapy is a more distant possibility. Various approaches to thrombolysis will be tested, including the use of tissue-type plasminogen activator. An ultimate goal is production of a completely synthetic substance that could promote the removal of tissue cholesterol, including that in the arterial wall, and facilitate its transport to the liver, where the cholesterol may be excreted as sterol or bile acid. The use of synthetic peptides mimicking the proteins of HDL represents an approach of this kind.

In the next 20 years, we will surely see more emphasis and effort given to prevention, with particular emphasis on the young. Prevention should become a part of every health education, science, and biology class. Perhaps the greatest impact can be made by altering the habits and beliefs of our young people. It is much more difficult to affect the lifestyle of the adult population, which will probably be more reluctant to give up the dietary and other habits to which they have become accustomed. It is possible to have restaurants that provide foods that are both a culinary delight and healthy for your heart. Government and volunteer organizations such as the American Heart Association must play a leadership role in the future if effective prevention is to become a reality.

In the field of arteriosclerotic disease, we continue to see changes in the patterns of disease. As the incidence of syphilitic and rheumatic heart disease has greatly diminished, so should the incidence of coronary heart disease by the close of this century. The coronary care unit of the year 2000 may be as deserted as the tuberculosis sanitorium of today. I believe that the disappearance of arteriosclerosis will require a major new breakthrough in therapy, but I believe that there is a good likelihood of this happening. Cardiovascular surgeons will not be put out of business by the disappearance of atherosclerosis, but they will be replacing worn out vessels rather than doing bypasses.

After all forms of heart disease, lung disease, and cancer have been cured, we will be left to face the process of aging. An English actuary by the name of Benjamin Gompertz made an interesting statement in this regard. Gompertz lived in Northampton and published his findings about 1825. His writings lay dormant until recent years when investigators in the field of cancer biology found that his mathematical formula could predict the growth of cancer cells during certain stages of their development. The curve plotted by this equation shows that beyond a certain age the risk of death increases geometrically[15] (figure 12). The implication is that if one reaches a certain age, beyond that point the likelihood of dying becomes more a function of having reached that age than it is of any specific disease entity. Thus, aging itself becomes the critical factor and if you do not die of one thing, you will die of another.

One of the exciting avenues of the future is the intersection of different disease entities at the level of basic science; for example, pulmonary disease and arteriosclerosis may merge at the level of the study of changes in collagen, endothelial cells, or prostaglandins. Studies of arteriosclerosis and neoplasms could have in common investigations of the proliferation of the capillary, as in the vasa vasorum around an atherosclerotic plaque, and of the role of the PDGF or other growth factors in stimulating cell growth. Cancer and arteriosclerosis may also merge in the study of the cell surface and of cell membranes. For example, the ratio of cholesterol to phospholipid and the degree of saturation and unsaturation of phospholipid in the membrane of a cell may alter the fluidity of the membrane, its physiologic properties, and its likelihood of the formation of a malignant clone or an atherosclerotic plaque.

In this panoramic view of arteriosclerosis, I have tried briefly to span a time just under 2000 years. I am optimistic about the future of medicine in the United States, and am especially optimistic over the prospects of conquering arteriosclerosis. With the applications of molecular biology and of basic science to the problems of arteriosclerosis and cardiovascular disease, I believe that we are poised to make discoveries over the next 50 years that rival the importance of those of the Italian Renaissance. At that remarkable time, some of the finest minds of Europe, including William Harvey, came to the universities of Northern Italy for advanced education. The social atmosphere was cosmopolitan and the intellectual climate was receptive of new ideas, new discoveries, and change. It was here that the term Renaissance man was most appropriately applied. William Harvey stood at the crossroads of a great breakthrough in understanding the circulation. The beauty of his work is an inspiration to all of us as we contemplate the past, study the present, and dream of the future.

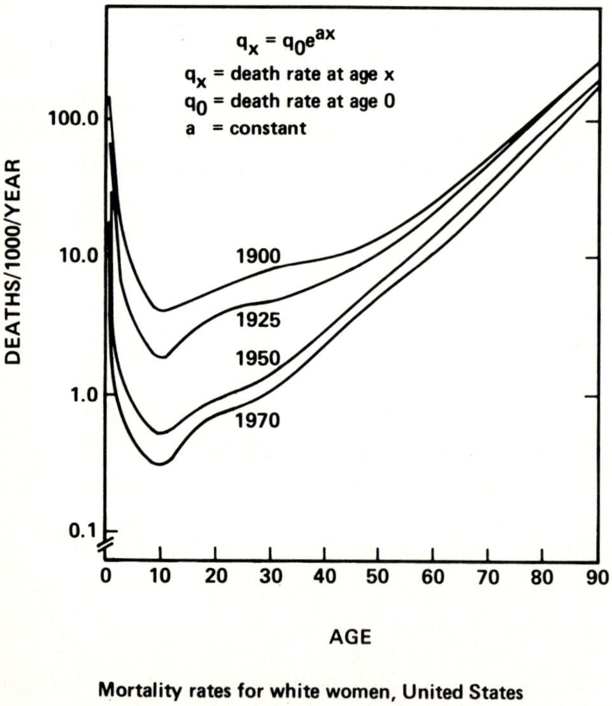

FIGURE 12. The Gompertzian curve and equation. (Adapted from McGill.[8])

References

1. Wilson LG: Erasistratus, Galen, and the pneuma. Bull Hist Med **33:** 293, 1959
2. Leibowitz JO: The history of coronary heart disease. Berkeley, 1970, University of California Press
3. Willius FA, Dry TJ: A history of the heart and the circulation. Philadelphia, 1948, W.B. Saunders Co.
4. Arcieri GP: Circulation of the blood. Andrea Cesalpino of Arezzo. New York, 1945, S.F. Vanni
5. Whitteridge G: William Harvey and the circulation of the blood. New York, 1971, Neale Watson Academic Publications, Inc.
6. Katz LN, Stamler J: Experimental atherosclerosis. Springfield, 1953, Charles C. Thomas
7. Ross R, Glomset JA: The pathogenesis of atherosclerosis. N Engl J Med **295:** 369; 420, 1976
8. McGill HC Jr: Persistent problems in the pathogenesis of atherosclerosis. The George Lyman Duff Memorial Lecture. Arteriosclerosis **4:** 443, 1984
9. Faggiotti A, Ross R, Harker L: Studies of hypercholesterolemia in the non-human primate. I. Changes that lead to fatty streaks. Arteriosclerosis **4:** 323, 1984
10. Faggiotto A, Ross R: Studies of hypercholesterolemia in the non-human primate. II. Fatty streak conversion to fibrous plaque. Arteriosclerosis **4:** 341, 1984
11. Stary HC: Macrophages in coronary artery and aortic intima and in atherosclerotic lesions of children and young adults up to age 29. *In* Schettler FG, Gotto AM, Middelhoff G, Habenicht AJR, Jurutka

KR, editors: Sixth International Symposium of Atherosclerosis. Berlin, 1982, Atherosclerosis IV. New York, 1983, Springer-Verlag, pp 462–466
12. Stary HC: Evolution of atherosclerotic plaques in the coronary arteries of young adults. Arteriosclerosis **3:** 471a, 1983
13. Lipid Research Clinics Program: The Lipid Research Clinics Coronary Primary Prevention Trial results. I. Reduction in incidence of coronary heart disease. JAMA **251:** 351, 1984
14. Lipid Research Clinics Program: The Lipid Research Clinics Coronary Primary Prevention Trial results. II. The relationship of reduction in incidence of coronary heart disease to cholesterol lowering. JAMA **251:** 365, 1984
15. Bearn AG, Hiatt HH, Katchadourian HA, Goldman R: Human growth and development. *In* Beeson PB, McDermott W, Wngaarden JB, editors: Cecil's textbook of medicine. 1978, Philadelphia, W.B. Saunders Co., vol I

EDITORIAL

Human tissue-type plasminogen activator: from the laboratory to the bedside

D. Collen, M.D., Ph.D.

IN AUGUST 1983, it was anticipated from biochemical observations and physiologic results in experimental animals that human tissue-type plasminogen activator (t-PA) held considerable promise as a clot-specific, coronary thrombolytic agent for patients with acute myocardial infarction.[1] This anticipation has been fulfilled remarkably promptly by clinical research.[2–5] Recently reported results from several randomized clinical trials[3–5] punctuate a long series of antecedent laboratory, preclinical, and clinical investigations. Accordingly, research focused on t-PA serves as a particularly good example of productive, sequential developments and collaborations involving investigators from disparate disciplines in academe and industry. This report summarizes some of the seminal studies in the development and characterization of native t-PA and the recombinant DNA–produced t-PA used in multicenter trials reported recently.[3–5]

Although t-PA was identified in the 1940s, its isolation and characterization were hampered by inadequate sources and purification procedures. In 1980, an attractive procedure for the isolation of human t-PA was developed by Rijken et al.,[6] yielding approximately 1 mg of t-PA from 5 kg of human uterine tissue. Subsequent development of t-PA and its application to coronary thrombolysis has progressed along four main lines: (1) isolation and characterization of t-PA from the Bowes melanoma cell line, (2) cloning and expression of the human t-PA gene, (3) delineation of the efficacy of purified t-PA in experimental animals with induced coronary thrombosis, and (4) evaluation of the coronary thrombolytic efficacy of t-PA in patients with acute myocardial infarction.

Isolation and characterization of t-PA from the Bowes melanoma cell line. The Bowes melanoma cell line was provided to us by Dr. D. B. Rifkin, New York University Medical School, toward the end of 1978. It had been obtained originally from pulmonary, metastatic melanoma cells from a patient named Bowes by Dr. G. Moore in 1974 and was maintained and exchanged among investigators because it secreted large amounts of plasminogen activator activity. However, the nature of the activity had not been elucidated. In collaboration with Dr. A. Billiau in the Laboratory of Virology at the University of Leuven, we introduced the Bowes cell line in our laboratory to study the spectrum of inhibition of plasminogen activators of malignant cells by synthetic inhibitors. In retrospect, selection of this cell line was fortuitous. Most malignant cell lines in culture produce urokinase-like plasminogen activators. Some produce mixtures of urokinase and an activator that does not react with urokinase antibodies.[7] Cell lines that secrete t-PA primarily or exclusively are quite rare. The Bowes cell line is unusually, if not uniquely, efficient in this regard. This explains why, after our initial description of t-PA isolated from the Bowes line, this source became the standard one for most investigators in the field.

When we sought initially to purify the plasminogen activator from Bowes melanoma cell culture fluid in 1979, we observed that the activator, like uterine t-PA but unlike urokinase, had a specific affinity for fibrin. When mixtures of fibrinogen and plasminogen activator were clotted, the activator remained associated with the clot but could be eluted with potassium isothiocyanate.

Thus the melanoma plasminogen activator resembled t-PA. However, with the use of purification methods developed previously for t-PA, no homogeneous, final product was obtainable initially.

In October 1979, Dr. D. C. Rijken joined us from the Gaubius Institute in The Netherlands. He had developed a method for the purification of the plasminogen activator from human uterus in which adsorption of the activator to surfaces was prevented by the use of Tween 80 and in which zinc-chelate agarose was used in the first chromatographic step. With a modified version of this purification procedure we were soon

From the Center for Thrombosis and Vascular Research, University of Leuven, Leuven, Belgium.

Address for correspondence: D. Collen, M.D., Ph.D., Center for Thrombosis and Vascular Research, Department of Medical Research, Campus Gasthuisberg-K.U., Leuven, Herestraat 49, B-3000 Leuven, Belgium.

able to purify melanoma cell culture fluid plasminogen activator material shown to be homogeneous by sodium dodecyl sulfate gel electrophoresis and to be immunologically identical to the uterine plasminogen activator (t-PA).[8] Subsequently, the purification procedure was scaled upward to produce a total amount of approximately 2 g of t-PA,[9] facilitating systematic characterization of its biochemical, biological, and physiologic properties.

With Dr. Matsuo from Miyazaki University in Japan who joined us in September 1979, thrombolytic effects of t-PA in plasma in vitro and thrombolytic effects in rabbits with experimental pulmonary embolus in vivo were demonstrated. With Drs. Rijken, M. Hoylaerts, H. R. Lijnen, I. Juhan-Vague, and C. Korninger, the kinetics of plasminogen activator were clarified and immunoassays for t-PA in plasma were developed.

In collaboration with Dr. W. Weimar in 1981, we treated two patients with renal vein thrombosis after kidney transplantation with intravenous infusions of 5 and 7.5 mg of t-PA over 24 hr.[10] Despite the fact that lysis occurred, the dose was probably too low for general use judging from the results of analogous patients (unpublished observations) and from extensive information acquired later in studies of coronary thrombolysis in animals and patients (see below).

Cloning and expression of the human t-PA gene. At the Fifth Congress on Fibrinolysis in Malmo, Sweden, where our first results with t-PA were presented, I met a scientist from the Department of Molecular Biology in the Genentech Corporation. Collaboration devoted to the cloning and expression of the t-PA gene ensued, with results reported at the Sixth Congress on Fibrinolysis in Lausanne, Switzerland, in 1982 and published in January 1983.[11] Building on the successful cloning and expression of t-PA, Genentech made a profound commitment to developing recombinant human t-PA (rt-PA). With the approval of the FDA, rt-PA was first administered to a patient on February 11, 1984. The rapid progress was possible only because of the efforts of many scientists at Genentech and concomitant investigations elsewhere characterizing some of the biological and thrombolytic properties of the material. We were able to demonstrate that the turnover of the rt-PA in rabbits is similar to that of melanoma cell t-PA and that its thrombolytic properties in a rabbit jugular vein thrombosis preparation are indistinguishable from those of the plasminogen activator of melanoma origin.[12]

Delineation of coronary thrombolysis by natural t-PA and rt-PA in experimental animals. Late in 1981 at an NIH workshop on coronary thrombolysis, Dr. B. E. Sobel from Washington University initiated a collaboration in which our two groups explored the use of t-PA for thrombolysis in the treatment of acute myocardial infarction. The work focused also on the impact of the coronary thrombolytic effects of t-PA on myocardial metabolism and perfusion assessed with positron emission tomography. Within a short time the utility of this approach was demonstrated in closed-chest dogs with coronary thrombosis induced by advancing a copper coil into the left anterior descending coronary artery (LAD). Intravenous infusion of human t-PA purified from melanoma cell culture fluid resulted in prompt coronary recanalization without systemic activation of the fibrinolytic system. Furthermore, it restored myocardial blood flow and intermediary metabolism in the region at risk demonstrated tomographically with ^{11}C-labeled palmitate and $H_2{}^{15}O$ given intravenously.[13] These results demonstrated that administration of native, human t-PA to animals with induced coronary thrombosis elicited prompt thrombolysis without predisposition to systemic bleeding attributable to a systemic lytic state. Subsequently, the observations were extended to rt-PA. In a collaborative study between the Cardiology Divisions of the University of Leuven, Belgium, and Washington University, the clot-specific coronary thrombolytic properties of rt-PA were demonstrated with the same experimental animal preparation.[14] In a concurrent collaborative study with Dr. H. K. Gold, Massachusetts General Hospital, coronary thrombosis was produced between two ligatures of the LAD in open-chest dogs. Infusion of t-PA elicited clot lysis and myocardial salvage in this preparation as well.[15] Subsequently, in a collaborative study with Dr. W. Flameng at the University of Leuven, the coronary thrombolytic properties, clot-specificity, and myocardial protection achievable with rt-PA were confirmed in baboons.[16]

Administration of t-PA to patients with acute myocardial infarction. The first study in which t-PA was administered to patients with acute myocardial infarction was performed between February and September 1983 with purified t-PA obtained from the Bowes cell line. Participants included Dr. F. van de Werf and co-workers at the University of Leuven and Dr. Sobel and co-workers at Washington University.[2] Intravenously administered t-PA in doses of 20,000 to 40,000 IU/min (200 to 400 μg) recanalized completely occluded coronary arteries within 30 to 60 min in six of seven patients without inducing a systemic, fibrinolytic state in any. These initial observations with native t-PA served as a template and stimulated initiation of a multicenter, blinded, randomized trial with rt-PA provided by Genentech. Fifty patients were studied between February 11 and June 20, 1984, at Washington University with Dr. Sobel and co-workers, at the Massachuetts General Hospital with Dr. Gold and co-workers, and at Johns Hopkins University with Dr. M. Weisfeldt and co-workers. Intravenous infusion of 0.5 mg/kg body weight rt-PA over 60 min or of the same dose followed by 0.25 mg/kg over an additional 60 min resulted in recanalization of occluded coronary arteries in 75% of patients. Fibrinogenolysis was absent or modest in most but not all of the patients.[3] Characterization of a subset of patients[17] indicated that therapeutic plasma levels of t-PA were achievable in a dose-dependent fashion despite individual variation. These t-PA levels affected the fibrinolytic system in a fashion consistent with the kinetics of the participating biochemical reactions.[17, 18] The results obtained in this initial study of rt-PA in patients with acute myocardial infarction provided a foundation for the design of both the recently implemented NIH Thrombolysis in Acute Myocardial Infarction (TIMI) trial in the United States and the European Cooperative trial in Belgium, France, West Germany, and The Netherlands.

In the TIMI trial thus far, rt-PA has been infused over 3 hr (40 mg for 1 hr and 20 mg for each of the next 2 hr). After an initial open-label phase carried out in 87 patients in June and July 1984, a double-blind comparison with 1.5 million U of streptokinase infused over 1 hr was performed in 316 patients between August 1984 and February 1985. rt-PA was found to be approximately twice as effective as streptokinase for recanalization and to be associated with substantially less fibrinogenolysis.[4]

In the European Cooperative trial, rt-PA was infused at a rate of 0.75 mg/kg over 90 min. Results were compared with those in patients given 1.5 million U of streptokinase over 1 hr. In 129 patients studied between July and December 1984, rt-PA was found to be more effective than streptokinase and to induce substantially less fibrinogenolysis.[5]

The concordant conclusions of the three prospective, randomized clinical trials with rt-PA from which results are available to date,[3-5] coupled with the extensive, antecedent biochemical, physiologic, and biological observations in experimental animals and patients, constitute a firm basis for the further evaluation of thrombolysis induced by t-PA in the management of patients with acute myocardial infarction. The relative safety and thrombolytic potential of t-PA appear to be well established. The ultimate benefit of coronary thrombolysis remains to be elucidated.

The author appreciates preparation of the typescript in the Departments of Biochemistry and Medicine at the College of Medicine, University of Vermont.

References

1. Collen D, Verstraete M: Systemic thrombolytic therapy of acute myocardial infarction? Circulation **68:** 462, 1983
2. Van de Werf F, Ludbrook PA, Bergmann SR, Tiefenbrunn AJ, Fox KAA, de Geest H, Verstraete M, Collen D, Sobel B: Clot-selective coronary thrombolysis with tissue-type plasminogen activator in patients with evolving myocardial infarction. N Engl J Med **310:** 609, 1984
3. Collen D, Topol EJ, Tiefenbrunn AJ, Gold HK, Weisfeldt ML, Sobel BE, Leinbach RE, Brinker JA, Ludbrook PA, Yasuda T, Bulkley BH, Robison AK, Hutter AM, Bell WR, Spadaro JJ, Khaw BA, Grossbard EB: Coronary thrombolysis with recombinant tissue-type plasminogen activator: a prospective, randomized, placebo-controlled trial. Circulation **70:** 1012, 1984
4. The TIMI Study Group: Special Report: The Thrombolysis in Myocardial Infarction (TIMI) Trial. N Engl J Med **312:** 932, 1985
5. Verstraete M, Bernard R, Bory M, Brower RM, Collen D, de Bono DP, Erbel R, Huhmann W, Lennane RJ, Lubsen J, Matthey D, Meyer J, Michels HR, Rutsch W, Schartl M, Schmidt W, Uebis R, von Essen R: Randomized trial of intravenous recombinant human tissue-type plasminogen activator versus intravenous streptokinase in acute myocardial infarction. Lancet **1:** 842, 1985
6. Rijken DC, Wijngaards G, Zaal-DeJong M, Welbergen J: Purification and partial characterization of plasminogen activator from human uterine tissue. Biochim Biophys Acta **580:** 140, 1979
7. Wilson EL, Becker MLB, Hoal EG, Dowdle EB: Molecular species of plasminogen activators secreted by normal and neoplastic human cells. Cancer Res **40:** 933, 1980
8. Rijken DC, Collen D: Purification and characterization of the plasminogen activator secreted by human melanoma cells in culture. J Biol Chem **156:** 7035, 1981
9. Collen D, Rijken DC, Van Damme J, Billiau A: Purification of human extrinsic (tissue-type) plasminogen activator in centigram quantities from a human melanoma cell culture fluid and its conditioning for use in vivo. Thromb Haemost **48:** 294, 1982
10. Weimar W, Stibbe J, van Seyen AJ, Billiau A, De Somer P, Collen D: Specific lysis of an iliofemoral thrombus by administration of extrinsic (tissue-type) plasminogen activator. Lancet **2:** 1018, 1981
11. Pennica D, Holmes WE, Kohr WJ, Harkins RN, Vehar GA, Ward CA, Bennet WF, Yelverton E, Seeburg PH, Heyneker HL, Goeddel DV, Collen D: Cloning and expression of human tissue-type plasminogen activator cDNA in *E. coli.* Nature **201:** 214, 1983
12. Collen D, Stassen JM, Marafino BJ Jr, Builder S, De Cock F, Ogez J, Tajiri D, Pennica D, Bennett WF, Salwa J, Hoyng CF: Biological properties of human tissue-type plasminogen activator obtained by expression of recombinant DNA in mammalian cells. J Pharm Exp Ther **231:** 146, 1984
13. Bergmann SR, Fox KAA, Ter-Pogossian MM, Sobel BE, Collen D: Clot-selective coronary thrombolysis with tissue-type plasminogen activator. Science **220:** 1181, 1983
14. Van de Werf F, Bergmann SR, Fox KAA, de Geest H, Hoyng CF, Sobel BE, Collen D: Coronary thrombolysis with intravenously administered human tissue-type plasminogen activator produced by recombinant DNA technology. Circulation **69:** 605, 1984
15. Gold HK, Fallon JT, Yasuda T, Khaw BA, Newell JB, Leinbach RC, Guerrero JL, Vislosky FM, Hoyng CF, Grossbard E, Collen D: Coronary thrombolysis with recombinant human tissue-type plasminogen activator. Circulation **70:** 700, 1984
16. Flameng W, Van de Werf F, Vanhaecke J, Verstraete M, Collen D: Coronary thrombolysis and infarct size reduction following intravenous infusion of recombinant tissue-type plasminogen activator in non-human primates. J Clin Invest **75:** 84, 1985
17. Tiefenbrunn AJ, Robison AK, Kurnik PB, Ludbrook PA, Sobel BE: Clinical pharmacology in patients with evolving myocardial infarction of tissue-type plasminogen activator produced by recombinant DNA technology. Circulation **71:** 110, 1985
18. Hoylaerts M, Rijken DC, Lijnen HR, Collen D: Kinetics of the activation of plasminogen by human tissue plasminogen activator: role of fibrin. J Biol Chem **257:** 2912, 1982

Cardiology in 1885

W. BRUCE FYE, M.D.

IT IS IMPOSSIBLE to ignore the dramatic developments that have occurred in the diagnosis and treatment of heart disease in recent years.[1] Borrowing heavily from the physical sciences, new diagnostic instruments have been invented that allow earlier and more precise identification of cardiac disease. Pharmacologic therapy of angina pectoris, dormant for nearly a century after the discovery that nitrates were effective in relieving this distressing symptom, has blossomed recently with the introduction of β-blockers, calcium antagonists, and long-acting nitroglycerin preparations. Surgical approaches to many forms of congenital and acquired heart disease have been developed. Julius Comroe asked, "How many patients who have undergone open heart surgery know of the tremendous efforts of many scientists through the years that provided the basic and practical knowledge which was essential for their successful operation?"[2] Indeed, how many physicians appreciate the enormous amount of multidisciplinary basic and clinical research necessary for the development of the present state of cardiology and cardiac surgery? Many of our senior colleagues remember the practice of cardiology before cardiac catheterization, echocardiography, or nuclear cardiology, and before there was "CPR" or coronary care units. I will describe the practice of cardiology a century ago to emphasize the dramatic advances in this field that have occurred as a result of millions of hours of observation and experiment by countless physicians and basic and clinical scientists.

The medical context. The average life expectancy for Americans born in 1885 was about 45 years, and infections were the leading cause of morbidity and mortality. Tuberculosis was responsible for the greatest number of deaths, but other communicable diseases took tens of thousands of lives annually.[3] Although significant advances in public health and sanitation had taken place since the 1850s, major obstacles remained, and many of the residents of the increasingly crowded cities were at great risk for contracting a potentially fatal infectious disease. In the cities wealthy patients received care in their homes or in the offices of private physicians and were admitted to a hospital only as a last resort. The urban working class and the poor received their care at dispensaries where one or two full-time employees, usually a resident physician and an apothecary, cared for dozens of patients a day.[4, 5] Hospitals had not yet become a major institution for the evaluation and treatment of the sick; this would soon change, however. Between 1875 and 1925 the number of hospitals in America rose dramatically from about 150 to nearly 7000.[6]

In the mid 19th century several discoveries were made that had major implications for the diagnosis and treatment of disease. Perhaps the most dramatic of these was the discovery of anesthesia in 1846. Equally important was the recognition of the role of microorganisms in the causation of disease, and the introduction of antiseptic, and ultimately, aseptic techniques of surgery. With the microscopic demonstration of bacteria in the 1870s and 1880s and the continued research of Koch, Pasteur, Lister, and others, the remaining skeptics of the germ theory of disease were silenced.

The practitioners. What did Americans do when they became ill a century ago? As is true today, many cared for themselves using home medical guides or "family recipes" rather than seeking formal medical evaluation.[7] For those who wanted to see a medical practitioner several options existed. Numerous medical sects thrived in America during the middle of the 19th century.[8] In addition to "regular" physicians, patients could choose homeopaths, botanics, eclectics, hydropaths, electrotherapists, phrenologists, or other sectarians. The American Medical Association was founded in 1847 in large part to attempt to elevate the standards of medical education, but another goal was to protect the regular physicians from the growing influence of "irregular" practitioners. In 1885 there were approximately 4200 medical graduates, of whom 85% were

Dr. Fye is Chairman of the Cardiology Department at the Marshfield Clinic in Marshfield, Wisconsin, Adjunct Assistant Professor of the History of Medicine and Clinical Assistant Professor of Medicine at the University of Wisconsin in Madison, and Clinical Assistant Professor at the Medical College of Wisconsin in Milwaukee. He has had a long-standing interest in the literature and history of medicine, the history of cardiology, and the development and implementation of advances in diagnostics and therapeutics.

Address for correspondence: W. Bruce Fye, M.D., Department of Cardiology, Marshfield Clinic, 1000 North Oak Ave., Marshfield, WI 54449.

regular physicians, 10% were homeopaths, and the remaining 5% were eclectics.[9] There were about 87,000 physicians of various schools, which represented one practitioner for 575 Americans. In 1980 this ratio was approximately one physician for 485 Americans. Concern about the "doctor glut" is not new. Writing in 1882 an editor observed, "We are so often asked concerning professional prospects by young men starting out in practice that we offer this as a general answer. It does not make much difference where he settles. Every place is full."[10]

Contemporary practitioners could not help but be impressed by the discoveries and inventions of European physicians, surgeons, and biomedical scientists. Nor could they ignore the trend toward specialization. Graduates who could afford it attempted to improve their chances of success in practice by traveling to the medical centers of Europe, Germany in particular, where the developing specialties were taught in the large university medical centers.[11, 12] A few medical schools and hospitals in America attempted to offer postgraduate training as well. The New York neurologist Edward Seguin claimed in 1880, "Of the many practical questions which present themselves to the minds of students of medicine, and even more forcibly to the minds of young graduates, few, I take it, are more interesting than the one: 'Shall I practice medicine in general, or become a specialist?' "[13] In this era the specialties were confined primarily to surgical subspecialties, dermatology, and neurology; cardiology did not exist as a distinct professional field. The debate about specialization continues despite the 1885 proclamation of the New York physician and medical editor, George Shrady, "Specialism is an established feature of modern medicine. . . . It is not an artificial addition to medicine, but a natural and inevitable development."[14]

The cardiac patient: history and cardiac physical examination. A century ago physicians relied heavily, as we do today, on the historical details of the present illness to determine the etiology and significance of a patient's complaints. However, they realized the difficulty of making an accurate diagnosis based on symptoms alone. Jacob DaCosta, a leading diagnostician, declared, "It is not easy to say what are and what are not the symptoms that belong to diseases of the heart."[15] The invention of the stethoscope in 1819 by the French physician and pathologist Laennec signaled the birth of modern physical diagnosis. Indeed, it has been claimed recently that this instrument "transformed the practice of medicine in the 19th century, altering the physicians's picture of disease and his relation to the patient."[16] Americans who studied in Paris during the middle third of the 19th century did much to popularize the use of the stethoscope in the United States. Austin Flint, "the American Laennec," was a strong advocate of auscultation and percussion. He published a popular textbook on cardiac physical diagnosis and the first monograph on heart disease written by an American.[17] The correlation of murmurs and abnormal heart sounds auscultated during life with autopsy results had led to a rather sophisticated understanding of the significance of these physical findings. Moreover, attempts were made, with reasonable success, to explain auscultatory abnormalities on the basis of physical principles.[18] Many cardiac conditions were "silent," however, and physicians of a century ago recognized their limited ability to diagnose nonvalvular diseases of the heart by physical examination.

Laboratory aids to diagnosis. Instruments designed to graphically record physiologic events became fundamental tools in physiologic laboratories during the second half of the 19th century, and some of these methods were applied to clinical practice. Carl Ludwig, the pioneering German physiologist, had invented the kymograph in 1847, and seven years later Karl Vierordt adapted this instrument to record the pulse in man. This "sphygmograph" enabled physicians and investigators to evaluate the character of the pulse objectively for the first time.[19] These recording instruments were combined with catheterization techniques developed by German and French physiologists to record intracardiac pressures in experimental animals nearly a century before these procedures were attempted in humans.[20] Another instrument "sometimes of considerable diagnostic value" was the cardiograph. This apparatus graphically recorded the apical impulse and was used primarily by physiologists to study the phases of the cardiac cycle. Clinical applications were recognized, however, and it was claimed, "By means of the cardiograph it is possible to clear up some obscure causes of cardiac disease, and to ascertain the exact relationship of murmurs (which it is difficult or impossible to 'time' in any other way) to the different periods of the cardiac cycle."[21]

Developments in the science of electricity were accompanied by growing interest in bioelectrical phenomena. By 1885 the electrical activity of the heart in intact animals had been recorded with a capillary electrometer. This instrument would be used by Augustus Waller in London two years later to record the first electrocardiogram in man.[22] However, electrocardiography would not become practical until the work of Einthoven, Lewis, and others in the early 20th century.

X-rays were not discovered until 1895, so, in 1885, physicians did not have access to two of the most important diagnostic tests for detecting cardiac disease.[23]

Ischemic heart disease. Although there was little insight into the pathophysiology of ischemic heart disease a century ago, there was no lack of enthusiasm for proposing various forms of therapy for angina pectoris.[24] In 1867, the British pharmacologist Lauder Brunton discovered that amyl nitrite administered during an attack of angina pectoris could abort the paroxysm or at least reduce its severity. William Murrell of London extended Brunton's studies on nitrates and reported the value of nitroglycerin in the treatment of angina in 1879. Then, as now, enthusiasm for advances in therapeutics overshadowed the response to reports of new insights into the pathophysiology of disease processes. Some observers, however, recognized the critical role of basic research in the discovery of these "breakthroughs." Referring to Brunton's discovery of the efficacy of amyl nitrite in angina, a reviewer exclaimed in 1883, "In few maladies are the improvements in our therapeutical resources more conspicuous. In the use of the most effective remedy for the relief of the paroxysm, an admirable illustration is given of the remarkable value of the contributions made to therapeutics by physiological investigations."[25]

The introduction of nitrates did not totally replace older therapies for angina for several decades, however. In addition to advocating the use of amyl nitrite and hypodermic morphine for the treatment of angina, the prominent Philadelphia physician Jacob DaCosta recommended arsenic, strychnine, and cannabis indica (marijuana) for this condition.[26] In 1885 empiric observation was the only means to assess the relative merits of the various therapeutic approaches to angina. It was nearly a century before it became possible to identify the existence of coronary artery lesions or evaluate their physiologic significance in the living patient.

Valvular heart disease. Diseases of the cardiac valves received great attention during the 19th century mainly because of the physician's ability to identify many valvular lesions with the stethoscope. It is likely that the prevalence of valvular heart disease was greater a century ago than today. Infectious diseases, notably streptococcal infections, could not be treated effectively in the preantibiotic era, and rheumatic heart disease was more common. Life expectancy was sufficiently short that degenerative diseases such as coronary artery disease and cancer were less prevalent. It was recognized by 1885 that valvular lesions could be congenital or acquired and that acute rheumatism often preceded the development of valvular heart disease in the older child or adult. The previous year Ernest Laseque had proclaimed, "Rheumatism is a disease which licks the joints . . . but it bites the heart."[27] Salicylates were first advocated for the treatment of acute rheumatism in 1876 by Thomas Maclagan, and the association of tonsillitis with this disease had been reported in 1880 by James Fowler.

Aortic valve disease was relatively easy to identify by careful auscultation. Alfred Loomis of New York claimed in 1885, "The treatment of aortic stenosis and of aortic regurgitation may be summed up under three heads — viz. rest, diet, and regimen. Rest is most important; it must be mental as well as physical; the appetite, emotions, and passions must be kept under perfect control. . . . The stomach also must have all the rest compatible with the most perfect nutrition . . . sugar, sweet vegetables, and animal fat must be sparingly indulged in. . . . The bowels should be gently moved once daily. That the cutaneous circulation may be active the body should be warmly clothed. Any prolonged exposure of the surface to cold is to be avoided."[28] If cardiac decompensation occurred, Loomis advocated the administration of digitalis, which had been introduced into medical practice a century earlier by William Withering. If syncope or vertigo supervened, Loomis suggested the administration of quinine and strychnine. "When the hepatic and gastric vessels are engorged," he advised, "three or four leeches over the liver or epigastrium . . . will afford temporary relief."[28]

The British physician Hilton Fagge claimed, "The diagnosis of mitral disease is far from resting on so satisfactory a footing as that of aortic obstruction and regurgitation."[29] Byrom Bramwell considered mitral insufficiency "a very common condition" and recognized that it "may result from a lesion of any part of the mitral valve apparatus (sphincter muscle, basal ring, valve segments, chordae tendineae, or papillary muscles)." He appreciated the variable natural history of mitral insufficiency and claimed, "In some cases, it neither interferes with the comfort of the patient, nor shortens life." It was well known, however, that this lesion could lead to progressive exertional dyspnea and ultimately to decompensation with anasarca (dropsy) and death. Bramwell advocated changes in life-style in the early stages of mitral insufficiency and claimed, "If the patient has been in the habit of following a laborious occupation he should be advised to give it up." Revealing concern for the patient's emotional response to the physician's prognostication, he warned that the patient "should not be allowed to take too serious a view of his own condition . . . [and] the fact that the disease has little or no tendency to cause sudden death should be impressed upon the patient; many of the laity, when they are told that their hearts are not quite sound, jump to the conclusion that they are affected with a disease which may at any moment prove fatal, and to persons of a nervous and anxious disposition this idea is often a source of perpetual and terrible anxiety." Alcohol, tobacco, tea, and coffee were to be used in a "strictly moderate" fashion, and mild exercise, a large amount of sleep, and fresh air were beneficial. Decompensation was treated with the same approach advocated for advanced aortic valve disease. Congestive heart failure was treated with digitalis, "by the internal administration of cardiac tonics and stimulants, diuretics and purgatives . . . [and] by local measures," including the use of Southey's trochars to physically drain fluid from edematous extremities.[21] To reduce pulmonary and systemic venous congestion, Fagge advocated "the removal of a portion of the venous blood by venosection, leeches, or cupping."[29] Agents used as diuretics included squill (*Urginea scilla*), juniper, broom (*Sarothamnus scoparius*), cream of tartar, and copaiba.[30]

Mitral stenosis was recognized as a complication of rheumatic fever, although a congenital form was acknowledged. The risk of embolization in the setting of mitral stenosis was recognized. Although the risk of thrombus formation was appreciated, emboli were most often attributed to detachment of vegetations from the diseased valve leaflets. If embolism occurred, the British physician Ernest Sansom advocated "the maintenance of rest and tranquility of the heart. The blood should be rendered as fluid and non-coagulable as possible, and to this end alkaline salts of ammonia or soda may be administered."[31]

Miscellaneous cardiac diseases. Endocarditis was attracting a great deal of attention a century ago and was the subject of William Osler's Gulstonian Lecture before the Royal College of Physicians of London in 1885. This disease had recently been attributed to microorganisms, and Osler commented that micrococci were invariably present in vegetations examined under the microscope. The predisposition of deformed valves for the development of endocarditis, the variable course of the illness, and the frequent predominance of systemic over cardiac symptoms were emphasized by Osler. He claimed, "Few diseases present greater difficulties in the way of diagnosis, difficulties which in many cases are practically insurmountable. . . . The protean character of the malady, the latency of the cardiac symptoms, and the close stimulation of other disorders, combine to render the detection peculiarly difficult."[32] In this preantibiotic era, infective endocarditis was invariably fatal, usually within a month of the onset of symptoms.

Cardiac arrhythmias were poorly understood in 1885 despite the long tradition of palpation of the pulse and the introduction of the sphygmograph. There was growing awareness of the role of the heart in sudden death, however, and William Osler claimed, "The cases of very rapid death are almost always due to affections of the heart, or of the great vessels."[33] Austin Flint recognized the risk of sudden death in patients with angina pectoris and warned, "A person subject to paroxysms of angina must be considered as in more or less danger of sudden death with the recurrence of each paroxysm. The physician should be sufficiently impressed with . . . this fact."[34] Although the risk of sudden cardiac death was recognized, its mechanism was obscure in 1885. Flint's explanation, "The immediate cause of sudden death in a paroxysm is probably an arrest of the heart's action in diastole," reflected contemporary attitudes regarding the pathophysiology of sudden cardiac death. In the late 1880s the Scottish physiologist John MacWilliam would propose that ventricular fibrillation was the usual mechanism of sudden cardiac death.[35]

Chronic irregularity of the pulse had been associated with mitral valve disease since the early 19th century, but atrial fibrillation was not recognized as the most common mechanism of this physical finding until the 20th century.[36] The identification of extrasystoles and attempts to understand their etiology and significance had to await the experiments and observations of Wenckebach, Mackenzie, and Lewis early in the present century. In 1885, palpitations were considered a functional disorder or "neurosis of the heart." It was recognized that alcohol, coffee, tea, and tobacco predisposed to palpitations and that certain types of individuals were more prone to this symptom. "The individuals most frequently affected are young adults and persons beyond middle age; females; nervous subjects; and fat, flabby people, who live highly and are habitually dyspeptic."[37] Although the mechanisms of cardiac irregularities were not understood, empiric observations made since the 18th century led physicians to prescribe digitalis for palpitations.

Although there was no understanding of the mechanism of palpitations and their significance was debated, contemporary practitioners prescribed a wide variety of remedies. Oliver Wendell Holmes proclaimed in 1860 that, with the exception of opium, anesthetics, and wine, "If the whole materia medica, as now used, could be sunk to the bottom of the sea, it would be all the better for mankind, — and all the worse for the fishes." This blunt plea for therapeutic nihilism had little effect on practitioners who Holmes admitted were responding, in part, to the public, "which insists on being poisoned" and exerts immense pressure on the physician, "tending to force him to active treatment of some kind."[38] A quarter of a century later, Frederick Roberts, a leading British practitioner, advocated a quiet calm environment for the treatment of an acute attack of palpitations as well as the administration of antispasmodics, sedatives, and stimulants "such as brandy, ether, ammonia, opium or morphia, hydrocyanic acid, bromide of potassium, tincture of henbane, musk, camphor, tincture of lavender, galbanum, or assafoetida, as well as medicines which act upon the heart directly, especially digitalis."[37] The treatment of palpitations was hardly scientific a century ago.

Many forms of congenital heart disease had been defined by 1885, due in large part to the detailed studies of European pathologists. A growing understanding of the origin of these anomalies had resulted from advances in embryology. Diagnosis during life was unusual, however, and rested upon the presence of certain characteristic murmurs and associated physical findings. Writing in 1891, Osler observed, "To the general practitioner congenital heart-disease has an extremely limited interest. A great majority of the cases are still-born, or do not survive many weeks or months. Instances which reach maturity are extremely rare. I do not call to mind more than one or two cases, in a some-what extended hospital practice, of subjects of congenital heart-disease in persons who had passed the age of puberty."[39]

Cardiac surgery. Although the introduction of anesthesia and antiseptic techniques led to important advances in surgical practice during the second half of the 19th century, surgery of the heart lagged because of problems posed by opening the thorax, to say nothing of opening the heart itself. By 1885, however, surgeons were experimenting on suturing wounds of the heart in experimental animals. The belief that this technique was incompatible with life was being dispelled by research. Nevertheless, it would be nearly a half century before there was a sustained effort directed at performing intracardiac surgery.[40] In 1885, the only "heart operation" performed in humans was pericardiocentesis, a procedure popularized in America by the innovative Philadelphia surgeon John Roberts. He concluded his 1880 monograph on the procedure by claiming, "Surely the record I have given supports the plea for the adoption of paracentesis of the pericardium into the family of accepted surgical procedures; surely it is noble to add three or four weeks to the life of a fellow-being. . . . Let the operation be palliative, if you will; but operate, and that before continuance of inflammation, maceration of the heart, and pressure of the distended sac have caused the tissues to assume pathological aspects of such a kind that a perfect return of function is impossible."[41]

The future. This review of the state of cardiology practice a century ago has revealed the limitations faced by practitioners when they attempted to diagnose and treat diseases of the heart. The development of "modern" cardiology and cardiovascular surgery depended on fundamental changes in the structure and philosophy of medical education and medical research. There was growing awareness of the importance of medical research among contemporary practitioners. In 1885, the New York ophthalmologist Henry Noyes observed, "During the year past, it has been permitted me to see many medical men and medical institutions in various parts of Europe. One gets a new impulse from such an opportunity, and one may be lifted to a wider horizon in the field of medicine. . . . The impression which, to me, has come uppermost, is that the line of advance must hereafter be through acute, exacting, and deep research." He continued,

> Our American physicians may be justly proud of their forwardness and energy in such efforts. The wonder is, that they do so much with the meagre facilities which are at their command. I pay willing tribute to men who sacrifice ease and health to pursuits of pure science; who must snatch time from bread-getting, who give public instruction, whose is the heroism of steadfastness and unshrinking labor, that they may contribute to the advance of scientific medicine. You will acquit me of any thought of belittling the achievements of aspirations of my brethren, if I venture to bring before you the need there is among us for better and more perfect methods of pursuing scientific medical research.[42]

Pursuing a similar theme, another writer claimed,

> The gulf between scientific and practical medicine is a wide one. The majority of the profession are practical men, while comparatively few have either the time or inclination to pursue the scientific aspects of medicine. . . . Unforunately, there is a certain amount of antagonism between these two classes [of scientific and practical men]. The practical men are much too apt to sneer at the teachings of the scientist, instead of carefully considering the practice value of their scientific investigations. Were the busy, every-day physician to carefully read, ponder over, and practically deduce from the laborious researches of the scientist, we would have a combination that would be very productive.[43]

During the second half of the 19th century, the emphasis placed on scientific research in the universities of Germany spread to Great Britain and finally to America. Philanthropic and ultimately governmental support of research led to the establishment of sophisticated research institutes and faculty positions in medical schools where original investigation was expected of the faculty members.[44] This fostered scientific research and ultimately led to great improvements in patient care. The development of cardiology as a distinct medical specialty began during the middle third of the 20th century as diagnostic and therapeutic techniques became increasingly specialized and time consuming.[45, 46] The empiricism that characterized cardiology practice a century ago has given way to a specialty deeply rooted in the biomedical and physical sciences. The precious "art" of medicine has been solidly framed in science and the benefactors have been our patients.

References

1. Comroe JH, Dripps RD: The top ten clinical advances in cardiovascular-pulmonary medicine and surgery 1945–1975. Washington, 1977, Government Printing Office
2. Comroe JH: Exploring the heart: discoveries in heart disease and high blood pressure. New York, 1983, W. W. Norton & Co.
3. Spink WW: Infectious diseases: prevention and treatment in the nineteenth and twentieth centuries. Minneapolis, 1978, University of Minnesota Press
4. Rosenberg CE: Social class and medical care in nineteenth-century America: the rise and fall of the dispensary. J Hist Med **29:** 32, 1974
5. Rosenberg CE: What it was like to be sick in 1884. Am Heritage **35:** 22, 1984
6. Rosen G: The hospital: historical sociology of a community institution. *In* From medical police to social medicine: essays on the history of health care. New York, 1974, Science History Publications, p 274
7. Risse GR, Numbers RL, Leavitt JW: Medicine without doctors: home health care in American history. New York, 1977, Science History Publications
8. Rothstein WG: American physicians in the nineteenth century: from sects to science. Baltimore, 1972, Johns Hopkins University Press
9. Medical education and the regulation of the practice of medicine in the United States and Canada. Chicago, 1884, W. T. Keener
10. Success in practice. Med Record **22:** 42, 1882
11. Bonner TN: American doctors and German universities: a chapter in international intellectual relations, 1870–1914. Lincoln, 1963, University of Nebraska Press
12. Hun H: A guide to American medical students in Europe. New York, 1883, William Wood & Co.
13. Seguin EC: The cultivation of specialties in medicine. Arch Med **4:** 280, 1880
14. Shrady G: A plea for the specialist. Med Record **27:** 183, 1885
15. DaCosta JM: Medical diagnosis with special reference to practical medicine, ed 6. Philadelphia, 1884, J. B. Lippincott & Co.
16. Reiser SJ: The medical influence of the stethoscope. Sci Am **240:** 148, 1979
17. Smith DC: Austin Flint and auscultation in America. J Hist Med Allied Sci **33:** 129, 1978
18. Keele KD: The application of the physics of sound to 19th century cardiology: with particular reference to the part played by J. B. Williams and James Hope. Clio Med **8:** 191, 1973
19. Schechter DC, Lillehei CW, Soffer A: History of sphygmology and of heart block. Dis Chest **55**(suppl 1): 535, 1969
20. Cournand A: Cardiac catheterization — development of the technique, its contributions to experimental medicine, and its initial applications in man. Acta Med Scand (suppl 579) 3, 1975
21. Bramwell B: Diseases of the heart and thoracic aorta. New York, 1884, D. Appleton & Co.
22. Burch GE, DePasquale NP: A history of electrocardiography. Chicago, 1964, Year Book Publishers
23. Reiser SJ: Medicine and the reign of technology. Cambridge, 1978, Cambridge University Press
24. Leibowitz JO: The history of coronary heart disease. London, 1970, Wellcome Institute of the History of Medicine
25. Forms and treatments of angina pectoris. Med News **43:** 433, 1883
26. Dunglison RJ: The present treatment of disease: an outline of the medical practice of the day. Philadelphia, 1886, William F. Fell & Co.
27. Murphy GE: The evolution of our knowledge of rheumatic fever: an historical survey with particular emphasis on rheumatic heart disease. Bull Hist Med **14:** 123, 1943
28. Loomis AL: Endocarditis and cardiac valvular diseases. *In* Pepper W, editor: A system of practical medicine. Philadelphia, 1885, Lea Brothers & Co., vol III, p 639
29. Fagge CH: Diseases of the valves of the heart. *In* Reynolds JR, editor: A system of medicine. Philadelphia, 1880, Henry C. Lea's Son & Co., vol II, p 706
30. Phillips CDF: Materia medica and therapeutics. New York, 1879, William Wood & Co.
31. Sansom AE: The Lettsomian lectures on the treatment of some of the forms of valvular disease of the heart. Philadelphia, 1883, P. Blakiston, Son & Co.
32. Osler W: The Gulstonian lectures on malignant endocarditis. Br Med J **1:** 467, 522, 577, 1885
33. [Osler W]: The causes of sudden death. Med News **47:** 630, 1885. This anonymous review is attributed to Osler by his bibliographer, Maude Abbott.
34. Flint A: Neuroses of the heart. *In* Pepper W, editor: A system of practical medicine. Philadelphia, 1885, Lea Brothers & Co., vol III, p 747
35. Fye WB: Ventricular fibrillation and defibrillation: historical perspectives with emphasis on the contributions of John MacWilliam, Carl Wiggers and William Kouwenhoven. Circulation **71:** 858, 1985
36. Bloomfield AL: Auricular fibrillation. *In* A bibliography of internal medicine: selected diseases. Chicago, 1960, University of Chicago Press, p 1
37. Roberts FT: The theory and practice of medicine, ed 5. Philadelphia, 1884, P. Blakiston, Son & Co.
38. Holmes OW: Currents and counter-currents in medical science. Boston, 1860, Ticknor & Fields
39. Osler W: Congenital affections of the heart. *In* Keating JM, editor: Cyclopaedia of the diseases of children. Philadelphia, 1891, J. B. Lippincott Co., vol II, p 747
40. Johnson SL: The history of cardiac surgery 1896–1955. Baltimore, 1970, Johns Hopkins Press
41. Roberts JB: Paracentesis of the pericardium. Philadelphia, 1880, J. B. Lippincott & Co.
42. Noyes HD: Pathfinding in medicine. Med Record **28:** 589, 1885
43. Science and practice. Med Surg Reporter **52:** 722, 1885
44. Shryock RH: American medical research past and present. New York, 1947, The Commonwealth Fund
45. Reichert P: A history of the development of cardiology as a medical specialty. Clin Cardiol **1:** 5, 1978
46. Bishop LF: The birth of a specialty: the diary of an American cardiologist 1926–1972. New York, 1977, Vantage Press

Fibrin formation and platelet aggregation in patients with severe coronary artery disease: relationship with the degree of myocardial ischemia

A. Gallino, M.D., A. Haeberli, Ph.D., H. R. Baur, M.D., and P. W. Straub, M.D.

ABSTRACT Fibrinopeptide A (FpA) concentrations in plasma and in 24 hr urine specimens as well as betathromboglobulin (BTG) in plasma were measured in 17 patients with severe angina pectoris, including both stable and unstable angina, and in 19 patients with acute myocardial infarction. Patients with unstable angina had plasma FpA and BTG levels of 5.2 ± 1.7 ng/ml and 91 ± 23 ng/ml, respectively. The corresponding concentrations of FpA in the 24 hr urine specimens were 8.2 ± 1.4 μg/24 hr. These values were similar to those measured in patients with acute myocardial infarction and higher than the corresponding levels in patients with stable angina ($p < .05$) and in normal control subjects ($p < .01$). The similarity of the platelet and coagulation findings in patients with unstable angina and in those with myocardial infarction favors the hypothesis that coronary thrombosis may play a major role in the pathogenesis of acute myocardial infarction.
Circulation 72, No. 1, 27–30, 1985.

CORONARY THROMBOSIS is frequently associated with acute myocardial infarction and with sudden death due to acute myocardial ischemia.[1-3] Elevated plasma levels of betathromboglobulin (BTG), reflecting enhanced platelet aggregation,[4] have been reported in patients with acute myocardial infarction.[5-8] We have recently found, in accordance with the results of other groups, that patients with acute myocardial infarction often present high plasma levels of fibrinopeptide A (FpA), a reliable index of fibrin formation in vivo.[7-13] Whether FpA is elevated in patients with coronary artery disease without acute myocardial infarction remains controversial. Two recent studies reported elevated plasma levels of BTG but normal FpA values,[6, 8] whereas previous reports indicated elevated FpA values in these patients.[14, 15]

We measured the plasma BTG and FpA levels in patients with severe coronary artery disease with stable and unstable angina pectoris and in the absence of acute myocardial infarction and compared them with the levels in patients with acute myocardial infarction. Since the course of patients with unstable angina is often complicated by acute myocardial infarction, particular attention was paid to the results in patients with unstable angina.

We also measured 24 hr urinary excretion of FpA in all patients with angina and in most of the patients with acute myocardial infarction, since urinary FpA excretion appears to be a reliable parameter for assessing the cumulative effect of thrombin action on fibrinogen.[16]

Methods

Patients

Patients with angina pectoris. A total of 17 patients with severe angina pectoris were admitted to the study. Criteria for admission were: (1) absence of acute myocardial infarction during the last 3 months, (2) absence of thromboembolic events or other factors predisposing to a coagulation disorder (neoplasia, severe infection, collagen disorder, glomerulonephritis), and (3) absence of anticoagulant drugs within the preceding 3 months. Nine of the 17 patients had chronic stable effort angina without rest pain, and eight had unstable angina with recent increase in frequency or severity of chest pain, frequent pain at rest, and progressive decrease in exercise tolerance during the preceding 3 months. A total of nine patients had a history of previous myocardial infarction. All patients had three-vessel disease documented by coronary angiograms obtained within 3 months before the study; seven of 17 patients had decreased ejection fractions between 40% and 60%. All patients were treated with propranolol and long- or short-acting nitrates. Patients with unstable angina also received nifedipine. No patient with stable angina complained of chest pain within 2 hr before blood sampling.

Patients with acute myocardial infarction. FpA and BTG levels were also measured on admission in a group of 19 patients with acute myocardial infarction. Criteria for admission in this group were: (1) history of typical chest pain, (2) electrocardiographic changes of Q waves and/or evolutionary ST-T changes,

From the Thrombosis Research Laboratory, Department of Medicine, University of Bern, Bern, Switzerland.

Address for correspondence: P. W. Straub, M.D, Department of Internal Medicine, University of Bern, Inselspital, CH-3010 Bern, Switzerland.

Received Feb. 19, 1985; accepted April 4, 1985.

(3) presence of elevated creatine kinase (CK) for 2 days, (4) absence of thromboembolic events or other diseases associated with coagulation abnormalities, and (5) absence of anticoagulant drugs within the preceding 3 months. All patients had electrocardiographic evidence of transmural myocardial infarction; nine of 19 had signs of anterior myocardial infarction, whereas the remaining 10 patients had inferior myocardial infarctions. Urinary FpA excretion in the first 24 hr after admission was also measured in 11 of 19 patients who did not receive anticoagulants during this period.

Platelet and coagulation tests. Blood samples were taken by careful venipuncture through an 18-gauge needle. All collections were done by the same investigator. For the BTG measurements 4.2 ml of blood was collected into Thrombotect tubes (Abbott Laboratories, Chicago), placed immediately on ice, and centrifuged within 1 hr at 2500 rpm for 60 min at 4° C. BTG was measured by radioimmunoassay.[5] For the FpA measurement 4.5 ml blood was collected into a plastic syringe containing 500 U of heparin and 500 U of aprotinin dissolved in 0.5 ml of physiologic saline. The samples were centrifuged within 1 hr for 30 min at 2500 rpm at 4° C. The plasma was stored at −25° C. FpA levels were measured by radioimmunoassay in plasma from which fibrinogen had been absorbed by bentonite.[13] Urine was collected over 24 hr periods from 15 normal individuals and from 28 patients. No preservatives were added. Volume and pH were recorded and the pH was adjusted to 8.5 before the assay; urine samples were tested for the presence of blood with the use of Combur 9-test-U (Boehringer, Mannheim, West Germany). Patients with more than five erythrocytes per milliliter were excluded from the study. Urine samples were stored at −25° C. FpA assay in urine samples was performed by radioimmunoassay without previous bentonite absorption or dialysis.

Data analysis. The measured values of FpA showed a skewness toward high values, therefore logarithmic transformation was required to obtain a normal distribution. Statistical analyses were therefore performed with the FpA data logarithmically transformed, and mean FpA levels are expressed as geometric means with standard deviations of the logarithmically transformed data. Statistical significance of changes in the same parameter was evaluated with Student's t test.

Results

Clinical course. Of the eight patients with unstable angina, three developed acute myocardial infarction within 2 days after blood collection, whereas an intracardiac thrombus was detected by angiography in one of them.

Of the nine patients with stable angina, none developed acute myocardial infarction and none had a cardiac thrombus as documented by the previously performed angiographic examination. Nine patients underwent elective aortocoronary bypass surgery and two underwent percutaneous transluminal angioplasty; six patients were treated medically.

Of the 19 patients with acute myocardial infarction, four died in the hospital (three anterior and one inferior myocardial infarction). Two-dimensional echocardiographic results showed a cardiac thrombus in only one patient with acute anterior myocardial infarction.

FpA in plasma and in 24 hr urine specimens (table 1, figures 1 and 2). Plasma and 24 hr urinary levels of FpA in patients with acute myocardial infarction were 5.3 ± 1.8 ng/ml and 6.2 ± 1.9 μg/24 hr and higher than those in patients with stable angina ($p < .05$) and in normal control subjects ($p < .01$). The concentrations of FpA in plasma and in the 24 hr urine specimens of patients with unstable angina were 5.2 ± 1.7 ng/ml and 8.2 ± 1.4 μg/24 hr and were similar to those measured in patients with acute myocardial infarction but were higher than the corresponding values in patients with stable angina ($p < .05$) and in normal control subjects ($p < .01$). Six of 17 patients with angina had normal plasma and urinary concentrations of FpA. All six had chronic stable effort angina without pain at rest (figures 1 and 2), whereas no patient with unstable angina had normal FpA concentrations in plasma or in the 24 hr urine samples. The highest plasma and urinary concentration of FpA were found in the only patient with left ventricular wall thrombus documented by echocardiography. When the values of FpA in plasma and in the 24 hr urine specimens were compared, a significant correlation was found ($r = .68$, $p < .01$, $n = 43$).

BTG in plasma (figure 3). BTG in patients with acute myocardial infarction (84 ± 25 ng/ml) was higher than

TABLE 1

Plasma and 24 hr urinary FpA and plasma BTG levels in control subjects and in different subgroups of patients

	Controls	Angina pectoris: Stable	Angina pectoris: Unstable	Myocardial infarction
n	15	9	8	19
Plasma FpA (ng/ml)	1.7±0.7	2.4±1.5	5.2±1.7^B	5.3±1.8^B
Urinary FpA (μg/24 hr)	1.9±0.9	2.4±1.9	8.2±1.4^B	6.2±1.9^B
Plasma BTG (ng/ml)	28±13	71±32^A	91±23^B	84±25^B
Urinary creatinine (g/24 hr)	1.4±0.4	2.1±1.2^C	1.7±0.9^D	2.0±0.9

^{A}Significantly different ($p < .01$) when compared with control subjects.
^{B}Significantly different ($p < .01$) when compared with patients with stable angina pectoris.
^{C}Significantly different ($p < .05$) when compared with control subjects.
^{D}n = 5.

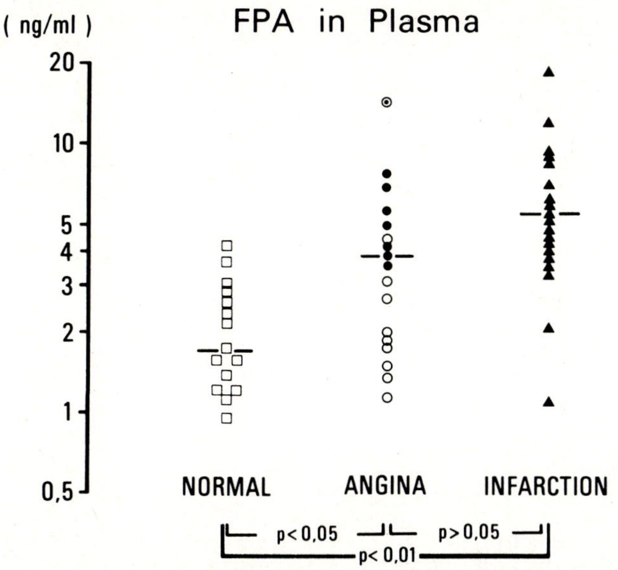

FIGURE 1. Plasma FpA concentrations in control subjects (□) and in patients with stable (○) and unstable angina (●), myocardial infarction (▲), and left ventricular thrombus (⊙) (n = 1).

that in normal control subjects ($p < .01$) but only slightly higher than that in patients with angina. The mean BTG levels of patients with unstable angina (91 ± 23 ng/ml) and acute myocardial infarction were comparable, but both were higher than the mean levels in patients with stable angina ($p < .05$). The patient with a cardiac thrombus had the highest BTG value (220 ng/ml).

Discussion

The elevated BTG and FpA levels in patients with unstable angina pectoris indicate that these patients may have enhanced platelet aggregation and fibrin formation similar to those in patients with acute myocardial infarction. Recent studies in patients with angina pectoris also reported elevated plasma levels of BTG but normal FpA.[6, 8] The discrepancy between these results and our data is probably due to the more severe degree of coronary artery disease but particularly to the presence of many cases with unstable angina in our group of patients. In fact, all our patients had three-vessel disease documented by a recent angiogram.

Our plasma FpA findings were furthermore supported by the results of the FpA concentrations found in the 24 hr urine specimens, which showed a good correlation with the plasma values. Urinary FpA excretion appears to represent a valid alternative to the measurement of FpA in plasma, because it should provide a cumulative measure of the overall thrombin action on fibrinogen.[16] Furthermore, urinary FpA is not influenced by technical factors like poor venipuncture. The observation that patients with unstable angina had significantly higher BTG and FpA values than those with stable angina despite a comparable extent of coronary obstructive disease suggest that the actual degree of ischemia at the time of the examination is a more important determinant of the amount of platelet activation and fibrin formation than the extent of anatomic obstruction.[15] This assumption is further supported by our findings that patients with unstable angina and patients with acute myocardial infarction showed comparable BTG and FpA elevations.

Acute myocardial infarction has often been associated with coronary thrombosis[1–3] and with a high rate of

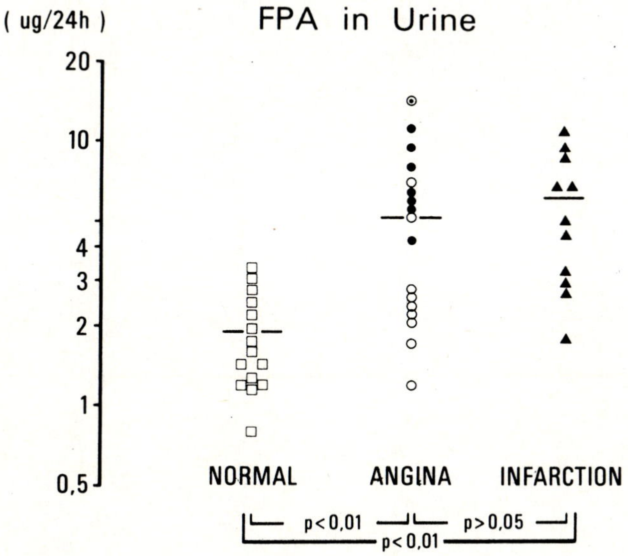

FIGURE 2. Twenty-four hour urinary FpA concentrations in control subjects (□) and in patients with stable (○) and unstable angina (●), myocardial infarction (▲), and left ventricular thrombus (⊙).

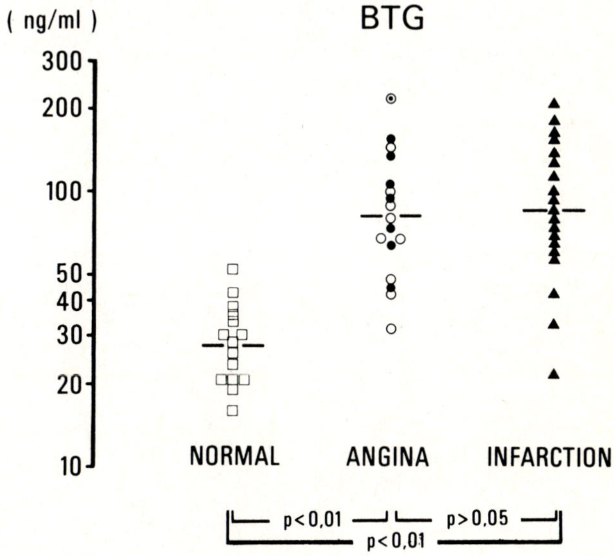

FIGURE 3. Plasma BTG concentrations in control subjects (□) and in patients with stable (○) and unstable angina (●), myocardial infarction (▲), and left ventricular thrombus (⊙).

fibrin formation and increased platelet aggregation in peripheral venous blood.[7–10] On the other hand, unstable angina is often complicated by the occurrence of acute myocardial infarction.[17] The finding in this study that unstable angina was associated with a comparable hypercoagulable state and a comparable increase in platelet aggregation as in acute myocardial infarction might favor the hypothesis that coronary thrombosis plays a major role in the pathogenesis of myocardial infarction.[1,2] Our results are also in agreement with the 12% incidence of intracoronary thrombus in patients with unstable angina pectoris[18] and with the recent observation that aspirin significantly reduces the incidence of myocardial infarction in such patients.[19] Our results do not prove a causal relationship between platelet aggregation, fibrin formation, and myocardial ischemia. It may be that the coagulation disorder represents a consequence rather than a cause of myocardial ischemia. Thus ischemia may transiently affect the integrity of the endocardial and/or the coronary endothelium to an extent that would explain the activation of both platelets and coagulation.

Further studies will be necessary to clarify the relationship between myocardial ischemia and the observed activation of both platelets and the plasmatic coagulation.[20]

We thank Miss Brigitte Rindlisbacher for her technical assistance and Dr. Giorgio Mombelli for valuable criticism of the manuscript.

References

1. Davies MJ, Woolf N, Robertson WB: Pathology of acute myocardial infarction with particular reference to occlusive coronary thrombi. Br Heart J **38:** 659, 1976
2. De Wood MA, Spores J, Notske R, Mouse LT, Burroughs R, Golden MS, Lang HT: Prevalence of total coronary occlusion during the early hours of transmural myocardial infarction. N Engl J Med **303:** 897, 1980
3. Davies MJ, Thomas A: Thrombosis and acute coronary artery lesions in sudden cardiac ischemic death. N Engl J Med **310:** 1137, 1984
4. Bolton AE, Ludlam CA, Moore S, Pepper DS, Cash JD: Three approaches to radioimmunoassay of betathromboglobulin. Br J Haematol **33:** 323, 1976
5. Kaplan KL, Owen J: Plasma levels of betathromboglobulin and platelet factor 4 as indices of platelet activation in vivo. Blood **57:** 199, 1981
6. Nichols AB, Owen J, Kaplan KL, Sciacca RR, Cannon PG, Nossel HL: Fibrinopeptide A, platelet factor 4 and betathromboglobulin levels in coronary heart disease. Blood **60:** 650, 1982
7. Rasi V, Ikkala E, Torstila I: Plasma betathromboglobulin in acute myocardial infarction. Thromb Res **25:** 203, 1982
8. Van Hulsteijn H, Kolff J, Briet E, van der Laarse A, Bertina R: Fibrinopeptide A and β-thromboglobulin in patients with angina pectoris and acute myocardial infarction. Am Heart J **107:** 39, 1984
9. Mombelli G, Im Hof V, Haeberli A, Straub PW: Effect of heparin on plasma fibrinopeptide A in patients with acute myocardial infarction. Circulation **69:** 684, 1984
10. Johnson H, Orinius E, Paul C: Fibrionopeptide A in patients with acute myocardial infarction. Thromb Res **16:** 255, 1979
11. Nossel HL: Radioimmunoassay of fibrinopeptides in relation to intravascular coagulation and thrombosis. N Engl J Med **295:** 428, 1976
12. Nossel HL, Yudelman I, Canfield RE, Butler VP Jr, Spanondis K, Wilner GD, Qureshi GD: Measurement of fibrinopeptide A in human blood. J Clin Invest **54:** 43, 1974
13. Hofmann V, Straub PW: A radioimmunoassay for the rapid measurement of human fibrinopeptide A. Thromb Res **11:** 171, 1977
14. Neri Serneri GG, Gensini GF, Abbate R, Laureano R, Parodi O: Is raised plasma fibrinopeptide A a marker of acute coronary insufficiency? Lancet **2:** 982, 1980
15. Sobel M, Salzman EW, Davies GC, Handin RI, Sweeney J, Ploetz J, Kurland G: Circulating platelet products in unstable angina pectoris. Circulation **63:** 300, 1981
16. Alkjaersig N, Fletcher AP: Catabolism and excretion of fibrinopeptide A. Blood **60:** 148, 1982
17. Gazes PC, Mobley EM, Farris HM, Duncan RC, Humphries GB: Preinfarction (unstable) angina — a prospective study — ten year follow-up. Circulation **48:** 331, 1973
18. Zack PM, Ischinger T, Aker UT, Dincer B, Kennedy HL: The occurrence of angiographically detected intracoronary thrombus in patients with unstable angina pectoris. Am Heart J **108:** 1408, 1984
19. Lewis HD Jr, Davies JW, Archibald DG: Protective effects of aspirin against acute myocardial infarction and death in men with unstable angina: results of Veteran Administration cooperative study. N Engl J Med **309:** 396, 1983
20. Mitchell JRA: Does thrombosis cause myocardial infarction or does myocardial infarction cause thrombosis? Acta Cardiol (Brux) **20** (suppl 1): 47, 1974

Risk factors for the development of prosthetic valve endocarditis

STEPHEN B. CALDERWOOD, M.D., LOIS A. SWINSKI, R.N., CHRISTINE M. WATERNAUX, PH.D., ADOLF W. KARCHMER, M.D., AND MORTIMER J. BUCKLEY, M.D.

ABSTRACT Risk factors for the development of prosthetic valve endocarditis (PVE) were analyzed in 2642 patients undergoing initial valve replacement at the Massachusetts General Hospital from 1975 to 1982. Follow-up was available for 2608 patients (98.7%); the mean length of follow-up was 39.8 months. PVE developed in 116 patients (4.4%). The actuarial risk of PVE was 3.1% at 12 months and 5.7% at 60 months. A Cox model was used to identify risk factors for PVE. Recipients of multiple valves had a higher risk of PVE than single valves ($p = .01$). There was no difference in the risk of PVE for patients receiving aortic valves vs those receiving mitral valves. Recipients of mechanical valves had a higher risk of PVE than recipients of porcine valves in the first 3 months after surgery ($p = .02$), but the risk of PVE was higher for porcine valve recipients 12 months or more after surgery ($p = .004$). Despite this difference in the time course of development of PVE, there was no significant difference in the cumulative risk of PVE by 5 years of follow-up between mechanical and porcine valve recipients. Male sex was a risk factor for PVE within 12 months of aortic valve replacement ($p = .008$) but not thereafter; sex did not influence the risk of PVE after mitral valve replacement. Older patients had a higher risk of late PVE after multiple ($p = .04$) or mitral valve replacement ($p = .08$), but not after aortic valve replacement.
Circulation 72, No. 1, 31–37, 1985.

PROSTHETIC valve endocarditis (PVE) is a serious but infrequent complication of cardiac valvular replacement. The incidence of PVE has been previously estimated at 1% to 4%.[1–6] However, several prior studies may have underestimated the true incidence of PVE because of the lack of comprehensive follow-up information on operated patients[2] or the use of nonactuarial methods of data analysis.[1] In other studies, the method of obtaining follow-up information and the number of patients lost to follow-up have not been detailed.[3, 5] Some reports have used "linearized rates" to quantify the risk of PVE, stated as a percentage incidence per unit time.[5, 7, 8] However, as confirmed in a recent study,[6] the risk of PVE is not constant with time but involves a higher risk period initially after surgery and a lower risk thereafter.

In this study, we wished to define the incidence of PVE over time in a large group of patients undergoing initial cardiac valvular replacement and to examine risk factors for the development of PVE. Identification of patients at higher risk of developing PVE should allow testing of new measures for prevention of infection in specific high-risk groups. In addition, clarification of risk factors for PVE may provide important insights into the pathogenesis of this infection.

Methods

Study population. All patients undergoing initial valve replacement at the Massachusetts General Hospital between January 1, 1975, and December 31, 1982, were studied; prior cardiac surgery other than valve replacement did not exclude patient entry. Information on each patient was entered into a computerized data base, preserving patient confidentiality. Data gathered included demographic information, preoperative cardiac diagnosis and findings of catheterization, and detailed information about the operation, including date, duration of cardiopulmonary bypass, duration of aortic cross-clamping, operative procedure, site and type of valve replacement(s), and concomitant procedures performed. Mechanical prostheses implanted during the study period included Starr-Edwards, Björk-Shiley, and St. Jude valves; porcine bioprostheses included Hancock and Carpentier-Edwards valves.[9]

All patients received perioperative antibiotic prophylaxis for a period of 2 to 7 days. The antimicrobial drugs used and the duration of therapy varied during the study period because of physician preference, patient allergy, and evolving concepts about optimal prophylaxis. In the first 2 years of the study, the most common prophylactic regimen was intravenous oxacillin or nafcillin, followed by oral cloxacillin or dicloxacillin for a

From the Infectious Disease and Cardiovascular Surgical Units, Massachusetts General Hospital, and Department of Biostatistics, Harvard School of Public Health, Boston.

Supported in part by grants from American Edwards Laboratories, Santa Anna, CA; Extracorporeal, Inc., King of Prussia, PA; and Shiley, Inc., Irvine, CA.

Address for correspondence: Stephen B. Calderwood, M.D., Infectious Disease Unit, Massachusetts General Hospital, Boston, MA 02114.

Received Nov. 26, 1984; revision accepted April 4, 1985.

total course of 5 to 7 days. In the later years of the study, a first-generation parenteral cephalosporin (cefazolin, cephalothin, or cephapirin) was frequently used for 2 to 5 days.

Follow-up of patients for the development of PVE was conducted between October 1, 1982, and October 1, 1983. Each patient or a relative was contacted by telephone to ascertain the current status of the valve recipient and to determine whether hospitalization had occurred in the interim since valve replacement. Physicians of patients were contacted if the patient could not be located or to verify the nature of subsequent hospital admissions. Detailed records of hospitalization, autopsy reports, or death certificates were examined as needed to substantiate the follow-up status of individual patients.

Patients who either died in the follow-up interval without PVE or who required a second valve replacement for reasons other than PVE were censored at the time of that event. The period of risk for PVE was calculated as the time between initial valve replacement and the earliest of the following: the date of death, the date of reoperation for reasons other than PVE, the date of telephone contact, or the date of onset of PVE.

Definitions. The diagnosis of PVE was accepted[2, 10] if at least two of the following three criteria were met: (1) a clinical illness compatible with bacterial endocarditis (two or more of: fever; new or changing heart murmur; presence of petechiae, splinter hemorrhages, Roth spots, Janeway lesions, or Osler nodes; unexplained emboli; unexplained anemia, elevated sedimentation rate, hematuria, or a positive test for rheumatoid factor); (2) two or more positive blood cultures for the same organism, either without an identifiable extracardiac source or, if associated with an identified extracardiac source, with evidence of valvular involvement by new or changing heart murmur, evidence of vegetations by echocardiogram or catheterization, or confirmation at surgery or autopsy; (3) histopathologic or microbiologic evidence of valvular infection at surgery or autopsy. Fifty-nine percent of our patients with PVE (68 of 116) were eventually proved pathologically.

The onset of PVE was taken as the earliest of: (1) the date of the first physician visit for an illness eventually proved to be PVE, (2) the date of the first positive blood culture for an organism eventually shown to be the causative pathogen of PVE, (3) the date of hospital admission for treatment of PVE.

Staphylococci were considered methicillin resistant if they were reported as resistant to methicillin or oxacillin by standard bacteriologic techniques or if they demonstrated the presence of methicillin heteroresistant subpopulations, as previously described.[11]

Data analysis. All statistical computations were performed with the Biomedical Programs statistical software (BMDP 1982). Two-way tables comparing the frequencies of categorical events without censoring were analyzed with the Pearson chi-square statistic. Life-table methods were used to compute the proportion of patients free of PVE at 3 month intervals, the corresponding monthly hazard rate and standard error, and the cumulative hazard function. The hazard rate at time t (in months) estimates the probability that a patient free of PVE at that time will develop PVE in the following month, and the cumulative hazard function estimates the cumulative probability of PVE over time. In this study, because the risk of PVE is relatively small, the mathematical expressions for the cumulative hazard function and the cumulative risk of PVE are virtually identical. Data in the figures are presented as the cumulative hazard function for PVE vs time. Actuarial estimates of the risk of PVE for two groups, without adjusting for any other risk factors or potentially confounding variables, were compared by the generalized Wilcoxon test.

Risk factors for the development of PVE were identified by means of a Cox regression model with a backward deletion algorithm. The following covariates were considered: sex, age, prior cardiac surgery, preoperative pulmonary capillary wedge pressure, position of valve(s) replaced, type of valve(s) implanted, duration of aortic cross-clamping and cardiopulmonary bypass, concomitant cardiac surgical procedures, and year of surgery. Cox regression models for the risk of early PVE (first 12 months after surgery) were fitted by censoring all patients free of PVE at 12 months. For analyzing the risk of late PVE, only patients who were free of PVE for more than 12 months were considered.

Results

During the study period, 2642 patients underwent initial valve replacement at the Massachusetts General Hospital; follow-up information was available after hospital discharge for 2608 patients (98.7%) and these constitute the study group. Thirty-four patients were lost to follow-up after valve replacement (21 male and 13 female; 19 aortic, nine mitral, and six multiple valve recipients). Duration of follow-up ranged from 0.5 to 103 months; mean follow-up was 39.8 months and the median was 38.0. The distribution by calendar year of patients operated on, lost to follow-up, and developing PVE is shown in table 1.

The age of the study group ranged from under 1 year to 86 years; the mean age was 59.2 years and the median was 61.0. Distribution by sex and by position of the implanted valve(s) is shown in table 2. Aortic valve replacement was more common in male patients and mitral valve replacement in female patients ($p < .001$). In the group with multiple valve replacements, 246 patients received aortic and mitral valves, 32 mitral and tricuspid, 17 aortic, mitral, and tricuspid, and one aortic and tricuspid. For single valve recipients, the type of valve inserted is shown by valve position in table 3.

The frequency of other surgical procedures done concomitantly with valve replacement was as follows:

TABLE 1

Distribution of patients by year of surgery, sex, completion of follow-up, and number with PVE

Year of operation	Sex: Female	Sex: Male	Total	Lost to follow-up	No. with PVE
1975	204	208	412	4	14
1976	177	175	352	1	22
1977	173	168	341	4	10
1978	159	186	345	6	24
1979	163	183	346	2	10
1980	136	153	289	6	12
1981	144	154	298	8	12
1982	120	139	259	3	12
Total	1276	1366	2642	34 (1.3%)	116 (4.4%)[A]

[A]Percentage of 2608 patients with follow-up who developed PVE.

TABLE 2
Distribution of study group and incidence of PVE by valve position and sex[A]

Sex	AVR	MVR	TVR	Multiple	Total
	Valve position				
Male	47/878	13/353	0/3	3/111	63/1345 (4.7%)
Female	8/419	28/657	0/2	17/185	53/1263 (4.2%)
Total	55/1297 (4.2%)	41/1010 (4.1%)	0/5	20/296 (6.8%)	116/2608 (4.4%)

AVR = aortic valve replacement; MVR = mitral valve replacement; TVR = tricuspid valve replacement.

[A]Numerator is the number of patients developing PVE in the follow-up interval; denominator is the number of patients with follow-up after hospital discharge. Percentage figures refer to incidence of PVE in each group.

coronary artery bypass surgery in 587 of 2608 patients (23%), other procedures using prosthetic material (such as repair of aortic aneurysms, patch closure of atrial or ventricular septal defects, repair of aortic coarctation) in 81 patients (3%), associated valve procedures without valve replacement (such as valvuloplasty or valvulotomy) in 69 patients (3%), and miscellaneous associated procedures in 151 patients (6%).

Incidence of PVE. During the follow-up interval, 116 of 2608 patients (4.4%) developed PVE. The incidence of PVE by valve position and sex is shown in table 2. The cumulative hazard function for PVE is shown in figure 1. The actuarial risk of PVE was 3.1% at 12 months and 5.7% at 60 months.

Bacteriology of infection. The distribution of cases of PVE by infecting organism and by time of onset after surgery is shown in table 4. The distribution of organisms was similar in patients with onset of infection within 2 months of surgery, between 2 and 6 months after surgery, and between 6 and 12 months after surgery. Coagulase-negative staphylococci caused 22 of 38 (58%) and 41 of 72 (57%) cases of PVE during the initial 2 months and 12 months after surgery, respectively. Patients with onset of PVE more than 12

TABLE 3
Distribution of single valve recipients by valve position and valve type

Valve type	AVR	MVR	TVR	Total
	Valve position			
Starr-Edwards	329	205	0	534
Björk-Shiley	134	113	0	247
Hancock	514	414	3	931
Carpentier-Edwards	319	275	2	596
St. Jude	1	3	0	4
Total	1297	1010	5	2312

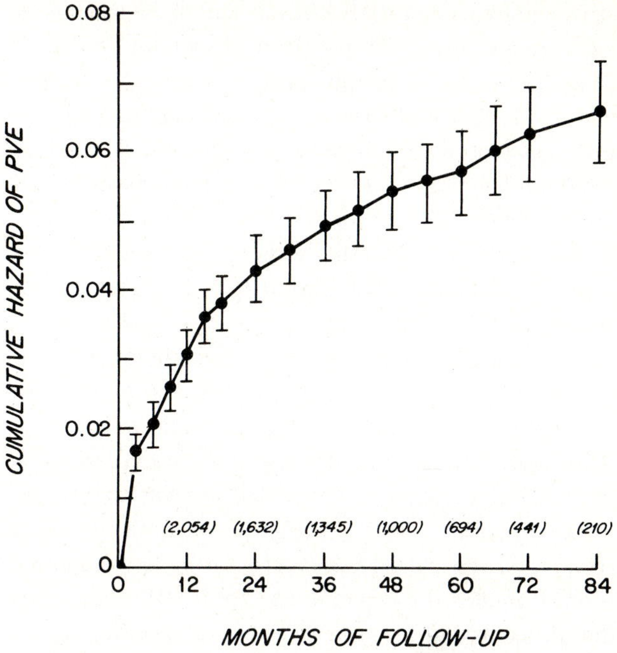

FIGURE 1. Cumulative hazard of PVE for all patients. Data points are mean values (± 1 SEM). Figures in parentheses along the abscissa refer to the number of patients being followed at the start of the subsequent interval.

months after valve replacement showed a different pattern of infecting organisms, with streptococci and the fastidious gram-negative coccobacilli (such as *Actinobacillus, Cardiobacterium,* and *Hemophilus spp*) predominating. The distribution of infecting organisms did not differ by valve position, valve type, or sex.

The majority of infections caused by coagulase-neg-

TABLE 4
Distribution of patients with PVE by time of onset after surgery and infecting organism

Infecting organism	<2 mo	2–6 mo	6–12 mo	>12 mo	Total
	Time of onset after surgery				
Coagulase-negative staphylococci	22	6	13	10	51
Gram-negative bacilli	2	0	1	1	4
Diphtheroids	4	0	0	1	5
Fungi	2	0	2	1	5
Staphylococcus aureus	2	1	2	5	10
Streptococci[A]	0	0	1	12	13
Enterococci	0	1	1	4	6
Fastidious gram-negative coccobacilli[B]	0	0	1	7	8
Other and mixed	3[C]	2[C]	0	1	6
Culture-negative	3	2	1	2	8
Total	38	12	22	44	116

[A]Excludes enterococci.
[B]*Actinobacillus, Cardiobacterium,* and *Hemophilus.*
[C]Includes one patient infected with coagulase-negative staphylococci plus a second organism.

ative staphylococci (81%) began within 12 months of valve replacement. Thirty-six of 43 strains (84%) of coagulase-negative staphylococci causing infection within 12 months of surgery were resistant to methicillin as compared with three of 10 strains (30%) causing infection later ($p = .001$). The frequency of methicillin resistance did not differ between strains from cases in the first 6 months after surgery (83%) and strains causing infection in the period 6 to 12 months after surgery (85%).

Incremental risk factors for PVE. Recipients of multiple valves had a higher risk of PVE throughout the follow-up interval than recipients of single valves ($p = .01$) (figure 2). This higher risk was particularly evident in female subjects ($p < .0001$) but was not present in male patients. Within the group of multiple valve recipients, significant risk factors for the development of PVE included advancing age ($p = .01$), concomitant procedure at the time of valve replacement ($p = .04$), and possibly female sex ($p = .08$). When patients with onset of PVE less than 12 months after surgery were analyzed separately from those with later onset, advancing age was a significant risk factor for late PVE ($p = .04$) but not for early onset.

The time course of development of PVE was different for recipients of mechanical valves as compared with those of porcine valves (figure 3). Recipients of mechanical valves had a higher risk of PVE in the 3 months after surgery ($p = .02$) but recipients of porcine valves had a higher risk of infection 12 months or more after surgery ($p = .004$). These differences in risk persisted unchanged when potentially confounding variables were accounted for in the Cox model. Although the time course of development of PVE was different between recipients of mechanical and porcine valves, the cumulative risk of PVE was not significantly different by 5 years of follow-up.

There was no difference overall in the risk of PVE between recipients of aortic and mitral prostheses or between male and female subjects (table 2). However, significant interactions occurred between these variables in the Cox model. For aortic valve recipients, risk factors for PVE included male sex ($p = .004$) and possibly prolonged cardiopulmonary bypass time ($p = .07$). When infections during the year after surgery were analyzed separately from those occurring later, male sex was a significant risk factor for the development of PVE within 12 months of surgery ($p = .008$) but not later. Recipients of porcine valves were at higher risk of PVE than those of mechanical valves 12 months or more after surgery ($p = .03$). In addition, prolonged cardiopulmonary bypass time was a significant risk factor for the later development of PVE ($p = .01$).

For mitral valve recipients, those with porcine valve

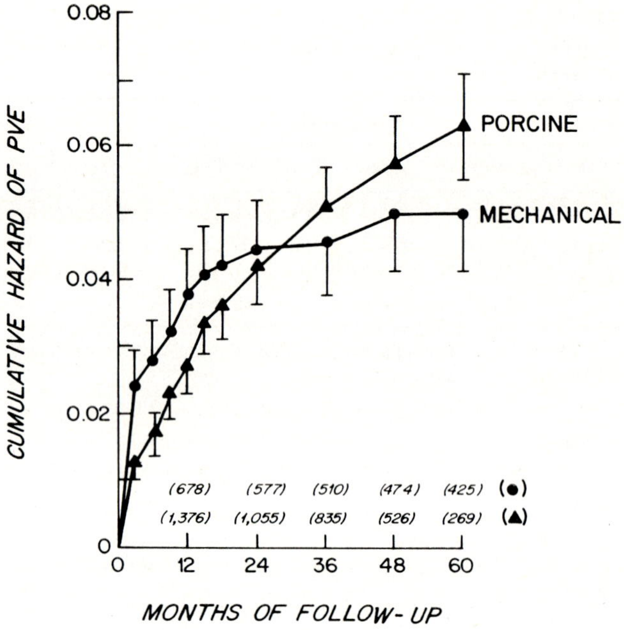

FIGURE 3. Cumulative hazard of PVE compared in recipients of mechanical prostheses and porcine prostheses. Data points are mean values (± 1 SEM). Figures in parentheses along the abscissa refer to the number of patients in each group being followed at the start of the subsequent interval.

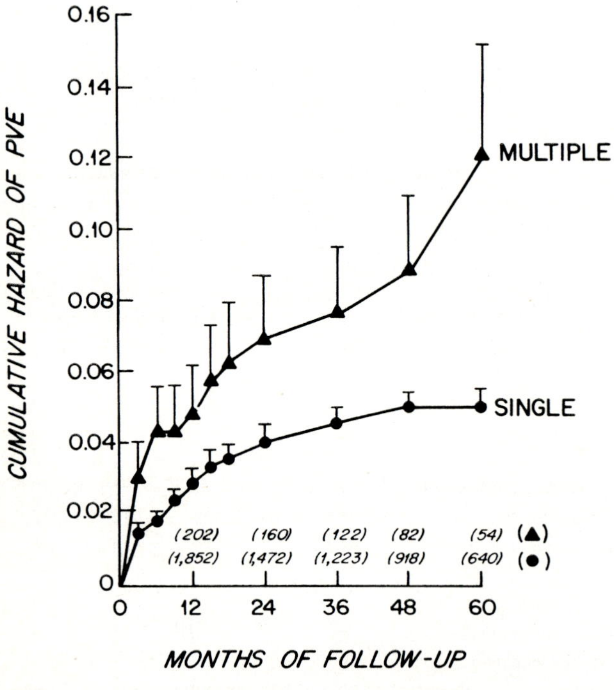

FIGURE 2. Cumulative hazard of PVE compared in multiple valve recipients and single valve recipients. Data points are mean values (± 1 SEM). Figures in parentheses along the abscissa refer to the number of patients in each group being followed at the start of the subsequent interval.

replacements had a lower incidence of PVE in the year after surgery than those with mechanical valves ($p = .02$) but had a higher incidence later ($p = .04$). In the period more than 12 months after surgery, there was a tendency toward higher risk of PVE with advancing age ($p = .08$).

Discussion

Despite major advances in cardiovascular surgical technique and postoperative care and routine use of prophylactic antimicrobial agents, PVE continues to complicate the course of a small percentage of patients after cardiac valve replacement. Further advances in the prevention of this infection will depend on a better understanding of its pathogenesis and on risk factors for its development.

PVE has been recognized to be a time-related event, with a higher risk in the months shortly after surgery and a lower risk thereafter. "Early onset" PVE has been arbitrarily defined as that occurring within 60 days of surgery[12, 13]; the pathogenesis of these infections has been attributed to events occurring either during or shortly after surgery.[12, 14] "Late onset" PVE has been defined as infection beginning 60 days or more after valve replacement.[12] These infections have been attributed to contamination of the valve during bacteremia that results from incidental infection or from trauma to body surfaces colonized with microorganisms.

Prior estimates of the incidence of PVE have frequently overlooked the time-related nature of this infection. Comprehensive follow-up of the operated group has either not been attempted[2] or the method and success of such follow-up has not been detailed.[3, 5] The use of nonactuarial methods to calculate the risk of PVE may lead to an underestimation of the true incidence because of a failure to recognize the importance of the duration of follow-up.[1] Calculation of "linearized rates," presented as incidence of infection per unit time, blurs the distinction between the higher risk period after surgery and the lower risk period later.[5, 7, 8]

In the present series, we sought to define carefully the incidence of PVE after initial valve replacement. We followed a large study population over an extended period of time and used a well-accepted definition[2, 10] for the presence of PVE. Using actuarial methods, we estimated the cumulative risk of PVE as 3.1% at 12 months and 5.7% at 60 months after surgery. Ivert et al.[6] have recently analyzed the incidence of PVE after initial valve replacement at the University of Alabama in Birmingham, using methods of data analysis similar to our own. They confirmed the higher risk of PVE in the first 6 to 12 months after surgery and the lower risk thereafter. Their actuarial estimates of the risk of PVE, 3.0% at 12 months and 4.1% at 48 months, are similar to the cumulative risks in the present study.

Among our patients with PVE, the distribution of infecting organisms with time after surgery (table 4) showed several interesting differences from previous studies. In the past, *Staphylococcus aureus*, enteric gram-negative bacilli, and coagulase-negative staphylococci were the most frequent pathogens causing PVE with onset in the first 2 months after surgery.[2, 13] Among patients with onset of PVE later than 2 months after surgery, streptococci were the predominant cause of PVE, with *S. aureus* and coagulase-negative staphylococci remaining prominent.[2, 13] In the present series, *S. aureus* and enteric gram-negative bacilli rarely caused PVE during the initial 2 months after surgery, while coagulase-negative staphylococci became the predominant causative organisms. In addition, among the organisms causing our cases of PVE, those bacteria considered likely to have caused infection acquired outside of the hospital (streptococci, enterococci, and fastidious gram-negative coccobacilli) did not appear prominently at 2 months after surgery but rather only after a year had elapsed from valve implantation. The spectrum of infecting organisms was quite similar throughout the first 12 months after surgery, suggesting these cases may share a similar pathogenesis. Support for this hypothesis derives from the high frequency of methicillin resistance (84%) among coagulase-negative staphylococci causing PVE throughout the initial 12 months after surgery, as contrasted with the significantly lower frequency of methicillin resistance (30%) among strains causing PVE thereafter. Karchmer et al.[11] have reported a similar distribution of methicillin resistance in coagulase-negative staphylococci from a multi-institutional study of PVE; they found methicillin resistance in 87% of strains from cases occurring within 1 year of surgery, as compared with 22% of strains from infections occurring later. Methicillin-resistant coagulase-negative staphylococci are infrequent isolates from cardiac surgical patients at the time of hospital admission but become common skin flora in these patients shortly after cardiac surgery,[15] suggesting that methicillin resistance is, to a degree, a marker for hospital-acquired strains of coagulase-negative staphylococci. The frequency of methicillin-resistant coagulase-negative staphylococci as causes of PVE throughout the initial year after surgery suggests the possible nosocomial origin of these cases. Thus the distribution of the organisms causing our cases of PVE suggests that 12 months may be a better break point for defining nosocomial (early onset) PVE than the previous definition of cases with onset within 2 months of surgery.

Several previous studies have examined risk factors for the development of PVE after valve replacement. Many of these studies had relatively small sample sizes or failed to analyze the differences found by statistical techniques. Recipients of multiple valves have been previously shown to be at higher risk for PVE than recipients of single valves.[5, 16] Some prior studies have suggested a higher incidence of infection in patients with aortic prostheses than in those with mitral prostheses,[2, 7, 8, 16, 17] although one study suggested the opposite[5] and two have shown no difference.[1, 6] One study suggested a higher risk of infection for porcine prostheses than for mechanical,[5] but two larger studies failed to find any difference.[7, 8]

Ivert et al.[6] carefully examined risk factors for PVE in a large study population with thorough follow-up. They found no difference overall in the incidence of PVE in patients with aortic or mitral prostheses. Patients with mechanical prostheses had a significantly higher risk of PVE than those with porcine prostheses in the initial 6 months after surgery, but the rates of infection were similar thereafter. These investigators identified four additional risk factors for the development of prosthetic valve infection: male sex, prolonged cardiopulmonary bypass time, antecedent native valve endocarditis, and black race.

The present series is the largest to date to examine incremental risk factors for the development of PVE by means of detailed statistical analysis. Our results confirm the enhanced risk of PVE among multiple valve recipients as compared with that of single valve recipients. This difference persisted when potentially confounding variables were taken into account in the Cox model. We found no difference overall between infection rates in patients with aortic and mitral prostheses, although the risk factors for infection within each group were different.

We confirmed the higher early risk of PVE in recipients of mechanical prostheses but showed that porcine valve recipients actually have a higher risk of late PVE. One possible explanation for the difference in our results compared with those of Ivert et al.[6] is the larger sample size in the present study, particularly the larger number of porcine valve recipients. The differing time course for the development of PVE in patients wih mechanical and porcine valves may indicate important differences in the pathogenesis of infection with these two valve types. Nevertheless, the absence of a significant difference between these two groups in the cumulative risk of PVE by 5 years of follow-up implies that the choice of a mechanical vs porcine prosthesis cannot be made at present on the basis of long-term risk of PVE.

We confirmed the influence of advanced age on the risk for PVE. However, we found that age predominantly affected the risk of PVE 12 months or more after surgery, particularly in recipients of multiple or mitral prostheses. Male sex was a risk factor for PVE on aortic prostheses in the 12 months after surgery but not thereafter; sex did not influence the risk of infection on mitral valve prostheses.

Explanations for the risk factors identified in the present study can only be speculative. More detailed analysis of the various groups will be necessary before the pathogenetic principles underlying the observed differences in the risk for PVE can be understood. Our results allow an accurate assessment of the risk for developing PVE at a major cardiovascular surgical center with current techniques and the identification of subgroups of patients at higher risk for PVE for whom new methods of infection prevention should be targeted.

We are indebted to John B. Newell, Director of Cardiac Computer Center, Massachusetts General Hospital, for expert assistance in analyzing the computerized data base and to Judy Feiner for the preparation of the manuscript.

References

1. Slaughter L, Morris JE, Starr A: Prosthetic valvular endocarditis: a 12-year review. Circulation **47:** 1319, 1973
2. Wilson WR, Jaumin PM, Danielson GK, Giuliani ER, Washington JA II, Geraci JE: Prosthetic valve endocarditis. Ann Intern Med **82:** 751, 1975
3. Masur H, Johnson WD Jr: Prosthetic valve endocarditis. J Thorac Cardiovasc Surg **80:** 31, 1980
4. Cohn LH, Mudge GH, Pratter F, Collins JJ Jr: Five to eight year follow-up of patients undergoing porcine heart-valve replacement. N Engl J Med **304:** 258, 1981
5. Turina M: Prosthetic valve endocarditis. Thorac Cardiovasc Surgeon **30:** 350, 1982
6. Ivert TSA, Dismukes WE, Cobbs CG, Blackstone EH, Kirklin JW, Bergdahl LAL: Prosthetic valve endocarditis. Circulation **69:** 223, 1984
7. Oyer PE, Stinson EB, Griepp RB, Shumway NE: Valve replacement with the Starr-Edwards and Hancock prostheses: comparative analysis of late morbidity and mortality. Ann Surg **186:** 301, 1977
8. Rossiter SJ, Stinson EB, Oyer PE, Miller DC, Schapira JN, Martin RP, Shumway NE: Prosthetic valve endocarditis: comparison of heterograft tissue valves and mechanical valves. J Thorac Cardiovasc Surg **76:** 795, 1978
9. McClung JA, Stein JH, Ambrose JA, Herman MV, Reed GE: Prosthetic heart valves: a review. Prog Cardiovasc Dis **26:** 237, 1983
10. Karchmer AW, Dismukes WE, Buckley MJ, Austen WG: Late prosthetic valve endocarditis: clinical features influencing therapy. Am J Med **64:** 199, 1978
11. Karchmer AW, Archer GL, Dismukes WE: *Staphylococcus epidermidis* causing prosthetic valve endocarditis: microbiologic and

clinical observations as guides to therapy. Ann Intern Med **98:** 447, 1983

12. Block PC, DeSanctis RW, Weinberg AN, Austen WG: Prosthetic valve endocarditis. J Thorac Cardiovasc Surg **60:** 540, 1970
13. Dismukes WE, Karchmer AW, Buckley MJ, Austen WG, Swartz MN: Prosthetic valve endocarditis: analysis of 38 cases. Circulation **48:** 365, 1973
14. Goldmann DA, Hopkins CC, Karchmer AW, Abel RM, McEnany MT, Akins C, Buckley MJ, Moellering RC Jr: Cephalothin prophylaxis in cardiac valve surgery: a prospective, double-blind comparison of two-day and six-day regimens. J Thorac Cardiovasc Surg **73:** 470, 1977
15. Archer GL, Tenenbaum MJ: Antibiotic-resistant *Staphylococcus epidermidis* in patients undergoing cardiac surgery. Antimicrob Agents Chemother **17:** 269, 1980
16. Mayer KH, Schoenbaum SC: Evaluation and management of prosthetic valve endocarditis. Prog Cardiovasc Dis **25:** 43, 1982
17. Oyer PE, Miller DC, Stinson EB, Reitz BA, Moreno-Cabral RJ, Shumway NE: Clinical durability of the Hancock porcine bioprosthetic valve. J Thorac Cardiovasc Surg **80:** 824, 1980

Participation of endogenous catecholamines in the regulation of left ventricular mass in progeny of hypertensive parents

BRUNO TRIMARCO, M.D., BRUNO RICCIARDELLI, M.D., NICOLA DE LUCA, M.D., ANTONIO DE SIMONE, M.D., ALBERTO CUOCOLO, M.D., MARIA D. GALVA, M.D., GIOVANNI B. PICOTTI, M.D., AND MARIO CONDORELLI, M.D.

ABSTRACT To investigate whether adrenergic activity is a determinant of left ventricular hypertrophy in human hypertension, in each of 10 normotensive subjects with two hypertensive parents we have examined the relationship between changes in echocardiographic parameters of left ventricular anatomy and those in circulating catecholamine levels induced by three, 3 week periods of different sodium and potassium intakes. A high sodium–normal potassium regimen induced a significant reduction in upright plasma norepinephrine (from 599 ± 89 to 379 ± 45 pg/ml, $p < .01$) and in posterior wall (PWT) and interventricular septal (IVST) thickness, as well as in the left ventricular mass index (LVMi). Changes in upright plasma norepinephrine concentrations correlated with those in IVST ($r = .822$, $p < .01$) and in LVMi ($r = .833$, $p < .01$). A low sodium–normal potassium diet resulted in increases in supine and upright plasma norepinephrine levels (from 356 ± 44 to 488 ± 89 pg/ml, $p < .001$; and from 565 ± 42 to 744 ± 33 pg/ml, $p < .01$) as well as increases in IVST and LVMi (from 97 ± 7 to 107 ± 7 g/m^2, $p < .001$). The changes in norepinephrine levels in supine and upright subjects correlated with changes in IVST ($r = .836$, $p < .01$ and $r = .796$, $p < .01$) and in LVMi ($r = .931$, $p < .001$ and $r = .947$, $p < .001$). No significant change in plasma catecholamine concentrations or in PWT, IVST, or LVMi was detected after a low sodium–high potassium regimen. Blood pressure was essentially unchanged throughout the study. Furthermore, an ancillary study was performed in another nine normotensive subjects with hypertensive parents who underwent a reduction in dietary salt intake combined with therapy with the β-adrenoreceptor–blocking agent atenolol. In these patients the increase in supine and upright plasma norepinephrine concentrations were not accompanied by any increase in IVST, PWT, or LVMi. These findings indicate that in hypertensive progeny catecholamines play a role in the physiologic regulation of left ventricular mass.
Circulation 72, No. 1, 38–46, 1985.

ALTHOUGH recent evidence that the degree of hypertensive left ventricular hypertrophy is closely related to blood pressure[1–6] seems to indicate that blood pressure levels are the main determinant of left ventricular mass (LVM), the possibility that other factors play a role in the control of LVM cannot be ruled out a priori. In spontaneously hypertensive rats, the participation of some humoral factors in the genesis of left ventricular hypertrophy has been supported by strong evidence.[7–10] Regarding the sympathetic nervous system, a number of experimental studies indicate that catecholamines can induce cardiac hypertrophy.[11, 12] On the other hand, in human beings there is only indirect evidence to suggest that the sympathetic system may be involved in the control of LVM. Corea et al.[13] reported that the increase in interventricular septal thickness (IVST) observed in borderline hypertensive subjects was not related to arterial pressure but rather to levels of plasma norepinephrine. More recently the same authors[5] found that arterial pressure and plasma norepinephrine levels were both related to the degree of left ventricular hypertrophy in patients with stable arterial hypertension. Finally, we have previously reported that the changes in LVM observed in hypertensive patients during antihypertensive therapy with acebutolol correlate with the changes in heart rate but not with those in arterial blood pressure.[14]

From I Clinica Medica, II Facoltá di Medicina, Napoli, and Dipartimento di Farmacologia, Chemioterapia e Tossicologia, Facoltá di Medicina, Milano, Italy.
Supported by C.N.R. (Progetto Finalizzato di Medicina Preventiva — Sottoprogetto Ipertensione Arteriosa).
Address for correspondence: Bruno Trimarco, M.D., I Clinica Medica, II Facoltá di Medicina, Via S. Pansini 5 — 80131 Napoli, Italy.
Received June 7, 1984; revision accepted Feb. 28, 1985.

This study was aimed at investigating whether in human hypertension changes in sympathetic activity and thus in catecholamine release[15] might induce changes in LVM. For this purpose, changes in dietary sodium intake were chosen as long-term influences on the sympathetic system to allow sufficient time for changes in LVM. Restriction of dietary sodium is known to increase plasma levels of norepinephrine,[15–17] while there is a trend toward lower plasma norepinephrine after excessive sodium intake.[16–18] Parallel changes in plasma epinephrine have also been reported.[19] In the present study, dietary sodium contents of 80 (low), 180 (normal), and 330 (high) meq/day were consumed.

Since in established hypertension, unlike in normotension, altered sodium intake is known to induce changes in blood pressure,[20] to study the effects of changes in sympathetic activity on LVM without interference from pressure changes, we chose young normotensive subjects with first-degree relatives who had essential hypertension. There is a very high incidence of hypertension later in life in such individuals.[21] Moreover, to exclude the possibility that changes in dietary sodium intake induce changes in LVM, if any, through mechanisms different from changes in sympathetic tone, we also attempted to reduce blood volume without increasing sympathetic tone by administering a low sodium–high potassium diet. Indeed, it has been shown that in the progeny of hypertensive patients a high potassium intake may prevent the increase in sympathetic activity induced by a low-sodium diet.[22, 23]

Subjects and methods

A group of 16 normotensive subjects, each with two parents with a history of essential hypertension and from 17 to 37 years old (mean age 27 ± 2 years) participated in the study. All subjects were fully informed about the procedure and the aim of the study, and written consent was obtained from each. None of the subjects had any abnormalities on admission screening that included physical examination, electrocardiography, M mode and two-dimensional echocardiography, chest x-ray and renography, hematologic profile, liver and renal function tests, tests for plasma aldosterone, plasma renin activity (supine and after 1 hr upright), and urinary vanillylmandelic acid and free catecholamine concentrations and a thyroid function test. Blood pressure was measured three times, at least a week apart, with the subjects in the supine position after 5 min of rest in a darkened room, with a mercury sphygmomanometer as recommended by the American Heart Association.[24] Blood pressures of all subjects were in the normal range. None of them had taken any medication for at least a month preceding the study and none received medication during the period of the study.

In the month preceding the study, as well as during the study, each subject consumed a daily diet containing 80 meq sodium, 70 meq potassium, 65 g protein, 50 g fat, 270 g carbohydrate, and 100 mg phosphorus as meat, eggs, bread, vegetables, and fruit (this was the low-sodium regimen). Personal food preferences were allowed as much as possible. Furthermore, while on this diet, which was designed to minimize changes in body weight due to changes in food intake, all subjects were also given 100 meq/day of NaCl divided in two doses of 50 meq each wrapped in wafers. Water intake was allowed as desired. Twenty-four hour urine specimens were obtained on the last 3 days of this period to determine diuresis, natriuresis, and kaliuresis. Moreover, on the last day of this month, the subjects were asked to abstain from tobacco, coffee, tea, chocolate, strenuous physical activity, and sexual intercourse for at least 24 hr, as well as to fast and abstain from fluids for 12 hr. At 9 A.M. they were weighed after voiding and their blood pressures were measured both while they were supine and after they had been upright for 2 min. An indwelling cannula was then inserted into a vein of the antecubital fossa of the arm of each and a blood sample was taken after the subjects had been supine for at least 2 hr to determine levels of hematocrit, serum electrolytes, creatinine, plasma renin activity, aldosterone, epinephrine, and norepinephrine. Additional blood samples for determination of plasma catecholamine levels were also taken after subjects had been standing for 5 min. A further blood sample was taken after the subjects had been standing for 1 hr and plasma renin activity and aldosterone levels were determined. Finally, M mode and two-dimensional echocardiograms were obtained for the assessment of LVM. After these measurements, the subjects continued on the diet but with different supplements of NaCl and potassium as follows: (1) 330 meq/day NaCl and 70 meq/day potassium (diet plus 250 meq of crystalline sodium chloride), (2) 80 meq/day NaCl and 70 meq/day of potassium (diet with no salt supplementation) and (3) 80 meq/day of NaCl and 150 meq/day potassium (diet plus 80 meq/day potassium). Each of the three regimens was followed for 3 weeks.

At the end of each period, all the measurements were repeated as previously described. The subjects were then given the standard diet supplemented with 100 meq of NaCl until the echocardiographic LVM returned to the basal level (about 3 weeks). A new set of measurements was then obtained and a different sodium regimen was instituted for 3 weeks. The order in which the diets were administered to each subject was according to a computer-based randomization scheme. The supplementation to the diet in period 1 was accomplished by adding five doses of 50 meq crystalline NaCl wrapped up by wafers and in period 3, 10 slow-release tablets of KCl containing 8 meq of potassium each, divided into five doses, were given.

To further investigate the relationship between catecholamines and LVM, we performed an ancillary study in 10 normotensive subjects (five men and five women), each with two parents with a history of essential hypertension, who were from 15 to 33 years old (mean 24 ± 3 years). They were asked to follow the same guidelines pertaining to diet, personal habits, and drug intake as those in the other group. The subjects were initially studied under control conditions. The same procedures were followed as in the previous study, both on the test day and on the days before the testing procedure. The daily supplement of 100 meq sodium chloride was then withdrawn and the subjects received 80 meq/day NaCl and 70 meq/day of potassium over 3 weeks. During this period they were also given the β-adrenoreceptor blocker atenolol (100 mg orally once a day). At the end of the 3 weeks the subjects were studied again.

Finally, the reproducibility of echocardiographic measurements was tested in a parallel series of 10 normal subjects studied three times with the same ultrasonic technique under the same conditions; an interval of 3 weeks was allowed between the first and second study and 2 months elapsed between the second and third study. Under these circumstances, the coefficient of variation for LVM was 4.1%.

Analyses. Blood pressure was measured by a standard sphygmomanometer. Urinary and serum electrolytes were measured with a flame photometer. Creatinine was measured by an automated technique. Epinephrine and norepinephrine were measured simultaneously in 50 μl of plasma by a sensitive and specific radioenzymatic method,[25] as previously described.[26] Plasma renin activity was measured by the method of Menard and Catt[27] (sensitivity 5 ± 0.4 pg/tube angiotensin I; i.e., PRA = 0.06 ng/ml/hr) and plasma aldosterone concentration by the method of McKenzie and Clements[28] (sensitivity 6 ± 1 pg/ml). M mode echocardiography was performed with standard techniques previously reported from this laboratory[14] and images were obtained under sector-scanning monitoring to detect the occurrence of any change in left ventricular shape and to avoid angulation of the ultrasonic beam.[29] Echocardiographic tracings were coded and read blind and in random order by two expert observers blinded to the protocol. End-diastolic measurements of IVST, left ventricular internal dimension (LVID), and posterior wall thickness (PWT) were made according to the Penn convention protocol to measure LVM.[30] This was calculated by the simple and anatomically validated formula $LVM = 1.04 ((IVST + LVID + PWT)^3 - LVID^3) - 13.6$. To minimize the impact of variation in body size on LVM, it was corrected for body surface area. End-diastolic and end-systolic measurements were also made according to the recommendations of the American Society of Echocardiography.[31]

Changes in plasma volume were estimated from the changes in peripheral microhematocrits with the formula: $P = 100/(100 - H_1) 100 (H_1 - H_2)/H_2$, in which P is the percent change in plasma volume and H_1 and H_2 are the initial and the final packed cell volumes.

Statistical analysis. The Student t test was used to compare prediet and postdiet values of the different parameters. The strength of the association between the changes in various parameters and those in LVM index (LVMi) and IVST was assessed by the product moment correlation coefficient and its test of significance.[32] Differences between the values for each parameter in the same subject under different circumstances were assessed by Student's t test for paired data.

Results

Six subjects were excluded from the study: two did not complete the protocol and in four urinary sodium and/or potassium excretion did not match the calculated intake. The data for the remaining 10 subjects are listed in tables 1 to 3. There were no differences in the basal values of the various parameters at any time in the study. The accuracy of the echocardiographic measurements was indicated by the observation that blind readings by two independent trained observers varied by 1 mm or less and also by comparing LVM at end-diastole and at end-systole in each echocardiographic tracing; the correlation coefficient varied between .9 and .98. No change in left ventricular shape was detected by two-dimensional echocardiography throughout the study.

Phase 1 (high sodium/normal potassium intake). During this phase serum sodium and potassium levels remained unchanged, while there were significant increases in urinary sodium output, body weight, and plasma volume (table 1). There was no change in systolic or diastolic blood pressure (table 2). Upright heart rate fell significantly (table 2): the response to standing was reduced from +12 ± 2 to +7 ± 2 beats/min ($p < .001$). Furthermore, there were significant decreases in both supine and upright plasma renin activity and plasma aldosterone concentrations (table 1). Upright plasma epinephrine and norepinephrine concentrations were also significantly reduced (table 3). LVMi decreased from 98 ± 6 to 88 ± 6 g/m^2 (p <

TABLE 1

Plasma volume, diuresis, body weight, serum and urinary electrolytes, plasma renin activity (PRA), and plasma aldosterone concentration before and after the three different sodium and potassium diets

	Phase					
	1		2		3	
Parameter	Before	After	Before	After	Before	After
Plasma volume (% change)		13.8±6.7^A		−9.8±4.6^A		−10.2±5.1^A
Diuresis (ml)	1372±168	1661±204^A	1235±160	990±99^A	1344±187	1673±251
Body weight (kg)	70.7±2.8	71.4±2.9^A	70.9±1.8	69.9±2.4^A	70.6±1	69.8±1^A
Serum Na$^+$ (meq/l)	144±2	147±1	147±1	146±2	145±2	148±2
Serum K$^+$ (meq/l)	4.2±0.1	4.4±0.2	4.3±0.2	4.4±0.2	4.4±0.1	4.7±0.1^A
Urinary Na$^+$ (meq/24 hr)	129±6	305±9^B	128±4	65±3^B	131±6	69±5^B
Urinary K$^+$ (meq/24 hr)	61±6	68±3	66±9	63±5	64±4	126±11^B
PRA supine (ng/ml/hr)	0.96±0.1	0.47±0.1^B	0.86±0.2	1.87±0.3^B	1.2±0.1	1.5±0.1^A
PRA upright (ng/ml/hr)	1.6±0.1^C	0.77±0.1^B	1.56±0.2^C	2.5±0.3^{B,C}	2.0±0.1^C	2.2±0.1^{A,C}
Aldosterone supine (pg/ml)	217±31	145±24^B	190±20	243±23^B	166±16	211±29^A
Aldosterone upright (pg/ml)	314±34^C	209±33^B	270±17^C	331±19^{B,C}	239±10^C	288±21^{A,C}

Means ± SE for 10 subjects.

^{A,B}p < .05 and p < .01, respectively, for values obtained before vs after each diet.

^{C}p < .05 for supine vs upright values.

TABLE 2
Supine and upright systolic and diastolic blood pressures (BPs) and heart rates, IVST and PWT, LVID and LVMi before and after three different sodium and potassium diets

	Phase					
	1		2		3	
Parameter	Before	After	Before	After	Before	After
Systolic BP supine (mm Hg)	128 ± 4	122 ± 3	128 ± 2	121 ± 6	123 ± 5	118 ± 6
Systolic BP upright (mm Hg)	133 ± 4	126 ± 3	127 ± 3	125 ± 5	126 ± 5	121 ± 6
Diastolic BP supine (mm Hg)	79 ± 1	81 ± 2	80 ± 1	78 ± 2	80 ± 2	75 ± 3
Diastolic BP upright (mm Hg)	87 ± 2	88 ± 2	88 ± 2	86 ± 3	85 ± 4	81 ± 4
Heart rate supine (bpm)	67 ± 3	63 ± 3	67 ± 2	74 ± 3^{A}	66 ± 4	68 ± 4
Heart rate upright (bpm)	79 ± 4^{C}	70 ± 3^{B}	76 ± 3^{C}	85 ± 4 ^{B,C}	78 ± 5^{C}	81 ± 3^{C}
IVST (cm)	0.81 ± 0.03	0.75 ± 0.03^{A}	0.803 ± 0.03	0.844 ± 0.03^{A}	0.813 ± 0.03	0.795 ± 0.02
PWT (cm)	0.79 ± 0.03	0.73 ± 0.03^{B}	0.822 ± 0.04	0.833 ± 0.04	0.791 ± 0.03	0.807 ± 0.03
LVID (cm)	5.19 ± 0.14	5.14 ± 0.15	5.0 ± 0.14	5.0 ± 0.10	5.11 ± 0.13	4.98 ± 0.11
LVMi (g/m^2)	98 ± 6	88 ± 6^{B}	97 ± 7	107 ± 7^{B}	97 ± 6	94 ± 6

Means ± SE for 10 subjects.
^{A,B}p < .05 and p < .01, respectively, for values obtained before vs after each diet.
^{C}p < .05 for supine vs upright values.

.01), IVST fell from 0.81 ± 0.03 to 0.75 ± 0.03 cm (p < .05), and PWT decreased from 0.79 ± 0.03 to 0.73 ± 0.03 cm (p < .01), while LVID remained unchanged (table 2). The changes in LVMi and IVST were significantly correlated with those in upright plasma norepinephrine concentration (figure 1).

Phase 2 (low sodium/normal potassium intake). In this phase also serum sodium and potassium levels remained unchanged, but we observed falls in sodium output, body weight, and plasma volume (table 1). No significant changes in systolic and diastolic blood pressures were seen, while heart rate increased in these subjects in both the supine and upright positions (table 2). Plasma renin activity and aldosterone concentrations and plasma norepinephrine increased significantly in both the supine and upright positions (tables 2 and 3). There were no significant changes in epinephrine plasma levels (table 3). In this phase there were significant increases in IVST (from 0.8 ± 0.03 to 0.84 ± 0.03 cm, p < .05) and LVMi (from 97 ± 7 to 107 ± 7 g/m^2, p < .001), but not in LVID (table 2).

These changes correlated wtih the changes in plasma norepinephrine levels in subjects in both the upright and supine positions (figures 2 and 3).

TABLE 3
Supine and upright plasma epinephrine and norepinephrine levels before and after the three different sodium and potassium diets

	Phase					
	1		2		3	
	Before	After	Before	After	Before	After
Epinephrine supine (pg/ml)	31 ± 4	29 ± 5	26 ± 5	30 ± 6	27 ± 6	20 ± 3
Epinephrine upright (pg/ml)	34 ± 3	20 ± 5^{B}	35 ± 6	35 ± 8	35 ± 6	37 ± 12
Norepinephrine supine (pg/ml)	306 ± 45	272 ± 38	356 ± 44	488 ± 49^{B}	298 ± 49	226 ± 20
Norepinephrine upright (pg/ml)	599 ± 89^{D}	379 ± 45^{B,C}	565 ± 42^{D}	744 ± 33^{B,C}	581 ± 113^{C}	571 ± 56^{D}

Means ± SE for 10 subjects.
^{A,B}p < .05 and p < .01, respectively, for values obtained before vs after each diet.
^{C,D}p < .05 and p < .01, respectively, for supine vs upright values.

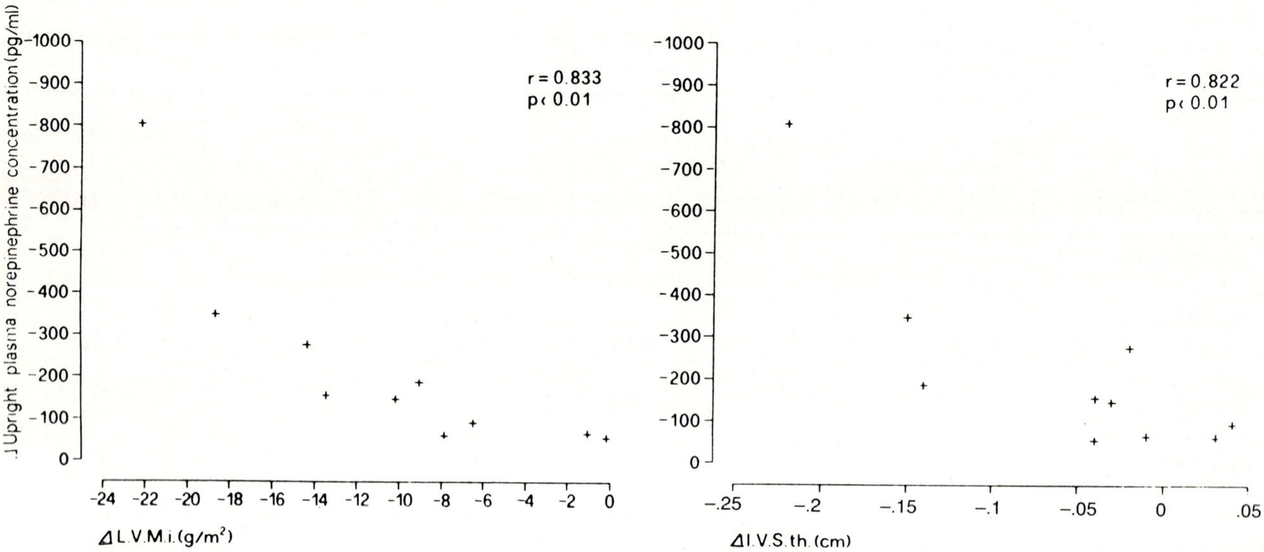

FIGURE 1. Relationship between changes in upright plasma norepinephrine concentration and LVMi (*left*) or interventricular septal thickness (IVSth) (*right*) with a high sodium–normal potassium diet.

Phase 3 (low sodium/high potassium intake). In this period we found a significant increase in serum potassium and in kaliuresis, a decrease in natriuresis, body weight, and plasma volume, and no change in serum sodium concentration (table 1). In this case the reduction in plasma volume was not accompanied by any significant increase in heart rate (table 2). Systolic and diastolic blood pressure remained unmodified, while plasma renin activity and plasma aldosterone concentration rose significantly (table 1). In this period we saw no significant change in plasma catecholamine levels (table 3) or in the echocardiographic parameters of left ventricular anatomy (table 2).

Study with atenolol. One subject was excluded from this study because his sodium excretion did not match the calculated intake. The data for the remaining nine subjects are listed in table 4. Under control conditions, no significant differences were detectable for any of the considered parameters between the subjects enrolled in this study and those participating in the study previously described. In the atenolol study, the effects of low sodium intake on blood pressure, sodium and

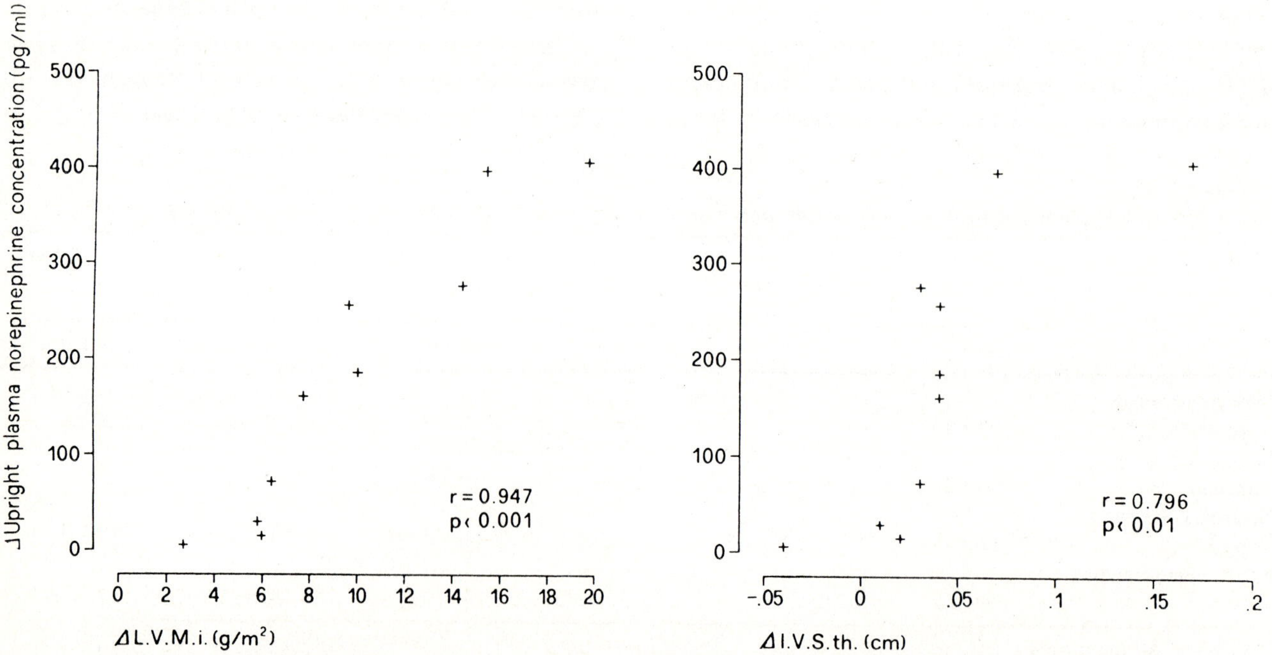

FIGURE 2. Relationship between changes in upright plasma norepinephrine concentration and LVMi (*left*) or interventricular septal thickness (IVSth) (*right*) with a low sodium–normal potassium diet.

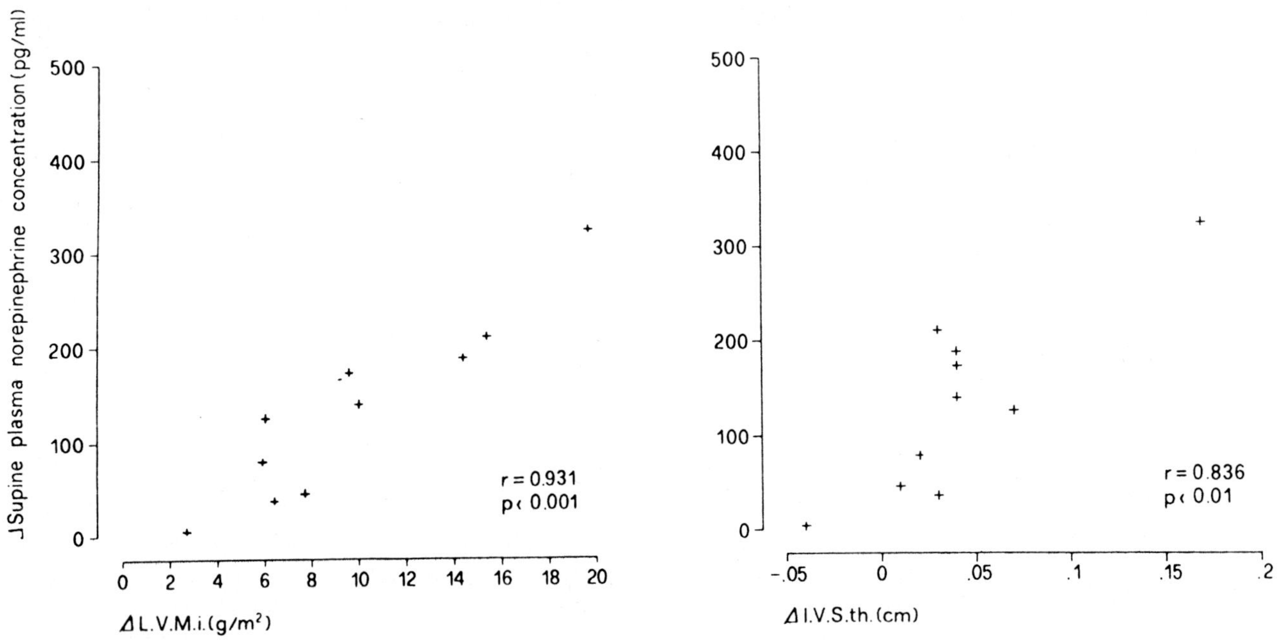

FIGURE 3. Relationship between changes in supine plasma norepinephrine concentration and LVMi (*left*) or interventricular septal thickness (IVSth) (*right*) with a low sodium–normal potassium diet.

potassium output, body weight, and plasma volume (−13.3 ± 4%, p < .01) were similar to those observed in phase 2 of the previous study (table 4). As expected, the changes in plasma renin activity and aldosterone concentrations induced by low sodium intake in subjects in both the supine and upright positions (data not shown), as well as the heart rate response to standing (table 4), were markedly blunted by atenolol. On the other hand, the pharmacologic blockade of β-adrenergic receptors did not modify the response of either epinephrine (supine, from 35 ± 6 to 40 ± 9 pg/ml, NS; upright, from 58 ± 15 to 46 ± 9 pg/ml, NS) or norepinephrine level (table 4) to dietary sodium restriction. Finally, no change in the echocardiographic parameters of left ventricular anatomy could be detected in this study (table 4).

TABLE 4

Effects of low sodium–normal potassium diet and atenolol (100 mg orally once a day) on physical, humoral, and echocardiographic parameters

	Before	After
Body weight (kg)	69 ± 3	68 ± 3^B
Urinary Na^+ (meq/24 hr)	131 ± 3.3	61 ± 2.6^B
Urinary K^+ (meq/24 hr)	69 ± 4.5	62 ± 4
MAP supine (mm Hg)	98 ± 3	97 ± 2
MAP upright (mm Hg)	103.6 ± 2.2	101.1 ± 2.1
Heart rate supine (bpm)	65 ± 6	57 ± 5^B
Heart rate upright (bpm)	82.4 ± 8.2^D	66.6 ± 7.8^B,C
Norepinephrine supine (pg/ml)	257 ± 36	356 ± 38^A
Norepinephrine upright (pg/ml)	395 ± 47^C	587 ± 35^B,D
IVST (cm)	0.83 ± 0.03	0.83 ± 0.05
PWT (cm)	0.87 ± 0.04	0.86 ± 0.04
LVID (cm)	5.22 ± 0.21	5.13 ± 0.21
LVMi (g/m^2)	102 ± 8.3	99 ± 9

Mean ± SE for nine subjects.

MAP = mean arterial pressure.

^A,B^p < .05 and p < .01, respectively, for values obtained before vs after each diet.

^C,D^p < .05 and p < .01, respectively, for supine vs upright values.

Discussion

Recent reports from several groups have shown that increased blood pressure is probably the main determinant of hypertension-induced left ventricular hypertrophy.[1-6] Therefore, when testing the possibility that other factors are involved in the control of LVM in human hypertension, it is necessary to keep arterial blood pressure constant when the variable being investigated changes. In this study, lasting changes in sympathetic activity without any blood pressure change were obtained by exposing normotensive offspring of hypertensive parents to different sodium intakes. Pressure changes would be anticipated if patients with established hypertension were exposed to analogous situations.[20] It should be noted that in animal experiments LVM has been shown to be greater in spontaneously hypertensive rats than in normotensive rats in which renal hypertension was produced by unilateral arterial obstruction when they were exposed to the same pressure load.[33] Although a similar finding has not been reported for humans, studies in normotensive subjects may not be suitable for investigating the mechanisms controlling LVM in hypertensive patients. However, it has been demonstrated[21] that the incidence of hypertension in offspring is 46% when both parents are hypertensive, 28% if one parent is hypertensive, and only 3% if neither parent is hypertensive. Therefore, normotensive subjects with two hypertensive parents, a population with a very high incidence of hypertension, offer the best opportunity for studying essential hypertension at its inception.

In our subjects, changes in dietary sodium intake did not induce any significant change in blood pressure, but did modify LVM.

Low sodium intake induced a 10% increase in LVM and high sodium intake was accompanied by a decrease in LVM of a similar magnitude. Both of these changes were reversed when sodium intake was returned to normal. In particular, the changes in LVM seem to be exclusively due to changes in left ventricular wall thickness since LVID remained unchanged throughout the study.

The first question raised by these results is the reliability of echocardiographic LVM measurement. It has been reported that echocardiography can repeatedly[34] and accurately[30] quantify the thickness of ventricular walls as well as the LVM. However, echocardiographic calculation of LVM requires many assumptions, the least well proved of which is that the longitudinal axis of the left ventricle is always twice as much as the anteroposterior or transverse diameter, which may not apply in hearts affected with a configuration-altering disease.[35] However, the present study includes relatively young patients with no history, symptoms, or signs of myocardial damage and who, therefore, can be assumed to have symmetrically contracting ventricles. Furthermore, in this study, changes in wall thickness and LVM were in the same direction, suggesting that the changes in LVM reflected changes in wall thickness more than changes in left ventricular volume.

The second consideration with regard to our results is that the magnitude of the changes in LVM, in both directions, were about 10% of the basal values. These are smaller than those obtained with antihypertensive therapy in patients with established hypertension.[5, 14, 29] However, this discrepancy is not surprising since the follow-up periods in those studies were longer than ours. Furthermore, hypertensive individuals have greater LVM than our subjects, who were still normotensive, and it has been demonstrated[29] that there is a significant correlation between the initial LVM and the magnitude of the change in this parameter induced by therapy.

In agreement with previous reports,[18, 20] low sodium intake was accompanied by an increase in plasma renin activity and plasma aldosterone and catecholamine concentrations, while opposite changes were observed during high sodium intake. Only the changes in plasma norepinephrine were found to be correlated with the changes in left ventricular anatomy, suggesting that the sympathetic system may play a role in the control of LVM in hypertensive patients. In fact, plasma norepinephrine concentration has been demonstrated to reflect the averaged contribution from the various vascular beds and, therefore, to be an index of overall sympathetic nervous activity.[36] The observation that the changes in plasma norepinephrine are accompanied by concomitant changes in heart rate documents the importance of catecholamine measurement as an index of the cardioadrenergic drive.

It should be noted that the correlation between changes in plasma norepinephrine and LVM does not allow us to rule out a direct effect of sodium per se on LVM.

The observation that a high potassium intake abolishes the increase in sympathetic tone induced by a low-sodium diet is in agreement with the findings of Parfrey et al.[23] in young subjects with a familial predisposition to hypertension. The mechanisms that underly this phenomenon are still unclear: both a genetically determined and specific effect of potassium on sympathetic activity[23] and an effect of external potassium concentration on the Na^+-K^+ pump[37] have been postulated. However it works, the observation that sodium restriction is unable to induce any change in LVM when the increase in sympathetic tone is prevented seems to corroborate the hypothesis that there is a cause-effect relationship between the changes in sympathetic nervous activity, as reflected by plasma norepinephrine concentration, and those in LVM induced by low sodium intake. The results obtained by administration of atenolol lend further support to this hypothesis. In fact, we were able to prevent the increase in left ventricular wall thickness and, consequently, in LVM induced by a reduction in dietary sodium intake by protecting the heart from the effects of an increased adrenergic drive. Although it has been previously reported that norepinephrine administered to dogs[38] and rats[39] in subhypertensive doses evokes myocardial hypertrophy, this study presents the first data showing that changes in norepinephrine levels within the physiologic range are related to changes in LVM in normotensive subjects who are first-degree relatives of patients with essential hypertension without changes in blood pressure. The present study does not, however, elucidate the precise role of the adrenergic influence of LVM. The observation that changes in sympathetic activity are always accompanied by concomitant changes in heart rate suggests that hemodynamic factors mediate the observed changes in LVM, as has been found in young spontaneously hypertensive rats[40] and in early phases of human hypertension.[41] However, changes in systemic hemodynamics might not be the only way whereby catecholamines are related to changes in ventricular weight, since catecholamines have been shown to facilitate the incorporation of amino acids into myocardial and vascular proteins.[42]

References

1. Dunn FG, Chandraratna P, De Carvalho JGR, Basta LL, Frohlich ED: Pathophysiologic assessment of hypertensive heart disease with echocardiography. Am J Cardiol **39:** 789, 1977
2. Savage DD, Drayer JIM, Henry WL, Mathews EC, Ware JH, Gardin JM, Cohen ER, Epstein SE, Laragh JH: Echocardiographic assessment of cardiac anatomy and function in hypertensive subjects. Circulation **59:** 623, 1979
3. Rowlands DB, Glover DB, Ireland MA, McLeay RA, Stellard DJ, Watson RD, Littler WA: Assessment of left ventricular mass and its response to antihypertensive treatment. Lancet **1:** 467, 1982
4. Devereux RB, Pickering TG, Harshfield GA, Kleinert HD, Denby LM, Clark L, Pregibon D, Jason M, Kleiner B, Borer J, Laragh JH: Left ventricular hypertrophy in patients with hypertension: importance of blood pressure response to regularly recurrent stress. Circulation **68:** 470, 1983
5. Corea L, Bentivoglio L, Verdecchia P: Echocardiographic left ventricular hypertrophy as related to arterial pressure and plasma norepinephrine concentration in arterial hypertension. Reversal by atenolol treatment. Hypertension **5:** 837, 1983
6. Drayer JIM, Weber MA, de Young JL: Blood pressure as a determination of cardiac left ventricular muscle mass? Arch Intern Med **143:** 90, 1983
7. Sen S, Tarazi RC, Khairallah PA, Bumpus FM: Cardiac hypertrophy in spontaneously hypertensive rats. Circ Res **35:** 775, 1974
8. Sen S, Bumpus FM: Chollagen synthesis in development and reversal of cardiac hypertrophy in spontaneously hypertensive rats. Am J Cardiol **44:** 954, 1979
9. Thomanek RJ, Davis JW, Anderson SC: The effects of alphamethyldopa on cardiac hypertrophy in spontaneously hypertensive rats: ultrastructural stereological and morphometric analysis. Cardiovasc Res **13:** 173, 1979
10. Frohlich ED, Tarazi RC: Is arterial pressure the sole factor responsible for hypertensive cardiac hypertrophy? Am J Cardiol **44:** 959, 1979
11. Barner BB, Jellinek M, Kaiser JC: Effects of isoproterenol infusion on myocardial structure and composition. Am Heart J **79:** 237, 1970
12. Gans JH, Cater MR: Norepinephrine induced cardiac hypertrophy in dogs. Life Sci **9:** 731, 1970
13. Corea L, Bentivoglio M, Verdecchia P, Motolese M: Left ventricular wall thickness and plasma catecholamines in borderline stable essential hypertension. Eur Heart J **3:** 164, 1982
14. Trimarco B, Ricciardelli B, De Luca N, Volpe M, Veniero AM, Cuocolo A, Condorelli M: Effects of acebutolol on left ventricular hemodynamics and anatomy in systemic hypertension. Am J Cardiol **53:** 791, 1984
15. Robertson D, Johnson GA, Robertson RM, Nies AS, Shand DG, Oates JA: Comparative assessment of stimuli that release neuronal and adrenomedullary catecholamines in man. Circulation **59:** 637, 1979
16. Luft FC, Ranklin LI, Henry DP, Bloch R, Grim CE, Weyman AE, Murray RM, Weinberger MH: Plasma and urinary norepinephrine values at extremes of sodium intake in normal man. Hypertension **1:** 261, 1979
17. Nicholls MG, Kiowsky W, Zweifler AJ, Julius S, Schork MA, Greenhouse J: Plasma norepinephrine variations with dietary sodium intake. Hypertension **2:** 29, 1980
18. Trimarco B, Volpe M, Ricciardelli B, Picotti GB, Galva MD, Petracca R, Condorelli M: Studies on the mechanisms underlying impairment of beta-adrenoreceptor-mediated effects in human hypertension. Hypertension **5:** 584, 1983
19. Fraser J, Nadeau J, Robertson D, Wood AJ: Regulation of human leukocyte betareceptors by endogenous catecholamine. J Clin Invest **67:** 1777, 1981
20. Masuo K, Ogihara T, Kumahara Y, Yamatodani A, Wada H: Plasma norepinephrine and dietary sodium intake in normal subjects and in patients with essential hypertension. Hypertension **5:** 767, 1983
21. Hyman D: Heredity in arteriolar (essential) hypertension: a clinical study of blood pressure in 1524 members of 277 families. Arch Intern Med **53:** 792, 1934
22. Holly JM, Goodwin FJ, Evans SJW, Vandenburg MJ, Ledingham JM: Re-analysis of data in two Lancet papers on the effects of dietary sodium and potassium on blood pressure. Lancet **2:** 1384, 1981
23. Parfrey PS, Wright P, Holly JMP, Evans SJW, Condon K, Vandenburg MJ, Goodwin FJ, Ledingham JM: Blood pressure and hormonal changes following alteration in dietary sodium and potassium in young men with and without a familial predisposition to hypertension. Lancet **1:** 113, 1981
24. Kirkendall WM, Burton MC, Epstein FM, Freis ED: Recommendation for human blood pressure determinations by sphygmomanometers. Circulation **36:** 980, 1967
25. De Prada M, Zurcher G: Simultaneous radioenzymatic determination of plasma and tissue adrenaline, noradrenaline and dopamine within the fentomole range. Life Sci **19:** 1161, 1976
26. Buhler HU, De Prada M, Haefley W, Picotti GB: Plasma adrenaline, noradrenaline and dopamine in man and different animal species. J Physiol (London) **276:** 311, 1978
27. Menard J, Catt KJ: Measurements of renin activity by radioimmunoassay of angiotensin I. Endocrinology **90:** 422, 1972
28. McKenzie JK, Clements SA: Simplified radioimmunoassay of serum aldosterone utilizing increased antibody specificity. J Clin Endocrinol Metabol **36:** 622, 1974
29. Fouad FM, Nakashima Y, Tarazi RC, Salcedo EE: Reversal of left ventricular hypertrophy in hypertensive patients treated with methyldopa. Lack of association with blood pressure control. Am J Cardiol **49:** 795, 1982
30. Devereux RB, Reichek N: Echocardiographic determination of left ventricular mass in man. Anatomic validation of the method. Circulation **55:** 613, 1977
31. Shan DJ, De Maria A, Kisslo J, Weyman A: Recommendations regarding quantitation in M-mode echocardiography: results of a survey of echocardiographic measurements. Circulation **58:** 1072, 1979
32. Armitage P: Statistics in medical research. New York, 1971, John Wiley & Sons Inc.
33. Lundgren Y, Hallback M, Weiss L, Folkow B: Rate and extent of adaptative cardiovascular changes in rats during experimental renal hypertension. Acta Physiol Scand **91:** 103, 1974
34. Wong M, Shan PM, Taylor RD: Reproducibility of left ventricular internal dimensions with M-mode echocardiography: effects of heart size, body position and transducer angulation. Am J Cardiol **47:** 1068, 1981
35. Falsetti HL, Carroll JR: Single plane angiography: current applications and limitations. *In* Harrison DC, Sandler H, Miller HA, editors: Cardiovascular imaging and image processing. Theory and practice. Palo Verde Estates, CA, 1975, The Society of Photooptical Instrumentations Engineers, p 123
36. Goldstein DS: Plasma catecholamines and essential hypertension. An analytical review. Hypertension **5:** 86, 1983
37. Iimura O, Kijima T, Kikucha K, Miyami A, Aredo T, Nakao T, Takigami J: Studies on the hypotensive effects of high postassium intake in patients with essential hypertension. Clin Sci **61:** 77s, 1981
38. Laks MM, Morady F, Swan HJC: Myocardial hypertrophy produced by chronic infusion of subhypertensive doses of norepinephrine in the dog. Chest **64:** 75, 1973

39. Cohen J: Role of endocrine factors in the pathogenesis of cardiac hypertrophy. Circ Res **34/35**(suppl II): 49, 1974
40. Pfeffer MA, Frohlich ED: Hemodynamic and myocardial function in young and old normotensive and spontaneously hypertensive rats. Circ Res **32/33**(suppl I): 28, 1972
41. Julius S, Shork MA: Borderline hypertension. A critical review. J Chron Dis **23:** 723, 1971
42. Kallfelt BJ, Hjalmareson AC, Isaksson OG: In vitro effects of catecholamines on protein synthesis in perfused rat heart. J Mol Cell Cardiol **8:** 787, 1976

Transient enhancement of sympathetic nervous system activity by long-term restriction of sodium intake

MASSIMO VOLPE, M.D., FRANCO B. MÜLLER, M.D., AND BRUNO TRIMARCO, M.D.

ABSTRACT To further investigate the relationship between salt intake and sympathetic nervous system activity, the short- and long-term effects of a low-salt diet (40 meq/day) were assessed in 10 normal subjects. Measurements of hemodynamic, hormonal, and other parameters were obtained on the day preceding institution of the low-salt diet (day 0) and on days 4, 7, 30, and 60 of the diet. Urinary sodium excretion was 178 ± 10 meq/24 hr on day 0 and 31 ± 4, 38 ± 4, 45 ± 6, and 47 ± 7 meq/24 hr on days 4, 7, 30, and 60, respectively (all $p < .001$ compared with day 0). Blood pressure, urinary potassium, serum electrolytes, and cardiac function (as assessed by echocardiography) were not modified by the 2 month low-salt diet. Plasma renin activity and plasma aldosterone were significantly elevated above control values throughout the entire period of the low-salt diet. In contrast, plasma norepinephrine concentration increased significantly only on days 4 and 7 (from 253 ± 20 pg/ml on day 0 to 495 ± 32 pg/ml, $p < .001$, and 347 ± 22 pg/ml, $p < .05$, respectively), returning to baseline at days 30 (280 ± 18 pg/ml) and 60 (262 ± 18 pg/ml). Changes in plasma epinephrine paralleled those observed for norepinephrine. Similarly, resting heart rate and the blood pressure response to isometric exercise were significantly increased only on days 4 and 7 of the low-salt diet. These results suggest that sympathetic nervous system activity is enhanced only transiently during a sustained reduction in sodium intake.
Circulation 72, No. 1, 47–52, 1985.

IT HAS LONG been hypothesized that the level of sodium intake affects sympathetic nervous system activity both in normal and in hypertensive subjects. There have been several reports that circulating catecholamines increase during dietary sodium restriction[1–8] and decrease upon sodium loading,[3, 6–9] although some conflicting data exist.[10–12] There have been contradictory reports on the influence of sodium intake on vascular reactivity and total peripheral resistance. Sullivan et al.[13] reported an increase in total peripheral resistance during sodium depletion in borderline hypertensive subjects, whereas Takeshita et al.[14] observed an increase in forearm vascular resistance during salt loading in subjects with hypertension. Other authors have reported that salt loading induces vasodilatation in normotensives[15, 16] and vasoconstriction in hypertensive subjects.[17] Finally, it has been reported that high sodium intake increases the vascular sensitivity to norepinephrine while it decreases the basal plasma concentration of norepinephrine,[18] but others have found no change in renal vascular reactivity to norepinephrine during acute sodium repletion.[19]

These discrepancies could be ascribed to differences in the experimental protocols used in the studies, such as differences in animal species used or clinical characteristics of the population studied (e.g., with respect to age, blood pressure) and differences in the duration and degree of the changes in salt intake.

The purpose of the present study was to assess the time course of the humoral and hemodynamic responses to a moderate reduction in sodium intake, particularly as related to sympathetic nervous system activity, in a homogeneous group of normal human subjects.

Methods

Twelve normal volunteer subjects from 23 to 39 years old (mean ± SEM = 35 ± 3.5 years) were enrolled in the study. As a group they had no history of serious illness and no family history of hypertension. Informed written consent was obtained from each and they took no drugs for the duration of the study. To achieve an equilibrium on a standardized diet for baseline measurements, the subjects were admitted to our metabolic

From Clinica Medica 1, 2 Facoltá di Medicina, Universitá di Napoli, Naples, Italy, and the Cardiovascular and Hypertension Center, Cornell University Medical Center, The New York Hospital, New York.

Address for correspondence: Massimo Volpe, M.D., Via Tasso 179, 80127 Napoli, Italy.

Received Feb. 20, 1985; accepted March 22, 1985.

ward and were maintained on a daily diet containing 200 meq sodium, 70 meq potassium, 60 g protein, 50 g fat, 280 g carbohydrate, and 400 mg calcium, for 1 week after their entry into the study. Each subject consulted with the research dietician before the study and personal food preferences were allowed as much as possible. After 7 days on this diet (day 0), the following baseline measurements were obtained: body weight, supine and upright heart rate and blood pressure, 24 hr urinary sodium and potassium excretion, 2 hr supine plasma renin activity, aldosterone, epinephrine and norepinephrine levels, peripheral venous hematocrit, creatinine clearance, and serum sodium and potassium. Resting M mode echocardiographic and blood pressure and heart rate responses to isometric exercise were determined after the humoral measurements. Blood samples for catecholamine measurement were drawn with the subject in the supine position on a comfortable bed at least 30 min after the insertion of a 20-gauge butterfly needle into a forearm vein. The room was kept quiet, darkened, and warm for the entire study. Subjects avoided caffeine, smoking, and strenuous physical exercise for the 24 hr preceding the sampling.

Subsequently, the subjects were prescribed a diet containing identical quantities of potassium, protein, fat, carbohydrate, and calcium, but only 40 meq of sodium, and were followed in the outpatient clinic for 60 days. The diet was reinforced periodically by reconsulting the dietician. Measurements of the above-mentioned parameters were repeated on days 4, 7, 30, and 60 of the diet. In addition, 24 hr urinary electrolytes were measured on day 1.

Plasma concentrations of norepinephrine and epinephrine were measured by a radioenzymatic method.[20] Plasma renin activity and aldosterone levels were measured by radioimmunoassay,[21, 22] and sodium and potassium concentrations in serum and urine were determined by flame photometry. Adequacy of 24 hr urine collection was evaluated by measurement of urinary creatinine. Blood pressure was measured by mercury sphygmomanometer according to the recommendations of the American Heart Association.[23]

The isometric muscular exercise consisted of sustained handgrip in the supine position on a hydraulic adjustable dynamometer. After the subjects had become familiar with the technique, maximum voluntary contraction of the dominant hand was assessed 15 min before the start of the actual experiment. After a 15 min period of supine rest, blood pressure and heart rate measurements were obtained each minute for 5 min in the nondominant arm and averaged to obtain the baseline value. The subjects then performed 75% maximum contraction handgrip for 1 min. Blood pressure and heart rate were measured during the last 15 sec of the effort. Percent changes in mean blood pressure and heart rate in response to handgrip were used for statistical comparisons.

M mode echocardiography was performed with the patient in left lateral position after 30 min of supine rest with use of an Irex system 2 echocardiograph with a 2.25 MHz, 15 mm diameter transducer. All tracings for left ventricular dimensions were recorded at the level of the tips of the mitral valve. The dimensions measured in each tracing, using the leading-edge technique and following the recommendations of the American Society of Echocardiography,[24] were ventricular septal thickness, left ventricular posterior wall thickness, and left ventricular diameter, with each dimension measured at both end-diastole and end-systole. The readings were performed by two observers in a double-blind fashion. Three beats were measured routinely; as many as 5 were measured if the recording was not easy to read. (Agreement between the two observers and reproducibility of the readings by the same observer were within 1 mm.) Heart rate values were obtained from a simultaneously recorded electrocardiogram. Echocardiographically measured volumes in end-diastole and end-systole were derived with the cube formula. Echocardiographic left ventricular mass index was calculated as the difference between total left ventricular end-diastolic volume (including muscle shell) and the inner left ventricular volume multiplied by effector 1.05 (the specific weight for heart muscle) and divided by body surface area.[25] Stroke volume was derived as the difference between end-diastolic and end-systolic volume, and cardiac output by multiplying stroke volume by heart rate. Mean blood pressure was obtained by adding one-third of the pulse pressure to diastolic blood pressure. Total peripheral resistance (dynes $\times$ sec $\times$ cm^{-5}) was calculated by dividing mean blood pressure by cardiac output and multiplying by 80. The mean velocity of circumferential fiber shortening (sec^{-1}) was calculated as the percent change in left ventricular dimension divided by the left ventricular ejection time.

Statistical analysis was performed by one-way analysis of variance (ANOVA). Differences were considered statistically significant at a level of $p < .05$. Data are expressed as mean $\pm$ SEM.

Results

Two of the 12 enrolled subjects were excluded during the course of the study because their 24 hr urine creatinine and sodium excretion indicated inaccuracy in urine collection and/or noncompliance with the low-sodium diet. Therefore, data from only 10 subjects were considered in further analysis.

Urinary sodium excretion was 178 $\pm$ 10 meq/24 hr on the last day of the normal sodium diet (day 0) and fell to 122 $\pm$ 20 meq/24 hr after 1 day on the low-sodium diet. Three more days were then allowed to achieve equilibrium on the new sodium regimen before the first humoral and hemodynamic measurements were obtained. Urinary sodium fell to 31 $\pm$ 4 meq/24 hr on day 4, to 38 $\pm$ 4 meq/24 hr on day 7, to 45 $\pm$ 6 meq/24 hr on day 30, and to 47 $\pm$ 7 meq/24 hr on day 60 ($p < .001$ for all as compared with the control value) (figure 1). There were no significant differences among the urinary sodium values obtained on days 4, 7, 30, and 60 of the low-sodium diet.

Table 1 shows the effects of the low-sodium diet on the different humoral and hemodynamic parameters. Blood pressure was not significantly altered. Both supine and upright heart rate increased modestly but significantly on days 4 and 7, returning to baseline thereafter. Supine plasma renin activity and aldosterone concentrations were significantly increased by day 4 of low sodium intake and remained significantly above baseline at days 7, 30, and 60. Body weight decreased significantly by day 7, whereas no significant change was detectable in urinary potassium excretion, creatinine clearance, or hematocrit.

Figure 1 illustrates the changes in plasma epinephrine and norepinephrine as related to the concurrent values for urinary sodium excretion. Plasma concen-

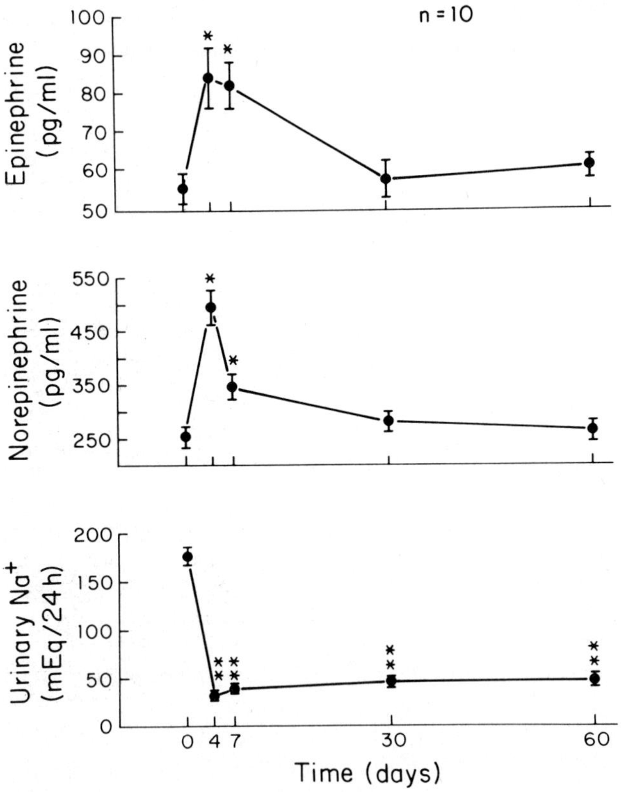

FIGURE 1. Time course of catecholamine plasma levels in subjects on the low-salt diet. *p < .05; **p < .001.

trations of both catecholamines were significantly increased on days 4 and 7 of the low-sodium diet, whereas by days 30 and 60 their values were no longer different from those obtained during the normal sodium diet.

The reliability of the catecholamine pattern found during the low-salt diet is supported by data obtained from four normal subjects given a 200 meq sodium diet identical to our control diet for 2 months. In these subjects, plasma norepinephrine and epinephrine concentrations measured on days 0, 4, 7, 30, and 60 were, respectively, 272 ± 20, 252 ± 21, 295 ± 26, 249 ± 18, and 279 ± 28 pg/ml for norepinephrine (all NS compared with 0 control) and 61 ± 17, 67 ± 15, 57 ± 8, 66 ± 10, and 54 ± 10 pg/ml for epinephrine (all NS compared with 0 control). No significant change from control in urinary sodium excretion could be detected during the 2 months of the diet in these subjects.

Table 2 summarizes the hemodynamic response to the low-salt diet as assessed by echocardiography and responses to isometric exercise. No significant change in any of the resting cardiovascular parameters was detected by echocardiography. In contrast, the percentage of increase in mean blood pressure induced by isometric exercise was significantly greater on days 4 and 7 compared with that under control conditions. This effect of sodium restriction was no longer apparent on days 30 and 60 of the diet. The heart rate response to exercise was not significantly affected by the low-salt diet.

Discussion

The evaluation of sympathetic nervous system activity has long been difficult and controversial. However, with the introduction of sensitive radioenzymatic assays for measurement of circulating catecholamines,

TABLE 1
Time course of effects of the low-salt diet (40 meq/day) on different hemodynamic and humoral parameters (n = 10)

	Days on diet				
	0	4	7	30	60
Supine BP					
Systolic (mm Hg)	128±7	125±4	124±4	120±4	120±6
Diastolic (mm Hg)	76±5	78±4	75±3	76±5	75±4
Upright BP					
Systolic (mm Hg)	136±4	126±3	129±5	122±5	124±5
Diastolic (mm Hg)	82±5	79±4	79±5	81±6	81±5
Supine HR (beats/min)	59±2	65±2[A]	65±2[A]	57±3	55±2
Upright HR (beats/min)	72±4	88±7[A]	80±3[A]	78±5	72±4
PRA (ng/ml/hr)	1.42±0.2	4.42±0.7[A]	2.95±0.5[A]	2.86±0.6[A]	2.62±0.6[A]
PAC (pg/ml)	130±9	260±35[A]	174±16[A]	191±16[A]	167±10[A]
UKV (meq/24 hr)	50±3	45±4	41±5	55±7	58±7
Hct (%)	42±0.8	43±0.8	43±0.8	44±0.9	44±0.3
Cr Cl (ml/min)	131±10	124±14	116±13	130±12	134±13
Weight (kg)	72±3	72±3	71±3[A]	71±2[A]	70±2[A]

BP = blood pressure; HR = heart rate; PRA = plasma renin activity; PAC = plasma aldosterone; UKV = urinary potassium excretion; Hct = hematocrit; Cr Cl = creatinine clearance.

[A]p < .05.

TABLE 2

Time course of effects of the low-salt diet (40 meq/day) on cardiac anatomy and hemodynamics and on cardiovascular response to isometric exercise (n = 10)

	Days on diet				
	0	4	7	30	60
Echocardiography					
LVID (cm)					
Diastole	5.0±0.2	5.0±0.2	5.0±0.2	5.1±0.1	5.1±0.2
Systole	3.4±0.2	3.5±0.2	3.5±0.2	3.6±0.2	3.6±0.2
LVV (cm^3)					
Diastole	126±10	127±11	127±10	130±12	130±12
Systole	49±6	50±6	51±6	50±7	52±8
LVMI (g/m^2)	96±4	96±5	97±5	98±5	98±5
VCF (sec^{-1})	1.1±0.05	1.08±0.05	1.08±0.05	1.03±0.04	1.05±0.05
CO (l/min)	6.6±0.7	6.4±0.6	6.6±0.3	6.3±0.3	6.3±0.3
TPR (dynes × sec × cm^{-5})	1240±208	1255±198	1200±78	1198±55	1241±85
Isometric exercise					
%Δ MBP	+22.3±4	+41±5[A]	+40±5[A]	+28±4	+23±3
%Δ HR	+42±10	+43±7	+52±8	+50±9	+40±7

LVID = left ventricular internal diameter; LVV = left ventricular volume; LVMI = left ventricular mass index; VCF = mean velocity of circumferential fiber shortening; CO = cardiac output; TPR = total peripheral resistance; HR = heart rate; MBP = mean blood pressure.

[A]$p < .05$.

a number of recent studies have indicated that such measurements can provide a reliable index of sympathetic activity under certain conditions,[1-12] particularly when factors such as body posture,[26] age,[27] smoking,[28] caffeine consumption,[29] stress,[30] exercise,[2] medications, salt intake,[1, 31] and blood pressure[8, 32] are taken into account. Much care was thus devoted in the present study to control of the blood sampling procedure, and only normal subjects falling into a restricted age range were studied. In addition, hemodynamic parameters that, at least in part, reflect neural sympathetic discharge were also monitored to further validate plasma catecholamine levels as a measure of sympathetic nervous system activity.

In keeping with most previous observations,[1-8] our results show that plasma catecholamine levels increase when sodium intake is decreased. However, in the present study, the increase in plasma catecholamines was detectable only in the early period of the low-salt diet. Measurements obtained after 30 and 60 days of a continuous low-salt diet showed that both plasma epinephrine and norepinephrine concentrations were no longer different from those obtained during the control period.

Consistent with the trend observed in plasma catecholamine levels are two additional findings of our study. First, the small but significant increases in heart rate (mostly in the upright position) paralleled those observed in plasma catecholamine levels, since they were restricted to the observations made on days 4 and 7. Similarly, the blood pressure response to isometric exercise was significantly enhanced only in the early period of the low-salt diet.

Taken together, these findings indicate that, in normotensive subjects, a sustained and protracted reduction in salt intake enhances sympathetic activity only transiently. A few earlier observations are consistent with our findings. For example, Carroll et al.[11] reported that long-term sodium depletion in dogs did not alter plasma catecholamine concentration despite a fourfold increase in plasma renin activity. Fujita et al.[4] reported that in salt-sensitive hypertensive patients switched from a low- to a high-salt diet, plasma norepinephrine decreased initially but then increased toward control values. These findings are compatible with the hypothesis that the catecholamine response to a change in sodium intake is transient.

Although we found that a transient increase in plasma catecholamines was associated with increases in heart rate and blood pressure responses to exercise, we failed to detect a significant effect of the low-salt diet on resting cardiac output or peripheral resistance, as evaluated by echocardiography. This contrasts in part with some earlier findings.[13] However, in most studies showing changes in local or systemic vascular resistance or contractility during a low-salt diet,[13-18] the responses to far more drastic sodium restriction were evaluated principally in patients with borderline or established hypertension who might have different hemodynamic responses than the normal subjects studied herein.

Another important finding of our study is that, unlike the parameters reflecting sympathetic function, both plasma renin activity and plasma aldosterone remained elevated for the duration of the low-salt diet. This is not surprising, given the known complexity of the control of renin secretion by the kidney. Thus, although the transient stimulation of sympathetic activity may have contributed to the initial rise in plasma renin, other mechanisms (such as stimulation via the macula densa) appear able to sustain the stimulation of the renin-angiotensin system despite waning of the sympathetic response. It must be pointed out that, since hormonal measurements were made only in the supine position, we may have underestimated the degree of stimulation of the renin-angiotensin system (as well as of the sympathetic nervous system) during long-term sodium depletion. It thus remains possible that some degree of sympathetic activation might persist in the upright posture, although our data on exercise responses are evidence against this. Whatever the case, the present findings demonstrate a dissociation between the long-term responses of the renin-angiotensin and sympathetic nervous systems.

The mechanisms responsible for the initial stimulation of sympathetic function induced by sodium restriction and for the waning of this response over the long term are not elucidated by the present study. It is, of course, possible that angiotensin II itself plays a role in stimulating the sympathetic nervous system, since several mechanisms have been proposed whereby this could occur.[33–37] If so, it is difficult to understand why the sympathetic response would fade despite maintained activation of the renin-angiotensin system; however, there is evidence that long-term angiotensin infusion appears to only transiently increase arterial epinephrine levels.[38] Other mechanisms are possible, such as initial changes in blood volume followed by redistribution of volume, but further work is needed to clarify this point.

In conclusion, our findings indicate that the duration of the change in salt intake has to be taken into account in evaluating the sympathetic nervous system responses to a reduction in sodium intake. They also support the hypothesis that long-term blood pressure homeostasis in normal subjects is accomplished mainly through the kidney and its control mechanisms, as indicated by the more sustained response of the renin-angiotensin system, whereas the autonomic nervous control of the circulation principally contributes to the short-term control of blood pressure homeostasis during long-term changes in sodium intake.

We thank Linda Stackhouse for preparation of the manuscript.

References

1. Robertson DH, Johnson GA, Brilis GM, Hill RE, Watson JT, Oates JA: Salt restriction increases serum catecholamines and urinary normetanephrine excretion. Fed Proc **36:** 956, 1977 (abst)
2. Robertson D, Johnson GA, Robertson RM, Nies AS, Shand DA, Oates JA: Comparative assessment of stimuli that release neuronal and adrenomedullary catecholamines in man. Circulation **59:** 637, 1979
3. Luft FC, Rankin LI, Henry DP, Block R, Grim CE, Weyman AE, Weinberger MH: Plasma and urinary norepinephrine values at extremes of sodium intake in normal man. Hypertension **1:** 261, 1979
4. Fujita T, Henry WL, Bartter FC, Lake CR, Delea CS: Factors influencing blood pressure in salt-sensitive patients with hypertension. Am J Med **69:** 334, 1980
5. Hong Tai Eng FW, Huber-Smith M, McCarm DS: The role of sympathetic activity in normal renin essential hypertension. Hypertension **2:** 14, 1980
6. Fraser J, Nadeau J, Robertson D, Wood AJJ: Regulation of the human leukocyte beta-receptor by endogenous catecholamines. J Clin Invest **67:** 1777, 1981
7. Campese VM, Romoff MS, Levitan D, Saglikes Y, Friedler RM, Massry SA: Abnormal relationship between sodium intake and sympathetic nervous system activity in salt-sensitive patients with essential hypertension. Kidney Int **21:** 371, 1982
8. Masuo K, Ogihara T, Kumahara Y, Yamatodari A, Wada H: Plasma norepinephrine and dietary sodium intake in normal subjects and patients with essential hypertension. Hypertension **5:** 767, 1983
9. Trimarco B, Volpe M, Ricciardelli B, Picotti GB, Galva MD, Petracca R, Condorelli M: Studies of the mechanisms underlying impairment of beta-adrenoceptor-mediated effects on human hypertension. Hypertension **5:** 584, 1983
10. Nicholls MG, Kiowski W, Zweifler AJ, Julius S, Schork MA, Greenhouse J: Plasma norepinephrine variations with dietary sodium intake. Hypertension **2:** 29, 1980
11. Carroll RG, Lohmeier TE, Brown AJ: Chronic sodium depletion does not alter plasma catecholamine concentration. The Physiologist **26:** 11, 1983 (abst)
12. Parfrey PS, Vanderburg MJ, Wright P, Holly JMP, Goodwin FJ, Evans SSW, Ledingham SM: Blood pressure and hormonal changes following alterations in dietary sodium and potassium in mild essential hypertension. Lancet **1:** 59, 1981
13. Sullivan JM, Ratts TE, Taylor JC, Kraus DH, Barton BR, Patrick DR, Reed SW: Hemodynamic effects of dietary sodium in man. A preliminary report. Hypertension **2:** 506, 1980
14. Takeshita A, Imaisumi T, Ashihara T, Nakamura M: Characteristics of responses to salt loading and deprivation in hypertensive subjects. Circ Res **51:** 657, 1982
15. Kirkendall WM, Connar WE, Abboud FM, Rastogi SP, Anderson TA, Fry M: The effect of dietary sodium on the blood pressure in normotensive man. *In* Genest J, editor: International Symposium on Renin-Angiotensin-Sodium in Hypertension. New York, Springer-Verlag, pp 360–373
16. Abboud FM: Effects of sodium, angiotensin, and steroids on vascular reactivity in man. Fed Proc **33:** 143, 1974
17. Mark AL, Lawton WJ, Abboud FM, Fitz AE, Connor WE, Heistad DD: Effects of high and low sodium intake on arterial pressure and forearm vascular resistance in borderline hypertension. Circ Res **36/37**(suppl I): I-194, 1975
18. Rankin LI, Luft FC, Henry DP, Gibbs PS, Weinberger MH: Sodium intake alters the effects of norepinephrine on blood pressure. Hypertension **3:** 650, 1981
19. Oliver JA, Cannon PJ: The effect of altered sodium balance upon renal vascular reactivity to angiotensin II and norepinephrine in dog. Mechanisms of variation in angiotensin responses. J Clin Invest **61:** 610, 1978
20. DaPrada M, Zürcher G: Simultaneous radioenzymatic determina-

tion of plasma and tissue adrenaline, noradrenaline and dopamine within the femtomole range. Life Sci **19:** 1161, 1976

21. Menard J, Catt KJ: Measurements of renin activity by radioimmunoassay of angiotensin I. Endocrinology **90:** 422, 1972
22. McKenzie JK, Clements SA: Simplified radioimmunoassay for serum aldosterone utilizing increased antibody specificity. J Clin Endocrinol Metab **36:** 622, 1974
23. Kirkendall WH, Burton HC, Epstein FH, Freis ED: Recommendations for human blood pressure determination by sphygmomanometers. Circulation **36:** 980, 1967
24. Sahn DJ, DeMaria A, Kisslo J, Weyman A: Recommendations regarding quantitation in M-mode echocardiography: results of a survey of echocardiographic measurements. Circulation **58:** 1072, 1979
25. Devereux RB, Reichek N: Echocardiographic determination of left ventricular mass in man: anatomic validation of the method. Circulation **55:** 613, 1977
26. Lake CR, Ziegler MG, Kopin IJ: Use of plasma norepinephrine for evaluation of sympathetic neuronal function in man. Life Sci **18:** 1315, 1976
27. Ziegler MG, Lake CR, Kopin IJ: Plasma noradrenaline increases with age. Nature **261:** 333, 1976
28. Cryer PE, Haymond MW, Santiago JV, Shah SD: Norepinephrine and epinephrine release and adrenergic mediation of smoking associated hemodynamic and metabolic events. N Engl J Med **295:** 573, 1976
29. Robertson D, Frohlich SC, Carr RK, Watson JT, Hollifield JW, Shand DG, Oates JA: Effects of caffeine on plasma renin activity, catecholamines, and blood pressure. N Engl J Med **298:** 181, 1978
30. Carruthers M, Conway N, Taggart P, Bates D, Somerville W: Validity of plasma-catecholamine estimations. Lancet **2:** 62, 1970
31. Romoff MS, Keusch G, Campese VM, Wang MS, Friedler RM, Weidmann P, Massry SG: Effect of sodium intake on plasma catecholamines in normal subjects. J Clin Endocrinol Metab **48:** 26, 1978
32. Henry DP, Luft FC, Weinberger MH, Fineberg NS, Grim CE: Norepinephrine in urine and plasma following provocative maneuvers in normal and hypertensive subjects. Hypertension **2:** 20, 1980
33. Samuels A, Johnson G, Peuler A: Physiologic effects of the renin angiotensin system on sympathetic nervous system activity in the conscious dog. *In* Buckley J, Ferrario CM, editors: Central actions of angiotensin and related hormones. New York, 1977, Pergamon, pp 135–144
34. Ferrario CM, Gildenberg PL, McCubbin JW: Cardiovascular effects of angiotensin mediated by the central nervous system. Circ Res **30:** 257, 1972
35. Zimmerman BG, Gomer SK, Liao JC: Action of angiotensin on vascular adrenergic nerve endings: facilitation of norepinephrine release. Fed Proc **31:** 1344, 1972
36. Zimmerman BG: Actions of angiotensin on adrenergic nerve endings. Fed Proc **37:** 199, 1978
37. Peach MJ, Cline WJ Jr, Watts DT: Release of adrenal catecholamines by angiotensin II. Circ Res **19:** 571, 1966
38. Carroll RG, Lohmeier TE, Brown AJ: Chronic angiotensin II infusion decreases renal norepinephrine overflow in conscious dogs. Hypertension **6:** 675, 1984

Is hypertension more benign when associated with obesity?

ELIZABETH BARRETT-CONNOR, M.D., AND KAY-TEE KHAW, M.B.

ABSTRACT To determine the effect of obesity on prognosis in hypertensive subjects, a population of 1727 men 50 to 79 years of age was dichotomized by baseline body mass index (<27 and ≥27 kg/m^2) and systolic blood pressure (<160 and ≥160 mm Hg). After 9 years of follow-up, age-adjusted all-cause, cardiovascular, and ischemic heart disease mortality rates were highest in the nonobese hypertensive subjects. The relative risk for mortality associated with a systolic blood pressure of 160 mm Hg or higher was significantly increased only in the nonobese group, with the largest difference in relative risk between obese and nonobese for ischemic heart disease. Results were consistent after separately excluding those with a history of heart disease, diabetes, current use of antihypertensive medication, and cigarette smoking, and those who died within 2 years of the baseline examination. When the independent effect of risk factors, including age, plasma cholesterol level, cigarette smoking, use of antihypertensive medication, and personal history of heart disease or diabetes was assessed with the Cox model, systolic blood pressure was a significant independent predictor of all-cause, cardiovascular, and ischemic heart disease death only in the nonobese subjects. We do not exclude an adverse effect of raised blood pressure in the obese. However, these data suggest that the prognosis is poorer in leaner hypertensive patients than in those who are overweight.
Circulation 72, No. 1, 53–60, 1985.

RAISED BLOOD PRESSURE is a well-established risk factor for cardiovascular disease. There is a considerable body of evidence showing a direct relationship between obesity and hypertension. Overweight subjects are more likely to be hypertensive and to develop hypertension; weight changes parallel blood pressure changes, and weight reduction reduces the blood pressure in overweight subjects with essential hypertension.[1-11]

Obesity is a weak but possibly independent predictor of cardiovascular disease.[12] On the other hand, high blood pressure is a strong predictor of cardiovascular disease; after controlling statistically for obesity, both systolic and diastolic blood pressure are predictive of cardiovascular disease independent of associated obesity.[13, 14] Although it has been stated that obese hypertensive subjects are at greater risk of ischemic heart disease and have higher mortality rates than nonobese hypertensive subjects,[2, 15] different cardiovascular phenomena in lean compared with obese hypertensive patients suggest that hypertension might have less clinical significance in obese subjects than in those of more normal weight.[16-18] For example, at a given level of blood pressure, leaner hypertensive subjects have more increased peripheral vascular resistance.[17, 19]

We tested the hypothesis that blood pressure is less predictive of ischemic heart disease death in obese subjects than in nonobese subjects by examining the mortality experience of a population of 1727 men 50 to 79 years of age who have been followed for 9 years. In this population, systolic blood pressure was independently predictive of ischemic heart disease death only in nonobese men.

Methods

Between 1972 and 1974, 82% of an adult upper-middle class Caucasian population in southern California was surveyed for heart disease risk factors (visit 1). Current cigarette smoking, the use of antihypertensive medication, and a personal history of heart disease and diabetes were ascertained by interview with the use of a standardized questionnaire. Patients' height and weight were measured while in light clothing and without shoes; obesity was estimated by the body mass index (weight in kilograms/height in meters squared). Systolic and diastolic blood pressures, first and fifth phase Korotkoff's sounds, were measured with a standard mercury sphygmomanometer and a 14 by 59 mm cuff after the participant had been seated for at least 5

From the Department of Community and Family Medicine and the Department of Medicine, School of Medicine, University of California San Diego, La Jolla.

Supported by NIH-NHLBI, Lipid Research Clinics Program, Contract No. NIH-NHLBI-HV-1-2160-L. Dr. Khaw was supported by the Wellcome Trust, London, England.

Address for correspondence: Elizabeth Barrett-Connor, M.D., Department of Community and Family Medicine (M-007), University of California, San Diego, School of Medicine, La Jolla, CA 92093.

Received Feb. 1, 1985; revision accepted April 18, 1985.

min. Any blood pressure greater than 160 mm Hg systolic or 90 mm Hg diastolic was repeated, and the lower of the two measurements was recorded. Total plasma cholesterol was measured in a standardized Lipid Research Clinic laboratory. Approximately 3 months after visit 1, one-third of this cohort (a 15% random sample and all those with hyperlipidemia) had a more extensive evaluation at visit 2. At this visit, blood pressure was measured twice after the subject had been seated for at least 5 min, and the mean of two measurements was used. Height and weight were again measured as above.

Vital status was determined annually for at least 9 years in 99.6% of the total cohort. Death certificates were obtained for all decedents and coded according to the 8th ICDA (International Classification of Diseases, Adapted) by a certified nosologist. All-cause, cardiovascular (codes 400 to 448), and ischemic heart disease (codes 410 to 414) mortality were recorded. In 30% of the study population, validation of death certificates with any mention of cardiovascular disease was attempted by interview with the next of kin and physician, and by review of hospital records. A panel of cardiologists determined that supporting data confirmed the death certificate diagnosis in approximately 85%.

For the present analysis, all 1727 men 50 to 79 years of age at visit 1 were dichotomized into those who were obese and nonobese. Obesity was defined as a body mass index in the top tertile for this population; this index of 27 or greater is at least 20% above the ideal for men of average build, according to recent Metropolitan Life tables.[20] Risk factor distribution by obesity category was determined. For univariate analyses of mortality rates, the cohort was further divided into systolic (≥160 mm Hg and <160 mm Hg) and diastolic (≥95 mm Hg and <95 mm Hg) blood pressure categories. Rates were age adjusted to this population by the direct method. The Mantel-Haenszel chi-square test was used to test the age-adjusted, 9 year mortality rates within each obesity category. This analysis was repeated with data obtained at visit 2. For the total cohort, age-adjusted rates and relative risks were also calculated after separately excluding those with a previous history of heart disease or diabetes, those who died within 2 years of follow-up, those who were currently using antihypertensive medication, and current cigarette smokers.

The Cox proportional hazards model[21] was used to determine the independent effect of blood pressure on all-cause, cardiovascular, and ischemic heart disease mortality within each obesity category, after adjusting for the effects of age, cholesterol level, cigarette smoking, history of diabetes, history of heart disease, and use of antihypertensive medication.

Finally, to determine whether extremely lean men were responsible for the higher mortality rate in the nonobese group or whether error in blood pressure measurement in the extremely obese[22-24] explained the lack of association in the obese, age-adjusted ischemic heart disease mortality rates by systolic blood pressure category were calculated by decile of body mass index. Overestimation of blood pressure in the obese[22-24] has been reported in some but not all studies. We also calculated age-adjusted all-cause, cardiovascular, and ischemic heart disease mortality rates in the obese for those with a systolic blood pressure greater than 170 mm Hg or a diastolic blood pressure greater than 105 mm Hg to examine the effects of overestimation of blood pressure of 10 mm Hg in the obese.

Results

One-third of the 1727 men 50 to 79 years of age were at least 20% above the ideal body mass index,[19] i.e., 27 kg/m^2 or more. Table 1 shows the distribution of selected risk factors in the obese (body mass index ≥27) and nonobese subjects (body mass index <27). Obese men were significantly more likely to have categorical hypertension and higher mean blood pressures and to be taking antihypertensive medication, but significantly fewer obese men had a past history of heart disease. Diabetes was slightly more common ($p < .07$) in the obese group. Other risk factors, including age, total plasma cholesterol level, and current cigarette smoking, did not differ significantly between the two groups. The proportion of former or heavy smokers did not differ between the obese and nonobese groups (now shown).

TABLE 1
Risk factor distribution by obesity category

	BMI < 27 (n = 1147)	BMI ≥ 27 (n = 580)
Age (yr)[A]	65.8±7.2	65.3±7.1
Systolic blood pressure (mm Hg)[A]	141.4±22.9	145.7±22.0[C]
Diastolic blood pressure (mm Hg)[A]	81.6±11.2	84.7±11.2[C]
Cholesterol (mg/dl)[A]	212.4±34.2	213.3±36.5
Obesity (kg/m^2)[A]	24.1±1.8	28.9±2.0[C]
Systolic blood pressure ≥ 160 mm Hg (%)	21.6	28.1[B]
Diastolic blood pressure ≥ 90 mm Hg (%)	12.9	19.5[B]
Current cigarette smokers (%)	20.5	17.6
Ex-smokers (%)	55.3	56.2
Diabetes by history (%)	6.1	9.0
Current use of antihypertensive drugs (%)	15.3	21.6[C]
Personal history of heart disease (%)	12.7	7.8[C]

BMI = body mass index (kg/m^2).
[A]Expressed as mean ± SD.
[B]$p < .01$.
[C]$p < .001$.

At the 9 year follow-up there were 393, 203, and 146 deaths from all-cause, cardiovascular, and ischemic heart disease, respectively. Table 2 shows age-adjusted all-cause, cardiovascular, and ischemic heart disease mortality rates by body mass index and systolic blood pressure at the 9 year follow-up. Mortality rates were significantly higher in the nonobese group with systolic blood pressure of 160 or higher compared with the rest of the cohort; the relative risks for mortality associated with a systolic blood pressure of 160 mm Hg or higher were significantly increased only in the nonobese group, with the largest relative risk differences between nonobese and obese in ischemic heart disease. Results were similar after separately excluding those with a history of heart disease or diabetes, those who died within 2 years of the baseline examina-

TABLE 2
Age-adjusted 9 year mortality rates (%) by obesity and systolic blood pressure category

		All cause		Cardiovascular disease		Ischemic heart disease	
		BMI < 27	BMI ≥27	BMI < 27	BMI ≥ 27	BMI < 27	BMI ≥ 27
No exclusions (n = 1727)[A]							
Rate/100	SBP < 160 mm Hg	20.6	21.4	9.2	10.4	6.5	8.1
Rate/100	SBP ≥ 160 mm Hg	32.7	27.8	20.3	14.1	14.7	8.8
Relative Risk		1.6[B]	1.3	2.2[C]	1.4	2.3[B]	1.1
Excluding all with a history of heart failure or heart disease (n = 1372)							
Rate/100	SBP < 160 mm Hg	19.2	21.3	7.7	9.5	5.1	6.9
Rate/100	SBP ≥ 160 mm Hg	30.1	27.2	16.9	12.5	10.9	7.4
Relative risk		1.6[B]	1.3	2.2[B]	1.3	2.1[B]	1.1
Excluding all who died within 2 yr of follow-up (n = 1649)							
Rate/100	SBP < 160 mm Hg	17.3	18.5	7.3	8.2	4.7	6.3
Rate/100	SBP ≥ 160 mm Hg	27.2	23.5	15.4	12.5	10.4	8.1
Relative risk		1.6[B]	1.3	2.1[C]	1.5	2.2[C]	1.3
Excluding all with a history of diabetes (n = 1605)							
Rate/100	SBP < 160 mm Hg	20.2	20.9	9.1	10.8	6.3	8.1
Rate/100	SBP ≥ 160 mm Hg	34.7	25.4	21.8	11.7	15.8	6.3
Relative risk		1.7[C]	1.2	2.4[C]	1.1	2.5[C]	0.8
Excluding all current smokers (n = 1390)							
Rate/100	SBP < 160 mm Hg	18.8	21.4	8.7	9.5	6.4	7.1
Rate/100	SBP ≥ 160 mm Hg	31.7	26.4	19.8	12.8	14.4	8.9
Relative risk		1.7[C]	1.2	2.3[C]	1.3	2.3[B]	1.3
Excluding all on antihypertensive medication (n = 1447)							
Rate/100	SBP < 160 mm Hg	19.0	21.6	8.2	9.1	5.7	7.4
Rate/100	SBP ≥ 160 mm Hg	28.4	21.4	17.6	10.9	12.7	7.2
Relative risk		1.5[B]	1.0	2.1[C]	1.2	2.2[B]	1.0

BMI = body mass index (kg/m^2); SBP = systolic blood pressure.
[A]The denominators are: SBP < 160, BMI < 27, n = 899; SBP < 160, BMI ≥ 27, n = 417; SBP ≥ 160, BMI < 27, n = 248; SBP ≥160, BMI ≥27, n = 163.
[B]$p < .01$; [C]$p < .001$.

tion, current cigarette smokers, and those taking antihypertensive medication. Table 3 shows adjusted mortality rates by body mass index and diastolic blood pressure at the 9 year follow-up. Trends were similar, although less marked, to those for systolic blood pressure with highest absolute death rates in the nonobese hypertensive group. Relative risks for all-cause and cardiovascular disease mortality for raised diastolic pressure were increased only in the nonobese group. Age-adjusted all-cause, cardiovascular, and ischemic heart disease mortality rates in the obese subjects who had systolic blood pressure greater than 170 mm Hg were 31.5%, 18.8%, and 12.3%, respectively, and rates in the obese subjects who had diastolic blood pressure greater than 105 mm Hg were 20.2%, 12.9%, and 0%, respectively. These rates were still lower than those in the nonobese subjects who had systolic blood pressure greater than 160 mm Hg or diastolic blood pressure greater than 95 mm Hg. Table 4 shows similar age-adjusted rates for the visit 2 sample.

The Cox model was used to assess the independent effect of risk factors on all-cause, cardiovascular, and ischemic heart disease mortality separately in the obese and the nonobese groups (table 5). Systolic blood pressure was a significant independent predictor of all-cause, cardiovascular, and ischemic heart disease mortality only in the nonobese subjects. The use of antihypertensive medication was also a significant mortality predictor only in the nonobese subjects. The independent predictive value of other risk factors also

TABLE 3
Age-adjusted 9 year mortality rates (%) by obesity and diastolic blood pressure category

		All cause		Cardiovascular disease		Ischemic heart disease	
		BMI < 27	BMI ≥27	BMI < 27	BMI ≥ 27	BMI < 27	BMI ≥ 27
No exclusions (n = 1727)							
Rate/100	DBP < 95 mm Hg	22.0	21.9	11.2	10.0	8.1	8.0
Rate/100	DBP ≥ 95 mm Hg	32.2	21.5	17.9	13.9	12.4	6.8
Relative risk		1.5[B]	1.0	1.6[C]	1.4	1.5	0.9
Excluding all with a history of heart failure or heart disease (n = 1372)							
Rate/100	DBP < 95 mm Hg	19.8	22.0	9.0	9.0	6.1	9.9
Rate/100	DBP ≥ 95 mm Hg	31.8	21.9	15.5	12.6	9.1	5.7
Relative risk		1.6[B]	1.0	1.7[A]	1.4	1.5	0.6
Excluding all who died within 2 yr of follow-up (n = 1649)							
Rate/100	DBP < 95 mm Hg	18.4	18.6	8.6	7.7	5.9	6.3
Rate/100	DBP ≥ 95 mm Hg	26.1	20.2	13.5	12.5	8.7	6.0
Relative risk		1.4[A]	1.1	1.6[A]	1.6	1.5	1.0
Excluding all with a history of diabetes (n = 1605)							
Rate/100	DBP < 95 mm Hg	21.7	28.1	11.2	9.8	8.0	7.7
Rate/100	DBP ≥ 95 mm Hg	34.8	21.5	18.9	13.3	13.1	5.7
Relative risk		1.6[B]	0.8	1.5[B]	1.4	1.6[A]	0.7
Excluding all current smokers (n = 1390)							
Rate/100	DBP < 95 mm Hg	20.3	22.2	10.6	9.7	8.1	7.6
Rate/100	DBP ≥ 95 mm Hg	31.5	20.1	17.3	12.1	11.2	6.1
Relative risk		1.6[A]	0.9	1.6	1.2	1.4	0.3
Excluding all on antihypertensive medication (n = 1447)							
Rate/100	DBP < 95 mm Hg	20.2	22.3	9.4	9.3	6.7	7.6
Rate/100	DBP ≥ 95 mm Hg	25.6	18.0	14.5	11.1	9.9	5.7
Relative risk		1.3[B]	8.0	1.5	1.2	1.5	0.8

BMI = body mass index (kg/m^2); DBP = diastolic blood pressure.
[A]$p < .05$; [B]$p < .01$; [C]$p < .001$.

differed in the obese and nonobese groups; smoking was predictive of all-cause mortality in the nonobese group and history of diabetes was predictive of mortality in the obese group. A history of heart disease was a stronger predictor of all-cause, cardiovascular, and ischemic heart disease mortality in the nonobese subjects.

As shown in figure 1, this excess ischemic heart

TABLE 4
Age-adjusted 9 year mortality rates (%) by obesity and systolic blood pressure category at visit 2 (n = 534)

	All causes		Cardiovascular disease		Ischemic heart disease	
	BMI < 27	BMI ≥ 27	BMI < 27	BMI ≥ 27	BMI < 27	BMI ≥ 27
SBP < 160 mm Hg	22.9	20.7	10.5	8.5	8.4	6.8
SBP ≥160 mm Hg	25.5	38.6	19.4	11.0	15.6	9.2
Relative risk	1.1	1.9	1.8[A]	1.3	1.9[A]	1.4
DBP < 95 mm Hg	22.0	23.8	11.3	9.1	9.4	7.0
DBP ≥ 95 mm Hg	36.7	19.2	22.4	7.9	14.3	7.9
Relative risk	1.7[A]	0.8	2.0[A]	0.9	1.5	1.1

BMI = body mass index (kg/m^2); SBP = systolic blood pressure; DBP = diastolic blood pressure.
[A]$p < .05$.

TABLE 5
Independent relative risks for mortality by obesity category (based on Cox regression model)

Risk factors	Relative risks (95% confidence limits) BMI < 27	BMI ≥ 27
All causes		
Age (per 10 yr)	2.4^D (1.9–3.0)	3.3^D (2.3–4.7)
Systolic blood pressure (per 20 mm Hg)^A	1.2^C (1.1–1.3)	1.1 (0.9–1.3)
Cholesterol (per 40 mg/dl)^A	1.1 (0.9–1.2)	1.2 (1.0–1.5)
Smoking (yes vs no)	1.8^C (1.2–2.7)	1.1 (0.6–2.0)
History of diabetes (yes vs no)	0.9 (0.5–1.2)	1.9^B (1.1–3.2)
History of heart disease (yes vs no)	2.0^D (1.5–2.7)	1.2 (0.6–2.2)
Antihypertensive medication (yes vs no)	1.6^C (1.2–2.2)	1.0 (0.7–1.6)
Cardiovascular disease		
Age (per 10 yr)	2.4^D (1.7–3.3)	2.8^D (1.7–4.4)
Systolic blood pressure (per 20 mm Hg)^A	1.3^C (1.1–1.5)	1.1 (0.8–1.4)
Cholesterol (per 40 mg/dl)^A	1.3^B (1.0–1.5)	1.3^B (1.0–1.8)
Smoking (yes vs no)	1.2 (0.7–2.2)	1.1 (0.5–1.3)
History of diabetes (yes vs no)	0.6 (0.3–1.4)	1.7 (0.7–3.7)
History of heart disease (yes vs no)	3.0^D (2.1–4.4)	2.3^B (1.2–4.6)
Antihypertensive medication (yes vs no)	2.0^D (1.4–3.0)	1.5 (0.9–2.6)
Ischemic heart disease		
Age (per 10 yr)	2.0^D (1.4–2.9)	2.5^D (1.5–4.2)
Systolic blood pressure (per 20 mm Hg)^A	1.3^C (1.1–1.5)	1.0 (0.8–1.4)
Cholesterol (per 40 mg/dl)^A	1.4^C (1.1–1.8)	1.2 (0.9–1.8)
Smoking (yes vs no)	0.8 (0.4–1.3)	0.8 (0.3–2.2)
History of diabetes (yes vs no)	0.6 (0.3–1.6)	1.9 (0.8–4.5)
History of heart disease (yes vs no)	4.3^D (2.8–6.6)	3.3^C (1.6–7.1)
Antihypertensive medication (yes vs no)	2.1^C (1.3–3.3)	1.4 (0.7–2.7)

^{A}For continuous variables except age, intervals approximate 1 SD.
$^B p < .05$; $^C p < .01$; $^D p < .001$.
BMI = body mass index (kg/m^2).

disease mortality rate in nonobese men was not limited to the leanest men. Mean diastolic and systolic blood pressure in those with systolic blood pressure of 160 mm Hg or higher or diastolic blood pressure of 95 mm Hg or higher did not differ significantly by decile of obesity or between the obese and nonobese groups, so the lower rates in hypertensive obese subjects were not due to lower mean blood pressures in this group.

Discussion

As previously reported, the mean body mass index in this male cohort was virtually identical to that in the National Health and Nutrition Survey.[25] In this population, hypertension was predictive of all-cause, cardiovascular, and ischemic heart disease death only in nonobese subjects, even though obese subjects had significantly more categorical hypertension and higher mean systolic and diastolic blood pressures overall. The increased mortality rate in nonobese hypertensive subjects did not appear to be a function of weight loss after manifest heart disease or diagnosed hypertension; exclusion of those with known cardiovascular disease and of those taking antihypertensive medications did not materially alter the results. Likewise, the higher mortality rates in nonobese hypertensive subjects is unlikely to have been caused by weight loss as a consequence of occult disease; results were similar after exclusion of all subjects who died within 2 years of the baseline examination. Exclusion of cigarette smokers, who might be expected to be leaner and have higher mortality rates, did not alter the results. Finally, exclusion of those with diabetes, a group at excess risk of obesity, hypertension, and cardiovascular death, did not significantly change the relationship. Results were also consistent when we repeated the analysis with blood pressure and obesity measurements at a second visit in a subsample of this cohort.

Both measured blood pressure and the use of antihypertensive medication were significant risk factors only in the nonobese subjects. The increased mortality risk associated with use of antihypertensive medication has been reported elsewhere,[26, 27] possibly reflecting selection bias; that is, subjects who were more ill or had more fixed hypertension are more likely to be given medication. However, the difference in predictive value of use of antihypertensive medication between obese and nonobese subjects in this population is unexplained.

In this older cohort, body mass index was significantly but weakly correlated with blood pressure (r = .15 for systolic blood pressure and .17 for diastolic; p

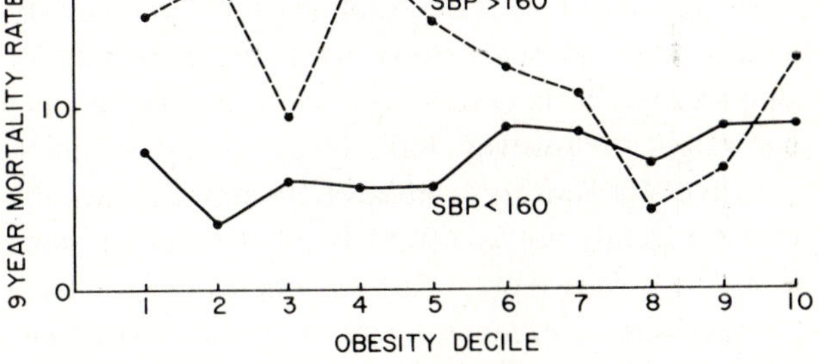

FIGURE 1. Nine year age-adjusted ischemic heart disease mortality rate by obesity decile and systolic blood pressure (SBP) category.

< .001). Others have noted that the correlation of obesity with blood pressure declines with age.[1, 28] Since this was a study of older men, we considered the possibility that survivorship bias produced these results. An analysis of the mortality rates in the 599 men 30 to 49 years of age in this population showed only 10 deaths from all causes, including two from ischemic heart disease; both of these men were hypertensive, one obese and one nonobese. Although based on a different birth cohort, these data do not suggest that obese hypertensive subjects are more likely to die than nonobese hypertensive subjects before reaching age 50.

Age-adjusted ischemic heart disease death rates by decile of obesity showed that the poorer prognosis in hypertensive nonobese men was not limited to those in the lowest decile of body weight. The relatively lower mortality in obese hypertensive men could have been caused by misclassification of blood pressure in obese subjects as a consequence of fixed cuff size. Although we cannot entirely exclude this possibility, this phenomenon should be more pronounced in men in the top decile of body mass, but men in the eighth and ninth decile were those with lower ischemic heart disease death rates. Furthermore, assuming a systematic 10 mm Hg overestimation of blood pressure in the obese subjects[22–24] we additionally compared age-adjusted death rates in the obese who had systolic blood pressure over 170 mm Hg or diastolic blood pressure over 105 mm Hg with nonobese subjects who had systolic blood pressure over 160 mm Hg or diastolic blood pressure over 95 mm Hg. The hypertensive obese group, so defined, still had lower rates than the hypertensive nonobese group.

These findings are contrary to the conventional wisdom that obese hypertensive subjects experience a greater risk of coronary artery disease than nonobese hypertensive subjects.[2] Data in support of this statement are in fact based largely on insurance company and military statistics, where the level of blood pressure is restricted at entry. Among the insured with levels of systolic blood pressure of 140 to 160 mm Hg, overweight curtails the expectation of life among individuals who are both overweight and hypertensive compared with "hypertensive" subjects who are not overweight.[15] However, individuals with blood pressures over 160 mm Hg systolic or 100 mm Hg diastolic were apparently not as adversely affected by the same degree of overweight. Among obese hypertensive Army officers, retirement related to cardiovascular-renal disease was more common in the obese or hypertensive groups alone[29]; cardiovascular deaths, however, were slightly more common in those who were not overweight.

Many case series of patients with more severe hypertension have found lower mortality rates in obese hypertensive subjects compared with those in nonobese hypertensive subjects. In the series of Frant and Groen,[30] obese hypertensive men had a lower 9 year mortality rate (26%) than nonobese hypertensive men (43%). After more than 25 years of follow-up of 1000 hypertensive patients, Bechgaard[31] reported that hypertensive men 40 to 59 years old who were 20 kg above normal weight had a lower mortality rate than patients with no excess weight. In a 10 year follow-up of hypertensive patients at the Mayo Clinic, Breslin et al.[32] found only a slightly greater mortality in individuals 30% overweight; in patients with retinal sclerosis or exudates, the prognosis was better in the obese group. Dimond[33] reported that obesity in a hypertensive group of 527 railway employees followed for up to 37 years was not related to the development of coronary disease; in fact, coronary heart disease rates were lowest in the heaviest (although data were not adjusted for age). Similarly, Sokolow and Perloff[34] reported that hypertensive patients who were obese had better prognosis than nonobese hypertensive patients.

The results of other studies are partially concordant with our data. In the 10 year follow-up of the Los Angeles Heart study,[13] hypertensive men under 50 years of age who had a higher index of relative weight had a lower incidence of coronary heart disease, although the reverse pattern was seen in older men. In the Framingham 18 year follow-up[35] the probability of developing coronary heart disease increased more steeply in men of moderate weight than in obese men; absolute probability rates were also greater in men of moderate weight compared with obese men at higher systolic blood pressure levels, although lean men had lower probability rates than the obese subjects at all levels of systolic blood pressure. However, the 26 year Framingham data reported no evidence of a blood pressure–obesity interaction.[12] Differences between the Framingham results and our data may reflect the greater proportion of men in the former study who were in extremely obese categories where mortality rates were very high. In the Chicago Peoples Gas Company Study,[36] the age-adjusted optimal weight increased when systolic blood pressure was taken into account, a finding consistent with our results. In the Western Collaborative Group Study,[37] in men 40 to 59 years old with diastolic blood pressure over 95 mm Hg, coronary heart disease rates in the lean were 1.5 times those in the overweight subjects. Results from the Australian therapeutic trial[38] also found a higher incidence of trial end points, mainly ischemic heart disease, in those with lower body mass index and apparent benefit from treatment was greater in those with lower body mass index.

Like the above studies, the results of the present analysis suggest that the detrimental effect of obesity on blood pressure–associated risk for cardiovascular disease is seen primarily in persons without categorical hypertension. Our data are compatible with an effect of obesity in normotensive subjects, where there was a nonsignificant but consistent slight excess in all-cause, cardiovascular, and ischemic heart disease death in those who were obese compared with those who were not (tables 2 and 3). In the presence of hypertension, however, obesity does not increase risk and, indeed, appears to be protective.

Is it biologically plausible that hypertension is less significant clinically in obese subjects than nonobese subjects? Both the etiology and the pathologic consequences of hypertension may differ in obese or nonobese subjects. Obesity may both potentiate and mitigate harmful cardiovascular effects of hypertension, as has been reviewed by Messerli and colleagues.[16–18] Raised total peripheral vascular resistance is the hallmark of essential hypertension and the major determinant of systemic hypertensive vascular disease.[39] As hypertension becomes established, total peripheral resistance increases and cardiac output reverts to normal.[18] With higher resistance there is contracted intravascular volume,[40–42] concentric left ventricular hypertrophy, and more restricted chamber volume.[43, 44] In obesity the increased stroke volume that augments cardiac output (in response to elevated metabolic requirements)[40, 45–48] is usually associated with an expansion of total blood volume.[48] Elevated preload gives rise to left ventricular dilatation and increasing ventricular volume. The compensatory increase in myocardial mass (eccentric left ventricular hypertrophy) remains proportional to chamber dilatation. As a consequence, at a given level of arterial pressure, total peripheral resistance is lower in an obese patient than a lean one.

These results should not be interpreted as an argument in favor of obesity. Obesity increases the risk of hypertension and extreme levels are associated with an increased risk of death. Neither do we exclude an adverse effect of raised blood pressure in the obese. These data do suggest that in the presence of high blood pressure, the prognosis may be poorer in the leaner subject. This observation may have important implications for interpreting the benefit of the treatment of hypertension.

Reference

1. Havlik RJ, Hubert HB, Fabsitz RR, Feinleib M: Weight and hypertension. Ann Intern Med **98** (part 2): 855, 1983
2. Chiang BN, Perlman LV, Epstein FH: Overweight and hypertension. Circulation **39:** 403, 1969
3. Tyroler HA, Heyden S, Hames CG: Weight and hypertension: Evans County studies of blacks and whites. *In* Paul O, editor: Epidemiology and control of hypertension. New York, 1975, Stratton Intercontinental Medical Book Corp., p 177
4. Stamler R, Stamler J, Riedlinger WF, Algera G, Roberts RH: Weight and blood pressure: findings in hypertension screening of 1 million Americans. JAMA **240:** 1607, 1978
5. Hypertension Detection and Follow-up Program Cooperative Group: Race, education and prevalence of hypertension. Am J Epidemiol **106:** 351, 1977
6. Reisin E, Frohlich ED: Effects of weight reduction on arterial pressure. J Chron Dis **35:** 887, 1982
7. Kannel WB, Brand N, Skinner JJ, Dawber TR, McNamara PM: The relation of adiposity to blood pressure and development of hypertension. Ann Intern Med **67:** 48, 1967
8. Ashley FW Jr, Kannel WB: Relationship of weight change to changes in atherogenic traits: The Framingham Study. J Chron Dis **27:** 103, 1974
9. Reed D, McGee D, Yano K: Biological and social correlates of blood pressure among Japanese men in Hawaii. Hypertension **4:** 406, 1982
10. Reisin E, Abel R, Modan M, Silverberg DS, Eliahou HE, Modan B: Effect of weight loss without salt restriction on the reduction of blood pressure in overweight hypertensive patients. N Engl J Med **298:** 1, 1978
11. Mann GV: The influence of obesity on health. N Engl J Med **291:** 178, 226, 1974
12. Hubert HB, Feinleib M, McNamara PM, Castelli WP: Obesity as an independent risk factor for cardiovascular disease: a 26 year followup of participants in the Framingham Heart Study. Circulation **67:** 968, 1983
13. Chapman JM, Massey FJ: The interrelationship of serum cholesterol, hypertension, body weight and risk of coronary disease. J Chron Dis **17:** 933, 1964
14. Gordon T, Kannel WB: Obesity and cardiovascular disease: The Framingham Study. Clin Endocrinol Metab **5:** 367, 1976
15. Lew EA: Blood pressure and mortality — life insurance experience. *In* Stamler J, Stamler R, Pullman TN, editors: The epidemiology of hypertension. New York, 1967, Grune and Stratton, p 392
16. Messerli FH: Cardiovascular effects of obesity and hypertension. Lancet **1:** 1165, 1982
17. Messerli FH, Christie B, DeCarvalho JGR, Aristimuno GG, Suarez DH, Dreslinski GR, Frohlich ED: Obesity and essential hypertension: hemodynamics, intravascular volume, sodium excretion and plasma renin activity. Arch Intern Med **141:** 81, 1981
18. Messerli FH, Ventura HO, Reisin E, Dreslinski GR, Dunn FG, MacPhee AA, Frohlich ED: Borderline hypertension and obesity: two prehypertensive states with elevated cardiac output. Circulation **66:** 55, 1982
19. Mujais SK, Tarazi RC, Dusrau HP, Fouad FM, Bravo GL: Hypertension in obese patients: hemodynamic and volume studies. Hypertension **4:** 84, 1982
20. Metropolitan Life Insurance Company: 1983 height and weight tables. New York, 1983, Health and Safety Education Division, Metropolitan Life Insurance Co.
21. Lee ET: Statistical methods for survival data analysis. Belmont, CA, 1980, Wadsworth, p 298
22. Karvonen MJ, Telivuo LJ, Jarvinen EJK: Sphygmomanometer cuff size and the accuracy of individual blood pressure measurement. Am J Cardiol **13:** 688, 1964
23. Nielsen PE, Janniche H: The accuracy of ausculatory measurement of arm blood pressure in very obese subjects. Acta Med Scand **195:** 403, 1974
24. Maxwell MH, Schroth PC, Waks AU, Karam M, Dornfeld LP: Error in blood pressure measurement due to incorrect cuff size in obese patients. Lancet **2:** 33, 1982

25. Barrett-Connor E: The prevalence of diabetes mellitus in an adult community as determined by history or fasting hyperglycemia. Am J Epidemiol **111:** 705, 1980
26. Multiple Risk Factor Intervention Trial: Risk factor changes and mortality results. JAMA **248:** 1465, 1982
27. Leren P, Helgeland A, Hjermann I, Holme I: MRFIT and the Oslo study. JAMA **249:** 893, 1983
28. Epstein FH, Francis T Jr, Hayner NS, Johnson BC, Kjelsberg MD, Napier JA, Ostrander LD Jr, Payne MW, Dodge HJ: Prevalence of chronic diseases and distribution of selected physiologic variables in a total community. Tecumseh, Michigan. Am J Epidemiol **81:** 307, 1965
29. Levy RL, White PD, Stroud WD: Overweight — its prognostic significance in relation to hypertension and cardiovascular-renal diseases. JAMA **131:** 951, 1946
30. Frant R, Groen J: Prognosis of vascular hypertension. Arch Intern Med **87:** 727, 1950
31. Bechgaard P: Arterial hypertension: a followup study of one thousand hypertonics. Acta Med Scand [Suppl] **172:** 13, 1946
32. Breslin DJ, Gifford RW, Fairbairn JF: Essential hypertension — a twenty year follow up study. Circulation **33:** 87, 1966
33. Dimond GE: Hypertension, body weight and coronary heart disease. Arch Intern Med **112:** 550, 1963
34. Sokolow M, Perloff D: The prognosis of essential hypertension treated conservatively. Circulaton **23:** 697, 1961
35. Kannel WB, Gordon T: Some determinants of obesity and its impact as a cardiovascular disease risk factor. *In* Howard A, editor: Recent advances in obesity research. I. Obesity, Proceedings of the 1st International Congress, Royal College of Physicians, London, England, October 1974. Technomic Publishing Co., Westport, CT, 1976, pp 14–27
36. Dyer AR, Stamler J, Berkson DM, Ludberg HA: Relationship of relative weight and body mass index to 14 year mortality in the Chicago Peoples Gas Company Study. J Chron Dis **28:** 108, 1975
37. Rosenman RH, Friedman M, Straus R, Jenkins CD, Zyzanski SJ, Wurm M: Coronary heart disease in the Western Collaborative Group Study. J Chron Dis **23:** 123, 1970
38. The Management Committee of the Australian National Blood Pressure Study: Prognostic factors in the treatment of mild hypertension. Circulation **69:** 668, 1984
39. Tarazi RC: Hemodynamics of hypertension. *In* Genest J, Kuchel O, Hamet B, Cantin M, editors: Hypertension: physiopathology and treatment, ed 2. New York, 1983, McGraw-Hill Book Co., Inc., p 15
40. Julius S, Pascual AV, Reilly K, London R: Abnormalities of plasma volume in borderline hypertension. Arch Intern Med **127:** 116, 1971
41. Messerli FH, deCarvalho JGR, Christie B, Frohlich ED: Essential hypertension in blacks and whites: hemodynamic findings and fluid volume state. Am J Med **67:** 27, 1979
42. Bauer JH, Brooks CS: Body fluid composition in normal and hypertensive man. Clin Sci **62:** 43, 1982
43. Dunn FG, Chandrarana PAN, deCarvalho JCR, Basta LL, Frohlich ED: Pathophysiological assessment of hypertensive heart disease with echocardiography. Am J Cardiol **39:** 789, 1977
44. Savage DD, Drayer JIM, Henry WL, Mathews EC, Ware JH, Gardin JM, Cohen ER, Epstein SE, Laragh JH: Echocardiographic assessment of cardiac anatomy and function in hypertensive patients. Circulation **59:** 623, 1979
45. Backman L, Freyschuss U, Hallberg D, Melcher A: Carciovascular function in extreme obesity. Acta Med Scand **193:** 437, 1973
46. Woodard CB, Quinones MA, Alexander JK: Pathogenesis of myocardial dysfunction in extreme obesity. Circulation **58** (suppl II): II-230, 1978
47. Kaltman AJ, Goldring RM: Role of circulatory congestion in the cardiorespiratory failure of obesity. Am J Med **60:** 645, 1976
48. Messerli FH, Sundgaard-Riise K, Reisin E, Dreslinski G, Dunn FG, Frolich ED: Disparate cardiovascular effects of obesity and hypertension. Am J Med **74:** 808, 1983

Characteristics of vascular hydraulic load in patients with heart failure

WARREN K. LASKEY, M.D., WILLIAM G. KUSSMAUL, M.D., JACK L. MARTIN, M.D., JOSEPH P. KLEAVELAND, M.D., JOHN W. HIRSHFELD, JR., M.D., AND SANJEEV SHROFF, PH.D.

ABSTRACT Aortic input impedance and hydraulic power were derived from simultaneous catheter recordings of ascending aortic pressure and velocity in eight normal subjects and 11 age-matched subjects with clinical heart failure secondary to idiopathic congestive cardiomyopathy. Resting data revealed the characteristic depression of cardiac output and elevation of systemic vascular resistance in patients with heart failure. The pulsatile component of vascular hydraulic load, characteristic impedance (Z_c), was similar in both groups (Z_c normal: 85 ± 30 dyne-sec-cm^{-5}; Z_c cardiomyopathy: 93 ± 33 dyne-sec-cm^{-5}). The oscillatory fraction of aortic input power in patients with heart failure (14 ± 4%) was also similar to that of normal subjects (11 ± 2%). The transition from rest to exercise in patients with heart failure was marked by a decrease in the steady component of arterial hydraulic load, although characteristic impedance did not change. A similar qualitative response occurred in normal subjects, although the systemic vascular resistance during exercise remained above normal in patients with heart failure. The modulus of the first harmonic of impedance significantly decreased during exercise in normal subjects but did not change significantly in patients with heart failure. Furthermore, the modulus of the first harmonic of the reflection coefficient decreased significantly during exercise in normal subjects but did not change in patients with heart failure in spite of systemic vasodilation. Exercise appears to impose no additional increase in vascular hydraulic load on the ejecting left ventricle. The similar aortic characteristic impedances in patients with heart failure and in normal subjects, at rest and during exercise, are consistent with a constant oscillatory fraction of input power.
Circulation 72, No. 1, 61–71, 1985.

ASSESSMENT of left ventricular function is incomplete without an understanding of the loading conditions during ejection. In particular, the failing left ventricle is markedly sensitive to alterations in afterload.[1] Exercise results in a constellation of hemodynamic alterations that represent a change in ventricular afterload. Therefore, exercise may impose an additional, and deleterious, hemodynamic burden on the failing left ventricle. Systemic vascular resistance represents the resistance to steady flow and, as such, is one component of left ventricular afterload. However, systemic vascular resistance does not take into account the pulsatile component of arterial hydraulic load.

Aortic input impedance represents the vascular hydraulic load encountered by the ejecting left ventricle.[2,3] The magnitude of impedance as well as the reflection characteristics of the arterial system completely define this hydraulic load.[4] Although it is generally agreed that the 0 Hz, or DC, component of impedance, systemic vascular resistance, is elevated in patients with congestive heart failure both at rest and during exercise,[5-9] there is conflicting evidence with regard to abnormalities in the pulsatile component of the vascular load.[10,11] Furthermore, experimental data suggest that arterial wave reflections decrease with systemic vasodilation and increase with vasoconstriction.[12] Reflected pressure waves during systole are additive and thus might augment afterload. Reflected flow waves, however, subtract from the forward flow pulse and thus may result in a diminished net forward flow. Both of these circumstances could be detrimental in patients with chronic heart failure and increased systemic resistance. Therefore an analysis of arterial wave reflections in patients with heart failure might provide additional insight into the effects of chronic systemic vasoconstriction on total hydraulic load as well as dynamic left ventricular performance.

Total aortic input power represents the external left ventricular hydraulic work per unit time required for

From the Cardiac Catheterization Laboratory, Hospital of the University of Pennsylvania and the University of Pennsylvania School of Medicine, Philadelphia, and the Cardiovascular Institute, Michael Reese Hospital and Medical Center, Chicago.

Address for correspondence: Warren K. Laskey, M.D., Cardiac Catheterization Laboratory, Hospital of the University of Pennsylvania, 3400 Spruce St., Philadelphia, PA 19104.

Received Dec. 17, 1984; revision accepted April 11, 1985.

steady and pulsatile forward flow. When pulsatile flow is considered, total hydraulic power exceeds mean power,[13] or the energy cost of discharging steady flow through a resistive load. Therefore an analysis of the pulsatile features of aortic pressure and flow provides for a more complete assessment of aortic hydraulic power. Additionally, whereas pulsatile hydraulic power is predominantly dependent on cardiac output, the pulsatile fraction of total hydraulic power is a function of aortic distensibility and aortic characteristic impedance.[14] A change in this fraction on exercise might therefore be the result of a disproportionate change in pulsatile power or vascular load, or both.

Accordingly, we derived external hydraulic power, aortic input impedance, and reflection coefficient spectra at rest and during exercise in eight normal subjects and 11 age-matched patients with heart failure secondary to idiopathic congestive cardiomyopathy. This analysis of impedance in patients with heart failure enabled us to examine changes in vascular load that are independent of ventricular performance and to determine whether distinct abnormalities in aortic stiffness exist in patients with heart failure.

Methods

Patients

Idiopathic congestive cardiomyopathy. Eleven patients (seven men, four women) 24 to 62 years old (mean 41 ± 10) constituted the study group. All 11 patients had clinical signs and symptoms of heart failure (New York Heart Association Class III to IV), and each had a dilated, diffusely hypokinetic left ventricle on M mode and cross-sectional echocardiogram. Patients were referred for diagnostic cardiac catheterization in most instances to rule out concomitant coronary artery disease. Ten of the 11 patients had structurally normal coronary arteries. The remaining subject was a 29-year-old man without anginal symptoms who had severe left ventricular dysfunction out of proportion to the demonstrated coronary atherosclerosis. All patients were in sinus rhythm. The angiographic and/or radionuclide left ventricular ejection fraction in these 11 subjects ranged from 14% to 39% with a mean of 27 ± 8%. No patient had significant mitral regurgitation. All patients were studied on a stable regimen of digitalis and a diuretic, which was continued through the time of study. No patient had significant peripheral edema.

Normal subjects. Eight subjects (seven men, one woman) 22 to 65 years old (mean 41 ± 15) were referred for diagnostic catheterization and angiographic examination because of chest pain syndromes. All had structurally normal coronary arteries, normal cardiac output, and normal angiographic left ventricular ejection fraction (range 56% to 79%, mean 71 ± 8%). No patient was receiving cardioactive medication at the time of study.

Informed consent was obtained in all patients on the day before the procedure.

Study protocol. Before angiographic examination, left ventricular and aortic pressures were measured by manometer-tipped catheters (Millar VPC-684D) inserted via brachial arteriotomy. The aortic pressure transducer was located 5 cm proximal to the tip (ventricular) pressure transducer. Both transducers were placed within the left ventricular cavity and balanced against a simultaneous pulmonary capillary wedge pressure obtained from a fluid-filled balloon flotation catheter in the pulmonary artery. The arterial catheter was then slowly withdrawn until an aortic pressure tracing was obtained from the proximal transducer. An electromagnetic flow probe mounted at the site of the aortic pressure transducer was used to derive instantaneous ascending aortic velocity. The probe was energized by a 500 Hz square wave electromagnetic flowmeter (Carolina Medical Electronics Inc., Model 501) whose frequency response was verified in our laboratory. Velocity signals were recorded at the 100 Hz filter setting (frequency response −3 dB at 100 Hz). At this setting, the phase lag was linear with frequency (2.5 msec at 100 Hz). The frequency responses of the pressure and velocity recording channels were flat from 0 to greater than 100 Hz. Cardiac output, obtained by thermodilution technique, was measured in triplicate along with aortic and pulmonary arterial blood oxygen saturation. The thermodilution cardiac output correlated well with direct Fick determinations in seven subjects ($r = .95$, $p < .001$).

All patients were studied in the resting supine state. Approximately 20 min after instrumentation, each subject's legs were passively elevated on a table-mounted bicycle ergometer (Quinton) and repeat measurements were obtained. This condition served as a control for all exercise measurements. After completion of the resting hemodynamic determinations, all subjects were exercised for 3 to 5 min at an external workload of 300 kg-m/min. Unchanging values of pulmonary arterial blood oxygen saturation 1 min apart confirmed a steady state, and at this point pressure and flow measurements were again obtained.

All subjects tolerated the exercise period well and there were no complications related to the procedure. After completion of the protocol all subjects underwent diagnostic coronary angiographic and left ventriculographic examinations.

Data analysis. Pressure and velocity signals were amplified and recorded on a Honeywell Meddars system. In addition, pressure and velocity signals were recorded continuously on FM magnetic tape at 3.75 ips. Pressure and velocity signals were taken directly from tape, low-pass filtered with corner frequency at 50 Hz (24 dB per octave), and automatically digitized at 250 Hz with a 12 bit analog-to-digital converter interfaced to a microcomputer. The velocity signal was scaled to volumetric flow by setting the integrated area beneath the velocity signal equal to the simultaneously determined cardiac output. This maneuver assumes that the ascending aortic velocity profile is flat and that there is little change in the aortic cross-sectional area over the cardiac cycle.

Ten to 30 beats were stored and subjected to analysis as follows: Only those beats with optimal velocity configuration (minimal early diastolic dip and a flat, late diastolic segment) were chosen for analysis. No postectopic beats were included and only beats with RR intervals within 5% of the mean value were analyzed. Beats were superimposed to verify similarity (figure 1, *A*). The computer-stored and signal-averaged pressure and velocity signals (figure 1, *B*) were then subjected to Fourier analysis. Computations were carried out, where possible, to the tenth harmonic. Pressure moduli less than 0.5 mm Hg and flow moduli less than 5 ml/sec were rejected from subsequent analysis since these values are within the noise level of our measuring system. The respective pressure (P_n) and flow (Q_n) moduli for each harmonic obtained from the Fourier series were used to derive the impedance modulus (Z_n) as P_n/Q_n while impedance phase (ϕ_n) is the difference of pressure and flow phase. The aortic input impedance spectrum was displayed as a plot of impedance modulus and phase vs frequency. The 0 Hz, or DC, term of the impedance spectrum corresponds to the

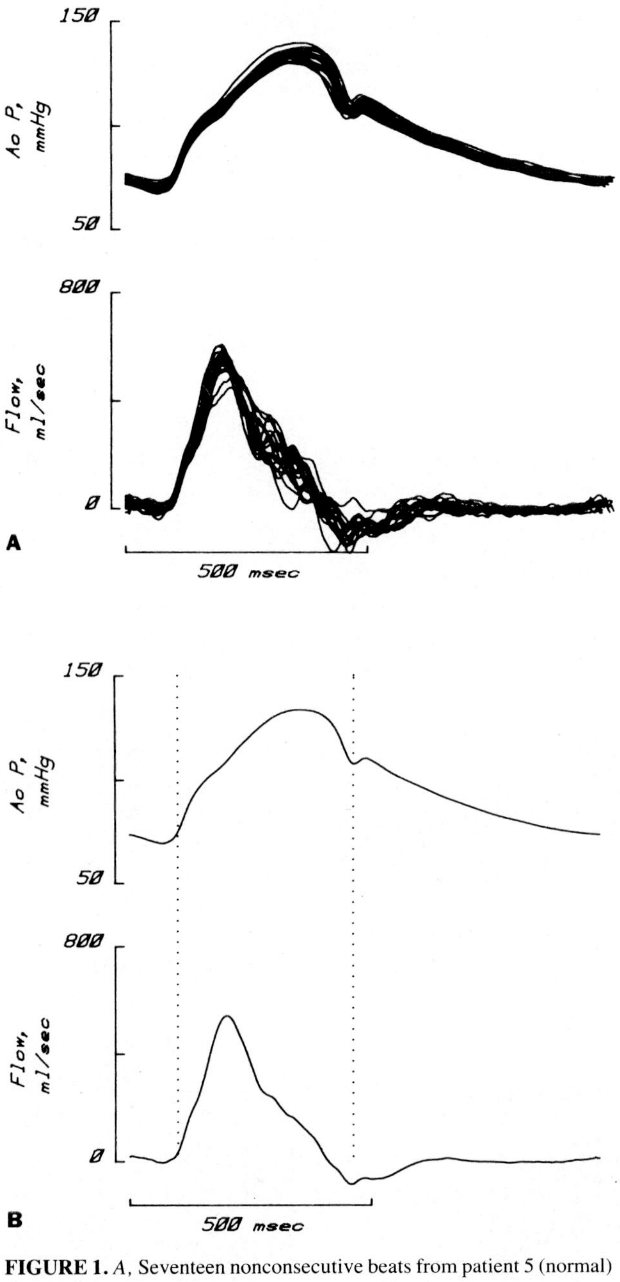

FIGURE 1. *A*, Seventeen nonconsecutive beats from patient 5 (normal) are shown superimposed to examine the beat-to-beat variability in pressure (top) and flow (bottom) signals. *B*, Computer-processed, signal-averaged composite pressure (top) and flow (bottom) wave derived from 17 beats shown in *A*. AoP = aortic pressure.

systemic vascular resistance. Characteristic impedance (Z_c) was taken as the average of impedance moduli from 4 to 12 Hz.

The modulus of the reflection coefficient was taken as RC = $(Z_n - Z_c)/(Z_n + Z_c)$, as described by Westerhof et al.[12] Reflection coefficient moduli were then plotted against frequency to describe the reflection coefficient spectrum.

Total aortic input pressure power (P_t) was computed as the summed product of instantaneous aortic pressure and flow over the cardiac cycle. Steady, or mean, aortic input pressure power (P_m) is the product of mean aortic pressure and cardiac output. The difference, $P_t - P_m$, represents the oscillatory (P_o), or pulsatile, component of power. Oscillatory power was also computed from impedance and flow moduli derived from Fourier analysis.[13] There was an excellent correlation between these two independent methods of computation (figure 2). The kinetic energy term is quantitatively a small component of total input power and therefore we deleted these computations from our analysis.

Statistics. All reported data are presented as mean ± SD. A paired t test was used to assess changes within individuals, and an unpaired t test was used in group comparisons. A p value less than .05 was considered statistically significant.

Results

Hemodynamic performance at rest and on exercise. Table 1 outlines individual hemodynamic determinations. In subjects with cardiomyopathy, mean aortic pressure was lower than normal. As expected, cardiac output was depressed whereas systemic vascular resistance and left ventricular end-diastolic pressure were elevated in patients with heart failure. The transition from rest to exercise in both normal subjects and patients with cardiomyopathy was marked by significant increases in heart rate and cardiac index, whereas systemic vascular resistance declined. However, cardiac index on exercise remained subnormal and systemic resistance remained elevated in patients with cardiomyopathy. Mean aortic pressure increased modestly in both groups, and left ventricular end-diastolic pressure did not change significantly during exercise in either group. Left ventricular stroke volume index increased significantly during exercise in normal subjects but did not change in the patients with cardiomyopathy.

Hydraulic load at rest and during exercise. Figures 3 and 4 depict input impedance spectra for each subject. There was considerable heterogeneity within each group in the appearance of the impedance spectrum. Group mean resting characteristic impedance in pa-

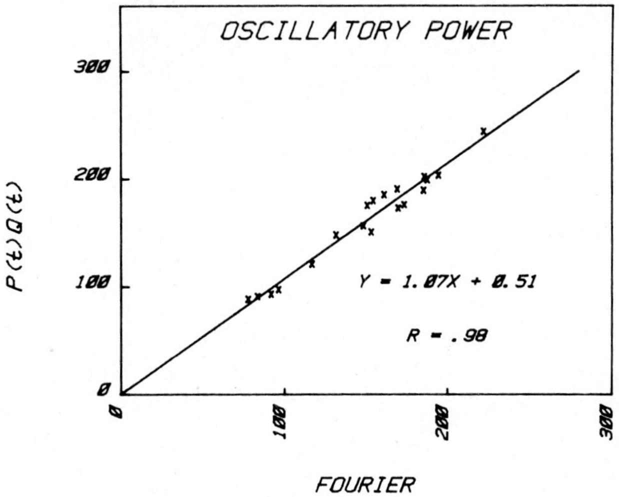

FIGURE 2. Oscillatory power derived from harmonic analysis of pressure and flow (Fourier) agree closely with the power computed from instantaneous aortic pressure and flow data ($P \times Q$).

TABLE 1
Hemodynamic performance at rest and during exercise

Patient	Age (yr)	HR (bpm) R	HR (bpm) E	AoP (mm Hg) R	AoP (mm Hg) E	LVEDP (mm Hg) R	LVEDP (mm Hg) E	CI (l/min/m²) R	CI (l/min/m²) E	SVI (ml/m²) R	SVI (ml/m²) E
Normal											
1	54	59	80	107	113	12	14	2.7	4.9	46	61
2	26	86	116	100	120	9	6	3.8	6.1	44	52
3	57	82	116	109	129	12	14	3.4	7.2	41	62
4	28	82	101	112	108	14	13	4.5	8.2	55	81
5	65	61	111	105	111	22	23	2.5	5.2	41	47
6	42	75	100	90	110	6	9	2.9	6.5	39	65
7	22	70	121	97	128	15	29	3.5	6.7	50	55
8	40	56	99	106	116	11	18	3.0	5.6	53	56
Mean	41	71	105^A	103	117^A	13	16	3.3	6.3^A	46	60
±SD	±15	±11	±13	±7	±8	±4	±7	±0.5	±1.1	±4	±10
Cardiomyopathy											
1	44	62	127	84	92	25	37	2.7	4.9	43	38
2	62	95	119	96	111	30	34	2.8	4.0	29	33
3	56	94	122	104	119	19	34	2.2	2.7	23	22
4	24	108	140	97	95	24	20	3.0	5.1	28	36
5	46	72	112	93	92	32	24	2.8	4.5	39	40
6	29	96	123	94	97	27	30	2.6	2.8	27	23
7	37	76	94	95	103	24	26	2.0	3.3	26	35
8	42	63	85	79	87	30	31	2.2	2.5	35	29
9	38	80	96	79	91	16	25	2.1	2.8	26	29
10	42	77	97	99	98	32	34	2.8	4.3	36	44
11	36	103	134	97	113	34	36	3.7	4.5	36	33
Mean	41	84	113^A	92^B	100^A,B	27^B	30^B	2.6^B	3.8^A,B	32^B	33^B
±SD	±10	±15	±17	±8	±10	±5	±5	±0.6	±0.8	±8	±9

AoP = mean aortic pressure; CI = thermodilution cardiac index; E = exercise; HR = heart rate; LVEDP = left ventricular end-diastolic pressure; R = rest; SVI = stroke volume index.

Statistical comparisons: $^{A}p < .005$ (R vs E); $^{B}p < .01$ (normal vs cardiomyopathy).

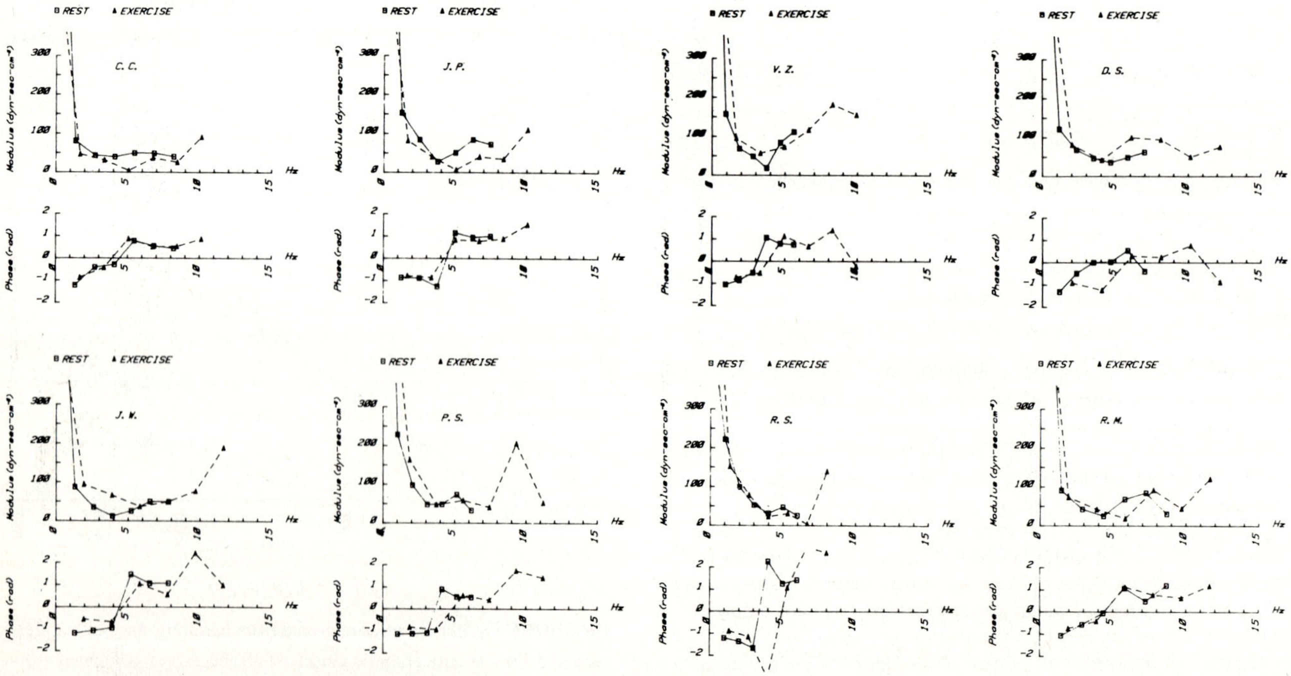

FIGURE 3. Aortic input impedance spectra in the eight normal subjects at rest (squares) and during exercise (triangles).

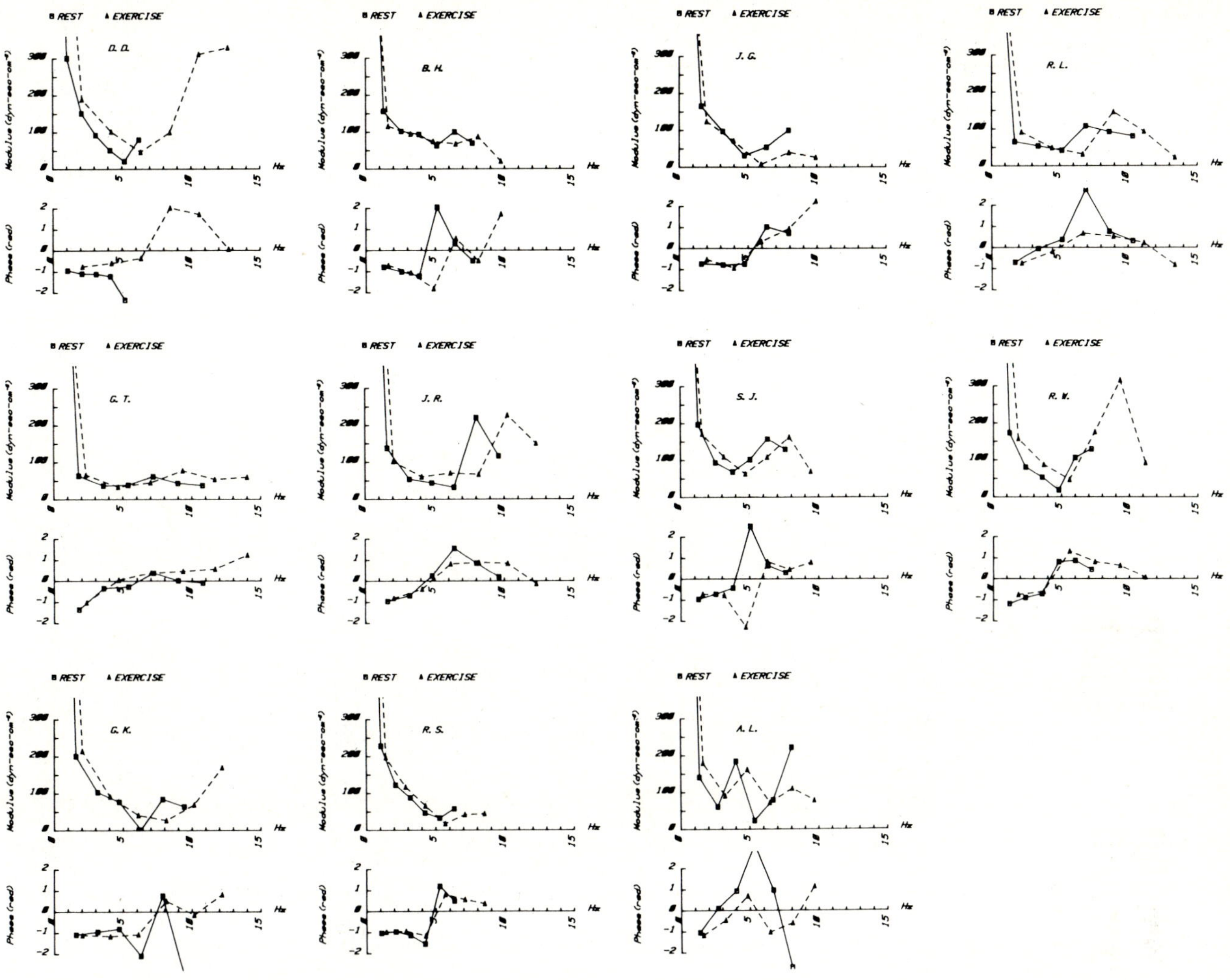

FIGURE 4. Aortic input impedance spectra at rest (squares), and during exercise (triangles) in the 11 subjects with heart failure.

tients with cardiomyopathy was not significantly different from normal (table 2). In addition, the interpolated first zero crossing of impedance phase (ϕ_0) was similar for both groups. The transition from rest to exercise was marked by the tendency for moduli and phase spectra in both groups to move to the right. Thus, ϕ_0 moved to higher frequencies as did the first minimum of the impedance spectrum. As previously noted, the DC component of input impedance, systemic vascular resistance, declined during exercise in both groups. Characteristic impedance, however, remained unchanged on exercise in both groups. The phase of the first harmonic of impedance consistently, and significantly, became less negative during exercise in both groups. The modulus of the first harmonic of the reflection coefficient declined significantly during exercise in normal subjects but not in patients with heart failure. Analysis of the individual reflection coefficient spectra at higher frequencies revealed no predictable change during exercise in either group. Figure 5 summarizes the changes in the moduli of the first and second harmonics of impedance and the reflection coefficient. The first harmonic of impedance significantly decreased during exercise in normal subjects. The response in the patients with heart failure did not reach statistical significance ($p = .09$), although a qualitative similarity to the response of normal subjects was seen. Of note, however, is the observation that impedance moduli during exercise in patients with heart failure were significantly higher than normal exercise levels. Furthermore, the first harmonic of the reflection coefficient significantly decreased during exercise in normal subjects but not in patients with heart failure, in spite of the drop in systemic resistance.

Hydraulic input power at rest and during exercise. As detailed in table 3, resting steady and oscillatory pressure power at the aortic root were significantly diminished in patients with cardiomyopathy. All subjects were able to augment both components of pressure power significantly during exercise, although at exer-

TABLE 2
Characteristics of hydraulic vascular load

Patient	Z_o (dyne-sec-cm^{-5}) R	Z_o E	Z_c (dyne-sec-cm^{-5}) R	Z_c E	ϕo (Hz) R	ϕo E	RC R	RC E	ϕ1 (radians) R	ϕ1 E
Normal										
1	1462	853	127	90	3.4	4.9	0.73	0.53	−1.21	−0.88
2	1032	584	69	68	4.4	4.4	0.60	0.39	−1.06	−0.74
3	1128	842	64	88	4.6	4.6	0.67	0.29	−1.15	−0.56
4	1062	553	52	53	4.4	3.9	0.71	0.46	−1.21	−0.86
5	1392	648	94	89	3.6	4.8	0.73	0.51	−1.14	−0.81
6	1059	682	105	52	4.4	4.2	0.49	0.46	−0.86	−0.77
7	1491	947	51	71	4.0	5.7	0.82	0.49	−1.31	−0.91
8	1389	816	121	131	3.1	3.8	0.58	0.41	−1.04	−0.72
Mean	1251	740^{A}	85	80	4.0	4.6	0.67	0.45^{A}	−1.12	−0.78^{A}
±SD	±198	±142	±30	±25	±0.5	±0.6	±0.1	±0.08	±0.14	±0.11
Cardiomyopathy										
1	1233	803	133	82	5.6	6.7	0.63	0.55	−0.94	−0.75
2	1622	1160	61	39	5.4	5.4	0.58	0.57	−0.73	−0.52
3	2092	1304	80	57	7.4	7.5	0.71	0.79	−1.08	−1.10
4	1700	1532	47	52	6.1	4.6	0.80	0.57	−1.35	−1.02
5	1319	912	89	157	4.2	4.3	0.72	0.39	−1.18	−0.75
6	2132	1822	126	106	4.3	4.7	0.52	0.42	−0.96	−0.81
7	1676	1098	139	111	3.9	5.8	0.54	0.42	−0.96	−0.71
8	1717	1659	55	59	4.8	5.1	0.78	0.72	−0.95	−0.98
9	1946	1661	126	114	2.5	3.8	0.57	0.69	−1.04	−1.16
10	1634	1019	81	75	4.3	6.1	0.51	0.42	−0.79	−0.70
11	961	716	80	79	3.6	4.9	0.38	0.39	−0.70	−0.73
Mean	1639^{B}	1244^{A,B}	93	85	4.7	5.4	0.62	0.54	−0.98	−0.84^{A}
±SD	±357	±378	±33	±34	±1.3	±1.1	±0.13	±0.14	±0.19	±0.20

RC = modulus of first harmonic of reflection coefficient; Z_c = characteristic impedance; Z_o = systemic vascular resistance; ϕo = first zero crossing of impedance phase; ϕ1 = phase of first harmonic of impedance. Other abbreviations and annotations as in table 1.

cise levels each component was again subnormal in patients with cardiomyopathy. The ratio P_o/P_t remained unchanged during exercise in both groups and did not differ between groups. The significant increase in power in the patients with cardiomyopathy is of interest in light of the attenuated stroke volume response to exercise.

Discussion

These findings indicate that there are substantial qualitative and quantitative similarities to normal behavior in the response of hydraulic load in patients with heart failure to submaximal supine exercise. However, not unexpectedly, significant differences also exist. Before consideration of these similarities and differences, a discussion of the technical limitations of this study is in order.

The use of catheter-mounted electromagnetic flow probes has been of great value in the study of the dynamic behavior of the circulation.[15-20] The advantage of a design facilitating placement of the catheter tip within the ventricular cavity, thereby providing a stabilizing effect, has allowed for use of these catheters in a wide variety of physiologic studies. Translation of the velocity of flow in the ascending aorta into volume flow is feasible if the velocity profile in the region studied is flat and if there is little change in aortic cross-sectional area over the cardiac cycle. Although neither of these assumptions has been rigorously evaluated in intact man, particularly during exercise, studies have shown that the velocity profile at rest in the ascending aorta is virtually flat.[21-24] Although small changes in aortic cross-sectional area do exist over the cardiac cycle,[25-27] these small displacements (±1% to 3%) should not preclude use of flow volume data obtained from velocity signals.

The quality of the velocity signal itself is a function of the probe and magnet size, the type of flowmeter, and the characteristics of the recording and amplification system. The velocity recordings in this study exhibit strong similarities to those illustrated in other reports.[15,16] Nevertheless, the signal-to-noise ratio is

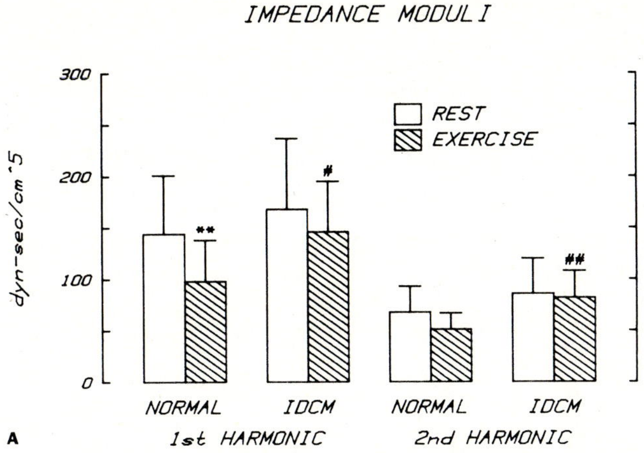

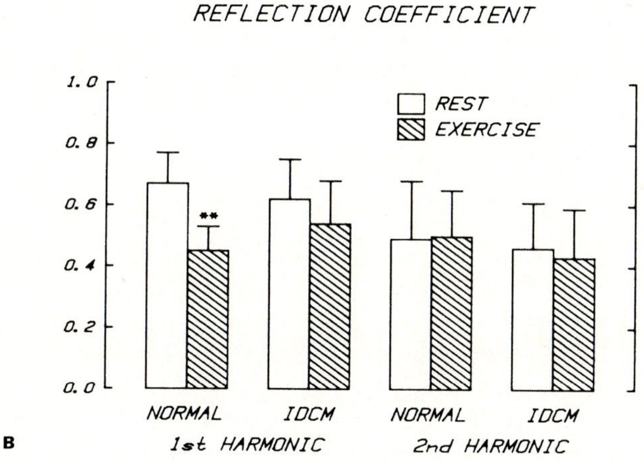

FIGURE 5. *A*, Moduli of the first two harmonics of aortic impedance at rest and during exercise. The first harmonic decreased significantly during exercise (**, $p < .01$) in normal subjects but not in patients with cardiomyopathy (IDCM). Additionally, the harmonics on exercise in cardiomyopathy are significantly elevated in comparison to normal (#, $p < .05$; ##, $p < .01$). *B*, Moduli of the first two harmonics of the reflection coefficient at rest and during exercise. In normal subjects only, the first harmonic significantly declined during exercise (**, $p < .01$). However, there is no difference in moduli between groups.

frequently lower than optimal. We therefore applied signal averaging techniques in our data analysis to optimize the information content of the velocity trace. Noise decreases as a root function of the number of analyzed beats, and therefore we processed multiple beats before entering the averaged velocity signal into the Fourier routine. In addition, we rejected flow moduli less than 5 ml/sec. The derived aortic input impedance moduli and phase spectra are qualitatively similar to those obtained in previous studies in man.[28, 29] In many patients, however, the descending portion of the impedance spectrum extended beyond 2 Hz and, for that reason, we chose to define characteristic impedance as the average of all moduli between 4 and 12 Hz. However, there would have been no significant difference in characteristic impedance if averaging had begun at 2 Hz (normal subjects at rest: 79 dyne-sec-cm^{-5}; patients with cardiomyopathy at rest: 92 dyne-sec-cm^{-5}). The limitation of the Fourier routine confines one to integral multiples of the fundamental frequency, and therefore the number of points available for averaging is less than ideal. Nevertheless, applying this method to both groups at rest and during exercise, we found no significant difference in characteristic impedance between normal subjects and those with heart failure secondary to cardiomyopathy. If characteristic impedance had been computed over the relatively flat frequency range from 4 to 8 Hz, again there would have been no significant difference between normal subjects at rest (70 ± 27 dyne-sec-cm^{-5}) and patients with heart failure at rest (86 ± 29 dyne-sec-cm^{-5}). Furthermore, there was no significant change during exercise when Z_c was computed in this manner. However, input resistance, or systemic vascular resistance, was elevated in patients with cardiomyopathy both at rest and during exercise.

Characteristic impedance of a vessel varies directly with the elastic modulus but inversely with the cross-sectional area of that vessel. It is well known that as a vessel is distended, its elastic modulus increases.[30, 31] The mean aortic pressure in the patients with heart failure was slightly, although significantly, lower than that in the normal subjects. Therefore one might wonder whether aortic characteristic impedance would be higher in patients with heart failure if their mean aortic pressure were identical to that of the normal subjects. However, several lines of evidence do not support this possibility. In a recent study of aortic impedance in subjects with cardiomyopathy, no significant difference in characteristic impedance was found in age- and mean aortic pressure–matched subjects.[11] Second, no significant relationship between aortic distending pressure and characteristic impedance was found in a previous study.[32] Similarily, we found no significant relationship between mean aortic pressure and characteristic impedance ($r = -.03$) in our study population, although the range of aortic pressures was rather narrow. Third, the velocity of wave propagation should reflect the material elastic properties of the aorta.[33] Although we did not directly measure the pulse wave velocity in this study, an indirect measure of wave velocity, the first zero crossing of impedance phase[34] was not significantly different between groups either in this study or in a previous study.[11] Moreover, phase velocity is only slightly dependent on distending pressure over the physiologic range of mean aortic pressure.[35–37] Finally, it might be questioned whether

TABLE 3
Hydraulic input power

	P_o (mW)		P_s (mW)		P_t (mW)		P_o/P_t	
Patient	R	E	R	E	R	E	R	E
Normal								
1	154	474	1190	2427	1344	2902	0.11	0.16
2	194	434	1802	3581	1996	4015	0.09	0.10
3	161	730	1667	4397	1829	5128	0.08	0.14
4	185	418	1964	3519	2150	3938	0.08	0.10
5	169	538	962	3022	1131	3561	0.15	0.15
6	173	486	1293	3072	1467	3558	0.11	0.13
7	150	275	1292	2772	1443	3048	0.10	0.09
8	187	383	1384	2847	1571	3231	0.11	0.11
Mean	172	467^A	1444	3205^A	1616	3673^A	0.11	0.13
±SD	±16	±132	±336	±613	±346	±708	±0.02	±0.03
Cardiomyopathy								
1	221	394	860	1865	1082	2259	0.26	0.17
2	185	457	1054	1335	1239	1793	0.15	0.25
3	83	102	583	799	667	902	0.12	0.11
4	96	278	1006	2019	1103	2297	0.08	0.12
5	131	333	912	1865	1043	2199	0.12	0.15
6	91	122	928	981	1020	1103	0.09	0.11
7	148	326	877	1642	1025	1969	0.14	0.16
8	114	123	632	839	746	962	0.15	0.13
9	77	79	343	734	421	813	0.18	0.09
10	153	220	990	1555	1143	1775	0.13	0.12
11	169	290	1303	1312	1473	1603	0.11	0.18
Mean	133^B	248^{A,B}	863^B	1359^{A,B}	996^B	1607^{A,B}	0.14	0.15
±SD	±46	±127	±259	±467	±288	±569	±0.04	±0.05

P_o = oscillatory pressure power; P_s = steady pressure power; P_t = total pressure power. Other abbreviations and annotations as in table 1.

differences in aortic root dimension might play a factor in the equality of characteristic impedance in our patient groups. The slightly lower distending pressure in the patients with heart failure might be compensated for by a smaller aortic root dimension, and thus impedance would appear normal. However, there was no significant difference in aortic root dimension, as measured from the opacified proximal aorta during angiographic examination (normal, 2.5 ± 0.3 cm; heart failure, 2.6 ± 0.4 cm).

The finding of similar characteristic impedance in our two patient groups differs from the findings of a previous study in which Z_c was elevated in patients with heart failure.[10] Although the normal mean characteristic impedance in that study was similar to our normal control group, mean Z_c in their patients with heart failure was significantly elevated at 131 ± 27 dyne-sec-cm^{-5}. In a more recent report, mean aortic characteristic impedance in subjects with heart failure and cardiomyopathy was quite similar to our mean data.[38] Unfortunately, normal control values for Z_c were not included in the latter study. Differences in the definition of characteristic impedance as well as differences in recording systems and data analysis (noise rejection criteria, etc.) may account for this discrepancy in reported values of Z_c in patients with heart failure. In a preliminary report from our group, we noted significant elevations in Z_c in comparison with that in normal control subjects,[39] although the patient population under study was more heterogeneous clinically than our group. We studied only patients with congestive cardiomyopathy and no history of hypertension or coronary artery disease. Furthermore, in our prior report the average age of the patients with heart failure was higher than that of the normal control group (50 vs 32 years, respectively). It has recently been shown that Z_c rises with increasing age,[40] and therefore we sought to control for age. Whether these differences completely account for the discrepancy with past studies is unclear. Nevertheless, the consistency of the data on exercise determinations tends to support the validity of our findings.

It has been previously reported that aortic characteristic impedance in normal subjects does not change during exercise.[41] However, no comparable data are available in patients with heart failure. In the present study, aortic characteristic impedance did not change during exercise in either group, although the spectra tended to move to the right (i.e., the first minimum of impedance modulus and ϕ_o tended toward higher frequency during exercise). This shift in ϕ_o suggests an increase in pulse wave velocity, which is a function of vessel elastic modulus.[42] The rise in aortic pressure was modest in both groups and is probably not sufficient to strongly alter characteristic impedance. It is also possible that slight increases in aortic cross-sectional area on exercise might tend to offset any change in aortic distending pressure, and thus characteristic impedance would remain at resting levels.[41]

Our findings indicate that no important change in aortic distensibility occurs in patients with heart failure, either at rest or during exercise. Because characteristic impedance reflects the material properties of the aortic wall, it is difficult to posit an a priori basis for a difference in elastic modulus or arterial distensibility in patients with heart failure secondary to cardiomyopathy. In a previous report it was noted that patients with coronary atherosclerosis and arterial hypertension had elevated characteristic impedances.[29] None of our patients had a history or clinical evidence of chronic systemic hypertension. Thus, whether elevation of Z_c in arterial hypertension reflects the presence of coexistent atherosclerotic aortic disease is open to question. All but one of our subjects were free of coronary atherosclerosis; thus it is unlikely that significant aortic atherosclerotic disease was present. In addition, the similarity of the pulsatile fraction of hydraulic power between groups would also suggest the absence of important differences in aortic distensibility.[14] Definitive conclusions as to the presence or importance of structural changes in the aortic wall in patients with heart failure must await histologic verification.

An anatomic basis for elevations in Z_c in patients with heart failure has been suggested.[10] The possibility of increased arterial wall sodium content with a secondary decrease in distensibility raises the intriguing possibility of altering arterial elastic properties in patients with heart failure with diuretic therapy. All of our patients with heart failure were studied after appropriate medical therapy and were in a clinically stable condition at the time of catheterization. All patients were free of peripheral edema as well. Whether different conclusions might have been reached had these patients been studied in an untreated state is open to question. Ethical considerations precluded us from studying patients before medical stabilization of their heart failure. Serial measures of impedance are technically and logistically difficult but may provide important data on the role of the salt-retention state in contributing to an elevated characteristic impedance.[43]

The transition from rest to exercise in both groups is marked by systemic vasodilation with a decrease in systemic vascular resistance. Vasodilation results in a decrease in low-frequency impedance phase, indicating a more in-phase relationship between pressure and flow. The low-frequency moduli of impedance decreased significantly on exercise in normal subjects, although the changes in the patients with heart failure, while qualitatively similar to those in normal subjects, failed to reach statistical significance. Moreover, low-frequency impedance moduli in patients with heart failure, while not significantly different from those of normal subjects at rest, were elevated in comparison with normal values during exercise. Vasodilation occurring at the termination of the arterial bed should also result in a decrease in the magnitude of wave reflection.[12, 34] However, a significant decrease on exercise in the modulus of the first harmonic of the reflection coefficient was observed only in the normal group. Reflection coefficient spectra at higher frequencies were less predictable and probably of little physiologic importance, since significant wave damping occurs at these higher frequencies. Thus, in spite of a decrease in input resistance, low-frequency impedance and reflection moduli in patients with heart failure fail to change with exercise as they do in normal subjects.

Instantaneous aortic pressure and flow are the determinants of aortic input power. A normal aortic characteristic impedance, in the absence of marked bradycardia or systemic vasodilation, suggests that the pulsatile fraction of total input power is also normal.[14] P_o/P_t, at rest and during exercise, was similar in both groups and was consistent with this lack of abnormal aortic distensibility in patients with heart failure. Total input power rises significantly on exercise in both groups, although total power remains below normal in patients with cardiomyopathy. The increase in power in the absence of significant changes in stroke volume in patients with cardiomyopathy reflects the fact that the cardiac output rises as a consequence of increased heart rate. Although oscillatory power should decline with an increased heart rate at constant flow,[13, 44] we observed that oscillatory power, but not P_o/P_t, increased on exercise. Since the first two harmonics of aortic power account for greater than 90% of the total power, an analysis of the harmonic components of impedance and flow yields some important distinctions in the development of hydraulic power in patients with heart failure. The increased flow allows for an increase in power in both groups. However, the higher moduli during exercise of the first and second harmonics of impedance in the patients with cardiomyopathy result in an increase in dissipated power because of elevations in both impedance and flow moduli (power $\alpha\ Q^2 Z\cos\phi$), whereas in normal subjects the dissipated power is the result of larger increases in flow at lower impedance moduli.

In summary, the steady component of vascular hydraulic load in patients with heart failure is greater than normal, although the pulsatile component of the load, or characteristic impedance, is similar to normal. The changes in vascular load on exercise in patients with heart failure are qualitatively similar to normal, although input resistance and low-frequency impedance moduli are significantly elevated. Characteristic impedance does not change during exercise. Consistent with an unchanging characteristic impedance during exercise, the oscillatory fraction of aortic input power is constant in spite of significant increases in both mean and pulsatile components of flow. Mild exercise in patients with heart failure appears to impose no additional increase in vascular hydraulic load on the ejecting left ventricle.

We are deeply indebted to Dr. Michael Simson for his time and efforts related to this project. We are also grateful to the technical staff of the cardiac catheterization laboratory without whom it would not have been possible to perform these studies. Finally, the expert secretarial assistance of Mrs. Nedra Ellis is greatly appreciated.

References

1. Ross J Jr: Afterload mismatch and preload reserve: a conceptual framework for the analysis of ventricular function. Prog Cardiovasc Dis **182:** 255, 1976
2. Milnor WR: Arterial impedance as ventricular afterload. Circ Res **36:** 565, 1975
3. Nichols WW, Pepine CJ, Geiser EA, Conti CR: Vascular load defined by the aortic input impedance spectrum. Fed Proc **39:** 196, 1980
4. Westerhof N, Elzinga G, Sipkema P, vanden Bos GC: Quantitative analysis of the arterial system and heart by means of pressure-flow relations. *In* Hwang NHC, Norman NA, editors: Cardiovascular flow dynamics and measurements. Baltimore, 1977, University Park Press, pp 403–438
5. Mason DT, Spann JF Jr, Zelis R, Amsterdam EA: Alterations of hemodynamics and myocardial mechanics in patients with congestive heart failure. Prog Cardiovasc Dis **12:** 507, 1970
6. Guyton AC, Jones CE, Coleman TG: Circulatory physiology: cardiac output and its regulation. Philadelphia, 1973, W. B. Saunders Co.
7. Epstein SE, Beiser GD, Stampfer M, Robinson BF, Braunwald E: Characterization of the circulatory response to maximal upright exercise in normal subjects and patients with heart failure. Circulation **35:** 1049, 1967
8. Kramer B, Massie B, Topic N: Hemodynamic differences between supine and upright exercise in patients with congestive heart failure. Circulation **66:** 820, 1982
9. Litchfield RL, Kerber RE, Benge JW, Mark AL, Sopko J, Bhatnagar RK, Marcus ML: Normal exercise capacity in patients with severe left ventricular dysfunction: compensatory mechanisms. Circulation **66:** 129, 1982
10. Pepine CJ, Nicholas WW, Conti CR: Aortic input impedance in heart failure. Circulation **58:** 460, 1978
11. Merillon JP, Fontenier G, Lerallut JF, Jaffrin HY, Chastre J, Assayag P, Motte G, Gourgon R: Aortic input impedance in heart failure: comparison with normal subjects and its changes during vasodilator therapy. Eur Heart J **5:** 447, 1984
12. Westerhof N, Sipkema P, vanden Bos GC, Elzinga G: Forward and backward waves in the arterial system. Cardiovasc Res **6:** 648, 1972
13. Milnor WR, Bergel DH, Bargainer JD: Hydraulic power associated with pulmonary blood flow and its relation to heart rate. Circ Res **19:** 467, 1966
14. O'Rourke MF: Steady and pulsatile energy losses in the systemic circulation under normal conditions and in simulated arterial disease. Cardiovasc Res **1:** 313, 1967
15. Murgo JP, Altobelli SA, Dorethy JF, Logsdon JR, McGranahan GM: Normal ventricular ejection dynamics in man during rest and exercise. AHA Monograph No. **46:** 92–101, 1975
16. Nichols WW, Pepine CJ, Conti CR, Christie LG, Feldman RL: Evaluation of a new catheter-mounted electromagnetic velocity sensor during cardiac catheterization. Cath Cardiovasc Diag **6:** 97, 1980
17. Mason DT, Gabe IT, Gault JH, Ross J Jr, Braunwald E, Shillingford JP: Applications of the catheter-tip electromagnetic velocity probe in the study of the central circulation in man. Am J Med **49:** 465, 1970
18. Gabe IT, Gault JM, Ross J Jr, Mason DT, Mills CJ, Shillingford JP, Braunwald E: Measurement of instantanteous blood flow velocity and pressure in conscious man with a catheter-tip velocity probe. Circulation **40:** 603, 1969
19. Bond RF, Barefoot CA: Evaluation of an electromagnetic catheter tip velocity-sentitive blood flow probe. J Appl Physiol **23:** 403, 1967
20. Mills CJ, Shillingford JP: A catheter-tip electromagnetic velocity probe and its evaluation. Cardiovasc Res **1:** 263, 1967
21. Atabek HB, Chang CC, Fingerson LM: Measurement of laminar oscillatory flow in the inlet length of a circular tube. Phys Med Biol **9:** 219, 1964
22. Freis ED, Heath WC: Hydrodynamics of aortic blood flow. Circ Res **14:** 105, 1964
23. Schultz DL, Tunstall-Pedhoe DS, Lee G, De J Gunning AJ, Bellhouse BJ: Velocity distribution and transition in the arterial system. *In* Circulatory and respiratory mass transport. Ciba Foundation Symposium, Boston, 1969, Little, Brown Co., pp 172–202
24. Seed WA, Wood NB: Velocity patterns in the aorta. Cardiovasc Res **5:** 319, 1971
25. Greenfield JC Jr, Patel DJ: Relation between pressure and diameter in the ascending aorta of man. Circ Res **10:** 778, 1962
26. Patel DJ, Defreitas F, Greenfield JC Jr, Fry DL: Relationship of radius to pressure along the aorta in living dogs. J Appl Physiol **18:** 111, 1963
27. Patel DJ, Greenfield JC Jr, Austen WG, Morrow AG, Fry DL: Pressure-flow relationships in the ascending aorta and femoral artery of man. J Appl Physiol **20:** 459, 1965
28. Murgo JP, Westerhof N, Giolma JP, Altobelli SA: Aortic input impedance in normal man: relationship to pressure wave forms. Circulation **62:** 105, 1980
29. Nichols WW, Conti CR, Walker WE, Milnor WR: Input impedance of the systemic circulation in man. Circ Res **40:** 451, 1977
30. Patel DJ, Janicki JS, Carew TE: Static anisotropic elastic properties of the aorta in living dogs. Circ Res **25:** 765, 1969
31. Bergel DH: Dynamic elastic properties of the arterial wall. J Physiol **156:** 458, 1961
32. Gundel W, Cherry G, Rajagopalan B, Tan L, Lee G, Schultz D: Aortic input impedance in man: acute response to vasodilator drugs. Circulation **63:** 1305, 1981
33. McDonald DA: Blood flow in arteries. London, 1974, Arnold, p 254
34. O'Rourke MF, Taylor MG: Input impedance of the systemic circulation. Circ Res **20:** 365, 1967
35. Dow P, Hamilton WF: An experimental study of the velocity of the

pulse wave propagated through the aorta. Am J Physiol **125:** 60, 1939
36. Patel DJ, Fry DL: In-situ pressure-radius-length measurements in ascending aorta of anesthetized dogs. J Appl Physiol **19:** 413, 1963
37. Cox RH, Pace JB: Pressure-flow relations in the vessels of the canine aortic arch. Am J Physiol **228:** 1, 1975
38. Yin FCP, Guzman PA, Brin KP, Maughan WL, Brinker JA, Traill TA, Weiss JL, Weisfeldt ML: Effect of nitroprusside on hydraulic vascular loads on the right and left ventricle of patients with heart failure. Circulation **67:** 1330, 1983
39. Laskey WK, Shroff SG, Kleaveland JP, Martin JL, Kussmaul WG, Hirshfeld JW, Weber KT: Arterial load at rest and exercise in chronic cardiac failure. Circulation **68**(suppl III): III-131, 1983 (abst)
40. Nichols W, Murgo J, O'Rourke M, Avolio A, Yaginuma T: Effect of age on aortic input impedance in normal man. Circulation **68**(suppl III): III-111, 1983 (abst)
41. Murgo JP, Westerhof N, Giolma JP, Altobelli SA: Effects of exercise on aortic input impedance and pressure wave forms in normal humans. Circ Res **48:** 334, 1981
42. Bramwell JC, Hill AV: The velocity of the pulse wave in man. Proc R Soc Biol **93:** 298, 1922
43. Avolio AP, Fa-Quan O, Wei-Keng L, Yao-Fei L, Zhen-Dong H, Lian-Fen X, O'Rourke MF: Effects of aging on arterial distensibility in populations with high and low prevalenace of hypertension: comparison between urban and rural communities in China. Circulation **71:** 202, 1985
44. Cox RH: Determinants of systemic hydraulic power in unanesthetized dogs. Am J Physiol **226:** 579, 1979

Effect of the sympathetic nervous system on limb circulation and metabolism during exercise in patients with heart failure

JOHN R. WILSON, M.D., NANCY FERRARO, R.N., AND DAVID H. WIENER, M.D.

ABSTRACT During exercise in patients with heart failure, activation of sympathetic vasoconstrictor nerves may impair vasodilation in active skeletal muscle and thereby interfere with skeletal muscle blood flow. To investigate this hypothesis, we examined the effect of acute α-adrenergic blockade with systemic administration of prazosin (10 patients) or regional administration of phentolamine (eight patients) on blood flow, vascular resistance, oxygen consumption ($\dot{V}O_2$), and lactate release in the leg during maximal bicycle exercise in patients with heart failure. During control exercise, systemic $\dot{V}O_2$ increased to 12.6 ± 4.3 ml/min/kg (normal > 20 to 25 ml/min/kg), leg blood flow to 2.8 ± 1.8 liters/min, and leg lactate release to 362 ± 256 mg/min. Prazosin decreased systemic vascular resistance (12.5 ± 3.2 to 9.7 ± 2.5 units; $p < .003$) and mean arterial pressure (101 ± 20 to 87 ± 22 mm Hg; $p < .002$) at maximal exercise, supporting the presence of substantial sympathetic vasoconstrictor nerve activity. Prazosin also decreased leg resistance during exercise. However, the magnitude of leg blood flow, leg oxygen extraction, and leg $\dot{V}O_2$ during exercise were unchanged, suggesting that vasodilation in the leg was produced by an autoregulatory response to the drop in blood pressure rather than by blockade of sympathetic vasoconstriction. Maximal systemic $\dot{V}O_2$ and leg lactate release were also not improved. Regional blockade with phentolamine did not substantially drop the arterial blood pressure and had no effect on vasodilation, blood flow, $\dot{V}O_2$, and lactate release in the leg during exercise. These data suggest that during exercise in patients with heart failure, the sympathetic nervous system helps to sustain arterial blood pressure and that this beneficial effect is not associated with adverse effects on blood flow to working skeletal muscle.
Circulation 72, No. 1, 72–81, 1985.

BLOOD FLOW to working skeletal muscle is frequently reduced during exertion in patients with heart failure.[1-3] This reduced perfusion of muscle is thought to be responsible, at least in part, for one of the major clinical symptoms experienced by such patients: exertional fatigue.[1,4,5] Therefore, to develop therapeutic strategies for alleviating exertional fatigue in patients with heart failure, it is important that the mechanism responsible for this reduced skeletal muscle blood flow be identified.

Previous observations suggest that impaired dilation of resistance vessels within working muscle may be an important contributor to this reduced muscle flow. We have noted that leg vascular resistance does not decrease normally during maximum upright bicycle exercise in patients with heart failure.[1] Zelis et al.[6] have reported that forearm vascular resistance does not decrease normally during forearm exercise in patients with heart failure. In an experimental canine preparation of heart failure, Higgins et al.[7] noted that iliac bed resistance did not decrease normally during exercise.

One potential mechanism responsible for impaired vasodilation in working muscle is activation of the sympathetic nervous system. In patients with heart failure, physical exertion usually produces earlier and more intense activation of the sympathetic nervous system than in normal subjects.[8,9] This activation produces vasoconstriction in inactive, nonessential vascular beds and thereby serves the useful purpose of supporting the systemic blood pressure and redistributing blood flow to vital organs. However, this activation also subjects the resistance vessels in active skeletal muscle to substantial vasoconstrictor influences. If

From the Cardiovascular Section, Department of Medicine, University of Pennsylvania, Philadelphia.

Supported in part by NIH Clinical Research Center Grant 5-M01-RR00040. Dr. Wilson is the recipient of New Investigator Award HL30665 from the NIH.

Address for correspondence: John R. Wilson, M.D., Cardiovascular Section, Hospital of the University of Pennsylvania, 943 W. Gates, 3400 Spruce St., Philadelphia, PA 19104.

Received Feb. 12, 1985; revision accepted April 18, 1985.

sufficiently intense, these influences could impair arteriolar vasodilation and thereby interfere with skeletal muscle blood flow.[10, 11]

This study was undertaken to investigate this specific hypothesis. In previous studies we have demonstrated that patients with heart failure have higher leg vascular resistance and lower leg blood flow during maximum upright bicycle exercise than do normal subjects.[4, 12] These hemodynamic abnormalities are accompanied by metabolic evidence of reduced nutritive flow to working muscles, including reduced maximum systemic and leg oxygen consumption ($\dot{V}O_2$), markedly increased leg oxygen extraction, and earlier than normal onset of leg lactate release.[1, 12] If sympathetic nerve activation reduces muscle flow by impairing vasodilation within working muscle, we hypothesize that α-adrenergic blockade should reduce leg vascular resistance during exercise, increase leg blood flow, and improve metabolic indexes of muscle nutritive flow.

Methods

Patients. Seventeen men with chronic left ventricular dysfunction (ejection fractions 21 ± 8%) were studied. The mean age was 56 ± 10 years. All patients had exertional breathlessness and/or fatigue despite administration of digoxin and diuretics and all were classified as New York Heart Association functional class II or III. None had peripheral edema, ascites, angina pectoris, intermittent claudication, or reduced pulses in their legs at the time of study. Before enrollment in this study, optimal diuresis was achieved in all patients by increasing diuretic dosage until evidence of fluid retention was gone or until mild prerenal azotemia was noted. All patients had maximum oxygen uptakes below the normal range for their ages, the average maximum oxygen uptake being 12.6 ± 4.3 ml/min/kg.[13] Left ventricular dysfunction was attributed to coronary artery disease in 11 patients and to idiopathic congestive cardiomyopathy in six patients. No patient had received any vasodilator for at least 1 week. The protocol was approved by the Committee on Studies Involving Human Subjects at the University of Pennsylvania. Written informed consent was obtained from all subjects.

Protocol. The protocol consisted of having each patient perform maximal upright bicycle exercise before and after α-adrenergic blockade. Systemic α-adrenergic blockade was accomplished with orally administered prazosin in 10 patients. In all of these patients, a control exercise test was performed first. Three or more hours later, the exercise test with prazosin was carried out. In eight patients regional α-adrenergic blockade of one leg was accomplished by injecting phentolamine into the femoral artery. In these patients the sequence of control exercise and exercise with phentolamine was alternated. In one of the four patients who performed exercise with phentolamine first, control exercise was followed by administration of prazosin and a third exercise test.

On the day before study, a trial maximal exercise test was performed to acquaint the patient with the exercise protocol. Exercise was performed on an upright, mechanically braked bicycle ergometer (Monarch), beginning at a workload of 20 W. Every 3 min the workload was increased by 20 W to symptomatic maximum. All exercise tests were performed at least 4 hr after meals.

The following morning, digoxin and diuretics were withheld. A Swan-Ganz catheter was inserted via an antecubital vein and positioned in the pulmonary artery. A No. 5F thermodilution catheter was inserted percutaneously into the left femoral vein and advanced 15 to 16 cm anterograde into the iliac vein. In the patients who received phentolamine, a 12 cm polyethylene catheter was inserted into the left femoral artery. In the remaining patients a short polyethylene catheter was inserted into a radial artery.

Thirty minutes after instrumentation, hemodynamic measurements were made and blood samples were obtained from the arterial and femoral venous catheters for measurement of oxygen saturation and lactate concentration. Femoral venous blood flow was measured in triplicate. Respiratory gases were measured with a Beckman Metabolic Cart equipped with oxygen and carbon dioxide analyzers and a turbine volume transducer. Phentolamine was then administered to four of the patients; the remaining subjects received no medication. Details of phentolamine administration and exercise are mentioned below. The patients not receiving medication mounted the bicycle and were allowed to equilibrate for 5 min, after which all measurements were repeated.

The patients then commenced exercise. Respiratory gas and hemodynamic measurements were made continuously. During each 3 min exercise stage, leg blood flow was measured every 30 sec starting at 30 sec and continuing until 2.5 min (total of five measurements). The average of these five measurements was then taken as the mean flow for the exercise stage. Blood sampling was performed during the last 30 sec of the stage. Leg flow was not measured during this period.

After exercise was terminated, the patients receiving prazosin were allowed to rest for 1 hr. One milligram of prazosin was then administered orally. Forty-five minutes later hemodynamic measurements were repeated. If the upright mean arterial blood pressure had decreased by 15 mm Hg or greater and/or the patient had orthostatic symptoms, no further prazosin was administered. If the upright mean blood pressure had decreased by 10 to 15 mm Hg, an additional 1 mg of prazosin was administered. If the decrease in upright blood pressure was less than 10 mm Hg, an additional 4 mg of prazosin was administered. Seven patients received a total of 5 mg, two received 2 mg, and one received 1 mg.

Three hours after control exercise, the exercise protocol was repeated. Hemodynamic and metabolic measurements were made at identical exercise times as during control exercise. If a patient exercised longer after drug administration, measurements were also made at the new maximum exercise level.

In the patients receiving phentolamine, four received phentolamine just before the first exercise test. Control exercise was then performed 3 hr later. In the other four patients, phentolamine was administered and exercise was repeated 3 hr after the control exercise test. In all patients, 1 mg of phentolamine was initially administered into the femoral artery and arterial blood pressure was monitored for 3 min to ensure that marked hypotension did not occur. An additional 1.5 mg was then administered. Three minutes later, resting measurements were made and exercise was then performed. All patients received a total of 2.5 mg of phentolamine. The timing of phentolamine administration and exercise was rigidly adhered to so as to minimize the time between administration of the test dose of phentolamine and the end of exercise. This time was 14 min in three subjects, 17 min in three, 20 min in one, and 24 min in one.

In one patient, leg blood flow was not measured during exercise because of technical difficulties. However, femoral venous effluent was measured in this patient both at rest and during exercise. In the patients receiving prazosin, supine lactate levels were not measured in general, since it was believed that upright lactate levels provided adequate resting data. During the phentolamine protocol, which followed the prazosin protocol, both supine and upright lactate measurements were made to ensure that this was the case. No significant difference between supine and upright measurements was noted.

Leg blood flow. Leg blood flow was determined by the thermodilution method described by Jorfeldt et al.[14-16] and previously used by this laboratory.[1, 12, 17] In brief, femoral vein flow was measured with a 50 cm No. 5F thermodilution catheter with the thermistor at 2 cm and injection port 12 cm from the tip. Flow was determined by rapid injection of a 2.5 ml iced dextrose bolus, with the aid of a commercially available thermodilution computer (Elecath). Output curves were displayed on a strip-chart recorder to ensure an exponential decay curve. Jorfeldt et al. have demonstrated that femoral venous flow measured by this technique agrees closely with leg flow determined by injection of indocyanine green into the femoral artery with sampling from the femoral vein.[14] Details of the evaluation of such flow measurements in our laboratory have been reported previously.[1, 12, 17]

Reproducibility studies. The period between exercise tests was 3 hr. To ensure that exercise results are reproducible when repeated at this interval, reproducibility measurements were made in six patients. At peak exercise, the following key measurements were found to be reproducible: systemic $\dot{V}O_2$ (1041 ± 553 vs 1000 ± 526 ml/min, first vs second exercise), arterial lactate (35.5 ± 9.4 vs 32.3 ± 9.5 mg/dl), leg flow (3.15 ± 1.40 vs 3.21 ± 1.57 liters/ min), femoral venous lactate (44.6 ± 11.5 vs 43.9 ± 16.4 mg/dl), and leg arteriovenous oxygen difference (13.23 ± 1.34 vs 12.94 ± 1.72 ml/dl).

Measured variables. Hemoglobin concentration was measured by Coulter counter; hemoglobin oxygen saturation was measured with a co-oximeter (Instrumentation Laboratories) precalibrated with human blood. Blood oxygen content was calculated as the product of hemoglobin, 1.34 ml oxygen/g hemoglobin, and percent oxygen saturation. Oxygen extraction was calculated as the ratio of the arteriovenous oxygen difference and arterial oxygen content. Cardiac output was calculated from the Fick principle as systemic oxygen uptake/systemic arteriovenous oxygen difference. Systemic vascular resistance was calculated as mean blood pressure/cardiac output.

Leg vascular resistance was calculated as (arterial pressure − femoral venous pressure)/leg flow. Leg oxygen consumption was calculated as the product of femoral flow and the arteriovenous oxygen difference across the leg. Blood for lactate determination was deproteinized with cold perchloric acid and assayed with a spectrophotometric technique.[18] Normal resting values for this technique in our laboratory are 3 to 12 mg/dl. Leg lactate release was calculated as: leg flow times (femoral venous − arterial lactate concentration). It should be noted that leg flow, oxygen extraction, and lactate data were not obtained simultaneously. Therefore calculation of leg oxygen uptake and lactate release assumes that leg flow remained relatively constant during exercise. In support of this assumption, we have observed that flow increases abruptly with the onset of exercise and stabilizes within 30 to 45 sec.

Statistical methods. Values are presented as mean ± SD. Submaximal exercise variables were quantified in each patient by averaging all data obtained during submaximal exercise. Differences between measurements at rest and during exercise were compared by the paired Student t test for all variables but leg resistance. The distribution of leg resistances was nonparametric. Therefore differences in this variable were compared by the rank sum test, the nonparametric analog of the paired t test. A probability of less than .05 was considered significant.

Results

The effects of α-adrenergic blockade on systemic and regional parameters are summarized in tables 1 to 4 and illustrated in figures 1 and 2. Submaximal exercise data were obtained in eight of the patients who received prazosin and in five of the patients who received phentolamine. The other patients did not exercise beyond the first workload.

Systemic α-adrenergic blockade with prazosin (tables 1 and 2). At supine rest before the administration of prazosin, cardiac output was 4.0 ± 1.1 liters/min, pulmonary wedge pressure was 19 ± 5 mm Hg, systemic vascular resistance was 22 ± 8 units, leg flow was 0.3 ± 0.1 liter/min, and leg resistance was 266 ±

TABLE 1

Effects of prazosin on systemic hemodynamic and metabolic responses to exercise

	HR (beats/min)	BP (mm Hg)	CO (l/min)	PWP (mm Hg)	$\dot{V}O_2$ (ml/min)	O_2 extraction (%)	Lactate (mg/dl)	SVR (units)
Control								
Lying (n = 10)	87±10	83±13	4.0±1.1	19±5	224±44	38±9	—	22.4±8.1
Bike (n = 10)	95±14	86±17	3.8±0.6	13±9	276±33	47±11	11.7±3.2	23.1±6.3
Submaximal exercise (N = 8)	115±14	97±19	7.4±1.1	24±7	778±137	66±7	21.7±4.2	13.3±3.4
Peak exercise (n = 10)[A]	129±20	101±20	8.4±1.9	30±7	1023±330	73±7	40.2±10.3	12.5±3.2
Prazosin								
Lying	89±7	77±13[C]	4.5±1.2[D]	13±5[D]	228±45	33±7[D]	—	18.1±4.9[D]
Bike	102±8	71±13[D]	4.4±1.0[D]	8±4[D]	289±37[C]	43±8[C]	13.8±6.2	17.0±4.9[D]
Submaximal exercise[B]	120±13	81±16[D]	8.4±1.1[C]	13±4[D]	839±179[C]	60±7[D]	24.1±6.3	9.5±1.4[D]
Peak exercise[A]	132±20	87±22[D]	9.4±2.6[C]	15±5[D]	1097±437	68±6[D]	37.7±10.1	9.7±2.5[D]

BP = blood pressure; CO = cardiac output; HR = heart rate; PWP = pulmonary wedge pressure; SVR = systemic vascular resistance.
[A]Values obtained at the highest identical work time achieved during both exercise tests.
[B]Measured at identical work times as during control exercise.
[C]p < .05 compared with control.
[D]p < .01 compared with control.

TABLE 2
Effects of prazosin on leg hemodynamic and metabolic responses to exercise

	Leg flow (l/min)	Leg $\dot{V}O_2$ (ml/min)	Leg resistance (units)	Leg O_2 extraction (%)	Femoral venous lactate (mg/dl)	Venous-arterial lactate difference (mg/dl)	Leg lactate release (mg/min)
Control							
Lying (n = 10)	0.3±0.1	16±5	266±76	38±12	—	—	—
Bike (n = 10)	0.3±0.1	24±8	289±69	55±16	12.8±4.3	1.1±2.4	4±8
Submaximal exercise (n = 8)	1.9±0.8	234±108	69±52	76±6	28.4±6.0	6.7±3.0	112±53
Peak exercise (n = 10)[A]	2.6±1.4	327±192	50±32	82±6	53.6±9.0	13.3±7.7	237±115
Prazosin							
Lying	0.3±0.1	17±6	212±72[C]	32±8	—	—	—
Bike	0.5±0.6	28±13	193±115[C]	52±7	15.7±3.7[C]	0.9±4.4	3±12
Submaximal exercise[B]	2.2±0.9[C]	240±111	44±24	72±7[C]	31±7[C]	6.5±3.5	134±61
Peak exercise[A]	2.8±1.6	344±205	35±17[C]	78±8[D]	51.3±9.4	13.7±7.2	389±247[C]

[A]Values obtained at the highest identical work time achieved during both exercise tests.
[B]Measured at identical work times as during control exercise.
[C]$p < .05$ compared with control.
[D]$p < .01$ compared with control.

76 units. During maximal exercise, patients exercised to a maximal $\dot{V}O_2$ of 1033 ± 322 ml/min, invariably terminating exercise because of leg fatigue. Exercise increased the cardiac output to 8.4 ± 1.9 liters/min and the pulmonary wedge pressure to 30 ± 7 mm Hg. Leg blood flow increased from 0.3 ± 0.1 to 2.6 ± 1.4 liters/min, leg $\dot{V}O_2$ from 16 ± 5 to 327 ± 192 ml/min, leg oxygen extraction from 38 ± 12% to 82 ± 6%, and leg lactate release from 4 ± 8 to 237 ± 115 mg/min.

Administration of prazosin decreased the resting systemic vascular resistance by 18 ± 8% to 18 ± 5 units ($p < .002$ vs control) and resting leg vascular resistance by 18 ± 24% to 212 ± 72 units ($p < .02$ vs control) (figure 1). The percentage change in systemic and regional resistance were not significantly different. This vasodilation was associated with an increase in the resting cardiac output from 4.0 ± 1.1 to 4.5 ± 1.2 liters/min ($p < .003$) and a decrease in the pulmonary wedge pressure from 19 ± 5 to 13 ± 5 mm Hg ($p < .001$) but no change in leg blood flow or leg oxygen extraction.

During maximal exercise testing after administration of prazosin there was no significant change in maximal $\dot{V}O_2$ (1033 ± 322 to 1105 ± 439 ml/min; p = NS) or exercise duration. Exercise duration was identical in eight patients, increased in one, and decreased in one.

To examine the effect of prazosin on exercise data, variables were compared at the highest identical peak exercise time achieved during both tests. At this peak exercise point, prazosin decreased systemic vascular resistance by 25 ± 14% associated with a substantial decrease in mean arterial blood pressure from 101 ± 20 to 87 ± 22 mm Hg ($p < .002$) (figure 1). Leg vascular resistance decreased by 23 ± 20%, from 50 ± 32 to 35 ± 17 units ($p < .04$) (figure 1). However, there was no significant change in leg blood flow (2.6 ± 1.4 to 2.8 ± 1.6 liters/min; p = NS) or leg $\dot{V}O_2$ (327 ± 192 to 344 ± 205 ml/min; p = NS) (figure 2). Leg lactate release actually increased from 237 ± 115 to 389 ± 247 mg/min ($p < .03$) (figure 2).

Regional α-adrenergic blockade with phentolamine (tables 3 and 4). At supine rest before the administration of phentolamine, cardiac output was 3.3 ± 0.8 liters/min, pulmonary wedge pressure was 25 ± 5 mm Hg, systemic vascular resistance was 29 ± 8 units, leg flow was 0.4 ± 0.1 liter/min, and leg resistance was 242 ± 64 units. During maximal exercise, patients exercised to a maximal $\dot{V}O_2$ of 754 ± 354 ml/min, invariably terminating exercise because of leg fatigue. Exercise increased the cardiac output to 6.0 ± 2.8 liters/min and the pulmonary wedge pressure to 28 ± 7 mm Hg. Leg flow increased from 0.4 ± 0.1 to 2.8 ± 2.0 liters/ min, leg $\dot{V}O_2$ from 26 ± 7 to 365 ± 276 ml/min, leg oxygen extraction from 45 ± 11% to 78 ± 9%, and leg lactate release from 4 ± 8 to 316 ± 212 mg/min.

Administration of phentolamine decreased the resting leg vascular resistance by 29 ± 18% (figure 1). Systemic vascular resistance decreased by 20 ± 16% (figure 1), significantly less than did leg resistance (p

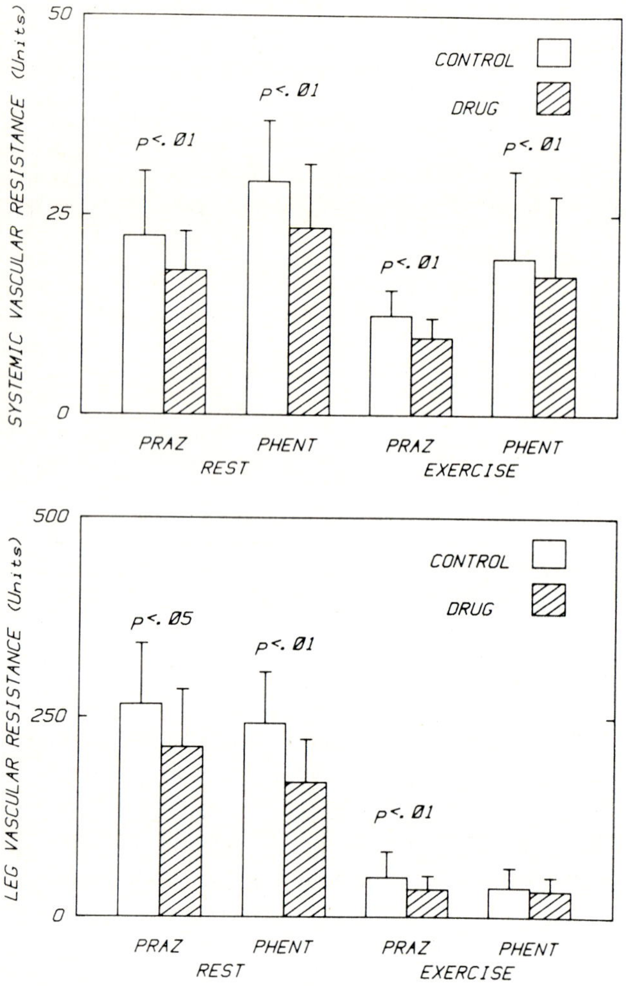

FIGURE 1. Effect of prazosin (PRAZ) and phentolamine (PHENT) on systemic and leg vascular resistance. Exercise data were obtained at the highest identical exercise time achieved during both tests.

$< .03$). Vasodilation was associated with an increase in the resting cardiac output from 3.3 ± 0.8 to 3.8 ± 1.1 liters/min and a decrease in the pulmonary wedge pressure from 25 ± 5 to 19 ± 10 mm Hg ($p < .05$). Leg blood flow increased from 0.4 ± 0.1 to 0.5 ± 0.2 liter/min ($p < .002$) while leg oxygen extraction decreased from 45 ± 11% to 25 ± 10% ($p < .002$).

During maximal exercise testing after administration of phentolamine, there was no significant change in maximal $\dot{V}O_2$ (754 ± 354 to 756 ± 365 ml/min; p = NS), with all patients discontinuing exercise within 30 sec of the control exercise duration. At maximal exercise, phentolamine decreased systemic vascular resistance by only 11 ± 10% (20 ± 11 to 18 ± 10 units; $p < .01$) (figure 1) associated with a modest drop in mean arterial blood pressure from 95 ± 11 to 90 ± 11 mm Hg ($p < .02$). Cardiac output, pulmonary wedge pressure, leg blood flow, leg vascular resistance, leg oxygen extraction, and leg lactate release were all unchanged (figures 1 and 2).

Discussion

Heart failure is accompanied by a reduction in blood flow to peripheral tissues both at rest and during exercise.[1, 4, 5] This reduced flow leads to the recruitment of a number of compensatory vasoconstrictor mechanisms designed to sustain the systemic blood pressure and redistribute blood flow to vital organs. The most important of these mechanisms is activation of the sympathetic nervous system.[8, 9]

At rest, when peripheral tissue oxygen demands are low, activation of the sympathetic nervous system is usually modest and largely beneficial. During exercise, however, it remains uncertain whether these va-

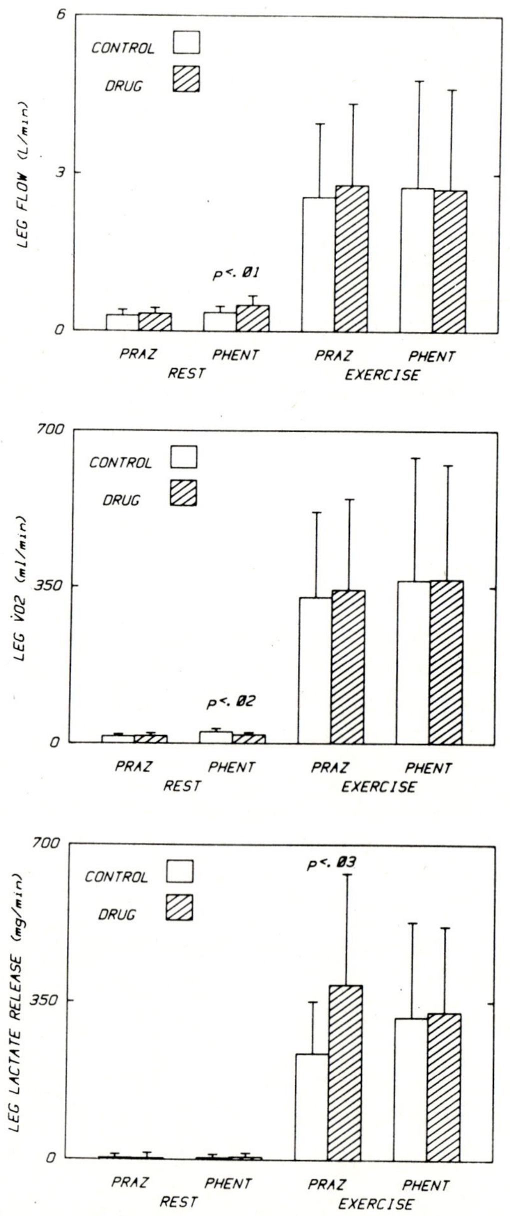

FIGURE 2. Effect of prazosin (PRAZ) and phentolamine (PHENT) on leg blood flow and metabolism. Exercise data were obtained at the highest identical exercise time achieved during both tests.

TABLE 3
Effects of phentolamine on systemic hemodynamic and metabolic responses to exercise

	HR (beats/min)	BP (mm Hg)	CO (l/min)	PWP (mm Hg)	$\dot{V}O_2$ (ml/min)	O_2 extraction (%)	Lactate (mg/dl)	SVR (units)
Control								
Lying (n = 8)	87 ± 12	91 ± 7	3.3 ± 0.8	25 ± 5	241 ± 60	44 ± 4	11.2 ± 2.9	29.3 ± 7.6
Bike (n = 8)	97 ± 15	89 ± 7	3.0 ± 0.9	24 ± 10	263 ± 57	53 ± 9	12.7 ± 2.9	32.3 ± 10.9
Submaximal exercise (n = 5)	116 ± 11	95 ± 11	5.3 ± 1.9	25 ± 7	620 ± 222	69 ± 5	23.6 ± 5.2	20.9 ± 10.6
Maximal exercise (n = 8)	123 ± 19	95 ± 11	6.0 ± 2.8	28 ± 7	754 ± 354	75 ± 7	30.7 ± 17.4	19.7 ± 11.1
Phentolamine								
Lying	88 ± 7	82 ± 6^C	3.8 ± 1.1^B	19 ± 10^B	234 ± 54	37 ± 5^C	10.5 ± 3.7	23.5 ± 8.0^C
Bike	94 ± 9	82 ± 8^C	3.3 ± 1.0	21 ± 10	268 ± 65	51 ± 3	10.6 ± 2.7^B	27.9 ± 11.8^B
Submaximal exercise^A	114 ± 9	86 ± 6^B	5.5 ± 2.0	24 ± 8	600 ± 193	67 ± 5^B	20.0 ± 3.5^B	19.0 ± 10.0
Maximal exercise^A	121 ± 12	90 ± 11^B	6.5 ± 3.3	27 ± 7	756 ± 365	70 ± 7^C	28.1 ± 12.4	17.5 ± 10.0^C

Abbreviations as in table 1.
^A Measured at identical work times as during control exercise.
^B $p < .05$ compared with control.
^C $p < .01$ compared with control.

soconstrictor mechanisms are beneficial or deleterious. In patients with heart failure, exercise activates the sympathetic nervous system much more intensively than at rest.[8, 9] From the standpoint of blood flow to working skeletal muscle, this activation on the one hand serves to sustain muscle perfusion pressure, a key determinant of muscle flow. However, this activation also exerts vasoconstrictor influences on arterioles in working muscle and thereby may interfere with the other key determinant of muscle flow, muscle vasodilation.

Determining which of these effects is dominant has major clinical as well as scientific importance. If activation of the sympathetic nervous system during exercise is detrimental, administration of α-adrenergic blocking agents to patients with heart failure should prove to be useful.

The extent to which vasodilation in active muscle is affected by sympathetic nervous activation is determined by the balance between local vasodilatory factors and vasoconstrictor influences. Studies in man and in experimental animals have shown that constrictor responses in muscle to sympathetic nerve activation and administration of norepinephrine are attenuated during exercise by local vasodilatory factors.[10, 11, 19, 20] In normal subjects and normal experimental animals,

TABLE 4
Effects of phentolamine on leg hemodynamic and metabolic responses to exercise

	Leg flow (l/min)	Leg $\dot{V}O_2$ (ml/min)	Leg resistance (units)	Leg O_2 extraction (%)	Femoral venous lactate (mg/dl)	Venous-arterial lactate difference (mg/dl)	Leg lactate release (mg/min)
Control							
Lying (n = 8)	0.4 ± 0.1	26 ± 7	242 ± 64	45 ± 11	12.1 ± 3.6	0.9 ± 2.2	4 ± 8
Bike (n = 8)	0.4 ± 0.1	32 ± 13	237 ± 62	58 ± 13	13.0 ± 3.0	0.3 ± 2.1	2 ± 7
Submaximal exercise (n = 5)	2.7 ± 1.7	358 ± 236	46 ± 25	78 ± 7	32.4 ± 5.0	8.9 ± 4.6	154 ± 158
Maximal exercise (n = 8)	2.8 ± 2.0	365 ± 276	37 ± 25	78 ± 9	43.9 ± 20.1	13.3 ± 4.4	316 ± 212
Phentolamine							
Lying	0.5 ± 0.2^C	20 ± 5^B	168 ± 55^C	25 ± 10^C	11.6 ± 3.1	1.1 ± 1.6	6 ± 9
Bike	0.5 ± 0.1^B	35 ± 8	174 ± 62^C	47 ± 12^C	12.7 ± 4.2	2.1 ± 2.2	11 ± 14
Submaximal exercise^A	2.6 ± 1.4	347 ± 187	36 ± 17	77 ± 5	28.3 ± 3.1^B	7.8 ± 1.8	164 ± 108
Maximal exercise^A	2.7 ± 1.9	367 ± 258	33 ± 18^B	77 ± 7	39.9 ± 16.6	11.9 ± 5.4	327 ± 191

^A Measured at identical work times as during control exercise.
^B $p < .05$ compared with control.
^C $p < .01$ compared with control.

the balance between these two competing influences is such that constrictor influences are markedly attenuated.[20-22] However, abnormally high levels of vasoconstrictor activity, as occur in heart failure, may be sufficient to interfere with metabolic vasodilation and thereby impair blood flow to working skeletal muscle.[10, 11]

In this study we sought to investigate this possibility by examining the effect of α-adrenergic blockade on vascular resistance, blood flow, and lactate release in the leg during maximal exercise in patients with heart failure. Leg resistance and blood flow were used as indexes of skeletal muscle resistance and flow, respectively; flow to nonmuscular tissue makes up only a small portion of leg blood flow during exercise.[23] Systemic and leg oxygen uptake and leg lactate release were used as indexes of the adequacy of oxygen delivery to working muscle.[24, 25] To evaluate changes in these variables during exercise, the variables were compared at identical work times. Exercise level influences muscle blood flow and metabolism. Therefore, comparison of data at different work times would leave uncertain whether any change that is observed is caused by α-adrenergic blockade or by differences in workload.

Two forms of α-adrenergic blockade were used: prazosin and phentolamine. Prazosin in the dosages used has previously been shown to produce α_1-adrenoceptor blockade.[26, 27] Phentolamine produces both α_1- and α_2-adrenoceptor blockade.[27] We chose a dose of phentolamine exceeding dosages previously shown to produce leg α-adrenergic blockade[6]; we considered it unreasonable to burden the patients with additional studies to titrate the dose in each patient. Regional phentolamine was used for several reasons. First, with this approach we sought to minimize the effect on arterial blood pressure during exercise so as to alter muscle perfusion pressure as little as possible. This goal was largely achieved, since mean blood pressure at peak exercise decreased only slightly with phentolamine from 95 $\pm$ 11 to 90 $\pm$ 11 mm Hg. In contrast, prazosin decreased mean blood pressure at peak exercise from 101 $\pm$ 20 to 87 $\pm$ 22 mm Hg. Second, we wished to block α_2-receptors because there is evidence that these receptors may also mediate vasoconstrictor influences.[28] Third, use of phentolamine permitted us to alternate control and interventional studies so as to avoid any bias that might result from obtaining all control studies first. Prazosin was used to examine blockade of the sympathetic nervous system with presynaptic α_2-receptors intact. In addition, phentolamine is relatively transitory in its effect; after a 5 mg bolus injection of phentolamine in normal subjects, hemodynamic variables often return to baseline within 30 min.[29] In this study, all measurements were made within 20 min of phentolamine administration in seven patients and by 24 min in the remaining patient. Nevertheless, it is possible that the degree of α-adrenergic blockade had begun to wane by the end of exercise. Use of prazosin avoided any concern with dissipation of blockade.

During control exercise, all patients developed metabolic changes suggesting impaired blood flow to working skeletal muscle. Specifically, patients were limited by fatigue at reduced maximum oxygen uptakes of 12.6 $\pm$ 4.3 ml/min/kg, the normal maximum oxygen uptake being in excess of 20 to 25 ml/min/kg.[13] The leg oxygen extraction and leg lactate release noted at maximum exercise were markedly increased above levels observed in normal subjects at comparable workloads.[30, 31] The limb vascular resistance noted at maximum exercise was also higher than levels observed by us in patients with normal exercise capacity,[1] suggesting reduced limb vasodilation.

α-Adrenergic blockade with both prazosin and phentolamine reduced systemic and limb vascular resistance at rest. With phentolamine, leg vasodilation exceeded systemic vasodilation, consistent with greater regional than systemic vasodilation. These findings serve to reinforce prior observations indicating that the sympathetic nervous system is an important mechanism in heart failure for sustaining resting arterial blood pressure.[32, 33] α-Adrenergic blockade was also accompanied by improved pump function at rest, as shown by a reduction in the pulmonary wedge pressure and an increase in the cardiac output.

Of greater interest, however, were the changes during exercise. At peak exercise, prazosin decreased systemic vascular resistance by 25 $\pm$ 14% accompanied by a substantial drop in mean arterial pressure. Phentolamine also decreased systemic resistance modestly. Thus the sympathetic nervous system also contributed importantly to sustaining blood pressure during exercise and therefore to optimizing muscle perfusion pressure.

Was this beneficial effect of sympathetic nerve activation offset by evidence of vasoconstriction in active muscle and consequent impaired muscle nutritive flow? Our finding that phentolamine had no effect on leg vascular resistance, leg blood flow, and leg oxygen extraction during exercise suggests that substantial α-adrenergic vasoconstriction was not present in the leg. Prazosin modestly decreased leg resistance. This is not inconsistent with the findings with phentolamine. Prazosin produced a major drop in arterial blood pressure and no change in leg blood flow or leg oxygen extraction. The accompanying decrease in leg resistance therefore most likely reflected an autoregulatory compensatory response on the part of resistance vessels to keep muscle flow constant.

The metabolic changes noted with α-adrenergic blockade further support the absence of significant vasoconstriction in active muscle. If sympathetic activity did interfere with muscle flow, one would expect that α-adrenergic blockade would increase muscle oxygen uptake and reduce muscle lactate release. In fact, neither prazosin nor phentolamine augmented leg $\dot{V}O_2$ during exercise or decreased leg lactate release. Prazosin actually increased leg lactate release at peak exercise, possibly because of adverse effect on muscle perfusion pressure caused by the substantial drop in mean arterial pressure. Maximal $\dot{V}O_2$, another variable thought to be determined by the adequacy of muscle oxygen delivery,[1, 5] was also unchanged by α-adrenergic blockade.

Therefore, the overall circulatory effect of sympathetic nerve activation during exercise in patients with heart failure is probably best viewed as beneficial. During exercise, this system helps to increase vascular resistance in nonexercising vascular beds and thereby to optimize the perfusion pressure of critical organs. In active skeletal muscle, sympathetic vasoconstrictor activity appears to be abolished by local metabolic factors.

This conclusion must be viewed within the context of several potential limitations. The use of skeletal muscle glycolysis as a marker of blood flow to working muscle is supported by prior observations that reducing muscle flow augments glycolysis.[24, 25] Nevertheless, glycolysis occurs normally in well-oxygenated working muscle and is affected by pH and substrate availability.[34, 35] We cannot totally exclude the possibility that changes in these other variables affected our results, but we doubt that such changes occurred. Second, the adequacy of α-adrenergic blockade was not directly established. To avoid marked hypotension, we chose to administer prazosin in sequential dosages depending on the blood pressure response. Hypotension would have precluded repeat exercise and, more importantly, might have offset a potentially beneficial regional effect of α-adrenergic inhibition by markedly reducing muscle perfusion pressure. It is therefore possible that α-adrenergic blockade was not complete in all patients. Nevertheless, the changes in systemic vascular resistance noted with prazosin suggest substantial blockade. Another possible criticism of our study is that we did not obtain plasma catecholamine levels. Prior studies have uniformly demonstrated higher than normal norepinephrine and epinephrine levels during exercise in similar patients with heart failure.[8, 9] Therefore it is likely that both sympathetic nerve activity and adrenal activation were increased in all of our patients.

A final limitation of this study is that it does not provide direct information about regional distribution of flow within skeletal muscle. Norepinephrine and sympathetic nerve activation not only produce α-adrenergically mediated vasoconstricton but also β_2-adrenergically mediated vasodilation after α-adrenergic blockade.[36, 37] The interaction between these two effects may play an important role in microcirculatory regulation during exercise.[37] For example, Nellis et al.[38] have demonstrated that α-adrenergic stimulation may actually enhance oxygen delivery to ischemic skeletal muscle by optimizing flow distribution. A comprehensive understanding of the impact of sympathetic activation on skeletal muscle in patients with heart failure must include attention to such issues. Other important related issues include the role of epinephrine in heart failure, a hormone with more pronounced β_2-adrenergic effects than norepinephrine, and the role of changes in vascular adrenergic receptors. From a clinical standpoint, it is important to address the effects of pharmacologic agents on the skeletal muscle vasculature. As an example, β-adrenergic blockade could exacerbate vasoconstriction in skeletal muscle by blocking β-adrenergically mediated vasodilation. However, these issues were beyond the scope of this study.

To our knowledge, this study represents the first to examine the effects of α-adrenergic blockade on limb flow and metabolism during maximal exercise in patients with heart failure. Nevertheless, our findings and conclusions are consistent with several prior observations. Zelis et al.[6] examined the effect of α-adrenergic blockade on forearm blood flow and forearm $\dot{V}O_2$ during forearm exercise in patients with heart failure. Blockade had no effect on either variable. Rubin et al.[39] examined the effect of prazosin on systemic lactate levels during upright maximal bicycle exercise in patients with heart failure. These investigators also failed to observe any change in either lactate levels or exercise duration with prazosin. Finally, our conclusion that local metabolic factors abolished sympathetic vasoconstriction in the active muscles of our patients is supported by a number of observations in normal human subjects and experimental animals indicating that the constrictor response to sympathetic nerve activation and/or norepinephrine administration in skeletal muscle is significantly attenuated during exercise.[10, 11, 19, 20]

The findings of this study have important clinical implications. The overall effect of sympathetic nerve activation during exercise in patients with heart failure appears to be beneficial when viewed from the standpoint of active skeletal muscle. This activation augments muscle perfusion pressure without affecting vasodilation in active muscle. Administration of α-adrenergic agents to such patients for the purposes of improving muscle blood flow and thereby relieving muscular fatigue is therefore not likely to be of value. This conclusion is consistent with the findings of two recent double-blind studies, which indicated that long-term prazosin therapy does not improve the maximal exercise capacity of patients with heart failure[40, 41]; maximal exercise capacity in such patients is thought to be determined by the adequacy of blood flow to working skeletal muscle.[1, 4, 5]

In summary, our results suggest that the sympathetic nervous system helps to sustain arterial blood pressure both at rest and during exercise in patients with chronic heart failure and that this beneficial effect is not associated with adverse effects on blood flow to working skeletal muscle.

We thank Drs. Robert Zelis and Nathaniel Reichek for critically reviewing the manuscript.

References

1. Wilson JR, Martin JL, Schwartz D, Ferraro N: Exercise intolerance in patients with chronic heart failure: role of impaired skeletal muscle nutritive flow. Circulation **69:** 1079, 1984
2. Zelis R, Longhurst J, Capone RJ, Mason DT: A comparison of regional blood flow and oxygen utilization during dynamic forearm exercise in normal subjects and patients with congestive heart failure. Circulation **50:** 137, 1974
3. Longhurst J, Gifford W, Zelis R: Impaired forearm oxygen consumption during static exercise in patients with congestive heart failure. Circulation **54:** 477, 1976
4. Wilson JR, Ferraro N: Exercise intolerance in patients with chronic left heart failure: relation to oxygen transport and ventilatory abnormalities. Am J Cardiol **51:** 1358, 1983
5. Weber KT, Kinasewitz GT, Janicki JS, Fishman AP: Oxygen utilization and ventilation during exercise in patients with chronic cardiac failure. Circulation **65:** 1218, 1982
6. Zelis R, Mason DT, Braunwald E: A comparison of the effects of vasodilator stimuli on peripheral resistance vessels in normal subjects and in patients with congestive heart failure. J Clin Invest **47:** 960, 1968
7. Higgins CB, Vatner SF, Franklin D, Braunwald E: Effects of experimentally produced heart failure on the peripheral vascular response to severe exercise in conscious dogs. Circ Res **31:** 186, 1972
8. Francis GS, Goldsmith SR, Ziesche SM, Cohn JN: Response of plasma norepinephrine and epinephrine to dynamic exercise in patients with congestive heart failure. Am J Cardiol **49:** 1152, 1982
9. Chidsey CA, Harrison DC, Braunwald E: Augmentation of the plasma norepinephrine response to exercise in patients with congestive heart failure. N Engl J Med **267:** 650, 1962
10. Thompson LP, Mohrman DE: Blood flow and oxygen consumption in skeletal muscle during sympathetic stimulation. Am J Physiol **245:** H66, 1983
11. Flaim SF, Crede W, Beech A, Nellis SH, Zelis R: The effects of norepinephrine on active hyperemia in the canine gracilis muscle. Circ Res **44:** 660, 1979
12. Wilson JR, Martin JL, Ferraro N: Impaired skeletal muscle nutritive flow during exercise in patients with congestive heart failure: role of cardiac pump dysfunction as determined by the effect of dobutamine. Am J Cardiol **53:** 1308, 1984
13. Bruce RA, Kusumi F, Hosmer D: Maximal oxygen intake and nomographic assessment of functional aerobic impairment in cardiovascular disease. Am Heart J **85:** 546, 1973
14. Jorfeldt L, Jublin-Dannefelt A, Pernow B, Wassen E: Determination of human leg blood flow: a thermodilution technique based on femoral venous bolus injection. Clin Sci Mol Med **54:** 517, 1968
15. Jorfeldt L, Wahren J: Leg blood flow during exercise in man. Clin Sci **41:** 459, 1971
16. Wahren J, Saltin B, Jorfeldt L, Pernow B: Influence of age on the local circulatory adaptation to leg exercise. Scand J Clin Lab Invest **33:** 79, 1974
17. Wilson JR, Martin JL, Ferraro N, Weber KT: Effect of hydralazine on perfusion and metabolism in the leg during upright bicycle exercise in patients with heart failure. Circulation **68:** 425, 1983
18. Weissman N, Pileggi VJ: Inorganic ions. *In* Henry RJ, editor: Clinical chemistry, principles and techniques. New York, 1974, Harper and Row, p 655
19. Burcher E, Garlick D: Antagonism of vasoconstrictor responses by exercise in the gracilis muscle of the dog. J Pharm Exp Ther **187:** 78, 1973
20. Strandell T, Shepherd JT: The effect in humans of increased sympathetic activity on the blood flow to active muscles. Acta Med Scand **472** (suppl 1): 146, 1967
21. Donald DE, Rowlands DJ, Ferguson DA: Similarity of blood flow in the normal and sympathectomized dog hindlimb during graded exercise. Circ Res **26:** 185, 1970
22. Hartling OJ, Trap-Jensen J: Haemodynamic and metabolic effects of α-adrenoceptor blockade with phentolamine at rest and during forearm exercise. Clin Sci **65:** 247, 1983
23. Rowell LB: Human cardiovascular adjustments to exercise and thermal stress. Physiol Rev **54:** 75, 1974
24. Walker PM, Idstrom J, Schersten T, Bylund-Fellenius A: Metabolic response in different muscle types to reduced blood flow during exercise in perfused rat hindlimb. Clin Sci **63:** 293, 1982
25. Bylund-Fellenius A, Walker PM, Elander A, Holm S, Holm J, Schersten T: Energy metabolism in relation to oxygen partial pressure in human skeletal muscle during exercise. Biochem J **200:** 247, 1981
26. Graham RM, Pettinger WA: Prazosin. N Engl J Med **300:** 232, 1979
27. Drew GM: Effects of α-adrenoceptor agonists and antagonists on pre- and postsynaptically located α-adrenoceptors. Eur J Pharmacol **36:** 313, 1976
28. Drew GM, Whiting SB: Evidence for two distinct types of postsynaptic α-adrenoceptors in vascular smooth muscle in vivo. Br J Pharmacol **67:** 207, 1979
29. Taylor SH, Sutherland GR, MacKenzie GJ, Staunton HP, Donald KW: The circulatory effects of intravenous phentolamine in man. Circulation **31:** 741, 1965
30. Pirnay F, Lamy M, DuJardin J, Deroanne R, Petit JM: Analysis of femoral venous blood during maximal muscular exercise. J Appl Physiol **33:** 289, 1972
31. Doll E, Keul J, Maiwald C: Oxygen tension an acid-base equilibria in venous blood of working muscle. Am J Physiol **215:** 23, 1968
32. Kluger J, Cody RJ, Laragh JH: The contributions of sympathetic tone and the renin-angiotensin system to severe chronic congestive heart failure: response to specific inhibitors (prazosin and captopril). Am J Cardiol **49:** 1667, 1982
33. Levine TB, Francis GS, Goldsmith SR, Simon AB, Cohn JN: Activity of the sympathetic nervous system and renin-angiotensin system assessed by plasma hormone levels and their relation to hemodynamic abnormalities in congestive heart failure. Am J Cardiol **49:** 1659, 1982
34. Connett RJ, Gayeski TEJ, Honig CR: Lactate accumulation in fully aerobic, working dog gracilis muscle. Am J Physiol **246:** H120, 1984

35. Holloszy JO, Booth FW: Biochemical adaptations to endurance exercise in muscle. Annu Rev Physiol **18:** 273, 1976

36. Viveros OH, Garlick DG, Renkin EM: Sympathetic beta adrenergic vasodilation in skeletal muscle of the dog. Am J Physiol **215:** 1218, 1968

37. Lundvall J, Jarhult J: Beta adrenergic dilator component of the sympathetic vascular response in skeletal muscle. Acta Physiol Scand **96:** 180, 1976

38. Nellis SH, Flaim SF, McCauley KM, Zelis R: α-Stimulation protects exercise increment in skeletal muscle oxygen consumption. Am J Physiol **238:** H331, 1980

39. Rubin SA, Chatterjee K, Parmley WW: Metabolic assessment of exercise in chronic heart failure patients treated with short-term vasodilators. Circulation **61:** 543, 1980

40. Markham RV, Corbett JR, Gilmore A, Pettinger WA, Firth BG: Efficacy of prazosin in the management of chronic congestive heart failure: a 6-month randomized, double-blind, placebo-controlled study. Am J Cardiol **51:** 1346, 1983

41. Higginbotham MB, Morris KG, Bramlet DA, Coleman RE, Cobb FR: Long-term ambulatory therapy with prazosin versus placebo for chronic heart failure: relation between clinical response and left ventricular function at rest and during exercise. Am J Cardiol **52:** 782, 1983

Transluminal, subselective measurement of coronary artery blood flow velocity and vasodilator reserve in man

ROBERT F. WILSON, M.D., DONALD E. LAUGHLIN, M.S.E.E., PETER H. ACKELL, M.D., WILLIAM M. CHILIAN, PH.D., MYRL D. HOLIDA, B.S., CRAIG J. HARTLEY, PH.D., MARK L. ARMSTRONG, M.D., MELVIN L. MARCUS, M.D., AND CARL W. WHITE, M.D.

ABSTRACT Assessment of coronary blood flow and the vasodilator reserve capacity of individual coronary arteries in the catheterization laboratory has been hampered by methodologic limitations. We have developed and validated a small Doppler catheter that can subselectively measure phasic coronary blood flow velocity (CBFV). In seven anesthetized calves, CBFV was varied from 0.1 to 5.7 times control CBFV. Changes in mean CBFV measured intraluminally by catheter in the left anterior descending and left circumflex arteries were similar to those measured simultaneously with an epicardial Doppler probe on the surface of the same vessel (n = 85, r = .95, slope = 1.04) and to changes in coronary sinus flow (n = 69, r = .97, slope = 1.06) measured with timed venous collections. Identical maximal coronary reactive hyperemic responses with the catheter present and absent in the artery being studied demonstrated that coronary obstruction by the catheter was minimal. Safety studies in six additional calves demonstrated that the catheter caused small changes in coronary endothelial permeability. Histologic studies revealed no endothelial denudation or thrombus formation. Stable phasic recordings of coronary blood flow velocity have been obtained in 58 of 70 patients studied. One of the 70 patients studied had abrupt coronary occlusion probably related to catheter-induced vasospasm. In 10 normal patients, intracoronary meglumine diatrizoate increased CBFV to 3.5 times that at rest (range 2.8 to 5.0). CBFV rose 5.0-fold after an intravenous infusion of dipyridamole (range 3.8 to 7.0). In each patient, dipyridamole produced greater vasodilation than meglumine diatrizoate. The time- and dose-response characteristics to dipyridamole infusion were heterogeneous, underscoring the advantage of continuous on-line measurement of CBFV in the measurement of vasodilator reserve. This method of measuring CBFV and assessing vasodilator reserve in the catheterization laboratory should facilitate studies of the coronary circulation in man.
Circulation 72, No. 1, 82–92, 1985.

MEASUREMENT OF phasic coronary blood flow velocity (CBFV) and the flow reserve capacity of individual coronary vessels has been hampered by methodologic limitations. Such data, if obtainable, could provide a means of assessing the physiologic significance of obstructive coronary artery disease at the time of cardiac catheterization.

Current methods of measuring coronary blood flow in conscious man have many limitations. Inert gas clearance techniques measure global myocardial blood flow but cannot detect rapid changes in flow.[1-3] Radionuclide techniques (e.g., ^{133}Xe clearance) measure regional blood flow, but do not permit on-line continuous assessment of coronary blood flow and are not accurate if blood flow is greater than 200 ml/min/100 g tissue.[4, 5] The coronary sinus thermodilution technique measures coronary venous effluent, but, except for that in the left anterior descending artery, cannot relate flow to an individual coronary artery. The technique is hampered further by catheter movement within the coronary sinus and inconsistencies in venous drainage patterns.[3, 6] These methodologic problems have prevented accurate measurements of coronary blood flow and the flow reserve capacity of individual vessels in conscious humans. Furthermore, the inability to obtain on-line flow measurements has prevented characterization of the time- and dose-response characteristics of coronary vasodilators.

From the Department of Internal Medicine and the Cardiovascular Center, University of Iowa Hospitals and Clinics, the Veterans Administration Hospital, Iowa City, and the University of Texas Health Science Center at Houston.

Supported by grants from the National Heart, Lung, and Blood Institute (HL 27633, 14388, and 29976), the Ischemic SCOR (HL 32295-01), and the Veterans Administration (MRIS 1100.2).

Address for correspondence: Robert F. Wilson, M.D., Department of Internal Medicine, University of Iowa Hospitals, Iowa City, IA 52240.

Received June 13, 1984; revision accepted March 28, 1985.

Previous techniques of measuring instantaneous phasic changes in coronary blood flow in conscious humans have used pulsed Doppler technology to measure CBFV. CBFV has been shown to correlate highly with volumetric measurements of coronary blood flow.[7] The Doppler technique of measuring flow velocity is advantageous because rapid changes in flow can be detected, on-line recordings can be obtained, and the method lends itself to miniaturization.

In 1974, Hartley and Cole[8, 9] developed a No. 5F (tip) Doppler catheter capable of measuring CBFV at the coronary ostium by placing a piezoelectric crystal at the tip of a Sones catheter. A major limitation of this and other coronary Doppler catheters available was that they were too large to place subselectively into coronary arteries. Furthermore, because the Doppler crystal is mounted on the catheter tip and the tip position is unstable, signal instability over time was a significant problem. Additionally, validation studies over a wide range of coronary flows have not been presented.

The purpose of our study was twofold: to develop and validate a coronary Doppler catheter that could be subselectively placed into individual coronary vessels to measure instantaneous changes in CBFV and to develop a method for determining subselective coronary vasodilator reserve at the time of cardiac catheterization.

Methods

The subselective coronary Doppler catheter was constructed by placing a 20 MHz piezoelectric crystal into the wall of a Rentrop reperfusion catheter (United States Catheter and Instrument, Co.) and used a 20 MHz pulsed Doppler meter (Bioengineering Department, University of Iowa) to measure blood flow velocity. The woven Dacron catheter is 120 cm in length and has a 1.6 mm outer diameter at the proximal end; the distal 20 cm tapers to 1.0 mm outer diameter (figure 1). This catheter has been approved for investigational use in humans by the U.S. Food and Drug Administration. Details of the catheter construction and specifications of the pulsed Doppler meter are contained in the Appendix.

To determine the relationship between mean flow velocity and Doppler frequency shift measured with the coronary Doppler catheter, the catheter was placed into the lumen of a 1.8 mm internal diameter polyethylene tube system filled with a mixture of water and laundry starch and connected to a roller pump (Sarns Co.). A windkessel chamber was used to minimize pulsatile flow. The starch has ultrasonic reflective characteristics similar to blood.[7] Mean flow velocity was calculated with the use of timed volume collections of tube flow. Paired measurements of flow velocity and Doppler frequency shift, obtained over a broad range of flows, were closely correlated (r = .99; figure 2).

Animal validation studies. Seven calves were anesthetized with ketamine (20 mg/kg im and iv) and pentobarbital sodium (10 mg/kg iv) and mechanically ventilated. A left thoractomy was performed and a 6.5 mm internal diameter catheter passed through the right atrial appendage into the proximal coronary sinus and secured with a ligature. Blood from the coronary sinus catheter could be returned to the jugular vein or diverted to a graduated cylinder for timed volume collections. Catheters were placed in the left femoral artery and both femoral veins for measurement of arterial pressure, withdrawal of blood samples, and drug infusions. A metal introducer was placed into the right

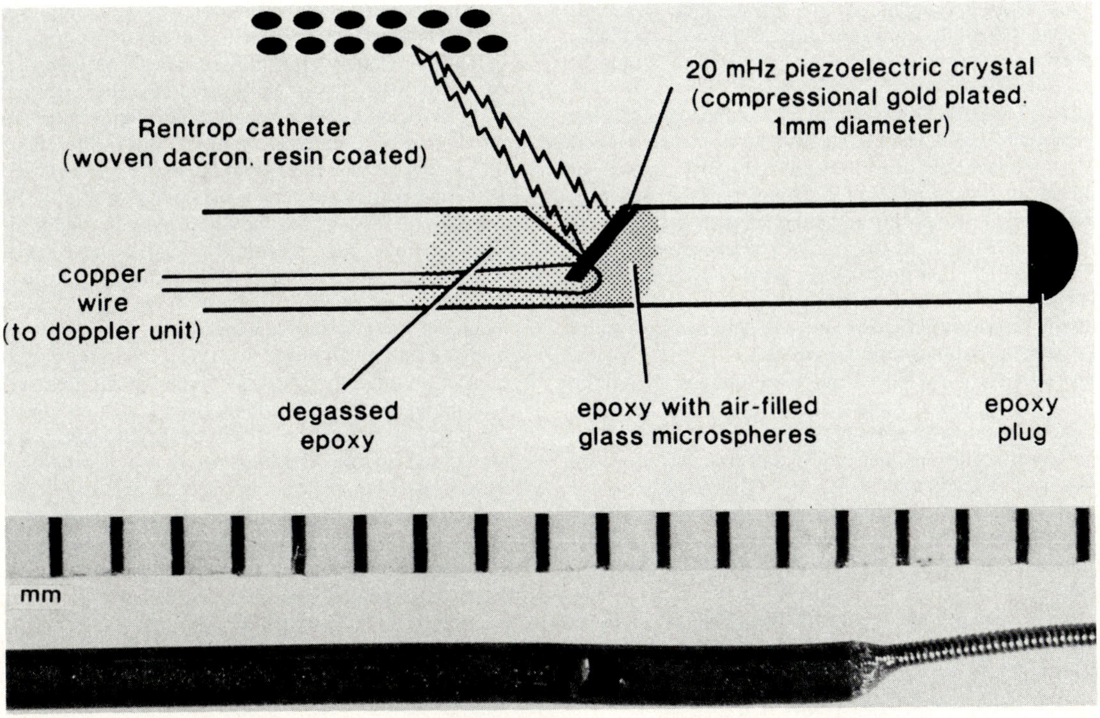

FIGURE 1. *Top*, Schematic diagram of the distal portion of the coronary Doppler catheter. The copper wires attached to the piezoelectric crystal exit from the proximal end of the catheter and are connected to a pulsed Doppler meter. *Bottom*, Photograph of the distal 3 cm of the catheter. A very flexible coiled wire has been attached to the tip to enhance safety in human studies.

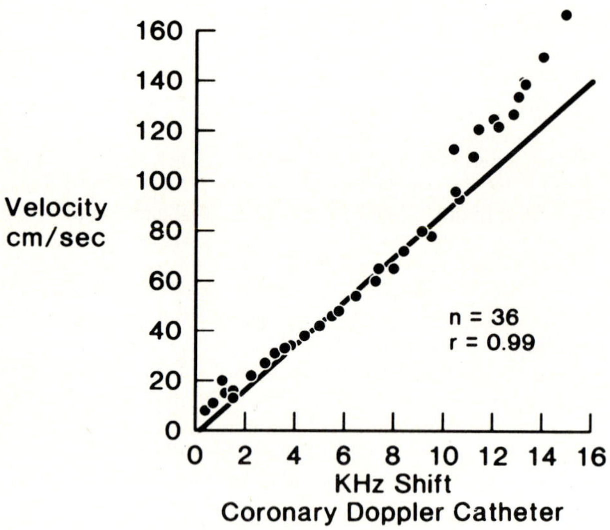

FIGURE 2. Validation of the coronary Doppler catheter in vitro in a rigid tube system with a flowing starch-water mixture. Changes in the Doppler frequency shift (kHz), assessed with the coronary Doppler catheter, were highly correlated with changes in mean tube flow velocities of up to 100 cm/sec.

internal carotid artery and positioned at the ostium of the left main coronary artery. Heparin sodium (15,000 units) was given intravenously. Under fluoroscopy, the coronary Doppler catheter was passed into the left anterior descending or circumflex coronary artery. The catheter position and range control were adjusted to obtain an audio signal of phasic CBFV. An acceptable phasic signal had the following qualities: the systolic signal was less than 25% of the diastolic signal, the CBFV in early systole approximated 0, the mean flow velocity with the artery occluded proximal to the catheter tip approximated 0, and the audio signal did not contain phasic low-frequency sounds caused by reflection of the ultrasonic pulse from the vessel wall. In all experiments the range control was adjusted to obtain the maximal frequency shift.

An epicardial suction Doppler probe[7] was then placed over the same coronary vessel distal to the catheter tip. Its signal was adjusted in a manner similar to the catheter signal. In each of three animals an epicardial suction Doppler probe was also placed over an artery in a perfusion field separate from the artery containing the catheter. Changes in CBFV measured with these epicardial suction Doppler probes have previously been shown to correlate highly with changes in myocardial perfusion measured with microspheres, timed volume collections of coronary sinus flow, and electromagnetic flowmeters.[7]

Alterations in coronary blood flow were produced by three methods. First, with use of a snare placed around the left main coronary artery, reactive hyperemic responses were obtained by 5 to 40 sec vessel occlusions. Second, global coronary flow was altered pharmacologically with adenosine (1 to 6 μM/kg/min iv) and epinephrine (0 to 3 μg/kg/min). Finally, hemorrhagic hypotension and the severe anemia following massive volume replacement with normal saline were also used to change coronary blood flow.

We compared results obtained with the coronary Doppler catheter with those by two standard techniques: measurement of CBFV with an epicardial Doppler probe and volumetric measurements of coronary sinus flow. If, during an experiment, the phasic CBFV signal from the catheter failed to meet criteria for an acceptable signal, the data collection was interrupted, the catheter was repositioned, and measurements resumed.

We assessed the extent and physiologic significance of flow obstruction resulting from the presence of the catheter in the vessel by two methods. First, using the epicardial Doppler probe, the maximal reactive hyperemic response with the catheter in the vessel was compared with that after removal of the catheter. Second, using pharmacologically induced global changes in CBFV, we compared simultaneous measurements of the change in blood flow velocity obtained with the epicardial Doppler probe and the Doppler catheter placed in separate perfusion fields.

Safety studies

Studies in vitro. Electrical isolation of the coronary Doppler catheter was evaluated by immersing the tip of the catheter in a beaker of saline and measuring the impedance between each lead and the saline. In the 10 catheters tested, the impedance was infinity.

Studies in vivo. To determine if the catheter produced changes in endothelial permeability, six calves (40 to 60 kg) were prepared in a manner similar to that described above. The coronary Doppler catheter was passed through the introducer into the mid left anterior descending or circumflex coronary artery with fluoroscopic guidance. Adjustments in catheter position were made and the catheter was left in the artery for 30 min. The catheter was withdrawn from the artery and inspected microscopically for thrombus. Evans blue dye (100 to 150 mg/kg) was then infused intravenously over 10 to 20 min. Thirty minutes after infusion of the dye, the animal was killed with intravenous KCl. The chest was opened and the heart removed. The epicardial coronary arteries were bluntly dissected from the heart, opened by a longitudinal incision, and carefully inspected for evidence of thrombus or staining. Sections were taken from any stained portion of the artery and also from arteries that had not come into contact with the catheter. Seven micron sections from these vascular segments were stained with hematoxylin and eosin or toluidine blue and microscopically examined for evidence of endothelial erosion by an observer blinded to the source of the sample.

Studies in dogs instrumented over the long term. We measured subselective coronary vasodilator reserve in many patients immediately after they received ergonovine maleate. To determine whether ergonovine maleate alters resting blood flow velocity or maximal coronary vasodilation after dipyridamole infusion, we studied five mongrel dogs (18 to 22 kg in weight) previously instrumented over the long term with indwelling left atrial and aortic catheters, a pneumatic arterial occluder placed circumferentially about the circumflex coronary artery, and a Doppler flow probe placed proximal to the occluder.

The animals were brought to the laboratory in an awake state. Recordings of the aortic pressure, heart rate, and phasic and mean circumflex flow velocity were obtained at rest. Arterial pressure and mean blood flow velocity were recorded during a 20 sec circumflex occlusion. Three 0.1 mg boluses of ergonovine maleate were infused into the left atrium. One minute after the final ergonovine bolus, the circumflex artery was occluded for 20 sec and the resultant reactive hyperemic response was measured. After a 2 min recovery, dipyridamole (0.56 mg/kg) was infused into the left atrium of each animal over 4 min and the increase in blood flow velocity was recorded. Ten minutes after the completion of the infusion, the 20 sec coronary occlusion was repeated and the reactive hyperemic response was measured.

The following day, animals were returned to the laboratory. The hyperemic response following a 20 sec circumflex occlusion was again recorded. After a 2 min recovery time, dipyridamole was infused as above. Ten minutes after completion of the infusion the 20 sec vessel occlusion was repeated.

An index of coronary resistance was calculated for each intervention as the quotient of (mean aortic pressure at peak flow/

peak blood flow velocity) and (resting aortic pressure/resting blood flow velocity).

Studies in humans. We studied 70 patients with the coronary Doppler catheter. All patients underwent cardiac catheterization and coronary angiography for the diagnosis of chest pain syndromes. In this article we report the measurement of coronary vasodilator reserve in 10 patients with angiographically normal or minimally stenosed (<25% luminal diameter narrowing) coronary vessels. A separate informed consent form for the Doppler studies was obtained from each patient. All clinical studies were approved by the Human Use Committee of the University of Iowa.

Patients were brought to the catheterization laboratory in a fasting state. Although a variety of sedatives were administered (table 1), no patient received atropine. After local anesthesia with 1% lidocaine, diagnostic coronary angiography was performed. After completion of the diagnostic catheterization, a Judkins No. 8F guiding catheter (United States Catheter and Instrument Co.) was positioned in the right or left coronary ostium of each patient. Heparin sodium (5 to 10,000 units iv) was given before intracoronary catheterization to increase the activated clotting time to at least twice control. The coronary Doppler catheter was passed through the guiding catheter into the coronary artery. The catheter position and Doppler meter range control were adjusted to obtain a good audio signal and phasic tracing of maximal resting CBFV. The catheter position and Doppler meter settings were not varied between measurements.

Measurement of vasodilator reserve. To assess vasodilator reserve, we measured changes in CBFV after intracoronary administration of meglumine diatrizoate and an intravenous infusion of dipyridamole. After baseline recordings of phasic and mean CBFV, 2 to 6 ml of meglumine diatrizoate was injected through the guiding catheter into the coronary ostium. The resultant changes in blood flow velocity were continuously recorded. After flow velocity returned to its baseline value, 0.56 mg/kg of dipyridamole was infused over 4 min by an infusion pump into the femoral vein. Recordings were continued until the increase in mean flow velocity appeared stable. In two patients, an additional dose of dipyridamole (0.4 mg/kg and 0.28 mg/kg) was given after the increase in mean flow velocity appeared stable for several minutes.

In six patients, arterial pressure was continuously recorded from the guiding catheter. Only mean arterial pressure could be accurately measured because of the marked damping of phasic pressure by the presence of the coronary Doppler catheter within

TABLE 1
Patient characteristics

Patient	Clinical diagnosis	Electrocardiogram	Medication	Vessel studied	ΔCBFV (× resting CBFV) Meglumine diatrizoate	ΔCBFV (× resting CBFV) Dipyridamole
D. S.	Atypical chest pain; hypertension; diabetes mellitus	Normal	Dipyridamole; ergonovine; nitroglycerin	Cx	—	4.2
C. C.	Atypical chest pain; hypertension	Normal	Ergonovine; nitroglycerin	RCA	3.5	6.2
C. B.	Atypical chest pain	Normal	Ergonovine; nitroglycerin	RCA	3.3	3.8
R. W.	Atypical chest pain; hypertension	Anterior ST-T changes	Ergonovine	Cx	3.1	4.5
N. B.	Angina pectoris; hypertension	Normal	Nitroglycerin; nifedipine; hydrochlorothiazide	LAD	4.2	5.3
F. Y.	6 months post LAD PTCA; asymptomatic Graves disease	Normal	Nifedipine; propranolol; dipyridamole; aspirin; hydrochlorothiazide	LAD	—	6.0
M. C.	Atypical chest pain	Nonspecific ST-T changes	Ergonovine; nitroglycerin	LAD	2.8	4.3
C. H.	Atypical chest pain; bronchitis	1° AV block; nonspecific ST-T changes	Ergonovine; nitroglycerin	RCA	2.9	3.8
C. F.	Atypical chest pain	Normal	Dipyridamole; aspirin; secobarbital; promethazine; atropine	RCA	5.0	7.0
K. M.	Atypical chest pain	Normal	Ergonovine; nitroglycerin	Cx	3.5	4.5

ΔCBFV = change in CBFV; Cx = circumflex coronary artery; LAD = left anterior descending coronary artery; RCA = right coronary artery; AV = atrioventricular; PTCA = percutaneous transluminal coronary angioplasty.

the guiding catheter lumen. After removal of the catheter, the catheter tip was examined microscopically for the presence of adherent thrombus.

For each intervention, an index of the change in coronary resistance was calculated as described above.

Results

Animal validation studies. Paired measurements of CBFV (peak frequency shift/resting frequency shift) obtained with the coronary Doppler catheter and with an epicardial Doppler probe placed immediately distal to the catheter correlated highly (r = .95, range = 0.1 to 5.7 times resting blood flow velocity, slope = 1.04). The correlation coefficients for studies done in individual animals varied from .90 to .99.

Changes in CBFV assessed with the coronary Doppler catheter were also highly correlated with changes in volumetric coronary sinus flow over a wide range (r = .97, range = 52 to 924 ml/min, slope = 1.06; figure 3).

Assessment of coronary obstruction produced by the catheter. The extent of coronary obstruction produced by the catheter was assessed by two approaches. Maximal reactive hyperemic responses after transient vessel occlusions with the catheter present and absent in the artery under study were measured by an epicardial Doppler probe. If any significant coronary obstruction was produced by the catheter, then the maximal flow response with the catheter present in the artery should have been less than when it was removed. We found, however, that the maximal flow responses were identical (n = 9, r = .99, slope = 1.03).

When global myocardial flow was altered pharmacologically, changes in CBFV assessed by the catheter were highly correlated with simultaneous measurements of flow velocity measured using an epicardial Doppler probe placed in a separate perfusion field (r = .94, n = 17, slope = 1.04; figure 4). These findings suggest that coronary obstruction produced by the catheter was minimal and of no physiologic significance.

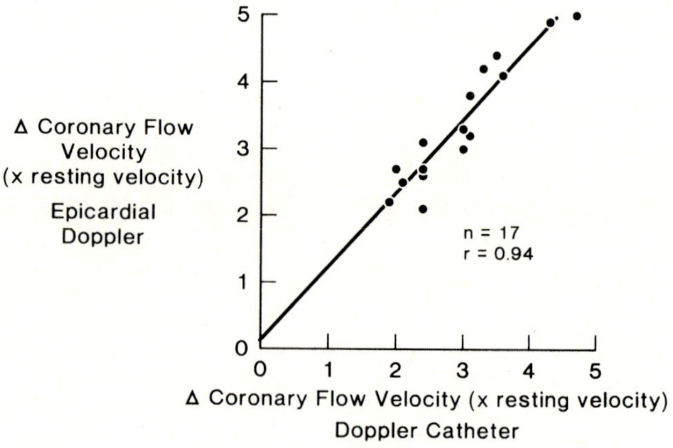

FIGURE 4. Effect of the coronary Doppler catheter on regional blood flow assessed by measuring changes in CBFV in two perfusion fields (one containing the catheter and an adjacent field with an epicardial Doppler probe). While flow was altered with systemic pharmacologic agents, changes in blood flow velocity assessed with the catheter in one field were equivalent to changes in velocity measured with an epicardial Doppler probe in an adjacent field.

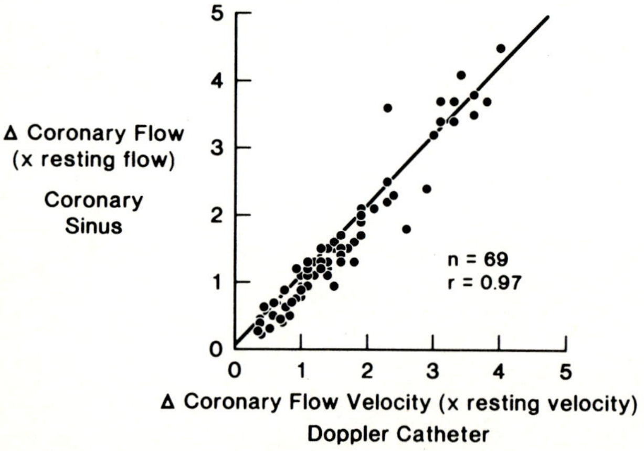

FIGURE 3. Validation of the coronary Doppler catheter in vivo with timed-volume collections of coronary sinus flow. Changes in CBFV assessed with the coronary Doppler catheter were highly correlated with simultaneously measured changes in coronary sinus blood flow over a wide range of flows.

Safety studies. We assessed the safety of this Doppler catheter system in several ways. First, we measured the amount of current leakage emanating from the catheter; we found none. Second, we looked for evidence of clot deposition in the artery or on the catheter after 30 min of intracoronary placement. We found no evidence of clot deposition in either the artery or on the catheter. Third, we looked for histologic evidence of endothelial erosion caused by the catheter. These studies revealed the endothelium to be intact without evidence of erosion. Fourth, we looked for changes in the permeability of coronary endothelium to Evans blue dye. In five of six animals, small linear streaks of endothelial staining were found in the artery containing the catheter. These streaks occurred in the proximal coronary artery and were not circumferential. The magnitude of staining was minimal compared with that seen in the aorta and coronary ostium resulting from coronary catheterization by the Seldinger technique and a Judkins diagnostic coronary catheter. These findings suggest that, although changes in endothelial permeability can be produced by the coronary Doppler catheter, the changes are minimal.

Studies in dogs instrumented over the long term. We studied five dogs instrumented over the long term to determine whether prior ergonovine administration

TABLE 2
Effect of ergonovine on vasodilator reserve

	HR (bpm)	MAP (mm Hg)	CBFV (× resting)	CVRI (× resting)
Day 1 (n = 5)				
Before ergonovine				
Rest	108±27	92±13	1.0	1.0
Reactive hyperemia	110±27	89±16	2.7±0.4	0.35±0.06
After ergonovine				
Rest	116±35	104±14	1.3±0.3	0.98±0.11[A]
Reactive hyperemia	122±24	109±17	3.2±0.7	0.38±0.06[B]
Dipyridamole	138±25	90±10	3.1±1.0	0.34±0.10[C]
Dipyridamole and reactive hyperemia	132±26	89±8	4.1±1.2	0.25±0.06[D]
Day 2 (n = 3)				
Rest	105±34	91±13	1.0	1.00
Reactive hyperemia	108±28	89±6	3.4±0.8	0.30±0.08
Dipyridamole	136±18	79±3	2.7±0.6	0.32±0.01
Dipyridamole and reactive hyperemia	135±14	75±4	3.3±0.8	0.26±0.07

All values are mean ± SEM.
HR = heart rate; MAP = mean arterial pressure; CVRI = coronary vascular resistance index.
[A]p = NS vs resting CVRI before ergonovine.
[B]p = NS vs CVRI after reactive hyperemia before ergonovine.
[C]p = NS vs CVRI after dipyridamole on day 2.
[D]p = NS vs CVRI after dipyridamole and reactive hyperemia on day 2.

might alter resting coronary flow velocity or change measurements of coronary vasodilator reserve (table 2). Resting blood flow velocity and coronary vascular resistance were unchanged after ergonovine. Similarly, vasodilator reserve, measured after transient vessel occlusion and after administration of dipyridamole, was not altered by ergonovine.

Studies in humans. Studies of 70 patients in the cardiac catheterization laboratory have shown that measurements of phasic CBFV could be readily obtained in 58 of 70 patients (figure 5). Inability to "steer" the catheter away from a small branch vessel accounted for most instances of poor signal quality. A stable signal was recorded for up to 30 min (the arbitrary length of the study). As expected, the ratio of systolic to diastolic CBFV was higher when measurements were obtained from the right coronary artery as compared with the left coronary artery (systolic/diastolic signal ratio of 0.67 ± 0.11 [±SEM] in the right coronary and 0.17 ± 0.05 in the left anterior descending coronary).

Subselective measurement of coronary vasodilator reserve in normal vessels. Intracoronary injection of meglumine diatrizoate resulted in a 3.5-fold increase in CBFV compared with control velocity (range 2.8 to 5.0 times resting blood flow velocity; figure 6). The average time from onset of injection to peak change in flow velocity was 17 sec (range 12 to 22 sec). Flow velocity returned to baseline within a mean of 50 sec (range 39 to 69 sec). The peak flow responses did not significantly vary with the coronary vessel studied.

Intravenous dipyridamole resulted in an average fivefold increase in resting flow velocity (range 3.8 to 7.0 times resting velocity; figure 7). Similarly, the coronary resistance index fell to 17% of baseline resistance (range 0.10 to 0.22 times resting coronary resistance index). In each patient, dipyridamole produced a greater rise in blood flow velocity and a greater fall in resistance than did meglumine diatrizoate.

Figure 8 depicts the time course of the change in

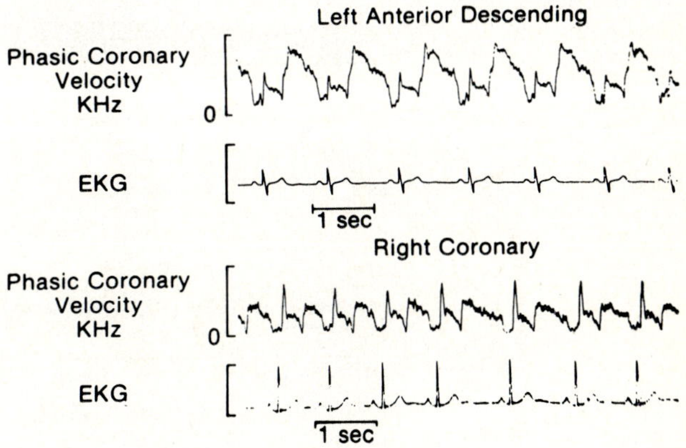

FIGURE 5. Phasic CBFV recordings obtained from two human subjects studied in the cardiac catheterization laboratory. *Top,* Left anterior descending artery; *bottom,* mid right coronary artery.

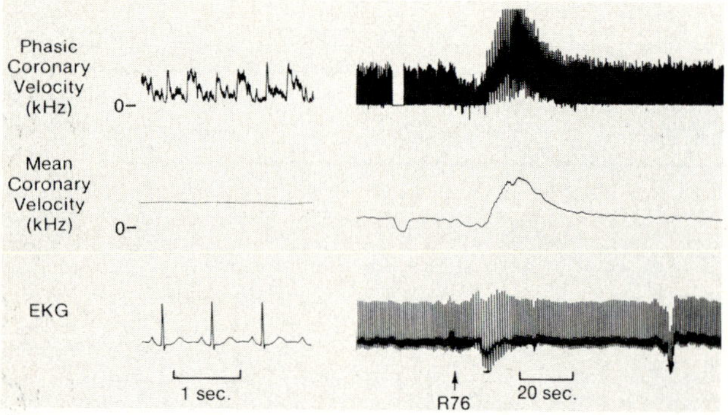

FIGURE 6. Effect of intracoronary injection of meglumine diatrizoate (3 ml) into the right coronary artery. *Top*, Phasic blood flow velocity; *middle*, mean blood flow velocity; *bottom*, electrocardiogram. After injection of meglumine diatrizoate, blood flow velocity rose to 3.5 times resting velocity.

flow velocity in each patient after infusion of dipyridamole. Although the mean time from onset of infusion to peak flow velocity was 6.5 min, the temporal course of the response was variable (range 2.5 to 8.7 min). Furthermore, at the end of the 4 min infusion, average mean flow velocity had increased to only 67% of the eventual peak velocity.

In nine of 10 patients, 0.56 mg/kg of dipyridamole increased CBFV to more than 3.8 times resting velocity. In one patient, however, 0.56 mg/kg dipyridamole increased flow velocity to only 2.3 times resting velocity. An additional 0.4 mg/kg of dipyridamole further increased flow velocity to 4.2 times resting velocity (figure 9). Thus, the conventional dose of dipyridamole did not produce maximal vasodilation in all patients.

Safety. Sixty-nine of 70 patients underwent subselective coronary catheterization and flow velocity measurement without adverse effects. One patient had abrupt occlusion of the left anterior descending coronary artery during flow velocity measurements. The occlusion was unresponsive to intracoronary streptokinase and balloon angioplasty. The patient had a history of chest pain suggestive of myocardial ischemia and a normal coronary angiogram. An ergonovine test to exclude vasospasm was not performed before the flow study. After coronary occlusion the catheter was immediately withdrawn and microscopically examined for adherent thrombus. None was found. The angiogram did not suggest dissection and the distal vessel was normal. The patient underwent emergency coronary artery bypass surgery. At surgery no visible changes in the arterial wall were observed. Although the patient sustained an anterior myocardial infarction, he recovered from surgery and at present is asymptomatic.

Discussion

In animal studies, we have shown that a No. 3F coronary Doppler catheter can accurately measure instantaneous changes in phasic CBFV in individual coronary arteries without producing physiologically significant coronary obstruction. In subsequent studies in awake patients, we have shown that phasic flow velocity and coronary vasodilator reserve can be measured at the time of cardiac catheterization. We have also demonstrated that dipyridamole produces a greater fall in coronary vascular resistance than does meglumine diatrizoate. More importantly, we have characterized the temporal characteristics of the coronary dilative responses to meglumine diatrizoate and dipyridamole in man.

Our No. 3F coronary Doppler catheter offers several advantages over existing methods of measuring CBFV. First, use of the Doppler technique permits continuous on-line recording of instantaneous phasic

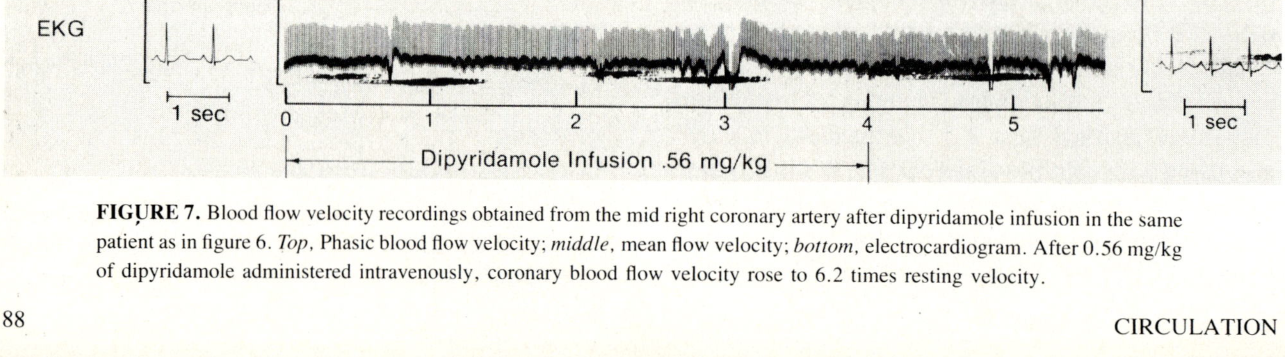

FIGURE 7. Blood flow velocity recordings obtained from the mid right coronary artery after dipyridamole infusion in the same patient as in figure 6. *Top*, Phasic blood flow velocity; *middle*, mean flow velocity; *bottom*, electrocardiogram. After 0.56 mg/kg of dipyridamole administered intravenously, coronary blood flow velocity rose to 6.2 times resting velocity.

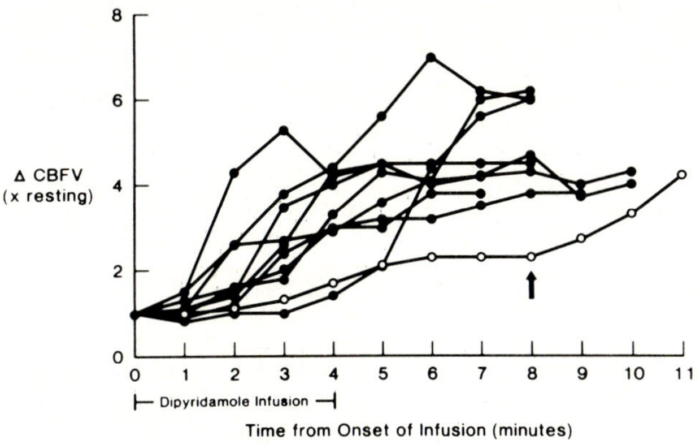

FIGURE 8. Time course of the change in blood flow velocity in each patient after infusion of dipyridamole. ↑ = additional 0.4 mg/kg dipyridamole infusion in a patient in whom maximal vasodilation did not occur after the initial infusion.

flow velocity. Consequently, transient changes in CBFV in response to neural or humoral stimuli can be readily measured. Second, because of its small diameter, the No. 3F coronary Doppler catheter can measure phasic flow velocity in individual coronary vessels well beyond the left main coronary artery without obstructing maximal coronary blood flow. Previous Doppler catheters have been unable to reproducibly measure flow beyond the coronary ostium without producing significant coronary obstruction. As a consequence, studies in patients with obstructions in the left anterior descending or circumflex coronary arteries were difficult to interpret. Third, signal stability over time has been improved.

The subselective pulsed Doppler coronary catheter methodology has several potential limitations. Movement of the catheter within the vessel could change the angle of the piezoelectric crystal relative to flow, thus artifactually changing the measured CBFV. When the quality of the phasic tracing remained intact, however, we found that changes in flow velocity correlated directly with coronary sinus flow. Since pulsed Doppler methodology measures flow velocity in only a small portion of the stream, movement of the catheter with myocardial contraction could change the sample window over the cardiac cycle. Previous studies, however, have shown that the velocity profile in the proximal coronary arteries is parabolic.[10, 11] Thus, small changes in the sample window could not be expected to result in significantly different velocity measurements unless the sample window was immediately adjacent to the vessel wall. In our validation studies, wall movement was easily recognized by a characteristic audio signal. The catheter might also change the blood flow velocity profile of the stream, producing velocities that may not linearly follow CBFV. Results of our study in normal vessels, however, confirm that changes in the maximal flow velocity in the stream parallel changes in both coronary sinus flow and CBFV measured in a vessel not containing the catheter. It is possible, however, that diffuse vascular disease could change the relationship between maximal flow velocity and mean flow velocity.

Changes in vessel caliber during interventions might alter the linear relationship between velocity and flow. In particular, large epicardial coronary vessels could dilate in direct response to agents producing vasodilation or to ascending dilation resulting from the increased coronary flow produced by vasodilation. Studies by Hintze and Vatner[12] in awake dogs suggest that the magnitude of large coronary dilation produced by dipyridamole (arterial cross-sectional area increased by 28%) might significantly alter the flow:flow velocity relationship. However, our studies and those by Marcus et al.[7] have shown a good correlation between maximal flow velocity and flow even at high flow rates. Other studies in animals and man suggest that dipyridamole produces only minor changes in large vessel size.[13, 14] Brown et al.[13] found that dipyridamole increased arterial cross-sectional area by only 4% in patients. Nonetheless, to compensate for changes in vessel size, arterial cross-sectional area could be measured with quantitative coronary angiography so that a relationship between flow velocity and flow could be determined.[15]

Another theoretical problem is that the catheter itself could cause partial coronary obstruction and result in distal arteriolar vasodilation. We showed that this does not occur in an animal with coronary vessels of slightly smaller diameter than those of an adult human with normal coronary vessels. Calculation of the magnitude of obstruction likely to be produced by the catheter in

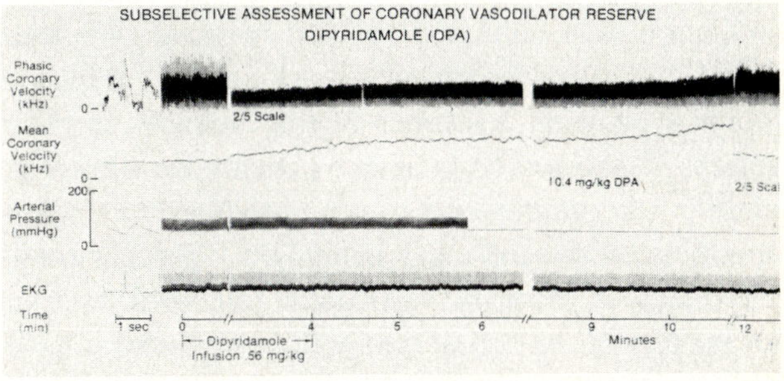

FIGURE 9. Recording of CBFV obtained from the circumflex coronary artery in a patient who did not achieve maximal vasodilation after a 0.56 mg/kg dipyridamole infusion. The *top* two panels show phasic and mean coronary blood flow velocity; the *bottom* panel displays the electrocardiogram. After a 0.56 mg/kg dipyridamole (DPA) infusion, blood flow velocity rose to 2.3 times resting flow velocity and remained stable. Another 0.4 mg/kg infused at 8.5 min increased flow velocity to 4.2 times resting flow velocity.

humans similarly suggested that significant obstruction would not result from the presence of the catheter in the proximal or middle portion of normal major epicardial coronary arteries. The cross-sectional area of the distal catheter (less than 0.8 mm^2) is less than 7% of the cross-sectional area of a normal human proximal left anterior descending artery and less than 22% of the area of a normal left anterior descending artery in its mid course.[16] Since maximal coronary blood flow is not diminished until at least 36 ± 10% luminal area narrowing is present,[17] physiologically significant coronary obstruction in normal human coronary arteries is unlikely. However, if diffuse luminal narrowing were present, then the additional obstruction produced by the catheter could restrict maximal flow. Determination of the cross-sectional area of the artery containing the catheter would provide a means of estimating the likelihood of flow restriction by the catheter in diffusely narrowed vessels.

Measurement of coronary vasodilator reserve. Measurement of vasodilator reserve with the coronary Doppler catheter has many advantages over currently available techniques. Unlike coronary sinus thermodilution or the inert gas methods, the coronary Doppler catheter can measure vasodilator reserve in individual coronary vessels. This subselective measurement of reserve is essential in measuring the impairment in flow reserve caused by an individual coronary stenosis. Another advantage, the ability to measure instantaneous changes in blood flow velocity, enables investigation of the time-response characteristics of a variety of agents used to unmask vasodilator reserve in man. This information should enhance the use of these drugs in noninvasive testing, in which time to maximal drug response and dosing must be approximated.

Our study confirms previous reports in animals and man that dipyridamole produces greater coronary vasodilation than iodinated contrast material. We also found that dipyridamole increased coronary flow velocity to at least 3.8 times resting velocity in each patient. These results in awake patients are similar to those in other studies of coronary vasodilator reserve in anesthetized patients[7] and animals.[17, 18] Recent measurements of coronary vasodilator reserve in normal awake patients by digital subtraction angiography have found only a 1.9-fold increase in flow after intracoronary administration of radiographic contrast material.[19, 20] This small rise in flow is inconsistent with that observed in studies in animals and our studies in patients. Several methodologic problems may account for these inconsistencies. Since the time at which peak flow is measured must be approximated with the digital subtraction method, peak flow velocity could be missed. Furthermore, the time required for measurement of flow (several seconds) reduces the frequency response of the system, potentially underestimating the effects of short-acting vasodilators. Finally, methodologic problems related to contrast injection and streaming may impair measurements of high coronary flows with currently available digital subtraction angiographic methods.

Many investigators have assumed that dipyridamole produces maximal coronary vasodilation in a predictable fashion.[21–23] Noninvasive studies with dipyridamole (e.g., ^{201}Tl-dipyridamole scintigraphy) are based on the premise that near maximal vasodilation will occur in all patients after a single dose of dipyridamole. We found, however, that the response to dipyridamole varied among patients (figure 8). On average, more than 2 min elapsed from the completion of the drug infusion into the femoral vein until 90% of the eventual peak/flow velocity was reached. In three of 10 patients, 90% of the eventual peak/resting flow velocity was not reached for 3 min after completion of the infusion. One of our patients had only a 2.3-fold rise in resting velocity after 0.56 mg/kg of dipyridamole. After an additional 0.4 mg/kg infusion of dipyridamole, flow velocity rose an additional 170% to 4.2 times control velocity. This heterogeneity in the response to dipyridamole underscores the advantage of instantaneous on-line measurements of blood flow velocity in measuring vasodilator reserve in man.

Several potential problems are inherent in this method of measuring vasodilator reserve. They include changes in resting blood flow velocity, changes in arterial pressure between measurements, prolonged effects of vasodilator agents, concomitant exposure to drugs that may effect vasodilator reserve, and, as previously discussed, dilation of large coronary vessels. First, since a ratio of peak to resting flow velocity is measured, an elevated resting velocity could falsely suggest a diminished vasodilator reserve. This is unlikely, however, in the absence of conditions that increase myocardial oxygen demand (e.g., tachycardia, hypertension, thyrotoxicosis) or diseases associated with high resting flow rates (e.g., severe anemia).[24–27] Second, changes in arterial pressure between measurements of resting and peak velocities could change the ratio of peak to resting flow. Calculation of an index of resistance can compensate for the changes in coronary perfusion pressure and better reflect the true change in coronary resistance.

Third, the prolonged increase in coronary flow after infusion of dipyridamole makes repeat measurements or studies of other vessels during the same procedure impossible. This represents a major disadvantage to the routine use of dipyridamole in measuring coronary vasodilator reserve. Use of other agents with shorter lasting effects, such as papaverine, may be more advantageous. The time- and dose-response characteristics of any potential agent, however, will need to be thoroughly studied in man before it can be used routinely.

Fourth, many of the patients we studied had immediate prior exposure to ergonovine. Theoretically, ergonovine could have altered resting flow or limited maximal vasodilation. Our studies in dogs instrumented over the long term, however, show that ergonovine does not change the maximal vasodilator response to dipyridamole or resting flow.

Safety considerations. There are several potential dangers when this Doppler catheter is used to measure CBFV. First, the catheter could act as a stimulus for clot formation. In animal and human studies we found no evidence of clot formation in the artery containing the catheter or on the catheter itself. Second, the catheter could cause serious endothelial injury. By light microscopy, we found no evidence of endothelial injury in arteries containing the catheter. We did find that the catheter produced a change in endothelial permeability in small areas of the coronary artery containing the catheter. Previous studies by others and in our laboratory have shown that the technique we used (endothelial staining with Evans blue dye) is a very sensitive technique in detecting even minor changes in endothelial permeability[28] and that endothelium disruption need not be present to produce a change in endothelial permeability to the dye.

A third potential problem is that the catheter could cause coronary vasospasm or dissection. Prior experience has demonstrated that intracoronary cannulation very infrequently results in vasospasm or dissection of angiographically normal vessels.[29] Nevertheless, one patient of the 70 patients we have studied developed coronary occlusion at a site where the catheter was present and required emergency coronary bypass surgery. We presume this was related to vasospasm, as opposed to dissection or thrombosis. To minimize the likelihood of this complication in future studies, the possibility of coronary vasospasm should be excluded before intracoronary cannulation in all patients without significant obstructive coronary artery disease. The need for excellent radiographic visualization and an operator experienced in techniques of subselective coronary catheterization is self evident. The incidence of coronary occlusion in standard catheterization laboratory procedures varies from 0.25% with routine coronary angiography to 3% to 8% during coronary angioplasty.[29, 30] Additional experience with the coronary Doppler catheter will need to be obtained to determine if the complication rate we observed (1.3%) is reflective of the true incidence of complications resulting from this procedure.

Future applications. Measurements of CBFV in individual coronary vessels of conscious humans should facilitate studies of the coronary circulation in man. We anticipate that use of this coronary Doppler catheter system will enable direct measurement of coronary vasodilator reserve and permit characterization of the physiologic significance of coronary artery stenoses during routine coronary angiography. Furthermore, instantaneous on-line coronary flow velocity recordings should be of great value in studying neural and humoral control of the coronary circulation.[31]

We wish to thank Tom Drews, B.S., B.M.E., Tim Schurman, B.S., and Mark Coppess, B.S., for their work on the Doppler catheter system, and Jill Christy for her enduring secretarial assistance.

Appendix

Doppler catheter construction. Two insulated copper wires (38 G) were passed through the length of the catheter and brought out through a V-shaped notch cut into the catheter wall 7 to 10 mm from the catheter tip (figure 1). To give the terminal ends of the two conductors more flexibility, the distal ends of these wires were tinned and soldered to a 1 cm length of 48-gauge insulated gold-plated copper wire. These short wires were then pulse-dot soldered to either side of a 0.7 to 1.0 mm × 0.7 to 1.0 mm fine-ground compressional piezoelectric 20 mHz crystal that was gold-plated on either side (Valpey-Fischer, Inc.). The back of the crystal was coated with an 180 degree lens of epoxy (No. 795-Hy-Sol) mixed with air-filled glass beads (FT 102, Emerson and Cumings). The beads provided insulation so that the ultrasound pulse was unidirectional. The crystal assembly was pulled into the notch in the catheter wall and placed at a 30 to 45 degree angle to the long axis of the lumen so that the insulated side of the crystal faced toward the tip of the catheter. Using this configuration, the ultrasonic pulse was projected at a 30 to 45 degree angle toward the proximal portion of the catheter. A lens of vacuum-degassed epoxy was placed about both sides of the crystal to fill the unoccupied space within the notch of the catheter. An epoxy plug (No. 795-Hy-Sol) was placed into the tip of the catheter lumen. To harden the epoxy, the distal end of the catheter was heated to 70° C for 30 min. The rough edges of the crystal were then filed and polished so that the catheter profile was similar to its "native" state.

To provide greater flexibility for human studies, we attached a 15 mm flexible guidewire 0.016 inch in diameter (United States Catheter and Instrument Co., angioplasty spring guide tip) to the catheter tip.

Doppler meter. The pulsed Doppler meter is a modification of a circuit described by Hartley[9] and has been described in detail elsewhere.[7] Briefly, a 20 MHz carrier frequency is provided by a crystal-controlled oscillator. A digital integrated circuit divides the basic frequency by 320 to produce a pulse repetition frequency of 62.5 kHz. A gate of 0.8 msec duration passes 16 cycles of 20 MHz to the transmitter, which amplifies the signal and couples it to a transducer. Energy returning to the transmitter is detected, amplified by the receiver, and passed to a dual-face detector. There, two reference signals locked to the transmitted frequency and separated in phase by 90 degrees are compared with the returning signal. During each 16 msec receiver cycle, the phase difference between the received and transmitted signals is converted to a voltage. The time during each received cycle at which this voltage is sampled is variable. By adjusting the range control the operator can move the sample window over a distance of 1 to 10 mm from the crystal face. Sample and hold circuits are used to extract the Doppler audiosignal from the phase detector outputs. The signals are then filtered to remove the pulse repetition frequency component. Thereafter the audio signals are passed to a dual-polarity frequency-to-voltage converter that is phase sensitive. The output of the converter, a voltage corresponding to the instantaneous velocity, is displayed on a strip-chart recorder. The audiosignal is amplified and fed to a speaker. The audiosignal is used to initially position the catheter.

References

1. Kochsiek K, Cott L, Tauchert M, Neubaur J, Larbig D: Measurement of coronary blood flow in various conditions using the argon technique. *In* Kaltenbach M, Lichtlen P, editors: Coronary heart disease. 1970, London, Thieme, p 137
2. Klocke FJ, Bunnell IL, Greene DG, Wittenberg SM, Visco JP: Average coronary blood flow per unit weight in patients with and without coronary artery disease. Circulation **50:** 547, 1974
3. Klocke FJ: Measurements of coronary blood flow and degree of stenosis: Current clinical implications and continuing uncertainties. J Am Coll Cardiol **1:** 31, 1983
4. Holman BL: Measuring regional myocardial blood flow with 133 Xe and the Anger camera. Radiology **112:** 99, 1974
5. Engel HJ: Assessment of regional myocardial blood flow by precordial 133 xenon clearance technique. *In* Schaper W, editor: The pathophysiology of myocardial perfusion. Amsterdam, 1979, Elsevier/North Holland Biomedical Press, p 58
6. Mathey DG, Chatterjee K, Tyberg JV, Likven J, Bruntage B, Parmley WW: Coronary sinus reflux: a source of error in the measurement of thermodilution coronary sinus flow. Circulation **57:** 778, 1978
7. Marcus ML, Wright C, Doty D, Eastham C, Laughlin D, Krumm P, Fastenow C, Brody M: Measurements of coronary velocity and reactive hyperemia in the coronary circulation of humans. Circ Res **49:** 877, 1981
8. Cole JS, Hartley CJ: The pulsed Doppler coronary artery catheter; preliminary report of a new technique for measuring rapid changes in coronary artery flow velocity in man. Circulation **56:** 18, 1977
9. Hartley CJ, Cole JS: An ultrasonic pulsed Doppler system for measuring blood flow in small vessels. J Appl Physiol **37:** 626, 1974
10. Nerem RM, Rumberger JA, Gross DR, Muir WW, Geiger GL: Hot film coronary artery velocity measurements in horses. Cardiovasc Res **10:** 301, 1976
11. Wells MK, Winter DC, Nelson AW, McCarthy TC: Blood velocity patterns in coronary arteries. Transactions of the ASME. J Mech Engin, 1977, p 26
12. Hintze TH, Vatner SF: Dipyridamole dilates large coronary arteries in conscious dogs. Circulation **68:** 1321, 1983
13. Brown BG, Josephson MA, Petersen RB, Pierce CD, Wong M, Hecht HS, Bolson E, Dodge HT: Intravenous dipyridamole combined with isometric handgrip for near maximal acute increase in coronary flow in patients with coronary artery disease. Am J Cardiol **48:** 1077, 1981
14. Noguchi K, Tomoike H, Ootsubo H, Sakai K, Nakamura M: Difference in the site and time course of coronary dilating effects of Trapidil, Nitroglycerin and Dipyridamole in anesthetized dogs. J Pharmacol Exp Ther **219:** 809, 1981
15. Brown BG, Bolson E, Frimer M, Dodge HT: Quantitative coronary angiography. Estimation of dimensions, hemodynamic resistance, and atheroma mass of coronary artery lesions using the arteriograms and digital computation. Circulation **55:** 329, 1977
16. Vieweg WVR, Alpert JS, Hagan AD: Caliber and distribution of normal coronary arterial anatomy. Cathet Cardiovasc Diagn **2:** 269, 1976
17. Folts JD, Gallagher K, Rowe GG: Hemodynamic effects of controlled degrees of coronary artery stenosis in short-term and long-term studies in dogs. J Thorac Cardiovasc Surg **73:** 722, 1977
18. Gould KL, Lipscomb K, Hamilton GW: Physiologic basis for assessing critical coronary stenosis. Am J Cardiol **33:** 87, 1974
19. O'Neill W, Vogel R, Lefvee M, Bates E, Kirlin P, Beauman G, Pitt B: Digital coronary radiographic assessment of relative regional coronary blood flow. Circulation **66**(suppl II): II-229, 1982
20. Averon F, Gruentzig A, Vogel MA, King S, Douglas J, Meier B, O'Neill WW, Bates E, LeFree M: Effects of successful percutaneous transluminal coronary angioplasty (PTCA) on acute and chronic coronary flow reserve. Circulation **68**(suppl III): III-31, 1983
21. Opherk D, Mall G, Zebe H, Schwarz F, Weihe E, Manthey J, Kubler W: Reduction of coronary reserve: a mechanism for angina pectoris in patients with arterial hypertension and normal coronary arteries. Circulation **69:** 1, 1984
22. Opherk D, Schwarz F, Mall G, Manthey J, Buller D, Kubler W: Coronary dilator capacity in idiopathic dilated cardiomyopathy: analysis of 16 patients. Am J Cardiol **51:** 1657, 1983
23. Leppo J, Boucher C, Okada RD, Newell JB, Strauss HW, Pohost GM: Serial thallium-201 myocardial imaging after dipyridamole infusion: diagnostic utility in detecting coronary stenoses and relationship to regional wall motion. Circulation **66:** 649, 1982
24. Strauer B: Ventricular function and coronary hemodynamics in hypertensive heart disease. Am J Cardiol **44:** 999, 1979
25. Rubio R, Berne RM: Regulation of coronary blood flow. Prog Cardiovasc Dis **18:** 105, 1975
26. Rowe GG, Huston JH, Weinstein AB, Tuchman H, Brown JF, Crumpton CW: The hemodynamics of thyrotoxicosis in man with special reference to coronary blood flow and myocardial oxygen metabolism. J Clin Invest **35:** 272, 1956
27. von Restorff W, Hofling B, Holtz J, Bassenge E: Effect of increased blood fluidity through hemodilution on coronary circulation at rest and during exercise in dogs. Pflugers Arch **357:** 15, 1975
28. Stemerman MB, Spaet TH, Pitlick F, Cintron J, Lejnieks I, Tiell ML: Intimal healing: the pattern of re-endothelialization and intimal thickening. Am J Pathol **87:** 125, 1977
29. Dorros G, Cowley MJ, Simpson J, Bentvoglio LG, Block PC, Bourassa M, Detre K, Gosselin AJ, Gruntzig AR, Kelsey SF, Kent KM, Mock MB, Mullin SM, Myler RK, Passamani ER, Stertzer SH, Williams DO: Percutaneous transluminal angioplasty: Report of complications from the National Heart, Lung and Blood Institute PTCA Registry. Circulation **67:** 723, 1983
30. Davis K, Kennedy JW, Kemp HG, Judkins MP, Gosselin AJ, Killip T: Complications of coronary arteriography from the collaborative study of coronary artery surgery (CASS). Circulation **59:** 1105, 1979
31. Wilson RF, Marcus ML, Laughlin DE, Hartley CJ, White CW: The pulmonary inflation reflex: Its physiologic significance in conscious humans. Fed Proc **43:** 1003, 1984 (abst)

The ratio of plasma high-density lipoprotein cholesterol to total and low-density lipoprotein cholesterol: age-related changes and race and sex differences in selected North American populations

The Lipid Research Clinics Program Prevalence Study*

MANFRED S. GREEN, M.D., PH.D., GERARDO HEISS, M.D., PH.D., BASIL M. RIFKIND, M.D., GERALD R. COOPER, M.D., PH.D., O. DALE WILLIAMS, PH.D., AND H. A. TYROLER, M.D.

ABSTRACT The distribution of the ratios of plasma high-density lipoprotein cholesterol (HDL-C) to total cholesterol (TC) and of HDL-C to low-density lipoprotein cholesterol (LDL-C) are presented for 6900 white and 495 black examinees greater than 4 years old. Measurements were obtained during the visit 2 survey of the Lipid Research Clinics (LRC) Program Prevalence Study, and correspond to a 15% random sample of 60,502 participants screened during the LRC visit 1 survey. Age-specific means, medians, and selected percentiles are given by sex and by gonadal hormone use in white women. Apparent in these cross-sectional data was a consistent age-related decline in the ratio of HDL-C to TC for white male participants, from a mean of 0.360 in the age group 5 to 9 to a mean of 0.211 in the age group 50 to 54. Thereafter the mean ratio increased slightly. In white women not using gonadal hormones the age-related decline in the ratio was only evident starting at the age group 35 to 39, from which it declines from 0.329 to 0.258 in the age group 55 to 59. White women using gonadal hormones showed very minor age-related changes in the HDL-C/TC ratio, varying around a mean of 0.300. The number of blacks examined was low and thus the racial comparisons must be interpreted with caution. For each gender, age-related trends were similar in black and white study participants. Black men, however, had a higher percentage of TC carried as HDL-C than white men in all age groups examined. Black women had a higher percentage of TC in HDL-C than white women only below age 20; in the adult age range no appreciable differences were seen. Pearson correlation coefficients between the lipid, lipoprotein, and lipoprotein ratios are presented. The ratio HDL-C/TC correlated highly with the ratio HDL-C/LDL-C (greater than 0.92 for all groups) and the former may be a more conveniently determined surrogate for the latter. Although not exhaustive regarding the information it conveys about a lipid pattern, the ratio HDL-C/TC has the advantage of summarizing complex associations into a single numerical approximation.

Circulation 72, No. 1, 93–104, 1985.

SINCE the late 1940s considerable epidemiologic evidence has accumulated in support of a strong association between elevated blood concentrations of total cholesterol (TC) and the subsequent development of ischemic heart disease (IHD). This association has been described as being the result largely of the atherogenic effect of the cholesterol carried in the low-density lipoprotein (LDL).[1] In 1951, Barr et al.[2] reported the results of a case-control study in which it was found that patients with IHD had lower blood concentrations of high-density lipoprotein (HDL) than healthy control subjects. This initial suggestion that the blood concentrations of the lipoprotein cholesterol fractions may be more sensitive predictors of IHD risk than the TC concentration was confirmed in 1966 when Gofman et al.[3] published the results of a cohort study with a 10 year follow-up in which lower plasma HDL cholesterol (HDL-C) levels were demonstrated among men who subsequently developed IHD.

A recent article[4] provides a comprehensive review

From the Departments of Epidemiology and Biostatistics, University of North Carolina, Chapel Hill, the Lipid Metabolism–Atherogenesis Branch, National Heart, Lung, and Blood Institute, National Institutes of Health, Bethesda, and the Clinical Chemistry Division, Centers for Disease Control, Atlanta.

Supported by NHLBI contracts NO1-HV1-2156-L, NO1-HV1-2160-L, NO1-HV2-2914-L, YO1-HV3-0010-L, NO1-HV2-2913-L, NO1-HV1-2158-L, NO1-HV1-2161-L, NO1-HV2-2915-L, NO1-HV2-2932-L, NO1-HV2-2917-L, NO1-HV1-2157-L, NO1-HV1-2243-L, NO1-HV1-2159-L, NO1-HV3-2961-L, and NO1-HV6-2941-L.

Address for correspondence: Basil M. Rifkind, M.D., Lipid Metabolism–Atherogenesis Branch, NHLBI, Federal Building, Room 401, NIH, Bethesda, MD 20205.

Received July 12, 1984; revision accepted April 11, 1985.

*Members of committees involved in this study are listed before the references.

of the various reported case-control and cohort studies designed to evaluate the association between blood concentration of HDL-C and IHD. The studies have been remarkably consistent in finding reduced blood HDL-C levels associated with increased IHD risk, and several investigators have found that the plasma concentration of HDL-C is a superior predictor of IHD risk compared with the blood TC concentration.[5, 6] Nonetheless it is clear that the use of blood HDL-C concentrations as the sole lipid parameter in assessing IHD risk excludes other potentially valuable information. The low-density lipoprotein cholesterol (LDL-C) concentration in the blood, which is highly correlated with the TC concentration,[7] has also been found in most epidemiologic studies to be strongly and positively associated with IHD risk. Furthermore, whereas the association between blood HDL-C concentration and IHD risk has been studied relatively recently, there is long-standing evidence of increased IHD risk with increasing blood TC levels, and this phenomenon has been demonstrated both within and between populations.[8]

The experimental evidence on the association between blood lipoprotein cholesterol fractions and atherosclerotic disease is also substantial. Atherosclerosis can be induced in laboratory animals by significantly increasing the serum TC.[9, 10] The Lipid Research Clinics (LRC) Coronary Primary Prevention Trial findings demonstrate that a plasma TC reduction achieved by lowering LDL-C can reduce the incidence of IHD morbidity and mortality in men with high LDL-C levels.[11] Also, an inverse relationship was found in the NHLBI Type II Coronary Intervention Study between coronary artery disease (CAD) progression and the combination of an increase in HDL-C and a decrease in LDL-C. The best predictors of changes indicative of CAD were changes in the ratios HDL-C/TC and HDL-C/LDL-C.[12]

Thus, both epidemiologic and experimental evidence tend to suggest that an index that combines the blood concentrations of HDL-C and LDL-C may adequately represent the joint contribution of the lipoproteins to IHD risk. A simple index that reflects the relative concentrations of HDL-C to LDL-C is the ratio of HDL-C to LDL-C (or the inverse). In practice, since TC is more easily measured than LDL-C and since the two are very highly correlated with one another,[7] the ratio of HDL-C to TC may be a more convenient index than the ratio of HDL-C to LDL-C, and may contain essentially the same information.

While there is clearly a need for more analytic evidence to substantiate the use of these ratios in IHD risk profiles, at this stage it is believed that descriptive data on these ratios in free-living populations would be useful to researchers, to clinicians, and to public health workers. The prevalence studies of the LRC program provide a unique data base for this purpose; studies were conducted as population surveys performed by a common protocol and rigorously standardized laboratories. In this communication we present a description of the distributions of the ratios of HDL-C to LDL-C and TC, and their association with sex, age, and sex hormone use by women, in the 10 North American populations studied by the LRC program. It is the aim of this report to provide a reference guide for use in the clinical context and as a basis for comparison with other populations.

Methods

The population studies component of the LRC program has been described in detail elsewhere.[13, 14] Briefly, 10 LRCs in the United States and Canada completed a series of population surveys between 1971 and 1976. The LRCs selected their study populations to ensure wide ethnic, geographic, socioeconomic, and age variation; the collaborative LRC data are not, however, representative of the Canadian or U.S. populations. All clinics used a common protocol[14] and highly standardized methods.[15]

A total of 13,852 participants of both sexes were examined during the LRC visit 2 survey. Of these, 7733 constitute a 15% randomly sampled subset of LRC visit 1 participants. Data presented in this report are from 3535 white male, 3365 white female, 228 black male, and 267 black female participants who were part of the random sample at visit 2. Criteria for exclusion from the analyses were fasting less than 12 hr before blood sampling, missing data for HDL-C, TC (for the analyses on HDL-C/TC), or LDL-C (for the analyses on HDL-C/LDL-C), pregnancy, or age less than 5 years. These criteria excluded a total of 153 observations. Also, two grossly unusual LDL-C values were regarded as missing values. The number of black women reporting the use of gonadal hormones was insufficient for the descriptive analyses presented in this report. The data from these 25 women are not presented here but are available on request.

The sampling frames and number of study participants for the LRCs have been reported elsewhere.[13] Overall participation rates were 74% for visit 1 and 85% for visit 2.

The data are presented as arithmetic means and SDs. In addition, where the sample sizes were adequate several percentiles are provided. For small sample sizes only the median is given. Correlation coefficients were only computed for the variables measured in the white participants, and since the sample sizes were large, Pearson correlation coefficients were considered adequate despite the skewed distributions of some of the variables.

Laboratory methods. A detailed description of the laboratory processing procedures is provided in the LRC Laboratory Methods Manual.[15] Briefly, plasma cholesterol and triglyceride levels were determined in each LRC core laboratory by use of Technicon Autoanalyzer I (AA-I) or Autoanalyzer II (AA-II), adapted by the LRC program. On frozen serum pools the AA-I instruments produced cholesterol values 2.1% higher than the manual Abell-Kendell target values; the AA-II instruments gave values 1.3% lower than target values.[16] For plasma triglyceride concentrations the individual instrument biases varied from

4.9% below to 1.0% above reference values. Between-run variability was often less than within-run variabilty and interlaboratory variation was considerably less than intralaboratory variation.[16] All study determinations were done on fresh samples and the comparative data indicate instrument differences even less than the values ascertained for frozen samples.[16–18]

Lipoproteins were separated by ultracentrifugal flotation at saline density (d = 1.006 g/ml) to yield a supernatant fraction containing very low-density lipoprotein cholesterol (VLDL-C) and an infranatant fraction containing both LDL-C and HDL-C.

HDL-C was estimated in total plasma after precipitation of the apo B–containing lipoproteins by means of heparin–manganese chloride. After direct estimation of HDL-C, LDL-C was computed by subtracting the HDL-C from the cholesterol in the 1.006 infranatant. Concentrations of VLDL-C were determined by subtracting the cholesterol in the 1.006 infranatant from the TC. In instances of incomplete precipitation of VLDL-C and LDL-C, the procedure was repeated on the infranatant fraction after ultracentrifugation.[19]

To ensure interlaboratory comparability of ultracentrifugal results on lipoproteins, 53 "freshly" collected frozen plasma pools were distributed quarterly, over a 3½ year period, to each laboratory. The average coefficients of interclinic variability in lipoprotein-cholesterol analyses in these samples were 5% for LDL-C and 10% to 15% for HDL-C.[20]

Results

The distributions of plasma lipids and lipoprotein cholesterol fractions in the LRC participants examined by the North American LRCs have been published elsewhere.[13, 20–22] The distributions of the ratio of HDL-C to TC by age, sex, and hormone use for the white participants in the LRC visit 2 random sample are shown in tables 1 to 3. The means, medians, and 10th and 90th percentiles of the ratio of HDL-C to TC are plotted by age, sex, and hormone use in figures 1 to 3, and the means are compared by age, sex, and hormone use in figure 4.

In these cross-sectional data there was apparent a consistent age-related decline in the percentage of TC

TABLE 1

Mean and percentile values for the ratio of plasma HDL-C to TC by age in white male participants, 5 to 70+ years old (visit 2 random sample)

Age group (years)	n	Mean	SD	Percentile				
				5th	10th	50th	90th	95th
5–9	141	0.360	0.073	0.240	0.265	0.359	0.443	0.475
10–14	293	0.344	0.073	0.235	0.261	0.341	0.433	0.464
15–19	298	0.307	0.082	0.193	0.214	0.295	0.407	0.452
20–24	118	0.287	0.081	0.169	0.189	0.282	0.393	0.432
25–29	253	0.259	0.078	0.156	0.171	0.246	0.365	0.401
30–34	403	0.242	0.070	0.135	0.157	0.237	0.335	0.369
35–39	371	0.224	0.069	0.125	0.144	0.213	0.300	0.351
40–44	383	0.221	0.066	0.126	0.149	0.210	0.304	0.336
45–49	325	0.218	0.062	0.133	0.148	0.210	0.291	0.335
50–54	338	0.211	0.059	0.126	0.144	0.206	0.283	0.320
55–59	257	0.227	0.074	0.133	0.150	0.215	0.311	0.357
60–64	131	0.242	0.073	0.138	0.163	0.235	0.330	0.370
65–69	105	0.234	0.070	0.124	0.148	0.228	0.344	0.359
70+	119	0.244	0.081	0.140	0.159	0.238	0.333	0.383
Total	3535							

Fifth and 95th percentiles not given if n < 100; 10th and 90th percentiles not given if n < 75. Where n < 50, the mean and median should be interpreted with caution.

TABLE 2

Mean and percentile values for the ratio of plasma HDL-C to TC by age in white female participants not on hormones and from 5 to 70+ years old (visit 2 random sample)

Age group (years)	n	Mean	SD	Percentile				
				5th	10th	50th	90th	95th
5–9	123	0.328	0.073	0.207	0.239	0.323	0.425	0.450
10–14	246	0.330	0.065	0.237	0.252	0.329	0.421	0.442
15–19	270	0.334	0.079	0.214	0.244	0.332	0.442	0.473
20–24	95	0.324	0.075	0.203	0.216	0.323	0.419	0.448
25–29	170	0.329	0.079	0.194	0.224	0.329	0.428	0.459
30–34	216	0.326	0.078	0.200	0.223	0.321	0.422	0.448
35–39	220	0.300	0.088	0.164	0.188	0.296	0.427	0.455
40–44	224	0.294	0.085	0.165	0.194	0.284	0.414	0.459
45–49	221	0.287	0.089	0.167	0.188	0.275	0.394	0.452
50–54	155	0.275	0.080	0.153	0.176	0.268	0.377	0.409
55–59	153	0.258	0.079	0.132	0.150	0.260	0.353	0.396
60–64	95	0.266	0.072	—	0.171	0.261	0.360	—
65–69	83	0.252	0.092	—	0.135	0.248	0.383	—
70+	104	0.266	0.076	0.150	0.164	0.259	0.367	0.418
Total	2375							

Fifth and 95th percentiles not given if n < 100; 10th and 90th percentiles not given if n < 75. Where n < 50, the mean and median should be interpreted with caution.

TABLE 3

Mean and percentile values for the ratio of plasma HDL-C to TC by age in white female participants on hormones and from 5 to 70+ years old (visit 2 random sample)

Age group (years)	n	Mean	SD	Percentile				
				5th	10th	50th	90th	95th
5–9	—	—	—	—	—	—	—	—
10–14	1	—	—	—	—	—	—	—
15–19	24	0.330	0.110	—	—	0.336	—	—
20–24	102	0.317	0.092	0.187	0.196	0.311	0.441	0.485
25–29	143	0.306	0.086	0.183	0.204	0.297	0.436	0.477
30–34	114	0.310	0.090	0.178	0.197	0.299	0.427	0.460
35–39	77	0.294	0.095	—	0.172	0.291	0.429	—
50–54	101	0.320	0.086	0.179	0.198	0.324	0.420	0.463
55–59	96	0.314	0.091	—	0.203	0.309	0.449	—
60–64	49	0.310	0.086	—	—	0.299	—	—
65–69	47	0.329	0.091	—	—	0.323	—	—
70+	38	0.297	0.094	—	—	0.291	—	—
Total	990							

Fifth and 95th percentiles not given if n < 100; 10th and 90th percentiles not given if n < 75. Where n < 50, the mean and median should be interpreted with caution.

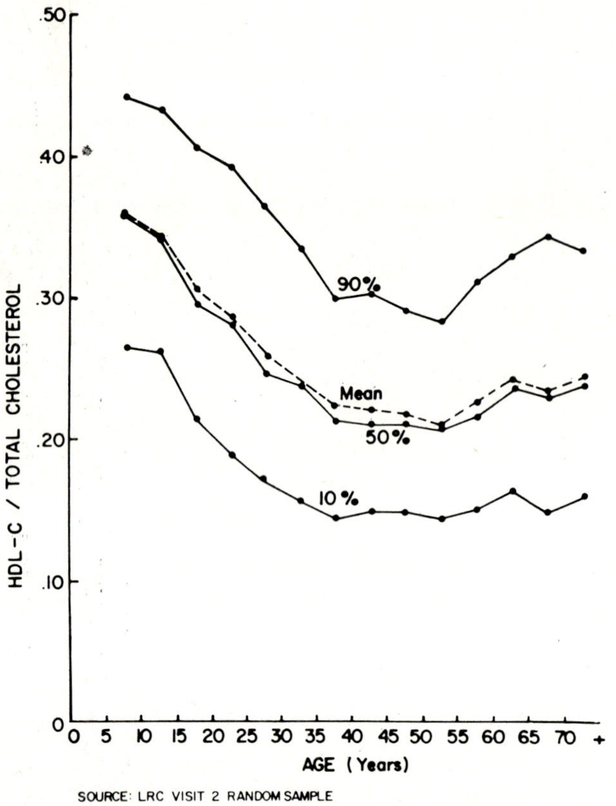

FIGURE 1. Mean and percentile values for the ratio of plasma HDL-C to TC by age: white male participants 5 to 70+ years old. LRC visit 2 random sample.

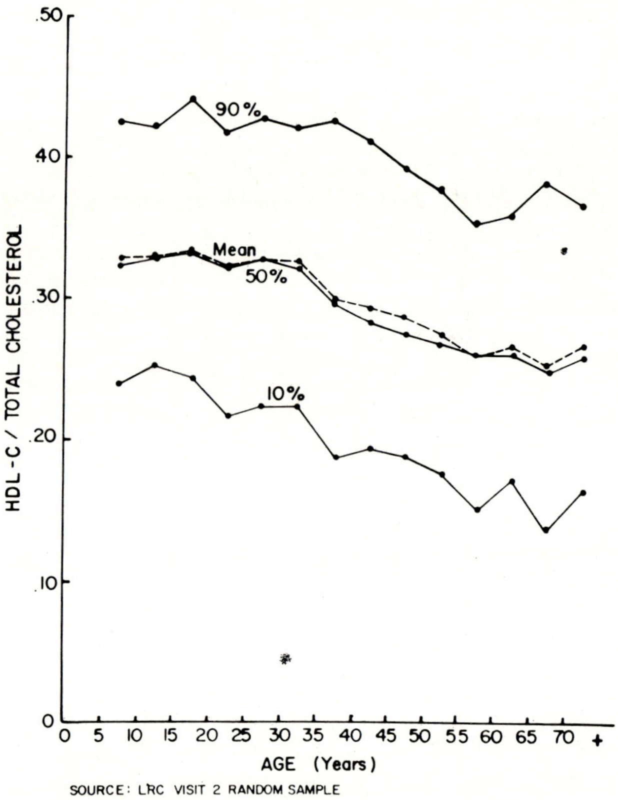

FIGURE 2. Mean and percentile values for the ratio of plasma HDL-C to TC by age: white female participants not on hormones and from 5 to 70+ years old. LRC visit 2 random sample.

carried by the HDL fraction in male participants (table 1, figure 1) from a mean of 36% in the age group 5 to 9 to a mean of 21.1% in the age group 50 to 54. Thereafter the percentage increased to a mean of 24.2% in the age group 60 to 64 and appeared to stabilize around this value.

In female participants not taking hormones (table 2, figure 2) the percentage of TC carried by HDL remained stable in the range of means from 32.4% to 33.4% for the age groups 5 to 9 to 30 to 34. Only in the age group 35 to 39 was there evidence of a decline from a mean of 32.6% to 30.0% and this value gradually declined to a mean of 25.8% in the age group 55 to 59. Thereafter there was a slight increase that appeared to stabilize around the value of 25% to 26%.

In women taking hormones (table 3, figure 3) the results were more difficult to interpret in view of the change from hormone use in the form of oral contraceptives (OC) to the use of replacement estrogen compounds. This changeover is likely to take place between the ages of 40 and 49 and as a result the values given for this age range include a mixed group of OC users and those taking replacement estrogens. (The results for this age range are shaded and indicated by a broken line in the graph in figures 3 and 4). Contrary to the pattern displayed by women not taking hormones, the decline in the percentage of TC carried by HDL was already evident in the age group 15 to 19, in which it constituted a mean of 33.0%, to the age group 20 to 24, in which it dropped to a mean of 30.6%. In women 30 to 39 years old, it appeared to stabilize around 30.0%, a value achieved by the nonhormone users only in the age range of 35 to 39.

As previously indicated, the perimenopausal age group of 40 to 49 includes both OC users and those on replacement estrogens. In the age range 50 to 69 the percentage of TC in HDL varied between 31% and 33%; women on hormones in this age group had a mean value of 25%. The mean value of 29.7% for hormone users was computed with data from a small sample (38 women).

Distributions of the ratio of HDL-C to LDL-C are shown in tables 4 to 6. Although the ratio of HDL-C to LDL-C is considered to represent the ratio of the antiatherogenic to the atherogenic lipoprotein cholesterol fractions, the ratio of HDL-C to TC may be more useful in practice. HDL-C/TC is bounded since HDL-C is contained in the TC and the values of HDL-C/TC must lie between 0 and 1. On the other hand, HDL-C/LDL-C is not bounded, and thus the distribution of

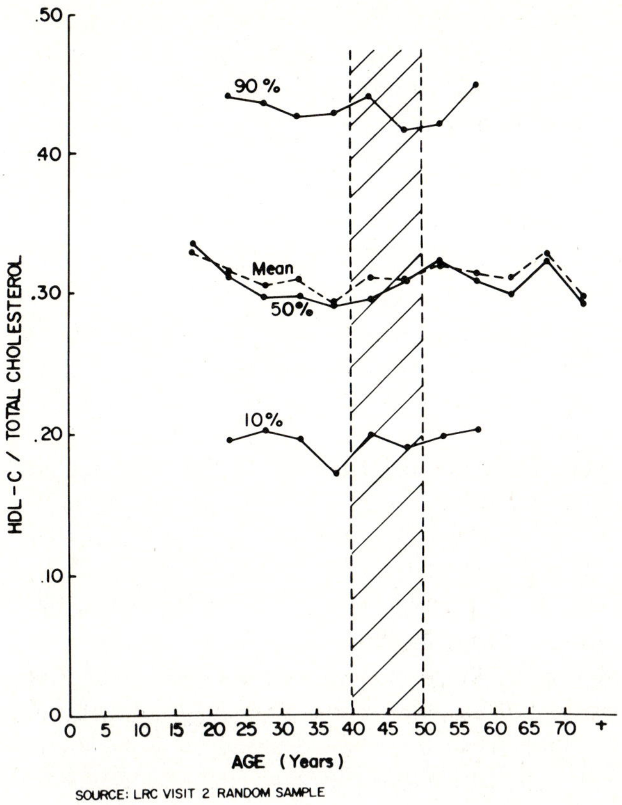

FIGURE 3. Mean and percentile values for the ratio of plasma HDL-C to TC by age: white female participants on hormones and from 5 to 70+ years old. LRC visit 2 random sample.

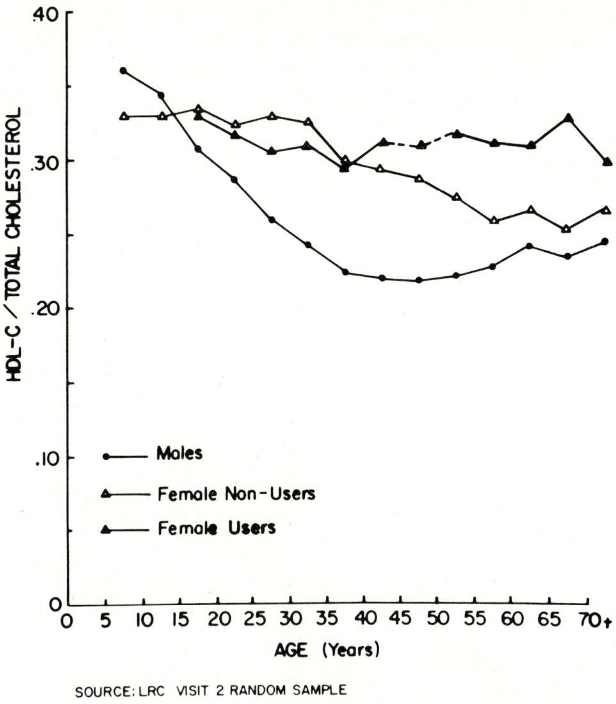

FIGURE 4. Mean values for the ratio of plasma HDL-C to TC by age and sex-hormone use: white participants from 5 to 70+ years old. LRC visit 2 random sample.

HDL-C/TC tends to be more symmetrical than that of HDL-C/LDL-C and is therefore a more convenient form for statistical analysis. Moreover, the results for the HDL-C/LDL-C ratio and its surrogate HDL-C/TC proportion parallel one another and they are essentially very similar. It should be noted, however, that the HDL-C/TC ratio is more likely to misrepresent the lipid profiles of individuals who are hypertriglyceridemic and have substantial amounts of VLDL-C.

Tables 7 to 9 display the Pearson correlation coefficients between the various lipids and lipoproteins and selected lipoprotein ratios. Since little variation was observed in the magnitude of the correlation coefficients between different age groups, the tables list data from participants 5 years old and above combined. The HDL-C/TC ratio correlated highly with HDL-C/LDL-C (from .923 for men to .956 for women on hormones), suggesting that TC may serve as an adequate surrogate for LDL-C in the ratio of HDL-C/LDL-C. Consequently, the ratio of HDL-C to TC is the one described in detail in this report. Since LDL-C is often approximated by the formula LDL-C* = TC − HDL-C − Triglycerides/5, the ratio of HDL-C/LDL-C* has been included in the correlation matrixes. As can be observed in tables 7 to 9, the correlations between HDL-C/LDL-C and HDL-C/LDL-C* were very high (.979 to .984) and thus the use of LDL-C* in place of LDL-C in the ratios should yield essentially the same results.

The distributions of the ratio of HDL-C to TC and

TABLE 4

Mean and percentile values for the ratio of plasma HDL-C to LDL-C by age in white male participants from 5 to 70+ years old (visit 2 random sample)

Age group (years)	n	Mean	SD	Percentile				
				5th	10th	50th	90th	95th
5–9	128	0.639	0.231	0.337	0.373	0.593	0.873	1.120
10–14	284	0.606	0.249	0.343	0.391	0.565	0.829	0.966
15–19	297	0.531	0.258	0.284	0.311	0.481	0.787	0.940
20–24	118	0.478	0.211	0.229	0.264	0.441	0.725	0.817
25–29	253	0.419	0.186	0.221	0.240	0.378	0.667	0.765
30–34	403	0.386	0.153	0.194	0.224	0.355	0.575	0.663
35–39	371	0.350	0.144	0.184	0.215	0.319	0.499	0.626
40–44	383	0.348	0.159	0.185	0.211	0.318	0.508	0.584
45–49	325	0.333	0.121	0.188	0.211	0.312	0.474	0.546
50–54	338	0.326	0.120	0.183	0.205	0.306	0.483	0.559
55–59	257	0.353	0.181	0.179	0.201	0.316	0.504	0.600
60–64	131	0.377	0.172	0.188	0.224	0.346	0.547	0.643
65–69	105	0.355	0.127	0.181	0.214	0.337	0.547	0.587
70+	119	0.380	0.248	0.192	0.214	0.342	0.549	0.620
Total	3512							

Fifth and 95th percentiles not given if n < 100; 10th and 90th percentiles not given if n < 75. Where n < 50, the mean and median should be interpreted with caution.

TABLE 5
Mean and percentile values for the ratio of plasma HDL-C to LDL-C by age in white female participants not on hormones and from 5 to 70+ years old (visit 2 random sample)

Age group (years)	n	Mean	SD	Percentile				
				5th	10th	50th	90th	95th
5–9	110	0.553	0.190	0.300	0.343	0.515	0.796	0.919
10–14	243	0.563	0.167	0.343	0.369	0.547	0.808	0.870
15–19	268	0.595	0.207	0.315	0.363	0.559	0.879	0.977
20–24	95	0.563	0.203	—	0.308	0.536	0.820	—
25–29	170	0.570	0.211	0.268	0.329	0.541	0.823	0.942
30–34	216	0.548	0.196	0.278	0.315	0.515	0.794	0.884
35–39	221	0.503	0.213	0.232	0.264	0.473	0.803	0.901
40–44	224	0.487	0.231	0.230	0.267	0.443	0.805	0.909
45–49	219	0.484	0.256	0.245	0.270	0.434	0.730	0.916
50–54	155	0.445	0.221	0.218	0.246	0.413	0.657	0.768
55–59	153	0.409	0.162	0.194	0.215	0.390	0.640	0.693
60–64	95	0.419	0.146	—	0.240	0.403	0.610	—
65–69	83	0.394	0.191	—	0.179	0.351	0.674	—
70+	104	0.415	0.156	0.203	0.256	0.385	0.605	0.771
Total	2358							

Fifth and 95th percentiles not given if n < 100; 10th and 90th percentiles not given if n < 75. Where n < 50, the mean and median should be interpreted with caution.

Two outliers excluded (LDL ≤12).

HDL-C to LDL-C for the black participants are presented by gender in tables 10 and 11. As indicated earlier, small sample sizes precluded the presentation of these data for black women reporting gonadal hormone use. Also, because of the smaller numbers of black examinees in the adult age range, wider age groupings have been used in tables 10 and 11. Similar to the trend observed for white males, black male participants showed a decline in the percentage of TC carried in HDL-C with age, from a mean of 38% at ages 5 to 9, to a mean of 24% in the decade 50 to 59 years. A slightly higher value of this ratio was observed in the group of examinees 60 and older. The last two values were calculated with data from small numbers of participants in each age stratum. It is of note that in every age group black male participants had a higher proportion of TC carried in HDL-C than white male participants. In black female participants not taking hormones the percentage of TC carried as HDL-C varied little by age between the ages 5 to 9 and 20 to 29. The magnitude of the HDL-C to TC ratio declined progressively in the older women. Whereas the age trend appeared to be similar in black and white women, the black women exhibited a higher percentage of TC in HDL-C than white women between ages 5 to 9 and 15 to 19. Thereafter, no appreciable differences in the magnitude of the ratio of HDL-C to TC could be seen between black and white women of comparable age. As in the white study participants, the correlation between the ratios HDL-C/TC and HDL-C/LDL-C in black male and female participants was approximately .90.

Discussion

While the literature attests to increasing use of lipoprotein ratios of various forms to reflect the lipoprotein cholesterol contribution to an IHD risk profile, information on the behavior of these ratios in the general population is lacking. The purpose of this report is to provide a description of the distribution of a selected lipoprotein ratio viz HDL-C/TC by age, sex, and hormone use in a large population sample of residents of the U.S. and Canada. The choice of the ratio HDL-C/TC for detailed descriptive analyses was based on its relative ease of determination, computational simplicity, ease of interpretation and, perhaps most important, frequency of use in reports in the literature. Since HDL-C/TC is not just a ratio but actually a proportion, its range of values is bounded and its distribution is more symmetrical and thus more convenient for statistical analysis. It is also highly correlated with the ratio HDL-C/LDL-C and may possibly be regarded as a more conveniently determined surrogate for that ratio.

Previous descriptive studies of lipoprotein cholesterol levels in North American populations have generally been limited to the individual lipoproteins considered separately. However, there is now considerable

TABLE 6
Mean and percentile values for the ratio of plasma HDL-C to LDL-C by age in white female participants on hormones and 5 to 70+ years old (visit 2 random sample)

Age group (years)	n	Mean	SD	Percentile				
				5th	10th	50th	90th	95th
5–9	—	—	—	—	—	—	—	—
10–14	—	—	—	—	—	—	—	—
15–19	24	0.601	0.064	—	—	0.575	—	—
20–24	102	0.574	0.028	0.254	0.273	0.529	0.930	1.175
25–29	143	0.525	0.019	0.257	0.286	0.475	0.854	1.035
30–34	111	0.527	0.021	0.249	0.272	0.503	0.809	0.901
35–39	77	0.511	0.028	—	0.245	0.460	0.857	—
50–54	101	0.566	0.023	0.249	0.280	0.561	0.868	1.008
55–59	96	0.561	0.025	—	0.307	0.507	0.938	—
60–64	49	0.515	0.029	—	—	0.458	—	—
65–69	47	0.576	0.039	—	—	0.512	—	—
70+	38	0.483	0.038	—	—	0.439	—	—
Total	986							

Fifth and 95th percentiles not given if n < 100; 10th and 90th percentiles not given if n < 75. Where n < 50, the mean and median should be interpreted with caution.

TABLE 7
Pearson correlation coefficients between selected lipids, lipoproteins, and lipoprotein ratios in white male participants from 5 to 70+ years old (visit 2 random sample)

	HDL-C/ TC	HDL-C/ LDL	HDL-C/ LDL-C*	TC	VLDL-C	TRIG	LDL-C	HDL-C	LDL-C*
HDL-C/TC	1.000								
HDL-C/LDL-C	.923	1.000							
HDL-C/LDL-C*	.943	.984	1.000						
TC	−.582	−.508	−.531	1.000					
VLDL-C	−.494	−.255	−.382	.436	1.000				
TRIG	−.599	−.433	−.418	.479	.814	1.000			
LDL-C	−.665	−.679	−.676	.893	.105	.349	1.000		
HDL-C	.749	.677	.680	.047	−.337	−.381	−.121	1.000	
LDL-C*	−.703	−.673	−.693	.939	.303	.319	.973	−.141	1.000

TRIG = triglyceride; LDL-C* = TC−HDL-C−TRIG/5.

epidemiologic and experimental evidence to suggest that both HDL-C and LDL-C levels are independently associated with the risk of IHD. Since both are lipid fractions that are postulated to participate in the atherogenic process via cholesterol transport and metabolism, it is intuitively appealing and appears scientifically sound to consider a single function to reflect the combined contribution of these lipoproteins to the risk of atherosclerotic disease.

In the pioneering work of Barr et al.,[2] both the mean HDL concentration and the mean percentage of HDL in the total blood lipoproteins were shown to differ in patients with and those without IHD. Brunner et al.[23] reported in 1962 that the percentage of TC carried by HDL was an index that effectively separated two ethnic groups, one with high and one with very low rates of IHD. By contrast, Sievers and Fisher[24] and Howard et al.[25] observed that there was a lower ratio of HDL-C to LDL-C in Southwestern American Indians than in non-Indians, although the IHD incidence is considerably lower in the former than the latter.

In reporting on the role of HDL-C in IHD risk, Gordon et al.[5] of the Framingham Study found that the ratio of HDL-C to LDL-C or TC emerged as strong predictors of IHD in multiple logistic regression analysis. However, at the time they cautioned against the use of these ratios because of uncertain biological interpretation. Goldbourt and Medalie[6] of the Israeli Ischemic Heart Disease Study described the distribution of the percentage of HDL-C in TC in their sample without commenting on the usefulness of this index.

Investigators from the Framingham Studies have advocated the use of the ratio of blood HDL-C to LDL-C or TC as the most convenient expression of their joint contribution to IHD risk.[26, 27, 78] In the Framingham Offspring Study, Wilson et al.[27] found that the ratio of blood TC to HDL-C was strongly associated with IHD risk, but that its use in analysis was not superior to use of the two lipoprotein fractions separately. Recently Castelli et al.[78] reported their findings in the evaluation of two specific ratios, namely TC/HDL-C and LDL-C/HDL-C, as predictors of CHD. Their main conclu-

TABLE 8
Pearson correlation coefficients between selected lipids, lipoproteins, and lipoprotein ratios in white female participants not on hormones and 5 to 70+ years old (visit 2 random sample)

	HDL-C/ TC	HDL-C/ LDL	HDL-C/ LDL-C*	TC	VLDL-C	TRIG	LDL-C	HDL-C	LDL-C*
HDL-C/TC	1.000								
HDL-C/LDL-C	.953	1.000							
HDL-C/LDL-C*	.960	.984	1.000						
TC	−.523	−.492	−.488	1.000					
VLDL-C	−.488	−.298	−.390	.364	1.000				
TRIG	−.590	−.465	−.436	.506	.744	1.000			
LDL-C	−.692	−.696	−.674	.933	.216	−.465	1.000		
HDL-C	.671	.615	.621	.237	−.291	−.279	−.014	1.000	
LDL-C*	−.715	−.695	−.699	.942	.347	.438	.982	−.333	1.000

Abbreviations are as in table 7.

TABLE 9
Pearson correlation coefficients between selected lipids, lipoproteins, and lipoprotein ratios in white female participants on hormones and 15 to 70+ years old (visit 2 random sample)

	HDL-C/ TC	HDL-C/ LDL	HDL-C/ LDL-C*	TC	VLDL-C	TRIG	LDL-C	HDL-C	LDL-C*
HDL-C/TC	1.000								
HDL-C/LDL-C	.956	1.000							
HDL-C/LDL-C*	.949	.979	1.000						
TC	−.369	−.346	−.334	1.000					
VLDL-C	−.428	−.241	−.273	.331	1.000				
TRIG	−.386	−.267	−.196	.373	.733	1.000			
LDL-C	−.660	−.675	−.656	.878	.161	−.265	1.000		
HDL-C	.779	.727	.719	.254	−.263	−.158	−.132	1.000	
LDL-C*	−.681	−.677	−.693	.858	.204	.168	.971	−.164	1.000

Abbreviations are as in table 7.

sion was that these ratios were useful summary estimates of the information contained in the lipoprotein cholesterol fractions and were strong predictors of coronary heart disease.

Either because lipoprotein ratios are regarded as a conceptually useful synthesis of a lipoprotein-cholesterol profile, or because of their potential use as an index of IHD risk, the literature reflects a rapidly growing use of these ratios. Ratios relating HDL-C to TC or LDL-C have been used to characterize dyslipoproteinemias,[28–32] myocardial infarction survivors and their relatives,[33–35] angiographically defined coronary artery disease,[29, 36–39] and other morbid conditions such as hypertension,[40, 41] diabetes,[40, 42] obesity,[41, 43, 44–48] and thyroid dysfunction.[49] Lipoprotein ratios have also been reported with regard to gonadal hormone use,[50] liver histology and disease,[51] drug therapy,[52–54] plasma exchange,[55] and jejunileal bypass.[56] An association between lipoprotein ratio values and age has been addressed by several authors in diverse study designs and selected populations.[33, 41, 57–59, 60–62] Various forms of lipoprotein ratios have been reported for populations defined by geographic and ethnic criteria, such as Southwestern American Indian,[24, 25] African,[63] Israeli,[6] Chinese,[50] and Japanese,[57, 64] and Caucasian populations in various countries. Investigators have also described the association between certain risk factors of IHD and the lipoprotein cholesterol ratio, such as physical activity and smoking habits,[18, 19] alcohol consumption,[65] modified fat diets,[66] vegetarian diets,[67, 68] and dietary fiber.[42]

It is apparent from the literature that not only are lipoprotein ratios often used, but they are being used in a diversity of forms reflecting different choices of numerators and denominators. Recent publications have used the ratios HDL-C/TC[A] and TC/HDL-C,[B] HDL-C/LDL-C,[34, 44, 57, 59] LDL-C/HDL-C,[49, 50, 52, 71, 74] HDL-C/VLDL-C + LDL-C,[53, 75, 76] and VLDL-C + LDL-C/HDL-C.[38] The ratio HDL-phospholipid/TC also has been used.[39] This variety of formulations for the lipo-

[A]References 28, 29, 33–35, 39, 40, 42, 43, 45, 50, 51, 53, 54, 58, 61, 63–65, 69, 70–72.
[B]References 36, 37, 41, 46, 55, 56, 60, 66, 73.

TABLE 10
The distribution of the ratio of plasma HDL to TC and HDL to LDL-C (mg/dl) by age in black male participants (visit 2 random sample)

Age group (years)	Ratio of HDL to TC: n	Mean	SD	Median	Ratio of HDL to LDL-C: n	Mean	SD	Median
5–9	40	0.379	0.073	0.367	39	0.687	0.248	0.625
10–14	56	0.348	0.085	0.357	56	0.623	0.255	0.598
15–19	58	0.345	0.080	0.343	58	0.616	0.275	0.562
20–29	15	0.313	0.073	0.318	15	0.569	0.242	0.542
30–39	29	0.299	0.094	0.280	29	0.513	0.229	0.467
40–49	14	0.278	0.086	0.270	14	0.465	0.222	0.413
50–59	7	0.237	0.077	0.262	7	0.382	0.076	0.381
60+	7	0.256	0.073	0.224	7	0.391	0.133	0.317
Total	228				227			

TABLE 11
The distribution of the ratio of plasma HDL to TC and HDL to LDL-C (mg/dl) by age in black female participants (visit 2 random sample)

Age group (years)	Ratio of HDL to TC				Ratio of HDL to LDL-C			
	n	Mean	SD	Median	n	Mean	SD	Median
5–9	45	0.346	0.079	0.329	43	0.605	0.231	0.548
10–14	59	0.333	0.065	0.333	59	0.558	0.155	0.553
15–19	56	0.345	0.066	0.340	56	0.612	0.215	0.559
20–29	15	0.324	0.077	0.311	15	0.544	0.195	0.507
30–39	43	0.317	0.104	0.324	43	0.552	0.306	0.529
40–49	25	0.283	0.081	0.256	25	0.450	0.194	0.375
50–59	16	0.236	0.055	0.238	16	0.372	0.103	0.378
60+	6	0.314	0.070	0.321	6	0.513	0.158	0.517
Total	267				264			

protein ratios, as well as some heterogeneity in the rationale for their use, is indicative of the absence of common guidelines and conventions in the use of a measurement that researchers in a diversity of disciplines find appealing. One such deficiency is addressed in this study by the provision of population levels and distributional characteristics of a commonly used form of lipoprotein cholesterol ratio reflecting rigorous and standardized lipid laboratory measurements and well-defined samples of free-living populations.

While the lipoprotein ratios appear to be attractive measures of the joint contribution of the lipoprotein cholesterol fractions to IHD risk, several inconsistencies have not been resolved. At very low TC levels, it is possible that IHD risk may be low regardless of HDL-C levels. On the other hand, excessively high levels of TC may produce high risk of IHD even in the presence of elevated HDL-C levels.[77] The ratio of the lipoprotein fractions may not reflect this effect and may have little predictive power at the extremes of the blood TC distribution. Nonetheless, over the intermediate range of plasma TC concentrations the various ratios of the lipoprotein cholesterol fractions are frequently used as indexes of the lipid component of IHD risk, and in at least one large study, they have been found to be strongly predictive of IHD mortality.[5]

Certain qualifications are necessary for the interpretation of the analyses presented here. The descriptions of the distributions of selected lipoprotein cholesterol ratios in themselves do not address the issue of IHD risk. No attempt has been made (nor can be made on the basis of these data) to determine "optimal" or "abnormal" lipoprotein cholesterol ratios. Our analyses merely describe the distributions of the ratios in a broadly based sample of North Americans. It is hoped that this report will be useful as a reference guide for researchers and clinicians in evaluating their own populations.

The concept of a lipoprotein cholesterol ratio being somehow indicative of the atherogenic potential of the blood lipids may not be applicable to individuals with genetic disorders of lipid metabolism. The ratio distributions presented here are based on a population not selected on the basis of blood lipid levels, and only relatively few individuals with genetic lipid metabolism disorders are likely to have been included. Thus, the significance of lipoprotein cholesterol ratios in individuals with disorders such as familial dyslipoproteinemias may be quite different than that in a general population in which they may vary largely as a result of environmental factors.

Our results show that certain demographic and behavioral characteristics are of relevance in the evaluation of the HDL-C/TC index. The data presented in this report demonstrate profound effects of gonadal hormone use on the levels of the HDL-C/TC and HDL-C/LDL-C ratios. Of singular importance are the observed black-white differences in these ratios, e.g., the higher proportion of TC carried as HDL-C in the black compared with the white juveniles and adult men. These findings add to the evidence of racial differences in plasma lipid distributions[4, 25] and are noteworthy because of the limited population-based data available on non-Caucasians. Further, the age-related changes in the HDL-C/TC and HDL-C/LDL-C ratios observed for male and female participants are both somewhat different and more marked than those observed in the individual lipoproteins or in TC. This is a reflection of the combined effect of the changes in the individual lipoproteins. This observation has far-reaching implications if, as much epidemiologic and experimental evidence suggests, the risk of atherosclerotic disease depends on the combined, independent effects of HDL-C and LDL-C.

For white women using gonadal hormones, the mean HDL-C values increased substantially between the ages of 20 and 59. However, the mean HDL-C/TC ratio did not show any obvious change over that age range. These data should be interpreted with caution since the composition of the gonadal hormone used is not uniform over this age range; hormone use is likely to consist of both progestogen and estrogen in those under 40 and primarily of estrogen in the older group.

As a summary index of the lipid profile the HDL-C/TC proportion has considerable potential for simplifying a variety of functions in clinical practice and public health, such as risk assessment, screening, therapeutic decisions, and follow-up. Although not exhaustive regarding the information it conveys about a lipid pattern and concentration, the expression HDL-C/TC has the advantage of summarizing complex associations into a single numerical approximation. With the proviso that the absolute concentrations of the lipid measurements on which this index is based may contribute additional information by themselves, this summary index constitutes a meaningful statistic for individuals as well as for population groups.

LRC Committees

Epidemiology Analysis Executive Committee. William Insull, M.D.; John C. LaRosa, M.D.; Robert B. Wallace, M.D.; Henry L. Taylor, Ph.D.; Jack Medalie, M.D.; Carl Rubenstein, M.D.; L. Thomas Sheffield, M.D.; Fred Mattson, Ph.D.; Gerardo Heiss, M.D., Ph.D.; Richard Mowery, Ph.D.; H.A. Tyroler, M.D. (Chairman); O. Dale Williams, Ph.D.; Manning Feinleib, M.D.; Basil M, Rifkind, M.D.; Kathe Kelly.

LRC Epidemiology Committee. H.A. Tyroler, M.D. (Chairman); Paul Anderson, Ph.D.; Elizabeth Barrett-Connor, M.D.; Mary Brockway, Ph.D.; Gary Chase, Ph.D.; Linda Cowan, Ph.D.; Bobbe Christensen, Ph.D.; Michael Criqui, M.D.; Michael Davies, M.D.; Alexander Deev, Ph.D.; Ido deGroot, M.P.H.; Manning Feinleib, M.D.; Marian Fisher, Ph.D.; Igor Glasunov, M.D.; Gaetan Godin, M.S.; S.T. Halfon, M.D.; Robin Harris, M.P.H.; William Haskell, Ph.D.; Gerardo Heiss, M.D., Ph.D.; David Hewitt, M.A.; Judith Hill, M.S.; Joanne Hoover, M.D.; Donald Hunninghake, M.D.; David Jacobs, Ph.D.; Kathe Kelly; J. Alick Little, M.D.; Arden Mackenthun, Ph.D.; Irma Mebane, M.S.; J. Medalie, M.D.; Richard Mowery, Ph.D.; John A. Morrison, Ph.D.; John B. O'Sullivan, M.D.; Basil M. Rifkind, M.D.; Carl Rubenstein, M.D.; William J. Schull, Ph.D.; Pearl Van Natta, Ph.D.; Robert B. Wallace, M.D.; O. Dale Williams, Ph.D.

LRC Directors Committee. Francois Abboud, M.D.; Stewart Agras, M.D.; Edwin Bierman, M.D.; Reagan Bradford, M.D., Ph.D.; Virgil Brown, M.D.; Marilyn Buzzard, Ph.D.; William Connor, M.D.; Gerald Cooper, M.D., Ph.D.; John Farquhar, M.D.; Ivan Frantz, M.D.; Charles Glueck, M.D.; Elena Gerasimova, M.D.; Antonio Gotto, M.D., Ph.D.; James Grizzle, Ph.D.; William R. Hazzard, M.D.; Donald Hunninghake, M.D.; Frank Ibbott, Ph.D.; William Insull, M.D.; Anatoli Klimov, M.D.; Robert Knopp, M.D.; Peter Kwiterovich, M.D.; John C. LaRosa, M.D.; J. Alick Little, M.D.; Fred Mattson, Ph.D.; Maurice Mishkel, M.D.; Basil M. Rifkind, M.D.; Gustav Schonfeld, M.D.; Helmut Schrott, M.D.; Yechezkiel Stein, M.D.; Daniel Steinberg, M.D.; George Steiner, M.D.; O. Dale Williams, Ph.D.

References

1. Kannel WB, Castelli WP, Gordon T, McNamara PM: Serum cholesterol, lipoproteins and the risk of coronary heart disease. Ann Intern Med **74:** 1, 1971
2. Barr DP, Russ EM, Eder HA: Protein-lipid relationships in human plasma II. In atherosclerosis and related conditions. Am J Med **2:** 480, 1951
3. Gofman JW, Young W, Tandy R: Ischemic heart disease, atherosclerosis and longevity. Circulation **34:** 679, 1966
4. Heiss G, Johnson NJ, Reiland S, Davis CE, Tyroler HA. The epidemiology of plasma high density lipoprotein cholesterol levels. Circulation **62**(suppl IV): IV-116, 1980
5. Gordon T, Castelli WP, Hjortland MC, Kannel WB, Dawber TR: High density lipoprotein as a protective factor against coronary heart disease. Am J Med **62:** 707, 1977
6. Goldbourt U, Medalie JH: High density-lipoprotein cholesterol and incidence of coronary heart disease — The Israeli Ischemic Heart Disease Study. Am J Epidemiol **109:** 296, 1979
7. Davis CE, Gordon D, LaRosa J, Wood PDS, Halperin M: Correlations of plasma high density lipoprotein cholesterol levels with other plasma lipid and lipoprotein concentrations. Circulation **62** (suppl IV): IV-24, 1980
8. Blackburn H: Workshop report: epidemiological section. Conference on the health effects of blood lipids: optimal distributions for populations. Prev Med **8:** 612, 1979
9. Ross R, Glomsett JA: The pathogenesis of atherosclerosis (I). N Engl J Med **295:** 369, 1976
10. Ross R, Glomsett JA: The pathogenesis of atherosclerosis (II). N Engl J Med **295:** 420, 1976
11. Lipid Research Clinics Program: The Lipid Research Clinics Coronary Primary Prevention Trial Results. I. Reduction in incidence of coronary heart disease. JAMA **251:** 351, 1984
12. Levy RI, Brensike JF, Epstein SE, Kelsey SF, Passamani ER, Richardson JM, Loh IK, Stone NJ, Aldrich RF, Battaglini JW, Moriarty DJ, Fisher ML, Friedman L, Friedewald W, Detre KM: The influence of changes in lipid values induced by cholestyramine on progression of coronary artery disease: Results of the NHLBI Type II Coronary Intervention Study. Circulation **69:** 325, 1984
13. Lipid Research Clinics Program: Plasma lipid distributions in selected North American populations: The Lipid Research Clinics Program Prevalence Study. Circulation **60:** 427, 1979
14. The Lipid Research Clinics Program: Protocol of the Lipid Research Clinics Program Prevalence Study. Central Patient Registry and Coordinating Center, Department of Biostatistics, University of North Carolina at Chapel Hill, 1976
15. Lipid Research Clinics Program: Manual of Laboratory Operations, Vol. 1, Lipid and lipoprotein analysis. DHEW Publication No. (NIH) 75-628, Washington, D.C., Government Printing Office, 1974
16. Lippel K, Ahmed S, Albers JJ, Bachorik P, Cooper G, Helms R, Williams J: Analytical performance and comparability of the determination of cholesterol by twelve Lipid Research Clinics. Clin Chem **23:** 1744, 1977
17. Ahmed S, Lippel K, Bachorik P, Albers J, Williams J, Cooper G: Analytical performance and comparability of the determination of triglyceride by twelve Lipid Research Clinics. Clin Chem **24:** 330, 1978
18. Bachorik PS, Wood PDS, Williams J, Kuchmak M, Ahmed S, Lippel L, Albers J: Automated determination of total plasma cholesterol: a serum calibration technique. Clin Chim Acta **96:** 145, 1979
19. Warnick GR, Albers JJ: A comprehensive evaluation of the heparin-manganese precipitation procedure for estimating high density lipoprotein cholesterol. J Lipid Res **19:** 65, 1978
20. Tamir I, Heiss G, Glueck GJ, Christensen B, Kwiterovich P, Rif-

kind BM: Lipid and lipoprotein distributions in white children ages 6 to 19 years. The Lipid Research Clinics Program Prevalence Study. J Chron Dis **34:** 27, 1981
21. Christensen B, Glueck C, Kwiterovich P, DeGroot I, Chase Y, Heiss G, Mowery R, Tamir I, Rifkind B: Plasma cholesterol and triglyceride distributions in 13,665 children and adolescents. The Prevalence Study of the Lipid Research Clinics Program. Pediatr Res **14:** 194, 1980
22. Heiss G, Tamir I, Davis CE, Tyroler HA, Rifkind BM, Schonfeld Y, Jacobs D, Frantz ID: Lipoprotein-cholesterol distributions in selected North American populations. The Lipid Research Clinics Program Prevalence Study. Circulation **61:** 302, 1980
23. Brunner D, Altman S, Loebl K, Schwartz S: Alpha-cholesterol percentages in coronary patients with and without increased total serum cholesterol levels and in healthy controls. J Athero Res **2:** 424, 1962
24. Sievers ML, Fisher JR: Increasing rate of acute myocardial infarction in southwestern American Indians. Arizona Med **36:** 739, 1979
25. Howard BV, Davis MP, Pettitt DJ, Krowler WC, Bennett PH: Plasma lipoprotein cholesterol and triglyceride concentrations in the Pima Indians: distributions differing from those of Caucasians. Circulation **68:** 716, 1983
26. Gordon T: HDL and coronary heart disease. Lancet **2:** 1139, 1980
27. Wilson PW, Garrison RJ, Castelli WP, Feinleib M, McNamara PM, Kannel WB: Prevalence of coronary heart disease in the Framingham offspring study: role of lipoprotein cholesterols. Am J Cardiol **46:** 649, 1980
28. Sale JL, Johnstone JH: Pre- and post-treatment values of HDL cholesterol and total: HDL cholesterol ratio in hyperlipoproteinaemic subjects. Ann Clin Biochem **19:** 71, 1981
29. Moberg B, Wallentin L: High density lipoprotein and other lipoproteins in normolipidemic and hypertriglyceridemic (type IV) men with coronary heart disease. Eur J Clin Invest **2:** 433, 1981
30. Toth L, Koenig W: Hypoalpha-hyperbeta-lipoproteinemia in a patient with coronary artery disease and occlusive peripheral arterial disease. Atherosclerosis **42:** 121, 1982
31. Franceschini G, Sirtori CR, Caputso A Jr, Weisgraber KH, Mahley RW: A-1 Milano apoprotein. Decreased high density lipoprotein cholesterol levels with significant lipoprotein cholesterol levels with significant lipoprotein modifications and without clinical atherosclerosis in an Italian family. J Clin Invest **66:** 892, 1980
32. Shore V, Salen G, Cheng FW, Forte T, Shefer S, Tint GS, Lindgren FT: Abnormal high density lipoproteins in cerebrotendinous xanthomatosis. J Clin Invest **68:** 1295, 1981
33. DeBacker G, Rosseneu M, Deslypere JP: Discriminative value of lipids and lipoproteins in coronary heart disease. Atheroslerosis **43:** 197, 1982
34. Oberhansli I, Pometta D, Micheli H, Raymond L: High-density lipoproteins in children with coronary disease. Helv Paediatr Acta **36:** 135, 1981
35. Kaukola S, Manninen V, Halonen DI: Serum lipids with special reference to HDl cholesterol and triglycerides in young male survivors of acute myocardial infarction. Acta Med Scand **208:** 41, 1980
36. Swanson IO, Pierpont G, Adicott A: Serum high density lipoprotein cholesterol correlation with presence but not severity of coronary artery disease. Am J Med **71:** 235, 1981
37. Uhl GS, Troxler RG, Hickman JR Jr, Clark D: Relation between high density lipoprotein cholesterol and coronary artery disease in asymptomatic men. Am J Cardiol **48:** 903, 1981
38. Gasilin US, Kurdanov KH A, Perova NV, Torkhovskaya TI, Polessky VA, Matveeva LS: The peculiarities of lipid and protein components of the high- and low-density lipoproteins in patients suffering from coronary atherosclerosis with different number of affected coronary arteries. Cor Vasa **23:** 248, 1981
39. Naito HK, Greenstreet RL, David JA, Sheldon WL, Shirey EK, Lewis RC, Proudfit WL, Gerrity RG: HDL-cholesterol concentration and severity of coronary atherosclerosis determined by cineangiography. Artery **8:** 101, 1980
40. Bihari-Varga M, Szekely J, Gruber E: Plasma high density lipoproteins in coronary, cerebral, and peripheral vascular disease. The influence of various risk factors. Atherosclerosis **40:** 337, 1981
41. Anger E, Morck HI, Brendstrup T, Hollnagel H, Schroll M, Gyntelberg F: Cholesterol, high-density lipoprotein-cholesterol (HDL) and cholesterol/HDL ratio versus arterial blood pressure. Acta Med Scand **646**(suppl): 25, 1981
42. Yamashita S, Yamashita K: Effect of high-fiber diet on plasma high density lipoprotein (HDL) cholesterol level in streptozotocin-induced diabetic rats. Endocrinol Jpn **27:** 671, 1980
43. Thorland WG, Gilliam TB: Comparison of serum lipids between habitually high and low active pre-adolescent males. Med Sci Sports Exerc **13:** 316, 1981
44. Brownell KD, Stunkard AJ: Differential changes in plasma high-density lipoprotein cholesterol levels in obese men and women during weight reduction. Arch Intern Med **141:** 1142, 1981
45. Hartung GH, Squires WG, Gotto AM Jr: Effect of exercise training on plasma high-density lipoprotein cholesterol in coronary disease patients. Am Heart J **101:** 181, 1981
46. Garrison RJ, Wilson PW, Castelli WP, Feinleib M, Kannel WB, McNamara PM: Obesity and lipoprotein cholesterol in the Framingham offspring study. Metabolism **29:** 1053, 1980
47. Phillips NR, Havel RJ, Kane JP: Levels and interrelationships of serum and lipoprotein cholesterol and triglycerides. Association with adiposity and the consumption of ethanol, tobacco, and beverages containing caffeine. Atherosclerosis **1:** 13, 1981
48. Nakazawa K, Murata K: Epidemiological study of serum high density lipoprotein cholesterol with respect to risk factors against ischemic heart disease and atherosclerosis. Tokoho J Exp Med **133:** 197, 1981
49. Aviram A, Luboshitzky R, Brook JG: Lipids and lipoprotein pattern in thyroid dysfunction and the effect of therapy. Clin Biochem **15:** 62, 1982
50. Cai H-J, Li Z-X, Yang S-M: Serum high density lipoprotein cholesterol leads in Chinese healthy subjects and patients with certain diseases. Atherosclerosis **43:** 197, 1982
51. Luoma PV, Arranto AJ, Ehnholm C, Sotaniemi EA: Liver histological changes and plasma high density lipoproteins in man. Res Commun Chem Pathol Pharmacol **33:** 163, 1981
52. Hunninghake DB, Bell CP, Olson L: Effect of probucol on plasma lipids and lipoproteins in type IIb hyperlipoproteinemia. Atherosclerosis **37:** 469, 1980
53. Kibata M, et al: Clinical study of niceritrol on serum lipids in the treatment of hyperlipidemia. Atherosclerosis **37:** 333, 1980
54. O'Neill B, Callaghan N, Stapleton M, Molloy W: Serum elevation of high density lipoprotein (HDL) cholesterol in epileptic patients taking carbamazepine or phenytin. Acta Neurol Scand **65:** 104, 1980
55. van de Wiel A, Kruiswijk T, Inhof JW, Hart HC, Holtkamp HC, Szakaly M: Effects of plasma exchange on serum cholesterol levels in heterozygous familial hypercholesterolemia. Acta Med Scand **210:** 461, 1982
56. Dobrea GM, Wieland RG, Johnson MW: The effect of rapid weight loss due to jejunileal bypass on total cholesterol and high-density lipoprotein. Am J Clin Nutr **34:** 1994, 1981
57. Nakai T, Tamai T, Yamada S, Kobayashi T, Hayashi T, Kutsumi Y, Oida K, Takeda R: Plasma lipids and lipoproteins of Japanese adults and umbilical cord blood. Artery **9:** 132, 1981
58. Pentila IM, Voutilainen E, Laitinen P, Juutilainean P: Comparison of different analytical and precipitation methods for direct estimation of serum high-density lipoprotein cholesterol. Scand J Clin Lab Invest **41:** 353, 1981
59. Richter V, Rassoul F, Senger H, Rotzsch W: HDL/LDL cholesterol, arteriosclerosis, and age. Z Alteruforschung (Dresden) **35:** 359, 1980
60. Makurati D, Hordynska-Kremont B, Kuzmaiaki D, Woch-Bialk Z, Przybylska J: Qualitative value of the total cholesterol of HDL cholesterol ratio of healthy persons of different age. Pol Tyg Lek **36:** 441, 1981
61. Nebieridze DU, Zhukovoski GS, Akhmeteli MA, Gerasimova EN, Deev AD: Mortality in men 40 to 59 years old from coronary and cerebral arteriosclerosis with varying cholesterol and triglyceride levels in the blood. Biull Vsesoiuznogo Kardiol Nauchn Tsentra **4:** 78, 1981
62. Epstein FH: Role of HDL in individual prediction and community prevention of coronary heart disease. *In* Gotto AM, editor: Atherosclerosis V. International Symposium on Atherosclerosis, Houston, 1979. New York, 1980, Springer-Verlag, p 484–487
63. Walker ARP, Walker BF, Mngomezuu QN: Serum high density

lipoprotein cholesterol levels in African school children living near or very far from school. Atherosclerosis **41:** 35, 1982
64. Kukita H, Imamara Y, Hamada M, Joh T, Kokubuk T: Plasma lipids and lipoproteins in Japanese male patients with coronary artery disease and in their relatives. Atherosclerosis **42:** 21, 1982
65. Williams P, Robinson D, Bailey A: High density lipoprotein and coronary risk factors in normal men. Lancet **2:** 72, 1979
66. Craig IH, Philips PJ, Lloyd JV, Watts S, Bracken A, Read R: Effects of modified fat diets on LDL/HDL ratio. Lancet **2:** 799, 1980 (letter)
67. Knuiman JT, West CF: The concentration of cholesterol in serum and in various serum lipoproteins in macrobiotic, vegetarian and non-vegetarian men and boys. Atherosclerosis **43:** 71, 1982
68. Castelli WR: Individual vs group response. *In* Beecher GR, editor: Beltsville Symposia in Agriculture Research. Human Research Meeting, Beltsville, MD, May 1979. Totowa, NJ, 1979, Allanheld, Osmiea and Co, vol IV, p 113–120
69. Knuiman JT, West CE, Hautvast JG: Role of diet to HDL-cholesterol and coronary disease: serum total and HDL-cholesterol in boys and men from developing and developed countries. Am Heart J **103:** 447, 1982 (letter)
70. Berg A, Keul J, Ringwald G, Stippig J, Deus B: Serum lipoprotein cholesterol in sedentary and trained male patients with coronary heart disease. Clin Cardiol **4:** 233, 1981
71. Kerttula Y, Weber TH, Tanner P: Effect of immune complexes on plasma HDL cholesterol in rabbits. Atherosclerosis **38:** 395, 1981
72. Schnabel A, Kindermann W: Effect of maximal oxygen uptake and different forms of physical training on serum lipoproteins. Eur J Applied Physiol **48:** 263, 1982
73. Adner MM, Castelli WP: Elevated high-density lipoprotein levels in marathon runners. JAMA **243:** 534, 1980
74. Schaefer EJ, Levy RI, Ernst ND, Van Sant FD, Brewer HB Jr: The effects of low cholesterol, high polyunsaturated fat, and low fat diets on plasma lipid and lipoprotein cholesterol levels in normal and hypercholesterolemic subjects. Am J Clin Nutr **34:** 1758, 1981
75. Schatz C, Jeanblanc B, Offner M: Cholesterol in serum high density lipoprotein fraction. Nouv Presse Med **9:** 3339, 1980
76. Ginsburg BE, Zetterstrom R: Serum cholesterol concentrations in newborn infants with gestational ages of 28–42 weeks. Acta Paediatr Scand **69:** 587, 1980
77. Wiklund O, Wilhelmsen L, Elmfeldt D, Wedel H. Valek J, Gustafson A: Alpha-lipoprotein cholesterol concentration in relation to subsequent myocardial infarction in hypercholesterolemic men. Atherosclerosis **37:** 47, 1980
78. Castelli WP, Abbott RD, McNamara PM: Summary estimates of cholesterol used to predict coronary heart disease. Circulation **67:** 730, 1983

Quantitative analysis of the high-frequency components of the signal-averaged QRS complex in patients with acute myocardial infarction: a prospective study

JOSEPH A. GOMES, M.D., RAHUL MEHRA, PH.D., PHILIP BARRECA, B.S., NABIL EL-SHERIF, M.D., ROBERT HARIMAN, M.D., AND RONALD HOLTZMAN, M.S.

ABSTRACT We performed a prospective study of the high-frequency components of the terminal portion of the QRS complex in 50 patients with acute myocardial infarction (AMI) (mean age 63 ± 10 years) within 3.25 ± 2.45 days of the acute event. Signal averaging (400 beats) at a filter setting of 80 to 300 Hz was performed and the duration of the low-amplitude signals of less than 40 μV in the terminal portion of the QRS, the root-mean-square (RMS) voltage of the terminal 40 msec of the QRS complex, and the total duration of the signal-averaged QRS vector complex were measured. The low-amplitude signals were abnormally prolonged in 22 of 50 patients (44%); the RMS-V was abnormal (<20 μV) in 21 of 50 patients (58%), and the signal-averaged vector complex was abnormal (>120 msec) in 15 of 46 patients (33%) without bundle branch block. There was no significant correlation between any of the signal-averaged parameters and site of AMI or total creatine kinase (CK) and CK-MB values. On the basis of the occurrence of spontaneous ventricular tachycardia in the acute and postcoronary care phase of AMI, the patients were divided into two groups. Group I consisted of 31 patients (62%) who had no documented ventricular tachycardia and group II consisted of 19 patients (38%) who had one or more runs of ventricular tachycardia. Fourteen of the 19 patients in group II (73.6%) had nonsustained ventricular tachycardia and five patients (26.3%) suffered sustained ventricular tachycardia/ventricular fibrillation or sudden death. The low-amplitude signals and the signal-averaged QRS complex duration were significantly longer in group II than group I. The RMS voltage was significantly lower in group II than group I. In addition, in five of the patients (10%) who had sustained ventricular tachycardia/fibrillation and/or sudden death the low-amplitude signals were 50 msec or greater and the RMS voltage was 13 μV or less; the signal-averaged QRS vector complex was greater than 120 msec in four of these patients. We conclude the following: (1) Abnormal signal-averaged parameters are seen in 33% to 58% of patients with AMI. (2) There is no correlation between any of the signal-averaged parameters and site of AMI or CK and CK-MB values. (3) Low-amplitude signals and the duration of the signal-averaged QRS complex are significantly longer and the RMS voltage significantly lower in patients with AMI who have spontaneous ventricular tachycardia in the acute and postcoronary care phase of AMI. (4) Signal-averaged parameters may be valuable in predicting arrhythmic events in patients with AMI.
Circulation 72, No. 1, 105–111, 1985.

EXPERIMENTAL AND CLINICAL STUDIES in recent years have demonstrated that reentry plays a major role in the genesis of most ventricular arrhythmias.[1–11] The conditions that favor the occurrence of reentry are slow conduction, unidirectional block, and recovery of excitability. The demonstration of delayed fractionated electrical activity during diastole in regions of experimental myocardial infarction and in patients with ventricular tachycardia and left ventricular aneurysm during endocardial catheterization and intraoperative mapping has provided evidence for slow conduction in the ventricular myocardium. Furthermore, delayed fractionated electrical activity in diastole has been closely correlated with the genesis of reentrant ventricular arrhythmias.[2, 3, 6, 10] Recently, several investigators using high-gain amplification and signal-averaging techniques demonstrated diastolic

From the Clinical Electrophysiology Laboratory, Department of Cardiology, Brooklyn VA Medical Center and SUNY Downstate Medical Centers, New York.
Supported by the Veterans Administration Medical Research Funds.
Address for correspondence: Joseph A. Gomes, M.D., Director, Electrophysiology and Electrocardiography Section, EKG Department The Mount Sinai Medical Center, One Gustave L. Levy Pl., New York, NY 10029.
Received July 24, 1984; revision accepted April 11, 1985.
Presented in part at the 56th Scientific Session of the American Heart Association, Anaheim, CA, November 1983.

electrical activity in experimental myocardial infarction and in patients with recurrent ventricular tachycardia and left ventricular aneurysm.[12-17] Furthermore, Simson et al.,[18,19] using quantitative analysis, have demonstrated low-amplitude signals in the terminal portion of the QRS complex in patients with recurrent sustained ventricular tachycardia.

Most previous signal-averaging studies have been done in patients with recurrent ventricular tachycardia with or without ventricular aneurysm and in dogs with experimental acute myocardial infarction.[12-19] The purpose of this prospective study was (1) to assess the occurrence of low-amplitude signals in the terminal portion of the QRS complex from body surface recordings in patients with an acute myocardial infarction (AMI), (2) to determine whether the occurrence of low-amplitude signals is related to the size and location of the infarct, and (3) to attempt to correlate the occurrence of low-amplitude signals with the occurrence of spontaneous ventricular tachyarrhythmias in the early phase of myocardial infarction.

Materials and methods

A total of 50 male patients with AMI were studied. In all patients the diagnosis of AMI was confirmed by (1) clinical, (2) electrocardiographic, and (3) total creatine kinase (CK) and CK-MB values. Signal averaging was not attempted in patients in pulmonary edema or cardiogenic shock. In addition a total of 20 normal male subjects underwent signal averaging of the body surface QRS complex for determination of normal signal-averaged parameters.

Signal-averaging technique. All patients with AMI underwent signal averaging within 3.25 ± 2.45 days (mean ± SD, range 1 to 10 days) of the acute event. None of the patients were on antiarrhythmic agents during the signal-averaging procedure and none had arrhythmias, including ventricular ectopic activity, during the signal-averaging procedure. In those patients who had been receiving antiarrhythmic therapy, including prophylactic lidocaine, these agents were withheld for at least five half-lives before the signal-averaging procedure. Signal averaging was done with the subjects lying comfortably supine in an "electrically quiet" but not specifically shielded environment after the experimental nature of the procedure had been explained to them and they had given informed signed consent. After each subject's skin was prepared with a mildly abrasive pad and washed with alcohol, seven self-adhesive silver/silver chloride electrodes were attached: the horizontal (X) electrodes in the right and left midaxillary lines at the fourth intercostal space, the vertical (Y) electrodes on the suprasternal notch and V_3 position, and the sagittal (Z) electrodes in the V_2 position anteriorly and at the corresponding position posteriorly. The seventh, indifferent, electrode was placed on the eighth rib in the right midaxillary line. The signal-processing system, hardware, and methods used in our laboratory have been described in detail previously.[20,21] After connecting the electrodes to the corresponding preamplifier inputs the three low-gain outputs (gain of 1000) were viewed simultaneously to select the channel with the largest QRS complex for triggering the signal averager. Bipolar X, Y, and Z lead signals were then filtered at filter frequencies of 80 to 300 (24 dB/octave) Hz and then underwent further (gain 250) amplication before being digitized and averaged with a 3001 Norland signal-processing system. Approximately 400 beats were signal averaged. Ten-bit resolution was used for analog-to-digital conversion. The data were stored on magnetic diskettes for subsequent measurement and photography.

The occurrence of ventricular arrhythmias in the coronary care unit was assessed by use of a Hewlett-Packard model 5600A Patient Management System with an arrhythmia monitoring option 78220A/B, which provides a special 9 hr trend display. The system has recall capabilities over 24 hr and editing and monitor strip recording capabilities over 9 hr trend display. Human validation of the rhythm disturbances on the monitoring system was done for every patient by the nursing staff using recall and editing capabilities and the rhythm was confirmed by the senior investigator. In the postcoronary care phase a 24 hr ambulatory Holter recording was obtained within 24 hr of the signal-averaging procedure. All patients were monitored in the coronary care unit for a period of 3 to 5 days and in the intermediate coronary care unit for an additional 10 days.

Definition of terms and calculations. A vector magnitude was calculated for each point of the averaged wave as

$$V = \sqrt{X^2 + Y^2 + Z^2}$$

The durataion of the low-amplitude signals was measured from the end of the signal-averaged QRS vector complex to the first point at which signals reached 40 μV. The end of the QRS vector complex was defined as the point at which the signals were more than twice the peak-to-peak noise amplitude as measured from the TP interval. Root-mean-square (RMS) voltage was measured for the terminal 40 msec of the QRS vector complex. The signal-averaged QRS vector complex was measured from the onset to the end of the QRS vector complex. All signal-averaged parameters were measured with a Norland 3001 computer. Electrocardiographic QRS complex was measured on the surface electrocardiogram obtained on the same day and within 1 hr of the signal-averaging procedure. Nonsustained ventricular tachycardia was defined as 3 or more successive beats of ventricular origin at a rate of 120 beats/min or greater that lasted for 30 sec or less and terminated spontaneously. Sustained ventricular tachycardia was defined as spontaneous tachycardia of ventricular origin that lasted for more than 30 sec or was associated with hemodynamic compromise. Sudden cardiac death was defined as death occurring within 1 hr of the onset of symptoms. Statistical analysis of the data was done by use of the χ^2 and Student's t test for unpaired and paired data. All data are expressed as mean ±SD.

Results

Clinical features. The patients with AMI ranged in age from 45 to 83 years (mean 63 ± 10 years). Twenty-four patients (48%) had an anterior wall AMI, 21 patients (42%) had an inferior wall AMI, and five patients (10%) had a subendocardial AMI. A total of four patients had bundle branch block. In these patients the duration of the electrocardiographic QRS complex and the signal-averaged QRS vector complex was not used to calculate the means and differentiate abnormal from normal values.

Signal-averaged parameters

Normal subjects. Normal ranges of values for signal-averaged parameters were determined by performing signal-averaging studies in 20 male subjects (age 32 ± 6 years) with no evidence of ischemic or other forms of organic heart disease. The duration of low-amplitude signals ranged from 7 to 37 msec and were less than 42 msec in all subjects (100%). The RMS voltage of the terminal 40 msec ranged from 14.1 to 81 μV and was greater than 20 μV in 19 of 20 subjects (95%). The signal-averaged QRS duration ranged from 76 to 103 msec and was less than 120 msec in all 20 subjects (100%).

Patients with AMI. The low-amplitude signals ranged from 11.5 to 98.5 msec (mean 42 ± 10 msec) in duration in the patients. Twenty-two of 50 patients (44%) had abnormally prolonged low-amplitude signals of greater than 42 msec (upper limit of normal for our laboratory +2 SDs). The RMS voltage of the terminal 40 msec of the signal-averaged complex QRS vector ranged from 2.38 to 68.2 μV (mean 24 ± 17 μV). Twenty-one of 50 patients (58%) had abnormal RMS voltage of less than 20 μV (upper limit of normal for our laboratory). The duration of the signal-averaged QRS vector complex ranged from 91 msec to 144.5 msec (mean 114 ± 16 msec) in patients without bundle branch block and was significantly longer ($p < .0001$) than the electrocardiographic QRS complex duration, which measured 95 ± 10 msec. In 15 of 46 patients (33%) without bundle branch block the mean signal-averaged QRS vector complex was greater than 120 msec.

Correlation between signal-averaged parameters and other clinical variables. There was no significant correlation between total CK and low-amplitude signals ($r = .218$), total CK and RMS voltage ($r = .0915$), or total CK and signal-averaged QRS vector complex ($r = .206$). No correlation was found between peak CK-MB fraction and low-amplitude signals ($r = .249$), peak CK-MB fraction and RMS voltage ($r = .136$), or peak CK-MB fraction and the signal-averaged vector complexes ($r = .165$). Similarly, no correlation was noted between the day of study, site of AMI, and the various signal-averaged parameters.

Ventricular tachyarrhythmias. On the basis of the occurrence of spontaneous ventricular tachyarrhythmias in the acute and immediate postcoronary care phase of AMI the patients were divided into two groups. Group I consisted of 31 patients (62%) who had no documented ventricular tachycardia and group II of 19 patients (38%) who had one or more runs of spontaneous ventricular tachycardia. Three patients from group I and one patient from group II had bundle branch block. Of the 19 patients in group II, 14 (73.6%) had nonsustained ventricular tachycardia and five (26.3%) suffered sustained ventricular tachycardia/ventricular fibrillation and/or sudden cardiac death. In 11 of the 19 patients in group II, ventricular arrhythmias occurred 2 to 30 days (mean 11 ± 9 days) after the signal-averaging procedure; in six patients the ventricular arrhythmias occurred 1 to 3 days (mean 2.0 ± 1.0 days) before the procedure and in two ventricular arrhythmias were noted on the day of the procedure. In 12 of the 19 patients (63%) the ventricular arrhythmias were noted after the first 3 days of AMI, whereas in the remaining seven patients (37%) arrhythmias were noted within the first 3 days after AMI. Of the five patients who developed sustained ventricular tachycardia, fibrillation, and/or sudden death, ventricular arrhythmias occurred on days 2, 15, 15, and 30 after the signal-averaging procedure in four patients and 3 days before the procedure in the remaining patient. Ventricular arrhythmias occurred within the first 3 days of AMI in only one of these five patients. None of the patients were on antiarrhythmic therapy when they experienced spontaneous ventricular arrhythmias.

Clinical differences between the two groups. Table 1 demonstrates the clinical differences between the two groups. There were no significant differences with respect to age, day of study, peak total CK and CK-MB, or site of AMI, although the mean values for total peak CK and CK-MB and the incidence of anterior wall AMI was slightly higher in group II than in group I patients. The incidence of inferior wall and subendocardial AMI was higher in group I when compared with group II, but these differences did not reach statistical significance.

Differences in signal-averaged parameters in the two groups. The data on the signal-averaged parameters for

TABLE 1
Clinical features of patients in the two study groups

Group	Age (yr)	Day of study (days after AMI)	CK (IU/l)	CK-MB	Site of AMI (% of patients) AWMI	IWMI	SEMI
I	63±11	3.25±2.42	1498±752	182±129	42	45	13
II	63±8	3.52±2.66	1527±894	201±130	53	37	10
p value	NS	NS	NS	NS	NS	NS	NS

AWMI = anterior wall MI; IWMI = inferior wall MI; SEMI = subendocardial MI.

TABLE 2
Signal-averaged parameters

Group	LAS (msec)	RMS-voltage (μV)	Signal-averaged QRS complex duration (msec)
I	30.42±9.8	26.91±15	109±12
II	50.31±24.11	17.66±15	120±19
p value	<.01	<.05	<.05

LAS = low-amplitude signals.

the two groups are shown in table 2 and figure 1. The low-amplitude signals were significantly longer ($p < .01$) in group II compared with group I. Whereas 10 of 31 patients (32%) from group I had low-amplitude signals of greater than 42 msec, 12 of 19 patients (63%) from group II had signals this long. The RMS voltage of the terminal 40 msec of the signal-averaged QRS vector complex was significantly lower ($p < .05$) in group II than group I. Fifteen of the 31 patients (48%) in group I had an RMS voltage less than 20 μV whereas 16 of the 19 patients (84%) in group II had an RMS voltage less than 20 μV. The signal-averaged QRS vector complex was significantly longer ($p < .05$) in group II than group I. Whereas five of the 28 patients (18%) from group I without bundle branch

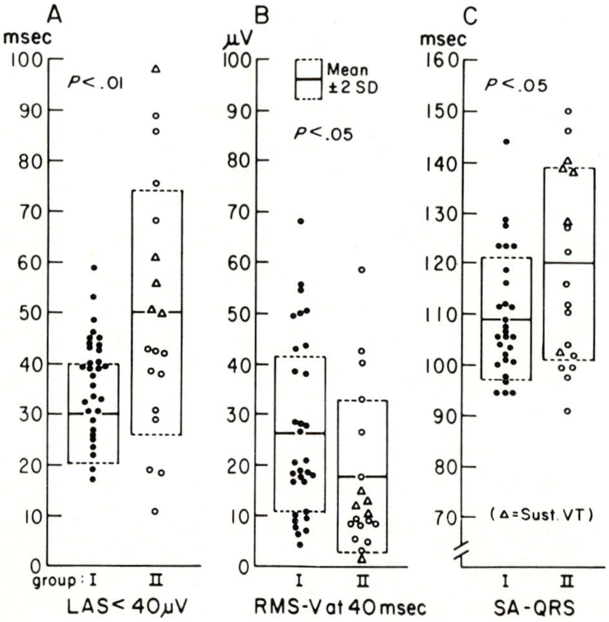

FIGURE 1. Individual signal-averaged QRS complex parameters for patients in groups I and II. *A*, Distribution of low-amplitude signals in group I (solid circle) and group II (open circle). *B*, Distribution of RMS voltages in group I (solid circle) and group II (open circle). *C*, Distribution of durations of signal-averaged QRS vector complexes in group I (solid circle) and group II (open circle). Data from patients wtih sustained ventricular tachycardia/fibrillation are represented by open triangles (group II).

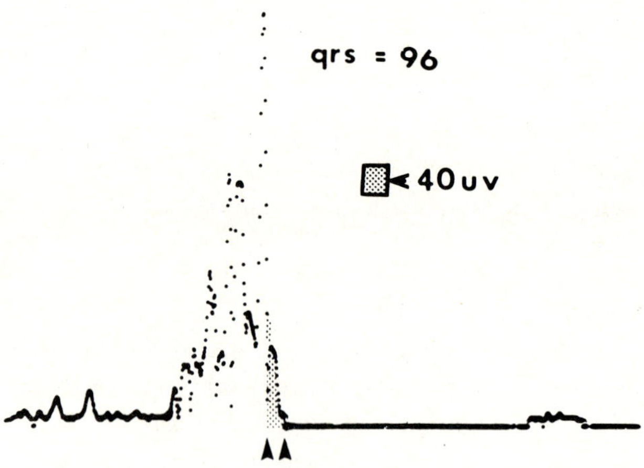

FIGURE 2. Signal-averaged QRS complex obtained 1 day after AMI in a patient in group I. The amplitude of the last 40 msec was 54.32 μV, the duration of the low-amplitude signal was 17 msec (hatched area), and the signal-averaged vector complex was 96 msec.

block had a QRS vector complex of greater than 120 msec in duration, eight of the 18 patients (44%) in group II without bundle branch block had a QRS vector complex greater than this. Examples of data from patients in groups I and II are shown in figures 2 and 3. All the five patients with sustained ventricular tachycardia/fibrillation and/or sudden death had low-amplitude signals of greater than 42 msec; all also had an RMS voltage of < 20 μV in the terminal 40 msec and four of five patients had a signal-averaged QRS vector complex of greater than 120 msec. An example from one of these patients is shown in figure 3. This patient underwent signal averaging 4 days after AMI

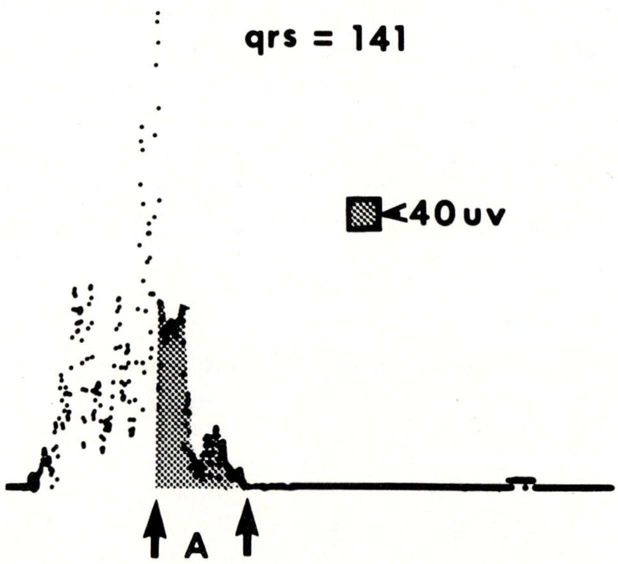

FIGURE 3. Signal-averaged QRS complex obtained 4 days after AMI in a patient in group II who 2 days later developed sustained ventricular tachycardia. The low-amplitude signal (hatched area) was 56 msec in duration, the RMS voltage was 13.05 μV, and the signal-averaged vector complex was 141 msec in duration.

and the results revealed abnormal parameters: low-amplitude signals were 56 msec in duration, the RMS voltage of the terminal 40 msec of the QRS complex was 13.05 μV, and the signal-averaged QRS vector magnitude was 141 msec. Two days after discharge from the coronary care unit the patient complained of palpitations and dizziness associated with profuse diaphoresis. An electrocardiogram was recorded at this time and revealed sustained ventricular tachycardia.

Specificity and sensitivity of signal-averaged parameters. The sensitivity and specificity of signal-averaged parameters in separating patients without ventricular arrhythmias (group I) from those with them (group II) and in separating patients with sustained ventricular tachycardia/fibrillation and or sudden death from those without are shown in table 3. The sensitivity and specificity of signal-averaged parameters ranged from 44% to 84% and from 52% to 84%, respectively, in separating patients with from those without ventricular tachyarrhythmias. The sensitivity and specificity of signal-averaged parameters ranged from 80% to 100% and from 42% to 88%, respectively, in separating patients with sustained ventricular tachycardia/fibrillation and/or sudden death from those without.

Discussion

In recent years several investigators have attempted to record late diastolic potentials wih high-gain amplification and signal averaging in patients with ventricular tachycardia and with and without left ventricular aneurysm.[14–16] These studies have demonstrated a high prevalence of late diastolic potentials in patients with recurrent sustained ventricular tachycardia. In addition a good correlation has been noted between the presence of late potentials and left ventricular wall motion abnormalities.[16] The majority of these studies, however, have assessed the presence of late potentials qualitatively. Qualitative assessment of late potentials can be frought with significant error since it is often difficult to decipher the end of the signal-averaged QRS complex and the onset of the late potentials. To obviate these limitations, Simson[18] proposed quantitative analysis of the high-frequency components of the terminal portion of the QRS complex by computer analysis. Using a 25 Hz filter, Simson observed that 92% of the patients with recurrent ventricular tachycardia had less than 25 μV of high-frequency voltage in the last 40 msec of the QRS complex and in 72% of the patients the QRS duration was longer than 120 msec. Denes et al.[22] have also recently demonstrated that high-frequency analysis of the signal-averaged body surface QRS is a reliable, reproducible method for distinguishing patients with recurrent ventricular tachycardia from those without it. Using a 40 Hz filter and a definition of normal of greater than 20 μV for the amplitude of the last 40 msec, 90% of patients without ventricular tachycardia and 83% of patients with ventricular tachycardia were correctly identified. Furthermore, these investigators found that the use of a 40 Hz filter markedly improved the separation between those with and without ventricular tachycardia and reduced the degree of variability resulting from use of a 25 Hz filter. Other investigators[16] have used 100 Hz filtering. In contrast to the method of Simson[18] and Denes et al.,[22] we used 80 Hz filtering to record low-amplitude signals. Although our method is not comparable to that of Simson or Denes et al., we, like the latter investigators, who used 40 Hz filtering, found that use of 20 μV as the normal value for amplitude of the last 40 msec resulted in good separation of normal from abnormal values. Simson, on the other hand, using 25 Hz filtering, found that use of 25 μV provided a separation between patients with and without ventricular tachycardia. Since the optimal bandpass is still unknown, in the future standardization of the use of specific filter frequencies will be needed for comparative purposes.

Myocardial infarction in man offers a unique setting in which to study the high-frequency components of the terminal portion of the signal-averaged QRS complex, to detect abnormal low-amplitude signals, and to determine their significance because the occurrence of these signals and clinically significant ventricular arrhythmias in the acute, subacute, and chronic phase of myocardial infarction can be correlated. In this study abnormally prolonged low-amplitude signals of greater than 42 msec in duration were seen in 44% of patients with an AMI. In addition, the low-amplitude signals in the terminal portion of the QRS vector com-

TABLE 3
Sensitivity and specificity of signal-averaged parameters

	Group I vs group II		Sustained VT/VF/SD vs no sustained VT/VF/SD	
Parameter	Sensitivity (%)	Specificity (%)	Sensitivity (%)	Specificity (%)
Low-amplitude signals	63	68	100	62
RMS Voltage	84	52	100	42
Signal-averaged QRS vector duration	44	82	80	88

VT = ventricular tachycardia; VF = ventricular fibrillation; SD = sudden death.

plex were less than 20 μV in 58% of patients with AMI. These observations probably reflect regional slow ventricular activation in the border zone of an acute infarct. In 33% of patients the signal-averaged QRS vector complex was greater than 120 msec when the surface electrocardiogram was normal in duration. Again, this observation probably reflects delay in ventricular activation since in this study the delayed potentials were assessed as part of the signal-averaged QRS vector complex rather than as a separate entity. It is not unreasonable to expect abnormal signal-averaged QRS complexes in patients with AMI. However, the detection of these abnormalities may be dependent on one or more of the following factors: (1) The size of the ischemic mass of ventricular myocardium in the border zone of the infarct, rather than the location or the size of the infarct. The latter is suggested by the observation that there was no correlation between any of the signal-averaged parameters and the location of the infarct or the peak total CK and CK-MB values. These findings are in agreement with the preliminary observations of Abdollah et al.[22] (2) Heart rate. Whereas late potentials may not be evident at resting heart rates, they may be evident and more pronounced during atrial pacing at rapid heart rates.[12] (3) The occurrence of Wenckebach-like conduction block in one or more areas of the ischemic border zone. This block may not be detectable by signal-averaging techniques.[6, 21]

Of considerable importance was our finding that the duration of the low-amplitude signals and the signal-averaged QRS vector complex was significantly longer, whereas the RMS voltage of the terminal 40 msec of the QRS complex was significantly lower, in patients with AMI and ventricular tachyarrhythmias, in contrast to those without tachyarrhythmias. Furthermore, in five patients with sustained ventricular tachycardia/fibrillation and/or sudden death the RMS voltage of the terminal 40 msec was less than 13 μV, the low-amplitude signals were 50 msec or more, and, in four of the five, the signal-averaged QRS vector complex was more than 120 msec. These observations suggest that patients with AMI who have ventricular tachyarrhythmias, particularly sustained ventricular tachycardia/fibrillation and/or sudden death, in the early phase of myocardial infarction demonstrate a greater degree of ventricular myocardial conduction delay, which could provide the substrate for reentrant ventricular tachyarrhythmias. These findings are in disagreement with the preliminary observations of Abdollah et al.,[23] who found that low-amplitude signals failed to predict the occurrence of in-hospital ventricular tachycardia in patients with AMI. However, it should be noted that whereas approximately 44% to 84% of our patients with ventricular arrhythmias had one or more abnormal signal-averaged parameter values, 18% to 48% of our patients without ventricular arrhythmias had one or more abnormal values. Thus, the sensitivity (42% to 84%) and specificity (52% to 84%) of signal-averaged parameters were not strong in separating patients with ventricular arrhythmias from those without. However, when patients with sustained ventricular tachycardia/fibrillation and/or sudden death were compared with those without, low-amplitude signals of greater than 42 msec and RMS voltage of less than 20 μV were the most sensitive (100% each) but lacked specificity (62% and 42%, respectively), whereas the duration of the signal-averaged QRS complex was both specific (88%) and sensitive (80%). The low specificity of the duration of low-amplitude signals and the RMS voltage of the terminal 40 msec of the QRS complex may be related to the following: (1) the presence of delayed ventricular activation in ischemic myocardium that was not sufficient to result in reentrant ventricular arrhythmias, (2) the presence of delayed ventricular activation within areas of exit block, and (3) a mechanism of ventricular arrhythmias other than reentry (e.g., triggered automaticity).[24, 25] In the last case the presence of delayed ventricular activation would be independent of the spontaneous ventricular arrhythmia.

A preliminary report by Haerten et al.[26] suggested that the presence of late potentials and inducibility of repetitive ventricular responses help to identify patients at risk of sudden death or ventricular tachycardia after myocardial infarction. More recently Kanovsky et al.[27] found that the signal-averaged electrocardiogram provided independent information in identifying patients with ventricular tachycardia after myocardial infarction. However, their study consisted of patients who were referred for electrophysiologic studies because of repeated episodes of ventricular tachycardia. They did not prospectively follow patients with AMI to determine whether signal averaging identified a group of patients at future risk of developing ventricular tachycardia and/or sudden death. Thus, the role of signal-averaging techniques in predicting future arrhythmic events in the postmyocardial infarction patient remains to be defined. Long-term prospective follow-up and sequential signal-averaging studies in a large number of postinfarction patients will be needed before this important and crucial question can be answered since the dynamic nature of myocardial infarction and the healing process could result in changes in late potential parameters.

We acknowledge Alma Lucus and Maxine Wright for their secretarial assistance.

References

1. Durrer D, Van Lier AA, Briller J: Epicardial and intramural excitation in chronic myocardial infarction. Am Heart J **64:** 765, 1964
2. Boineau JP, Cox JL: Slow ventricular activation in acute myocardial infarction. A source of reentrant premature ventricular contraction. Circulation **48:** 702, 1973
3. Waldo AL, Kaiser GA: A study of ventricular arrhythmias associated with acute myocardial infarction in the canine heart. Circulation **47:** 1222, 1973
4. Witt AL, Cranefield PF, Hoffman BF: Slow conduction and reentry in the ventricular conduction system II. Single and sustained circus movement in networks of canine and bovine purkinje fibers. Circ Res **30:** 11, 1972
5. Scherlag BJ, El-Sherif N, Hope RR, Lazzara R: Characterization and localization of ventricular arrhythmias due to myocardial ischemia and infarction. Circ Res **35:** 372, 1974
6. El-Sherif N, Scherlag BJ, Lazzara R, Hope RR: Reentrant ventricular arrhythmias in the late myocardial infarction period I. Conduction characteristics in the infarction zone. Circulation **55:** 686, 1974
7. El-Sherif N, Smith RA, Evans K: Canine ventricular arrhythmias in the late myocardial infarction period. 8 Epicardial mapping of reentrant circuits. Circ Res **49:** 255, 1981
8. Witt AL, Alessie MA, Bonke FIM, Lammers W, Smeets J, Fenoglio JJ: Electrophysiologic mapping to determine the mechanism of experimental ventricular tachycardia initiated by premature stimulation. Experimental approach and initial results demonstrating reentrant excitation. Am J Cardiol **49:** 166, 1982
9. Mehra R, Zeiler RH, Gough WB, El-Sherif N: Reentrant ventricular arrhythmias in the late myocardial infarction period. Electrophysiologic — anatomic correlation of reentrant circuits. Circulation **67:** 11, 1983
10. Josephson ME, Horowitz LN, Farshidi A: Continuous local electrical activity; a mechanism of recurrent ventricular tachycardia. Circulation **57:** 659, 1978
11. Horowitz LN, Harken AH, Kastor JA, Josephson ME: Ventricular resection guided by epicardial and endocardial mapping for the treatment of recurrent ventricular tachycardia. N Engl J Med **302:** 589, 1980
12. Berbari EJ, Scherlag BJ, Hope RR, Lazzara R: Recording from the body surface of arrhythmogenic ventricular activity during the ST segment. Am J Cardiol **41:** 697, 1978
13. Simson MB, Enle D, Michaelson EL, Falcone RA, Spear JF, Moore EN: Detection of delayed ventricular activation of the body surface in dogs. Am J Physiol **241:** H-363, 1981
14. Fontaine G, Frank R, Gallais-Hamonno F, Allali I, Phan-Thuc H, Grosgogeat Y: Electrocardiographie des potentials tardifs du syndrome de post-excitation. Arch Mal Coeur **71:** 854, 1978
15. Rozanski JJ, Mortara D, Myerburg RJ, Castellanos A: Body surface detection of delayed depolarizations in patients with recurrent ventricular tachycardia and left ventricular aneurysm. Circulation **63:** 1172, 1981
16. Breithardt G, Borgraffe M, Karbenn A, Abendroth RR, Yey HL, Seipel L: Prevalence of late potentials in patients with and without ventricular tachycardia: Correlation with angiographic findings. Am J Cardiol **49:** 1932, 1982
17. Hombach M, Braun V, Happ HW, Gil-Sanchez D, Schodl H, Behrenbeck DW, Tranchert M, Higler HH: The application of signal averaging technique in clinical cardiology. Clin Cardiol **5:** 107, 1982
18. Simson MG: Identification of patients with ventricular tachycardia after myocardial infarction from signals in the terminal QRS complex. Circulation **64:** 235, 1981
19. Simson MB, Untereker WJ, Spielman SR: Relation between late potentials on the body surface and directly recorded fragmented electrograms in patients with ventricular tachycardia. Am J Cardiol **57:** 105, 1983
20. Mehra R, Kelen G, Zeiler R, Zephirnan D, Fried P, Gomes JAC, El-Sherif N: Noninvasive His bundle electrogram: value of three vector lead recordings. Am J Cardiol **49:** 344, 1982
21. El-Sherif N, Mehra RA, Gomes JAC, Kelen G: Appraisal of a low noise electrocardiogram. J Am Coll Cardiol **1:** 2, 456, 1983
22. Denes P, Santarelli O, Houser RG, Uritz UF: Quantitative analysis of the high frequency components of the terminal portion of the body surface QRS in normal subjects and in patients with ventricular tachycardia. Circulation **67:** 1129, 1983
23. Abdollah H, Richards DA, Dool A, Dassen WRM, Bratt S, de Zwann C, Wellens HJJ: Signal averaged ECG in post myocardial infarction patients. Circulation **68** (suppl III): III-172, 1983 (abst)
24. Rosen MR, Reder RF: Does triggered activity have a role in the genesis of cardiac arrhythmias? Ann Intern Med **94:** 794, 1981
25. El-Sherif N, Gough WB, Zeiler RH, Mehra R: Triggered ventricular rhythms in 1-day-old myocardial infarction in the dog. Circ Res **52:** 566, 1983
26. Haerten K, Borgraffe M, Breithardt G: Repetitive ventricular response and late potential in patients early after myocardial infarction. Circulation **68** (suppl III): III-174, 1983 (abst)
27. Kanovsky MS, Falcone RA, Dresden CA, Josephson ME, Simson ME: Identification of patients with ventricular tachycardia after myocardial infarction: signal averaged electrocardiogram, Holter monitoring, and cardiac catheterization. Circulation **70:** 264, 1984

Lysis of left ventricular thrombi with urokinase

PETER KREMER, M.D., RAINER FIEBIG, M.D., VOLKMAR TILSNER, M.D., WALTER BLEIFELD, M.D., AND DETLEF G. MATHEY, M.D.

ABSTRACT In 16 patients with recent myocardial infarction (3 to 12 week old) and with large left ventricular thrombi systemic thrombolysis with urokinase was performed. Left ventricular thrombi were diagnosed by two-dimensional echocardiography; in all patients the mural thrombus was located in the area of recent myocardial infarction. Each of three patients suffered an embolic episode before the initiation of thrombolytic therapy and the episode caused a stroke in one. Urokinase was infused intravenously at a rate of 60,000 U/hr for 2 to 8 days in combination with intravenous heparin (200 units/kg × 12 hr). Left ventricular thrombi were successfully lysed in 10 of 16 patients, as determined by two-dimensional echocardiography. In four of the six remaining patients only partial thrombolysis was achieved and in two thrombolytic treatment failed. There was no evidence of embolic events during thrombolysis in any of the 16 patients. The success of thrombolysis seemed to depend on the age of the thrombus: the thrombus was dissolved in eight of nine patients undergoing thrombolysis within 4 weeks of the acute myocardial infarction vs in two of seven patients receiving treatment later (p = .057). The presence of a left ventricular aneurysm or depressed left ventricular function also appeared to reduce the likelihood of successful thrombolysis. All patients were discharged on oral anticoagulants. At 6 months follow-up (n = 9) no recurrence of left ventricular thrombus was found. These results show that left ventricular thrombi can be safely lysed by intravenous urokinase. However, for better definition of the risk and benefit of this new therapy further investigation is necessary.
Circulation 72, No. 1, 112–118, 1985.

MURAL LEFT VENTRICULAR thrombi are common in patients with acute myocardial infarction.[1–4] As calculated from autopsy reports, the incidence of mural thrombi in patients who died of myocardial infarction ranged from 14% to 68%.[5–9] Thrombi are more common in patients with large than in those with small infarcts.[1, 2, 4, 10] Although a mural thrombus adheres to the endocardium, it can produce systemic emboli. The incidence of embolism varies considerably depending on whether the mural thrombus is detected during life or at autopsy. Autopsy studies[5, 8, 10–14] have reported a 22% to 64% incidence of embolism in patients with cardiac thrombus, whereas in clinical studies, in which the left ventricular thrombus was diagnosed by angiography, two-dimensional echocardiography, or at operation, a lower incidence (0 to 36%) has been described.[2, 4, 15–22] In one study, half of the emboli were cerebral.[23]

Left ventricular thrombi are commonly found by two-dimensional echocardiography in patients in the early stages of acute myocardial infarction, especially those with an extensive anterior infarction.[1, 2, 4, 22, 24–28] However, no generally accepted therapy for patients with left ventricular thrombi has been found. Some authors advise use of anticoagulation[2, 3, 29, 30] or antithrombotic[29, 30] therapy in the presence of a left ventricular thrombus; in some patients with large, protruding thrombi surgery is recommended because of the high risk of embolization.

In this report, thrombolytic therapy with urokinase as an alternative therapeutic method is described in a series of 16 patients with large, protruding left ventricular thrombi developing early after infarction.

Methods

Patients. In 16 patients (age 40 to 69 years) with left ventricular thrombi systemic thrombolysis with urokinase was performed. The clinical characteristics of the patients are summarized in table 1. All patients had their first myocardial infarction 3 weeks to 3 months before study entry. Selection criteria for inclusion in the study were (1) large, protruding left ventricular thrombi located in the area of myocardial infarction, (2) time after acute myocardial infarction of 3 weeks to 3 months, and (3) no contraindications to systemic thrombolytic therapy with urokinase.

Immediately before initiation of thrombolytic therapy five patients were on heparin (three on low-dose heparin [100 units/kg body weight sc every 12 hr], two on full-dose heparin [200

From the Departments of Cardiology and Blood Coagulation Disorders, University Hospital Eppendorf, Hamburg.

Address for correspondence: Peter Kremer, M.D., Department of Cardiology, University Hospital Eppendorf, Martinistr. 52, D-2000 Hamburg 20, West Germany.

Received Aug. 29, 1984; revision accepted April 4, 1985.

TABLE 1
Patient characteristics

Patient No.	Age/sex	Infarct location	Time between MI and urokinase therapy	Anticoagulation before urokinase therapy	^{99m}Tc platelet scan	LV EF (%)	Effect of thrombolytic therapy on LV thrombus	Duration of thrombolytic therapy (days)	Complications: Before thrombolysis	Complications: During thrombolysis
1	62/M	A (aneur)	4 wk	Dicumarol	Pos.	32	↓	7		
2	63/M	A	3 mo	None	Neg.	46	+ (late)	8		
3	57/F	A (aneur)	2 mo	Aspirin		38	↓	5		Hematuria requiring discontinuation
4	40/M	A	4 wk	None	Neg.	52	+ (late)	8	Stroke	
5	69/M	I (aneur)	2 mo	None	Pos.	60	+	2		
6	53/F	A	3 wk	Full-dose heparin	Neg.	33	+	7		
7	68/F	A	3 mo	Dicumarol	Neg.	38	↓	8		
8	50/M	A	3 wk	Low-dose heparin		57	+	3	Systemic embolus: A. tibialis anterior	
9	63/M	I	4 wk	None	Equivocal	55	+	3		
10	55/M	A (aneur)	3 mo	Dicumarol	Neg.	29	−	8		
11	52/M	A	4 wk	Full-dose heparin		35	+	8	Systemic embolus: A. tibialis posterior	Mild hematuria
12	45/M	A (aneur)	5 wk	Low-dose heparin		30	−	7		
13	49/M	A	4 wk	Dicumarol		49	+	4		
14	59/M	A	4 wk	Dicumarol		34	+	7		
15	61/M	A	4 wk	Low-dose heparin		37	+	3		
16	54/F	A	2.5 mo	Dicumarol		50	↓	8		

A = anterior; I = inferior; aneur = left ventricular aneurysm; LV = left ventricular; EF = ejection fraction; ↓ = reduction in thrombus size; + = resolution of thrombus; − = no change.

units/kg in over 12 hr]), six were on dicumarol, and one was on aspirin (500 mg tid). Four patients received no anticoagulants or antithrombotic drugs. Dicumarol and aspirin were discontinued before the initiation of thrombolytic therapy.

Three patients had clinical evidence of systemic emboli before the institution of thrombolytic therapy; one patient (No. 4) suffered a stroke resulting in temporary right-sided hemiparesis. The two other patients (Nos. 8 and 11) had systemic emboli in the left A. tibialis anterior and the left A. tibialis posterior, respectively, resulting in temporary numbness and paresthesia of the affected areas. All patients were fully informed of the benefits and risks associated with thrombolytic therapy and of the investigational nature of this procedure. They all gave their consent to participate in the study.

The first case of successful lysis of a left ventricular thrombus was incidental. The patient (No. 6) had undergone bypass surgery and afterward had suffered an anterior myocardial infarction. Two weeks later a large left ventricular thrombus was seen on two-dimensional echocardiographic examination despite continuous heparin therapy.

Three weeks after bypass surgery and while still on a full dose of heparin, the patient experienced deep-vein thrombosis resulting in massive swelling of the right leg. To resolve the venous thrombosis intravenous urokinase therapy was initiated. To our surprise, not only the venous thrombosis, but also the left ventricular thrombus had disappeared after 7 days of therapy; there was no evidence of systemic or pulmonary embolization.

In a next step we performed intravenous thrombolysis in three patients who had a large mobile left ventricular thrombi despite heparin therapy and who were considered candidates for surgical thrombectomy. Because two of the patients had undergone bypass surgery in the weeks before and had poor left ventricular function, reoperation carried a major risk. In these patients thrombolysis resulted in complete dissolution of the left ventricular thrombus with no complications.

After these positive experiences we were encouraged to perform thrombolysis in patients with large, mobile left ventricular thrombi likely to embolize. In most of the patients these had developed despite use of anticoagulant therapy.

Two-dimensional echocardiography. Two-dimensional echocardiograms were obtained with a Diasonics 3400 R phased-array sector scanner. A standard two-dimensional echocardiographic examination consisting of parasternal short- and long-axis views and apical two- and four-chamber views was performed in all patients; additionally, multiple tangential views from the apex were recorded to measure maximal thrombus size.

In all patients thrombus size was such that the two-dimensional echocardiographic study was considered definitely positive for left ventricular thrombus by three different observers.

A thrombus was defined as an echo-dense mass adjacent to an asynergic left ventricular segment protruding into the left ventricular cavity. As described by Stratton and Ritchie,[30] maximal thrombus thickness was estimated by measuring the distance between the thrombus-blood interface and the thrombus-endocardial interface. Between a first and second analysis intraobserver reproducibility was as follows: mean thickness of the left ventricular thrombus was 3.8 ± 1.3 and 3.7 ± 1.2 cm, respectively, with a correlation coefficient between the two analyses of r = .97. Interobserver reproducibility was assessed by having a second observer (3.5 ± 1.1 cm) analyze the same echocardiograms. The correlation coefficient between these two observer measurements was r = .96. To assess the reproducibility of thrombus thickness measurements over time eight patients with long-standing left ventricular thrombi were restudied after 6 to 9 months by two-dimensional echocardiography. In close concordance with data published by Stratton et al.,[30] thrombus thickness neither increased nor decreased more than 8 mm on serial studies. Thus, a reduction of greater than 8 mm in thrombus thickness was considered a reduction in thrombus size.

An aneurysm was defined echocardiographically as a well-circumscribed bulging segment of myocardium demonstrating dyskinesis or akinesis.

Global left ventricular ejection fraction was estimated from the apical two- and four-chamber view by tracing the endocardium of the left ventricle (excluding the left ventricular thrombus) at end-diastole (peak R wave) and end-systole (smallest left ventricular area in both views) with a Philips light-pen unit. Global ejection fraction was calculated separately for the two- and four-chamber views; the average between the two measurements was used in the analysis. A significant left ventricular dysfunction was defined as a global ejection fraction of less than 40%.

Two-dimensional echocardiographic examination was performed before starting thrombolytic treatment, every day during intravenous urokinase therapy, and 2 days and 1 week after termination of thrombolytic therapy.

Follow-up studies by two-dimensional echocardiography were performed 3, 6, and 12 months after thrombolysis.

^{99}Tc-platelet imaging. Eight patients underwent ^{99m}Tc-platelet scintigraphy immediately before initiation of thrombolytic therapy. The mean injected dose for all eight patients was 8 ± 2 mCi. Images were obtained in the anterior, 30 degree left anterior oblique, and the left lateral position for 200 to 300,000 counts/view at 3 to 5 hr after injection of labeled platelets with use of a standard field-of-view gamma scintillation camera (Pho/Gamma, L.E.M., Searle) with a parallel-hole high-resolution low-energy collimator. The camera was interfaced with a dedicated nuclear medicine computer system (PDP 11-34, Gamma-11). A scintigraphic scan was considered positive when a discrete area of intracardiac activity was clearly greater than the background blood pool in at least two of three views. A study result was defined as equivocal when the area of intracardiac activity was only slightly greater than the background in one or more views. Scintigraphic images were evaluated by two different observers who were in agreement as to the results in all eight cases.

Thrombolytic therapy. After an initial intravenous bolus injection of 250,000 U urokinase (Ukidan R, Serono Pharmaceutical Company, Freiburg, West Germany), the drug was infused intravenously at a rate of 60,000 U/hr for 2 to 8 days in combination with heparin (mean dosage 200 units/kg iv over 12 hr). After termination of thrombolytic therapy dicumarol was administered and heparin was withheld as soon as dicumarol was effective. All patients were discharged on dicumarol.

Results

Effects of thrombolysis. Left ventricular thrombi were successfully lysed in 10 of 16 patients as evidenced by the absence of residual thrombus visible on the two-dimensional echocardiogram (figures 1 to 4). In four patients only partial thrombolysis was achieved, i.e., there was a reduction in thrombus size of greater than 8 mm as compared with the initial echocardiogram. In two patients no reduction in thrombus size was seen

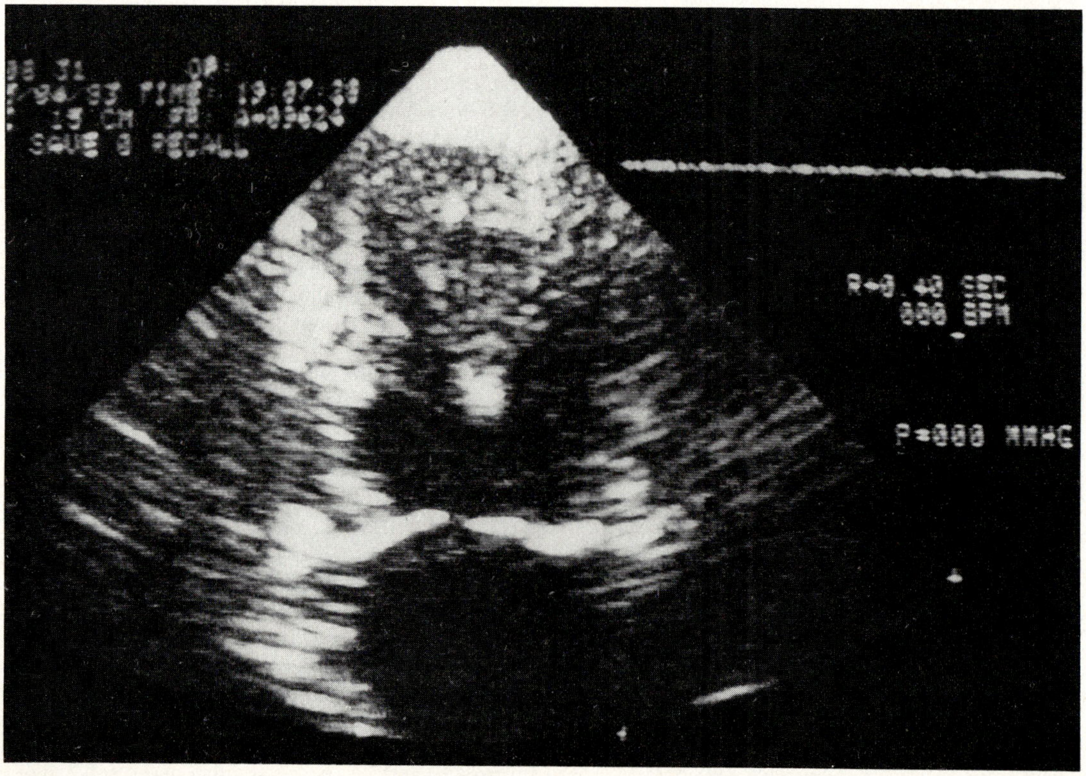

FIGURE 1. Echocardiogram from the two-chamber view demonstrating a large left ventricular thrombus protruding into the left ventricular outflow tract.

after thrombolytic therapy. The time required for thrombolysis differed considerably: in eight patients in whom the left ventricular thrombus disappeared completely, thrombolysis occurred within 2 to 8 days of urokinase therapy. In two patients (Nos. 2 and 4) with residual thrombus after 8 days of urokinase the thrombus had completely disappeared by 1 week after termination of urokinase therapy. In the four patients in whom only partial thrombolysis could be demonstrated infusion of urokinase was maintained for 8 days, as in the two patients who failed to respond.

On follow-up, nine of the 10 patients in whom thrombolysis was successful were restudied by two-dimensional echocardiography 6 months after treatment. In no case was there evidence of reoccurrence of thrombus.

The follow-up to this point dates back 12 months in five patients: reexamination by two-dimensional echocardiography in this subset also did not reveal reformation of left ventricular thrombus.

Determination of successful thrombolysis. On retrospective analysis patient data revealed some differences concerning the efficacy of thrombolytic therapy. The chances for successful thrombolysis were best when the age of the thrombus was 4 weeks or less. In eight of nine patients undergoing thrombolytic therapy 3 to 4 weeks after acute myocardial infarction left ventricular thrombi were successfully dissolved by systemic urokinase. However, thrombolysis was successful in only two of seven patients with a myocardial infarction between 5 and 12 weeks old ($p = .057$).

Left ventricular ejection fraction estimated by two-dimensional echocardiography was moderately or severely depressed in all but one of the six patients in whom thrombolysis was partial or did not occur ($36 \pm 8\%$, $n = 6$); only four of 10 patients in whom thrombolysis was successful had evidence of significant left ventricular dysfunction, whereas the remaining six patients had a normal or mildly depressed left ventricular ejection fraction ($46 \pm 10\%$, $n = 10$).

In each of five patients a left ventricular aneurysm was demonstrated by two-dimensional echocardiography; four patients had a left ventricular apical aneurysm after acute myocardial infarction and one patient had a posterior wall aneurysm. In all four patients with an apical aneurysm thrombolytic therapy was unsuccessful, in contrast to the case in the one patient with a posterior wall aneurysm in whom thrombolysis was successful.

Immediately preceding thrombolytic therapy ^{99m}Tc-platelet imaging was performed in eight patients. At the time the platelet scan was performed four patients were on anticoagulants, three were on dicumarol, and one was on full-dose heparin. Four patients received

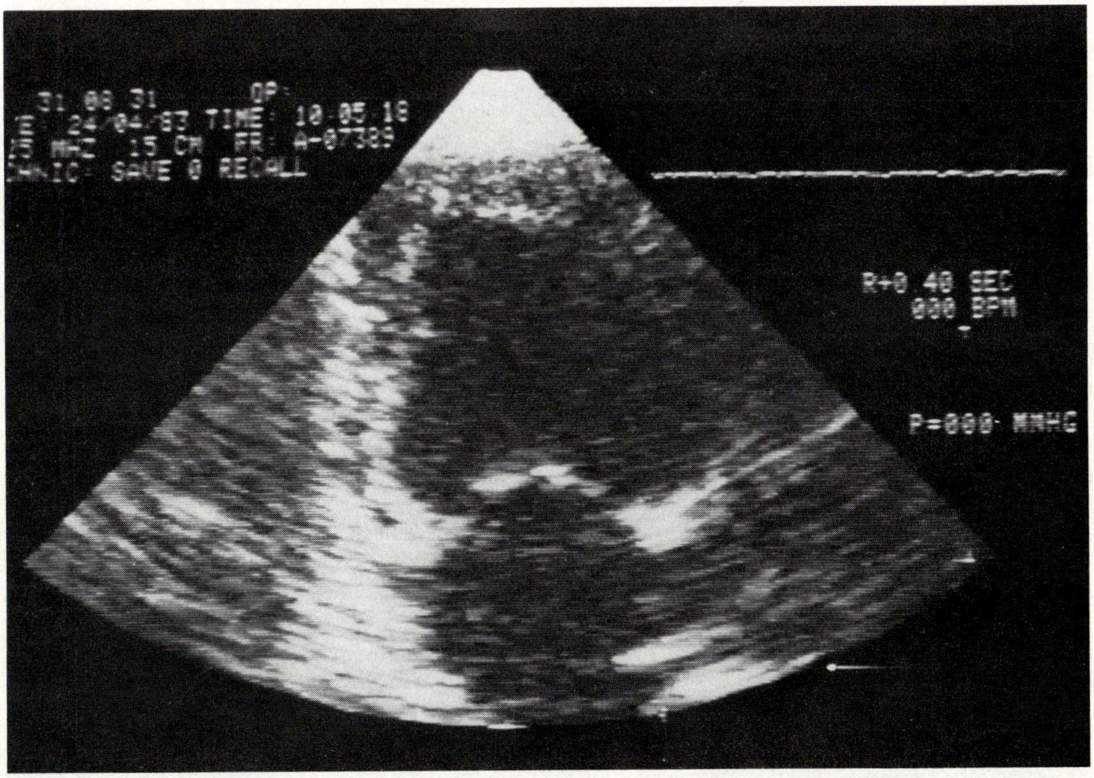

FIGURE 2. Image for same patient as in figure 1. After 7 days of intravenous urokinase the left ventricular thrombus had completely disappeared.

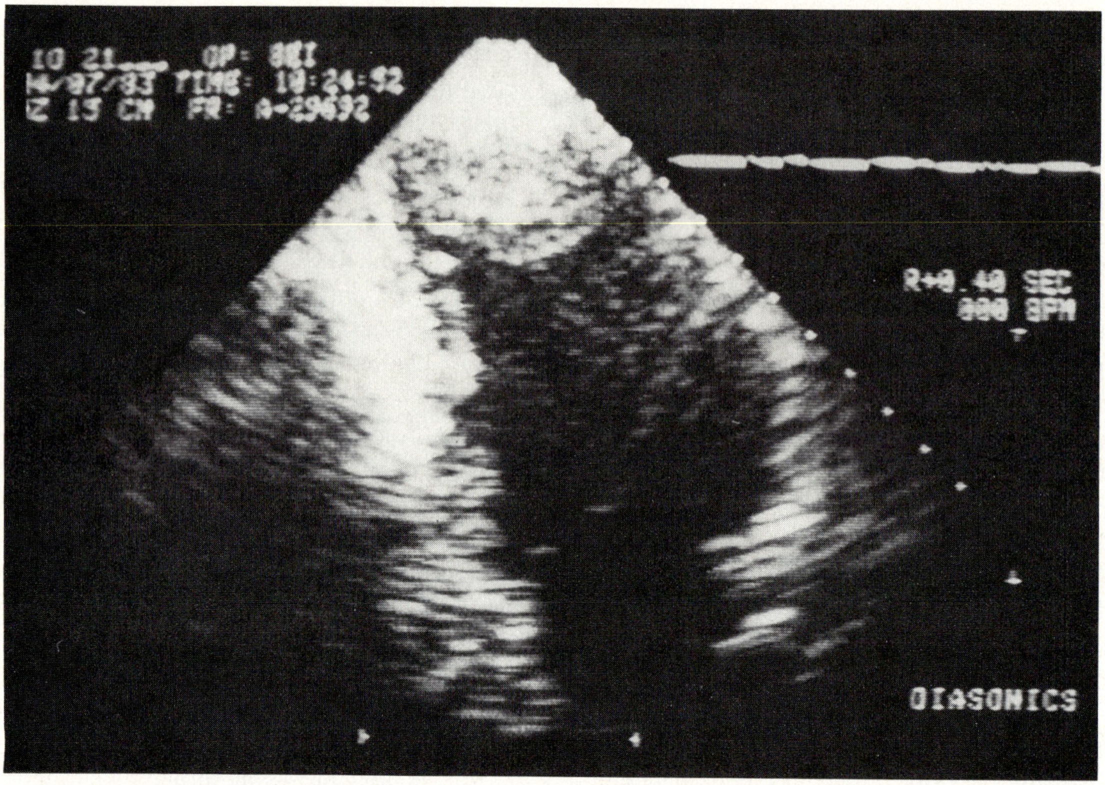

FIGURE 3. Large apical left ventricular thrombus in a patient after acute myocardial infarction.

no antithrombotic or anticoagulant drugs. Only two patients, one of them on dicumarol, demonstrated ongoing platelet deposition on the ^{99m}Tc-platelet scan. Despite demonstration of thrombus activity, thrombolysis was effective in only one of the two patients; in the other patient (No. 1), who had an apical aneurysm, thrombus size decreased slightly during therapy, but the larger part of the apical clot remained unchanged.

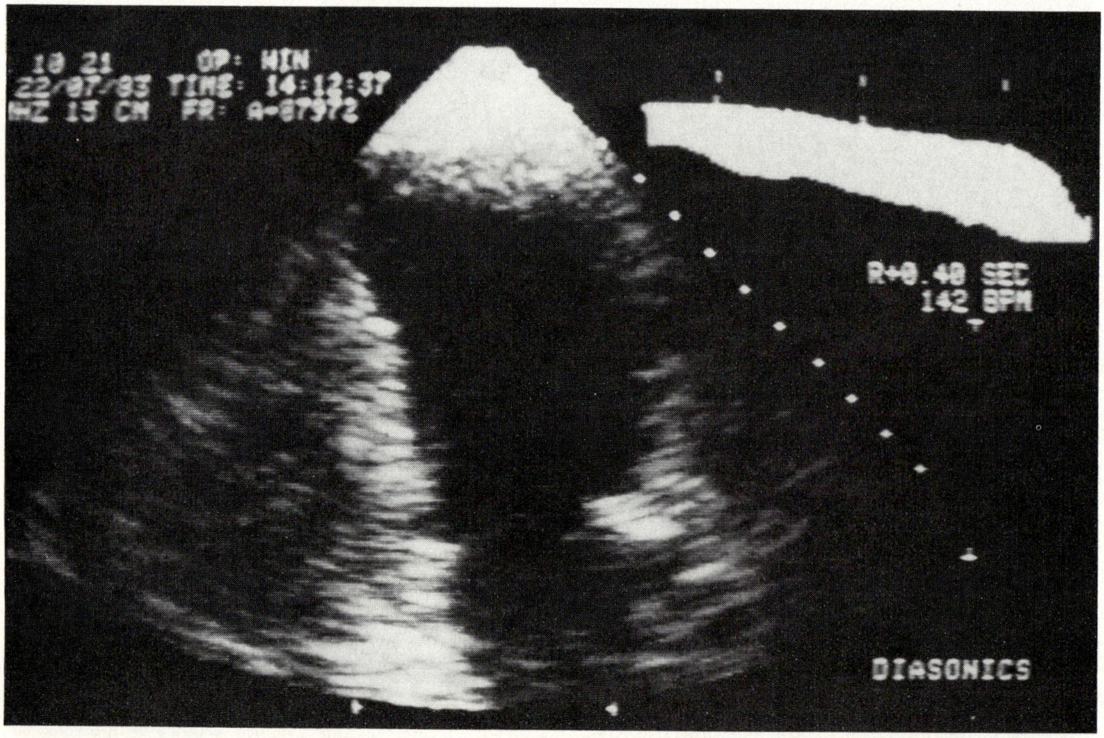

FIGURE 4. Same patient as in figure 3. Thrombus resolved after 8 days of thrombolytic treatment with intravenous urokinase.

Five patients had negative platelet scans; despite the failure to demonstrate thrombus activity by this technique thrombolysis was successful in three patients. Additionally, successful thrombolysis was achieved in one patient with an equivocal scan.

Complications. During thrombolytic therapy and at follow-up there was no clinical evidence of embolic events in any of 16 patients. One patient developed hematuria during thrombolytic therapy, which required discontinuation of the therapy after 5 days of treatment. At that time, the left ventricular thrombus had been partially dissolved. Reexamination by two-dimensional echocardiography 1 week and 6 months later revealed no further reduction in thrombus size. Another patient developed only mild hematuria after 3 days of therapy with intravenous urokinase. Thrombolytic treatment was continued and resulted in complete thrombolysis of a large left ventricular thrombus that initially protruded into the left ventricular outflow tract.

Discussion

Systemic embolic are a well-known complication of mural thrombi in patients with transmural myocardial infarction.[4, 15, 20–22] Since left ventricular mural thrombi can now easily be diagnosed by two-dimensional echocardiography,[1, 2, 22, 24] patients at risk of systemic embolism can be identified. The question arises, however, as to how these patients should be treated to prevent embolization. Long-term anticoagulation is considered by many a method of diminishing the risk of embolization after myocardial infarction.[31–35] However, to our knowledge no prospective studies are available demonstrating a lower incidence of emboli with anticoagulant therapy in patients with proven left ventricular thrombi. Anticoagulation is thought to prevent further apposition of the thrombus by enhancing organization and endothelialization. Edwards,[36] however, reports that thrombi larger than 5 mm are rarely organized, regardless of their age.

Recently published data suggest that full-dose heparin or warfarin anticoagulation may lead to thrombus resolution in the setting of acute myocardial infarction.[2, 3, 29, 30] According to the report of Visser et al.,[1] oral anticoagulant therapy resulted in thrombus resolution in only two of 15 patients within a period of 4 months. In contrast, Asinger et al.[2] reported that in six of seven patients on oral anticoagulants left ventricular thrombi were found to be resolved 9 ± 5 months after acute myocardial infarction. These authors also found that resolution of thrombus occurred in some patients without anticoagulation or with antithrombotic drugs.

In seven of 10 patients on coumarin therapy Tramarin et al.[29] observed the disappearance of left ventricular thrombi within 5 weeks after myocardial infarction.

However, in contrast to our patient population, the patients of Tramarin et al. did not begin anticoagulant therapy until their left ventricular thrombi were observed by two-dimensional echocardiography. Since the left ventricular thrombi in our patients had developed despite anticoagulation in the majority of cases, it appears unlikely that they would have been dissolved by the same medication.

If recurrent systemic emboli develop despite adequate anticoagulation surgical removal of the thrombus becomes necessary. This may also be true for large protruding and mobile thrombi that are likely to embolize.[37–39]

In this report we introduce an alternative method of treatment of mural left ventricular thrombi, i.e., systemic thrombolysis with urokinase. By use of this method left ventricular thrombi less than 3 months old that were adherent to an area of myocardial infarction were dissolved in two of three of patients. All patients were fully heparinized during the acute stage of myocardial infarction, i.e., they received heparin for at least 72 hr or until they were ambulatory. Half of the patients (eight of 16) were on oral anticoagulants or were fully heparinized before thrombolysis.

Left ventricular thrombi of patients in this study were remarkably large, with an average maximal diameter of 3.7 ± 1.2 cm. Nevertheless, it took only several days of thrombolytic therapy to completely resolve them. Although some of the thrombi were attached to the left ventricular wall with a stalk, no emboli occurred during or after thrombolysis independent of the result. During a follow-up period of 6 months, no recurrence of thrombus or embolism was noted.

These data suggest that intravenous lysis with urokinase is an effective and probably safe method of dissolving large left ventricular thrombi. In our opinion, lysis should be attempted (1) in patients being considered for surgical removal of thrombus, (2) in patients with peripheral recurrent emboli despite adequate anticoagulation, and (3) possibly in patients with large protruding thrombi likely to embolize.

The potential benefit of thrombolysis has to be weighed against the risks of urokinase-induced bleeding and embolization.[40, 41] In the small series of 16 patients reported here bleeding complications in the form of hematuria was seen in two and required termination of urokinase therapy in one. Urokinase-induced embolization was not noted at all. However, the number of patients is too small to provide conclusive evidence concerning the risk related to urokinase-induced thrombolysis of left ventricular thrombi. Additionally, since this study had no control group, the likely behavior of the left ventricular thrombi in the absence of thrombolytic treatment cannot be judged. Therefore, the suggestions above should be considered preliminary. For a definite answer regarding the benefit and risks of the new method a prospective randomized trial is required.

References

1. Visser CA, Kan G, Lie KI, Durrer D: Left ventricular thrombus following acute myocardial infarction: A prospective serial echocardiographic study of 96 patients. Eur Heart J **4:** 333, 1983
2. Asinger RW, Mikell FL, Elsperger J, Hodges M: Incidence of left-ventricular thrombus after acute transmural myocardial infarction. N Engl J Med **305:** 297, 1981
3. McEntee CW, Van Reet RE, Winters WL, Nelson JG, Waggoner AD, Miller RR, Quinones MA: Incidence and natural history of mural thrombi in acute myocardial infarction by two-dimensional echocardiography. Circulation **64**(suppl IV): IV-93, 1981 (abst)
4. Johannessen KA, Nordrehang JE, von der Lippe G: Left ventricular thrombus and cerebrovascular accident in acute myocardial infarction. Br Heart J **51:** 553, 1981
5. Dunow MH, Burchell HB, Titus JL: Postinfarction ventricular aneurysm: a clinicomorphologic and electrocardiographic study of 80 cases. Am Heart J **70:** 753, 1965
6. Schlichter J, Hellerstein HK, Katz LN: Aneurysm of the heart: a correlative study of one hundred and two proved cases. Medicine (Baltimore) **33:** 43, 1954
7. Abrams DL, Edelist A, Luria MH, Miller AJ: Ventricular aneurysm: a reappraisal based on a study of sixty-five consecutive autopsied cases. Circulation **27:** 164, 1963
8. Phares WS, Edwards JE, Burchell HB: Cardiac aneurysms: clinicopathologic studies. Proc Staff Meet Mayo Clin **28:** 264, 1953
9. Jordan RA, Miller RD, Edwards JE, Parker RL: Thrombo-embolism in acute and in healed myocardial infarction. I. Intracardiac mural thrombosis. Circulation **6:** 1, 1952
10. Yater WM, Welsh PP, Stapleton JF, Clark ML: Comparison of clinical and pathologic aspects of coronary artery disease in men of various age groups: a study of 950 autopsied cases from the Armed Forces Institute of Pathology. Ann Intern Med **34:** 352, 1951
11. Miller RD, Jordan RA, Parker RI, Edwards JE: Thrombo-embolism in acute and in healed myocardial infarction. II. Systemic and pulmonary arterial occlusion. Circulation **6:** 7, 1952
12. Hellerstein HK, Martin JW: Incidence of thrombo-embolic lesions accompanying myocardial infarction. Am Heart J **33:** 443, 1947
13. Foord AG: Embolism and thrombosis in coronary heart disease. JAMA **138:** 1009, 1948
14. Berman B, McGuire J: Cardiac aneurysm. Am J Med **8:** 480, 1950
15. Reeder GS, Lengyel M, Tayjik AJ, Seward JB, Smith HC, Danielson GK: mural thrombus in left ventricular aneurysm-incidence, role of angiography, and relation between anticoagulation and embolization. Mayo Clin Proc **56:** 77, 1981
16. Cooley DA, Hallmann GL: Surgical treatment of left ventricular aneurysm: experience with excision of postinfarction lesions in 80 patients. Prog Cardiovasc Dis **11:** 222, 1968
17. Favaloro RG, Effler DB, Groves LK, Westcott RN, Snarez E, Lozada J: Ventricular aneurysm: clinical experience. Ann Thorax Surg **6:** 227, 1968
18. Loop FD, Effler DB, Navia JA, Sheldon WC, Groves LK: Aneurysms of the left ventricle: survival and results of a ten-year surgical experience. Ann Surg **178:** 399, 1973
19. Kluge TH, Ullal SR, Hill JD, Kerth WJ, Gerbode F: Dyskinesia and aneurysm of the left ventricle: surgical experience in 36 patients. J Cardiovasc Surg **12:** 273, 1971
20. Stratton JR, Ritchie JL, Hammermeister KE, Kennedy JE, Hamilton GW: Detection of left ventricular thrombi by radionuclide angiography. Am J Cardiol **48:** 565, 1981
21. Hamby RI, Wisoff BG, Davidson ET, Hartstein ML: Coronary artery disease and left ventricular mural thrombi: clinical, hemodynamic, and angiocardiographic aspects. Chest **66:** 488, 1974
22. Stratton JR, Lightly GW, Pearlman AS, Ritchie JL: Detection of left ventricular thrombus by two-dimensional echocardiography: sensitivity, specificity, and causes of uncertainty. Circulation **66:** 156, 1982
23. Davies MJ, Woolf N, Robertson WB: Pathology of acute myocardial infarction with particular reference to occlusive coronary thrombi. Br Heart J **38:** 659, 1976
24. Reeder GS, Tajik AJ, Seward JB: Left ventricular mural thrombus: two dimensional echocardiographic diagnosis. Mayo Clin Proc **56:** 82, 1981
25. Ezekowitz MD, Wilson DA, Smith EO, Burow RD, Harrison LH, Parker DE, Elkins RC, Peyton M, Taylor FB: Comparison of indium-111 platelet scintigraphy and two-dimensional echocardiography in the diagnosis of left ventricular thrombi. N Engl J Med **306:** 1509, 1982
26. Ports TA, Cogan J, Schiller NB, Rapaport E: Echocardiography of left ventricular masses. Circulation **58:** 528, 1978
27. DeMaria AN, Bommer W, Newmann A, Grehl T, Weinart L, DeNardo S, Amsterdam EA, Mason DT: Left ventricular thrombi identified by cross-sectional echocardiography. Ann Intern Med **90:** 14, 1979
28. Meltzer RS, Guthaner D, Rakowski H, Popp RL, Martin RP: Diagnosis of left ventricular thrombi by two-dimensional echocardiography. Br Heart J **42:** 261, 1979
29. Tramarin R, Pozzoli M, Febo O, Opasich C, Cobelli F, Specchia G: Echocardiographic assessment of therapy efficacy in left ventricular thrombosis post myocardial infarction. Circulation **68** (suppl III): III-331, 1983 (abst)
30. Stratton JR, Ritchie JL: The effects of antithrombotic drugs in patients with left ventricular thrombi: assessment with indium-111 platelet imaging and two-dimensional echocardiography. Circulation **69:** 561, 1984
31. VA Cooperative Clinical Study Group: Anticoagulants in acute myocardial infarction. JAMA **225:** 724, 1973
32. Drapkin A, Merskey C: Anticoagulant therapy after acute myocardial infarction: relation of therapeutic benefit to patient's age, sex and severity of infarction. JAMA **222:** 541, 1972
33. Reports on the working party on anticoagulant therapy in coronary thrombosis to the medical research council. Assessment of short term anticoagulant administration after cardiac infarction. Br Med J **1:** 335, 1969
34. Wright IS, Marple CD, Beck DF: Myocardial infarction: its clinical manifestation and treatment with anticoagulants: a study of 1031 cases. New York, Grune & Stratton, 1954
35. Harvald B, Hilden T, Lund E: Long-term anticoagulant therapy after myocardial infarction. Lancet **2:** 626, 1962
36. Edwards WD: Aneurysms and mural thrombi of the left ventricle. Mayo Clin Proc **56:** 129, 1981
37. Cabin HS, Robert WC: Left ventricular aneurysm, intraaneurysmal thrombus and systemic embolus in coronary heart disease. Chest **77:** 5, 586, 1980
38. Meltzer RS, Visser CA, Kan G, Roelandt J: Two-dimensional echocardiographic appearance of left ventricular thrombi with systemic emboli after myocardial infarction. Am J Cardiol **53:** 1511, 1984
39. Haugland JM, Asinger RW, Mikell FL, Elsperger J, Hodges M: Embolic potential of left ventricular thrombi detected by two-dimensional echocardiography. Circulation **70:** 588, 1984
40. Bell WR, Meek AG: Guidelines for the use of thrombolytic agents: N Engl J Med **301:** 1266, 1979
41. Urokinase-Streptokinase embolism trial: phase 2 results: a cooperative study. JAMA **229:** 1606, 1974

Left ventricular systolic and diastolic function in coronary artery disease: effects of revascularization on exercise-induced ischemia

JOHN D. CARROLL, M.D., OTTO M. HESS, M.D., HEINZ O. HIRZEL, M.D., MARKO TURINA, M.D., AND HANS PETER KRAYENBUEHL, M.D.

ABSTRACT Left ventricular systolic and diastolic function were studied before and after surgical revascularization in a group of 24 patients with stable angina who all had an excellent clinical response to surgery. With use of micromanometer left ventricular pressure measurements and ventricular volumes, calculated from biplane cineangiograms, left ventricular function at rest and during exercise before and after surgery was compared. Before surgery all patients had exercise-induced ischemia with new asynergy, a fall in ejection fraction from 57% to 49% ($p < .001$), and a rise in left ventricular end-diastolic pressure from 23 to 37 mm Hg ($p < .001$). Postoperative exercise resulted in no new asynergy and ejection fraction rose from 59% to 61% ($p < .05$). Left ventricular end-diastolic pressure still rose from 17 to 25 mm Hg ($p < .01$). Left ventricular pressure decay during exercise was greatly improved after revascularization and allowed maintenance of reduced early diastolic pressures. The early diastolic pressure nadir before surgery rose from 9 to 21 mm Hg ($p < .001$); the postoperative nadir was 5 mm Hg at rest and 6 mm Hg during exercise. All patients had an upward shift in the diastolic pressure-volume relationship during preoperative exercise. After revascularization there was no upward shift in some patients and a much smaller shift in others. The postoperative increase in left ventricular end-diastolic pressure was due to increased end-diastolic volume, not altered compliance. There was an increase in mean right atrial pressure during exercise either before (6 to 11 mm Hg) or after surgery (4 to 10 mm Hg). These increases were quite variable, suggesting no consistent role of pericardial restraint during exercise. Early diastolic peak filling rate during exercise was greater after surgery (1260 vs 950 ml/sec, $p < .001$). In fact, during postoperative exercise early diastolic filling rates were greater than normal, reflecting the persistence of abnormally high atrial pressures for filling. As at preoperative study, late diastolic filling during exercise was restricted after revascularization when compared with that in a control group. Postoperatively patients undergoing bypass procedures with a good clinical result showed significantly improved left ventricular diastolic and systolic function. Persistent elevation of end-diastolic and atrial pressures and other abnormalities of diastolic function may reflect chronic structural changes and need to be taken into account when evaluating patients after bypass surgery.
Circulation **72, No. 1, 119–129, 1985.**

BYPASS SURGERY dramatically alters the symptomatic status of many patients and prolongs life in some. An increasing number of patients with prior surgery are undergoing clinical and hemodynamic evaluation. It has not been clear to what extent surgery alters the left ventricular dysfunction often associated with exercise, and misinterpretation of hemodynamic abnormalities may lead to incorrect clinical decisions. Therefore, this study was designed to investigate not only the degree to which "complete revascularization" alters hemodynamics, but also to contrast the postoperative results with those in a group of control patients without significant cardiac disease.

The pathophysiology of ischemic mechanical dysfunction, particularly of the left ventricle, has been extensively studied. Animal preparations have provided important insights into the nature of regional dysfunction.[1-4] Yet, the human coronary circulation is clearly different from those of all other species because of the presence of collaterals and the diffuse and varied manifestations of atherosclerosis. Thus, human studies

From the Department of Internal Medicine, University of Chicago, and the Medical Policlinic, Cardiology and Surgical Clinic A, University Hospital, Zurich.
Supported by a grant from the Swiss National Science Foundation.
Address for correspondence: Hans Peter Krayenbuehl, M.D., Med. Poliklinik, Kardiologie, Universitatsspital Zurich, 8091, Zurich, Switzerland.
Received Nov. 7, 1984; revision accepted March 15, 1985.

of the pathophysiology of ischemia have been of paramount importance. The induction of ischemia in man by pacing has provided the initial human model of left ventricular ischemic dysfunction. New asynergy, impaired pressure decay, elevated diastolic pressures, and the upward diastolic pressure-volume shift are some of the typical manifestations of ischemia.[5-9] We have described the nature of left ventricular dysfunction in man during ischemia induced by exercise.[10-15] These studies have emphasized the complex interplay of exercise-induced changes in function and ischemia-related abnormalities.

It has been well documented that after revascularization exercise tolerance improves even when antianginal medications are reduced.[16-18] There have been other studies showing that global and regional systolic left ventricular function during exercise improve with successful bypass grafting of significantly stenosed, major epicardial coronary arteries.[18-23] Much less has been published regarding the reversibility of ischemia-related alterations in left ventricular relaxation, diastolic filling dynamics, and diastolic pressure-volume relationships. Therefore, for this study we selected patients who had exercise-induced ischemia before surgery, subsequently had an uncomplicated bypass operation (with bypass of all major stenotic lesions), and were symptomatically improved after surgery. This approach provides unique data concerning left ventricular function after a clinically optimal surgical result in patients with definite preoperative functional abnormalities.

Methods

Patient population. Characteristics of the patients studied are summarized in table 1. Twenty-four patients with coronary artery disease between the ages of 34 and 68 years old (mean = 56) had stable angina refractory to medical therapy. Six had two-vessel disease (greater than 50% diameter narrowing) and the remainder had three-vessel disease. At the time of preoperative catheterization all had exercise-induced ischemia defined as new asynergy (table 2). All patients underwent coronary artery bypass surgery at the Surgical Clinic A at the University Hospital, Zurich, between June 1981 and October 1983. A total of 83 distal anastomoses were placed: 81 were patent at postoperative catheterization. All patients improved symptomatically after surgery, with a reduction in mean New York Heart Association class of from 2.5 to 1.2 and with only five patients having any angina with strenuous exertion. This was despite a reduction in the number of antianginal medications being taken (nitrates, β-blockers, calcium antagonists) from an average of 2.3 to 0.4 per patient, with 14 patients taking no antianginal medications postoperatively. In 12 patients there was a preoperative history of hospitalization for myocardial infarction documented by cardiac enzyme levels and electrocardiography. In seven of these Q waves had developed on the electrocardiogram.

Five patients with no or minimal cardiovascular disease and a rise in ejection fraction with exercise served as a control group.

TABLE 1
Patient characteristics

No. of patients studied before and after surgery	24
Mean age (yr)	56 (range 34–68)
Mean No. of major (3) epicardial vessels diseased	2.7 (range 2–3)
Clinical history of past infarction (n)	12
Mean No. of daily cardiac medications	
Before surgery	2.3 (range 0–3)
After surgery	0.4 (range 0–1)
Mean NYHA functional class	
Before surgery	2.5 (range 2–3)
After surgery	1.2 (range 1–2)
Mean maximum exercise level achieved at catheterization (W)	90 (range 50–140)
Mean total duration of exercise (min)	3.6 (range 1.5–7)
No. of patients with angina during exercise	
Before surgery	16
After surgery	0
No. of distal bypass anastamoses	83 (mean 3.5, range 1–7)
No. of patent anastomoses at postoperative catheterization	81

All were undergoing catheterization because of atypical chest pain.

Cardiac catheterization. Informed consent was obtained from all patients. All 29 patients underwent right and left heart catheterization and biplane cineangiography at rest and during supine bicycle exercise. The 24 patients undergoing postoperative catheterization were studied an average of 7.7 months after surgery (range 3 to 18 months). Cardiovascular medications were withheld for 12 to 24 hr before catheterization. Premedication consisted of 10 mg of chlordiazepoxide given orally 1 hr before catheterization. Left ventricular pressure was measured with a Millar pigtail angiographic micromanometer catheter introduced from the femoral artery. Pressures were recorded at a paper speed of 250 mm/sec (Electronics for Medicine VR16), along with the first derivative of pressure (dP/dt), (dP/dt)/instantaneous pressure, and an intracardiac electrocardiogram from the right-sided catheter (figure 1). Before resting and exercise recordings were obtained the pressure was calibrated against a fluid-filled system.

Biplane left ventricular cineangiograms were obtained in the right anterior oblique (30 degrees) and left anterior oblique (60 degrees) projections at a filming rate of 50 frames/sec. Volumes were calculated by the area-length method. Each angiographic frame had a digital time corresponding to time marks on the pressure recordings.

Exercise protocol. All patients underwent bicycle exercise testing before preoperative catheterization to determine achieved workload and exercise limitations. At catheterization, pressures were recorded before and after each patient's feet were strapped to the bicycle device. All resting data presented here are from the first angiogram, which was obtained with the patient's legs in this elevated position. As previously shown, this accounts, in the majority of the patients, for the elevation in end-diastolic pressures at rest.[10] After the resting angiogram and subsequent 12 to 15 min pause, patients began to exercise to a low level. Preoperatively patients exercised at progressively higher workloads until either angina or other limiting symptoms occurred or until they achieved a submaximal heart rate predicted by sex, height, and age. After surgery patients followed the

TABLE 2
Effect of revascularization on ventricular function

	Before surgery (n = 24)		After surgery (n = 24)		Before vs after	
	Rest	Exercise	Rest	Exercise	Rest	Exercise
HR (beats/min)	67 ± 12	115 ± 11^C	75 ± 16	129 ± 19^C	$p<.05$	$p<.001$
EF (%)	57 ± 9	49 ± 9^C	59 ± 11	61 ± 11^A	NS	$p<.001$
ESVI (ml/m^2)	49 ± 14	64 ± 19^C	44 ± 18	46 ± 21	NS	$p<.001$
EDVI (ml/m^2)	114 ± 24	125 ± 23^B	108 ± 25	115 ± 27^B	NS	$p<.05$
LVEDP (mm Hg)	23 ± 6	37 ± 8^C	17 ± 4	25 ± 10^B	$p<.001$	$p<.001$
P_L (mm Hg)	9 ± 4	21 ± 8^C	5 ± 3	6 ± 3	$p<.001$	$p<.001$
Peak LVP (mm Hg)	149 ± 23	156 ± 19	144 ± 21	177 ± 20^C	NS	$p<.001$
Max +dP/dt (mm Hg/sec)	1530 ± 274	2210 ± 512^C	1637 ± 370	3314 ± 113^C	NS	$p<.001$
Max −dP/dt (mm Hg/sec)	1546 ± 284	1873 ± 419^C	1589 ± 297	2653 ± 555^C	NS	$p<.001$
T (msec)	54 ± 9	37 ± 9^C	52 ± 11	30 ± 9^C	NS	$p<.01$
P_B (mm Hg)	-9 ± 8	10 ± 9^C	-10 ± 10	-7 ± 12	NS	$p<.001$

HR = heart rate; EF = ejection fraction; ESVI = end-systolic volume index; EDVI = end-diastolic volume index; LVEDP = left ventricular end-diastolic pressure; Max +dP/dt = maximum rate of left ventricular pressure rise; Max −dP/dt = maximum rate of left ventricular pressure decline.

$^A p < .05$, rest vs exercise; $^B p < .01$, rest vs exercise; $^C p < .001$, rest vs exercise.

same exercise protocol they had followed before surgery to match external workloads. Exercise duration and maximal workload for each patient were therefore identical for both studies. At the point of peak exercise, pressures were again recorded and simultaneous cineangiography was completed. Coronary arteriograms by the Judkins technique were obtained after exercise.

Data analysis. Methods of analysis have previously been described in detail.[10–13] In summary, resting and exercise data were derived from well-opacified sinus beats that were not immediately postextrasystolic. Pressure tracings were digitized. The characteristics of isovolumetric pressure decay were derived from a linear regression of pressure and dP/dt coordinates as shown in figure 2. Thus two variables, T, representing the negative reciprocal of the slope, and P_B, representing the pressure axis intercept, were derived for each patient at rest and during exercise.

Ventricular volumes were calculated from frame-by-frame analysis of biplane angiograms. End-diastole was taken as the beginning of the rapid rise in left ventricular pressure after the onset of the QRS complex. End-systole was taken as the smallest volume at the end of ejection with the aid of the intracardiac phonocardiogram to identify aortic valve closure. To describe filling dynamics (figure 3) the time of mitral valve opening was noted as 20 msec before the time of the first frame showing the entry of unopacified blood into the left ventricle. The time from mitral valve opening to end-diastole is referred to as the filling time. This filling time was divided into halves, the midpoint being mid-diastole. The average filling rates were calculated for the first and second halves of diastole. In addition, the peak early diastolic filling rate was derived from three-point smoothing of frame-by-frame volume calculations. The total filling volume was taken as the volume entering the ventricle from mitral valve opening to end-diastole.

Left atrial pressure is a major determinant of filling.[24] Since left atrial pressure was not measured, we recorded the pressure at the time at which unopacified blood first entered the ventricle. This pressure is termed the opening pressure and is an index of the left atrial pressure responsible for mitral valve opening, i.e., the driving pressure for early diastolic filling.

Diastolic pressure-volume relationships for resting and exercise data were constructed as in figure 4.[5–8] To permit compari-

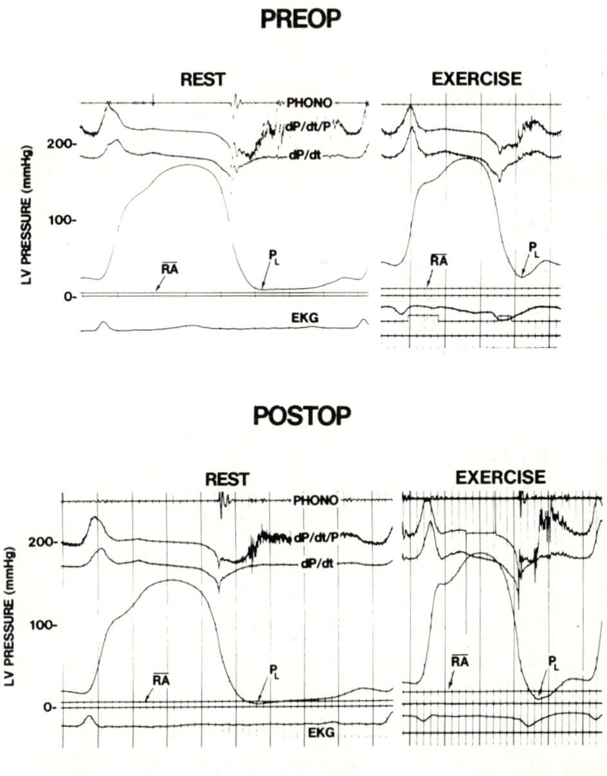

FIGURE 1. Left ventricular pressure tracings at rest and during exercise-induced ischemia from one patient with severe triple-vessel disease. Before surgery, there was a dramatic rise in the early diastolic pressure nadir, P_L, from 6 to 18 mm Hg during ischemia. Right atrial mean pressure ($\overline{RA}$) also increased during ischemia. Simultaneous cineangiography showed the development of severe anterior wall ischemia with exercise. The same patient also underwent exercise testing 4 months after complete revascularization. P_L did not rise with exercise but left ventricular end-diastolic pressure increased to 30 mm Hg. Simultaneous cineangiography revealed no new asynergy with exercise and there was no angina. Right atrial pressure increased with exercise in the absence of significant left ventricular ischemia.

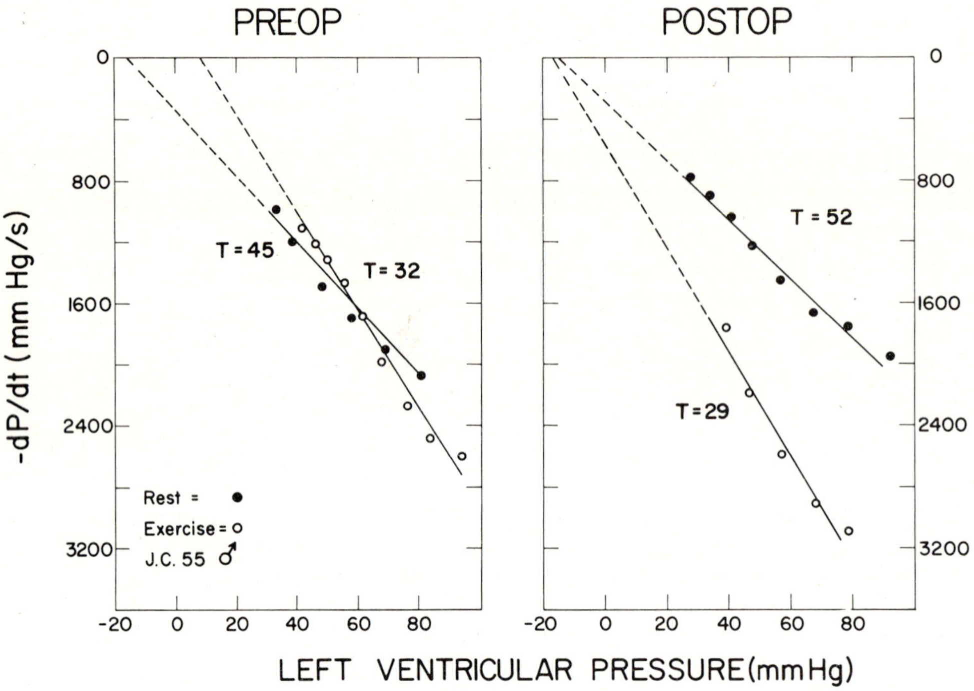

FIGURE 2. The characteristics of left ventricular pressure decay during the isovolumetric relaxation period for the same patient as in figure 1. The time constant (T, in msec) of pressure decay is the negative reciprocal of the slope of the linear regression of dP/dt and pressure coordinates. The regression line's pressure axis intercept is termed the baseline pressure (P_B, in mm Hg). During preoperative exercise, ischemia occurred and T decreased and P_B rose. After revascularization the characteristics of pressure decay during exercise were nearly normal. See text for details.

sons of preoperative and postoperative data and that from control subjects we derived mean pressure-volume relationships for each group at rest and during exercise. Three diastolic pressure-volume coordinates were used, including the early diastolic pressure nadir, mid-diastole, and end-diastole (figure 5).

Resting and exercise data within groups and preoperative and postoperative results were tested for significant differences by use of the paired t test. Differences between the control group and the patients were tested with an unpaired t test. Data on figures are mean ± SEM while those in tables and text are mean ± SD.

Results

A summary of hemodynamic and angiographic data is presented in table 2. During exercise before surgery, when all patients developed new asynergy, ejection fraction fell from 57% to 49% as end-systolic and end-diastolic volumes increased. During exercise after surgery ejection fraction rose from 59% to 61% due to an increased end-diastolic volume, but there was no significant change in end-systolic volume. This was in contrast to the case in the control group, in which ejection fraction increased from 64 ± 3 to 73 ± 4 ($p < .01$) and end-systolic volume decreased (35 ± 5 to 28 ± 6, $p < .05$) and there was no significant increase in end-diastolic volume (96 ± 6 to 102 ± 11). Only six patients had a 5% or more increase in ejection fraction during exercise, and end-systolic volume decreased in only six as well.

Peak left ventricular systolic pressure did not rise significantly during preoperative exercise. Eight of 25 patients experienced an exercise-induced drop of 5 mm Hg or more. Postoperatively, there was a significant rise in peak pressure (from 144 to 177 mm Hg) and no patient experienced a fall in pressure during exercise. This appeared to be due, in part, to improved generation of left ventricular pressure. Preoperatively maximum positive dP/dt was 2210 mm Hg/sec during exercise; postoperatively it was 3314 mm Hg/sec ($p < .001$). In the control group maximum positive dP/dt with exercise increased from 1418 ± 374 to 2894 ± 558 ($p < .01$). The increase in heart rate in the control group was slightly smaller (70 to 119 beats/min) than that in the postoperative patients.

Diastolic pressures became greatly elevated during preoperative exercise. The early diastolic pressure nadir rose from 9 to 21 mm Hg and end-diastolic pressure rose from 23 to 37 mm Hg. During exercise after surgery the early diastolic pressure nadir remained low (6 mm Hg), but end-diastolic pressure still rose from 17 to 25 mm Hg. In 20 of 24 patients, after surgery end-diastolic pressure rose during exercise by 5 mm Hg or more. During exercise in the control group there was a fall in the early diastolic pressure nadir from 11 ± 6 to 4 ± 5 mm Hg and no significant rise in end-

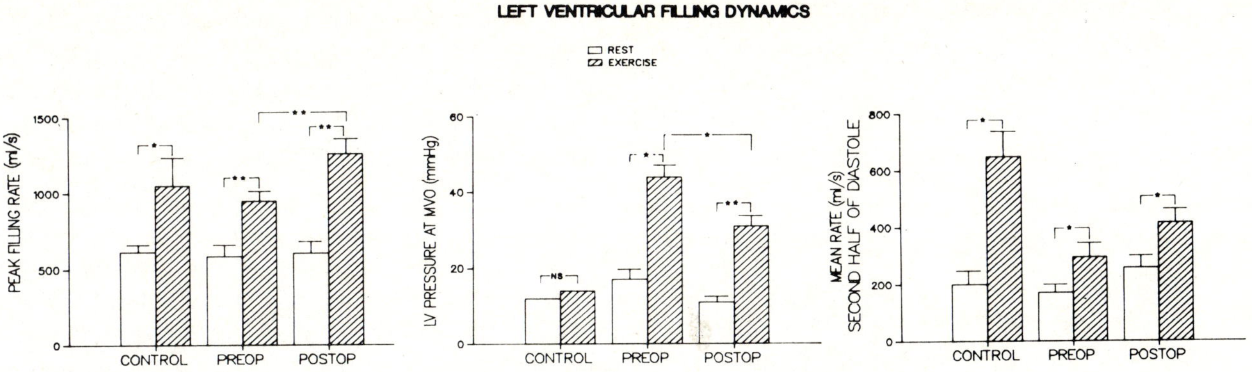

FIGURE 3. Left ventricular filling dynamics for three groups of patients: a control group with normal exercise hemodynamics, a preoperative group (n = 13) of patients who developed exercise-induced ischemia, and a postoperative group (the patients in the preoperative group after successful revascularization). *Left,* Mean values for early diastolic peak filling rate are shown at rest and during exercise. Despite abnormal pressure decay, the patients in the preoperative group had peak filling rates during exercise similar to those in the control subjects. After revascularization, peak filling increased to a greater extent during exercise. *Middle,* Mean values for the left ventricular pressure at which mitral valve opening occurred. This index of the left atrial driving pressure for filling did not change with exercise in the control group but greatly increased during exercise-induced ischemia before surgery. After revascularization the driving pressure was not as great but still increased during exercise. The combination of accelerated pressure decay and high driving pressures probably produced the high peak filling rates seen during postoperative exercise. Mean filling rates for the second half of diastole are shown on the *right.* Mean filling rates for the second half of diastole were significantly lower than control during preoperative exercise, and did not statistically increase after revascularization. Chronic, passive chamber properties may have restricted late filling during postoperative exercise. See text for details. *p < .05; **p < .01.

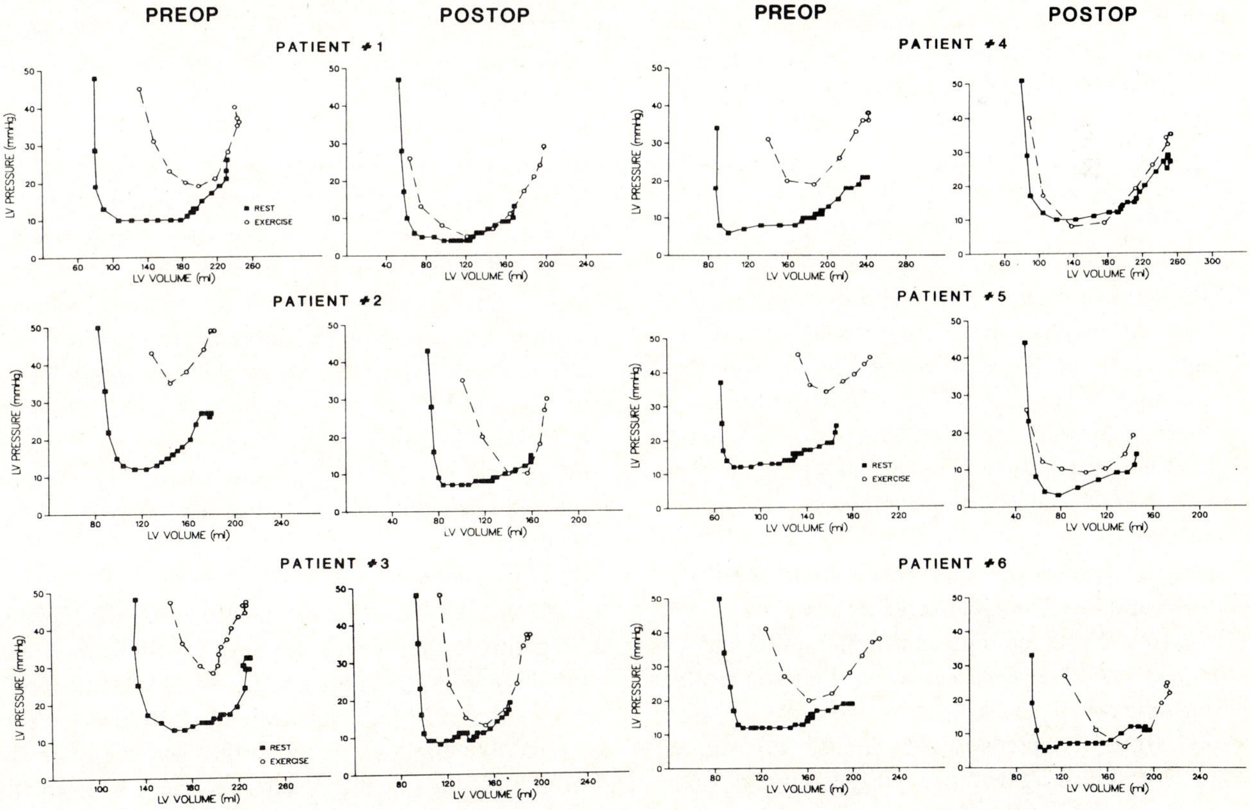

FIGURE 4. The preoperative and postoperative diastolic pressure-volume relationships for six patients. During preoperative exercise there was an upward shift composed of an increased end-systolic volume, abnormal isovolumetric pressure decay, and an increased pressure at which mitral valve opening occurred. After revascularization there were no or minimal shifts during exercise. There was an increased left ventricular end-diastolic pressure during exercise, but it appeared on the same pressure-volume curve as at rest.

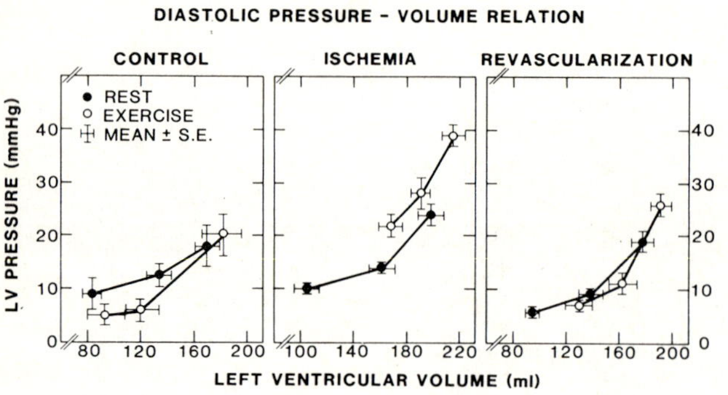

FIGURE 5. Resting and exercise diastolic pressure-volume relationships in the three groups. Coordinates of pressure are averages at three diastolic points: the early diastolic pressure nadir, mid-diastole, and end-diastole. *Left*, The control group had a downward shift in the early diastolic pressure-volume relationship. *Middle* and *right*, Data from 13 patients before (Ischemia) and after surgery (Revascularization). During preoperative exercise an upward shift developed that was reversed by revascularization. Despite the lack of ischemia during exercise, left ventricular end-diastolic pressure was significantly elevated during postoperative exercise.

diastolic pressure (18 ± 8 to 20 ± 9 mm Hg). The high resting values reflect, in large part, leg elevation.[10]

The characteristics of isovolumetric pressure decay were clearly altered by exercise-induced ischemia and, subsequently, by revascularization (figure 2). The time constant of isovolumetric relaxation, T, decreased during preoperative exercise from 54 to 37 msec, while in the control group it fell to a greater extent (49 ± 15 to 22 ± 2 msec, $p < .01$). Postoperatively, T fell from 52 to 30 msec, which was significantly different from before surgery, with nine of 24 patients having a value less than 25 msec during exercise. The second characteristic describing isovolumetric pressure decay, P_B, increased during preoperative exercise from −9 to 10 mm Hg, but postoperatively it did not change during exercise. This postoperative response was similar to that in the control group, in which P_B did not change during exercise (0 ± 1 to 3 ± 11 mm Hg).

The seven patients who had Q wave infarction had a fall in ejection fraction with exercise of from 49 ± 8% to 45 ± 10%. Postoperatively ejection fraction was 49 ± 9 at rest and 49 ± 9 with exercise. Left ventricular end-diastolic pressure rose from 24 ± 7 to 38 ± 9 mm Hg ($p < .01$) during preoperative exercise and from 13 ± 4 to 27 ± 4 mm Hg ($p < .01$) postoperatively. End-diastolic volume increased during preoperative (115 ± 24 to 127 ± 26 ml/m^2, $p < .05$) and postoperative exercise (116 ± 28 to 127 ± 31 ml/m^2, $p < .01$). Left ventricular pressure generation improved with revascularization. Preoperatively left ventricular systolic pressure did not rise significantly (143 ± 13 to 155 ± 14 mm Hg), while during postoperative exercise it did (137 ± 19 to 169 ± 15 mm Hg, $p < .01$). Maximum +dP/dt also increased from 1365 ± 159 to 2033 ± 394 mm Hg/sec ($p < .001$) during preoperative exercise and from 1586 ± 264 to 3102 ± 800 mm Hg/sec ($p < .001$) during postoperative exercise. As in the whole group of 24 patients, the seven with prior Q wave infarctions had a greater exercise heart rate after surgery despite a similar workload. Preoperative heart rate increased from 66 ± 9 to 115 ± 14 beats/min ($p < .001$) and after surgery it increased from 77 ± 15 to 135 ± 15 ($p < .001$).

The seven patients with Q wave infarction had more impressive improvement in early diastolic pressures during exercise after revascularization. The early diastolic pressure nadir, P_L, increased from 11 ± 4 to 24 ± 11 mm Hg ($p < .01$) during preoperative exercise, but did not change significantly during postoperative exercise (5 ± 3 to 8 ± 1 mm Hg, NS). Pressure decay improved with revascularization: T had fallen from 60 ± 12 to 40 ± 12 msec ($p < .05$) before surgery, but fell to 31 ± 9 msec during postoperative exercise from a resting value of 55 ± 10 msec ($p < .01$). Before surgery P_B rose from −8 ± 7 to +11 ± 16 mm Hg ($p < .05$), but was unchanged during postoperative exercise (−9 ± 5 to −4 ± 9 mm Hg, NS).

In a subgroup of 13 patients in whom all four ventriculograms were of the highest quality frame-by-frame analysis was completed for diastole. These 13 patients were representative of all the patients in terms of the previously presented angiographic and pressure data at rest and during exercise. For example, ejection fraction fell during preoperative exercise from 58 ± 10% to 47 ± 9% ($p < .001$) and after surgery it rose from 57 ± 12% to 59 ± 12% ($p < .05$). Diastolic filling data are presented for these patients in table 3. Before surgery, the filling time fell during exercise from 486 to 185 msec and the total filling volume decreased from 110 to 89 ml. In contrast, during postoperative exercise filling volume increased from 102 to 112 ml despite a greater abbreviation of diastolic filling time. The greater decrease in filling time was probably due to the higher heart rate during postoperative exercise. Filling rates were also altered by revascularization, particularly in early diastole (figure 3). The peak filling rate increased before surgery from 585 to 950 ml/sec during exercise and after surgery it increased from 604 to 1260 ml/sec. The mean filling rate for the first half of diastole showed a similar trend. Neither filling rate at rest was significantly increased by revascularization, but during exercise both rates

TABLE 3
Effect of revascularization on left ventricular filling dynamics

	Before surgery (n = 13)		After surgery (n = 13)		Before vs after	
	Rest	Exercise	Rest	Exercise	Rest	Exercise
Diastolic filling time (msec)	486±81	185±47[C]	391±121	165±30[C]	p<.05	NS
Filling volume (ml)	110±24	89±20[C]	102±29	112±25	NS	p<.01
Peak filling rate (ml/sec)	585±210	950±185[C]	604±235	1260±319[C]	NS	p<.001
Mean filling rate 1 (ml/sec)	296±93	693±174[C]	336±134	946±288[C]	NS	p<.001
Mean filling rate 2 (ml/sec)	171±72	296±188[A]	258±164	414±161[B]	NS	NS
LVP at MVO (mm Hg)	17±6	44±10[C]	11±4	31±9[C]	p<.01	p<.01
T (msec)	55±11	38±11[B]	52±11	29±7[C]	NS	p<.05
P_B (mm Hg)	−7±6	10±11[C]	−9±10	−7±10	NS	p<.001

LVP at MVO = left ventricular pressure at mitral valve opening.
[A]p < .05, rest vs exercise; [B]p < .01, rest vs exercise; [C]p < .001, rest vs exercise.

were significantly increased after surgery. A major determinant of early filling rates, the left atrial pressure, was estimated by the left ventricular pressure at mitral valve opening. Left ventricular pressure at mitral opening increased during preoperative exercise from 17 to 44 mm Hg (figure 3). At postoperative exercise it increased from 11 to 31 mm Hg, which was significantly ($p < .01$) less than the preoperative exercise value. All postoperative patients, including those with apparently normal systolic function, had a 9 mm Hg or greater increase in left ventricular pressure at mitral opening during exercise. In the control group left ventricular pressure at mitral opening was 12 ± 7 at rest and 14 ± 10 with exercise and peak filling rate increased from 615 ± 163 to 1050 ± 318 ml/sec during exercise ($p < .05$). Mean filling rate for the first half of diastole increased from 358 ± 104 to 649 ± 244 ml/sec during exercise ($p < .05$). The early diastolic filling rates in the control group were actually less than those in the postoperative patients during exercise, but these differences did not achieve statistical significance.

Mean filling rates during the second half of diastole were likewise altered by revascularization, yet remained clearly different from those in the control group (figure 3). Before surgery the mean rate increased from 171 to 296 ml/sec during exercise and the postoperative mean rate was 258 ml/sec at rest and 414 ml/sec during exercise. The increased rates at rest and during exercise after surgery were not significantly different from preoperative values. The control group had a mean rate of filling for the second half of diastole of 199 ± 111 ml/sec at rest and 649 ± 244 ml/sec during exercise. The control group's exercise value was significantly greater than the preoperative value ($p < .05$), but not the postoperative one.

Mean diastolic pressure-volume relationship data are presented in figure 5. There was an upward shift in the relationship in all patients during preoperative exercise and no clear shifts during postoperative exercise. Results in six typical patients are presented in figure 4 and show not only the improvement after revascularization, but the heterogeneity of the preoperative upward shifts.

There was a great inconsistency in changes in mean right atrial pressure during exercise both before and after surgery. In nine patients right atrial pressure recordings were available for both periods. There was a preoperative increase in right atrial pressure from 6 ± 2 to 11 ± 4 mm Hg ($p < .001$) and a similar postoperative change (4 ± 2 to 10 ± 4 mm Hg, $p < .001$). The degree of right atrial pressure elevation was not a major, consistent determinant of the left ventricular diastolic pressure-volume relationship.

Discussion

The results of this study support the hypothesis that revascularization significantly improves both left ventricular systolic and diastolic function during exercise. Several key issues require discussion. First, to what extent does left ventricular function, both systolic and diastolic, return to normal after revascularization? What is the nature of the persistent abnormalities and their possible causes? What are the implications of these findings for patient care?

Systolic dynamics. The development of a transient regional wall motion abnormality is a classic manifestation of systolic dysfunction due to ischemia. By study design, all patients had exercise-induced asynergy at the preoperative study, and none had it after revascularization. There was a postoperative improvement in both the shortening characteristics and pressure generation capability of the left ventricle. There was also a small increase in ejection fraction during postoperative exercise, which is in agreement with results of other studies. The mechanism of this augmentation of ejection fraction was the significant increase in end-diastolic volume and preload, not a reduction in end-systolic volume as occurs in normal individuals. Thus, an increase in stroke volume during exercise does occur and combines with the tachycardia to allow a clear increase in exercise cardiac output, which is blunted before surgery.[12] The inability of most of the patients to reduce end-systolic volume with exercise may not only limit the rise in ejection fraction, but has potential implications for subsequent pressure decay and diastolic events (see below).

The increase in pressure generation during exercise after revascularization is shown by maximum positive dP/dt. Achievement of an increased exercise heart rate and the greater degree of synchrony are two factors that influence the maximum value of dP/dt. In addition, muscle that before surgery had greatly reduced contractile strength because of ischemia was capable after surgery of contributing to pressure generation. This resulted in a significant rise in peak left ventricular pressure during exercise. The reversal of preoperative exercise-induced fall in systolic pressure has also been described by other investigators.[25, 26]

Left ventricular pressure decay and early diastolic pressures. The abnormal systolic dynamics of ischemia, including asynchrony and increased end-systolic volume, are probably major factors that combine with direct disruption of muscle relaxation by ischemia to produce abnormal pressure decay. In man both pacing and exercise induction of ischemia have been shown to alter pressure decay in the left ventricle.[9, 10, 27, 28] We have previously stressed the importance of the abnormalities in pressure decay that contribute to increased early diastolic pressures.[10] These data show that abnormal pressure decay in the left ventricle can be greatly improved by revascularization. Subsequently, early diastolic pressures maintain a low level. The enhancement in relaxation is probably due to the correction of multiple biochemical and mechanical abnormalities that occur during preoperative ischemia.[29] β-Blockers could have blunted the preoperative heart rate response to exercise and, thus, the catecholamine-mediated enhancement of relaxation. In addition, a heightened sympathetic state occurs postoperatively, although none of our patients were restudied before 3 months after surgery. The role of preoperative β-blocker therapy was probably an unimportant one in the pressure decay abnormalities during exercise. First, all cardiac medications were held for 12 to 24 hr before catheterization. Second, the gross abnormalities produced by exercise-induced ischemia probably greatly overshadowed any effects of medication. And finally, the medications that were taken before surgery would be expected to lessen hemodynamic abnormalities because of their anti-ischemic effects.[30]

As with other parameters, the mean values for pressure decay parameters clearly showed improvement during postoperative exercise. These mean values were obtained from data in the majority of patients who had some persistent abnormalities and the few who were indistinguishable from the control group. The exercise-induced abnormalities in a group of patients with prior infarction but no ischemia with exercise, a scar group, have been previously reported.[10–12] Many of the postoperative patients with similar pressure decay abnormalities during exercise had prior infarctions, although only six had resting ejection fractions of 50% or less and only seven had Q waves on their electrocardiograms. It appears that revascularization converts the exercise hemodynamics of many patients from those typical of ischemia to those typical of chronic infarction without acute ischemia. Yet even patients without clinical histories or signs of transmural infarction have increased fibrotic content of the myocardium served by stenotic arteries.[14] Recurrent bouts of ischemia may produce permanent structural changes with long-term hemodynamic sequelae similar to those abnormalities in patients with classic infarctions.

Diastolic pressure-volume relations. In individual patients (figure 4) and for groups (figure 5), the data show the reversibility of one of the classic manifestations of ischemia, the upward shift in diastolic pressure-volume relationship in the left ventricle. Few postoperative patients have totally normal diastolic pressure-volume relationships during exercise. As illustrated in figure 5, the control subjects had a reduction in the early diastolic pressure nadir, P_L, with a downward shift in the early diastolic pressure-volume relationship. It has been suggested that during exercise in individuals without heart disease, intense catecholamine stimulation produces a significant reduction in end-systolic chamber size, which may lead to a physiologically significant degree of internal restoring forces within the left ventricle.[31] This could create diastolic suction.[32] Whether this mechanism is present in our control subjects or postoperative patients cannot be determined from these data. As discussed above, very few of our patients experienced a reduction in end-systolic volume during postoperative exercise. This, combined with data showing that pressure decay normalization is infrequently achieved, may explain why the diastolic pressure-volume relationship during exercise rarely normalizes despite clinically successful revascularization.

The complexity of the diastolic pressure-volume relationship has been discussed in several reviews.[33–35] Previous experimental studies have shown that severe ischemia directly alters myocardial stress-strain characteristics.[4] It has also been suggested that a component of the upward shift seen during ischemia is related to acute pericardial restraint. Janicki and Weber[36] have shown that the pericardium can enhance ventricular interaction and mediate upward shifts in the left ventricle's diastolic pressure-volume relationship. This problem was addressed in pacing-induced angina by Mann et al.,[7] who measured right ventricular end-diastolic pressure during ischemia, a time when there was a left ventricular diastolic pressure-volume shift. They found no significant increase in right ventricular end-diastolic pressure. Likewise, Momomura et al.[37] recently presented data from a dog preparation that also showed that right ventricular compression of the left ventricle is not likely to be responsible for the upward shift during ischemia. We did see increases in right atrial mean pressure in many of our patients during exercise-induced ischemia and when upward shifts in the left ventricular diastolic pressure-volume relationship occurred, but there was no consistency in the degree of increase in right atrial pressure or the degree or type of upward shift.[13] In some patients right atrial pressure rose by only several millimeters of mercury when large left ventricular upward shifts were seen. On the other hand, in many postoperative patients there were persistent gross elevations in right atrial pressures during exercise, but no upward shift was present in the left ventricle. We conclude that in exercise-induced ischemia there is no consistent effect of pericardial restriction. Other factors may elevate right atrial pressures during exercise. In some patients the pericardium may play a role in determining left ventricular diastolic properties during exercise, but this remains to be proven. Although the pericardium was left open postoperatively, some constricting effect cannot categorically be excluded. Alterations in intrapleural pressures may also play a role in altered diastolic function.

An unexpected finding of this study was the degree to which left ventricular end-diastolic pressure increased during postoperative exercise. The increase in pressure was less than that before surgery and was not associated with clear signs of ischemia, i.e., new asynergy. The postoperative increase in end-diastolic pressure was related to a parallel increase in end-diastolic volume. This suggests that there was no significant acute change in compliance. During postoperative exercise heart rate increased more than before surgery. This increase should have tended to lower, not increase, end-diastolic pressure. The difference in the early diastolic pressure, P_L, is striking, since it failed to rise during postoperative exercise. This can be seen in the example of figure 1. The increase in end-diastolic pressure may reflect the abnormally stiff ventricle frequently seen in coronary artery disease. Even in the absence of clinical infarction intraoperative transmural biopsies have shown the frequent occurrence of increased interstitial fibrosis and myocardial hypertrophy in these patients.[14]

The steep pressure-volume relationship with the increased end-diastolic pressure during postoperative exercise is probably a major reason mitral valve opening pressures were still elevated postoperatively in our patients, but other factors can contribute to the determination of left atrial pressure, e.g., the chamber's own pressure-volume relationship and systolic performance. This could not be evaluated by our data. Significant mitral regurgitation was not present in any of our patients.

Filling dynamics. As seen in figure 3, filling dynamics are altered after revascularization, allowing an increased amount of blood to enter the left ventricle despite an even greater reduction in filling time during postoperative exercise. Left ventricular filling is a dynamic process involving the interaction of active and passive properties of the atria and ventricles. The rate of left ventricular pressure decay and the subsequent atrial-ventricular gradient are major factors determining early diastolic filling.[24] The operative stiffness of the left ventricle becomes increasingly important as filling progresses.[38, 39] The strength and timing of atrial systole determines the end-diastolic "kick" to ventricular filling.[40–42] We have previously shown that during exercise-induced ischemia filling dynamics are altered in a characteristic fashion.[11] Despite the abnormalities in pressure decay, early filling rates are maintained during exercise by the gross elevation of the atrial driving force. Recent experimental data have also shown how changes in atrial pressure may increase filling rates despite alterations in relaxation that would tend to decrease filling.[43] Unlike in the normal ventricle, filling in the later portion of diastole during exercise is restricted both before and after surgery. During ischemia with the acute increase in end-systolic volume, the ventricle begins to fill on a rightward, and thus steeper, portion of the diastolic pressure-volume curve. This is in addition to an acute stiffening of the

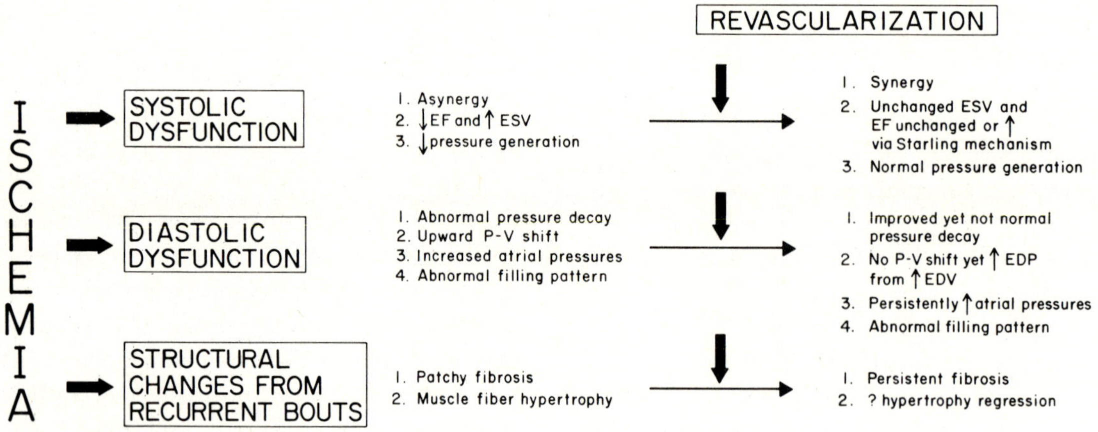

FIGURE 6. A schematic summary of left ventricular function during exercise-induced ischemia and after revascularization. Chronic structural changes, even in the absence of clinical infarction, may occur with repetitive bouts of ischemia and persist after revascularization. Many of the persistent diastolic abnormalities during postoperative exercise can be explained by chronic, passive changes in compliance in the left ventricle that may be related to the structural alterations.

ventricle due to the ischemia itself.[44] Despite the lack of significant upward diastolic pressure-volume shifts during postoperative exercise, late filling still shows some restriction compared with that in normal subjects. A useful analogy is provided by the filling profiles of patients with constrictive pericarditis in the study of Tyberg et al.[45] Those with constriction had very rapid filling during the first half of diastole compared with normal and, subsequently, filling during the second half of diastole virtually stopped. The gross elevations in atrial driving pressures, small end-systolic volumes, probably near-normal pressure decay, and a stiff left ventricle (in this case due to the pericardium) produce a similar combination of filling parameters, as in our postoperative patients during exercise. Their study, like ours, also highlights the observation that rapid filling rates cannot be given qualitative labels such as "good" or "normal." The elevation in atrial pressures required to produce these rates is clearly not normal.

Influence of chronic structural changes. The abnormalities in diastolic function that are observed during post-revascularization exercise may reflect increased amounts of interstitial fibrosis and myocardial hypertrophy. The structural changes may be gross (postinfarction scars) or more subtle (patchy fibrosis). Revascularization may prevent or minimize acute, exercise-induced ischemia with the acute stiffening of the left ventricular chamber. However, the chronic changes in chamber compliance would not be expected to be altered by revascularization. In figure 6 a summary of our functional data and the effect of revascularization is outlined.

Hess et al.[46] studied the effect of myocardial structure on ventricular function in a group of postoperative patients with aortic valve disease. Residual abnormalities in diastolic stiffness were shown to be accompanied by a relative increase in interstitial fibrosis and regression of myocardial hypertrophy. In patients with coronary artery disease repetitive bouts of ischemia may induce hypertrophy and increase interstitial fibrosis[14] and there is some evidence of a reduction in left ventricular mass after revascularization.[47] Further clarification of the interrelationship of myocardial structure and function in this group of patients is needed.

We thank Brenda Cochran and Joyce Bolden in Chicago for typing the manuscript and Petrit Alibali for the graphics. Mafalda Hegetschweiler and Rosy Hug in Zurich are thanked for their technical assistance.

References

1. Tomoike H, Franklin D, McKown D, Kemper WS, Guberek M, Ross J Jr: Regional myocardial dysfunction and hemodynamic abnormalities with strenuous exercise in dogs with limited coronary flow. Circ Res **42:** 487, 1978
2. Horwitz LD, Peterson DF, Bishop VS: Effect of regional myocardial ischemia on cardiac pump performance during exercise. Am J Physiol **234:** H157, 1978
3. Paulus WJ, Serizawa T, Grossman W: Altered left ventricular diastolic properties during pacing-induced ischemia in dogs with coronary stenoses. Circ Res **50:** 218, 1982
4. Hess OM, Osakada G, Lavelle JF, Gallagher KP, Kemper WS, Ross J Jr: Diastolic myocardial wall stiffness and ventricular relaxation during partial and complete coronary occlusions in the conscious dog. Circ Res **52:** 387, 1983
5. Dwyer EM: Left ventricular pressure-volume alterations and regional disorders of contraction during myocardial ischemia induced by atrial pacing. Circulation **42:** 1111, 1970
6. Barry WH, Brooker JZ, Alderman EL, Harrison DC: Changes in diastolic stiffness and tone of the left ventricle during angina pectoris. Circulation **49:** 255, 1974
7. Mann T, Goldberg S, Mudge GH, Grossman W: Factors contributing to altered left ventricular diastolic properties during angina pectoris. Circulation **49:** 255, 1974
8. Mann T, Brodie BR, Grossman W, McLaurin LP: Effect of angina on the left ventricular diastolic pressure-volume relationship. Circulation **55:** 761, 1977

9. Grossman W, Serizawa T, Carabello BA: Studies of the mechanisms of altered left ventricular diastolic pressure-volume relations during ischemia. Eur Heart J **1** (suppl A): 141, 1980
10. Carroll JD, Hess OM, Hirzel HO, Krayenbuehl HP: Exercise-induced ischemia: the influence of altered relaxation on early diastolic pressures. Circulation **67:** 521, 1983
11. Carroll JD, Hess OM, Hirzel HO, Krayenbuehl HP: Dynamics of left ventricular filling at rest and during exercise. Circulation **68:** 59, 1983
12. Carroll JD, Hess OM, Studer NP, Hirzel HO, Krayenbuehl HP: Systolic function during exercise in patients with coronary artery disease. J Am Coll Cardiol **2:** 206, 1983
13. Carroll JD, Hess OM, Hirzel HO, Krayenbuehl HP: Inconsistency of changes in right atrial pressure during exercise-induced left ventricular ischemia. Circulation **68** (suppl III): III-102, 1983 (abst)
14. Hess OM, Schneider J, Carroll JD, Eqloff L, Turina M, Krayenbuehl HP: Myocardial structure of LV segments with and without exercise-induced wall motion abnormalities in patients with coronary artery disease. J Am Coll Cardiol **1:** 734, 1983 (abst)
15. Carroll JD, Hess OM, Hirzel HO, Krayenbuehl HP: Determinants of left ventricular diastolic function during ischemia. Eur Heart J **5:** 352, 1984 (abst)
16. Frick MH, Harjola PT, Valle M: Persistent improvement after coronary bypass surgery: ergometric and angiographic correlations at 5 years. Circulation **67:** 491, 1983
17. McIntosh HD, Garcia JA: The first decade of aortocoronary bypass grafting, 1967–1977. A review. Circulation **57:** 405, 1978
18. Rahimtoola SH: Postoperative exercise response in the evaluation of the physiologic status after coronary bypass surgery. Circulation **65** (suppl II): II-106, 1982
19. Chesebro JH, Ritman EL, Frye RL, Smith HC, Vlietstra RE, Pluth JR: Left ventricular performance before and after aortocoronary artery bypass surgery. Circulation **65** (suppl II): II-98, 1982
20. Kent KM, Borer JS, Green MV, Bacharach SL, McIntosh CL, Conkle DM, Epstein SE. Effects of coronary-artery bypass on global and regional left ventricular function during exercise. N Engl J Med **298:** 1434, 1978
21. Bussmann WD, Mayer V, Kober G, Kaltenbach M: Ventricular function at rest, during leg raising and physical exercise before and after aortocoronary bypass surgery. Am J Cardiol **43:** 488, 1979
22. Campeau L, Elias G, Esplugas E, Lesperance J, Bourassa MG, Grondin CM: Left ventricular performance during exercise before and one year after aortocoronary bypass surgery for angina pectoris. Circulation **50** (suppl II): II-103, 1974
23. Barry WH, Pfeifer JF, Lipton MJ, Tilkian AG, Hultgren HN: Effects of coronary artery bypass grafting on resting and exercise hemodynamics in patients with stable angina pectoris: a prospective, randomized study. Am J Cardiol **37:** 823, 1976
24. Yellin EL, Sonnenblick EH, Frater RWM: Dynamic determinants of left ventricular filling: an overview. *In* Baan J, Arntzenius AC, Yellin EL, editors: Cardiac dynamics. The Hague, 1980, Martinus Nijhoff, pp 145–158
25. Morris SN, Phillips JF, Jordan JW, McHenry PL: Incidence and significance of decreases in systolic blood pressure during graded treadmill exercise testing. Am J Cardiol **41:** 211, 1978
26. Thompson PD, Keleman MH: Hypotension accompanying the onset of exertional angina. A sign of severe compromise of left ventricular blood supply. Circulation **52:** 28, 1975
27. Thompson DS, Waldron CB, Juul SM, Naqvi N, Swanton RH, Coltart DJ, Jenkins BS, Webb-Peploe MM: Analysis of left ventricular pressure during isovolumic relaxation in coronary artery disease. Circulation **65:** 690, 1982
28. Brown DL, Craig WE, Layton SA, Rubal BJ, Murgo JP: Exercise induced abnormalities of left ventricular relaxation in coronary artery disease. Circulation **64** (suppl IV): IV-77, 1981
29. Brutsaert DL, Rademakers FE, Sys SU: Triple control of relaxation: implications in cardiac disease. Circulation **69:** 190, 1984
30. Kumada T, Gallagher KP, Shirato K, McKown D, Miller M, Kemper WS, White F, Ross J Jr: Reduction of exercise-induced regional myocardial dysfunction by propranolol. Studies in a canine model of chronic coronary artery stenosis. Circ Res **46:** 190, 1980
31. Sonnenblick EH: The structural basis and importance of restoring forces and elastic recoil for the filling of the heart. Eur Heart J **1** (suppl A): 107, 1980
32. Sabbah HN, Stein PD: Pressure-diameter relations during early diastole in dogs. Incompatibility with the concept of passive left ventricular filling. Circ Res **45:** 357, 1982
33. Glantz SA, Parmley WW: Factors which affect the diastolic pressure-volume curve. Circ Res **42:** 171, 1978
34. Mirsky I, Rankin JS: The effects of geometry, elasticity, and external pressure on the diastolic pressure-volume and stiffness-stress relations. How important is the pericardium? Circ Res **44:** 601, 1979
35. Grossman W, Barry WH: Diastolic pressure-volume relations in the diseased heart. Fed Proc **39:** 148, 1980
36. Janicki JS, Weber KT: The pericardium and ventricular interaction, distensibility, and function. Am J Physiol **238:** H494, 1980
37. Momomura S, Bradley AB, Grossman W. Left ventricular diastolic pressure-segment length relations and end-diastolic distensibility in dogs with coronary stenoses. Circ Res **55:** 203, 1984
38. Gaasch WH, Levine HJ, Quinones MA, Alexander J: Left ventricular compliance: mechanisms and clinical implications. Am J Cardiol **38:** 645, 1976
39. Grossman W, McLaurin LP: Diastolic properties of the left ventricle. Ann Intern Med **84:** 316, 1976
40. Noble MIN, Milne EN, Goerke RJ, Carlsson E, Domenesch RJ, Saunders KB, Hoffman JIE: Left ventricular filling and diastolic pressure-volume relations in the conscious dog. Circ Res **24:** 269, 1969
41. Skinner NS, Mitchell JH, Wallace AG, Sarnoff ST: Hemodynamic effects of altering the time of atrial systole. Am J Physiol **205:** 499, 1963
42. Hammermeister KE, Warbasse JR: The rate of change on left ventricular volume in man. II. Diastolic events in health and disease. Circulation **49:** 739, 1974
43. Ishida Y, Meisner JS, Tsujioka K, Gallo J, Yoran C, Frater R, Yellin E: Peak rapid filling rate may not reflect left ventricular relaxation properties when left atrial pressure compensates for changes in loading conditions. Circulation **70** (suppl II): II-349, 1984 (abst)
44. Bourdillon PD, Lorell BH, Mirsky I, Paulus WJ, Wynne J, Grossman W: Increased regional myocardial stiffness of the left ventricle during pacing-induced angina in man. Circulation **67:** 316, 1983
45. Tyberg TI, Goodyer AVN, Hurst VA, Alexander J, Langou RA: Left ventricular filling in differentiating restrictive amyloid cardiomyopathy and constrictive pericarditis. Am J Cardiol **47:** 791, 1981
46. Hess OM, Ritter M, Schneider J, Grimm J, Turina M, and Krayenbuehl HJP: Diastolic stiffness and myocardial structure in aortic valve disease before and after valve replacement. Circulation **69:** 855, 1984
47. Meester GT, Brower RW, Hugenholtz PG: Regression of left ventricular wall mass index after coronary artery bypass surgery in a group of patients with stable angina pectoris. Eur Heart J **3** (suppl A): 155, 1982

Results of triple valve replacement in 91 patients: perioperative mortality and long-term follow-up

BERNARD J. GERSH, M.B.,CH.B., D. PHIL., HARTZELL V. SCHAFF, M.D., PIERCE J. VATTEROTT, M.D., GORDON K. DANIELSON, M.D., THOMAS A. ORSZULAK, M.D., JEFFREY M. PIEHLER, M.D., FRANCISCO J. PUGA, M.D., JAMES R. PLUTH, M.D., AND DWIGHT C. MCGOON, M.D.

ABSTRACT Between 1961 and 1984, 91 patients underwent simultaneous triple valve replacement at the Mayo Clinic. Of the 273 prosthetic valves used, 77% were Starr-Edwards. Perioperative (30 day) mortality was 24% to 27% between 1962 and 1974 and 7% between 1975 and 1983 ($p = .17$). In patients with NYHA class IV symptoms, perioperative mortality was 44%, and in those with milder symptoms, it was 8% ($p < .0001$). The median follow-up was 7.5 years (range, 6 weeks to 20 years). Cumulative survival, which was calculated taking into consideration perioperative mortality, was 64% at 1 year, 55% at 5 years, 40% at 10 years, and 25% at 15 years. Multivariate analysis identified preoperative functional class and age as predictors of late survival. Among causes of late mortality were sudden death in 32.5%, congestive heart failure in 15%, thromboembolism in 12.5%, prosthetic valve dysfunction in 7.5%, and infective endocarditis in 5%. Late complications included systemic emboli in 42% (embolic rate, 12.3 events per 100 patient-years), bleeding in 22%, myocardial infarction in 16%, and infective endocardititis in 6%. Eight patients required reoperation for prosthetic valve dysfunction, and 12 patients had permanent pacemakers. Of the 29 patients still alive, 79% are in NYHA class I or II. In summary, perioperative mortality after triple valve replacement appears to be declining; long-term survival in 30 day survivors is similar to that after single valve replacement and excellent symptomatic improvement can be obtained, although morbidity is high.
Circulation 72, No. 1, 130–137, 1985.

OVER the past 10 years, reports from many centers have defined the early and late results of cardiac valve replacement for most categories of patients.[1–9] The outcome of triple valve replacement (aortic, mitral, and tricuspid valve replacement) is less well defined, primarily because of the relatively small numbers of patients who have undergone the operation. With the trend toward conservative tricuspid valve surgery coupled with the development of more predictable methods of valve repair and the declining incidence of rheumatic heart disease in the United States, triple valve replacement is less frequently required than it was previously. Nonetheless, rheumatic heart disease with involvement of multiple valves remains a serious problem in many countries.[10] Accordingly, we report our experience in 91 consecutive patients with rheumatic heart disease who underwent simultaneous triple valve replacement at the Mayo Clinic. This is the largest reported series and is particularly notable for the long follow-up period, which spanned 20 years (median duration of follow-up, 7.5 years in perioperative survivors). During this period, major changes in the preoperative, intraoperative, and postoperative practice of valve surgery have occurred. Particular attention has been focused on factors influencing operative risk and late survival, on the causes of late death and late complications, and on the accumulated knowledge derived from this prolonged learning experience. Our earlier experience with triple valve replacement has been reported.[11, 12]

From the Mayo Clinic and Mayo Foundation, Rochester, MN.
Address for correspondence: Bernard J. Gersh, M.B.,Ch.B., D.Phil., Mayo Clinic, 200 First St. SW, Rochester, MN 55905.
Received Nov. 12, 1984; revision accepted March 22, 1985.
Presented in part at the 32nd Annual Scientific Session, American College of Cardiology, New Orleans, March 20 to 24, 1983.

Material and methods

We reviewed the records of all 91 patients with rheumatic heart disease who underwent aortic, mitral, and tricuspid valve replacement during a single operation at the Mayo Clinic from 1962 through 1984. For perspective, this cohort represents only 1% of the total 8359 patients who underwent cardiac valve replacement during the same period. At our institution, the frequency of triple valve replacement has progressively declined: 78 operations were performed from 1962 through 1974, whereas only 14 triple valve replacements were done on 13 patients from 1975 through 1984. One patient had undergone triple-valve replacement in 1970, but all three cloth-covered Starr-Edwards valves were replaced in 1984 because of hemolysis.

Clinical data on the 91 patients are summarized in table 1. The severity of preoperative symptoms appears to have changed. Between 1962 and 1974, 50% of patients were in New York Heart Association (NYHA) class IV before surgery and 50% were in NYHA class II or III; of those undergoing operation from 1975 through 1984, only 8% were in NYHA class IV and 92% were in class II or III ($p = .024$). The predominant valve lesion was classified according to clinical findings, preoperative and intraoperative intracardiac pressure recordings, and operative inspection (table 2). Preoperatively 86% of patients were in atrial fibrillation, one patient was in paced rhythm, and one patient had episodic sinus arrest. The remaining patients (14%) were in sinus rhythm.

All patients had rheumatic heart disease, and 23 patients had 35 previous cardiac operations. Eight prior operations involved the aortic valve, 24 involved the mitral valve (21 mitral commissurotomies), and three were performed for tricuspid valve disease. Four patients had undergone previous valve replacements (including the patient with a prior triple valve replacement). During the interval of this study, a variety of prosthetic heart valves were used, and these are listed in table 3. Most (77%) were Starr-Edwards prostheses.

Surgical techniques. Methods of extracorporeal circulation and surgical techniques evolved throughout the two decades of this study. All operations were performed through a median sternotomy, and high-flow (2.0 to 2.4 liters/min/m^2) hypothermic extracorporeal circulation was used. For the first 84 patients in this series, myocardial protection was achieved by continuous coronary artery perfusion; in the last seven patients, cold potassium cardioplegia was used during aortic cross-clamping. Anticoagulation with sodium warfarin was begun in all patients as soon as possible after operation, generally on the second or third postoperative day.

Follow-up. Current information on all patients was obtained by questionnaires to both patients and referring physicians, by telephone contact, or, in patients who had been seen before the end of the present review, by Mayo Clinic records. If possible, the cause of death was ascertained from copies of death certificates or from information supplied by the patient's physician or family.

The diagnosis of thromboembolism was made by a history of stroke, transient cerebrovascular ischemic attacks, or myocardial infarction in patients younger than 45 years or in those with documented normal coronary arteries. Splenic, renal, and pulmonary emboli were diagnosed in a few patients in whom adequate documentation was present, including those in whom a diagnosis was made at autopsy. All patient contacts included specific questions related to possible thromboembolic episodes.

TABLE 1
Preoperative characteristics of patients

	n	%
Total	91	
Male	23	25
Female	68	75
NYHA class		
II	3	3
III	47	52
IV	41	45

Mean age of the patients was 48 years, range 19 to 68.

TABLE 2
Predominant valvular lesions

Valve	Stenosis	Insufficiency	Mixed
Aortic	10	33	57
Mitral	22	12	66
Tricuspid	1	49	50

Values are percentages of patients with each lesion.

The amount of data available regarding the adequacy of anticoagulation was insufficient for further analysis.

Statistical analysis

Perioperative mortality. Univariate analysis of discrete variables was performed by means of a chi-square test or, when needed, Fisher's exact test, and continuous variables were analyzed by the two-sample t test or Wilcoxon rank-sum test. Multivariate analysis of prognostic variables related to perioperative death was by a logistic multiple regression model.

Late survival. Survival was calculated actuarially by the Kaplan-Meier method. Univariate analysis of discrete variables was by the log-rank test or Gehan-Wilcoxon test. Both univariate and multivariate analyses of continuous variables were performed with the Cox proportional-hazards model.

Results

Perioperative mortality. Perioperative (30 day or hospital) mortality was 24% (22 patients). There was a trend toward improved mortality in recent years. Among the 14 operations between 1975 and 1984, there was only one perioperative death (mortality 7%; $p = .17$). This death occurred in a patient who had undergone a previous mitral commissurotomy and subsequent mitral and tricuspid valve replacement. At the time of triple valve replacement, she underwent replacement of her malfunctioning tricuspid prosthesis, replacement of a malfunctioning mitral prosthesis, and an additional replacement of a stenotic native aortic valve.

The following factors were analyzed by univariate and multivariate logistic multiple regression analysis to evaluate their influence on perioperative mortality: sex, age, NYHA class, presence of atrial fibrillation (pure tricuspid insufficiency as opposed to mixed stenosis and insufficiency), previous surgery, duration of aortic cross-clamping, duration of cardiopulmonary bypass, use of cardioplegia, and year of operation. Univariate analysis identified only preoperative NYHA class, duration of cardiopulmonary bypass, and pure tricuspid insufficiency as significant predictors of hospital mortality ($p < .0001$, $< .002$, and $< .01$). By the multiple regression model, the only significant variable influencing hospital mortality was preoperative NYHA class IV ($p < .02$). Perioperative mortality was 44% among patients with class IV disability but was only 8% in patients with milder symp-

TABLE 3
Types of prostheses used in 91 patients undergoing simultaneous replacement of three valves

Type	Aortic valve n	Aortic valve %	Mitral valve n	Mitral valve %	Tricuspid valve n	Tricuspid valve %
Starr-Edwards	71	78	72	79	69	76
Björk-Shiley	6	7	7	8	5	5.5
Braunwald-Cutter	5	5.5	5	6	6	6.5
Smeloff-Cutter	0	0	4	4	2	2
Bioprosthesis	3	3	2	2	9	10
Magovern-Cromie	5	5.5	0	0	0	0
Hall-Medtronic	1	1	1	1	0	0

toms ($p < .0001$). Preoperative catheterization data and measurements of ejection fraction were available in insufficient numbers of patients to enable those variables to be subjected to statistical analysis. Cardioplegia was used in only seven patients during triple valve replacement.

Causes of perioperative death. Low cardiac output was the principal cause of perioperative death in the patients, including seven patients who could not be weaned from cardiopulmonary bypass and died in the intraoperative period. Four died in the early postoperative period because of inadequate myocardial function. Multiorgan failure, hemorrhage, and arrhythmia accounted for the hospital deaths of the remaining 11 patients.

Long-term survival. Figure 1 illustrates the cumulative survival of all patients and all 30 day perioperative survivors. The high attrition rate in the first year was not sustained, so that between years 1 and 10 the rate was about 3.5% per year. Overall survival was 64% at 1 year, 55% at 5 years, 40% at 10 years, and 25% at 15 years. For 30 day survivors, late survival was 54% at 10 years and 33% at 15 years. In perioperative (30 day) survivors, the median duration of follow-up was 7.5 years (range, 6 weeks to 20 years). The longest survivor is alive and well (NYHA class II) 20 years after operation, and one patient (previously reported) had a successful pregnancy after triple valve replacement.[13] In patients with class II or III disability before surgery, overall 5 and 10 year survival rates were 73% and 54%, respectively; in contrast, survival rates for patients with preoperative class IV disability were 33% and 25%, respectively (figure 2). As expected, most of the difference between the two groups formed according to preoperative disability were noted in early mortality. In perioperative survivors 5 and 10 year survival rates were 80% and 59% in those with class II or III disability before surgery compared with 59% and 45% in those with class IV disability.

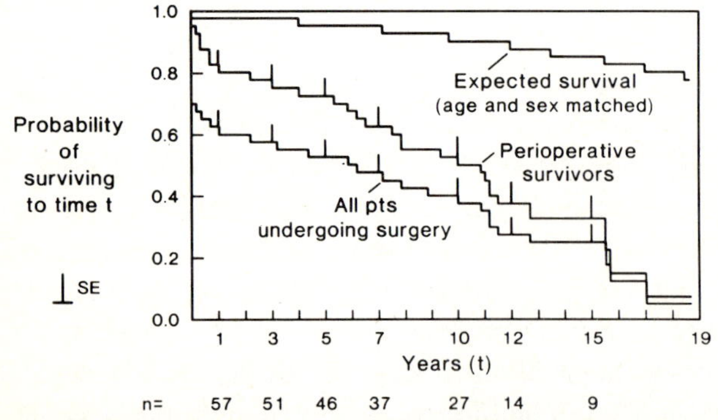

FIGURE 1. Cumulative survival of all patients undergoing simultaneous triple valve replacement and that of perioperative survivors. Number of patients at risk is shown below the horizontal axis. Expected survival, determined on the basis of age and sex distribution, is from the 1970 life table for the West North Central states.

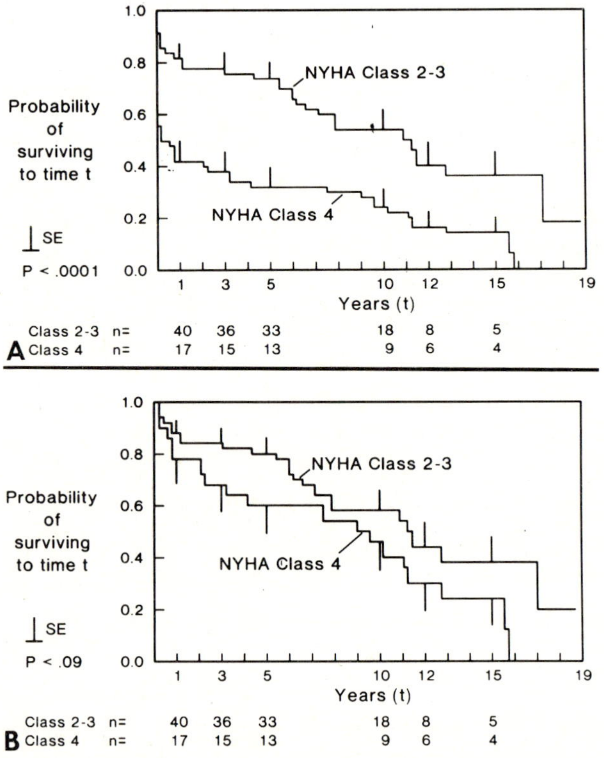

FIGURE 2. Cumulative survival of patients, stratified by preoperative functional class, undergoing simultaneous triple valve replacement. *A*, Entire series. *B*, Perioperative survivors. Number of patients at risk is shown below horizontal axis.

We compared the late survival of patients discharged from the hospital after triple valve replacement between 1962 and 1971 with that of a previously reported group of patients at the Mayo Clinic who underwent single valve replacement during the same period (figure 3).[7] The survival curves are remarkably similar during the first 10 to 15 postoperative years. For 11 patients undergoing triple valve replacement since 1975, the cumulative 5 year survival rate was 81%; in comparison, the rate was 52% for patients who underwent triple valve replacement before 1975.

With use of the Cox proportional-hazards model, only preoperative NYHA class IV symptoms and advanced age were related to poor survival ($p < .0002$ and $p < .01$, respectively).

Causes of late death. Causes of late death among 67 perioperative survivors are listed in table 4. The most common cause was sudden death (death within 1 hr of symptoms). Three patients had fatal strokes, one patient died of pulmonary embolism presumed to be related to the Starr-Edwards tricuspid prosthesis, and one patient had thrombosis of a Starr-Edwards aortic valve and extension of the thrombus to the left main coronary artery. Progressive congestive heart failure was believed to be the cause of death in 15% of patients, and three other patients died as a result of prosthetic valve dysfunction (including reoperation in one patient). Two patients died of infective endocarditis.

Late complications. Major late complications are listed in table 5. Thromboembolism and hemorrhagic complications of anticoagulation produced serious morbidity during the follow-up period. Eight patients required reoperation on 11 cardiac valves. One patient underwent successful replacement of all three cloth-covered Starr-Edwards valves (6300 series) because of cloth wear and severe hemolysis. Isolated tricuspid valve malfunction requiring reoperation developed in two patients with Starr-Edwards prostheses and in one patient with a Björk-Shiley prosthesis. One patient required replacement of both Starr-Edwards aortic and tricuspid prostheses, and two patients underwent reoperation for mitral periprosthetic leaks, which required valve replacement in one patient and suture repair in the other. The remaining patient underwent reoperation for a malfunctioning Braunwald-Cutter aortic valve. The actuarially determined risk of reoperation due to valve malfunction or periprosthetic leak was 4% at 5 years, 12% at 10 years, and 17% at 12 years.

Thromboembolism occurred in 29 patients, and 12 of these had multiple episodes of thromboembolism (table 6). The thromboembolic rate (reflecting all thromboembolic episodes, regardless of severity) was 12.3 per 100 patient-years. The central nervous system was the most commonly involved site, and in three patients, cerebrovascular thromboembolism was fatal. Most episodes (30 of 43) were not associated with permanent neurologic deficits. Figure 4 illustrates the actuarially determined survival free of thromboembolism. Only the first thromboembolic event was considered in the actuarial analysis, but all first episodes were included, regardless of severity. Embolism-free survival rates were 86% at 1 year, 70% at 5 years, and 43% at 10 and 12 years after surgery.

Twelve patients in this series required permanent

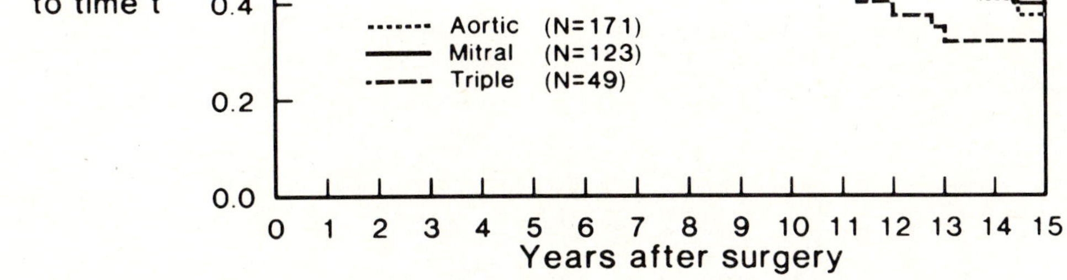

FIGURE 3. Cumulative survival of patients undergoing simultaneous triple valve replacement between 1962 and 1971 compared with a previously reported group of patients undergoing single valve replacement for isolated aortic or mitral insufficiency at the Mayo Clinic between 1962 and 1971. [Modified from McGoon MD, Fuster V, McGoon DC, Pumphrey CW, Pluth JR, Elveback LR: Aortic and mitral valve incompetence: long-term follow-up (10 to 19 years) of patients treated with the Starr-Edwards prosthesis. J Am Coll Cardiol **3:** 930, 1984. By permission of the American College of Cardiology.]

TABLE 4
Causes of late death in 40 of 69 perioperative survivors

Cause of death	n	%
Sudden death	13	32.5
Congestive heart failure	6	15
Thromboembolism	5	12.5
Prosthetic valve dysfunction (including reoperation in one patient)	3	7.5
Unknown	3	7.5
Infective endocarditis	2	5
Other	5	12.5
Hemorrhage	3	
Septicemia	1	
Myocardial infarction	1	
Acute pulmonary edema (cause unknown)	1	2.5
Noncardiac death	2	5

pacemakers. In two patients, permanent pacemaker implantation was performed in the perioperative period. In the other 10 patients, permanent pacemakers were required for symptomatic bradyarrhythmias, and the most frequent indication was atrial fibrillation with complete heart block or symptomatic pauses. In these patients, the interval from operation to pacemaker implantation ranged from 3 to 18 years (mean, 9.4 years) after initial valve replacement.

Functional outcome. Figure 5 illustrates the functional class of the 29 patients (32% of the total population) still alive at the end of follow-up. The median duration of follow-up was 10.7 years. Clinical improvement was striking. Before surgery 96% of patients were NYHA class III or IV, and at the time of last follow-up 79% of patients were NYHA class I or II.

Discussion

At our institution, the frequency of triple valve replacement has decreased markedly during the past decade. This may be explained by a decrease in the incidence of rheumatic heart disease and by recent trends toward conservative reparative procedures for patients with functional tricuspid valve insufficiency. Between 1975 and 1984, 59 patients have undergone aortic and mitral valve replacement with additional tricuspid annuloplasty at our institution.

Early mortality. The reported risk of triple valve replacement varies widely — from 10.5% to 50%.[11, 12, 14–25] This probably reflects the lack of uniformity in operative techniques, choice of prostheses, and patient selection criteria over the past 20 years as well as the small number of patients in most published series. In our own experience, operative mortality appears to have declined since 1975. It is likely that the relatively small number of patients undergoing this procedure since 1975 precludes statistical significance in comparisons of mortality, but many improvements in the management of patients with triple valve disease are believed to have been implemented during this experience. Most important is the improved preoperative clinical status of patients referred for operation. The higher operative risk for patients with class IV

TABLE 5
Late complications in 69 perioperative survivors

Complication	n	%	No. in whom complication was fatal
Embolism	29	42	5
Bleeding	15	22	3
Myocardial infarction	11	16	1
Cerebrovascular episode	11	16	5[A]
Reoperation	8	11.5	1
Permanent pacemaker implantation	10	14	
Infective endocarditis	4	6	2

Some patients had more than one complication.
[A]Including two with hemorrhage.

TABLE 6
Thromboembolic events occurring more than 30 days after triple valve replacement in 69 perioperative survivors[A]

Site of emboli	n	%
Total central nervous system	43	67
Fatal	3	4
Permanent deficit	10	16
Transient deficit	30	47
Cardiac (fatal in one patient)	10	16
Pulmonary (fatal in one patient)	7	11
Other, total	4	6
Spleen	3	
Peripheral	1	

[A]Number with emboli = 29 (42%); 12 patients experienced multiple episodes.

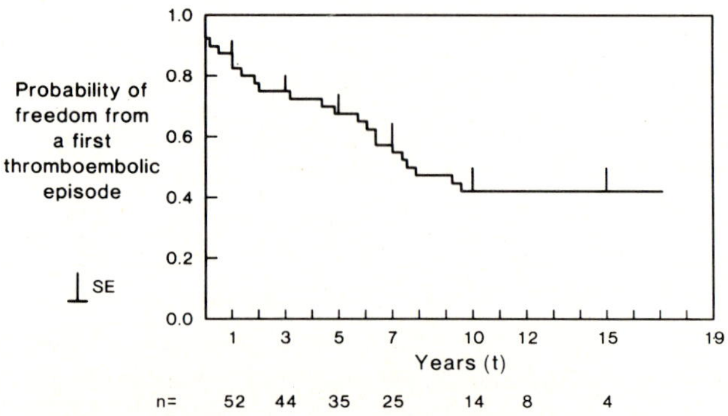

FIGURE 4. Cumulative survival free of a first thromboembolic event in perioperative survivors after triple valve replacement. Number of patients at risk is shown below horizontal axis.

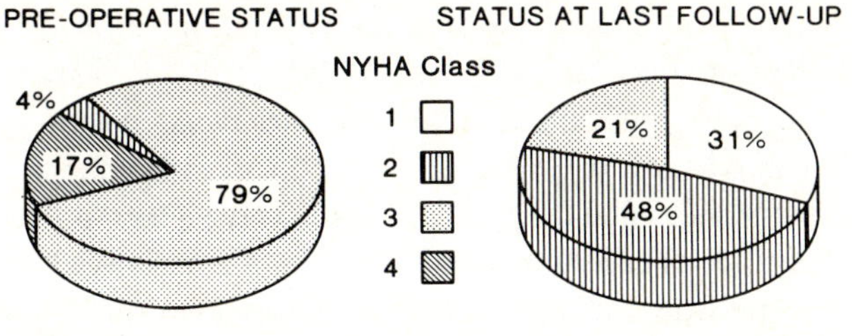

FIGURE 5. Functional outcome as defined by severity of symptoms in the 29 patients still alive after simultaneous triple valve replacement. Severity of symptoms before surgery is shown on *left*, and status at last follow-up is depicted on *right*. Median length of follow-up was 10.8 years, and range was 7 months to 20 years. Data from the 62 patients who died (perioperative and late deaths) are excluded from the analysis illustrated in this figure.

disability before surgery is similar to findings in other reports,[17, 20, 22, 24, 26] and is emphasized in our study by the results of the univariate and multivariate analyses, which show that preoperative functional status is the most powerful predictor of perioperative mortality. It is relevant that the percentage of patients with preoperative class IV disability decreased from 50% in the period before 1975 to 8% in the 1975 through 1984 period ($p < .02$).

Significant changes in surgical techniques occurred during the latter part of our experience. Although the small numbers of patients undergoing triple valve replacement since 1975 precluded further statistical analysis, the reduction in perioperative mortality could also reflect improved methods of intraoperative protection (only seven patients had cardioplegia) and subtle technical advances, including those in the areas of methods for suturing prosthetic valves, methods for removing intracardiac air at the conclusion of extracorporeal circulation, and routine placement of epicardial temporary pacing electrodes for control of postoperative arrhythmias. Before 1975, temporary pacing was used in 24% of patients; this rate increased to 54% from 1975 onward.

Operative mortality was 34% in patients with pure tricuspid insufficiency, which is significantly higher than the 13% in patients with mixed tricuspid valve disease. In some of the former group, tricuspid insufficiency might have been functional and a manifestation of poor right ventricular function and pulmonary hypertension,[27] whereas in patients with mixed disease, tricuspid valve involvement presumably was organic.

Late mortality. Late attrition — that after the first postoperative year — is relatively small but consistently observed. The overall 5, 10, and 15 year survival rates in this series are similar to rates in other studies. Five year survival rates were reported to range from 42% to 67%,[17, 19–21, 23] 10 year rates from 37% to 55%,[2, 23] and a 15 year survival rate of 23% was reported by Teply et al.[2] Again, patients with advanced heart failure and class IV disability have a much higher long-term mortality. This fact and the relatively good results of triple valve replacement in our patients with milder symptoms (all but three of whom were NYHA class III) argue strongly for earlier operation. Five year survival in perioperative survivors operated on since 1975 is 90% and is at least partially related to their better preoperative status; only one patient had class IV symptoms. Furthermore, the date of surgery did not appear as an independent predictor of long-term mortality.

For perspective, we compared the long-term results of triple valve replacement with those of single valve replacement over a similar time span (figure 3). Other authors have emphasized that late survival after triple valve replacement is significantly worse than that noted in patients who have undergone single valve replacement.[2–6, 8] However, most of this difference relates to the high *perioperative* mortality in the multiple valve replacement group. For example, our data (figure 3) indicate that the outcome for perioperative survivors after triple valve replacement is similar to that of patients surviving single valve replacement.[7, 9] Since the severity of symptoms is such an important predictor of perioperative mortality, the case for earlier operation is further strengthened.

Causes of late death. Approximately one-third of the late deaths in this series were determined to be related to thromboembolism, bleeding, or prosthetic valve dysfunction. This incidence of valve-related deaths is similar to the 43% reported by Macmanus et al.[19] after triple valve replacement and higher than that noted after single valve replacement.[2]

The high frequency of late sudden deaths after triple valve replacement is disturbing. In other long-term follow-up series of patients undergoing surgery for valvular heart disease, sudden death was the primary cause of late mortality in 20% to 43%.[2, 4, 7, 17, 19, 20, 28] Some of the deaths in this study were due to documented ventricular arrhythmias. The frequency of complex ventricular arrhythmias after tricuspid and triple valve replacement has been alluded to previously but not systematically evaluated.[16, 29, 30] Other possible causes of sudden death are thromboembolism, intracerebral hemorrhage, sudden prosthetic valve dysfunction, and intracardiac conduction disease.[31–33] Sudden death after valve replacement is clearly a cause for concern; the scope of the problem and the approach to management, however, need further evaluation.

An important finding of this review was the significant incidence of bradyarrhythmias requiring permanent pacemaker implantation. The causes are multifactorial, including intraoperative damage to the conduction system, fibrosis secondary to chronic compressive effects of the rigid mitral and tricuspid sewing ring, and rheumatic heart disease. During the course of this experience, indications for permanent pacing have become more liberal, and this change could have contributed to the late incidence of permanent pacemaker implantation. Nonetheless, all the patients undergoing pacemaker implantation, except one in whom implantation was performed intraoperatively, did have symptoms of major conduction disease.

Our data suggest that late survivors after valve replacement should be regularly evaluated (including Holter monitoring) for ventricular arrhythmias and conduction disturbances.[34] A high index of suspicion should be maintained, since the presentation of conduction disease and arrhythmias may be subtle.

Currently, we advocate implantation of permanent epicardial leads at the time of triple valve replacement to avoid a pacemaker lead being placed across the prosthetic tricuspid valve.

Thromboembolism. Comparing the incidence of thromboembolism in different series is difficult.[35, 36] The incidence varies widely and depends on criteria used to define a thromboembolic event, frequency and accuracy of follow-up data, type of valve used, and the inherent limitations of retrospective analyses.[35] Clearly, thromboembolism is a frequent cause of serious morbidity and mortality after triple valve replacement; the embolic rate of 12.3 events per 100 patient-years in this study is similar to the 11.4 events per 100 patient-years reported by Macmanus et al.[19] Embolism-free survival at 5 years is 70%, similar to that in other *early* series of single valve replacements with Starr-Edwards valves.[2, 4, 7–9, 34–38] The 10 year embolism-free rate is lower and the overall embolic rate higher in patients with three valves than in those with single or double valves.[2, 5, 7, 9, 35, 37–39] Several reports have documented a recent reduction in incidence of thromboembolism after valve replacement.[2, 3, 5, 6] This may be related to improved methods of maintaining anticoagulation, the addition of antiplatelet agents, earlier operation, improved prosthetic valve design, or a combination of these.

Valve durability. The durability of the Starr-Edwards valve is underscored by the relatively low incidence of reoperation or death due to prosthetic valve dysfunction. The vulnerability of the mechanical prosthesis (particularly tilting-disk prostheses) in the tricuspid position to thrombosis and sudden malfunction has been noted by others.[12, 23, 40–43] Five of the 11 valves requiring replacement were in the tricuspid position, and two deaths were due to tricuspid valve thrombosis, an indication that the Starr-Edwards valve is also prone to dysfunction in this position. There are lessons to be derived from this experience. The use of certain prosthetic valves subsequently found to be associated with a high incidence of problems, for example, the Braunwald-Cutter valve and the cloth-covered Starr-Edwards valve, was discontinued later. Improved techniques for tricuspid annuloplasty have undoubtedly diminished the requirement for tricuspid valvular replacement, and when replacement is still found to be necessary, the knowledge that mechanical prostheses tend to do less well in the tricuspid position than in the mitral or aortic position has led to our current policy of using tissue valves for tricuspid valve replacement.

Symptomatic status. The symptomatic status of patients currently alive is encouraging, and the results of comparisons with preoperative status are quite striking. That 79% of patients after a median duration of follow-up of almost 11 years should be in NYHA class I or II is indicative of the value of the procedure, but these results must be construed in light of the fact that 68% were dead at the time of last follow-up. Furthermore, the impact of surgery on these patients is not confined to the procedure of triple valve replacement. Twenty-three patients had had prior cardiac surgical procedures, and some of these patients were still alive and well more than 30 years after an initial mitral commissurotomy.

In conclusion, in our experience operative mortality for patients undergoing triple valve replacement appears to have been reduced. The frequency of use of the procedure has declined markedly in parallel with an increase in the number of patients undergoing double valve replacement and tricuspid annuloplasty. Early and late results can be expected to improve further if operative intervention is carried out before the onset of class IV symptoms. The frequency of late sudden death is of concern, and periodic evaluation for ventricular arrhythmias and conduction disturbances is recommended. The increased rate of thromboembolism and the significant incidence of bleeding after triple valve replacement with mechanical prostheses mandate meticulous anticoagulation for life.

Because most late mechanical prosthetic failures were of valves in the tricuspid position, the use of tricuspid annuloplasty when possible is recommended; if tricuspid valve replacement is required, a biologic prosthesis should be considered.

In patients who survive the perioperative period, the favorable long-term outcome and excellent symptomatic relief after triple valve replacement establish a continued role for the procedure in patients with severe multivalvular rheumatic heart disease.

We thank Duane M. Ilstrup and Mrs. Chu-Pin Chu of the Department of Medical Statistics and Epidemiology at the Mayo Clinic for statistical assistance.

References

1. Chaffin JS, Daggett WM: Mitral valve replacement: a nine-year follow-up of risks and survivals. Ann Thorac Surg **27:** 312, 1979
2. Teply JF, Grunkemeier GL, Sutherland HD, Lambert LE, Johnson VA, Starr A: The ultimate prognosis after valve replacement: an assessment at twenty years. Ann Thorac Surg **32:** 111, 1981
3. Cheung D, Flemma RJ, Mullen DC, Lepley D Jr, Anderson AJ, Weirauch E: Ten-year follow-up in aortic valve replacement using the Björk-Shiley prosthesis. Ann Thorac Surg **32:** 138, 1981
4. Barnhorst DA, Oxman HA, Connolly DC, Pluth JR, Danielson GK, Wallace RB, McGoon DC: Long-term follow-up of isolated replacement of the aortic or mitral valve with the Starr-Edwards prosthesis. Am J Cardiol **35:** 228, 1975
5. Marshal WG Jr, Kouchoukos NT, Karp RB, Williams JB: Late results after mitral valve replacement with the Björk-Shiley and porcine prostheses. J Thorac Cardiovasc Surg **85:** 902, 1983
6. Karp RB, Cyrus RJ, Blackstone EH, Kirklin JW, Kouchoukos NT, Pacifico AD: The Björk-Shiley valve: intermediate-term follow-up. J Thorac Cardiovasc Surg **81:** 602, 1981
7. McGoon MD, Fuster V, McGoon DC, Pumphrey CW, Pluth JR, Elveback LR: Aortic and mitral valve incompetence: long-term follow-up (10 to 19 years) of patients treated with the Starr-Edwards prosthesis. J Am Coll Cardiol **3:** 930, 1984
8. Sala A, Schoevaerdts JC, Jaumin P, Ponlot R, Chalant CH: Review of 387 isolated mitral valve replacements by the Model 6120 Starr-Edwards prosthesis. J Thorac Cardiovasc Surg **84:** 744, 1982
9. Miller DC, Oyer PE, Stinson EB, Reitz BA, Jamieson SW, Baumgartner WA, Mitchell RS, Shumway NE: Ten to fifteen year reassessment of the performance characteristics of the Starr-Edwards Model 6120 mitral valve prosthesis. J Thorac Cardiovasc Surg **85:** 1, 1983
10. Stollerman GH: Global strategies for the control of rheumatic fever. JAMA **249:** 931, 1983 (editorial)
11. Duvoisin GE, Wallace RB, Ellis FH Jr, Anderson MW, McGoon DC: Late results of cardiac-valve replacement. Circulation **37/38**(suppl II): II-75, 1968
12. Sanfelippo PM, Giuliani ER, Danielson GK, Wallace RB, Pluth JR, McGoon DC: Tricuspid valve prosthetic replacement: early and late results with the Starr-Edwards prosthesis. J Thorac Cardiovasc Surg **71:** 441, 1976
13. Nagorney DM, Field CS: Successful pregnancy 10 years after triple cardiac valve replacement. Obstet Gynecol **57:** 386, 1981
14. Kittle CF, Dye WS, Gerbode F, Glenn WWL, Julian OC, Morrow AG, Sabiston DC Jr, Weinberg M: Factors influencing risk in cardiac surgical patients: cooperative study. Circulation **39/40** (suppl I): I-169, 1969
15. Midell AI, DeBoer A: Multiple valve replacement: an analysis of early and late results. Arch Surg **104:** 471, 1972
16. Shanahan MX, Windsor HM: Triple valve replacement. Med J Aust **1:** 636, 1973
17. Stephenson LW, Kouchoukos NT, Kirklin JW: Triple-valve replacement: an analysis of eight years' experience. Ann Thorac Surg **23:** 327, 1977
18. Rhodes GR, McIntosh CL, Redwood DR, Itscoitz SB, Epstein SE: Clinical and hemodynamic results following triple valve replacement: mechanical vs porcine xenograft prostheses. Circulation **56**(suppl II): II-122, 1977
19. Macmanus Q, Grunkemeier G, Starr A: Late results of triple valve replacement: a 14-year review. Ann Thorac Surg **25:** 402, 1978
20. Heck HA, Wright CB, Doty DB, Rossi NP, Ehrenhaft JL: Combined multiple-valve procedures: a five-year experience with 125 patients. Ann Thorac Surg **27:** 320, 1979
21. Piekarski A, Dewilde J, Dumoulin P, Farah E, Bourthoumieux A, Slama R, Acar J: Les triples remplacements valvulaires. Arch Mal Coeur **72:** 1196, 1979
22. Péterffy A, Jonasson R, Björk VO: Ten years' experience of surgical management of triple valve disease: early and late results in thirty-four consecutive cases. Scand J Thorac Cardiovasc Surg **13:** 191, 1979
23. Thorburn CW, Morgan JJ, Shanahan MX, Chang VP: Long-term results of tricuspid valve replacement and the problem of prosthetic valve thrombosis. Am J Cardiol **51:** 1128, 1983
24. West PN, Ferguson TB, Clark RE, Weldon CS: Multiple valve replacement: changing status. Ann Thorac Surg **26:** 32, 1978
25. Bourezak SE, Chauvaud S, Romano M, Carpentier A, Blondeau Ph, Mostefai MC, Dubost Ch: Triple replacement valvulaire: bilan de 90 opérés. Arch Mal Coeur **77:** 724, 1984
26. Livi U, Bortolotti U, Rissoli G, Valfré C, Mazzucco A, Gallucci V: Surgical treatment of patients with triple heart valve disease: results and analysis of factors affecting the surgical outcome. Thorac Cardiovasc Surg **30:** 288, 1982
27. King RM, Schaff HV, Danielson GK, Gersh BJ, Orszulak TA, Piehler JM, Puga FJ, Pluth JR: Surgery for tricuspid regurgitation late after mitral valve replacement. Circulation **70**(suppl I): I-193, 1984
28. Santinga JT, Kirsh MM, Flora JD Jr, Brymer JF: Factors relating to late sudden death in patients having aortic valve replacement. Ann Thorac Surg **29:** 249, 1980
29. Starr A, Herr R, Wood J: Tricuspid replacement for acquired valve disease. Surg Gynecol Obstet **122:** 1295, 1966
30. Herr R, Starr A, McCord CW, Wood JA: Special problems following valve replacement: embolus, leak, infection, red cell damage. Ann Thorac Surg **1:** 403, 1965
31. Schoen FJ, Titus JL, Lawrie GM: Autopsy-determined causes of death after cardiac valve replacement. JAMA **249:** 899, 1983
32. Gabbay S, Factor SM, Strom J, Becker R, Frater RW: Sudden death due to cuspal dehiscence of the Ionescu-Shiley valve in the mitral position. J Thorac Cardiovasc Surg **84:** 313, 1982
33. Maroñas JM, Such M, Sánchez P, González-Pont G, Caffarena JM: Fatal coronary obstruction due to cloth-wear of a cloth-covered Starr-Edwards aortic valve prosthesis. Chest **82:** 645, 1982
34. Gradman AH, Harbison MA, Berger HJ, Geha AS, Shaw RK, Crocco CJ, Stoterau S, Pytik L, Zaret BL: Ventricular arrhythmias late after aortic valve replacement and their relation to left ventricular performance. Am J Cardiol **48:** 824, 1981
35. Edmunds LH Jr: Thromboembolic complications of current cardiac valvular prostheses. Ann Thorac Surg **34:** 96, 1982
36. McGoon DC: The risk of thromboembolism following valvular operations: how does one know? J Thorac Cardiovasc Surg **88:** 782, 1984 (editorial)
37. Fuster V, Pumphrey CW, McGoon MD, Chesebro JH, Pluth JR, McGoon DC: Systemic thromboembolism in mitral and aortic Starr-Edwards prostheses: a 10-year follow-up. Circulation **66** (suppl I): I-157, 1982
38. Isom OW, Spencer FC, Glassman E, Teiko P, Boyd AD, Cunningham JN, Reed GE: Long-term results in 1375 patients undergoing valve replacement with the Starr-Edwards cloth-covered steel ball prosthesis. Ann Surg **186:** 310, 1977
39. Starr A, Grunkemeier G, Lambert L, Okies JE, Thomas D: Mitral valve replacement: a 10-year follow-up of non-cloth-covered vs cloth-covered caged-ball prostheses. Circulation **54**(suppl III): III-47, 1976
40. Samaan HA, Murali R: Acute tricuspid valve obstruction following the use of tricuspid ball valve prosthesis. Thorax **25:** 334, 1970
41. VanderVeer JB Jr, Rhyneer GS, Hodam RP, Kloster FE: Obstruction of tricuspid ball-valve prostheses. Circulation **43/44**(suppl I): I-62, 1971
42. Bache RJ, From AHL, Castaneda AR, Jorgensen CR, Wang Y: Late thrombotic obstruction of Starr-Edwards tricuspid valve prosthesis. Chest **61:** 613, 1972
43. Bourdillon PDV, Sharratt GP: Malfunction of Björk-Shiley valve prosthesis in tricuspid position. Br Heart J **38:** 1149, 1976

Improved graft patency in patients treated with platelet-inhibiting therapy after coronary bypass surgery

B. GREG BROWN, M.D., PH.D., RAMON A. CUKINGNAN, M.D., TIMOTHY DEROUEN, PH.D., LACY V. GOEDE, B.S., MAYLENE WONG, M.D., HENRY J. FEE, M.D., JACK A. ROTH, M.D., AND JOSEPH S. CAREY, M.D.

ABSTRACT One hundred forty-seven consecutive coronary bypass patients were enrolled in a randomized, double-blind, risk-stratified, placebo-controlled prospective trial evaluating the effect on graft patency of 325 mg tid aspirin (ASA) plus 75 mg tid dipyridamole (DP) or ASA alone. One hundred twenty-seven patients (399 total grafts) underwent surgery, initiation of drug therapy 67 ± 27 (SD) hr postoperatively, five clinic visits, and repeat angiography at 1 year. A logistic regression statistical model was used to determine the effects of 28 different measured variables on graft patency and to adjust for these effects in determining the relationship between antiplatelet therapy and graft occlusion. No patient-specific variable contributed significantly to the prediction of occlusion in either the placebo or the treated group. Six graft-specific variables (arterial diameter, severity of stenosis, graft flow, reactive hyperemia, presence or absence of collaterals, and graft type) did contribute and were included in the model. Twenty-one percent of placebo-treated grafts became occluded. Compared with placebo, the relative risk of graft occlusion with ASA was 0.47 ($p = .04$); with ASA + DP, it was 0.50 ($p = .04$). This benefit was principally due to reduction of occlusion in the most common and presumably most important groups of grafts, those in which flow exceeded 40 ml/min, or supplying arteries having luminal diameters greater than 1.5 mm. Grafts lacking reactive hyperemia had a 32% occlusion frequency in placebo-treated patients; relative risk of their occlusion averaged 0.26 ($p < .01$) with platelet-inhibiting therapy. Therapy is most effective if started on or before the second postoperative day. ASA and the combination of ASA and DP given after surgery were equally effective in maintaining graft patency. Thus, early postoperative ASA appears to be a simple, inexpensive, and effective form of therapy for most bypass patients. We question the need for the addition of preoperative or postoperative DP to this ASA regimen.
Circulation 72, No. 1, 138–146, 1985.

EACH YEAR in the United States, over 100,000 patients undergo coronary bypass surgery,[1] and approximately 300,000 saphenous vein grafts are implanted. Since the clinical success of this operation is found to depend on the completeness of revascularization,[2–4] measures to improve the patency of bypass grafts are of potential value.

Graft patency declines with time after the operation. About 10% of all grafts are occluded after the first 1 or 2 weeks,[5–8] as are about 17% and 20% after 6 and 12 months, respectively.[5–9] The occlusion rate is 2% to 4% per year in those still patent at 1 year.[10–12] The early graft patency rate is reported to depend also on the experience of the surgeon,[5] the sex of the patient,[13] the artery grafted,[14] the operative graft flow,[15] the severity of the proximal arterial stenosis,[16, 17] the size of the grafted artery,[16, 18] and the presence of reactive hyperemia.[16] The great majority of occlusive episodes in the first 2 months are thrombotic, after which thrombosis usually combines with accelerated intimal fibromuscular hyperplasia to obstruct the graft.[19, 20] Beyond 1 year, grafts usually occlude with progressive atherosclerosis.[19, 20]

Thrombus formation in the arterial circulation is retarded by drugs that inhibit platelet function.[21] Intimal fibromuscular hyperplasia is accelerated by a mitogenic substance released from the α-granules of the

From the Medicine and Research Departments, Cardiology Section and Thoracic Surgery Section, Wadsworth Veterans Administration Hospital, UCLA School of Medicine, Los Angeles, and the Departments of Medicine and Biostatistics, University of Washington, Seattle.

Supported in part by VA project No. 1102-01, in part by Dr. Brown's Clinical Investigator Award from the Veterans Administration, and in part by an Established Investigator Award from the American Heart Association.

Address for correspondence: B. Greg Brown, M.D., Ph.D., Division of Cardiology, RG-22, University of Washington School of Medicine, Seattle, WA 98125.

Received Sept. 6, 1983; revision accepted April 11, 1985.

platelet,[22, 23] and is retarded, experimentally, by platelet-inhibiting therapy.[24] Because of the implied role of the platelet in these two mechanisms of graft occlusion, therapy designed to limit adhesion and aggregation of platelets and their release of α-granules would hypothetically improve graft patency. We investigated this hypothesis in a randomized, double-blind, risk-stratified comparison of aspirin (ASA), aspirin plus dipyridamole (ASA + DP), and placebo in a sufficiently large group of consecutive patients to confirm a 50% drug benefit, if present, at $p < .05$ with a power of 0.90. We have found that there is a substantial benefit with respect to graft patency from early postoperative platelet-inhibiting therapy, particularly for the most important and common groups of grafts — those with moderate or high graft flow perfusing moderate or large arteries.

Methods

Patients. One hundred forty-seven consecutive eligible male coronary bypass patients, ages 34 to 70 years, were enrolled in a prospective study of platelet-inhibiting therapy during the year after surgery. Forty-four of 191 patients (23%) undergoing elective coronary bypass surgery during the 3 year enrollment period were excluded from the study because of ASA intolerance (n = 4), ASA requirement (n = 3), history of peptic ulcer disease (n = 9), prohibitive travel distance (n = 5), refusal (n = 19), or insufficient time for preoperative interview (n = 4). One hundred twenty-seven completed the protocol, which included surgery, clinical monitoring for 1 year, and readmission for postoperative evaluation. Patients were enrolled between catheterization and the operation after fully informed written consent was obtained. Preoperative data collected included that obtained by history, physical examination, laboratory screening, electrocardiography, and exercise testing (Bruce protocol) and pertinent information from the catheterization.

Surgery. After pentothal and nitrous oxide induction and ethrane inhalation anesthesia and midsternal thoracotomy, cardiopulmonary bypass was initiated in each patient with 2.4 liters of balanced electrolyte and albumin pump prime and a bubble oxygenator. Over the course of the 3½ year enrollment period (1976 to 1980), three techniques for myocardial preservation were used: (1) normothermic intermittent cross-clamping, (2) hypothermic intermittent cross-clamping with cold arrest, and (3) cold potassium cardioplegia.[25] Three hundred ninety-nine saphenous vein grafts were placed to previously unoperated arteries with 50% or more stenosis; of these, 39 veins (80 grafts) were the continuity type anastomosed side-to-side to one or more diseased arteries and end-to-side to another.

Veins were resected with gentle handling and, if small, were distended with blood at moderate pressure. Sites of possible injury by traumatic clamps were resected; only broad "nontraumatic" bulldog clamps were used during graft placement. When the distal anastomosis was nearly complete, a series of olive-tip probes calibrated in 0.5 mm diameter increments was passed proximally and distally into the grafted artery to estimate vessel caliber and to ensure the patency of the anastomosis. Just before chest closure, flow was measured electromagnetically* in each leg of the grafts. Reactive hyperemia was determined as the percent increase above baseline flow after temporary graft occlusion for 15 sec.

Study protocol. Therapy was assigned before surgery to patients in a fully randomized, double-blind fashion. Protocol treatment groups were as follows: (1) ASA + DP: 325 mg ASA plus 75 mg DP to be taken three times daily, 1 hr before meals, (2) ASA: 325 mg ASA plus a DP placebo taken three times a day before meals, and (3) placebo: double placebo taken three times a day as above.

The randomized drug assignment was stratified for preoperative cigarette smoking and fasting serum cholesterol levels to balance the distribution of these two presumed risk factors in each group. For the first 78 patients, protocol drug was scheduled to start on the third postoperative day unless bleeding or thrombocytopenia occurred. Because no complications occurred, the next 49 consecutive patients were started on therapy on the second postoperative day. On the average, therapy was initiated 67 ± 27(SD) hr after the patient left the operating room. The first dose was given by the principal investigator. Subsequent doses were given by the nursing staff in compliance with written orders. In-hospital drug compliance was checked daily by the project administrative assistant using patient interviews and review of the charted medications. Drug instructions were reviewed with the patient at the time of hospital discharge.

After discharge, patients were seen in the clinic as needed, routinely at week 1 and 4 and then at 3, 6, and 9 months after surgery. Follow-up was conducted by the principal investigator. Patients were instructed to avoid platelet-active medications and were given acetaminophen for analgesia. Hypertension was treated with thiazide diuretics and α-methyldopa. Patients' drug supplies were renewed at each 3 month clinic visit. Compliance was assessed by count of the returned pills and by urine salicylate and Ivy bleeding time measured and recorded by independent technicians at the 6 month visit and the 12 month readmission. At 1 year, evaluation included history, physical examination, laboratory screening, treadmill testing, and catheterization.

Catheterization data. Aortic and left ventricular pressures were measured, the latter at high gain with zero level at a measured midchest position. Ejection fraction was computed from the 30 degree right anterior oblique angiogram.[26] The native coronary arteriograms were performed in a defined sequence of projections, which was the same in both studies. A detailed map of the coronary anatomy documented the distribution and size of all important branches, the location and severity of focal narrowing, the collateral anatomy, and the direction of flow. At the 1 year recatheterization, native vessel arteriograms were repeated. All grafts were selectively catheterized, guided by surgically implanted metal markers, and were opacified and filmed in three or four of the original projection angles. Grafts (distal anastomoses) fully visualized to supply the distal artery during selective injection were called "patent"; otherwise they were considered "occluded." The details of the original vascular map were confirmed by review of both sets of films, which were projected simultaneously at fivefold magnification on two parallel overhead projectors. The anatomy and patency of each graft and changes in native vessel disease were then added to the vascular map in color code. Arterial diameter at each point of anastomosis was estimated from the preoperative arteriogram by caliper comparison with the catheter.

Data analysis. Patient-specific and graft-specific variables were prospectively defined and measured to determine the utility of each as a predictor of graft occlusion and to allow adjustments for them, if necessary, in evaluating the effect of the platelet-inhibiting therapy. Preoperative, intraoperative, and postoperative measurements were included.

*Gould-Statham, Model SP2204, Oxnard, CA.

The analysis of the effect of the antiplatelet therapy was performed by logistic regression[27] in which the dependent variable was the occlusion or nonocclusion (y = 1 or 0) of a graft at 1 year. Independent variables included graft-specific and patient-specific measurements, as well as a dichotomous variable that indicated whether the therapy administered was ASA alone (1 = yes, 0 = no) or ASA + DP. When both therapy variables were equal to zero, the therapy was placebo. Thus, these two dichotomous variables specified the therapy group for each graft.

Logistic regression is a nonlinear analog of multiple linear regression, and can be used to relate the probability of the occurrence of a dichotomous outcome (occlusion, nonocclusion) to several independent variables, which can be categorical or continuous.[28, 29]

The logistic model is of the form

$$P_i = \text{Prob (occlusion in the i}^{th}\text{ graft)} = \frac{\exp(\beta_o + \beta_1 X_1 + \ldots + \beta_k X_k)}{1 + \exp(\beta_o + \beta_1 X_1 + \ldots + \beta_k X_k)}$$

or, equivalently

$$\ln(P_i/1 - P_i) = \beta_o + \beta_1 X_1 + \ldots + \beta_k X_k$$

Using maximum likelihood techniques, one can estimate β_j, the coefficient of independent variable X_j in the model, which measures the effect of X_j on the probability of occlusion. The test of $\beta_j = 0$ is the test of whether variable X_j (for example, the administration of ASA + DP) has a significant effect on the probability of occlusion.

The use of logistic regression was necessary because the experimental unit of interest is the occlusion or nonocclusion of an individual graft, yet it is not possible to randomize individual grafts to therapy. This presents a dilemma in the analysis of the data. An analysis that used the patient as the observational unit of interest (e.g., comparing the proportions of patients who had all grafts patent) was deemed inappropriate because it ignored the fact that certain graft-specific variables such as graft flow and arterial diameter were important determinants of occlusion and it also reduced the effective sample size considerably. A precise evaluation of the effect of therapy on graft occlusion should include adjustments for imbalances among the treatment groups of variables predictive of occlusion. Since the variables predictive of occlusion were graft specific, and since individual grafts were not randomized, the randomization procedure itself could not be expected to achieve balance among the groups with respect to graft-specific variables. The logistic model used the graft as the observational unit and allowed adjustment for graft-specific variables, although the analysis became "observational" in nature since the grafts were not randomized. Use of this model avoided the assumption of independent behavior of two grafts in the same patient by assuming that any dependence of two such grafts could be modeled by including appropriate patient-specific and graft-specific variables.

As a first step, univariate logistic regression analyses were performed with use of each of the 28 variables as a single independent variable to determine which were significantly related to occlusion and should, therefore, be included as covariates in evaluating the effect of therapy. Analyses were performed separately in the placebo and the drug-treated groups to avoid the designation of a variable as related to occlusion merely because it correlated with drug administration. No patient-specific and six graft-specific variables were identified as significantly related to occlusion in either the placebo or platelet-inhibition group or both. The six graft-specific variables were included as covariates in the subsequent analysis that evaluated the effects of therapy.

Measurements were obtained for all grafts for four of the six independent covariates. Flow and reactive hyperemia were measured in virtually every individual graft. However, these data could not always be obtained for each anastomosis of continuity-type grafts. As a consequence, direct measurements were missing for 53 of the 2394 covariate values essential to the logistic regression analysis. However, graft flow was significantly predicted by proximal stenosis and vessel size, and reactive hyperemia was predicted by proximal stenosis and receipt of collaterals. By use of these predictive relationships, missing flow and hyperemia values were estimated for inclusion in the logistic analysis.

The tests for the significance of the effects of ASA or ASA + DP were performed by fitting a logistic model with the six covariates plus the dichotomous therapy group variables. The estimated coefficient of a variable in this model divided by its standard error follows a standard normal distribution, and allows one to test whether the variable contributes a significant amount of information toward predicting graft occlusion while adjusting for the effect of other variables in the model. For grafts in the ASA or ASA + DP groups, the risk of occlusion relative to that in the placebo group, with all other covariates held constant, is estimated by the odds ratio, the exponential of the coefficient of the therapy variable (e^{β}). A significant odds ratio is one that differs significantly from 1.0.

In further testing the results (e.g., in looking at the numbers of occluded grafts as a determinant of postoperative ischemia), some simple comparisons of proportions and means were made. In these, the χ^2 test for contingency tables was used for categorical data, and one-way analysis of variance was used to compare means for continuous data. All p values computed were based on two-sided tests.

Results

Enrollment and dropout. One hundred forty-seven patients were enrolled and began protocol therapy in the early postoperative period. One hundred twenty-seven patients completed the protocol, including the catheterization procedure at 1 year. Table 1 summarizes the reasons for failure to complete the protocol. There were no significant differences among therapeutic groups with respect to number enrolled or dropouts.

TABLE 1
Patient enrollment and reasons for dropout

	Placebo	ASA	ASA + DP
Patients entering study (n)	51	47	49
Reasons for dropping out (n)			
Died during study	1	1	1
Refused second angio	3	1	0
Side effects	0	3	1
Lack of interest	2	2	1
Warfarin became necessary	0	1	1
Cerebrovascular accident	1	1	0
Patients completing study (n)	44	38	45
Total grafts	147	114	138
Grafts/patient	3.3	3.1	3.1

Compliance: pill count. Medications were taken regularly, under supervision, by all patients during their initial 7 to 12 day hospital stay, starting 67 ± 27(SD) hr after surgery. Unused protocol drugs were returned at the 3 month clinic visits and were counted. Sixty-one percent of patients had average pill-count compliance of greater than 90%. A scoring system awarded two points to those taking at least 75% of the specified doses during the first 3 month period and one point for 75% or greater compliance during each of the three succeeding 3 month periods. Maximum score was thus five points. A compliance score of five was attained by 72% of patients, that of at least four by 88%, and that of at least three by 94%. Unannounced urine samples were obtained at 6 and 12 months and tested with Trindler's solution for salicylate. These tests were positive 73% of the time in patients on ASA + DP and 72% of the time in patients on ASA. Results of both tests were negative in only three patients in each group. Positive test results indicative of casual ASA use were obtained 4% of the time in patients on placebo. Ivy bleeding time was measured at 6 and 12 months. It averaged 2.7 ± 1.6 min in placebo patients, and was significantly increased at 5.1 ± 2.6 min ($p < .001$) in the ASA + DP group and at 4.9 ± 2.7 min ($p < .001$) in the ASA group.

Factors predictive of graft occlusion. Twenty-eight variables, continuous and dichotomous, were screened in preliminary logistic regression analysis for their predictive value. Dichotomous variables (e.g., presence or absence of collaterals) were entered as 1 or 0. For purposes of this screening, a variable was called predictive if the logistic regression indicated that it was significantly ($p < .05$) associated with occlusion in either the placebo or the drug-treated groups.

None of the preoperative clinical variables tested were significantly related to graft occlusion, including age, cigarette smoking, cholesterol, triglycerides, serum creatinine, fasting glucose, angina functional class, and previous myocardial infarction. Nonpredictive variables from the preoperative catheterization were aortic mean pressure, left ventricular end-diastolic pressure, ejection fraction, and the presence of collaterals originating from the grafted vessel. Intraoperative determinations of little value in predicting graft occlusion were the presence of moderate or severe arterial disease at the anastomotic site, the surgeon (there were two attending surgeons, R. C. and J. C.), and the type of myocardial preservation used. Postoperatively, cigarette smoking, blood pressure, postoperative ejection fraction, and outpatient compliance with therapy were not predictive of occlusion. Graft occlusion was strongly associated with left ventricular end-diastolic pressure of 12 mm Hg or greater at the postoperative catheterization (22% vs 9%; $p < .01$). This was most likely an *effect* of graft occlusion rather than a cause, because an elevated preoperative left ventricular end-diastolic pressure had no predictive value. Consequently, postoperative left ventricular end-diastolic pressure was not included as one of the covariates in the logistic regression analysis. Similarly, bleeding time, significantly altered by therapy, was not included as a predictive covariate. Finally, anastomotic luminal diameter measured from the preoperative arteriogram correlated highly with the operative estimate, and therefore was not included.

The six variables significantly associated with graft occlusion in either the placebo or the drug-treated subsets are listed in table 2. For purposes of illustration, these graft risk factors were dichotomized into high-risk and low-risk categories. For example, if operative luminal diameter at the site of graft anastomosis was greater than 1.5 mm, graft occlusion in the ASA and ASA + DP groups was 8% vs 29% ($p < .001$) for smaller vessels in the same therapy group.

Effectiveness of therapy: overall graft patency. Fifty-nine percent of 44 patients taking placebo had all grafts patent, compared with 67% of 45 taking ASA + DP and 74% of 38 taking ASA.

Results of the logistic regression analysis testing the effects of therapy are given in table 3. The statistical model estimated the probability of graft occlusion in each of the treatment groups at comparable levels of the other covariates. The odds ratio, defined above, provides an estimate of the risk of occlusion in the treated group relative to that in the placebo group with all other significant covariates being equal. The data in table 3 indicate statistically significant overall therapeutic benefit for the group receiving ASA (odds ratio = 0.47, $p = .04$) and for the group receiving ASA + DP (odds ratio = 0.50, $p = .04$). A test comparing the two treatment groups indicated no significant difference ($Z = 0.18$, $p = .86$). This beneficial effect of therapy is demonstrated in the simple proportion of grafts occluded, which was 21% in the placebo group, 14% in the ASA + DP group, and 12% in the ASA group. The odds ratios are not exactly equal to the ratios of simple proportions because of small differences in distributions of the six covariates biasing in favor of placebo and against ASA + DP (see table 2). Adjustments were made for this in the logistic model.

Although the traditional coronary risk factors (age, cigarette smoking, diastolic blood pressure, cholesterol, and fasting glucose) were not found to be signifi-

TABLE 2
Variables significantly predictive of graft occlusion in placebo and PIT[A] groups, and their distribution among the three treatment groups

		% of grafts occluded in each subgroup			% of grafts in each group having specified "high risk" values		
Predictive variable	Scoring system	Placebo (total 21%; n = 147)	PIT (total 13%; n = 252)	Relative risk of occlusion	Placebo (n = 147)	ASA+DP (n = 138)	ASA (n = 114)
Continuation	Yes	6 (33)[B]	19 (48)	Low			
graft	No	25 (114)	12 (204)	High	78	80	82
% proximal	≥70%	15 (97)	11 (163)	Low			
stenosis	<70%	32 (50)	18 (89)	High	34	39	31
Operative	>1.5 mm	19 (113)	8 (184)	Low			
luminal diameter	≤1.5 mm	29 (34)	29 (68)	High	23	28	26
Collateral	Yes	22 (50)	8 (80)	Low			
recipient	No	21 (97)	16 (172)	High	66	73	62
Reactive	≥10%	9 (69)	10 (122)	Low			
hyperemia	<10%	32 (78)	17 (130)	High	47	48	47
Graft flow	>40 ml/min	21 (101)	9 (174)	Low			
	≤40 ml/min	22 (46)	23 (78)	High	25	27	26

[A]PIT subgroup includes patients on ASA and those on ASA + DP.
[B]Values in parentheses are the numbers of grafts at risk of occlusion in each subgroup.

cantly related to graft occlusion, they were included with the above six graft-specific covariates in a larger logistic regression analysis that tested for effects of therapy. The results were virtually identical with those of the above analysis (relative risk for ASA = 0.41, p = .03; and for ASA + DP = 0.44, p = .02).

Initiation of therapy. Data relating graft patency to the time of initiation of platelet-inhibiting therapy appear in figure 1. Forty-nine patients began therapy on the second postoperative day (≤60 hr after surgery). Among these, 13 of 56 (23%) grafts in patients in the placebo group, three of 39 (8%, p < .05) in those in

TABLE 3
Logistic regression analysis of data for all grafts comparing groups receiving placebo, ASA, and ASA + DP, adjusting for six covariates

Variable	Coefficient (β_i)	Standard error	p value	Odds ratio[A]
Constant	4.290	1.190	<.001	
Graft type C[B]	−0.107	0.488	.826	
Operative diameter	−1.790	0.496	<.001	
Collateral recipient	−0.092	0.424	.826	
% stenosis	−0.014	0.0094	.121	
Graft flow	−0.013	0.0054	.016	
% reactive hyperemia	−0.011	0.0062	.082	
ASA	−0.759	0.372	.041	0.47
ASA + DP	−0.688	0.341	.043	0.50

[A]Ratio of odds of occlusion, in comparison with placebo group.
[B]Any of the two or more distal anastomoses in a continuation-type vein graft.

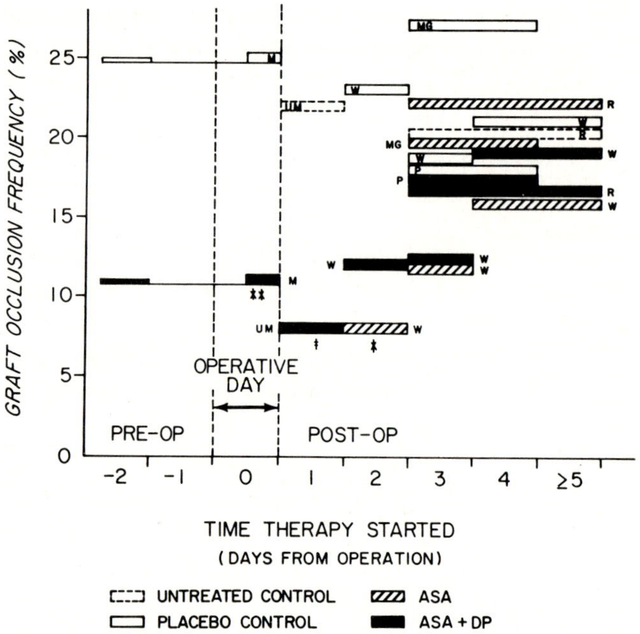

FIGURE 1. Relationships among therapy, time of its initiation, and frequency of graft occlusion for this and five other randomized clinical trials. M = Dipyridamole, 100 mg qid, begun 2 days preoperatively and continued immediately postoperatively as DP (75 mg tid) in combination with ASA (325 mg tid).[41] UM = Dipyridamole, 50 mg bid, and aspirin, 650 mg bid, begun on the first postoperative day.[39] W = ASA or ASA + DP started between the second and the fifth postoperative day (data from this report). P = ASA + DP started on the third or fourth postoperative day.[9] MG = Aspirin, 325 mg bid, started on the third or fourth postoperative day.[38] R = Aspirin or aspirin plus dipyridamole started on third, fourth, or fifth postoperative day.[42] χ^2 statistical comparison of treated grafts vs same-day controls: *p < .05, ≠ <.02; **p < .001.

the ASA group, and seven of 59 (12%, NS) in those in the ASA + DP group were occluded. Seventy-eight patients began therapy on the third postoperative day or later. Among these, 18 of 91 (20%) grafts in patients in the placebo group, 11 of 75 (15%, NS) in those in the ASA group, and 13 of 79 (16%, NS) in those in the ASA + DP group were occluded. All 34 grafts were patent in 11 patients starting ASA or ASA + DP less than 48 hr after surgery; 19 of 26 grafts were patent in seven comparable patients on placebo ($p < .001$).

Effect of therapy: occlusion in certain important graft subsets. Is the observed beneficial effect of therapy uniform or is it selective for certain subgroups? To address this question, separate logistic analyses were conducted in each of three particularly important graft subgroups to estimate the effects in the therapy groups while adjusting for the effects of the six covariates previously identified. In the following discussion, graft flow is designated as "good" if it was greater than 40 ml/min and "low" if it was less. Arteries are called "small" if luminal diameter at the point of anastomosis was 1.5 mm or less, and "larger" if it was greater than that. Reactive hyperemia is called present if it was at least 10% above baseline flow and absent if it was less.

Figure 2 demonstrates that 74% of the 399 grafts studied were to larger arteries; in this subset a 69% reduction in the odds of occlusion was obtained with platelet-inhibiting therapy. There was no difference in the odds ratio with ASA (0.32; $p < .05$) or ASA + DP (0.31; $p < .05$). Sixty-nine percent of grafts had good flow; in this subset a mean 65% reduction in the odds of occlusion was obtained with either ASA (0.30; $p < .01$) or ASA + DP (0.39; $p < .05$). Forty-eight percent of grafts lacked reactive hyperemia.[30] In this subset a mean 74% reduction in the odds of occlusion was obtained with either ASA (0.27; $p < .01$) or ASA + DP (0.25; $p < .01$).

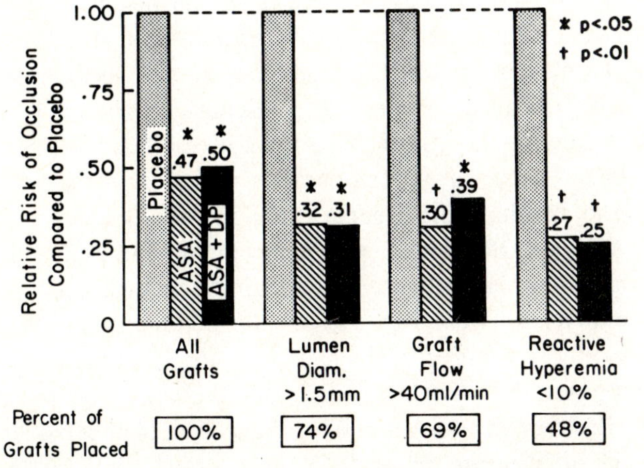

FIGURE 2. Effect of therapy on overall graft occlusion and in certain subgroups: results of the logistic regression analysis. The relative risk of occlusion compared with the unit risk with placebo was significantly reduced by treatment with ASA alone or with ASA + DP. Certain large subsets of the graft population obtained an even greater relative benefit from therapy, as shown. Conversely, treatment had no significant effect on the relative risk of occlusion for grafts to arteries with luminal diameters of 1.5 mm or less (relative risk: ASA = 0.77; ASA + DP = 0.90), grafts with flow of 40 ml/min or less (ASA = 0.89; ASA + DP = 1.09), and those with reactive hyperemia 10% or more above baseline flow (ASA = 0.89; ASA + DP = 1.35).

Clinical benefit. Does graft patency correlate with clinical benefit? To address this question, we measured changes in certain objectively defined indexes of the surgical benefit and correlated them with graft occlusion. Table 4 summarizes this analysis. Sixty-six patients had angina during their preoperative treadmill test; an additional 19 had spontaneous resting angina with ST-T changes and did not undergo exercise testing preoperatively. Of these, 19 (22%) had some degree of angina during the postoperative exercise stress. Table 4 shows that only 13% of these patients with all grafts patent had persistent pain, compared with 25% of patients with one occluded graft and 54% of those with two or more occluded ($p < .02$). Similar observations were made for two other signs of myocardial ischemia: exercise-induced ST segment abnormalities and left ventricular compliance abnormalities. Thus, impressive clinical, electrocardiographic, and hemodynamic improvements resulted from coronary bypass surgery and, in all cases, lack of improvement in these three indexes of myocardial ischemia was significantly related to the number of occluded grafts.

TABLE 4

Number of occluded grafts as a determinant of ischemia at postoperative evaluation

	No. of occluded grafts			Significance of trends
	None	1	≥2	
% of patients with angina on postop. ETT[A] (No. of patients in subset)	13 (52)	25 (20)	54 (13)	$p < .02$
% of patients with abnormal ST segment response on postop. ETT[B] (No. of patients in subset)	27 (55)	30 (20)	75 (12)	$p < .01$
Average postop. improvement in LVEDP[C] in mm Hg (No. of patients in subset)	6.3 (59)	4.4 (18)	1.5 (18)	$p < .025$

ETT = Bruce protocol exercise tolerance test.

[A]Subset of patients with angina on preop. ETT, or with resting angina.

[B]Patients with abnormal (≥0.1 mV) ST segment shift on preop. ETT.

[C]Patients with abnormal left ventricular end-diastolic pressure (LVEDP) (≥12 mm Hg) at preop. catheterization.

Discussion

Although ASA and DP appear to be appropriate agents to test the hypothesis that platelet-inhibiting therapy can improve aortocoronary graft patency,[21, 24, 31–37] contradictory conclusions have been reached in published studies[9, 38–41] and preliminary reports[42] of the use of these drugs after bypass surgery. While a number of considerations may help to account for these discrepancies, the time of initiation of drug therapy may be the most important. Chesebro and Fuster and their colleagues[40, 41] have emphasized the importance of starting therapy early; they report a convincing benefit from DP begun 48 hr before surgery and continued in combination with ASA soon after operation. Rate of graft occlusion at 1 year in their placebo-treated patients was 25%; in ASA + DP patients, it was 11%. The relationships among therapy, the time of its initiation, and graft occlusion are illustrated in figure 1, in which data from this trial are compared with those from five other trials.[9, 38, 39, 41, 42] Substantial benefits are associated with initiation of therapy before surgery or on the first or second postoperative day. Unfortunately, in many of the previously reported studies therapy was begun on the third to fifth postoperative day — too late to realize the potential benefits.

It may not be necessary to pharmacologically inhibit platelet function in the immediate perioperative period, because platelet counts[43] and adhesiveness[44] are acutely suppressed by the trauma of cardiopulmonary bypass. Indeed, among 91 of our 127 patients for whom adequate data were available, the mean platelet count was 229,000 ± 75,000(SD) before surgery, 105,000 immediately after surgery, 122,000 on the first postoperative day, and 101,000 in 30 of these patients for whom samples were considered clinically indicated on the second postoperative day. Dewanjee et al.[45] found no difference between treated and untreated dogs with respect to platelet adhesion to autologous saphenous vein grafts on the first postoperative day, although platelet-inhibiting drugs suppressed adhesion on postoperative days 3 to 30.

The data in table 2 and figure 2 provide insight into the mechanisms of graft occlusion. Arterial size appears to be an independent determinant of the risk of occlusion, presumably for technical reasons. While good operative flow was predictive of graft patency, our data suggest that reactive hyperemia correlates with patency even more strongly. The absence of reactive hyperemia appears to indicate that the distal coronary bed is graft independent in patients in the resting state. Eighty-four percent of grafts with 10% or less reactive hyperemia were associated with either moderate (<70%) proximal stenosis or with a developed collateral supply to the distal bed. Thus, grafts that are necessary for perfusion at rest appear to have a built-in safeguard against occlusion, but grafts that compete with the native vessel or with well-developed collaterals in the resting postoperative state lack this safeguard. In this latter setting, platelet-inhibiting therapy appears to alter the delicate dynamic balance to preserve patency in 74% of such grafts that would otherwise progress to occlusion. Therefore, as surgeons begin to bypass an increasing number of moderately diseased arteries in multigraft procedures, use of platelet-inhibiting therapy will help to avoid undesirably high occlusion rates.

Clinical implications. Overall graft patency, particularly of those grafts without reactive hyperemia, those with good flow, and those to larger arteries, was clearly improved by platelet-inhibiting therapy in this study. All but one of our patients had at least one graft with at least one of these characteristics. Therefore, if intraoperative measurements have identified such a graft, or in the absence of these measurements, we recommend that platelet-inhibiting therapy be initiated, unless contraindicated, no later than 48 hr after operation.

What is the "best" platelet-inhibiting regimen? The data of this study support the position that, postoperatively, ASA is as effective as ASA + DP. Additional data are not available; there has been no other graft patency trial comparing ASA with combined therapy and placebo in which therapy was started sufficiently early to expect a benefit. In particular, no clinical trial to date has examined the comparative efficacy of preoperative vs early postoperative initiation of therapy. The data in figure 1 support the position that ASA or ASA + DP, started on the first or second postoperative day, is as effective as a regimen requiring preoperative dipyridamole. Despite its popularity and experimentally predicted superiority, the combined drug regimen has not been clinically proven to be more effective than ASA alone for preventing thrombosis in the arterial circulation.[46, 47]

In conclusion, this study adds to information emerging from other such trials. This is the second largest of the six controlled studies to date. It uses appropriate statistical methods to adjust for imbalances in the nondrug determinants of graft occlusion; it demonstrates a substantial overall therapeutic benefit, and an even greater benefit to several clinically important graft subsets; it supports and extends current understanding of the need for early initiation of therapy; and its results permit a plausible mechanistic interpretation of the importance of graft reactive hyperemia. We believe that available data support the position that therapy with 325 mg of oral ASA three times a day, begun within 48 hr of operation, provides a substantial benefit with respect to graft patency, particularly in patients with grafts with good flow supplying larger arteries. Although we did not find that additional DP further improved graft patency, this study does not directly exclude the possibility of added benefit from preoperative DP continued postoperatively with ASA.[40, 41] Furthermore, use of DP may be considered because of the small advantage of combined therapy over ASA alone in preventing perianastomotic arterial stenosis at the graft site,[48] or because of the possible,[24] but currently unproved,[49] advantage of use of combined therapy in retarding the progression of native coronary or graft atherosclerosis. The minimum daily dose[50] and minimum required period of treatment are unknown, and further studies are necessary for their definition.

We are indebted to Mr. Al Skulsky, Ms. Easter Moon, and Ms. Clara Pruitt for their attention to the details of the catheterization laboratory and film processing. Drs. Sylvia Mansour, Abrahim Helmyi, Michael Brawer, and Andrew Stemar assisted in the analysis. Drs. Wilbur Benson and Alan Ranhosky of Boehringer-Ingelheim, Ltd., provided the drug for this study and Russell Post of Wadsworth VA Pharmacy Service supervised its dispensation. We are grateful to Dr. Ellis Rolett and Dr. Laurence Harker for their guidance in developing the study protocol and their editorial comments. We thank Sue Schaefer and Sarah Wilson for preparation of the manuscript.

References

1. Cohn PF, Braunwald E: Chronic coronary artery disease. *In* Braunwald E, editor: A textbook of cardiovascular medicine. Philadelphia, 1980, W.B. Saunders, p 1418
2. Assad-Morell JL, Frye RL, Connolly DC, Davis GD, Pluth JR, Wallace RBG, Barnhorst DA, Elveback LR, Danielson GK: Aortocoronary artery saphenous vein bypass surgery: Clinical and angiographic results. Mayo Clin Proc **50:** 379, 1975
3. Hartman CW, Kong Y, Margolis JR, Warren SG, Peter RH, Behar VS, Oldham HN: Aortocoronary bypass surgery: correlation of angiographic, symptomatic, and functional improvement at one year. Am J Cardiol **37:** 352, 1976
4. Cukingnan RA, Carey JS, Wittig JR, Brown BG: Influence of complete coronary revascularization on relief of angina. J Thorac Cardiovasc Surg **79:** 188, 1980
5. Campeau L, Crochet D, Lesperance J, Bourassa MG, Grondin CM: Postoperative changes in aortocoronary saphenous vein grafts revisited: Angiographic studies at two weeks and at one year in two series of consecutive patients. Circulation **52:** 369, 1975
6. Fitzgibbon GM, Burton JR, Leach AJ: Coronary bypass graft fate: angiographic grading of 1400 consecutive grafts early after operation and of 1132 after one year. Circulation **57:** 1070, 1978
7. Lawrie GM, Lie JT, Morris GC Jr, Beazley HL: Vein graft patency and intimal proliferation after aortocoronary bypass: early and long-term angiopathologic correlations. Am J Cardiol **38:** 856, 1976
8. Marco JD, Barner HB, Kaiser GC, Codd JE, Mudd JG, Willman V: Operative flow measurements and coronary bypass graft patency. J Thorac Cardiovasc Surg **71:** 545, 1976
9. Pantely GA, Goodnight SH Jr, Rahimtoola SH, Harlan BJ, DeMots H, Calvin L, Rösch J: Failure of antiplatelet and anticoagulant therapy to improve patency of grafts after coronary artery bypass. A controlled, randomized study. N Engl J Med **301:** 962, 1979
10. Grondin CM, Campeau L, Lesperance J, Solymoss BC, Vouhé P, Castonguay YR, Meere C, Bourassa MG: Atherosclerotic changes in coronary vein grafts six years after operation. Angiographic aspect in 110 patients. J Thorac Cardiovasc Surg **77:** 24, 1979
11. Kouchoukos NT, Karp RB, Oberman A, Russell RO Jr, Alison HW, Holt HI Jr: Long-term patency of saphenous veins for coronary bypass grafting. Circulation **58** (suppl I): I-96, 1978
12. Seides SF, Borer JS, Kent KM, Rosing DR, McIntosh CL, Epstein SE: Long-term anatomic fate of coronary artery bypass grafts and functional status of patients 5 years after operation. N Engl J Med **298:** 1213, 1978
13. Bolooki H, Vagas A, Green R, Kaiser GA, Ghahramani A: Results of direct coronary artery surgery in women. J Thorac Cardiovasc Surg **69:** 271, 1975
14. Higginbotham M, Hunt D, Stuckey J, Sloman G: Prospective angiographic assessment of factors affecting early patency of saphenous vein-coronary artery bypass grafts. Aust NZ J Med **10:** 295, 1980
15. Grondin CM, LePage G, Castonguay Y: Aortocoronary bypass graft: Initial blood flow through the graft and early postoperative patency. Circulation **44:** 815, 1971
16. Roth JA, Cukingnan RA, Brown BG, Gocka E, Carey JS: Factors influencing patency of saphenous vein grafts. Ann Thorac Surg **28:** 1976, 1979
17. Rees S: The watershed: a factor in coronary vein graft occlusion. Br Heart J **38:** 197, 1976
18. Grondin CM, Castonguay YR, Lesperance J, Bourassa MG, Campeau L, Grondin P: Attrition rate of aorto-to-coronary artery saphenous vein bypass grafts after 1 year: A study in a consecutive series of 96 patients. Ann Thorac Surg **14:** 223, 1972
19. Vlodaver Z, Edwards JE: Pathologic analysis in fatal cases following saphenous vein coronary arterial bypass. Chest **64:** 555, 1973
20. Unni KK, Kottke BA, Titus JL, Frye RL, Wallace RB, Brown AL: Pathologic changes in aortocoronary saphenous vein grafts. Am J Cardiol **34:** 526, 1974
21. Harker LA, Slichter SJ: Arterial and venous thromboembolism: kinetic characterization and evaluation of therapy. Thromb Diath Haemorrh **31:** 188, 1974
22. Ross R, Glomset J, Kariya B, Harker L: A platelet-dependent serum factor that stimulates the proliferation of arterial smooth muscle cells in vitro. Proc Natl Acad Sci USA **71:** 1207, 1974
23. Witte LD, Kaplan KL, Nossel H, Lages BA, Weiss HG, Goodman DS: Studies of the release from human platelets of the growth factor for cultured human arterial smooth muscle cells. Circ Res **42:** 402, 1978
24. Metke MP, Lie JT, Fuster V, Josa M, Kaye MP: Reduction of intimal thickening in canine coronary bypass vein grafts with dipyridamole and aspirin. Am J Cardiol **43:** 1144, 1979
25. Follette DM, Mulder DG, Maloney JV Jr, Buckberg GD: Advantages of blood cardioplegia over continuous coronary perfusion or intermittent ischemia. J Thorac Cardiovasc Surg **76:** 604, 1978
26. Dodge HT, Kennedy JW, Petersen JL: Quantitative angiographic methods in the evaluation of valvular heart disease. Prog Cardiovasc Dis **16:** 1, 1973
27. Cox DR: The analysis of binary data. London, 1970, Methue & Co., Ltd.
28. Breslow NE, Day NE: Statistical methods in cancer research. Volume I: The analysis of case-control studies. Lyon, France, 1980, International Agency for Research on Cancer, pp 192–246
29. Schlesselman JJ: Case-control studies: design, conduct, analysis. New York, 1982, Oxford University Press, pp 227–290
30. Brower RW, Serruya PW, Bos E, Nauta J: Regional myocardial shortening in relation to graft reactive hyperemia and flow after coronary bypass surgery. J Thorac Cardiovasc Surg **77:** 92, 1979
31. Fuster V, Dewanjee MK, Kaye MD, Josa M, Metke MP, Chesebro JM: Noninvasive radioisotopic technique for detection of platelet deposition in coronary artery bypass grafts in dogs and its reduction with platelet inhibitors. Circulation **60:** 1508, 1979
32. Steele P, Rainwater J, Vogel R, Genton E: Platelet-suppressant therapy in patients with coronary artery disease. JAMA **240:** 228, 1978

33. Ritchie JL, Harker LA: Platelet and fibrinogen survival in coronary atherosclerosis. Am J Cardiol **39:** 595, 1977
34. Moncada S, Korbut R: Dipyridamole and other phosphodiesterase inhibitors act as antithombotic agents by potentiating endogenous prostacyclin. Lancet **1:** 1286, 1978
35. Roth GJ, Majerus PW: The mechanism of the effect of aspirin alone on human platelets. I. Acetylation of the particulate fraction protein. J Clin Invest **56:** 624, 1975
36. Harker LA, Hanson SA: Experimental arterial thromboembolism. Mechanism, quantitation and pharmacologic prevention. J Clin Invest **64:** 559, 1979
37. Honour AJ, Hockaday TDR, Mann JI: The synergistic effect of aspirin and dipyridamole upon platelet thrombi in living blood vessels. Br J Exp Pathol **58:** 268, 1977
38. McEnany MT, Salzman EW, Mundth ED, DeSanctis RW, Harthorne JW, Weintraub RM, Gates S, Austen WG: The effect of antithrombotic therapy on patency rates of saphenous vein coronary artery bypass grafts. J Thorac Cardiovasc Surg **83:** 81, 1982
39. Mayer JE Jr, Lindsay WG, Casteneda W, Nicoloff DM: Influence of aspirin and dipyridamole on patency of coronary artery bypass grafts. Ann Thorac Surg **31:** 204, 1981
40. Chesebro JH, Clements IP, Fuster V, Elveback LR, Smith HC, Bardsley WT, Frye RL, Holmes DR Jr, Vlietstra RE, Pluth JR, Wallace RB, Puga JR, Orszulak TA, Piehler JM, Schaff HV, Danielson GK: A platelet-inhibitor drug trial in coronary-artery bypass operations. Benefit of perioperative dipyridamole and aspirin therapy on early post-operative vein graft patency. N Engl J Med **307:** 74, 1982
41. Chesebro JH, Fuster V, Elveback LR, Clements IP, Smith HC, Holmes DR, Bardsley WT, Pluth JR, Wallace RB, Puga JR, Orszulak TA, Piehler JM, Dannielson GK, Scnaff HV, Frye RL: Effect of dipyridamole and aspirin on late vein-graft patency after coronary bypass operations. N Engl J Med **310:** 210, 1984
42. Sharma GV, Skuri SF, Folland ED, Josa M, Parisi AF: Lack of benefit from aspirin-dipyridamole therapy in aorto-coronary vein graft patency. Circulation **66** (suppl II): II-94, 1982 (abst)
43. van den Dungen JJ, Karliczek GF, Brenken U, Homan van der Heide JH, Wildevuur CH: Clinical study of blood trauma during perfusion with membrane and bubble oxygenators. J Thorac Cardiovasc Surg **83:** 108, 1982
44. Harker LA, Malpass TW, Branson HE, Hessel EA, II, Slichter SJ: Mechanisms of abnormal bleeding in patients undergoing cardiopulmonary bypass. Acquired transient platelet dysfunction associated with selective alpha-granule release. Blood **56:** 824, 1980
45. Dewanjee MK, Tago M, Josa M, Fuster V, Kaye MP: Quantification of platelet retention in aortocoronary femoral vein bypass graft in dogs treated with dipyridamole and aspirin. Circulation **69:** 350, 1984
46. The Persantine-Aspirin Reinfarction Study Research Group: Persantine and aspirin in coronary heart disease. Circulation **62:** 449, 1980
47. Bousser MG, Eschwege E, Haguenau M, Lefaucconnier JM, Thibult N, Touboul D, Touboul PJ: "AICLA" Controlled Trial of Aspirin and Dipyridamole in the Secondary Prevention of Athero-Thrombotic Cerebral Ischemia. Stroke **14:** 5, 1983
48. Brown BG, Cukingnan RA, Petersen RB, Pierce CD, Bolson EL, Dodge HT: Perianastomotic arteriosclerosis in grafted human coronary arteries. Prevention with platelet-inhibiting therapy. Am J Cardiol **47:** 968, 1982 (abst)
49. Brown BG, Bolson EL, Pierce CD, Petersen RB, Wong M, Dodge HT: The progression of native coronary atherosclerosis is not altered by aspirin plus dipyridamole. Circulation **68** (suppl III): III-398, 1983
50. Lorenz RL, Weber M, Kolzun J, Theisen K, Schacky CV, Meistes W, Reichardt B, Weber PC: Improved aortocoronary bypass patency by low-dose aspirin (100 mg daily). Lancet **2:** 1261, 1984

Periodic procainamide for paroxysmal tachycardia

D. Woodrow Benson, Jr., M.D., Ph.D., Ann Dunnigan, M.D., Thomas P. Green, M.D., David G. Benditt, M.D., and Shanda P. Schneider, R.N.

ABSTRACT We evaluated the efficacy of a single oral dose of procainamide to terminate paroxysmal tachycardia, when procainamide was taken shortly after onset of tachycardia, a regimen we have termed "periodic procainamide." In 12 patients (mean age 15 years) with non–life-threatening tachycardia (orthodromic reciprocating tachycardia, 8/12; ventricular tachycardia, 3/12; atrial flutter, 1/12) in whom intravenously administered procainamide (15 mg/kg at 1 mg/kg/min) terminated tachycardia, efficacy of a single oral dose of procainamide (25 mg/kg) to terminate tachycardia was tested during electrophysiologic study. After oral administration of procainamide, tachycardia was terminated and could not be reinitiated in 11 of 12 patients (9/12 < 75 min, 2/12 > 120 min after administration). Time of tachycardia termination approximately coincided with the time of peak serum concentration of procainamide after the single oral dose. Delayed response or failure of procainamide to terminate tachycardia was associated with delayed and diminished peak serum procainamide concentration. After evaluation, 10 responders were instructed to take a single dose of procainamide when tachycardia occurred. During a mean follow-up of 9 months (range 2 to 17) seven of 10 patients had an opportunity to use periodic procainamide on one to more than 100 occasions; four of 10 patients have not had recurrence of tachycardia. Tachycardia was successfully terminated in six of seven patients using the periodic regimen and could not be terminated on the first out-of-hospital use in one of seven patients. Success of periodic procainamide was predicted during evaluation by rapid termination of tachycardia after oral administration.
Circulation 72, No. 1, 147–152, 1985.

TRADITIONAL treatment of patients with paroxysmal tachycardia has been long-term oral prophylaxis with antiarrhythmic drugs to prevent recurrences. With a prophylactic drug regimen, one or more antiarrhythmic drugs are taken on a scheduled basis, one or more times a day, to prevent paroxysmal tachycardia, which may occur relatively infrequently. The risk of adverse side effects and the cumulative expense of medication are recognized disadvantages of long-term prophylactic therapy, especially in young patients with paroxysmal tachycardias. Margolis et al.[1] proposed use of intermittent drug therapy in which a combination of antiarrhythmic drugs in the form of a "cocktail" was taken only after the onset of an episode of tachycardia. Their study established the feasibility of this approach, and they reported success in 24 of 32 patients with supraventricular or ventricular tachycardias.

We evaluated the ability of a single oral dose of procainamide to terminate tachycardia, when procainamide was taken shortly after the onset of tachycardia, a regimen we have termed "periodic procainamide." Procainamide was selected because, among available antiarrhythmic drugs, it is effective for a variety of tachycardias, it is available for both parenteral and oral administration, and it is well absorbed after oral administration in most patients. We attempted to minimize the influence of interpatient variation in pharmacodynamic properties or "drug effects" by administering the drug orally only to patients in whom the intravenous preparation terminated paroxysmal tachycardia; thereby we hoped to evaluate the pharmacokinetic basis for success or failure of the periodic regimen.

From the Department of Pediatrics, Pharmacology, and Medicine, University of Minnesota, Minneapolis.

This work was supported in part by grant 83 898 from the American Heart Association and was completed during Dr. Benditt's tenure as an Established Investigator of the American Heart Association.

Address for correspondence: D. Woodrow Benson, Jr., M.D., Ph.D., Box 94 Mayo, Pediatric Cardiology, University of Minnesota, Minneapolis, MN 55455.

Received Jan. 11, 1985; revision accepted April 4, 1985.

Methods

Patient selection. During electrophysiologic study, we administered procainamide intravenously to 27 patients (17 male, 10 female; ages 0.6 to 38 years) with recurrent paroxysmal tachycardia. Before all procedures, written informed consent was obtained. Each patient had had electrocardiographic (ECG) documentation of paroxysmal tachycardia on more than one occasion. In these patients, recurrences of tachycardia usually exceeded 3 hr and often necessitated an emergency visit for termination of the arrhythmia. During spontaneous tachycardia, no patient had syncope and each had demonstrated an ability to tolerate tachycardia for 3 hr or longer.

During electrophysiologic study with either transvenous[2, 3] or transesophageal catheters,[4] all patients had inducible tachycardia (orthodromic reciprocating tachycardia, 14/27; ventricular tachycardia, 7/27; and atrial flutter, 6/27). In each case, ECG features of induced tachycardia were identical to those that had occurred spontaneously.

After initiation of tachycardia, procainamide was administered intravenously by infusion pump (15 mg/kg at a rate of 1 mg/kg/min). During infusion, patients were questioned for symptoms, and blood pressure was measured frequently by sphygmomanometer or continuously by an indwelling arterial line. In 12 patients tachycardia was terminated during the infusion and could not be reinitiated by a stimulation protocol similar to that used before drug infusion. The results of these 12 responders form the basis of this report.

Description of procainamide responders. Of the 12 patients responding to the intravenous preparation of procainamide, eight were male and four female (ages 0.6 to 33 years, mean 15) (table 1). Patient 5 had levo transposition of the great arteries with mild Ebstein's anomaly of the left-sided atrioventricular valve. Patients 3, 4, 6, 9, 11, and 12 exhibited ECG features of Wolff-Parkinson-White syndrome. No patient had other recognized heart disease. No patient had evidence of hepatic or renal dysfunction.

The past history of tachycardia was varied among the 12 procainamide responders. Each had been admitted to the hospital or emergency room for conversion of tachycardia on one or more occasions (mean 3.4, range 1 to 5). Only four patients or their parents acknowledged that tachycardia had ever converted spontaneously without treatment. Three patients had never taken antiarrhythmic drugs except under emergency circumstances; however, nine patients had previously used an average of 2.2 (range 1 to 3) antiarrhythmic drugs (digoxin, propranolol, verapamil, and quinidine sulfate) alone or in combination in an effort to prevent recurrence of tachycardia.

Initial electrophysiologic evaluation of procainamide responders. Each patient underwent electrophysiologic study in the fasting state on two occasions. Before each study written informed consent was obtained. During the initial assessment the response to the intravenous preparation of procainamide was assessed. At the second study, the response of tachycardia to oral administration of procainamide was assessed. The techniques used in this laboratory during transvenous[2, 3] or transesophageal[4] electrophysiologic study have been previously described but are reviewed here briefly.

At the initial study, nine patients underwent transvenous electrophysiologic evaluation. In brief, after percutaneous cannulation of the right femoral and left median basilic or subclavian veins, four No. 6F quadripolar electrode catheters were positioned in the high right atrium, right ventricular apex, across the tricuspid valve to record the His electrogram, and within the coronary sinus by fluoroscopic guidance. Patients were medicated with lidocaine for local anesthesia and diazepam (1.0 to 2.5 mg) as needed for sedation. Atrioventricular and ventriculoatrial conduction and refractoriness were assessed by incremental pacing and extrastimulus testing in the right atrium, right ventricle, and coronary sinus. Additionally, in patients with evidence of accessory atrioventricular connection, short bursts (four to 10 stimuli) at cycle lengths of 200 to 70 msec were delivered in the right atrium and coronary sinus in an effort to initiate atrial fibrillation. Finally, in patients without evidence of accessory atrioventricular connection, efforts were made to induce ventricular tachycardia by a previously described protocol.[3] No patient required more than three extra stimuli for initiation of ventricular tachycardia.

In all nine patients undergoing catheter electrophysiologic study, tachycardia with ECG features identical to spontaneously observed tachycardia was initiated. In patients 2, 8, and 10, ventricular tachycardia was present.[5] In these three patients, the ECG pattern of right bundle branch block with left axis deviation suggested ventricular tachycardia similar to that described by Lin et al.[6] Patients 4, 6, 9, 11, and 12 had ECG features of ventricular preexcitation during sinus rhythm, and during elec-

TABLE 1
Clinical features

Patient	Arrhythmia	Age (yr)	Height (cm)	Weight (kg)	Oral dose (mg)	Follow-up time (mo)	Use (No.)	Comment
1	ORT	5	110	18	500 (27.8)[A]	17	>50	
2	VT	13	152	42	1000 (23.8)	1	5	B
3	ORT	2	94	15	375 (25.0)	14	>100	D
4	ORT	18	152	45	1125 (25.0)	14	0	D
5	ORT	0.6	73	8.3	250 (30.0)	—	—	
6	ORT	10	147	41	1000 (24.4)	11	1	D
7	AF	33	185	110	2500 (22.7)	7	1-Fail	
8	VT	14	157	44	1125 (25.6)	—	—	
9	ORT	23	165	67	1750 (26.1)	8	1	D
10	VT	11	152	55	1375 (25.0)	4	1	
11	ORT	24	178	71	2000 (28.2)	2	0	C,D
12	ORT	22	178	82	2250 (27.4)	2	0	D

AF = atrial flutter; ORT = orthodromic reciprocating tachycardia; VT = ventricular tachycardia.

[A]Data in parentheses are expressed as mg/kg.

[B]Switched to long-term prophylaxis after 1 month.

[C]Concomitant therapy with long-term propranolol.

[D]Wolff-Parkinson-White syndrome.

trophysiologic study they were determined to have accessory atrioventricular connections with bidirectional conduction that participated in orthodromic tachycardia. Patient 7 had no evidence of accessory atrioventricular connection or ventricular tachycardia, but he did have inducible atrial flutter.

Patients 1, 3, and 5 underwent transesophageal electrophysiologic study. A silicone rubber–coated bipolar catheter with 22 mm interelectrode spacing (Medtronic Inc, 6904-A) was inserted through the nares to the minimum pacing threshold site in the distal esophagus.[4] Patients were sedated with meperidine (1 to 2 mg/kg) as needed for sedation. Atrioventricular conduction and refractoriness were assessed by incremental pacing and extrastimulus testing from the esophageal pacing site. Additionally, short bursts (four to 10 stimuli) at cycle lengths of 200 to 70 msec were delivered in an effort to initiate atrial fibrillation. Based on ventriculoatrial intervals during tachycardia with a normal QRS complex and during transient, rate-related bundle branch block, patients 1, 3, and 5 were thought to have orthodromic reciprocating tachycardia.[7] Patient 3 demonstrated preexcitation during normal sinus rhythm.

During initial electrophysiologic study, each patient received procainamide intravenously (15 mg/kg at 1 mg/kg/min) after initiation of tachycardia. In each patient serum concentration was documented at the completion of the infusion (time 0), and in eight patients serum concentrations were determined at 30, 60, 120, 180, 270, and 360 min after cessation of the procainamide infusion.

Characteristics of tachycardia in procainamide responders. In eight patients with orthodromic reciprocating tachycardia the cycle lengths ranged from 240 to 350 msec (mean 281). During induced atrial fibrillation the minimum interval between preexcited QRS complexes in any patient was 240 msec. During ventricular tachycardia in patients 2, 8, and 10, the cycle length ranged from 270 to 290 msec (mean 278). In patient 7 the ventricular response was irregular during atrial flutter and averaged 390 msec.

Oral administration of procainamide to procainamide responders. At a second electrophysiologic study, performed more than 36 hr after intravenous administration of procainamide and after a fast of 6 hr or longer, tachycardia was reinitiated with a single transvenous (seven patients) or transesophageal (five patients) catheter by a stimulation protocol that had previously initiated tachycardia. Procainamide was administered orally in a dose of approximately 25 mg/kg with available capsule sizes of 250, 375, and 500 mg 15 min after initiation of tachycardia. In the two youngest patients, the contents of the capsule were added to applesauce at the time of ingestion. The oral doses ranged from 250 mg for the smallest patient (8.3 kg) to 2500 mg for the largest patient (110 kg). The average oral dose was 25.9 mg/kg, with a range of 22.7 to 30.0 (table 1). After oral administration of procainamide, patients were monitored for 3 hr, during which blood pressure was monitored frequently with a sphygmomanometer. If tachycardia was terminated, efforts were made to reinitiate tachycardia by a stimulation protocol similar to that which had previously initiated tachycardia in each individual in the untreated state. After oral administration of procainamide (time 0), serum concentrations were determined at approximately 30, 60, 120, 180, 270, and 360 min. If the time of tachycardia conversion did not coincide with a concentration determination, the procainamide concentration at the time of tachycardia conversion was estimated by linear interpolation from measured values.

Pharmacologic studies. Procainamide and *N*-acetyl procainamide (NAPA) concentrations were determined in separate assays by means of the Abbott TDx System, an immunoassay that uses fluorescent polarization.[8] The sensitivity of this method is 1 mg/liter for procainamide and 1 mg/liter for NAPA. Model-independent pharmacokinetic analysis[9] was used to determine procainamide elimination half-life and total systemic procainamide clearance. Bioavailability of oral vs intravenous administration of procainamide was determined as the ratio of the areas under the respective procainamide concentration-time curves.

Results

Pharmacokinetic analysis. Pharmacokinetic data from individual patients are presented in table 2. The mean values of procainamide elimination half-life and clearance in patients we studied are similar to those reported by Singh et al.[10] in young patients but different than those reported by Lima et al.[11] in older patients. The bioavailability of oral vs intravenous administration of procainamide was similar to that observed by Manion et al.[12] in young patients.

Results in patient 6 deserve special comment. After oral administration of procainamide, the serum concentration in this patient never exceeded 1 mg/liter, the lower sensitivity of our analysis system. Thus bioavailability could not be determined. However, the area under the concentration-time curve after intravenous administration of procainamide was lower than that for any other patient (6.8 mg hr/liter). Thus the bioavailability in patient 6 may be similar to that observed in other patients.

Intravenous administration of procainamide. In the 12 responders, tachycardia was terminated within 6 to 15 min (mean 12.4) after initiation of the infusion (15 mg/kg at 1 mg/kg/min). At termination of the infusion, the peak procainamide concentration ranged from 6.6 to 29.6 mg/liter (mean = 17.9). After infusion of procainamide, NAPA serum concentrations were always less than 2.0 mg/liter, and the area under the serum NAPA concentration-time curve was 9.2 ± 11.6% of the area under the procainamide concentration-time curve. There were no complications from this infusion regimen.

Oral administration of procainamide. All patients had immeasurable serum concentrations of procainamide and NAPA before oral administration of procainamide. After oral administration, tachycardia was terminated and could not be reinitiated in 11 of 12 responders to intravenous therapy. Tachycardia converted within 75 min of ingestion of procainamide (mean 41, range 23 to 74) in nine patients (Nos. 1, 3, 4, 6, 7, and 9 to 12) (table 2). Tachycardia in patient 6 converted despite a procainamide serum concentration that never exceeded 1 mg/liter. In the remaining eight patients, peak serum procainamide concentration (10.5 ± 3.4 mg/liter, mean ± SD) occurred in less than 120 min, and procainamide concentration estimated by linear interpolation at the time of tachycardia

TABLE 2
Pharmacokinetic features

	T½β (hr)	Cl (l/kg/hr)	F (%)	Cmax (mg/l)	Tmax (min)	Cconv (mg/l)	Tconv (min)
1	1.85[A]	—	—	6.9	30	6.7	55
2	1.68	1.21	123	5.1	180	3.7	155
3	1.49	1.18	87	6.9	30	6.6	35
4	1.82	1.03	156	14.4	60	14.4	60
5	2.12	0.69	62	5.4	125	5.4[C]	>180
6	1.84	2.15	B	<1.0	—	<1.0	30
7	2.95	0.36	85	15.3	60	9.6	74
8	2.96	1.71	92	7.3	270	3.2	175
9	1.1	0.56	77	12.9	60	11.1	53
10	2.6[A]	—	—	11.3	75	1.9	33
11	3.1[A]	—	—	7.7	110	6.0	43
12	3.5[A]	—	—	8.5	45	4.2	23
Mean	2.25	1.11	97				
SD	0.75	0.6	32				

T½β = elimination half-life; Cl = total systemic clearance (intravenous study); F = bioavailability; Cmax = maximum measured serum concentration after oral dose; Tmax = time at which Cmax was measured; Cconv = estimated serum concentration at time of conversion to sinus rhythm; Tconv = time of conversion.

[A]From oral study.

[B]Could not determine.

[C]Tachycardia not converted; concentration at 180 min.

conversion was 7.5 ± 3.9 mg/liter. In patients 2 and 8, ventricular tachycardia terminated in 155 and 175 min, and in patient 5 orthodromic reciprocating tachycardia failed to terminate within 180 min (table 2). In these three patients, the peak procainamide serum concentration (5.9 ± 1.2 mg/liter) occurred more than 120 min after administration of procainamide, and the procainamide concentration estimated at the time of conversion was 4.1 ± 1.2 mg/liter. After administration of procainamide the NAPA serum concentrations were less than 2.0 mg/liter during the first 2 hr. After 2 hr the peak NAPA concentration never exceeded 3.6 mg/liter. The area under the concentration-time curve for NAPA was 30 ± 15% of that for procainamide.

Figures 1 and 2 demonstrate examples of procainamide kinetics in two patients. Procainamide concentrations in figure 1 were obtained from a 2-year-old child with orthodromic reciprocating tachycardia. Tachycardia was terminated 11 min after onset of the intravenous infusion of procainamide. After termination of the infusion, the procainamide concentration rapidly fell during drug redistribution. After oral administration of procainamide, the peak concentration was recorded at 30 min. In this patient, tachycardia was terminated 35 min after oral administration of procainamide and could not be reinitiated.

Figure 2 illustrates the results from a 14-year-old patient with recurrent ventricular tachycardia. During intravenous infusion of procainamide, tachycardia terminated in 8 min. After termination of the intravenous infusion, the kinetics appeared to be similar to those in figure 1. After oral administration, the serum concentration of procainamide rose slowly, and the peak was not recorded until 180 min after ingestion. Tachycardia was terminated at 155 min and could not be reinitiated. The shape of the concentration-time curve with its marked delay in the time of peak concentration and its reduced peak concentration was quite different than that shown in figure 1.

Observations at the time of tachycardia conversion. At the time of tachycardia conversion by the intravenous or oral preparation of procainamide, each patient, except for the two youngest ones, acknowledged an abrupt change in heart rate. No patient had any other symptoms. In each case, sinus rhythm promptly resumed. The longest sinus pause after tachycardia conversion was 1.3 sec. In the eight patients with orthodromic tachycardia, procainamide-induced termination of tachycardia occurred after ventricular depolarization (i.e., block in the retrograde limb). After termination, tachycardia episodes exceeding 10 sec could not be induced. Shortly after administration of procainamide, nonsustained orthodromic reciprocating tachycardia was always terminated with ventricular depolarization. Atrial fibrillation exceeding 10 sec could not be induced in the eight patients with accessory connections. In the remaining four patients, the tachycardia rate gradually slowed before termination.

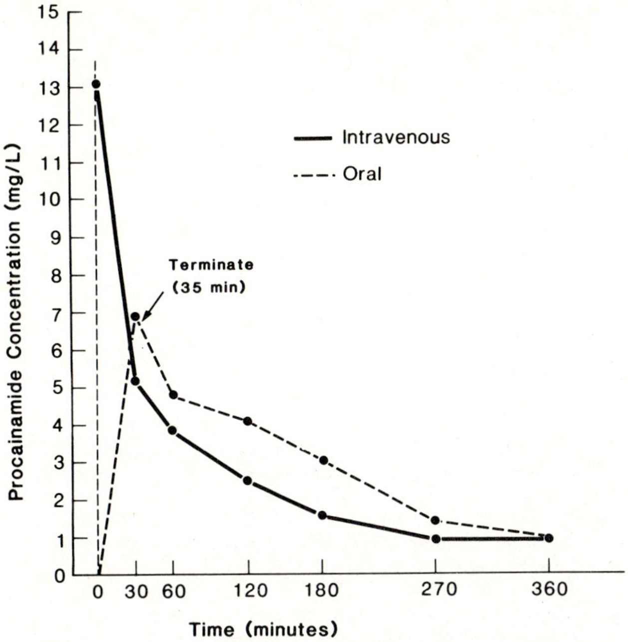

FIGURE 1. Time vs procainamide concentration in a 2-year-old child (patient 3). During intravenous infusion, orthodromic reciprocating tachycardia was terminated in 11 min. After oral administration, procainamide peak concentration was measured at 30 min. Tachycardia was terminated 35 min after ingestion. Curves have been approximated by connecting adjacent points with straight lines. In this graph, time 0 denotes both the termination time of the 15 min intravenous infusion and the time of ingestion of the oral dose.

Tachycardia episodes exceeding 10 sec could not be induced after procainamide-induced termination of tachycardia.

Follow-up. Ten of 12 patients were discharged and advised to take procainamide orally at the onset of an episode of tachycardia (i.e., periodic procainamide therapy). The dose selected was that demonstrated to be effective during evaluation. Patient 5, in whom conversion could not be achieved after oral administration of procainamide, and patient 8, who required 175 min for termination of tachycardia, were not discharged on the periodic regimen. Patient 11 takes propranolol on a daily basis in addition to using periodic procainamide. During follow-up of 2 to 17 months (mean 9) seven of 10 patients had an opportunity to use periodic procainamide. Patients 1, 2, 3, 6, 9, and 10 have successfully used periodic procainamide on one to more than 100 occasions. Patient 2 opted for long-term therapy within 1 month because of frequent recurrences and the relatively long time (155 min) required for procainamide to terminate tachycardia. In patient 7, the only patient with atrial flutter and the patient with the lowest dose per weight (table 1), the periodic regimen failed in the first out-of-hospital use. Three of 10 patients have not had an opportunity to use the regimen out of the hospital since they have not had recurrence of tachycardia.

Discussion

The principal finding of this study is that in selected patients with paroxysmal tachycardia, procainamide administered orally after onset of tachycardia resulted in termination. The time course of this action is rapid enough to be of practical benefit in some patients with paroxysmal tachycardia. Selection of patients for successful application of the periodic regimen appears to be relatively straightforward: non–life-threatening paroxysmal tachycardia, tachycardia termination by intravenous administration of procainamide, and relatively rapid absorption of procainamide after oral administration. Extrapolation of results in the young patients we evaluated to older patients or those with serious associated cardiac disease should be done cautiously.

The response to an antiarrhythmic drug in a periodic regimen is dependent on both the pharmacodynamic and pharmacokinetic properties of the drug.[13] We selected patients for periodic treatment who had a pharmacodynamic response of tachycardia termination during intravenous administration of procainamide. The oral, single-dose regimen appeared promising in nine of 12 patients; the principal cause of failure of the periodic procainamide regimen in three patients appeared to be pharmacokinetic and was related to de-

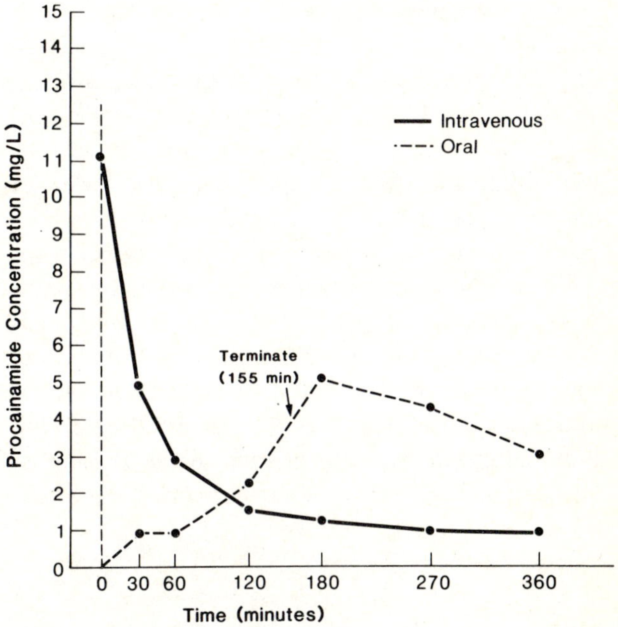

FIGURE 2. Time vs procainamide concentration in a 14-year-old boy (patient 2). The format is similar to that shown in figure 1. During intravenous infusion, ventricular tachycardia terminated in 8 min. After oral administration, procainamide peak concentration is measured at 180 min. Tachycardia terminated 155 min after ingestion.

layed absorption with diminished peak serum concentration of procainamide. However, in one patient with atrial flutter, the regimen failed in out-of-hospital use in spite of pharmacokinetic features that appeared favorable. Failure in this patient may be related to variation in the pharmacodynamic effect of procainamide on atrial flutter or to intraindividual variation in the pharmacokinetics of procainamide.

The intravenous infusion protocol of 15 mg/kg administered over 15 min has been a regimen used in our laboratory for several years for procainamide loading during electrophysiologic study, and in patients without congestive heart failure significant hypotension requiring a change in the infusion rate has not been a problem. Similarly, the oral dose of 25 mg/kg is our usual initial loading dose for patients beginning long-term oral therapy; we have encountered no complications from this oral dose. In these short-term studies, the principal antiarrhythmic effect is probably due to procainamide, since the serum concentrations of NAPA were quite low, especially at the time of tachycardia conversion.

In the application of periodic procainamide for termination of tachycardia we attempted to exploit the well-known pharmacokinetic features of rapid oral absorption and short half-life of procainamide, which are usually considered undesirable features when the drug is administered for purposes of long-term prophylaxis. Factors affecting oral absorption of procainamide have been incompletely defined.[12, 14] None of the patients we studied was chronically ill, none had congestive heart failure, and at the time of study all had fasted for 6 hr or longer. The cause for the relatively poor absorption seen in three patients is not apparent.

In a recently published study, Yeh et al.[15] demonstrated in young patients (mean age 34 years) that a single dose combining diltiazem with propranolol was effective in terminating tachycardia caused by reentry within the atrioventricular node or orthodromic reciprocating tachycardia when the drugs were taken shortly after the onset of tachycardia. As emphasized by Yeh et al.,[15] the benefits of periodic compared with long-term multiple daily dosing of antiarrhythmic drugs are considerable. Increased convenience and reduced cost of treatment is of substantial benefit in young patients who may require treatment for decades. In the case of procainamide, we are optimistic that periodic treatment will avoid some of the complications of long-term use.[14, 16]

References

1. Margolis B, DeSilva RA, Lown B: Episodic drug treatment in the management of paroxysmal arrhythmias. Am J Cardiol **45:** 621, 1980
2. Benditt DG, Klein GJ, Kriett JM, Dunnigan A, Benson DW Jr: Enhanced atrioventricular nodal conduction in man: electrophysiologic effects of pharmacologic autonomic blockade. Circulation **69:** 1088, 1984
3. Benson DW Jr, Benditt DG, Anderson RW, Dunnigan A, Pritzker MR, Kulik TJ, Zavoral JH: Cardiac arrest in young, ostensibly healthy patients: clinical, hemodynamic and electrophysiologic findings. Am J Cardiol **52:** 65, 1983
4. Benson DW Jr, Dunnigan A, Benditt DG, Schneider SP: Transesophageal cardiac pacing: history, application, technique. Clin Prog Pacing Electrophysiol **2:** 360, 1984
5. Benson DW Jr, Smith WM, Dunnigan A, Sterba R, Gallagher JJ: Mechanisms of regular, wide QRS tachycardia in infants and children. Am J Cardiol **49:** 1778, 1982
6. Lin FC, Finley CD, Rahimtoola SH, Wu D: Idiopathic paroxysmal ventricular tachycardia with a QRS pattern of right bundle branch block and left axis deviation: a unique clinical entity with specific properties. Am J Cardiol **52:** 95, 1983
7. Gallagher JJ, Smith WM, Kasell J, Smith WM, Grant AO, Benson DW Jr: Use of the esophageal lead to the diagnosis of mechanisms of reciprocating supraventricular tachycardia. PACE **3:** 440, 1980
8. Jolley ME: Fluorescence polarization immunoassay for determination of therapeutic drug levels in human plasma. J Anal Toxicol **5:** 236, 1981
9. Wagner JG: Linear pharmacokinetic equations allowing direct calculation of many needed pharmacokinetic parameters from the coefficients and exponents of polyexponential equations which have been fitted to the data. J Pharmacokinet Biopharm **4:** 443, 1976
10. Singh S, Gelband H, Mehta AV, Kessler K, Casta A, Pickoff A: Procainamide elimination kinetics in pediatric patients. Clin Pharmacol Ther **32:** 607, 1982
11. Lima JJ, Conti DR, Goldfarb AL, Tilstone WJ, Golden LH, Jusko WJ: Clinical pharmacokinetics of procainamide infusions in relation to acetylator phenotype. J Pharmacokinet Biopharm **7:** 69, 1977
12. Manion CV, Lalka D, Baer DT, Meyer MB: Absorption kinetics of procainamide in humans. J Pharm Sci **66:** 981, 1977
13. Galeazzi RL, Benet LZ, Sheiner LB: Relationship between the pharmacokinetics and pharmacodynamics of procainamide. Clin Pharmacol Ther **20:** 278, 1976
14. Lima JJ: Procainamide. *In* Evans WF, Schentage JJ, Jusko WJ, editors: Applied pharmacokinetics. San Francisco, 1980, Applied Therapeutics, Inc., p 404
15. Yeh SJ, Lin FC, Chou YY, Hung JS, Wu D: Termination of paroxysmal supraventricular tachycardia with a single dose of diltiazem and propranolol. Circulation **71:** 104, 1985
16. Lahita R, Kluger J, Drayer DE, Koffler D, Reidenberg MM: Antibodies to nuclear antigens in patients treated with procainamide or acetyl procainamide. N Engl J Med **301:** 1382, 1979

Comparative efficacy of transvenous cardioversion and pacing in patients with sustained ventricular tachycardia: a prospective, randomized, crossover study

SANJEEV SAKSENA, M.D., PRATHAP CHANDRAN, M.D., YOGESH SHAH, M.D., ROBERTO BOCCADAMO, M.D., DEMETRIS PANTOPOULOS, M.E., AND STEPHEN T. ROTHBART, M.D.

ABSTRACT We performed a prospective, randomized crossover study to evaluate the comparative efficacy of transvenous cardioversion and rapid ventricular pacing for termination of induced ventricular tachycardia in patients with spontaneous ventricular tachycardia and organic heart disease. Sixty-two episodes of ventricular tachycardia were induced in 15 patients, mean age 60 ± 10 years, during electrophysiologic studies. All patients underwent a preselected electrical therapy protocol in a randomized crossover sequence. Transvenous cardioversion was performed by an incremental protocol of three sequential shocks (0.5, 1.1, and 2.7 J). Six asynchronous sequential bursts of rapid ventricular pacing (10 and 15 paced stimuli at 90%, 75%, and 65% of ventricular tachycardia cycle length) were used. Mean cycle length of ventricular tachycardia for the study population was 391 ± 85 msec. The morphology of the tachycardia was left bundle branch block in 27, right bundle branch block in 32, and indeterminate in three. Characteristics of ventricular tachycardia terminated by the two techniques were comparable. Rate of success for termination of tachycardia with the two methods was also comparable (transvenous cardioversion 83%, rapid ventricular pacing 80%; $p > .1$) and these responses were concordant in 78%. The modes of termination of ventricular tachycardia were similar. The incidence of acceleration of ventricular tachycardia per episode with these preselected protocols was also comparable (transvenous cardioversion 11%, rapid ventricular pacing 6%; $p > .2$). Transient supraventricular tachyarrhythmias were more frequent after transvenous cardioversion (23%) than after rapid ventricular pacing (3%). Significant patient discomfort occurred only after transvenous cardioversion (incidence of 57%). We conclude that transvenous cardioversion and rapid ventricular pacing have comparable and usually concordant efficacy for termination of ventricular tachycardia. Transvenous cardioversion results in a higher incidence of postcardioversion arrhythmias and poorer patient tolerance than does rapid ventricular pacing.

Circulation 72, No. 1, 153–160, 1985.

TERMINATION of sustained ventricular tachycardia by the use of different techniques of internal electrical cardiac stimulation has been reported.[1] The comparative efficacy and safety of each technique and its potential role in clinical practice remain to be defined. Bursts of rapid ventricular pacing have been used to terminate sustained ventricular tachycardia in man for over a decade.[2] More recently the efficacy of intracavitary cardioversion of ventricular tachycardia with a transvenous electrode catheter has been documented during experimental studies and uncontrolled clinical trials.[3, 4] We have recently examined its clinical efficacy and safety in a controlled prospective randomized study.[5] However, there has been no controlled prospective study of the comparative efficacy of transvenous cardioversion and rapid ventricular pacing in terminating sustained ventricular tachycardia in the same patient population. In this report we examined the comparative clinical efficacy and safety of these two modes of electrical termination of tachycardia using a prospective randomized crossover study design.

From the Section of Cardiac Electrophysiology, Division of Cardiology, Newark Beth Israel Medical Center, and University of Medicine and Dentistry of New Jersey–New Jersey Medical School, Newark.

Address for correspondence: Sanjeev Saksena, M.D., Co-Director, Division of Cardiology, Newark Beth Israel Medical Center, 201 Lyons Ave., Newark, NJ 07112.

Received Dec. 31, 1984; revision accepted April 4, 1985.

Presented in part at the 57th Scientific Sessions, American Heart Association, Miami Beach, 1984.

Methods

Patient selection. Patients entering this study fulfilled the following criteria: (1) They had recurrent sustained ventricular tachycardia. Patients were undergoing clinically indicated electrophysiologic studies (EPSs). For purposes of this study "recurrent" was defined as three or more spontaneous episodes and "sustained" was defined as ventricular tachycardia of greater than 30 sec duration or requiring termination because of hemodynamic compromise. (2) They had not suffered recent (less than 30 days) myocardial infarction. (3) They had undergone reproducible induction of sustained ventricular tachycardia during EPS. (4) They gave informed consent for the cardioversion and electrophysiologic procedure.

Fifteen consecutive consenting patients (12 men and three women) with ages ranging from 36 to 73 (mean 60 ± 10) years and satisfying all entry criteria were enrolled in this study. Twelve patients had coronary artery disease. Of these, four had experienced a prior myocardial infarction and one had undergone coronary artery bypass surgery and aortic valve replacement. Two patients had congestive cardiomyopathy and one had documented mitral valve prolapse. The mean left ventricular ejection fraction of the study population ranged from 17% to 50% (mean 27 ± 13%). Thirty-five EPSs were performed in these patients (2.3 per patient). At the time of EPS, eight patients were undergoing control and 14 patients were undergoing serial drug EPS.

Study design. Patients were prospectively randomized into two study groups (see figure 1). All patients underwent EPS and programmed electrical stimulation for induction of sustained ventricular tachycardia. After its induction, electrical termination of the sustained ventricular tachycardia was attempted. Group A patients were initially treated with a preselected incremental transvenous cardioversion protocol and group B patients were initially treated with a preselected rapid ventricular burst pacing protocol. If termination of ventricular tachycardia was accomplished with this initial treatment the arrhythmia was then reinduced by the same technique and the other mode of electrical therapy was applied. Thus, group A patients were subsequently treated with the preselected rapid ventricular pacing protocol and group B patients subsequently underwent the preselected transvenous cardioversion protocol. If ventricular tachycardia could not be terminated with the initial selected mode of electrical treatment, the other mode of electrical treatment was applied. If ventricular tachycardia could not be terminated by either form of electrical treatment, pharmacologic interventions and/or transthoracic electrical cardioversion were used for termination of arrhythmia.

Electrophysiologic procedures. Patients underwent the initial EPS in the drug-free, nonsedated, postabsorptive state. Multipolar catheters were inserted by the standard percutaneous introducer techniques. A Medtronic 6880 temporary electrode catheter was used for transvenous cardioversion and pacing. This is a tripolar electrode catheter with a pair of bipolar electrodes at its distal end that are used for electrogram sensing and pacing. During cardioversion the electrodes become electrically common and form the cathode. A proximal electrode 125 mm from the distal electrodes functions as the anode during cardioversion. Intracardiac electrograms were monitored at the high and midright atrium, the His bundle, and the right ventricular apex. Surface electrocardiographic leads I, aVF, and V_1 were recorded simultaneously. Arterial blood pressure was monitored by an indwelling femoral artery sheath connected to a Statham P23 transducer. A multichannel display recorder (Electronics for Medicine VR-16, White Plains, NY) was used to amplify and display the electrograms. Hard copy recordings were obtained at paper speeds of 50 to 250 mm/sec. Programmed electrical stimulation and rapid pacing were performed with a programmable stimulator (Bloom Associates, Ltd., Narbeth, PA) that delivered rectangular pulses of 1 or 2 msec duration at twice diastolic threshold. Programmed stimulation was performed with a standard protocol from our laboratory, as previously described.[6] Transvenous cardioversion was performed with a Medtronic 5350 external cardioverter/defibrillator. This is a battery-operated external device that is capable of delivering truncated exponential electrical discharges with graded energies ranging from 0.03 to 28.0 J. Different energy waveforms controlled by tilt settings can be selected. The cardioverter/defibrillator is capable of synchronization with the patient's QRS complex. The modes of operation of this device have been previously described in detail.[5] The external cardioverter/defibrillator was interfaced with the programmable stimulator for rapid application of both forms of electrical therapy.

After sustained ventricular tachycardia was induced, rapid ventricular pacing or transvenous cardioversion, depending on the randomization status, was first attempted. The entire protocol was attempted unless successful termination of ventricular tachycardia was achieved or tachycardia accelerated or degenerated into ventricular fibrillation when it was aborted and the arrhythmia was terminated by transthoracic cardioversion or defibrillation. Subsequently patients were restudied one or more times during serial electrophysiologic testing while they were on antiarrhythmic drugs. The entire randomization process was repeated for serial studies to avoid selection bias. However, in view of the need for repeated induction and termination of hemodynamically unstable ventricular tachycardia in this study, the multiple inductions and terminations required to establish reproducibility of each technique were not performed.

Electrical therapy protocol. Preselected incremental electrical treatment protocols were used for transvenous cardioversion and rapid ventricular pacing. The transvenous cardioversion protocol consisted of three synchronized sequential shocks of 0.5, 1.1, and 2.7 J. All shocks were delivered at a tilt of 63%. The rapid ventricular pacing protocol consisted of two asynchronous trains of 10 and 15 paced stimuli applied sequentially at 90%, 75%, and finally 65% of the cycle length of the induced ventricular tachycardia.

Study parameters. The parameters analyzed in this study were demographic factors (age, sex), disease and functional status, standard electrocardiographic intervals (RR interval, PR interval, QRS duration, corrected QT interval), intracardiac intervals, left ventricular ejection fraction, characteristics of ventricular tachycardia (cycle length, morphology, induction mode), ventricular effective refractory period, lead threshold, and the presence or absence of antiarrhythmic drugs. Tolerance of each form of therapy was classified on the basis of the patient's subjective perception of the procedure as painless or minimally uncomfortable, moderately painful but tolerable, or severely and intolerably painful.

Results

Comparison of study groups. The study design exposed all patients to both types of electrical therapy in a randomized fashion. Thus there was no difference in the demographic, disease, functional, or electrophysiologic characteristics of the study groups exposed to the two techniques. In addition, the characteristics of the induced ventricular tachycardia (morphology, frontal plane axis, and cycle length) were similar for both forms of treatment (table 1). The randomized study groups A and B were also comparable with respect to these factors, as shown in table 2.

Clinical efficacy of rapid ventricular pacing and transvenous cardioversion. Sixty-two episodes of ventricular

TABLE 1

Characteristics of arrhythmias in patients with sustained ventricular tachycardia (VT) before application of transvenous cardioversion and rapid ventricular pacing

	Transvenous cardioversion	Rapid ventricular pacing
No. of patients	15	15
VT characteristics		
No. of episodes	35	35
Control EPS	8	8
Drug EPS	27	27
Mean cycle length (range)	392±93 msec (230–620)	397±87 msec (280–620)
QRS complex morphology		
RBBB	18	17
LBBB	15	16
Indeterminate	2	2

RBBB = right bundle branch block; LBBB = left bundle branch block.

tachycardia were induced in 15 patients during the course of this study. Each mode of electrical therapy was applied to 35 episodes of ventricular tachycardia. Eight episodes were unresponsive to attempted termination with the first mode of electrical therapy and the patients were subsequently exposed to the second mode of electrical therapy.

Twenty-nine episodes of ventricular tachycardia were successfully terminated with transvenous cardioversion, with an overall efficacy rate of 83%. Fifty-five transvenous cardioversion shocks were required (mean 1.6 per episode of tachycardia). Rapid ventricular pacing terminated 28 episodes, with an overall efficacy rate of 80%. A total of 85 attempts at rapid ventricular pacing were rquired (mean 2.4 per episode of ventricular tachycardia). Figure 1 illustrates the electrophysiologic effects of termination of ventricular tachycardia with both methods in the same patient during an electrophysiologic procedure. Induced ventricular tachycardia of an identical morphology and cycle length was immediately and rapidly terminated by a transvenous cardioversion shock of 1.08 J (figure 1, *A*) and rapid ventricular pacing (figure 1, *B*) at 396 msec (90% of ventricular tachycardia cycle length). Successful pacing modes and transvenous cardioversion shock energies in this study group are listed in table 3. Rapid ventricular pacing was successful at 90% and 75% of ventricular tachycardia cycle length at both stimulus train durations. Transvenous cardioversion was often successful at 0.5 J, but intermediate and high energies were needed in some patients. There was a high degree of concordance with respect to successful interruption of ventricular tachycardia by the two methods (figure 2), with a total of 25 of 32 successfully terminated episodes (78%) of ventricular tachycardia being terminated by both methods. There were seven of 35 episodes that did not terminate with rapid ventricular pacing (20%), and six of 35 that did not terminate with transvenous cardioversion (17%). Three episodes did not terminate with either, so that unsuccessful termination often demonstrated discordance between the two methods (figure 2).

Influence of antiarrhythmic therapy and ventricular tachycardia characteristics on the efficacy of both techniques for termination of ventricular tachycardia. The effects of specific factors such as antiarrhythmic therapy and characteristics of the tachycardia on the comparative efficacy of either technique for termination of ventricular tachycardia are examined in table 4. Efficacy of either technique was not affected by the presence or absence of antiarrhythmic therapy or specific characteristics of the arrhythmia, except in the case of transvenous cardioversion, which was more effective in ventricular tachycardia with longer cycle lengths ($p < .05$). Failure of either technique also could not be correlated with any of these factors.

Mechanism of termination of ventricular tachycardia with transvenous cardioversion and rapid ventricular pacing. Immediate termination of ventricular tachycardia was the most common mechanism of termination with both methods (transvenous cardioversion 88%, rapid

TABLE 2

Electrocardiographic, electrophysiologic, and ventricular tachycardia (VT) characteristics in patients in groups A and B before application of transvenous cardioversion or rapid ventricular pacing

	Group A (n = 7)	Group B (n = 8)	p value
ECG and EP parameters			
Mean QRS duration (msec)	118±31	133±44	NS
Mean corrected QT interval (msec)	469±53	472±71	NS
Mean RV ERP (msec)	273±29	268±24	NS
VT characteristics			
No. VT episodes	17	18	NS
Control EPS	3	4	NS
Drug EPS	14	14	NS
Mean cycle length (msec)	388±73	403±101	NS
Morphology (n)			
RBBB	9	8	NS
LBBB	7	9	
Indeterminate	1	1	

ECG = electrocardiographic; EP = electrophysiologic; RV ERP = right ventricular effective refractory period; other abbreviations are as in table 1.

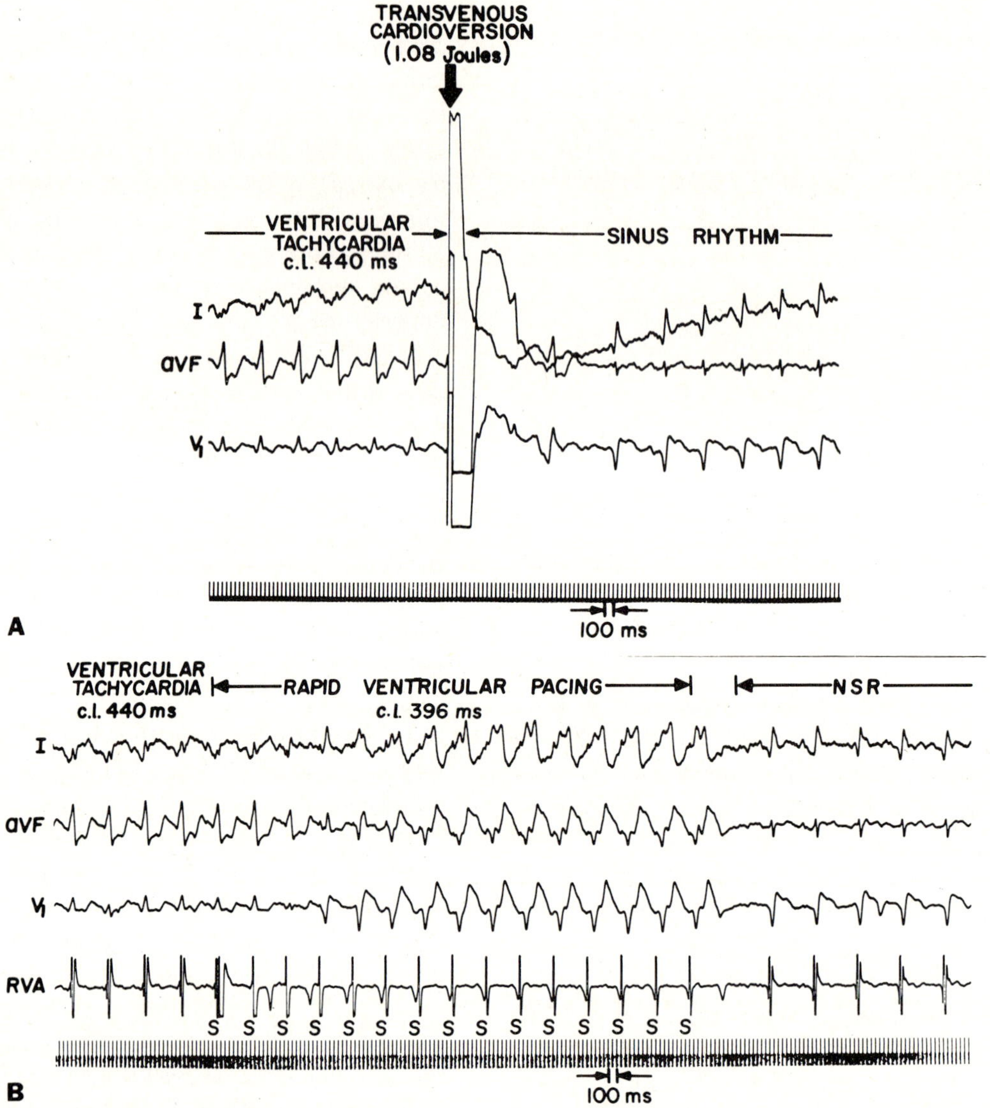

FIGURE 1. *A*, Termination of sustained ventricular tachycardia by a single transvenous cardioversion shock of 1.1 J. *B*, Termination of sustained ventricular tachycardia by a train of rapid ventricular pacing at 90% of the cycle length of the tachycardia.

ventricular pacing 96%). Change in morphology of ventricular tachycardia before termination was observed during two episodes after transvenous cardioversion (6%) and in one episode after rapid ventricular pacing (4%). Acceleration of ventricular tachycardia before termination was observed only during two episodes (6%) in which transvenous cardioversion was attempted.

Safety of transvenous cardioversion and rapid ventricular pacing

Sustained acceleration of ventricular tachycardia or ventricular fibrillation (figure 3). Sustained acceleration of induced ventricular tachycardia was observed during four episodes in three patients who underwent transvenous cardioversion (incidence per shock 7%, incidence per episode 11%), and during two episodes in two patients who underwent rapid ventricular pacing (incidence per burst 2%, incidence per episode 6%). There was no overlap between patients experiencing acceleration of tachycardia with both methods. The differences between the two methods were not statistically significant ($p > .2$). Induction of ventricular fibrillation was not encountered with either method. However, a substantial proportion of patients in whom termination failed with both techniques developed accelerated ventricular tachycardia.

Supraventricular tachyarrhythmias. Transient supraventricular tachycardias were observed after termination of ventricular tachycardia by both methods. Termination with transvenous cardioversion was followed by atrial fibrillation (five episodes), atrial flutter (two episodes), and sinus tachycardia (one episode), for an

TABLE 3
Successful modes of termination of ventricular tachycardia (VT) with transvenous cardioversion and rapid ventricular pacing

Transvenous cardioversion			Rapid ventricular pacing		
Shock energy (J)	No. of VT episodes (No. of patients) cardioverted	Percentage of total success/ VT episode	Pacing mode	No. of VT episodes (No. of patients) cardioverted	Percentage of total success/ VT episode
0.5	22 (12)	76	90% VT CL, 10 stimuli	16 (11)	57
1.1	4 (4)	14	90% VT CL, 15 stimuli	7 (5)	25
2.7	3 (3)	10	75% VT CL, 10 stimuli	3 (2)	11
			75% VT CL, 15 stimuli	2 (2)	7
			65% VT CL, 10 stimuli	0 (0)	—
			65% VT CL, 15 stimuli	0 (0)	—

CL = cycle length.

overall incidence of tachyarrhythmia of 23%. These arrhythmias were usually nonsustained, although sustained atrial flutter/fibrillation was observed in two episodes (6%) in two patients. One episode terminated spontaneously and the other was terminated by infusion of procainamide. Sustained sinus tachycardia was observed after termination of ventricular tachycardia with rapid ventricular pacing during one episode (incidence 3%).

Electrode catheter dislodgement. Catheter dislodgement was not observed with either technique in this study.

Patient tolerance. Subjective patient discomfort during episodes of ventricular tachycardia treated with transvenous cardioversion was reported to be severe by seven (20%), moderate by 13 (37%), mild by 11 (31%), and absent by four patients (12%). Rapid ventricular pacing was painless in all instances. This difference was highly significant ($p < .001$).

Discussion

Efficacy. The efficacy of programmed ventricular extrastimuli and rapid ventricular pacing for termination of sustained ventricular tachycardia has been previously documented.[2, 7–10] Long-term therapy by this approach with implantable devices has been reported.[11–16] Zipes et al.[4] documented successful termination of ventricular tachycardia using intracavitary countershocks delivered with a transvenous electrode catheter. Recently the same investigators reported their early experience with an implantable low-energy cardioversion device for termination of sustained tachycardia.[17]

The efficacy rates of pacing techniques for termination of ventricular tachycardia have varied depending on the mode used. Uncontrolled studies have suggested that bursts of rapid ventricular pacing have superior efficacy when compared with programmed ventricular extrastimuli.[2, 18] Whereas overall efficacy rates for one or two extrastimuli vary from 42% to 50%, these have varied from 60% to 89% for bursts of rapid ventricular pacing.[2, 18] The major factor determining efficacy was the cycle length of the tachycardia and antiarrhythmic drug therapy increased efficacy only if it prolonged the cycle length. The efficacy of different transvenous cardioversion protocols for termination of ventricular tachycardia has been recently examined in our laboratory with the use of a prospective randomized study design.[5] The overall efficacy of this technique in unselected patients was 62%. Factors influencing efficacy included (1) cycle length of ventricular tachycardia, (2) energy of delivered shock, (3) tilt of energy waveform, (4) time to initial cardioversion, and (5) QRS duration in sinus rhythm.[5, 19]

The present study compared the efficacy of these two methods with the use of a prospective randomized crossover study design. In comparing the efficacy of the two methods it was necessary to select an optimal protocol for each method. We have previously demonstrated that 83% of all successful transvenous cardioversion of ventricular tachycardia is achieved at energies up to 2.0 J.[5] Since patient tolerance rapidly

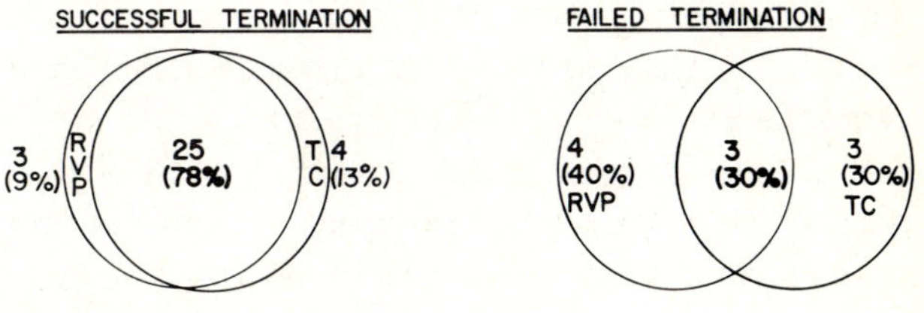

FIGURE 2. Concordance and discordance of results with transvenous cardioversion and rapid ventricular pacing in successful and unsuccessful attempts at termination of ventricular tachycardia.

TABLE 4
Comparative efficacy of transvenous cardioversion (TC) and rapid ventricular pacing (RVP) as related to specific factors

	Successful termination of VT			Unsuccessful termination of VT		
	TC	RVP	p (TC vs RVP)	TC	RVP	p (TC vs RVP)
Drug therapy						
Control EPS (%)	78	89	NS	22	11	NS
Drug EPS (%)	85	77	NS	15	23	NS
VT characteristics						
Mean VT cycle length (msec)	408±90	390±72	NS	318±76	421±145	NS
VT morphology (n)						
RBBB	14	15	NS	4	3	NS
LBBB	14	11		1	4	
Indeterminate	1	2		1	0	

VT = ventricular tachycardia; other abbreviations are as in tables 1 and 2.

declines at energies beyond this, an upper limit of 2.7 J was selected in this study. Retrospective analysis by Fisher et al.[2] of bursts of rapid ventricular pacing resulting in successful termination of ventricular tachycardia indicated that rates between 70% to 90% of cycle length of the tachycardia have the highest success rates. At extremely short pacing cycle lengths one-to-one ventricular capture cannot be achieved. In addition, up to 5 to 10 captured paced beats are usually needed. Therefore pacing rates of 90%, 75%, and 65% of cycle length were selected with pacing trains of 10 and 15 beats to allow a sufficient number of pacing captures during asynchronous pacing.

Our observations indicate that these two methods of electrical therapy have comparable efficacy for termination of sustained ventricular tachycardia when the protocols used in this study are applied. The mechanisms of successful termination of ventricular tachycardia by both techniques appear to be similar. Prior studies in which endocardial catheter mapping was applied during transvenous cardioversion suggest that it can either interrupt or reset and destabilize the ventricular tachycardia circuit.[5] Entrainment and interruption of ventricular tachycardia with rapid ventricular pacing has also been demonstrated.[20] Pacing termination of ventricular tachycardia can be explained either by penetration of the tachycardia circuit by the impulse with both antegrade and retrograde block or by development of instability due to resetting of the circuit and appearance of new areas of conduction block.[20-22] Similar mechanisms could explain the efficacy of transvenous cardioversion and rapid ventricular pacing in termination of ventricular tachycardia. Systematic cardiac mapping studies will be needed to further clarify these mechanisms.

Safety. Earlier studies have estimated the incidence of acceleration of ventricular tachycardia with rapid ventricular pacing to vary from 4% to 18%.[2, 17] However, a preselected systematic protocol was not used in these studies. On the basis of previous data, we used a controlled preselected incremental pacing protocol and noted a low incidence (2%) of this complication, the mechanisms of which include reinduction of the tachycardia after termination by late pacing-captured beats. These tachycardias can use alternative reentrant pathways as a result of modification of electrophysiologic parameters in the conducting tissues in the circuit.[22] Further modification of our protocol could conceivably minimize or eliminate this complication. Acceleration of tachycardia was also observed during transvenous cardioversion. While the mechanisms of this

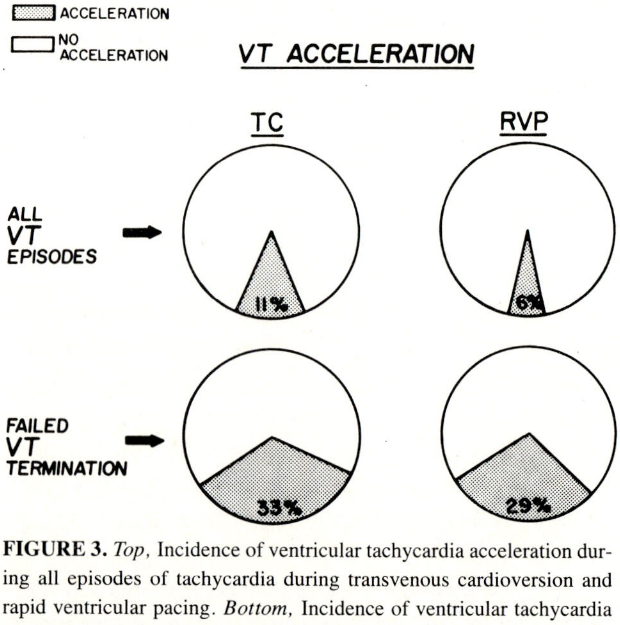

FIGURE 3. *Top,* Incidence of ventricular tachycardia acceleration during all episodes of tachycardia during transvenous cardioversion and rapid ventricular pacing. *Bottom,* Incidence of ventricular tachycardia acceleration during transvenous cardioversion and rapid ventricular pacing in unsuccessful attempts at termination of tachycardia.

phenomenon have not been systematically examined, they could be similar to those postulated for rapid pacing. We have previously reported an incidence of 8% per shock in unselected patients.[5] However, drug therapy may reduce the frequency of this complication. In this study the incidence of acceleration in drug-treated patients was lower (7%).

Transient arrhythmias after termination of ventricular tachycardia were more frequent after transvenous cardioversion than after rapid ventricular pacing. While these were usually nonsustained, we have observed sustained supraventricular arrhythmias after transvenous cardioversion in this and prior studies.[5] These may have considerable importance with reference to reestablishing hemodynamic stability after termination of ventricular tachycardia as well as for sensing algorithms of implantable cardioversion devices.[17] Also, patient tolerance of rapid ventricular pacing was clearly superior to transvenous cardioversion. Stability of the electrode catheter was demonstrated with both methods in this report.

Limitations of current study. Reproducibility of our results with regard to the efficacy and safety of the two methods used has not been established by our observations. This is an important issue since repeated demonstration of the efficacy and safety of the electrical therapy mode is necessary before implantation of permanent devices.[14, 15] Furthermore, differences between the cycle lengths of induced ventricular tachycardia and spontaneous clinical ventricular tachycardia remain a major problem in attempting to predict results of long-term use of these therapeutic devices. The time interval between the initiation of ventricular tachycardia and the application of therapy also remains an important issue. We have previously reported that successful transvenous cardioversion of ventricular tachycardia is associated with a shorter time interval between onset of tachycardia and delivery of shock.[5] A systematic analysis of this issue for both transvenous cardioversion and rapid ventricular pacing was not performed as a result of the constraints imposed by the need to deliver multiple therapies during the study. A systematic controlled study of this issue is clearly warranted.

Potential roles of rapid ventricular pacing and transvenous cardioversion in electrical therapy of ventricular tachycardia. Available information suggests that both of the techniques we studied have limited efficacy in unselected patients with ventricular tachycardia, but that this can be increased by careful patient selection.[2, 5, 18] The higher degree of efficacy observed in this study as compared with prior reports could be due to the longer cycle lengths of ventricular tachycardia we observed in drug-treated patients. Both methods have comparable and usually concordant efficacy, indicating that in many cases they are competitive, but rapid ventricular pacing has significant advantages with respect to patient tolerance and postcardioversion arrhythmias. With the delineation of a preselected pacing protocol some of the cumbersome aspects of selection of rapid ventricular pacing protocols can be eliminated. Both methods carry a small but definite hazard of acceleration of ventricular tachycardia and should only be used, both in short- and long-term therapy, when high-energy cardioversion/defibrillation capability is available.

We can visualize the use of pacing methods as a complement to, and preceding the application of, low- or high-energy countershock for termination of ventricular tachycardia. When carefully and systematically applied, this would, in our opinion, substantially reduce the number of patients exposed to the unpleasant and traumatizing experience of high-energy electrical countershock and would be ideal for temporary use, for example in an intensive care unit. For long-term treatment of ventricular tachycardia with implanted electrical devices rapid ventricular pacing techniques may offer superior patient tolerance and easier differentiation of postcardioversion rhythms with currently available sensing algorithms. They should, in our opinion, be considered as the first line of electrical therapy by an implanted unit before proceeding to cardioversion techniques. However, the discordance between transvenous cardioversion and rapid ventricular pacing with respect to the episodes of ventricular tachycardia failing to terminate with either technique suggests that transvenous cardioversion may play a complementary role in treatment of some patients. This may particularly apply to patients with tachycardias of longer cycle lengths. In such a case the optimum electrical therapy may be pacing with low-energy cardioversion as sequential therapy and with high-energy cardioversion on standby.

We express our appreciation for the assistance of Ms. Ruth Harrison in the preparation of this manuscript.

References

1. Fisher JD, Matos JA, Kim SG: The sparkling joules of internal cardiac stimulation: Cardioversion, defibrillation and ablation. Am Heart J **104:** 177, 1982
2. Fisher JD, Mehra R, Furman S: Termination of ventricular tachycardia with bursts of rapid ventricular pacing. Am J Cardiol **41:** 94, 1978
3. Jackman WM, Zipes DP: Low-energy synchronous cardioversion of ventricular tachycardia using a catheter electrode in a canine model of subacute myocardial infarction. Circulation **66:** 187, 1982

4. Zipes DP, Jackman WM, Heger JJ, Chilson DA, Brown KF, Naccarelli GV, Rahilly GT, Prystowsky EN: Clinical transvenous cardioversion of recurrent life threatening ventricular tachyarrhythmias: low energy synchronized cardioversion of ventricular tachycardia and termination of ventricular fibrillation in patients using a catheter electrode. Am Heart J **103:** 789, 1982
5. Ciccone JM, Saksena S, Shah Y, Pantopoulos D: A prospective randomized study of the clinical efficacy and safety of transvenous cardioversion for termination of ventricular tachycardia. Circulation **71:** 571, 1985
6. Saksena S, Rothbart ST, Cappello G, Bernstein A, Somani P: Clinical and electrophysiologic effects of chronic lorcainide therapy in patients with refractory ventricular tachycardia. J Am Coll Cardiol **2:** 538, 1983
7. Escher DJW, Furman S: Emergency treatment of cardiac arrhythmias. JAMA **214:** 2028, 1970
8. Wellens HJJ, Schuilenberg RM, Durrer D: Electrical stimulation of the heart in patients with ventricular tachycardia. Circulation **46:** 216, 1972
9. Spurrell RAJ, Sowton E, Deuchar DC: Ventricular tachycardia in 4 patients evaluated by programmed electrical stimulation of heart and treated in 2 patients by surgical division of anterior radiation of left bundle branch. Br Heart J **35:** 1014, 1973
10. Denes P, Wu D, Dhingra RC, Amat-y-leon F, Wyndham CRC, Mautner RK, Rosen KM: Electrophysiological studies in patients with chronic recurrent ventricular tachycardia. Circulation **54:** 229, 1976
11. Bennet MA, Pentecost BL: Reversion of ventricular tachycardia by pacemaker stimulation. Br Heart J **33:** 922, 1971
12. Moss AJ, Rivers RJ, Jr: Termination and inhibition of recurrent tachycardias by implanted pervenous pacemakers. Circulation **50:** 942, 1974
13. Ruskin JN, Garan H, Parkin F, Havthorne JW: Permanent radiofrequency ventricular pacing for management of drug resistant ventricular tachycardia. Am J Cardiol **46:** 317, 1980
14. Hartzler GO, Holmes DR, Osborn MJ: Patient activated transvenous cardiac stimulation for the treatment of supraventricular and ventricular tachycardia. Am J Cardiol **47:** 903, 1981
15. Saksena S, Pantopoulos D, Parsonnet V, Rothbart ST, Hussain SM, Gielchinsky I: Clinical evaluation of an implantable antitachycardia system. PACE **7:** 476, 1984
16. Ferguson D, Saksena S, Greenberg E, Craelius W: Management of recurrent ventricular tachycardia: Economic impact of therapeutic alternatives. Am J Cardiol **53:** 531, 1984
17. Zipes DP, Heger JJ, Miles WM, Mahomed Y, Brown JW, Spielman SR, Prystowsky EN: Initial experience with an implantable cardioverter. N Engl J Med **311:** 485, 1984
18. Naccarelli GV, Zipes DP, Rahilly GT, Heger JJ, Prystowsky EN: Influence of tachycardia cycle length and antiarrhythmic drugs on pacing termination and acceleration of ventricular tachycardia. Am Heart J **105:** 1, 1983
19. Shah Y, Saksena S, Ciccone JM, Rothbart ST, Tranotti K: Determinants of success and failure during transvenous cardioversion for ventricular tachycardia. PACE **7:** 464, 1984
20. Maclean WAH, Plumb VJ, Waldo AL: Transient entrainment and interruption of ventricular tachycardia. PACE **4:** 358, 1981
21. Waldo AL, Hawthorn RW, Plumb VJ, Maclean WAH: Demonstration of the mechanism of transient entrainment and interruption of ventricular tachycardia with rapid atrial pacing. J Am Coll Cardiol **3:** 422, 1984
22. El-Sherif H, Gough WB, Hariman R, Zeiler R, Restivo M, Kowtha V: Mechanisms of termination or acceleration of reentrant tachycardia by burst pacing. Circulation **70** (suppl II): II-91, 1984

Atrial fibrillation in patients with Wolff-Parkinson-White syndrome: incidence after surgical ablation of the accessory pathway

A. D. SHARMA, M.D., G. J. KLEIN, M.D., G. M. GUIRAUDON, M.D., AND S. MILSTEIN, M.D.

ABSTRACT The effect of surgical ablation of atrioventricular accessory pathways on the incidence of atrial fibrillation in patients with Wolff-Parkinson-White syndrome was examined and the results of preoperative electrophysiologic testing were studied to determine factors predictive of outcome. Among 50 consecutive surgical cases, 19 patients were identified with a past history of at least one episode of spontaneous atrial fibrillation documented by electrocardiogram before surgery. The mean number of episodes of atrial fibrillation was 1.97/patient/year during a mean symptomatic period of 6.9 years before surgery. These patients were compared with 19 consecutive patients undergoing surgery during the same time period who had a history of only reciprocating tachycardia. Patients with atrial fibrillation had a significantly shorter antegrade accessory pathway effective refractory period (270 ± 39 vs 330 ± 107 msec; $p < .05$) and much faster ventricular rates during induced atrial fibrillation (shortest RR interval 219 ± 73 vs 294 ± 60 msec, $p < .005$; average RR interval 324 ± 109 vs 405 ± 127 msec, $p < .01$). Patients with atrial fibrillation also had longer PA intervals (47 ± 13 vs 37 ± 7 msec; $p < .02$). At preoperative electrophysiologic testing, 18 patients with atrial fibrillation had atrial fibrillation induced and 14 sustained the arrhythmia for longer than 10 min. In contrast, atrial fibrillation, although induced in 14 of 19 patients with reciprocating tachycardia, was not sustained in any. Thus electrophysiologic testing suggested that both accessory pathway properties and atrial vulnerability may predispose to atrial fibrillation. There were five episodes of atrial fibrillation in three patients (0.3/patient) during the first month after surgery. During a mean follow-up of 1.9 years, only one patient with an associated cardiomyopathy has had recurrent atrial fibrillation. We conclude that surgical ablation of the accessory pathway in patients without organic heart disease prevents further atrial fibrillation. This suggests that reciprocating tachycardia or ectopy mediated by the accessory pathway is the mechanism of induction of spontaneous atrial fibrillation in the majority of patients with Wolff-Parkinson-White syndrome.
Circulation 72, No. 1, 161–169, 1985.

ATRIAL FIBRILLATION occurring in patients with Wolff-Parkinson-White syndrome is a potentially life-threatening arrhythmia because it may lead to ventricular fibrillation.[1] Accordingly, the pathogenesis of atrial fibrillation in these patients has been the subject of a number of investigations. Electrophysiologic testing of patients has revealed that atrioventricular (AV) reciprocating tachycardia can be induced in the majority of patients who have a past history of atrial fibrillation.[2, 3] Furthermore, the spontaneous degeneration of AV reciprocating tachycardia to atrial fibrillation has been observed during electrophysiologic testing.[2, 4–6] These findings suggest that atrial fibrillation can occur secondary to AV reentry by means of the accessory pathway and that the accessory pathway directly participates in the induction of atrial fibrillation.

However, only a minority of patients with a past history of atrial fibrillation are observed to have spontaneous degeneration of AV reciprocating tachycardia to atrial fibrillation during electrophysiologic testing.[2, 4, 7] In patients in whom extrastimulus techniques have been required to induce atrial fibrillation,[2, 7, 8] the induction of atrial fibrillation by a single extrastimulus has suggested primary atrial vulnerability to fibrillation.[7] In these patients the accessory pathway would not be an obligatory link in the initiation of atrial fibril-

From the Clinical Electrophysiology Laboratory, University Hospital, University of Western Ontario, London, Ontario.

This work was supported by grants from the Ontario Heart Foundation and the Ontario Ministry of Health.

Address for correspndence: A. D. Sharma, M.D., University Hospital, Box 5339, Station A, London, Ontario, Canada N6A 5A5.

Received Dec. 19, 1984; revision accepted April 11, 1985.

Presented in part to the Canadian Cardiovascular Society, October 1984.

lation, and atrial fibrillation would be expected to recur even after the surgical ablation of the accessory pathway.

To determine the role of the accessory pathway in the pathogenesis of atrial fibrillation, we first compared the electrophysiologic properties of patients with atrial fibrillation to those with only reciprocating tachycardia. Second, we studied the effects of surgical ablation of the accessory pathway on the incidence of atrial fibrillation in patients with a past history of atrial fibrillation.

Methods

Patient selection. The records of 50 consecutive patients undergoing surgical ablation of an atrioventricular accessory pathway between August 1981 and February 1984 were examined. Indications for surgery included prior cardiac arrest, arrhythmias refractory to pharmacologic therapy, or intolerable side effects from pharmacologic therapy. Nineteen patients were identified with a past history of at least one episode of atrial fibrillation that had been documented by 12-lead electrocardiograms. Although a number of patients described irregular palpitations suggestive of atrial fibrillation, for the purposes of this study only electrocardiographically documented episodes of atrial fibrillation were included. Efforts were made to obtain all electrocardiographic tracings from referring physicians. This study group was compared with 19 consecutive patients undergoing surgical ablation of an accessory pathway during the same period who had no past history of atrial fibrillation documented by electrocardiogram.

Clinical evaluation. All patients provided their medical history and underwent physical examination, chest roentgenography, 12-lead electrocardiography, 24 hr Holter monitoring, exercise testing, and two-dimensional echocardiography. Male patients over the age of 40 and patients with clinical evidence of significant organic heart disease underwent coronary angiography and left ventriculography.

Study protocol. All patients underwent a standard protocol that consisted of a preoperative electrophysiologic study, intraoperative epicardial AV ring mapping, and a limited electrophysiologic study carried out 1 week after surgery using epicardial wires implanted during the operation. Written informed consent was obtained for each of these procedures. All patients underwent continuous electrocardiographic monitoring for 24 to 48 hr immediately after surgery. Patients were reviewed 6 weeks after surgery and a 12-lead electrocardiogram was obtained at that time. All patients were contacted at the end of the study period and any patients with symptoms of palpitation or documented irregularity of pulse on physical examination were asked to forward copies of electrocardiograms.

Electrophysiologic testing. Electrophysiologic evaluation was carried out with patients in the postabsorptive, nonsedated state after all antiarrhythmic medication had been discontinued for five half-lives. The protocol for the preoperative electrophysiologic study has been previously described.[9] Briefly, this consists of the recording of basic intervals, sinoatrial conduction time, sinus node recovery time, atrial extrastimulus testing at cycle lengths 400 and 600 msec, antegrade incremental pacing to AV block, ventricular refractory periods at cycle length 400 and 600 msec, and ventricular incremental pacing to ventriculoatrial block. In all patients a quadripolar catheter was positioned in the coronary sinus. In cases where there was evidence to suggest a right-sided accessory pathway, the right atrial catheter was replaced by a bipolar atrial mapping catheter for tricuspid AV ring mapping. Standard criteria for the participation of an accessory pathway in atrioventricular reciprocating tachycardia were used.[10] In patients in whom atrial fibrillation was not induced before this, rapid atrial pacing at rates of 400 to 500 beats/min was performed until atrial fibrillation was induced. The pacing stimuli used throughout the study were square-wave pulses of 2 msec duration at an amplitude two times diastolic threshold.

Surgical technique. The surgical approach to the ablation of accessory pathways has been previously described. During the study period the technique varied and included both open[11] and closed[12] techniques for ablating left-sided accessory pathways. Intraoperatively, ventricular activation at the AV ring was determined during right atrial pacing. Retrograde atrial activation at the AV ring was determined during ventricular pacing or reciprocating tachycardia. In each case the findings of the previous electrophysiologic study were confirmed. At the conclusion of the procedure, epicardial wires were sutured to the right atrium and right ventricle for use during postoperative electrophysiologic testing.

Postoperative electrophysiologic testing. One week after surgery, all patients underwent repeat electrophysiologic testing. This included atrial incremental pacing to the point of AV block and ventricular incremental pacing to the point of ventriculoatrial block. When necessary, atrial and ventricular extrastimulus testing were used to clarify the absence of conduction characteristic of accessory pathways.

Statistical analysis was performed with the Student t test for unpaired data, chi square analysis, and the Wilcoxon signed-rank test to compare preoperative and postoperative incidence of atrial fibrillation.

Results

Patient characteristics. Nineteen patients were identified with a past history of atrial fibrillation among the 50 consecutive patients who underwent surgical ablation of an AV accessory pathway. The mean age was 28.9 years (range 12 to 58). Fourteen patients were male and five were female. Sixteen patients had no evidence of cardiac disease other than Wolff-Parkinson-White syndrome, and one had Ebstein's anomaly, one mitral valve prolapse, and one patient an idiopathic congestive cardiomyopathy. There was no evidence for coronary artery disease in this group of patients. Two of these patients had a past history of cardiac arrest. The onset of atrial fibrillation was related to various factors, including exercise ($n = 8$), sleep ($n = 2$), emotion ($n = 1$), alcohol ingestion ($n = 1$), and no known factors ($n = 7$).

The study group was compared with 19 consecutive patients who underwent surgical ablation of an accessory pathway during the same period. None of these patients with only reciprocating tachycardia had organic heart disease. Patient characteristics are summarized in table 1.

Electrophysiologic testing. At the initial electrophysiologic study, both groups of patients were characterized in terms of accessory pathway location and properties, functional properties of the normal AV conduction

TABLE 1
Patient characteristics

	AF (n = 19)	RT (n = 19)
Age (yr)	28.9	32.1
Sex (M/F)	14/5	7/12
Heart disease		
Normal	16	19
Ebstein's anomaly	1	0
Mitral valve prolapse	1	0
Cardiomyopathy	1	0
Accessory pathway location		
Left lateral	11	11
Posteroseptal	9	5
Right anteroseptal	6	5
Right free wall	0	2

AF = patients with a documented history of atrial fibrillation; RT = patients with no history of atrial fibrillation but with AV reciprocating tachycardia.

system, and ventricular response to atrial fibrillation.

Accessory pathway characteristics. In patients with paroxysmal atrial fibrillation, accessory pathways were located in the left lateral position in 11, the posteroseptal region in nine, and the right anteroseptal location in six. Seven of 19 patients had multiple accessory pathways, five had dual AV nodal pathways, and one had a nodoventricular Maheim pathway. Thus, 11 of 19 patients had either dual AV nodal pathways or multiple accessory pathways (58%) that could contribute to multiple sites for retrograde atrial activation. Among the patients without atrial fibrillation, significantly fewer subjects (n = 4) had either multiple accessory pathways (n = 2) and/or dual AV nodal pathways (n = 3) ($p < .025$). No other differences were noted in location of accessory pathways. However, all patients with atrial fibrillation had ventricular preexcitation, whereas only 14 patients without atrial fibrillation had antegrade accessory pathway conduction ($p < .05$). That is, no patient with a concealed accessory pathway had atrial fibrillation.

The results of electrophysiologic testing are summarized in table 2. Patients with paroxysmal atrial fibrillation had significantly shorter antegrade accessory pathway effective refractory period (drive cycle length 600 msec) ($APERP_{600}$ 270 ± 39 msec) compared with patients with only reciprocating tachycardia (330 ± 107 msec) ($p < .05$). Consistent with this observation, when atrial fibrillation was induced during electrophysiologic testing, patients with paroxysmal atrial fibrillation had more rapid ventricular rates. The group mean of the shortest interval between consecutive preexcited beats (SRR) was 219 ± 73 msec, and the mean of the average interval between preexcited beats (ARR)[13] was 334 ± 109 msec. In patients with only reciprocating tachycardia, the mean SRR was 294 ± 60 msec ($p < .005$) and the mean ARR was 405 ± 127 msec ($p < .01$). The differences between the two patient groups were greater than the means indicated because one patient with atrial fibrillation and a cardiomyopathy had a very slow ventricular rate during atrial fibrillation. In the remaining 18 patients with atrial fibrillation, the mean SRR was 205 ± 45 msec.

AV reciprocating tachycardia of the orthodromic type was induced in 37 patients. In addition, five patients had antidromic tachycardia and two patients had AV nodal reentrant tachycardia. No differences were observed between the two groups of patients in the ease of initiation of reciprocating tachycardia, tachycardia mechanism, or tachycardia cycle length. There were no differences in retrograde effective refractory period of the accessory pathway.

Functional properties. No differences were observed between the two patient groups in spontaneous sinus node cycle length, AH interval, sinus node recovery time, sinoatrial conduction time, or atrial and ventricular functional and effective refractory periods. The PA interval was significantly longer in patients with atrial fibrillation (47 ± 13 msec) compared with patients with only reciprocating tachycardia (37 ± 7 msec; $p < .02$). Ten patients with atrial fibrillation had a PA greater than 45 msec, and in eight of these patients the left atrium was adequately visualized echocardiographically. The left atrial dimensions were normal

TABLE 2
Electrophysiologic parameters in patients with atrial fibrillation compared with patients with only reciprocating tachycardia

	AF (n = 19) (msec ± SD)	RT (n = 19) (msec ± SD)	
$APERP_{600}$	270 ± 39	330 ± 107	$p < .05$
$APERP_{600}$ (retrograde)	268 ± 40	261 ± 26	NS
SRR (AF)	219 ± 73	294 ± 60	$p < .005$
ARR (AF)	324 ± 109	405 ± 127	$p < .01$
RTCL	307 ± 61	333 ± 34	NS
$AERP_{600}$	199 ± 36	209 ± 27	NS
PA interval	47 ± 13	37 ± 7	$p < .02$
AH interval	65 ± 35	75 ± 19	NS
WCL (postop)	290 ± 61	338 ± 98	NS
Multiple AP or dual AVN	11	4	$p < .025$
Antegrade preexcitation	19	14	$p < .05$

APERP = accessory pathway effective refractory period at designated cycle length; SRR = shortest RR interval in atrial fibrillation; ARR = average interval during atrial fibrillation; RTCL = cycle length of AV reciprocating tachycardia; AERP = atrial effective refractory period; WCL = Wenckebach cycle length; AP = accessory pathway; AVN = AV node; other abbreviations as in table 1.

(<40 mm) in seven, with one patient (with cardiomyopathy) having an enlarged left atrium. Thus slowing of intra-atrial conduction was rarely associated with structural abnormality in these patients. AV nodal conduction could be assessed only in the minority of patients, but antegrade (254 ± 41 vs 262 ± 43 msec) and retrograde AV nodal effective refractory periods (322 ± 117 vs 371 ± 145 msec) did not differ in those patients where it could be measured. We therefore compared the AV nodal Wenckebach cycle length in all patients postoperatively and observed no differences between the two groups of patients. However, among patients with paroxysmal atrial fibrillation, nine of 19 patients had an AH interval less than or equal to 60 msec and a postoperative Wenckebach cycle length less than 300 msec, consistent with "enhanced" AV nodal conduction. Only two patients with reciprocating tachycardia had similarly rapid AV nodal conduction.

Atrial fibrillation during electrophysiologic testing. Induction of atrial fibrillation was attempted during the preoperative electrophysiologic study in all but one patient. This patient had a documented past history of rapid atrial fibrillation and refused to be studied off medication. The modes of induction of atrial fibrillation are described in table 3. All patients with a past history of atrial fibrillation had atrial fibrillation induced only during electrophysiologic testing and the atrial fibrillation was sustained more than 10 min in 14 of 18. When clinically indicated, these patients were given disopyramide (n = 9) or procainamide (n = 3) intravenously, and if atrial fibrillation failed to terminate, a transthoracic cardioversion shock was used to restore sinus rhythm (n = 4). In contrast, atrial fibrillation could be induced only in 14 of the patients who had no past history of atrial fibrillation, and in only one of these patients was atrial fibrillation sustained more than 10 min.

The modes of induction of atrial fibrillation suggested that the arrhythmia was easier to induce in those patients who had documented spontaneous episodes of atrial fibrillation. These patients frequently developed atrial fibrillation inadvertently during atrial or coronary sinus catheter placement (n = 6) or after a single atrial extrastimulus (n = 3) (figure 1). In the latter episodes, the onset of atrial fibrillation was not associated with AV reentry. The preceding modes of induction were rarely observed in patients with a past history of only reciprocating tachycardia. The latter patients usually required rapid atrial pacing (n = 10) to initiate a brief period of atrial fibrillation (figure 2). Among all 38 patients, only four (10.5%) were observed to have spontaneous degeneration of reciprocating tachycardia to atrial fibrillation (figure 3). One patient with a history of only reciprocating tachycardia was observed to rapidly revert to sinus rhythm after reciprocating tachycardia degenerated to atrial fibrillation. This rapid, spontaneous cardioversion could have accounted for the lack of documentation of spontaneous atrial fibrillation.

TABLE 3
Induction of atrial fibrillation during electrophysiologic testing

	AF (n = 19)	RT (n = 19)
Induction of AF	18/18[A]	14/19
AF sustained 10 min	14/18	0/14[B]
Method of induction		
Single extrastimulus	3	3
RT to AF	3	1
Rapid atrial pacing	6	10
Mechanical stimulation	6	0

AF = atrial fibrillation; other abbreviations as in table 1.
[A]Atrial fibrillation induction not attempted in one patient with documented rapid atrial fibrillation.
[B]$p < .001$.

Some of the modes of onset of atrial fibrillation are illustrated in figures 1 to 4. In these examples, earliest spontaneous atrial activity was observed to occur at a site removed from the accessory pathway, usually the high right atrium. This suggests that onset of atrial fibrillation was related to intra-atrial factors rather than to an abnormality of the atrium at the site of the atrial insertion of the accessory pathway. The induction of atrial fibrillation during ventricular pacing (figure 4) indicates that patients with concealed accessory pathways may potentially be at risk for the development of atrial fibrillation.

Incidence of atrial fibrillation (table 4). A past history of atrial fibrillation was determined by electrocardiographic documentation. An arbitrary upper limit of 10 episodes of atrial fibrillation was allowed per patient for purposes of analysis. This was done to prevent the results of a few patients with many episodes from skewing the data. In addition, as the episodes of atrial fibrillation became more frequent, it was increasingly difficult to obtain accurate histories and electrocardiographic documentation. All patients had an episode of atrial fibrillation during the year before surgery and this frequently precipitated referral for surgery. During a mean preoperative symptomatic period of 6.9 ± 5.8 years there were 89 episodes of atrial fibrillation in 19 patients. The incidence of atrial fibrillation in each patient was determined with a resultant average incidence of 1.97 ± 2.5/patient/year. This is undoubtedly

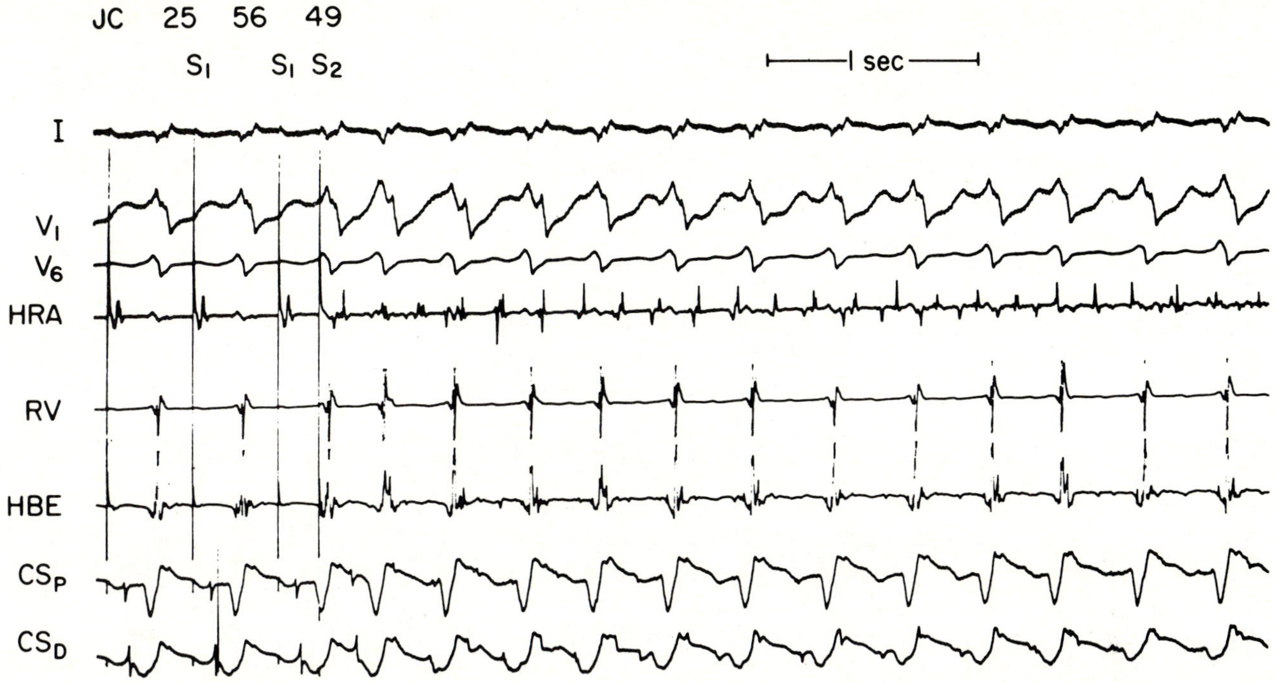

FIGURE 1. Induction of atrial flutter by a single atrial extrastimulus. After a drive of 8 beats at cycle length 400 msec, a premature stimulus at coupling interval 190 msec induces atrial flutter with 2:1 antegrade conduction via an accessory pathway. In this patient with a single left lateral atrioventricular accessory pathway, earliest spontaneous atrial activity is observed in the His bundle recording (HBE), at a site distant from the atrial insertion of the accessory pathway. The onset of atrial flutter is not related to atrioventricular reentry. Atrial flutter rapidly degenerated to atrial fibrillation. HRA = high right atrium; RV = right ventricle; CS_P = proximal coronary sinus; CS_D = distal coronary sinus.

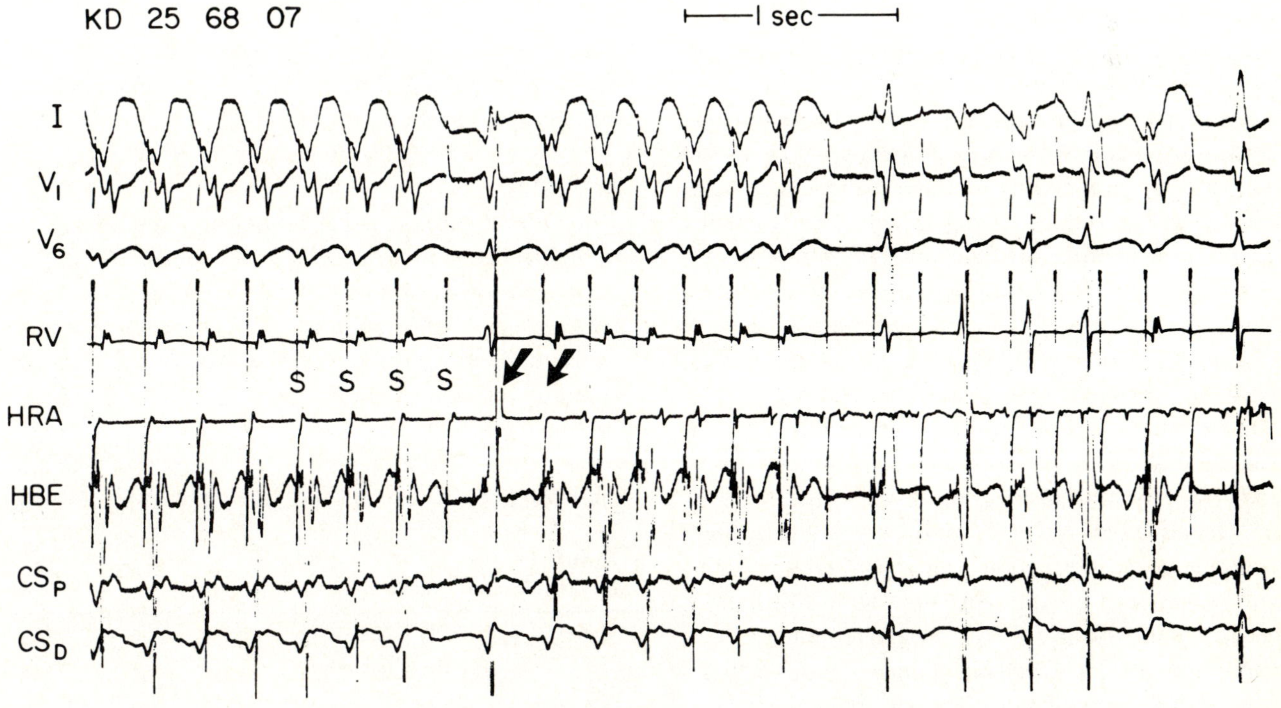

FIGURE 2. Induction of atrial fibrillation during atrial incremental pacing. After antegrade block in the accessory pathway, an alteration is observed in the high right atrial electrogram (first arrow). On the second cycle after block, activity in the high right atrium is observed to precede the stimulus artifact (second arrow). Organized repetitive atrial activity arising in the high right atrium continues for a further six cycles before degenerating to atrial fibrillation, which was sustained when the pacing was terminated. Abbreviations as in figure 1.

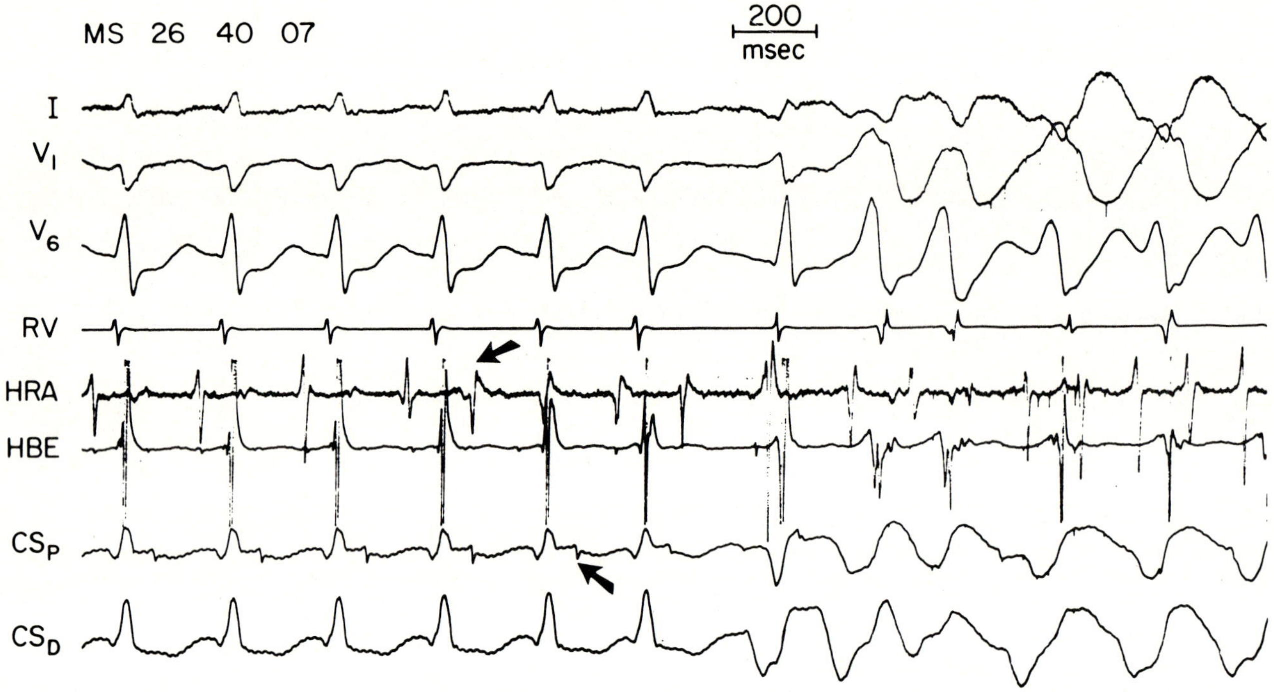

FIGURE 3. Spontaneous degeneration of AV reciprocating tachycardia to atrial fibrillation. Orthodromic AV reciprocating tachycardia used a left lateral accessory pathway in this patient. At the point indicated by the first arrow, spontaneous premature activation is observed in the high right atrium. Repetitive atrial activity follows. However, reciprocating tachycardia continues for a further two cycles before atrial activation at the coronary sinus is altered. After this, rapid antegrade conduction via the accessory pathway is observed during atrial fibrillation. Abbreviations as in figure 1.

a conservative estimate because of the requirement for documentation, and the upper limit of fibrillation episodes set per patient. Two patients had only one episode of atrial fibrillation.

Surgical results in this group of 38 patients include successful ablation of accessory pathways in all but two patients, no mortality, and one patient with heart block. Surgical failures occurred with the use of the open heart technique[11] in patients with multiple accessory pathways. During the first month after surgery there were five episodes of atrial fibrillation in three patients (0.3/patient). These early episodes of atrial fibrillation may have been related to postoperative inflammation. No episodes of atrial fibrillation were induced at the 1 week postoperative electrophysiologic study. During a mean long-term follow-up of 1.9 ± 0.7 years (range 0.8 to 3.2), only one patient has had recurrent atrial fibrillation. This particular patient, with a history of preoperative slow atrial fibrillation, has a cardiomyopathy. His ventricular response is well controlled and he has been maintained without medication. With the following exceptions, all patients have been maintained without medication. One patient with unsuccessful surgical ablation of the accessory pathway has been treated with amiodarone successfully. One patient had AV nodal reentrant tachycardia 1 year after surgery. This patient has been treated with propafenone and has had no further episodes of tachycardia. Preoperatively, this patient had reciprocating tachycardia and atrial fibrillation using an accessory pathway despite medical therapy.

Discussion

Recurrent paroxysmal atrial fibrillation has been reported to occur in up to 32% of patients with Wolff-Parkinson-White syndrome.[4] Atrial fibrillation in these patients may be potentially life threatening when it leads to rapid ventricular rates that may ultimately result in ventricular fibrillation. When pharmacologic management fails to control these arrhythmias, surgical ablation of the accessory pathway is a suitable alternative. However, it is not known whether surgical

TABLE 4
Incidence of atrial fibrillation

	Duration of symptoms (yr)	Episodes	Patients	Incidence (/patient/yr)
Preoperative	6.9 ± 5.8	89	19	1.97 ± 2.54^{A}
1 month postop	0.08	5	3	—
Follow-up	1.9 ± 0.7	5	1	0.098 ± 0.42^{A}

$^{A}p < .01$.

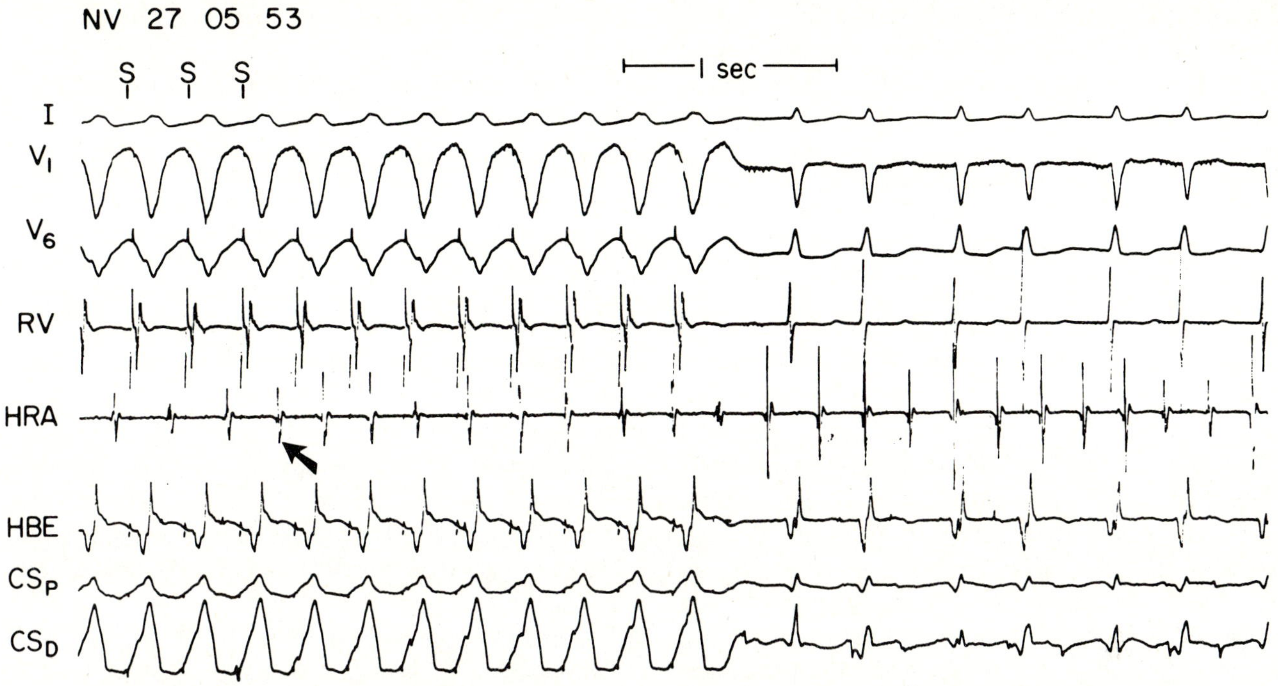

FIGURE 4. Induction of atrial flutter during ventricular incremental pacing. The arrow points to the first complex of atrial flutter. This patient had two atrioventricular accessory pathways, in the posteroseptal and left lateral region, both capable of conducting retrogradely. The presence of multiple pathways may lead to atrial activation from multiple sites during spontaneous ventricular ectopy. A collision of multiple atrial activation fronts may have provided the substrate for intra-atrial reentry. Atrial flutter rapidly degenerated to sustained atrial fibrillation in this case.

ablation of the accessory pathway will merely result in continued atrial fibrillation without preexcitation or whether it will actually alter the incidence of atrial fibrillation. Our study attempted to determine the effect of surgical ablation of the accessory pathway on the incidence of recurrent atrial fibrillation and to determine whether there are certain electrophysiologic parameters that identify patients in whom surgery is more likely to prevent recurrent atrial fibrillation.

Patients with a past history of recurrent, spontaneous atrial fibrillation are characterized by the presence of antegrade preexcitation, the frequent presence of multiple accessory pathways, and the presence of an accessory pathway with a relatively short antegrade effective refractory period. This combination of factors contributes to the excessively rapid ventricular rates that may occur in this group of patients when atrial fibrillation develops.[1, 14] A major difference observed between patients with a past history of atrial fibrillation and those with only reciprocating tachycardia was that the atrial fibrillation tended to be sustained when it was induced in the laboratory. In contrast, patients with reciprocating tachycardia had nonsustained atrial fibrillation in the electrophysiology laboratory and even this required more aggressive stimulation techniques. Two potential differences between these groups of patients may have contributed to atrial fibrillation being sustained. First, rapid ventricular responses to atrial fibrillation may result in hemodynamic deterioration and hypotension,[15] with a resultant reflex increase in sympathetic neural activity.[16] This increased sympathetic neural activity may predispose to the maintenance of atrial fibrillation and the development of more rapid ventricular response rates. This phenomenon has been observed in the electrophysiology laboratory in response to isoproterenol.[17] Second, the PA interval was observed to be significantly longer in patients with a past history of atrial fibrillation. This measurement may provide an index of intra-atrial conduction time.[18] Thus, in patients with potentially slower right intra-atrial conduction, there may be a predisposition to developing sustained atrial fibrillation. Therefore the results of the electrophysiologic study suggested a multifactorial etiology for sustained atrial fibrillation, including factors related to both the accessory pathway and slow conduction in the atrium.

The mode of initiation of atrial fibrillation in the laboratory more frequently suggested the presence of primary atrial vulnerability to atrial fibrillation. We observed spontaneous degeneration of AV reciprocating tachycardia to atrial fibrillation in only 16% of our patients, which is similar to the 26% observed by

Bauernfeind et al.[2] and 19% observed by Sung et al.[6] It is not clear to what extent this mode of induction of atrial fibrillation reflects primary atrial vulnerability. In the majority of patients, extrastimulus techniques or mechanically induced extrastimuli induced atrial fibrillation. Examination of the onset of atrial flutter and fibrillation by these modes did not indicate that the accessory pathway participated. We and others[7] have observed that sustained atrial fibrillation is rarely induced in normal patients during catheter placement or extrastimulus testing. This suggests that patients with atrial fibrillation induced by catheter placement or extrastimulus testing very likely have a primary atrial vulnerability to the development of atrial fibrillation.

On the basis of results of electrophysiologic testing, we could not determine whether recurrent atrial fibrillation was purely a function of the accessory pathway properties or whether there was indeed primary atrial vulnerability to the development of atrial fibrillation. We hypothesized that if recurrent atrial fibrillation is due entirely to the presence of the accessory pathway, then surgical ablation of the accessory pathway should prevent recurrent atrial fibrillation. In contrast, if there is primary atrial vulnerability then atrial fibrillation may continue to occur after surgery. Indeed, one might expect atrial fibrillation to occur more frequently in the immediate postoperative phase.

A total of 89 episodes of atrial fibrillation had been documented in 19 patients during a mean preoperative period of 6.9 years. This produced a conservative estimate of 1.97 episodes of atrial fibrillation per patient/year. During a mean follow-up of 1.9 years, only one patient had recurrent atrial fibrillation ($p < .01$). On the basis of this dramatic reduction in the recurrence of atrial fibrillation, we conclude that the accessory pathway is of prime importance in the induction of spontaneous atrial fibrillation and that any intraatrial abnormalities are of secondary importance and may contribute only to sustaining atrial fibrillation once initiated. This finding is of considerable significance because it allows us to maintain this group of patients without antiarrhythmic drug therapy after surgery. Recurrent atrial fibrillation after surgery could still be potentially dangerous in a high percentage of our patients. We observed that nine of 19 patients had AV nodal properties consistent with enhanced AV nodal conduction and might be able to sustain relatively rapid ventricular rates in the event of recurrent atrial fibrillation. Thus it is of considerable importance that atrial fibrillation does not recur after surgery. It will be of importance to determine whether this group of young patients with apparent atrial vulnerability will develop a high incidence of atrial fibrillation as they age.

It might be argued that the duration of follow-up is inadequate to determine the precise effects of surgery. However, among our patients, all had had at least one episode of atrial fibrillation during the year before surgery. In addition, only two patients had had a single episode of atrial fibrillation. Thus the great majority of our patients had multiple episodes of atrial fibrillation during their preoperative period. In addition, most patients showed a trend toward increasing frequency and severity of episodes of atrial fibrillation despite pharmacologic management. Only two of our patients required pharmacologic therapy after surgery, and thus, in the absence of antiarrhythmic drug therapy, we might have expected to have seen an even greater incidence of recurrent atrial fibrillation in the absence of a surgical effect.

Certain insights were provided by the single patient who continued to have recurrent atrial fibrillation. This patient was markedly different from the remaining population of patients with atrial fibrillation. This particular patient had a cardiomyopathy and thus was one of the few patients with organic heart disease in our patient population. In addition, the shortest RR interval during induced atrial fibrillation in this patient was 450 msec. This patient was therefore distinctly different in that his ventricular rate during atrial fibrillation was generally slow even in the absence of pharmacologic therapy. The observation that the occurrence of atrial fibrillation in patients with Wolff-Parkinson-White syndrome and organic heart disease may have different substrates than patients without heart disease is consistent with previous findings. Bauernfeind et al.[2] demonstrated that a subgroup of patients with Wolff-Parkinson-White syndrome without inducible AV reentrant tachycardia frequently had organic heart disease (86%). Thus organic heart disease may lead to atrial fibrillation even in the absence of AV reciprocating tachycardia. Our patient with a cardiomyopathy did have AV reciprocating tachycardia, but one would expect that this would only make the patient more likely to have atrial fibrillation in the presence of organic heart disease.

We conclude that patients with Wolff-Parkinson-White syndrome who have no organic heart disease but have antegrade preexcitation and develop rapid ventricular response rates during atrial fibrillation are not likely to have recurrent atrial fibrillation after surgical ablation of their accessory pathways. In contrast, patients with a history of paroxysmal atrial fibrillation who have organic heart disease, absent antegrade conduction via an accessory pathway, or slow ventricular rates during induced atrial fibrillation may be likely to have recurrent atrial fibrillation after ablation of their accessory pathways. This latter group may require continued antiarrhythmic therapy after surgery.

We express our appreciation to A. MacDonald, R.N., and N. Smith, R.N., for assistance in the electrophysiology laboratory, and to Mrs. D. Vigna for secretarial work.

References

1. Klein GJ, Bashore TM, Sellers TB, Pritchett ELC, Smith WM, Gallagher JJ: Ventricular fibrillation in the Wolff-Parkinson-White syndrome. N Engl J Med **301:** 1080, 1979
2. Bauernfeind RA, Wyndham CR, Swiryn SP, Palileo EV, Strasberg B, Lam W, Westveer D, Rosen KM: Paroxysmal atrial fibrillation in the Wolff-Parkinson-White syndrome. Am J Cardiol **47:** 562, 1981
3. Denes P, Wu D, Amat-y-Leon F, Dhingra R, Wyndham C, Kehoe R, Ayres BF, Rosen KM: Paroxysmal supraventricular tachycardia induction in patients with Wolff-Parkinson-White syndrome. Ann Intern Med **90:** 153, 1979
4. Campbell RWF, Smith RA, Gallagher JJ, Pritchett ELC, Wallace AG: Atrial fibrillation in the preexcitation syndrome. Am J Cardiol **40:** 514, 1977
5. Wellens HJJ: The electrophysiological properties of the accessory pathway in the Wolff-Parkinson-White syndrome. *In* Wellens HJJ, Lie KI, Janse MJ, editors: The conduction system of the heart: structure, function and clinical implications. Philadelphia, 1976, Lea and Febiger, p 567
6. Sung RJ, Castellanos A, Mallon SM, Bloom MG, Gelband H, Myerburg RJ: Mechanisms of spontaneous alternation between reciprocating tachycardia and atrial flutter-fibrillation in the Wolff-Parkinson-White syndrome. Circulation **56:** 409, 1977
7. Bauernfiend RA, Swiryn SP, Strasberg B, Palileo E, Scagliotti D, Rosen KM: Electrophysiologic drug testing in prophylaxis of sporadic paroxysmal atrial fibrillation: technique, application and efficacy in severely symptomatic preexcitation patients. Am Heart J **103:** 941, 1982
8. Morady F, Sledge C, Shen E, Sung RJ, Gonzales R, Scheinman MM: Electrophysiologic testing in the management of patients with the Wolff-Parkinson-White syndrome and atrial fibrillation. Am J Cardiol **51:** 1623, 1983
9. Klein GJ, Prystowsky EN, Pritchett ELC, Davis D, Gallagher JJ: Atypical patterns of retrograde conduction over accessory atrioventricular pathways in the Wolff-Parkinson-White syndrome. Circulation **60:** 1477, 1979
10. Gallagher JJ, Pritchett ELC, Sealy WC, Kasell J, Wallace AG: The preexcitation syndromes. Prog Cardiovasc Dis **20:** 285, 1978
11. Sealy WC, Gallagher JJ, Wallace AG: The surgical treatment of Wolff-Parkinson-White syndrome: evolution of improved methods for identification and interruption of the Kent bundle. Ann Thorac Surg **22:** 443, 1976
12. Klein GJ, Guiraudon GM, Perkins DG, Jones DL, Yee R, Jarvis E: Surgical correction of the Wolff-Parkinson-White syndrome in the closed heart using cryosurgery: a simplified approach. J Am Coll Cardiol **3:** 405, 1984
13. Watt JH, Donner AP, McKinney CM, Klein GJ: Atrial fibrillation: minimal sampling interval to estimate average rate. J Electrocardiol **17:** 153, 1984
14. Wellens HJJ, Durrer D: Wolff-Parkinson-White syndrome and atrial fibrillation: relation between refractory period of accessory pathway and ventricular rate during atrial fibrillation. Am J Cardiol **34:** 777, 1974
15. McIntosh HD, Kong Y, Morris JJ: Hemodynamic effects of supraventricular arrhythmias. Am J Med **37:** 712, 1964
16. Waxman MB, Sharma AD, Cameron DA, Huerta F, Wald RW: Reflex mechanisms responsible for early spontaneous termination of paroxysmal supraventricular tachycardia. Am J Cardiol **49:** 259, 1982
17. Wellens HJJ, Brugada P, Roy D, Weiss J, Bar FW: Effect of isoproterenol on the anterograde refractory period of the accessory pathway in patients with Wolff-Parkinson-White syndrome. Am J Cardiol **50:** 353, 1982
18. Josephson ME, Scharf DL, Kastor JA, Kitchen JG III: Atrial endocardial activation in man: electrode catheter techniques for endocardial mapping. Am J Cardiol **39:** 972, 1977

Efficacy and safety of transcatheter ablation of posteroseptal accessory pathways

FRED MORADY, M.D., MELVIN M. SCHEINMAN, M.D., STUART A. WINSTON, M.D., LORENZO A. DICARLO, JR., M.D., JESSIE C. DAVIS, M.D., JERRY C. GRIFFIN, M.D., MICHAEL RUDER, M.D., JOSEPH A. ABBOTT, M.D., AND MICHAEL ELDAR, M.D.

ABSTRACT Eight patients with a posteroseptal accessory pathway and symptomatic atrial fibrillation and/or orthodromic reciprocating tachycardia underwent attempted transcatheter ablation of the accessory pathway. A quadripolar electrode catheter was positioned within the coronary sinus such that the proximal pair of electrodes straddled the os. This proximal pair of electrodes was made electrically common and connected to the cathodal output of a defibrillator. A patch electrode placed over the midthoracic spine was connected to the anodal sink of the defibrillator. Two to three transcatheter shocks were delivered, with a cumulative energy of 600 to 900 J. Immediately after the shocks were delivered, retrograde accessory pathway conduction was absent in each patient. Anterograde conduction through the posteroseptal accessory pathway was absent in six patients and could not be assessed in two patients who each had a second right-sided accessory pathway. Long-term results were assessed in seven patients 4 to 11 months after delivery of the shocks. Anterograde and retrograde conduction through the posteroseptal accessory pathway was absent in five patients. In one patient, retrograde accessory pathway conduction was absent and anterograde conduction was present but was slower than at baseline. In this patient, orthodromic tachycardia was no longer inducible and the ventricular rate during induced atrial fibrillation was 150 beats/min, compared with 220 beats/min before the attempted ablation. He has remained asymptomatic without antiarrhythmic drug therapy for 18 months. In one patient, the transcatheter shocks had no long-term effect on accessory pathway conduction. The shocks delivered at the os of the coronary sinus were well tolerated. There was no long-term effect on anterograde conduction through the atrioventricular junction. Retrograde conduction through the atrioventricular junction was impaired in three patients. In four patients who underwent direct or angiographic visualization of the coronary sinus, no abnormalities were seen. Transcatheter ablation of posteroseptal accessory pathways has a long-term success rate of at least 75% and a low morbidity rate. Closed-chest catheter ablation of posteroseptal accessory pathways is an attractive alternative to surgical ablation of these pathways.
Circulation 72, No. 1, 170–177, 1985.

EXPERIENCE in more than 150 patients with supraventricular tachycardia refractory to pharmacologic treatment has indicated that catheter ablation of the atrioventricular junction results in good or excellent arrhythmia control in approximately 90% of patients.[1, 2] Catheter ablation of accessory pathways has also been attempted, but with less overall success. Attempts at ablation of left-sided accessory pathways by shocks delivered within the coronary sinus have generally been unsuccessful and, moreover, have resulted in perforation of the coronary sinus.[3] Catheter ablation of right-sided accessory pathways has been limited by difficulty in precisely localizing these pathways.[4–6] Attempts at transcatheter ablation of posteroseptal accessory pathways have met with some degree of success but, to date, the total published experience with this technique has consisted of only six patients.[7–10] The posteroseptal accessory pathway was successfully ablated in four of these six patients, and no complications were reported. However, only two cases in which the procedure was successful were reported in detail.[7, 10] Although encouraging, the results reported to date are clearly too preliminary to allow valid conclusions regarding the efficacy or safety of the catheter ablation technique in the treatment of patients who have a posteroseptal accessory pathway.

The purpose of this report is to present the results of

From the Department of Medicine and Cardiovascular Research Institute, University of California, San Francisco, and Division of Cardiology, Department of Internal Medicine, University Hospitals, University of Michigan, Ann Arbor.

Address for correspondence: Fred Morady, M.D., Division of Cardiology, W-11511, Box 55, University Hospitals, University of Michigan, 1405 E. Ann St., Ann Arbor, MI 48109.

Received March 5, 1985; revision accepted April 11, 1985.

attempted catheter ablation of a posteroseptal accessory pathway in a series of eight patients to help define the efficacy and safety of this new alternative to surgical ablation of posteroseptal accessory pathways.

Methods

Patient characteristics. The subjects of this report were five men and three women who had recurrent, symptomatic orthodromic reciprocating tachycardia. Their mean age was 31 ± 10 years (mean ± SD). Seven patients had the Wolff-Parkinson-White syndrome and a documented history of between one and six episodes of atrial fibrillation at an average rate varying between 220 and 300 beats/min. One patient (No. 4) had a concealed bypass tract and no history of atrial fibrillation. Seven patients had been treated with a mean of 2.3 ± 1.4 antiarrhythmic drugs that were either ineffective or not tolerated because of side effects. One patient did not undergo a clinical trial of antiarrhyhmic drug treatment before the attempt at catheter ablation. Patient 1 was the subject of a prior report.[7]

Baseline electrophysiologic study. Before catheter ablation, each patient underwent an electrophysiologic study while in the fasting, unsedated state, at least four half-lives after discontinuation of antiarrhythmic drugs. Quadripolar electrode catheters were introduced through a femoral or subclavian vein and positioned within the right atrium, right ventricle, coronary sinus, and across the tricuspid valve for recording the His bundle electrogram. The baseline accessory pathway conduction properties and refractory periods are listed in table 1. When determination of the anterograde or retrograde effective refractory period of the accessory pathway was limited by atrial or ventricular refractoriness, the accessory pathway effective refractory period was considered to be equal to or less than the atrial functional refractory period or the ventricular effective refractory period.

Orthodromic reciprocating tachycardia was induced in each patient. Participation of an accessory pathway as the retrograde limb of the tachycardia circuit was proven with use of standard criteria.[11]

Mapping of the accessory pathway was performed by recording atrial electrograms during orthodromic reciprocating tachycardia at various locations in the coronary sinus and around the tricuspid anulus. A posteroseptal accessory pathway was thought to be present if the earliest atrial activation during orthodromic reciprocating tachycardia was recorded at the os of the coronary sinus. Six patients were found to have a single posteroseptal accessory pathway, whereas two patients (Nos. 7 and 8) had both a posteroseptal and a right anterior accessory pathway. The interval between the onset of ventricular activation and the atrial electrogram recorded at the os of the coronary sinus during orthodromic reciprocating tachycardia varied from 77 to 130 msec (table 1).

In five patients, 1 to 1.5 g of intravenous procainamide (mean serum level 8.2 ± 3.1 mg/ml) was administered and found not to have any appreciable effects on accessory pathway conduction or refractoriness. Electropharmacologic testing was not performed in patient 3 or 4.

Catheter ablation protocol. The patients were offered the options of treatment with an investigational or, if appropriate, a conventional antiarrhythmic drug, surgical accessory pathway ablation, or catheter ablation. The two patients who had dual accessory pathways chose to undergo an attempt at catheter ablation of the posteroseptal accessory pathway in hopes of improving symptoms or as a prelude to surgical ablation of the right anterior accessory pathway. Before undergoing the catheter ablation procedure, each patient provided informed consent under a protocol approved by the Committee on Human Research at the University of California, San Francisco, or the University of Michigan.

Patients were brought to the electrophysiology laboratory while they were in the fasting, unsedated state. Blood pressure was monitored with a No. 5F cannula inserted into a femoral artery. An electrode catheter was inserted into a femoral vein and positioned against the right ventricular apex for pacing, if needed.

A No. 6F or 7F central lumen catheter was inserted into a subclavian vein and positioned in the coronary sinus under fluoroscopic guidance. After injection of contrast material to visualize the location of the os of the coronary sinus, this catheter was removed and replaced with a No. 6F or 7F quadripolar electrode catheter with 1 cm interelectrode distance (USCI, Billerica, MA). This catheter was positioned in the coronary sinus such that the proximal pair of electrodes straddled the os (figure 1). This proximal pair of electrodes was made electrically common and connected to the cathodal output of a defibrillator (Physio-Control, Redmond, WA). A 16 cm patch electrode (R-2 Corp., Skokie, IL) was placed over the midthoracic spine and connected to the anodal sink of the defibrillator. The patients were then anesthetized with sodium thiopental or sodium methohexital, and two or three 200 to 400 J discharges synchronized to the QRS were delivered within a 30 min period.

Atrial and ventricular stimulation were performed 5 to 10 min after each shock to assess their short-term effects on the accessory pathway.

After the ablation procedure, serial creatine kinase and creatine kinase–MB fraction levels were measured and the patients underwent continuous electrocardiographic monitoring for at least 4 days. A technetium pyrophosphate scintigram was obtained in each of five patients. A 24 hr continuous ambulatory electrocardiographic recording was obtained 4 to 7 days after delivery of the shocks.

A follow-up electrophysiologic study was performed 4 to 8 months after the attempt at catheter ablation in each of the six

TABLE 1

Accessory pathway characteristics before catheter ablation

Patient No.	1:1 anterograde conduction (msec)[A]	Anterograde ERP (msec)	1:1 retrograde conduction (msec)[B]	Retrograde ERP (msec)	VA at os of CS (msec)[C]
Patients with a single posteroseptal accessory pathway					
1	275	≤320	<250	≤200	90
2	300	≤280	300	290	126
3	250	≤280	225	≤230	100
4	CBT	CBT	275	260	85
5	250	250	250	≤230	77
6	275	≤250	300	310	115
Patients with a posteroseptal and right-sided accessory pathway					
7	275	260	300	ND	100
8	400	330	250	310	130

ERP = effective refractory period; VA = ventriculoatrial interval; CS = coronary sinus; CBT = concealed bypass tract; ND = not determined.

[A]Minimum atrial paced cycle length associated with 1:1 anterograde accessory pathway conduction.

[B]Minimum ventricular paced cycle length associated with 1:1 retrograde accessory pathway conduction.

[C]Ventriculoatrial interval recorded at the os of the coronary sinus during orthodromic reciprocating tachycardia.

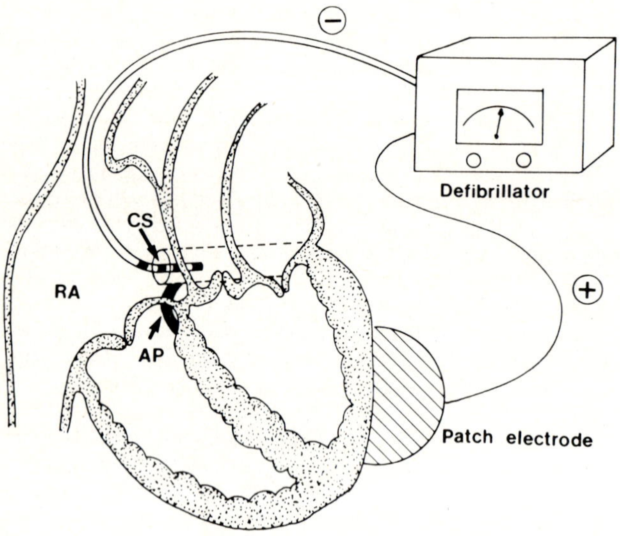

FIGURE 1. A schematic illustration of the technique used to ablate posteroseptal accessory pathways with transcatheter shocks. A quadripolar electrode catheter is positioned in the coronary sinus such that the proximal pair of electrodes straddles the os. This pair of electrodes is made electrically common and connected to the cathodal output of a defibrillator. A patch electode positioned over the midthoracic spine is connected to the anodal sink of the defibrillator. Not shown is an electrode catheter that is placed into the right ventricle for backup pacing if needed. A transcatheter shock is delivered after the patient is anesthetized. AP = accessory pathway; CS = coronary sinus; RA = right atrium.

patients who had an isolated posteroseptal accessory pathway. In patient 8, the effect of the intracardiac shocks on the posteroseptal accessory pathway was assessed by direct epicardial mapping 11 months later, at the time of surgical ablation of the right anterior accessory pathway. Patient 7 has not undergone follow-up electrophysiologic testing.

In three patients (Nos. 1, 5, and 6) coronary angiography was performed and the coronary sinus was visualized during the venous phase 4 months after the catheter ablation procedure. In patient 8, the coronary sinus was inspected directly at the time of surgical ablation of a right-sided accessory pathway 11 months after the catheter ablation procedure.

Results

Immediate results (table 2). The initial shock was either 300 or 400 J in strength. The immediate effect of this initial shock was to abolish anterograde conduction through the posteroseptal accessory pathway in four of the seven patients in whom the bypass tract was not concealed. In patient 6, anterograde conduction was not abolished after an initial shock of 300 J, but was abolished after a second shock of 400 J. In the two patients with dual accessory pathways (patients 7 and 8), the short-term effect of the shocks on anterograde conduction through the posteroseptal accessory pathway was indeterminate because of the presence of ventricular preexcitation via the right anterior accessory pathway. No change in the delta wave pattern during sinus rhythm or incremental atrial pacing was noted in these two patients.

In seven patients, retrograde conduction through the posteroseptal accessory pathway was abolished after the first shock; in patient 6, retrograde conduction over the accessory pathway was abolished only after the second shock.

After anterograde and/or retrograde conduction was abolished by the first or second shock, each patient received an additional 200 to 400 J discharge. The cumulative stored energy used was 600 to 900 J (mean 762 ± 106 J).

Late results (table 2). The long-term effects of the transcatheter shocks on conduction through the posteroseptal accessory pathway were assessed after 4 to 11 months of follow-up in seven patients. In five patients, there was no evidence of anterograde or retrograde conduction through the posteroseptal accessory pathway (figures 2 and 3). Each of these patients has remained asymptomatic over a follow-up period of 5 to 22 months (mean 11.4 ± 7.3 months).

Delta waves reappeared on the electrocardiogram between 1 and 6 weeks after delivery of the transcatheter shocks in patient 2. He remained asymptomatic without antiarrhythmic medications, and an electrophysiologic study 8 months later demonstrated one-to-one anterograde accessory pathway conduction to a minimum atrial paced cycle length of 350 msec, and an anterograde accessory pathway effective refractory period of less than 210 msec. However, there was no evidence of retrograde accessory pathway conduction,

TABLE 2
Effects of transcatheter shocks on posteroseptal accessory pathway conduction

Patient No.	No. of shocks	Cumulative energy (J)	Immediate results: Ant cond	Immediate results: Retro cond	Late results (4–11 mo): Ant cond	Late results (4–11 mo): Retro cond
1	2	800	0	0	0	0
2	2	800	0	0	+[A]	0
3	2	800	0	0	+	+
4	2	600	CBT	0	CBT	0
5	2	600	0	0	0	0
6	3	900	0	0	0	0
7	2	800	Indet[B]	0	ND	ND
8	2	800	Indet[B]	0	0	0

0 = No conduction; + = conduction present; Ant = anterograde; cond = conduction; CBT = concealed bypass tract; Indet = indeterminate; ND = not determined; Retro = retrograde.

[A]Conduction present, but markedly diminished from baseline.

[B]Effect on conduction indeterminate because of ventricular preexcitation via right anterior accessory pathway.

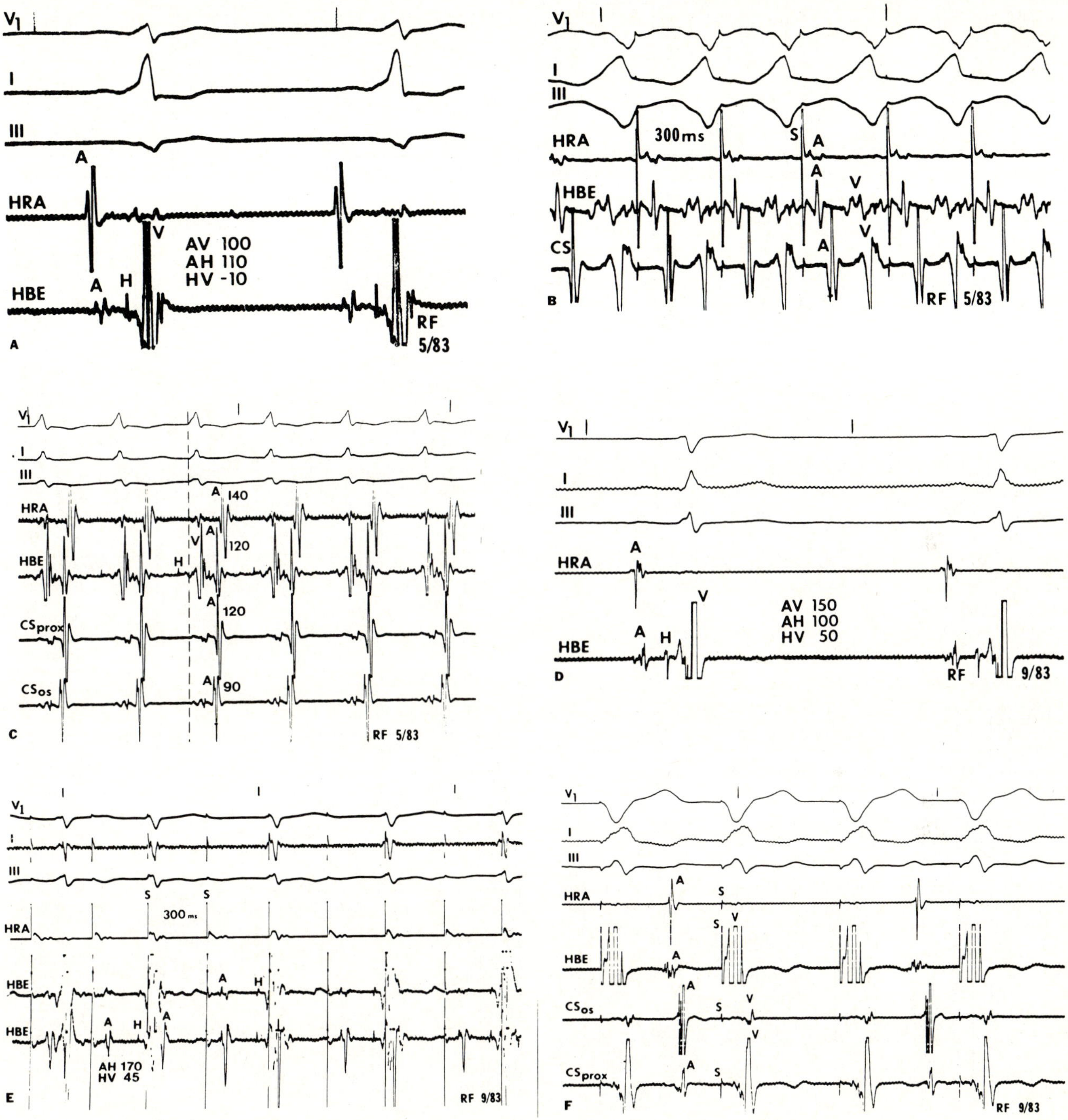

FIGURE 2. Results of electrophysiologic testing before and 4 months after transcatheter ablation of a posteroseptal accessory pathway in patient 1. *A*, Baseline His bundle electrogram (HBE) demonstrated ventricular preexcitation, with an HV of −10 msec and an atrioventricular interval (AV) of 100 msec. A = atrial electrogram; H = His bundle depolarization; HRA = high right atrial electrogram. Time lines in this and subsequent figures represent 1 sec intervals. *B*, Atrial pacing at a cycle length of 300 msec resulted in 1:1 conduction through the accessory pathway. The AV interval remained constant at 100 msec. CS = coronary sinus electrogram. *C*, During orthodromic reciprocating tachycardia, the shortest ventriculoatrial (VA) interval (90 msec) was recorded at the os of the coronary sinus (CS_{os}), consistent with retrograde conduction over a posteroseptal accessory pathway during the tachycardia. The number over each electrogram refers to the VA interval in msec recorded in that electrogram. CS_{prox} = proximal coronary sinus. *D*, Four months after the delivery of two 400 J shocks at the os of the coronary sinus, there is no ventricular preexcitation during sinus rhythm. The HV has increased to 50 msec, and the AV to 150 msec. *E*, Atrial pacing at a cycle length of 300 msec resulted in 2:1 atrioventricular nodal block, with an HV of 45 msec and no ventricular preexcitation. S = stimulus. *F*, Ventricular pacing at a cycle length of 600 msec resulted in 2:1 retrograde conduction through the atrioventricular junction. Note that the low septal right atrial electrogram (recorded in the HBE) now precedes the atrial electrogram recorded at the coronary sinus os. In this patient, anterograde and retrograde conduction over the posteroseptal accessory pathway were completely eliminated by the transcatheter shocks.

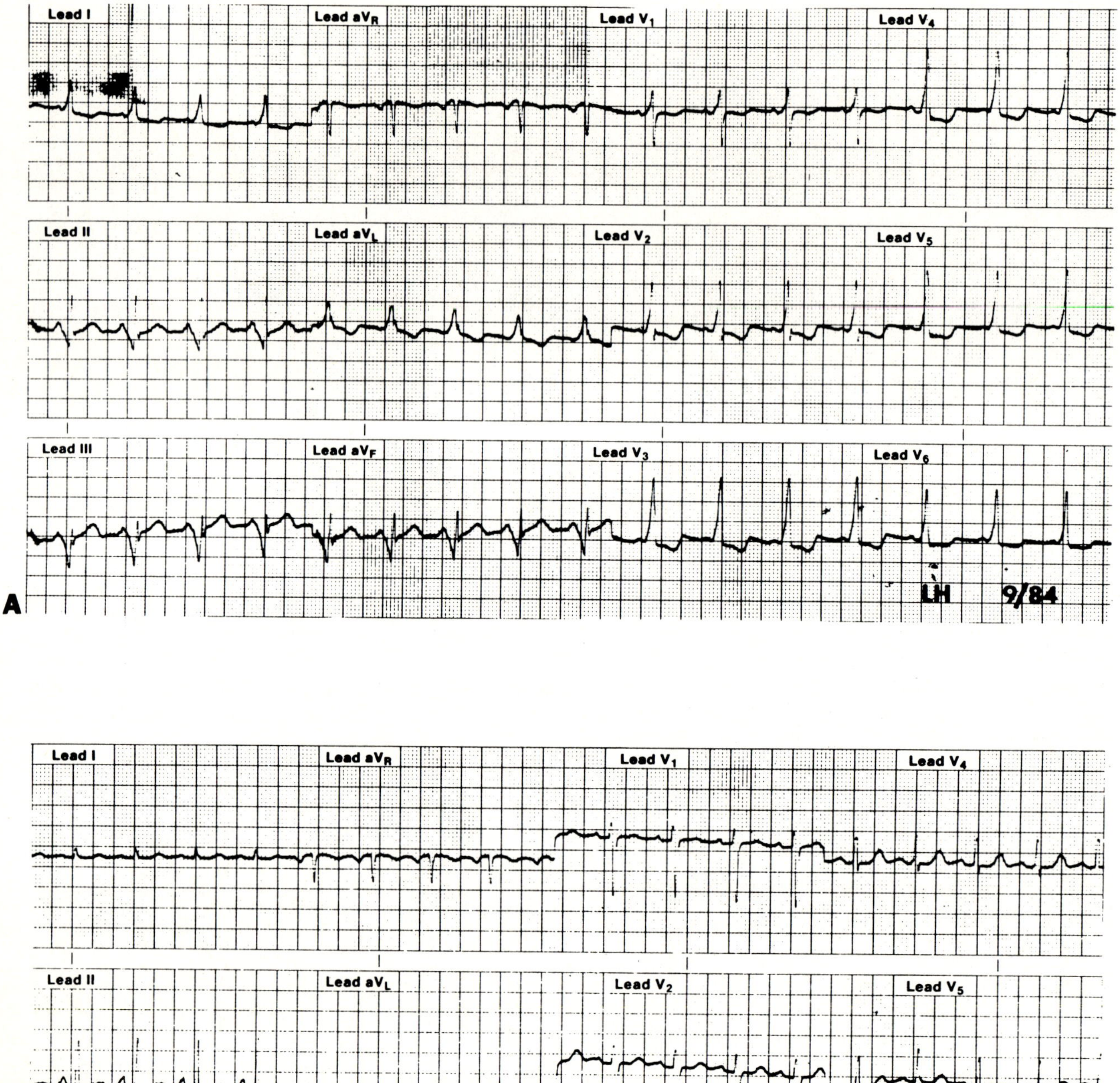

FIGURE 3. Electrocardiograms before and 4 months after transcatheter ablation of a posteroseptal accessory pathway in patient 5. *A*, The baseline electrocardiogram demonstrated inverted delta waves in leads II, III, and aVF, and upright delta waves in leads I, aVL, and V_1–V_6. This pattern of delta waves and the transition from a small to large R wave between V_1 and V_2 is characteristic of ventricular preexcitation over a posteroseptal accessory pathway. *B*, Four months after the delivery of two 300 J shocks at the coronary sinus os, there is a normal PR interval and delta waves are not present. Electrophysiologic testing demonstrated the absence of anterograde or retrograde accessory pathway conduction.

and orthodromic reciprocating tachycardia was not inducible. When atrial fibrillation was induced, the average ventricular rate was 150 beats/min, and the shortest preexcited RR interval was 320 msec (vs 220 beats/min and 200 msec, respectively, at baseline). This patient has remained asymptomatic without drug treatment over a follow-up period of 18 months.

In patient 3, delta waves reappeared on the electrocardiogram on the sixth day after delivery of the transcatheter shocks. An electrophysiologic study 1 day later demonstrated that both anterograde and retrograde accessory pathway conduction were present, without a change from baseline. He was treated with quinidine and nadolol and experienced no symptomatic arrhythmia. After 9 months, drug therapy was temporarily discontinued and an electrophysiologic study demonstrated that the conduction and refractoriness properties of the accessory pathway were not changed from baseline. He was treated with procainamide and has remained asymptomatic over a total follow-up period of 17 months.

Effects on the atrioventricular junction. A transient junctional rhythm lasting several seconds to several minutes occurred in each patient immediately after delivery of the transcatheter shocks. Atrioventricular nodal Wenckebach block occurred for several minutes in one patient. Continuous ambulatory electrocardiographic monitoring 4 to 7 days after delivery of the shocks demonstrated sinus rhythm without atrioventricular block in all patients.

The effects of the transcatheter shocks on the atrioventricular junction were assssed in six patients during a follow-up electrophysiologic study 4 to 9 months after delivery of the transcatheter shocks (table 3). The atrioventricular nodal conduction time (AH) was 75 to 100 msec (mean 87 ± 11 msec) and in each patient was within 5 msec of the baseline AH (mean 88 ± 12, $p > .05$). The infranodal conduction time (HV) was 40 to 50 msec (mean 45 ± 4 msec) in the absence of ventricular preexcitation during sinus rhythm (patients 1, 4 to 6), after 700 mg of intravenous procainamide (patient 2), and during orthodromic reciprocating tachycardia (patient 3).

During incremental atrial pacing there was one-to-one conduction through the atrioventricular junction to a mimimum paced cycle length of 275 to 400 msec (mean 380 ± 54 msec). In patient 3, the presence of ventricular preexcitation during atrial pacing prevented assessment of conduction through the atrioventricular junction. The mean atrioventricular nodal effective refractory period was 305 ± 54 msec (range 240 to 370 msec).

TABLE 3

Effects of transcatheter shocks delivered at the os of the coronary sinus on the atrioventricular junction at 4 to 9 months of follow-up

Patient No.	AH (msec)	HV (msec)[A]	1:1 anterograde cond (msec)[B]	Ant AVN ERP (msec)	1:1 retro cond (msec)[C]	Retro ERP (msec)
1	100	50	400	280	700	340
2	100	50	400	370	VAD	—
3	85	45	Preex	240	ND[D]	ND[D]
4	80	40	400	370	VAD	—
5	75	45	275	300	350	220
6	80	40	375	270	350	260

Ant = anterograde; cond = conduction; ERP = effective refractory period; Preex = preexcited; VAD = ventriculoatrial dissociation.

[A]In the absence of ventricular preexcitation.

[B]Minimum paced atrial cycle length associated with 1:1 conduction.

[C]Minimum paced ventricular cycle length associated with 1:1 conduction.

[D]Not determined, because of retrograde accessory pathway conduction.

Incremental ventricular pacing demonstrated that ventriculoatrial dissociation was present in two patients (Nos. 2 and 4). One-to-one retrograde conduction through the atrioventricular node was present to a minumum paced cycle length of between 350 and 700 msec (mean 467 ± 202 msec) in four patients. The retrograde effective refractory period could be determined in four patients and varied between 220 and 340 msec (mean 273 ± 61). In patient 3, the presence of retrograde accessory pathway conduction prevented the measurement of retrograde conduction or refractoriness in the atrioventricular junction.

Other effects of the transcatheter shocks. The mean peak creatine kinase serum level after delivery of the shocks was 364 ± 360 IU/liter, and the mean peak MB fraction was 31 ± 28 IU/liter. A technetium pyrophosphate scintigram showed no myocardial uptake in four patients and focal lateral ventricular uptake suggestive of a myocardial infarction in one patient.

Occasional multiform ventricular premature depolarizations were noted in patient 3 during the first 4 days after the catheter ablation procedure. Ventricular or supraventricular tachycardia was not observed in any patient.

In three patients (Nos. 1, 5, and 6) coronary angiography demonstrated a normal left and right coronary artery and a normal coronary sinus. In patient 8, the coronary sinus and right atrium appeared grossly normal on direct visual inspection at the time of surgical ablation of a right-sided accessory pathway 11 months after delivery of the transcatheter shocks.

Discussion

The results presented herein suggest that the delivery of transcatheter shocks at the os of the coronary sinus is an effective and safe technique by which posteroseptal accessory pathways can be ablated on a long-term basis. Evaluation at 4 or more months of follow-up demonstrated that accessory pathway conduction was completely eliminated, or at least modified so that potentially life-threatening tachyarrhythmias no longer occurred, in a minimum of six of eight patients (75%). Because the ablation procedure may have been effective in patient 7 (who did not undergo a follow-up electrophysiologic study) the success rate may have been as high as 88% (seven of eight patients). The catheter ablation technique therefore appears to be an attractive alternative to surgical bypass tract ablation in patients with a posteroseptal accessory pathway who are appropriate candidates for nonpharmacologic therapy. The catheter ablation technique obviates the need for a thorocotomy and is associated with less expense, less discomfort, and a considerably shorter convalescence period than is surgical accessory pathway ablation.

There have been few detailed histologic studies of posteroseptal accessory pathways. In a recent report by Critelli et al.[12] postmortem histologic analysis in a patient who had a posteroseptal accessory pathway demonstrated that the fibers of the accessory pathway originated from the lower rim of the coronary sinus. The close proximity of posteroseptal accessory pathways to the os of the coronary sinus provides the anatomic basis for the effectiveness of the technique used in the present report, in which transcatheter shocks are applied at the coronary sinus os. Although the reason that the ablation procedure was not successful in patient 3 is unclear, it may be that the posteroseptal accessory pathways do not always originate at the rim of the coronary sinus os.

A prior study on the effects of transcatheter shocks delivered within the coronary sinus in patients with left-sided accessory pathways demonstrated that perforation of the coronary sinus and cardiac tamponade was possible with two shocks of 100 and 150 J.[3] Although the shocks used in the present report were as high as 400 J in strength, no patient developed signs of coronary sinus perforation or cardiac tamponade. However, great care was taken to deliver these high-energy shocks at the os, where there is atrial myocardium, instead of within the coronary sinus, which is a thin-walled vein. The risk of cardiac tamponade induced by transcatheter shocks delivered within the coronary sinus emphasizes the importance of visualizing the os by contrast injection and positioning the electrode catheter such that the proximal two electrodes straddle the os and are not actually within the coronary sinus when the transcatheter shocks are delivered.

Because posteroseptal accessory pathways may lie in close proximity to the atrioventricular node–His bundle axis, surgical ablation of these pathways is associated with approximately a 10% risk of creating high-degree atrioventricular block.[13] Our results indicate that although transcatheter shocks at the os of the coronary sinus may temporarily impair atrioventricular conduction, persistent atrioventricular block is unlikely to occur. Although transient junctional rhythm or atrioventricular nodal block occurred in several patients, persistent high-degree atrioventricular nodal block was never induced by the transcatheter shocks. The only long-term effect on the atrioventricular junction observed was impaired retrograde conduction in three patients. A study on the effects of transcatheter shocks on the atrioventricular junction in dogs demonstrated that even when shocks are delivered in close proximity to the atrioventricular node, histologic damage to the atrioventricular junction may be associated with only minimal changes in atrioventricular conduction[14]; this observation suggests that there is a large safety margin for atrioventricular conduction. It is therefore unlikely that high-degree atrioventricular block would occur from shocks applied at the coronary sinus os. However, because of the possibility of inducing transient atrioventricular block, a temporary ventricular pacemaker should be in place before catheter ablation of a posteroseptal accessory pathway is attempted.

Prior reports have demonstrated an association between posteroseptal and right-sided accessory pathways in patients with and those without Ebstein's anomaly.[15, 16] Accordingly, two patients in this report (Nos. 7 and 8) had a posteroseptal and right-sided acccessory pathway. Although an effect of the transcatheter shocks on retrograde conduction through the posteroseptal accessory pathway was apparent based on a dramatic change in the atrial activation sequence during orthodromic reciprocating tachycardia, the effect on anterograde conduction was obscured by the presence of ventricular preexcitation via the right-sided accessory pathway. It is interesting to note that both patients had inverted delta waves in the inferior leads on their baseline electrocardiograms, consistent with ventricular activation through a posteroseptal accessory pathway. In neither patient was there a change in the delta wave pattern after the transcatheter shocks had been delivered. Although this suggested that there was persisting anterograde conduction over the posteroseptal accessory pathway, direct epicardial mapping at the time of surgical ablation of the right-sided accessory pathway in patient 8 demonstrated no evidence of anterograde or retrograde conduction through a posteroseptal accessory pathway. The reason that the delta wave pattern did not change despite complete conduction block in the posteroseptal accessory pathway is unclear.

As would be expected, transcatheter shocks of 200 to 400 J resulted in some degree of myocardial injury, as evidenced by release of creatine–kinase MB fraction. However, technetium pyrophosphate scintigrams demonstrated either no myocardial uptake or a small area of focal uptake, suggesting that the injury was very localized. Although ventricular premature depolarizations occurred transiently in one patient, no patient experienced a malignant ventricular arrhythmia as a complication of the transcatheter shocks.

Coronary angiography in three patients demonstrated that the transcatheter shocks did not cause any damage to the coronary arteries. Whereas shocks within the coronary sinus frequently result in coronary sinus obstruction or stenosis,[3, 17] no coronary sinus abnormalities were observed as a result of transcatheter shocks to the coronary sinus os in the four patients in the present series in whom the coronary sinus was visualized either directly or during angiography.

Approximately one-third of accessory atrioventricular connections are posteroseptal in location.[13] In the past, if the patient with a posteroseptal pathway was an appropriate candidate for nonpharmacologic therapy, the definitive form of treatment was surgical ablation of the accessory pathway. However, even in the best of hands, surgical ablation of posteroseptal accessory pathways is more difficult than ablation of free-wall accessory pathways, and is associated with approximately a 10% risk of complete atrioventricular block.[13] Our results suggest that catheter ablation of posteroseptal accessory pathways may be a viable alternative to surgical ablation. Although confirmation in a larger number of patients is needed, the long-term success rate of the catheter ablation technique described herein appears to be at least 75% and the morbidity rate appears to be acceptably small.

We gratefully acknowledge the secretarial assistance of Mrs. Lisa Hackbarth.

References

1. Scheinman MM, Evans-Bell T, and the Executive Committee of the Percutaneous Cardiac Mapping and Ablation Registry: Catheter ablation of the atrioventricular junction: a report of the percutaneous mapping and ablation registry. Circulation **70:** 1024, 1984
2. Nathan AW, Bennett DH, Ward DE, Bexton RS, Camm AJ: Catheter ablation of atrioventricular conduction. Lancet **I:** 1280, 1984
3. Fisher JD, Brodman R, Kim SG, Matos JA, Brodman LE, Wallerson D, Waspe LE: Attempted nonsurgical electrical ablation of accessory pathways via the coronary sinus in the Wolff-Parkinson-White syndrome. J Am Coll Cardiol **4:** 685, 1984
4. Kunze KP, Kuck KH: Transvenous ablation of accessory pathways in patients with incessant atrioventricular tachycardia. Circulation **70**(suppl II): II-412, 1984
5. Weber H, Schmitz L: Catheter technique for closed-chest ablation of an accessory atrioventricular pathway. N Engl J Med **308:** 653, 1983
6. Weber H, Schmitz L, Hellberg K: Pacemaker-mediated tachycardias: a new modality of treatment. Pace **7:** 1010, 1984
7. Morady F, Scheinman MM: Transvenous catheter ablation of a posteroseptal accessory pathway in a patient with the Wolff-Parkinson-White syndrome. N Engl J Med **310:** 705, 1984
8. Jackman WM, Friday KJ, Scherlag BJ, Dehning MM, Schechter E, Reynolds DW, Olson EG, Berbari EJ, Harrison LA, Lazzara R: Direct endocardial recording from an accessory atrioventricular pathway: localization of the site of block, effect of antiarrhythmic drugs, and attempt at nonsurgical ablation. Circulation **68:** 906, 1983
9. Nathan AW, Davies DW, Creamer JE, Butrous GS, Camm AJ: Successful catheter ablation of abnormal atrioventricular pathways in man. Circulation **70**(suppl II): II-99, 1984
10. Bardy GH, Poole JE, Coltorti F, Ivey TD, Block TA, Trobaugh GB, Greene HL: Catheter ablation of a concealed accessory pathway. Am J Cardiol **54:** 1366, 1984
11. Josephson ME, Seides SF: Clinical cardiac electrophysiology. Philadelphia, 1979, Lea & Febiger, p 225
12. Critelli G, Gallagher JJ, Monda V, Coltorti F, Scherillo M, Rossi L: Anatomic and electrophysiologic substrate of the permanent form of junctional reciprocating tachycardia. J Am Coll Cardiol **4:** 601, 1984
13. Gallagher JJ, Sealy WC, Cox JL, Kasell JH: Results of surgery for preexcitation in 200 consecutive cases. *In* Levy S, Scheinman MM, editors: Cardiac arrhythmias from diagnosis to treatment. New York, 1984, Futura, p 540
14. Scheinman MM, Bharati S, Wang YS, Shapiro WA, Lev M: Electrophysiologic and anatomic changes in the atrioventricular junction of dogs after direct-current shocks through tissue fixation catheters. Am J Cardiol **55:** 194, 1985
15. Smith WM, Gallagher JJ, Kerr CR, Sealy WC, Kasell JH, Benson DW Jr, Reiter MJ, Sterba R, Grant AO: The electrophysiologic basis and management of symptomatic recurrent tachycardia in patients with Ebstein's anomaly of the tricuspid valve. Am J Cardiol **49:** 1223, 1982
16. Morady F, Scheinman MM, DiCarlo LA Jr, Winston SA, Davis JC, Baerman JM, Krol RB, Crevey BJ: Coexistent posteroseptal and right-sided atrioventricular bypass tracts. J Am Coll Cardiol **5:** 640, 1985
17. Brodman R, Fisher JD: Evaluation of a catheter technique for ablation of accessory pathways near the coronary sinus using a canine model. Circulation **67:** 923, 1984

A comparison of the thrombolytic and hemorrhagic effects of tissue-type plasminogen activator and streptokinase in rabbits

GIANCARLO AGNELLI, M.D.,** MICHAEL R. BUCHANAN, PH.D., FRANCOISE FERNANDEZ, D.UN.PH., BERNARD BONEU, M.D.,** JOANNE VAN RYN, B.SC., JACK HIRSH, M.D., AND DÉSIRÉ COLLEN, M.D.

ABSTRACT Tissue-type plasminogen activator (t-PA) is a promising thrombolytic agent because it can produce thrombolysis without inducing a plasma proteolytic state. It is uncertain if this potentially important feature renders t-PA less hemorrhagic than other plasminogen activators. We have compared the hemorrhagic and thrombolytic effects of t-PA and streptokinase in rabbits. Streptokinase, 4000 U/kg/hr over 4 hr, failed to produce significant thrombolysis and 8000 U/kg/hr streptokinase over 4 hr produced only 28 ± 6% thrombolysis. Both streptokinase regimens were associated with a plasmin-mediated plasma proteolytic state and both streptokinase regimens produced a significant increase in hemorrhage that was evident within 15 min of beginning the infusion and was progressive over the 4 hr of drug administration. In contrast, t-PA in a dose of 7500 U/kg/hr produced 35 ± 6% thrombolysis, but it did not produce a plasmin-mediated plasma proteolytic state or a significant increase in hemorrhage over the 4 hr of infusion. t-PA in a dose of 15,000 U/kg/hr produced 85 ± 4% thrombolysis but was associated with a plasmin-mediated proteolytic state and produced significant bleeding which, in contrast to streptokinase-induced bleeding, was delayed in onset. Therefore, t-PA induced less hemorrhage than streptokinase at doses that produced more effective thrombolysis. Bleeding with both thrombolytic agents was associated with a plasmin-mediated proteolytic state.
Circulation 72, No. 1, 178–182, 1985.

THROMBOLYTIC THERAPY with streptokinase and urokinase is gaining increasing acceptance as a treatment for venous thrombosis and pulmonary embolism and is presently being reevaluated for the treatment of acute myocardial infarction.[1-5] The major side effect of thrombolytic therapy is hemorrhage. Bleeding is caused by a combination of lysis of fibrin in wounds and of a systemic hemostatic defect that occurs as a consequence of plasmin-mediated proteolysis of plasma coagulation factors. The systemic hemostatic defect is characterized by hypofibrinogenemia, a reduction in the levels of factors V and VIII, an increase in fibrinogen-split products (which causes defective fibrin polymerization),[6] and possibly by a platelet function defect.[7]

In recent years, a new plasminogen activator has been developed that has potential advantages over streptokinase and urokinase because it can produce fibrinolysis without inducing a generalized hemostatic defect. This enzyme, known as extrinsic tissue plasminogen activator (t-PA), is a serine protease that has been isolated from a human melanoma cell line[8] and has been produced for clinical uses by recombinant DNA technology.[9] t-PA binds to fibrin with a greater affinity than either urokinase or streptokinase and when bound to fibrin, it is activated and converts plasminogen to plasmin on the fibrin surface.

Investigations in animals and in humans have demonstrated that the infusion of melanoma cell–derived t-PA is associated with thrombolysis without a significant generalized coagulation defect.[10-16] These findings have recently been confirmed in studies of DNA-recombinant t-PA.[17-19]

The potential advantages of use of t-PA rather than

From the Departments of Medicine and Pathology, McMaster University, Hamilton, Ontario, and Centre for Thrombosis and Vascular Research, University of Leuven, Belgium.

Supported by a grant from the Ontario Heart and Stroke Foundation.

Address for correspondence: Dr. M. R. Buchanan, Room 3N10, Department of Pathology, McMaster University Medical Centre, 1200 Main St. West, Hamilton, Ontario, Canada L8N 3Z5.

Received Oct. 30, 1984; revision accepted Feb. 28, 1985.

*Present address: Istituto di Clinica Medica, Universita di Perugia, Policlinico Monteluce, 06100, Perugia, Italy.

**Present address: Centre Regionale de Transfusion Sanguine, Laboratoire Central d'Hematologie et de Genetique, Hopital Purpan, 31052 Toulouse, France.

urokinase and streptokinase as a thrombolytic agent is predicated by its ability to induce fibrinolysis without inducing a plasma proteolytic state. The importance of this potential advantage is critically dependent on the following relative contributions to bleeding associated with therapeutic thrombolysis: (1) local fibrinolysis in hemostatic plugs and (2) the plasmin-induced generalized coagulation defect. To date, the relative contributions of these mechanisms to hemorrhage caused by thrombolytic therapy has not been defined. We have performed a study in which the hemorrhagic effects of equivalent thrombolytic concentrations of streptokinase and t-PA were compared in rabbits.

Materials and methods

Materials. t-PA was derived from the culture fluid of human melanoma cells according to the method of Rijken and Collen.[8] Its specific activity was determined by assessing its dose-related fibrinolytic effects on plasminogen-enriched bovine fibrin plates and was expressed as international units as compared with known amounts of urokinase. Streptokinase (Streptase; lot No. 0180A) was obtained from Behringwerke AG, Marburg, F.D.R. The chromogenic substrate (S2251, lot No. 85794 51) and the human plasmin (25 caesin U/bottle; lot No. 6728951) used in the α_2-antiplasmin activity assays were obtained from Kabi Diagnostica, Stockholm, Sweden. ^{125}I (Na^{125}I, 610 mCi/ml, carrier free) was obtained from New England Nuclear, Boston. Sodium pentobarbital was obtained from MTC Pharmaceuticals, Hamilton, Ontario. Fibrinogen (>90% clottable) was prepared from pooled rabbit plasma and labeled with ^{125}I by the iodine/monochloride method.[20] All animal studies were performed with New Zealand white rabbits and conformed to the guiding principles of the American Physiological Society.

Method of preparation of radioactive jugular vein thrombi. Standard-sized, preformed ^{125}I-labeled thrombi were produced in the external jugular veins of rabbits (2.3 to 3.5 kg). The procedure used to produce radiolabeled thrombi was as follows: Both external jugular veins were exposed through a paramedial incision in the neck. Each vein was cleared over a distance of 2 cm and small side branches were ligated. A 3-0 Ti-Cron braided polyester thread, presoaked in a collagen solution, was then introduced lengthwise in the lumen of the jugular vein. After 30 min the vein was clamped both proximally and distally to isolate the vein segment. Then 0.15 ml of rabbit blood containing 5 μl of ^{125}I-labeled rabbit fibrinogen (approximately 500,000 cpm) was aspirated in a 1 ml syringe containing 1 U of thrombin and 10 μl of $CaCl_2$ (0.25M). This mixture was quickly injected in the isolated jugular vein with the use of a 25-gauge needle. In all instances the thrombus formed quickly and it was allowed to age for 30 min before both vessel clamps were removed. The restoration of blood flow was checked.

Characteristics of jugular vein thrombi

Urea solubility. Radioactive jugular vein thrombi were prepared as described above. The thrombi were removed and the solubility in 5M urea was tested. The thrombi were washed in saline and then immersed in 5 ml 5M urea and the supernatant was assayed for radioactivity at 0, 30, 60, 120, 240, and 360 min and 24 hr. Less than 1% of the radioactivity appeared in the supernatant over the 24 hr incubation period.

Release of radioactivity during thrombolysis in vitro. To determine whether the thrombi were uniformly labeled with ^{125}I, jugular vein thrombi were recovered and incubated in rabbit platelet-poor plasma containing streptokinase in a final concentration of 300 U/ml. The experiment was performed with eight thrombi. Two thrombi were removed at 1, 2, 3, and 4 hr, respectively, they were weighed, and the total radioactivity measured. There was a parallel decrease in weight and total radioactivity over the 4 hr period (r = .998).

Assessment of thrombolysis in vivo. Rabbits were infused through the marginal ear vein with streptokinase (4000, 8000 or 16,000 U/kg/hr) or t-PA (7500 and 15,000 U/kg/hr) or an equivolume of suspending vehicle (saline). Ten percent of the total dose of both fibrinolytic agents was administered as a bolus loading dose and the remaining 90% of the total dose was infused over the next 4 hr. (This dosage regimen was designed to simulate regimens that have been successful in inducing thrombolysis in patients with acute vein thrombosis and pulmonary embolism.[1, 2]) At the end of the infusion, the thrombi remaining in the vessels were removed and their size was determined by measuring the amount of residual ^{125}I-labeled fibrinogen remaining in the thrombi and by measuring their wet weight and comparing the results with those of the saline controls.

Assessment of hemorrhagic side effects. Other rabbits were injected with 1 ml of ^{51}Cr-labeled red cells (2×10^6, 200,000 cpm). One hour later, the rabbits were anesthetized and given either 4000 or 8000 U/kg/hr of streptokinase, 7500 or 15,000 U/kg/hr of t-PA, or an equivolume of saline. At the highest dose of streptokinase (16,000 U/kg/hr), profuse bleeding occurred at all wound sites, including ear puncture wounds, neck incisions, and sites of venous cannulation. It was therefore not technically possible to accurately quantitate the blood loss from the ear puncture sites. As in the studies of thrombolysis, 10% of the dose was administered as a bolus loading dose and 90% was infused over the next 4 hr. Three minutes after the loading bolus dose was administered and immediately before the continuous infusion commenced, each rabbit's ear was pierced five times with a Bard-Parker No. 11 scalpel to produce five standard 9 mm full-thickness incisions. Each ear was then immersed in a 950 ml saline bath that was constantly stirred and maintained at 37° C. The amount of ^{51}Cr-labeled red cells lost into the saline bath from the puncture wound sites over the initial 15 min was determined and expressed as initial blood loss. Further blood loss into the saline bath was measured at 30 min intervals over the next 4 hr. This method and reproducibility of its results have been previously reported.[21]

Assessment of systemic fibrinolysis. The effect of streptokinase and t-PA on plasma proteolysis was determined by measuring the level of α_2-antiplasmin by the method of Teger-Nielsson et al.[22] in which the chromogenic substrate S2251 was used and by determining the thrombin clotting time (TCT).[23] Blood was withdrawn from the rabbit carotid artery directly into 3.8% sodium citrate (9/1, vol/vol). All samples were collected before and 30, 60, 120, 180, and 240 min after the infusion began.

Statistical methods. Data were analyzed by one- or two-way analysis of variance or by the normal difference test, when appropriate. The blood loss data were log-transformed to accommodate increasing variation with increasing values.[24, 25]

Results

The size of thrombus in saline-treated rabbits was 44 $\pm$ 3 μl (volume, based on ^{125}I radioactivity) and 34 $\pm$ 4 mg (wet weight) (mean $\pm$ SEM, n = 18). The size of thrombus measured 4 hr later was unchanged (101 $\pm$ 8% of initial size). For each set of experiments, the size of thrombus was measured in the control animals (saline infusion) and in the t-PA– and streptokinase-treated animals. The size of thrombus in the animals treated with t-PA and streptokinase was expressed as a percent of the size of thrombus at 4 hr in saline-treated controls (i.e., the thrombus in saline controls at 4 hr was considered to be 100%). Streptokinase and t-PA produced a dose-related decrease in size of thrombus both when measured as volume based on radioactivity and as wet weight. Streptokinase, 4000, 8000, and 16,000 U/kg/hr, produced zero, 28 ± 6%, and 57 ± 4% thrombolysis, respectively, whereas 7500 and 15,000 U/kg/hr t-PA produced 35 ± 6% and 85 ± 4% thrombolysis, respectively (figure 1).

The effects of t-PA and streptokinase on initial and continuous blood loss are shown in figure 2. Streptokinase in doses of 4000 and 8000 U/kg/hr produced a significant increase in initial blood loss compared with that in saline-treated controls ($p < .001$). In addition, both lower streptokinase doses caused a progressive increase in bleeding that continued throughout the 4 hr of infusion ($p < .0001$). t-PA (7500 U/kg/hr) produced neither a significant increase in initial blood loss nor a progressive increase in continuous blood loss throughout the 4 hr of infusion. The larger dose of t-PA (15,000 U/kg/hr) had no effect on initial blood loss, but like streptokinase, produced a progressive increase in bleeding over the 4 hr of infusion ($p < .0001$). There were, however, a number of differences in the kinetics of bleeding in the animals treated with streptokinase and t-PA (15,000 U/kg/hr). Excessive bleeding was

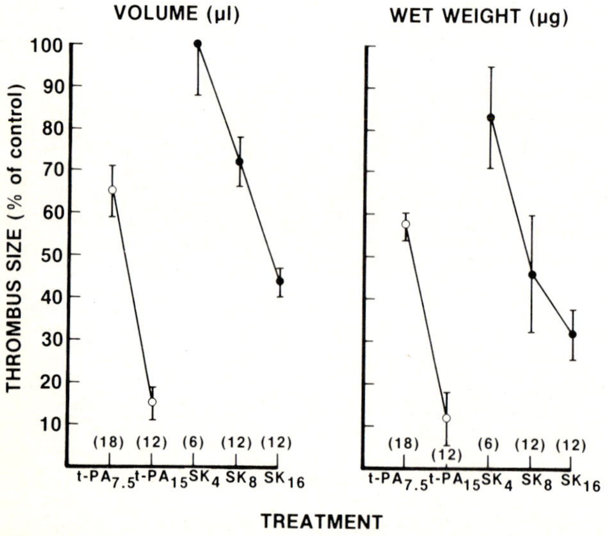

FIGURE 1. Thrombolytic effects of 4 hr infusions of t-PA and streptokinase (SK). Thrombolysis was expressed as thrombus size (% of thrombus in saline controls), measured both in volume (based on amounts of ^{125}I fibrinogen) and wet weight. Doses: t-PA$_{7.5}$ = 7500 U/kg/hr; t-PA$_{15}$ = 15,000 U/kg/hr; SK$_4$ = 4000 U/kg/hr; SK$_8$ = 8000 U/kg/hr; SK$_{16}$ = 16,000 U/kg/hr. Data are expressed as mean ± SEM. Numbers in parentheses are n values.

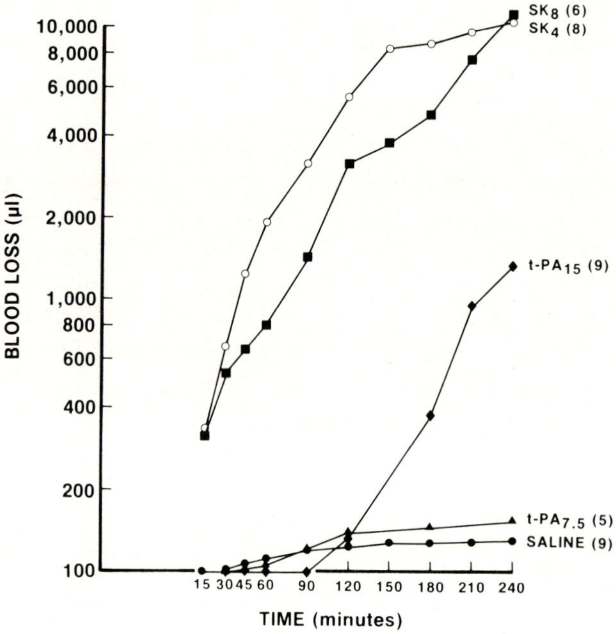

FIGURE 2. Effect of saline, t-PA, and streptokinase on blood loss from punctured ear wound sites during the 4 hr of infusion. Data are expressed as geometric means due to increasing variation with increasing blood loss. Doses: t-PA$_{7.5}$ = 7500 U/kg/hr; t-PA$_{15}$ = 15,000 U/kg/hr; SK$_4$ = 4000 U/kg/hr; SK$_8$ = 8000 U/kg/hr. Numbers in parentheses are n values.

evident after both doses of streptokinase within 15 min of commencing the infusion, whereas bleeding was observed with t-PA only after 90 min of infusion. At 4 hr, blood loss with the two lower doses of streptokinase was 10,500 μl (range 600 to 14,200 μl) and 11,000 μl (range 400 to 23,000 μl); blood loss was 1400 μl (range 0 to 8100 μl) in the animals treated with 15,000 U/kg/hr of t-PA ($p < .001$; figure 2). With the lowest dose of t-PA (7500 U/kg/hr) blood loss was 144 μl (range 3 to 244 μl).

The effect of streptokinase and t-PA on α_2-antiplasmin levels and the prolongation of the TCT are shown in figure 3. Streptokinase, 4000 and 8000 U/kg/hr, produced a significant decrease in α_2-antiplasmin levels ($p < .001$) and a significant prolongation of the TCT ($p < .001$). t-PA, 7500 U/kg/hr, had no effect on either the α_2-antiplasmin level or the TCT, but the 15,000 U/kg/hr dose produced a significant decrease in α_2-antiplasmin level and a significant prolongation of the TCT. These effects were significant after 120 min of infusion ($p < .01$).

Discussion

Investigations in animals and in humans have demonstrated that the infusion of t-PA can produce thrombolysis without inducing a plasmin-mediated plasma proteolytic state.[10–19] The results of our study confirm

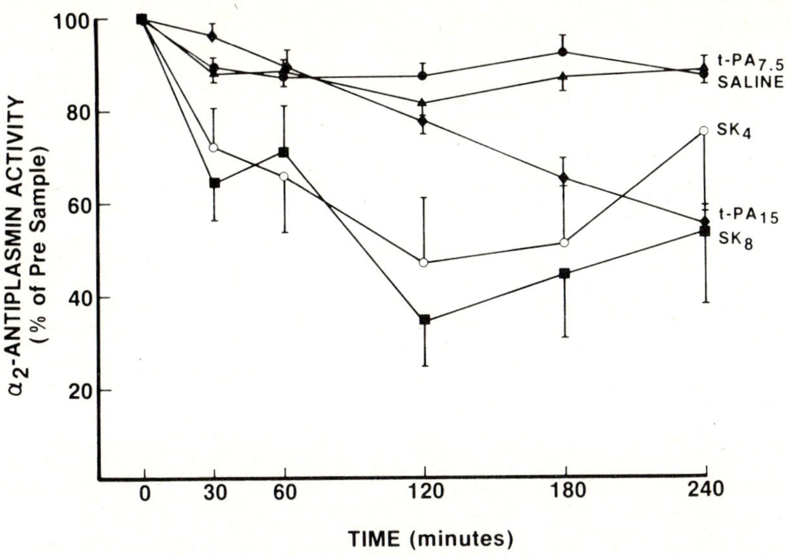

FIGURE 3. Time-related effects of saline, t-PA, and streptokinase on α_2-antiplasmin levels and the prolongation of the TCT. Data are expressesd as mean ± SEM, n ≥ 6. Doses: t-$PA_{7.5}$ = 7500 U/kg/hr; t-PA_{15} = 15,000 U/kg/hr; SK_4 = 4000 U/kg/hr; SK_8 = 8000 U/kg/hr.

these observations since we demonstrated that t-PA, infused over 4 hr in a dose of 7500 U/kg/hr, produced thrombolysis without inducing a decrease in α_2-antiplasmin level or a prolongation of the TCT. The thrombolytic effect of the lower dose of t-PA was not associated with an increase in blood loss when this was measured with a sensitive method that has been shown to be responsive to the hemorrhagic effect of heparin and thrombocytopenia.[26] In contrast streptokinase produced an increase in blood loss at doses of 4000 and 8000 U/kg/hr, both of which induced less thrombolysis than t-PA in a dose of 7500 U/kg/hr. The higher dose of t-PA (15,000 U/kg/hr) given for 4 hr produced evidence of a plasmin-mediated proteolytic state, as demonstrated by a fall in α_2-antiplasmin and a prolongation of the TCT. This finding is in keeping with predictions made by Sobel et al.[27] that very high concentrations of t-PA are likely to induce a plasma proteolytic state. t-PA–induced proteolysis was associated with excessive bleeding. The pattern of this bleeding differed from that observed after streptokinase in that it was delayed for up to 90 min after the infusion began. The onset of bleeding coincided with a fall in α_2-antiplasmin and a prolongation of TCT and therefore with the effects of a plasmin-mediated proteolytic state. However, blood loss in the rabbits treated with 15,000 U/kg/hr of t-PA was only 1400 μl compared with the mean 10,500 μl blood loss over 4 hr in the two groups of streptokinase-treated animals. Thus, when compared with streptokinase, t-PA had a greater thrombolytic effect but was less likely to produce hemorrhage according to blood loss measured both in the first 15 min and throughout the 4 hr of infusion.

The reason for the differences in bleeding observed with roughly equivalent thrombolytic effects of streptokinase and t-PA (8000 U/kg/hr and 7500 U/kg/hr, respectively) is not readily apparent. Excessive bleeding observed with streptokinase cannot be explained solely on the basis of a streptokinase-induced coagulation defect, since excessive bleeding was present 15 min after starting the infusion at a time when there was not a significant prolongation of TCT. It is possible, however, that the hyperplasminemic state induced by streptokinase produced bleeding by other mechanisms.

Recently, Adelman et al.[7] reported that streptokinase produced a plasmin-mediated defect in platelet membrane glycoproteins. It is possible, therefore, that the bleeding mediated by streptokinase is caused by a combination of lysis of fibrin in the hemostatic plug and a plasmin-induced platelet function defect. This proposed mechanism could also explain the bleeding observed with the higher dose of t-PA since it also produced a plasmin-mediated plasma proteolytic state. Alternatively, it is possible that fibrin present in the platelet-rich hemorrhagic plug is relatively resistant to lysis by t-PA because of high concentrations of platelet-derived fibrinolytic inhibitors. This hypothesis is supported by the results of recent studies that demonstrated that platelet thrombospondin combines with plasminogen and inhibits its activation.[28]

The reason that bleeding was not induced by t-PA in a concentration that was able to produce approximately 35% lysis is less clear. It is possible that fibrin present in the hemostatic plug is more resistant to lysis by t-PA than fibrin in thrombi. Alternatively, the instability of the hemostatic plug during streptokinase therapy may be contributed to by a plasmin-mediated platelet function defect that is not produced in the animals treated with t-PA (7500 U/kg/hr). Whatever its mechanism, the absence of significant bleeding with thrombolytic concentrations of t-PA suggests that this plasminogen activator has considerable clinical potential.

References

1. Goldhaber SZ, Buring JE, Lipnick RJ, Hennekens CH: Pooled analysis of randomized trials of streptokinase and heparin in phlebographically documented acute deep vein thrombosis. Am J Med **76:** 393, 1984
2. A cooperative study: urokinase-streptokinase embolism trial. Phase II results. JAMA **229:** 1606, 1974
3. Stampfer MJ, Goldhaber SZ, Yusuf S, Peto R, Hennekens CH: Effect of intravenous streptokinase on acute myocardial infarction: pooled results from a randomized trial. N Engl J Med **307:** 1180, 1982
4. Anderson JL, Marshall HW, Bray BE, Lutz JR, Frederick PR, Yanowitz FG, Datz FL, Klausner SC, Hagan AD: A randomized trial of intracoronary streptokinase in the treatment of acute myocardial infarction. N Engl J Med **308:** 1312, 1983
5. Kennedy JW, Ritchie JL, Davis KB, Fritz JJ: Western Washington trial of intracoronary streptokinase in acute myocardial infarction. N Engl J Med **309:** 1477, 1983
6. Collen D, Verstraete M: α_2-Antiplasmin consumption and fibrinogen breakdown during thrombolytic therapy. Thromb Res **14:** 631, 1979
7. Adelman B, Loscatzo J, Michelson AD, Handin RI: Fibrinolytic therapy inhibits platelet/von Willebrand factor interactions. Blood **62** (suppl): 296a, 1983
8. Rijken DC, Collen D: Purification and characterization of the plasminogen activator secreted by human melanoma cells in culture. J Biol Chem **256:** 7035, 1981
9. Pennica D, Holmes WE, Kohr WH, Harkins RN, Vehar GA, Ward CA, Bennett WF, Yelverton E, Seeburg PH, Heyneker HL, Goeddel DV, Collen D: Cloning and expression of human tissue-type plasminogen activator cDNA in E. coli. Nature **301:** 214, 1983
10. Korniger C, Matsuo O, Suy R, Stassen JM, Collen D: Thrombolysis with human extrinsic (tissue-type) plasminogen activator in dogs with femoral vein thrombosis. J Clin Invest **69:** 573, 1982
11. Matsuo O, Rijken DC, Collen D: Thrombolysis by human tissue plasminogen activator and urokinase in rabbits with experimental pulmonary embolus. Nature **291:** 590, 1981
12. Weimar W, Stibbe J, VanSeyen AJ, Billau A, DeSomer P, Collen D: Specific lysis of an iliofemoral thrombus by administration of extrinsic (tissue-type) plasminogen activator. Lancet **2:** 1018, 1981
13. Collen D, Stassen JM, Verstraete M: Thrombolysis with human extrinsic (tissue-type) plasminogen activator in rabbits with experimental jugular vein thrombosis. J Clin Invest **71:** 368, 1983
14. Bergmann SR, Fox KAA, Ter-Pogossian MM, Sobel BE, Collen D: Clot-selective thrombolysis with tissue-type plasminogen activator. Science **220:** 1181, 1983
15. Sobel BE, Geltman EM, Tiefenbrunn AJ, Jaffe AS, Spadaro JJ, Ter-Pogossian MM, Collen D, Ludbrook PA: Improvement of regional myocardial metabolism after coronary thrombolysis induced with tissue-type plasminogen activator or streptokinase. Circulation **69:** 983, 1984
16. Van De Werf F, Ludbrook PA, Bergmann SR, Tiefenbrunn AJ, Fox KAA, DeGeest H, Verstraeta M, Collen D, Sobel BE: Coronary thrombolysis with tissue-type plasminogen activator in patients with evolving myocardial infarction. N Engl J Med **310:** 609, 1984
17. Gold HK, Fallon JT, Yasuda T, Khaw BA, Guerrero JL, Vislowsky JM, Leinbach RC, Harper R, Hoying C, Grossbard E, Collen D: Coronary thrombolysis with recombinant human tissue plasminogen activator. Circulation **68**(suppl III): III-150, 1983
18. Van De Werf F, Bergmann SR, Fox KAA, DeGeest H, Hoying CF, Sobel B, Collen D: Coronary thrombolysis with intravenously administered human tissue-type plasminogen activator produced by recombinant DNA technology. Circulation **69:** 605, 1984
19. Topol EJ, Ciuffo AA, Pearson TA, Dillman J, Builder S, Grossbard E, Bulkeley BH, Weisfeldt ML: Thrombolysis with recombinant activator in atherosclerotic thrombotic occlusion. Clin Res **32:** 212a, 1984
20. Regoeczi E: Fibrinogen catabolism: kinetics of catabolism following sudden elevation of the pool with exogenous fibrinogen. Clin Sci **38:** 111, 1970
21. Carter CJ, Kelton JG, Hirsh J, Cerskus A, Santos AV, Gent M: The relationship between the hemorrhagic and antithrombotic properties of low molecular weight heparin in rabbits. Blood **59:** 1239, 1982
22. Teger-Nilsson AC, Fibergen P, Gyzander E: Determination of a new rapid plasmin inhibitor in human blood by means of a plasmin specific tripeptide substrate. Scand J Clin Lab Invest **37:** 403, 1977
23. Fletcher AP, Alkjaersig N, Sherry S: The maintenance of a sustained thrombolytic state in man. 1. Induction and effects. J Clin Invest **38:** 1096, 1959
24. Bruning JL, Kintz BL: Computational handbook of statistics. Glenview, IL, 1977, Scott, Foresman and Company, p 18
25. Colton T: Statistics in medicine. Boston, 1974, Little, Brown and Company, p 151
26. Carter CJ, Kelton JG, Gent M, Hirsh J: The relationship between haemorrhagic and antithrombotic effects of standard and low molecular weight (LMW) heparins. Circulation **62**(suppl III): III-51, 1980
27. Sobel BE, Gross RW, Robison AK: Thrombolysis, clot selectivity, and kinetics. Circulation **70:** 160, 1984
28. Silverstein RL, Leung LLK, Harpel PC, Nachman RL: Complex formation of platelet thrombospondin with plasminogen. Modulation of activation by tissue activator. J Cli Invest **74:** 1625, 1984

The dependence of myocardial ultrasonic integrated backscatter on contractile performance*

SAMUEL A. WICKLINE, M.D., LEWIS J. THOMAS III, PH.D., JAMES G. MILLER, PH.D., BURTON E. SOBEL, M.D., AND JULIO E. PÉREZ, M.D.

ABSTRACT We have recently shown that the cardiac cycle–dependent variation in myocardial ultrasonic integrated backscatter is blunted with regional ischemia in dogs. To determine if global and intramural regional myocardial contractile performance can be quantified by integrated backscatter, we analyzed ultrasonic responses after induction of increased and decreased contractility in five dogs. A recently developed analog data-acquisition system for measuring integrated backscatter in real time was used to sample radiofrequency signals gated from subepicardial or subendocardial regions. Baseline recordings of integrated backscatter, left ventricular pressure, left ventricular dP/dt, and wall thickness were made at 12 left ventricular sites for both intramural regions. Contractility was modified subsequently by either paired pacing or propranolol to produce significantly elevated or depressed values for maximum left ventricular dP/dt compared with baseline (1083 ± 289 to 1868 ± 398 to 3001 ± 570 mm Hg/sec; $p < .01$ for all). The amplitude of the cyclic variation of integrated backscatter was 50% greater (arithmetically) in subendocardial than in subepicardial regions for all treatments (7.6 ± 0.3 vs 6.0 ± 0.5 dB, $p < .001$). The maximum rate of change in integrated backscatter waveforms during isovolumetric contraction was faster with paired pacing and slower with propranolol than at baseline for all regions (56 ± 6 to 74 ± 6 to 82 ± 5 dB/sec, $p < .005$). The maximum rate of change in integrated backscatter also was greater in subendocardial than subepicardial regions ($p < .001$). Thus, both regional and global differences in myocardial contractile performance are manifest quantitatively in integrated backscatter waveforms. We propose that the physiologic determinants of these differences may depend on regional and global variations in myofibril elastic characteristics.
Circulation **72, No. 1, 183–192, 1985.**

CHARACTERIZATION OF MYOCARDIUM based on quantitative ultrasonic integrated backscatter measurements may permit noninvasive elucidation of cardiac pathology.[1-3] The physical basis for ultrasonic tissue differentiation of pathologic properties of the heart is reflected by the variation in intrinsic scattering properties among individual tissue types. For the heart, the scattering properties are determined in part by the local variations in density and compressibility of discrete intramural regions, and may vary throughout a selected volume of tissue.[4-8] Ultrasonic backscatter parameters are modified substantially by pathologic changes. We have previously shown that irreversible morphologic changes accompanying experimental myocardial infarction or cardiomyopathy are associated with significant elevations in time-averaged ultrasonic integrated backscatter measurements.[7-11] Furthermore, we found recently that physiologic myocardial contraction and relaxation are associated with a parallel, cyclic variation in integrated backscatter.[12] The magnitude of this cardiac cycle–dependent variation in integrated backscatter is reduced greatly with even brief ischemia in dogs and recovers with reperfusion.[13, 14] However, the temporal association between segmental akinesis and blunted cyclic variation in backscatter does not establish that the magnitude of cyclic variation reflects myocardial contractile function quantitatively.

The purpose of this study was to determine the dependence of ultrasonic integrated backscatter measurements on global and intramural regional myocardial contractile performance by analysis of ultrasonic responses after induced increased or decreased con-

From the Department of Medicine, Cardiovascular Division, and Department of Physics, Washington University, St. Louis.

Supported in part by National Institutes of Health grants HL17646 (SCOR in Ischemic Heart Disease), HL28998, a Squibb Cardiovascular Research Fellowship (Dr. Pérez), and NASA grant NSG-1601.

Address for correspondence: Julio E. Pérez, M.D., Box 8086, Cardiovascular Division, Washington University School of Medicine, 660 South Euclid Ave., St. Louis, MO 63110.

Received Nov. 26, 1984; revision accepted April 4, 1985.

*All editorial decisions for this article, including selection of reviewers and the final disposition, were made by a guest editor. This procedure applies to all manuscripts with authors from the Washington University School of Medicine.

tractility in dogs. A new analog data acquisition system that we described recently for measurement of integrated backscatter in real time[15] permitted instantaneous beat-to-beat collection of integrated backscatter waveforms and enabled more discriminating analysis of these signals than was possible previously. The study was also designed to define quantitatively the relationships between integrated backscatter and myocardial contractile performance to facilitate development of a real-time, noninvasive, clinically applicable technique for assessment of regional contractile properties by direct interrogation of the tissue rather than by assessment of pump function.

Methods

Animal preparation. Five mongrel dogs (15 to 30 kg) were anesthetized with intravenous pentobarbital (20 to 30 mg/kg), and ventilated with room air supplemented with oxygen with the use of a volume respirator adjusted to maintain physiologic concentrations of arterial blood gases. A femoral artery cannula was inserted in each dog to monitor blood gases and aortic pressure. A right thoracotomy was performed. Pacing wires were sutured to the right ventricular epicardium low in the pulmonary outflow tract area and attached to a Grass stimulator. The atrioventricular node was injected with 1 to 2 ml of formalin through the right atrial wall to induce complete heart block, yielding a ventricular escape rate of less than 60 beats/min. The heart was paced with 3 msec square-wave pulses at a voltage of 1.5 times threshold (6 to 9 V). Adequate hemostasis was ensured and the pericardium and right thoracotomy were closed. A left thoracotomy was performed and a pericardial cradle was created to expose the left ventricular anterior free wall. A short, fluid-filled cannula was inserted into the left ventricular cavity through the apex for monitoring left ventricular pressure. A 2.5 × 2.5 cm region of the anterior free wall was demarcated approximately two-thirds down from the circumflex artery toward the apex and midway between the anterior descending coronary artery and the major marginal branch of the circumflex artery. Twelve readily identifiable sites approximately 0.6 cm apart (3 rows × 4 columns) were specified for ultrasonic data collection. A Honeywell monitoring system was used to amplify and record physiologic signals. Femoral artery and left ventricular pressures were obtained with Statham strain-gauge transducers calibrated with a mercury manometer. The first derivative of the left ventricular pressure (dP/dt) was obtained with an analog differentiator calibrated by determining the average maximum positive and negative slopes of the left ventricular pressure wave and comparing the slopes to the average peak positive and negative dP/dt values on high-speed paper recordings. The use of this method to determine maximum dP/dt (dP/dt_{max}) values allowed a clear separation of conditions of normal, reduced, and improved contractile performance in response to the negative and positive inotropic interventions (see Results). Standard limb-lead electrocardiograms were also recorded.

Ultrasonic data acquisition system. Our procedure for measuring ultrasonic integrated backscatter in real time has been described recently.[15] In brief, a standard two-dimensional/M mode imaging system (Honeywell Ultra-Imager) was used to drive a focused piezoelectric transducer (Panametrics V309, 5 MHz center frequency, 1.3 cm diameter, 5 cm focal length) to produce broadband ultrasonic pulses. The hand-held transducer was mounted on a Plexiglas water column fitted with a latex tip and applied directly to the epicardium to position the focal point within the myocardium. Two portions of the backscattered radiofrequency (rf) signal (3 μsec each, representing a tissue sample length of 2.25 mm each) were gated sequentially from two regions of myocardium with the use of a programmable timing device. The gates were contiguous, with front boundaries located 2 mm (2.7 μsec) and 4.25 mm (5.7 μsec) below the epicardial specular reflection. The latter was reliably detectable as a large amplitude transition in the rf signal from the water path to the epicardium. The gates were always located at the same point in time and space below the epicardial specular echo throughout the cardiac cycle. The use of this gating procedure ensured the exclusion of both epicardial and endocardial specular echoes. The transducer focal point was located at the border between the two gates. These gated regions defined subepicardial and subendocardial zones in diastole. In systole the positions of both gates shifted relative to total wall thickness into more subepicardial zones throughout the course of wall thickening as a consequence of the electronic gating system, which positions the gates relative to the epicardial specular echo. At end-systole, the subendocardial gate lay well within the midmyocardial region. Accordingly, we will refer to the two regions as proximal and distal with respect to the epicardial surface.

The gated signal was fed to an acoustoelectric energy detector, yielding a peak output voltage directly proportional to the average energy contained in the signal over the frequency band of interest. The output was sampled at 5 msec intervals and thus constituted integrated backscatter at single instants in the heart cycle. For calibration, a reference value was obtained for integrated backscatter from a flat stainless steel reflector positioned at the focal point. Changes in the reference value around the focal point (a measure of ultrasonic beam diffraction from proximal to distal gates) were insignificant due to the substantial depth of field of the transducer. The ratio of the intensity of integrated backscatter from the myocardium to that from the reflector was expressed in decibels. The time-varying integrated backscatter values, sampled every 5 msec throughout the cardiac cycle, were recorded with accompanying left ventricular dP/dt waveforms on magnetic tape for analysis later. The signals were fed simultaneously to an analog integrator with a 5 sec time constant to provide a cumulative display of time-averaged integrated backscatter. The backscatter waveforms along with simultaneous M mode scans, left ventricular dP/dt, and electrocardiographic signals were displayed in real time on the imager screen and recorded on ½ inch videotape (figure 1). Optimal orientation of the ultrasonic transducer over the epicardium (perpendicular) was defined according to the following qualitative criteria: (1) the brightest specular reflection from both endocardium and epicardium observed in M mode scans, (2) the sharpest M mode scan of the myocardial wall, thinnest at end-diastole, with appropriate thickening during systole, and (3) the smoothest integrated backscatter signals with the greatest amplitude of cyclic variation. These criteria were applied to avoid inadvertent motion artifact of the hand-held transducer and to minimize the potential influence of either ventricular fiber angle or ultrasonic anisotropy on the results. The stability of both M mode traces and integrated backscatter signals notable in figure 1 was typical of all recordings.

Data collection. Data sets were recorded consecutively under three sets of conditions with respect to contractile performance: baseline, increased contractile performance in response to paired pacing, and decreased performance in response to β-blockade with propranolol. Initially, basal contractile performance was measured with the heart paced at a rate of 80 beats/min and subsequently at 110 beats/min. At each heart rate 5 sec of continuous time-varying backscatter and dP/dt waveforms were

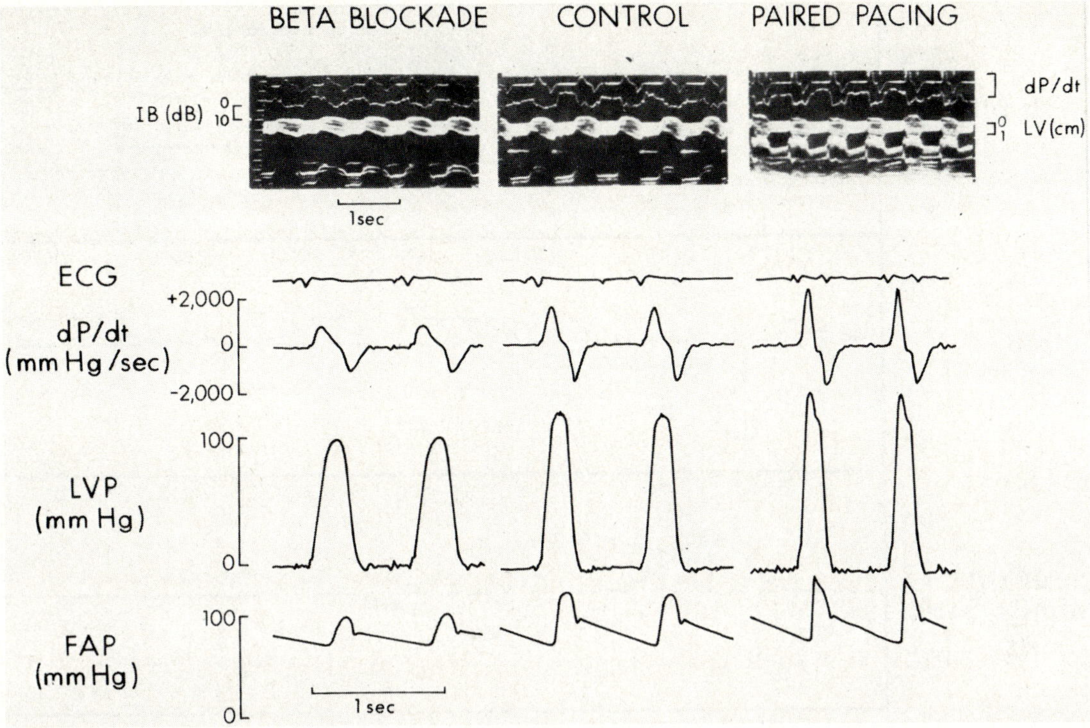

FIGURE 1. Responses to altered contractile performance. The upper panels represent *Top*, Real-time displays of left ventricular (LV) dP/dt, integrated backscatter (IB), and M mode echocardiograms of the left ventricular anterior wall. *Bottom*, Physiologic parameters for corresponding states of contractile performance. ECG = electrocardiogram; LVP = left ventricular pressure; FAP = femoral arterial pressure.

recorded at each of 12 sites for proximal and then distal regions. The value for time-averaged backscatter, determined by analog integration over the 5 sec period, was recorded also. Physiologic parameters were recorded at each heart rate as were videotaped M mode scans and simultaneous left ventricular dP/dt, electrocardiographic, and backscatter waveforms for proximal and distal regions (figure 1).

After basal measurements had been obtained paired pacing was initiated, first at a heart rate of 80 beats/min and then at a rate of 110 beats/min. A substantial elevation of peak left ventricular dP/dt was noted after the first several beats. Each stimulus pair produced only a single observable mechanical contraction. The S_1-S_2 intervals at the rates of 80 (approximately 240 msec) and 110 (approximately 200 msec) were adjusted to achieve maximal left ventricular dP/dt. Data sets equivalent to those for the basal state were recorded at each rate. Paired pacing was then discontinued and the heart was allowed to recover from the expected rebound depression of performance.[16]

Subsequently, *d,l*-propranolol (2 mg/kg) was infused intravenously over 15 min and then data sets were recorded within 15 min as described at both heart rates. Adequate β-blockade was reflected by left ventricular chamber dilation and wall thinning evident on the displayed M mode echocardiogram and a gradual decline in peak left ventricular dP/dt to a stable but low level. Data were collected with heart rate maintained at 80 or 110 beats/min.

Data analysis. At each of the sites interrogated with ultrasound seven to 10 consecutive RR intervals were recorded during the 5 sec interval of collection of integrated backscatter and left ventricular dP/dt waveform data. The integrated backscatter and left ventricular dP/dt recordings were averaged to produce single waveforms for each site. The waveforms at each site were subsequently averaged into a regional composite waveform for each set of conditions and region (example: paired pacing, heart rate = 80 beats/min, proximal site with respect to the epicardium). The positive peaks of the left ventricular dP/dt signals were used as timing references for the alignment of phasic integrated backscatter waveforms. The signal-averaging procedure improved signal-to-noise ratios and provided reformatted information that could be treated by more conservative statistical analysis on a dog-to-dog basis, rather than simply a site-to-site basis, for assessment of cardiac cycle–dependent variation of backscatter.

Ultrasonic parameters were delineated from the regional composite waveforms as depicted in figure 2. The *amplitude* of the time-varying integrated backscatter signals was computed as the maximum peak-to-trough excursion. The first derivative of the composite integrated backscatter curves was determined digitally, and the maximum negative value ($-dIB/dt_{max}$) was calculated from the nadir of this curve. The *time-averaged* value for integrated backscatter was obtained by analog integration of the unprocessed signals. The *phase shift* of the integrated backscatter waveforms relative to the "zero point" (end-diastole) of the left ventricular pressure waveform was determined in two ways. For the first, a "digital" method, Fourier transforms were performed on regional composite waveforms and the fundamental frequency and phase shift were determined. For the second, an "analog" method, a lock-in detector was used to identify phase shifts in integrated backscatter signals at individual sites relative to the left ventricular pressure waveform that served as a reference.[15] By comparing results obtained with these two methods of phase analysis, potential effects of signal averaging on the shapes of the composite waveforms could be determined.

Myocardial wall thickness was calculated off-line from the videotaped M mode scans with the use of a Microsonics analyz-

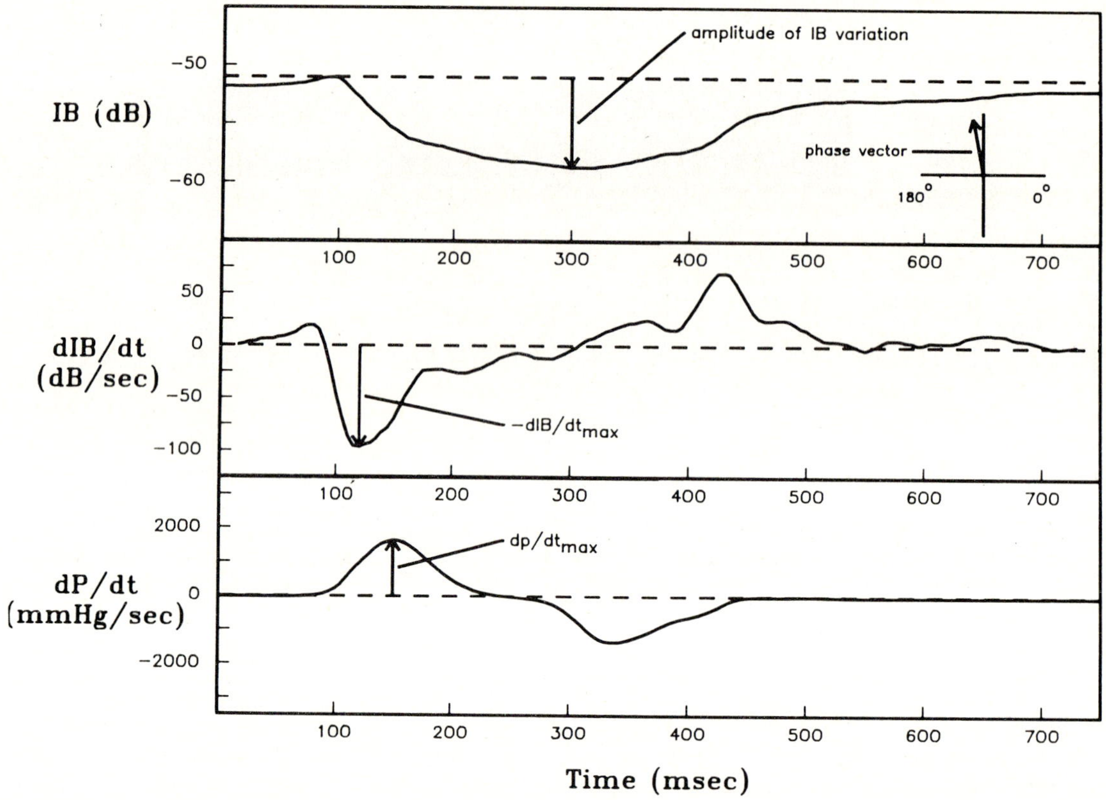

FIGURE 2. Ultrasonic parameters for data analysis obtained from composite waveforms. *Top*, Amplitude of integrated backscatter (IB) variation, determined peak-to-trough and measured in decibels. The phase vector represents the displacement of the nadir of the IB waveform with respect to end-diastole. Angles lying within 90 to 180 degrees indicate systolic decreases in IB. *Middle*, The first derivative of IB in time; the maximal rate of decrease is determined. *Bottom*, Left ventricular dP/dt_{max} measurement.

er. Thickness was measured at end-diastole and at end-systole. The simultaneously recorded left ventricular dP/dt signal was used for timing with reference to the zero-point and peak negative left ventricular dP/dt values, respectively.[17, 18]

Statistical methods. The major objective of this study was to determine if parameters derived from ultrasonic backscatter (rate of change in integrated backscatter, amplitude of cyclic variation in integrated backscatter, and time-averaged integrated backscatter) manifest differences in contractile performance, intramural region, and heart rate. A 3 × 4 factorial analysis of variance was used to compare treatments (propranolol, normal, and paired pacing) against different substrates (proximal regions paced at 80 or 110 beats/min; distal regions paced at 80 or 110 beats/min). The overall significance of differences among the three states of contractile performance and among the rates and regions was assessed by the F test. In addition, a limited number (10) of independent comparisons were planned a priori to contrast specific linear combinations of means.[19] The significance of differences was determined by two-tailed independent t test procedures for these planned comparisons. Although conventional alpha levels are appropriate for determining the significance of differences for these "planned" comparisons,[19] p values corrected by the Bonferroni technique are also reported. The Bonferroni adjustment for multiple comparisons is made by dividing the conventional alpha level (.05) by the number of comparisons made to produce the minimum acceptable alpha level (.005 for 10 comparisons). The test criterion (t value) must exceed the value under the corrected alpha level (i.e., .005) to be considered significant at the reported level ($p < .05$). Both "planned" and "Bonferroni" p values are listed for the appropriate comparisons to demonstrate that the choice of statistical approach does not affect the conclusions. Among treatments, six comparisons were planned: (1) all normals vs all β-blockade, (2) all normals vs all paired pacing, (3) normals in distal regions vs β-blockade in distal regions (each at 80 and 110 beats/min), (4) normals in distal regions vs paired pacing in distal regions (each at both rates), (5) normals in proximal regions vs β-blockade in proximal regions (each at both rates), and (6) normals in proximal regions vs paired pacing in proximal regions (each at both rates). Between regions, two comparisons were planned: (1) all distal regions vs all proximal regions, and (2) normals in distal regions vs normals in proximal regions (each at both rates). Between heart rates, two comparisons were planned: (1) all recordings at 80 beats/min vs all recordings at 110 beats/min, and (2) normals at 80 beats/min vs normals at 110 beats/min. Linear regressions and other t tests were used as noted. Data are reported in the text as mean ± SD.

Results

Physiologic responses. Ventricular paired pacing elevated left ventricular pressure and left ventricular dP/dt_{max} significantly from control values of 114 ± 18 to 131 ± 19 mm Hg and 1868 ± 398 to 3001 ± 570 mm Hg/sec (p for both < .01). Infusion of propranolol significantly reduced ventricular pressure and left ventricular dP/dt values to 94 ± 13 mm Hg and 1083 ± 289 mm Hg/sec (p for both < .01). End-systolic wall

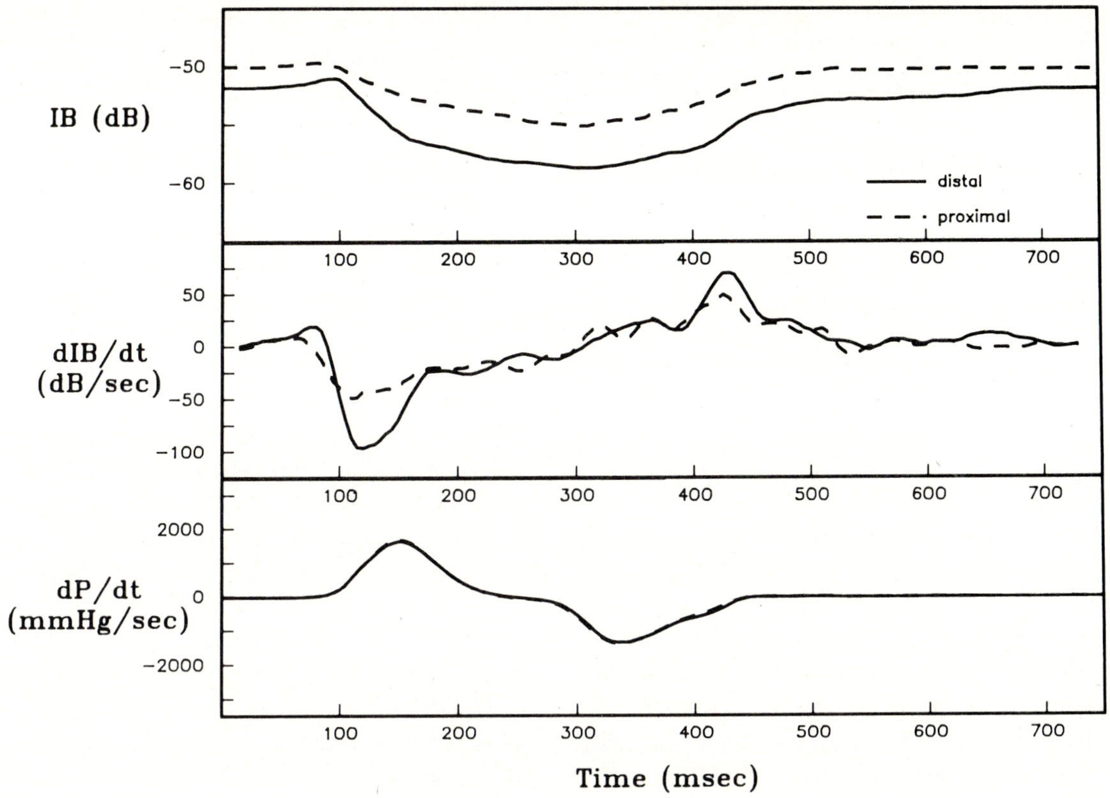

FIGURE 3. Distal and proximal regional backscatter waveforms from an animal paced at a heart rate of 80 beats/min. The left ventricular dP/dt curves for the two different regions overlap. The format is similar to that of figure 2.

thickness increased by 15 ± 8% over the normal value with paired pacing ($p < .005$) and decreased by 27 ± 7% with β-blockade ($p < .001$). Representative recordings are shown in figure 1.

Changes in cardiac cycle–dependent variation of ultrasonic backscatter.

Control state. Typical responses in proximal and distal regions of myocardium associated with basal contractile performance are shown in figure 3 and the data are summarized in tables 1 and 2. The $-dIB/dt_{max}$ was greater in distal than in proximal regions ($p < .005$, planned; $p < .05$, Bonferroni). In addition, distal regions exhibited greater amplitudes of cyclic variation than did proximal regions ($p < .01$, planned; $p = .07$, Bonferroni). Neither $-dIB/dt_{max}$ nor amplitude measurements were influenced significantly by differences in heart rate ($p > .40$ and $p > .10$, respectively, for planned comparisons between rates). The average phase of integrated backscatter signals determined from Fourier transforms was greater when heart rate was 110 than when it was 80 beats/ min (135 ± 18 vs 116 ± 18 degrees; $p < .005$).

Paired ventricular pacing and β-blockade. Changes in the cardiac cycle–dependent variation of integrated backscatter with paired pacing or β-blockade are summarized in tables 1 and 2. Representative waveforms from a distal region are shown in figure 4 and compared with responses obtained under control conditions. In distal regions of myocardium rates of change and amplitudes of waveforms appeared to exceed those in proximal regions under both conditions. Comparisons between groups demonstrated significantly faster $-dIB/dt_{max}$ values under control conditions compared with under conditions of β-blockade ($p < .005$, planned; $p < .05$,

TABLE 1
Influence of contractile performance on $-dIB/dt_{max}$

	β-Blockade	Control	Paired pacing
Distal regions			
80 beats/min	63±16	93±22	93±13
110 beats/min	64±28	78±16	88±23
Proximal regions			
80 beats/min	49±9	58±11	73±15
110 beats/min	43±15	60±18	71±12

All values (±SDs) are in $-dB/sec$; n = 5.

F ratio = 7.5 ($p < .005$) by analysis of variance for differences between rows (regions and heart rates).

F ratio = 12.1 ($p < .005$) by analysis of variance for differences between columns (states of contractile performance).

Row-column interactions were nonsignificant (F ratio = 0.37).

TABLE 2
Influence of contractile performance on the amplitude of cyclic variation of integrated backscatter

	β-Blockade	Control	Paired pacing
Distal regions			
80 beats/min	8.0±1.9	8.3±1.5	7.8±0.6
110 beats/min	6.9±1.3	7.3±1.7	7.1±0.7
Proximal regions			
80 beats/min	5.8±1.6	6.4±1.4	6.1±1.6
110 beats/min	5.9±1.9	5.9±1.5	5.8±0.9

All values (±SDs) are in dB; n = 5.

F ratio = 6.8 (p < .005) for differences between rows (regions and heart rates).

Differences between columns (states of contractile performance) were nonsignificant (F ratio = 0.35).

Row-column interactions were nonsignificant (F ratio = 0.07).

Bonferroni) and marginally, but not significantly, faster values during paired pacing as compared with during control (p > .10, planned). No apparent differences in the amplitude of cyclic variation of integrated backscatter were observed across the treatment groups. Under all conditions tested $-dIB/dt_{max}$ occurred an average of 6 ± 20 msec before dP/dt_{max}.

Comparative effects of the interventions tested. The relationship between left ventricular dP/dt_{max} and the cycle-dependent variation in ultrasonic backscatter parameters evaluated under different conditions are depicted in figures 5 and 6. With respect to $-dIB/dt_{max}$ (figure 5), progressively greater rates of change in the backscatter waveforms accompanied increasing contractile performance. A linear regression trend analysis, performed by fitting a line for individual animals to the three intervention points at each region and rate, revealed an average slope of −0.01 dB/sec/mm Hg/sec (p < .005 for slope ≠ 0). As indicated in table 1, analysis of variance confirmed the significance of overall differences between interventions and control conditions (p < .005 for F ratio). Significant overall differences were also found among rates and regions (p < .005 for F ratio). The lack of significant row-column interactions suggests that the effects of different treatments on $-dIB/dt_{max}$ were independent of the myocardial region or the heart rate at which measurements were obtained. Distal regions exhibited significantly greater rates of change in integrated backscatter than did proximal regions (p < .001, planned; p < .05, Bonferroni). Differences in the rate of change between the heart rates were not significant (p > .30, planned).

With respect to the amplitude of cyclic variation of integrated backscatter (figure 6), the analysis of variance summarized in table 2 confirms the significance

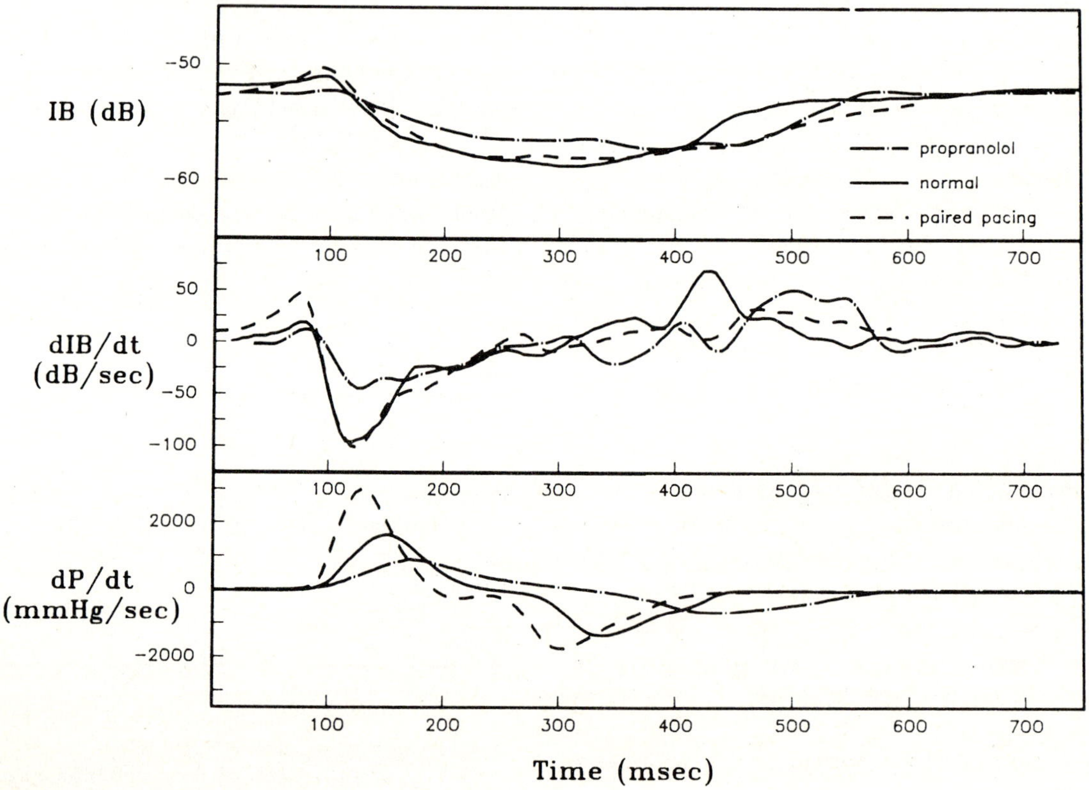

FIGURE 4. Composite waveforms for different contractile states in the distal region of an animal paced at 80 beats/min. The format is similar to that of figure 2.

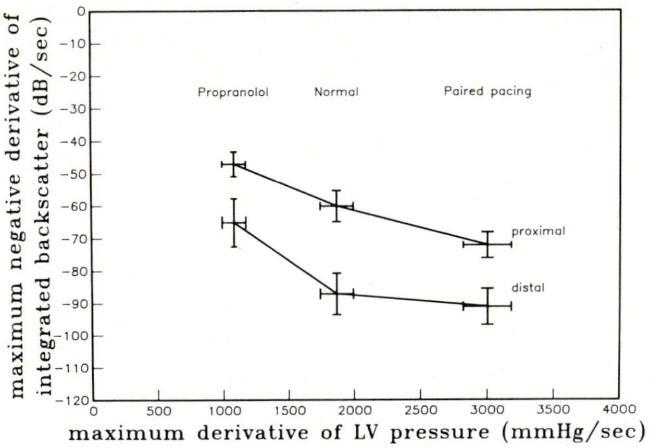

FIGURE 5. Effects of alterations in contractile performance on the maximal rate of change in IB measured in two regions for all animals. Significant differences were demonstrated among the three contractile states and between the two intramural regions by analysis of variance. Error bars represent SEM.

of overall differences between rates and regions ($p < .005$ for F ratio). However, the amplitude was not affected significantly overall by the conditions modifying contractile performance (p = NS for F ratio). Distal regions of myocardium exhibited significantly greater amplitudes compared with proximal regions ($p < .001$, planned; $p < .05$, Bonferroni). Differences in amplitude between the heart rates were not significant ($p > .05$, planned).

Time-averaged integrated backscatter values (averaged across all sites in a region) were slightly higher in proximal than in distal regions of myocardium (-53.8 ± 2.7 vs -54.8 ± 2.3 dB; $p < .005$, planned; $p < .05$, Bonferroni). However, no overall significant differences were demonstrated in time-averaged backscatter for different conditions, or for different combined heart rates and regions, judging from analysis of variance (p = NS for all F ratios). Smaller distal time-averaged backscatter values might be expected because additional ultrasonic attenuation is encountered as the beam propagates further into the tissue, but such small differences may be obscured by the width of the range of normal values.

The phase values determined from Fourier transforms of normal regional composite waveforms differed significantly for heart rates of 80 and 110 beats/min ($p < .005$). However, values were similar for different regions and for different interventions. The average phase values determined by the lock-in analyzer at individual sites were not significantly different from the composite phases determined by Fourier analysis for an entire region. The average standard deviation for the single-site lock-in analysis was 4.3 degrees (n = 120 sites), which is indicative of a uniform grouping of phases across all sites, regions, rates, and interventions. Because regional composite waveforms were composed of individual site data with intrinsically similar phases, these results indicate that the fundamental components of waveform shape were not distorted significantly by signal averaging.

Discussion

One objective of myocardial tissue characterization is acquisition of real-time quantitative ultrasonic correlates of fundamental pathologic and physiologic processes. Results of this study suggest several promising ultrasonic criteria. The $-dIB/dt_{max}$ appears to change in parallel with global contractile function. Both the amplitude of the cyclic variation of the backscatter waveform and the maximum rate of change appear to change in parallel with previously reported intrinsic regional intramural differences in contractile performance.[20–28] The time average of backscatter signals is a less sensitive index than the other parameters studied with respect to contractile performance. This result may reflect the obfuscation of subtle differences in dynamic information in backscatter waveforms by the wide range of normal values for time-averaged integrated backscatter. Nevertheless, the time average of integrated backscatter signals discriminates normal from pathologic tissue architecture.[7–11] The phase of the cyclic variation of integrated backscatter waveforms, determined from the fundamental frequency of Fourier transforms, is relatively constant for all levels of contractile performance at the rates used in this study. This finding suggests that changes in contractile state may be manifest in more subtle, or higher frequency, components of the backscatter waveforms.

One potential source of the observed differences in

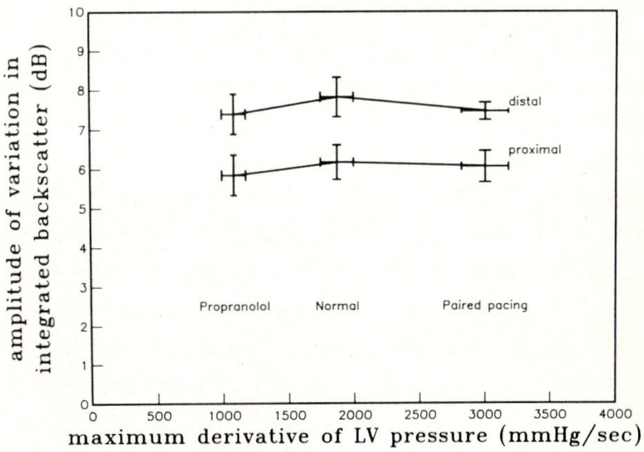

FIGURE 6. Effects of alterations in contractile performance on the amplitude of cyclic variation in IB measured in two regions for all animals. Significant differences were demonstrated between regions by analysis of variance. Error bars represent SEM.

regional intramural cyclic variation in integrated backscatter is the difference in sarcomere function throughout the myocardial wall. Yoran et al.[20] showed that diastolic sarcomere length increases progressively from the outer to the inner wall, except in the penultimate subendocardium where decreased lengths occur.[20] With the use of implanted ultrasonic crystals LeWinter et al.[21] and Sabbah et al.[22] found that inner wall segments contract more than outer wall segments. Streeter and Hanna[23] calculated that sarcomere shortening increases from outer to inner wall zones, except in the subendocardial zone. Stein et al.[24] have reported greater measured intramural dP/dt_{max} values in subendocardial than in subepicardial regions. Computations by Chadwick[25] support the concept of transmural gradients for diastolic sarcomere length, extent of sarcomere shortening, and systolic fiber tension from epicardium to endocardium, as do calculations by others using different models.[26–28]

The greater amplitudes of cyclic variation in integrated backscatter waveforms for distal compared with proximal regions (figure 6) suggest that the cardiac cycle–dependent backscatter variation depends, at least in part, on the absolute extent of sarcomere shortening. If distal sarcomeres shorten more than proximal sarcomeres in the same interval, their average velocity of shortening must be greater. Our observation of greater rates of change for waveforms in distal compared with proximal regions (figure 5) therefore also suggests a dependence of cyclic backscatter variation on the velocity of sarcomere shortening.

These observations, together with prior reports from our laboratory, may provide a foundation for a hypothetical physiologic model of the behavior of cardiac cycle–dependent integrated backscatter. The complete constitutive elements of such a model include both active and passive cardiac mechanical components, tissue anisotropy, myocardial fiber arrangement, and determinants of attenuation. In this report we will limit the description of the proposed model to the active components.

The hypothesis that sacomere shortening in some way determines the cardiac cycle–dependent variation in backscatter is consistent with several considerations. In general, the magnitude of ultrasonic energy scattered by inhomogeneities smaller than the insonifying wavelength is determined by local variations in material density and compressibility. If one limits consideration to investigation of 180 degree scatter (i.e., backscatter), the backscattered energy is approximately proportional to local variations in acoustic impedance. This approximation is highly accurate under conditions in which variations in density and compressibility are relatively modest, such as the case of soft tissue. Consequently, the magnitude of backscatter is related to local differences in impedance, which are the products of the square root of the mass density and the appropriate elastic modulus. If we invoke the simple Maxwell-type model for cardiac cell mechanical behavior, then the activated myofibril assembly may be visualized as a contractile element in series with an elastic element.[29] As sarcomeres shorten auxotonically, the series elastic element is stretched. Because the series elastic element exhibits non-Hookian behavior with elongation, its stiffness, or elastic modulus, increases with progressive force development.[29–31] This change in elastic modulus during sarcomere shortening could directly affect local acoustic impedance values. If so, measurements of backscattered acoustic energy would reflect the impedance changes in a time-varying manner throughout the active state. Because backscatter occurs at the boundaries between zones of soft tissue (such as myocardium) that exhibit different basal acoustic impedances, the magnitude of the acoustic impedance mismatch at these boundaries will determine the magnitude of backscatter. From the work of O'Donnell et al.[8] and Schung and Reid,[32] myocardial scatterers appear to be comparable in size to cardiac cells. We thus tentatively assign the time-varying acoustic impedance of the intracellular myofibril-sarcomere assembly to one of the two interfacing zones that are hypothetically responsible for backscatter. We propose that the other zone is extracellular, that it possesses a larger basal acoustic impedance than the time-varying medium, and that its impedance changes minimally throughout the cardiac mechanical cycle. Thus, we hypothesize that sarcomere shortening would cause a relative increase in intracellular acoustic impedance and a reduction in the impedance mismatch between the two interfacing media. As a consequence, backscattered energy would decrease during systole, consistent with what has been observed experimentally.

The observed differences between backscatter waveforms in distal compared with proximal sites may arise from the more rapid development of greater fiber stresses and elastic moduli in the inner wall in systole. The greater rates of change for backscatter waveforms with increasing contractile performance may reflect more rapid increases in local elastic moduli as a consequence of greater sarcomere shortening velocities. We suspect that the flattening of dIB/dt response to paired pacing in distal regions (figure 5) may represent the limited capacity of subendocardial fibers to augment their contractile performance. An interesting hypothetical corollary is that the major portion of myocardial contractile reserve is contributed by outer wall fibers.

The lack of any significant effect of interventions affecting contractile performance on the amplitude of the cyclic variation in integrated backscatter initially appears to be inconsistent with the observed increases in wall thickening. The principal factor responsible for this apparent paradox involves the method for gating the backscattered rf signal. Because of the use of the epicardial specular echo as a gating reference, the studied regions are always located 2 and 4.25 mm below the epicardial surface (see Methods). Despite absolute increases in wall thickening, both gates necessarily reflect contractile events occurring at more subepicardial loci in regions in which fibers may develop less stress.[25] Hence, local elastic moduli change less than expected and smaller cyclic variations in backscatter result. Thus, despite the development of an increased transmural stress gradient, the regions in which measurements are made may not represent those with maximally increased local contractile performance in terms of amplitude. With our present gating technique it is not possible to follow precisely the same volume of tissue throughout systole. However, this limitation does not vitiate conclusions regarding regional intramural differences that depend on stress and velocity gradients.

Because the maximal rate of change in backscatter waveforms occurs at the time of peak left ventricular dP/dt, $-dIB/dt_{max}$ provides an index of contractile performance that is approximately isovolumetric. Like other indexes of this sort, it exhibits substantial variability among "normals." Although left ventricular dP/dt_{max} is used as a comparative measure of contractile performance, this index does not define a range of normal values for the potentially corresponding ultrasonic parameter. Additionally, because open-chest dogs were studied, artifactual heterogeneity may have been introduced into measurements of "normal" contractility. The trend analyses provide evidence that ultrasonic parameters are sensitive to changes in contractile performance for groups of animals. The capacity of these parameters to discriminate normal contractility in individual animals and their applicability to individual subjects remain undefined.

The potential clinical utility of the backscatter parameters identified in this study remains to be elucidated. Two difficulties may confront clinical implementation and assessment: the necessity for taking measurements through the chest wall, and the need for attenuation corrections. The geometric constraints imposed by the closed chest may be overcome by adjusting signal gating so that any myocardial region observable with a standard two-dimensional M mode imaging system can be studied. With respect to the second difficulty, we have demonstrated that myocardial integrated backscatter data obtained through the closed chest wall of dogs can be compensated for attenuation losses to characterize ischemic myocardial tissue.[33] If we presume that the attenuation of chest wall remains constant throughout the cardiac mechanical cycle, myocardial backscatter values require correction for attenuation encountered as the ultrasonic beam traverses the intervening tissue. Fortunately, this correction is not required for the rate of change, the amplitude of cyclic variation, or the phase of the integrated backscatter, but it is necessary to determine the absolute value of time-averaged integrated backscatter.

We thank Delbert McGraw for his skillful technical assistance and Joyce Kalayeh for patience in preparation of this manuscript.

References

1. Miller JG, Sobel BE: Cardiac ultrasonic tissue characterization. Hosp Pract **1:** 143, 1982
2. Miller JG, Pérez JE, Mottley JG, Madaras EI, Johnston PH, Blodgett ED, Thomas LF, Sobel BE: Myocardial tissue characterization: an approach based on quantitative backscatter and attenuation. *In* Proceedings of the 1983 IEEE Ultrasonics Symposium. 1983, vol 83, CH1947-1, p 782–793
3. Miller JG, Pérez JE, Sobel BE: Ultrasonic characterization of myocardium. Prog Cardiovasc Dis (in press)
4. O'Brien WD, Olerud J, Shung KK, Reid JM: Quantitative acoustical assessment of wound maturation with acoustic microscopy. J Acoust Soc Am **69:** 575, 1981
5. Chivers RC: Tissue characterization. Ultrasound Med Biol **7:** 1, 1981
6. Reid JM: The scattering of ultrasound by tissues. *In* Proceedings of Seminar on Ultrasonic Tissue Characterization (1975). Washington, D.C., 1976, National Bureau of Standards Special Publication, vol 453, p 29
7. Mimbs JW, O'Donnell M, Bauwens D, Miller JG, Sobel BE: The dependence of ultrasonic attenuation and backscatter on collagen content in dog and rabbit hearts. Circ Res **47:** 49, 1980
8. O'Donnell M, Mimbs JW, Miller JG: Relationship between collagen and ultrasonic backscatter in myocardial tissue. J Acoust Soc Am **62:** 580, 1981
9. Mimbs JW, Bauwens D, Cohen RD, O'Donnell M, Miller JG, Sobel BE: Effects of myocardial ischemia on quantitative ultrasonic backscatter and identification of responsible determinants. Circ Res **49:** 89, 1981
10. Mimbs JW, O'Donnell M, Miller JG, Sobel BE: Detection of cardiomyopathic changes induced by doxorubicin based on quantitative analysis of ultrasonic backscatter. Am J Cardiol **47:** 1056, 1981
11. Pérez JE, Barzilai B, Madaras EI, Glueck RM, Saffitz JE, Johnston P, Miller JG, Sobel BE: Application of ultrasonic tissue characterization for longitudinal assessment and differentiation of calcification and fibrosis in cardiomyopathy. J Am Coll Cardiol **4:** 88, 1984
12. Madaras EI, Barzilai B, Pérez JE, Sobel BE, Miller JG: Changes in myocardial backscatter throughout the cardiac cycle. Ultrasonic Imaging **5:** 229, 1983
13. Barzilai B, Madaras EI, Sobel BE, Miller JG, Pérez JE: Effects of

myocardial contraction on ultrasonic backscatter before and after ischemia. Am J Physiol **247:** H478, 1984
14. Glueck RM, Mottley JG, Miller JG, Sobel BE, Perez JE: Effects of coronary artery occlusion and reperfusion on cardiac cycle-dependent variation of myocardial ultrasonic backscatter. Circ Res (in press)
15. Thomas LJ, Wickline SA, Perez JE, Sobel BE, Miller JG: A real-time integrated backscatter measurement system for quantitative tissue characterization. IEEE Trans Sonics Ultrasonics (in press)
16. Ross J Jr, Sonnenblick EH, Kaiser GA, Frommer PL, Braunwald E: Electroaugmentation of ventricular performance and oxygen consumption by repetitive application of paired electrical stimuli. Circ Res **16:** 332, 1965
17. Abel FL: Maximal negative dP/dt as an indicator of end of systole. Am J Physiol **240:** H676, 1981
18. Wildenthal K, Mierzwiak DS, Mitchell JH: Effect of sudden changes in aortic pressure on left ventricular dP/dt. Am J Physiol **216:** 185, 1969
19. Snedecor GW, Cochran WG: Statistical methods, ed 7. Ames, Iowa, 1980, Iowa State University Press
20. Yoran C, Covell JW, Ross J Jr: Structural basis for the ascending limb of left ventricular function. Circ Res **32:** 297, 1973
21. LeWinter MM, Kent RS, Kroener JM, Carew JW: Regional differences in myocardial performance in the left ventricle of the dog. Circ Res **37:** 191, 1975
22. Sabbah HN, Marzilli M, Stein PD: The relative role of subendocardium and subepicardium in left ventricular mechanics. Am J Physiol **240:** H920, 1981
23. Streeter DD Jr, Hanna WT: Engineering mechanics for successive states in canine left ventricular myocardium. II. Fiber angle and sarcomere length. Circ Res **33:** 656, 1973
24. Stein PD, Marzilli M, Sabbah HN, Lee T: Systolic and diastolic pressure gradients within the left ventricular wall. Am J Physiol **238:** H625, 1980
25. Chadwick RS: Mechanics of the left ventricle. Biophys J **39:** 279, 1982
26. Pierce WH: Body forces and pressures in elastic models of the myocardium. Biophys J **34:** 35, 1981
27. Streeter DD, Vaishnav RN, Patell DJ, Spotnik HM, Ross J Jr, Sonnenblick EH: Stress distribution in the canine left ventricle during systole and diastole. Biophys J **10:** 345, 1970
28. Ghista DN, Sandler H: An analytic elastic-viscoelastic model for the shape and the forces in the left ventricle. J Biomechan **2:** 35, 1969
29. Braunwald E, Ross J Jr, Sonnenblick EH: Mechanics of contraction of the normal and failing heart, ed 2. Boston, 1976, Little, Brown and Co.
30. Sonnenblick EH: Series elastic and contractile elements in heart muscle: changes in muscle length. Am J Physiol **207:** 1330, 1964
31. Brady AJ, Tan ST, Ricchiuti NV: Perturbation measurements of papillary muscle elasticity. Am J Physiol **241:** H155, 1981
32. Shung KK, Reid RM: Ultrasonic scattering from tissue. *In* Proceedings of the 1977 Ultrasonic Symposium of the IEEE. 1977, Cat 77CH12364-ISV, p 230
33. Cohen RD, Mottley JG, Miller JG, Kurnik PB, Sobel BE: Detection of ischemic myocardium in vivo through the chest wall by quantitative ultrasonic tissue characterization. Am J Cardiol **50:** 838, 1982

Ultrasonic tissue characterization: detection of acute myocardial ischemia in dogs

INGELA SCHNITTGER, M.D., AUGUST VIELI, PH.D., JOSEPH E. HEISERMAN, PH.D., BRUCE A. DIRECTOR, M.S., MARGARET E. BILLINGHAM, M.D., STEPHEN G. ELLIS, M.D., ROBERT S. KERNOFF, M.S., TOSHIHIKO TAKAMOTO, M.D., AND RICHARD L. POPP, M.D.

ABSTRACT Ultrasonic tissue characterization is a new area of investigation in the field of cardiac ultrasound. The amplitude and frequency of the ultrasound signal are normally altered as the signal penetrates through tissue. It is assumed that the amplitude distribution and frequency shift of diseased or edematous tissue are different than those of normal tissue. A statistical approach to the analysis of the unprocessed radiofrequency signal in the amplitude domain was used to study the effect of acute myocardial ischemia on the parameter mean amplitude/standard deviation of the amplitude (MSR). Ten dogs were anesthetized and underwent left lateral thoracotomy. Baseline mean MSR from the interventricular septum was 1.99 ± 0.05, but increased by 30 min after coronary artery occlusion and started to plateau at 1 hr (mean 2.24 ± 0.06). Reproducibility in noninfarcted myocardium (left ventricular inferoposterior wall) was good, with a mean MSR of 2.00 ± 0.05 at baseline and 1.98 ± 0.04 3 to 4 hr later. There was no difference in mean MSR when data were obtained through chest wall and when they were obtained directly from the surface of the heart. We conclude that statistical analysis in the amplitude domain of the unprocessed radiofrequency signal can detect acute myocardial ischemia within 30 min after coronary artery occlusion, provides reproducible measurements, and is unaffected by chest wall filtering.
Circulation 72, No. 1, 193–199, 1985.

DETECTION OF early acute myocardial ischemia in man is currently suboptimal. The electrocardiogram may not always reveal acute ischemia because it may demonstrate only nonspecific changes. The technetium pyrophosphate scintigram usually requires a delay of 24 hr before it can be interpreted as positive for myocardial injury. The information obtained from serum creatine kinase–MB levels is also delayed. A history of angina pectoris may be the only evidence of ongoing myocardial infarction in these patients. It would be highly desirable to have a noninvasive tool available for diagnosis and localization of early acute myocardial injury.

Echocardiography has traditionally been used as an imaging device. Recent work by several investigators suggests that interactions between the ultrasound energy and tissue can be analyzed to characterize the histologic state of tissue, both in vitro[1, 2] and in vivo.[3–6] However, several quite different approaches to ultrasonic tissue characterization have been pursued. Miller, Mimbs, and Cohen and their colleagues[1, 2, 4] have measured quantitated integrated backscatter from the unprocessed radiofrequency (rf) signal. In vivo, lack of an absolute calibration standard and the presence of the chest wall, with its variable acoustic characteristics, have been problems. Skorton et al.[3, 5] have analyzed the rf signal after it has been processed and displayed on the traditional image, applying various texture algorithms to extract information about the tissue. The potential disadvantage of image analysis is its dependence on the transducer and machine used to collect and process data and on the position of the region of interest within the scan field.[7] We have previously worked with a statistical approach to the study of the unprocessed rf signal[8] in which we analyzed the amplitude domain.[9,10] We have shown that the measured parameter is independent of the measurement site when tested in a tissue-mimicking phantom. In the phantom there was no statistically significant difference in the parameter mean amplitude/standard deviation of the amplitude (MSR) whether it was sampled at a depth of 1 to 2, 5 to 6, or 9 to 10 cm.[9] This

From the Cardiology Division, Stanford University School of Medicine, Stanford, CA.
Supported in part by contract No. 15534-01-00 from Hewlett-Packard, Andover, MA.
Address for correspondence: Richard L. Popp, M.D., Cardiology Division, Stanford University Medical Center, Stanford, CA 94305.
Received Sept. 24, 1984; revision accepted April 18, 1985.

approach is unaffected by time-gain compensation (mean amplitude) over the range of 16% to 50% of the full scale of the A/D converter.[9]

Using ultrasonic tissue characterization, Cohen et al.[4] reported an increase in integrated backscatter within 2 hr of coronary artery occlusion but used a constant factor to compensate for chest wall–dependent attenuation of the signal. Although their results indicate that myocardial backscatter could be quantified in the intact dog when chest wall attenuation was compensated for, humans are more likely to have a wider variation in chest wall thickness than the five dogs reported in that study. Skorton et al.,[5] using texture algorithm on the processed rf signal, could detect myocardial injury 2 days after coronary artery occlusion in closed-chest dogs. Parisi et al.[11] have described serial changes in tissue characteristics of myocardial injury in vivo starting 24 hr after coronary occlusion. They used a color-encoded two-dimensional echocardiographic image technique. Rasmussen et al.,[12] using computer enhancement and a mathematically defined integrated backscatter ratio, found changes in backscatter within 12 min of coronary artery occlusion in open-chest dogs. However, a calibration measurement using internal landmarks such as endo-myo-epicardium in an area close to the infarcted region was also required for this study. The need for such internal calibration requires normal reference tissue.

In the present protocol we investigated the possibility of use of our statistical amplitude analysis of the unprocessed rf signal as a noninvasive "biopsy" in the detection of early acute ischemic injury in the dog. Our hypothesis was that the measurements would be unaffected by chest wall characteristics even without external or internal calibration.

Methods

Tissue characterization: statistical analysis of rf. A volume of healthy myocardium can be modeled as a large number of independent scatterers. Ultrasound scattered from such a volume will show a particular distribution of amplitudes, called a Rayleigh distribution. Disease processes such as collagen formation, calcium deposits, and edema may cause the scatterers to become correlated (i.e., dependent). A situation in which some fraction of the scatterers are dependent and some are independent leads to a different, non-Rayleigh, amplitude distribution. The ratio MSR is a computationally simple way to distinguish between Rayleigh and non-Rayleigh distributions. The MSR for a Rayleigh distribution is 1.91 and is expected to increase above this value for tissue that contains some fraction of correlated scatterers.[13]

Data acquisition. Two-dimensional echocardiograms were obtained with a commercially available sector scanner (Hewlett-Packard 77020A) with a focused phased-array 3.5 MHz transducer. The region of suspected infarct or presumed normal tissue was imaged in the parasternal short-axis view and the M mode cursor (one scan line) was directed through the area of interest. The gain settings (transmit power and time-gain compensation controls) were adjusted to obtain an optimal image. The unprocessed rf signal from the cursor-selected scan line was sampled at 20 MHz and digitized with a Biomation 8100 transient recorder (8 bits) under microprocessor control (Cromemco, Z-2 Mountain View, CA). One repetition consisted of 40 M mode scan lines sampled sequentially over 40 msec. The first five to 10 ultrasonic scan lines were used to calculate a MSR for that repetition. An average MSR was then calculated from 10 such repetitions. This averaged MSR represented a single measurement at a given point in time. All data were acquired in mid-diastole to minimize any potential cyclic variation in MSR such as that reported for integrated backscatter.[14] Each scan line contained 1000 data points corresponding to 4 cm. The data were stored on a nine-track magnetic tape and later transferred to a Hewlett-Packard HP1000 F-series minicomputer for processing. For the last two animal experiments in this series we used a different acquisition system. This system consisted of a Hewlett-Packard A-series computer with a Hewlett-Packard model 5180 waveform recorder. The signal was digitized at 20 MHz and stored on the computer's disk.

Data analysis. The unprocessed rf signal was displayed as amplitude vs tissue depth (figure 1). The operator selected the depth corresponding to the anatomic region of interest. The computer derived a histogram (figure 1) representing the number of occurrences of rectified peak amplitudes of the digitized signal on the y axis and the amplitudes on the x axis. In each window of interest, the amplitude of the peaks of the rectified signal were calculated. The ratio of the mean to the standard deviation of these amplitudes was described by the MSR value. Considerable care was taken in the setting of the data window within the rf tracing. The window width was kept constant at approximately half a centimeter and adjusted as needed in the middle of the myocardial wall to avoid high-amplitude endocardial or epicardial reflections. In a tissue-mimicking phantom and in human blood we have previously shown that gate size does not significantly alter MSR if kept at 0.5 to 1 cm.[9] To assess problems with improper gate settings, the window was automatically shifted 15 points (1.2 mm) to each side of the original position to ensure that specular interfaces were not included in the window. If the MSR changed more than 3% as the window shifted, the primary window was moved, if possible, to find an area that did not show this change. If such a window could not be found, then the rf was rejected.

Animal preparation. Ten mongrel dogs were sedated with morphine sulphate (2 mg/kg, im) and anesthetized with intravenous chloralose (85 mg/kg) and urethane (625 mg/kg). Ventilation was provided by a Harvard pump, which delivered room air through a cuffed endotracheal tube. Depth and rate of respiration were adjusted to maintain arterial pH between 7.35 and 7.45, Po_2 between 80 and 110 mm Hg, and Pco_2 between 35 and 45 mm Hg. A large-bore catheter was inserted into the left femoral artery of each dog to monitor the systemic arterial pressure with a Statham P23Db transducer. A second catheter was placed in the right femoral vein for administration of additional anesthetic agent, which was given to maintain deep anesthesia throughout the experiment. The right jugular vein was catheterized for infusion of antiarrhythmic drug. The chest of each dog was opened by means of a left lateral thoracotomy and the heart was exposed and supported in a pericardial sling. A bipolar pacemaker electrode was attached to the right ventricle. Ventricular pacing rate was maintained at 150 beats/min with one channel of a WPI 800 series stimulator.

The left anterior descending coronary artery (LAD) was dissected free and a snare was placed around the artery at the level of the mid-LAD (beyond the first large diagonal branch). Before

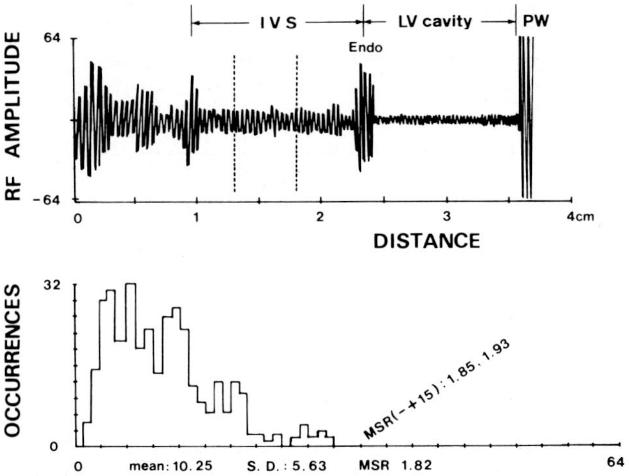

FIGURE 1. *Top,* One sample of unprocessed rf signal displaying amplitude (RF AMP) on the y axis and distance on the x-axis. The rf signal was obtained from a closed-chest measurement with the cursor cutting slightly obliquely through the septum. A definable window (dashed verticle lines) was set in the septum, within the myoardium, for further analysis with use of a histogram of the data. Endo = endocardium; IVS = interventricular septum; PW = posterior wall. *Bottom,* Histogram constructed with data from 10 samples such as those in the *top* panel and displaying the number of occurrences of a certain amplitude plotted on the y axis and amplitudes on the x axis. The mean amplitude, standard deviation of amplitudes, and MSR are automatically derived by the computer. Gates that were too close to specular interfaces were detected by comparing the MSR values for the selected window with the ones obtained when the window was shifted by a predetermined amount to the left or the right. In this study, the gate was shifted 15 points (1.2 mm) and the corresponding MSR values are displayed to the right in this panel.

occlusion of the artery, 16.7 μg/kg/min diltiazem was infused for 30 min as antifibrillatory drug therapy (total dose of diltiazem, 0.5 mg/kg). At the completion of this infusion the artery was tied off to create an infarct in the LAD distribution.

Open-chest measurements. The dog was placed supine on its right side in a specially constructed wooden cradle. Open-chest measurements were obtained by placing the transducer directly on the interventricular sulcus angling steeply toward the left ventricular apex. The transducer was hand held and a very light pressure was applied on the heart to ensure contact between the transducer and the beating heart. No gel or stand-off device was used. An image from the parasternal short-axis view was obtained at the level of the papillary muscles.

Radiofrequency data were collected in all 10 dogs from the midinterventricular septum and left ventricular inferoposterior wall before occlusion of the coronary artery. After occlusion, data were sampled from the septum at 30 and 60 min after occlusion and then hourly for 4 hr. Data from the left ventricular inferoposterior wall were again obtained at 4 hr. Although there was no absolute way to determine that data were being sampled from the same area before and after occlusion, the level of the papillary muscles was imaged similarly at all times and a conscientious effort was made to sample rf from the same area throughout the study.

Closed-chest measurements. The closed-chest measurements were obtained with the animal in the same position as described for the open-chest measurements. Data were collected with the transducer placed under the wooden cradle in a specially built opening to allow images to be obtained from

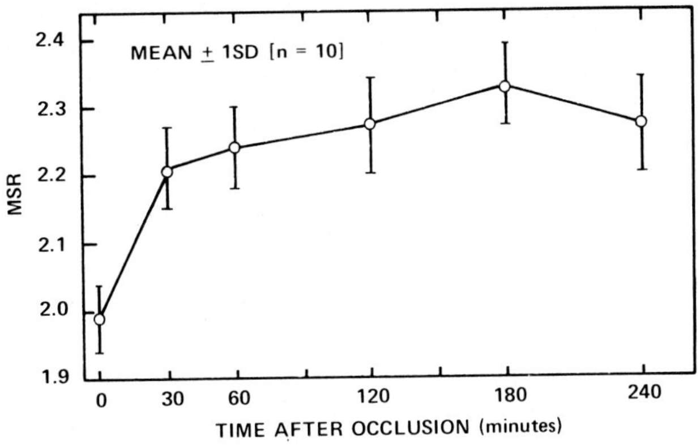

FIGURE 2. MSR as a function of time after occlusion of the LAD in 10 dogs. All error bars are expressed as mean ± SD.

underneath the dog. The ultrasound beam then passed through the right chest wall, right ventricle, and finally the left ventricle. A short-axis parasternal view was obtained at the level of the papillary muscles. Radiofrequency data from the midinterventricular septum were obtained through the right chest wall at the same time intervals as for the open-chest measurements.

Histology. A biopsy sample was obtained from the infarcted area at the time each dog was killed. To ensure that samples were from the area of ultrasonic sampling, a long needle was passed through the interventricular sulcus and into the midseptum along the direction of the ultrasound beam. Tissue was analyzed by light and electron microscopy to allow examination of the ultrastructure of the tissue after occlusion that reflected the change observed in the ultrasonic parameter.

Statistical analysis. The MSR obtained for each point in time for each animal was the result of averaging 10 MSRs. The unpaired Student t test was used to compare posterior wall measurements at different times. Two-factor analysis of variance was used to compare open- and closed-chest measurements and MSRs at baseline and after coronary occlusion. Multiple simultaneous comparisons were done to determine if baseline MSR was different from MSR after coronary occlusion.

Results

MSR as a function of time after occlusion of the LAD in 10 dogs is illustrated in figure 2. The data used in the following analyses are listed in table 1. All MSRs are mean ± SD. A two-factor analysis of variance was done with one factor being the measurement of the interventricular septum in a closed or open position and the other time after occlusion.

Table 2 represents the results of the analysis of variance. The F statistic for open vs closed chest was 0.41, which was not statistically significant ($p > .5$). The comparison of MSR at baseline and at five intervals after occlusion yielded a F statistic of 23.0, $p < .0001$.

A set of multiple comparisons of the differences between the baseline MSR and each MSR after occlusion is shown in table 3. The 99% confidence interval did not overlap zero, so the baseline MSR was significantly different from each postocclusion ratio.

Reproducibility of MSR in noninfarcted tissue of

TABLE 1
Mean (±SD) MSRs

	Time after occlusion (min)					
	0	30	60	120	180	240
Septum open	1.99±0.05	2.21±0.06	2.26±0.11	2.24±0.07	2.32±0.17	2.29±0.09
Septum closed	2.01±0.07	2.22±0.07	2.22±0.05	2.30±0.05	2.34±0.06	2.28±0.06
Posterior wall	2.00±0.05					1.98±0.04

TABLE 2
Two-factor analysis of variance with unequal replication

Source of variation	Sum of squares	d.f.	Variance	F ratio	p value
Open vs closed chest	0.0031	1	0.0031	0.41	>.5
Time after occlusion	0.8683	5	0.1737	23.0	<.0001
Residual	0.3393	45	0.0075		

d.f. = degrees of freedom.

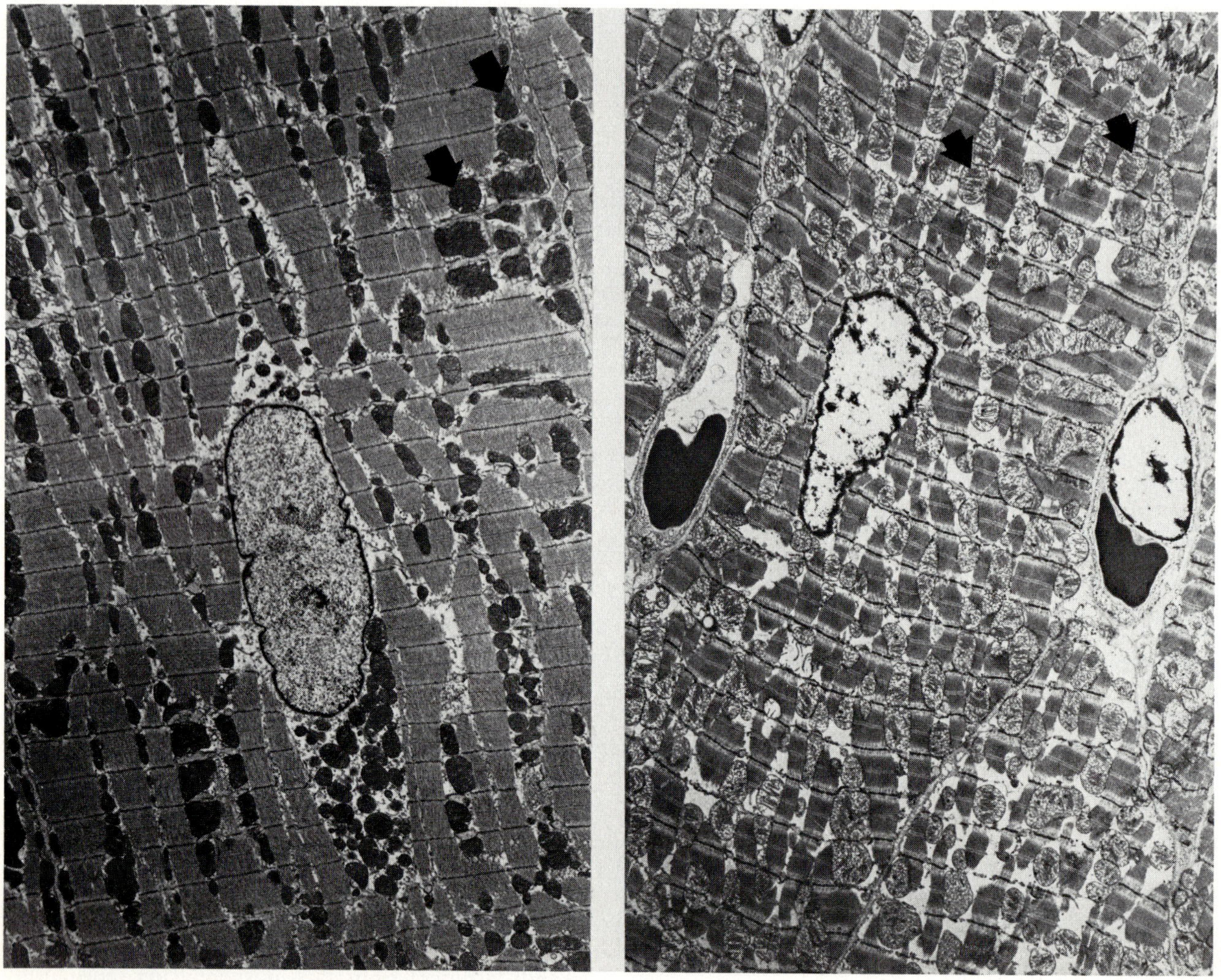

FIGURE 3A. Electron microscopic slide of swelling of mitochondria with cristal stacking (arrows, to the *right*) compared with normal tissue (*left*).

TABLE 3
Difference in MSR at baseline vs after occlusion

Time (min)	Difference from baseline	99% simultaneous confidence interval
30	0.198	0.067
60	0.249	0.067
120	0.252	0.067
180	0.335	0.067
240	0.285	0.067

open-chest dogs (left ventricular inferoposterior wall), tested in six animals, was 2.00 ± 0.05 at baseline and 3 to 4 hr later it showed no significant change by unpaired Student's t test (1.98 ± 0.04; $p = .49$).

Electron microscopy releaved swelling of the sarcotubular system, mitochondrial swelling, and "cristal stacking" (figure 3A), as well as swelling of the capillary endothelium (figure 3B), at 3 to 4 hr after coronary occlusion. At this time light microscopy showed only minimal changes associated with ischemic contraction (figure 4).

Discussion

Ultrasonic tissue characterization is a new and potentially exciting field of cardiac ultrasound. Several different approaches to ultrasonic tissue characterization have been tested and it is not yet clear which, if any, is superior. We have worked with the statistical approach to ultrasonic tissue characterization and found that we can detect ischemia as early as 30 min after coronary artery occlusion in this study. This is in agreement with what some others have found using very different techniques.[4, 12] Although the current data are expressed as mean ± SD, and our method required a fair amount of averaging of data, the measurement 30 min after coronary artery occlusion was statistically significantly different from baseline. There may be several reasons for the relatively large spread in indi-

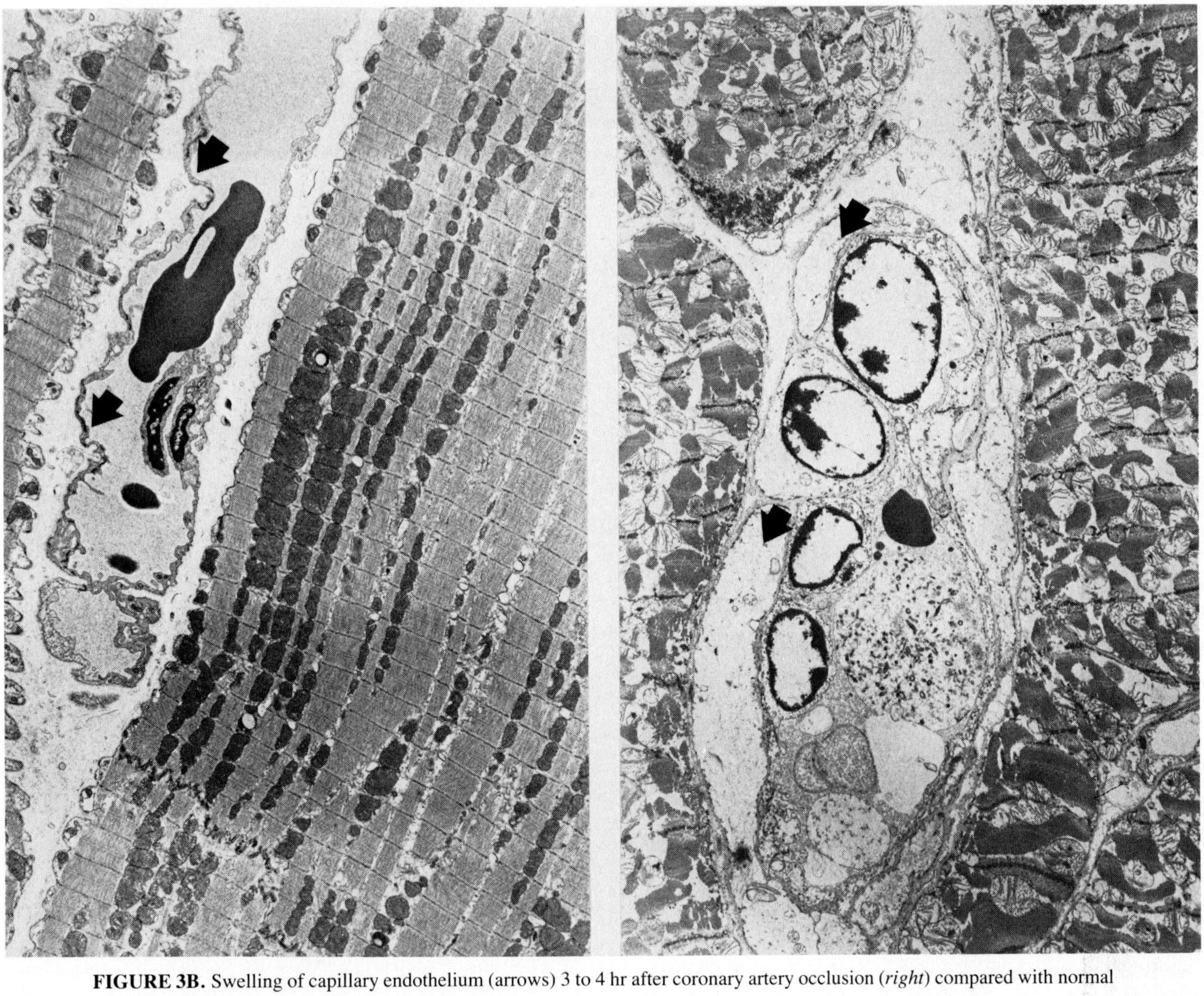

FIGURE 3B. Swelling of capillary endothelium (arrows) 3 to 4 hr after coronary artery occlusion (*right*) compared with normal tissue (*left*).

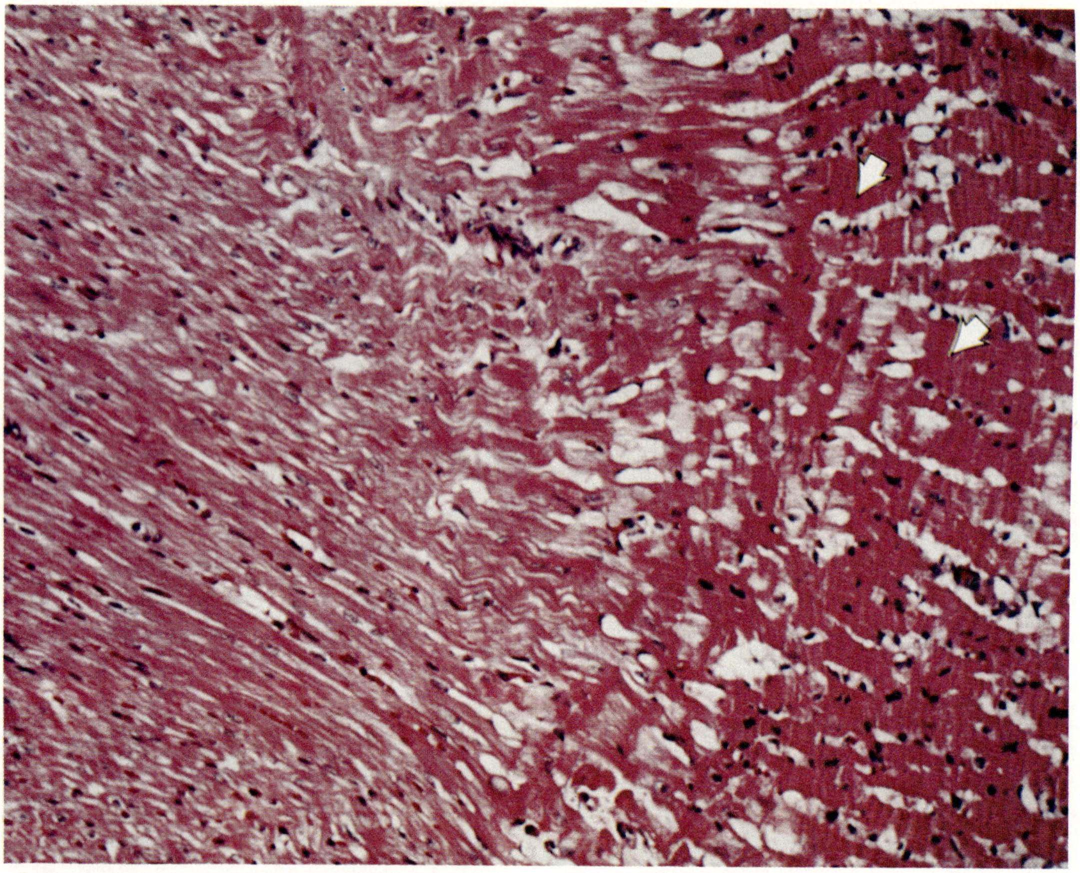

FIGURE 4. Light microscopic slide illustrating only very minimal changes associated with ischemic contraction (arrows) at 3 to 4 hr after coronary artery occlusion.

vidual measurements of MSR. First, the myocardium sampled may not have been homogeneously ischemic from epicardium to endocardium and this may be a patchy process. Second, there is most likely a degree of variation inherent in the method itself. Third, our method is extremely sensitive to any inclusion of high-amplitude signals in analysis of the window of interest, since such a specular reflector immediately will markedly increase the standard deviation of amplitudes and thereby decrease the MSR. Nevertheless, in contrast to that of Cohen et al.,[4] our method of analysis was independent of acoustic filtering by the chest wall and did not require any external or internal calibration such as that reported by Cohen and by Rasmussen et al.[12] This is a very important feature since the method therefore becomes potentially applicable in humans. Our amplitude analysis showed excellent reproducibility over time in nonischemic myocardium when tested in the left ventricular inferoposterior myocardium.

The explanation for the altered rf signal in early ischemia, as reflected in the MSR, is not entirely clear. Our MSR parameter did not increase as a matter of increased echogenicity alone (higher mean amplitude) since we also registered a decrease in the standard deviation of the amplitude. The electron microscopic analysis suggests there are changes in tissue structures at the subcellular level and this may alter scattering properties. Although we have not proven that the changes seen on the electron microscopic slides can account for the observed changes in MSR, it is important to know there are changes in the tissue at this early point in time after coronary occlusion. Myocardial cells or bundles of cells can be looked upon as individual scatterers, and as found by others using erythrocytes,[15] when the density of scatterers changes, the backscatter may change. Despite the uncertainty about why the MSR measurement changes with acute myocardial ischemia, we believe the results reported here, obtained with this statistical approach to the study of unprocessed rf data analysis and ultrasonic tissue characterization, are encouraging and warrant further work to better understand and utilize the technique.

References

1. O'Donnell M, Mimbs JW, Miller JG: Relationship between collagen and ultrasonic backscatter in myocardial tissue. J Acoust Soc Am **69:** 580, 1981

2. Mimbs JW, O'Donnell M, Miller JG, Sobel BF: Detection of cardiomyopathic changes induced by Doxorubicin based on quantitative analysis of ultrasonic backscatter. Am J Cardiol **47:** 1056, 1981
3. Skorton DJ, Collins SM, Nichols J, Pandian NG, Beau JA, Kerber RE: Quantitative texture analysis in two-dimensional echocardiography: application to the diagnosis of experimental myocardial contusion. Circulation **68:** 217, 1983
4. Cohen RD, Mottley JG, Miller JG, Kurnik PB, Sobel BE: Detection of ischemic myocardium in vivo through the chest wall by quantitative ultrasonic tissue characterization. Am J Cardiol **50:** 838, 1982
5. Skorton DJ, Melton HE, Pandian NG, Nichols J, Koyanagi S, Marcus ML, Collins SM, Kerber RE: Detection of acute myocardial infarction in closed-chest dogs by analysis of regional two-dimensional echocardiographic gray level distributions. Circ Res **52:** 36, 1983
6. Allen LD, Joseph MC, Tynan M: Clinical value of echocardiographic colour image processing in two cases of primary cardiac tumor. Br Heart J **49:** 154, 1983
7. Skorton DJ, Collins SM, Melton HE Jr, Woskoff SD: Texture in two-dimensional echocardiograms: regional variability. J Am Coll Cardiol **1:** 669, 1983 (abst)
8. Joynt L: A stochastic approach to ultrasonic tissue characterization, doctoral thesis. Stanford University Technical Report No. G557-4, 1979
9. Vieli A, Heiserman J, Schnittger I, Popp RL: An improved stochastic approach to rf amplitude analysis in ultrasonic tissue characterization. Ultrasonic Imaging **6:** 139, 1984
10. Green S, Joynt L, Fitzgerald PJ, Rubenson D, Popp RL: In vivo ultrasonic tissue characterization of human intracardiac masses. Am J Cardiol **51:** 231, 1983
11. Parisi AF, Nieminen M, O'Boyle JE, Moynihan PF, Khuri S, Kloner RA, Folland ED, Schoen FJ: Enhanced detection of the evolution of tissue changes after acute myocardial infarction using color-encoded two-dimensional echocardiography. Circulation **66:** 764, 1982
12. Rasmussen S, Lovelace DE, Knoebel SB, Ransbury R, Corya BC: Echocardiographic detection of ischemia and infarcted myocardium. J Am Coll Cardiol **3:** 733, 1984
13. Beckman P: Probability in communication engineering. New York, 1967, Harcourt, Brace & World, Inc.
14. Gluech RM, Mottley JG, Miller JG, Sobel BE, Perez JE: Cyclic variation of myocardial backscatter: an ultrasonic index of contractile function. Circulation **68**(suppl III): III-330, 1983 (abst)
15. Yaun YW, Shung KK, Fei DY: Effects of flow disturbance and erythrocyte aggregation on ultrasonic backscatter from blood. J Acoust Soc Am **75:** 1265, 1984

Day-to-day variations in inducibility of ventricular tachyarrhythmias during the late postmyocardial infarction phase in conscious dogs

STUART M. COBBE, M.D., M.R.C.P.,* ELLEN HOFFMANN, ANDREAS RITZENHOFF, JOHANNES BRACHMANN, M.D., WOLFGANG KÜBLER, M.D., AND JOCHEN SENGES, M.D.

ABSTRACT The inducibility of ventricular tachyarrhythmias was studied daily on days 3 through 8 after experimental myocardial infarction in 15 conscious dogs. Although a sustained ventricular tachyarrhythmia was produced on one or more occasions in 11 of 15 dogs (73%), there was marked daily variation in the results of programmed stimulation. Ventricular fibrillation or sustained ventricular tachycardia was elicited in six dogs on day 3 after infarction. In two of these dogs, no sustained tachycardia could be induced by day 7. In nine dogs sustained ventricular arrhythmias were not inducible on day 3. By day 6 to 7, sustained ventricular tachycardia was inducible in five of these dogs. In clinical practice similar variation in the inducibility of sustained ventricular arrhythmias may conceivably complicate the use of results of programmed ventricular stimulation as determinants of risk of sudden death after myocardial infarction.
Circulation 72, No. 1, 200–204, 1985.

THERE HAS BEEN considerable recent interest in the possibility of identifying patients at risk of sudden death after recovery from acute myocardial infarction. An invasive approach to prognostic evaluation involves the use of programmed ventricular extrastimulation 1 to 4 weeks after recovery to determine whether ventricular arrhythmias are inducible.[1–3] Inducible ventricular tachycardia appears to require a substrate of areas of electrophysiologically depressed, slowly conducting myocardium, usually at the border of the infarcted area.[4, 5] These areas confer chronic "electrical instability," with its attendant risk of malignant arrhythmias. We have studied the day-to-day variability in the results of programmed ventricular stimulation in conscious dogs after experimental myocardial infarction to determine whether major changes in the inducibility of ventricular arrhythmias are to be expected in the early postinfarction period. We have also investigated the possible influence of resting sinus cycle length and ventricular effective refractory period on the outcome of programmed stimulation.

From the Abteilung Innere Medizine III (Kardiologie), Universitätsklinik Heidelberg, West Germany.
Supported under SFB 90 der Deutschen Forschungsgemeinschaft.
Address for correspondence: Dr. S. M. Cobbe, Cardiac Department, John Radcliffe Hospital, Headington, Oxford, England.
Received March 12, 1984; revision accepted Feb. 28, 1985.
*Current address: Cardiac Department, John Radcliffe Hospital, Headington, Oxford, England. Dr. Cobbe is a recipient of a Fellowship of the Alexander von Humboldt Foundation.

Methods

Mongrel dogs (11 to 24 kg) were premedicated with morphine and chlorpromazine and anesthetized with pentobarbital (15 mg/kg). After induction of anesthesia, 1 megaunit benzyl penicillin and 30 mg/kg methylprednisolone were given intravenously.[6] The surgical technique of two-stage proximal ligation of the left anterior descending coronary[7] and implantation of atrial and ventricular bipolar stimulating electrodes and subcutaneous electrocardiographic electrodes has recently been described in detail.[8]

Fifteen dogs were studied with programmed stimulation over 3 to 8 days after infarction. They had been trained to stand unsedated in a sling. Bipolar electrograms (30 to 500 Hz, 1 mV/cm) were recorded from the left atrial appendage and noninfarcted area of the left ventricle except when the electrodes were being used for stimulation. The subcutaneous electrocardiographic signal (direct current to 500 Hz, 1 mV/cm) corresponded to an orthogonal Z lead. After each animal had settled in the sling, resting sinus cycle length was recorded.

Pacing protocol for induction of tachycardia. Pacing was performed with a Medtronic programmable constant-current stimulator with the use of square-wave stimuli of 2 msec duration at 3 times diastolic threshold. The stimulation protocol was as follows: (1) Atrial pacing frequency series at cycle lengths of 400 to 160 msec. (2) Premature ventricular stimulation with single (V_2) and double (V_2V_3) extrastimuli after every 8 ventricular paced beats at basic cycle lengths of 350, 300, and 250 msec. The effective refractory period to single ventricular extrastimuli (VERP) was measured during ventricular drive pacing at a cycle length of 300 msec. (3) Ventricular pacing frequency series at cycle lengths of 400 to 160 msec. (4) Bursts of four to five ventricular extrastimuli at cycle lengths of 200 to 130 msec, with 10 attempts at each cycle length. Bursts were not synchronized to the R wave.

The pacing protocol was performed in an identical manner on each day of the study. The end point of the stimulation on each occasion was development of sustained ventricular tachycardia or ventricular fibrillation, or completion of the full pacing protocol. Unless cardioversion had been necessary, the reproducibility of induction of each tachycardia was confirmed three times.

Sustained ventricular tachycardia was defined as a stable tachycardia with a uniform QRS pattern that required termination by overdrive pacing or, if necessary, by cardioversion. Nonsustained ventricular tachycardia was defined as any self-terminating response of 4 or more pleomorphic ventricular beats.

Repeat study. At the end of each programmed stimulation series, the dogs were returned to the animal quarters. Programmed ventricular stimulation to the same end point was repeated on a daily basis until day 7 or 8.

Statistical methods. Results are expressed as mean ± SD. Differences between groups were assessed by Student's t test. Two-tailed p values <.05 were considered indicative of a significant difference.

Results

Ventricular tachyarrhythmias. A total of 57 programmed stimulations was performed (mean 3.8 per dog). Stimulation produced ventricular fibrillation in four (7%), sustained ventricular tachycardia in 18 (32%), nonsustained ventricular tachycardia in 28 (49%), and no ventricular tachycardia in seven (12%) studies. A sustained tachyarrhythmia (tachycardia or fibrillation) was produced on one or more occasions in 11 of 15 dogs (73%), and at least nonsustained ventricular tachycardia was produced in each dog.

Ventricular fibrillation occurred immediately after stimulation in two cases, accompanied by appearance of continuous chaotic electrical activity in the surface electrocardiogram and ventricular electrogram. In two other cases 7 to 12 beats of rapid polymorphic ventricular tachycardia, cycle lengths 116 and 155 msec, were noted before the onset of ventricular fibrillation. In two other cases rapid but monomorphic ventricular tachycardia (cycle lengths 119 and 121 msec) degenerated to ventricular fibrillation after 15 to 30 sec; these two were considered examples of secondary fibrillation. Excluding these two instances the mean cycle length of stable sustained ventricular tachycardia was 188 ± 27 msec. The mean number of unstimulated beats during nonsustained ventricular tachycardia was 8.1 ± 7.2, with a cycle length of 142 ± 7 msec. This cycle length was significantly shorter than that recorded during stable sustained ventricular tachycardia ($p < .001$).

Daily variation in results of programmed stimulation. The results of the first programmed stimulation study on day 3 were used to divide the dogs into two groups according to whether a sustained tachyarrhythmia was induced or not. Group 1 comprised two dogs with primary ventricular fibrillation and four with stable monomorphic ventricular tachycardia. Of the nine dogs in group 2, eight had nonsustained ventricular tachycardia and in one no tachycardia was induced. The results of programmed stimulation in dogs in groups 1 and 2 on subsequent days are shown in figures 1 and 2.

The two dogs that showed primary ventricular fibrillation on day 3 could not be resuscitated. Of the four that had stable sustained ventricular tachycardia on day 3, two developed ventricular fibrillation on day 4. One dog was successfully defibrillated and produced no further sustained tachycardias on subsequent testing. Two dogs had stable sustained ventricular tachycardia on 4 consecutive days, although the cycle length varied on a day-to-day basis from 185 to 235 msec in one and from 169 to 203 msec in the other. One dog died on day 6 as a result of ventricular fibrillation produced by overpacing in an attempt to end the tachycardia, while the other dog showed no further sustained arrhythmias on days 7 and 8. Figure 2 shows the results of the daily stimulation in group 2. Of eight dogs with nonsustained ventricular tachycardia on day 3, five had developed sustained tachycardia by day 6 or 7.

Mode of initiation of tachyarrhythmias. No tachyarrhythmias were induced by rapid atrial pacing. Ventricular fibrillation was induced by double ventricular

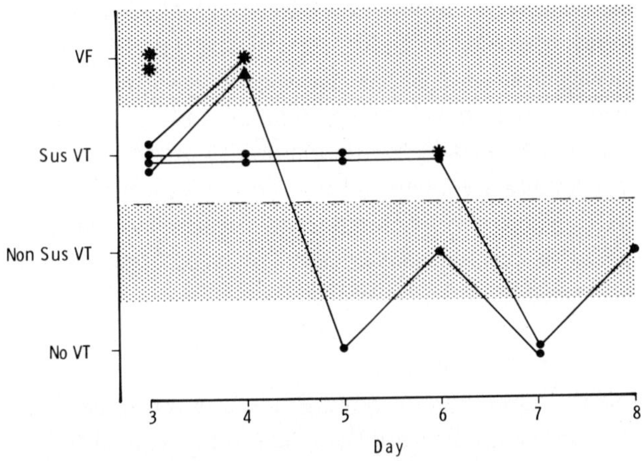

FIGURE 1. Result of programmed stimulation in six dogs that developed ventricular fibrillation or sustained ventricular tachycardia on day 3. Of the four dogs that showed sustained ventricular tachycardia, two developed ventricular fibrillation on day 4 and two had stable sustained ventricular tachycardia on 4 consecutive days. Two dogs eventually became "stable"; no sustained tachyarrhythmia was inducible. Each symbol represents one programmed stimulation. Episodes of use of direct-current shock in an attempt to terminate arrhythmias are represented as follows: ▲ = successful cardioversion/defibrillation; * = unsuccessful defibrillation.

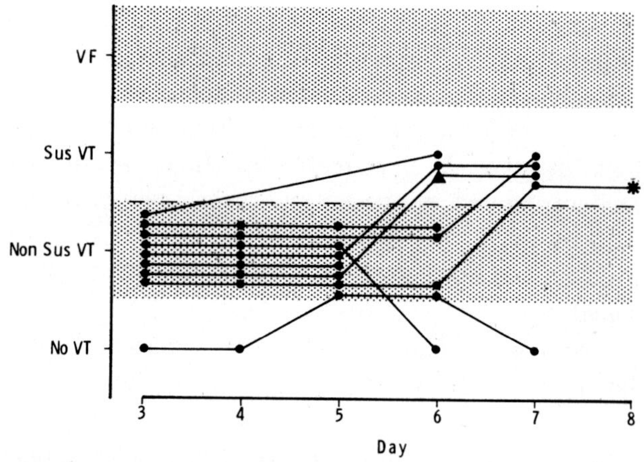

FIGURE 2. Results in nine dogs that did not show ventricular fibrillation or sustained ventricular tachycardia on day 3. By day 6 or 7, five of the nine had progressed from nonsustained to sustained ventricular tachycardia. Each symbol represents one programmed stimulation. Symbols are as in figure 1.

premature stimuli ($V_1V_2V_3$) in one instance, and by ventricular burst pacing in three. Sustained monomorphic ventricular tachycardia was induced by V_1V_2 stimulation in three studies (17%), by $V_1V_2V_3$ in three studies (17%), and by ventricular burst pacing in 12 studies (67%). Nonsustained ventricular tachycardia was induced by V_1V_2 stimulation in four experiments (14%), by $V_1V_2V_3$ in 20 (71%), and burst pacing in four (41%). No consistent pattern of change in the mode of induction of tachycardia from day to day was noted.

VERP. Diastolic pacing thresholds varied from 1 to 3 mA during the study, with no discernable consistent trend. Mean VERP for all dogs was 148 ± 13 msec on day 3, and fell to 121 ± 9 msec on day 6 ($p < .001$). Mean VERP in the six dogs that had sustained ventricular tachycardia or fibrillation on day 3 was 154 ± 12 msec, compared with 144 ± 13 msec in the nine others (NS). There was a general trend towards shortening of VERP with time, irrespective of the outcome of programmed stimulation (figure 3).

Sinus cycle length (SCL). Mean SCL in all dogs was 414 ± 55 msec on day 3 and 376 ± 38 msec on day 6 (NS). There was no significant difference between SCL in the group 1 dogs and that in the others (441 ± 46 vs 397 ± 55 msec). The mean SCL in the five dogs in group 2 that progressed from nonsustained to sustained ventricular tachycardia during the study was 404 ± 18 msec on day 3 and 401 ± 41 msec on the day of onset of sustained tachycardia.

Discussion

Our results demonstrate a considerable daily variation in the inducibility of ventricular tachyarrhythmias in the early postinfarction period. We used a pacing protocol that was similar to that in previous studies of chronic canine infarction.[9, 10] Although double extrastimuli may produce ventricular fibrillation in the noninfarcted heart under open-chest conditions,[11] there is a low incidence of false-positive induction of fibrillation, and none of sustained ventricular tachycardia, in conscious closed-chest dogs.[12] The variation in inducibility of ventricular tachyarrhythmias after experimental myocardial infarction has received little attention, since most groups have used anesthetized open-chest dogs in which serial studies were impracticable.

Karagueuzian et al.[13] studied induction of ventricular tachycardia in conscious dogs 2 to 9 days after infarction. Only two of 10 dogs that underwent permanent left anterior descending occlusion developed sustained ventricular tachycardia, each of these on one occasion only. Sustained ventricular tachycardia was induced on day 3 in 11 of 16 dogs that had undergone occlusion and reperfusion. Of the dogs showing sustained ventricular tachycardia on day 3, none had in-

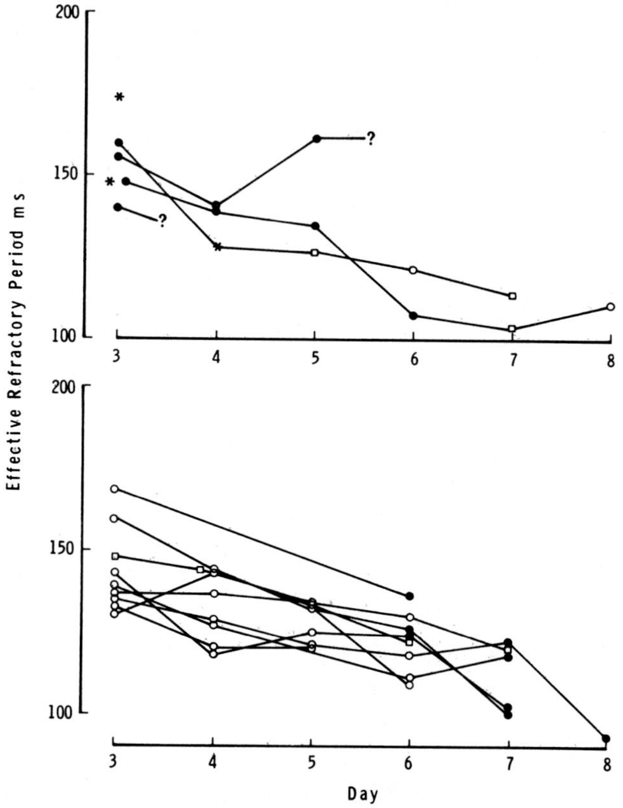

FIGURE 3. Changes in VERP over time in dogs of group 1 (*top*) and group 2 (*bottom*). There was a trend toward shortening of VERP with time in most dogs, irrespective of the outcome of programmed stimulation. Symbols designate outcome of programmed stimulation as follows: * = ventricular fibrillation; ● = sustained ventricular tachycardia; ○ = nonsustained ventricular tachycardia; □ = no ventricular tachycardia; ? = VERP inadvertently not recorded.

ducible sustained or nonsustained ventricular tachycardia by day 6, and no dog progressed from nonsustained to sustained ventricular tachycardia as they did in our study. Some major differences between the study of Karagueuzian et al. and the present work must be pointed out. The previous investigators used an occlusion/reperfusion preparation that produces a heterogeneous area of infarction unlike the uniform infarct produced by permanent occlusion, and they did not use methylprednisolone, which has been shown empirically to favor ventricular tachycardia induction.[6] We used a pacing protocol involving $V_1V_2V_3$ and burst pacing, while Karagueuzian et al. used only V_1V_2 stimulation. In a later study of conscious dogs subject to the same occlusion/reperfusion protocol,[10] the same group showed that V_1V_2 stimulation on days 3 to 5 produced sustained ventricular tachycardia in 14% of dogs, and ventricular burst pacing produced tachycardia in 26%, giving an overall incidence of 29%. Our success rate for induction of sustained tachyarrhythmias (ventricular tachycardia and ventricular fibrillation) was 22 of 57 studies (39%) in 11 of 15 dogs (73%).

Echt et al.[14] reported a study of multiple programmed ventricular stimulation performed once or twice weekly in 13 dogs that had undergone 2 hr occlusion and reperfusion of the left anterior descending artery. Sustained ventricular tachycardia, defined as a cycle length greater than 180 msec, occurred in only two of 178 programmed stimulation studies, with ventricular flutter in 25, primary ventricular fibrillation in 128, and flutter degenerating into fibrillation in 23. A number of dogs finally underwent open-chest electrophysiologic study, but the results were not significantly different from those in the closed-chest conscious preparation. The high incidence of ventricular fibrillation in their study may be the result of the use of triple extrastimuli. We did not use this technique, and were not able to continue our study beyond day 8, so we cannot comment on the late changes in inducibility of ventricular tachycardia in our preparation. There are differences in cellular electrophysiologic properties between the time periods of 3 to 5 days and 8 to 15 days after infarction,[15] with recovery of membrane potential, action potential amplitude, and rate of phase O depolarization. Thus, the early postinfarction period is one of changing electrophysiologic properties, although cellular electrophysiologic abnormalities are still demonstrable weeks to months after infarction in both experimental animals[16] and man.[17]

Our study was of course confined to induced rather than spontaneous tachyarrhythmias. We used implanted stimulating electrodes to provide a consistent site for stimulation, and did not observe major changes in stimulation threshold. We were, however, unable to investigate multiple sites of stimulation, particularly at the border of the infarcted area, where the inducibility of ventricular tachycardia may vary considerably.[9]

The ability to induce a sustained tachyarrhythmia may depend critically on the invasion of an area of potential reentrant activity by a sufficiently premature stimulus.[9] It was therefore of interest to note that the mean VERP was not significantly different in the dogs that developed sustained ventricular tachycardia or fibrillation on day 3 than in the others. The values for VERP at a cycle length of 300 msec were similar to those previously reported.[9, 13] Unlike Karagueuzian et al.,[13] we observed a general trend toward shortening of VERP with time. However, this did not appear to be a critical factor in the inducibility of sustained ventricular tachyarrhythmias at any stage. One possible explanation for the shortening of VERP with time might be an increase in sympathetic tone. This might have occurred as a result of psychological stress, which is known to reduce the threshold for repetitive ventricular responses.[18] We did not measure plasma catecholamine levels, but we also did not observe a significant increase in basal heart rate during the study, despite the decreases in VERP. Furthermore, shortening of VERP did not occur only in dogs that had experienced sustained ventricular tachycardia or cardioversion. On the basis of this indirect evidence, at least, there appeared to have been no major change in sympathetic activity.

In conclusion, we have shown in this experimental study that there is considerable day-to-day variation in the inducibility of sustained ventricular tachyarrhythmias in the early postinfarction period. Similar variation in inducibility of tachyarrhythmias may occur in the early postinfarction period in man, and may be of relevance to the optimal timing of electrophysiologic studies for prognostic evaluation.

References

1. Greene HL, Reid PR, Schaeffer AH: The repetitive ventricular response in man. A predictor of sudden death. N Engl J Med **299:** 730, 1978
2. Hamer A, Vohra J, Hunt D, Sloman G: Prediction of sudden death by electrophysiological studies in high risk patients surviving acute myocardial infarction. Am J Cardiol **50:** 223, 1982
3. Richards DA, Cody DV, Denniss AR, Russell PA, Young AA, Uther JB: Ventricular electrical instability: a predictor of death after myocardial infarction. Am J Cardiol **51:** 75, 1983
4. Klein H, Karp RB, Kouchoukos NT, Zorn GL, James TN, Waldo AL: Intraoperative electrophysiologic mapping of ventricles during sinus rhythm in patients with a previous myocardial infarction. Identification of the electrophysiologic substrate of ventricular arrhythmias. Circulation **66:** 847, 1982
5. Simson MB, Untereker WJ, Spielman SR, Horowitz LN, Marcus NH, Falcone RA, Harken AH, Josephson ME: Relation between late potentials on the body surface and directly recorded fragmented

electrograms in patients with ventricular tachycardia. Am J Cardiol **51:** 105, 1983
6. Kabell G, Scherlag BJ, Hope RR, Lazzara R: Patterns of interectopic activation recorded during pleomorphic ventricular tachycardia after myocardial infarction in the dog. Am J Cardiol **49:** 56, 1982
7. Harris AS: Delayed development of ventricular ectopic rhythms following experimental coronary occlusion. Circulation **1:** 1318, 1950
8. Cobbe SM, Hoffmann E, Ritzenhoff A, Brachmann J, Kübler W, Senges J: Action of sotalol on potential re-entrant pathways and ventricular tachyarrhythmias in conscious dogs in the late post-myocardial infarction phase. Circulation **68:** 865, 1983
9. Michelson EL, Spear JF, Moore EN: Initiation of sustained ventricular tachyarrhythmias in a canine model of myocardial infarction: Importance of the site of stimulation. Circulation **63:** 776, 1981
10. Davis J, Glassman R, Wit AL: Method for evaluating the effects of antiarrhythmic drugs on ventricular tachycardias with different electrophysiologic characteristics and different mechanisms in the infarcted canine heart. Am J Cardiol **49:** 1176, 1982
11. Wetstein L, Michelson EL, Simson MB, Moore EN, Harken AH: Initiation of ventricular tachyarrhythmia with programmed stimulation: sensitivity and specificity in an experimental canine model. Surgery **92:** 206, 1982
12. Hamer AW, Karagueuzian HS, Sugi K, Zaher CA, Mander WJ, Peter T. Factors related to the induction of ventricular fibrillation in the normal canine heart by programmed stimulation. J Am Coll Cardiol **3:** 751, 1984
13. Karagueuzian HS, Fenoglio JJ, Weiss MB, Wit AL: Protracted ventricular tachyarrhythmias induced by premature stimulation of the canine heart after coronary artery occlusion and reperfusion. Circ Res **44:** 833, 1979
14. Echt DS, Griffin JC, Ford AJ, Knutti JW, Feldman RC, Mason JW: Nature of inducible ventricular tachyarrhythmia in a chronic canine myocardial infarct model. Am J Cardiol **25:** 1127, 1983
15. Spear JF, Michelson EL, Moore EN: Cellular electrophysiologic characteristics of chronically infarcted myocardium in dogs susceptible to sustained ventricular tachyarrhythmias. J Am Coll Cardiol **1:** 1099, 1983
16. Myerburg RJ, Gelband H, Nilsson K, Sung RY, Thurer RJ, Morales AR, Bassett AL: Long-term electrophysiological abnormalities resulting from experimental myocardial infarction in cats. Circ Res **41:** 73, 1977
17. Spear JF, Horowitz LN, Hodess AB, MacVaugh N, Moore EN: Cellular electrophysiology of human myocardial infarction. 1. Abnormalities of cellular activation. Circulation **59:** 247, 1979
18. Lown B, Verrier R, Corbalan R: Psychological stress and threshold for repetitive ventricular response. Science **182:** 834, 1974

An enzyme histochemical study of human sinus node, coronary sinus, and mitral valve muscle

CLAUDE THÉRY, M.D., IVAN KRIVOSIC, M.D., PHILIPPE ASSEMAN, M.D. AND
A. E. F. HUGO MEIJER, M.D.

ABSTRACT An enzyme histochemical study of the sinoatrial node, the coronary sinus, and the atrial muscle extending into the anterior mitral valve was performed on human hearts. Investigation of the activity and localization of the structurally bound enzymes was performed by conventional histochemical techniques. Determination of the activity of nonstructurally or weakly structurally bound enzymes was performed by histochemical techniques in which leakage of enzymes during the incubation period was reduced by the application of semipermeable membranes. The sinoatrial node is characterized by a high degree of anaerobic enzyme capacity and a relatively low degree of aerobic enzyme capacity. The discriminatory nature of these reactions allows examination of the structure of the sinoatrial node and its approaches. The presence of transitional cells was confirmed; isolated clusters of nodal cells were found in the atrial myocardium around the sinoatrial node, but no evidence of specialized tissue forming the beginning of an internodal pathway was found by this technique. The specific histochemical reactions that characterize the sinoatrial node also occur in the atrial muscle, extending into the anterior mitral valve, the anterior wall of the coronary sinus, and the atrial tissue near the orifice of the coronary sinus. These observations seem to corroborate the hypothesis that arrhythmic ectopic foci can arise in these regions.
Circulation 72, No. 1, 205–213, 1985.

A THOROUGH knowledge of the structure and physiology of the automatic and conductive cells involved in generating and propagating electrical impulses in the heart is fundamental to the understanding of the origins of cardiac rhythm disorders. Enzyme histochemical study of these cells supplies both anatomic and physiologic information. However, with conventional techniques nonstructurally bound, partially structurally bound, or weakly structurally bound enzymes diffuse out of sections during the histochemical incubation period. With the development of histochemical semipermeable membrane techniques,[1] studies that could not be performed by conventional histochemical techniques are now possible. In these techniques a semipermeable membrane is interposed between the incubating solution and the tissue section. Because only molecules with a molecular weight of 20,000 can penetrate the membrane,[2] diffusion of enzymes out of the sections is prevented, whereas substrate molecules and other components necessary for the staining reaction diffuse through the membrane. Membrane techniques are therefore indeed suitable for metabolic studies because they prevent the leakage of the enzymes by the membranes.[2]

Conventional or semipermeable membrane techniques have already been used to study the Purkinje system,[3–14] and to a lesser degree the atrioventricular node and the bundle of His.[8–14] Thusfar however, the sinus node has only been studied by conventional enzyme histochemical methods[10–12, 15, 16] and therefore data on the histochemical features of the human sinoatrial node are still incomplete.

It has already been shown that mitral valve muscle[17, 18] and the coronary sinus region[19] are capable of giving rise to automatic electrical activity and that they have electrophysiologic characteristics that closely resemble pacemaker cells: a weak resting potential, a low action potential amplitude, and spontaneous diastolic depolarization. The purpose of this study was to examine the human sinoatrial node, as well as the coronary sinus and the mitral valve muscle, which

From the Service de Soins Intensifs, Hôpital Cardiologique, Lille, and The Laboratoire d'Anatomie Pathologique, Université de Lille, France, and the Laboratory of Experimental Neurology, University of Amsterdam.

Supported by D.G.R.S.T., contract No. 79-7-1009.

Address for correspondence: Dr. Claude Théry, Service de Soins Intensif, Hôpital Cardiologique, Boulevard du Professeur Leclercq, 59037 Lille, France.

Received Oct. 24, 1984; revision accepted April 4, 1985.

have electrophysiologic characteristics strongly resembling pacemaker cells, with recently developed histochemical semipermeable membrane techniques.

Material and methods

Material. Hearts from six subjects were used in the study (four men, two women; mean age 32 years, range 21 to 42). None of the subjects had known heart disease. The human hearts were all removed within the first hour after death. Pathologically the hearts were normal.

In all cases two specimens were studied. The first tissue sample was taken from the superior one-third of the right atrium and contained the superior vena cava up to the point of pericardial reflection, the crest of atrial appendage, and the upper third of the right atrium. A posterior vertical incision was then made, opening the cone-shaped structure and allowing us to roll it out flat. The second sample consisted of a rectangular portion of myocardium, the boundaries of which were the orifice of the coronary sinus in back, the posterior half of the membranous septum in front, the inferior border of the fossa ovalis on top, and the insertion of the mitral and tricuspid valves on the bottom. This fragment contained part of the septal tricuspid valve on the right, and on the left the anterior mitral valve and a fragment of the posterior mitral valve.

The tissue samples were rapidly frozen in isopentane cooled to $-150°$ C with liquid nitrogen (the total time between death and freezing never exceeded 75 min) and stored in a freezer at $-70°$ C before sections were cut at 10 μm in a cryostat adjusted to $-30°$ C. The right atrial tissue was sliced vertically (parallel to the axis of the superior vena cava), and the second sample was sliced perpendicular to the mitral and tricuspid valve rings. Localization of the section of interest of each specimen was done by rapid staining with methyl green pyronin dye. After this region was identified, sections were cut off for histochemical study and were occasionally stained with standard hematoxylin and eosin dye for permanent reference. Whenever it seemed necessary to examine a specific structure more closely, serial slices were cut and examined after staining.

Enzyme histochemistry. To study the nonstructurally bound or weakly structurally bound enzymes, histochemical semipermeable membrane techniques were used. Briefly, these techniques use membrane type 36/32 (Visking Co and Cenco, Chicago) with a thickness of 0.018 mm. Only substances with a molecular weight of less than 20,000 can pass through the membrane.[20] The membranes are stretched across the end of a plastic cylinder 3 cm in diameter, and an incubation medium solidified with 4% agar gel is poured into the tube. The tissue sample section is then placed flat against the outside of the semipermeable membrane. The presence of the membrane prevents nontightly bound enzymes from moving into the incubation medium, while the substrate molecules as well as other molecules used in the staining reactions are free to move through the membrane and the subsequent reaction can be histochemically evaluated. Using the semipermeable membrane principle, we were able to study the anaerobic part of carbohydrate metabolism by use of the technique for lactate dehydrogenase (EC 1.1.1.27)[21] and glucose-6-phosphate isomerase (EC 5.3.1.9).[22] The activity of the pentose phosphate pathway enzymes 6-phosphogluconate dehydrogenase (EC 1.1.1.44) and glucose-6-phosphate dehydrogenase (EC 1.1.1.49) was demonstrated according to the method of Meijer and de Vries,[23] as was the activity of isocitrate:NADP+ oxidoreductase (EC 1.1.1.42) and malate:$NADP^+$ oxidoreductase (EC 1.1.1.40).[24]

To study the structurally bound enzymes, the following conventional histochemical reactions were used: succinate dehydrogenase (a flavoprotein-bound mitochondrial dehydrogenase) activity (EC 1.3.99.1) was demonstrated according to the method of Nachlas et al.[25] The activity of cytochrome C oxidase (EC 1.9.3.1) was demonstrated by the technique of Seligman et al.[26] with or without the addition of supplemental (0.5 mg/ml) cytochrome C to the incubation medium. NADH:tetrazolium oxidoreductase (EC 1.6.99.3) activity was demonstrated with the method of Dubowitz and Brooke,[27] and choline esterase I activity (EC 3.1.1.7) was determined by Gomori's method.[28]

The intensity of histoenzymatical reactions is proportional to the amount of staining deposited at the site of the reaction. These reactions are therefore quantitative.[29] To measure the intensity of these reactions we have used a microscope (Polyvar Reichert-Jung) linked to a photometer (Reichert type 6526-01). The intensity of the lighting in the microscopic studies was set at a constant value. The area of the preparation under study was focused on with use of an oil immersion lens that allowed the study of a field measuring 250 μm in diameter. The intensity of light on the area under study was measured by the photometer first with a nonstained preparation for reference (measurement M1) and then with the specimen to be tested (measurement M2). The optical density (OD) of the specimen was expressed as $OD = 10 \cdot \log M1/M2$. The density gradation ranged from zero for the nonstained preparation to nine for the darkest preparation. The meaurements were recorded independently by two different observers.

Results

Enzyme activity. Table 1 shows the intensity of the staining reactions of the enzymes present in the different structures studied. The intensity of the reactions observed in the atrioventricular node and the bundle of His are listed to allow comparison of the metabolic activities of automatic and conductive cardiac tissue with that of working myocardial tissue.

The sinoatrial node. Anaerobic enzyme (lactate dehydrogenase and glucose-6-phosphate isomerase) activity was found to be greater in the sinoatrial node than in working myocardial tissue. Moreover, the levels of activity of both oxidative enzymes of the pentose phosphate pathway were higher. On the other hand, the activity levels of malate:$NADP^+$ oxidoreductase and of the aerobic enzymes succinate dehydrogenase, isocitrate:$NADP^+$ oxidoreductase, cytochrome C oxidase, and NADH diaphorase were lower than inside working myocardial tissue. Tests for activity of choline esterase were strongly positive in nerves and ganglion cells; the sinoatrial node cells showed circumferential choline esterase activity, tests of atrial cells were only weakly positive, and those in ventricular myocardial cells were negative (figure 1).

Mitral valve muscle. In comparison with working myocardial fibers, the activity of isocitrate:$NADP^+$ oxidoreductase, succinate dehydrogenase, NADH diaphorase, and cytochrome C oxidase was low in myocardial fibers of the proximal region of the anterior mitral cusp as well as in atrial myocardium surrounding the mitral annular fibrosis. The opposite was true for glucose-6-phosphate isomerase, 6-phosphoglucon-

TABLE 1
Distribution of enzyme activities

Enzyme	Sinus node	Working atrial muscle	Coronary sinus	Mitral valve muscle	AV node	His bundle	Ventricular muscle
Glucose-6-phosphate isomerase	5	1	3	5	5	3	1
6-Phosphogluconate dehydrogenase	3	0	2	2	3	2	0
Glucose-6-phosphate dehydrogenase	5	0	4	5	5	4	0
Lactate dehydrogenase	3	1	3	4	3	3	0
Malate:NADP$^+$ oxidoreductase	1	3	3	3	5	5	2
Isocitrate:NADP$^+$ oxidoreductase	3	9	4	2	3	3	9
Succinate dehydrogenase	1	5	3	3	1	1	6
Cytochrome C oxidase	2	7	4	4	4	4	7
NADH:tetrazolium oxidoreductase	3	6	4	4	3	3	6
Choline esterase	8	2	8	8	8	8	0

Grading system for enzymatic activity: A measurement of the optical density was made for each section. The density gradations ranged from 0 for a nonstained preparation to 9 for the darkest preparation (see text).
AV = atrioventricular.

ate dehydrogenase, and especially choline esterase activity (figure 2).

Coronary sinus. The same pattern of activity was observed in the wall of the coronary sinus, especially in its left anterior wall, in and around the Thebesian valve, and in the atrial fibers around the anterior-inferior part of the orifice of coronary sinus near the insertion of the tricuspid valve. Conversely, malate: NADP$^+$ oxidoreductase and lactate dehydrogenase activity was the same in these specialized regions as it was in working myocardial tissue (figure 3).

Enzyme distribution. Histochemical reactions observed for the anaerobic and especially aerobic (mitochondrial) enzymes showed architectural differences in the muscle fibers within the various structures studied. Cross sections of working atrial cells showed a wheel-spoke pattern of dye deposits outlining the myofibrils. Small dye deposits could be seen peripherally on the internal surface of the sarcolemma. In the central part of the sinoatrial node, the pattern was quite different: there were very few dye deposits (two to three per cell cross section) with poorly defined boundaries, and they were separated by wide, seemingly open spaces. Moving toward the outside of the sinoatrial node, the cells became progressively larger, the dye deposits became more numerous, and the cells acquired some of the morphologic characteristics of working myocardial cells. There seemed to be a continuous gradation from nodal cells to working cells with all types of intermediary forms between the two (figure 4).

This progression was visible throughout the peripheral area of the sinoatrial node, but was especially notable in the inferior segment in the crista terminalis (the cauda of the sinus node). Isolated clusters of sinoatrial nodal cells could be found in the atrial myocardium near the sinoatrial node, but in the serial sections studied (which contained the sinoatrial node and the upper third of the right atrium) we did not find any continuous tracts in connection with sinoatrial node made of cells histochemically different from working atrial myocardial fibers. In several locations the intranodal artery was found to be surrounded by a ring of atrial working–like cells.

Discussion

While a number of studies of the histochemical properties of human and animal Purkinje fibers have already been done, there have been relatively few comprehensive studies published concerning the atrioventricular node, the His bundle, and the sinoatrial node. Moreover, the results are conflicting. Some of the results of Schiebler,[3] Otsuka et al.,[4] and Snijder and Meijer[5] fail to support the hypothesis concerning the metabolic differences between conducting cells and common myocardial cells. Gossrau[10] found that the conducting cells in the hearts of birds were characterized by relatively low activity of the glycolytic enzymes aldolase and glycerophosphate dehydrogenase. However, the possibility that the discrepant results of Gossrau reflect species-dependent differences in metabolism cannot be excluded. Another cause of these conflicting results may be the use of enzyme histochemical techniques that are not suitable for metabolic studies.

To our knowledge, the semipermeable membrane

technique has not yet been used to study the enzymatic properties of the sinoatrial node, the coronary sinus, and the heart valve muscles in man.

The semipermeable membrane techniques are more precise than the conventional enzyme assay methods for the study of nonstructurally bound enzymes. These techniques also provide a good indication of low-grade enzyme activity. It has been demonstrated that the levels of enzyme activity detected by semipermeable membrane techniques are very close to the levels obtained with biochemical assays.[29] We found the techniques especially useful in the identification of activity

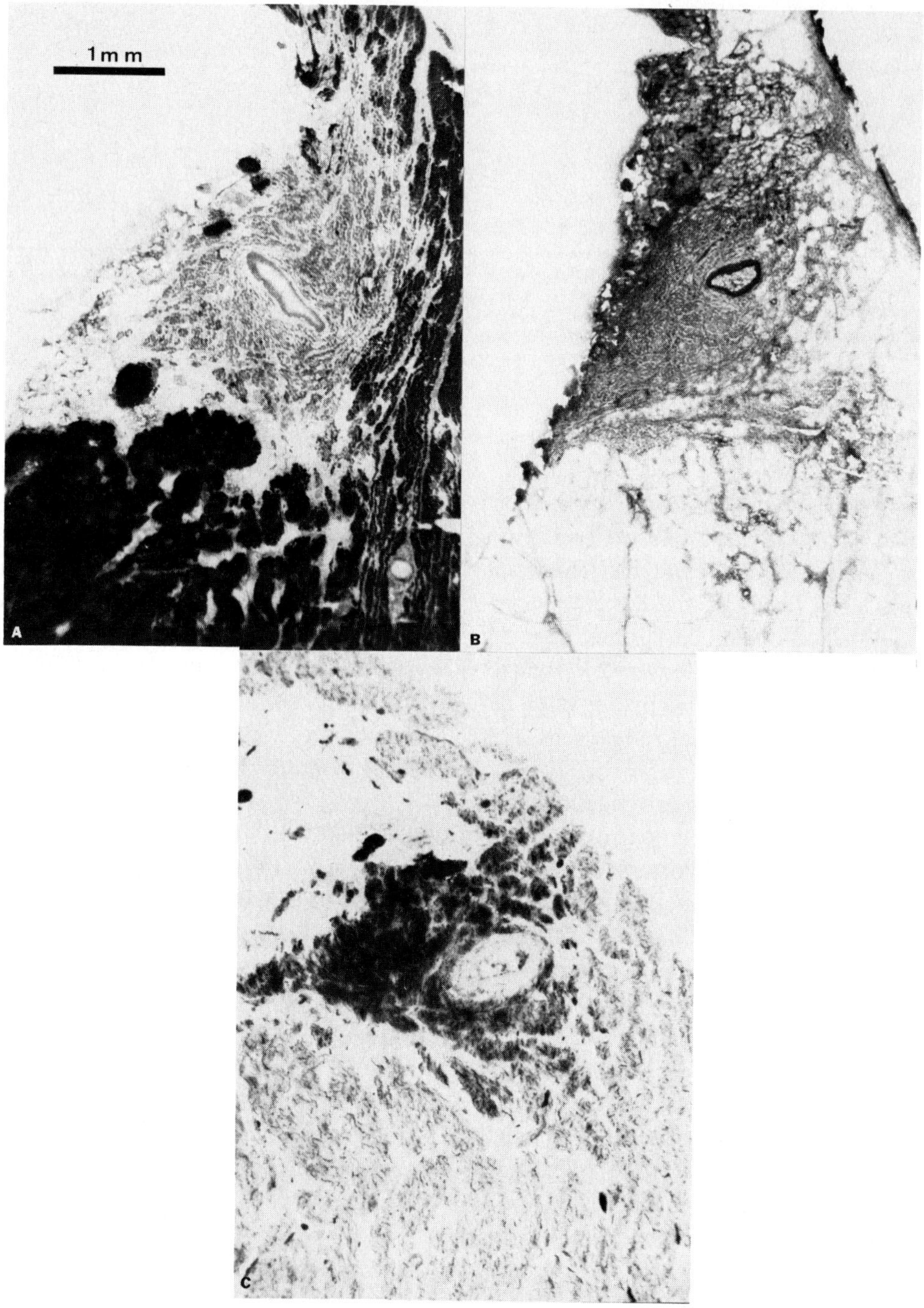

FIGURE 1. Sinus node histoenzymology. At the top of each panel is the superior vena cava, on the left the epicardium, on the right the endocardium and in the middle the sinoatrial node with it's artery in the center. *A*, Isocitrate:NADP$^+$ oxidoreductase reaction. The reaction is much less strong in the sinoatrial node (light area) than in the surrounding atrial working cells. *B*, Glucose 6-phosphate dehydrogenase reaction. The reaction is positive in the sinoatrial node and negative in the atrial myocardium (the positive zones in the atrium and superior vena cava are zones of fatty tissue, blood vessels, or conjunctive tissue). *C*, Choline esterase reaction. The intensity of the reaction is much greater in the sinoatrial node than in surrounding atrial myocardium.

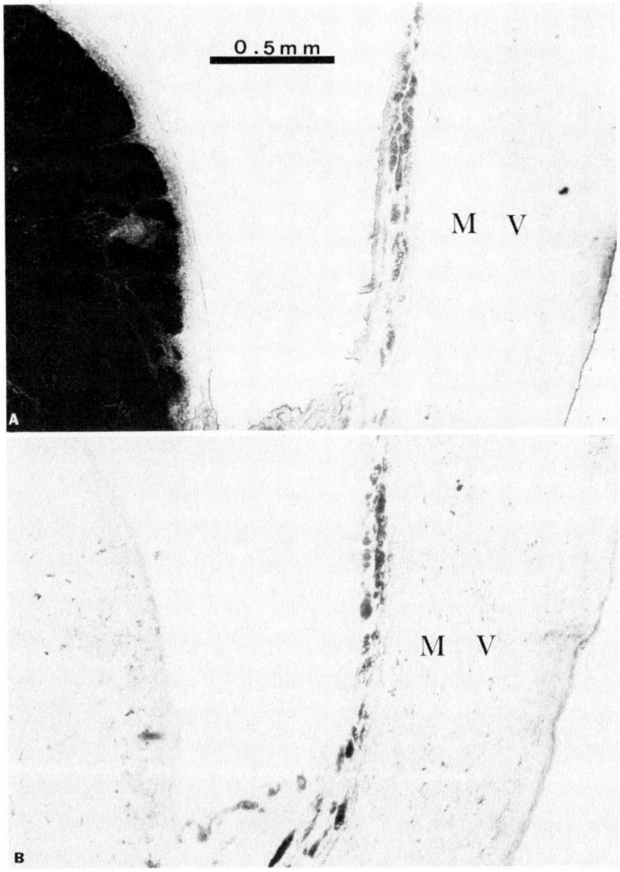

FIGURE 2. Histoenzymatic reactions in the anterior mitral valve muscle. In each panel the mitral valve (MV) is on the right and the left atrium is on the left. *A*, Isocitrate:NADP$^+$ oxidoreductase. The reaction is less strong in the mitral valve muscle than in the atrial myocardium. *B*, Glucose-6-phosphate isomerase reaction. The reaction is positive in the mitral valve muscle and negative in the atrial myocardium.

of nonstructurally bound dehydrogenases because use of the conventional histochemical methods causes nonstructurally bound enzymes to diffuse out of the sections during the incubation period causing unreliable staining results.[2]

The overall enzymatic activity in the carbohydrate metabolic pathways is low in the sinoatrial node compared with working myocardial tissue (figure 1). There is a very low level of aerobic enzyme activity, a relatively moderate level of activity of anaerobic glycolytic enzymes, and a high level of activity of pentose phosphate pathway dehydrogenases. These observations indicate that the sinoatrial node can function more efficiently under anaerobic circumstances than working myocardial tissue. This is in accord with studies that have shown that the sinoatrial node is, electrophysiologically, one of the longest enduring structures under conditions of prolonged anoxia.[30]

The fibers of the sinoatrial node therefore enzymatically strongly resemble type II skeletal muscles, which are also predominently anaerobic muscles. There is however one important difference between the two: the level of activity of malic enzyme (malate:NADP$^+$ oxidoreductase) in the sinoatrial node is low, even lower than in the atrioventricular node or in the His bundle. This enzyme plays a role in the synthesis of glycogen from pyruvate through the NADPH-transferring malate shuttle. This shuttle connects the extramitochondrial carbohydrate metabolism with the mitochondrial part of the carbohydrate metabolism.[24]

The center of the sinoatrial node is made up of small cells that James et al.[31] have called P cells. Structurally, these cells have been found to have very few randomly distributed myofibrils and mitochondria, in direct contrast with working myocardial tissue, in which myofibrils and the mitochondria packed between them are abundant.[31] The distribution of enzymatic activities of mitochondrial and sarcoplasmic enzymes observed in our study corresponds to this architectural structure (figure 4).

The sinoatrial node cells that are in contact with the sinoatrial node artery form a sort of ring around the artery in numerous places, and the cells that make up this ring strongly resemble working atrial myocardium. It is possible that the pulsations of this artery provoke a modification of these cells. The modified cells, which are subjected to constant stretching, assume working cell characteristics.

A positive reaction to choline esterase has been observed in the sinoatrial node of many different species of animals.[11, 12, 15, 32–34] In man, the reaction is positive as early as the sixth week of embryonic life.[35] In our experience, both the nerves and the cells of sinoatrial nodal tissue were choline esterase positive, with the

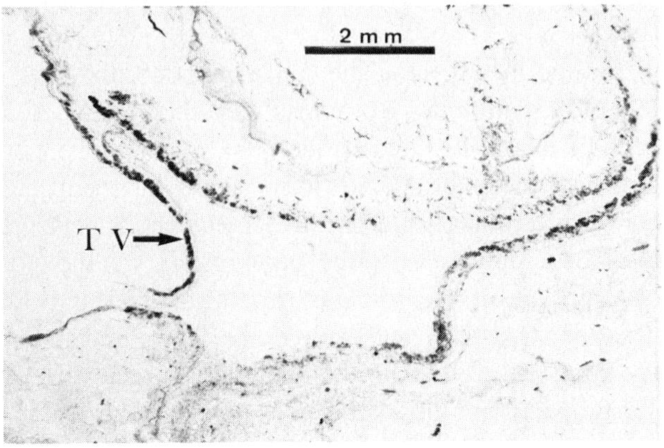

FIGURE 3. Choline esterase reaction in the coronary sinus. The coronary sinus, cut longitudinally here, opens into the right atrium (on the left in the figure). The wall of the coronary sinus and the Thebesian valve (TV) react strongly to choline eterase, whereas the atrial myocardium reacts weakly.

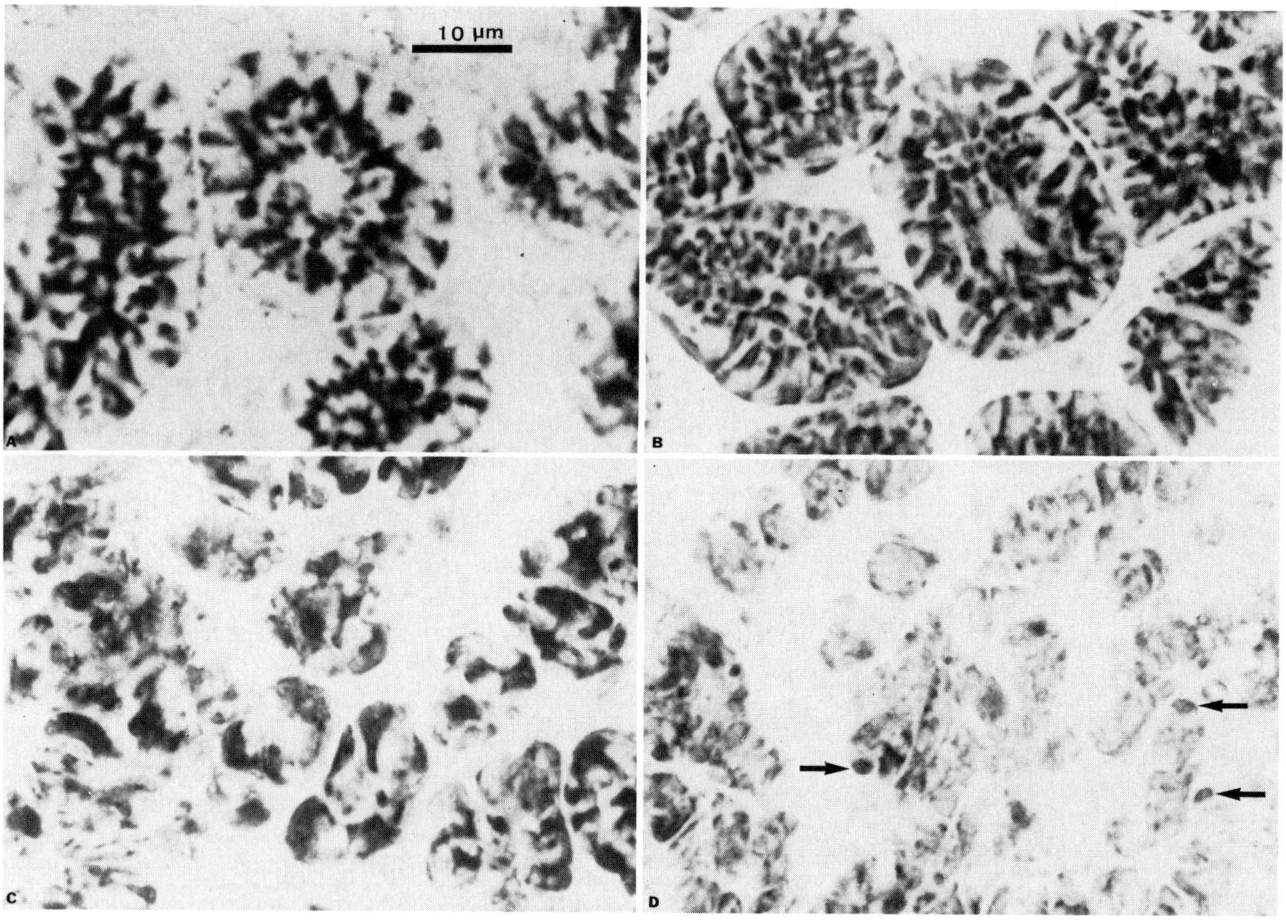

FIGURE 4. Enzyme distribution. Isocitrate:NADP$^+$ oxidoreductase reaction (*A*) and cytochrome C oxidase reaction (*B*) in working atrial cells. The deposits of dye form a reticular pattern. *C*, Transitional cells (cytochrome C oxidase rection). At the edge of the sinoatrial node, the cells become larger and the dye deposits more numerous. *D*, Central sinus node region (cytochrome C oxidase reaction). Only a few dye patches (arrows) are seen in the pale and small nodal cells.

periphery of nodal cells showing the most activity. Similar activity is seen in the Purkinje fibers, the His bundle, and the compact portion of the atrioventricular node. According to Anderson et al.[35] this is sarcolemmal activity, whereas Kent et al.[6] consider it neural activity.

Around the edges of the sinoatrial node, the structure of the cells change progressively: the stain patches become thread-like and arrayed in a wheel-spoke pattern. All the intermediate forms between nodal and contractile cells are present, as James[36] and Bleeker et al.[37] also reported. On the other hand, we did not observe any of the so-called intercalated clear cells described by Viragh and Porte,[38] nor did we find any of the large pale cells reported by Truex.[39] According to Tranum-Jensen[40] these large cells may have an artifactual origin.

The existence of internodal conduction pathways has long been a subject of controversy. Anatomic arguments in favor of their existence have been put forward by some authors,[41–44] while some argue against their existence.[33, 37, 38, 45] Histochemical studies using conventional techniques have been performed. In the ferret Truex[46] has described the existence of tracts that differ from the rest of the myocardium with respect to their choline esterase content. On the other hand, Anderson,[13, 33] using various species, has been unable to demonstrate the existence of any internodal tracts by use of conventional histochemical techniques, including those in which choline esterase histochemical reactions are observed. To our knowledge no study has been done with semipermeable membranes. Using electrophysiologic techniques of mapping,[47, 48] microelectrode studies,[49] or altered ionic milieu,[50] some authors have put forward arguments in favor of the existence of conducting tracts within the atrial tissues, but their results have not been confirmed by others.[37, 51, 52] (For reviews see Sherf and James,[44] Janse and Anderson,[45] Chuaqui.[53])

In our study no histochemical differences were found between the perisinus region and working myocardial tissue. We studied only the superior third of the right atrium, including the upper part of the crista terminalis and the approaches of the atrioventricular node. In these regions, we found only working myocardium, which contained no continuous tracts with histochemical characteristics that might correspond to the beginning of internodal pathways. If such tracts exist they possess no histochemical characteristics enabling them to be differentiated from surrounding atrial tissue at the periphery of the sinoatrial node. We did find several small clusters of cells near the sinoatrial node that had the same characteristics as central node cells, but they were not organized in a proper pathway. They were not found at a distance from the sinoatrial node on serial slices. The role of these cells is not yet clear, but this zone of cellular nonhomogeneity may be responsible for the phenomenon of sinus echo.[54]

The atrial myocardial fibers along the mitral valve (figure 2) and those just above the insertions of this valve have histoenzymatic characteristics similar to those of the sinoatrial node (table 1).

Wit et al.[17, 18] have shown that the muscle of mitral valves of rabbits, dogs, monkeys, and men have transmembrane potentials that differ greatly from those of atrial myocardium, despite the fact that their ultrastructures are identical. The weak resting potential and slow rate of depolarization of mitral valve muscle resemble the transmembrane potentials of nodal cells. These fibers are capable of spontaneous slow rhythm activity, which is set off or quickened by stretching or by the presence of catecholamines, and is slowed down or stopped by acetylcholine. Conduction is very slow and both sympathetic and parasympathetic innervation are abundant.

There are therefore both histoenzymatic and electrophysiologic similarities between tissue in the mitral valve muscle and sinoatrial and atrioventricular nodal tissue.

The coronary sinus (figure 3), especially the anterior wall, the layer of atrial fibers that forms the inferior lip, and the Thebesian valve, show a strong positive reaction to choline esterase in both the nerves and the peripheral part of the cells. The histochemical reactions of aerobic and anaerobic enzymes and both dehydrogenases of the pentose phosphate pathway are similar, as in mitral valve muscle and sinus node. Working with dog hearts, Wit and Cranefield[19] found spontaneous electrical activity and provoked rhythmic activity in this zone, as well as a specific zone that presented a pacemaker type of activity. We found the coronary sinus to be histoenzymatically homogeneous, with the exception of the anterior border in which a stronger reaction was observed. There was a zone of atrial muscle around the exterior orifice in which sinus node–like histochemical reactions were observed. This zone seems to correspond to the zone of atrial tissues outside the orifice, where Wit and Cranefield[19] found that an automatic activity could be unveiled by the presence of noradrenaline.

A specialized type of extranodal tissue adjacent to the atrioventricular junction was described by Truex et al.[55] and Gossrau.[11, 12] Paes de Carvalho[56] found electrophysiologically specialized tissue in the annexes of rabbit heart valves. Working with rats, rabbits, guinea pigs, and human embryos, Anderson[33, 34] found specialized tissue around the atrial margins of the entire circumference of the atrioventricular valves. This seems to be the remainder of the atrioventricular ring of the primitive heart tube that is squeezed into the atrial myocardium and extends down the base of the valves. Anderson[34] found that in rats, this specialized tissue is made up of small cells that have a strong positive reaction to choline esterase, and which, under the electron microscope, have a clear cytoplasm and peripheral myofibrils. It is possible that the histochemical characteristics that we noted in the atrial tissue around the mitral valve and in the mitral valve itself were the expression of this specialized tissue.

As early as 1907, Erlanger and Blackmann (cited by Wit and Cranefield[19]) reported that the coronary sinus region of rabbits possessed a "high degree of rhythmicity." The destruction of the sinus node may result in atrial rhythm originating from the coronary sinus region.[57] Based on this, the hypothesis that arrhythmias originate in this region has often been put forth, but never proven. Likewise, the hypothesis that left atrial ectopic foci are responsible for certain arrhythmias has been suggested, and is still under discussion.[58, 59] It could be that the stretching of the mitral valve muscle in mitral valve prolapse provokes the firing of an ectopic focus.[60]

In conclusion, the fact that both zones with known electrophysiologic features similar to those of the sinoatrial node also demonstrated the same histoenzymatic profile, which was different from that of the atrial myocardium, suggests that electrophysiologic and histoenzymatical properties may be linked, although no single study has yet correlated these two properties.

References

1. McMillan PJ: Differential demonstration of muscle and heart type lactic dehydrogenase of rat muscle and kidney. J Histochem Cytochem **15:** 21, 1967
2. Meijer AEFH: Semipermeable membrane techniques in quantitative enzyme histochemistry. *In* Evered D, O'Connor M, editors:

Trends in enzyme histochemistry and cytochemistry. Amsterdam, 1973, Excerpta Medica, pp 103–120
3. Schiebler TH: Über den histochemischen Nachweis von Atmungsfermenten im Reizleitungssystem. Anat Anz **111** (Erg-Heft): 103, 1962
4. Otsuka N, Hara T, Okamoto H: Histotopochemische Untersuchungen am Reizleitungssystem des Hundeherzens. Histochemistry **10:** 66, 1967
5. Snijder J, Meijer AEFH: Enzyme histochemical studies on the Purkinje fibres of canine, bovine and porcine hearts. Histochem J **2:** 395, 1970
6. Kent FM, Epstein SE, Cooper T, Jacobowitz DM: Cholinergic innervation of the canine and human ventricular conducting system: Anatomic and electrophysiologic correlation. Circulation **50:** 948, 1974
7. Meijer AEFH, DeVries GP: Enzyme histochemical studies on the Purkinje fibres of the atrioventricular system of the bovine and porcine hearts. Histochem J **10:** 399, 1978
8. Alcini E, Lageron A, Wegmann R: Etude histoenzymologique du metabolism glucidique du faisceau de His (à différents niveaux) et du myocarde ventriculaire chez le rat. Ann Histochem **10:** 127, 1965
9. Isaacson R, Boucek RJ: The atrioventricular conduction tissue of the dog. Histochemical properties; influence of electric shock. Am Heart J **75:** 206, 1968
10. Gossrau R: Über das Reizleitungssystem der Vögel. Histochemische und elektronenmikroskopische Untersuchungen. Histochemie **13:** 111, 1968
11. Gossrau R: Histochemische, fluoreszenzmikroskopische und experimentelle Untersuchungen am Reizleitungssystem von Goldhamster, Maus and Ratte. Histochemie **26:** 44, 1971
12. Gossrau R: Über zusätzliches Reizleitungsgewebe im Goldhamsterherzen. Z Zellforsch **115:** 587, 1971
13. Anderson RH: Histologic and histochemical evidence concerning the presence of morphologically distinct cellular zones within the rabbit atrioventricular node. Anat Rec **173:** 7, 1972
14. Chomette G, Le Charpentier Y, Auriol M, Tranbaloc P: Les cellules des voies de conduction dans le faisceau de His humain. Etude histoenzymologique et ultrastructurale. Arch Mal Coeur **74:** 373, 1981
15. James TN, Spence CA: Distribution of cholinesterase within the sinus node and AV node of the human heart. Anat Rec **155:** 151, 1966
16. Schiebler TH, Gossrau R, Von Mohrenschild H: Zur Histochemie und Kapillarversorgung des Sinusknotens. Histochemie **30:** 181, 1972
17. Wit AL, Fenoglio HH Jr, Wagner BM, Bassett AL: Electrophysiological properties of cardiac muscle in the anterior mitral valve leaflet and adjacent atrium in the dog. Possible implications for the genesis of atrial dysrythmias. Circ Res **32:** 731, 1973
18. Wit AL, Fenoglio JJ Jr, Hordof AJ, Reemtsma K: Ultrastructure and transmembrane potentials of cardiac muscle in the human anterior mitral valve leaflet. Circulation **59:** 1284, 1979
19. Wit AL, Cranefield PF: Triggered and automatic activity in the canine coronary sinus. Circ Res **41:** 435, 1977
20. Craig LC, Koningsberg W: Dialysis studies. III. Modification of pore size and shape in cellophane membranes. J Phys Chem **65:** 166, 1961
21. Meijer AEFH: Semipermeable membranes for improving the histochemical demonstration of enzyme activities in tissue sections. III. Lactate dehydrogenase. Histochemie **35:** 165, 1973
22. De Vries GP, Meijer AEFH: Semipermeable membranes for improving the histochemical demonstration of enzyme activities in tissue sections. VI. D-glucose 6-phosphate isomerase and phosphoglucomutase. Histochemistry **50:** 1, 1976
23. Meijer AEFH, de Vries GP: Semipermeable membrane for improving the histochemical demonstration of enzyme activities in tissue sections. IV. Glucose 6-phosphate dehydrogenase and 6-phosphogluconate dehydrogenase (decarboxylating). Histochemistry **40:** 349, 1974
24. Meijer AEFH, de Vries GP: Semipermeable membranes for improving the histochemical demonstrtion of enzyme activities in tissue sections. V. Isocitrate: $NADP^+$ oxidoreductase (decarboxylating) and malate:$NADP^+$ oxidoreductase (decarboxylating). Histochemistry **43:** 225, 1975
25. Nachlas MM, Tsou KC, De Souza E, Cheng CS, Seligman AM: The cytochemical demonstration of succinate dehydrogenase by the use of a new P-nitrophenyl substituted ditetrazole. J Histochem Cytochem **5:** 420, 1957
26. Seligman AM, Karnowsky MJ, Wasserkrug HL, Hanker JS: Non droplet ultrastructural demonstration of cytochrome oxidase activity with a polymerizing osmophilic reagent, diaminobenzidine (DAB). J Cell Biol **38:** 1, 1968
27. Dubowitz V, Brooke MM: Muscle biopsy: a modern approach. London, 1973, W.B. Saunders, p 29
28. Gomori G: Microscopic histochemistry — principles and practice. Chicago, 1952, University of Chicago Press
29. Meijer AEFH, Israel DE: Evaluation of histochemical observations of activity of acid hydrolases obtained with semipermeable membrane techniques: a combined histochemical and biochemical investigations. Histochemistry **57:** 23, 1978
30. Puech P: L'activité électrique auriculaire normale et pathologique. Paris, 1956, Masson, p 148
31. James TN, Sherf L, Fine G, Morales AR: Comparative ultrastructure of the sinus node in man and dog. Circulation **34:** 139, 1966
32. Bojsen-Moller F, Tranum-Jensen J: Whole mount demonstration of cholinesterase-containing nerves in the right atrial wall, nodal tissue, and atrioventricular bundle of the pig heart. J Anat **108:** 375, 1971
33. Anderson RH: The disposition, morphology and innervation of cardiac specialized tissue in the guinea pig. J Anat **111:** 453, 1972
34. Anderson RH: The disposition and innervation of atrio-ventricular ring specialized tissue in rats and rabbits. J Anat **113:** 197, 1972
35. Anderson RH, Becker AE, Wenink ACG, Janse MJ: The development of the cardiac specialized tissue. *In* Wellens HJJ, Lie KI, Janse MJ, editors: The conduction system of the heart. Leiden, 1976, Stenfert Krose BV, p 3
36. James TN: The sinus node. Am J Cardiol **40:** 965, 1977
37. Bleeker WK, Mackaay AJC, Masson-Pevet M, Bouman LN, Becker AE: Functional and morphological organization of the rabbit sinus node. Circ Res **46:** II, 1980
38. Viragh SZ, Porte A: The fine structure of the conduction system of the monkey heart (Macaca mulatta). I. The sino atrial node and the internodal connections. Z Zellforch **145:** 191, 1973
39. Truex RC: The sino atrial node and its connections with the atrial tissue. *In* Wellens HJJ, Lie KI, Janse MJ, editors: The conduction system of the heart. Leiden, 1976, Stenfert Kroes BV, p 209
40. Tranum-Jensen J: The fine structure of the atrial and atrioventricular (AV) junctional specialized tissues of the rabbit heart. *In* Wellens HJJ, Lie KI, Janse MJ, editors: The conduction system of the heart. Leiden, 1976, Stenfert Kroes BV, p 55
41. James TN: Connecting pathways between the sinus node and A-V node and between the right and the left atrium in the human heart. Am Heart J **66:** 498, 1963
42. Merideth J, Titus JL: The anatomical atrial connections between sinus and A-V node. Circulation **37:** 566, 1968
43. Emberson JW, Challice CR: Studies on the impulse conducting pathways in the atrium of the mammalian heart. Am Heart J **79:** 653, 1970
44. Sherf L, James TN: Fine structure of cells and their histologic organization within internodal pathways of the heart: clinical and electrocardiographic implications. Am J cardiol **44:** 435, 1979
45. Janse MJ, Anderson RH: Specialized internodal atrial pathways-fact or fiction? Eur J Cardiol **2:** 117, 1974
46. Truex RC: Structural basis of atrial and ventricular conduction. Cardiovasc Clin **6**: 1, 1974
47. Holsinger JW, Wallace AG, Sealy WC: The identification and surgical significance of the atrial internodal conduction tracts. Ann Surg **167:** 447, 1968
48. Waldo AL, Bush HL Jr, Gelband H, Zorn GL, Vitikai-Nen KJ, Hoffman BF: Effects on the canine P wave of discrete lesions in the specialized atrial tracts. Circ Res **29:** 452, 1971
49. Hogan PM, Davis LD: Electrophysiological characteristics of canine atrial plateau fibers. Circ Res **28:** 62, 1971
50. Vassalle M, Hoffman BF: The spread of sinus activation during potassium administration. Circ Res **17:** 285, 1965
51. Goodman D, Van Der Steen ABM, Van Dam RT: Endocardial and epicardial activation pathways of the canine right atrium. Am J Physiol **220:** 1, 1971
52. Spach MS, Lieberman M, Scott EA, Kootsen JM: Excitation se-

quences of the atrial septum and AV node in isolated hearts of the dog and the rabbit. Circ Res **29:** 156, 1971
53. Chuaqui B: Über die Ausbreitungsbundel des Sinusknoten. Eine kritische Analyse der wichtigsten Arbeiten. Virchows Arch **355:** 179, 1972
54. Narula OS: Sinus node reentry: a mechanism for supraventricular tachycardia. Circulation **50:** 1114, 1974
55. Truex RC, Bishof JK, Hoffman EL: Accessory atrioventricular muscle bundles of the developing human heart. Anat Rec **131:** 45, 1958
56. Paes De Carvalho A: Cellular electrophysiology of the atrial specialized tissues. *In* Paes De Carvalho AP, de Mello WC, Hoffman BF, editors: The specialized tissues of the heart. New York, 1961, Elsevier, p 115
57. Sealy WC, Bache RJ, Seaber AV, Bhattacharga SK: The atrial pacemaking site after surgical exclusion of the sinoatrial node. J Thorac Cardiovasc Surg **65:** 841, 1973
58. Mirowski M: Ectopic rhythms originating in the left atrium. Am Heart J **74:** 299, 1967
59. Lau SH, Cohen SI, Stein E, Haft JI, Rosen KM, Damato AN: P waves and P loops in coronary sinus and left atrial rhythms. Am Heart J **79:** 201, 1970
60. Swartz MH, Teichholz LE, Donoso E: Mitral valve prolapse. A review of associated arrhythmias. Am J Med **62:** 377, 1977

The effects of premature stimulation of the His bundle on epicardial activation and body surface late potentials in dogs susceptible to sustained ventricular tachyarrhythmias

JOSEPH F. SPEAR, PH.D., DAVID A. RICHARDS, M.D., GEORGE J. BLAKE, PH.D., MICHAEL B. SIMSON, M.D., AND E. NEIL MOORE, D.V.M.

ABSTRACT Experiments were performed on 20 anesthetized dogs to determine the effects of premature stimulation of the His bundle on epicardial conduction and late potentials recorded on the body surface. Fifteen dogs underwent occlusion of the left anterior descending coronary for 2 hr followed by reperfusion, and five that did not undergo operation served as controls. Animals were studied 2 to 52 weeks after the induction of infarction, and four animals with infarction and four control animals exhibited no sustained arrhythmias in response to programmed ventricular extrastimulation. Five dogs with infarction and one control dog had ventricular fibrillation while the six remaining dogs had inducible sustained ventricular tachycardia. All animals with ventricular tachycardia had late potentials in the terminal portion of the signal-averaged body surface QRS complexes during sinus rhythm and QRS durations in the animals were 64 msec or greater. The voltage in the last 20 msec of the QRS complex was 13.5 μV or less and the duration of late activity below 30 μV was 18.2 msec or more. These values did not overlap values in animals with no inducible arrhythmias. Ventricular fibrillation was a nonspecific end point in these experiments and values overlapped those in animals with no arrhythmias and those with ventricular tachycardia. All animals with infarction and late potentials associated with their QRS complexes also had delayed and prolonged epicardial electrograms that extended into the time of the late potentials recorded from 45 standard sites in the infarcted regions. A single premature beat evoked by His bundle pacing (coupling interval of 192 to 270 msec) had no significant effect on late potentials or their relationship to epicardial activation in the area of infarct. However, changes in the durations of electrograms in response to premature beats were different in animals with infarction and ventricular tachycardia than in those with ventricular fibrillation. In animals with ventricular tachycardia, electrograms at 15 of 210 sites increased in duration by more than 10 msec while those at 61 of 210 sites decreased in duration. In animals with ventricular fibrillation, electrograms at 40 of 207 sites were of increased duration while those at 26 of 207 decreased. The decreases in duration were usually due to components of fractionated electrograms "dropping out" and likely represent local conduction block near the recording electrode. Thus, the present studies demonstrate that delayed and prolonged activation in the infarcted epicardium correlates with late potentials on the body surface and that single premature His bundle beats have no significant effect on either late potentials or on their relationship with epicardial activation. Animals with ventricular tachycardia could be distinguished from those with no arrhythmias based on signal-averaged QRS criteria defining late potentials.
Circulation 72, No. 1, 214–224, 1985.

STUDIES IN MAN in which high-resolution techniques were used to record body surface potentials have shown that low-energy high-frequency late potentials occur during the terminal portion of the QRS complex in many postmyocardial infarction patients susceptible to sustained ventricular tachyarrhythmias.[1-6] Studies correlating ventricular activation with body surface potentials suggest that late potentials re-

From the Department of Animal Biology, School of Veterinary Medicine, University of Pennsylvania, Philadelphia.

Supported by grants HL-23071, HL-25213, HL-28393, HL-33593, and HL-27925 from the National Heart, Lung, and Blood Institute and by a grant from the W. W. Smith Charitable Trust.

Address for correspondence: Dr. Joseph F. Spear, Department of Animal Biology, School of Veterinary Medicine, University of Pennsylvania, 3800 Spruce St., Philadelphia, PA 19104.

Received Jan. 14, 1985; revision accepted April 18, 1985.

Dr. Simson is the Samuel Bellet Associate Professor of Medicine and Cardiology.

sult from abnormal delayed conduction within the infarcted region.[7] This abnormal conduction may also provide the substrate for the reentrant arrhythmias in these patients.[8,9] Thus, the presence of late potentials on the electrocardiogram can be used as a noninvasive marker for patients at risk of developing ventricular arrhythmias.

Acute occlusion of the left anterior descending coronary artery in dogs causes delayed activity in the ischemic zone and produces late potentials on the body surface.[10] Changes in the degree of delay associated with the evolution of ischemia are accurately reflected by similar changes in the timing of the late potentials.[10] During the early stage of infarction (3 to 6 days) premature atrial beats slow conduction through the infarct and cause a corresponding delay in late potentials on the body surface.[11] The effect of premature activation on late potentials in the setting of chronic, stable infarction at a time when inducible sustained ventricular arrhythmias occur has not been investigated in either animals or man. Since late potentials are not recorded in all patients with ventricular tachycardia,[3] it was thought that premature activation might provide a method for exaggerating late potentials and therefore increase their manifestation on the body surface as well as provide additional insight into their mechanisms.

In the present studies we used a canine preparation of infarction in which both delayed epicardial conduction in the infarcted region and pacing-induced ventricular tachyarrhythmias occur chronically after coronary artery occlusion and reperfusion.[12] Our objectives were first to establish that delayed conduction in the infarcted region produces late potentials on the body surface and second to determine if criteria similar to those described for late potentials in man can be used to identify animals prone to inducible ventricular tachycardia. In addition, we evaluated the effect of premature supraventricular beats on epicardial conduction and body surface late potentials to determine if premature beats could enhance the sensitivity and specificity of the technique.

Methods

Animal preparation. Experiments were performed on 20 mongrel dogs weighing between 8 and 16 kg. Fifteen animals were studied 2 to 56 weeks after experimental anterior myocardial infarction, and five animals that did not undergo operation served as controls. The technique for producing infarction has been described previously.[13] Briefly, animals were anesthetized with sodium pentobarbital (30 mg/kg) and through a limited left lateral thoracotomy, the anterior descending coronary artery was occluded in two stages for 2 hr followed by complete reperfusion.

Body surface potentials. At the time of study, body surface electrocardiographic potentials were recorded in each animal with signal-averaging procedures and computer-based analyses described by Simson.[3] The animals were anesthetized with 30 mg/kg sodium pentobarbital and before thoracotomy bipolar x, y, and z leads were recorded. The x lead was recorded between the right and left lateral chest wall at the fifth intercostal space, the y lead between the superior manubrium and the left leg, and the z lead between the anterior chest wall over the sternum and a corresponding posterior position over the vertebral column. The analog signals from each lead were sequentially analog-to-digital converted at 1000 Hz to 12-bit accuracy and stored on a Winchester hard disk (Hewlett-Packard 9834A) with a Hewlett-Packard 9836 microcomputer. Between 100 and 200 QRS complexes were stored for each lead. The digital signals for each lead were passed through a template recognition program to eliminate noisy or ectopic beats. The x, y, and z QRS complexes were averaged and then filtered with use of a bidirectional digital filter set at a high-pass of 50 Hz. This value was chosen to eliminate low-frequency signals that are present in the ST segment of the dog.[10] The filtered signals for the three leads were combined into a vector magnitude and the QRS onset and termination were determined by a computer algorithm.

In the experiments involving premature His bundle stimulation, digital conversion of x, y, and z lead analog data was triggered to begin 20 msec before the premature His stimulus and was terminated 256 msec later. During the bidirectional digital filtering of the averaged QRS complexes, the forward digital filter was gated to begin 5 msec after the termination of the stimulus artifact to prevent filter ringing from obscuring the beginning of the QRS complex.

Pacing and recording. His bundle stimulation was chosen as the mode for introducing premature beats since this permitted coupling intervals shorter than those attained by atrial stimulation to be induced and also prevented the obscuring of late potentials by ventricular pacing.

To pace the bundle of His, a bipolar catheter was introduced into the root of the aorta by way of the left carotid artery. The catheter had an interelectrode distance of 10 mm and was positioned to obtain a stable His bundle electrogram. The catheter was then connected to a constant-current stimulus isolation unit with use of the distal electrode as the cathode. The current intensity was increased until effective His pacing occurred. His pacing was confirmed by noting that the stimulus artifact–to–Q wave interval was comparable to the His bundle electrogram–to–Q wave interval recorded before stimulation and by the same QRS and T wave configurations as during sinus rhythm. After every 8 basic His pacing beats a premature His bundle stimulus was introduced as early as possible without causing aberration in the QRS complex. To prevent retrograde atrial activation or atrial echo beats from obscuring the terminal portion of the premature His QRS complex, the atrium was paced with a second catheter introduced into the right atrium by way of the left jugular vein. For the 8 basic drive beats, the atrial stimulation was coincident with His bundle pacing. For the premature His beat, the atrium was preexcited such that it would be refractory during the time of the premature QRS complex.

The signal-averaging procedure was first carried out in the dogs during sinus rhythm with the pacing catheters in place. The mean cycle length during sinus rhythm was 396 msec and ranged between 307 and 507 msec in the experiments. After the sinus rhythm sequence, signal averaging was repeated for the premature His beat. The coupling interval for the premature His stimulus relative to the last basic His stimulus ranged from 192 to 270 msec, mean 224 msec.

After the signal-averaging procedures each animal's chest was opened with a midsternal incision and the heart was exposed and supported in a pericardial sling. In animals that had undergone the occlusion-reperfusion procedure, the infarcted region was located visually on the anterior left ventricle and a 45-site plastic template was oriented in a standard way and sutured over the infarcted region (figure 1). In animals without infarcts the template was applied in a corresponding region with the same orientation. Electrograms were sequentially recorded at the 45 positions with a hand-held roving electrode array in dogs in sinus rhythm and during premature His bundle stimulation at the same coupling intervals as in the signal-averaging procedures. Bipolar plunge-wire electrodes were inserted subepicardially in normal areas of the right and left ventricles for recording reference electrograms and for stimulation during the arrhythmia induction protocol. The roving electrode array consisted of two orthogonally arranged bipolar leads (figure 1, *insert*). Each pole was 0.3 mm in diameter and the center-to-center distance between pairs was 0.6 mm. The bipolar axes of the electrode pairs are indicated in figure 1, *insert*, by the lines and are designated as x and y. The positive poles of each bipole are also indicated. During all recording procedures, the orientation of the array was maintained with the axis of the x bipolar electrode parallel to the longitudinal axis of the 45-position template. An orthogonal array was used for recording electrograms to decrease the possibility of activity not being recorded at a site due to a wavefront simultaneously intercepting both poles of a single bipolar electrode. The electrograms were filtered with a band pass of 40 to 1000 Hz. The electrocardiogram, both orthogonal electrograms, and the right and left reference electrograms were displayed simultaneously on a memory oscilloscope (Tektronix D-15) and recorded on a Gould electrostatic strip-chart recorder at a paper speed of 250 mm/sec.

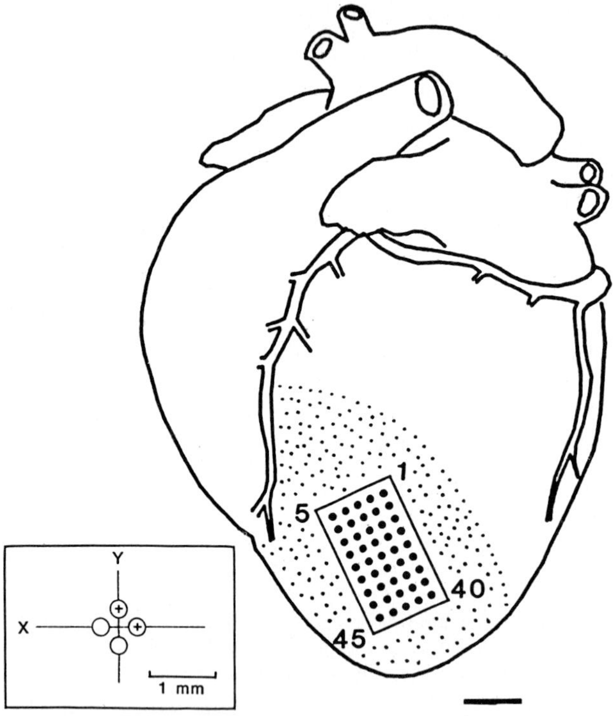

FIGURE 1. A schematic representation of the standard location of a 45-site template applied over the infarcted region (stippled area) of the anterior left ventricle and used to guide the mapping electrode. Each site was separated from its neighbors by 2.5 mm. The numbering system for the sites is indicated. *Inset,* The arrangement and dimensions of the poles of the orthogonal dual bipolar electrode used to record activity at each site. The poles were insulated except at the surface in contact with the heart.

After the experimental procedures, all animals were evaluated for their susceptibility to ventricular tachyarrhythmias by a previously described pacing protocol.[12] After basic drive at cycle lengths of 350 and 300 msec, single, double, and triple ventricular extrastimuli were introduced. The stimulation protocol was first performed with right and then left ventricular stimulation at an intensity of twice diastolic threshold. If tachyarrhythmias were not induced, the entire procedure was repeated with a current of four times diastolic threshold. Once an arrhythmia was reproducibly induced the protocol was terminated.

At the end of the experiments the animals were killed, their hearts were removed, and the area of infarction was verified by gross inspection.

Data analysis. Dogs were separated into three groups. Group I had no inducible ventricular tachyarrhythmias, group II had inducible ventricular fibrillation, and group III had inducible sustained (greater than 10 sec) ventricular tachycardia during electrophysiologic testing.

All 45 electrograms recorded during the mapping procedure were referenced to the beginning of the QRS complex and parameters were manually digitized with a Hewlett-Packard 9836 computer system. The system had a resolution of 0.002 mV and 0.1 msec. The orthogonal bipolar electrode array was considered to be at a nonactivated epicardial site when the largest component in both electrograms did not exceed 0.1 mV.[12] The onset of activity at a site was taken as the point on the electrogram at which the signal deviated from the baseline by greater than 0.1 mV and the termination of the signal was taken as the latest deflection exceeding 0.1 mV. Local activation time was measured to the peak or baseline crossing of the largest fast deflection in the electrograms. Electrogram duration was measured as the difference between the termination and onset of the electrogram. Electrogram amplitude was measured as the vector sum of the peak amplitude of the largest fastest deflections in the orthogonal electrograms x and y.

Late potentials were characterized by parameters that are similar to those used in man[3, 4] and were calculated from the signal-averaged and filtered body surface QRS potentials. Parameters included the total QRS duration, the total root-mean-square (RMS) voltage in the QRS, the RMS voltage in the last 20 msec of the QRS complex, and the duration of activity in the terminal portion of the QRS complex below the 30 μV level.

Statistical methods. Electrographic data are presented for each experiment as the mean and SD for the 45 electrode sites. Mean and SD pooled data from all experiments within a group are also presented. Significant differences between groups for a given parameter were determined by analysis of variance. Differences in electrographic parameters recorded during sinus rhythm and His premature stimulation for the 45 sites were analyzed by Student's paired t test for each animal. Body surface QRS data were compared between groups by analysis of variance. A p value of less than or equal to .05 was considered to indicate a significant difference. QRS parameters during sinus rhythm and His bundle stimulation were compared by linear regression analysis.

Results

The characteristics of the arrhythmias for each animal are presented in table 1. Four of the control animals and four of the animals with infarction had no inducible ventricular arrhythmias. Six animals, one of which was a control dog, had inducible ventricular fibrillation. The six remaining dogs with infarction exhibited inducible sustained ventricular tachycardia

TABLE 1
Characteristics of arrhythmias

		Tachycardia		Induction parameters			
Experiment No.	Weeks after infarct	Type	Cycle length (msec)	Site of stimulation	Basic cycle length (msec)	Number of extrastimuli	Current (× diastolic)
Group I							
1	—			LV	300	3	4
2	—			LV	300	3	4
3	—			LV	300	3	4
4	—			LV	300	3	4
5	24			LV	300	3	4
6	2			LV	300	3	4
7	2			LV	300	3	4
8	2			LV	300	3	4
Group II							
1	—			LV	350	3	4
2	24			LV	350	3	2
3	24			LV	350	3	2
4	2			LV	350	3	2
5	2			LV	300	3	4
6	56			RV	300	3	4
Group III							
1	24	Poly	160	LV	350	3	2
2	24	Mono	160	LV	300	2	2
3	3	Mono	176	LV	350	2	4
4	20	Mono	152	RV	350	3	2
5	24	Mono	152	LV	300	3	2
6	2	Mono	136	RV	350	3	2

LV = left ventricle; RV = right ventricle; Poly = polymorphic sustained ventricular tachycardia; Mono = monomorphic sustained ventricular tachycardia.

with cycle lengths ranging between 136 and 176 msec. With the exception of experiment 1, the type of ventricular tachycardia induced was monomorphic. The polymorphic ventricular tachycardia in experiment 1, although reproducibly induced and sustained for greater than 10 sec, eventually degenerated to ventricular fibrillation.

Body surface QRS complex in sinus rhythm. Table 2 summarizes the characteristics of the filtered body surface QRS complexes recorded during sinus rhythm. It was noted when group I animals with no arrhythmias and group III dogs exhibiting ventricular tachycardia were compared that all animals with ventricular tachycardia had QRS durations of 64 msec or greater. The voltage in the last 20 msec of the QRS complex was 13.5 μV or less and the duration of activity below 30 μV was 18.2 msec or more in the group III animals. These values did not overlap with those in animals with no arrhythmias. Therefore, animals having inducible ventricular tachycardia had low-amplitude, high-frequency late potentials on the terminal portion of the filtered QRS complex that clearly distinguished them from animals having no arrhythmias.

In the group II animals with ventricular fibrillation mean values for these parameters fell between those in groups I and III. However, values for individual animals with ventricular fibrillation ranged across those for animals with no arrhythmia and those with ventricular tachycardia. Therefore, the group II animals were a mixed population and could not be distinguished from those in groups I and III based on the filtered QRS complex.

Epicardial activation during sinus rhythm. In table 3 the characteristics of the ventricular electrograms from dogs in sinus rhythm are presented for each parameter. Animals without arrhythmia (group I) differed from those with ventricular tachycardia (group III), with electrogram amplitudes being significantly depressed and the local activation time and duration of the electrograms being significantly prolonged in group III. These findings are similar to those previously reported for another series of experiments in which different recording techniques were used.[10] The coefficients of variance (SD divided by the mean times 100) for the local activation times were significantly greater in the group III than in group I animals, indicating a greater

TABLE 2
Characteristics of the signal-averaged QRS complex during sinus rhythm

Experiment No.	QRS duration (msec)	Vt (μV)	V20 (μV)	D30 (msec)
Group I				
1	57	288.0	28.5	14.9
2	55	254.1	17.6	14.9
3	55	438.8	53.8	12.8
4	54	278.7	48.3	12.8
5	57	166.0	59.3	16.1
6	62	282.9	21.8	14.9
7	49	259.7	82.5	8.5
8	57	188.1	38.3	11.7
Mean ± SD	55.8 ± 3.7	269.5 ± 81.9	43.8 ± 21.7	13.3 ± 2.4
Group II				
1	55	375.6	17.3	14.3
2	82	162.0	1.5	43.2
3	86	309.8	3.7	41.9
4	55	203.9	52.1	11.5
5	53	201.0	13.4	17.4
6	63	199.3	10.9	18.9
Mean ± SD	65.7 ± 14.7	241.9 ± 82.2	16.5 ± 18.4	24.5 ± 14.2
p value	NS	NS	.03	.047
Group III				
1	64	209.9	13.5	18.2
2	69	261.0	3.3	28.9
3	71	168.4	7.6	37.6
4	69	204.8	12.4	20.5
5	68	221.4	5.5	22.1
6	72	291.3	2.1	26.9
Mean ± SD	68.8 ± 2.8	226.1 ± 43.7	7.4 ± 4.7	25.7 ± 7.1
p value	<.001	NS	<.002	<.001

p value by analysis of variance versus group I.
Vt = total RMS voltage in the QRS; V20 = RMS voltage in the last 20 msec of the QRS; D30 = Duration of late activity below 30 μV.

degree of disparity in the times of activation among the 45 sites for animals with ventricular tachycardia. As was the case for the filtered QRS parameters, individual animals with ventricular fibrillation (group II) had electrographic characteristics that ranged between values for animals with ventricular tachycardia and those for dogs with no arrhythmias.

The relationship between epicardial activation and the filtered QRS for each experiment is graphically displayed in figures 2, 3, and 4. Sinus rhythm results are shown at the left in each case. The timing of onset and termination of the electrograms relative to the beginning of the QRS complex are displayed as horizontal lines for each of the 45 sites, with the time of local activation of each site indicated by an open circle. Sites are displayed in sequence from 1 through 45 from bottom to top with each nonactivated site being indicated by an x at the beginning of the QRS complex. The three vertical lines on the abscissa, from left to right, indicate the time of onset of the QRS complex, the time at which the voltage dropped below the 30 μV level, and the end of the QRS complex. The area of the QRS complex between the time at which the voltage dropped below 30 μV to the end of the complex is emphasized by the dark shading.

In group I animals epicardial local activation occurred within the high-voltage region of the QRS complex (figure 2; table 4). With the exception of in experiment 6, electrograms tended to be of short duration and few extended into the terminal portion of the QRS. In contrast, group III animals (figure 4) had prolonged or delayed electrograms that extended into the terminal portion of the QRS complex (table 4). Group II animals (figure 3) displayed patterns that ranged between those observed in group I and group III dogs.

Figures 2 to 4 and table 4 demonstrate that animals with delayed or prolonged activation also had late potentials and prolonged QRS durations. However, the correlation between epicardial activation and late potentials was not perfect. There were epicardial sites the activity of which extended beyond the end of the QRS and did not appear to contribute potentials on the body surface. It is probable that there is some vector cancellation of epicardial activity involved and also that there is an energy "threshold" that must be exceeded to allow activity to be detected on the body surface. The latter point is supported by experiment 2 in figure 3 and experiment 1 in figure 4. In these cases, there were a considerable number of sites on the epicardial surface activated beyond the end of the QRS complexes and this late activity was not detected on the body surface. In these two experiments the lowest mean electrogram amplitudes were noted (table 3), suggesting that the total energy was insufficient for detection.

The effect of premature His bundle pacing. Technically acceptable His bundle stimulation was not accomplished in seven of the 20 animals (figures 2 to 4, table 3). Inspection of the records after the experiments revealed the following problems. In experiment 1 in the group I animals His bundle pacing was confounded by simultaneous ventricular septal activation during the epicardial mapping procedure. This occurred also during the signal-averaging procedure in experiments 4, 5, and 8. In experiment 7, a retrograde p wave obscured the terminal portion of the QRS complex during signal averaging of the premature His beat. In the group II animals (figure 3, table 3), ventricular septal pacing occurred in experiment 6. For the group III animals (figure 4, table 3) ventricular septal stimulation occurred in experiment 4 and a retrograde p wave

TABLE 3
Characteristics of the electrograms during sinus rhythm and premature stimulation of the His

Experiment	Amplitude (mV)		Local activation time (msec)		Duration (msec)		Activation coefficient of variance (%)	
No.	Sinus	His	Sinus	His	Sinus	His	Sinus	His
Group I								
1	6.2±3.8	—	27.4±3.6	—	16.6±4.3	—	13.1	—
2	3.0±1.0	2.7±1.7	21.9±3.8	23.6±3.0	23.1±5.2	22.6±4.5^{A}	17.4	12.7
3	5.3±3.0	5.6±3.2	24.6±2.7	18.1±2.9	16.0±3.8	16.6±3.0^{A}	11.0	16.0
4	8.6±3.4	—	27.9±4.0	—	16.5±3.0	—	14.7	—
5	5.0±3.0	—	22.5±2.6	—	16.3±3.5	—	11.6	—
6	3.8±2.2	3.5±2.0^{A}	26.2±4.0	24.8±3.4	36.9±18.2	29.6±6.2	15.3	13.7
7	3.2±1.6	3.1±1.7^{A}	22.2±3.4	22.5±3.7^{A}	22.5±7.3	23.5±7.1^{A}	15.3	16.4
8	5.3±2.5	—	29.4±4.5	—	20.8±4.3	—	15.3	—
Mean±SD	5.0±3.2	3.8±2.5	25.2±4.5	22.2±4.1	21.2±10.1	23.1±8.1	14.2±2.1	14.7±1.8
Group II								
1	11.1±4.7	10.2±4.2^{A}	23.8±3.0	19.1±3.0	22.0±5.6	22.8±5.9^{A}	12.6	15.7
2	0.5±0.4	0.4±0.6^{A}	53.9±39.9	51.4±36.7^{A}	71.1±37.3	79.8±45.3^{A}	74.1	71.4
3	2.4±1.8	2.2±1.3^{A}	53.1±23.6	57.9±38.0^{A}	65.2±24.2	70.0±33.8^{A}	44.4	65.8
4	2.8±2.5	3.1±2.8	40.1±6.8	42.5±8.6	58.3±19.5	57.2±17.5^{A}	16.9	20.2
5	6.5±2.5	6.8±2.4	29.9±4.5	26.9±5.0	20.0±3.9	20.9±4.1	15.1	18.6
6	3.3±1.5	—	28.1±2.5	—	17.1±5.5	—	8.9	—
Mean±SD	4.6±4.4	4.9±4.4	37.4±21.1	38.4±26.7	40.9±29.4	47.7±34.1	28.7±25.6	38.3±27.7
p value	NS	.003	<.001	<.001	<.001	<.001	NS	NS
Group III								
1	1.0±0.8	0.9±0.7	50.4±12.7	66.8±17.4	50.8±20.3	45.8±13.8^{A}	25.2	26.0
2	1.7±1.5	1.7±1.2^{A}	42.9±19.7	30.5±17.6	44.1±26.0	28.8±21.4	45.9	57.8
3	4.2±3.8	4.0±3.4	51.6±24.5	45.2±19.5	40.8±28.0	31.9±15.7	47.4	43.1
4	1.7±0.8	—	45.9±6.5	—	41.9±18.3	—	14.2	—
5	4.7±3.3	5.6±4.1	30.4±6.9	33.1±9.5	31.2±13.0	28.2±10.8	22.7	28.7
6	2.5±2.6	2.8±3.2	34.8±16.0	31.5±15.9	39.3±16.5	33.9±16.0	45.9	50.5
Mean±SD	2.6±2.8	3.0±3.3	42.4±17.2	41.2±21.2	41.3±21.4	33.8±17.0	33.6±14.6	41.2±13.7
p value	<.001	.010	<.001	<.001	<.001	<.001	.004	.007

p value by analysis of variance.
^{A}Not significant by paired t test.

obscured the terminal QRS in experiment 5. In some experiments the end of the p wave from the atrial preexcitation obscured the beginning of the premature His complex (for example, experiments 1 and 2, figure 4). In these cases the beginning of the QRS was estimated by overlaying the sinus complex.

In animals in which premature His bundle stimulation was successful there were no significant differences in the QRS duration (figure 5, *A*), the voltage in the last 20 msec of the QRS (panel *B*), or in the duration of activity below 30 μV (panel *C*) during the premature His beats compared with sinus rhythm.

Premature stimulation of the His bundle had a variable effect on the characteristics of electrograms recorded from the infarcted epicardial surface (table 3 and figures 2 to 4). In individual experiments, premature stimulation of the His bundle increased, decreased, or caused no significant change in the parameters measured. The effect of prematurity on the electrogram duration was different in the group II and group III animals. Table 4 lists electrographic data that indicate changes in duration greater than 10 msec for each experiment. Group II animals had a larger percentage of electrograms showing an increase in duration than group III dogs. The opposite was true for the group III animals, in which duration was more often decreased in response to a premature beat. This difference was significant by chi-square analysis. In these cases a decrease in the duration of a fractionated electrogram was usually due to components of the electrogram dropping out in response to the premature beat (figure 6). The likely mechanism of this effect involves local block of conduction near the recording electrode.

Discussion

Arrhythmias and late potentials. All animals with inducible sustained ventricular tachycardia (group III) had well-defined infarcts, prominent delays in epicar-

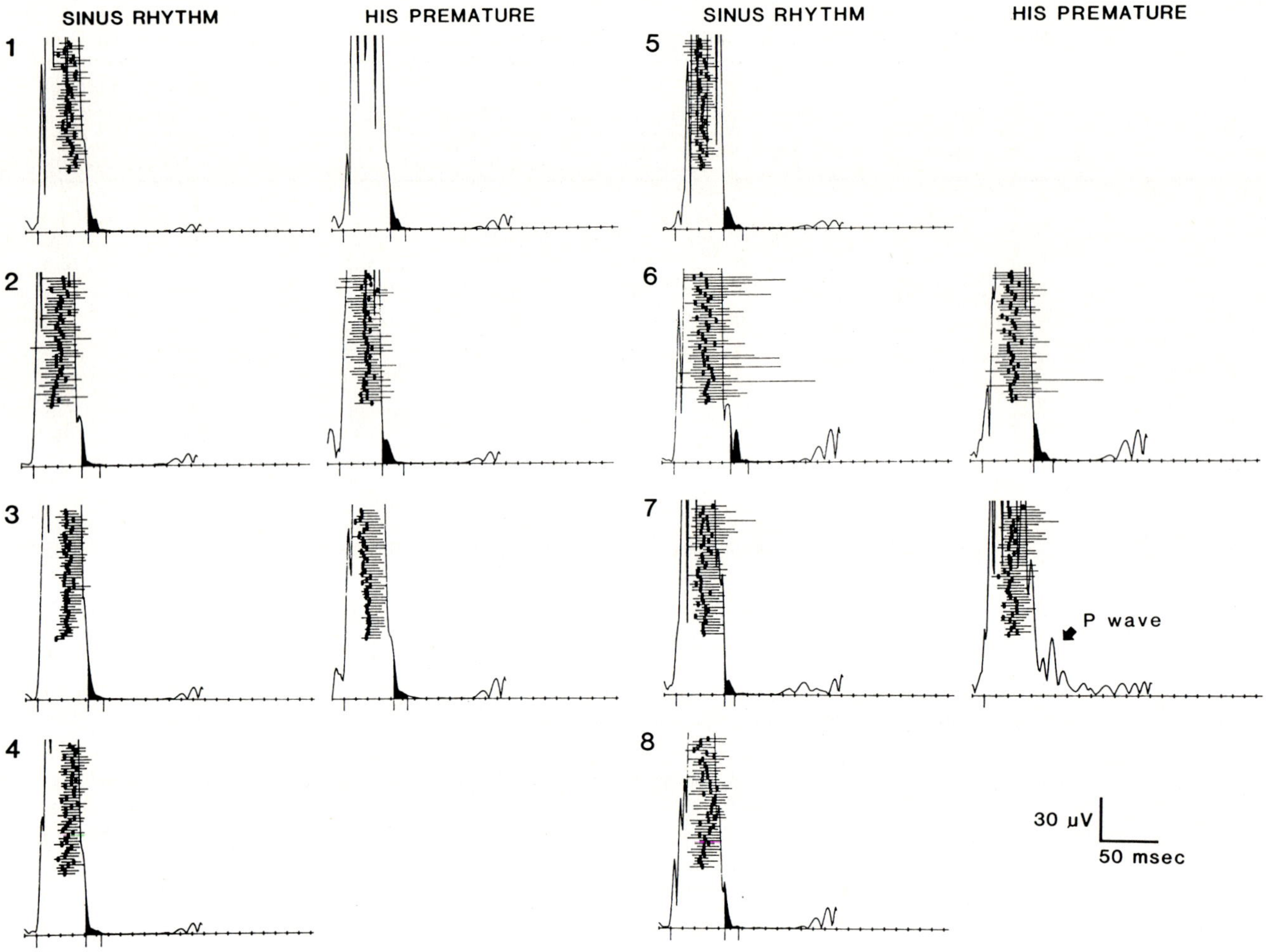

FIGURE 2. Signal-averaged, filtered QRS complexes and epicardial electrographic parameters for eight animals without inducible arrhythmias. Experiments 1 through 4 were controls, and dogs in experiments 5 through 8 underwent infarction. Data obtained during sinus rhythm are shown at the *left* and those obtained during premature His bundle stimulation at the *right*. See text for discussion.

dial activation, prolonged and fractionated electrograms, and late potentials in the filtered body surface QRS. These findings are in marked contrast to those in group I animals in which no arrhythmias could be induced. Group II animals, in which ventricular fibrillation was induced, included those animals with infarcts and delayed and prolonged epicardial activation and late potentials (experiments 2 and 3) as well as those without late potentials and minor or moderate abnormalities in epicardial activation (experiments 4, 5, and 6). Included in this group was a control dog (experiment 1). In this animal, induction of ventricular fibrillation required 3 premature beats delivered to the left ventricle at four times diastolic threshold after pacing at a basic cycle length of 350 msec. Before ventricular fibrillation ensued, there were no extra beats induced by the premature stimuli. Induction of ventricular fibrillation in normal dogs by aggressive stimulation protocols have been reported by others.[14, 15] In experiments 5 and 6 in group II fibrillation also was induced by similar aggressive pacing and was not preceded by nonsustained runs of ventricular beats (table 1). Thus, because ventricular fibrillation was a nonspecific end point in these experiments, group II must be considered a mixed population of animals. The range of values for the filtered QRS and electrographic parameters in group II extended across values obtained in group I and in group III.

In contrast, all animals with inducible ventricular tachycardia could be distinguished from those with no arrhythmia based on abnormal activation in the infarct and the following body surface QRS criteria: a QRS duration of 64 msec or greater, a RMS voltage in the last 20 msec of the QRS complex of 13.5 μV or less, and a duration of terminal activity below 30 μV of 18.2 msec or greater. The similarity between these data and the findings in humans[1–6, 8, 9] further supports this animal preparation as a useful analog for studying

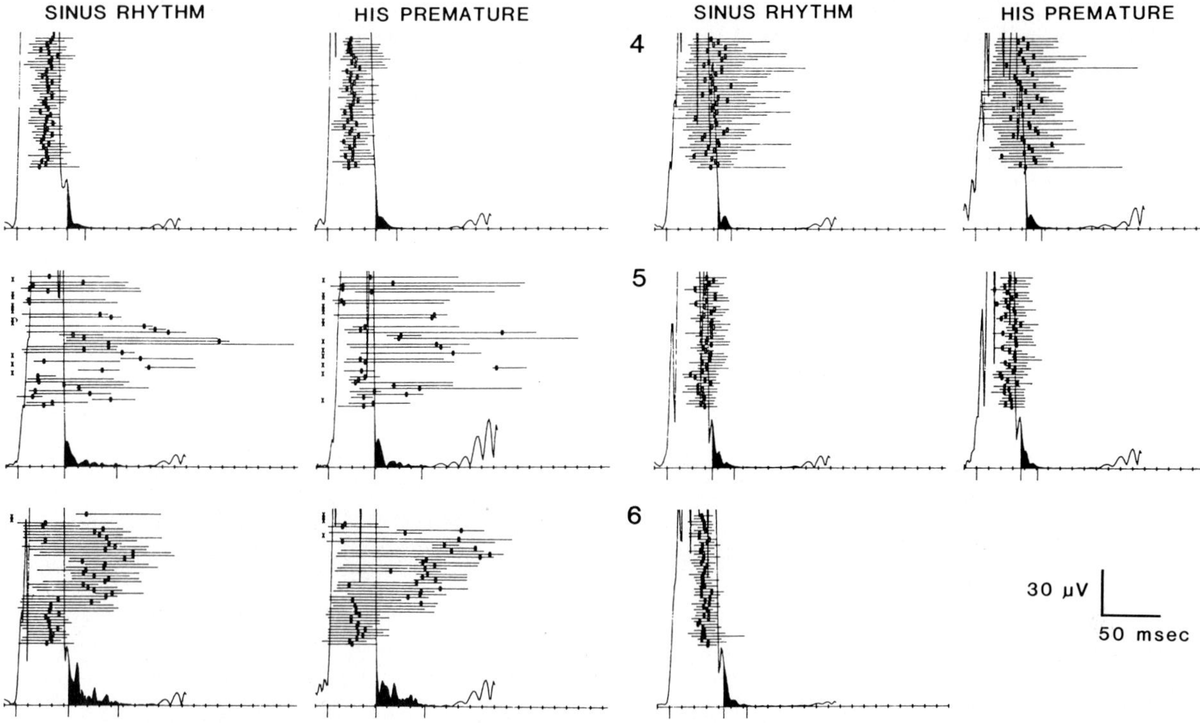

FIGURE 3. Signal-averaged, filtered QRS complexes and epicardial electrographic parameters for six animals with inducible ventricular fibrillation. Experiment 1 was from a control animal. The data are arranged as in figure 2.

the mechanisms of sustained ventricular tachycardia.

Epicardial activation and late potentials. A consistent finding in all experiments was that animals with late potentials had delayed and fractionated epicardial electrograms that persisted into the time of the late potentials (table 4). Although all regions of the infarct were not sampled and some epicardial activity extended beyond the end of the QRS, these correlations suggest

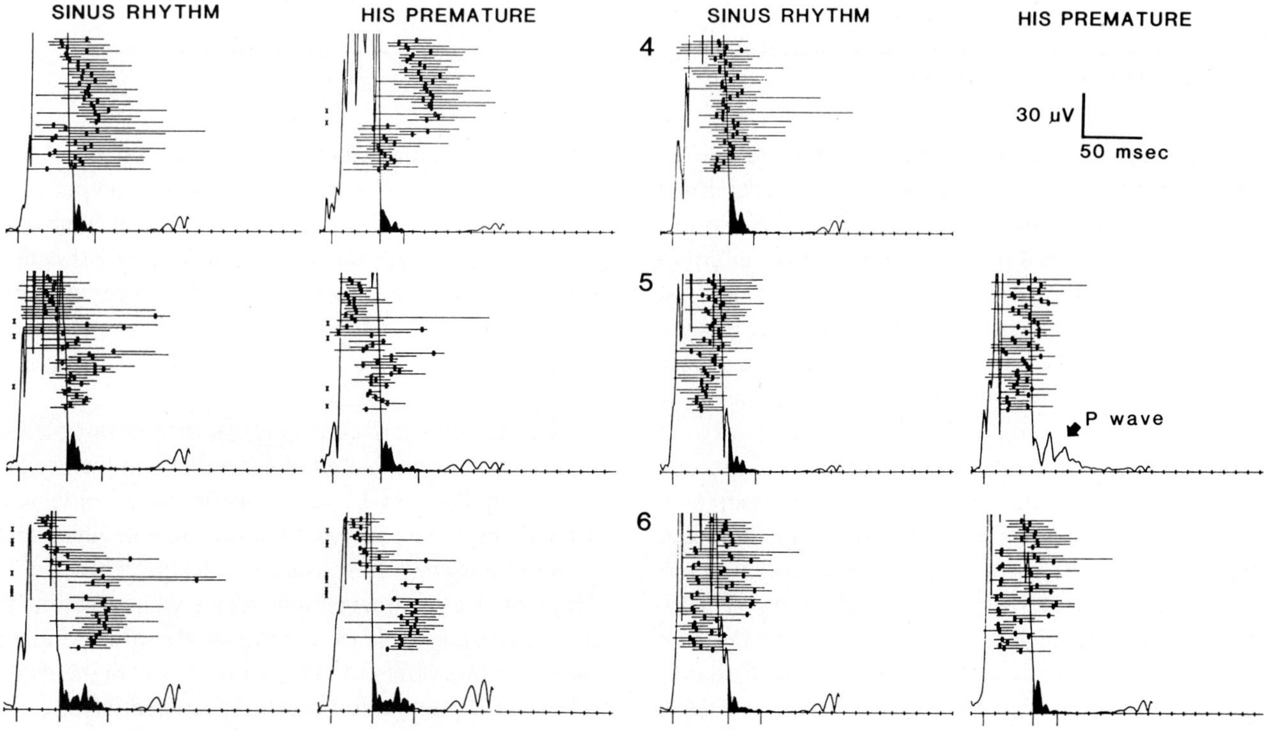

FIGURE 4. Signal-averaged, filtered QRS complexes and epicardial electrographic parameters for six infarcted animals in which ventricular tachycardia was inducible. The data are arranged as in figure 2.

TABLE 4
Effect of premature stimulation of the His on electrogram local activation and duration

Experiment No.	Proportion of local activations occurring after the onset of D30		Proportion of electrograms extending into D30		Changes in electrogram duration >10 msec	
	Sinus	His	Sinus	His	Increasing	Decreasing
Group I						
1	0/45	—	5/45	—	—	—
2	0/45	0/45	6/45	15/45	1/45	1/45
3	0/45	0/45	1/45	1/45	0/45	0/45
4	0/45	—	6/45	—	—	—
5	0/45	—	0/45	—	—	—
6	0/45	0/45	21/45	26/45	0/45	0/45
7	0/45	—	11/45	—	0/45	0/45
8	0/45	—	8/45	—	—	—
Total	0/360 (0.0%)	0/135 (0.0%)	58/360 (16.1%)	42/135 (31.1%)	1/180 (0.6%)	11/180 (6.1%)
Group II						
1	0/45	0/45	5/45	11/45	2/45	2/45
2	19/34	13/34	31/34	26/31	15/31	5/31
3	25/43	22/41	34/43	38/41	17/41	8/41
4	11/45	20/45	45/45	44/45	6/45	11/45
5	5/45	0/45	41/45	39/45	0/45	0/45
6	0/45	—	3/45	—	—	—
Total	60/257 (23.3%)	55/207 (26.6%)	159/257 (61.9%)	158/207 (76.3%)	40/207 (19.3%)	26/207 (12.6%)
Group III						
1	32/45	39/43	44/45	43/43	12/43	11/43
2	21/42	11/41	39/42	25/41	0/41	24/41
3	26/38	24/38	36/38	33/36	0/36	8/36
4	15/45	—	44/45	—	—	—
5	0/45	—	23/45	—	1/45	7/45
6	12/45	13/45	29/45	30/45	2/45	11/45
Total	106/305 (34.8%)	87/165 (52.7%)	215/305 (70.5%)	131/165 (79.4%)	15/210 (7.1%)	61/210 (29.1%)

Abbreviations are as in table 2.

that abnormal conduction within the infarcted epicardium contributes to the late potentials on the body surface. The low mean electrogram amplitude in experiment 2 in group II dogs and experiment 1 in group III animals and the poorer correlation between delayed epicardial activation and late potentials in these cases emphasizes that there is an energy threshold below which delayed activity is not detected on the body surface.

The findings of the present studies contrast in one respect with data derived from similar studies in humans. In patients with ventricular tachycardia and late potentials, fragmented electrograms are seen primarily at endocardial sites.[7] The focus of the arrhythmia is also usually localized to the endocardium in these patients.[16] In the animal preparation the epicardium appears to be the preferential region for these phenomena.[12]

Effects of premature beats. The effect of premature stimulation of the His bundle on late potentials was minimal. While the configuration of the late potentials in the filtered signal was visibly changed in some cases (for example, experiment 3, figure 3; experiment 1, figure 4), the criteria used to define their presence were not significantly altered (figure 5). In the present experiments a single premature beat did not facilitate identification of late potentials.

The degree of effect of a premature beat on epicardial activation was also relatively minor. In the group II and group III animals, some sites showed prolongation of activation time and/or duration while in others these values shortened or showed no change. However, in individual experiments, the mean values during the His premature beat were comparable to those during sinus rhythm (table 3). This correlates with the lack of effect of a premature beat on late potentials.

The present study does not address the question of the effects of multiple His bundle or ventricular extra-

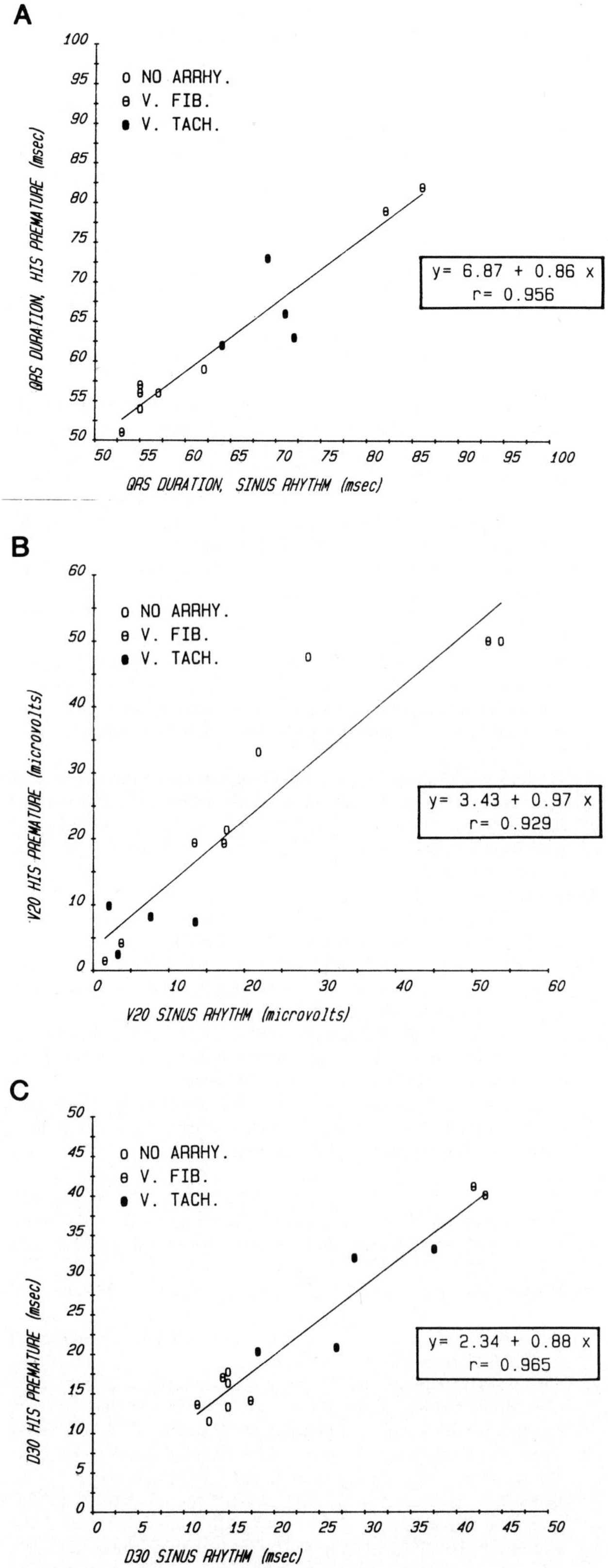

FIGURE 5. A comparison of the signal-averaged QRS complexes during sinus rhythm and during premature stimulation of the His bundle. *A*, The duration of the QRS complex, *B*, The amplitude in the last 20 msec of the QRS (V20). *C*, The duration of late activity below 30 μV (D30). Also shown are the equations for the regression lines and their r values.

stimuli on the above parameters. At least two ventricular extrastimuli were required to induce ventricular tachycardia in the group III animals (table 1). Since these were delivered at shorter coupling intervals than the His bundle extrastimuli their effects on conduction would be expected to be more severe. However, the effects of the single premature His beat on individual electrograms does provide some insight into the mechanisms underlying the induction of tachycardia by premature beats.

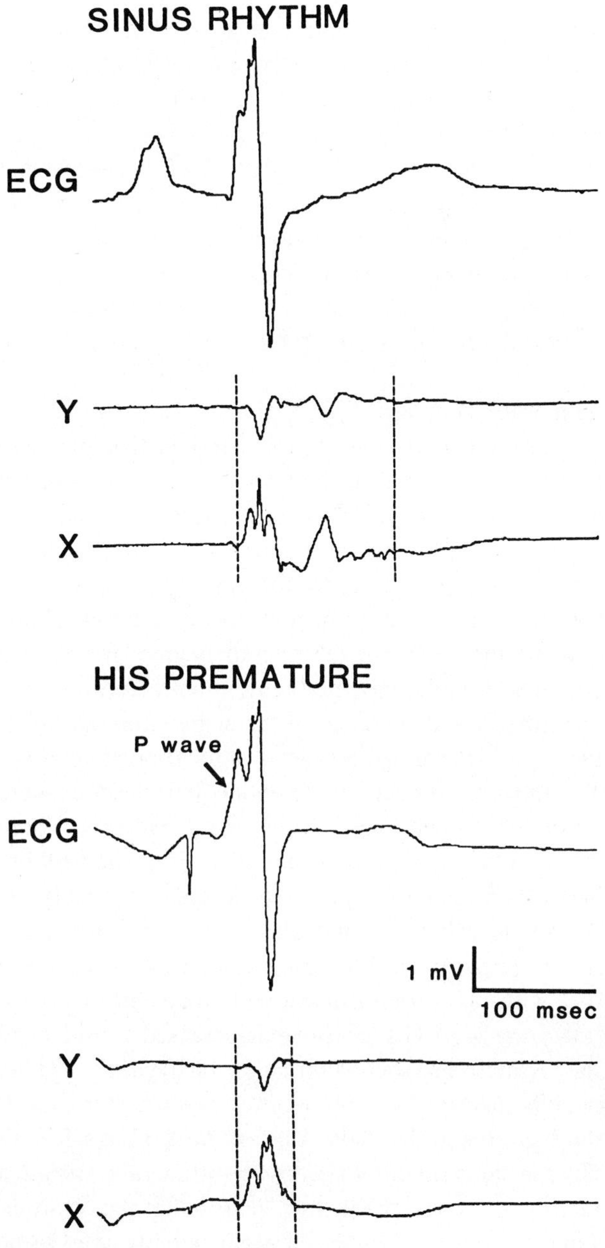

FIGURE 6. Analog records demonstrating the shortening of the duration of electrograms at a site within the infarcted region during premature stimulation of the premature His. The cycle length during sinus rhythm was 467 msec and the coupling interval of the premature His beat was 220 msec.

The shortening of some electrogram durations in response to a premature His beat (figure 6) can be explained by local block in part of the conducting path responsible for the fractionated electrogram in the region of the recording electrode. In this regard, block of conduction in the infarcted region seems analogous to what occurs in normal fast-conducting tissue such as muscle or the His-Purkinje system, where relatively little prolongation in conduction time occurs in response to the premature beat before the coupling interval that induces the block. This is in contrast to conduction in earlier infarcts,[11] where a premature beat delays both activation and late potentials. These tissues behave like the atrioventricular node, where beats of increasing prematurity cause progressive delays in conduction before the point of block is reached. The sudden local block in the present experiments was not unanticipated since previous studies have shown that action potential depolarizations are relatively normal in the infarcted tissues beyond 2 weeks.[17, 18] At that time the major mechanism of the abnormal discontinuous conduction in the infarct is probably disruption in cell-to-cell electrical continuity[19] and not depression in membrane depolarization.

More epicardial sites of group III dogs than of group II dogs exhibited electrogram shortening in response to a premature beat (table 4). In the infarcts of animals capable of sustaining ventricular tachycardia, conduction seems more prone to undergo local block in response to a premature beat. One implication of this may be that it is not the overall degree of delay in conduction in the infarcted region that determines the inducibility and character of the arrhythmia but rather these are determined by the way local areas interact. The most prominent late potentials in this series were observed in experiment 3 of figure 3. However, only eight of the 41 viable epicardial sites showed decreased duration in response to a premature beat (table 4) and the arrhythmia in this dog was ventricular fibrillation. Experiment 2 of figure 4 illustrates results in a dog with less prominent late potentials. In this case, however, 24 of 41 sites showed decreased duration and the arrhythmia was ventricular tachycardia. Thus, delayed and dissociated conduction sufficient to produce prominent late potentials on the body surface in dogs in sinus rhythm may not be sufficient to sustain a reentrant circuit producing ventricular tachycardia. This is consistent with clinical findings that some patients with late potentials do not have ventricular tachycardia.[3]

We ackowledge the expert technical assistance of Ralph Iannuzzi, William Moore, Bejay Moore, and Charles Prood.

References

1. Uther JB, Dennett CJ, Tan A: The detection of delayed activation signals of low amplitude in the vectorcardiogram of patients with recurrent ventricular tachycardia by signal averaging. *In* Sandoe E, Julian DG, Bell JW, editors: Management of ventricular tachycardia — role of mexiletine. Amsterdam, 1978, Excerpta Medica, p 80
2. Rozanski JJ, Mortara D, Myerburg RJ, Castellanos A: Body surface detection of delayed depolarizations in patients with recurrent ventricular tachycardia and left ventricular aneurysm. Circulation **63:** 1172, 1980
3. Simson MB: Use of signals in the terminal QRS complex to identify patients with ventricular tachycardia after myocardial infarction. Circulation **64:** 235, 1981
4. Breithardt G, Becker R, Seipel L, Abendroth R, Ostermeyer J: Non-invasive detection of late potentials in man — a new marker for ventricular tachycardia. Eur Heart J **2:** 1, 1981
5. Denes P, Santarelli P, Hauser RG, Uretz EF: Quantitative analysis of the high-frequency components of the terminal portion of the body surface QRS in normal subjects and in patients with ventricular tachycardia. Circulation **67:** 1129, 1983
6. Cain ME, Ambos HD, Witkowski FX, Sobel BE: Fast-fourier transform analysis of signal-averaged electrocardiograms for identification of patients prone to sustained ventricular tachycardia. Circulation **69:** 711, 1984
7. Simson MB, Untereker WJ, Spielman SR, Horowitz LN, Marcus NH, Falcone RA, Harken AH, Josephson ME: Relation between late potentials on the body surface and directly recorded fragmented electrograms in patients with ventricular tachycardia. Am J Cardiol **51:** 105, 1983
8. Wellens HJJ, Durrer DR, Lie KI: Observations on mechanisms of ventricular tachycardia in man. Circulation **54:** 237, 1976
9. Josephson ME, Horowitz LN, Farshidi A, Spielman SR, Michelson EL, Greenspan AM: Sustained ventricular tachycardia. Evidence for protected localized reentry. Am J Cardiol **42:** 416, 1978
10. Simson MB, Euler D, Michelson EL, Falcone RA, Spear JF, Moore EN: Detection of delayed ventricular activation on the body surface in dogs. Am J Physiol **241:** H363, 1981
11. Berbari EJ, Scherlag BJ, Hope RR, Lazzara R: Recording from the body surface of arrhythmogenic ventricular activity during the S-T segment. Am J Cardiol **41:** 697, 1978
12. Richards DA, Blake GJ, Spear JF, Moore EN: Electrophysiologic substrate for ventricular tachycardia: correlation of properties in vivo and in vitro. Circulation **69:** 369, 1984
13. Michelson EL, Spear JF, Moore EN: Electrophysiologic and anatomic correlates of sustained ventricular tachyarrhythmias in a model of chronic myocardial infarction. Am J Cardiol **45:** 583, 1980
14. Wetstein L, Michelson EL, Simson MB, Moore EN, Harken AH: Initiation of ventricular tachyarrhythmia with programmed stimulation: sensitivity and specificity in an experimental canine model. Surgery **92:** 206, 1982
15. Hamer AW, Karagueuzian HS, Sugi K, Zaher C, Mandel WJ, Peter T: Factors related to the induction of ventricular fibrillation in the normal canine heart by programmed electrical stimulation. J Am Coll Cardiol **3:** 751, 1984
16. Marcus NH, Falcone RA, Harken AH, Josephson ME, Simson MB: Body surface late potentials: effects of endocardial resection in patients with ventricular tachycardia. Circulation **70:** 632, 1984
17. Spear JF, Michelson EL, Moore EN: Cellular electrophysiologic characteristics of chronically infarcted myocardium in dogs susceptible to sustained ventricular tachyarrhythmias. J Am Coll Cardiol **1:** 1099, 1983
18. Gardner P, Ursell PC, Fenoglio JJ, Allessie MA, Bonke FIM, Wit AL: Structure of the epicardial border zone in canine infarcts is a cause of reentrant excitation. Circulation **64:** 320, 1981 (abst)
19. Spear JF, Michelson EL, Moore EN: Reduced space constant in slowly conducting regions of chronically infarcted canine myocardium. Circ Res **53:** 176, 1983

Collateral conductance changes during a brief coronary occlusion in awake dogs

SUSAN BRAZZAMANO, PH.D., JOHN M. FEDOR, M.D., JUDITH C. REMBERT, PH.D., AND JOSEPH C. GREENFIELD, JR., M.D.

ABSTRACT Function of the coronary collateral circulation during the course of a single abrupt coronary occlusion was evaluated in awake dogs instrumented over the long term. Studies were performed approximately 2 weeks after collateral development had been stimulated in the dogs by partial stenosis of the proximal left circumflex coronary artery. The pressure drop from the central aorta to the distal circumflex coronary artery was measured continuously. Under control conditions and at 30 sec and 4 min of a single abrupt complete circumflex occlusion, myocardial blood flow was determined by a radioactive microsphere technique. Coronary collateral conductance was calculated as mean collateral blood flow divided by the mean drop in pressure. The following was noted in dogs that developed collateral vessels: during the coronary occlusion, mean distal circumflex coronary pressure increased from 42 ± 9 to 49 ± 10 mm Hg ($p \leq .01$); mean collateral flow increased from 0.78 ± 0.30 to 0.84 ± 0.33 ml/min/g ($p \leq .05$); the endocardial/epicardial flow ratio increased from 0.77 ± 0.36 to 1.04 ± 0.25 ($p \leq .01$); and the coronary collateral conductance increased significantly from 0.017 ± 0.017 to 0.021 ± 0.021 (ml/min/g)/mm Hg ($p \leq .005$). These data suggest that during a brief occlusion of a major coronary artery, immature coronary collateral channels do not reach maximal function immediately after the occlusion. Rather, coronary collateral conductance increases with time and may be associated with improved transmural perfusion of the myocardium.
Circulation 72, No. 1, 225–232, 1985.

SIGNIFICANT AREAS of viable myocardium often are dependent on coronary collateral channels for blood supply when advanced occlusive coronary artery disease is present. During periods of coronary spasm or acute occlusion of a major coronary artery, the degree of myocardial ischemia that develops is dependent in part on the availability of coronary collateral channels and the rate at which these channels begin to function. A native and usually marginally functional collateral circulation exists in both dogs and humans. Collateral channels develop rapidly after an appropriate stimulus in dogs, but do not become as functional as native arteries until approximately 6 months; thus, during development they are characterized as immature. Studies in which Khouri et al.[1] measured coronary pressure in dogs suggested that previously well-formed collateral channels may open gradually. Greenfield et al.[2] observed in patients undergoing coronary artery bypass surgery that reactive hyperemia was present after an acute 10 sec interruption of flow in the vein graft. However, reactive hyperemia largely disappeared if the occlusion was maintained for up to 1 min. This observation suggests that existing collateral channels may not fully open immediately after an acute interruption of antegrade blood flow but may begin to function over several minutes. Brazzamano et al.[3] observed in dogs that when immature collaterals were present, repeated coronary artery occlusions of 5 min duration augmented collateral flow above that during the initial coronary occlusion.

The purpose of the present study was to determine the rapidity with which immature coronary collateral channels begin to function during a brief occlusion of a major coronary artery. An awake animal preparation was used in which coronary collateral development had been stimulated by the placement of a partial stenosis on the left circumflex coronary artery. In this preparation a region of myocardium was perfused by both the partially stenosed circumflex coronary artery and from immature but developing coronary collateral channels. The change of the pressure drop across the

From the Department of Medicine, Division of Cardiology, Duke University Medical Center, and the Medical Service, Cardiology Section, Veterans Administration Medical Center, Durham.

This study was supported in part by the National Institutes of Health grant HL 18468 and the Medical Research Service of the Veterans Administration.

Address for correspondence: Joseph C. Greenfield, Jr., M.D., Box 3246, Duke University Medical Center, Durham, NC 27710.

Received Feb. 5, 1985; revision accepted April 11, 1985.

collateral network as well as transmural myocardial flow was determined during a brief interruption in circumflex coronary flow. These measurements allowed an estimation of the time course of the changes in conductance across the collateral network independent from conductance changes occurring in the distal myocardial circulation. These observations have not been made previously and are important to the understanding of the physiology of the coronary collateral circulation.

Methods

Thirty-eight mongrel dogs of both sexes weighing from 30 to 40 kg were instrumented and studied. They were free of signs of ill health and were suited in temperament to the laboratory environment.

Surgical preparation. Surgical anesthesia was induced with sodium thiamylal (30 to 40 mg/kg iv). A left thoracotomy was performed via the fourth intercostal space under sterile conditions. Small supplemental doses of sodium thiamylal were given throughout the operative procedure as required. The heart was suspended in a pericardial cradle. Heparin-filled polyvinylchloride catheters (3.0 mm outside diameter [OD]) were introduced into the arch of the aorta via the internal mammary artery, into the left ventricle through the apex, and into the left atrium via the atrial appendage. The catheters were secured with purse-string sutures. The left circumflex coronary artery was dissected free from its origin proximal to the first large marginal branch. A pneumatic coronary artery occluder, constructed in our laboratory, was placed on the circumflex coronary artery. In 25 of the 38 dogs, an electromagnetic flow probe (Howell Instruments, Inc.) was placed just proximal to the occluder. Since results of the study are based on the condition that zero antegrade coronary flow was maintained during coronary occlusion, the flow probe was used specifically to verify zero flow at that time. A specially constructed Teflon sleeve 4 mm in length was placed proximal to the occluder and the electromagnetic flow probe. The internal diameter of the Teflon sleeve was chosen to produce an approximate 85% reduction in the luminal area of the coronary artery.

A Teflon coronary pressure catheter that could be inserted into the coronary artery was constructed in our laboratory. This catheter was designed as a modification of the method described by Gould.[4] The catheter was 1.00 mm OD, 0.80 mm inside diameter (ID) in the first 2 cm of length, and 1.25 mm OD, 1.00 mm ID in the remaining 4 cm of length. The distal end was tapered to aid with insertion. Three polyvinylchloride rings 1 mm in length and of 1.25 mm ID were placed on the distal end of the pressure catheter to prevent movement of sutures used in securing the catheter to the myocardium. Figure 1 shows the phasic coronary pressure tracings. The frequency response of the coronary catheter system and other pressure catheters were evaluated with use of a pop test.[5] The natural frequency was approximately 11 cycles/sec with a damping coefficient of 0.4 for the coronary pressure catheter system. The natural frequency of the aortic and left ventricular catheters was approximately 60 cycles/sec with a damping coefficient of 0.3.

Gould[4] has evaluated the degree of difference expected between a downstream as compared with a sidearm coronary pressure determination and found that this difference was approximately 1 to 2 mm Hg. This should have been consistent throughout our study and therefore should have had a negligible effect on the observed data. The lengths of the coronary, aortic, and left ventricular catheters were 25 to 30 cm. The distances

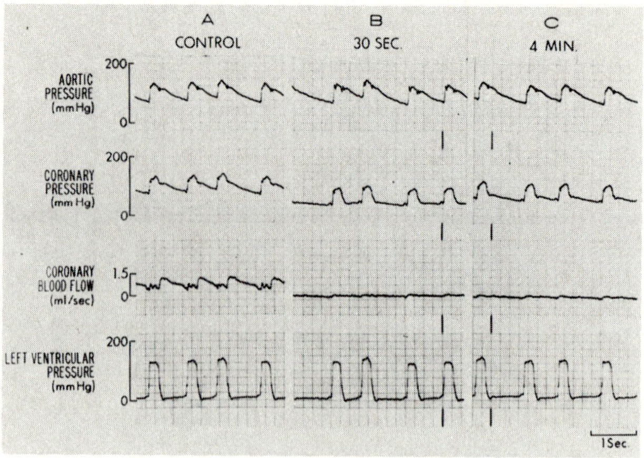

FIGURE 1. Typical examples of pressure and flow tracings from a group I dog. Coronary pressure was measured in the distal circumflex coronary artery. Coronary blood flow was measured in the circumflex coronary artery proximal to the coronary pressure catheter. Note the fidelity of the coronary pressure tracings. *A*, Control, resting conditions. *B*, Thirty seconds after the onset of an abrupt circumflex occlusion. *C*, Four minutes into the same circumflex occlusion.

from the distal end of coronary and aortic catheters to the orifice of the left coronary artery were similar. The catheter was inserted into the coronary artery with the aid of a metal needle stylet. A needle puncture was made through the arterial wall with the needle stylet and the Teflon catheter was advanced into the left circumflex coronary artery facing downstream just distal to the balloon occluder. The inner stylet was removed and the Teflon catheter was connected to a 20 cm length of clear polyvinylchloride tubing, 1.5 mm OD, 1.25 mm ID. The Teflon pressure catheter was secured to the fascia and the connective tissue surrounding the coronary artery with a 4-0 silk suture. Since no arteriotomy had been performed, there was no bleeding at the site of insertion. The distal end of the coronary catheter was secured to the myocardium.

The catheters, balloon snare occluder, and electromagnetic flow probe leads were tunneled dorsally and exteriorized individually at the base of the neck. The coronary pressure catheter was fitted with a rubberized heparin well. The heparin well was secured to the skin with a purse-string suture. The coronary catheter then could be flushed percutaneously via a needle puncture through the rubber membrane. The dogs were treated with antibiotics for 7 days. The coronary pressure catheter was flushed daily for 5 days with 1000 units of heparin, and then every 2 days until the time of study. Postmortem evaluation indicated that the coronary pressure catheter obstructed the left circumflex vessel by 10% to 20%. This measurement was obtained in five dogs by planimetry of a cross-sectional area of the barium-filled circumflex vessel, which contained the coronary pressure catheter.

Study protocol. All animals were brought to the laboratory approximately 7 to 14 days after the surgical procedure and were evaluated to be sure that they were fully recovered, afebrile, had normal hematocrits, and had resting pulse rates less than 90 beats/min. They were premedicated with 10 mg im morphine for analgesic purposes at least 1 hr before the study. Aortic, atrial, left ventricular, and coronary pressure catheters were connected to Statham P23Db pressure transducers and adjusted to the same zero pressure reference at the midchest level. The transducers were calibrated equally by simultaneous standardization with a mercury column. Coronary flow was measured with a Howell electromagnetic flowmeter. Before the study, flowmeter calibrations were performed in vitro by collecting measured amounts of normal saline through the probes within a known amount of time; both high and low flow rates were measured to test linearity. The coronary probe calibrations remained within ±4% throughout the series of experiments. In this report coronary flow refers to antegrade blood flow through the left circumflex coronary artery.

Lead II of the electrocardiogram was monitored. Hemodynamic data were recorded both on a Hewlett-Packard direct-writing oscillograph (model 7700), and an FM magnetic tape recorder (model 3520B.) After the instrumentation was connected, hemodynamic data were monitored continuously to ensure that steady-state conditions had been obtained. After recording of control pressure and myocardial flow measurements a single coronary occlusion lasting approximately 5 min was performed in all dogs. Regional myocardial blood flow determinations were made at 30 sec and then again at 4 min during this single coronary occlusion. The occluder was released and the animals were allowed to recover. Blood flow was measured by injection of carbonized radioactive microspheres 9 ± 1 μm in diameter, labeled with one of seven gamma-emitting nuclides (^{125}I, ^{141}Ce, ^{51}Cr, ^{95}Nb, ^{113}Sn, ^{103}Ru, or ^{46}Sc; New England Nuclear). The microsphere method, tissue counting, and flow calculations used in our laboratory have been described previously by others.[6, 7]

At the end of the study all animals were killed with a lethal dose of sodium thiamylal followed by potassium chloride. Each heart was removed and the circumflex artery was cannulated at the orifice. Methylene blue dye was injected into the proximal circumflex coronary artery during an occlusion of the balloon occluder to verify the completeness of the coronary occlusion in the 13 dogs without flow probes. The heart was then placed in buffered formalin. The left ventricle was sectioned into four transverse rings and six anatomic regions as described previously.[7] Each region was divided into four transmural layers, epicardium (layer 1) to endocardium (layer 4), each 0.5 to 2 g of myocardial tissue. If myocardial infarction or fibrosis exceeded 15% of the surface in any one of the four transmural myocardial layers, or if fibrosis was found in more than one layer, the data from the animal were rejected. In five dogs these changes were observed in the collateral-dependent myocardium and therefore the data were excluded from the analysis.

For purposes of this study, the collateral-dependent region was defined as the region of most severe ischemia as determined by radioactive microsphere measurements and was most often the posterior papillary muscle. The anterior region was defined as the control, noncollateral-dependent region.

Data analysis. Collateral coronary conductance was calculated as the mean myocardial blood flow in the collateral-dependent area divided by mean aortic pressure minus mean circumflex coronary arterial pressure. The systolic, diastolic, and mean aortic-circumflex pressure gradients were not significantly different. Thus, the mean gradient was used in the calculation of conductance. Distal coronary conductance was calculated as mean myocardial blood flow in the collateral-dependent area divided by mean coronary pressure minus left ventricular end-diastolic pressure.

$$\text{Collateral coronary conductance} = \frac{\text{Mean collateral blood flow}}{\text{Mean aortic} - \text{mean circumflex pressure}}$$

$$\text{Distal coronary conductance} = \frac{\text{Mean collateral blood flow}}{\text{Mean circumflex} - \text{left ventricular end-diastolic pressure}}$$

The nonparametric Wilcoxon two-sample signed-rank test was used for statistical comparisons within each group. Comparisons between groups were done with Student's t test for unpaired data. Linear regression analysis was used to evaluate trends and relationships between parameters. All data presented are expressed as mean ± SD.

Results

Studies were performed in 38 dogs. Data from 14 dogs were excluded from the analysis: five dogs were excluded because of the development of significant myocardial fibrosis and nine dogs were excluded because of technical difficulties. The 24 dogs in which complete studies were performed were separated into two groups according to their circumflex coronary pressure 30 sec after circumflex coronary occlusion at the time of study. Group I consisted of 16 dogs with evidence of collateral development at the time of study and circumflex diastolic pressure greater than 17 mm Hg at 30 sec. This value represents 1 SD above the mean of the diastolic coronary pressure observed in five dogs in which distal coronary pressure during occlusion was measured at the time of the initial surgical instrumentation. This pressure is similar to pressures observed by Khouri et al.,[1] who studied awake dogs before collateralization. Group II consisted of eight dogs without evidence of collateral development and diastolic circumflex pressures of less than 17 mm Hg at 30 sec.

The hemodynamic and myocardial blood flow data for both groups are summarized in table 1. During control resting conditions in group I dogs the myocardial blood flow was 0.83 ± 0.34 ml/min/g in the collateral-dependent posterior papillary region and 0.82 ± 0.36 ml/min/g in the noncollateral-dependent anterior region. The transmural blood flow was distributed so that endocardial/epicardial blood flow ratios were 1.13 ± 0.19 and 1.39 ± 0.24, respectively. In group II dogs under control resting conditions, similar myocardial blood flows and distributions were observed in collateral- and in noncollateral-dependent areas.

Thirty seconds after the onset of a complete circumflex occlusion in group I dogs, mean circumflex coronary pressure was 42 ± 9 mm Hg. At 4 min, mean circumflex coronary pressure had increased significantly to 49 ± 10 mm Hg ($p \leq .01$). The minimal coronary pressure was usually reached within the first 15 sec. The subsequent increase in pressure was gradual over the course of the duration of occlusion. No significant changes occurred in heart rate or aortic or left ventricular pressure. From 30 sec to 4 min after onset of circumflex occlusion mean myocardial flow in the collateral-dependent region increased slightly from

TABLE 1
Hemodynamic data

	Heart rate (beats/min)	Pressure (mm Hg): Aortic	Pressure (mm Hg): Circumflex coronary	Pressure (mm Hg): Mean aortic circumflex gradient	Pressure (mm Hg): Left ventricular end-diastolic	Myocardial flow (ml/min/g): Posterior papillary: Flow	Myocardial flow (ml/min/g): Posterior papillary: Endo/epi	Myocardial flow (ml/min/g): Anterior: Flow	Myocardial flow (ml/min/g): Anterior: Endo/epi
Group I (n = 16)									
Circumflex occlusion									
30 sec	82 ± 17	120 ± 11/78 ± 7	70 ± 14[B]/28 ± 7	50 ± 11[B]	7 ± 3	0.78 ± 0.30	0.77 ± 0.36[B]	0.81 ± 0.30	1.35 ± 0.24
4 min	79 ± 17	119 ± 12/79 ± 7	80 ± 11[A,B]/34 ± 9	42 ± 11[A,B]	6 ± 2	0.84 ± 0.33[A]	1.04 ± 0.25[A]	0.79 ± 0.26	1.37 ± 0.31
Control	77 ± 13	118 ± 12/79 ± 8	107 ± 12/67 ± 12	12 ± 8	6 ± 2	0.83 ± 0.34	1.13 ± 0.19	0.82 ± 0.36	1.39 ± 0.24
Group II (n = 8)									
Circumflex occlusion									
30 sec	98 ± 14[B]	116 ± 5/81 ± 7	36 ± 11[B]/12 ± 2	72 ± 3[B]	8 ± 3[B]	0.12 ± 0.06[B]	0.17 ± 0.10[B]	0.90 ± 0.24	1.37 ± 0.23
4 min	110 ± 35[A,B]	113 ± 9/78 ± 11	40 ± 13[B]/16 ± 7	65 ± 5[B]	10 ± 4[B]	0.15 ± 0.09[B]	0.14 ± 0.10[B]	1.11 ± 0.70[A]	1.31 ± 0.17
Control	79 ± 12	119 ± 7/76 ± 10	114 ± 8/73 ± 13	3 ± 3	5 ± 1	0.82 ± 0.29	1.30 ± 0.37	0.87 ± 0.46	1.38 ± 0.10

Values are mean ± SD.
[A]p ≤ .05 comparing the observations made at 30 sec and at 4 min during the same circumflex occlusion; [B]p ≤ .05 comparing observations at 30 sec and 4 min with control.

0.78 ± 0.30 to 0.84 ± 0.33 ml/min/g (p ≤ .05). The transmural blood flow distribution improved, resulting in a significant increase in mean endocardial/epicardial flow ratio from 0.77 ± 0.36 to 1.04 ± 0.25 (p ≤ .01). No significant changes were observed in myocardial flow or in the transmural flow distribution in the noncollateral-dependent anterior region. In group II dogs, from 30 sec to 4 min after coronary occlusion no significant changes in mean myocardial flow or in the transmural flow distribution were observed in the collateral-dependent area. Mean circumflex coronary pressure increased slightly but significantly (p ≤ .05) from 20 ± 5 to 24 ± 8 mm Hg.

Conductance changes from 30 sec to 4 min during coronary occlusion are shown for all 24 dogs in figure 2. Collateral conductance for group II dogs changed minimally from 0.001 ± 0.001 to 0.002 ± 0.002 (ml/min/g)/mm Hg (p ≤ .02). Only one of the dogs in group II had collateral conductance changes of more than 0.002 (ml/min/g)/mm Hg. In group I dogs, however, mean collateral conductance was 0.017 ± 0.017 (ml/min/g)/mm Hg at 30 sec and significantly increased to 0.021 ± 0.021 (ml/min/g)/mm Hg at 4 min (p ≤ .005) (figure 2, *A*). In 11 of 16 group I dogs, collateral conductance increased by greater than 0.002 (ml/min/g)/mm Hg. The change in distal conductance was quite variable and did not reach statistical significance (figure 2, *B*).

The relationship between initial collateral conductance and the change in collateral conductance during coronary occlusion was examined (figure 3). In dogs with low levels of collateral development (group II), little change in conductance was observed during coronary occlusion. In dogs with evidence of collateral development (group I), variable increases of collateral conductance were observed during the occlusion, but a trend indicating a relationship between the magnitude of the initial conductance and the change was apparent. The overall correlation was r = .69.

The transmural flow distribution (endocardial/epicardial) at 30 sec and 4 min of circumflex occlusion are compared in figure 4. In group II dogs no significant trend in coronary pressure or in the endocardial/epicardial flow ratio was apparent during the occlusion. In group I dogs the endocardial/epicardial flow ratio increased as coronary pressure increased. In three group I dogs coronary pressure increased despite the fact that the endocardial/epicardial flow ratios were greater than unity at 30 sec.

The reproducibility of the change in collateral conductance during coronary occlusion was evaluated in eight dogs (four from each group). These dogs under-

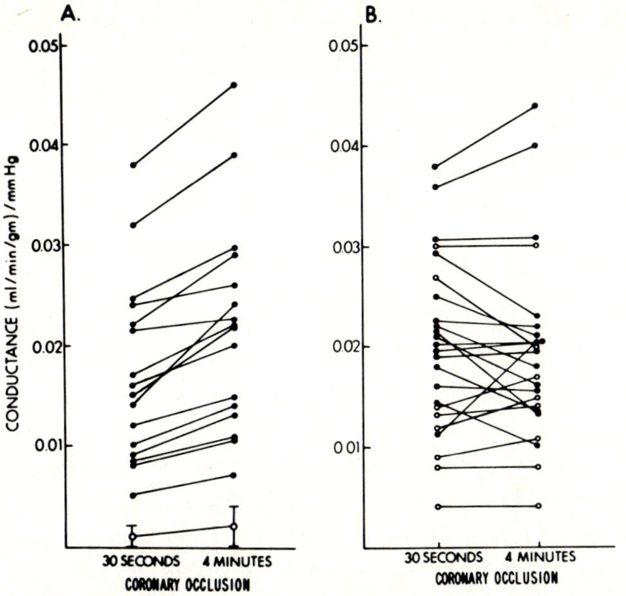

FIGURE 2. Conductance changes in each dog at 30 sec and 4 min of circumflex coronary occlusion. Closed circles represent data from dogs in group I; open circles represent data from dogs in group II. *A*, Changes in the collateral conductance. Open circles are the average data of all eight group II dogs. *B*, Conductance changes in the distal myocardial bed.

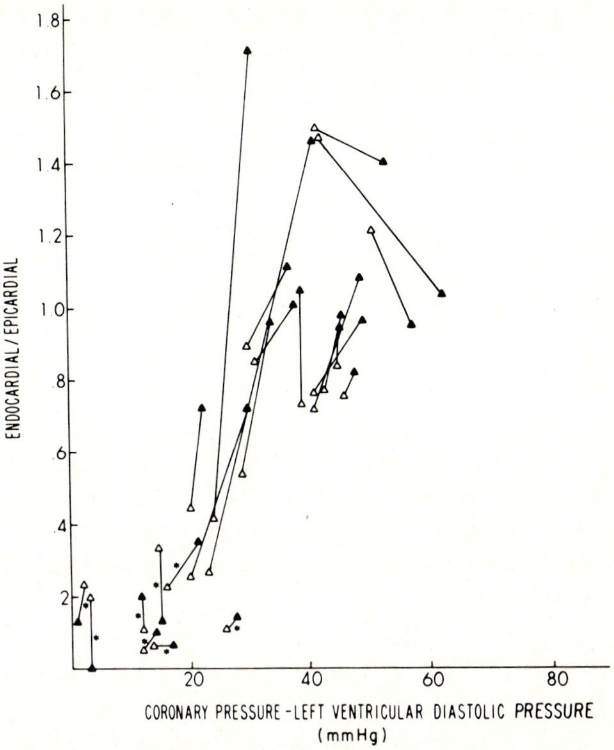

FIGURE 4. The transmural flow distribution estimated by the endocardial/epicardial flow ratio at 30 sec (open triangles) and 4 min (closed triangles) compared with mean circumflex minus left ventricular end-diastolic pressure. Each line connects the response at 30 sec (open triangles) and 4 min (closed triangles) for each dog. Data from both group I and group II dogs are shown. Asterisks represent data from group II.

went two circumflex coronary occlusions separated by 2 hr to allow baseline conditions to return. The change in conductance was not significantly different during the first and the second occlusions in dogs in either group. Hemodynamic parameters were also similar during each of the occlusions.

When differences between group I and group II were examined under control conditions, hemodynamics were similar as were blood flows to the posterior papillary and anterior regions and endocardial/epicardial blood flow ratios ($p \geq .15$) (table 1). Under control conditions the only difference between groups was in the aortic-coronary pressure drop ($p \leq .02$). Differences were found between groups at both 30 sec and 4 min during coronary occlusion in heart rate, posterior papillary blood flow, and the endocardial/epicardial blood flow ratio ($p \leq .02$). The change in coronary collateral conductance from 30 sec to 4 min was significantly greater for group I, 0.004 ± 0.002 (ml/min/g)/mm Hg, than group II, 0.001 ± 0.000 (ml/min/g)/mm Hg ($p \leq .04$). The separation of dogs into groups I and II was something of an artificial one since they represent a continuum. A certain amount of collateral vasculature was present in all the animals and appeared to respond in a similar manner during the two occlusions. It is clear, however, that the magnitude of the changes in collateral conductance were a function of the degree of collateralization and thus were greater in group II (figure 3).

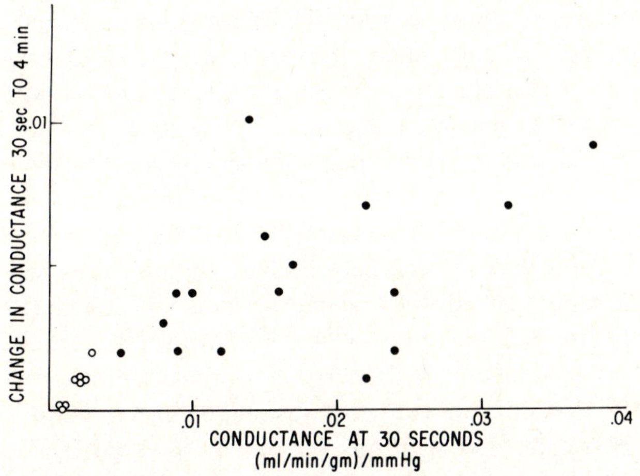

FIGURE 3. The initial collateral conductance at 30 sec during coronary occlusion compared with the change in collateral conductance from 30 sec to 4 min of the occlusion. Each closed circle represents one group I dog and each open circle represents one group II dog. The correlation coefficient for data from all dogs was r = .69.

Discussion

The primary purpose of this research was to evaluate coronary collateral function during brief occlusion of a major coronary artery. Previous investigators have described an experimental preparation of partial coronary stenosis[3, 8–10] that often results in rapid collateral development over a period of approximately 2 weeks. This preparation produces an area of myocardium that has a dual blood supply. The resting mean circumflex coronary flow in 11 dogs with flow probes in group I was 27 ± 15 ml/min. Data from our laboratory indicate that the mean circumflex flow in dogs without coronary stenosis studied in the awake state is in the range of 34 ml/min.[11] Also, the aortic-to-coronary pressure gradient was small under control conditions compared with during occlusion (table 1). Thus, under resting conditions the segment of myocardium is perfused primarily by flow through the stenotic vessel rather than the collateral vessels. These studies provided an opportunity to observe how rapidly immature collateral channels function after a brief coronary occlusion. The experimental preparation is analogous to spasm or thrombus occurring in the setting of partial coronary stenosis, which may result in coronary occlusion with a brief interruption of antegrade blood flow.

Blood flow into a region of myocardium perfused by collateral channels may be regulated by a number of factors including the resistance in (1) the collateral vessels themselves, (2) the arteriolar or precapillary and the penetrating vessels in the distal myocardial bed, or (3) a combination of both. The data obtained in these dogs can be used to compute separately the conductance at the level of the collateral channels and that occurring in the distal myocardial bed. To make this distinction, the pressure drop across the collateral network and a measurement of collateral blood flow must be obtained. During coronary occlusion, it was assumed that the pressure drop from the central aorta to the distal circumflex coronary artery represented the pressure drop across the collateral network. Previous studies have indicated that in the absence of coronary stenosis the gradient along the epicardial coronary artery is small.[12] The current study supports these data in that group II dogs had only a 3 mm Hg resting aortic-circumflex pressure gradient. This suggests that the major amount of change in pressure gradient occurred over the collateral network rather than from the aorta to the point of origin of the collateral vessels. The precise location and determinants of the pressure gradient across the distal myocardial bed is uncertain. For the purpose of this study it was assumed that the difference between distal circumflex coronary pressure and left ventricular end-diastolic pressure would at least provide a directional estimate of this pressure gradient. It is likely that this is at best a very gross estimate since evidence points to the existence of a "vascular waterfall" occurring in the distal myocardial bed.[13, 14] It is likely that the conductance of the distal myocardial bed as calculated here is a rather insensitive index of the dynamics occurring at the level of the penetrating vessels or the distal arterioles. No correlations of distal bed conductance with collateral conductance change during coronary occlusion or with the extent of collateral stimulation were apparent. However, the lack of correlation may be due to the limitations inherent in the computation of distal bed conductance as an index of vasomotion in the distal bed.

The dogs with evidence of collateral development invariably had an increase in collateral conductance from 30 sec to 4 min during occlusion of the circumflex coronary artery. These conductance changes were not associated with significant changes in heart rate, arterial pressure, or left ventricular end-diastolic pressure. At 4 min the endocardial/epicardial flow ratio, mean myocardial flow, and distal coronary pressure were significantly increased as compared with 30 sec. Furthermore, the improvement in collateral conductance during occlusion correlated with the initial level of conductance during coronary occlusion. These observations suggest that immature collateral channels do not function maximally at the onset of a coronary occlusion but may gradually improve function during the occlusion.

Thirty seconds was chosen as the time of the initial measurement because contraction of the ischemic muscle has ceased by this time and the coronary pressure is at a reliable steady state. The time of 4 min was chosen because it was believed that this would allow sufficient time for a detectable change in collateral function to have occurred. The observation that collateral conductance increases from 30 sec to 4 min during coronary occlusion is consistent with previous findings in the peripheral circulation.[15, 16] Rosenthal and Guyton[16] found in the dog that with occlusion of the femoral artery, peripheral conductance of collateral blood flow increased 277% during the first 70 sec, suggesting that the collateral network may not reach maximal function immediately but may increase function rapidly after femoral artery occlusion. The overall increase in distal pressure in the peripheral circulation observed by Rosenthal and Guyton was approximately 30 mm Hg, compared with the 7 mm Hg observed in the coronary circulation in the present study. These differences may relate to differences in the anatomy, physiology, or the degree of collateralization of the leg as compared with the heart in dogs.

The mechanism of the increase in collateral conductance after coronary occlusion is uncertain. Several possible mechanisms could explain this phenomenon: ischemic, hemodynamic, myogenic, or neural mechanisms could be involved. Ischemia could effect an improvement in perfusion of the collateral-dependent myocardium in at least two ways. First, a potent humoral effect on the collateral vessels could be produced by release of a vasoactive metabolite from inadequately perfused myocardium. Improved collateral conductance correlated with improved transmural perfusion during the occlusion, suggesting that collateral conductance changes may be related in some way to the recovery from subendocardial underperfusion.

Second, hypokinesis of the collateral-dependent region during occlusion could result in decreased systolic wall forces. Theoretically, the collateral-dependent myocardium might benefit in this situation by allowing collateral blood flow during both diastole and systole.

Arguing against the hypothesis that subendocardial ischemia is responsible for the increase in collateral conductance after circumflex occlusion is the fact that in three of our dogs in which there was no evidence of subendocardial underperfusion after 30 sec of occlusion collateral conductance increased over the course of the occlusion. It would appear, then, that the observed increase in collateral conductance during coronary occlusion cannot be explained as a consequence of release of a vasoactive substance from underperfused myocardium.

There are several ways in which physical forces may effect a change in the collateral vessels. One possible mechanism is that changes in the distending pressure may have resulted in a dilatation or opening of collateral channels. Pressure was not measured directly inside the collateral vessels, but was measured in the distal circumflex coronary artery. This pressure fell during coronary occlusion, suggesting that pressure inside collateral vessels was lower during coronary occlusion than under control conditions. It would seem unlikely, therefore, that an increase in distending pressure occured during the coronary occlusion and "popped" the collaterals open.

A physical force acting on the collateral vessels that potentially could be increased during coronary occlusion is the collateral flow velocity. The mean pressure gradient under control conditions was relatively low across the collateral network, suggesting that little collateral flow occurred at rest. During occlusion, the pressure gradient across the collateral network markedly increased, suggesting that the collateral flow velocity also increased. Increased flow velocity across the collateral channels would be expected to result in an increase in the shearing stress exerted on the luminal wall of the collateral vessel. In small vessels shearing stress, even under conditions of moderate changes in flow velocity, could conceivably become quite high.[17] It is possible that increased flow velocity may alter the endothelial lining of the vessel wall to cause a release of a vasodilating substance such as prostacyclin.

A possible myogenic mechanism[18] must be considered. According to the myogenic hypothesis the vasculature tone of the collateral vessel would be regulated in response to changes in a force applied by the distending pressure. If pressure fell in the collateral vessel then it would dilate, resulting in a decrease in collateral vasculature resistance or enhanced collateral conductance. However, the poor correlation ($r = .57$) between the degree of pressure drop during the occlusion and the change in conductance perhaps indicates that myogenic factors were not of paramount importance.

Evidence from the present study against both release of a vasodilator substance and a myogenic mechanism is the fact that the immature collateral vessels do not have well-developed vascular smooth muscle. Without the presence of smooth muscle both responses would seem improbable. The vessels develop smooth muscle as part of the vessel growth process but it is not known whether these cells respond as mature vascular smooth muscle. The distal and proximal connections of collaterals to large arteries probably do contain smooth muscle.[19] The amount these vessels contribute to collateral conductance is unknown. The possible involvement of neural influences was not investigated.

The data obtained in these studies may have important implications for the mechanism of the relief of angina pectoris in patients with significant coronary artery disease. If collateral vessels are present, the rapidity with which they open and become functional may be highly significant during coronary artery spasm or with the increased need for flow in a stenosed vessel during exercise. The data obtained in these studies clearly demonstrate that collateral conductance increases over a 4 min period during total occlusion of a partially stenosed coronary artery. Thus, it seems reasonable to conclude that these collateral vessels did not function at maximal capacity immediately. If minutes are required to achieve the maximal collateral flow, this finding may explain the relief of ischemic pain that occurs after several minutes in patients with resting angina or the "walk through" phenomena, which occurs in some patients with exercise-induced angina.

We gratefully acknowledge support from the following located at the Durham Veterans Administration Medical Center:

Dianne Higginbotham and Cynthia Mills for preparation of the manuscript, Kirby Cooper and Eric Fields for surgical expertise, Mike Taylor and the staff of the Animal Care Facility, and the Medical Media Production Service.

References

1. Khouri EM, Gregg DE, McGranahan GM Jr: Regression and reappearance of coronary collaterals. Am J Physiol **220:** 655, 1971
2. Greenfield JC Jr, Rembert JC, Young WG Jr, Oldham HM Jr, Alexander JA, Sabiston DC Jr: Studies of blood flow in aorta-to-coronary venous bypass grafts in man. J Clin Invest **51:** 2724, 1972
3. Brazzamano S, Mays A, Rembert JC, Greenfield JC Jr: Increase in collateral blood flow following repeated coronary artery occlusion and nitroglycerine administration. Circ Res **54:** 204, 1984
4. Gould LK: Pressure-flow characteristics of coronary stenosis in unsedated dogs at rest and during coronary vasodilation. Circ Res **43:** 242, 1978
5. Glantz SA, Tyberg JV: Determination of frequency response from step response: application to fluid filled catheters. Am J Physiol **236:** H376, 1979
6. Cobb FR, Bache RJ, Greenfield JC Jr: Regional myocardial blood flow in awake dogs. J Clin Invest **53:** 1618, 1974
7. Swain JL, Parker JP, McHale PA, Greenfield JC Jr: Effects of nitroglycerine and propanolol on the distribution of transmural myocardial blood flow during ischemia in the absence of hemodynamic changes in the unanesthetized dog. J Clin Invst **63:** 947, 1979
8. Cohen MV, Yipintsoi T: Myocardial performance and collateral flow after transient coronary occlusion in exercising dogs. Am J Physiol **237:** H520, 1979
9. Schwartz F, Wagner HO, Sesto M, Hoffman M, Schaper W, Kubler W: Native collaterals in the development of collateral circulation after chronic coronary stenosis in mongrel dogs. Circulation **66:** 303, 1982
10. Wüsten B: The Degree of Coronary Stenosis as a Determinant of Collateral Development. *In* Shaper W, editor: Pathophysiology of myocardial perfusion. Amsterdam, 1980, Biomedical Press, pp 453–457
11. Rembert JC, Boyd LM, Watkinson WP, Greenfield JC Jr: Effect of adenosine on transmural myocardial blood flow in the awake dog. Am J Physiol **239:** H7, 1980
12. Kelly KO, Feigl EO: Segmental α-receptor-mediated vasoconstriction in the canine coronary circulation. Circ Res **43:** 908, 1979
13. Riley RL, Permutt S: Hemodynamics of collapsible vessels with tone: The vascular waterfall. J Appl Physiol **18:** 924, 1963
14. Rouleau J, Boerboom LE, Surjadhana A, Hoffman JE: The role of autoregulation and tissue diastolic pressures in the transmural distribution of left ventricular blood flow in anesthetized dogs. Circ Res **45:** 804, 1979
15. Eckstein RW, Gregg DE, Pritchard WH: The magnitude and time of development of the collateral circulation in occluded femoral, carotid and coronary arteries. Am J Physiol **132:** 351, 1941
16. Rosenthal SL, Guyton AC: Hemodynamics of collateral vasodilatation following femoral artery occlusion in anesthetized dogs. Circ Res **23:** 239, 1968
17. Fry DL: Acute vascular endothelial changes associated with increased blood velocity gradients. Circ Res **22:** 168, 1968
18. Bayliss WM: On the local reactions of the arterial wall to changes in internal pressure. J Physiol **28:** 220, 1902
19. Schaper J, Borgers M, Schafer W: Structure of the ischemia induced changes in the precapillary anastomatic network of the heart. Am J Cardiol **29:** 851, 1972

Effect of the combination of diltiazem and atenolol on exercise-induced regional myocardial ischemia in conscious dogs

Masunori Matsuzaki, M.D., Brian Guth, Ph.D., Tsukasa Tajimi, M.D., W. Scott Kemper, M.S.E.E., and John Ross, Jr., M.D.

ABSTRACT The effect of combination therapy with diltiazem and atenolol on the regional myocardial blood flow–function relationship was studied in eight conscious dogs with chronic coronary artery stenosis. An ameroid constrictor and hydraulic occluder were placed around the left circumflex coronary artery, sonomicrometers were implanted for measuring wall thickness in control and ischemic regions, and regional myocardial blood flow was measured with the microsphere method. Eighteen days (average) after surgery, resting regional myocardial function and blood flow were normal, but treadmill exercise induced severe regional myocardial dysfunction in the posterior wall (wall thickening during systole reduced from 25.5% to 2.7%, a 90% reduction). Subendocardial blood flow decreased by 68% from the control standing value, while subepicardial flow increased. An identical exercise bout was performed 3 hr after administration of atenolol (1.0 mg/kg orally) and 15 min after administration of diltiazem (0.3 mg/kg iv). Heart rate during running was significantly lower as were left ventricular peak systolic pressure, end-diastolic pressure, and peak dP/dt. Wall thickening in the control region was not augmented during exercise after atenolol and diltiazem. There was less dysfuncion in the ischemic region (35% reduction) and the improved performance was accompanied by a substantial increase in subendocardial perfusion (0.31 $\pm$ 0.14 vs 0.61 $\pm$ 0.30 ml/min/g, a 36% reduction from rest). Epicardial flow was unchanged, and the endocardial/epicardial ratio increased (0.27 $\pm$ 0.13 vs 0.62 $\pm$ 0.29). Recovery time for regional wall thickening also improved. The beneficial effects of the combination of atenolol and diltiazem in a preparation of single-vessel chronic coronary stenosis were shown to be significantly greater than those of either drug alone.
Circulation 72, No. 1, 233–243, 1985.

β-ADRENERGIC BLOCKADE is effective in improving exercise tolerance in patients with angina pectoris but sometimes optimum results are not achieved when the drugs are used alone.[1–3] A second drug is therefore sometimes added to therapy, such as a long-acting nitrate,[4] a calcium blocker,[5–7] or occasionally digitalis.[8] Calcium channel–blocking drugs, which inhibit the influx of calcium ions during cell depolarization in both smooth and cardiac muscle, are highly effective in the therapy of vasospastic myocardial ischemia and stable angina pectoris.[9–15] The efficacy of calcium antagonists in patients receiving propranolol has been studied clinically,[5, 6] but little is known about how the combination of β-adrenergic blockade with a calcium antagonist acts in man or experimental animals. Also to be determined is whether exercise-induced maldistribution of regional myocardial blood flow and contractile dysfunction are modified by the therapy. Diltiazem is a calcium channel–blocking drug that has been reported in clinical and experimental studies to have smaller negative inotropic and chronotropic properties than verapamil and less inotropic and vasodilator action than nifedipine.[16, 17] Accordingly, in conscious exercising dogs with chronic coronary artery stenosis we have investigated the effects of diltiazem in combination with the cardioselective β-blocking drug atenolol.

From the Division of Cardiology, Department of Medicine, University of California, San Diego School of Medicine, La Jolla.

Supported by a National Institutes of Health (Specialized Center for Research on Ischemic Heart Disease) grant HL-17682.

Address for correspondence: John Ross, Jr., M.D., Head, Division of Cardiology, Department of Medicine, M-013, University of California, San Diego School of Medicine, La Jolla, CA 92093.

Received July 30, 1984; revision accepted April 11, 1985.

Methods

Animal preparation. Eight adult mongrel dogs weighing 19 to 30 kg (mean 24.7 kg) were anesthetized with sodium pentobarbital (25 mg/kg iv) and ventilated with a Harvard respirator. A left lateral thoracotomy was performed by a sterile technique through the fifth intercostal space. A miniature pressure transducer (Konigsberg P7) and a Tygon fluid-filled catheter (2.2 mm internal diameter) were introduced into the left ventricle through the apex. Left ventricular pressure measured through the fluid-filled catheter (Statham P23Db) was used to calibrate the Konigsberg gauge, zero reference being taken at the estimated level of the right atrium while each dog lay on its right side. Tygon catheters were inserted into the left atrium for injection of microspheres, and into the descending aorta to withdraw reference blood samples.

A 2.5 cm section of the proximal left circumflex coronary artery was dissected free and a single crystal (10 MHz) Doppler flowprobe was placed around the coronary artery. An ameroid constrictor was positioned distal to the flowprobe, and a hydraulic occlusive cuff was placed beyond the constrictor. The ameroid constrictor was encased in a slotted stainless steel ring (5 mm wide, external dimension 8 mm, lumen 2.5 to 3.0 mm). The constrictor was designed to produce gradual constriction of the coronary artery[18] and is known to stimulate development of collateral vessels.[19-21]

Two pairs of miniature ultrasonic dimension gauges (5 MHz) were implanted in the left ventricular wall for measuring regional myocardial wall thickness as previously described.[22] One pair was positioned in the posterior free wall supplied by the circumflex artery to measure posterior (ischemic) wall thickness, and the other was placed in the distribution of the anterior descending artery to measure anterior (control) wall thickness. In brief, one crystal (2 mm diameter) of each pair was inserted obliquely through the myocardium to the subendocardium. The second crystal (8 mm diameter) was sewn on the epicardial surface where the ultrasonic transit time between the crystals was shortest. The pericardium was left open and all wires and catheters were tunneled subcutaneously to the back of the dog and brought out through the skin between the scapulae. The chest was then closed, the pneumothorax evacuated, and an antibiotic (ampicillin, 300 mg/day) was administered intramuscularly for 3 days after surgery. The position of all crystal pairs was carefully determined and recorded at the time of necropsy to verify correct alignment. Of the 16 available pairs of crystals (eight dogs), data from 15 were considered acceptable. Eleven subendocardial crystals (six in the ischemic area and five in the control area) were positioned just inside the endocardial surface spanning nearly all of the wall, while the remaining four inner crystals were found within 2 mm of the endocardial surface, spanning approximately 80% of the full wall thickness. One pair of crystals that was to be used to measure control wall thickness was not usable because of improper alignment. There was no gross indication of infarction, and the crystals were surrounded by fibrous connective tissue (approximately 1 mm), as described previously.[22]

Regional myocardial blood flow. The reference withdrawal method was used to measure regional myocardial blood flow with 15 μm diameter radionuclide-labeled microspheres (^{57}Co, ^{114}In, ^{113}Sn, ^{103}Ru, ^{95}Nb, or ^{46}Sc; New England Nuclear). The microspheres were diluted in 10% low–molecular weight dextran with Tween 80 added. Details of the methods of regional myocardial blood flow determination in this laboratory have been described previously.[23] Left ventricular pressure, wall dimensions, coronary blood flow velocity, and subendocardial electrograms in the ischemic area were monitored continuously during the reference sample withdrawal period and the microsphere injection. If arrhythmias or signifiant changes in heart rate and left ventricular pressure were observed during the withdrawal period, the measurement in question was discarded. Immediately after the final experiment, each dog was anesthetized with intravenous sodium pentobarbital and killed with a lethal dose of potassium chloride. The heart was removed, the left and right coronary arteries were flushed gently with saline followed by formalin, and the heart was placed in 10% formalin for 3 to 5 days to facilitate sectioning by techniques previously described.[23] Histologic examination of the tissue between crystal pairs was performed,[23] and the extent of necrosis was determined with a point-counting technique.[24]

The radioactivity of myocardial and reference blood samples was counted in a Packard Autogamma Spectrometer (Model 5912) at window settings corresponding to the primary energy peak of each isotope with a matrix inversion technique for resolving the various isotope windows.[25] The myocardial blood flow to each sample was calculated by a standard method.[26] Flow was divided by the sample weight and expressed in milliliters per minute per gram (wet weight) of myocardium.

Data are reported from only the samples of the tissue containing the crystal pairs, but the entire slice (eight full-thickness samples) was counted and results confirmed that the tissue containing the crystal pair was always representative of the central ischemic zone.

Experimental protocol. Before operation, all dogs were familiarized with the laboratory and trained to run on a motorized treadmill. Starting 7 days after surgery, all eight dogs studied were evaluated every 2 to 3 days. The conscious, unsedated dog rested quietly on its right side, and after basal control recordings of hemodynamics, coronary blood flow velocity, and dimensions were obtained, temporary circumflex coronary artery occlusion was abruptly induced by inflating the hydraulic cuff. Complete coronary occlusion was maintained for 10 sec followed by full release of the cuff; the subsequent reactive hyperemia was recorded for at least 5 min. Seven days after surgery, mean basal blood flow velocity in the circumflex coronary artery was 40.2 ± 10.0 cm/sec (mean ± SD), and mean peak hyperemic flow velocity was 107.4 ± 20.1 cm/sec (268% of resting value). On the first evaluation day (7 days after surgery), brief coronary occlusion caused severe dysfunction in the ischemic area, but as time passed dysfunction of the ischemic wall during coronary occlusion gradually diminished and reactive hyperemia also decreased progressively, indicating collateral development. When peak reactive hyperemic flow velocity was reduced to less than approximately 130% of the preocclusion value treadmill exercise evaluation was performed, and if ischemic dysfunction was produced during this brief evaluation run (for approximately 1 min), the experiment was carried out on the same day. If the exercise-induced dysfunction during control exercise was not severe (systolic wall thickening reduced by less than 50% of standing value), the study was delayed. At an average of 18 ± 4 days after surgery (range 14 to 27 days), the exercise studies were performed. All eight dogs exhibited normal activity, were afebrile, showed normal hematocrits (range 39.0% to 45.5%), and were capable of repeated exercise on the treadmill.

On the study day, in four of eight dogs circumflex coronary artery blood flow velocity at rest was decreased, averaging 28.2 ± 4.6 cm/sec ($p < .01$ compared with 7 days after surgery), and peak reactive hyperemic flow velocity was also significantly decreased to 36.2 ± 6.6 cm/sec (128% of rest, $p < .01$ compared with at 7 days). In the remaining four dogs, blood flow through the circumflex coronary artery was absent because of complete obstruction by the ameroid constrictor. As previously noted,[27, 28] dogs with occluded arteries were not different from the other dogs with respect to the responses of regional function at rest or during exercise before or after drugs; the average subendocardial blood flow during exercise after drugs tended to be lower in dogs with occluded arteries, but numbers were too small for statistical analysis.

Control recordings and the first microsphere injection were made while the dog stood quietly on the treadmill. Each dog was then run on the treadmill at a speed and grade sufficient to substantially decrease systolic wall thickening in the ischemic area (average 9.6 ± 1.5 km/hr, 5% grade). All treadmill runs were performed for 3.2 to 4.2 min (average 3.6 ± 0.4 min) with microspheres injected between 2 and 2.5 min into the run when a steady state was apparent.[27] Data were recorded and taped during running, for 5 min after the end of the exercise period, and then intermittently for the next ½ hr. At least ½ hr after full recovery from control exercise was confirmed, atenolol (1 mg/kg) was administered orally. Approximately 3 hr after atenolol was given, data were recorded and diltiazem (0.3 mg/kg) was administered via the left atrial catheter over 5 min. Ten to fifteen minutes later, control data for the second exercise period were recorded with the dog standing quietly on the treadmill. The treadmill exercise was then repeated at exactly the same speed and grade, and for the same running time. The third microsphere injection was made when steady-state conditions were achieved (approximately 2 to 2.5 min into the run), as characterized by stable regional function and hemodynamics.

As reported previously, we have found that maximum effect on suppression of exercise-induced tachycardia by atenolol occurs at 3 to 4 hr after oral administration.[27] We have previously reported a high degree of reproducibility in sequential runs performed 3 hr apart in this animal preparation without intervention, with very similar responses of regional blood flow, hemodynamics, and regional wall thickening in both ischemic and normal zones.[27]

Data analysis. Recordings during each experiment were made on a Brush forced-ink recorder and on magnetic tape for subsequent analysis. The variables analyzed were wall thickness at end-diastole (identified at the point just before the onset of the positive dP/dt signal) and end-systole (defined as the maximum systolic thickening occurring at or within 20 msec of peak negative dP/dt), extent of systolic wall thickening, left ventricular peak and end-diastolic pressures, mean and phasic blood flow velocities in the circumflex coronary artery, and heart rate. The extent of wall thickening was calculated as the difference (in mm) between end-diastolic and end-systolic dimensions and was also expressed as the percentage change from end-diastolic wall thickness. The values for wall thickness were normalized to a 10 mm initial end-diastolic thickness by dividing the end-diastolic and end-systolic wall thickness by the control standing end-diastolic wall thickness and multiplying by 10.[24–29] The absolute values of end-diastolic wall thickness in the ischemic and control areas during control standing conditions ranged from 8.21 to 11.67 mm (average 10.35 ± 1.21 mm) and from 8.44 to 11.61 mm (average 9.75 ± 1.28 mm), respectively. Mean ejection phase wall thickening velocity (mWThV) of the ischemic and control walls was calculated by the following equation: mWThV = (ESWTh − EDWT)/ET, where ESWTh = end-systolic wall thickness; EDWTh = end-diastolic wall thickness; and ET = left ventricular ejection time (defined as the interval between the time of maximum left ventricular positive dP/dt and 20 msec before left ventricular peak negative dP/dt). Hemodynamic, dimensional, and coronary flow velocity data were digitized from magnetic tape with use of a computer system (PDP/11/03). Twenty consecutive cardiac cycles (10 consecutive cardiac cycles at the initial phase of exercise) were sampled and averaged.

Statistical analysis of the difference between control exercise and exercise with the combination of atenolol and diltiazem and comparison of mean values during exercise with those in the resting state were done with a multifactor analysis of variance for repeated measures.[30] When an overall difference was detected, Tukey's least significant difference test was used to determine which means differed significantly. Blood flow data were analyzed with a single-factor (repeated measures) analysis of variance, and multiple analysis of variance was used to analyze differences between blood flow in each layer in the ischemic and control areas.[30] An analysis of variance for repeated measures was also used to compare heart rate, left ventricular pressures, and peak left ventricular dP/dt values obtained in the present study with those observed in previous studies in which atenolol[27] and diltiazem[28] were used alone. In addition, points on the myocardial blood flow-function relationship comparing atenolol and diltiazem combined with values observed in the previous studies using atenolol or diltiazem alone were analyzed by Hotelling's multivariate t test for two variables.[30] Data are reported as mean ± SD; $p < .05$ was considered indicative of a significant difference.

Results

Hemodynamic responses. Hemodynamic data are summarized in figure 1. Representative tracings showing hemodynamic variables and dimensions during control exercise and during exercise after administration of atenolol and diltiazem are illustrated in figure 2.

Within 10 sec of the beginning of control exercise, heart rate increased abruptly and remained elevated throughout the run, whereas left ventricular peak systolic pressure and peak (+) dP/dt initially increased, fell somewhat during the first minute, and then stabilized (figures 1 and 2). Left ventricular end-diastolic pressure gradually increased and was significantly elevated by 1 min into the control run. At the time of microsphere injection (approximately 2.5 min into the run), heart rate was increased from 103 ± 14 (standing rest) to 227 ± 31 beats/min ($p < .01$). Left ventricular peak systolic pressure and left ventricular peak (+) dP/dt were also significantly increased (figure 1). During recovery from control exercise, these values (except for heart rate) returned to near the control standing values within 5 min (figure 1).

Fifteen minutes after diltiazem (3 hr and 15 min after administration of atenolol), left ventricular peak (+) dP/dt in dogs standing at rest was significantly decreased (by 10% from that before control exercise), while resting heart rate, left ventricular peak systolic pressure, and left ventricular end-diastolic pressure were unchanged. During the exercise period after drugs, the initial rapid response of hemodynamic parameters was absent and subsequent increase of those variables was markedly attenuated (figures 1 and 2). Heart rate and left ventricular diastolic pressure increased significantly, but the increases were greatly reduced throughout the entire exercise period (both different, $p < .01$, compared with control exercise). Left ventricular peak systolic pressure and left ventricular peak (+) dP/dt during exercise with atenolol and diltiazem were not different from resting values before exercise.

In four of the eight dogs, the circumflex coronary artery was still open throughout the studies. Blood flow velocity was 28.2 ± 4.6 cm/sec (at rest) before

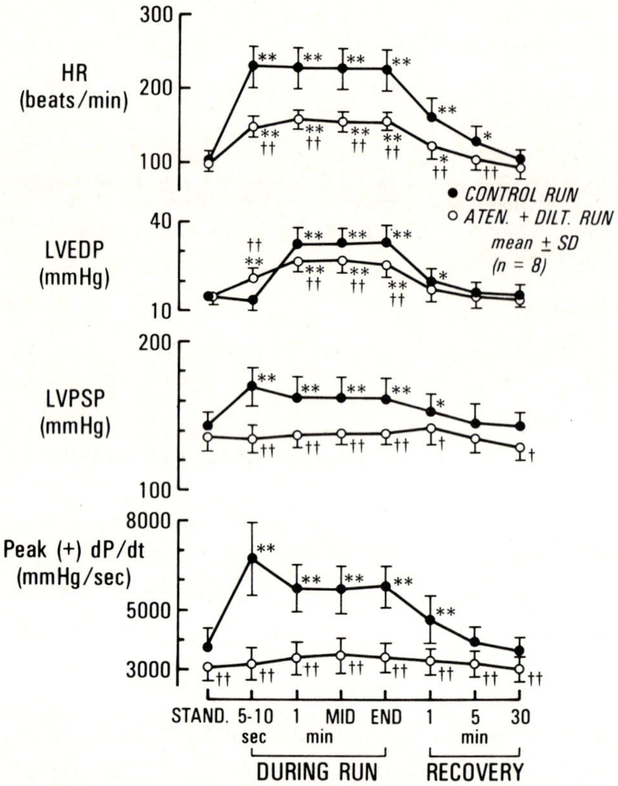

FIGURE 1. Hemodynamic responses to exercise and subsequent recovery before (closed circles) and after (open circles) administration of atenolol and diltiazem. All parameters, heart rate (HR), left ventricular end-diastolic pressure (LVEDP), left ventricular peak systolic pressure (LVPSP), peak positive left ventricular dP/dt, were reduced during the run after administration of atenolol and diltiazem.

control exercise and it was 33.4 ± 6.9 cm/sec at the time of exercise microsphere injection (NS). After atenolol and diltiazem were given, flow velocity in the circumflex coronary artery in dogs at rest was 25.7 ± 5.7 cm/sec (change NS) and it remained unchanged during exercise.

Myocardial blood flow. Average blood flow data at standing control, control exercise, and exercise with atenolol and diltiazem in ischemic and control areas, along with subendocardial to subepicardial flow ratios, are presented in table 1. The transmural flow distributions are summarized graphically in figure 3. At standing rest, mean transmural, subendocardial, midmyocardial, and subepicardial blood flows were not significantly different in the ischemic and the control areas.

Control area. During control exercise, the blood flow in the normal area increased uniformly in each layer (figure 3), and subendocardial to subepicardial blood flow ratios in the control area were similar at rest and during exercise (table 1). During exercise after drugs myocardial blood flow was higher in the control area than during control standing (except for epicardial blood flow), but it was markedly reduced in all layers compared with that during control exercise (figure 3).

Ischemic area. During control exercise, blood flow distribution in the ischemic area was markedly changed. Subendocardial and midmyocardial blood flows decreased by 68% and 38%, respectively, from the standing values, while subepicardial flow exceeded the standing value by 48% (table 1, figure 3). The subendocardial to subepicardial flow ratio in the ischemic area decreased from 1.17 to 0.27 (table 1).

In the ischemic area during exercise after atenolol and diltiazem subendocardial blood flow decreased by 36% from the control standing level, but this value was significantly higher than that during control exercise (approximately twice the control exercise value) (figure 3). Midmyocardial blood flow was slightly higher and subepicardial blood flow slightly lower, but these values were not significantly different from those at rest or during control exercise (figure 3). After atenolol

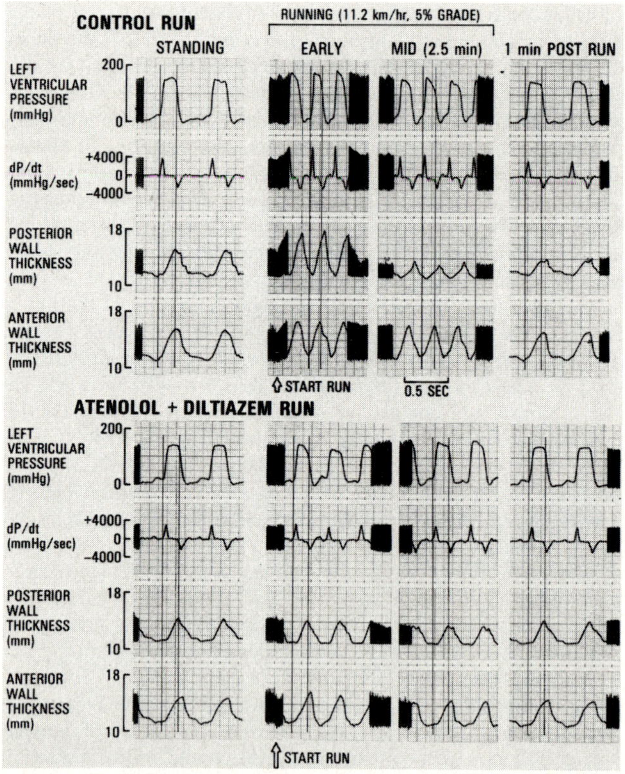

FIGURE 2. Tracings obtained during a control run *(top)* and during a run with atenolol and diltiazem *(bottom)* from one dog. Early into the run, heart rate, ventricular pressure, dP/dt, and wall thickening in both regions increased. Systolic wall thickening in the posterior wall soon decreased progressively to a steady-state level of severe dysfunction, at which time microspheres were injected (MID). During the run with atenolol and diltiazem, the initial increases in all parameters were absent and the deterioration of wall thickening in the posterior wall was less. Also, wall thickening in the ischemic zone returned to control after 1 min of recovery, whereas dysfunction persisted for a longer period after the control run.

TABLE 1
Regional myocardial blood flow during control exercise and exercise after atenolol and diltiazem (mean ± SD ml/min/g)

	Standing	Control exercise	A + D exercise
Ischemia area (n = 8)			
ENDO	0.96±0.16	0.31±0.14^{B}	0.61±0.30^{B,C}
MID	0.96±0.14	0.60±0.24^{B}	0.82±0.26
EPI	0.83±0.13	1.23±0.42^{A}	0.99±0.27
Mean	0.92±0.13	0.71±0.20	0.81±0.23
ENDO/EPI	1.17±0.15	0.27±0.13^{B}	0.62±0.29^{B,C}
Control area (n = 8)			
ENDO	0.99±0.15	2.28±0.35^{B}	1.23±0.36^{A,C}
MID	0.94±0.16	2.28±0.57^{B}	1.31±0.41^{B,C}
EPI	0.79±0.16	2.04±0.40^{B}	1.04±0.33^{C}
Mean	0.90±0.15	2.18±0.43^{B}	1.19±0.36^{A,C}
ENDO/EPI	1.26±0.20	1.13±0.17	1.20±0.13

ENDO = subendocardium; MID = midmyocardium; EPI = subepicardium.

$^{A}p < .05$, $^{B}p < .01$ compared with standing; $^{C}p < .01$ compared with control exercise.

and diltiazem, the subendocardial to subepicardial flow ratio in the ischemic area during exercise increased significantly from that during control exercise (0.27 to 0.62; table 1).

Normalized blood flow data in the ischemic area (expressing flow as a decimal fraction of blood flow in the control area) are graphically presented in figure 4. Normalized subendocardial, midmyocardial, epicardial, and mean transmural blood flows in the ischemic zone during exercise after drugs were greatly improved compared with those during control exercise (all p < .01) (figure 4). Subepicardial blood flow in the ischemic area during exercise with atenolol and diltiazem was not significantly different from that in the control area (figure 4). Normalized subendocardial flow during exercise after drug administration was reduced by less than 50% (control decrease 84%), and midmyocardial flow was 33% below the control area value (control decrease 70%).

Regional myocardial function. Dimension data during control exercise and exercise with atenolol and diltiazem are summarized in figure 5, and the recordings in figure 2 illustrate changes in these measurements during exercise without and with atenolol and diltiazem in a single dog.

Control wall. During control exercise, average end-diastolic wall thickness significantly increased by 4.2% over the control standing value. This was accompanied by significant augmentation of systolic wall thickening at steady state from 27.7 ± 5.6% to 32.9 ± 4.9% (figure 5).

After the administration of atenolol and diltiazem, resting sysolic wall thickening was somewhat reduced (24.1 ± 5.1%), but it was not significantly different from the standing value before control exercise. However, increases in systolic wall performance during exercise were abolished after atenolol and diltiazem (figure 5); there was no significant increase in percent change in wall thickness during exercise and it was significantly less than that during control exercise.

Ischemic wall. During control exercise, the ischemic wall exhibited severe dysfunction in all dogs (figures 2 and 5). End-diastolic wall thickness increased abruptly during the initial phase of exercise but was not different from the control standing value in later phases of exercise or recovery. Percent change in wall thickness decreased from 25.5% during standing rest to 2.7% at the time of microsphere injection, a 90% reduction (figure 5). Mean systolic wall thickening velocity was initially increased (16.6 ± 3.6 to 25.7 ± 8.1 mm/sec, p < .01), but then decreased by 1 min of exercise to 2.3 ± 1.9 mm/sec (p < .01). During control exercise, the values for percent change in wall thickness and mean systolic wall thickening velocity were not significantly different at 1 min, the midpoint, and late

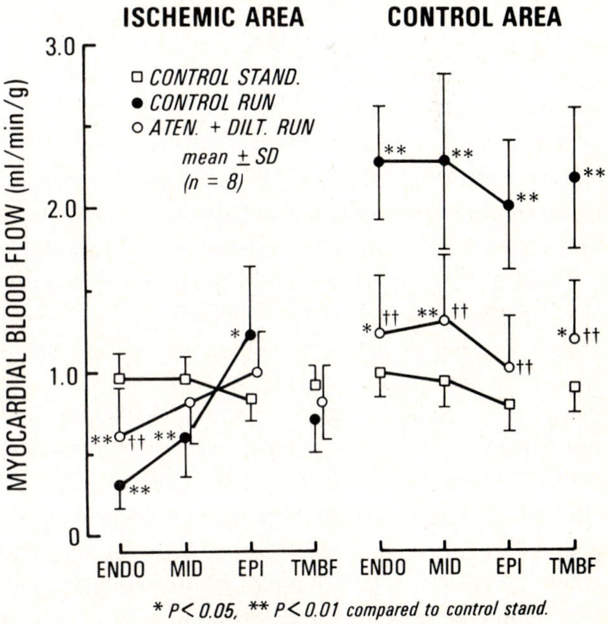

FIGURE 3. Transmural distribution of regional blood flow in the ischemic area *(left)* containing the ischemic wall thickness crystals and in the control area *(right)*. Blood flow was measured in subendocardium (ENDO), midmyocardium (MID), and subepicardium (EPI); average transmural blood flow (TMBF) is also presented. During control standing (open squares), myocardial blood flow distribution in the ischemic area was the same as that in the control area. Values during the control run (closed circles) and after atenolol and diltiazem (open circles), are also shown.

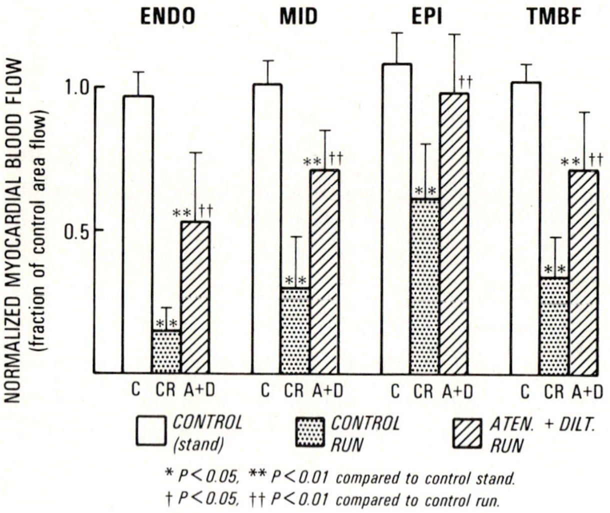

FIGURE 4. Distribution of blood flow in the ischemic zone expressed as a fraction of control area flow to emphasize the heterogeneity of blood flow during running. During control standing (C, open bars), there was homogeneous flow in the left ventricle; i.e., ischemic zone blood flow was similar to control zone flow across the wall. The control run (CR; stippled bars) was characterized by a large perfusion differential between the ischemic and control areas in each transmural layer. During the run with atenolol and diltiazem (A + D, striped bars), the heterogeneity was less with improved normalized blood flow in both the ventricular subendocardium (ENDO) and midwall (MID), and the subepicardium (EPI) showed no perfusion abnormality.

during exercise, indicating that a steady state of regional myocardial dysfunction had been achieved. Percent change in wall thickness during systole in the ischemic area remained depressed at 5 min after the end of control exercise ($p < .05$), but was not significantly different from the control standing value by 30 min (76% of control standing value, NS) (figure 5).

At rest after drug administration, the wall was slightly thinner at end-diastole, but the small decrease in percent systolic wall thickening was not significant (figure 5). During exercise after atenolol and diltiazem there was significant improvement in ischemic wall function (figures 2 and 5). End-diastolic wall thickness was less than that during control exercise, and remained unchanged during exercise. Percent systolic wall thickening decreased compared with the standing value (22.6% to 13.7%), but the systolic wall performance was significantly improved compared with that during control exercise, being reduced by 39% from the resting value (figure 5). Mean wall thickness velocity was improved at steady state from 2.3 ± 1.9 to 9.6 ± 4.3 mm/sec ($p < .002$).

After exercise with atenolol and diltiazem, recovery of systolic wall function from exercise-induced dysfunction was much faster than after control exercise. One minute after the end of exercise, percent change in wall thickness and mean systolic wall thickening velocity had recovered to 90% and 98%, respectively, of standing values before the second exercise bout (differences from control NS) and were significantly improved from those after control exercise (figure 5).

Comparison of combination of atenolol and diltiazem with either drug alone. The findings in the present study were compared with closely similar exercise runs previously reported in which either atenolol[27] or diltiazem[28] alone was used.

The hemodynamic conditions during control running were nearly identical, the heart rates at steady state exercise averaging 228 ± 30 and 227 ± 33 beats/min in the two previous studies and 227 ± 31 beats/min in the present study, and the peak left ventricular systolic pressures were not significantly different in the three control runs. After administration of atenolol alone, heart rate during running averaged 181 beats/min vs 204 beats/min after diltiazem alone ($p <$

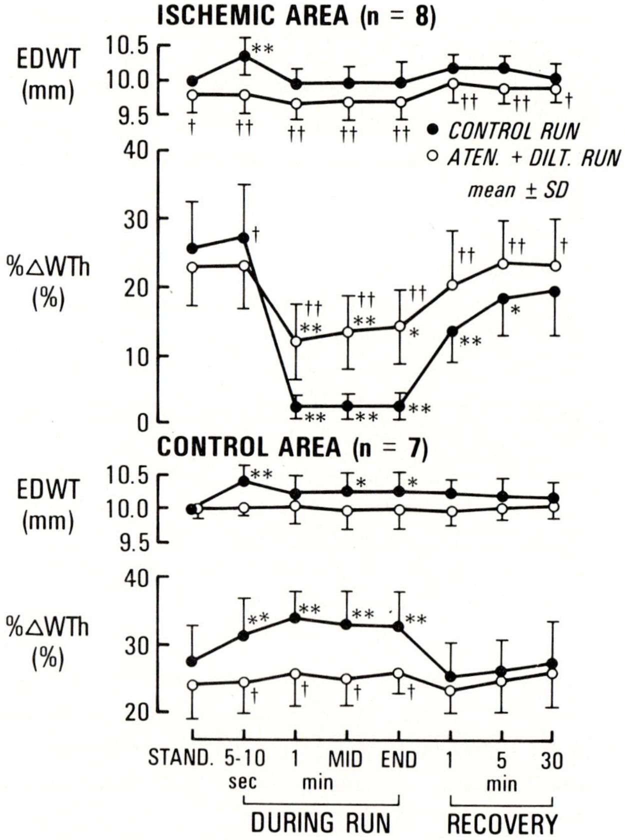

FIGURE 5. Changes in end-diastolic wall thickness (EDWT) and systolic wall thickening (%ΔWTh) in ischemic *(top)* and control *(bottom)* regions during exercise before and after administration of atenolol and diltiazem. During the run with atenolol and diltiazem, %ΔWTh was improved compared with that during control exercise and recovery of thickening from the exercise-induced dysfunction was faster. In the control area after atenolol and diltiazem %ΔWTh did not increase during the exercise.

.01), values significantly different from those obtained in the present combined drug experiment (155 beats/min) ($p < .01$). With diltiazem alone, peak systolic pressure was not different from that during control exercise, whereas with atenolol alone it was lower; the difference between exercise with atenolol alone (144 mm Hg) and atenolol plus diltiazem (139 mm Hg) was small but significant ($p < .01$). Peak (+) dP/dt with exercise after diltiazem alone was not different from that during the control run (5982 mm Hg/sec), but was higher than that after atenolol alone (3787 mm Hg/sec, $p < .01$); with running after atenolol plus diltiazem, peak (+) dP/dt was 3496 mm Hg/sec, which was not significantly different from that after atenolol alone.

The relationship between normalized regional systolic wall thickening (expressed as a percentage of the resting systolic wall thickening) and the normalized subendocardial blood flow (expressed as a percentage of the control area flow) for all three control runs, the runs with atenolol and diltiazem alone, and the combined atenolol and diltiazem study, are summarized in figure 6. The points in the three control runs are not significantly different. The flow-function points during running after atenolol or diltiazem alone were significantly different from those during control running, but not significantly different from each other ($p = .90$). Comparison of running after atenolol alone with running after atenolol plus diltiazem revealed a highly significant difference ($p < .02$). The difference between running with diltiazem alone and running after atenolol and diltiazem was also highly significant ($p = .025$). Therefore, the improvement of the flow-function relationship observed in the present study after administration of atenolol and diltiazem was significantly greater than with either drug alone.

Histologic examination. At autopsy, there was no gross ischemic damage between crystals. Microscopically, myocardial ischemic damage constituted 2.1 ± 2.9% (range 0 to 7.8%) of the inner one-third layer of the wall, and 1.7 ± 2.2% (0 to 5.8%) of the midmyocardium between the crystals in the ischemic wall. There was no ischemic damage in the outer third of the myocardium in the ischemic area. In the ischemic wall section, scar information around the subendocardial crystals was 7.6 ± 4.6% (range 2.3% to 15.1%) of the inner third of the myocardium.

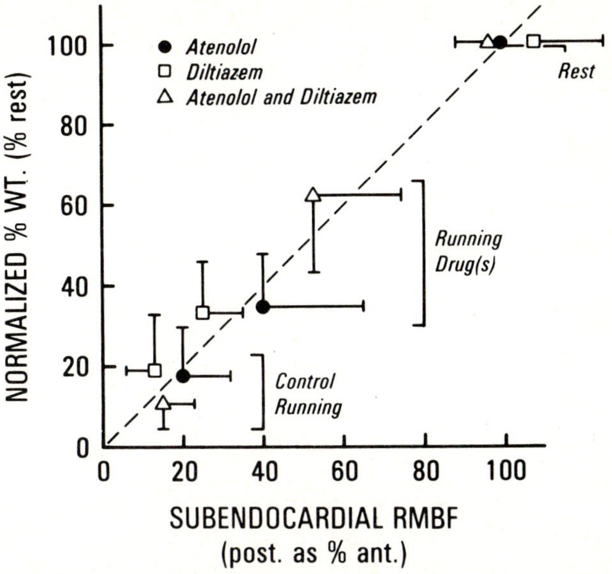

FIGURE 6. Regional myocardial blood flow-function relationship during exercise-induced regional ischemia in the present study (atenolol and diltiazem) compared with results of previous studies in which atenolol[27] or diltiazem alone was used.[28] Data from control runs are not different among groups, but results of drug studies show that combined therapy was more effective than either atenolol or diltiazem alone. The percent systolic wall thickening (%WT) during running is expressed as a fraction of the resting value before each run, and the subendocardial regional myocardial blood flow (RMBF) in the posterior (post.) ischemic zone is expressed as a percent of that in the normal anterior (ant.) wall. Dashed line = hypothetical linear reduction in subendocardial flow and wall thickening with progressive ischemia.

Discussion

In many patients, severe coronary artery stenosis is associated with normal ventricular function at rest, but exercise produces myocardial ischemia and regional myocardial dysfunction. The canine preparation used in the present study was developed previously by our laboratory to simulate the setting in patients with single-vessel coronary artery disease.[20, 27, 28] Exercise in these dogs induces regional myocardial dysfunction and allows measurements of regional myocardial blood flow with radiolabeled microspheres together with determinations of regional wall thickening dynamics. Additionally, in a prior study we demonstrated that regional blood flow and function during exercise-induced ischemia in this preparation are reproducible in runs performed 3 hr apart without interventions.[27] Thus, our preparation permits study of the effects of running before and after pharmacologic intervention. The combination of β-adrenergic blockade with calcium-channel blockade has been used successfully clinically, yet little was known about the interaction of these agents with respect to how they may affect the regional myocardial blood flow-function relationship during exercise.

In four of the eight dogs used in this study, the circumflex coronary artery was open on the day of the study but exhibited decreased blood flow velocity compared with that measured 1 week after surgery. The other four dogs had no antegrade flow on the study day. However, no regional myocardial ischemia at rest was detected either by microspheres or by regional myocardial dysfunction in the eight dogs. Therefore, at rest all animals had adequate myocardial perfusion either through a combination of limited antegrade flow with some collateral flow or solely through collateral channels. The induction of collateral development in this preparation is readily detected with use of serial, transient occlusions of the coronary artery after operation by demonstrating progressively less regional myocardial dysfunction and reduced reactive hyperemia after release of the occluder. These observations are similar to those reported previously from this laboratory and others.[20, 21, 28, 31, 32]

In this preparation, the control exercise period produced profound dysfunction in the posterior left ventricular wall perfused by the circumflex artery. This hypokinesia, found during steady-state exercise, was preceded by a transient phase of increasing and then decreasing regional function in the collateral-dependent zone over the first minute of exercise. The onset of exercise was associated with an abrupt increase in heart rate, left ventricular peak systolic pressure, and left ventricular (+)dP/dt in the initial 5 to 10 sec. Likewise, mean systolic wall thickening velocity in the ischemic zone initially increased and percent change in wall thickness was not reduced. Soon, however, regional wall performance declined in the ischemic zone such that by 1 min into the exercise bout, wall thickening in the posterior wall was reduced and steady at 2.5% (from a resting value of 25.5%). Mean coronary blood flow velocity in the circumflex coronary artery did not increase in the four dogs with a patent vessel, confirming the existence of critical stenosis.

During this control exercise bout, regional myocardial blood flow to the ischemic zone exhibited a marked perfusion abnormality, with an absolute reduction in regional myocardial perfusion to the subendocardium and midwall, and a mild increase in subepicardial flow. The importance of subendocardial perfusion to maintenance of systolic wall thickening has been reported by Gallagher et al.[33] and Roan et al.[34] in preparations of acute myocardial ischemia. Roan et al., using conscious dogs, showed a relationship between subendocardial blood flow and systolic wall thickening in zones in and around a region supplied by an occluded vessel.[34] Vatner[35] has described an exponential relationship between regional subendocardial flow and regional segmental function in conscious dogs with various degrees of ischemia. Gallagher et al.[33] found the correlation between subendocardial flow and systolic wall thickening to be high and nearly linear in anesthetized and conscious dogs[36] during graded coronary stenosis, and this correlation was also shown during exercise.[37, 38] Redistribution of flow away from the subendocardium to the subepicardium (transmural "steal") has been produced previously in exercising dogs with acute partial coronary stenosis[35, 39] and it was theorized that this phenomenon relates to the limitation of diastolic perfusion time in the subendocardium with metabolic vasodilation in the subepicardium during exercise.[39] Responses during the control run in the present experiments in the presence of chronic coronary stenosis were similar.

After the administration of atenolol and diltiazem, the effect of exercise on regional myocardial blood flow in the ischemic zone was substantially altered, with improvement of the distribution of flow across the ventricular wall. This improvement in ischemic zone blood flow was characterized by an increase in the absolute subendocardial blood flow (compared with control exercise), failure of the subepicardial flow to rise significantly, and a large increase in the endocardial/epicardial ratio. This enhancement of ischemic zone perfusion was associated with significant increases in ischemic zone wall thickening and thickening velocity during exercise after administration of atenolol and diltiazem. Although a regional wall thickening abnormality still occurred during this exercise bout, it should be recognized that resting function in the ischemic zone was somewhat reduced after the drugs and that exercise function in the normal zone was also attenuated. Thus, regional wall function during exercise after drugs decreased by only 39% of the resting value (compared with 90% during the control run) and function in the ischemic zone during exercise after drugs was 55% of that in the normal area, whereas it was only 8% of normal function during control exercise.

Figure 6 illustrates the magnitude of the improvement observed with combined therapy compared with that observed previously when diltiazem and atenolol were used separately. In all three studies, the amount of exercise-induced dysfunction that occurred during control exercise as well as the perfusion to the subendocardium of the ischemic zone were closely similar (ischemia during the control run for the combined study being slightly more severe). Since results of repeat runs 3 hr apart in the same dog without drug intervention are highly reproducible,[27] this finding supports the validity of comparing the effects of the combined study with those of the two previous experiments. The magnitude of the effects on the normalized subendocardial flow-function points during running with atenolol or diltiazem alone were similar (figure 6), although the hemodynamic actions of the two drugs during exercise differed markedly. Thus, exercise after diltiazem alone mildly lowered the heart rate and did not affect peak left ventricular pressure, peak left ventricular dP/dt, or percent change in wall thickness in the normal zone,[28] whereas atenolol further lowered exercise heart rate, markedly reduced peak left ventricular pressure and dP/dt, and diminished percent change in wall thickness in the normal zone during exercise.[27] The hemodynamic responses after the combination of the two drugs resembled those after atenolol alone, although the heart rate was lowered significantly further (155 beats/min), suggesting that the heart rate effect of combined therapy may be the main factor causing the enhanced improvement, although the peak left ventricular pressure was 5 mm Hg lower as well. The combination of these two drugs appears approximately additive (figure 6), and it is interesting to note that the data from all three studies appear to fall close to a linear relationship between subendocardial perfusion and transmural wall thickening. This suggests the existence of a close relationship between subendocardial blood flow and wall thickening during exercise-induced ischemia,[38] as has been found with acute coronary stenosis,[36] even when points on the relationship are modified by different pharmacologic interventions.

Numerous mechanisms may be involved in the beneficial effect of atenolol and diliazem on the regional blood flow-function relationship during exercise-induced regional myocardial ischemia. Atenolol can be presumed to substantially reduce the myocardial oxygen consumption of the left ventricle, thereby reducing an imbalance between regional oxygen supply and demand. The reduction of myocardial oxygen requirements at steady state by atenolol can be predicted from the substantial decreases in exercise heart rate, left ventricular systolic pressure, and contractility (dP/dt); this lowering of oxygen consumption is reflected in the significant reduction in blood flow in the nonischemic zone during exercise after administration of atenolol and diltiazem (figure 3).

We have hypothesized that "relative ischemia" does not exist in the steady-state condition and that regional function will closely follow the amount of absolute ischemia in the subendocardium.[38] Thus, the concept of "relative ischemia" may be applicable only during the initial transient phase of exercise, when regional function exceeds that predicted on the basis of regional perfusion. Consequently, this is necessarily a transient phase until regional function can stabilize at a lower steady-state level, which can be supported by the available regional subendocardial blood flow.

The decrease in heart rate after atenolol and diltiazem caused improved blood flow per beat because of the increase in diastolic perfusion time.[27] Therefore, while mean transmural blood flow was not affected by atenolol and diltiazem, more flow was available per minute and per beat to the subendocardium to support improved contraction, and the transmural flow distribution was improved with an increase in endocardial/epicardial ratio. This was related not only to increased subendocardial blood flow, but also to reduced subepicardial flow because of the decreased myocardial oxygen requirements after the drugs were given. Thus, transmural steal may have been reduced, further supporting enhanced regional performance. This sequence places emphasis on reduced heart rate in explaining the beneficial effect of atenolol on regional perfusion and, consequently, regional function. However, Tomoike et al.,[40] studying the effect of propranolol during acute coronary arterial stenosis, found improved ischemic zone shortening and an improved coronary blood flow pattern that was only partially lost by cardiac pacing at the same rate observed before propranolol. Whether or not such an effect might exist during exercise will require further study.

Of the commonly used calcium antagonists, diltiazem has a relatively minimal negative inotropic effect.[15, 16] When studied alone in a preparation identical to the one used in this study, the reduction in heart rate was smaller than that reported for atenolol, and no negative inotropic effect on the normal region was evident.[28] While the contribution of diltiazem to improved regional perfusion of the ischemic zone may include its modest negative chronotropic effects, other mechanisms may be more important. Specifically, the vasodilative action of diltiazem could have increased perfusion to the ischemic zone, either directly or through an increase in blood flow in the coronary collateral vessels supplying that zone.[28] Diltiazem alone also results in a lower left ventricular end-diastolic pressure during exercise-induced ischemia, which could enhance subendocardial perfusion.[28] In addition, the transmural maldistribution of blood flow could have been reduced by diltiazem. Bache and Tockman[41] have reported that nifedipine limits reactive hyperemia after coronary occlusion and inhibits the redistribution of blood flow away from the subendocardium during coronary arterial stenosis. Therefore, diltiazem could act primarily to augment absolute blood flow to the ischemic zone and improve its distribution within that region.

The possibility exists that, in addition to increased perfusion, reduced afterload during exercise also could have contributed to improved wall motion in the ischemic zone, since left ventricular peak systolic pressure was 22 mm Hg lower during exercise after drug administration than during control exercise. However, regional function in the normal zone was substantially reduced during running after the drugs compared with during the control run, suggesting lack of a major role of reduced afterload per se in the increase in wall motion.

In conclusion, we have demonstrated a substantial improvement in the regional myocardial blood flow-function relationship during exercise-induced ischemia by combined use of a β-blocker and a calcium channel–blocking drug. The improved regional myocardial performance observed in the ischemic zone appears to relate to a more favorable blood flow distribution within the ischemic zone, with an increase in absolute and relative subendocardial blood flow, and a reduction in subepicardial flow. The additive effect of atenolol and diltiazem, compared with that of either drug alone, probably relates to differing mechanisms for augmenting flow to the ischemic zone. Our finding of significant improvements in both perfusion and performance in zones subject to ischemia during exercise stress in a conscious canine preparation may provide an objective basis for the use of these agents in combination clinically for the treatment of patients with exercise-induced angina pectoris.

References

1. Harrison DC: Circulatory effects and clinical uses of beta-adrenergic–blocking drugs. Amsterdam, 1972, Excerpta Medica
2. Alderman EL, Davies RO, Crowley JJ, Lopes MG, Brooker JZ, Friedman JP, Graham AC, Matlof HM, Harrison DC: Dose response effectiveness of propranolol for the treatment of angina pectoris. Circulation **51:** 964, 1975
3. Thadani U, Parker JO: Propranolol in the treatment of angina pectoris. Comparison of duration of action in acute and sustained oral therapy. Circulation **59:** 571, 1979
4. Danahy DT, Burwell DT, Aronow WS, Prakash R: Sustained hemodynamic and antianginal effect of high dose oral isosorbide dinitrates. Circulation **55:** 381, 1977
5. Packer M, Meller J, Medina N, Yushak M, Smith H, Holt J, Guererro J, Tood GD, McAlister RG, Gorlin R: Hemodynamic consequences of combined beta-adrenergic and slow calcium channel blockade in man. Circulation **65:** 660, 1982
6. Bassan M, Weiler-Ravell D, Shalev O: The additive antiangina action of oral nifedipine in patients receiving propranolol. Magnitude and duration of effect. Circulation **66:** 710, 1982
7. Kieval J, Kirseten EB, Kessler KM, Mallon SM, Myerburg RJ: The effects of intravenous verapamil on hemodynamic status of patients with coronary artery disease receiving propranolol. Circulation **65:** 653, 1982
8. Crawford MH, LeWinter MM, O'Rourke RA, Karliner JS, Ross J Jr: Combined propranolol and digoxin therapy in angina pectoris. Ann Intern Med **83:** 449, 1975
9. Nakarmua M, Koiways Y: Beneficial effect of diltiazem, a new antianginal drug, on angina pectoris at rest. Jpn Heart J **20:** 613, 1979
10. Yasue H, Omote S, Takizawa A, Nagao M, Miwa K, Tanaka S: Exertional angina pectoris caused by coronary artery spasm: effects of various drugs. Am J Cardiol **43:** 647, 1979
11. Waters DD, Szlachcic J, Theroux P, Dauwe F, Mizgala HF: Ergonovine testing to detect spontaneous remissions of variant angina drug longterm treatment with calcium antagonist drugs. Am J Cardiol **47:** 179, 1981
12. Sandler G, Clayton GA, Thornicroft SG: Clinical evaluation of verapamil in angina pectoris. Br Med J **3:** 224, 1968
13. Moskowitz RM, Piccini PA, Nacarelli GW, Zelis R: Nifedipine therapy for stable angina pectoris: preliminary results of effects on angina frequency and treadmill exercise response. Am J Cardiol **44:** 811, 1979
14. Hossack KF, Bruce RA: Improved exercise performance in persons with stable angina pectoris receiving diltiazem. Am J Cardiol **47:** 95, 1981
15. Strauss WE, McIntyre KM, Parisi AF, Sharpiro W: Safety and efficacy of diltiazem hydrochloride for the treatment of stable angina pectoris: report of a cooperative clinical trial. Am J Cardiol **49:** 560, 1982
16. Henry PD: Comparative pharmacology of calcium antagonists: nifedipine, verapamil and diltiazem. Am J Cardiol **46:** 1047, 1980
17. Nakaya H, Schwartz A, Millard RW: Reflex chronotropic and inotropic effects of calcium channel-blocking agents in conscious dogs. Diltiazem, verapamil, and nifedipine compared. Circ Res **52:** 302, 1983
18. Vineburg A, Mahanti B, Litvak J: Experimental gradual coronary artery constriction by ameroid constrictor. Surgery **47:** 765, 1960
19. Elliott EC, Jones EL, Bloor CM, Leon AS, Gregg DE: Day to day changes in coronary hemodynamics secondary to constriction of circumflex branch of left coronary artery in conscious dogs. Circ Res **22:** 237, 1968
20. Kumada T, Gallagher KP, Shirato K, McKown D, Miller M, Kemper WS, White F, Ross J Jr: Reduction of exercise-induced regional myocardial dysfunction by propranolol. Studies in a canine model of chronic coronary artery stenosis. Circ Res **46:** 190, 1980
21. Tomoike H, Inoh T, Watanabe K, Mizukami M, Kikuchi Y, Nakamura M: Functional significance of collaterals during ameroid-induced coronary stenosis in conscious dogs. Interrelationships among regional shortening, regional flow and grade of coronary stenosis. Circulation **67:** 1001, 1983
22. Sasayama S, Franklin D, Ross J Jr, Kemper WS, McKown D: Dynamic changes in left ventricular wall thickness and their use in analyzing cardiac function in the conscious dog. Am J Cardiol **38:** 870, 1976
23. Matsuzaki M, Gallagher KP, Kemper WS, White F, Ross J Jr: Sustained regional dysfunction produced by prolonged coronary stenosis: gradual recovery after reperfusion. Circulation **68:** 170, 1983
24. White FC, Sanders M, Peterson T, Bloor CM: Ischemic myocardial injury after exercise stress in the pressure overloaded heart. Am J Pathol **97:** 473, 1979
25. Schosser R, Argos KE, Messmer K: Mic-II — a program for the determination of cardiac output, arteriovenous shunt, and regional blood flow using the radio microsphere method. Comput Program Biomed **9:** 19, 1979
26. Heyman MA, Payne BD, Hoffman KIE, Rodolph AM: Blood flow measurements with radionuclide labelled particles. Prog Cardiovasc Dis **20:** 55, 1977
27. Matsuzaki M, Patritti J, Tajimi T, Miller M, Kemper WS, Ross J Jr: Effects of beta blockade on regional myocardial flow and function during exercise. Am J Physiol **16:** H52, 1984
28. Matsuzaki M, Gallagher KP, Patritti J, Tajimi T, Kemper WS, White FC, Ross J Jr: Effects of a calcium-entry blocker (diltiazem) on regional myocardial fow and function during exercise in conscious dogs. Circulation **69:** 801, 1984
29. Theroux P, Franklin D, Ross J Jr, Kemper WS: Regional myocardial function during acute coronary occlusion and its modification by pharmacologic agents in the dog. Circ Res **35:** 896, 1974
30. Winer BJ: Statistical principles in experimental design. New York, 1962, McGraw-Hill, pp 185–196; 514–603
31. Scheel KW, Rodriguez RJ, Ingram LA: Directional coronary growth with chronic circumflex occlusion in the dog. Circ Res **40:** 384, 1977

32. Lambert PR, Hess DS, Bache RJ: Effect of exercise on perfusion of collateral-dependent myocardium in dogs with chronic coronary artery occlusion. J Clin Invest **59:** 1, 1977
33. Gallagher KP, Kumada T, Koziol JA, McKown MD, Kemper WS, Ross J Jr: Significance of regional wall thickening abnormalities relative to transmural myocardial perfusion in anesthetized dogs. Circulation **62:** 1266, 1980
34. Roan PG, Buja LM, Izquierdo C, Hashimi H, Saffer S, Willerson JT: Interrelationships between regional left ventricular function, coronary blood flow, and myocellular necrosis during the initial 24 hours and 1 week after experimental coronary occlusion in awake, unsedated dogs. Circ Res **49:** 31, 1981
35. Vatner SF: Correlation between acute reductions in myocardial blood flow and function in conscious dogs. Circ Res **47:** 201, 1980
36. Gallagher KP, Matsuzaki M, Koziol JA, Kemper WS, Ross J Jr: Regional myocardial perfusion and wall thickening during ischemia in conscious dogs. Am J Physiol **16:** H727, 1984
37. Gallagher KP, Osakada G, Matsuzaki M, Kemper WAS, Ross J Jr: Myocardial blood flow and function with critical coronary stenosis in exercising dogs. Am J Physiol **243:** H698, 1982
38. Gallaher KP, Matsuzaki M, Osakada G, Kemper WS, Ross J Jr: Effect of exercise on the relationship between myocardial blood flow and systolic wall thickening in dogs with acute coronary stenosis. Circ Res **52:** 716, 1983
39. Ball RM, Bache RJ: Distribution of myocardial blood flow in the exercising dog with restricted coronary artery flow. Circ Res **38:** 60, 1976
40. Tomoike H, Ross J Jr, Franklin D, Crozatier B, McKown D, Kemper WS: Improvement by propranolol of regional myocardial dysfunction and abnormal coronary flow pattern in conscious dogs with coronary narrowing. Am J Cardiol **41:** 689, 1978
41. Bache RJ, Tockman BA: Effect of nitroglycerin and nifedipine on subendocardial perfusion in the presence of a flow limiting coronary stenosis in the awake dog. Circ Res **50:** 678, 1982

For many patients

POST-MI PROTECTION

Regardless of:

Heart size[1]

Infarction site[1]

Transmural or nontransmural MI[1]

Risk group[1]

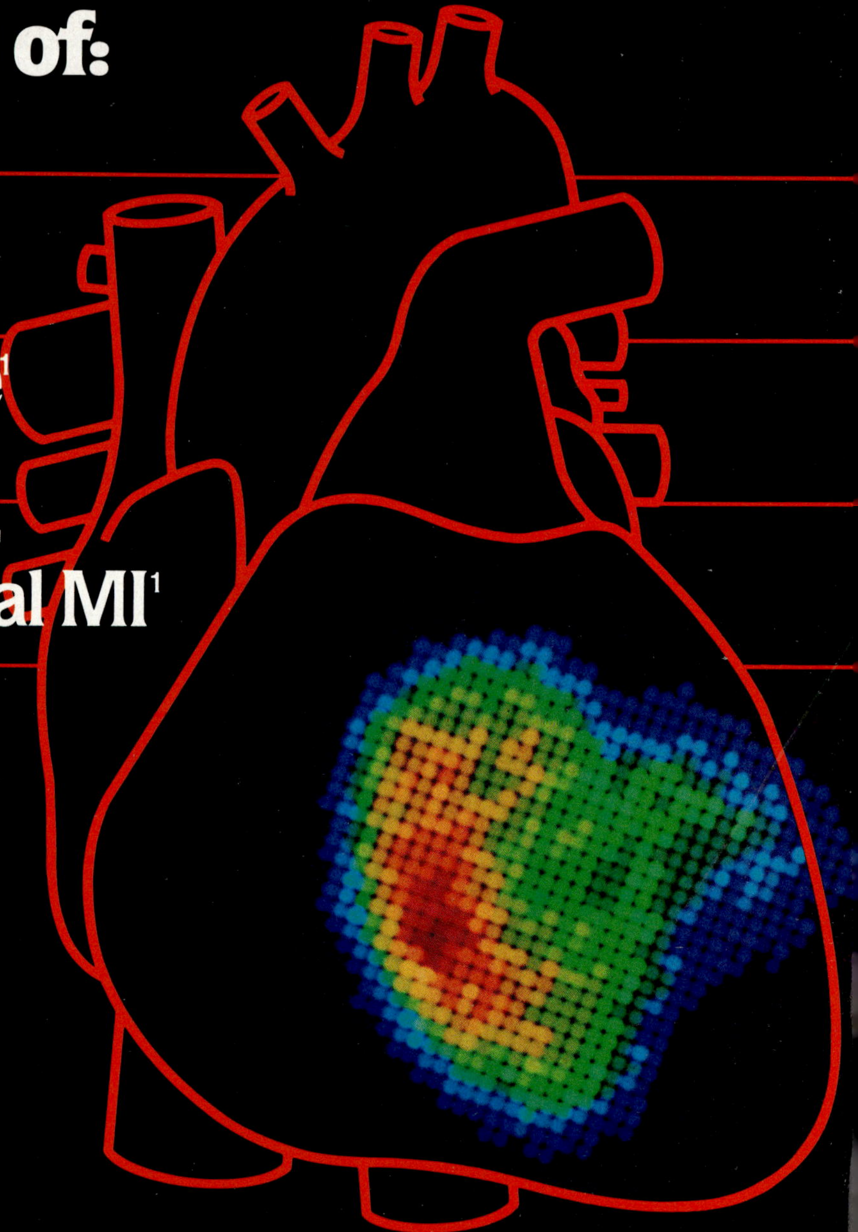

Radionuclide scan of an infarcted heart.

BLOCADREN® (Timolol Maleate, MSD) is contraindicated in patients with bronchial asthma, a history of bronchial asthma, or severe chronic obstructive pulmonary disease (see below); sinus bradycardia; second- and third-degree atrioventricular block; overt cardiac failure (see below); cardiogenic shock; and hypersensitivity to this product. Although beta blockers should be avoided in overt congestive heart failure, they can be used, if necessary, with caution in patients with a history of failure who are well compensated. In patients without a history of cardiac failure, continued depression of the myocardium with beta-blocking agents over a period of time can, in some cases, lead to cardiac failure.

Exacerbation of Ischemic Heart Disease following Abrupt Withdrawal—Hypersensitivity to catecholamines has been observed in patients withdrawn from beta-blocker therapy; exacerbation of angina and, in some cases, myocardial infarction have occurred after *abrupt* discontinuation of such therapy. When discontinuing chronically administered timolol maleate, particularly in patients with ischemic heart disease, the dosage should be gradually reduced over a period of one to two weeks, and the patient should be carefully monitored. If angina markedly worsens or acute coronary insufficiency develops, timolol maleate administration should be reinstituted promptly, at least temporarily, and other measures appropriate for the management of unstable angina should be taken. Patients should be warned against interruption or discontinuation of therapy without the physician's advice. Because coronary artery disease is common and may be unrecognized, it may be prudent not to discontinue timolol maleate therapy abruptly even in patients treated only for hypertension.

In patients with nonallergic bronchospasm or with a history of nonallergic bronchospasm (e.g., chronic bronchitis, emphysema), BLOCADREN should be administered with caution.

For a Brief Summary of Prescribing Information, please see last page of this advertisement.

Circulation

VOL 72 AUGUST NO 2 1985

An Official Journal of the American Heart Association, Inc.®

FEATURES

Dopamine receptors: applications in clinical cardiology

LEON I. GOLDBERG, M.D., PH.D., AND SOL I. RAJFER, M.D.

THE DISCOVERY of the renal vasodilating action of dopamine more than 20 years ago led to extensive research that demonstrated other unusual actions of this endogenous catecholamine.[1-3] Investigators using traditional pharmacologic models and modern biochemical techniques have documented the existence of distinct dopamine receptor subtypes that mediate these responses. Appreciation of the structure-activity requirements of these receptors has led to the synthesis of drugs that may have a profound influence on the management of the patient with heart disease.

Taxonomy of dopamine receptors. Rigid criteria must be met to prove the existence of a new receptor by classical pharmacologic methods, including construction of a unique potency series of agonists and demonstration of specific antagonism.[4, 5] In contrast, biochemical techniques are applied to tissue homogenates, and different standards are frequently used to classify receptors.[6, 7]

After many years of research, two distinct dopamine receptor subtypes, DA_1 and DA_2, were identified conclusively by classical criteria in physiologic preparations.[5] DA_1 receptors are located postsynaptically and subserve vasodilation in renal, mesenteric, coronary, and cerebral blood vessels (figure 1). DA_1-induced vasodilation can be observed in other vascular beds, but the response is less prominent, probably because of the lower density of dopamine receptors. The molecular structure required for activation of DA_1 receptors is very strict.[4] Currently, all active compounds have two hydroxyl groups in positions analogous to the 3- and 4-positions on the benzene ring of the dopamine molecule, and a limited distance exists between the hydroxyl groups and the amino group.

From the Committee on Clinical Pharmacology, Departments of Pharmacological and Physiological Sciences and Medicine, Section of Cardiology, The University of Chicago.

Address for correspondence: Leon I. Goldberg, M.D., Ph.D., Committee on Clinical Pharmacology, The University of Chicago, 947 E. 58th St., Chicago, IL 60637.

Supported in part by National Institutes of Health grant GM-22220 and HL-00872. Dr. Rajfer is the recipient of a National Institutes of Health Clinical Investigator award HL-00872.

DA_2 receptors are located on postganglionic sympathetic nerves and autonomic ganglia, and when these receptors are activated, norepinephrine release from sympathetic nerve endings is inhibited (figure 1). DA_2 receptors are also located in the emetic center of the area postrema and in the anterior lobe of the pituitary gland. Activation of these receptors results in emesis and inhibition of prolactin release, respectively. The structural requirements for DA_2 agonists are much less restrictive than those for DA_1 agonists. Indeed, the structures of DA_2 agonists are so diverse that it is difficult to determine molecular requirements for activity.[4]

Major advances have been made in the synthesis of new dopamine agonists, and compounds are now available with spectra of receptor activity different from that of dopamine. Of significance, the benzazepine derivative, fenoldopam, proved to be a selective DA_1 agonist.[8] Selective DA_2 agonists have been available for several years. Examples include piribedil and ergot derivatives, which are used for the treatment of Parkinson's disease, and LY 17155, an ergoline derivative.[4]

The first dopamine antagonists used to classify dopamine receptors were the neuroleptics, haloperidol and chlorpromazine.[2] Although these agents made it possible to distinguish dopamine receptors from other receptors, the dose range in which they are specific antagonists for dopamine receptors is very narrow. Furthermore, these antagonists cannot be used to differentiate dopamine receptor subtypes. Recently, selective antagonists that discriminate between DA_1 and DA_2 receptors have been synthesized. An example of a selective DA_1 antagonist is the benzazepine, SCH 23390, which is chemically related to fenoldopam.[9] Domperidone, a butyrophenone derivative related to haloperidol, is an example of a selective DA_2 antagonist.[10]

Availability of selective dopamine agonists and antagonists has aided in the determination of whether dopamine subtypes classified on the basis of cardio-

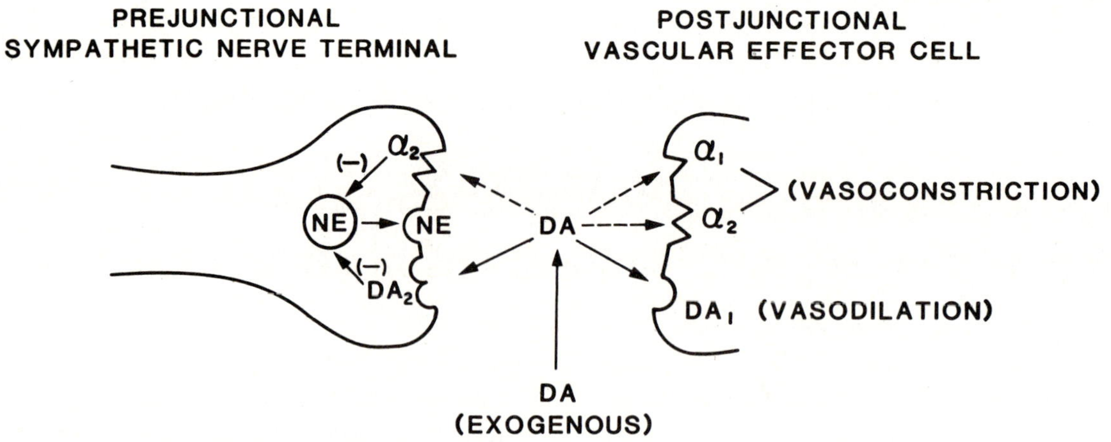

FIGURE 1. Location of DA_1 receptors, α_1- and α_2-adrenoceptors on postganglionic vascular effector cells, and DA_2 receptors and α_2-adrenoceptors on the prejunctional sympathetic nerve terminal. When dopamine is administered, activation of DA_1 receptors causes vasodilation and activation of DA_2 receptors causes inhibition (−) of norepinephrine (NE) release from storage granules. A larger dose of dopamine activates α_1- and α_2-adrenoceptors on the postjunctional effector cells to cause vasoconstriction and on α_2-adrenoceptors on the prejunctional sympathetic terminal to inhibit release of norepinephrine. Norepinephrine released from the prejunctional sympathetic terminal also acts on α_1- and α_2-adrenoceptors.

vascular responses are similar to those receptors identified in brain and endocrine tissues by biochemical techniques. In one biochemical method, dopamine receptors are subdivided according to the effects of agonists on the enzyme, adenylate cyclase. Activation of D_1 receptors results in stimulation of adenylate cyclase; activation of D_2 receptors either results in inhibition of adenylate cyclase or has no effect on that enzyme.[6] In a second biochemical method, dopamine receptors are subdivided according to the pattern of displacement of radioactive ligands by dopamine agonists or antagonists.[7] The radioligand binding assays have been extremely controversial because of the many inconsistencies in the dopamine receptor subtypes "identified" by these assays.[6, 7] It appears that many of the early ligand-binding investigations yielded increased numbers of receptor subtypes because the ligands used were not selective or because strict criteria required to characterize receptors were not fulfilled.[4, 6] Recent studies conducted with more selective ligands have identified only two dopamine subtypes similar to D_1 and D_2.[6] Comparison of the DA_1 and DA_2 classification with the revised D_1 and D_2 classification suggests that the same receptors are identified by the two methods. However, a few significant discrepancies in the potency series of agonists and antagonists remain, and further studies are needed to determine the reasons for these differences.[4]

Pharmacologic actions of dopamine. The activation of adrenoceptors and dopamine receptors by dopamine is the basis for its diverse clinical applications.[2, 3] Because of extreme individual variations in the infusion rates of dopamine required to activate the different receptors, patients must be monitored carefully to achieve the desired hemodynamic profile. DA_1 and DA_2 receptors are activated at the lowest infusion rates, resulting in a decline in peripheral vascular resistance and modest increments in renal blood flow, urine volume, and sodium excretion. At these low rates of infusion (usually 0.5 to 2 μg/kg/min) dopamine may initiate a diuresis in patients refractory to furosemide.[11] As the infusion rate is increased (usually above 2 μg/kg/min), β_1-adrenoceptors are activated and cardiac output begins to increase, typically with little change in heart rate. This is the hemodynamic response sought in the treatment of heart failure. The infusion rate may then be gradually increased until recruitment of α_1- and α_2-adrenoceptors occurs as manifested by an increase in vascular resistance or until excessive β_1-adrenoceptor activity leads to tachycardia or ventricular arrhythmias. Higher infusion rates can be used if the undesirable vasoconstriction is eliminated by simultaneous administration of a vasodilating agent.[3] With such concurrent administration, caution must be exercised to avoid excessive reduction in arterial pressure. Indeed, unmasking of the vasodilating effects of dopamine in the presence of phenoxybenzamine was the first demonstration of its potential use in the treatment of hypertension.[12] A different hemodynamic pattern may be achieved by conjoint administration of dopamine and dobutamine. This combination provides greater β_1-adrenoceptor activity, maintenance of the beneficial renal effects of dopamine, and avoidance of α-adrenoceptor–mediated vasoconstriction seen with high doses of dopamine.[3]

Orally active pro-drugs. Poor oral bioavailability of

dopamine stimulated the development and investigation of orally active pro-drugs with dopamine activity. Two oral pro-drugs, levodopa and ibopamine, have been studied in the treatment of congestive heart failure.

After oral administration of the biochemical precursor of dopamine, levodopa, dopamine is generated by the action of aromatic amino acid decarboxylase in the liver and other tissues. Investigations in patients with Parkinson's disease demonstrated that oral administration of levodopa in doses of 1 to 1.5 g produces cardiac and natriuretic effects approximating the responses observed with intravenous infusions of dopamine at rates of 2 to 4 μg/kg/min.[2] On this basis, levodopa was studied recently in patients with severe congestive heart failure. After ingestion of levodopa (1.5 to 2.0 g), significant improvement in cardiac performance was observed. Furthermore, the beneficial hemodynamic effects were sustained during long-term therapy for 3 or more months. The lack of tolerance to levodopa is in sharp contrast to the findings of previous studies conducted with pirbuterol, which was ineffective after sustained therapy.[13] This difference could be explained by the partial agonist activity of pirbuterol and the full agonist activity of dopamine. Down-regulation of β_1-adrenoceptors with continuous therapy should decrease activity of partial agonists to a much greater extent than that of full agonists.[14]

No serious adverse effects were observed in this initial study with levodopa. However, levodopa can produce nausea and vomiting unless the dose is gradually increased. Accordingly, the dose was increased from 250 mg qid to 1.5 to 2.0 g qid over a 5 to 7 day period. In addition 50 mg of pyridoxine was administered daily, since previous studies have shown that this vitamin is required for the decarboxylation of levodopa.

In addition to the trial of levodopa in congestive heart failure, the pro-drug has also been used to help wean patients from long-term intravenous infusion of dopamine.[3]

Ibopamine is the diisobutyric ester of *N*-methyl dopamine (epinine). When ibopamine is absorbed, it is acted upon by esterases in the plasma to release *N*-methyl dopamine (epinine). Epinine resembles dopamine pharmacologically. Several studies in Europe and the United States have shown that oral ingestion of 100 to 300 mg of ibopamine produces beneficial hemodynamic effects in patients with congestive heart failure.[15, 16] Ibopamine has recently been approved for clinical use in Italy.

New dopamine agonists. The possibility that several receptors may be responsible for the beneficial hemodynamic effects of dopamine, levodopa, and ibopamine is supported by the results of studies which demonstrate that dopamine agonists lacking β_1-adrenergic activity elicit beneficial responses in patients with severe congestive heart failure. Propylbutyl dopamine (an agonist of DA_1 and DA_2 receptors) was administered intravenously to patients with severe congestive heart failure.[17] Cardiac index increased while pulmonary capillary wedge pressure and systemic vascular resistance were significantly reduced. No change in heart rate was observed. Mean arterial pressure decreased in a dose-related manner, declining 20 mm Hg when infused at a rate of 20 μg/kg/min. Vasodilation caused by activation of DA_1 and DA_2 receptors by propylbutyl dopamine appeared to be responsible for the hemodynamic responses observed. Renal hemodynamics were not measured in these patients, but studies in normal subjects and hypertensive patients demonstrated that propylbutyl dopamine produces pronounced increments in renal blood flow.[12]

Hemodynamic improvement was also observed in patients with severe congestive heart failure when the ergot derivative, bromocriptine, was administered orally in a dose of 2.5 mg.[18] Bromocriptine has been shown to act as a DA_2 agonist in peripheral nerves but also may decrease sympathetic activity via a central nervous system mechanism. Heart rate, mean arterial pressure, left ventricular end-diastolic pressure, and mean right atrial pressure decreased while stroke volume increased. Cardiac index did not increase, possibly because of the decrease in heart rate. A decline in plasma norepinephrine concentrations accompanied these hemodynamic changes.

Hemodynamic actions of the selective DA_1 agonist, fenoldopam, were evaluated in a pilot study in patients with congestive heart failure.[19] Oral administration of fenoldopam (200 mg) resulted in a decline in pulmonary capillary wedge pressure and systemic vascular resistance and an increase in cardiac index. Heart rate did not change. The renal effects of fenoldopam were not studied in these patients, but increments in renal blood flow and sodium excretion were observed when the drug was administered to normal subjects and hypertensive patients.[12] The natriuresis induced by DA_1 agonists is unusual for vasodilating agents.

The availability of orally effective dopamine congeners has greatly expanded the potential clinical indications for these agonists. Of particular significance, fenoldopam, propylbutyl dopamine, and bromocriptine have been found to be effective in lowering blood pressure in hypertensive patients.[12] Another possible new use for dopamine agonists is in the treatment of arrhythmias. A study in the anesthetized dog has shown that bromocriptine is effective in the prevention of digitalis-induced arrhythmias.[20] The mechanism responsible for this antiarrhythmic effect appears to be decreased sympathetic activity.

In summary, the results of studies with orally effective dopamine agonists have suggested new approaches to the management of patients with cardiovascular disease. The safety and efficacy of these agents during long-term therapy remains to be established. Athough the results of preliminary investigations are encouraging, only a limited number of patients have been observed for prolonged periods. Regardless of the results of these studies, future research will undoubtedly lead to the development of new dopamine agonists with greater bioavailability, different spectra of receptor activity, and fewer adverse effects. A new and exciting era of dopamine research has begun.

References

1. McDonald RH Jr, Goldberg LI, McNay JL, Tuttle EP Jr: Effects of dopamine in man: augmentation of sodium excretion, glomerular filtration rate, and renal plasma flow. J Clin Invest **43:** 1116, 1964
2. Goldberg LI: Cardiovascular and renal actions of dopamine: potential clinical applications. Pharmacol Rev **24:** 1, 1972
3. Goldberg LI, Hsieh YY, Resnekov L: Newer catecholamines for treatment of heart failure and shock: an update on dopamine and a first look at dobutamine. Prog Cardiovasc Dis 4: 327, 1977
4. Goldberg LI, Kohli JD: Differentiation of dopamine receptors in the periphery. *In* Kaiser C, Kebabian JW, editors: American Chemical Society Symposium Series No. 224. Dopamine receptors. Washington, DC, 1983, American Chemical Society, pp 101–113
5. Goldberg LI, Kohli JD: Peripheral pre- and post-synaptic dopamine receptors: are they different from dopamine receptors in the central nervous system? Commun Psychopharmacol **3:** 447, 1979
6. Stoof JC, Kebabian JW: Two dopamine receptors: biochemistry, physiology, and pharmacology. Life Sci **35:** 2281, 1984
7. Seeman P: Brain dopamine receptors. Pharmacol Rev **32:** 230, 1981
8. Hahn RA, Wardell JR Jr, Sarua HM, Ridley PT: Characterization of the peripheral and central effects of SK&F 82526, a novel dopamine receptor agonist. J Pharmacol Exp Ther **223:** 305, 1982
9. Goldberg LI, Glock D, Kohli JD, Barnett A: Separation of peripheral dopamine receptors by a selective DA_1 antagonist, SCH 23390. Hypertension **6** (suppl 1): I-25, 1984
10. Kohli JD, Glock D, Goldberg LI: Selective DA_2 versus DA_1 antagonist activity of domperidone in the periphery. Eur J Pharmacol **89:** 137, 1983
11. Henderson IS, Beattie TJ, Kennedy AC: Dopamine hydrochloride in oliguric states. Lancet **2:** 827, 1980
12. Goldberg LI: Dopamine receptors and hypertension: physiological and pharmacological implications. Am J Med **77:** 37, 1984
13. Rajfer SI, Anton AH, Rossen J, Goldberg LI: Beneficial hemodynamic effects of oral levodopa in heart failure: relationship to the generation of dopamine. N Engl J Med **310:** 1357, 1984
14. Kenakin TP, Ferris RM: Effects of in vivo beta-adrenoceptor down-regulation on cardiac responses to prenalterol and pirbuterol. J Cardiovasc Pharmacol **5:** 90, 1983
15. Dei Cas L, Bolognesi R, Cucchini F, Fappani A, Riva S, Visioli O: Hemodynamic effects of ibopamine in patients with idiopathic congestive cardiomyopathy. J Cardiovasc Pharmacol **5:** 249, 1983
16. Ren JH, Unverferth DV, Leier CV: The dopamine congener, ibopamine, in congestive heart failure. J Cardiovasc Pharmacol **6:** 748, 1984
17. Fennell WH, Taylor AA, Young JB, Brandon TA, Ginos JZ, Goldberg LI, Mitchell JR: Propylbutyldopamine: hemodynamic effects in conscious dogs, normal human volunteers, and patients with heart failure. Circulation **67:** 829, 1983
18. Francis GS, Parks R, Cohn JN: The effects of bromocriptine in patients with congestive heart failure. Am Heart J **106:** 100, 1983
19. Leon CA, Suarez JM, Aranoff RD, Murray MJ, Pratt CM, Young JB: Fenoldopam: efficacy of a new orally active dopamine analog in heart failure. Circulation **70** (suppl II): II-307, 1984
20. Kao A, Kriett JM, Tobler HG, Detloff BLS, Pritzker MR, Benson DW Jr, Benditt DG: Bromocriptine treatment of digitalis-induced ventricular tachyarrhythmias: studies in a canine model. J Am Coll Cardiol **4:** 1188, 1984

Atrial flutter: a synthesis of concepts

JOHN P. BOINEAU, M.D.

ATRIAL FLUTTER (AFL) is the designation applied to a group of tachyarrhythmias with atrial rates of from 240 to 360 beats/min. Distinctive in this group of arrhythmias is typical AFL, characterized by a unique consistency of atrial rate (300 ± 10 beats/min) and an electrocardiographic pattern demonstrating undulating F waves without isoelectric intervals in leads II, III, and aVF. This article attempts to identify the salient factors relevant to AFL and integrate them into a comprehensive concept. This synthesis is not intended to catalogue all or refute any of the factors that might operate in AFL. The purpose is to identify a minimal set of readily demonstrable factors that, through interaction, could cause spontaneous AFL. The present discussion concerns AFL, but the same concepts are also applicable to reentrant ventricular arrhythmias.

There have been many different mechanisms proposed to explain AFL. In many studies, complex mechanisms have been incompletely elucidated because the focus was on only those aspects readily revealed by a single technique. Also, most experimental studies of AFL have been conducted in animals without spontaneous flutter and therefore the principal factors involved in this tachyarrhythmia may not have been discovered. Although endocardial potentials have been recorded in some patients,[1] there have been no detailed activation sequence mapping studies carried out in patients with AFL. Even given the opportunity to record the activation in spontaneous AFL, if a fundamental factor happened to be an abnormality in atrial structure, then the true basis of the altered electrical state might not be recognized. The result is that either very diffuse or very specific and singular mechanisms have been postulated, none of which explains all of the unique characteristics of spontaneous AFL, which very likely is the result of a complex multifactorial process. In the absence of comprehensive data in man, an alternative preparation for study would be an animal with *spontaneous* AFL. In 1975, we discovered such an animal. The combined electrical and anatomic observations in that animal, as well as in subsequent studies on experimentally induced flutter-like tachycardias, have suggested that the mechanism of human AFL is a multifactorial one.[2]

Types of AFL can be categorized either descriptively or mechanistically. A useful classification would distinguish between different mechanisms and also relate each mechanism to the unique clinical and electrocardiographic features of the specific arrhythmia. It is the high degree of consistency of atrial rate and electrocardiographic pattern, occurring throughout a large population of individual patients, that implies a common substrate of relatively constant location in this specific form of the arrhythmia. A classification of types of AFL for this presentation, with emphasis on their mechanisms, might be: (1) focal (or automatic) flutter, (2) obstacle AFL (also termed macroreentrant, or circus motion AFL), and (3) intramyocardial (also termed microreentrant) AFL. This discussion is limited to the reentry concept which, in this investigator's opinion, is the most likely mechanism of AFL. This thesis is supported by our findings in spontaneous and experimental canine AFL,[2,3] by data on experimental flutter-like tachycardias described by Allessie et al.,[4-6] and by results of clinical electrophysiologic studies in patients.[1]

One might summarize the causal factors of reentrant AFL by grouping them into the following three categories: (1) the anatomic, or geometric, substrate, (2) the functional substrate, and (3) the initiating agent, or trigger. All three categories seem to be important in AFL. The principal substrate is an anatomic abnormality in atrial myocardium, which combines with the natural orifices of the vena cava to create a discontinuity in conduction; together they shape the potential reentrant pathway. The dimensions of this discontinuity are critical in determining the length of the surrounding pathway and the potential for sustained and stable reentry. The functional substrate is a nonuniform duration of repolarization of myocardium within or adjacent to the potential reentrant pathway. The triggering event is represented by one or more atrial premature depolarizations.

From the Section of Cardiology, Medical Service, Veterans Administration Medical Center, Downtown Division, and Department of Medicine, Medical College of Georgia, Augusta.

Address for correspondence: John P. Boineau, M.D., Division of Cardiothoracic Surgery, Washington University School of Medicine, 660 S. Euclid Ave., Box 8109, St. Louis, MO 63110.

These general components of the reentry model were apparent to Mines, Rosenbleuth and Garcia-Ramos, Wiener and Rosenbleuth, Kimura, and others. What is lacking is knowledge of the precise configurations and interactions of these fundamental components and how they may bring about spontaneous AFL. For atrial reentry, the key factors can be reduced to a two-dimensional problem and are therefore more readily identified than in the case of reentrant ventricular tachyarrhythmias, for which a three-dimensional exposition is required. However, once identified in the atrium,[2] similar mechanisms can be sought in a three-dimensional distribution in the ventricles.[8] There are other factors important in other reentrant arrhythmias that may also be important in AFL, such as depressed excitability, directional differences in cell-to-cell coupling, and others. Some of these factors are discussed below.

Obstacle flutter and circus motion (macro) reentry. The classic studies of Mayer, Mines, Garrey, Lewis et al., Rosenbleuth and Garcia-Ramos, Kimura et al., and Hayden et al.[7] have demonstrated conclusively that circulating depolarization waves can be forced to propagate around artificial obstacles and natural orifices in excitable tissue or cardiac muscle. The primary focus of attention of many of these studies was on whether the circumference of the separate or combined orifices of the superior and inferior venae cavae represented a long enough pathway to sustain a stable circus motion. The other factors involved in this model of sustained circus motion were the conduction velocity of the circulating wave and the duration of repolarization of the tissue. For circus motion to occur, the tissue ahead of the return wave must repolarize, i.e., the wavefront cannot run into the "wave rear." This could result from either a sufficiently large obstacle or orifice, a small orifice along with slow conduction of the circus wave in the circuit, or a short wave length due to a uniformly short repolarization time. In certain of the studies it was necessary to damage the intercaval tissue to create the conditions under which flutter could occur. These studies have been summarized in a classic review by Rytand.[7]

Repolarization inhomogeneity and intramyocardial (micro) reentry. To create the conditions necessary for one-way circus motion around the loop in obstacle flutter, nonuniform repolarization, in which an interface between repolarized and unrepolarized tissue intersects the boundary between the obstacle and its surrounding myocardium, must be present. Additionally, for the atrial premature depolarization to initiate one-way circus conduction in the loop, it must originate at a critical time and in close proximity to the junction between the two (functional and anatomic) boundaries. This represents an interaction between nonuniform repolarization and gross myocardial discontinuity.

The experimental studies of Allessie et al.[4, 5] have demonstrated that a flutter-like tachycardia can result from a form of intramyocardial reentry and that anatomic obstacles are not an essential component of the circuit. Activation maps obtained illustrated that the reentry resulted from regional differences in conduction of premature impulses within small zones of atrial myocardium between or distal to the natural orifices. In their studies, the critical or active reentrant circuit was quite small and the wavefronts appeared to move about a very small barrier to conduction. Thus, the spread of activation throughout the atrium had a vortical, rather than circular, pattern. The unidirectional block and one-way conduction of the revolving wavefront could be correlated with regional differences in the atrial effective refractory period or repolarization inhomogeneity. They proposed that a small functional barrier to conduction existed near the center of the vortex and was maintained in the refractory state by the continuous flow of current resulting from the depolarization and repolarization of adjacent tissue. They referred to this proposed mechanism of vortical reentry as "the leading circle theory."[6]

My co-workers and I[2] examined the role of repolarization inhomogeneity in the genesis of intra-atrial reentry tachycardias in dogs. Using programmed extrastimuli, we observed a rapid repetitive tachycardia and recorded activation sequence maps in several animals. Repolarization inhomogeneity exists during the early phases of recovery of excitability, when adjacent regions are both repolarized and unrepolarized. As shown in figure 1, if a critically timed and located atrial premature depolarization invades such a region, it will be asymmetrically conducted, delayed, blocked, and shaped by the unevenly repolarizing tissue. Given a particular distribution in which short and long repolarization times coexist in close proximity, a form of intramyocardial reentry can result. The activation blocks along boundaries approximating the regions of longer repolarization time. These boundaries were subsequently referred to by El-Sherif as "arcs of conduction block" in his studies of ventricular tachycardia.[8]

It is important to note that, as in Allessie's studies and our experimental studies on repolarization inhomogeneity reentry (figure 1), the actual reentrant circuit is confined to a relatively small field, measuring less than 1 cm. However, the wavefront spreads outward to envelop the rest of the atrium. No gross anatomic obstacles such as the cavae are required for this type of reentry and orifices are involved only secondarily, depending on their location in relation to the primary microreentry circuit. However, smaller discontinuities due to normal geometric complexities at the macroscopic and microscopic levels may play a role in the shorter reentrant pathways presently ascribed solely to repolarization inhomogeneity.[9]

Ultimately, it must be concluded that reentry resulting from repolarization inhomogeneity differs from spontaneous AFL in that the circuit is too small and the

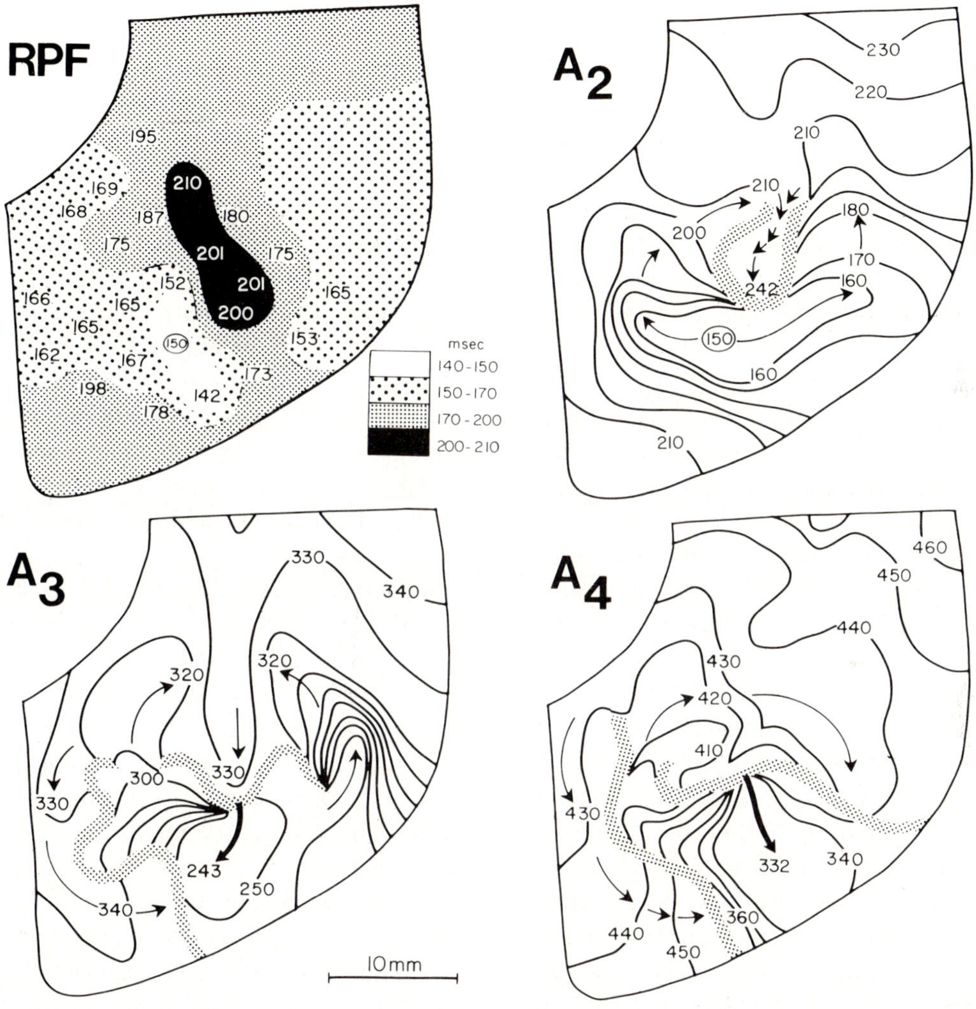

FIGURE 1. Reentry due to repolarization inhomogeneity. The effect of repolarization inhomogeneity on the conduction of a single atrial premature depolarization resulting in two subsequent reentrant cycles. The repolarization field map (RPF) illustrates the effective refractory period distribution determined from a single S_2 applied at each of the 24 points indicated after a series of S_1 stimuli were always delivered at the encircled point (150). The refractory times indicated for each of the S_2 include both the activation time from the S_1 site and the individual repolarization times. The RPF map represents the actual repolarization field encountered by the A_2. Note that the repolarization field is bimodal with close proximity of the zones of short and long repolarization times. The activation sequence maps of an atrial premature depolarizaton (A_2) delivered at 150 msec at the encircled site and two subsequent reentrant cycles (A_3 and A_4) were constructed from 72 electrode points. In comparing the sequence maps of the A_2 with the RPF maps note that activation propagates rapidly in regions with short repolarization times (light zones) and blocks on the adjacent boundary created by the zone of long repolarization duration (dark zone). Thus, the premature wavefront is kept from entering the zone of long repolarization time until after 210 msec. Note that in the A_2 the arcs of block are related to the longer repolarization times seen in the RPF map but are not perfectly superimposable. Subsequently the later A_2 wave turns back to activate the region of late repolarization within the cul-de-sac at 242 msec. Because of the proximity of the late depolarizing site to the site of initial activation and earliest recovery, the impulse reenters this zone and begins A_3. Reentry actually occurs closer to the point of earliest repolarization time slightly below the point of initial stimulation.

The first reentrant cycle (A_3) is followed by a second reentrant cycle (A_4), which blocks. Note that the effect of this bimodal repolarization inhomogeneity is to mold the wavefront and nonuniformly shape the activation pathway by uneven block and conduction, routing the wavefront back to the zone of earlier recovery causing reentry.

rate too fast in the former. As a consequence of the extremely rapid cycle time (60 to 140 msec), the activation pattern changes from cycle to cycle and is unstable. These arrhythmias either terminate spontaneously or degenerate into atrial fibrillation as secondary wavelets occur when activation encounters tissue in different stages of repolarization due to the short cycle time or blocks at small discontinuities as a result of the progressively diminishing efficacy of the stimulation by dissociated depolarizations. The arrhythmias therefore represent prefibrillatory tachycardia that is an intermediate stage between flutter and fibrillation. Allessie et al.[5] were able to stabilize repetitive cycles of intramyocardial reentry tachycardia by infusing aetylcholine to shorten the duration of repolarization. However, as important as repolarization inhomogeneity is to the *initiation* of a reentrant flutter-like tachycardia, this factor alone does not seem to be a sufficient substrate for spontaneous sustained AFL.

Role of myocardial discontinuity in slow conduction and block. Another mechanism for reentry is slow, or decremental, conduction and failure of impulse transmission unassociated with repolarization. The significance of abnormal conduction and its mechanisms have received limited attention and will require more definitive elucidation before certain forms of reentry can be explained.

The traditionally accepted form of cell-to-cell conduction is explained on the basis of the flow of intracellular current across low-resistance, specialized junctions between adjacent cells. These mechanisms derive from microelectrode studies of transmembrane potentials, ionic currents, and dV/dt max, among other things, which are generally presumed to be the principal factors determining normal and abnormal cardiac conduction. Slowing or failure of impulse propagation is ascribed to elevated resting potential, inactivation of sodium-channel conductance, depressed $\dot{V}_{max}$, and so on.

In contrast to the aforementioned membrane mechanisms, Spach et al.[10] showed theoretically and experimentally that geometric factors related to fiber orientation and directional differences in cell coupling accounted for marked variations in conduction velocity. Their studies indicated that geometric anisotropies could be more important than membrane factors in determining differences in conduction velocity. They demonstrated that fast propagation in the long axis of cells was associated with slow upstrokes of action potentials and that slower propagation was associated with faster upstrokes in a direction perpendicular to the fiber axes. This was just opposite of the expected relationship between action potential upstroke velocity and wavefront propagation. In their model, differences in resistive coupling parallel and perpendicular to the long axis of the fibers were related to marked differences in velocity in the two directions. These directional differences in coupling resistances associated with anisotropic myocardial geometry would be amplified in areas of discontinuity where wide gaps of unexcitable tissue were interposed between fibers.

Another possible mechanism relating macroscopic and gross myocardial discontinuities to slow conduction and block could be failure of extracellular, or ephaptic, conduction. As mentioned above, until recently, most studies of cardiac conduction and block have focused upon local circuit cell-to-cell spread of current. Little attention has been given to the possibility of rapid, synchronous propagation via the extracellular space with recruitment of adjacent fibers as a result of high voltages and current densities outside the cells. Based on data demonstrating slow conduction, we have previously considered the possibility that extracellular conduction might be a mechanism of fast normal propagation.[11] This hypothesis was proposed to account for the finding of a simultaneous loss of extracellular potential amplitude and increased duration and fragmentation of local electrograms associated with regional slowing in conduction velocity and failure of impulse transmission. This occurred as wavefronts approached areas of anatomic or functional myocardial discontinuity.[12, 13] Suenson[14] presented evidence in support of extracellular propagation as a mechanism in cardiac muscle. He demonstrated that extracellular transmission could occur between two cylindrical myocardial structures in close apposition due to a high extracellular resistance and extracellular potentials exceeding 30 mV. He further hypothesized that the obligatory high extracellular resistance might be accomplished if the extracellular space were reduced to narrow clefts between tightly packed cells. This would result in a very high current density within the normally restricted extracellular space. Assuming it has a role, the resulting effect of ephaptic conduction would be a mutually enhanced interaction such that the extracellular field, sustained at a high level by the nearly simultaneous depolarization of upstream fibers, would provide the necessary stimulation to maintain synchronous propagation in the normal geometrically discontinuous matrix of fibers. The electrical field surrounding the fibers might be quite intense due to the summation of multiple small extracellular currents resulting from the simultaneous depolarization of numerous cells. The effect of this external summation could take place through a capacitive interaction among tightly packed fibers with extracellular recruitment of adjacent resting cells via depolarization of their neighbors. A beneficial consequence of this extracellular field summation might be to bring all fibers within a specific spatial range into action together, ensuring coordinated propagation. Extracellular conduction might fail in fibrotic or dysplastic regions in which electrically viable fibers are widely separated due to loss of ephaptic mechanisms. The presence of wide gaps between excitable fibers would diminish the effects of extracellular electrical summation and result in loss of synchronous recruitment and propagation. Whether the dissociation of activation observed in the presence of normal and abnormal myocardial discontinuity is due only to increased resistivity of intercellular connections[10] or whether ephaptic-capacitive coupling is also involved is an intriguing question.

Finally, normal conduction might occur at several different levels, including by cell-to-cell spread via low-resistance junctions, by asymmetric conduction due to geometric anisotropies at both microscopic and macroscopic levels, and by a component of extracellular, or ephaptic, conduction. It seems apparent that abnormal conduction after repolarization is basic to the reentrant process in many arrhythmias. Also, it is apparent that the basic mechanisms of normal and slow conduction and block have not been completely elucidated. Specific questions are as follows: (1) How does the cardiac geometry affect conduction? (2) Why are slow conduction and propagation decrement and failure frequently associated with myocardial discontinuity? (3) What, if any, is the role of extracellular conduction?

Spontaneous canine AFL. In 1975, we serendipitously discovered a dog with spontaneous AFL.[2] The results of the activation and anatomic studies in this dog are directly relevant to human AFL for the following reasons: (1) The AFL was spontaneous and not experimentally produced by surgery, drugs, or programmed stimulation. (2) The AFL was stable and longlasting. (3) There was a consistent and reproducible rate and electrocardiographic pattern for each episode. (4) The cycle length of the flutter was longer than in experimental AFL. (5) Two forms of AFL were observed in the same dog. One mimicked the classic electrocardiographic pattern of typical human AFL and the other a form of atypical human AFL. (6) Both forms of AFL resulted from circus motion reentry, one type due to clockwise and the other to counterclockwise motion in the right atrium. (7) The basic substrate for both forms of reentry was a region of myocardial band discontinuity in the right atrium that combined with the contiguous vena cava to form a large anatomic obstacle creating a pathway sufficiently long to permit stable AFL. (8) Slow, decremental conduction was present in the zone of myocardial discontinuity.

In the dog with AFL (figure 2) there was discontinuity consisting of almost complete disruption of connections between the upper and lower crista terminalis and between the upper crista and the intercaval band muscle. In addition, there was discontinuity between the pectinate muscle bridges linking the posterior crista with the anterior tricuspid ring structures. Following from the assumptions relating myocardial discontinuity and geometric complexities to conduction, it is proposed that this disruption between the major connecting muscle bands produces a zone of slow conduction and propagation failure and that this region simultaneously serves as an added area of discontinuity in the conduction circuit. This region of electrical discontinuity, slow conduction, and block is designated zone S in the model of AFL illustrated in figure 2, *C* and *D*.

As a result of this study, we defined the form of AFL resembling the typical human form as type 1 flutter and that resembling the atypical human form as type 2 flutter.[2] The two forms of flutter observed in the dog demonstrated different reentrant activation patterns that accounted for the differences in rate and electrocardiographic morphology. Wells et al.[1] subsequently described two forms of AFL differentiated by their rates in patients. In their study, type 2 was faster than type 1 and it is tempting to speculate that this may have been due to a shorter reentrant pathway in their second group of subjects.

Two pathways of circus motion reentry with nonuniform conduction velocities. In the type 1 flutter (figure 2, *C*) in our previous study, the wavefront (viewed posteriorly) moved clockwise around the combined regions of discontinuity in the superior and inferior venae cavae, returning medially to the site of origin between the two cavae. The cycle time over that pathway was 175 msec, resulting in an atrial rate of 343 beats/min. In type 2 flutter (figure 2, *D*), the wavefront moved counterclockwise around the superior vena cava and spread through the intercaval region to return to its point of origin over a shorter pathway. This resulted in a shorter cycle length (151 msec) and a faster atrial rate (397 beats/min). Both forms of flutter were associated with circus motion within a zone of fast conduction (zone F) and slow conduction within an area of myocardial discontinuity contiguous with the superior vena cava (zone S). In type 2 flutter, there was definite propagation failure in zone S and an excitable gap of

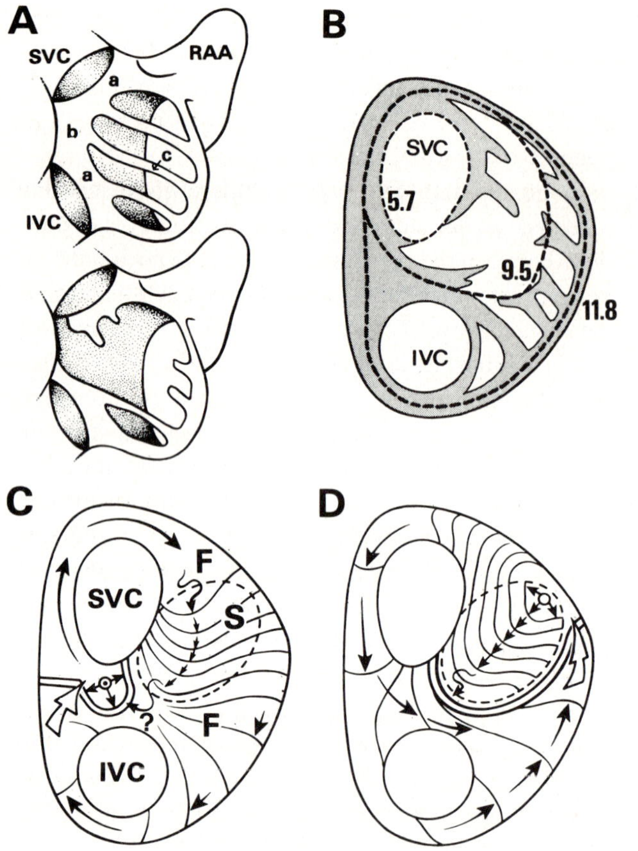

FIGURE 2. Model of atrial flutter: interaction between multiple factors. *A,* Schema of a three-dimensional lateral view of the normal dog's right atrium (upper diagram) and the right atrium of the dog with atrial flutter (lower diagram). Emphasized are the major right atrial conduction bands and connections, the upper and lower crista terminalis (a), the intercaval band (b), and the pectinate muscles (c). Although not shown, the walls of the superior and inferior venae cavae (SVC and IVC) and spaces between the pectinate muscles contain normal thin myocardium. In the normal atrium, the crista terminalis and septal bundles join with the intercaval band to form a "figure 8" around the venae cavae. This posterior ring structure about the cavae is connected to an anterior tricuspid valve ring structure by the pectinate muscle bridges laterally and by septal bands medially. In the dog with AFL note the discontinuity of the upper crista terminalis with the intercaval band and lower crista and also the hypoplastic pectinate musles causing disruption of lateral connections between the anterior and posterior right atrial rings. The actual reentrant structure is a two-dimensional circular surface, bordered anteriorly by the tricuspid anulus and posteriorly by the combined discontinuities of superior vena cava and hypoplastic myocardium. These edges represent the long and short pathways that, via directionally determined preferential conduction in one or the other, result in either type 1 or type 2 AFL. For simplicity, a two-dimensional diagram of these right atrial pathways is presented in *B, C,* and *D,* by flattening the anteroposterior axis shown in *A*. The anterior atrioventricular annular structures are represented at the perimeter, whereas the SVC, IVC, and contiguous posterior structures are represented centrally. *B,* The areas of discontinuity in the dog with AFL. Also indicated are the circumferential distances (broken lines) around the SVC (5.7 cm) and around the shortest (9.2 cm) and longest (11.8 cm) components of the flutter wave pathway. *C* and *D,* Types 1 and 2 AFL, respectively. Zone F represent the zone of normal fast conduction and zone S the area of discontinuity and zone of slow conduction. A further interacting factor needed to explain the initiation of the first reentrant beat is repolarization inhomogeneity indicated by the double solid line. *C,* Type 1 or typical AFL with clockwise rotation of the circus wave in the longer pathway of zone (F) created by both the SVC and IVC orifices plus the zone of myocardial discontinuity (S). Question marks indicate a questionable source of late depolarization and reentry from zone S. *D,* Type 2 or atypical AFL with countercockwise rotation of the circus wave in the shorter pathway of zone (F), which does not include the IVC and is therefore associated with a shorter cycle length. There is antegrade block in zone S and reentry is from the fast pathway. Symbols:

- ➔ (heavy arrow) = direction and pathway of circus wavefront in normal myocardium, zone F;
- → (light arrow) = direction of slow conduction in abnormal dysplastic myocardium, zone S;
- ∼→ (wavy arrow) = entry and ? exit of depolarization in zone S;
- ⇨ (open arrow) = reentry of return wavefront;
- ═ (double line) = arc of block, representing boundary between repolarized and unrepolarized muscle;
- ------ = boundary between zones F and S.

50 msec was present before the return wave encountered the boundary of previous antegrade block. Thus, in type 2, the major circus wave in zone F was its own source of reentry as it propagated around the combined discontinuitics of the superior vena cava and zone of slow conduction. In type 1 flutter, because of the similar directions of wavefronts in the zones of slow and fast conduction resulting in a vortex-likc motion of the wavefront, we considered that there might have been continuity of activation wavefronts across the boundary (dotted line). Also, we could not discern whether the reentry resulted from the fast component in zone F returning over the larger caudal pathway around the inferior vena cava, or from a delayed component exiting zone S in the short pathway. However, because of the existence of block in zone S in type 2 AFL, which might also be expected to occur in type 1, and because of the exact correlation between the flutter cycle length and the arrival time of the faster wavefront in the larger circuit (zone F), we presumed that zone F was also the source of the reentry in type 1 AFL. If this is correct, then the region of slow conduction and propagation failure (zone S) serves only as a passive area of discontinuity in both forms of AFL by preventing rapid conduction of the circus wave in a shorter pathway encircling only the superior vena cava. From this analysis, it would appear that the normal superior vena caval orifice alone does not provide a long enough circus pathway to permit stable AFL. However, the addition of the bordering region of slow conduction (zone S) may result in type 1 flutter over a longer pathway by linking the superior and inferior venae cavae area of discontinuity, or may result in the more rapid type 2 flutter if there is rotation of the wave about a slightly

shorter pathway formed only by the superior vena cava and continguous zone S.

A relatively wide region of myocardium (zone F) lies between the posterior areas of discontinuity of the superior vena cava and zone S and the anterior area of the tricuspid anulus. These geometric conditions create a circular surface with critical size discontinuities of different dimensions at both anterior and posterior boundaries. The resulting reentrant pathway is therefore a two-dimensional one. Within zone F, the minimal pathway length bordering the posterior area of discontinuity was 9.5 cm (figure 2, *B*). This compares with 5.7 cm, which was the circumference of the superior vena caval orifice alone. The maximum length of the anterior aspect of the circus pathway was 11.8 cm. The velocity of the circus wavefront varied as a function of the distance from zone S in both forms of AFL. Thus, the wave traveling in the short posterior portion of the reentrant pathway was slowest and the velocity of that portion of the wave traveling in the longer anterior pathway was fastest so that, in zone F, there was a continuum of conduction velocity between these two limits and a fanlike rotation of the wavefronts. The mechanism for this difference in conduction velocity in the anterior and posterior pathways is not known. It could be due to preferential conduction in the continuous, thicker anterior pathway adjacent to the atrioventricular anulus, where the direction of the wavefront parallels the direction of continuity.

Since the circuit with the longest conduction time receives depolarization from the circuit with the shortest conduction time, only the velocity of the latter pathway can be calculated. In type 1 AFL the conduction time around the longer anterior circuit was shorter than that around the shorter posterior pathway. The conduction velocity in the anterior circuit during clockwise (type 1) depolarization was 0.67 m/sec. In type 2 flutter, the conduction time in the shorter posterior pathway was less than in the longer anterior path and the conduction velocity during the counterclockwise depolarization was 0.63 m/sec. Even though the conduction velocity in the anterior pathway seemed faster in type 2 AFL (estimated to be 0.78 m/sec based on the cycle time of 151 msec), the combination of the shorter path and slightly slower velocity of the posterior circuit resulted in its having the fastest cycle time. Thus, the pathway with the shortest cycle time becomes the effective reentrant circuit and is first to deliver the return wave back to the site of reentry. Conduction velocity was also nonuniform along the axis of propagation, as evidenced by the segmental differences in areas where the isochrones are close together during slow and further apart during faster conduction.

In summary, the factors that result in two different atrial rates in types 1 and 2 AFL are (1) the two reentrant pathways of different length, or more precisely, the two circumferences of the anterior and posterior aspects of the reentrant circuit (figure 2), (2) the different conduction velocities associated with the long and short pathways, and (3) the different conduction velocities in association with clockwise and counterclockwise rotation of the wavefront in each of the two pathways. Therefore, in comparison with the classic one-dimensional model of circus motion, which has only one path length and a uniform conduction velocity, the actual flutter pathway is more complex, at least two-dimensional, has major and minor circumferences, and exhibits a range of conduction velocities. It remains to be determined whether it is also a two-dimensional, two-pathway reentrant structure that determines the different atrial rates in patients exhibiting two forms of AFL.

Preferential conduction in AFL. Apart from the semantic dilemma, there is a conceptual difference between specialized and preferential conduction in the atrium. Maximum atrial conduction velocity is between 0.7 to 1.3 m/sec and this velocity is confined to the large myocardial bands or trunks that have been anatomically identified as the crista terminalis, pectinate muscles, Bachmann's bundle, and certain septal muscle bands.[15] Activation in thin areas of atrial muscle, like that associated with the venae cavae and other sparse transparent tissue between pectinate muscles, is slower (between 0.3 to 0.7 m/sec).[15, 16] Although there are several different types of cell in the atrium, there is no anatomic or electrical evidence that a collection of any of these special cell types are arranged in continuous structure that represent specialized tracts that conduct atrial impulses faster than 1.3 m/sec. There is, however, ample evidence that the larger trunks not only conduct faster than the thin atrium, but also maintain conduction, in spite of increased extracellular potassium concentration, when other thin areas of atrial muscle fail to exhibit propagation.[17]

Our observations suggest that the right atrial myocardium is arranged to form a preferential conduction system. Because the larger bands consist of parallel and tightly packed fiber bundles, conduction velocity in the long axis of these structures is fast (0.7 to 1.3 m/sec), or preferential. As illustrated in figure 2, *A*, the right atrial bands form a tridimensional fast-conducting myocardial skeleton in which all of the major trunks are connected. Rapid craniocaudal conduction is through the crista terminals. Rapid conduction between the posterior muscle bands (crista, etc.) and the anterior pathways encircling the tricuspid orifice is through the pectinate muscles.

Pastelin et al.[17] produced intra-atrial reentrant arrhythmias and experimental AFL in dogs and observed that activation continued to circulate in loops of atrial muscle during increased potassium concentrations and after disruption of specific muscle bundles. They concluded that AFL occurs via preferential conduction through anterior and posterior interatrial tracks. Given the limited number of recording electrodes in their studies, their observations on preferential conduction of the flutter wave in the major atrial muscle bundles can be readily incorporated into the model of AFL shown in figure 2, *B* and *C*. Our findings indicate that it is the absence of preferential conduction in certain pathways that leads to the preferential reentrant conduction in others. The diagram illustrates that conduction is faster in the intact longer atrial pathway associated with the tricuspid anulus. However, a more complete representation is that there is preferential, or faster, conduction in this pathway because of the impediment to access of the circus wavefront to shorter preferential routes blocked by the myocardial discontinuity of zone S. Also, the atrial muscle of the tricuspid anulus is thicker and manifests uninterrupted circumferential continuity. Preferential conduction is also illustrated by the differences in which pathway (long or short) becomes the effective reentrant circuit in the clockwise and counterclockwise circus rhythms associated with the two forms of AFL in the dog. Also, as indicated by the activation data,[2] depolarization in AFL is not restricted to the thicker preferential routes, but is continuous, with wavefronts present in adjacent thin areas if there is no impediment to conduction.

AFL model and synthesis of concepts. Figure 2 defines the interaction of the major components resulting in AFL, and emphasizes the synthesis of previous and present concepts.

The anatomic substrate is fundamental to the existence of AFL. It determines that an otherwise abortive series of short reentrant cycles will become AFL. The structural substrates of the caval orifices and the contiguous zone of myocardial discontinuity and slow conduction, which together form the principal obstacle about which the flutter wave circulates, are most important. The superior or inferior vena cava alone are not large enough orifices to allow a circulating wave to become established. It seems evident that the caval openings and the contiguous zone of myocardial discontinuity are positioned such that the reentrant wavefront is forced into a longer pathway, resulting in a stable pattern of repetition. In the adult dog, a critical pathlength of 9 to 10 cm seems to be required. Smaller loops could sustain circus motion if the effective refractory period was uniformly of short duration. The tricuspid anulus forms an integral anterior component of the circular reentrant surface. If these data apply to patients, it is the dimensions, spatial position, and orientation of this annular structure that represent a structural constant that is reflected in the consistent atrial rate and electrocardiographic patterns found in type 1 AFL. However, of greater causal significance is the posterior discontinuity that determines the minimal necessary loop size needed to sustain reentry in the adult dog. Zone S eliminates fast-conduction "shortcuts" that would minimize the effective lengths of potential reentrant loops and prevent the establishment of AFL.

Repolarization inhomogeneity is a salient factor and is important in the initiation of the reentrant process when coupled with a critically timed and located atrial premature depolarization. However, unlike the anatomic substrate, it is dynamic and unstable due to changes in autonomic input or changing intrinsic sensitivity to the autonomic agonists.[18] Intra-atrial reentrant cycles will occur only with certain refractory field distributions (figure 1), and AFL may require a particular spatiotemporal superposition of geometric and functional substrates and atrial premature depolarization. Consider that a bimodal field of uneven repolarization is positioned so close to the zone of myocardial discontinuity that a cycle of intramyocardial reentry is forced into the AFL circuit, where it is entrapped in a continuous motion.[7] Once the reentry starts, it is the basic anatomic substrate of myocardial discontinuity and the location of this region in relationship to the natural orifices of the atrium that determine the unique features of AFL, including rate, activation pattern, and electrocardiographic morphology.

The atrial premature depolarization is the triggering event that, when combined with repolarization inhomogeneity, initiates the reentrant depolarizations (figure 1). Not only is the timing of the atrial premature depolarization (A_2) important, but the site of origin is also crucial. For intramyocardial reentry to occur, the wavefront must encounter both repolarized and nonrepolarized myocardium existing in close proximity. If repolarization inhomogeneity is not optimally distributed for the occurrence of reentry, then multiple spontaneous or programmed atrial premature depolarizations may be required to set up a particularly vulnerable distribution of repolarization.

I am grateful for the efforts of Anita Wylds, Margaret Beasley and Dawn Schuessler in preparing the manuscript, and to the Medical Media Production Service of the Veterans Administration Medical Center for their photographic assistance.

References

1. Wells JL Jr, MacLean WAH, James TN, Waldo AL: Characterization of atrial flutter. Studies in man after open heart surgery using fixed atrial electrodes. Circulation **60:** 66, 1979
2. Boineau JP, Schuessler RB, Mooney CR, Miller CB, Wylds AC, Hudson RD, Borremans JM, Brockus CW: Natural and evoked atrial flutter due to circus movement in dogs. Am J Cardiol **45:** 1167, 1980
3. Boineau JP, Wylds AC, Autry LJ, Schuessler RB, Miller CB: Mechanisms of atrial flutter as determined from spontaneous and experimental models. *In* Josephson ME, Wellens HJJ editors: Tachycardias: mechanisms, diagnosis, treatment. Philadelphia, 1984, Lea & Febiger, pp 91–111
4. Allessie MA, Bonke FIM, Schopman FJG: Circus movement in rabbit atrial muscle as a mechanism of tachycardia. II. The role of nonuniform recovery of excitability in the occurrence of unidirectional block, as studied with multiple microelectrodes. Circ Res **39:** 168, 1976
5. Allessie MA, Lammers WJEP, Bonke FIM, Hollen J: Intra-atrial reentry as a mechanism for atrial flutter induced by acetylcholine and rapid pacing in the dog. Circulation **70:** 123, 1984
6. Allessie MA, Bonke FIM, Schopman FJG: Circus movement in rabbit atrial muscle as a mechanism of tachycardia. III. The "leading circle" concept: a new model of circus movement in cardiac tissue without the involvement of an anatomical obstacle. Circ Res **41:** 9, 1977
7. Rytand DA: Circus movement (entrapped circuit wave) hypothesis and atrial flutter. Ann Intern Med **65:** 125, 1966
8. El-Sherif N, Smith RA, Evans K: Canine ventricular arrhythmias in the late myocardial infarction period. 8. Epicardial mapping of reentrant circuits. Circ Res **49:** 255, 1981
9. Spach MS: The electrical representation of cardiac muscle based on discontinuities of axial resistivity at a microscopic and macroscopic level. In Paes de Carvalho A and Hoffman BF, editors: Normal and abnormal conduction in the heart. Mt. Kisco, NY, 1982, Futura Publishing Co, pp 145 –179
10. Spach MS, Miller WT III, Geselowitz DB, Barr RC, Kootsey JM, Johnson EA: The discontinuous nature of propagation in normal canine cardiac muscle. Evidence for recurrent discontinuities of intracellular resistance that affect the membrane currents. Circ Res **48:** 39, 1981
11. Boineau JP, Mooney CR, Hudson RD, Hughes DG, Erdin RA Jr, Wylds AC: Observations on re-entrant excitation pathways and refractory period distributions on spontaneous and experimental atrial flutter in the dog. *In* Kulbertus HE, editor: Re-entrant arrhythmias. Mechanisms and treatment. Lancaster, 1977, MTP Press Limited, pp 72–98
12. Boineau JP, Cox JL: Slow ventricular activation in acute myocardial infarction. Circulation **48:** 702, 1973
13. Walston A, Boineau JP, Alexander JA, Sealy WC: Dissociation and delayed conduction in the canine right bundle branch. Circulation **53:** 605, 1976
14. Suenson M: Ephaptic impulse transmission between ventricular myocardial cells in vitro. Acta Physiol Scand **120:** 445, 1984
15. Boineau JP, Schuessler RB, Hackel DB, Miller CB, Brockus CW, Wylds AC: Widespread distribution and rate differentiation of the atrial pacemaker complex. Am J Physiol **239**(Heart Circ Physiol 8): H406, 1980
16. Hayashi H, Lux RL, Wyatt RF, Burgess MJ, Abildskov JA: Relation of canine atrial activation sequence to anatomic landmarks. Am J Phyiol **242**(Heart Circ Physiol 11): H421, 1982
17. Pastelin G, Mendez R, Moe GK: Participation of atrial specialized conduction pathways in atrial flutter. Circ Res **4:** 386, 1978
18. Corr PB, Shayman JA, Kramer JB, Kipnis RJ: Increased alpha-adrenergic receptors in ischemic cat myocardium. J Clin Invest **67:** 1232–1236, 1981

EDITORIAL

Cardiology at a precipice

ROBERT A. O'ROURKE, M.D.

THE LOVE AFFAIR between the American public and American medicine, extant since World War II, has come to an inevitable end. This is not surprising, considering that the increase in the cost of health care delivery has been eight times greater than the inflationary rise in the gross national product (GNP) since 1950. National health expenditures accounted for 4.4% of the GNP in 1950 and now account for almost 12% of the total GNP.[1] Part of the increase in health care costs is the result of an oversupply of physicians. In 1950 there were 141 physicians per 100,000 population. Presently there are about 220 per 100,000.[2] There are several indications that the increase in the quantity of physicians and health care resources is occurring faster than any increment in the demand for physician services.[3] Although people are living longer, which will eventually result in a greater number of elderly patients, the maximum effect of this increase in the aged patient population will not take place until the beginning of the 21st century. Moreover, in recent years there has been a decline in the number of hospitals and an even greater reduction in the quantity of hospital beds; as a consequence, the number of hospital beds per physician decreased from 5.2 in 1970 to 3.1 in 1980.[4] In the near future, the further increase in the number of physicians and coincident reduction in hospital beds will lower this ratio to an even greater extent. Furthermore, as specialists continue to locate in nonmetropolitan areas and small cities, referral patterns for specialized care are changing. With certain specialties in medicine being overcrowded, some physicians may have to change or add specialties to maintain economically viable medical practices.

The federal government has adopted an interventional approach to alter the economic performance of the health care sector, and third-party payors have become more aggressive in containing health care costs to reduce the rate of increase in health insurance premiums. At the same time, hospitals have become more active in containing costs, competition among physicians for access to hospital resources has grown considerably, and actual competition between physicians and hospitals in the primary medical care market is evolving. Big business is developing its own health care delivery plans, and the number of health maintenance organizations and preferred-provider organizations are increasing rapidly. Medicine is truly at a crossroads.

Factors affecting cardiology training programs. These problems affecting general medicine have a great impact on cardiologists and cardiology training programs. The available data suggest that there is an overabundance of cardiologists in the United States today, at least in private practice. From 1970 to 1980, there was an increase in the number of specialists in cardiovascular disease of between 51% and 66%.[5–7] Furthermore, as might be anticipated, cardiology was specifically identified as an overcrowded specialty by many physician respondents to an American Medical Association attitudinal survey on physician manpower in 1982. On the other hand, the data concerning the probable surplus of cardiologists are "soft." Many physicians who are neither board-eligible nor board-certified in cardiovascular diseases call themselves "cardiologists." Whether or not there are too many qualified cardiologists in 1985 is a matter of some speculation. There certainly appears to be too few academic cardiologists with adequate training in clinical and/or basic science research.[8]

There are currently between 240 and 270 cardiology training programs in the United States and somewhat over 1700 cardiology trainees.[9, 10] The number of cardiology trainees increased greatly from 1970 to 1975, rose by a small increment between 1976 and 1981, and then underwent a second important growth phase between 1981 and 1985.[11–14] The number of trainees in cardiology is more than twice the number of trainees in either of the two next most popular medical subspecialty training programs, gastroenterology and pulmonary diseases. It is of interest that the latest increment in the number of trainees correlates with the widespread use of interventional coronary angiography in the practice of cardiology.

From the Division of Cardiology, Department of Medicine, University of Texas Health Science Center, San Antonio.

Address for correspondence: Robert A. O'Rourke, M.D., Division of Cardiology, Department of Medicine, University of Texas Health Science Center, San Antonio, TX 78284.

Presently, the subspecialty programs in internal medicine are undergoing their first individual evaluations for accreditation over a three year cycle that will end in October 1986. Subsequently, a list of accredited programs in cardiovascular disease as judged by the Residency Review Committee–Internal Medicine (RRC-IM) for the Accreditation Committee on Graduate Medical Education will be published and eventually only physicians trained in accredited programs will be allowed to take the American Board of Internal Medicine (ABIM) subspecialty examination in cardiovascular diseases. Accreditation criteria in cardiovascular diseases include well-rounded training in all aspects of clinical cardiology, including a major training component in cardiovascular research. Although only two years of training in cardiovascular disease are currently required, information is being collected by the RRC-IM relative to a third year of training from those programs in which that option exists or in which three years of training are required.

At the last two meetings of the Association of University Cardiologists and of the American College of Cardiology Program Directors, there was considerable discussion concerning the optimal structure of training programs in cardiovascular diseases, the certifying examination in the subspecialty of cardiology, and the dwindling federal support of clinical cardiovascular research. In addition, these organizations have conducted several written surveys of cardiologists relating to problems facing our subspecialty. The majority of attendees at these meetings and survey respondents indicated that a minimum of three years of training should be required to provide well-rounded experience in clinical cardiology, including competence in noninvasive and invasive cardiac techniques, minimal to more extensive experience in cardiovascular research, and sufficient background in patient-related activities to become a cardiac consultant. Two years of training are inadequate to obtain sufficient clinical skills in cardiology; to receive appropriate training in electrocardiography, echocardiography, cardiac catheterization and angiography, nuclear cardiology, and clinical electrophysiology; and to participate in meaningful cardiovascular research. In many cases, four years of training may be optimal, especially for the academic cardiologist developing expertise in basic research who will need to compete for cardiovascular research funding on a regular basis during his or her professional career. Most cardiology program directors agree that there are too few truly academic cardiologists and that current programs are not developing a sufficient number of cardiologists interested in long-term academic careers with a major component of their activities related to clinical or basic research.

Potential solutions. There are several potential methods for reducing the number of cardiovascular trainees if there is agreement that the number of "cardiologists" is excessive for the health care delivery needs of the United States in 1985. The first method is to reduce, voluntarily, the number of programs and/or the number of cardiology trainees. Although this has been initiated in certain medical centers, it is unlikely to happen in great numbers. Cardiology trainees provide a "double-edged sword" for the program director. On one hand their manpower is required to support the multiple clinical, teaching, and research activities of the typical cardiology division, and additional well-trained academic cardiologists are needed. On the other hand, many, if not most, of the trainees eventually enter the private practice of cardiology and often end up in competition with the cardiology program where they were trained. Perhaps this manpower problem could be resolved if monies used for trainee support could be allocated to fund additional full-time cardiovascular scientists, research nurses, and cardiology technicians.

Second, the number of cardiology training programs may be reduced by the firm application of strict accreditation criteria. However, many pre-reviewers participating in the current subspecialty accreditation process estimate that less than 20% of cardiology training programs will be refused accreditation by the criteria applied. These primarily will be small, private hospital–based programs where one to four trainees care for the hospitalized patients of private-practice cardiologists, who appropriately spend most of their time in their practices.

A third approach is to reduce the percentage of cardiologists passing the certification examination in cardiovascular disease. In the past, the rate of successful candidates has been relatively high, averaging 67% overall, with United States medical schools first-time candidates having a passing rate of greater than 80%.[15] Specific action by the Subspecialty Board in Cardiovascular Diseases and the parent ABIM will be required to exercise this approach.

A fourth method for reducing the number of trainees completing fellowship programs each year is to increase the required duration for training in cardiology fellowship programs to three years. If the latter approach is applied and the number of available stipends is kept constant, the number of cardiology fellows completing training each year can be reduced by one-third. As discussed above, the trend toward three year programs is consistent with the criteria for accreditation of subspecialty programs in cardiology, particularly considering the need for each program to have a research component. Recently, the American Board of Clinical Pathology and the Pediatric Subspecialty Board of Hematology-Oncology each increased by one year the duration of training required for board certification. The Pediatric Subspecialty Board of Pulmonology started with a three year training requirement and the Pediatric Subspecialty Board of Nephrology has requested another year of required training before certification. The ABIM would have to approve any additional training requirement for certification in adult cardiology as would the American Board of Medical Specialists, but precedence certainly exists.

Recent changes in cardiology. During the past decade there have been important basic and clinical research developments that have reduced the morbidity and mortality due to cardiovascular disease in the United States. As a result there are better diagnostic and therapeutic options for patients with cardiovascular disease. Many of these advances have resulted from the application of new high-technology procedures to the practice of cardiology. Many cardiology trainees desire to learn these special techniques and almost every practicing cardiologist wants to have them available for his or her patients. The further development and more frequent use of cardiac transplantation, electrophysiologic testing, implantable cardiac defibrillators, Doppler echocardiography, nuclear cardiology techniques, early postinfarction coronary thrombolysis, and percutaneous transluminal coronary angioplasty have been major achievements in cardiology. However, the expense of providing these options for large segments of the American public is staggering. Furthermore, there is great potential hazard to individual patients when some of the more complex techniques and procedures are performed by physicians with inadequate training and experience in their use, as many patients become part of the operator's "learning curve."

Most cardiovascular trainees and practicing cardiologists want to be trained in all income-generating cardiovascular procedures. It is reasonable to assume that a trained cardiologist will probably not be used as a cardiac consultant unless he or she can perform all diagnostic and therapeutic procedures that are available in other parts of the community. Moreover, because of the large number of cardiologists in private practice and the large number of trainees in cardiology, there is considerable competition for cardiovascular patients who require these procedures. Many believe that this results in the more frequent use of expensive cardiovascular procedures. Many cardiologists, including those at academic centers, believe that if they do not perform a procedure with borderline or questionable indications, the referring physician will find another "cardiologist" who will. This approach has a deleterious effect on the cost of health care delivery and has nearly exhausted the capacity of the American patient population to absorb increasing cardiovascular health care expenses.

Presently, cardiovascular trainees too frequently neglect their research activities or their experience in less dramatic aspects of clinical cardiology so they may be present at interventional diagnostic or therapeutic studies performed within their cardiology divisions. Recent test results suggest that the general clinical ability of those taking the cardiology subspecialty examinations has declined as the need and desire to provide training in an increasing number of high-technology procedures during the usual two years of experience have grown. For example, the performance of candidates in the electrocardiography portion of the most recent subspecialty examination in cardiovascular diseases was mediocre at best.

Implications for cardiology. These considerations lead to the important question of whether or not all "cardiologists" should be trained to perform "interventional cardiology." Should there be special certification for specific procedures, with additional training requirements and assessment of competency for cardiologists who perform percutaneous transluminal coronary angioplasty or clinical electrophysiologic testing? There are no generally accepted standards for training in these areas. Standards have been proposed for training in echocardiography and in nuclear cardiology, but neither have been rigidly applied.[16, 17] There are no cardiology procedures that have been designated to be reimbursed only when performed by board-eligible or board-certified cardiologists, let alone procedures earning monies only for cardiologists with additional documented training and expertise in highly specialized procedures and in interpretation of their results. This designation would be a new posture for the health care community.

Nevertheless, hospital administrators and chairmen of departments of medicine of the current era are cognizant of the large number of cardiologists in relation to the quantity of hospital beds and to the number of testing facilities. Therefore they are likely to respond to guidelines indicating requirements for performing specialized procedures by permitting only cardiologists who meet the stated criteria to use their hospital facilities for performing such studies. For similar reasons, third-party payors might also reimburse only cardiologists who meet the stated criteria.

There are many problems facing cardiology and cardiology training programs. Considering the state of cardiology manpower, the inadequate federal funding of clinical and research activities, the cost of cardiology health care delivery, and the number of high-technology cardiac procedures available, the time for action is now. Cardiology is at a precipice. Whether or not it falls into the abyss of complete federal control depends on whether the leaders in academic centers, members of cardiology professional societies, and practitioners of cardiology in general are willing to modify their self-interests and interact with other elements in the health care delivery sector to produce the reasonable changes necessary for continuing excellence in the delivery of cardiovascular health care to the American public.

References

1. Freeland MS, Schendler CE: National health expenditure growth in the 1980s: an aging population, new technologies, and increasing competition. Health Care Financing Review, March 1983, pp 1–58
2. Tarlov AR: Special report: Shattuck lecture. The increasing supply of physicians, the changing structure of the health-service system, and the future practice of medicine. N Engl J Med **308:** 1235, 1983
3. The American Medical Association: The environment of medicine. Report of the Council on Long Range Planning and Development. December, 1983
4. American Hospital Association: Hospital statistics, 1982 edition, 1982
5. Haug JN, Robach GA, Martin BC: Distribution of physicians in the United States. Chicago, 1971, American Medical Association
6. Bidese KA, Danias DG: Physician characteristics and distribution in the United States, 1981 edition. Chicago, 1982, American Medical Association
7. Physician characteristics and distribution, 1983 edition. Department of Data Release Services, Division of Survey and Data Resources, American Medical Association, 1984
8. Positions available in medical school facilities. Clin Res **33:** 12, 1985
9. National Study of Internal Medicine Manpower: Directory of training programs in internal medicine: residency and subspecialty fellowships. 1982–1983. Prepared by National Study of Internal Medicine Manpower, The University of Chicago
10. Education Update: Adult cardiovascular training programs in the United States. J Am Coll Cardiol **3:** 455, 1984
11. Tarlov AR, Weil PA, Schleiter MK, and the Association of Professors of Medicine Task Force on Manpower: National study of internal medicine manpower. 1. Residency training 1976–1977. Ann Intern Med **88:** 413, 1978
12. Tarlov AR, Schleiter MK, Weil PA and the Association of Professors of Medicine Task Force on Manpower: National study of internal medicine manpower. IV. Residency and fellowship training 1977–1978 and 1978–1979. Ann Intern Med **91:** 295, 1979
13. Schleiter MK, Tarlov AR, Weil PA and the Association of Professors of Medicine Task Force on Manpower: National study of internal medicine manpower. VII. Residency and fellowship training 1976–1977 through 1980–1981. Ann Intern Med **95:** 762, 1981
14. Schleiter MK, Tarlov AR and the Association of Professors of Medicine Task Force on Manpower: National study of manpower. VIII. Internal medicine residency and fellowship training: 1983 update. Ann Intern Med **99:** 380, 1983
15. Hancock EW: Report from the American Board of Internal Medicine. Proceedings of the 10th Annual Symposium for Directors of Adult Cardiovascular Training Programs. American College of Cardiology. Dallas, March 1984
16. Martin RP, Kisslo J, Quinones MA, Popp RL, Feigenbaum H, Tajik AJ, Hagan AD: Report of the American Society of Echocardiography Committee on Physician Training in Adult M-Mode and Two-Dimensional Echocardiography. April 1982
17. Zaret BL, Buttler A, Berger JH, Bodenheimer MM, Borer JS, Brochier M, Hugenholtz PG, Neufeld HN, Pfisterer ME: Report of the Joint International Society and Federation of Cardiology/World Health Organization Task Force on Nuclear Cardiology. Circulation **70:** 768A, 1984

The delayed diagnosis of myocardial infarction: it took half a century!

W. BRUCE FYE, M.D.

IN 1940 the physiologist Carl Wiggers claimed, "Delayed recognition of important physiological discoveries frequently continues untenable and wrong points of view. . . . Greater mutual efforts ought to be made by clinicians and physiologists for better dissemination, digestion and absorption of important physiological discoveries."[1] Although angina pectoris had been described by William Heberden in the 18th century, and some 19th century physicians recognized an association between this symptom and sclerosis of the coronary arteries found at autopsy, the syndrome of acute myocardial infarction was not recognized until the 20th century.[2–5] The "wrong point of view" that led to the long delay in the recognition of acute myocardial infarction was the belief that sudden coronary occlusion was invariably fatal. This view predominated until 1912 when James Herrick proposed that myocardial infarction in man was not always fatal and could be recognized during life. Additional factors that contributed to this delay included: (1) the inconstant relationship of symptoms to pathological findings in ischemic heart disease, (2) the excessive reliance on auscultation as an indicator of cardiac disease, (3) the failure to routinely examine the coronary arteries or the myocardium at autopsy, (4) the reluctance or tardiness of clinicians to incorporate new pathophysiologic discoveries into medical practice, (5) a willingness to accept theories of disease without scientific evidence to support them, (6) the preoccupation with the new field of bacteriology, which distracted clinicians and biomedical scientists from the more traditional organ-centered approach to disease, and (7) the lack of any diagnostic techniques with which to objectively identify coronary artery obstruction or its consequences during life. Nevertheless, during the second half of the 19th century many discoveries were made that ultimately led to an understanding of the clinical and pathologic sequelae of coronary occlusion. Most of the important observations were made by individuals who combined extensive experience in pathology with clinical practice.

In the 1840s several British physicians became interested in the coronary circulation. John Erichsen studied the relationship of cardiac arrest and experimental coronary occlusion, Joseph Swan attempted to demonstrate coronary anastomoses using injection techniques, and Richard Quain initiated a detailed study of "fatty diseases of the heart." Quain received his medical training at University College, London, where he studied physiology under William Sharpey, one of the first in Britain to use the microscope in medical teaching. Quain was appointed assistant physician to the Brompton Hospital for diseases of the chest in 1848.[6] His thorough scientific training and clinical experience equipped him to investigate the clinical and pathologic features of heart disease. Quain's attention had been drawn to this subject in 1845 "by the sudden death of a gentleman, in whose body no sufficient explanation of that event could be found. A peculiar fatty condition of the heart was observed and recorded during the examination. The occurrence, soon afterwards, of two similar cases, led to the conclusion, that the presence of this fatty matter in the heart's texture bore some important relations to the structure and functions of the organ."[7]

In 1850 Quain published a comprehensive review on fatty diseases of the heart based on a study he had undertaken with Charles Williams who had reported the association of coronary artery sclerosis with myocardial scars more than a decade earlier. Williams, professor of medicine at University College, had studied under Hope, Magendie, Laennec, and other leaders of the scientific study of heart disease and was later characterized by Quain as ". . . the principal founder of our modern school of Pathology . . ."[8] Quain reviewed the histories and cardiac pathologic findings in

Dr. Fye is Chairman of the Cardiology Department at the Marshfield Clinic in Marshfield, Wisconsin, Adjunct Assistant Professor of the History of Medicine and Clinical Assistant Professor of Medicine at the University of Wisconsin in Madison, and Clinical Assistant Professor at the Medical College of Wisconsin in Milwaukee. He has had a long-standing interest in the literature and history of medicine, the history of cardiology, and the development and implementation of advances in diagnostics and therapeutics.

Address for correspondence: W. Bruce Fye, M.D., Department of Cardiology, Marshfield Clinic, 1000 North Oak Ave., Marshfield, WI 54449.

83 patients with fatty disease of the heart he or his colleagues had seen or whose cases had been previously published. He differentiated epicardial fat from the circumstance in which "the muscle fibre itself *degenerates* into molecular fatty matter," a condition he denoted "fatty degeneration." Quain believed this process had been overlooked in the past because the microscope was rarely used in studying the heart at autopsy. He sought to prove "that the molecular fatty matter in the fibre is the result of a chemical or physical change in the composition of the muscular tissue itself independent of those processes which we call vital."[7] Quain rejected the "vitalism" that had dominated medical and scientific thought for generations and sought to establish scientific truths through accurate observation.[9]

His study revealed the "close relation which exists between this condition [ossification of the coronary arteries] and fatty degeneration." In every heart with fatty degeneration examined, Quain found "the coronary arteries were more or less ossified or obstructed. . . . I have seen the coronary artery extremely ossified, going directly to the only part of the heart affected." Despite these important observations, Quain failed to appreciate the subtleties of the pathophysiology of coronary artery disease. He felt that the "degenerated condition of the heart's fibres is a very sufficient source in itself of the several phenomena (viz. breathlessness, faintness, and pain), which are recognized under the name of *angina pectoris,* or *syncope anginosa.*" In a recent review, the British pathologist A. D. Morgan concluded 52 of Quain's 83 cases probably represented ischemic heart disease.[10] Although Quain's report was enthusiastically reviewed it had little impact on clinical practice; microscopic examination of the myocardium and careful assessment of the patency of the coronary arteries would not become routine in autopsies for several decades.

Some mid-19th century writers recognized that coronary occlusion could result in fatty degeneration and cardiac rupture. Duben, a Swedish pathologist, reported this in 1859. A decade later the German pathologist Rindfleisch attributed fatty degeneration to "atheromatous degeneration of the coronary arteries with plugging of one of their larger branches by a thrombus . . . in every instance. . . ."[11] The American physician Austin Flint accepted Quain's theory of the causal relationship between coronary occlusion and "fatty degeneration" of the myocardium, but believed that other "general" rather than "local" causes could also account for this pathologic finding.[12] Flint recognized the serious nature of fatty degeneration and observed in 1870, "Fatty degeneration is . . . especially attended with notable disorder and danger. . . . It may prove fatal, by leading to rupture. Sudden death is liable to occur in an attack of syncope." Flint claimed the diagnosis of fatty degeneration "was not difficult" if the symptoms of feebleness, dyspnea on exertion, palpitations, and precordial distress were present "especially if the patient have passed the middle period of life, if his habits have been luxurious and indolent . . . if he have the *arcus senilis,* or if there be a tendency to obesity." Although Flint identified several "risk factors" for the development of coronary artery disease, it would be a mistake to credit him with the insight into ischemic heart disease this quotation might suggest. The symptoms he attributted to fatty degeneration of the heart are not specific for coronary artery disease and the antemortem diagnosis of coronary thrombosis had not yet been made.

The first reported case of coronary thrombosis recognized during life was published in 1878 by Adam Hammer. Hammer received his medical training in Germany, but emigrated to America in 1848 and settled in St. Louis where he became a successful practitioner and medical teacher.[13] Before his return to Europe in 1877, he discussed his case at a meeting of the German Medical Society of New York, but ". . . even the most learned Dr. [Abraham] Jacobi, who might well be called a walking dictionary of medicine, knew nothing of the disease."[14–16] After his return to Germany Hammer discovered that several prominent physicians, including Adolf Kussmaul, were unaware of a similar case. It is clear from the history and gross pathologic findings (there is no mention of a microscopic examination of the heart) that Hammer's was not a case of atherosclerotic coronary artery disease. An aortic valve vegetation with an attached thrombus had obstructed the coronary artery. Indeed, Hammer's explanation of how he reached the antemortem diagnosis of coronary thrombosis, and his brief description of the heart, fail to reveal any true insight into the relationship of acute coronary obstruction to myocardial necrosis. Nevertheless, Hammer hoped his case would stimulate interest among clinicians who might also recognize the condition before the death of the patient and experimental pathologists who "we would also expect . . . to study this matter in the near future."

Important advances in our understanding of the pathophysiology of ischemic heart disease can be traced to the pathology laboratory of Julius Cohnheim at the University of Leipzig.[17] Cohnheim had studied under Rudolf Virchow and continued his mentor's studies on thrombosis and embolism. William Osler, after a visit to Cohnheim's laboratory in 1884, characterized him as an experimental pathologist without rival in Europe. Another pupil of Virchow's, Carl Weigert, became Cohnheim's assistant in 1874 and made important contributions to the study of histology of thrombosis and embolism and these Cohnheim incorporated into the second edition of his pathology textbook that appeared in 1882.[18] When Cohnheim and Weigert arrived at Leipzig from the University of Breslau in 1878, they brought a new perspective according to Adolf Strümpell, assistant in the medical clinic at the time. He claimed, "For the first time the question of the etiology of disease was placed in the foreground."[19]

Weigert extended Virchow's and Cohnheim's studies on tissue injury and proposed the theory of coagulation necrosis, a term coined by Cohnheim. In an 1880 article Weigert discussed the pathologic appearance of infarcts in several organs including the heart. Based upon more than ten years of experiments, he claimed that passive tissue injury was the fundamental mechanism of cellular proliferation in inflammation. He applied his theory to the poorly understood histologic finding of "chronic myocarditis" and claimed,

> . . . with atheromatous changes of the coronary arteries thrombotic or embolic occlusions of their branches not infrequently occur. If the closures result slowly, or, more important still, in such a way that collateral channels, even though insufficient for nourishment, exist, there ensues a slower atrophy with disappearance of the muscle fibers, but without injury to the connective tissue. These destroyed muscle fibers are then replaced by fibrous tissue, and the so-called chronic myocarditis is nothing else but such a process. If, however, a very sudden complete cutting off of the blood supply occurs in certain parts of the heart, yellow dry masses entirely similar to coagulated fibrin result. Here also, however, microscopic examination reveals almost no fibrous exudate, but often an apparently quite normal tissue (even the cross-striations of the muscle fibers often recognizable) but all muscle fibers and all connective tissue are devoid of nuclei. A reactive infiltration of round cells and spindle cells is present in the vicinity.[20, 21]

Two years later, Carl Huber, Weigert's clinical colleague at Leipzig, published the histories of the patients who were found at autopsy to have had myocardial infarctions. Based upon Weigert's studies, Huber declared that angina pectoris and myocardial infarction were both manifestations of coronary artery disease.

Weigert's research led Cohnheim to claim, "It is now known that the very great majority of the myocarditic indurations . . . are due to an advanced sclerosis . . . of the coronary arteries supplying the affected part. . . . Furthermore, most pathologists are probably now unanimous in regarding numerous cases of fatty degeneration as the sequelae simply of severe coronary sclerosis. . . . The degeneration usually affects first the papillary muscles, next the subendocardial layer of muscle fibres, and finally, in extreme cases, the whole thickness of the muscular wall." Although Cohnheim believed, based on his experiments and those of others, that sudden occlusion of a coronary artery was usually fatal, he acknowledged that death was not inevitable. He wrote in 1882, "The occlusion of a coronary artery — in case it does not prove fatal . . . leads to the destruction of the contractile substance of that portion of the heart which is fed by the affected artery, and afterwards to the formation there of so-called myocarditic indurations."[22]

The pathologic observations of the Leipzig group had little impact on medical practice in the 1880s. The clinical event we now call acute myocardial infarction was occasionally described, but it was not distinguished from angina. The pathologic features of myocardial infarction were sometimes discovered at autopsy and were found to be associated with coronary occlusion, but the relationship of symptoms to pathologic findings remained obscure. Skilled diagnosticians still debated the pathophysiology of angina pectoris. An example is provided in the 1880 case report of a 62-year-old obese merchant who for two and a half years had "an oppression and constriction in the carotid regions, with a sense of *dread* while walking up hill." Dr. Frederick Winsor, a Harvard graduate, diagnosed "temporary exhaustion of the nervous centres" and advised rest. After a severe episode the patient was seen by the prominent Boston physician Henry Bigelow, who suggested the possibility of angina pectoris. The patient was kept in bed but had a three and one-half hour episode of precordial discomfort associated with irregularity of the pulse and pallor. The patient was treated with amyl nitrite and morphine and was thought to be recovering when, four days later, "he quietly died without pain or distress." At autopsy an apical aneurysm with cardiac rupture was found and "in the vicinity of the rent . . . the characteristic appearance of the muscle was lost, the muscular fibres being here filled with a granular material and in many places with minute fat drops." The coronary arteries were atherosclerotic and a thrombus occluded the left anterior descending artery. "The portion of the heart in which the rupture had occurred and in which the fibres were found degenerated corresponded to the territory supplied by the branches of this artery." Winsor and his consultants were surprised at these findings since they had "detected nothing wrong in the heart or lungs" the day after the severe episode and believed the patient would recover. Winsor observed, "I cannot see . . . how the diagnosis, prognosis, or treatment could have been improved on in light of our present knowledge. The case, however, goes to increase one's distrust of the accuracy of physical examination of the chest." In discussing the case, Dr. Richard Hodgdon "said that he considered angina pectoris a symptom or group of symptoms, and not a disease . . . and thought it 'unscientific to dignify with the name of a disease some symptoms which, between 1763 and 1832, received fifteen different names, implying nearly as many different origins of the symptoms.' "[23] It is clear that the pathophysiology of ischemic heart disease was poorly understood by practitioners a century ago.[24]

A major factor that made it difficult for physicians to distinguish the various ischemic heart disease syndromes we now recognize was the inconstant relationship of symptoms and pathologic findings. Samuel West, a British physician who had studied in Vienna and Berlin, wrote several articles on coronary artery disease in the 1880s and studied coronary anastamoses using injection techniques. He observed in 1883, "It is very remarkable how large an amount of obstruction there may be to both coronary arteries without any cardiac symptoms during life, or any gross pathological change recognisable in the muscle of the heart after death."[25] Cohnheim also noted the poor correlation of anatomy and symptoms, and wrote, "Now it is quite true, that in individuals who have suffered during life from *angina pectoris,* or perhaps succumbed to an attack, there has repeatedly been found *post mortem* a more or less extensive and advanced rigidity and sclerosis of the coronary arteries. Nevertheless, a true causal relationship need not therefore exist, especially as it often happens that no trace of disease is to be found in the coronary arteries of such subjects, and — what is still more common — that a very high degree even of coronary sclerosis is met with in persons who have never had an attack of angina." Cohnheim anticipated the eventual recognition of coronary artery spasm and spontaneous recanalization of a coronary thrombus when he claimed, "Even if the statistics telling in favour of a connection between both processes were more satisfactory than is really the case, this would be little to the purpose. It would always be open to suppose that the circulation through the coronaries, being already impeded, had been still further impaired by some transient accidental circumstance or other; such a supposition, however, is incapable of proof."[22, 26] Cohnheim's assessment was realistic in an era before electrocardiography and coronary arteriography. Only when techniques became available to objectively identify narrowing of the coronary arteries and myocardial ischemia would it be possible to correlate the symptoms of the various ischemic heart disease syndromes with the underlying anatomic and physiologic abnormalities.[27]

Other Europeans further elucidated the pathophysiology of ischemic heart disease in the 1880s. Ernst Ziegler, a Swiss pathologist, proposed the term "myomalacia cordis" for the pathologic changes that result from coronary occlusion. He described the evolution of histologic changes as the age of the infarction increased and declared that myocardial infarction was not invariably fatal. Ziegler wrote, "When the destructive process has gone a certain length, and death does not ensue, processes of repair are set up." The British physician Donald MacAlister, who translated Ziegler's text, claimed, "myomalacia cordis has hitherto received but little attention as an integral process; it has been treated under many and various partial names. Clinical observers generally confound it with myocarditis or with fatty degeneration; though it agrees in strictness with neither. The affection is really anaemic necrosis. . . . It is not a rare affection, and when at all extensive it brings about death by failure or rupture of the heart."[28, 29]

A valuable report that synthesized contemporary concepts of ischemic heart disease was published in 1884 by Ernst von Leyden, a Berlin physician and pathologist. He explained that while the emphasis on physical diagnosis had led to significant advances in the area of valvular heart disease, this approach was of limited value in myocardial disease. He encouraged his readers to pay more attention to the pathologic and physiologic alterations underlying the various ischemic heart disease syndromes. Leyden separated coronary artery sclerosis into four groups based on the pathologic findings and divided the clinical manifestations into acute, subacute, and chronic types.[30]

The Scottish physician and pathologist John Steven had studied with Weigert and Huber and was perplexed that their observations had received so little attention. Speaking of Byrom Bramwell's comprehensive monograph on heart disease published in 1884, Steven remarked, "in the long account of the etiology and pathology of the condition [fibroid degeneration], not a hint is given of the possible direct connexion which this lesion may have with disease of the coronary arteries or obstruction of these vessels."[31] Despite Quain's admonition a generation earlier, the heart was rarely carefully examined at autopsy. Samuel West observed in 1884 that "the coronary arteries are frequently overlooked in making an ordinary *post-mortem* examination."[25] Moreover, localized areas of myocardial scarring were "very likely to be overlooked unless all parts of the organ are completely sliced up" according to Hilton Fagge, a British physician and pathologist.[32] Fagge claimed to "have met with an exceptionally large number of instances of the localized fibroid disease" in the autopsy room of Guy's Hospital, although he claimed, "Clinically, fibroid disease and aneurism of the heart can very seldom, if ever, be diagnosed." These comments support the recent claim of pathologist A. D. Morgan: "Although ischaemic heart disease may have masqueraded in the nineteenth century as angina pectoris, fatty degeneration, rupture of the heart, cardiac aneurysm, fibroid degeneration or chronic myocarditis, there would seem to have been . . . quite a lot of it about."[10]

The publication of Stevens' review of coronary artery disease and the appearance of English translations of the pathology texts of Ziegler and Cohnheim in the late 1880s provided contemporary clinicians with summaries of the recent scientific observations on the pathophysiology of ischemic heart disease. The concept of myocardial infarction from a pathologic point of view was gradually making its appearance in the clinical literature of Europe, Great Britain, and America. William Osler discussed the pathophysiology of ischemic heart disease and suggested the possibility of short-term survival after coronary occlusion in 1889. He claimed

> The local disturbances of nutrition caused by the blocking of a terminal branch of a coronary artery produce the condition known as infarct of the heart. . . . The danger is not alone at the period of preliminary softening, but time gradually effects a transformation of the softened areas into fibrous tissue, which yield and lead in many cases to aneurism of the cardiac wall and rupture. . . . In a number of cases death occurs suddenly, without any premonition; in other cases, precordial distress, pain in the left side, and signs of cardiac trouble have preceded the fatal illness for days or even weeks.[33, 34]

In 1892 Osler declared, "A knowledge of the changes produced in the myocardium by diseases of the coronary vessels gives a key to the understanding of many problems in cardiac pathology."[35] Still, confusion about the causal relationship of pathologic findings to symptoms is apparent in contemporary publications. The American pathologist William Welch, who had studied with Cohnheim and Weigert in the mid-1880s, presented a specimen "in which a thrombus had formed in the apex of the left ventricle, a portion breaking off obstructed the anterior coronary artery completely, thus causing anaemia of the wall, coagulation necrosis, and a white infarction."[36] The pathologic observations were undoubtedly accurate, but the sequence of events described reveals a lack of understanding of the pathophysiology of myocardial infarction and its sequelae.

Pathologists continued to bemoan the lack of interest among clinicians in coronary artery disease. In 1893 Steven complained before the members of the British Medical Association, "Of late years the etiology and morbid anatomy of the lesions of the myocardium have been much studied, but it may well be doubted whether these important, and in many cases suddenly fatal, affections have received the attention they deserve from the clinical side." He emphasized the value of the recent discoveries reported at the International Medical Congress held the previous year in Berlin and claimed, "The wealth of pathological observation and experiment then recorded [on the disturbances of the myocardium] gave promise of abundant and early fruit in the fields of clinical research and practical medicine."[37] This congress was attended by 5000 representatives including 500 from the United States. Although von Recklinghausen delivered an important talk on myocardial diseases and there were other sessions devoted to heart disease, the topic that attracted the most attention was bacteriology, with its implications for public health and the practice of medicine and surgery.[38] The preoccupation of physicians with bacteriology in the closing years of the 19th century almost certainly contributed to the long delay between the important observations of Weigert, Cohnheim, Leyden, and others in the 1880s and the appreciation of the clinical relevance of their findings a generation later. Some individuals continued to focus on the heart, however, and studies on sudden death and experimental coronary occlusion by John MacWilliam, William Porter, and others ultimately led to the recognition of the spectrum of syndromes associated with coronary artery disease and myocardial ischemia.[39, 40]

One of the first antemortem diagnoses of myocardial infarction was reported in 1896 by George Dock, who had studied in Germany with Weigert, Huber, and Leyden after his graduation from the University of Pennsylvania School of Medicine in 1884. Dock claimed, "The epoch-making discovery of mediate auscultation engrossed the attention and diverted the minds of physicians especially toward the examination of the valves of the heart, and away from the muscle itself."[41] He attributed the renewed interest in the coronary arteries to the growing awareness of their significance in cases of sudden death and claimed, "From an early period physiologists and pathologists investigated the subject experimentally, with great advantage." Dock ascribed the tardy recognition of the importance of coronary artery disease among clinicians "to a peculiarity of the disease or diseases in question. From the nature of the cases hospital physicians see but a part of their course, and that not always the most important for a successful diagnosis." Dock anticipated the role Herrick would ultimately play when he declared, "It must, therefore, remain for those physicians in general practice who have an oversight of patients for long periods, and who at the same time have the sort of scientific zeal that influenced a Jenner to give the final touches to the pictures of coronary disease."

In 1896 William Osler delivered a series of lectures on angina pectoris in which he recounted recent experiments that were shedding light on the pathophysiology of ischemic heart disease. Although the theme of his lecture series was angina, Osler's comment that "the effect of plugging of the [coronary] artery is the production of what is known as an anaemic infarct, a well-recognized pathological condition, the consideration of which need not detain us" is revealing. He made no mention of the *clinical* counterpart of the "pathological condition" of myocardial infarction. The clinical features of what we recognize as acute myocardial infarction were described as part of a broad spectrum of angina pectoris. Osler was aware of the occurrence of coronary thrombosis, but believed this was fatal in virtually all instances; he characterized the left anterior descending artery as "artery of sudden death."[42] There was, however, a growing awareness that coronary occlusion was not invariably fatal. William Welch, Osler's colleague at Johns Hopkins and America's leading pathologist, declared in 1889, "Thrombosis of the coronary arteries is . . . an affection of great clinical importance."[43] After summarizing recent publications Welch claimed, "The main trunk of one of the two coronary arteries may be plugged by a thrombus without causing sudden death. . . . If the patient lives long enough, the usual, but not absolutely imperative, anatomical result . . . is infarction in the area supplied by the occluded artery." Although Welch believed "the symptoms associated with coronary thrombosis are those of the angiosclerotic heart, so that it is hardly possible to make a positive diagnosis of thrombotic occlusion of the coronary arteries," he proclaimed, "cardiac infarction . . . is more common than would appear from the meagre attention usually given to the subject in text-books, and is of much anatomical and clinical interest." Although at first reading the 1900 statement of a pragmatic Minnesota physician seems overly pessimistic, his conclusion was quite true. He claimed, "As regards diagnosis, there appears to be nothing characteristic in the symptoms nor physical signs in a case of thrombosis of the coronary arteries which would enable us to distinguish it from the heart in a case of general arteriosclerosis. We can here however console ourselves with the fact that could we diagnosticate the condition nothing could be done to avert the inevitable fatal termination of these cases."[44] It would be several decades before research would lead to the development of means to identify and treat the arrhythmias that are often the fatal event in ischemic heart disease.[39]

Ludwig Hektoen, a Chicago pathologist and Herrick's colleague, was almost certainly the author of an 1899 editorial, "Infarction of the Heart." Referring to the recent work of Porter and Baumgarten at Harvard, the writer claimed, "These experimental studies are very interesting, because they show more in detail what must happen in occlusion of the coronary arteries in the human heart. From the experience of pathologists cardiac infarction seems to be much more frequent than is indicated by the small amount of attention given to the subject in text-books of clinical medicine." Hektoen's concluding sentence reveals his understanding of the pathophysiology of coronary occlusion: "While cardiac infarction may be caused by embolism, it is caused much more frequently by thrombosis, and thrombosis again is usually secondary to sclerotic changes in the coronaries. . . ."[45, 46] The growing recognition that coronary occlusion was not invariably fatal led to a renewed interest in the debate over the functional significance of coronary anastomoses. Porter and several European investigators began studying this subject.[27] Two decades of research were finally resulting in a shift from the concept of inflammation to ischemia as the underlying mechanism of many of the symptoms and pathologic findings in cases of myocardial disease. A Philadelphia physician observed in 1906, "The comparative importance of myocarditis to other pathological changes in the heart muscle steadily diminish as knowledge increases. . . ."[47] The New York physician and pioneer electrocardiographer Alfred Cohn claimed in 1912, "While up to five or six years ago we concerned ourselves with valvular lesions . . . now we have come to regard the heart as a whole, and to lay more stress on its working muscular portions and less on its automatically acting valves."[48]

The European and American studies of the pathophysiology of ischemic heart disease were known to two Russian physicians, Obrastzow and Straschesko, when they published an article on coronary thrombosis in 1910. Obrastzow was a pathologist who had visited several European laboratories, including Virchow's.

After presenting cases with autopsy correlation, these authors concluded, "The differential diagnosis of coronary thrombosis from angina pectoris is made by the presence of status anginosus with coronary thrombosis and its absence with isolated attacks of angina pectoris. Although cardiac dysfunction occurs with angina pectoris, in the presence of coronary thrombosis, it does not remit with the termination of an angina attack but persists quosque ad finem vitae."[49, 50] The views of the Russians were known to, and shared by, James Herrick. Herrick matriculated at Rush Medical College in Chicago in 1885 and, after an internship at Cook County Hospital, entered private practice. He was appointed attending physician at Cook County, where he was actively involved in medical teaching. Herrick spent the summer of 1894 in Europe "to do some practical work in pathology and clinical diagnosis," and worked primarily with the pathologist Hans Chiari in Prague.[51] Writing from Europe, Herrick claimed, "It is somewhat comforting to find that we, in America, are not the only ones who sometimes err in matters of diagnosis. I have seen here the best of the teachers make mistakes. Perhaps the most instructive feature of it all is to see the interest the diagnostician takes in the autopsy, and his eagerness and readiness to profit by his errors. The European teachers certainly have a great advantage in having their mistakes corrected by autopsy."[52]

In 1910 Herrick complained to members of the American Medical Association that the image of an attack of angina pectoris and its subsequent course was so "fixed in the minds of many physicians that they are unable to admit any deviation from its details as consistent with this disease." He proposed that the attitude toward angina was "two narrow" and that, although it generally carried a grave prognosis, "the fatal termination may be deferred for years and, exceptionally, complete recovery seems to ensue." Herrick closed his presentation with the suggestion, "closer observation of the atypical cases, with collocation of the results with those of anatomic and experimental studies will lead to unifying knowledge concerning the pathogenesis of this disease, to greater precision in its recognition, and to more appropriate treatment."[53] Elsewhere, I have discussed the fact that Herrick was familiar with the experimental studies of coronary occlusion performed by Porter and extended by Joseph Miller of Chicago.[40] Miller, who was present during the reading of Herrick's 1910 report, commented that his recent experimental studies had demonstrated that pharmacologic interventions might alter the outcome of acute coronary occlusion. Like Herrick, Miller was an attending physician at Cook County Hospital so it is probable that the two discussed their mutual interest in ischemic heart disease. Through Miller, Herrick had a personal link to basic research on coronary occlusion. Moreover, the pathologist who performed autopsies on several of Herrick's patients, including the case in which Herrick first made the diagnosis of coronary thrombosis during life, was Ludwig Hektoen who had been interested in coronary artery disease for two decades. Herrick undoubtedly benefitted from his colleagues' experiences and counsel.

Herrick later claimed there were two lessons to be learned from his experiences leading to the widespread clinical recognition of coronary thrombosis: "the first was that all medicine needs periodic overhauling. We should avoid the paralyzing influence of the dead hand of tradition. . . . The second lesson was . . . that there was still room for sane, careful, bedside observation. Neither the all-time hospital clinician nor the laboratory worker had a just claim to proprietary ownership of productive, healthy doubt and skepticism. There was a place for all types of investigation. The laboratory, the ward, the library should all be regarded as workshops for observation, experiment, and logical thinking. The watchword should be cooperation."[54] Herrick admitted that when he initially presented his first case of coronary thrombosis in 1910 he "did not at once grasp the full significance" of it. By 1912, however, he had synthesized his views and presented them before the Association of American Physicians. His address was widely circulated when it was republished in the *Journal of the American Medical Association*. The purpose of Herrick's report was to "prove that sudden obstruction [of a coronary artery] is not necessarily fatal. Such proof is afforded by a study of the anatomy of the normal as well as the diseased heart, by animal experiment and by bedside experience." After a concise synopsis of the relevant European and American literature Herrick claimed, "experimentally, then, sudden death, even late death, is not a necessary consequence of obstruction of even large branches, such as the descending branch of a coronary artery." Herrick deduced from the work of others and from his own experience that survival after coronary thrombosis was a distinct possibility. It is this declaration that makes Herrick's achievement notable. Others had provided the experimental, clinical, and pathologic data that enabled Herrick to conclude "from a consideration of the clinical histories of numerous cases in which there has been careful autopsy control, from animal experiments and from anatomic study, that there is no inherent reason why the stoppage of a large branch of a coronary artery, or even of a main trunk, must of necessity cause sudden death. Rather may it be concluded that while sudden death often does occur, yet at times it is postponed for several hours or even days, and in some instances a complete, i.e., functionally complete, recovery ensues."

Clinicians had long complained of the difficulty of diagnosing coronary sclerosis during life. Herrick provided a pathophysiologic explanation of the broad spectrum of symptoms that might accompany coronary thrombosis: "The clinical manifestations of coronary obstruction will evidently vary greatly, depending on the size, location and number of vessels occluded. The symptoms and end-results must also be influenced by blood-pressure, by the condition of the myocardium not immediately affected by the obstruction, and by the ability of the remaining vessels properly to carry on their work, as determined by their health or disease. No simple picture of the condition can, therefore, be drawn." Herrick included two cases of his own and a description of the various symptoms he believed might accompany coronary thrombosis. He advocated absolute bed rest for patients thought to have suffered acute coronary thrombosis and claimed, "The hope for the damaged myocardium lies in the direction of securing a supply of blood through friendly neighboring vessels so as to restore so far as possible its functional integrity."[55] Earlier observers had come close to recognizing the syndrome of coronary thrombosis, but it remained for Herrick to synthesize the clinical observations and experimental results of more than half a century and thereby delineate the clinical manifestations of myocardial infarction.

Herrick recalled that his presentation on coronary thrombosis before the leading internists of the day "fell like a dud" and the publication of his manuscript "aroused no more comment than it did when it had been read six months before."[54] He claimed, "The fate of that early paper was a surprise to me and a keen disappointment. I did not realize, as I do now [1936], that in medical history, as in the history of the growth of ideas in general, while some new facts are accepted as soon as announced, or at least attract enough attention to be subjects for discussion, very often others are passed unnoticed or unapproved until again brought forward in more striking form or with more convincing proof and at a time when the medical world is more ready to listen."[56]

The application of the relatively new technique of electrocardiography to coronary artery disease provided Herrick with "more convincing proof" of the clinical event we call acute myocardial infarction. The electrocardiograph, developed by William Einthoven and Thomas Lewis, was introduced into America in 1909 at Mt. Sinai Hospital in New York by Alfred Cohn.[57] Cohn had studied with Thomas Lewis, as had another New Yorker, Bernard Oppenheimer, who with Lewis used the electrocardiograph to determine the origin of the heartbeat in the dog in 1910.[58] For the first decade after the electrocardiograph was introduced into clinical practice it was used almost exclusively to investigate cardiac arrhythmias.[59] Working at Mt. Sinai, Oppenheimer extended the scope of electrocardiographic studies to include abnormalities of the wave forms independent of cardiac arrhythmias.[60] When Oppenheimer reported his results in 1917, Emanuel Libman, who had made the only comment after Herrick's 1912 presentation on coronary thrombosis, mentioned the difficulty of recognizing coronary thrombosis clinically. Libman remarked, "An electrocardiograph examination might be of value in confirming the diagnosis." Herrick, also present for Oppenheimer's report, revealed to the audience that he and his colleagues in Chicago had been investigating the electrocardiographic manifestations of experimental coronary occlusion in dogs. Moreover, Herrick recognized a similarity between the electrocardiogram recorded from one of Oppenheimer's patients found at autopsy to have coronary thrombosis and "that which we got in dogs by ligating the left branch of the coronary artery."

Fred Smith, a recent graduate of Rush Medical College and Herrick's assistant, published the results of an electrocardiographic study of experimental coronary ligation in 1918.[61] This investigation was suggested by Herrick who observed,

> There is some hope that the work may assist in interpreting abnormal human electrocardiograms. The thought has been that if it can be proved that with a certain artery obstructed there is a definite lesion in the heart muscle or in the conducting system, and if with that lesion there is a definite electrocardiogram, may we not, when we encounter that abnormal electrocardiogram in the human being, particularly if he has had symptoms suggestive of coronary thrombosis, be able to state with a reasonable degree of certainty that the patient has had obstruction in a particular portion of the coronary system?[62]

After the publication, in 1918, of Smith's and Herrick's articles on coronary thrombosis and its recognition with the aid of the electrocardiogram, Herrick claimed, "There was a veritable flood of articles on this topic."[56] During the 1920s physicians made the diagnosis of coronary thrombosis with increasing frequency.[63] Through Herrick's efforts, they were more aware of the clinical features of this event, and the growing availability of the electrocardiograph allowed them to confirm the diagnosis. Herrick's perseverance had paid off; the impediments to the recognition of acute myocardial infarction outlined in the introduction to this article had been overcome.

It may seem hard to understand why it took clinicians more than half a century to incorporate the important scientific observations of European pathologists into clinical practice. The recent "discovery" of mitral valve prolapse is quite analogous to the delayed recognition of acute myocardial infarction. The new techniques of angiography and echocardiography were critical in identifying the source of the auscultatory abnormalities that had been recorded for decades but were poorly understood. Once there was a means to diagnose this condition it was possible to study the various manifestations of the syndrome and delineate its natural history. In each instance new technology provided the critical link between the observations of clinicians and pathologists. Only when there was a means to identify a pathologic condition during life could clinicians and pathologists begin a meaningful dialogue and systematically study the "new disease."

The diagnostic instruments employed by clinicians are the result of countless basic scientific discoveries, which further reveals the reliance of clinical medicine on basic research. The electrocardiogram was not developed as an aid to the diagnosis of myocardial infarction, but evolved from instruments designed to quantitate electric currents. Its potential value in the diagnosis of myocardial infarction was first appreciated by clinicians with thorough training in, and great respect for, pathology. Herrick provided clinicians with a new approach to the diagnosis of coronary thrombosis and an intellectual framework for conceptualizing survival after this event. When his colleagues failed to respond to his masterful description of the clinical manifestations of acute myocardial infarction, he was not deterred. He applied new techniques to the study of ischemic heart disease and helped establish the critical role of electrocardiography in identifying acute coronary occlusion. His intellectual curiosity and pragmatism led him to accept new experimental evidence to "avoid the paralyzing influence of the dead hand of tradition."[54, 64]

References

1. Wiggers CJ: Pathways of medical progress. Science **91:** 25, 1940
2. Leibowitz JO: The history of coronary heart disease. London, 1970, Wellcome Institute of the History of Medicine
3. Bloomfield AL: Coronary occlusion and myocardial infarction. *In* Bloomfield AL, editor: A bibliography of internal medicine: selected diseases. Chicago, 1961, University of Chicago Press, p 16
4. Willius FA: The historic development of knowledge relating to the coronary circulation and its disease: the nineteenth century. Mayo Clin Proc **21:** 77, 1946
5. Wrigley PFM: Ischaemic heart disease in the nineteenth century. Oxford Med Sch Gaz **14:** 158, 1962
6. Power D: Sir Richard Quain. *In* The compact edition of the dictionary of national biography. Oxford, 1975, Oxford University Press, p 2455
7. Quain R: On fatty diseases of the heart. Med Chirg Trans **33:** 121, 1850
8. Williams CJB: Memoirs of life and work. London, 1884, Smith, Elder, & Co.
9. Goodfield GJ: The growth of scientific physiology: physiological method and the mechanist-vitalist controversy, illustrated by the problems of respiration and animal heat. London, 1960, Hutchinson
10. Morgan AD: Some forms of undiagnosed coronary disease in nineteenth-century England. Med Hist **12:** 344, 1968
11. Rindfleisch E: A manual of pathological histology to serve as an introduction to the study of morbid anatomy (translated by Baxter EB). London, 1872, New Sydenham Society
12. Flint A: A practical treatise on the diagnosis, pathology, and treatment of diseases of the heart, ed 2. Philadelphia, 1870, Henry C. Lea
13. Ball JM: Dr. Adam Hammer, surgeon and apostle of higher medical education. J MO Med Assoc **6:** 155, 1909
14. Hammer A: Ein Fall von Thrombotischem Verschlusse Einer der Kranzarterien des Herzens. Weiner Med Wochenschr **28:** 97, 1878
15. Hammer A: Thrombosis of one of the coronary arteries of the heart diagnosed during life (translated by Workman J). Can J Med Sci **3:** 353, 1878
16. Lie JT: Centenary of the first correct antemortem diagnosis of coronary thrombosis by Adam Hammer (1818–1878): english translation of the original report. Am J Cardiol **42:** 848, 1978
17. Malkin HM: Julius Cohnheim (1839–1884): his life and contributions to pathology. Ann Clin Lab Sci **14:** 335, 1984
18. Cohnheim J: Vorlesungen über Allgemeine Pathologie, ed 2. Berlin, 1882, August Hirschwald
19. Morrison H: Carl Weigert. Ann Med Hist **6:** 163, 1924
20. Weigert C: Ueber die Pathologischen Gerinnungsvorgänge. Arch Pathol Anat (Virchow) **79:** 87, 1880
21. Benson RL: The present status of coronary arterial disease. Arch Pathol Lab Med **2:** 876, 1926
22. Cohnheim J: Lectures on general pathology (Translated from the German ed 2 by McKee AB). London, 1889, New Sydenham Society
23. Putney GE: Extracts from the records of the Middlesex East District Medical Society. Boston Med Surg J **103:** 398, 1880
24. Fye WB: Cardiology in 1885. Circulation **72:** 21, 1985
25. West S: Cases of complete obliteration of one coronary artery, with remarks upon the coronary circulation. Trans Pathol Soc London **35:** 110, 1884
26. MacAlpin RN: Coronary arterial spasm: a historical perspective. J Hist Med Allied Sci **35:** 288, 1980
27. Fye WB: Coronary arteriography — it took a long time! Circulation **70:** 781, 1984
28. Ziegler E: A text-book of pathological anatomy and pathogenesis (translated and edited by Macalister D). New York, 1887, William Wood & Co
29. Manion WC: Myocarditis: a review of the development of the concept. Med Ann D C **35:** 405, 1966
30. Leyden E: Ueber die Sclerose der Coronar-Arterien und die davon Abhängigen Krankheitszustände. Z Klin Med **7:** 459; 539, 1884
31. Steven JL: Lectures on fibroid degeneration and allied lesions of the heart, and their association with diseases of the coronary arteries. Lancet **2:** 1153; 1205; 1255; 1305, 1887
32. Fagge CH: The principles and practice of medicine. Philadelphia, 1886, P. Blakiston, Son & Co.
33. Osler W: Rupture of the heart. Med News **54:** 129, 1889 (This unsigned editorial is attributed to Osler by his bibliographer Maude Abbott).
34. Dock G: Historical notes on coronary occlusion: from Heberden to Osler. JAMA **113:** 563, 1939
35. Osler W: The principles and practice of medicine. New York, 1892, D. Appleton & Co.
36. Welch W: Diseases of the coronary arteries and alterations in the muscular walls of the heart. Proc Trans Pathol Soc Toronto **1:** 8, 1889

37. Stevens JL: The pathology of fibroid degeneration (fibrous transformation) of the heart, with twenty-one cases. J Pathol Bacteriol **2:** 190, 1894
38. Foster WD: A history of medical bacteriology and immunology. London, 1970, Heinemann
39. Fye WB: Ventricular fibrillation and defibrillation: historical perspectives with emphasis on the contributions of John MacWilliams, Carl Wiggers, and William Kouwenhoven. Circulation **71:** 858, 1985
40. Fye WB: Acute Coronary Occlusion Always Results in Death — or Does It? The Observation of William T. Porter. Circulation **71:** 4, 1985
41. Dock G: Notes on the coronary arteries. Ann Arbor, 1896, Inland Press
42. Osler W: Lectures on angina pectoris and allied states. New York, 1897, D. Appleton & Co.
43. Welch WH: Thrombosis and embolism. *In* Allbutt C, editor: A system of medicine. London, 1899, MacMillan & Co., VII, p 155
44. Rothrock JL: Thrombosis of the coronary arteries, with sudden death. St Paul Med J **2:** 515, 1900
45. Infarction of the heart. JAMA **33:** 919, 1899
46. Hektoen L: Embolism of the left coronary artery; sudden death. Med News **61:** 210, 1892
47. Daland J: Pathology and diagnosis of myocardial inflammations and degenerations. NY Med J **83:** 12, 1906
48. Cohn AE: Recent advances in anatomy and pathology of the heart from a clinical point of view. Am J Med Sci **142:** 558, 1911
49. Obrastzow WP, Straschesko ND: Zur Kenntnis der Thrombose der Koronararterien des Herzens. Z Klin Med **71:** 116, 1910
50. Muller JE: Diagnosis of myocardial infarction: historical notes from the Soviet Union and the United States. Am J Cardiol **40:** 269, 1977
51. Herrick JB: Memories of eighty years. Chicago, 1949, University of Chicago Press
52. Herrick JB: Letter[s] from Europe. JAMA **22:** 928; 999 and **23:** 120; 318, 1894
53. Herrick JB: Certain popular but erroneous notions concerning angina pectoris. JAMA **55:** 1421, 1910
54. Herrick JB: An intimate account of my early experience with coronary thrombosis. Am Heart J **27:** 1, 1944
55. Herrick JB: Clinical features of sudden obstruction of the coronary arteries. JAMA **59:** 2015, 1912
56. Herrick JB: Historical note. *In* Levy RL, editor: Diseases of the coronary arteries and cardiac pain. New York, 1936, The MacMillan Co., p 17
57. Burch GE, DePasquale NP: A history of electrocardiography. Chicago, 1964, Year Book Publishers
58. Lewis T, Oppenheimer BS, Oppenheimer A: The site of origin of the mammalian heart-beat; the pacemaker in the dog. Heart **2:** 147, 1910
59. Howell JD: Early perceptions of the electrocardiogram: from arrhythmia to infarction. Bull Hist Med **58:** 83, 1984
60. Oppenheimer BS, Rothschild MA: Electrocardiographic changes associated with myocardial involvement with special reference to prognosis. JAMA **69:** 429, 1917
61. Smith FM: The ligation of coronary arteries with electrocardiographic study. Arch Intern Med **22:** 8, 1918
62. Herrick JB: Thrombosis of the coronary arteries. JAMA **72:** 387, 1919
63. Wearn JT: Thrombosis of the coronary arteries, with infarction of the heart. Am J Med Sci **165:** 250, 1923
64. Harvey AM: Classics in clinical science: from horse and buggy doctor to clinical investigation: the story of James Bryan Herrick. Am J Med **68:** 639, 1980

Local changes in myosin types in diseased human atrial myocardium: a quantitative immunofluorescence study

PATRICE BOUVAGNET, M.D., JOCELYNE LÉGER, PH.D., CLAUDE A. DECHESNE, GEORGES DUREAU, M.D.,* MONIQUE ANOAL, AND JEAN J. LÉGER, PH.D.

ABSTRACT Two monoclonal antibody groups were prepared from adult human atrial and ventricular myosin heavy chains. Using these two groups, we were able to identify two myosin variants in human atria and to classify human atrial fibers into α-, mixed, or β-fibers according to the reactivity of the two monoclonal antibody groups to α- and β-myosin heavy chains of normal young and hypothyroid rat ventricles, respectively. The α-fiber percentage of the left atria in two normal human hearts was 15% higher than in the right atria. The auricles contained two to three times more α-fibers than β-fibers, whereas the proportion was reversed in the crista terminalis. The mean fiber diameter of the α- and β-fibers was 13.6 ± 3 μm. A complete α- to β-fiber transition was observed in all atrial regions of two hearts with severe ventricular myocardial infarction; a moderate α- to β-fiber transition was observed only in the left atria of two hearts with primary congestive cardiomyopathy. The mean diameters of the two fiber types were significantly increased in all diseased hearts (19 ± 3.8 μm). We hypothesize that pressure overload and increased wall tension successively induce an enlargement of the fiber diameter and an α- to β-myosin transition.
Circulation **72, No. 2, 272–279, 1985.**

AT LEAST TWO molecular variants of myosin heavy chains have been identified in normal human atrial myocardium by histochemical and indirect immunofluorescence studies involving polyclonal and monoclonal antibodies.[1-4] We have referred to the human atrial myosin, which reacts strongly with one set of our monoclonal antibodies, as "β-like" atrial myosin since this set of monoclonal antibodies strongly reacts with ventricular β-myosin in hypothyroid rats.[3] This human atrial β-like myosin variant has been separated from the other myosin form by immunochromatography, and it has been shown that each form of human atrial myosin has a different primary structure but the same high enzymatic activity in vitro.[5] No direct evidence concerning any immunologic cross-reactivity of the other human atrial myosin with rat ventricular α-myosin is available at present. The fibers containing either β-like myosin or the other myosin form are not randomly distributed within the different regions of the atria in normal hearts, and marked changes in their local distributions have been described in diseased human hearts.[2, 3] Neither the distribution of the two fiber types in the different atrial regions nor their pathologic modifications have ever been quantified.

In this study we used, for the first time, two groups of monoclonal antibodies that specifically detect each atrial myosin variant in the rat heart as well as in the human heart. We also quantified the fiber type distributions within different regions of the atria in two normal and four diseased human hearts. In the latter, different isomyosin distributions were shown to be related to different pathologic conditions.

Materials and methods

Patients. Four adult human hearts were obtained from three recipients of cardiac transplants (denoted as hearts A, B, and C) (Cardiological Hospital of Lyon) and from a patient who died at the coronary care unit (denoted as heart D) (Cardiological Department, St. Eloi Hospital, Montpellier). The atria from these hearts were compared with the atria from two 16-year-old boys who died in traumatic accidents (denoted as hearts N1 and N2) (Nephrology and Urology Departments, Hospital St. Charles, Montpellier). Informed consent was obtained from the patients or from the patients' families.

Patients A and B had primary congestive cardiomyopathies.

From the Institut National de la Santé et de la Recherche Medicale, Montpellier et Lyon, France.

Supported in part by "L'Institut de la Recherche Medicale" and by "la Fondation de la Recherche Medicale."

Address for correspondence: Patrice Bouvagnet, M.D., INSERM U249. LPM2, Institut de Biologie, Bld. Henri IV, 34000 Montpellier, France.

Received Oct. 15, 1984; revision accepted April 11, 1985.

*Present address: INSERM U37. 18, avenue du doyen Lépine, 69500 Bron, France.

They underwent heart transplantation because of progressive heart failure despite maximum dosages of digitalis, diuretics, and vasodilators. Patient C had two myocardial infarctions (13 years and 1 year before transplantation) involving, as seen on gross examination, the posterior basal wall and the posterior papillary muscle of the left ventricle. While waiting for a suitable donor, patient C developed a congestive heart failure that was treated with digoxin, a diuretic, and a vasodilator, but his health continued to deteriorate rapidly. No cardiac catheterization was performed before heart transplantation. Patient D had a massive anterior apical myocardial infarction at the age of 47. A ventricular aneurysmectomy was performed 11 years after infarction. He died at the hospital from heart failure. His medications included digoxin, furosemide, isosorbide dinitrate, and amiodarone. The last medication was required because of numerous premature ventricular beats. Shortly before death, a hyperthyroid function was diagnosed. Clinical data for the four patients are summarized in table 1.

Preparation of tissue. Hearts from patients A, B, and C were immediately weighed and examined after their removal. The three other hearts were obtained within 2 hr after death. If available, at least seven different tissue samples were excised from the following areas of the atria: three samples from the right atrium (auricle, anterior trabeculated wall, and crista terminalis), three samples from the left atrium (auricle, posterior and superior free wall), and a sample from the interatrial septum. Because of cardiac transplantation requirements, only four atrial samples were excised from each of the three recipients' hearts (hearts A, B, and C) and compared with homologous regions of the heart obtained at necropsy (heart D) and with the two normal hearts (hearts N1 and N2). All atrial samples were frozen within 3 hr after death.

Experimental model. Normal Wistar rats (6 weeks old) and hypothyroid rats from the same strain (5 mg of propylthiouracil forcibly fed daily for 4 weeks) were killed by a sharp blow on the neck. The hearts were rapidly removed, and the samples were excised and processed like the human samples. These animals were chosen because, according to Hoh et al.,[6] the normal young rat ventricle is mainly composed of α-myosin heavy chain, whereas the hypothyroid rat ventricle is mainly composed of β-myosin heavy chain.

Monoclonal antibodies. Human ventricular myosin and one of the human atrial myosins were successively used as immunogens to obtain different populations of antimyosin monoclonal antibodies. The ventricular myosin used as an immunogen for the first generation of monoclonal antibodies was extracted from the left ventricle of a 53-year-old woman who had a hypertrophic obstructive cardiomyopathy. Mice immunization, fusion, screening, and cloning of the hybridoma cell cultures have been described in detail elsewhere.[3] By indirect immunofluorescence, it has been observed that some of these antiventricular myosin monoclonal antibodies react heterogeneously with the atrial fibers of normal human hearts.[3] Furthermore, a few of them react strongly with the ventricular fibers of hypothyroid rat hearts, which mainly contain the β-type ventricular myosin heavy chain,[3] and react weakly or not at all with the ventricular fibers of normal young rat hearts. This set of monoclonal antibodies, which are specific for the β-type rat ventricular myosin and react with one of the human atrial myosins, are hereafter referred to as anti-β Mab. To further check the specificity of the antibodies, total muscle extracts of normal and hypothyroid rat ventricles were first purified by sodium dodecyl sulfate polyacrylamide gel electrophoresis and then blotted on nitrocellulose paper. After incubation with anti-β Mab, the immune band was revealed by rabbit antimouse immunoglobulin G coupled with peroxidase.[3–5]

Atrial myosin was prepared from a fraction of the left atrium of a normal patient (N1) and applied on affinity columns with one of the anti-β Mab.[5] The atrial myosin fraction that did not react with the anti-β Mab did not fix to the column and was used as an immunogen to produce the second population of monoclonal antibodies. The same procedures as above[3] were used for production of hybridoma. A few of the resulting antibodies were selected according to their cross-reactivity with the ventricular fibers of a normal rat, which mainly contain α-type ventricular myosin heavy chains; these monoclonal antibodies are hereafter referred to as anti-α Mab (see Results). The specificity of this group of antibodies was also verified by immunoblots.

Immunofluorescence. Tissue samples were kept frozen at $-80°$ C until used. Sections (4 to 6 μm) were cut in a cryostat at $-20°$ C. Indirect immunofluorescence was performed according to the method of Gorza et al.[7] with fluorescein- or rhodamine-labeled rabbit antimouse IgG specially prepared to avoid nonspecific cross-reaction with human tissue (Nordic Immunological Laboratories, Tilburg, The Netherlands). Some anti-β Mab were coupled to fluorescein isothiocyanate[8] (FITC) (Nordic Immunological Laboratories). For indirect/direct immunofluorescence labeling, sections were processed for indirect immunofluorescence as usual, then the sections were adsorbed with 1/10 diluted nonimmune mouse serum for 30 min at 37° C. After a 5 min wash with phosphate-buffered saline (PBS), an FITC-coupled monoclonal antibody was added and sections were incubated for 30 min at 37° C. The sections were rinsed 10 min with two changes of PBS, then 10 min with 2% PBS-formaldehyde, and were finally mounted. The incubation with nonimmune mouse serum was performed to block excess rabbit antimouse binding sites.[9]

Sections were examined under a Leitz Orthoplan microscope with epifluorescence optics equipped with Ploemopak filter sets containing specific filter combinations for fluorescein and rhodamine. Controls of immunofluorescence were performed by successively omitting one of the steps in the procedures or by incubating sections with a cell culture supernatant either without monoclonal antibodies or containing an antibody to renin (a generous gift from B. Pau). These controls enabled us to verify the absence of any contaminating cross-reactions.

Fiber counting. To quantitate variations in the proportion of the different fiber types detected by each population of monoclonal antibodies within the different regions of the normal

TABLE 1
Cardiac characteristics of patients

	Patients			
	A	B	C	D
Age (yr)	43	50	55	62
Sex	M	M	M	M
Auscultation	GR	GR	MI	GR MI
Echocardiographic data				
Left atrial diameter (mm)	40	40	60	55
Left ventricular diameter (mm)	82/74	75/69	80/73	74/60
Hemodynamic data				
LVEDP (mm Hg)	36	12	—	35
Heart weight (g)	560	640	440	480
Diagnosis	PCC	PCC	IHD	IHD

GR = gallop rhythm; IHD = ischemic heart disease; LVEDP = left ventricular end-diastolic pressure; MI = mitral insufficiency; PCC = primary congestive cardiomyopathy.

atria, we arbitrarily formed three groups of fibers according to their isomyosin content: α-fibers, mixed, and β-fibers (see Results). A point-counting method with a test grid[10] was carried out on photomicrographs of randomly selected areas within well-defined atrial regions. We counted the different fiber-type contents in 10 to 20 nonserial sections of the same tissue region. This method was repeated on each sample from the normal and diseased hearts. The difference between the percentages of each fiber group on repeated measurements by two trained observers was less than 10%.

Morphometry. The fiber diameter of atrial cells was measured on photomicrographs of cross and oblique sections of myocardial cells (magnification ×200). When oblique sections were used, the shortest diameter of the fiber profile was measured. Fiber diameters were measured on four to 10 nonserial sections of each tissue sample. More sections were needed for α-fibers in the auricles of hearts C and D because these fibers were extremely rare.

Statistical analysis. Student's t test for unpaired data was used. Data are expressed as mean ± SD.

Results

Specificity of monoclonal antibodies. The two groups of monoclonal antibodies were raised in mice injected either with adult human ventricular myosin[3] or with one of the adult human atrial myosins purified by affinity chromatography with an antihuman ventricular myosin monoclonal antibody.[5] Preliminary immunoreplicate or immunofluorescence experiments were made to select, from among the numerous monoclonal antibodies available after each fusion, those that differentially reacted on normal young rat ventricles mainly containing α-myosin heavy chain, as opposed to hypothyroid rat ventricles mainly containing β-myosin heavy chains. This classification corresponds to the terminology adopted by Hoh et al.[6] for designating the two types of myosin heavy chains present in rat ventricles. Thus, according to the results of immunoblotting experiments, monoclonal antibodies strongly reacting with normal young rat myosin heavy chains and reacting poorly or not at all with hypothyroid rat myosin heavy chains were selected and referred to as anti-α Mab. Similarly, the monoclonal antibodies strongly reacting with hypothyroid rat myosin heavy chains and reacting poorly or not at all with normal young rat myosin heavy chains were selected and referred to as anti-β Mab[3,5] (data not shown). The group of anti-α Mab used in the immunofluorescence experiments reacted strongly and homogeneously with the ventricular fibers of normal young rat hearts but poorly and heterogeneously with those of hypothyroid rat hearts (figure 1, *a* and *c*); the group of anti-β Mab reacted in a complementary way with the anti-α Mab group in both types of rat ventricle (figure 1, *b* and *d*). At all antibody dilutions, many fibers in the hypothyroid rat ventricle did not react at all with the anti-α Mab (figure 1, *c*), whereas many fibers in the normal young rat hearts did not react at all with the anti-β Mab (figure 1, *b*). These results indicate that the anti-α and the anti-β Mab did not cross-react with either the β- or the α-myosin heavy chains, respectively. Any fiber strongly stained with the anti-α Mab but not reacting with the anti-β Mab consequently does not contain β-myosin heavy chains and is referred to here as an α-fiber. Similarly, any fiber strongly stained with the anti-β Mab but not reacting with the anti-α Mab is referred to here as β-fiber. Some other fibers in the hypothyroid rat ventricles and in the normal young rat ventricles were stained at various immunofluorescent levels with either the anti-α or the anti-β Mab, respectively, whereas they were all strongly stained with either the anti-β or the anti-α Mab, respectively; these fibers are referred to here as mixed fibers since they apparently contained variable amounts of α- and β-myosin heavy chains (if not other).

Normal human atria. Most of the monoclonal antibodies so selected in each hybridoma group reacted in a heterogeneous way with transverse sections of normal human atrial fibers in regions previously known for their myosin heterogeneity.[3] The specificity of the two groups of antibodies permitted a classification of human atrial fibers according to their myosin content. Figure 2 shows an atrial section of the posterior free wall of a normal human left atrium (patient N1), indirectly stained with an anti-α Mab and rhodamine then further stained with an anti-β Mab coupled to fluorescein. As with the rat ventricles, the human atrial fibers that were intensely stained with the anti-α Mab (arrowhead in figure 2, *a*) but not with the anti-β Mab (arrowhead in figure 2, *b*), were called α-fibers since they presumably contained only the α-like type of human atrial myosin. Conversely, the human atrial fibers that were not reactive with the anti-α Mab (arrow in figure 2, *a*) but were intensely stained with the anti-β Mab (arrow in figure 2, *b*) were called β-fibers since they presumably contained only β-like human atrial myosin. Besides these extreme situations, a significant number of human atrial fibers were intermediately stained with both antibody groups. These atrial fibers, hereafter denoted as mixed fibers, presumably contained a mixture of the α- and β-like human atrial myosin. It should be noted that some fibers that were strongly and equally stained with one type of antibody (see fibers in the top left corner of figure 2, *a*) exhibited different degrees of intermediate staining with the other type of antibody (figure 2, *b*). This was observed repeatedly on sections from different samples of normal atria.

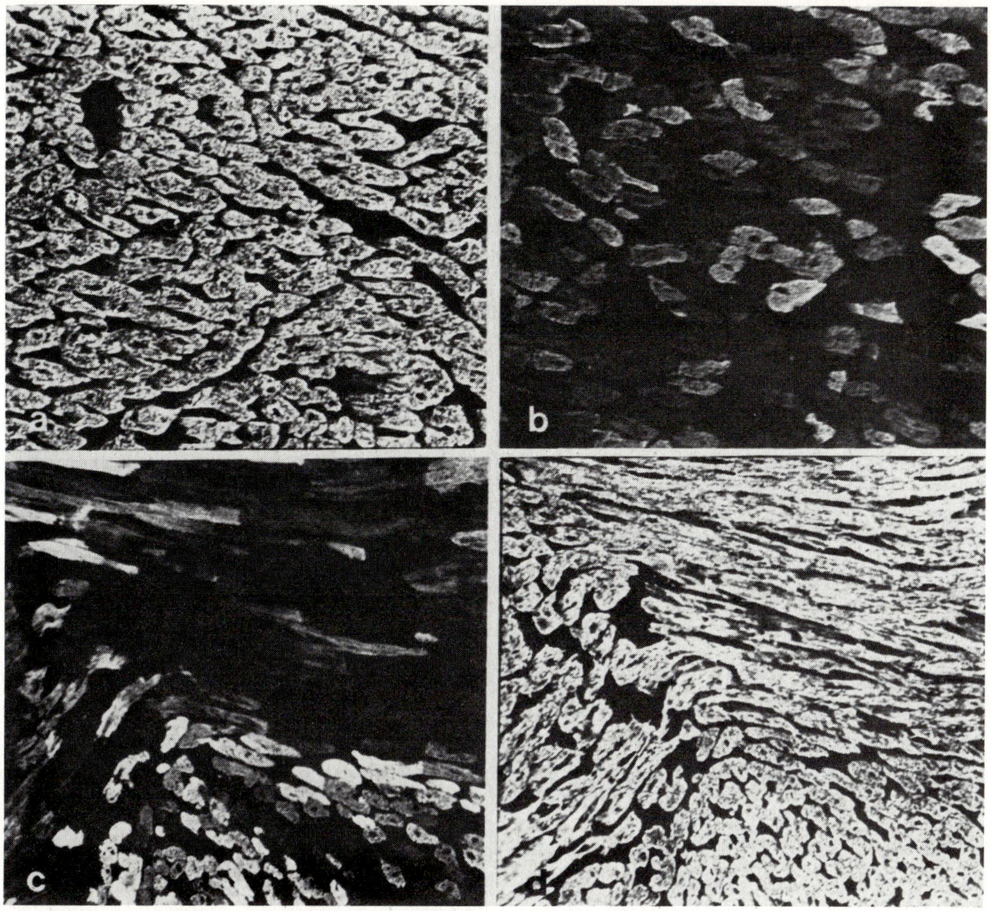

FIGURE 1. Serial sections of the left ventricle of a normal young rat (*a* and *b*) and of a hypothyroid rat (*c* and *d*) stained with an anti-α Mab (*a* and *c*) or with an anti-β Mab (*b* and *d*) (see Materials and methods).

The anatomic description of atrial myosin distribution in normal human hearts, previously made with the anti-β Mab,[3] was corroborated in this study by the anti-α Mab. We also attempted a quantification of the percentages of α- and β-fibers contained in limited areas randomly selected within the atria, using a point-counting method.[10] Of the total fibers in the atrial areas studied in the two normal hearts, 20% to 35% were mixed and at present are not classifiable as either α- or β-fiber types. Within this limitation and the 10% margin of error observed for the quantitation measurements, a mean fiber distribution corresponding to a

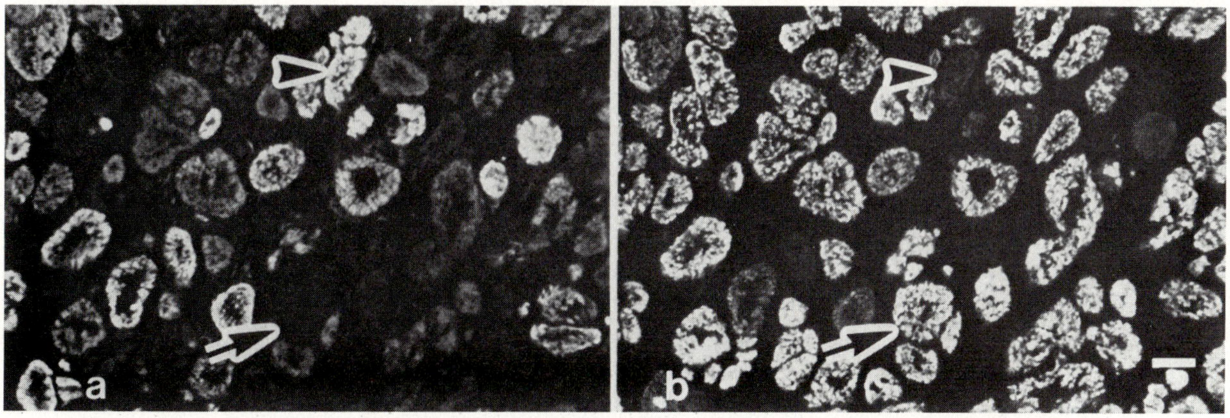

FIGURE 2. Section of the posterior wall of a normal human left atrium stained simultaneously with an anti-α Mab (*a*) and with an anti-β Mab (*b*). The reactivity of each fiber with these two types of monoclonal antibody allowed a classification into α- (arrowhead), mixed, and β-fibers (arrow). (Bar = 20 μm.)

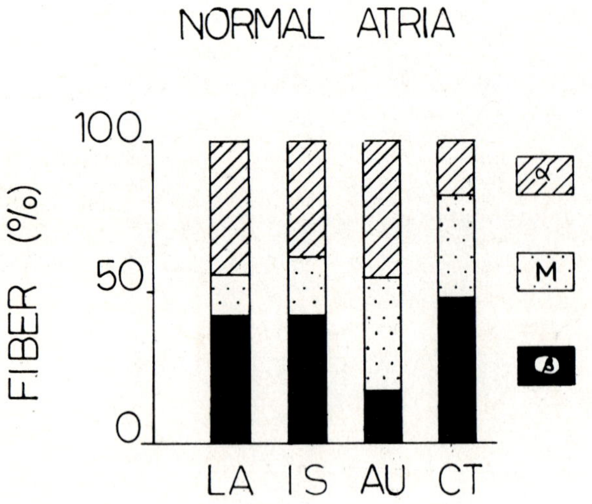

FIGURE 3. Percentage of each fiber type evaluated on sections from four atrial regions in the two normal hearts. α = α-fiber; M = mixed fiber; β = β-fiber; LA = left atrium; IS = interatrial septum; AU = auricle; CT = crista terminalis.

balanced number of α- and β-fibers, roughly 40% each, was observed over large regions of normal left and right atria. Slight variations around this mean fiber distribution were observed in some regions in the left and right atria and in the interatrial septa. The total number of α-fibers was about 15% less in the right atria than in the left, and no significant individual variation was observed. The most extreme fiber distributions were observed in both auricles and in the crista terminalis of the right atrium; the β-fiber content in both auricles was about 18%, whereas the α-fiber content was more than 45%. The β-fiber content of the crista terminalis in the right atrium was about 50%, while the α-fiber content was 20%. Figure 3 and table 2 present these "typical" fiber distributions. The measurements of the mean fiber diameter indicated that the diameters of the α- and β-fibers were roughly the same in all atrial regions (table 3).

Diseased human hearts. The same two groups of monoclonal antibodies applied to atrial sections from the four diseased human hearts allowed the same fiber classification into α-, mixed, and β-fibers as in the normal hearts. The same method of quantitating the different fibers indicated a significant increase in the percentages of the β-fibers in the atria of the four diseased hearts. Moreover, the diseased hearts could be separated into two groups according to their fiber distributions and according to their pathologic history. The left atria from hearts A and B with primary congestive cardiomyopathy showed a significant and similar increase in their β-fiber content. Their mean fiber distribution roughly corresponded to an α-fiber content of 25%, mixed fibers 15%, and β-fibers 60%, which was significantly different from the mean distributions observed in both normal hearts (figure 4 and table 2). The interatrial septa also showed this shift to an increased β-fiber content. Curiously, the left auricles and the anterior walls of the right atria of hearts A and B contained the same fiber distributions as the corresponding atrial regions in both normal hearts. Atria from the ischemic hearts C and D exhibited a dramatic shift in their fiber distribution, since all atrial regions had fiber distributions corresponding to 98% to 100% β-fibers (figure 4 and table 2). For example, the fiber most reactive with the anti-α Mab (figure 5, *a*, arrow) is the unique weakly reactive fiber on the serial section processed with the anti-β Mab (figure 5, *b*, arrow). Surprisingly, some of these atrial fibers still exhibited various degrees of fluorescence after labeling with the anti-α Mab, although they did not differ with respect to brightness after labeling with the anti-β Mab. The mean fiber diameters were the same in the four diseased hearts and did not differ between the α- and β-fibers. However, the fiber diameters of the diseased atria were significantly larger than those of the atrial fibers in the two normal hearts (table 4).

Discussion

On the basis of the results presented here and in three recent articles,[3-5] one can postulate that normal human atria contain at least two types of structurally

TABLE 2
Percentage of α-, mixed, and β-fibers evaluated in four different atrial regions of two normal and four diseased hearts

	Left atrium			Interatrial septum			Auricle			Crista terminalis		
Hearts	α	M	β	α	M	β	α	M	β	α	M	β
N1	45	20	35	38	25	37	47	33	20	16	31	53
N2	44	18	38	39	23	38	44	40	16	27	30	43
A	22	12	66	20	16	64	44	27	29	21	28	51
B	24	15	61	16	16	68	41	36	23	22	20	58
C	1	1	98	0	1	99	3	5	92	0	1	99
D	1	0	99	0	1	99	2	2	96	0	0	100

TABLE 3
Comparison of the mean fiber diameters of α- and β-fibers in three regions of normal atrium (mean ± SD)

Fiber types	Left atrium: Posterior wall (n = 60)	Left atrium: Auricle (n = 60)	Right atrium: anterior wall (n = 60)	Mean[A] (n = 180)
α (μm)	15.8±3.8	12.0±1.7	13.2±2.2	13.8±3
β (μm)	14.4±3.5	12.1±3.1	13.2±2.2	13.4±2.9

n values refer to the number of measurements made on each atrial specimen.

[A]Mean diameter of α- and β-fibers in all regions together.

different myosin heavy chains, each immunologically related to the α- and β-myosin heavy chains detected in the ventricular myocardia of normal young and hypothyroid rats,[6] respectively. This α- and β-like classification of myosin heavy chains within human atria clearly results from the specificity of the two groups of monoclonal antibodies used; these results extend the previous histochemical and immunologic observations of myosin heterogeneity within human atria.[1, 2] We know that human atrial and ventricular β-myosins have different light and heavy chains and different enzymatic activities in vitro.[5] The relationship between the structures of the α-myosin heavy chains present in human atria and ventricles is still unknown, although the two human cardiac myosins have different light chains.[5] To summarize, in human atria as well as in human ventricles,[1–5, 11] and more generally in the atria and ventricles of most mammalian hearts (for a review see refs. 12 and 13), two different genes that code for α- and β-myosin heavy chains can be expressed.

The availability of monoclonal antibodies that react specifically to each atrial myosin heavy chain type makes it feasible to classify at least 70% of the total atrial fibers into pure α- or β-myosin–containing fibers and to study isomyosin transition within human hearts. With both sets of antibodies it is possible to detect the simultaneous presence of the two types of atrial myosin heavy chains within a fiber on serial sections and to evaluate its content in terms of myosin types. As previously suggested by Schiaffino et al.[14] and demonstrated here, the strong reactivity of an atrial fiber with an antibody specific for the α- or β-heavy chain, for example, cannot be taken as an indication that this particular fiber contains only the α- or β-heavy chain. Our use of antibodies specific for α-myosin heavy chain shows that the same fibers in fact contain some amounts of α-myosin heavy chain (see figure 5). The availability of two specific populations of monoclonal antibodies, together with the high sensitivity of immunofluorescence in detecting myosin components, finally enables us to monitor isomyosin transition within individual muscle fibers. The presence of a third myosin heavy chain, immunologically related to the previously described human atrial α- and β-myosin heavy chains, cannot be totally excluded by the present experiments. This situation has already been described in normal rat[15, 16] and human ventricles.[3] Additional experiments are needed to verify this hypothesis.

The second conclusion of our study concerns the quantification of local fiber changes. These regional fiber variations with regard to their myosin content have already been demonstrated within human and bovine atria by polyclonal or monoclonal sera specific for the β-myosin heavy chains.[2, 3, 7] However, the fiber distributions observed in the two human atrial studies differ in large regions of the left atrium and interatrial septum. With our dual monoclonal antibody system, we observed that a very balanced mixture of α- and β-fibers characterizes the overall mean fiber distribution in both atria and in the interatrial septa of normal human hearts, whereas the right atrium contains roughly 15% more β-fibers than the left atrium. In contrast, Gorza et al.,[2] using polyclonal antibodies that did not detect atrial α-fibers in normal human hearts, indicated that atrial fibers staining for the β-myosin heavy chains were rare in the left atrium and particularly abundant in the right atrium and the interatrial septum. These apparent quantitative discrepancies with respect to the regional distributions of myosin types in the human atrium could be caused by the complexity of

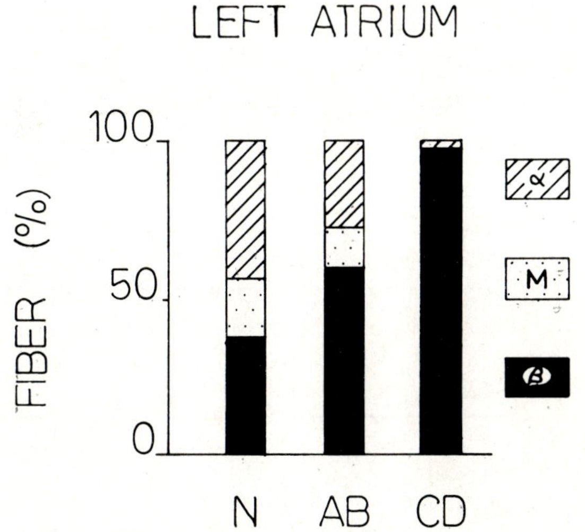

FIGURE 4. Percentage of each fiber type evaluated on sections of the left atria of normal (N) and diseased hearts (A, B, C, and D). Abbreviations as in figure 3.

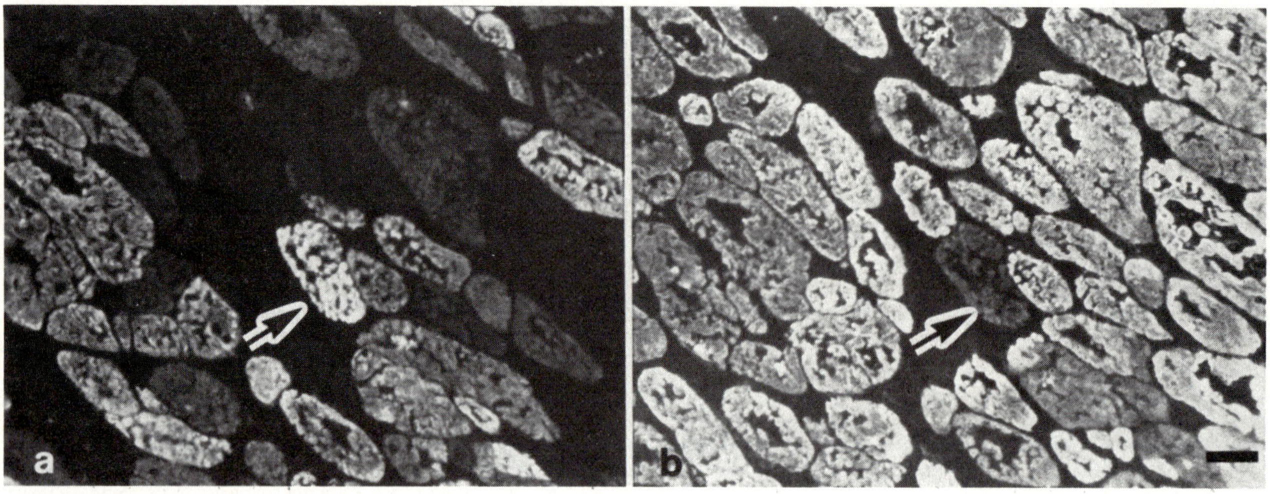

FIGURE 5. Two serial sections of the left atrium of heart C processed for immunofluorescence with anti-α Mab (*a*) and anti-β Mab (*b*). Note that the α- to β-myosin transition is nearly complete in all fibers except one (arrow). (Bar = 20 μm.)

the mixture of polyclonal immunoglobulins; the mixture was raised from myosin prepared from human skeletal pectoralis muscle and absorbed on bovine left atrial myosin, and both myosin preparations were a mixture of different myosin types.[7, 17] In our study, additional cross-reactivities resulting from the use of different animal species or muscles as immunogens have been partially avoided in each antibody group, since the antibodies were prepared from human ventricular myosin or from a purified fraction of human atrial myosin. Only a quantitative determination of the myosin content within each fiber would resolve these discrepancies.

The local changes in distribution of atrial fiber types and their quantification within four diseased human hearts provide new information on the possible physiologic meaning of the local expression of atrial α- and β-myosin genes. These four atria, all of which had a hemodynamic pressure overload, contained significantly more β-fibers than did the normal human atria. This transition from α- to β-myosin heavy chains has been described previously in the hypertrophic ventricles of many animal hearts that have been experimentally submitted to a volume-pressure overload, and recently in diseased human hearts.[2] Curiously, this myosin-type transition in response to sustained mechanical or hormonal stress has not, to date, been detected in animal atria.[18] In our study the levels and the localizations of the atrial myosin transitions in hearts A and B were different from those in hearts C and D. The α- to β-fiber transition was nearly complete in all atrial regions of hearts C and D, which sustained ventricular myocardial infarctions. In contrast, a moderate but significant increase in the β-fiber content, compared with that of normal atria, was observable only in the left atria (minus the left auricles), and not in the right atria of hearts A and B, which had congestive cardiomyopathies. These differences in the myosin gene expression are presumably related to pathologic differences between the four hearts. Patients A and B differed in cardiac characteristics from patients C and D; patients C and D had murmurs from mitral insuffi-

TABLE 4
Comparison of the diameters of α- and β-fibers (mean ± SD) in the auricles of the normal (N1 and N2) and diseased hearts (A, B, C, and D)

	Hearts				
Fiber types	N1 and N2 (n = 60)	A (n = 60)	B (n = 60)	C (n = 60)	D (n = 60)
α (μm)	12.0±1.7	20.5±4.1	19.8±3.2	18.5±3.1	17.6±3.2
β (μm)	12.1±3.1	18.4±3.5	18.5±4.1	19.7±2.9	17.6±3.7
Mean (μm)[A]	12.1±2.4	19.5±3.9[B]	19.2±3.8[B]	19.1±3.0[B]	17.6±3.5[B]

n values refer to the number of measurements made on each atrial sample.
[A]Value obtained when α- and β-fiber diameters of each auricle were pooled.
[B]$p < 10^{-4}$.

ciency and their left atria were larger, as observed by echocardiography. On the other hand, patients A and B had heavier hearts. The difference in the pathogenesis of cardiac overload explains the heavier hearts in patients A and B; the large scars of ventricle necrosis in hearts C and D were responsible for the relatively smaller increase in heart weight. The difference in pathogenesis is presumably not involved in the β-fiber transition; the atria of hearts C and D as well as those of hearts A and B were free of necrosis. The main pathologic difference between the atria of the hearts A and B and those of hearts C and D is presumably a difference in the tension of the atrial walls. Considering that wall tension increases with the diameter of the cavity, at constant pressure, we can assume that the tension of the atrial walls in hearts C and D was higher than that in hearts A and B (table 1). We finally hypothesize that the local increase in the expression of the atrial β-myosin gene results from the difference in the tension of the atrial wall. We have already proposed the same hypothesis to explain the low β-fiber content observed in the auricles of normal human hearts that had the same inner pressure as the rest of the atrium but a smaller diameter.[3] Patient D, who underwent long-term therapy with amiodarone and had hyperthyroidism, had the same atrial fiber pattern as patient C. Although no data are available on the effect of dysthyroidism or amiodarone on isomyosin distribution in human hearts, we could expect an effect since these features can modify the myosin gene expression in animal ventricles.[6, 19]

Finally, it is interesting to note that the atrial myosin transition observed in the diseased human hearts did not coincide with the increase in diameter observed in the corresponding fibers. Under hemodynamic pressure overload, atrial fibers, like ventricular fibers, increase in size; this increase in intracellular organelles corresponds in part to an increase in the production of myofibrils.[20] The absence of significant differences in the mean atrial fiber diameter in the four diseased hearts supports the view that a maximum adaptation of this feature had been reached. However, hearts C and D, which sustained greater increases in wall tension, exhibit a larger α- to β-fiber transition than hearts A and B. Thus, one can hypothesize that among the many adaptive processes induced by cardiac overload, there is a quantitative adaptation, i.e., an increase in the production of myofibrils, followed by a qualitative adaptation, i.e., a transition from α- to β-myosin heavy chains. For this reason, it is impossible to predict the isomyosin composition of a fiber according to its diameter. The increase in fiber diameter preceding the myosin-type transition in the diseased human hearts suggests a further concomitant use of these two markers in evaluating the timing of the adaptive process involved in these cardiac diseases.

We thank Dr. J. Demaille and P. Puech for valuable discussion, the unit of Pathology of the hospital of Lyon of excellent cooperation, and Dr. R. Volpilière for friendly and efficient cooperation. We are grateful to Dr. B. Pau and collaborators for the support given by the "Service d'Immunodiagnostic" of the Clin Midy firm.

References

1. Thornell LE, Forsgren S: Myocardial cell heterogeneity in the human heart with respect to myosin ATPase activity. Histochem J **14:** 479, 1982
2. Gorza L, Mercadier JJ, Schwartz K, Thornell LE, Sartore S, Schiaffino S: Myosin types in the human heart: an immunofluorescence study of normal and hypertrophied atrial and ventricular myocardium. Circ Res **54:** 694, 1984
3. Bouvagnet P, Leger Joc, Pons F, Dechesne C, Leger JJ: Fiber type and myosin types in human atrial and ventricular myocardium: an anatomical description. Circ Res **55:** 794, 1984
4. Léger Joc, Dechesne C, Bouvagnet P, Pons F, Léger JJ: Characterisation and distribution of myosin variants in normal and pathological human hearts. Eur Heart J **5**(suppl F): 111, 1984
5. Dechesne C, Léger Joc, Bouvagnet P, Claviez M, Léger JJ: Fractionation and characterization of two molecular variants of myosin from adult human atrium. J Mol Cell Cardiol (in press)
6. Hoh JFY, McGrath PA, Hale PT: Electrophoretic analysis of multiple forms of rat cardiac myosin: effects of hypophysectomy and thyroxine replacement. J Mol Cell Cardiol **10:** 1053, 1978
7. Gorza L, Sartore S, Schiaffino S: Myosin types and fiber types in cardiac muscle. II. Atrial myocardium. J Cell Biol **95:** 838, 1982
8. Cebra JJ, Goldstein G: Chromatographic purification of tetramethylrhodamine-immune globulin conjugates and their use in the cellular localization of rabbit gamma-globulin polypeptide chains. J Immunol **95:** 230, 1965
9. Hynes RD, Destree A: Relationships between fibronetin (LETS protein) and actin. Cell **15:** 875, 1978
10. Weibel ER, Kistler GS, Scherle WF: Practical stereological methods for morphometric cytology. J Cell Biol **30:** 23, 1966
11. Mercadier JJ, Bouveret P, Gorza L, Schiaffino S, Clark WA, Zak R, Swinghedauw B, Schwartz K: Myosin isozymes in normal and hypertrophied human ventricular myocardium. Circ Res **53:** 52, 1983
12. Alpert NR: Myocardial hypertrophy and failure. New York, 1983, Raven Press
13. Zak R: Growth of the heart in health and disease. New York, 1984, Raven Press
14. Schiaffino S, Gorza L, Sartore S: Distribution of myosin types in normal and hypertrophic hearts: an immunological approach. *In* Alpert NR, editor: Perspectives in cardiovascular research. Vol. 7: Myocardial hypertrophy and failure. New York, 1983, Raven Press
15. Watras J: Changes in rat cardiac myosin during development and in culture. J Mol Cell Cardiol **13:** 1011, 1981
16. Mahdavi V, Periasamy M, Nadal-Ginard B: Molecular characterization of two myosin heavy chain genes expressed in the adult heart. Nature **297:** 659, 1982
17. Billeter R, Heizmann CW, Howald H, Jenny E: Analysis of myosin light chain types in single human skeletal muscle fibers. Eur J Biochem **116:** 389, 1981
18. Barnejee SK: Comparative studies of atrial and ventricular myosin from normal, thyrotoxic, and thyroidectomized rabbits. Circ Res **52:** 131, 1983
19. Wiegand V, Oberschmidt R, Henniges A, Kreuzer H: Hypothyroid like effect of amiodarone on myosin isozymes of the ventricular myocardium of the rat. J Mol Cell Cardiol **16** (suppl 2): 137, 1984
20. Schwarz F, Schaper J, Kittstein D, Flameng W, Walter P, Schaper W: Reduced volume fraction of myofibrils in myocardium of patients with decompensated pressure overload. Circulation **63:** 1299, 1981

Left ventricular aneurysm and the prediction of left ventricular enlargement studied by two-dimensional echocardiography: quantitative assessment of aneurysm size in relation to clinical course

MASAYUKI MATSUMOTO, M.D., FUMIKO WATANABE, M.D., AKIRA GOTO, M.D., YUTAKA HAMANO, M.D., KIYOSHI YASUI, TAKAZO MINAMINO, M.D., HIROSHI ABE, M.D., AND TAKENOBU KAMADA, M.D.

ABSTRACT A retrospective study was performed to elucidate the process of left ventricular aneurysm formation and its influence on left ventricular enlargement based on serial two-dimensional echocardiographic observations from 150 consecutive patients with first acute anterior myocardial infarction. Echocardiograms were available and interpretable through the entire period of observation in 68 patients. Because of early death in 13 patients, echocardiograms of 55 patients, 22 with and 33 without aneurysm, were analyzed from 1 to 28 days after infarction. Patients with aneurysms were separated into two groups with large (group 1, 11 patients) and small aneurysms (group 2, 11 patients) on the basis of ratios of aneurysm to overall left ventricular circumferential length [Lcf-LV(RAO)] and area [Area-LV(RAO)], i.e., Lcf(An/LV)-RAO and Area(An/LV)-RAO, respectively, in the right anterior oblique equivalent view at the time of aneurysm formation, with reference to Forrester's subset. Group 1 consisted of patients with Lcf(An/LV)-RAO of 0.4 or greater or Area(An/LV)RAO of 0.3 or greater while group 2 included patients with Lcf(An/LV)-RAO less than 0.4 or Area(An/LV)-RAO less than 0.3. In the test for time trend in these groups with a one-way analysis of variance, Lcf-LV in RAO equivalent and apical four-chamber views and Area-LV in apical four-chamber view effectively separated group 1 from groups 2 and 3 (without aneurysm) with significance ($p < .005$, $p < .01$, and $p < .01$). In group 1 the incidence of heart failure was significantly higher than that in groups 2 and 3 (77.8% vs 0% and 21.1%; $p < .001$, $p < .001$), and the mortality was high compared with that of the other two groups (38.7% vs 8.3% and 13.2%) showing statistical significance only with group 3 ($p < .05$). The present criteria for separating patients with left ventricular aneurysm seem useful in predicting future left ventricular enlargement and developing clinical prognosis even at the time of aneurysm formation.

Circulation 72, No. 2, 280–286, 1985.

LEFT VENTRICULAR aneurysm is a frequent complication associated with acute myocardial infarction and is often the cause of heart failure, intractable arrhythmias, and mural thrombus of the left ventricle.[1,2] Early diagnosis of this aneurysm is important for the management of the disease, including preload and afterload reduction and surgical intervention.[3] Although there are several reports on two-dimensional echocardiographic detection of left ventricular aneurysms,[4-6] only Eaton et al.[7] provided data on the process of left ventricular aneurysm formation. They studied 28 patients with acute transmural myocardial infarction during the first 2 weeks after infarction by serial two-dimensional echocardiography, but quantitative analysis was not performed with regard to the degree of expansion of infarct. A clinical review of over 150 patients with first acute anterior myocardial infarction indicated the necessity of a tight retrospective and chronologic analysis of the left ventricular size of these patients with regard to the presence and especially to the size of the left ventricular aneurysm. The consensus was that large left ventricular aneurysms affected successive dilatation of the left ventricle in these pa-

From the Division of Cardiology, The First Department of Medicine, Osaka University Medical School, and Divisions of Cardiology, Sakurabashi Watanabe Hospital, Osaka National Hospital, and Ohtemae General Hospital, Osaka, and Department of Gerontology, Kanazawa Medical University, Kanazawa, Japan.

Address for correspondence: Masayuki Matsumoto, M.D., Department of Gerontology, Kanazawa Medical University, 1-1, Daigaku, Uchinada-cho, Kahoku-gun, Ishikawa Prefecture, 920-02, Japan.

Received Jan. 25, 1984; revision accepted April 11, 1985.

tients. Therefore two-dimensional echocardiographic observations of the left ventricle were performed in patients with first acute anterior myocardial infarction from days 1 to 28 after infarction. Based on these observations, the study continued toward quantitative estimation of the size of the left ventricular aneurysm and its influence on left ventricular enlargement and clinical prognosis.

Materials and methods

Patients. Two-dimensional echocardiographic examinations during the period from January 1, 1980, to January 1, 1983, were reviewed in 150 consecutive patients with first acute transmural myocardial infarction, who were admitted within 24 hr of the onset of symptoms. Interpretable two-dimensional echocardiographic recordings were obtained through the entire period of observation in 68 patients. Thirteen of these 68 died within 28 days of infarction; thus serial two-dimensional echocardiography covering all five stages of examination was performed in 55 patients. Forty-eight of these 55 patients and 105 of the total 150 patients underwent left ventriculography in the right anterior oblique (RAO, 30 degrees) and left anterior oblique (LAO, 60 degrees) projections approximately 40 days after infarction.

Two-dimensional echocardiography. Serial two-dimensional echocardiograms were recorded on days 1, 3, 7, 14, and 28 after infarction. On each day two-dimensional echocardiograms in the RAO equivalent view (in 55 cases), the short-axis view at the papillary muscle level (in 51 cases), and the apical four-chamber view (in 33 cases) were recorded on 8 mm movie film with a Hitachi 10-A, 72 degree phased-array echocardiograph. The smaller number in studies in the apical-four chamber view was due to the late inclusion of this view in the examination. In this study an echocardiographic aneurysm was defined as an outward bulging of the left ventricular wall with hinge points occurring during both systole and diastole (BCD in the left panel of figure 1).[4, 5] The presence of left ventricular aneurysm and its extent were examined on each day of examination.

Quantitative measurement of sizes of the left ventricle and left ventricular aneurysm. For a quantitative assessment of sizes of the overall left ventricle and left ventricular aneurysm, six indexes as shown in the left panel of figure 1 were obtained by tracing the endocardial contour of the RAO equivalent view of the left ventricle in end-diastole. Left ventricular circumferential length [Lcf-LV(RAO)] was measured around the left ventricle from the aortic root to the posterior mitral valve ring (ABCDE in the left panel of figure 1) with a curvemeter. In patients with aneurysms the circumferential length of the aneurysm [Lcf-An(RAO)] was measured around the aneurysm between two hinge points in end-diastole (BCD in the left panel of figure 1) and the ratio of Lcf-An(RAO) to Lcf-LV(RAO) [Lcf(An/LV)-RAO] was calculated.

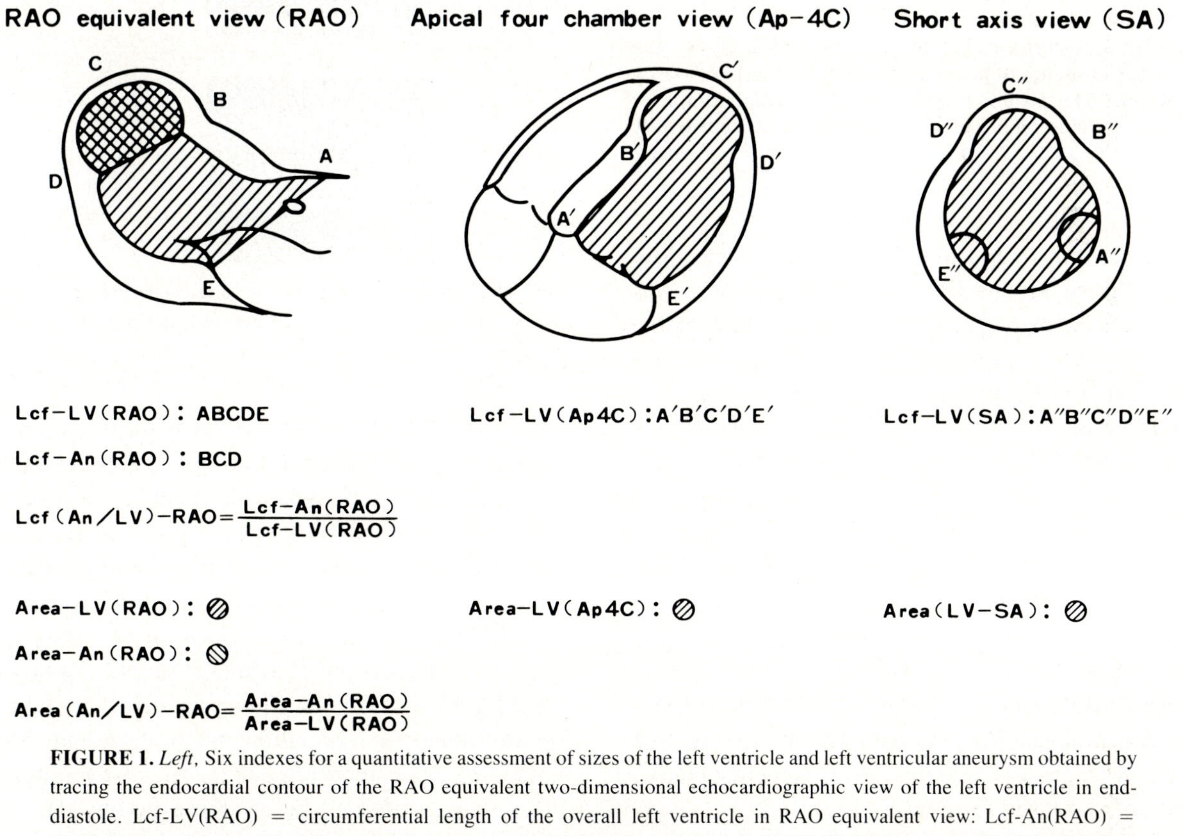

FIGURE 1. *Left*, Six indexes for a quantitative assessment of sizes of the left ventricle and left ventricular aneurysm obtained by tracing the endocardial contour of the RAO equivalent two-dimensional echocardiographic view of the left ventricle in end-diastole. Lcf-LV(RAO) = circumferential length of the overall left ventricle in RAO equivalent view: Lcf-An(RAO) = circumferential length of the left ventricular aneurysm in RAO equivalent view; Lcf(An/LV)-RAO = ratio of Lcf-An(RAO) to Lcf-LV(RAO); Area-LV(RAO) = area of the overall left ventricle in RAO equivalent view; Area-An(RAO) = area of the left ventricular aneurysm in RAO equivalent view; Area(An/LV)-RAO = ratio of Area-An(RAO) to Area-LV(RAO). *Center*, Lcf-LV and Area-LV in apical four-chamber view. Lcf-LV(Ap4C) = circumferential length of the overall left ventricle in apical four-chamber view; Area-LV(Ap4C) = area of the overall left ventricle in apical four-chamber view. *Right*, Lcf-LV and Area-LV in short-axis view. Lcf-LV(SA) = circumferential length of the overall left ventricle in short-axis view; Area-LV(SA) = area of the overall left ventricle in short-axis view.

Areas of the left ventricle [Area-LV(RAO)] and left ventricular aneurysm [Area-An(RAO)] were also measured with a Digisonic Echo Computer by tracing the endocardium of the left ventricle and left ventricular aneurysm as shown in the left panel of figure 1, and their ratio [Area(An/LV)-RAO] was calculated. In apical four-chamber and short-axis views, the circumferential length and area of the overall left ventricle were measured similarly to those in the RAO equivalent view as shown in the center and right panels of figure 1.

Statistical analysis. All measurements were performed by two independent observers and each observer made duplicate readings. Interobserver and intraobserver variabilities were examined for measurements in the RAO equivalent view. Testing for interobserver variability of the qualitative assessment of the presence or absence of aneurysm was done by the McNemar test on each day of examination (5 points). The judgment of the two observers coincided well and no significant difference was found. Interobserver and intraobserver variability in the quantitative assessment of circumference and area measurements of the left ventricle and aneurysm were examined by the paired Student t test for duplicate reading on each day examined by each observer [5 points of Lcf-LV(RAO) and Area-LV(RAO) and 5 points of Lcf-An(RAO) and Area-An(RAO), 20 points in total], and no significant difference was observed in interobserver or intraobserver variabilities.

Statistical comparison over time for each group with large aneurysm, with small aneurysm, and without aneurysm was performed with three different echocardiographic views by a one-way analysis of variance.[8]

Statistical comparisons for age and cumulated release of creatine kinase were performed by the unpaired Student t test, and those for sex, presence of heart failure, and short-term mortality by Fisher's exact probability test because of the small sample of patients. A p value of .05 or less was considered statistically significant.

Results

Frequency, time, and site of left ventricular aneurysm formation. Formation of left ventricular aneurysm was observed in 30 of 68 patients in whom interpretable echocardiograms were available (44.1%). The incidence of aneurysm was much lower by contrast left ventriculography (23 patients, 21.9%), which was performed in 105 of 150 patients. Aneurysm formation was observed in seven patients on the first day after infarction, in nine on day 3, in nine on day 7, and in five on day 14. As for the site of aneurysm, eight patients developed aneurysm in the apical region, 16 in the apical and anterior region, and six in the extensive anterior region and inferior wall up to the posterior papillary muscle. Serial recordings of RAO equivalent view, two-dimensional echocardiograms at the five designated stages of examination in a representative patient are shown in figure 2.

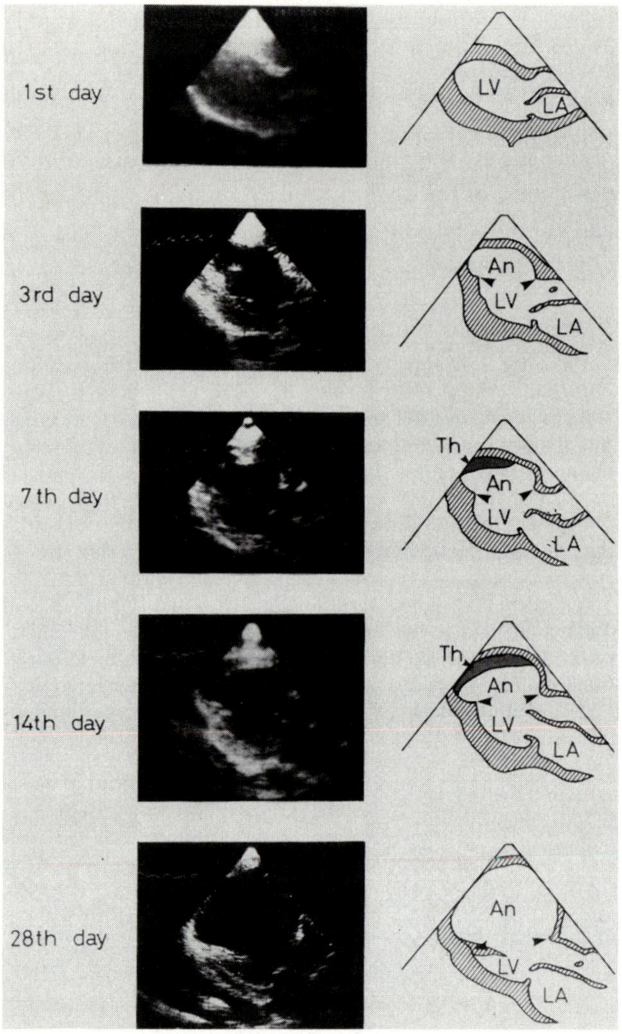

FIGURE 2. Serial recordings of two-dimensional echocardiograms in end-diastole at the five designated stages of examination in a representative patient. LV = left ventricle; LA = left atrium; An = left ventricular aneurysm; Th = thrombus. Arrows indicate hinge points.

Relationship between the presence or size of aneurysm and temporal change in circumferential length and area of the left ventricle. The relationship between the presence or size of left ventricular aneurysm and temporal change in overall left ventricular size was analyzed in surviving patients with (n = 22) and without (n = 33) aneurysm. Patients with aneurysm were divided into two groups by referring to Forrester's subset on day 28 in 17 patients in whom measurements of cardiac index and pulmonary capillary wedge pressure were available. As shown in table 1, when the ratio of aneurysm size to overall left ventricle in circumferential length in the RAO equivalent view [Lcf(An/LV)-RAO] was smaller than 0.4 and that in area in the RAO equivalent view [Area(An/LV)-RAO] was smaller than 0.3 at the time of aneurysm formation, none of the patients belonged to Forrester's classes II, III, and IV and only class I was observed below these points. The mean values of serial measurements for Lcf-LV and Area-LV at five stages of examination in RAO equivalent, apical-four chamber, and short-axis views in groups 1 and 2 and in group 3 without aneurysm are shown in figure 3, and those on days 1 and 28 after infarction are shown in table 2.

TABLE 1

Correlation of the ratios of aneurysm size to the overall left ventricular circumferential length [Lcf(An/LV)-RAO] and area [Area(An/LV)-RAO] at aneurysm formation with Forrester's subset 28 days after infarction in 17 patients

	Aneurysm size: Lcf(An/LV)-RAO			
	Group 2		Group 1	
Forrester's subset	0.2–0.3	0.3–0.4	0.4–0.5	0.5–0.6
Class I	2	6	3	0
Class II	0	0	0	0
Class III	0	0	1	3
Class IV	0	0	1	1
	Aneurysm size: Area(An/LV)-RAO			
	Group 2		Group 1	
	0.1–0.2	0.2–0.3	0.3–0.4	0.4–0.5
Class I	4	4	2	1
Class II	0	0	0	0
Class III	0	0	1	3
Class IV	0	0	0	2

Data are number of patients.

Analysis of the temporal pattern of enlargement was performed by a one-way analysis of variance on indexes of Lcf-LV and Area-LV in three echocardiographic views for three groups (table 3). As shown, a significant statistical difference in trend was observed specifically for group 1 in Lcf-LV in the RAO equivalent view and in Lcf-LV and Area-LV in the apical four-chamber view. In Area-LV in the RAO equivalent view and Area-LV in the short-axis view a significant difference was observed between groups 1 and 3. In Lcf-LV in the short-axis view all groups showed statistically significant differences.

Clinical comparison of three groups with and without aneurysm. Age, sex, cumulated release of creatine kinase, presence of heart failure, and short-term mortality were compared for the three groups of patients (table 4). A statistically significant difference was observed between groups 1 and 3 for age ($p < .05$), sex ($p < .05$), presence of heart failure ($p < .001$), and mortality ($p < .05$). Between groups 1 and 2 a significant difference was observed for the presence of heart fail-

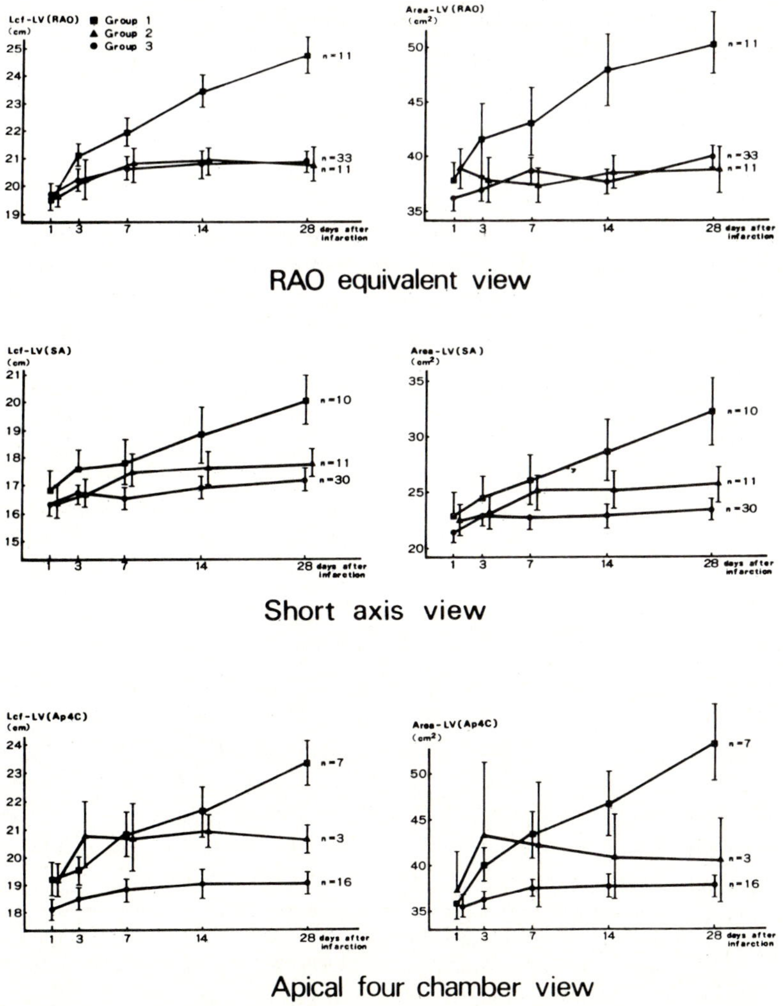

FIGURE 3. Temporal changes during 28 days of observation. Left column, Lcf-LV; right column, Area-LV; top panels, RAO equivalent view; center panels, short-axis view; bottom panels, apical four-chamber view.

TABLE 2
Means and SEs of left ventricular circumferential length and area on days 1 and 28 after infarction in three echocardiographic views

		Lcf-LV (cm)		Area-LV (cm^2)	
Group[A]	n	Day 1	Day 28	Day 1	Day 28
Group 1					
RAO	11	19.5±0.4	24.7±0.7	37.7±1.6	50.2±2.8
SA	10	16.8±0.7	20.1±0.9	22.8±2.1	32.1±3.1
Ap4C	7	19.2±0.6	23.3±0.8	35.8±1.6	52.9±4.1
Group 2					
RAO	11	19.6±0.4	20.7±0.6	38.8±1.8	38.7±2.1
SA	11	16.4±0.6	17.8±0.5	22.4±1.3	25.6±1.6
Ap4C	3	19.2±0.6	20.6±0.5	37.4±4.1	40.3±4.5
Group 3					
RAO	33	19.7±0.4	20.8±0.4	36.2±1.2	39.8±1.0
SA	30	16.3±0.4	17.2±0.4	21.3±0.9	23.2±1.0
Ap4C	16	18.1±0.4	19.0±0.4	35.6±1.3	37.5±1.1

Lcf-LV = circumferential length of the overall left ventricle; Area-LV = area of the overall left ventricle; RAO = right anterior oblique equivalent view; SA = short-axis view; Ap4C = apical four-chamber view.

[A]Group 1, patients with large aneurysm with Lcf(An/LV)-RAO ≧ 0.4 and Area(An/LV)-RAO ≧ 0.3; group 2, patients with small aneurysm with Lcf(An/LV)-RAO < 0.4 and Area(An/LV)-RAO < 0.3; group 3, patients without aneurysm.

ure ($p < .001$). Clinical comparison of the group of 13 patients who died within 28 days of infarction is also included in table 4 and data are listed individually in table 5. The possibility of the above listed clinical parameters as contributors to mortality was analyzed between surviving and nonsurviving patients in groups 1 and 3 (there was only one nonsurviving patient in group 2). In group 3 a significant difference was observed between surviving and nonsurviving patients in cumulated release of creatine kinase (1090 ± 96 vs 3693 ± 871 IU; $p < .001$) and presence of heart failure (12.1% vs 80.0%; $p < .005$).

Discussion

Eaton et al.[7] studied 28 patients early after acute transmural myocardial infarction and recognized disproportionate dilatation of the infarct zone in 29% of them by sequential two-dimensional echocardiograms, with a cutpoint of 2 SDs above the mean for a normal value. They observed that eight patients with infarct expansion showed a significant overall left ventricular dilatation of 25.3%, and 20 patients without infarct expansion showed an insignificant dilatation of 5.2%. However, they did not perform a quantitative study with regard to the degree of expansion of infarct. We have performed a quantitative study based on the relative size of echocardiographically determined left ventricular aneurysm. In this study the process of left ventricular aneurysm formation and especially the influence of size of left ventricular aneurysm on left ventricular enlargement were analyzed quantitatively by serial observation of two-dimensional echocardiograms from days 1 to 28 after infarction.

An effort has been made to quantitate the size of ventricular aneurysm by Barret et al.[5] using an echocardiographic technique of calculating residual myocardium. In our study Lcf(An/LV)-RAO and Area (An/LV)-RAO were used as indexes to represent the relative size of aneurysm against the overall size of the left ventricle and to investigate the influence of aneurysm size on left ventricular size. The degree of left ventricular enlargement was found to be influenced by the size of left ventricular aneurysm at the time of its formation.

In the test for trend, group 1 patients showed significant differences in all indexes measured. Group 2 patients showed no significant differences in these indexes except in Lcf-LV in the short-axis view. Group 3 patients showed significant differences in Area-LV in the RAO equivalent view and Lcf-LV and Area-LV in the short-axis view. Group 1 was separated best from the other groups by the apical four-chamber view followed by the RAO equivalent view. These two echocardiographic views were suitable for detecting the temporal enlargement of left ventricular aneurysm be-

TABLE 3
Analysis of temporal enlargement performed by one-way analysis of variance on Lcf-LV and Area-LV in three echocardiographic views[A]

Index	Group	n	F value	Significance
Lcf-LV (RAO)	1	11	19.5	<.005
	2	11	2.46	NS
	3	33	1.22	NS
Area-LV (RAO)	1	11	20.4	<.005
	2	11	0.532	NS
	3	33	6.29	<.05
Lcf-LV (SA)	1	10	11.1	<.01
	2	11	6.64	<.05
	3	30	5.33	<.05
Area-LV (SA)	1	10	9.89	<.05
	2	11	4.09	NS
	3	30	4.96	<.05
Lcf-LV (Ap4C)	1	7	14.4	<.01
	2	3	1.74	NS
	3	16	4.17	NS
Area-LV (Ap4C)	1	7	18.1	<.01
	2	3	1.23	NS
	3	16	0.642	NS

Abbreviations as in table 2.

[A]Degree of freedom for test, 1 and n-1 were used instead of (5-1) and (5-1)(n-1).

TABLE 4
Clinical comparison of the patient groups (mean ± SE)

	Group 1 (n = 18)	Group 2 (n = 12)	Group 3 (n = 38)	Statistically significant difference	
Age (yr)					
S	n=11 60.5±3.9	n=11 62.2±3.6	n=33 55.8±2.0		
D	n=7 70.6±5.2	n=1 60	n=5 54.0±7.1		
S+D	n=18 64.4±3.2	n=12 62.0±3.3	n=38 55.5±1.9	1-3^{A}	
Sex (M/F)					
S	7/4	8/3	30/3	1-3^{A}	
D	4/3	1/0	4/1		
S+D	11/7	9/3	34/4	1-3^{A}	
ΣCK(IU)					
S	n=7 1694±669	n=11 1061±191	n=29 1090±96		
D	n=5 1671±390	n=1 1233	n=4 3693±871^{E}		
S+D	n=12 1685±406	n=12 1076±175	n=33 1406±195		
Heart failure (%)					
S	72.7 (8/11)	0 (0/11)	12.1 (4/33)^{D}	1-2^{B}	1-3^{B}
D	85.7 (6/7)	0 (0/1)	80.0 (4/5)		
S+D	77.8 (14/18)	0 (0/12)	21.1 (8/38)	1-2^{C}	1-3^{C}
Mortality					
S+D	38.7 (7/18)	8.3 (1/12)	13.2 (5/38)	1-3^{A}	

ΣCK = cumulated release of creatine kinase; S = surviving patients; D = nonsurviving patients.
Group differences: $^{A}p < .05$; $^{B}p < .01$; $^{C}p < .001$.
Significant differences between S and D in each group: $^{D}p < .005$; $^{E}p < .001$.

cause they were suitable for visualizing the main portion of the aneurysm that enlarged toward the apex of the left ventricle.

In this study of 150 patients, left ventriculography was performed in 105 patients and aneurysm formation was observed in 23 (21.9%). This frequency of aneurysm formation was within the range reported by other investigators.[1, 2, 9, 10] In 68 patients for whom serial echocardiographic studies were possible, left ventricular aneurysm formation was observed in 30 (44.1%). This frequency seems biased by the fact that there was a greater chance for patients with aneurysm to be included in the present serial echocardiographic study because of the large acoustic window produced by the aneurysm near the apical region. The risk period for aneurysm formation ranged from day 1 to day 14 after infarction. Although Eaton et al.[7] reported that expansion began approximately 3 days after infarction, in our observation seven patients had evidence of aneurysm on the first day, nine on the third, nine on the seventh, and five on the fourteenth day.

Parmley et al.[11] carried out a study to elucidate the expandable nature of surgically removed human ventricular aneurysms. In established fibrous and stiff aneurysms examined more than 9 months after myocardial infarction, an average increase of only 2.4% in circumference in systole was observed. In muscular, compliant aneurysms examined less than 6 days after infarction, however, an average increase of 14.6% in circumference in systole was observed. This extensibility is consistent with our observations that left ven-

TABLE 5
Clinical comparison of 13 nonsurviving patients in three groups who were excluded from the serial study

	Age (yr)/ sex	Day of death after infarct	Cause of death	ΣCK (IU)	Forrester's subset on the first day
Group 1					
1	85/M	3	Arrhythmia	1471	III
2	79/M	24	Apoplexy	—	III
3	68/F	3	Cardiac rupture	2013	III
4	44/M	6	Cardiac rupture	1929	I
5	78/M	28	Heart failure	2643	IV
6	76/F	25	Heart failure	300	III
7	64/F	14	Arrhythmia	—	II
Group 2					
8	60/M	7	Cardiac rupture	1233	I
Group 3					
9	59/M	1	Arrhythmia	—	—
10	51/M	2	Heart failure	1240	IV
11	31/M	12	Heart failure	3777	II
12	54/M	15	Arrhythmia	5247	IV
13	75/F	24	2nd infarction	4508	III

ΣCK = cumulated release of creatine kinase.

tricular aneurysms developed within 2 weeks after infarction and that these aneurysms expanded gradually through our observation end point of 28 days after infarction. The overall enlargement of the left ventricle was caused by the selective topographic dilatation of the aneurysm itself as observed by us and Eaton et al.[7] Even in our study, with a larger number of patients compared with that of Eaton et al.,[7] no statistically significant difference was observed between infarct size, estimated from the cumulated release of creatine kinase, and aneurysm formation.

With the advent of real-time two-dimensional echocardiography, serial noninvasive observation of early pathophysiologic changes of acute myocardial infarction has become possible. We were able to determine time of left ventricular aneurysm formation and the influence of aneurysm size on overall left ventricular enlargement, which had been indeterminable in the surviving patients. With reference to the hemodynamic classes of Forrester's subset, the present indexes for quantitative representation of aneurysm size proved useful in predicting left ventricular enlargement even at the time of aneurysm formation. The patients with large left ventricular aneurysm assigned to group 1 showed a significantly high presence of heart failure compared with those with small or no aneurysm. Thus the cutpoints of 0.4 and 0.3 for the ratio of aneurysm size against total left ventricular circumference and area were found to be useful for identifying patients with aneurysms. However, because these points for separating patients with large and small aneurysms were chosen retrospectively, the values of these points for separation should be further confirmed. Our results may provide a basis for altering conventional management of patients with left ventricular aneurysms and will contribute to the improvement of prognosis.

We are deeply indebted to Dr. Hideo Kusuoka for his valuable advice in the statistical analysis.

References

1. Cabin HS, Roberts WC: True left ventricular aneurysm and healed myocardial infarction. Am J Cardiol **46:** 754, 1980
2. Schlichter J, Hellerstein HK, Katz LN: Aneurysm of the heart: a correlative study of one hundred and two proved cases. Medicine **33:** 43, 1954
3. Swan HC, Magnusson PT, Buchbinder NA, Matloff JM, Gray RJ: Aneurysm of the cardiac ventricle: its management by medical and surgical intervention. West J Med **129:** 26, 1978
4. Weyman AE, Peskoe SM, Williams ES, Dillon JC, Feigenbaum H: Detection of left ventricular aneurysms by cross-sectional echocardiography. Circulation **54:** 936, 1976
5. Barrett MJ, Charuzi Y, Corday E: Ventricular aneurysm: cross-sectional echocardiographic approach. Am J Cardiol **46:** 1133, 1980
6. Chiang BN, Yeh PSH, Chen YT, Lee SS, Wang SJ: Detection of postinfarction ventricular aneurysms by cross-sectional echocardiography and radionuclide ventriculography. Prog Cardiol **9:** 43, 1980
7. Eaton LW, Weiss JL, Bulkley BH, Garrison JB: Regional cardiac dilatation after acute myocardial infarction: recognition by two-dimensional echocardiography. N Engl J Med **300:** 57, 1979
8. Wallenstein S, Zucker CL, Fleiss JL: Some statistical methods useful in circulation research. Circ Res **47:** 1, 1980
9. Cheng TO: Incidence of ventricular aneurysm in coronary artery disease: an angiographic appraisal. Am J Med **50:** 340, 1971
10. Abrams DL, Edilist A, Luria MH, Miller AJ: Ventricular aneurysm: a reappraisal based on a study of sixty-five consecutive autopsied cases. Circulation **27:** 164, 1963
11. Parmley WW, Chuck L, Kivowitz C, Matloff JM, Swan HJC: In vitro length-tension relations of human ventricular aneurysms: relation of stiffness to mechanical disadvantage. Am J Cardiol **32:** 889, 1973

Factors that modify the flow response to intracoronary injections

HÅKAN EMANUELSSON, M.D., STIG HOLMBERG, M.D., KJELL SELIN, M.D., AND JAN WALLIN, M.D.

ABSTRACT Coronary sinus flow (CSF) was measured in seven patients with normal coronary arteries (group A) during intracoronary injections of 6 ml arterial blood, 6 ml blood from the coronary sinus, 3 and 6 ml isotonic saline, 3 and 6 ml hypertonic glucose, and 6 ml of a contrast agent (sodium metrizoate). In 10 patients with coronary artery disease (group B), CSF was measured after administration of 6 ml isotonic saline, 6 ml sodium metrizoate, and 6 ml of another contrast medium (iohexol). In group A, arterial blood did not affect CSF, while coronary sinus blood induced a 33% increase. After 6 ml isotonic saline, there was a 35% increase in flow and after hypertonic glucose an increase of 70%. Metrizoate induced a rise in flow of 109%. In group B, the increase in CSF after intracoronary injection of saline, metrizoate, and iohexol was 30%, 83%, and 67%, respectively. Blood from the coronary sinus, in contrast to arterial blood, induced a marked rise in peak flow, suggesting a role for reactive hyperemia secondary to myocardial hypoxia in this response. A similar mechanism might have been operative after injection of isotonic saline, as well as after the hyperosmolar contrast agents. However, additional mechanisms mediated by the high osmotic pressure of these substances, such as induction of the Bezold-Jarisch reflex, which will induce coronary vasodilation, may have played a role. Finally, when hyperosmolar agents are used, the possibility of some direct vasodilating properties of the agents cannot be excluded.
Circulation 72, No. 2, 287–291, 1985.

AN INTRACORONARY INJECTION of a substance will in most cases lead to a change in coronary blood flow. Factors other than the pharmacologic properties of the injectate can affect the flow response. Such factors include the chemical composition and physical properties of the compound, such as its hyperosmolality and oxygen content. When contrast media are injected in a coronary artery, there is a marked increase in flow that is dependent on the hyperosmolality but not on the iodine content of the agent.[1] The actual mechanisms of the increase in flow are not well known. The present study was conducted to try to evaluate factors influencing the flow response to intracoronary injections. Various amounts of different substances were therefore injected into the left coronary arteries of 17 patients during continuous measurement of coronary sinus blood flow (CSF).

From the Division of Cardiology, Department of Medicine I, and Department of Radiology I, Sahlgrenska Hospital, S-413 45 Göteborg, Sweden.

Address for correspondence: Dr. Håkan Emanuelsson, Division of Cardiology, Department of Medicine I, Sahlgrenska Hospital, S-413 45 Göteborg, Sweden.

Received Nov. 26, 1984; revision accepted April 18, 1985.

Material and methods

Patients. Seventeen patients who had been admitted to the hospital for coronary angiographic examination due to angina-like chest pain were investigated. Seven patients (group A) had angiographically normal coronary arteries. Two were women and five men, and their median age was 57 years (range 39 to 62). Group B consisted of 10 patients, all of whom proved to have significant coronary artery disease with narrowing of at least one vessel of more than 70%. There were two female and eight male patients in this group and their median age 57 years (range 48 to 62). No cardiac medication was given for 12 hr before the study. Informed consent was obtained from each patient and the Hospital Ethics Committee approved the study.

Catheterization. A Judkins catheter was used to engage the ostium of the left coronary artery of each patient. A thermodilution pacing catheter (Wilton-Webster Lab.) was positiond in the coronary sinus. The position of the catheter was confirmed by injection of radiopaque dye and was adjusted during flow measurement until there was a stable baseline flow curve. With a bolus injection of 10 ml of isotonic saline in the right atrium during temperature recording in the coronary sinus, the presence of reflux as a source of measurement error[2] could be detected and was eliminated when necessary by changing the position of the catheter.

Measurements. The CSF was determined with the continuous-infusion thermodilution method.[3] Isotonic saline solution at room temperature was infused into the coronary sinus at a rate of 44 ml/min by infusion pump. Blood oxygen saturation was determined by a photometric method[4] and the erythrocyte volume fraction (EVF) was estimated after 10 min centrifugation of

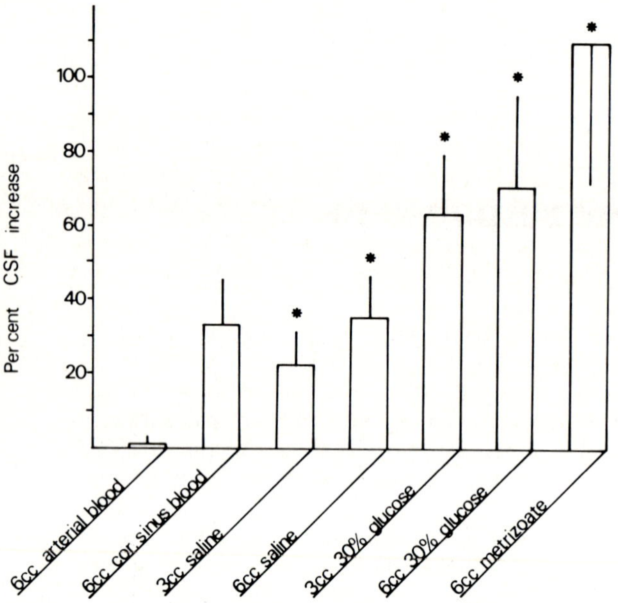

FIGURE 1. Changes in CSF after intracoronary injections in group A. Values are mean ± SEM *p < .007 compared with control value, which is the p value necessary for statistical significance after adjustment for the multiplicity of testing (see text).

the blood sample. The electrocardiogram was continuously recorded with a bipolar chest lead with one electrode in the V_5 position and the other in the right subclavicular region.

Procedure. Coronary sinus temperature and the electrocardiogram were recorded continuously before, during, and after the intracoronary injections. All substances were administered by injection by the same person throughout the study, and the injection rate was 2 ml/sec. In group A, the following injections were given: 6 ml arterial blood (drawn from the coronary artery catheter), 6 ml coronary venous blood (obtained via the coronary sinus catheter), 3 and 6 ml isotonic saline, 3 and 6 ml hypertonic glucose (30% solution, which corresponds to 1400 mOsm/kg), and 6 ml sodium metrizoate (Isopaque Coronar 370, Nyegaard & Co A/S), which is an ionic contrast medium with calcium added and with an osmolality of 2100 mOsm/kg.

There was an interval of at least 5 min between the injections. Two injections of each substance were given and the mean difference in the increase in flow between duplicate measurements was 8 ± 3% and did not exceed 15% for any of the agents. In the first three patients, repeat injections were also given of solutions (saline and contrast medium) at body temperature. Since the flow response was within the limits of the variation in the duplicate measurements mentioned above, only solutions at room temperature were used in the remaining patients.

In group B, all injections were given during atrial pacing to a rate 20% above resting heart rate. Three different substances were injected: 6 ml isotonic saline, 6 ml sodium metrizoate, and 6 ml iohexol (Omnipaque 350, Nyegaard & Co). The latter is a new nonionic and low osmolar (700 mOsm/kg) contrast agent. At least 5 min were allowed between the injections. Two injections of each substance were given. The coronary flow was measured during the first injection, and blood samples for analysis of oxygen saturation and EVF were collected at 0, 30, 120, and 300 sec after the second injection. Atrial pacing was performed throughout the procedure in group B patients.

Calculations. CSF was calculated with the formula $Fb = Fi \times k\,(Tb-Ti)/(Tb-Tm)-1$, where Fb = blood flow in the coronary sinus (ml/min); Fi = infusion rate of saline (ml/min); Tb, Ti, Tm = temperature of blood, injectate, and mixture of blood and injectate, respectively; k = a constant derived from the density and specific heat of saline solution and blood.

Statistical methods. In group A, the effects on CSF of seven substances were investigated, and a double-sided test was performed for each substance. To adjust for testing multiplicity, Bonferroni's method was used.[5] According to this technique, the alpha error of an individual test is reduced to 0.05/7, which approximates 0.007. This value corresponds to the probability of one or more of the seven individual hypotheses being erroneously rejected. Thus, only a p value below .007 was considered to indicate statistical significance. In group B, multiple comparisons of results with each substance at different time intervals after intracoronary injections were performed (Wilcoxon matched-pairs signed-ranks test). In accordance with the discussion above, Bonferroni's method was used, and thus only p values less than .0167 (0.05/3) were considered to indicate statistical significance. In addition, the reactions to the individual substances were tested against each other at the different time intervals, and the p value was similarly corrected.

Results

Group A. All patients were in sinus rhythm before and during the intracoronary injections and the mean heart rate was not significantly changed after any of the injections. Figure 1 illustrates the reaction of CSF to injection of the various substances. This parameter was not affected by the injection of arterial blood. Blood from the coronary sinus, on the other hand, did produce a 33 ± 12% increase after intracoronary injection. After 3 and 6 ml isotonic saline, the CSF rose

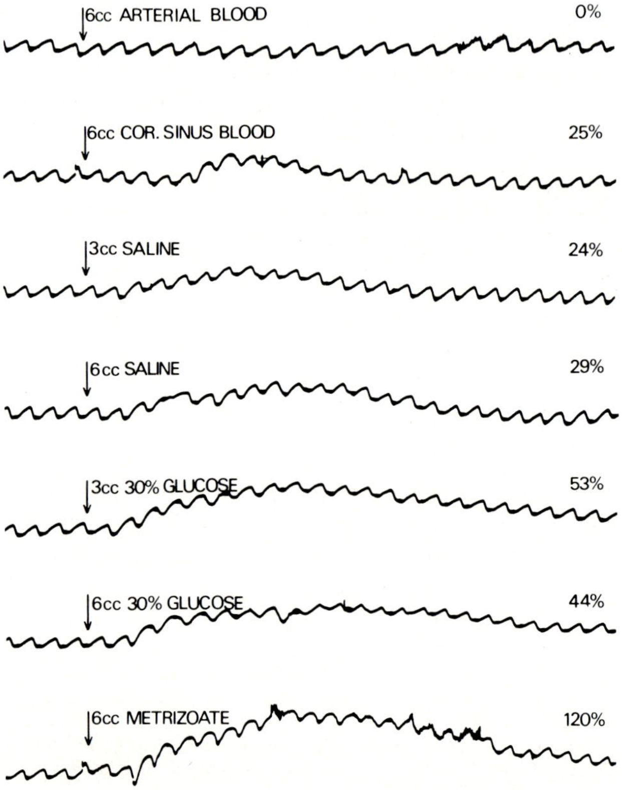

FIGURE 2. CSF recordings in one patient in group A.

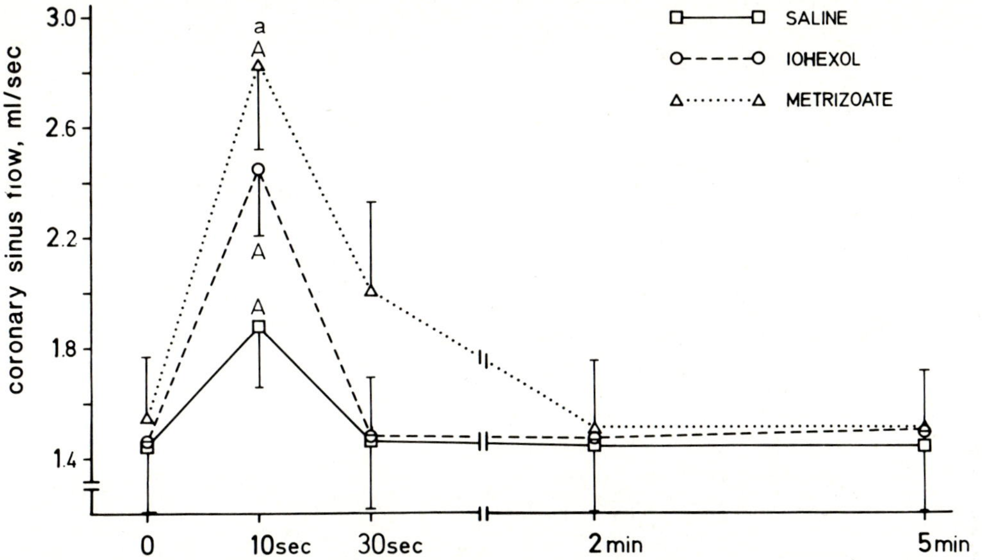

FIGURE 3. CSF in group B after intracoronary injections of isotonic saline, sodium metrizoate, and iohexol. Values are mean ± SEM. [A]$p < .0167$ compared with zero values. [a]$p < .0167$ for metrizoate values compared with iohexol and saline values. The p value of .0167 is the highest accepted for obtaining statistical significance after adjusting for testing multiplicity (see text).

22 ± 9% and 35 ± 11%, respectively. Hypertonic glucose induced increments in flow that were two to three times greater than those induced with isotonic saline. The most pronounced increase in CSF was seen after sodium metrizoate (109 ± 38%). Figure 2 shows typical responses of flow to various intracoronary substances in one patient.

Group B. Figure 3 illustrates the effects on CSF of intracoronary saline, iohexol, and sodium metrizoate. The peak increase was most pronounced after metrizoate (83%). The corresponding values for iohexol and saline were 67% and 30%, respectively. The same pattern was noted regarding the oxygen saturation of CSF and EVF, i.e., metrizoate produced the most marked increase in oxygen saturation and the greatest fall in EVF (figures 4 and 5).

Discussion

Injection of all but one of the various substances tested into the left coronary artery elicited a transient

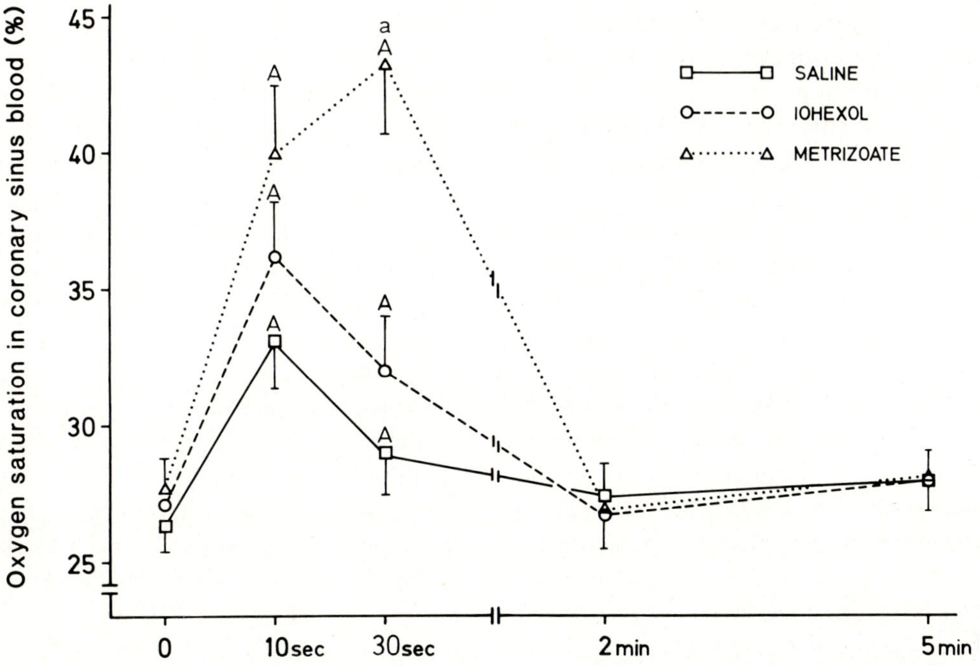

FIGURE 4. Changes in oxygen saturation of coronary sinus blood in patients in group B. Values are mean ± SEM. Symbols of significance are as in figure 3.

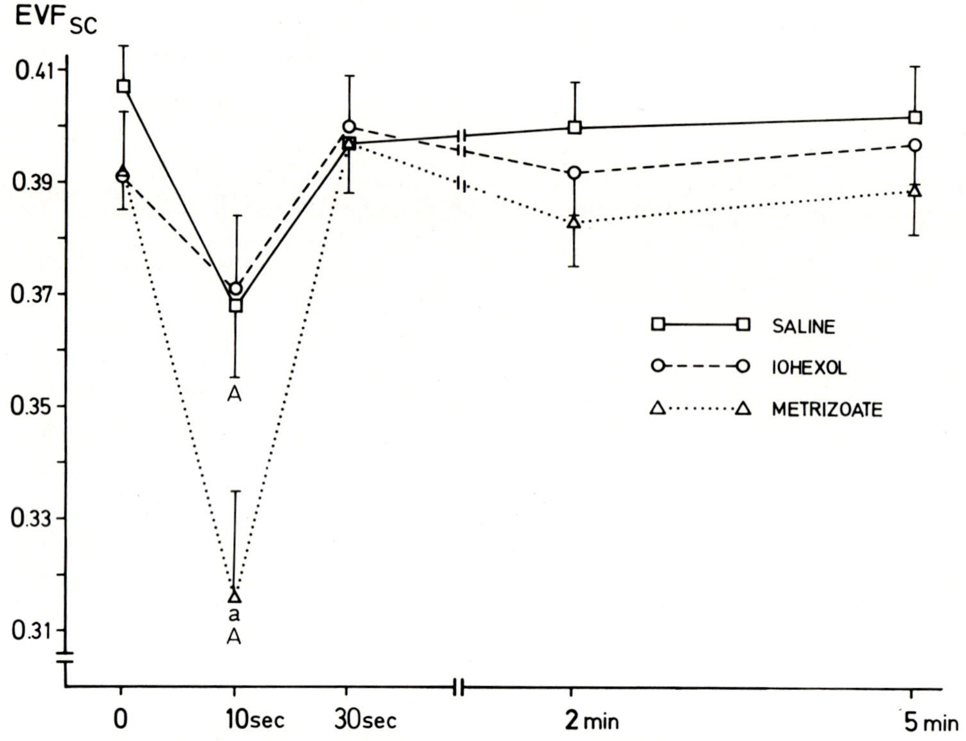

FIGURE 5. Changes in EVF in group B. Values are mean ± SEM. Symbols of significance are as in figure 3.

increase in CSF. The exception was arterial blood, which did not induce any significant alteration in flow. This implies that the injection per se was not a stimulus for a change in coronary blood flow.

In group A patients, the increase in CSF varied markedly depending on the substance injected. There was a 20% to 30% rise in flow after injection of isotonic saline or coronary venous blood. Injection of hypertonic glucose solution resulted in 60% increase and after metrizoate the flow more than doubled. It was also noted that the coronary flow response was more marked when a larger volume of the same substance was injected.

The time sequence of the increase in blood flow after injection of isotonic saline, iohexol, and metrizoate was demonstrated in more detail in the group B patients. The maximal flow occurred at about 10 sec after the injection and in these patients as well as in those in group A, the most marked increase was seen after metrizoate. At the time of increase in coronary flow there was also a significant increase in oxygen saturation of the coronary sinus blood. Again, the most pronounced response was noted after metrizoate injection. The increase in oxygen saturation was short-lasting and returned to the baseline level at 20 sec after saline and iohexol, while the reaction to metrizoate lasted somewhat longer.

The observed changes in coronary hemodynamics after intracoronary injections in this study resemble the reactive hyperemia seen after a brief coronary artery occlusion, when an increase in coronary sinus oxygen saturation is regularly seen and there is an overpayment of flow as well as of oxygen debt.[6]

A similar flow response can be elicited by hypoxia.[7, 8] The mechanism of hypoxic vasodilation is not known in detail. Local release of adenosine, increased extracellular potassium concentration, or local prostaglandin synthesis are proposed but not proved mechanisms for vasodilation.[9, 10] The most likely cause is a direct action of lowered P_{O_2} on the coronary vasculature causing vasodilation. Experimentally, coronary flow has been demonstrated to vary inversely with the arterial oxygen content.[11] Since the intracoronary injection of all substances except arterial blood produced a short period of myocardial hypoxia in the present study, this mechanism may be an important factor in the reactive hyperemia observed in our patients.

There was a progressively increasing hyperemic response to the same amount of saline, hypertonic glucose, and metrizoate. This suggests gradually increasing hypoxic stress on the coronary circulation, which might be explained by different degrees of hyperosmolality. The change in EVF, which was most marked after metrizoate, suggests a varying degree of hemodilution for the different substances. If the hyperosmolar solution causes diffusion of water from extravascular to intravascular space, the volume of fluid with low oxygen content passing the vascular bed will increase. This will cause a more marked hypoxic stimulus of reactive hyperemia. However, exact interpretation of these changes cannot be made since dehydration of erythrocytes in a hyperosmolar solution also could contribute to changes in EVF.

Additional mechanisms might partly explain the changes in coronary flow. For example, it has been demonstrated that the intracoronary injection of contrast material induces bradycardia and peripheral vasodilatation (the so-called Bezold-Jarisch reflex).[12, 13] The explanation for this reaction is probably that mechanoreceptors in the coronary arteries are activated by injection of hyperosmolar agents. Thus, coronary vasodilation due to this mechanism might contribute to the increase in flow after injection of hypertonic glucose solution, iohexol, and metrizoate. On the other hand, the increase in coronary flow caused by injection of isotonic saline and coronary venous blood is not explained by this type of reflex.

Direct vascular actions of the injected substances, i.e., pharmacologic vasodilatation, could also have a hyperemic effect. However, it seems improbable that isotonic saline could have such an effect.

In conclusion, several factors seem to influence the degree of reactive hyperemia after an intracoronary injection. The hypoxic stimulus of the injection, direct and/or indirect effects of hyperosmolarity, and pharmacologic properties of the substances injected seem to be some of the most important determinants of the response.

References

1. Grainger RG: Osmolality of intravascular radiological contrast media. Br J Radiol **53:** 739–746, 1980
2. Mathey DG, Chatterjee K, Tyberg JV, Lekven J, Brundage B, Parmley WW: Coronary sinus reflux. A source of error in the measurement of thermodilution coronary sinus flow. Circulation **57:** 778, 1978
3. Ganz W, Tamura K, Maracus HS, Donoso R, Yoshida S, Swan HJC: Measurement of coronary sinus blood flow by continuous thermodilution in man. Circulation **64:** 181, 1971
4. Siggard-Andersen O: Experiences with a new direct reading oxygen saturation photometer using ultrasound for hemolyzing the blood. Scand J Clin Lab Invest **37:** 45, 1977
5. Snedecor GW, Cochran WG: Statistical methods. Ames, Iowa, 1980, The Iowa State University Press, pp 115–117
6. Schwartz GG, McHale PA, Greenfield JC: Hyperemic response of the coronary circulation to brief diastolic occlusion in the conscious dog. Circ Res **50:** 28, 1982
7. Gellai M, Norton JM, Detar R: Evidence for direct control of coronary vascular tone by oxygen. Circ Res **32:** 279, 1973
8. Gellai M, Detar R: Evidence in support of hypoxia but against high potassium and hyperosmolarity as possible mediators of sustained vasodilation in rabbit cardiac and skeletal muscle. Circ Res **35:** 681, 1974
9. Katori M, Berne RM: Release of adenosine from anoxic hearts. Relationship to coronary flow. Circ Res **19:** 420, 1966
10. Rubio R, Berne RM: Regulation of coronary blood flow. Prog Cardiovasc Dis **18:** 105, 1975
11. Bache RJ, Dymek DJ: Local and regional regulation of coronary vascular tone. Prog Cardiovasc Dis **24:** 191, 1981
12. Zelis R, Caudill CC, Baggette K, Mason DT: Reflex vasodilation induced by coronary angiography in human subjects. Circulation **53:** 490, 1976
13. Perez-Gomez F, Garcia-Aguado A: Origin of ventricular reflexes caused by coronary arteriography. Br Heart J **39:** 967, 1977

Coronary anatomy and left ventricular function in the first 12 hours of acute myocardial infarction: the Western Washington Randomized Intracoronary Streptokinase Trial

MICHAEL L. STADIUS, M.D., CHARLES MAYNARD, M.S., JAMES K. FRITZ, M.D., KATHRYN DAVIS, PH.D., JAMES L. RITCHIE, M.D., FLORENCE SHEEHAN, M.D., AND J. WARD KENNEDY, M.D.*

ABSTRACT The relationships among clinical variables, coronary anatomy, and left ventricular function during the early hours of acute myocardial infarction (AMI) were evaluated from data acquired in the Western Washington Intracoronary Streptokinase Trial. All patients had symptoms and electrocardiographic changes typical of AMI. All data were obtained before treatment with streptokinase. Mean time to catheterization was 4.1 hr after onset of symptoms. Coronary angiograms (n = 245) were analyzed for location of infarct-related occlusion and collateral flow to the infarct bed. Left ventricular ejection fraction and regional left ventricular function were quantitated in 227. Sixty-two percent of occlusions were in the most proximal segment of the involved coronary artery. Collateral circulation was seen in 42% overall, in 31% with left anterior descending artery (LAD) occlusion, and in 52% with right coronary artery (RCA) occlusion ($p < .005$). Left ventricular ejection fraction was lowest and regional function was most abnormal in the group with proximal LAD occlusion. Hyperkinesis was present in 32%; in those with hyperkinesis, hyperkinetic segment length was longest in those with RCA or circumflex occlusion. Multivariate analysis identified proximal LAD occlusion as the factor most closely associated with left ventricular ejection fraction and with measures of left ventricular regional hypofunction. We conclude that (1) AMI is usually caused by occlusion or subtotal occlusion in the most proximal portion of the involved coronary artery, (2) collateral circulation is more frequent with RCA than with LAD occlusion, and (3) location of the infarct-related occlusion is the most important determinant of global and regional left ventricular function in the early hours of AMI.
Circulation 72, No. 2, 292–301, 1985.

THERAPY of acute myocardial infarction (AMI) has undergone a series of revolutionary changes in the past 12 years. With the realization that cardiac catheterization can be performed in the early hours of the acute event with minimal additional risk,[1, 2] aggressive therapies for the treatment of AMI have evolved. Emergency coronary artery bypass surgery,[3, 4] intracoronary infusion of thrombolytic agents,[1, 5–7] and percutaneous transluminal coronary angioplasty[8, 9] are all being used in attempts to improve mortality after AMI. Each of these therapies is dependent on knowledge of coronary artery anatomy. Despite the recent widespread use of these different therapies, systematic description of coronary anatomic findings during the early hours of AMI has not yet been reported. Furthermore, the relationships among baseline clinical characteristics, left ventricular function, and coronary anatomy has not been widely studied in man.

Our objective in this report was to describe the angiographic findings in patients in the Western Washington Intracoronary Streptokinase Trials, to define coronary anatomy and global and regional left ventricular function, and to study the relationships among coronary anatomy, left ventricular function, and clinical features of these patients.

From the Department of Medicine, Division of Cardiology, and the Department of Biostatistics, University of Washington School of Medicine, and the Seattle Veterans Administration Medical Center, Seattle.
Supported in part by the W. M. Keck Foundation and the Medical Research Service of the Veterans Administration. Dr. Stadius was supported in part by a research fellowship from the Washington Affiliate of the American Heart Association.
Address for correspondence: J. Ward Kennedy, M.D., Division of Cardiology, RG-22, University Hospital, Seattle, WA 98195.
Received April 3, 1985; accepted May 9, 1985.
*Principal investigators and their associates are listed in an appendix to this article.

Methods

The protocol and early results of the Western Washington Intracoronary Streptokinase Trial, patient selection, and exclusion criteria have been published in detail previously.[7,10] Patients were eligible for enrollment if they had symptoms of AMI of less than 12 hr duration, were 75 years of age or less, and had electrocardiographic changes typical of AMI.[7] Criteria for exclusion were: (1) presence of disease or conditions other than coronary disease involving a substantial increased risk of death (e.g., cancer, severe liver or kidney disease, coma, etc.), (2) failure to give informed consent, (3) prior exposure to streptokinase, (4) any contraindication to anticoagulation therapy, and (5) any treatment for congestive heart failure before the onset of AMI.

After giving informed consent, all patients were taken to the cardiac catheterization laboratory. Clinical variables, including cardiac history before the event and clinical status at the time of catheterization, were recorded. Left heart catheterization with left ventricular angiography in the 30 degree right anterior oblique projection was performed first, followed by coronary arteriography. The noninvolved coronary artery was studied before the infarct-related artery. If a partially or totally occluded vessel serving the region of the suspected infarct was identified, 0.2 mg of nitroglycerin was infused into the artery followed by repeat arteriography to detect coronary artery spasm. Patients with total occlusion or subtotal occlusion with thrombosis were randomly assigned to the treatment or control group.

All available angiograms were reviewed in the central laboratory by a panel of cardiologists. The site of the infarct-related occlusion was recorded according to the Coronary Artery Surgery Study coronary anatomy map (figure 1).[11] The severity of the initial occlusion and the response to contrast agent and intracoronary nitroglycerin were evaluated. Stenosis less than 90% diameter reduction was measured with hand-held electronic calipers.[12] More severe stenosis was estimated visually. The extent of collateral flow to the infarct bed was graded as none, 1+, 2+, or 3+. Collateral flow of 1+ represented very faint opacification of a small portion of the distal infarct vessel, while 2+ collateral flow was faint opacification of a substantial portion of the infarct vessel, and 3+ collateral flow was good opacification of the substantial portion of the infarct-related vessel.

For quantitative determination of global and regional left ventricular function, angiograms were reviewed in a blinded fashion by an experienced technician and ventricular contours were drawn if the ventricle was adequately opacified during a cardiac cycle not preceded by a premature contraction. End-systole and end-diastole were identified visually. The end-systolic and end-diastolic contours were digitized into a computer and the ejection fraction was calculated by the area-length method developed in this laboratory.[13] Regional wall motion was measured at 100 equally spaced chords perpendicular to a centerline constructed midway between the end-systolic and end-diastolic contours (figure 2).[14,15] Motion at each chord was normalized for heart size by dividing by the end-diastolic perimeter length. Comparison of motion among different chords requires that motion be expressed in comparable units; therefore, the normalized motion of a given chord was converted into units of standard deviation (SD) from the mean motion for that chord as determined in a group of 64 normal patients. This method of normalization allows direct comparison of wall motion between different chords in the same ventricle and chords in different ventricles.[15]

Chord motion expressed in units of SD was plotted for each

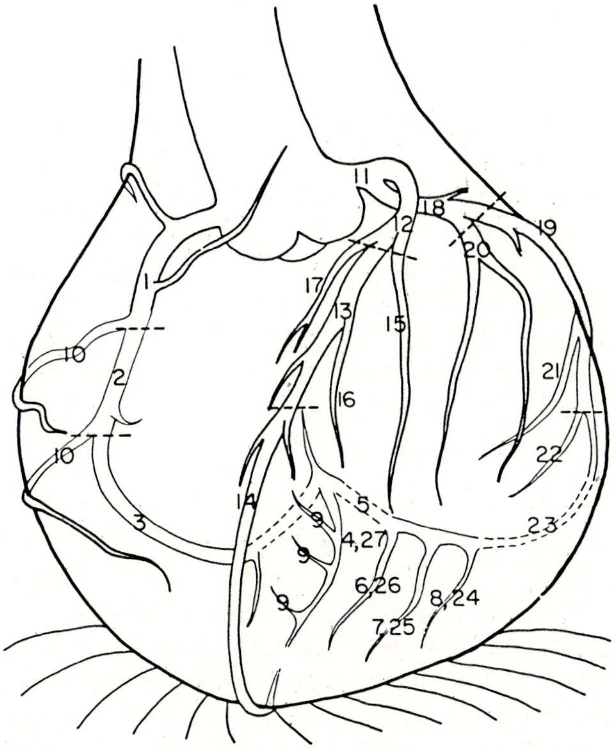

FIGURE 1. Location of the infarct-related occlusion was classified according to this coronary artery anatomy map (from Killip T and the Principal Investigators of the Coronary Artery Surgery Study. Circulation **63** (suppl I): I-59, 1981. Reprinted with permission of the authors and the American Heart Association, Inc.).

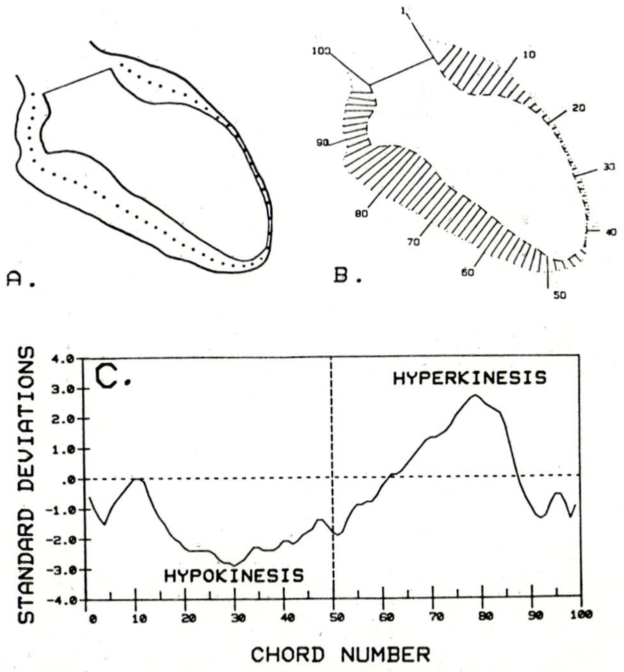

FIGURE 2. *A*, End-systolic and end-diastolic contours with location of centerline indicated. *B*, One hundred equidistant chords constructed perpendicular to the centerline. *C*, Motion at each chord is measured, corrected for end-diastolic perimeter length, then compared with normal expected motion for that chord as previously determined in a group of normal patients. The difference between observed and expected motion is expressed in units of standard deviation from normal mean value and plotted as shown in this N standard plot.

patient (figure 2). Analysis of regional wall motion was carried out between chord numbers 10 and 80. Chords 1 to 9 and 81 to 100 were not analyzed because they reflect motion related to the aortic and mitral valves. For each patient, hypokinetic segment length, abnormally contracting segment length, and hyperkinetic segment length were determined. The hypokinetic segment represents chords with hypokinetic, akinetic, or dyskinetic motion; chord motion was hypokinetic if it was −2.00 SD or less (i.e., equal to or more depressed than 2 SD below normal). The hyperkinetic segment length includes chords with motion 2.00 SD or greater above the normal (see figure 3). The abnormally contracting segment represents chords with akinetic or dyskinetic motion and includes those with absolute motion of 0 or less. Hypokinetic segment length, hyperkinetic segment length, and abnormally contracting segment length each included all chords between 10 and 80 that met criteria for inclusion; that is, chords did not have to be contiguous to be included in a given segment length. Each segment length was expressed as the percentage of the total left ventricular perimeter for each patient. To derive a single numerical value describing all possible forms of abnormal regional function, the "regional function score" was calculated as hypokinetic segment length − hyperkinetic segment length.

Statistical methods. Differences between patient groups were determined with the chi-square statistic for discrete variables and the t and F tests for continuous variables. The t test was used when two groups were compared, the F test when more than two groups were examined. Stepwise multiple regression was used to select clinical and angiographic variables related to key indexes of left ventricular function, namely left ventricular ejection fraction, hypokinetic segment length, abnormally contracting segment length, and hyperkinetic segment length. Variables with F values of 4.0 or greater ($p < .05$) are included in this report. Values are expressed as the mean ± 1 SD.

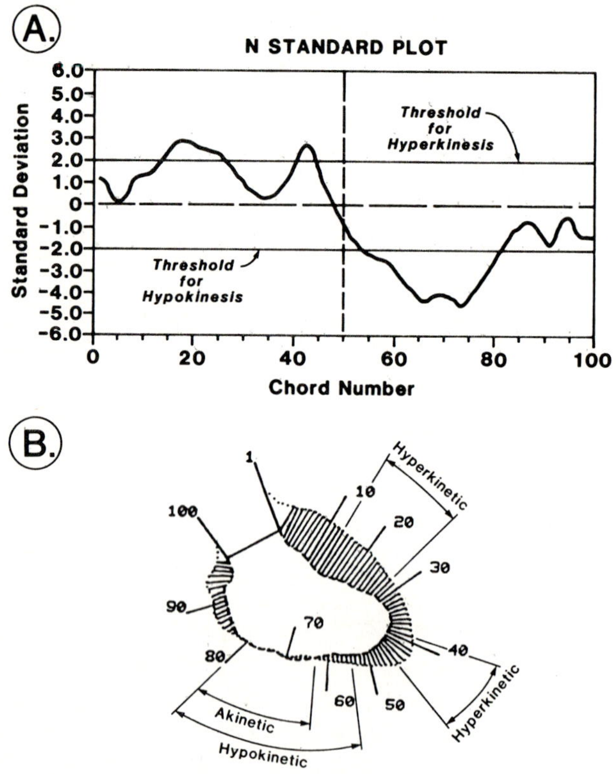

FIGURE 3. *A*, N standard plot from a patient with inferior AMI. Thresholds for hyperkinetic and hypokinetic motion are indicated by solid lines. *B*, End-systolic and end-diastolic contours from N standard plot above. Akinetic, hypokinetic, and hyperkinetic segments determined from analysis of the N standard plot are indicated. The akinetic segment corresponds to the abnormally contracting segment described in the text.

Results

Left ventricular and coronary cineangiograms were available for review in 245 of the 250 patients. Men composed 86.1% of this group. The mean age was 56.5 ± 10.6 years and the mean time from onset of symptoms to randomization was 4.6 ± 2.1 hr. Cardiac catheterization preceded randomization and is estimated to have taken about 30 min to perform. Therefore the mean time to onset of angiography is estimated to be 4.1 hr. Thirteen percent of the patients had a history of prior MI.

Coronary anatomy. The locations of the infarct-related occlusions according to the Coronary Artery Surgery Study anatomy map are listed in table 1. The infarct-related vessel was the left anterior descending artery (LAD) in 114 patients (47%), the right coronary artery (RCA) in 111 patients (45%), and the circumflex artery in 20 patients (8%). In patients with LAD infarct-related occlusions, the occlusion was in the proximal vessel (segment 12) in 67.5%, in the mid-LAD (segment 13) in 30.7%, and in the first diagonal artery in 1.8%. In patients with RCA infarct-related occlusions, the occlusion was proximal to the first acute marginal branch (segment 1) in 57.7%, between the first acute marginal branch and the posterior descending artery (segments 2 and 3) in 38.7%, and more distal (segments 4 and 5) in 3.6%. Of the 20 patients with infarct-related occlusion in the circumflex artery, five had left dominant coronary circulations. The infarct-related occlusion was in the circumflex vessel in 16 patients, and in the obtuse marginal arteries in four patients. Two hundred eight patients (84.9%) demonstrated total occlusion of the infarct-related vessel on initial injection of that vessel. The rate of total occlusion did not vary when analyzed by vessel (84.7% for the RCA, 90.0% for the circumflex, and 84.2% for the LAD).

Hand injection of contrast agent and bolus infusion of intracoronary nitroglycerin had little effect on the severity of the infarct-related occlusions. Only nine patients (3.7%) showed any improvement in the infarct-related occlusion after hand injection of contrast agent (change in mean stenosis from 100% to 94%) and 12 patients (4.9%) showed improvement after bolus intracoronary administration of nitroglycerin (from 99% to 89%). In two patients the response to nitroglyc-

TABLE 1
Site of infarct-related occlusion

Artery	CASS segment number	n	% of total by artery
RCA			
Proximal to AM_1	1	64	57.7
AM_1 to AM_2 or to acute angle	2	31	27.9
AM_2 to PDA	3	12[A]	10.8
PDA	4	1	0.9
LV extension	5	3	2.7
LAD			
Proximal to S_1 and D_1	12	77	67.5
S_1 or D_1 to S_3 or D_3	13	35	30.7
D_1	15	2	1.8
Circumflex artery			
Proximal to OM_1	18	11	55
OM_1 to OM_2	19	5	25
OM_1	20	3	15
OM_2	22	1	5

CASS = Coronary Artery Surgery Study; AM = acute marginal artery; PDA = posterior descending artery; LV = left ventricular; S = septal perforator artery; D = diagonal artery; OM = obtuse marginal artery; subscript numerals refer to branch number.

[A]One patient in this group had occlusion of a saphenous vein bypass graft to segment 3 of the RCA.

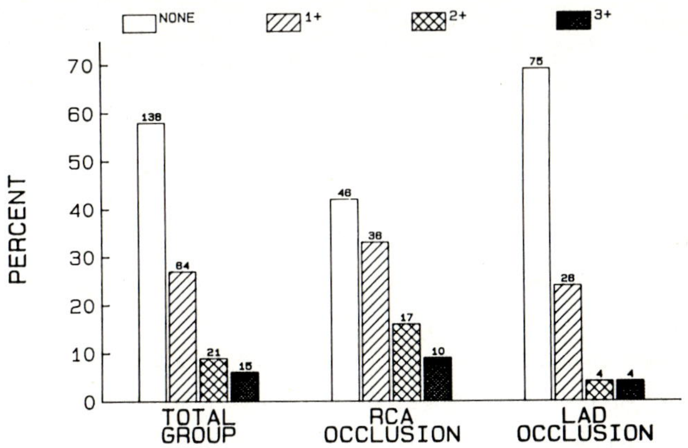

FIGURE 4. Distribution of patients according to assessment of collateral flow to the infarct bed. The grading system used for classification of collateral is discussed in the Methods section. Collateral flow was more prevalent in those with RCA occlusion compared with LAD occlusion ($p < .001$).

erin was dramatic, with a change from total occlusion to 55% diameter stenosis in one and from total occlusion to 70% diameter stenosis in the other.

Adequate coronary angiograms for assessment of collateral blood flow to the infarct bed were available in 238 patients. At least some degree of collateralization was present in 100 patients (42%) (figure 4). Only 34 of the 109 patients (31%) with LAD occlusion had visible collateral flow, while 63 of 109 patients (58%) in the group with RCA occlusion demonstrated collateral flow ($p < .005$). The higher frequency of collateral flow in patients with RCA occlusions persisted when patients with prior AMI were excluded (57% vs 34%; $p < .001$). Collateral flow of 3+ was rare (present in only 15 of the 238 patients, 6%).

Left ventricular function. Left ventricular angiography was performed in 236 of these 245 patients. In nine the angiograms were not suitable for quantitative analysis because of premature contractions or faint opacification. Global left ventricular ejection fraction and regional left ventricular function correlated significantly with the location of the infarct-related occlusion (table 2). Patients with proximal LAD occlusion had the lowest left ventricular ejection fraction, the longest abnormally contracting segment and hypokinetic segment lengths, and the shortest hyperkinetic segment length. Akinesis was present in 94% of patients with LAD

TABLE 2
Global and regional left ventricular function according to the site of the infarct-related occlusion

Location[A]	n	Ejection fraction	Abnormally contracting segment: % of LV perimeter	Abnormally contracting segment: n, % by location	Hypokinetic segment: % of LV perimeter	Hypokinetic segment: n, % by location	Hyperkinetic segment: % of LV perimeter	Hyperkinetic segment: n, % by location
Proximal LAD (segment 12)	68	41.3±10.7	22.0±11.6	64,94%	43.5±12.1	68,100%	7.0±9.0	17,25%
Mid-LAD (segment 13)	30	51.0±11.4	17.3±11.1	28,93%	31.3±14.5	30,100%	5.9±3.1	13,43%
Proximal RCA (segments 1 to 3)	104	53.3±10.0	8.3±6.5	53,51%	21.5±10.6	100,96%	14.5±10.3	38,37%
Proximal circumflex (segments 18 to 20)	17	48.4±11.0	12.2±6.0	6,35%	19.8±10.3	17,100%	17.3±17.9	3,18%
		$p < .0001$	$p < .0001$	$p < .001$	$p < .0001$	p = NS	$p < .01$	p = NS

LV = left ventricular.

[A]Data from eight patients fell outside this classification scheme: four had distal RCA (segments 4 or 5) occlusions, two had diagonal (segment 15) occlusions, one had distal obtuse marginal (segment 23) occlusion, and one had occlusion of a bypass graft to the distal RCA.

occlusion, while only 53% with RCA occlusion and 35% with circumflex occlusion had akinesis ($p < .001$).

Because global left ventricular function can be influenced by a number of variables related to the patient's history and coronary anatomy, stepwise multiple regression was performed to evaluate the relationship of these variables with left ventricular ejection fraction. The following variables were considered in this analysis: patient age, sex, history of prior myocardial infarction, time to randomization (randomization immediately followed cardiac catheterization), severity (% diameter reduction) of infarct occlusion on initial angiographic view, extent of collateral flow to infarct bed, number of vessels with 70% or greater stenosis, and location of infarct-related occlusion. The result of the analysis is presented in table 3. Occlusion in the proximal LAD was the variable most closely related to left ventricular ejection fraction. Other variables that were significantly related to ejection fraction were (in order of decreasing importance): severity of the initial infarct-related occlusion, number of coronary arteries with 70% or greater diameter stenosis reduction, and history of prior AMI. Stepwise multiple regression analysis with the variables listed above was also performed for measures of regional left ventricular function as well. Only proximal and mid-LAD location of the infarct-related occlusion and patient age were significantly related to the abnormally contracting segment length (table 4). These same three variables were also significantly related to the hypokinetic segment length (table 4). Surprisingly, longer hypokinetic segment lengths were associated with absence of prior history of AMI and with higher degrees of collateral blood flow to the infarct bed. The correlation between abnormally contracting segment length and left ventricular ejection fraction was fair ($r = -.52$), while the correlation between hypokinetic segment length and left ventricular ejection fraction was good ($r = -.78$). The left ventricular ejection fraction correlated best with "regional function score" ($r = -.83$).

TABLE 3

Significant variables identified by multiple regression analysis relating global ejection fraction to clinical and angiographic variables

Variable	F value	p value
Proximal LAD occlusion	54.403	<.001
Severity of infarct-related occlusion on initial injection of contrast	7.905	<.01
No. of vessels with ≥ 70% stenosis	6.211	<.01
History of prior MI	4.207	<.05

MI = myocardial infarction.

TABLE 4

Significant variables identified by multiple regression analysis relating regional wall motion parameters to clinical and angiographic variables

Variable	F value	p value
Abnormally contracting segment		
Proximal LAD occlusion	144.1	<.0001
Mid-LAD occlusion	30.3	<.001
Age	7.2	<.01
Hypokinetic segment		
Proximal LAD occlusion	183.8	<.0001
Mid-LAD occlusion	16.3	<.001
Age	11.3	<.01
History of prior MI	8.8	<.01
Extent of collateral flow	4.8	<.05
Hyperkinetic segment		
Proximal RCA occlusion	6.8	<.05
Age	5.7	<.05

MI = myocardial infarction.

Hyperkinesis was seen in 72 (32%) of the patients. When patients with hyperkinesis were compared with those without, there was no significant difference in age, sex, history of prior AMI, time from onset of symptoms to cardiac angiography, initial infarct-related occlusion (percent diameter reduction), and left ventricular end-diastolic pressure (table 5). The incidence of hyperkinesis was similar when analyzed by infarct-related artery (RCA, 35% with hyperkinesis; LAD, 31%; circumflex, 17%; $p = .29$). In those with hyperkinesis, the length of the hyperkinetic segment was related to the location of the infarct-related occlusion. Patients with infarct-related occlusion in the proximal RCA or proximal circumflex artery had long-

TABLE 5

Baseline characteristics in patients with and without hyperkinesis[A]

	Hyperkinesis present (n = 72)	Hyperkinesis absent (n = 155)
Age	56±10	58±10
Sex (% male)	79	88
History of prior MI (% positive)	7	16
Time to randomization from onset of symptoms (hr)[B]	4.7±2.0	4.6±3.6
LV end-diastolic pressure	21±7	22±9
Infarct-related occlusion (% diameter reduction)	99±6	97±10

MI = myocardial infarction; LV = left ventricular.

[A]There were no statistically significant differences between the two groups.

[B]Catheterization preceded randomization and is estimated to have taken about 30 min.

er hyperkinetic segment lengths than those with occlusion in the LAD (table 2).

Global left ventricular ejection fraction was significantly higher in the group of patients with hyperkinesis than in the group without hyperkinesis (56.8 ± 9.6 vs 45.3 ± 10.5; $p < .0001$). Likewise, the hypokinetic segment length was shorter in the groups with hyperkinesis; however, there was no difference in akinetic segment length between these two groups (table 6). When analyzed by infarct-related vessel, left ventricular ejection fraction remained significantly higher and hypokinetic segment length was shorter in patients with hyperkinesis (table 6).

Discussion

Coronary anatomy. Thrombosis is the proximate cause of AMI in patients presenting with ST segment elevation on their initial electrocardiograms.[2] The majority of patients in our series had thrombotic occlusion or subtotal occlusion with thrombosis in the most proximal segment of the involved coronary vessel. Interestingly, involvement of the circumflex artery was uncommon. Only 20 patients (8.1%) had involvement of the circumflex artery; furthermore, five of these 20 had left dominant coronary distributions. Thus only 6.1% of this group had infarction limited to the lateral left ventricular wall. One explanation for this finding is that elevation of the ST segment, a criteria for entry in this study, is an uncommon finding in those with circumflex disease leading to AMI. Other explanations are more speculative. Certainly, from pathologic series, significant atherosclerosis appears to be evenly distributed among the three coronary beds.[16, 17] However, whether thrombosis occurs with similar frequency in all three coronary beds remains open to question.

Our observations on the frequency of collateral flow to the infarct bed are consistent with the findings and conclusions of prior reports.[18, 19] Extensive collateral flow in the early hours of AMI was very common (present in only 6% of the patients). On the other hand, lesser collateral circulation was present in an additional 36% of this group. Presence of collateral flow had no beneficial effect on global or regional left ventricular function in these short-term studies. However, angiographically detectable collateral flow in the early hours of AMI may be associated with evolution of smaller infarctions. Schwartz et al.[20] reported in a small series of patients that resting thallium defects late after AMI appeared to be smaller in patients with faint collaterals present early in the infarction compared with resting defect size in patients without early collateral flow. Nitzberg et al.[19] likewise reported that presence of early collateral circulation was associated with improved left ventricular ejection fraction in late follow-up studies. These two reports at least raise the possibility that the presence of faint collateralization early in AMI may provide some protective effect to the infarct zone. If this is true, then some protective effect from collateral flow may be present in a third or more of patients with AMI.

At this time, we can only offer speculation as to why collateral flow is more frequent in those with RCA occlusion compared with those with LAD occlusion. The LAD and circumflex arteries serve only left ventricular myocardium, a relatively high-resistance bed. The RCA, on the other hand, serves both left and right ventricular myocardium and the latter is a relatively low-resistance bed. It is likely that the resistance in the RCA bed remains lower in the presence of an occlusion proximal to the acute marginal branches. The presence of the two different myocardial resistance beds in the RCA may well explain why collateral circulation is more common with RCA than with LAD or circumflex occlusion.

Left ventricular function. This study illustrates the im-

TABLE 6
Relationship of hyperkinesis to other measures of left ventricular function

	HYPO	ACS	LVEF
Total group			
Hyperkinesis absent (n = 155)	30.7±15.7	10.5±11.7	45.3±10.5
Hyperkinesis present (n = 72)	25.3±14.7	11.2±12.5	56.8±9.6
	p < .05	p = NS	p < .0001
LAD occlusion			
Hyperkinesis absent (n = 70)	41.4±13.9	19.0±11.8	40.8±10.3
Hyperkinesis present (n = 31)	35.9±13.4	19.5±13.4	52.2±10.8
	p < .05	p = NS	p < .0001
RCA occlusion			
Hyperkinesis absent (n = 70)	22.1±11.5	3.5±5.3	49.5±9.2
Hyperkinesis present (n = 38)	17.5±9.9	5.2±7.5	60.2±6.8
	p < .05	p = NS	p < .0001
Circumflex artery occlusion			
Hyperkinesis absent (n = 15)	21.1±10.2	4.5±7.2	45.9±9.2
Hyperkinesis present (n = 3)	15.0±11.1	2.3±4.0	60.3±10.7
	p = NS	p = NS	p < .05

HYPO = hypokinetic segment length; ACS = abnormally contracting segment length; LVEF = left ventricular ejection fraction.

portant relationship between coronary anatomy and global and regional left ventricular function in the setting of AMI. The location of the infarct-related occlusions was identified as the single most important variable related to every measure of left ventricular function. Proximal LAD occlusion (segment 12) was associated with the lowest mean ejection fraction (41.3%) and was identified by multiple regression analysis as the variable most closely associated with left ventricular ejection fraction. Likewise, proximal LAD occlusion was associated with the longest mean abnormally contracting segment and hypokinetic segment lengths, and in both cases was identified by multiple regression analysis as the best predictor of these measures of regional left ventricular function. On the other hand, in patients with hyperkinesis, location of the infarct occlusion in the RCA or circumflex artery was associated with longer (but not more frequent) hyperkinetic segment lengths.

This very strong relationship between location of the infarct-related occlusion in the coronary bed and left ventricular function has not been emphasized in the past. Pathologic study has demonstrated a somewhat predictable relationship between a coronary artery and the size of its myocardial perfusion bed in man.[21] By injecting coronary arteries with contrast medium then serially slicing the left ventricular myocardium (free wall and whole interventricular septum), it was possible to determine the relative size of the three coronary perfusion beds in a series of 171 postmortem heart specimens. Approximately two-thirds of the left ventricular myocardium received its blood supply from the LAD in this analysis. Our observations provide the physiologic correlate to these anatomic observations. Location of the infarct-related occlusion in the LAD was associated with the greatest decrease in ejection fraction and with the longest hypokinetic and abnormally contracting segment lengths.

The relationship between location of the infarct-related occlusion and ventricular function has implications for the design of interventional trials in AMI. If serial studies of left ventricular function are selected as an end point for evaluation of a proposed intervention, then the intervention should have the same success rate in all coronary beds before measures of left ventricular function from all patient studies can be grouped together. If the intervention varies in rate of success according to location of infarct-related occlusion or if distribution of locations of the infarct-related occlusions vary in treatment and control groups, then measures of left ventricular function would need to be evaluated by location of the infarct-related occlusion.

Factors other than location of the infarct-related occlusion were related to measures of left ventricular function. For left ventricular ejection fraction, three other variables were identified. Percent diameter obstruction of the infarct-related vessel on initial injection of contrast agent presumably influences function within the infarct zone. The other two factors, history of prior AMI and number of noninfarct zone vessels with 70% or greater diameter stenoses, influence ventricular function outside the infarct zone. Patient age and sex, collateral flow to the infarct bed, and time from onset of symptoms to study were not related to ejection fraction in our study. Animal studies have shown that the major portion of myocardial dysfunction occurs within several minutes of coronary occlusion.[22, 23] Thus the angiographically determined ejection fraction at 3 to 6 hr is probably very similar to that a few minutes after occlusion. Although age was not related to left ventricular ejection fraction, it was related to each of the measures of regional left ventricular function. Older age was associated with longer abnormally contracting segment and hypokinetic segment lengths and shorter hyperkinetic segment length. This effect of age is not well understood, but the results of the multivariate analysis suggest that it is not related in a simple manner to more advanced coronary disease or prior AMI.

In this analysis, we have described three measures of regional left ventricular function. The abnormally contracting segment has been described previously.[24] Hypokinetic and hyperkinetic segment lengths are analogous to the abnormally contracting segment. They represent our attempts to measure quantitatively hypokinesis and hyperkinesis in addition to akinesis and dyskinesis. Each is based on the statistical nature of the centerline method for regional wall motion analysis[14, 15]; that is, motion at a given point is classified as abnormal if it is 2.00 SD or greater from the expected normal mean value for that point. As with any measure of function based on the 30 degree right anterior oblique contrast angiogram, some caution must be used in interpretation of the data. The anterior wall and apex are well represented in this single-plane image, but lateral, septal, and some parts of the posterobasal aspects of the left ventricle are not represented in the image. Realignment of end-systolic and end-diastolic contours further complicate regional wall motion analysis.[25, 26] The relatively low percentage of patients with RCA and circumflex occlusions who have akinesis may be explained in part by these limitations of the 30 degree right anterior oblique angiogram.

Sheehan et al.[27] and Stack et al.[28] have previously

demonstrated that global left ventricular ejection fraction in the setting of AMI is a relatively poor indicator of potential for salvage of regional function in the infarct zone. The global ejection fraction was in many cases influenced by hyperkinesis in the nonischemic myocardium outside the infarct zone. These authors concluded that the best measure of functional recovery was assessment of the regional function in the infarct zone, not evaluation of serial changes in the global ejection fraction. Our observations also illustrate the important disparity between function in the infarct zone and left ventricular ejection fraction. In the absence of prior AMI, the abnormally contracting segment length should be closely correlated with infarct size. However, the correlation between abnormally contracting segment length and ejection fraction here was only fair ($r = -.52$). On the other hand, correlation between ejection fraction and the "regional function score" ($r = -.83$) was much better. This regional function score represented all possible types of regional dysfunction, including dyskinesis, akinesis, hypokinesis, and hyperkinesis.

Because abnormally contracting segment length has been used in prior investigations[24, 29, 30] in patients several days to 12 months after AMI, a comparison of findings can be made. Feild et al.[24] found no significant difference in the abnormally contracting segment length when they compared patients with anterior and inferior myocardial infarction. However, their report included only 17 patients in the analysis. Rigaud et al.[29] studied 62 patients and found a significant difference in abnormally contracting segment length between groups with anterior and inferior infarction at 2 to 6 days after AMI (anterior, 34 ± 14%; inferior, 28 ± 7%; $p < .02$). Likewise, Bertrand et al.,[30] in patients 7 to 21 days after AMI, found that the abnormally contracting segment length was 39 ± 2% in those with anterior AMI and 28 ± 2% in those with inferior AMI ($p < .001$). When our data for abnormally contracting segment length from the groups with proximal LAD and proximal RCA occlusion are compared with the data of Rigaud et al. and Bertrand et al., it is clear that the abnormally contracting segment length recorded 2 to 21 days after AMI is substantially longer than that recorded in the first hours of AMI, particularly in patients with inferior AMI. Some of these differences may be due to technique. Our computer-based method for measuring abnormally contracting segment length included all points with the criteria for akinesis or dyskinesis but did not include points with hypokinetic wall motion within the akinetic region. Planimetry by hand, as was done in prior studies, would tend to include hypokinetic points within the akinetics region, thus leading to longer abnormally contracting segment lengths. We also excluded chords 81 to 100 because they corresponded to motion of the mitral valve apparatus and not to myocardial wall motion. Inclusion of these chords would decrease the discrepancy in the abnormally contracting segment length at the different intervals, particularly in the group with inferior AMI. However, it is doubtful that these methodologic differences account for all the discrepancy between our early abnormally contracting segment lengths and those reported by others from later in the course of AMI. Thus it is quite possible that the abnormally contracting segment continues to enlarge between 4 and 5 hr after onset of AMI and 2 to 21 days later. Only serial studies in the same patients will provide definite answers on this issue.

Hyperkinesis in AMI has been reported previously.[27, 28, 31, 32] However, factors potentially related to hyerkinesis have not been evaluated in detail. In this series, 32% of patients had evidence of at least some amount of hyperkinesis. Patient age, sex, history of prior AMI, time from onset of symptoms to study, left ventricular end-diastolic pressure, and severity of occlusion on initial injection of contrast agent appear unrelated to the ability of the left ventricle in a given patient to mount a hyperkinetic response. We could not evaluate any potential relationships between medications and hyperkinesis because of lack of detailed data about medications given between presentation and study. Importantly, global left ventricular ejection fraction was significantly higher in the group of patients with hyperkinesis than in the group without hyperkinesis. Whether presence of hyperkinesis has important clinical implications for the patient remains unclear. Only Nieminen et al.[32] have explored the relationship between occurrence of hyperkinesis (defined by echocardiography) and clinical status of the patients at the time of study. They concluded that hyperkinetic function was seen only in patients with uncomplicated or "moderately" complicated AMIs. Hyperkinesis was absent in those with complicated infarction and cardiogenic shock. These findings have yet to be confirmed; furthermore, the long-term implications of occurrence of hyperkinesis have not been evaluated.

In summary, the following clinical implications can be drawn from this analysis: (1) anterior infarction results in lower left ventricular ejection fraction and larger measures of regional left ventricular dysfunction than inferior infarction; (2) collateral flow to the infarct bed is common but has no beneficial effect on global or regional left ventricular function in the early hours of

AMI; (3) hyperkinesis is common and, when present, results in improved ejection fraction; and (4) involvement of the circumflex artery is rare when patients with AMI are selected because of ST segment elevation.

We thank Carol Alcock and Lorelle Lambert for technical assistance and Sylvia Duncan for manuscript preparation.

Appendix

The principal investigators and their associates of the Western Washington Intracoronary Streptokinase Trial (italics denote investigators administratively responsible for the trial at their institutions): J. W. Kennedy, Director; J. L. Ritchie, Co-Director; K. B. Davis, Investigator; J. K. Fritz, Investigator. Angiographic Analysis Committee: J. W. Kennedy, J. K. Fritz, M. L. Stadius. Policy Board: S. Rubenstein, Chairman; P. B. Beeson, T. S. Inui, L. Fisher. Data Coordinating Center: K. B. Davis, C. Maynard. Technicians: C. Alcock, A. Coleman, K. Gaines. Nurses: D. Erickson, K. McFadden. Clinical Associates: Overlake Hospital (Bellevue, WA), *C. E. Hansing,* K. M. Hynes, R. E. Haynes, D. B. Ferrin, J. S. Schneider, J. T. Holder; St. Joseph Hospital (Bellingham, WA), *R. S. Trenouth,* D. C. Brown, D. D. McAfee; Everett General Hospital (Everett, WA), *J. P. Nolan,* D. J. Stewart, W. J. MacDonald, K. H. Prindle, N. D. Smith, J. Schmitt; Providence Hospital (Seattle), *G. A. Logan, F. M. Tobis,* T. A. Block, J. G. Doces, M. T. English, P. C. Albro, A. L. Sytman, R. A. Crone, C. G. Hale, B. Green; Swedish Hospital (Seattle), *F. A. Short,* W. E. Samson, R. J. Westcott, J. L. Peterson; University Hospital (Seattle), *D. K. Stewart,* J. A. Murray, K. F. Hossack, J. A. Werner, G. Frank, B. G. Brown, D. W. Weaver, G. B. Trobaugh; Veterans Administration Hospital (Seattle), *J. W. Kennedy, J. L. Ritchie,* J. H. Caldwell, J. Stratton; Virginia Mason Hospital (Seattle), *R. R. Johnston;* Madigan Army Hospital (Tacoma, WA), *J. L. Hill,* T. Steudel, R. Chamusco; Tacoma General Hospital (Tacoma, WA), *E. Lapin,* T. Reagan; St. Joseph's Hospital (Tacoma, WA), *J. R. McDonough,* M. Henry; Vancouver General Hospital (Vancouver, BC), *R. R. Ricci;* Wenatchee Valley Hospital (Wenatchee, WA), *D. Larson,* J. Gorham; St. Elizabeth Hospital (Yakima, WA), *D. A. Monick,* R. D. Twiss, A. B. Preacher, R. K. Spiegel.

References

1. Rentrop P, Blanke H, Karsch KR, Kaiser H, Kostering H, Leitz K: Selective intracoronary thrombolysis in acute myocardial infarction and unstable angina pectoris. Circulation **63:** 307, 1981
2. DeWood MA, Spores J, Notske R, Mouser LT, Burroughs R, Golden MS, Lang HT: Prevalence of total coronary occlusion during the early hours of transmural myocardial infarction. N Engl J Med **303:** 897, 1982
3. Pifarre R, Spinazzola A, Nemickas R, Scanlon PJ, Tobin JR: Emergency aorto-coronary bypass for acute myocardial infarction. Arch Surg **103:** 525, 1971
4. DeWood MA, Spores J, Notske RN, Long HT, Shields JP, Simpson CS, Rudy LW, Grunwald R: Medical and surgical management of myocardial infarction. Am J Cardiol **44:** 1356, 1983
5. Ganz W, Buchbinder N, Marcus H, Mondkar A, Maddahi J, Charuzi Y, O'Connor L, Shell W, Fishbein MC, Kass R, Miyamoto A, Swan HJC: Intracoronary thrombolysis in evolving myocardial infarction. Am Heart J **101:** 4, 1981
6. Mathey DG, Kuck K-H, Tilsner V, Krebber H-J, Bleifeld W: Nonsurgical coronary artery recanalization in acute transmural myocardial infarction. Circulation **63:** 489, 1981
7. Kennedy JW, Ritchie JL, Davis KB, Fritz JK: Western Washington Randomized Trial of Intracoronary Streptokinase in Acute Myocardial Infarction. N Engl J Med **309:** 1477, 1983
8. Erbel R, Pop T, Meinertz T, Kaspar W, Ruckel A, Schreiner G, Pfeiffer C, Meyer J: Combined medical and mechanical recanalization in acute myocardial infarction. Circulation **68** (suppl III): III-326, 1983 (abst)
9. Prida XE, Feldman RL, Hill JA, Pepine CJ: Coronary angioplasty of totally occluded vessels in acute myocardial infarction. Circulation **70** (suppl II): II-107, 1984 (abst)
10. Kennedy JW, Fritz JK, Ritchie JL: Streptokinase in acute myocardial infarction. Western Washington Randomized Trial: protocol and progress report. Am Heart J **104:** 899, 1982
11. Killip T and the Principal Investigators: The National Heart Lung, and Blood Institute Coronary Artery Surgery Study (CASS). Circulation **63** (suppl I): I-59, 1981
12. Scoblionko DP, Brown BG, Mitten S, Caldwell JH, Kennedy JW, Bolson EL, Dodge HT: A new digital electronic caliper for measurement of coronary arterial stenosis: comparison with visual estimates and computer-assisted measurements. Am J Cardiol **53:** 689, 1984
13. Kasser IS, Kennedy JW: Measurement of left ventricular volumes in man by single plane cineangiography. Invest Radiol **4:** 83, 1969
14. Bolson EL, Kliman S, Sheehan F, Dodge HT: Left ventricular segmental wall motion — a new method using local direction information. IEEE Comput Cardiol 245, 1980
15. Sheehan FH, Stewart DK, Dodge HT, Mitten S, Bolson EL, Brown BG: Variability in the measurement of regional left ventricular wall motion from contrast angiograms. Circulation **68:** 550, 1983
16. Arnett EN, Isner JM, Redwood DR, Kent KM, Baker WP, Ackerstein H, Roberts WC: Coronary artery narrowing in coronary heart disease: comparison of cineangiographic and necropsy findings. Ann Intern Med **91:** 350, 1979
17. Roberts WC, Jones AA: Quantification of coronary arterial narrowing at necropsy in acute transmural myocardial infarction. Am J Cardiol **61:** 786, 1980
18. Schwartz H, Leiboff RH, Bren GB, Wasserman AG, Katz RJ, Varghese PJ, Sokil AB, Ross AM: Temporal evaluation of the human coronary collateral circulation after myocardial infarction. J Am Coll Cardiol **4:** 1088, 1984
19. Nitzberg WD, Nath HP, Rogers WJ, Hood WP Jr, Whitlow PL, Reeves RC, Baxley WA: Change in collateral blood flow supply during evolving acute myocardial infarction. J Am Coll Cardiol **3:** 575, 1984 (abst)
20. Schwartz F, Schuler G, Hofmann M, Kubler W: Recruitment of collaterals following acute coronary occlusion reduces infarct size in man. J Am Coll Cardiol **1:** 591, 1983 (abst)
21. Kalbfleisch H, Hort W: Quantitative study on the size of coronary artery supplying areas postmortem. Am Heart J **94:** 183, 1977
22. Theroux P, Franklin D, Ross J Jr, Kemper WS: Regional myocardial function during acute coronary artery occlusion and its modification by pharmacologic agents in the dog. Circ Res **35:** 896, 1974
23. Walens SO, DaLuz PL, Wyatt HL, Swan HJC, Forrester JS: Early changes in regional and global left ventricular function induced by graded reductions in regional coronary perfusion. Am J Cardiol **39:** 537, 1977
24. Feild BJ, Russell RO, Dowling JT, Rackley CE: Regional left ventricular performance in the year following myocardial infarction. Circulation **46:** 679, 1972
25. Chaitman BR, Bristow JD, Rahimtoola SH: Left ventricular wall motion assessed by using fixed external reference systems. Circulation **48:** 1043, 1973
26. Sheehan FH, Stewart DK, Dodge HT, Mitten S, Bolson EL, Brown BG: Variability in the measurement of regional left ventricular wall motion from contrast angiograms. Circulation **68:** 550, 1983
27. Sheehan FH, Mathey DG, Schofer J, Krebber H-J, Dodge HT: Effects of interventions in salvaging left ventricular function in acute myocardial infarction: a study of intracoronary streptokinase. Am J Cardiol **52:** 431, 1983
28. Stack RS, Phillips HR III, Grierson DS, Behar VS, Kong Y, Peter RH, Swain JL, Greenfield JC Jr: Functional improvement of jeopardized myocardium following intracoronary streptokinase infusion in acute myocardial infarction. J Clin Invest **72:** 84, 1983
29. Rigaud M, Rocha P, Boschat J, Farcot JC, Bardet J, Bourdaris JP: Regional left ventricular function assessed by contrast angiography in acute myocardial infarction. Circulation **60:** 130, 1979
30. Bertrand ME, Rousseau MF, Lablanche JM, Corre AG, Lekieffre

JP: Cineangiographic assessment of left ventricular function in the acute phase of transmural myocardial infarction. Am J Cardiol **43:** 472, 1979
31. Theroux P, Ross J Jr, Franklin D, Covell JW, Bloor CM, Sasayana S: Regional myocardial function and dimensions early and late after myocardial infarction in the unanesthesized dog. Circ Res **40:** 158, 1977
32. Nieminen M, Heikkila J: Echoventriculography in acute myocardial infarction. III. Clinical correlations and implication of the noninfarcted myocardium. Am J Cardiol **38:** 1, 1976

Mildly dilated congestive cardiomyopathy

ANDRE KEREN, M.D., MARGARET E. BILLINGHAM, M.D., DOMINIQUE WEINTRAUB, M.D., EDWARD B. STINSON, M.D., AND RICHARD L. POPP, M.D.

ABSTRACT Five patients with only mildly dilated ventricles but other features typical of congestive cardiomyopathy underwent cardiac transplantation for class IV NYHA heart failure. The findings of clinical studies, cardiac catheterization, endomyocardial biopsy, and pathologic examination of the removed hearts in this group with mildly dilated congestive cardiomyopathy (MDCM) were compared with similar data in four patients with idiopathic restrictive cardiomyopathy (IRCM) and in 10 patients with typical dilated congestive cardiomyopathy (DCM). In comparison with the other groups, patients with MDCM had a higher incidence of familial cardiomyopathy ($p = .02$) and a shorter symptomatic period than patients with IRCM ($p < .02$). Patients with both MDCM and DCM had globular hearts (with predominant left ventricular dilatation), congestive hemodynamics and poor left ventricular contractility (ejection fraction 12% to 19%), and high incidence of ventricular thrombi. Patients with IRCM showed normal ventricular size, marked atrial dilatation, restrictive hemodynamics, mild-to-moderate decrease in left ventricular contractility (ejection fraction 29% to 55%), and absence of ventricular thrombi. Cardiac index, ventricular wall thickness, and light microscopic findings were similar in the three groups of patients. Electron microscopy showed no myofibrillar loss in patients with IRCM but mild (partial) or moderate-to-severe (almost total) myofibrillar loss in those with MDCM and DCM, respectively. We conclude that (1) end-stage congestive cardiomyopathy may occur without significant ventricular dilatation and (2) patients with MDCM have heart sizes intermediate between those found in IRCM and DCM but their clinical, hemodynamic, and pathologic findings are virtually identical to those of patients with typical DCM.
Circulation **72, No. 2, 302–309, 1985.**

CONGESTIVE and restrictive cardiomyopathies represent distinct entities with different hemodynamic and morphologic features.[1] Congestive cardiomyopathy is characterized by ventricular dilatation and poor systolic function with greatly reduced ejection fraction.[1–4] Dilatation of the ventricles usually occurs earlier than heart failure and is considered the most important manifestation of the disease.[3, 5] For this reason, the terms "dilated"[2, 6] or "dilated congestive"[3, 4] cardiomyopathy are currently preferred. Light and electron microscopic assessment show major but nonspecific abnormal changes.[1, 3, 6]

Restrictive cardiomyopathy is characterized by normal or near normal ventricular size and systolic function but compromised ventricular relaxation leading to distinctive hemodynamic findings.[3, 4] The term restrictive (nondilated) cardiomyopathy is preferred by some authors to emphasize the absence of ventricular dilatation.[4] Infiltrative processes or endomyocardial fibrosis, with or without eosinophilia, usually represent its pathologic basis.[1, 6] Rarely has a primary[7] or idiopathic[8] form of the disease been reported in which histologic examination did not reveal specific changes.[7–9]

This study presents the clinical and morphologic data of patients who underwent cardiac transplantation in whom the characteristic features of congestive cardiomyopathy occurred without significant ventricular dilatation. For better characterization of these patients, with what we tentatively term "mildly dilated" congestive cardiomyopathy (MDCM), the findings of this group were compared with those of heart transplant recipients with idiopathic restrictive cardiomyopathy (IRCM) and with typical dilated congestive cardiomyopathy (DCM).

Methods

Patients. Review of the pathologic findings in 103 consecutive patients with idiopathic cardiomyopathy who underwent cardiac transplantation revealed normal ventricular size or bor-

From the Cardiology Division, Stanford University Medical Center, Stanford, CA.

Supported in part by Fogarty Fellowship Grant FO5 TWO 3416-01-B1 from the National Institutes of Health, by the Israeli Heiden Fellowship, and by Clinical Heart and Heart-Lung Transplantation Grant HL-13108-15 from the National Heart, Lung, and Blood Institute.

Address for correspondence: Richard L. Popp, M.D., Cardiology Division, Stanford University Medical Center, Stanford, CA 94305.

Received April 10, 1985; accepted May 16, 1985.

derline ventricular enlargement in 10 patients. Of these, eight patients were included in the study by fulfilling the following additional criteria: (1) normal or slightly enlarged left and right ventricular diameter (no more than 10% to 15% above normal range after correction for body surface area) on preoperative echocardiogram and/or angiogram, (2) well preserved recipient heart specimens suitable for current analysis, and (3) available preoperative clinical charts and catheterization data. Based on data from clinical, hemodynamic, and echocardiographic studies and from the results of pericardial biopsy (two patients), the preoperative diagnosis was IRCM in three patients and congestive cardiomyopathy with mild ventricular dilatation (MDCM) in five. We also included a nonconsecutive patient who was recently admitted to the heart transplantation program and in whom angiography, echocardiography, right ventricular endomyocardial biopsy, and hemodynamic study proved the presence of IRCM. The clinical, hemodynamic, and pathologic data in these two categories of patients were compared with similar data recorded in 10 contemporaneous patients with typical DCM.

Echocardiography. Two-dimensional and M mode echocardiograms were obtained 2 to 80 days (32 ± 17 days) before surgery with a Hewlett-Packard model 77020A imaging system and a 2.5 or 3.5 MHz medium- or short-focused tranducer. All studies included at least the standard parasternal, apical, and subcostal views.[10] Echocardiographic measurements were performed in a standard way.[11] The right ventricular and right atrial diameters were measured from the apical four-chamber view, as previously described.[10] Both M mode and two-dimensional echocardiographic measurements (corrected for body surface area) were compared with normal values obtained in our laboratory.[10, 12] The range of normal values (expressed in cm/m^2) are: left ventricular diastolic diameter, 2.0 to 3.2; left atrial systolic diameter, 1.1 to 2.3[12]; right ventricular diastolic minor axis, 1.0 to 2.8; right atrial systolic minor axis, 1.7 to 2.5.[10]

Cardiac catheterization and angiography. Left and right heart catheterization were performed with standard transducers and fluid-filled catheters. Pressure tracings were specifically analyzed for presence or absence of restrictive patterns.[3, 4] Left ventricular angiograms were obtained in the 30 degree right anterior oblique projection. The parameters measured during these tests (table 1) represented the major preoperative criteria for classifying the patients into the groups with restrictive or congestive cardiomyopathy. The results of coronary arteriography were normal in all patients.

Pathology. Pathologic assessment included morphologic examination of the removed hearts and microscopic evaluation of preoperative and postoperative endomyocardial biopsy specimens. The presence of atrial thrombi and characteristics of the pericardium were evaluated during operation and, when indicated, pericardial biopsy specimens were taken.

Collection of heart specimens. Immediately after excision the recipient heart was collected, weighed, and photographed, and a gross description was made. Wall thickness measurements were made in the pulmonary outflow tract for the right ventricle (normal range 0.2 to 0.3 cm) and in the left ventricular wall opposite the caudal tip of the anterolateral papillary muscle (normal range 1 to 1.2 cm). The heart was then placed in 10% formalin for fixation. Because the atria are partially left within the patient, it was not possible to inflate the hearts; whenever possible, however, the ventricles were packed with wadding before fixation to maintain their shape. After fixation, the heart

TABLE 1
Clinical and hemodynamic findings in all patients

	IRCM (n = 4)	MDCM (n = 5)	DCM (n = 10)	p value
Age (yr)	30.2±2.1	32.8±16.0	28.2±12.7	NS
Family history	0[C]	4	2[C]	<.02
Symptomatic period (mo)	65.2±17.4[C]	34.0±18.0	27.4±14.2	<.01
Atrial fibrillation[A]	4	2	4	NS
AV block (3°)	2	1	1	NS
VT/VF	2	2	6	NS
LVDI (cm/m^2)[B]	2.6±0.3[C]	3.4±0.1	4.5±0.5[C]	<.001
LVSI (cm/m^2)	2.1±0.3[C]	3.1±0.2	4.1±0.6	<.001
RVDI (cm/m^2)	2.6±0.2	2.6±0.5	2.5±0.7	NS
LASI (cm/m^2)	3.0±0.3	2.8±0.2	2.9±0.3	NS
RASI (cm/m^2)	2.8±0.1	2.7±0.7	2.5±0.6	NS
LVFS (%)	21.5±2.7[C]	8.8±2.7	9.1±3.9	<.001
RAP (mean, mm Hg)	20.3±5.4	15.8±5.5	16.8±5.3	NS
PCWP (mean, mm Hg)	25.2±4.3	28.3±7.0	30.0±11.0	NS
RVDP (mm Hg)	19.0±4.5	15.4±6.9	15.3±5.8	NS
LVDP (mm Hg)	22.8±5.5	25.2±5.9	27.0±4.0	NS
Ejection fraction (%)	39.0±6.6[C]	17.0±4.0	15.0±3.3	<.001
Cardiac index (l/min/m^2)	1.7±0.4	1.4±0.2	1.5±0.3	NS

AV = atrioventricular; LVFS = left ventricular fractional shortening; LASI = left atrial systolic index; LVDI = left ventricular diastolic index; LVDP = left ventricular end-diastolic pressure; LVSI = left ventricular systolic index; PCWP = pulmonary capillary wedge pressure; RAP = right atrial pressure; RASI = right atrial systolic index; RVDI = right ventricular diastolic index; RVDP = right ventricular end-diastolic pressure; VT/VF = ventricular tachycardia/ventricular fibrillation.

[A]Paroxysmal and/or chronic atrial fibrillation.

[B]Echocardiographic measurements of cavity sizes and left ventricular fractional shortening not performed in one patient with IRCM.

[C]Statistically significant difference found as compared with mildly dilated cardiomyopathy (MDCM).

was opened and visual and photographic descriptions of the interior of the ventricles were made. The presence of thrombi and endocardial fibrosis was noted. The extent of endocardial fibrosis was analyzed in the three ventricular portions (inflow, outflow, and trabeculated area) and graded from 0 (no fibrosis found) to 3 (fibrosis present in all three ventricular portions).

Light microscopy. After fixation, sections were taken from the left and right ventricles and interventricular septum. These sections were embedded in paraffin, sectioned at 4 to 6 μm thickness, stained routinely with hematoxylin and eosin for cellular and nuclear morphologic examination, and stained with Masson's trichrome for evaluation of fibrous tissue. The degree of myocyte hypertrophy was measured at a level that included the myocyte nucleus, in approximately 100 myocytes in random fields with a micrometer scale built into the microscope eyepiece. A mean myocyte width of less than 30 μm, between 30 and 50 μm, and greater than 50 μm was estimated for each sample. On hematoxylin and eosin sections, the myocyte nuclei were estimated visually for size, hyperchromaticity, and bizarre shape as compared with normal myocytes (figure 1). Fibrosis was assessed as present in a fine pattern or in coarse bands (figure 2). Morphometric estimations were not made.

Electron microscopy. Tissue for ultrastructural evaluation was taken by endomyocardial biopsy from the right ventricular septum just before cardiac transplantation and/or from the beating heart within minutes of being explanted. The tissue fragments were minced to 1 to 3 mm and placed in a cold solution of 2% paraformaldehyde, 2.5% glutaraldehyde, and 0.1M sodium cacodylate buffer for fixation. The samples were then postfixed in 2% osmium tetroxide and stained with uranyl acetate en bloc. After dehydration and infiltration, in LX epoxy resin, thin sections were cut on an LKB III ultramicrotome, stained with lead citrate, and screened with a Phillips 201 electron microscope.

At the ultrastructural level, myocyte hypertrophy and nuclear configuration were assessed and compared with normal (figure 3). Myofibrillar loss was assessed at both the 1 μm (thick plastic) sections as well as by ultrastructural examination of the tissue. Myofibrillar loss was assessed as partial (figure 4, *A*) or total (figure 4, *B*). All available tissue was screened (never fewer than five blocks) and electron micrographs were made of all the myocytes showing myofibrillar loss. Severe and diffuse myofibrillar loss (more than 20% of all the cells in five plastic blocks) was graded as 3+, many affected myocytes (10% to 15% of all myocytes in five plastic blocks) were graded 2+, and less than 10% of all myocytes affected in five plastic blocks was graded as 1+, similar to techniques used in grading anthracycline cardiotoxicity.[13]

Statistical analysis was performed by analysis of variance, chi square, and the two-tailed Student t test for equal and unequal variances where indicated.

Results

Some of the clinical and laboratory findings are summarized in table 1. All patients suffered from symptoms of congestive heart failure (class IV NYHA) and were free of systemic diseases, as required by the cardiac transplantation protocol.[14] Symptoms of congestive heart failure occurred 2 months postpartum in a 28-year-old patient with MDCM. None of the patients

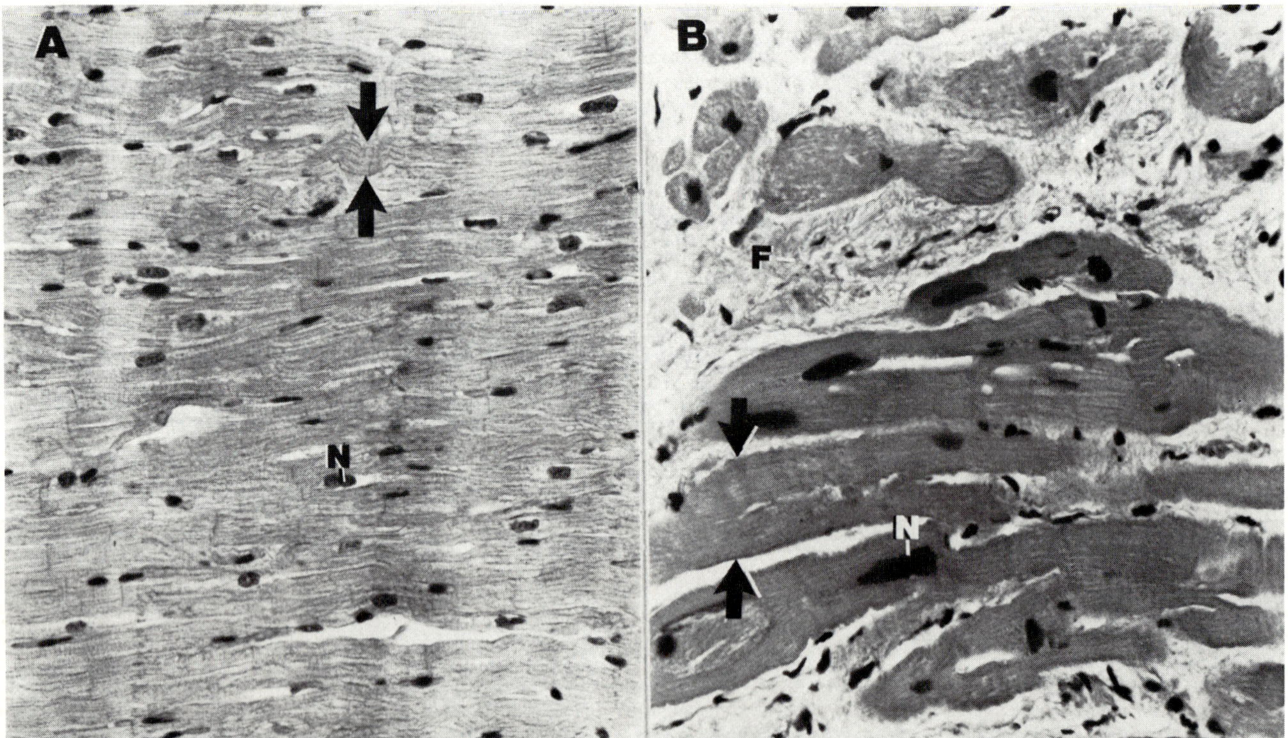

FIGURE 1. *A*, Normal myocardium showing the normal width (arrows) of the myocytes, with normal shape and size of the nuclei (N). *B*, Myocardium showing myocyte hypertrophy (arrows), with large hyperchromic nuclei (N) and coarse interstitial fibrosis (F) from a patient with end-stage DCM. (Hematoxylin and eosin, original magnification × 320 [both panels].)

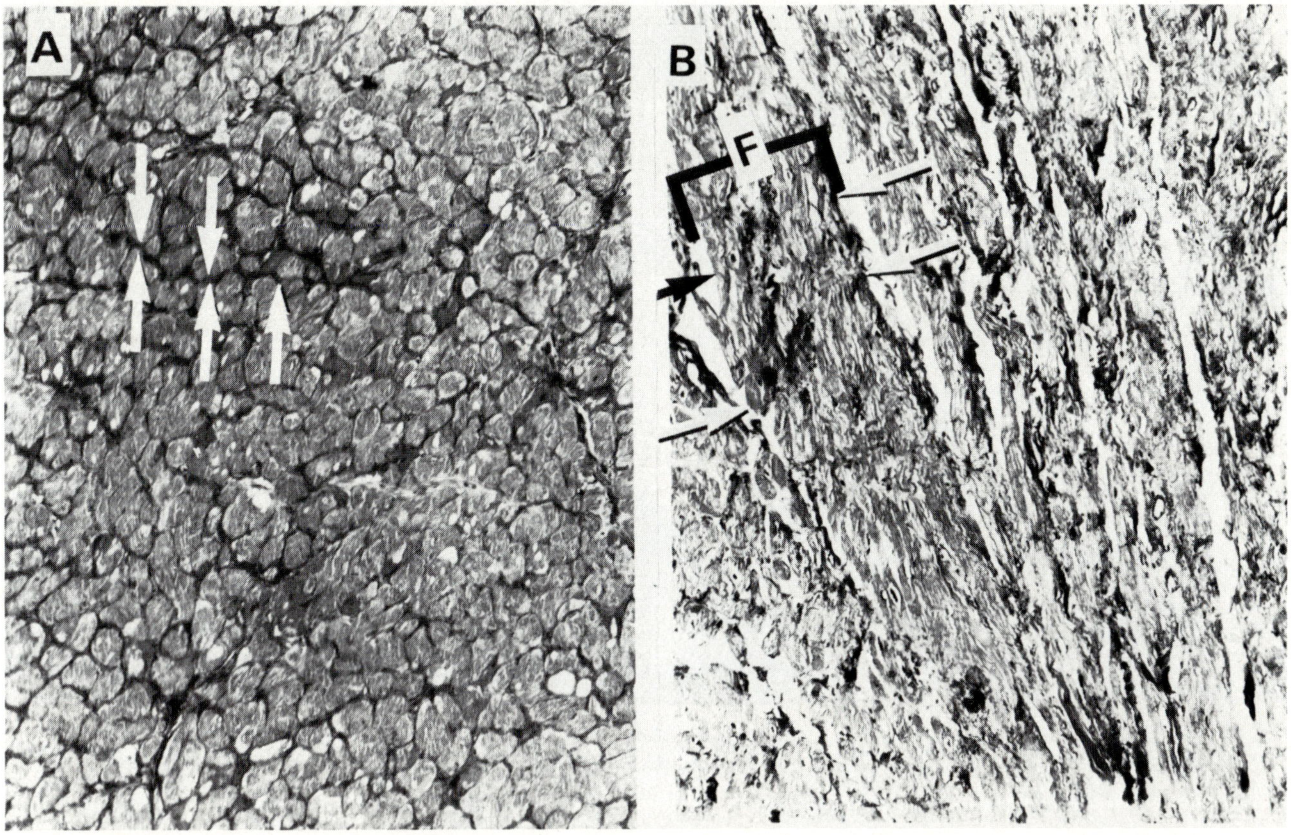

FIGURE 2. *A*, Section of myocardium from a patient with IRCM showing fine perimyocytic fibrosis (arrows, darker areas). *B*, Section from a patient with DCM showing a coarse fibrosis (arrows, bracket, F). (Both panels Masson's trichrome, original magnification × 100).

had a previous history of arterial hypertension or alcohol abuse. In all six patients with positive family history, the siblings suffered from typical DCM, although four of these six propositi had MDCM.

The physical findings were similar in the three groups except for the apical impulse, which was markedly displaced in patients with DCM. Left atrial lift was found in two patients with DCM. A third or fourth heart sound was present in all patients and a systolic murmur was found in 14 of 17 patients in whom a specific record was made of this finding.

The electrocardiogram showed nonspecific findings in all three groups of patients: ST-T wave changes, left ventricular hypertrophy, and left or biatrial enlargement. Arrhythmias and conduction disturbances were found in all three groups of patients. Sustained ventricular tachycardia was documented in 10 of the 19 patients (52%), whereas ventricular fibrillation needing cardiopulmonary resuscitation was present in two of five patients with MDCM.

The preoperative chest roentgenograms were not available in all patients so we reviewed the original radiologists' readings. These reports noted congestive heart failure and varying degrees of cardiac enlargement in all patients with MDCM and DCM. Mild cardiomegaly was read in three of the four patients with IRCM, and the fourth patient's results were variably interpreted (see figure 5).

M mode and two-dimensional echocardiographic recordings were not available in one patient with IRCM. At the time of echocardiographic evaluation, six patients had atrial fibrillation and four patients had implanted ventricular pacemakers. The size of cardiac chambers and other data are summarized in table 1. Patients with MDCM and DCM showed globular hearts with preponderant left ventricular dilatation, whereas in patients with IRCM only dilatation of the atria was found. A left atrial/left ventricular diameter ratio was less than 0.8 in all patients with MDCM and DCM and was 1.0 or greater in all patients with IRCM. The percent systolic thickening of the interventricular septum was significantly higher in patients with IRCM (30.3 ± 12.0%) than in those with MDCM (2.5 ± 2.0%) or DCM (2.0 ± 0.8%; $p < .001$). The mitral valve E-point septal separation index[15] was normal in only one patient with IRCM, who had a 55% angiographic ejection fraction. Segmental wall motion analysis by both echocardiography and angiography dem-

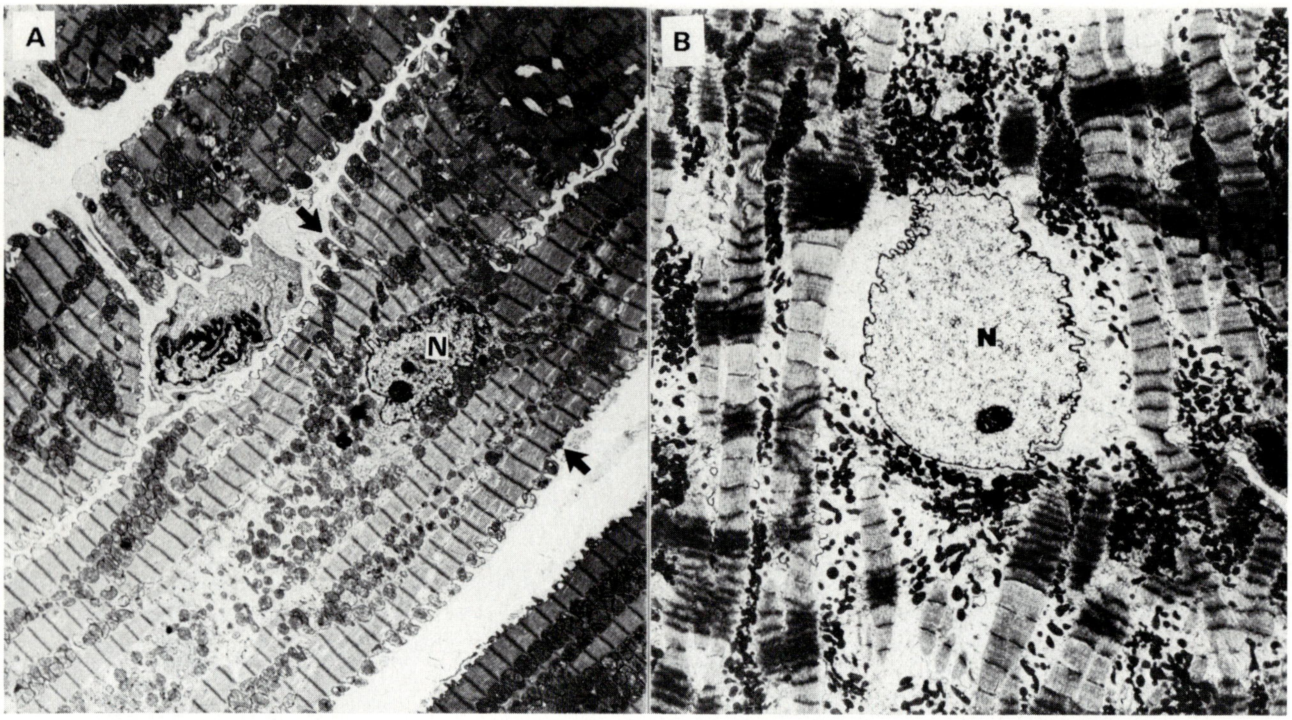

FIGURE 3. *A*, Electron micrograph showing normal myocyte width (arrows) and normal nucleus (N). *B*, Section from a patient with DCM showing a hypertrophied myocyte (edges beyond the border of this field) with a large nucleus (N). (Both panels original magnification × 4500.)

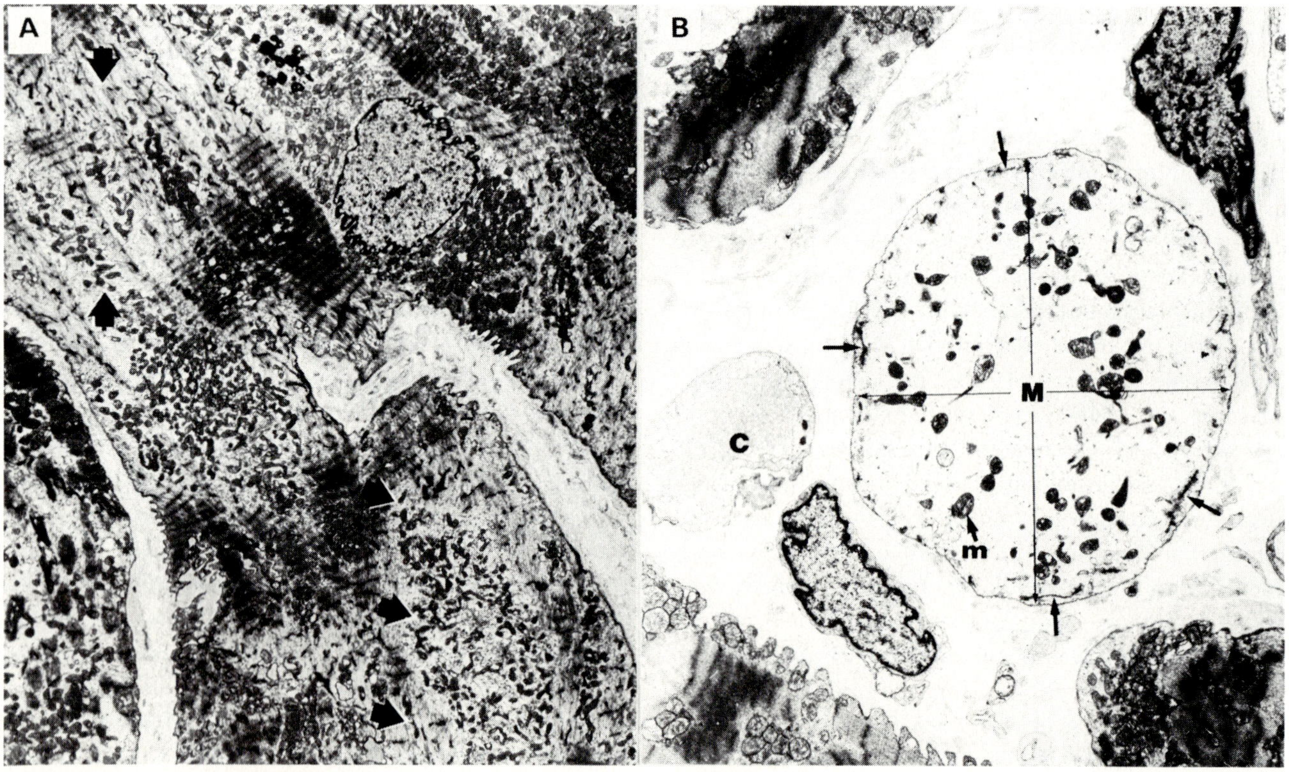

FIGURE 4. *A*, Electron micrograph showing a myocyte from a patient with MDCM with only partial myofibrillar loss (arrows). (Original magnification × 4000). *B*, Myocyte (M) from a patient with DCM with severe, almost total, myofibrillar loss (represented by the pale area). Only peripheral Z-bands (large arrows) remain. See text for explanation of grading. C = capillary; m = mitochondria. (Original magnification × 6500.)

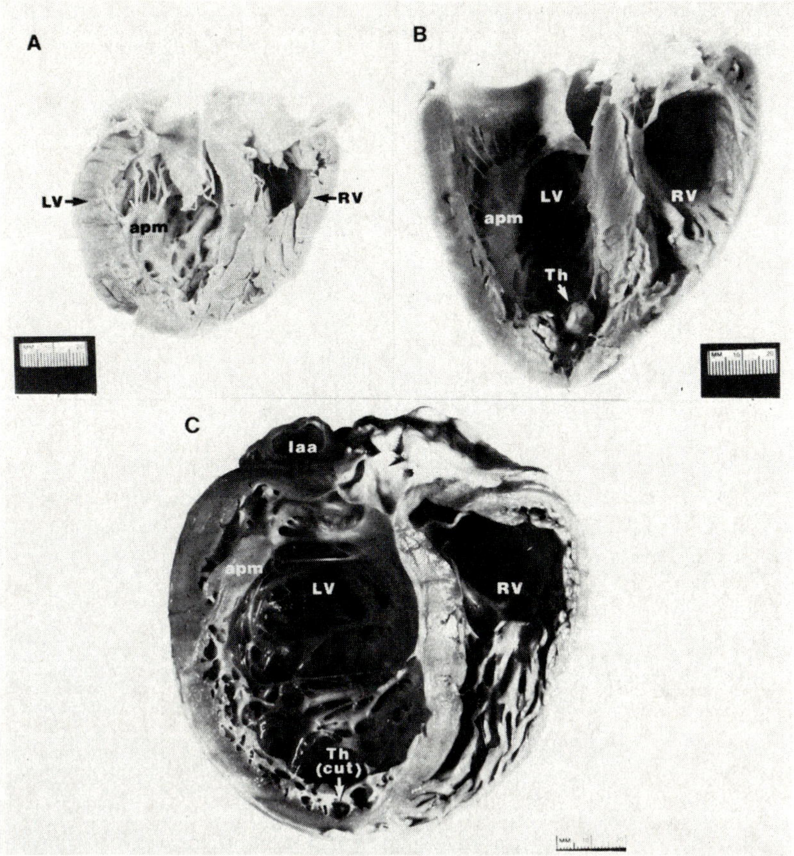

FIGURE 5. Longitudinally sectioned cardiac specimens removed at transplantation, fixed in the physiologic shape (see text), and photographed at equal scale from our patients with IRCM (*A*), MDCM (*B*), and DCM (*C*). The specimen in panel *A* is the smallest heart in the series, but the shape and size of the specimens in panels *B* and *C* are typical of their respective categories. Note the apical thrombi (Th) in the hearts in panels *B* and *C*. The majority of the atria are absent because of our surgical technique of transplantation. apm = anterolateral papillary muscle; laa = left atrial appendage; LV = left ventricle; RV = right ventricle.

onstrated diffuse mild-to-moderate hypokinesis in patients with IRCM, whereas the patients with MDCM and DCM had severe hypokinesis or akinesis.

Hemodynamic findings also are summarized in table 1. All patients had increased end-diastolic pressure, but a square root sign and equalization of right and left ventricular diastolic pressures were present only in patients with IRCM. The pulmonary arterial pressures and pulmonic and systemic vascular resistances were similar in the three groups of patients. Mitral regurgitation was present in 14 patients; its degree was mild to moderate in those IRCM and MDCM and mild to severe in those with DCM.

Pathologic findings are summarized in table 2 and

TABLE 2
Morphologic findings in all patients

	IRCM (n = 4)	MDCM (n = 5)	DCM (n = 10)	p value
Macroscopic[A]				
Residual weight (g)	223.7 ± 101.20^C	350.0 ± 39.6	505.0 ± 133.1^C	<.005
LVW thickness (cm)	1.7 ± 0.20	1.4 ± 0.4	1.4 ± 0.5	NS
RVW thickness (cm)	0.9 ± 0.01	0.7 ± 0.4	0.6 ± 0.2	NS
LV endocardial fibrosis	3	5	10	NS
LV endocardial score	1.67 ± 0.06	1.2 ± 0.5	2.4 ± 0.3^C	<.001
RV endocardial fibrosis	3	3	4	NS
Thrombi	0	2	4	NS
Light microscopy[B]				
Nonspecific changes	4	5	10	NS
Electron microscopy				
Myofibrillar loss	0^C	4	10	<.001

LVW = left ventricular wall; RVW = right ventricular wall.
[A]Macroscopic evaluation not performed in one patient with IRCM.
[B]For types of changes, see text.
[C]Statistically significant difference as compared with MDCM.

figures 1 to 5. Macroscopic evaluation of the heart specimens showed increased interventricular wall thickness in all patients with IRCM examined, three of five with MDCM, and six of 10 with DCM. Patchy or diffuse left ventricular endocardial fibrosis was present in all patients. Endocardial fibrosis scores were similar in patients with IRCM (1.67 ± 0.58) and MDCM (1.2 ± 0.5) (see Methods). The extent of fibrosis in patients with DCM (2.4 ± 0.3) was significantly higher than that found in patients with IRCM ($p < .05$) or MDCM ($p < .001$). Right ventricular endocardial fibrosis was found in all patients with IRCM but in only two of five with MDCM and three of 10 with DCM. When present, the fibrosis was patchy in patients with MDCM and DCM and more diffuse in those with IRCM. Pathologic pericardial thickening was not found in any of the patients. Light microscopic assessment of endomyocardial biopsy specimens showed similar findings in the three groups of patients. All patients had myocyte hypertrophy (mostly in the range of 30 to 50 μm), bizarre-shaped nuclei, and hyperchromatism (figure 1, *B*). Fine, perimyocytic fibrosis (figure 2, *A*) was found in all patients with IRCM and MDCM and in eight of 10 with DCM. Coarse interstitial fibrosis (figures 1, *B*, and 2, *B*) was present in the remaining two patients with DCM. Coarse fibrosis was found in addition to the fine fibrosis in one patient with IRCM and two with MDCM.

Electron microscopy showed myocyte hypertrophy in all patients (figure 3, *B*). Myofibrillar loss was not detected in any patient with IRCM and in only one with MDCM. Four of the five patients with MDCM showed partial myofibrillar loss (graded +1, or mild form of cardiomyopathy) (figure 4, *A*). Five of 10 patients with DCM showed predominantly partial myofibrillar loss (graded +2, or moderate form of cardiomyopathy) and the other five had predominantly total myofibrillar loss (graded +3, or severe form of cardiomyopathy) (figure 4, *B*). Compared with MDCM, the degree of myofibrillar loss was significantly higher in patients with DCM ($p < .001$).

Discussion

We have described five patients in whom clinical, hemodynamic, and morphologic features typical of DCM occurred in the absence of significant ventricular dilatation (10% to 15% above normal range corrected for body surface area). In describing these patients we have used the term MDCM based on the findings discussed below.

Characteristic features. The major findings in patients with MDCM were: (1) severe clinical congestive heart failure (class IV NYHA), (2) mild left ventricular dilatation associated with similar or lesser degree of enlargement of the other cardiac chambers (globular heart), (3) lack of the square root sign or diastolic pressure equalization and presence of diffusely poor left ventricular contractile motion (ejection fraction 12% to 19%), and (4) nonspecific changes on light microscopic examination and only partial myofibrillar loss documented in the hearts of four of five patients examined by electron microscopy. The groups with MDCM with DCM could not be well segregated by most of the variables included in tables 1 and 2. However, the degree of myofibrillar loss was greater ($p < .001$) in patients with DCM. Left ventricular endocardial fibrosis was present in all patients with DCM and MDCM, but it was scored as more extensive in patients with DCM as compared to those with MDCM ($p < .001$) or with IRCM ($p < .05$). Some clinical, hemodynamic, and morphologic criteria showed significant differences between patients with MDCM and those with IRCM. Patients with IRCM showed a longer symptomatic period, smaller (normal sized) and only mild-to-moderately hypocontractile left ventricles, atrial dilatation, restrictive hemodynamic pattern, more extensive right ventricular endocardial fibrosis, and lack of myofibrillar loss. In contrast to patients with MDCM, none of those with IRCM and only two of 10 with DCM had a positive family history of cardiomyopathy.

Restrictive or congestive cardiomyopathy? Congestive cardiomyopathy may represent the "final common path of many differing conditions that insult the ventricular myocardium."[1] Therefore it is debatable whether MDCM represents one of the final stages of IRCM. This hypothesis cannot be discarded with certainty. Given the rarity of IRCM, very little is known about the natural history. The small number of cases reported in the literature[7, 9, 16] and our four cases seem to suggest that patients with end-stage IRCM usually retain the characteristic restrictive hemodynamic pattern with or without associated impairment of left ventricular contractility. Tei et al.[17] recently described a type of "minimally dilated cardiomyopathy" of alcoholic etiology, in which severe decrease in left ventricular contractility was associated with typical restrictive hemodynamics. Until more data are accumulated about the natural history of IRCM, the inclusion of our patients among other "atypical" types of congestive cardiomyopathy seems justified.[18]

Correlation between length of survival and degree of ventricular dilatation. Most previous studies reported a negative correlation or inverse relationship between the degree of ventricular dilatation and length of survival of patients with congestive cardiomyopathy,[1, 4–6] but some failed to find such a correlation.[19, 20] Benjamin et al.[20] examined the hearts of 30 patients with DCM at necropsy. The authors state that all hearts had "biventricular enlargement," although left ventricular diameters ranged 3.5 to 8.0 cm. The degree of left ventricular dilatation was similar in short- and long-term survivors, but long-term survivors had more hypertrophy in proportion to dilatation.[20] Two-thirds of these patients died from causes other than congestive heart failure. Roberts and Ferrans[6] also noted among patients with dilated cardiomyopathy that "some have relatively thick ventricular walls and only mildly dilated cavities." Because the attention in these previous studies[6, 20] was not focused specifically on patients with mildly dilated ventricles, the degree of functional impairment, hemodynamic findings, and cause of death were not specified.

The value and limitations of pathologic evaluation. This study supports previous observations attesting to the lack of specificity of pathologic findings in patients with DCM and IRCM and the lack of correlation between the degree of hemodynamic impairment and extent of pathologic changes.[1, 3, 6, 21] Except for size and individual heart weight, inspection of the removed hearts and light microscopic examination did not reveal major differences among these different types of cardiomyopathy. Findings described in patients with IRCM, such as increased wall thickness and fine endocardial and interstitial fibrosis,[7–9, 16] also were documented in patients with mildly or grossly dilated congestive cardiomyopathy. The presence of myofibrillar loss in patients with congestive cardiomyopathy and its absence, even in advanced forms of IRCM, suggest a correlation between ventricular dilatation and myofibrillar loss. This finding can be considered an interesting preliminary observation that needs future confirmation. Evaluation at the structural and ultrastructural levels are important, however, to exclude specific etiologies in patients with restrictive and congestive cardiomyopathy.[1, 6]

Conclusions. Congestive cardiomyopathy is an "enigmatic disease"[21] in which, usually, "the size of the left ventricular cavity appears to be roughly proportional to the severity and duration of symptomatic congestive heart failure."[6] We call attention to a group of patients with end-stage heart disease, not an "early" form of cardiomyopathy, whose hearts are only mildly dilated and who display nonrestrictive hemodynamics. Such patients either have not been noted or have been given only passing acknowledgment in prior series. The ultrastructural features in these cases are interesting, and there is an intriguing trend toward finding a family member with DCM.

We thank Corrie Naasz, Marjorie Pittman, Virginia Briskin, and Stephen Hill for their technical assistance in performing the echocardiograms. We also thank Dr. D. K. Ahn for his help in statistical evaluation of the data and Gretchen Houd for preparation of the manuscript.

References

1. Goodwin JF: Prospects and predictions for the cardiomyopathies. Circulation **50:** 210, 1974
2. Report of the WHO/ISFC task force on the definition and classification of cardiomyopathies. Br Heart J **44:** 672, 1980
3. Goodwin JF: The frontiers of cardiomyopathy. Br Heart J **48:** 1, 1982
4. Johnson RA, Palacios I: Dilated cardiomyopathies of the adult. N Engl J Med **307:** 1051, 1982
5. Fuster V, Gersh BJ, Giuliani ER, Tajik AJ, Brandenburg RO, Frye RL: The natural history of idiopathic dilated cardiomyopathy. Am J Cardiol **47:** 525, 1981
6. Roberts WC, Ferrans VJ: Pathologic anatomy of the cardiomyopathies. Idiopathic dilated and hypertrophic types, infiltrative types, and endomyocardial disease with and without eosinophilia. Human Pathol **6:** 287, 1975
7. Arbustini E, Buonanno C, Trevi G, Pennelli N, Ferrans VJ, Thiene G: Cardiac ultrastructure in primary restrictive cardiomyopathy. Chest **84:** 236, 1983
8. Siegel RT, Shah PK, Fishbein MC: Idiopathic restrictive cardiomyopathy. Circulation **70:** 165, 1984
9. Benotti JR, Grossman W, Cohn PF: Clinical profile of restrictive cardiomyopathy. Circulation **61:** 6, 1980
10. Schnittger I, Gordon EP, Fitzgerald PJ, Popp RL: Standardized intracardiac measurements of two-dimensional echocardiography. J Am Coll Cardiol **2:** 934, 1983
11. Sahn DJ, DeMaria A, Kisslo J, Weyman A — The committee on M-Mode Standardization of the American Society of Echocardiography: Recommendations regarding quantitation in M-mode echocardiography: results of a survey of echocardiographic measurements. Circulation **58:** 1072, 1978
12. Valdez RS, Motta JA, London E, Martin RP, Haskell WL, Farquhar JW, Popp RL, Horlick L: Evaluation of the echocardiogram as an epidemiologic tool in an asymptomatic population. Circulation **60:** 921, 1979
13. Billingham ME, Mason J, Bristow M, Daniels J: Anthracycline cardiomyopathy monitored by morphological changes. Cancer Treat Rep **62:** 865, 1978
14. Hunt SA, Harrison DC, Stinson EB: Cardiac transplantation. In Willerson J, Saunders I, editors: Clinical cardiology. New York, 1977, Grune & Stratton, p 613
15. Massie BM, Schiller NB, Ratshin RA, Parmley WW: Mitral-septal separation: new echocardiographic index of left ventricular function. Am J Cardiol **39:** 1008, 1977
16. Dubost C, Durand M, Camilleri JP, Deloche A: Deux cas de myocardiopathies restrictives primitives. Bull Acad Natl Med (Paris) **164:** 251, 1980
17. Tei C, Boltwood CM, Shah PM: Minimally dilated cardiomyopathy: a distinct subset of severe systolic dysfunction. Circulation **68**(suppl III): III-336, 1983 (abst)
18. Fitchett DH, Sugrue DD, MacArthur CG, Oakley CM: Right ventricular dilated cardiomyopathy. Br Heart J **51:** 25, 1984
19. Convert G, Delaye J, Beaune T, Biron A, Gonin A: Prognosis of primary nonobstructive cardiomyopathies. Arch Mal Coeur **73:** 227, 1980
20. Benjamin IJ, Schuster EH, Bulkley BH: Cardiac hypertrophy in idiopathic dilated congestive cardiomyopathy: a clinicopathologic study. Circulation **64:** 442, 1981
21. Baandrup U, Florio RA, Reholm M, Richardson PJ, Olsen ECJ: Critical analysis of endomyocardial biopsies from patients suspected of having cardiomyopathy. II. Comparison of histology and clinical/haemodynamic information. Br Heart J **45:** 487, 1981

Diastolic abnormalities in patients with hypertrophic cardiomyopathy: relation to magnitude of left ventricular hypertrophy

PAOLO SPIRITO, M.D., BARRY J. MARON, M.D., FRANCESCO CHIARELLA, M.D., PAOLO BELLOTTI, M.D., ROBERTO TRAMARIN, M.D., MASSIMO POZZOLI, M.D., AND CARLO VECCHIO, M.D.

ABSTRACT To investigate the relationship between diastolic abnormalities and left ventricular hypertrophy, 52 patients with hypertrophic cardiomyopathy (HCM) and 22 normal subjects were studied with digitized M mode echocardiography and two-dimensional echocardiography. Echocardiographic indexes of diastolic function were compared in patients with different extent of left ventricular hypertrophy. Time interval from minimum left ventricular internal dimension to mitral valve opening and time to peak rate of increase in left ventricular internal dimension were significantly prolonged (80 ± 31 and 100 ± 37 msec, respectively) in patients with HCM and the most extensive left ventricular hypertrophy compared with those in patients with mild left ventricular hypertrophy (59 ± 25 and 74 ± 34 msec, respectively; $p < .01$). Furthermore, peak rate of posterior wall diastolic excursion was significantly reduced in those patients with HCM and posterior wall hypertrophy (8.3 ± 4.0 cm/sec) compared with that in patients with HCM but normal posterior wall thickness (11.2 ± 3.4 cm/sec; $p < .002$). However, abnormal M mode echocardiographic indexes of diastolic function were also identified in a substantial proportion of patients (i.e., 73%) with HCM and only mild left ventricular hypertrophy. In these patients, time interval from minimum left ventricular internal dimension to mitral valve opening (59 ± 25 msec), peak rate (12 ± 4 cm/sec), and time to peak rate of increase in left ventricular internal dimension (74 ± 34 msec) were significantly different from normal (25 ± 12 msec, 21 ± 3 cm/sec, and 49 ± 12 msec, respectively; $p < .01$). Furthermore, in 32 patients with HCM who had normal posterior wall thickness, peak rate of posterior wall diastolic excursion was significantly reduced (11.2 ± 3.4 cm/sec) compared with normal (16.7 ± 2.4 cm/sec; $p < .001$). In conclusion, our findings show a relationship, in patients with HCM, between magnitude of left ventricular hypertrophy and extent of diastolic wall motion abnormalities. However, our results also show that diastolic wall motion abnormalities are common in patients with HCM and mild localized left ventricular hypertrophy and may even be identified in segments of the left ventricle that are of normal thickness. These data suggest that the primary cardiomyopathic process in HCM may not be limited to areas of gross wall thickening, and nonhypertrophied regions of the left ventricle may contribute to impairment of diastolic function in patients with this disease.
Circulation 72, No. 2, 310–316, 1985.

HYPERTROPHIC CARDIOMYOPATHY (HCM) is characterized by both increased ventricular wall thickness[1–6] and impairment of left ventricular filling.[7–14] However, the interrelation between these two pathologic features of the disease is not well understood. For example, it is not known whether left ventricular diastolic dysfunction is solely the consequence of hypertrophy, or if diastolic abnormalities may also be present in ventricles with only mild left ventricular hypertrophy. The purpose of the present investigation was to define the relationship, in patients with HCM, between the magnitude of left ventricular hypertrophy (LVH) as assessed with M mode and two-dimensional echocardiography and the impairment in left ventricular diastolic wall motion evaluated with digitized M mode echocardiography.

From the Divisione di Cardiologia, Ente Ospedaliero Ospedali Galliera, Genoa, Italy; the Echocardiography Laboratory of the Cardiology Branch, National Heart, Lung, and Blood Institute, Bethesda; and the Divisione di Cardiologia, Fondazione Clinica del Lavoro, Montescano, Pavia, Italy.

Address for correspondence: Dr. Paolo Spirito, Cardiology Branch, National Heart, Lung, and Blood Institute, Building 10, Room 7B-15, Bethesda, MD 20205.

Received Jan. 3, 1985; revision accepted May 16, 1985.

Methods

Selection and characterization of patients. Fifty-two patients with HCM comprise the study population; 30 were evaluated at the National Heart, Lung, and Blood Institute, and 22 were evaluated at the Ente Ospedaliero Ospedali Galliera. The diagnosis of HCM was established by typical clinical findings,[2, 3, 5] and by two-dimensional echocardiographic demonstration of localized or diffuse hypertrophy in a nondilated left ventricle, in absence of another cardiac or systemic disease that could produce LVH.[15] Patients were selected for this study on the basis of the following criteria: (1) a high-quality M mode echocardiogram, with optimal visualization of the ventricular septum and the left ventricular posterior wall sufficient to allow clear identification of the borders of these structures, and (2) a technically satisfactory two-dimensional echocardiogram, with clear recognition of the endocardial and epicardial borders of the left ventricular wall in the parasternal short-axis and long-axis views permitting reliable identification of the distribution and extent of LVH.[6]

The 52 study patients with HCM ranged in age from 9 to 70 years (mean 37); 39 (75%) were male patients. Thirty-two patients were asymptomatic, 13 had mild functional limitation (New York Heart Association functional class II), and seven had moderate functional limitation (class III). Echocardiographic studies were performed at least 48 hr after cessation of all cardiac medications; all patients were in normal sinus rhythm.

Magnitude of left ventricular outflow tract obstruction under basal conditions was assessed at cardiac catheterization in 12 patients and estimated from the M mode echocardiogram based on the magnitude and duration of systolic anterior motion of the mitral valve in the other 40.[16, 17] Left ventricular outflow tract obstruction under basal conditions (gradient $\geq$30 mm Hg) was considered to be present in 10 patients and was absent or less than 30 mm Hg in the other 42.

Twenty-two normal volunteers without evidence of cardiovascular disease served as control subjects. They ranged in age from 15 to 55 years (mean 30); 15 (64%) were male subjects.

Echocardiography. An Advanced Technology Laboratory (ATL) Mark 300 or Mark 500 mechanical sector scanner with a 3 MHz transducer was used to perform the echocardiographic studies. M mode echocardiographic recordings were made while the cardiac anatomy was visualized with two-dimensional echocardiography. The M mode echocardiographic cursor was positioned at the level of the mitral valve, where the ventricular septum, the left ventricular posterior wall, and the point of separation of the mitral leaflets were best imaged. Because the diastolic slope of the left ventricular posterior wall may vary considerably depending on the angulation of the M mode beam, care was taken to obtain the echocardiographic recordings with the beam perpendicular to the posterior wall where the maximum diastolic slope of the posterior wall was visualized.[18] Thickness of ventricular septum and left ventricular posterior wall was measured at mitral valve level, according to the criteria of the American Society of Echocardiography.[19] M mode echocardiograms were recorded at a paper speed of 100 mm/sec.

The two-dimensional echocardiographic examination, performed to identify the extent and distribution of LVH, included the imaging of a number of cross-sectional planes through the heart.[6] Serial short-axis views of the left ventricle were obtained by maintaining the transducer in a fixed location on the chest wall and slowly angling the image plane from aorta to apex. The long-axis view was obtained by orienting the sector plane at a 90 degree angle to the short-axis plane and parallel to the longitudinal axis of the left ventricle. The apical four-chamber view was obtained with the transducer positioned at the left ventricular apex, and the image plane was directed perpendicular to the ventricular and atrial septa. Finally, the transducer was rotated clockwise from the apical four-chamber view so that the ultrasound beam was approximately parallel to the ventricular septum, permitting simultaneous visualization of the aorta and left ventricular outflow tract. Two-dimensional echocardiographic images were recorded on 1 inch reel-to-reel Sony videotape or on Panasonic NV-8200 videotape.

Digitized M mode echocardiography. Measurement of indexes of diastolic function were obtained with digitized M mode echocardiography. In each patient, two to five (an average of four) consecutive cardiac cycles with clearly identifiable left septal and posterior wall endocardial echoes were digitized and the values were averaged. Contours of the left side of the septum and the endocardium of the posterior wall were traced, and the point of initial opening of the mitral valve was identified. Digitization was performed with a hand-controlled cursor (Hewlett-Packard Graphic Tablette 9111A) and processed by a Hewlett-Packard 1000 computer system that provided a continuous plot of change in left ventricular internal dimension, its first derivative, and the first derivative of the posterior wall endocardial excursion.

The following echocardiographic parameters of diastolic function were derived from this computer analysis: time interval from minimum left ventricular internal dimension to mitral valve opening, peak rate of increase in left ventricular internal dimension, time to peak rate of increase in left ventricular internal dimension (measured as the time interval from minimum left ventricular internal dimension to maximal rate of increase in left ventricular internal dimension,[20] and peak rate of posterior wall diastolic excursion.[21]

Assessment of LVH

Overall extent and distribution of LVH. The pattern of LVH was assessed in a semiquantitative fashion from the two-dimensional echocardiogram. This analysis primarily utilized the parasternal short-axis planes. However, the parasternal long-axis view was also useful in evaluating the extent of LVH in the anterior ventricular septum, and the apical views were used primarily to exclude the presence of hypertrophy in the apical portion of the left ventricle.

The location and extent of LVH was defined with respect to the short-axis cross-sectional plane (figure 1).[6] The ventricular septum was divided into two approximately equal segments (anterior and posterior); the left ventricular free wall was divided into lateral and posterior segments. Hypertrophy of the anterior ventricular septum and the posterior free wall was considered to be present if the wall was at least 15 mm in thickness. The posterior portion of septum and lateral free wall are visual-

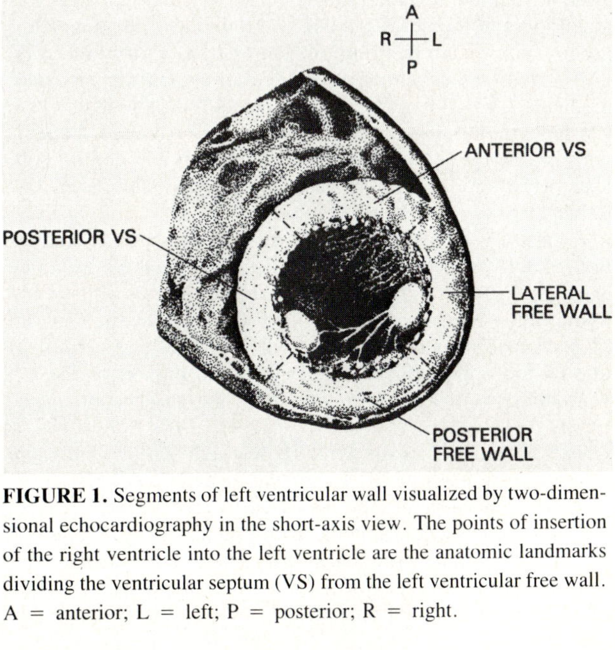

FIGURE 1. Segments of left ventricular wall visualized by two-dimensional echocardiography in the short-axis view. The points of insertion of the right ventricle into the left ventricle are the anatomic landmarks dividing the ventricular septum (VS) from the left ventricular free wall. A = anterior; L = left; P = posterior; R = right.

TABLE 1

Clinical data and digitized parameters of diastolic function in control subjects and in three subgroups of patients with HCM and different magnitudes of LVH

	Age (yr)	Sex (% male)	Heart rate (beats/min)	VS thickness[A] (mm)	PW thickness[A] (mm)	VS/PW[A]	Symptoms (% patients)	dD/dt (cm/sec)	T max dD/dt (msec)	T to MVO (msec)
Normal subjects (n = 22)	30 (15–55)	64	75 ± 15	9 ± 2[B]	8 ± 2	1.1	0	21 ± 3[B]	49 ± 12[B]	25 ± 12[B]
HCM										
Mild LVH (n = 15)	40 (9–70)	87	68 ± 12	16 ± 4	11 ± 3	1.5	33	12 ± 4	74 ± 34	59 ± 25
Moderate LVH (n = 10)	31 (13–45)	60	67 ± 11	20 ± 8	11 ± 2	1.8	30	12 ± 4	108 ± 33[C]	73 ± 32
Severe LVH (n = 27)	37 (9–67)	74	72 ± 14	25 ± 8[C,D]	12 ± 3	2.3	44	11 ± 4	100 ± 37[C]	80 ± 31[C]

dD/dt = peak rate of increase in left ventricular internal dimension; PW = posterior wall; T to MVO = time from minimum left ventricular internal dimension to mitral valve opening; T max dD/dt = time to peak rate of increase in left ventricular internal dimension; VS = ventricular septum; VS/PW = ratio of ventricular septal to posterior wall thickness.

[A]Obtained by M mode echocardiography at mitral valve level, according to the criteria of the American Society of Echocardiography.[19]

[B]For each of these parameters, values for normal subjects were significantly different from each of the subgroups of patients with HCM ($p < .005$).

[C]Each of these parameters was significantly different when compared to the subgroup of patients with HCM and mild LVH ($p < .01$).

[D]This parameter was significantly different when compared to the subgroup of patients with HCM and moderate LVH ($p < .02$).

ized in the lateral regions of the sector (in the short-axis plane) where resolution is less than optimal. Therefore, to ensure that the frequency with which hypertrophy in these segments was identified would not be overestimated, the posterior septum and lateral free wall were considered hypertrophied only if the wall was judged to be at least 17 mm in thickness.[6] Wall thickness was assessed directly from the television monitor with the aid of calipers and with the use of a calibration scale produced by the instrument. Location of endocardial and epicardial borders was identified by viewing the pertinent portions of videotape in slow-motion and real-time modes. In some instances, wall thickness was also measured in the stop-action mode at end-diastole from the television monitor.

On the basis of these two-dimensional echocardiographic criteria, the number of hypertrophied left ventricular segments was identified and the study patients were divided into three subgroups with regard to overall extent of LVH as follows: mild LVH, involving only one left ventricular segment (15 patients); moderate LVH, involving two segments (10 patients); severe LVH, involving three or four segments (27 patients). Patients with HCM and different magnitudes of LVH and control subjects were similar with respect to age, sex, and heart rate (table 1).

Posterior wall hypertrophy. In patients with HCM, the portion of left ventricular posterior wall identified by M mode echocardiography may be of normal or increased thickness.[6] Therefore, we considered this region of the left ventricular wall of particular interest in the present investigation, because it offered the opportunity to assess diastolic motion of the left ventricular wall in the presence or in the absence of hypertrophy.

The 52 study patients with HCM were divided into two groups on the basis of left ventricular posterior wall thickness. M mode echocardiography was used to assess posterior wall thickness because the M mode beam visualizes this region with greater ultrasound resolution than does two-dimensional echocardiography. The posterior wall was normal ($\leq$11 mm)[22, 23] in 32 patients, and hypertrophied (>11 mm) in the remaining 20 patients. Patients with HCM (with or without posterior wall thickening) did not differ from the control subjects with respect to age, sex, or heart rate (table 2).

Reproducibility of the study measurements. Intraobserver and interobserver reproducibility of the digitized echocardiographic measurements was assessed in 31 study patients (14 with HCM and 17 controls). To assess intraobserver variability, one investigator digitized two different sets of four cardiac cycles in each patient. Values from the four cardiac cycles were averaged. To assess interobserver variability, two investigators digitized two different sets of four cardiac cycles in each patient. Values from the four cardiac cycles were averaged. The coefficients of variation for these digitized measurements were obtained for each of the 31 patients and the intraobserver and interobserver mean coefficients of variation were calculated.[24] Values for intraobserver and interobserver reproducibility (expressed as mean coefficient of variation) were, respectively, 8.8% and 10.7% for time interval from minimum left ventricular internal dimension to mitral valve opening, 5.6% and 5.1% for peak rate of increase in left ventricular internal dimension,

TABLE 2

Clinical data in control subjects and in patients with HCM and either normal or increased posterior wall thickness

	Age (yr)	Sex (% male)	Heart rate (beats/min)	PW thickness (mm)
Normal subjects (n = 22)	30 (15–55)	64	75 ± 15	8 ± 2 (6–11)
HCM with PW ≤11 mm (n = 32)	34 (9–67)	78	68 ± 13	10 ± 1 (6–11)
HCM with PW >11 mm (n = 20)	41 (15–70)	70	72 ± 13	14 ± 2 (12–18)

PW = posterior wall.

15.0% and 12.1% for time to peak rate of increase in left ventricular internal dimension, and 6.8% and 5.3% for peak rate of posterior wall diastolic excursion.

Intraobserver agreement on the determination of overall extent of LVH, as assessed from two-dimensional echocardiography, was evaluated in the first 16 patients with HCM who entered the study. Two interpretations of the same echocardiographic study, obtained by one observer 5 months apart, were compared. There was complete agreement regarding the number of hypertrophied segments in 14 of the 16 patients (88%).

Statistical methods. Data were expressed as mean ± SD. Differences between means were determined by the one-way analysis of variance. Differences between proportions were determined with the chi-square test.

Results

Relationship between overall extent and distribution of LVH and digitized echocardiographic indexes of diastolic function. Patients with HCM were classified according to the distribution and extent of LVH and then compared with respect to the echocardiographic indexes of diastolic function. Time interval from minimum left ventricular internal dimension to mitral valve opening and peak rate and time to peak rate of increase in left ventricular internal dimension were significantly different in each of the three morphologic subgroups of patients with HCM when compared with normal (table 1). When echocardiographic parameters of diastolic function were analyzed with regard to individual patients, 45 (87%) of the 52 patients with HCM showed diastolic impairment, defined as the coexistence of at least two abnormal echocardiographic parameters of diastolic function. Both the time interval from minimum left ventricular internal dimension to mitral valve opening and peak rate of increase in left ventricular internal dimension were prolonged in patients with severe LVH (80 ± 31 and 100 ± 37 msec), compared with those in patients with mild LVH (59 ± 25 and 74 ± 34 msec, respectively; $p < .01$) (figures 2 and 3). In patients with moderate LVH, time interval from minimum left ventricular internal dimension to mitral valve opening and peak rate of increase in left ventricular internal dimension were intermediate and not significantly different from those in the other two groups; time to peak rate of increase in left ventricular internal dimension was significantly prolonged in patients with moderate LVH (108 ± 33 msec) compared with that in patients with mild LVH (74 ± 34 msec; $p < .01$).

Of note, echocardiographic diastolic abnormalities were common in patients with mild LVH. Values for peak rate of increase in left ventricular internal dimension were below the lower limit of normal in 12 (80%) of the patients with mild LVH; time to peak rate of increase in left ventricular dimension and time from minimum left ventricular dimension to mitral valve

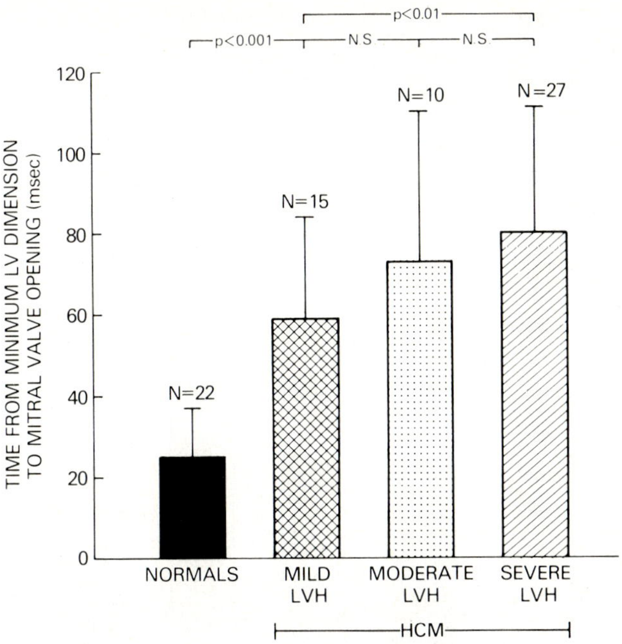

FIGURE 2. Comparison of the time interval from minimum left ventricular internal dimension to mitral valve opening in normal subjects and in patients with HCM having mild, moderate, or severe LVH. LV = left ventricular.

opening also exceeded the upper limit of normal in seven (47%) and nine (60%) of the patients, respectively. In these patients with mild LVH, each of these three parameters was significantly different from normal (table 1).

Relationship between posterior wall thickness and posterior wall diastolic dynamics. Peak rate of diastolic posterior wall excursion was significantly reduced in the 20 patients with HCM and increased left ventricular posterior wall thickness (8.3 ± 4.0 cm/sec) compared with that in the 32 patients with HCM but normal left ventricular posterior wall thickness (11.2 ± 3.4 cm/sec; $p < .002$) (figure 4).

Peak rate of posterior wall diastolic excursion was also significantly reduced in the 32 patients with HCM and normal posterior wall thickness (11.2 ± 3.4 cm/sec) compared with that in control subjects (16.7 ± 2.4 cm/sec; $p < .001$) (figures 4 and 5), and in 19 (59%) of these 32 patients it was below the lower limit measured in the control subjects.

Discussion

Previous studies have demonstrated that diastolic function is impaired in most patients with HCM.[7–14] Prolonged isovolumetric relaxation[9–12] and diminished rapid diastolic filling[7–14] have been identified with digitized echocardiography, radionuclide angiography, and with measurements obtained at cardiac catheterization. Diastolic impairment, as assessed with digi-

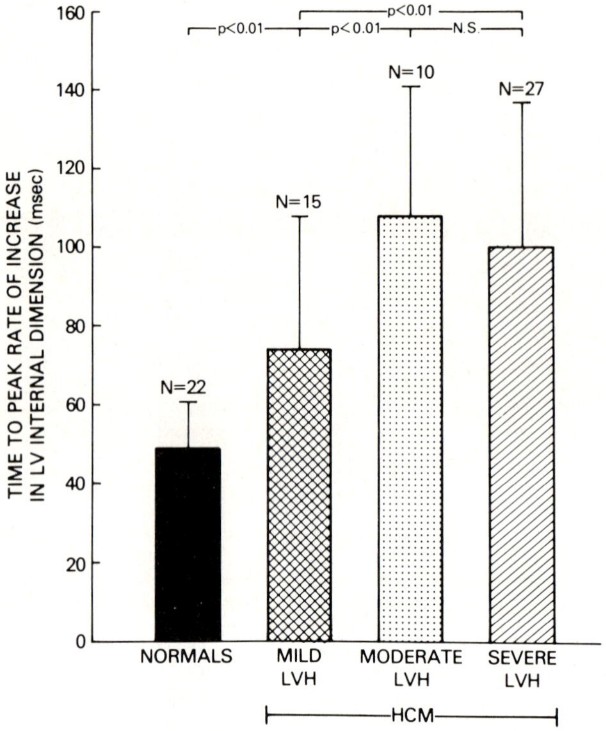

FIGURE 3. Comparison of time to peak rate of increase in left ventricular (LV) internal dimension in normal subjects and in patients with HCM having mild, moderate, or severe LVH.

tized M mode echocardiography, was detected in over 80% of our study patients with HCM.

Unlike previous studies,[7-14] in the present investigation of patients with HCM we analyzed the relationship between the magnitude of LVH and the severity of diastolic abnormalities. Both the time interval from minimum left ventricular internal dimension to mitral valve opening and the time to peak rate of increase in left ventricular internal dimension were significantly prolonged in patients with the most extensive LVH compared with those in patients with mild LVH. Furthermore, peak rate of diastolic posterior wall excursion was significantly reduced in patients with posterior wall hypertrophy compared with that in patients with HCM but normal posterior wall thickness. Hence, our findings suggest that more severe diastolic abnormalities, as detected with digitized M mode echocardiography, are present in patients with the most extensive hypertrophy of the left ventricle.

On the other hand, we also identified diastolic abnormalities in patients with HCM and only mild LVH, i.e., with LVH limited to no more than one left ventricular segment. For example, in patients with mild LVH, time from minimum left ventricular internal dimension to mitral valve opening, as well as peak rate and time to peak rate of increase in left ventricular internal dimension, were significantly different from normal, and at least two of these indexes were impaired in more than 70% of these patients. Furthermore, diastolic wall motion abnormalities were frequently identified in nonhypertrophied segments of the left ventricle of patients with HCM. For example, peak rate of posterior wall diastolic excursion was significantly reduced in patients with normal posterior wall thickness compared with that in control subjects, and the values for this parameter fell below the lower limit of normal in about 60% of these patients.

These findings raise certain conceptual issues regarding the relationship between hypertrophy and the cardiomyopathic process in HCM. Most investigators agree that the thickened, noncompliant left ventricle constitutes the primary morphologic and functional expression of the cardiomyopathic process in the majority of patients with HCM.[4, 7-14] However, while our data show an association between marked hypertrophy and impaired left ventricular diastolic wall motion, we also found that diastolic abnormalities were common in left ventricles with only mild hypertrophy and were also present in nonhypertrophied left ventricular seg-

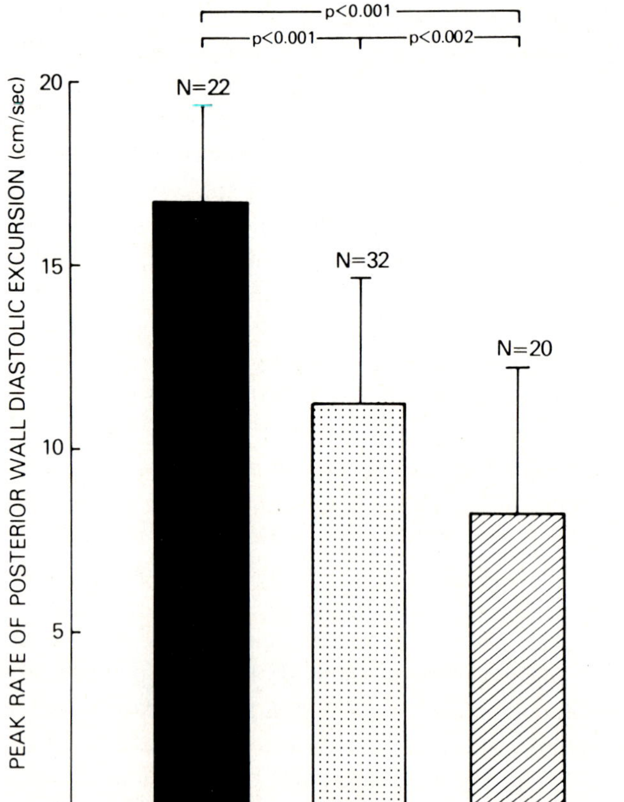

FIGURE 4. Comparison of peak rate of posterior wall diastolic excursion in normal subjects, in patients with HCM and normal (≤11 mm) posterior wall thickness, and in patients with HCM and increased (>11 mm) posterior wall thickness. PW = posterior wall.

ments. These findings suggest that gross wall thickening may not be a sine qua non of impaired diastolic function in patients with HCM. Although the observations reported here do not provide an explanation for the mechanism of abnormal diastolic wall motion in nonhypertrophied segments of the left ventricle, previous necropsy studies have shown myocardial fibrosis[25] and intramural coronary artery abnormalities[26] to be common in patients with HCM. It is possible that such structural alterations may be partially responsible for diastolic abnormalities in nonhypertrophied (as well as hypertrophied) segments of the left ventricle.

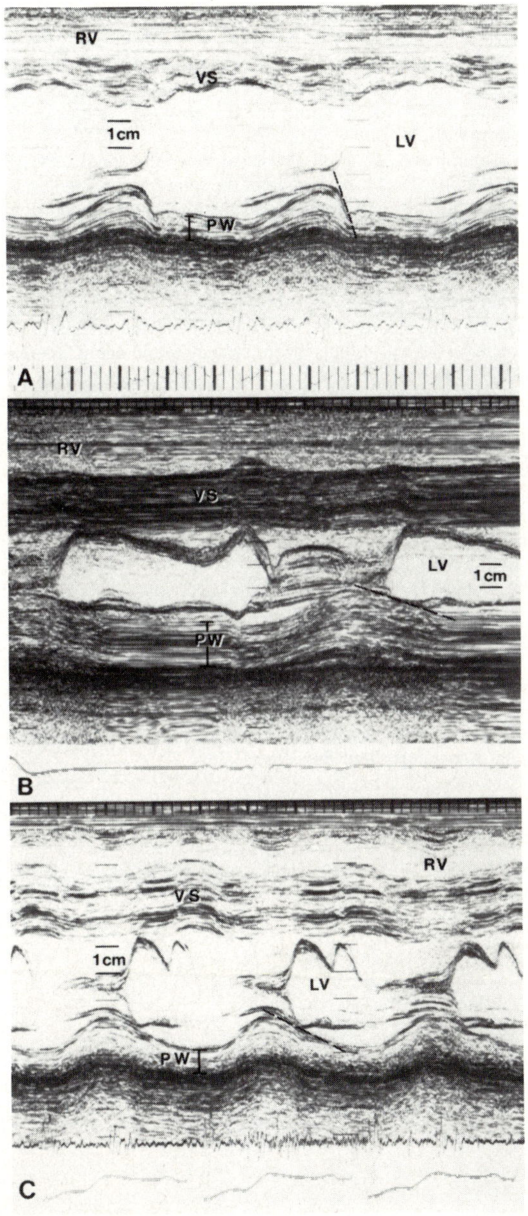

FIGURE 5. M mode echocardiograms obtained from a normal subject (*A*), and from patients with HCM having either left ventricular posterior wall (PW) hypertrophy (*B*) or normal PW thickness (*C*). Broken lines indicate diastolic slope of PW. In the normal subject (*A*), the slope of PW is steep; in patients with HCM and either increased (*B*) or normal (*C*) PW thickness, the slope is substantially reduced compared with that in the normal subject. Peak rate of PW diastolic excursion is 16.7 cm/sec in *A*, 4.1 cm/sec in *B*, and 4.8 cm/sec in *C*. LV = left ventricle; PW = posterior wall; RV = right ventricle; VS = ventricular septum.

In the present study, we used digitized echocardiography, in a manner similar to other investigators,[10-13] to assess left ventricular diastolic dynamics. We acknowledge that the indexes of diastolic function measured with this technique are not solely influenced by left ventricular wall thickness and by the intrinsic properties of the left ventricular wall, but are also dependent on the loading conditions of the ventricle.[27-29] Therefore, changes in left atrial driving pressure or in residual left ventricular volume from the preceding systole may alter these diastolic indexes independent of left ventricular wall thickness. In addition, cardiac motion (relative to the fixed position of the echo transducer on the chest) may influence echocardiographic measurements of wall motion such as the excursion of the posterior wall endocardium. Because hemodynamic measurements were not obtained in the present investigation, the influence of wall thickness on diastolic wall motion could not be separated, in the individual patient, from the potential influence of loading conditions. However, our observations that diastolic wall motion abnormalities were more severe in patients with diffuse LVH, and were also common in patients with mild localized LVH, were based on analysis of group data. While in individual patients such diastolic abnormalities could conceivably be explained as the consequence of variables other than wall thickness, this interpretation is unlikely for our patient subgroups that were segregated exclusively on the basis of the magnitude of LVH.

In conclusion, our data show a relationship, in patients with HCM, between magnitude of LVH and severity of diastolic wall motion abnormalities. Our results also show that diastolic wall motion abnormalities may be identified in patients with HCM and mild LVH (i.e., hypertrophy involving only one segment of the left ventricle) and that impaired diastolic wall motion may also be present in nonhypertrophied left ventricular segments. The pathogenesis of diastolic wall motion abnormalities in patients with HCM and mild localized LVH remains to be determined.

We are grateful to Gianni Pinna, Ph.D., for his assistance in obtaining the computerized data.

References

1. Goodwin JF, Hollman A, Cleland WP, Teare RD: Obstructive cardiomyopathy simulating aortic stenosis. Br Heart J **22:** 403, 1960

2. Wigle ED, Heimbecker RO, Gunton RW: Idiopathic ventricular septal hypertrophy causing muscular subaortic stenosis. Circulation **26:** 325, 1962
3. Braunwald E, Lambrew CT, Rockoff SD, Ross J Jr, Morrow AG: Idiopathic hypertrophic subaortic stenosis. I. A description of the disease based upon an analysis of 64 patients. Circulation **30**(suppl IV): IV-3, 1964
4. Goodwin JF: Congestive and hypertrophic cardiomyopathies. A decade of study. Lancet **1:** 731, 1970
5. Epstein SE, Henry WL, Clark CE, Roberts WC, Maron BJ, Ferrans VJ, Redwood DR, Morrow AG: Asymmetric septal hypertrophy. Ann Intern Med **81:** 650, 1974
6. Maron BJ, Gottdiener JS, Epstein SE: Patterns and significance of distribution of left ventricular hypertrophy in hypertrophic cardiomyopathy. A wide angle, two dimensional echocardiographic study of 125 patients. Am J Cardiol **48:** 418, 1981
7. Stewart S, Mason DT, Braunwald E: Impaired rate of left ventricular filling in idiopathic hypertrophic subaortic stenosis and valvular aortic stenosis. Circulation **37:** 8, 1968
8. Goodwin JF, Oakley CM: The cardiomyopathies. Br Heart J **34:** 545, 1972
9. Sanderson JE, Gibson DG, Brown DJ, Goodwin JF: Left ventricular filling in hypertrophic cardiomyopathy: an angiographic study. Br Heart J **39:** 661, 1977
10. Sanderson JE, Traill TA, St. John Sutton MG, Brown DJ, Gibson DG, Goodwin JF: Left ventricular relaxation and filling in hypertrophic cardiomyopathy: an echocardiographic study. Br Heart J **40:** 596, 1978
11. St. John Sutton MG, Tajik AJ, Gibson DG, Brown DJ, Seward JB, Giuliani ER: Echocardiographic assessment of left ventricular filling and septal and posterior wall dynamics in idiopathic hypertrophic subaortic stenosis. Circulation **57:** 512, 1978
12. Hanrath P, Mathey DG, Siegert R, Bleifeld W: Left ventricular relaxation and filling in different forms of left ventricular hypertrophy: an echocardiographic study. Am J Cardiol **45:** 15, 1980
13. Lorell BH, Paulus WJ, Grossman W, Wynne J, Cohn PF: Modification of abnormal left ventricular diastolic properties by nifedipine in patients with hypertrophic cardiomyopathy. Circulation **65:** 499, 1982
14. Bonow RO, Rosing DR, Bacharach SL, Green MV, Kent KM, Lipson LC, Maron BJ, Leon MB, Epstein SE: Effects of verapamil on left ventricular systolic function and diastolic filling in patients with hypertrophic cardiomyopathy. Circulation **64:** 787, 1981
15. Maron BJ, Epstein SE: Hypertrophic cardiomyopathy: a discussion of nomenclature. Am J Cardiol **43:** 1242, 1979
16. Henry WL, Clark CE, Glancy DL, Epstein SE: Echocardiographic measurement of left ventricular outflow gradient in idiopathic hypertrophic subaortic stenosis. N Engl J Med **288:** 989, 1973
17. Pollick C, Rakowski H, Wigle DE: Muscular subaortic stenosis: the quantitative relationship between systolic anterior motion and pressure gradient. Circulation **69:** 43, 1984
18. Pollick C, Fitzgerald P, Popp RL: Variability of digitized echocardiography: size, source, and means of reduction. Am J Cardiol **51:** 576, 1983
19. Sahn DJ, DeMaria A, Kisslo J, Weyman A: The Committee on M mode Standardization of the American Society of Echocardiography: Recommendations regarding quantitation in M mode echocardiography. Results of a survey of echocardiographic measurements. Circulation **58:** 1072, 1978
20. TenCate FJ, Serruys PW, Mey Simon, Roelandt J: Effects of short-term administration of verapamil on left ventricular relaxation and filling dynamics measured by a combined hemodynamic-ultrasonic technique in patients with hypertrophic cardiomyopathy. Circulation **68:** 1274, 1983
21. O'Rourke RA, Hanrath P, Henry WN, Hugenholtz PG, Pisa Z, Roelandt J, Tanaka M: Report of the Joint International Society and Federation of Cardiology/World Health Organization task force on recommendations for standardization of measurements from M mode echocardiograms. Circulation **69:** 854A, 1984
22. Feigenbaum H: Echocardiography, ed 3. Philadelphia, 1981, Lea and Febiger, p 550
23. Henry WL, Gardin JM, Ware JH: Echocardiographic measurements in normal subjects from infancy to old age. Circulation **62:** 1054, 1980
24. Colton T: Statistics in medicine. Boston, 1974, Little, Brown and Company, p 39
25. Roberts WC, Ferrans VJ: Pathological aspects of certain cardiomyopathies. Circ Res **34/35**(suppl II): II-238; II-144, 1974
26. Maron BJ, Wolfson JK, Epstein SE, Roberts WC: Intramural "small vessel" coronary artery disease in hypertrophic cardiomyopathy: prevalence and potential significance. Am J Coll Cardiol **5:** 395, 1985 (abst)
27. Gamble WH, Shaver JA, Alvares RF, Salerni R, Reddy PS: A critical appraisal of diastolic time intervals as a measure of relaxation in left ventricular hypertrophy. Circulation **68:** 76, 1983
28. Carroll JD, Hess OM, Hirzel HO, Krayenbuehl HP: Dynamics of left ventricular filling at rest and during exercise. Circulation **68:** 59, 1983
29. Grossman W, McLaurin LP: Diastolic properties of the left ventricle. Ann Intern Med **84:** 316, 1976

Validation of attenuation-corrected equilibrium radionuclide angiographic determinations of right ventricular volume: comparison with cast-validated biplane cineventriculography

LOUIS J. DELL'ITALIA, M.D., MARK R. STARLING, M.D., RICHARD A. WALSH, M.D., FREDERICK R. BADKE, M.D., JOHN C. LASHER, M.D., AND RALPH BLUMHARDT, M.D.

ABSTRACT To determine the accuracy of attenuation-corrected equilibrium radionuclide angiographic determinations of right ventricular volumes, we initially studied 14 postmortem human right ventricular casts by water displacement and biplane cineventriculography. Biplane cineventriculographic right ventricular cast volumes, calculated by a modification of Simpson's rule algorithm, correlated well with right ventricular cast volumes measured by water displacement (r = .97, y = 8+0.88x, SEE = 6 ml). Moreover, the mean volumes obtained by both methods were no different (73 ± 28 vs 73 ± 25 ml). Subsequently, we studied 16 patients by both biplane cineventriculography and equilibrium radionuclide angiography. The uncorrected radionuclide right ventricular volumes were calculated by normalizing background corrected end-diastolic and end-systolic counts from hand-drawn regions of interest obtained by phase analysis for cardiac cycles processed, frame rate, and blood sample counts. Attenuation correction was performed by a simple geometric method. The attenuation-corrected radionuclide right ventricular end-diastolic volumes correlated with the cineventriculographic end-diastolic volumes (r = .91, y = 3+0.92x, SEE = 27 ml). Similarly, the attenuation-corrected radionuclide right ventricular end-systolic volumes correlated with the cineventriculographic end-systolic volumes (r = .93, y = −1+0.91x, SEE = 16 ml). Also, the mean attenuation-corrected radionuclide end-diastolic and end-systolic volumes were no different than the average cineventriculographic end-diastolic and end-systolic volumes (160 ± 61 and 83 ± 44 vs 170 ± 61 and 86 ± 43 ml, respectively). Comparison of the uncorrected and attenuation-corrected radionuclide right ventricular volumes demonstrated narrower 95% confidence intervals for the attenuation-corrected right ventricular volume determinations over a wide range of cineventriculographic volumes. Thus we conclude that: (1) attenuation-corrected radionuclide right ventricular end-diastolic and end-systolic volumes compare closely with those obtained by a cast-validated biplane cineventriculographic method and (2) attenuation-corrected radionuclide right ventricular volumes correspond more closely to determinations of biplane cineventriculographic right ventricular volumes and are thus likely to be more accurate than uncorrected radionuclide right ventricular volumes.
Circulation 72, No. 2, 317–326, 1985.

SEVERAL invasive and noninvasive techniques have been used successfully for the measurement of right ventricular ejection fraction.[1-9] However, precise estimates of right ventricular volumes are more difficult to obtain because of the complex configuration of the right ventricle. Nonetheless, several geometric models have been used to calculate right ventricular volumes from biplane cineventriculograms.[1-6] Two-dimensional echocardiography and radionuclide angiography have also been used to obtain estimates of right ventricular volumes.[7-10] However, two-dimensional echocardiographic determinations of right ventricular volume are also dependent on geometric assumptions, and echocardiograms of the right ventricle are difficult to obtain in all patients because of technical limitations.[7-9] In contrast, good-quality radionuclide angiographic images of the right ventricle can be obtained in nearly all patients. More importantly, calculation of

From the University of Texas Health Science Center, San Antonio.
Supported in part by NIH New Investigator Research Awards R23 HL27508 and R01-HL32845, Research Training Grant T32-HL07350 from the NHLBI, and a grant-in-aid from CGR Medical Corp. Dr. Starling is supported by NIH Research Career Development Award K04-HL01446 from the NHLBI.
Address for correspondence: Louis J. Dell'Italia, M.D., Department of Medicine/Cardiology, The University of Texas Health Science Center, 7703 Floyd Curl Dr., San Antonio, TX 78284.
Received Oct. 24, 1984; revision accepted May 2, 1985.

right ventricular volumes can be obtained from chamber count rate, which is relatively independent of simplifying assumptions regarding chamber geometry. Dehmer et al.[10] reported that radionuclide right ventricular stroke volumes that were not corrected for photon attenuation correlated with thermodilution stroke volumes. Radionuclide stroke volumes were obtained by regression equation correction of the uncorrected stroke volumes. Theoretically, right ventricular volumes obtained by this method may be imprecise in an individual patient because photon attenuation is dependent on two variables: the constitution of the intervening body tissue and the distance between the gamma camera and the right ventricular center of mass. Because these variables differ for each patient, radionuclide methods that assume constant attenuation for all patients may produce inexact determinations of right ventricular volumes.

Recently, we reported accurate estimates of left ventricular volumes from equilibrium radionuclide angiographic count data by means of a simple geometric method for attenuation correction,[11] and we demonstrated its improved precision over uncorrected radionuclide left ventricular volumes for estimating left ventricular volumes.[12] The objectives of the present investigation were to apply this approach to the right ventricle in a consecutive series of patients (1) to validate attenuation-corrected radionuclide right ventricular volumes compared with cast-validated biplane cineventriculographic right ventricular volumes and (2) to determine whether this radionuclide method of determining right ventricular volumes is more accurate than that using radionuclide right ventricular volumes that were not corrected for photon attenuation.

Methods

Validation of the biplane cineventriculographic volume determinations. Fourteen postmortem human heart specimens were obtained in normal saline within 24 hr of death. The semilunar and atrioventricular valves were oversewn to prevent leakage. Radiopaque latex was infused simultaneously into the right and left ventricles to a distending pressure of 15 mm Hg. The casts were allowed to harden and were then removed from the heart. Excess muscle tissue was stripped away from trabeculations, the base of the heart, and the right and left ventricular outflow tracts. Right ventricular cast volumes were obtained from an average of five measurements by water displacement. The right ventricular casts were placed on the catheterization table in a position which closely approximated the orientation of the right ventricle in a patient lying in the supine position. Biplane cineventriculograms (CGR, Double Angiomax) of the casts were obtained at 60 frames/sec in the 30 degree right anterior oblique and 60 degree left anterior oblique/20 degree cranial angulations. The biplane cineventriculographic right ventricular cast images were outlined with a sonic digitizer (Science Accessories) mounted on a cine projector (Vanguard Instrument Co.) by two blinded experienced angiographers on separate occasions. The right ventricular long axes (ℓ) in both planes were determined from a line drawn from the midpoint of the pulmonic valve to the right ventricular base. The digitized data were processed with an on-line minicomputer (IBM PC), and volumes were calculated by a modification of Simpson's rule algorithm developed in our laboratory (see Appendix). Correction for magnification and pincushion distortion was performed with correction factors obtained by filming NAMIC grids at the center of mass of the casts in both planes.

Patients. The study group consisted of 16 patients, eight male and eight female, who gave written informed consent on a form approved by our Institutional Review Board. Their ages ranged between 17 and 67 years with a mean of 37 years. Clinical indications for cardiac catheterization included atrial septal defect (n = 2), biventricular heart failure (n = 2), postsurgical repair of Tetrology of Fallot (n = 3), mild pulmonic stenosis (n = 2), severe subpulmonic stenosis (n = 1), inferior myocardial infarction (n = 2), mitral stenosis (n = 2), severe aortic regurgitation (n = 1), and atypical chest pain (n = 1). All patients were in sinus rhythm. Equilibrium radionuclide angiography was performed 18 to 24 hr after the cardiac catheterization in 15 of the 16 patients and 24 hr before cardiac catheterization in one patient. During this period cardiac medications and clinical status in all patients was unchanged.

Cardiac catheterization. Right and left heart catheterization was performed in the 16 patients by the brachial or femoral approach. Right ventricular biplane cineventriculography was performed at 60 frames/sec in the 30 degree right anterior oblique and 60 degree left anterior oblique/20 degree cranial angulations. A No. 8F Berman catheter was positioned in the right ventricular apex where ventricular ectopic beats were minimal. Forty to 50 ml of meglumine diatrizoate (Renografin 76) were injected over 4 sec at 450 psi. Analysis was conducted on one of the first 3 sinus beats when the effect of iodinated contrast material is minimal.[13] Ventricular ectopic and postventricular ectopic beats were rejected from analysis. Correction factors from each image intensifier to the right ventricular geometric center of mass were recorded for correction of magnification and pincushion distortion.

Right ventricular end-diastolic and end-systolic images were defined as the maximum and minimum silhouette areas observed on stop frame analysis of the cineventriculogram. The right ventricular long axes in the 30 degree right anterior oblique and 60 degree left anterior oblique/20 degree cranial angulations were determined by a line drawn from the midpoint of the pulmonic valve to the right ventricular base. The right ventricular volumes were then calculated from the end-diastolic and end-systolic images by means of the computer program. The calculated cineventriculographic right ventricular volumes were then corrected to absolute volumes by the regression equation calculated for our laboratory from the right ventricular cast data.

Equilibrium radionuclide angiography. Equilibrium radionuclide angiography was performed with a 37 photomultiplier tube single crystal gamma scintillation camera equipped with an all-purpose parallel-hole collimator. Red blood cell labeling in vivo was accomplished by intravenous administration of stannous pyrophosphate followed in 15 min by 20 to 25 mCi of technetium-99m pertechnetate. In the anterior camera position a point source of technetium-99m was placed over the right ventricle midway between the inferior border of the right ventricle and the pulmonic valve and in line with the right ventricular outflow tract and pulmonary artery (figure 1, *A*). This point was marked on the chest and the left anterior oblique position was selected that best separated the right and left ventricles in the plane of the interventricular septum. In our patient population, this angle (θ) ranged between 20 and 60 degrees. The point source was then placed over the right ventricular

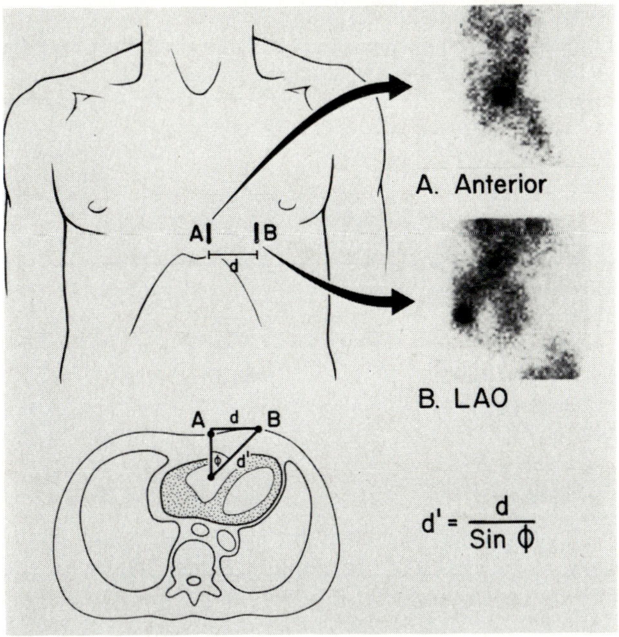

FIGURE 1. Method of obtaining the horizontal distance (d) for use in calculating the distance (d') from the right ventricular center of mass to the camera in the left anterior oblique (LAO) projection. With the camera in the anterior (*A*) and LAO (*B*) projections, the technetium-99m point source was placed over the right ventricle and marks were placed on the anterior chest (*left*). The horizontal distance (d) between the two marks was measured and the distance (d') was calculated by a simple geometric method (*lower right*).

cavity midway between the septum and lateral wall and equidistant from the apex and the pulmonic valve (figure 1, *B*). The horizontal distance (d) between the two marks was measured in centimeters and averaged for three measurements. The maximum difference between individual marks did not exceed 4 mm on three separate measurements. The distance (d) was inserted into the formula:

$$d' = \frac{d}{\sin \theta}$$

where θ = the angulation of the camera in the left anterior oblique projection. This is a simple geometric method, applied to the right ventricle, which calculates the distance (d') from the right ventricular center of mass to the gamma camera. Ten degrees of caudal angulation added to the left anterior oblique position increases slightly the calculated d' and subsequently produces a 1.63% increase in the attenuation correction factor (A). This amounts to only a small increase in the attenuation corrected volumes and therefore has been neglected in this investigation. However, the effect on the attenuation correction factor (A) increases exponentially as larger caudal angles are used, as other investigators have done.[10] Therefore, if caudal angulation of greater than 10 degrees is used, then d' should be corrected appropriately because this may result in a significant underestimation of right ventricular volume.

Radionuclide images were acquired in the same left anterior oblique position described above with 10 degrees of caudal tilt. R wave–gated 30 msec frames were acquired consecutively throughout the cardiac cycle into 64 × 64 byte matrix images until the count information from 1000 RR intervals had been processed. Information was stored in the computer memory (A^2, Medical Data Systems, Inc.) for later analysis. Midway through the radionuclide acquisition, a 2 ml blood sample was drawn and later counted on the collimator for 2 min. The time (t) delay from drawing to counting the blood sample was recorded for radioisotope decay correction.

Right ventricular end-diastolic and end-systolic counts were obtained by a hand-drawn region-of-interest method similar to that described by Maddahi et al.[14] To facilitate selection of regions of interest, a commercially available phase-analysis program (MDS A^2) was used to delineate the pulmonic valve plane and right atrial-right ventricular border in the left anterior oblique projection. The end-diastolic frame determined from the semiautomated variable time-activity curve was displayed. Background was obtained manually from a left ventricular end-diastolic paraventricular region of interest 2 pixels wide placed inferior and lateral to the left ventricle and 2 to 3 pixels away from the left ventricular border. After the end-diastolic background was subtracted and the image had undergone nine point spatial smoothing, the operator manually outlined a right ventricular end-diastolic region of interest that totally encompassed the right ventricle with the pulmonic valve as the superior border. In a similar manner, the right ventricular end-systolic image was recalled, the image was background subtracted and smoothed, and the operator manually outlined a right ventricular end-systolic region of interest. From these right ventricular hand-drawn regions of interest, the right ventricular end-diastolic and end-systolic counts were obtained. Finally, the static blood sample image was displayed, and the operator positioned a 10 × 15 pixel rectangular region of interest around the image to obtain blood sample counts. Since background around the blood sample image averaged 0 counts/pixel, no background subtraction was considered necessary.

Right ventricular end-diastolic and end-systolic volumes were calculated as:

$$\frac{\text{background corrected RV counts}}{\text{blood sample counts}} \times A$$

where background corrected right ventricular (RV) counts are right ventricular end-diastolic or end-systolic counts that had been normalized in the following manner:

$$\frac{\text{background corrected RV counts} \times 60\ \text{sec/min;}}{1000\ \text{beats} \times 0.03\ \text{sec/beat}}$$

where 1000 beats is the total number of RR intervals processed, 0.03 sec/beat is the frame rate during acquisition, and 60 sec/min converts counts per second to counts per minute. The blood sample counts in counts per 2 minutes per 2 milliliters obtained on the collimator were corrected for decay by:

$$e^{\lambda t}$$

where $\lambda = 0.693/t_{1/2}$ ($t_{1/2}$ is 360 min for technetium-99m) and t is the time in minutes from drawing the blood sample until the blood sample was counted. This results in uncorrected right ventricular end-diastolic and end-systolic volumes. This value can be multiplied by A to correct for photon attentuation, where A is:

$$e^{ud'}$$

where $u = 0.15\ cm^{-1}$ represents the linear attenuation coefficient for the 140 keV photon of technetium-99m in water[11] and d' represents the distance in centimeters calculated from the gamma scintillation camera in the left anterior oblique position to the right ventricular center of mass. After multiplying by A, the result is attenuation-corrected radionuclide right ventricular end-diastolic and end-systolic volumes in milliliters.

Statistics. Comparisons of right ventricular volumes determined by water displacement and biplane cineventriculography in casts and of those determined by radionuclide and biplane cineventriculography in patients were performed by least squares linear regression analysis to determine correlation coefficients, regression equations, 95% confidence intervals, and standard errors of the estimate. Correlation coefficients for uncorrected and attenuation-corrected radionuclide right ventricular volume determinations were compared by Fischer's Z-transformation. Group data were expressed as a mean ± 1 SD and were compared by a paired t test or an analysis of variance where indicated. A significant difference was considered present when a p value of .05 or less was observed.

Results

Biplane cineventriculographic right ventricular volumes. The right ventricular volumes obtained by biplane cineventriculography correlated with the right ventricular cast volumes (average of five measurements by water displacement) (r = .97, y = 8+0.88x, SEE = 6 ml; figure 2). Moreover, the mean right ventricular volumes obtained by both methods did not differ significantly (73 ± 25 vs 73 ± 28 ml, respectively). Biplane cineventriculograms of the right ventricular casts and patient studies were traced independently by two experienced angiographers on separate occasions in a blinded fashion. Intraobserver and interobserver correlations and differences are listed in table 1. In addition, the mean values for the cast and patient right ventricular volumes for observers 1 and 2 did not differ significantly.

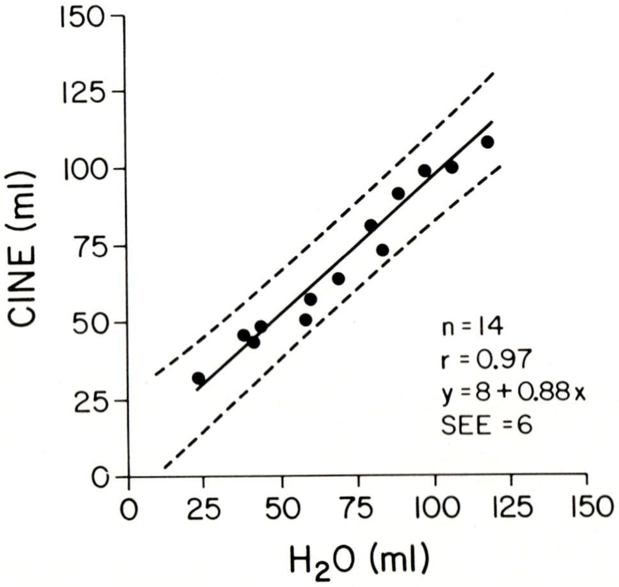

FIGURE 2. Comparison of right ventricular cast volumes measured by water displacement (H_2O) and biplane cineventriculography (CINE). The individual points, regression line, 95% confidence intervals, correlation coefficient (r), regression equation, and standard error of the estimate are shown.

TABLE 1

Intraobserver and interobserver correlations and differences for biplane cineangiographic right ventricular volumes

	r	Mean absolute difference between observations[A]
Intraobserver		
Casts (n = 14)	.97	1
Patients (n = 16)		
End-diastole	.98	1
End-systole	.96	1
Interobserver		
Casts (n = 14)	.97	5
Patients (n = 16)		
End-diastole	.96	3
End-systole	.97	4

[A]Expressed as a percent of observer 1's first determinations.

Radionuclide and biplane cineventriculographic right ventricular end-diastolic volumes. Attenuation-corrected radionuclide right ventricular end-diastolic volumes correlated with the cast-validated biplane cineventriculographic right ventricular end-diastolic volumes (r = .91, y = 3+0.92x, SEE = 27 ml; figure 3). Moreover, the average right ventricular end-diastolic volumes by radionuclide angiography and biplane cineventriculography did not differ significantly (160 ± 61 vs 170 ± 61 ml, respectively).

Radionuclide and biplane cineventriculographic right ventricular end-systolic volumes. Attenuated-corrected radionuclide right ventricular end-systolic volumes correlated with the end-systolic volumes obtained by

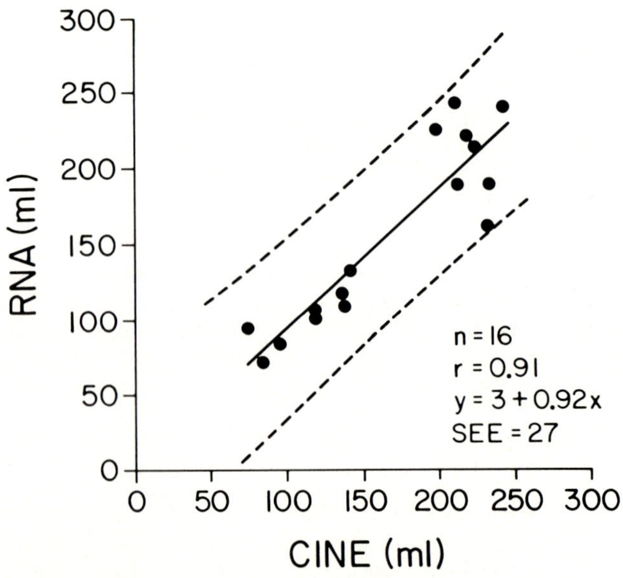

FIGURE 3. Comparison of right ventricular end-diastolic volumes measured by radionuclide angiography (RNA) and biplane cineventriculography (CINE) in 16 patients.

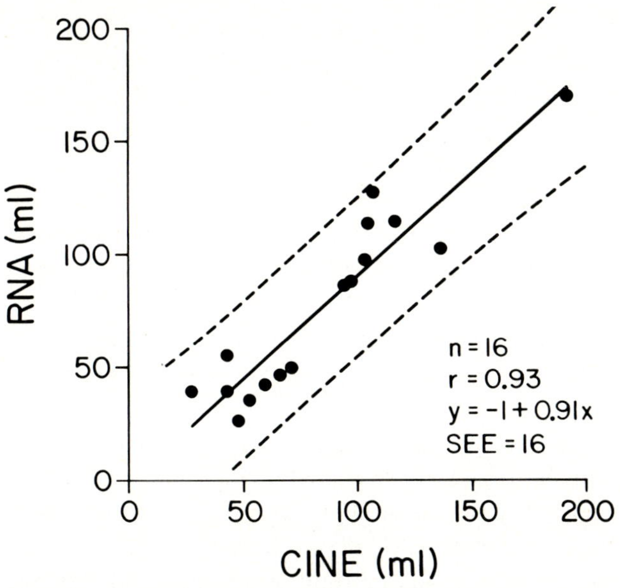

FIGURE 4. Comparison of right ventricular end-systolic volumes measured by radionuclide angiography (RNA) and biplane cineventriculography (CINE) in 16 patients.

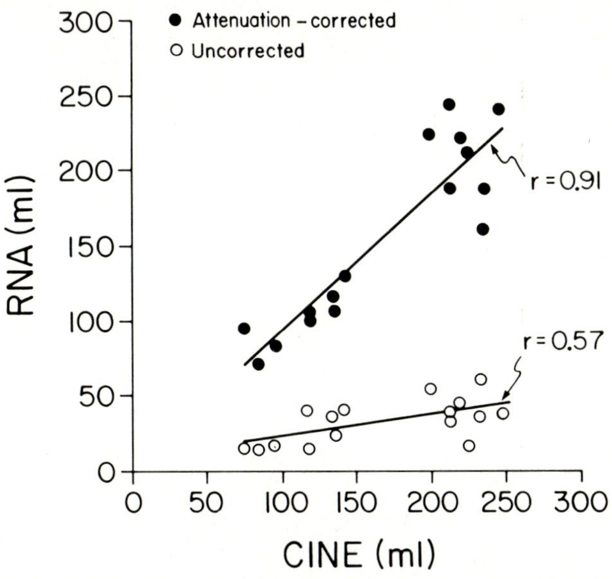

FIGURE 5. Relationship between uncorrected and attenuation-corrected right ventricular radionuclide angiographic (RNA) end-diastolic volumes and biplane cineventriculographic (CINE) volumes.

biplane cineventriculography (r = .93, y = −1 + 0.91x, SEE = 16 ml; figure 4). In addition, the mean right ventricular end-systolic volumes by both methods did not differ significantly (83 ± 44 vs 86 ± 43 ml, respectively).

Reproducibility of radionuclide volume data. The attenuation-corrected radionuclide right ventricular volumes were highly reproducible. Intraobserver and interobserver correlations and differences are listed in table 2. In addition, the mean values for the radionuclide end-diastolic and end-systolic right ventricular volumes for observers 1 and 2 did not differ significantly.

Accuracy of right ventricular volume determinations: uncorrected vs attenuation-corrected radionuclide volumes. Radionuclide right ventricular end-diastolic and end-systolic volumes that were not corrected for photon attenuation correlated with the biplane cineventriculographic right ventricular volumes (r = .57, y = 2.2x + 91 and r = .71, y = 3.2x + 20, SEE = 31 ml, respectively; figures 5 and 6, table 3). Attenuation-corrected radionuclide right ventricular end-diastolic and end-systolic volumes demonstrated an improved correlation with the biplane cineventriculographic end-diastolic and end-systolic volumes (p = .02).

With biplane cineventriculographic volumes as the standard for comparison, the relative accuracy of uncorrected and attenuation-corrected radionuclide right ventricular volumes were evaluated with the 95% confidence intervals for the uncorrected and attenuation-corrected radionuclide data. Regression equation correction of the uncorrected and attenuation-corrected radionuclide right ventricular volumes for a range of biplane cineventriculographic volumes (50 to 450 ml) demonstrated that the calculated ranges for the attenuation-corrected right ventricular end-diastolic and end-systolic volumes were substantially narrower than those obtained from the uncorrected radionuclide right ventricular volumes (figures 7 and 8). Despite this fact, attenuation-corrected right ventricular end-diastolic volumes still yielded an SEE of 27 ml compared with cast-validated biplane cineventriculographic volumes. However, when 150 ml was used as the approximate upper limit of normal for cineventriculographic right ventricular end-distolic volume,[2, 6] the attenuation-corrected radionuclide method appropriately separated patients with normal from those with en-

TABLE 2
Intraobserver and interobserver correlations and differences for attenuation-corrected radionuclide right ventricular volume determinations

	r	Mean absolute difference between observations[A]
Intraobserver		
End-diastole	.99	5
End-systole	.97	5
Interobserver		
End-diastole	.97	6
End-systole	.97	1

[A]Expressed as a percent of observer 1's first determinations.

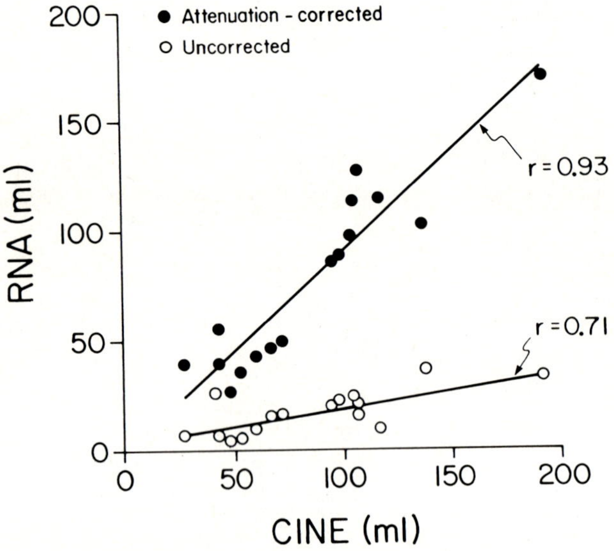

FIGURE 6. Relationship between uncorrected and attenuation-corrected right ventricular radionuclide angiographic (RNA) end-systolic volumes and biplane cineventriculographic (CINE) volumes.

larged right ventricles. In addition, the normal right ventricles yielded a better correlation between the attenuation-corrected radionuclide and biplane cineventriculographic end-diastolic volumes than did the enlarged right ventricles.

Discussion

Biplane cineventriculography. Several investigators have shown that biplane cineventriculography of right ventricular casts yield calculated right ventricular volumes that correlate with cast volumes measured by water displacement.[1-6] Ferlinz et al.[1,2] reported an excellent correlation between right ventricular cast and biplane cineventriculographic volumes using a pyramid on a triangular base as the geometric model to calculate right ventricle volumes. Fisher et al.[3] also demonstrated a good correlation with right ventricular cast volumes using a similar geometric model, a prism on a triangular base, to calculate biplane cineventriculographic right ventricular volumes. Arcilla et al.[4] and Slutsky et al.,[5] using biplane cineventriculography of right ventricular casts, showed that a simple area-length method for the calculation of right ventricular volumes produced a reasonable correlation with actual cast volumes measured by water displacement. All of these studies used right ventricular casts that were in the normal range for right ventricular end-diastolic volumes by water displacement. Thus various geometric approximations may produce accurate volume calculations when the right ventricle is of normal size. However, as the right ventricle enlarges secondary to a volume load or becomes hypertrophic secondary to a pressure load, its intracavitary configuration may become deformed and may no longer aproximate a simple geometric model.

Genzler et al.[6] imaged right ventricular casts with biplane cineventriculography and demonstrated a high correlation between cast volumes calculated by a Simpson's rule algorithm and cast volumes measured by water displacement. These same investigators sub-

TABLE 3
Individual cineangiographic right ventricular volumes compared with uncorrected and attenuation-corrected radionuclide angiographic volumes

	Cine		Uncorrected RNA		A	Corrected RNA	
Patient	RVEDV	RVESV	RVEDV	RVESV	($e^{ud'}$)	RVEDV	RVESV
1	237	95	37	20	4.42	163	86
2	201	98	55	21	4.16	230	88
3	86	43	18	10	4.05	74	39
4	121	53	18	6	6.13	110	35
5	238	137	72	38	2.66	192	102
6	248	192	46	32	5.34	245	169
7	215	107	40	21	6.16	249	127
8	76	27	17	7	5.70	97	39
9	228	117	17	9	13.01	217	114
10	97	48	22	7	3.97	87	26
11	137	72	38	16	3.15	120	49
12	215	109	35	18	5.45	192	97
13	223	105	46	23	4.88	226	113
14	138	60	25	10	4.42	111	42
15	144	67	42	14	3.21	134	46
16	120	43	47	25	2.24	105	55

CINE = cineangiography; RNA = radionuclide angiography; RVEDV = right ventricular end-diastolic volume; RVESV = right ventricular end-systolic volume; A = attenuation correction factor ($e^{ud'}$).

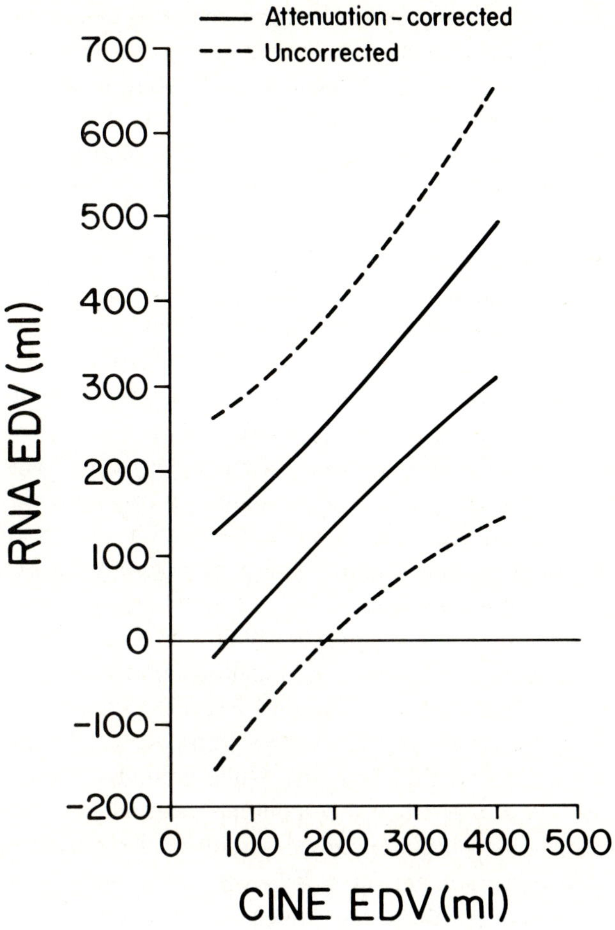

FIGURE 7. Comparison of the range of 95% confidence intervals for the uncorrected and attenuation-corrected radionuclide angiographic (RNA) right ventricular end-diastolic volumes (EDV) after regression equation correction. The range of attenuation-corrected volumes is significantly smaller for predicting individual cineventriculographic (CINE) volumes.

sequently used this method to obtain right ventricular volumes in 32 patients, 16 of whom had enlarged right ventricles with end-diastolic volumes in excess of 100 ml/m². All other reports[1-5] in which right ventricular volumes were calculated in patients described end-diastolic volumes of less than 100 ml/m². Use of a Simpson's rule algorithm should provide a more accurate estimate of volume in normal as well as enlarged right ventricles, since this mathematical model for the estimation of volume minimizes errors that arise from geometric assumptions because the cardiac chamber is divided into multiple subunits.

In our investigation biplane cineventriculographic right ventricular cast volumes calculated by a Simpson's rule algorithm produced an excellent correlation with cast volumes measured by water displacement. The right ventricle was imaged in a 30 degree right anterior oblique and 60 degree left anterior oblique/20 degree cranial angulations. Previously, biplane right ventricular cineventriculography had been performed either in the anteroposterior and lateral or 30 degree right anterior oblique and 60 degree left anterior oblique projections.[1-6] Cranial angulation of the 60 degree left anterior oblique projection allowed for a longer axial view of the interventricular septum. This projection is minimally influenced by foreshortening of the right ventricle in the left anterior oblique projection, thereby improving the evaluation of right ventricular regional wall motion and anatomy without compromising the accuracy of the calculated right ventricular volumes by a Simpson's rule algorithm.

Noninvasive studies. Biplane cineventriculography is an accurate method for determining right ventricular volumes; however, it is an invasive procedure that poses some risk to the patient. Moreover, it cannot be used when serial long-term studies are needed to evaluate the effects of drug therapy or progression of disease. Noninvasive techniques such as two-dimensional

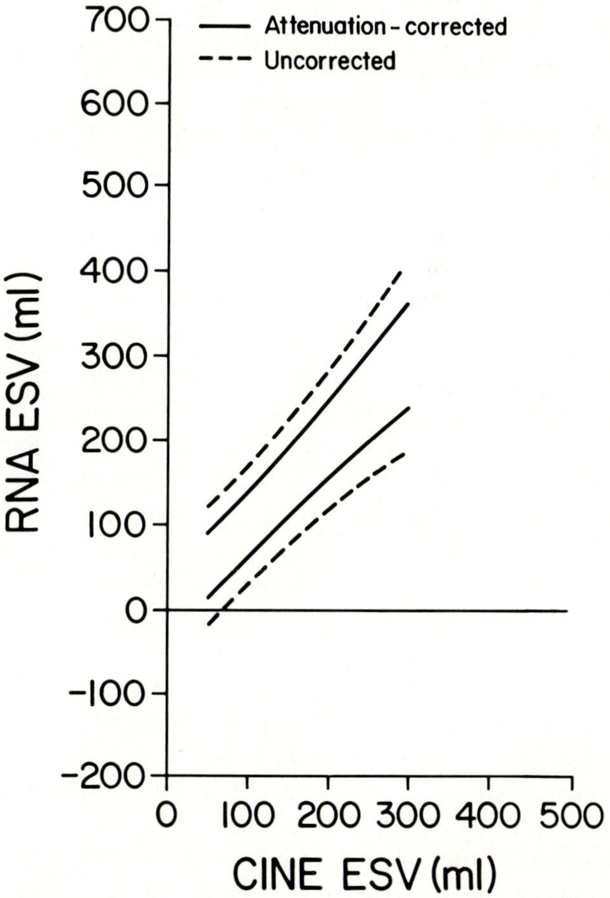

FIGURE 8. Comparison of the range of 95% confidence intervals for the uncorrected and attenuation-corrected radionuclide angiographic (RNA) right ventricular end-systolic volumes (ESV) after regression equation correction. The range of attenuation-corrected volumes is smaller for predicting individual cineventriculographic (CINE) volumes.

echocardiography have been used to obtain estimates of right ventricular volumes.[7-9] However, radionuclide angiography offers significant advantages over two-dimensional echocardiography in that adequate studies may be obtained in nearly all patients, and volume estimates that are relatively independent of geometry may be obtained on the basis of chamber count rates.

In a study that compared geometric methods to a count-based approach for determining left ventricular volume by radionuclide angiography, Massie et al.[15] demonstrated that both techniques yielded high correlation coefficients with single-plane cineventriculographic left ventricular volumes. However, the standard errors of the estimate for the geometric radionuclide techniques were higher, and consequently the 95% confidence intervals were wider than those for the count-based radionuclide technique. Therefore a count-based equilibrium radionuclide method appears to yield more accurate determinations of left ventricular volumes.

Dehmer et al.[16] and Slutsky et al.[17] used count-based methods to obtain left ventricular volumes by equilibrium radionuclide angiography. Their methods yielded uncorrected left ventricular volumes derived from the ratio of left ventricular counts to peripheral blood sample counts. Left ventricular volumes were obtained by regression equation correction of the corresponding volumes that were not corrected for photon attenuation. Theoretically, a method that is highly dependent on regression equation correction may yield estimates of left or right ventricular volumes that are imprecise, since each patient has variable technetium-99m photon attenuation because of the composition of the intervening body tissue and the distance between the left and right ventricular centers of mass and the gamma camera. Therefore the assumption of a constant photon attenuation may result in highly variable radionuclide left and right ventricular volume estimates in individual patients.

Links et al.[18] obtained attenuation-corrected equilibrium radionuclide left ventricular volumes that correlated highly with single-plane cineventriculographic volumes. A computer-assisted method was used to calculate the distance from the camera to the left ventricular center of mass, and attenuation correction was made for each patient by means of the calculated distance and the linear attenuation coefficient for a beam of technetium-99m photons in water. We recently reported an excellent correlation between attentuation-corrected radionuclide left ventricular volumes and biplane cineventriculographic volumes.[11] A simple geometric method was used to obtain the distance from the camera to the left ventricular center of mass, and attenuation correction was performed with this distance and the linear attenuation coefficient of technetium-99m photons in water.[11,12] Attenuation correction produced more accurate left ventricular volumes with narrower 95% confidence intervals than comparable volumes obtained from uncorrected radionuclide left ventricular volumes when both values were compared with biplane cineventriculographic volumes.[12]

Using a count-based radionuclide method similar to their method for the calculation of left ventricular volumes, Dehmer et al.[10] reported that uncorrected radionuclide right ventricular stroke volumes correlated with thermodilution stroke volumes. Again, radionuclide right ventricular stroke volumes were highly dependent on regression equation correction of the radionuclide stroke volumes that were not corrected for photon attenuation. In this investigation, we used a simple geometric method to obtain the distance from the camera to the right ventricular center of mass. The measured distance was used to calculate attenuation-corrected radionuclide right ventricular volumes. These radionuclide right ventricular volumes correlated highly with the corresponding cast-validated biplane cineventriculographic volumes. As was previously demonstrated for the left ventricle, attenuation correction produced more accurate radionuclide right ventricular volumes compared with uncorrected radionuclide right ventricular volumes.

Limitations. Although this method has advantages over previously reported techniques, there are several potential sources of error. The choice of u as the linear attenuation coefficient of a beam of technetium-99m photons in water may not represent the true physiologic condition in the body. Nonetheless, Links et al.[18] used this value in clinical studies with excellent results. In the same study these investigators constructed a phantom model using 50 to 250 ml flasks of a known concentration of technetium-99m in water. They arrived at a measured value of u that ranged from 0.14 to 0.15 cm^{-1}. In contrast, Maurer et al.[19] corrected for tissue photon attenuation by positioning an esophogeal point source behind the left atrium and calculating a transmission factor for each patient, while the distance from the left ventricular center of mass to the gamma camera was assumed to be constant. These radionuclide left ventricular volume determinations also correlated highly with biplane cineventriculographic volumes.

The accuracy of radionuclide right ventricular volumes is also dependent on the reproducibility of the following variables: (1) blood sample counts, (2) measurement of the distance d, and (3) right ventricular end-diastolic and end-systolic counts. First, the counts obtained from the 2 ml blood sample could have affected the right ventricular volumes. The blood sample counts were corrected for decay to obviate problems with the time delay from drawing to counting the sample. We chose to count the blood sample on the camera face, since collimator efficiency for a point source in air is independent of the source to collimator distance.[20] Furthermore, we have shown that accurate left ventricular volumes can be obtained with a 2 ml blood sample irrespective of the distance at which blood sample counts are acquired from the camera, and the blood sample counts are highly reproducible.[11] Second, the distance d on the chest used to calculate d′ for attenuation correction was obtained from the average of three measurements. Interobserver variability for these measurements differed by only 4 mm or less in all instances; therefore, it accounted for very little variation in the radionuclide right ventricular volumes calculated by each observer. Finally, right ventricular counts are highly dependent on hand-drawn regions of interest at both end-diastole and end-systole. This can present a potential problem in the left anterior oblique projection for the right ventricle when one attempts to find the right atrial–right ventricular border and pulmonic valve plane. However, by phase analysis, the borders of the right ventricle in the area of the right atrium and pulmonic valve were clearly defined. This eliminated a great deal of ambiguity and subjectivity when attempting to draw right ventricular end-diastolic and end-systolic regions of interest. Thus the intraobserver and interobserver reproducibility was high for both the radionuclide right ventricular end-diastolic and end-systolic volumes.

Another potential problem was the selection of a left paraventricular region of interest for background. As Maddahi et al.[14] described, there are several possible sources of background activity that may contribute to right ventricular counts: overlying right atrium, scatter from the left ventricle, and the pulmonary vascular bed. A left paraventricular region of interest includes the latter two sources. The right atrial source may account for a high contribution to right ventricular counts, particularly at end-systole, when this structure increases in size. In this study, several patients had both right atrial and right ventricular enlargement. However, there was a tendency for underestimation of right ventricular volumes by radionuclide angiography. Seiderer et al.[21] have demonstrated that a parabolic background correction provided a better correlation between radionuclide left ventricular volumes and single-plane cineventriculographic volumes, while a uniform left paraventricular background correction consistently yielded an underestimate of the cineventriculographic volumes. Therefore, our choice of background correction may not have accounted for the effects of right ventricular blood self-absorption, which is taken into account by a parabolic background correction, and thus it might have resulted in lower total right ventricular counts and lower right ventricular volumes when compared with biplane cineventriculographic volumes. Because the majority of our patients had mild-to-markedly enlarged right ventricular volumes, this factor may have played a greater role in the underestimation of the larger right ventricular volumes.

Conclusions. These results demonstrate that radionuclide right ventricular volumes can be obtained by a method that incorporates attenuation correction with a distance measurement derived from a simple geometric method in each patient. In patients with a wide variety of cardiac problems and right ventricular volumes, attenuation-corrected radionuclide right ventricular volumes were more accurate than those obtained from uncorrected right ventricular volumes, which assume a constant attenuation. Thus this radionuclide count-based method of measuring right ventricular volumes may be useful in serial clinical studies to evaluate therapeutic interventions or to follow the progression of right ventricular disease processes.

Appendix

Briefly, the computer program provides x-y-z coordinate data for segmentation of each of the two orthogonal images into 100 elliptical segments. The diameters are calculated in each view as the vector distance between points on opposite sides of the endocardial outline that lie on a line perpendicular to the long axis. The true long axis L_T is derived mathematically in three-dimensional space using the measured long axis in each projection by triangulation: If ℓ_x and ℓ_y are the coordinate lengths of the measured long axis in the right anterior oblique view (L_{RAO}) and ℓ_z is the z coordinate length in the left anterior oblique view (L_{LAO}), then

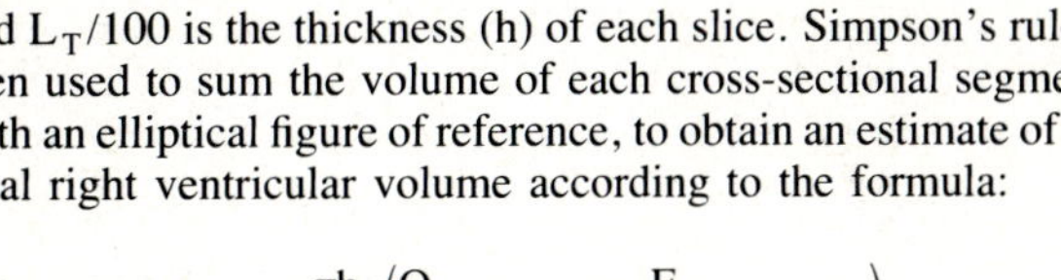

Since the y axis is common to both films, ℓ_y should be equal in the RAO and LAO projections. Then $\sqrt{(\ell_y)^2 + (\ell_x)^2} = L_{RAO}$ and $L_T = \sqrt{(L_{RAO})^2 + (\ell_z)^2}$, thus $L_T = \sqrt{(\ell_y)^2 + (\ell_x)^2 + (\ell_z)^2}$ and $L_T/100$ is the thickness (h) of each slice. Simpson's rule is then used to sum the volume of each cross-sectional segment, with an elliptical figure of reference, to obtain an estimate of the total right ventricular volume according to the formula:

$$V = \frac{\pi h}{3}\left(\sum^{O} D_R \cdot D_L + \sum^{E} \tfrac{1}{2} D_R \cdot D_L\right)$$

where D_R and D_L represent the right and cranially angulated left anterior oblique diameters, respectively. E are even and O odd numeral diameters.

References

1. Ferlinz J, Delvicario M, Gorlin R: Incidence of right ventricular asynergy in patients with coronary artery disease. Am J Cardiol **38:** 557, 1976
2. Ferlinz J, Gorlin R, Cohn PF, Herman MV: Right ventricular performance in patients with coronary artery disease. Circulation **52:** 608, 1975
3. Fisher EZ, DuBrow IW, Hastreiter AR: Right ventricular volume in congenital heart disease. Am J Cardiol **36:** 67, 1975
4. Arcilla RA, Tsai P, Thilenius O, Ranniger K: Angiographic method for volume estimation of right and left ventricles. Chest **60:** 446, 1971
5. Slutsky R, Bhargava V, Dittrich H, Costello D: Comparison of single-plane and biplane contrast analyses of right ventricular function and size. Am Heart J **104:** 100, 1982
6. Gentzler RD, Briselli MF, Gault JH: Angiographic estimation of right ventricular volume in man. Circulation **50:** 324, 1974
7. Bommer W, Weinert L, Neumann A, Neef J, Mason DT, DeMaria A: Determination of right atrial and right ventricular size by two-dimensional echocardiography. Circulation **60:** 91, 1979
8. Watanabe T, Katsume H, Matsukobo H, Furukawa K, Ijichi H: Estimation of right ventricular volume with two-dimensional echocardiography. Am J Cardiol **49:** 1946, 1982
9. Starling MR, Crawford MH, Sorenson SG, O'Rourke RA: A new two-dimensional echocardiographic technique for evaluating right ventricular size and performance in patients with obstructive lung disease. Circulation **66:** 612, 1982
10. Dehmer GJ, Firth BG, Hillis LD, Nicod P, Willerson JT, Lewis SE: Nongeometric determination of right ventricular volumes from equilibrium blood pool scans. Am J Cardiol **49:** 78, 1982
11. Starling MR, Dell'Italia LJ, Walsh RA, Little WC, Benedetto AR, Nusynowitz ML: Accurate estimates of absolute left ventricular volumes from equilibrium radionuclide angiographic count data using a simple geometric attenuation correction. J Am Coll Cardiol **3:** 789, 1984
12. Starling MR, Dell'Italia LJ, Nusynowitz ML, Walsh RA, Little WC, Benedetto AR: Estimates of left-ventricular volumes by equilibrium radionuclide angiography: importance of attenuation correction. J Nucl Med **25:** 14, 1984
13. Karliner JS, Bouchard RJ, Gault JH: Hemodynamic effects of angiographic contrast material in man. Br Heart J **34:** 347, 1972
14. Maddahi J, Berman DS, Matsuoka DT, Waxman AD, Stankus KE, Forrester JS, Swan HJC: A new technique for assessing right ventricular ejection fraction using rapid multiple-gated equilibrium cardiac blood pool scintigraphy. Circulation **60:** 581, 1979
15. Massie BM, Kramer BL, Gertz EW, Henderson SG: Radionuclide measurement of left ventricular volume: comparison of geometric and counts-based methods. Circulation **65:** 725, 1982
16. Dehmer GJ, Lewis SE, Hillis LD, Twieg D, Falkoff M, Parkey RW, Willerson JT: Nongeometric determination of left ventricular volumes from equilibrium blood pool scans. Am J Cardiol **45:** 293, 1980
17. Slutsky R, Karliner J, Ricci D, Kaiser R, Pfisterer M, Gordon D, Peterson K, Ashburn W: Left ventricular volumes by gated equilibrium radionuclide angiography: a new method. Circulation **60:** 556, 1979
18. Links JM, Becker LC, Shindledecker JG, Guzman P, Burow RD, Nickoloff EL, Alderson PO, Wagner HN: Measurement of absolute left ventricular volume from gated blood pool studies. Circulation **65:** 82, 1982
19. Maurer AH, Siegel JA, Denenberg BS, Carabello BA, Gash AK, Spann JF, Malmud LS: Absolute left ventricular volume from gated blood pool imaging with use of esophageal transmission measurement. Am J Cardiol **51:** 853, 1983
20. Sorenson JA, Phelps ME: Physics in nuclear medicine. New York, 1980, Grune & Stratton, Inc.
21. Seiderer M, Bohn I, Buell U, Kleinhans E, Strauer BE: Influence of background and absorption correction on nuclear quantification of left ventricular end-diastolic volume. Br J Radiol **56:** 183, 1983

Quantification of myocardial infarction: a comparison of single photon–emission computed tomography with pyrophosphate to serial plasma MB–creatine kinase measurements*

DONALD E. JANSEN, M.P.H., M.D., JAMES R. CORBETT, M.D., CHRISTOPHER L. WOLFE, M.D., SAMUEL E. LEWIS, M.D., GREGORY GABLIANI, M.D., NEIL FILIPCHUK, M.D., GREGORY REDISH, M.D., ROBERT W. PARKEY, M.D., L. MAXIMILIAN BUJA, M.D., ALLAN S. JAFFE, M.D., ROBERT RUDE, M.D., BURTON E. SOBEL, M.D., AND JAMES T. WILLERSON, M.D.

ABSTRACT Single photon–emission computed tomography (SPECT) with ^{99m}Tc-pyrophosphate (PPi) has been shown to estimate size of myocardial infarction accurately in animals. We tested the hypothesis that SPECT with ^{99m}Tc-PPi and blood pool subtraction can provide prompt and accurate estimates of size of myocardial infarction in patients. SPECT estimates are potentially available early after the onset of infarction and should correlate with estimates of infarct size calculated from serial measurements of plasma MB–creatine kinase (CK) activity. Thirty-three patients with acute myocardial infarction and 16 control patients without acute myocardial infarction were studied. Eleven of the patients had transmural anterior myocardial infarction, 16 had transmural inferior myocardial infarction, and six had nontransmural myocardial infarction. SPECT was performed with a commercially available rotating gamma camera. Identical projection images of the distribution of ^{99m}Tc-PPi and the ungated cardiac blood pool were acquired sequentially over 180 degrees. Reconstructed sections were color coded and superimposed for purposes of localization of infarct. Areas of increased PPi uptake within myocardial infarcts were thresholded at 65% of peak activity. The blood pool was thresholded at 50% and subtracted to determine the endocardial border for the left ventricle. Myocardial infarcts ranged in size from 1 to 126 gram equivalents (geq) MB-CK. The correlation of MB-CK estimates of size of infarct with size determined by SPECT (both in geq) was good (r = .89 with a regression line of y = 13.1 + 1.5x). Close correlations were found between values in patients with anterior transmural infarction (r = .93), those with inferior transmural infarction (r = .85), and those with nontransmural myocardial infarction (r = .91). We conclude that the estimation of size of infarction with SPECT and ^{99m}Tc-PPi in patients is accurate and that the results correlate well with MB-CK estimates of size of infarction.
Circulation **72, No. 2, 327–333, 1985.**

PROTECTION AND SALVAGE of ischemic myocardium in the early stages of acute myocardial infarction has been a goal of several recent studies.[1–3] The measurement of size of myocardial infarction is critical in the assessment of interventions to limit that size. Recent work has shown that ^{99m}Tc-pyrophosphate (PPi) with single photon–emission computed tomography (SPECT) can be used to measure size of infarction in animals, and SPECT with ^{99m}Tc-PPi has been used to size myocardial infarction in patients.[4–6] However, the measurement of myocardial infarction with SPECT using ^{99m}Tc-PPi has not previously been validated by comparison with currently accepted alternative methods. The level of creatine kinase isoenzyme (MB-CK) has been used extensively for detection and quantification of myocardial infarcts.[7–9] Therefore, the purpose of this study was to test the hypothesis that SPECT with ^{99m}Tc-PPi and blood pool subtraction can accurately measure size of infarction in patients with acute

From the University of Texas Health Science Center at Dallas and Parkland Memorial Hospital, Dallas, and Washington University School of Medicine, St. Louis.

This study is an ancillary study from the Multicenter Investigation of Limitation of Infarct Size "MILIS" (NHLBI NO1-HV72942) and was supported in part by NHLBI Ischemic SCOR grants HL17646 and HL17669, and the Moss Heart Fund, Dallas.

Address for correspondence: Donald E. Jansen, M.P.H., M.D., Division of Cardiology, Room L5.134, U. T. Health Science Center, 5323 Harry Hines Bvd., Dallas, TX 75235.

Received Oct. 13, 1984; revision accepted May 9, 1985.

*All editorial decisions for this article, including selection of reviewers and the final disposition, were made by a guest editor. This procedure applies to all manuscripts with authors from the Washington University School of Medicine.

myocardial infarcts by comparing results with this method with estimates made from serial plasma MB-CK measurements.

Methods

Study population. Thirty-three patients admitted to Parkland Memorial Hospital, Dallas, between April 1981 and June 1983 with acute myocardial infarction and enrolled in the Multicenter Investigation of Limitation of Infarct Size (MILIS) were studied. The diagnosis of acute myocardial infarction was confirmed by history, electrocardiographic data, and serial enzyme determinations. There were 11 patients with transmural anterior myocardial infarctions, 16 patients with transmural inferior myocardial infarctions, and six patients with nontransmural myocardial infarctions. The average age of the patients studied was 51.3 ± 10.4 (mean ± 1 SD) years. The group included 25 male and eight female subjects.

A control group of 16 patients underwent imaging. This group included patients with stable angina, unstable angina, and chest pain of uncertain cause. The control patients were studied between November 1981 and June 1983; several were described in a previous report from our institution.[5] No control patients had enzymatic or electrocardiographic evidence of acute myocardial infarction.

SPECT imaging. SPECT was performed 3.3 ± 1.8 days after admission. Imaging began 2 to 4 hr after the intravenous injection of 25 mCi of ^{99m}Tc-PPi. Patients underwent imaging while supine with the left arm positioned beside the head. Thirty-two projection images were acquired over 180 degrees from 60 degrees right anterior oblique to 30 degrees left posterior oblique at a zoom of 1.3 to 1 with a rotating wide-field-of-view gamma camera (GE 400T) equipped with a low-energy, general-purpose, parallel-hole collimator. Projection images were stored as 64 × 64 matrixes in the memory of a dedicated nuclear medicine computer system (MDS; Ann Arbor, MI). Projection images were acquired for a preset time of 15 to 20 sec each, and contained 100,000 to 200,000 counts per image (total activity approximately 4.8 × 10^6 counts). The radius of rotation ranged from 21 to 27 cm and was selected to minimize the distance from detector to the chest wall. Immediately after the acquisition of the last ^{99m}Tc-PPi projection image, 20 mCi of ^{99m}Tc-labeled autologous red blood cells labeled in vitro were injected. Five minutes later, 32 identical ungated cardiac blood pool projection images were acquired in the same manner. Projections were acquired for a preset time interval of 10 to 20 sec each and contained 300,000 to 600,000 counts per projection. Total

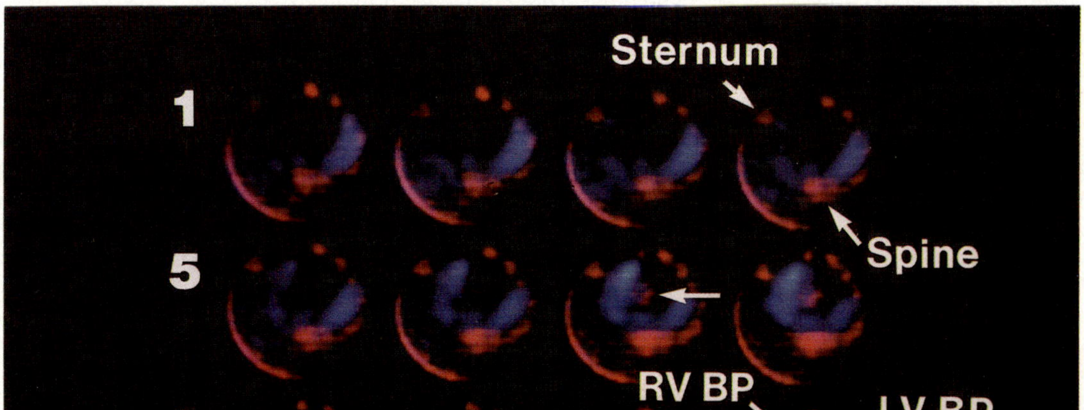

FIGURE 1A. Color-coded overlay of PPi (in orange) on the ungated blood pool (in blue). Images are of transaxial sections through the volume of the thorax including the heart. Sections 1 to 16 begin caudal to the heart and progress cephalad through the thorax. Sections are in standard computed tomographic format, i.e., head in face up, except that the sections have been rotated counterclockwise so that the ventricular apex is at 12 o'clock. Note the sternum at 10 o'clock and the spine at 4 o'clock. An intense area of ^{99m}Tc-PPi uptake (→) along the posterior segment of the left ventricle can be seen in images 7 to 12.

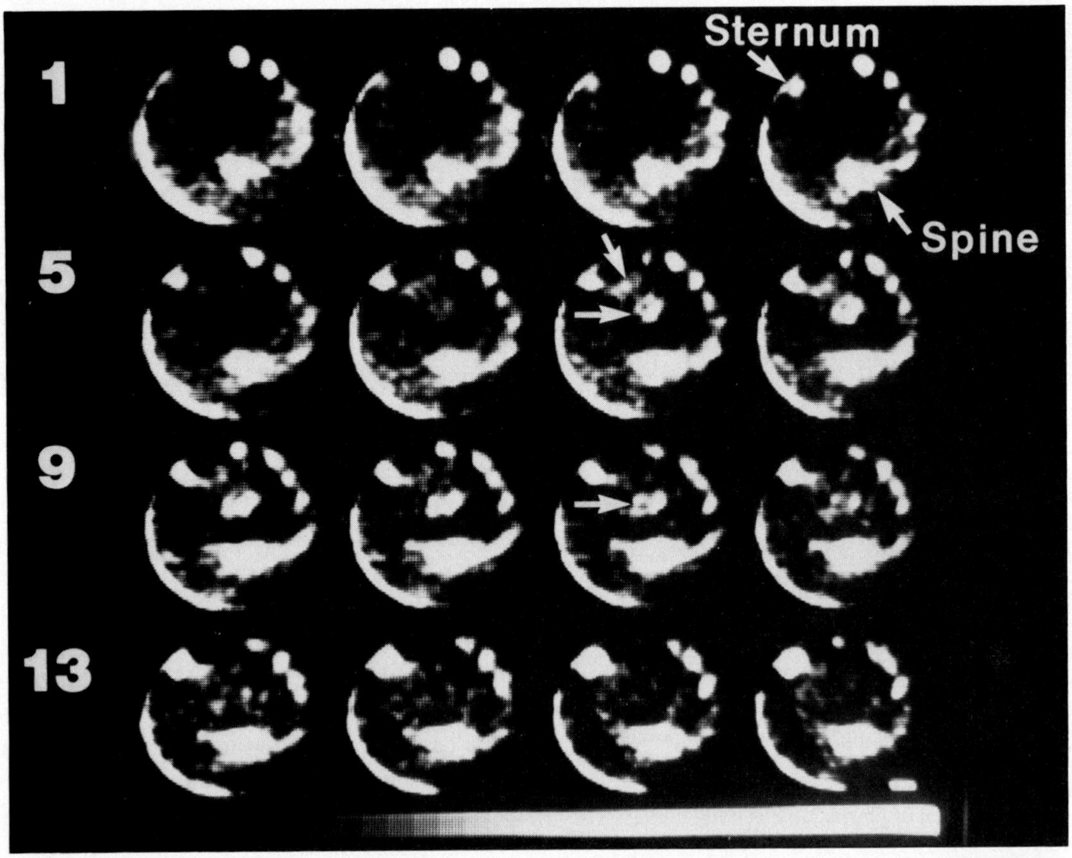

FIGURE 1B. PPi transaxial sections generated by filtered backprojection. Sections are in the same format as in figure 1A and are used for masking. Note sternum and spine. There is an intense area of ^{99m}Tc-PPi uptake (→) along the posterior segment of the left ventricle in images 7 to 12. Faint right ventricular uptake (→) can be seen just behind the sternum in sections 6 to 8.

imaging time for the two SPECT studies was 20 to 30 min. The resolution in the reconstructed volume of the imaging system at 140 keV was 15.7 mm full width half maximum measured in a water-filled cylinder of 10 cm radius positioned at the center of rotation with an orbit radius of 20 cm.

All projection images were corrected for field nonuniformity and for center of rotation. Transverse sections of one-pixel thickness were reconstructed by filtered backprojection. The filter used for reconstruction was the product of a Hanning low-pass filter with a frequency cutoff of 0.75 and a ramp filter. The digital resolution of reconstructed slices was 64 × 64. Attenuation correction was not attempted. Voxel dimensions were 0.476 cm × 0.476 cm × 0.476 cm.

Infarct localization: overlay technique. The distribution of myocardial uptake of ^{99m}Tc-PPi was determined on a slice-by-slice basis with a color-coded overlay of PPi on the ungated blood pool (figure 1A). With a dedicated nuclear medicine computer system equipped with an array processor (Technicare 560; Solon, OH), sectional images were count normalized and the pixel values were mapped into a range of 0 to 512. A bichromic color table was generated with blood pool images monochromatic in blue over the range 0 to 512 and PPi images monochromatic in orange over the range 513 to 1023. PPi images were placed in the orange range by adding 512 to each pixel. Each slice was viewed as a static slice-for-slice overlay.

Infarct sizing procedure: SPECT. All measurements were made prospectively by two independent observers who were blinded to the enzyme determinations and to each others results. The localization and distribution of myocardial infarction were determined subjectively by each observer from the acute PPi uptake identified from the overlaid blood pool and PPi tomograms (see above). Noncardiac activity was removed from the respective PPi tomographic and blood pool slices by widely masking around the areas of myocardial uptake (figure 1B) and areas of the cardiac blood pool on a slice-by-slice basis. Myocardial uptake was determined from the activity remaining in the ^{99m}Tc-PPi transaxial sections by a simple three-dimensional thresholding procedure at 65% of the peak voxel value within the infarct volume (figure 1C). Blood pool regions were determined with the use of a threshold of 50% of the peak voxel value within the blood pool volume. The blood pool regions were used to define the endocardial border within the PPi tomogram, which resulted in removal of any residual blood pool activity. Blood pool regions were subtracted slice for slice from the corresponding ^{99m}Tc-PPi regions of interest (figure 1D). The "infarct voxels" were then summed, and size of infarction was determined by multiplying the infarct voxels by 0.1078 cm^3/voxel and 1.05 g/cm^3 muscle. A previous investigation at our institution has shown that subtraction of blood pool activity provides a significantly better identification of myocardial infarcts and estimate of their relative size than does measurement without blood pool subtraction.[5]

Thresholds were determined from phantom studies in which a 25 g infarct and a 100 ml left ventricular blood pool were simulated. A 25 ml ^{99m}Tc-filled balloon was applied to the surface of a 100 ml cone-shaped vial. This was suspended eccentrically in a 20 cm diameter water-filled cylinder and imaged as previously described. Imaging was repeated with the balloon removed and the vial filled with ^{99m}Tc to simulate a labeled 100 ml left ventricular blood pool.

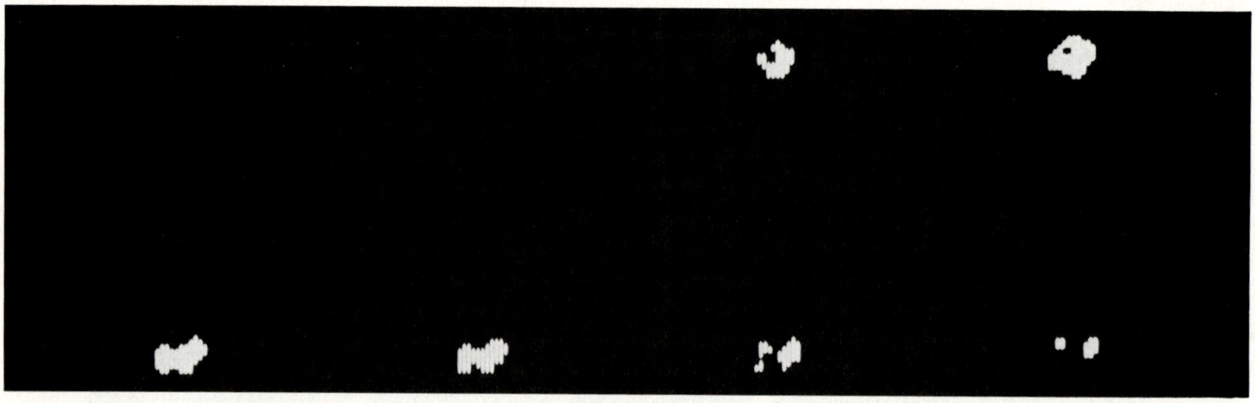

FIGURE 1C. PPi uptake after masking and thresholding. Format is as in figure 1B.

Infarct sizing procedure: MB-CK determinations. Plasma MB-CK determinations were made in samples drawn from each patient at the time of admission, hourly for 4 hr, every 2 hr for the next 4 hr, and every 4 hr until completion of a 72 hr interval from the time of the initial sample. Serial samples were then drawn every 8 hr for the next 48 hr, and every 12 hr for the next 9 days. MB-CK was measured by both radioimmunoassay and batch absorption on glass beads. The radioimmunoassay provided a quality control for the adequacy of sampling and protection of each sample during freezing, storage, and shipping to the CK laboratory at Washington University School of Medicine in St. Louis. MB-CK values determined by the glass-bead method were used for construction of plasma time-activity curves. Size of infarction was calculated based on measured MB-CK appearing in plasma, the distribution volume of MB-CK, and the amount of MB-CK activity contained in myocardium and lost in association with irreversible injury, as previously described.[9] Results were expressed in gram equivalents of MB-CK.

Statistical methods. Comparison of MB-CK–determined size of infarction with that determined by SPECT was by regression equations calculated by least squares methods. The correlation coefficients reported are Pearson r values calculated by regression analysis. All means are reported ±1 SD. Intraobserver and interobserver reproducibility are reported as percent variability or as the Pearson r value.

Results

In the control group, two of 16 patients had abnormal tomographic ^{99m}Tc-PPi uptake suggestive of myocardial infarction. One had unstable angina with a history of an extensive anterior myocardial infarction 3 months previously, and infarct size in this patient was 9 g. The second patient had chest pain, no previous history of cardiac disease, and an infarct size of 8 g.

Of the 33 patients with known acute myocardial infarction, analysis of electrocardiograms revealed that 11 patients had transmural anterior myocardial infarctions, 16 patients had transmural inferior myocardial infarctions, and six patients had nontransmural myocardial infarction. The PPi estimate of size of infarction ranged from 6 to 81 geq, with a mean of 33.7 ± 18.5 geq. The mean size of anterior transmural infarcts was 41.4 ± 20.6 geq; that of inferior transmural infarcts, 34 ± 15.9 geq; and that of nontransmural infarcts, 18.7 ± 13.1 geq. The MB-CK estimates of infarct size ranged from 1 to 126 geq, with a mean of 37.9 ± 31.4 geq. The mean size of anterior transmural infarcts was 51.8 ± 32.1 geq; that of inferior transmural infarcts, 36.2 ± 32.2 geq; and that of nontransmural infarcts, 16.8 ± 13.7 geq. The correlation between MB-CK– and SPECT-determined infarct size was good, with a correlation coefficient of .89 ($p < .001$) and an SEE of 14.5 geq (regression line by least squares method $y = -13.13 + 1.52x$; figure 2). Values for patients with transmural anterior myocardial infarctions were $r = .93$ ($p < .001$) and SEE = 12.8 geq (figure 3); those for patients with transmural inferior myocardial infarctions, $r = .85$ ($p < .001$) and SEE = 17.6 geq (figure 4); and those for patients with nontransmural myocardial infarctions, $r = .91$ ($p = .01$) and SEE = 6.3 geq (figure 5).

Interobserver and intraobserver determinations were made in a blinded manner and 6 months was allowed to elapse between determinations by the same observer. The intraobserver variability by mean percent difference was 10.7 ± 9.6% and the interobserver variability was 15.8 ± 15.2%. The intraobserver correlation was represented by $r = .97$ ($p < .001$) and SEE = 4.7 geq, with a regression line of $y = 1.67 + 0.95x$. The interobserver correlation was represented by $r = .96$ ($p < .001$) and SEE = 5.4 geq, with a regression line of $y = 3.38 + 0.94x$.

Discussion

These data demonstrate a close correlation between size of myocardial infarction calculated from serial plasma MB-CK measurements and values calculated with SPECT with ^{99m}Tc-PPi. Previous studies have shown that size of infarct determined with the latter method correlates well with prognosis.[5,6] Our data suggest that SPECT with PPi imaging permits accurate

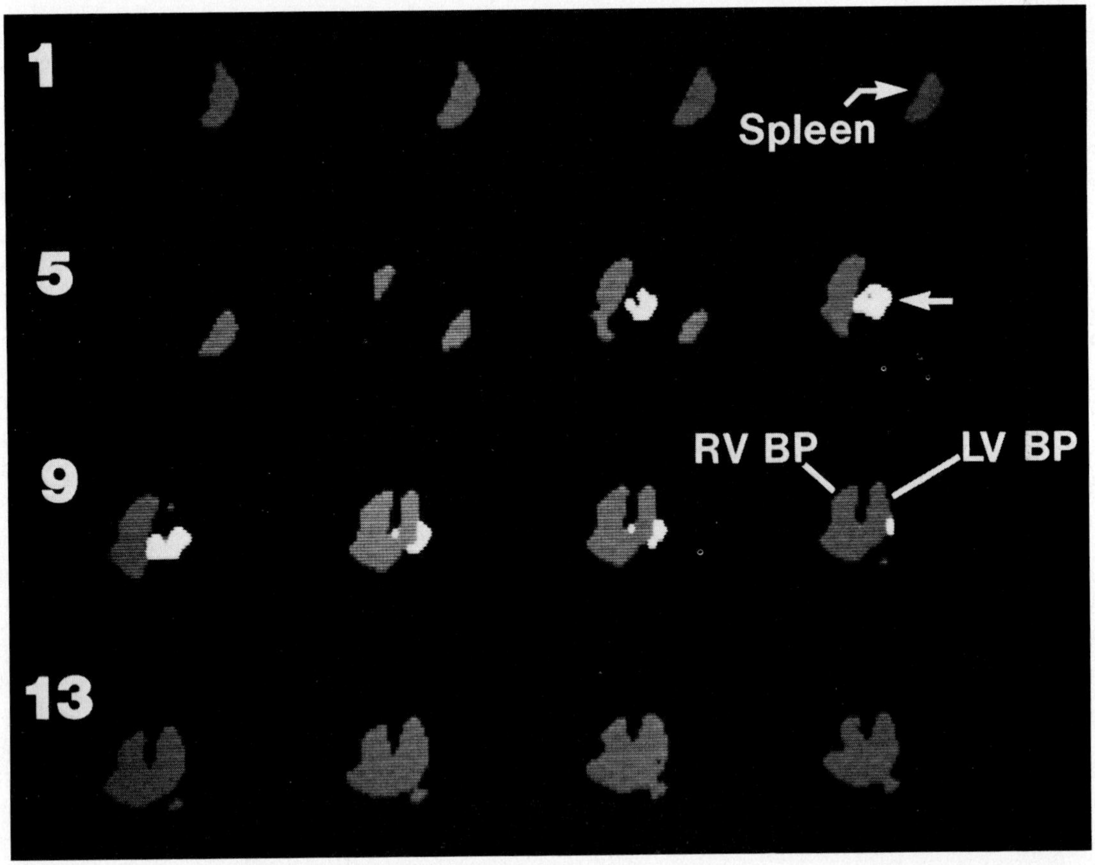

FIGURE 1D. PPi uptake (in white) after masking and thresholding. Subtraction of blood pool (in grey) results in determination of final infarct areas of interest. The format is as in figures 1B and 1C.

estimation of size of infarct in patients with transmural (Q wave) and nontransmural (non-Q wave) myocardial infarctions.

SPECT is superior to planar imaging because of the three-dimensional nature of tomographic reconstructed images.[5, 6] Previously, poor correlations have been found between size of infarct on planar PPi images and postmortem size in dogs with nontransmural and inferior/posterior infarcts.[4, 10, 11] Thus, the present study confirms our previous work and that of others in dogs that SPECT with ^{99m}Tc-PPi provides an excellent means of sizing myocardial infarcts irrespective of infarct location[4, 12] and extends these observations to patients.

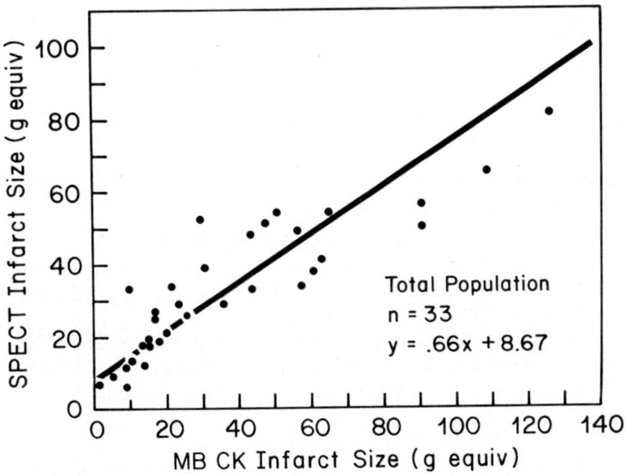

FIGURE 2. Comparison of size of infarction by SPECT and that by MB-CK analysis in all patients with myocardial infarctions.

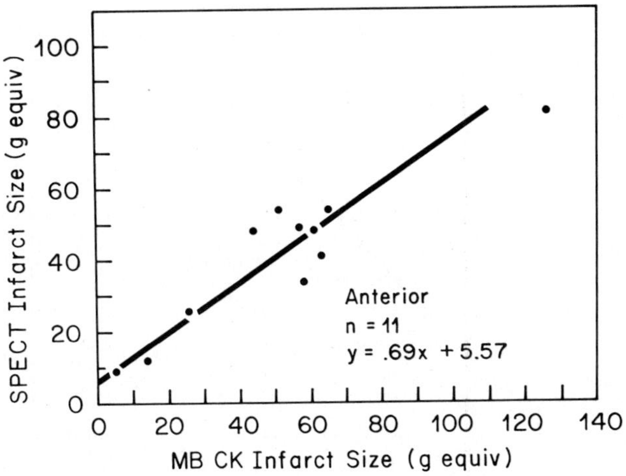

FIGURE 3. Comparison of size of infarction by SPECT and that by MB-CK analysis in patients with transmural anterior myocardial infarctions.

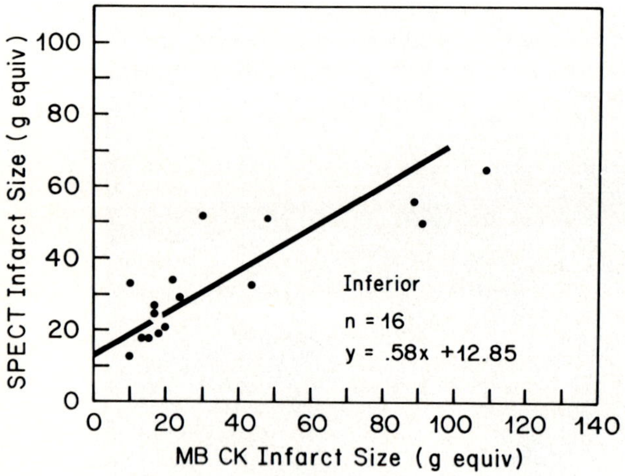

FIGURE 4. Comparison of size of infarction by SPECT and that by MB-CK analysis in patents with transmural inferior myocardial infarctions.

The correlation between size of myocardial infarction determined by SPECT and that by MB-CK analyis was close despite the presence of several potential sources of error associated with SPECT measurements.[13] First, some patients underwent imaging at less than ideal times after myocardial infarction: in the present study, seven patients underwent imaging 5 to 10 days after the onset of chest pain. Second, attenuation correction was not attempted in the present study and projections were acquired over 180 degrees. We suspect that attenuation correction, which requires 360 degree projection image sets, might be a useful addition to our methods. Large myocardial infarcts may have been underestimated because no correction for attenuation was made. Third, the simple edge detector used in this study might include high-intensity apical uptake at the expense of lower intensity basal activity. Furthermore, the limited resolution of our system may result in overestimation of small infarcts. Improved tomographic imaging systems and more accurate edge detection programs should help eliminate some of these potential problems.

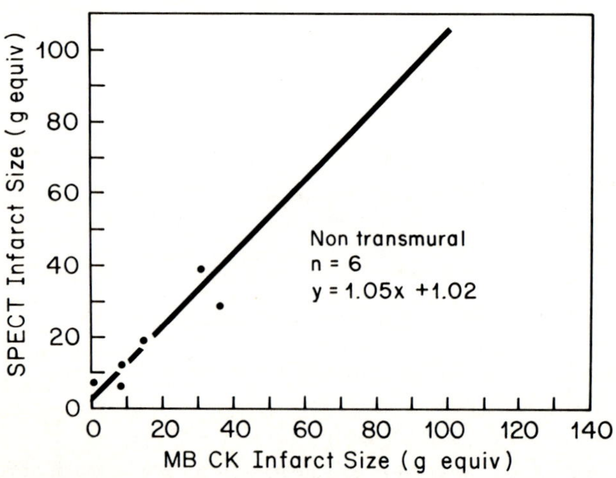

FIGURE 5. Comparison of size of infarction by SPECT and that by MB-CK analysis in patients with nontransmural myocardial infarctions.

SPECT with PPi imaging allows accurate localization and determination of size of acute infarction in patients. The method can be useful in patients when repetitive blood sampling is not possible or if timing of the patient's myocardial infarction prohibits proper serial MB-CK sampling for purposes of estimating infarct size. Furthermore, some institutions do not have the necessary equipment for MB-CK curve analysis and SPECT provides an alternative method for infarct sizing. Patients in our study did not undergo thrombolytic therapy or other early reperfusion therapies. Rapid reperfusion with thrombolytic therapy or angioplasty affects MB-CK release and may limit the usefulness of MB-CK curve analysis for determination of size of infarction after early reperfusion. Early reperfusion has been shown to allow earlier detection of myocardial infarcts by PPi imaging,[14, 15] although the ability to size infarcts after early reperfusion with SPECT and PPi imaging is an area of ongoing research.

In summary, our data suggest that SPECT with ^{99m}Tc-PPi can accurately size myocardial infarcts in patients. Previous studies have shown that infarct sizes determined by ^{99m}Tc-PPi tomography correlate with patient prognosis.[5, 6] The present study demonstrates that the SPECT measurements correlate closely with those by an established clinically useful method, i.e., measurement of serial plasma MB-CK levels. Although further correlations with other measurements of size of infarction in patients may be necessary, our data suggest that SPECT imaging with PPi is useful in estimating size of acute myocardial infarction in patients.

We appreciate the skilled technical assistance of Mr. Marvin Akers and Miss Loretta Ressler; the cooperation and help of the nurses, medical house officers, and Cardiology fellows in the medical intensive care unit at Parkland Memorial Hospital in Dallas, and the secretarial assistance of Nancy Dickey.

References

1. Rude RE, Muller JE, Braunwald E: Efforts to limit the size of myocardial infarcts. Ann Intern Med **95:** 736, 1981
2. Norwegian Multicenter Study Group: Timolol-induced reduction in mortality and reinfarction in patients surviving acute myocardial infarction. N Engl J Med **304:** 801, 1981
3. Stampfer MJ, Goldhaber SZ, Yusuf S, Peto R, Hennekens CH: Effect of intravenous streptokinase on acute myocardial infarction: pooled results from randomized trials. N Engl J Med **307:** 1180, 1982
4. Lewis SE, Devous MD, Corbett JR, Izquierdo C, Nicod P, Wolfe CL, Parkey RW, Buja LM, Willerson JT: Measurement of infarct size in acute canine myocardial infarction by single photon emission tomography with technetium-99m pyrophosphate. Am J Cardiol **54:** 193, 1984

5. Corbett JR, Lewis SE, Wolfe CL, Jansen DE, Lewis M, Rellas JS, Parkey RW, Rude RE, Buja LM, Willerson JT: Measurement of myocardial infarct size by technetium pyrophosphate single photon tomography. Am J Cardiol **54:** 1231, 1984
6. Holman BL, Goldhaber SZ, Kirsch CM, Polak JF, Friedman BJ, English RJ, Wynne J: Measurement of infarct size using single photon emission computed tomography and technetium-99m pyrophosphate: a description of the method and comparison with patient prognosis. Am J Cardiol **50:** 503, 1982
7. Sobel BE, Bresnahan GF, Shell WE, Yoder RD: Estimation of infarct size in man and its relationship to prognosis. Circulation **46:** 640, 1972
8. Shell WE, Kjeksus JK, Sobel BE: Quantitative assessment of the extent of myocardial infarction in the conscious dog by means of analysis of serial changes in creatinine phosphokinase activity. J Clin Invest **50:** 2614, 1971
9. Roberts R, Henry PD, Sobel BE: An improved basis for enzymatic estimates of infarct size. Circulation **52:** 743, 1975
10. Poliner LR, Buja LM, Parkey RW, Stokely EM, Stone MJ, Harris R, Saffer SW, Templeton GH, Bonte FJ, Willerson JT: Comparison of different noninvasive methods of infarct sizing during experimental myocardial infarction. J Nucl Med **18:** 517, 1977
11. Willerson JT, Parkey RW, Stokely EM, Bonte FJ, Lewis SE, Harris RA, Blomqvist CG, Poliner L, Buja LM: Infarct sizing with technetium-99m stannous pyrophosphate scintigraphy in dogs and man: the relationship between scintigraphic and precordial mapping estimates of infarct size in patients. Cardiovasc Res **11:** 291, 1977
12. Keyes JW Jr., Leonard PF, Brody SL, Svetkoff DJ, Rogers WL, Lucchesi BR: Myocardial infarct quantification in the dog by single photon emission computed tomography. Circulation **58:** 227, 1978
13. Budinger TF, Gulberg GT, Huesman RH: Emission computed tomography. *In* Herman GT, editor: Topics in applied physics. Image reconstruction from projections, implementation, and applications. Berlin, 1979, Springer-Verlag
14. Parkey RW, Kulkarni P, Lewis S, Datz F, Gutekunst D, Dehmer G, Buja L, Bonte F, Willerson JT: Effect of coronary blood flow and site of injection on Tc-99m-PPi detection of early canine myocardial infarcts. J Nucl Med **22:** 133, 1981
15. Wheelan K, Wolfe C, Corbett J, Rude RE, Winniford M, Parkey RW, Buja LM, Willerson JT: Early positive technetium-99m stannous pyrophosphate images as a marker of reperfusion after thrombolytic therapy for acute myocardial infarction. Am J Cardiol (in press)

The effects of coronary angioplasty and reperfusion on distribution of myocardial flow

D. W. Wahr, M.D., T. A. Ports, M.D., E. H. Botvinick, M.D., M. Dae, M.D., N. Schechtmann, M.D., J. Huberty, M.D., R. S. Hattner, M.D., J. W. O'Connell, M.D., and K. Turley, M.D.

ABSTRACT To assess the effects of angioplasty (PTCA) and intracoronary streptokinase (ICSK) on relative myocardial perfusion, we administered ^{99m}Tc-macroaggregated albumin (MAA) to the uninvolved coronary artery before successful PTCA in 33 patients and before successful infusion of ICSK in eight patients and of ^{111}In-MAA into the same vessel after the intervention. In 10 patients who underwent PTCA, MAA was injected into the involved, instrumented coronary artery. Computer-processed images were acquired in registry and compared. Similar scintigraphic studies were performed in six control patients and in 11 in whom planned interventions were not performed or were unsuccessful. Distribution of MAA was also compared with angiographic results and with the distribution of ^{201}Tl on images obtained in patients at rest or on redistribution images obtained before and soon after intervention in 22 patients. In control patients and those studied after aborted or unsuccessful intervention, scintigraphic results showed excellent correlation with the angiographic anatomy and were without serial change. When MAA was injected into the uninvolved vessel, the scintigram revealed evidence of collateral perfusion with retraction of the perfusion zone from that of the involved coronary in 19 of 33 patients undergoing PTCA and in three of eight of those receiving ICSK. When MAA was injected into the involved artery, a relative increase in perfusion was seen in eight of 10 patients after PTCA. Although 30 patients demonstrated scintigraphic evidence of collateral vessels, only 10 patients had angiographic evidence of collateral circulation before intervention. The distribution of ^{201}Tl demonstrated little change in its global pattern and regions previously supplied by collaterals were generally well perfused after intervention. Coronary collateral perfusion may be inapparent angiographically and regress rapidly after angioplasty or reperfusion. Native perfusion is generally and quickly restored after successful PTCA or ICSK infusion, which obviates the need for collaterals. After intervention, the distribution of total perfusion may not change, but its regional source may demonstrate beneficial alterations, shifting from collateral to native circulation.
Circulation 72, No. 2, 334–343, 1985.

THE IMPORTANCE of the coronary collateral circulation in patients with ischemic heart disease is controversial.[1] Some studies have demonstrated that it is important,[2–7] while others have suggested that it is not.[8–10] The specific stimuli to collateral formation and their exact role in the preservation of myocardial viability and function in patients with severe coronary artery disease are only suspected. Two important factors contributing to our incomplete understanding of coronary collaterals relate to the relative insensitivity of coronary angiography for visualization of collaterals and our prior inability to make instantaneous alterations in the pattern of coronary blood flow. To increase the sensitivity of detection of collateral flow, intracoronary injections of radiolabeled microspheres or macroaggregated albumin particles (MAA) can be used.[11–20] Recent developments in interventional cardiology, including percutaneous transluminal coronary angioplasty (PTCA)[21–23] and the intracoronary infusion of streptokinase (ICSK)[24–28] in the setting of acute myo-

From the Departments of Medicine, Cardiovascular Division, and Radiology, Section of Nuclear Medicine, and the Cardiovascular Research Institute of the University of California, San Francisco.

Supported in part by a grant-in-Aid from the California Heart Association, with funds contributed by local heart associations, and by a grant from the Fannie Ripple Foundation, Madison, NJ.

Address for correspondence: Elias Botvinick, M.D., Associate Professor of Medicine and Radiology, 1186 Moffitt Hospital, University of California, San Francisco, CA 94143.

Received Dec. 11, 1984; revision accepted May 16, 1985.

Dr. Botvinick is an Established Investigator of the American Heart Association, with funds contributed by local heart associations, and is supported in part by a grant from the George D. Smith Fund, San Francisco.

This work was performed while Dr. Schechtman worked as a Research Associate at the University of California, San Francisco.

cardial infarction, now provide a cohort of patients who undergo controlled and immediate dynamic changes in their coronary circulation and a new opportunity to study coronary collateral blood flow. The purpose of this study was to assess the effects of PTCA and ICSK on relative myocardial perfusion and the coronary collateral circulation with the use of sequential MAA injections.

Methods

Patient population. All stable patients selected for elective single-vessel PTCA to reduce a significant obstruction, or selected for emergency thrombolytic therapy with ICSK to restore patency to a totally and acutely occluded coronary artery were considered candidates for the protocol. All patients gave informed consent. The protocol could be technically implemented in 70 patients, representing a nearly complete and random sampling of patients presenting for these procedures over a 6 month period. Image data was complete and technically adequate in 62 patients, 52 of those undergoing PTCA and 10 of those receiving ICSK. There were 45 men and 17 women, with a mean age of 54 years. To document the reliability of the imaging method, its validity as a reflection of the distribution of coronary perfusion, and its safety as performed in our laboratory, MAA particles were administered sequentially into the right and left coronary arteries of four patients with normal coronary anatomy. MAA was also administered sequentially into the uninstrumented stenotic coronary arteries of six "control" patients not undergoing intervention. Cardiac catheterization and coronary angiography were performed in all cases.

Procedures. Coronary anatomy was defined by selective coronary angiography performed in multiple projections by the Judkins technique. A significant coronary lesion was considered one creating greater than 50% diameter stenosis in orthogonal projections, or greater than 75% diameter stenosis in any single projection, equivalent to greater than 75% area stenosis of a major coronary artery or primary branch vessel. Two experienced readers graded the severity of stenosis in 5% increments up to total occlusion. The presence and distribution of collateral vasculature was noted. Biplane left ventriculography was also performed.

According to the established method,[14, 17, 18] 50,000 MAA particles of 10 to 40 μm diameter each, with a mean diameter of 25 μm, were labeled with 1.0 mCi of ^{99m}Tc or 0.3 mCi of ^{111}In and used for study in each patient. In patient subsets 1, 2, and 3 below, in which the vascular bed under study was expected to demonstrate some retraction of the perfusion zone after intervention, the lower energy ^{99m}Tc-MAA was first injected into the coronary artery under study. An intervention was performed and ^{111}In-MAA particles were injected into the same artery. In cases in which the vascular bed under scrutiny was expected to expand after intervention, as in subset 4 below, radionuclide administration was performed in the opposite order. Care was taken to ensure that both the ^{99m}Tc and ^{111}In particles were injected with exactly the same technique and with similar catheter placement. A minimum of 3 min was allowed to elapse between any injection of contrast and subsequent particle injection to avoid any potential changes in coronary blood flow induced by the contrast agent. Injections of particles were given according to the following patient subsets: (1) into the left coronary artery (LCA) before and after PTCA of a right coronary artery (RCA) stenosis (n = 18), (2) into the RCA before and after PTCA of a left anterior descending coronary artery (LAD) (n = 19) or circumflex (LCX) stenosis (n = 3), (3) into the uninvolved uninstrumented RCA or LCA before and after administration of ICSK (n = 10), and (4) into the LCA before and after PTCA of the LAD (n = 10) or LCX (n = 2).

^{111}In-MAA was also administered into the RCA and ^{99m}Tc-MAA was injected sequentially into the LCA in four patients with normal vessels. Six control patients, three with RCA and three with LAD stenoses, were studied serially according to sequence 1 and 2, respectively, in the absence of intervention.

Images of the distribution of both radionuclides in each projection were obtained in registry by maintaining camera position and varying the energy window. Thus, the different MAA species injected into the same coronary artery sequentially were imaged "simultaneously" after the procedure. In addition to visual assessment of relative radionuclide distribution, a color composite image was constructed in each projection to delineate zones of distribution of each radionuclide. Owing to the variable territorial dominance and regional overlap in perfusion zones expected, angiographic results and MAA distribution were first evaluated separately and blindly by different observers. The final relationship between particle distribution and coronary anatomy was then assessed by comparison of angiographic and scintigraphic findings.

MAA particle imaging was performed within 2 hr of completion of the catheterization procedure with an Ohio Nuclear Series 120 or Siemens LEM portable scintillation camera equipped with a high-resolution medium-energy collimator. Acquisitions were conducted for 5 min in anterior, left anterior oblique 30 or 40 degree, and left anterior oblique 70 degree projections. The specific projection of the image obtained with the mild left obliquity was taken as that which appeared to best separate and display the ventricular distribution of particles. ^{99m}Tc images were obtained with a 20% energy window focused on the 140 keV photopeak, while for ^{111}In images a 20% window was used for the middle 273 keV energy peak and a 15% window was used for the lower 173 keV energy peak. Phantom studies showed no visually appreciable evidence of down scatter from the 273 and 173 keV energy peaks into the 140 keV photo peak when the distribution of the higher energy peaks were imaged in the lower energy window. When this method was applied to imaging-superimposed offset linear grids filled with ^{99m}Tc- and ^{111}In-MAA, respectively, in amounts proportional to that administered in patients, complete resolution of the distribution of each radionuclide could be demonstrated in the presence of the other.

Native coronary distribution was defined as that expected based on the distribution of angiographic territories in each case. The safety and reliability of the method performed in our laboratory and the relationship between coronary distribution and the scintigraphic pattern was documented in the four patients without coronary disease studied, as shown in figure 1, and in six coronary patients not undergoing intervention. After independent and blinded analysis of scintigraphic and angiographic studies, the two were correlated to definitively assess the presence of scintigraphically detectable collaterals. Collateral blood flow was defined as the presence of radioactivity in territory other than that of the vessel receiving the injection, as judged by the angiographic distribution. Any sequential change in the pattern and area of distribution of labeled MAA particles was also taken to represent an alteration in collateral blood flow.

Stress perfusion scintigraphy with ^{201}Tl was performed in 12 patients before and after PTCA, as clinically indicated. Rest perfusion scintigraphy and blood pool studies were also performed in all patients 48 hr to 1 week after they received ICSK to assess global myocardial viability. Here, normal relative perfusion on images obtained in patients at rest or on redistribution images and persistent contraction of the affected region indicated myocardial preservation. Particulate scintigrams were

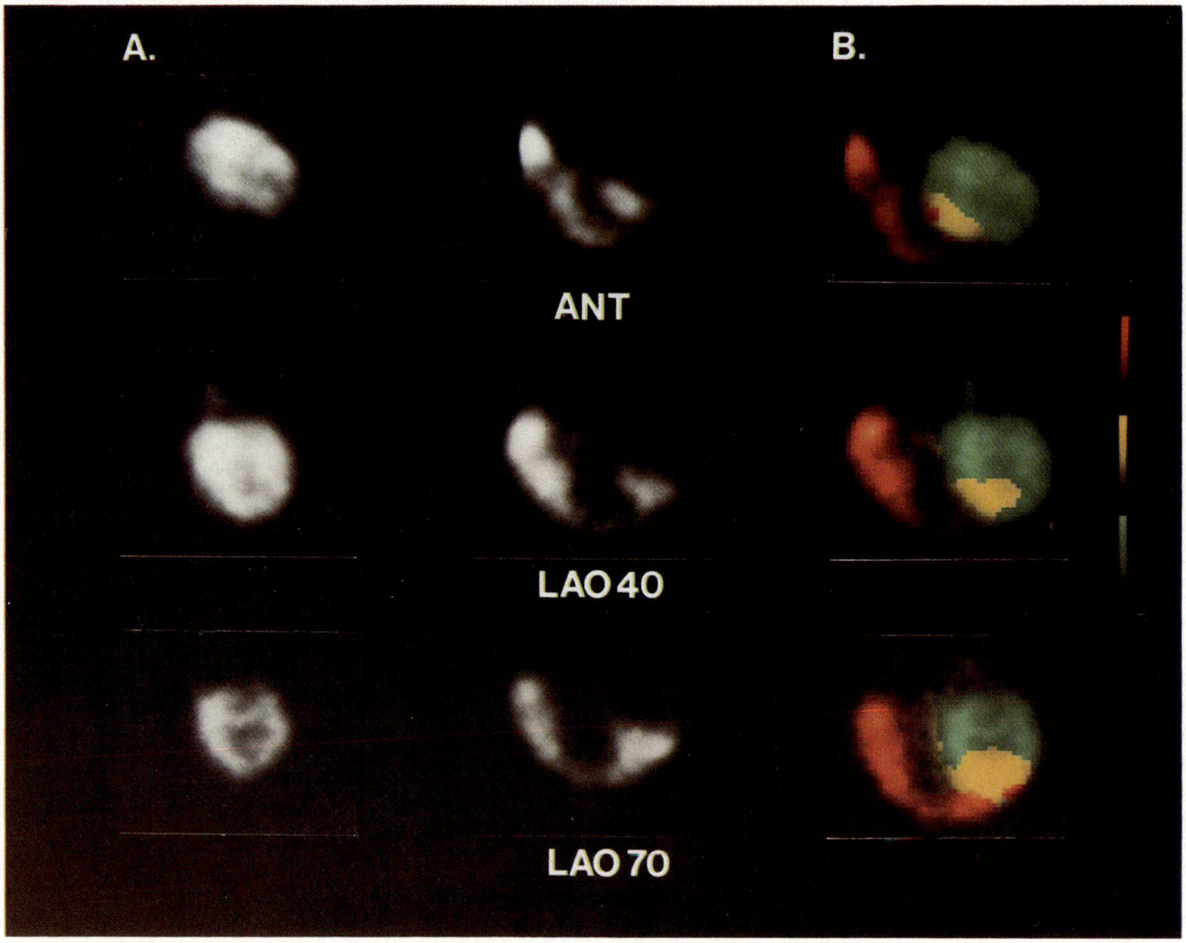

FIGURE 1. Normal distribution of MAA. Black and white (*A*, left and center columns) and color composite (*B*) images of MAA distribution obtained in registry after injection of ^{99m}Tc into the LCA (*A*, left column and *B*, green area) and ^{111}In into the RCA (*A*, right column and *B*, red area) in the anterior (ANT) and 40 and 70 degree left anterior oblique (LAO) projections. Note the region of overlap (*B*, yellow area) in septal and inferoapical segments in all projections, indicating dual perfusion of this region. Alternatively, the regional overlap, especially when seen in a single projection, could simply relate to a spatial superimposition of different vascular areas. These alternatives can be differentiated by use of multiple projections and the color display applied to our imaging protocol. The differentiation between dual blood supply and coronary collateralization can also be made by the observation of change in the perfusion pattern after intervention. Normal patients were studied only to demonstrate the relationships between angiographic and scintigraphic perfusion patterns and to demonstrate the reliability and safety of the method in our laboratory.

interpreted blindly by three observers who agreed on image findings in all but seven cases in which interpretation was made by consensus. Perfusion scintigrams and results of blood pool studies were also interpreted blindly without knowledge of other study results.

Successful PTCA was defined that resulting in a reduction of coronary stenosis to less than 20% or total abolition of the "crossing" gradient measured at the time of catheterization. Successful infusion of ICSK was defined as the restoration of coronary patency documented angiographically. PTCA and ICSK were successful in 43 and eight patients, respectively.

Results

In 33 patients who underwent successful PTCA, MAA was administered serially to the uninstrumented vessel. Nineteen of these patients with scintigraphic evidence of collaterals showed immediate postintervention regression. Figure 2 illustrates these serial scintigraphic changes. Among these 19 patients only six had angiographic evidence of collaterals (table 1). Of the 10 patients undergoing successful PTCA who received serial injections into the instrumented vessel, eight showed evidence of collaterals with immediate scintigraphic evidence of extension of the perfusion zone after the intervention (table 2). Angiographic collaterals were present in only three of these patients. Figure 3 illustrates related serial scintigraphic changes. Among those patients undergoing PTCA who underwent serial perfusion imaging, the relative pattern of resting global perfusion seen on ^{201}Tl images was not significantly altered regardless of the demon-

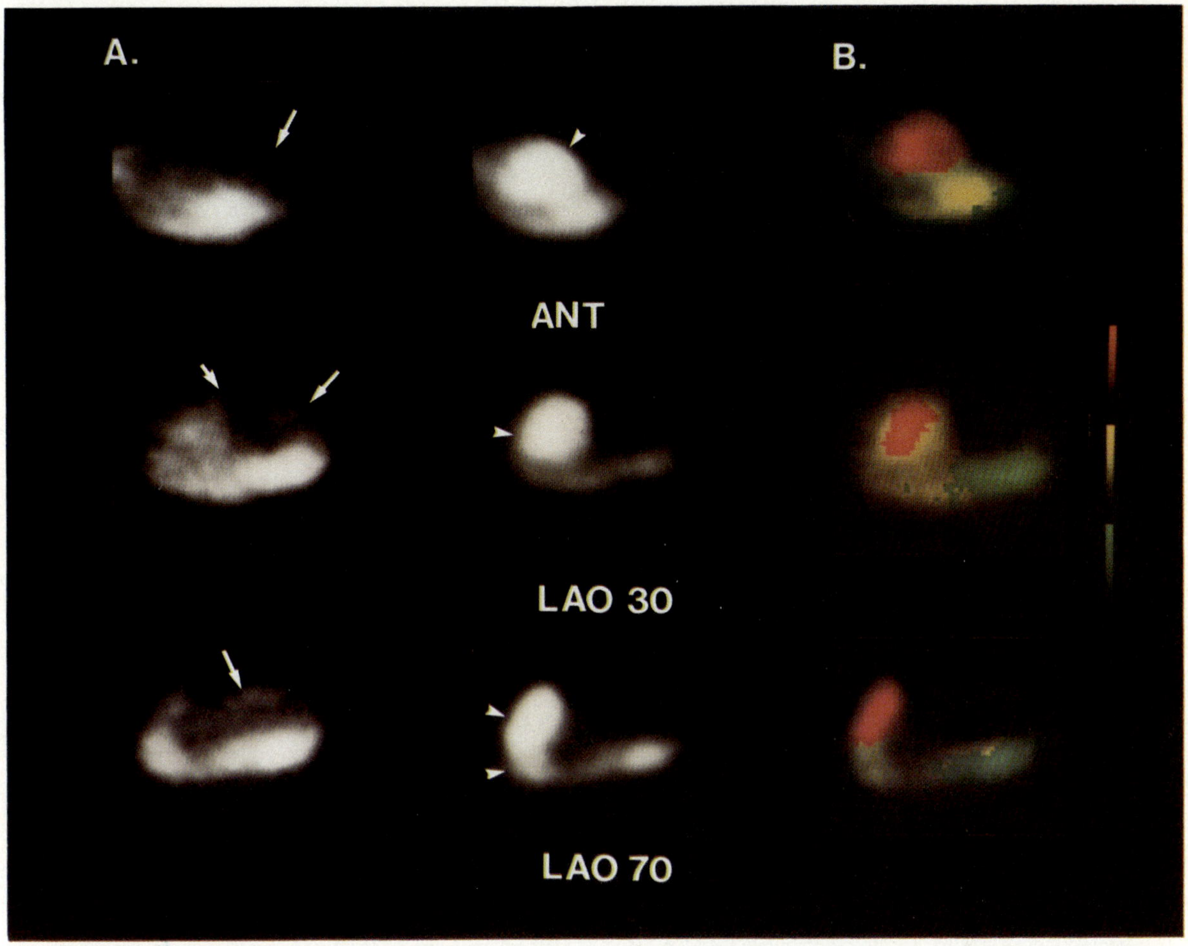

FIGURE 2. LAD PTCA. Black and white (*A*, left and center columns) and color composite (*B*) images of MAA distribution obtained in registry after injection of ^{99m}Tc into the RCA before (*A*, left column) and ^{111}In into the same vessel after (*A*, center column) successful PTCA of the LAD. In the color composite image, the distribution of perfusion primarily determined by the initial administered radionuclide is shown in green, while that primarily determined by the radionuclide administered last is shown in red. Areas in common are shown in yellow. Evidence of initial anterior and lateral left ventricular radioactivity (*A*, left, arrows and *B*, faint green areas) indicate right-to-left collaterals. These are no longer evident after PTCA since elements of the injected RCA perfusion territory are enhanced (*A*, center column arrow points and *B*, red area).

stration of collateral blood flow on the sequential MAA image. Serial stress scintigrams demonstrated resolution or improvement in the defect noted before intervention when the patient was reevaluated after successful PTCA at the same or increased double product. Although a trend was noted between severity of stenosis and the presence of collaterals, there was no definite relationship between these factors in the vessels assessed here.

TABLE 1
Evaluation of angiographic and scintigraphic findings in patients undergoing successful PTCA

Instrumented vessel	n	Injected vessel	Angiographic collaterals[A]	Scintigraphic collaterals[A]
RCA	14	LCA	3	7
LAD	16	RCA	3	9
LCX	3	RCA	0	3
LAD	8	LCA	2	7
LCX	2	LCA	1	1

[A]The presence of angiographic or scintigraphic evidence of coronary collaterals could not be directly related to the severity of stenosis beyond 75% narrowing.

Of the eight patients studied after successful infusion of ICSK, three had scintigraphic evidence of collateral blood flow, although only one of these had angiographic evidence of collateral flow (table 2). All had remnant significant stenosis. Particulate imaging studies revealed a retraction of the perfusion zone of the injected uninstrumented vessel in each of these three patients. Evidence of myocardial preservation was suggested by preserved regional wall motion in the affected area and the improved relative perfusion seen on serial ^{201}Tl images in two of the patients. In the remaining patient, ^{201}Tl perfusion was maintained

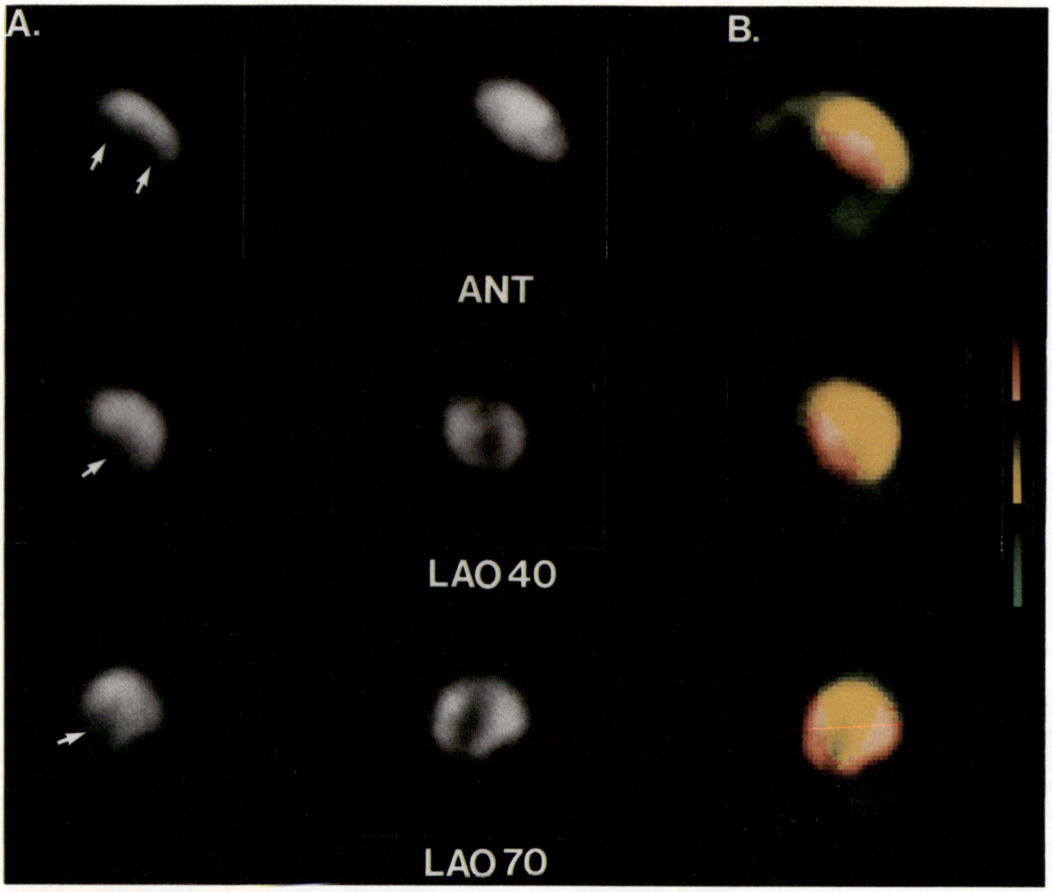

FIGURE 3. Improved perfusion after PTCA. Black and white (*A*, left and center columns) and color composite (*B*) MAA images obtained in registry after injection of ^{111}In into the LCA before (*A*, left column) and ^{99m}Tc after (*A*, center column) successful PTCA of the LAD. The apical and septal regions were defective initially (*A*, left column arrows) but normalized after PTCA (*B*, red area).

without change, suggesting a restoration of native coronary supply to a region previously supported, possibly adequately, by collateral flow. Images from this patient are illustrated in figure 4.

Serial scintigraphic studies were performed in 11 patients in whom PTCA was unsuccessful (two patients) or was not performed owing to clinical factors or the anatomic unsuitability of the lesion (seven patients), or in whom ICSK therapy was unsuccessful (two patients). Serial scintigraphic changes were not evident in these 11 patients, six of whom had scintigraphic evidence of collaterals, nor were they evident in the six "control" patients. There were also no serial scintigraphic changes in those 21 patients studied in whom PTCA or ICSK was successful but in whom there was no evidence of collaterals. Figure 5 illustrates such an example.

There was no patient with angiographic evidence of collaterals who did not also have supporting scintigraphic evidence. Each of 10 patients with angiographic evidence of collaterals before a successful intervention demonstrated a retracted distribution or absence of collaterals on the angiogram obtained after the intervention.

TABLE 2
Evaluation of angiographic and scintigraphic findings in patients receiving successful treatment with ICSK

Occluded vessel	Angiographic collaterals	Scintigraphic collaterals	Restoration of patency	Scintigraphic evidence of myocardial preservation
RCA	+	+	+	+
LAD	−	+	+	+
LAD	−	+	+	+
RCA	−	−	+	−
CIRC	−	−	+	−
LAD	−	−	+	−
RCA	−	−	+	−
RCA	−	−	+	−

Discussion

The current study confirms prior observations demonstrating that coronary collateral perfusion, unappar-

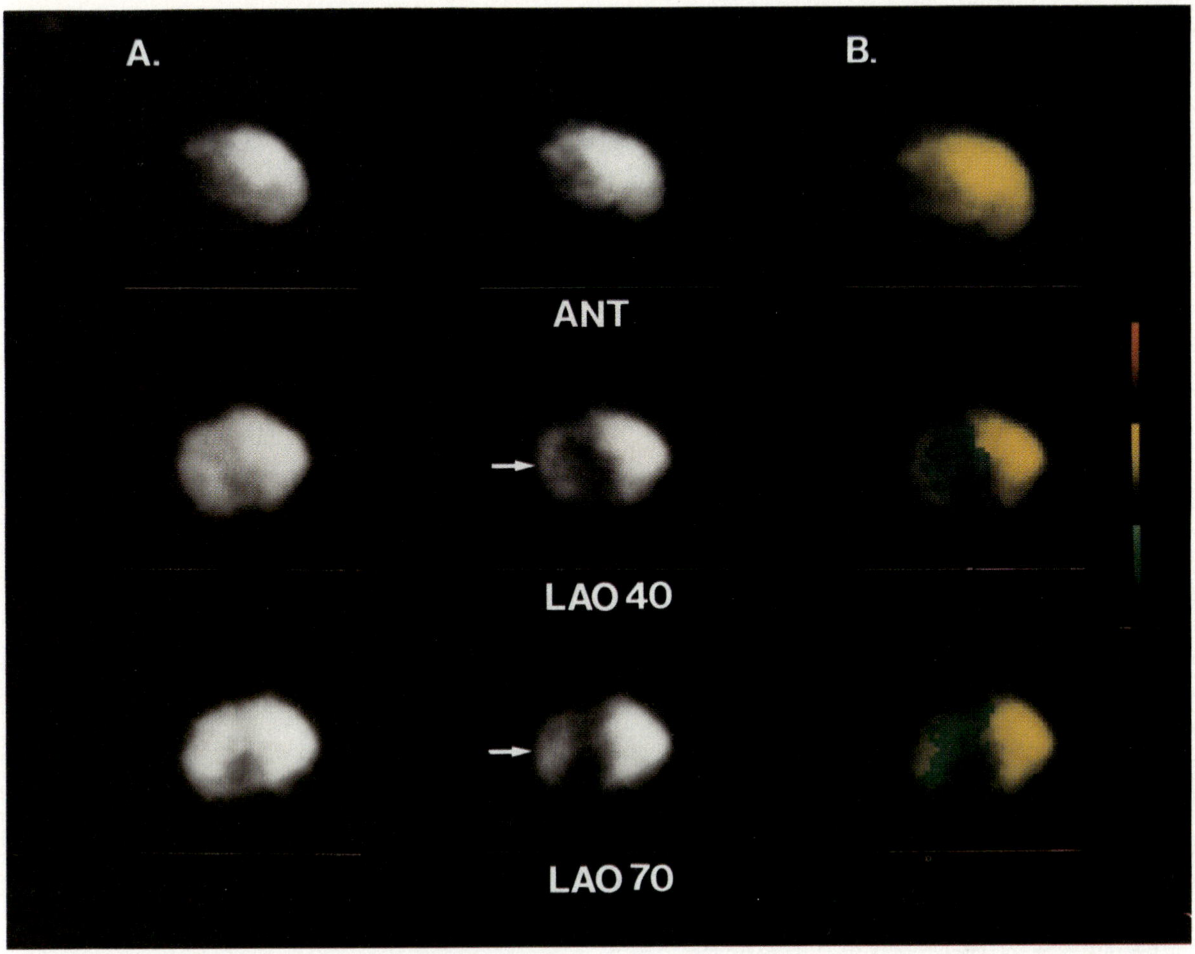

FIGURE 4. Images obtained before and after ICSK. Black and white (*A*, left and center columns) and color composite (*B*) images of MAA distribution obtained in registry after injection of ^{99m}Tc into the LCA before (*A*, left column) and ^{111}In after (*A*, center column) successful ICSK infusion of the occluded RCA. Relative septal radioactivity is seen to decrease (*A*, center column arrow) and green area, representing ^{99m}Tc, predominates in the color image (*B*), indicating a retraction of left-to-right septal collaterals and the restoration of a dual septal blood supply. Resting ^{201}Tl images after ICSK showed relatively normal and unchanged septal perfusion and the septum revealed preserved motion on radioangiographic examination.

ent angiographically, may be well demonstrated scintigraphically.[22, 29] The prior studies, however, were performed in patients undergoing conventional coronary angiography and serial studies[23] before and after intervention were not possible. The scintigraphic method, the comparison of sequential images acquired in registry, and the color display increased our ability to detect collateral blood flow in a high percentage of patients (table 1). This is not surprising when the method is analyzed. Particle sizes ranged from 10 to 40 μm in diameter[11] and were labeled with different radionuclides, the varying energies of emission of which permitted individual imaging despite their simultaneous presence in the myocardium. While collateral channels as small as 10 μm could potentially be detected with this technique, angiographic visualization is estimated to require a vessel diameter of greater than 150 μm. The particle technique provides excellent image resolution owing to the high ratio of myocardial-to-background radioactivities. Also, right ventricular perfusion, scintigraphically quite difficult to image, can be very well defined[14] and infarcted myocardium does not seem to be perfused by MAA.[11, 17, 26, 30] However, such particulate imaging is not quantitative and can only yield information regarding distribution and serial change in patterns of coronary perfusion.

In spite of numerous prior studies testifying to the reliability of the method, we sought to confirm our findings by evaluating technical aspects of our method in studies performed in four patients with normal coronary arteries and a group of patients with coronary lesions who were not undergoing intervention. Although imaging was performed as much as 2 hr after injection, previous studies have demonstrated the stability of particle localization.[12, 15] Images revealed essentially absent background radioactivity, indicating

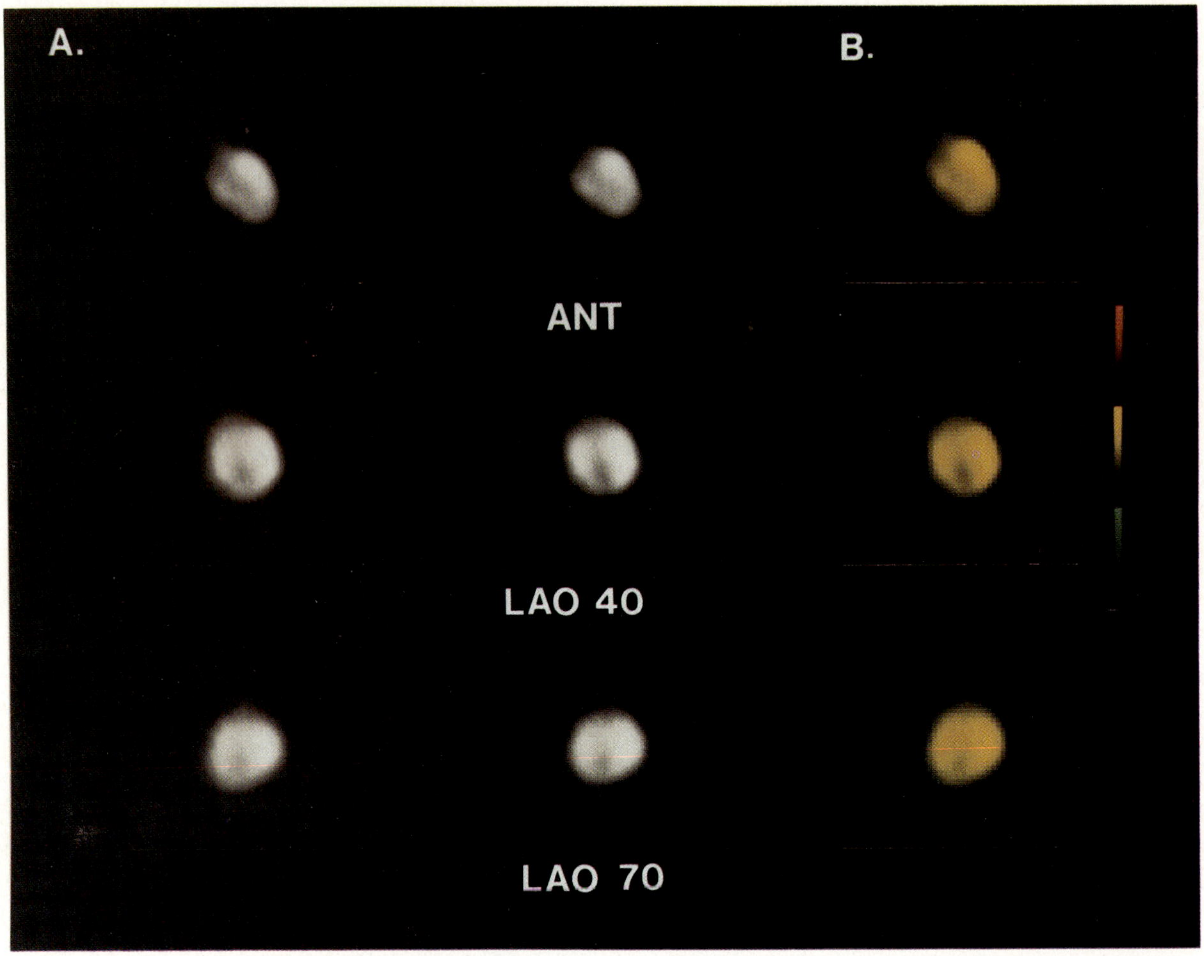

FIGURE 5. PTCA of the RCA. Shown according to the same format as Figure 2 are the black and white (*A*, left and center columns) and color composite (*B*) images of MAA distribution obtained in registry after injection of ^{99m}Tc into the LCA before (*A*, left column) and ^{111}In after (*A*, center column) successful PTCA of the RCA in the absence of collaterals. Images in *A* are unchanged and the color code in *B* represents a mixed distribution.

the absence of general radionuclide distribution, and the coronary distribution pattern was always confined to the appropriate region relating to the injection site. Furthermore, localization was unchanged in controls and in patients studied serially who were without collaterals or without sequential alteration in coronary anatomy, again supporting the stability of particle localization. Results in the 11 patients who underwent angiographic and scintigraphic study in the setting of an aborted or unsuccessful intervention also demonstrate the reproducibility of the imaging method and the reproducibility of sequential intracoronary injections. Phantom studies demonstrate our ability to separate the distribution of the two radionuclides and the order of their administration further ensures the reliability of the results. Regional overlap of injected radionuclides can be troublesome. However, the added information obtained in multiple projections and the separation of regional distribution of individual injections provided by the imaging protocol and color display made interpretation quite objective and reproducible. Subsequent studies applying tomographic imaging methods may be helpful. It should be noted that patients with normal coronary arteries and controls were only studied to demonstrate the safety and reliability of the method in our laboratory and to demonstrate the close correlation between angiographic and scintigraphic patterns. The data base was formed, however, by those patients imaged before and after instrumentation.

The inability to definitely correlate the observed severity of stenosis in vessels with greater than 75% area stenosis with the presence of coronary collaterals could relate to many factors. These include the recognized difficulty in assessing the percentage stenosis, the difference between anatomic and pathophysiologic measures of significance of stenosis, the inability to assess length of narrowing and serial lesions, and the suspected individual variability in vascular reactivity. Of course, pathophysiologic evidence of significance of stenosis is best garnered during stress. Studies during stress could not be performed in this protocol, but the initial pathophysiologic significance of all lesions was documented with presenting symptoms and electrocardiographic or diagnostic test results.

We observed evidence of rapid collateral regression after successful PTCA and infusion of ICSK (table 1). At this time, we can conclude that native perfusion is restored after successful PTCA or ICSK, and these procedures appear to relieve the need for collateral perfusion. The study does not comment on the ability to recruit these collaterals subsequently, nor on their potential protective value. However, rest and redistribution perfusion scintigrams demonstrated no significant change in patients after PTCA, suggesting that total global perfusion was unchanged. Among those patients studied in association with administration of ICSK, three, each with evidence of collaterals, demonstrated evidence of myocardial preservation. While in two of these patients there was actual improvement in relative thallium distribution and perfusion in the involved area, the third showed no serial changes in global thallium distribution in association with a shift in septal perfusion from collateral to native vessel (figure 4).

These cases suggest the importance of collaterals as a determinant of myocardial preservation after ICSK. They also point to a potential dual benefit from reperfusion, the known direct benefit of flow restoration and the less frequently mentioned shift from collateral to native perfusion. The latter may not result in prevention of infarction, since the areas appeared relatively well perfused both before and after ICSK, but the alteration in pattern demonstrates the return of the collateral circulation to a reserve status, restoring a potential "safety net" to regional perfusion. Although we cannot comment on absolute flow and the distribution of perfusion may not change, its source may demonstrate an apparently beneficial alteration of a shift from collateral to native circulation. This native source may be generally tenuous, however, and could pose a renewed clinical threat for subsequent reobstruction.

It has been suggested that improvement apparent on perfusion scintigrams obtained serially during and immediately after infusion of ICSK may not relate to restored myocardial viability. However, maintained or restored regional perfusion demonstrated on rest or redistribution scintigrams performed days after the intervention generally support myocardial viability. Evidence of such viability was further supported by preserved regional wall motion, a generally accepted criterion. While changed metabolic demands could explain scintigraphic evidence of altered perfusion in damaged regions after revascularization with ICSK, the altered pattern most likely relates to beneficial effects of restored patency. Several investigators have demonstrated that ICSK can potentially salvage jeopardized mycardium if given quickly.[31-35] Time is clearly an important factor,[32] but the potential protective value of collateral flow has also been suggested.[34] Although the number of patients was small, only those patients with demonstrated collateral coronary blood flow also demonstrated evidence of preservation of myocardium in this study.

The apparent importance of collateral perfusion is especially well demonstrated in the subset of patients in whom myocardial viability was maintained or restored even though they received ICSK late after the onset of symptoms. Schaper and Pasyk[35] have demonstrated in dogs that myocardial salvage and reperfusion are possible after prolonged ischemia if even a small amount of collateral flow is present and Gold et al.[36] have demonstrated the same principle in patients with the use of electrocardiographic data. Revascularization in acute infarction may, in fact, provide the greatest benefit by preserving ischemic "infarcting" myocardium, which is prophylactically supported by collaterals. In those more stable patients undergoing PTCA, the importance of collaterals is apparently related to stress but is difficult to demonstrate at rest.

Particle scintigraphy is valuable in studying collateral perfusion, but is a purely qualitative technique. Furthermore, the method does not evaluate total coronary blood flow, but only relative regional perfusion. The method also cannot always be used to determine myocardial viability as can ^{201}Tl imaging, although absence of particle localization is related to presence of infarction. The technique does increase the capability of detecting collateral flow, yet its functional importance can only be surmised. While regression of collaterals can be assessed, the complete absence of collaterals could not be so readily evaluated, and may persist to some degree in the presence of significant remaining stenoses. Also, the scintigraphic assessment of coronary collaterals could not be performed with confidence in the initial preintervention particle study or in association with unchanging serial studies without correlation with angiographic findings. Here, angiographically apparent collaterals supported scintigraphic findings. However, in the frequent absence of collaterals, scintigraphic particle distribution to areas possibly representing collateral distribution was confirmed only by the angiographic evidence. Here, coronary obstruction or stenosis in the distribution of the uninvolved, contralateral, frequently noninjected vessel supported the scintigraphic evidence of collateralization.

There was careful attention to quality control in this study to ensure the position and timing of sequential intracoronary injections. Since contrast agents can independently increase coronary flow,[37] there was a delay between contrast and particle injection. All injections were made slowly and short left main coronary arteries were avoided to ensure successful and reproducible radionuclide administration. Again, absence of MAA regional uptake may relate simply to perfusion by the noninjected vessel and the significance of absent or reduced particle localization must be, and was, assessed in relation to the known coronary anatomy.

This study has again confirmed that coronary collateral flow is more easily demonstrated with the MAA technique than by angiography alone and has also shown that coronary collateral perfusion regresses rapidly after successful PTCA or infusion of ICSK. In this subset of patients, the restoration of native perfusion with regression of collateral flow after PTCA resulted in no apparent change in total relative global perfusion, as demonstrated by intravenous ^{201}Tl injection, while offering apparent great symptomatic benefit. This suggests the importance, yet insufficiency, of collateral perfusion. In other cases, collaterals may serve as important determinants of myocardial preservation after administration of ICSK. The understanding of new interventional techniques in cardiology and their relationship with the collateral circulation may be substantially benefitted by the application of methods of particulate radionuclide imaging by which scintigraphic alterations are determined.

References

1. Sheldon W: On the significance of coronary collaterals. Am J Cardiol **24:** 303, 1969
2. Levin D: Pathways and functional significance of the coronary collateral circulation. Circulation **50:** 831, 1974
3. Williams D, Amsterdam E, Miller R, Mason D: Functional significance of coronary collateral vessels in patients with acute myocardial infarction: Relation to pump performance, cardiogenic shock and survival. Am J Cardiol **37:** 345, 1976
4. Banka V, Bodenheimer M, Helfant R: Determinants of reversible asynergy: Effects of pathologic Q waves, coronary collaterals and anatomic location. Circulation **50:** 714, 1974
5. Betriu A, Castaner A, Sanz G, Pare J, Roig E, Col S, Magrina J, Navarro-Lopez F: Angiographic findings 1 month after myocardial infarction: A prospective study of 259 survivors. Circulation **65:** 1105, 1982
6. Kolibash A, Bush C, Wepsic R, Schroeder D, Tetalman M, Lewis R: Coronary collateral vessels: Spectrum of physiologic capabilities with respect to providing rest and stress myocardial perfusion, maintenance of left ventricular function and protection against infarction. Am J Cardiol **50:** 230, 1982
7. Schwartz F, Wagner H, Sesto M, Hofmann M, Schaper W, Kubler W: Native collaterals in the development of collateral circulation after chronic coronary stenosis in mongrel dogs. Circulation **66:** 303, 1982
8. Carroll R, Verani M, Falsetti H: The effect of collateral circulation on segmental left ventricular contraction. Circulation **50:** 709, 1974
9. Ferguson R, Petitclerc R, Choquette G, Chaniotis L, Gauthier P, Huot R, Allard C, Jankowski L, Campeau L: Effect of physical training on treadmill exercise capacity, collateral circulation and progression of coronary disease. Am J Cardiol **34:** 764, 1974
10. Eng C, Patterson R, Horowitz S, Halgash D, Pichard A, Midwall J, Herman M, Gorlin R: Coronary collateral function during exercise. Circulation **66:** 309, 1982
11. Kolibash A, Tetalman M, Olsen J, Schen J, Bush C, Lewis R: Intracoronary radiolabeled particulate imaging. Semin Nucl Med **10:** 178, 1980
12. Wagner H, Rhodes B, Sasaki Y, Ryan J: Studies of the circulation with radioactive microspheres. Invest Radiol **4:** 374, 1969
13. Ritchie J, Hamilton G, Williams D, Kennedy J: Myocardial imaging with radionuclide-labeled particles. Radiology **121:** 131, 1976
14. Hamilton G, Ritchie J, Allen D, Lapin E, Murray J: Myocardial perfusion imaging with ^{99m}Tc or ^{113m}In: Macroaggregated albumin: correlation of the perfusion image with clinical angiographic, surgical and histologic findings. Am Heart J **89:** 708, 1975
15. Ashburn W, Braunwald E, Simon A, Peterson K, Gault J: Myocardial perfusion imaging with radioactive-labeled particles injected directly into the coronary circulation of patients with coronary artery disease. Circulation **44:** 851, 1971
16. Quinn J, Serratto M, Kezdi P: Coronary artery bed photoscanning using radioiodine albumin macroaggregates. J Nucl Med **7:** 107, 1966
17. Kirk G, Adams R, Jansen C, Judkins M: Particulate myocardial perfusion scintigraphy: Its clinical usefulness in evaluation of coronary artery disease. Semin Nucl Med **7:** 67, 1977
18. Kolibash A, Call T, Tetalman M, Bush C, Schev J: Comparison of resting intracoronary particulate imaging and stress thallium-201 studies. Radiology **135:** 439, 1980
19. Kolibash A, Lewis R, Goodenow J, Bush C, Tetalman M: Extensive myocardial blood flow distribution through individual coronary artery bypass grafts. Chest **77:** 17, 1980
20. Kolibash A, Call T, Bush C, Tetalman M, Lewis R: Myocardial perfusion as an indicator of graft patency after coronary artery bypass surgery. Circulation **61:** 882, 1980
21. Gruentzig AR, Senning A, Siegenthaler WE: Nonoperative dilatation of coronary artery stenoses: percutaneous transluminal coronary angioplasty. N Engl J Med **301:** 61, 1979
22. David PR, Waters DD, Scholl JM, Crepeau J, Szlachcic J, Lesperance J, Hudon G, Bourassa MG: Percutaneous transluminal coronary angioplasty in patients with variant angina. Circulation **66:** 695, 1982
23. Douglas JS Jr, Gruentzig AR, King SB III, Hollman J, Ischinger P, Meier B, Craver JM, Jones EL, Waller JL, Bone DK, Guyton R: Percutaneous transluminal coronary angioplasty in patients with prior coronary bypass surgery. J Am Coll Cardiol **2:** 745, 1983
24. Rentrop P, Blancke H, Karsch K, Kaiser H, Lostering H, Leitz K: Selective intracoronary thrombolysis in acute myocardial infarction and unstable angina pectoris. Circulation **63:** 307, 1981
25. Ganz W, Buchbinder N, Marcus H, Mondkar A, Maddahi J, Charuzi Y, O'Connor L, Shell W, Fishbein M, Kass R, Miyamoto A, Swan H: Intracoronary thrombolysis in evolving myocardial infarction. Am Heart J **101:** 4, 1981
26. Markis J, Malagold M, Parker A, Silverman K, Barry W, Als A, Paulin S, Grossman W, Braunwald E: Myocardial salvage after intracoronary thrombolysis with streptokinase in acute myocardial infarction. N Engl J Med **305:** 777, 1981
27. Schwartz F, Schuller G, Katus H, Mehmel H, VonOhlshausen K, Hofmann M, Hermann HJ, Kubler W: Intracoronary thrombolysis in acute myocardial infarction: correlations among serum enzyme, scintigraphic and hemodynamic findings. Am J Cardiol **50:** 32, 1982

28. Khaja F, Walton JA Jr, Brymer JF, Lo E, Osterberger L, O'Neill WW, Colfer HT, Weiss R, Lee T, Kurian P, Goldberg AD, Pitt B, Goldstein S: Intracoronary fibrinolytic therapy in acute myocardial infarction. Report of a prospective randomized trial. N Engl J Med **308:** 1305, 1983
29. Schelbert HR, Ashburn WL, Covell JW: Feasibility and hazards of the intracoronary injection of radioactive serum albumin macroaggregates for external myocardial perfusion imaging. Invest Radiol **6:** 379, 1971
30. Kolibash AJ, Tetelman MR, Olsen JO, Scheu JB, Bush CA, Lewis RP: Intracoronary radiolabeled particulate imaging. Semin Nucl Med **10:** 178, 1980
31. Schuler G, Schwartz F, Hofmann M, Mehmel H, Manthey J, Maurer W, Rauch B, Herrmann HJ, Kubler W: Thrombolysis in acute myocardial infarction using intracoronary streptokinase: assessment by thallium-201 scintigraphy. Circulation **66:** 658, 1982
32. Schwartz F, Schulker G, Katus H, Hofmann M, Manthey J, Tillmanns H, Menmel H, Kubler W: Intracoronary thrombolysis in acute myocardial infarction: duration of ischemia as a major determinant of late results after recanalization. Am J Cardiol **50:** 933, 1982
33. Rentrop P, Merx W, Mathey D, Blanke H, Rutsch W, Karsch KR: Functional results of streptokinase — reperfusion in relation to collaterals and duration of symptoms. Circulation **64**(suppl IV): IV-129, 1981 (abst)
34. Rogers WJ, Hood WP Jr, Mantle JA, Baley WA, Kirklin JK, Zorn GL, Nath HP: Return of left ventricular function after reperfusion in patients with myocardial infarction: importance of subtotal stenosis or intact collaterals. Circulation **69:** 338, 1984
35. Schaper W, Pasyk S: Influence of collateral flow on the ischemic tolerance of the heart following acute and subacute coronary occlusion. Circulation **53**(suppl I): I-57, 1976
36. Gold HK, Leinbach RC, Maroko PR: Propranolol induced reduction of signs of ischemic injury during acute myocardial infarction. Am J Cardiol **58:** 689, 1976
37. Kloster FE, Friesen WG, Green GS, Judkins MP: Effects of coronary arteriography on myocardial bloods flow. Circulation **46:** 438, 1972

Frequency-dependent effects of verapamil on atrioventricular nodal conduction in man

KENNETH A. ELLENBOGEN, M.D., LAWRENCE D. GERMAN, M.D., WILLIAM G. O'CALLAGHAN, M.B., PAUL G. COLAVITA, M.D., ANNE C. MARCHESE, M.D., MARCEL R. GILBERT, M.D., AND HAROLD C. STRAUSS, M.D., C.M.

ABSTRACT We sought to determine if verapamil induces frequency-dependent prolongation of atrioventricular nodal conduction in 10 consecutive patients studied in the electrophysiology laboratory. We used a maintenance infusion of verapamil designed to produce plasma concentrations of verapamil in the "therapeutic" range and that did not alter heart rate or blood pressure significantly. Frequency-dependent prolongation of atrioventricular nodal conduction (AH interval) was demonstrated in all 10 patients ($p < .001$), and no change in HV conduction time with decreasing cycle length was noted in any patient while receiving verapamil. Two patterns of use-dependent response were seen. In four patients frequency-dependent prolongation of the $\Delta(AH)$ interval [$\Delta(AH) = AH_{verapamil} - AH_{control}$ at a given cycle length] was seen with each decrement in pacing cycle length. In six patients frequency-dependent prolongation of the $\Delta(AH)$ interval was not manifest until the fifth to eighth pacing cycle length tested. There was no association between the pattern observed and the initial heart rate or AH interval. After an abrupt change in pacing cycle length, the kinetics of $\Delta(AH)$ interval prolongation were rapid; equilibrium was achieved by five to eight pulses in all patients. There was no correlation between the magnitude of prolongation of the AH interval noted at a particular cycle length and the concentration of verapamil during the maintenance infusion. These results indicate that verapamil causes use-dependent prolongation of atrioventricular nodal conduction in man.
Circulation 72, No. 2, 344–352, 1985.

A DESIRABLE GOAL of antiarrhythmic drug therapy is to terminate or suppress tachycardia without affecting impulse initiation or propagation at physiologic heart rates.[1, 2] Ideally, a drug used to treat reentrant tachycardia will demonstrate maximal effects on conduction and refractoriness during tachycardia, but will have minimal effects at slower heart rates after its termination. The extent of a drug's effects on conduction velocity can be inferred from its effects on phase 0 maximum upstroke velocity ($\dot{V}_{max}$) of the action potential.[3] In 1957, Johnson and McKinnon[4] showed that quinidine decreased $\dot{V}_{max}$ progressively as the driving rate was increased. Observations similar to this have been made with other local anesthetic types of antiarrhythmic drugs in nerve and cardiac muscle.[1, 2] Subsequent studies in nerve and cardiac muscle have characterized the use- or frequency-dependent action of local anesthetic agents, leading to the evolution of the modulated receptor hypothesis.[5, 6] Experiments in vitro have demonstrated use-dependent block for a variety of sodium channel–blocking agents, including disopyramide, flecainide, mexiletine, and lidocaine.[7–10] Recently, preliminary reports have appeared describing frequency-dependent prolongation of conduction time in the human heart with procainamide, amiodarone, lidocaine, and mexiletine.[11, 12]

Use-dependent block has also been demonstrated for calcium-channel blockers in vitro. Wit and Cranefield[13] studied the effects of verapamil on isolated rabbit atrioventricular nodes and were able to demonstrate frequency-dependent prolongation of atrioventricular nodal conduction. In 1975, while studying the effect of verapamil on cat papillary muscle, Bayer et al.[14, 15] were also able to infer that the drug caused frequency-dependent blockade of the slow inward current. Later, Ehara and Kaufman[16] and McDonald et al.[17] directly demonstrated frequency-dependent block of the calcium current with verapamil and its cogener, methoxy-

From the Division of Cardiology, Department of Medicine, and Department of Pharmacology, Duke University Medical Center, Durham, NC 27710.

Supported in part by grants 19216, 17670, and 07101 from the National Heart, Lung, and Blood Institute.

Address for correspondence: Harold C. Strauss, M.D., C.M., Division of Cardiology, Box 3845, Duke University Medical Center, Durham, NC 27710.

Received Feb. 22, 1985; revision accepted April 25, 1985.

verapamil. Excitation and, as a result, conduction in the atrioventricular node, are dependent on the slow inward (calcium) current.[18] Extrapolation of these findings in vitro to man would predict that the effect of verapamil on atrioventricular conduction should be frequency dependent. Demonstration of this action would represent a significant advance in our understanding of the relevance of these findings in vitro to man.

Methods

The study group consisted of 10 consecutive adult patients referred for electrophysiologic evaluation of symptomatic or suspected cardiac arrhythmias. Patients were excluded from this study if they demonstrated manifest preexcitation on the electrocardiogram, atrioventricular block on Holter or electrocardiographic monitoring, an ejection fraction less than 30% as determined by radionuclide angiography, two-dimensional echocardiography, or cardiac catheterization, or if they had symptomatic congestive heart failure. Patients taking calcium antagonists (nifedipine, diltiazem, verapamil), β-blockers, or digoxin were also excluded from this study. All cardioactive medications were withheld for at least five half-lives before the study. Informed consent was obtained from all patients.

Electrophysiologic study protocol. The studies were performed in nonsedated, fasting patients. Three multipolar catheters were introduced percutaneously and positioned in the heart under fluoroscopic guidance in the right atrial appendage, across the tricuspid valve to record a His bundle potential, and in the right ventricular apex in each patient.

Stimulation was performed with a custom-designed, programmable stimulator with an optically isolated current source producing 2 msec pulses at twice diastolic threshold. Bipolar intracardiac electrograms were recorded with five surface electrocardiographic leads (I, II, III, V_1, and V_6) and were displayed on an oscilloscope. Graphic records were obtained on-line with a multichannel ink-jet recorder (Siemens Mingograph) at 200 mm/sec. A 10 msec time code was generated with the data during all recordings.

The following routine intracardiac electrophysiologic studies were performed on all patients: (1) Incremental atrial pacing was performed beginning at rates just above the sinus rate to the point at which atrioventricular block occurred. (2) Right atrial refractory period was determined by the extrastimulus technique at a driven cycle length of 600 msec. In each of six patients, atrial pacing was performed for 2 min at a driven cycle length of 50 to 100 msec shorter than the patient's spontaneous cycle length and was then suddenly decreased by 100 to 150 msec. Continuous recordings were obtained during pacing. Each patient then underwent incremental atrial pacing for 1 min at each cycle length, starting at cycle lengths just below the sinus cycle length and decreasing stepwise (25 msec steps) until atrioventricular block occurred. Graphic records were obtained during the last 10 sec at each pacing cycle length for data analysis.

All patients then received 10 mg of verapamil (Isoptin, Knoll Pharmaceutical, Whippany, NJ) in 4 ml of saline administered intravenously over 2 min. Blood pressure was monitored by an external continuous monitor (Infrasonde model D4000), and rhythm was monitored continuously during the verapamil infusion. Each patient then received a rapid loading infusion of verapamil, 0.375 mg/min for 30 min, followed by a maintenance infusion at 0.125 mg/min via an IVAC pump through an 18-gauge Teflon cannula inserted into a superficial arm vein. Plasma for verapamil assay was obtained from a vein in the opposite arm after the maintenance infusion was begun. The plasma was placed in heparinized glass tubes and immediately centrifuged, separated, frozen, and stored at −20° C until assay. Plasma samples were extracted in diethyl ether after addition of an internal standard solution of D517-HC1. Peak height ratios of drug concentration vs internal standard were measured by high-pressure liquid chromotography with use of a fluorometric detection assay as previously described.[19] Verapamil concentrations were based on three calibration curves, the average correlation coefficient of which was .997 ± .001. Five minutes after the establishment of a maintenance infusion, the electrophysiologic protocol was repeated.

Data analysis. The AH and HV intervals were measured with use of criteria previously defined.[20] The AH interval was measured between the earliest reproducible rapid atrial deflection and the onset of the earliest deflection from baseline on the His bundle catheter recording. The AH interval was measured for 3 to 5 beats, and an average value was obtained (incremental atrial pacing). If the AH interval varied more than 5 msec in sequential beats, the patient was excluded from the study. Two patients were excluded from this study because of excessive variation in AH conduction times. The HV interval was measured from the onset of the His bundle deflection to the onset of ventricular depolarization. During incremental atrial pacing the HV interval was measured for 3 to 5 beats and an average value was obtained (incremental atrial pacing). All data were recorded at 200 mm/sec. It has been reported that the accuracy of measurements made at 100 mm/sec is approximately ±5 msec.[20] Δ(AH) interval was defined as the difference between the AH interval measured during the infusion of verapamil and that during the control study at the same cycle length.

Statistical methods. Changes in heart rate and blood pressure after the bolus dose of verapamil were analyzed with the Wilcoxon signed-rank test. Trends in heart rate and blood pressure during the loading and maintenance infusions were analyzed by computing the slope of the measurement vs time separately for each patient, and then testing for whether the slopes had a mean value that was significantly different from zero with the Wilcoxon signed-rank test. Frequency dependence was analyzed with the sign test based on divergence of Δ(AH) interval with decreasing cycle length. The AH interval vs cycle length curves were assessed separately for each patient to determine if the difference in AH interval between drug and control curves was greater for the shorter cycle lengths tested. The sign test determined whether the proportion of divergent curves was significantly greater than one half. Linear regression analysis was used to correlate verapamil concentration with the magnitude of Δ(AH) intervals at a given cycle length over the entire range of cycle lengths tested.

Results

Patients studied. The clinical and electrocardiographic characteristics of the patient population are shown in table 1. Nine of the 10 patients had normal ejection fractions, and one patient (No. 2) had an ejection fraction of 32%. The baseline descriptors of atrioventricular nodal function in the patients are shown in table 2. All refractory periods were determined at a cycle length of 600 msec unless otherwise indicated. In four patients the functional refractory period of the atrium precluded determination of the effective refractory period of the atrioventricular node.

TABLE 1
Clinical and electrocardiographic descriptors of patients

Patient No.	Age/sex	Reason for study	Heart disease	PR (sec)	QRS (sec)
1	42/F	VE	None	0.10	0.08
2	46/M	VT	CM	0.16	0.08
3	31/F	Syncope	None	0.14	0.10
4	69/F	Syncope	None	0.18	0.10
5	57/M	SVT	None	0.18	0.08
6	30/M	SVT	None	0.16	0.08
7	54/F	Palpitations	None	0.10	0.08
8	29/F	Palpitations	None	0.16	0.08
9	49/M	VT	CAD	0.16	0.08
10	46/F	VE	None	0.16	0.09

VT = ventricular tachycardia; SVT = supraventricular tachycardia; CAD = coronary artery disease; CM = cardiomyopathy; VE = complex ventricular ectopy (on Holter monitoring).

Plasma verapamil concentration. The verapamil level was determined 2 min after the beginning of the maintenance infusion (0.125 mg/min). The levels ranged from 37 to 125 ng/ml (mean ± SD, 85 ± 35 ng/ml).

Hemodynamics. Analysis of measurements of blood pressure showed a 12% decrease in mean systolic blood pressure at 2 min during the bolus phase of drug administration, which was a significant decrease ($p < .05$). There was no significant change in mean diastolic blood pressure at 2 min ($p > .05$). Mean heart rate (82 beats/min) increased significantly at 2 min (90 beats/min, $p < .05$). There was no significant change in mean heart rate, systolic pressure, or diastolic pressure during the loading and maintenance phases of the verapamil infusion ($p < .05$). These results are presented in figure 1.

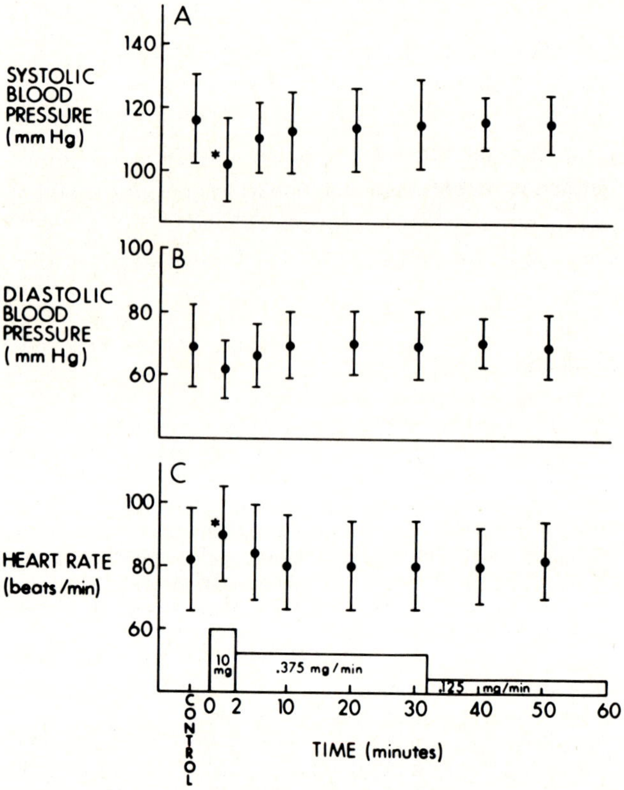

FIGURE 1. Changes in heart rate and systolic and diastolic blood pressure before and during the verapamil infusion protocol for all 10 patients (mean ± SD) Protocol for infusion of verapamil is indicated in boxes. * $p < .05$ for comparison of control and verapamil.

Kinetics. To determine the kinetics of change in AH interval during incremental pacing, pacing at a cycle length of 500 or 750 msec for 2 min was followed by an abrupt 100 to 150 msec cycle length decrease, and the number of beats needed for the AH interval to reach

TABLE 2
Electrophysiologic descriptors of patients

Patient No.	AH/CL (msec)		AVN ERP (msec)		AVN FRP (msec)		Minimum CL with 1:1 AV conduction (msec)	
	Control	Verapamil	Control	Verapamil	Control	Verapamil	Control	Verapamil
1	42/870	58/840	293	490	435	523	450	550
2	70/640	90/580	<263[A,B]	DNM	<383[A,B]	DNM	270	375
3	75/920	80/800	299	391	369	482	340	500
4	52/880	120/860	<292	<400	<412	<550	340	500
5	57/880	100/845	338	549	425	620	450	550
6	35/640	40/700	<258	<320	<270	<340	230	400
7	62/625	80/600	<265[B]	<326[B]	<280[B]	<418[B]	260	350
8	96/630	122/620	268	316	371	399	240	350
9	68/810	92/840	341	480	421	540	360	525
10	75/1000	100/1040	300	433	450	548	425	575

DNM = did not measure; CL = cycle length (measured in msec); AVN = atrioventricular nodal; ERP = effective refractory period; FRP = functional refractory period.

[A]Refractory period terminated because of nonsustained atrial flutter/atrial fibrillation.

[B]Refractory period determined at 500 msec.

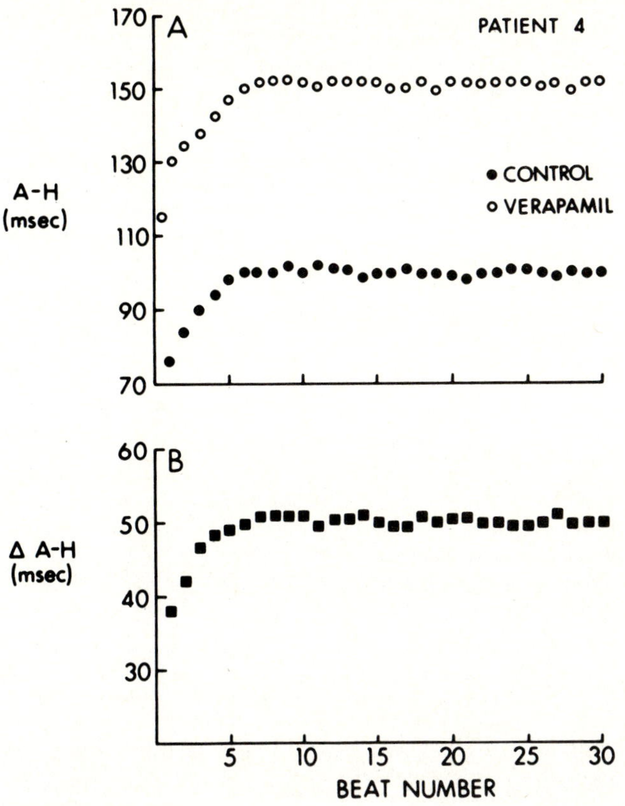

FIGURE 2. Kinetic data for patient 4. Atrial pacing at a cycle length of 750 msec for 2 min preceded a sudden decrement in atrial pacing cycle length to 600 msec. *A*, Sequential AH intervals (msec) during pacing (600 msec), the control period, and the infusion of verapamil. *B*, Δ(AH) (AH verapamil − AH control) for each beat. In this patient, equilibrium was reached by beat number 7.

a steady-state level was determined in six of the 10 patients. This was performed both before and during the maintenance infusion of verapamil. The results in a sample patient (No. 4) are illustrated in figure 2. In the patients studied in the control state, equilibrium was reached in a mean of 6 (range 4 to 8) beats. During infusion of verapamil, an equilibrium value for the Δ(AH) interval was reached in a mean of 6 (range 5 to 8) beats.

Electrophysiologic variables. Descriptors of atrioventricular nodal function determined during the maintenance infusion of verapamil are listed in table 2. In each patient in whom the effective and functional refractory periods of the atrioventricular node could be determined, there was an increase in these parameters during the infusion of verapamil of approximately 30% (range 10% to 60%). The minimum cycle length at which 1:1 atrioventricular conduction was present increased by 100 to 175 msec after infusion of drug.

Frequency dependence of atrioventricular nodal conduction time. In the baseline electrophysiology study, as the pacing cycle length was decreased, the AH interval increased. The curves relating AH interval to atrial pacing cycle length were similar to those previously reported in the literature and seen in other patients studied in our electrophysiology laboratory for a variety of arrhythmias.[20, 21]

In each patient studied, during the infusion of verapamil evidence of use-dependent prolongation of the Δ(AH) interval was evident as the pacing cycle length was decreased ($p < .001$). Analog data from patient 9 are shown in figure 3. Two patterns of frequency-dependent prolongation of the AH interval were seen. In six patients (Nos. 1, 3, 4, 6, 9, and 10) there was no change in the Δ(AH) interval for the initial four to seven cycle lengths tested; however, at subsequent shorter cycle lengths, there was a nonlinear increase in this interval. In two patients, prolongation of the Δ(AH) interval was absent for the first four cycle lengths tested, in one patient it was absent for the initial five pacing cycle lengths, in one patient it was absent for the initial six pacing cycle lengths tested, and in two patients it was absent for the initial seven pacing cycle lengths. For these six patients the Δ(AH) interval between the first and second cycle lengths tested ranged from 0 to 2 msec (mean ± SD, 1 ± 0.5 msec).

In four patients (Nos. 2, 5, 7, and 8) there was a progressive increase in the Δ(AH) interval noted with each decrement in pacing cycle length. In these patients the Δ(AH) interval between the first and second cycle lengths tested ranged from 5 to 11 msec (mean ± SD, 7 ± 2 msec).

There was a wide spectrum of baseline heart rates and AH intervals observed in patients demonstrating each pattern of frequency dependence. These two patterns of frequency dependence are shown in figure 4 with sample data from patients 4, 6, and 7.

In six patients, atrial pacing was begun at a cycle length of 800 msec. The mean data for these six patients are shown in figure 5, *A*. There was a progressive increase in the mean Δ(AH) interval as the cycle length was decreased. At a cycle length of 600 msec, the mean Δ(AH) interval was 44 msec.

Frequency dependence of HV conduction time. Since verapamil has been shown to decrease phase 0 $\dot{V}_{max}$ in polarized ventricular muscle cells, we also examined the effects of verapamil on conduction time of the HV interval. There was no change in the mean HV conduction time as the cycle length was decreased at control or during the infusion of verapamil. This is illustrated in figure 5, *B*, for the six patients in which atrial pacing was begun at a cycle length of 800 msec.

Concentration-response relationship. There was no

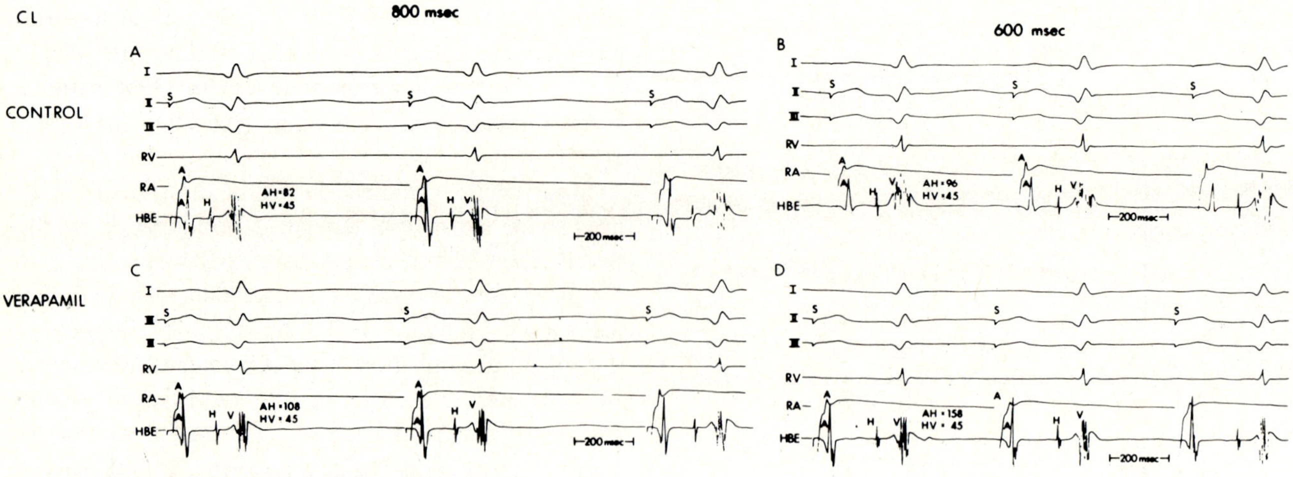

FIGURE 3. Analog data from patient 9, demonstrating use dependence. When pacing cycle length decreased from a cycle length of 800 to 600 msec (*A* and *B*) the AH interval increased from 82 to 96 msec, an increase of 14 msec, while HV interval remained constant. During verapamil (*C* and *D*), after a decrease in atrial pacing cycle length from 800 to 600 msec, the AH interval increased from 108 to 158 msec, an increase of 50 msec, and HV interval remained constant. The surface electrocardiographic leads are I, II, III; intracardiac recordings are from the right ventricle (RV), right atrium (RA), and His bundle. S = stimulus artifact; A = atrial electrogram; HBE = His bundle electrogram; V = ventricular electrogram. AH and HV intervals expressed in msec.

correlation between the verapamil level during the maintenance infusion and the Δ(AH) intervals observed at cycle lengths of 800 msec ($n = 6$, $r = -.7$, $p > .05$), 600 msec ($n = 5$, $r = -.02$, $p > .05$), 500 msec ($n = 4$, $r = -.8$, $p > .05$), and 400 msec ($n = 4$, $r = -.7$, $p > .05$).

Discussion

The most important finding of this study is the demonstration of verapamil's frequency-dependent prolongation of AH conduction time in man. After an abrupt change in atrial pacing cycle length, the AH interval rapidly reached a new equilibrium value within 8 beats. On the other hand, verapamil had no effect on the HV interval at any pacing cycle length tested. We could not establish any correlation between verapamil concentration and the magnitude of the Δ(AH) interval at any cycle length tested.

One of the most intriguing findings to emerge from studies of use- or frequency-dependent block of local anesthetic type antiarrhythmic drugs has been that these drugs preferentially slow conduction during tachycardia, but have relatively little effect on conduction at normal heart rates. These studies have also led to the evolution of the modulated receptor hypothesis that states that local anesthetic types of antiarrhythmic drugs diffuse to a binding site in the aqueous pore of the ionic channel through either an aqueous (hydrophilic) or membrane (hydrophobic) pathway.[5,6] Since most antiarrhythmic agents have pK_as in the 7 to 10 range, they exist as a combination of the neutral and the charged forms of the drug. Receptor affinity or access of drugs to the binding site is believed to vary with the state of the channel.[5,6,22] For example, with depolarization of a Purkinje fiber, the majority of the sodium channels will be transiently shifted to the open or activated state. In this state, both charged and uncharged forms of the drug can access the sodium channel through the hydrophilic pathway from the inside of the cell and the uncharged form can access the channel through the hydrophobic pathway in the membrane. During the plateau phase of repolarization, the majority of sodium channels are in the inactivated state, and now access to the sodium-channel binding site is restricted to the uncharged form of the drug via the membrane (hydrophobic) path. Association of drug with the ionic channel occurs predominantly during the upstroke and plateau phase of the action potential, while dissociation occurs predominantly during diastole.[1,2,22] When the drug is bound to its receptor site in the channel, that channel can no longer conduct. Thus, as the driving rate of a preparation is increased, the rest (diastolic) interval becomes shortened, and there is less time for the drug to dissociate from the channels and to completely recover from block. Frequency-dependent block of sodium channels as deduced from measurement of the sodium current of phase 0 $\dot{V}_{max}$ has been demonstrated in vitro for all the commonly used antiarrhythmic agents as well as for many investigational antiarrhythmic drugs.[1,2]

Less information is available about the function

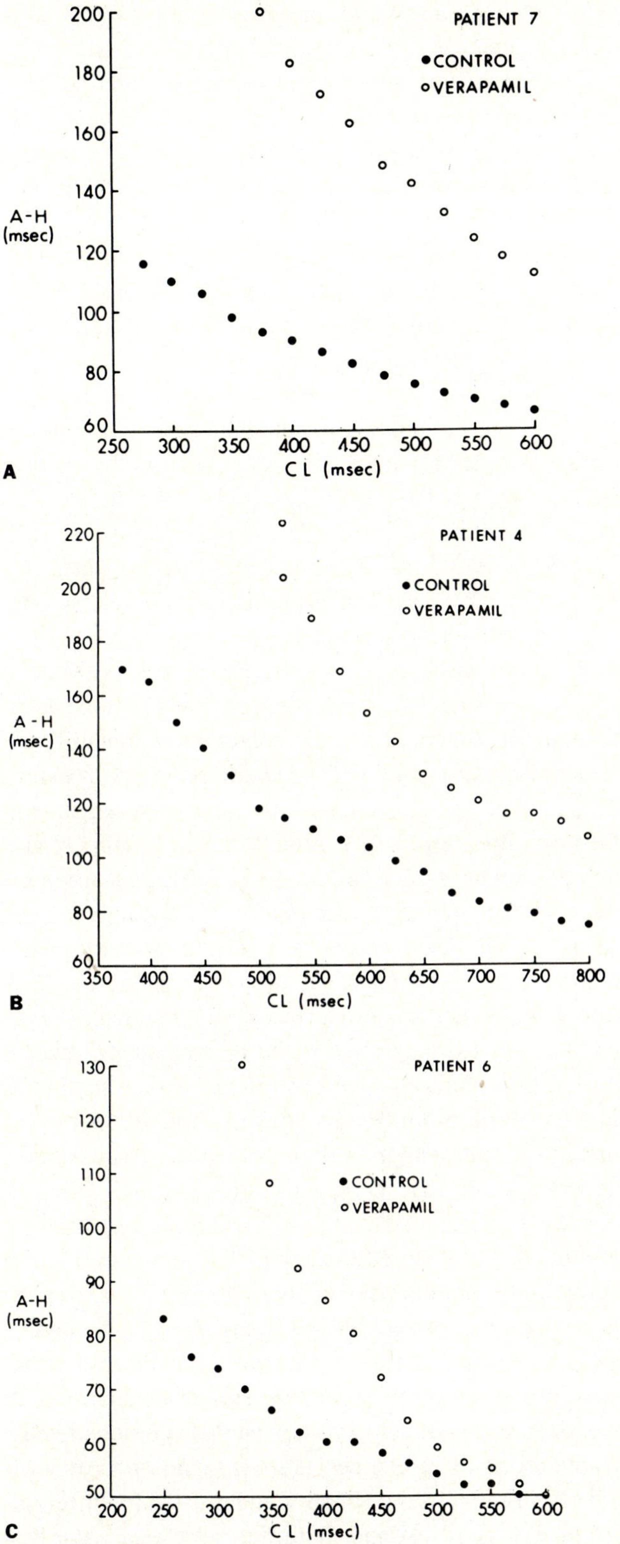

FIGURE 4. Two patterns of frequency (use) dependence. In patient 7 (*A*) use dependence was demonstrated by an increase in AH interval during verapamil infusion at every cycle length (CL) tested. A second pattern is shown in *B* and *C*. In patient 4 (*B*), AH interval during verapamil infusion was relatively constant over the first four CLs tested. Over the next nine CLs, the AH interval progressively increased in magnitude. A similar pattern was seen in patient 6 (*C*), despite the small baseline increment in the AH interval during the infusion of verapamil.

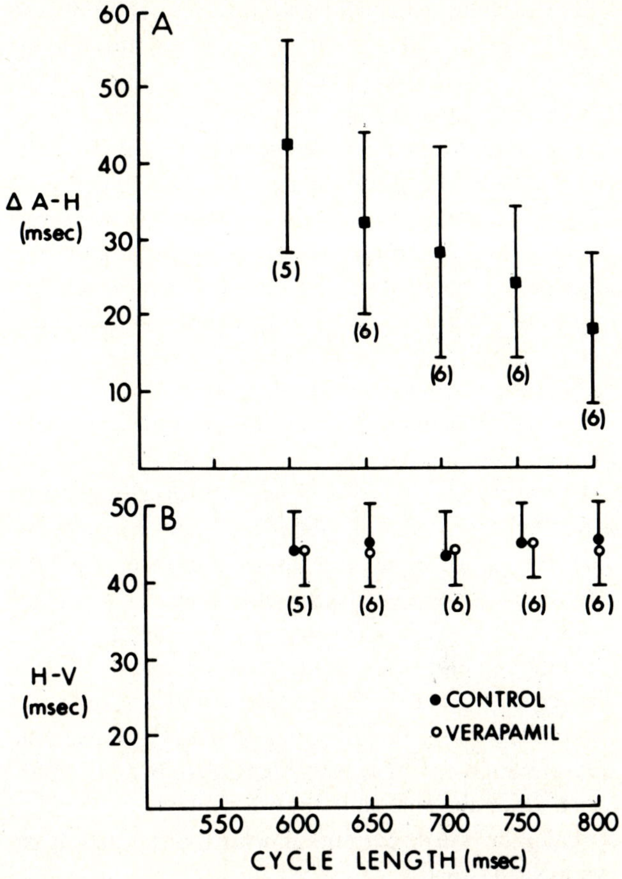

FIGURE 5. Data for the six patients in whom testing was begun at a cycle length of 800 msec. *A*, The mean Δ(AH) interval increased from 18 msec at a cycle length of 800 to 44 msec at a cycle length of 600 msec. *B*, There was no increase in HV interval (ΔHV = 0) at any of the cycle lengths tested.

of the calcium channel because of the greater variability in its molecular structure and function in different species as well as in different tissues of the same species.[23, 24] Although information about gating of calcium channels is still incomplete, there is evidence to suggest that there are many similarities between the sodium and calcium channels. For example, an inactivation as well as an activation process controls channel permeability.[23, 24] Furthermore, similarities exist between calcium- and sodium-channel blockers.[1, 2, 17, 23, 25] For example, the calcium-channel blockers that show use dependence have a pK_a in the 7 to 10 range. As in the case of sodium-channel blockers, permanently charged derivatives of calcium-channel antagonists do not induce frequency-dependent block when applied to the outer surface of the membrane, but do induce block when applied to the inner surface of the membrane.[25] This implies that the pathways by which the channel binding site is accessed are similar for calcium- and sodium-channel blocking drugs.

The calcium-dependent slow inward current plays a major role in transmission of impulses through the atrioventricular node. Studies performed in the 1970s demonstrated that the calcium current is primarily responsible for the action potential upstroke in N and NH cells of the atrioventricular node.[18] Verapamil is known to depress calcium current in voltage-clamped preparations of atrioventricular node obtained from mammalian myocardium.[27] Since propagation velocity in the atrioventricular node is dependent on the underlying calcium current as well as passive membrane properties, a drug-induced decrease in ionic current should be reflected in a prolongation of atrioventricular nodal conduction time.

Unfortunately, there is a scarcity of clinical evidence indicating that use-dependent blockade may occur in humans. Evidence for its presence could be inferred from the observation of frequency-dependent changes in propagation velocity or conduction time. Recently, preliminary observations have suggested that type I antiarrhythmic drugs will cause cycle length–dependent prolongation of the HV interval or QRS duration.[11, 12] However, there have been no studies in which the possibility of use-dependent blockade by calcium- (slow-current) blocking drugs has been examined in man.

In our study, frequency-dependent prolongation of the AH interval was demonstrated in each patient. Two patterns of prolongation of the AH interval were noted. One pattern showed a constant Δ(AH) interval for the first four to seven pacing cycle lengths tested, followed by progressively increasing Δ(AH) intervals at the remaining pacing cycle lengths. The second pattern demonstrated a nonlinear increase in Δ(AH) interval that was noted by the second cycle length tested. There was no correlation between the pattern of use dependence seen and the baseline heart rate or AH interval. Furthermore, there was no correlation between hemodynamic response to the infusion of verapamil and the pattern of frequency dependence observed. There are several other factors that would be expected to modulate the magnitude and pattern of frequency-dependent prolongation of the AH interval. Cellular phenomena, such as changes in diastolic membrane potential, may cause different degrees of tonic block.[2, 22] Catecholamines have been shown to augment the calcium-channel current, and changing catecholamine levels could modulate the degree of prolongation of the AH interval seen with rapid atrial pacing.[28] Finally, atrioventricular nodal conduction reflects a wide spectrum of atrioventricular nodal physiology, and interindividual differences in baseline properties could contribute to the different responses we observed with incremental atrial pacing.[29]

The kinetics of equilibration of the AH interval with abrupt changes in atrial pacing cycle length in man were studied to compare our observations on conduction time in vivo with observations on calcium current in vitro. Earlier work with different mammalian myocardial preparations has shown that after onset of a pulse train, verapamil induces steady-state block of the calcium current by 10 to 15 pulses.[17, 26] A comparison such as this presumes a relatively linear relationship between propagation velocity and available calcium conductance. In all six patients studied, equilibrium values for Δ(AH) intervals were obtained by 5 to 8 beats, which is similar to the number of impulses required to attain equilibrium in vitro. From a practical viewpoint, this justifies our assumption that data obtained 45 sec after a change in pacing cycle length represented steady-state values.

Although verapamil is primarily considered to be a calcium-channel blocker, previous investigations have demonstrated that the (+) isomer of verapamil decreases $\dot{V}_{max}$ of phase 0 of the action potential in mammalian ventricular myocardium in a rate-dependent fashion, presumably by blocking the sodium channel.[30, 31] Since verapamil exists as a racemic mixture, the (+) isomer might also cause rate-dependent prolongation of HV conduction time. In our study, no evidence of rate-dependent prolongation of the HV interval was seen during the infusion of verapamil. The most likely explanation for the discrepancy between our findings and observations in vitro is that the levels of verapamil produced by the infusion are approximately tenfold less than those shown to cause a rate-dependent decrease in $\dot{V}_{max}$ in vitro.

We also attempted to show a concentration-response relationship. We predicted that the concentration of verapamil would be higher in a patient with a greater Δ(AH) interval at a given cycle length. This, however, was not the case. There are several explanations for the lack of correlation between the level of verapamil and the degree of frequency dependence demonstrated. Unquantifiable influences are the wide spectrum of atrioventricular nodal function manifested by different AH intervals at rest and the different responses of the AH interval to incremental pacing in each patient. In addition, differing degrees of change in autonomic tone may have contributed to the variable degrees of frequency dependence noted in individual patients. To minimize this complication, we excluded patients with heart failure in whom verapamil might have caused hypotension and a subsequent change in autonomic tone.[32] For the maintenance infusion, we used an infusion protocol that Reiter et al.[33] have shown to result in constant plasma concentrations of verapamil. This protocol did not cause a significant change in heart rate or blood pressure during the loading or maintenance phase of the infusion in our patients, implying that changes in autonomic tone were minimal.[33]

Verapamil administered intravenously is the agent of choice for terminating acute episodes of paroxysmal supraventricular tachycardia without hemodynamic compromise.[34] Its efficacy approaches 90% for termination of reentrant supraventricular tachycardia, regardless of the mechanism of the tachycardia. The infusion of verapamil studied produced drug levels similar to those reported in patients taking 80 mg of oral verapamil every 6 hr.[35] The changes in effective and functional refractory periods of the atrioventricular node and in cycle length sustaining 1:1 atrioventricular conduction during the maintenance infusion of verapamil were similar to those reported in several other clinical studies.[35-39] The magnitude of use dependence we observed [Δ(AH) at final cycle length tested $-$ Δ(AH) at initial cycle length tested] varied from 25 to 70 msec (mean $\pm$ SD, 51 $\pm$ 17 msec). This additional increase in AH interval resulting from frequency-dependent prolongation of atrioventricular nodal conduction is of the same order of magnitude as the increase in AH intervals seen just before termination of tachycardia in many patients receiving intravenous or oral verapamil.[35, 37, 40] Thus, these data suggest that the frequency- or rate-dependent effects demonstrated in this study are of sufficient magnitude to be of therapeutic significance in the termination of paroxysmal supraventricular tachycardia.

In conclusion, the results of this study demonstrate use-dependent blockade of atrioventricular nodal conduction with verapamil in man. The kinetics of block are rapid and were achieved in five to eight pulses. There was no evidence of use-dependent prolongation of His-Purkinje conduction (HV interval). The degree of use dependence observed in this study did not correlate with the verapamil concentration.

We thank Thorir Bjornsson, M.D., Director, Clinical Pharmacology Laboratory, for the performance of the verapamil assays and Frank Harrell, Ph.D., for advice on the statistical analysis. We also thank Steffani Webb and Mary Holben for preparation of this manuscript, and Laura Cook, R.N., Rose Smith, R.N., and Ineke Philippo, R.N., for providing excellent patient care.

References

1. Hondeghem LM, Katzung BG: Antiarrhythmic agents: the modulated receptor mechanism of action of sodium and calcium channel-blocking drugs. Ann Rev Pharmacol Toxicol **24:** 387, 1984
2. Grant AO, Starmer CF, Strauss HC: Antiarrhythmic drug action: Blockade of the inward sodium current. Circ Res **55:** 427, 1984
3. Fozzard HA: Conduction of the action potential. *In* Berne RM, editor: Handbook of physiology: the cardiovascular system, section 2, volume I. Bethesda, 1979, American Physiological Society, p 335
4. Johnson EA, McKinnon MG: The differential effect of quinidine and pyrilamine on the myocardial action potential at various rates of stimulation. J Pharmacol Exp Ther **120:** 460, 1957
5. Hille B: Local anesthetics: hydrophilic and hydrophobic pathways for the drug-receptor reaction. J Gen Physiol **69:** 497, 1977
6. Hondeghem LM, Katzung BG: Time- and voltage-dependent interactions of antiarrhythmic drugs with cardiac sodium channels. Biochim Biophys Acta **472:** 373, 1977
7. Kojima M, Ban T, Sada H: Effects of disopyramide on the maximum rate of rise of the potential (V_{max}) in guinea pig papillary muscles. Jpn J Pharmacol **32:** 91, 1983
8. Campbell TJ, Vaughan Williams EM: Voltage- and time-dependent depression of maximum rate of depolarisation of guinea-pig ventricular action potentials by two new antiarrhythmic drugs, flecainide and lorcainide. Cardiovasc Res **17:** 251, 1983
9. Courtney KR: Comparative actions of mexiletine on sodium channels in nerve, skeletal and cardiac muscle. Eur J Pharmacol **74:** 20, 1975
10. Chen CM, Gettes LS, Katzung BG: Effect of lidocaine and quinidine on steady state characteristics and recovery kinetics of (dv/dt) max in guinea pig ventricular myocardium. Circ Res **37:** 20, 1975
11. Mercer AB, Foster JR, Simpson RJ, Gettes LS: Use-dependency of antiarrhythmic drugs in the human heart. Circulation **68**(suppl III): III-296, 1983
12. Gang E, Denton T, Oseran D, Mandel W, Peter T: Procainamide-induced prolongation of the HV interval is heart rate dependent. Circulation **70**(suppl II): II-445, 1984
13. Wit AL, Cranefield PF: Effect of verapamil on the sinoatrial nodes and atrioventricular nodes of the rabbit and the mechanism by which it arrests reentrant atrioventricular nodal tachycardia. Circ Res **35:** 413, 1974
14. Bayer R, Hennekes R, Kaufmann R, Mannhold R: Inotropic and electrophysiological actions of verapamil and D600 in mammalian myocardium. I. Pattern of inotropic effects of the racemic compounds. Naunyn-Schmeidebergs Arch Pharmacol **290:** 49, 1975
15. Bayer R, Kaufmann R, Mannhold R: Inotropic and electrophysiological actions of verapamil and D600 in mammalian myocardium. II. Pattern of inotropic effects of the optical isomers. Naunyn-Schmeidebergs Arch Pharmacol **290:** 69, 1975
16. Ehara T, Kaufman R: The voltage- and time-dependent effects of (−)-verapamil on the slow inward current in isolated cat ventricular myocardium. J Pharmacol Exp Ther **207:** 49, 1978
17. McDonald TF, Pelzer D, Trautwein W: Basic features of the frequency and voltage dependent block by D600 of calcium channels in ventricular muscle. *In* Sperelakis N, Caulfield JB, editors: Calcium antagonists. Mechanisms of action on cardiac muscle and vascular smooth muscle. Hingham, MA, 1984, Martinus Nijhoff Publishing, p 118
18. Zipes DP, Fischer JC: Effect of agents which inhibit the slow channel on sinus node automaticity and atrioventricular conduction in the dog. Circ Res **34:** 184, 1974
19. Harapat SR, Kates RE: Rapid high-pressure liquid chromatographic analysis of verapamil in blood and plasma. J Chromatogr **170:** 385, 1979
20. Josephson ME, Seides SF: Clinical cardiac electrophysiology: techniques and interpretations. Philadelphia, 1979, Lea and Febiger, p 23
21. Damato AN, Lau SH, Helfant RH, Stein E, Berkowitz WD, Cohen SI: Study of atrioventricular conduction in man using electrode catheter recordings of His bundle activity. Circulation **39:** 287, 1969
22. Starmer CF, Grant AO, Strauss HC: Mechanisms of use-dependent block of sodium channels in excitable membranes by local anesthetics. Biophys J **46:** 15, 1984
23. Reuter H: Properties of two inward membrane currents in the heart. Ann Rev Physiol **41:** 413, 1979
24. Tsien RW: Calcium channels in excitable cell membranes. Ann Rev Physiol **45:** 341, 1983

25. Hescheler J, Pelzer D, Trube G, Trautwein W: Does the organic calcium channel blocker D600 act from inside or outside on the cardiac cell membrane. Pflugers Arch **393:** 287, 1982
26. Lee KS, Tsien RW: Mechanisms of calcium channel blockade by verapamil, D600, diltiazem and nitrendipine in simple dialyzed heart cells. Nature **302:** 790, 1983
27. Noma A, Irisawa H, Kokobun S, Kotake H, Nishimura M, Watanabe Y: Slow current systems in the A-V node of the rabbit heart. Nature **285:** 228, 1980
28. Reuter H: Calcium channel modulation by neurotransmitters, enzymes and drugs. Nature **301:** 569, 1983
29. Jackman WM, Prystowsky EN, Naccarelli GV, Fineberg NS, Rahilly GT, Heger JJ, Zipes DP: Reevaluation of enhanced atrioventricular nodal conduction evidence to suggest a continuum of normal atrioventricular nodal physiology. Circulation **67:** 441, 1983
30. Bayer R, Kalusche D, Kaufmann R, Mannhold R: Inotropic and electrophysiological actions of verapamil and D600 in mammalian myocardium. III. Effects of optical isomers on transmembrane action potentials. Naunyn-Schmeidebergs Arch Pharmacol **290:** 81, 1975
31. Raschack M: Relationship of antiarrhythmic to inotropic activity and antiarrhythmic qualities of the optical isomers of verapamil. Naunyn-Schmeidebergs Arch Pharmacol **294:** 285, 1976
32. Singh BN, Roche AHG: Effects of intravenous verapamil on hemodynamics in patients with heart disease. Am Heart J **94:** 593, 1977
33. Reiter MJ, Shand DG, Aaronsen LM, Wagoner R, McCarthy E, Pritchett ELC: Pharmacokinetics of verapamil: experience with a sustained intravenous infusion regimen. Am J Cardiol **50:** 716, 1982
34. Hung JS, Yeh SJ, Lin FC, Rose J, Wu D: Calcium channel blockers in the management of paroxysmal supraventricular tachycardia. Clin Prog Pacing Electrophysiol **2:** 325, 1984
35. Wu D, Kou HC, Yeh SJ, Lin FC, Hung JS: Effects of verapamil in patients with atrioventricular reentrant tachycardia incorporating an accessory pathway. Circulation **67:** 426, 1983
36. Mitchell LB, Schroeder JS, Mason JW: Comparative clinical electrophysiologic effects of diltiazem, verapamil and nifedipine: a review. Am J Cardiol **49:** 629, 1982
37. Sung RJ, Elser B, McAllister RG: Intravenous verapamil for termination of re-entrant supraventricular tachycardia. Intracardiac studies correlated with plasma verapamil concentrations. Ann Intern Med **93:** 682, 1980
38. Mangiardi LM, Hariman RH, McAllister RG, Bhargava V, Surawicz B, Shabetai R: Electrophysiologic and hemodynamic effects of verapamil. Correlation with plasma drug concentration. Circulation **57:** 366, 1978
39. Husaini MM, Kvasnicka J, Ryden L, Holmberg S: Action of verapamil on sinus node, atrioventricular and intraventricular conduction. Br Heart J **35:** 734, 1973
40. Rinkenberger RL, Prystowsky EN, Heger JJ, Troup PJ, Jackman WM, Zipes DP: Effects of intravenous and chronic oral verapamil administration in patients with supraventricular tachyarrhythmias. Circulation **62:** 996, 1980

Improvement in regional wall motion and left ventricular relaxation after administration of diltiazem in patients with coronary artery disease

HAROLD DASH, M.D., GARY L. COPENHAVER, B.S., AND SUSAN ENSMINGER, B.A.

ABSTRACT To assess the effect of diltiazem on left ventricular systolic regional wall motion and diastolic function in patients with coronary artery disease (CAD), 22 patients underwent biplane left ventricular cineangiography before and after intravenous diltiazem (plasma concentration 154 ± 12 ng/ml). Left ventricular and right ventricular pressures were measured by micromanometer-tipped catheters. Regional wall motion was assessed quantitatively with an area ejection fraction technique. Diltiazem decreased mean arterial pressure 11.5% ($p < .0001$) and heart rate 6.8% ($p < .005$); it increased cardiac index 8.8% ($p < .025$) and global ejection fraction 9.1% ($p < .0001$). However, left ventricular end-diastolic pressure increased 14.2% ($p < .001$) and the left ventricular end-systolic pressure-volume (P-V) ratio decreased 8.8% ($p < .02$). Diltiazem decreased the time constant of left ventricular relaxation by 14.3% ($p < .002$), despite lack of change in the left ventricular diastolic P-V relationship, in 16 patients. Diltiazem caused a significant increase in area ejection fraction in 53% of hypokinetic areas supplied by diseased arteries compared with 13% of normokinetic areas supplied by diseased arteries ($p < .0001$). Response of ejection fraction to diltiazem in areas supplied by normal coronary arteries was less ($p < .05$) than that in hypokinetic areas supplied by arteries affected by disease. In conclusion, diltiazem improves regional wall motion abnormalities in patients with CAD and the improvement is associated with better left ventricular relaxation but not with a change in the diastolic P-V relationship. Global indexes of left ventricular systolic performance are favorably influenced by diltiazem, despite a mild negative inotropic effect.
Circulation 72, No. 2, 353–363, 1985.

DILTIAZEM HYDROCHLORIDE is a calcium-channel blocker that is effective in the therapy of exertional[1, 2] and variant[3] angina pectoris. Like other calcium-channel blockers, it has complex cardiovascular effects[4–6]: it dilates peripheral and coronary arteries, is a negative inotropic agent, and depresses conduction in the atrioventricular and sinus nodes. The primary hemodynamic effect of intravenous or oral diltiazem is peripheral vasodilation, usually occurring without reflex sympathetic stimulation so that there is no change or a decrease in heart rate.[6, 7] The consequent decrease in the rate-pressure product is thought to be a major mechanism by which diltiazem exerts its protective effect in patients with exercise-induced angina pectoris.[1, 7] Other mechanisms that might protect the myocardium from ischemia have not been demonstrated conclusively. Measurements of total coronary blood flow have shown little change after diltiazem,[7, 8] and it has not been possible to demonstrate a clinically apparent negative inotropic effect of the drug[4, 9, 10] except during acute myocardial ischemia[5] or in an animal preparation of high-output congestive heart failure.[11]

Early in the course of coronary artery disease (CAD), patients develop abnormalities of regional left ventricular contraction[12, 13] and alterations in diastolic function,[14, 15] even in the absence of myocardial infarction. Given the critical role that calcium plays in the processes of cardiac contraction and relaxation, one might expect that the calcium-channel blockers might affect these abnormalities of systolic and diastolic function seen in patients with CAD. Studies[2, 16, 17] have shown that diltiazem improves resting left ventricular global ejection fraction and attenuates the hemodynamic and global ejection fraction abnormalities that develop during exercise-induced angina, but there has been no comprehensive evaluation of the effects of

From the Division of Cardiology, Department of Medicine, Pennsylvania State University College of Medicine, The Milton S. Hershey Medical Center, Hershey, PA.

Supported in part by grants from The South Central Pennsylvania Chapter of the American Heart Association and from Marion Laboratories, Inc.

Address for correspondence: Harold Dash, M.D., The Everett Clinic, Colby at 39th, Everett, WA 98201.

Received May 30, 1984; revision accepted April 30, 1985.

diltiazem on systolic and diastolic ventricular function in patients with CAD. We designed this investigation to assess the effects of diltiazem on left ventricular systolic regional wall motion, left ventricular relaxation, and diastolic compliance in patients with CAD.

Methods

Patient population. Twenty-two patients undergoing cardiac catheterization for the evaluation of chest pain syndromes comprised the study population. All were men and their mean age was 56.5 ± 8.6 (range 41 to 71) years. Criteria for exclusion from the study were presence of unstable angina, acute myocardial infarction within 3 months of catheterization, severe congestive heart failure or hypotension, valvular heart disease, atrial fibrillation, uncontrolled arrhythmias, and second- or third-degree atrioventricular block. All cardioactive medications except long-acting nitrates were discontinued at least 48 hr before catheterization. Long-acting nitrates were discontinued at least 12 hr before the study. The experimental protocol was approved by the Clinical Investigation Committee of The Milton S. Hershey Medical Center, and all patients participating gave informed consent.

Experimental protocol. All patients underwent catheterization, while they were in the fasting state and without premedication, from the femoral approach. Arterial pressure was measured with a cannula inserted into the left radial artery. Baseline right heart pressures were measured with a flow-directed pulmonary artery catheter inserted percutaneously into the right femoral vein. Cardiac output was measured by indicator-dilution technique. The flotation catheter was then exchanged for a No. 7F micromanometer-tipped catheter (Millar Instruments, Inc.), which was positioned in the right ventricle. A No. 8F micromanometer-tipped pigtail injection catheter was then inserted percutaneously into the right femoral artery and advanced to the left ventricle.

Both micromanometer-tipped catheters were calibrated to external transducers, and the calibration was checked at intervals throughout the study. The 0 mm Hg reference level for the external transducer was at the midchest level. All measurements were made during a held, gentle, submaximal inspiration. When performed properly, such a respiratory maneuver results in stable intracardiac pressures.[18] We confirmed that each patient performed the maneuver properly by observing respiratory motion fluoroscopically and intracardiac pressures during pressure recordings. We collected the pressure data on an Electronics for Medicine VR12 recorder set at a 2500 Hz filter and interfaced with an Electronics for Medicine Catheterization Laboratory Computer with a sampling rate of 200 Hz.

After measuring baseline intracardiac pressures, we performed biplane 30 degree right anterior oblique/60 degree left anterior oblique left ventricular cineangiography with 40 ml of 66% diatrizoate meglumine and 10% diatrizoate sodium (Renografin-76) injected at a rate of 12 ml/sec. Film speed was 60 frames/sec. Pressures were measured during the left ventricular cineangiographic examination, and an electrically triggered cine tracer marked the x-ray film and sent a timing signal to the VR12 recorder to allow for simultaneous measurement of pressure and volumes.

After a rest period of 15 to 20 min, intracardiac pressures were again measured to confirm that hemodynamics had returned to baseline. Previous studies[18–20] have documented that such a rest period eliminates any effects of the radio-iodinated contrast agent from the first left ventricular cineangiogram on the systolic and diastolic left ventricular function as determined at the second cineangiographic examination. We then administered diltiazem intravenously as an initial bolus of 0.25 mg/kg followed by a continuous infusion of 0.0014 mg/kg/min for 10 min. The continuous infusion was increased every 2 min by 0.0014 mg/kg/min as necessary to maintain a fall in mean arterial pressure of approximately 10% from baseline. Plasma diltiazem levels were measured before and after the infusion. At the end of 10 min, when systemic arterial pressure was stable, we repeated intracardiac pressure measurements and then obtained a second biplane left ventricular cineangiogram with the use of an identical dose of contrast agent.

After the completion of the protocol, all patients underwent selective coronary angiographic examination by the femoral approach.

Data analysis. We analyzed hemodynamic and volumic data from the first adequately opacified sinus beat within the first five cardiac cycles after injection of contrast agent and did not use postpremature beats. Left ventricular cineangiographic film frames were projected with a Vanguard XR-35 projector and the left ventricular silhouettes were digitized with a Graf-Pen ultrasonic digitizer interfaced with a PDP 11/05 computer. Right and left anterior oblique grids obtained at the time of each study were also digitized to correct for x-ray magnification and distortion. For each patient, the two left ventricular cineangiograms were projected in random order and the investigator was blinded as to their order and identity. Volumes were determined by the biplane area-length method. We measured volumes serially every 33.3 msec.

The digitized pressure data were stored on a magnetic disk for analysis by the PDP 11/05 computer. Simultaneous left ventricular pressures and volumes from the time of minimal diastolic pressure to end-diastolic (post–a wave) pressure were fitted to the polynomial equation

$$P = aV + bV^2 + cV^3 + dV^4 + e \quad (1)$$

where P = left ventricular pressure (mm Hg) and V = left ventricular volume index (ml/m^2). We used multiple linear analysis[21] of the control and diltiazem diastolic pressure-volume (P-V) relationships to assess the adequacy of the P-V fits for each experimental condition. To determine the short-term effect of diltiazem on the left ventricular P-V relationship, we then performed a multiple linear regression analysis of the combined data with the following equation:

$$P = aV^4 + bV^3 + cV^2 + dV + e + f(DTZ) + g(DTZ \times V) \quad (2)$$

where DTZ = 0 during the control state and DTZ = 1 during the drug study. The coefficients a, b, c, d, and e in equation 1 are not necessarily identical to those in equation 2. This type of P-V analysis is a modification of that described by Glantz.[22] Linear regression analysis can tell us whether the terms f(DTZ) and g(DTZ × V) contribute significantly to the diastolic P-V relationship. If f(DTZ) is statistically significant, then diltiazem causes a significant shift in the intercept of the P-V fit; if g(DTZ × V) is statistically significant, then diltiazem causes a significant shift in the slope of the diastolic P-V fit.

The polynomial relationship is an empiric fit between pressure and volume during diastole and thus makes no assumptions about the physiologic interaction of pressure and volume. As a consequence, the coefficients of the equation do not represent indexes of ventricular chamber stiffness. We used such an approach rather than the more traditional exponential analysis because we wanted to evaluate the effect of diltiazem on the entire period of left ventricular filling. The left ventricular diastolic P-V relationship approximates an exponential function only during passive filling when elastic properties of the left ventricle are of paramount importance.[22, 23] Deviation from the exponential occurs during rapid filling and at end-diastole,

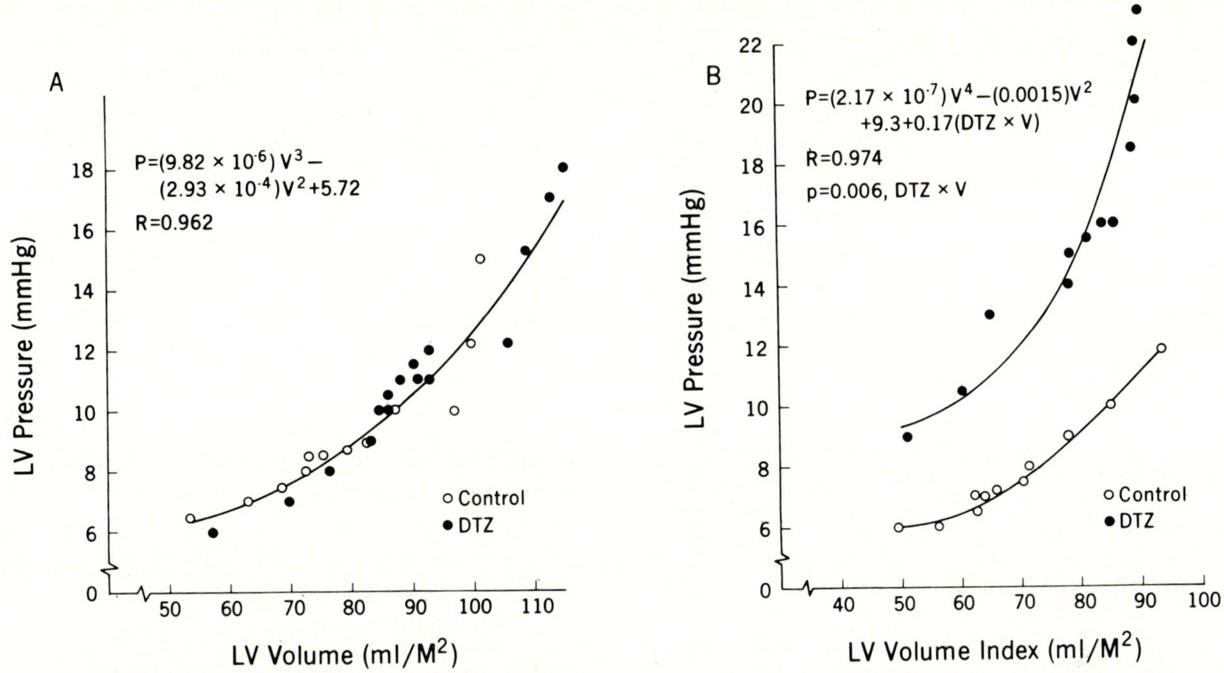

FIGURE 1. *A*, Left ventricular (LV) diastolic pressure volume fit (R = .962) in a patient with no change in compliance after diltiazem (DTZ) despite an increase in LV diastolic pressure (P) and volume (V). *B*, LV diastolic pressure volume fit (R = .974) in a patient with a decrease in LV compliance after diltiazem. DTZ = 0 for the control study and DTZ = 1 for the diltiazem study. The change in slope after DTZ is reflected by the inclusion of the term "DTZ × V" in the equation with p = .006.

when viscous properties of the left ventricle are apparent.[24] Using the polynomial fit we were able to quantify the shifts in the overall left ventricular diastolic P-V relationship caused by diltiazem and using linear regression analysis we were then able to determine whether shifts in the left ventricular diastolic P-V relationship in individual patients were statistically significant (figure 1). This contrasts to previous studies of left ventricular diastolic function in which investigators used grouped data[25–27] to evaluate the effects of an intervention on left ventricular diastolic P-V relationships or assessed the individual P-V fits visually.[28–30] The advantages of the polynomial approach have been discussed previously.[22]

To assess the effect of diltiazem on left ventricular relaxation, we measured the time constant (T) of the negative monoexponential pressure decay during isovolumetric left ventricular relaxation. T was derived according to the method suggested by Craig and Murgo[31] and verified by Thompson et al.[32] Pressure was measured during isovolumetric relaxation every 5 msec from maximum negative dP/dt to a pressure that was 5 mm Hg above the left ventricular end-diastolic pressure of the next beat and fit to the equation

$$P(t) = (P_0 - P_B)\, e^{-t/T} + P_B$$

where P = pressure; t = time; P_0 = pressure at t = 0; P_B = base pressure if isovolumetric left ventricular pressure decay continued indefinitely (t = ∞); T = time constant. By taking the derivative, the equation is transformed to

$$dP(t)/dt = P(t)/T + P_B/T$$

resulting in a linear relationship between dP/dt and P with a slope that is the negative reciprocal of T. T is then derived by linear regression analysis. The validity of such a model depends on how well the model describes the physiologic system. Others have reported that isovolumetric left ventricular relaxation is not exactly a negative monoexponential decay.[33] Consequently, for each beat analyzed we determined the correlation coefficient of the linear relationship between T and left ventricular negative dP/dt. We also used least squares analysis to reconstruct the original equation (the monoexponential equation) from the calculated T. The SEE of such an analysis indicates how closely the mathematic model actually fits the raw pressure data. We measured at least 25 beats in every patient. In all cases an R value greater than .953 and an SEE less than 1.7 mm Hg were obtained, indicating that in our patients, T accurately described the time constant of left ventricular relaxation. Because recent work has suggested that T is load dependent,[33] we assessed the effects of diltiazem-induced changes in load on T by linear regression analysis. The other index of left ventricular relaxation measured was maximum negative dP/dt.

We evaluated left ventricular systolic function by measuring the ejection phase indexes of global ejection fraction and mean velocity of circumferential fiber shortening (Vcf), the isovolumetric index of maximum positive dP/dt, and the left ventricular end-systolic P-V ratio.[34]

In addition to global left ventricular systolic function, we assessed regional wall motion with a quantitative area ejection fraction technique.[35] The left ventricle was divided into eight areas. End-diastolic and end-systolic left ventricular silhouettes were identified with use of frame-by-frame analysis. For each area

$$\text{Area EF} = \frac{\text{End-diastolic area} - \text{end-systolic area}}{\text{End-diastolic area}}$$

where EF is ejection fraction. Normokinesis was considered to be present when the area ejection fraction was within 1 SD of the normal mean value for our laboratory; hypokinesis was defined as an area ejection fraction of less than 1 SD of the normal mean value. A statistically significant change in area ejection fraction caused by diltiazem was defined as a change beyond the 95% confidence intervals of random variability in this value as determined in our laboratory.[36] Such an approach allowed us to quantitate significant changes in regional wall motion not only in individual patients, but also in individual left ventricular regions.

Significant CAD was defined as a coronary stenosis of greater than 70% of luminal diameter. For each patient, the relationship between regional CAD and myocardial area was documented. Those areas jeopardized by CAD were defined as CAD areas. The effect of diltiazem on area ejection fraction and its relation to CAD areas was determined by chi-square analysis.

To assess the influence of baseline left ventricular function on the results, we divided the patients into two groups according to the presence or absence of baseline left ventricular dysfunction, as defined by the range of normal values for our laboratory. The criteria used were an elevated left ventricular end-diastolic volume index (≥100 ml/m^2), elevated left ventricular end-diastolic pressure (≥17 mm Hg when measured during ventriculography), or a depressed global ejection fraction (<0.54).

To compare data obtained at control and after diltiazem in individual patients, we used the paired t test. Group comparisons of continuous data were evaluated with the t test for differences between group means or, when multiple comparisons were made, analysis of variance. All data are mean ± SEM.

Results

Clinical characteristics. Twenty of the 22 patients had CAD. All had stable angina pectoris and 14 had suffered prior myocardial infarction. Multivessel CAD was common: 13 patients had three-vessel disease, four had two-vessel disease, and three had one-vessel disease. Left ventricular asynergy was present in 19 of the 20 patients with CAD and in neither of the patients with normal coronary arteries. The amount of left ventricle jeopardized by CAD averaged 65.9 ± 6.2%. The two patients with normal coronary arteries had atypical chest pain and normal resting left ventricular function. They have been included in the study because eliminating their data from the analysis did not alter the results.

Effect of diltiazem on hemodynamics and left ventricular volume. Table 1 shows that diltiazem caused significant decreases in mean arterial pressure (11.5%), left ventricular systolic pressure (13.5%), calculated systemic vascular resistance (20.8%), and heart rate (6.8%). Cardiac output increased 8.8% and left ventricular stroke volume index increased 16.7%. Significant changes in the ejection phase indexes of left ventricular function indicated an improvement in left ventricular systolic performance: Global ejection fraction increased 9.1% from 0.55 ± 0.02 to 0.60 ± 0.02 and left ventricular mean Vcf increased 10.3%. In addition, left ventricular end-systolic volume index decreased by 7.6%. The findings indicate that diltiazem given intravenously reduced afterload acutely and improved global left ventricular systolic performance. The extent of improvement in left ventricular systolic function as assessed by percentage increase in global ejection fraction correlated with the percentage decrease in left ventricular systolic pressure ($R = .564$, $p < .01$).

Despite the improvement in global left ventricular systolic performance, diltiazem had some intrinsic negative inotropic effects (table 1). The significant fall

TABLE 1
Hemodynamics and left ventricular volumes and function before and after diltiazem (n = 22)

	C	D	% Change	p value
Heart rate (beats/min)	68.7±3.3	64.0±2.6	−6.8	<.005
Mean systemic arterial pressure (mm Hg)	101.3±2.6	89.6±2.0	−11.5	<.0001
LV systolic pressure (mm Hg)	141.2±4.2	122.1±3.9	−13.5	<.0001
LV end-diastolic pressure (mm Hg)	17.6±1.1	20.1±1.0	+14.2	<.001
LV maximum positive dP/dt (mm Hg/sec)	1470±66	1315±53	−10.5	<.001
LV maximum negative dP/dt (mm Hg/sec)	−1782±87	−1655±88	−7.1	<.02
T (msec)	68.5±7.3	58.7±5.5	−14.3	<.002
P_B (mm Hg)	−14.2±2.8	−7.7±2.3	+45.8	<.0001
RV systolic pressure (mm Hg)	29.0±1.8	30.7±1.6	+5.9	<.03
RV end-diastolic pressure (mm Hg)	9.3±0.7	10.0±0.6	+7.5	NS
Cardiac index (l/min/m^2)	3.20±0.14	3.48±0.12	+8.8	<.025
Systemic vascular resistance (dynes-sec-cm^{-5})	1290±52	1022±39	−20.8	<.0001
LV end-diastolic volume index (ml/m^2)	86.9±3.3	91.8±3.3	+5.6	<.005
LV end-systolic volume index (ml/m^2)	39.7±2.6	36.7±2.4	−7.6	<.002
LV stroke volume index (ml/m^2)	47.2±1.9	55.1±2.5	+16.7	<.001
LV global EF	0.55±0.02	0.60±0.02	+9.1	<.0001
LV mean Vcf (circ/sec)	1.07±0.09	1.18±0.08	+10.3	<.025
LV end-systolic P-V ratio	3.29±0.24	3.00±0.20	−8.8	<.02

All data are mean ± SEM.

C = control; D = diltiazem; LV = left ventricular; RV = right ventricular; EF = ejection fraction.

of 10.5% in left ventricular maximum positive dP/dt may have reflected the decrease in afterload rather than negative inotropy, but the left ventricular end-systolic P-V ratio also decreased by 8.8% after diltiazem. Diltiazem increased left ventricular end-diastolic pressure significantly (14.2%) from 17.6 ± 1.1 to 20.1 ± 1.0 mm Hg. This increase in pressure was paralleled by a mild increase in right ventricular systolic pressure, but occurred without any significant change in end-diastolic pressure in the right ventricle. In addition to the increase in left ventricular end-diastolic pressure, diltiazem also significantly increased the left ventricular end-diastolic volume index by 5.6%.

Effect of diltiazem on the left ventricular diastolic P-V relationship and left ventricular relaxation. We were able to generate left ventricular diastolic P-V fits in 20 of the 22 patients. In the other two patients, the cine tracer failed, preventing us from correlating simultaneous left ventricular pressures and volumes. In the 20 patients, the diastolic P-V fits to polynomial equation 1 for both control and diltiazem P-V curves were excellent, with the correlation coefficients ranging from .955 to .996. The mean correlation coefficient for these left ventricular diastolic P-V relationships was .976 ± .002. When the data obtained at control and after diltiazem were combined and analyzed with polynomial equation 2, the correlation coefficients ranged from .956 to .988, with a mean of .972 ± .002. Thus, combining the two sets of data to create a single polynomial equation did not degrade the "goodness" of fit of the diastolic P-V analysis.

In 16 of the 20 patients there was no change in the left ventricular diastolic P-V relationship after diltiazem (figure 1, *A*). In three patients there was an upward shift after diltiazem caused by a change in slope in two patients (figure 1, *B*) and a change in intercept in one patient. In none of these three patients did right ventricular end-diastolic pressure increase more than 1 mm Hg after diltiazem. In one patient there was a downward shift in the intercept of the left ventricular diastolic P-V relationship after diltiazem. This patient experienced no change in right ventricular end-diastolic pressure after diltiazem. Thus, in most patients diltiazem had no effect on the left ventricular diastolic P-V relationship, despite increasing left ventricular end-diastolic pressure and volume.

Diltiazem improved left ventricular relaxation significantly (table 1), shortening T by 14.3% ($p < .002$). T decreased in 18 of the 22 patients. The improvement in relaxation rate was not accompanied by an increase in left ventricular maximum negative dP/dt, perhaps because of the load dependency of maximum negative

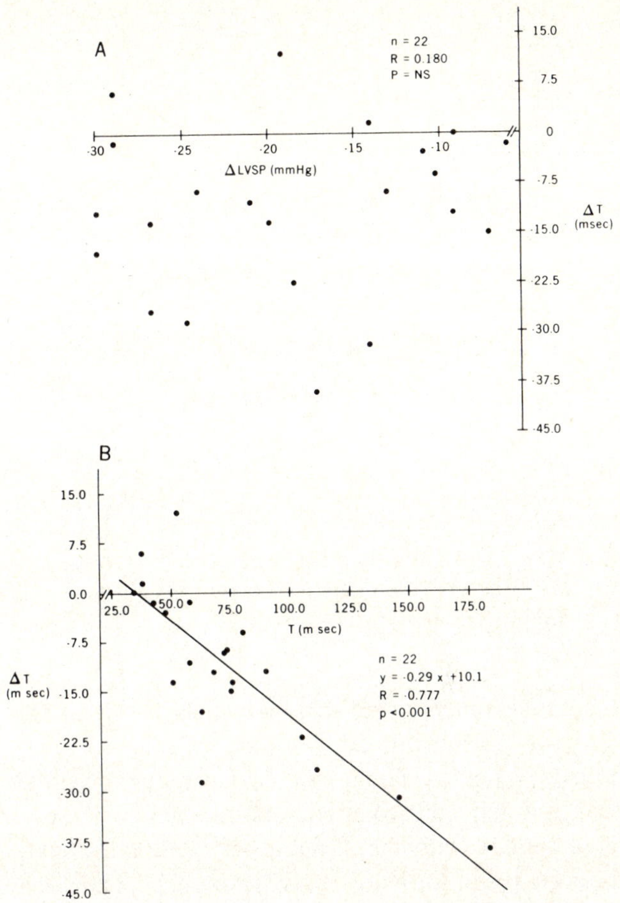

FIGURE 2. *A*, Lack of correlation between the change in left ventricular systolic pressure (ΔLVSP) after diltiazem and the change in relaxation rate (ΔT). *B*, Correlation (R = −.777) between the baseline relaxation rate (T) and the change in ΔT after diltiazem.

dP/dt. The effect of load on T is illustrated in figure 2, *A*; the changes in T did not correlate with changes in left ventricular pressure ($R < .200$). We obtained similar results when T was compared with left ventricular end-diastolic pressure or end-systolic volume. P_B, the asymptote of the monoexponential equation describing isovolumetric relaxation, was negative in patients at rest ($P_B = -14.2 \pm 2.8$ mm Hg) and became less negative (by 45.8%) after diltiazem. Changes in P_B were unrelated to changes in left ventricular end-systolic volume (R = .294).

Influence of baseline left ventricular function on the effects of diltiazem. Thirteen patients had abnormal and nine normal baseline left ventricular function. There were no significant differences in the effects of diltiazem on hemodynamic variables, left ventricular volumes, global left ventricular systolic function, or left ventricular relaxation in the two groups of patients. However, the three patients in whom there was an upward shift in the left ventricular diastolic P-V relationship after diltiazem all had normal baseline left

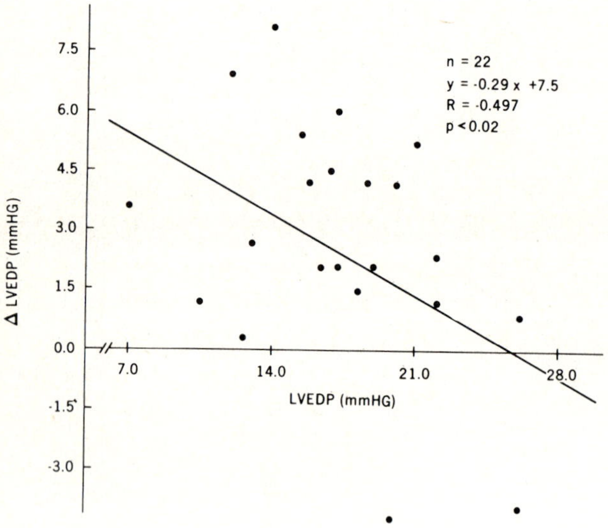

FIGURE 3. There was a weak correlation (R = −.497) between resting left ventricular end-diastolic pressure (LVEDP) and the change in end-diastolic pressure (ΔLVEDP) after diltiazem.

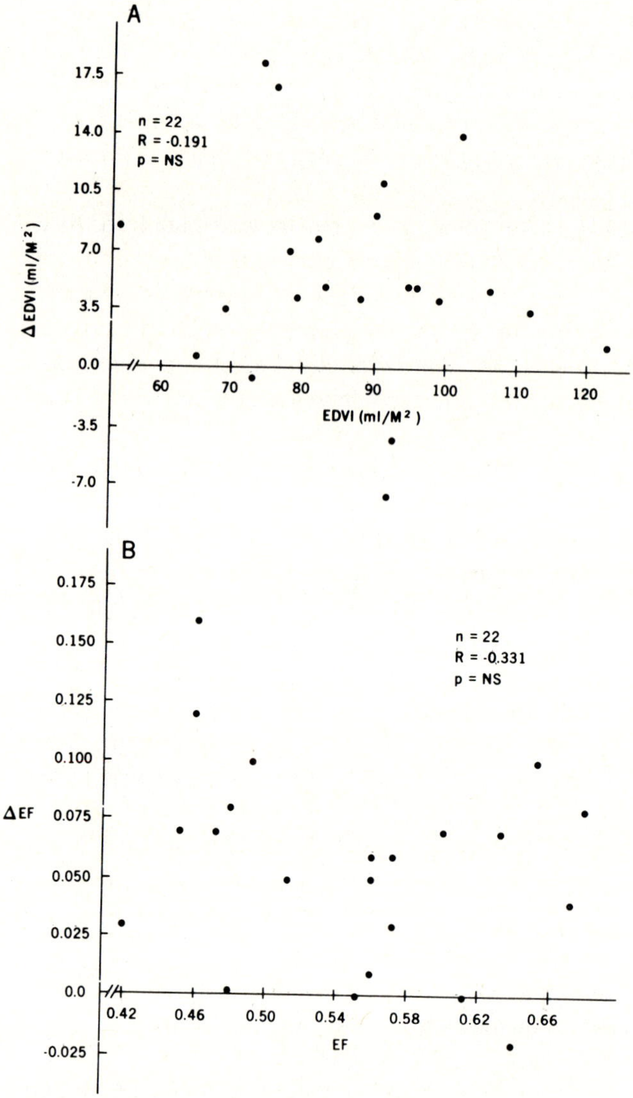

FIGURE 4. *A*, Lack of correlation between resting left ventricular end-diastolic volume index (EDVI) and the change in end-diastolic volume index (ΔEDVI) after diltiazem. *B*, Lack of correlation between resting global ejection fraction (EF) and the change in ejection fraction (ΔEF) after diltiazem.

ventricular function and the one patient in whom the shift was downward had abnormal baseline left ventricular function. Figure 3 demonstrates that the change in left ventricular end-diastolic pressure correlated weakly with the baseline left ventricular end-diastolic pressure ($R = -.497$, $p < .02$). Thus, the negative inotropic effect of diltiazem was somewhat less apparent at higher baseline levels of left ventricular end-diastolic pressure. On the other hand, figure 4 illustrates that changes in left ventricular end-diastolic volume and global ejection fraction were completely unrelated to the baseline values. Figure 2, *B*, shows that the effect of diltiazem on left ventricular relaxation was strongly correlated with the baseline relaxation rate ($R = -.777$, $p < .001$). Diltiazem improved left ventricular relaxation the most when baseline T was markedly prolonged.

Effect of diltiazem on left ventricular systolic regional wall motion. We were able to analyze regional wall motion in 21 of the 22 patients. One patient shifted his position between cineangiograms, preventing evaluation of comparable areas for the control and diltiazem studies. There were 47 areas supplied by normal coronary arteries or in which CAD was nonocclusive and there were 121 areas supplied by arteries with significant CAD. Response of area ejection fraction was unrelated to regional CAD in general: there was significant improvement in area ejection fraction in 40 (33%) CAD areas after diltiazem compared with 13 (28%) areas supplied by normal arteries ($p =$ NS). A significant decrease in area ejection fraction after diltiazem was noted in only four areas: two CAD areas with resting hypokinesis and two areas supplied by normal coronary arteries with resting normokinesis.

Of the 121 CAD areas, baseline contraction was normal in 60 and hypokinetic in 61. After diltiazem, there was a significant increase in area ejection fraction in 32 (53%) hypokinetic CAD areas compared with only eight (13%) normokinetic CAD areas ($p < .001$). This is reflected in the magnitude of the area ejection fraction response to diltiazem, as depicted in figure 5. In the normokinetic CAD areas, area ejection fraction increased from 0.51 ± 0.015 to 0.53 ± 0.017 after diltiazem, a small but statistically significant ($p < .02$) improvement. In the hypokinetic CAD areas there was a larger increase in area ejection fraction from $0.33 \pm$

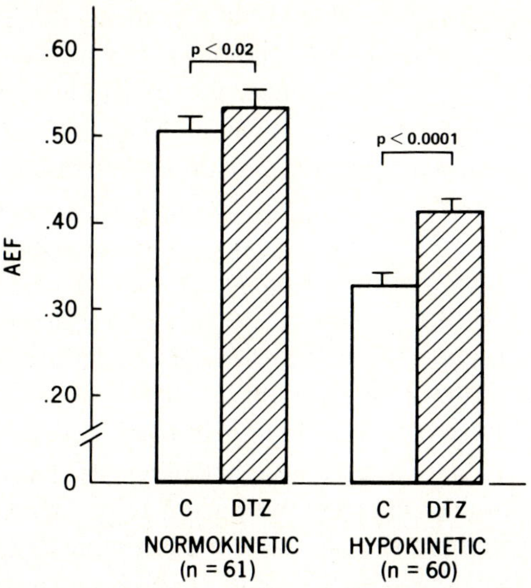

FIGURE 5. Response of area ejection fraction (AEF) to diltiazem in areas supplied by coronary arteries with significant disease. Areas with normokinesis at baseline are on the left; areas with hypokinesis at baseline are on the right. C = control; D = diltiazem.

0.014 to 0.42 ± 0.014 ($p < .0001$). When both regional CAD and resting wall motion abnormalities were taken into consideration, the percent increase in area ejection fraction in the hypokinetic CAD areas after diltiazem was significantly greater than the percent increases in the hypokinetic areas supplied by normal arteries or the normokinetic CAD and "non-CAD" areas (figure 6). Figure 7 illustrates the effect of diltiazem on regional wall motion abnormalities in a patient with a 90% stenosis of the proximal right coronary artery. The inferior wall hypokinesis (areas 4 and 5) that was present at baseline improved significantly after diltiazem.

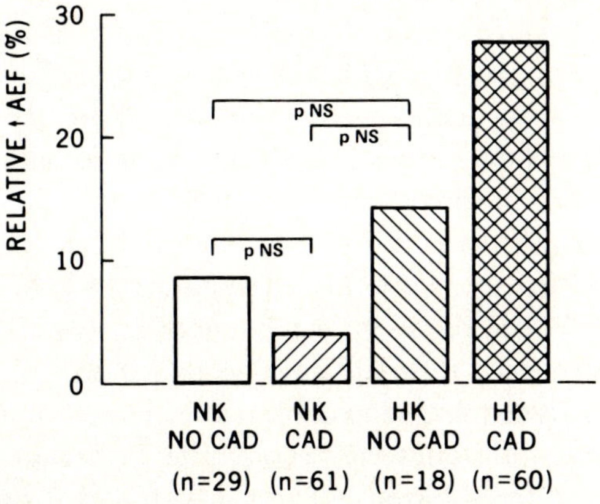

FIGURE 6. Percent increase in area ejection fraction (↑ AEF) after diltiazem compared with at baseline. NK, NO CAD = normokinetic areas supplied by normal coronary arteries; NK, CAD = normokinetic areas supplied by coronary artery disease; HK, NO CAD = hypokinetic areas supplied by normal coronary arteries; HK, CAD = hypokinetic areas supplied by coronary artery disease.

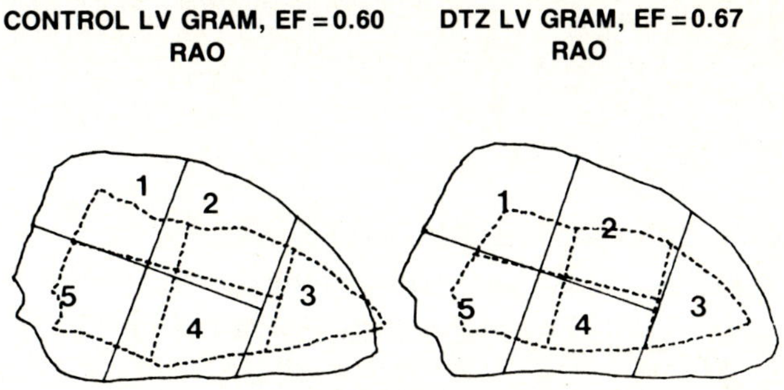

FIGURE 7. Control left ventricular cineangiogram (LV Gram) and LV Gram obtained after diltiazem (DTZ) in the right anterior oblique (RAO) projection with the ventricle divided into five areas. The solid line is the end-diastolic LV tracing and the dashed line is the end-systolic LV tracing. The patient had single-vessel coronary artery disease with a severe proximal right coronary stenosis. There was baseline inferior hypokinesis (ejection fraction [EF] of area 4 = 0.28 and of area 5 = 0.27). After diltiazem, there was a significant increase in EF to 0.44 in both areas.

Plasma diltiazem levels. No patient had a measurable level of diltiazem during the control study. At the time of the postdiltiazem left ventricular cineangiographic study the mean plasma diltiazem level was 154 ± 12 ng/ml.

Discussion

Effects of diltiazem on global left ventricular systolic function. The results of this study indicate that diltiazem has complex effects on cardiac function in patients with CAD. The plasma diltiazem levels achieved in our patients were similar to those reported in studies[37] of patients taking oral diltiazem for the therapy of angina pectoris. Thus, the hemodynamic effects that we have documented here are probably comparable to those that can be expected in clinical practice.

Our data confirm the results of others[2, 16, 17] that diltiazem improves such afterload-dependent indexes of global left ventricular systolic performance as ejection fraction, cardiac index, and stroke volume index. On the other hand, we found in our patients that diltiazem did have some intrinsic negative inotropic effects, causing a decrease in the left ventricular end-systolic P-V ratio in conjunction with an increase in left ventricular end-diastolic pressure and volume. In addition, it is possible that the slower heart rate after diltiazem, by lengthening the diastolic filling period, resulted in some increase in left ventricular end-diastolic volume. Our findings are in contrast to those reported recently by Walsh et al.[10] in a group of patients with congestive heart failure. In their patients, left ventricular filling pressure decreased after diltiazem and a negative inotropic effect was not demonstrable. Differences in both method and patient populations most likely account for the discrepant results. Walsh's patients had a greater decrease in arterial pressure than our patients and their baseline left ventricular function was much worse. Of interest, therefore, is our finding that the negative inotropic effect of diltiazem tended to be least apparent in those patients with the highest resting left ventricular end-diastolic pressures (figure 3).

Effect of diltiazem on abnormalities of diastolic function in patients with CAD. Previous investigations have demonstrated that left ventricular relaxation is often slowed[15] and left ventricular compliance diminished[14] in patients with CAD. Although abnormalities are most marked during episodes of acute myocardial ischemia when the left ventricular diastolic P-V relationship shifts upward acutely and left ventricular relaxation is prolonged,[25, 28, 38] they are also present at rest. In some cases, myocardial scarring may account for the resting abnormalities in diastolic function; in others, the pathophysiologic mechanism is uncertain. It has been suggested that chronic ischemia is present; however, no myocardial lactate production is noted in patients with stable angina pectoris when they are studied in the asymptomatic state. Braunwald and Kloner[39] recently hypothesized the concept of the "stunned myocardium," in which postischemic myocardium is depleted of ATP reserves and calcium metabolism is deranged, to account for the left ventricular systolic regional wall motion abnormalities that occur in patients with CAD in the absence of myocardial infarction or active ischemia. Because left ventricular relaxation depends on calcium sequestration in the sarcoplasmic reticulum of myocardial fibers and is an energy-dependent process, the stunned myocardium may not only result in abnormalities of contraction but also those of relaxation.

The beneficial effect of diltiazem on diastolic function in our patients was confined to early diastolic events, with a significant improvement in left ventricular relaxation rate as measured by T. Diltiazem may have influenced relaxation in several ways. First, relaxation is a process often dependent on load.[40] In our patients, the effects of dilatiazem on load were variable, with a decrease in afterload and an increase in load at end-diastole. Although we found no relationship between T and systolic or end-diastolic pressure, it is possible that had we measured a more sensitive index of load, such as wall stress, we might have found a relationship. Second, impairment of calcium sequestration[41] may prolong the myocardial inactivation process in patients with CAD, leading to delayed relaxation. Although the effects of diltiazem on intracellular calcium metabolism are unknown, it is possible that the drug improved left ventricular relaxation by direct effects on myocardial inactivation. Third, left ventricular relaxation rate depends on the degree of uniformity of contraction throughout the ventricle.[40] In patients with CAD, Gibson et al.[42] have demonstrated localized delays in left ventricular relaxation with resting asynergy. Thus, the improvement in systolic regional wall motion after diltiazem may have led to an increase in left ventricular relaxation rate.

In contrast to our results with diltiazem, Ludbrook et al.[27] found that nifedipine did not affect left ventricular relaxation. The differing results may in part be related to the different methods used for calculating T, different mechanisms of action of the two drugs,[4] or to the different patient populations in the two studies. Most of our patients had left ventricular asynergy, whereas most patients in the previous study did not. The effect of diltiazem on left ventricular relaxation in our patients was greatest in those with the most abnormal baseline left ventricular relaxation rate (figure 2, *B*). Therefore, the difference between the previous study and ours may in part be one of degree. It is of interest to note that nifedipine did improve left ventricular relaxation in patients with hypertrophic cardiomyopathy,[29] a condition in which left ventricular relaxation is seriously deranged.

We found that, in addition to its effect on T, diltiazem also significantly altered P_B, but how P_B is related to left ventricular relaxation is uncertain. Yellin et al.[43] have reported that left ventricular pressure becomes negative if the mitral valve orifice is occluded transiently and left ventricular relaxation is allowed to continue uninterrupted by left ventricular filling. They reported that the extent of left ventricular relaxation correlated inversely with left ventricular end-systolic volume, with more negative pressure at smaller end-systolic volumes. Our finding that P_B is usually less than zero is in agreement and is supported by the work of Thompson et al.[44] However, we found no correlation between P_B and left ventricular end-systolic volume. If P_B did represent the extent of left ventricular relaxation, then it should have become more negative as T shortened and relaxation rate increased. Our results with diltiazem were the opposite: P_B became less negative after diltiazem. Others have reported similar directional changes in P_B and T.[44, 45] It is therefore probable that P_B does not represent the extent of left ventricular relaxation but rather is a theoretic term that contributes to the mathematic description of left ventricular pressure decay during isovolumetric relaxation. The interaction of left ventricular filling with left ventricular relaxation most likely invalidates any direct calculation of the extent of left ventricular relaxation in the intact heart.

The lack of effect of diltiazem on the left ventricular diastolic P-V relationship was unexpected given the drug's beneficial effect on left ventricular relaxation. In our patients, left ventricular relaxation may not have been sufficiently impaired in the resting state to affect the left ventricular diastolic P-V relationship. Other factors that may shift the left ventricular diastolic P-V relationship acutely, such as right ventricular diastolic dynamics[26] and coronary perfusion,[46] were probably not affected by diltiazem. Diltiazem did not alter right ventricular diastolic pressure in our patients; therefore, ventricular interaction was not important. This is in contrast to studies of nifedipine[27] and nitroglycerin[26] in which downward shifts in the left ventricular diastolic P-V relationship occurred in conjunction with decreases in right heart pressures. We did not measure coronary perfusion, but two recent studies[7, 8] have suggested that total coronary sinus flow does not change after intravenous diltiazem in patients with CAD. The upward shifts in the left ventricular diastolic P-V relationship in three patients with normal baseline left ventricular function remain unexplained. These three patients had no clinical characteristics or hemodynamic responses to diltiazem that distinguished them from the other patients with normal left ventricular function at baseline. Similarly, the reason for the downward shift in the left ventricular diastolic P-V relationship after diltiazem in one patient with abnormal baseline left ventricular function is unknown, since he had hemodynamic responses to the drug similar to those of the other patients with abnormal baseline function.

Systolic regional wall motion response to diltiazem. Given the beneficial effect of diltiazem on global left ventricular relaxation and the known association between abnormalities of relaxation and contraction in patients with CAD, it is not surprising that the drug significantly improved area ejection fraction in hypokinetic areas supplied by diseased arteries (figures 5 to 7). The increase in area ejection fraction in hypokinetic areas did not occur at the expense of normokinetic areas because the latter did not decrease area ejection fraction after diltiazem. Reversal of resting systolic regional wall motion abnormalities has been reported previously after administration of nitroglycerin,[13] but not after the administration of other calcium-channel blockers. Vliestra et al.[47] reported no change in regional wall motion after administration of intravenous verapamil. Two studies[48, 49] have shown that nifedipine did not alter resting wall motion abnormalities in patients with CAD, although it did prevent exercise-induced abnormalities. The differences reported here may relate to varying mechanisms of action of the three agents, methodologic differences among various studies, and the differing patient populations.

Several mechanisms may have contributed to the favorable effect of diltiazem on left ventricular systolic regional wall motion. The improvements in regional systolic contraction may have correlated with more rapid local left ventricular relaxation. Ludbrook et al.[50] noted improvement in regional left ventricular relaxation associated with reversal of regional wall motion abnormalities after administration of nitroglycerin in patients with CAD. We did not measure regional relaxation and this must be considered a limitation of our study, but the increase in global left ventricular relaxation rate after diltiazem that was associated with improvement in regional left ventricular systolic function does support the concept that in our patients, relaxation and contraction abnormalities in CAD areas were interrelated.

The arterial vasodilating effect of diltiazem contributed to the improvement in global left ventricular systolic function and may have played a role in increasing regional contraction as well. Our analysis of regional left ventricular systolic contraction suggests that other factors were also important, because clinically evident increases in area ejection fraction occurred primarily in left ventricular areas that were supplied by stenosed coronary arteries and were hypokinetic at rest. If the improvements were secondary only to afterload reduction, area ejection fraction would be expected to increase similarly in all regions. Mechanisms that might account for the ability of diltiazem to improve regional contraction selectively in asynergic areas of the left ventricle supplied by diseased arteries include effects on regional coronary blood flow, calcium metabolism, and ATP utilization. Although intravenous diltiazem does not alter total myocardial blood flow,[7, 8] Bache and Dymek[51] have shown that it partially corrects the derangement in the subendocardial/subepicardial flow ratio that occurs in a dog preparation of acute myocardial ischemia. Moreover, Malacoff et al.[52] showed that another calcium-channel blocker, nifedipine, improves regional myocardial flow distal to stenosed coronary arteries. Nifedipine also prevents the accumulation of intracellular calcium that occurs during acute myocardial ischemia.[41] Of note, therefore, is the observation of Weishaar et al.[53] in a dog preparation of regional ischemia that diltiazem reduces ATP depletion, diminishes lactate production, and improves contractility in the ischemic area of the left ventricle. No studies have been performed to evaluate the effects of a calcium-channel blocker on regional left ventricular function in a preparation that simulates the stunned myocardium, which was likely present in the patients studied here. But if the stunned myocardium does represent a postischemic state in which coronary flow is marginal, ATP is depleted, and calcium metabolism is deranged, then diltiazem might potentially exert its beneficial effects through any of the mechanisms described above.

In conclusion, intravenous diltiazem in a dose that provided a plasma level comparable to that reported for effective therapy of angina pectoris improved global left ventricular systolic performance, regional wall motion, and left ventricular relaxation rate in patients with CAD. The favorable effects of diltiazem on left ventricular performance occurred despite evidence of a mild negative inotropic effect. The improvement in regional contraction was confined to areas supplied by diseased arteries in which there was resting hypokinesis. The increase in left ventricular relaxation rate occurred without any overall effect on the left ventricular diastolic P-V relationship.

We could not have completed this study without the assistance of the technicians and nurses in the Cardiac Catheterization Laboratory. We are grateful to Lori Skalland for providing biostatistical assistance and to Susan Landucci and Verna Ebersole for typing the manuscript. Robert Zelis provided helpful suggestions during the preparation of the manuscript.

References

1. Hossack KF, Pool PE, Steele P, Crawford MH, DeMaria AN, Cohen LS, Ports TA: Efficacy of diltiazem in angina of effort: a multicenter trial. Am J Cardiol **49:** 567, 1982
2. Petru MA, Crawford MH, Sorenson SG, Chaudhuri TK, Levine S, O'Rourke RA: Short- and long-term efficacy of high-dose oral diltiazem for angina due to coronary artery disease: a placebo-controlled, randomized, double-blind crossover study. Circulation **68:** 139, 1983
3. Schroeder JS, Feldman RL, Giles TD, Friedman MJ, DeMaria AN, Kinney EL, Mallon SM, Pitt B, Meyer R, Basta LL, Curry RC Jr, Groves BM, MacAlpin RN: Multiclinic controlled trial of diltiazem for Prinzmetal's angina. Am J Med **72:** 227, 1982
4. Millard RW, Grupp G, Grupp IL, DiSalvo J, DePover A, Schwartz A: Chronotropic, inotropic, and vasodilator actions of diltiazem, nifedipine, and verapamil: A comparative study of physiological responses and membrane receptor activity. Circ Res **52**(suppl I): I-29, 1983
5. Urquhart J, Patterson RE, Bacharach SL, Green MV, Speir EH, Aamodt R: Comparative effects of verapamil, diltiazem, and nifedipine on hemodynamics and left ventricular function during acute myocardial ischemia in dogs. Circulation **69:** 382, 1984
6. Mitchell LB, Schroeder JS, Mason JW: Comparative clinical electrophysiologic effects of diltiazem, verapamil and nifedipine: a review. Am J Cardiol **49:** 629, 1982
7. Joyal M, Cremer KF, Feldman RL, Pieper JA, Pepine CJ: Is coronary vasodilation due to diltiazem responsible for relief of stress-induced angina? Circulation **68**(suppl III): III-18, 1983 (abst)
8. Bertrand ME, Dupuis BA, Lablanche JM, Tilmant PY, Thieuleux FA: Coronary hemodynamics following intravenous or intracoronary injection of diltiazem in man. J Cardiovasc Pharmacol **4:** 695, 1982
9. Walsh RA, Badke FR, O'Rourke RA: Differential effects of systemic and intracoronary calcium channel blocking agents on global and regional left ventricular function in conscious dogs. Am Heart J **102:** 341, 1981
10. Walsh RW, Porter CB, Starling MR, O'Rourke RA: Beneficial hemodynamic effects of intravenous and oral diltiazem in severe congestive heart failure. J Am Coll Cardiol **3:** 1044, 1984
11. Porter CB, Walsh RA, Badke FR, O'Rourke RA: Differential effects of diltiazem and nitroprusside on left ventricular function in experimental chronic volume overload. Circulation **68:** 685, 1983
12. Herman MV, Heinle RA, Klein MD, Gorlin R: Localized disorders in myocardial contraction: asynergy and its role in congestive heart failure. N Engl J Med **277:** 222, 1967
13. McAnulty JH, Hattenhauer MT, Rosch J, Kloster FE, Rahimtoola SH: Improvement in left ventricular wall motion following nitroglycerin. Circulation **51:** 140, 1975
14. Diamond G, Forrester JS: Effect of coronary artery disease and acute myocardial infarction on left ventricular compliance in man. Circulation **45:** 11, 1972
15. Papatietro SE, Coghlan HC, Zissermann D, Russell RO Jr, Rackley CE, Rogers WJ: Impaired maximal rate of left ventricular relaxation in patients with coronary artery disease and left ventricular dysfunction. Circulation **59:** 984, 1979
16. Hossack KF, Bruce RA, Ritterman JB, Kusumi F, Trimble S: Divergent effects of diltiazem in patients with exertional angina. Am J Cardiol **49:** 538, 1982
17. Hung J, Lamb IH, Connolly SJ, Jutzy KR, Goris ML, Schroeder JS: The effect of diltiazem and propranolol, alone and in combination, on exercise performance and left ventricular function in patients with stable effort angina: a double-blind, randomized, and placebo-controlled study. Circulation **68:** 560, 1983
18. Ludbrook PA, Byrne JD, Kurnik PB, McKnight RC: Influence of reduction of preload and afterload by nitroglycerin on left ventricular diastolic pressure-volume relations and relaxation in man. Circulation **56:** 937, 1977
19. Friesinger GC, Schaffer J, Criley JM, Gaertner RA, Ross RS: Hemodynamic consequences of the injection of radiopaque material. Circulation **31:** 730, 1965
20. Cohn PF, Levine JA, Bergeron GA, Gorlin R: Reproducibility of the angiographic left ventricular ejection fraction in patients with coronary artery disease. Am Heart J **88:** 713, 1974
21. Dixon WJ, Brown MB, editors: Biomedical computer programs P-Series. Berkeley, 1979, University of California Press, p 380–417
22. Glantz SA: Computing indices of diastolic stiffness has been counterproductive. Fed Proc **39:** 162, 1980
23. Noble MIM, Milne ENC, Goerke RJ, Carlsson E, Domenech RJ, Saunders KB, Hoffman JIE: Left ventricular filling and diastolic pressure-volume relations in the conscious dog. Circ Res **24:** 269, 1969
24. Rankin JS, Arentzen CE, McHale PA, Ling D, Anderson RW: Viscoelastic properties of the diastolic left ventricle in the conscious dog. Circ Res **41:** 37, 1977
25. Barry WH, Brooker JZ, Alderman EL, Harrison DC: Changes in diastolic stiffness and tone of the left ventricle during angina pectoris. Circulation **49:** 255, 1974
26. Ludbrook PA, Byrne JD, McKnight RC: Influence of right ventricular hemodynamics on left ventricular diastolic pressure-volume relations in man. Circulation **59:** 21, 1979
27. Ludbrook PA, Tiefenbrunn AJ, Reed FR, Sobel BE: Acute hemodynamic responses to sublingual nifedipine: Dependence on left ventricular function. Circulation **65:** 489, 1982
28. Dwyer EM Jr: Left ventricular pressure-volume alterations and regional disorders of contraction during myocardial ischemia induced by atrial pacing. Circulation **42:** 1111, 1970
29. Lorell BH, Paulus WJ, Grossman W, Wynne J, Cohn PF: Modification of abnormal left ventricular diastolic properties by nifedipine in patients with hypertrophic cardiomyopathy. Circulation **65:** 499, 1982
30. Mann T, Brodie BR, Grossman W, McLaurin LP: Effect of angina on the left ventricular diastolic pressure-volume relationship. Circulation **55:** 761, 1977
31. Craig WE, Murgo JP: Evaluation of isovolumic relaxation in nor-

mal man during rest, exercise and isoproterenol infusion. Circulation **62**(suppl III): III-92, 1980 (abst)
32. Thompson DS, Waldron CB, Coltart DJ, Jenkins BS, Webb-Peploe MM: Estimation of time constant of left ventricular relaxation. Br Heart J **49:** 250, 1983
33. Raff GL, Glantz SA: Volume loading slows left ventricular isovolumic relaxation rate: Evidence of load-dependent relaxation in the intact dog heart. Circ Res **48:** 813, 1981
34. Grossman W, Braunwald E, Mann T, McLaurin LP, Green LH: Contractile state of the left ventricle in man as evaluated from end-systolic pressure-volume relations. Circulation **56:** 845, 1977
35. Gelberg HJ, Brundage BH, Glantz S, Parmley WW: Quantitative left ventricular wall motion analysis: A comparison of area, chord and radial methods. Circulation **59:** 991, 1979
36. Dash H, Wint RM: Quantitative variability in regional wall motion during serial left ventricular cineangiography: Guidelines for assessing changes in segmental function with intervention studies. Am J Cardiol **53:** 1148, 1984
37. Subramanian VB, Khurmi NS, Bowles MJ, O'Hara M, Raftery EB: Objective evaluation of three dose levels of diltiazem in patients with chronic stable angina. J Am Coll Cardiol **1:** 1144, 1983
38. Mann T, Goldberg S, Mudge GH Jr, Grossman W: Factors contributing to altered left ventricular diastolic properties during angina pectoris. Circulation **59:** 14, 1979
39. Braunwald E, Kloner RA: The stunned myocardium: prolonged, postischemic ventricular dysfunction. Circulation **66:** 1146, 1982
40. Brutsaert DL, Rademakers FE, Sys SU: Triple control of relaxation: implications in cardiac disease. Circulation **69:** 190, 1984
41. Henry PD, Schuchleib R, Davis J, Weiss ES, Sobel BE: Myocardial contracture and accumulation of mitochondrial calcium in ischemic rabbit heart. Am J Physiol **233:** H677, 1977
42. Gibson DG, Prewitt TA, Brown DJ: Analysis of left ventricular wall movement during isovolumic relaxation and its relation to coronary artery disease. Br Heart J **38:** 1010, 1976
43. Yellin EL, Yoran C, Hori M, Sonnenblick EH, Frater RWM: Time constant of left ventricular relaxation in the filling and transiently non-filling (completely isovolumic) intact canine heart. Circulation **62**(suppl III): III-205, 1980 (abst)
44. Thompson DS, Waldron CB, Juul SM, Naqvi N, Swanton RH, Coltart DJ, Jenkins BS, Webb-Peploe MM: Analysis of left ventricular pressure during isovolumic relaxation in coronary artery disease. Circulation **65:** 690, 1982
45. Carroll JD, Hess OM, Hirzel HO, Krayenbuehl HP: Exercise-induced ischemia: The influence of altered relaxation on early diastolic pressures. Circulation **67:** 521, 1983
46. Vogel WM, Apstein CS, Briggs LL, Gaasch WH, Ahn J: Acute changes in left ventricular diastolic chamber stiffness: Role of the "erectile" effect of coronary arterial pressure and flow in normal and damaged hearts. Circ Res **51:** 465, 1982
47. Vliestra RE, Farias MAC, Frye RL, Smith HC, Ritman EL: Effect of verapamil on left ventricular function: A randomized, placebo-controlled study. Am J Cardiol **51:** 1213, 1983
48. Zacca NM, Verani MS, Chahine RA, Miller RR: Effect of nifedipine on exercise-induced left ventricular dysfunction and myocardial hypoperfusion in stable angina. Am J Cardiol **50:** 689, 1982
49. Pfisterer M, Glaus L, Burkart F: Comparative effects of nitroglycerin, nifedipine and metoprolol on regional left ventricular function in patients with one-vessel coronary disease. Circulation **67:** 291, 1983
50. Ludbrook PA, Byrne JD, Tiefenbrunn AJ: Association of asynchronous protodiastolic segmental wall motion with impaired left ventricular relaxation. Circulation **64:** 1201, 1981
51. Bache RJ, Dymek DJ: Effect of diltiazem on myocardial blood flow. Circulation **65**(suppl I): I-19, 1982
52. Malacoff RF, Lorell BH, Mudge GH Jr, Holman BL, Idoine J, Bifolck L, Cohn PF: Beneficial effects of nifedipine on regional myocardial blood flow in patients with coronary artery disease. Circulation **65**(suppl I): I-32, 1982
53. Weishaar R, Ashikawa K, Bing RJ: Effect of diltiazem, a calcium antagonist, on myocardial ischemia. Am J Cardiol **43:** 1137, 1979

Systemic and regional hemodynamic effects of captopril and milrinone administered alone and concomitantly in patients with heart failure

THIERRY H. LEJEMTEL, M.D., CAROL S. MASKIN, M.D., DONNA MANCINI, M.D., LAWRENCE SINOWAY, M.D., HARRY FELD, M.D., AND BRIAN CHADWICK, R.N.

ABSTRACT The effects of milrinone and captopril on ventricular performance, renal blood flow, and femoral vein oxygen content were compared in 11 patients with severe chronic heart failure. The increase in stroke volume index was greater with milrinone than with captopril (28 ± 7 vs 24 ± 7 ml/m^2; $p < .05$), while pulmonary capillary wedge pressures fell similarly (19 ± 10 vs 21 ± 7 mm Hg). Mean systemic arterial pressure decreased significantly from 84 ± 10 to 73 ± 11 mm Hg ($p < .05$) with captopril but did not with milrinone. Neither drug changed heart rate significantly. Although milrinone produced a greater improvement in ventricular performance than captopril, renal blood flow increased similarly with both drugs from 289 ± 78 to 417 ± 111 ml/min ($p < .05$) and from 278 ± 77 to 441 ± 115 ml/min ($p < .05$), respectively. Femoral vein oxygen content was increased by milrinone from 7.9 ± 2.6 to 9.8 ± 3.0 ml/100 ml ($p < .05$) and was not changed by captopril. In seven additional patients, intravenous milrinone, administered at the peak effect of captopril, further augmented stroke volume index from 24 ± 6 to 32 ± 6 ml/m^2 ($p < .05$) and tended to reduce pulmonary capillary wedge pressure further from 20 ± 8 to 18 ± 9 mm Hg (p = NS). The addition of intravenous milrinone to captopril did not reduce mean systemic arterial pressure (71 ± 8 vs 71 ± 8 mm Hg) or significantly increase heart rate (89 ± 17 vs 92 ± 18 beats/min) when compared with captopril alone. Although renal blood flow was not further increased by the addition of intravenous milrinone to captopril, femoral vein oxygen content increased from 6.8 ± 1.9 to 9.9 ± 1.8 ml/100 ml ($p < .05$). Thus simultaneous administration of captopril and milrinone has synergistic effect on cardiac performance and complementary effects on the peripheral circulation.

Circulation 72, No. 2, 364–369, 1985.

RECENTLY, angiotensin-converting enzyme inhibition with captopril has been shown not only to improve short-term left ventricular performance but also to enhance long-term exercise tolerance in patients with chronic congestive heart failure during long-term therapy.[1-4] Accordingly, therapy with captopril has gained wide acceptance for the treatment of congestive heart failure not controlled by digitalis glycosides and diuretics. However, in addition to the fact that some patients fail to benefit or have side effects from long-term captopril therapy that limit its efficacy, some patients with advanced heart failure also become increasingly symptomatic despite this therapy and thus may benefit from further inotropic support.[5] Milrinone, a newly synthesized, selective phosphodiesterase inhibitor that exerts both positive inotropic and vasodilatory properties, can produce sustained improvement in cardiac performance in patients with refractory heart failure.[6-9] In contrast to its precursor amrinone, milrinone, when administered over the long term, has not been complicated by side effects and thus may be more promising for the treatment of patients with congestive heart failure. This study was undertaken to compare the short-term effects of captopril and milrinone on cardiac performance and regional hemodynamics and to assess the hemodynamic safety and possible synergistic benefits of combined administration of captopril and milrinone in patients with severe heart failure.

From the Department of Medicine, Division of Cardiology, The Albert Einstein College of Medicine, Bronx, NY.

Address for correspondence: Thierry H. LeJemtel, M.D., Department of Medicine, Albert Einstein College of Medicine, 1300 Morris Park Ave., Forchheimer Bldg., G-42, Bronx, NY 10461.

Received March 19, 1985; revision accepted May 16, 1985.

Materials and methods

Patients. Sixteen men and two women with severe chronic congestive heart failure were studied (mean age 60 years, range 32 to 79). Ten had ischemic heart disease as documented on the basis of past myocardial infarctions or coronary arteriograms. Eight had cardiomyopathy of unknown origin. No patients had hypertension, recent myocardial infarction, or primary valvular disease. All patients were restricted in activity by fatigue and/or dyspnea, and not by angina, despite therapy with digitalis, diuretics, and long-acting nitrates. Mean digoxin level was 0.9 ng/ml (range 0.3 to 1.9). All patients were in functional class III or IV of the New York Heart Association for at least 3 months. All were in sinus rhythm except one patient, who was in atrial fibrillation. Their maximal oxygen uptake averaged 9.9 ml/kg/min (range 6.1 to 15.4). Left ventricular ejection fraction measured under resting conditions by gated nuclear scanning was below 20% in all patients.

The patients were admitted to the coronary care unit at least 24 hr before the hemodynamic evaluation. Long-acting nitrates were discontinued and a 2 g sodium diet was prescribed. The patients continued to receive their usual daily doses of digitalis glycosides and diuretics during the study. The nature, potential benefits, and possible risks of the study were explained to all patients, who then gave written informed consent. The study protocol was approved in advance by the Committee on Clinical Investigations of the Albert Einstein College of Medicine.

Hemodynamic measurements. After 24 hr of bedrest, patients underwent right heart catheterization performed with flow-directed, balloon-tipped, thermodilution catheters (Edwards Laboratories). Mean pulmonary arterial, pulmonary wedge, and right atrial pressures were recorded on a photographic recorder (Electronics for Medicine). Cardiac output was determined by the thermodilution technique with 5% dextrose in water and obtained in triplicate with less than 10% variation. Systemic arterial pressure was measured via an indwelling artery catheter. Mean systemic arterial pressure was obtained by electronic integration. Derived hemodynamic variables, including cardiac index, stroke volume index, and systemic vascular resistance, were calculated from standard formulas. An electrocardiographic lead was monitored throughout the study.

Renal blood flow. Renal blood flow was determined as the left renal venous blood flow by the continuous thermodilution technique and a No. 7F dual thermistor catheter (Webster Laboratories).[10–13] The injection orifice is located 15 mm proximal to the distal end and on the concavity of the bend to prevent vascular wall contact with the opening obliquely oriented at 30 to 40 degrees against the blood stream to increase turbulence and to ensure optimal indicator/blood admixture. The external "dilution" thermistor is located 10 mm proximal to the injection orifice and the second "indicator" thermistor is within the catheter just proximal to the orifice. The catheter was introduced into the femoral vein via the Seldinger technique and advanced into the left renal vein under fluoroscopy. Optimal positioning within the renal vein was confirmed by injection of meglumine diatrizoate (Renografin) through the catheter, and determination of oxygen saturation of renal vein blood was done with samples withdrawn from the catheter. At the end of the study, the position of the catheter was reconfirmed by fluoroscopy. For each determination of blood flow, 5% dextrose at room temperature was infused through the catheter with a Harvard Pump (Model 921) at a constant rate of 50 ml/min until the resistance deflections of both termistors were stable. A standard three-channel thermodilution Wheatstone Bridge (Webster Laboratories) was used to convert the resistance changes into calibrated voltages, which were recorded on photographic paper. Blood flow was then calculated with the formula derived by Ganz et al.,[12] with a modification to correct for thermotransport within the Webster catheter at blood flow rate ranging from 300 to 1500 ml/min.[14] Each measurement of left renal vein blood flow was made at least five times, and three determinations within 10% were averaged.

Femoral vein oxygen content. Retrograde catheterization of the femoral vein was also performed with an 18 gauge angiographic catheter introduced percutaneously and advanced 10 cm distally into the femoral vein. The catheter was used to withdraw blood samples while the patient was resting in a supine position. All samples were evaluated in triplicate for oxygen content (ml/100 ml) with a Lex O_2-Con-TL oxygen analyzer (Lexington Instruments).

Drug administration. In the first 11 patients, evaluated in the postprandial state, 7.5 mg of milrinone and 12.5 mg of captopril were administered orally in variable order. Six patients received milrinone and then captopril, and five received captopril and then milrinone. Milrinone or captopril was first administered after two similar sets of control measurements were obtained 30 min apart. Systemic hemodynamic measurements were repeated at 30 min intervals for 2 hr and hourly thereafter until values returned to baseline levels. Renal blood flow and femoral vein oxygen content were measured at 30, 60, and 90 min. One of these measurements corresponded to peak increase in cardiac index in all patients. Two hours after return of the hemodynamic parameters to baseline levels, captopril or milrinone was administered and measurements were repeated as previously described. Renal and femoral vein catheters were removed immediately after completion of the study.

During the first day of the study, the remaining seven patients received an intravenous bolus of 25 μg/kg milrinone. Three patients who failed to demonstrate an increase in cardiac index of at least 20% received a second bolus of 50 μg/kg milrinone administered 3 hr after the initial one. On the second day of the study, captopril was administered after renal and femoral vein catheters had been inserted. Systemic hemodynamic measurements, renal blood flow, and femoral vein oxygen content were measured at 30, 60, and 90 min, with the last measurement corresponding to the peak increase in cardiac index in all patients. Milrinone was then administered intravenously at a dose identical to that given the day before. Ten minutes later, all measurements were repeated and femoral and renal vein catheters were removed.

Statistical analysis. The results are expressed as mean $\pm$ SD and were considered significant at $p < .05$. Comparison of the hemodynamic and metabolic effects of milrinone and captopril were made with a two-factor repeated measures analysis of variance. Comparisons of hemodynamic and metabolic parameters under the three treatment conditions (milrinone, captopril, and captopril plus milrinone) were performed with analysis of covariance.

Results

Milrinone, which was administered orally to 11 patients at a dose of 7.5 mg, produced a greater improvement in cardiac performance than did 12.5 mg of captopril, as documented by a greater stroke volume index (28 $\pm$ 7 vs 24 $\pm$ 7 ml/m^2; $p < .05$) and similar decrements in pulmonary capillary wedge pressures (19 $\pm$ 10 vs 21 $\pm$ 7 mm Hg; p = NS) (figure 1). Mean systemic arterial pressure was significantly reduced by captopril from 84 $\pm$ 10 to 73 $\pm$ 11 mm Hg ($p < .05$) but was only modestly decreased by milrinone from 84 $\pm$ 10 to 80 $\pm$ 10 mm Hg (p = NS). Heart rate tended to decrease after captopril from 94 $\pm$ 15 to 91 $\pm$ 17 beats/min (p = NS) and was not changed by milrinone (93 $\pm$ 15 vs 94 $\pm$ 15 beats/min). Systemic vascular resistance significantly decreased with both captopril and milrinone from 1981 $\pm$ 416 to 1406 $\pm$ 251 dyne-

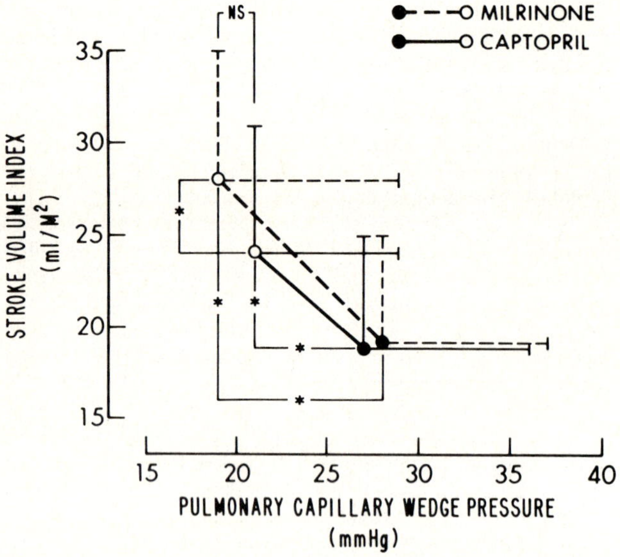

FIGURE 1. Stroke volume index and pulmonary capillary wedge pressure in 11 patients during the control period (closed circles) and at maximum response (open circles). Values are mean ± SD at an oral dose of 7.5 mg of milrinone and 12.5 mg of captopril. *p < .05.

sec-cm^{-5} (p < .05) and from 1929 ± 367 to 1269 ± 199 dyne-sec-cm^{-5} (p < .05), respectively.

Captopril, which at peak effect did not augment cardiac index as much as milrinone at peak effect (2.0 ± 0.4 vs 2.5 ± 0.4 liters/min/m^2; p < .05), increased renal blood flow from 278 ± 77 to 441 ± 115 ml/min (p < .05) (figure 2). Milrinone increased renal blood flow from 289 ± 78 to 417 ± 111 ml/min (p < .05). The increase in renal blood flow after milrinone tended to be lower than that produced by captopril, although it did not reach statistical significance.

Of note was the observation that resting femoral oxygen content was unchanged by captopril (8.0 ± 2.8 vs 8.1 ± 2.4 ml/100 ml) but was increased by milrinone (7.9 ± 2.6 to 9.8 ± 3.0 ml/100 ml; p < .05).

An intravenous bolus of milrinone administered to seven patients at a mean dose of 36 μg/kg (range 25 to 50) increased stroke volume index from 20 ± 4 to 27 ± 4 m/m^2 (p < .05) and decreased pulmonary capillary wedge pressure from 26 ± 7 to 20 ± 6 mm Hg (p < .05) (figure 3). Systemic vascular resistance decreased significantly from 1874 ± 389 to 1332 ± 129 dyne-sec-cm^{-5} (p < .05). The changes in systemic arterial pressure from 83 ± 12 to 84 ± 13 mm Hg and in heart rate from 89 ± 15 to 94 ± 18 beats/min were not statistically significant. In the same seven patients, captopril at an oral dose of 12.5 mg increased stroke volume index from 19 ± 5 to 24 ± 6 mm Hg (p < .05) and decreased pulmonary capillary wedge pressure from 29 ± 9 to 20 ± 8 mm Hg (p < .05). Systemic arterial pressure and vascular resistance decreased significantly from 82 ± 9 to 71 ± 8 mm Hg (p < .05) and from 1926 ± 418 to 1392 ± 362 dyne-sec-cm^{-5} (p < .05), respectively. An identical intravenous bolus of milrinone administered at the peak hemodynamic effect of captopril increased stroke volume index further from 24 ± 6 to 32 ± 6 ml/m^2 (p < .05) and tended to decrease pulmonary capillary wedge pressure further

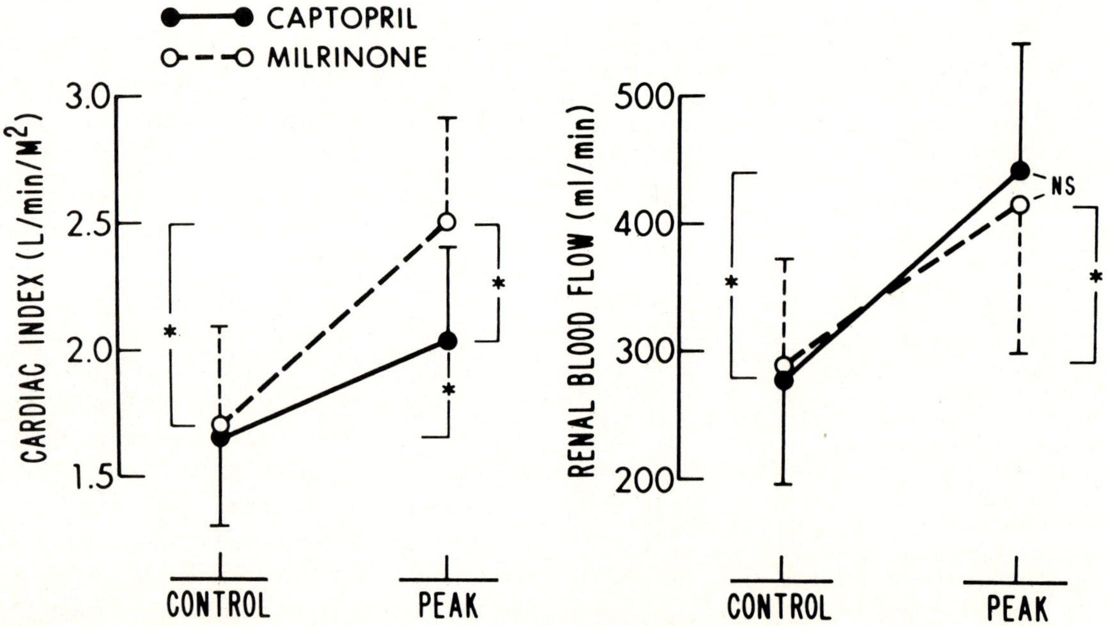

FIGURE 2. Maximal changes in cardiac index and renal blood flow after an oral dose of 7.5 mg of milrinone and 12.5 mg of captopril in 11 patients. Values are mean ± SD. *p < .05.

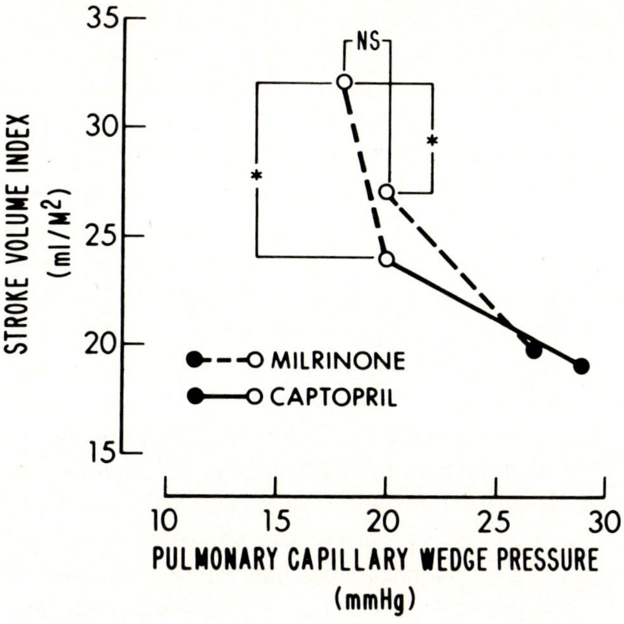

FIGURE 3. Maximal changes in stroke volume index and pulmonary capillary wedge pressure during control period (closed circles) and at maximum response (open circles) to 12.5 mg of captopril and to an intravenous bolus of 36 μg/kg milrinone administered alone and at peak hemodynamic effect of captopril in seven patients. Values are mean ± SD. *$p < .05$.

from 20 ± 8 to 18 ± 9 mm Hg (p = NS). Systemic vascular resistance also decreased further after concomitant intravenous administration of milrinone from 1392 ± 362 to 1071 ± 283 dyne-sec-cm^{-5} ($p < .05$) when compared with captopril alone. Systemic arterial pressure and heart rate did not change (71 ± 8 vs 71 ± 8 mm Hg and 89 ± 17 vs 92 ± 18 beats/min). When compared with intravenous milrinone alone, the concomitant administration of captopril and intravenous milrinone also resulted in a greater stroke volume index (32 ± 6 vs 27 ± 4 ml/m^2; $p < .05$), while pulmonary capillary wedge pressure tended to be lower (18 ± 9 vs 20 ± 6 mm Hg; p = NS).

Resting femoral vein oxygen content and renal blood flow were measured before oral administration of captopril, at peak effect of captopril, and after intravenous administration of milrinone (figure 4). Femoral vein oxygen content was unchanged by captopril (7.1 ± 1.5 vs 6.8 ± 1.9 ml/100 ml), but was increased by milrinone (9.3 ± 1.8 ml/100 ml; $p < .05$). Renal blood flow, which was increased by captopril (278 ± 63 to 403 ± 110 ml/min; $p < .05$), was not further enhanced by concomitant administration of milrinone (437 ± 123 vs 403 ± 110 ml/min; p = NS).

Discussion

In this study, milrinone produced a greater improvement in cardiac performance than captopril for a similar increase in renal blood flow. Resting limb blood flow was increased by milrinone but not by captopril. In addition, concomitant administration of captopril and milrinone was safe and resulted in synergistic effects on cardiac performance and complementary effects on the peripheral circulation.

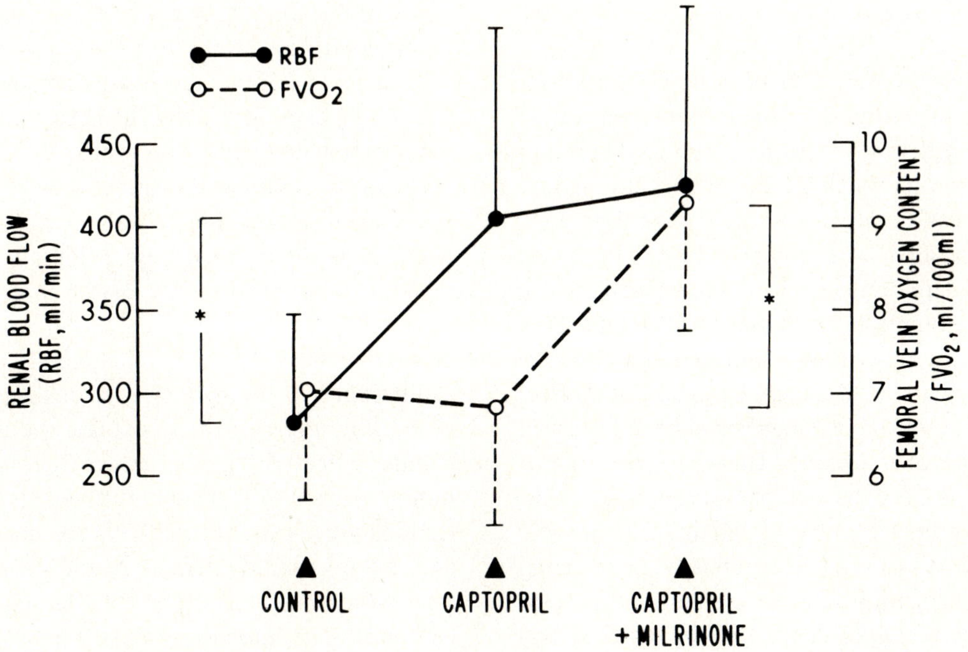

FIGURE 4. Renal blood flow (RBF) and femoral vein oxygen content (FVO_2) during control, at maximal response to 7.5 mg of captopril, and after concomitant intravenous administration of milrinone at a mean dose of 36 μg/kg in seven patients. Values are mean ± SD. *$p < .05$.

After administration of 12.5 mg of captopril, our patients demonstrated an improvement in cardiac performance similar to that reported previously.[2-4] In view of the flat dose-response curve to captopril, administration of higher doses would not have improved ventricular performance further, although the duration of action may have been prolonged.[15] With oral milrinone, 7.5 mg now represents the starting dose and, as was demonstrated by Kubo et al.,[16] a dose of 10 or 12.5 mg probably would have produced greater improvement in cardiac performance. Despite the relatively low dose used in this study, milrinone increased stroke volume index substantially more than angiotensin-converting enzyme inhibition with short-term administration of captopril, while left ventricular filling pressures were reduced to a similar extent by both pharmacologic interventions.

Milrinone improves cardiac performance by enhancing myocardial contractility and directly lowering cardiac afterload.[7, 9, 17] The positive inotropic action of milrinone seems to be mediated by selective inhibition of a fraction III of cardiac phosphodiesterase that is specific for cyclic AMP.[18] The vasodilating properties of milrinone most probably result from phosphodiesterase inhibition in the smooth muscle. In contrast, captopril improves cardiac performance only by lowering arterial impedance through inhibition of the production of angiotensin II and perhaps by additional mechanisms.[19] The substantial fall in systemic arterial pressure that was observed only with captopril supports the potent arteriolar vasodilator effects of the latter drug.

The hemodynamic safety of short-term intravenous administration of milrinone at the peak hemodynamic effect of captopril was documented by the absence of further reduction in systemic arterial pressure and by the lack of excessive fall in left ventricular filling pressure when compared with captopril alone. The synergistic hemodynamic effect was demonstrated by the rise in stroke volume index, which was greater than that derived with either drug administered alone. We did not determine whether a similar synergistic effect of captopril and milrinone would have been observed at a higher dose of milrinone. This study has significant implications for the use of inotropic agents vs vasodilators for the treatment of patients with chronic congestive heart failure. Theoretically, enhancing myocardial contractility may have adverse effects on the rate of progression of the underlying disease[20] and may have the potential for increasing malignant ventricular arrhythmias.[21] Thus one might prefer to reduce arterial impedance with specific vasodilators such as captopril before mobilizing the entire contractile reserve available with higher doses of milrinone.[17] In addition, the complementary effects of captopril and milrinone on the peripheral circulation further support combining the two agents.

Captopril did not alter resting femoral oxygen content. In patients lying supine, in whom lower limb oxygen consumption was presumably constant, an increase in femoral oxygen content would have occurred if captopril had increased blood flow to the limbs. Our findings corroborate with those of Faxon et al.,[22] who found that captopril did not alter calf vascular resistance over the short term. In contrast, milrinone increased femoral vein oxygen content and thus presumably lowered limb vascular resistance flow at rest. Whether milrinone can cause short-term increased limb blood flow during maximal exercise is as yet not known. However, an increase in resting blood flow may have contributed to the delay in anaerobic metabolism induced by short-term administration of amrinone (the precursor of milrinone) during submaximal exercise.[23] Such short-term improvement in submaximal exercise may explain the immediate clinical benefit noted during therapy with milrinone.[7]

Both captopril and milrinone increased renal blood flow in our patients. However, the increase tended to be greater with captopril. Thus the ratio of the increase in renal blood flow and cardiac index was substantially higher for captopril as compared with milrinone (2.7 vs 0.9). In experimental preparations, short-term inhibition of the converting enzyme consistently increases renal blood flow.[19, 24, 25] In patients with chronic congestive heart failure, the results are more controversial. Creager et al.[26] showed that captopril increased renal blood flow by 60%, which is identical to our findings. In contrast, Powers et al.[27] failed to demonstrate an increase, and Mujais et al.[28] even noted a decrease in renal blood flow at initiation of captopril therapy. As pointed out by Blythe,[29] an excessive fall in systemic arterial pressure may, in certain instances, be responsible for a fall in renal blood flow. However, a difference in the methods used to determine renal blood flow may also help explain the discrepancy in results. Although the continuous thermodilution technique, as used in this study, allows instantaneous determination, clearance methods are not instantaneous and require a steady hemodynamic state for 60 to 160 min, which may not be present after administration of captopril. The increase in renal blood flow produced by milrinone is consistent with our prior data with amrinone[30] but is at variance with the lack of changes in renal blood flow measured after 1 month of therapy with milrinone.* The lack of additional improvement in renal blood flow despite the further improvement in cardiac performance produced by intravenous administration of milrinone at the peak hemodynamic effect of captopril cannot be readily explained. The renal vasculature, which was already dilated by angiotensin-converting enzyme inhibition, may have been less sensitive to the vasodilating effect of milrinone. Consequently, the increase in cardiac output produced by milrinone may have been shunted to vascular beds where conductance could be improved, i.e., skeletal muscle. Such complementary redistribution of the increased cardiac output may be an important therapeutic benefit of combining therapy with captopril and milrinone.

References

1. Davis R, Ribner HS, Keung E, Sonnenblick EH, LeJemtel TH: Treatment of chronic congestive heart failure with captopril, an oral inhibitor of angiotensin-converting enzyme. N Engl J Med **301:** 117, 1979
2. Dzau VJ, Colucci WS, Williams GH, Curfman G, Meggs L, Hollenberg NK: Sustained effectiveness of converting enzyme inhibition in patients with severe congestive heart failure. N Engl J Med **302:** 1373, 1980
3. Levine BT, Franciosa JA, Cohn JA: Acute and long-term response to an oral converting enzyme inhibitor, captopril, in congestive heart failure. Circulation **62:** 35, 1980
4. Ader R, Chatterjee K, Ports T, Brundage B, Hiramatsu B, Parmley W: Immediate and sustained hemodynamic and clinical improvement in chronic heart failure by an oral angiotensin-converting enzyme inhibitor. Circulation **61:** 931, 1980
5. Applefeld MM, Newman KA, Grove SR, Sutton FJ, Roffman DS, Reid WP, Linzberg SE: Intermittent, continuous outpatient dobutamine infusion in the management of congestive heart failure. Am J Cardiol **51:** 455, 1983
6. Maskin CS, Sinoway L, Chadwick B, Sonnenblick EH, LeJemtel TH: Sustained hemodynamic and clinical effects of a new cardiotonic agent WIN 47203 in patients with severe congestive heart failure. Circulation **67:** 1065, 1983
7. Baim DS, McDovell AV, Cherniles J, Monrad ES, Parker JA, Edelson J, Braunwald E, Grossman W: Evaluation of a new bipyridine inotropic agent — milrinone — in patients with severe congestive heart failure. N Engl J Med **309:** 748, 1983
8. Sinoway L, Maskin CS, Chadwick B, Forman R, Sonnenblick EH, LeJemtel TH: Long-term therapy with a new cardiotonic agent WIN 47203: drug dependent improvement in cardiac performance and progression of the underlying disease. J Am Coll Cardiol **2:** 327, 1983
9. Jaski BE, Fifer MA, Wright RF, Braunwald E, Colucci WS: Positive inotropic and vasodilator actions of milrinone in patients with severe congestive heart failure: dose response relationship and comparison with nitroprusside. J Clin Invest **75:** 623, 1985
10. Hornych A, Brod J, Sclechta V: The measurement of the renal venous outflow in man by the local thermodilution method. Nephron **8:** 17, 1971
11. Warembourg H, Ketellers JY, Lekieffre J, Bertrand M, Houdas Y, Carre A: La mesure du debit sanguin renal par la methode de thermodilution. Arch Mal du Coeur **65:** 218, 1972
12. Ganz W, Tamura K, Marcus HS, Donoso R, Yoshida S, Swan HJC: Measurement of coronary sinus blood flow by continuous thermodilution in man. Circulation **54:** 181, 1971
13. Sato Y, Matsuzawa H: Comparative study of effects of adrenaline, dobutamine and dopamine on systemic hemodynamics and renal blood in patients following open heart surgery. Jpn Circ J **46:** 1059, 1982
14. Haggmark S, Biber B, Sjodin JG, Winso O, Gustarsson B, Reiz S: The continuous thermodilution method for measuring high blood flows. Scand J Clin Lab Invest **42:** 315, 1982
15. Brunner HR, Gavras H, Walber B, Kersharr GR, Turini GA, Vakovich RA, McKinstry DN, Gavras I: Oral angiotensin-converting enzyme inhibitor in long-term treatment of hypertensive patients. Ann Inten Med **90:** 19, 1979
16. Kubo SH, Cody RG, Chatterjee K, Simonton C, Ruttman H, Leonard D: Acute dose range study of milrinone in congestive heart failure. Am J Cardiol **155:** 726, 1985
17. Borow KM, Come P, Newmann A, Baim DS, Braunwald E, Grossman W: Milrinone (WIN 47203): differentiation of its inotropic and vasodilator effects in humans. J Am Coll Cardiol **3:** 472, 1984 (abstr)
18. Bristol JA, Sircar I, Moos WH, Evans DB, Weishaar RE: Cardiotonic agents 1,4,5-dihydro-6-{4-1H-imidazol-l-yl) phenyl}-3 (2H)-pyridazones: novel positive inotropic agents for the treatment of congestive heart failure. J Med Biochem **27:** 1099, 1984
19. Hollenberg NK: Renal response to angiotensin-converting enzyme inhibition. Am J Cardiol **49:** 1425, 1982
20. Katz AM: Biochemical "defect" in the hypertrophied and failing heart: deleterious or compensatory. Circulation **47:** 1076, 1973
21. Dobmeyer DJ, Stine RA, Leier CV, Greenberg R, Schaal SF: The arrhythmogenic effects of caffeine in human beings. N Engl J Med **308:** 814, 1983
22. Faxon DP, Halperin JL, Creager MA, Gavras H, Schick EC, Ryan TJ: Angiotensin inhibition in severe heart failure: acute central and limb hemodynamic effects of captopril with observation on sustained oral therapy. Am Heart J **101:** 548, 1981
23. Siskind SJ, Sonnenblick EH, Forman R, Scheuer J, LeJemtel TH: Acute substantial benefit of inotropic therapy with amrinone on exercise hemodynamics and metabolism in severe congestive heart failure. Circulation **64:** 966, 1981
24. Gavras H, Liang C, Brunner HR: Redistribution of regional blood flow after inhibition of the angiotensin-converting enzyme. Circ Res **43**(suppl I): I-59, 1978
25. Heyndrickx GR, Baettcher DH, Vatner SF: Effects of angiotensin, vasopressin and methoxamine on cardiac function and blood flow distribution in conscious dogs. Am J Physiol **231:** 1579, 1976
26. Creager MA, Halperin JL, Bernard DB, Faxon DP, Melidossian CD, Gavras H, Ryan TJ: Acute regional circulatory and renal hemodynamic effects of converting enzyme inhibition in patients with congestive heart failure. Circulation **64:** 483, 1981
27. Powers ER, Bannerman KS, Stone J, Reison DS, Escala EL, Kalisher A, Weiss MB, Sciacca RR, Cannon PJ: The effect of captopril on renal, coronary and systemic hemodynamics in patients with severe congestive heart failure. Am Heart J **104:** 1203, 1982
28. Mujais SK, Fouad FM, Textor SC, Tarazi RC, Bravo EL, Hart N, Gifford RW: Transient renal dysfunction during initial inhibition of converting enzyme in congestive heart failure. Br Heart J **52:** 63, 1984
29. Blythe WB: Captopril and renal autoregulation. N Engl J Med **308:** 390, 1983
30. LeJemtel TH, Keung E, Ribner HS, Davis R, Wexler J, Blaufox DM, Sonnenblick EH: Sustained beneficial effects of oral amrinone on cardiac and renal function in patients with severe congestive heart failure. Am J Cardiol **45:** 123, 1980

*Cody RG: Personal communication.

Dispersion of ventricular repolarization and arrhythmia: study of two consecutive ventricular premature complexes

CHIEN-SUU KUO, M.D., HIROTSUGU ATARASHI, M.D., C. PRATAP REDDY, M.D., AND BORYS SURAWICZ, M.D.

ABSTRACT The effect of two consecutive ventricular premature stimuli (S_1S_2) during atrial pacing on dispersion of repolarization and inducibility of ventricular arrhythmias was studied in 16 dogs under control conditions and in four dogs in the presence of an increased dispersion of repolarization during atrial pacing induced by general hypothermia and regional warm blood perfusion via selective cannulation of the distal branch of left anterior decending coronary artery. Dispersion of repolarization was measured as the maximal difference between the ends of six simultaneously recorded monophasic action potentials (MAPs) from anterior ventricular surface, and consisted of MAP duration difference and activation time difference. Dispersion of repolarization during atrial pacing at control was 29 ± 7 msec (activation time difference 4 ± 6 msec, MAP duration difference 25 ± 8 msec), that after S_1 at paraseptal the site was 81 ± 8 msec (activation time difference 73 ± 12 msec, MAP duration difference 8 ± 5 msec), and that after S_1S_2 was 148 ± 27 msec (activation time difference 103 ± 21, MAP duration difference 44 ± 26 msec). Neither S_1 nor S_1S_2 induced ventricular arrhythmia. Hypothermia and regional warm blood reperfusion increased dispersion of repolarization during atrial pacing to 70 ± 22 msec (activation time difference 9 + 3 msec, MAP duration difference 61 ± 19 msec). During hypothermia and regional warm blood reperfusion, S_1 produced a dispersion of repolarization of 149 ± 29 msec (activation time difference 85 ± 8 msec, MAP duration difference 64 ± 23 msec) and did not induce ventricular arrhythmia. However, S_1S_2 at the paraseptal site induced ventricular fibrillation in all four dogs. At the time of induction of fibrillation, the S_2-induced activation time difference increased while the MAP duration difference decreased. Our results show the following: (1) S_1S_2 of 2 msec duration and up to 10 times diastolic threshold strength does not induce ventricular arrhythmia in normal myocardium, but does induce arrhythmia in the presence of increased dispersion of repolarization during atrial pacing; (2) S_1 does not induce ventricular arrhythmia but facilitates induction of arrhythmia by S_2 by increasing activation time difference distal to the stimulation site; (3) Increased MAP duration difference facilitates induction of ventricular arrhythmia by increasing activation time difference, but is no longer essential in perpetuation of ventricular arrhythmia after the onset of arrhythmia. Our results imply that S_1S_2, i.e., an equivalent of a ventricular couplet, does not create sufficient MAP duration difference and activation time difference for induction of ventricular arrhythmia in normal ventricular myocardium.
Circulation 72, No. 2, 370–376, 1985.

IN A PREVIOUS STUDY, we have shown that a single ventricular premature simulus (S_1) of 2 msec duration and of up to 40 mA strength applied during atrial pacing did not induce arrhythmia in open-chest anesthetized dogs.[1] The dispersion of repolarization after the earliest S_1 averaged 89 ± 16 msec on the ventricular surface, and consisted of a 23 ± 13 msec difference in monophasic action potential (MAP) duration and a 66 ± 11 msec difference in activation time. When we increased the dispersion during atrial pacing (basic dispersion) from an average of 32 ± 10 to 111 ± 16 msec,[1] S_1 produced an additional dispersion averaging 75 msec and induced arrhythmia.

In this study, we tested the effect of two consecutive ventricular premature stimuli (S_1 and S_2) during atrial pacing. The purpose of this study was to determine the

From the Department of Medicine, University of Kentucky, College of Medicine, Lexington, and Indiana University School of Medicine and Krannert Institute of Cardiology, Indianapolis.

Supported by NHLBI grant HL 21929 and by The American Heart Association, Kentucky Affiliate.

Address for correspondence: Chien-Suu Kuo, M.D., Department of Medicine, Division of Cardiology, Room MN670, University of Kentucky Medical Center, Lexington, KY 40536.

Received Dec. 17, 1984; revision accepted April 18, 1985.

magnitude and the components of dispersion induced by S_1 and S_2, and their relation to the inducibility of the arrhythmia by this procedure, under control conditions and in the presence of increased basic dispersion of repolarization.

Methods

Studies were done in sixteen open-chest, artificially ventilated mongrel dogs weighing 20 to 33.5 kg, anesthetized with intravenous pentobarbital sodium (30 mg/kg). The heart rate was kept constant after sinus node crush by atrial pacing with rates ranging from 109 to 120 beats/min (average 114 ± 7). The details of the method have been previously described.[1,2] Six suction electrodes were applied to record MAPs at the following locations: (1) on the anterior surface of the right ventricle, (2) on the anterior surface of the left ventricle between the second diagonal branch and the distal branch of the left anterior descending coronary artery (LAD), (3) on the anterior surface of left ventricle between the first and the second diagonal branches of the LAD, (4) on the anterior surface of the left ventricle either medial or lateral to the first diagonal branch of the LAD, and (5) and (6) on the anterolateral surface near the obtuse margin of the left ventricle. The interelectrode distance was 2 to 4 cm between electrodes at sites 1 and 2 and 1 to 2 cm between the remaining electrodes. Local electrograms were recorded with six bipolar plunge electrodes placed at subepicardial locations within 5 mm of the sites of MAP recording. The signals were recorded with a Gould universal preamplifier and amplifier (Model 13-4614-56); the frequency response was set at 0.05 to 1 kHz for MAPs, 30 to 300 Hz for local electrograms, and 0.05 to 300 Hz for the electrocardiogram. The electrograms were recorded simultaneously with the MAPs and an electrocardiographic orthogonal Y lead of the system designed for the dog by McFee and Parungao[3] with Gould Brush 2800 and Honeywell 1858 fiberoptic recorders at paper speed of 200 mm/sec.[1] The criteria for acceptance of the MAPs and the methods of measuring MAP duration and activation time were described previously.[1,2,4,5]

For pacing and programmed premature stimulation, one bipolar pacing electrode was attached to the right atrium and two electrodes were attached to the left ventricle, one within 5 mm of electrode 2 (paraseptal side) and the other within 5 mm of electrode 6 (lateral site). The stimulus during atrial pacing was a rectangular pulse of 2 msec duration and of two times diastolic threshold strength. Programmed ventricular premature stimulation was performed during atrial pacing by applying a single premature stimulus (S_1) to one of the two (paraseptal or lateral) stimulation sites. A premature stimulus of two times diastolic threshold scanned diastole at intervals decreasing by 10 to 20 msec until the effective refractory period (ERP) was reached. After reaching the ERP, the stimulus strength was increased to four times diastolic threshold and premature stimulation was repeated, scanning early diastole at intervals decreasing by 10 msec. The procedure was then repeated with progressively stronger stimuli of six, eight, and 10 times diastolic threshold strength. After the completion of this program, S_1 of two times diastolic threshold was applied at the paraseptal site at a coupling interval 10 msec longer than ERP. Keeping this stimulation site as well as the strength and the coupling interval of S_1 constant, a second premature stimulus (S_2) was applied and the scanning procedure was repeated at each of the two stimulation sites. The threshold of diastolic excitability of the ventricle measured 0.07 ± 0.02 mA at the paraseptal site and 0.10 ± 0.13 mA at the lateral site (p = NS), and remained stable throughout each experiment.

In four of 16 dogs the basic dispersion of repolarization was increased by altering action potential duration with a combination of general hypothermia and selective perfusion of a branch of the LAD with heated blood (regional warm blood perfusion).[1] The blood was cooled with ice water to 30° to 31° C, measured in the left atrium, and warmed to 39° to 40° C, measured at the outlet of the shunt before entering the LAD. This temperature range was selected to introduce an increase basic dispersion of repolarization at a lower level than the previously established critical value for induction of arrhythmia by S_1 alone.[1] Programmed premature stimulation was performed after hypothermia and regional warm blood perfusion by the protocol described above. The threshold of diastolic excitability of the ventricle in this group of dogs measured 0.08 ± 0.03 mA at the paraseptal site and 0.07 ± 0.03 mA at the lateral site (p = NS) and remained stable throughout each experiment.

Dispersion of repolarization was measured directly as the greatest temporal difference between the ends of simultaneously recorded MAPs. Each value of dispersion could result from MAP duration difference alone, activation time difference alone, or added contributions of both. A negative contribution of activation time or MAP duration difference means that at the site of maximum dispersion, the activation time, or the MAP duration difference detracted from the difference created by one of the other component. In the earlier studies, we have shown that under these experimental conditions the dispersion of repolarization faithfully reflects the dispersion of recovery of excitability.[1,2] The basic dispersion refers to the dispersion of repolarization during atrial pacing, and the premature dispersion to that during S_1 or S_2 premature stimulation. The magnitude of the premature dispersion changed with changing coupling interval. The results reported are the maximum values obtained during each scanning procedure. In those experiments in which S_2 induced ventricular fibrillation, ventricular arrhythmia leading to fibrillation started before completion of the preceding repolarization; this prevented accurate measurement of the MAP duration difference and the maximum dispersion. In these experiments, we measured the maximum dispersion and its two components in the ventricular premature complex induced by the earliest S_2 that caused no arrhythmia.

The statistical probability of differences between means was calculated with paired t test, and by analysis of variance when more than two groups of data were compared.

Results

Premature ventricular stimulation (S_1 and S_2) in the absence of increased basic dispersion (table 1 and figure 1). In 16 dogs QRS duration during atrial pacing averaged 50 ± 4 msec (range 45 to 57) and MAP duration averaged 238 ± 18 msec (range 185 to 280). Table 1 shows the dispersion of repolarization and its two components, MAP duration and activation time difference, during atrial pacing and ventricular premature stimulation. The basic dispersion of repolarization averaged 29 ± 7 msec (range 15 to 40) and consisted of 4 ± 6 msec (range −5 to 15) of activation time difference and 25 ± 8 msec (range 10 to 35) of MAP duration difference. The latter represented the difference between an MAP duration of 250 ± 16 msec and one of 225 ± 15 msec. The dispersion induced by S_1 was significantly greater than that during atrial pacing due to the significantly greater contribution of activation time differ-

TABLE 1

Basic and premature dispersion of repolarization and its components at control and during general hypothermia (H) and regional warm blood perfusion (RWBP)

Experimental condition	Pacing type	No. of observations	Dispersion (msec)	AT difference (msec)	MAP duration difference (msec)
Control	Atrial	16	29±7	4±6	25±8
Control	Atrial + VPS-PS	16	81±18	73±12	8±15
Control	Atrial + VPS-PS_1 VPS-PS_2	16	148±27	103±21	44±26
Control	Atrial + VPS-PS_1 VPS-L_2	16	112±24	77±19	35±20
H + RWBP	Atrial	4	70±22	9±3	61±19
H + RWBP	Atrial + VPS-PS_1	4	149±29	85±8	64±23
H + RWBP	Atrial + VPS-PS_1 VPS-L_2	4	123±10	91±3	31±11
H + RWBP	Atrial + VPS-PS_1 VPS-PS_2 (before VF)	4	133±34	109±20	24±21
H + RWBP	Atrial + VPS-PS_1 VPS-PS_2 (at induction of VF)	4	—	138±5	—

VF = ventricular fibrillation; AT = activation time; VPS-PS_1 = ventricular premature stimulation with first premature stimulus at the paraseptal site; VPS-PS_2 = ventricular premature stimulation with second premature stimulus at the paraseptal site; VPS-L_2 = ventricular premature stimulation with second premature stimulus at the lateral site.

$^A p < .001$; $^B p < .005$; $^C p < .01$; $^D p < .05$.

ence; the contribution of MAP duration difference decreased. The average MAP duration difference of 8 ± 15 msec represented the difference between an MAP duration of 220 ± 19 msec and one of 212 ± 20 msec.

The dispersion induced by S_2 at both the paraseptal site and the lateral site was significantly greater than that induced by S_1 (table 1 and figure 1) due to the significantly greater MAP duration difference at both stimulation sites and the greater activation time difference at the paraseptal site. The average MAP duration difference of 44 ± 26 msec during S_2 stimulation at the paraseptal site represented the difference between an MAP duration of 189 ± 19 msec and one of 145 ± 24 msec. The average MAP duration difference of 35 ± 20 msec during S_2 stimulation at the lateral site represented the difference between an MAP duration of 221 ± 21 msec and one of 186 ± 20 msec.

No ventricular arrhythmia was induced by S_1 or S_1 + S_2 at either the paraseptal or the lateral site.

Premature ventricular stimulation (S_1 and S_2) in the presence of increased basic dispersion (table 1 and figure 2). Basic dispersion was increased in four of 16 dogs in which hypothermia and regional warm blood perfusion were used. The magnitude of this dispersion was about 25% to 30% smaller than that critical for induction of arrhythmia by S_1 alone at the paraseptal site in the previous study.[1] In these animals, the control measurements before hypothermia and regional warm blood perfusion were not significantly different from the corresponding control values in the other 12 dogs.

Hypothermia and regional warm blood perfusion caused no significant change in QRS duration (51 ± 5 msec) but increased significantly the basic dispersion of repolarization to 70 ± 22 msec (range 40 to 90) ($p < .01$). This was due to an increase in the MAP duration difference from 21 ± 10 to 61 ± 19 msec ($p < .01$) and an insignificant increase in the activation time difference from 4 ± 5 to 9 ± 3 msec (p = NS). The average MAP duration difference represented the difference between an MAP duration of 245 ± 7 msec and one of 184 ± 13 msec. The maximum dispersion induced by S_1 during hypothermia and regional warm blood perfusion was significantly greater than at control ($p < .001$) due to significantly greater contribution of the MAP duration difference, which averaged 64 ± 23 msec and represented the difference between an MAP duration of 238 ± 13 msec and one of 174 ± 18 msec.

During hypothermia and regional warm blood perfusion, ventricular arrhythmia did not occur spontaneously and was not induced by S_1. However, S_1 and S_2 induced ventricular arrhythmia when both stimuli were applied at the paraseptal site (figure 2, *C*). In all four dogs the induced ventricular arrhythmia progressed to

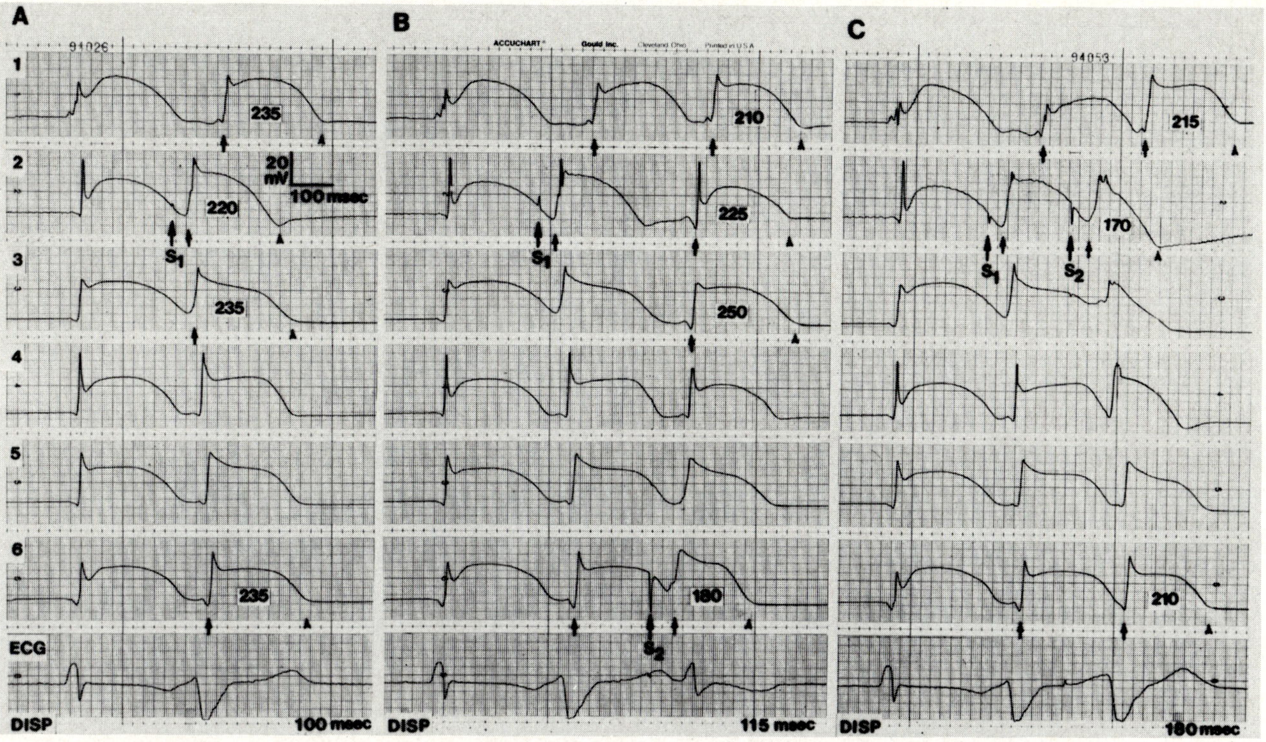

FIGURE 1. Dispersion of repolarization induced by S_1 and S_2 in one control dog. Shorter arrows indicate the onset and arrow heads the end of MAPs. Longer arrows indicate the artifacts of S_1 and S_2. Number within MAPs indicates MAP duration in milliseconds. MAP duration during atrial pacing was 255 msec at recording site 1, 240 msec at site 2, 265 msec at site 3, 245 msec at site 4, 250 msec at site 5, and 255 msec at site 6. The maximum basic dispersion during atrial pacing (15 msec) was between sites 2 and 3, and resulted from an MAP duration difference of 25 msec minus 10 msec activation time difference. In other words, the site of the longer MAP (No. 3) was activated 10 msec earlier than the site of the shorter MAP (No. 2). The maximum dispersion induced by S_1 (*A*) was between site 2 and 1 and equaled 100 msec, resulting from an MAP duration difference of 15 msec and an activation time difference of 85 msec. *B*, Two ventricular premature complexes, the first induced by S_1 as in *A*, and the second induced by S_2 at the lateral site. The maximum dispersion induced by the second premature stimulus was between site 6 and 1 and equaled 115 msec, resulting from an MAP duration difference of 30 msec and an activation time difference of 85 msec. *C*, Two ventricular premature complexes, the first induced by S_1 as in *A*, and the second induced by S_2 at the paraseptal site. The maximum dispersion induced by the second premature stimulus was between site 2 and 1 and equaled 180 msec, resulting from an MAP duration difference of 45 msec and an activation time difference of 135 msec. See text.

ventricular fibrillation. The strength of the stimulus that induced the arrhythmia was two times diastolic threshold in two, four times diastolic threshold in one, and six times diastolic threshold in one dog. No arrhythmia was induced in any of the four dogs when S_1 was applied at the paraseptal site and S_2 was applied at the lateral site (figure 2, *B*).

The maximum dispersion induced by S_2 at the lateral site was 123 ± 10 msec (table 1). It consisted of activation time difference of 91 ± 3 msec and an MAP duration difference of 31 ± 11 msec, which represented the difference between an MAP duration of 237 ± 23 msec and one of 206 ± 14 msec. The maximum dispersion induced by the earliest S_2 that did not induce ventricular fibrillation at the paraseptal site was 133 ± 34 msec. It consisted of an activation time difference of 109 ± 20 msec and an MAP duration difference of 24 ± 21 msec (the difference between an MAP duration of 175 ± 11 msec and one of 150 ± 25 msec). The premature dispersion and each of its two components at two stimulation sites were not significantly different from one another. The maximum activation time difference of ventricular premature contractions induced by S_2 at the paraseptal site and resulting in ventricular fibrillation was 138 ± 5 msec. This value was significantly greater than the maximum activation time difference induced by S_2 at the lateral site, by S_1 at the paraseptal site ($p < .001$), or by S_2 at either the paraseptal or lateral site under control conditions ($p < .02$ for paraseptal and $p < .001$ for lateral site).

During propagation of the ventricular complex induced by S_2, the earliest activation was recorded at the site of electrode 2 in all four dogs, but during propagation of the first nonstimulated ventricular complex leading to ventricular fibrillation, the earliest acti-

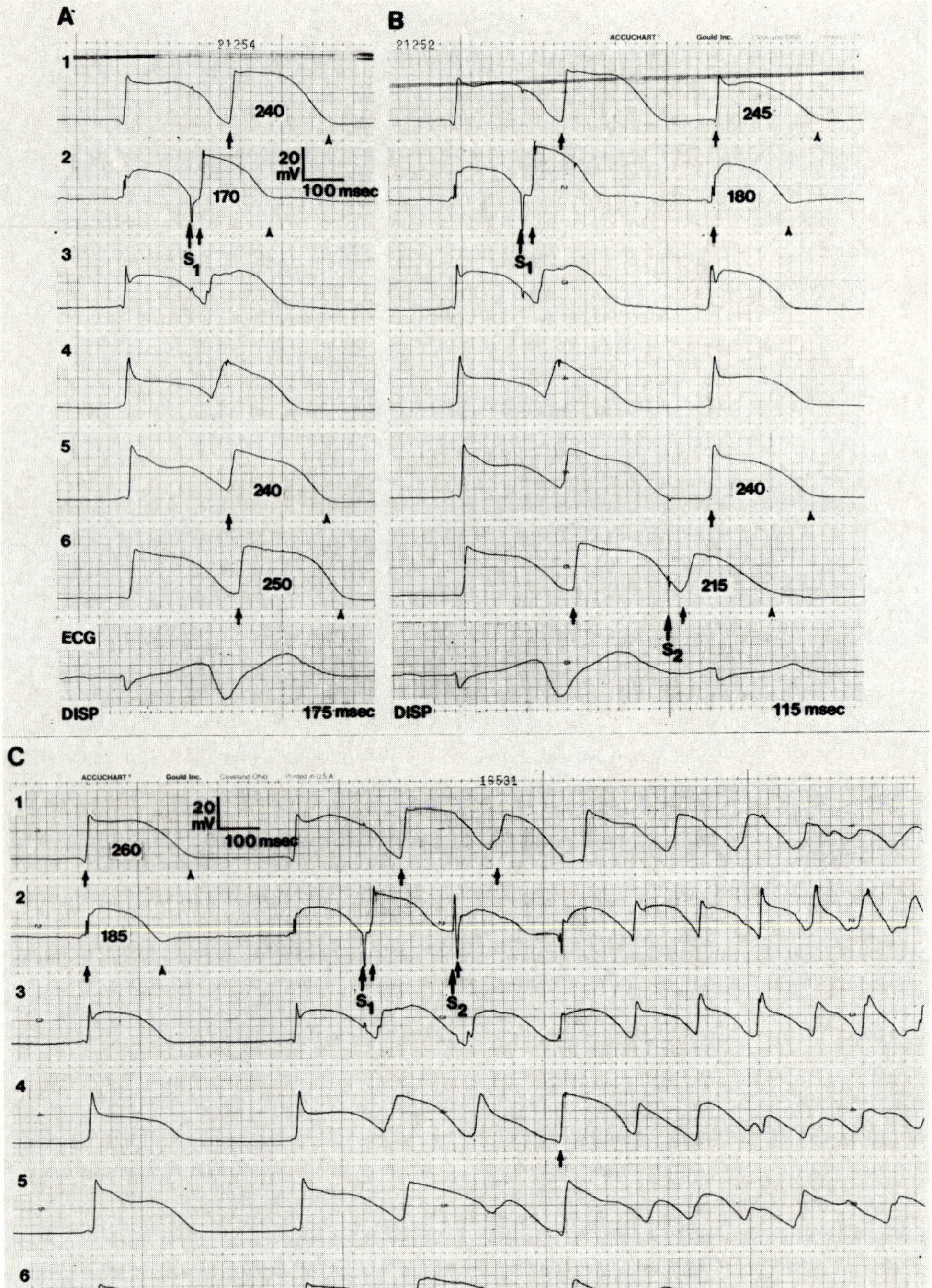

FIGURE 2. Dispersion of repolarization of ventricular premature complexes induced by S_1 and S_2 during hypothermia combined with regional warm blood perfusion in one dog. The dispersion during atrial pacing was 80 msec (*C*), and resulted from an MAP duration difference of 70 msec and an activation time difference of 10 msec. The dispersion induced by the first premature stimulus (*A*) was 175 msec, and resulted from an MAP duration difference of 80 msec and an activation time difference of 95 msec. The dispersion induced by S_2 at the lateral site (*B*) was 115 msec, and resulted from an MAP duration difference of 30 msec and an activation time difference of 85 msec. The S_2 at the paraseptal site resulted in ventricular fibrillation (*C*). The dispersion induced by S_2 at the paraseptal site could not be accurately measured, but the maximal activation time difference between sites 2 and 6 was 135 msec. Symbols are as in figure 1. The arrow below the fifth action potential of site 4 in *C* indicates the earliest activation of the complex initiating sustained ventricular arrhythmia. See text.

vation was recorded at the site of electrode 3 in two, and at the site of electrode 4 in the other two dogs (figure 2, *C*).

Discussion

Our results show that the application of two ventricular premature stimuli during atrial pacing did not induce ventricular arrhythmia under normal conditions but did induce arrhythmia in the presence of increased dispersion of repolarization caused by increased difference in action potential durations. Although we measured the dispersion only on the ventricular surface, we believe that by cooling and warming the blood rather than the cardiac surface, we avoided large transmural temperature gradients, and thus sampled the representative regions with short and long MAPs.

Mechanism of induced arrhythmia

Role of S_1 in the presence of an increased dispersion. Induction of arrhythmia by S_1S_2 required a lesser magnitude of critical basic dispersion than that needed for induction of arrhythmia by a single premature stimulus.[1] This suggests that S_1 introduced additional electrophysiologic disturbances that, in the presence of a less than critical dispersion, facilitated the induction of arrhythmia by S_2. One of the mechanisms that has been proposed to explain the increased yield of arrhythmia induction with an increasing number of premature stimuli is the shortening of refractoriness that is induced by the first premature stimulus at the site of stimulation, which allows the subsequent premature impulse to be applied earlier and penetrate the reentry circuit.[6]

Although under some conditions the operation of the above mechanism is plausible, our results suggest that in this preparation the role of S_1 in the induction of arrhythmia was not limited to the shortening of refractory period at the site of stimulation. We found that S_1 not only shortened MAP at the site of stimulation but also increased the activation time difference at the sites distal to the site of stimulation and that activation time difference was further augmented by S_2 at the time of induction of arrhythmia. In our preparation of increased dispersion resulting from increased MAP duration difference, the induction of presumed reentrant arrhythmia by S_1 was attributed to conduction block and slow conduction resulting from an activation front reaching the still refractory, or incompletely repolarized regions of myocardium with prolonged MAP.[1] We assume that in this study S_1 had a similar effect. However, because of a less pronounced MAP duration difference S_1 did not induce arrhythmia but created conditions for completion of reentry of premature impulse induced by S_2. Such mechanism of arrhythmia induction by S_1S_2 may not be limited to the setting in which the unidirectional block and the slow conduction are attributed to the differences between action potential durations. Mehra et al.[7] proposed a similar mechanism of arrhythmia induction in an infarction preparation in which reentrant arrhythmias were induced by S_1S_2 but not by S_1 alone. The induction of arrhythmia by S_2 was attributed to a long propagation time of the second premature impulse that allowed the dissipation of functional block at the site of reentry. However, S_1 failed to create reentry even though the S_1- induced impulse reached the site of reentry circuit.[7]

Role of MAP duration difference. S_1 decreased MAP duration difference at control but did not change this parameter during hypothermia and regional warm blood perfusion. S_2 increased MAP duration difference at control, but decreased it during hypothermia and regional warm blood perfusion. This confirms our earlier observation that when the basic MAP duration difference is already increased, premature stimulation causes no further increase.[1] The decrease in MAP duration difference induced by S_2 during hypothermia and regional warm blood perfusion can be attributed to the operation of two mechanisms that control the noncycle length–dependent premature action potential duration in the ventricular myocardium, namely the proximity of the premature action potential to the preceding basic action potential and the duration of the preceding basic action potential.[8] The duration of premature action potential decreases with increasing proximity to the preceding basic potential, but at each diastolic interval (proximity) is proportional to the duration of the preceding basic potential. In our study, these two factors interacted as follows: At short coupling intervals, the proximity of the premature MAP to the basic MAP tended to be similar at all sites (figure 2 *A*), while at longer coupling intervals the premature MAP tended to be in closer proximity to the long preceding basic MAP than to the short preceding basic MAP (figure 2, *B*, second premature MAP). In both instances, the absolute shortening of premature MAP was greater after a longer than after a shorter preceding basic MAP. Thus, we found that, in contrast to the increasing activation time difference, the MAP duration difference during S_2 decreased before the induction of arrhythmias. This suggests that in this animal preparation, the increased basic MAP duration difference is needed to delay conduction of the first premature impulse, which in turn leads to further conduction disturbance during propagation of the second premature impulse and initiation of arrhythmia. It appears that after the initiation of arrhythmia an increased MAP duration difference is no longer needed for its perpetuation.

Strength of premature stimuli. The study of Spear et al. suggests that a significant increase in the dispersion of recovery of excitability at the site of stimulation occurs when the strength of premature stimuli exceeds 2.0 mA. In our study, the strength of the conditioning S_1 and S_2 that induced ventricular fibrillation was less than 1.0 mA. This suggests that the arrhythmia induced in our study was probably not due to the "destabilizing" effect of S_1 in the vicinity of the stimulation site, a conclusion supported by the finding that the arrhythmia originated at some distance from the site of premature stimulation.

Site of premature stimulation. We confirmed the previously established importance of the site of stimulation in the induction of arrhythmia.[1] The arrhythmia was induced only when S_2 was applied at the same site as S_1, i.e., at a site with short MAP duration. The S_2 applied at this site produced greater activation time difference than that applied at a site different from that of S_1, i.e., a site with a long MAP duration. This suggests that the second premature impulse propagated more slowly when it originated from the site at which repolarization was completed early.

Implications of the study. Ventricular couplet has been classified as high-grade ventricular arrhythmia.[10] A significant association between ventricular couplet and ventricular tachycardia was noted in patients recovering from myocardial infarction,[11, 12] but not in patients without heart disease.[13] Couplets have been found to account for a large proportion of the complex but clinically "benign" ventricular arrhythmias observed during ambulatory electrocardiographic recording in individuals without heart disease.[14, 15] These observations suggest that the prognostic significance of couplets depends on the clinical setting.

It has been shown that in experimental myocardial infarction in dogs, two premature ventricular stimuli of 10 times diastolic threshold or less induce ventricular tachyarrhythmia in the presence of infarction but not under control conditions.[16–18] Our study provides additional experimental evidence that the effect of two consecutive premature stimuli depends on the electrophysiologic homogeneity of the underlying myocardium. Thus, both the clinical and the experimental observations imply that the decisions based on the grading of complexity of ventricular arrhythmia require the consideration of the characteristics of the population at risk.

We acknowledge the secretarial assistance of Ms. Kate Bowns and Ms. Anna Wells in the preparation of this manuscript.

References

1. Kuo CS, Munakata K, Reddy CP, Surawicz B: Characteristics and possible mechanism of ventricular arrhythmia dependent on the dispersion of action potential duration. Circulation **67:** 1356, 1983
2. Kuo CS, Amlie JP, Munakata K, Reddy CP, Surawicz B: Dispersion of monophasic action potential durations and activation times during atrial pacing, ventricular pacing, and ventricular premature stimulation in canine ventricles. Cardiovasc Res **17:** 152, 1983
3. McFee R, Parungao A: An orthogonal lead system for clinical electrocardiography. Am Heart J **62:** 93, 1961
4. Autenrieth G, Surawicz B, Kuo C: Sequence of repolarization on the ventricular surface in the dog. Am Heart J **89:** 463, 1975
5. Autenrieth G, Surawicz B, Kuo C, Arita M: Primary T-wave abnormalities caused by uniform and regional shortening of ventricular monophasic action potential in dogs. Circulation **51:** 668, 1975
6. Waxman HL, Josephson ME: Ventricular tachycardia in man: mechanisms. *In* Surawicz B, Reddy CP, Prystowsky EN, editors: Tachycardia. Boston, 1984, Matimis Nijhoff, p 263
7. Mehra R, Zeiler RH, Gough WB, El-Sherif N: Re-entrant ventricular arrhythmias in the late myocardial infarction period. 9. Electrophysiologic-anatomic correlation of re-entrant circuits. Circulation **67:** 11, 1983
8. Amlie JP, Kuo C, Munakata K, Reddy CP, Surawicz B: Duration of premature action potential in canine ventricle: Effect of basic ation potential duration and proximity. Circulation **64** (suppl IV): IV-217, 1981
9. Spear JF, Moore EN, Horowitz LN: Effect of current pulses delivered during the ventricular vulnerable period upon the ventricular fibrillation threshold. Am J Cardiol **32:** 814, 1973
10. Lown B, Wolf M: Approaches to sudden death from coronary heart disease. Circulation **44:** 130, 1971
11. Anderson KP, DeCamilla J, Moss AJ: Clinical significance of ventricular tachycardia (3 beats or longer) detected during ambulatory monitoring after myocardial infarction. Circulation **57:** 890, 1978
12. Bigger JT, Weld FM, Rolnitzky LM: Prevalence, characteristics and significance of ventricular tachycardia (three or more complexes) detected with ambulatory electrocardiographic recording in the late hospital phase of acute myocardial infarction. Am J Cardiol **48:** 815, 1981
13. Kuo C, Surawicz B: Coexistence of ventricular parasystole and ventricular couplets: Mechanisms and clinical significance. Am J Cardiol **44:** 435, 1979
14. Kennedy HL, Underhill SJ: Frequent or complex ventricular ectopy in apparent healthy subjects. A clinical study of 25 cases. Am J Cardiol **38:** 141, 1976
15. Kennedy HL, Pescarmona JE, Bouchard RJ, Goldberg RJ: Coronary artery status of apparently healthy subjects with frequent and complex ventricular ectopy. Ann Intern Med **92:** 179, 1980
16. Hamer AW, Karagueuzian HS, Sugi K, Zaher CA, Mandel WJ, Peter T: Factors related to the induction of ventricular fibrillation in the normal canine heart by programed electrical stimulation. Am Coll Cardiol **3:** 751, 1984
17. Echt DS, Griffin JC, Ford AJ, Knutti JW, Feldman RC, Mason JW: Nature of inducible ventricular tachyarrhythmias in a canine chronic myocardial infarction model. Am J Cardiol **52:** 1129, 1983
18. Fisher JD, Cohen HL, Mehra R, Altschuler H, Escher DJW, Furman S: Cardiac pacing and pacemakers. II. Serial electrophysiologic–pharmacologic testing for control of recurrent tachyarrhythmias. Am Heart J **93:** 658, 1977

A Doppler–two-dimensional echocardiographic method for quantitation of mitral regurgitation

KATHRYN J. ASCAH, M.D., WILLIAM J. STEWART, M.D.,* LENG JIANG, M.D.,** J. LUIS GUERRERO, JOHN B. NEWELL, B.S., LINDA D. GILLAM, M.D., AND ARTHUR E. WEYMAN, M.D.

ABSTRACT A noninvasive method to accurately quantitate the severity of mitral insufficiency would be of major clinical value. In theory, in the absence of confounding variables, regurgitant mitral flow should represent the difference between forward mitral blood flow and aortic blood flow. Since Doppler–two-dimensional echocardiographic (D2DE) methods for measuring transvalvular mitral and aortic flow have been validated, it should be possible to use mitral and aortic flows derived by this method to calculate regurgitant mitral flow. To assess the validity and accuracy of this combined approach for quantitation of regurgitant flow, we developed an open-chest canine preparation in which we could simulate, vary, and accurately measure degrees of mitral regurgitation. Seven animals were anesthetized and prepared to allow controlled right heart output. Mitral regurgitation was then simulated by placing a flexible conduit incorporating a one-way valve and electromagnetic flowmeter between the left ventricular apex and left atrium. Flow through the tube (effective mitral regurgitation) was varied between 0.2 and 1.8 liters/min and forward cardiac output ranged between 0.5 and 4 liters/min. Transmitral and transaortic flows were calculated by previously reported Doppler methods. Doppler-derived estimates of forward flow through the aortic valve correlated well with the flow measured by flowmeter (r = .92), and regurgitant flow and regurgitant fraction calculated by the D2DE approach also compared well with those measured by flowmeter (r = .84 and .83, respectively). This study demonstrates that mitral regurgitant flow and regurgitant fraction calculated by the D2DE method provide an acceptable measure of both absolute regurgitant flow and the regurgitant fraction in the experimental setting.
Circulation 72, No. 2, 377–383, 1985.

AN ASSESSMENT of the severity of mitral regurgitation is often important in the management of patients with mitral valvular disease.[1] The degree of mitral regurgitation may be gauged angiographically with the use of the degree of left atrial opacification, as suggested by Sellers et al.[2] Unfortunately, this approach is subject to considerable interobserver variability and the inherent qualitative nature of the data makes it difficult to assess changes in the degree of mitral regurgitation over time. The more rigorous Sandler-Dodge method, in which the regurgitant volume is calculated as the difference between the angiographic left ventricular output and forward cardiac output by the thermodilution, Fick, or dye-dilution technique is thus usually used to provide quantitative information.[3] The accuracy of this approach, however, is limited by the nonsimultaneous acquisition of the angiographic and forward cardiac outputs, the errors inherent in each of the cardiac output measurements, and the presence of associated regurgitant lesions and arrhythmias. Finally, both the Sandler-Dodge and Sellers methods may provide somewhat misleading information in that changes in loading conditions and contractility induced by the catheterization procedure may lead to underestimation or overestimation of the basal severity of the lesion.

Several noninvasive techniques for assessing mitral regurgitation have also been reported. With M mode and cross-sectional echocardiography, the presence of regurgitation may be inferred from a large left ventricle and atrium, in association with abnormalities of mitral valve structure and/or function.[4] An increased left-to-right ventricular stroke volume ratio on the radionuclide angiogram is suggestive of left-sided valvular

From the Cardiac Ultrasound Laboratory, Division of Cardiology, Massachusetts General Hospital, and Harvard Medical School, Boston.

Address for correspondence: Arthur E. Weyman, M.D., Cardiac Ultrasound Laboratory, Massachusetts General Hospital, Boston, MA 02114.

Received Feb. 22, 1985; revision accepted May 9, 1985.

Dr. Ascah is a fellow of the Canadian Heart Association.

*Current address: Department of Cardiology, Cleveland Clinic Foundation, Cleveland, OH 44106.

**Current address: Department of Cardiology, Shanghai Cardiovascular Institute, Shanghai, People's Republic of China.

insufficiency.[5] More recently, Doppler echocardiographic assessment of the spatial extent of systolic frequency dispersion within the left atrium has been shown to provide a semiquantitative measure of the severity of mitral regurgitation.[6-9] Although use of these methods has the advantages of being noninvasive and providing information about function in the basal state, none provide truly quantitative data. Thus, to date, there is no completely satisfactory means, invasive or noninvasive, of quantitating mitral insufficiency.

Combined Doppler–two-dimensional echocardiographic (D2DE) techniques for measuring flows at specific points within the heart have recently been validated[10-13] and the relationship of Doppler-derived systemic and pulmonic flows has been successfully used to quantitate intracardiac shunting.[14-18] Since regurgitant flow through the mitral valve theoretically equals the difference between forward mitral and aortic flows, it should, likewise, be possible to calculate regurgitant volume as the difference between the Doppler–two-dimensional echocardiographically calculated flows through these valves.

The purpose of this study was to test the validity of this combined D2DE approach to the quantitation of mitral regurgitation with use of an open-chest canine preparation of mitral insufficiency in which both forward cardiac output and mitral regurgitant flow could be precisely controlled.

Methods

Experimental preparation. To create a preparation of effective mitral regurgitation, a preparation of controlled right heart cardiac output previously employed in our laboratory was modified by the addition of a valved conduit between the left ventricle and left atrium.[11, 19]

Seven mongrel dogs weighing 16 to 23 kg were studied. The dogs were anesthetized with sodium pentobarbital (35 mg/kg) and mechanically ventilated with a pressure-cycled respirator (Bird Corporation, Palm Springs, CA). The chest was opened through a midline sternotomy, and the heart suspended in a pericardial cradle. The superior and inferior venae cavae were cannulated to collect systemic venous return, and then severed proximal to the site of the cannula. A third cannula was inserted through the inferior vena caval stump into the coronary sinus and sutured in place to collect coronary sinus return. All three venous cannulae emptied into a bubble oxygenator and roller pump, which had been calibrated with use of a stopwatch and graduated cylinder. The output of the roller pump was returned to the right atrium through the stump of the superior vena cava (figure 1). Total forward cardiac output could thus be precisely controlled by the roller pump by regulating the amount of oxygenated blood infused into right atrium. Respiration was then suspended for the remainder of the experiment. To maintain a constant heart rate, the sinus node was crushed and atrial pacing was established with right atrial epicardial electrodes. An electromagnetic flow probe was placed snugly around the ascending aorta and calibrated to the roller pump. The femoral arteries

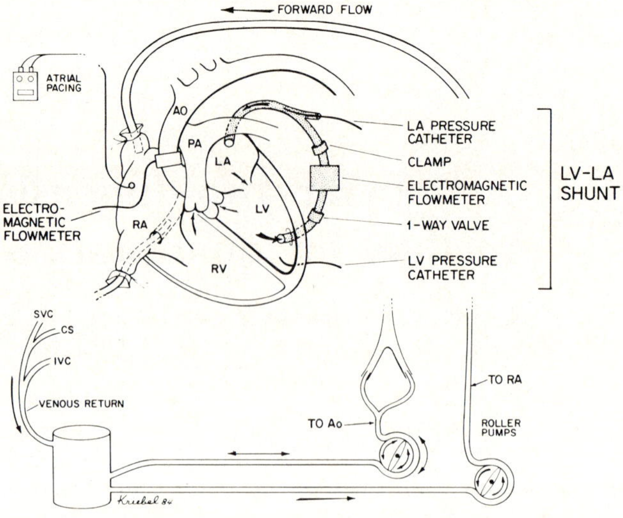

FIGURE 1. Diagram of the preparation. Systemic venous return is collected and directed to a membrane oxygenator, and returned to the right heart at a controlled rate. A second roller pump infuses or withdraws blood from the femoral arteries to alter aortic impedence. The heart is paced via atrial electrodes. An electromagnetic flowmeter is placed on the ascending aorta (Ao). A flexible tube, in which a flowmeter and one-way valve are incorporated, is sutured in place between the left ventricle (LV), left atrium (LA), such that blood passes from the LV to the LA simulating mitral insufficiency. RA = right atrium; RV = right ventricle.

were cannulated and the cannulae were attached to a second roller pump that permitted blood to be infused into or withdrawn from the aorta. This permitted maintenance of a constant aortic pressure (mean 75 mm Hg) at low flows, as well as variation of aortic impedence and therefore shunt flow during the experimental studies (see below). Left ventricular and central aortic pressure were continuously monitored with fluid-filled polyethylene catheters connected to Statham P-23 PD pressure transducers positioned at the mid-thoracic level.

To simulate regurgitant flow, a flexible polyethylene conduit (½ inch diameter) into which a one-way valve and electromagnetic flow probe were incorporated was inserted through stab wounds in the left ventricular lateral wall near the apex and the posterior left atrial wall and sutured in place (figure 1). The conduit valve permitted flow only from the left ventricle to the left atrium. The shunt flowmeter was calibrated before insertion against timed volumes measured by graduated cylinder. Flow through the shunt was regulated by variable occlusion of the tubing with an adjustable clamp as well as by varying aortic impedence throughout the infusion or withdrawal of blood from the aorta through the roller pump attached to the femoral arteries. A fluid-filled catheter was positioned in the left atrium through the shunt to monitor left atrial pressure. Aortic, left atrial, and left ventricular pressures, a monitoring (modified chest lead) electrocardiogram, and aortic and shunt electromagnetically measured flows were recorded on a multichannel recorder.

Echocardiographic imaging and acquisition of Doppler data. All D2DE studies were performed with a combined two-dimensional echocardiographic/range-gated Doppler instrument, ATL MK600 (Advanced Technology Laboratories, Bellevue, Washington), equipped with a mechanical transducer using a 3.0 MHz carrier frequency. Doppler velocity spectra, echocardiographic images, and simultaneous single-lead electrocardiograms were recorded on ½ inch videotape with VHS format on a Panasonic NV8200 Omnivision II recording system.

A saline bath was suspended over the heart to optimize the interface between the transducer and the heart. Care was taken throughout the study not to apply direct pressure to the heart or to distort cardiac anatomy. Complete exposure of the anterior surface of the heart allowed the transducer to be positioned appropriately so as to allow optimal structural imaging and Doppler velocity recordings.

Echocardiographic image acquisition. Calculation of cardiac output by the Doppler technique requires knowledge of the cross-sectional area of the vessel or valve through which blood is flowing and the linear velocity of flow. In this study, the aortic cross-sectional area was calculated from the vessel diameter, assuming a circular configuration. This diameter was measured from a long-axis recording of the aorta in which the scan plane was aligned to include the aortic valve and proximal ascending aorta (figure 2).

Calculation of the effective mitral valve flow area was more complex due to the normal variation in size of the mitral orifice during diastole. A mean diastolic mitral valve area was therefore computed, as illustrated in figure 3, following the method of Fisher et al.[10]

Doppler velocity recordings. Aortic flow velocities were recorded with the transducer placed directly over the cardiac apex. The scan plane was directed toward the base of the heart and rotated to include the left ventricular outflow tract and ascending aorta. The Doppler cursor was positioned as nearly parallel to flow in the left ventricular outflow tract as possible and the sample volume was placed superior to the aortic valve. From this starting point, the system was switched to the Doppler mode and the beam scanned in a tight radial pattern with slight changes in the axial depth of sampling until the velocity profiles with the largest Doppler shifts were recorded (see figure 2).

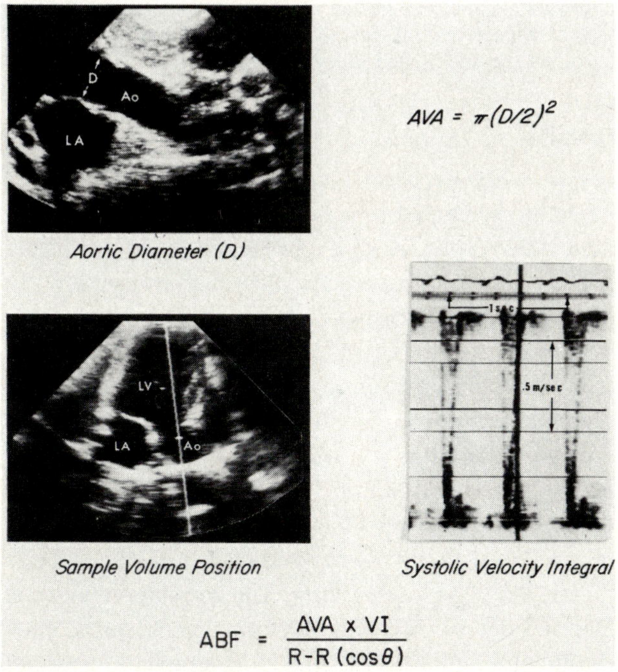

FIGURE 2. Aortic valve calculation of cardiac output with Doppler echocardiography. *Top left*, Measurement of the aortic diameter at the aortic valve anulus. *Top right*, Formula used to calculate area of the aortic valve. *Bottom left*, Positioning of sample volume for recording of aortic velocity integral. *Bottom*, Formula for calculation of cardiac output through the aortic valve.

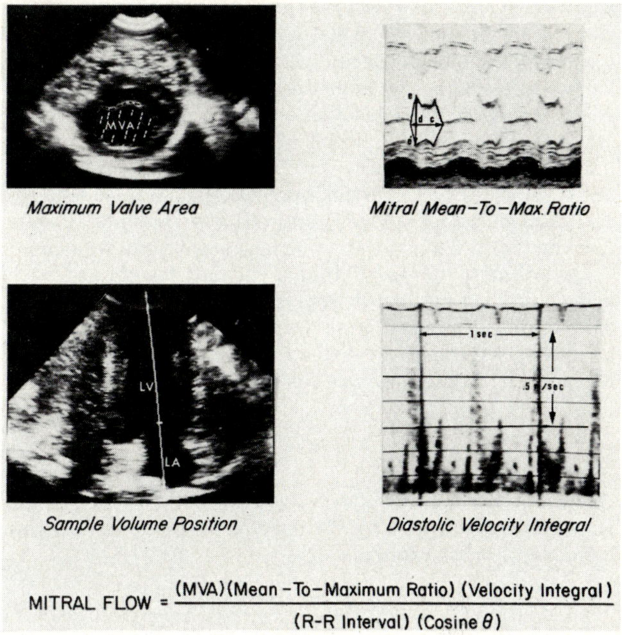

FIGURE 3. Mitral valve calculation of cardiac output with Doppler echocardiography. *Top left*, Measurement of the mitral valve area at the tips of the leaflets. *Top right*, Measurement of the diastolic mitral area, e-e′, and d-c lengths from the M mode echocardiogram of the mitral valve. *Bottom left*, Positioning of sample volume for recording mitral velocity integral. *Bottom*, Formula for calculation of cardiac output through the mitral valve.

Mitral inflow velocity recordings were obtained from the equivalent of the standard apical four-chamber or apical two-chamber view. The Doppler cursor was initially aligned parallel to the apparent direction of flow and the sample volume was positioned at the depth of the mitral anulus in diastole. In Doppler mode, the flow profile with the highest apparent velocities was searched for in a manner analogous to that described for the aortic valve (see figure 3). At the end of each flow recording, a careful search was made to exclude native mitral and aortic valvular insufficiency.

Echocardiographic/Doppler analysis. All measurements were made with an off-line computer graphics system (Easy View II, Microsonics, Indianapolis). Each echocardiographic and Doppler measurement was obtained in nine different cardiac cycles, and the average was used in subsequent analysis.

The systolic diameter of the aortic valve was measured at the point of insertion of the valve leaflets, in the field immediately following valve opening, from inner edge to inner edge. The mitral valve area was measured in short axis from the frame showing maximal diastolic opening by tracing the midpoint of the leaflet echoes. The e-e′ distance, the d-c interval, and the total area between the anterior and posterior leaflets during diastole were measured from the M mode echocardiogram. The mean leaflet separation (area between the leaflets divided by the d-c interval) was divided by the maximal leaflet separation (e-e′) to give the "mean-to-max" ratio. To determine a mean diastolic area of valve orifice, the maximal valve area derived from the two-dimensional study was then multiplied by this ratio.

Doppler measurements were made directly from the velocity spectra with the computer graphics system. The Doppler spectra chosen for analysis were those that demonstrated the greatest velocities and that had profiles with a narrow frequency bandwidth (representative of undisturbed "laminar" flow). The area under the systolic (aortic) or diastolic (mitral) velocity profile was traced through the modal components of the frequency spectrum. The modal velocity, which is determined visually as the brightest component of the spectral display (highest amplitude), represents the velocity at which the greatest number of red cell scatterers are traveling. The enclosed area (velocity integral), in units of distance (cm), is the integral of the instantaneous velocities over time and is proportional to stroke volume. The cardiac cycle length (RR interval) was measured directly from the video tracing of the simultaneous electrocardiogram.

Quantitative flow calculations. Forward flow through each valve was then calculated from the product of the effective cross-sectional area and mean linear velocity. Mean linear velocity was determined by dividing the velocity integral by the RR interval. Aortic flow was calculated with the formula

$$\text{Flow} = \pi \left(\frac{D}{2} \right)^2 \times \frac{SVI}{RR}$$

where D = the diameter of the valve anulus; SVI = the systolic velocity integral; RR = the RR interval. Mitral valve flow was calculated from the formula

$$\text{Flow} = MVO_{(max)} \times \frac{D_{mean}}{D_{max}} \times \frac{DVI}{RR}$$

where $MVO_{(max)}$ = the maximal area of the mitral valve orifice; (D_{mean}/D_{max}) = ratio of mean to maximal M mode valve diameter. Since the flows resulting from these calculations were in cubic centimeters per second they were converted to liters per minute by multiplying 60 sec/min × 1 liter/1000 cc.

In all velocity recordings, the angle between the Doppler cursor and the apparent direction of flow on the two-dimensional echocardiographic image was negligible, and no correction was made for the effect of angle on the recorded flow velocity.

Doppler-determined regurgitant volume was calculated as the difference between mitral (DMF) and aortic flow (DAF) as follows:

$$DRV = DMF - DAF$$

The Doppler-determined regurgitation fraction (DRF) was calculated as

$$DRF = (DMF - DAF)/DMF \times 100\%$$

In cases in which the aortic blood flow was calculated to be greater than the mitral flow by the D2DE method (n = 7), the regurgitant volume and regurgitant fraction were set to zero, since this situation is not physiologically possible.

Analysis of hemodynamic data. Forward flow through the aortic valve and shunt flow were also determined directly with the aortic and shunt electromagnetic flowmeters. Total mitral valve flow, MF_{emf}, was taken as the sum of the shunt flow (SF_{emf}) and aortic flow (AF_{emf}). Regurgitant fraction was calculated as $RF_{emf} = (SF_{emf}/(SF_{emf} + AF_{emf})) \times 100\%$.

Experimental protocol. To test the ability of the Doppler method to record consistently accurate control flows through the mitral and aortic valves in this preparation, as well as to assess the ability of this method to quantitate varying levels of shunt flow, aortic and mitral flows were determined by Doppler echocardiography according to the following general protocol: (1) Control flows were recorded in all animals at roller pump flows of 1.5 to 2 liters/min, with aortic pressure maintained constant and the shunt closed. (2) With forward flow maintained constant, the shunt was opened. (3) With forward flow constant and the shunt opened, flow into the aorta was increased by the femoral artery roller pump to increase aortic impedance. The rate of aortic inflow was increased until an obvious increase in shunt flow was noted on the electromagnetic shunt flow recording. (4) The shunt was then closed, aortic inflow was reduced to return aortic pressure to the control level, and roller pump output was increased to from 2.5 to 4.0 liters/min; and a second series of control values was then recorded at the higher forward flow. (5) At an increased forward flow (between 2.5 and 3.5 liters/ min, depending on the size of the animal), the shunt was reopened to permit the highest flow the animal could tolerate without developing left ventricular failure (visibly apparent left ventricular dilatation with increasing left ventricular end-diastolic pressure). Fine adjustments in both forward and shunt flows were then made to stabilize the preparation. (6) When possible, aortic pressure was again increased to increase shunt flow. (7) Finally, to create the highest possible regurgitant fraction, forward output was reduced to 0.75 to 1 liter/min, the shunt was fully opened, and aortic impedance was increased. The experiment was then terminated and the animal was killed with an overdose of pentobarbital. In applying this protocol, it was necessary to adjust actual forward and shunt flows according to size of the animal and the ability of the left ventricle to tolerate the resulting volume load. This resulted in a wide range of forward and shunt flows across animals.

Reproducibility of measurements. Interobserver and intraobserver variations in measurements of mitral and aortic flows by Doppler echocardiography for our laboratory have been previously examined and reported.[11] The relative correlations for two observers with a roller pump were r = .99 and .94 (n = 10) for the aortic valve and r = .97 and .96 (n = 10) for the mitral valve. The experimental design precludes meaningful assessment of observer variation for the regurgitant volume and regurgitant fraction.

Statistical analysis. Correlations between Doppler-derived flows and those recorded by electromagnetic flow probe were made by the least squares method of linear regression. The expected error for the derived mitral regurgitant volume was calculated as $V_e = V_m + V_a$, where V_e is the expected variance, and V_m and V_a are the variance of the mitral and aortic flows, respectively. A first-order approximation was used to calculate the anticipated mitral regurgitant fraction error.

Results

Forward flows. Aortic and mitral flows were measured by the Doppler method and with the electromagnetic flow probe at 35 experimental stages with and without the shunt open. As illustrated in figure 4, an excellent correlation was observed between the two flow measurements over a range of forward outputs from 0.5 to 4 liters/min (r = .92, y = 1.06x + 0.16). Doppler-determined mitral valve flow recorded with the shunt closed at 10 experimental stages showed an equally good correlation with forward cardiac output determined by electromagnetic flowmeter (r = .92, y = 1.05x + 0.08; figure 5). In each case, the slope of regression was close to unity. The correlation between Doppler-determined and electromagnetic mitral flow (aortic plus shunt flow by electromagnetic flow probe) was similar with the shunt open and closed (y = 0.88x + 0.59 vs y = 1.05x + 0.08, respectively, p = NS).

Regurgitant flows. Effective mitral regurgitant flow measured by the shunt flowmeter ranged from 0.2 to 1.8 liters/min. The relationship between directly mea-

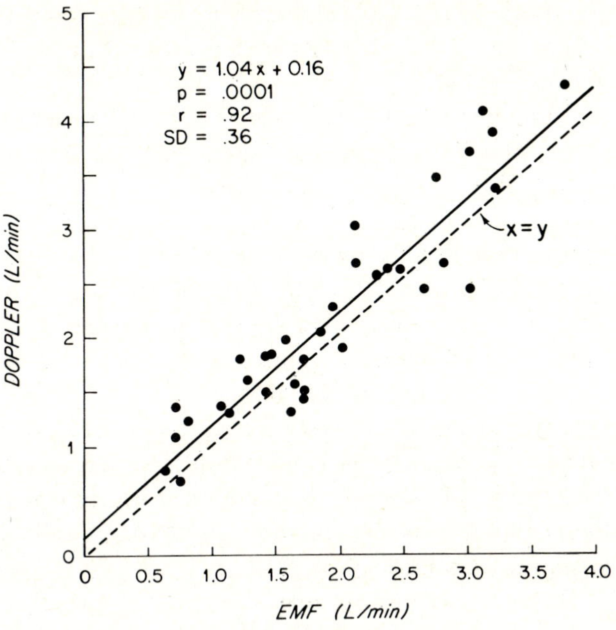

FIGURE 4. Comparison of Doppler-determined aortic cardiac output with that measured by electromagnetic flowmeter.

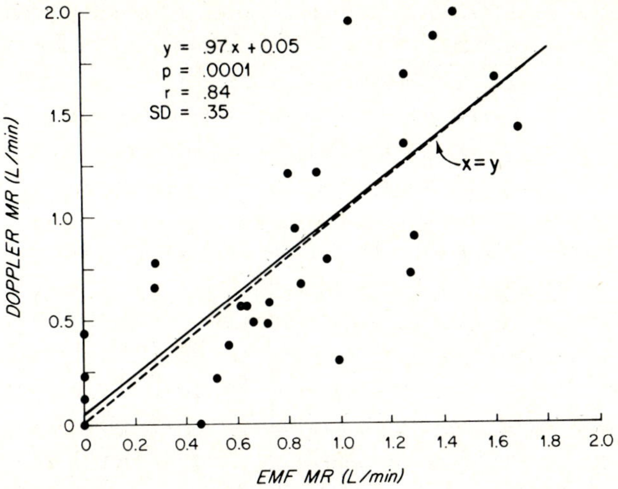

FIGURE 6. Regurgitant flow measured by the D2DE method vs that measured by electromagnetic flowmeter.

sured shunt flow and regurgitant volume calculated by the Doppler method is illustrated in figure 6. Despite the relatively small range of shunt flows achievable in this preparation, a good correlation between the two methods was still apparent ($r = .84$, $y = 0.97x + 0.05$). The regurgitant fraction derived from the D2DE data likewise showed a good correlation with that calculated with the flows measured by electromagnetic flowmeter ($r = .83$, $y = 0.75x + 5.25$).

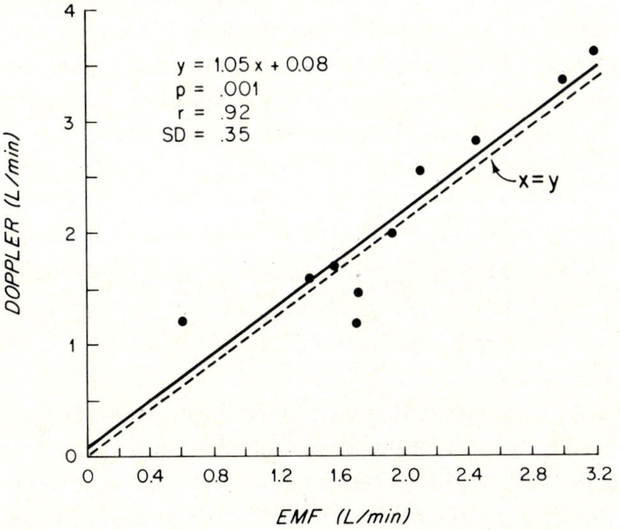

FIGURE 5. Comparison of Doppler-determined mitral cardiac output, in the absence of mitral regurgitation, with aortic cardiac output determined by electromagnetic flowmeter.

Discussion

Doppler echocardiography is uniquely able to noninvasively measure volumetric flow at multiple locations within the heart and great vessels. In the normal flow state, this capability permits the determination of forward cardiac output from flow data derived from each of the four cardiac valves. When flow is disturbed as a result of shunt or valvular regurgitation, quantitation of the disturbance should theoretically also be possible by comparison with flow volumes at serial points along the path of normal blood flow through the heart.

The accuracy of the Doppler method in defining forward cardiac output,[10, 13] the effects of sampling site on these measurements,[3] and its accuracy in assessing shunt flow[14–18] have been extensively studied. Less attention, however, has been given to the use of this technique for quantifying regurgitant flow.[20]

We have recently presented preliminary clinical data suggesting that a significant correlation ($p = .001$) exists between the Doppler-derived regurgitant fraction and the hemodynamic/angiographic mitral regurgitant fraction calculated by the method of Sandler and Dodge.[3] The clinical method of Sandler and Dodge, however, is based on the difference between forward cardiac output as measured by thermodilution, Fick, or dye-dilution techniques and the angiographic stroke volume. Each of these measurements contains significant inherent sources of error.[21] Furthermore, although this method is theoretically attractive, it has not to our knowledge been independently validated. Therefore, we believed that to properly interpret and understand our clinical data, it was important to define the accuracy of the Doppler method of calculating regurgitant fraction in a more rigidly controlled experimental preparation in which forward and regurgitant flows could be precisely measured.

Our preparation was a modification of one with controlled right heart output that we had previously used to study the accuracy and sources of variability in Doppler flow measurements through the mitral, aortic, and pulmonic valves.[11] To simulate mitral regurgitation, the basic preparation was modified by placing a valved conduit between the left ventricular apex and left atrium. To exclude the possibility that the addition of the conduit would alter left ventricular or mitral valve geometry in a manner that would adversely affect flow measurements, we initially compared the Doppler-determined aortic flow and mitral (shunt closed) measurements to those obtained with the aortic electromagnetic flow probe. As noted, the correlation between the Doppler- and electromagnetically determined aortic flow was good and similar to that obtained in a previous study in which no valved conduit was used.[11] Likewise, the baseline mitral flows with the shunt closed correlated well with simultaneous electromagnetically measured aortic flows. Finally, since flow through the conduit should alter the pattern, volume, and pressure of return to the left atrium, we compared electromagnetically calculated absolute mitral flow (conduit plus aortic) when the shunt was open with absolute Doppler-determined mitral flow. Again, the correlation was good (r = .82), and the line of best fit did not differ significantly from that observed with the shunt closed.

Having validated the accuracy of the basic Doppler measurements in this preparation of modified flow, we then tested the accuracy of the D2DE quantitation of mitral regurgitant flow, which was calculated as the difference between total left ventricular inflow and forward cardiac output. In this study a good correlation (r = .84) was obtained between D2DE and electromagnetic estimates of regurgitant flow and the slope of the line of best fit approximated unity (0.97). These data therefore suggest that this method can accurately measure regurgitant volume in the ideal experimental setting. The fact that the correlation coefficient between Doppler- and electromagnetically based calculations of regurgitant volume was weaker than that between the "raw" aortic and mitral valve flows determined by the two methods may simply reflect the relatively narrow range of regurgitant volumes (0 to 1.8 liters/min) obtainable in this experimental preparation as opposed to the broader range of forward cardiac outputs (0.5 to 4.0 liter/min). For example, if electromagnetic and D2DE estimates of aortic flow are compared over a range comparable to that in the regurgitant volume study (i.e., 2 to 4 liters/min), the r value falls between .92 and .78.

While one might expect that the errors in the raw data would be compounded in the regurgitant volume and fraction correlations, the variance for both these calculated variables is less than predicted from the errors in the directly measured variables (observed = .35, 11%; predicted = .50, 27%). Thus, it appears that some of the inherent error is canceled in the calculation of the regurgitant volume or fraction.

In seven instances, Doppler-derived aortic blood flow was greater than Doppler-calculated mitral blood flow by an average of 175 ml. This difference is within the error of the method. In all but one case, in which the shunt flow was 0.45 liter/min, the shunt was closed when this occurred.

"The application to disease states of data derived from acute canine experiments which simulate such states, is necessarily limited."[19] Despite this, when testing any new technology, it is important first to define its capabilities and limitations in an ideal setting where it can be tested against established standards of known accuracy. Experimental validation of a new technique is particularly important in areas in which the clinical "gold standard" has significant inherent sources of error. The information derived from the validation studies provides the framework that is necessary to interpret the results from clinical studies in which few physiologic parameters can be controlled. Thus, our preparation, while admittedly different from the human situation in which the mitral valve itself is responsible for the regurgitant flow, hemodynamically simulates mitral insufficiency while allowing regulation and precise measurement of both forward and effective regurgitant flow. In addition, in this preparation, all valves are intrinsically normal and the open-chest setting provides optimum conditions for Doppler recording and echocardiographic imaging. This ensures any that errors due to intrinsic valvular regurgitation or difficulty in measurement of valve orifices or velocity integrals are minimized. Thus, we were able to validate our method of calculating regurgitant flow and evaluate its accuracy in the absence of confounding variables.

When applying these results to the clinical environment, a number of problems can be expected. First, in patients with mitral regurgitation, the mitral and aortic valves are frequently deformed, making measurement of valve areas and velocity integrals more difficult. Second, coexisting aortic insufficiency may cause an overestimation of the true forward flow and may affect the measurement of mitral valve area and velocity integral as a result of impingement of the regurgitant aortic jet on the mitral valve. Third, differences in heart rate may make measurement more complex. All of our studies were performed at a paced heart rate of 120 beats/min to maintain a constant cardiac output during acquisition of the D2DE data. Since our method for calculation of cardiac output does include the effects of heart rate, the results for individual measurements should not be significantly influenced by the rate. However, large variations in heart rate or changes in rhythm may affect both forward flow and regurgitant volume, and if there is an interval between the measurement of aortic and mitral flows it may affect the calculation of regurgitant volume.

Finally, there appear to be species-specific differences in the geometry of the mitral valve anulus that have produced conflicting opinions as to the appropriate method for measuring mitral flow. In the dog, the method of Fisher et al.[10] has been extensively validated and its accuracy has been demonstrated. When applied to human studies, however, others have found this approach less accurate and several alternative methods for measuring the effective mitral orifice in the clinical setting have been suggested. Although this methodologic point is of major importance, it can be assumed that once the optimal clinical method for measuring mitral valve area is determined, the concepts and methods validated in this study can be easily adapted to the derived clinical formula.

In conclusion, we have described a method for the noninvasive measurement of regurgitant mitral flow. This method employs combined D2DE techniques to measure aortic outflow and mitral inflow and is based on the theory that the difference between total mitral inflow and forward flow through the aortic valve equals the regurgitant flow. We have demonstrated that this method can provide accurate quantification of regurgitant mitral flow in the experimental setting. This technique, being noninvasive, repeatable, and accurate has significant advantages over angiography and may prove to be the method of choice in the clinical assessment of mitral regurgitation.

We gratefully acknowledge the secretarial assistance of Kathleen Lundgren.

References

1. Braunwald E: Heart disease: a textbook of cardiovascular medicine. Philadelphia, 1980, W.B. Saunders and Company, p 1117
2. Sellers RD, Levy MJ, Amplatz K, Lillehei CW: Left retrograde cardioangiography in acquired cardiac disease. Am J Cardiol **14:** 437, 1964
3. Sandler H, Dodge HT, Hay RE, Rackley CE: Quantitation of valvular insufficiency in man by angiography. Am Heart J **65:** 501, 1963
4. Weyman AE: The left ventricular inflow tract, part 1: the mitral valve. *In* Weyman AE, editor: Cross-sectional echocardiography. Philadelphia, 1982, Lea and Febiger, pp 139–192
5. Rigo P, Alderson PO, Robertson RM, Becker LC, Wagner HN Jr: Measurement of aortic and mitral regurgitation by gated cardiac blood pool scans. Circulation **60:** 306, 1979
6. Patel AK, Rowe GG, Thomsen JH, Dhanani SP, Kosolcharoen P, Lyle LE: Detection and estimation of rheumatic mitral regurgitation in the presence of mitral stenosis by pulsed Doppler echocardiography. Am J Cardiol **51:** 986, 1983
7. Abbassi AS, Allen MW, DiCristofaro D, Ungar I: Detection and estimation of the degree of mitral regurgitation by range-gated pulsed Doppler echocardiography. Circulation **61:** 143, 1980
8. Quinones M, Young JB, Waggoner AD, Ostojic MC, Ribeiro LGT, Miller RR: Assessment of pulsed Doppler echocardiography in detection and quantification of aortic and mitral regurgitation. Br Heart J **44:** 612, 1980
9. Veyrat C, Ameur A, Bas S, Lessana A, Abitbol G, Kalmanson D: Pulsed Doppler echocardiographic indices for assessing mitral regurgitation. Br Heart J **51:** 130, 1984
10. Fisher DC, Sahn DJ, Friedman MJ, Larson D, Valdes-Cruz LM, Horowitz S, Goldberg SJ, Allen HD: The mitral valve orifice method for non-invasive two-dimensional Doppler determination of cardiac output. Circulation **67:** 872, 1983
11. Stewart WJ, Jiang L, Guerrero JL, Weyman AE: Variable effects of changes in flow rate through the aortic, pulmonic, and mitral valves on valve area and flow velocity: Impact on quantitative Doppler flow calculations. J Am Coll Cardiol (in press)
12. Freidman MJ, Sahn DJ, Larson D, Flint A: Two-dimensional echo-range gated Doppler measurements of cardiac output and stroke volume in open-chest dogs. Circulation **62:** 101, 1980
13. Fisher DC, Sahn DJ, Freidman MJ, Larson D, Valdes-Cruz LM, Horowitz S, Goldberg SJ, Allen HD: The effect of variations on pulsed Doppler sampling site an calculation of cardiac output: An experimental study in open chest dogs. Circulation **67:** 370, 1983
14. Valdes-Cruz LM, Horiwitz S, Mesel E, Sahn DJ, Fisher DC, Larson D, Goldberg SJ, Allen H: A pulsed Doppler echocardiographic method for calculation of pulmonary and systemic flow: accuracy in a canine model with ventricular septal defect. Circulation **68:** 597, 1983
15. Meijboom EJ, Valdes-Cruz LM, Horowitz S, Sahn DJ, Larson DF, Young KA, Lima CO, Goldberg SJ, Allen HD: A two-dimensional Doppler echocardiographic method for calculation of pulmonic and systemic blood flow in a canine model with variable-sized left-to-right extracardiac shunt. Circulation **68:** 437, 1983
16. Sanders SP, Yaeger S, Williams RG: Measurement of systemic and pulmonary and QP/QS ratio using Doppler and two-dimensional echocardiography. Am J Cardiol **51:** 952, 1983
17. Goldberg SJ, Sahn DJ, Allen HD, Valdes-Cruz LM, Hoenecke H, Carnahan Y: Evaluation of pulmonary and systemic blood flow by two-dimensional Doppler echocardiography using fast Fourier transform spectral analysis. Am J Cardiol **50:** 1398, 1982
18. Barron JV, Sahn DJ, Valdes-Cruz LM, Lima CO, Goldberg SJ, Grenadier E, Allen HD: Clinical utility of two-dimensional Doppler echocardiographic techniques for estimating pulmonary to systemic blood flow ratios in children with left to right shunting atrial septal defect, ventricular septal defect or patent ductus arteriosis. J Am Coll Cardiol **3:** 169, 1984
19. Braunwald E, Welch GH Jr, Sarnoff SJ: Hemodynamic effects of quantitatively varied experimental mitral regurgitation. Circ Res **5:** 539, 1957
20. Nichol PM, Boughner DR, Persaud S: Non-invasive assessment of mitral insufficiency by transcutaneous Doppler ultrasound. Circulation **54:** 956, 1976
21. Grossman W, Dexter L: Profiles in valvular heart disease. In: Grossman W, editor: Cardiac catheterization and angiography. Philadelphia, 1980, Lea and Febiger, p 315

Coronary thrombolysis in dogs with intravenously administered human pro-urokinase

D. COLLEN, M.D., PH.D., D. STUMP, M.D., F. VAN DE WERF, M.D., I. K. JANG, M.D., M. NOBUHARA, PH.D., * AND H. R. LIJNEN, PH.D.

ABSTRACT Coronary thrombolysis was induced by infusion of highly purified human pro-urokinase isolated from a transformed kidney cell line (ACHN) or by infusion of urokinase of urinary origin in anesthetized dogs with 1-hr-old clots in the left anterior descending coronary artery. The clots were induced with a copper coil and thrombolysis was detected by repeat coronary angiography. Intravenous infusion of pro-urokinase at a rate of 10 μg/kg/min for 30 min in two dogs did not induce thrombolysis, which was only obtained after 8 and 15 min of its subsequent intracoronary administration. Intravenous infusion of pro-urokinase at a rate of 20 μg/kg/min for 30 min in four dogs induced coronary thrombolysis within 23 ± 2 min (mean ± SEM). This was not associated with systemic fibrinolytic activation because the α_2-antiplasmin and fibrinogen levels did not decrease. Intravenous infusion of urokinase at a rate of 10 μg/kg/min for 30 min elicited thrombolysis in four of seven dogs within an average of 19 ± 2 min. In the other three dogs thrombolysis was only obtained within 11 ± 3 min of its subsequent intracoronary infusion. Administration of urokinase was associated with systemic fibrinolytic activation as evidenced by a decrease of α_2-antiplasmin to about 10% and of fibrinogen to 43 ± 13% of the preinfusion value. It is concluded that intravenous infusion of pro-urokinase at a sufficiently high rate produces coronary thrombolysis without systemic fibrinolysis in dogs.
Circulation 72, No. 2, 384–388, 1985.

CORONARY THROMBOLYSIS has been widely investigated as a means to abort the evolution of acute transmural myocardial infarction. Several attempts have also been made to develop fibrin-specific thrombolytic agents that would be more effective than streptokinase and would induce less systemic fibrinolysis. Thrombolytic agents with anticipated fibrin selectivity now include human tissue-type plasminogen activator (t-PA),[1] acylated plasminogen-streptokinase complex,[2] and pro-urokinase.[3]

Pro-urokinase is a precursor of urokinase, first identified in tissue-culture media[4, 5] and later purified from urine,[6] plasma,[7] conditioned cell culture media,[8–11] and transformed bacteria.[12] Although the mechanism of action of pro-urokinase remains to be established, recent reports have provided evidence that it can indeed induce more clot-selective thrombolysis in animal preparations than urokinase.[3, 11, 13]

In this study we used a well-characterized preparation for the study of thrombolysis after coronary occlusion in dogs[14] to evaluate the relative fibrinolytic effects of pro-urokinase as compared with urokinase.

Methods

Thirteen dogs weighing approximately 20 kg were anesthetized with 10 to 15 mg/kg sodium pentobarbital and artificially ventilated. Coronary thrombosis was induced by advancing a 3 to 5 mm long copper coil attached to an intracoronary catheter via the carotid artery 3 to 5 cm into the left anterior descending coronary artery distal to the first main diagonal branch, as previously described.[14] An occlusive thrombus formed within 5 to 10 min and was confirmed angiographically in all dogs. All of the animals studied developed electrocardiographic signs typical of ischemia. One hour after induction of the coronary thrombus, pro-urokinase or urokinase was infused via a peripheral vein at a rate of 10 μg/kg/min for 30 min. Whenever complete thrombolysis had not occurred after 30 min of infusion, the agents were administered immediately thereafter at the same rate but via the intracoronary route for an additional 15 min. This was the case in the two dogs treated with pro-urokinase and in three of the seven dogs treated with urokinase. In four dogs given pro-urokinase intravenously at a rate of 20 μg/kg/min for 30 min, complete thrombolysis was observed before the end of the infusion in three dogs and near complete thrombolysis in one. In the latter dog, reocclusion occurred within 10 min after

From the Center for Thrombosis and Vascular Research, Department of Medical Research, and Laboratory of Experimental Cardiology, Department of Pathophysiology, University of Leuven, Belgium.

Supported by the Geconcerteerde Onderzoeksactie (project 80-85-3) and grants from the University of Leuven, Belgium. D. Stump is the recipient of NHLBI Clinical Investigator Award HL 01176.

Address for correspondence: D. Collen, M.D., Center for Thrombosis and Vascular Research, Department of Medical Research, Campus Gasthuisberg–University of Leuven, Herestraat 49, B-3000 Leuven, Belgium.

Received Jan. 30, 1985; revision accepted April 18, 1985.

*Permanent address: Mochida Pharmaceutical Co., Research Laboratory of Cell Science, Tokyo, 115 Japan.

the end of the infusion and recanalization was obtained by intracoronary infusion.

Thrombolysis was generally heralded by the onset of reperfusion arrhythmia and was confirmed in each animal by angiography performed at 10 min intervals. Heparin was administered via intravenous injections of 1000 U at the onset of the infusion of the thrombolytic agents and 15 and 30 min later to prevent reocclusion.[14]

To measure the turnover rate of pro-urokinase and the extent of systemic activation of the fibrinolytic system, blood samples were collected in citrate before and 2, 5, 10, 20, and 30 min after the onset of intravenous infusion, at the end of intracoronary infusion if one was administered, and at 2, 5, 10, 20, 30, 40, and 50 min after completion of the infusion of thrombolytic agents. Samples were cooled immediately on ice and centrifuged for immediate analysis of fibrinogen and α_2-antiplasmin activity, as described previously.[14] Circulating levels of pro-urokinase were measured on frozen plasma samples by a classic radioimmunoassay with a rabbit antibody against human urinary urokinase. Titration curves of urokinase and pro-urokinase with this antibody were superimposable.

Pro-urokinase, highly purified from a transformed human kidney cell line (ACHN), was provided by Mochida Chemical Co. The material migrated as a single band (over 90% homogeneity) with M_r 54,000 on sodium dodecyl sulfate gel electrophoresis. The material could be fully activated by plasmin and displayed a specific activity of 95,000 IU/mg protein as measured on fibrin plates. The pro-urokinase preparation used in this study contained approximately 5% of activated molecules as measured by amidolytic assay. This concentration of urokinase is far below the minimum level necessary to measure any fibrinolytic effects in vivo. In addition, we have shown that the activation of plasminogen by pro-urokinase is not dependent on the presence or formation of activated urokinase.[15]

Urokinase (Winkinase) was a gift from Dr. G. Murano, Bureau of Biologics, Bethesda, MD.

Results

Pro-urokinase did not induce thrombolysis within 30 min when administered intravenously at a rate of 10 μg/kg/min in two dogs. Subsequent intracoronary infusion at the same rate produced recanalization after 8 and 15 min, respectively (table 1). Intravenous infusion of pro-urokinase at a rate of 20 μg/kg/min in four dogs resulted in complete reperfusion in three dogs within 20, 21, and 22, min, respectively, as demonstrated by coronary angiography (figure 1). In one dog recanalization was nearly complete after 30 min and reocclusion occurred within 10 min after the end of the infusion. In this dog recanalization was obtained within 8 min by intracoronary infusion of pro-urokinase at the same rate.

Intravenous infusion of urokinase at a rate of 10 μg/kg/min in seven dogs produced recanalization in four of them within 19 ± 2 min. In the three other dogs recanalization was obtained within 11 ± 3 min of intracoronary infusion of urokinase at the same rate.

Analysis of the plasma levels of fibrinogen and α_2-antiplasmin (figure 2) indicated that intravenous infusion of pro-urokinase at a rate of 20 μg/kg/min did not cause systemic fibrinolytic activation, whereas infusion of urokinase at half this rate caused extensive α_2-antiplasmin consumption and significant fibrinogen breakdown.

TABLE 1
Coronary thrombolysis in dogs

Agent	Dose (μg/kg/min)	Number	Infusion	Recanalization Number	Recanalization Time (min)
Pro-urokinase	10	2	IV	0	
			IV + IC	2	37 and 45
	20	4	IV	4	23±2[A]
			IV + IC	1	38[B]
Urokinase	10	7	IV	4	19±2
			IV + IC	3	41±3

IV = intravenous infusion for 30 min; IV + IC = intravenous infusion for 30 min followed by intracoronary infusion for 15 min.

[A]Time to complete reperfusion in three dogs and near complete reperfusion in 1 dog (mean ± SEM).

[B]The reoccluded coronary artery in the dog with near complete reperfusion was recanalized within 8 min of intracoronary administration of pro-urokinase.

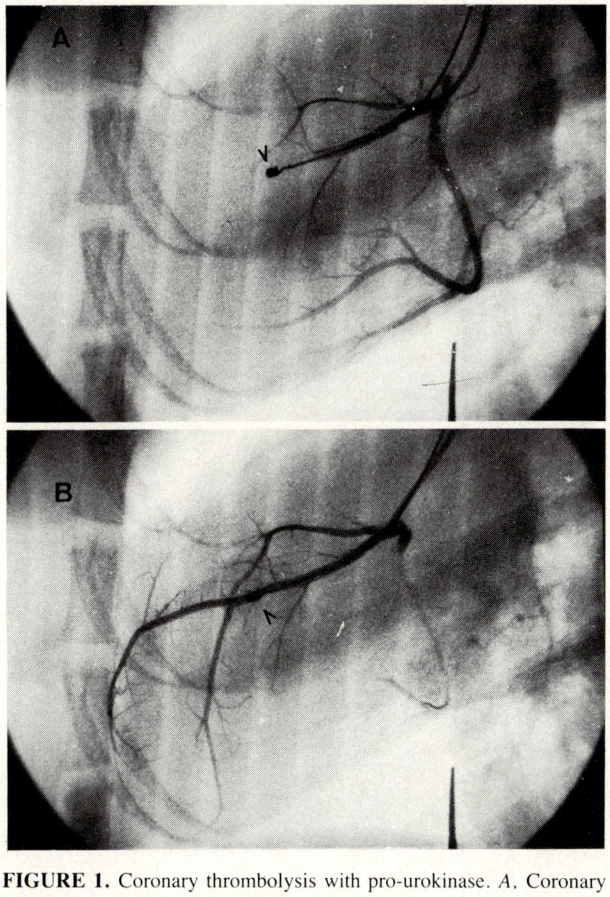

FIGURE 1. Coronary thrombolysis with pro-urokinase. *A*, Coronary angiogram after introduction of the copper coil (arrow), showing occlusive thrombosis extending proximally over a segment of 2 cm. *B*, Coronary angiogram after intravenous infusion of pro-urokinase, showing complete reperfusion.

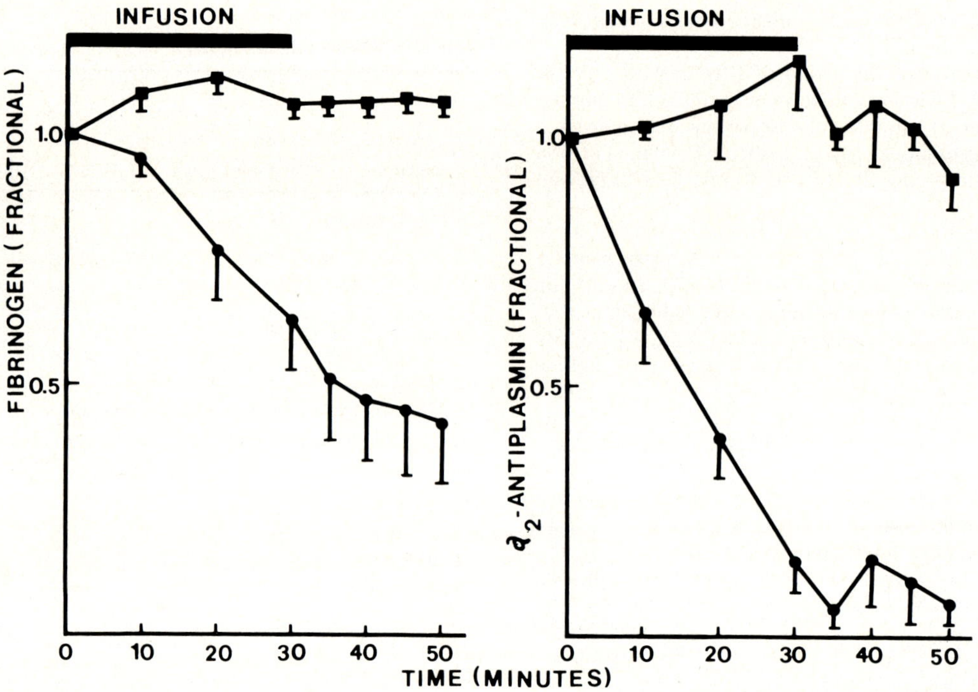

FIGURE 2. Changes in fibrinogen and α_2-antiplasmin levels in plasma during intravenous infusion of pro-urokinase or urokinase in dogs with acute myocardial infarction. ■, Pro-urokinase (20 μg/kg/min for 30 min); ●, urokinase (10 μg/kg/min for 30 min). Results are mean ± SD. The measurements were performed on fresh blood samples.

The pharmacokinetics of pro-urokinase after its intravenous infusion at a rate of 20 μg/kg/min for 30 min, as measured by radioimmunoassay, are summarized in figure 3. A gradual increase of the plasma level was observed to reach a plateau level of 3.5 μg/ml. After the end of the infusion, the pro-urokinase antigen disappeared from plasma with an initial t½ of 7 min, but the disappearance curve was not monotone.

In contrast to the measured plasma levels of pro-urokinase for which dilution curves were uniformly linear, those for samples containing urokinase were nonlinear when serially diluted. This observation was unexpected in view of the identical titers of the antibody to each agent as measured in buffer systems and must reflect interference with the measurement of urokinase by plasma factors such as antiproteinases,

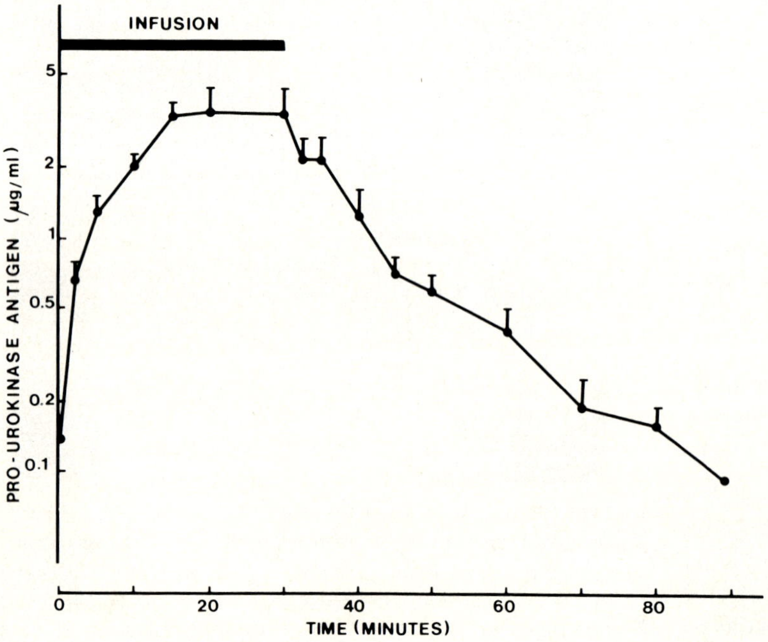

FIGURE 3. Pro-urokinase associated antigen levels in plasma during and after intravenous infusion of pro-urokinase at a rate of 20 μg/kg/min for 30 min. Results are mean ± SD. The disappearance rate after cessation of the infusion occurs with a t½ of 7 min.

which react with urokinase but not with pro-urokinase.[3]

Discussion

The results of this study indicate that pro-urokinase, when administered intravenously at a sufficiently high rate (20 μg/kg/min), can cause dissolution of occlusive coronary clots in dogs without systemic fibrinolytic activation. Urokinase, although causing coronary thrombolysis with at least equal potency, does so only in the presence of significant systemic fibrinolysis as reflected by decreased levels of fibrinogen and α_2-antiplasmin. This confirms and extends previous observations that natural[3, 11] and recombinant[13] pro-urokinase cause thrombolysis with increased fibrin specificity relative to their two-chain counterparts. Our observation that urokinase effects thrombolysis at relatively similar doses as pro-urokinase is contrary to those of previous studies.[3, 11, 13] The reason is not readily apparent, although all of these previous reports used preparations of venous thrombosis, while we have made the first comparison between pro-urokinase and urokinase in arterial thrombosis.

Although t-PA was not used directly in this study, our preparation of coronary thrombolysis has been applied previously to the study of fibrinolysis induced by recombinant t-PA. Coronary reperfusion was achieved regularly within 13.7 $\pm$ 1.9 min without systemic fibrinolysis by an infusion of 10 μg/kg/min t-PA with control values from urokinase comparable to those obtained in this study. Although clearly not a controlled comparison, it would nonetheless appear that the specific thrombolytic activity of t-PA is at least twofold higher than that of pro-urokinase. Similar results were noted in a controlled comparison between the two in rabbits with jugular vein thrombosis,[13] although the rabbit is a relatively urokinase-resistant species and might constitute a less-than-optimal animal preparation for such a comparison.

Pro-urokinase is rapidly removed from the circulation, with a postinfusion t½ in plasma of 7 min. This clearance rate is comparable to that of t-PA in dogs, which has a t½ of 5 min.[14] The clearance rate of pro-urokinase is also comparable with that of urokinase in man (t½ 16 min),[16] considering the inverse relationship between body weight and turnover. The similar turnover rate of recombinant pro-urokinase and active urokinase was also established in rabbits.[17] Therefore the maintenance of a therapeutic level of pro-urokinase in plasma will most likely, as is the case for t-PA and for urokinase, require continuous infusion.

Because of the large interspecies variability of the response to thrombolytic agents, the results obtained in dogs cannot as such be extrapolated to man. Using a system composed of a radioactive plasma clot immersed in plasma,[18] we have previously confirmed this large interspecies variability but have observed comparable relative thrombolytic effects of t-PA, pro-urokinase, and urokinase within the same species. On the basis of the finding that the fibrinolytic system of man is more responsive to activation by t-PA and urokinase than that of most other mammalian species, it may be anticipated that the human fibrinolytic system may be more responsive to pro-urokinase than that of the dog.

In conclusion, this study confirms the results of previous reports that natural and recombinant pro-urokinase are more clot-selective thrombolytic agents than active urokinase in animals with venous thrombosis. We have now extended this observation to an experimental preparation of arterial thrombosis, which may be relevant for acute myocardial infarction. Whether pro-urokinase might constitute an alternative to t-PA for coronary thrombolysis in man remains to be further investigated.

References

1. Collen D, Topol EJ, Tiefenbrunn AJ, Gold HK, Weisfeldt ML, Sobel BE, Leinbach RC, Brinker JA, Ludbrook PA, Yasuda I, Bulkley BH, Robison AK, Hutter AM Jr, Bell WR, Spadaro JJ Jr, Khaw BA, Grossbard EB: Coronary thrombolysis with recombinant human tissue-type plasminogen activator: a prospective, randomized, placebo-controlled trial. Circulation **70:** 1012, 1984
2. Smith RAG, Dupe RJ, English PD, Green J: Fibrinolysis with acyl-enzymes: a new approach to thrombolytic therapy. Nature **290:** 505, 1981
3. Gurewich V, Pannell R, Louie S, Kelley P, Suddith RL, Greenlee R: Effective and fibrin-specific clot lysis by a zymogen precursor form of urokinase (pro-urokinase): a study in vitro and in two animal species. J Clin Invest **73:** 1731, 1984
4. Bernik MB: Increased plasminogen activator (urokinase) in tissue culture after fibrin deposition. J Clin Invest **52:** 823, 1973
5. Nolan C, Hall L, Barlow G, Tribby IIE: Plasminogen activator from human embryonic kidney cell cultures: evidence for a proactivator. Biochim Biophys Acta **496:** 384, 1977
6. Husain S, Gurewich V, Lipinski B: Purification and partial characterization of a single-chain high-molecular-weight form of urokinase from human urine. Arch Biochem Biophys **220:** 31, 1983
7. Wun TC, Schleuning WD, Reich E: Isolation and characterization of urokinase from human plasma. J Biol Chem **257:** 3276, 1982
8. Wun TC, Ossowski L, Reich E: A proenzyme form of human urokinase. J Biol Chem **257:** 7262, 1982
9. Nielsen LS, Hansen JG, Skriver L, Wilson EL, Kaltoft K, Zeuthen J, Danø K: Purification of zymogen to plasminogen activator from human glioblastoma cells by affinity chromatography with monoclonal antibody. Biochemistry **21:** 6410, 1982
10. Kohno T, Hopper P, Lillquist JS, Suddith RL, Greenlee R, Moir DT: Kidney plasminogen activator: a precursor form of human urokinase with high fibrin affinity. Biotechnology **2:** 628, 1984
11. Sumi H, Maruyama M, Matsuo O, Mihara H, Toki N: Higher fibrin-binding and thrombolytic properties of single polypeptide chain–high molecular weight urokinase. Thromb Haemost **47:** 297, 1982
12. Heyneker HL, Holmes WE, Vehar GA: Preparation of functional human urokinase proteins. European Patent Application No. 83103629.8, Publication No. 0092182A2, European Patent Office, Munich, West Germany, 1983

13. Collen D, Stassen JM, Blaber M, Winkler M, Verstraete M: Biological and thrombolytic properties of proenzyme and active forms of human urokinase. III. Thrombolytic properties of natural and recombinant urokinase in rabbits with experimental jugular vein thrombosis. Thromb Haemost **52:** 27, 1984
14. Van de Werf F, Bergmann SR, Fox KAA, De Geest H, Hoyng CF, Sobel BE, Collen D: Coronary thrombolysis with intravenously administered human tissue-type plasminogen activator produced by recombinant DNA technology. Circulation **69:** 605, 1984
15. Lijnen HR, Zamarron C, Collen D: Pro-urokinase: kinetics and mechanism of action. Thromb Haemost (1985, in press)
16. Alkjaersig N, Fletcher A: Metabolism of urokinase. *In* Paoletti R, Sherry S, editors: Thrombosis and urokinase. New York, 1977, Academic Press Inc., p 129
17. Collen D, De Cock F, Lijnen HR: Biological and thrombolytic properties of proenzyme and active forms of human urokinase. II. Turnover of natural and recombinant urokinase in rabbits and squirrel monkeys. Thromb Haemost **52:** 24, 1984
18. Lijnen HR, DeWreede K, Demarsin E, Collen D: Biological and thrombolytic properties of proenzyme and active forms of human urokinase. IV. Variability in fibrinolytic response of plasma of several mammalian species. Thromb Haemost **52:** 31, 1984

The effect of cyclooxygenase inhibition on vasomotion of proximal coronary arteries with endothelial damage

GARY E. LANE, M.D., AND ALFRED A. BOVE, M.D., PH.D.

ABSTRACT Vasomotion of the proximal branches of the left coronary artery was studied in an intact anesthetized canine preparation after injury to the endothelium of the left anterior descending branch of the left coronary artery (LAD) with a balloon angioplasty catheter. The dimensions of the left coronary artery were examined by quantitative angiography and LAD flow was measured by determining intracoronary ^{133}Xe washout. Thirty minutes after endothelial damage alone dimensions of the LAD remained unchanged. In five dogs continued observation for a total of 120 min revealed no significant change in dimensions of the LAD. In another group of five dogs, after the administration of 5 mg/kg indomethacin there was a progressive reduction in cross-sectional area of the LAD by 60, 90, and 105 min (37%, 42%, and 50%, respectively, $p < .05$). No significant change in the dimensions of the undamaged left circumflex artery was noted after the administration of indomethacin. The effect of another cyclooxygenase inhibitor (4 mg/kg meclofenamate) on endothelial damage to the LAD in an additional four dogs was also examined. Again significant reduction of the cross-sectional area of the LAD was seen at 60 and 120 min (40% and 44%, respectively, $p < .05$). Heart rate and blood pressure were unchanged throughout the experiment in control and indomethacin-treated dogs. Mean blood pressure rose slightly after administration of meclofenamate (from 80 ± 5 to 98 ± 7 at 120 min, $p < .05$). These data indicate that the combination of endothelial injury and cyclooxygenase inhibition with indomethacin or meclofenamate results in proximal coronary artery vasoconstriction. This phenomenon may have important implications regarding the complications of coronary angioplasty and in focal spasm of diseased coronary arteries.
Circulation 72, No. 2, 389–396, 1985.

THE ENDOTHELIUM has been demonstrated in vitro to have an important role in mediating relaxation of vascular smooth muscle.[1] Recently, we used an intact canine preparation to demonstrate an enhanced response to vasoconstrictor agents of proximal coronary arteries with endothelial damage,[2] but factors influencing these phenomena have not been specifically defined. The products of arachidonic acid metabolism may play a role in modulating the vasomotor response, considering the potent effects that such metabolites have been shown to exert on the coronary circulation.[3]

Isolated coronary arteries have been demonstrated to contract in response to disruption of arachidonic acid metabolism by cyclooxygenase inhibition.[4-7] In addition, balloon catheter–induced damage of canine carotid arteries resulted in a reduction in vasodilator metabolites prostaglandin (PG) I_2 and PGE_2, while vasoconstrictor metabolites of the lipoxygenase pathway were increased.[8]

The clinical importance of these concepts may be reflected in the complications of balloon coronary angioplasty and the spontaneous vasomotion (spasm) of atherosclerotic coronary arteries. In this study we hypothesized that endothelial damage in the setting of cyclooxygenase blockade would result in significant vasoconstriction of proximal coronary arteries.

Methods

Experimental preparation. Ten adult mongrel dogs were anesthetized with Innovar-vet (0.2 ml/kg im) and ventilated with 70% nitrous oxide in oxygen via a Harvard respirator (model 807). This form of anesthesia produces minimal effects on the coronary circulation.[9, 10]

A No. 6F Lehman catheter and a No. 5F bipolar pacing catheter were advanced under fluoroscopic monitoring through branches of the right external jugular vein into the coronary sinus for blood sampling and pacing. Blood samples for Po_2,

From the Cardiovascular Division, Mayo Clinic, Rocheter, MN.
Supported in part by a grant from the PepsiCo Foundation.
Dr. Lane is a postdoctoral fellow supported by NIH training grant NO. HL07111.
Address for correspondence: Alfred A. Bove, M.D., Ph.D., Cardiovascular Division, Mayo Clinic, Rochester, MN 55905.
Received Oct. 4, 1984; revision accepted May 9, 1985.

oxygen saturation, and hemoglobin were obtained throughout the experimental period.

A coronary guide catheter was advanced under fluoroscopy retrograde through the left carotid artery to the ascending aorta. After engagement of the ostium of the left coronary artery, as determined by test injections of radiopaque contrast medium (meglumine diatrizoate [Renografin-76]), a G20-20 or 20-25S balloon dilatation catheter (USCI) was advanced into the proximal portion of the left anterior descending branch of the left coronary artery (LAD). Statham P23DG pressure transducers were balanced and calibrated for monitoring pressure from the coronary guide catheter, balloon dilatation catheter, and a cannula inserted in the left femoral artery. The pressures and electrocardiogram were monitored continuously and recorded during each stage of the experiment.

Data analysis. Coronary blood flow was determined by injection of 0.25 mCi of ^{133}Xe through a No. 4F infusion catheter positioned subselectively in the proximal LAD. Radioisotope washout was monitored with a single crystal detector positioned over the left chest at the midventricular level. Count data were processed by a PDP 11/34 computer (Digital Equipment Corp.) and the first 60 sec of the washout curve was used to determine the slope (K) by a monoexponential log-linear least squares calculation. Coronary blood flow was calculated as

$$\text{Flow (ml/min·g)} = 0.72\ K/1.05$$

where 0.72 = myocardium-blood partition coefficient; 1.05 = density of the myocardium.

Coronary vascular resistance (mm Hg/ml/g·min) was calculated from the ratio

$$\frac{\text{Mean arterial pressure}}{\text{LAD flow}}$$

Dimensions of the left coronary artery were quantitated with a computerized angiographic analysis system.[11] Angiographic examination was performed by injection of 4 to 5 ml of meglumine diatrizoate through the guide catheter into the left main coronary artery. Spot x-ray films were obtained at 85 kV for 35 msec during mid-diastole with an electrocardiographic trigger system. Angiograms were acquired in a constant right anterior oblique projection in each animal. The opacified luminal edges of the coronary artery were manually traced and digitized with a quantitative angiography program in a PDP 11/34 computer (Digital Equipment Corp.). The program calculated luminal diameter and cross-sectional area at 1 mm intervals along the artery measured. A representative 5 mm section of each scanned artery was used to evaluate the results. The method of analysis has been previously tested and described.[12]

Arteriovenous oxygen differences (ml/dl) were calculated by taking the difference between arterial and coronary sinus blood oxygen content. Oxygen content was calculated as (hemoglobin g/100 ml) × 1.35 ml O_2/g × oxygen saturation.

Experimental procedure. After positioning of the catheters, the baseline heart rate, blood pressure, and coronary blood flow were measured and recorded. Subsequently, an angiogram of the left coronary artery was obtained. After the control measurements, balloon endothelial damage was performed. The balloon dilatation catheter was advanced under fluoroscopic and pressure monitoring to the midportion of the LAD. The balloon was then inflated with a 50% contrast solution under low pressure. While inflated the catheter was withdrawn to the proximal portion of the artery. This procedure was repeated four to five times, during which the fluoroscopic image was recorded on videotape to localize the region of balloon endothelial damage. This method has previously been shown to reliably induce endothelial damage as identified by scanning electron microscopy.[2] Microscopic evaluation of arteries damaged in these experiments revealed findings similar to those of our previous studies. A 2.0 mm balloon was selected for use in arteries with luminal diameters of between 2.0 and 3.0 mm to avoid a myogenic response or possible medial damage.

After endothelial injury, a 30-min period was allowed to eliminate any transient responses. At the end of ths 30 min-period, the heart rate, pressures, LAD coronary blood flow, and angiographic dimensions were obtained. All animals in the experimental groups sustained endothelial damage as described. In the control group (n = 5), after the stabilization period, serial recording of pressures, heart rate, and coronary dimensions were obtained every 15 min for 90 min. Coronary blood flow measurements were taken at 30 min intervals. In one treated group (n = 5) 5 mg/kg iv indomethacin was administered and pressure, coronary blood flow, and coronary angiographic measurements were recorded as described. In the other treated group (n = 4), 4 mg/kg iv meclofenamate was administered and the same measurements were obtained.

Statistical analysis. Results are reported as mean ± SEM. Data were analyzed with Student's t test for paired variables and by two-way analysis of variance.

Results

Hemodynamic parameters. The arterial pressure and heart rate did not change significantly throughout the study in the control animals (table 1). The indomethacin-treated animals demonstrated a slight, but nonsignificant, increase in arterial pressure and heart rate after the administration of indomethacin (table 2). In the meclofenamate-treated animals there was a significant increase in arterial pressure from the 30 min measurement until the end of the experiment, and heart rate was unchanged (table 3).

Coronary blood flow and resistance. In the control animals (endothelial damage only) there was a significant decrease in coronary blood flow (−21% at 90 min, $p < .05$). However, the calculated coronary vascular resistance revealed only a slight, statistically nonsignificant, increase (table 1).

In the indomethacin-treated animals there was a decrease in coronary blood flow and an increase in coronary vascular resistance to values that were not significantly different from initial control values (table 2).

A small but significant rise in coronary blood flow was seen after the endothelial damage procedure was performed in the meclofenamate group (+34% after endothelial damage, $p < .05$). The coronary vascular resistance decreased slightly at this point, and increased significantly (+19%, $p < .05$) at 90 min after the administration of meclofenamate.

Hemoglobin levels were 9.3 ± 1.6 g/dl in the control group, 10.6 ± 1.4 g/dl in the indomethacin group, and 11.1 ± 3 g/dl in the meclofenamate group. There were no significant changes in myocardial arteriovenous oxygen difference throughout the experimental period in either group of animals. Arterial oxygen saturation was 95% to 96% throughout the experiment.

TABLE 1
Hemodynamic parameters in control animals with endothelial damage only

	Heart rate (bpm)	Mean arterial pressure (mm Hg)	LAD coronary blood flow (ml/min·g)	LAD coronary vascular resistance (mm Hg/ml/g·min)	Myocardial arteriovenous oxygen difference (ml O_2/dl)
Control	78±7	82±5	1.66±0.09	50±5	5.98±0.70
15 min	73±7	82±7	—		
30 min	77±6	82±4	1.40±0.08	59±4	6.37±0.84
45 min	74±7	82±5	—		
60 min	77±6	80±5	1.66±0.26	57±11	5.84±0.62
75 min	76±5	84±7	—		
90 min	75±7	81±6	1.31±0.08^	62±5	6.59±0.80
105 min	76±7	82±7	—		
120 min	77±7	83±7	1.38±0.07^	58±4	5.69±0.57

Data are mean ± SEM.
^p < .05 vs control.

Dimensions of the left coronary artery. Figure 1 illustrates a typical coronary angiogram of the dog left coronary artery after endothelial injury and indomethacin. The midportion of the LAD is narrowed compared with control.

In dogs from the control group (endothelial damage only) the portion of the LAD that sustained endothelial damage did not change significantly in diameter or cross-sectional area for 120 min after the injury (figure 2).

In the dogs in the indomethacin-treated group, there were no significant changes in diameter of cross-sectional area of the undamaged left circumflex coronary artery either before or after drug. In addition, after endothelial damage of the LAD no change in luminal dimensions occurred for 30 min. However, the administration of indomethacin produced a significant reduction in the luminal diameter of the LAD at 60, 90, and 105 min (21%, $p < .02$; 25%, $p < .01$; and 30%, $p < .01$, respectively) vs initial baseline diameter (figure 3). Cross-sectional area was concurrently reduced at 60, 90, and 105 min (37%, $p < .02$; 42%, $p < .02$; and 50%, $p < .02$, respectively) vs initial baseline area (figure 4).

TABLE 2
Hemodynamic parameters in animals with endothelial damage receiving indomethacin

	Heart rate (bpm)	Mean arterial pressure (mm Hg)	LAD coronary blood flow (ml/min·g)	LAD coronary vascular resistance (mm Hg/ml/g·min)	Myocardial arteriovenous oxygen difference (ml O_2/dl)
Control	73±8	86±8	2.12±0.59	48±8	6.07±0.28
Endothelial damage					
15 min	65±5	85±5			
30 min	73±8	85±7	1.81±0.18	49±5	7.15±0.40
Indomethacin					
15 min	70±5	87±6			
30 min	70±4	90±5	1.90±0.17	48±5	7.0±0.52
45 min	70±6	94±4			
60 min	74±6	89±5	1.63±0.2	55±4	6.99±0.57
75 min	78±6	94±3			
90 min	78±7	91±3	1.69±0.24	59±8	7.5±0.60
105 min	76±6	96±4			

Data are mean ± SEM.

TABLE 3
Hemodynamic parameters in animals with endothelial damage receiving meclofenamate

	Heart rate (bpm)	Mean arterial pressure (mm Hg)	LAD coronary blood flow (ml/min·g)	LAD coronary vascular resistance (mm Hg/ml/g·min)	Myocardial arteriovenous oxygen difference (ml O_2/dl)
Control	72±15	80±5	2.03±0.43	48±14	6.76±0.49
Endothelial damage					
30 min	80±14	91±6	2.73±0.47[A]	35±5	6.86±0.64
Meclofenamate					
15 min	72±13	94±3	2.09±0.56	51±11	7.35±0.26
30 min	71±10	92±3[A]	2.07±0.46	51±11	7.12±0.33
60 min	71±8	94±5[A]	2.27±0.47	47±9	7.44±0.69
90 min	74±11	96±5[A]	2.04±0.50	57±15[A]	7.14±0.30
120 min	71±10	98±7[A]	2.18±0.49	55±17	7.90±0.51[A]
NTG	72±9	96±6[A]			7.76±0.39

Data are mean ± SEM.
NTG = nitroglycerin.
[A]$p < .05$.

Analysis of the dimensions of the LAD in the group treated with meclofenamate (n = 4) also revealed a significant reduction in diameter at 60, 90, and 120 min (21%, 18%, and 27%, respectively, all $p < .05$). Cross-sectional area (figure 5) was concurrently reduced at 60 and 120 min (40% and 49%, respectively, $p < .05$). After the administration of 200 μg of intracoronary nitroglycerin the dimensions of the LAD returned to baseline in both the indomethacin and meclofenamate groups.

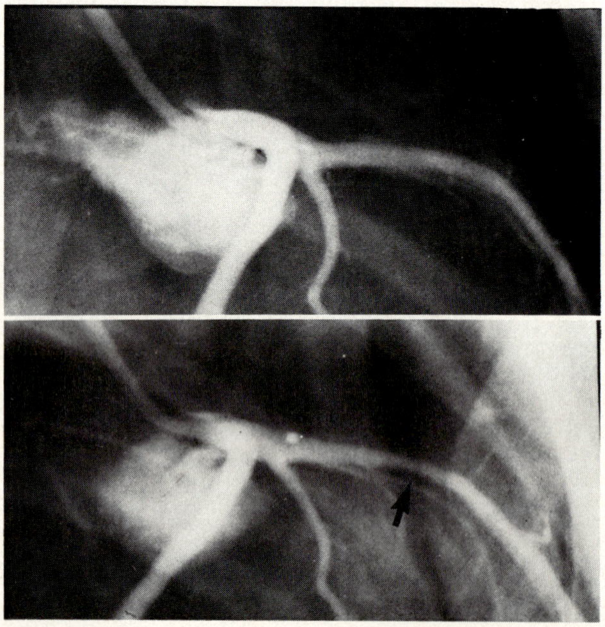

FIGURE 1. Right anterior oblique left coronary angiogram from an intact dog before (*top*) and after combined indomethacin and endothelial injury (*bottom*). There is a focally narrowed area in the mid portion of the LAD (arrow).

Discussion

We have demonstrated significant vasoconstriction of endothelial-damaged proximal LADs in the setting of cyclooxygenase inhibition. Indomethacin did not affect the dimensions of the undamaged left circumflex coronary artery, and control animals with endothelial damage alone did not have significant constriction. Significant vasoconstriction of damaged LADs was also seen in a group of meclofenamate-treated dogs. The similar effect of indomethacin and meclofenamate

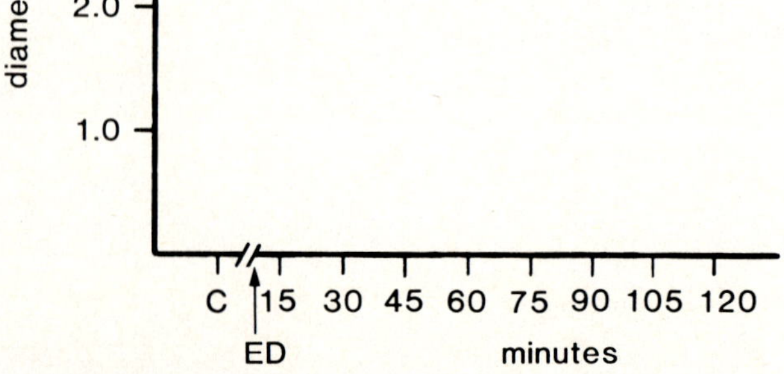

FIGURE 2. Diameter of mid portion of LAD measured by quantitative coronary angiography over a 120 min period after endothelial damage (ED). Data expressed as mean ± SEM.

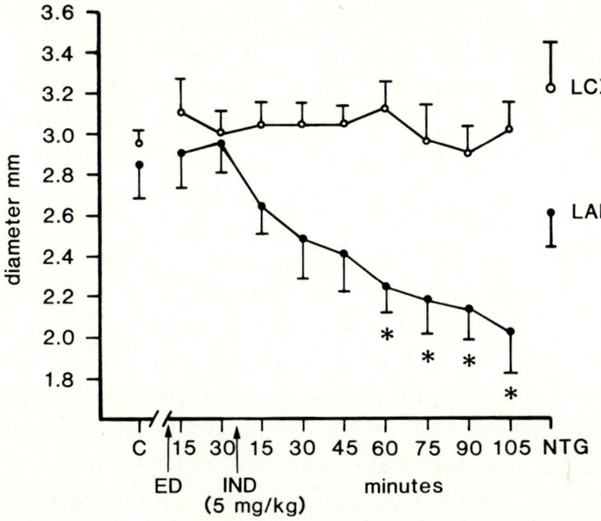

FIGURE 3. Diameter of mid portion of LAD and circumflex (LCX) coronary arteries measured by quantitative angiography over 105 min after endothelial damage (ED) to the LAD and intravenous indomethacin (IND). The LAD showed a progressive focal narrowing in the endothelial-damaged segment. NTG = nitroglycerin. Data expressed as mean ± SEM.

on the damaged LAD would support a shared mechanism of action such as cyclooxygenase inhibition.

The reduction in the dimensions of the damaged coronary arteries in the group treated with indomethacin or meclofenamate could not be explained by a

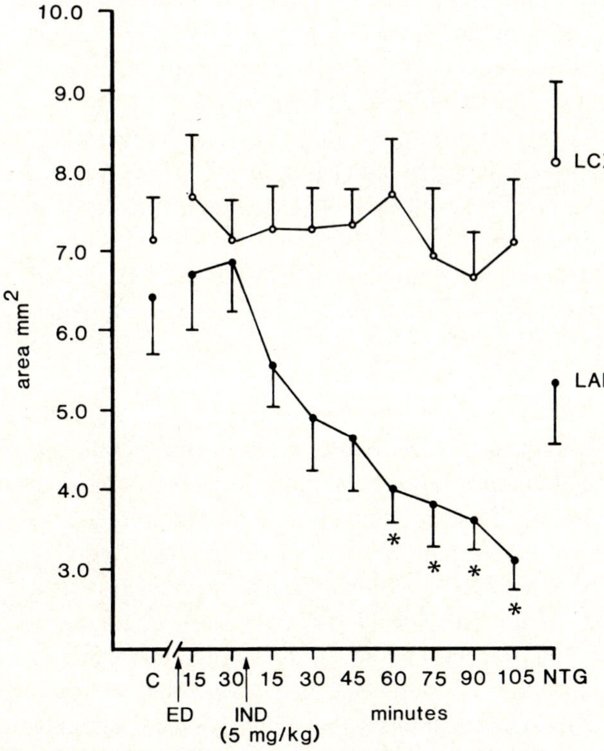

FIGURE 4. Cross-sectional area of LAD, and circumflex (LCX) coronary arteries after endothelial damage (ED) to the LAD and indomethacin (IND). NTG = nitroglycerin. Data expressed as mean ± SEM.

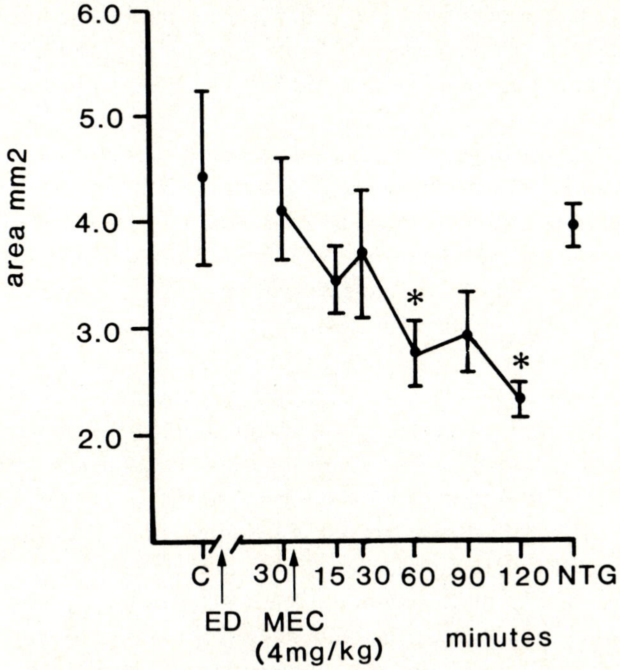

FIGURE 5. Cross-sectional area of the LAD after endothelial damage (ED) and meclofenamate (MEC). NTG = nitroglycerin. Data are expressed as mean ± SEM.

decrease in myocardial metabolic demands,[13] since the heart rate and blood pressure actually increased slightly during the experiment.

There was also no significant alteration of coronary blood flow or coronary vascular resistance in the group treated with indomethacin. A small but significant increase in coronary vascular resistance was noted 90 min after the administration of meclofenamate. These measurements were made in dogs in the resting state and no attempt was made to determine the coronary flow reserve during the vasoconstriction. It is probable that the degree of vasoconstriction seen in this experiment would result in a serious limitation to nutrient flow through a coronary arterial lumen previously compromised to a moderate degree by an atherosclerotic stenosis.

Intravenous indomethacin has been shown to slightly decrease resting coronary blood flow[4, 14] and in some experiments to diminish the reactive hyperemic response in open-chest or isolated heart canine preparations.[15] However, in other anesthetized animal preparations a significant alteration of resting coronary blood flow or coronary vascular resistance has not been observed.[16–18] Indomethacin causes contraction of isolated coronary artery strips in vitro.[4, 6, 7] In addition, isolated balloon-dilated canine carotid arterial segments exhibit an enhanced contractile response to norepinephrine after the addition of indomethacin.[16] The principal action of indomethacin is to inhibit the enzyme cyclooxygenase.[20] Another cyclooxygenase inhibitor, acetylsalicylic acid, has also been shown to contract isolated coronary arterial preparations.[5, 7] In man, Freidman et al.[21] have demonstrated a substantial fall in coronary blood flow (181 to 111 ml/min) and a rise in coronary vascular resistance (+73%) in response to the administration of intravenous indomethacin (0.5 mg/kg) to patients with coronary artery disease. The exact mechanism underlying this response has not been elucidated. In particular, it is unknown whether this elevation of coronary resistance occurs because of vasoconstriction within the distal resistance vasculature or at the level of proximal conductance in coronary arteries with significant stenoses.

Recently, extensive investigation in vitro has documented the importance of the endothelium in the regulation of vasomotion.[1] The responses (especially relaxation) of vascular smooth muscle to many neurohumoral mediators are endothelium-dependent. The endothelium is susceptible to many toxic or mechanical injury processes. For example, coronary transluminal balloon angioplasty causes a loss of endothelium and platelet adhesion to the denuded arterial wall.[22] Also, endothelial damage has been postulated to be an important feature in the evolution of an atherosclerotic stenosis.[23] These examples illustrate how endothelial-damaged vessels may potentiate abnormal vasoconstrictor responses of proximal coronary arteries.

Derivatives of arachidonic acid have been demonstrated to produce impressive effects on the coronary circulation. Prostacyclin plays an important role in controlling platelet aggregation on vascular endothelium.[24] In addition, it is a potent coronary vasodilator.[25] Infusion of thromboxane A_2 into coronary arteries will result in vasoconstriction.[26] Recently, products of the alternative pathway of arachidonic acid metabolism (via lipoxygenase) have also been demonstrated to exert impressive effects on the coronary circulation.[27, 28] Leukotrienes C_4, D_4, and E_4 (originally described as slow-reacting substance of anaphylaxis or SRS-A) have been shown to provoke potent coronary vasoconstriction resulting in significant ischemia in several animal preparations.[28–32]

Trauma induced by the angioplasty balloon catheter does result in an alteration of arachidonic acid metabolism, which in turn results in a decrease in vasodilator PGs such as prostacyclin and an increase in lipoxygenase products.[8] Coronary arteries that sustained endothelial damage alone in our experiments did not manifest vasoconstriction. Intervention into the metabolic pathway of arachidonic acid by inhibition of the enzyme cyclooxygenase with indomethacin did result in significant vasoconstriction. Experimental evidence has demonstrated enhanced release of anaphylatic mediators (SRS-A) from lung, enhancement of antigen-induced tracheal contraction,[33] and increased production of chemotatic factors in the presence of cyclooxygenase inhibitors.[34] These findings suggest that inhibition of cyclooxygenase may result in preferential metabolism of arachidonic acid via the lipoxygenase pathway with the production of vasoconstrictor leukotrienes.[35] This shift in metabolism may accentuate the production of lipoxygenase products as previously described in balloon catheter–traumatized canine carotid arteries.[8] Alternatively, a reduction in the amount of prostacyclin present in the arterial wall caused by a combination of trauma and cyclooxygenase inhibition could result in vasoconstriction. The precise alteration in arachidonic acid metabolism responsible for the results cannot be specified with the available data.

A direct vasoconstrictor action of indomethacin on endothelial-damaged arteries could be postulated. However, the temporal course of the vasoconstrictor would suggest an action requiring time for alteration of a biosynthetic pathway. Further experimentation should allow for a more accurate explanation of the vasoconstrictor response. Kalsner[7] has demonstrated contraction of coronary artery preparations in vitro by aspirin and indomethacin. Addition of one inhibitor followed by the other did not potentiate the vasoconstriction, suggesting a similar mechanism of action for the two agents in these experiments in vitro. In addition, vasoconstriction induced by meclofenamate in the present study would also support the importance of cyclooxygenase inhibition in mediating the vasoconstrictor response.

Methodologic considerations. The procedure of balloon catheter–induced endothelial injury used in these experiments has been previously shown to reliably result in extensive endothelial loss with platelet aggregation.[2] The technique described was used after consideration of several factors, including the significance of endothelial damage in modulating vasomotor responses. The importance of avoiding a myogenic response, and possibly overdistending the artery resulting in paralysis of the muscular media was considered.[36] Although possibly not completely analogous to clinical coronary angioplasty, this preparation does reproduce the common occurrence of endothelial injury. In addition, it is unlikely that extensive medial damage occurs often during clinical coronary angioplasty, in view of the relatively common occurrence of spasm in this setting.[37]

Isolated artery preparations have been described to undergo indomethacin-induced vasoconstriction even when no procedures are performed to induce endothelial injury.[4–7] It is possible that inadvertent endothelial injury occurred in these preparations or that the dose of indomethacin responsible for the effects seen was not analogous to the dose used in our experiments. Use of acetylcholine as a spasmogen in some of these experiments[6, 37] would support the former possibility. Also, interaction between blood and the vessel wall is not allowed for in the experiments in vitro.

The doses of indomethacin and meclofenamate used in our experiments were selected because they have been shown to be effective in inducing cyclooxygenase inhibition in the canine coronary circulation.[14] It should also be noted that neither indomethacin or meclofenamate prevented a proximal coronary artery vasodilator response to intracoronary nitroglycerin.

Clinical importance of findings. Percutaneous transluminal coronary angioplasty results in extensive endothelial damage.[22] Coronary artery spasm occurs in 4% to 5% of the coronary angioplasty procedures.[38] One third of these episodes of spasm are associated with major complications such as myocardial infarction, emergency coronary artery bypass surgery, or death. There are data to suggest that coronary artery spasm plays a major role in the development of acute occlusion after percutaneous coronary angioplasty.[39] Many patients undergoing this procedure receive cyclooxygenase inhibitors for their antiplatelet effects. Our work suggests that the interaction of endothelial injury and cyclooxyenase inhibition may lead to a propensity for vasoconstriction of the proximal coronary artery. However, the dose of cyclooxygenase inhibitor used in our study was equivalent to doses used for treatment of inflammatory disorders and platelet-inhibitory doses are generally lower.

As mentioned previously, the study of Freidman et al.[21] demonstrated a substantial elevation of coronary vascular resistance by indomethacin in patients with atherosclerotic coronary artery disease. The anatomic site of this vasoconstrictor effect has not been localized. It is possible that the diseased proximal coronary arteries of these patients provided a setting for the vasoconstrictor action of indomethacin at the site of atherosclerotic stenoses. This could explain the decrease in coronary blood flow noted in these patients.

In concluson, we have demonstrated an important interaction of endothelial injury of normal coronary arteries and cyclooxygenase inhibition that resulted in a coronary vasoconstrictor response in an intact anesthesized canine preparation. Further study of this phenomenon should allow for greater understanding of the role of PGs and leukotrienes in the pathogenesis of abnormal coronary vasomotion.

We thank Messers. J. Dewey, C. Grabau, and R. Owen for technical assistance and Mrs. L. Schwieder for preparing the manuscript.

References

1. Furchgott RF: Role of endothelium in responses of vascular smooth muscle. Circ Res **53:** 557, 1983
2. Brum JM, Sufan QW, Lane GE, Bove AA: Increased vasoconstrictor activity of endothelial-damaged proximal coronary arteries in intact dogs. Circulation **70:** 1006, 1984
3. Dusting GJ, Moncada S, Vane JR: Prostaglandins, their intermediates and precursors: cardiovascular actions and regulatory roles in normal and abnormal circulatory systems. Prog Cardiovasc Dis **21:** 405, 1979
4. Sakanashi M, Araki H, Yonemura K: Indomethacin induced contractions of dog coronary arteries. J Cardiovasc Pharmacol **2:** 657, 1980
5. Sakanashi M, Araki H, Furukawa T, Rokutanda M, Yonemua K: A study on constrictor responses of dog coronary arteries to acetylsalicylic acid. Arch Int Pharmacodyn Ther **252:** 86, 1981
6. Cornish WJ, Goldie RG, Krstew EU, Miller RC: Effect of indomethacin on responses of sheep isolated coronary artery to arachadonic acid. Clin Exp Pharmacol Physiol **10:** 171, 1983
7. Kalsner S: Endogenous prostaglandin release contributes directly to coronary artery tone. Can J Physiol Pharmacol **53:** 560, 1975
8. Cragg A, Einzig S, Castaneda-Zuniga W, Amplatz K, White J, Ruo GHR: Vessel wall arachidonate metabolism after angioplasty: possible mediators of post-angioplasty vasospasm. Am J Cardiol **51:** 1441, 1983
9. Altura MD, Altura BT, Cavella A, Turlpaty DDUM, Weinbert J: Vascular smooth muscle and general anesthetics. Fed Proc **39:** 1584, 1980
10. Rorie DK, Muldoon SM, Tyce GM: Effects of fentyl on adrenergic function in canine arteries. Anesth Analg **60:** 21, 1981
11. Owen RM, Dewey JD, Bove AA: Evaluation of dimensions and steady-state hydraulic properties of coronary arteries. Biomed Sci Instrum **19:** 43, 1983
12. Bove AA, Dewey JD: Effects of serotonin and histamine on proximal and distal coronary vasculature in dogs: comparison with alpha adrenergic stimulation. Am J Cardiol **52:** 1333, 1983
13. Macho P, Hintze TH, Vatner SF: Regulation of large coronary arteries by increases in myocardial metabolic demands in conscious dogs. Circ Res **49:** 594, 1981
14. Hintze TH, Kaley G: Prostaglandins and the control of blood flow in the canine myocardium. Circ Res **40:** 313, 1977
15. Alexander RW, Kent KM, Pisano JJ, Keiser HR, Cooper T: Regulation of post-occlusive hyperemia by endogenously synthesized prostaglandins in the dog heart. J Clin Invest **55:** 1174, 1975
16. Harlan DM, Rooke TW, Belloni FL, Sparks HV: Effect of indomethacin on coronary vascular response to increased myocardial oxygen consumption. Am J Physiol **235:** H372, 1978
17. Owen TL, Ehrhart IC, Weidner WJ, Scott JB, Haddy FJ: Effects of indomethacin on local blood flow regulation in canine heart and kidney. Proc Soc Exp Biol Med **149:** 871, 1975
18. Block AJ, Feinberg H, Herbacynska-Cedro K, Vane JR: Anoxia-induced release of prostaglandins in rabbit isolated hearts. Circ Res **36:** 34, 1975
19. Zollikofer CL, Cragg AH, Einzig S, Castenda-Zuniga WR, Castenda F, Rysavy J, Bruhlmann WF, Shebuski RJ, Amplatz K: Prostaglandins and angioplasty. Radiology **149:** 681, 1983
20. Shea T, Winter CA: Chemical and biological studies on indomethacin, sulindac, and their analogs. Adv Drug Res **12:** 89, 1977
21. Freidman PL, Brown ZJ, Gunther S, Alexander RW, Barry WH, Mudge GH, Grossman W: Coronary vasoconstrictor effect of indomethacin in patients with coronary artery disease. N Engl J Med **305:** 1171, 1982
22. Pasternak RC, Baughman KL, Fallon JT, Block PC: Scanning

electron microscopy after coronary transluminal angioplasty of normal canine coronary arteries. Am J Cardiol **45:** 591, 1980
23. Ross R, Glomset JA: The pathogenesis of atherosclerosis: N Engl J Med **295:** 420, 1976
24. Moncada S: Prostacyclin and arterial wall biology. Arterioclerosis **2:** 193, 1982
25. Pitt B, Shea MJ, Romson JL, Lucchesi BR: Prostaglandins and prostaglandin inhibitors in ischemic heart disease. Ann Intern Med **99:** 83, 1983
26. Bove AA, Safford RE, Dewey JD: Vasomotor response to U46619 and endothelial damage in canine proximal coronary arteries. Eur Heart J (suppl 1): 21, 1984 (abst)
27. Lewis RA, Austin FA: The biologically active leukotrienes. J Clin Invest **73:** 889, 1984
28. Feuerstein G: Leukotrienes and the cardiovascular system. Prostaglandins **27:** 781, 1984
29. Michelassi F, Landa L, Hill RD, Lewenstein E, Watkins WD, Petaku AJ, Zapol WM: Leukotriene D_4: a potent coronary artery vasoconstrictor associated with impaired ventricular contraction. Science **217:** 841, 1982
30. Pazenbeck MJ, Kaley G: Leukotriene D_4 reduces coronary blood flow in the anesthetized dog. Prostaglandins **25:** 661, 1983
31. Ezra D, Boyd LM, Feuerstein G, Goldstein RE: Coronary constriction by leukotriene C_4, D_4, and E_4 in the intact pig heart. Am J Cardiol **51:** 1451, 1983
32. Roth DH, Lefer AM: Studies on the mechanism of leukotriene induced coronary artery constriction. Prostaglandins **26:** 573, 1983
33. Burka JF, Paterson NAM: Enhancement of antigen-induced tracheal contraction by cyclo-oxygenase inhibition. *In* Samuelsson B, Ramwell PW, Paoletti R, editors: Advances in prostaglandin and thromboxane research. New York, 1980, Raven Press, vol VIII, p 1755
34. Higgs GA, Eakins KE, Mugridge KC, Moncada S, Vane JR: The effects of nonsteroid antiinflammatory drugs on leukocyte migration in carrageenin-induced inflammation. Eur J Pharmacol **66:** 81, 1980
35. Mitchell HW: The effect of mixed inhibitors of cyclo-oxygenase and lipoxygenase on indomethacin-induced hyper-reactivity in the isolated trachea of the pig. Br. J Pharmacol **77:** 701, 1982
36. Castaneda-Zuniga WR, Laerum F, Rysavy J, Rusnak B, Amplatz K: Paralysis of arteries by intraluminal balloon dilatation. Radiology **144:** 75, 1982
37. Kalsner S: Prostaglandin mediated relaxation of coronary artery strips. Prostaglandins Med **1:** 231, 1978
48. Cowley MS, Dorros G, Kelsey SF, Van Raden M, Detre KM: Acute coronary events associated with percutaneous transluminal coronary angioplasty. Am J Cardiol **53:** 12C, 1984
39. Hollman J, Gruentzig AR, Douglas JS, King S, Ischinger T, Meier B: Acute occlusion after percutaneous transluminal angioplasty — a new approach. Circulation **68:** 725, 1983

Cyclic blood flow variations induced by platelet-activating factor in stenosed canine coronary arteries despite inhibition of thromboxane synthetase, serotonin receptors, and α-adrenergic receptors

P. APPRILL, M.D., J. M. SCHMITZ, M.D., W. B. CAMPBELL, PH.D., G. TILTON, M.D., J. ASHTON, PH.D., S. RAHEJA, M.D., L. M. BUJA, M.D., AND J. T. WILLERSON, M.D.

ABSTRACT The phospholipid platelet-activating factor (PAF) stimulates platelet aggregation and coronary vasoconstriction. In this study we determined whether PAF alters coronary flow patterns in vivo in a canine preparation with concentric coronary artery stenosis. This preparation is characterized by cyclic flow variations in coronary blood flow associated with transient platelet aggregation at the site of the coronary constriction. Thirty-nine male mongrel dogs were used in three protocols. In protocol 1, PAF (10^{-9} or 10^{-8} mol/min) was infused into the coronary artery proximal to the stenosis to determine (1) whether PAF induces cyclic flow variations and (2) whether PAF has an effect on systemic hemodynamics. Cyclic flow variations were induced in three of six dogs; in these animals, mean arterial pressure decreased by 5.5% and 42.1% 10 min after infusion of the lower and higher dose of PAF. In protocol 2, cyclic flow variations were abolished with either the thromboxane synthetase inhibitor UK38485 (mean dose 2.2 mg/kg iv), the serotonin antagonist ketanserin (0.5 mg/kg iv), or the α_2-adrenergic antagonist yohimbine (2 mg/kg iv). Subsequent administration of PAF restored the frequency of cyclic flow variations to the preantagonist levels. Thromboxane (Tx) B_2 and 6-keto-$PGF_{1\alpha}$, the stable metabolites of TxA_2 and prostacyclin, respectively, were measured in blood obtained distal to the coronary stenosis. TxB_2 levels increased substantially during cyclic flow variations and were returned to control values with the thromboxane synthetase inhibitor UK38485. Infusion of PAF subsequently restored cyclic flow variations without altering coronary arterial TxB_2 levels. Furthermore, although PAF-induced platelet aggregation in vitro was associated with an increase in platelet thromboxane release, thromboxane synthetase inhibition did not alter PAF-induced platelet aggregation. Taken together, these data indicate that PAF may initiate and/or restore cyclic flow variations after their abolition with either a thromboxane synthetase inhibitor or a serotonin or α_2-receptor antagonist. These data support previous studies in vitro demonstrating an action of PAF on platelet aggregation that is independent of thromboxane, serotonin, or α_2-adrenergic agonists.
Circulation 72, No. 2, 397–405, 1985.

THE CLINICAL SYNDROME of unstable angina pectoris may occur in association with decreases in myocardial oxygen supply.[1] This may be caused by factors that reduce coronary blood flow. Some of these factors include (1) coronary arterial spasm, (2) hemorrhage into a nonocclusive plaque, (3) platelet aggregation over areas of plaque or endothelial denudation, and (4) natural progression of coronary atherosclerosis. Platelet aggregates may mechanically obstruct an artery or may synthesize and release vasoactive agents such as thromboxane (Tx) A_2, which has vasoconstrictor properties. Hirsh et al.[2] found elevated coronary sinus-to-aortic ratios of TxB_2, the stable metabolite of TxA_2, in patients with unstable angina pectoris.

Folts et al.[3] developed an experimental preparation of a concentrically stenosed canine coronary artery. In this preparation there are episodic, spontaneous decreases in coronary blood flow interrupted by restorations of blood flow. These alterations in coronary blood flow have been called cyclic flow variations, which are associated with microscopic thrombi composed of platelets, erythrocytes, and leukocytes[3, 4] and

From the Departments of Internal Medicine (Cardiology Division), Pharmacology, and Pathology, University of Texas Health Science Center, Dallas.

Supported in part by NIH Ischemic SCOR 17669, HL-25471, and the Moss Fund, Dallas. Dr. Campbell is the recipient of NIH Research Career Development Award KO4-HL00801.

Address for correspondence: James T. Willerson, M.D., Room L5.134, University of Texas Health Science Center, 5323 Harry Hines Blvd., Dallas, TX 75235.

Received Jan. 8, 1985; revision accepted May 2, 1985.

with endothelial damage at the site of coronary arterial narrowing.[4,5] We have shown that TxB_2 concentrations increase in the distal portion of the stenosed coronary artery and that an inhibitor of thromboxane synthetase, dazoxiben, abolishes cyclic flow variations and decreases the TxB_2 concentration measured distal to the stenosis.[4] Similarly, serotonin or α_2-adrenergic antagonists attenuate the frequency of cyclic flow variations.[6] Taken together, these data suggest that platelet-derived agents that alter platelet aggregation and vascular tone may mediate cyclic flow variations either alone or in concert. It is possible that thromboxane, serotonin, and α_2-adrenergic receptor mechanisms are only some of the mediators of platelet activation in this experimental preparation; other agents may also influence platelet aggregation in the coronary circulation with resulting changes in coronary vascular tone and cyclic flow variations.

In this study we evaluated the recently isolated phospholipid 1-0-hexadecyl-2-acetyl-sn-glyceryl-phosphorylcholine, or platelet-activating factor (PAF). PAF stimulates human platelet aggregation in vitro[7-9] and is released by human platelets[10] and leukocytes.[11] It is a potent peripheral vasodilator[12] and decreases coronary blood flow when given by intracoronary injection in the pig.[13] Because of these physiologic effects, we wished to determine (1) whether PAF is capable of inducing cyclic flow variations in a stenosed canine coronary artery and (2) whether its effect is mediated through thromboxane, serotonin, or α_2-adrenergic mechanisms.

Materials and methods

Surgical preparation. Male mongrel dogs weighing 16 to 32 kg were anesthetized with 30 mg/kg pentobarbital and ventilated on room air with a Harvard ventilator. Temperature was controlled with a heating pad and monitored by measuring rectal temperature. Jugular venous and carotid arterial catheters were inserted, and a left thoracotomy was performed. The heart was exposed via a pericardial sling, and a left atrial catheter was placed. A Konigsberg pressure transducer (P23) was placed in the left ventricular apex for measurement of left ventricular pressure and dP/dt. Next, a 1 cm segment of the left anterior descending coronary artery (LAD) was cleared and small branches were ligated. A Doppler flow probe[14] and a small cylindric plastic constrictor were placed around the artery[4] (figure 1). A branch of the distal LAD below the flow probe was isolated, and a small polyethylene catheter (id 0.034 inch, od 0.050 inch) was placed for monitoring coronary pressure and for blood collection.[9] Next, either a small right ventricular branch of the LAD or a diagonal branch immediately above the Doppler flow probe was isolated and cannulated with a polyethylene catheter of similar size for infusion of the drug. The carotid catheter and both coronary arterial polyethylene catheters were kept heparinized with bovine heparin. Hemodynamic variables were monitored continuously on a Honeywell Electronics for

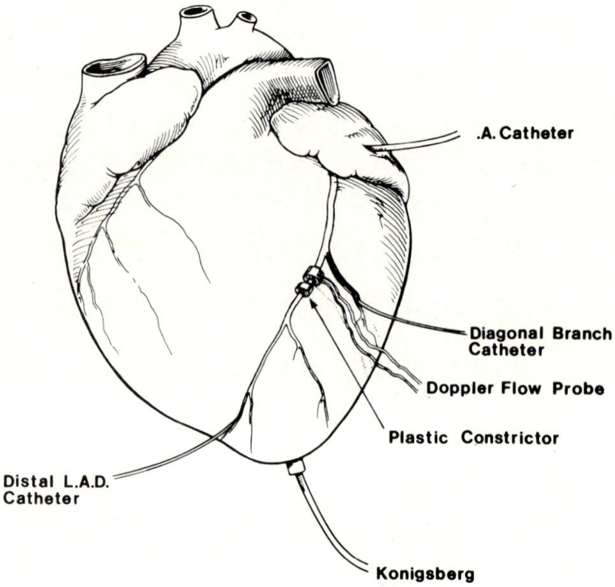

FIGURE 1. The experimental preparation includes a Doppler flow probe and plastic constrictor on a 1 cm segment of isolated coronary artery, distal coronary and diagonal branch catheters and left atrial (A) catheter, and a Konigsberg pressure transducer.

Medicine VR12 recorder and recorded on a Hewlett-Packard 7758A eight-channel recorder.

Protocol 1. Six male dogs were used to determine the systemic and coronary hemodynamic effects produced by an intracoronary infusion of PAF. After completion of the above surgical preparation, a small plastic constrictor was placed on the LAD to decrease resting phasic coronary blood flow by approximately 50% and to abolish the hyperemic response of a brief coronary occlusion.[4] Aortic pressure, heart rate, left ventricular pressure, left ventricular dP/dt, distal LAD pressure, and LAD phasic and mean blood flow by Doppler flow probe were measured. PAF, dissolved in 0.9% sodium chloride containing 1% bovine serum albumin, was infused into a catheter placed in the diagonal LAD branch proximal to the constrictor. Initially, 10^{-9} mol/min at 0.1 ml/min was infused with a Harvard infusion pump. The dose was increased to 10^{-8} mol/min after 30 min.

Protocol 2. To determine the mechanism of action of PAF on cyclic flow variations, the same experimental animal preparation was used. Hemodynamics were measured. Simultaneous blood samples were collected on ice in 15 ml Vacutainer tubes (Becton-Dickinson) with 2000 U of bovine heparin sodium and 40 μg of indomethacin from the heparinized carotid arterial and the distal LAD catheters from four animals. These samples were analyzed subsequently as a group for TxB_2 and 6-keto-$PGF_{1\alpha}$, the stable metabolic products of TxA_2 and prostacyclin, respectively. After placement of the plastic constrictor on the LAD, cyclic flow variations were quantitated for at least 1 hr. To decrease coronary arterial thromboxane levels and to abolish cyclic flow variations, the thromboxane synthetase inhibitor UK38485 was administered (2 to 6 mg/kg iv). Hemodynamics were monitored for at least 30 min after cyclic flow variations were abolished and blood samples were obtained again for measurement of prostaglandin levels. Five dogs received an intracoronary infusion of the vehicle only, 1% bovine serum albumin in 0.9% saline at 0.1 ml/min, and 12 dogs received PAF (10^{-9} or 10^{-8} mol/min). An aortic constrictor was placed above the aortic arch to maintain systolic blood pressure at approximately 100 mm Hg. Hemodynamics were monitored, cyclic flow variations were quantitated, and blood was collected at the nadir of coronary flow for prostaglandin measurement before and during infusion of PAF in four dogs.

Protocol 3. Ten dogs were used in two variations of protocol 2. Dogs were instrumented as described. Cyclic flow variations were produced in the LAD with the plastic constrictor and were quantitated. After 1 hr, either the serotonin antagonist ketanserin was given in a dose of 0.5 mg/kg iv[15] or yohimbine, an α_2-adrenergic antagonist, was given in a dose of 1 to 3 mg/kg iv. Previous studies[6] have shown that ketanserin and yohimbine usually abolish or reduce cyclic flow variations, respectively, in this preparation. Cyclic flow variations were abolished in every dog given ketanserin and in approximately half of the dogs given yohimbine. In those animals in which cyclic flow variations were abolished by ketanserin or yohimbine, PAF was infused into the LAD as described above and cyclic flow variations were quantitated.

In all animals the placement of the catheter was checked with the infusion of 2 ml of monastral blue dye in 10 ml of saline through the diagonal branch catheter. Dogs in which the dye did not stain the area of coronary constriction and the distal LAD bed were excluded from subsequent analysis.

PAF-induced platelet aggregation in vitro. To further evaluate the mechanism of PAF-induced platelet aggregation, studies were performed on blood from seven of the dogs instrumented as described in the above protocols. After instrumentation but before any drugs, 45 ml of blood was obtained from the jugular venous catheter and transferred to a tube containing 5 ml of 3.5% sodium citrate, pH 7.4. The blood samples were centrifuged at 100 *g* for 20 min, resulting in a plasma suspension of platelets containing 300,000 to 500,000 platelets/mm^3. After removing the platelet-rich plasma, the remaining blood was centrifuged at 1500 *g* for 10 min to obtain platelet-poor plasma. Platelet aggregation was measured in vitro with a Sienco (Model DP 247-E) dual-channel aggregometer by the turbidometric method of Born.[16] The rate and extent of aggregation in response to various concentrations of PAF were measured in a reaction volume of 500 μl of platelet-rich plasma. Five minutes after the addition of PAF, a 50 μl sample was removed from the aggregation cuvette and diluted into 450 μl of ice-cold distilled water containing indomethacin 10^{-5}M. These samples were subsequently assayed for TxB_2. In a separate set of experiments, platelet-rich plasma was preincubated with UK38485 (10^{-5}M) for 3 min before the addition of PAF.

Prostaglandin measurements. TxB_2 and 6-keto $PGF_{1\alpha}$ were measured by the method of Dray et al.[17] as modified by Campbell et al.[18] and Hirsh et al.[2]

Statistical methods. All values are expressed as mean ± SEM. A p value of < .05 was considered significant. All hemodynamic variables were analyzed with general linear models procedure and Duncan's multiple range test developed by SAS Institute, Inc.[19] Data involving the frequency of cyclic flow variations and the nadir of coronary arterial pressure during cyclic flow and platelet aggregation were analyzed by analysis of variance and Newman-Keuls multiple comparisons procedure.

Materials. 1-0-Hexadecyl-2-acetyl-sn-glyceryl-phosphorylcholine (PAF) was supplied by Dr. John Pike of Upjohn Co., Kalamazoo, MI. UK38485 was a gift of Dr. Pedro Urquilla of Pfizer, Inc., Groton, CT. Dr. J. M. van Neuten of Jaunsen Pharmaceutical supplied the ketanserin. The indomethacin, yohimbine, and bovine serum albumin were purchased from Sigma Chemical Co., St. Louis. Pentobarbital was purchased from Abbott Laboratories, North Chicago, IL, and bovine heparin from Organon, West Orange, NJ. ^{3}H-TxB_2 and ^{3}H-6-keto $PGF_{1\alpha}$ were obtained from Amersham and TxB_2 and 6-keto $PGF_{1\alpha}$ were obtained from the Upjohn Co.

Results

Hemodynamic data. PAF (10^{-8} mol/min) produced a significant decrease in aortic systolic, diastolic, and mean blood pressures (all p < .001) (table 1). After 10 min of infusion of PAF 10^{-8} mol/min, the systolic, diastolic, and mean pressures were 59.9 ± 8.5, 43.7 ± 5.6, and 49.0 ± 6.5 mm Hg, respectively, compared with control values of 97.7 ± 7.0, 80.1 ± 6.7, and 86.0 ± 6.7 mm Hg (figure 2). Because of the marked changes in systemic blood pressure, no attempt was made to evaluate coronary blood flow. Subsequent studies were performed with aortic pressure controlled by an aortic constrictor (table 2).

There were no major hemodynamic effects of the thromboxane synthetase inhibitor UK38485 (table 2). In the dogs given ketanserin, control blood pressure was reduced (p < .05) compared with the pretreatment value. Treatment with ketanserin had no other major hemodynamic effects (table 3). In the yohimbine-treated dogs there were no significant changes in systolic blood pressure (table 4). There were no other consistent changes in any hemodynamic variable in the yohimbine-treated dogs.

Cyclic flow variations. Cyclic flow variations developed in three of six dogs in protocol 1, in which PAF was infused into a stenosed coronary artery. No cyclic flow variations had occurred in these animals before the infusion. In protocol 2 cyclic flow variations occurred spontaneously in 22 of 23 dogs. In three of these

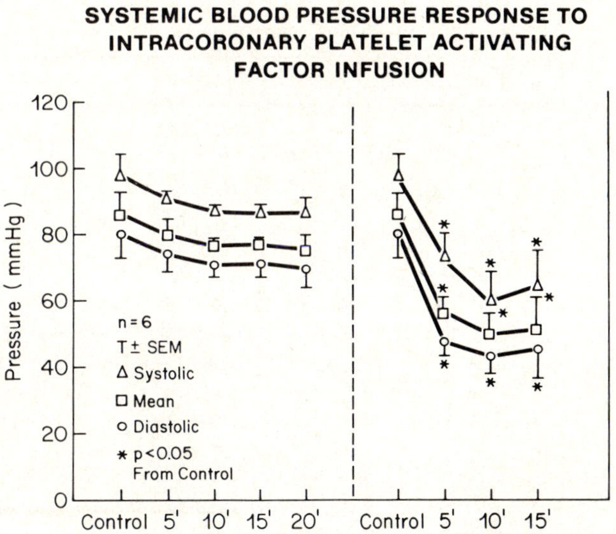

FIGURE 2. Systemic blood pressure response to intracoronary infusion of PAF in dogs in protocol 1. Significant decreases in aortic systolic, diastolic, and mean pressures occurred during infusion of PAF 10^{-8} mol/min. Values are mean ± SEM.

TABLE 1
Hemodynamic data for dogs in protocol 1 (n = 6) (mean ± SEM)

		PAF 10^{-9} mol/min				PAF 10^{-8} mol/min		
	Control	5 min	10 min	15 min	20 min	5 min	10 min	15 min
HR (beats/min)	143±13.7	140±16	140±22	142±17	129±18^A	—	126±22^A	139±4
AOS (mm Hg)	97.7±7.0	90.8±3.3	87.4±1.8	86.5±2.8	86.1±4.9	72.5±7.3^A	59.9±8.5^A	64.1±10.9^A
AOD (mm Hg)	80.1±6.7	74.4±5.4	70.8±2.9	71.8±3.8	69.1±5.8	47.7±4.0^A	43.7±5.6^A	45.6±8.8^A
AOM (mm Hg)	86.0±6.7	79.8±4.6	76.3±2.5	76.6±3.5	74.7±5.2	55.9±5.1^A	49.0±6.5^A	51.7±9.5^A
LV dP/dt (mm Hg/sec)	1143±310	1118±272	996±206	975±192	1085±276	816±263^A	732±228^A	848±356^A
−dP/dt (mm Hg/sec)	−1084±267	−989±185	−1015±135	−958±201	−1021±279	−813±221	−645±211^A	−717±239^A

HR = heart rate; AOS = systolic blood pressure; AOD = diastolic blood pressure; AOM = mean aortic blood pressure; dP/dt = rate of rise of left ventricular pressure; −dP/dt = rate of fall of left ventricular pressure.
^A $p < .05$ vs control value.

22 animals, UK38485 in doses up to 6 mg/kg did not abolish the cyclic flow variations; therefore these three dogs were not used in the protocol. One dog died of ventricular fibrillation before infusion of PAF. In another dog the dye through the diagonal branch catheter did not stain the LAD but perfused a branch of the diagonal, and the dog was excluded from analysis. Therefore 17 dogs were available for treatment with PAF or the vehicle. Figure 3 illustrates a typical tracing of the results found in protocol 2. During the initial period, coronary flow declined slowly and then increased only to fall again. Treatment with UK38485 inhibited these cyclic flow variations. The infusion of PAF restored the cyclic declines in coronary flow, and the cyclic flow variations resembled those observed during the initial period. The frequency of cyclic flow variations in dogs in protocol 2 was standardized to the number of cyclic flow variations over 30 min for each of three time periods: (1) the initial period of cyclic flow variations, designated "control"; (2) the 30 min after the thromboxane synthetase inhibitor; and (3) the final treatment time (figures 3 and 4). This procedure

TABLE 2
Hemodynamic data for dogs in protocol 2 (mean ± SEM)

Variable	Treatment	Control	CFV 60 min	UK38485 30 min	Treatment 20 min
HR	BSA (N = 5)	146±12^A	135±10^A,B	118±10^A	110±9^A
	PAF (N = 12)	146±7	143±10	142±12	145±12^B
AOS	BSA	102.8±3^B	98.1±6.3	87.5±9.0^B	87.0±4.5^B
	PAF	119.3±5.0^B	107.1±7.3	113.6±4.3^B	113.2±3.8^B
AOD	BSA	86.5±3.9	84.6±6.7	67.2±9	70.3±5.3^B
	PAF	98.9±4.8^A	82.8±6.1^A	85.7±4.3^A	84.5±5.6^A,B
AOM	BSA	91.9±3.5	89.1±6.6	73.9±9.0	75.8±4.9^B
	PAF	105.6±4.7	90.8±6.4	94.9±3.9	93.9±4.7^B
dP/dt	BSA	1,719±195	1,499±197	1,505±223	1,285±172^B
	PAF	1,761±104	1,564±96	1,589±72	1,468±92^B
−dP/dt	BSA	−1,437±95^A	−1,249±177^A	−1,063±144^A,B	−977±78^A,B
	PAF	−1,732±78^A	−1,402±84^A	−1,562±93^A,B	−1,409±62^A,B
PROD	BSA	15,120±1,490^A	13,320±1,430^A	10,460±2,050^A	9,690±1,190^A,B
	PAF	17,440±1,370	15,100±1,350	15,820±1,160	16,200±1,370^B

CFV = cyclic flow variations; BSA = bovine serum albumin; PROD = AOS × HR; other abbreviations as in table 1. The units for each of the hemodynamic variables are the same as in table 1.
^A $p < .05$ difference between different time periods within one treatment group.
^B $p < .05$ between groups at a given time period.

TABLE 3
Hemodynamic data for ketanserin-treated dogs (n = 6) (mean ± SEM)

	Control	CFV 60 min	Ketanserin 10 min	Ketanserin 30 min	PAF 20 min
HR	145±14	152±14	138±15	149±14	159±17
AOS	125.6±6.4[A]	103.9±2.6[B]	95.3±2.7[A]	97.0±1.9[A]	99.3±2.2[A]
AOD	101.7±7.0[A]	80.5±4.5[A]	65.5±3.9[A]	69.6±3.6[A]	71.2±2.6[A]
AOM	109.5±6.7[A]	88.2±3.7[A]	75.3±3.4[A]	78.6±2.8[A]	80.5±2.2[A]
dP/dt	1,631±104	1,465±103	1,438±98	1,493±142	1,475±132
−dP/dt	−1,557±67	−1,364±24	−1,241±114	−1,273±64	−1,259±95
PROD	18,010±1,580[A]	16,050±1,860[A]	13,250±1,640[A]	14,430±1,420[A]	15,870±1,980[A]

CFV = cyclic flow variation; other abbreviations as in tables 1 and 2. The units for each of the hemodynamic variables are the same as in table 1.

[A]$p < .05$ difference between times.

TABLE 4
Hemodynamic data for yohimbine-treated dogs (n = 4) (mean ± SEM)

	Control	CFV 60 min	Yohimbine 10 min	Yohimbine 30 min	PAF 20 min
HR	154±8	155±12	142±14	152±14	165±17
AOS	115.7±2.8	124.3±10.1	110.0±5.3	100.7±9.3	104.3±4.3
AOD	94.3±3.7	97.4±6.7	84.5±7.2	76.2±7.1	74.9±3.5
AOM	101.4±3.2	106.3±7.4	92.9±6.5	84.3±7.8	84.6±3.7
dP/dt	−1,780±59	−1,760±142	1,581±172	1,482±92	1,414±175
−dP/dt	−1,576±59	−1,650±190	−1,236±92	−1,196±67	−1,362±126
PROD	17,800±1,080	19,490±2,940	15,460±980	15,030±800	18,310±1,590

CFV = cyclic flow variation; other abbreviations as in tables 1 and 2. The units for each of the hemodynamic variables are the same as in table 1.

was used to quantitate the cyclic flow variations for the different times involved in the three phases of the protocol. Dogs were grouped according to the final treatment they received, i.e., the vehicle or PAF. The frequency of cyclic flow variations during control was identical in the two treatment groups (5.6 ± 0.6 vs 5.6 ± 0.4 cyclic flow variations over 30 min) (figure 4). The frequency of cyclic flow variations after treatment with the thromboxane synthetase inhibitor was zero in all groups because only dogs in which cyclic flow variations were abolished were used. As shown in figures 3 and 4, PAF (but not its vehicle) restored cyclic flow variations after the thromboxane synthetase inhibitor from 0 to 5.0 ± 1.0 cyclic flow variations over 30 min. This value was not different from those observed initially.

To evaluate potential hemodynamic differences between the initial and PAF-induced cyclic flow variations, the mean coronary blood flows at the nadir of flows were averaged during the initial cyclic flow variations and after the infusion of UK38485. The nadir of coronary blood flow during the initial cyclic flow variations was similar in the two groups and averaged 30.9 ± 2.6% of control for all dogs (figure 5). The thromboxane synthetase inhibitor increased blood flow to 77.1 ± 6.9% of control values and cyclic flow variations were abolished. The mean nadir of coronary flow decreased in PAF-treated dogs to 28.4 ± 6.0% of control as cyclic flow variations were restored. The mean flow in dogs receiving only the vehicle and in which cyclic flow variations were not restored was 69.9 ± 12.5% ($p = .002$ difference by analysis of variance).

Cyclic flow variations were produced in 10 dogs in protocol 3 (table 5). In six dogs, there were 6.2 ± 0.6 cyclic flow variations over 30 min in the control period. Ketanserin abolished these cyclic flow variations, but they were restored in all dogs by PAF (table 5). In four dogs, the initial cyclic flow variations were abolished with yohimbine (during the control period), and PAF at least partially restored them to a frequency comparable to that present during the control period.

Prostaglandin data. TxB_2 and 6-keto-$PGF_{1\alpha}$ concentrations in aortic and distal coronary blood were determined in four animals in protocol 2 receiving PAF with control of blood pressure. Distal coronary arterial

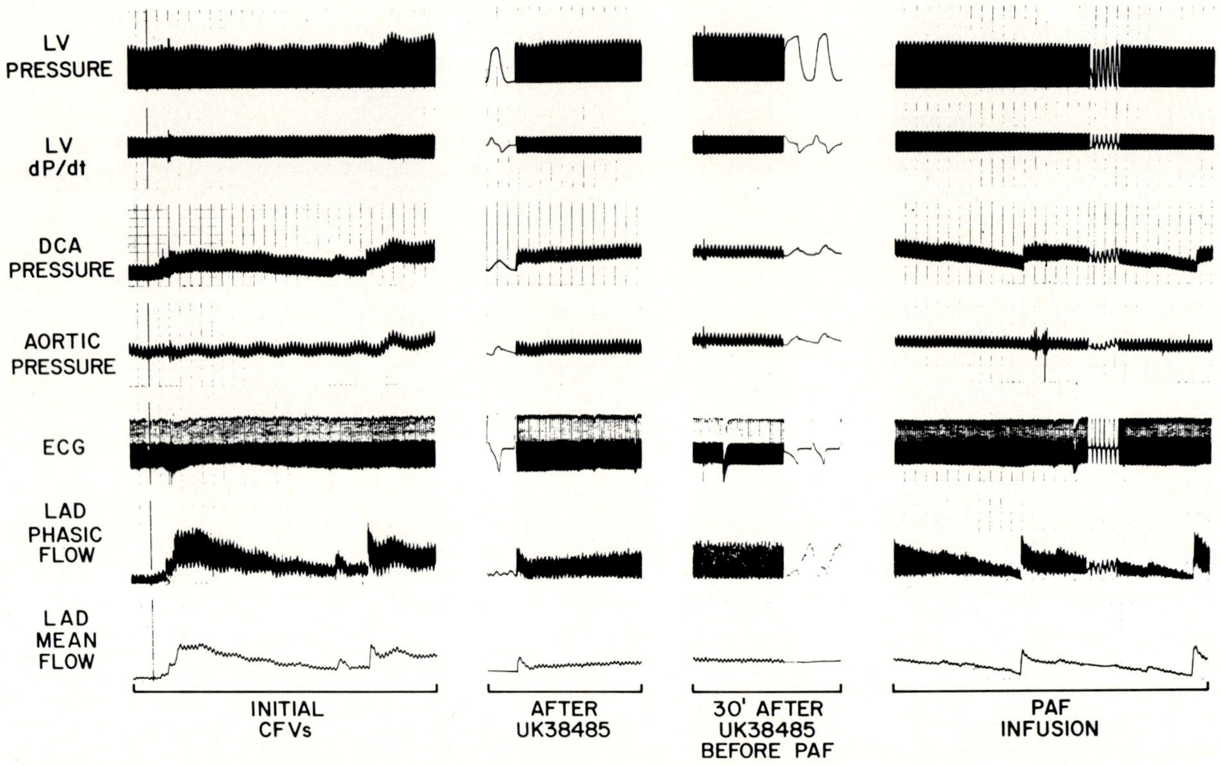

FIGURE 3. Typical tracing from a single dog receiving PAF by intracoronary infusion with an aortic constrictor to control blood pressure. Shown are initial cyclic flow variations (CFVs) (*left panel*), after UK38485 (*middle panels*), and during infusion of PAF (*right panel*) with CFVs restored. DCA = distal coronary artery pressure.

TxB_2 concentrations increased from 51.5 ± 19.3 to 148.5 ± 60.9 during cyclic flow variations (table 6); the thromboxane synthetase inhibitor decreased these elevated values to 55.7 ± 40.2 in association with abolition of the cyclic flow variations. During infusion of PAF the cyclic flow variations were restored. However, the TxB_2 concentrations in the distal coronary artery did not increase. There was no change in aortic TxB_2 concentrations. Both aortic and distal coronary arterial 6-keto-$PGF_{1\alpha}$ concentrations increased over time (table 5). Neither UK38485 nor PAF altered the release of 6-keto-$PGF_{1\alpha}$ into the coronary blood.

Platelet aggregation in vitro. As shown in figure 6,

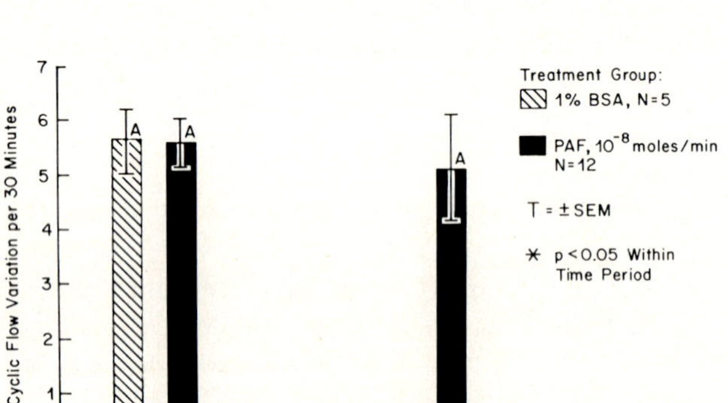

FIGURE 4. Frequency of cyclic flow variations in dogs in protocol 2 during control cyclic flow variations (CFVs), after UK38485, and during each treatment period according to the final treatment group. A and B signify p < .05 difference within a treatment group. PAF restored CFVs after the thromboxane synthetase inhibitor UK38485. BSA = bovine serum albumin.

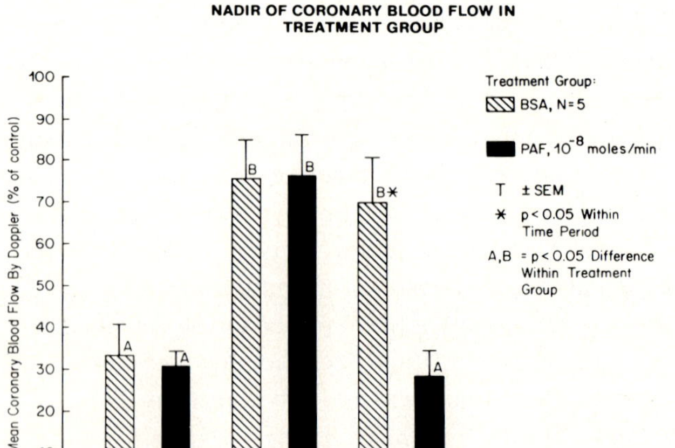

FIGURE 5. Mean coronary blood flow in dogs in protocol 2 during initial cyclic flow variations (CFVs), after UK38485, and during the treatment period, separated according to final treatment group. UK38485 increased coronary blood flow by abolishing CFVs. The nadir of flow was similar during the initial CFVs and the PAF-induced CFV's. BSA = bovine serum albumin.

TABLE 5
Cyclic flow variations with PAF after ketanserin and yohimbine[A]

	Control	Nadir of CBF	Drug	Nadir of CBF	PAF	Nadir of CBF
Ketanserin	6.2 ± 0.6 (n = 6)	$25.8 \pm 7.6\%$	0	$107.3 \pm 14.2\%$[B]	4.4 ± 1.0 (NS)	$41.3 \pm 12.3\%$
Yohimbine	9.0 ± 0.9 (n = 4)	$21.8 \pm 12.7\%$	0	$82.6 \pm 16.5\%$[B]	4.5 ± 1.2 (p = .049)	$16.6 \pm 6.0\%$

[A]Data expressed as number of cyclic flow variations over 30 min.
[B]$p < .05$ compared with control and after PAF.

TABLE 6
Alterations in TxB_2 and 6-keto $PGF_{1\alpha}$ levels (mean ± SEM)[A]

	Control	During CFVs	After UK38485	With PAF and return CFVs
Aortic TxB_2 (pg/ml)	48.2 ± 15.2	37.5 ± 7.5	46.7 ± 15.7	27.5 ± 9.7
DCA TxB_2 (pg/ml)	51.5 ± 19.3	148.5 ± 60.9	55.7 ± 40.2	22.7 ± 13.2
Aortic 6-keto-$PGF_{1\alpha}$ (pg/ml)	96.7 ± 22.2	255 ± 73.5	310.5 ± 97.8	348.2 ± 81.4
DCA 6-keto-$PGF_{1\alpha}$ (pg/ml)	105.2 ± 15.4	320.0 ± 79.6	278 ± 111.8	492.75 ± 93.9

CFVs = cyclic flow variations; DCA = distal coronary artery.
[A]Protocol 2 (n = 4).

PAF-induced aggregation of canine platelets in vitro at concentrations between 10^{-8} and 10^{-6}M. With the platelet aggregation there was stimulation of the synthesis of TxB_2, which was also concentration related. In the platelet-rich plasma suspensions preincubated with UK38485 at 10^{-5}M, platelet aggregation still occurred with PAF, but there was no detectable increase in thromboxane synthesis.

Discussion

PAF is a member of a recently described phospholipid family with potent hypotensive[12] and platelet-aggregating properties.[8,9] PAF causes bronchospasm in the guinea pig[20] and its release is postulated to be a mechanism for inducing asthma.[21] Human leukocytes release PAF[11] when stimulated by immune complexes. Human and rabbit platelets form PAF when stimulated with the calcium ionophore A23187,[10] as do human endothelial cells in culture.[22] Previous histologic studies of canine coronary arteries with concentric stenosis have demonstrated the presence of platelets and polymorphonuclear leukocytes at the site of the constriction.[3,4] Since PAF may be released from the white blood cells or platelets, the potential for the local generation of PAF is present at the site of an experimental coronary arterial stenosis. This investigation was designed to determine the effect of PAF on coronary blood flow in such a preparation.

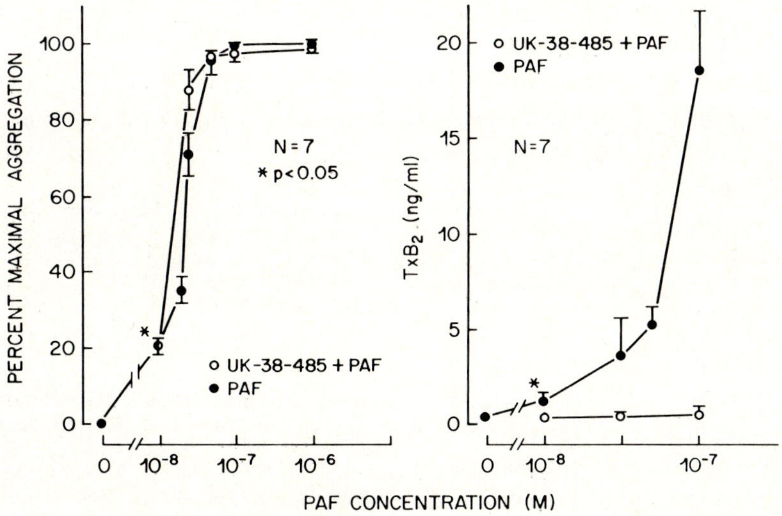

FIGURE 6. Effect of increasing the concentration of PAF on percentage platelet aggregation (*left*) and TxB_2 concentration (*right*). Complete aggregation was noted at concentrations between 10^{-8}M and 10^{-7}M.

The results of our study indicate that PAF, when given by an intracoronary infusion, may cause or restore cyclic flow variations in a stenosed canine coronary artery. Specifically, PAF restores cyclic flow variations in spite of the inhibition of thromboxane synthesis by UK38485 or pretreatment with antagonists for serotonin or α_2-adrenergic receptors. Furthermore, PAF induces aggregation of canine platelets in vitro, and PAF-induced platelet aggregation is not prevented by inhibition of thromboxane synthesis.

Since the initial description of this preparation and of the cyclic declines in coronary blood flow called cyclic flow variations,[3] much attention has been directed to defining mechanisms and developing methods for altering or abolishing cyclic flow variations. Folts[23] initially described the ability of aspirin and indomethacin, both inhibitors of cyclooxygenase, to abolish cyclic flow variations. Aiken et al.[24] have used prostacyclin to prevent cyclic flow variations. We have found that TxB_2 levels increase during cyclic flow variations and that a thromboxane synthetase inhibitor, dazoxiben, decreases coronary arterial thromboxane levels and abolishes or markedly attenuates cyclic flow variations.[4] Therefore, previous data have implicated thromboxane in the generation of cyclic flow variations in this experimental preparation.

The question arises, however, as to whether increased TxA_2 concentration is the major cause of cyclic flow variations or whether thromboxane is only one of several factors that might potentially cause these variations. In this regard, we wished to determine whether cyclic flow variations could be produced in the absence of an elevated TxA_2 level within the coronary artery. Our data demonstrate that PAF causes platelet aggregation and cyclic flow variations despite thromboxane synthetase inhibition.

The mechanism by which PAF aggregates platelets is controversial. However, most data suggest that PAF induces primary platelet aggregation in spite of inhibitors of cyclooxygenase or thromboxane synthetase[25] or removal of ADP with the scavenging system, creatine phosphate/creatine phosphokinase. The lipoxygenase pathway has been implicated by some investigators as the mediator of PAF effects.[20] Currently, PAF is postulated to represent a "third pathway" of platelet aggregation.[25]

We do not know whether release of endogenous PAF plays a significant role in causing cyclic flow variations in this preparation. However, it is interesting that if cyclic flow variations were abolished with various inhibitors, the infusion of PAF usually restored the cyclic flow variations to a value similar to that before the administration of the inhibitors. This lends support to the premise that cyclic flow variations may be due at least in part to platelet aggregates and thrombi.[3, 4, 23, 24, 26] Others have shown that PAF, when given as an intracoronary bolus in the pig, decreases coronary blood flow.[13] Whether PAF causes direct coronary constriction in the dog with a partial coronary stenosis is not clear from our data, but such an effect may have contributed to the restoration of cyclic flow variations in our studies. Cyclic flow variations are associated with an elevated coronary arterial TxB_2 concentration in blood distal to the stenosis, and a thromboxane synthetase inhibitor usually abolishes cyclic flow variations in this preparation.[4] Ketanserin and yohimbine abolish or reduce the frequency of cyclic flow variations, respectively.[6] PAF induces cyclic flow variations in spite of the presence of each of these drugs. Therefore, with spontaneous cyclic flow variations it appears that thromboxane and serotonin release are important and that inhibition of either agent's synthesis or agonist effects reestablishes normal coronary blood flow. PAF may not occupy a role as central as that of thromboxane or serotonin, but when given at sufficient concentrations it can cause cyclic flow variations. However, the final determination of the significance of PAF in causing dynamic alterations in coronary blood flow will await the development of a suitable assay for measuring the PAF concentration and production during cyclic flow variations in preparations with partial coronary stenosis and the development of specific antagonists.

In summary, PAF given by intracoronary infusion at 10^{-9} and 10^{-8} mol/min causes a decrease in systemic blood pressure. PAF can induce cyclic flow variations in a stenosed canine coronary artery. It can also restore cyclic flow variations that have been abolished by a thromboxane synthetase inhibitor (UK38485), a serotonin$_2$ receptor antagonist (ketanserin), or an α_2-adrenergic receptor antagonist (yohimbine). Therefore, the ability of PAF to restore cyclic flow variations is not dependent on thromboxane, serotonin, or α_2-adrenergic mechanisms.

We thank Janice McNatt, Judy Ober, and Mary Beth Santowski for their technical assistance, Nancy Dickey for her secretarial assistance, and Dr. J. E. Pike of the Upjohn Co. for providing the PAF.

References

1. Willerson JT, Hillis LD, Buja LM: Ischemic heart disease: clinical and pathophysiological aspects. New York, 1982, Raven Press, p 18
2. Hirsh PD, Hillis LD, Campbell WB, Firth BG, Willerson JT: Release of prostaglandins and thromboxane into the coronary circu-

lation in patients with ischemic heart disease. N Engl J Med **304:** 685, 1981

3. Folts JD, Crowell EB, Rowe GG: Platelet aggregation in partially obstructed vessels and its elimination with aspirin. Circulation **54:** 365, 1976
4. Bush LR, Campbell WB, Tilton GD, Buja LM, Willerson JT: Effects of the selective thromboxane synthesis inhibitor dazoxiben on cyclic blood flow variations in stenosed canine coronary arteries. Circulation **69:** 1161, 1984
5. Gertz SD, Uretsky G, Wajnberg RS, Navot N, Gotsman MS: Endothelial cell damage and thrombus formation after partial arterial constriction: relevance to the role of coronary artery spasm in the pathogenesis of myocardial infarction. Circulation **63:** 476, 1981
6. Bush LR, Campbell WB, Kern K, Tilton GD, Apprill P, Ashton J, Schmitz J, Buja LM, Willerson JT: The effects of $alpha_2$ adrenergic and serotoninergic receptor antagonists on cyclic blood flow alterations in stenosed canine coronary arteries. Circ Res **55:** 642, 1984
7. Chesney CM, Pifer DD, Byers LW, Muirhead EE: Effect of platelet-activating factor (PAF) on human platelets. Blood **59:** 582, 1982
8. McManus LM, Hanahan DJ, Pinckard RN: Human platelet stimulation by acetyl glyceryl ether phosphorylcholine. J Clin Invest **67:** 903, 1981
9. Marcus AJ, Safier LB, Ullman HL, Wong KTH, Brockman MJ, Weksler BB, Kaplan KL: Effects of acetyl glyceryl ether phosphorylcholine on human platelet function *in vitro*. Blood **58:** 1027, 1981
10. Alam I, Smith JB, Silver MJ: Human and rabbit platelets form platelet-activating factor in response to calcium ionophore. Thromb Res **30:** 71, 1983
11. Virella G, Lopes-Virella MFL, Schuler C, Sherwood T, Espinoza GA, Winocour P, Colwell JA: Release of PAF by human polymorphonuclear leukocytes stimulated by immune complexes bound to sepharose particles and human erythrocytes. Immunology **50:** 43, 1983
12. Smith KA, Prewitt RL, Byers LW, Muirhead EE: Analogs of phosphatidylcholine: alpha-adrenergic antagonists from the renal medulla. Hypertension **3:** 460, 1981
13. Feuerstein G, Boyd LM, Ezra D, Goldstein RE: Effect of platelet-activating factor on coronary circulation of domestic pig. Am J Physiol **246:** H466, 1984
14. Hartley CJ, Hanley HG, Lewis RM, Cole JS: Synchronized pulsed Doppler blood flow and ultrasonic dimension measurement in conscious dogs. Ultrasound Med Biol **4:** 99, 1978
15. Jansen PAJ: 5-HT_2 receptor blockade to study serotonin-induced pathology. Trends Pharmacol Sci **4:** 198, 1983
16. Born GVR: Aggregation of blood platelets by adenosine diphosphate and its reversal. Nature **194:** 927, 1962
17. Dray F, Charbonnel B, Maclouf J: Radioimmunoassay of prostaglandins $F_{\alpha 1}$, E_1, and E_2 in human plasma. Eur J Clin Invest **5:** 311, 1975
18. Campbell WB, Gomez-Sanchez CE, Adams BV: Role of prostaglandin in angiotensin-induced steroidogenesis: absence of an effect by prostaglandin E_2. Hypertension **2:** 471, 1980
19. SAS Institute, Inc.: SAS users guide: statistics. 1982 edition. Cary, NC, SAS Institute, 1982
20. Bonnet J, Thibadeau P, Bessin P: Dependancy of the PAF-acether induced bronchospasm on the lipoxygenase pathway in the guinea pig. Prostaglandins **26:** 457, 1983
21. Vargaftig BB, Chignard M, Benveniste J: Present concepts on the mechanisms of platelet aggregation. Biochem Pharmacol **30:** 263, 1981
22. Camussi G, Aglietta M, Malavassi F, Tetta C, Piacibello W: The release of platelet activating factor from human endothelial cells in culture. J Immunol **131:** 2397, 1983
23. Folts JD: Experimental arterial platelet thrombosis, platelet inhibitors, and their possible clinical relevance. Cardiovasc Rev Rep **3:** 370, 1982
24. Aiken JW, Gorman RR, Shebuski RJ: Prevention of blockage of partially obstructed coronary arteries with prostacyclin correlates with inhibition of platelet aggregation. Prostaglandins **17:** 483, 1974
25. Vargaftig BB, Fouque F, Benveniste J, Odiot J: Adrenaline and PAF-acether synergize to trigger cyclooxygenase independent activation of plasma-free human platelets. Thromb Res **28:** 557, 1982
26. Folts JD, Gallagher K, Rowe GG: Blood flow reductions in stenosed canine coronary arteries: vasospasm or platelet aggregation? Circ Res **65:** 248, 1982

Survival after an experimental myocardial infarction: beneficial effects of long-term therapy with captopril

MARC A. PFEFFER, M.D., PH.D., JANICE M. PFEFFER, PH.D., CYNTHIA STEINBERG, B.S., AND PETER FINN, M.D.

ABSTRACT Although vasodilator therapy has been shown to improve functional capacity in patients with congestive heart failure, there is no evidence that such therapy can prolong survival. Coronary artery ligation in the rat was used to produce a wide range of myocardial infarct sizes and a resultant spectrum of left ventricular dysfunction. To determine the relationship between size of myocardial infarction and long-term survival and to test the hypothesis that long-term therapy with captopril could improve survival after myocardial infarction, 302 rats were randomly assigned to either placebo or captopril therapy 14 days after coronary artery ligation. The animals were kept in a laminar flow unit and followed daily for a 1 year period or until spontaneous death. Size of myocardial infarction was determined by planimetry of serial histologic sections of the left ventricle. One year survival in placebo-treated rats decreased markedly in direct relation to increasing size of infarction (from 71% in noninfarcted rats to only 8% in rats with large infarcts). Long-term captopril therapy prolonged the survival of rats with infarcts ($p < .02$). The most marked improvement in survival was noted in the animals with infarcts of moderate size, in which 1 year survival was 21% in the placebo-treated rats and 48% in the captopril-treated rats. Thus, in this experimental preparation of myocardial infarction and left ventricular dysfunction, survival was inversely related to size of infarction. Long-term therapy with captopril, which we had previously shown to improve left ventricular function and lessen dilatation in the chronic phase of infarction, also had a pronounced effect on prolonging survival in this preparation of chronic infarction.
Circulation 72, No. 2, 406–412, 1985.

THE DIAGNOSIS of congestive heart failure has a grave prognosis.[1,2] In the Framingham Study, the 5 year mortality rate was greater than 50% for individuals newly diagnosed as having congestive heart failure.[1] In more recent studies, the median survival of patients with less clearly defined durations of ventricular dysfunction was often measured in months, not years.[3–5] Although congestive heart failure is a syndrome that encompasses multiple etiologies, the severity of the cardiac dysfunction appears to have greater prognostic significance than does the specific cause of disease.[4] The use of vasodilators, especially the angiotensin-converting enzyme inhibitors, in the treatment of patients with severe heart failure has led to an improvement in functional capacity.[6–11] However, there is no evidence that these therapeutic interventions result in a prolongation of life in individuals with rather advanced congestive heart failure.[12–14]

Coronary artery ligation in the rat provides an animal preparation of myocardial infarction in which a wide range of infarct sizes and left ventricular dysfunction can be produced.[15,16] Since we have shown that captopril improves ventricular performance in this preparation of heart failure,[17] the present study was designed (1) to determine the relationship between size of infarction and long-term survival, and (2) to test the hypothesis that a therapeutic agent that has a beneficial effect on ventricular performance can prolong survival after experimental myocardial infarction.

Methods

Study design. Commercially obtained virgin female Wistar rats (West Jersey Biological Supply), ranging in age from 16 to 20 weeks, were housed in our animal facility for at least 2 weeks before operation. Left coronary artery ligation or a sham operation was performed in each by a previously described method.[15,16] Since this study was concerned with the chronic phase

From the Cardiovascular Division, Department of Medicine, Harvard Medical School and Brigham and Women's Hospital, Boston.

Supported in part by a grant from The Squibb Institute for Medical Research.

Address for correspondence: Marc A. Pfeffer, M.D., Ph.D., Department of Medicine, Cardiovascular Division, Brigham and Women's Hospital, 75 Francis St., Boston, MA 02115.

Received March 5, 1985; revision accepted May 2, 1985.

Dr. J. Pfeffer is the recipient of a Research Career Development Award HL 01186 from the NHLBI of the National Institutes of Health. Dr. M. Pfeffer is the recipient of an Established Investigatorship of the American Heart Association.

of myocardial infarction, 14 days after the operative procedure all survivors (302) were briefly anesthetized with ether and electrocardiograms were obtained with a previously described nine-lead system.[18] At the time of anesthesia a metal identification tag was affixed to the nape of the neck of each rat. A balanced-block randomization process was used to allocate animals to either placebo or captopril therapy groups. This randomization process was stratified according to three arbitrary electrocardiographic groups. The first group had a normal QRS complex without evidence of a pathologic Q wave in limb leads I or aVL; the second group had a Q wave ($\geq$ 1 mV) in either of leads I or aVL, yet maintained a precordial R wave total of 10 mV or greater; and the third group had both abnormal limb-lead Q waves and a sum of precordial R waves that was 10 mV or less. This electrocardiographic classification system was used only in an attempt to maintain a balance of rats with and without infarction in the placebo and captopril groups, and not for the subsequent survival analysis, which was performed with the histologic determinations of the size of myocardial infarction only.

Animals were housed in clear polyethylene cages (up to a maximum of four rats per cage) and placed according to therapy assignment and time of entry into the study. All animals were allowed free access to food and the assigned therapy (water or captopril, 2 g/liter of drinking water). The room was temperature and humidity controlled and had a 12 hr light-dark cycle. The cages were maintained on two racks, each of which abutted one side of a double-sided laminar flow unit (Germ Free Laboratories). Cages with animals assigned to placebo or captopril were alternately placed on the rack. An additional 39 rats in which no operation was performed were selected from the same shipments used for this study and maintained concurrently with the study animals. Each animal was followed until death or for up to 1 year after the operative procedure.

Cages were inspected for dead animals twice daily on weekdays and daily on weekends and holidays. The date of each death was noted and the carcass was weighed and a gross postmortem examination was performed. The thoracic contents were removed en bloc and placed in formalin along with the metal identification tag. This identification number, which in itself did not discriminate between the therapy groups, was used in all subsequent pathologic processing. All survivors at 1 year after infarction were anesthetized with ether and the heart of each was arrested with intravenous KCl. The same coded pathologic evaluation was performed on these animals as was conducted on all spontaneous deaths.

Pathology. The formalin-fixed lungs were dissected from the heart and examined for areas of consolidation. The following scoring system for thoracic infections was applied to each specimen: grade 1, no gross infection; grade 2, small area(s) of consolidation involving less than one-third of the estimated lung volume; and grade 3, large area(s) of consolidation involving more than one-third of the estimated lung volume or diffuse thoracic infection without localization. The heart was examined and the atria and great vessels were trimmed from the ventricles. The right ventricular free wall was dissected from the left ventricle and both ventricles were weighed separately. The left ventricle was dehydrated in alcohol, cleared in xylene, and embedded in paraffin. Transverse 50 μm sections were cut from the apex to the base of the left ventricle, every twentieth section of which (representing 1 mm intervals) was mounted and stained with Masson's trichrome from which hematoxylin was omitted to provide a clearer discrimination between fibrous scar and muscle.

A slide of each section then was projected onto a screen for the planimetric measurement (Numonics Corp.) of size of infarction. The endocardial and epicardial circumferences as well as the lengths of scar for each of these surfaces were measured for each section. The lengths of scar and of circumference were summed separately for each of the epicardial and endocardial surfaces and the sums were expressed as a ratio of scar length to ventricular circumference for each surface. These two ratios were then averaged and expressed as a percentage to define size of infarction. Since serial sections of the entire left ventricle were evaluated, the size of infarction determined represents the percent of the left ventricular endocardial and epicardial surface areas occupied by fibrous scar tissue.

Statistical analysis. The following four previously determined classifications of size of infarction were used in the analysis: noninfarcted, 4.99% or less; small, 5% to 19.99%; moderate, 20% to 39.99%; and large, 40% or more of the left ventricular surface area occupied by fibrous scar tissue. A one-way analysis of variance was used to determine whether the randomization process resulted in groups that were matched for age and body weight at the time of operation. The t test was used to test for matched treatment (water to captopril) groups within each of the four categories of size of infarction with respect to these variables. Log-rank tests were conducted to determine whether size of infarction altered 1 year survival in the untreated group. In these untreated rats, the effect of size of infarction also was analyzed as a continuous variable using the Cox model to calculate the relative risk of 1 year mortality with increasing infarct size.

Comparisons of survival in untreated and captopril-treated rats were also performed separately by log-rank tests for all of the rats with and without infarction. Similar analyses were performed for each of the three groups based on size of infarction. Since potential differences in rates of thoracic infections could have contributed to a possible alteration in group survival, results in animals with a thoracic infection score of grade 3 were treated as censored observations and the log-rank tests for comparisons between treatment groups were repeated as a separate analysis. An additional log-rank analysis of 1 year survival in the rats without infarction that either did or did not undergo operation was also conducted.

Results

Seven (three untreated and four captopril-treated) of the 302 animals entered into the study were excluded. One rat died during the brief interval between randomization and placement into the therapy cage, and in six other animals the determination of size of infarction was not possible because of postmortem cannibalization.

The randomization process produced a balance between the therapy groups with respect to both the sample size and the distribution of infarct sizes in each classification (table 1). At the time of operation there were no significant differences in age between the therapy groups for any of the infarct size classifications or among the untreated rats with infarcts of different sizes. However, among the groups of captopril-treated rats with infarction there was a significant difference in age (of about 1 week) that was of questionable biologic significance. There were no significant differences in body weight among the groups for any of the infarct size classifications (table 1).

TABLE 1
Physical characteristics and distribution of rats with and without infarcts in the various groups

	No infarct	Infarct		
		Small	Moderate	Large
Sample size (No.)				
H_2O	62	15	29	40
CAP	63	13	35	37
Infarct size (%)				
H_2O	0	12.7±1.3	33.4±0.8	47.3±0.7
CAP	0	12.7±1.4	33.1±0.9	46.4±0.7
Age (weeks)				
H_2O	20.5±0.3	20.6±0.6	20.0±0.4	19.6±0.2
CAP	20.7±0.3	20.8±0.6	20.0±0.4	19.4±0.2[A]
Body weight (g)				
H_2O	295±4	298±5	294±5	304±5
CAP	295±4	282±6	296±4	304±3

Results are expressed as mean ± SEM.
H_2O = untreated rats; CAP = captopril-treated rats.
[A]$p < .05$ compared with "no infarct" group.

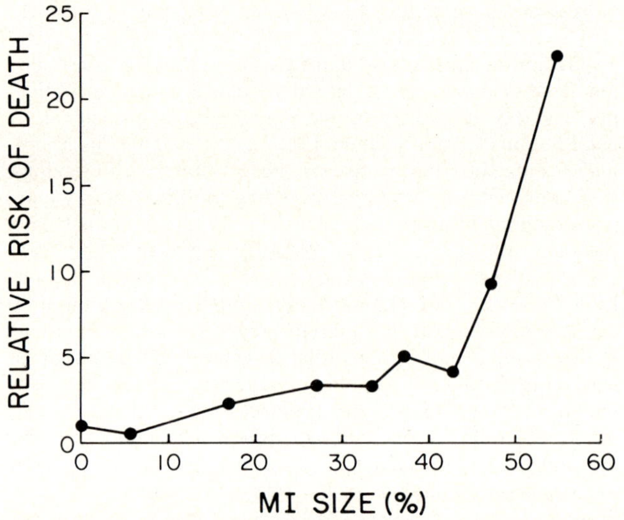

FIGURE 2. Risk of death for untreated rats with infarction relative to operated rats without infarction (infarct size, 0%). The median value of eight categories of size of infarction was used to define the relative risk of death for animals with infarcts.

Within either treatment group the 1 year mortality for the sham-operated rats was not significantly different than that for rats that did not undergo operation. The "all causes," 1 year mortality for the rats assigned to water only was increased ($p < .0001$) as a function of size of infarction (figure 1). The median survival for the animals without infarction was greater than the 365 day observation period and was therefore undefined. Animals with small, moderate, and large infarctions demonstrated reduced median survival durations of 360, 228, and 146 days, respectively. In these animals, the relative risk of death increased progressively with increasing size of infarction (figure 2). Untreated rats with infarcts of between 20% and 29.9% formed the smallest infarct size group to have a relative risk that was significantly greater ($p < .01$) than that in rats without infarction. The risk of death increased steeply as infarct size increased and became 22.6 times greater in untreated rats with extensive (≥50%) infarctions than in those without infarction.

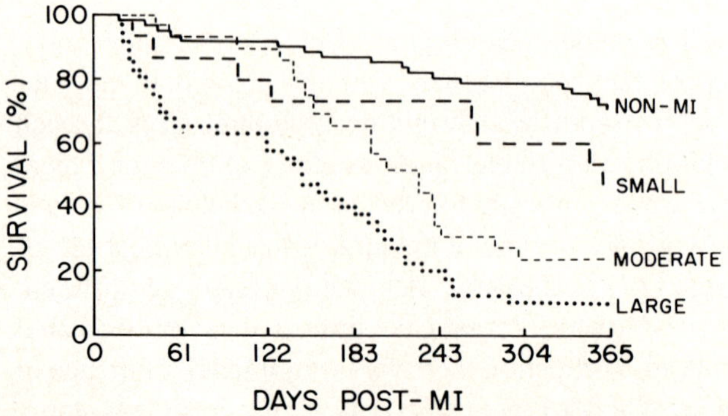

FIGURE 1. Survival of untreated animals without infarction and of those in the three predetermined infarct size groups (small, 5% to 19.99%; moderate, 20% to 39.9%; and large ≥40% of left ventricular surface).

In the rats without infarction receiving captopril, survival was quite similar to that in the untreated rats without infarction (figure 3, *A*). In contrast, all captopril-treated rats with infarctions demonstrated a reduced 1 year mortality rate ($p = .01$) compared with untreated rats with infarction (figure 3, *B*). The median survival for the entire group of rats with infarction was 197 days for the untreated animals and 260 days for the captopril-treated group. This improved survival of the captopril-treated rats was observed uniformly across all infarct size groups, although the difference was not always statistically significant within each subgroup (figure 4). The overall 1 year mortality for rats with small (5% to 19.9%) infarctions did not differ ($p = .23$) in treated and untreated groups (figure 4, *A*). In contrast, rats with moderate (20% to 39.9%) infarctions treated with captopril exhibited a marked improvement ($p = .02$) in 1 year survival compared with untreated rats (figure 4, *B*). Although there was an initial trend toward improved survival in rats with large (≥40%) infarctions receiving captopril, a long-term beneficial effect was not sustained ($p = .24$) (figure 4, *C*).

Censoring of results in rats with thoracic infections was performed to reduce the confounding influence of a potential noncardiac cause of mortality. The incidence of grade 3 infections (an infection likely to account for death) did not differ between treatments or infarct size groups. Indeed, censoring for high-grade

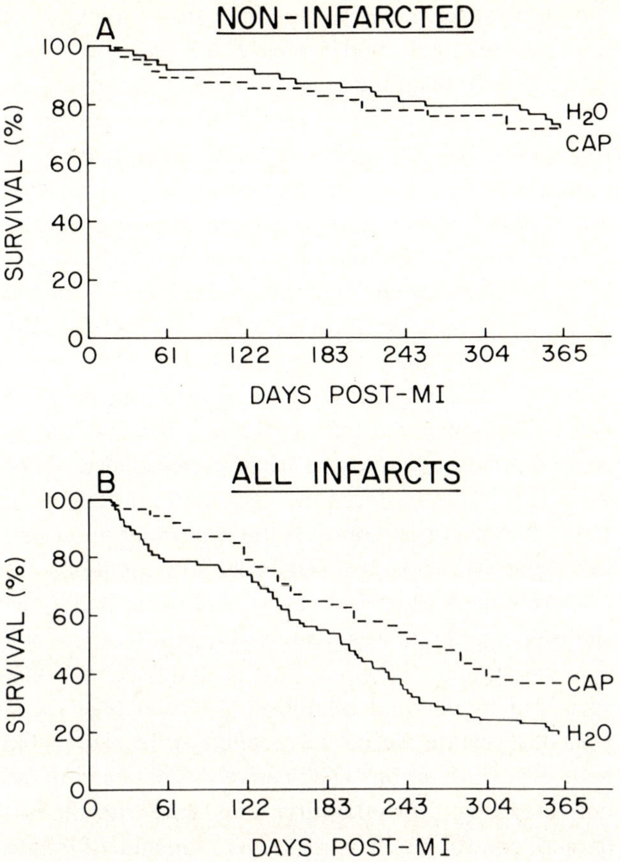

FIGURE 3. *A*, Survival of untreated (H_2O) and captopril-treated (CAP) animals that underwent operation but did not sustain myocardial infarction. No differences were observed between therapy groups. The median survival for both groups was undefined since it was greater than the 365 day observation period. *B*, Survival of all untreated (H_2O) and captopril-treated (CAP) animals that sustained myocardial infarction. Survival for infarcted animals receiving captopril was prolonged compared with that in untreated rats ($p < .02$). The median survival for the untreated rats was 187 days and that in CAP animals was 260 days.

thoracic infections actually reinforced the relationship between increasing size of infarction and reduced mortality and the beneficial effects of captopril therapy in rats with chronic myocardial infarctions. With the use of this censored analysis the median survival for rats without infarcts and those with small infarcts in both therapy groups was undefined (greater than the 365 day observation period). In rats with moderate infarcts the median survival was 228 days for the untreated rats and greater than 365 for the captopril-treated rats. The median survival for rats with large infarcts was unchanged by therapy (untreated 184 days and captopril-treated 205 days).

Discussion

Therapy for heart failure has focused on the relief of symptoms of congestion by the restriction of physical activity and dietary sodium intake and the use of pharmacologic agents such as diuretics. Cardiac glycosides are also widely used for the treatment of heart failure, although their efficacy in patients with sinus rhythm has been questioned. Vasodilating drugs recently have been introduced as adjunctive therapy in patients with congestive heart failure because of the hemodynamic improvements observed during their short-term administration. Although long-term beneficial hemodynamic responses to vasodilators have not been observed uni-

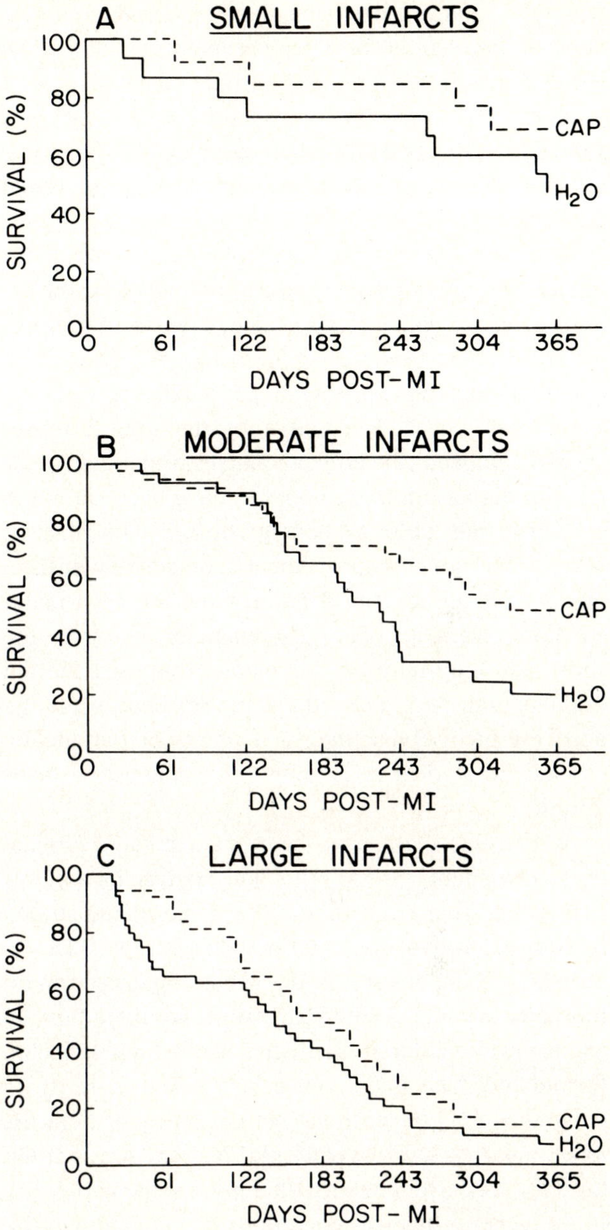

FIGURE 4. Survival of untreated (H_2O) and captopril-treated (CAP) rats with small (*A*), moderate (*B*), or large (*C*) infarctions. In the small infarct groups the median survival was 360 days and that in the untreated and CAP groups was undefined (greater than the 365 day observation period). In the moderate infarct group the median survivai was 228 and 329 days for the untreated and CAP rats, respectively. In the large infarct groups the median survival was 146 and 181 days for the untreated and captopril-treated rats, respectively.

formly,[19] captopril has been shown to produce a sustained improvement in objective measures of cardiac performance in patients with chronic congestive heart failure.[6-11] In a placebo-controlled trial, captopril was shown to have a benefit both in reducing the symptoms of congestive heart failure and in improving functional capacity.[11]

Although the observed improvement in hemodynamics was the rationale for the initial use of vasodilating agents in patients with congestive heart failure, recently it has become apparent that the short-term hemodynamic response to a particular vasodilating agent may not be predictive of the long-term response.[20] Indeed, the clinical courses of patients treated with the vasodilator minoxidil have been shown to be worse than those of patients treated with placebo despite a sustained improvement in objective measurements of baseline hemodynamics and left ventricular ejection fraction.[21] The discrepancies between the short- and long-term hemodynamic responses and the findings with regard to clinical course underscore the need for precisely defined end points of therapeutic efficacy in studies in patients with congestive heart failure.[22]

At present, there have been no extensive clinical trials in patients or experimental studies in animals with congestive heart failure that have demonstrated prolonged survival due to vasodilator therapy.[14] Determination of the effect of a therapeutic intervention on mortality in patients with heart failure would require an extensive clinical trial, the logistics of which would be formidable. The major obstacles to such a study in patients are (1) the extreme heterogeneity of both the level and duration of ventricular dysfunction, (2) the need for concurrent medical therapy, (3) the variability in the general medical conditions of patients and the presence of concurrent illnesses, and (4) the relatively short-term follow-up that is usually possible. However, the rat preparation of experimental myocardial infarction provides a homogeneous population in which graded left ventricular dysfunction, from minimal impairment to overt heart failure, is the only discriminating factor that could potentially alter survival.[15, 16] In the chronic phase of experimental infarction in the rat, left ventricular function and cavitary size are closely related to the extent of the myocardial infarction.[15-17] Another important feature of this preparation of heart failure is the ability to produce, maintain, and treat large numbers of these animals under uniform conditions for relatively protracted periods of time.

In the present study we used mortality as the single end point for determining the relationship between long-term survival and size of myocardial infarction in this experimental model. Since we had previously demonstrated that long-term (3 months) captopril therapy resulted in an improvement in ventricular pump function and an attenuation of ventricular dilatation in comparison with untreated rats with infarcts of comparable sizes,[17] in this study a similar regimen of captopril (2 g/liter of drinking water) was initiated 2 weeks after coronary artery ligation to determine whether such therapy would improve survival in these rats with experimentally induced left ventricular dysfunction. This dose of captopril was chosen since our previous study[17] demonstrated that it resulted in reductions in arterial pressure and total peripheral resistance in rats with and without infarction. The long-term effects of other dosages of captopril or those of other vasodilating agents was not assessed in the present study.

During the 1 year observation period survival in the sham-operated rats was similar to that in their cohorts not undergoing operation. In the untreated rats that sustained myocardial infarction, survival over the 1 year observation period was related to the size of the myocardial infarction. The relative risk of death for the untreated rats with infarction compared with the untreated, control group increased as a function of infarct size (figure 2). Rats with infarcts of between 20% and 29.9% were the first group to have a relative risk of death that was significantly greater than that in the population without infarction. Of importance, a dramatic rise in the relative risk was observed for rats with infarcts of between 40% and 50%. In our previous studies of left ventricular function in rats with myocardial infarction, this latter range of infarct sizes was associated with the occurrence of overt left ventricular dysfunction, as manifested by a marked elevation of ventricular filling pressures, a reduction in cardiac output, and a marked dilatation of the left ventricular cavity.[15-17] It was therefore demonstrated in the untreated rats in this study that survival during the 1 year observation period was closely related to the size of the myocardial infarction and therefore the extent of chronic left ventricular dysfunction.

Although the survival of patients with large myocardial infarctions has been shown to be poorer than that of patients with less extensive infarctions,[23] it is not possible to use size of infarction as the sole discriminating variable in clinical trials. In the present study, the relationship between survival during the observation period and size of myocardial infarction was not confounded by differences in baseline status of coexisting coronary artery disease. Indeed, in this protocol rats were not entered into the study until 14 days after coronary artery ligation. By this time the acute inflammatory process of infarction is over and scar formation is complete.[24] None of the deaths within the observation period was associated with hemothorax, an indicator of myocardial rupture.

An excellent balance of infarct sizes between the untreated and captopril-treated groups was achieved by the randomization process. The survival of the rats without infarction from both treatment groups was identical (figure 3, *A*). When all infarcted animals were pooled separately for each treatment, the survival of the captopril-treated group was superior to that of the untreated cohort (figure 3, *B*). Subclassification according to size of infarction revealed that this prolongation of survival was not distributed uniformly across all infarct size groups. The rats with small infarcts made up the smallest number of animals with infarction and a log-rank test did not reveal a difference in survival between the treatment groups. In contrast, in the rats classified as having moderate infarctions there was a prolongation of survival in the animals allocated to the captopril group (figure 4, *B*). Of note is the fact that this difference in survival was observed primarily in the late period after the experimental infarction: the captopril-treated animals did not demonstrate the late mortality that was observed in the untreated group. In the rats with large myocardial infarctions there was no overall difference in survival during the 1 year observation period and, although there appeared to be an early prolongation of survival in the captopril-treated animals, this trend was not sustained over the predetermined observation period.

This study was designed with total mortality as the single end point; however, a second analysis was performed in which results in animals with overt thoracic infections were censored. The elimination of these data from the analysis only served to strengthen all of the above conclusions.

This study demonstrates that survival is related to size of myocardial infarction and that long-term captopril therapy can prolong the survival of animals with healed myocardial infarction and left ventricular dysfunction. The most benefit from drug therapy with respect to survival was noted in animals with infarctions of moderate size. This is in agreement with results of our prior study of the effects of long-term captopril therapy on ventricular performance and cavitary size, in which rats with extensive infarctions demonstrated minimal hemodynamic benefit from long-term therapy. The implication of these results is that in severe heart failure it may be unrealistic to anticipate that captopril therapy will prolong survival. However, this animal study underscores the need for a clinical evaluation of captopril in patients with less severe ventricular dysfunction. Indeed, an important implication of this study is that captopril therapy may be effective in prolonging life if instituted early in the course of left ventricular dysfunction after myocardial infarction and possibly in patients with other forms of early congestive heart failure.

We thank Professor Eugene Braunwald for his thoughtful review of the manuscript. The statistical consultation provided by Dr. James Anderson and Ms. Harriet F. Peterson, M.S., of the Harvard School of Public Health is gratefully acknowledged. Data organization and analysis was assisted by the CLINFO data management and analysis system at Brigham and Women's Hospital, Boston, supported by GCRC No. 5 M01 RR00888-10 CLR. We thank Mrs. Angela Perry for her secretarial assistance in the preparation of this manuscript. Captopril was generously supplied by Drs. John C. Alexander and Zola P. Horovitz of the Squibb Institute for Medical Research.

References

1. McKee PA, Castelli WP, McNamara PM, Kannel WB: The natural history of congestive heart failure: The Framingham Study. N Engl J Med **285:** 1441, 1971
2. Smith WF: Epidemiology of congestive heart failure. Am J Cardiol **55:** 3A, 1985
3. Cohn JN, Levine TB, Olivari MT, Garberg V, Lura D, Francis GS, Simon AB, Rector T: Plasma norepinephrine as a guide to prognosis in patients with chronic congestive heart failure. N Engl J Med **311:** 819, 1984
4. Wilson JR, Schwartz JS, St. John Sutton M, Ferraro N, Horowitz LN, Reichek N, Josephson ME: Prognosis in severe heart failure: relation to hemodynamic measurements and ventricular ectopic activity. J Am Coll Cardiol **2:** 403, 1983
5. Franciosa JA, Wilen M, Ziesche S, Cohn JN: Survival in men with severe chronic left ventricular failure due to either coronary heart disease or idiopathic dilated cardiomyopathy. Am J Cardiol **51:** 831, 1983
6. Chatterjee K, Parmley WW: Vasodilator therapy for acute myocardial infarction and chronic congestive heart failure. J Am Coll Cardiol **1:** 133, 1983
7. Awan NA, Mason DT: Vasodilator therapy of severe congestive heart failure: the special importance of angiotensin-converting enzyme inhibition with captopril. Am Heart J **104:** 1127, 1982
8. Creager MA, Faxon DP, Halperin JL, Melidossian CD, McCabe CH, Schick EC, Ryan TJ: Determinants of clinical response and survival in patients with congestive heart failure treated with captopril. Am Heart J **104:** 1147, 1982
9. Massie BM, Kramer BL, Topic N: Lack of relationship between the short-term hemodynamic effects of captopril and subsequent clinical responses. Circulation **69:** 1135, 1984
10. Dzau VJ, Colucci WS, Williams GH, Curfman G, Meggs L: Sustained effectiveness of converting enzyme inhibition in patients with severe congestive heart failure. N Engl J Med **302:** 1373, 1980
11. The Captopril Multicenter Research Group: A placebo-controlled trial of captopril in refractory chronic congestive heart failure. J Am Coll Cardiol **2:** 755, 1983
12. Cohn JN: Vasodilators: rationale, application, and future prospects. *In* Braunwald E, Mock MB, Watson J, edtiors: Congestive heart failure: current research and clinical applications. New York, 1982, Grune and Stratton, Inc., p 279
13. Braunwald E: Heart failure: evaluation of therpay based on a consideration of natural history. *In* Braunwald E, Sonnenblick EH, Chakrin LW, Schwarz RP, editors: Milrinone: investigation of new inotropic therapy for congestive heart failure. New York, 1984, Raven Press, p 1
14. Furberg CD, Yusuf S: Effect of vasodilators on survival in chronic congestive heart failure. Am J Cardiol **55:** 1110, 1985

15. Pfeffer MA, Pfeffer JM, Fishbein MC, Fletcher PJ, Spadaro J, Kloner RA, Braunwald E: Myocardial infarct size and ventricular function in rats. Circ Res **44:** 503, 1979
16. Fletcher PJ, Pfeffer JM, Pfeffer MA, Braunwald E: Left ventricular diastolic pressure-volume relations in rats with healed myocardial infarction. Effects on systolic function. Circ Res **49:** 618, 1981
17. Pfeffer JM, Pfeffer MA, Braunwald E: Influence of chronic captopril therapy on the infarcted left ventricle of the rat. Circ Res (in press)
18. Dunn FG, Pfeffer MA, Frohlich ED: ECG alterations with progressive left ventricular hypertrophy in spontaneous hypertension. Clin Exp Hypertens **1:** 67, 1978
19. Packer M: Vasodilator and inotropic therapy for severe chronic heart failure: passion and skepticism. J Am Coll Cardiol **2:** 841, 1983
20. Franciosa JA, Dunkman WB, Leddy CL: Hemodynamic effects of vasodilators and long-term response in heart failure. J Am Coll Cardiol **3:** 1521, 1984
21. Franciosa JA, Jordan RA, Wilen MM, Leddy CL: Minoxidil in patients with chronic left heart failure: contrasting hemodynamic and clinical effects in a controlled trial. Circulation **70:** 63, 1984
22. Oberman A, Cutter GR, Rogers WJ, Mantle JA: Clinical end points. *In* Braunwald E, Mock MB, Watson J, editors: Congestive heart failure: current research and clinical applications. New York, 1982, Grune and Stratton, Inc., p 341
23. Geltman EM, Ehsani AA, Campbell MK, Schechtman K, Roberts R, Sobel BE: The influence of location and extent of myocardial infarction on long-term ventricular dysrhythmia and mortality. Circulation **60:** 805, 1979
24. Fishbein MC, Maclean D, Maroko PR: Experimental myocardial infarction in the rat. Am J Pathol **90:** 57, 1978

Effects of propranolol and diltiazem alone and in combination on the recovery of left ventricular segmental function after temporary coronary occlusion and long-term reperfusion in conscious dogs

LARRY R. BUSH, PH.D., L. MAXIMILIAN BUJA, M.D., GREGORY TILTON, M.D., MARK WATHEN, M.D., PHILLIP APPRILL, M.D., JULIET ASHTON, PH.D., AND JAMES T. WILLERSON, M.D.

ABSTRACT We evaluated the ability of propranolol and dilitazem alone and in combination to enhance the recovery of left ventricular (LV) segmental function during 1 month of reperfusion after two temporary occlusions of the left anterior descending coronary artery (LAD) in conscious dogs instrumented with ultrasonic crystals for the measurement of regional net systolic wall thickening (NET). LV segments were classified according to their contractile function after 1 hr of LAD occlusion: class 1, greater than 67% of preocclusion (control) NET; class 2, 0% to 66.9%; class 3, less than 0% (paradoxical systolic wall thinning). Propranolol (1 mg/kg iv) or diltiazem (20 μg/kg/min) was given 65 min after LAD occlusion in dogs that had 2 (group I) or 4 hr (group II) of LAD occlusion. Diltiazem plus propranolol (same doses) were given to another group of dogs that underwent 4 hr (but not 2) of LAD occlusion. Untreated control dogs received 25 ml of saline and underwent 2 or 4 hr of LAD occlusion. The NET of class 2 and 3 segments in group I control dogs increased significantly during 1 month of reperfusion, from 32 ± 5% and −43 ± 6% to 66 ± 9% and 26 ± 9%, respectively ($p < .05$). Neither diltiazem nor propranolol enhanced the long-term recovery of these segments in group I dogs. However, diltiazem prevented further deterioration of contractile dysfunction observed in control dogs immediately after reperfusion in both segment classes. The NET of class 2 segments in group II control dogs after 4 weeks of reperfusion remained at levels observed during LAD occlusion: 30 ± 4% to 37 ± 12%. Class 3 NET increased from −33 ± 5% to 12 ± 12% with 1 month of reperfusion, but these segments were essentially akinetic. Propranolol or diltiazem alone did not produce significant overall increases in NET, but diltiazem again prevented further declines in NET of class 2 and 3 segments during early reperfusion. However, the combination of diltiazem and propranolol significantly enhanced overall recovery of class 2 NET in group II dogs (44 ± 3% to 88 ± 7%) and prevented the worsening of NET associated with early reperfusion. Compared with untreated dogs, propranolol plus diltiazem also significantly decreased the extent of histologic necrosis in class 2 and 3 segments as well as the macrohistochemically determined infarct size in group II dogs. Propranolol alone caused significant declines in heart rate and LV dP/dt_{max}; diltiazem alone lowered aortic pressure significantly; aortic pressure and LV dP/dt were lowered by combined propranolol and diltiazem. Thus we conclude that (1) diltiazem alone prevents further deterioration of LV segmental function early after reperfusion following 2 to 4 hr of occlusion, but neither diltiazem nor propranolol alone enhances segmental functional recovery, and (2) the combination of propranolol and diltiazem results in significantly improved recovery of systolic segmental function and a significant reduction in the extent of necrosis in moderately dysfunctional segments after 4 hr of temporary LAD occlusion followed by 1 month of reperfusion. These data demonstrate that combined therapy with diltiazem and propranolol together extends the "window" for preserving segmental ventricular function from 2 to 4 hr of temporary LAD occlusion in this experimental preparation.

Circulation 72, No. 2, 413–430, 1985.

From the Departments of Internal Medicine (Cardiology Division) and Pathology, University of Texas Health Science Center, Southwestern Medical School, Dallas.

Supported by the National Institutes of Health Ischemic (SCOR) Grant HL-17669, the American Heart Association (Texas Affiliate), and the Moss Heart Fund, Dallas. Dr. Bush was an NIH Postdoctoral Fellow (HL 070360-04) during the period in which this work was performed.

Address for correspondence: James T. Willerson, M.D., Room L5.134, University of Texas Health Science Center, 5323 Harry Hines Blvd., Dallas, TX 75235.

Received Jan. 11, 1985; revision accepted May 16, 1985.

THE EFFICACY of thrombolytic therapy and surgical methods for revascularizing ischemic myocardium during evolving myocardial infarction and growing interest in these techniques have raised several important questions regarding the salvage of myocardial tissue and preservation of contractile function.[1-3] Previously we[4] and others[5] have demonstrated in conscious dogs that temporary, proximal occlusion of a major coronary artery for longer than 2 hr results in persistent impairment of segmental contractile function at sites of previous moderate and severe dysfunction. Accordingly, we tested the hypothesis that a carefully selected pharmacologic intervention may extend this "window of time," or the period of coronary occlusion after which reperfusion may still provide a beneficial influence by preserving segmental contractile function and reducing the extent of myocardial necrosis.

Many studies have suggested that several different β-adrenergic antagonists may limit ischemic injury.[6-9] Slow-channel calcium (Ca^{2+}) antagonists have also been demonstrated to protect ischemic myocardium in some experimental preparations.[10-16] The potential mechanisms by which these drugs may exert their protective actions include (1) reduced myocardial energy demand, secondary to declines in heart rate or afterload[10]; (2) an increase in collateral blood flow to ischemic myocardium[11]; and (3) direct protection from myocellular Ca^{2+} overload[12, 13, 15, 16] or catecholamine-induced myocyte damage.[6-8] In this study, the effects of a β-adrenergic and a calcium-channel blocker were evaluated alone and in combination to assess their efficacy in protecting left ventricular segmental function during temporary coronary occlusion and reperfusion in awake, chronically instrumented dogs. We believed that β-adrenergic antagonism with propranolol might prevent the reflex increase in heart rate and contractility caused by the reduction in peripheral vascular resistance with administration of a Ca^{2+} channel blocker. Diltiazem was chosen as the slow-channel calcium antagonist because it alters heart rate and blood pressure in a desirable manner in the intact animal[11, 12] and in man,[14, 17] and it has been previously shown to exert beneficial effects in a variety of experimental preparations of myocardial ischemia.[11-13, 16] Data from our previous study, in which we compared the long-term recovery of regional myocardial function after 2 or 4 hr of coronary occlusion, were used for our control, saline-treated groups.[4]

Materials and methods

Surgical preparation. Mongrel dogs (22 to 30 kg) of either sex were anesthetized with sodium pentobarbital (30 mg/kg iv) and artificially ventilated with room air delivered by a Harvard respirator via a cuffed endotracheal tube. Under sterile conditions, a left thoracotomy was performed and the heart was suspended in a pericardial cradle. A Konigsberg pressure transducer was inserted in the left ventricular apex and polyethylene catheters were inserted into the left atrium and descending aorta for monitoring pressure was well as for injecting microspheres and collecting reference blood samples. A proximal segment of the left anterior descending coronary artery (LAD) was gently dissected away from the epicardium and an inflatable balloon occluder, described previously[4, 18] was placed around the artery. Epicardial crystals attached to small (1 cm^2) dacron patches were sutured to the epicardial surface, and smaller endocardial crystals were inserted into the subendocardium obliquely so as not to disturb the intervening myocardium between the crystal pairs. Final placement of the endocardial crystals was guided by observing their radiofrequency signals, which were displayed on an oscilloscope, and the crystal wire was secured with a purse-string suture on the epicardial surface. All wires and catheters were tunneled between the scapulae and exteriorized through two small incisions at the base of the neck. The chest was closed in layers and any air in the thorax was evacuated by suction-drainage. Dogs were allowed to recover for at least 1 week before experimental study.

Study protocol. After a sufficient recovery period and acclimatization to a standing sling, dogs were studied awake and unsedated. Control measurements of aortic left ventricular (LV), and left atrial pressures, and a lead II electrocardiogram were recorded on an Electronics for Medicine (Model VR-12) physiologic recorder. The maximum rate of LV pressure development (peak LV dP/dt) was obtained by electronic differentiation of the LV pressure pulse. Left ventricular wall thickness measurements were recorded on a Hewlett-Packard eight-channel recorder interfaced with a Tektronix (Model 465) oscilloscope. Regional myocardial blood flow was measured with carbonized microspheres (9 to 15 μm diameter) labeled with ^{125}I, ^{46}Sc, ^{113}Sn, ^{85}Sr, ^{95}Nb, and ^{57}Co, which were suspended in 0.05% polysorbate 80 (Tween-80) and agitated vigorously by vortexing just before each injection. One to 2 million microspheres were injected into the left atrium over 8 to 10 sec. Starting 10 sec before and continuing for 90 sec after microsphere injection, reference arterial blood was withdrawn from the carotid artery at a constant rate of 7.8 ml/min with a Harvard infusion/withdrawal pump. The order of isotope administration was changed randomly.

Dogs underwent two (group I) or 4 hr (group II) of proximal LAD occlusion produced by inflating the pneumatic balloon occluder around the LAD. Dogs were excluded from the study if (1) infusion of the occluder caused no change at any site at which wall thickness was measured or (2) large, spontaneous improvements in wall thickening in akinetic or dyskinetic segments occurred soon after LAD occlusion, suggesting unsuccessful or incomplete occlusion. Hemodynamic and wall thickness measurements were recorded at hourly intervals after LAD occlusion as well as 5, 30, 75, and 90 min after LAD occlusion; blood flow was measured either 2 (group I) or 4 hr (group II) after LAD occlusion. Sixty-five minutes after LAD occlusion and immediately after hemodynamic and wall thickness measurements were obtained, subgroups of dogs in groups I and II received saline (1.0 ml/kg), d,l-propranolol HCl (1 mg/kg, single iv bolus), or diltiazem HCl (20 μg/kg/min, infusion rate 0.19 to 0.38 ml/min). In group II animals, an additional subgroup of dogs received both propranolol and diltiazem at the same doses used when the agents were administered singly. Diltiazem was given as a constant infusion and continued until 2 hr after reperfusion. Propranolol-treated dogs that underwent 4 hr of LAD occlusion received an additional 0.5 mg/kg 1 hr after reperfusion (4 hr after the initial dose). In group I, 11 dogs received saline, nine received propranolol, and seven received diltiazem. In group II, 15 dogs received saline, nine received propranolol, 10 received diltiazem, and 11 received propranolol and diltiazem.

In our previous study,[4] data from 13 group I and 14 group II dogs were described. In the present study, we report data from 11 group I and 15 group II saline-treated control dogs. One group I dog, whose wall thickening signals were of marginal quality before occlusion, was later omitted from data analyses. A second animal in this group was also omitted from subsequent data analyses because, after elimination of several segments due to poor signal quality (which was also done in the original study), this dog provided wall thickening data from only one LV site. Other hemodynamic and blood flow alterations in this animal led us to conclude that it had not been studied in a relaxed, unaroused state. Thus the blood flow data and one regional signal were also eliminated from this animal in the final data analyses. Data from an additional group II saline-treated control animal have been included in the present analyses. Because of the large numbers of regional segments involved in the analysis of regional systolic function in this study, the subtraction of two dogs and the addition of one dog in groups I and II, respectively, have had a trivial impact on the final mean values.

Ten minutes before the LAD occlusion was released and just after hemodynamic, wall thickness, and blood flow measurements were obtained, dogs were given an intravenous bolus injection of lidocaine (25 mg) followed by an infusion of 0.5 mg/min for 20 min (10 min each before and after coronary reperfusion) to minimize the risk of reperfusion-induced arrhythmias. Reflow was produced by deflating the balloon occluder. Thus dogs actually were subjected to 130 or 250 min of LAD occlusion; for simplicity, these periods of LAD occlusion will be referred to as "2 hr" and "4 hr," respectively.

If resistance to further inflation of the occluder at the end of the occlusive period was absent at this time, dogs were excluded from study for reasons similar to those cited above. Deflation of the balloon occluder was ensured by applying additional vacuum to the catheter, and coronary reperfusion was confirmed by dramatic upward shifts in LV wall thickness by hypokinetic or akinetic segments.[4, 18–20]

Hemodynamic and wall thickness recordings were obtained just before and 5 min after discontinuation of the lidocaine infusion and at 1 and 2 hr after reperfusion. Regional myocardial blood flow was measured at the latter time, after which dogs were returned to their quarters. Dogs were returned to the laboratory and studied at 24 hr and at weekly intervals for 4 weeks. Regional myocardial blood flow also was measured again at 4 weeks after reperfusion.

Autopsy procedure. At the conclusion of the study, dogs were given sodium heparin (5000 U iv) followed 5 min later by a lethal overdose of sodium pentobarbital. The hearts were excised quickly and rinsed under cold tap water. The balloon occluder around the LAD was examined and the patency of the coronary artey was determined by expelling heparinized blood or saline from a No. 7F polyethylene catheter positioned in the LAD proximal to the occlusion site and observing the anterograde run-off in the epicardial vessels of the distal LAD bed. Next, to determine the size of the occluded bed (or "anatomical risk region"), we mounted the heart on a perfusion apparatus similar to that described previously.[4, 21] The aorta was cannulated and perfused with a warm solution of 0.5% (vol/vol) monastral blue dye (DuPont) in normal saline, and the LAD was cannulated and perfused simultaneously with a warm 1% solution of phosphate-buffered triphenyltetrazolium chloride,[4, 22] both at a perfusion pressure of 100 to 120 mm Hg. Thus this method identified the area at risk as well as the extent of infarction therein.

After removal of the subendocardial crystals, the heart was sliced into five or six transverse sections. The epicardial crystals were left sutured to the myocardium so that crystal pairs could be identified later by color coding. The heart slices were fixed in 10% buffered formalin, weighed, and photographed on both sides to measure the extent of infarction and the size of the occluded bed. Transmural sections (approximately 1 cm along the epicardial circumference) encompassing the segment between pairs of endocardial and epicardial crystals were dissected, trimmed of epicardial fat and large blood vessels, and divided into epicardial, midwall, and endocardial thirds. These sections were weighed and placed in scintillation vials containing 10% formalin. Myocardium from the posterior free wall, representing nonischemic control tissue, was sampled for blood flow measurements and, when possible, blocks also were taken from myocardium exhibiting the maximal extent of transmural necrosis and termed "infarct center." Samples were counted for radioactivity in a Packard Autogamma scintillation spectrometer for 5 min with window settings adjusted appropriately for each isotope.[23] Regional myocardial blood flow was calculated by a computer-assisted program (ml/min/g).

Quantification of segmental necrosis, area at risk, and infarct size. After radioactivity for blood flow determinations was counted, epicardial, midwall, and endocardial tissue samples were embedded in paraffin en bloc, sectioned, mounted, and stained with hematoxylin and eosin. Each section was photographed under magnification and the areas comprising granulation tissue and fibrosis were interpreted as evidence of prior necrosis and thus termed "necrotic." The boundaries of necrotic area were traced on photomicrographs, while the same histologic sections were examined by light microscopy. The area of necrosis (relative to total cross-sectional area) was outlined and later measured by planimetry with a digitizing tablet (Talos) coupled with a PDP 11/05 (Digital Equipment) computer, as described previously.[4, 24] The term "total necrosis" represents the weighted average of the transmural segment; that is, it takes into account differences in the areas of the three layers of tissue. These determinations were made without knowledge of the contractile, hemodynamic, or blood flow data.

The sizes of myocardial infarcts and areas at risk were measured planimetrically, similar to the technique described above. The bed at risk was defined as myocardium not stained by the blue dye, which was injected via the aorta into all branches of the right and left coronary system proximal to the occlusion site in the LAD. Since the bed at risk was perfused simultaneously with tetrazolium solution, this region possessed stained (uninfarcted) and unstained (infarcted) tissue. Color slides of both sides of transverse slices were illuminated on a translucent digitizing table, and the outlines of infarcted, jeopardized (area at risk), and total LV myocardium were digitized. The fractions of total LV area representing the bed at risk and the infarcted tissue were multiplied by the weight of each left ventricular slice to obtain the percentage, by weight, of total LV that was infarcted and at risk.

Measurements of LV segmental function. Segmental LV wall thickness was measured in millimeters, assuming the speed of sound through myocardium to be 1.5 mm/μsec.[24, 25] To correct for the variation in initial separation of crystal pairs, as well as the regional performance of the nonischemic ventricle,[26] wall thickness measurements are expressed as a percent of preocclusion control values.[4, 18, 24]

Three measurements of wall thickness were made, from which four variables describing regional segmental function were calculated. Left ventricular end-diastolic wall thickness (EDWTh) was determined immediately before the rapid upstroke of the LV pressure tracing and at the nadir of wall thinning caused by atrial contraction. This was also defined as the

TABLE 1
Hemodynamic changes in dogs that underwent 2 hr of coronary occlusion and 4 weeks of reperfusion (mean ± SEM)

			Occlusion			Reperfusion		
	n	Control	5 min	1 hr	2 hr	1 hr	2 hr	24 hr
HR (bpm)								
S	11	105±9	120±6[B]	118±7	111±7	106±4	114±5	141±5[A]
P	9	104±6	121±8[B]	114±8	99±4	99±8	105±8	115±10
D	7	103±4	117±6[B]	113±5	125±5[A]	117±5	116±6	115±6
AOS (mm Hg)								
S	11	142±4	139±5	146±5	141±4	131±3	132±3	128±4[A]
P	9	148±9	147±8	154±8	149±8	142±8	141±8	149±11
D	7	147±8	141±6	144±7	135±6	125±5[A]	129±5	129±7
AOD (mm Hg)								
S	11	100±5	98±4	107±4	100±3	97±5	95±3	96±4
P	9	91±3	92±3	99±4	98±6	93±5	91±4	91±5
D	7	96±5	95±4	98±4	85±4	84±4	83±3	85±4
AOM (mm Hg)								
S	11	118±4	117±5	123±4	118±4	111±3	110±3	109±4
P	9	113±3	112±3	117±4	118±5	108±5	106±4	110±4
D	7	119±5	115±4	121±5	102±4[A]	102±3[A]	103±3[A]	103±5[A]
ATM (mm Hg)								
S	11	9.5±1.1	12.8±2.0[B]	12.2±1.2	11.8±1.3	12.6±1.6	12.3±1.4	13.5±1.5[A]
P	9	10.5±11	12.6±1.1	11.2±1.1	14.1±0.9	12.8±1.0	12.6±1.3	12.3±1.2
D	7	8.6±1.1	11.3±1.3[B]	11.8±1.4	12.9±1.2	10.9±1.3	13.2±1.5	13.2±1.9
LV dP/dt (mm Hg/sec)								
S	11	3196±89	2913±117[B]	2987±96	2938±119	2747±110	2665±101[A]	2644±142
P	9	3058±49	2874±50[B]	3110±90	2632±64	2539±91	2540±42	2520±31
D	7	2961±136	2830±97	2869±93	2899±135	2475±200	2468±167	2357±173
HR × AOS (×10^3)								
S	11	15.1±0.9	16.9±1.2	17.3±1.1	15.7±1.1	13.9±0.6	15.2±0.9	17.9±0.8
P	9	15.2±0.9	17.6±1.2	17.6±1.6	14.8±1.6	14.2±1.5	14.9±2.8	17.7±2.8
D	7	15.0±0.6	16.4±0.9	16.3±1.0	17.0±1.2	14.7±1.0	15.1±1.2	15.0±1.4

S = saline; P = propranolol; D = diltiazem; HR = heart rate; AOS = aortic systolic pressure; AOD = aortic diastolic pressure; AOM = aortic mean pressure; ATM = atrial mean pressure; LV dP/dt = peak rate of change in LV pressure; HR × AOS = double product.

[A]Variable within a treatment group that is significantly different from control ($p < .05$ by analysis of variance and Duncan's multiple range test).

[B]Significantly different from control value by paired t test.

The brackets join values significantly different between two treatment groups at one time point (Duncan's multiple range test and $p < .05$ by one-way analysis of variance).

point immediately before the upstroke of the LV dP/dt signal.[18, 24] The maximal extent of LV segmental wall thickening was defined between peak positive and negative LV dP/dt, which corresponds closely to aortic valve opening and closure, respectively. When appropriate, the maximal extent of wall thinning (paradoxical wall motion) also was measured during this interval. The variable net systolic wall thickening (NET), as defined previously,[18] equals the difference between maximal systolic wall thickness and EDWTh, minus any paradoxical wall thinning if present. Analog wall thickness tracings and hemodynamic recordings were digitized with a Graf/Pen (Science Accessories Corp.) coupled to a DEC 10 computer.

Calculations. In the analysis of regional LV contractile function, segments were classified according to their severity of dysfunction 1 hr after LAD occlusion: class 1 segments displayed minimal ischemic dysfunction, possessing 67% or greater of their preocclusion values for NET; class 2 consisted of segments that displayed moderate dysfunction, defined as those with NET values of 0% to 66.9% of control NET; class 3 segments showed severe contractile dysfunction, manifested by paradoxical systolic wall thinning. Segments in this class had NET values less than 0% of their control values.

Statistical methods. All values are expressed as the mean ± SEM. Comparisons between time points and with segment classes or treatment groups were made with a two-way analysis of variance,[27] and multiple comparisons within classes over time or between classes within a time period were performed with Duncan's multiple range test.[28] Statistical significance was achieved when p values were less than .05. Comparisons with preocclusion control for segmental function data were made with a one-sample t test. Since the control value was constant, based on the number of comparisons, p was considered to be statistically significant if less than .005.[29]

Results

Hemodynamic changes. The saline-treated dogs in groups I and II, which we have described previously,[4] provided the basis for comparison of the three treatment regimens. Thus these two groups were studied sequentially, relative to the other five drug-treated groups, which were mixed randomly. Of a total of 99

TABLE 1
(Continued)

Reperfusion			
1 wk	2 wk	3 wk	4 wk
113±6	112±7	114±7	107±8
128±8	107±10	102±11	97±5
139±6	129±7^{A}	121±9^{A}	118±10
144±4	136±4	150±7	144±7
136±5	144±9	134±8	131±8
128±4	137±6	134±11	134±6
98±5	94±6	102±7	96±4
92±3	90±7	92±6	83±12
95±4	92±5	98±12	98±7
113±3	111±4	123±7	115±5
107±2	110±5	110±6	103±6
103±3^{A}	114±5	112±11	114±4
13.3±1.8^{A}	13.4±1.8^{A}	13.8±1.3^{A}	11.1±1.1
9.1±1.2	9.2±2.1	8.0±1.1	8.7±0.7
10.5±1.3	9.8±1.2	10.5±1.9	9.3±1.2
2922±222	3318±168	3460±237	3241±172
2786±95	2330±21	2762±32	2939±37
2285±109	2876±136	2751±318	3309±21
16.4±1.2	15.1±1.3	17.2±2.0	15.4±1.4
17.0±0.8	16.1±2.4	14.6±1.8	12.5±1.4
17.7±0.8	17.6±1.3	15.5±0.6	19.7±0.5

dogs studied, 27 died before completion of the 4 week study period. These were distributed among the five treatment groups as follows: six group I dogs treated with saline (one 30 min after occlusion, one within the first hour of reperfusion, and four between 24 hr and 2 weeks after reperfusion); five group I dogs treated with propranolol (one within the first hour after coronary occlusion; four between 24 hr and 2 weeks after reperfusion); five group I dogs treated with diltiazem (one 90 min after LAD occlusion and four between 24 hr and 1 week after reperfusion); three group II dogs treated with saline (one less than 1 hr after occlusion, one 75 min after occlusion, and one at 1 week after reperfusion); five group II dogs treated with diltiazem (two less than 1 hr after LAD occlusion, one 45 min after coronary reperfusion, and two between 24 hr and 1 week after reperfusion); two group II dogs treated with propranolol (both of which developed ventricular fibrillation less than 1 hr after LAD occlusion); and one group II dog treated with propranolol plus diltiazem (which died 3 weeks after reperfusion). Dogs that died either during the short-term study or before the end of the 1 month after reperfusion were not included in data analysis. Most dogs that died between 24 hr and 3 weeks were found dead. Thus, because of autolysis and clotting, perfusion staining and histologic analysis of their hearts were impossible.

Group I dogs. Short-term LAD occlusion caused a sinus tachycardia in all dogs, which persisted for the duration of LAD occlusion in control dogs (table 1), but caused little or no change in aortic pressure. Mean left atrial pressure also increased over the short-term with LAD occlusion in saline- and diltiazem-treated animals. LV dP/dt usually declined with LAD occlusion. In dogs that received saline or propranolol alone, this decline was significantly different from the preocclusion value.

Figure 1 demonstrates the short-term hemodynamic effects of propranolol and diltiazem during LAD occlusion. Propranolol lowered heart rate and LV dP/dt. Diltiazem lowered aortic pressure significantly, which resulted in a 10 to 15 beat/min elevation in heart rate that was significantly higher than the value at 1 hr after

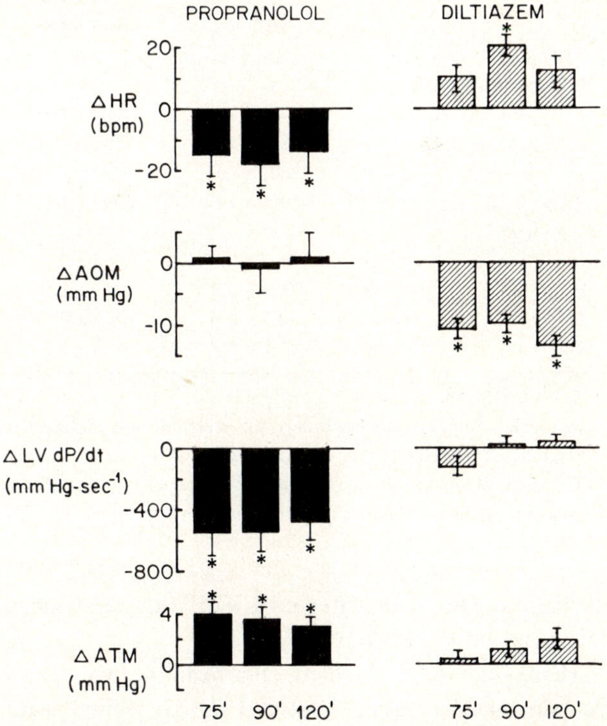

FIGURE 1. Short-term hemodynamic effects of propranolol or diltiazem during LAD occlusion in group I dogs. Values shown represent the change in each variable relative to the value before drug administration (60 min after occlusion) as measured 75, 90, and 120 min after occlusion. *Significant difference ($p < .05$) vs 60 min after occlusion (based on analysis of variance, Duncan's multiple range test of actual mean values at 60 through 120 min after occlusion). HR = heart rate; AOM = mean aortic pressure; ATM = mean left atrial pressure.

TABLE 2
Hemodynamic changes in dogs that underwent 4 hr of coronary occlusion and 4 weeks of reperfusion (mean ± SEM)

	n	Control	Occlusion 5 min	1 hr	2 hr	3 hr	4 hr
HR (bpm)							
S	15	110±3	117±4	108±5	104±5	102±4	101±6
P	9	107±4	120±6^B	118±7	97±4	94±5	89±2
D	10	105±4	122±5^B	116±4	123±5^C	116±4	121±6
P&D	11	100±4	128±7^B	116±5	99±6	105±7	113±10
AOS (mm Hg)							
S	15	141±5	138±5	138±4	132±6	136±5	133±4
P	9	145±4	141±3	140±3	138±3	134±3	137±5
D	10	137±4	132±4	134±4	124±4^A	118±3	117±3^A
P&D	11	128±6	129±5	129±5	120±2	116±3	114±3
AOD (mm Hg)							
S	15	89±2	88±4	90±3	87±3	87±3	86±3
P	9	99±4	101±3	102±4	101±4^C	97±4	95±5
D	10	91±3	90±4	90±3	80±4	76±3^A	75±4^A
P&D	11	87±4	91±4	90±3	82±2	78±3^A	75±3^A
AOM (mm Hg)							
S	15	109±3	107±4	111±3	106±4	109±4	105±2
P	9	114±4	114±3	114±3	113±3	109±3	109±5
D	10	106±3	104±4	105±3	95±4^A	90±3^A	89±3^A
P&D	11	104±4	104±3	97±3	91±3	88±2^A	86±3^A
ATM (mm Hg)							
S	15	9.3±1.2	11.1±1.5	10.3±1.4	10.4±1.5	10.9±1.2	11.7±1.2
P	9	9.7±1.3	11.4±1.5^B	11.0±1.6	12.8±1.2	13.7±1.5	13.6±1.8
D	10	9.0±1.1	10.5±1.4^B	10.6±1.2	11.5±1.9	12.3±2.0	13.7±2.4^A
P&D	11	9.4±1.1	10.3±2.8	9.7±1.4	14.6±3.4	15.7±3.0	15.5±3.1
LV dP/dt (mm Hg/sec)							
S	15	3050±191	2780±150^B	2869±170	2699±128	2736±168^C	2657±146
P	9	2535±150	2485±178	2564±187	2149±175	2114±151^A	2103±176
D	10	2607±103	2402±110	2447±103	2367±121	2304±102	2256±110^B
P&D	11	2986±174	2793±192	2689±204	2207±143	2126±145	2072±152^A
HR × AOS							
S	15	15.7±0.9	16.2±0.6	14.9±0.8	13.8±1.0	13.9±0.6	13.4±0.8
P	9	15.6±0.9	16.9±1.0	16.5±1.2	13.5±0.9	12.6±0.8	12.2±0.6
D	10	14.4±0.6	16.2±0.9	15.4±0.6	15.2±0.7	13.8±0.6	14.2±1.0
P&D	11	13.6±0.8	16.8±1.6	14.8±0.6	11.8±0.7^C	12.2±0.9	12.9±1.1

Abbreviations as in table 1.

^A Variable within a treatment group that is significantly different from control ($p < .05$ by analysis of variance).

^B Significantly different from control value by paired t test.

The brackets join values significantly different between treatment groups at one time point (Duncan's multiple range test and $p < .05$ by one-way analysis of variance). ^C Significantly different from all other treatment groups.

occlusion. Diltiazem affected LV dP/dt_{max} and mean left atrial pressure trivially.

Heart rate was elevated significantly (141 ± 5 beats/min) 24 hr after short-term LAD occlusion-reperfusion in saline-treated dogs, caused primarily by arrhythmias, which crested at 24 hr and were usually characterized as regular junctional or unifocal ventricular rhythms.

Aortic pressure returned to control levels in all groups by 1 week after reperfusion. Mean left atrial pressure also returned to control levels in propranolol- and diltiazem-treated dogs by 1 week but remained significantly elevated in the control dogs until 3 weeks after reperfusion. Neither LV dP/dt nor the double product differed significantly from control values during early or late reperfusion.

Group II dogs. The hemodynamic changes produced by short-term LAD occlusion and reperfusion resembled those observed in group I dogs (table 2). Heart rate rose, aortic pressure changed trivially, mean left atrial pressure increased consistently, and LV dP/dt and double product did not generally change signifi-

TABLE 2
(Continued)

Reperfusion						
1 hr	2 hr	24 hr	1 wk	2 wk	3 wk	4 wk
135 ± 6[A]	142 ± 7[A]	128 ± 4[A]	114 ± 8	110 ± 6	110 ± 6	104 ± 5
128 ± 11	127 ± 12	128 ± 9	119 ± 8	113 ± 12	118 ± 9	120 ± 10
128 ± 7[A]	130 ± 8	136 ± 13[A]	111 ± 5	108 ± 11	114 ± 5	115 ± 6
131 ± 10[A]	117 ± 10	110 ± 11	111 ± 9	106 ± 11	106 ± 8	103 ± 8
128 ± 5	130 ± 4	127 ± 3[A]	148 ± 5	138 ± 7	129 ± 10	138 ± 7
120 ± 5[A]	124 ± 6[A]	125 ± 6[A]	140 ± 7	127 ± 2[A]	118 ± 9[A]	129 ± 11[A]
112 ± 4[A]	114 ± 4[A]	126 ± 7	124 ± 3[A]	135 ± 11	129 ± 8	125 ± 6
110 ± 5	106 ± 4[A]	120 ± 5	129 ± 6	126 ± 7	131 ± 4	129 ± 6
92 ± 3	94 ± 3	88 ± 3	96 ± 3	94 ± 6	79 ± 0.3	94 ± 3
92 ± 5	94 ± 6	96 ± 6	102 ± 5	89 ± 3	81 ± 10[A]	92 ± 8
76 ± 4[A]	76 ± 3[A]	91 ± 5	80 ± 4	95 ± 13	86 ± 6	85 + 5
74 ± 2[A]	74 ± 3[A]	88 ± 4	84 ± 4	85 ± 6	87 ± 2	86 ± 4
105 ± 3	106 ± 3	101 ± 3	116 ± 3	114 ± 6	108 ± 9	114 ± 4
101 ± 5	103 ± 6	105 ± 6	114 ± 6	102 ± 2[A]	93 ± 10[A]	105 ± 8
88 ± 4[A]	89 ± 3[A]	102 ± 6	95 ± 3	108 ± 12	100 ± 6	99 ± 5
84 ± 3[A]	98 ± 4	99 ± 4	99 ± 6	102 ± 3	102 ± 3	100 ± 5
9.9 ± 1.4	10.7 ± 1.2	9.5 ± 1.4	9.9 ± 1.1	10.7 ± 1.9	9.2 ± 1.2	8.4 ± 1.4
11.7 ± 1.3	13.0 ± 1.7	15.3 ± 2.8[A]	13.3 ± 2.3	11.4 ± 1.6	11.0 ± 1.8	7.0 ± 1.4
12.5 ± 2	11.9 ± 2.1	8.9 ± 1.3	8.0 ± 0.9	10.2 ± 2.1	8.0 ± 0.5	8.0 ± 1.7
13.0 ± 2.2	14.5 ± 1.8	9.6 ± 1.7	9.9 ± 0.9	8.0 ± 1.8	7.2 ± 0.7	9.7 ± 0.6
2471 ± 173[A]	2317 ± 155[A]	2517 ± 167[A]	2772 ± 232	2920 ± 473	2142 ± 110	2715 ± 179
1838 ± 142[A]	1818 ± 135[A]	2053 ± 213[A]	2510 ± 159	2600 ± 93	2714 ± 61	2635 ± 209
2233 ± 139[B]	2156 ± 140[A]	2256 ± 200	2304 ± 298	2566 ± 184	2400 ± 305	2420 ± 110
1983 ± 137	1827 ± 76[A]	2453 ± 143	2947 ± 210	2709 ± 210	3123 ± 210	3064 ± 241
17.2 ± 0.9	18.5 ± 1	16.1 ± 0.5	17.2 ± 0.9	15.9 ± 1.9	14.5 ± 1.2	14.3 ± 1.4
15.4 ± 1.5	15.7 ± 1.7	16.2 ± 1.6	16.9 ± 1.7	14.5 ± 2.0	15.3 ± 1.9	15.8 ± 2.3
14.3 ± 0.9	14.8 ± 0.9	16.8 ± 1.4	13.7 ± 0.7	14.7 ± 3.3	14.4 ± 1.1	15.2 ± 1.0
14.1 ± 0.8	12.2 ± 0.8	12.9 ± 1.1	14.2 ± 1.2	13.0 ± 0.7	13.8 ± 0.8	13.1 ± 0.8

cantly. LV dP/dt was significantly decreased after coronary occlusion in some dogs.

Figure 2 shows the short-term hemodynamic effects of propranolol and diltiazem alone and in combination. Propranolol lowered heart rate and LV dP/dt significantly and caused significant elevations in mean left atrial pressure. Diltiazem lowered mean aortic pressure significantly but did not change heart rate or mean left atrial pressure significantly. Diltiazem infusion decreased LV dP/dt by 4 hr after coronary occlusion. Propranolol and diltiazem together significantly decreased mean arterial pressure and LV dP/dt.

Arrhythmias again caused a significant elevation in heart rate in two of the four treatment groups 2 to 24 hr after reperfusion. After 1 week heart rate was not significantly different from control. By 1 week after reperfusion, mean left atrial pressure, LV dP/dt, and the double product also had returned to control values.

Changes in LV segmental function during LAD occlusion and reperfusion. Table 3 shows the mean control (preocclusion) values for EDWTh and NET. The number of dogs providing LV segments to each functional class is indicated in the legend. EDWTh averaged 9.51 ± 0.24 and 9.29 ± 0.20 mm in all group I and II dogs, respectively. These values are in close agreement with previously reported values.[25] NET averaged 2.04 ± 0.10 and 1.96 ± 0.11 mm in groups I and II dogs, respectively. Thus the fractional increase in segmental wall thickness during systole ranged from 0.19 ± 0.05 to 0.25 ± 0.02. These values are also in close agree-

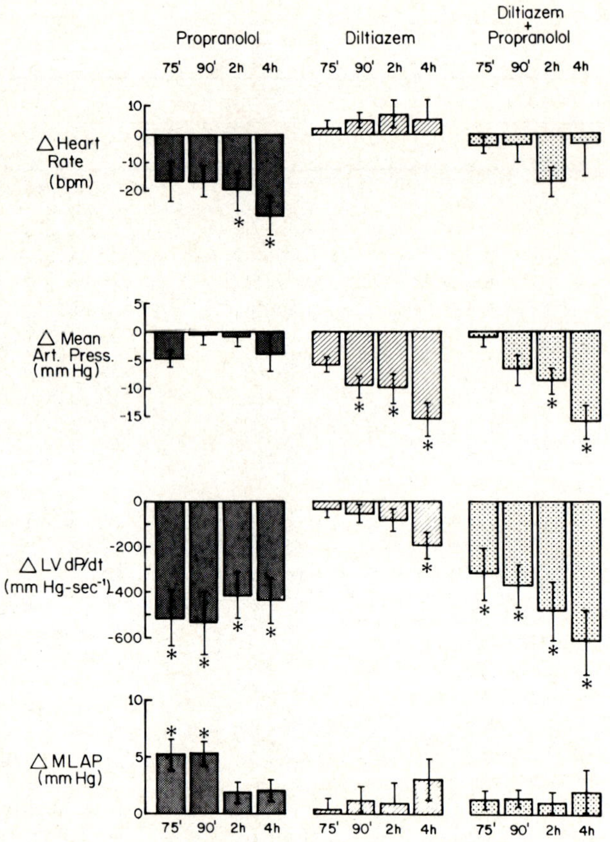

FIGURE 2. Short-term hemodynamic effects of propranolol, diltiazem, and propranolol plus diltiazem during LAD occlusion in group II dogs. Values shown represent the mean (± SE) change in each variable relative to values at 60 min after occlusion as measured 75 and 90 min and 2 and 4 hr after occlusion. *Significantly different from 60 min after occlusion. MLAP = mean left atrial pressure.

ment with values reported by Sasayama et al.[25] and Heyndrickx et al.[19] There were no significant differences between any of the treatment groups in any of these variables.

Figure 3 shows a representative LV wall thickness tracing from a saline-treated control dog with 4 hr of LAD occlusion followed by 1 month of reperfusion. LAD occlusion produced abrupt and variable declines in both EDWTh and the extent of systolic wall thickening in ischemic LV segments. Within 5 to 10 min, no further spontaneous changes in EDWTh or NET occurred. Segments that demonstrated moderate or severe dysfunction during LAD occlusion regained little or no functional recovery after long-term reperfusion. Figure 4 shows similar short-term changes in segmental function during LAD occlusion in a propranolol- and diltiazem-treated dog with 4 hr of temporary LAD occlusion but a lack of worsening of segmental function during reperfusion and the recovery of function in most segments with long-term reperfusion.

TABLE 3
Control (preocclusion) values of EDWTh, NET, and percentage increase in systolic wall thickening

	n	EDWTh (mm)	NET (mm)	NET/EDWTh
Group I dogs				
Control	46[A]	9.75 ± 0.23	2.09 ± 0.12	0.21 ± 0.03
Propranolol	43[B]	9.12 ± 0.21	1.94 ± 0.10	0.22 ± 0.01
Diltiazem	39[C]	9.63 ± 0.27	2.09 ± 0.09	0.22 ± 0.01
Group II dogs				
Control	60[D]	9.70 ± 0.24	1.83 ± 0.09	0.19 ± 0.05
Propranolol	38[E]	9.35 ± 0.22	1.87 ± 0.12	0.22 ± 0.02
Diltiazem	40[F]	9.08 ± 0.29	2.10 ± 0.12	0.23 ± 0.01
Propranolol + Diltiazem	38[G]	8.83 ± 0.23	2.14 ± 0.13	0.25 ± 0.02

[A]Ten class 1 segments (nine dogs), 12 class 2 segments (eight dogs), and 24 class 3 segments (10 dogs).

[B]Fifteen class 1 (six dogs), 13 class 2 (seven dogs), and 15 class 3 (eight dogs).

[C]Thirteen class 1 (seven dogs), 11 class 2 (six dogs), and 15 class 3 segments (seven dogs).

[D]Eighteen class 1 (10 dogs), 24 class 2 (13 dogs), and 18 class 3 (14 dogs).

[E]Eight class 1 (seven dogs), seven class 2 (seven dogs), and 23 class 3 (nine dogs).

[F]Eleven class 1 (nine dogs), 13 class 2 (eight dogs), and 16 class 3 (10 dogs).

[G]Nine class 1 (six dogs), 16 class 2 (eight dogs), and 13 class 3 (seven dogs).

Changes in NET during LAD occlusion and long-term reperfusion: group I dogs. The changes in NET that occurred in dogs subjected to 2 hr of LAD occlusion and 1 month of reperfusion are summarized in figure 5. The NET of class 1 segments 5 min after LAD occlusion were 87 ± 8%, 79 ± 10%, and 88 ± 4% of control in saline-, propranolol-, and diltiazem-treated dogs, respectively. Small, insignificant increases in NET of these segments occurred spontaneously between 5 min and 1 or 2 hr after occlusion. Reperfusion caused an approximately 10% decrease in NET in saline- and propranolol-treated segments, which lasted approximately 24 hr in the saline-treated dogs; however, these values still did not differ significantly from control values. These segments in diltiazem-treated dogs did not show a significant decrease in NET with reperfusion. After 1 month of reperfusion, class 1 segments in the three treatment groups had NET values between 75% and 95% of control. Values of NET did not differ significantly between the three treatment groups at any time during LAD occlusion or reperfusion.

The NET of moderately dysfunctional class 2 segments declined promptly and significantly with LAD occlusion (figure 5, *middle panel*); mean (± SE) val-

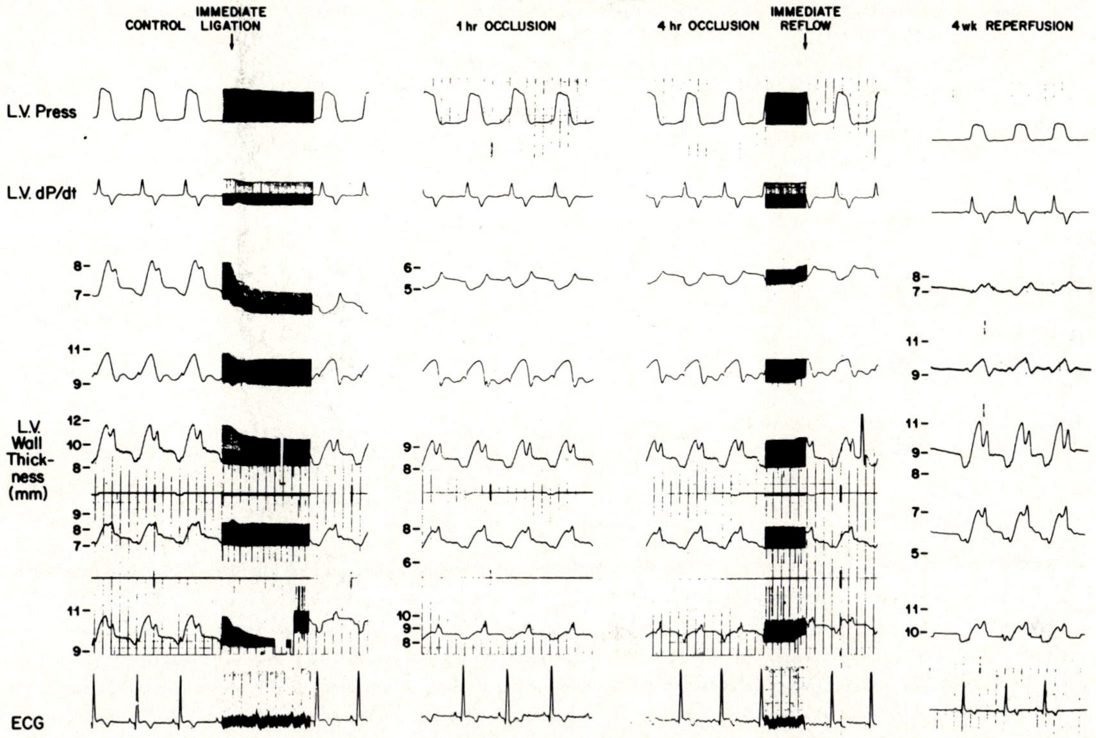

FIGURE 3. Actual physiologic recording from a control (saline-treated) dog that underwent 4 hr of LAD occlusion and 1 month of reperfusion. Recording shows (from top down) analog signals of LV pressure, LV dP/dt, and wall thickness at five LV segments, and the electrocardiogram (ECG). Several segments undergo sudden decline in EDWTh and NET with short-term LAD occlusion and display minimal NET or paradoxical systolic wall thickening, which persists throughout LAD occlusion and early reperfusion. Even after 1 month of reperfusion, previously moderately dysfunctional LV segments display persistent contractile dysfunction.

ues for NET 5 min after coronary occlusion in saline-, propranolol-, and diltiazem-treated dogs were 31 ± 5%, 22 ± 11%, and 35 ± 6% of control, respectively. One hour later, when segments were classified according to their severity of dysfunction, NET values were practically unchanged (32 ± 5%, saline; 25 ± 4%, propranolol; 39 ± 6%, diltiazem). One hour later, just before coronary reperfusion, class 2 segmental NET was 36 ± 6%, 28 ± 7%, and 36 ± 5% of control (no significant differences) in saline-, propranolol-, and diltiazem-treated dogs, respectively. Initially, reperfusion caused a further significant decline in NET in class 2 segments, which persisted for at least 24 hr in saline-treated control animals. This reperfusion-induced exacerbation of contractile dysfunction was less pronounced in propranolol-treated dogs and was prevented by diltiazem. In fact, class 2 segmental NET increased immediately after reperfusion in the diltiazem-treated dogs; NET values in this group exceeded those in untreated segments signficantly at 1, 2, and 24 hr. Values of NET did not differ significantly between treatment groups from 1 week to 1 month after reperfusion (figure 5), nor did the average changes in NET between 1 hr after occlusion and 1 month after reperfusion. One month after coronary reperfusion, the NET in saline-, propranolol-, and diltiazem-treated segments was 66 ± 9%, 76 ± 12%, and 75 ± 6% of control, respectively.

Class 3 segments in all treatment groups underwent rapid, severe declines in contractile function with LAD occlusion (figure 5, *bottom panel*); systolic wall thickening in these segments was replaced by holosystolic wall thinning (figure 5). After 2 hr of occlusion, NET remained the same in diltiazem and control dogs but increased to −19 ± 5% in propranolol-treated dogs. Early reperfusion was also associated with worsening of contractile function in class 3 segments. Diltiazem again prevented the exacerbation of segmental dysfunction with reperfusion in these segments; the extent of systolic wall thinning diminished from a postocclusion NET of −39 ± 9% to −22 ± 7% 1 hr after reflow and to −10 ± 7% 1 hr later. Twenty-four hours later these segments were essentially akinetic (NET −4 ± 13%). In contrast, NET in class 3 segments declined to −27 ± 9% and −32 ± 10% 1 and 2 hr after reperfusion in propranolol-treated segments and from −36 ± 6% to −57 ± 7% and −52 ± 5% at the same time in control dogs. Over the ensuing

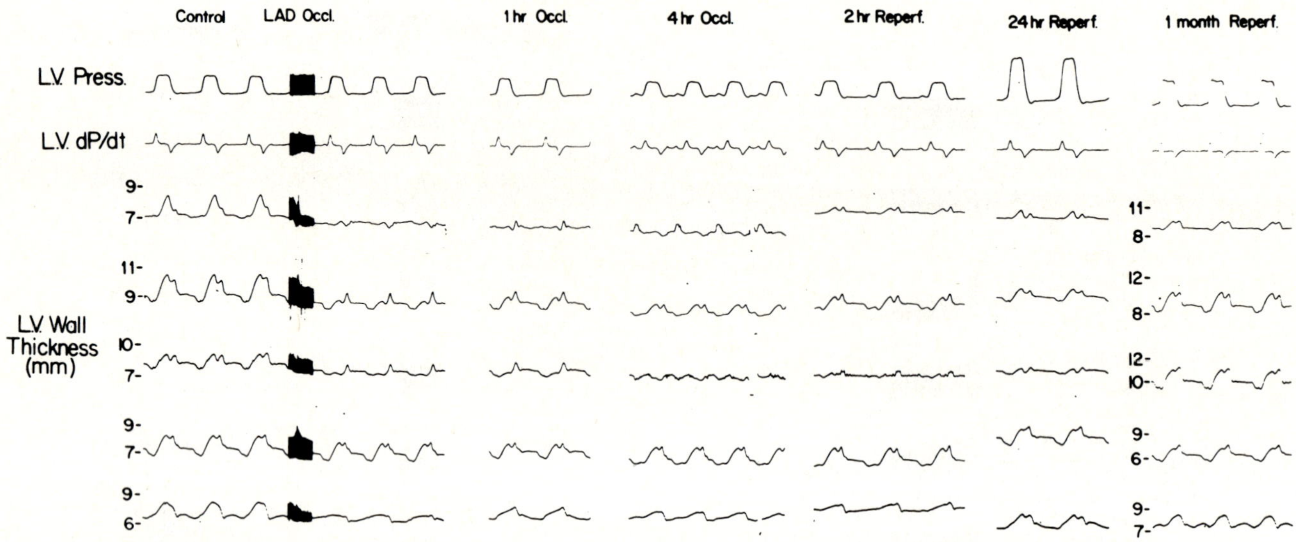

FIGURE 4. Actual recordings of LV pressure, LV dP/dt, and regional LV wall thickening in a dog that underwent 4 hr of LAD occlusion and received propranolol (1 mg/kg) plus diltiazem (20 μg/kg/min) 1 hr after LAD occlusion. The first and third LV segments (from the top), which are dyskinetic and akinetic, regain significant contractile function during 1 month of reperfusion. The second and fifth segments, which are moderately dysfunctional during LAD occlusion, also regain active systolic wall thickening with long-term reperfusion. The fourth LV segment from the top, which is minimally dysfunctional during LAD occlusion, is a class 1 segment. LV pressure 24 hr after reperfusion was not elevated; the gain in this signal was increased in this dog at this time point.

month after reperfusion, NET increased progressively and significantly, reaching a value of 26 ± 9% of preocclusion values in control animals. Neither propranolol nor diltiazem significantly improved the overall recovery of NET in these segments.

Short-term effects of propranolol and diltiazem on NET during LAD occlusion: group I dogs. Neither diltiazem nor saline affected NET in any segment class during LAD occlusion. NET declined significantly immediately (75 and 90 min vs 60 min) in class 2 segments in propranolol-treated dogs. The extent of systolic wall thinning was diminished significantly in propranolol-treated class 3 segments from a predrug level (at 60 min after ligation) of −32 ± 4% to −19 ± 5% and 16 ± 5% at 75 and 120 min, respectively.

Changes in NET during LAD occlusion and long-term reperfusion: group II dogs. The changes in NET in class 1 segments during 4 hr of LAD occlusion and 1 month of reperfusion in the four groups of dogs are shown in figure 6 (*top panel*.) NET declined 14% immediately after LAD occlusion and remained near this value throughout the period of LAD occlusion in the saline-treated control animals. Class 1 segmental NET changed similarly in dogs that received diltiazem alone or in combination with propranolol; the NET of class 1 segments in propranolol-treated dogs rose insignificantly (106 ± 10%) with LAD occlusion. NET declined immediately after coronary reperfusion in the control (−18%) and propranolol-treated dogs (−11%), whereas diltiazem alone, or in combination with propranolol, prevented this decline in NET. Within the next 24 hr the NET of class 1 segments in the control group returned to near control values after 1 week and remained at this level for the next 3 weeks. NET returned to near control levels more promptly in the three remaining groups. Between 1 and 4 weeks after reperfusion, NET was not significantly different from control levels in any group.

Immediately after (5 min) LAD occlusion, the NET of class 2 segments was 24 ± 6%, 38 ± 9%, 37 ± 7%, and 33 ± 6% in control, propranolol-, diltiazem-, and propranolol plus diltiazem–treated dogs, respectively (figure 6, *middle panel*). These values changed trivially within the next hour after LAD occlusion. No further changes in NET occurred between 1 and 4 hr in any group except in dogs receiving propranolol alone (see below). There were no significant differences in the values of NET between the four treatment groups during the entire occlusive period.

NET declined significantly (compared with end-occlusion values) with reperfusion in the control (−18%) and propranolol-treated dogs (−23%); this decline in NET was prevented in dogs receiving diltiazem alone or in combination with propranolol. Compared with values recorded at the end of 4 hr of LAD occlusion, no significant increases in NET occurred after 24 hr of reperfusion in all treatment groups. No further recovery of NET (30 ± 6% [at end-occlusion]

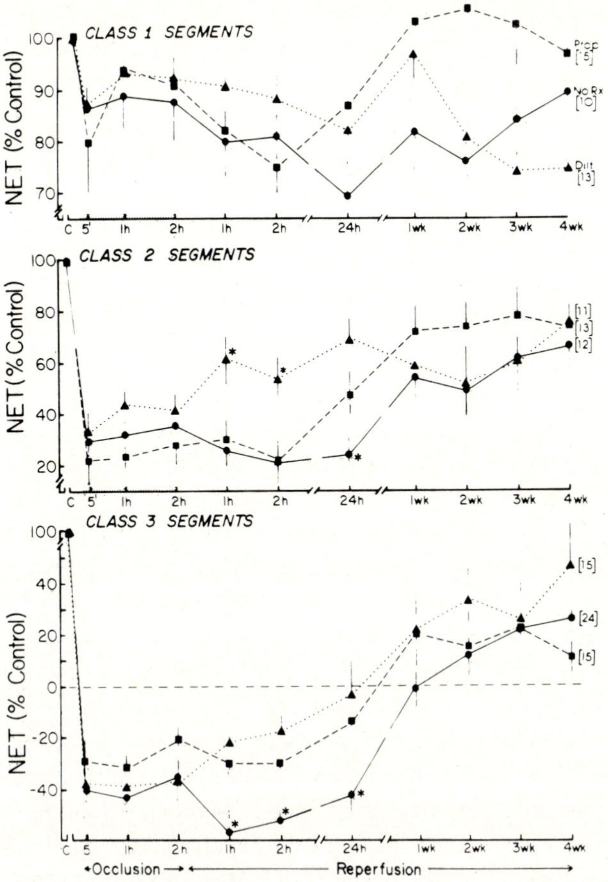

FIGURE 5. Changes in NET expressed as a percentage of control value during 2 hr of LAD occlusion and 1 month of reperfusion in group I dogs. *Significant difference vs other two treatment groups ($p < .05$ analysis of variance, Duncan's multiple range test). The numbers in parentheses represent the number of segments in each class and treatment group.

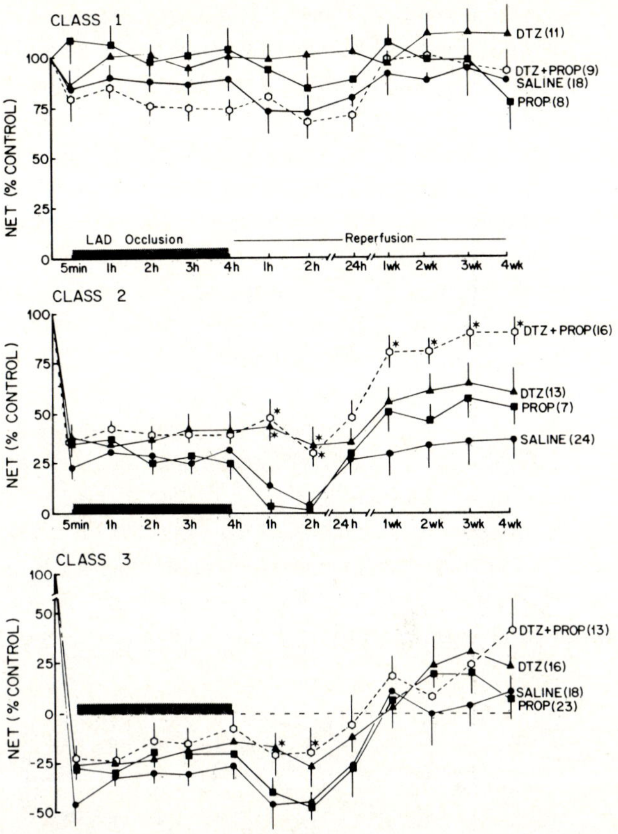

FIGURE 6. Changes in NET during 4 hr of LAD occlusion and 1 month of reperfusion in group II dogs. Asterisks during early reperfusion in class 2 segments denote significance vs other two treatment groups. Asterisks at 1 to 4 weeks after reperfusion denote a significant difference between propranolol plus diltiazem vs saline-treated groups only. In class 3 segments, asterisks denote that the value for diltiazem-treated dogs alone was significantly different compared with the propranolol- or saline-treated dogs at 1 hr after reperfusion and for propranolol plus diltiazem dogs alone at 2 hr after reperfusion. DTZ = diltiazem; PROP = propranolol.

to 37 ± 10% [4 weeks]) was observed after 1 month of reperfusion in control dogs. The NET of class 2 segments in dogs that received propranolol or diltiazem alone increased during the ensuing month of reperfusion, but their NET was not significantly different than that of the control group. However, the ultimate recovery of NET in group II dogs that received propranolol plus diltiazem (NET 88 ± 7% at 4 weeks) was significantly greater than that of the control group. Moreover, the average changes in NET between either 1 or 4 hr after occlusion and 1 month after reperfusion (46.5 ± 6.9% and 51.7 ± 7.5%, respectively) of propranolol plus diltiazem–treated dogs significantly exceeded those in control dogs (6.6 ± 9.2% and 7.1 ± 10.9%, respectively).

The NET of class 3 segments declined severely with LAD occlusion (figure 6, *bottom panel*). Values of NET 1 hr after LAD occlusion did not differ significantly between the four treatment groups. After 1 hr of LAD occlusion, NET was −33 ± 5%, −31 ± 4%, −25 ± 4%, and −26 ± 6% in control, propranolol-, diltiazem-, and propranolol plus diltiazem–treated dogs, respectively. NET did not change significantly during the next 3 hr of LAD occlusion in dogs receiving saline and diltiazem, whereas the extent of ischemia-induced systolic wall thinning diminished slightly in dogs that received either propranolol alone or in combination with diltiazem. Diltiazem alone, or in combination with propranolol, prevented the exacerbation of contractile dysfunction associated with the early reperfusion period. Again, 24 hr appeared to be the minimum period required for NET to return to end-occlusion values. The ultimate recovery of NET did not differ significantly between groups nor did the average changes in NET between either 1 or 4 hr after occlusion and 1 month after reperfusion. However, a trend toward improved recovery of contractile function was displayed by class 3 segments in dogs that received propranolol plus diltiazem.

Short-term effects of propranolol, diltiazem, or propranolol plus diltiazem on NET during LAD occlusion: group II dogs. Similar to results obtained in group I dogs, diltiazem did not affect the NET of any segment class during LAD occlusion, whereas propranolol caused slight declines in NET of class 1 and 2 segments. Propranolol alone and in combination with diltiazem also caused a diminution of systolic wall thinning of class 3 segments during the period of drug administration. No change in NET in class 1, 2, or 3 segments occurred during this interval in the saline-treated dogs.

Changes in EDWTh

Group I dogs. The time-dependent changes in segmental EDWTh during LAD occlusion and 1 month of reperfusion are shown in figure 7. The EDWTh of minimally dysfunctional class 1 segments declined 1% to 2% with LAD occlusion over the short-term. The administration of propranolol caused a further decline in EDWTh (significantly different from preocclusion

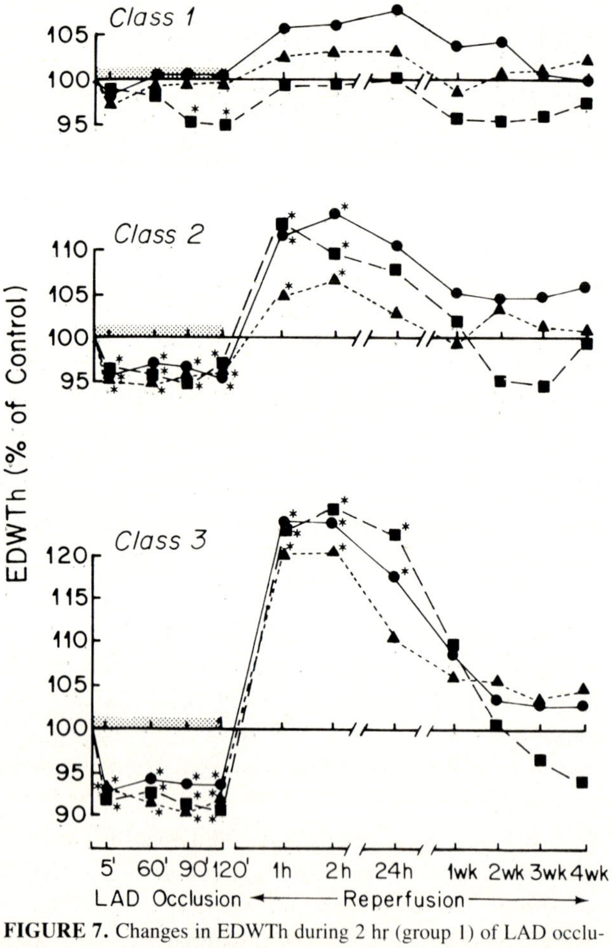

FIGURE 7. Changes in EDWTh during 2 hr (group I) of LAD occlusion and 1 month of reperfusion in saline- (filled circles), propranolol- (filled squares), diltiazem- (filled triangles), or propranolol plus diltiazem–treated dogs (filled circles, broken lines). *Significantly different from control values (100%) at a $p < .005$ level (see text, Bonferroni's method).

control, $p < .005$), probably reflecting the lowered heart rate and inotropic state plus an elevation in wall tension (figure 7). Reperfusion caused a slight (5% to 7%) increase in EDWTh, which crested between 2 and 24 hr after reperfusion and returned to control values in the ensuing month.

LAD occlusion produced more consistent and dramatic declines in EDWTh in both class 2 and 3 segments in all treatment groups. One hour after LAD occlusion, EDWTh of class 2 and 3 segments in control dogs averaged 96.9 ± 1.1% and 93.0 ± 0.9% of control, respectively. The EDWTh of segments in other treatment groups declined similarly; there were no significant differences in this variable between treatment groups.

Class 2 and 3 segmental EDWTh increased dramatically immediately after reperfusion, with values remaining elevated for at least 2 hr in class 2 segments and for 24 hr in propranolol- and saline-treated class 3 segments. The overshoot in EDWTh above control values was even more pronounced in class 3 segments; EDWTh exceeded control values by 24.0 ± 3.2% and 17.7 ± 3.4% early (1 and 2 hr) and 1 day after reperfusion in saline-treated animals. Similar elevations in EDWTh occurred during early reperfusion in the other treatment groups. In the month after short-term reperfusion, EDWTh returned to near control levels in all segmental classes.

Group II dogs. The changes in segmental EDWTh during 4 hr of LAD occlusion and 1 month of reperfusion were nearly identical to those seen in group I dogs (not shown). The only salient difference between group I and II dogs related to the ability of all three interventions to cause elevations of class 2 segmental EDWTh between 2 and 4 hr after occlusion. EDWTh returned to values not differing significantly from control values by 1 month after reperfusion.

Changes in regional myocardial blood flow

Group I dogs. The changes in blood flow to ischemic segments as well as nonischemic and infarcted myocardium during coronary arterial ligation and reperfusion are shown in figure 8, *A*. After 2 hr of LAD occlusion, endocardial blood flow to class 1 segments was reduced 34 ± 6%, 35 ± 7%, and 17 ± 19% in saline-, propranolol-, and diltiazem-treated dogs, respectively (not statistically different from control). Blood flow to these segments increased variably 2 hr after reperfusion but did not exceed their respective control values significantly at this time or at 4 weeks.

Endocardial blood flow to moderately dysfunctional class 2 segments declined 49 ± 18% below control levels in saline-treated control dogs after 2 hr of LAD

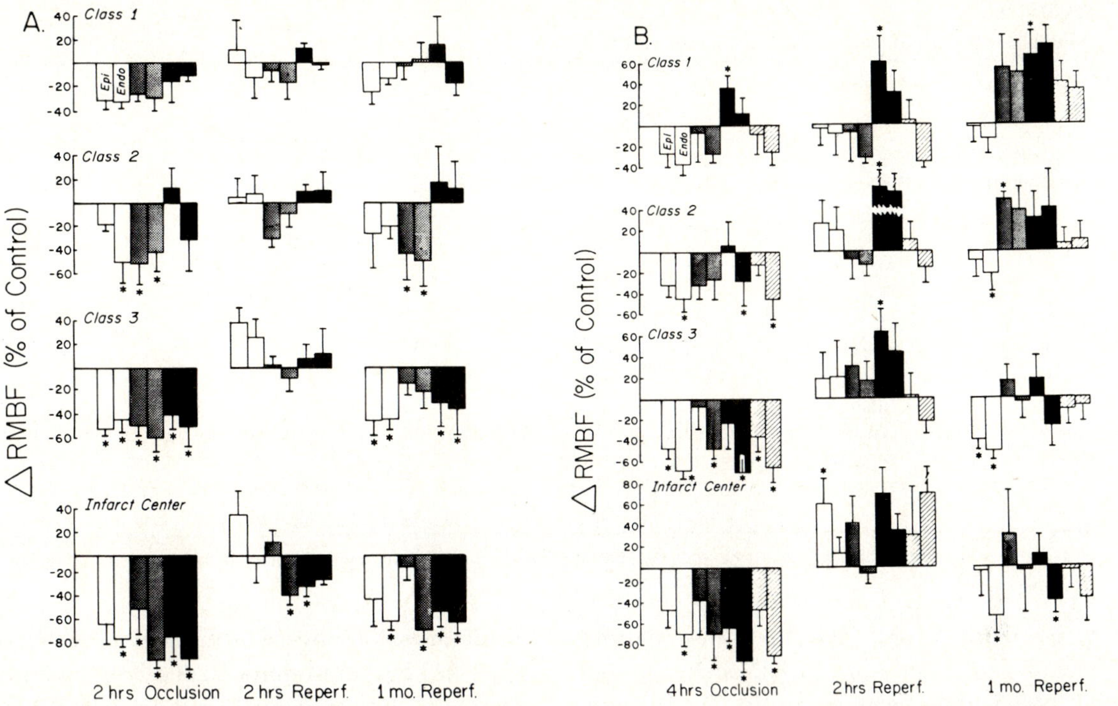

FIGURE 8. Changes (relative to control [before occlusion]) in regional myocardial blood flow (RMBF) in class 1 through 3 LV segments and myocardium sampled from the infarct center in saline- (open bars), propranolol- (stippled bars), diltiazem- (solid bars), and propranolol plus diltiazem–treated dogs (striped bars). *A*, group I; *B*, group II. *Significant difference ($p < .05$; analysis of variance plus Duncan's multiple range test, based on actual values of RMBF [ml/min per g]) vs control time point. See figure for number of segments in each class. The first and second bars for each treatment group represent subepicardial and subendocardial layers, respectively (see class 1, 2 hr occlusion).

occlusion. Epicardial flow declined approximately 19 ± 30% in these segments (not significantly different from control values). Both epicardial and endocardial blood flow to class 2 segments in propranolol-treated dogs underwent significant declines in flow (−53% and 46%, respectively) after LAD occlusion. After 2 hr of LAD occlusion, epicardial blood flow of class 2 segments in dogs that received diltiazem increased above control values, whereas endocardial blood flow declined 33 ± 27%, reflecting perhaps a drug-induced increase in collateral blood flow to the subepicardial layer in these segments. Blood flow to these segments reached or exceeded control values 2 hr after coronary reperfusion in control and diltiazem-treated groups, but remained below control values in propranolol-treated dogs. Blood flow to endocardial layers of class 2 segments after 4 weeks of reperfusion was depressed significantly in saline- and propranolol-treated dogs but not in dogs that received diltiazem.

Blood flow to class 3 segments declined transmurally in all treatment groups after 2 hr of LAD occlusion. Early after reperfusion (2 hr), blood flow to these segments exceeded (not significantly) or returned to control values in saline- and diltiazem-treated dogs. After 2 hr of reperfusion, blood flow to these segments in propranolol-treated dogs remained below control levels. After 4 weeks of reperfusion, transmural blood flow to class 3 segments was depressed significantly in dogs that received saline and diltiazem; endocardial blood flow was significantly lower in the propranolol-treated group at this time.

Blood flow in nonischemic LV myocardium changed trivially during short-term LAD occlusion and reperfusion in saline-treated or diltiazem-treated groups (not shown). Blood flow to ischemic myocardium in propranolol-treated dogs declined (significantly in the epicardial layers) during short-term LAD occlusion and reperfusion, probably secondary to lowered metabolic demands, since heart rate and LV dP/dt were lowered significantly by this drug.

The alterations in blood flow to myocardium displaying the greatest extent of transmural necrosis at 4 weeks (infarct center) were similar qualitatively but more severe than those in class 3 segments. Similar restorations or overshoots in blood flow early (2 hr) after reperfusion and later (4 weeks) persistent declines were observed in tissue taken from these regions.

Group II dogs. The changes in blood flow with 4 hr of LAD occlusion and long-term reperfusion in group II dogs followed a pattern similar to that in group I dogs

TABLE 4
Macrohistochemically determined infarct size (g/100 g)

Hours of occlusion	Variable	Saline	Propranolol	Diltiazem	Propranolol and diltiazem
2 (group I)	Risk / Total LV	19.7±1.5	23.8±2.3	18.4±1.9	
	Infarct / Risk	22.7±4.9	23.0±5.8	22.0±4.1	
	Infarct / Total LV	5.0±0.9 (n = 13)	5.1±1.3 (n = 6)	4.8±1.1 (n = 7)	
4 (group II)	Risk / Total LV	19.8±2.4	19.3±2.1	18.9±1.8	28.0±3.9
	Infarct / Risk	29.2±7.4	21.3±3.6	15.7±4.9	8.9±5.4
	Infarct / Total LV	7.1±1.7^{A} (n = 11)	4.3±0.8^{A,B} (n = 9)	2.9±0.9^{B} (n = 9)	2.1±1.0^{B} (n = 8)

Values with different superscripts are significantly different from one another by one-way analysis of variance and Duncan's multiple range test.

(figure 8, *B*). Class 1 segmental blood flow did not decline significantly after 4 hr of LAD occlusion, but epicardial blood flow was increased significantly above control values in the diltiazem-treated dogs throughout LAD occlusion as well as early and late after coronary reperfusion.

Four hours after LAD occlusion, endocardial blood flow in class 2 segments had declined 45%, 25%, 28%, and 46% in saline-, propranolol-, diltiazem-, and propranolol plus diltiazem–treated groups, respectively. During early reperfusion, blood flow returned to or exceeded control levels in all but the propranolol-treated groups. After 1 month of reperfusion, endocardial blood flow was significantly lower compared with preocclusion levels only in the saline-control dogs.

Endocardial blood flow to severely dysfunctional class 3 segments declined significantly after 4 hr of LAD occlusion in all treatment groups (range $-68 \pm 9\%$ in saline-treated dogs to $-48 \pm 8\%$ in propranolol-treated dogs). Blood flow returned to or exceeded control levels early after reperfusion. Transmural blood flow was depressed significantly 1 month later in saline-treated dogs.

Gross infarct size. There was no significant difference in the extent of infarction or in the size of the bed at risk between treatment groups in group I dogs (table 4). The ratio of infarcted to total left ventricle was significantly reduced in group II dogs that received diltiazem, either alone or in combination with propranolol, compared with saline-treated control dogs. Comparisons between all animals in groups I and II (for effects of duration of occlusions) did not reveal significant differences in any variable relating to estimation of infarct size or area at risk.

Segmental necrosis. Postmortem inspection of hearts revealed a layer of fibrotic adhesions covering the epicardium, but epicardial crystals themselves caused

TABLE 5
Extent of histologic necrosis in left ventricular segments: group I

Wall region	Saline	Propranolol	Diltiazem
Class 1			
Epi	3.8±2.0	5.4±1.9	3.8±2.5
Mid	1.9±1.0	5.4±2.3	1.9±1.1
Endo	5.3±2.1	8.2±3.0	3.9±1.8
Total	3.8±1.2 (n = 8)	6.1±1.9 (n = 14)	3.1±1.5 (n = 11)
Class 2			
Epi	8.6±2.5	5.8±2.1	1.6±1.0
Mid	15.2±5.9	10.5±4.1	5.7±1.7
Endo	22.6±7.1	16.3±5.4	6.8±3.0
Total	15.6±4.8 (n = 9)	10.7±3.4 (n = 14)	4.6±1.5 (n = 8)
Class 3			
Epi	17.6±2.9^{A}	9.9±3.0^{A,B}	3.9±1.1^{B}
Mid	33.1±4.7^{A}	21.3±5.5^{A,B}	13.2±6.6^{B}
Endo	34.0±7.0	37.5±9.2	20.2±7.1
Total	28.8±4.3^{A} (n = 21)	22.5±5.3^{A,B} (n = 12)	12.0±3.2^{B} (n = 12)

Data expressed as percent necrosis (mean ± SEM), with number of segments in which necrosis was quantified in parentheses.

For each class and level, values with different superscripts are significantly different from one another by one-way analysis of variance and Duncan's multiple range test. In some instances, the number of segments available for functional assessment and histologic estimate of the extent of necrosis were different because of loss of functional signal at some point in the course of the study or an unsatisfactory specimen for histologic analysis.

Epi, Mid, Endo = necrosis in epicardial, midwall, and endocardial layers; total = weighted transmural average.

TABLE 6
Extent of histologic necrosis in left ventricular segments: group II

Wall region	Saline	Propranolol	Diltiazem	Propranolol and diltiazem
Class 1				
Epi	6.3 ± 2.2^{A}	$3.9 \pm 3.9^{A,B}$	$1.8 \pm 0.5^{A,B}$	0 ± 0^{B}
Mid	8.7 ± 3.2	3.1 ± 2.0	5.2 ± 2.3	0 ± 0
Endo	12.6 ± 6.6	7.0 ± 4.7	10.0 ± 3.6	0.5 ± 0.5
Total	8.6 ± 2.9	4.5 ± 1.9	4.7 ± 1.4	0.1 ± 0.1
	(n = 13)	(n = 5)	(n = 26)	(n = 7)
Class 2				
Epi	17.1 ± 4.1^{A}	$11.3 \pm 8.1^{A,B}$	6.6 ± 1.9^{B}	1.5 ± 0.7^{B}
Mid	16.7 ± 5.8	28.0 ± 13.0	21.5 ± 5.5	4.8 ± 1.8
Endo	23.7 ± 6.2^{A}	26.8 ± 12.7^{A}	$17.2 \pm 4.7^{A,B}$	4.3 ± 1.7^{B}
Total	18.8 ± 4.6^{A}	22.4 ± 10.8^{A}	$14.0 \pm 3.5^{A,B}$	3.0 ± 0.8^{B}
	(n = 19)	(n = 6)	(n = 26)	(n = 21)
Class 3				
Epi	19.9 ± 4.9^{A}	$14.3 \pm 4.2^{A,B}$	$13.3 \pm 3.2^{A,B}$	3.6 ± 1.5^{B}
Mid	28.2 ± 6.5^{A}	23.6 ± 5.7^{A}	23.3 ± 3.9^{A}	7.1 ± 1.8^{B}
Endo ($p = .07$)	34.6 ± 6.8^{A}	35.1 ± 6.9^{A}	32.7 ± 5.7^{A}	14.1 ± 3.7^{B}
Total	27.2 ± 5.6^{A}	23.7 ± 4.9^{A}	23.5 ± 4.2^{A}	7.8 ± 2.2^{B}
	(n = 17)	(n = 20)	(n = 24)	(n = 16)

Data expressed as percent necrosis (mean ± SEM), with number of segments in which necrosis was quantified in parentheses. Abbreviations and other notations as in table 5.

minimal additional necrosis. Endocardial crystals were surrounded by a thin rim (≈0.5 mm thick) of fibrosis. The extent of histologic necrosis in group I and II dogs is shown in tables 5 and 6, respectively. No significant effects of occlusive interval were observed for class 1 segmental necrosis.

Signifcant differences between group I and II dogs were observed in class 2 segments only in diltiazem- and propranolol-treated dogs. In group I dogs no differences between treatment groups existed; however, in group II dogs, the extent of class 2 segmental necrosis in epicardial and endocardial layers, as well as "total" transmural necrosis, was significantly lower in dogs that received propranolol plus diltiazem, compared with saline- and propranolol-treated control animals. Propranolol alone and diltiazem alone also significantly reduced the extent of necrosis in selected tissues.

No significant effect of occlusive interval on extent of class 3 segmental necrosis was observed, although a tendency toward greater epicardial necrosis ($p < .06$) was present in the group II dogs. In group I dogs significantly less necrosis in the epicardium and midwall layers and in total segments was found in diltiazem- vs saline-treated dogs. In group II dogs there was significantly less necrosis in the epicardial, midwall, and endocardial layers as well as less "total necrosis" of class 3 segments in dogs that received propranolol plus diltiazem compared with the other animals. Propranolol and diltiazem alone also reduced necrosis in the epicardium of class 3 segments.

Discussion

We have previously shown that in the conscious dog severely dysfunctional (class 3) LV segments have a limited capacity for physiologically important recovery of contractile function, whereas moderately dysfunctional (class 2) segments retain contractile reserve and a potential for recovery of NET with reperfusion after 2 hr of coronary arterial occlusion.[4] In the absence of pharmacologic intervention, these segments do not regain important contractile function if the occlusive interval is lengthened to 4 hr. Significant recovery of contractile segmental function at sites of moderate dysfunction occurs over several weeks after coronary reperfusion, also in agreement with previous studies by Constantini et al.[30] and Theroux et al.[31]

Reperfusion after 2 or 4 hr of LAD occlusion exacerbates contractile dysfunction, an effect that lasts for several hours. Diltiazem attenuated or abolished this worsening of segmental function with reperfusion, but prevention of this phenomenon (by diltiazem alone) did not translate into enhanced ultimate recovery of contractile function, suggesting a dissociation between early and late contractile dysfunction after ischemia and reperfusion. However, the combined administration of propranolol and diltiazem enhanced ultimate recovery of contractile function of class 2 segments after 4 hr of LAD occlusion to levels that equaled the recovery in saline-treated, group I dogs, which underwent 2 hr of coronary occlusion. Thus the "window of time" of coronary occlusion after which irreversible contractile dysfunction occurs can be lengthened by appropriate pharmacologic intervention. Important salvage of function appears to require aggressive therapy, since neither agent alone significantly enhanced the ultimate recovery of function nor diminished segmental necrosis.

Approximately one quarter of all dogs that died before completion of the 1 month study did so of ventricular fibrillation (six dogs) or cardiogenic shock (one dog), occurring in all instances except one within the first hour after LAD occlusion. Thus these deaths bear no relationship to drug treatment or lack thereof. Another 59% of the dogs dying prematurely died between 24 hr and 3 weeks. These dogs were divided evenly between five of the treatment groups. The major beneficial drug effect in this study was evident in the group II dogs that received propranolol plus diltiazem and diltiazem alone. One dog that received propranolol plus diltiazem died prematurely and three of the five group II diltiazem-treated dogs died during the short-term study (two of these before the drug was to be given). Thus within the two treatment groups that displayed the greatest overall recovery of LV segmental function and the least amount of gross or histologic (segmental) necrosis, only three dogs died between 24 hr and 3 weeks after reperfusion (compared with 21 survivors in these two groups). Therefore it is unlikely that the beneficial effects of propranolol plus diltiazem were enhanced by elimination of data from nonsurvivors, who might have had larger infarcts and less recovery of contractile function. In the treatment group to which these two were compared (group II, saline-treated), only one late death (of three) occurred. The other two occurred within the first hour after occlusion or reperfusion. Thus, although we cannot discount the rate of a selection phenomenon in the results of this study, we are unable to identify any protocol or animal survival differences that might explain the data.

The mechanism(s) by which propranolol plus diltiazem produced these beneficial effects is not known. Propranolol alone, by reducing heart rate and contractility — two important determinants of myocardial oxygen consumption — would be expected to protect ischemic myocardium; however, it also increased mean left atrial pressure, reflecting increased LV filling pressure and wall tension, which would tend to oppose its beneficial effects. In group I and II dogs, propranolol depressed the NET of class 1 and 2 segments and caused a diminution of class 3 systolic wall thinning, consistent with observations by Vatner et al.,[32] who also reported a favorable redistribution of blood flow to moderately or severely ischemic segments by propranolol. Based on results in this study, early beneficial effects on regional LV function may not predict or translate into significant reduction of ultimate necrosis and long-term improvement in LV function.

In contrast to propranolol, diltiazem alone, which lowered aortic pressure and increased heart rate, did not affect NET in any segment class during coronary arterial occlusion, but it did prevent the worsening of segmental dysfunction during early reperfusion. Considerable experimental evidence supports the notion that Ca^{2+} overload of ischemic-reperfused myocytes plays an important role in this phenomenon.[33-35] An impaired ability to replete high-energy phosphates after reperfusion of ischemic myocardium may also contribute.[36] Bush et al.[21] have demonstrated that diltiazem decreased infarct size in anesthetized dogs undergoing temporary coronary occlusion, the extent of calcification in injured LV myocardium, and ischemia-induced losses of contractile function in isolated blood-perfused cat hearts.[13]

Interestingly, diltiazem's prevention of worsening of contractile segmental dysfunction associated with early reperfusion did not translate ultimately into improved recovery of segmental function. One possible explanation is that myocellular Ca^{2+} overload in moderately dysfunctional segments is reversible after 2 hr of coronary occlusion and that ultimate recovery is not linked obligatorily to early segmental dysfunction. Alternatively, perhaps diltiazem *delayed* reperfusion-associated contractile dysfunction and Ca^{2+} overload, since by 24 hr after reperfusion differences between diltiazem- and saline- or propranolol-treated groups were minimal. Intracellular Ca^{2+} overload has also been implicated in LV diastolic abnormalities associated with cardiomyopathies or ischemic heart disease.[37, 38] Studies from our laboratory by Tilton et al.[39] as well as others[40] have demonstrated beneficial effects of Ca^{2+} entry blockers on regional and global diastolic function during experimental myocardial infarction.

Diltiazem, by lowering aortic pressure, may have reduced myocardial energy demands by reducing afterload or impedance. Although it cannot be excluded conclusively, it seems unlikely that diltiazem's ability to prevent the exacerbation of contractile dysfunction during early reperfusion is attributable exclusively to afterload reduction, since one would expect this influence to be manifested during coronary occlusion and not only 1 and 3 hr after reperfusion in groups I and II, respectively.

Several investigators have shown that diltiazem and other Ca^{2+} entry blockers can augment (collateral) blood flow to ischemic myocardium in various experimental preparations.[11, 41] The enhanced recovery of class 2 segmental NET and reduction of ultimate necrosis in dogs that received diltiazem plus propranolol may also be attributable, in part, to the complementary hemodynamic effects of these two agents. As with β-blockers and nitrates, the reflex tachycardia that accompanies reduced aortic pressure caused by diltiazem was abolished or reversed by propranolol; diltiazem appeared not to aggravate propranolol's ability to raise preload. Reduced myocardial energy demands probably contributed to the beneficial effects of propranolol and diltiazem; however, compared with propranolol alone, reductions in heart rate, LV dP/dt, and double product were not significantly lower in animals that received propranolol plus diltiazem. However, there may also have been direct cellular protection from catecholamine- and Ca^{2+}-mediated injury by the combination of propranolol and diltiazem.

Measuring wall thickening as an index of LV segmental function is potentially subject to spurious increases in this variable due to translational or rotational ("shear") movements of the LV wall. However, using a triangulation technique for studying segmental wall thickness, Osakada et al.[20] have shown that careful placement of the endocardial crystal minimizes the contribution of these factors to segmental wall thickness measurements. In this study, we removed endocardial crystals before the heart was sliced, precluding confirmation of the crystal pairs' exact alignment. It is likely that some segments were not aligned exactly parallel to the small axis of the heart. However, because we related changes in segmental wall thickening to each segment's preocclusion function, it was more critical that the crystals remained in their original positions. Therefore we excluded crystal pairs with poor signal quality, those that did not display normal, uninterrupted systolic wall thickening before LAD occlusion, and those that underwent large, spontaneous changes in EDWTh after the initial 24 hr of reperfusion, suggesting that misalignment of crystal pairs had occurred.

LAD occlusion caused prompt and significant declines in EDWTh of both class 2 and 3 LV segments. Previous studies have demonstrated that marginally ischemic segments undergo an increase in end-diastolic length, combined with a decline in systolic segmental shortening.[41] Decreases in EDWTh that reflect regional LV wall dilatation may have increased local wall stress in class 2 and 3 segments; this may have allowed class 2 segments to exploit the Frank-Starling relationship. With reperfusion, the EDWTh of class 2 and 3 segments exceeded values before or during LAD occlusion to an extent that appeared to be related inversely to the extent of occlusion-associated alterations in wall thinning.

Measurements of segmental histologic necrosis, infarct size, and area at risk revealed that increasing segmental contractile dysfunction was associated with increased histologic necrosis. Also, increasing the duration of LAD occlusion from 2 to 4 hr resulted in significantly greater transmural necrosis in class 2 segments in the epicardial and midwall layers. Comparable infarct sizes were found between saline-treated groups I and II, regardless of whether this variable was expressed as a percentage of the entire left ventricle or anatomic area at risk. The average areas at risk were not significantly different between any of the seven groups of dogs. The tendency toward larger area at risk in dogs that received propranolol plus diltiazem would, if anything, increase the extent of infarction in this group, since Lowe et al.[42] and Jugdutt et al.[43] have shown that the extent of ischemic injury is related to the size of the occluded coronary bed. Diltiazem alone in class 3 segments in group I dogs and in group II dogs in combination with propranolol significantly reduced the extent of histologic necrosis in class 2 and 3 segments. Thus the beneficial effects of pharmacologic intervention seem to be attributable at least in part to salvage of myocardium from ultimate necrosis.

In summary, administration of the Ca^{2+} entry blocker diltiazem 1 hr after LAD occlusion prevents the worsening of segmental contractile dysfunction early after coronary reperfusion following 2 or 4 hr of LAD occlusion, but it does not significantly enhance the ultimate segmental recovery of contractile function. The combined administration of propranolol and diltiazem improves segmental contractile function during early and later reperfusion and decreases the extent of histologic necrosis in moderately and severely dysfunctional LV segments in dogs with temporary LAD occlusion for 4 hr followed by 1 month of reperfusion. Thus the combination of selected β-adrenergic and Ca^{2+} entry blocking agents can lengthen the "window of time" of short-term coronary occlusion after which important recovery of contractile function occurs with reperfusion in this experimental preparation.

We gratefully acknowledge the expert technical assistance of Michael Deguchi, Cora Marsaw, Janice McNatt, Judy Ober,

David Perry, Gifford Ramsey, Donna Buja, and Dorothy Thomas, and the statistical assistance of Rebecca Lundswick, Kent Dana, and Nancy Wilson. We also thank Nancy Dickey and Laurie Christian for secretarial assistance in preparing this manuscript.

References

1. Rentrop P, Blanke H, Karsch KR, Kaiser H, Kostering H, Leitz K: Selective intracoronary thrombolysis in acute myocardial infarction and unstable angina pectoris. Circulation **63:** 307, 1981
2. DeWood MA, Spores J, Notske RN, Long HT, Shields JP, Simpson CS, Rudy LW, Grunwald R: Medical and surgical management of myocardial infarction. Am J Cardiol **44:** 1356, 1979
3. Phillips SJ, Kongtahworn C, Zeff RN, Benson M, Iannone L, Brown T, Gordon DF: Emergency coronary artery revascularization: a possible therapy for acute myocardial infarction. Circulation **60:** 241, 1979
4. Bush LR, Buja LM, Samowitz W, Rude RE, Wathen M, Tilton GD, Willerson JT: Recovery of left ventricular segmental function after long-term reperfusion following temporary coronary occlusion in conscious dogs. Circ Res **53:** 248, 1983
5. Lavallee M, Cox D, Patrick TA, Vatner SF: Salvage of myocardial function by coronary artery reperfusion 1, 2, and 3 hours after occlusion in conscious dogs. Circ Res **53:** 235, 1983
6. Reimer KA, Rasmussen MM, Jennings RB: Reduction by propranolol of myocardial necrosis following temporary coronary occlusion in dogs. Circ Res **33:** 353, 1973
7. Mueller HS, Ayres SM, Religa A, Evans RG: Propranolol in the treatment of acute myocardial infarction: effects on myocardial oxygenation and hemodynamics. Circulation **49:** 1978, 1974
8. Gold HK, Leinbach RC, Maroko PR: Propranolol-induced reduction in signs of ischemic injury during acute myocardial infarction. Am J Cardiol **38:** 689, 1976
9. Cutler JA: A review of ongoing trials of beta blockers in the secondary prevention of coronary heart disease. Circulation **67** (suppl I): I-62, 1983
10. Nagao T, Sato M, Nakajima H, Kyomoto A: Studies on a new 1,5-benzothiazepine derivative (CRD-401) II, vasodilator actions. Jpn J Pharmacol **22:** 467, 1972
11. Clozel JP, Theroux P, Bourassa MG: Effects of diltiazem on experimental myocardial ischemia and on left ventricular performance. Circ Res **52** (suppl I): I-120, 1983
12. Weishaar R, Ashikawa K, Bing R: Effect of diltiazem, a calcium antagonist on myocardial ischemia. Am J Cardiol **43:** 1137, 1979
13. Bush LR, Li YP, Shlafer M, Jolly SR, Lucchesi BR: The protective effects of diltiazem during global ischemia in isolated cat hearts. J Pharmacol Exp Ther **218:** 653, 1981
14. Henry PD: Comparative pharmacology of calcium antagonists: nifedipine, verapamil and diltiazem. Am J Cardiol **46:** 1047, 1980
15. Nagao T, Matlib MA, Franklin D, Millard RW, Schwartz A: Effects of diltiazem, a calcium antagonist, on regional myocardial function and mitochondria after brief coronary occlusion. J Mol Cell Cardiol **12:** 29, 1980
16. Schwartz A, Grupp G, Millard RW, Lathrup DA, Matlib MA, Vaghy PL, Valle JR: Calcium-channel blockers: possible mechanisms of protective effects on the ischemic myocardium. *In* Weiss EB, editor: New perspectives on calcium antagonists. Bethesda, MD, 1981, American Physiological Society, pp 191–210
17. Zelis RF, Kinney EL: The pharmacokinetics of diltiazem in healthy American men. Am J Cardiol **49:** 529, 1982
18. Roan PG, Scales F, Saffer S, Buja LM, Willerson JT: Functional characterization of left ventricular segmental responses during the initial 24H and 2 WK after experimental canine myocardial infarction. J Clin Invest **63:** 1974, 1979
19. Heyndrickx GR, Millard RW, McRitchie RJ, Maroko PR, Vatner SF: Regional myocardial functional and electrophysiological alterations after brief coronary artery occlusion in conscious dogs. J Clin Invest **56:** 978, 1978
20. Osakada G, Sasayama S, Kawai C, Hirahawa A, Kemper WS, Franklin D, Ross J Jr: The analysis of left ventricular wall thickness and shear by an ultrasonic triangulation technique in the dog. Circ Res **47:** 173, 1980
21. Bush LR, Romson JL, Ash JL, Lucchesi BR: Effects of diltiazem on extent of myocardial injury resulting from temporary coronary artery occlusion in dogs. J Cardiovasc Pharmacol **4:** 285, 1982
22. Lie JT, Pairolero PC, Holly KE, Titus JL: Macroscopic enzyme-mapping verification of large homogeneous experimental myocardial infarcts of predictable size and location in dogs. J Thorac Cardiovasc Surg **69:** 599, 1975
23. Heymann MA, Payne BD, Hoffman JIE, Rudolph AM: Blood flow measurements with radionuclide-labeled particles. Prog Cardiovasc Dis **20:** 55, 1977
24. Roan PG, Buja LM, Izquierdo C, Hashimi H, Saffer S, Willerson JT: Interrelationship between regional left ventricular function, coronary blood flow, and myocellular necrosis during the initial 24 hours and 1 week after experimental coronary occlusion in awake, unsedated dogs. Circ Res **49:** 31, 1981
25. Sasayama S, Franklin D, Ross J Jr, Kemper WS, McKown D: Dynamic changes in left ventricular wall thickness and their use in analyzing cardiac function in the conscious dog. Am J Cardiol **38:** 870, 1976
26. LeWinter MM, Kent RS, Kroener JM, Careu TE, Covell JW: Regional differences in myocardial performance in the left ventricle of the dog. Circ Res **37:** 191, 1975
27. SAS Statistical Package: Raleigh, NC, 1976, SAS Institute, pp 127–144
28. Duncan DB: Multiple range and multiple t tests. Biometrics **11:** 1, 1955
29. Miller RG: Simultaneous statistical influence. New York, 1966, McGraw-Hill Book Co., Inc., pp 67–70
30. Constantini C, Corday E, Lang TW, Meerbaum S, Brasch J, Kaplan L, Rubins S, Gold H: Revascularization after 3 hours of coronary arterial occlusion: effects on regional cardiac metabolic function and infarct size. Am J Cardiol **36:** 368, 1975
31. Theroux P, Ross J Jr, Franklin D, Kemper WS, Sasayama S: Coronary arterial reperfusion. III. Early and late effects on regional myocardial function and dimensions in conscious dogs. Am J Cardiol **38:** 599, 1976
32. Vatner SF, Baig H, Manders WT, Ochs H, Pagoni M: Effects of propranolol on regional myocardial function, electrograms, and blood flow in conscious dogs with myocardial ischemia. J Clin Invest **60:** 353, 1977
33. Shen AC, Jennings RB: Kinetics of calcium accumulation in acute myocardial ischemic injury. Am J Pathol **67:** 441, 1972
34. Henry PD, Schuchleib R, Davis J, Weiss ES, Sobel BE: Myocardial contracture and accumulation of mitochondrial calcium in ischemic rabbit heart. Am J Physiol **233:** H677, 1977
35. Opie LH: Myocardial infarct size I. Basic considerations. Am Heart J **100:** 355, 1980
36. Reimer KA, Jennings RB, Tatum AH: Pathobiology of acute myocardial ischemia: metabolic, functional, and ultrastructural studies. Am J Cardiol **52:** 72A, 1983
37. Bourdillon PD, Lovell BH, Mirsky I, Paulus WJ, Wynne J, Grossman W: Increased regional myocardial stiffness of the left ventricle during pacing-induced angina in man. Circulation **67:** 316, 1983
38. Hess OM, Ritter M, Schneider J, Grimm J, Turina M, Krayenbruhl HP: Diastolic stiffness and myocardial structure in aortic valve disease before and after valve replacement. Circulation **69:** 855, 1984
39. Tilton GD, Bush LR, Apprill PG, Buja LM, Willerson JT: Effect of diltiazem and propranolol on left ventricular segmental relaxation during temporary coronary arterial occlusion and 1 month of reperfusion in conscious dogs. Circulation **71:** 165, 1985
40. Theroux P, Franklin D, Ross J Jr, Kemper WS: Regional myocardial function during acute coronary artery occlusion and its modification by pharmacologic agents in the dog. Circ Res **35:** 896, 1974
41. Matsusaki M, Gallagher KP, Patritt J, Tajimi T, Kemper WS, White FC, Ross J: Effects of a calcium entry blocker (diltiazem) on regional myocardial blood flow and function during exercise in conscious dogs. Circulation **69:** 801, 1984
42. Lowe JA, Reimer KA, Jennings RB: Experimental infarct size as a function of the area at risk. Am J Pathol **90:** 363, 1978
43. Jugdutt BI, Hutchins GM, Bulkley BH, Becker LC: Myocardial infarction in the conscious dog: three-dimensional mapping of infarct, collateral flow, and region at risk. Circulation **60:** 1141, 1979

Immediate functional recovery and avoidance of reperfusion injury with surgical revascularization of short-term coronary occlusion

J. Vinten-Johansen, Ph.D., T. Arthur Edgerton, M.D., Harold R. Howe, M.D., Pamela A. Gayheart, B.A., Stephen A. Mills, M.D., George Howard, M.P.H.S., and A. Robert Cordell, M.D.

ABSTRACT Functional recovery with surgical revascularization of acutely ischemic myocardium has not been compared with its nonsurgical counterpart in experimental preparations of coronary occlusion. This study compares the functional and metabolic recovery of ischemic (1 hr coronary occlusion) segments revascularized either by restoration of coronary patency (simulating nonsurgical recanalization, e.g., angioplasty) or by surgical revascularization with multidose hypothermic potassium blood cardioplegic solution. Twenty-two anesthetized open-chest dogs were instrumented with Millar micromanometer-tip catheters to measure left ventricular and aortic pressures. Piezoelectric ultrasonic dimension gauges were implanted in the subendocardium supplied by the left anterior descending coronary artery to measure segmental contractile function. In five dogs, only biopsy samples were obtained for control measurements of ATP, creatine phosphate, and tissue water content. In the remaining 17 dogs, the left anterior descending artery and collaterals were ligated for 1 hr. The ligatures were removed in eight dogs and coronary perfusion continued for 2 hr, simulating nonsurgical reperfusion. The remaining nine dogs were placed on cardiopulmonary bypass and the hearts were arrested for 1 hr with multidose (every 20 min) blood cardioplegic solution enhanced with glutamate and aspartate, simulating surgical revascularization (coronary artery bypass grafting). The coronary ligatures were not released until the second cardioplegic infusion, simulating graft placement. One hour of coronary occlusion placed 39.4 ± 2.5% of the left ventricle at risk, and converted active systolic shortening to persistent paradoxical bulging (25.2 ± 2.2% to −5.8 ± 1.2% systolic shortening). Surgical revascularization resulted in greater recovery of postischemic systolic shortening (7.95 ± 1.90% vs −6.90 ± 2.01% systolic shortening; $p < .05$), lower subendocardial water content (79.36 ± 0.50% vs 81.14 ± 0.53%; $p < .05$), and less gross histochemically apparent (triphenyltetrazolium chloride) tissue damage (4.2 ± 4.2% vs 30.9 ± 6.8% of area at risk; $p < .05$) compared with hearts reperfused nonsurgically. There were no differences in regional ATP and creatine phosphate levels between surgically and nonsurgically revascularized hearts despite the marked differences in functional recovery. We conclude that (1) myocardium subjected to 1 hr of coronary occlusion is potentially recoverable depending on the modality of the early phase of reperfusion and (2) surgical revascularization avoids reperfusion injury resulting in immediate postischemic functional recovery.
Circulation 72, No. 2, 431–439, 1985.

THE GOALS of revascularization of acute myocardial infarcts are to arrest the progression of damage and restore morphologic integrity and functional capacity to the involved segment. The nonsurgical approach of pharmacologic thrombolysis and percutaneous transluminal coronary angioplasty (PTCA) is a strong and popular alternative to restoring coronary patency and perfusion to the previously ischemic segment. However, equivocal success in restoring systolic function globally as well as in the involved segment[1, 2] has tempered enthusiasm for this approach. Experimental studies have shown that restoration of blood flow after a period of transient coronary occlusion produces myocardial hemorrhage,[3, 4] advances mitochondrial deterioration,[5–8] and produces discrete areas of "no-reflow."[9, 10] Several studies suggest that many of these manifestations of tissue damage may occur or be exac-

From the Section of Cardiothoracic Surgery, Department of Surgery, and the Biostatistics Division of the Department of Neurology, Bowman Gray School of Medicine, Wake Forest University, Winston-Salem, NC.

Supported in part by a grant-in-aid from the American Heart Association, North Carolina Affiliate (No. 84-85-A7), and by NIH grant RR-05404.

Address for correspondence: J. Vinten-Johansen, Ph.D., Section of Cardiothoracic Surgery, Bowman Gray School of Medicine, 300 South Hawthorne Rd., Winston-Salem, NC 27103.

Received April 16, 1985; accepted May 16, 1985

erbated during the reperfusion period itself (reperfusion injury).[7, 11, 12] Whatever the pathophysiologic mechanisms involved, restoration of blood flow after transient occlusion (15 min to 4 hr) fails to fully restore wall motion in the ischemic segment, even after prolonged periods of recovery.[13–15]

On the other hand, results of experiments with surgical revascularization of globally ischemic hearts emphasize that the consequences of ischemia and reperfusion can be reversed or avoided, resulting in recovery of aerobic metabolism, limitation of intramyocardial edema, preservation of the ultrastructural integrity, and substantial recovery of immediate postischemic function.[16–18] In contrast to nonsurgical recanalization techniques, the surgical approach affords complete control of the conditions (unloaded ventricle, coronary perfusion pressure) and composition (cardioplegia) of the reperfusate during the initial phases of reperfusion. This study tests the hypothesis that appropriate modification of the reperfusion phase during surgical revascularization of short-term (1 hr) coronary occlusion reverses or avoids reperfusion damage. We will show that appropriate management of reperfusion allows less edema formation, less histochemically apparent tissue damage, and immediate functional recovery compared with nonsurgical revascularization.

Methods

Experimental procedures complied with the "Guiding Principles in the Use and Care of Animals" approved by the Council of the American Physiological Society as well as with state and federal regulations.

Twenty-two dogs weighing between 14 and 24 kg were anesthetized with 30 mg/kg iv sodium pentobarbital (Nembutal), supplemented as necessary to maintain deep anesthesia. After endotracheal intubation, positive-pressure ventilation was initiated (Harvard volume cycle respirator) with 100% oxygen. The dogs were then divided into two groups: those receiving unmodified reperfusion by restoring coronary patency and those revascularized by surgical procedures with blood potassium cardioplegic solution.

Nonsurgical reperfusion group. In eight dogs the chest was opened in the fifth left intercostal space. A No. 7.5F thermodilution catheter (Critikon, Inc.) was introduced into the right external jugular vein and manipulated into the pulmonary artery for measurement of pulmonary arterial wedge pressure and cardiac output in triplicate (3 ml iced saline), and for volume and pharmacologic management. The dogs were given 2 to 3 mg/kg sodium heparin.

Surgical revascularization group. In nine dogs the chest was opened by median sternotomy and the pericardium was tented. After systemic heparinization (2 to 3 mg/kg), cardiopulmonary bypass with right heart bypass capability (to generate Sarnoff function curves) was established by cannulating the inferior and superior venae cavae and directing the venous return to a Shiley S-100A bubble oxygenator through which flowed oxygen and carbon dioxide mixed appropriately for adequate blood gases. Oxygenated blood was returned by a cannula either in the left subclavian artery (total bypass) or in the main pulmonary artery (right heart bypass). Cannulas were placed in the left ventricle and the left atrium via the left atrial appendage to either vent the heart during total bypass or measure mean left atrial pressure, respectively. Total coronary effluent was drained continuously by a cannula in the right ventricle.

In all dogs, Millar MPC-500 pressure transducers were placed into the aortic arch via the right carotid artery or the left internal mammary artery (aortic pressure) and through the apical dimple to measure left ventricular intracavitary pressure. A segment of the left anterior descending coronary artery (LAD) distal to the first diagonal branch was dissected free and a ligature was placed loosely around it for subsequent occlusion. A pair of 2.5 mm diameter ultrasonic piezoelectric dimension transducers were implanted in the subendocardium of the myocardium served by the LAD to measure segmental systolic shortening with a Triton Model 120 Sonomicrometer (Triton Technology, Inc., San Diego).

All measurements were recorded on a Hewlett Packard 7758B thermal recorder and simultaneously digitized and printed by a Buxco Datalogger (Buxco Electronics, Sharon, MA). The end-diastolic and end-systolic segment lengths from the ultrasonic crystals were timed off the upstroke of the instantaneous left ventricular pressure trace and the dicrotic notch of the aortic pressure pulse, respectively. The percent systolic shortening was calculated as $100 \times (EDL - ESL)/EDL$ where EDL and ESL are end-diastolic and end-systolic segment lengths in millimeters, respectively. A positive value indicates active shortening and a negative value represents passive bulging (paradoxical wall motion) during systole.

Protocol. In dogs receiving normal blood reperfusion (nonsurgical reperfusion), hemodynamic and functional data were obtained in the control state with the LAD patent. In the surgical revascularization group, Sarnoff function curves[17] were obtained in the control state by incrementally increasing cardiac output from 1.5 to 5.0 liters/min while maintaining mean arterial pressure at 80 mm Hg via the subclavian cannula. The cardiac workload was then adjusted to 100 ml/kg cardiac output and a pressure of 100 mm Hg.

In all dogs, 2 to 3 mg/kg lidocaine was administered as a bolus while 0.5 mg/kg/hr was continuously provided as an intravenous drip. The obvious collateral arteries encroaching on the LAD territory and finally the LAD were ligated for a total of 1 hr. Hemodynamic and segmental function data were recorded every 20 min. Blood gases were maintained at a pH between 7.38 and 7.42 and at P_{CO_2} 30 to 40 mm Hg. Arrhythmias were treated with lidocaine as necessary. Ventricular fibrillation, when encountered, was electrically converted; data were not accepted if (1) the ischemic segment was not dyskinetic for the entire hour, (2) ventricular fibrillation persisted for more than 3 min, or (3) the cardioplegic solution was not within ranges stipulated.

In nonsurgically revascularized dogs receiving normal blood reperfusion, all ligatures were removed after the 1 hr ischemic period and reperfusion continued for a total of 2 hr. In dogs in which revascularization was accomplished surgically, total cardiopulmonary bypass and ventricular decompression was established after the 1 hr occlusion period. Thermistor probes were placed in ischemic (anterior) and nonischemic (posterior) zones. The aorta was cross-clamped and blood cardioplegic solution enriched with glutamate (13 mM) and aspartate (13 mM) (table 1) was delivered with a Buckberg-Shiley Cardioplegia Delivery device (4:1 blood to cardioplegia components ratio) in the aortic root through a preplaced double-lumen catheter (inner lumen for measurement of cardioplegic infusion pressure, outer lumen for delivery of cardioplegic solution) at 50 mm Hg for a total of 10 min. The first 5 min of this period was normothermic (37° C) and the final 5 min hypothermic (4° C).[18]

TABLE 1
Composition of amino acid–enhanced cardioplegic solution

Principle	Component	Values
Oxygenation	Blood	C_aO_2 11.84±0.4 Hct 17.6±1.2
Buffer acidosis	Tromethamine	8.028±0.067
Appropriate pH		@4°–8° C
Substrates	Glutamate, aspartate	13 mM each
Reduce calcium	CPD chelation	0.80±0.02 meq
Avoid edema	Hyperosmolarity	381±3 mOsm
	Low pressure	50 mm Hg
Reduce O_2 demands		
Immediate arrest	Hyperkalemia	22.1±2.3 meq K^+
Hypothermia		4°–8° C delivery

CaO_2 = cardioplegia oxygen content in ml O_2/100 ml (volume percent); CPD = citrate-phosphate-dextrose; Hct = hematocrit.

Simultaneous with the delivery of hypothermic cardioplegic solution, systemic temperature was decreased to 28° C. Intermittent infusions of 4° C blood cardioplegic solution were given at 20 and 40 min for a total arrest time of 60 min. The coronary ligatures were removed just before the 20 min infusion, simulating delivery of cardioplegic solution down a graft with distal anastomosis complete or infusion into the aortic root of cardioplegic solution after completion of both proximal and distal anastomoses in a single graft.[19] After 1 hr of cardioplegia, systemic temperature was raised to 37° C and reperfusion cardioplegia was administered for 3 min at 50 mm Hg and 9° C above septal temperature.[20] Systemic pressure was lowered to 50 mm Hg and the cross-clamp was removed. When electromechanical activity was visible, systemic pressure was gradually raised to 100 mm Hg over 3 min. The heart was maintained in the beating empty state for 30 min and was subsequently placed in the working (right heart bypass) state at 100 ml/kg cardiac output and 100 mm Hg systemic pressure for an additional 30 min. Postischemic hemodynamics and regional and global function were then determined.

After each experiment, transmural biopsy specimens were taken by high-speed drill from the nonischemic and ischemic zones, divided into subepicardial (EPI) and subendocardial (ENDO) halves, and quick-frozen in liquid nitrogen for later analysis of tissue ATP and creatine phosphate (CP).[21] Parallel biopsy specimens were also taken from each zone for analysis of tissue water content (percent water = 100 [1 − (dry tissue weight/wet tissue weight)]. Biopsy sites were repaired with pledgeted sutures and all coronary ligatures were replaced. Gentian violet stain (0.2 ml/kg) was infused either into the left atrium (normal blood reperfusion group) or into the aortic root cardioplegia cannula (surgical revascularization group) to demarcate normally perfused from ischemic myocardium. Hearts were arrested with KCl, excised, and cut into 5 mm thick transverse slices, and the ischemic (unstained) and normally perfused (stained) areas were determined by planimetry. The area placed at risk by coronary occlusion was calculated as 100 × (unstained area/total left ventricular area). The slices were incubated in triphenyltetrazolium chloride (TTC) at 37° C for 15 to 20 min.[22] TTC stains normal myocardium brick red while leaving damaged or necrotic myocardium pale. The "area of necrosis" was determined by planimetry and calculated as 100 × (TTC unstained area/total left ventricular area). The left ventricular tissue damage is expressed as the ratio of the area of necrosis/area at risk, expressed in percent.

Five dogs used to obtain control biopsy samples were instrumented as in the medical reperfusion group for the purpose of obtaining measurements of myocardial ATP, CP, and water content in the control state.

Data were analyzed with the Statistical Analysis System (Cary, NC) biostatistical package. Differences with respect to time, myocardial region, and group were analyzed by the general linear model multivariate analysis followed by Wilk's lambda test.

Results

Ligation of the LAD and encroaching collateral vessels placed 39.9 ± 4.3% of the left ventricular mass at risk in the nonsurgical group and a similar value of 39.0 ± 2.6% of the left ventricle in the surgically revascularized group.

Hemodynamic data for both groups during control, 1 hr of coronary occlusion (ischemia), and reperfusion are summarized in table 2. Ischemia was accompanied by modest decreases in heart rate and systolic pressure whereas left ventricular end-diastolic pressure increased significantly. In the nonsurgical reperfusion group, cardiac output decreased by 20% during ischemia and by 33% during reperfusion from control levels ($p < .05$). At the end of 2 hr of reperfusion, cardiac output in the nonsurgical reperfusion group was 16% ($p < .05$) below that in the surgical revascularization group, in which cardiac output was held constant by the extracorporeal bypass circuit.

End-diastolic length and systolic shortening were similar in both groups during the control period (table 3). Ligation of the LAD immediately replaced active contractile shortening with paradoxical systolic bulging, which persisted for the entire ischemic period. The degree of paradoxical segmental wall motion was equivalent in both groups and averaged −25.3% of control systolic shortening for all hearts.

Hearts revascularized surgically arrested within 1.5 min of initiation of cardioplegia. As expected, the anterior ischemic border zones showed fine fibrillation up to 1.5 min into the cardioplegic period while the posterior segment arrested within 45 sec. This persistence of asynchronous electromechanical activity in the ischemic segment is most likely a result of maldistribution of cardioplegic solution beyond the total occlusion; the anterior ischemic segment remained warmer by 13.9° C than the posterior segment, which received unimpeded flow at 4° to 8° C (figure 1).

With 2 hr of reperfusion initiated by simple release of the ligature (nonsurgical), there was no significant restoration of systolic function in the previously ischemic segment. In sharp contrast, those hearts given amino acid–enriched blood cardioplegic solution surgically as the initial reperfusate showed recovery of immediate systolic shortening averaging 32.8% of its

TABLE 2
Hemodynamic variables during control, coronary occlusion, and reperfusion

	HR	LVSP (mm Hg)	LVEDP (mm Hg)	Arterial pressure (mm Hg) Systolic	Diastolic	Mean	Cardiac Output (l/min)
Blood reperfusion (n = 8)							
Control	158±7	132±4	6.6±0.8	134±4	107±6	117±5	2.79±0.25
Ischemia	150±7	129±5	9.6±1.1^A	133±5	111±5	117±5	2.22±0.17^A
Reperfusion	157±6	115±6	9.2±1.2	122±6^A	96±7	105±7^B	1.86±0.11^A,B
Surgical revascularization (n = 9)							
Control	180±7	133±4	5.1±0.8	129±4	90±5	100±5	2.21±0.19
Ischemia	169±5^A	126±5^A	7.7±1.0^A	123±5	85±5	97±5	2.21±0.12
Reperfusion	164±4^A	131±5	6.6±1.2	131±6	82±6	95±6	2.21±0.08

Data expressed as mean ± SEM.
HR = heart rate; LVSP = left ventricular systolic pressure; LVEDP = left ventricular end-diastolic pressure.
^A Significantly different from group control values.
^B Significantly different from group ischemic values.

preischemic level (figure 2). This segmental shortening was significantly greater than postischemic wall motion in hearts reperfused nonsurgically ($p = .00008$).

High-energy phosphates. ATP and CP levels in control hearts were similar between EPI and ENDO regions ($p = .67$ and $.71$, respectively) in both anterior and posterior walls. ATP levels were depleted comparably in the nonsurgical reperfusion group (EPI = 61.8%, ENDO = 30.4% of control) and the surgical revascularization group (EPI = 52.0% and ENDO = 42.8% of control) (figure 3) despite differences in their functional recovery. A slight "overshoot" in CP levels was observed in both groups. No significant changes in high-energy phosphate levels occurred in the posterior, normally perfused myocardium.

Tissue water content. Myocardial water content in control hearts averaged 78.18 ± 0.12% and 78.60 ± 0.14% in anterior EPI and ENDO regions and averaged 78.10 ± 0.08% and 78.44 ± 0.12% in posterior EPI and ENDO regions, respectively. There were no differences between anterior and posterior wall or between EPI and ENDO regions. With nonsurgical reperfusion, anterior myocardial water content rose significantly by 2.76% in the EPI and 2.70% in the ENDO region (figure 4). There was no significant tissue water accumulation in the posterior wall, with the EPI value averaging 78.40 ± 0.50% and the ENDO value averaging 78.54 ± 0.53%. With surgical revascularization in which the conditions and composition of the initial reperfusate were controlled, there was a 1.95% gain in EPI water content that was not different from the value in the nonsurgical group. However, edema in the ENDO

TABLE 3
Segmental length data during control, ischemia, and reperfusion

Group/time	End-diastolic (mm)	End-systolic (mm)	% Shortening
Nonsurgical			
Control	11.55±1.06	8.40±0.78	26.28±3.36
Ischemia	12.72±1.44	13.30±1.56^A	−4.50±1.68^A
Reperfusion	12.09±1.27	12.94±1.44^A	−6.90±2.01^A
Surgical			
Control	14.03±1.00	10.61±0.73	24.24±3.16
Ischemia	17.53±1.36^A	18.76±1.47^A	−6.99±1.59^A
Reperfusion	15.31±1.20^A	14.23±1.35^A	7.95±1.90^B

Data expressed as mean ± SEM.
^A Significantly different from group control values.
^B Significantly different from group ischemic values.

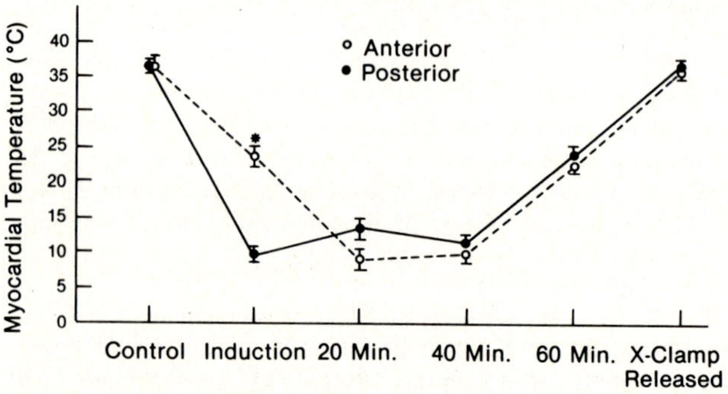

FIGURE 1. Myocardial temperatures in the anterior (ischemic) and posterior (nonischemic) zones after each infusion of cardioplegic solution. Myocardial temperature was significantly higher in the ischemic zone during the induction phase when its distribution was impaired by the ligature. Thereafter, myocardial temperatures were identical in ischemic and nonischemic zones. *$p < .05$.

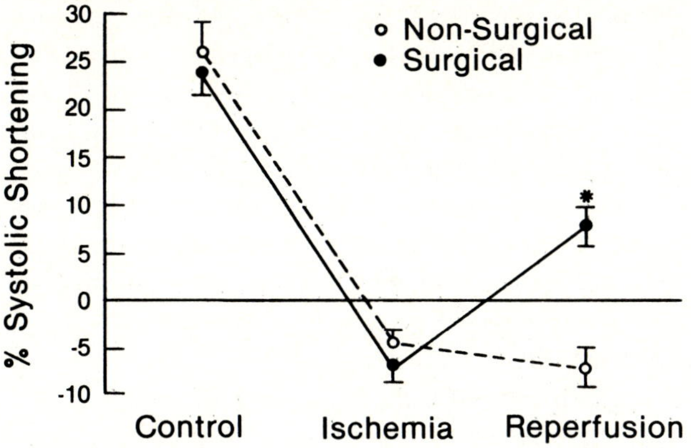

FIGURE 2. Systolic shortening in the myocardium perfused by the LAD is shown at control, after 1 hr of coronary occlusion (ischemia), and after reperfusion. Negative values indicate paradoxical bulging during systole. Paradoxical bulging persisted in the nonsurgical revascularization group in contrast to the 32.8% of control active systolic shortening regained in the surgical revascularization group. $*p < .05$.

region was significantly less marked (0.76% increase) than that in nonsurgically revascularized segments and was indistinguishable from control ENDO tissue water content (figure 4). Despite the global ischemia experienced during the 1 hr cardioplegic period in the surgical revascularization group, there was no significant alteration in posterior myocardial water content (EPI = 78.01 ± 0.35% and ENDO = 77.62 ± 0.67%).

Macroscopic tissue damage. Tissue damage expressed as the area of necrosis demarcated by TTC staining relative to the area involved in the coronary occlusion (area at risk) averaged 30.9 ± 6.8% in nonsurgically revascularized hearts. The apparent tissue damage ranged from confluent involvement of the ENDO region to a diffuse transmural "patchy" appearance with islands of stained (normal) tissue interdigitating closely with large discrete nonstained (damaged) areas. In contrast, segments revascularized surgically showed significantly less damage (4.2 ± 4.2%), with seven of the eight hearts histochemically analyzed demonstrating no area of TTC-sensitive damage.

Discussion

We examined the benefits of surgical revascularization using modification of conditions and composition of the initial reperfusate in restoring metabolism, morphologic integrity, and function in the involved segment. The results emphasize that the eventual fate of myocardium exposed to ischemia is not only related to the duration and severity of the occlusion but is also dependent on the initial reperfusion phase. The severity and duration of ischemia was identical in both groups before reperfusion. This "reperfusion injury" is

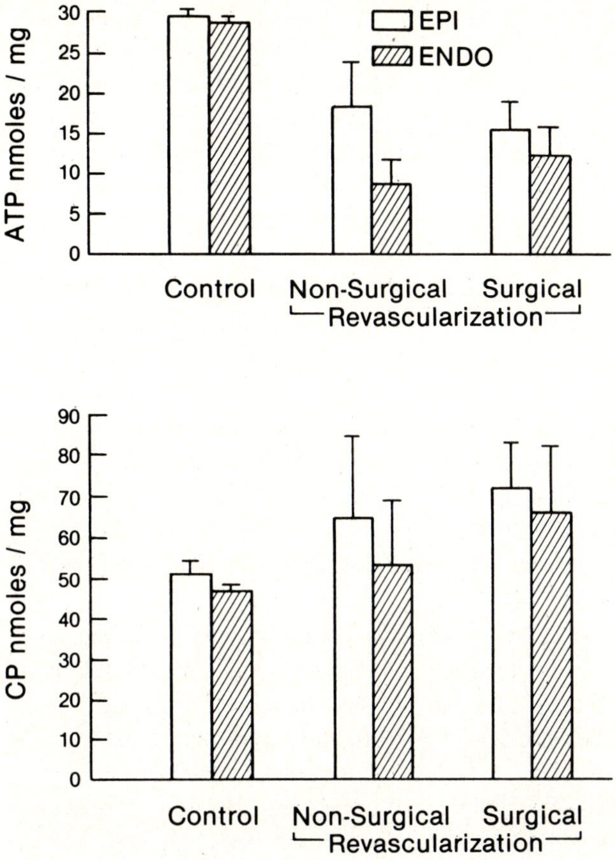

FIGURE 3. ATP (*top panel*) and CP levels (*bottom panel*), in EPI and ENDO regions of the anterior (ischemic) zone. Control values were obtained from the anterior zone in five dogs not subjected to coronary occlusion. ATP was significantly depleted in EPI and ENDO regions in both nonsurgical and surgical groups relative to controls.

avoidable when appropriate management of the reperfusion phase is observed. Avoidance or reversal of reperfusion injury, by modification of the conditions and composition of reperfusate as is possible during

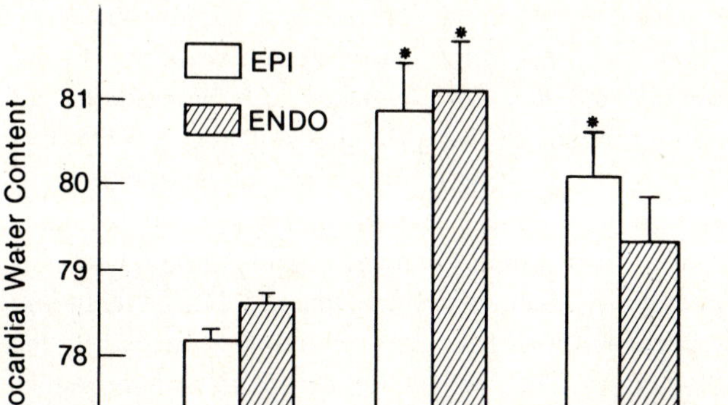

FIGURE 4. Tissue water content in the anterior (ischemic) EPI and ENDO regions. *Significant ($p < .05$) differences from controls in comparable regions.

coronary artery bypass grafting, leads to immediate recovery in tissue that was previously thought to be metabolically and functionally "stunned." Although we could not identify the factor or factors responsible for myocardial stunning in this study, our findings emphasize that this delay or failure in recovery may be overcome by modification of the reperfusate.

We chose the model of 1 hr of ischemia on the basis of the total lack of recovery obtained when unmodified blood was the reperfusate and the subtotal recovery shown with surgical revascularization when blood cardioplegic solution was the initial reperfusate. The clinical correlate of an occlusion of such a short duration is a short-term occlusion occurring either spontaneously in the hospital or during attempted angioplasty. Studies currently in progress in this laboratory have extended the duration of this ischemic period to 3 hr.

Ischemia caused by total coronary occlusion initiates a cascade of biochemical and morphologic changes, the severity of which has been related to the duration and degree of flow inadequacy. Contractile function and high-energy phosphate pools are rapidly lost,[23, 24] and with more prolonged periods of occlusion glycogen stores are depleted,[25] ionic and cell volume homeostasis are lost,[26, 27] and sarcolemmal integrity and subcellular architecture deteriorate.[25] Cell damage and eventual death begin first in the more vulnerable subendocardium and progress with time to the outer, subepicardial tissue in a "wavefront" pattern.[28] These alterations in cellular integrity and metabolism predispose the involved myocardium to further deleterious changes that occur with the resumption of coronary blood flow, specifically (1) the influx and accumulation of calcium in the contractile apparatus and mitochondria[7, 25] resulting in further deterioration of contractile and metabolic capacity, (2) peroxidation of membrane structures by oxygen radicals,[29, 30] (3) washout of metabolic precursors and metabolites of high-energy phosphates, and (4) intramyocardial hemorrhage[3, 4] and edema. Therefore, myocardium that is potentially reversibly damaged and salvageable before reperfusion may become irreversibly damaged by the deleterious sequelae just outlined. Although the pathophysiologic factors involved in determining the transition from reversibly injured to irreversibly injured myocardium are not yet clear and the limits of cell viability not defined, myocardium made transiently ischemic for relatively short durations (15 min to 4 hr) remain metabolically[24] and functionally[13–15] "stunned" for up to 4 weeks of reperfusion. The major thrust of research effort has been directed toward the reduction of infarct size and severity by altering the oxygen supply-demand balance pharmacologically. Relatively few studies have addressed the issue of reperfusion injury and how this specific injury after a given duration of ischemia can be minimized. Our results from this study confirm the concept of reperfusion injury as a separate entity and show that this injury can be avoided or reversed, resulting in immediate restoration of contractile function by specifically modifying the reperfusion phase appropriately.

The principles of appropriate modification of the initial reperfusate have evolved from studies of myocardial protection with potassium cardioplegic solution during global ischemia encountered in cardiac surgery. The basic tenets of reperfusate modification developed by proponents of blood cardioplegia are summarized in table 1. These principles may apply as well to the setting of regional ischemia produced by coronary occlusion. First, immediate cardiac arrest and subsequent hypothermia reduce myocardial energy requirements to allow channeling of available energy to reparative processes. This may be important in the setting of coronary occlusion, since studies suggest that the oxygen demands of the ischemic segment exhibiting paradoxical motion are high by virtue of passive wall tension during systolic bulging although active tension (contraction) is absent.[31] Second, the accumulation of protons (H^+) during ischemia is buffered by the relative alkalosis created by tromethamine,[16, 19] while the gradient favoring calcium influx from the extracellular space is reduced by chelation with citrate-phosphate-dextrose. The deleterious effects of tissue acidosis and calcium accumulation on myocardial oxidative metabolism, glycolysis, and the cellular oxidation-reduction state are well known.[7, 32, 33] Third, the amino acids glutamate and asparate provide substrates for anaerobic metabolism during global arrest and replace Krebs cycle intermediates metabolized oxidatively once sufficient oxygen is restored.

The addition of the amino acids L-glutamate and L-aspartate to the blood cardioplegic solution was based on previous results in global models of ischemia and reperfusion where postischemic recovery of function and oxygen utilization were improved in hearts given amino acid–enhanced blood cardioplegic solution.[17, 34] Oxygen utilization is characteristically impaired in hearts damaged by ischemia and reperfusion.[9, 17, 18] Other studies have substantiated the depletion of these amino acids during ischemia[35] and their uptake and incorporation when exogenously supplied.[36–38] The salutary effects of glutamate and aspartate in hearts subjected to cardioplegia may be exerted by three possible mechanisms. First, during ischemia these amino acids may be anaerobically metabolized ultimately to succinate to yield two additional moles of high-energy phosphate each, independently of glycolysis.[36, 38–40] Second, glutamate and aspartate incorporated into the cell replenish Krebs cycle intermediates lost during ischemia.[40] Third, glutamate and aspartate participate directly in the malate-aspartate shuttle.[37, 41] This shuttle is the primary mechanism by which reducing equivalents (protons) are transported from the cytosol to the mitochondria, thereby maintaining the normal intracellular oxidation-reduction state. The malate-aspartate shuttle is tightly linked to and coordinates glycolysis and the Krebs cycle to maintain a balanced oxidation-reduction state.[37] We suspect that glutamate and aspartate provided a better metabolic environment during cardioplegia, which allowed better cellular repair and functional recovery. Others have also found amino acid supplementation to improve postischemic myocardial function.[42] However, the salutary effects of amino acid supplementation could not be assessed independent of the other modifications in this study.

The normothermic induction of cardioplegia was designed to maximize the rate of cellular repair by maintaining the basal metaboic rate (cell maintenance and repair) while avoiding the additional energy requirements of mechanical work. Normothermic induction of cardioplegia in globally ischemic hearts was associated with a greater oxygen uptake during the induction period and improved postischemic oxygen utilization and function.[18] However, the efficacy of this phase depends on the distribution of cardioplegic solution to the involved myocardium. Coronary occlusion offers a significant impediment to the adequate delivery of cardioplegic solution to the myocardium distal to the occlusion.[19] This maldistribution is inferred from figure 1 by the significant temperature gradient demonstrated between the ischemic and normally perfused segment. Therefore the ischemic segment did not receive the benefit of the initial warm phase of cardioplegia and in reality did not receive adequate cardioplegia until the ligation was relieved before the second (hypothermic) infusion. The importance of this initial normothermic phase on postischemic recovery is emphasized by the results of a previous experiment in which an ischemic segment demonstrated greater (55%) recovery of segmental function when given the benefit of the normothermic infusion despite an additional hour (2 hr total) of coronary occlusion.[43] We suspect that greater postischemic recovery could have been gained in the present study if the segment was initially normothermically perfused. Perhaps a clinical strategy could be developed to ensure the distribution of a normothermic infusion of cardioplegic solution subsequent to completion of distal anastomosis to optimize postischemic recovery.

Tissue levels of high-energy phosphates have in the past been considered an index of the adequacy of myocardial protection.[23] Therefore, cardioplegic techniques and formulations that result in higher ATP levels are considered to be superior in myocardial protection than techniques and formulations resulting in lower ATP levels. Several studies have shown a critical level of ATP below which cell survival is doubtful,[28, 44–46] and failure of ATP levels to be restored has been speculated in the etiology of myocardial stunning.[15, 24] However, our results contradict this correlation of tissue ATP levels with cell viability and adequacy of myocardial protection. We found no differences in ATP and CP levels between myocardial segments showing functional recovery, less marked edema, and little or no morphologically apparent damage than those exhibiting no functional restoration and gross edema. A similar lack of correlation has been reported by others.[17, 47, 48] Static levels of ATP and CP are only a measure of the size of the pool and do not reflect the turnover rate, which may be independent of the ATP pool size. Oxygen consumption may be a more sensitive index of metabolic rate than static ATP levels. Previous studies have shown a good correlation between oxygen consumption and the functional recovery of myocardium after global ischemia of various durations.[17, 18]

Surgical revascularization of acutely ischemic myocardium has been shown to be feasible.[49–52] However, quantitative substantiation of the functional and metabolic restoration of ischemic myocardium as well as the mechanisms involved with surgical revascularization are lacking. This study represents our initial efforts to understand the potential mechanisms underlying salvage of myocardium with surgical techniques so that methods may be designed to optimize recovery from more prolonged durations of ischemia.

We are grateful for the expert assistance provided by A. C. Shircliffe and the Surgery Research Unit, and by Kevin S. Harbourne, B.S. Appreciation is extended to Robin Tesh for meticulous preparation of the manuscript and to William E. Johnston, M.D., for his thoughtful comments. Oxygenators and cardioplegia delivery devices were kindly donated by Shiley, Inc., through the efforts of Danny Daniel.

References

1. Rentrop KP, Feit F, Blanke H, Stecy P, Schneider R, Rey M, Horowitz S, Goldman M, Karsch K, Meilman H, Cohen M, Siegel

S, Sander J, Slater J, Gorlin R, Fox A, Fagerstrom R, Calhoun WF: Effects of intracoronary streptokinase and intracoronary nitroglycerin infusion on coronary angiographic patterns and mortality in patients with acute myocardial infarction. N Engl J Med **311:** 1457, 1984
2. Khaja F, Walton JA, Brymer JF, Lo E, Osterberger L, Oneill WW, Colfer HT: Intracoronary fibrinolytic therapy in acute myocardial infarction: report of a prospective randomized trial. N Engl J Med **308:** 1305, 1983
3. Bresnahan GF, Roberts R, Shell WE, Ross J Jr, Sobel BE: Deleterious effects due to hemorrhage after myocardial reperfusion. Am J Cardiol **33:** 82, 1974
4. Mathey DG, Schoffer J, Kuck KH, Beil U, Kloppel G: Transmural hemorrhagic myocardial infarction following intra-coronary streptokinase: clinical, angiographic and autopsy findings. Br Heart J **48:** 546, 1982
5. Kloner RA, Ganote CE, Whalen D, Jennings RB: Effect of a transient period of ischemia on myocardial cell. II. fine structure during the first few minutes of reflow. Am J Pathol **74:** 399, 1974
6. Jennings RB, Reimer KA: Factors involved in salvaging ischemic myocardium effects of reperfusion of arterial blood. Circulation **68** (suppl I): I-25, 1983
7. Ferrari R, Williams A, DiLisa F: The role of mitochondrial function in the ischaemic and reperfused myocardium. *In* Caldarera CM, Harris P, editors: Advances in studies on heart metabolism. Bolgna, 1982, Cooperativa Libraria Universitaria Editrice, pp 245–255
8. Sharma GP, Varley KG, Kim SW, Barwinsky J, Cohen M, Dhalla NS: Alterations in energy metabolism and ultrastructure upon reperfusion of the ischemic myocardium after coronary occlusion. Am J Cardiol **36:** 234, 1975
9. Rosenkranz ER, Buckberg GD: Myocardial protection during surgical coronary reperfusion. J Am Coll Cardiol **1:** 1235, 1983
10. Smith HJ, Kent KM, Epstein SE: Contractile damage from reperfusion after transient ischemia in the dog. J Thorac Cardiovasc Surg **75:** 452, 1978
11. Darsee JR, Kloner RA: The no reflow phenomenon: a time-limiting factor for reperfusion after coronary occlusion? Am J Cardiol **46:** 800, 1980
12. Schofer J, Montz DG: Scintigraphic evidence of the "no-reflow" phenomen in human beings after coronary thrombolysis. J Am Coll Cardiol **5:** 593, 1985
13. Bush LR, Buja MI, Samowitz W, Rude RE, Wathen M, Tilton GE, Willerson JT: Recovery of left ventricular segmental function after long-term reperfusion following temporary coronary occlusion in conscious dogs: comparison of 2 and 4 hour occlusions. Circ Res **53:** 248, 1983
14. Lavallee M, Cox D, Patrick TA, Vatner SF: Salvage of myocardial function by coronary artery reperfusion 1, 2, and 3 hours after occlusion in conscious dogs. Cir Res **53:** 235, 1983
15. Braunwald E, Kloner RA: The stunned myocardium: prolonged, postischemic ventricular dysfunction. Circulation **66:** 1146, 1982
16. Follette DM, Fey K, Buckberg GD, Helly JJ Jr, Steed DL, Foglia RP, Maloney JV Jr: Reducing postischemic damage by temporary modification of reperfusate calcium, potassium, pH, and osmolarity. J Thorac Cardiovasc Surg **82:** 221, 1981
17. Rosenkranz ER, Okamoto F, Buckberg GD, Vinten-Johansen J, Robertson JM, Bugyi H: Safety of prolonged aortic clamping with blood cardioplegia. II. glutamate enrichment in energy-depleted hearts. J Thorac Cardiovasc Surg **88:** 402, 1984
18. Rosenkranz ER, Vinten-Johansen J, Buckberg GD, Okamoto, Edwards H, Bugyi HI: Benefits of normothermic induction of blood cardioplegia in energy-depleted hearts with maintenance of arrest by multidose cold blood cardioplegia infusions. J Thorac Cardiovasc Surg **84:** 667, 1982
19. Becker H, Vinten-Johansen J, Buckberg GD, Follette DM, Robertson JM: Critical importance of ensuring cardioplegic delivery with coronary stenosis. J Thorac Cardiovasc Surg **81:** 507, 1981
20. Robertson JM, Vinten-Johansen J, Buckberg GD, Rosenkranz ER, Maloney JV Jr: Safety of prolonged aortic clamping with blood cardioplegia. I. glutamate enrichment in normal hearts. J Thorac Cardiovasc Surg **88:** 395, 1984
21. Lowry OH, Passoneau JV: A flexible system of enzymatic analysis. New York, 1972, Academic Press, Inc., pp 151–156
22. Lie JT, Pairolero PC, Holley KE, Titus JL: Macroscopic enzymatic-mapping verification of large, homogenous, experimental myocardial infarcts of predictable size and location in dogs. J Thorac Cardiovasc Surg **69:** 599, 1975
23. Hearse DJ: Oxygen deprivation and early myocardial contractile failure: a reassessment of the possible role of adenosine triphosphate. Am J Cardiol **44:** 1115, 1979
24. Kloner RA, DeBoer LWV, Darsee JR, Ingwall JS, Hale S, Tumas J, Braunwald E: Prolonged abnormalities of myocardium salvaged by reperfusion. Am J Physiol **241:** H591, 1981
25. Schaper J, Schaper W: Reperfusion of ischemic myocardium: ultrastructural and histochemical aspects. J Am Coll Cardiol **4:** 1037, 1983
26. Reimer KA, Jennings RB, Hill ML: Total ischemia in dog hearts in vitro. 2. high energy metabolism, cell volume regulation, and sarcolemmal integrity. Cir Res **49:** 901, 1981
27. DiBona DR, Powell J Jr: Quantitative correlation between cell swelling and necrosis in myocardial ischemia in dogs. Circ Res **47:** 653, 1980
28. Reimer KA, Lowe JE, Rasmussen MM, Jennings RB: The wavefront phenomenon of ischemic cell death. I. myocardial infarct size vs duration of coronary occlusion in dogs. Circulation **56:** 786, 1977
29. Jolly SR, Kane WJ, Baile MB, Abrams GD, Lucchesi BR: Canine myocardial reperfusion injury: its reduction by the combined administration of superoxide dismutase and catalase. Circ Res **54:** 277, 1984
30. Scott JA, Khaw BA, Locke E, Haber E, Homcy C: The role of free radical-mediated processes in oxygen-related damage in cultured murine myocardial cells. Circ Res **56:** 72, 1985
31. Allen BS, Rosenkranz ER, Buckberg GD, Vinten-Johansen J, Okamoto F, Leaf J: Influence of high O_2 demands of dyskinetic segments on recovery during reperfusion. J Am Coll Cardiol **3:** 592, 1984
32. Rovetto MJ, Lamberton WF, Neely JR: Mechanisms of glycolytic inhibition in ischemic rat hearts. Circ Res **37:** 742, 1975
33. Williamson JR, Schaffer SW, Ford C, Safer B: The cellular basis of ischemia and infarctions: contribution of tissue acidosis to ischemic injury in the perfused rat heart. Circulation **53** (suppl I): I-3, 1976
34. Lazar HL, Buckberg GD, Manganaro AJ, Becker H, Maloney JV Jr: Reversal of ischemic damage with amino acid substrate enhancement during reperfusion. Surgery **88:** 702, 1980
35. Thomassen AR, Nielsen TT, Bagger JP, Hansen P: Myocardial exchanges of glutamate, alanine and citrate in controls and patients with coronary artery disease. Clin Sci **64:** 33, 1983
36. Sanborn T, Gavin W, Berkowitz S, Perille T, Lesch M: Augmented conversion of aspartate and glutamate to succinate during anoxia in rabbit heart. Am J Physiol **237:** H535, 1979
37. Safer B: The metabolic significance of the malate-aspartate cycle in heart. Circ Res **37:** 527, 1975
38. Taegtmeyer H: Metabolic responses to cardiac hypoxia: increased production of succinate by rabbit papillary muscles. Cirs Res **43:** 808, 1978
39. LaNoue KF, Walajtes EI, Williamson JR: Regulation of glutamate metabolism and interactions with citric acid cycle in rat heart mitochondria. J Biol Chem **248:** 7171, 1973
40. Wilson MA, Cascarano J: The energy-yielding oxidation of NADH by fumarate in submitochondrial particles of rat tissue. Biochim Biophys Acta **216:** 54, 1970
41. Safer B, Smith CM, Williamson JR: Control of the transport of reducing equivalents across the mitochondrial membrane in perfused rat heart. J Mol Cell Cardiol **2:** 111, 1971
42. Rau EE, Shine KI, Gervais A, Douglas AM, Amos EC III: Enhanced mechanical recovery of anoxic and ischemic myocardium by amino acid perfusion. Am J Physiol **236:** H873, 1979
43. Vinten-Johansen J, Okamoto F, Rosenkranz E, Buckberg GD, Bugyi H, Leaf J: Superiority of surgical vs non-surgical revascularization after coronary occlusion. Circulation **68** (suppl III): III-157, 1983
44. Reibel DK, Rovetto MJ: Myocardial ATP synthesis and mechanical function following oxygen deficiency. Am J Physiol **234:** H620, 1978
45. Hearse DJ, Garlick PB, Humphrey SM: Ischemic contracture of the myocardium: mechanisms and prevention. Am J Cardiol **39:** 986, 1977
46. Jennings RB, Hawkins HK, Lowe JE, Hill ML, Klotman S,

Reimer KA: Relation between high energy phosphate and lethal injury in myocardial ischemia in the dog. Am J Pathol **92:** 187, 1978
47. Okamoto F, Rosenkranz ER, Buckberg GD, Vinten-Johansen J, Bugyi H: Failure of myocardial ATP levels to predict functional recovery. Circulation **58** (suppl III): III-250, 1983
48. Rosenkranz ER, Okamoto F, Vinten-Johansen J, Buckberg GD, Bugyi HI, Leaf J: Improved adenosine triphosphate recovery in energy-depleted hearts treated with 5-amino-4-imidazole carboxamide riboside (AICAR). Surg Forum **34:** 330, 1983
49. DeWood MA, Berg R Jr: The role of surgical reperfusion in myocardial infarction. Cardiol Clin **2:** 113, 1984
50. Berg R Jr, Selinger SL, Leonard JJ, Grunwald RP, O'Grady WP: Immediate coronary artery bypass for acute evolving myocardial infarction. J Thorac Cardiovasc Surg **81:** 493, 1981
51. Cohn LH, Gorlin R, Herman MV, Collins JJ Jr: Aorto-coronary bypass for acute coronary occlusion. J Thorac Cardiovasc Surg **64:** 503, 1972
52. DeWood MA, Spores J, Berg R Jr, Kendall RW, Grunwald RP, Selinger SL, Hensley GR, Sutherland KI, Sheilds JP: Acute myocardial revascularization: a decade of experience with surgical reperfusion in 701 patients. Circulation **68** (suppl II): II-8, 1983

Accuracy of volume measurement by conductance catheter in isolated, ejecting canine hearts

DANIEL BURKHOFF, ENNO VAN DER VELDE, DAVID KASS, M.D., JAN BAAN, PH.D., W. LOWELL MAUGHAN, M.D., AND KIICHI SAGAWA, PH.D.

ABSTRACT We evaluated the accuracy of the recently reported technique of estimating intraventricular volume by measurement of intracavitary electrical conductance in six isolated, ejecting, canine left ventricles. Left ventricular volumes were measured directly by a previously validated servosystem that employed an electroconductive balloon placed in the left ventricular cavity. The volume measured continuously by the balloon method (V_{bal}) was compared with that estimated by the conductance method (V_{cath}). For this test, the hearts were made to eject and fill physiologically by the use of a previously described computer-simulated arterial loading system. Complex ejection and filling patterns were created by stimulating the atrium mechanically, which resulted in irregular arrhythmatic contractions spanning a wide range of volumes. We found that there was a highly linear relationship ($r^2 = .982 \pm .014$) between V_{bal} and V_{cath}: $V_{cath} = 0.82 (\pm .05) V_{bal} + 26.7 (\pm 11.8)$ ml. Despite the wide variation in the offset term of this relationship among the different hearts, the offset within a given heart was predicted within 3.5 ml by a previously detailed "dilution" method that is applicable to the heart in situ within a closed thorax. Thus, since the offset term is obtainable in situ, the conductance method provides a signal that is proportional to the actual volume. To determine whether right ventricular volume influenced the accuracy of left ventricular measurement, we compared the relationship between V_{cath} and V_{bal} obtained with right ventricular volumes of 0 and 30 ml. Increasing the right ventricular volume shifted the relationship upward by less than 3 ml in the working range. Finally, with the left ventricle constrained to contract isovolumetrically, there was less than ± 2 ml variation about a mean value in the conductance signal, indicating that the geometric rearrangements occurring during contraction do not significantly influence the accuracy of this method. We conclude that the conductance method of left ventricular volume measurement provides a continuous signal that is proportional to the actual chamber volume and may therefore prove to be useful in the assessment of ventricular performance in patients and in laboratory animals.
Circulation 72, No. 2, 440–447, 1985.

INSTANTANEOUS ventricular pressure and volume are the fundamental variables essential for understanding and assessing ventricular contraction. Whereas semiconductor catheter–tip transducers provide high-fidelity continuous measurement of ventricular pressure, techniques for measuring instantaneous ventricular volume of the heart in vivo accurately and continuously throughout the cardiac cycle have not been available. Recently, however, a method was introduced by Baan et al.[1] whereby ventricular volume could be estimated by measurement of intraventricular conductance with a specially designed catheter. In previous studies, the accuracy of this method for determining stroke volume and cardiac output has been evaluated in dogs with an electromagnetic flow probe,[1] and in humans with the thermodilution technique.[2, 3] The accuracy of absolute left ventricular volume and ejection fraction measurements obtained with this catheter was tested in vitro in isolated canine hearts,[4] in intact dogs using ferromagnetic fluid dilution,[3] and in humans by cineventriculography.[2, 3] The results of all these studies have generally shown good correlations between the volume measured by the conductance technique (V_{cath}) and those by other methods, but the correlation data obtained in vivo showed significant scatter. Because each of the methods against which the conductance catheter method was compared in vivo

From the Department of Biomedical Engineering, The Johns Hopkins University School of Medicine, Baltimore, and Department of Pediatrics, The University of Leiden, The Netherlands.

Supported by USPHS NIH research grant HL 14903, by grants from the Netherlands Organization for the Advancement of Pure Research through the Foundation for Technical Sciences, and by grants from the Netherlands Heart Foundation.

Address for correspondence: Daniel Burkhoff, Department of Biomedical Engineering, The Johns Hopkins University School of Medicine, Traylor Bldg., Rm. 223, 720 Rutland Ave., Baltimore, MD 21205.

Received April 9, 1985; accepted May 16, 1985.

has limited accuracy in measuring ventricular volume, the scatter could have been caused, at least in part, by inaccuracies in the other methods rather than those in the conductance catheter method.

The purpose of the present study, therefore, was to reevaluate the accuracy of the conductance catheter method more reliably than in previous studies by use of an isolated, beating left ventricular preparation in which left ventricular volume could be measured accurately by use of a balloon fitted to its cavity. To our knowledge, the balloon method yields the most accurate measurement of the ventricular cavity volume in isolated hearts.[5] Furthermore, in this preparation it is possible to produce physiologic changes in ventricular volume with the use of a specially designed computer-simulated arterial loading system.[6] Thus, the evaluation was made in physiologically ejecting left ventricles of isolated canine hearts.

Methods

Conductance catheter. The technique used to estimate ventricular volume by measuring electrical conductance in the cavity has been described in detail by Baan et al.[1, 3] Briefly, a catheter with eight electrodes equidistantly placed along the end of a No. 7F catheter was positioned inside the ventricular cavity (figure 1). To match the electrode spacing on the catheter to the size of the left ventricle of a 20 kg dog, we used a catheter in which the distance between the first and the last electrode was 6 cm. An alternating current, with a constant amplitude (20 kHz, 30 μA) was passed between electrodes 1 (in the apex) and 8 (at the base) to set up an electrical field inside the ventricular chamber. The five potential differences, $\Phi_i(t)$, between each successive pairs of remaining electrodes (i.e., electrode pairs 2–3, 3–4, 4–5, 5–6, and 6–7) were measured continuously. Dividing the current by each of the $\Phi_i(t)$ signals results in five conductances [$G_i(t)$; i = 1 to 5)]. Summing the $G_i(t)$s gives an overall signal, G(t), which is linearly related to ventricular volume, V(t), by the following equation[3]:

$$V(t) = (1/\alpha)\,(L^2/\sigma)\,G(t) - V_c \qquad (1)$$

where α is a dimensionless slope constant, L is the distance between adjacent electrodes, σ is the conductivity of the fluid in the cavity, and V_c is a correction term that accounts for the conductance of the tissues surrounding the cavity. V_c will be discussed in detail below. The current is delivered by a signal conditioner-processor (Leycom Model Sigma-5, The Netherlands). In addition, this signal processor is equipped with the means to measure the resistivity (rho) of the blood, which it displays on a digital readout panel. Rho is simply equal to the reciprocal of the conductivity, σ, in equation 1 (rho = $1/\sigma$). Since the device provides a direct readout of this quantity, we will report the value of rho rather than that of σ. Finally, the Leycom device measures the voltages $\Phi_i(t)$ and performs the necessary analog computations to obtain V(t) *not* accounting for the correction terms V_c and α of equation 1. The output signal of the processor [i.e., $(L^2/\sigma)\,G(t)$] will be referred to as the (uncorrected) catheter volume, $V_{cath}(t)$.

V_c is linearly related to the parallel conductance of the surrounding structures, G^p, by[3]

$$V_c = (1/\alpha)\,(L^2/\sigma)\,G^p \qquad (2)$$

which follows from the condition that, when cavity volume is zero [V(t) = 0 in equation 1], all current passes through the surrounding structures. In the isolated heart preparation, G^p is composed of the conductances of the balloon used to measure cavity volume (see below), the ventricular wall, and the contents of the right ventricle. Two methods have been described previously for determination of the value of αV_c for the heart in situ,[3] one of which was used in the present study.

We used the so-called dilution method to obtain αV_c, which is applicable to the heart in situ within a closed thorax. Briefly, a bolus (1 to 2 ml) of saturated saline solution (conductivity = 75 S/m in contrast to that of blood, which is approximately 0.7 S/m) is injected into the hydraulic system while end-systolic and end-diastolic volumes are held constant. As the bolus mixes with the fluid in the ventricular cavity, its conductivity (σ in equation 1) increases, causing the overall conductance signal, G(t), to increase while the parallel component, G^p, remains constant. In practice then, end-systolic overall conductance, G_{es}, is plotted as a function of end-diastolic overall conductance, G_{ed}, during the mixing of the bolus; linear regression analysis is applied to the G_{es}-G_{ed} data points, and G^p is equal to the intersection point between the regression line and the line of identity.[3] In our study (see figure 4) we plotted V_{cath} (= $[L^2/\sigma]G$) at end-systole vs end-diastole rather the G, while considering the factor L^2/σ constant and equal to its original value before the bolus injection. Thus, the value determined by the intersection of the regression line with the line of identity was equal to αV_c (= $[L^2/\sigma]G^p$). This procedure will be described in detail below.

The value for αV_c obtained by the dilution method was compared with a more direct measure of this offset volume that was determined by plotting V_{cath} against actual balloon volume

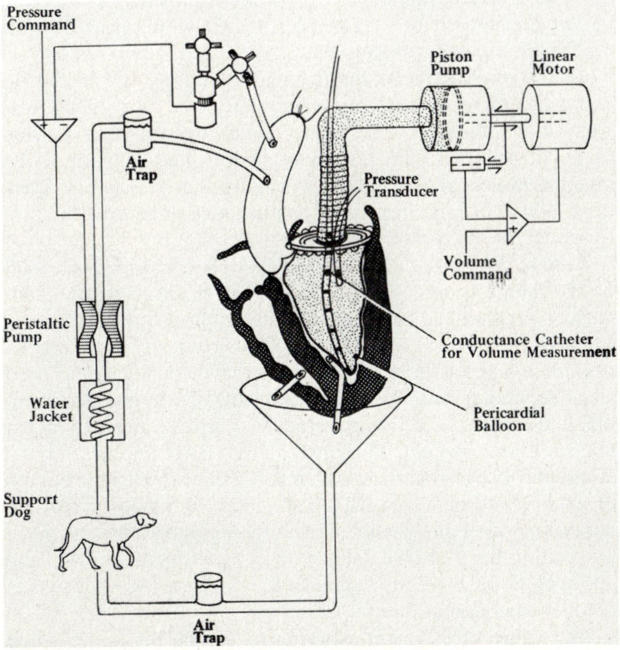

FIGURE 1. Schematic diagram of the isolated heart preparation indicating the positions of the conductance catheter and pressure sensor relative to the left ventricular chamber. Electrode 1, situated near the apex, and electrode 8, at the level of the base, are used to apply alternating current. Remaining electrodes (2 through 7) are used to measure voltage drops, which are converted to segmental volume. Note that the balloon placed inside the left ventricle was made out of pericardial tissue.

(V_{bal}) as measured directly by the servosystem (see below). Applying linear regression analysis to the data over a wide range of volumes, we obtained

$$V_{cath} = m\,V_{bal} + b \qquad (3)$$

in which, from comparison to equation 1, it is evident that the y intercept, b, provides an estimate of αV_c, while the slope, m, gives an estimate of α.

No independent experimental way to estimate the slope factor α has been devised yet, but theoretical studies[4,7,8] have addressed this problem by consideration of a possible relationship between α and G^p, as discussed below.

Surgical preparation. The procedures used to isolate and support the canine hearts were similar to those described by Suga and Sagawa.[5] Six pairs of mongrel dogs were anesthetized with sodium pentobarbital (30 mg/kg iv). The femoral arteries and veins of one dog of each pair (support dog) were cannulated and connected to a perfusion system (figure 1) used to supply oxygenated blood to the heart isolated from the second dog (donor dog). The chest of the donor dog was opened under artificial respiration. The left subclavian artery was cannulated with the arterial line of the perfusion system. The brachiocephalic artery was cannulated to monitor the coronary perfusion pressure. The azygos vein, superior and inferior venae cavae, descending aorta, and lung hili were ligated. The heart was then removed from the donor dog and coronary perfusion was provided by the support dog via a constant-pressure perfusion pump. The left atrium was opened and all the chordae tendineae were freed from the mitral valve leaflets. A plastic adapter that holds the isolated heart to the ventricular volume servopump system (see below) was sutured to the mitral ring. When the surgical preparation was complete, this mitral ring adaptor was connected to the pump system so that a specially made saline-filled pericardial balloon (described below) could be fitted inside the left ventricular cavity (figure 1).

The conductance catheter was positioned in the intraventricular balloon so that the most distal electrode was in the apex and the most proximal electrode would lie between 3 and 7 mm outside the balloon, the exact distance being dependent on the size of the heart studied.

In all experiments the coronary perfusion pressure was maintained between 80 and 100 mm Hg by a servocontrolled finger pump. The temperature of the perfusate was maintained between 35° and 37° C.

Ventricular volume servosystem. A servosystem, depicted in the upper right portion of figure 1, was used to control ventricular volume. Details of its design and performance have been reported by Sunagawa et al.[9] A linear motor controlled the position of the piston within a double rolling–diaphragm cylinder. A specially made pericardial balloon was secured to a tube connected to the outflow tract of the cylinder. The cylinder, connecting tube, and balloon were all filled with water made conductive by adding sodium chloride. The position of the piston was sensed by a linear displacement transducer attached to the shaft of the piston, thus producing a signal proportional to the V_{bal} and therefore ventricular cavity volume. This signal was used in a negative feedback loop for comparison with a volume command signal that represented the desired instantaneous volume. The error signal resulting from this comparison was supplied to a power amplifier (Crown DC-300), which in turn drove the linear motor.

The accuracy of ventricular volume thus measured is expected to be within less than 1 ml of the actual ventricular volume as long as the balloon is tightly fitted to the endocardial surface.[10]

Simulated arterial loading system. The volume signal for the volume servosystem was generated by the interaction between the left ventricular pressure signal, measured by a semiconductor tip transducer (Miller, model 380), and a specially designed loading system that has previously been described in detail by Sunagawa et al.[6] The afterloading circuit was the three-element modified windkessel model, which has been shown to be a reasonable respresentation of the aortic hydraulic input impedance,[11] and a diode that functioned as the aortic valve. Using this system, the isolated heart can be made to eject physiologically. The ventricle was also filled in diastole by the computer-simulated venous filling circuit, which consisted of a pressure source and a resistance to filling.

Pericardial balloon. Because the myocardium is electrically conductive (σ of approximately 0.25 S/m[12]), although less so than blood (σ of approximately 0.70 S/m), some of the excitation current delivered by the catheter passes through the ventricular wall and therefore the conductance method overestimates the volume of the ventricular lumen by an amount αV_c (equation 1), as explained above. To avoid elimination of this offset by the use of standard nonconductive rubber balloon within the isolated heart, we made balloons out of pericardial tissue, which is highly conductive (surface conductance >2 S/m^2). This provided electrical continuity between the fluid inside the balloon and the myocardial tissue. In addition, the conductivity, σ, of the fluid inside the balloon was adjusted to be comparable to that of blood, i.e., approximately 0.70 S/m (resistivity, rho = $1/\sigma$, of blood approximately 140 $\Omega\cdot$cm).

Protocol and data analysis.

Pericardial balloon study. Before performing studies on the isolated heart, we evaluated the ability of the catheter to measure the volume of the balloon alone. The catheter was positioned inside a pericardial balloon, as described above. This balloon was filled with saline solution with a resistivity of 135 $\Omega\cdot$cm, which is comparable to that of canine blood. The balloon was then completely submersed in fluid contained within a Plexiglass tank, which created a parallel conductance. V_{bal} was varied sinusoidally at a frequency of 1 Hz with a peak-to-peak amplitude of approximately 35 ml. V_{cath} and volume measured by the servosystem were digitized at a sampling rate of 200 Hz and a quantitative comparison between these two signals was performed off-line by computer. After investigating a wide range of volumes, the resistivity of the fluid outside of the chamber was changed and the procedure was repeated to determine how a change in parallel conductance influences the performance of the volume catheter.

Isolated heart studies. Experiments were performed on a total of six canine hearts. Each ventricle was made to pump under various preload and afterload conditions producing ventricular volumes over a wide range from approximately 15 to 50 ml. To provide a rigorous test for the conductance catheter, the right atrial appendage was stimulated mechanically to produce irregular and complex ejection patterns. V_{cath} and V_{bal} were digitized at a sampling rate of 200 Hz and analyzed off-line by a digital computer. In each heart approximately 30 sec (6000 data points) of continuous data obtained under a wide range of loading conditions were analyzed in each run. A comparison was made by plotting the digitized data for V_{cath} as a function of V_{bal} and applying linear regression analysis to obtain the regression coefficients of equation 3.

The value of αV_c was determined by the dilution method outlined above in five of the hearts. This value was compared with the value of b determined directly by applying linear regression to the V_{cath} and V_{bal} data as outlined above.

The influence of right ventricular volume on left ventricular V_{cath} was determined in three hearts by placing a second pericardial balloon inside the right ventricle and repeating the measurements outlined above with the right ventricle filled with a constant volume of 30 ml of saline of the same conductivity as the fluid in the left ventricle.

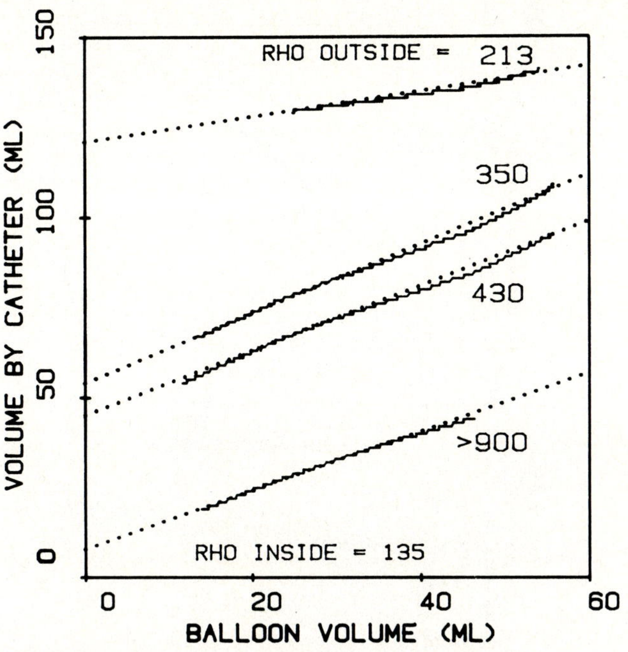

FIGURE 2. Isolated pericardial balloon study: relationship between actual V_{bal} and V_{cath} when the resistivity of the surrounding fluid is varied. See text and table 1 for details.

Finally, the influence on the conductance signal of changes in ventricular shape that occur during the cardiac cycle[13] was investigated. This was accomplished by recording the V_{cath} signal during forced isovolumetric contraction of the left ventricle at different volume settings.

Results

Pericardial balloon studies. The result of the studies with the pericardial balloon, filled with saline solution with resistivity of 135 Ω·cm and submersed in fluids with different resistivities, are presented in figure 2. The V_{cath} is plotted as a function of the actual V_{bal} imposed by the servosystem. As is evident in these graphs, the catheter provided a signal that was linearly related to the actual volume inside the balloon. The results of the quantitative analysis of these data are summarized in table 1. When the resistivity of the surrounding fluid was high (rho > 900 Ω·cm), the relationship between V_{bal} and V_{cath} had a slope of 0.80 and a y intercept of 8.4 ml, which is close to the line of identity. When the resistivity of the surrounding fluid was decreased, the y intercept increased, and at very low resistivities (rho = 213 Ω·cm) the slope decreased significantly. The linearity of the relationship, however, was not altered, as judged by the linear correlation coefficients which were always high (table 1). The situation in which the external-internal resistivity ratio was 350:135 (3 in table 1) closely mimics conditions in the left ventricle in situ.

TABLE 1
Influence of surrounding resistivity on the performance of the conductance catheter

	Surrounding resistivity (Ω·cm)	m	b (ml)	r^2
1.	>900	0.80	8.4	.998
2.	430	0.90	44.7	.999
3.	350	0.95	54.3	.997
4.	213	0.36	120.6	.981

Resistivity of fluid in balloon 135 Ohm-cm.
m = slope; b = y axis intercept.

TABLE 2
Results of linear regression analysis V_{cath} and V_{bal} data (n = 5 hearts)

Heart No.	m	b (ml)	r^2	αV_c (ml)	Error in αV_c (ml)
1	0.75	11.0	.963	7.5	−3.5
2	0.81	22.9	.972	23.1	0.2
3	0.83	25.0	.987	22.9	−2.1
4	0.89	43.3	.998	45.2	1.9
5	0.80	31.1	.992	28.7	−2.4

Abbreviations are as in table 1.
αV_c was determined by the dilution method (error in $\alpha V_c = \alpha V_c - b$).

Isolated heart studies. Simultaneous ventricular volume tracings obtained in an isolated heart by the balloon method and by the conductance catheter are presented in figure 3. The resistivity of the fluid inside the pericardial balloon was 120 Ω·cm. The right atrial appendage of the heart was stimulated mechanically to produce an irregular ejection pattern, as is depicted in the two panels at the top of the figure. As is shown, V_{cath} closely tracked the V_{bal} throughout this series, except for small deviations during isovolumetric pauses, and V_{cath} computed by conductance was linearly related to V_{bal}: in the example in figure 3, in which instantaneous V_{cath} is plotted as a function of V_{bal}, $V_{cath} = 0.76\ V_{bal} + 26.5$ ($r^2 = .987$).

In five experiments we evaluated the dilution method of determining $\alpha V_c{}^2$ (see Methods). The procedure is depicted in figure 4. First, a comparison between actual V_{bal} and V_{cath} was obtained by a method similar to that shown in figure 3. In the example of figure 4, *A*, the value of the y intercept is 31.1 and the slope is 0.8. Next, the conductivity of the fluid inside the chamber was increased by the infusion of hypertonic saline solution. As depicted in the original recordings in figure 4, *B*, the actual end-systolic and end-diastolic volumes, as recorded by the balloon method, were constant during this run, while the catheter signal increased in magnitude as the hypertonic saline mixed with the fluid in the pericardial balloon. As explained

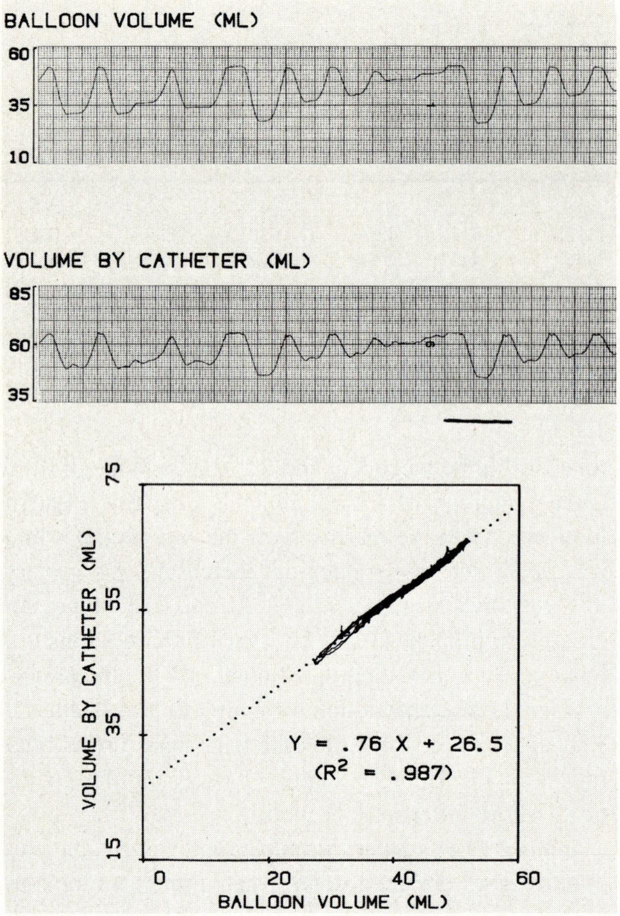

FIGURE 3. Simultaneous recordings from the conductance catheter and from the servosystem obtained from a typical isolated heart experiment while mechanically stimulating the right atrial appendage to produce a complex ejection pattern. Solid line below *middle* panel is 1 sec marker. The relationship between V_{cath} and V_{bal} is illustrated at the *bottom*. Dotted line represents the line of regression between the two.

in Methods, end-systolic values for V_{cath} were plotted as a function of end-diastolic V_{cath} for several of the beats during the transient period, as depicted in panel *C*. The αV_c was then estimated by applying linear regression analysis to the data and determining the point of intersection of that regression line with the line of identity. A value of 28.7 ml was obtained for αV_c, which compared favorably with the 31.1 ml y intercept value determined directly (figure 4, *A*).

The results of this analysis in five isolated hearts are summarized in table 2, where the slope, intercept, and correlation coefficient of the linear regression between V_{cath} and V_{bal} are presented along with αV_c obtained by changing intracavitary conductivity. These results indicate a highly linear relationship between V_{cath} and the actual volume measured by the servosystem. The error in the dilution method–estimated αV_c is small in each experiment.

Influence of the right ventricle. The influence of right ventricular volume on the performance of the conductance catheter was assessed in three ventricles. The left ventricles filled and ejected as described above, and the volume of the right ventricular pericardial balloon was kept constant at either 0 or 30 ml. The results from the three hearts are presented in table 3. On average, increasing right ventricular volume from 0 to 30 ml did not influence the correlation coefficient significantly,

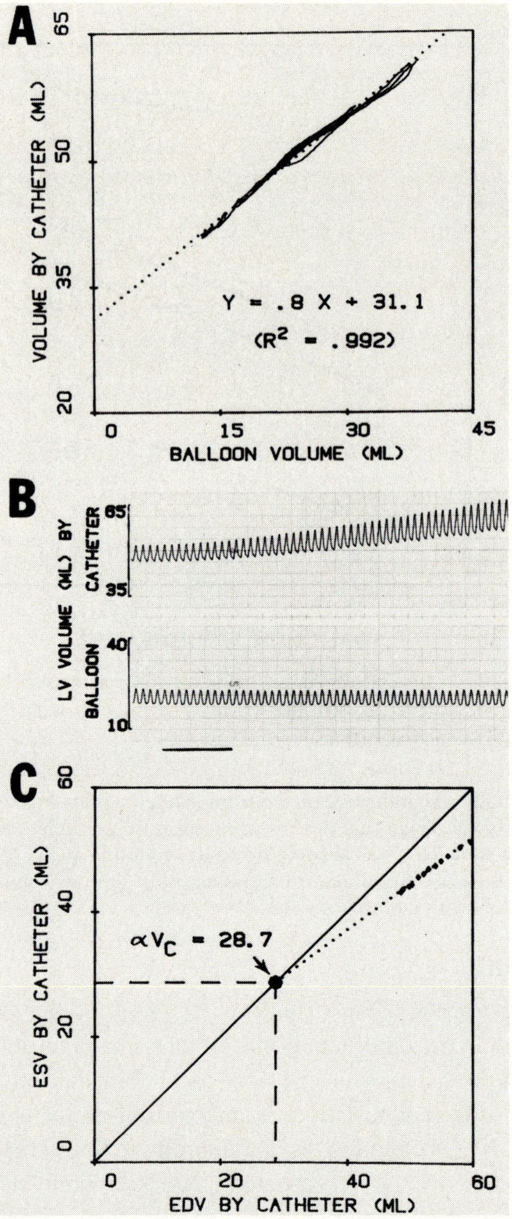

FIGURE 4. *A*, Relationship between V_{bal} and V_{cath} obtained over a wide range of volumes. By linear regression the slope, m = 0.8, estimates α while the offset, b = 31.1, estimates αV_c. *B*, While maintaining ventricular end-systolic and end-diastolic volumes constant, the resistivity of the fluid inside the balloon was decreased by infusion of hypertonic saline. V_{cath} gradually increased to a new steady level as this hypertonic fluid mixed with the fluid in the balloon. Solid line at the bottom is a 5 sec marker. *C*, End-systolic V_{cath} plotted as a function of end-diastolic V_{cath} during the transient in *B*. The intersection of the line of regression (dotted line) with the line of identity (solid line) estimated αV_c as 28.7, which is very close to that determined directly in *A*.

TABLE 3
Influence of right ventricular volume on left ventricular V_{cath}

	Experiment No.								
	1			2			3		
RVV	m	b (ml)	r^2	m	b (ml)	r^2	m	b (ml)	r^2
0	0.83	12.1	.984	0.77	26.0	.983	0.81	31.1	.970
30	0.82	15.0	.985	0.84	24.7	.983	0.79	32.3	.990

RVV = right ventricular volume (ml); other abbreviations are as in table 1.

while the influence on the slope, and the offset were small. Theoretically, the increase in right ventricular volume should hardly affect slope and should increase the value of the offset (see Discussion), which was indeed the case in experiments 1 and 3. The very slight changes in the slope (0.01 and 0.02, respectively) in experiments 1 and 3 are not statistically significant. The 0.07 increase in slope in experiment 2, and the accompanying slight decrease in offset, are somewhat anomalous.

Isovolumetric contractions. The influence of the geometric changes brought about by isovolumetric contractions on the conductance signal were evaluated in three ventricles. Original recordings from one typical experiment are illustrated in figure 5. The ventricle was made to contract isovolumetrically at 10, 15, 20, 25, 30, and 35 ml. Peak isovolumetric pressure increased from 40 to greater than 180 mm Hg over this range of volumes. The V_{cath} fluctuated by at most ±2 ml around the mean level during the cardiac cycle. The amount of fluctuation in the catheter signal was a function of ventricular volume, which suggests that ventricular volume modulates the influences of contraction on chamber geometry. Minimal fluctuations (<0.5 ml) were observed at a volume of 25 ml and they were maximal at 35 ml. The results of the other experiments were essentially identical. Similar conclusions regarding the influence of volume on geometry in an ejecting ventricle may be drawn from the pressure-volume loops shown in figure 6 obtained by balloon and by conductance catheter. (The V_{cath}-V_{bal} correlation data corresponding to these tracings are presented in figure 4). The overall similarity between the two panels is striking. However, closer inspection reveals that the isovolumetric relaxation phases show some differences. Those in figure 6, *A*, obtained by balloon, display a slight but uniform skewness, while the isovolumetric relaxation parts of the conductance loops in panel *B* show a reversal in skewness for end-systolic volumes larger than 23 ml.

Discussion

The accuracy of the conductance catheter has been assessed previously by comparison of V_{cath} with volume measured by cineventriculography and with thermodilution and electromagnetic flow determinations of stroke volume. However, none of these techniques

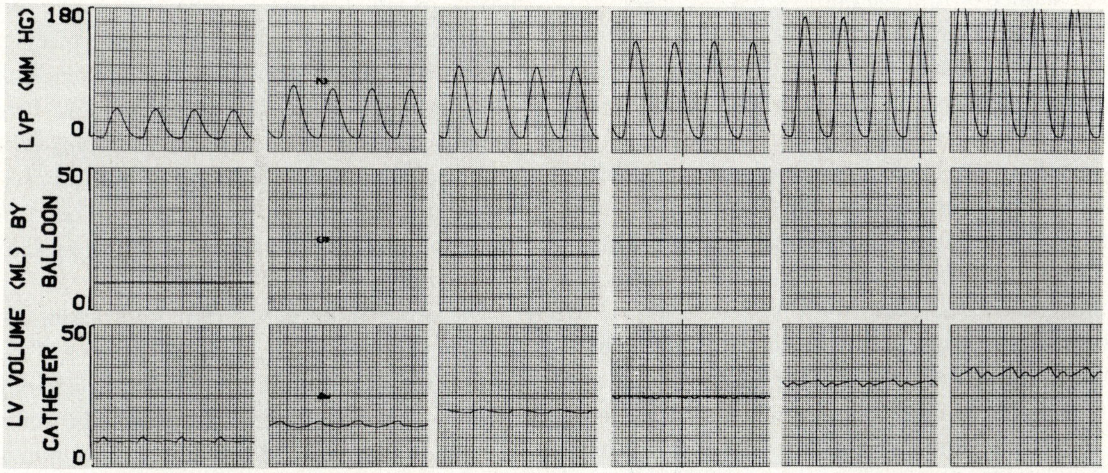

FIGURE 5. Measurement of left ventricular volume by balloon (*middle*) and by conductance catheter (*bottom*) during isovolumetric contractions at, from left to right, 10, 15, 20, 25, 30, and 35 ml. Left ventricular pressure (LVP, *top*) increased from 40 to more than 180 mm Hg. V_{cath} fluctuated by a maximum of ±2 ml around the mean level during the cardiac cycle.

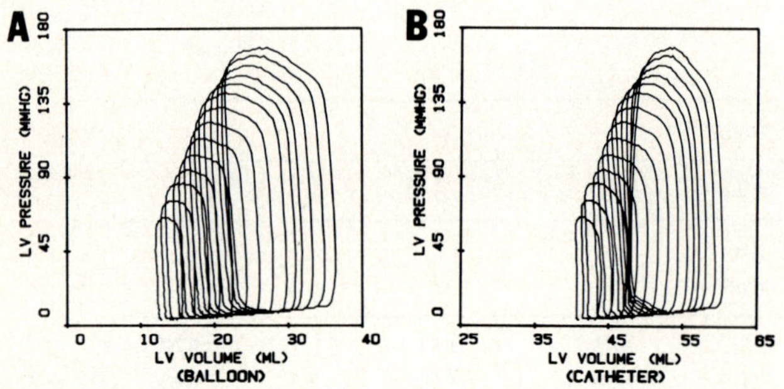

FIGURE 6. Pressure-volume loops obtained by changing preload volume in the servosystem with volume measured simultaneously by the balloon method in *A*, and by the conductance catheter in *B*. See figure 4, *A* for the relationship between V_{bal} and V_{cath}. V_{cath} as shown is directly from the Leycom signal processor, and is not corrected for the offset αV_c determined by the dilution method.

has been thoroughly validated against a truly reliable method and shown to provide precise measures of (changes in) ventricular volume throughout the cardiac cycle. In the present study the "gold standard" of ventricular volume measurement to which the conductance catheter measurements were compared was provided by the intraventricular balloon method, which has been previously validated. In this method, the volume of fluid inside the balloon is accurately measured by a carefully calibrated linear displacement transducer coupled to the shaft of a piston pump that controls the balloon value. The balloon, in principle, completely fills the ventricular lumen, thereby providing a precise measure of ventricular volume. In a previous study[10] it has been shown that this assumption is valid to within less than 1 ml, one likely source of error being that the balloon does not fill all the intertrabecular cavities in the wall. Also, in the isolated heart preparation used in this study the small amount of volume contained within the outflow tract beneath the aortic valve and above the plane of the mitral valve (where the plastic holder was sutured) is not included in the balloon measurement of ventricular volume. The extent to which this "pocket" of volume is measured by the conductance catheter depends on whether it is filled by air or by blood as provided by Thebesian vessel drainage. We were unable to determine this, but the pocket volume is probably 2 ml at most, and constant throughout the cardiac cycle.

Measurements of changes in ventricular volume by the balloon method are likely to be more precise than measurements of absolute volume since the errors discussed above are relatively constant in a given heart and independent of the ventricular volume. With knowledge of the magnitude of the potential errors in balloon method, we consider it to be the best method available at present for measuring absolute ventricular volume in an ejecting heart and therefore an appropriate gold standard for evaluation of the accuracy of the conductance catheter.

We first studied the influence of changes in the parallel conductance on the performance of the conductance catheter by changing the resistivity of the fluid surrounding the pericardial balloon without a heart. From figure 2 and table 1 it is clear that this maneuver does not influence the linearity of the measurement, but the value of the y intercept clearly increases with decreasing fluid resistivity (rho), as expected from equation 2. In fact, plotting the y intercept data against the 1/rho data in table I yielded a linear relationship ($r = .996$), which, theoretically, should be the case (see equation 2). The substantial decrease in slope when rho is lowered is also expected: in the hypothetical and extreme case in which the resistivities of the fluids inside and outside the balloon would be equal and the balloon material would have the same rho, no variation in V_{cath} (slope $= 0$) should be observed despite changes in the actual V_{bal}.

Results obtained with the isolated heart indicated a highly correlated, linear relationship between the volume measured by the servosystem and that measured by the catheter over a wide range of volumes and under different loading conditions, including arrhythmic contraction. The offset in the regression between V_{cath} and V_{bal} was predicted rather accurately (<3.5 ml error, table 2) by the dilution method, which estimates αV_c by increasing the conductivity (decreasing resistivity) of the fluid inside the cavity by infusion of hypertonic saline.

The variation in offset between different hearts is quite large, an observation that has also been made in hearts in situ.[3] Much less heart-to-heart variation is observed for the slope constant (range of from 0.75 to 0.89, which roughly covers the same range observed in situ).[3] In studies in a theoretical model,[7,8] the values for α were predicted by the (measurable) value of G^p, but the present results (table 2) do not fully support the model predictions in this respect. Therefore, more work to elucidate the factors influencing the slope is warranted.

The observed effect of right ventricular volume on V_{cath} is in accordance with the predictions of theory. An increase of right ventricular volume by a fixed quantity of well-conducting fluid increases the amount and overall conductivity of the tissue surrounding the left ventricular cavity, and thus increases G^p and, per equation 2, the y axis intercept. An increase in G^p should also result in a small decrease in slope constant.[7,8]

Generally, the observed influences on slope and offset of adding fluid to the right ventricle are quite small and are likely caused in part by statistical uncertainties.

The influence of changes in ventricular shape occurring during contraction were assessed by making conductance measurements of volume during isovolumetric ventricular contractions. In this rigorous test, only relatively small effects (less than ± 2 ml from the mean) were observed.

A potential limitation in the applicability of the results of the present study to the situation in situ arises from the fact that the conductance catheter was placed through the mitral valve and not through the aortic valve as would normally be the case in patients and intact animals. First, we could not assess the possible influences of left atrial volume on catheter measurements. This is a potentially important factor since the mitral valve is very conductive and the catheter excitation current may pass into the left atrium. Second, the influence of right ventricular volume may be slightly different in situ since, when the catheter is positioned through the aortic valve, the geometric relationship between the axis of the electrical field and the right ventricular cavity would be slightly different than in the present study. These questions should be addressed in more detailed theoretical models or in postmortem studies of hearts. Preliminary studies with the latter preparation in Baan's laboratory show that the effect of left atrial volume on conductance in the left ventricle is very small.*

The advantage of the use of the conductance catheter over other methods of measurement of ventricular volume is that it provides a continuous measure of ventricular volume. It is therefore highly suitable for making on-line measurements of ventricular pressure-volume loops, such as those shown in figure 6, and thus facilitates the assessment of ventricular performance in vivo in such terms. The volume signal used in figure 6, *B* was generated in real time by the Leycom signal processor; in practice, the offset volume determined by the dilution method (28.7 ml in this case, as in figure 4, *C*) would be subtracted from this signal, resulting in a signal proportional to volume determined by the balloon method.

In summary, the conductance method of estimating continuous left ventricular volume was highly linearly correlated with volume determined by the balloon method over a wide volume range and under a large variety of loading conditions and contraction modes. The value of the offset of the regression, αV_c, was predictable with reasonable accuracy by the dilution method. The slope of the regression was constant for a given heart, and varied between 0.75 and 0.89 among hearts. The influences of right ventricular volume and geometric changes occurring during the cardiac cycle on the catheter measurements were minimal. We conclude that the intracavitary conductance method of measurement of ventricular volume provides a continuous signal throughout the cardiac cycle that is essentially proportional to actual ventricular volume. Further work is needed to determine ways of estimating the exact magnitude of the proportionality factor, α, for a given heart in situ. The conductance method of continuous volume estimation is likely to facilitate the assessment of ventricular contractile state by providing crucial information about ventricular volume.

*Baan J, et al: Unpublished observation.

We are grateful to Dr. Hiroyuki Suga, who suggested the use of pericardial balloons for this study. We also thank Mr. Kenneth Rent for his excellent technical assistance.

References

1. Baan J, Aouw Jong TT, Kerkhof PLM, Moene RJ, Van Dijk AD, Van der Velde ET, Koops J: Continuous stroke volume and cardiac output from intra-ventricular dimensions obtained with impedance catheter. Cardiovasc Res **15:** 328, 1981
2. Baan J, De Bruin HG, Van der Velde ET, Senden PJ, Sedney M, Buis B: Absolute LV volume in man by conductance catheter, compared to angiography and thermal dilution. Circulation **68** (suppl III): III-135, 1983 (abst)
3. Baan J, Van der Velde ET, De Bruin HG, Smeenk GJ, Koops J, Van Dijk AD, Temmerman D, Senden J, Buis B: Continuous measurement of left ventricular volume in animals and humans by conductance catheter. Circulation **70:** 812, 1984
4. Mur G, Baan J: Computation of the input impedances of a catheter for cardiac volumetry. IEEE Trans Biomed Eng **31:** 448, 1984
5. Suga H, Sagawa K: Instantaneous pressure-volume relationships and their ratio in the excised, supported canine left ventricle. Circ Res **35:** 117, 1974
6. Sunagawa K, Burkhoff D, Lim K, Sagawa K: Impedance loading servo pump system for excised canine ventricle. Am J Physiol **243:** H346, 1982
7. DeBruin HG, Mur G, Van der Velde ET, Homan J, Baan J: Measurement of LV blood volume by conductance catheter (CC): further assessment of properties in the analytic prolate spheroid model. Fed Proc (in press)
8. De Bruin HG, Mur G, Van der Velde ET, Baan J: Measurement of left ventricular blood volume by eight-electrode catheter: models for electrical conductance of the heart. *In* Bajzer Z, Franconi C, editors: Applications of physics to medicine and biology. Singapore, 1984, Workday Medical Publisher, p 50
9. Sunagawa K, Lim KO, Burkhoff D, Sagawa K: Microprocessor control of a ventricular volume servo-pump. Ann Biomed Eng **10:** 145, 1982
10. Suga H, Sagawa K: Accuracy of ventricular lumen volume measurement by intraventricular balloon method. Am J Physiol **236:** H505, 1979
11. Westerhof N, Elzinga G, Sipkema P: An artificial system for pumping hearts. J Appl Physiol **31:** 776, 1971
12. Rush S, Abildskov JA, McFee R: Resistivity of body tissue at low frequencies. Circ Res **12:** 40, 1963
13. Rankin JS, McHale PA, Arentzen CE, Ling D, Greenfield JC, Anderson RW: The three dimensional dynamic geometry of left ventricle in the conscious dog. Circ Res **39:** 304, 1976

For many patients

POST-MI PROTECTION

Regardless of:

Heart size[1]

Infarction site[1]

Transmural or nontransmural MI[1]

Risk group[1]

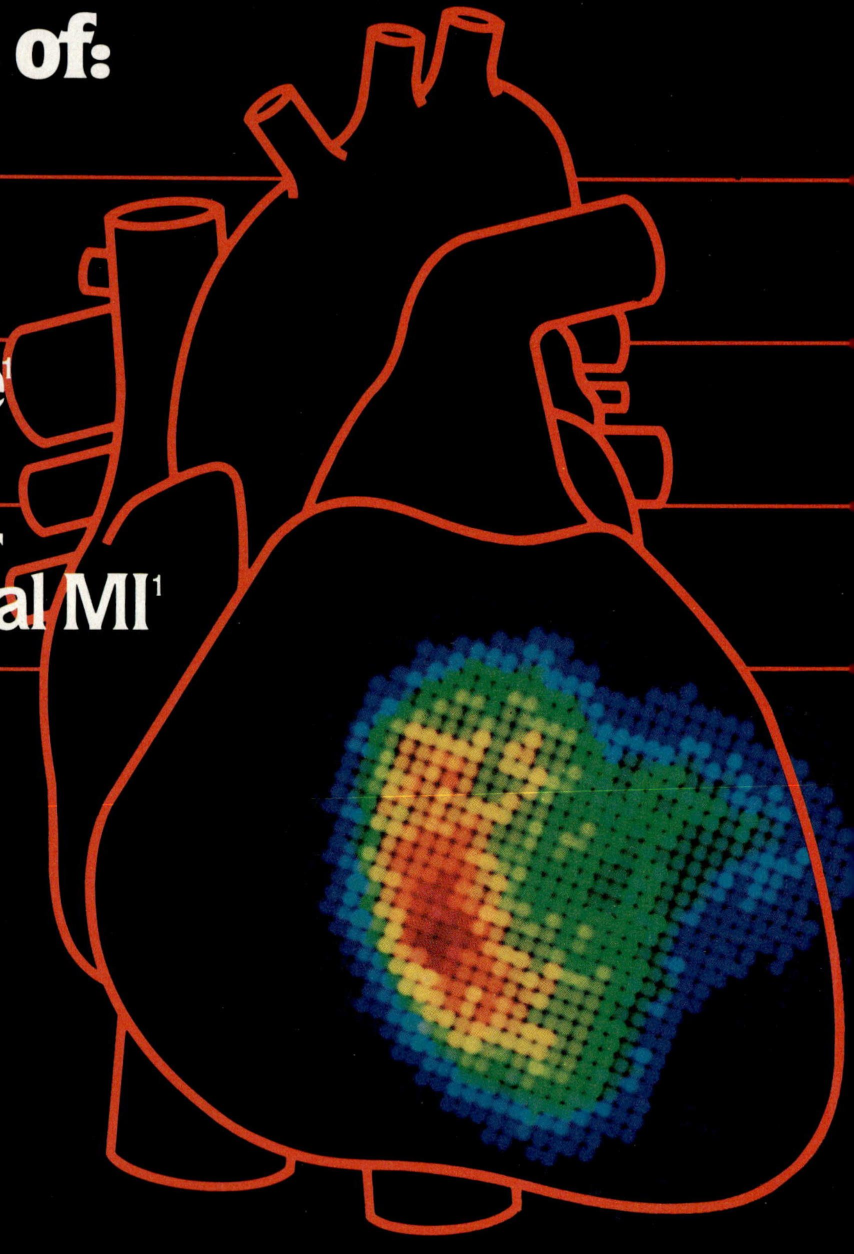

Radionuclide scan of an infarcted heart.

BLOCADREN® (Timolol Maleate, MSD) is contraindicated in patients with bronchial asthma, a history of bronchial asthma, or severe chronic obstructive pulmonary disease (see below); sinus bradycardia; second- and third-degree atrioventricular block; overt cardiac failure (see below); cardiogenic shock; and hypersensitivity to this product. Although beta blockers should be avoided in overt congestive heart failure, they can be used, if necessary, with caution in patients with a history of failure who are well compensated. In patients without a history of cardiac failure, continued depression of the myocardium with beta-blocking agents over a period of time can, in some cases, lead to cardiac failure.

Exacerbation of Ischemic Heart Disease following Abrupt Withdrawal—Hypersensitivity to catecholamines has been observed in patients withdrawn from beta-blocker therapy; exacerbation of angina and, in some cases, myocardial infarction have occurred after *abrupt* discontinuation of such therapy. When discontinuing chronically administered timolol maleate, particularly in patients with ischemic heart disease, the dosage should be gradually reduced over a period of one to two weeks, and the patient should be carefully monitored. If angina markedly worsens or acute coronary insufficiency develops, timolol maleate administration should be reinstituted promptly, at least temporarily, and other measures appropriate for the management of unstable angina should be taken. Patients should be warned against interruption or discontinuation of therapy without the physician's advice. Because coronary artery disease is common and may be unrecognized, it may be prudent not to discontinue timolol maleate therapy abruptly even in patients treated only for hypertension.

In patients with nonallergic bronchospasm or with a history of nonallergic bronchospasm (e.g., chronic bronchitis, emphysema), BLOCADREN should be administered with caution.

For a Brief Summary of Prescribing Information, please see last page of this advertisement.

Circulation

VOL 72 NO 3
SEPTEMBER 1985

An Official Journal of the American Heart Association, Inc.®

FEATURES

Some unexpected lessons from large multicenter randomized clinical trials

SHAHBUDIN H. RAHIMTOOLA, M.B., F.R.C.P.

RANDOMIZATION is considered to have started[1] with the report of Fisher and MacKenzie in 1923 on agricultural experiments carried out by T. Eden on the effect of manure on the crops of different potato varieties.[2] Feinstein states, "The modern era of biostatistically planned randomized trials occurred in 1947, when streptomycin was evaluated in the treatment of tuberculosis."[1] Other subsequent triumphs of randomized trials — for example, penicillin for prevention of recurrences of rheumatic fever and the Veterans Administration study of drug treatment of hypertension[3, 4] — led to an unbounded enthusiasm for these trials. In the 1960s and 1970s it was increasingly proposed without proof that randomized clinical trials were the best way or the only correct way to evaluate new therapies. This euphoric phase (Phase 1, figure 1) is predictably leading to a phase of doubt and uncertainty (Phase 2), as we recognize the many problems of randomized clinical trials, particularly those of large multicenter trials.[1, 5–12] The period of doubt and uncertainty is likely to be followed by disillusionment (Phase 3) and reflection (Phase 4), until finally we arrive at a balanced perspective (Phase 5, reality). It is the purpose of this editorial to suggest midcourse corrective action while we are still in the early part of phase 2 in the evolution of large multicenter trials by highlighting some of the unexpected lessons learned from these trials so that we may abbreviate the process and move quickly to phase 5. Therefore, the expected findings and other positive findings that have been discussed elsewhere[1, 5–19] will not help in the goal of this editorial and will not be reviewed here.

Therapeutic modalities: role of industry. Although randomized clinical trials have proved to be a great success in the short-term evaluation of pharmaceutical agents, their application to procedures and other therapeutic modalities has not been entirely successful. Industry support of studies is very important, but industry control of data is potentially a major problem and source of serious concern and misgiving.[20–24]

Importance of small, short-lived clinical trials. The two randomized trials of coronary bypass surgery for unstable angina provide an illustrative example. The Portland Veterans Administration Study was designed as a 4 month randomized trial from a single institution to evaluate whether "urgent" bypass surgery was superior to medical therapy in the short term. A small number of patients underwent randomization; in 1975, patient entry was completed and the data were published.[25] The results showed that "urgent" coronary bypass surgery was not superior to medical therapy with regard to short-term survival and prevention of myocardial infarction but was much better for relief of symptoms and relief of ischemia that was documented objectively.[9] In the National Cooperative Study (a large multicenter trial), patient entry was completed in 1976; initial data published in 1978[26] confirmed the findings of the Portland VA Study. Preliminary 5 year follow-up data from the National Cooperative Study were presented in 1982[27] but have not yet been published, 9 years after patient entry was completed. The crossover rate from the medical to surgical therapy in this multicenter trial was more than 40%, and therefore there is concern about the true clinical value of its long-term findings. Both trials likely excluded the high-risk patient,[9] limiting their clinical applicability only to patients at comparatively low risk. Thus, in certain circumstances most of the useful information can be obtained from small, short-lived, low-cost randomized clinical trials.

Importance of subsidiary results. It appears likely that the Multicenter Investigation of Limitation of Infarct

From the Section of Cardiology, Department of Medicine, LAC-USC Medical Center, University of Southern California School of Medicine, Los Angeles.

Address for correspondence: S. H. Rahimtoola, M.B., Chief, Section of Cardiology, University of Southern California, 2025 Zonal Ave., Los Angeles, CA 90033.

Common Time Course of
Ideas, Diagnostic Procedures, Therapies, etc.

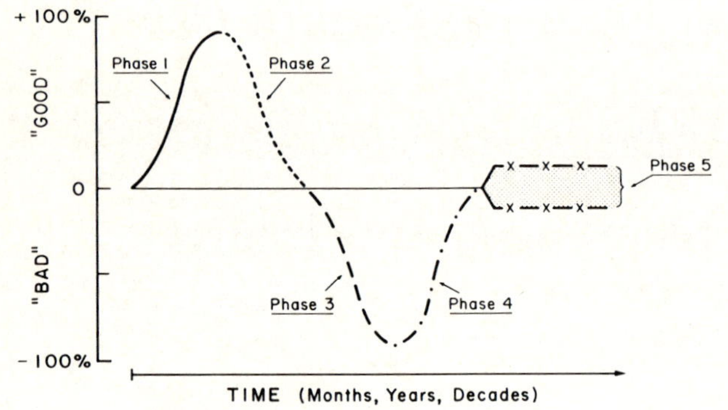

Phase 1: Euphoria
Phase 2: Doubt and Uncertainty
Phase 3: Disillusionment
Phase 4: Reflection
Phase 5: Reality

FIGURE 1. Frequently observed course after introduction of procedures, therapies, ideas, etc.

Size (MILIS) trial will not demonstrate a beneficial effect of interventions that are being evaluated.[28] However, it has already demonstrated that estimation of infarct size by creatine kinase levels correlated well with infarct size estimated at autopsy,[29] emphasizing the importance of well-planned trials that increase the likelihood of yielding at least some valuable information.

Importance of hypotheses not tested. The great enthusiasm with which the results of the trials of coronary bypass surgery for chronic stable angina have been publicized has brought at least three issues regarding "medical" therapy of angina into sharp focus:

(1) Are we administering optimal medical therapy? The incidence of various risk factors such as hypertension, hypercholesterolemia, and overweight in both the medically and surgically assigned groups in the Coronary Artery Surgery Study (CASS) was similar before randomization and 5 years later,[30] suggesting that medical therapy in these research studies left a great deal to be desired; similar data are not available from other trials of bypass surgery.[10] How is it that research studies provided such a low level of excellence of therapy? It is likely that in routine clinical practice medical therapy may not be much better. Should we not be emphasizing our deficiencies in this regard and working to improve the situation?[11]

(2) What is the evidence that pharmacologic therapy of angina improves long-term survival? There are no randomized trials, to my knowledge, that demonstrate that pharmacologic therapy of angina improves survival at 1, 5, or 10 years in patients with stable angina.[10] It is likely that pharmacologic therapy does not improve survival in patients with unstable angina.[9] In fact, the secondary prevention trials (for example, the Beta-Blocker Heart Attack Trial [BHAT]) have demonstrated no benefit of the trial pharmacologic agents in the low-risk group.[31] Thus, in some subgroups of patients treated with pharmacologic agents, the patients are exposed to the complications of such drugs with no demonstrable beneficial effects; pharmacologic therapy cannot be considered to be without risk. I guess the "genie" of the pharmacologic therapy of angina has been "out of the bottle"[32, 33] for so long that we have failed to notice it. Again, should we not be working to correct the situation?

(3) If the above are correct perceptions, namely that risk-factor control in randomized trials of coronary bypass surgery were inadequate and pharmacologic therapy of angina is of unproven value in prolonging life, then the possibility exists that survival data in randomized trials of bypass surgery were a comparison of surgery with placebo.[10]

In view of all of the above, the extremists who state that the benefits of coronary bypass surgery can be shown *only* by randomized clinical trials exposes all of us to the risk of being accused of practicing a double standard, one for surgical therapy and another for therapy administered by internists and cardiologists.

Inappropriate conclusions and extrapolations. Inappropriate conclusions and extrapolations are the major clinical problem of the large multicenter randomized trials. Many conclusions and extrapolations are inappropriate because of problems in study design, data analysis, and presentation.[10, 34]

Biostatistical tenets. Biostatisticians state, without experimental proof, that the correct way to analyze data from randomized trials is by therapy assigned rather than by therapy administered. In trials of bypass surgery that have a significant crossover problem[10] (and that have demonstrated better relief of pain and ischemia, less need of pharmacologic therapy, and better survival in subgroups assigned to surgery[9, 10]), analysis by therapy assigned results in: (1) improving the results of "medical" therapy, (2) changing the hypothesis actually tested (figure 2), and (3) reducing the clinical relevance of the findings. In clinical practice, the patient and physician are interested in therapy administered and not in therapy assigned; analysis by therapy assigned is of great interest to biostatisticians, but they do not have the responsibility of providing clinical care. Should not biostatisticians do experimental studies to prove their tenets are correct?[10]

Arbitrary p values. P values estimate the probability of the observed findings being due to chance; considering

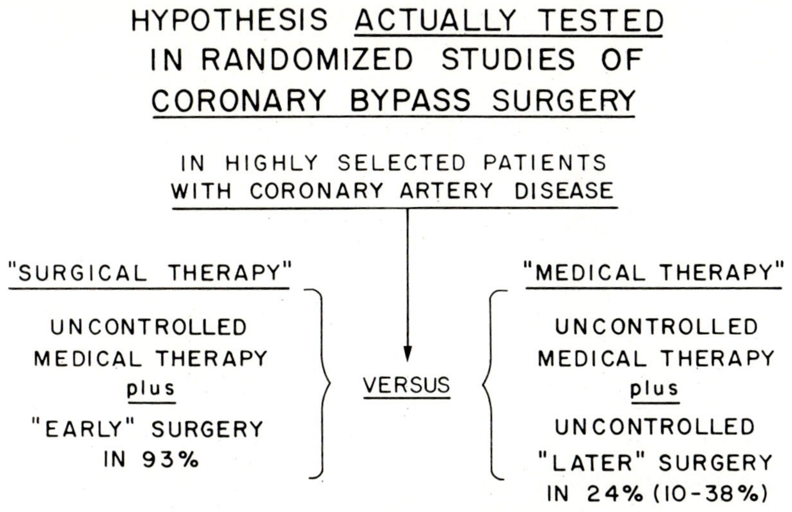

FIGURE 2. Analysis of results of randomized clinical trials by therapy assigned changes the hypothesis actually tested. Since 10% to 38% of patients in the medical group received coronary bypass surgery, this group cannot be called "medical group" or "medical therapy." Likewise, 7% of patients in the "surgical group" did not receive bypass. Therefore these groups should be called by their correct names, "medically assigned group" and "surgically assigned group."

only p values of ≤ .05 as significant is arbitrary.[35] This has been carried too far[10] where a p value of .057 is now considered nonsignificant.[36] We need to move away from such extreme positions. P values of ≥ .5 are clearly nonsignificant and those of ≥ .33 are probably nonsignificant, but where do we draw the line, or can we draw the line, between .33 and .05? We need to come to a reasonable position on this matter or the expression "statistically nonsignificant" may eventually lose its value. P values should be published and the readers should make up their minds about significance.[37] I suggest that journal editors insist the authors provide p values up to .1.

The problem of bias. The major advantage of a randomized trial is the exclusion of bias in the assignment of therapy, and these trials are indeed free of bias at the moment of randomization.[10] However, in practice the large multicenter trials have not been free of bias before and also after randomization because they have not included many, and in some instances the majority of,[36, 38] eligible patients and have allowed a high percentage of patients to cross over in an uncontrolled, subjective manner.[10]

Moreover, the goals of the study and biostatistical methods have at times been altered as the study progresses and also when the final data analysis becomes available.[12] In some studies, methods of data analysis follow the protocol of the study in some instances[30, 36] but not in others.[39] Both of these actions demonstrate additional sources of bias.

The inhomogeneity of patients undergoing randomization. An idealized situation is one in which all patients undergoing randomization are homogeneous with regard to all major factors known to influence the end points of the study. This reduces the numbers of patients available for study at any one center. The large multicenter trial has been the answer to this problem, but it has the problem of uneven quality of diagnostic and therapeutic procedures between the centers participating in the trial; moreover, even the large multicenter trials have failed to recruit enough patients, particularly in many of the subgroups.[10]

To overcome these disadvantages, "epidemiologic" multicenter trials that have huge numbers of patients has been considered the answer. However, in these studies the patients are not characterized in adequate detail because it is not practical or feasible to study so many patients with the more appropriate clinical tests that require high levels of skill and expertise and are also more expensive; therefore, their findings are difficult to extrapolate in clinical practice to an individual patient. Moreover, these studies also enter only a small fraction of patients (for example, the BHAT enrolled 23% of patients after myocardial infarction)[38]; therefore their findings cannot be extrapolated "epidemiologically" to all patients with that particular disorder without proof.

Presentation of data. In the Lipid Research Center–Coronary Primary Prevention Trial (LRC-CPPT)[40] and the BHAT,[38] the beneficial effect of cholestyramine and propranolol was presented as a percent reduction in percent of coronary deaths and total deaths, respectively (figure 3). Percent of a percent is an interesting but dubious mathematical calculation! The actual difference by life-table analysis in the two studies at the end of 7 and 2 years, respectively, was 1.6% in cardiac mortality[40] and 2.1% in total deaths.[38] In CASS,[36] the improvement in mortality in the surgically assigned group of patients with mild angina and left ventricular ejection fraction of 0.35 to 0.49 was 11% at 5 years and represented a 73% reduction in mortality, but the data were not presented in a manner similar to the

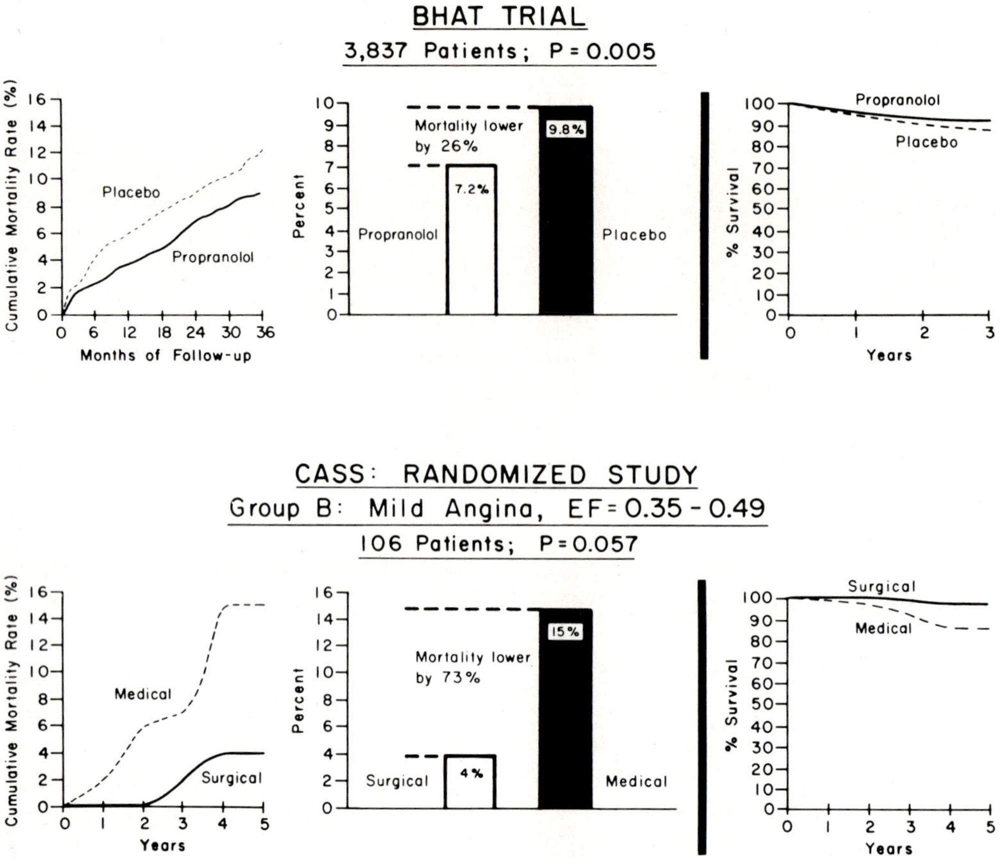

FIGURE 3. Data from the BHAT[38] and CASS[36] are redrawn so that they are presented uniformly. EF = ejection fraction.

LRC-CPPT and the BHAT studies (figure 3). The magnitude of the improvement in the CASS was not emphasized,[36] perhaps because the p value for the difference was .057. It is not unusual for investigators to present data in a manner that best supports their beliefs and conclusions. However, it is important that the National Institutes of Health not be a party to such biases; journal reviewers and editors should be especially vigilant and take appropriate corrective action. If we do not do so in a timely manner, we run the risk of building a significant credibility problem with the people of the United States because such manipulations and hyperbole will eventually become known to them and they will react adversely to the whole medical profession.

For reasons cited above, it is especially important that we be very careful about conclusions and extrapolations of the findings from large multicenter trials.[10] For example, it is inappropriate to conclude from the BHAT study that propranolol is indicated for all patients after myocardial infarction. In fact, as discussed earlier, the low-risk group that may constitute 50% or more of patients who have recovered from acute myocardial infarction[31] would be at risk for complications of β-blocker therapy[38] without any benefit[31] if they were treated with β-blockers. In CASS, low-risk patients underwent randomization,[10, 34] and in the group of patients with left ventricular ejection fractions of 0.35 to 0.49 there were only 19, 63, and 78 randomized patients with one-, two-, and three-vessel disease, respectively.[10] Therefore it is important that results of the CASS not be applied to patients at higher risk,[34] and special note should be made that the numbers of patients in many of the subgroups were inadequate to prove or disprove the benefit of surgery.[10] It is inappropriate to claim from the results of the LRC-CPPT that reduction of serum cholesterol by diet in patients with mild-to-moderate hypercholesterolemia will reduce mortality due to coronary heart disease.[11, 12]

Investigators and administrators who participate in long-term clinical trials have put in an enormous amount of effort and want to be recognized for their efforts. It is difficult for them to view objectively their product, which had a gestation of 10 years or more. We must have compassion for the investigators and administrators of these trials of long gestation; however, their unbridled enthusiasm must be controlled and kept in perspective. Should they be allowed to comment on their own studies?[41] Probably not[12]; others should do so.[2, 8–19, 42, 43] Investigators and administrators of large multicenter trials often hold important positions in volunteer and federally funded health agencies and in medical societies. They should be especially careful not to comment or participate in discussions of the relevant clinical trials in their role as spokespersons of health agencies and medical societies to abort suggestions of conflict of interest.

Monitoring of clinical trials. It is customary for a policy board and/or monitoring committee to be set up that is supposed to monitor a multicenter trial.[36] The BHAT study was stopped because of a statistically significant beneficial effect of propranolol, many months after the results of the timolol study[44] were published; therefore, time was available for thought. Before the BHAT study was stopped, the treated group could have been randomized into continued treated and placebo subgroups, which would have provided information on the benefits, if any, of continued β-blocker treatment. This would have provided valuable clinical information about the required duration of therapy. A golden research opportunity that may never arise again was missed, probably because committees are a poor mechanism for innovative thought.[11, 45] In view of the multitude of problems with clinical trials, one has to question whether the formation, function, and authority of monitoring boards is adequate?

The young investigator. Perhaps the most important lesson and one that causes the greatest concern is the negative impact of the large randomized trials on the young investigator. The clinical investigator is considered to be an endangered species.[45, 46] These trials represent an enormous commitment of time, patients, and resources; as a result, they stifle creativity and ongoing research. They also provide the wrong training about how to do research. Traditional training about the mechanics of research is as follows: (1) formulate a hypothesis, (2) design studies to answer the question(s), (3) perform the study and collect data meticulously and precisely, (4) analyze the data, (5) present the findings at scientific meetings, and (6) publish the study in a peer-reviewed journal. The investigators then receive credit for their work from their peers. In multicenter trials, the young investigator(s) recruits the patients, does the studies, collects the data, and sends it to the data coordinating center, all of which represents a major commitment of their time and effort. Others (advisory committees, principal investigators, data coordinating center, steering committees, policy boards, and funding agency staff) do the rest. In one trial the chairman of the steering committee and in another a staff member authored a large number of publications, but most of the (young) investigators authored none; if these "administrators" want to do research, should they not become investigators and compete with other scientists? It is worth remembering that promotions committee(s) at universities correctly assign no academic credit to the (young) investigator for being a cog in the wheel of a clinical trial and for publications that have 10 or more authors.

I am deeply concerned about another entirely pernicious attitude toward clinical research that has been germinated and is being fostered, albeit unintentionally. This is the approach of entering a huge amount of data into the data bank of a multicenter trial or of registries with the aim of asking questions in the future or just seeing what turns out to be significant. There is no study design in such approaches, which are anti-intellectual. Are such efforts research? Registry data have provided a lot of useful information[47, 48] but their limitations (in spite of good study design) must always be kept in mind.[49, 50] If a study is not well designed, it is wishful thinking to believe that computers and statistics will provide solutions to errors of study design (for example, bias of patient entry into study, bias in allocation of therapy, bias in changing therapy, bias in data analysis, and evaluation of outcomes between groups that were not identical in most if not all major and relevant characteristics at the start of the study) by complex statistical adjustments,[51, 52] e.g., by control of covariates.

Summary and recommendations. Large multicenter randomized clinical trials are very useful and have provided important information. They are most easily applied to assessing efficacy of short-term therapy, particularly of pharmacologic agents. Industry control of the data is potentially a major problem.

Multicenter trials are clearly beset with many problems. They are not scientifically innovative and usually provide no real "new" information. Many recent trials have only stirred more controversy rather than provide clinically meaningful answers.[1] Clinical trials are slow, ponderous, and expensive.[1] Frequently, rapid evolution leads to obsolescence of treatments and of hypotheses that are being tested; moreover, declining incidence of morbidity and mortality often precludes the ability to prove or disprove the hypotheses that are being tested.

Inappropriate conclusions and extrapolations are the greatest clinical danger of large clinical trials, which combined with the untempered enthusiasm of those involved with the study may eventually lead to a significant credibility gap for the whole profession. Investigators and administrators must meticulously avoid conflicts of interest. Randomized trials are contributing to the plight of the young investigator, albeit unintentionally, which is the single most important problem of these studies.

It is better for us to think "small." We need to dissect out questions of interest and do research studies and, if necessary, perform small randomized trials to answer these questions. We should bank on innovative ideas, high-quality original investigators, and proven scientifiic leaders who continue to be innovative and productive, and let them perform studies that are of interest. We must protect the young investigator.

The large multicenter randomized clinical trials should be considered a last resort to obtaining answers; they are needed in carefully selected circumstances and should follow the following guidelines:

(1) The hypothesis to be tested should be clearly stated in writing at the outset. It should be determined whether the hypothesis is important and that the only way to test the hypothesis is to perform a clinical trial. The feasibility of such a trial successfully answering the questions that need resolution must be critically evaluated.

(2) The final protocol of the trial should undergo the same rigorous, independent scientific review as other research grant applications.

(3) This final protocol should be published rapidly so that it is available for review when the results are eventually published.

(4) The monitoring of the multicenter trial must be improved and strengthened. Those monitoring the trial should be held accountable and therefore must be given appropriate authority.

(5) Only the young investigators (those 45 years old or younger?) should present the design, protocol, and results of clinical trials at scientific and other meetings and should author the publications. Older investigators, members, and chairmen of policy and/or monitoring boards, staff, and chairmen of steering committees should be explicitly and strictly excluded from these functions.

(6) Data should be first presented at scientific meetings and in peer-reviewed journals. Scientific sessions program committees should select young investigators for invited presentations; investigators and administrators should avoid possible conflict of interest. "Hoopla,"[45] hyperbole, and inappropriate conclusions and extrapolations must be assiduously avoided.

(7) Data storage, analysis, and presentation should not be under the control of industry.

References

1. Feinstein AR: Current problems and future challenges in randomized clinical trials. Circulation **70:** 767, 1984
2. Fisher RA, MacKenzie WA: Studies in crop variation. II. The manurial response to different potato varieties. J Agric Sci **13:** 315, 1923
3. Kohn KH, Milzer A, Maclean H: Prophylaxis of recurrence of rheumatic fever with penicillin given orally: final report of a five-year study. JAMA **151:** 347, 1953
4. Veterans Administration Cooperative Study Group on Antihypertensive Agents: Effects of treatment on morbidity in hypertension: results in patients with diastolic blood pressure averaging 115 through 129 mm Hg. JAMA **202:** 1028, 1967
5. Feinstein AR: An additional basic science for clinical medicine. II. The limitations of randomized trials. Ann Intern Med **99:** 544, 1983
6. Feinstein AR, Horwitz RJ: Double standards, scientific methods, and epidemiologic research. N Engl J Med **307:** 1611, 1982
7. Comstock GW: Reviews and commentary: Uncontrolled ruminations on modern controlled trials. Am J Epidemiol **108:** 81, 1978
8. Rahimtoola SH: Coronary bypass surgery for chronic angina — 1981. A perspective. Circulation **65:** 225, 1982
9. Rahimtoola SH: Coronary bypass surgery for unstable angina. Circulation **69:** 842, 1984
10. Rahimtoola SH: A perspective on the three large multicenter (VA, ECSS, CASS) randomized clinical trials of coronary bypass surgery for chronic stable angina. Circulation (in press; suppl to Dec. 1985 issue)
11. Rahimtoola SH: Cholesterol and coronary heart disease: a perspective. JAMA **253:** 2094, 1985 (Editorial)
12. Kronmal R: Commentary on the published results of the Lipid Research Clinics Coronary Primary Prevention Trial. JAMA **253:** 2091, 1985
13. Braunwald E: Coronary artery surgery at the crossroads. N Engl J Med **297:** 661, 1977
14. Harland WR, Stross JK: An educational view of a national initiative to lower plasma lipid levels. JAMA **253:** 2087, 1985
15. Feinstein AR: The scientific and clinical tribulations of randomized clinical trials. Clin Res **26:** 241, 1978
16. Chalmers TC, Smith H Jr, Ambroz A, Reitman D, Schroeder BJ: In defense of the VA randomized control trial of coronary artery surgery. Clin Res **26:** 230, 1978
17. Braunwald E: Effects of coronary artery bypass grafting on survival: implications of the randomized Coronary Artery Surgery Study. N Engl J Med **309:** 1181, 1983
18. Braunwald E: Treatment of the patient after myocardial infarction: the last decade and the next. N Engl J Med **302:** 290, 1980 (Editorial)
19. Braunwald E, Muller JE, Klones RA, Maroko PR: Role of beta-adrenergic blockade in the therapy of patients with myocardial infarction. Am J Med **74:** 113, 1983
20. The Anturane Reinfarction Trial Research Group: Sulfinpyrazone in the prevention of sudden death after myocardial infarction. N Engl J Med **302:** 250, 1980
21. Temple R, Pledger GW: The FDA's critique of the Anturane Reinfarction Trial. N Engl J Med **303:** 1488, 1980
22. Relman AS: Sulfinpyrazone after myocardial infarction: no decision yet. N Engl J Med **303:** 1476, 1980 (Editorial)
23. The Anturane Reinfarction Trial Policy Committee: The Anturane Reinfarction Trial: reevaluation of outcome. N Engl J Med **306:** 1005, 1982
24. Hood WB Jr: More on sulfinpyrazone after myocardial infarction. N Engl J Med **306:** 988, 1982 (Editorial)
25. Selden R, Neill WA, Ritzmann LW, Okies JE, Anderson RP: Medical vs. surgical therapy for acute coronary insufficiency: a randomized study. N Engl J Med **293:** 1329, 1975
26. Unstable angina pectoris: National cooperative study group to compare surgical and medical therapy. II. Inhospital experience and initial follow-up results in patients with one-, two-, and three vessel disease. Am J Cardiol **42:** 839, 1978
27. Conti R, Becker L, Biddle T, Hutter A, Resnekov L, Rosati R, Russell R, Schroeder R, Wolk M, Louis T, Mock M: Unstable angina: NHLBI Cooperative Study Group to compare medical and surgical therapy: long-term morbidity and mortality. Am J Cardiol **49:** 1007, 1982 (abst)
28. Muller J, Roberts R, Stone P, Rude R, Raabe D, Gold H, Jaffe A, Strauss W, Turi Z, Hartwell T, Poole K, Passamani E, Willerson J,

Sobel B, Braunwald E and MILIS Group: Failure of propranolol administration to limit infarct size in patients with acute myocardial infarction. Circulation **68**(suppl III). III-294, 1983 (abst)
29. Hackel DB, Reimer KA, Idekar RE, Mikat AM, Hartwell TD, Parker CB, Braunwald EB, Buja M, Gold HK, Jaffe AS, Muller JE, Raabe DS, Rude RE, Sobel BE, Stone PH, Roberts R, and the MILIS Study Group: Comparsion of enzymatic and anatomic estimates of myocardial infarct size in man. Circulation **70:** 824, 1984
30. CASS Principal Investigators and their Associates: Coronary Artery Surgery Study (CASS): a randomized trial of coronary artery bypass surgery. Quality of life in patients randomly assigned to treatment groups. Circulation **68:** 951, 1983
31. Furberg C, Hawkins CM, Lichstein E: Effect of propranolol in postinfarction patients with mechanical or electrical complication. Circulation **69:** 761, 1984
32. Braunwald E: Direct coronary revascularization: a plea not to let the genie escape from the bottle. Hosp Pract **6:** 9, 1971
33. Muller JE, Stone PH, Markis JE, Braunwald E: Let's not let the genie escape from the bottle — again. N Engl J Med **304:** 1294, 1981
34. Rahimtoola SH: Are the findings from the randomized Coronary Artery Surgery Study (CASS) of value in the management of high-risk patients soon after acute myocardial infarction? Am J Cardiol July 1985 (Editorial)
35. Fisher RA: The design of experiments, ed 8. London, 1966, Oliver and Boyd, p 13
36. CASS Principal Investigators and their Associates: Coronary Artery Surgery Study (CASS): a randomized trial of coronary artery bypass surgery. Survival data. Circulation **68:** 939, 1983
37. Mather K: Statistical analysis in biology, ed 5. London, 1966, Meuthaen & Co. Ltd., p 21.
38. β-Blocker Heart Attack Trial Research Group: A randomized trial of propranolol in patients with acute myocardial infarction. I. Mortality results. JAMA **247:** 1707, 1982
39. CASS Principal Investigators and their Associates: Myocardial infarction and mortality in the Coronary Artery Surgery Study (CASS) Randomized Trial. N Engl J Med **310:** 750, 1984
40. Lipid Research Clinics Program: The Lipid Research Clinics coronary primary prevention trial results. JAMA **251:** 351, 1984
41. Killip T, Ryan TJ: Randomized trials in coronary bypass surgery. Circulation **71:** 418, 1985
42. Roberts WC, Manning DM: The Coronary Artery Surgery Study (CASS): do the results apply to your patient? Am J Cardiol **54:** 440, 1984
43. Gunnar RM, Loeb HS: An alternative interpretation of the results of the coronary artery surgery study. Circulation **71:** 193, 1985
44. The Norwegian Multicenter Study Group: Timolol-induced reduction in mortality and reinfarction in patients surviving acute myocardial infarction. N Engl J Med **304:** 801, 1981
45. Rahimtoola SH: The twenty-fifth anniversary of valve replacement: a time for reflection. Circulation **71:** 1, 1985
46. Wyngaarden JB: The clinical investigator as an endangered species. Presidential address. Association of American Physicians, May 1979. N Engl J Med **301:** 1254, 1979
47. Kannel WB, Sorlie P, McNamara PH: Prognosis after initial myocardial infarction: The Framingham Study. Am J Cardiol **44:** 53, 1979
48. Pell S, Fayerweather WE: Trends in the incidence of myocardial infarction and in associated mortality and morbidity in a large employed population, 1957–1983. N Engl J Med **312:** 1005, 1985
49. McAnulty JH, Rahimtoola SH, Murphy E, DeMots H, Ritzman L, Kanarek PE, Kauffman S: Natural history of "high-risk" bundle branch block: final report of a prospective study. N Engl J Med **307:** 137, 1982
50. Bhandari AK, Rahimtoola SH: Indications for cardiac pacing in patients with bradyarrhythmias: do we know all the answers? JAMA **252:** 1327, 1984 (Editorial)
51. Alderman EL, Fisher LD, Litwin P, Kaiser GC, Myers WO, Maynard C, Levine F, Schloss M: Results of coronary artery surgery in patients with poor left ventricular function (CASS). Circualtion **68:** 785, 1983
52. Hammermeister KE, DeRouen TA, Dodge HT: Comparison of survival of medically and surgically treated coronary disease patients in Seattle Heart Watch: a nonrandomized study. Circulation **65**(suppl II): II-53, 1982

PERSPECTIVE

Atherosclerosis, calcium, and calcium antagonists

PHILIP D. HENRY, M.D.

ALTHOUGH it has been generally recognized that atherosclerosis is associated with a deposition of calcium in the arterial wall, the pathogenic significance of this calcification remains unclear. In recent years, a number of calcium-chelating agents, lanthanum chloride, and organic calcium antagonists have been shown to exert antiatherogenic effects in animals with dietary hypercholesterolemia. This brief review discusses possible interrelations between arterial calcification and atherogenesis, and summarizes some of the data in the literature on the effects of chelating and calcium antagonistic agents.

Deposition of calcium salts in the walls of human arteries begins in childhood and progresses with age. Electron microscopic studies of human atherosclerotic arteries have shown that calcification in the media and intima is associated with extracellular membranous vesicles structurally resembling matrix vesicles in bone and other calcifying tissues.[1] These vesicles contain noncristalline particles and needle-shaped crystals that have the diffraction patterns of apatite.[1] The membranous structures occur in the vicinity of degenerating cells that enclose similar vesicular formations. This suggests that calcifying vesicles represent the debris of mitochondria and other organelles from degenerating medial and intimal cells. The biochemical composition of the membranes has not yet been determined, but it appears likely that phospholipids constitute an important component. It is of interest that atheromatous lesions contain a vitamin K–dependent (γ-carboxyglutamic acid–containing) calcium-binding protein that appears to be functionally analogous but structurally dissimilar to osteocalcin.[2] Like γ-carboxyglutamic acid–containing proteins of the blood clotting system, this protein may bind calcium and phospholipid and play a role in regulating the calcification of atherosclerotic plaques. Results of the studies cited above are based on analysis of material obtained at autopsy and prepared by conventional histologic techniques, a procedure that does not satisfactorily preserve the physical state and localization of electrolytes in soft tissues. Additional investigations in which rapidly frozen (frozen-hydrated) samples and electron-probe microanalysis are used are needed, since with these techniques it would be possible to determine if calcium in degenerating macrophages and smooth muscle cells accumulates in the mitochondria, as has been demonstrated in other syndromes associated with cell necrosis.

Blumenthal et al.[3] were among the first to point out that in the human aorta medial calcification (or other processes altering vascular elastance, such as syphylitic aortitis) is a structural alteration always preceding the development of intimal plaques. A similar sequence of events is observed in rabbits and swine fed vitamin D in doses inducing little or no hypercalcemia.[4] In these normolipidemic animals atherosclerotic lesions appear only months after fibromuscular changes, cell necrosis, and calcifications have developed. Recent findings with regard to the influence of mechanical factors on atherogenesis suggest that arterial stiffness may play a role in the localization and development of atheromas.[5] The relationship between the physical properties of arteries, fluid mechanics, and atherogenesis will require further investigative attention. In addition, the possibility must be considered that crystalline deposits alter the deformability of atheromatous lesions. In coronary arteries, vessels subjected to continual bending movements, crystalline bodies could be traumatic to surrounding soft tissues and cause acute structural changes such as plaque hemorrhage or rupture. It has been recently reemphasized that the dense neovascularization of atheromas may render the artery susceptible to intramural hemorrhage, a possible mechanism of coronary thrombosis.[6]

Recently, evidence has accumulated indicating that calcium antagonists may protect muscle and nonmuscle cells by a variety of pathophysiologic processes. Protective effects have been reported in ischemic, cytotoxic, and degenerative syndromes involving skeletal muscle, myocardium, brain, liver, kidney, intes-

From the Section of Cardiology, Baylor College of Medicine, Houston.

Supported in part by grants HL31487 and HL31488 from the National Institutes of Health, Bethesda.

Address for correspondence: Philip D. Henry, M.D., Section of Cardiology, The Methodist Hospital, Suite F-905, Baylor College of Medicine, 6535 Fannin St., Houston, TX 77030.

tine, and the eye.[7] The fact that calcium antagonists have a protective effect supports the notion that excessive calcium uptake, in particular mitochondrial calcium overload, plays a role in mediating cell death after various insults. An important question is whether there are membrane physiologic alterations in atherosclerosis that might favor an excessive uptake of calcium. It is well established that modest changes in membrane lipids may alter the functional characteristics of membrane proteins such as ion channels, ion transporters, and receptors. The importance of the abundance of membrane cholesterol in regulating the functional characteristics of membranes has been well demonstrated in red blood cells and platelets. Certain membrane enzymes, such as ATPase transporters, appear to be particularly sensitive to changes in membrane cholesterol.[8, 9] Recently Locher et al.[9] have demonstrated in human red blood cells that increases in membrane cholesterol augment the entry of calcium through a channel that can be blocked with a dihydropyridine calcium antagonist. Inspired by experiments relating changes in membrane lipids to calcium uptake we performed experiments with isolated canine coronary arteries incubated in a high-cholesterol environment.[8] Arteries exposed to low concentrations of cholesterol in aqueous solution (10^{-12}M) or to human low-density lipoprotein underwent slow contractions and preincubation of arteries with cholesterol sensitized the arteries to the constrictor effects of calcium over a wide range of external calcium concentrations. The uptake of radioactive cholesterol associated with these changes in arterial reactivity was very low. The fact that the constrictor effects of cholesterol were blocked by calcium antagonists and that sterols structurally closely related to cholesterol were ineffective suggested to us that cholesterol did not act by a simple detergent effect. Our findings support the hypothesis that physiologic changes in membranes caused by a high-cholesterol environment may favor calcium uptake by arterial smooth muscle.

Interrelations between membrane lipids, calcium uptake, and cell necrosis may be relevant to atherogenesis. Necrosis of arterial cells may play a pivotal role in the initiation, progression, and regression of atherosclerotic lesions.[10] Results of studies of coronary arteries of children and young adults support the view that cell death and accumulation of cellular debris in the intima are important features distinguishing early fibrotic plaques from the pure foam cell lesions (fatty streaks).[11] Cell death also results in the release of cytotoxic substances such as polar lipids and lytic enzymes, a process that may amplify cell necrosis and contribute to the stimulation of a fibroproliferative response.

If cell necrosis is an important process in the formation of atheroma and if cell death is mediated in part by changes in membranes that facilitate the intracellular accumulation of calcium, drugs capable of reducing calcium uptake might exert antiatherogenic effects. Almost 20 years ago, Wartman et al.[12] treated cholesterol-fed rabbits with subcutaneous injections of magnesium EDTA and concluded that this chelating agent suppressed the deposition of collagen and elastin in the arteries. Unfortunately, Wartman's experiments have to my knowledge never been repeated, but other chelating agents were subsequently tested for their antiatherogenic effects. Kramsch et al.[13] administered diphosphonic acid and thiophene derivatives to rabbits fed a high-cholesterol diet. The treatments did not influence serum cholesterol or triglycerides, but inhibited calcification, lipid accumulation, and plaque formation in arteries. In addition, these investigators demonstrated that $LaCL_3$ exerted antiatherogenic effects in rabbits and monkeys.[13]

In view of our considerations concerning altered calcium uptake in atherosclerosis and the therapeutic results obtained with chelating agents, we evaluated the effects of nifedipine, a calcium antagonist, on atherogenesis in rabbits with diet-induced atherosclerosis.[14] Rabbits were fed a 2% cholesterol diet for 8 weeks with or without treatment with oral nifedipine (40 mg/rabbit/day). High-dose oral nifedipine was well tolerated and produced modest transient hypotensive effects. Compared with rabbits receiving placebo, treated animals exhibited highly significant reductions in sudanophilic lesions, aortic total cholesterol, and aortic calcium. As with the chelating agents, the drug did not influence the hyperlipidemic response to the diet. Our findings were subsequently confirmed by Willis et al.,[15] who demonstrated that high-dose nicardipine and nifedipine produced substantial reductions in aortic lesions, aortic total cholesterol, and aortic triglyceride in cholesterol-fed rabbits. In another study, low-dose nifedipine (2 mg/rabbit/day) was reported to exert antiatherogenic effects in rabbits, although the number of animals studied was small.[16] Subsequently, calcium antagonists structurally unrelated to nifedipine, such as verapamil, diltiazem, and flunarizine, were demonstrated to exert antiatherogenic effects in cholesterol-fed rabbits.[17–19]

Two groups of investigators have failed to demonstrate that calcium antagonists exert antiatherogenic effects in cholesterol-fed rabbits. In the first study,[20] however, high-dose nifedipine was administered by the sublingual route, which may evoke severe hypotensive episodes and trigger a sympathetic discharge. The reflex release of catecholamines, agents that stimulate the uptake of calcium, may have promoted the intracellular accumulation of calcium. Such an effect would oppose the therapeutic action of calcium antagonists. There is evidence that antiadrenergic drugs such as reserpine, guanethidine, and propranolol suppress atherogenesis in cholesterol-fed rabbits.[21] In the second study,[22] in which calcium antagonists were found ineffective in suppressing atherogenesis in cholesterol-fed rabbits given antiadrenergic drugs, plaques of the whole aorta were approximately one-tenth to one-fifth of those reported in the literature.[13–19] Moreover, in two control groups receiving the same cholesterol diet, plaque areas expressed as a percent of the intimal area varied by more than 300% (4.4% vs 13.9%), a variation that would make the detection of significant effects in drug-treated groups difficult if not impossible.

The mechanism of action of chelating agents and calcium antagonists remains unclear. Calcium antagonists might exert antiatherogenic effects by reducing arterial pressure. In conscious normotensive rabbits, however, nifedipine administered by the oral route exerts only modest transient hypotensive effects.[14] Blumlein et al.[19] concluded that the antiatherogenic action of verapamil was unrelated to lowering of arterial pressure. Nakao et al.[23] have reported that the calcium antagonist nicardipine inhibits the migration of cultured vascular smooth muscle from rat aorta, an effect that might play a role in inhibiting atherogenesis. Recently Stein et al.[24] demonstrated that high concentrations of verapamil enhanced the receptor-mediated uptake and disposal of low-density lipoprotein (LDL) by aortic cells in culture. They proposed that verapamil-induced stimulation of receptors might aid in the removal of LDL cholesteryl esters from the aortic interstitium. An action of calcium antagonists via LDL receptors might explain why the Watanabe rabbit, an animal that lacks LDL receptors, does not respond favorably to nifedipine.[25] However, studies in Watanabe rabbits should be repeated in larger groups of animals receiving drug under controlled conditions. Recently, Etingin and Hajjar[26] demonstrated that nifedipine produced a 50% loss of cholesterol and cholesteryl esters from lipid-laden rabbit aortic smooth muscle in culture. They concluded that nifedipine decreased cholesterol and cholesteryl ester accumulation in arterial smooth muscle by increasing cholesteryl ester hydrolysis.

In summary, current evidence indicates that calcium-chelating (anticalcifying) agents and calcium antagonists (calcium-channel blockers) have antiatherogenic effects in rabbits and monkeys. The drugs exert their effects without reducing dietary hypercholesterolemia. Therefore, the mechanism of action differs from that of hypolipidemic interventions.

Clinical implications. For many years it has been claimed by some that the chelating agent EDTA exerts beneficial effects in patients suffering from coronary and peripheral artery disease. Unfortunately, treatment with EDTA has never been subjected to a controlled trial and no statement can be made regarding the efficacy of this controversial therapy. On the other hand, several controlled studies with calcium blockers have recently been initiated in North America and Europe. To my knowledge, the ongoing trials are all based on the evaluation of sequential coronary arteriograms of patients undergoing catheterization for symptomatic coronary disease. For such trials to be successful, patients in placebo groups will have to be kept off calcium antagonists, and patient groups will have to be matched with respect to antiadrenergic manipulations (β-adrenergic blockade), which may influence the progression of atherosclerosis.

The excellent assistance of Patricia Farrell in the preparation of this manuscript is gratefully acknowledged.

References

1. Tanimura A, McGregor DH, Anderson HC: Matrix vesicles in atherosclerotic calcification. Proc Soc Exp Biol Med **172:** 173, 1983
2. Levy RJ, Lian JB, Gallop PM: Atherocalcin, a γ-carboxyglutamic acid containing protein from atherosclerotic plaque. Biochem Biophys Res Commun **71:** 41, 1979
3. Blumenthal HT, Lansing AI, Wheeler PA: Calcification of the media of the human aorta and its relation to intimal arteriosclerosis, ageing, and disease. Am J Pathol **20:** 665, 1944
4. Toda T, Leszczynski DE, Kummerow FA: The role of 25-hydroxy-vitamin D_3 in the induction of atherosclerosis in swine and rabbit by hypervitaminosis D. Acta Pathol Jpn **33:** 37, 1983
5. Stehbens WE: Fluid dynamic approaches to atherosclerosis. In: Schettler G, Nerem RM, Schmid-Schoenbein H, Moerl H, Diehm C, editors: Fluid dynamics as a localizing factor for atherosclerosis. Berlin, 1983, Springer-Verlag, p 3
6. Barger AC, Beeuwkes R, Lainey LL, Silverman KJ: Hypothesis: vasa vasorum and neovascularization of human coronary arteries — a possible role in the pathophysiology of atherosclerosis. N Engl J Med **310:** 175, 1984
7. Henry PD, Perez JE: Clinical pharmacology of calcium antagonists. *In* Conti C, Brest AN, editors: Cardiac drug therapy. Philadelphia, 1984, F. A. Davis Co, p 93
8. Yokoyama M, Henry PD: Sensitization of isolated canine coronary arteries to calcium ions by exposure to cholesterol. Circ Res **45:** 479, 1979
9. Locher R, Neyses L, Stimpel M, Kueffer B, Vetter W: The cholesterol content of the human erythrocyte influences calcium influx through the channel. Biochem Biophy Res Commun **124:** 822, 1984
10. Thomas WA, Imai H, Florentin RA, Reiner JM, Scott RF: Smooth muscle and endothelial cell deaths in atherogenesis studied by autoradiography. Prog Biochem Pharmacol **14:** 234, 1977
11. Stary HC: Macrophages in coronary artery and intima and in

atherosclerotic lesions of children and young adults up to age 29. *In* Schettler FG, Gotto AM, Middelhoff G, Habenicht AJR, Jurutka KR, editors: Atherosclerosis VI. Berlin, 1983, Springer-Verlag, p 462
12. Wartman A, Lampe TL, McCann DS, Boyle AJ: Plaque reversal with MgEDTA in experimental atherosclerosis: elastin and collagen metabolism. J Atherosclerosis Res **7:** 331, 1967
13. Kramsch DM, Aspen AJ, Rozler LJ: Atherosclerosis: Prevention by agents not affecting abnormal levels of blood lipids. Science **213:** 1511, 1981
14. Henry PD, Bentley KL: Suppression of atherogenesis in cholesterol-fed rabbit treated with nifedipine. J Clin Invest **68:** 1366, 1981
15. Willis AL, Nagel B, Churchill V, Whyte MA, Smith DL, Mahmud I, Puppione D: Anti-atherosclerotic effects of nicardipine and nifedipine in cholesterol-fed rabbits. Arteriosclerosis **5:** 250, 1985
16. Panagiotopoulos S, Nayler WG: Calcium antagonists and the suppression of atherosclerosis. J Mol Cell Cardiol **16:** XIV, 1984
17. Rouleau JL, Parmley WW, Stevens J, Wikman-Coffelt J, Sievers R, Mahley RW, Havel RJ: Verapamil suppresses atherosclerosis in cholesterol-fed rabbits. J Am Coll Cardiol **1:** 1453, 1983
18. Ginsburg R, Davis K, Bristow MR, McKennet K, Kodsi SR, Billingham ME, Schroeder J: Calcium antagonists suppress atherogenesis in aorta but not in the intramural coronary arteries of cholesterol-fed rabbits. Lab Invest **49:** 154, 1983
19. Blumlein SL, Sievers R, Kidd P, Parmley WW: Mechanism of protection from atherosclerosis by verapamil in the cholesterol-fed rabbit. Am J Cardiol **54:** 884, 1984. Stender S, Stender I, Nordestgaard B, Kjeldsen K: No effect of nifedipine on atherogenesis in cholesterol-fed rabbits. Arteriosclerosis **4:** 389, 1984
20. Stender S, Stender I, Nordestgaard B, Kjeldsen K: No effect of nifedipine on atherogenesis in cholesterol-fed rabbits. Arteriosclerosis **4:** 389, 1984
21. Whittington-Coleman PJ, Carrier O, Douglas BH: The effects of propranolol on cholesterol-induced atheromatous lesions. Atherosclerosis **18:** 337, 1973
22. Naito M, Kuzuya F, Asai K, Shibata K, Yoshimine N: Ineffectiveness of Ca^{2+}-antagonists nicardipine and diltiazem on experimental atherosclerosis in cholesterol-fed rabbits. Angiology **35:** 622, 1984
23. Nakao J, Ito H, Oyama T, Chang WC, Murota S. Calcium dependency of aortic smooth muscle cell migration induced by 12-1-hydroxy-5, 8, 10, 14-eicosatetraenoic acid — effects of A23187, nicardipine, and trifluorperazine. Atherosclerosis **46:** 309, 1983
24. Stein O, Leitersdorf E, Stein Y: Verapamil enhances receptor-mediated endocytosis of low density lipoproteins by aortic cells in culture. Arteriosclerosis **5:** 35, 1985
25. Van Niekerk JLM, Hendriks T, De Boer HHM, Van't Laar A: Does nifedipine suppress atherogenesis in WHHL rabbits? Atherosclerosis **53:** 91, 1984
26. Etingin OR, Hajjar DP: Nifedipine increases cholesteryl ester hydrolytic activity in lipid-laden rabbit arterial smooth muscle cells: a possible mechanism for its anti-atherogenic effect. J Clin Invest **75:** 1554, 1985

PERSPECTIVE

The radiographic assessment of coronary blood flow parameters

ROBERT A. VOGEL, M.D.

TO HAVE a complete understanding of coronary artery disease, a clinician must be able to evaluate coronary anatomy, ventricular function, and coronary blood flow. Selective coronary arteriography and left ventriculography remain the standard means for obtaining information on the first two factors. Although visual analysis of percent diameter coronary stenosis suffers from significant intraobserver and interobserver variability, quantitative analysis of arteriographic images provides accurate and objective measurements of arterial geometry. The third factor, coronary blood flow, is rarely measured directly. Most often, alterations in blood flow are inferred clinically from the coronary anatomy. This inference is based on the close correlation between percent diameter stenosis and coronary flow reserve found in experimental animals, coronary flow reserve being defined as the ratio of maximal hyperemic-to-baseline blood flow in a coronary artery.[1] Contrary to these experimental observations are data suggesting that human coronary flow reserve correlates poorly with percent diameter stenosis and only moderately with absolute measurements of stenosis geometry.[2]

Recent developments in radiographic technology have therefore rekindled an interest in measuring coronary blood flow and flow reserve in the catheterization laboratory, with the intention of providing an independent means for their assessment. Results of preliminary trials suggest that this is possible, although contrast media cannot be used to measure coronary blood flow by traditional approaches. Early data also suggest that many factors in addition to epicardial arterial stenosis need to be considered in the clinical interpretation of blood flow parameters.

From the Cardiology Section, Veterans Administration Medical Center, and the Department of Medicine, University of Michigan Medical Center, Ann Arbor.

Supported in part by research funds of the Veterans Administration, Washington, DC, and the American Heart Association of Michigan, Lathrup Village, MI.

Address for correspondence: Robert A. Vogel, M.D., Chief, Cardiology Section, Veterans Administration Medical Center, 2215 Fuller Rd., Ann Arbor, MI 48105.

Technical aspects of measuring coronary blood flow. Direct measurements by electromagnetic flowmeter and radionuclide particle distribution can be made only in experimental animals. Most clinical methods for measuring regional blood flow or perfusion are based on one of the following principles: indicator-dilution (Stewart-Hamilton), inert substance washout (Kety-Schmidt), or first-pass distribution (Sapirstein).[3] Coronary sinus thermodilution, xenon-133 myocardial washout, and thallium-201 scintigraphy are representative examples of application of these three methods. However, none of these general principles can be used directly for the radiographic measurement of coronary blood flow largely because of the effects of the contrast medium on the coronary circulation and the method by which it is injected. Primarily, all of these methods require that the indicator substance does not affect the regional flow being measured.

Unlike the substances used in the traditional clinical methods, all contrast media have substantial vascular effects, although nonionic media may disturb blood flow less than ionic agents. The effects of a selectively injected bolus of ionic contrast medium on baseline and already hyperemic coronary blood flow are shown in figure 1.[4] Flow was measured by electromagnetic flowmeter and hyperemic flow was induced by a previously injected bolus of contrast medium given 10 sec before the period depicted. Even in the presence of free reflux of contrast into the sinus of Valsalva, a small increase in blood flow (usually $<10\%$) is often observed during the injection period. After this period of relatively constant flow, which lasts about 1.5 sec, a $54 \pm 10\%$ decrease in flow ensues, probably caused by the viscosity and hyperosmolality of the contrast medium as the bolus transits the microcirculation. The widely recognized hyperemic response then follows, raising baseline flow approximately threefold and already hyperemic flow by about 20%. Both curves peak at about 10 sec after contrast injection. The magnitude of the transient decrease in coronary flow after contrast injection is independent of the initial flow, which makes the early baseline-to-hyperemic flow ratio ap-

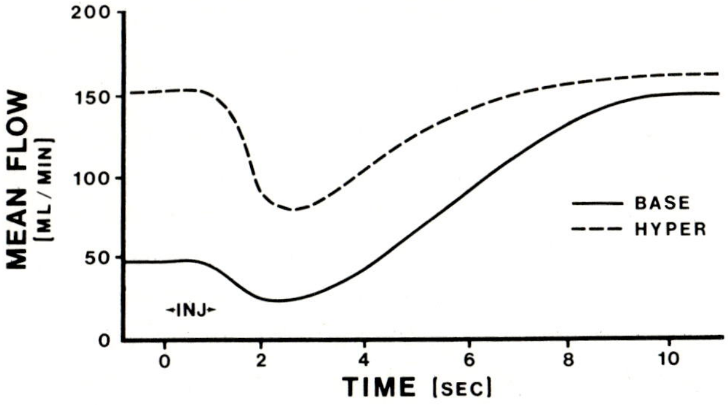

FIGURE 1. Mean baseline (BASE) and contrast-induced hyperemic (HYPER) coronary blood flow in a canine preparation after a selective injection of a 3 ml bolus of contrast medium (INJ).

proximately constant during this period. Thus radiographic measurements of absolute blood flow and relative flow ratios should be made during the first 1.5 and 5 sec contrast injection, respectively. This is analogous to the practice of measuring ventriculographic parameters soon after contrast injection to exclude the ventriculographic effects of the contrast medium.

Other problems exist with the use of contrast media as blood flow indicators. The Stewart-Hamilton principle requires administration of a fixed or known amount of an indicator, which must remain intravascular and detectable quantitatively downstream. Contrast media cannot be administered easily in fixed or known amounts without subselective injection to prevent reflux. Moreover, contrast media increase peripheral coronary intravascular volume as part of their vasodilator effect. This affects downstream contrast medium quantification by effectively increasing the vascular volume under study. Because of the complexities of contrast media diffusion, surface adherence, capillary sludging, and vasoreactivity, the requirement of tracer inertness necessary for application of the Kety-Schmidt principle is not fulfilled. Lastly, the factors of minimal first-pass uptake and regional variability of image intensifier veiling glare and radiation scatter and absorption make the use of the Sapirstein principle problematic.

Videodensitometry. Using alternative geometric approaches, Rutishauser et al.[5] and Smith and colleagues developed the first successful radiographic techniques for assessing regional coronary blood flow. These similar approaches measure the density of contrast medium at two sequential locations in a proximal coronary artery to determine the transit time of the contrast bolus between the two points. The volume of the arterial segment between the chosen points is then determined geometrically from the segment's mean diameter and length. The flow traversing the arterial segment is calculated from the segment's volume and the bolus' transit time with the following equation:

$$\text{Regional flow} = \text{Vascular volume/transit-time} \qquad (1)$$

This approach cannot be applied to branching, distal, or circuitous arterial segments. For segments that cannot be positioned parallel to the plane of the image intensifier, multiple radiographic projections must be used. Although it requires precise determinations of transit time and arterial diameter, this technique does measure absolute blood flow (ml/min). Using current technology, Spiller et al.[6] have recently reported excellent correlations between data obtained by electromagnetic flowmeter and mean and phasic blood flow measurements obtained by a similar approach. The reported technique uses determinations of wavefront transit time in opposition to the measurements of mean transit time used by the previous investigators. Use of measurements obtained during this earliest phase of contrast transit, before blood flow is perturbed by the contrast itself, gives this approach a theoretical advantage.

An indicator-dilution videodensitometric method, which measures relative coronary flow ratios rather than absolute blood flow, was reported by Foerster et al.[7] A fixed amount of contrast medium is injected, and indicator-dilutional analysis is performed on videodensitometric data obtained over an arterial region of interest. This approach eliminates the need for precise measurements of arterial diameter and length and can be applied to more distal arterial segments. It is complicated, however, by streaming and reflux of contrast medium. Using subselective contrast injection and linearized contrast density detection, Nissen and colleagues recently found this method to be valid.

Digital techniques. In an attempt to increase the detection of very low concentrations of contrast material, the technique of digital radiography was introduced during the last few years. This method consists of conversion of analog radiographic or fluoroscopic video images into digital arrays, with contrast enhancement being achieved through subsequent application of one of several arithmetic operations. The simplest enhancement operation is mask-mode subtraction, which is accomplished by subtracting a radiographic image obtained just before injection of contrast medium (mask) from each of the subsequent contrast-containing images. This eliminates densities common to the mask and subsequent frames, ideally leaving visualization of only the contrast-containing structures. With this approach, arterial structures can be visualized by either intravenous or reduced-dose intra-arterial administration of contrast medium. The quality of mask-mode subtraction images is very sensitive to subject motion, which alters the superposition of the mask and contrast-containing images and produces registration artifact. Because of the cyclic cardiac motion, registration artifact can be minimized by use of electrocardiogram (ECG)-synchronized mask selection.

The use of ECG-synchronized mask-mode subtraction for the purpose of measuring regional blood flow was first proposed by Robb and colleagues. These investigators demonstrated that digital substraction results in a significant increase in the ability to visualize contrast medium transit in its myocardial phase after selective coronary injection. Our laboratory has combined this approach with a modification of the vascular volume/transit time analysis of Rutishauser and Smith. We use color- and intensity-coded parametric images to depict the timing and density of a selectively injected bolus of contrast medium as it transits the coronary circulation.[8] *Relative* coronary flow ratios are assessed in myocardial regions of interest by quantitatively comparing parametric images obtained at baseline and during the hyperemic condition.

Regional time-density curves that serve as the basis for an understanding of this technique are shown in figure 2. Mean mask-mode subtracted radiographic time-density curves are shown for regions-of-interest over a proximal coronary artery, mid-to-distal myocardium perfused by this artery, and noncardiac background. These representative curves were obtained in a canine preparation with selective, ECG-synchronized power injections of contrast media under baseline and contrast-induced hyperemic conditions. The electromagnetic flowmeter ratio of hyperemic-to-baseline flow was approximately 3:1. Proximal arterial time-density curves are similar, suggesting accurate injection timing and complete displacement of the arterial blood with contrast medium. A significant level of background density is seen after about 5 sec, most likely caused by transit of contrast medium into the right heart circulation. This factor and the effects of contrast media on blood flow detailed above favor the use of data obtained within the first 5 sec after injection of contrast.

Measurement of relative regional coronary blood flow by means of the principle summarized in equation 1 requires independent assessment of both transit time and vascular volume.[8] Relative contrast medium transit time to myocardial regions of interest can be analyzed within the initial 5 sec period by application of a threshold criterion. Absolute transit-time probably cannot be measured with this approach because of perturbation of the contrast medium wavefront. Use of such a threshold criterion results in calculation of transit times T_b and T_h for the two myocardial curves shown. Considering equation 1, the fact that the transit time ratio for these values (1.6:1) is less than the flow ratio (3:1) suggests that the hyperemia-inducing stimulus does in fact increase the vascular volume.[8] As a first-order approximation, vascular volume can be estimated by the following radiographic relationship:

$$\text{Vascular volume} = k\ (\text{integrated contrast medium density}) / (\text{contrast medium concentration}) \qquad (2)$$

where k represents the primary radiographic imaging system transfer function. Assuming that the vascular space has been filled with contrast medium but that additional vasodilation or substantial diffusion has not yet occurred, vascular volume is then proportional to mask-mode subtracted density. Relative flow ratios can then be calculated by substitution of density data for vascular volume in equation 1. With use of density measurements at a time thought to meet these criteria (D_b and D_h) and transit times T_b and T_h, a 2.7:1 hyperemic-to-baseline flow ratio is calculated for the given case. Despite the difficulties associated with the use of contrast media and the densitometric rather than geometric assessment of relative vascular volume employed, a good correlation (r = .92) between electromagnetic flowmeter and digital radiographic determinations of relative regional coronary blood flow was found with the above method of analysis.[8] This approach does not appear to underestimate high flow ratios and was found to have adequate reproducibility (13%) and observer variability (r = .98). However, the interpretation of individual ratio values must

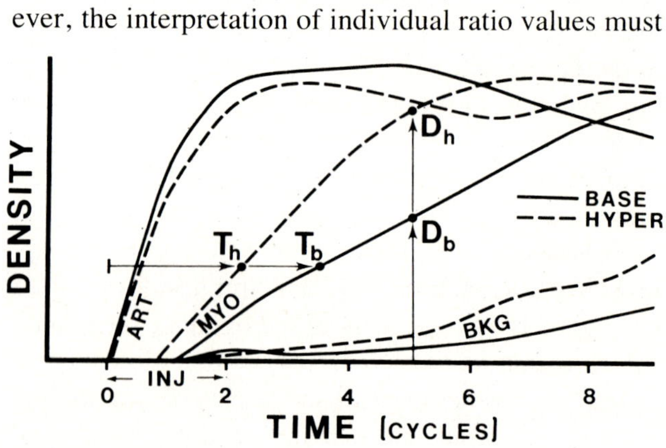

FIGURE 2. Mask-mode subtracted contrast medium time-density curves over proximal arterial (ART), mid-to-distal myocardial (MYO), and noncardiac background (BKG) regions of interest after selective injection of contrast medium (INJ) in a canine preparation under baseline (BASE) and contrast-induced hyperemic (HYPER) conditions. T_h and T_b = transit times; D_h and D_b = density values.

be performed with consideration to the ±0.7 ratio units 95% confidence limits found.

This approach can be implemented on a pixel-by-pixel basis with parametric images in which individual pixel color and intensity are modulated according to the transit-time and density values calculated for that pixel. Region-of-interest density/transit time values are then calculated as the mean of the individual pixel ratios, thus increasing precision by averaging several thousand ratios. Parametric images have the advantages of providing simultaneous visualization of the entire arterial bed undergoing analysis and recognition of problems in injection of contrast medium, such as streaming. Two clinical examples of parametric images obtained under baseline and contrast-induced hyperemic conditions are shown in figure 3. The color of each pixel is coded according to the number of cardiac cycles required for contrast medium transit: red, yellow, white, and green denote appearance within the first through the fourth cardiac cycles after injection, respectively. The intensity of each pixel is coded by information on contrast medium density.

An alternative digital radiographic method that measures relative coronary flow by the washout (Kety-Schmidt) principle has been suggested. Resultant washout ratios vary with severity of coronary stenosis, but their correlation with actual flow ratios has been reported to be of variable accuracy. This may be the result of reactive hyperemia occurring concomitantly with contrast washout. Within the limitations of application of the Kety-Schmidt principle detailed above, this technique may be clinically useful for assessing

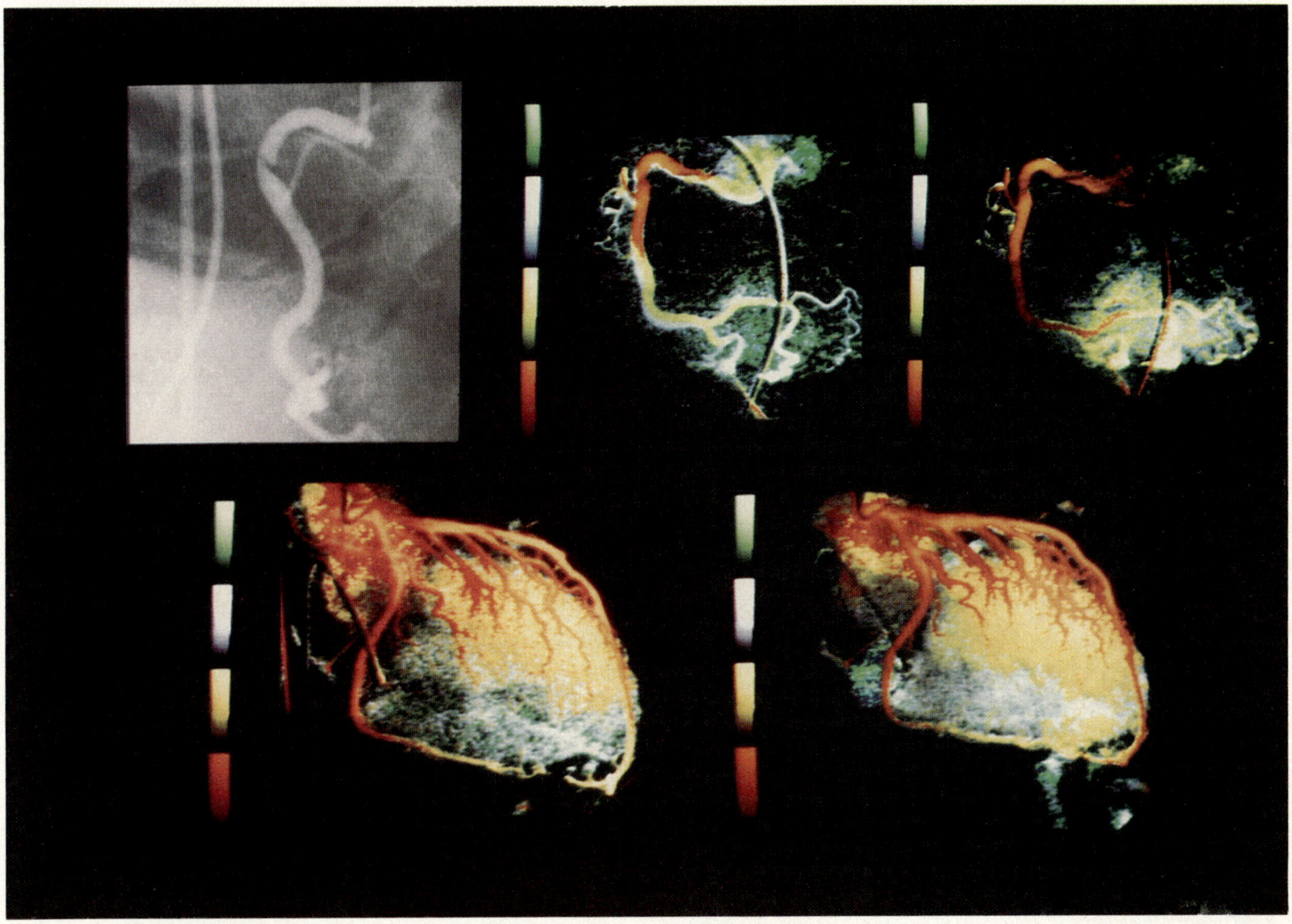

FIGURE 3. *Top,* Right anterior oblique projection arteriogram obtained in a patient with a proximal right coronary artery stenosis (left). Left anterior oblique projection parametric images of this arterial distribution acquired under baseline (center) and contrast-induced hyperemic conditions (right) demonstrate greater hyperemic than baseline flow. This is visualized as a faster transit time and an increased density of the arterial perfusion bed in the hyperemic state. Coronary flow reserve was calculated as 2.1. *Bottom,* Right anterior oblique projection parametric images of a left coronary artery in a patient with angina pectoris and normal coronary arteries under baseline (left) and contrast-induced hyperemic conditions (right). Little change between the two images is seen, suggesting a very low coronary flow reserve. Coronary flow reserve was calculated as 1.2.

the physiologic significance of stenoses or other factors that limit maximal blood flow. The washout approach does have the advantage of not requiring precise timing or volume of contrast medium administration.

Clinical applications and limitations. Several centers are gaining clinical experience with the parametric imaging and washout techniques for measuring relative blood flow. The parametric imaging technique can be performed rapidly during cardiac catheterization, although atrial pacing, ECG-synchronized power injection of contrast media, digital radiographic equipment capable of direct digital storage, and fixed patient positioning need to be added to the routine technique. Atrial pacing and power injection of contrast media have not resulted in problems to date. Patient motion has proved to be the most prevalent problem, however, necessitating the repetition of many studies. In our catheterization laboratory, this type of parametric imaging has proved helpful for the determination of the physiologic significance of intermediate coronary artery stenoses. Even though a 50% diameter stenosis value seems to be the best criterion for determining the physiologic significance of the stenosis, about a quarter of stenoses in the 25% to 75% range will be incorrectly assessed by this criterion. As an example, assessment of coronary flow reserve in a right coronary artery with a 60% diameter stenosis is shown in the upper panels of figure 3. Despite the anatomic narrowing, normal flow reserve, normal stress thallium-201 scintigraphic results, and no translesional pressure gradient were found. At present none of the parameters for determining the significance of individual lesions, i.e., arterial stenosis, flow reserve, stress scintigraphy, and translesional gradient, have sufficient accuracy to be used alone. The clinician must use concordance of test results to perform this important assessment.

It should be emphasized that coronary flow reserve can be reduced by many factors other than epicardial coronary stenosis, including myocardial hypertrophy, hypertension, prior myocardial infarction, collateralization, coronary spasm and intrinsic vasoreactivity, syndrome X, prolonged ischemia, early angioplasty, and vasoactive drugs. Arterial, ventricular end-diastolic, and intrathoracic pressures, which can vary during arteriographic techniques, also affect flow reserve.[9] Changes in coronary flow in one artery may affect flow in other arteries. Lastly, as a relative parameter, flow reserve ratios are altered by changes in resting blood flow. These factors need to be considered in using flow reserve to clinically determine physiologic severity of lesions and may explain, in part, conflicting anatomic and physiologic data. An example of the difficulty with the use of coronary flow reserve to predict the physiologic significance of individual coronary stenosis is illustrated in the lower panels of figure 3. In this case of a patient with angina pectoris, hypertension, and normal coronary arteries, a very low flow reserve is evident, from the small color and intensity differences between the baseline and hyperemic studies. Abnormal results of stress radionuclide ventriculography tended to confirm a functional abnormality. This example suggests that abnormally low flow reserve cannot be directly ascribed to a specific coronary stenosis without consideration of the above factors.

Higher levels of hyperemic coronary flow can be achieved with agents other than contrast media, which are currently used for reasons of clinical safety. The parametric technique described appears to assess papaverine- and contrast-induced flow changes with approximately equivalent accuracy. However, early data suggest that contrast is equivalent to more potent stimuli in differentiating normal from abnormal coronary physiology, and the peak of contrast-induced hyperemia has been reported to be at about 10 sec after injection in both normal and abnormal coronary vessels. Clinical studies have also shown close associations between coronary flow reserve data and the results of stress scintigraphy.[10] Moreover, contrast-induced coronary flow reserve has been shown to correlate closely with increases of blood flow between resting conditions and pacing-induced angina. These findings support the clinical utility of radiographic methods that can measure coronary blood flow. Ultimately, clinical techniques capable of measuring absolute blood flow may be useful for differentiating the specific cause of abnormal flow ratios. Implementation of rapid, simple catheterization methods for assessing coronary blood flow is likely, as imaging technology and an understanding of the effects of contrast media improve.

I wish to express my gratitude to Michael LeFree, B.S., Fred Aueron, M.D., John Hodgson, M.D., and Victor LeGrand, M.D., for their assistance in the development and validation of the parametric imaging technique, to Diane Bauer for her help in preparing this manuscript, and to my many colleagues whose ideas and data contributed to this review but could not be referenced because of limitations of space.

References

1. Gould KL, Lipscomb K, Hamilton GW: Physiologic basis for assessing critical coronary stenosis: instantaneous flow response and regional distribution during coronary hyperemia as measures of coronary flow reserve. Am J Cardiol **33:** 87, 1974
2. Harrison DG, White CW, Hiratzka LF, Doty DB, Barnes DH, Eastham CL, Marcus ML: The value of lesion cross-sectional area

determined by quantitative coronary angiography in assessing the physiologic significance of proximal left anterior descending arterial stenoses. Circulation **69:** 1111, 1984

3. Klocke FJ: Measurements of coronary blood flow and degree of stenosis: current clinical implications and continuing uncertainties. J Am Coll Cardiol **1:** 31, 1983
4. Hodgson JM, Mancini GBJ, LeGrand V, Vogel RA: Characterization of changes in coronary blood flow during the first six seconds after intracoronary contrast injection. Invest Radiol (in press)
5. Rutishauser W, Bussman W-D, Noseda G, Meier W, Wellauer J: Blood flow measurement through single coronary arteries by roentgen densitometry. Part I. A comparison of flow measured by a radiologic technique applicable in the intact organism and by electromagnetic flowmeter. Am J Roentgenol **109:** 12, 1970
6. Spiller P, Schmiel FK, Politz B, Block M, Fermor U, Hackbarth W, Jehle J, Korfer, Pannek H: Measurements of systolic and diastolic flow rates in the coronary artery system by x-ray densitometry. Circulation **68:** 337, 1983
7. Foerster J, Link DP, Lantz BMT, Lee G, Holcroft JW, Mason DT: Measurement of coronary reactive hyperemia during clinical angiography by video dilution technique. Acta Radiol **22:** 209, 1981
8. Hodgson JM, LeGrand V, Bates ER, Mancini GBJ, Aueron FM, O'Neill WW, Simon SB, Beauman GJ, LeFree MT, Vogel RA: Validation in dogs of a rapid digital angiographic technique to measure relative coronary blood flow during routine cardiac catheterization. Am J Cardiol **55:** 188, 1985
9. Hoffman JIE: Maximal coronary flow and the concept of vascular reserve. Circulation **70:** 153, 1984
10. LeGrand V, Aueron FM, Hodgson JM, Mancini GBJ, Bates ER, Smith JS, O'Neill WW, Gross MD, Vogel RA: What decrease in coronary flow reserve results in an abnormal functional test? Circulation **70**(suppl II): II-124, 1984 (abst)

Effects of β-adrenoreceptor–blocking drugs in patients with Raynaud's phenomenon

JAY D. COFFMAN, M.D., AND HELEN M. RASMUSSEN, R.D.M.S.

ABSTRACT Digital vasospastic phenomena have been reported to result from use of nonselective and cardioselective β-adrenoreceptor–blocking drugs. The effects of 80 mg/day propranolol and 100 mg/day metoprolol on finger hemodynamics and clinical responses were compared with those of placebo in 16 patients with Raynaud's phenomenon. A double-blind, 2 week crossover study design was used with a 2 week washout placebo period between drugs. Total fingertip blood flow (FBF) as determined by venous occlusion plethysmography, fingertip capillary flow (FCF) as determined by radioisotope disappearance rate, and finger systolic blood pressure (FSP) were measured in a 28.3° and a 20° C room at the end of each period. Subjects kept diaries to record vasospastic attacks. There were no significant changes in FBF, FCF, or FSP in the warm or cool environment during drug treatment as compared with during the placebo period. A decrease in pulse rate occurred with both drugs and there was a decrease in blood pressure with metoprolol. There were no significant changes in the number of vasospastic attacks or in the patients' overall evaluation of their conditions while they were receiving the drugs. It is concluded that the presence of Raynaud's phenomenon is not a contraindication to the use of β-adrenoreceptor–blocking drugs in the normotensive population.
***Circulation* 72, No. 3, 466–470, 1985.**

USE OF β-adrenoreceptor–blocking drugs has been associated with the development of Raynaud's phenomenon, cold extremities, and intermittent claudication. The mechanism of action is unknown. Unopposed stimulation of vascular α-adrenoreceptors, decreased cardiac output and blood pressure resulting in lower perfusion pressure and blood flow, a decreased blood volume, or increased reflex sympathetic vasoconstriction by the central cardiovascular depressant effects of β-blockade have been suggested.[1–4] β-Adrenoreceptors have been shown to be present in the arteriovenous anastomoses of the fingers. They are only responsive to humoral agents and not to neurogenic stimulation, but could be involved in the development of Raynaud's phenomenon.[5] Vasospastic phenomenon have been described with use of both nonselective and cardioselective agents[2, 6] and cardioselective agents have been shown to affect the peripheral circulation.[7] Since these agents must sometimes be used in patients with Raynaud's phenomenon and coronary artery disease, we investigated the effect of a cardioselective and a nonselective β-blocking drug in equivalent doses on fingertip hemodynamics and clinical symptoms in patients with Raynaud's phenomenon.

From the Peripheral Vascular Section, Evans Memorial Department of Clinical Research, Department of Medicine, University Hospital, Boston University Medical Center.

Supported by National Institutes of Health grant HL 26320 and Ciba-Geigy Pharmaceuticals, Summit, NJ.

Address for correspondence: Jay D. Coffman, M.D., University Hospital, 75 E. Newton St., Boston, MA 02118.

Received April 1, 1985; revision accepted May 23, 1985.

Methods

Subjects gave informed consent and the institutional committee on human research approved the study protocol. Sixteen women who had had Raynaud's phenomenon for 3 to 29 years were studied. Their average age was 35 years (range 24 to 59). Raynaud's phenomenon was diagnosed in the presence of episodic attacks of well-demarcated color changes (to white or blue) of the fingers on both hands on exposure to cold. Fourteen patients were classified as having idiopathic disease because of negative history, normal physical examination, and laboratory results; two subjects were classified as having collagen vascular disease on the basis of positive antinuclear antibodies.

Total fingertip blood flow (FBF) was measured by venous occlusion plethysmography and fingertip capillary flow (FCF) was measured by the disappearance rate of a radioisotope after a fingertip injection. The hand and arm were elevated slightly above heart level. The plethysmograph was attached by a fingercup sealed to the fingertip beyond the distal interphalangeal joint with caulking compound. A 2.5 cm pneumatic cuff was applied proximal to the fingercup. The lowest venous occlusion pressure required to obtain the maximal rate of increase in fingertip volume was determined at the beginning of each experiment and averaged 57 mm Hg. Changes in fingertip blood volume were detected by a Validyne low-pressure transducer (MP 45-14) connected by stiff plastic tubing to the outlet of the fingercup and recorded by a Hewlett-Packard 8805B preamplifier and recorder. The recording system was calibrated after equilibration for 1 hr at 28.3° and 20° C room temperature by introducing known quantities of air into the system. Fingertip blood volume within the fingercup was determined by water displacement to express blood flow in milliliters per min per 100 ml of tissue. Arm blood pressure was determined by the sphygmomanometric method. The mean blood pressure was calculated by adding one-third of the pulse pressure to the diastolic pressure. Finger vascular resistance was calculated by dividing the mean arm blood pressure by total FBF and was expressed as millimeters mercury per minute per 100 ml of tissue. This is only an estimate of the finger vascular resistance because the finger blood pressure may be smaller than the brachial artery pressure in the warm environment.[8] Finger systolic pressure (FSP) was measured by inflating the finger pneumatic cuff to suprasystolic pressure and then slowly releasing the pressure. The cuff pressure at which the first increase in fingertip volume occurred was recorded as the systolic pressure.

The disappearance rate of a radioactive isotope from a local injection in an adjacent fingertip was used as a measure of FCF. Approximately 0.01 ml $Na^{131}I$ in saline solution (0.9%) was injected with a 27-gauge needle into the skin of the pad of one fingertip. Disappearance rate was monitored by a scintillation probe, rate meter (time constant set at 5 sec), and linear recorder. The scintillation probe contained a thallium-activated sodium iodide crystal. Dose of the isotope used was about 2 μCi. Disappearance rates were plotted on semilogarithmic paper after subtraction of the background counts and were expressed as half-times. Disappearance rates were also converted into an estimated blood flow in milliliters per minute per 100 ml of tissue by dividing the natural logarithm of 2 by the half-time and multiplying by the tissue-to-blood coefficient (0.5) times 100.

The randomized, double-blind, crossover design consisted of a 2 week placebo run-in period, a 2 week drug period, a 2 week washout placebo period, and a 2 week alternate drug period. Finger hemodynamic studies were performed at the end of the placebo run-in and after each drug period. Measurements at each session were obtained after 1 hr in a warm (28.3° C) room and after 1 hr in a cool (20° C) room. Subjects took their medication at the beginning of the experiment. In the warm room, subjects were covered with a blanket, while in the cool room they wore only a hospital gown. The setting of the 20° C room with the patient in a short gown was chosen since previous experience has shown that lower temperatures may induce shivering. FBF and isotope disappearance rates were followed for 8 min in each environment. Arm blood pressure and FSP were also determined in the warm and cool rooms.

Metoprolol (50 mg), propranolol (40 mg), and placebo in identical tablets were supplied by Ciba-Geigy Pharmaceuticals Division and pills were taken two times a day. Blood samples for determination of chemistry profiles and complete blood count and urine samples were collected at the beginning of the study and on each of the measurement days. Antinuclear antibodies and sedimentation rates were measured on the first visit. Subjects kept daily diaries of the frequency of their vasospastic attacks. They also gave an overall evaluation of their condition at the end of each period, rating their response as worse, unchanged, or as 25% to 50%, 50% to 75%, or 75% to 100% improved. The daily mean temperature in the Boston area was also recorded.

Hemodynamic data from the first placebo period and the two drug periods were analyzed and compared; similar evaluations were performed for the diaries and overall evaluations for all four periods. Since there was a large variation in the FBFs and the number of vasospastic attacks between patients, $\log_{10}$-transformed data were also analyzed. A Latin square analysis was used to determine the effect of the order of administration of drugs.[9] An analysis of variance for a crossover design with repeated measures was then used (Program SPSS-X). Where appropriate the Newman-Keuls test was applied to determine significance at the $p < .05$ level. Data were expressed as mean ± SE.

Results

There were no significant differences in the finger hemodynamic measurements between drug and placebo periods or between the two drug periods in the warm or cool rooms (table 1). In the cool room, the mean FBF tended to be smaller with both drugs than with placebo, but three patients had large blood flows in this environment (figure 1). One other patient had a large blood flow only while on metoprolol. When the values in these three patients were excluded, average FBF was very similar during the three periods: 2.1 ± 0.4 ml/100 ml tissue/min for placebo, 2.0 ± 0.3 ml/100 ml tissue/min for metoprolol, and 2.1 ± 0.4 ml/100 ml tissue/min for propranolol. With the exception of FSP, differences in parameter values recorded in the warm and cool rooms from patients on both

TABLE 1

Hemodynamic measurements in the finger during drug and placebo periods

	FBF (ml/100 ml tissue/min)	FVR (mm Hg/100 ml tissue/min)	FCF (ml/100 ml tissue/min)	FSP (mm Hg)
Warm room (28.3° C)				
Placebo	50.1±9.2	4.8±2.1	6.3±0.4	94.0±3.0
Metoprolol	44.0±7.8	6.1±2.9	6.3±0.6	90.5±3.8
Propranolol	46.4±7.4	3.2±0.8	6.5±0.7	95.0±4.8
Cool room (20° C)				
Placebo	9.1±3.8	38.0±6.6	2.5±0.4	104.8±5.0
Metoprolol	6.4±2.5	38.3±7.2	3.2±0.5	98.9±4.9
Propranolol	3.8±1.4	53.3±12.3	2.3±0.3	105.6±4.1

Data are mean ± SE. There were no significant differences between drug and placebo periods for any of the variables.

FVR = fingertip vascular resistance.

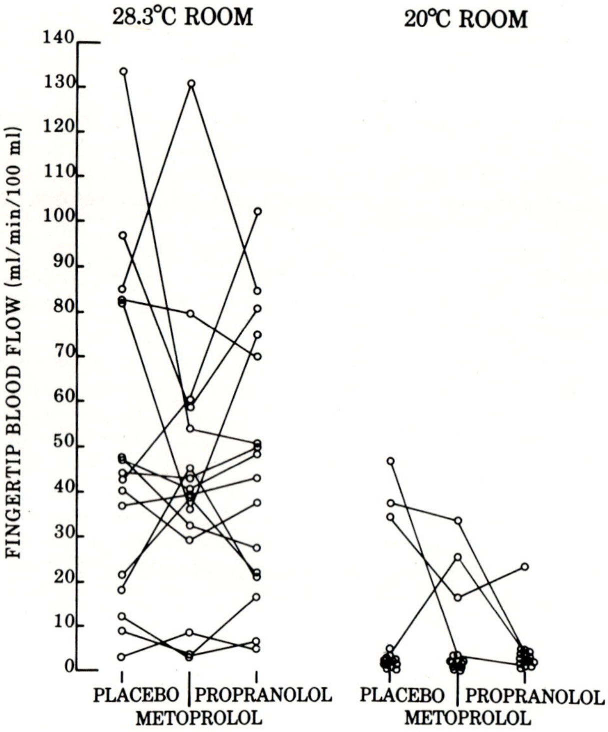

FIGURE 1. FBFs during placebo, metoprolol, and propranolol periods in the warm and cool environments.

drugs and placebo were significantly different. The FSP did not increase significantly in the cool room during either drug period (metoprolol $p < .1$; propranolol $p < .06$).

No significant differences were found with respect to number of vasospastic attacks per 2 week period or to the patients' overall evaluations of their symptoms between the two drug periods or between drug and placebo periods (tables 2 and 3).

After both metoprolol and propranolol there was a significant decrease in pulse rate compared with after placebo in both the warm and cool rooms (table 4). Pulse rate was not significantly different during the two drug periods in either environment. Mean blood pressure after metoprolol in both the warm and cool rooms was significantly lower than that during the placebo period. In the cool room blood pressure was

TABLE 2
Number of vasospastic attacks per 2 week period

Period	No. of attacks
Placebo	15.3±4.0
Metoprolol	14.3±3.8
Placebo	15.8±5.3
Propranolol	14.5±4.0

Data are mean ± SE. There were no significant differences between the four 2 week periods.

TABLE 3
Patients' subjective evaluations

Period	Score[A]
Placebo	2.0±0.1
Metoprolol	2.4±0.3
Placebo	2.1±0.3
Propranolol	2.4±0.2

Data are mean ± SE. There were no significant differences between the four 2 week periods.

[A]1 = worse; 2 = unchanged; 3 = 25% to 50% improved; 4 = 50% to 75% improved; 5 = 75% to 100% improved.

significantly lower with metoprolol than propranolol ($p = .01$).

Average daily temperature in the Boston area was 5.9 ± 1.2° C during the first placebo period, 6.9 ± 2.0° C during the metoprolol period, 8.1 ± 1.6° C during the second placebo period, and 8.6 ± 2.2° C during the propranolol period; these were not significantly different.

Side effects with the medications were few and did not cause any patient to discontinue or decrease dosage of medication. Two patients on placebo reported lethargy and a third had depression. Two patients had lightheadedness, one had lethargy, one had nausea, and one had diarrhea while taking metoprolol. Two patients reported nausea, one lightheadedness, and one headaches while on propranolol. No abnormal blood test results or urinalyses were obtained during placebo or drug periods.

Discussion

In this study, 80 mg/day propranolol or 100 mg/day metoprolol for 2 weeks did not significantly alter FBF, FCF, or FSP in a warm or cool environment when compared with placebo. There were no significant

TABLE 4
Pulse rate and blood pressure during drug and placebo periods

	Pulse rate (beats/min)	Mean blood pressure (mm Hg)
Warm room (28.3° C)		
Placebo	69.0±3.4	78.8±2.2
Metoprolol	61.9±3.1[A]	72.7±2.5[A]
Propranolol	61.8±3.0[A]	75.9±2.0
Cool room (20° C)		
Placebo	65.4±2.8	83.8±2.9
Metoprolol	56.9±3.4[A]	78.3±2.3[A]
Propranolol	55.9±2.4[A]	83.0±2.9

Data are mean ± SE.

[A]$p = .01$ for differences between drug and placebo.

changes in the number of vasospastic attacks recorded by diary or in the patients' overall evaluations of their conditions while they were receiving the drugs. The decrease in pulse rate with both drugs and the decrease in blood pressure with metoprolol indicate a degree of β-adrenoreceptor blockade was produced. A greater decrease in blood pressure in normal subjects has previously been reported with metoprolol compared with propranolol and placebo.[10] We were therefore unable to demonstrate a significant change in the digital circulation or an aggravation of Raynaud's phenomenon in patients taking a nonselective or a cardioselective β-blocking agent with objective tests or subjective evaluations. It is possible that higher doses of the drugs may have produced different results, but Marshall et al.[2] found no association between vasospastic symptoms and dose.

In a previous study, we have shown that patients with Raynaud's phenomenon had significantly smaller FBFs and FCFs than normal subjects in a warm or cool environment.[11] However, the overlap in flow values did not distinguish between patients and normal subjects on an individual basis. The average total flow measured in the warm room in this study was larger than that in our previous report, but the patients were not covered with blankets in the latter study. The cool room total and capillary flows are comparable; in the previous study they were significantly less than those in the normal subjects. In studying patients with primary or secondary Raynaud's phenomenon, we usually find a few patients with large FBFs in the cool room.[11, 12] The three patients with large values in this study represented patients with primary and secondary disease and numbers of vasospastic attacks ranging from one to 53 per week. Furthermore, number of attacks did not increase during drug treatment in these patients. Apparently, they do not represent a special subset of the disease. Although the study group of 16 patients is rather small to allow generalization of results to the population at large, these patients represented a broad spectrum of the disease.

McSorley and Warren[13] reported a decrease in skin temperature and skin and muscle blood flow in normal subjects on 80 mg propranolol daily, and 100 mg metoprolol daily also decreased skin flow in hypertensive patients. Nielsen and Nielsen,[14] using a technique of finger cooling during ischemia, found increased digital arterial tone at low temperatures after administration of 120 to 240 mg propranolol daily but not after metoprolol (100 to 150 mg daily) in hypertensive patients. However, they also reported the development of vasospastic attacks in one patient on a cardioselective drug. Holti presents some evidence that patients with long-standing Raynaud's disease and hypertension fared worse on 160 mg of long-acting propranolol than on 400 mg acebutolol.[15] However, Steiner et al.[16] reported no difference in finger temperature or symptoms in 14 hypertensive patients with Raynaud's phenomenon during propranolol or labetalol treatment.

Almost all studies reporting the development of Raynaud's phenomenon or cold extremities with β-blocking drugs concern patients with hypertension. Nielsen et al.[17] have demonstrated that digital arterial tone during cooling is significantly greater among hypertensive subjects than among normotensive controls. Feleke et al.[18] have commented that hypertension may predispose to vasospastic reactions.

It is unclear why there is such a marked variation in results of studies of the incidence of Raynaud's phenomenon, cold extremities, or even intermittent claudication in patients on β-blockers or in the reported effects of these agents on skin and muscle blood flow in normal individuals or hypertensive patients.[7, 19] The incidence of this side effect varies from as low as 4.1% to as high as 41% in studies of patients with hypertension[2, 6]; both cardioselective and nonselective agents have been implicated. None of the patients in our study were hypertensive. In fact, patients with Raynaud's disease tend to have a significantly lower blood pressure than normal subjects[20, 21]; average mean blood pressure was only 79 mm Hg in our group. Therefore, our results cannot be applied to hypertensive patients. Vasospastic phenomena do occur in nonhypertensive patients treated with β-blockers; eight of the 21 patients reported by Eliasson et al.[4] did not have high blood pressure.

From our study and evidence in the literature, it may be concluded that the presence of Raynaud's phenomenon is not a contraindication to the use of β-adrenoreceptor–blocking drugs. Zacharias[22] reported that only 3% of their hypertensive patients required withdrawal of the drug or reduction of the dose due to severe Raynaud's phenomenon. This is especially important for the patient with coronary artery disease and Raynaud's phenomenon for whom therapy with β-blocking agents may be a necessity. It is probably prudent to avoid use of β-blocking drugs in patients with hypertension and Raynaud's phenomenon.

References

1. White C deB, Udivadia BP: β-Adrenoceptors in the human dorsal hand vein, and the effects of propranolol and practolol on venous sensitivity to noradrenaline. Br J Clin Pharmacol **2:** 99, 1975
2. Marshall AJ, Roberts CJC, Barritt DW: Raynaud's phenomenon as a side effect of beta-blockers in hypertension. Br Med J **1:** 1498, 1976

3. Julius S, Pascual AV, Abbrecht PH, London R: Effect of beta-adrenergic blockade on plasma volume in human subjects. Proc Soc Exp Biol Med **140:** 985, 1972
4. Eliasson K, Lins L-E, Sundqvist K: Vasospastic phenomena in patients treated with beta-adrenoceptor blocking agents. Acta Med Scand **628**(suppl): 39, 1979
5. Cohen RA, Coffman JD: β-Adrenergic vasodilator mechanism in the finger. Circ Res **49:** 1196, 1981
6. Vandenburg MJ, Evans SJW, Cooper WD, Bradshaw F, Currie WJC: Is the feeling of cold extremities experienced by hypertensive patients due to their disease or their treatment. Eur J Pharmacol **27:** 47, 1984
7. Smith RS, Warren DJ: Effect of acute oral beta-adrenergic blockade on muscle blood flow in man. Cardiovasc Res **16:** 205, 1982
8. Krahenbuhl B, Nielsen SL, Lassen NA: Closure of digital arteries in high vascular tone states as demonstrated by measurement of systolic blood pressure in fingers. Scand J Clin Lab Invest **37:** 71, 1977
9. Snedecor GW, Cochran WG: Statistical methods, ed 6. Ames, Iowa, 1967, Iowa State University Press, p 312
10. Hiatt WR, Fradl DC, Zerbe GO, Byyny RL, Nies AS: Selective and nonselective β-blockade of the peripheral circulation. Clin Pharmacol Ther **35:** 12, 1984
11. Coffman JD, Cohen AS: Total and capillary fingertip blood flow in Raynaud's Phenomenon. N Engl J Med **285:** 259, 1971
12. Coffman JD, Rasmussen HM: Effect of thromboxane synthetase inhibition in Raynaud's phenomenon. Clin Pharmacol Ther **36:** 369, 1984
13. McSorley PD, Warren DJ: Effects of propranolol and metoprolol on the peripheral circulation. Br Med J **2:** 1598, 1978
14. Nielsen PE, Nielsen SL: Digital arterial tone in hypertensive subjects treated with cardioselective and nonselective beta-adrenoreceptor blocking agents. Dan Med Bull **28:** 76, 1981
15. Holti G: A comparison of two beta-blocking drugs in patients with Raynaud's phenomenon. Practitioner **226:** 781, 1982
16. Steiner JA, Cooper R, Gear JS, Ledingham JGG: Vascular symptoms in patients with primary Raynaud's phenomenon are not exacerbated by propranolol or labetol. Br J Clin Pharmacol **7:** 401, 1979
17. Nielsen SL, Olsen N, Nielsen PE: Increased digital arterial tone in hypertensive subjects indicated by local cooling and propranolol treatment. Clin Physiol **1:** 21, 1981
18. Feleke E, Lyngstam O, Rastam L, Ryden L: Complaints of cold extremities among patients on antihypertensive treatment. Acta Med Scand **213:** 381, 1983
19. Jensen K, Skagen K, Henriksen O, Kjoller E: Local blood flow regulation in normotensive man during prolonged treatment with propranolol. Eur J Pharmacol **24:** 723, 1983
20. Thulesius O: Methods for evaulation of peripheral vascular function in the upper extremities. Acta Chir Scand Suppl **465:** 53, 1976
21. Cohen RA, Coffman JD: Reduced transmural systolic pressure promotes arterial closure in Raynaud's disease. Clin Res **30:** 179A, 1982
22. Zacharias FJ: Patient acceptability of propranolol and occurrence of side effects. Postgrad Med J **52**(suppl 4): 87, 1976

Abnormal distribution of pulmonary blood flow after the Glenn shunt or Fontan procedure: risk of development of arteriovenous fistulae

ALAIN CLOUTIER, M.D., JUDITH M. ASH, M.D., JEFFREY F. SMALLHORN, M.D., WILLIAM G. WILLIAMS, M.D., GEORGE A. TRUSLER, M.D., RICHARD D. ROWE, M.D., AND MARLENE RABINOVITCH, M.D.

ABSTRACT Since the Fontan procedure results in low pulsatile pulmonary blood flow similar to that seen in patients with a Glenn shunt, it may also be associated with abnormal distribution of flow to the lower lung lobes and with the development of pulmonary arteriovenous fistulae (PAVF). In 12 patients 0.8 to 4.5 years after Fontan procedure and in 20 patients 0.2 to 18 years after receipt of Glenn shunts we assessed ventilation (with ^{133}Xe) and perfusion (after a peripheral injection of ^{99m}Tc-macroaggregated albumin) to compare upper to lower lobe distribution of blood flow with that in a control group. The presence of PAVF was assessed by radionuclide activity in kidneys and the brain and by a two-dimensional echocardiographic contrast study. A decreased upper/lower lobe perfusion ratio was noted in 13 of 20 patients with Glenn shunts (65%) and correlated with the time after surgery ($p < .05$). Despite the shorter follow-up period, two of 12 (16%) patients who had undergone the Fontan procedure also had a decreased upper/lower lobe perfusion ratio, and one of these developed right heart failure. Brain and kidney radionuclide counts above control values were observed in all patients with Glenn shunts and in 11 of 12 patients who had the Fontan operation. However, in only five of 20 (25%) patients with Glenn shunts were PAVF confirmed by the two-dimensional echocardiographic contrast study. Three of the five patients with PAVF had Glenn shunts of long duration. While only two of five patients with PAVF had a decreased upper/lower lobe perfusion ratio at the time of the study, this abnormality may have been present in the other three at an earlier stage. Our data suggest that a decreased ratio of upper/lower lobe perfusion may be one of several factors associated with the development of PAVF after a Glenn shunt. Also, longer follow-up of patients who have had a Fontan procedure will be necessary to determine whether they are also a group at risk.
Circulation 72, No. 3, 471–479, 1985.

THE FONTAN procedure,[1] which establishes a right atrial–to–pulmonary arterial (RA-PA) communication, and its modification, which incorporates the right ventricle (RA-RV communication), result in low pulsatile pulmonary blood flow. This hemodynamic state is similar to the one observed after creation of a Glenn shunt (superior vena cava–to–pulmonary arterial anastomosis).[2] It is well established that the Glenn shunt favors distribution of pulmonary flow to the lower lobe[3] and that with increasing duration of shunt time, pulmonary arteriovenous fistulae (PAVF) can occur in the same area.[4] Whether these PAVF result from the low pulsatile pulmonary blood flow or from the maldistribution of flow or are associated with other factors such as pulmonary hypertension in the unshunted lung[5] is still unclear. If indeed low pulsatile pulmonary flow leads to maldistribution and the potential to develop PAVF, then patients who have had Fontan's procedure represent a group at risk.

We therefore performed ventilation/perfusion lung scans to determine the distribution of pulmonary blood flow in patients after the Fontan procedure (RA-PA and RA-RV). We assessed the presence of PAVF by the scintigraphic appearance of ^{99m}Tc-macroaggregated albumin (MAA) in the brain and kidneys after a peripheral intravenous injection and by two-dimensional echocardiographic contrast studies. Our findings were compared with those obtained in patients with Glenn shunts and in normal subjects.

From the Departments of Cardiology and Cardiovascular Surgery and the Division of Nuclear Medicine, The Hospital for Sick Children, and from the departments of Pediatrics, Surgery, and Radiology, The University of Toronto, Ontario.

Address for correspondence: Marlene Rabinovitch, M.D., Department of Cardiology, The Hospital for Sick Children, 555 University Ave., Toronto, Ontario, Canada M5G 1X8.

Received Oct. 22, 1984; revision accepted May 23, 1985.

Methods

Patient population. We reviewed the records of the cardiac patients who received a Glenn shunt or underwent Fontan procedure between June 1965 and August 1983 at the Hospital for Sick Children, Toronto. Twenty-nine patients were available and consented to participate in our study. In 20, a Glenn shunt had been created; three of these patients and nine others had undergone Fontan procedure. Of those 12 with a Fontan procedure, six had RA-RV and six RA-PA communication. This represents a random group of 22% of all patients in whom these procedures had been performed. The age range was similar in the Fontan and Glenn groups (table 1), but the duration after surgery was shorter in the Fontan (0.08 to 4.5 years, mean 2.4) than in the Glenn group (0.02 to 18 years, mean 8.8). Six volunteers from 28 to 32 years old served as normal control subjects. All studies were carried out after approval of the protocol and the method of obtaining informed consent by our Clinical Investigation Committee.

Radionuclide assessment. The ventilation/perfusion lung scan was performed with a Picker gamma camera (Dynacamera 4/15) interfaced to a Medical Data System A^2 computer. Ventilation was assessed from a posterior view of the lungs, with the patient in the sitting position, with ^{133}Xe as the radionuclide tracer. The patient breathed until equilibrium, then washout of the substance was allowed. For assessment of perfusion, the patient and camera position remained unchanged. In control subjects and in those with a Glenn shunt or Fontan procedure only, a dose of 0.05 mCi/kg (1.85 MBq) of ^{99m}Tc-MAA was injected in an arm vein. In patients who had undergone a Fontan procedure and had a previous Glenn shunt, half the dose was injected in a leg vein for determination of perfusion of the left lung supplied by the Fontan anastomosis, and the other half dose was injected in an arm vein to image perfusion of the right lung supplied by the Glenn shunt. After each injection, the camera was also positioned over the opposite lung and over the kidneys and brain to detect radionuclide activity at these sites.

The ^{133}Xe ventilation study was used to determine the height of the lung on the scintigram and from this, the lung was divided into three equidistant segments from base to apex. Radionuclide perfusion counts (^{99m}Tc-MAA) were measured in each of these regions. An upper-to-lower lobe perfusion ratio was then calculated.

The presence of right-to-left shunting was detected by the appearance of ^{99m}Tc-MAA in the kidneys and brain and contralateral lung of patients with Glenn shunts. These large radionuclide particles (10 to 50 μm) should otherwise lodge and remain in the capillaries of the lung.[6] For control subjects and patients who underwent a Fontan procedure, we calculated the ratio of brain + kidney counts/right and left lung counts; for patients with a Glenn shunt, brain + kidney + left lung counts/right lung counts was calculated. (For the one patient with a left-sided Glenn shunt, the lung counts were reversed.) For patients who had Fontan procedure and a previous Glenn shunt, we used the following formula: brain + kidney + right lung counts/left lung counts for the Fontan (peripheral leg injection) and brain + kidney + left lung counts/right lung counts for the Glenn (peripheral arm injection). Since the arm injection was given after the leg injection, the residual counts from the latter were subtracted before counting the ratio for the former.

Echocardiographic contrast study. A two-dimensional contrast study was performed the same day as the radionuclide scan. The heart was visualized in the precordial four-chamber view. Ten milliliters of normal saline mixed with approximately

TABLE 1
Clinical details on patients studied

Group	Patients (n)	Mean age in years (range)	Years postop. (range)	Diagnosis (n)	Previous palliative surgery (n)
Glenn	20	14.5 (4.2–22.9)	8.8 (0.02–18.0)	Tricuspid atresia (6)	Blalock-Taussig (3), Potts (3), central shunt (1)
				Single ventricle (7), Pulmonary atresia (7)	PA band (2), Blalock-Taussig (2), Waterston (1), Potts (2), RVOT reconstruction (2)
				TGA with small right ventricle (1)	PA banding (1)
				TGA with pulmonary stenosis (1), DORV with mitral atresia (1)	Rastelli procedure (1), PA banding (1)
				DORV with common atrioventricular valve (2)	PA banding (1), Waterston (1), Azygols continuation of IVC to RPA (1)
Fontan	6	15.8	1.5	Tricuspid atresia (4)	Blalock-Taussig (2), Glenn (1)[A]
RA-PA		(6.9–20.9)	(0.08–3.5)	Single ventricle (2)	Potts (1)
					PA band (1), Glenn (1)[A]
Fontan RA-RV	6	15.3 (10.4–19.7)	3.25 (2.5–4.5)	Tricuspid atresia (6)	PA band (2), Blalock-Taussig (2), Potts (1), Glenn (1)[A]
Control	6	30 (29–32)	—	—	—

TGA = transposition of the great arteries; RVOT = right ventricular outflow tract; DORV = double-outlet right ventricle; IVC = inferior vena cava; RPA = right pulmonary artery.

[A]Also included in the Glenn shunt group.

5 ml of CO_2 was injected through the same peripheral intravenous site used for the radionuclide tracer. Normally, after a right-sided injection,[7] the echo quality of the bolus is lost in the passage through the pulmonary capillary bed and therefore no "bubbles" should be observed in the left heart. In patients with a Glenn shunt bubbles observed in the pulmonary veins and left atrium suggest the presence of PAVF, and bubbles in the right atrium indicate the presence of a systemic venous collateral. In patients who had undergone the Fontan procedure, the contrast bolus was followed from its first appearance in the right atrium. After disappearance of the bolus in the lung, attention was directed to the pulmonary veins and left atrium to identify any return suggestive of PAVF. In the patients with a Glenn shunt who had also undergone a Fontan procedure, separate injections in an arm and leg vein were performed.

Cardiac catheterization study. During the period of this study cardiac catheterization was carried out in nine patients in whom it was clinically indicated; six had Glenn shunts and three a Fontan procedure (all RA-RV communication). Angiographic findings were correlated with features of PAVF suggested by the radionuclide scan and by the two-dimensional echocardiographic contrast study.

Analysis of data. Multiple linear regression analysis was used to correlate distribution of pulmonary blood flow (upper/lower lobe ratio) as well as radionuclide and two-dimensional echocardiographic contrast evidence of PAVF with age at surgery and time after surgery in patients with a Glenn shunt or who had undergone Fontan procedure (RA-PA and/or RA-RV communication). A p value $<.05$ was considered indicative of a significant difference.

Results

Ventilation. In all control subjects and patients, the scintigraphic appearance of homogeneous distribution of ^{133}Xe through both lung fields suggested normal ventilation.

Distribution of pulmonary perfusion. In control subjects the upper/lower lobe radionuclide count perfusion ratio was 0.07 to 0.29 in the right lung and 0.10 to 0.28 in the left. Four of five patients with Glenn shunts whose upper/lower lobe perfusion ratios fell within this "normal" range had received the shunts less than 4 years before, whereas 12 of 13 patients with a decreased ratio were studied at a later time postoperatively ($p < .05$) (figures 1 and 2). In the remaining two Glenn patients the upper/lower lobe perfusion ratio was increased: one had surgery less than 4 years before, the other more than 4 years before the study. There was no correlation between upper/lower lobe perfusion ratio and the age at which the Glenn shunt was received nor was there any correlation with the presence, type, or duration of a previous surgically created systemic-to-pulmonary arterial shunt. In one patient with a Glenn shunt and a decreased upper/lower lobe perfusion ratio (0.005), the creation of an axillary-to-pulmonary arterial fistula resulted in an increase of the ratio to 0.51.

Eight of 12 patients who had undergone the Fontan procedure had a normal upper/lower lobe perfusion ratio. All were studied less than 4 years after surgery. Two patients had a decreased ratio; one with a RA-RV communication was studied 4.5 years after repair and the other, with a RA-PA communication, only 1 year later. The latter patient developed severe congestive heart failure, perhaps as a result of pulmonary vasoconstriction secondary to ventilation/perfusion mismatch. An increased ratio of upper/lower lobe perfusion was observed in the remaining two patients (both RA-RV) (figure 3). One of us (G. T.) independently scored the patients in the RA-RV Fontan group as to size of the right ventricle and pulmonary valve. We could not correlate these features with either an increased or a decreased upper/lower lobe perfusion ratio. We could not detect any influence on the ratio in the left lung after the Fontan operation if a previous Glenn shunt had been created in the right lung. Of three patients who had undergone both procedures, all had decreased ratios in the right (Glenn) lung, but only one had a decreased ratio in the left lung; the other two were normal.

Radionuclide detection of right-to-left shunt. In control subjects the ratio of brain + kidney/right + left lung radionuclide counts ranged from 0.003 to 0.005. In all patients with a Glenn shunt or who had Fontan procedure the ratio was higher (0.02 to 1.30). In eight of 20 patients in the Glenn group and in 11 of 12 of those in

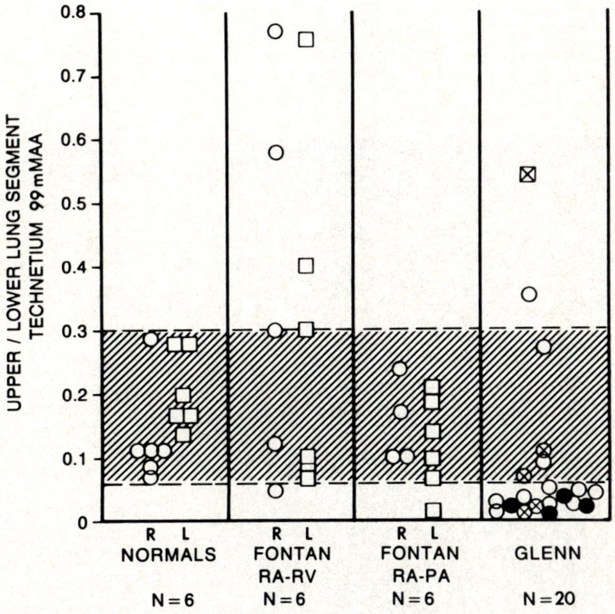

FIGURE 1. Upper/lower lobe perfusion ratios in patients and control subjects. Hatched area represents the range of control values. Open circle = right lung; open square = left lung; circle or square with x = PAVF confirmed by two-dimensional echocardiographic contrast study; closed circle = systemic venous collateral.

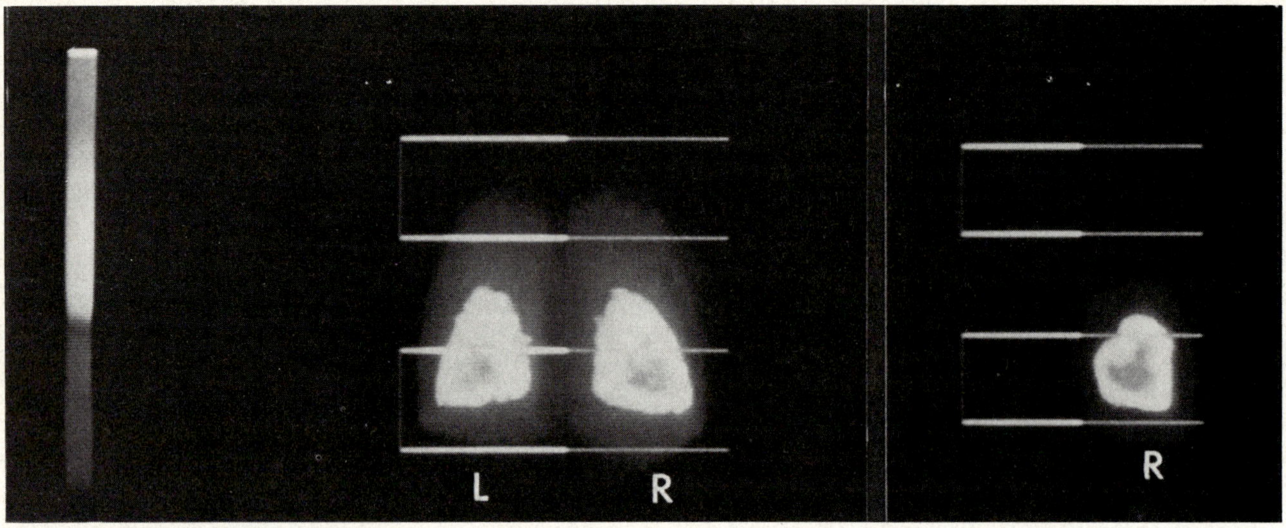

FIGURE 2. *Left,* Radionuclide lung scan from control subject. Both right (R) and left (L) lungs are visualized. *Right,* Lung scan from a patient with a previous Glenn shunt. The horizontal lines represent the three equidistant lung segments based on the ventilation study. Note the decreased perfusion to the upper and middle lobes in the patient with the Glenn shunt.

the Fontan group, the ratio was 0.03 to 0.06, but in the others it was 0.07 to 1.30.

Detection of PAVF with radionuclide scanning and two-dimensional echocardiographic contrast. In no patient with a radionuclide shunt ratio of less than 0.07 did an echocardiographic contrast bolus appear in the right atrium (Glenn group) or in the pulmonary veins or left atrium (Glenn and Fontan group), suggesting that the degree of right-to-left shunting was trivial. Of 12 Glenn patients with a shunt ratio of 0.07 or greater, the echocardiographic contrast study confirmed the presence of PAVF in five and identified systemic venous collaterals in four (figures 4 and 5). Two of the remaining three patients with Glenn shunts had anatomic characteristics that could explain the discrepancy between the positive radionuclide results and the negative echocardiographic contrast study. In one, an end-to-side Glenn shunt had been performed so the right pulmonary artery was in continuity with the left, and in the other, an anomalous pulmonary vein was draining into an innominate vein. Hence there was a high brain + kidney + left lung/right lung count but echocardiographic contrast bubbles did not appear in the left atrium. The third patient did not undergo cardiac catheterization to clarify the reason for the discrepancy between the two noninvasive studies, but we believe the bolus of contrast in the echocardiographic study was inadequately injected. In the one patient in the

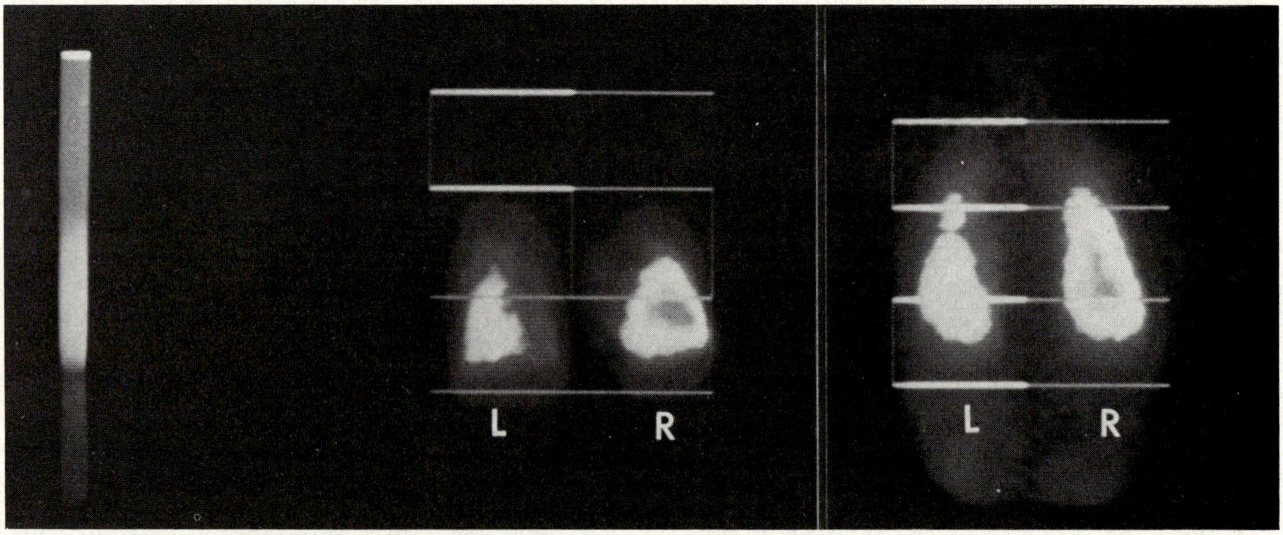

FIGURE 3. *Left,* Radionuclide lung scan from a patient with decreased flow to the upper lobes after Fontan procedure (RA-PA). *Right,* Patient with increased flow to the upper lobes after Fontan procedure (RA-RV). Incidentally noted are increased counts in the kidneys, suggesting some right-to-left shunting.

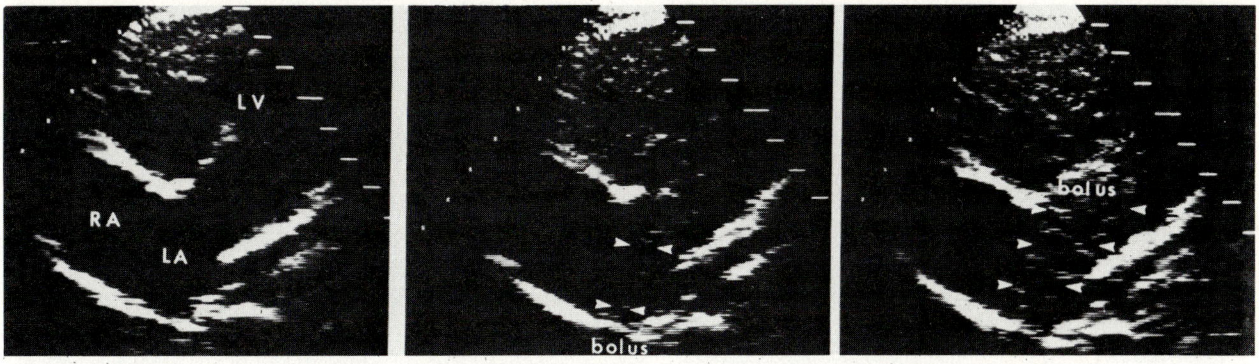

FIGURE 4. Two-dimensional echocardiogram from a patient with pulmonary atresia and straddling atrioventricular valve and a Glenn shunt. The appearance of contrast bolus in the right atrium is suggestive of a venous collateral. The venous collateral originates near the anastomotic site of the Glenn shunt and empties into the right atrium.

Fontan group with a radionuclide ratio of greater than 0.07, right-to-left shunting at the atrial level was observed on two-dimensional echocardiogram.

Cardiac catheterization study and PAVF. In two of the six patients with Glenn shunts who underwent cardiac catheterization there were findings consistent with PAVF on both the radionuclide scan and the two-dimensional echocardiogram. In one patient, PAVF were confirmed, but in the other, they were not apparent angiographically. However, since pulmonary venous saturations were not obtained, we could not exclude the presence of small communications in the latter patient. The positive catheterization study was obtained in the patient with the highest radionuclide shunt ratio (1.3), while the negative study was obtained in the patient with a much lower value (0.08). In the patient with the positive catheterization study, the PAVF were embolized; on subsequent radionuclide study, the shunt ratio had decreased from 1.3 to 0.43 (figure 6).

Cardiac catheterization confirmed the presence of systemic venous collaterals in two patients. The absence of venous collaterals as well as PAVF was confirmed in another and, in the remaining patient, the anatomic source of right-to-left shunting was identified as an anomalous pulmonary vein. The absence of venous collaterals or PAVF was also confirmed in the three patients in the Fontan group that underwent cardiac catheterization.

Duration of Glenn shunt, distribution of pulmonary blood flow, and PAVF. Three of the five patients with PAVF had Glenn shunts of long duration (13 to 16 years). Two of these had decreased ratios of upper/lower lobe perfusion: radionuclide ratios were 0.07 and 0.08. The third patient had an increased upper/lower lobe perfusion ratio, probably because severe right-to-left shunting through PAVF (radionuclide ratio = 1.3) caused impaired trapping of radionuclide material in the lower lobe. Two patients with PAVF and Glenn shunts of only 2 to 4 years duration had normal upper/lower lobe perfusion ratios. Both were severely cyanotic and in both, perfusion to the left lung was decreased. In one patient this was due to a thrombosed left pulmonary artery, in the other, to an obstructed left Blalock-Taussig shunt. Both conditions favor distribution of flow to the right lung and may have accelerated the formation of PAVF. Only one of these patients, however, had more severe right-to-

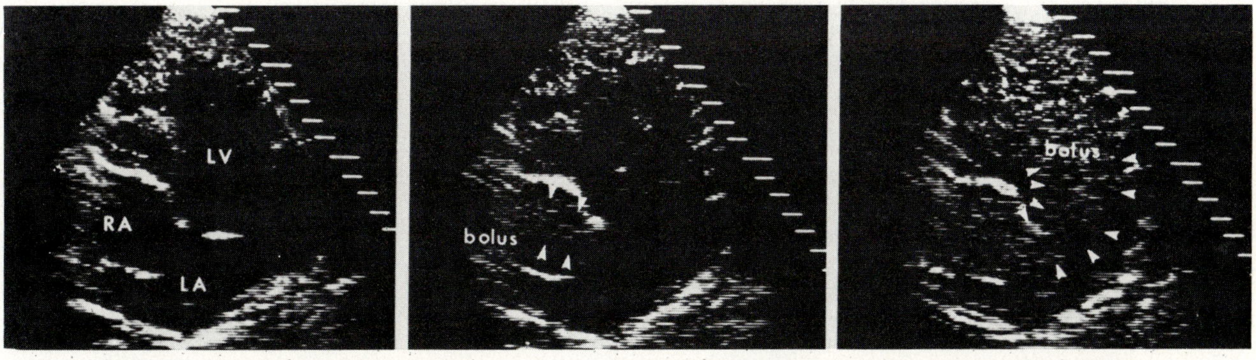

FIGURE 5. Two-dimensional echocardiogram from a patient with tricuspid atresia and a Glenn shunt. The appearance of contrast bolus in the pulmonary veins is suggestive of PAVF.

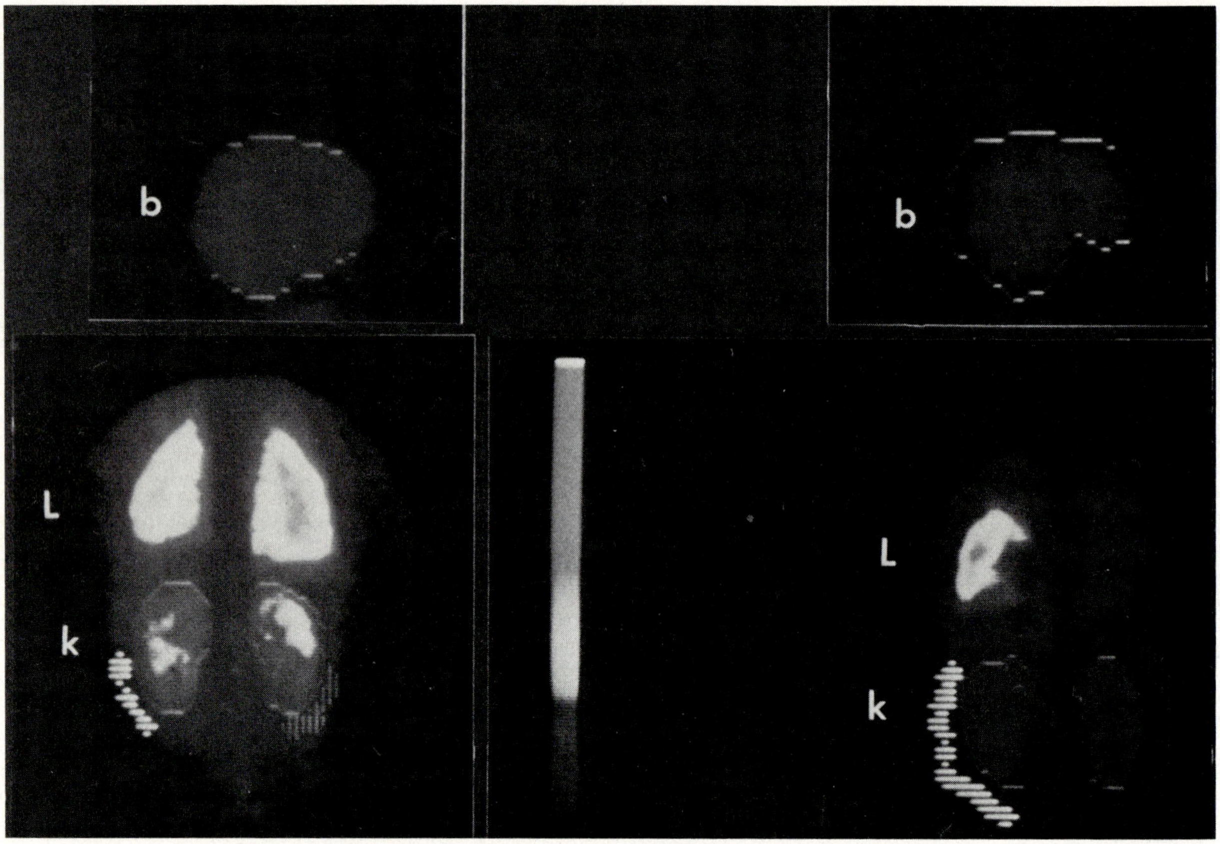

FIGURE 6. *Left,* Radionuclide shunt study from a patient with a Glenn shunt and large PAVF (on echocardiogram and angiogram). Note the appearance of radionuclide counts in lungs (L), brain (B), and kidneys (K). *Right,* The same study repeated after embolization of the fistula. There are fewer counts at all three sites.

left shunting (radionuclide ratio of 0.28), and presumably less trapping of radionuclide material, than the patients with decreased upper/lower lobe perfusion ratios (table 2).

Discussion

Methodology. Abnormal distribution of pulmonary blood flow in patients with Glenn shunts has been described qualitatively,[3, 8, 9] but its quantification and relationship to development of PAVF has not been determined. Moreover, we are aware of comparisons in only four patients who have had Fontan's procedure after placement of a Glenn shunt and these are all qualitative descriptions.[8, 9] The pulmonary blood flow was reported to be evenly distributed in the left (Fontan) lung, whereas the right lung had the characteristic maldistribution observed with a Glenn shunt. The time after surgery at which the patients were studied was not mentioned. Our study is the first to quantify distribution of pulmonary blood flow in right and left lungs in

TABLE 2
Results in patients in the Glenn group

		Radionuclide data on left-to-right shunting		2D echo data	
Ratio of upper/lower lobe perfusion	n	≥0.07[A] (n)	Value in PAVF pt(s)	PAVF (n)	Venous collateral (n)
>.28 (increased)	2	1	1.3	1	0
≥0.07, ≤0.28 (normal)	5	2	0.08, 0.23	2	0
<0.07 (decreased)	13	9[B]	0.07, 0.08	2	4
Total (%)	20 (100)	12 (60)		5 (25)	4 (20)

2D echo = two-dimensional echocardiographic.
[A]Brain + kidney + left lung/right lung.
[B]Includes two patients with other anatomic sources of right-to-left shunting.

patients after placement of a Glenn shunt and after the Fontan procedure, to combine the use of radionuclide scans and two-dimensional echocardiographic contrast studies to detect right-to-left shunting, and to determine the source of this shunting.

Our method of assessing radionuclide distribution of pulmonary flow differs from that described by Friedman et al.[10] and accounts for the lower values for upper/lower lobe perfusion ratio we obtained. We used ^{133}Xe to measure the lung height, whereas they took this measurement from the perfusion study. Use of our method is advantageous in patients in whom there is impaired segmental perfusion that may make determination of lung boundaries inaccurate. The nature of the radionuclide studies required that our control volunteers be young adults. The mean age of our patients was 15 years. Previous investigations suggest that children of normal height who are more than 10 years of age should have the same distribution of perfusion as adults.[11] Younger children may be expected to have more flow to the apeces. Since the latter constituted 18% of our group (five patients) we may have underinterpreted as normal a decreased upper/lower lobe perfusion ratio in three patients in the Glenn and one patient in the Fontan group and overinterpreted as high a normal value in another patient with a Glenn shunt. This, however, could not be determined with certainty.

Detection of PAVF by radionuclide scanning in patients with other conditions,[12, 13] as well as in patients with Glenn shunt,[4, 8, 9, 14] has depended largely on a qualitative assessment. In a quantitative study by Glenn et al.,[5] the presence of PAVF was inferred by decreased uptake of ^{99m}Tc-MAA in the right lung. Our method has the added advantage of quantifying the distribution of isotopes in peripheral organs and should therefore be more sensitive.

The echocardiographic contrast method used also had advantages over the one described previously in patients with this condition.[4] A greater contrast was added by the use of CO_2 and use of the two-dimensional rather than the M mode echocardiographic approach allowed simultaneous visualization of all four cardiac chamber and pulmonary veins, as well as easier differention of venous collateral vessels from PAVF.

Abnormal distribution of perfusion. Our findings are in agreement with those of Boruchow et al.[15] who observed increased perfusion to the lower lung lobes, the amount of which correlated with duration after placement of a Glenn shunt. In our study, the increase was observed consistently when the patient was studied 4 years or more after surgery. These changes occur before there is any clinical evidence of shunt failure,[16–19] which is uncommon until 10 years after surgery. The exact cause of the maldistribution is unknown and, while it most likely results from the inability of low pulsatile pulmonary blood flow to counteract the effect of gravity, it is difficult to understand why it takes years to become manifest. Presumably the upper lobe vessels constrict and the lower ones dilate to accommodate the preferential direction of flow. A change in distribution of perfusion may not be readily apparent on a lung scan until the vessels become altered structurally and the discrepancy is more severe. The only patient in the Fontan group who had undergone surgery more than 4 years before this study had preferential flow to lower lung lobes. He was asymptomatic but had a RA-RV communication. The other patient developed preferential flow to the lower lobes only 1 year after surgery along with concomitant right-sided congestive heart failure. He also had a RA-PA communication, so we can speculate that since he lacked the ancillary pump a right ventricular chamber might provide,[20] he could tolerate less well the pulmonary vasoconstriction that may have resulted from ventilation/perfusion mismatch. Alternatively, other factors that contributed to congestive heart failure might also have resulted in a decreased ratio of upper/lower lobe perfusion. This seems unlikely since right-sided congestion, particularly if associated with a rise in pulmonary arterial pressure, would tend to favor distribution toward the upper lung.[21]

We cannot readily explain the fact that two patients who had undergone Fontan procedure (RA-RV) had increased flow to the upper lung lobes. They could not be distinguished from the others with respect to age, duration after surgery, nature of previous palliative procedures, or anatomic or hemodynamic characteristics.

PAVF and abnormal distribution of flow. The 25% incidence of PAVF in patients with Glenn shunts that we observed is similar to that previously reported.[5] Increased perfusion to lower lung lobes was only present in two of five patients with PAVF, and both of these had had Glenn shunts for more than 13 years. The two patients in whom PAVF were associated with normal perfusion were studied only 2 and 4 years after surgery, respectively. Both were symptomatic and each had an anatomic abnormality causing decreased perfusion to the left lung. In these patients it is possible that there was diversion of flow from the lower extremities to the superior vena cava (via the azygous vein) and this accelerated the formation of PAVF. In patients with severe right-to-left shunting through PAVF, less trapping of radiopharmaceutical material in the lower lobes may result in a normal or increased ratio of upper/lower lobe perfusion. Thus, the formation of PAVF may result from several interrelated factors that could include an abnormally increased distribution of flow to the lower lobes, increased time after surgery, and decreased perfusion or increased resistance in the contralateral lung.[5] Degree of hypoxemia or polycythemia may be additional contributing factors, but this could not be determined from our small series.

Clinical implications. We do not know why patients who had undergone Fontan procedure or had received a Glenn shunt had higher radionuclide counts in peripheral organs when compared with control subjects. Perhaps it is a feature common to other patients after thoracotomy or perhaps it is low pulsatile pulmonary blood flow that induces the formation of small arteriovenous communications. We speculate that with increasing time after surgery and in response to preferential distribution of pulmonary flow to lower lung lobes, these communications, regardless of their cause, may enlarge to form true fistulae. There is no experimental basis for this speculation, but studies of the response of the microcirculation to nonpulsatile flow are certainly feasible[22] and could be carried out.

The radionuclide scan indicated the presence of a right-to-left shunt and the two-dimensional echocardiographic contrast study localized the site of shunting in almost every patient. In two patients there was an anatomic reason for the apparent right-to-left shunt that was clarified by results of cardiac catheterization. In one patient there was still a discrepancy but the bolus of contrast material may have been inadequately injected or visualized. PAVF may be missed by catheterization studies[4, 12, 18] unless, as suggested by Glenn et al.,[5] selective pulmonary venous saturations and angiograms are obtained, but this may not always be technically feasible.

On the basis of our findings we propose that when a surgical procedure such as creation of a axillary arteriovenous fistula or a Fontan operation is being considered in patients with a Glenn shunt, radionuclide scan and two-dimensional echocardiographic contrast studies should be performed and analyzed, according to the method presented, as part of the preoperative evaluation. If, on the basis of these studies, PAVF are suspected, cardiac catheterization should be directed at localizing them and evaluating their hemodynamic significance. Embolization may be of great benefit in selective cases.[23]

Patients who have undergone the Fontan procedure may be at risk for the development of PAVF. All patients in this group in our series had at least trivial right-to-left shunting identified on their radionuclide scans (as did all Glenn patients), and two demonstrated maldistribution of flow. It is possible that when the length of the follow-up period for patients who have had a Fontan procedure reaches that for patients with a Glenn shunt, a similar incidence of fistulae will be found. If maldistribution of flow causes hypoxic pulmonary vasoconstriction resulting from ventilation perfusion mismatch it may be poorly tolerated in post-Fontan patients, particularly those with RA-PA communications, who lack whatever contribution to cardiac output the small right ventricle may provide.[20]

We gratefully acknowledge the help of the cardiology fellows Drs. Brian Craig, Neil Adelman, Chander Bhagraith, Hersch Rosenberg, and Rob Gow, the technical assistance of Ms. Maria Green, Rosie Puntillo, Daniela Filice, Bernadette Lisico, and Mr. Paul Denhartog in performing and analyzing the radionuclide studies, and the secretarial assistance of Ms. Pamela Longley. We also thank Ms. Eva Struthers and Mr. Ray Caesar for their help in preparing the illustrations.

References

1. Fontan F, Baudet E: Surgical repair of tricuspid atresia. Thorax **26:** 240, 1971
2. Glenn WW: Circulatory bypass of the right side of the heart IV. Shunt between superior vena cava and distal right pulmonary artery — report of clinical application. N Engl J Med **259:** 117, 1958
3. Samanek M, Oppelt A, Kasalicky J, Voriskova M: Distribution of pulmonary blood flow after cava pulmonary anastomosis (Glenn operation). Br Heart J **31:** 511, 1969
4. McFaul RC, Tajik AJ, Mair DD, Danielson GK, Seward JB: Development of pulmonary arteriovenous shunt after superior vena cava-right pulmonary artery (Glenn) anastomosis. Circulation **55:** 212, 1977
5. Glenn WW, Hellenbrand WE, Henisz A, Laks H, Kope G, Stansel HC Jr, Talner NS: Superior vena cava–right pulmonary artery anastomosis: present status. *In* Tucker BL, Luiseswiter GG, Tarahashi M, editors: Obstructive lesion of the right heart. Baltimore, 1984, University Park Press, p 121–134
6. Tow DE, Wagner HN Jr, Lopez-Masano V, Smith EM, Migita T: Validity of measuring regional pulmonary arterial flow with macro aggregates of human-serum albumin. J Roentgenol Radium Ther Nucl Med **96:** 664, 1966
7. Seward JB, Tajik AJ, Spangler JG, Ritter DG: Echocardiographic contrast studies, initial experience. Mayo Clin Proc **50:** 163, 1975
8. Laks H, Midd JG, Slandeven JW, Fagan L, Willman VL: Long-term effect of the superior vena cava — pulmonary artery anastomosis on pulmonary blood flow. J Thorac Cardiovasc Surg **74:** 253, 1979
9. Pennington PG, Nouri S, Ho J, Secker-Walker R, Patel B, Swakoff M, William VL: Glenn shunt: long-term results and current role in congenital heart operations. Ann Thorac Surg **31:** 532, 1980
10. Friedman WF, Braunwald E, Morrow AG: Alterations in regional pulmonary blood flow in patients with congenital heart disease studied by radioisotope scanning. Circulation **37:** 747, 1968
11. O'Brodovich HM, Mellins RB, Mansell AL: Effects of growth on the diffusion constant for carbon monoxide. Am Rev Respir Dis **125:** 670, 1982
12. Keren G, Biochis H, Zwas TS, Frand M: Pulmonary arteriovenous fistulae in hepatic cirrhosis. Arch Dis Child **58:** 302, 1983
13. Genovesi MG, Tierney DF, Taplin GV, Eisenberg H: An intravenous radionuclide method to evaluate hypoxemia caused by abnormal alveolar vessels. Am Rev Respir Dis **114:** 58, 1976
14. Van den Bogaert-Van Heesvelde AM, Derom F, Kunnen M, Van-

egmond H, Devloo-Blangquaert A: Surgery for arteriovenous fistulas and dilated vessels in the right lung after the procedure. J Thorac Cardiovasc Surg **76:** 195, 1978
15. Boruchow IB, Swenson EW, Elliot LP, Wheat MW, Schiebler GL: Study of the mechanisms of shunt failure after superior vena cava right pulmonary artery anastomosis. J Thorac Cardiovasc Surg **60:** 532, 1970
16. Martin SP, Anabtawi IN, Selmonosky CA, Folger GM, Ellison LT, Ellison RG: Long-term follow-up after superior vena cava — right pulmonary artery anastomosis. Ann Thorac Surg **9:** 339, 1970
17. Bargeron LM, Karp RB, Barcia A, Kirklin JW, Hunt D, Deverall PB: Late deterioration of patients after superior vena cava to right pulmonary artery anastomosis. Ann J Cardiol **30:** 211, 1982
18. DiCarlo D, Williams WG, Freedom RM, Trusler GA, Rowe RD: The role of cava-pulmonary (Glenn) anastomosis in the palliative treatment of congenital heart disease. J Thorac Cardiovasc Surg **83:** 437, 1982
19. Stanton RE: Experience with the cava-pulmonary artery (Glenn) anastomosis at Children's Hospital of Los Angeles. *In* Tucker BL, Lindesmith GG, Tardhashi M, editors: Obstructive lesions of the right heart. Baltimore, 1984, University Park Press, p 111
20. Bull C, de Leval MR, Stark J, Taylor JFN, Macartney FJ, McGoon D: Use of a subpulmonary ventricular chamber in the Fontan circulation. J Thorac Cardiovasc Surg **85:** 21, 1983
21. Daly W, Giammona S, Ross J, Feigenbaum H: Effects of pulmonary vascular congestion on postural changes in the perfusion and filling of the pulmonary vascular bed. J Clin Invest **43:** 68, 1964
22. Davis MJ, Joyner WL, Gilmore JP: Microvascular pressure distribution and responses of pulmonary allografts and cheek pouch arterioles in the hamster to oxygen. Circ Res **49:** 125, 1981
23. Gomes A, Benson L, George B, Laks H: Management of pulmonary arteriovenous fistulas after superior vena cava-right pulmonary artery (Glenn) anastomosis. J Thorac Cardiovasc Surg **87:** 636, 1984

The effects of overdrive pacing and lidocaine on atrioventricular junctional rhythm in man: the role of abnormal automaticity

JÓZSEF TENCZER, M.D., LÁSZLÓ LITTMANN, M.D., MIKLÓS ROHLA, M.D., AND TAMÁS FENYVESI, M.D.

ABSTRACT The effects of overdrive pacing and lidocaine were studied in 22 patients with atrioventricular (AV) junctional rhythms. Based on the responses to cardiac pacing and lidocaine, patients were divided into two groups. AV junctional rhythms in group I (17 patients) were suppressed by overdrive pacing, and their rates were decreased by lidocaine. Lidocaine also prolonged the junctional recovery time in these patients. AV junctional rhythms in group II (five patients) were not suppressed by overdrive pacing. In contrast, the rate increased after overdrive pacing. Lidocaine did not alter the basic cycle lengths or the recovery times of the AV junctional rhythms in this group of patients. The data suggest that AV junctional rhythms in group I were caused by normal automaticity, while those in group II were probably due to abnormal automaticity.
Circulation 72, No. 3, 480–486, 1985.

IN RECENT YEARS there has been a considerable increase in our understanding of the mechanisms of clinical arrhythmias. As a result of clinical electrophysiologic studies, arrhythmias in man are usually diagnosed as being reentrant or automatic.[1] For some years, however, it has been recognized that mechanisms other than reentry or overdrive suppressible automaticity may be operative in the genesis of arrhythmias.[2] These electrophysiologic mechanisms include triggered activity resulting from early and delayed afterdepolarization[3, 4] and abnormal automaticity due to partial membrane depolarization.[5, 6] Although there have been some attempts to identify clinical arrhythmias based on these mechanisms, the results have not been entirely convincing.[7–9] The purpose of this study was to analyze the effects of overdrive pacing and lidocaine on atrioventricular (AV) junctional rhythms (AV junctional escape rhythms and accelerated AV junctional rhythms) in an attempt to reveal the mechanisms responsible for these arrhythmias.

Material and methods

The study group consisted of 22 patients, 14 men and eight women, with ages ranging from 41 to 81 years (mean 66 years). The patients were admitted because of acute myocardial infarction, unstable angina, or clinically suspected digitalis intoxication. Three patients had complete AV block with junctional escape rhythm, five had high-grade AV block with junctional escape rhythm, four had accelerated AV junctional rhythm, four had AV junctional escape beats revealed by premature atrial impulses, and six had junctional rhythm due to sinus bradycardia. Pertinent clinical, electrocardiographic, and electrophysiologic data are summarized in tables 1 and 2.

After informed consent was obtained, right heart catheterization was performed in the patients while in the postabsorptive state. A bipolar pacing electrode was introduced percutaneously through the right subclavian or femoral vein and advanced to the right atrium and the right ventricle. AV junctional recovery time was measured by overdrive atrial and/or ventricular pacing at several cycle lengths ranging from 1500 to 300 msec. Junctional recovery time was defined as the interval between the last paced QRS complex and the first junctional beat after cessation of pacing. Each stimulation period was 15 sec in duration, and each stimulus was tested twice. After control measurements were taken, the same stimulation program was repeated after lidocaine was administered as a 100 mg intravenous bolus injection over 5 min. AV junctional cycle length was also measured before and after administration of lidocaine. AV junctional origin of the escape rhythm was confirmed by His bundle electrocardiography in three cases.

Statistical methods. The effects of increasing driving rates on junctional recovery times before and after lidocaine were analyzed by two-way analysis of variance (ANOVA).[10, 11] In this study the hypothesis of no variation over different driving heart rates is rejected if the F statistic formed by the ratio of the mean square for different treatments to the mean square for residual exceeds the critical value with degrees of freedom (j–l) and (j–l) (i–l), where j is the number of different conditions and i is the number of patients. For the intercomparison of data points before and after lidocaine we computed a two-way ANOVA

From the Third Department of Medicine, Semmelweis University Medical School, Budapest, Hungary.

Address for correspondence: József Tenczer, M.D., Third Department of Medicine, Semmelweis University Medical School, Eötvös utca 12, Budapest 1121, Hungary.

Received July 18, 1984; revision accepted May 2, 1985.

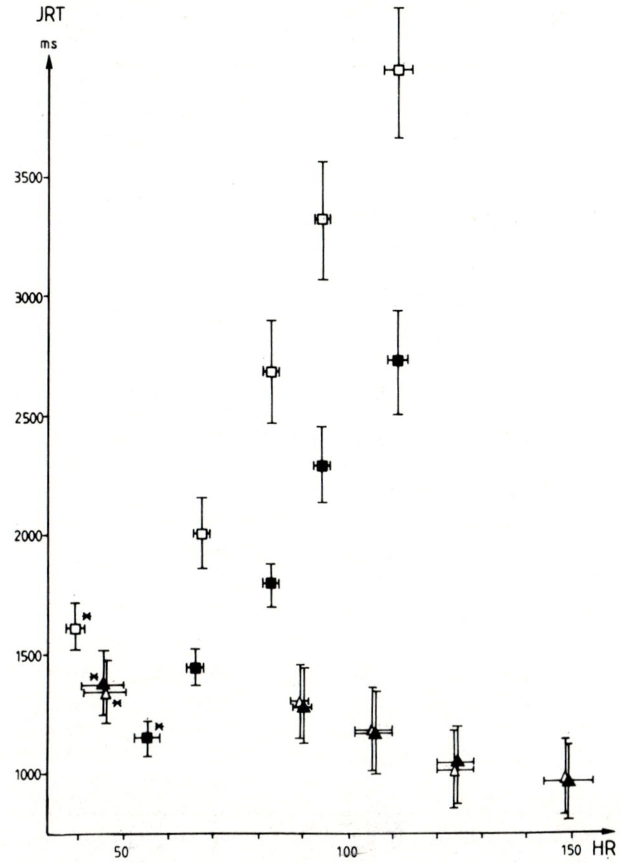

from the differences between corresponding data points ($X_{i,j\ after} - X_{i,j\ before}$), and calculated the t values from the formula

$$t = \frac{\text{mean difference}_j}{\sqrt{\text{mean square residual}}} \times \sqrt{i}$$

Since five sets of data were intercompared (the initial junctional cycle length and four junctional recovery times), we used a critical t value at $p < .01$, that is, .05/5.

Results

Based on the responses to overdrive pacing and lidocaine, two patient groups were identified. Pertinent electrophysiologic findings in groups I and II are listed in tables 1 and 2 and are graphically summarized in figure 1. When asystole after overdrive pacing was longer than 5 sec, ventricular demand pacing was initiated (patients 5, 6, 9, and 12) (table 1). In these patients junctional recovery time was 5000 msec or more. In two patients (Nos. 3 and 13), junctional escape beats occurred only after premature stimulation. After lidocaine, the compensatory pauses were not

FIGURE 1. The effects of increasing driving rates (HR) on AV junctional recovery times before (open symbols) and after lidocaine (closed symbols). Squares and triangles denote group I and group II patients, respectively. Initial cycle lengths are marked by asterisks.

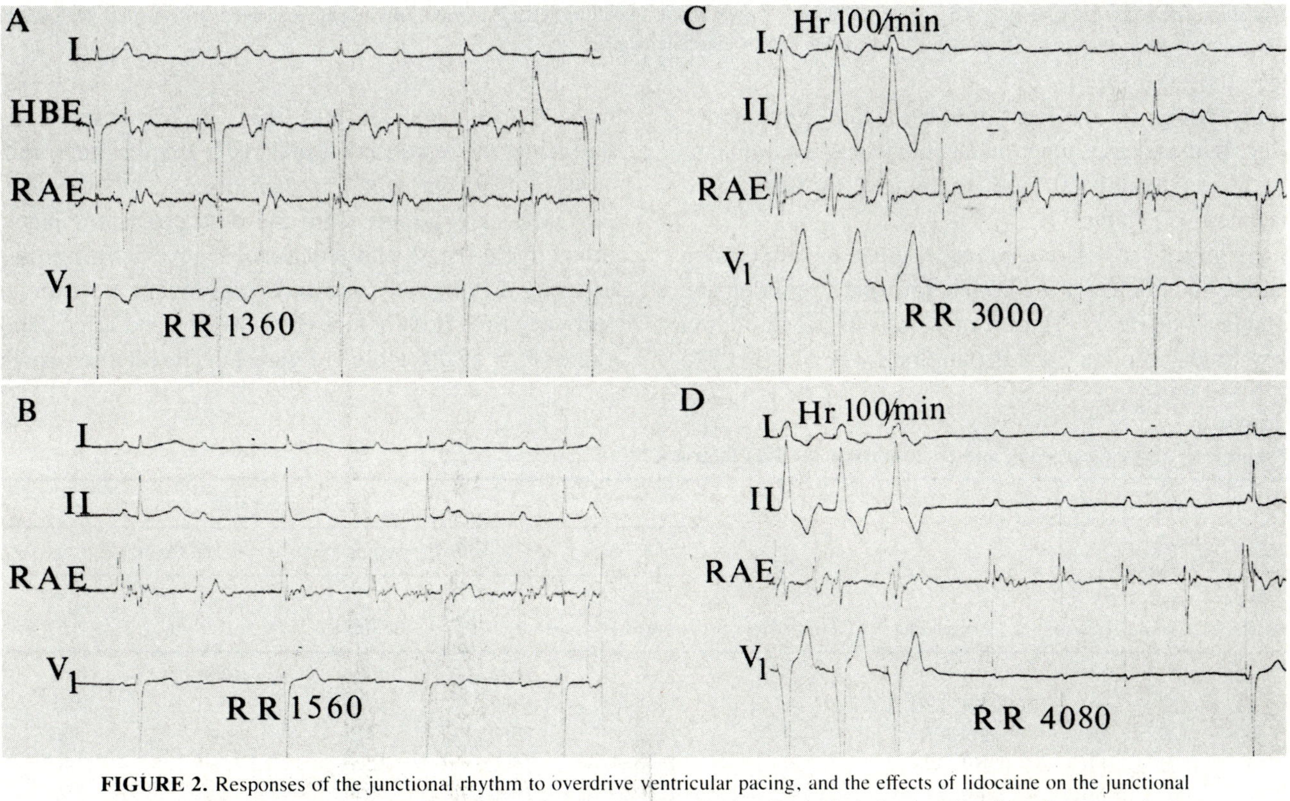

FIGURE 2. Responses of the junctional rhythm to overdrive ventricular pacing, and the effects of lidocaine on the junctional cycle length and junctional recovery time in patient 16. *A* and *B*, Junctional cycle lengths before and after lidocaine, respectively. *C* and *D*, Junctional recovery times before and after lidocaine, respectively. I, II, V_1 = surface electrocardiographic leads; RAE = right atrial electrogram; HBE = His bundle electrogram; Hr = paced heart rate. RR represent the junctional cycle lengths in *A* and *B*, and the junctional recovery times in *C* and *D*.

TABLE 1
Clinical, electrocardiographic, and electrophysiologic data in group I

					Before lidocaine				
						JRT (msec) at mean ± SE HR (bpm) of:			
Patient No.	Age (yr)	Diagnosis	Arrhythmia	DSBP (mm Hg)	JCL (msec)	65.9±1.8	82.5±0.9	94.4±1.1	110.9±2.9
1	59	MI	CAVB, JER	20	1000	1320	1600	1760	2040
2	77	DI	AJR	—	800	1080	1200	1360	1480
3	67	UA	ES JER	—	1440	1800	1960	2200	2480
4	70	DI	AJR	—	840	1000	1120	1200	1400
5	41	MI	HAVB, JER	—	1100	1440	1520	3000	4500
6	77	MI	CAVB, JER	20	1320	1800	2120	2680	3360
7	79	DI	AJR	—	840	1300	1600	1640	1700
8	73	DI	AJR	—	900	1000	1640	1920	2000
9	71	UA	HAVB, JER	30	1500	1680	1920	2040	2760
10	45	MI	HAVB, JER	—	1000	1900	2160	2800	3000
11	61	MI	HAVB, JER	—	1200	1320	1980	2720	3220
12	50	DI	HAVB, JER	—	1240	1560	2900	3200	3700
13	81	UA	ES JER	20	960	1080	1160	1360	1520
14	53	MI	SB, JER	—	1080	1360	1900	2960	3800
15	60	MI	SB, JER	—	1200	1560	1680	2800	3040
16	63	UA	CAVB, JER	—	1360	1600	2040	2400	3000
17	72	UA	SB, JER	—	1600	1800	1920	3000	3440
Mean					1140	1447	1789	2296	2732
±SE					59	72	105	160	223

AJR = accelerated junctional rhythm; CAVB = complete AV block; DI = digitalis intoxication; DSBP = the maximum drop in systolic blood pressure (cuff sphygmomanometer) observed during pacing or lidocaine; ES JER = junctional rhythm revealed by extrasystoles; HAVB = high-grade AV block; HR = driving heart rate; JCL = junctional cycle length; JER = junctional escape rhythm; JRT = junctional recovery time; L = lidocaine; MI = myocardial infarction; SB = sinus bradycardia; UA = unstable angina.

long enough for the junctional beats to become manifest. In these cases junctional cycle length was equal to or longer than 1600 msec (patient 3) or 1200 msec (patient 13) (table 1).

In group I, overdrive pacing resulted in suppression of the junctional rhythm both before and after lidocaine (table 1, figure 1). The mean ± SE junctional recovery time at the maximal driving rate was 2732 ± 223 msec before lidocaine and 3831 ± 276 msec after lidocaine; the respective initial cycle lengths measured 1140 ± 59 and 1641 ± 102 msec. The two-way ANOVA calculations from the data points for junctional cycle length and junctional recovery time at increasing driving rates showed a significant increase in recovery time both before ($F = 47.18$) and after lidocaine ($F = 57.2$) (table 1, figure 1). The intercompari-

TABLE 2
Clinical, electrocardiographic, and electrophysiologic data in group II

					Before lidocaine				
						JRT (msec) at mean ± SE HR (bpm) of:			
Patient No.	Age (yr)	Diagnosis	Arrhythmia	DSBP (mm Hg)	JCL (msec)	91.0±1.9	106.0±4.0	124.0±4.0	149.0±5.6
18	72	MI	SB, JER	—	1200	1080	1000	1000	880
19	65	MI	SB, JER	—	1760	1760	1700	1600	1480
20	69	DI	ES JER	—	1040	960	720	640	560
21	71	MI	SB, JER	30	1640	1600	1520	1280	1160
22	72	MI	ES JER	—	1260	1000	920	880	820
Mean					1380	1280	1148	1080	980
±SE					137	166	177	166	157

Abbreviations are as in table 1.

TABLE 1
(Continued)

	After lidocaine			
	JRT (msec) at mean ± SE HR (bpm) of:			
JCL (msec)	64.7±1.6	82.6±0.9	93.8±1.0	111.5±3.2
1320	1520	1900	2080	2400
1040	1400	1600	1720	1920
>1600	1920	2520	2900	2920
2200	2480	2600	2600	2840
1360	1680	2180	3600	>5000
2360	2880	3960	4440	>5000
1400	1780	1780	2200	2680
1100	1360	1440	1800	2120
2500	3000	4000	4720	>5000
1900	2120	2800	3200	4040
1600	1880	2600	3000	3600
1440	1720	2960	3800	>5000
>1200	1600	3000	3840	5000
1600	1920	3400	4400	4600
1440	1680	2000	3600	3920
1560	1800	2600	3600	4080
1800	3520	4400	5000	5000
1614	2015	2691	3324	3831
102	147	209	246	276

son of data points before and after lidocaine showed a significant increase in cycle length and recovery time after drug. Mean differences are summarized in table 3.

Responses of junctional rhythms to overdrive pacing and lidocaine were quite different in group II patients. Junctional rhythm in group II was not suppressed by overdrive; the first postpacing interval shortened after overdrive pacing (table 2, figure 1). In this group, the mean ± SE recovery time corresponding to the highest driving rate was shortened from 1380 ± 137 (initial cycle length) to 980 ± 157 msec before, and from 1364 ± 142 (initial cycle length) to 984 ± 155 msec after lidocaine. The two-way ANOVA calculations showed a significant decrease in junctional recovery time both before ($F = 30.12$) and after lidocaine ($F = 20.05$). In this group lidocaine alone did not have any effect (table 3, figure 1).

TABLE 2
(Continued)

	After lidocaine			
	JRT at mean ± SE HR (bpm) of:			
JCL (msec)	90.0±1.6	106.0±4.0	124.0±4.0	149.0±5.6
1140	1160	1080	920	920
1760	1800	1700	1640	1460
1040	1000	680	640	560
1640	1600	1540	1200	1180
1240	960	920	840	800
1364	1304	1172	1048	984
142	168	185	173	155

Representative tracings demonstrating the effects of overdrive pacing and lidocaine on the junctional rhythms in group I and II patients are shown in figures 2 to 4. The electrocardiograms in figure 2 were taken from a group I patient with complete AV block (patient 16). Lidocaine prolonged the junctional cycle length from 1360 to 1560 msec (figure 2, *A* and *B*). Overdrive ventricular pacing at a rate of 100 beats/min resulted in suppression of the junctional escape rhythm both before and after lidocaine. Junctional recovery time before and after lidocaine measured 3000 and 4080 msec, respectively (figure 2, *C* and *D*). Electrocardiograms in figures 3 and 4 were obtained from a group II patient (No. 22). Figure 3 illustrates results of a stimulation study before lidocaine. A junctional escape interval was induced by ventricular stimuli (figure 3, first panel). On increasing the atrial pacing rate from 85 to 165 beats/min, shortening of the postpacing interval from 1000 to 820 msec occurred (figure 3, second through fifth panels). After lidocaine, a similar time relation to that observed in figure 3 existed between the pacing rate and junctional recovery time (figure 4). At an atrial pacing rate of 165 beats/min junctional recovery time was 800 msec. The tracings clearly demonstrate that as the driving cycle lengths diminished, so did the coupling intervals of the AV junctional rhythms.

Discussion

In this report we present effects of overdrive pacing and lidocaine on AV junctional rhythms in 22 patients. Based on responses to overdrive pacing, two types of junctional rhythms were identified, namely one that could be suppressed by overdrive (group I) and one that was not overdrive suppressible (group II). Because of the relatively small number of patients, further classification according to clinical diagnosis did not seem to be reasonable.

AV junctional rhythms that are depressed by overdrive stimulation are conventionally thought to result from a normal automatic mechanism (group I), but the overdrive acceleration seen in group II patients cannot be explained by normal automaticity. This system of classification of the mechanism of arrhythmia, which is based solely on responses to pacing, has certain limitations. First, abnormal automaticity may be over-

TABLE 3
The effects of lidocaine on junctional cycle length and junctional recovery time in groups I and II

	Group I					Group II				
	JCL	JRT	JRT	JRT	JRT	JCL	JRT	JRT	JRT	JRT
Mean difference	474.1	584.7	901.2	1027.1	1098.8	−16	20	24	−32	4
t value	4.44	5.48	8.45	9.63	10.3	−0.82	1.02	1.23	−1.65	0.21
Critical value of t			2.6549					2.92		

JCL = junctional cycle length; JRT = junctional recovery time.

drive suppressible if it occurs at a slightly decreased membrane potential. It cannot therefore be ruled out that certain patients in group I, e.g., those with digitalis intoxication, had overdrive suppressible abnormal automaticity. Second, entrance block to the junctional pacemaker may theoretically be responsible for absence of overdrive suppression. A junctional recovery time, however, which is shorter than the cycle length is not likely to occur with this mechanism. Moreover, in three of five group II patients junctional recovery time was determined and was found to be essentially identical after atrial and ventricular stimulation. This strongly suggests that in at least these three patients entrance block to the pacemaker was probably not an important factor. Third, normal automaticity may exhibit overdrive acceleration under certain conditions, e.g., under the effects of catecholamine. Although in one of the group II patients (No. 21), in whom overdrive stimulation resulted in a fall in blood pressure, a sympathetic discharge–induced increase in junctional rate could not be ruled out with certainty, such a simple mechanism would not account for the linear relationship of the first postpacing interval to the pacing rate observed in each of the group II patients.

Experimental observations indicate that overdrive enhancement as seen in group II may be consistent with two cellular electrophysiologic phenomena, namely delayed afterdepolarization and abnormal automaticity. The role of delayed afterdepolarization and abnormal automaticity in human arrhythmias has not been clarified. Castellanos, Lown, Wittenberg, and Zipes and their colleagues[12–15] have demonstrated in the intact canine heart that toxic levels of digitalis can induce ventricular escape rhythms that progressively accelerate after a progressive increase in driving rate. By microelectrophysiologic techniques, delayed afterdepolarization was demonstrated to be the mechanism responsible for accelerated ectopic rhythms resulting from toxic levels of digitalis.[3, 4] Arrhythmias due to delayed afterdepolarization were also shown to occur in the absence of digitalis intoxication in fibers of the atrioventricular valves,[16] of the coronary sinus region,[17] and of the atrial muscle.[18] In a recent publication a set of rules was outlined that was considered to be useful in recognizing some of the clinical characteristics of delayed afterdepolarization–induced arrhythmias.[2] It seems that an arrhythmia that is induced and terminated by electric stimulation might be the result of either reentrant excitation or delayed afterdepolarization. If overdrive pacing at increasing rates or extra-

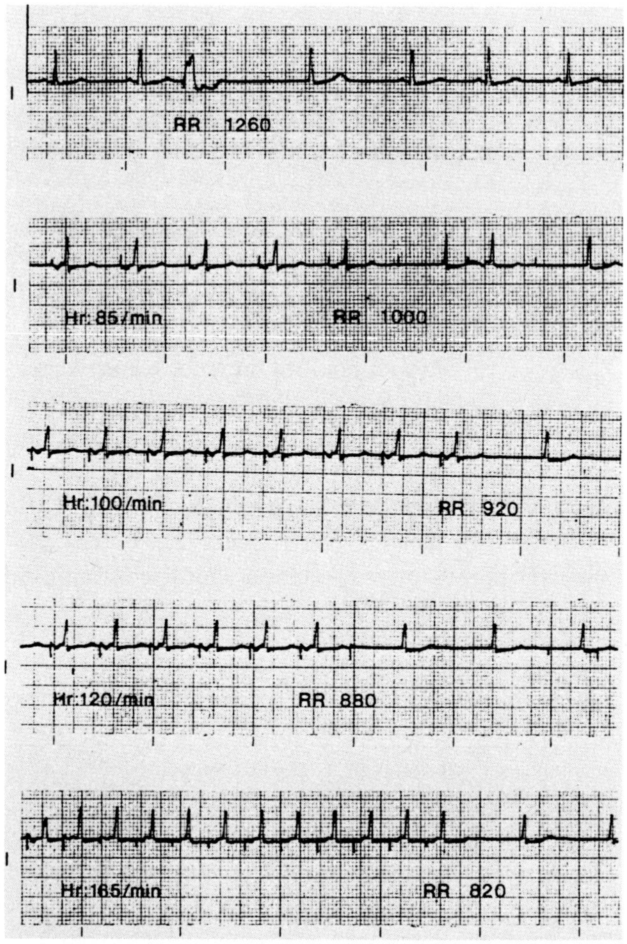

FIGURE 3. Responses of junctional rhythm to overdrive atrial pacing in patient 22. On increasing the pacing rate, shortening of the junctional recovery time occurred. Some ineffective pacing stimuli are seen in the second and fourth panels. RR represents the basic junctional cycle length in the first panel and the junctional recovery times in the others. Hr = paced heart rate.

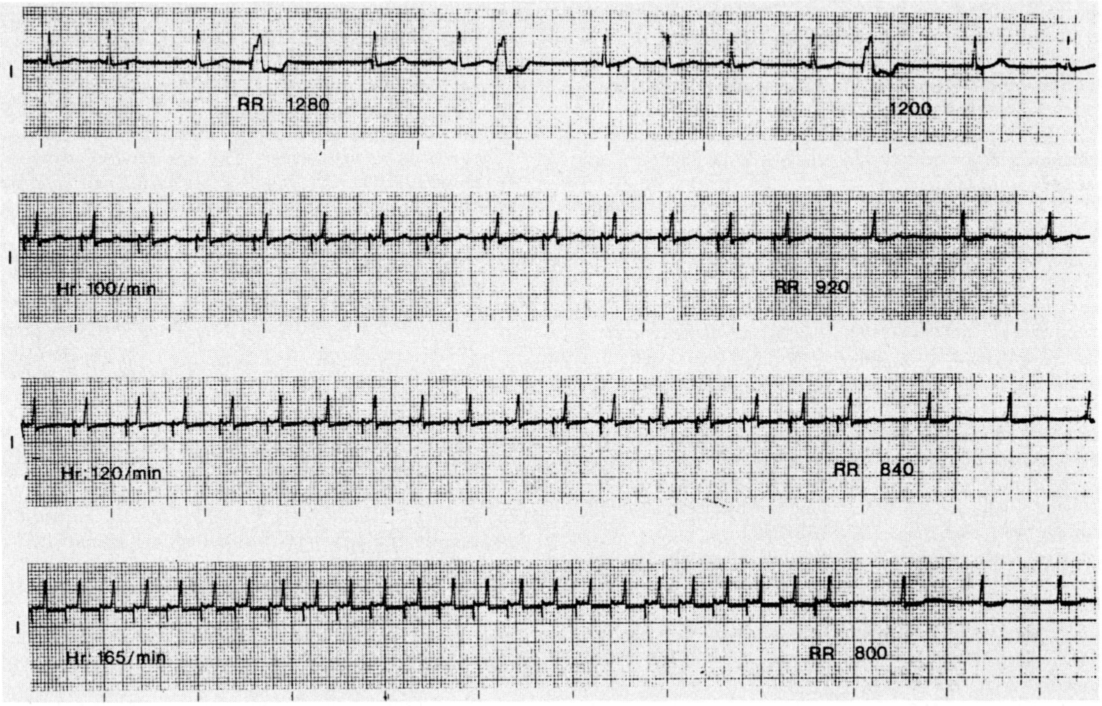

FIGURE 4. The effects of lidocaine on the junctional cycle length and recovery time in patient 22. Junctional recovery time and cycle length were not significantly altered by lidocaine. Abbreviations as in figure 3.

stimulation with increasing prematurity results in shortening of the first postpacing interval, the mechanism is more likely to be delayed afterdepolarization.

The role of abnormal automaticity in human arrhythmogenesis is also not clear. Abnormal automaticity shows characteristics of both normal automaticity and delayed afterdepolarization. Like normal automaticity, its occurrence does not depend on the presence of a previous impulse. On the other hand, it is not depressed by overdrive stimulation of brief duration (10 to 20 sec). In contrast, the rate of the abnormal automatic rhythm may increase after overdrive pacing, and premature stimulation may also result in abbreviation of cycle length.[6, 19] Because of these features, it is difficult to differentiate clinical arrhythmias resulting from delayed afterdepolarization from those resulting from abnormal automaticity. Various pharmacologic agents may be useful in recognizing the underlying electrophysiologic mechanism.[19–21]

In our study, which is a clinical extension of the experimental work of Ilvento et al.,[19] we have used lidocaine for this purpose. It must be stressed that while Ilvento's study dealt with idioventricular rhythms, our study deals with AV junctional rhythms. Lidocaine has been shown to have varying effects on AV junctional rhythms in man,[22] but the underlying electrophysiologic mechanisms have not been analyzed. Under experimental conditions and with use of the microelectrode technique, lidocaine has been shown to depress the normal automatic mechanism[23] and delayed afterdepolarization[24, 25] in Purkinje fibers, but it has no or very little effect on abnormal automaticity.[26] As far as these experimental observations can be extrapolated to AV junctional rhythms in man, our study with lidocaine confirmed the observations obtained during stimulation procedures in that junctional rhythms in group I showed characteristics of normal automaticity. In the patients in whom junctional rhythms were not overdrive suppressible (group II), responses to lidocaine seemed to favor abnormal automaticity rather than delayed afterdepolarization.

In conclusion, despite limitations of clinical electrophysiologic methods in delineating the cellular mechanisms of AV junctional rhythms, our results seem to be consistent with the suggestion that some junctional rhythms in man are probably caused by abnormal automaticity.

References

1. Wellens HJJ: Value and limitations of programmed electrical stimulation of the heart in the study and treatment of tachycardias. Circulation **57:** 845, 1978
2. Rosen MR, Reder RF: Does triggered activity have a role in the genesis of cardiac arrhythmias? Ann Intern Med **94:** 794, 1981
3. Cranefield PF: Action potentials, afterpotentials, and arrhythmias. Circ Res **41:** 415, 1977
4. Rosen MR, Gelband H, Merker C, Hoffman BF: Mechanisms of digitalis toxicity: effects of ouabain on phase 4 of canine Purkinje fiber transmembrane potentials. Circulation **47:** 681, 1973

5. Dangman KH, Hoffman BF: Effects of nifedipine on electrical activity of cardiac cells. Am J Cardiol **46:** 1059, 1980
6. Dangman KH, Hoffman BF: Effects of overdrive and premature stimuli on abnormal automaticity in canine cardiac Purkinje fibers. Circulation **63**(suppl III): III-55, 1980 (abst)
7. Zipes DP, Foster PF, Troup PJ, Pedersen DH: Atrial induction of ventricular tachycardia: reentry versus triggered automaticity. Am J Cardiol **44:** 1, 1979
8. Rosen MR, Fisch C, Hoffman BF, Danilo P, Lovelace ED, Knoebel SB: Can accelerated atrioventricular junctional escape rhythms be explained by delayed afterdepolarizations? Am J Cardiol **45:** 1272, 1980
9. Tenczer J, Littmann L, Rohla M: Atrioventricular junctional rhythm induced by atrial stimulation: a suspected clinical manifestation of "triggered" activity. Am J Cardiol **53:** 631, 1984
10. Armitage P: Statistical methods in medical research. Oxford, 1971, Blackwell
11. Wallenstein S, Zucker CL, Fleiss JL: Some statistical methods useful in circulation research. Circ Res **47:** 1, 1980
12. Castellanos A, Lemberg L, Centurion MJ, Berkovits EE: Concealed digitalis induced arrhythmias unmasked by electrical stimulation of the heart. Am Heart J **73:** 484, 1967
13. Lown B, Cannon RL, Rossi MA: Electrical stimulation and digitalis drugs: Repetitive response in diastole. Proc Soc Exp Biol Med **126:** 698, 1967
14. Wittenberg SM, Streuli F, Klocke FJ: Acceleration of ventricular pacemakers by transient increases in heart rate in dogs during ouabain administration. Circ Res **26:** 705, 1970
15. Zipes DP, Arbel E, Knope RF, Moe GK: Accelerated cardiac escape rhythms caused by ouabain intoxication. Am J Cardiol **33:** 248, 1974
16. Wit AL, Cranefield PF: Triggered activity in cardiac muscle fibers of the simian mitral valve. Circ Res **38:** 85, 1976
17. Wit AL, Cranefield PF: Triggered and automatic activity in the canine coronary sinus. Circ Res **41:** 435, 1977
18. Saito T, Otoguro M, Matsubara T: Electrophysiological studies of the mechanism of electrically induced sustained rhythmic activity in the rabbit right atrium. Circ Res **42:** 199, 1978
19. Ilvento JP, Provet J, Danilo P, Rosen MR: Fast and slow idioventricular rhythms in the canine heart: a study of their mechanism using antiarrhythmic drugs and electrophysiologic testing. Am J Cardiol **49:** 1909, 1982
20. Klevans LR, Kelly RJ: Effect of autonomic neural blockade on verapamil-induced suppression of the accelerated ventricular escape beat in ouabain treated dogs. J Pharmacol Exp Ther **206:** 259, 1978
21. Foster A, King RM, Nicoli AB, Zipes DP: Suppression of ouabain induced ventricular rhythms with aprindine HCL: a comparison with other antiarrhythmic agents. Circulation **53:** 315, 1976
22. Kuo C, Reddy CP: Effect of lidocaine on escape rate in patients with complete atrioventricular block. B. Proximal His bundle block. Am J Cardiol **47:** 1315, 1981
23. Davis LD, Temte JV: Electrophysiological actions of lidocaine on canine ventricular muscle and Purkinje fibers. Circ Res **24:** 639, 1969
24. Eisner DA, Lederer WJ: A cellular basis for lidocaine's antiarrhythmic action. J Physiol **295:** 25, 1979
25. Rosen MR, Danilo P: Effects of tetrodotoxin, lidocaine, verapamil and AHR-266 on ouabain-induced delayed afterdepolarizations in canine Purkinje fibers. Circ Res **46**: 117, 1980
26. Brennan FJ, Cranefield PF, Wit AL: Effects of lidocaine on slow response and depressed fast response action potentials of canine Purkinje fibers. J Pharmacol Exp Ther **204:** 312, 1978

Programmed ventricular stimulation in survivors of an acute myocardial infarction

DENIS ROY, M.D., ETIENNE MARCHAND, M.D., PIERRE THÉROUX, M.D.,
DAVID D. WATERS, M.D., GUY B. PELLETIER, M.D., AND MARTIAL G. BOURASSA, M.D.

ABSTRACT The prognostic significance of programmed ventricular stimulation and its usefulness in relation to other forms of invasive and noninvasive testing was evaluated in 150 survivors of acute myocardial infarction. Ventricular tachyarrhythmias of 6 beats or more were induced in 35 (23%) patients. No significant differences existed between patients with inducible ventricular tachyarrhythmias and those without inducible ventricular tachycardia with respect to occurrence of spontaneous ventricular arrhythmias in the acute and early recovery phase of infarction or predischarge exercise-induced ischemia or arrhythmias, severity of coronary artery disease, or degree of left ventricular dysfunction. A higher incidence of inferior myocardial infarction was observed in patients with inducible ventricular tachycardia when compared with those without inducible ventricular tachycardia (66% vs 41%, $p < .01$). During a mean follow-up of 10 ± 5 months (range 2 to 19), there were two sudden deaths, three nonsudden deaths, and two additional patients developed sustained ventricular tachyarrhythmias. There was no significant difference between patients with and those without inducible ventricular tachyarrhythmias with respect to the occurrence of these events . In this study population, a lower mean ejection fraction ($p < .01$), the presence of a ventricular aneurysm ($p < .05$), and exercise-induced ventricular premature contractions ($p < .05$) were predictors of sudden death and of spontaneous ventricular tachycardia. Thus, the findings of this study do not support the hypothesis that the induction of ventricular tachyarrhythmias in patients recovering from acute myocardial infarction identifies a group at high risk for sudden cardiac death.
Circulation 72, No. 3, 487–494, 1985.

SURVIVORS OF MYOCARDIAL INFARCTION represent a large and easily identifiable population of patients at risk for sudden cardiac death and considerable efforts have been made to identify in this group those patients at highest risk for subsequent fatal arrhythmic events. Although it has been demonstrated that frequent and repetitive ventricular premature complexes during ambulatory electrocardiographic monitoring are associated with increased mortality,[1–9] the predictive accuracy of this marker of risk for sudden death and its relationship to left ventricular dysfunction are still somewhat controversial.[10–16] Furthermore, trials of class I antiarrhythmic drug therapy after myocardial infarction have produced discouraging results.[17, 18]

Programmed electrical stimulation has been used effectively in the diagnosis and management of patients with life-threatening ventricular arrhythmias.[19–24] More recently, it has been suggested that this technique could accurately predict patients at risk for sudden death after myocardial infarction.[25, 26] However, this finding has not been substantiated by other investigators,[27] and the relationship between the information obtained by electrophysiologic testing and other prognostic indicators has not yet been evaluated.

This prospective study was undertaken to evaluate the prognostic significance of programmed ventricular stimulation in patients with recent myocardial infarction. In addition, the prognostic value of results of programmed ventricular stimulation was compared with that of the site and size of myocardial infarction, the incidence of spontaneous arrhythmias observed during both the acute and early recovery phase of infarction, the severity of coronary artery disease, and the degree of left ventricular dysfunction.

Methods

Patient population. The study population was selected from 320 patients admitted to the coronary care unit of the Montreal Heart Institute between May 1983 and October 1984 for acute

From the Department of Medicine, Montreal Heart Institute and the University of Montreal Medical School, Montreal, Quebec, Canada.
Supported by the Montreal Heart Institute Research Fund, Montreal, Quebec, Canada.
Address for correspondence: Denis Roy, M.D., Montreal Heart Institute, 5000 East Belanger St., Montreal, Quebec H1T 1C8, Canada.

myocardial infarction and who satisfied the following criteria: (1) age 65 years or less, (2) absence of uncontrolled angina or heart failure, (3) absence of sustained ventricular tachycardia 72 hr or more after the onset of infarction, and (4) absence of significant nonischemic heart disease. Of these patients, 150 gave written informed consent to undergo treadmill exercise testing, 24 hr ambulatory electrocardiographic monitoring, coronary angiography, left ventricular radionuclide angiography, and programmed ventricular stimulation.

Clinical evaluation. A detailed clinical history and physical examination were obtained from each patient. On admission, patients were assigned by clinical criteria to Killip classes I through IV.[28] Serum creatine kinase and MB isoenzyme levels were measured at 8 hr intervals for the first 24 hr and then daily for the next 48 hr. The criteria for acute myocardial infarction included at least two of the following: myocardial ischemic pain lasting more than 30 min, serum levels of creatine kinase elevated at least twice above the upper limit of normal with presence of the MB fraction, and Minnesota code–electrocardiographic criteria[29] for acute infarction.

Programmed ventricular stimulation. All patients underwent programmed ventricular stimulation while in the postabsorptive state and while receiving no antiarrhythmic medication for at least 72 hr before the study. The tests were performed a mean of 12 ± 2 days (range 8 to 20) after myocardial infarction. A quadripolar electrode catheter was inserted percutaneously and positioned at the right ventricular apex under fluoroscopic guidance. Stimulation was performed with a programmable stimulator and an isolated constant current source. The stimuli were rectangular pulses 1.5 msec in duration at twice diastolic threshold (0.3 to 1.4 mA). The following protocol of programmed stimulation was used: (1) A single ventricular extrastimulus (S_2) was introduced in late diastole during two paced ventricular cycle lengths (S_1-S_1 = 600 and 400 msec) and moved earlier until ventricular refractoriness was encountered. (2) Double ventricular extrastimuli were then introduced starting at an S_1-S_2 interval 50 msec longer than the ventricular refractory period and an S_2-S_3 equal to S_1-S_2. S_2-S_3 was shortened in 10 msec decrements until S_3 failed to capture the ventricle and S_1-S_2 was then shortened until S_3 evoked a response. This was continued until both S_2 and S_3 reached refractoriness. (3) The entire sequence was then repeated at the right ventricular outflow tract. The protocol was terminated prematurely if a sustained ventricular tachycardia or ventricular fibrillation occurred.

Repetitive ventricular responses were defined as one to five ventricular complexes in response to a ventricular stimulus. Ventricular tachycardia was defined as nonsustained if it persisted for six complexes or more but terminated spontaneously within 30 sec. Ventricular tachycardia was considered sustained if it lasted more than 30 sec or if it required immediate termination because of hemodynamic collapse.

Electrocardiographic monitoring. All patients were observed with continuous visual electrocardiographic monitoring assisted by rate alarms for the first 4 days in the coronary care unit. A two-channel 24 hr Holter recording was obtained in 147 patients a mean of 11 ± 9.5 days (range 5 to 90) after myocardial infarction. Counts were made of the total number of ventricular premature complexes during each hour and the arrhythmias were also graded according to the system devised by Lown and Wolf.[30]

Exercise testing. Exercise testing was performed as previously described[31] in 148 patients a mean of 9 ± 2 days (range 6 to 17) after myocardial infarction by the Naughton protocol.[32] End points were 70% of age-predicted maximal heart rate, workload of 5 mets, appearance of limiting symptoms, severe ventricular arrhythmias, and greater than 5 mm of ST segment depression. A test result was considered abnormal if 1 mm or more of ST segment depression developed compared with the baseline tracing and with the use of a minimum of three and in most instances 12 electrocardiographic leads.

Catheterization and angiographic procedures. Selective coronary arteriography was performed as previously described[33] in all patients a mean of 10 (range 7 to 19) days after myocardial infarction. Each patient was classified as having one-, two-, or three-vessel coronary artery disease based on the presence of a 75% or more reduction of the internal vessel diameter of the main arteries or branches. Left ventricular ejection fraction was calculated in each patient from a radionuclide-gated scan obtained with the use of technetium perchlorate.

Follow-up. Patients were followed up to 19 months at 3 to 6 month intervals. No patient was lost to follow-up and follow-up data were complete in all patients. A clinical history, physical examination, and electrocardiogram were obtained during each visit. For the purpose of this report, January 31, 1985 was determined a common termination date and follow-up information was obtained in all patients during the 6 weeks preceding this date.

The end points of the study were death or the development of documented sustained ventricular tachyarrhythmias. Death was defined as sudden if it occurred within 1 hr of the onset of symptoms.

Although the results of the programmed ventricular stimulation study were available to the treating physician, they did not influence treatment since this technique was considered as a research procedure. Only one patient was discharged on antiarrhythmic drug therapy. This patient, who had inducible sustained ventricular tachycardia, did not undergo stimulation-guided antiarrhythmic therapy and drug therapy had been discontinued at the time of last follow-up.

Differences among continuous variables were analyzed by the unpaired Student t test. Discrete variables were compared with the chi-square test. For 2 × 2 tables with cell frequencies of less than 5, analysis was performed with Fisher's exact probability test. All values are expressed as mean ± 1 SD. A p value of less than .05 was considered indicative of a significant difference.

Results

Response to programmed ventricular stimulation (table 1). Ventricular fibrillation during programmed ventricular stimulation occurred in two patients. Sustained ventricular tachycardia was induced in 16 patients. The arrhythmia had a right bundle branch block morphology in 10 patients and a left bundle branch block morphology in six. The mean cycle length of the tachycardia was 246 msec (range 200 to 330) and its mean duration was 40 sec (range 13 to 180). Nonsustained ventricular tachycardia was initiated in 17 patients. The tachycardia was polymorphic in 13 patients and had a right bundle branch block morphology in four. The mean cycle length of the tachycardia was 214 msec (range 175 to 300) and its duration was 16 complexes (range 6 to 43). Two ventricular extrastimuli were required to initiate all sustained and nonsustained ventricular tachyardias. External countershock was required to terminate sustained ventricular tachyarrhythmia in 10 patients.

TABLE 1
Response to programmed ventricular stimulation

Response	n
Group A (n = 35)	
Ventricular fibrillation	2
Sustained ventricular tachycardia	16
Nonsustained ventricular tachycardia	17
Group B (n = 115)	
Repetitive ventricular responses	85
No response	30

Repetitive ventricular responses were induced in 85 patients. Thirty patients had no extra response to programmed ventricular stimulation.

On the basis of programmed stimulation, the patients were divided into two groups. Group A consisted of the 35 patients (23%) with inducible ventricular tachycardia or ventricular fibrillation. Group B comprised the remaining 115 patients (77%), who had either one to five repetitive ventricular responses or no extra response to programmed ventricular stimulation at all.

Seventeen patients belonging to group A and 56 patients in group B were receiving β-blockers at the time of programmed ventricular stimulation (p = NS). The mean stimulation threshold was 0.71 ± 0.18 among patients in group A and 0.62 ± 0.24 in group B ($p < .05$). However, ventricular refractory periods were similar between the two groups (252 ± 20 vs 259 ± 22 msec; p = NS).

The ventricular stimulation studies caused no deaths. All sustained ventricular tachyarrhythmias were converted promptly to sinus rhythm, although conversion was complicated by persistent neurologic sequelae in one patient.

Clinical characteristics. The clinical characteristics of the patients in the two groups are summarized in table 2. The average age of all patients was 52 years; 87% were men and 26% had suffered a previous myocardial infarction. The location of acute infarction was anterior in 45% of the patients and inferior in 47% of patients. Thirty percent of patients had non–Q wave infarction. The mean peak creatine kinase level for all patients was 1989 IU/liter. Most patients had no evidence of left ventricular failure at the time of admission. The incidence of inferior infarction was significantly higher in the patients in group A (66%) compared with those in group B (41%, $p < .01$) and anterior infarctions were more frequent in group B (51%) than in group A (26%, $p < .01$). There was no significant difference in age, sex distribution, incidence of prior myocardial infarction, incidence of non–Q wave infarction, peak creatine kinase levels, or Killip class between the two groups.

Comparison of the spontaneous ventricular arrhythmias in the acute (≤72 hr) phase of myocardial infarction and response to programmed ventricular stimulation (table 3). Thirty-eight (25%) of the 150 patients suffered from ventricular tachycardia or fibrillation in the first 72 hr after myocardial infarction. Twelve (8%) patients had a sustained ventricular tachyarrhythmia requiring cardioversion and 26 (17%) patients had nonsustained ventricular tachycardia. The proportion of patients having these arrhythmias was not significantly different between group A and group B.

Comparison of the arrhythmias recorded during 24 hr ambulatory electrocardiographic monitoring and response to programmed ventricular stimulation. The mean number of ventricular premature complexes per hour recorded during 24 hr Holter monitoring was 4.3 ± 10.9 among patients of group A compared with 2.4 ± 6.5 in patients of group B. Although a trend was present this difference was not significant and, as illustrated in figure 1, the number of ventricular premature complexes per hour was evenly distributed between the two groups. Only 11 (7%) patients in this study had more than 10 ventricular premature complexes per hour.

There was also no significant difference in Lown grade classification between patients in group A and group B. Thirteen patients (38%) in group A and 32 patients (28%) in group B had grade 3 or 4 arrhythmias.

Correlation of results of exercise testing with results of programmed ventricular stimulation (table 4). Forty-eight (32%) of the 148 patients who underwent exercise testing developed 1 mm or more ST segment depres-

TABLE 2
Clinical characteristics

	Group A (n = 35)	Group B (n = 115)	Total (n = 150	p value
Age (years)	52	52	52	NS
Sex (men)	32 (91%)	99 (86%)	131 (87%)	NS
Prior MI	9 (26%)	30 (26%)	39 (26%)	NS
Location of acute MI				
Anterior	9 (26%)	59 (51%)	68 (45%)	<.01
Inferior	23 (66%)	47 (41%)	70 (47%)	<.01
Undetermined	3 (8%)	9 (8%)	12 (8%)	NS
Non–Q wave MI	8 (23%)	37 (32%)	45 (30%)	NS
Peak creatine kinase (IU/L)	2546±3458	1727±1503	1989±2277	NS
Killip class ≥2	7 (20%)	13 (11%)	20 (13%)	NS

MI = myocardial infarction.

TABLE 3
Comparison of the arrhythmias recorded in the coronary care unit with the results of programmed ventricular stimulation

	Group A (n = 15)	Group B (n = 115)	Total (n = 150)	p value
Sustained VT/VF	5 (14%)	7 (6%)	12 (8%)	NS
Nonsustained VT	5 (14%)	21 (18%)	26 (17%)	NS
VT/VF	10 (28%)	28 (24%)	38 (25%)	NS

VT = ventricular tachycardia; VF = ventricular fibrillation.

sion. Sixty-two (42%) patients developed either exercise-induced angina or ST segment depression. Ventricular premature complexes during or after exercise were observed in 14 patients (9%). Again the incidence of these findings was not significantly different between the two groups.

Coronary angiography and radionuclide ventriculography. As shown in table 5, no significant differences existed between the two groups with respect to the number of coronary vessels with a stenosis of 75% or more (1.5 ± 0.8 vs 1.6 ± 0.8), the mean ejection fraction measured by predischarge radionuclide gated scan (45 ± 12% vs 46 ± 12%), and the number of patients with a left ventricular aneurysm (three vs nine patients).

Follow-up. In table 6, the results of programmed ventricular stimulation are correlated with clinical outcome during the 10 ± 5 months (range 2 to 19) of follow-up evaluation. There were seven (5%) fatal or near-fatal cardiac events. Four of these seven events occurred within 3 months of infarction. There were two sudden deaths. One group A patient with inducible sustained ventricular tachycardia died suddenly at 15

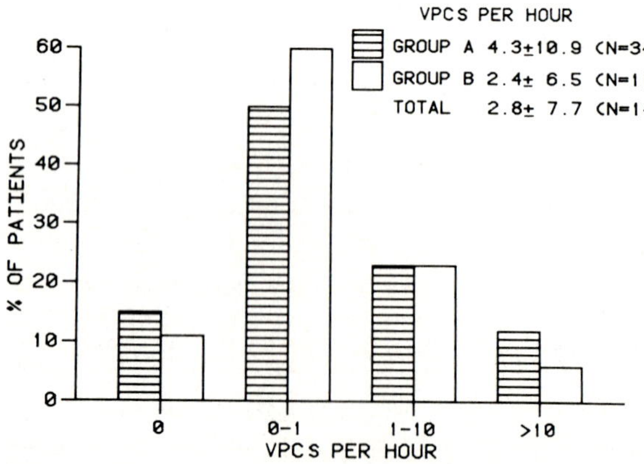

FIGURE 1. Relationship between the number of ventricular premature contractions (VPCs) per hour during 24 hr ambulatory electrocardiographic monitoring and the response to programmed ventricular stimulation.

TABLE 4
Correlation between results of exercise testing and those of programmed ventricular stimulation

	Group A (n = 34)	Group B (n = 114)	Total (n = 148)	p value
ST segment depression (≥1 mm)	10 (29%)	38 (33%)	48 (32%)	NS
Angina or ST segment depression	14 (41%)	48 (42%)	62 (42%)	NS
VPCs	3 (9%)	11 (10%)	14 (9%)	NS

VPCs = ventricular premature contractions.

months of follow-up and one patient belonging to group B died suddenly 15 days after hospital discharge. Three patients belonging to group B suffered nonsudden cardiac deaths. All three deaths were due to cardiogenic shock, two secondary to recurrent myocardial infarction and one related to coronary bypass surgery. Two patients, one in each group, were resuscitated from spontaneous sustained ventricular tachycardia. The arrhythmia occurred 1 week after hospital discharge in the patient in group A with inducible sustained ventricular tachycardia and developed in the late hospital course of a recurrent myocardial infarction in the patient in group B. There were no significant differences in the occurrence of sudden death, nonsudden death, and/or spontaneous sustained ventricular tachycardia between the two groups. There was also no significant difference in the occurrence of these events when the 18 patients with inducible sustained ventricular tachyarrhythmias were compared with the 132 patients without inducible sustained arrhythmias at the time of programmed ventricular stimulation. Patients with inducible sustained tachyarrhythmias had a lower mean ejection fraction than

TABLE 5
Response to programmed ventricular stimulation related to the results of coronary angiography and radionuclide ventriculography

	Group A (n = 35)	Group B (n = 115)	Total (n = 150)	p value
No. of coronary vessels with ≥75% stenosis	1.5±0.8	1.6±0.8	1.5±0.8	NS
Left ventricular ejection fraction (%)	45±12	46±12	46±12	NS
Left ventricular aneurysm (pts)	3	9	12	NS

TABLE 6
Correlation between results of programmed ventricular stimulation and clinical outcome (mean follow-up 10 ± 5 months)

	Group A (n = 35)	Group B (n = 115)	Total (n = 150)	p value
Deaths	1	4	5	NS
Sudden	1	1	2	NS
Nonsudden	0	3	3	NS
Spontaneous sustained VT	1	1	2	NS
Recurrent MI	0	6	6	NS
Therapy at end of follow-up				
β-Blockers	15	51	66	NS
Coronary bypass surgery or coronary angioplasty	4	17	21	NS
Antiarrhythmic drugs	2	3	5	NS

MI = myocardial infarction; VT = ventricular tachycardia.

those without inducible sustained arrhythmias (40 ± 12% vs 46 ± 11%, p < .05). There were no significant differences between patients with and those without inducible sustained tachyarrhythmias with respect to other clinical characteristics.

Six patients, all belonging to group B, experienced recurrent nonfatal myocardial infarction.

At the end of follow-up, 15 group A and 51 group B patients were receiving the pharmacologic equivalent of propranolol, 160 mg/day or less (p = NS). Four patients in group A and 17 patients in group B underwent coronary bypass surgery or coronary angioplasty for control of angina (p = NS). Two patients in group A and three patients in group B were receiving antiarrhythmic drug therapy (p = NS). Of these five patients, two were being treated for paroxysmal atrial fibrillation and antiarrhythmic therapy was initiated for premature ventricular complexes in three patients.

To determine if other factors could accurately identify high-risk patients, the subjects who died or experienced spontaneous sustained ventricular tachyarrhythmias were compared with those who did not experience these events during the follow-up period with respect to clinical characteristics and results of all available tests. The mean ejection fraction was significantly lower in the seven patients who died or had sustained ventricular tachyarrhythmias when compared with the remaining 143 patients (35 ± 14% vs 46 ± 11%, p < 0.01). Ventricular arrhythmias occurred during exercise testing in three of the seven patients suffering end point events (43%) as compared with 11 of 141 (8%) survivors (p < .05). When the analysis compared only the four patients who died suddenly or had sustained ventricular tachyarrhythmias with the patients who did not experience an arrhythmic event, the differences still attained statistical significance: the mean ejection fraction was 29 ± 12% in these four patients as compared with 46 ± 11% in the remaining 146 patients (p < .01) and exercise-induced ventricular arrhythmias were observed in two of four patients (50%) who died suddenly or later developed sustained ventricular tachyarrhythmias as compared with 12 of 144 patients (8%) who did not experience these events during follow-up (p < .05). Furthermore, the incidence of sudden death or spontaneous sustained ventricular tachyarrhythmias was significantly greater in patients with a left ventricular aneurysm than in patients without an aneurysm (17% vs 1%, p < .05). No statistically significant difference could be detected between survivors and patients who died and/or had spontaneous ventricular tachyarrhythmias in terms of history of prior myocardial infarction, site and extension of acute infarction, Killip class at admission, peak creatine kinase level, occurrence of ventricular arrhythmias in the acute phase of infarction, mean ventricular premature contractions per hour or Lown grade during Holter monitoring, exercise-induced angina or ST segment depression, two- or three-vessel coronary artery diseases, or medication at the time of follow-up.

The 170 nonassessed patients underwent a follow-up similar to that in the 150 assessed patients. There were eight (5%) deaths during a mean follow-up of 9 ± 5 months: four were nonsudden, two were sudden, and two were due to undetermined causes.

Discussion

This study was designed to test the hypothesis that the induction of ventricular tachyarrhythmias soon after a myocardial infarction could identify those patients at risk for subsequent serious arrhythmic events. In this prospective study, patients also underwent 24 hr Holter monitoring, exercise testing, coronary angiography, and radionuclide ventriculography before hospital discharge. There are three major findings: first, the response to programmed ventricular stimulation was unrelated to the indexes of infarct size or the severity of coronary artery disease, or to the occurrence of spontaneous ventricular arrhythmias in the acute and early recovery phase of myocardial infarction; second, the initiation of a ventricular tachyarrhythmia by electrophysiologic testing was a poor marker of risk for the occurrence of sudden death or spontaneous ventricular tachycardia during the 10 month follow-up period; third, prognosis was more related to ejection fraction, exercise-induced ventricular premature contractions, and presence of a left ventricular aneurysm.

Comparison with previous studies. The ability to sustain reentrant circuits in areas of ischemic or infarcted ventricular tissue is believed to be a major mechanism causing sudden arrhythmic death. Programmed ventricular stimulation has been validated as a method of reproducing clinically occurring ventricular tachyarrhythmias.[20–24] Because the capacity for such arrhythmias may exist in survivors of myocardial infarction, programmed ventricular stimulation has been proposed as a method for assessing electrical instability and for predicting sudden arrhythmic death after myocardial infarction. Green et al.[34] reported that the induction of repetitive responses in postinfarction patients was predictive of future serious arrhythmias. However, the significance of repetitive responses has since been questioned and several studies have demonstrated that they are unrelated to outcome.[35–38]

Two recent reports[25, 26] have shown a correlation between the elicitation of sustained or nonsustained ventricular tachyarrhythmias and the occurrence of sudden death after myocardial infarction. Hamer et al.[25] studied 70 patients with myocardial infarction complicated by heart failure or arrhythmia and found that four of 12 patients with inducible ventricular tachycardia of 5 beats or more died suddenly while only one of 25 patients without ventricular tachycardia after maximal provocation died suddenly ($p < .05$). Richards et al.[26] evaluated 165 survivors of a myocardial infarction and found that 12 of 38 patients with electrical instability died suddenly or had spontaneous ventricular tachycardia compared with only two of the 127 stable patients. Our findings differ from these observations but extend those of Marchlinski et al.,[27] who studied 46 patients after myocardial infarction and reported one sudden death among their 10 patients with inducible arrhythmias (≥4 beats) compared with five sudden deaths in the remaining 36 patients.

It is difficult to compare results between studies because methods of assessment differ. Our stimulation protocol consisted of up to two extrastimuli at twice diastolic threshold but did not include the high current intensities (up to 20 mA) tested by Hamer et al.[25] and Richards et al.[26] However, these latter two studies did not describe the relationship between the high current used and the induction of arrhythmias. We chose this stimulation protocol because its sensitivity and specificity have already been established for patients with clinically documented arrhythmias.[39, 40] The specificity of use of high current strength has yet to be determined and it has been shown that aggressive stimulation protocols can result in elicitation of ventricular tachyarrhythmias in patients without documented or suspected clinical arrhythmias.[41] Furthermore, we were able to induce a ventricular tachyarrhythmia of 6 beats or more in a sizable proportion (23%) of patients. This rate of inducibility is similar to that obtained in the previous studies of patients after myocardial infarction.[25–27] Therefore, it is unlikely that our results are due to the use of inadequate stimulation techniques.

End points and definitions of abnormal responses to programmed ventricular stimulation have also varied between studies. The end point of testing in our study was the induction of a sustained arrhythmia. We could not identify a specific response to programmed ventricular stimulation that could predict the subsequent occurrence of sudden death. Eighteen of our patients had electrical instability as defined by Richards et al.[26] (ventricular arrhythmia lasting at least 10 sec). Sixteen of these patients (89%) have survived to follow-up without an arrhythmic event. None of 17 patients with nonsustained ventricular tachycardia died or experienced an arrhythmic event. One of the 85 patients with repetitive ventricular responses developed sustained ventricular tachycardia and one of the 30 patients with no extra response to programmed ventricular stimulation died suddenly.

Limitations. The overall prognosis for this study population was good: only seven patients (5%) suffered a fatal or near-fatal cardiac event during the 10 month follow-up period. Although programmed ventricular stimulation resulted in initiation of ventricular tachyarrhythmias in a significant proportion of patients (23%), the power of the study may have been decreased by the small numbers of patients who experienced either sudden death or serious arrhythmias. The exclusion of patients with severe heart failure and unstable angina undoubtedly accounts for the low mortality. In studies of nonselected postinfarction patients a 19% 1 year mortality has been reported.[42] However, our rate is comparable to the 2% to 6% mortality in recent studies of more highly selected patients.[43–47] Therefore, our data may not be applicable to the very high-risk subpopulation of survivors of myocardial infarction in whom no further tests may be necessary because their high risk is already clinically obvious.

The outcome in our patients may also have been influenced by information obtained from exercise testing or coronary angiography and the current attitudes about medical and surgical therapy of survivors of myocardial infarction. At the final review over 40% of patients in both groups were being treated with β-blocking agents, which may also account for the low mortality and may have contributed to the lack of a significant difference in the incidence of cardiac events in the two groups. However, no attempt was made to suppress the arrhythmias induced by programmed ventricular stimulation and only five patients were receiving antiarrhythmic therapy at the end of follow-up.

Clinical implication. The findings of this study suggest that the induction of ventricular tachyarrhythmias in postinfarction patients does not identify a subgroup at high risk for sudden cardiac death. Because this invasive technique is associated with some morbidity and potential mortality, we do not recommend it for routine clinical risk stratification of patients recovering from an acute myocardial infarction.

We acknowledge the excellent technical assistance of Emma Lemire and Richard Cartier.

References

1. Kotler MN, Tabatznik B, Mower MM, Tominaga S: Prognostic significance of ventricular ectopic beats with respect to sudden death in the late post-infarction period. Circulation **47:** 959, 1973
2. Vismara LA, Amsterdam EA, Mason DT: Relation of ventricular arrhythmias in the late hospital phase of acute myocardial infarction to sudden death after hospital discharge. Am J Med **59:** 6, 1975
3. Ruberman W, Weinblatt E, Goldberg JD, Frank CW, Shapiro S: Ventricular premature beats and mortality after myocardial infarction. N Engl J Med **297:** 750, 1977
4. Rehnqvist N, Lundman T, Sjogren A: Prognostic implications of ventricular arrhythmias registered before discharge and one year after acute myocardial infarction. Acta Med Scand **204:** 203, 1978
5. Moss AJ, Davis HT, DeCamilla J, Bayer LW: Ventricular ectopic beats and their relation to sudden death and nonsudden cardiac death after myocardial infarction. Circulation **60:** 998, 1979
6. Ruberman W, Weinblatt E, Goldberg JD, Frank CW, Chaudhary BS, Shapiro S: Ventricular premature complexes and sudden death after myocardial infarction. Circulation **64:** 297, 1981
7. Bigger JT Jr, Weld FM, Rolnitzky LM: Prevalence, characteristics and significance of ventricular tachycardia (three or more complexes) detected with ambulatory electrocardiographic recording in the late hospital phase of acute myocardial infarction. Am J Cardiol **48:** 815, 1981
8. Bigger JT Jr, Fleiss JL, Kleiger R, Miller JP, Rolnitzky LM, and the Multicenter Post-Infarction Research Group: The relationship among ventricular arrhythmias, left ventricular dysfunction, and mortality in the 2 years after myocardial infarction. Circulation **69:** 250, 1984
9. Mukharji J, Rude RE, Poole WK, Gustafson N, Thomas LJ Jr, Strauss HW, Jaffe AS, Muller JE, Roberts R, Raabe DS Jr, Croft CH, Passamani E, Braunwald E, Willerson JT and the Milis Study Group: Risk factors for sudden death after acute myocardial infarction: two-year follow-up. Am J Cardiol **54:** 31, 1984
10. Anderson KP, DeCamilla J, Moss AJ: Clinical significance of ventricular tachycardia (3 beats or longer) detected during ambulatory monitoring after myocardial infarction. Circulation **57:** 890, 1977
11. Schulze RA Jr, Strauss HW, Pitt B: Sudden death in the year following myocardial infarction: relation to ventricular premature contractions in the late hospital phase and left ventricular ejection fraction. Am J Med **62:** 192, 1977
12. de Soyza N, Bennett FA, Murphy ML, Bisset JK, Kane JJ: The relationship of paroxysmal ventricular tachycardia complicating the acute phase and ventricular arrhythmia during the late hospital phase of myocardial infarction to long-term survival. Am J Med **64:** 377, 1978
13. Moss AJ: Factors influencing prognosis after myocardial infarction. Curr Probl Cardiol **4:** 1, 1979
14. Taylor GJ, Humphries JO, Mellits ED, Pitt B, Schulze RA, Griffith LSC, Achuff SC: Predictors of clinical course, coronary anatomy and left ventricular function after recovery from acute myocardial infarction. Circulation **62:** 960, 1980
15. Baird MG, Williams WL, Nair R, Allan K, Higginson LA, Beanlands DS: The limited prognostic value of ventricular ectopy recorded early after myocardial infarction. Circulation **64**(suppl IV): IV-306, 1981 (abst)
16. Califf RM, McKinnis RA, Burks J, Lee KL, Harrell FE Jr, Behar VS, Pryor DB, Wagner GS, Rosati RA: Prognostic implications of ventricular arrhythmias during 24 hour ambulatory monitoring in patients undergoing cardiac catheterization for coronary artery disease. Am J Cardiol **50:** 23, 1982
17. May GS, Eberlein KA, Furberg CD, Passamani ER, DeMets DL: Secondary prevention after myocardial infarction: a review of long term trials. Prog Cardiovasc Dis **24:** 331, 1982
18. Furberg CD: Effect of antiarrhythmic drugs on mortality after myocardial infarction. Am J Cardiol **52:** 32C, 1983
19. Fisher JD, Cohen HL, Mehra R, Altschuler H, Escher DJW, Furman S: Cardiac pacing and pacemakers. II. Serial electrophysiologic-pharmacologic testing for control of recurrent tachyarrhythmias. Am Heart J **93:** 658, 1977
20. Josephson ME, Horowitz LN, Farshidi A, Kastor JA: Recurrent sustained ventricular tachycardia. I. Mechanisms. Circulation **57:** 431, 1978
21. Mason JW, Winkle RA: Electrode-catheter arrhythmia induction in the selection and assessment of antiarrhythmic drug therapy for recurrent ventricular tachycardia. Circulation **58:** 971, 1978
22. Horowitz LN, Josephson ME, Farshidi A, Spielman SR, Michelson EL, Greenspan AH: Recurrent sustained ventricular tachycardia. 3. Role of the electrophysiologic study in the selection of antiarrhythmic regimens. Circulation **58:** 986, 1978
23. Ruskin JN, DiMarco JP, Garan A: Out-of-hospital cardiac arrest: electrophysiologic observations and selection of long-term antiarrhythmic therapy. N Engl J Med **303:** 607, 1980
24. Roy D, Waxman HL, Kienzle MG, Buxton AE, Marchlinski FE, Josephson ME: Clinical characteristics and long-term follow-up in 119 survivors of cardiac arrest: relation to inducibility at electrophysiologic testing. Am J Cardiol **52:** 969, 1983
25. Hamer A, Vohra J, Hunt D, Sloman G: Prediction of sudden death by electrophysiologic studies in high risk patients surviving acute myocardial infarction. Am J Cardiol **50:** 223, 1982
26. Richards DA, Cody DV, Denniss AR, Russell PA, Young AA, Uther JB: Ventricular electrical instability: a predictor of death after myocardial infarction. Am J Cardiol **51:** 75, 1983
27. Marchlinski FE, Buxton AE, Waxman HL, Josephson ME: Identifying patients at risk of sudden death after myocardial infarction: Value of the response to programmed stimulation, degree of ventricular ectopic activity and severity of left ventricular dysfunction. Am J Cardiol **52:** 1190, 1983
28. Killip T, Kimball JT: Treatment of myocardial infarction in a coronary care unit: a two year experience with 250 patients. Am J Cardiol **20:** 457, 1967
29. Blackburn H, Keys A, Simonson E, Rautaharju P, Punsar S: The electrocardiogram in population studies. A classification system. Circulation **21:** 1160, 1960
30. Lown B, Wolf M: Approaches to sudden death from coronary heart disease. Circulation **44:** 130, 1971
31. Théroux P, Waters DD, Halphen C, Debaisieux JC, Mizgala HF: Prognostic value of exercise testing soon after myocardial infarction. N Engl J Med **301:** 341, 1979
32. Naughton J, Sevelius G, Balke B: Physiologic responses of normal and pathological subjects to a modified work capacity test. J Sport Med **3:** 201, 1963
33. Bourassa MG, Lespérance J, Campeau L, Bois M, Saltiel J: Selective coronary angiography using a percutaneous femoral technique. Can Med Assoc J **102:** 170, 1970
34. Green HL, Reid PR, Schaeffer AH: The repetitive ventricular response in man — a predictor of sudden death. N Engl J Med **299:** 729, 1978
35. Mason JW: Repetitive beating after single ventricular extrastimuli:

incidence and prognostic significance in patients with recurrent ventricular tachycardia. Am J Cardiol **45:** 1126, 1980
36. Farshidi A, Michelson EL, Greenspan AM, Spielman SR, Horowitz LN, Josephson ME: Repetitive responses to ventricular extrastimuli: incidence, mechanism and significance. Am Heart J **100:** 59, 1980
37. Gomes JAC, Kang PS, Khan R, Kelen G, El-Sherif N: Repetitive ventricular response: its incidence, inducibility, reproducibility, mechanism and significance. Br Heart J **46:** 159, 1981
38. Ruskin JN, DiMarco JP, Garan H: Repetitive responses to single ventricular extrastimuli in patients with serious ventricular arrhythmias: incidence and clinical significance. Circulation **63:** 767, 1981
39. Vandepol CJ, Farshidi A, Spielman SR, Greenspan AM, Horowitz LN, Josephson ME: Incidence and clinical significance of induced ventricular tachycardia. Am J Cardiol **45:** 725, 1980
40. Livelli FD, Bigger JT Jr, Reiffel JA, Gang ES, Patton JN, Noethling PM, Rolnitzky LM, Gliklich JI: Response to programmed ventricular stimulation: sensitivity, specificity and relation to heart disease. Am J Cardiol **50:** 452, 1982
41. Brugada P, Abdollah H, Heddle B, Wellens HJJ: Results of a ventricular stimulation protocol using a maximum of 4 premature stimuli in patients without documented or suspected ventricular arrhythmias. Am J Cardiol **52:** 1214, 1983
42. Bigger JT Jr, Heller CA, Wenger TL, Weld FM: Risk stratification after acute myocardial infarction. Am J Cardiol **42:** 202, 1978
43. Davis HT, DeCamilla J, Bayer LW, Moss AJ: Survivorship patterns in the post-hospital phase of myocardial infarction. Circulation **60:** 1252, 1979
44. DeFeyter PJ, Van Eenige MJ, Dighton DH, Visser FC, De Jong J, Roos JP: Prognostic value of exercise testing, coronary angiography and left ventriculography 6-8 weeks after myocardial infarction. Circulation **66:** 527, 1982
45. Gibson RS, Watson DD, Craddock GB, Crampton RS, Kaiser DL, Denny MJ, Beller GA: Prediction of cardiac events after uncomplicated myocardial infarction: a prospective study comparing predischarge exercise thallium-201 scintigraphy and coronary angiography. Circulation **68:** 321, 1983
46. DeBusk RF, Kraemer HC, Nash E, Berger WE, Lew H: Stepwise risk stratification soon after myocardial infarction. Am J Cardiol **52:** 1161, 1983
47. Abraham RD, Roubin GS, Harris PJ, Bernstein L, Kelly DT: Coronary and left ventricular angiographic anatomy and prognosis of survivors of first acute myocardial infarction. Am J Cardiol **52:** 257, 1983

Change in ventricular cavity size: differential effects on QRS and T wave amplitude

TED FELDMAN, M.D., RORY W. CHILDERS, M.D., KENNETH M. BOROW, M.D., ROBERTO M. LANG, M.D., AND ALEX NEUMANN, B.S.

ABSTRACT Although many factors have been reported to change the R wave amplitude of the electrocardiogram (ECG), few observations have been made of the associated changes in T wave amplitude. We hypothesized that changes in R and T wave amplitude should parallel each other. To test this hypothesis, R and T wave amplitudes were measured in 15 normal subjects during increased and decreased left ventricular dimensions induced by infusion of methoxamine and by Valsalva maneuver, respectively, as well as during changes in the proximity of the left ventricle to the chest wall (i.e., shift in patient position from supine to left lateral position). Simultaneous nine-lead ECGs and two-dimensional–guided M mode echocardiograms of the left ventricle were recorded at rest and under each experimental condition. R wave amplitude increased as the left ventricular lateral wall moved closer to the V_5 and V_6 electrodes. Alterations in R wave amplitude seen with changes in left ventricular chamber size were primarily caused by radial movement of the left ventricle in relation to the chest wall. Proximity of the left ventricle to the chest wall was therefore a major determinant of R wave amplitude. In contrast, T wave amplitude varied directly with alterations in left ventricular chamber size but was unaffected by changes in proximity to the recording electrode on the chest wall. Left ventricular chamber size, and possibly the associated alteration in endocardial-to-epicardial surface area ratio, appeared to be the major determinants of T wave amplitude.
Circulation 72, No. 3, 495–501, 1985.

CHANGES in ST-T wave morphology are commonly used to evaluate clinical problems such as electrolyte disturbances, drug intoxications, myocardial ischemia, and infarction. Although many factors modify QRS amplitude, there are few studies examining the factors determining concomitant change in the T wave.[1]

Many significant influences on the amplitude of the electrocardiographic QRS complex have been described. Changes have been noted during dynamic exercise,[2,3] in pericardial effusion, during myocardial ischemia,[4,5] with QRS axis shifts,[6] and with changes in intramyocardial conduction.[7] Conditions causing changes in left ventricular chamber size cause alterations in electrocardiographic waveform amplitude in humans.[8–15] In left ventricular volume overload states, increases in both T and R wave amplitude have been observed, but no explanation has been proposed for the finding.[16] Using a mathematical model, Brody[9] suggested that intracardiac blood, a highly conductive mass, augments the electrocardiographic surface potential if the progress of myocardial excitation is radial to the blood mass. In contrast, we have recently shown that increases in R wave amplitude, associated with increases in left ventricular chamber size, are primarily a function of changes in the proximity of the left ventricular lateral wall to the chest wall rather than of an increase in left ventricular blood volume.[17]

We hypothesized that variations in T wave amplitude should parallel those of R wave amplitude. To test this hypothesis, R and T wave amplitudes were measured during alterations in left ventricular chamber size and in position of the left ventricle in the chest.

Methods

The study population consisted of 15 healthy male subjects 21 to 33 years old (mean ± SD 26 ± 4). All subjects had normal intracardiac anatomy and left ventricular performance on two-dimensional echocardiographic study as well as a normal scalar electrocardiogram (ECG). The experimental protocol was approved by the University of Chicago Clinical Investigation Committee; written informed consent was obtained from each subject.

Nine-lead ECGs were recorded during held end-expiration on

From the Cardiology Section, Department of Medicine, University of Chicago Hospitals and Clinics, Chicago.

Supported in part by NHLBI Training Grant 2-T32-HL07381.

Address for correspondence: Ted Feldman, M.D., University of Chicago Hospitals and Clinics, 950 E. 59th St., Box 250, Chicago, IL 60637.

Received April 16, 1985; accepted May 23, 1985.

a Marquette Electronics MAC II (Microcomputer Augmented Cardiograph). Leads V_2, V_3, and V_4 were not recorded to permit echocardiographic imaging during the electrocardiographic recording. The electrocardiographic recorder was programmed to write out the median QRS-T complex averaged over 10 sec from all the complexes in a given lead. In this manner variations in amplitude during any single recording were minimized. R wave amplitude was measured as the vertical distance from the PR segment to the peak of the R wave. T wave amplitude was measured from the PR segment to the peak of the T wave. T wave area was planimetered from computer-stored records magnified to twice the usual amplitude at a paper speed of 50 mm/sec.

The experimental protocol used for echocardiographic recordings in this study has been described previously.[19] Scalar ECGs and two-dimensional and targeted M mode echocardiograms were recorded simultaneously from 10 subjects. Recordings were made under resting conditions, during Valsalva maneuver to decrease left ventricular dimensions,[18] and at peak pressor effect induced by the specific α_1-adrenergic agonist methoxamine to increase left ventricular dimensions.[19] Systemic blood pressure was monitored throughout these studies by the Dynamap 1846P Vital Signs Monitor (Critikon Inc., Tampa, FL). In eight subjects simultaneous targeted M mode echocardiograms and ECGs were recorded at end-expiration with subjects in the supine and then in the left lateral decubitus positions to vary the proximity of the left ventricle to the lateral chest wall. These tracings were made under baseline resting conditions without other interventions. Simultaneous recordings of the targeted left ventricular M mode echocardiogram and ECG were performed at held end-expiration under control conditions. Recordings were repeated during the strain phase of the Valsalva maneuver when the left ventricular end-diastolic dimension was smallest. After returning to control status, all subjects received an intravenous bolus of atropine sulfate (0.01 mg/kg). This was followed by an infusion of methoxamine hydrochloride (1 mg/min). When peak systolic blood pressure had increased 30 to 60 mm Hg above control, the methoxamine infusion was discontinued. The peak pressor effect lasted 2 to 5 min, during which time another set of end-expiratory echocardiographic and electrocardiographic recordings was made. A 20 degree left lateral position was used during the control phase, Valsalva maneuver, and methoxamine phase to facilitate echocardiographic recording.

Left ventricular dimensions and wall thicknesses were measured as previously described[19] from targeted M mode echocardiograms recorded on a Hewlett-Packard Ultrasound Imaging System model 77020A (Andover, MA). In addition, the distances from the chest wall to the leading edge of the right septal surface and from the chest wall to the leading edge of the posterior epicardial surface were measured. Distance between the chest wall adjacent to the V_5 electrocardiographic electrode and the left ventricular endocardium was measured from targeted M mode echocardiograms obtained with the transducer in the apical four-chamber position. This distance was measured from the first chest wall echo to the leading edge of the left ventricular apical endocardium.

To further characterize geometric differences between the baseline, decreased, and augmented left ventricular volume conditions, the surface area of the endocardium and that of the epicardium were computed. The short-axis echocardiographic dimension was used as the minor diameter of a prolate ellipse; the major diameter was assumed to be twice the minor diameter. Twice the left ventricular end-diastolic wall thickness was then added to the endocardial end-diastolic dimension to approximate epicardial diameter. The endocardial or epicardial radius of curvature (r) was calculated as the left ventricular dimension divided by 2. These assumptions have previously been shown to be reasonable in normal subjects without regional wall motion abnormalities.[20, 21] Endocardial and epicardial surface areas (S) were derived as follows. The volume of an ellipse is:

$$V = 4/3\ \pi\ (r_1)\ (r_2)\ (r_3)$$

where r_1 = the major axis and r_2 and r_3 = the minor axes of the ellipse. The two minor axes of a prolate ellipse are equal, so $r_2 = r_3$:

$$V = 4/3\ \pi\ (r_1)\ (r_2)^2$$

In a normal left ventricle the major axis is approximately twice the minor axis, therefore

$$V = 4/3\ \pi\ (2)\ (r_2)^3$$

or

$$V = 8/3\ \pi\ r^3$$

The surface area is the first derivative of the volume:

$$S = 8\ \pi\ r^2$$

All echocardiographic measurements were taken as the average of three to five cardiac cycles. Echocardiographic tracings and electrocardiographic T wave areas were digitized and analyzed on a Franklin Quantic 1200 analog-to-digital computer (Bruce Franklin, Inc., Seattle WA).

Statistical analysis. Paired t tests were performed to compare control values with data obtained at peak effects of Valsalva maneuver and methoxamine and supine vs left lateral positions. A p value $<.05$ was considered statistically significant. To test the relationship between two variables, correlation coefficients were calculated by least-squares linear regression analysis. Group data are expressed as mean ± SD.

Results

Relationship between R wave amplitude and left ventricular chamber size and position. In all subjects, left ventricular dimension decreased at peak Valsalva maneuver and increased at peak methoxamine effect relative to baseline values ($p < .001$). R wave amplitude did not change consistently in electrocardiographic leads I, II, III, aVR, aVL, aVF, or V_1 (table 1). As seen in figure 1, *A*, changes in left ventricular size were associated with significant changes in R wave amplitude in leads V_5 and V_6. For each subject the lead showing the greatest change was used in this analysis. There was a 21% increase in R wave amplitude with increased left ventricular size and a 17% decrease with decreased size ($p < .001$). In every instance interventions resulted in directionally similar changes in R wave amplitude and left ventricular end-diastolic dimension ($p < .001$). When the percent change in R wave amplitude vs the change in end-diastolic dimension was considered, the correlation coefficient was .81.

The correlation coefficient between distance from the chest wall to the left ventricular wall and change in R wave amplitude was .79. Thus as the left ventricular chamber expanded radially toward the posterior and lateral chest wall, R wave amplitude increased. Simi-

TABLE 1

Effect of changes in left ventricular chamber size and proximity to the chest wall on R and T wave amplitudes and the T/R ratio

	Frontal leads			Lateral precordial leads	
	I	II	III	V_5	V_6
R wave amplitude (mV)					
Valsalva	0.39±0.34	1.15±0.27	1.15±0.61	2.04±0.66	1.80±0.64
Control	0.46±0.23	1.14±0.28	1.02±0.54	2.18±0.77	2.07±0.79
Methoxamine	0.41±0.19	1.06±0.32	1.02±0.48	2.66±0.85	2.32±0.82
		A		A	B
Supine	0.70±0.34	1.48±0.17	1.09±0.80	2.02±0.57	1.53±0.41
Left lateral	0.42±0.37	1.38±0.51	1.26±0.75	2.64±0.58	2.02±0.46
	B			B	B
T wave amplitude (mV)					
Valsalva	0.16±0.09	0.18±0.10	0.03±0.10	0.36±0.20	0.24±0.14
Control	0.21±0.07	0.21±0.08	0.06±0.11	0.45±0.18	0.35±0.17
Methoxamine	0.24±0.08	0.32±0.13	0.10±0.10	0.80±0.21	0.64±0.30
	A	B	A	B	B
Supine	0.30±0.06	0.38±0.12	0.11±0.08	0.48±0.19	0.36±0.14
Left lateral	0.19±0.10	0.33±0.10	0.15±0.12	0.61±0.14	0.49±0.17
	A	A		B	B
T/R amplitude ratio					
Valsalva	0.42±0.29	0.16±0.10	0.01±0.22	0.19±0.13	0.13±0.08
Control	0.54±0.29	0.19±0.07	0.03±0.17	0.23±0.13	0.17±0.08
Methoxamine	0.69±0.27	0.29±0.11	0.12±0.15	0.33±0.11	0.27±0.08
	B	B		B	B
Supine	0.48±0.17	0.28±0.10	0.11±0.08	0.24±0.08	0.24±0.08
Left lateral	0.53±0.12	0.27±0.12	0.06±0.23	0.24±0.05	0.25±0.08

Data expressed as mean ± SD.

Statistical comparisons (Valsalva vs methoxamine or supine vs left lateral): $^{A}p < .05$; $^{B}p < .01$.

larly, R wave amplitude decreased as the heart moved away from the chest wall. R wave amplitude in leads V_5 and V_6 also changed when the subject was moved from the supine to the left lateral position. With this maneuver, the left ventricular endocardium moved an average of 9 ± 2 mm ($p < .001$) closer to the V_5 and V_6 electrodes. This was associated with a 42% increase in R wave amplitude ($p < .001$). There was no concomitant change in left ventricular end-diastolic dimension.

Relationship between T wave amplitude and left ventricular chamber size and position. As left ventricular chamber size increased with infusion of methoxamine, T wave amplitude increased in the frontal leads as well as in lateral precordial leads V_5 and V_6 ($p < .05$ leads I and II; $p < .01$ leads II, V_5 and V_6). Similarly, T wave amplitude decreased as chamber size decreased during Valsalva maneuver (table 1). With movement of the subject from the supine to the left lateral position, T wave amplitude increased in leads V_5 and V_6 ($p < .01$) but not in the frontal leads (figure 1 *B*). The planimetered area under the T wave paralleled T wave amplitude in leads V_5 and V_6 in all cases (r = .85 for V_5 and .83 for V_6). Changes in T wave amplitude occurred without associated changes in mean frontal R or T wave axis under any condition (table 2). To evaluate the mean T wave vector in the horizontal plane, the precordial lead in which T wave amplitude was greatest in a given patient was examined. There was no change in that lead under any condition. T wave morphology changed in only one subject, with flattening during the Valsalva maneuver. There were no differences in QT or corrected QT intervals under any condition (table 2). Heart rate, which was 64 ± 12 beats/min under control conditions, increased with Valsalva maneuver to 85 ± 13 beats/min and with methoxamine infusion (after atropine) to 76 ± 13 beats/min ($p < .01$ and $p < .05$ vs control, respectively). Heart rate did not change when subjects were shifted from supine to left lateral position.

Relationship between changes in T wave and R wave amplitudes. To distinguish between primary and parallel changes in T and QRS amplitude, the T/R ratio was calculated for each of the experimental conditions (table 1). On the shift from supine to left lateral positions, the relative increase in T wave amplitude was similar

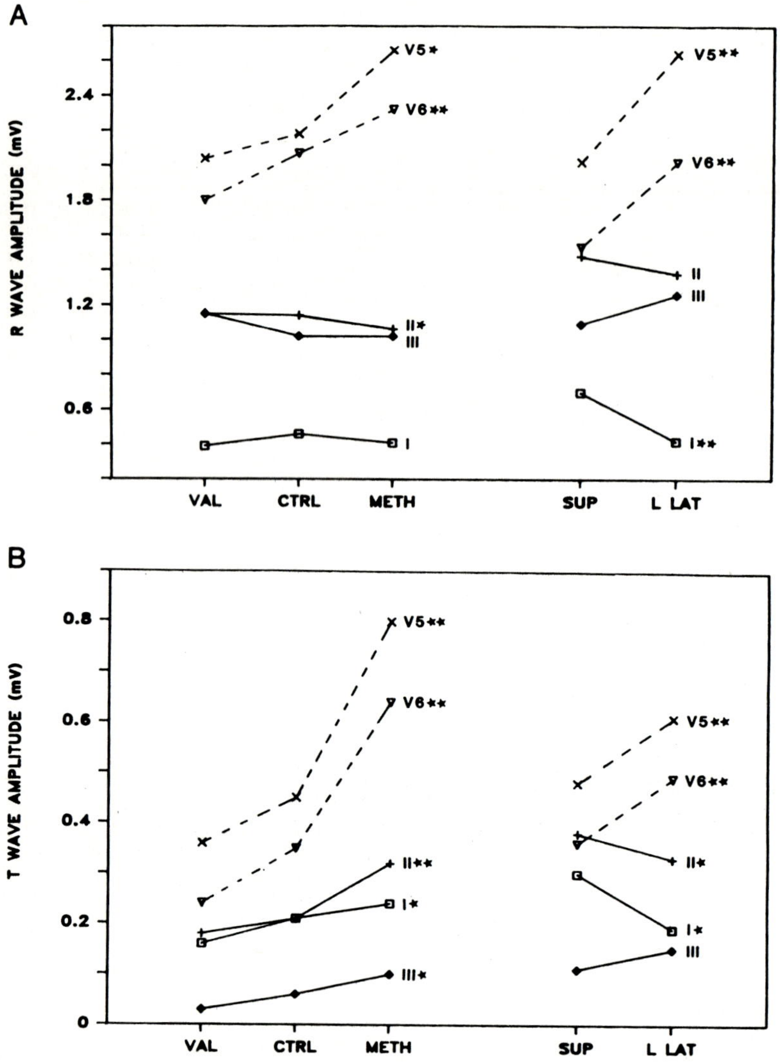

FIGURE 1. *A*, Factors influencing R wave amplitude. Effects of changes in left ventricular chamber size with Valsalva maneuver (VAL) and methoxamine infusion (METH) are compared with effects of increased proximity of the left ventricle to the chest wall (movement from supine [SUP] to left lateral [L LAT] positions). R wave amplitude changes consistently in the lateral precordial leads (dashed lines) but not in the frontal leads (solid lines). *B*, T wave amplitude increases in both frontal and lateral precordial leads as left ventricular dimension increases. T wave amplitude increases only in the lateral precordial leads with changes in position. This change in leads V_5 and V_6 parallels the associated increase in R amplitude. CTRL = control. *p < .05; **p < .01 Valsalva vs methoxamine.

to the associated R wave amplitude increase (R and T in lead V_5 increased 30% and 29%, respectively; R and T in lead V_6 increased 32% and 34%, respectively). In the left lateral position, frontal plane R and T wave mean axes shifted to the right. Although the change was not statistically significant, it was associated with decreases in QRS and T amplitude in the relevant leads, as has been previously described.[8] In contrast, the T/R ratio increased with alteration in ventricular dimensions (figure 2). Moreover, this primary effect registered on the T wave of the frontal as well as the lateral precordial leads.

Change in endocardial/epicardial surface area ratio. Endocardial surface area decreased 21% and epicardial 9% with Valsalva maneuver. With methoxamine infusion there was a 14% increase in endocardial surface area and a 7% increase in epicardial surface area. The increase in the ratio of calculated endocardial-to-epi-

TABLE 2
Electrocardiographic axis, heart rate, and QT interval under conditions of varying R wave amplitude

	QRS axis (degrees)	T wave axis (degrees)	HR (beats/min)	QT (msec)	QT_c (msec)
Valsalva	79±36	45±32	85±13[B]	364±40	417±44
Control	77±25	39±20	64±12	401±38	412±21
Methoxamine	78±23	48±13	76±16[A]	397±47	425±20
Supine	62±26	42±15	62±7	401±25	407±12
Left lateral	79±26	50±21	62±7	406±21	408±10

QT_c = corrected QT interval; HR = heart rate.
Statistical comparisons (vs control): [A]p < .05; [B]p < .01.

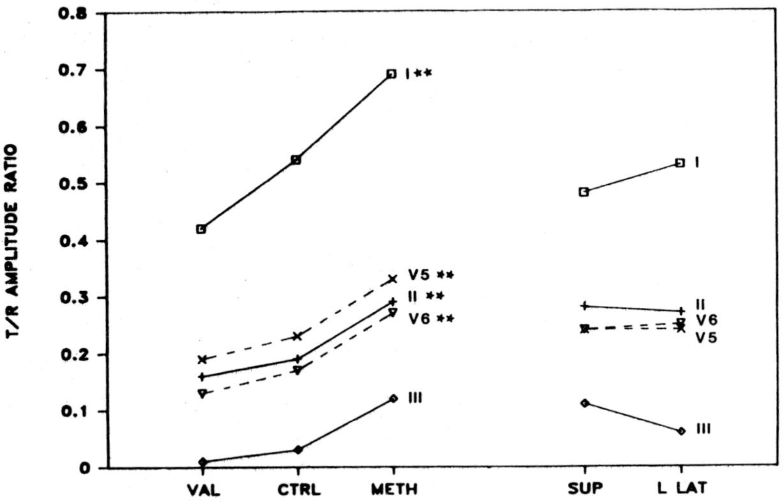

FIGURE 2. Plot showing the effects of various interventions on T/R amplitude ratio. T/R amplitude ratio varied with left ventricular chamber size but not with changes in position when left ventricular volume remained constant. Similar changes in T/R amplitude ratio were seen in the frontal and precordial leads. Abbreviations as in figure 1. $^{**}p < .01$ Valsalva vs methoxamine.

cardial surface area with increasing left ventricular dimension, from smallest to largest, was 23% ($p < .01$). This paralleled the increase in T wave amplitude (see figure 4 and table 3).

Discussion

Determinants of T and R wave amplitude. In this study we found that a major determinant of T wave amplitude is left ventricular cavity size, while R wave amplitude is influenced more by the proximity of the left ventricle to the chest wall. R wave amplitude changes were noted consistently only in the lateral precordial leads, where proximity of the left ventricle to the chest wall varies with both left ventricular volume and changes in left ventricular position (figure 1). In contrast, T/R amplitude ratio changed with left ventricular chamber size but not with change in position (figure 3). Changes in T wave amplitude and T/R ratio were also seen in both the frontal and precordial leads. Thus it appears that the T wave is a more convincing substrate for the "Brody effect" than the QRS complex, since alternative explanations for change in QRS amplitude are available.[17]

Although the R wave is largely an expression of the ordered, sequential activation of myocardial fibers, the orientation of the T wave is dependent both on the sequence of repolarization and the comparative local durations of this recovery process.[1, 22–24] Fundamental in this respect is the gradient of action potential duration from endocardium to epicardium.[25, 26] The duration of the endocardial action potential normally exceeds that of the epicardium. Although recently challenged,[27] the explanation for this difference has long been attributed to the electrotonically expanding influence of Purkinje fibers on the endocardial action potentials.[28] When the difference is substantial and exceeds the transmural propagation time, the T wave is positive in overlying unipolar surface leads, particularly those near the cardiac apex. Conditions that enhance the endocardial/epicardial gradient without rearranging the relationship of the various regional (base, apex, etc.) recovery times can similarly augment the amplitude of positive T waves.[25]

Alteration in plasma levels of sympathetic amines may cause changes in T wave amplitude.[29] However, these changes consist of a flattening of the T wave, a finding opposite to that found in this study. T wave changes caused by sympathetic agonists have almost

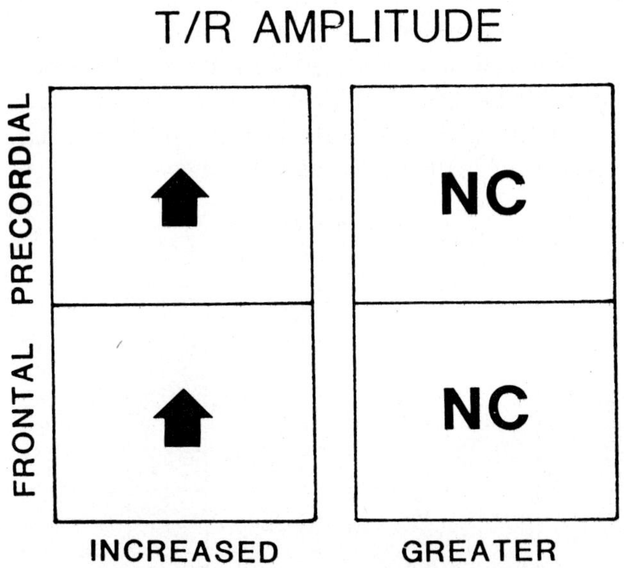

FIGURE 3. Schematic diagram of the relative changes in R and T wave amplitude. With altered left ventricular chamber size the ratio of T to R wave amplitude increases, while with variation in proximity of the left ventricle to the chest wall there is no change (NC).

invariably been associated with changes in QT interval.[29, 30] None of our subjects demonstrated significant change in QT or corrected QT intervals. It is therefore unlikely that variations in autonomic tone played a part in the changes in T wave amplitude observed in this investigation.

Endocardial/epicardial surface area ratio. According to solid angle theory, the major determinants of the voltage of an electrocardiographic deflection at any given moment include the area subtended by the boundary separating areas of differing voltage and the gradient of voltage difference across this boundary.[31] If reduction or expansion of cavity size does not alter the endocardial/epicardial gradient, there is a change in the relationship between the total available areas at the two surfaces. Assuming the cavity is an ellipse, it expands at the expense of epicardial surface area. In this study the endocardial/epicardial ratio increases by 23% (figure 4 and table 3). We believe that this augmentation of endocardial influence may explain why the amplitude of the T wave, unlike that of the QRS complex, is altered directly by changes in cavity size. With respect to T wave amplitude it is possible that this alteration in the endocardial/epicardial area rather than a change in intracavitary blood volume is the explanation of the "Brody effect" as it applies to the T wave.[9] If the thinning of the ventricular wall found with left ventricular cavity expansion caused a reduction in the endocardial-to-epicardial propagation time, this also would exaggerate the transmural gradient of recovery times, favoring augmentation of T wave amplitude.

Clinical implications of the T wave/R wave relationship. Many of the causes of altered ventricular size have associated primary T wave changes specific to the cause itself, such as left ventricular hypertrophy with

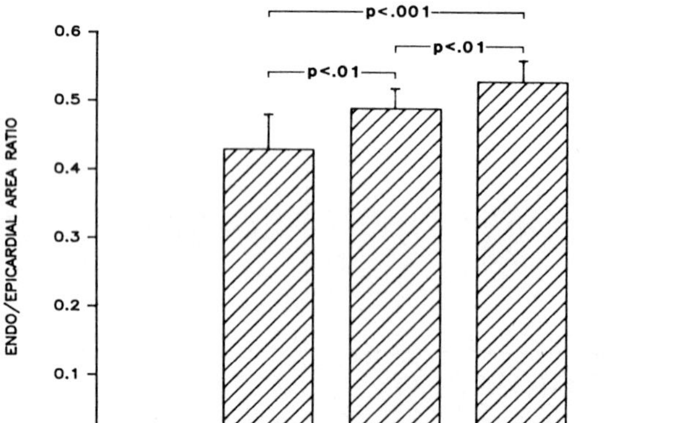

FIGURE 4. Ratio of calculated endocardial-to-epicardial surface area increases as left ventricular size increases, paralleling the associated increase in T/R amplitude ratio. VAL = Valsalva; CTRL = Control; METH = methoxamine.

TABLE 3
Relationship between endocardial and epicardial surface areas and left ventricular dimensions

	Valsalva	Control	Methoxamine
D_{ed} (cm)	4.23 ± 0.36^B	4.74 ± 0.28	5.06 ± 0.36^A
h_{ed} (cm)	1.12 ± 0.14	1.10 ± 0.11	0.96 ± 0.12^A
$Area_{endo}$ (cm^2)	112 ± 18^B	142 ± 18	162 ± 22^A
$Area_{epi}$ (cm^2)	262 ± 34	288 ± 40	308 ± 50
Surface endo/epi	0.43 ± 0.05^B	0.49 ± 0.03	0.53 ± 0.03^B

D_{ed} = end-diastolic dimension; h_{ed} = end-diastolic wall thickness; endo = endocardial; epi = epicardial.

Statistical comparisons (vs control): $^Ap < .05$; $^Bp < .01$.

strain or ischemic heart disease with T wave inversion. Changes in the T wave/R wave relationship are also seen in exercise testing.[32–34] This study demonstrates that changes in T wave size may result from alterations in both left ventricular dimension and R wave amplitude per se. In the interpretation of T wave changes in clinical settings, the effect of left ventricular expansion on T wave amplitude must be considered in conjunction with the underlying condition.

We thank Morton F. Arnsdorf, M.D., for his review of the manuscript and helpful comments and Dina Janzen for preparation of graphics.

References

1. Abildskov JA, Burgess MJ, Urie PM, Lux RL, Wyatt RF: The unidentified information content of the electrocardiogram. Circ Res **40:** 3, 1977
2. Berman JL, Wynne J, Cohn PF: Multiple lead QRS change with exercise testing: diagnostic value and hemodynamic implications. Circulation **61:** 53, 1980
3. Greenberg PS, Ellestad MH, Berge R, Johnson K, Hayes M, Bible M, Morales-Ballejo H: Radionuclide angiographic correlation of the R wave, ejection fraction, and volume responses to upright exercise. Chest **80:** 459, 1981
4. David D, Kitchen JG, Michelson EL, Naito M, Sawin HS, Chen CC: R wave amplitude responses to rapid atrial pacing: a marker for myocardial ischemia. Am Heart J **107:** 53, 1984
5. Schick EC, Weiner DA, Hood WB, Ryan TJ: Increase in R-wave amplitude during transient epicardial injury (Prinzmetal type). J Electrocardiol **13:** 259, 1980
6. Watanabe K, Bhargava V, Froelicher VF: The relationship between exercise induced R wave amplitude changes and QRS vector loops. J Electrocardiol **14:** 129, 1981
7. David D, Naito M, Michelson E, Watanabe Y, Chen CC, Morganroth J, Shaffenburg M, Blenko T: Intramyocardial conduction: a major determinant of R wave amplitude during acute myocardial ischemia. Circulation **65:** 161, 1982
8. Lepeschkin E, Wilson FN: Modern electrocardiography. Baltimore, 1955, Williams & Wilkins, pp 234, 397
9. Brody DA: A theoretical analysis of intracavitary blood mass influence on the heart-lead relationship. Circ Res **4:** 731, 1956
10. Rudy Y, Plonsey R, Leibman J: The effects of variations in conductivity and geometrical parameters on the electrocardiogram, using an electrical spheres model. Circ Res **44:** 104, 1979
11. Daniels S, Iskandrian AS, Hakki AH, Kane SA, Bemis CE, Horowitz LN, Greenspan AM, Segal BL: Correlation between changes in R wave amplitude and left ventricular volume induced by rapid atrial pacing. Am Heart J **107:** 711, 1984
12. Ellestad MH: The mechanism of exercise induced R wave ampli-

tude changes in coronary heart disease: still controversial. Arch Intern Med **142:** 963, 1982
13. Deanfield JE, Davies G, Mongiadi F, Savage C, Selwyn AP, Fox KM: Factors influencing R wave amplitude in patients with ischaemic heart disease. Br Heart J **49:** 8, 1983
14. Battler A, Froelicher V, Slutsky R, Ashburn W: Relationship of QRS amplitude changes during exercise to left ventricular function and volumes and the diagnosis of coronary artery disease. Circulation **60:** 1004, 1979
15. Lekven J, Chatterjee K, Tyberg JV, Parmley WW: Reduction in endocardial and epicardial potentials during acute increments in left ventricular dimensions. Am Heart J **98:** 200, 1979
16. Cabrera E, Monroy JR: Systolic and diastolic loading of the heart. II. Electrocardiographic data. Am Heart J **43:** 669, 1952
17. Feldman T, Borow KM, Neumann A, Lang RM, Childers RW: Relation of electrocardiographic R wave amplitude to changes in left ventricular size and position in normal subjects. Am J Cardiol **55:** 1168, 1985
18. Parisi AF, Harrington JJ, Askenazi J, Pratt RC, McIntyre KM: Echocardiographic evaluation of the Valsalva maneuver in healthy subjects and patients with and without heart failure. Circulation **54:** 921, 1976
19. Borow KM, Green LH, Grossman W, Braunwald E: Left ventricular end-systolic stress-shortening and stress-length relations in humans: normal values and sensitivity to the inotropic state. Am J Cardiol **50:** 1301, 1982
20. Kronik G, Slany J, Mosslacher H: Comparative value of eight M-mode echocardiographic formulas for determining left ventricular stroke volume. Circulation **60:** 1308, 1979
21. Tiechholz LE, Kreulin T, Herman MV, Gorlin R: Problems in echocardiographic volume determinations: echocardiographic-angiographic correlations in the presence or absence of asynergy. Am J Cardiol **37:** 7, 1976
22. Abildskov JA, Burgess MJ, Lux RL, Wyatt R, Vincent M: The expression of normal ventricular repolarization in the body surface distribution of T potentials. Circulation **54:** 901, 1976
23. Higuchi T, Nakaya Y: T wave polarity related to the repolarization process of epicardial and endocardial ventricular surfaces. Am Heart J **108:** 290, 1984
24. Lux RL, Urie PM, Burgess MJ, Abildskov JA: Variability of the body surface distributions of QRS, ST-T, and QRST deflection areas with varied activation sequence in dogs. Cardiovasc Res **14:** 607, 1980
25. Burgess MJ: Ventricular repolarization and electrocardiographic T wave form and arrhythmia vulnerability. *In* Levy MN, Vassalle M, editors: Excitation and neural control of the heart. Bethesda, MD, 1982, American Physiological Society, p 181
26. Spach MS, Barr RC: Origin of epicardial ST-T wave potentials in the intact dog. Circ Res **39:** 475, 1976
27. Veenstra RD, Joyner RW, Rawling DA: Purkinje and ventricular activation sequences of canine papillary muscle: effects of quinidine and calcium on the Purkinje-ventricular conduction delay. Circ Res **54:** 500, 1984
28. Mendez C, Mueller WJ, Merideth J, Moe GK: Interaction of transmembrane potentials in canine Purkinje fibers and at Purkinje fiber-muscle junctions. Circ Res **22:** 361, 1969
29. Daoud FS, Surawicz B, Gettes LS: Effect of isoproterenol on the abnormal T wave. Am J Cardiol **30:** 810, 1972
30. Browne KF, Zipes DP, Heger JJ, Prystowsky EN: Influence of the autonomic nervous system on the Q-T interval in man. Am J Cardiol **50:** 1099, 1982
31. Holland RP, Arnsdorf MF: Solid angle theory and the electrocardiogram. Prog Cardovasc Dis **19:** 431, 1977
32. Hakki AH, Iskandrian AS, Kutalek S, Hare TW, Sokoloff NM: R wave amplitude: a new determinant of failure of patients with coronary heart disease to manifest ST segment depression during exercise. J Am Coll Cardiol **3:** 1155, 1984
33. Gerson MC, Morris SN, McHenry PL: Relation of exercise induced physiologic S-T segment depression to R wave amplitude in normal subjects. Am J Cardiol **46:** 778, 1980
34. Hollenberg M, VanDyke DC, Massie BM, Gertz EW, Wisneski JA: The magnitude of exercise-induced ST depression is influenced by QRS amplitude. J Am Coll Cardiol **1:** 736, 1983 (abst)

Are right and left ventricular ejection fractions equal?

Ejection fractions in normal subjects and in patients with first acute myocardial infarction

JENS MARVING, M.D., POUL F. HØILUND-CARLSEN, M.D., BENT CHRÆMMER-JØRGENSEN, M.D., AND NIELS GADSBØLL, M.D.

With the technical assistance of Birte Hjort Jensen

ABSTRACT Right and left ventricular ejection fractions (RVEF and LVEF) were determined by radionuclide imaging in 37 normal subjects and 37 patients by means of (1) the traditional way of calculating ejection fraction from first-pass time-activity curves of each ventricle generated from a single fixed ventricular region of interest, (2) dual first-pass time-activity curves generated from the end-diastolic and end-systolic regions, respectively, and (3) the multigated equilibrium method, also applying separate regions in end-diastole and end-systole for each ventricle. Values for RVEF measured by method 2 were significantly higher than values obtained by methods 1 and 3. In normal subjects, the values for RVEF measured by method 2 were equal to the values for LVEF determined by either this method or the equilibrium technique. Methods 1 and 3 had a tendency for underestimation of RVEF, probably because of inclusion of right atrial activity into the right ventricular region of interest. Methods 2 and 3 were applied to measure RVEF and LVEF, respectively, in 153 patients in the second week after first acute myocardial infarction. Among these, 25% had normal ejection fractions, 47% had a decrease in only LVEF, 8% a decrease in only RVEF, and 20% a decrease in both RVEF and LVEF.
Circulation 72, No. 3, 502–514, 1985.

IN A RECENT textbook of cardiovascular medicine, it is stated that "in man, the end-diastolic volumes of the two ventricles are approximately equal, and therefore the ejection fractions of the two ventricles are normally similar as well."[1] In the literature, however, the matter seems not quite settled, since some investigators have reported equal or nearly equal size of the ventricular volumes,[2–6] whereas the majority of recent reports support the view that the right ventricle is larger than the left.[7–18]

With the last years' increasing interest in the function of both ventricles and their interdependence,[19, 20] it has become relevant to have access to methods — preferably noninvasive — that can reliably quantify right and left ventricular function. Because of different chamber geometry and pattern of contraction of the two ventricles, dedicated methods of analysis should be applied to describe their function. Using radionuclide techniques, we have compared traditional with more elaborate, and in our opinion conceptually more correct, methods of analysis for calculation of right and left ventricular ejection fraction (RVEF and LVEF) in healthy human subjects and in patients with cardiac disease. Applying the same elaborate methods, we have also examined the incidence of abnormal values for RVEF and LVEF in a group of patients with first acute myocardial infarction (AMI).

From the Department of Clinical Physiology and Nuclear Medicine, Department of Anesthesia, and Department of Cardiology, Glostrup Hospital, Copenhagen, Denmark.

Supported by the Danish Heart Association.

Address for correspondence: Poul Flemming Høilund-Carlsen, M.D., Department of Clinical Physiology and Nuclear Medicine, Glostrup Hospital, DK-2600 Glostrup, Denmark.

Received Feb. 12, 1985; revision accepted May 9, 1985.

Methods

The study population comprised three groups. Groups I and II, including 37 healthy and 37 diseased subjects, respectively, were investigated to compare three different radionuclide methods for determination of RVEF and LVEF: (1) the first-pass fixed area (fpFA) method, (2) the first-pass separate areas (fpSA) method, and (3) the multigated equilibrium (muga) approach. (These methods are described in detail below.) To examine the interobserver variation, two independent observers calculated "blindly," by means of the three methods of radionuclide analysis, six ejection fraction values in each of the 74 subjects: three values for RVEF ($RVEF_{fpFA}$, $RVEF_{fpSA}$,

$RVEF_{muga}$) and three values for LVEF ($LVEF_{fpFA}$, $LVEF_{fpSA}$, $LVEF_{muga}$).

In group III, comprising 153 patients with first AMI, RVEF and LVEF were determined only once by a single observer using the fpSA method for calculation of RVEF and the muga technique to determine LVEF.

All subjects investigated were in stable sinus rhythm as required for multigated radionuclide imaging. Details concerning the three groups were as follows:

Group I. Thirty-seven healthy volunteers, 14 women (mean age 38 years, range 29 to 50) and 23 men (mean age 38 years, range 25 to 66), gave informed consent to participate in this part of the study, which was approved by the regional Scientific-Ethical Committee. All had a history without cardiopulmonary diseases and all had normal findings on physical examination, electrocardiogram and chest roentgenogram.

Group II. To compare the interobserver variation in normal and diseased subjects, 37 radionuclide studies from 37 patients were selected so as to cover a wide range of values for RVEF. There were 10 women (mean age 64 years, range 47 to 81) and 27 men (mean age 57 years, range 40 to 78). Their diagnoses were AMI (n = 29), heart failure caused by ischemic heart disease and/or previous myocardial infarction (n = 5), cardiomyopathy (n = 2), and endocarditis (n = 1).

Group III. This group included 153 consecutive patients fulfilling the following criteria: (1) first myocardial infarction, (2) hospitalization within 24 hr after the onset of symptoms, and (3) radionuclide examination carried out in the second week (eighth to fifteenth day inclusive) after the onset. There were 38 women (mean age 65 years, range 45 to 81) and 115 men (mean age 58 years, range 35 to 78).

The diagnosis of AMI was based on previously described criteria,[21] defined by the occurrence of a temporary, significant rise (>30 U/liter) in serum creatine kinase (CK)-MB levels in patients presenting with symptoms and/or electrocardiographic changes indicative of this disease. In five patients with maximal CK-MB levels between 18 and 30 U/liter the diagnosis was sustained by positive myocardial scintigraphic results with ^{99m}Tc-pyrophosphate. (Scintigraphy is the hospital routine procedure in patients with equivocal electrocardiographic changes and CK-MB levels between 15 and 60 U/liter).

If the characteristic electrocardiographic changes (decreasing or disappearing R wave and/or increasing Q waves together with typical development of ST-T changes) occurred in the precordial leads, infarcts were classified as anterior. Posteroinferior location meant appearance of the same changes in leads II and III and/or the reverse changes in precordial leads $V_{1-(2)}$.[22] Cases in which characteristic electrocardiographic changes could not be detected, e.g., because of the presence of bundle branch block, were also included and considered indeterminate.

Radionuclide imaging. All investigations were performed with subjects in the resting supine position. Red blood cells were labeled by a modified in vivo/in vitro technique[23] with methylene-diphosphonate (Ostelite, NEN) and 30 mCi ^{99m}Tc. Approximately 5 ml of labeled blood was placed in a saline-filled nylon line connected to an indwelling plastic cannula, preferably in a right medial cubital vein. An initial first-pass study was performed in a standard 30 degree right anterior oblique (RAO) view after flushing with 20 ml of saline. Data were collected in list mode during continuous recording of the electrocardiogram for later dynamic and/or gated reframing (see below). Subsequently, gated equilibrium imaging was undertaken in a left anterior oblique (LAO) view, giving optimal separation of the left ventricle from other chambers of the heart. A total of 5 million counts were collected in a 64 × 64 word matrix, with 20 frames per RR interval, the acquisition lasting typically 6 to 8 min.

Data processing

First-pass studies

FPFA METHOD. After dynamic reframing (20 frames/sec, i.e., frame duration 50 msec), frames were added to create pictures of the right and left ventricles. Because the activity in the two ventricles will reach maximum successively, pictures of each can be obtained without disturbing overlap of the other ventricle, despite the definite anatomic overlap in this projection (RAO). The outlines of the ventricles were drawn manually with a joystick on each picture, and the respective time-activity curves were generated (figure 1). RVEF was determined without background correction as the mean of a few successive (typically 2 or 3) beats, starting with the beat at the top of the curve, with the formula EF = (end-diastolic counts − end-systolic counts)/end-diastolic counts. LVEF was determined similarly, but with correction for background activity with use of an area near the apex of the ventricle (figure 1) and normalization of this area to the area of the left ventricular region of interest.

FPSA METHOD. From the curves generated from the right and left ventricular regions with method 1, the frame numbers representing diastole and systole could be read. The diastolic frames were added to make a composite end-diastolic picture (figure 2, *A* and *E*), and similarly, systolic frames were summed to create an end-systolic picture (figure 2, *B* and *F*). On these new pictures the outline of each ventricle was redrawn to generate the corresponding time-activity curves (figure 2, *C* and *G*). Subse-

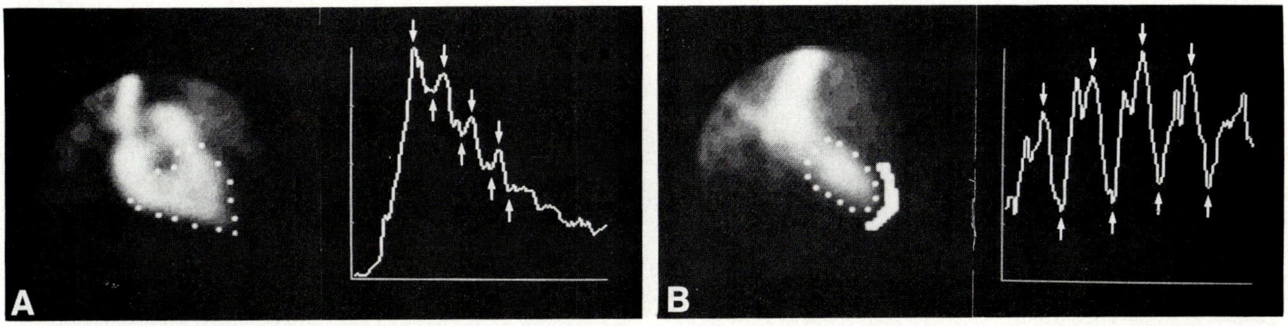

FIGURE 1. Traditional method of calculating RVEF (*A*) and LVEF (*B*) from a first-pass study performed in the 30 degree RAO view (fpFA). For each ventricle only a single region of interest is drawn on a composite picture, often representing one or several seconds of acquisition to improve image quality. Time-activity curves from this fixed area are recorded and ejection fraction is calculated as the mean of a few successive beats — on the left side after proper background subtraction. The arrows denote the beats used for calculation in the examples chosen.

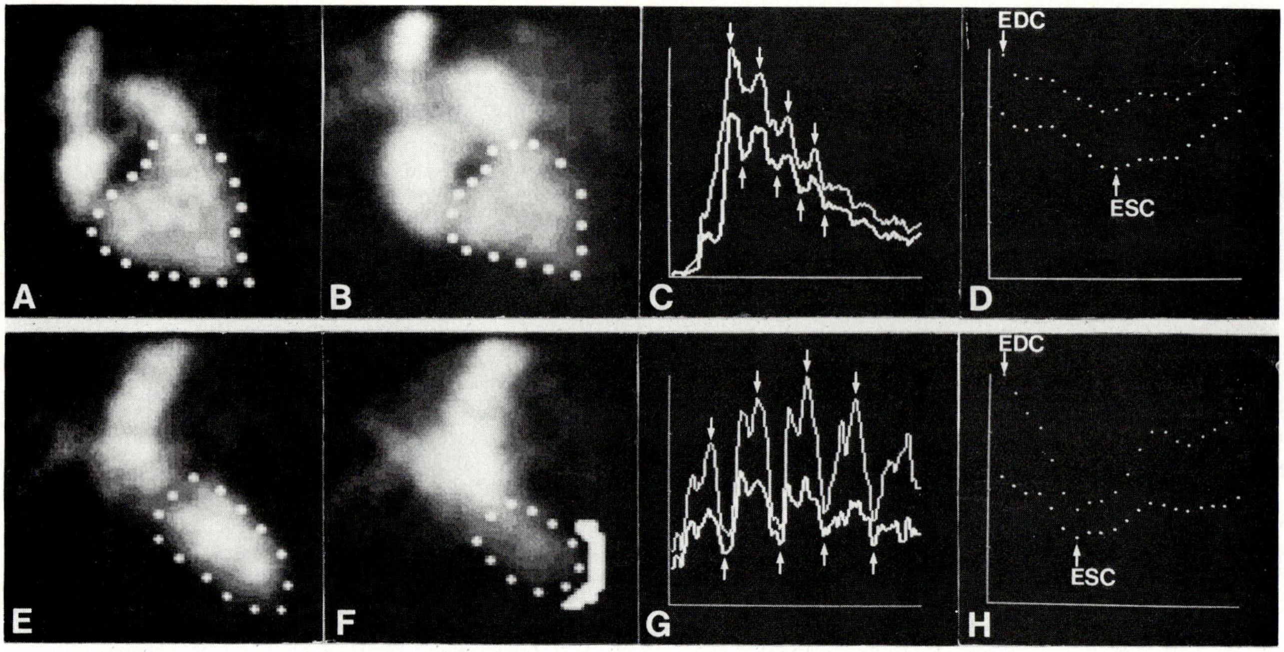

FIGURE 2. Calculation of RVEF (*top panel*) and LVEF (*bottom panel*) by fpSA. The outline of each ventricle is drawn in diastole (*A* and *E*) and systole (*B* and *F*) on pictures composed of selected diastolic and systolic frames, respectively (see text). For background correction, a systolic area along the apical border of the ventricles is used (only shown for the left ventricle [*F*]). Resulting dual dynamic time-activity curves are displayed in *C* and *G*. Ejection fractions are calculated with the peaks (↓) of the upper (diastolic area) curve and the troughs (↑) of the lower (systolic area) curve. In *D* and *H* are shown the corresponding average curves obtained when gated instead of dynamic reframing is used (20 frames/cycle used in these examples). Ejection fraction is calculated from the end-diastolic (EDC) and end-systolic counts (ESC).

quently, ejection fraction was calculated from the peaks of the diastolic area-curve and the troughs of the systolic area-curve. A crescent-shaped region for background correction was drawn at the apex of the right and left ventricles.

Because this procedure is time-consuming and cumbersome and because the same data could be obtained more easily by gated reframing of appropriate sections of the original list mode sequence, we chose instead to reframe sections representing the right and left ventricular passage with 16 frames per RR interval. At an average heart rate of 75 beats/min this would result in a frame duration of 50 msec. The end-diastolic and end-systolic frames, typically frames 1 and 7, respectively, were identified, and separate diastolic and systolic ventricular regions of interest were drawn as above. Often, a few frames adjacent to the end-diastolic and end-systolic frames, e.g., frames 2 and 15 + 16 or frames 6 and 8, were added to improve the quality of the two images. The corresponding geminate curves were generated, and the peak of the average diastolic area-curve and the troughs of the average systolic area-curve were used for calculation of ejection fraction (figure 2, *D* and *H*). Background correction by area normalization was carried out with use of a region near the apex of each ventricle (figure 2, *F*).

Because the quantitative information is essentially the same whether the list mode data are reframed in the dynamic or gated mode, the latter procedure was used throughout the entire investigation. (Slight differences between the two modes of reframing are mainly caused by variation in frame duration with the gated approach because of the different heart rates of the patients.)

Equilibrium studies. These were collected in 20 frames. $RVEF_{muga}$ was determined manually after identification of the frames representing right ventricular end-diastole and end-systole (which, in accordance with early reports on this matter,[24–26] were not always identical to those representing the same phases of left ventricular contraction). The outline of the ventricle was drawn with a joystick on the two frames, and RVEF was calculated from the background-corrected counts included in the two areas. An area with the same location as applied for correction of the left ventricular activity was drawn for background correction (see below).

$LVEF_{muga}$ was determined by a semiautomatic program for calculation of LVEF from operator-defined end-diastolic and background regions of interest. The latter was invariably placed in the inferolateral vicinity of the left ventricle, encompassing the pixels with lowest activity in the end-systolic frame. Whenever inaccuracies in the automated computer analysis were noted, the outline of the left ventricle was drawn manually in both end-diastole and end-systole. This method of determining the LVEF had previously been validated by comparison with cineangiographic measurements.[27]

Statistical evaluation. Comparisons between sets of values for ejection fractions were carried out by correlation analysis, the paired t test, and Pratt's nonparametric test for paired data.[28] For these comparisons, we used either the mean of the values obtained by the two observers (i.e., in case there was no statistically significant difference between their values) or the single values obtained by the two observers (i.e., in case such a difference [indicated by + in table 1] was present). The Bonferroni method[29] was used to decrease the chance of mistakenly declaring significance due to multiple comparisons.

In the patients with AMI, linear regression analyses were carried out according to the least-squares principle.[30] Differences between values for the serum CK-MB concentration were tested for by the unpaired t test.

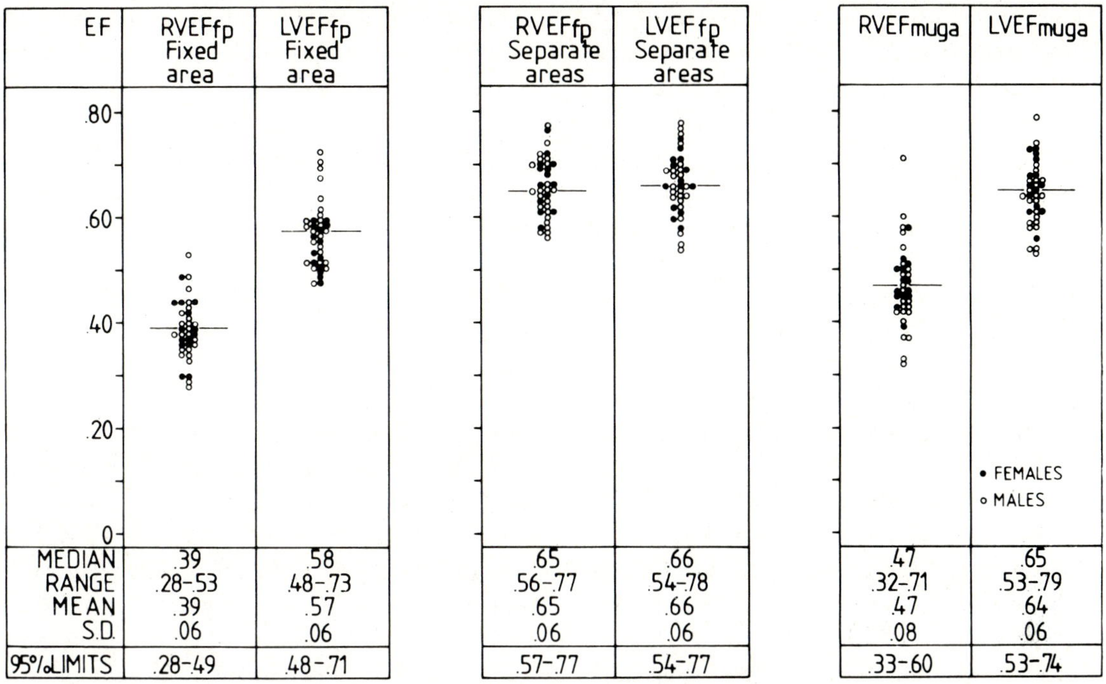

FIGURE 3. Ejection fractions obtained in the 37 healthy individuals (each point is the mean of two observers' values). Because the 95% confidence limits were defined by the 2.5 and 97.5 percentiles by removing the lowest and highest values in each of the six columns, this meant that a little more than 5% of the population (i.e., 2/37, 5.43%) was discarded. For compensation, the next highest and next lowest figures in each column were rounded up and down, respectively, whenever possible. This procedure accounts for the apparent discrepancy between the respective 95% limits given at the bottom of the figure and the next lowest points in columns 1, 4, and 6 (from the left) and the next highest point in column 3.

Results

Comparison of the different methods of radionuclide analysis. Results obtained in the 37 normal subjects are shown in figure 3, and in table 1 with the values from the 37 patients.

In the normal subjects, women and men were comparable in age. We failed to identify any differences between values for ejection fraction recorded in the two sexes. The 95% confidence limits of normal, defined by the 2.5 and 97.5 percentiles, are given at the bottom of figure 3.

The following relationships were observed between the ejection fractions recorded with various methods of analysis.

RVEF. In the normal subjects, values obtained by the fpSA method were significantly higher (mean 18 ejection fraction units, range 0 to 46; $p < .001$) than values determined by the muga technique, which again were higher (mean 8 units, range -8 to 21; $p < .001$) than the values calculated by the fpFA method (figure 3).

In the 37 patients the fpSA values were also lying at a clearly higher level than the fpFA and muga values for RVEF, which were of similar size (p in both instances $< .001$) (table 1).

The interobserver variation, expressed by the co-

TABLE 1

Values for ejection fraction obtained by 2 observers (A and B) in 37 normal and 37 diseased subjects with different methods of calculation

Method	Ejection fraction[A] A	Ejection fraction[A] B	Correlation coefficient	Coefficient of variation (%)
Normals (n = 37)				
$RVEF_{fpFA}$	40 (29–53)	37 (27–53)[B]	.88	7
$LVEF_{fpFA}$	56 (48–70)	58 (45–75)[B,C]	.78	6
$RVEF_{fpSA}$	65 (54–75)	66 (54–79)	.85	4
$LVEF_{fpSA}$	65 (51–77)	67 (53–79)[B]	.88	4
$RVEF_{muga}$	47 (35–70)	46 (26–71)	.27	18
$LVEF_{muga}$	64 (53–79)	64 (52–79)	.91	3
Patients (n = 37)				
$RVEF_{fpFA}$	38 (17–71)	38 (15–70)	.98	6
$LVEF_{fpFA}$	35 (14–77)	37 (15–78)[B]	.97	7
$RVEF_{fpSA}$	53 (20–88)	52 (18–85)[B,C]	.99	4
$LVEF_{fpSA}$	37 (9–73)	37 (13–73)	.98	6
$RVEF_{muga}$	36 (15–68)	39 (11–72)	.80	19
$LVEF_{muga}$	37 (13–74)	36 (12–77)	.99	6

[A]Values (mean and ranges) are given in "ejection fraction units" (0–100); i.e., an ejection fraction of 0.37 = 37.

[B]Denotes significant ($p < .05$) difference between A and B.

[C]Not significant after applying the Bonferroni correction for multiple comparisons.[29]

efficient of variation, was somewhat lower with the fpSA (4% in normal subjects and 4% in patients) than with the fpFA method (7% and 6%) but was very much higher with the muga technique (18% and 19%) (table 1).

LVEF. In the normal subjects, ejection fractions obtained by the fpSA method were on an average 9 units (range -6 to 24) higher ($p < .001$) than those recorded with the fpFA method, against only 2 units (range -5 to 9) higher ($p < .001$) than the values determined by the muga technique (table 1).

In the patients, the sets of values for LVEF obtained by the three different methods were at the same level (table 1).

The interobserver variation was slightly lower with the fpSA method (4% in normal subjects and 6% in patients) than with the fpFA method (6% and 7%) and approximately of the same size as with the muga technique (3% and 6%).

RVEF vs LVEF. Remarkable was the finding in normal subjects that the values for $RVEF_{fpSA}$, $LVEF_{fpSA}$, and $LVEF_{muga}$ were similar (figure 3), with no statistically significant differences between them, except for the slightly higher values for $LVEF_{fpSA}$ than for $LVEF_{muga}$ (mentioned above).

In each of the normal subjects the difference between $RVEF_{fpSA}$ and $LVEF_{fpSA}$ or $LVEF_{muga}$ was less than 10 units (RVEF − LVEF: mean 1 unit, range -9 to 9).

Comparisons between values for RVEF and LVEF in diseased subjects were not relevant for the purpose of method evaluation (but of course pertinent when studying the nature of disease, as done below in the patients with AMI).

The influence of background correction on $RVEF_{fpSA}$ values was studied in the 37 patients. With correction, RVEF was on an average 1 unit (range 0 to 3) higher than when background correction was omitted.

RVEF and LVEF in patients with first AMI. Corresponding values for $RVEF_{fpSA}$ and $LVEF_{muga}$ measured in normal subjects and in the 153 patients with AMI are plotted in figure 4. Values for RVEF and LVEF were not significantly different in women and men.

Infarct location was anterior in 80 patients (52%), posteroinferior in 64 patients (42%), both anterior and posteroinferior in four patients (3%), and indeterminate in five (3%). Thirty-eight patients (25%) had normal ejection fractions in both ventricles, 72 (47%) had a decrease in LVEF only, 13 (8%) a decrease in RVEF only, and 30 (20%) had a decrease in both RVEF and LVEF.

Of the patients with a decrease in LVEF only, 69% (50/72) had anterior infarction, whereas 85% (11/13) of those with an isolated decrease in RVEF had posteroinferior infarction. This difference was highly significant (χ^2-test, $p < .001$). Patients with decreased ejection fraction in both ventricles had equally frequent anterior and posteroinferior infarction. Conversely, of the patients with an isolated anterior infarction, 80% (64/80) had a decrease in LVEF and only 20% (16/80) had a decrease in RVEF. Of those with posteroinferior

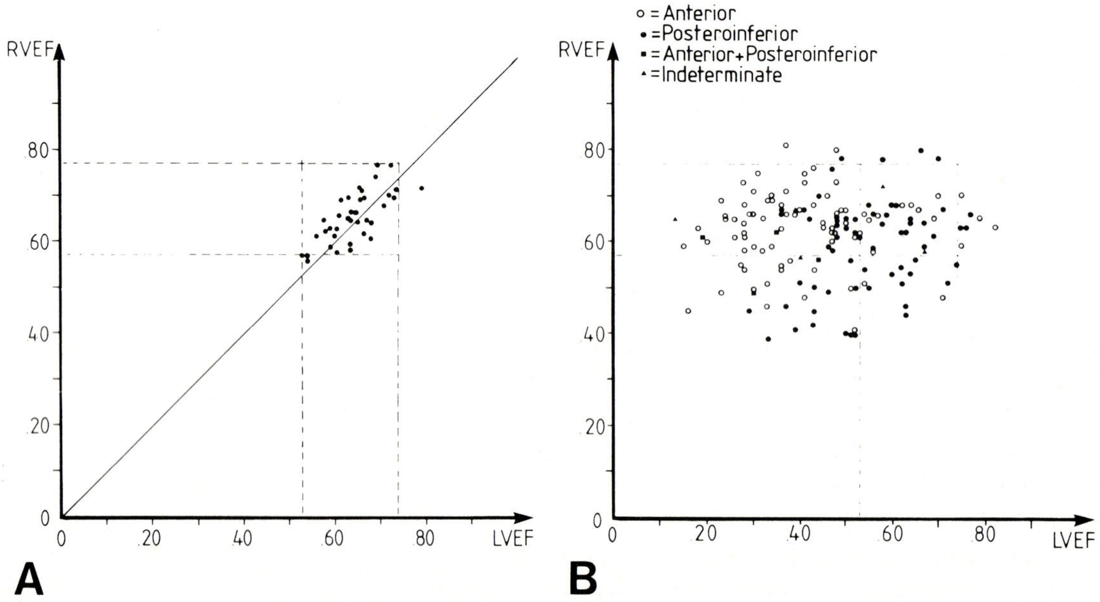

FIGURE 4. Relationship between RVEF and LVEF in 37 normal subjects (*A*) and 153 patients with first AMI (*B*). The unbroken line in *A* is the line of identity; the broken lines indicate the 95% confidence limits. The various symbols in *B* indicate the infarct locations.

infarction, 39% (25/64) had a decrease in RVEF and 48% (31/64) had a decrease in LVEF.

The serum concentrations of CK-MB were significantly lower in patients with normal ejection fractions (mean 138 U/liter, range 18 to 428) than in patients with a decreased ejection fraction (p for all comparisons $< .005$). CK-MB levels were about the same whether there was a decrease in RVEF only (mean 262 U/liter, range 53 to 413), LVEF only (mean 251 U/liter, range 24 to 1090), or both (mean 285 U/liter, range 36 to 1381). There was a poor but significant inverse correlation between CK-MB levels and both RVEF ($r = -.17$; $p < .05$) and LVEF ($r = -.28$; $p < .01$).

Discussion

The occurrence of minor beat-to-beat fluctuations in stroke volume (and ejection fraction) is probably a normal phenomenon.[31, 32] Sudden disturbance of the function of one ventricle can induce transient divergencies (lasting a few cycles) between the stroke volumes of the two ventricles,[26, 33] but a state of balanced outputs must occur if systemic or pulmonary venous congestion is to be avoided.[34] In the resting supine subject, the stroke volumes of the right (RV) and left ventricle (LV) must be practically identical, except in the presence of valve insufficiency or an intracardiac shunt. Since the ejection fraction is defined as stroke volume (SV) divided by end-diastolic volume (EDV), RVEF and LVEF are the same only if the end-diastolic volumes of the ventricles are equal:

$$SV_{RV} = SV_{LV} = EF_{RV} \cdot EDV_{RV} = EF_{LV} \cdot EDV_{LV}$$

and hence

$$\frac{EF_{RV}}{EF_{LV}} = \frac{EDV_{LV}}{EDV_{RV}}$$

Different methods based on various physical principles have been used to estimate ventricular volumes and ejection fractions. By means of an electric conductivity indicator dilution technique, Holt et al.[35] measured the end-diastolic volume of both ventricles in nine species of mammals varying 1790-fold (rat to horse) in body weight. They found that the end-diastolic volumes of mammals were linear functions of body weight and not of body surface, an observation that was later confirmed by data reported in a cineangiographic study by Graham et al.[3] Further, Holt et al.[35] observed that the end-diastolic volume of the right ventricle was on an average slightly smaller than that of the left when expressed in relation to body weight (right ventricular, 2.0 ml/kg; left ventricular 2.3 ml/kg), whereas the opposite was found when expressed in relation to body surface (right ventricular, 109 ml/m^2; left ventricular, 93 ml/m^2). However, the most widely applied methods in man are the cineangiographic and the radionuclide techniques (tables 2 and 3).

Cineventriculography. Table 2 summarizes data from cineventriculographic studies in human beings.[2–5, 36–41] Although single-plane cineventriculography has been successfully used to measure right ventricular volume and ejection fraction,[42] only studies applying the biplane technique have been included here. Even with the latter approach the geometric assumptions upon which the calculations rest might not always be fulfilled, especially not in the right ventricle with its complex and highly variable shape.[36, 38, 43, 44] Of the different principles of calculation, Simpson's rule may provide the safest way of calculation, although it is difficult to ensure with these techniques that a measured length or diameter is obtained without distortion. Most of the studies cited in table 2 were carried out in children with normal hemodynamic findings on heart catheterization. With the exception of a single study,[37] it was found that the end-diastolic volumes and the ejection fractions of the two ventricles were equal or nearly equal.

Radionuclide studies. Radionuclide techniques are widely used for noninvasive determination of both RVEF and LVEF. In the beginning, RVEF was measured only by first-pass techniques, but in recent years determination by gated equilibrium imaging has also been reported. Table 3 summarizes data from radionuclide investigations including values for RVEF obtained in either normal subjects or control patients.[6–18, 45–49]

First-pass studies. With this approach the RAO view can be used to separate the right ventricle from the right atrium. The position of the tricuspid valve plane is shifted anteriorly and to the left during ventricular contraction. Therefore a fixed ventricular region of interest will not represent a reliable demarcation of the atrioventricular border in both diastole and systole (figure 5). Inclusion during systole of even a small portion of atrial activity within the ventricular region of interest will result in substantial underestimation of calculated RVEF because the atrium is in the process of being filled in this phase of the cardiac cycle. This tendency is particularly apparent in normal hearts and less pronounced in enlarged ventricles with poor contraction, because in the latter the change in ventricular size from diastole to systole is reduced and the shift of the tricuspid valve plane relatively less marked (figure 5).

Fixed regions of interest have been used by most investigators (table 3), and RVEF has generally been found to be lower than LVEF in normal subjects with this method of analysis. Various kinds of background correction have been applied, resulting in different influence of atrial bias (overlap) on the calculated ejection fraction values. During the first passage of the radioactive bolus through the right ventricle there should be only negligible activity adjacent to it, except for the activity in the right atrium and the pulmonary artery. If proper delineation of the ventricle can be obtained in both diastole and systole, then background correction of the dual time-activity curves (figure 2, *C* and *D*) might well be unnecessary. In this respect, our study confirmed the findings of Winzelberg et al.,[6] who stressed the importance of using separate areas and found insignificant effect of background correction and normal values for RVEF in the same range, as we did.

Previously, we too have used the fpFA method for calculation of RVEF[50] and found lower values for RVEF than for LVEF. However, visual inspection of gated equilibrium studies obtained in the same persons did not confirm that the right ventricle was bigger than

TABLE 2

Data from articles concerning radiologic determination (biplane cineangiography) of right ventricular volume and/or ejection fraction in intact human hearts[A]

Author, year	No. of patients	Age (yr)	RVEDV ml	RVEDV ml/m²	LVEDV ml	LVEDV ml/m²	RVEDV/LVEDV	RVEF	LVEF	RVEF/LVEF	Comments[B]
Carlsson et al.[2] 1971	4	5–17	75	69	73	66	1.04	0.62	0.64	0.97	Values are calculated means of values given in table 1; AP and lateral views, modified Simpson's rule and two other methods
Graham et al.[3] 1973	7	< 1	11	39	11	39	1.01	0.66	0.63	1.04	Values from table 1. AP and lateral views. Simpson's rule and two-chamber method
	9	4–14	75	70	74	69	1.01	0.64	0.65	0.99	
Gentzler et al.[36] 1974	9	Adults		81(63–101)				0.51 (0.40–0.66)			Frontal and lateral views; Simpson's rule method; no LV data
Thilenius et al.[37] 1974	7	≦ 1		64		43	1.49	0.52	0.79	0.66	Values from table 2; frontal and lateral views; "parallelepiped method" of Arcilla et al.[41]
	9	2–10		78		66	1.18	0.61	0.74	0.82	
Ferlinz et al.[38] 1975	8	32–57		76(63–99)				0.66 (0.59–0.79)			Values from table 1; RAO 30° and LAD 60° views; pyramid method; no LV data
Fisher et al.[4] 1975	70	0.5–22		64		59	1.08	0.61	0.68	0.90	Values from table 2; frontal and lateral views; Simpson's rule
Nakazawa et al.[5] 1976	40/87	0–16	75.1	$BSA^{1.43}$	72.5	$BSA^{1.43}$	1.02	0.61	0.63	0.97	Values from table 2; AP and lateral views; Simpson's rule method
Lange et al.[39,40] 1978	100	0–16	73.1	$BSA^{1.219}$			1.12	0.63		0.88	Values from table 5 in two successive articles; AP and lateral views; Simpson's rule method with corrections
	83	0–19			65.1	$BSA^{1.219}$			0.72		

RV = right ventricular; LV = left ventricular; EDV = end-diastolic volume; EF = ejection fraction; AP = anteroposterior; BSA = body surface area.

[A]All listed figures were obtained in "normal" patients, i.e., control patients with normal hemodynamic findings.

[B]The table numbers given refer to tables in the cited articles, not to tables in the present work.

the left; rather, the two ventricles appeared to be of equal size. This observation led to the elaboration of the fpSA method and the finding of equal RVEF and LVEF in normal subjects.

Values for LVEF calculated from the first-pass studies by either the fpFA or fpSA method differed less because the aortic valve plane is relatively fixed and because the left atrium interferes minimally in the RAO view. The slightly higher values for LVEF with the fpSA method than with the muga technique might be caused by differences in background correction. With the first-pass approach the background activity is coming mainly from the pulmonary vascular bed, varying with time. After equilibrium the activity from labeled blood cells in many different tissues contributes to the background activity in a much more complex fashion. "True" background cannot be determined accurately with either method.

Some investigators have proposed the use of stroke volume images to define the ventricular region of interest.[7, 18] In our experience, this also results in underestimation of RVEF because of the omission of diastolic ventricular activity near the tricuspid valve plane. Stroke volume counts in this area are counterbalanced and thereby abolished by atrial activity appearing in the same region during ventricular systole. This undesirable effect will be even greater if the anterior projection is used,[7–10, 16] since there is greater overlap between right atrium and right ventricle in this view. Subtraction of the activity in a narrow area in this transitional zone[7–10, 16] is an arbitrary way of solving the problem of overlap, resulting in higher but not necessarily correct RVEF values.

Multigated equilibrium studies. Maddahi et al.[11, 47] were the first to report determination of RVEF by gated equilibrium imaging. They recognized the problems with overlap between the right atrium and the right ventricle in the LAO view necessary for equilibrium studies and clearly demonstrated that if RVEF is calculated by means of a fixed diastolic region of interest, right atrial activity will become included in this region resulting in underestimation of RVEF. Using a procedure comparable to that of Maddahi et al.,[11] including the fpSA method, Winzelberg et al.[6] and we found similar RVEF values in normal subjects by gated equilibrium imaging, but these values were substantially lower than those obtained by the fpSA method (table 3). In 20 patients, Maddahi et al.[11] compared values for RVEF obtained by both gated first-pass and gated equilibrium imaging. They found a good agreement between the two methods, probably because they performed the first-pass studies in the anterior position with consequent overlap between the right atrium and the right ventricle and corresponding underestimation of RVEF.

Stroke volume images have also been used with the gated equilibrium principle in an attempt to overcome the problems in defining the right ventricular region of interest.[15, 17, 49] However, the right atrium is often completely hidden behind the right ventricle in diastole and clear of it to an unknown degree in systole, depending on the size of both the ventricle and the atrium itself and on the individual degree of rotation of the heart. Under these circumstances it is therefore unclear what the stroke volume image represents.

Because of these reservations, we find it difficult to believe in the accuracy of the multigated equilibrium method for the determination of RVEF, even if separate areas are applied in diastole and systole. We would also be reluctant to measure relative changes in RVEF with this approach because of the poor reproducibility we have found in another investigation.[51]

It seems that these problems with separation of right atrial and right ventricular activity have not been recognized as serious in most previous studies because comparisons were often made between values for RVEF measured by two different methods, each with their individual tendency for underestimation. Such comparisons may result in apparent agreement, especially if only diseased patients are investigated. The lower half of table 1 illustrates this. Except for the higher values for RVEF measured by the fpSA method, all other values seem to be almost equal with similar ranges. However, in the individual patients, RVEF (or LVEF) measured by either the fpFA method or the muga technique differed by up to 22 units in both directions. The reason for these divergences was clearly exposed in the first-pass studies from normal subjects, in whom the overlap between right atrium and right ventricle has a relatively greater influence on the size of the calculated ejection fraction (figure 5).

Conclusions on determination of RVEF. From a review of the literature and on the basis of our own results, we believe that reasonably accurate determinations of RVEF by radionuclide methods can be made only in an RAO view, in which right atrial and right ventricular activity can be reliably separated by first-pass techniques. Other projections will introduce overlap of right atrial and right ventricular activity, which cannot be properly corrected for. For this reason, muga equilibrium studies should not be used for determination of RVEF.

Our values for RVEF obtained in normal subjects by the fpSA method were similar to those measured by

TABLE 3
Data from articles concerning radionuclide determination of RVEF[A]

Author, year	Method(s)	Subjects	No. of patients	Age (yr)	RVEF	LVEF	RVEF/LVEF	Comments[B]
Steele et al.[45] 1976	First pass	Controls	14	Adults	0.57(0.51–0.64)	0.66(0.57–0.74)	0.86	RAO 40°; slant hole collimator; Swan-Ganz catheter; "multiplied" background curve; fpFA method
Berger et al.[7] 1978	First pass	Normals	50	27–66	0.55(0.45–0.71)	0.69(0.58–0.70)	0.80	Anterior view, supine; background correction by area at tricuspid valve region; region of interest defined by stroke volume image; upper limit for LVEF a misprint?
Berger et al.[8] 1979	First pass	Controls & normals	6 8	—	0.54	0.67	0.81	Same method as ref. 7; upright position
Berger et al.[9] 1979	First pass	Controls & normals	6 13	27–59	0.55	0.67	0.82	Anterior view; upright position; same procedure as in refs. 7 and 8
Tobinick et al.[46] 1978	First pass	Normals	22	17–73	0.52(0.44–0.60)	0.60(0.52–0.73)	0.87	RAO 30°; background correction; fpFA method
Johnson et al.[10] 1979	First pass	Controls & normals	3 8	25–69	0.47(0.43–0.55)	0.68(0.52–0.78)	0.69	Anterior view; same method as ref. 7
Maddahi et al.[11] 1979	Muga	Normals	15	28–66	0.48(0.39–0.57)	0.63(0.54–0.79)	0.76	LAO 40°–50°; separate areas in diastole and systole; systolic background correction; comparison with gated first-pass studies (fpSA method, anterior view) in 20 patients
Maddahi et al.[47] 1980	Muga	Controls & normals	2 8	28–66	0.49(0.42–0.55)			Same procedure as in ref. 11
Slutsky et al.[12] 1980	First pass (1) Muga (2)	Controls & normals	5 15	24–52	(1)0.53(0.46–0.83) (2)0.49(0.39–0.77)	(2)0.61	0.87 0.80	(1) RAO 30°, supine; fpFA method; same as ref. 46 (2) LAO 45°, supine; fixed area for right ventricular, variable for left ventricular
Holman et al.[13] 1980	Muga	Controls	11	—	0.59(0.49–0.74) 0.45(0.35–0.61) 0.59(0.42–0.88)	0.68(0.52–0.76)		Three different methods of calculating RVEF, all using fixed areas; LAO 35°–40°; slant-hole collimator; background region along right side of heart

RV = right ventricular; LV = left ventricular; EF = ejection fraction.

[A]The listed figures were obtained in either control patients (controls), i.e., patients with normal hemodynamic findings, or in healthy individuals (normals). Ejection fractions are mean values with ranges in parentheses.

[B]The table numbers given refer to tables in the cited articles, not to tables in the present work.

TABLE 3
(Continued)

Author, year	Method(s)	Subjects	No. of patients	Age (yr)	RVEF	LVEF	RVEF/LVEF	Comments[B]
Winzelberg et al.[6] 1981	First pass (1) Muga (2)	Controls	13	13–81	(1)0.60 (2)0.47	(2)0.62	0.97 0.76	(1) RAO 30°, supine; fpSA method; gated first pass; no background subtraction. (2) Muga ad modum Maddahi[11]
Marmor et al.[14] 1981	Muga	Normals	10	38–64	0.43(0.34–0.67)	0.64(0.49–0.80)	0.67	LAO 30–45°; automatic edge detection for both ventricles, i.e., variable regions. Background: minimum activity lateral to ventricular edges
Franquiz et al.[48] 1982	Muga (1) Muga (2)	Normals	28	18–55	(1)0.56(0.44–0.66) (2)0.36(0.26–0.48)	0.63(0.47–0.75) 0.64(0.51–0.76)	0.89 0.56	LAO 30°–45°; two muga methods, one with various image filtering (1), and one without (2). fpFA method
Korr et al.[15] 1982	Muga	Controls	20	33–62	0.53(0.42–0.67)	0.71(0.55–0.85)	0.75	LAO view; slant-hole collimator; separate areas defined by combining stroke volume image and the reciprocal image
Peter et al.[16] 1983	First pass	Normals	10	24–28	0.44	0.61	0.72	Same method as in ref. 7
Legrand et al.[17] 1983	Muga	Normals	10	23–54	(1)0.48 (2)0.59	0.70	(1)0.69 (2)0.84	LAO view, supine. (1) fpFA method. (2) Separate areas method ad modum Maddahi et al.[11] Four special images to define RV region of interest
Konstam et al.[49] 1983	Muga	Controls	16	27–71	0.47			LAO view; slant-hole collimator; method similar to ref. 12, but using stroke volume image
Hurwitz et al.[18] 1984	First pass	Normals	74/72	0.2–20	0.53(0.43–0.73)	0.68(0.49–0.86)	0.78	RAO view, supine; slant-hole collimator; region of interest defined by stroke volume image

Winzelberg et al.[6] by the same methods as well as those in the majority of the previous studies applying biplane cineangiography (table 2). On this basis, it seems fair to assume that the end-diastolic volume of the right ventricle in normal subjects is close to that of the left ventricle and that RVEF under normal conditions is approximately the same as LVEF with only small individual differences between them.

Ejection fractions in patients with AMI. Many have measured LVEF by radionuclide imaging in the initial stages of AMI[14, 52–58] or within the first days.[46, 59] Some have done it serially,[60–64] others at the time of hospital discharge[65–68] or during the ensuing months,[69] sometimes in combination with submaximal exercise testing.[65–67, 69–71] Several have also measured RVEF in these patients,[14, 46, 62, 64, 72–77] either serially,[62, 64] or more often in the initial stage and on a later occasion.[14, 56, 73, 74, 77]

To our knowledge, our study population comprises the largest reported number of patients with first AMI

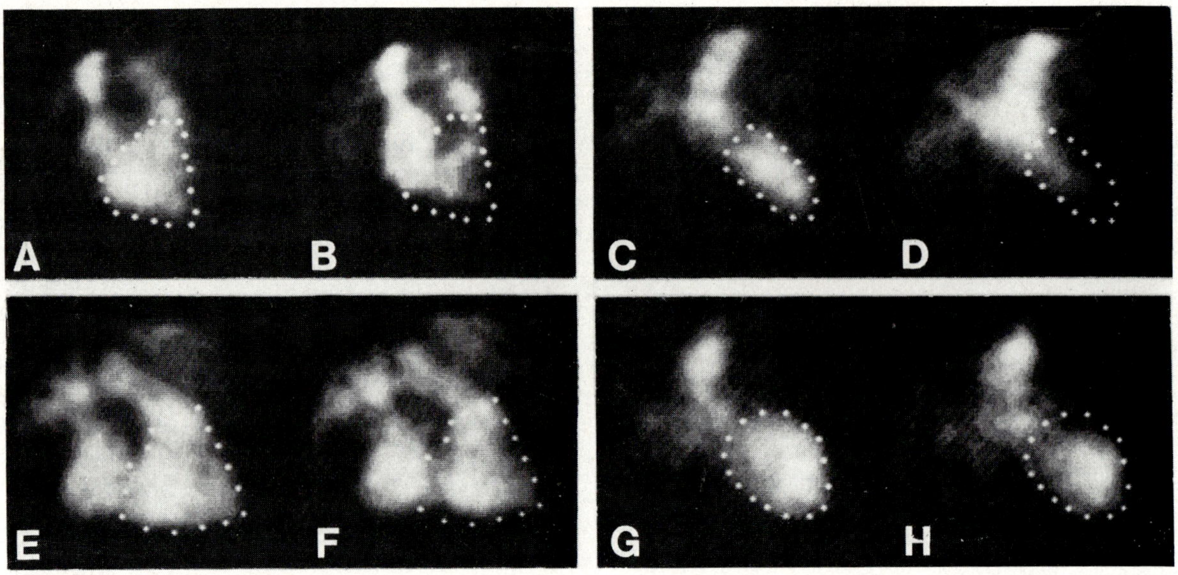

FIGURE 5. First-pass studies (30 degree RAO view) of a normal (*top panel*) and a diseased heart (*bottom panel*) showing (*left*) the right ventricle in diastole (*A* and *E*) and systole (*B* and *F*) and (*right*) the left ventricle in diastole (*C* and *G*) and systole (*D* and *H*). Respective diastolic regions of interest are superimposed on the systolic pictures to illustrate possible inclusion during systole of extraventricular activity into the fixed ventricular regions of interest. As demonstrated, this effect is particularly pronounced for the right ventricle and especially in normal hearts. To prevent consequent underestimation of the ejection fraction, time-activity curves for each ventricle should be generated from separate diastolic and systolic regions of interest (c.f., figure 2). The only "true" points in the resulting dual time-activity curves are the peaks of the diastolic region-of-interest curve and the troughs of the systolic region-of-interest curves. Only these points should be used for calculation of the ejection fraction.

in whom both RVEF and LVEF have been systematically measured. Radionuclide investigations were performed in the second week after infarction, at a time when the clinical condition of most patients was relatively stable. The prognostic significance of the combined determination of RVEF and LVEF in these patients will be dealt with separately.

Applying our method of measuring RVEF together with determination of LVEF by current radionuclide principles, we found that about one-fourth of the patients had entirely normal ejection fractions. Almost one-half had a decreased LVEF with a normal RVEF, less than one-tenth had a decrease in RVEF only, and one-fifth had a decrease in both ejection fractions.

Clinical implications. If RVEF and LVEF are almost equal in normal subjects, divergences between them (e.g., exceeding 10 units or more) might be an indication of beginning cardiac disease, even if both RVEF and LVEF are within the normal limis. This might be worth studying in patients with chronic pulmonary disease, in whom early depression of right ventricular function may be difficult to reveal. Berger et al.[7] found, by their (rather) arbitrary first-pass method, depressed RVEF in a substantial number of patients with chronic obstructive pulmonary disease, even in those who did not present with any clinical symptoms of cor pulmonale. Furthermore, they demonstrated abnormal right ventricular reserve during exercise in patients with normal RVEF at rest.[9] In contrast to this, Pop et al.[78] could not demonstrate decreased RVEF in any patients unless they had clinical signs of either compensated or decompensated cor pulmonale.

In patients with AMI, measurement of both RVEF and LVEF may be clinically relevant, not only because this may reveal involvement of both ventricles, but also because it might aid in characterizing certain subgroups with prognostic and/or clinical implications.

We gratefully acknowledge the technical assistance and advice of Harald Lønborg-Jensen, MSc. We thank the staffs of the Department of Anesthesia, the Coronary Care Unit, and the Department of Clinical Physiology and Nuclear Medicine for their ready collaboration. We also thank secretaries Lone Jørgensen and Jonna Mouritsen for preparing the manuscript.

References

1. Braunwald E, Sonnenblick EH, Ross J Jr: Contraction of the normal heart. *In* Braunwald E, editor: Heart disease: a textbook of cardiovascular medicine, ed 2. Philadelphia, 1984, W. B. Saunders Co., p 429
2. Carlsson E, Keene RJ, Lee P, Goerke RJ: Angiocardiographic stroke volume correlation of the two cardiac ventricles in man. Invest Radiol **6:** 44, 1971
3. Graham TP Jr, Jarmakani JM, Atwood GF, Canent RV Jr: Right ventricular volume determinations in children. Circulation **47:** 144, 1973
4. Fisher EA, DuBrow IW, Hastreiter AR: Right ventricular volume in congenital heart disease. Am J Cardiol **36:** 67, 1975
5. Nakazawa M, Marks RA, Isabel-Jones J, Jarmakani JM: Right and left ventricular volume characteristics in children with pulmonary

stenosis and intact ventricular septum. Circulation **53:** 884, 1976

6. Winzelberg GG, Boucher CA, Pohost GM, McKusick KA, Bingham JB, Okada RD, Strauss HW: Right ventricular function in aortic and mitral valve disease: relation of gated first-pass radionuclide angiography to clinical and hemodynamic findings. Chest **79:** 520, 1981
7. Berger HJ, Matthay RA, Loke J, Marshall RC, Gottschalk A, Zaret BL: Assessment of cardiac performance with quantitative radionuclide angiocardiography: right ventricular ejection fraction with reference to findings in chronic obstructive pulmonary disease. Am J Cardiol **41:** 897, 1978
8. Berger HJ, Johnstone DE, Sands JM, Gottschalk A, Zaret BL: Response of right ventricular ejection fraction to upright bicycle exercise in coronary artery disease. Circulation **60:** 1292, 1979
9. Berger HJ, Matthay RA, Davies RA, Zaret BL, Gottschalk A: Comparison of exercise right ventricular performance in chronic obstructive pulmonary disease and coronary artery disease: noninvasive assessment by quantitative radionuclide angiocardiography. Invest Radiol **14:** 342, 1979
10. Johnson LL, McCarthy DM, Sciacca RR, Cannon PJ: Right ventricular ejection fraction during exercise in patients with coronary artery disease. Circulation **60:** 1284, 1979
11. Maddahi J, Berman DS, Matsuoka DT, Waxman AD, Stankus KE, Forrester JS, Swan HJC: A new technique for assessing right ventricular ejection fraction using rapid multigated equilibrium cardiac blood pool scintigraphy. Circulation **60:** 581, 1979
12. Slutsky R, Hooper W, Gerber K, Battler A, Froelicher V, Ashburn W, Karliner J: Assessment of right ventricular function at rest and during exercise in patients with coronary heart disease: a new approach using equilibrium radionuclide angiography. Am J Cardiol **45:** 63, 1980
13. Holman BL, Wynne J, Zielonka JS, Idoine JD: A simplified technique for measuring right ventricular ejection fraction using the equilibrium radionuclide angiocardiogram and the slant-hole collimator. Radiology **138:** 429, 1981
14. Marmor A, Geltman EM, Biello DR, Sobel BE, Siegel BA, Roberts R: Functional response of the right ventricle to myocardial infarction: dependence on the site of left ventricular infarction. Circulation **64:** 1005, 1981
15. Korr KS, Gandsman EJ, Winkler ML, Shulman RS, Bough ES: Hemodynamic correlates of right ventricular ejection fraction measured with gated radionuclide angiography. Am J Cardiol **49:** 71, 1982
16. Peter CA, Bowyer K, Jones RH: Radionuclide analysis of right and left ventricular response to exercise in patients with atrial and ventricular septal defects. Am Heart J **105:** 428, 1983
17. Legrand V, Chevigne M, Foulon J, Rigo P: Evaluation of right-ventricular function by gated blood-pool scintigraphy. J Nucl Med **24:** 886, 1983
18. Hurwitz RA, Treves S, Kuruc A: Right ventricular and left ventricular ejection fraction in pediatric patients with normal hearts: first-pass radionuclide angiocardiography. Am Heart J **107:** 726, 1984
19. Bove AA, Santamore WP: Ventricular interdependence. Prog Cardiovasc Dis **23:** 365, 1981
20. Weber KT, Janicki JS, Shroff S, Fishman AP: Contractile mechanics and interaction of the right and left ventricles. Am J Cardiol **47:** 686, 1981
21. Grande P, Christiansen C, Pedersen A, Christensen MS: Optimal diagnosis in acute myocardial infarction: a cost-effectiveness study. Circulation **61:** 723, 1980
22. Schamroth L: The electrocardiology of coronary artery disease, ed 2. Oxford, 1984, Blackwell Scientific Publications, pp 31–131
23. Callahan RJ, Froelich JW, McKusick KA, Leppo J, Strauss HW: A modified method for the in vivo labeling of red blood cells with Tc-99m: concise communication. J Nucl Med **23:** 315, 1982
24. Braunwald E, Fishman AP, Cournand A: Time relationship of dynamic events in the cardiac chambers, pulmonary artery and aorta in man. Circ Res **4:** 100, 1956
25. Guz A, Hoffman JIE, Charlier A, Wierich WR, Zanger L, Benke J: Simultaneous observations of right and left ventricular stroke volumes in conscious dog. Fed Proc **20:** 133, 1961
26. Franklin DL, Van Citters RL, Rushmer RF: Balance between right and left ventricular output. Circ Res **10:** 17, 1962
27. Høilund-Cralsen PF, Rasmussen S, Hesse B, Dige-Petersen H, Folke K, Godtfredsen J, Jensen G, Fabricius J: Determination of left ventricular ejection fraction by radionuclide angiocardiography. Ugeskr Laeger **144:** 3234, 1982
28. Rahe AJ: Tables of critical values for the Pratt matched pair signed rank statistic. J Am Stat Assoc **69:** 368, 1974
29. Wallenstein S, Zucker CL, Fleiss JL: Some statistical methods useful in circulation research. Circ Res **47:** 1, 1980
30. Hald H: Statistical theory with engineering applications. New York, 1952, John Wiley, pp 522–584
31. Camargo EE, Harrison KS, Wagner HN JR, Bourguignon MH, Reid PR, Anderson PO, Baxter RH: Noninvasive beat to beat monitoring of left ventricular function by a nonimaging nuclear detector during premature ventricular contractions. Am J Cardiol **45:** 1219, 1980
32. Steingart RM, Meller J, Barowick J, Patterson R, Herman MV, Teichholz LE: Pulsed Doppler echocardiographic measurement of beat-to-beat changes in stroke volume in dog. Circulation **62:** 542, 1980
33. Hoffman JIE, Guz A, Charlier AA, Wilcken DEL: Stroke volume in conscious dogs: effect of respiration, posture, and vascular occlusion. J Appl Physiol **20:** 865, 1965
34. Weber KT, Janicki JS, Shroff S, Fishman AP: Contractile mechanics and interaction of the right and left ventricles. Am J Cardiol **47:** 686, 1981
35. Holt JP, Rhode EA, Kines H: Ventricular volumes and body weight in mammals. Am J Physiol **215:** 704, 1968
36. Gentzler RD, Briselli MF, Gault JH: Angiographic estimation of right ventricular volume in man. Circulation **50:** 324, 1974
37. Thilenius OG, Arcilla RA: Angiographic right and left ventricular volume determination in normal infants and children. Pediatr Res **8:** 67, 1974
38. Ferlinz J, Gorlin R, Cohn PF, Herman MV: Right ventricular performance in patients with coronary artery disease. Circulation **52:** 608, 1975
39. Lange PE, Onnasch D, Farr FL, Heintzen PH: Angiographic left ventricular volume determination: accuracy, as determined from human casts, and clinical application. Eur J Cardiol **8:** 449, 1978
40. Lange PE, Onnasch D, Farr FL, Heintzen PH: Angiographic right ventricular volume determination: accuracy, as determined from human casts, and clinical application. Eur J Cardiol **8:** 477, 1978
41. Arcilla RA, Tsai P, Thilenius O, Ranninger K: Angiographic method for volume estimation of right and left ventricles. Chest **60:** 446, 1971
42. Ferlinz J: Measurements of right ventricular volumes in man from single plane cineangiograms: a comparison to the biplane approach. Am Heart J **94:** 87, 1977
43. Berger HJ, Matthay RA: Noninvasive radiographic assessment of cardiovascular function in acute and chronic respiratory failure. Am J Cardiol **47:** 950, 1981
44. Ferlinz J: Right ventricular function in adult cardiovascular disease. Prog Cardiovasc Dis **25:** 225, 1982
45. Steele K, Kirch D, LeFree M, Battock D: Measurement of right and left ventricular ejection fractions by radionuclide angiocardiography in coronary artery disease. Chest **70:** 51, 1976
46. Tobinick E, Schelbert HR, Henning H, LeWinter M, Taylor A, Ashburn WL, Karliner JS: Right ventricular ejection fraction in patients with acute anterior and inferior myocardial infarction assessed by radionuclide angiography. Circulation **57:** 1078, 1978
47. Maddahi J, Berman DS, Matsuoka DT, Waxman AD, Forrester JS, Swan HJC: Right ventricular ejection fraction during exercise in normal subjects and in coronary artery disease patients: assessment by multiple-gated equilibrium scintigraphy. Circulation **62:** 133, 1980
48. Franquiz JM, Cardenas R, Lord E, Garcia-Barreto D: Measurement of right and left ventricular ejection fractions by gated equilibrium scintigraphy using Fourier functional images. Nucl Med **21:** 131, 1982
49. Konstam MA, Idoine J, Wynne J, Grossman W, Cohn L, Beck JR, Kozlowski J, Holman BL: Right ventricular function in adults with pulmonary hypertension with and without atrial septal defect. Am J Cardiol **51:** 1144, 1983
50. Høilund-Carlsen PF, Marving J: Determination of right ventricular ejection fraction by radionuclide angiocardiography. Ugeskr Laeger **144:** 3247, 1982
51. Høilund-Carlsen PF, Marving J, Hjort Jensen B, Rasmussen S, Gadsbøll N, Chræmmer-Jørgensen B, Lauritzen SL: Reliability of

determination of right ventricular ejection fraction by radionuclide cardiography. (Manuscript in preparation)
52. Rigo P, Murray M, Strauss HW, Taylor D, Kelly D, Weisfeldt M, Pitt B: Left ventricular function in acute myocardial infarction evaluated by gated scintiphotography. Circulation **50:** 678, 1974
53. Ramanathan KB, Bodenheimer MM, Banka VS, Helfant RH: Severity of contraction abnormalities after acute myocardial infarction in man: response to nitroglycerin. Circulation **60:** 1230, 1979
54. Shah PK, Pichler M, Berman DS, Singh BN, Swan HJC: Left ventricular ejection fraction determined by radionuclide ventriculography in early stages of first transmural myocardial infarction. Am J Cardiol **45:** 542, 1980
55. Sanford CF, Corbett J, Nicod P, Curry GL, Lewis SE, Dehmer GJ, Anderson A, Moses B, Willerson JT: Value of radionuclide ventriculography in the immediate characterization of patients with acute myocardial infarction. Am J Cardiol **49:** 637, 1982
56. Croft CH, Nicod P, Corbett JR, Lewis SE, Huxley R, Mukharji J, Willerson JT, Rude RE: Detection of acute right ventricular infarction by right precordial electrocardiography. Am J Cardiol **50:** 421, 1982
57. Becker LC, Silverman KJ, Bulkley BH, Kallman CH, Mellits ED, Weisfeldt M: Comparison of early thallium-201 scintigraphy and gated blood pool imaging for predicting mortality in patients with acute myocardial infarction. Cirulation **67:** 1272, 1983
58. Nicod P, Corbett JR, Sanford CF, Mukharji J, Dehmer GJ, Croft CH, Rude RE, Lewis S, Willerson JT: Comparison of the influence of acute transmural and nontransmural myocardial infarction on ventricular function. Am Heart J **107:** 28, 1984
59. Battler A, Slutsky R, Karliner J, Froelicher V, Ashburn WL, Ross J Jr: Left ventricular ejection fraction and first third ejection fraction early after acute myocardial infarction: value for predicting mortality and morbidity. Am J Cardiol **45:** 197, 1980
60. Kostuk WJ, Ehsani AA, Karliner JS, Ashburn WL, Petersen KL, Ross J Jr, Sobel BE: Left ventricular performance after myocardial infarction assessed by radioisotope angiocardiography. Circulation **47:** 242, 1973
61. Schelbert HR, Henning H, Ashburn WL, Verba JW, Karliner JS, O'Rourke RA: Serial measurements of left ventricular ejection fraction by radionuclide angiography early and late after myocardial infarction. Am J Cardiol **38:** 407, 1976
62. Reduto LA, Berger HJ, Cohen LS, Gottschalk A, Zaret BL: Sequential radionuclide assessment of left and right ventricular performance after acute transmural myocardial infarction. Ann Intern Med **89:** 441, 1978
63. Rodger JC, Railton R, Young KC, Lakhani AK, Ghouri MAK: Nuclear angiography in convalescent phase of myocardial infarction: serial study of left ventricular performance. Br Heart J **43:** 499, 1980
64. Nemerovski M, Shah PK, Pickler M, Berman DS, Shellock F, Swan HJC: Radionuclide assessment of sequential changes in left and right ventricular function following first acute transmural myocardial infarction. Am Heart J **104:** 709, 1982
65. Corbett JR, Dehmer GJ, Lewis SE, Woodward W, Henderson E, Parkey RW, Blomquist CG, Willerson JT: The prognostic value of submaximal exercise testing with radionuclide ventriculography before hospital discharge in patients with recent myocardial infarction. Circulation **64:** 535, 1981
66. Dewhurst NG, Muir AL: Prognostic value of radionuclide ventriculography after first acute myocardial infarction. Br Heart J **45:** 611, 1981 (abst)
67. Corbett JR, Nicod P, Lewis SE, Rude RE, Willerson JT: Prognostic value of submaximal exercise radionuclide ventriculography after myocardial infarction. Am J Cardiol **52:** 82A, 1983
68. Olson HG, Lyons KP, Troop P, Butman S, Piters KM: The high-risk acute myocardial infarction patient at 1-year follow-up: identification at hospital discharge by ambulatory electrocardiography and radionuclide ventriculography. Am Heart J **107:** 358, 1984
69. Nicod P, Corbett JR, Firth BG, Lewis SE, Rude RE, Huxley R, Willerson JT: Prognostic value of resting and submaximal exercise radionuclide ventriculography after acute myocrdial infarction in high-risk patients with single and multivessel disease. Am J Cardiol **52:** 30, 1983
70. Croft CH, Rude RE, Lewis SE, Parkey RW, Poole WK, Parker C, Fox N, Roberts R, Strauss HW, Thomas LJ, Raabe DS Jr, Sobel BE, Gold HK, Stone PH, Braunwald E, Willerson JT, MILIS Study Group: Comparison of left ventricular function and infarct size in patients with and without persistently positive technetium-99m pyrophosphate myocardial scintigrams after acute myocardial infarction: analysis of 357 patients. Am J Cardiol **53:** 421, 1984
71. Pulido JI, Doss J, Twieg D, Blomqvist GC, Faulkner D, Horn V, DeBates D, Tobey M, Parkey RW, Willerson JT: Submaximal exercise testing after acute myocardial infarction: myocardial scintigraphic and electrocardiographic observations. Am J Cardiol **42:** 19, 1978
72. Steele P, Kirch D, Ellis J, Vogel R, Battock D: Prompt return to normal of depressed right ventricular ejection fraction in acute inferior infarction. Br Heart J **39:** 1319, 1977
73. Dunn RF, Botvinick EH, Benge W, Chatterjee K, Parmley WW: The significance of nitroglycerin-induced changes in ventricular function after acute myocardial infarction. Am J Cardiol **49:** 1719, 1982
74. Klein HO, Tordjman T, Ninio R, Sareli P, Oren V, Lang R, Gefen J, Pauzner C, Segni ED, David D, Kaplinsky E: The early recognition of right ventricular infarction: diagnostic accuracy of the electrocardiographic V_4R lead. Circulation **67:** 558, 1983
75. Baigrie RS, Haq A, Morgan CD, Rakowski H, Drobac M, McLaughlin P: The spectrum of right ventricular involvement in inferior wall myocardial infarction: a clinical, hemodynamic and noninvasive study. J Am Coll Cardiol **1:** 1396, 1983
76. Starling MR, Dell'Italia LJ, Chaudhuri TK, Boros BL, O'Rourke RA, Heyl B, Patrick-Fischer S: First transit and equilibrium radionuclide angiography in patients with inferior transmural myocardial infarction: criteria for the diagnosis of associated hemodynamically significant right ventricular infarction. J Am Coll Cardiol **4:** 923, 1984
77. Dell'Italia LJ, Starling MR, Crawford MH, Boros BL, Chaudhuri TK, O'Rourke RA: Right ventricular infarction: identification by hemodynamic measurements before and after volume loading and correlation with noninvasive techniques. J Am Coll Cardiol **4:** 931, 1984
78. Pop T, Boydan M, Cinteza M, Dumitrache D, Toroiman E, Gherasim L: Right and left ventricular ejection fraction in chronic cor pulmonale disease. Eur J Nucl Med **8:** A37, 1983 (abst)

Altered left ventricular mechanics in patients with valvular aortic stenosis and coarction of the aorta: effects on systolic performance and late outcome

KENNETH M. BOROW, M.D., STEVEN D. COLAN, M.D., AND ALEXANDER NEUMANN, B.S.

ABSTRACT Despite similar degrees of left ventricular systolic hypertension shortening characteristics are usually greater in patients with congenital valvular aortic stenosis (VAS) than in patients with coarctation of the aorta (CoA). We hypothesized that these dissimilarities were caused by differences in myocardial mechanics rather than by alterations in contractile state. Eleven patients with VAS (ages 6 to 41 years) and 11 with CoA were matched for age, body surface area, and peak systolic ejection gradient. Results were compared with data from 22 normal subjects matched for age and body surface area. Echocardiographic tracings of the left ventricle were recorded in conjunction with left ventricular pressure measurements (VAS) or calibrated carotid pulse tracings (CoA and normal subjects). Peak and end-systolic wall stresses as well as left ventricular shortening fraction (%ΔD) and rate-corrected velocity of fiber shortening (Vcf_c) were calculated. No differences for left ventricular dimensions, heart rate or peak wall stress were present. Ventricular peak systolic pressures and wall mass were higher for the patients with VAS or CoA than for the normal subjects ($p < .001$). These parameters did not differ between the VAS and CoA groups. The patients with VAS had higher %ΔD and Vcf_c than either the CoA or normal groups ($p < .01$). Afterload, as quantified by end-systolic stress, was 41% lower than normal for the patients with VAS ($p < .001$) and 13% higher than normal for those with CoA ($p < .05$). Left ventricular contractility as assessed by load-independent indexes (i.e., end-systolic stress/%ΔD and end-systolic stress/Vcf_c relationships) was depressed in three of 11 patients with CoA. All of these patients were over 20 years of age. In contrast, the increased systolic performance noted in the patients with VAS was caused by reduced afterload at end-systole rather than by altered contractile state. Thus the extent and velocity of left ventricular shortening is lower in patients with CoA than in those with VAS because of disadvantageous afterload conditions and/or an age-related depression in contractile state.

Circulation **72, No. 3, 515–522, 1985.**

PATIENTS wth congenital valvular aoartic stenosis (VAS) or coarctation of the aorta (CoA) have left ventricular pressure overload resulting in concentric ventricular hypertrophy. The stimulus for hypertrophy in both of these lesions is believed to be the peak forces (i.e., wall stress) acting on the myocardial fibers during systole.[1-7] The ventricle responds by increasing wall thickness until peak systolic wall stress is normalized.[2, 3] Despite a similar hypertrophic response to long-term pressure overload, the left ventricle in patients with VAS is frequently hyperkinetic when compared with that in patients with CoA.[7-11] Indeed, children and young adults with VAS often demonstrate a progressive increase in the extent and velocity of myocardial shortening associated with increasing left ventricular peak systolic pressures and transvalvular pressure gradients.[7, 8, 11] This response appears to contradict the usual inverse relationship between left ventricular shortening characteristics and afterload.[12-14] Recently, we showed that afterload, as measured by end-systolic wall stress, is an important determinant of the extent and velocity of left ventricular fiber shortening in humans.[15-18] This study explores the hypothesis that differences in ventricular afterload rather than differences in left ventricular contractility could account for many of the dissimilarities in ventricular shortening characteristics found in patients with VAS or CoA. This issue was examined by means of load-independent left ventricular end-systolic indexes of contractility in age- and body surface area–matched patients with VAS or CoA and normal subjects.

From the Cardiology Section, Department of Medicine, The University of Chicago Medical Center, Chicago, and the Department of Cardiology, The Children's Hospital, Harvard Medical School, Boston.

Address for correspondence: Kenneth M. Borow, M.D., Department of Medicine, The University of Chicago Medical Center, 950 E. 59th St., Box 44, Chicago, IL 60637.

Received Jan. 28, 1985; revision accepted May 30, 1985.

Methods

Study population. The study population consisted of 11 patients with isolated congenital VAS and 11 age-matched patients with uncomplicated CoA (table 1). Ages ranged from 6 to 40 years and 6 to 41 years, respectively. None of the patients with CoA had evidence of VAS on physical examination or by two-dimensional echocardiographic study. All patients were well compensated with no history of congestive heart failure and no findings of diminished cardiac output at the time of study.

Comparisons between the patients with VAS or CoA were made with 22 normal subjects matched for age and body surface area. These subjects were free of known cardiovascular disease and none was a competitive athlete. All subjects had normal two-dimensional echocardiograms without evidence of valvular heart disease, regional wall motion abnormalities, or increased left ventricular wall thickness.

Experimental design. All of the patients with VAS underwent routine right and left heart catheterizations performed from the femoral vessels. Left ventricular and aortic pressures were recorded with fluid-filled catheters attached to Statham P23Db transducers zeroed at the midchest level. Simultaneous left ventricular pressure as well as high-frequency phonocardiographic, M mode echocardiographic, and electrocardiographic tracings were obtained. Echocardiographic data were recorded with either a 2.25 or 3.5 MHZ transducer on an Irex Systems II or Hewlett-Packard ultrasound module. Ultrasound images of the left ventricle were obtained above the level of the papillary muscles just off the tip of the anterior leaflet of the mitral valve. Patients with left ventricular regional wall motion abnormalities or evidence of coronary artery disease on coronary angiography were excluded from the study. Peak systolic ejection gradient across the aortic valve was measured by catheter pullback from the left ventricle to the aorta. Left ventricular end-diastolic dimension and wall thickness were measured at the beginning of the Q wave of the electrocardiogram while end-systolic dimension, wall thickness, and pressure were measured at the first high-frequency component of the aortic second heart sound. Values for each of the above were taken as the mean of five cardiac cycles.

Patients with CoA as well as normal subjects had simultaneous electrocardiogram, phonocardiogram, left ventricular M mode echocardiogram, carotid pulse, and systemic blood pressures recorded. Peak pressure gradients across the site of CoA were measured as the difference between systolic pressures recorded simultaneously from the right leg and right arm. The carotid pulse tracing was recorded from the right carotid artery and calibrated with the Dinamap 845 Vital Signs Monitor (Critikon, Tampa, FL). This method of calibration involves assignment of systolic blood pressure to the peak of the tracing and diastolic pressure to the nadir.[15-20] This device has been shown to estimate central aortic pressures accurately over a wide range of values in children and adults.[19, 20] Echocardiographic measurements were performed as described for the patients with VAS. The pressure tracings as well as the left ventricular echocardiograms for the patients with CoA were analyzed with the Quantic 1200 (Bruce Franklin, Inc., Seattle). This instrument is programmed to correct the carotid pulse tracing for pulse transmission time by aligning the discrotic notch with the first high-frequency component of A_2.

The left ventricular ejection time (LVET) was measured from the central aortic pressure tracing in the patients with VAS and from the carotid pulse tracing in the patients with CoA and in control subjects. The LVET was rate-corrected to a heart rate of 60 beats/ min, with left ventricular rate-corrected ejection time (ET_c) = LVET/$\sqrt{\text{RR interval}}$. Ventricular percent fractional shortening (%ΔD) was calculated as (end-diastolic dimension-end-systolic dimension)/end-diastolic dimension. The mean velocity of left ventricular fiber shortening (Vcf), which is sensitive to changes in RR interval, was rate corrected and normalized to the end-diastolic dimension by the following formula[16]:

$$Vcf_c = \frac{D_{ed} - D_{es}}{D_{ed}} \frac{1}{LVET_c} = \frac{\%\Delta D}{LVET_c}$$

where Vcf_c is the rate corrected Vcf, D_{ed} is the end-diastolic dimension, and D_{es} is the end-systolic dimension. Instantaneous left ventricular meridional wall stress (σ) was calculated throughout ventricular ejection by the Quantic 1200 equipped with a digitizing pad that has a sampling rate of 80/cm or approximately 400/sec. The following angiographically validated formula was used[3, 21]:

$$\sigma = \frac{(P)\,(D)\,(1.35)}{(h)\left(1 + \frac{h}{D}\right)(4)}$$

where P = left ventricular pressure (mm Hg), D = left ventricular dimension (cm), h = left ventricular wall thickness (cm), and 1.35 is the factor used to convert mm Hg to g/cm^2. The left ventricular mean systolic wall stress was calculated as the average of instantaneous wall stresses during ejection. The left ventricular shortening load was defined as the integral of the time-stress plot from the onset to the end of ventricular ejection.[22] Left ventricular wall mass was calculated by adapting the formula of Devereux et al.[23]:

$$LVM = 1.04\left[\,[D_{ed} + 2\,(h_{ed})]^3 - (D_{ed})^3\right] - 14\text{ g}$$

where LVM = left ventricular wall mass (g), 1.04 = specific gravity of myocardium, D_{ed} = left ventricular end-diastolic dimension (cm), and h_{ed} = left ventricular posterior wall thickness at end-diastole (cm).

Data analysis. Unless otherwise noted, the data are presented as mean ± SD. The hemodynamic data are compared among the groups by an unpaired t test for two means with a $p < .05$ considered statistically significant. The left ventricular end-systolic stress/%ΔD and end-systolic stress/Vcf_c relationships were determined for all patients with VAS or CoA. Previously reported normal values for these relationships were used to define data points statistically different from the normal population.[15, 16]

TABLE 1
Profile of study population

	Control (n = 22)	VAS (n = 11)	CoA (n = 11)
Age (yr)			
Range	6–40	6–40	6–41
Mean ± SD	16±10	16±10	15±10
BSA (m^2)	1.41±0.47	1.35±0.43	1.43±0.40

BSA = body surface area.

Results

Table 2 summarizes the hemodynamic data for the three study groups. Left ventricular peak systolic pressure, peak systolic ejection gradient, end-diastolic wall thickness, and wall mass were higher for the patients with VAS or CoA than for the age-matched

TABLE 2
Hemodynamic data

	Control	VAS	CoA	Control vs VAS	Control vs CoA	VAS vs CoA
HR (bpm)	79±16	83±19	76±18			
P_{ps} (mm Hg)	112±10	149±32	137±19	<.001	<.001	
PSEG (mm Hg)	0	44±28	45±32	<.001	<.001	
P_{es} (mm Hg)	90±10	86±9	104±13		<.01	<.01
D_{ed} (cm)	4.25±0.75	4.05±0.55	4.55±1.00			
D_{es} (cm)	2.85±0.55	2.60±0.40	3.10±0.85			
h_{ed} (cm)	0.80±0.15	1.05±0.20	0.95±0.20	<.001	<.05	
h_{es} (cm)	1.30±0.25	1.65±0.30	1.40±0.25	<.01		
LVM (g)	114±21	160±30	167±35	<.001	<.001	
ET_c (msec)	310±14	322±27	325±16			
%ΔD	33.0±2.1	36.3±2.5	31.8±4.6	<.01		<.01
Vcf_c	1.01±0.07	1.13±0.06	0.98±0.11	<.01		<.01
σ_{ps} (g/cm^2)	148±17	149±21	141±28			
σ_{es} (g/cm^2)	46±7	27±10	53±10	<.001	<.05	<.001
σ_m (g/cm^2)	92±14	89±11	103±17			
SL (g-sec/cm^2)	26±5	24±4	30±7			<.05

HR = heart rate; P_{ps} = left ventricular peak systolic pressure; PSEG = peak systolic ejection gradient; P_{es} = left ventricular end-systolic pressure; D_{ed} = left ventricular end-diastolic dimension; D_{es} = left ventricular end-systolic dimension; h_{ed} = left ventricular end-diastolic wall thickness; h_{es} = left ventricular end-systolic wall thickness; LVM = left ventricular wall mass; ET_c = rate corrected left ventricular ejection time; σ_{ps} = left ventricular peak systolic wall stress; σ_{es} = left ventricular end-systolic wall stress; σ_m = left ventricular mean systolic wall stress; SL = left ventricular shortening load.

control subjects. These parameters did not differ between the VAS and CoA groups. There were no significant differences for heart rate, left ventricular end-diastolic dimension, end-systolic dimension, rate-corrected ejection time, or peak or mean wall stress between the three groups. Nineteen of the 22 patients with VAS or CoA had peak stress values within the 95% confidence limits generated from our control subjects (figure 1). Despite normal values of peak stress, the mean values for %ΔD and Vcf_c were higher for the patients with VAS than for either the patients with CoA or the control subjects ($p < .01$). There were no

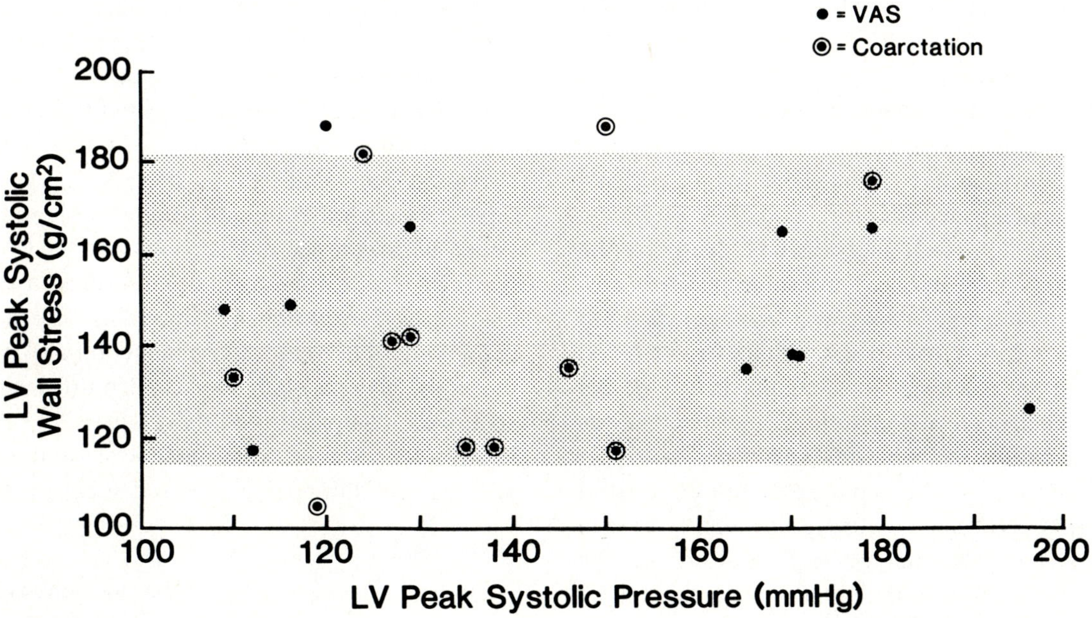

FIGURE 1. Plot of left ventricular peak systolic wall stress vs peak systolic pressure. The shaded area represents the 95% confidence limits for peak stress generated from the normal subjects in this study. Nineteen of 22 patients with VAS or CoA had normal peak stress values.

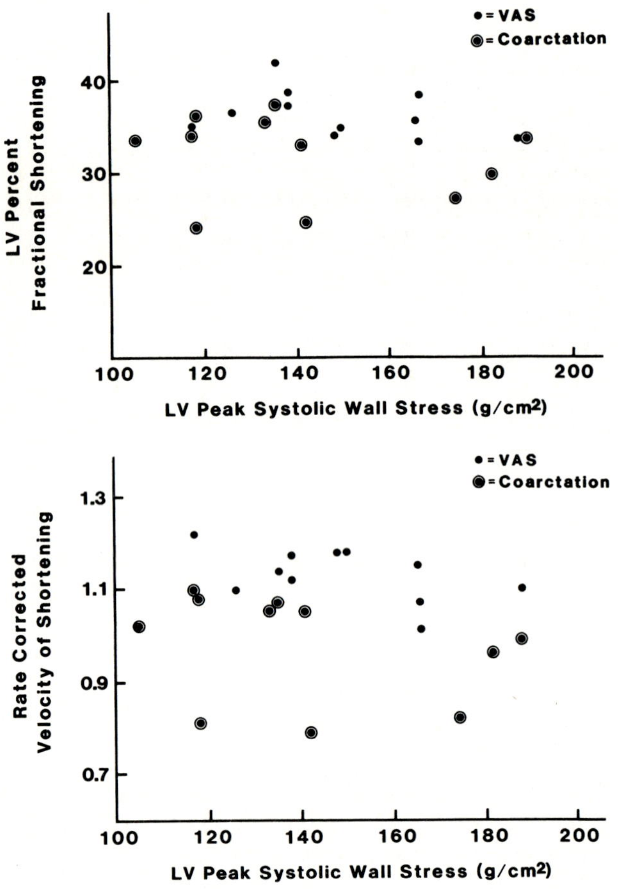

FIGURE 2. Plot of left ventricular percent fractional shortening *(top)* and rate-corrected velocity of shortening *(bottom)* against left ventricular peak systolic wall stress. There was a poor correlation between peak stress and both the extent and velocity of left ventricular shortening in the patients with VAS or CoA.

differences in these values between the patients with CoA and control subjects. There was no significant correlation between peak stress and either %ΔD or Vcf_c for either patient group (figure 2).

When compared with control values, end-systolic pressure was within the normal range for the patients with VAS and elevated for those with CoA. Left ventricular end-systolic wall thickness was greater for the patients with VAS than for control subjects. There was a trend for greater end-systolic wall thickness values in the patients with VAS compared with those with CoA, but this did not reach statistical significance. The net result was an average end-systolic stress value that was 41% lower for the patients with VAS and 13% higher for those with CoA when compared with the control subjects ($p < .001$ and $p < .05$, respectively). As seen in figure 3, the lowest end-systolic stress values for the patients with VAS occurred in those patients with the highest left ventricular peak systolic pressures. In addition, end-systolic stress was lower for the patients with VAS than for those with CoA at all levels of left ventricular peak systolic pressure. The left ventricular shortening load (i.e., integral of the time-stress plot during ejection) was similar for the control group as compared with both the VAS and CoA groups. However, shortening load was significantly higher ($p < .05$) for the patients with CoA than for those with VAS (table 2, figure 4).

In figure 5, the data from the 22 patients with VAS or CoA are plotted against the normal values for the left ventricular end-systolic stress/%ΔD and end-systolic stress/Vcf_c relationships. These plots include the normal values (mean ± 2 SD) for %ΔD and Vcf_c over a wide range of afterload (i.e., end-systolic stress). Values above the normal range indicate augmented contractility, while values below the normal range suggest depressed contractile state. The use of the end-systolic stress/%ΔD relationship as an index of left ventricular contractility is predicated on the fact that there are no differences in preload between the groups. This was indeed the case in our study if left ventricular end-diastolic dimension is used as a measurement of preload status. It is therefore possible to distinguish afterload-related alterations in left ventricular shortening from those caused by altered contractility. Despite high individual values for %ΔD, 10 of the 11 patients with VAS fell within the normal range for end-systolic stress/%ΔD. All 11 demonstrated normal end-systolic stress/Vcf_c relationships. This suggests that the increased left ventricular performance that is characteristic of young patients with moderate-to-severe congenital VAS is caused by reduced afterload at end-systole (i.e., end-systolic stress) rather than by augmented contractile state. In contrast, patients with CoA have higher end-systolic wall stress values and lower values for %ΔD and Vcf_c. Although eight of the patients with CoA fell within the normal limits for both end-systolic stress/%ΔD and end-systolic stress/Vcf_c relationships, three patients fell below these limits. These three patients, who were the oldest patients in the CoA group (i.e., 20, 25, and 41 years of age), demonstrated depressed left ventricular shortening characteristics caused by abnormal ventricular contractility. When the eight patients with CoA and normal contractile state were compared with the 11 patients with VAS, the differences in left ventricular systolic function and afterload conditions remained statistically significant.

Discussion

Complex changes in cardiovascular physiology occur in the presence of long-term left ventricular pressure overload.[24–26] Because of the inability of traditional measures of left ventricular performance to separate

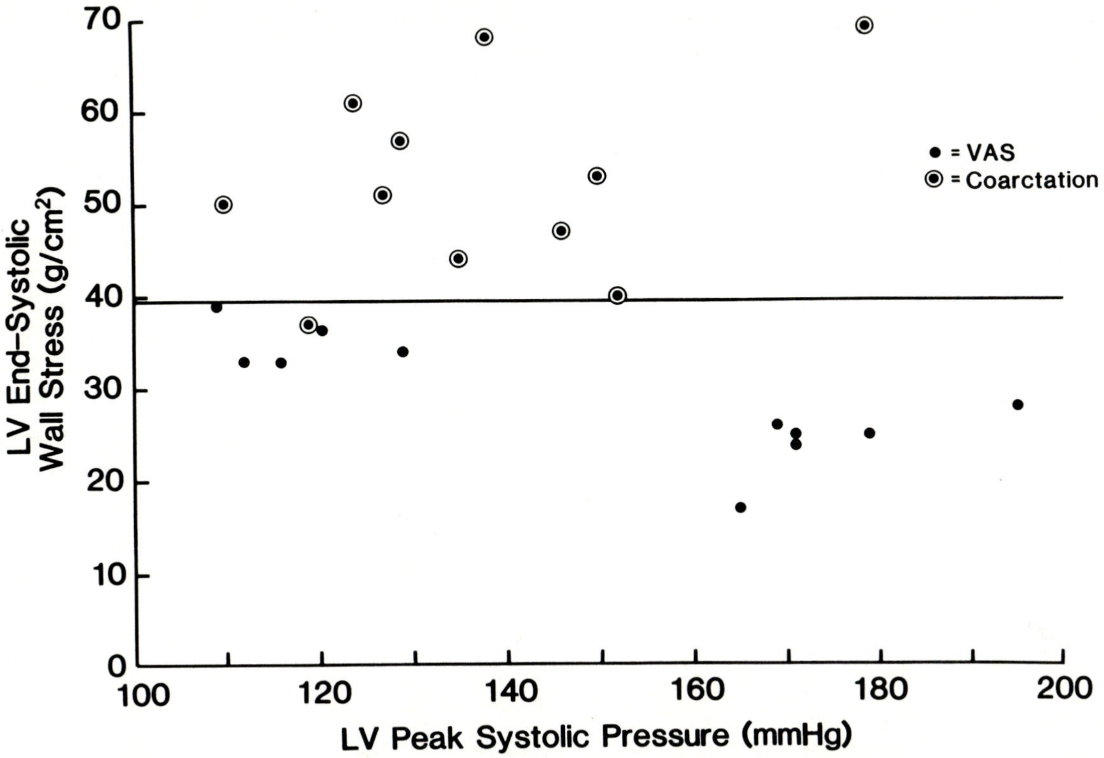

FIGURE 3. Relationship between left ventricular end-systolic wall stress and left ventricular peak systolic pressure. End-systolic wall stress was lower for the patients with VAS than for those with CoA at all levels of peak systolic pressure. For the VAS group, the lowest end-systolic stress values occurred in patients with the highest peak systolic pressures.

derangements in afterload and preload from alterations in contractility,[14, 27] it remains controversial whether the left ventricle in these patients has normal inotropic properties.[5–9, 28, 29] In an attempt to better address this issue, ventricular mechanics have been defined in

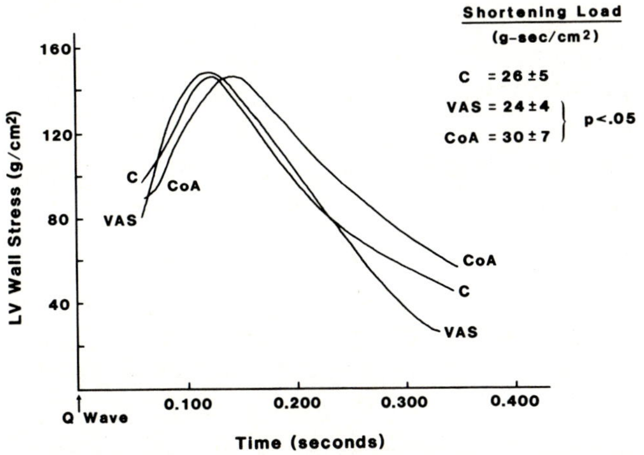

FIGURE 4. Comparison of the time course of left ventricular wall stress during the ejection phase of the cardiac cycle in patients with CoA or VAS and in control subjects (C). Although peak systolic wall stress values are comparable, marked disparities exist at end-systole. The left ventricular shortening load was similar for the control group as compared with the VAS and CoA groups. However, shortening load was significantly higher ($p < .05$) for the patients with CoA than for those with VAS.

terms of force-shortening-velocity characteristics.[12, 16, 18] In our patients with congenital VAS or CoA, increases in left ventricular peak systolic pressure were associated with increases in left ventricular wall thickness over the entire cardiac cycle. This resulted in normalization of peak stress, a finding in agreement with many previous studies of long-term left ventricular pressure overload.[1–7] Although peak stress values were similar for all groups, the patients with VAS demonstrated decreased end-systolic stress. This was caused by normal end-systolic pressure in association with increased end-systolic wall thickness. In these patients the increased left ventricular wall thickness that is appropriate to normalize peak stress (which occurs during early systole) is excessive for the much lower left ventricular pressure in the ventricle at end-systole. This decreased end-systolic pressure in conjunction with increased end-systolic wall thickness resulted in low end-systolic wall stress values. The left ventricle at end-systole therefore acted as if it were afterload reduced. In contrast, the patients with CoA had significantly elevated end-systolic pressure with normal end-systolic wall thickness. This resulted in slightly increased values for end-systolic wall stress. It should be noted that in this study, meridional wall stress was used to quantitate afterload. Although cir-

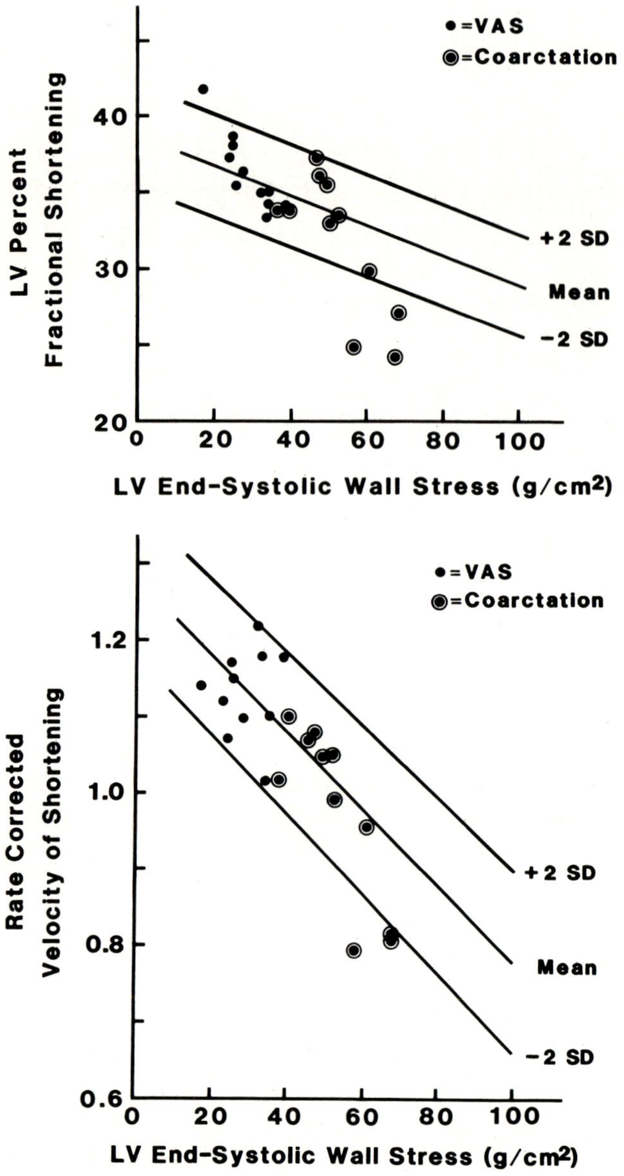

FIGURE 5. Data from the VAS and CoA groups plotted against normal values for the left ventricular end-systolic stress/%ΔD *(top)* and end-systolic stress/Vcf_c *(bottom)* relationships. All of the patients with VAS and eight of 11 patients with CoA had normal left ventricular contractile state. The three patients with CoA with depressed left ventricular contractility were all over 20 years of age.

cumferential wall stress may be a more ideal measure of ventricular load because it incorporates both minor and major axis dimensions, studies of patients with VAS have shown that these two wall stresses correlate well.[30, 31] It has been previously reported that in patients with VAS, the heart maintains a relatively normal size and shape throughout most of the course of the disease and thus the minor-to-major axis ratio is relatively unaltered.[32] This would appear to be true in our study, since there were no differences in end-diastolic or end-systolic dimensions between the control, VAS, and CoA groups. In addition, we have previously demonstrated the clinical utility of end-systolic meridional wall stress as a measure of left ventricular afterload.[15–18] Thus the use of meridional rather than circumferential wall stress seems reasonable and should not alter the interpretation of the data.

It is known that for any level of contractility, the end-systolic fiber length is linearly related to the end-systolic force (i.e., wall stress).[33, 34] Thus the myocardium continues to shorten until the force generated by the myocardium equals the maximal force generating capacity at that fiber length. The active state then ends and ventricular shortening is terminated. By relating end-systolic stress to the extent and velocity of left ventricular fiber shortening, important information about left ventricular mechanics can be obtained. In our study, the end-systolic stress/%ΔD and end-systolic stress/Vcf_c relationships were used to assess contractile state. Although both of these indexes incorporate afterload and are sensitive to contractility, only the end-systolic stress/Vcf_c relationship is independent of left ventricular preload conditions.[16] Although left ventricular performance by traditional indexes was significantly augmented in the VAS group, 10 of 11 end-systolic stress/%ΔD and all end-systolic stress/Vcf_c points fell within our previously reported normal range of values for these relationships (figure 5). In all cases there was an appropriate physiologic response to decreased end-systolic stress with upward and leftward movement along the normal force-shortening-velocity curve. Thus children and young adults with congenital VAS have normal left ventricular contractility. In contrast, our younger patients with CoA demonstrated elevations in end-systolic stress, resulting in %ΔD and Vcf_c values that were appropriately lower for a normal left ventricular contractile state. The three oldest CoA patients, who were all over 20 years of age, had inappropriately low %ΔD and Vcf_c values for their level of end-systolic stress. Left ventricular contractile state was depressed in these patients. Because the end-systolic stress/%ΔD and end-systolic stress/Vcf_c relationships differ with respect to preload dependency, the concordance of data for these two relationships within the VAS and CoA groups suggests that preload was not a hemodynamically important determinant of differences in left ventricular performance in these resting measurements.

The age-related differences in the contractility data in our VAS and CoA groups are in agreement with the previously described natural history of these two conditions.[10, 24, 29, 32, 35, 36] Patients with congenital VAS usually maintain compensated left ventricular performance for many years.[24, 32, 36] Excluding infants with critical aortic stenosis, only in the very late stages of congenital VAS does left ventricular failure occur.[24, 32, 36] It is unclear whether this long latency period reflects progressively increasing obstruction to left ventricular ejection or rather a period of stable hemodynamics after adolescence, which only becomes compromised late in life when fibrosis or calcification of the valve occurs. In contrast, patients with CoA have congestive heart failure as an acquired complication second in frequency only to systemic hypertension.[10, 35] In Campbell's review[35] of 304 autopsy cases of unrepaired CoA, 25% of patients died before age 20, 50% by age 32, 75% by age 46, and 90% by age 58. Twenty-six percent of all deaths were caused by congestive heart failure; the mean age at the time of death of these patients was 39 years.[35] In a more recent review of 234 cases of CoA, 67% of patients older than age 40 years had symptoms of congestive heart failure.[10]

Throughout the latter two-thirds of ejection, the reduction in ventricular dimension and increase in wall thickness result in a progressive decline in instantaneous wall stress. This ability of the myocardium to "unload" itself is greater in the normal ventricle than in the dilated failing ventricle.[27] As illustrated in figure 4, the heart with VAS has a greater than normal fall in load (i.e., wall stress) by end-systole. In contrast, CoA is characterized by less "unloading" than normal and high end-systolic wall stress values. The resultant mechanical disadvantage in CoA has several implications. First, although hypertrophy in patients with CoA results in normalization of peak systolic wall stress so that the maximum force per unit cross-sectional area is not elevated, the left ventricular shortening load (i.e., integral of wall stress over ejection time) is higher for patients with CoA than for these with VAS. This suggests that myocardial oxygen consumption was increased in the patients with CoA, since shortening load and oxygen consumption are linearly related.[22] This could well play a role in the accelerated myocardial deterioration typical of this disease. Second, as we and others have reported,[37] for an equivalent degree of hypertrophy both systolic shortening and myocardial thickening relate directly to early diastolic function. Thus elevated late systolic load and the consequent reduction in systolic function result in impaired early diastolic function.[37] This would be expected to be of greatest importance during exercise. Combined left ventricular diastolic and systolic dysfunction in conjunction with an inability to increase blood flow maximally to the lower extremities may contribute to the decreased exercise capacity reported in patients with CoA relative to normal subjects or patients with VAS.[38, 39] Finally, coarctation of the aorta, unlike VAS, is characterized by impaired arterial function relative to its ability to accept pulsatile blood flow from the left ventricle.[40, 41] This is caused by a marked reduction in central arterial capacitance leading to alterations in the pulsatile properties of the proximal aorta and upper body arteries.[42] This disadvantage is even more hemodynamically significant during exercise when cardiac output is higher.[42] Studies of aortic impedance as well as pulsatile and steady-state power in patients with CoA and VAS may give important information regarding the physiologic differences between two seemingly similar left ventricular hypertensive conditions. Thus the worse prognosis and decreased contractile state found in older patients with CoA relative to age-matched patients with VAS may be caused by differences in internal and external left ventricular mechanical factors.

References

1. Sandler H, Dodge HT: Left ventricular tension and stress in man. Circ Res **13:** 91, 1963
2. Hood WP, Rackley CE, Rolett EL: Wall stress in the normal and hypertrophied human left ventricle. Am J Cardiol **22:** 550, 1958
3. Grossman W, Jones D, McLaurin LP: Wall stress and patterns of hypertrophy in the human left ventricle. J Clin Invest **56:** 56, 1975
4. Gould KL, Kennedy JW, Fremer M, Pollack GH, Dodge HT: Analysis of wall dynamics and directional components of left ventricular contraction in man. Am J Cardiol **38:** 322, 1976
5. Grossman W: Cardiac hypertrophy: useful adaptation or pathologic process. Am J Med **69:** 576, 1980
6. Glanz S, Hellenbrand WE, Berman MA, Talner NS: Echocardiographic assessment of the severity of aortic stenosis in children and adolescents. Am J Cardiol **38:** 620, 1976
7. Aziz KU, van Grondelle A, Paul MH, Muster AJ: Echocardiographic assessment of the relation between left ventricular wall and cavity dimensions and peak systolic pressure in children with aortic stenosis. Am J Cardiol **40:** 775, 1977
8. Johnson GL, Meyer RA, Schwartz DC, Korfhagen J, Kaplan S: Left ventricular function by echocardiography in children with fixed aortic stenosis. Am J Cardiol **38:** 611, 1976
9. Sasayama S, Franklin D, Ross J Jr: Hyperfunction with normal inotropic state of the hypertrophied left ventricle. Am J Physiol **232:** H418, 1977
10. Liberthson RR, Pennington DG, Jacobs ML, Daggett WM: Coarctation of the aorta: review of 234 patients and clarification of management problems. Am J Cardiol **43:** 835, 1979
11. Donner R, Carabello BA, Black I, Spann JF: Left ventricular wall stress in compensated aortic stenosis in children. Am J Cardiol **51:** 946, 1983
12. Sonnenblick EH, Parmley WW, Urschel CW: The contractile state of the heart as expressed by force-velocity relations. Am J Cardiol **23:** 488, 1969
13. Weber KT, Janicki JS: The dynamics of ventricular contraction: force, length and shortening. Fed Proc **39:** 188, 1980
14. Braunwald E, Ross J: Control of cardiac performance. *In* Berne RM, Sperclakis N, Geiger SR, editors: Handbook of physiology. The cardiovascular system. Baltimore, 1979, Williams & Wilkins, p 533
15. Borow KM, Green LH, Grossman W, Braunwald E: Left ventricular end-systolic stress-shortening and stress-length relations in humans: normal values and sensitivity to inotropic state. Am J Cardiol **50:** 1301, 1982
16. Colan SD, Borow KM, Neumann A: The left ventricular end-

systolic wall stress-velocity of fiber shortening relation: a load independent index of myocardial contractility. J Am Coll Cardiol **4:** 715, 1984
17. Borow KM, Neumann A, Arensman FW, Yacoub MH: Left ventricular contractility and contractile reserve in humans after cardiac transplantation. Circulation **71:** 866, 1985
18. Lang RM, Borow KM, Neumann A, Feldman T: Adverse cardiac effects of acute alcohol ingestion in young adults. Ann Intern Med **102:** 742, 1985
19. Borow KM, Newburger J: Noninvasive estimation of central aortic pressure using the oscillometric method for analyzing systemic artery pulsatile blood flow: comparative study of indirect systolic, diastolic, and mean brachial artery pressure with simultaneous direct ascending aortic pressure measurements. Am Heart J **103:** 879, 1982
20. Colan SD, Fujii A, Borow KM, MacPherson D, Sanders S: Noninvasive determination of systolic, diastolic, and end-systolic blood pressure in neonates, infants and young children: comparison with central aortic pressure measurements. Am J Cardiol **52:** 867, 1983
21. Brodie BR, McLaurin LP, Grossman W: Combined hemodynamic-ultrasonic method for studying left ventricular wall stress: comparison with angiography. Am J Cardiol **37:** 864, 1976
22. Weber KT, Janicki JS: Myocardial oxygen consumption: the role of wall force and shortening. Am J Physiol **233:** H421, 1977
23. Devereux RB, Reichek N: Echocardiographic determination of left ventricular mass in man: anatomic validation of method. Circulation **55:** 613, 1976
24. Rapaport E: Natural history of aortic and mitral valve disease. Am J Cardiol **35:** 221, 1975
25. Gunther S, Grossman W: Determinants of ventricular function in pressure-overload hypertrophy in man. Circulation **59:** 679, 1979
26. Carabello BA, Green LH, Grossman W, Cohn LH, Koster JK, Collins JJ Jr: Hemodynamic determinants of prognosis of aortic valve replacement in critical aortic stenosis and advanced congestive heart failure. Circulation **62:** 42, 1980
27. Weber KT, Janicki JS: The heart as a muscle-pump system and the concept of heart failure. Am Heart J **98:** 371, 1979
28. Smith N, McAnulty JH, Rahimtoola SH: Severe aortic stenosis and impaired left ventricular function and clinical heart failure: results of valve replacement. Circulation **58:** 255, 1978
29. Graham TP: Ventricular performance in adults after operation for congenital heart disease. Am J Cardiol **50:** 612, 1982
30. DePace NL, Ren JF, Iskandrian AS, Kotler MN, Hakki AH, Segal BL: Correlation of echocardiographic wall stress and left ventricular pressure and function in aortic stenosis. Circulation **67:** 854, 1983
31. Gould KL, Lipscomb K, Hamilton GW, Kennedy JW: Relation of left ventricular shape, function and wall stress in man. Am J Cardiol **34:** 627, 1974
32. Fischl SJ, Gorlin R, Herman MV: Cardiac shape and function in aortic valve disease: physiologic and clinical implications. Am J Cardiol **39:** 170, 1977
33. Suga H, Kitabatake A, Sagawa K: End-systolic pressure determines stroke volume from fixed end-diastolic volume in the isolated left ventricle under a constant contractile state. Circ Res **44:** 238, 1979
34. Weber KT, Janicki JS, Hefner LL: Left ventricular force-length relations of isovolumic and ejecting contractions. Am J Physiol **231:** 337, 1976
35. Campbell M: Natural history of coarctation of the aorta. Br Heart J **32:** 633, 1970
36. Rotman M, Morris JJ Jr, Behar VS, Peter RH, Kong Y: Aortic valve disease: comparison of types and their medical and surgical management. Am J Med **51:** 241, 1971
37. Colan SD, Borow KM, Neumann A: Effects of loading conditions and contractile state on left ventricular early diastolic function. Am J Cardiol **55:** 790, 1985
38. Alpert BS, Moses DM, Durant RH, Strong WB, Flood NL: Hemodynamic response to ergometer exercises in children and young adults with left ventricular pressure or volume overload. Am J Cardiol **52:** 563, 1983
39. Cumming GR: Maximal exercise capacity of children with heart defects. Am J Cardiol **42:** 613, 1978
40. O'Rourke MF, Cartmill TB: Influence of aortic coarctation on pulsatile hemodynamics in the proximal aorta. Circulation **44:** 281, 1971
41. Covell JW, Pouleur H, Ross J Jr: Left ventricular wall stress and aortic input impedance. Fed Proc **39:** 202, 1980
42. Nichols WW, Pepine CJ: Left ventricular afterload and aortic input impedance: implications of pulsatile blood flow. Prog Cardiovasc Dis **24:** 293, 1982

A new approach to noninvasive evaluation of aortic regurgitant fraction by two-dimensional Doppler echocardiography

AKIRA KITABATAKE, M.D., HIROSHI ITO, M.D., MICHITOSHI INOUE, M.D., JUN TANOUCHI, M.D., KEN ISHIHARA, M.D., TOSHIO MORITA, M.D., KENSHI FUJII, M.D., YUTAKA YOSHIDA, M.D., TOHRU MASUYAMA, M.D., HIDEO YOSHIMA, M.D., MASATSUGU HORI, M.D., AND TAKENOBU KAMADA, M.D.

ABSTRACT The aortic regurgitant fraction was estimated noninvasively in 20 patients with aortic regurgitation from systolic aortic and pulmonary volume flow determined by duplex Doppler echocardiography. By assuming that an excess of the aortic volume flow (AF) compared with the pulmonary volume flow (PF) is due to aortic regurgitant flow, the aortic regurgitant fraction (RF) was calculated as follows: $RF(\%) = (AF - PF)/AF \times 100$. The aortic and pulmonary volume flows were determined as products of systolic integrals of ejection flow velocities and cross-sectional areas of the left and right ventricular outflow tracts, respectively. The Doppler estimate of the regurgitant fraction was compared by semiquantitative grading (1+ to 4+) by cineaortography and with the measurement of regurgitant fraction by catheter technique. The mean Doppler-determined aortic regurgitant fraction was 2.4% for normal subjects, 28.0% for the patients with 1+, 32.6% for the patients with 2+, 53.3% for the patients with 3+, and 62.4% for the patients with 4+. A fair correlation was found between Doppler estimates of regurgitant fraction and semiquantitative cineaortographic grades ($r = .80$, $p < .01$). In the patients without associated mitral regurgitation, a close correlation was observed between Doppler and catheter estimates of regurgitant fraction ($r = .96$, $p < .01$; $y = 1.0x - 0.08$). In the patients with associated mild mitral regurgitation, however, Doppler estimates of regurgitant fraction substantially underestimated those determined by the conventional catheter technique, which cannot separately quantitate the aortic regurgitant fraction in the presence of mitral regurgitation. These observations indicate that the proposed Doppler technique provides a useful method to evaluate the aortic regurgitant fraction specifically regardless of the presence of associated mitral lesions.
Circulation 72, No. 3, 523–529, 1985.

A PULSED DOPPLER technique has been used to evaluate semiquantitatively the severity of aortic regurgitation based on the extent of the distribution of the flow disturbances in the left ventricle.[1-5] Although this method is simple in clinical use, some problems have been identified in its use in the assessment of severity in the presence of other pathologic lesions. On the other hand, previous studies have demonstrated the clinical utility of the Doppler technique in investigating aortic flow velocity patterns for the quantitative evaluation of the severity of aortic regurgitation.[6-8] However, these investigations were based only on the planimetric analysis of the aortic flow velocity traces, not on the actual measurement of the regurgitant flow volume, so that their results would suffer from several practical problems such as the differences in cross-sectional area between systole and diastole and loss of blood flow to the brain, upper extremities, and coronary arteries.[7]

Recent studies have demonstrated the accuracy and reliability of two-dimensional Doppler echocardiography in measuring aortic and pulmonary flow under normal circulatory conditions[9-11] and even in the presence of intracardiac or extracardiac shunt.[12-15] Because the Doppler technique provides net forward flow volume through the valves, Doppler measurement of the systolic aortic flow in the presence of aortic regurgitation is thought to be the sum of effective forward and

From the First Department of Internal Medicine, Osaka University School of Medicine, Osaka, Japan.

Address for correspondence: Akira Kitabatake, M.D., The First Department of Internal Medicine, Osaka University School of Medicine, 1-1-50 Fukushima, Fukushima-ku, Osaka 553, Japan.

Received Feb. 1, 1985; revision accepted May 2, 1985.

Presented in part at the 57th Scientific Sessions of the American Heart Association.

regurgitant flow, whereas that of the systolic pulmonary flow equals only the effective forward flow.

This study was designed to estimate the aortic regurgitant fraction from the Doppler measurements of systolic aortic and pulmonary flows by assuming that an excess of the aortic flow compared with the pulmonary flow is caused by aortic regurgitant flow. The accuracy and clinical utility of Doppler estimates of regurgitant fraction were examined by comparing them with catheter measurements and cineaortographic grades of regurgitation.

Material and methods

Study population. The study population comprised 20 patients with chronic aortic regurgitation either isolated or in association with other valvular abnormalities (13 male and seven female patients, ages 14 to 75 years, mean 42) who underwent diagnostic cardiac catheterization. Ten normal subjects (eight men and two women, ages 37 to 59 years, mean 49) served as control subjects. All patients met the following criteria: (1) the presence of aortic regurgitation of any origin confirmed by a cineaortogram, (2) left ventriculograms of good quality (the difference in heart rate during cineangiography and Doppler examination was within 10 beats/min), (3) the absence of intracardiac or extracardiac shunt lesions and absence of significant mitral regurgitation (more than 1+ by Sellers classification) and pulmonary regurgitation (regurgitant signal detected more than 1 cm from the pulmonary valve in the right ventricular outflow tract by the Doppler examination), and (4) absence of aortic stenosis (all patients had transvalvular gradients less than 10 mm Hg).

The distribution of valvular diseases was as follows: 10 patients with isolated aortic regurgitation, seven with associated mild mitral regurgitation, one with associated mild mitral and pulmonary regurgitation, one with associated mitral stenosis-insufficiency and pulmonary regurgitation, and one with associated pulmonary and tricuspid regurgitation. The interval between the cardiac catheterization and Doppler examination was within 24 hr in 12 patients, within 1 week in four, within 1 month in two, and within 6 months in two. The clinical status of these patients did not change during the interval.

Apparatus. We used a duplex Doppler echocardiograph (either Hitachi EUB-10B or Toshiba SDS-21A with SSH-40A). Two-dimensional echocardiographic images, M mode echocardiographic tracings, and Doppler-determined flow velocity data were obtained with the same transducer array (2.5 MHz for EUB-10B and 2.4 MHz for SDS-21A). Any cursor line could be interrogated for Doppler recording and simultaneous M mode echocardiography. The Doppler sample volume could be positioned at any depth along the cursor line, which permitted the precise location of the sample volume on the two-dimensional echocardiographic image. The sample volume was a cylinder with a diameter of 3 mm and a length of 2 mm at a depth of 7.5 cm for the EUB-10B and with a diameter of 5 mm and a length of 2 mm at a depth of 10 cm for SDS-21A. In Doppler mode, for the former, the pulse repetition rate was 5.4 kHz for sampling at a depth within 12 cm; for the latter, the pulse repetition rate was 6 kHz for sampling at a depth within 12 cm and 4 kHz for a depth between 12 and 18 cm. In measuring blood flow parallel to the Doppler beam, the maximum detectable velocity within the Nyquist limit is 81 cm/sec for the former, 96 cm/sec within a depth of less than 12 cm, and 64 cm/sec for a depth between 12 and 18 cm for the latter. Doppler signals derived from the structures were minimized by a high-pass filter of 200 Hz. All sampled signals were analyzed in real time by the chirp-Z transform for the EUB-10B and by the fast-Fourier transform for the SDS-21A and were simultaneously displayed at a paper speed of 100 cm/sec on a strip chart recorder along with lead II of the electrocardiogram and phonocardiogram.

A continuous-wave Doppler device was also used in five patients (Sonacolor CD, Carolina Medical Electronics Inc.). Doppler sampling was performed with a 2.5 MHz interrogation frequency. The device allowed the detection of a maximum velocity of 6.0 m/sec. The quadrature Doppler signals were processed by the fast-Fourier transform; a 200 Hz filter was used to minimize the contamination of lower velocities from the cardiac structures. Doppler frequency outputs and simultaneous lead II electrocardiogram were recorded on a video recorder.

Doppler protocol

Measurements in the right ventricular outflow tract. Each patient rested in a supine position and breathed in a relaxed manner during Doppler examination. The transducer was placed in the third intercostal space on the left sternal border and was aimed to depict the long-axis view of the right ventricular outflow tract (figure 1, *A*). When a suitable image was achieved, the Doppler sample volume was positioned at the center of the pulmonary orifice and the ejection flow velocity was recorded. The Doppler incident angle and the orifice diameter were measured from a two-dimensional echocardiographic image gated in midsystole. The Doppler incident angle was measured as an angle of Doppler beam against the long axis of the structure of the outflow tract. In the measurement of the orifice diameter, we asked the patient to rest in a left decubitus position so as to obtain the echocardiogram on which the pulmonary orifice was depicted as parallel to the ultrasound beam as possible (figure 1, *A*) and the orifice diameter was measured as a distance between inner borders.

Measurements in the left ventricular outflow tract. The transducer was placed on the cardiac apex and was aimed medially and superiorly to depict the left ventricular outflow tract on the left anterior oblique equivalent view (figure 1, *B*). The sample volume was positioned at the center of the aortic orifice and ejection flow velocity was recorded. When we encountered frequency aliasing, in which Doppler shift was greater than a half of pulse repetition frequency, we tried to record total Doppler shifts within a pulse repetition frequency by increasing the Doppler incident angle against the flow direction; therefore, the part of waveform exhibiting aliasing was successfully depicted without overlapping with the part of waveform under the baseline (figure 2, *A*). The Doppler incident angle was determined as an angle of Doppler beam against the long axis of the outflow tract on the midsystolic gated frozen image. The aortic orifice was measured as an inner diameter on the midsystolic gated frozen image of the parasternal long-axis view of the left ventricle.

In five patients, left ventricular ejection flow velocity was also measured with a continuous-wave Doppler technique and was compared with that obtained by the pulsed Doppler technique for examining the reliability of measuring the high flow velocity from the ambiguous waveform. The transducer was placed on the cardiac apex and was angulated medially and superiorly until maximum velocity was identified by listening to the audio outputs and by observing the Doppler outputs on the color monitor. The maximum velocity was identified by the highest and most uniform pitch of audio signals.

Analysis of Doppler recordings

Reconstruction of total Doppler waveform from ambiguous spectrum. Although all Doppler shifts of the right ventricular ejection flow were always within the Nyquist frequency, those of the left ventricular ejection flow exceeded the Nyquist frequency in 18 of 20 patients. In these patients, the flow deflection began with directional character, extending inferiorly as a tapering waveform, being cut off at the negative Nyquist frequency with the top of the waveform exhibiting aliasing, and appearing from the positive Nyquist frequency, as if in the opposite direction (figure 2). We obtained the total waveform of the Doppler shifts by taking the higher part and putting it on the flat top of the lower spectrum. The feasibility of this procedure has been theoretically confirmed by Hale et al.[16] and Stevenson et al.[17]

The reliability and accuracy of this procedure was examined by comparing the reconstructed waveform with the paired recording of the unambiguous waveform by the continuous-wave technique in five patients (figures 2 and 3). The shapes of these two waveforms were similar. Figure 3 shows the comparison of peak flow velocities (*A*) and systolic velocity integrals (*B*) between these two waveforms. Good coincidence was observed both in peak velocities and in systolic velocity integrals between the two. These results indicate that we can reliably obtain the total waveform of the Doppler shifts even from the ambiguous waveform by summing positive and negative velocity components. We then applied this procedure in the remaining 13 patients who underwent only pulsed Doppler examination.

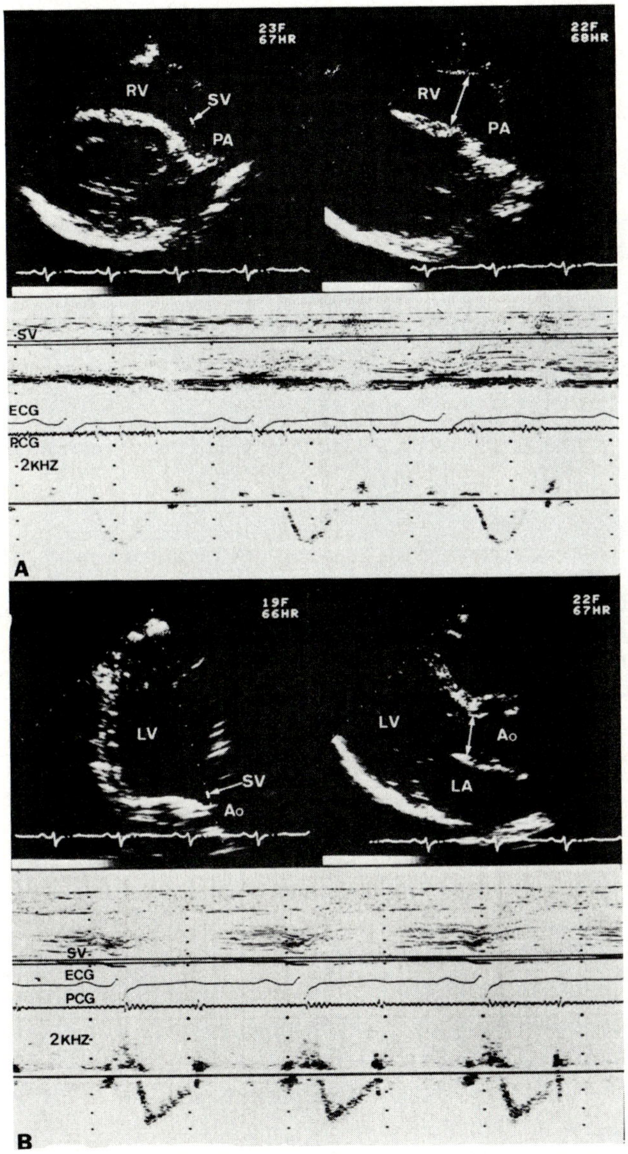

FIGURE 1. Measurements of flow velocity and diameter in the right (*A*) and left (*B*) ventricular outflow tracts in a patient with aortic regurgitation. The Doppler beam and the sample volume are shown as a white cursor line and a white dot on the line, respectively, on the midsystolic gated frozen images (upper left panels of *A* and *B*), from which the Doppler incident angle against the flow vector is determined. The diameter of the pulmonary orifice is axially measured as an interval between inner walls (solid white line in the upper right panel of *A*). The diameter of the aortic orifice is measured from a midsystolic gated frozen image of the parasternal view of the left ventricle. Bottom panels of *A* and *B* are Doppler recordings obtained. Ao = aorta; ECG = lead II electrocardiogram; LV = left ventricle; PA = pulmonary artery; PCG = phonocardiogram; RV = right ventricle; SV = Doppler sample volume.

Doppler estimation of regurgitant fraction. Right and left ventricular stroke volumes (RSV and LSV) were obtained as products of semilunar orifice areas and systolic integrals of angle-corrected flow velocity according to the following equations:

$$R(L)SV = \pi\ (D/2)^2 \times \int_{Es}^{Ee} Vmax(t)dt$$

$$Vmax(t) = fd \times c/(2 \times fo \times \cos\theta)$$

where Es = start of ejection, Ee = end of ejection, D = diameter of the pulmonary or aortic orifice, fd = Doppler shift frequency, fo = carrier frequency, c = sound velocity in biological material (1500 m/sec), θ = Doppler incident angle against the flow direction, and Vmax(t) = instantaneous maximum blood flow velocity.

Systolic velocity integral was obtained as an area under the envelope of the native or reconstructed Doppler spectrum with a digitizer (Cardio 80, Kontron Co., Ltd.). Correction for the Doppler incident angle was performed when the angle was greater than 20 degrees. Both right and left ventricular stroke volumes were obtained as averages of five to seven consecutive cardiac cycles. By regarding the right ventricular stroke volume as an effective forward output and the left as a total forward output, the regurgitant fraction was determined as the ratio of the difference between the left and right ventricular stroke volumes against the left ventricular stroke volume:

$$\text{regurgitant fraction (\%)} = (LSV - RSV)/LSV \times 100.$$

To test the reliability of this method, we randomly selected 10 patients from the 20 and calculated the regurgitant fraction by one observer on two occasions (intraobserver variability). Another observer independently performed the determination for the same 10 patients (interobserver variability). The observers were blinded to each other's results as well as to the results of cardiac catheterization. Mean absolute differences between observations (expressed as a percentage of the first observer's first observation) were 4.5% (intraobserver) and 7.6% (interobserver).

Catheterization. All patients underwent diagnostic right and left heart catheterization, left ventriculography, and cineaortography. Effective forward cardiac output was measured by the thermodilution method before the administration of the contrast materials. Left ventricular volumes were determined from the right anterior oblique projection of the single-plane left ventriculogram by the area-length method. The regurgitant fraction was calculated as the ratio of the difference between angiographic left ventricular output and forward output against the angiographic output. Cineaortographic findings were graded on a 1+ to 4+ scale on the following findings: 1+ = slight

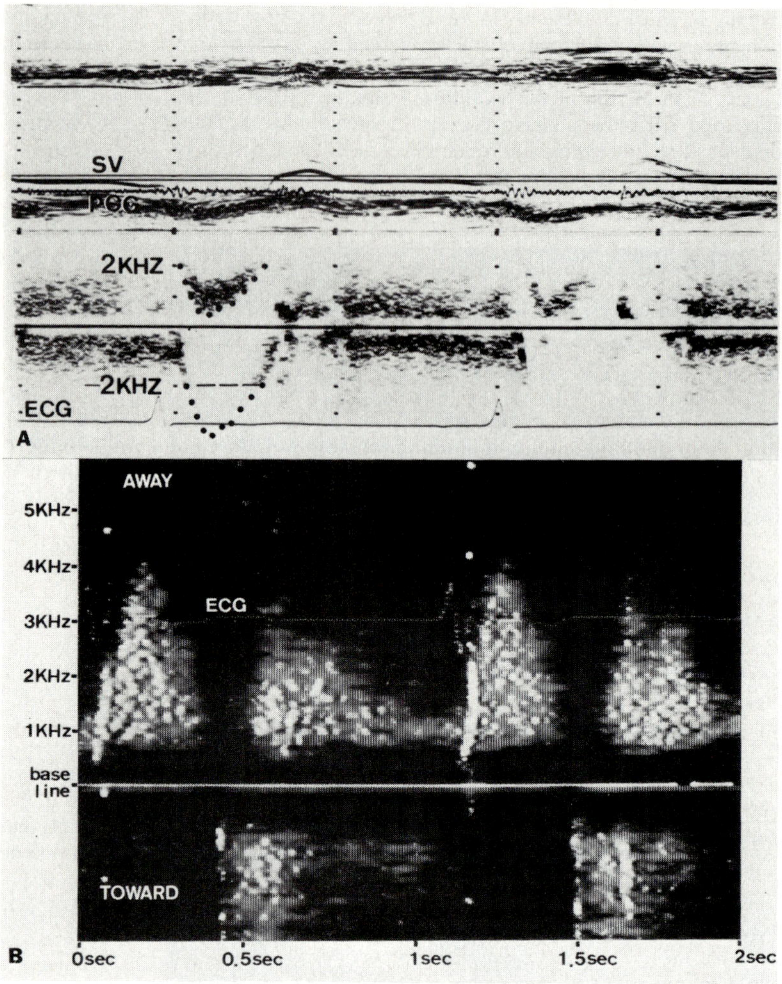

FIGURE 2. Ambiguous Doppler waveform obtained by the pulsed Doppler technique (*A*) and an unambiguous waveform obtained by the continuous-wave Doppler technique (*B*) at the left ventricular outflow tract are shown. Direction of flow deflection by the continuous-wave Doppler technique is depicted in a reverse fashion to that by the pulsed Doppler method. We reconstructed total peak Doppler shifts by taking the higher part and putting it on the flat top of the negative spectrum as shown in *A*. Good resemblance was found between reconstructed and unambiguous waveforms. Abbreviations as in figure 1.

opacification of the left ventricle clearing completely in one cycle, 2+ = moderate opacification of the left ventricle not completely clearing in one cycle but without progressive opacification, 3+ = progressive opacification of the left ventricle over three or more cycles, 4+ = total opacification of the left ventricle within one or two cycles.

Statistical analysis. All results were described as mean ± SD. The Doppler estimate of regurgitant fraction was compared with the cineaortographic grade in the patients with the aortic regurgitation. The significance of the differences found among mean values was assessed with an analysis of variance and Student's t test. The estimates of regurgitant fraction by the Doppler and catheter techniques were compared by linear regression analysis.

Results

Doppler estimates of regurgitant fraction in normal subjects. In 10 normal subjects, the calculated value for the Doppler estimate of regurgitant fraction was 2.4 ± 5.0% and always less than 10%. These data demonstrate that the Doppler estimates of regurgitant fraction approximate zero in normal subjects and the upper limit of the normal range for these Doppler estimates is about 10%.

Comparison with semiquantitative angiography in patients with aortic regurgitation. In the patients with aortic regurgitation, Doppler estimates of regurgitant fraction were significantly greater than those for normal subjects ($p < .01$) and were greater than 10%. The relationship of the semiquantitative cineaortographic grades to the Doppler estimates of regurgitant fraction is shown in figure 4. The Doppler estimate of regurgitant fraction was 28.0 ± 9.2% in two patients with 1+, 32.6 ± 10.0% in four patients with 2+, 53.3 ± 8.6% in 10 patients with 3+, and 62.4 ± 5.5% in four patients with 4+ regurgitation. Even though there was significant overlap among different groups, the regurgitant fraction tended to increase with higher grade of severity ($r = .80$, $p < .01$). The regurgitant fraction for the patients with 3+ and 4+ regurgitation was significantly greater than that for patients with 2+ and 1+ regurgitation ($p < .05$).

Comparison of regurgitant fractions measured by Doppler and catheter techniques. Doppler estimates of regurgitant fraction were compared with those obtained by left ventriculography and the thermodilution method (figure 5). On the whole, a fair correlation was found

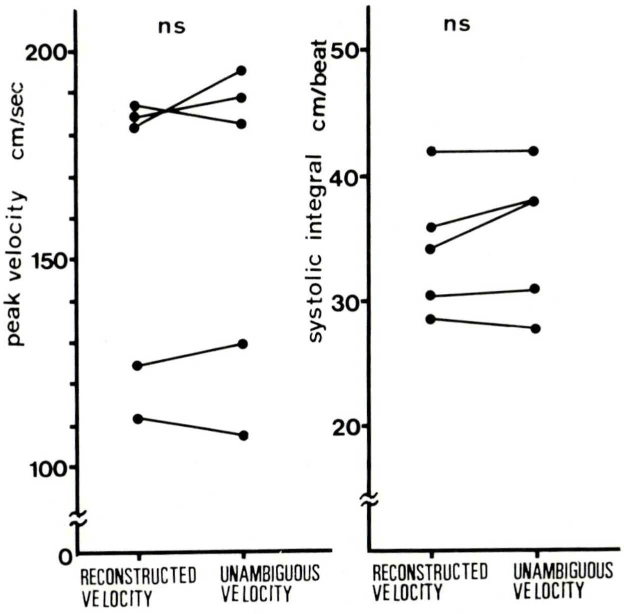

FIGURE 3. Comparison of peak flow velocity (*left*) and systolic velocity integrals (*right*) of the reconstructed and unambiguous Doppler waveforms. Good coincidence was observed both in peak velocities and in systolic velocity integrals between these two waveforms.

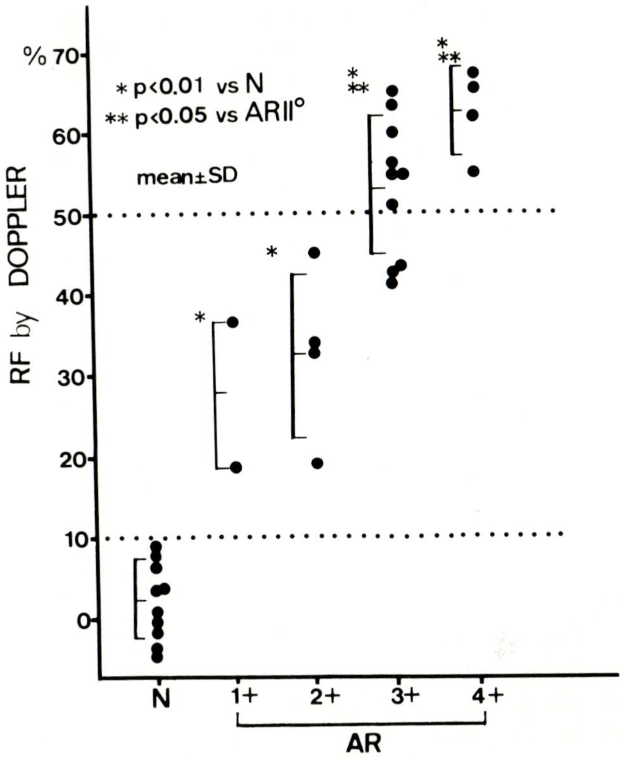

FIGURE 4. Comparison of Doppler estimates of regurgitant fraction (RF) with cineaortographic grades. In normal subjects, the Doppler-determined regurgitant fraction approximated zero, whereas the values for the patients with aortic regurgitation (AR) were significantly greater than those for normal subjects (N). Although there was variation in the values for the regurgitant fraction within each group, the regurgitant fraction increased with higher grade of the severity ($r = .80$, $p < .01$).

between these two variables with a correlation coefficient of .94 ($p < .01$; $y = 1.0x + 4.1$). If the patients with associated mitral regurgitation were excluded, a close correlation was demonstrated between these two measurements ($r = .96$, $p < .01$; $y = 1.0x - 0.08$) and a good coincidence was found between the two variables especially in the higher range. On the other hand, although the correlation was significant, catheter measurements of the regurgitant fraction in the patients with associated mild mitral regurgitation tended to substantially overestimate the Doppler estimates ($r = .93$, $p < .01$; $y = 0.84x + 15.5$). The differences between Doppler- and catheter-determined regurgitant fractions would reflect the contribution of the mitral regurgitant flow, which cannot be differentiated from aortic regurgitant flow by a conventional catheter method.

Discussion

The unique feature of this study was that the aortic regurgitant fraction was determined noninvasively from the Doppler measurements of the aortic and pulmonary flows by assuming that an excess of the aortic flow compared with pulmonary flow is caused by the regurgitant flow in the presence of aortic regurgitation. Our results indicate that this quantitative Doppler method provides a specific and accurate estimation of the aortic regurgitant fraction.

In measuring flow velocity by a pulsed Doppler

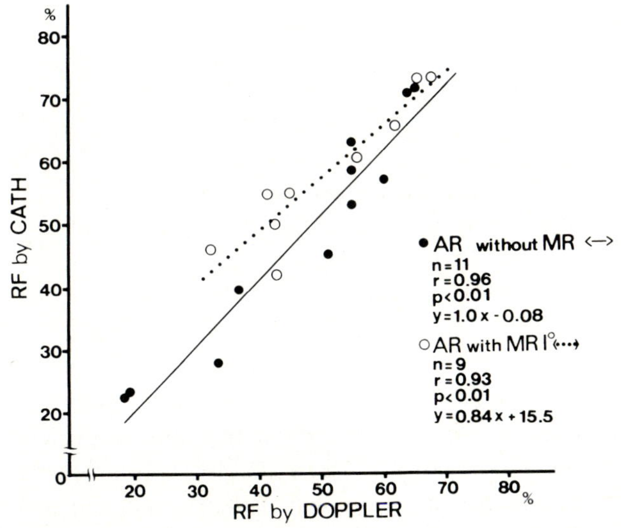

FIGURE 5. Doppler estimates of regurgitant fraction (RF) plotted against those obtained by catheter technique. A fair correlation was found between the two variables with a correlation coefficient of .94. A close correlation was found between the two variables in the patients without mitral regurgitation (MR) ($r = .96$, $p < .01$; $y = 1.0x - 0.08$). On the other hand, in the patients with associated mild mitral regurgitation, catheter measurements substantially overestimated the regurgitant fraction compared with Doppler estimates ($r = .93$, $p < .01$; $y = 0.84x + 15.5$). AR = aortic regurgitation.

technique, the frequency aliasing has been thought to be one of the factors that might obscure the accurate recognition of the total flow velocity pattern and it was recommended that the Doppler shifts be recorded within the Nyquist limit. In this study, however, we could not record the left ventricular ejection flow velocity within the Nyquist limit in 18 of 20 patients with aortic regurgitation. When the transmitted frequency is fixed, maximal detectable velocity within the Nyquist frequency is proportional to the pulse repetition frequency, which is inversely proportional to the sampling depth because of the finite transit time of the pulsed signal. In the patients with aortic regurgitation, Doppler recordings of the left ventricular ejection flow velocity often suffer from the frequency aliasing phenomenon because of the augmented flow velocity due to the increase in total forward output and because of the deep location of the sample volume due to the dilated left ventricle. Even when the frequency aliasing was observed, we could successfully obtain the total Doppler wave form by summing the positive and negative velocity components, as Hatle et al.[16] and Stevenson et al.[17] suggested. This procedure can be reliably performed only when the flow deflection is directional and the continuity of the envelope of the positive and negative waveform is easily recognizable. In this study, we examined the reliability of this reconstruction procedure by comparing the reconstructed total waveform of the left ventricular ejection flow velocity with the corresponding unambiguous waveform by the continuous-wave technique in five patients with aortic regurgitation. Good coincidence was found both in peak velocities and in systolic velocity integrals between these two waveforms. These results indicate that we can determine the total waveform of the Doppler shift even from the ambiguous waveform with high reliability. When a Doppler device with an electronic zero shifter is available, this reconstruction process is performed automatically.

In the patients with isolated aortic regurgitation, a close correlation was found between Doppler- and catheter-determined regurgitant fractions. Especially in the higher range of regurgitant fraction, Doppler estimates agreed closely with catheter measurements. These results indicate that our proposed Doppler method allows the accurate quantitation of regurgitant fraction in the patients with mild-to-severe aortic regurgitation. However, in the patients with associated mild mitral regurgitation, catheter measurements of regurgitant fraction substantially overestimated those determined by Doppler method. Hunt et al.[18] demonstrated that any conventional catheter procedure cannot separately quantify the amount of mitral regurgitant flow from that of aortic regurgitant flow, since both aortic and mitral regurgitation contributed to the regurgitant flow, which is obtained as the difference between angiographic output and that by the thermodilution method. In the present Doppler method, the aortic regurgitant flow was estimated as the difference between Doppler measurements of the aortic and pulmonary flows, so that it would not be affected by the presence of associated mitral regurgitation. Thus the proposed Doppler technique provides a novel and specific means of estimating the aortic regurgitant fraction regardless of the presence of associated mitral regurgitation. The differences between Doppler- and catheter-determined regurgitant fractions in the patients with associated mitral regurgitation would reflect the extent of the contribution of mitral regurgitation to the total regurgitant fraction by the catheter method.

The Doppler estimates of regurgitant fraction for normal subjects never exceeded 10%, which seemed to be the upper limit of the normal range, whereas those for the patients with aortic regurgitation were significantly greater than those for the normal subjects. In comparison with cineangiographic grades, although the Doppler estimates of regurgitant fraction increased progressively with increasing degrees of aortic regurgitation, some overlapping occurred in the range of those values in each cineaortographic grade of regurgitation. The Doppler estimates of regurgitant fraction for the patients with 3+ and 4+ regurgitation were significantly greater than those for the patients with 2+ and 1+, whereas no significant difference was found between those values for patients with 1+ and 2+ nor for patients with 3+ and 4+ regurgitation. The cineaortographic grading is semiquantitative and dependent on the visual inspection, so that it may be influenced not only by the amount of regurgitation but also by other factors, such as the size and the contractile function of the left ventricle and the presence or absence of mitral regurgitation.[18–20] Even if the amount of regurgitation were the same, the low contractile state of the left ventricle and concomitant mitral regurgitation might lead to the long persistence of regurgitated contrast material in the chamber, which would lead to the overestimation in the severity of the cineaortographic grade.

Limitations. Outflow obstructions, intracardiac or extracardiac shunts, and pulmonary regurgitation limit the use of this pulsed Doppler method. Extreme high velocity and associated flow disturbances caused by stenotic lesion introduce difficulties in the recognition of true velocity deflection by a pulsed Doppler technique. A continuous-wave Doppler technique may have the potential to overcome this limitation. Pulmonary regurgitation is also thought to modify the Doppler estimates of regurgitant fraction according to the severity of regurgitation, since Doppler measurement of pulmonary flow is not effective but total forward flow through the pulmonary valve. The results of our previous study demonstrated that the mild pulmonary regurgitation, in which the regurgitant flow signals are detected within 1 cm from the pulmonary valve in the right ventricular outflow tract, did not cause a significant error in the quantitation of the pulmonary to systemic flow ratio in the patients with atrial septal defects.[15] In this study, three of 20 patients had mild pulmonary regurgitation revealed by the additional Doppler examination, in whom significant discrepancy was not found between Doppler- and catheter-determined regurgitant fractions. Intracardiac or extracardiac shunts also limit the use of this technique, since a shunt lesion itself causes the unequal Doppler measurements of pulmonary and aortic flow. Thus the presence or absence of shunt lesions should be evaluated with additional and careful Doppler and echocardiographic examinations before the application of this proposed Doppler technique.

Conclusion. Our proposed Doppler method provides the accurate estimation of regurgitant fraction in patients with aortic regurgitation. This technique is noninvasive and can be performed repeatedly without deleterious effects, so that it may be promising in the initial screening examination, the assessment of serial changes in hemodynamics, and the evaluation of the response to drugs and surgical interventions.

We are deeply indebted to Drs. Kenji Ohnishi and Yoshio Kobayashi of the Osaka Prefectural Hospital for allowing their patients to enter in this study. We are grateful to Dr. Michihiko Tada for his critical review of this manuscript, to Drs. Hiroshi Abe and Masato Asao for their helpful comments and to Ms. Reiko Matsuo for her assistance in preparing the manuscript.

References

1. Brubakk AO, Angelsen BAJ, Hatle J: Diagnosis of valvular heart disease using transcutaneous Doppler ultrasound. Cardiovasc Res **11:** 461, 1977
2. Quinones MA, Young JB, Waggoner AD, Ostojic MC, Ribeiro LGT, Miller RR: Assessment of pulsed Doppler echocardiography in detection and quanification of aortic and mitral regurgitation. Br Heart J **44:** 612, 1980
3. Esper RJ: Detection of mild aortic regurgitation by range-gated pulsed Doppler echocardiography. Am J Cardiol **50:** 1037, 1982
4. Ciobanu M, Abbasi AS, Allen M, Hermer A, Spellberg R: Pulsed Doppler echocardiography in the diagnosis and estimation of severity of aortic insufficiency. Am J Cardiol **49:** 339, 1982
5. Veyrat C, Lessana A, Abitol G, Ameur A, Benaim R, Kalmanson D: New indexes for assessing aortic regurgitation with two-dimensional Doppler echocardiographic measurement of the regurgitant aortic valve area. Circulation **68:** 998, 1983
6. Boughner DR: Assessment of aortic insufficiency by transcutaneous Doppler ultrasound. Circulation **52:** 874, 1975
7. Hatteland K, SEmb BKH: Assessment of aortic regurgitation by means of Doppler ultrasound. Ultrasound Med Biol **8:** 1, 1982
8. Pernneau BDP, Blanchard D, Colonna G, Guermonprez JL, Forman J, Seller P, Maurice P: Non-invasive quantification of aortic regurgitation by Doppler echocardiography. Br Heart J **49:** 167, 1983
9. Magnin PA, Stewart JA, Myers S, Ramm O, Kisslo JA: Combined Doppler and phased-array echocardiographic estimation of cardiac output. Circulation **60:** 388, 1981
10. Gisvold SE, Brubakk AO: Measurement of instantaneous blood flow velocity in the human aorta using pulsed Doppler ultrasound. Cardiovasc Res **16:** 26, 1982
11. Goldberg SJ, Sahn DJ, Allen HD, Valdes-Cruz LM, Hoenecke H, Carnahan Y: Evaluation of pulmonary and systemic blood flow by 2-dimensional Doppler echocardiography using fast Fourier transform spectral analysis. Am J Cardiol **50:** 1394, 1982
12. Sanders SP, Yeager S, Williams RG: Measurement of systemic and pulmonary blood flow and Qp/Qs ratio using Doppler and two-dimensional echocardiography. Am J Cardiol **51:** 952, 1983
13. Barron JV, Sahn DJ, Valdes-Cruz LM, Lima CO, Goldberg SJ, Grenadier E, Allen HD: Clinical utility of two-dimensional Doppler echocardiographic techniques for estimating pulmonary to systemic blood flow ratios in children with left to right shunting atrial septal defect, ventricular septal defect or patent ductus arteriosus. J Am Coll Cardiol **3:** 169, 1984
14. Valdes-Cruz LM, Horowitz S, Mesel E, Sahn DJ, Fisher DC, Larson D: A pulsed Doppler echocardiographic method for calculating pulmonary and systemic blood flow in atrial level shunts: validation in animals and initial human experience. Circulation **69:** 80, 1984
15. Kitabatake A, Inoue M, Asao M, Ito H, Masuyama T, Tanouchi J, Morita T, Hori M, Yoshima H, Ohnishi K, Abe H: Noninvasive evaluation of the ratio of pulmonary to systemic flow in atrial septal defect by duplex Doppler echocardiography. Circulation **69:** 73, 1984
16. Hatle L, Angelsen B: Clinical significance of velocity ambiguity in PW mode. *In* Hatle L, Angelsen B, editors: Doppler ultrasound in cardiology. Philadelphia, 1982, Lea & Febiger, ch 3.6, pp 51–57
17. Stevenson J, Kawabori K: Noninvasive evaluation of pulmonary stenosis by high repetition frequency pulse Doppler technique. Am J Cardiol **52:** 352, 1984
18. Hunt D, Baxley WA, Kennedy JW, Judge TP, Williams JE, Dodge HT: Quantitative evaluation of cineaortography in the assessment of aortic regurgitation. Am J Cardiol **31:** 696, 1973
19. Cohn LH, Mason DT, Ross J Jr, Morrow AS, Braunwald E: Preoperative assessment of aortic regurgitation in patients with mitral valve disease. Am J Cardiol **19:** 177, 1967
20. Mennel RG, Joyner CR Jr, Thompson PD, Pyle RR, MacVaugh H III: The preoperative and operative assessment of aortic regurgitation. Am J Cardiol **29:** 360, 1972

Influence of intimal dissection on restenosis after successful coronary angioplasty

PIERRE P. LEIMGRUBER, M.D.,* GARY S. ROUBIN, M.B., PH.D., H. VERNON ANDERSON, M.D., CLAYTON E. BREDLAU, M.D., HALL B. WHITWORTH, M.D., JOHN S. DOUGLAS, JR., M.D., SPENCER B. KING III, M.D., AND ANDREAS R. GREUNTZIG, M.D.

ABSTRACT We studied 986 patients who underwent follow-up angiography after successful percutaneous transluminal coronary angioplasty (PTCA) to determine the influence of uncomplicated intimal dissection on restenosis rate. Angiographic evidence of intimal dissection after PTCA was present in 248 patients or 25%. After a mean follow-up time of 7 ± 5 months (SD) the restenosis rate in patients without intimal dissection was 30% compared with 24% in patients with intimal dissection ($p = .08$). Patients with available transstenotic pressure gradients were divided according to the hemodynamic result into two subgroups: those with final gradients at the conclusion of PTCA of 15 mm Hg or less ($n = 638$) and those with gradients greater than 15 mm Hg ($n = 244$). Patients with intimal dissection had a significantly lower restenosis rate than patients without intimal dissection if the final gradient was 15 mm Hg or less (19% vs 28%; $p < .05$). If the final gradient was greater than 15 mm Hg, the presence or absence of intimal dissection had no significant influence on restenosis rate, which was 35% and 39%, respectively ($p =$ NS). We conclude that an uncomplicated intimal dissection after a successful coronary angioplasty has no adverse influence on angiographic restenosis. An excellent angiographic long-term outcome can be expected if the intimal dissection is associated with a favorable hemodynamic result.
Circulation 72, No. 3, 530–535, 1985.

PERCUTANEOUS transluminal coronary angioplasty (PTCA) is now an accepted revascularization procedure in the treatment of selected patients with coronary artery disease. The increase in vessel lumen is brought about partially by compression of soft atheromatous material.[1, 2] However, stretching of the arterial wall and disruption of intima and media are thought to be the most important contributors in increasing the arterial lumen.[3–6] This process is recognized arteriographically as an intimal tear or intimal dissection. During the healing process, arteriographic irregularities usually regress[7, 8] and either improvement (figure 1) or deterioration in luminal narrowing can occur.

The precise relationship between intimal dissection and restenosis after coronary angioplasty, however, is unclear.[4, 9] Some investigators have suggested that intimal dissection promotes restenosis,[4, 10] while others have indicated that it is a benign arteriographic finding.[7] Still others associate intimal dissection with an improved long-term outcome.[11]

The purpose of this study was to define the hemodynamic importance of an intimal dissection after uncomplicated, successful PTCA and its relationship to arteriographic restenosis.

From Emory University School of Medicine, Atlanta.

Dr. Roubin is a National Heart Foundation of Australia Overseas Research Scholar.

Address for correspondence: Andreas R. Greuntzig, M.D., Interventional Cardiovascular Medicine, Emory University Hospital, 1364 Clifton Rd., Atlanta, GA 30322.

Received April 2, 1985; revision accepted June 13, 1985.

Presented in part at the 57th Scientific Sessions of the American Heart Association, Miami Beach, 1984.

*Present address: Deaconess Medical Bldg., Spokane, WA 99204.

Methods

Patients. Between July 1980 and January 1984, 1880 patients underwent first, single-vessel PTCA to native coronary arteries. According to a combination of angiographic (>20% reduction in diameter stenosis)[12] and clinical criteria (no electrocardiographic or enzymatic evidence of myocardial infarction, no need for emergency bypass surgery, and no in-hospital death), the procedure was successful in 1650 patients (88%). Of these, the 986 patients (60%) who had angiographic follow-up form the study population. All patients underwent PTCA in accordance with a standard protocol that has been previously described.[13] Clinical and angiographic data were prospectively recorded on standard data collection sheets and stored in a relational data base by means of a VAX-750 computer.

Coronary intimal dissection was defined according to the NHLBI PTCA Registry by (1) the presence of angiographically evident intimal damage producing an intraluminal filling defect, (2) extraluminal extravasation of contrast material, (3) linear luminal density or luminal staining.[14] Evidence of intimal dis-

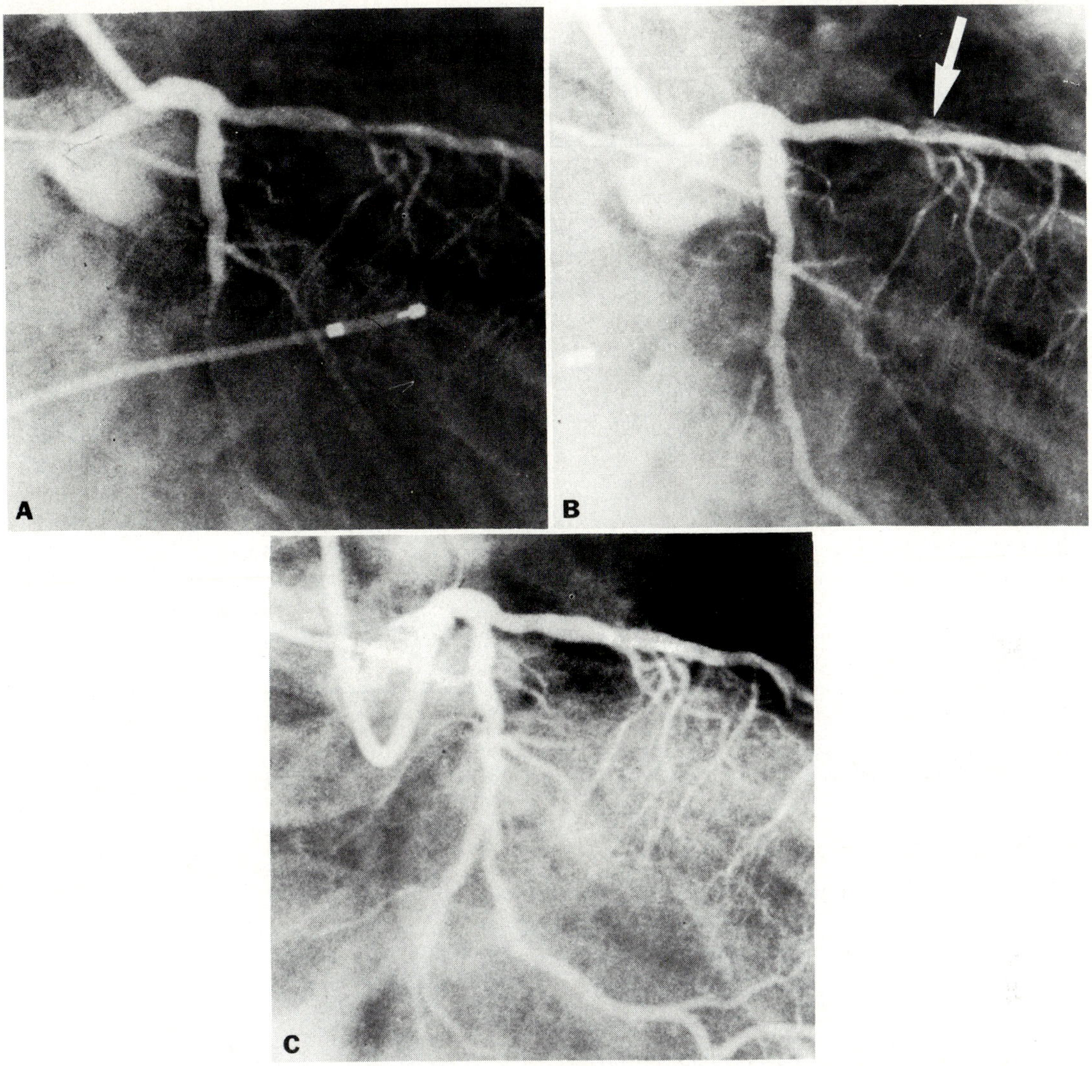

FIGURE 1. Angiogram of the left coronary artery in the right anterior oblique projection before PTCA of a subtotally occluded circumflex coronary artery (Cx) and of a moderately stenosed proximal anterior descending coronary artery (LAD) (*A*). The Cx shows an excellent result and the LAD demonstrates an intimal dissection (arrow) immediately after PTCA (*B*). Both arteries are widely patent 6 months after PTCA and the intimal dissection has healed (*C*).

section was present in 248 patients (25%). The prevalence of dissection in patients without available follow-up angiograms was not significantly different, 190 of 664 patients (29%). The degree of arterial obstruction was measured in percent diameter with a digital electronic caliper. This method has been previously validated.[15] An individual stenosis was expressed as the mean of the stenoses measured in at least two different orthogonal projections.

A transstenotic pressure gradient was defined as the difference in mean arterial pressure between the tip of the guiding catheter proximal to the stenosis and the tip of the balloon catheter distal to the stenosis undergoing PTCA. Because of technical difficulties in obtaining satisfactory measurements, pressure gradients were not available in all patients (table 1). Follow-up angiograms were available at a mean of 7 ± 5 months (SD). Restenosis was defined as a loss of 50% or more of the initial gain in luminal diameter achieved at PTCA.[1,6] Long-term gain was defined as the difference between the stenosis before angioplasty and residual stenosis at the time of follow-up angiography.

Patients with intimal dissection were not routinely treated with a prolonged heparin infusion. Discharge medications, which included aspirin and a calcium antagonist, were also similar in patients with dissection as compared with patients without dissection.

Statistical analysis. Statistical analysis was performed with the SPSS-X Program with the chi-square test to assess differences in categorical variables. A one-way analysis of variance was used to assess differences in continuous variables between groups.

In a subset of 882 patients with available transstenotic pressure gradient at the conclusion of PTCA (final gradient), a stepwise linear discriminant analysis was performed to determine the independent influence of uncomplicated intimal dissection and final gradient on restenosis.[17] P values less than .05 were considered statistically significant.

Results

Patient characteristics and intimal dissection (table 1). Intimal dissection was identified in 248 patients, or 25% of the study population. The dissection group

TABLE 1
Patient characteristics

	No intimal dissection (n = 738)	Intimal dissection (n = 248)	p value
Male	596 (81%)	177 (71%)	<.01
Female	142 (19%)	71 (29%)	<.01
Age (yr ± SD)	54.4±9.6	53.5±10	NS
New-onset angina (≤ 2 mo)[A]	247/657 (33%)	78/221 (35%)	NS
History of previous MI	193 (26%)	63 (25%)	NS
History of diabetes mellitus	63 (9%)	26 (10%)	NS
PTCA–vessel			
LM	2 (0.3%)	1 (0.4%)	NS
LAD	439 (59.5%)	142 (57.3%)	NS
RCA	203 (27.5%)	61 (24.6%)	NS
LCx	94 (12.7%)	44 (17.7%)	NS
Mean % stenosis (± SD)			
Pre-PTCA	74±12	74±12	NS
Post-PTCA	25±12	24±11	NS
Transstenotic gradient (mm Hg ± SD)[B]			
Pre-PTCA	50±14 (n = 695)	53±13 (n = 220)	<.05
Post-PTCA	12±7 (n = 666)	14±8 (n = 216)	<.001
Time of follow-up angiogram (mo ± SD)	7±5	7±4	NS

[A]Of 878 patients with typical angina.
[B]When available.
MI = myocardial infarction; LM = left main; LAD = left anterior descending; RCA = right coronary artery; LCx = left circumflex.

contained more women than the group without dissection (29% vs 19%; p < .01). Other clinical characteristics were similar; there were no significant differences in age, presence of new-onset angina, and history of myocardial infarction or diabetes mellitus. The distribution of coronary vessels dilated and the mean diameter stenosis before and after PTCA were also not significantly different. Transstenotic pressure gradients both before and after dilatation were slightly higher in the group with intimal dissection.

Restenosis rate and intimal dissection. The overall restenosis rate in the study population was 29%. Restenosis rate in the group with intimal dissection was lower (24%) than that in the group with no dissection (30%), but the difference did not reach statistical significance (p = .08; figure 2).

Mean percent stenosis (±SD) at follow-up in patients with dissection, however, was lower than that in the group with no dissection (34 ± 23% vs 38 ± 23%; p = .01). Conversely, the long-term gain in lumen diameter was greater (40 ± 25% vs 35 ± 26%, p = .01) in the group with dissection (figure 3).

Intimal dissection and transstenotic pressure gradient. Patients with intimal dissection had slightly higher transstenotic pressure gradients both before and after PTCA (table 1). Stepwise discriminant analysis revealed that the final gradient and the presence of intimal dissection were both strongly and independently

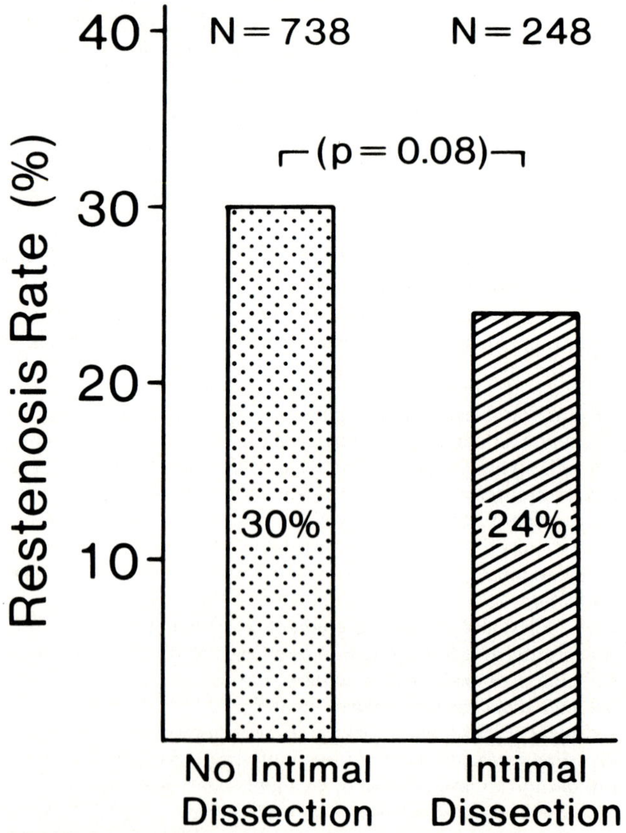

FIGURE 2. Angiographic restenosis rate of 738 patients without intimal dissection and 248 patients with evidence of intimal dissection after successful PTCA. There was a trend towards a lower restenosis rate in the group with intimal dissection.

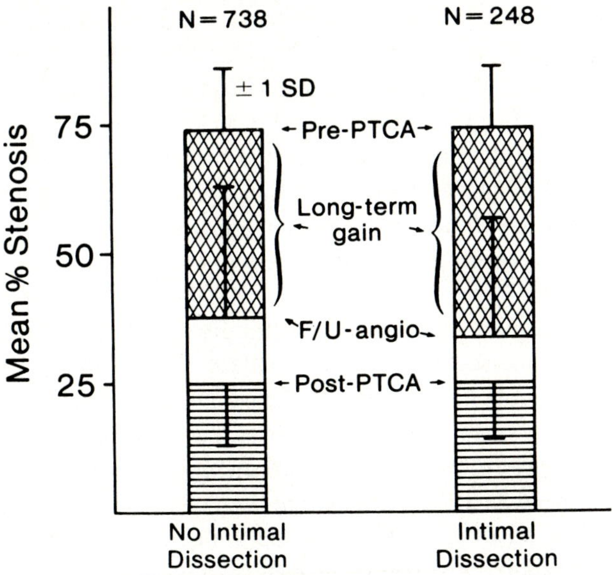

FIGURE 3. Mean percent stenosis (±SD) in patients without intimal dissection and in patients with intimal dissection before angioplasty (pre-PTCA), immediately after angioplasty (post-PTCA), and at the time of follow-up angiography (F/U-angio). The long-term gain was 35 ± 26% in patients without intimal dissection and 40 ± 25% in patients with intimal dissection (p = .01).

related to restenosis. Final gradient appeared to be most significant (table 2).

To determine a final gradient that would best predict restenosis, we analyzed the restenosis rate in subgroups with final gradients 5 or less vs greater than 5 mm Hg, 10 or less vs greater than 10 mm Hg, 15 or less vs greater than 15 mm Hg, 20 or less vs greater than 20 mm Hg, and 25 or less vs greater than 25 mm Hg. There was a significant relationship to restenosis when a final gradient of less or greater than 10, 15, and 20 mm Hg was used. The relationship was strongest ($p < .001$) when restenosis rate was analyzed in patients with final gradients of 15 or less vs greater than 15 mm Hg. We therefore examined the influence of intimal dissection on restenosis rate in the two subgroups: those with final gradients of 15 mm Hg or less (n = 638) and those with final gradients greater than 15 mm Hg (n = 244; figure 4).

In the subgroup with final gradients of 15 mm Hg or less the group with intimal dissection had a slightly higher mean final gradient (±SD) than the group without intimal dissection (9 ± 4 vs 8 ± 4 mm Hg; $p < .05$). In the subgroup with final gradients greater than 15 mm Hg the mean final gradient was 21 ± 5 mm Hg in patients without intimal dissection, which was not significantly different from 22 ± 7 mm Hg in the intimal dissection group.

Patients with intimal dissection had a significantly lower restenosis rate than patients without intimal dissections when the final gradient was 15 mm Hg or less (19% vs 28%; $p < .05$). If, on the other hand, the final gradient was greater than 15 mm Hg, the restenosis rate was not significantly different whether an intimal dissection was present or absent (35% vs 39%; p = NS). The restenosis rate of all patients with final gradients of 15 mm Hg or less was 26% and significantly lower than the restenosis rate of patients with final gradients greater than 15 mm Hg (38%; $p < .001$).

TABLE 2

Multivariate discriminant analysis of final gradient and intimal dissection as predictors of restenosis

	Canonical discriminant function coefficient	p value	Low restenosis rate
Final gradient	0.1228	.0007	Low gradient after PTCA
Intimal dissection	−1.2549	.0104	Presence of intimal dissection
	Constant 0.06546		

Discussion

Intimal disruption, seen as vascular irregularities on the immediate postangioplasty arteriogram, have been reported to be present in up to 70% of arteries dilated.[18] Although most patients with this finding have an uneventful hospital course, intimal dissection represents a risk factor for major complications.[14] The NHLBI PTCA Registry reported major complications in 30%

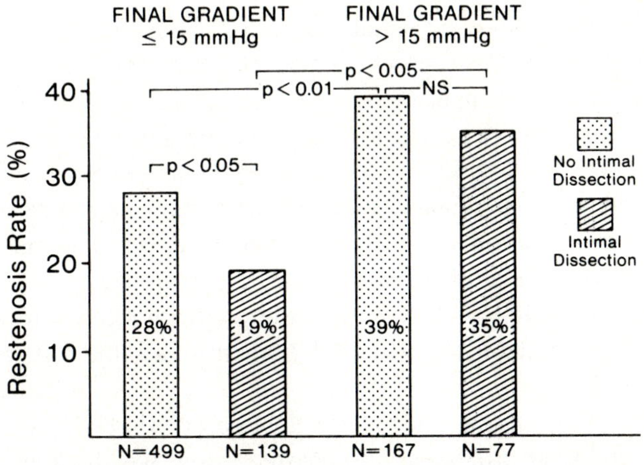

FIGURE 4. Restenosis rate in subgroups of patients with post-PTCA (final) transstenotic pressure gradient of 15 mm Hg or less or greater than 15 mm Hg. Patients with intimal dissection had a signficantly lower restenosis rate than patients without intimal dissection in the subgroup with final gradients of 15 mm Hg or less. Intimal dissection had no significant influence on restenosis rate when the final gradient was greater than 15 mm Hg.

of patients with intimal tears or dissections when compared with an overall complication rate of 9.4%.[14] It must be emphasized therefore that data presented in this study refer only to patients with an angiographically and clinically successful PTCA. Patients with intimal dissection leading to major complications (myocardial infarction, bypass graft surgery, or death) are not included.

Concern has been expressed that an intimal dissection during PTCA may contribute to accelerated restenosis.[4, 10, 19] In this study we found no increase in restenosis rate and, in fact, observed an overall trend toward a lower restenosis rate in patients with intimal dissection.

Our results further demonstrate the importance of considering the final gradient when evaluating the significance of an intimal dissection. Similarly, transstenotic pressure gradients have been correlated with improved thallium perfusion abnormalities and coronary vasodilatory flow reserve after PTCA, emphasizing its clinical usefulness.[20, 21]

The mechanism of PTCA in improving blood flow was originally thought to represent compression and compaction of soft atheromatous material.[1, 2, 22] Increasing evidence from experimental and human studies suggests that luminal enlargement of stenosed arteries may also be related to splitting of intima and media and stretching of adventitial tissues.[3, 5, 6, 9, 23–26] The favorable long-term results seen in our patients with intimal dissection further corroborate these findings. The intimal dissection described in our study is probably anatomically and angiographically different from the classic intramural dissection that occurs within the media and results in a propagating intramural hematoma and subsequent occlusion of the artery.[26] This process appears to occur unpredictably in a small proportion of patients having angiographic evidence of intimal dissection.[6, 14, 27] A low final gradient associated with an intimal dissection may therefore indicate that the intramural hematoma is small and of no hemodynamic significance. This would explain the low restenosis rate of 19% in the subgroup with intimal dissection and associated final gradient of 15 mm Hg or less.

There was a significantly higher proportion of women in our group with intimal dissection, which agrees with the NHLBI PTCA Registry findings.[14] The higher incidence of coronary dissection and intimal tear in women may be related to differences in plaque composition, structural characteristics of the vessel wall, and differences in vessel size.[28] Although women have smaller coronary vessels than men,[29] the same balloon size (3 mm diameter) tended to be used most commonly in both men and women. It is possible that the higher balloon/artery ratio in women induced a higher incidence of intimal dissection. Because a larger balloon size may favorably influence the recurrence rate after PTCA,[30] one is tempted to conclude that the higher incidence of intimal dissection produced by larger balloons may explain the lower restenosis rate reported in women.[28]

Although there was no angiographic evidence of intimal dissection in 75% of patients in this study, we cannot conclude that PTCA did not produce small fractures of plaque and intima. It is therefore likely that some patients had small intimal disruptions not evident on the post-PTCA angiogram. Conclusions from this study must therefore be limited to patients having angiographic evidence of intimal disruptions.

The accuracy of luminal diameter measurements after PTCA, especially if the vascular wall is irregular because of intimal dissection, has been questioned.[21] To minimize this problem, we averaged the stenosis from at least two orthogonal projections. This is important because the definition of restenosis used in this study is based on luminal gain achieved immediately after PTCA. Given this limitation, however, we believe that taking the mean of stenosis measurements in several projections represents the best currently available technique for assessing the anatomic severity of coronary artery stenosis in most patients.[31]

The accurate measurements of transstenotic pressure gradients with a balloon catheter have also been questioned.[32] Because of the relatively large cross-sectional area of the deflated balloon, the gradients could be artifactually increased. Even the smallest catheter across a stenosis will interfere with blood flow and the true gradient may be difficult to measure. A large final gradient after an otherwise successful PTCA may therefore be artifactually elevated. In the absence of significant collateral flow, however, a small final gradient (<15 mm Hg) measured with a balloon catheter should indicate that the true gradient across the residual stenosis is less than 15 mm Hg. These problems notwithstanding, the strong relationship between final gradient and restenosis mentioned earlier emphasizes the clinical usefulness of transstenotic pressure measurements.

Our study population represents only 60% of all patients with successful PTCA (n = 1650) and therefore these results cannot be used to determine overall restenosis rate. However, the restudy rate of all patients with successful PTCA and evident intimal dissection was 57% (248/438), and not significantly different than that of patients without intimal dissection (61%, 738/1112; p = NS). Because patients who are symptomatic are more likely to have a repeat angiogram, the overall restenosis rate could be expected to be lower than we found in this population.[16]

It is possible that heparinization for 12 to 18 hr after PTCA, used more commonly in patients with intimal dissection, may have had an influence on restenosis. The effect of short-term heparinization after PTCA on restenosis, however, is not known and should be determined in a controlled study. Further studies will also be required to define ways to control vessel injury during PTCA, optimizing initial results while keeping short-term complications low and improving long-term success.

In summary, patients with intimal dissection who have an uncomplicated post-PTCA course did not have an increased risk of restenosis. The presence of an intimal dissection appeared to have a beneficial effect on restenosis rate if the final transstenotic pressure gradient was favorable.

We thank Johnny Tate and George Cotsonis for computer programming and statistical assistance. We also thank Linda Greene, Allyson Bakewell, Diana Nelson, Claire Rice, and Eileen Ball for technical assistance and Diana Williams for typing the manuscript.

References

1. Gruentzig A, Hopff H: Perkutane Rekanalisation chronischer arterieller Verschluesse mit einem neuen Dilatationskatheter. Dtsch Med Wochenschr **99:** 2502, 1974
2. Dotter CT, Judkins MP: Transluminal treatment of arteriosclerotic obstruction: description of a new technic and a preliminary report of its application. Circulation **30:** 654, 1964
3. Castaneda-Zuniga WR, Formanek A, Tadavarthy M, Vlodaver Z, Edwards JE, Zollikofer C, Amplatz K: The mechanism of balloon angioplasty. Radiology **135:** 565, 1980
4. Cowley MJ, Vetrovec GW, Wolfgang TC: Efficacy of percutaneous transluminal coronary angioplasty: technique, patient selection, salutary results, limitations and complications. Am Heart J **101:** 272, 1981
5. Block PC, Baughman KL, Pasternak RC, Fallon JT: Transluminal angioplasty: correlation of morphologic and angiographic findings in an experimental model. Circulation **61:** 778, 1980
6. Block PC, Myler RK, Stertzer S, Fallon JT: Morphology after transluminal angioplasty in human beings. N Engl J Med **305:** 382, 1981
7. Dorros G, Spring DA: Healing of coronary artery intimal dissection after percutaneous transluminal angioplasty. Am J Cardiol **45:** 423, 1980 (abst)
8. Zarins CK, Lu CT, Gewertz BL, Lyon RT, Rush DS, Glagov S: Arterial disruption and remodeling following balloon dilatation. Surgery **92:** 1086, 1982
9. Holmes DR, Vlietstra RE, Mock MB, Reeder GS, Smith HC, Bove AA, Bresnahan JF, Piehler JM, Schaff HV, Orszulak TA: Angiographic changes produced by percutaneous transluminal coronary angioplasty. Am J Cardiol **51:** 676, 1983
10. Essed CE, Van den Brand M, Becker AE: Transluminal coronary angioplasty and early restenosis: fibrocellular occlusion after wall laceration. Br Heart J **49:** 393, 1983
11. David PR, Renkin J, Moise A, Dangoisse V, Val PG, Bourassa MG: Can patient selection and optimization of technique reduce the rate of restenosis after percutaneous transluminal coronary angioplasty? J Am Coll Cardiol **3:** 470, 1984 (abst)
12. Gruentzig AR, Senning A, Siegenthaler WE: Nonoperative dilatation of coronary-artery stenosis: percutaneous transluminal coronary angioplasty. N Engl J Med **301:** 61, 1979
13. Gruentzig AR: Technique of percutaneous transluminal coronary angioplasty. *In* Hurst JW, editor: The heart. New York, 1982, McGraw-Hill Book Co., Inc., p 1904
14. Cowley MJ, Dorros G, Kelsey SF, Van Raden M, Detre KM: Acute coronary events associated with percutaneous transluminal coronary angioplasty. Am J Cardiol **53:** 12C, 1984
15. Scoblionko DP, Brown BG, Mitten S, Caldwell JH, Kennedy JW, Bolson EL, Dodge HT: A new digital electronic caliper for measurement of coronary arterial stenosis: comparison with visual estimates and computer-assisted measurements. Am J Cardiol **53:** 689, 1984
16. Thornton MA, Gruentzig AR, Hollman J, King SB, Douglas JS: Coumadin and aspirin in prevention of recurrence after transluminal coronary angioplasty: a randomized study. Circulation **69:** 721, 1984
17. Lachenbruch PA: Discriminant analysis. New York, 1975, Hafner Press
18. Roth FJ, Cappius G, Fingerhut E: Radiological pattern at and after angioplasty. *In* Dotter CT, Gruentzig A, Schoop W, Zeitler E, editors: Percutaneous transluminal angioplasty. Berlin, 1983, Springer Verlag, p 73
19. Waller BF: Early and late morphologic changes in human coronary arteries after percutaneous transluminal coronary angioplasty. Clin Cardiol **6:** 363, 1983
20. Wijns W, Serruys PW, Reiber JHC, Van den Brand M, Simoons ML, Kooijmans CJ, Balakumaran K, Hugenholtz PG: Quantitative angiography of the left anterior descending coronary artery: correlations with pressure gradient and results of exercise thallium scintigraphy. Circulation **71:** 273, 1985
21. O'Neill WW, Walton JA, Bates ER, Colfer HT, Aueron FM, LeFree MT, Pitt B, Vogel RA: Criteria for successful angioplasty as assessed by alterations in coronary vasodilatory reserve. J Am Coll Cardiol **3:** 1382, 1984
22. Leu HJ: Percutaneous transluminal angioplasty: mechanism and morphology: The morphological concept of percutaneous transluminal angioplasty. *In* Dotter CT, Gruentzig A, Schoop W, Zeitler E, editors: Percutaneous transluminal angioplasty. Berlin, 1983, Springer Verlag, p 46
23. Block PC: Percutaneous transluminal coronary angioplasty. Am J Radiol **135:** 955, 1980
24. Hoffman MA, Fallon JT, Greenfield AJ, Waltman AC, Athanasoulis CA, Block PC: Arterial pathology after percutaneous transluminal angioplasty. Am J Radiol **137:** 147, 1981
25. Castaneda-Zuniga WR, Tadavarthy SM, Laerum F, Amplatz K: "Pseudo" intramural injection following percutaneous transluminal angioplasty. Cardiovasc Intervent Radiol **7:** 104, 1984
26. Kinney TB, Chin AK, Rurik GW, Finn JC, Shoor PM, Hayden WG, Fogarty TJ: Transluminal angioplasty: a mechanical-pathophysiological correlation of its physical mechanisms. Radiology **153:** 85, 1984
27. Wood WG: Transluminal coronary angioplasty. N Engl J Med **306:** 1055,1982
28. Cowley MJ, Mullin SM, Kelsey SF, Kent KM, Gruentzig AR, Detre KM, Passamani ER: Sex differences in early and long-term results of coronary angioplasty in the NHLBI PTCA Registry. Circulation **71:** 90, 1985
29. Roberts CS, Roberts WC: Cross-sectional area of the proximal portions of the three major epicardial coronary arteries in 98 necropsy patients with different coronary events: relationship to heart weight, age and sex. Circulation **62:** 953, 1980
30. Schmitz HJ, von Essen R, Meyer J, Effert S: The role of balloon size for acute and late angiographic results in coronary angioplasty. Circulation **70**(suppl II): II-295, 1984 (abst)
31. Meier B, Gruentzig AR, Goebel N, Pyle R, von Gosslar W, Schlumpf M: Assessment of stenoses in coronary angioplasty: inter- and intraobserver variability. Int J Cardiol **3:** 159, 1983
32. Feldman RC, Anderson DJ: Gradients at PTCA: physiological or artifactual? J Am Coll Cardiol **5:** 525, 1985 (abst)

Improvement in symptoms and exercise tolerance by metoprolol in patients with dilated cardiomyopathy: a double-blind, randomized, placebo-controlled trial

RICHARD S. ENGELMEIER, M.D., JOHN B. O'CONNELL, M.D., RONALD WALSH, D.O., NANCY RAD, R.N., PATRICK J. SCANLON, M.D., AND ROLF M. GUNNAR, M.D.

ABSTRACT It has been suspected that the increased sympathetic activity seen in patients with chronic congestive heart failure from dilated cardiomyopathy may be harmful. We therefore tested the long-term effect of metoprolol on eight patients in a double-blind, randomized protocol and 12 patients in an unblinded, crossover protocol who were treated for 12 months (range 10 to 24), and compared them with 16 similar subjects who were treated with placebo for 10 months (range 6 to 12) in a double-blind, randomized protocol. Patients were followed by serial clinical assessment, treadmill testing, radionuclide ventriculography, and echocardiography. Metoprolol-treated patients had an improvement in mean exercise capacity by 3 mets ($p < .0001$) while experiencing a significant improvement in functional classification ($p < .001$) during both the double-blind and open-label crossover studies and had an improved ejection fraction during the double-blind study ($p < .02$). These improvements were not seen in matched control subjects receiving placebo. Seven of 20 patients receiving long-term metoprolol therapy had resolution of nearly all symptoms of heart failure, doubled their exercise capacity, and had progressive improvement in resting radionuclide left ventricular ejection fraction ($12.6 \pm 3\%$ to $26.9 \pm 6\%$) and echocardiographic left ventricular end-diastolic dimension (7.7 ± 0.5 to 6.5 ± 0.5 cm). Only one of 21 patients treated was intolerant of metoprolol. We conclude that metoprolol can be given safely to a select group of patients with dilated cardiomyopathy in doses that substantially reduce both resting and exercise heart rates. Long-term β-blockade improved functional class and exercise capacity in 14 of 20 patients while producing an exceptional clinical response in seven that was accompanied by improved resting parameters of left ventricular function.
Circulation 72, No. 3, 536–546, 1985.

DILATED CARDIOMYOPATHY is a disease of heart muscle characterized by left ventricular dilatation and congestive heart failure.[1] It affects a younger population than does ischemic heart disease and frequently results in functional impairment and premature death. The reflex neurohumoral responses that accompany the syndrome of congestive heart failure are useful in maintaining short-term compensation of cardiac function.[2,3] Norepinephrine is released from sympathetic nerve endings to activate myocardial β-receptors that increase both the heart rate and force of ventricular contraction.[4] Stimulation of α-receptors results in peripheral vasoconstriction to help maintain critical end-organ perfusion.[5] With time these compensatory mechanisms fail to prevent clinical deterioration and may actually contribute to the progressive downward course that characterizes this disease.[3] Although elevated plasma norepinephrine levels may be only an indirect indicator of generalized sympathetic activation in patients with dilated cardiomyopathy, a direct correlation exists between these levels and the severity of heart failure as well as prognosis.[6,7] Therapy directed at reducing these humoral alterations may be beneficial in altering the natural history of dilated cardiomyopathy. This was suggested by Waagstein et al.[8,31] and Swedberg et al.,[9,10] who demonstrated improved symptoms, left ventricular function, and survival in uncontrolled trials of long-term β-blockade in patients with dilated cardiomyopathy. Recent placebo-controlled studies have not confirmed the Swedish experience but differed in that heterogenous populations and only 4 week treatment periods were used.[11,12]

This trial was designed to evaluate the effect of

From the Department of Medicine, Section of Cardiology, Loyola University Medical Center, Maywood, IL.

Address for correspondence: Richard S. Engelmeier, M.D., Section of Cardiology, Loyola University Medical Center, Room 0001, 2160 S. First Ave., Maywood, IL 60153.

Received Jan. 11, 1985; revision accepted May 23, 1985.

Presented in part at the 57th Annual Scientific Sessions of the American Heart Association, Miami Beach, November 1984.

long-term sympathetic β-blockade with metoprolol on symptoms, exercise tolerance, and noninvasive indexes of left ventricular function in prospective, double-blind, placebo-controlled, and crossover studies of dilated cardiomyopathy. Our results confirm the safety and efficacy of metoprolol when given to patients with symptoms of dilated cardiomyopathy receiving conventional medical therapy.

Materials and methods

Patient selection. Consecutive patients referred to our institution from October 1981 through September 1983 and diagnosed as having idiopathic dilated cardiomyopathy by criteria established by the WHO/ISFC[13] task force on dilated cardiomyopathy were considered for the study. Symptomatic but not rapidly deteriorating patients with radiographic cardiomegaly (cardiothoracic ratio >0.5), radionuclide left ventricular impairment (ejection fraction <.49), or echocardiographic evidence of left ventricular enlargement and dysfunction were considered. Thirty-one patients were referred but four were not enrolled: two had postpartum cardiomyopathy, one had refractory ventricular tachycardia as the primary diagnosis, and the final patient lived too far from Chicago, making follow-up impossible. Twenty-seven were enrolled but two improved spontaneously during the 6 week observation period and were rejected. Therefore 25 patients underwent randomization. All were clinically stable but remained symptomatic despite the use of digoxin and furosemide in 24 and of vasodilators in 10. Cardiac catheterization and coronary angiography were performed in all patients over 35 years of age or in the presence of atherosclerotic risk factors. Endomyocardial biopsy was done in all patients with a clinical history compatible with myocarditis or recently acquired symptoms of heart failure. Coronary artery disease was excluded in all 24 patients studied and myocarditis was excluded in all 22 patients who underwent biopsy. Electrocardiography, chest radiography, radionuclide ventriculography, multistage treadmill testing, M mode echocardiography, and 24 hr ambulatory electrocardiography were performed before enrollment into the study. Those patients with histories of active alcoholism, obstructive lung disease, and advanced atrioventricular block were excluded from the study. After informed consent was obtained, patients were randomly assigned to receive placebo or metoprolol in blinded fashion for 1 year. After 1 year, or earlier if clinical deterioration requiring hospitalization occurred, the code was broken and both groups were to cross over to the other treatment in a single-blind study. Interruption of metoprolol therapy precipitated a marked worsening of heart failure symptoms and ventricular tachyarrhythmias in the first two patients to cross over, and all subsequent metoprolol-treated patients were continued uninterrupted on the drug. Hence, the crossover group consisted of patients initially assigned to receive placebo who either remained stable for 1 year or deteriorated early and were then treated with metoprolol. All three groups were similar in baseline demographic, clinical, hemodynamic, and noninvasive parameters (table 1).

Study design

Double-blind, randomized study. Written informed consent was obtained from each patient before enrollment. After a 6 week stabilization and observation period, all patients were randomly assigned to receive placebo or metoprolol in a double-blind fashion. Patients were started on 6.25 mg (one-quarter tablet) once daily and then were given 6.25 to 12.5 mg increments of placebo or metoprolol (Lopressor 25 mg tablets, kindly supplied by Ciba-Geigy, Summit, NJ) that were increased once or twice weekly over 4 to 6 weeks. They were evaluated before each dose increase and then observed for bradycardia, hypotension, or clinical decompensation for 2 hr after administration of the drug. The therapeutic end point was 100 mg. Patients received less than 100 mg if their systolic blood pressure was less than 90 mm Hg or if their resting heart rate was less than 60 beats/min.

During drug maintenance, patients were reevaluated every 3 months. The NYHA guidelines were used for functional classification, which was aided by a questionnaire filled out at each visit that requested information regarding the patient's ability to perform routine daily activities.[14] Compliance was ensured by careful questioning and tablet counts. Serial noninvasive testing included left ventricular radionuclide ejection fraction and echocardiographic left ventricular end-diastolic determinations every 3 months, and maximal oxygen consumption estimated by multistage exercise treadmill testing (met score) every 6 months. Clinically stable patients were to remain blinded to the medication for 1 year. All practical attempts were made to prevent biasing of follow-up studies, which could be affected by knowledge of heart rate responses during titration of the study drug. These efforts included having treadmill tests, radionuclide ventriculography, and echocardiography supervised and interpreted as data were generated by blinded physicians not associated with the study. Functional classification and management decisions were usually made by a blinded study physician who did not participate in the drug titration.

Crossover study. The second part of the trial was a crossover study designed to evaluate the effects of metoprolol on the symptoms, exercise tolerance, and noninvasive parameters of left ventricular function of patients initially assigned to receive placebo. During this phase, neither the patients nor investigators were blinded. Metoprolol was administered and patients were serially investigated as previously described. Treadmill

TABLE 1

Baseline clinical and hemodynamic features of patients in placebo and metoprolol groups[A]

	Placebo (n = 16)	Metoprolol (n = 9)	Placebo to metoprolol crossover (n = 12)
Age (yr)	49.1 ± 11	51.2 ± 8.2	47.4 ± 8.1
Sex, n (%) male	9 (56)	7 (78)	4 (40)
Symptomatic period (mo)	26 ± 24	21 ± 32	24.9 ± 27
Functional class (NYHA)	2.4 ± 0.8	2.4 ± 0.9	2.5 ± 0.6
Systolic blood pressure (mm Hg)	121 ± 22	120 ± 18	118 ± 23
Pulse (beats/min)	92 ± 12	92 ± 15	93 ± 15
Cardiothoracic ratio by x-ray >0.5, n (%)	15 (94)	9 (100)	9 (90)
Cardiac index (l/min/m²)	2.3 ± 0.4	2.2 ± 0.6	2.4 ± 0.4
Pulmonary capillary wedge (mm Hg)	16.7 ± 11	14.3 ± 6.9	16.1 ± 12
RNV EF (%)	18.6 ± 11	15.8 ± 9.2	18 ± 12
LVEDD (cm)	6.9 ± 1.1	7.2 ± 0.8	6.7 ± 0.8
Exercise tolerance (met score)	6.6 ± 2.8	4.4 ± 2.2	5.4 ± 2.4

LVEDD = left ventricular end-diastolic dimension; met score = metabolic equivalent utilization units from multistage treadmill testing; RNV EF = radionuclide left ventricular ejection fraction.

[A]p = NS in all categories.

tests, radionuclide ventriculograms, and echocardiograms were interpreted as data were generated by blinded physicians not associated with the study. Twelve patients have been followed for 12 months on metoprolol (range 10 to 24 months) after crossing over from placebo and comprise the crossover group. Four patients did not cross over from placebo: two died, one improved significantly, and the other experienced normalization of ejection fraction, although his other clinical, treadmill, and noninvasive parameters did not change.

This study was approved by the Institutional Review Board for the Protection of Human Subjects of Loyola University Medical Center.

Noninvasive and treadmill testing. Radionuclide ventricular ejection fraction was obtained by the electrocardiogram-gated equilibrium method[15]; 25 mCi of 99m-technetium-labeled red blood cells were used after labeling in vivo. Imaging was performed in multiple views by an Anger scintillation gamma camera and collected at 20 frames/cycle. Left ventricular ejection fraction was calculated from a MDS A-3 computer–derived, background-corrected time-activity curve, using the left anterior oblique projection. An arrhythmia filtration technique was used in the two patients with atrial fibrillation and in 18 patients with repetitive ventricular arrhythmias (Lown grade 4). A wide individual variability in ejection fraction was attributed to the high frequency of arrhythmias in all groups. A significant change in ejection fraction was therefore defined as a progressive increase or decrease terminating at least seven percentage points above or below the pretreatment control value.

Echocardiographic left ventricular end-diastolic dimension was determined on a commercially available ATL recorder and a 2.25 MHz transducer. Measurements were obtained at end-diastole on the R wave of the electrocardiogram-derived QRS complex, just below the mitral leaflets, by means of the standard left parasternal or subcostal windows.[16] Transducer position was aided by cross-sectional echocardiographic analysis. Good-quality echocardiograms were obtained in 24 of 25 patients. Less individual variability was observed in left ventricular end-diastolic dimension than in ejection fraction. A significant change was defined as a progressive increase or decrease in left ventricular end-diastolic dimension, terminating at least 0.5 cm above or below the pretreatment control value. All calculations of left ventricular end-diastolic dimension were made as data were generated by a blinded cardiologist not associated with the study.

Maximal oxygen consumption (met score) was estimated with patients in the postabsorptive state by multistage exercise testing carried out according to a standard Naughton or Bruce protocol.[17, 18] The procedure was selected by a cardiologist blinded to the treatment group after a preliminary assessment of the patient's exercise capability. Both exercise protocols used 3 min stages and continuous three-channel electrocardiographic monitoring. Blood pressure was obtained after 2 min of each stage. Patients exercised to exhaustion and usually terminated exercise because of leg symptoms, fatigue, or dyspnea. No test was terminated for chest pain, heart rate criteria, ST segment abnormalities, or exercise-induced hypotension. One patient had exercise terminated before exhaustion because of nonsustained ventricular tachycardia that occurred before and after metoprolol was started. Exercise-induced arrhythmias were common but no patient experienced morbidity or mortality as a result of the exercise test. Because two exercise protocols of differing grades and speeds were used, duration of exercise was converted to metabolic energy utilization units (met score) based on a nomogram described by Fox et al.,[19] enabling comparison of exercise capacity for both protocols. A change in met score greater than 2 was considered significant, which was based on our experience with patients with dilated cardiomyopathy who performed both treadmill protocols as part of an independent study.

Statistical analysis. Comparison of change in NYHA functional class from the pretreatment control to serial evaluations was made by Friedman's two-way analysis of variance. Comparison of change in met score, ejection fraction, and left ventricular end-diastolic dimension from pretreatment control to serial investigations was made by analysis of variance for multiple observations. Comparison of percent change was made by Student's t test for unpaired variables. Heart rate response to exercise at the last follow-up on metoprolol compared with the pretreatment control value was evaluated for significance by covariance. Stepwise discriminant analysis was performed on data from all metoprolol-treated patients to analyze parameters predictive of a favorable response to the drug. Results are expressed as mean ± SD unless otherwise specified; $p < .05$ rejected the null hypothesis.

Results

Double-blind, randomized study

Changes in clinical status and functional class with placebo. Sixteen patients were randomly assigned to receive placebo. Ten clinically stable patients remained blinded for 12 months while another crossed over at 6 months after no improvement on the blinded protocol at the request of the referring physician. Four deteriorating patients were hospitalized for progressive heart failure at 6 months, with one of the four succumbing to refractory congestive heart failure. The three survivors were stabilized on intravenous diuretic therapy. The final patient died suddenly at 3 months. The clinically stable patients had no changes in medications.

Functional classification was assessed quarterly. The mean NYHA functional class did not change significantly during the first 6 months or at the last follow-up of patients on placebo when compared with the pretreatment control. The minor improvement at 9 months reflects the drop-out of the deteriorating patients. Thirteen individuals had the same or worse functional class at all follow-up intervals. Three had minor amelioration of symptoms that represented less than one full class improvement (table 2, figure 1).

Serial treadmill tests and noninvasive studies with placebo. Thirteen patients had at least one and eight had two follow-up treadmill tests while on placebo. Reasons for failure of a 6 month study included one death, one case of severe incapacitation from progressive heart failure, and one refusal. Five additional patients did not have a 12 months study because of one death, three cases of deterioration and removal from placebo, and one refusal. There was no significant difference in mean met score at the 6 month and last follow-up interval when compared with the pretreatment control value. Two individuals showed improvement in met score at 6 and 12 months. One of these experienced

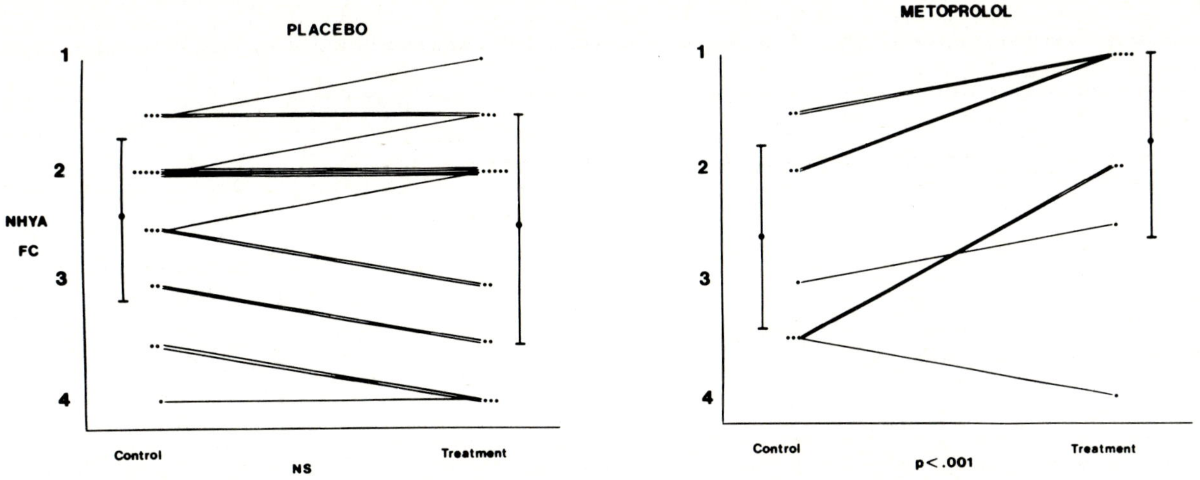

FIGURE 1. Individual and mean changes in functional classification (NYHA FC) in placebo and metoprolol groups, comparing baseline (Control) with completion of the blinded trial (Treatment).

normalization of her mildly abnormal ejection fraction and left ventricular end-diastolic dimension, while the other probably benefited from a self-motivated conditioning regimen undertaken without change in noninvasive parameters of left ventricular function. Four individuals had decreases in met score at the 6 month study that persisted in the two undergoing a 12 month study. Seven individuals had no change noted at 6 months as well as four individuals at 12 months (table 2, figure 2).

Mean ejection fraction and left ventricular end-diastolic dimension did not change significantly at the quarterly evaluations of patients on placebo when compared with the pretreatment control values. Only one patient had an improvement in both parameters (ejection fraction 32% to 56%, left ventricular end-diastolic dimension 5.7 to 4.8 cm), which accompanied improved symptoms and met score. Another patient had an improvement in ejection fraction (23% to 53%) that was not accompanied by change in symptoms, exercise capacity, or left ventricular end-diastolic dimension. Three patients had echocardiographic progression of left ventricular enlargement: one died, one had decompensation from heart failure, and the third was stable (table 2, figures 3 and 4).

Changes in clinical status and functional class with metoprolol. Nine patients were randomly assigned to metoprolol therapy. One with atrial fibrillation acquired a slow ventricular response during low-dose titration and was removed from the study within 4 weeks. Because he lacked follow-up studies, he was not evaluated with the metoprolol treatment group. Therefore only patients tolerant of 100 mg of metoprolol or whose heart rates were limited to less than 60 beats/min or systolic blood pressures to less than 90 mm Hg by β-blockade are considered in the subsequent discussion. Eight patients tolerated an average metoprolol dose of 92 mg (range 63 to 100). Seven clinically stable patients re-

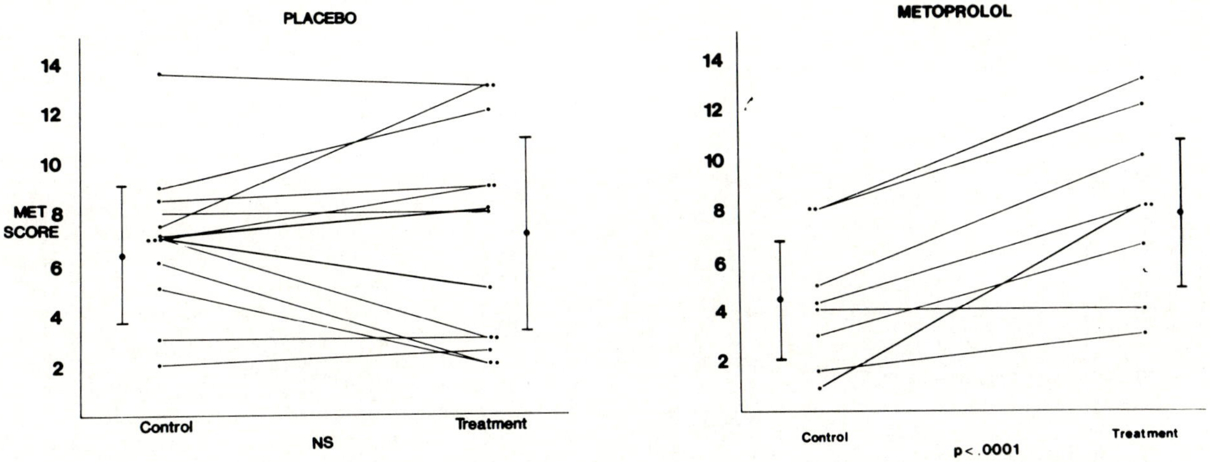

FIGURE 2. Individual and mean changes in exercise capacity (met score) in placebo and metoprolol groups, comparing baseline (Control) with completion of the blinded trial (Treatment).

TABLE 2

Serial changes in mean functional class, treadmill results, and noninvasive studies with placebo and metoprolol: double-blind, randomized study

	Placebo					Metoprolol	
	Control	3 mo	6 mo	9 mo	Last F/U[A]	Control	3 mo
NYHA FC	2.40±0.7 (16)	2.34±0.7 (16)	2.43±0.9 (14)	2.1±0.9 (13)	2.47±1 (16)	2.56±0.8 (8)	1.9±0.6[D] (8)
Exercise tolerance (met score)	6.9±2.7 (13)		6.3±3.9 (13)		6.9±4 (13)	4.4±2.3 (8)	
RNV EF (%)	18.2±10 (16)	19.6±9 (16)	21.6±11 (12)	21.6±13 (8)	21.9±14 (16)	13.1±6 (8)	18.2±5[E] (8)
LVEDD (cm)	6.7±0.9 (15)	6.9±1 (14)	7.2±1.2 (14)	7.0±1.4 (8)	6.9±1.1 (15)	7.3±0.6 (8)	7.2±0.6 (7)

Results are expressed as mean ± SD, with number of tests averaged in parentheses.

LVEDD = echocardiographic left ventricular end-diastolic diameter; met score = maximal oxygen consumption estimated by treadmill test; NYHA FC = New York Heart Association functional classification; RNV EF = radionuclide left ventricular ejection fraction.

[A]Last follow-up on placebo: 10 ± 3 months.

[B]Last follow-up on metoprolol: 12 ± 0.7 months.

Comparing serial investigations to pretreatment control: [C]$p < .0001$; [D]$p < .001$; [E]$p < .02$.

mained blinded to the medication for 12 months, and the final patient was unblinded after 7 months because of progressive heart failure. Diuretic dosage was increased but he continued to deteriorate and required hospitalization, where metoprolol was discontinued. He died 2 weeks later from refractory heart failure. No other metoprolol-treated patient received additional medication during the blinded period.

Mean functional class was assessed quarterly. By 3 months the mean was significantly improved and continued to improve in subsequent evaluations when compared with the pretreatment control ($p < .001$). Four individuals had a full class improvement by 3 months, with three of four showing sustained improvement for the subsequent 9 months. The fourth patient had decompensation at 6 months, requiring hospitalization for congestive heart failure at 9 months and died 2 weeks later while off metoprolol. One patient improved one full class at 9 months, and the remaining three patients had less than one full class improvement (table 2, figure 1).

Serial treadmill tests and noninvasive studies with metoprolol. All eight patients had 6 month treadmill tests and all seven survivors had 12 month treadmill tests. Mean met score improved significantly at 6 months (4.4 to 7.4 mets; $p < .0001$) and at 12 months (8.4 mets; $p < .0001$) in the seven survivors when compared with the pretreatment control values. The last follow-up mean result in all eight patients likewise was significantly improved (7.9 mets; $p < .0001$). Six individuals improved with three of them doubling their exercise capacity by 6 months, which was sustained through 12

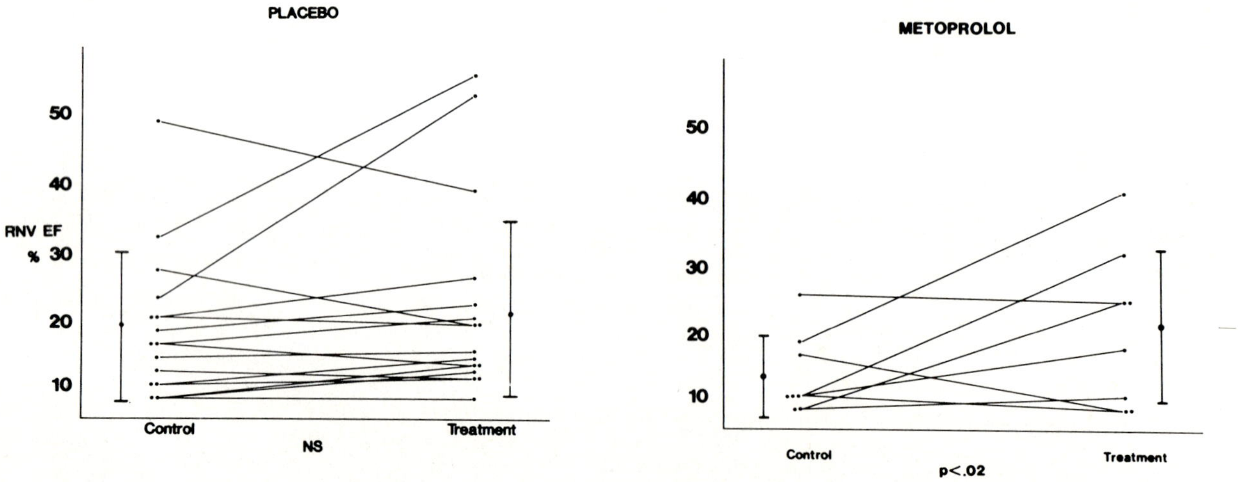

FIGURE 3. Individual and mean changes in radionuclide left ventricular ejection fraction (RNV EF) in placebo and metoprolol groups, comparing baseline (Control) with completion of the blinded trial (Treatment).

TABLE 2
(Continued)

Metoprolol			
6 mo	9 mo	12 mo	Last F/U[B]
1.88 ± 0.8^D (8)	1.81 ± 0.8^D (8)	1.50 ± 0.6^D (7)	1.75 ± 0.9^D (8)
7.4 ± 3.3^C (8)		8.4 ± 3^C (7)	7.9 ± 2.9^C (8)
20.5 ± 8^E (7)	21 ± 10^E (8)	20.7 ± 10^E (7)	19.1 ± 10^E (8)
7.1 ± 0.5 (8)	7.1 ± 0.6 (8)	6.8 ± 0.6 (6)	6.9 ± 0.5 (8)

months. Of the two who did not by definition improve, one had increased exercise capacity from 1.6 to 3 mets and the other had no change at 6 months and ultimately died from progressive heart failure (table 2, figure 2).

The mean ejection fraction improved by 3 months and was sustained at all subsequent follow-up intervals when compared with the pretreatment control value ($p < .02$). Mean left ventricular end-diastolic dimension did not change significantly with metoprolol from the pretreatment control value. Three patients had progressive, simultaneous improvements in ejection fraction (12.4% to 29 ± 7%) and left ventricular end-diastolic dimension (7.7 ± 0.6 to 6.6 ± 0.7 cm) while returning to functional class I and II and doubling their exercise capacity over the 12 month blinded period. One patient who died had progressive deterioration of ejection fraction beginning at 3 months, and another stable patient had progressive enlargement of left ventricular end-diastolic dimension. Two other patients had no changes (table 2, figures 3 and 4).

Changes in mean functional class, met score, and results of noninvasive studies. Percent change in mean NYHA functional class, met score, ejection fraction, and left ventricular end-diastolic dimension at the last follow-up compared with the pretreatment control values was evaluated in the placebo and metoprolol groups. The percent change in functional class and met score was significantly better ($p < .001$) in the metoprolol group, whereas the percent change in ejection fraction and left ventricular end-diastolic dimension favored neither group (figure 5).

Crossover trial (table 3)

Changes in clinical status and functional class with placebo and metoprolol. Twelve patients randomly assigned to receive placebo crossed over and received open-label metoprolol. Eight clinically stable patients remained blinded on placebo for 1 year, and one crossed over at 6 months at the request of the referring physician because she showed no improvement on the blinded drug. Three patients experienced acute decompensation from congestive heart failure while on placebo, requiring hospitalization, and were stabilized on intravenous diuretics. All 12 patients were stable and have been followed for at least 10 months on metoprolol (range 10 to 24 months). One was hospitalized for syncope and newly diagnosed diabetes mellitus, and another died at 15 months from metabolic acidosis and respiratory failure of unknown cause. Diuretic dosages were increased in one patient, and vasodilator and digitalis therapy was discontinued in two patients receiving metoprolol.

Mean functional classification did not change in patients on placebo at quarterly evaluations but did improve at 3 months in patients on metoprolol; this improvement was sustained through the last follow-up

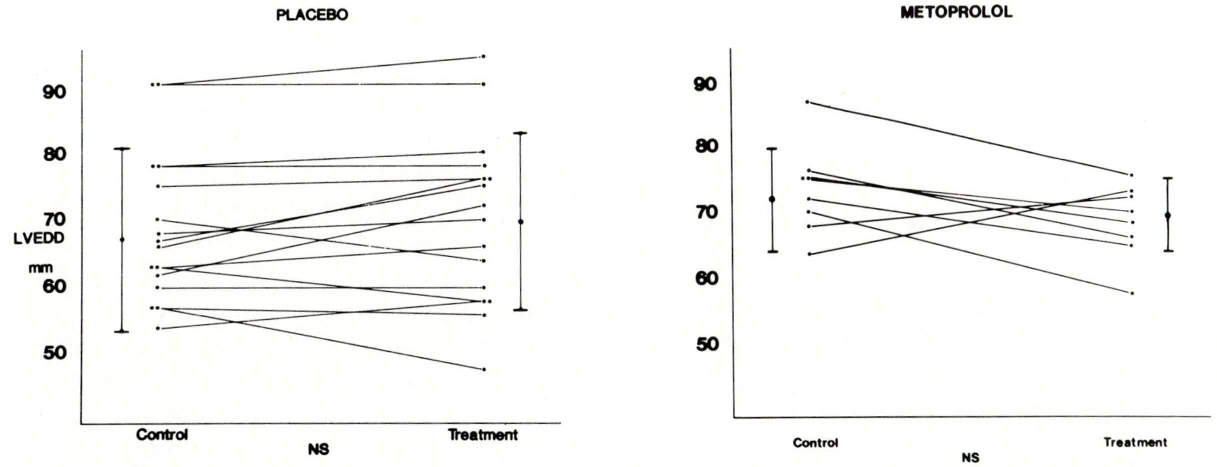

FIGURE 4. Individual and mean changes in echocardiographic end-diastolic dimension (LVEDD) in placebo and metoprolol groups, comparing baseline (Control) with completion of the blinded trial (Treatment).

TABLE 3
Serial changes in mean functional class, treadmill results, and noninvasive studies with placebo and metoprolol: crossover study

	Placebo					Metoprolol	
	Control	3 mo	6 mo	9 mo	Last F/U[A]	Control	3 mo
NYHA FC	2.38±0.7 (12)	2.33±0.7 (12)	2.36±0.7 (11)	2.1±0.8 (9)	2.42±0.9 (12)	2.42±0.9 (12)	1.92±0.7[C] (12)
Exercise tolerance (met score)	7.3±2.5 (10)		7.0±3.5 (10)		7.3±3.8 (10)	6.7±3.8 (12)	
RNV EF (%)	17.5±11 (12)	17.3±7 (12)	17.9±8 (10)	19.3±12 (7)	17.3±8 (12)	17.2±8 (12)	22.8±11[E] (11)
LVEDD (cm)	6.9±1.0 (12)	7.1±1.0 (12)	7.5±1.0 (11)	7.2±1.0 (7)	7.2±1.0 (12)	7.2±1.0 (12)	7.0±1.0 (12)

Results are expressed as mean ± SD, with number of tests averaged in parentheses. Abbreviations as in table 2.
[A]Last follow-up on placebo: 10 ± 3 months.
[B]Last follow-up on metoprolol: 15 ± 3 months.
Comparing serial investigations to pretreatment control: [C]$p < .001$; [D]$p < .05$; [E]$p < .06$.

when compared with the last follow-up value in placebo-treated patients ($p < .001$). No patient had a full class improvement on placebo, but two at 3 months, three at 6 months, and one at 9 months improved while on metoprolol.

Treadmill tests and noninvasive studies with placebo and metoprolol. The mean met score did not change at 6 months or at last follow-up in 10 patients who underwent serial studies while on placebo. After 6 months, the 12 patients on metoprolol showed an improvement in mean met score (6.7 to 9.3 mets; $p < .05$) that was sustained through the last follow-up (9.6 mets; $p < .05$) when compared with the last follow-up value in placebo-treated patients. Seven individuals improved by 6 months, and six had sustained improvement in met score at 12 months. Three of six doubled their exercise capacity while on metoprolol.

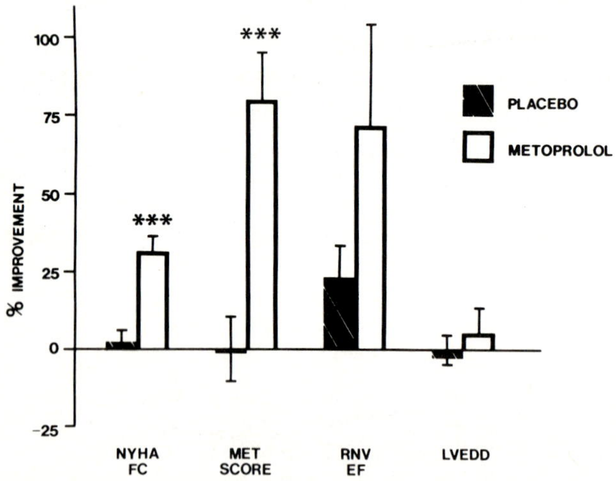

FIGURE 5. Percent improvement in mean functional class, exercise capacity, and noninvasive studies in placebo and metoprolol groups. The last follow-up study was expressed as a percent improvement of the pretreatment control value for each patient and then averaged in the placebo and metoprolol groups. Results expressed as mean ± SE. LVEDD = left ventricular end-diastolic dimension; MET Score = maximal oxygen consumption estimated by treadmill test; NYHA FC = New York Heart Association functional classification; RNV EF = radionuclide left ventricular ejection fraction. ***$p < .001$.

The mean ejection fraction and left ventricular end-diastolic dimension did not change significantly with placebo but the mean change in ejection fraction bordered on significance with metoprolol at 3 months; this value was sustained through the last follow-up ($p < .06$). Four individuals had progressive simultaneous improvement in ejection fraction (13 ± 2% to 25 ± 2%) and left ventricular end-diastolic dimension (7.6 ± 0.3 to 6.5 ± 0.4 cm) with metoprolol. These changes were accompanied by a return to NYHA functional class I and II, a doubling of exercise capacity in three, and an improvement by 5 mets in the fourth.

Changes in mean functional class, met score, and results of noninvasive studies. Percent change in mean NYHA functional class, met score, ejection fraction, and left ventricular end-diastolic dimension at last follow-up compared with control was evaluated during placebo and metoprolol therapy. The percent changes in NYHA functional class and met score were significantly better ($p < .01$, $p < .05$) with metoprolol in these 12 patients as compared with placebo. No difference was observed in percent change in noninvasive parameters with placebo or metoprolol (figure 6).

Stepwise discriminant analysis. Stepwise discriminant analysis was used to evaluate which clinical parameters would predict a favorable response to metoprolol in patients with dilated cardiomyopathy. The following baseline variables times the corresponding coefficient was 78% accurate in predicting a favorable clinical response if the sum was greater than zero: −1.33

TABLE 3
(Continued)

Metoprolol		
6 mo	9 mo	Last F/U[B]
1.67±0.6[C] (12)	1.59±0.5[C] (11)	1.42±0.4[C] (12)
9.3±2.8[D] (12)		9.6±2.9[D] (12)
21.4±10[E] (12)	21.4±10[E] (11)	23.4±10[E] (12)
7.0±1.0 (12)	6.7±0.7 (10)	6.7±0.9 (12)

+ (HR × .04) + (sex × .84) + (DOS × (−.001)) + (RNV EF × (−.01)), where HR = heart rate, male sex = 0, female sex = 1, DOS = duration of symptoms (in months), and RNV EF = radionuclide left ventricular ejection fraction.

Heart rate responses to metoprolol. The resting heart rate did not change with placebo, remaining at 92 ± 14 beats/min. With metoprolol, however, it decreased from 91 ± 16 to 75 ± 14 beats/min ($p < .001$). The mean heart rate response to exercise with placebo did not change from the pretreatment control value, but with metoprolol it was suppressed at all levels of exercise compared with the pretreatment control value (figure 7) ($p < .001$). The mean peak heart rate with metoprolol was identical to that at baseline control or with placebo, with the major difference being that it occurred after significantly more exercise in the metoprolol-treated patients.

Adverse effects of metoprolol. Twenty patients received an average maintenance dose of 92 ± 21 mg/day metoprolol. During the dosing phase, patients occasionally experienced mild worsening of heart failure symptoms, weakness, fatigue, mild nausea, and depression that usually responded favorably to prolongation of the dosing interval or rarely to intermittent addition of diuretics. Only one patient had a serious side effect requiring dismissal from the study (bradyarrhythmia). During the maintenance phase, one patient with a history of bipolar illness suffered an episode of severe depression that improved when atenolol replaced metoprolol. Another with peripheral vascular disease had worsening of claudication during maximal treadmill exercise, although his functional classification actually improved. Serious exacerbation of heart failure or cardiovascular collapse did not result from our protocol of metoprolol administration and patient selection.

Discussion

The rationale for treating patients with severe chronic congestive heart failure from dilated cardiomyopathy with metoprolol, a β_1 selective blocking agent, may appear misguided and likely to worsen heart failure. The latter may occur if this agent is administered in standard dosage or during acute cardiac decompensation.[20] We administered metoprolol in an ambulatory

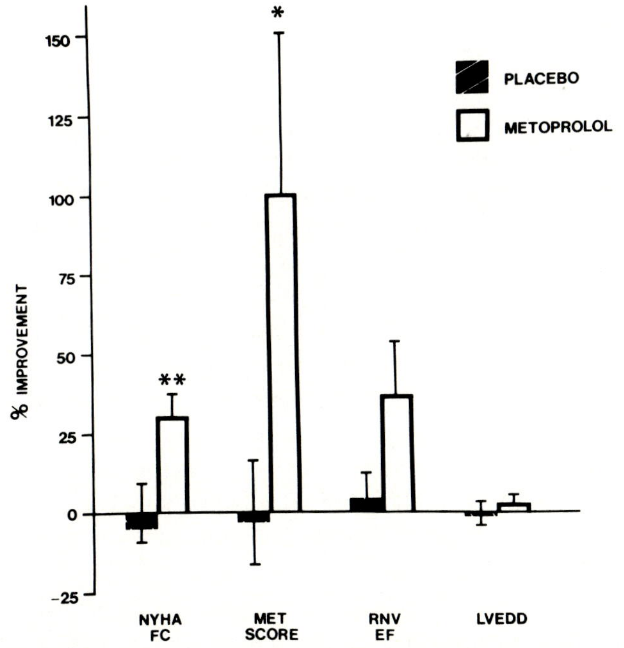

FIGURE 6. Percent improvement in mean functional class, exercise capacity, and noninvasive studies with placebo or metoprolol in crossover study. The last follow-up study was expressed as a percent improvement of the pretreatment control value for each patient and then averaged for placebo and metoprolol. Results expressed as mean ± SE. Abbreviations as in figure 5. **p < .01; *p < .05.

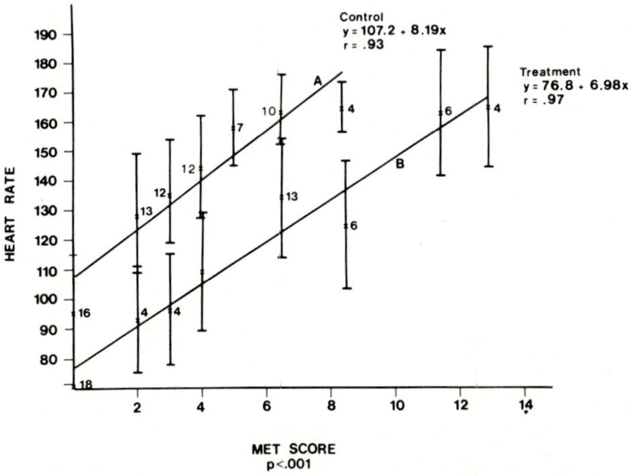

FIGURE 7. Heart rate response to exercise before and after metoprolol. The heart rates were averaged for all patients (number under line) at each level of exercise (line A) before administration of metoprolol and were then compared with the same patients' averaged heart rates at similar levels of exercise with metoprolol (line B). Significant suppression of heart rate response was observed at all levels of exercise.

setting to relatively stable, incapacitated patients with dilated cardiomyopathy, beginning with small doses and increasing the dose only after prolonged intervals under close supervision. This dosing phase frequently required 6 weeks, since patients occasionally experienced mild worsening of heart failure symptoms after each increment. Only one of 21 patients was intolerant of metoprolol, which was obvious during the first few weeks, and he was quickly removed without serious consequence. Once reaching a stable dose of 100 mg or having heart rates of 60 beats/min or systolic blood pressure of 90 mm Hg after β-blockade, 14 out of 20 had improved exercise tolerance and less symptomatic impairment, usually noted within 3 months. Seven of 20 patients had an exceptional response to the drug, which was characterized by returning to functional class I or II, doubling exercise tolerance, and progressively improving ejection fraction and left ventricular end-diastolic dimension.

The only plausible explanation for the improvements seen was the addition of long-term sympathetic β-blockade. There were minimal changes in other medications with doses of diuretics more frequently increased in the placebo group. Vasodilators and inotropic agents were not added after randomization. Alcohol consumption was carefully scrutinized at all follow-up visits and was not a factor. Ischemic cardiomyopathy and myocarditis were ruled out by invasive procedures in all 18 of 20 metoprolol-treated patients that were studied. Spontaneous improvement of myocardial function is also an unlikely explanation because the metoprolol patients were symptomatic for an average of 2 years and the exceptional responders were symptomatic for 37 months (range 3 to 108) before randomization. Additionally, only one of 16 patients randomly assigned to receive placebo improved spontaneously. This patient was minimally symptomatic for 12 months with mild left ventricular impairment at entry (ejection fraction 32%, left ventricular end-diastolic dimension 5.7 cm), which contrasts sharply with 20 of 25 of our study patients, including all eight who were tolerant of metoprolol and all seven exceptional responders who had an ejection fraction less than 20% and a left ventricular end-diastolic dimension greater than 6.3 cm. These patients undoubtedly had end-stage dilated cardiomyopathy that did not improve spontaneously, nor did they receive other medications that could account for their status changes.

There was no degree of left ventricular impairment that prevented the safe administration of metoprolol as long as patients were clinically stable. The three patients who required hospitalization for progressive heart failure were stabilized with intravenous diuretics before receiving metoprolol. The most favorable response occurred in patients with higher resting heart rates and poorer noninvasive indexes of left ventricular function. With these parameters, stepwise discriminant analysis was 78% accurate in predicting a favorable clinical response to metoprolol.

Significant changes in resting ejection fraction and left ventricular end-diastolic dimension correlated well with the clinical outcome in all groups and frequently preceded overt clinical changes. Seven of eight patients with improved ejection fraction and left ventricular end-diastolic dimension had the greatest symptomatic and exercise responses, while both patients with worsened ejection fraction died, and two of four with worsened left ventricular end-diastolic dimension developed more severe congestive heart failure with one dying. These results demonstrate the utility of serial noninvasive studies in patients with dilated cardiomyopathy in defining prognosis and may allow consideration of earlier interventions, such as transplantation, that may not be indicated solely on clinical grounds.

This study was not designed to explain how patients with moderate-to-severe heart failure from dilated cardiomyopathy improve after metoprolol. We suspect that several mechanisms may be responsible, including blocking the cardiotoxic effect of catecholamines,[21, 22] restoring the down-regulated β-adrenergic pathway to normal,[23–26] suppressing an inappropriate exercise-induced tachycardia,[27] inhibiting ventricular tachyarrhythmias,[28, 29] or altering renin-angiotensin activity.[30] These mechanisms need to be addressed by a multicenter study designed to explore the cardiovascular sympathetic response to long-term sympathetic β-blockade in patients with dilated cardiomyopathy.

Our results are in agreement with those of the Swedish group.[8–10, 31] The patients in both studies were comparable except that ours had better functional classification at entry (2.6 ± 0.9 vs 3.2 ± 0.5), which may be a result of improved conventional therapy and use of vasodilators. Eighteen of 23 patients with hemodynamic measurements had a pretreatment pulmonary capillary wedge pressure below 20 mm Hg, with a mean of 11.5 ± 4.9 mm Hg. Most of our patients achieved symptomatic improvement by 3 months, with the maximal improvement noted at 5.6 ± 3.8 months. Sixty percent of the patients studied by Swedberg and colleagues improved by 3 months, with their maximal improvement occurring at 7.4 ± 5.9 months. We discontinued metoprolol in only the first two patients completing 1 year. Similar to the Swedish experience, both had profound worsening of symptoms and ventricular tachyarrhythmias within 2 weeks. We therefore did not discontinue metoprolol in any other patients. There were similar numbers of patients experiencing improvements in exercise capacity in our study (14 of 20) compared with theirs (13 of 22).

Anderson et al.[32] demonstrated improved survival and functional class in a randomized study of 25 patients treated with long-term, low-dose β-blockade. They did not, however, document the improved exercise tolerance that was seen in our study. Possible explanations for this lack of improvement include a lower dose of metoprolol (61 vs 92 mg) used in patients with less left ventricular impairment (ejection fraction 27% vs 16%) with lower baseline resting heart rates (82 vs 91 beats/min). Only one-half of their patients underwent treadmill exercise testing. The best response in our study occurred in patients with higher resting heart rates and poorer left ventricular function.

Two placebo-controlled trials have shown no benefit from β-blocker therapy. In one study, 40% of subjects had significant double- or triple-vessel coronary artery disease, and in the other 70% of subjects had alcoholic heart disease. Both studies followed patients for only 4 weeks.[10, 11] Although we did not systematically reassess our patients at 4 weeks, only six of 15 patients improved in the series of Swedberg and associates by 1 month. Three of these improved further several months later, implying that benefit from β-blockade is delayed and usually occurs after 1 month of therapy. These studies are therefore limited by heterogenous patient populations and short follow-up periods, and the findings must be interpreted with caution.

Our study was limited by insufficient patient numbers and a relatively short follow-up in any single treatment group, making it impossible to predict the effect of metoprolol on survival in patients with moderate-to-severe degrees of dilated cardiomyopathy. Our experience is limited only to metoprolol, and the favorable results cannot be extrapolated to other β_1-blocking agents with varying degrees of β_2-blockade, and β_1-agonist, or α-antagonist properties. An explanation for the clinical improvement, effects on survival, and efficacy in other forms of heart failure are unknown and need to be addressed by a larger, multicenter trial.

In summary, metoprolol improves the symptoms and exercise tolerance of most patients with dilated cardiomyopathy. A subset of these patients will become nearly free of symptoms and have improved noninvasive indexes of resting left ventricular function. Most patients will tolerate the drug when selected and treated by our protocol. We suggest that metoprolol be considered as a therapeutic option for patients with dilated cardiomyopathy who remain symptomatic despite conventional therapy. Metoprolol must be administered cautiously and patients selected carefully to avoid worsening of already impaired left ventricular function. Further studies are necessary to evaluate the effect of metoprolol on survival and determine its mechanism of action.

We are indebted to Kimberly Treckler for help in preparing the manuscript.

References

1. O'Connell JB, Gunnar RM: Dilated-congestive cardiomyopathy: prognostic features and therapy. Heart Transplant **2:** 7, 1982
2. Chidsey CA, Harrison DC, Baunwald E: Augmentation of the plasma norepinephrine response to exercise in patients with congestive heart failure. N Engl J Med **267:** 650, 1962
3. Francis GS, Goldsmith SR, Olivari MT, Levine TB, Cohn JN: The neurohumoral axis in congestive heart failure. Ann Intern Med **101:** 370, 1984
4. Sonnenblick EH: Implication of muscle mechanics in the heart. Fed Proc **21:** 975, 1962
5. Kramer RS, Mason DT, Braunwald E: Augmented sympathetic neurotransmitter activity in the peripheral vascular bed of patients with congestive heart failure and cardiac norepinephrine depletion. Circulation **38:** 629, 1968
6. Thomas JA, Marks BH: Plasma norepinephrine in congestive heart failure. Am J Cardiol **41:** 233, 1978
7. Cohn JN, Levine TB, Olivari MT, Garberg V, Lura D, Francis GS, Simon AB, Rector T: Plasma norepinephrine as a guide to prognosis in patients with chronic congestive heart failure. N Engl J Med **311:** 819, 1984
8. Waagstein F, Hjalmarson A, Varnauskas E, Wallentin I: Effect of chronic beta-adrenergic receptor blockade in congestive cardiomyopathy. Br Heart J **37:** 1022, 1975
9. Swedberg K, Hjalmarson A, Waagstein F, Wallentin I: Beneficial effects of long-term beta-blockade in congestive cardiomyopathy. Br Heart J **44:** 117, 1980
10. Swedberg K, Hjalmarson A, Waagstein F, Wallentin I: Adverse effects of beta-blockade withdrawal in patients with congestive cardiomyopathy. Br Heart J **44:** 134, 1980
11. Currie PJ, Kelly MJ, McKenzie A, Harper RW, Lim YL, Federman J, Anderson ST, Pitt A: Oral beta-adrenergic blockade with metoprolol in chronic severe dilated cardiomyopathy. J Am Coll Cardiol **3:** 203, 1984
12. Ikram H, Fitzpatrick D: Double-blind trial of chronic oral beta blockade in congestive cardiomyopathy. Lancet **1:** 490, 1981
13. Report of the WHO/ISFC Task Force on the definition and classification of cardiomyopathies. Br Heart J **44:** 672, 1980
14. The Criteria Committee of the New York Heart Association, Inc: Diseases of the heart and blood vessels: nomenclature and criteria for diagnosis, ed 6. Boston, 1964, Little, Brown and Co.
15. Pavel DG, Zimmer AM, Patterson VN: In vivo labelling of red blood cells with ^{99}Tc: a new approach to blood pool acquisition. J Nucl Med **18:** 305, 1977
16. Feigenbaum H: Echocardiography. Philadelphia, 1976, Lea and Febiger
17. Bruce RA, Kusumi F, Hosmer D: Maximal oxygen intake and nomographic assessment of functional aerobic impairment in cardiovascular disease. Am Heart J **85:** 546, 1973
18. Patterson JA, Naughton J, Pietras RJ, Gunnar RM: Treadmill exercise in assessment of the functional capacity of patients with cardiac disease. Am J Cardiol **30:** 757, 1972
19. Fox SM, Naughton JP, Haskell WL: Physical activity and the prevention of coronary heart disease. Ann Clin Res **3:** 404, 1971
20. Hoffbrand BI: Beta adrenergic blockade in congestive cardiomyopathy. Lancet **1:** 1031, 1980

21. Yates JC, Bernish RE, Dhalla NS: Ventricular dysfunction and necrosis produced by adrenochrome metabolites of epinephrine: relation to pathogenesis of catecholamine cardiomyopathy. Am Heart J **102:** 210, 1981
22. Tanaka M, Tsuchihashi Y, Katsumi H, Ijichi H, Ibata Y: Comparison of cardiac lesions induced in rats by isoproterenol and by repeated stress of restraints and water immersion with special reference to etiology of cardiomyopathy. Jpn Circ J **44:** 971, 1980
23. Bristow MR, Ginsburg R, Minobe W, Cubicciotti RS, Sageman WS, Lurie K, Billingham ME, Harrison DC, Stinson EB: Decreased catecholamine sensitivity and beta-adrenergic receptor density in failing human hearts. N Engl J Med **307:** 205, 1982
24. Ginsburg R, Esserman JL, Bristow MR: Myocardial performance and extracellular ionized calcium in a severely failing human heart. Ann Intern Med **98:** 603, 1983
25. Fowler MB, Bristow MR, Lasser JA, Ginsburg R, Scott LB, Schroeder JS: Beta blocker therapy in severe heart failure: improvement related to beta-1 adrenergic receptor up regulation? Circulation **70**(suppl II): II-112, 1984
26. Wilson JR, Martin JL, Schwartz D, Ferraro N: Exercise intolerance in patients with chronic heart failure: role of impaired nutritive flow to skeletal muscle. Circulation **69:** 1079, 1984
27. Weber KT, Likoff MJ, McCarthy D: Low-dose beta blockade in the treatment of chronic cardiac failure. Am Heart J **104:** 877, 1982
28. Pratt CM, Yepsen SC, Bloom MG, Taylor AA, Young JB, Quinones MA: Evaluation of metoprolol in suppressing complex ventricular arrhythmias. Am J Cardiol **52:** 73, 1983
29. Anderson JL, Rodier HE, Green LS: Comparative effects of beta-adrenergic blocking drugs on experimental ventricular fibrillation threshold. Am J Cardiol **51:** 1196, 1983
30. Michelalis AM, McAllister RG: The effect of chronic adrenergic blockade on plasma renin activity in man. J Clin Endocrinol Metab **34:** 386, 1972
31. Waagstein F, Hjalmarson A, Swedberg K, Wallentin I: Beta-blockers in dilated cardiomyopathies: they work. Eur Heart J **4**(suppl A): 173, 1983
32. Anderson JL, Lutz JR, Gilbert EM, Sorenson SG, Yanowitz FG, Menlove RL, Bartholomew M: A randomized trial of low dose beta-blockade therapy for idiopathic dilated cardiomyopathy. Am J Cardiol **55:** 471, 1985

Retraction

The authors of the following manuscript have requested that it be retracted. An excerpt from the authors' letter requesting the retraction follows:

> We wish to retract our paper previously published in *Circulation* entitled "Increased circulating bradykinin during hypothermia and cadiopulmonary bypass in children" (*Circulation* **60:** 1503, 1979). We have been unable to repeat the results with respect to bradykinin.

Leila M. Pang, M.D.
S. Alex Stalcup, M.D.
Joel S. Lipset, M.S.
Constance J. Hayes, M.D.
Frederick O. Bowman, Jr., M.D.
Robert B. Mellins, M.D.

The interaction of verapamil and norverapamil with β-adrenergic receptors

ROSS D. FELDMAN, M.D., GLEN D. PARK, PHARM.D., AND CHEIN-YU CYNTHIA LAI, B.SC.

ABSTRACT To determine the effect of calcium-channel blockers on β-adrenergic receptors, we studied the interactions of verapamil, diltiazem, and nifedipine with both human lymphocyte β_2-adrenergic receptors and rat myocardial β_1-adrenergic receptors by means of radioligand binding assays. We also determined the functional consequences of these interactions by measuring adenylate cyclase activity. Radioligand binding studies in vitro demonstrated a K_i of verapamil for the lymphocyte β_2-receptor of 32 ± 4 μM. Diltiazem and nifedipine were much less potent. In studies of adenylate cyclase activity, verapamil was shown to act as a competitive β-receptor antagonist. Also, norverapamil, the active metabolite of verapamil, had the highest affinity for the β-receptor of any of the calcium-channel blockers studied (K_i = 4.2 ± 0.8 μM). After 1 week of verapamil administration in six normal subjects, isoproterenol-stimulated adenylate cyclase activity in lymphocytes was increased from 60 ± 4% to 83 ± 10% over basal activity ($p < .05$). This was associated with an increase in lymphocyte β-receptor affinity for agonist as represented by the decrease in the IC_{50} for isoproterenol inhibition of [^{125}I] iodocyanopindolol binding from 240 ± 20 to 170 ± 10 nM ($p < .05$). Additionally, plasma norepinephrine levels were reduced from 206 ± 58 to 92 ± 18 pg/ml with 1 week of verapamil treatment ($p < .05$). Our data suggest that verapamil affects lymphocyte β-receptors in vitro and with long-term administration regulates lymphocyte β-receptor function either directly or indirectly via a reduction in plasma catecholamine levels.
Circulation 72, No. 3, 547–554, 1985.

IMPORTANT differences in clinical effects are apparent between the Food and Drug Administration–approved calcium-channel blockers verapamil, diltiazem, and nifedipine. This difference is evident in the pharmacologic effects of these agents. For example, both nifedipine and verapamil reduce blood pressure in hypertensive subjects. However, nifedipine is associated with an increase in heart rate and stroke index,[1] whereas verapamil may cause a reduction in heart rate and stroke index.[2] The reason for these differences is not clear but is not surprising considering the marked structural differences between these agents. It has been suggested that these agents may act at different calcium channels (reviewed in ref. 3). Additionally, it has been appreciated that verapamil and related compounds may interact at sites other than calcium channels, including opiate and α-adrenergic receptors,[3–5] and this interaction may be of therapeutic significance.[6]

Because many of the effects of verapamil are similar to those seen with β-adrenergic receptor blockers, we have studied the possible interactions of verapamil with β_1- and β_2-adrenergic receptor systems by means of radioligand binding techniques and assays of β-adrenergic–mediated adenylate cyclase activity. We have also compared the effects of verapamil in vitro with those of diltiazem, nifedipine, and norverapamil, the primary active metabolite of verapamil. Additionally, to determine the effect of verapamil on β-receptor regulation in vivo, we have studied human leukocyte β-receptors from normal subjects before, during, and after long-term oral administration of verapamil.

From the Departments of Internal Medicine and Pharmacology, College of Medicine and the Division of Clinical/Hospital Pharmacy, College of Pharmacy, University of Iowa, Iowa City.

Supported by USPHS grants HL 32501-01, AM 25295, and RR59. Dr. Feldman is the recipient of the George Morris Piersol Teaching and Research Scholarship from the American College of Physicians.

Address for correspondence: Ross D. Feldman, M.D., Department of Internal Medicine, University of Iowa Hospitals and Clinics, Iowa City, IA 52242.

Received Feb. 27, 1985; revision accepted May 30, 1985.

Methods

Materials. The following drugs were gifts from the manufacturers: verapamil hydrochloride and norverapamil bioxalate from Dr. Siebeneick, Knoll Pharmaceutical Co.; diltiazem hydrochloride from Marion Laboratories; nifedipine hydrochloride from Pfizer Laboratories. [α^{32}P]ATP, [^{3}H]cyclic AMP, and [^{125}I]iodocyanopindolol (ICYP) were purchased from New England Nuclear, Ltd. All other compounds were obtained from Sigma Chemical Co.

Tissue preparation. Whole blood was taken from healthy volunteers according to a modification of previously described methods.[7] Lymphocytes were isolated from ethylenediamine tetra-acetate acid (EDTA)-anticoagulated blood according to the method of Boyum.[8] Fresh blood (100 ml) was centrifuged at 300 *g* for 14 min at room temperature, the platelet-rich plasma was aspirated, and the buffy coats were collected into two 50 ml tubes and diluted approximately fourfold with 30 ml of phosphate-buffered saline (pH 7.6). A Ficoll (6%) Hypaque (10%) solution was carefully subfused and the samples centrifuged at 400 *g* for 40 min at room temperature. After careful removal of the saline/plasma layer, thc lymphocyte band was harvested by aspiration. The mononuclear cells isolated by this procedure were at least 80% small lymphocytes.

The lymphocytes were washed with ice-cold buffer containing 100 mM NaCl, 15 mM $MgCl_2$, 3 mM EDTA, 6 mM sucrose, and 20 mM Tris-HCl (pH 7.9 at room temperature) and centrifuged at 37,000 *g* for 10 min. The supernatant was discarded and the pellet was resuspended in an ice-cold "lysing" buffer of 3 mM EDTA and 2 mM Tris-HCl (pH 7.9 at room temperature) and homogenized with a Polytron, setting 7, for 10 sec. The homogenate was centrifuged at 37,000 *g* for 10 min. The pellet from this centrifugation was demonstrated morphologically to contain no intact cells. For binding studies, the preparations were resuspended in 20 mM Tris-HCl, 15 mM $MgCl_2$, 3 mM EDTA, and 100 mM NaCl (pH 7.9 at 25° C) at a concentration of 200 to 300 μg protein/ml and frozen and stored at −80° C. Storage for up to 10 days did not alter binding characteristics. For adenylate cyclase studies, preparations were suspended in 75 mM Tris-HCl and 25 mM $MgCl_2$ (pH 7.9 at 25° C) and assayed immediately.

Rat ventricular cell homogenates were prepared from primary cell cultures of heart cells from neonatal rats according to the methods of Marvin et al.[9] Membranes were prepared from cell cultures as follows: growth medium was removed and adherent cells were washed twice with a cold lysis buffer containing 3 mM Tris-HCl (pH 7.4 at 4° C), 2 mM EDTA, and 2 mM $MgCl_2$. Cell lysis was achieved by incubating the cells in lysis buffer for 15 min on ice. This resulted in cell swelling. The cells then lysed when the plates were scraped with a rubber policeman. The resulting lysate was pelleted at 37,000 *g* for 10 min at 4° C, then resuspended in 20 mM Tris-HCl (pH 7.5 at 37° C), 100 mM NaCl, 15 mM $MgCl_2$, 6 mM sucrose, and 3 mM EDTA.

Radioligand binding studies. β-Receptor binding studies were performed according to modifications of previously described methods,[7] with use of ICYP (2.2 Ci/μmol, New England Nuclear Corp.). ICYP and other drugs were prepared in 1.25 mM ascorbic acid as an antioxidant with 10 μg/ml bovine serum albumin.

Aliquots of the lymphocyte or cardiac cell preparations containing 10 to 20 μg of protein were incubated with various concentrations of ICYP in a final volume of 250 μl containing 0.5 mM ascorbic acid, 1.0 μg bovine serum albumin, 12 mM Tris-HCl (pH 7.9, 24° C), 60 mM NaCl, 9 mM $MgCl_2$, 1.8 mM EDTA, and 3.6 mM sucrose. Samples were incubated in disposable polypropylene tubes at 37° C for 100 min, at which time steady state had been reached at all concentrations. Incubations were stopped by the addition of 10 ml of 0.9% NaCl with 10 mM Tris-HCl and 15 mM $MgCl_2$ (pH 7.9 at 25° C) to each assay tube followed by separation of membrane-bound and "free" ICYP by rapid filtration through Whatman GF/C filters. Each filter was washed with an additional 10 ml of buffer and radioactivity was determined in a gamma counter. Protein concentration was determined by the method of Lowry et al.,[10] with bovine serum albumin as a standard.

ICYP bound selectively to β-adrenergic receptors in both cardiac and lymphocyte membrane preparations. Specific binding of ICYP was reversible and saturable, and linear Scatchard plots were obtained consistent with antagonist binding to a single class of receptors. Nonspecific binding was determined by the amount of ICYP bound in the presence of 100 μM isoproterenol and accounted for less than 20% of total binding at concentrations of ICYP approximating its K_D. By means of competition binding techniques, binding was shown to be stereoselective. The order of potency for agonists (determined by comparing the concentrations required to inhibit 50% of specific ICYP binding [IC_{50}]) in lymphocyte membranes was isoproterenol > epinephrine > norepinephrine, consistent with binding to a β_2-receptor subtype. In cardiac membranes the order of potency was isoproterenol > epinephrine = norepinephrine, consistent with binding to a β_1-receptor subtype.

Receptor affinity for calcium-channel blockers was derived from the inhibition of ICYP competition binding with varying concentrations of verapamil, norverapamil, diltiazem, or nifedipine. The former three drugs were dissolved in ethanol to a final concentration of 0.2%. Nifedipine was dissolved in 2% ethanol. Studies in which nifedipine was used were conducted under dim light to prevent the drug from degrading. Concentrations of ethanol up to 2% did not alter binding.

In studies of the effect of verapamil treatment on β-receptors in vivo, affinity for the agonist isoproterenol was determined from competition curves in the absence and presence of guanylimidodiphosphate [Gpp(NH)p, a hydrolysis-resistant analog of GTP], as previously described.[7]

For each competition curve, specific binding was analyzed by a nonlinear curve-fitting procedure with a generalized model for complex ligand receptor systems.[11] This procedure, based on the law of mass action, provides estimates of the dissociation constants for the competitor. Fitted estimates of receptor affinity for the competitors were obtained assuming one and two affinity states. The two affinity state model was accepted only if it significantly improved ($p < .05$) the "fit" of the data over the one affinity state model. Additionally, for isoproterenol competition curves, the IC_{50} for isoproterenol was calculated by logit analysis to determine a measure of β-receptor affinity for agonist, independent of a particular model for agonist-receptor interactions.

We demonstrated that competition curves for the agonist isoproterenol in the absence of added guanine nucleotides were "shallow," with a slope factor less than 1, and were best fit to a two affinity state model. These data suggest heterogeneous binding of agonists to the leukocyte β-receptor. This is not caused by the presence of multiple β-receptor subtypes, since the lymhocyte β-receptor population is primarily of the β_2-subtype. These data are consistent with the ternary complex model of the β-receptor, i.e., that the receptor binds agonists with two affinities, high and low.[12, 13] According to this model, formation of the "high affinity complex" is a prerequisite for β-receptor–mediated adenylate cyclase activity. An impaired ability to form the high-affinity complex has been correlated with reduced β-adrenergic adenylate cyclase activity (so-called uncoupling of the β-receptor complex) as in the phenomenon of desensitization.[13] Changes in the ability to form the high-affinity complex can be inferred from changes in the competition curves for agonists (e.g., isoproterenol).[13] By means of computerized fitting of isoproterenol competition curves, an impaired ability to form the high-affinity state has been correlated with reductions in the computer-derived estimates for the proportion of receptors binding agonist with a high affinity (%R_H) and for the ratio of the dissociation constants of the high- and low-affinity states (K_L/K_H).[13] Therefore, to study the effect of verapamil treatment on the ability to form the high-affinity complex of the β-receptor, we performed agonist competition curves with lymphocyte membranes from subjects given verapamil.

With the addition of Gpp(NH)p the fit of isoproterenol competition curves was not significantly improved by assuming a two-affinity state model. This is consistent with the results of previous studies, suggesting that addition of guanine nucleotides in vitro converts the receptor population to a homogeneous low-affinity state.[13] Therefore the IC_{50} for isoproterenol competition in the presence of added guanine nucleotides solely represents the low-affinity state of the receptor for agonists.

In initial studies we showed that competition curves for the antagonist propranolol were steeper (slope factor approaching 1) and were best explained by a one affinity site model. This suggests that for the lymphocyte β-receptor, as in other model systems, an antagonist binds with one homogeneous affinity, not dependent on guanine nucleotides.[13]

Receptor density and K_D for the antagonist radioligand ICYP were determined from saturation curves of specific ICYP binding at six concentrations of ICYP from 5 to 30 pM. Receptor density and K_D were determined by computerized nonlinear curve fitting analysis.

Adenylate cyclase assay. Adenylate cyclase activity was measured in lymphocyte membrane preparations by a modification of the method of Salomon et al.[14] Enzyme activity was inferred by the ability of membranes to mediate conversion of [α^{32}P] ATP to [α^{32}P] cyclic AMP (cAMP). One hundred to 200 μg of membranes suspended in 75 mM Tris-HCl and 25 mM $MgCl_2$ (pH 7.9, 25° C) was added to give a final incubation volume of 150 μl with 1 μCi [α^{32}P] ATP (New England Nuclear), 0.3 mM ATP, 10 mM $MgCl_2$, 0.1 mM cAMP, 5 mM phosphoenolpyruvate, 40 μg/ml pyruvate kinase, and 20 μg/ml myokinase. GTP (100 μM) was added to samples incubated with isoproterenol. Maximal activity of adenylate cyclase (non–β-receptor mediated) was determined by the addition of NaF (3 mM) in the absence of GTP. Incubations were carried out at 37° C for 8 min and were terminated by the addition of 1 ml of a solution containing 100 μg ATP, 50 μg cAMP, and 15,000 counts/min [^{3}H] cAMP (New England Nuclear). cAMP was isolated by sequential Dowex and Alumina chromatography as described by Salomon et al.[14] and corrected for recovery with [^{3}H] cAMP as the internal standard. NaF and isoproterenol-stimulated adenylate cyclase activity were expressed as the percentage increase in activity compared with basal and GTP stimulated activity, respectively. Adenylate cyclase activity was linear with time and protein concentration over the range studied.

Schild plots for verapamil and norverapamil inhibition of isoproterenol-stimulated adenylate cyclase activity were constructed from concentration-response curves, each with six concentrations of isoproterenol either with no inhibitor or at three concentrations of each inhibitor. The EC_{50} was determined from logit analysis of the dose-response curves of isoproterenol-stimulated adenylate cyclase activity. The dose ratio was determined at each concentration of verapamil or norverapamil, i.e., the EC_{50} for isoproterenol-stimulated adenylate cyclase activity at each concentration of the inhibitor was divided by the EC_{50} for isoproterenol in the absence of inhibitor. From the plot of log dose ratio-1 vs log inhibitor concentration, the antilog of the x-intercept is the A_2, a measure of how potently the drug inhibits isoproterenol-stimulated adenylate-cyclase activity.

All experiments described were performed on three to six different occasions.

Subject protocol. To determine the effect of verapamil on leukocyte β-receptor regulation in man, we studied six healthy male subjects before, during, and after treatment with verapamil.

Subjects were between 20 and 33 years of age and had no abnormality on routine history and physical examination and were normotensive. All were drug free for at least 3 days before study. Subjects were studied on three occasions: before treatment, after 1 week of verapamil treatment (120 mg three times daily), and at least 4 days after discontinuing verapamil. All subjects remained in bed overnight in the University of Iowa Clinical Research Center. Before 7 A.M. and before rising, an indwelling catheter was inserted; 20 min later a 100 ml blood sample was drawn.

Blood samples were analyzed for plasma norepinephrine by high-performance liquid chromatography–electrochemical detection and for verapamil and norverapamil by high-performance liquid chromatography–fluorescence detection (Bio-Science, Bellwood, IL). Radioligand binding studies and assays for adenylate cyclase activity were performed as described above. Maximal β-adrenergic–mediated adenylate cyclase activity was determined at a 100 μM concentration of isoproterenol. Maximal nonreceptor-stimulated activity was determined with 3 mM NaF.

The statistical significance of differences between study periods was determined by analysis of variance followed by Student's t test for paired data or Wilcoxon signed ranks test (where appropriate); $p < .05$ in a two-sided test was taken as the minimum level of significance.

Results

In the lymphocyte broken cell preparation, verapamil inhibited specific ICYP binding with a K_i of 32 ± 4 μM. In contrast, diltiazem was considerably less potent and nifedipine showed essentially no affinity for β-adrenergic receptors (table 1).

To further characterize the nature of verapamil competition for ICYP binding, saturation binding studies were performed in the presence and absence of 100 μM verapamil. The addition of verapamil resulted in a 155 ± 2% increase in the K_D of ICYP with virtually no change in receptor concentration (B_{max}) consistent with the effect of a competitive inhibitor (figure 1).

To determine by radioligand binding techniques whether verapamil might be a β-receptor agonist or antagonist, we analyzed verapamil competition curves. In the absence of Gpp(NH)p, competition curves were best fit by a model of verapamil binding to

TABLE 1

Inhibition of ICYP binding by calcium-channel blockers: results of competition curve studies

	K_i (μM)	
Drug	Lymphocyte β_2-receptor	Cardiac β_1-receptor
Norverapamil	4.2±0.8	26±11
Verapamil	32±4	115±15
Diltiazem	137±21	131±14
Nifedipine	> 300	> 300

The K_i (mean ± SEM) for each drug was determined from competition curve experiments performed on three separate occasions except for the K_i of verapamil for the β_2-receptor, which was determined from six experiments.

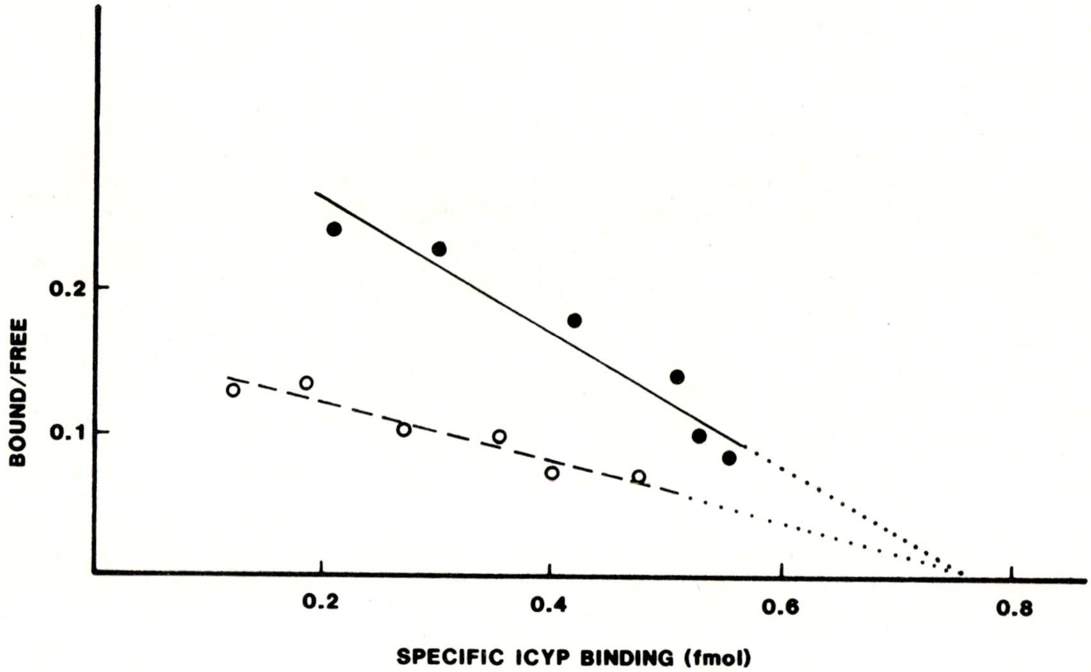

FIGURE 1. Alterations in ICYP saturation binding curves by verapamil in the lymphocyte preparation: Scatchard analysis. The addition of 100 μM verapamil (○) resulted in a reduction in apparent K_D for ICYP binding. This is demonstrated by the more shallow slope as compared with control (●). However, total binding (B_{max}) was unaltered, as shown by the virtually identical x-intercepts of the plots. Actual B_{max} and K_D were determined by computer curve fitting analysis of saturation binding curves. Each point is the mean of triplicate determinations (representative of three identical experiments).

the β-receptor with a single affinity. Also, verapamil competition curves were not altered by the addition of Gpp(NH)p. The homogeneous binding of verapamil and the lack of effect of guanine nucleotides are characteristic of a β-receptor antagonist.

The possibility that verapamil inhibited isoproterenol-stimulated adenylate cyclase activity by competitive interactions at the β-receptor was studied using a Schild plot analysis. The EC_{50} of dose-response curves for isoproterenol-stimulated adenylate cyclase activity with each of three concentrations of verapamil were determined by logit analysis and dose ratios were calculated. Verapamil inhibited isoproterenol-stimulated adenylate cyclase activity in a dose-dependent fashion. The calculated A_2 value from the Schild plot for verapamil inhibition of isoproterenol-stimulated adenylate cyclase activity was 48 μM (figure 2). This closely approximated the affinity derived from radioligand binding assays. Verapamil demonstrated no effect on basal or NaF-stimulated activity.

The effects of calcium-channel blockers on ICYP binding were measured in rat myocyte β_1-receptors. The K_i of verapamil for the myocyte β_1-receptor was almost 4 fold higher (115 $\pm$ 15 μM) than that in the lymphocyte β_2-receptor and closely approximated that for diltiazem (table 1).

Effects of norverapamil. We studied the effects of norverapamil (the major metabolite of verapamil) in both lymphocyte β_2-adrenergic and myocyte β_1-adrenergic receptor systems and compared the effects of norverapamil with those of the parent compound. In the lym-

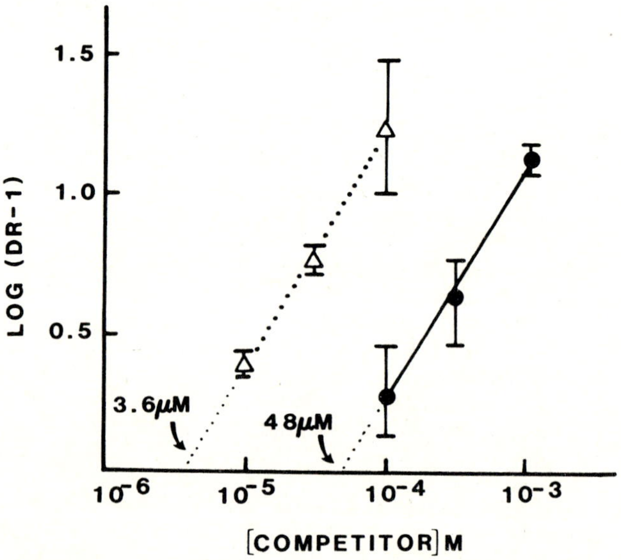

FIGURE 2. Verapamil and norverapamil inhibition of isoproterenol-stimulated adenylate cyclase activity in the lymphocyte preparation: Schild plot. Each point represents the mean $\pm$ SEM determined from triplicate determinations from each of three separate experiments. The x-intercept, A_2, is a measure of the potency of verapamil (●) or norverapamil (△) for the inhibition of β-receptor–mediated adenylate cyclase activity.

phocyte β_2-adrenergic receptor system, norverapamil was approximately eightfold more potent than verapamil in competing for ICYP binding (K_i norverapamil = 4.2 ± 0.8 μM) (figure 3). The addition of norverapamil bioxalate (10 μM) to saturation binding studies resulted in an increase in apparent K_D for ICYP (188 ± 25% of control) with no change in B_{max} (107 ± 4% of control). Norverapamil inhibited isoproterenol-stimulated adenylate cyclase activity with an A_2 of 3.6 μM (figure 2) but had no effect on basal or NaF-stimulated activity. To rule out the possibility that the oxalate salt independently affected adenylate cyclase activity we studied the effect of sodium oxalate. The addition of sodium oxalate up to a concentration of 1 mM had no demonstrable effect on basal or isoproterenol-stimulated adenylate cyclase activity.

In the cardiac β_1-receptor system, the potency of norverapamil in inhibiting ICYP binding was lower (K_i = 26 ± 11 μM) than that in the β_2-receptor system. However, norverapamil still demonstrated a higher potency for the cardiac β-receptor than verapamil (K_i = 115 ± 15 μM).

Effect of oral verapamil treatment on lymphocyte β-receptors. Our study of the effect of oral verapamil treatment on lymphocyte β-receptor regulation was based on the following hypothesis: if verapamil or norverapamil were acting as β-receptor antagonists in vivo, we would expect that long-term administration of verapamil would result in β-receptor "up-regulation" analogous to that observed with long-term administration of propranolol.[15–17] Oral therapy with verapamil in human subjects resulted in plasma concentrations of verapamil and norverapamil comparable to those previously reported.[18, 19] Plasma concentrations were 128 ± 21 ng/ml (0.28 ± 0.05 μM) for verapamil and 155 ± 21 ng/ml (0.35 ± 0.05 μM) for norverapamil 5 to 7 hr after drug administration after 1 week of treatment.

Verapamil treatment was associated with significant alterations in leukocyte β-receptor properties as determined by assays of adenylate cyclase activity and by radioligand binding studies. Isoproterenol-stimulated adenylate cyclase activity increased from 60 ± 4% to 83 ± 10% (over basal activity) after 1 week of verapamil treatment ($p < .05$, see figure 4). After withdrawal of verapamil, isoproterenol-stimulated adenylate cyclase activity decreased to a level not different from the initial control values (figure 4). Neither basal adenylate cyclase activity nor NaF-stimulated activity was altered by treatment with verapamil (table 2).

The increase in β-adrenergic–mediated adenylate

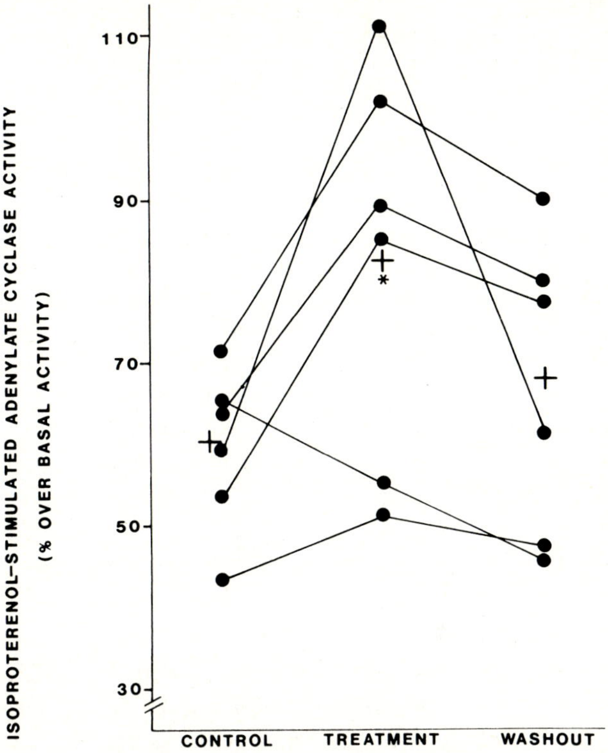

FIGURE 4. Alterations in β-adrenergic–mediated adenylate cyclase activity with verapamil administration. Isoproterenol-stimulated adenylate cyclase activity was expressed as the percentage increase in activity compared to GTP-stimulated activity. + = mean in six subjects. *$p < .05$ compared with pretreatment control and posttreatment washout periods.

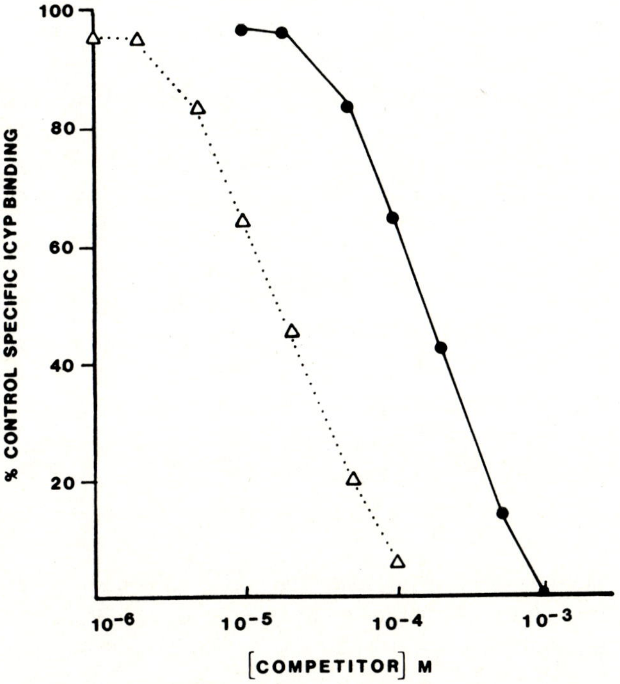

FIGURE 3. Verapamil and norverapamil competition for ICYP binding in the lymphocyte β_2-receptor system. Each point is the mean of triplicate determinations. The verapamil (●) and norverapamil (△) curves are representative of three experiments.

TABLE 2
Alterations in adenylate cyclase activity with verapamil treatment

Period	NaF-stimulated activity (%)	Basal activity (pmol cAMP/min·mg)
Control	367±47	83±11
Treatment	393±34	89±8
Washout	314±34	96±11

Adenylate cyclase activity is represented as the mean ± SEM of triplicates from each of six subjects studied before, during, and after treatment with verapamil 120 mg three times daily for 1 week.

cyclase activity after verapamil treatment was associated with an increase in β-receptor affinity for the agonist isoproterenol as determined in radioligand binding studies. Thus the IC_{50} of isoproterenol in competing for ICYP binding in the absence of Gpp(NH)p was reduced from 240 ± 20 to 170 ± 10 nM ($p < .05$), representing a 41% increase in affinity (figure 5). Withdrawal of verapamil was associated with a return of the IC_{50} of isoproterenol to pretreatment levels (270 ± 50 nM). Computer analysis of competition curves with a two-site model for agonist binding demonstrated no significant changes with treatment in either the ratio of high-affinity sites/low-affinity sites (R_H/R_L) or the ratio of dissociation constants for the high- and low-affinity sites (K_L/K_H). A reduction in the IC_{50} for isoproterenol in the presence of Gpp(NH)p was also demonstrated with treatment (control, 719 ± 169 nM; treatment, 373 ± 63 nM; washout, 680 ± 142 nM; $p < .05$ between treatment and either control or washout periods) (figure 5). However, neither receptor density (B_{max}) nor affinity for the radioligand (K_D of ICYP) was altered after 1 week of verapamil treatment.

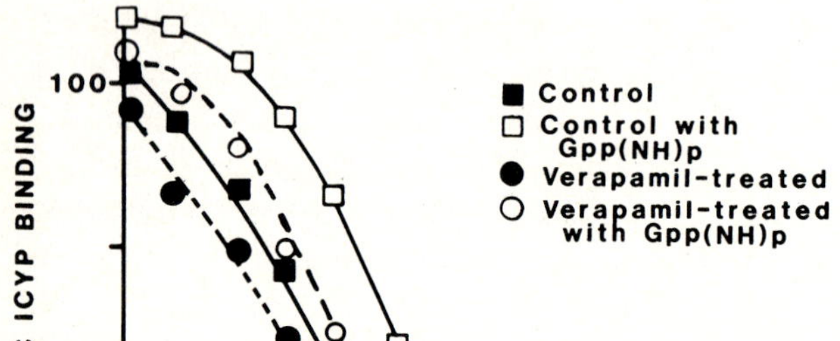

FIGURE 5. Alterations in β-receptor affinity for agonist with verapamil administration. After 1 week of verapamil treatment, isoproterenol competition curves either in the absence or presence of Gpp(NH)p are shifted to the left, as compared with competition curves from samples taken during the control period. The curves are representative of studies in six subjects.

For all six subjects, plasma norepinephrine levels from supine blood samples were decreased from 206 ± 58 to 92 ± 18 pg/ml ($p < .05$) during treatment and returned to baseline levels after treatment (236 ± 58 pg/ml). In contrast, plasma epinephrine and dopamine levels were unaltered with treatment. No significant correlations were demonstrated between plasma norepinephrine levels and either isoproterenol-stimulated adenylate cyclase activity or β-receptor affinity for agonist.

Discussion

Initial studies in the 1960s suggested verapamil acted as a β-adrenergic antagonist based on its hemodynamic effects and antagonism of β-agonist stimulated effects.[20] Subsequently, its effect as a calcium-channel blocker was elucidated and its primary pharmacologic action was attributed to this mechanism (for reviews see refs. 3 and 21 to 23).

Our radioligand binding data demonstrate that verapamil in vitro acts competitively to inhibit β-receptor–specific ICYP binding. Verapamil's effect as a β-adrenergic antagonist is shown by the insensitivity of verapamil to the guanine nucleotide Gpp(NH)p in radioligand competition binding curves and by verapamil inhibition of isoproterenol-stimulated adenylate cyclase activity. It should be pointed out, however, the potency ($1/K_i$) of verapamil at the human lymphocyte β-receptor is more than 100 times lower than its reported potency at calcium channels in other tissues.[21, 22]

In the two β-receptor systems studied, verapamil showed a much higher potency at the lymphocyte β_2-receptor than at the cardiac β_1-receptor, where verapamil and diltiazem were virtually identical in their potency for β-receptor interactions. Although the actual K_i estimates between different tissue preparations are not necessarily comparable, it is interesting that nifedipine and diltiazem exhibit similar K_i values in both leukocyte and myocardial β-receptor systems. Of the three drugs, only verapamil showed a difference in potency between β_1- and β_2-receptor systems. Therefore these data suggest some degree of β_2-adrenergic selectivity for verapamil. This is consistent with the results of previous studies by Karliner et al.,[5] which demonstrated that cardiac β_1-receptor affinity for verapamil was very low.

We also found that norverapamil, the major metabolite of verapamil, had a much higher affinity for the β-receptor than the parent compound. Norverapamil is partially active as a calcium-channel blocker,[24] appears rapidly in the plasma after oral administration of verapamil, and achieves comparable plasma concentrations to the parent drug (up to 1 μM).[18, 19] Our data obtained in vitro demonstrate that norverapamil is a competitive β_2-receptor antagonist with a K_i in the low micromolar range. In the studies in vivo, plasma norverapamil levels 5 to 7 hr after oral administration of verapamil were 0.35 ± 0.05 μM, much lower than the K_D of norverapamil for the β-receptor as determined from studies in vitro. This might suggest that norverapamil could not act as a β-blocker in vivo. However, tissue levels for verapamil and norverapamil have been found to be up to 10-fold higher than corresponding plasma levels.[25] Assuming that the effect of verapamil on the lymphocyte β-receptor was representative of its effect on β_2-receptors in other tissues (e.g., vascular smooth muscle), at the dosage of verapamil studied (360 mg/day), tissue concentrations of norverapamil could be within the range where we would expect significant β_2-receptor blockade.

In vivo, long-term verapamil administration was associated with increased lymphocyte β-adrenergic–mediated adenylate cyclase activity. This appears to be related to an increase in receptor affinity for agonists without a corresponding increase in antagonist binding (that is, an increase in the B_{max} or a decrease in the K_D for ICYP). It is notable that the increase in β-receptor affinity for isoproterenol was not associated with an increase in R_H/R_L or in K_L/K_H and was also demonstrated in the presence of Gpp(NH)p. Thus the increase in affinity of the recognition site of the receptor for isoproterenol is caused by a shift of both the high- and low-affinity states of the receptor for agonist. Therefore the associated increase in β-adrenergic–mediated adenylate cyclase activity cannot be caused simply by an increased ability to form the high-affinity complex (according to the ternary complex model[12, 13]). Alterations in the low-affinity state have been reported in other studies of human leukocyte β-receptor regulation.[26, 27] However, the molecular explanation for these changes is unclear. The increase in receptor affinity for agonist with verapamil treatment is not caused by persistent verapamil in the membrane preparation, since this would have caused an artifactual reduction in receptor affinity for isoproterenol.

The reduction in plasma norepinephrine levels seen with verapamil administration was unexpected. Theoretically, verapamil might have been expected to mediate an increase in plasma norepinephrine through its effect as a presynaptic α_2-adrenergic receptor antagonist.[4, 28] However, we have found the reverse situation. Assuming the reduction in plasma norepinephrine levels does represent a decrease in central sympathetic outflow, this observation may explain why verapamil treatment does not cause the reflex increase in heart rate and contractility seen with other vasodilators.

One interpretation of our data is that the increase in lymphocyte β-receptor responsiveness with verapamil administration is related to the β-receptor–blocking effect of verapamil (or norverapamil) in vivo. This interpretation is made by analogy to the effect of propranolol on lymphocyte β-receptor regulation. Long-term administration of propranolol has been shown to result in up-regulation of lymphocyte β-receptors presumably by blocking the long-term desensitizing effects of circulating catecholamine hormones.[15–17] In fact, the proportional increase in leukocyte β-receptor responsiveness seen with verapamil is comparable to that seen after treatment with the β-blocker propranolol.[15–17] However, it is notable that the increase in lymphocyte β-adrenergic responsiveness with propranolol therapy is primarily thought to be caused by increased receptor density.[16, 17] In contrast, we saw no changes in lymphocyte β-receptor density with verapamil but instead noted an increase in β-receptor affinity for agonists.

Alternatively, enhanced β-receptor responsiveness with verapamil administration could be secondary to the reduction in plasma norepinephrine levels. As we have previously demonstrated, small changes in plasma catecholamines within the physiologic range have been associated with regulation of human lymphocyte β-adrenergic responsiveness and β-receptor affinity for agonist.[7] The reduction in plasma norepinephrine levels associated with verapamil treatment is within the range over which reciprocal increases in β-adrenergic responsiveness might be anticipated. Hopefully future studies will resolve which of the two mechanisms, i.e., β-blockade vs reduction in plasma catecholamine levels, is primarily responsible for the effect of verapamil treatment on human lymphocyte β-receptors in vivo.

We are indebted to Dr. William Marvin for supplying neonatal rat myocytes for this study and to Drs. Lee Limbird and Harvey Motulsky for their constructive comments in the preparation of this manuscript. In addition, we thank Doris Lewis, Rita Yeggy, and Ann Aschoff for their expert preparation of the manuscript.

References

1. Olivari MT, Bartorelli C, Polese A, Fiorentini C, Moruzzi P, Guazzi MD: Treatment of hypertension with nifedipine, a calcium antagonistic agent. Circulation **59:** 1056, 1979

2. Lewis BS, Mitha AS, Gotsman MS: Immediate hemodynamic effects of verapamil in man. Cardiology **60:** 366, 1975
3. Triggle DJ, Swamy VC: Calcium antagonists: some chemical-pharmacologic aspects. Circ Res **52**(suppl I): I-17, 1983
4. Motulsky HJ, Snavely MD, Hughes RJ, Insel PA: Interaction of verapamil and other calcium channel blockers with α_1- and α_2-adrenergic receptors. Circ Res **52:** 226, 1983
5. Karliner JS, Motulsky HJ, Dunlap J, Brown JA, Insel PA: Verapamil competitively inhibits α_1-adrenergic and muscarinic but not β-adrenergic receptors in rat myocardium. J Cardiovasc Pharmacol **4:** 515, 1982
6. Maisel AS, Motulsky HJ, Insel PA: Hypotension after quinidine plus verapamil: possible additive competition at alpha-adrenergic receptors. N Engl J Med **312:** 167, 1985
7. Feldman RD, Limbird LE, Nadeau J, Fitzgerald GA, Robertson D, Wood AJJ: Dynamic regulation of leukocyte beta adrenergic receptors by physiological changes in circulating catecholamines. J Clin Invest **72:** 164, 1983
8. Boyum A: Isolation of mononuclear cells and granulocytes from human blood. Scand J Clin Lab Invest **21** (suppl 97): 77, 1968
9. Marvin WJ, Robinson RB, Hermsmeyer K: Correlation of function and morphology of neonatal rat and embryonic chick cultured cardiac and vascular tissue. Circ Res **45:** 528, 1979
10. Lowry OH, Rosebrough NJ, Farr AL, Randall RJ. Protein measurement with Folin phenol reagent. J Biol Chem **193:** 265, 1951
11. Hancock AA, DeLean AL, Lefkowitz RJ: Quantitative resolution of beta-adrenergic receptor subtypes by selective ligand binding: application of a computerized model fitting technique. Mol Pharmacol **16:** 1, 1979
12. DeLean A, Stadel J, Lefkowitz RJ: A ternary complex model explains the agonist-specific binding properties of the adenylate cyclase-coupled β-adrenergic receptor. J Biol Chem **255:** 7108, 1980
13. Kent RS, DeLean A, Lefkowitz RJ: A quantitative analysis of beta-adrenergic receptor interactions: resolution of high and low affinity states of the receptor by computer modelling of ligand binding data. Mol Pharmacol **17:** 14, 1980
14. Salomon YC, Londos C, Rodbell M: A highly sensitive adenylate cyclase assay. Anal Biochem **58:** 541, 1974
15. Lima DR, Turner P: Propranolol increases reduced beta-receptor function in severely anxious patients. Lancet **2:** 1505, 1983
16. Aarons RD, Niew AS, Gal J, Hegstrand LR, Molinoff PB: Elevation of β-adrenergic receptor density in human lymphocytes after propranolol administration. J Clin Invest **65:** 949, 1980
17. Fraser J, Nadeau J, Robertson D, Wood AJJ: Regulation of human leukocyte beta receptors by endogenous catecholamines: relationship of leukocyte beta receptor density to the cardiac sensitivity to isoproterenol. J Clin Invest **67:** 1777, 1981
18. Shand DG, Hammil SC, Aanonsen L, Pritchett ELC: Reduced verapamil clearance during long-term oral administration. Clin Pharmacol Ther **30:** 701, 1981
19. Freeman SB, Richmond DR, Ashley JJ, Kelly DT: Verapamil kinetics in normal subjects and patients with coronary artery spasm. Clin Pharmacol Ther **30:** 644, 1981
20. Melville KI, Benfey BG: Coronary vasodilatory and cardiac adrenergic blocking effects of ipoveratril. Can J Physiol Pharmacol **43:** 339, 1965
21. Antman EM, Stone PH, Muller JE, Braunwald E: Calcium channel blocking agents in the treatment of cardiovascular disorder. I. Basic and clinical electrophysiological effects. Ann Intern Med **93:** 875, 1980
22. Schwartz A, Triggle DJ: Cellular action of calcium channel blocking drugs. Annu Rev Med **35:** 325, 1984
23. Janis RA, Scriabine A: Sites of action of Ca^{2+} channel inhibitors. Biochem Pharmacol **32:** 3499, 1983
24. Neugebauer G: Comparative cardiovascular actions of verapamil and its major metabolites in the anesthetized dog. Cardiovasc Res **12:** 247, 1978
25. Kates RE, Keefe D, Schwartz J, Harapat S, Harrison D, Kirsten E, Johnson SM: Disposition kinetics of verapamil and norverapamil. Clin Pharmacol Ther **29:** 257, 1981 (abst)
26. Davies AO, Lefkowitz RJ: Agonist-promoted high affinity state of the β-adrenergic receptor in human neutrophils: modulation by corticosteroids. J Clin Endocrinol Metab **53:** 703, 1981
27. Feldman RD, Limbird LE, Nadeau J, Robertson D, Wood AJJ: Alterations in leukocyte β-receptor affinity with aging: a potential explanation for altered β-adrenergic sensitivity in the elderly. N Engl J Med **310:** 815, 1984
28. Galzin AM, Langer SZ: Pre-synaptic alpha 2-adrenoceptor antagonism by verapamil but not by diltiazem in rabbit hypothalamic slices. Br J Pharmacol **78:** 571, 1983

Erratum

Reardon MF, et al: Lipoprotein predictors of the severity of coronary artery disease in men and women. Circulation **71:** 881, 1985

There is a discrepancy between the values given in table 1 and figure 2 in the above article. The correct values are found in table 1.

Electrophysiologic and antiarrhythmic effects of sotalol in patients with life-threatening ventricular tachyarrhythmias

KOONLAWEE NADEMANEE, M.D., GREGORY FELD, M.D., JOANN HENDRICKSON, B.S., PRAMIL N. SINGH, AND BRAMAH N. SINGH, M.D., D.PHIL.

ABSTRACT Sotalol is a unique β-blocker that lengthens cardiac repolarization and effective refractory period (ERP). Its efficacy after intravenous (1.5 mg/kg) and oral (160 to 480 mg bid) administration was therefore evaluated in 37 patients with refractory recurrent ventricular tachycardia/fibrillation (VT/VF). Thirty-five patients, 33 with inducible VT/VF, underwent electrophysiologic testing. Intravenous sotalol lengthened the ERP in the atrium (+24.6%, $p < .01$), atrioventricular node (+24.9%, $p < .01$), and ventricle (+14.9%, $p < .01$). It also significantly lengthened sinus node recovery time, corrected QT interval (QTc), and the AH interval, but not the HV interval. Sotalol prevented reinduction of VT/VF in 15 patients (45.5%). Twenty-five of the 33 patients (15 with positive results of electrophysiologic tests; 10 with negative results) were given oral sotalol. The drug was ineffective in seven (26.9%) and aggravated arrhythmia in one (3.8%). In four patients sotalol was withdrawn because of side effects; arrhythmias recurred late in two (7.7%). Eleven patients (42.3%) have continued on oral sotalol over a mean follow-up period of 9.2 ± 8.6 months. Sotalol reduced ($n = 21$) total premature ventricular complex (PVC) count on the Holter electrocardiogram by 73% ($p < .01$), paired PVCs by 89% ($p < .01$), and beats of ventricular tachycardia by 95% ($p < .01$). In 52% ($n = 11$), total reduction in PVCs was at least 85%, and incidence of paired and tachycardiac beats was reduced at least 90% (group A). In the remainder ($n = 10$), PVC suppression was not significant (group B). Group A included nine patients with nonreinducible VT/VF and two in whom it was reinducible; in group B, eight of 10 patients had reinducible VT/VF. The difference between the two groups (Fisher exact test) was significant ($p < .01$). The prevention of reinduction of VT/VF by intravenous sotalol and suppression of spontaneously occurring arrhythmias by the oral drug were both predictive of long-term drug efficacy. Sotalol is a significant advance in the short- and long-term management of life-threatening ventricular tachyarrhythmias.
Circulation 72, No. 3, 555–564, 1985.

ALTHOUGH SOTALOL was introduced as a specific β-blocking drug 24 years ago,[1] interest in it as a broad-spectrum antiarrhythmic compound has been relatively recent.[2-4] In 1970 Singh and Vaughan Williams,[5] and subsequently Strauss et al.,[6] showed that in concentrations somewhat greater than those required to produce significant β-blocking activity in isolated cardiac muscle, sotalol consistently lengthened the action potential duration without effect on the upstroke velocity of phase 0 of the action potential. The drug, administered intravenously, was found to prolong the corrected QT interval (QTc) of the surface electrocardiogram in anesthetized guinea pigs in which the compound prevented the onset of ventricular fibrillation due to ouabain toxicity.[5] Since these overall electrophysiologic and antiarrhythmic actions differed from those of either the quinidine-like drugs or other β-antagonists, sotalol was thought to act by homogeneously lengthening cardiac repolarization and refractoriness.[5]

Subsequent studies in patients have confirmed that sotalol administered over the both the short and long term lengthens repolarization and refractoriness in the heart.[7-9] Its so-called class III[5] antiarrhythmic actions have also been confirmed from the direct recordings of monophasic action potentials via suction electrodes in

From the Department of Cardiology, Wadsworth Veterans Administration Hospital and the Department of Medicine, UCLA School of Medicine, Los Angeles.
Supported by grants from the Medical Research Service of the Veterans Administration and The American Heart Association of the Greater Los Angeles Affiliate (789 G1-1) and by a grant-in-aid from the Bristol-Myers Company, Evansville, IN.
Address for correspondence: Koonlawee Nademanee, M.D., Department of Cardiology 691/111E, Wadsworth VA Hospital, Wilshire and Sawtelle Blvds., Los Angeles, CA 90073.
Received April 1, 1985; revision accepted June 6, 1985.

man.[7-9] However, there remains a paucity of data dealing with the effect of sotalol on cardiac arrhythmias.[10-14] The purpose of the the present study was to evaluate the efficacy and safety of sotalol in patients with symptomatic, sustained, life-threatening ventricular tachyarrhythmias. The study was conducted in two parts. In the first, the effects of the intravenously administered drug on the inducibility of ventricular tachycardia by programmed electrical stimulation of the heart relative to the electrophysiologic actions of the compound were determined. In the second, the effects of the orally administered drug on spontaneously occurring tachyarrhythmias documented on 24 hr ambulatory electrocardiographic recordings relative to the dose and plasma concentrations of the drug were evaluated.

Materials and methods

Patients. The study population consisted of 37 patients who had clinically manifest sustained symptomatic recurrent ventricular tachycardia and/or ventricular fibrillation (VT/VF). There were 36 male and one female patient with a mean age of 58 (range 25 to 72) years. None had an identifiable reversible cause of the ventricular arrhythmia or recent myocardial infarction (i.e., in the 4 weeks immediately before the study). Except for one patient who had sarcoidosis, all others had coronary artery disease. The mean ejection fraction measured either by contrast or radionuclide ventriculography for 23 patients was 33.0 ± 14.0%. Patients in whom there was a contraindication to β-blockade or who had evidence of decompensated cardiac failure were excluded from the study. Data from two patients in whom ventricular tachycardia could not be induced during the control study were excluded from analysis (see below). All patients except one had failed on or had not tolerated one or more (mean number, 2.76 ± 1.3) conventional antiarrhythmic drugs. In two patients with recurrent and frequent VT/VF that had not responded to intravenous lidocaine, procainamide, and bretylium tosylate, intravenous sotalol was given but electrophysiologic studies were not done either before or after the drug was given because of clinical exigencies. These patients were both men, and were 55 and 67 years old.

Protocol. All patients were admitted to the coronary care unit for continuous electrocardiographic monitoring. Previously prescribed antiarrhythmic drugs were discontinued for at least five elimination half-lives of these agents. Whenever possible a 24 hr ambulatory electrocardiographic recording was obtained at a time the patients were not taking any other antiarrhythmic drugs. This recording served as a baseline with respect to the spontaneously occurring tachyarrhythmias and was subsequently used for gauging the efficacy of drug therapy. Thirty-five patients underwent electrophysiologic studies for the evaluation of the effects of 1.5 mg/kg iv sotalol hydrochloride (Bristol-Myers, Evansville, IN), administered over a period of 5 to 10 min, on the inducibility of ventricular tachycardia relative to the electrophysiologic effects and plasma concentrations of the drug. Oral sotalol was started if the intravenous drug prevented the inducible VT/VF. However, a patient was started on the oral regimen even if the intravenous drug failed to prevent the inducible tachyarrhythmia, provided the baseline 24 hr Holter recording demonstrated significant ventricular ectopy so that the changes in the severity of the spontaneously occurring arrhythmias could be used as an index for judging the effects of the oral drug. Oral sotalol was not given to any patient in whom ventricular tachycardia was induced while he was on the intravenous drug and who did not exhibit frequent ventricular arrhythmias on 24 hr Holter recordings.

The initial oral dosage was 160 mg bid. In some patients the dose was increased in a stepwise fashion to 320 or 480 mg bid, respectively, if ventricular tachycardia was not controlled at the lower dose or if the goal of therapy was not met according to the Holter recordings. This goal was 85% suppression of the mean premature ventricular complexes (PVCs) and 90% suppression of paired PVCs and beats of ventricular tachycardia (three or more PVCs in a row exceeding a rate of 100 beats/min). The criterion for drug failure was the occurrence of VT/VF or cardiac arrest on oral sotalol. Oral sotalol was discontinued when clinical VT/VF occurred or side effects precluded the continuation of the drug therapy. The patients in whom sotalol was not effective were subsequently treated with amiodarone empirically, beginning with a loading dose followed by a maintenance regimen.

After the in-hospital stabilization period and control of the ventricular arrhythmias, the patients were discharged on sotalol and their clinical progress was followed at 3 month intervals in the arrhythmia clinic. The protocol was reviewed and approved by the Wadsworth Hospital Research Committee for the Protection of Human Subjects.

Electrophysiologic studies. Studies were performed in the electrophysiologic laboratory in patients in the preabsorptive state who had not received premedication. Electrode catheters were inserted percutaneously and positioned at multiple cardiac sites under fluoroscopic control. The recording sites included the high right atrium, His bundle, and right ventricular apex. Standard quadripolar electrode catheters with 1 cm interelectrode distance (USCI, Billerica, MA) were used for stimulation and recording from specific sites. Surface electrocardiographic leads I, aVF, and V_1 were displayed simultaneously with the intracardiac signals and were recorded on a VR-12 (Electronics for Medicine) recorder at a paper speed of 100 mm/sec. Cardiac stimulation was performed with a programmable constant-current stimulator (Medtronic 5325) that delivered rectangular pulses of 2 msec duration at twice the diastolic threshold. Intracardiac electrograms were filtered at 30 to 500 Hz. The right atrial, right ventricular, and atrioventricular nodal (when possible) refractory periods were obtained with the extrastimulus method.[15] Sinus node recovery time was determined by pacing the right atrium at incrementally higher fixed pacing rates at 1 min intervals to a maximum of 170 beats/min or until atrioventricular nodal Wenckebach block developed.

Ventricular tachycardia induction protocol. VT/VF was induced by programmed electrical stimulation (PES) with the following protocol: (1) Premature right ventricular stimulation with single (S_2) or double (S_2S_3) extrastimuli was used during ventricular pacing or sinus rhythm. The S_2S_3 technique was used when S_2 during scanning from late diastole to ventricular refractoriness did not induce tachycardia. S_2S_3 extrastimuli were introduced at an S_1S_2 interval 50 msec longer than the ventricular refractory period, with the S_2S_3 interval being equal to the S_1S_2 interval. The S_2S_3 interval was progressively shortened, and when S_3 failed to elicit a V_3, the S_1S_2 interval was decreased until S_3 did evoke a response or until tachycardia developed. This technique was used until both S_2 and S_3 reached ventricular refractoriness. At least three cycle lengths (sinus and 600, 500, and 400 msec) were used sequentially in every patient. (2) If ventricular tachycardia could not be elicited in this way, brief bursts of rapid ventricular pacing at the cycle length close to the ventricular refractory period were undertaken for 10 beats. If no inducible tachycardia resulted from use of either technique, the right ventricular outflow tract was stimulated by a technique identical to that used for the stimulation of the right ventricular apex. (3) Repeat electrophysiologic studies after 10 min of sotalol infusion were performed in the same manner as those during the baseline period. The protocol for ventricular stimulation was identical to that described above and we went through at least three cycle lengths sequentially before considering that ventricular tachycardia was not inducible (see below for the definition of inducible ventricular tachycardia). We stimulated only the right ventricular site at which tachycardia was produced before sotalol was tested. (4) During ventricular tachycardia, programmed single or double extrastimuli and rapid ventricular pacing were used to terminate the arrhythmia: cardioversion was used in refractory cases or for hemodynamic deterioration.

Definition of sustained vs nonsustained ventricular tachycardia. A sustained tachycardia was defined as one that persisted for at least 30 sec and required pacing or external defibrillation for termination. Nonsustained tachycardia was defined as that which persisted for at least 6 beats and reverted to sinus rhythm spontaneously within 30 sec.

Analysis of Holter electrocardiographic intervals. The electrocardiogram was analyzed for alterations in PR, QRS, and QT intervals before and after the drug was given. The QTc interval was obtained from the formula: $QTc = QT/\sqrt{RR}$. The 24 hr Holter tapes were analyzed commercially (Cardio-Data, Inc, Haddonfield, NJ) for mean heart rates, total number of PVCs per 24 hr, and paired and total beats of ventricular tachycardia per 24 hr.

Measurement of sotalol plasma levels. Plasma levels were determined by high-performance liquid chromatography by the method described by Karkkainen and Neuovonen.[16] The blood samples were obtained shortly after intravenous injection of sotalol and during long-term administration of drug.

Data and statistical analysis. The data are presented as mean ± SD. Student's t test for paired data (two-tailed) was used to evaluate the significance of the changes in various parameters at baseline and during sotalol therapy. The Fisher exact test was used when appropriate. A probability less than .05 was accepted as the limit of statistical significance.

Results

Electrophysiologic effects of intravenously administered sotalol. Of the 37 patients enrolled in the study, 35 patients underwent electrophysiologic studies. The effects of 1.5 mg/kg iv sotalol could be evaluated in 33. The time course of change in the mean plasma levels of sotalol measured in 14 patients is shown in figure 1. The range of plasma levels of sotalol at 10 min after administration of the drug was 982 to 12,096 ng/ml (the latter high value was recorded in only one patient, the remainder having levels lower than 4000 ng/ml), 1208 to 3123 ng/ml after 20 min, and 917 to 1685 ng/ml after 30 min.

The mean data on the effects of sotalol on various electrophysiologic parameters are summarized in table 1. The effects of the drug were characterized essentially by a prolongation in the effective refractory (ERP) period in all tissues, with an increase in the intranodal conduction time. Intravenous sotalol reduced the heart rate by 29.4% ($p < .01$) and lengthened the intranodal

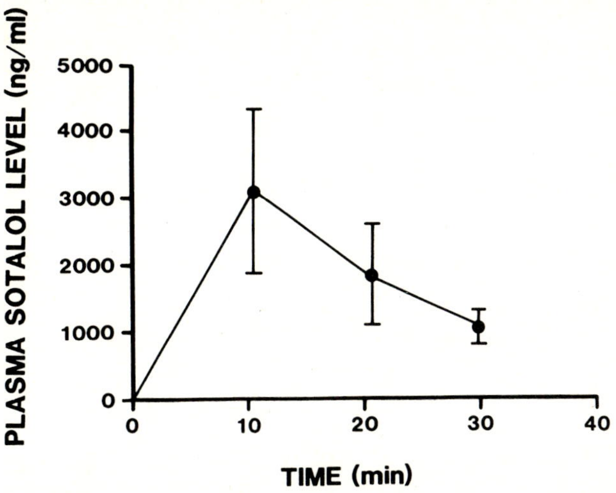

FIGURE 1. The time course of plasma sotalol levels after intravenous injection of 1.5 mg/kg of the drug in patients undergoing electrophysiologic studies. The data points represent means ± SD for 14 patients.

(AH) conduction time by 17.8% ($p < .01$), but it had no significant effect on infranodal conduction (HV interval). Sotalol did, however, increase the QTc interval (+10.8%, $p < .01$), as well as the ERP in the atrium (+24.6%, $p < .01$), atrioventricular node (+24.9%, $p < .01$), and ventricle (+14.9%, $p < .01$). In the case of the ventricle, the ratio QTc/ERP was 1.65 before sotalol was given and 1.59 after the drug. The difference was not statistically significant.

Effects of intravenous sotalol on inducibility of ventricular arrhythmias (tables 2 and 3). Electrophysiologic studies were not undertaken in two of the 37 patients. These patients (Nos. 25 and 26) had incessant VT/VF in the coronary care unit; they were given intravenous sotalol intermittently for control of arrhythmias (figure 2). While the control of VT/VF was achieved, one of the patients died of anoxic brain damage because of recurrent cardiac arrests suffered before institution of sotalol therapy, and the other died from acute myocardial infarction. Of the remaining 35 patients, ventricular tachycardia could not be induced in two patients and their data were excluded from the final analysis. Therefore the effect of sotalol on the clinical outcome could be assessed in a homogeneous group of 33 patients in whom VT/VF could be provoked by PES. Of these 33 patients, 24 had inducible sustained ventricular tachycardia, eight had nonsustained tachycardia, and one had ventricular fibrillation. Intravenous sotalol prevented the induction of VT/VF in 15 patients (45.5%), but did not prevent it in 18 (in nine induced ventricular tachycardia was sustained and in nine it was nonsustained). Sotalol converted a sustained tachycardiac response to a nonsustained one in three patients (9.1%; see table 2). However, the latter was not

TABLE 1
Electrophysiologic effects of intravenously administered sotalol in patients with life-threatening ventricular tachycardia

Electrophysiologic parameters (msec)	Baseline	After sotalol	Percentage change from control	Significance of change from control
RR interval	738.2±163	955±182	+29.4	p < .01
AH	85.7±20.0	101±24.36	+17.8	p < .01
HV	59.6±18.2	60.9±19.8	+2.2	NS
QTc	397±50	440±40	+10.8	p < .05
Atrial ERP	248.4±39.0	309.4±52.3	+24.6	p < .01
AVN ERP (anterograde)	345.5±59.0	431.4±61.4	+24.9	p < .01
AVN Wenckebach cycle length	371.1±65.4	466.1±84.1	+25.6	p < .01
Ventricular ERP	240.6±29.1	276.6±27.5	+14.9	p < .01
SNRT	870.4±275.4	1149.5±405.2	+32.0	p < .01

The data represent mean ± SD data from 33 patients to whom sotalol (1.5 mg/kg iv) was given during electrophysiologic study. The significance of the difference between the control value of a particular parameter and that after sotalol was tested by Student's paired (two-tailed) t test.

AVN = atrioventricular node; SNRT = sinus node recovery time.

considered to be a "protective" response. In those patients in whom the drug did not suppress ventricular tachycardia, the cycle length of the inducible tachycardia increased from 256 ± 65 to 306 ± 77 msec (+19.5%, $p < .05$). No systemic relationship was found between the lengthening of the ERP by sotalol and its effect on the inducibility of ventricular tachycardia by PES of the heart. However, the possibility of such a relationship is not excluded by the data because of the limited number of patients studied in this series.

The clinical outcome in patients with inducible vs noninducible VT/VF after intravenous sotalol relative to the subsequent administration of oral sotalol was as follows. Of the patients in whom intravenous sotalol prevented inducible VT/VF (n = 15), the arrhythmia could be controlled in 13 (86.7%) by oral sotalol; the drug failed early (within the first month) in one and appeared to aggravate the condition of another. During long-term therapy (longer than 1 month), arrhythmia recurred in two patients (at 8 and 8.4 months), and side effects precluded the continued use of the drug in an additional two patients. Eight patients remain free of arrhythmias and without side effects during a mean follow-up period of 14.5 ± 7.5 (range 2 to 23) months. Of 18 patients in whom sotalol failed to suppress VT/VF, oral sotalol was given to 10; in the other eight it was not given because they did not have significant PVCs on baseline ambulatory electrocardiographic recordings. Of the 10 patients who were given oral sotalol even though they had inducible ventricular tachycardia after intravenous sotalol, six had recurrent VT/VF and one had a limiting side effect. The remaining three patients have been free of arrhythmias (mean follow-up 8.6 months, range 8 to 9). In the patients treated with 160 mg bid oral sotalol the mean plasma levels were 2.3 ± 0.8 μg/ml (n = 6) and levels of 3.1 ± 0.4 μg/ml (n = 3) were found in those treated with 320 mg bid.

Effects of orally administered sotalol on spontaneously occurring ventricular tachyarrhythmias. This could be evaluated in 21 of 25 patients on oral sotalol in whom baseline 24 hr ambulatory electrocardiographic recordings (obtained while they were off all antiarrhythmic drugs and showing high-density PVCs exceeding 30 beats/hr) were obtained under control conditions and when a steady-state level of sotalol was reached during oral administration. The overall data relative to the inducibility of VT/VF and clinical outcome are presented in table 2.

The mean data showed that sotalol reduced the total PVC count by 73% ($p < .01$), paired PVCs by 89% ($p < .01$), and beats of ventricular tachycardia by 95% ($p < .01$). In 11 of the 21 patients, sotalol reduced total PVCs by at least 85%, and paired PVCs and tachycardiac beats by at least 90% (group A). In the other 10 patients, sotalol did not significantly suppress spontaneously occurring arrhythmias (group B). There was no systematic relationship between changes in heart rate and the degree of PVC suppression by sotalol.

As is evident in table 2 and figure 3, *A*, group A (11 patients) included nine patients in whom ventricular tachycardia could not be reinduced and two in whom it remained inducible. By contrast, ventricular tachycardia remained inducible in eight of 10 patients in group B. Analysis by Fisher exact test showed that group A included a significantly greater number of patients with noninducible ventricular tachycardia than did group B ($p < .01$). Moreover, in group A (figure 3, *B*) there were only two patients (18%) who had recurrent VT/VF whereas there were seven patients in group B with recurrent VT/VF (70%, $p < .06$). Two patients in group A and one patient in group B had significant side effects necessitating discontinuation of drug therapy.

Adverse reactions. During the intravenous administration of sotalol there were no significant hemodynamic disturbances in the patients. In four patients, distal atrioventricular block developed transiently: the details on this effect will be reported elsewhere.[17] During oral administration, lethargy, weakness, and fatigue developed in four patients and there was depres-

TABLE 2
Effects of long-term sotalol therapy on spontaneous ventricular arrhythmias in patients with life-threatening ventricular tachyarrhythmias: relation to effect on induction of tachycardia and clinical outcome

Patient	PVC/hr		Paired PVC's/24 hr		VT/24 hr		Dose	VT induction		Clinical	Duration of therapy
No.	Control	Sotalol	Control	Sotalol	Control	Sotalol	(mg bid)	Control	Sotalol	outcome	(months)
1	49	83	20	22	12	0	320	yes	yes	VT recurrence; given Am	0.3
2	311	402	76	120	54	37	160	yes	yes	VT recurrence; given Am	0.4
3	1138	1347	NA	1678	208	1982	320	yes	no	Arrhythmia aggravation? well on Am	1
4	514	421	1260	666	1343	59	320	yes	no	VT recurrence; given Am	8.4
5	272	52	1518	68	88	3	320	yes	yes[A]	Arrhythmia free; no side effects	4
6	1858	807	954	4417	1226	58	160	yes	yes	VT recurrence; well on Am	0.2
7	201	54	226	16	25	0	320	yes	yes[A]	Sotalol discontinued; severe bradycardia Am	0.2
8	320	77	1034	82	210	12	480	yes	yes	VT recurrence; given Am	0.4
9	53	9	2	0	0	0	160	yes	yes[A]	Arrhythmia free; no side effect	9
10	589	88	1842	186	1229	69	480	yes	no	Arrhythmia free; no side effect	6
11	84	12	220	6	46	0	160	yes	no	Sotalol discontinued; aggravation of CHF Am	0.8
12	336	44	682	18	34	0	320	yes	no	Arrhythmia free; no side effects	0.6
13	84	9	146	0	3	0	160	yes	yes[A]	VT recurrence; death on flecainide	1.3
14	710	74	520	VF	24	VF	160	yes	yes	Sotalol discontinued; death on Am	0.2
15	542	40	2296	10	293	0	320	yes	no	Arrhythmia free; no side effects	12
16	596	42	972	28	189	4	320	yes	no	Arrhythmia free; no side effects	21
17	148	9	40	0	12	0	160	yes	no	Arrhythmia free; no side effects	19
18	1088	58	3548	3	576	0	320	yes	yes	Arrhythmia free; no side effects	9
19	40	1	8	0	0	0	160	yes	no	Arrhythmia free; no side effects	7
20	916	3	3270	0	13123	0	320	yes	no	VT recurrence; well on Am	9
21	309	.5	6	0	2995	0	160	yes	no	Sotalol discontinued; β-blocking side effects	1.4
Mean	484	179	1893	202	2947	430					
± SD	446	323	1291	417	1242	118					
p value[B]	< .01		< .001		< .001						

VT = ventricular tachycardia; Am = amiodarone; CHF = congestive heart failure.
[A]Conversion of sustained VT to nonsustained VT.
[B]The level of significance refers to the difference between control and sotalol periods.

TABLE 3
Clinical outcome in patients in whom baseline Holter recordings showed infrequent spontaneous ventricular arrhythmia or could not be obtained

Patient No.	VT induction: Control	VT induction: Sotalol	Therapy with sotalol	Clinical outcome
22	yes	no	Oral sotalol (160 mg bid)	Arrhythmia free; no side effects at 23 months
23	yes	no	Oral sotalol (160 mg bid)	Arrhythmia free; no side effects at 22 months
24	yes	no	Oral sotalol (160 mg bid)	Recurrence of VT/VF; sotalol discontinued; on Am
25[A]	No EP study		Given iv sotalol to control recurrence of VF resistant to bretylium, lidocaine, and procainamide	Arrhythmia controlled by sotalol but death occurred due to brain damage
26	No EP study		Recurrent VT treated successfully by iv sotalol	Death occurred from subsequent acute infarction
27	yes	no	10 days (oral therapy)	On Am; alive and well, sotalol discontinued due to side effects
28	yes	yes	—	On Am; alive and well
29	yes	yes	—	On Am; alive and well
30	yes	yes	—	On Am; alive and well
31	yes	yes	—	On Am; alive and well
32	yes	yes	—	On Am; alive and well
33	yes	yes	—	On Am; alive and well
34	yes	yes	—	On Am; alive and well Am failed; had surgery with successful outcome
35	yes	yes	—	Died suddenly on Am

VF = ventricular fibrillation; all other abbreviations are as in table 2.
[A]Patient had coronary artery disease and previous myocardial infarction with a left ventricular ejection fraction of 26%. He had over 100 episodes of fibrillation in the cardiac care unit before he was given sotalol. The possibility that the recurrence of fibrillation was caused by antiarrhythmic drugs was ruled out.

sion in one, aggravation of heart failure in one, severe bradycardia in two, decreased libido and impotence in two, and dry mouth in one patient. In four patients, the side effects were sufficiently severe to necessitate discontinuation of drug therapy. The left ventricular ejection fraction determined by radionuclide ventriculography in 10 patients before oral sotalol was given was 33.1 ± 14.0% (range 11.0% to 55.0%); on sotalol it was 42.6 ± 16.0% (range 17% to 46%).

Summary of overall clinical outcome. Thirty-three patients who had inducible ventricular tachycardia during the control period were followed to determine clinical outcome. Of the 33 patients, 25 (15 with positive results of electrophysiologic tests; 10 with negative results) were given oral sotalol. Arrhythmia was aggravated early in one (3.8%) and in seven (26.9%) the drug was not effective during the dose adjustment period (over the first month). In four patients the drug was withdrawn because of side effects (three early and one late); late occurrence of the arrhythmia supervened in two (7.7%). Eleven patients (42.3%) currently continue on oral sotalol without significant side effects or recurrence of arrhythmia over a mean follow-up period of 9.2 ± 8.6 months.

Of the 22 patients who were either not initially given oral sotalol (n = 8) or did not respond to or tolerate sotalol (n = 14), one was subsequently treated with flecainide and 21 were given amiodarone in the manner previously described.[18] The patient given flecainide developed incessant VT/VF in-hospital and could not be resuscitated. In the remaining patients, during a minimum follow-up period of 6 months, there have been two cases of sudden death. Another patient failed to respond to amiodarone and underwent successful surgical treatment for his ventricular tachycardia. Eighteen patients continue to be treated with amiodarone and remain free of arrhythmias and limiting side effects.

Discussion

Although the β-blocking properties of sotalol have been recognized for about two decades, interest in its clinical antiarrhythmic actions resulting from its non–β-blocking activity has been relatively re-

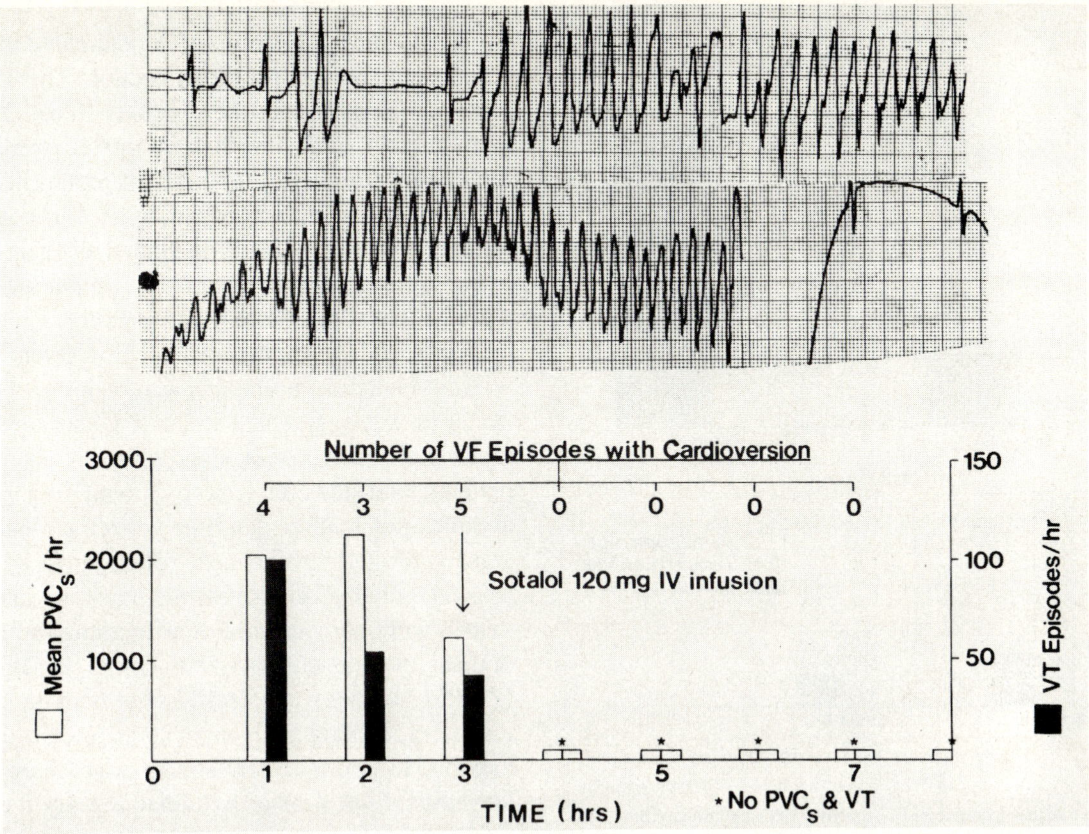

FIGURE 2. Effects of intravenous sotalol in a patient with recurrent VT/VF resistant to lidocaine, procainamide and bretylium. *Top*, The characteristic patterns of incessant ventricular tachyarrhythmias uncontrolled by conventional antiarrhythmic therapy. *Bottom*, The changes in the total PVC count and number of episodes of ventricular tachycardia before and after the intravenous injection of sotalol. Note that after sotalol was given, there were no further recurrences of VT/VF.

cent.[2, 4, 12–14, 19] It has followed in the wake of reports that have demonstrated the unusually potent actions of amiodarone, a drug that is thought to act, at least in part, by lengthening cardiac repolarization. This prolongation of the action potential duration and the corresponding increase in refractoriness is also produced by sotalol.[5–9] Thus, there has always been a sound theoretical basis for significant electrophysiologic and antiarrhythmic actions of sotalol in man. In recent years, there have been experimental[20] and clinical reports that have indicated that such effects of sotalol differ from those of conventional β-blocking drugs.[14, 19] Our data clearly establish the broad-spectrum electrophysiologic effects produced by the drug after intravenous administration in man. They also provide further confirmatory evidence of the efficacy of the drug in the control of life-threatening ventricular tachyarrhythmias, both in terms of preventing the inducibility of VT/VF and in suppressing spontaneously occurring arrhythmias documented on baseline Holter recordings.

Electrophysiologic effects. It is now well established that sotalol, unlike other β-adrenergic–blocking drugs,[21] lengthens the duration of the cardiac action potential,[2, 4–9] and hence the QTc interval, of the surface electrocardiogram.[5, 22] The electrophysiologic effects noted in our study in man are consistent with these observations. Our data confirm and extend the earlier clinical reports that the drug significantly lengthens the effective refractory period of all cardiac tissues[2, 4] and, as in patients on long-term amiodarone treatment,[18] it prolongs the monophasic cardiac action potentials as recorded by suction electrodes placed in intracardiac chambers.[7–9] In our studies, the intravenously administered drug increased the ERP more in the atria than in the ventricle. There was also a significant increase in this parameter corresponding to an increase in the QTc interval and the slowing of the ventricular tachycardia cycle length in patients in whom the drug did not prevent the induction of the arrhythmia. The drug had no effect on the HV interval, its depressant effect on conduction being confined to intranodal conduction. Such an aggregate of electrophysiologic effects is not the result of calcium antagonism, inhibition of the myocardial sodium channel, or β-blockade alone. Instead, these effects suggest that

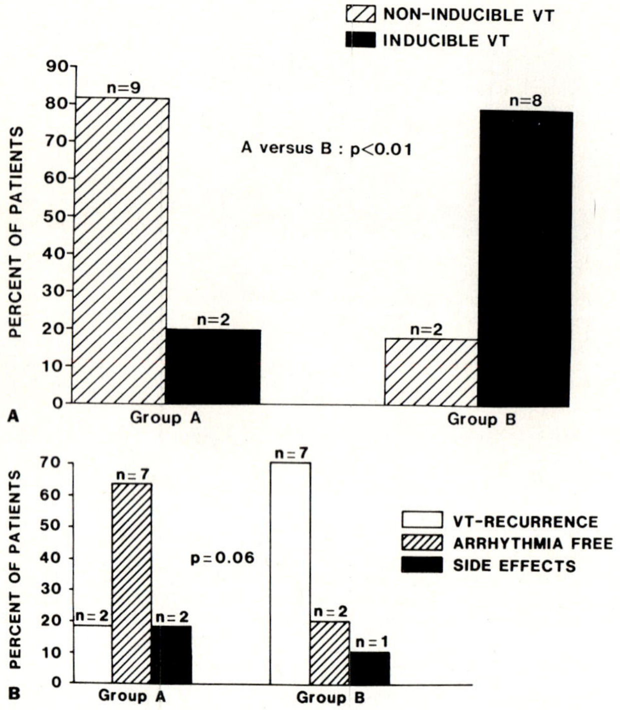

FIGURE 3. *A*, The relationship between the effects of intravenous sotalol on the inducibility of VT/VF and the degree of suppression by the oral drug of the spontaneously occurring ventricular arrhythmias in the same patients. Group A patients: administration of sotalol resulted in 85% suppression of total PVCs and 90% suppression of paired PVCs and beats of ventricular tachycardia. Group B: sotalol did not have these effects. Note that the number of patients in whom sotalol prevented reinduction of VT/VF was significantly higher in group A than in group B. *B*, The differences in the clinical outcome in patients relative to the degree of suppression of spontaneously occurring arrhythmias during Holter monitoring. The separation of patients into groups A and B is by the same criteria as in *A*. The difference between the two groups is of borderline significance. The data presented in this figure suggest that the prevention of inducible VT/VF by intravenous sotalol and the suppression of spontaneously occurring arrhythmias by oral sotalol are both predictive of long-term clinical outcome of prophylactic sotalol therapy in patients with ventricular tachyarrhythmias.

the somewhat unique electrophysiologic properties of the drug are due to the combined effects of β-blockade and the lengthening of the cardiac action potential.

Antiarrhythmic efficacy. In our study,intravenous sotalol prevented the reinduction of VT/VF in 45.5% of the patients, a figure that is generally higher than those reported for the so-called membrane-active or class I compounds.[21] There is little data on this issue for other class III agents, with the exception of amiodarone, which has been reported to prevent reinduction of VT/VF after long-term therapy in 8% to 50%[23] of patients. However, Senges et al.[14] recently showed that in their hands, intravenous sotalol prevented reinduction of VT/VF in 12 of 18 patients (67%), which is a somewhat higher success rate than that in our own series in which VT/VF became noninducible in 15 of 33 patients after intravenous sotalol. The VT/VF of nine of 12 patients in the previous study, who were subsequently treated with oral sotalol over the long term, was completely or partially controlled over a mean follow-up period of 16 months. Our own data on long-term oral therapy is in line with their observations. For example, in 13 of the 15 patients (85.7%) in whom intravenous sotalol had prevented reinduction of VT/VF, early control of arrhythmia was achieved with oral sotalol; in one of the remaining two the arrhythmia was aggravated and in the other there was no effect. Late arrhythmias occurred in only two of the 13 patients, and side effects necessitating drug withdrawal developed in three at a time when their arrhythmias were controlled. Over a mean follow-up of 14.5 (range 6 to 24) months, eight patients have continued to be treated without recurrence of arrhythmias or the development of side effects. Thus, in 11 of 15 patients (73.3%), sotalol was effective over both the short and long term, although only eight could tolerate long-term therapy. In contrast, oral sotalol was effective in the long-term control of arrhythmias in only three of 10 (30%) of those in whom the intravenous drug had failed to prevent induction of VT/VF. Although the number of patients in our series has been limited, there appears to be a trend indicating the clinical utility of electrophysiologic testing in predicting long-term effectiveness of oral sotalol in controlling VT/VF. Our data, as well as those of Senges et al.,[14] have dealt with the predictive value of the response to intravenous sotalol and do not exclude the possibility that a greater predictive accuracy with respect to the inducibility of VT/VF might be attained by the use of oral drug testing.

Our data also demonstrate that orally administered sotalol is moderately effective in suppressing PVCs, particularly complex and repetitive forms. In over 50% of patients, the drug was found to suppress at least 85% of total PVC counts and nearly abolish complex forms (paired PVCs and tachycardia beats), a feature that was concordant with drug-induced prevention of induction of VT/VF by PES of the heart when evaluated in the same patients (table 2 and figure 3). Furthermore, 70% of the patients in whom sotalol was found to be effective in suppressing spontaneously occurring ventricular arrhythmias on Holter recordings have continued to do well clinically and to remain free of their arrhythmias. In contrast, only 20% of the patients in whom sotalol did not suppress PVCs on Holter recordings remained free of arrhythmias; the remaining 70% had recurrence of arrhythmias or side effects. It was noteworthy that no systematic relationship could be established between the magnitude of heart rate reduction and the degree of PVC suppression induced by sotalol. However, the reduction in resting heart rate is a crude index of β-blockade and the contribution of β-antagonism to the observed suppression of PVCs by sotalol cannot be excluded as a possibility. A comparison of the effects of sotalol demonstrated here with those of conventional β-blockers[21] nevertheless suggests that the major antiarrhythmic effects of the drug in patients with life-threatening VT/VF might be mediated through its nonadrenergic properties. Further resolution of this issue is likely to be accomplished by a direct comparison of the antiarrhythmic effects of the dextroisomer of the compound with those of the racemate.

Our study was not specifically designed to compare the relative merits of the techniques of prevention of inducible VT/VF by PES and of suppression of spontaneously occurring arrhythmias in predicting the outcome of long-term drug therapy of ventricular arrhythmias. However, our limited data on sotalol suggest that both techniques may be equally effective in this regard. The data thus raise the possibility that the removal of the "trigger" for the initiation of VT/VF may be a significant mechanism by which this drug exerts its salutary antiarrhythmic actions in patients with life-threatening ventricular arrhythmias.

Arrhythmogenicity and other adverse reactions. Previous reports have suggested that torsade de pointes in association with QTc prolongation may complicate the course of sotalol therapy.[24–28] However, most such cases have occurred in the context of drug overdose or of significant hypokalemia. Neither in our series nor in that of Senges et al.[14] was torsade de pointes encountered. In one of our patients, there was a marked increase in the frequency of all categories of PVCs and nonsustained runs of ventricular tachycardia. Fibrillation in another patient who had previously experienced this arrhythmia while on sotalol was documented.

The remainder of the side effects noted in our study, as in those of Senges et al.,[14] could be attributed to β-blockade, but it is noteworthy that heart failure was exacerbated in only one patient despite the mean low ventricular ejection fraction in the group given oral sotalol. This is in line with the report by Brooks et al.,[29] who showed that the intravenous drug, unlike other β-blockers, had little or no depressant effect on systemic hemodynamics in patients with heart failure. It would therefore appear that lengthening of the action potential duration induced by the drug augments contractility, a phenomenon that has been demonstrated in isolated cardiac muscle.[5, 30] Such an effect may, in part, offset the depressant effect of β-blockade in the patient with cardiac decompensation, a feature that distinguishes sotalol from conventional β-blocking drugs.

In summary, our data show that sotalol is an effective antiarrhythmic compound for a significant number of patients with life-threatening VT/VF refractory to conventional antiarrhythmic drugs. Our preliminary data suggest that sotalol has a lower order of potency than amiodarone, another class III antiarrhythmic drug, but that it has a more predictable side effect profile. Sotalol appears to have low arrhythmogenic potential and since it has a rapid onset of action with a predictable long-term outcome, as determined by electrophysiologic testing after intravenous administration, it appears to represent a significant advance in the short-term and prophylactic management of ventricular tachyarrhythmias.

We are indebted to Lawrence Kimble for secretarial assistance and to Earle Lockhart, M.D., for advice and encouragement during the early stages of this study. We are grateful to Cindy Ansbro, R.N., for her help, support, and for data collation, and to Dr. M. Bartek and Dr. J. A. La Budde (of Bristol-Myers) for serum drug determinations. The assistance of the Medical Media for illustrations and photography is acknowledged. This study would not have been possible without the help of the cardiac catheterization and electrophysiology laboratories.

References

1. Lish PM, Weikel JH, Dungan KW: Pharmacological and toxicological properties of two new beta-adrenergic receptor antagonists. J Pharmacol Exp Ther **149:** 161, 1965
2. Ward DE, Camm AJ, Spurrell RAJ: The acute cardiac electrophysiological effects of intravenous sotalol hydrochloride. Clin Cardiol **2:** 185, 1979
3. Julian DG, Jackson FS, Prescott RJ, Szekely P: Controlled trial of sotalol for one year after myocardial infarction. Lancet **2:** 1142, 1982
4. Nathan W, Hellestrand KJ, Bextan RS, Ward DE, Spurrell RAJ, Camm AJ: Electrophysiological effects of sotalol — just another beta-blocker? Br Heart J **47:** 515, 1982
5. Singh BN, Vaughan Williams EM: A third class of anti-arrhythmic action: effects on atrial and ventricular intracellular potentials, and other pharmacologic actions on cardiac muscle, of MJ 1999 and AH 3474. Br J Pharmacol **39:** 675, 1970
6. Strauss HC, Bigger JT, Hoffman BF: Electrophysiological and beta-receptor blocking effects of MJ 1999 on dog and rabbit cardiac tissue. Circ Res **26:** 661, 1970
7. Edvardsson N, Hirsch I, Emanuelsson H, Ponten J, Olsson SB: Sotalol-induced delayed ventricular repolarization in man. Eur Heart J **1:** 335, 1980
8. Edvardsson N, Olsson SB: Effects of acute and chronic beta-receptor blockade on ventricular repolarisation in man. Br Heart J **45:** 628, 1981
9. Echt DS, Bert LE, Clusin WT, Samuelsson RG, Harrison DC, Mason JW: Prolongation of the human cardiac monophasic action potential by sotalol. Am J Cardiol **50:** 1088, 1982
10. Prakash R, Parmley WW, Allen HN, Matloff JM: Effect of sotalol on clinical arrhythmias. Am J Cardiol **29:** 397, 1972
11. Fogelman F, Lightman SL, Sillett RW, McNicol MW: The treatment of cardiac arrhythmias with sotalol. Eur J Clin Pharmacol **5:** 72, 1972

12. Simon A, Berman E: Long-term sotalol therapy in patients with arrhythmias. J Clin Pharmacol **19:** 547, 1979
13. Myburgh DP, Goldman AP, Cartoon J, Schamroth JM: The efficacy of sotalol in suppressing ventricular ectopic beats. Afr Med J **56:** 295, 1979
14. Senges J, Lengfelder W, Jauernig R, Czyfan E, Brachmann J, Rizos I, Cobbe S, Kubler W: Electrophysiologic testing of therapy with sotalol for sustained ventricular tachycardia. Circulation **69:** 577, 1984
15. Durrer D, Schoo L, Schuilenburg RM, Wellens HJJ: The role of premature beats in the initiation and termination of supraventricular tachycardia in the Wolff-Parkinson-White Syndrome. Circulation **36:** 644, 1967
16. Karkkainen S. Neuvonen PJ: Effects of oral charcoal and urine pH on sotalol pharmacokinetics. Int J Clin Pharmacol Ther Toxicol **22:** 441, 1984
17. Nademanee K, Feld G, Noll E, Hendrickson JA, Singh BN: Effect of sotalol, class III antiarrhythmic agent, on conduction and refractoriness of the His Purkinje system in man. J Am Coll Cardiol **5:** 438, 1985
18. Nademanee K, Singh BN, Hendrickson J, Intarachot V, Lopez B, Feld G, Cannom DS, Weiss JN: Amiodarone in refractory life-threatening ventricular arrhythmias. Ann Intern Med **98:** 577, 1983
19. Rizos I, Senges J, Jauernig R, Lengfelder W, Czygan E, Brachmann J, Kubler W: Differential effects of sotalol and metoprolol on induction of paroxysmal supraventricular tachycardia. Am J Cardiol **53:** 1022, 1984
20. Cobbe SM, Hoffman E, Ritzenhoff A, Brachmann J, Kubler W, Senges J: Action of sotalol on potential re-entrant pathways and ventricular tachyarrhythmias in conscious dogs in the late postmyocardial infarction phase. Circulation **68:** 865, 1983
21. Horowitz LN, Josephson ME, Kastor JA: Intracardiac electrophysiologic studies as a method for the optimization of drug therapy in chronic ventricular arrhythmia. Prog Cardiovasc Dis **23:** 81, 1980
22. Castro M, DesCamps R, Thomas JA: Electrocardiographic changes after long-term treatment with sotalol in hypertensive patients. Int J Clin Pharmacol Toxicol **20:** 88, 1982
23. Horowitz LN, Spielman SR, Greenspan AM, Webb CR, Kay HR: Ventricular arrhythmias: Use of electrophysiologic studies. Am Heart J **106:** 881, 1983
24. Laakso M, Pentikainen PH, Lampainen E: Sotalol, Prolonged Q-T interval, and ventricular tachyarrhythmias. Ann Clin Res **13:** 439, 1981
25. Laakso M, Pentikainen PH, Pyorola K, Neuvonen PJ: Prolongation of the Q-T interval caused by sotalol-possible association with ventricular tachyarrhythmias. Eur Heart J **2:** 355, 1981
26. Nauvonen PH, Elonen E, Tanskanen A, Tuomilehto J: Sotalol prolongation of the QTc interval in hypertensive patients. Clin Pharmacol Ther **32:** 25, 1982
27. Neuvonen PJ, Elonen E, Vuorenmaa T, Laakso M: Prolonged Q-T interval and ventricular tachyarrhythmias; common features of sotalol intoxication. Eur J Clin Pharmacol **20:** 85, 1981
28. McKibben JK, Pocock WA, Barlow JB, Miller RNS, Obel IWP: Sotalol, hypokalemia, syncope and torsade de pointes. Br Heart J **51:** 157, 1984
29. Brooks H, Banas J, Meister S, Szues M, Dalen J, Dexter L: Sotalol-induced beta-blockade in cardiac patients. Circulation **42:** 99, 1970
30. Kaumann AJ, Olson CB: Temporal relationship between longlasting aftercontractions and action potentials in cat papillary muscles. Science **163:** 293, 1968.

Metabolic fate of radioiodinated heptadecanoic acid in the normal canine heart

FRANS C. VISSER, M.D., MACHIEL J. VAN EENIGE, PH.D., GERRIT WESTERA, PH.D., WIM DEN HOLLANDER, PH.D., CASPAR M. B. DUWEL, M.D., ERNST E. VAN DER WALL, M.D., GUIDO A. K. HEIDENDAL, M.D., AND JAN P. ROOS, M.D.

ABSTRACT To clarify the metabolic fate of radioiodinated heptadecanoic acid in myocardium, the time course and distribution of the radioactivity over ^{131}I-heptadecanoic acid, free radioiodide, and various lipids (with incorporated iodoheptadecanoic acid) were determined in normal canine myocardium. In 10 dogs seven biopsy specimens were taken over 30 min after injection of ^{131}I-heptadecanoic acid. The radioactivity in the specimens increased until the fifth minute and decreased thereafter, with a half-time of 36 min. In the fifth minute, 61% of the radioactiviy was free iodide, and its curve paralleled the curve of the total radioactivity. As early as the first minute ^{131}I-heptadecanoic acid activity was reduced to 14% and decreased further. Activity of radioiodinated phospholipids, (mono, di, tri)-glycerides, and cholesterol-esters remained constant after an initial increase. These results indicate that immediately after uptake, ^{131}I-heptadecanoic acid is either metabolized, liberating the radioiodide, or stored in lipids. Because the activity of radiolabeled lipids remained constant during the study period and because iodide activity paralleled the total activity in biopsy specimens, it is concluded that in normal myocardium, washout of free radioiodide determines the elimination rate as observed during a scintigraphic study. Thus the elimination rate cannot be related to the β-oxidation rate as previously supposed.
Circulation 72, No. 3, 565–571, 1985.

THE HEART uses a variety of substances like glucose, free fatty acids, and lactate as an energy source for its metabolism. Under normal physiologic conditions, 60% to 80% of energy-rich phosphate bonds are derived from oxidation of long-chain free fatty acids.[1–7] Therefore long-chain free fatty acids labeled with a radioisotope were proposed as indicators of cardiac metabolism in vivo. One of these radiolabeled free fatty acids was heptadecanoic acid (HDA) labeled with ^{123}I in the omega position.

It was found that after administration of radiolabeled HDA, regional elimination of the radioactivity differed under various pathophysiologic conditions of the myocardium. In ischemic myocardium the elimination rate was found to be lower than that in comparable normal myocardium.[8–10] In some patients with a recently sustained infarction, a higher elimination rate was found.[11] Patients with congestive cardiomyopathy showed a diffuse, inhomogeneous pattern of elimination.[12] The rate of elimination was also influenced by simultaneous administration of glucose and insulin.[13] These results suggested a potential use of radioiodinated HDA as metabolic tracer.

Two hypotheses have been developed to explain the observed differences in elimination rates. Both hypotheses are related to cardiac metabolism of radioiodinated free fatty acids. After uptake in the myocyte, radioiodinated long-chain free fatty acids are degraded by β-oxidation[14] in the mitochondria. Radioiodine is split off and leaves the cell.

In the first hypothesis the elimination rate is related to the β-oxidation rate of the radioiodinated fatty acids[15] in the mitochondria. In the second hypothesis the elimination rate is related to the diffusion rate of radioiodide from the myocardial mitochondria into the systemic circulation.[16]

Because knowledge of the underlying mechanism is important for interpretation of scintigraphic data, this study was undertaken to ascertain which of the two hypotheses is correct. From normal canine myocardi-

From the Departments of Cardiology and Nuclear Medicine, Free University Hospital, Amsterdam, The Netherlands, and Abteilung Nuklearmedizin, Universitätsspital, Zürich, Switzerland.

Address for correspondence: F. C. Visser, M.D., Department of Cardiology, Free University Hospital, De Boelelaan 1117, 1007 MB Amsterdam, The Netherlands.

Received July 10, 1984; revision accepted May 16, 1985.

um serial biopsy specimens were taken after administration of ^{131}I-HDA. Distribution of the radioactivity over ^{131}I-HDA, over its metabolite free radioiodide, and over various lipids was measured in these specimens.

Materials and methods

Preparation of ^{131}I-HDA. ^{131}I-HDA was prepared by nonisotopic halogen exchange, with 17-bromo-HDA as the parent compound.[17] ^{131}I-HDA was dissolved in a minimal volume of ethanol and diluted with physiologic saline and 20% human serum albumin. After purification over Sephadex A25 the final solution contained less than 5% ethanol.

Animal experiments. Ten mongrel dogs (22 to 36 kg) were studied after 24 hr of fasting. After premedication with atropine (0.5 mg), droperidol (5 mg), and fentanyl (0.1 mg), dogs were anesthetized with sodium pentobarbital (30 mg/kg iv). After intubation, pulmonary ventilation was maintained with a Pulmonat positive-pressure respirator. Two different types of anesthesia were used: In dogs 1 to 6 anesthesia was maintained with nitrous oxide and oxygen in combination with 2% trifluoroethane. Because of low blood pressure, anesthesia in dogs 7 to 10 was maintained with nitrous oxide, oxygen, and 0.2% to 0.4% halothane in combination with fentanyl. Except for the anesthesia, all experimental conditions were the same in both groups.

A polyethylene catheter was placed in a carotid artery. Under fluoroscopy a second catheter was placed through a jugular vein into the coronary sinus. Catheters were used for pressure recording and blood sampling. Electrocardiograms were monitored continuously.

The chest was opened by an incision through the fifth left intercostal space. The pericardium was opened widely and fixed to the chest to form a pericardial cradle. Three to 10 mCi (111 to 370 MBq) ^{131}I-HDA was rapidly injected into the left atrium. Serial biopsy specimens were taken from the myocardial area perfused by the anterior descending branch of the left coronary artery. With a fast-spinning hollow needle (bore of 2.4 mm), cylindrical biopsy specimens were obtained, ranging in length between 5 and 15 mm. Mean weight of the specimens was 48 ± 18 mg (n = 66). Specimens were taken at 1, 2, 3, 5, 10, 20, and 30 min after injection of the ^{131}I-HDA and immediately stored in liquid nitrogen. At the same time 2 ml blood samples were drawn from the arterial and coronary sinus catheters. The blood samples were stored in melting ice.

Myocardial biopsy. Samples were allowed to thaw at 6°C and were blotted free of blood, weighed, and refrozen in liquid nitrogen. Thereafter samples were counted for 1 min in a gamma well counter (LKB Ultrogamma 1280) with a suitable window setting for the isotope. After counting, specimens were refrozen in liquid nitrogen.

The specimens were ground in a mortar. One milliliter of a mixture of methanol and chloroform 1/2 v/v[18] was added during pulverization. After addition of a sufficient amount of HCl to keep the medium acidic and 1 ml of 40% urea, samples were centrifuged at 2000 rpm, 4°C, for 10 min. Three fractions were obtained: an aqueous fraction containing the free radioiodide,[19] a pellet, and an organic fraction containing ^{131}I-HDA and various radioiodinated lipids. The solvent of the organic fraction was evaporated under a stream of nitrogen until a volume of about 200 μl was left. To separate the various lipid fractions, thin-layer chromatography was performed over silica gel (Merck 60 F-254 Alufolien) with hexane/ether/acetic acid (80/20/1 v/v) as the solvent.[20] On the chromatography plates, ^{131}I-HDA and radioiodinated triglycerides were identified by comparison with standards under fluorescence after spraying with di-chloro fluorescein (30 mg/10 ml ethanol). The other lipid fractions were identified by R_f values (^{131}I-phospholipids, 0.0; ^{131}I-HDA, 0.5; radioiodinated [mono, di, tri]-glycerides, between 0.7 and 0.9; ^{131}I-cholesterol-esters, 0.95). All bands were isolated by cutting the chromatography plates in appropriate strips. The separate chromatography strips, the pellet, and the aqueous fraction were counted in the gamma well counter and corrected for decay. Counting time was 3 min.

Blood samples. After centrifugation, 200 μl of plasma was eluted over Sephadex A25, separating free radioiodide from ^{131}I-HDA. Total plasma activity, the Sephadex column containing the free ^{131}I, plasma containing the ^{131}I-HDA, chromatography strips, and the aqueous fraction of the myocardial biopsy specimens were counted in one counting series.

Data analysis. Biopsy count rates were expressed as counts per minute (cpm) per milligram. The fractions of radioiodinated HDA, free iodide, phospholipids, (mono, di, tri)-glycerides, and cholesterol-esters were expressed as a percentage of the total activity of a specimen obtained before pulverization.

To determine the time course of radiolabeled components, count rates of biopsy specimens and fractions were also expressed as a percentage of the activity of the specimen with the highest count rate.

Both arterial and coronary sinus plasma activity was expressed as a percentage of the arterial plasma sample with the highest count rate in a dog. In all dogs the arterial sample with the highest count rate was obtained at the first minute after injection of ^{131}I-HDA.

For slight differences in sampling time of biopsy specimens and blood samples, interpolation was applied: a linear curve was fitted between two count rate data of adjacent sampling times. The count rates on the exact sampling moment as mentioned above was calculated from this linear curve.

Scintigraphic study. In three dogs (Nos. 7, 8, and 10) a mobile gamma camera (Elscint Dymax MB) with a medium energy collimator was placed under the chest and scintigraphy was performed over 30 min. One minute frames were obtained in a matrix of 64 × 64 pixels. A region of interest was drawn over the myocardial area and the time-activity curve was displayed. Background correction for circulating free iodide in blood was performed as described previously[21] between the fifth and thirtieth frame. In short, correction is based on subtraction of a constant background value from the myocardial count rates. The background activity in a myocardial region to be subtracted is determined by extrapolating a monoexponential curve through the myocardial time-activity curve and subtracting the calculated value at 60 min uniformly from the uncorrected curve. A monoexponential curve is fitted through the corrected count rates and half-time values are derived. This background procedure was validated by comparing the results of intravenous and intracoronary studies.[22] The corrected time-activity curve and the course of the radioactivity in biopsy specimens were compared.

Results

Before myocardial biopsy specimens were taken, systolic blood pressure in dogs 1 to 6 was 82 ± 14 mm Hg and diastolic blood pressure was 60 ± 13 mm Hg. At the end of the experiment, systolic and diastolic blood pressures were 75 ± 15 and 54 ± 16 mm Hg, respectively. Heart rate increased from 137 ± 13 to 145 ± 28 beats/min. In dogs 7 to 10 initial systolic blood pressure was 102 ± 5 mm Hg and diastolic blood pressure was 70 ± 5 mm Hg. At the end of the study, systolic and diastolic blood pressures were 98 ± 7 and 63 ± 6 mm Hg, respectively. Heart rate increased from 103 ± 34 to 124 ± 20 beats/min.

Myocardial biopsy. During pulverization and analysis, an average of 13% of the radioactivity was lost. Tables 1 to 3 show the radioactivity data in myocardial biopsy specimens and the distribution of the radioactivity originating from ^{131}I-HDA, free ^{131}I, and the various radioiodinated lipids. Although anesthesia and blood pressure differed between dogs 1 to 6 and 7 to 10, no difference in the course of radioactivity was observed and all data are presented together. ^{131}I-HDA activity decreased from 19.7% in the first minute to 4.2% at 30 min. The relative contribution of radioiodide, radiolabeled phospholipids, and cholesterol-esters remained constant during the study. Activity of ^{131}I-glycerides increased from 6.8% to 16%.

Table 4 and figure 1 show the mean biopsy data expressed as a percentage of the specimen with the highest count rate. After injection of ^{131}I-HDA, total count rates of the biopsy specimens increased until the fifth minute; thereafter a decrease was observed. Half-time calculated by linear regression analysis of semilogarithmic plots from the fifth until the thirtieth minute was 36 min.

Of the analyzed metabolites, free ^{131}I contributed most to the curve of the total count rate, running parallel to this curve. The half-time of radioiodide calculated the same way as for total radioactivity was 25 min. As early as the first minute after administration, ^{131}I-HDA activity had decreased to 13.5% of total radioactivity and diminished rapidly thereafter. Cholesterol-esters remained a negligible fraction throughout the study, accounting for less than 1% of the radioactivity. After an initial increase during the first minutes, activity of phospholipids and glycerides remained constant during the study, reaching maximal values of 19% and 13%, respectively.

TABLE 1
Total count rates (cpm/mg) in myocardial biopsy specimens

	Time (min)						
Dog	1	2	3	5	10	20	30
1	—	—	704	737	520	392	—
2	2689	2802	3512	3829	3107	2363	—
3	753	868	1041	1086	1041	971	922
4	1819	2018	1993	2254	2208	1930	1752
5	1931	2520	2445	2672	2345	1632	1343
6	2763	3358	3558	3959	4058	3261	3079
7	373	533	537	462	522	399	209
8	688	793	821	448	642	536	428
9	477	1530	1322	1358	923	736	529
10	492	501	462	599	563	488	402

TABLE 2
Free radioiodide (percentage of total count rate of a biopsy specimen)

	Time (min)						
Dog	1	2	3	5	10	20	30
1	—	—	75.5	70.3	58.6	48.4	—
2	85.9	84.0	87.4	91.4	95.9	87.3	—
3	42.5	29.5	32.0	39.6	36.9	25.4	42.1
4	50.7	64.5	66.2	61.9	54.6	45.5	32.7
5	77.2	82.1	80.1	75.9	63.8	59.7	54.5
6	65.3	72.2	70.5	67.1	59.7	49.0	71.6
7	55.4	40.2	59.2	71.9	46.3	72.2	76.8
8	72.1	81.5	69.3	49.7	56.5	38.8	80.6
9	48.0	44.0	54.6	70.5	51.0	48.9	63.4
10	30.1	50.1	44.9	71.0	70.8	66.7	47.5
Mean	58.6	60.9	64.0	66.9	59.4	54.2	58.6
SD	17.9	20.5	16.7	14.2	15.8	17.8	17.3

Blood analysis. In the first 10 min, both arterial and coronary sinus plasma activity decreased rapidly. Thereafter a plateau phase was reached (table 5 and figure 2). In the first minutes, the major component in plasma was ^{131}I-HDA, which then fell rapidly to low levels. The half-time of arterial ^{131}I-HDA was 2.1 min. After 30 min almost 90% of the radioactivity in plasma was radioiodide.

Figure 3 shows the averaged extraction fraction of ^{131}I-HDA on a sample-by-sample basis. The extraction fraction decreased significantly from 43 ± 8% in the first minute to 30 ± 13% at the tenth minute ($p < .01$, Student's t test for unpaired data). At 20 min ^{131}I-HDA activity in blood was too low for reliable calculation of the extraction fraction.

The ratio of free iodide activity in biopsy specimens vs blood was 9.2 ± 5.4 at 5 min and 3.6 ± 1.9 at 30 min after administration of ^{131}I-HDA.

Scintigraphy. In figure 4 the course of radioactivity in biopsy specimens and the corrected time-activity curve derived from the scintigram are shown. The half-time values of the scintigraphic curve were 20, 21, and 25 min in dogs 7, 8, and 10.

Discussion

Radiolabeled long-chain free fatty acids are used as noninvasive indicators of myocardial fatty acid metabolism.[23] Although palmitic acid labeled with an isotope of a natural element has been used successfully to quantify the pathophysiologic state of myocardial metabolism,[24, 25] high costs for production and detection

TABLE 3
^{131}I-Lipids (percentage of total count rate of a biopsy specimen)

	Time (min)						
	1	2	3	5	10	20	30
Phospholipids	14.7	17.9	15.8	16.3	22.1	26.9	20.4
	±5.8	±10.3	±4.8	±7.9	±9.7	±13.7	±14.3
Glycerides	6.8	8.4	11.6	10.7	15.1	15.8	16.0
	±4.7	±8.8	±12.0	±10.0	±10.0	±6.8	±10.6
HDA	19.7	12.5	8.4	5.7	3.0	2.6	4.2
	±15.6	±10.0	±5.8	±3.8	±2.1	±2.7	±5.7
Cholesterol-esters	0.3	0.3	0.2	0.3	0.4	0.6	0.8
	±0.1	±0.2	±0.2	±0.2	±0.3	±0.4	±0.9

Data expressed as mean ± SD.

facilities limit the general use of these positron-emitting nuclides. Radioiodinated HDA was proposed as an alternative. Because iodide structurally resembles a methyl group, biological properties of radioiodinated free fatty acids are almost identical to the natural analogs. Analysis of washout of radioactivity has indicated a metabolic behavior of ^{131}I-HDA.[8–10, 13, 26]

Because of this important concept to measure lipid — and especially oxidative lipid — metabolism noninvasively, the aim of this study was to establish whether the elimination rate of ^{131}I-HDA was specifically related to the rate of oxidation of the fatty acids or to washout of free radioiodide, split off from the carbon chain during β-oxidation.[27]

Analysis of myocardial tissue. Uptake of ^{131}I-HDA in normal myocardium is homogeneous.[17] As seen in tables 1 to 3 and figure 1, total count rates of the biopsy specimens increased until the fifth minute; thereafter radioactivity decreased, with a half-time of 36 min. The increase in the first 5 min was caused by uptake of ^{131}I-HDA from the arterial circulation, since in this period the major part of the blood radioactivity consists of ^{131}I-HDA (figure 2 and table 5).

Analysis of the components of the total activity curve (tables 1 to 4 and figure 1) shows that ^{131}I-HDA activity is less than 14% in the first minute and decreases during the study. Activity of radioiodinated glycerides and phospholipids remains constant after an initial increase during the first 5 min, and cholesterol esters remain a negligible fraction. The major part of the radioactivity consists of free radioiodide, and its curve runs parallel to that of the total radioactivity.

The results indicate that immediately after uptake, ^{131}I-HDA is partly stored in lipids — mainly phospholipids and glycerides — or is oxidized, during which process iodide is split off.[14] Thus the radioiodinated free fatty acids show behavior similar to that of the natural analogs in terms of distribution into lipid and oxidative pools. When the data are compared with the results of studies with ^{14}C-palmitate,[28] a higher per-

TABLE 4
Count rates and distribution over metabolites (percentage of biopsy specimen with highest count rate)

	Time (min)						
	1	2	3	5	10	20	30
Total	68.6	87.5	89.7	90.8	84.6	68.7	59.2
	±15.7	±9.6	±7.2	±13.9	±13.1	±14.2	±18.5
Free radioiodide	39.7	52.9	56.1	61.1	50.2	36.9	32.4
	±16.1	±18.1	±17.0	±17.7	±14.4	±12.5	±9.1
Phospholipids	11.2	15.9	16.2	14.6	18.8	18.8	13.6
	±6.0	±9.7	±6.0	±6.3	±9.4	±11.8	±16.4
Glycerides	4.1	7.3	10.3	9.8	12.9	11.1	10.7
	±2.1	±7.3	±11.5	±10.0	±9.6	±6.7	±9.4
HDA	13.5	11.1	7.0	5.0	2.3	1.6	2.0
	±13.0	±9.4	±3.8	±3.2	±1.2	±1.3	±1.8
Cholesterol-esters	0.2	0.3	0.2	0.3	0.4	0.4	0.4
	±0.1	±0.2	±0.2	±0.2	±0.3	±0.3	±0.5

Data expressed as mean ± SD.

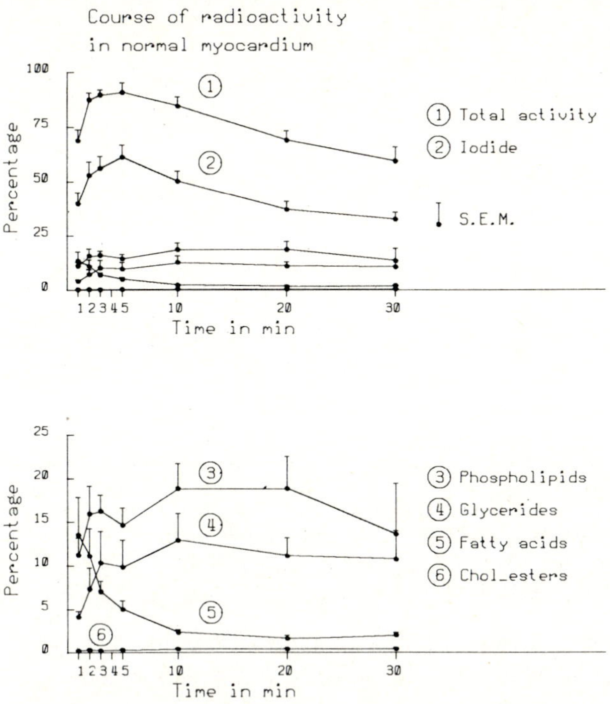

FIGURE 1. Course of radioactivity, normalized to peak count rate (100%), and distribution over ^{131}I-HDA, free radioiodide, and various lipids with incorporated ^{131}I-HDA ([mono,di,tri]-glycerides, phospholipids, and cholesterol-esters).

centage of ^{131}I-HDA activity is recovered in the phospholipid fraction and less in the triglyceride fraction. Although the same observation was made by Bontemps et al.,[29] an acceptable explanation has not been proposed.

Because lipid activity remains constant, the decrease of total myocardial activity is based on the decrease of free radioiodide. Thus it is concluded that in normal myocardium, washout of free radioiodide from the myocyte into the circulation determines the elimination rate as observed during a scintigraphic study.

As a result of release of iodide into the circulation, a high blood activity is built up, possibly interfering with washout of iodide from myocardium. Free iodide activity in biopsy specimens will not be influenced significantly by iodide in blood, as indicated by the iodide specimen-blood ratios of 9.2 and 3.6 at 5 and 30 min, respectively. Furthermore, Machulla et al.[30] found that after intravenous injection of ^{131}I-NaI, activity of free iodide was maximally 10% of free iodide after injection of ^{131}I-HDA.

Relationship between biopsy specimens and scintigraphic results. In three dogs scintigraphy was performed in the same period biopsy specimens were taken. Background-corrected half-time values were slightly higher, as reported previously.[26] Possibly the higher half-time values are related to the prolonged halothane anesthesia.[13] Because of differences in data collection, only a qualitative comparison can be made between biopsy and scintigraphic data. In these dogs the course of total radioactivity from the biopsy specimens is comparable with the time-activity curve.

Based on the results of this study, changes in the scintigraphic elimination rate might be explained by two factors: (1) Alterations in the diffusion rate of free radioiodide might have been caused by alterations in the porosity of mitochondrial and cellular membranes under ischemia or metbolic interventions. (2) In a previous study,[31] the distribution of radioactivity in nor-

TABLE 5
Arterial and coronary sinus plasma activity as a percentage of the first minute arterial sample

	Time (min)						
	1	2	3	5	10	20	30
Arterial							
Total	97.9	63.6	45.5	26.3	13.3	11.7	11.0
	±3.7	±16.0	±12.3	±7.6	±5.6	±4.0	±4.1
^{131}I-HDA	92.4	58.0	38.7	17.5	4.3	1.5	1.4
	±4.9	±15.5	±12.2	±7.2	±2.4	±1.1	±1.1
Free radioiodide	5.5	5.6	6.8	8.8	9.0	10.2	9.6
	±1.9	±2.7	±3.2	±3.5	±3.4	±3.9	±4.0
Coronary sinus							
Total	57.6	45.6	34.3	24.0	15.8	13.6	11.7
	±16.0	±12.6	±8.7	±6.5	±5.7	±5.2	±4.8
^{131}I-HDA	51.4	38.3	24.9	12.1	3.1	1.2	1.2
	±15.6	±12.7	±8.5	±5.8	±2.1	±0.9	±1.0
Free radioiodide	6.2	7.3	9.4	11.9	12.7	12.4	10.5
	±2.6	±3.9	±4.7	±5.7	±5.6	±5.1	±4.8

Data expressed as mean ± SD.

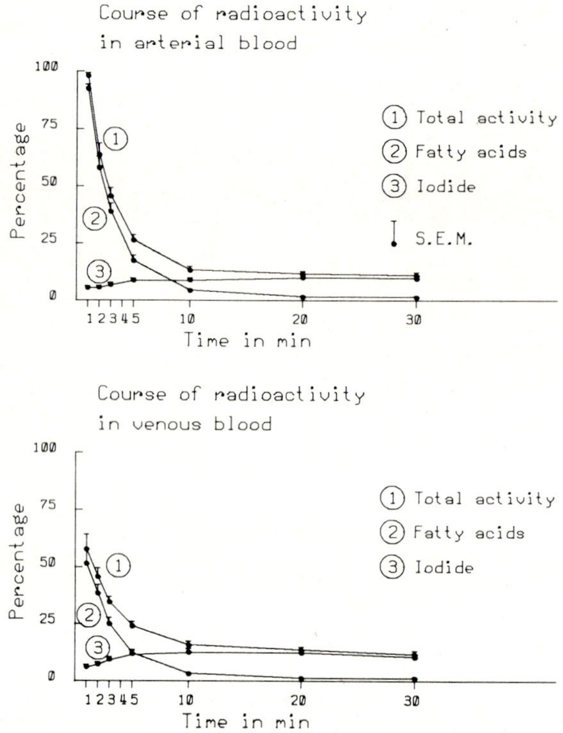

FIGURE 2. Course of radioactivity in arterial and coronary sinus blood after injection of ^{131}I-HDA. Data were normalized to the peak value of arterial blood found in the first minute. The distribution over ^{131}I-HDA and free radioiodide is given.

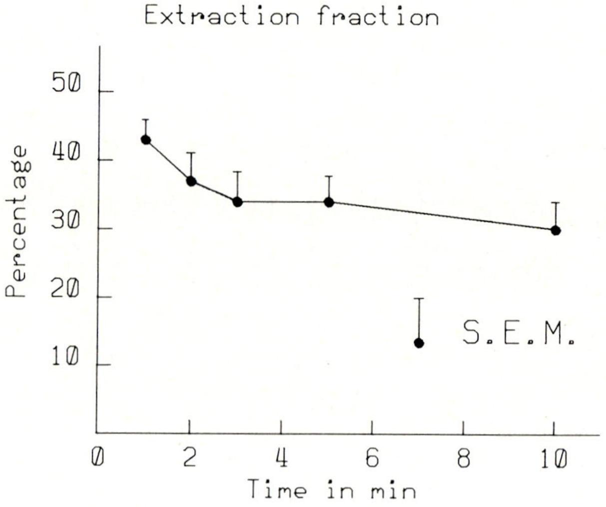

FIGURE 3. Extraction fraction on a sample-by-sample basis in the first 10 min. Extraction fraction = (^{131}I-HDA art. − ^{131}I-HDA cor. sin.)/^{131}I-HDA art.

mal and ischemic canine myocardium was analyzed 5 min after injection of ^{131}I-HDA. In normal myocardium 76% was free iodide, 5% was ^{131}I-HDA, and 19% was radioiodinated lipids. These data are comparable with our results. In contrast, in ischemic myocardium 40% was free iodide, 9% was ^{131}I-HDA, and 51% was radiolabeled lipids, indicating the preferential conversion of ^{131}I-HDA into lipid pools under ischemia. The altered conversion was also observed in rats during infusion of glucose.[32]

Because scintigraphy detects only the total decrease of radioactivity from different compartments, an increased incorporation into slow-turnover lipid pools can also decrease the externally observed elimination rate, even without changes in the elimination rate of various compartments.

Blood analysis. Arterial and venous blood samples showed a rapid decline of the radioactivity caused by uptake of ^{131}I-HDA in various organs (mainly liver). During the study there was a gradual increase of free radioiodide. These data are similar to those of previously published studies.[11, 26, 33]

The extraction fraction of ^{131}I-HDA was calculated from the arterial–coronary sinus difference (figure 4). In the first minute the extraction fraction was 43%, decreasing to 30% in the tenth minute. These extraction fractions are about half the values reported by Poe et al.[33] However, distinctly different methods were used, with the latter calculated by extrapolation of a time-activity curve. Our values are more in line with those reported by Schoen et al.[34] The 13% decrease in extraction fraction during the first 10 min can be explained by back-diffusion of unaltered ^{131}I-HDA into the coronary venous circulation.[35]

Conclusions. ^{131}I-HDA behaves like the natural ana-

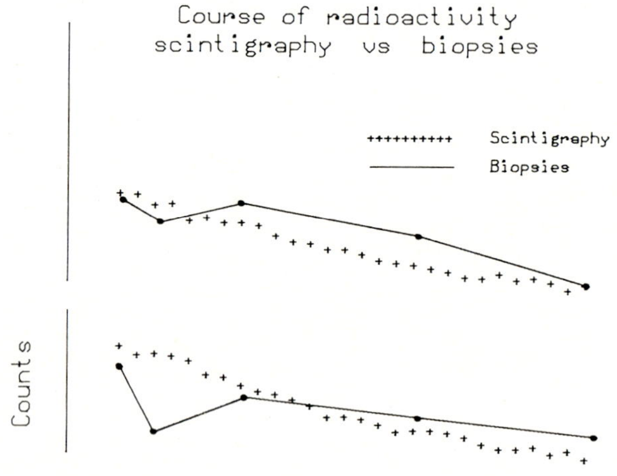

FIGURE 4. Comparison of time-activity curves from biopsy specimens and from simultaneously recorded scintigrams in three dogs. On the linear scale of the ordinate, the counts per minute of the biopsy specimens are plotted against the counts per minute per pixel in the same dog.

logs with regard to distribution. In normal myocardium the elimination rate of the radioactivity is not related to the β-oxidation rate but is governed by diffusion of free radioiodide, being split off during oxidation.

Alterations in elimination as observed during metabolic interventions and ischemia might be explained by a combination of altered conversion into various pools or changes in the diffusion rate of radioiodide, possibly caused by changes in membrane porosity.

We thank Dr. W. Horst, Head, Department of Nuclear Medicine, Universitaetsspital Zürich, for allowing one of us (G.W.) to participate in these experiments. Furthermore, we thank Andries Plu for his skillful technical assistance and Siny Scholtalbers and Margreet Koelemaij for their excellent secretarial assistance.

References

1. Neely JR, Rovetto MJ, Oram JF: Myocardial utilization of carbohydrate and lipids. Prog Cardiovasc Dis **15:** 289, 1972
2. Opie LH: Metabolism of the heart in health and disease. Part 1. Am Heart J **76:** 685, 1968
3. Evans JR: Importance of fatty acid in myocardial metabolism. Circ Res **14**(suppl II): II-96, 1964
4. Goodale WT, Hackel DB: Myocardial carbohydrate metabolism in normal dogs, with effects of hyperglycemia and starvation. Circ Res **1:** 509, 1953
5. Miller HI, Yum KY, Durham BC: Myocardial free fatty acid uptake in unanesthetized dogs at rest and during exercise. J Physiol **220:** 589, 1971
6. Most AS, Brachfeld N, Gorlin R, Wahren J: Free fatty acid metabolism of the human heart at rest. J Clin Invest **48:** 1177, 1969
7. Carlsten A, Hallgren B, Jagenburg R, Svanborg A, Werko L: Myocardial metabolism of glucose, lactic acid, amino acids and fatty acids in healthy human individuals at rest and at different work loads. Scand J Clin Lab Invest **13:** 418, 1961
8. Van der Wall EE, Heidendal GAK, Den Hollander W, Westera G, Roos JP: Metabolic myocardial imaging with I-123 labeled heptadecanoic acid in patients with angina pectoris. Eur J Nucl Med **6:** 391, 1981
9. Dudczak R: Myokardszintigraphie mit Jod-123-markierten Fettsaeuren. Wiener Klin Wochenschr **95:** 1, 1983
10. Vyska K, Freundlieb C, Hoeck A, Feinendegen LE, Machulla HJ, Stoecklin G: Myocardial imaging and measurement of myocardial fatty acid metabolism using omega-I-123-heptadecanoic acid. Adv Clin Cardiol **1:** 422, 1980
11. Van der Wall EE, Den Hollander W, Heidendal GAK, Westera G, Majid PA, Roos JP: Dynamic myocardial scintigraphy with I-123 labeled free fatty acids in patients with myocardial infarction. Eur J Nucl Med **6:** 383, 1981
12. Hoeck A, Freundlieb C, Vyska K, Loesse B, Erbel R, Feinendegen LE: Myocardial imaging and metabolic studies with [17-I-123]iodoheptadecanoic acid in patients with idiopathic congestive cardiomyopathy. J Nucl Med **24:** 22, 1983
13. Dudczak R, Kletter K, Frischauf H, Losert U, Angelberger P, Schmoliner R: The use of I-123-labeled heptadecanoic acid (HDA) as metabolic tracer: preliminary report. Eur J Nucl Med **9:** 81, 1984
14. Chatelain P, Luthy P, Buesslinger B, Moret P, Blaeustein P, Lerch R: Effect of reduced fatty acid metabolism on myocardial I-123 release from I-123-heptadecanoic acid. J Mol Cell Cardiol **16:** P72, 1984
15. Otto CA, Brown LE, Wieland DM, Beierwaltes WH: Radioiodinated fatty acids for myocardial imaging: effects of chain length. J Nucl Med **22:** 613, 1981
16. Kloster G, Stoecklin G, Smith EF, Schroer K: Omega-halofatty acids: a probe for mitochondrial membrane integrity. In vitro investigations in normal and ischaemic myocardium. Eur J Nucl Med **9:** 305, 1984
17. Westera G, Van der Wall EE, Heidendal GAK, Van den Bos GC: A comparison between terminally radioiodinated hexadecenoic acid (I-HA) and Tl-201-thallium chloride in the dog heart: implications for the use of I-HA for myocardial imaging. Eur J Nucl Med **5:** 339, 1980
18. Folch J, Lees M, Stanley GHS: A simple method for the isolation and purification of total lipids from animal tissues. J Biol Chem **226:** 497, 1957
19. Freundlieb C, Hoeck A, Vyska K, Feinendegen LE, Machulla HJ, Stoecklin G: Myocardial imaging and metabolic studies with [17-I-123]iodoheptadecanoic acid. J Nucl Med **21:** 1043, 1980
20. Malins DC, Mangold HK: Analysis of complex lipid mixtures by thin-layer chromatography and complementary methods. J Am Oil Chem Soc **37:** 576, 1960
21. Van Eenige MJ, Visser FC, Lingen van A, Van der Wall EE, Heidendal GAK, Roos JP: Evaluation of background correction methods. Eur Heart J (in press)
22. Visser FC, van Eenige MJ, van der Wall EE, Westera G, van Engelen CJ, van Lingen A, de Cock CC, den Hollander W, Heidendal GAK, Roos JP: The elimination rate of I-123-heptadecanoic acid after intracoronary and intravenous administration. Eur J Nucl Med (in press)
23. Schelbert HR, Henze E, Schoen HR, Keen R, Hansen H, Selin C, Huang SC, Barrio JR, Phelps ME: C-11 palmitate for the noninvasive evaluation of regional myocardial fatty acid metabolism with positron computed tomography. III. In vivo demonstration of the effects of substrate availability on myocardial metabolism. Am Heart J **105:** 492, 1983
24. Schoen HR, Schelbert HR, Robinson G, Najafi A, Huang SC, Hansen H, Barrio J, Kuhl DE, Phelps ME: C-11 labeled palmitic acid for the noninvasive evaluation of regional myocardial fatty acid metabolism with positron-computed tomography. I. Kinetics of C-11 palmitic acid in normal myocardium. Am Heart J **103:** 532, 1982
25. Weiss ES, Hoffman EJ, Phelps ME, Welch MJ, Henry PD, Ter-Pogossian MM, Sobel BE: External detection and visualization of myocardial ischemia with C-11-substrates in vitro and in vivo. Circ Res **39:** 24, 1976
26. Van der Wall EE, Westera G, Den Hollander W, Visser FC: External detection of regional myocardial metabolism with radioiodinated hexadecenoic acid in the dog heart. Eur J Nucl Med **6:** 147, 1981
27. Kloster G, Stoecklin G, Wutz W, Smith EF, Schroer K: Radioiodinated omega-halofatty acids: biochemical investigations in normal and ischemic isolated perfused hearts. *In* Adam WE, editor: Imaging of organ function and metabolism. Heidelberg, 1983, Brausdruck, vol 21, p 138
28. Scheuer J, Brachfeld N: Myocardial uptake and fractional distribution of palmitate-1-C-14 by the ischemic dog heart. Metabolism **15:** 945, 1966
29. Bontemps L, Damaison L, Keriel C, Pernin C, Matthieu JP, Marti-Battle D, Vidal M, Fabret D, Comet M, Cuchet P: Kinetics of (16-123-I) iodohexadecenoic acid metabolism in the rat myocardium, influence of glucose-concentration in the perfusate and comparison with (I 14C) palmitate. Eur Heart J (in press)
30. Machulla HJ, Stoecklin G, Kupfernagel C, Freundlieb C, Hoeck A, Vyska K, Feinendegen LE: Comparative evaluation of fatty acids labeled with C-11, Cl-34m, Br-77 and I-123 for metabolic studies of the myocardium: concise communication. J Nucl Med **19:** 298, 1978
31. Visser FC, Westera G, van Eenige MJ, Van der Wall EE, Den Hollander W, Roos JP: The myocardial elimination rate of radioiodinated heptadecanoic acid. Eur J Nucl Med **10:** 118, 1985
32. Comet M, Pilichowski P, Wolf JE, Busquet G, Dubois F, Mathieu JP, Pernin C, Riche F, Vidal M: Scintigraphie myocardique apres injection i.v. d'acide 15-[I-123] hexadecene 9-oique: etude de l'influence des concentrations plasmatiques des acides gras et du glucose. J Biophys Med Nucl **4:** 151, 1983
33. Poe ND, Robinson GD Jr, Graham LS, MacDonald NS: Experimental basis for myocardial imaging with I-123-labeled hexadecenoic acid. J Nucl Med **17:** 1077, 1976
34. Schoen HR, Senekowitsch R, Berg D, Schneidereith M, Moellenstaedt S, Kriegel H, Pabst HW, Bloemer H: Kinetics of I-123 heptadecanoic acid in normal myocardium. *In* Amsersham, editor: European Nuclear Medicine Congress, Helsinki. Heidelberg, 1984, Brausdruck, p 58
35. Fox KAA: The importance of back-diffusion on myocardial kinetics of C-11-palmitate. J Am Coll Cardiol **3:** 574, 1984

Angle dependence of ultrasonic backscatter in arterial tissues: a study in vitro

EUGENIO PICANO, M.D., LUIGI LANDINI, PH.D., ALESSANDRO DISTANTE, M.D., MARCO SALVADORI, FABIO LATTANZI, M.D., MICHELE MASINI, M.D., AND ANTONIO L'ABBATE, M.D.

ABSTRACT The object of this study was to obtain quantitative data on the angle dependence of reflected ultrasound signals in freshly excised normal human arterial walls and those with different degrees of atherosclerotic involvement (fatty, fibrofatty, fibrous, or calcified). Fifteen specimens were evaluated in each pathologic subset. The backscatter coefficient (BS, expressed as $cm^{-1} \times steradians^{-1}$), measured at the single frequency of 10 MHz, was evaluated at a normal angle of incidence of the interrogating beam to the tissue sample and over an angular span of 60 degrees (±30 degrees around normal incidence, 2 degree steps). BS measured at normal incidence separated normal ($10^{-2} \times 0.155 \pm 0.018$; mean ± SE) from fibrofatty ($10^{-1} \times 0.0103 \pm 0.008$), fibrous ($10^{-1} \times 0.182 \pm 0.016$), and calcified ($0.202 \pm 0.016$) specimens; normal and fatty ($10^{-3} \times 0.759 \pm 0.142$) and fibrofatty and fibrous samples could not be distinguished from each other in a statistically significant way. Angular scattering measurements identified two patterns: (1) A "directive" pattern, characterized by a strongly angle-dependent BS that falls abruptly when the beam is moved slightly away from normal incidence. This pattern was typical of calcified, fibrous, and less markedly, fibrofatty and normal samples. (2) A "nondirective" pattern, characterized by a BS that is not significantly angle dependent and fluctuates throughout the entire angular range. This was typical of fatty samples.
***Circulation* 72, No. 3, 572–576, 1985.**

ULTRASONIC tissue characterization has recently proved experimentally useful in different fields of cardiovascular pathology.[1-3] The usefulness of ultrasonic indexes — based either on backscatter[4] or on attenuation[5] — for characterization of atherosclerotic disease has also been demonstrated recently. In contrast to the echoes arising from the myocardium, which are relatively independent of the angle of incidence of the ultrasonic beam to the tissue, those arising from arterial walls are generally said to be of a "specular type."[6] This is a major limitation to any application based on a quantitative diagnostic approach in vivo, since specular reflectors give rise to a signal the amplitude of which is highly dependent on the angle of incidence of the ultrasonic beam to the tissue target. The purpose of this study was to obtain quantitative data on the angle dependence of reflected signals from normal arterial walls and those with different degrees of atherosclerotic involvement.

From the Istituto di Fisiologia Clinica, C.N.R., and the Facoltá di Ingegneria and the Istituto di Patologia Medica I, Universitá di Pisa, Italy.

Address for correspondence: Eugenio Picano, M.D., Istituto di Fisiologia Clinica, C.N.R., Via Savi, 8, 56100 Pisa, Italy.

Received January 16, 1985; revision accepted May 9, 1985.

Dr. Picano is a recipient of the A.R.MED. Research Fellowship for Ultrasonic Diagnosis of Atherosclerosis.

Materials and methods

Experimental procedure. Fresh specimens of arterial wall were taken from human aortas at autopsy and those with one of four distinct kinds of lesions (fatty, fibrofatty, fibrotic, and calcified) and with regions, whenever possible, of relatively normal tissue were chosen for study. To deal with potential problems of methodology, such as variation in time after death at which the tissue was obtained and examined by ultrasound or variation in the temperature of the tissue during examination,[7] samples were used only when the interval between death and excision ranged from 10 to 15 hr, and the ultrasonic examination was started immediately after excision and was performed while tissue was in a water bath at a constant temperature of 20° C.

Excised samples of aorta were cut down the anterior midline, opened flat, mounted on a sample holder (consisting of a rectangular metallic hollow rim with pins around its periphery), and placed on an angular scanning system in a distilled water bath at 20° C. This device enabled the aortic sample to be stabilized while maintaining it in the focus of the transducer, so avoiding interference with ultrasonic measurements. Once the ultrasonic studies were completed, the tissue was removed from the water bath and wall thickness was measured with a micrometer (at each site of ultrasonic study) before the tissue was prepared for histologic examination. Thickness values in each of the five groups studied were as follows: normal walls, 2.0 ± 0.9 mm (mean ± SD); fatty plaques, 2.6 ± 0.4 mm; fibrofatty plaques,

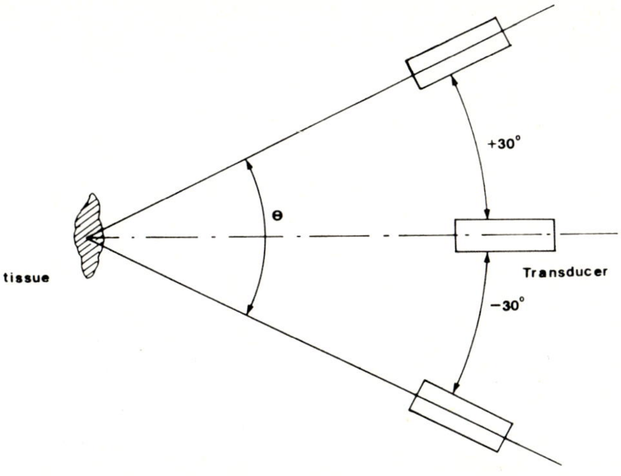

FIGURE 1. Experimental system used.

3.3 ± 0.3 mm; fibrotic plaques, 2.6 ± 0.4 mm; and calcific plaques, 3.8 ± 0.3 mm. For each pathologic subset, the first 15 consecutive values obtained were considered in the analysis.

Ultrasonic technique. Ultrasonic measurements were obtained with the system shown in figure 1. It comprises a single transducer (Aerotech, model gamma, 15 MHz nominal frequency, 0.5 cm diameter, 8.5 cm focal distance, 2 cm focal length) acting as both transmitter and receiver. The use of a small-diameter transducer reduces the phase cancellation artifacts caused by phase-sensitive transducers.[8, 9] The ultrasonic beam width (4 mm evaluated at −3 dB) was determined at 10 MHz (continuous-wave signal) by means of a metallic Rayleigh reflector. The transducer was excited with a broadband pulser/receiver (Panametric, model 5052 PR).

To evaluate the orientation dependence of tissue scattering, a single frequency from the incidental beam was analyzed.[10] Accordingly, the received signal was analyzed by fast-Fourier transform, in which frequency component of 10 MHz is derived by gating the broadband spectrum of the received signal in the frequency domain. The transducer was fixed on a half-crown scanning system; in this way the mechanical axis of the transducer was able to cross the geometric center of the crown, where the holder was placed, at all angles. For measurements of angular scattering, the transducer was rotated over an angle of ±30 degrees with respect to the perpendicular axis of the sample holder (0 degrees), moving in steps of 2 degrees (within a total range of 60 degrees). The received signal was captured with a transient recorder (Tektronik, model 7912 AD, conversion rate of 10 nsec, 9 bits of amplitude resolution).

Ultrasonic data analysis. The backscatter analysis involved a tissue volume approximately equal to the product of the beam area and the thickness of the specimen. During the acquisition, the gate length was fixed at 5 μsec, to allow digitization of the signal from the full thickness of the specimen. Before ultrasonic analysis, a masking operation was performed on each ultrasonic record under computer control so that echoes could be distinguished from water-tissue interfaces. The mask length was of 40 data points, corresponding to the time length of the transmitted pulse (about 400 nsec). Afterwards, a thickness normalization procedure was performed for each specimen. Thus, the measurement obtained was independent of biological variability in wall thickness. The backscatter coefficient (BS) was calculated in the frequency domain by squaring the amplitude of the spectral component at 10 MHz and by normalizing for the volume of insonated tissue; it was expressed as inverse centimeters times inverse steradians. A correction was performed with an almost perfect reflector (a stainless steel plate) placed in the focus of the transducer. A simple quantitative analysis of the angular distribution function was also performed. To express quantitatively the angular behavior of the integrated backscatter, a curve of BS as a function of the angle was derived: on the abscissa the range of values is 0 degrees (i.e., normal incidence) to 14 degrees; on the ordinate, BS values are displayed (see figure 3). The slope of the best-fitting straight line (S) was calculated from the data obtained from each specimen.

Pathologic characterization. After ultrasonic measurements each aortic region was studied histologically with Weigert-Van Gieson stain. As stated above, according to generally accepted criteria,[10] five pathologic subsets were identified: normal aortic walls, fatty plaques (characterized by the accumulation of lipids in the intima), fibrofatty plaques (usually characterized by a fibrous cap and a lipid core), fibrous plaques (i.e., wall thickened by connective tissue), and calcified plaques (walls in which the atheromata were calcified).

Statistical analysis. For each index the mean and the SEM were measured. Differences were tested for significance by analysis of variance, with subgroup analysis by the Newman-Keuls test.[11]

Results

The BS, measured at a normal angle of incidence, can differentiate normal specimens from fibrofatty, fibrous, and calcified specimens (table 1), although differences between normal and fatty and between fibrous and fibrofatty samples do not reach statistical significance. The BS value varies as a function of the angle differently in the various subsets. As shown in figure 2, the value falls steeply in normal, fibrofatty, fibrous, and calcified plaques when the beam departs from 0 degree (a behavior typical of the so-called directive or specular reflectors). Fatty plaques, however, have a peculiar "plateau-like" profile of angular scattering (typical of nonspecular or nondirective reflectors). When the data obtained for each subset at each angle of incidence are pooled (figure 3), it becomes apparent that a change of as little as a few degrees in the angle of incidence may completely blunt differences recorded at normal incidence. It is also apparent from figures 2 and 3 that the highest variation in the

TABLE 1

BS values recorded at a normal angle of incidence (mean ± SE)

	BS (cm^{-1} × $sterad^{-1}$)	Comparisons NL	FA	FF	FI	CL
NL	$(10^{-2}) \times 0.155 \pm 0.018$		NS	A	A	A
FA	$(10^{-3}) \times 0.759 \pm 0.142$			A	A	A
FF	$(10^{-1}) \times 0.103 \pm 0.008$				NS	A
FI	$(10^{-1}) \times 0.182 \pm 0.016$					A
CL	0.202 ± 0.016					

NL = normal wall; FA = fatty plaque; FF = fibrofatty plaque; FI = fibrous plaque; CL = calcified plaque.

[A]$p < .01$.

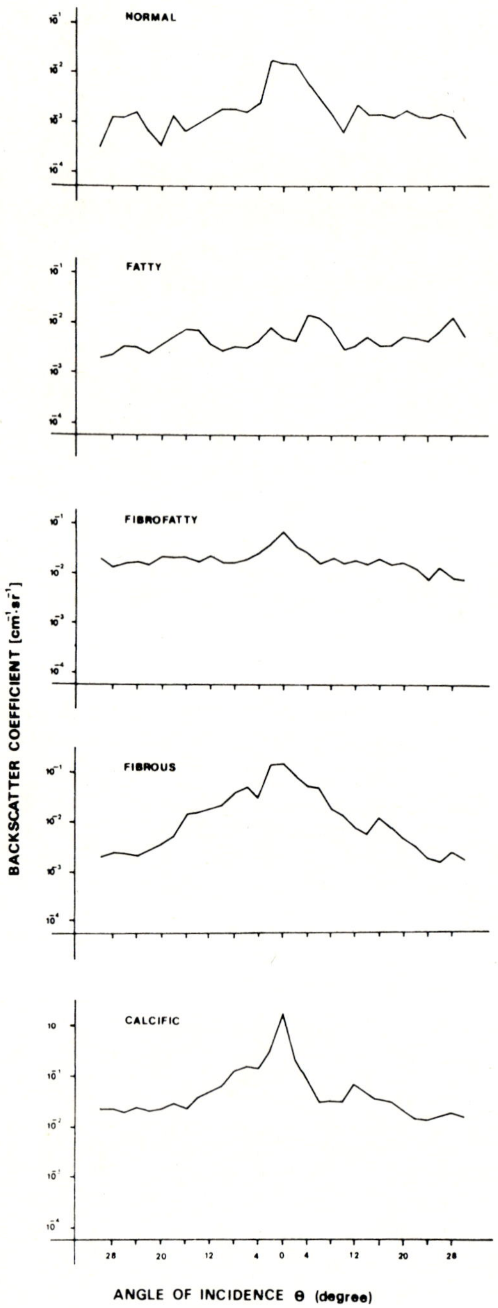

FIGURE 2. The angular scattering behavior in one specimen from each subset. In normal, fibrofatty, fibrous, and calcific specimens the BS value falls abruptly — with increasing steepness — when the beam is moved slightly away from the normal (θ = 0) angle of incidence (specular reflectors). The BS in the fatty plaque fluctuates throughout the entire angular range (non specular reflectors).

profile of angular scattering is recorded in the range of ±14 degrees around the normal incidence; the index S (previously described) was calculated in this angular span. This simple statistical parameter provided a further distinction within the groups not resolved by the normal incidence BS, permitting differentiation of fatty from normal and fibrofatty from fibrous walls (table 2). The backscatter decay was steeper (i.e., the S value was more negative) in fibrous and calcified walls, it was intermediate in fibrofatty and normal samples, and it was almost flat in fatty plaques.

Discussion

The angle of incidence between the ultrasonic beam and the tissue target is a critical factor in the quantitative characterization of atherosclerosis based on reflected signals. A change of as little as a few degrees in the angle of incidence may blunt the difference (recorded at a normal incidence, table 1) between noncalcified plaques and normal fatty specimens. However, such angle dependence is not a complete drawback: fatty components of the atherosclerotic plaque show a peculiar pattern of angle dependence that may be considered their acoustical "fingerprint," a potentially useful feature.

The histogram of angular scattering in normal, fibrofatty, fibrous, and calcified walls is clearly peaked, i.e., it falls abruptly when the beam departs from a normal angle of incidence. It appears more plateau-like (less angle dependent) in fatty plaques. Simple statistical indexes (such as the slope of the scattering decay as a function of the angle of incidence) can quantitatively discriminate these different shapes. The histologic architecture and biochemical composition of the arterial wall might be a reasonable morphologic substrate for the recorded difference in angular scattering, which is determined by size and orientation of the scatterers relative to the ultrasonic beam (figure 4).

A directive angular response may be due to simple planar organization of the targets within the tissue. Scatterers in the normal wall might be physically identified in the thin elastic membranes present within the normal media layer and oriented perpendicularly to the beam axis. They give rise to directional scattering typical of that in structures in which large plane interfaces exist within the scattering volume. In fibrous and calcified specimens, the scatterers might be physically identified in thick collagen bundles and calcium lam-

TABLE 2
Slopes of angular backscatter decay

		Comparisons				
	Mean ± SE	NL	FA	FF	FI	CL
NL	$-(10^{-5})\times$ 9.8 ± 0.6		A	A	A	A
FA	$(10^{-5})\times$ 0.3 ± 1.0			A	A	A
FF	$-(10^{-5})\times$ 46.1 ± 5.8				A	A
FI	$-(10^{-5})\times$ 102.1 ± 22.9					A
CL	$-(10^{-5})\times$ 636.9 ± 46.9					

$^{A}p < .01$.

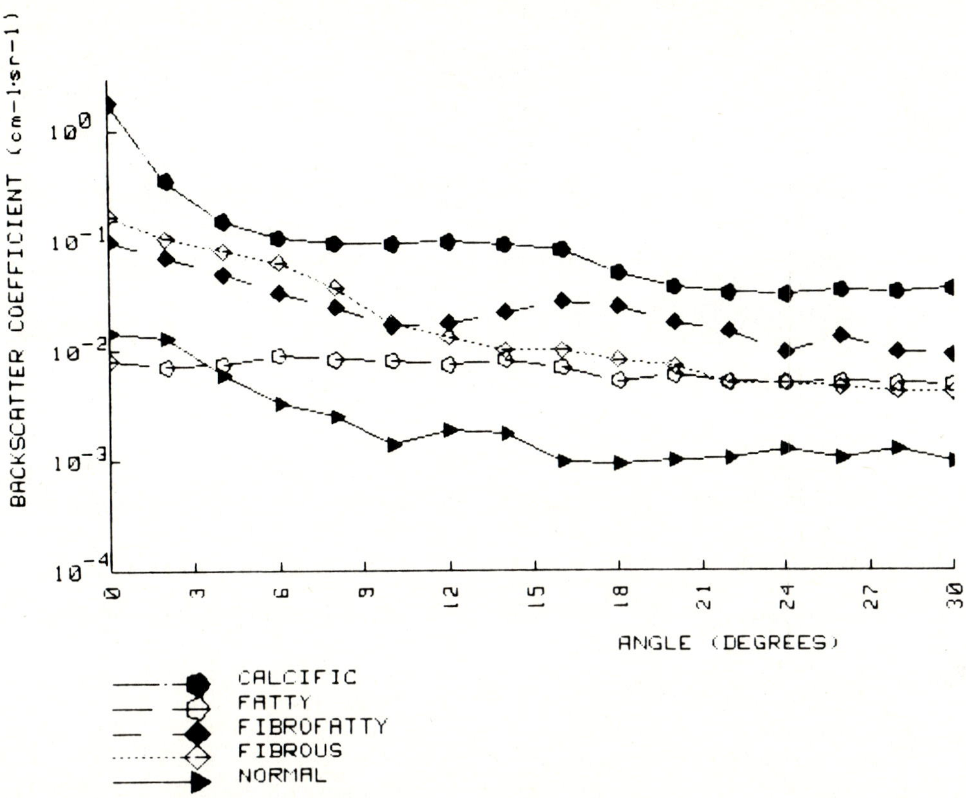

FIGURE 3. Graph illustrating the pooled data from all specimens in each subset. A variation of as little as a few degrees may completely blunt differences between noncalcified atherosclerotic and normal specimens recorded at a normal angle of incidence. Marked changes in angular scattering pattern are evident, especially in the ±14 degrees range.

inae, which are, like elastic membranes, oriented perpendicular to the beam (figure 4). This might explain the very high directivity of these plaques. In fatty plaques, lipids accumulate in the intima, mainly in the amorphous state but also as cholesterol crystals. Such crystals are comparable in size to the wavelength of the beam, and are spatially arranged in a random fashion (figure 4). The absence of a spatial orientation and the small size of the scatterers both contribute to the nondirective type of angular scattering in these plaques.

In the fibrofatty plaque the markedly directive response is probably due to the fibrous cap; however, the coexistence within the scattering volume of a nondirective structure (the fatty core, absent in the purely fibrous plaques) partially blunts the directivity of the angular response (which is substantially less than in the fibrous samples, as shown in figure 3 and table 2).

To evaluate the orientation dependence of tissue scattering, a single frequency was used for the incidental beam.[12] Since the angular scattering behavior is a function of the wavelength of the incidental beam, it is important to stress that in the present study a single 10 MHz fixed frequency was used. The chosen frequency was the one that was potentially most useful with respect to clinical applications. In fact, "an ideal, hypothetical carotid scanning device would be a B mode imaging system, functioning at 8 to 10 MHz".[13] Furthermore, coronary intraoperative imaging systems also work with either 9 or 12 MHz central frequency.[14] Since "any commercial device that is ultimately developed will probably have both conventional imaging and quantitative tissue characterization imaging built into the same basic hardware,"[1] the frequency chosen for the present study was the one most compatible with conventional imaging needs.

In conclusion, the angular dependence of arterial backscatter — potentially a considerable limitation to quantitative ultrasonic diagnosis — may itself become a tool for atherosclerosis characterization. The BS at a normal angle of incidence cannot distinguish normal from fatty or fibrous from fibrofatty samples. Such a distinction can be accomplished, however, if simple statistical parameters describing angular scattering are used. Lipid tissue deposition, which occurs in the atherosclerotic plaque without being spatially organized in specific geometric patterns, introduces a nonspecular component to the structure of the plaque, and gives a peculiar nondirective distribution to the angular scattering. On the basis of their angular responses, fatty plaques can be differentiated from normal walls

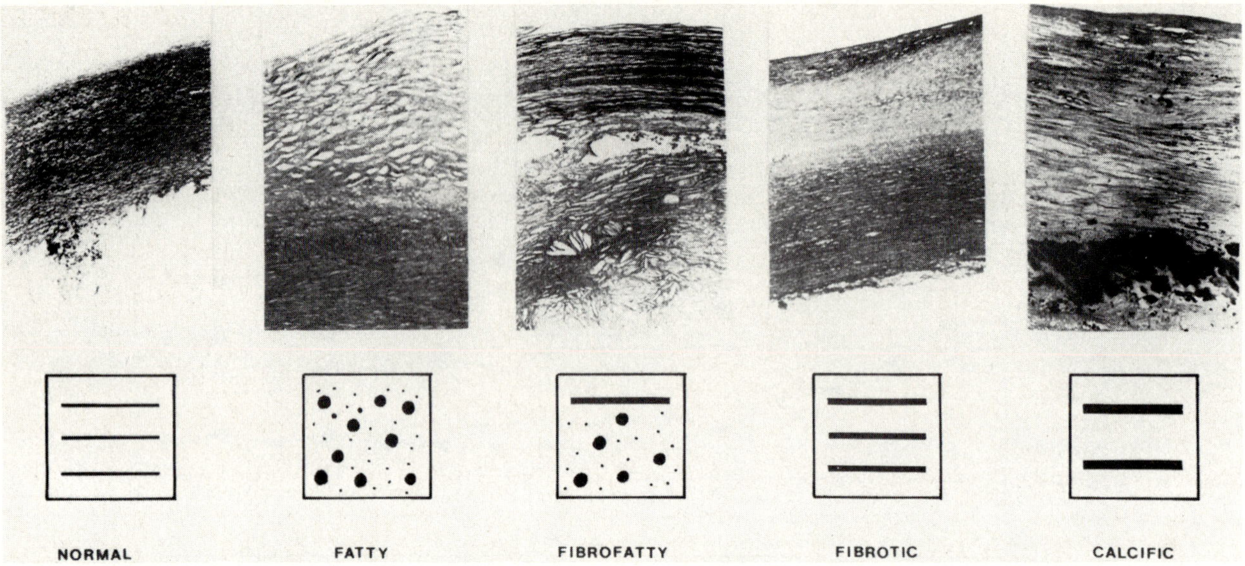

FIGURE 4. *Top,* Typical histologic appearance of a specimen from each subset (Weigert-Van Gieson stain, original magnification × 32). *Bottom,* Schematic representation of a specimen from each pathologic subset. Directive scatterers are represented by lines that indicate the planar organization of the target within the scattering volume. The width of the line is proportional to the echo value at a normal angle of incidence. Nondirective scatterers are represented by circles. In normal, fibrous, and calcific samples the scatterers can be physically identified in thin elastic membranes, thick collagen bundles, and calcium laminae, respectively. In all these cases the scatterers represent plane interfaces within the tissue, which are relatively large if compared with the wavelength, and which give rise to directional scattering. In fatty plaques, scatterers can be physically identified in amorphous lipid tissue and cholesterol crystals, which are spatially oriented at random and of various sizes, but which in many cases are smaller than the wavelength of the incidental beam (nondirective reflectors). In the fibrofatty plaque, both a fibrous cap (directive) and a lipidic core (nondirective) are present. The end product is a directive response, but a less marked one than in the purely fibrous plaque.

and fibrofatty plaques can be distinguished from fibrous samples.

We are grateful to Eng. Mimmo Iracá and Dr. Christopher Shaw for useful advice and to Dr. Felicita Andreotti for reviewing the manuscript.

References

1. Miller JG, Sobel BE: Cardiac ultrasonic tissue characterization. Hosp Pract **1:** 143, 1982
2. Miller JG, Perez JG, Mottley JG, Madaras EC, Johnston PH, Blodgett ED, Thomas III LJ, Sobel BE: Myocardial tissue characterization: an approach based on quantitative backscatter and attenuation. 1983 IEEE Ultrasonic Symposium Proceedings, IEEE Catalog No. 83CH1947-1, p 782
3. Skorton DJ, Collins SM: Digital computer image analysis in echocardiography. Echocardiogr Rev Cardiovasc Ulrasound **1:** 15, 1984
4. Picano E, Landini L, Distante A, Sarnelli R, Benassi A, L'Abbate A: Different degrees of atherosclerosis detected by backscattered ultrasound: an in vitro study on fixed human aortic walls. J Clin Ultrasound **11:** 375, 1983
5. Picano E, Landini L, Distante A, Benassi A, Sarnelli R, L'Abbate A: Fibrosis, lipids, and calcium in human atherosclerotic plaque: in vitro differentiation from normal aortic walls by ultrasonic attenuation. Circ Res **56:** 556, 1985
6. Hill RH: Ulrasonic attenuation and scattering by tissues. In de Vlieger M, editor: Clinical handbook of ultrasonics in medicine. New York, 1978, John Wiley & Sons, p 91
7. Mimbs JW, O'Donnell M, Miller JG, Sobel BE: Changes in ultrasonic attenuation indicative of early myocardial ischemic injury. Am J Physiol **236:** 340, 1979
8. Mimbs JW, Yuhas DE, Miller JG, Weiss AN, Sobel BE: Detection of myocardial infarction in vitro based on altered attenuation of ultrasound. Circ Res **41:** 192, 1977
9. Landini L, Picano E, Sarnelli R: Attenuation measurements in atherosclerotic tissues: problems with phase cancellation artifacts. Med Biol Eng Comput (in press)
10. Robbins SL, Cotran RS: Pathological basis of disease, ed 2. Philadelphia, 1979, W. B. Saunders, p 598
11. Wiener BJ: Statistical principles in experimental design, ed 2. New York, 1971, McGraw-Hill Publishing Co., p 196
12. Nicholas D: An introduction to the theory of acoustic scattering by biological tissues. *In* White DN, editor: Recent advances in ultrasound in biomedicine. Oregon, 1977, Research Study Press, p 1
13. Blankenhorn DH, Rooney JA, Curry PJ: Noninvasive assessment of atherosclerosis. Prog Cardiovasc Dis **26:** 295, 1983
14. Sahn DJ, Copeland JG, Temkin LP, Wirt DP, Mammana R, Glenn W: Anatomic-ultrasound correlations for intraoperative open-chest imaging of coronary artery atheroslerotic lesions in human beings. J Am Coll Cardiol **3:** 1196, 1984

The accuracy of Doppler ultrasound measurement of pressure gradients across irregular, dual, and tunnellike obstructions to blood flow

PAUL S. TEIRSTEIN, M.D., PAUL G. YOCK, M.D., AND RICHARD L. POPP, M.D.

ABSTRACT The accuracy of Doppler-estimated pressure gradients in the setting of irregular, multiple, and tunnellike stenoses was investigated. An in vitro model of the left ventricular outflow tract was designed to allow pulsatile flow of red cells in saline across valve orifices from 0.01 to 2.5 cm^2. Simultaneous pressure gradients were estimated by both Doppler and direct-pressure manometer techniques. Gradients obtained by the two methods correlated well for valve areas in the range of clinical stenoses at pressure gradients of 10 to 150 mm Hg (r = .97 to .99). Model valves were constructed with a large orifice (0.75 to 1.25 cm^2) placed beside a small orifice (0.02 to 0.25 cm^2) in the same outflow tract. A distinct jet was recorded when the Doppler transducer was aligned with each orifice. Doppler-estimated gradients for each pair of large and small orifices were identical and correlated well with those measured by manometer (r = .97 to .99). Irregularly shaped orifices also provided good correlation between the two methods (r = .98 to .99). Pulsatile flow was generated through long tunnellike obstructions with cross-sectional areas varying from 0.06 to 1.25 cm^2. Tunnel length varied from 0.1 to 4 cm. Tunnel areas above 0.25 cm^2 gave good Doppler-to-manometer correspondence at all tunnel lengths. Doppler underestimated manometer-determined values in the 0.25 cm^2 tunnel by 8% at 3 cm and by 15% at 4 cm. In the 0.06 cm^2 tunnel, Doppler underestimated manometer gradients by 12%, 15%, 32%, and 42% at lengths of 1, 2, 3, and 4 cm, respectively. We conclude that accurate Doppler estimation of transvalvular pressure gradients is possible in the setting of irregular or multiple valve orifices. Doppler-estimated pressure gradients across tunnellike obstructions are accurate under most geometric conditions seen in noncoronary stenoses. However, decreasing tunnel cross-sectional area and increasing tunnel length cause underestimation of manometer-derived values by Doppler. This underestimation becomes significant at tunnel areas below 0.25 cm^2 and tunnel lengths above 3 cm.
Circulation 72, No. 3, 577–584, 1985.

THE PRESSURE GRADIENT across an obstruction to blood flow can be estimted noninvasively by measuring the maximum velocity (V) beyond the obstruction with Doppler echocardiography and a simplified Bernoulli equation (pressure gradient = $4V^2$). The accuracy of this simplified Bernoulli equation has been validated both in vivo[1–5] and in vitro with models of valvular stenosis.[1, 6, 7] These models used discrete, round orifices of varying diameters to simulate stenotic lesions. Clinical obstructions to blood flow, however, are often irregular and nondiscrete. For example, calcific or rheumatic aortic valve deformities are usually asymmetric. Severe stenoses often contain multiple small orifices that produce multiple jets of blood.[8] Prosthetic valvular stenoses can also produce irregular or multiple orifices if a thrombus forms between the valve struts and the ball or disc. In other lesions, nondiscrete or tunnellike obstructions to blood flow are created. These include subpulmonic or infundibular pulmonic stenosis, some ventricular septal defects, and coarctation of the aorta. Coronary arterial stenoses represent another kind of tunnellike obstruction to blood flow. The adequacy of coronary angioplasty can be assessed by documenting the reduction of a pressure gradient across a coronary stenosis.[9, 10] Catheter-tipped Doppler ultrasonography has been suggested as an alternative method for measuring these changes in pressure gradient. In light of these geometric variations in clinically observed stenoses, we asked the following question: Does the simplified Bernoulli equation as

From the Cardiology Division, Stanford University School of Medicine, Stanford, CA.
Supported in part by grant 5 T 32 HL 07625 from the National Institutes of Health.
Address for correspondence: Richard L. Popp, M.D., Cardiology Division, Stanford University Medical Center, Stanford, CA 94305.
Received Feb. 5, 1985; revision accepted June 20, 1985.

applied to blood velocities measured by Doppler ultrasound accurately predict pressure gradients across irregular, multiple, and tunnellike orifices?

Methods

A model was designed to create pulsatile blood flow through stenoses of varying diameters and lengths in vitro. A pulse of blood was generated with a 60 ml plastic syringe (diameter 2.8 cm). The syringe tip was removed and the barrel connected directly to a lucite inlet chamber (figure 1). The inlet chamber was bolted to an outflow chamber of the same dimensions. Interchangeable lucite plates with a variety of orifice shapes and sizes were inserted between the inlet and outflow chambers as illustrated in figure 1. Multiple lucite plates were stacked in series to create tunnel obstructions. Blood leaving the outflow chamber entered a 500 ml reservoir. Circulation from the reservoir back to the inlet chamber was provided by a centrifugal pump (Biomedicus Inc., Minnetonka, MN).

Continuous-wave Doppler flow signals were recorded with a 2 MHz nonimaging transducer and an Irex Exemplar (Irex, Ramsey, NJ) ultrasonograph. This transducer has a beam diameter of 0.5 cm at its focal point of 4 cm. The beam diverges as it leaves its focal point. At 7 cm the beam diameter is 0.8 cm; at 11 cm it is 1.1 cm. The Doppler transducer was inserted through a rubber gasket into the inlet chamber and directed downstream toward the orifice. When directed at a single orifice the distance between the transducer and orifice was 6.5 cm. This distance was either 6.0 or 7.0 cm when the sound beam was moved across a dual-orifice plate. (Because of the angle inherent in the transducer head, when it is moved 3 cm horizontally it must also be moved 1 cm forward to maintain parallel alignment with the jet.)

While the centrifugal pump circulated blood at a constant velocity, the Doppler transducer was precisely aimed along the jet of blood flowing through the orifice. We found that continuous flow allowed accurate transducer alignment parallel to the jet. Position of the transducer was adjusted by both the audio and spectral signal of the frequency shift to obtain the highest blood velocities, indicating an angle of near zero degrees between the ultrasound beam and the flow stream caused by the stenosis. When the highest velocity was obtained, the transducer was clamped in position, the pump was stopped, and pulsatile flow was generated by manually depressing the syringe plunger.

Simultaneous direct pressure measurements were obtained from pressure ports provided both in the inlet and outflow chambers. The pressure ports were positioned 5 cm on either side of the obstruction. Pressure transducers (Microdot Inc., Industrial City, CA) were connected to these ports and recordings were made on a physiologic recorder (Hewlett-Packard, Palo Alto, CA). In addition to continuous recordings of inlet and outflow chamber pressures, a separate signal subtraction channel directly displayed the pressure difference between the two chambers. Pressure transducers were calibrated with a mercury manometer. The accuracy of pressure transducer measurement was initially verified by simultaneous measurement with manometer-tipped catheters (Millar Instruments, Houston), placed directly into the inlet and outflow chambers. Pressure waveforms generated during pulsatile flow were virtually identical in both measurement systems. Moving the manometer-tipped catheter to a variety of positions within the outflow chamber did not significantly alter the pressure measurements.

ABO- and Rh-compatible, outdated, banked human red blood cells were used as Doppler targets. Packed cells at room temperature were diluted with 0.9% saline. Blood was anticoagulated with 3000 U of heparin/liter. Hematocrits were measured with a Coulter Counter (Coulter Electronics, Hialeah, FL) and maintained between 33% and 36%.

Orifice preparation. Single-orifice obstructions were prepared by drilling holes in the center of thin lucite plates (thickness 1 mm). Orifice area varied from 0.01 to 2.5 cm^2. Sets of dual parallel orifices were prepared by drilling one large and one small hole in a single lucite plate. The holes were positioned equidistant from the center of the plate and separated by 3.0 cm (figure 1). Other irregular orifices, with a variety of shapes, were cut in lucite discs with a jeweler's saw. Tunnel obstructions were prepared by drilling holes through a stack of lucite plates (thickness 3 mm each). Tunnel cross-sectional area was 0.06, 0.25, 0.75, or 1.25 cm^2. The plates were aligned precisely between the inlet and outflow chambers with three guiding bolts to ensure a smooth tunnel surface (figure 1). Serial addition of plates provided tunnel lengths from 1 mm to 4 cm.

Measurements. Peak blood velocity (V) in meters per second was obtained from the hard copy of the Doppler waveform

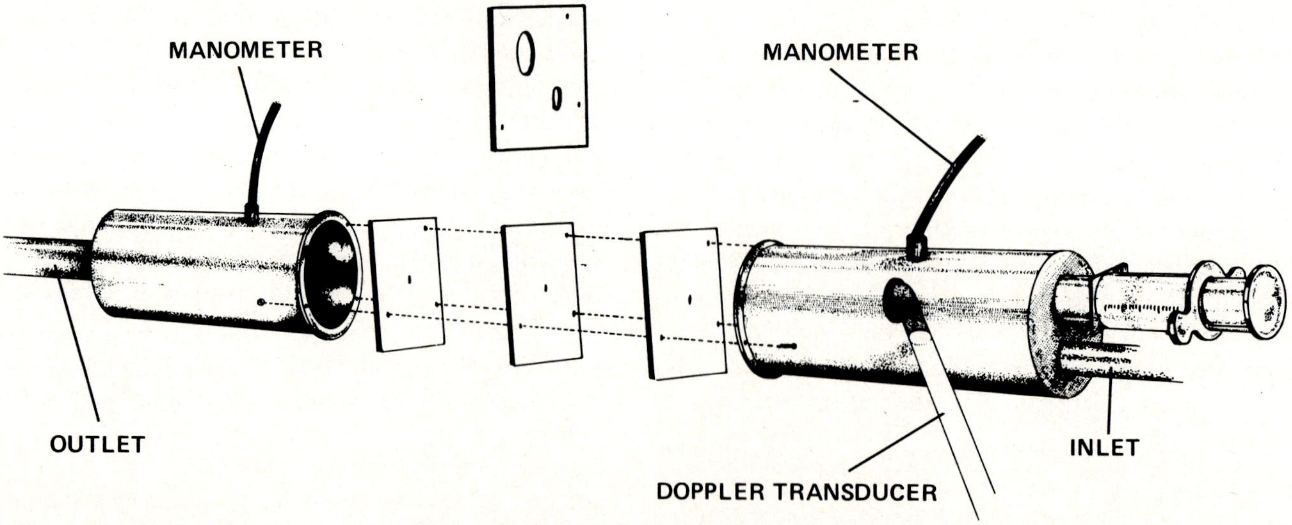

FIGURE 1. Diagram of experimental apparatus. Orifice plates are interchangeable. (A plate containing parallel dual orifices is shown at the top). Pulsatile flow is generated with the syringe mounted above the inlet (right). The Doppler transducer measures blood velocity while the pressure gradient is simultaneously recorded as the difference of the two manometers.

(paper speed 50 mm/sec). The highest coherent portion of the spectral display was designated as the maximum velocity (figure 2). Doppler-estimated pressure gradients (mm Hg) were calculated from the simplified Bernoulli equation (pressure gradient = $4V^2$).[1] Direct manometer-derived maximal pressure gradients (mm Hg) were obtained from the subtraction channel of the physiologic recorder (paper speed 50 mm/sec). For each orifice approximately 10 pulses of blood flow were analyzed. The pulses were generated by hand injections and the volume and speed of each injection were varied to provide a range of pressure gradients between 10 and 150 mm Hg.

Statistics. Statistical analysis was performed by a linear regression analysis. Correlation coefficient, standard deviation, y intercept, and slope of the regression line were obtained. A t test was performed to test the degree of doubt that the slope was not equal to 1. In the case of parallel dual orifices, the t test established the degree of doubt that the two slopes were not equal.

Results

Single round orifices (table 1). An example of simultaneous manometer and Doppler recordings is provided in figure 2. Of note, despite the use of continuous-wave Doppler, the tracings have a narrow spectral density. This indicates that most of the Doppler targets are moving at the same speed. Each pulse of blood is

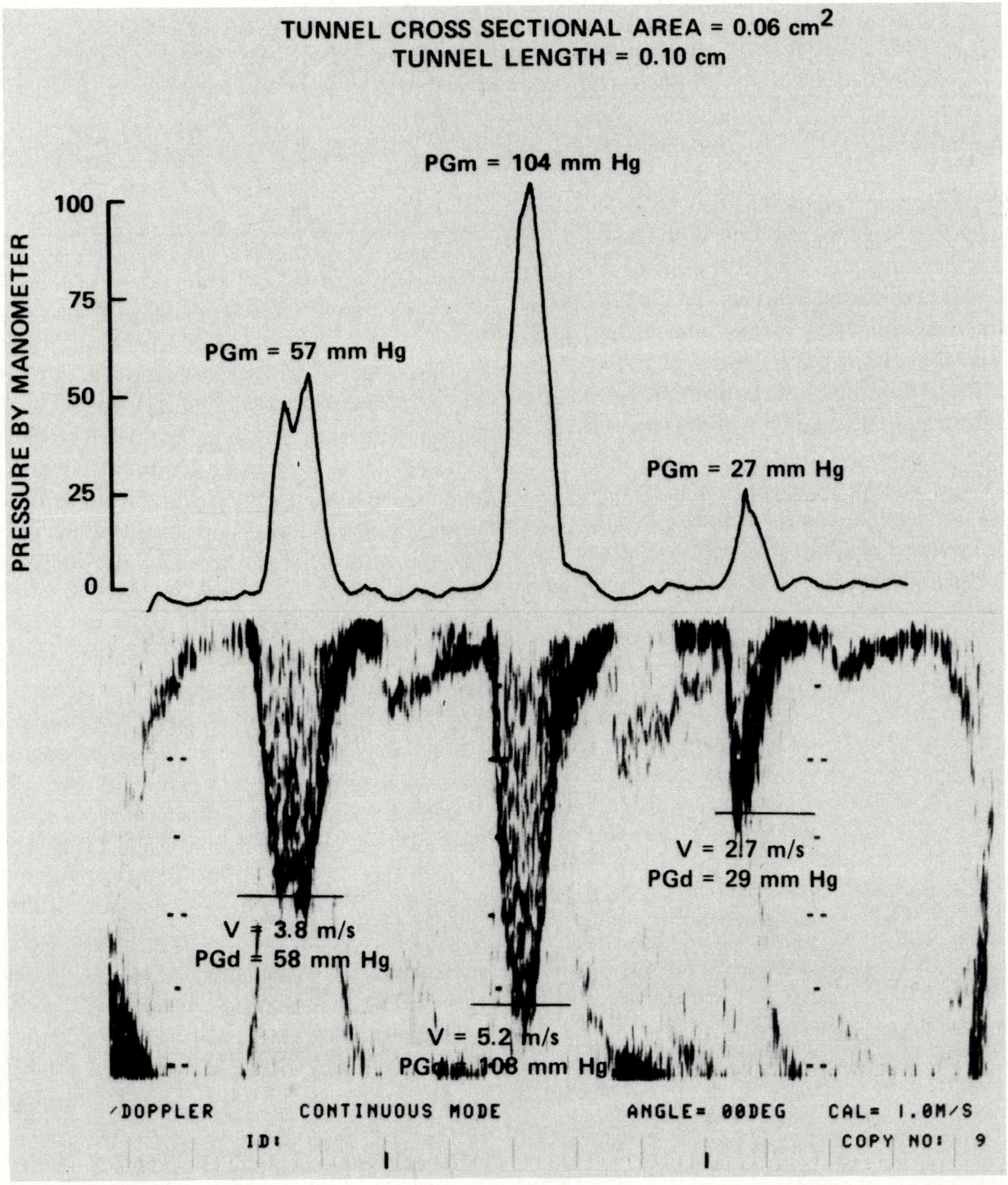

FIGURE 2. Example tracings of simultaneous manometer (PGm) and Doppler (PGd) pressure gradients with extreme variation in contour to demonstrate the nearly identical waveform pattern obtained with both techniques. Orifice area is 0.06 cm^2. Paper speed is 50 mm/sec. V = velocity.

TABLE 1
Single round orifices: Doppler-estimated vs manometer-measured gradients[A]

Orifice area (cm²)	y intercept	SD mm Hg	r	Slope
0.01	0.16	2.02	.98	.97
0.02	−0.78	1.80	.99	1.00
0.06	−2.36	2.88	.99	1.06
0.25	−0.43	2.66	.99	1.04
0.50	−0.71	2.15	.99	.99
0.75	−1.57	2.01	.99	1.00
1.0	3.23	0.66	.99	.97
1.25	−1.85	1.58	.99	1.00
1.50	0.19	1.01	.99	1.00
2.0	−0.55	0.98	.98	1.02
2.5	−0.57	0.79	.99	1.02

[A]p value (indicating degree of doubt that the slope is not equal to 1) is <.5 for each orifice tested.

TABLE 2
Parallel dual round orifices: Doppler-estimated vs manometer-measured gradients[A]

Orifice area (cm²)	y intercept	SD mm Hg	r	Slope
[0.75	−2.00	1.19	.98	.97]
0.02]	1.47	1.37	.98	.95]
[0.75	−0.62	1.18	.99	1.00]
0.06]	1.40	2.93	.98	1.02]
[0.75	−2.12	2.85	.99	1.01]
0.13]	−1.64	1.93	.99	.99]
[0.75	−3.35	4.29	.99	1.05]
0.25]	−1.19	3.99	.99	1.02]
[1.25	0.12	3.05	.98	.95]
0.02]	1.21	1.61	.99	.97]
[1.25	−0.55	2.06	.99	1.04]
0.06]	3.31	1.99	.99	.98]
[1.25	2.66	2.54	.99	1.00]
0.13]	−1.77	3.47	.97	1.06]
[1.25	4.19	3.28	.99	.99]
0.25]	3.66	1.85	.98	.94]

[A]Brackets enclose parallel orifices. p value (indicating degree of doubt that the two slopes derived from each pair of parallel orifices are not equal to each other) is <.5 for each pair of orifices tested.

generated by manual depression of a 60 cc plastic syringe. The jagged contour of some of the tracings is intentional. These nonphysiologic waveforms demonstrate the excellent correlation between Doppler and manometer measurements. In the first tracing, the Doppler signal shows a peak velocity of 3.8 m/sec, yielding a Doppler-estimated maximum pressure gradient of 58 mm Hg. The maximum manometer-derived gradient for the same pulse was 57 mm Hg. A representative plot of Doppler vs manometer gradients for a valve area of 1 cm² is shown in figure 3. The two methods correlated well at low pressure gradients (<50 mm Hg) with orifices of 0.01 to 2.5 cm² (r = .98 to .99, slope = .95 to 1.06). Correlation was good at high gradients (50 to 152 mm Hg) with orifices of 0.06 cm² or greater but 1.5 cm² or less. High gradients could not be generated across the 2.0 or 2.5 cm² orifices with our injection system. High gradients across smaller orifices (0.01 and 0.02 cm²) were difficult to interpret because of dispersion of the Doppler signal (see Discussion).

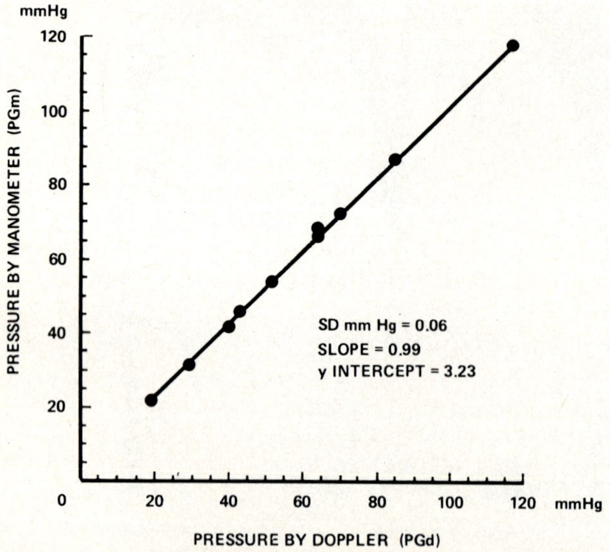

FIGURE 3. Plot of pressure gradient obtained by Doppler (PGd) vs pressure gradient obtained by manometer (PGm), with a single round orifice area of 1.0 cm² in the apparatus of figure 1. The slope is not significantly different from 1.0, indicating excellent correspondence between the two techniques.

Parallel dual round orifices (table 2). Parallel dual round orifices were separated from one another by 3 cm. The Doppler transducer produces a beam diameter of 8 mm at 6 to 7 cm (−60 dB). This provides ample resolution of the two distinct jets. Directing the transducer across the face of a plate with two orifices allowed recording of two distinct jets with an intervening area of low velocity in all cases. Each set of dual orifices had a large orifice (either 0.75 or 1.25 cm²) and a small orifice (0.02, 0.06, 0.13, or 0.25 cm²). Eight sets of dual orifices were tested. Doppler and manometer gradients correlated well with each orifice (r = .97 to .99, slope = .94 to 1.07).

Irregular orifices (figure 4). The irregularly shaped orifices (see table 3) all demonstrated good Doppler-to-manometer correlation (r = .98 to .99, slope = .99 to 1.06).

Tunnel obstructions (table 3). Tunnels with cross-sectional areas of 1.25 and 0.5 cm² resulted in good Doppler-to-manometer correlation at tunnel lengths of 1 mm to 4.0 cm (r = .98 to .99, slope = .94 to 1.07). The

Orifice Shape	y Intercept	SD mm Hg	r	Slope
	-1.99	5.59	0.98	0.99
	0.02	5.05	0.99	1.05
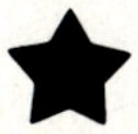	-1.20	1.12	0.99	1.04

FIGURE 4. Irregular orifices used in the apparatus of figure 1 are shown at left (approximate cross-sectional area of each orifice is 1.0 cm^2). Parameters of linear regression analysis of Doppler-estimated vs manometer-measured pressure gradients are listed for each orifice. The p value (indicating degree of doubt that the slope is not equal to 1) is <.5 for each orifice tested, indicating excellent correspondence between the two techniques.

two methods correlated well with the 0.25 cm^2 tunnel area at tunnel lengths of 1 mm to 2 cm (r = .99, slope = .98 to 1.05); t values for all the above tunnels indicated that the slope was not statistically different from 1. The 3 and 4 cm tunnel lengths demonstrated a slope of 1.08 (r = .99) and 1.15 (r = .99), respectively, indicating an 8% and 15% underestimation of manometer-derived gradients by Doppler; t values indicated the slope was statistically different from 1. The 0.06 cm^2 tunnel area demonstrated striking underestimation of manometer-derived gradients by Doppler that increased as tunnel length increased. The r values were .99 for all tunnel lengths. The slope was 1.12, 1.14, 1.30, and 1.42 for the 1 mm, 1 cm, 2 cm, and 4 cm tunnel lengths, respectively (figure 5). This indicates that Doppler underestimates manometer gradients by 42% at the 4 cm tunnel length.

Discussion

It is important to emphasize the nonphysiologic nature of this model of flow through a stenosis. For example, the orifice is not a valve and there is no leaflet motion. Moreover, no attempt is made to mimic the contractile characteristics of the left ventricle. However, this simplified model does provide an ideal setting to evaluate the accuracy of the simplified Bernoulli equation. Previous verification of Doppler estimated pressure gradients in vitro has been limited to stenoses with discrete, round orifices. Holen et al.,[1] using a model somewhat different from ours, found good correlation between Doppler-derived and manometer-derived pressure gradients for orifice areas greater than 0.10 cm^2. Requarth et al.[6] also found good correlation between Doppler-estimted vs manometer-measured gradients for valve areas ranging from 0.3 to 0.85 cm^2. Our experiments confirm the accuracy of Doppler gradient determinations with single round orifices. Doppler and manometer gradients were essentially identical for most orifices tested over a large range of pressure gradients. One unanticipated finding was that high gradients (>50 mm Hg) across small orifies (<0.06 cm) resulted in signal dispersion. The Doppler waveform lost definition and differentiation between signal and noise became difficult. This signal dispersion probably occurs as flow becomes non-

TABLE 3
Tunnel obstructions: Doppler-estimated vs manometer-measured pressure gradient

Tunnel length (cm)	y intercept	SD mm Hg	r	Slope
Cross-sectional area 1.25 cm^2				
0.10	1.85	1.58	0.99	1.00
1.00	−4.57	2.38	0.99	1.07
2.5	−0.25	2.62	0.98	0.95
4.0	0.94	2.22	0.99	0.98
Cross-sectional area 0.50 cm^2				
0.10	−2.36	3.34	0.99	0.94
1.0	−1.74	3.18	0.99	0.96
2.0	−1.74	4.76	0.99	1.01
3.0	−1.63	3.39	0.98	1.03
4.0	3.16	4.19	0.98	0.99
Cross-sectional area 0.25 cm^2				
0.10	0.42	1.85	0.99	1.03
1.0	−1.16	3.10	0.99	1.05
2.0	1.69	2.14	0.99	0.98
3.0	−7.59	1.01	0.99	1.08[A]
4.0	−1.15	1.61	0.99	1.15[A]
Cross-sectional area 0.06 cm^2				
0.10	1.43	1.49	0.99	1.01
1.0	1.41	3.44	0.99	1.12[A]
2.0	4.46	2.45	0.99	1.14[A]
3.0	2.38	3.04	0.99	1.30[A]
4.0	4.67	2.77	0.99	1.42[A]

[A]p value (indicating degree of doubt that the slope is not equal to 1) is <.01. All other p values are <.5.

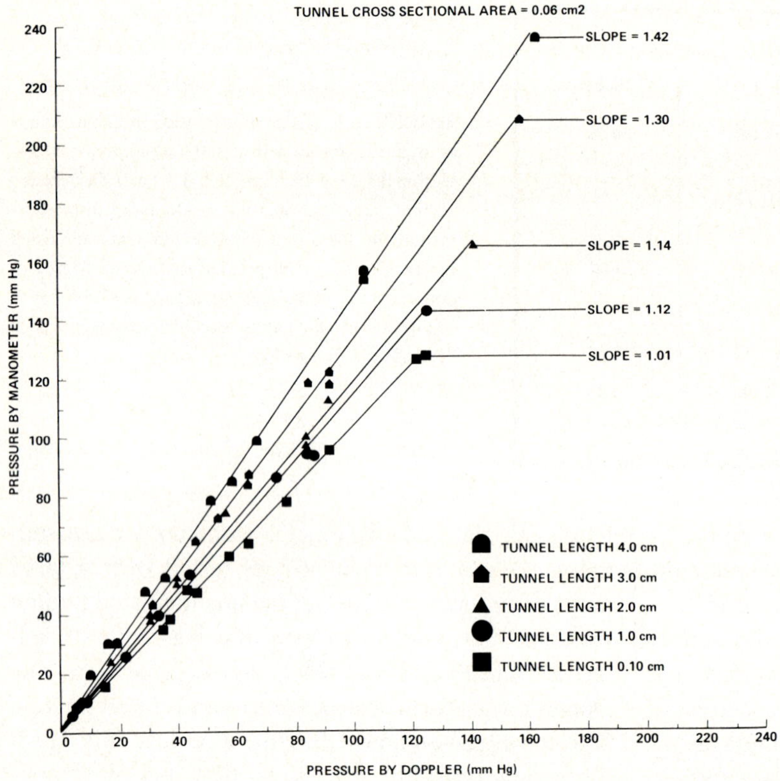

FIGURE 5. Plot of simultaneous manometer-measured pressure gradient and Doppler-estimated pressure gradient in five tunnels. All tunnels are 0.06 cm^2 in cross-sectional diameter. As tunnel length increases from 0.1 to 4.0 cm, the slope increases, indicating underestimation of manometer-measured gradients by the Doppler technique at longer tunnel lengths.

laminar and turns into a spray. Studies by Requarth et al.,[6] using flow systems with direct visualization of postobstructive jets, suggest that "spray" formation occurs at small orifice diameters. Spray formation could cause dispersion of the Doppler signal if blood flow becomes turbulent and no longer moves parallel to the transducer.

Our study is the first to demonstrate that the Doppler gradient technique can be applied to irregular stenoses, multiple orifices, and tunnel obstructions. We found Doppler measurement of jet velocities produced by various irregularly shaped orifices provided accurate estimations of pressure gradient. We also tested a more specific form of irregular stenosis, the presence of dual orifices.

When a smaller, secondary orifice was placed parallel to the large orifice, Doppler measurements remained accurate. Blood velocities were identical in both the small and large jets and both accurately reflected the pressure gradient. One might intuitively expect a higher velocity jet through the small orifice. This does not occur because the increased resistance offered by the small orifice in effect causes a shift of blood flow toward the low-resistance large orifice. The result is a net pressure drop between the upstream and downstream chambers, regardless of the geometry of the orifice. These results are best understood if one views the velocity of blood moving through an orifice as the direct result of the pressure gradient across that orifice. If the pressure gradients across two orifices are the same (and they must be if the two orifices are in parallel), the blood velocities generated by those pressure gradients must also be the same, as dictated by the Bernoulli equation. This should not be confused with the absolute quantity of blood flow (measured in ml/min), which is, of course, larger through the larger orifice. The velocity (measured in m/sec) refers to the speed of red blood cells as they move through the orifice. Thus more blood flows through the larger orifice but the velocity of red blood cells moving through each orifice is the same.

These results indicate that in severely distorted native and prosthetic valvular stenoses, where irregular flow or multiple jets are produced, Doppler estimation of pressure gradients is accurate. If the transducer is aimed parallel to one jet, the presence of other jets in different planes should not interfere with determination of Doppler pressure gradient.

Little data are available regarding the accuracy of Doppler measurements in tunnel obstructions in vivo.[4, 11] Our results in vitro indicate that Doppler-measured gradients are accurate within certain anatomic limitations. Tunnels with cross-sectional areas of 0.5 cm^2 or greater yielded accurate Doppler measurements, even at tunnel lengths of 4 cm. However, at tunnel areas of 0.25 cm^2 we found that Doppler underestimated pressures by 15% at the 4 cm tunnel length. This underestimation became severe in the 0.06 cm^2 tunnel area, where Doppler underestimation of the pressure gradient increased as the tunnel length increased. At the 4 cm length, Doppler underestimated manometer-measured gradients by as much as 42%.

One explanation for this underestimation is found in the Bernoulli equation[12]:

$$PG = 4\,V^2 + \text{flow acceleration} + \text{viscous resistance}$$

where PG is the pressure gradient and V is the maximum velocity.

The simplified Bernoulli equation omits the acceleration and resistance terms because in most clinically encountered stenoses they are negligible relative to the convective acceleration represented by the term $4V^2$.[1] This is supported by our data above. However, the pressure drop caused by viscous resistance can be calculated as described by Poiseuille's law[13]:

$$PGr = \frac{8 \times V \times \mu \times L}{r^2}$$

where PGr is the pressure drop along a tunnel caused by viscous resistance, V is the Doppler-measured velocity of blood, μ is the viscosity of blood (10^{-2} Pascal sec),[13] L is the tunnel length, and r is the tunnel radius.

It is apparent from this equation that with increases in tunnel length and decreases in tunnel diameter, viscous resistance produces a larger pressure drop. The pressure drop (mm Hg) attributable to viscous resistance can be calculated for each of our tunnel obstructions (see Appendix). For example, given a blood velocity of 5 m/sec through a 0.06 cm^2 tunnel that is 4 cm in length, the underestimation predicted by the Poiseuille equation is 38.7%. This is reasonably close to our observed 42% underestimation. Some differences are expected both because of assumptions in the calculation about blood viscosity and because of the application of the Poiseuille equation (based on constant flow) to our model (which uses pulsatile flow).

Our results indicate that Doppler-estimated pressure gradients are accurate in most clinically encountered stenoses (>0.25 cm^2 in cross-sectional area and <1.0 cm in length). Perhaps the most common clinical situation in which Doppler-estimated pressure gradients may prove inaccurate is in the setting of epicardial coronary artery disease. A 50% stenosis in the diameter of 6 mm coronary vessel results in a cross-sectional area of 0.068 cm^2, whereas a 75% diameter reduction gives an area of 0.018 cm^2. Thus coronary stenoses are in the range where our tunnel experiments demonstrate underestimation of pressure gradients by Doppler.

In summary, we found that Doppler ultrasound accurately estimates pressure gradients across a wide variety of clinically encountered obstructions to blood flow. As studied here, Doppler measurements are unaffected by eccentric or multiple orifices. The pressure gradient across most tunnel stenoses can be measured by Doppler but underestimation occurs in long, very narrow obstructions. Pressure drops along tunnels with cross-sectional areas less than 0.25 cm^2 are subject to significant underestimation by Doppler. This validates the accuracy of Doppler measurements in most clinical situations but raises serious questions about its use in determining gradients across coronary arteries.

Addendum

Since submission of this work, Wong et al.[14] have reported similar findings in a dual orifice flow model.

We appreciate the excellent technical assistance of Bruce Director, Cecil Profitt, Eben Kermit, James Johnston, Ph.D., and Arthur Casper, M.S. We also thank Helen Kramer, Ph.D., for her help with the statistical analysis and Gretchen Houd for her preparation of the manuscript.

Appendix

Calculation of the pressure drop caused by viscous resistance using Poiseuille's law

Using Poiseuille's equation to calculate the expected viscous resistance, we made the following assumptions: (1) Blood viscosity = 10^{-2} Pascal sec.[13] We did not measure the actual blood viscosity in our system. However, we suspect the viscosity will be somewhat less than 10^{-2} Pascal sec because we used only red blood cells diluted with saline. (Other components contributing to blood viscosity, i.e., platelets, white cells, and plasma proteins, are excluded). (2) The Reynold's number is less than 2000, indicating laminar flow. (3) Pousille's equation, derived for continuous flow, is applicable to pulsatile flow.

Poseuille's equation:

PG_r (pressure drop caused by viscous resistance)[13] in Pascals $= (8 \times V \times \mu \times L)/r^2$, where V = blood velocity (m/sec), μ = blood viscosity (Pascal sec), L = tunnel length (m), r = tunnel radius (m).

Examples:

(1) Tunnel area = 0.06 cm^2 (radius = 0.0014 m)
Tunnel length = 1.0 cm (0.01 m)
Blood velocity = 5 m/sec

$$\frac{8 \times 5\text{ m/sec} \times 10^{-2}\text{ Pascal sec} \times 0.01\text{ m}}{0.0014\text{m}^2} = 2105.26\text{ Pascals}$$

$$1\text{ Pascal} = 0.0075\text{ mm Hg (ref. 15)}$$

Therefore PG_r = 15.78 mm Hg.

(2) For the same conditions as in example 1, but with a tunnel area of 0.25 cm^2 (radius = 0.0028 m), PG_r = 3.85 mm Hg.

(3) For the same conditions as in example 1, but with a tunnel area of 0.5 cm^2 (radius = 0.004 m), PG_r = 1.88 mm Hg.

(4) For the same conditions as in example 1, but with a tunnel area of 1.25 cm^2 (radius = 0.0063 m), PG_r = 0.76 mm Hg.

In each of the above examples, blood velocity was 5 m/sec. With the simplified Bernoulli equation ($PG = 4V^2$), the expected pressure drop is 100 mm Hg. Our calculations, however, indicate that there is an additional pressure drop caused by viscous resistance. Without taking these resistive forces into account, the simplified Bernoulli equation will provide an underestimation of the actual pressure drop. In the 1.25 and 0.5 cm^2 tunnels, this additional pressure drop is small (0.76 and 1.88 mm Hg/cm tunnel length, respectively). Calculations for the 0.25 cm^2 tunnel indicate a pressure drop of 3.85 mm Hg/cm tunnel length. Therefore, in this tunnel, at the 3 and 4 cm lengths, we would expect underestimations of 11.55 and 15.4 mm Hg, respectively. When the tunnel cross-sectional area is reduced to 0.06 cm^2, the expected pressure drop caused by viscous resistance becomes quite significant. Here the calculated underestimation is 15.78 mm Hg/cm tunnel length. Therefore, in the 4 cm tunnel the Poiseuille equation predicts an underestimation of 63.12 mm Hg. This means that a pressure gradient of 163.12 mm Hg is required to generate a velocity of 5 m/sec (instead of the 100 mm Hg pressure gradient predicted by the simplified Bernoulli equation: $PG = 4V^2$). By not taking the resistive forces into account, the simplified Bernoulli equation has underestimated the actual pressure gradient by (163.62–100)/163.12 or 38.7%. Our experimentally observed underestimation was 42%.

Therefore, the resistive forces as calculated by the Poiseuille equation offer one possible explanation for the underestimation of pressure gradients by Doppler ultrasonography in long, narrow tunnellike obstructions.

References

1. Holen J, Aaslid R, Landmark K, Simonsen S, Ostrem T: Determination of effective orifice area in mitral stenosis from non-invasive ultrasound Doppler data and mitral flow rate. Acta Med Scand **201:** 83, 1977
2. Hatle L, Brubakk A, Tromsdal A, Angelsen B: Noninvasive assessment of pressure drop in mitral stenosis by Doppler ultrasound. Br Heart J **40:** 131, 1978
3. Hatle L, Angelsen BA, Tromsdal A: Non-invasive assessment of aortic stenosis by Doppler ultrasound. Br Heart J **43:** 284, 1980
4. Hatle L: Noninvasive assessment and differentiation of left ventricular outflow obstruction with Doppler ultrasound. Circulation **64:** 381, 1981
5. Lima CO, Sahn DJ, Valdes-Cruz LM, Allen HD, Goldberg SJ, Grenadier E, Barron JV: Prediction of the severity of left ventricular outflow tract obstruction by quantitative two-dimensional echocardiographic Doppler studies. Circulation **68:** 348, 1983
6. Requarth JA, Goldberg SJ, Vasko SD, Allen HD: In vitro verification of Doppler prediction of transvalve pressure gradient and orifice area in stenosis. Am J Cardiol **53:** 1369, 1971
7. Tomizuka F, Valdes-Cruz LM, Yoganathan A, Sahn DJ, Main J, Swensson RE, Jones M, Eidbo E: Comparison of continuous wave and high prf ultrasound Doppler velocities to laser Doppler anemometry in an *in vivo* pulsatile flow model of valve pulmonic stenosis: accuracy for gradient prediction. Circulation **70** (suppl II): II-116, 1984 (abst)
8. Roberts WC: The structure of the aortic valve in clinically isolated aortic stenosis: an autopsy study of 162 patients over 15 years of age. Circulation **42:** 91, 1970
9. O'Neill WW, Walton JH, Bates ER, Colfer HT, Aueron FM, LeFree MT, Pitt B, Vogel RH: Criteria for successful coronary angioplasty as assessed by alterations in coronary vasodilatory reserve. J Am Coll Cardiol **3:** 1382, 1984
10. Meir B, Gruentzig AR, Hollman J, Ischinger T, Bradford JM: Does length or eccentricity of coronary stenoses influence the outcome of transluminal dilatation? Circulation **67:** 497, 1983
11. Horowitz S, Valdes-Cruz LM, Sahn D, Larson D, Young KA, Mesel E: Estimation of gradients across aortic coarctations by continuous wave 2D echo Doppler: experimental canine studies and initial clinical experience. J Am Coll Cardiol **3:** 494, 1984 (abst)
12. Hatle L, Angelsen B: Doppler ultrasound in cardiology. Philadelphia, 1985, Lea & Febiger, p. 24
13. Hatle L, Angelsen B: Doppler ultrasound in cardiology. Philadelphia, 1985, Lea & Febiger, pp 17–18
14. Wong M, Vijayaraghaven G, Bae JH, Shah PM: In-vitro study of the pressure-velocity relationship across stenotic orifices. J Am Coll Cardiol **5:** 402, 1985 (abst)
15. Halliday D, Resnicke R: Physics. New York, 1978, John Wiley & Sons, Appendix G, p A-30

Effects of unilateral stellate ganglion stimulation and ablation on electrophysiologic changes induced by acute myocardial ischemia in dogs

MICHIEL J. JANSE, M.D., PETER J. SCHWARTZ, M.D., FRANCIEN WILMS-SCHOPMAN, RON J. G. PETERS, M.D., AND DIRK DURRER, M.D.†

ABSTRACT We recorded direct-current extracellular electrograms simultaneously from 60 left ventricular epicardial sites in 38 α-chloralose-anesthetized dogs during repeated, 5 min coronary arterial occlusions. In each dog recordings made during control occlusions were compared with those made in occlusions after, or during, the following interventions on the sympathetic nervous system: left stellate ganglion stimulation, left stellectomy, right stellectomy, and clamping the abdominal aorta with intact sympathetic nerves to induce a rise of blood pressure equal to that present during left stellate stimulation. Heart rate was kept constant. Measurements included determination of TQ segment potentials and times of local activation. After 2 min of ischemia, the degree of TQ segment depression was increased by left stellate ganglion stimulation and was decreased by both left stellectomy and clamping the aorta. Also, the area showing negative TQ potentials, indicating decreased resting membrane potentials, was enlarged by both left stellate stimulation and right stellectomy and reduced by left stellectomy. No differences were found in the results of experiments in which the left anterior descending coronary artery was occluded and those in which the circumflex branch was occluded. Left stellate stimulation significantly improved conduction within the ischemic zone. No evidence was found to suggest that the arrhythmogenic effects of left stellate stimulation and of right stellectomy, confirmed in the present study, resulted from an increased likelihood for reentry in the subepicardium of the ischemic zone.
Circulation 72, No. 3, 585–595, 1985.

IT IS generally accepted that the sympathetic nerves play an important role in the genesis of ventricular arrhythmias caused by acute myocardial ischemia.[1–3] Furthermore, studies employing unilateral denervation have shown that, by removing tonic activity or by preventing the occurrence of cardiocardiac reflexes,[4, 5] right and left sympathectomy are not equivalent and actually produce different results.[6] More specifically, left stellectomy has been found to exert an antiarrhythmic effect,[7] while right stellectomy has been found to have an arrhythmogenic effect.[8] However, the mechanisms underlying these findings have remained elusive.

In this study we attempted to gain insight into these effects by recording direct-current extracellular electrograms simultaneously from 60 epicardial sites on both ischemic and nonischemic myocardium during short-lasting and repeated coronary occlusions coupled with specific interventions on the stellate ganglia. We measured the direct-current potential at each electrode during the TQ segment of beats propagated from the atrium, and the time of local activation. The TQ segment potential was chosen because depolarization of resting membrane causes depression of the TQ segment in direct-current recordings. The amount of TQ segment depression and the delay in activation time both served as an index for the severity of ischemia-induced changes in electrical activity.

From the Department of Cardiology and Experimental Cardiology, Academisch Medisch Centrum, Amsterdam, and the Interuniversity Cardiology Institute, The Netherlands; and Unita di Studio delle Aritmie, Centro di Fisiologia Clinica, Istituto di Clinica Medica IV, CRN Ospedale Maggiore, Universita di Milano, Italy.

Address for correspondence: Dr. M. J. Janse, Department of Cardiology and Experimental Cardiology, Academisch Medisch Centrum, Meibergdreef 9, 1105 AZ Amsterdam, The Netherlands.

Received Nov. 4, 1983; revision accepted May 9, 1985.

†Deceased.

Methods

Thirty-eight dogs ranging in weight from 18 to 30 kg were anesthetized with a short-acting barbiturate (hypnodil 2 mg iv) followed by intravenous injection of α-chloralose (50 to 100 mg/kg). Administration of α-chloralose during the experiment was repeated as necessary. No measurements were made for at least 20 min after drug administration.

A carotid artery was cannulated to monitor arterial pressure, and a femoral vein was cannulated to administer anesthetics. The vagus nerves were isolated in the neck and cut. The chest was opened via a midsternal incision. The left or right stellate ganglion was isolated from the surrounding connective tissue and prepared for subsequent ablation or stimulation. Stimulation was carried out by a constant current stimulator, which delivered rectangular current pulses of 2 msec duration at a frequency of 10 to 20 Hz, with an intensity of 1.5 to 2 mA. Stimulation was always performed after decentralization, when the only connections of the stellate ganglion were the cardiac nerves and the ansae subclaviae, to avoid reflex activation of the contralateral stellate ganglion.[5] Ablation was performed after topical application of 1% lidocaine to avoid the effects of injury currents through the cardiac nerves.

After a pericardial cradle was constructed, stimulating bipolar electrodes were sutured on the right atrium. After a brief period of left stellate ganglion stimulation, the success of which was judged by noting an increase in average blood pressure of 20 to 40 mm Hg and which sometimes also resulted in a slight increase in heart rate, the atrium was paced at such a rate as to ensure a constant heart rate throughout the experiment. Basic cycle length varied in the different experiments from 290 to 490 msec but usually was in the range of 300 to 350 msec. The left anterior descending coronary artery (LAD) or circumflex branch was prepared free, and a ligature was placed around the artery. This ligature served as a guide to clamp the artery with a 3 mm broad clamp.

A very brief occlusion was performed to localize the ischemic area, visible as a cyanotic zone, and a multipolar electrode was then sutured onto the epicardial surface so as to have as many terminals as possible overlying the ischemic area. The electrode consisted of 60 polyethylene tubes filled with saline and containing cotton wicks.[9] The electrodes were arranged in five rows of 12, and interelectrode distance was 4 mm. In some experiments an electrode was used in which six rows of 10 terminals were arranged at intervals of 3 mm. The electrode tips were glued to a rubber sheet perforated by small holes (diameter 0.5 mm), with the wicks protruding slightly through the holes in the sheet. The sheet could easily be sutured onto the epicardial surface. Simultaneous recordings from 60 direct-current electrodes were made with respect to another cotton wick, attached to the tissue rostral to the split sternum, with a computer system (for a detailed description see refs 9 and 10). Briefly, after an initial 20-fold amplification in a high-impedance, low-pass (cut-off frequency 40 Hz), 60-channel amplifier, the signals were led into a high-speed multiplexing analog-to-digital converter (maximal sampling frequency 130 kilocycles/sec; Microconsultants VHF MOD 15). Samples were taken every 4 msec and written into a circular buffer. Signals of a 2 sec or a 1 sec period were transferred to a high-speed digital tape recorder (Kennedy 7300). Analysis of the data was performed with the same PDP-11-34 computer, by means of an interactive program in which the stored signals were displayed on a Megatek graphic display. The simultaneous recording of 60 direct-current electrograms allowed the construction of activation maps by measuring local activation times and of determining isopotential maps at any desired moment of the cardiac cycle, which in these experiments was the TQ segment of beats propagated from the atrium.

Electrograms were also printed continuously on an Elema Inkwriter to document the occurrence of arrhythmias.

Experimental protocol. In five experiments, repeated coronary arterial occlusions of 5 min duration were performed, separated by 15 to 20 min reperfusion intervals, to determine whether the electrophysiologic changes were reproducible. In one additional experiment, ventricular fibrillation was induced by application of direct current at the end of the third and fifth occlusions to determine whether fibrillation and defibrillation would affect the electrophysiologic changes during subsequent occlusions.

In 32 experiments, interventions with the stellate ganglia were performed during or before occlusion of either the LAD (19 dogs) or circumflex branch (13 dogs). In each experiment, two 5 min occlusions were performed without any intervention to the sympathetic nervous system, the second of which was used as a "control occlusion" (see Results).

Fourteen experiments (seven with occlusion of the LAD, seven with occlusion of the circumflex branch) were performed to evaluate the effects of stimulation of the decentralized left stellate ganglion (third occlusion) and ablation of the ganglion (fourth occlusion). In addition, in five experiments, only the effects of left stellate ganglion ablation were measured (four LAD, one circumflex); in four experiments, only the effects of left stellate ganglion stimulation were studied (two LAD, two circumflex). To evaluate whether the effects of left ganglion stimulation might have been caused by the increase in blood pressure, the abdominal aorta was partially clamped during eight coronary occlusions (four LAD, four circumflex) to obtain a similar increase in average blood pressure in the carotid artery (40 mm Hg) as during left stellate stimulation. In four animals, when four or five occlusions had been made, systolic blood pressure fell below 90 mm Hg, and measurements made at such low pressures were discarded. Sometimes, because of ventricular fibrillation, no recordings could be made after 4 or 5 min, since reperfusion and defibrillation had to be carried out immediately. Because electrical signals during the reperfusion period quickly returned to normal and because in one experiment with repeated occlusions fibrillation and defibrillation did not affect electrophysiologic changes in subsequent occlusions, these animals were not excluded from the study and measurements made in subsequent occlusions were used.

Finally, the effects of ablation of the right stellate ganglion were measured in nine occlusions (seven LAD, two circumflex).

Data analysis

TQ segment potentials. Zero potentials during the TQ segment were obtained from preocclusion recordings. During occlusions, measurements of TQ potentials in successive cycles were identical, and therefore TQ isopotential maps were constructed from measurements of one cycle only. In some instances, baseline shifts, or 50-cycle interference, did not allow accurate determination of TQ potentials, and these measurements had to be discarded. This never involved more than five of 60 extracellular recordings, and it occurred in seven experiments. Values for TQ potentials at each electrode during preocclusion and postocclusion recordings were printed out by the computer, and isopotential maps were made by hand. To quantify the effects of stellate ganglion ablation or stimulation on TQ potentials, the following procedure was used: only sites that recorded activity from ischemic myocardium were considered. These sites were chosen from the occlusion in which the largest number of recording sites showed negative values for the TQ potential. This was done because, for example, left stellate stimulation increased the area showing TQ depression, whereas left stellectomy decreased this zone. Thus the area showing ischemic changes such as TQ segment depression could not always be determined during the control occlusion. A ΔTQ value was obtained by subtracting the mean TQ level in the control occlusion from the mean TQ level during an intervention. In this way, a negative ΔTQ value signifies a greater TQ depression during the intervention compared with the TQ depression during the control occlusion; a positive value signifies less TQ depression. More TQ depression could mean an increase in the area showing ischemic changes or a greater degree of ischemic changes. The degree of ST segment elevation could not be easily quantified because the actual potential value depended greatly on the moment in the cardiac cycle when it was measured. Depending on slight changes in activation, ST potentials could, at a fixed moment of the cardiac cycle, be positive or negative, without reflecting changes in local intracellular action potential configuration.

Activation times. The signals were displayed in groups of five on the screen of a Megatek graphic display, and times of maximum negative dV/dt were indicated on the undifferentiated signal on the screen by the investigator using a joystick. Sites that failed to be activated during ischemia displayed monophasic potentials. Activation was manifest as an easily identifiable, sharp, large negative intrinsic deflection. Activation times were printed out by the computer, and isochronic activation maps were made by hand. In 28 experiments, two stimulation electrodes were placed in the nonischemic left ventricle, about 1 cm from the lateral edge of the recording electrode. Simultaneous pacing from these sites produced a broad wavefront that propagated more or less parallel to the long axis of the multipolar recording electrode. This allowed a more reliable interpretation of the changes in conduction than during propagation of impulses originating in the atria. However, because epicardial activation patterns sometimes indicated that, even with epicardial stimulation, epicardial sites were excited via unknown intramural pathways, no accurate determination of conduction velocity was possible. We therefore measured in each occlusion the "activation delay," which was the difference between the earliest and latest activated site (msec).

The paired Student t test was used to determine statistical significance in ΔTQ and in the differences in conduction delay.

Results

Reproducibility of changes in TQ segment potential with repeated occlusions. In three experiments, seven repeated occlusions of the left anterior descending artery were performed in the absence of any other intervention, and in two experiments five successive occlusions were made. Each occlusion lasted for 5 min, and a reperfusion period of 15 to 20 min was allowed before the next occlusion.

The extracellular potentials after a 5 min occlusion quickly returned to control values upon reperfusion, and after a 15 to 20 min reperfusion period, TQ potentials did not differ more than 1 mV from recordings made before the first occlusion.

In figure 1, direct-current electrograms from six epicardial sites are displayed during preocclusion recordings, and 5 min after occlusion in a series of five successive occlusions separated by a 20 min reperfusion period. The configuration of the complexes is not the same for the first and second occlusion, the ischemic changes tending to be more marked in the first occlusion. However, in agreement with earlier findings in isolated hearts,[10] the extracellular potentials during the second occlusion were very similar to those in subsequent occlusions. There was some variability in ΔTQ, but no significant differences in TQ depression in the second and subsequent occlusions were found (table 1). In particular, there was no specific trend in which, for example, TQ depression became less (or greater) in later occlusions. We always used the second occlusion as the "control occlusion," and all interventions concerning the sympathetic nervous system were performed only after two occlusions had been made.

In one additional experiment, six repeated occlusions were performed, but at the end of the third and fifth occlusion, ventricular fibrillation was induced by application of direct current. Reperfusion and defibrillation were carried out within seconds. No significant differences in TQ segment potentials and activation delays were found between second and all subsequent occlusions (after 2 min, average TQ potential in the second occlusion was -6.5 ± 0.3 mV, in the third -6.3 ± 0.25 mV, in the fourth -6.4 ± 0.3 mV, in the fifth -6.7 ± 0.3 mV, and in the sixth -6.2 ± 0.3 mV). Maximal conduction delays were 115, 109, 97, 120, and 114 msec in occlusions two to six, respectively.

In all experiments, before occlusions were performed recordings were made during a 2 min period of stimulation of the left stellate ganglion. No measurable effects on TQ potentials and activation patterns were observed. The only alterations in the local direct-current electrograms were those in the T wave. Usually, T waves became larger when positive or changed from negative to positive. In only one instance did the T wave become more negative, and in one heart no changes in T wave configuration were observed.

Effects of interventions on TQ potentials

Left stellate ganglion stimulation. In figure 2, TQ segment maps and selected electrograms are shown during the control occlusion and during an occlusion in which the left stellate ganglion was continuously stimulated. The degree of TQ depression is greater during left stellate ganglion stimulation, and the area showing TQ depression is also larger. In the control occlusion the 0 mV isopotential zone marks the lateral electrophysiologic border; during left stellate ganglion stimulation, TQ potentials in that region are in the order of -8 mV. Surprisingly, the other signs of ischemia are less marked during stellate stimulation. Sites that, during the control occlusion, show monophasic or nearly monophasic potentials, indicating absence of propagating responses, display a clear intrinsic deflection during stellate ganglion stimulation, indicating the presence of transmembrane action potentials with fairly large amplitudes.

In 16 of 18 experiments, left stellate ganglion stimulation caused a significant increase in TQ depression;

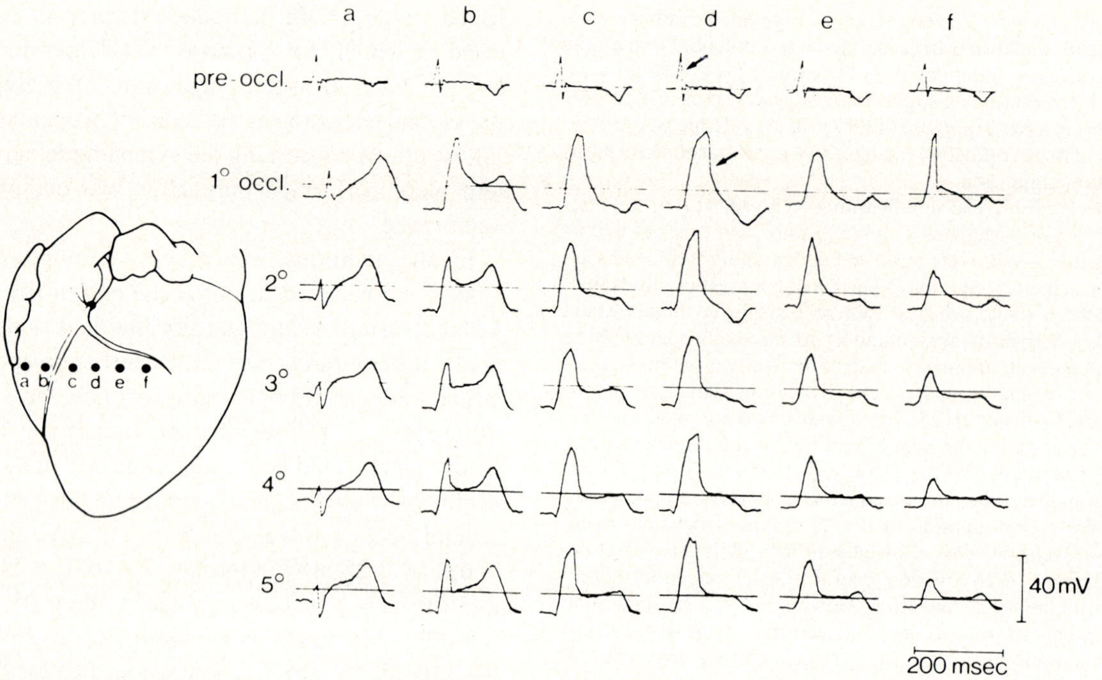

FIGURE 1. Reproducibility of electrophysiologic changes in repeated occlusions. Selected direct-current extracellular electrograms are shown (from sites a to f indicated in inset) before occlusion of the LAD (upper row) and 5 min after occlusion during five repeated occlusions. The horizontal line is the zero potential level. Coronary occlusion results in depression of the TQ segment, changes in the ST-T segment, and delayed activation (arrows mark the intrinsic deflection, which indicates the time of local activation). Note that the changes during the first and second occlusion are not identical but that the configuration and magnitude of changes during the second occlusion are very similar to those in subsequent occlusions.

with maintained stellate stimulation, this effect was less marked after 4 to 5 min of occlusion (see table 1 and figure 4).

Left stellectomy. In the majority of cases (14 of 19), left stellectomy resulted in a reduction of the degree of depression of the TQ segment. Figure 3 shows selected direct-current electrograms 2 min after the control occlusion and 2 min after a subsequent occlusion when the left stellate ganglion had been removed. Also shown are isopotential maps during the TQ segment in both instances. The extracellular complexes show much more marked ischemic changes during the control occlusion than during the occlusion after left stellectomy. For example, the complex recorded from site E is monophasic, indicating absence of local regenerative activity. After left stellectomy, the fairly large intrinsic deflection recorded at site E demonstrates that local excitation still occurs. In the signals from sites A through D, the intrinsic deflection is faster, larger, and earlier after left stellectomy than during the control occlusion, and the degree of TQ segment depression is clearly less marked. This is more completely shown in the isopotential maps from the TQ segment; during the control occlusion, a large part of the myocardium cov-

TABLE 1

Changes in average values for TQ depression and conduction delay after occlusion with and without manipulations with the stellate ganglion

	Δ TQ (mV)		Δ conduction delay
	2 min after occl	5 min after occl	4–5 min after occl (msec)
Repeated occlusions	+0.6 (±0.2) NS (n = 5)	+0.2 (±0.1) NS (n = 5)	−2.2 (±4.1) NS (n = 5)
Left stellate ganglion stimulation	−1.7 (±0.6)^A (n = 18)	−0.6 (±0.5) NS (n = 15)	−14.3 (±5.3)^A (n = 16)
Left stellectomy	+1.3 (±0.4)^A (n = 19)	+0.3 (±0.4) NS (n = 15)	−0.4 (±4.0) NS (n = 14)
Right stellectomy	−1.0 (±0.6) NS (n = 9)	−1.1 (±0.6) NS (n = 9)	−4.0 (±7.9) NS (n = 9)
Partial aortic clamp	+1.6 (±0.4)^A (n = 8)	+2.7 (±0.4)^A (n = 7)	−23.0 (±10.1) NS n = 7)

A minus sign indicates more TQ depression and less conduction delay compared with a control occlusion; a positive sign indicates less TQ depression.

^A $p < .05$.

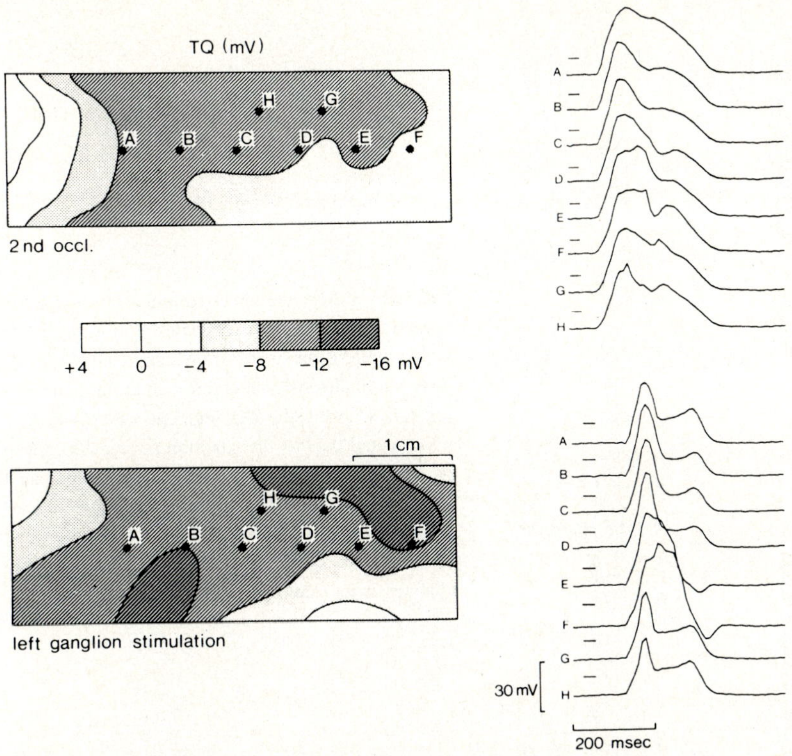

FIGURE 2. Selected direct-current electrograms from sites A to H recorded 5 min after the second (control) occlusion and during a subsequent occlusion in which the left stellate ganglion was stimulated. On the left, the area where 60 electrograms were simultaneously recorded is indicated and isopotentials during the TQ-segment are shown. Note that stimulation of the left stellate ganglion increased the TQ segment depression but that intrinsic deflections indicating local activity were larger and steeper compared with the complexes recorded during the control occlusion.

ered by the electrode has a TQ potential of −8 to −16 mV, whereas this same area has a TQ potential of −4 to −8 mV after the occlusion performed after left stellectomy.

The changes produced by left stellectomy were not always so clear; in some instances changes in the opposite direction were found. When all experiments were considered together, the reduction in TQ potential after 2 min was statistically significant; after 5 min, the differences were no longer statistically significant (see table 1 and figure 4).

Right stellectomy. The changes induced by right stellectomy were opposite to those caused by left stellectomy: the extracellular complexes recorded from the ischemic myocardium after right stellectomy usually showed ischemic changes to a far more advanced degree than during the control occlusion. The degree, and even the direction, of changes induced by right stellectomy, however, were variable (see figure 4). Both after 2 and 5 min of occlusion, an increase in the degree of TQ depression compared with the control occlusion was found in six of seven experiments in which the LAD was occluded. A decrease was found in one occlusion of the LAD and in two circumflex occlusions.

Increase in aortic pressure. Left sympathetic stimulation increased the average aortic pressure by about 40 mm Hg. The consequent increase in oxygen consumption might have accelerated the development of ischemic changes, whereas the increased perfusion pressure could have had opposite effects. To evaluate the effect of an increase in aortic pressure alone, we performed eight experiments in which the abdominal aorta was partially clamped in the presence of intact sympathetic nerves to achieve an average increase in pressure in the carotid artery of 40 mm Hg.

Compared with the control occlusion, the degree of ischemic changes was less marked when aortic pressure was thus increased and much less marked than during left stellate ganglion stimulation when similar increases in aortic pressure were produced (see table 1 and figure 4), suggesting that the increased perfusion pressure, in addition to a possible reflexly induced reduction in sympathetic activity, overcame the effects of increased oxygen consumption. In figure 4, the results of all experiments are summarized, as far as the effects on TQ potentials are concerned. From this figure, it cannot be determined whether, for example, an increase in TQ depression (negative ΔTQ) signifies a greater degree of TQ depression within the same area or an increase in the area showing TQ depression, and therefore shifts in the border zone will be discussed separately.

Shifts in the electrophysiologic border zone. The electrophysiologic border zone, defined as the area in which TQ potentials began to become negative, could

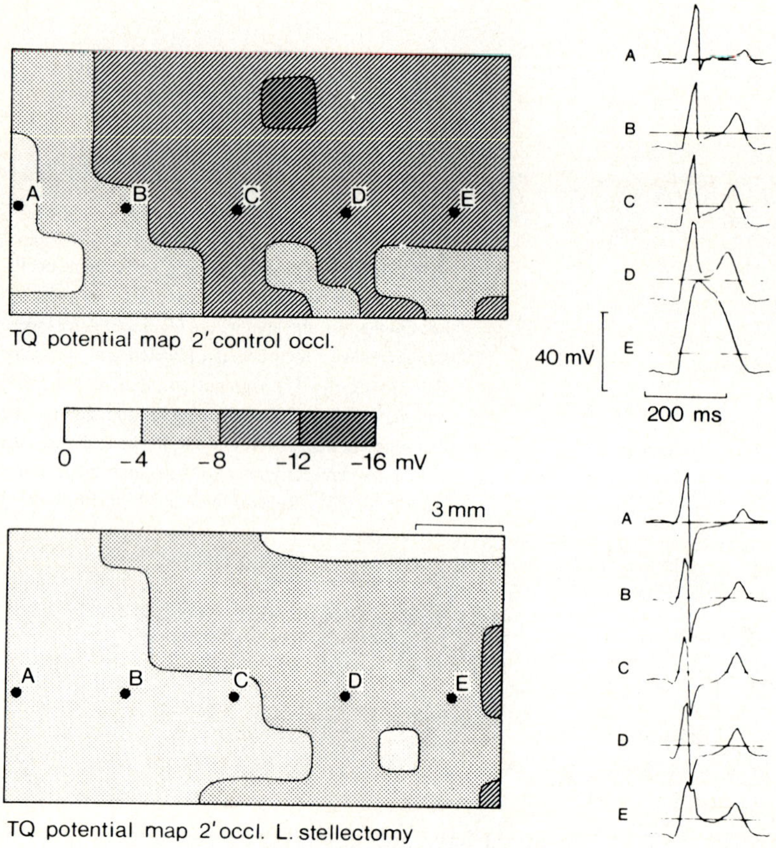

FIGURE 3. Selected direct-current electrograms recorded 2 min after coronary occlusion from sites A to E. On the left, the area from which 60 electrograms were simultaneously recorded is indicated, and isopotentials during the TQ segment are shown. The upper panel depicts the situation during the control occlusion (second occlusion), and the lower panel shows the situation 2 min after a subsequent occlusion was made when the left stellate ganglion had been removed. Note that the degree of ischemic changes is less marked after stellectomy.

be markedly shifted by stellate ganglion ablation or stimulation (see figures 2 and 3). In some experiments, the ischemic area was larger than the electrode, and most of the electrophysiologic border was outside the area covered by the electrodes. Therefore no quantitative assessment of the degree of shift in border zone can be given for all experiments. Of the 18 experiments in which left stellate ganglion stimulation was performed, a shift in border zone could be demonstrated in 10; in all cases the area showing ischemic changes became larger. In 13 of 19 experiments in which left stellectomy was performed, the electrophysiologic border was within the area covered by the electrode in the control occlusion. In eight experiments, the area showing negative TQ potentials became smaller after left stellectomy, and in five experiments no clear changes were seen. In seven experiments in which a shift of the border could be assessed after right stellectomy, the ischemic area became larger in four, while in three experiments no clear changes occurred. Partially occluding the abdominal aorta reduced the area showing TQ depression in five experiments; in three no distinct shift in the electrophysiologic border occurred.

Changes in conduction. The results on the differences in conduction delay are summarized in table 1. Because conduction within the ischemic zone was only minimally affected despite marked changes in TQ potentials after 2 min of occlusion, only findings after the fourth or fifth minute were analyzed. In repeated occlusions, no differences in conduction delay were found. In experiments in which either the right or the left stellate ganglion was removed, only minimal and nonsignificant changes were found. The improvement in conduction during left stellate ganglion stimulation is shown in figure 5. In this heart, the circumflex branch was occluded and the multipolar electrode was placed on the posterolateral aspect of the left ventricle. The ventricles were paced simultaneously from two electrodes, about 1 cm from the lateral edge of the recording electrode, so that in the preocclusion situation, activity propagated as a broad wavefront parallel to the long axis of the electrode. Isochrones separate areas activated within the same 10 msec interval, time zero being the moment of stimulation. No major differences between the activation patterns can be seen during the control occlusion, and in the occlusions during which the left stellate ganglion was either decentralized (third occlusion) or completely removed (fifth occlusion). In all three situations the wavefront invading the ischemic myocardium from the right meets an area of conduction block, and activity slowly bypasses

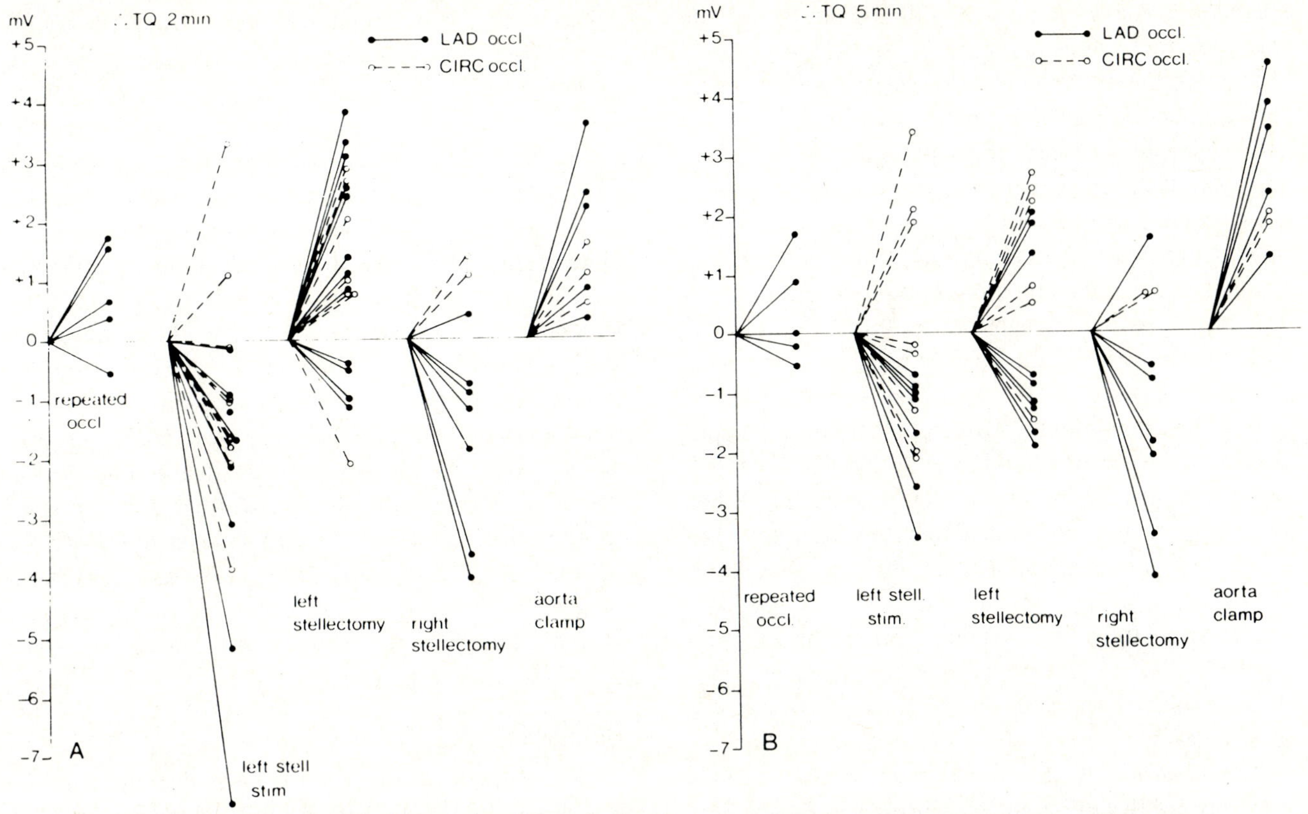

FIGURE 4. Effects on TQ segment potentials of repeated occlusions in the absence of manipulations to the stellate ganglion (first column), of left stellate ganglion stimulation (second column), of left stellectomy (third column), of right stellectomy (fourth column), and of partially clamping the abdominal aorta (fifth column) 2 min (*A*) and 5 min (*B*) after coronary occlusion. The data are represented as differences between the values obtained during the second (control) occlusion and subsequent occlusions. The means of the differences at each site are plotted on the ordinate. A change in the positive direction signifies less TQ depression than during the control (second) occlusion; a shift in the negative direction indicates more TQ depression. CIRC = circumflex branch.

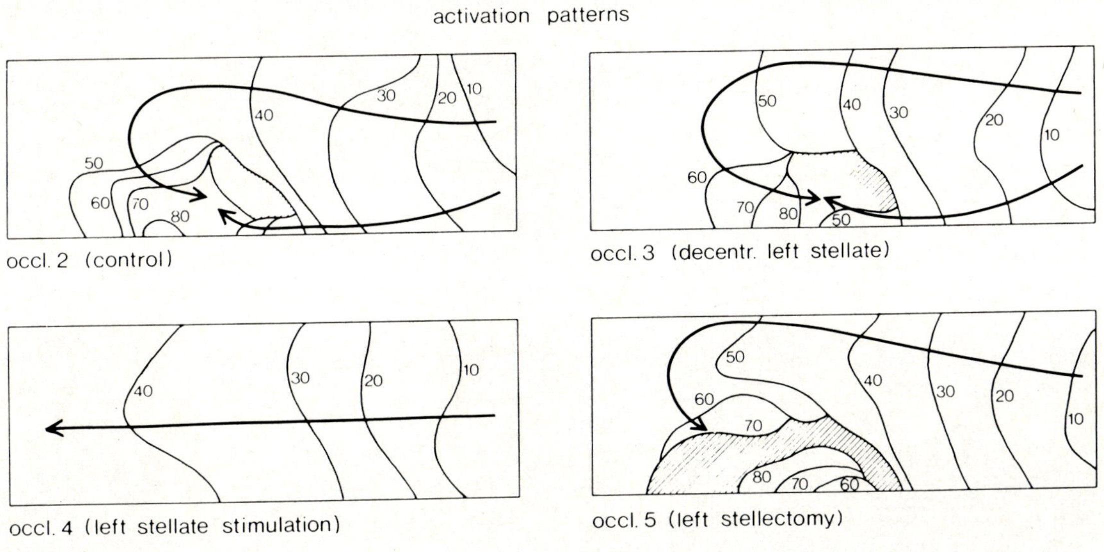

FIGURE 5. Effects of left stellate ganglion stimulation on conduction in ischemic myocardium. Isochrones separate areas activated within the same 10 msec interval; areas of conduction block are shaded. Activation patterns are shown 5 min after each of the following: control occlusion; the third occlusion, prior to which the left stellate ganglion was decentralized; the fourth occlusion, during which the left stellate ganglion was stimulated; and the fifth occlusion, after removal of the left stellate ganglion. Note improvement of conduction during stellate ganglion stimulation.

this area to make an unsuccessful attempt to reexcite the inexcitable zone retrogradely. In contrast, during left stellate stimulation, no conduction block occurs and conduction proceeds regularly and relatively fast at an apparent velocity of about 1 m/sec. (Since the intramural activation patterns are unknown, this figure must be interpreted with caution. Activation could spread partly from endocardium to epicardium and activate parts of the epicardium more or less simultaneously. This figure therefore almost certainly does not represent true conduction velocity.)

In 11 experiments (six occlusions of the LAD and five of the circumflex) a marked reduction of the conduction delay occurred, whereas in the five other experiments only minor changes were observed. When all experiments were considered together, this improvement of conduction was significant (see table 1). In the experiments in which the aorta was partially occluded, marked improvements in conduction occurred in five of seven experiments. However, standard deviations were too large to reach significance (see table 1).

Arrhythmias. The occurrence of ventricular arrhythmias during the different experiments is depicted in figure 6. An arbitrary classification was made into categories of increasing severity: (1) no arrhythmias, (2) ventricular premature beats whether single or in couplets, (3) ventricular tachycardia (three or more successive impulses), and (4) ventricular fibrillation. For each occlusion, the highest category was scored. In figure 6, for each set of experiments the maximal score during the second (control) occlusion is compared with the maximal score in subsequent occlusions. Because two occlusions were performed in some experiments during, for example left stellate stimulation, and since we could not "average" arrhythmias, we displayed the arrhythmias as they occurred per occlusion rather than in one experiment. It can be seen that in the experiments in which repeated occlusions were performed without interventions on the stellate ganglia, there is a tendency for arrhythmias to decrease in severity in later occlusions. In contrast, left stellate ganglion stimulation and right stellectomy are either without effect or increase the severity of arrhythmias. In three instances the score was lower when left stellate stimulation was performed than in the control occlusion. In most occlusions performed after left stellectomy the arrhythmias had the same severity as during the control occlusion of the experiment; however, both an increase and a decrease in severity was observed. Partially occluding the aorta reduced the severity of the arrhythmias in general.

Discussion

TQ potentials. These results show that the cardiac sympathetic nerves affect the electrophysiologic changes produced by coronary arterial occlusion in the same animal. Overall, stimulation of the left stellate ganglion increased the degree of TQ depression, whereas left stellate ganglion ablation and partially occluding the aorta (with possibly a baroreflex-induced reduced sympathetic activity) decreased the degree of TQ depression. These changes were statistically significant in the early phase of ischemia, i.e., 2 min

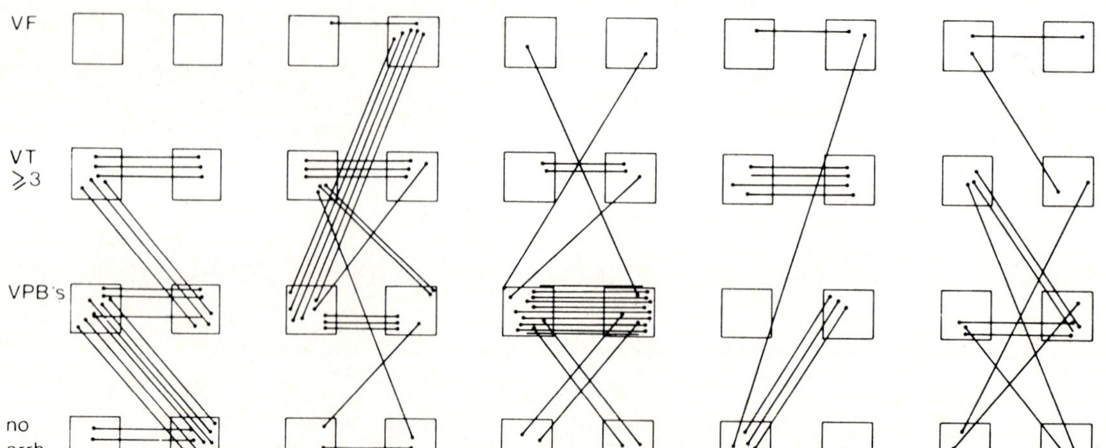

FIGURE 6. Effects of manipulations with the stellate ganglia on the occurrence of arrhythmias during a 5 min coronary occlusion. VPB = ventricular premature beats (single or couplets); VT = ventricular tachycardia (three or more consecutive VPBs); VF = ventricular fibrillation; LSS = left stellate ganglion stimulation; L- and R-ect = left or right stellectomy.

after coronary occlusion, but after 4 to 5 min statistical significance was lost. We have no explanation for this finding.

Depression of the TQ segment in local direct-current extracellular electrograms is caused by the decrease in resting potential and by the resulting local current circuit set up between the ischemic and the normally perfused cells.[9] An increase in TQ depression can therefore be interpreted as an increase in the degree of depolarization of ischemic cells. However, geometrical factors also play a role; in many experiments in which a sufficient number of electrodes were on both sides of the electrophysiologic border during control occlusions (i.e., the 0 mV isopotential line during the TQ segment), shifts in the position of this border could be demonstrated after manipulations with the sympathetic nerves. In general, the size of the ischemic area was increased by left stellate stimulation and reduced by left stellectomy. An increase in TQ depression could thus be interpreted either as an increase in the depolarization of ischemic cells or as an increase in the area in which a decrease in resting membrane potential occurs. Furthermore, a change in the geometry of the ischemic zone could alter TQ potentials. Because no intramural recordings were made, no information about the three-dimensional characteristics of the ischemic zone can be given. Finally, since the coupling resistance between ischemic and normal cells also determines the magnitude of TQ segment changes, possible effects of sympathetic nervous activity on cell coupling must be considered. If in the early phase of ischemia coupling resistance increases and sympathetic stimulation reverses the uncoupling, TQ depression would increase, even when resting membrane potentials remained the same. However, it is unlikely that sympathetic stimulation would decrease coupling resistance. Since catecholamines stimulate glycolysis, one could expect a further decrease in intracellular pH, which is known to cause uncoupling.[11]

Variability and the effects of collateral flow. A certain degree of variability was found in this study. Thus, although in most animals distinct effects were observed on TQ depression and conduction when the left or right stellate ganglion was removed, in some animals no effect was found or changes in the opposite direction occurred. This variability may have depended on several factors such as the anatomic distribution of the coronary arteries and the extent of their functional collaterals, the metabolic effects of changes in sympathetic activity, and the effects on blood pressure.

Sympathetic activation can cause coronary vasoconstriction, which may overcome metabolically induced vasodilatation.[12] Therefore, sympathetic stimulation may enlarge the area showing ischemic changes by constricting collateral vessels. In some dogs with abundant collateral connections, such effects may be large; in others, with few collaterals, shifts in the electrophysiologic border would be insignificant.[13] Indeed, it has been found that stellate stimulation during coronary occlusion could result in opposite electrophysiologic responses; in dogs in which regional myocardial blood flow increased, the amplitude of bipolar electrograms increased and their duration shortened. In animals in which regional flow decreased, the electrograms were prolonged and the amplitude became smaller.[14] The size of the ischemic zone per se may also be of influence. With a large ischemic area and with little or no collateral circulation, the ischemic changes may be so severe that a reduction of sympathetic tone will have little effect, nor will an increase in sympathetic activity do much to increase the already maximal electrophysiologic changes. With a small ischemic zone, the electrophysiologic alterations may be so discrete that a reduction in sympathetic tone will be without effect, whereas an increase in tone may induce a noticeable increase in the degree of ischemic changes.

An increased sympathetic activity could increase the degree of ischemic changes because of the increased oxygen consumption and the faster depletion of energy stores. The increased afterload, which also will increase oxygen consumption, does not in itself appear to be of great influence. When afterload was increased by clamping the aorta and sympathetic activity was presumably reduced via the baroreflexes, the changes in TQ potentials were opposite to those during left stellate stimulation, the effects being significant at both 2 and 5 min after coronary occlusion. Possibly, the increased perfusion pressure in the coronary arteries and the partial removal of vasoconstrictor tone overcame the extra workload imposed on the heart. The net effect of increased sympathetic activity on collateral flow, and thus on size of the ischemic area, will depend on the relative contribution of increased blood pressure on one hand and of coronary vasoconstriction on the other.

Right stellectomy vs left stellate ganglion stimulation. The changes induced by right stellectomy were in most experiments qualitatively similar to those produced by left stellate stimulation. Although at first glance it may seem difficult to conceive how a reduction in sympathetic activity on one side may induce the same kind of changes produced by augmented activity on the other side, this phenomenon has recently been described in a variety of experimental conditions.[6, 8, 15] There is evidence[16] that stellectomy interrupts afferent fibers that inhibit part of the sympathoexcitatory pathways located in the vicinity of the intermediolateral spinal nucleus; this results in increased sympathetic activity through the contralateral stellate ganglion.

Activation. In 11 of 16 experiments, left stellate stimulation markedly improved conduction within the ischemic zone at 4 or 5 min of occlusion; in four experiments there were no effects, and in one a slight increase in conduction delay occurred. An improvement in conduction in ischemic myocardium has also been reported during bilateral stellate ganglion stimulation.[17] It could be argued that the increase in blood pressure caused by sympathetic stimulation is responsible for the improvement in conduction by increasing perfusion of the ischemic zone. In that case, one would expect TQ depression to diminish. However, in the experiments in which conduction improved, TQ depression was increased. This seems paradoxical, since an increased TQ depression indicates a more advanced degree of depolarization of resting potential of ischemic cells. Action potential amplitude and upstroke velocity both decrease at lower resting membrane potential. Conduction velocity is partly determined by upstroke velocity, and in general the lower the rate of rise of action potential upstroke, the lower the conduction velocity. However, conduction velocity is also determined by the difference between resting potential and threshold potential, and action potentials elicited at a reduced membrane potential can indeed be conducted faster when threshold potential does not change.[18, 19] Also, the coupling resistance between cells determines conduction velocity, since conduction depends on local current circuits bringing adjacent cells to threshold. As argued before, it is unlikely that increased sympathetic activity would decrease coupling resistance. It is unknown whether catecholamines have an effect on threshold potential in ischemic cells.

In the very early phase of ischemia, the upstroke of the transmembrane action potential of myocardial cells is often separated into two components, the first of which is most likely caused by the depressed fast Na^+ inward current, the second to the slow inward current, carried mainly by Ca^{++} ions.[20] A similar separation of the upstroke is seen when isolated muscle preparations are exposed to elevated extracellular K^+ concentrations.[21, 22] The latter authors found that β-adrenergic stimulation has an inhibitory effect on the first component but increases the second component. The negative effect on conduction velocity caused by the decrease of the first component might be overcome by the simultaneous stimulation of the Ca^{++} inward current. However, detailed information on the relative contribution of both components of the action potential upstroke on conduction velocity is lacking. It should be emphasized that in this study, only the first 5 min of ischemia were considered. The effect of sympathetic stimulation on conduction in later phases might be quite different.

Arrhythmias. In agreement with the results of previous studies,[6, 8, 23] left stellate ganglion stimulation and right stellectomy increased the incidence of ventricular arrhythmias during the short-term occlusion in our study. Left stellectomy, however, did not result in a significant reduction of arrhythmias in this study, in contrast to other reports.[24] The reasons for this are not clear, but several factors can be considered.

First, it is known that the antiarrhythmic effect of short-term surgical denervation is much less marked than that produced by chronic denervation.[25] Second, the limiting effects of anesthesia on autonomic responses must be taken into account.[26] Indeed, the greatest antiarrhythmic efficacy of left stellectomy has been observed in long-term studies with conscious dogs.[7, 27]

Other parameters, apart from an increased or decreased left sympathetic tone, may determine whether arrhythmias will become manifest. One of these is the size of the ischemic area, which in our experiments was not determined accurately. Because the site of the occlusion was not the same in all dogs in our experiments, the size of the ischemic zone may have varied considerably from dog to dog. If the ischemic zone is very large, arrhythmias will occur regardless of a decreased sympathetic tone; if the zone is very small and arrhythmias do not occur in control occlusion, a reduction in sympathetic tone will also be without apparent effect. Moreover, since the effect of left stellectomy depends on the level of sympathetic tone before the stellectomy and since this could have varied from dog to dog, the number of experiments in this study may have been too small to uncover a protective effect of left sympathectomy.

Because reentry plays an important role in the genesis of ventricular arrhythmias in acute ischemia and because an increase in left sympathetic activity increases the likelihood for these arrhythmias to occur, it seems reasonable to expect that left stellate stimulation would induce electrophysiologic changes that would facilitate reentry. Slow conduction and the occurrence of areas of (unidirectional) block are factors that increase the likelihood of reentry, yet left stellate stimulation had effects in the opposite direction. Areas of conduction block were converted into zones of conduction, and conduction was more regular and faster than in control occlusion or in occlusions made after left stellectomy. Because we recorded electrograms only from the ischemic subepicardium, reentry in intramural or subendocardial sites cannot, of course, be ruled out. Previous studies indicated that although reentry is the predominant mechanism in the later phase of ventricular tachycardia and fibrillation, the initial ectopic premature impulses that initiate reentrant mechanisms are caused by a "focal" mechanism localized on the nonischemic side of the ischemic border.[9] Although the exact nature of this "focal" mechanism remains to be determined, one may speculate that it could be some form of abnormal automaticity or triggered activity, in which one of the triggers could be the current of injury.[9, 20] Since it is well known that both abnormal automaticity and delayed afterdepolarizations[28, 29] are enhanced by catecholamines, it may be that left sympathetic stimulation exerts its arrhythmogenic influence, not so much by promoting reentry but rather by enhancing the likelihood of the "focal" mechanism to become manifest.

References

1. Corr PB, Gillis RA: Autonomic neural influences on the dysrhythmias resulting from myocardial infarction. Circ Res **43:** 1, 1978
2. Lown B: Sudden cardiac death: the major challenge confronting contemporary cardiology. Am J Cardiol **43:** 313, 1979
3. Schwartz PJ, Stone HL: The role of the autonomic nervous system in sudden coronary death. Ann NY Acad Sci **382:** 162, 1982
4. Mailliani A, Schwartz PJ, Zanchetti A: A sympathetic reflex elicited by experimental coronary occlusion. Am J Physiol **217:** 703, 1969
5. Schwartz PJ, Pagani M, Lombardi F, Mailliani A, Brown AM: A cardio-cardiac sympatho vagal reflex in the cat. Circ Res **32:** 215, 1973
6. Schwartz PJ: Sympathetic imbalance and cardiac arrhythmias. *In* Randall WC, editor: Neural control of cardiovascular function. Oxford, 1984, Oxford University Press, pp 225–252
7. Schwartz PJ, Stone HL: Left stellectomy in the prevention of ventricular fibrillation caused by acute myocardial ischemia in conscious dogs with anterior myocardial infarction. Circulation **62:** 1256, 1980
8. Schwartz PJ, Stone HL, Brown AM: Effects of unilateral stellate ganglion blockade on the arrhythmias associated with coronary occlusion. Am Heart J **92:** 589, 1976
9. Janse MJ, van Capelle FJL, Morsink H, Kleber AG, Wilms-Schopman F, Cardinal R, Naumann d'Alnoncourt C, Durrer D: Flow of "injury" current and patterns of excitation during early ventricular arrhythmias in acute regional ischemia in isolated porcine and canine hearts: evidence for two arrhythmogenic mechanisms. Circ Res **47:** 151, 1980
10. Cardinal R, Janse MJ, van Eeden I, Werner G, Naumann d'Alnoncourt C, Durrer D: The effects of lidocaine on intracellular and extracellular potentials, activation and ventricular arrhythmias during acute regional ischemia in isolated porcine hearts. Circ Res **49:** 792, 1981
11. Weingart R, Reber W: Influence of internal pH on Ri of Purkinje fibers from mammalian heart. Experientia **35:** 929, 1979 (abst)
12. Mohrman DE, Feigl EO: Competition between sympathetic vasoconstriction and metabolic vasodilation in the canine coronary circulation. Cir Res **42:** 79, 1978
13. Janse MJ, Wilms-Schopman F: Effects of changes in perfusion pressure on the position of the electrophysiological border zone in acute regional ischemia in isolated perfused dog and pig hearts. Am J Cardiol **50:** 74, 1982
14. Ruffy R, Lovelace DE, Knoebel SB, Elharrar V, Zipes DP: Relationship between left ventricular electrograms and regional blood flow in acute myocardial ischemia with and without stellate stimulation. Circulation **56**(suppl III): III-137, 1977 (abst)
15. Schwartz PJ, Verrier RL, Lown B: Effect of stellectomy and vagotomy on ventricular refractoriness. Circ Res **40:** 536, 1977
16. McCall RB, Gebber GL, Barman SM: Spinal interneurons in the baroreceptor reflex arc. Am J Physiol **232:** H657, 1977
17. Millar K, Lux RL, Wyatt RF: Ischemia induced ventricular conduction delay: reversal by cardiac nerve stimulation. Circulation **53/54**(suppl II): II-131, 1977
18. Peon J, Ferrier GR, Moe GK: The relationship of excitability to conduction velocity in canine Purkinje tissue. Circ Res **43:** 125, 1978
19. Dominguez G, Fozzard HA: Influence of extracellular K^+ concentration on cable properties and excitability of sheep cardiac Purkinje fibers. Circ Res **26:** 565, 1970
20. Janse MJ, Kleber AG: Electrophysiological changes and ventricular arrhythmias in the early phase of regional myocardial ischemia. Circ Res **49:** 1069, 1981
21. Mascher D: Electrical and mechanical responses from ventricular muscle fibers after inactivation of the sodium carrying system. Pfluegers Arch **317:** 359, 1970
22. Windisch H, Tritthart HA: Isoproterenol, norepinephrine and phosphodiesterase inhibitors are blockers of the depressed fast Na^+-system in ventricular muscle fibers. J Mol Cell Cardiol **14:** 431, 1982
23. Vanoli E, Zaza A, Zuanetti G, Pappalettera M, Schwartz PJ: Reduction in infarct size produced by left stellectomy. *In* Proceedings of the Ninth World Congress of Cardiology, Moscow, 1982
24. Schwartz PJ, Stone HL: Left stellectomy in the prevention of ventricular fibrillation caused by acute myocardial ischemia in conscious dogs with anterior myocardial infarction. Circulation **62:** 1256, 1980
25. Ebert PA, Vanderbeek RB, Allgood RJ, Sabiston DC Jr: Effect of chronic cardiac denervation on arrhythmias after coronary artery ligation. Cardiovasc Res **4:** 141, 1970
26. Vatner SF, Braunwald E: Cardiovascular control mechanisms in the conscious state. N Engl J Med **293:** 970, 1975
27. Schwartz PJ, Billman GE, Stone HL: Autonomic mechanism in ventricular fibrillation induced by myocardial ischemia during exercise in dogs with healed myocardial infarction: an experimental preparation for sudden cardiac death. Circulation **69:** 790, 1984
28. Katzung BG, Hondegem LM, Grant AO: Cardiac ventricular automaticity induced by current of injury. Pfluegers Arch **360:** 193, 1975
29. Hoffman BF: Role of sympathetic nervous system in arrhythmias occurring after coronary artery occlusion and myocardial infarction. *In* Schwartz PJ, Brown AM, Malliani A, Zanchetti A, editors: Cardiac arrhythmias. New York, 1978, Raven Press, pp 155–166

Electrophysiologic and anatomic basis for fractionated electrograms recorded from healed myocardial infarcts

PHYLLIS I. GARDNER, M.D., PHILIP C. URSELL, M.D., JOHN J. FENOGLIO, JR., M.D., AND ANDREW L. WIT, PH.D.

ABSTRACT The electrophysiologic and anatomic basis for fractionated electrograms were investigated in superfused epicardial preparations from infarcted canine hearts. Fractionated bipolar electrograms were frequently recorded in preparations from infarcts 2 weeks to 18 months old but only rarely in preparations from 5-day-old infarcts. The fractionated electrograms were not caused by movement artifacts. They were not associated with depressed transmembrane resting or action potentials (which were found in the 5-day-old infarcts), but rather transmembrane potentials recorded in the vicinity of the bipolar electrodes were normal. Despite the normal transmembrane potentials, activation time in regions where fractionated electrograms occurred was prolonged. However, prolonged activation time by itself did not cause fractionation, since fractionated electrograms were not recorded from normal preparations in which conduction was markedly slowed by a superfusate containing 16 mM potassium and epinephrine. Unipolar electrograms recorded with glass microelectrodes (tip size 1 to 5 μm) showed that activation in regions where fractionated electrograms were recorded was inhomogeneous. Prepotentials were found preceding the upstrokes of some action potentials in regions where double potentials were recorded, suggesting the possibility of electrotonic transmission across high resistance or inexcitable gaps, but no electrotonic potentials were seen in regions with multicomponent fractionated electrograms. Fractionated electrograms were recorded in regions where infarct healing caused wide separation of individual myocardial fibers while distorting their orientation. The anatomic changes probably caused slow and inhomogeneous activation.
Circulation 72, No. 3, 596–611, 1985.

FRACTIONATED electrograms,[1–11] consisting of either two discrete deflections separated by an isoelectric interval (double potentials or split deflections[4, 7, 8, 12]) or comprised of many components[1, 2, 6, 7] have been recorded during mapping studies on patients with ischemic heart disease and a history of chronic ventricular tachycardia. These kinds of electrograms have been found during sinus rhythm[2, 6, 7, 9–11] as well as during tachycardia.[1–3]

It is important to determine why fractionated electrograms occur and what they mean. Their occurrence during sinus rhythm might sometimes assist in identifying patients who can develop ventricular tachycardia.[6, 8] The site at which these electrograms are recorded either during sinus rhythm or during tachycardia may indicate the site where a reentrant circuit is located.[2, 6–11] On the other hand, fractionated electrograms might sometimes be artifacts of recording techniques,[5] caused by such things as electrode movement,[13, 14] or distortions of the electrical signal by the filtering characteristics of the amplifiers.[14] Furthermore, since high amplification is often necessary to record fractionated activity in and around aneurysms, it is possible that the fractionated electrograms might sometimes represent activity originating in distant and possibly normal areas.[5, 13]

The studies to determine the value of fractionated electrograms for indicating those patients at risk of having ventricular tachycardia or for locating reentrant circuits must be done in humans.[9, 11] However, it will be difficult to determine the exact physiologic causes for such electrograms in clinical studies. To understand why fractionated electrograms occur, we have done electrophysiologic and anatomic investigations on areas where such activity is present in isolated

From the Departments of Pharmacology and Pathology, College of Physicians and Surgeons, Columbia University, New York, NY.
Supported by Program Project Grant HL-30557 and by a Cardiovascular Training Grant (HL-07271) from the National Heart, Lung, and Blood Institute. Also supported by BRSG SO7RR0539-24, NIH.
Address for correspondence: Andrew L. Wit, Ph.D., Department of Pharmacology, College of Physicians and Surgeons, Columbia University, 630 W. 168th St., New York, NY 10032.
Received Sept. 28, 1984; revision accepted June 13, 1985.

superfused preparations from canine infarcts. Preliminary reports of some of our results have been presented.[15, 16]

Methods

Surgical production of myocardial infarction. Myocardial infarction was caused in 50 mongrel dogs weighing 13 to 18 kg by a two-stage ligation of the left anterior descending coronary artery (LAD) 5 to 10 mm from its origin, with sterile techniques.[17, 18] Forty-five dogs survived the surgical procedure. In this report we include only data from the 36 transmural infarcts.

At various times after coronary occlusion the surviving dogs were reanesthetized with sodium pentobarbital (15 to 30 mg/kg iv) for the electrophysiologic and anatomic study. Ten animals were studied at 5 days, six at 15 days, seven at 2 months, six at 4 months, four at 8 months, two at 16 months, and one at 18 months. We chose these times because they represent periods during the subacute (5 days), healing (15 days), and healed (2 to 18 months) phases of myocardial infarction. We characterized the electrograms and the cellular electrophysiologic and microanatomic features of the muscle that survives on the epicardial surface of the transmural infarcts at each of these different stages. Five normal dogs that had not undergone coronary artery ligation served as controls.

Electrophysiologic studies in vitro. After induction of anesthesia, the chest was reopened and the infarcted region was visually identified by a mottled or pale appearance. A piece of myocardium approximately 20 × 20 × 3 mm was then excised rapidly with a sharp scalpel blade from the epicardial aspect of the infarcted left ventricle in situ. Whenever possible this piece was taken from a region devoid of large epicardial coronary arteries. It was immediately pinned to the waxed base of a 25 ml superfusion chamber, epicardial surface upward, and superfused with oxygenated Tyrode's solution (composition previously described[19]) at a rate of 50 ml/min. The solution was briskly bubbled with a 95% O_2/5% CO_2 gas mixture both in the reservoir and in the bath. The pH of the Tyrode's in the tissue bath under these conditions was 7.30 to 7.35. The temperature was maintained constant at 36.5 ± 0.5° C.

The preparations of epicardial muscle were stimulated through Teflon-coated, bipolar, silver-wire electrodes at basic stimulus cycle lengths of 800 to 1000 msec.[19] After an initial equilibration period of 60 min, extracellular electrograms and transmembrane action potentials were recorded from subepicardial fibers at multiple sites.[18, 19] Extracellular electrograms were recorded through electrodes made from Teflon-coated silver wire. The diameter of the electrode surface in contact with the tissue was 0.3 mm. Bipolar electrodes had a distance between recording poles (measured from the center of one pole to the center of the other) of 0.5 to 1.0 mm. When a unipolar electrode was used, the indifferent electrode was located in the bath approximately 30 mm from the recording electrode. Extracellular signals were amplified with a Tektronix 2A61 differential amplifier. The low and high bandpasses were 0.06 and 6000 Hz. We also used 3M KCl–filled glass capillary electrodes with tip diameters estimated to be about 1 to 5 μm to record unipolar electrograms. The signal recorded with these electrodes was led into the high-input impedance negative capacitance amplifier that was used for the transmembrane potential recordings.

Membrane potentials and electrograms were displayed on a Tektronix 565 oscilloscope and photographed with a Grass C-4 oscilloscopic camera. Action potential parameters were measured by methods described in other publications.[18, 19]

Histologic and morphometric analysis. We did not usually find fractionated electrograms in preparations from noninfarcted hearts or from 5-day infarcted hearts (see Results). Because electrograms in most regions had a similar configuration, it was not necessary to mark a specific recording site for anatomic study. Instead, the entire preparation of epicardium was fixed in 10% neutral buffered formaldehyde. After fixation, the tissue was sliced into five pieces and cut perpendicular to the LAD border and perpendicular to the plane of the epicardium. The slices were then processed for histologic study according to routine methods.[20] Each histologic section (5 μm thick), stained with hematoxylin-phloxine-saffron, showed the full thickness of the preparation, from the epicardial surface to the surface where the preparation was cut from the ventricular wall.

In the preparations from the healed infarcts, both fractionated and nonfractionated electrograms were found (see Results). Selected areas at which electrograms with different characteristics were recorded were marked with color-coded pins during the experiment, and then with India ink before fixation. These marked areas were then cut from the epicardial surface with a sharp razor blade and fixed in formaldehyde. The size of these pieces was approximately 2 × 4 mm and 1 to 2 mm thick. The remainder of each preparation was also fixed in the formaldehyde. The small, marked pieces were oriented in the paraffin embedding blocks so that the epicardial surface formed one margin of each section. These specimens were then serially sectioned (5 μm thick) and each section stained with hematoxylin-phloxine-saffron. The number of muscle fibers surviving at the recording sites was determined from the serial sections.

We also applied morphometric techniques to the histologic sections to determine the relative proportion of heart muscle to nonmuscular tissue in regions where different kinds of electrograms were recorded. Representative experiments from each age of infarct as well as noninfarcted hearts were selected for this analysis (two normal, four at 5 days, two at 15 days, two at 2 months, and four at 4 to 18 months). Morphometric analysis was done on blocks that were serially sectioned, yielding 50 to 150 5 μm thick sections. The sections were stained and mounted on glass slides in the usual manner. Tissue sections without folds were selected randomly (eight to 10 sections per experiment) and photographed. Each negative was enlarged and printed on 8 × 10 inch photographic paper (final magnification × 130 to 500). Morphometric analysis was confined to the region designated as the epicardial border zone.[19] This area extends from the layer of muscle cells immediately subjacent to the epicardium to the deepest surviving muscle layer overlying the infarct. Within the region we determined the amount of muscular tissue relative to nonmuscular tissue (including blood vessels, connective tissue, and inflammatory cells) using the point-counting method.[21] A grid composed of boxes no larger than the average muscle fiber diameter was superimposed on the photographs. If the tissue to be measured contained longitudinally oriented muscle fibers, the axis of the grid was placed at 19 degrees to the long axis of the fibers to counteract the bias introduced by anisotropy.[22] The appropriate density of points for each case was implied by the magnification of the photomicrograph.[21] Each cross point on the grid was evaluated to determine whether it lay over heart muscle or nonmuscular tissue. A ratio of heart muscle "hits" to nonmuscular "hits" was made. The mean and standard deviation of the ratio from all photographs from the experiments were determined.

Results

Characteristics of extracellular electrograms

Dependence on infarct age. Ventricular muscle survives on the epicardial surface of transmural canine infarcts.[19, 23, 24] We determined the characteristics of the extracellular waveforms recorded from this subepicar-

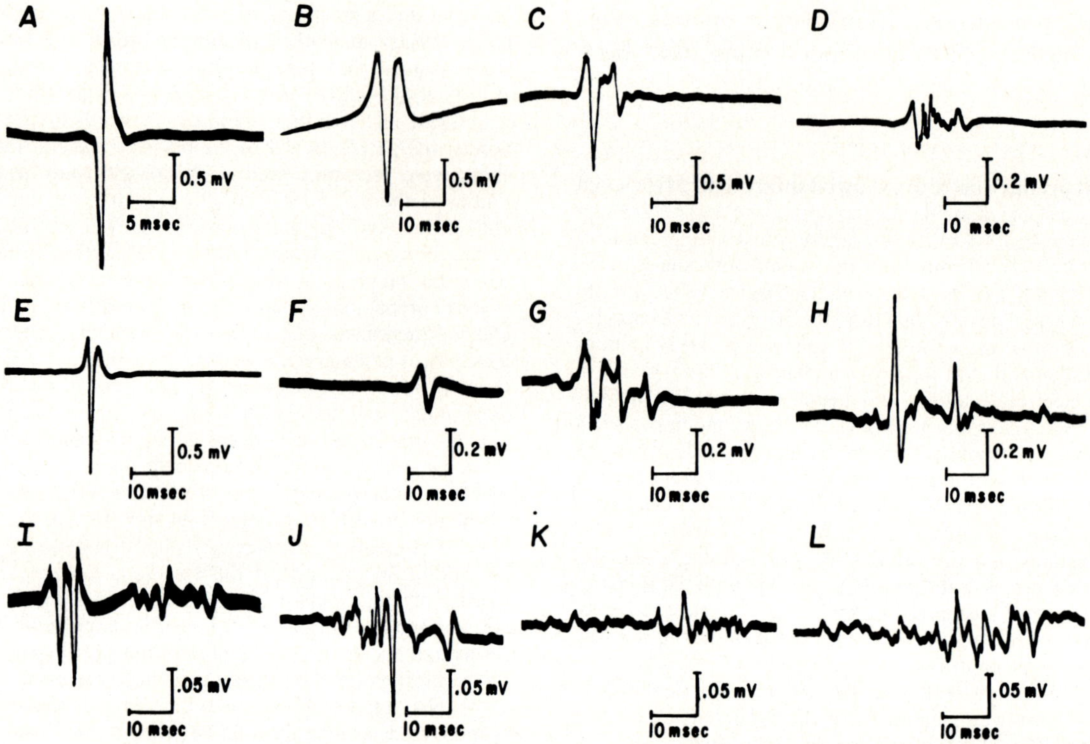

FIGURE 1. Representative bipolar electrograms recorded from superfused subepicardial preparations. Preamplifier filters were set at 0.06 to 6000 Hz. The electrogram shown in *A* was recorded from a noninfarcted preparation, the electrograms in *B* and *C* from 5-day-old infarcts, the electrograms in *D* and *G* from 2-week-old infarcts, the electrograms in *E, F, I,* and *J* from 16-month-old infarcts, and the electrograms in *H, K,* and *L* from 2-month-old infarcts.

dial muscle with bipolar electrodes and compared them with electrograms recorded from noninfarcted preparations. Bipolar recordings were used in much of this study because the clinical reports on fractionated electrograms have relied on this technique.[1-11] Thirty to 60 electrograms were recorded at approximately 2 mm intervals over the entire surface of each preparation. Extracellular waveforms recorded from subepicardial muscle in preparations from noninfarcted hearts consisted of smooth contour, biphasic, or triphasic deflections with amplitudes of 2 to 4 mV and durations of less than 5 msec (figure 1, *A*). Most of the bipolar electrograms recorded from preparations from hearts with 5-day-old infarcts had similar configurations (figure 1, *B*). The main difference between electrograms recorded from these infarct preparations and normal preparations was a decrease in the amplitude of the electrograms recorded from the infarcts (range from 500 μV to 2 mV) and a small increase in duration (up to 10 msec). Occasionally, electrograms were recorded from some preparations from 5-day-old infarcts, which had irregular waveforms, characterized by notching or multiple components (figure 1, *C*). The total duration of these electrograms was not longer than 10 msec.

Unlike the 5-day-old infarct preparations, fractionated electrograms were frequently recorded with bipolar electrodes from the 2-week- to 18-month-old infarcts (figure 1, *D* and *G* to *L*). In three of the preparations from healed infarcts (one 2 months old, one 16 months old, one 18 months old) all electrograms were fractionated. In the remaining preparations both fractionated electrograms and electrograms with normal contours were recorded (figure 1, *E* and *F*). Some of the fractionated electrograms had two or more discrete spikes separated by isoelectric intervals (see figures 5 and 10). Other electrograms consisted of multiple spikes, separated either by slower waveforms or isoelectric segments (figure 1, *G* to *L*). The duration of the fractionated electrograms was highly variable and, in general, there was an increase with infarct age. The duration of electrograms was greater in 2- to 18-month-old infarcts (20 to 70 msec duration) (figure 1, *H* to *L*) than in 2-week-old infarcts (10 to 20 msec duration) (figure 1, *D* and *G*). We did not notice any marked differences in duration among the 2- to 18-month-old infarcts. The amplitude of the signals also decreased with infarct age so that at 2 weeks, amplitudes were consistently between 200 μV and 1 mV (figure 1, *D* and *G*) while at 2 months and more they were often less than 200 μV (figure 1, *I* to *L*). In these healed infarcts electrograms that were not fractionated often had low amplitudes as well (figure 1, *F*).

Is fractionation caused by recording artifacts? It has been suggested that the fractionated nature of some electrograms might be artifactual, caused by contraction-induced electrode movement or by the filtering characteristics of the amplifier used to record them (see above). We recorded stable fractionated electrograms for 3 to 5 hr after the tissue was mounted in the superfusion chamber. Because these preparations had only a narrow surface rim of viable muscle fibers (see histologic results) there was often no visible contraction or movement of the electrodes even when the preparation was observed under the high-power optics of the dissection scope over the tissue chamber. Therefore the fractionated nature of the electrograms could not be attributed to artifacts generated by gross movement at the electrode-tissue interface. Nor was fractionation an artifact introduced by filtering out low-frequency components of a single broad electrogram. The electrograms shown in figure 1 were recorded at a bandpass of 0.06 to 6000 Hz, which permits most slow and fast components of extracellular activity to be recorded except for direct current potentials. The total duration of fractionated electrograms and number of components was influenced by changing the bandpass but we did not study these effects in detail. In general, increasing the high bandpass filter setting from 0.06 to 60 Hz decreased the amplitude of the electrograms and attenuated the slow components (compare right panels *A* and *B* in figure 2).

Effects of electrode configuration and direction of impulse propagation. The recording electrode configuration also influenced the characteristics of the fractionated electrograms. The electrograms shown in figure 1 were recorded with a bipolar electrode. Fractionated electrograms, however, were not caused by bipolar recording techniques per se. At all sites at which fractionated electrograms were recorded with bipolar electrodes we could also record fractionated activity with unipolar electrodes (figure 2, *left*). In experiments in which bipolar electrograms were first recorded and then unipolar electrograms recorded from each of the bipoles as shown in the figure, it appeared that the fractionated waveform of the bipolar electrogram resulted from summation of the fractionated unipolar waveforms (figure 2, *left*).

The direction of impulse propagation with relation to the orientation of the bipoles also affected the characteristics of the fractionated electrograms. Usually when the site of stimulation was changed to alter the propagation direction the number of components either increased or decreased (figure 3).

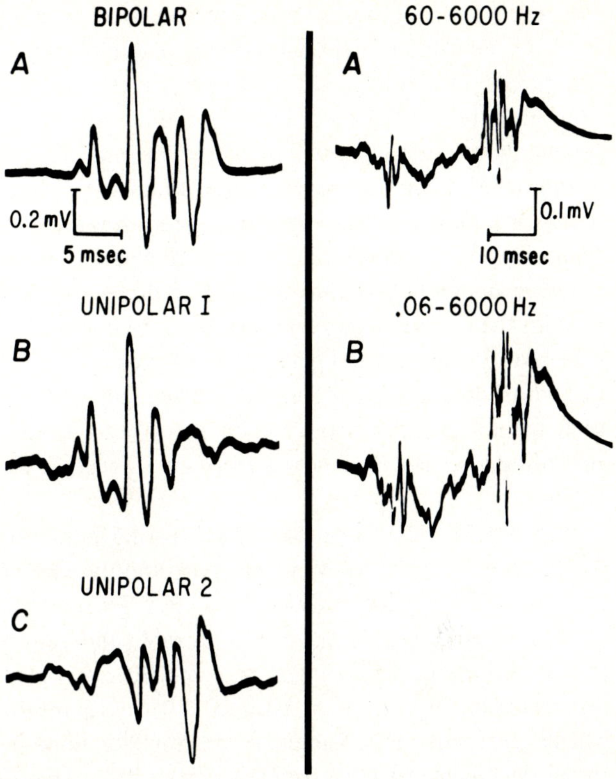

FIGURE 2. *Left,* Fractionated electrogram recorded with a bipolar electrode (panel *A*) and with each of the poles separately (panels *B* and *C*). *Right,* Fractionated electrogram recorded with different preamplifier filter settings.

Electrophysiologic basis for fractionated electrograms

Transmembrane potentials in regions of fractionation. We have shown that fractionated electrograms appear during infarct healing. The question then arises, are there special electrophysiologic properties of the healing infarct that cause them? Spach et al.[25] have indicated that complex polyphasic waveforms (fractionation) could arise from a peculiar shape of the transmembrane action potentials — from membrane currents associated with a complex or multicomponent phase of depolarization of individual cells. Fractionation might also be

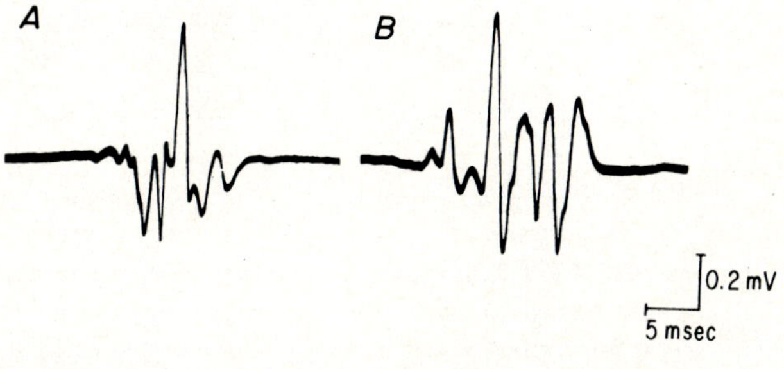

FIGURE 3. Effects of changing the direction of impulse propagation on a fractionated electrogram. Panels *A* and *B* show an electrogram recorded as the preparation was stimulated from two different sites.

the result of superposition of extracellular currents from asynchronous depolarizations in a number of functionally different cells with normally shaped action potentials.[25] We recorded transmembrane action potentials in regions from which fractionated electrograms were recorded and compared them with transmembrane potentials in regions where smooth, normally shaped electrograms were recorded to determine whether any particular characteristic could be correlated with the occurrence of fractionated activity. Action potentials were recorded from 10 to 30 sites within a 2 to 5 mm^2 area around the extracellular electrode and then from the region from which this electrode was recording after it was removed from the surface of the tissue.

In 5-day-old infarct preparations, resting potential (RMP) was −77 ± 7 mV, action potential maximum upstroke velocity ($\dot{V}$max) was 73 ± 9 V/sec, amplitude of phase 0 (APA) was 86 ± 8 mV, and action potential duration to 50% (APD_{50}) and 90% (APD_{90}) repolarization was 120 ± 10 and 170 ± 15 msec. These represent mean values ± SE for 348 impalements at electrogram recording sites in 10 preparations. All values are significantly less ($p < .05$) than values for muscle fibers in noninfarcted preparations where normal electrograms were recorded (RMP = −91 ± 4 mV, $\dot{V}$max = 102 ± 18 V/sec, APA = 103 ± 6 mV, APD_{50} = 175 ± 8 msec, APD_{90} = 210 ± 15 msec; 283 impalements in five preparations). A representative transmembrane potential recorded from a muscle fiber in a 5-day-old infarct is shown in the top left panel of figure 4. Similar results have been previously reported from other studies on transmembrane potentials of epicardial muscle surviving in infarcted regions at this period.[19, 26, 27] These alterations in the transmembrane potentials, however, were not associated with fractionated electrograms, which, as shown above, were not common in these preparations (figure 4, *top left*). In 2-week-old infarcts, resting potential (−88 ± 9 mV), $\dot{V}$max (104 ± 21 v/sec), and action potential amplitude (101 ± 8 mV) were not significantly different than normal, although action potential duration (APD_{50} = 92 ± 8 msec, APD_{90} = 115 ± 12 msec) was still short ($p < .05$; 169 impalements in six preparations). In the healed infarcts (2 months and older) where fractionated electrograms were most prominent, the transmembrane potentials of the muscle fibers were not significantly different from normal, including the time course for repolarization (RMP = −86 ± 5 mV, $\dot{V}$max = 101 ± 15 V/sec, APA = 98 ± 10 mV; APD_{50} = 160 ± 8 msec, APD_{90} = 205 ± 12 msec; mean values for 180 impalements in seven preparations). A representative action potential recorded at a site of fractionated activity in a healed infarct is

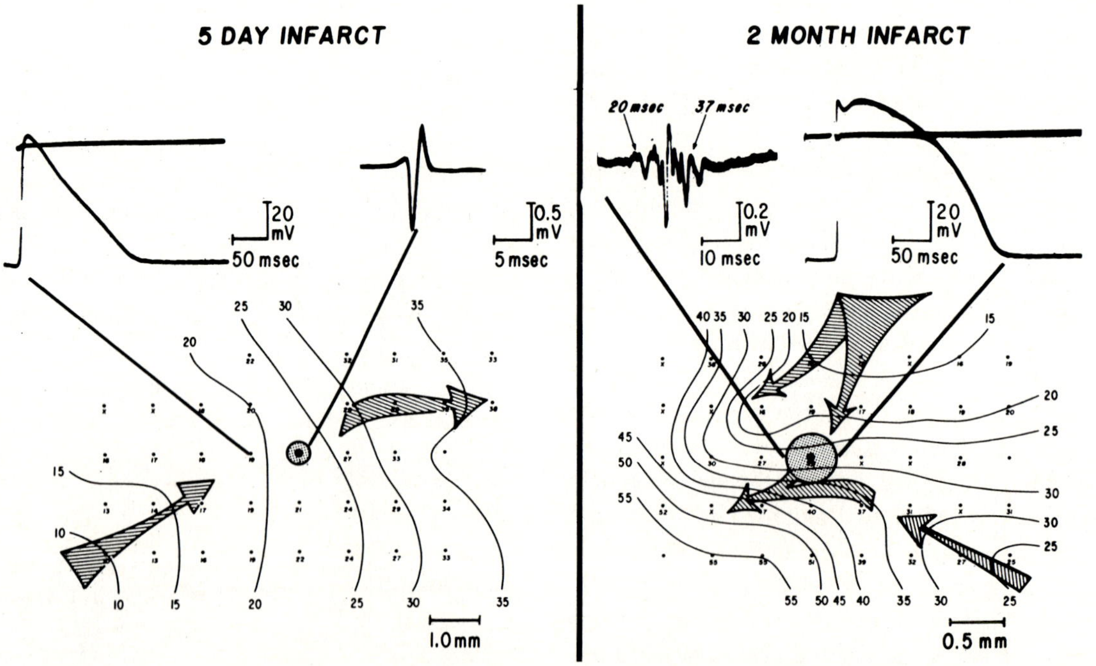

FIGURE 4. Activation maps of regions around bipolar electrodes in two different infarct preparations. The location and size of the electrodes are indicated by the stippled circle and the electrograms recorded in each experiment are shown above. The points at which action potentials were recorded in each panel are indicated by the dots. Representative action potentials are also shown. The arrows and isochrones show the direction of activation. The stimulus sites are not included in the maps. The distance scale for each panel is shown below; note that the scale is two times larger for the 5-day-old infarct preparation than for the 2-month-old infarct preparation.

shown in the top right panel of figure 4. In addition, in preparations from healed infarcts, transmembrane potentials recorded from regions where there were fractionated electrograms were no different from transmembrane potentials recorded from regions where electrograms had a normal contour.

In the experiments in which action potentials were recorded from regions with fractionated electrograms containing a large number of spikes (such as electrograms *K* and L in figure 1), the upstrokes were characterized by a normal smooth S-shaped curve. Fractionation, therefore, could not be caused by a complex action potential depolarization phase. In experiments in which action potentials were recorded from regions where "double potentials" were found, we sometimes saw low-amplitude prepotentials before the action potential upstroke (figure 5, *E* and *F*). Action potentials with two component upstrokes were also found, each component corresponding with an electrogram deflection (figure 5, *C* and *D*). For reasons described later, we do not attribute these multiple components of the upstroke to different active membrane processes but rather the evidence suggests that they are caused by electrotonic interactions among adjacent, poorly coupled fibers. Our conclusion from the data presented in this section is that fractionated electrograms are not necessarily related to depressed resting potentials or action potential upstroke velocities. Complex upstrokes of action potentials of individual muscle cells do not appear to cause multiple component fractionated electrograms, although they were sometimes found to be associated with double potentials.

Relationship of fractionation to characteristics of local activation. It has been suggested that fractionated electrograms recorded in acute myocardial infarction are caused by slow activation.[28] It was therefore surprising that the transmembrane action potentials at the sites where these electrograms were recorded in healed infarcts arose from normal resting potentials and had normal upstroke velocities, properties not usually associated with slow conduction.[29] To evaluate conduction characteristics in regions where electrograms were recorded, we also mapped impulse propagation. Action potentials were recorded from 20 to 50 sites within a 10 to 20 mm^2 area around the extracellular electrode. Activation maps were constructed for regions in which both normal and fractionated electrograms were recorded by using the beginning of the extracellular electrogram as a reference (where the potential first deviated from isoelectric) and determining the time of activation at each microelectrode recording site (measuring the time interval from the reference to the upstroke at 50% of its maximum amplitude). Normally shaped electrograms recorded from preparations from noninfarcted hearts and from some regions in preparations from infarcted hearts were found in areas where a broad wavefront propagated rapidly past the recording site (figure 4, *left*). The region around the bipolar recording electrode was activated in less than 5 msec. In the normal preparations and in these regions of preparations from healed infarcts 2 months and older, the apparent conduction velocity calculated in a direction normal to the isochrones and parallel to myocardial fiber orientation (verified by subsequent histologic study; see below) was 0.5 to 1.0 m/sec. In regions of 5-

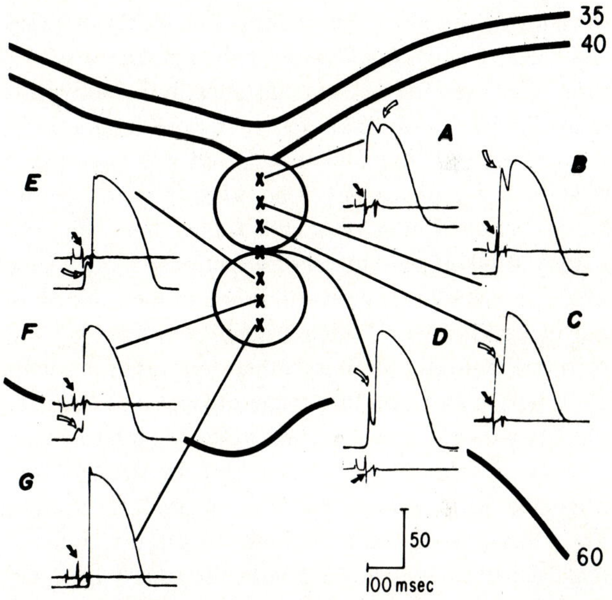

FIGURE 5. Action potentials in a region where a "double" potential was recorded. The two circles in the middle of the figure indicate the bipolar electrode. The x's show where action potentials were recorded. (The microelectrode was actually adjacent to the bipoles and not beneath them.) The thick dark lines are isochrones indicating activation times and the direction of propagation at this recording site. Panels *A* to *G* show simultaneous recordings of the action potentials and the extracellular electrogram. The solid arrows in each panel indicate the first component of the "double" potential. This component is preceded by a stimulus artifact. The upstroke of the action potentials in *A* and *B* occur simultaneously with the first electrogram deflection. The unfilled arrows indicate possible electrotonic influences on the plateau phase. The upstrokes of the action potentials in *C* and *D* have two components, one corresponding to the first electrogram deflection (unfilled arrow) and one corresponding to the second electrogram deflection. The upstrokes of the action potentials in *E* and *F* are simultaneous with the second electrogram deflection but are preceded by an electrotonic prepotential (unfilled arrows) that begins with the first electrogram deflection and spans the isoelectric segment between the two deflections. The upstroke of the action potential in *G* occurs just after the second electrogram deflection and is not preceded by a prepotential. In this experiment, no action potential upstrokes were found to occur in the isoelectric segment between electrogram deflections. Voltage calibration is for the transmembrane potential recording.

day-old infarcts where normally shaped electrograms were recorded, apparent conduction velocity calculated in the same manner was 0.2 to 0.4 m/sec (figure 4, *left*).

Activation of the regions in the vicinity of the electrodes recording fractionated electrograms took a much longer period of time. The prolonged activation time was particularly pronounced in the preparations from hearts with healed infarcts (2 to 18 months) despite the normal resting potentials and action potential upstroke velocities. In figure 4, *right,* the fractionated electrogram had a total duration of about 17 msec. In the region from which this electrogram was recorded it took more than 12 msec for the impulse to move a distance of about 0.5 mm between the electrode poles (indicated by the stippled circle) as compared with a time of 2 msec for the same distance in the activation map of a 5-day-old infarct shown in the left panel. If it is assumed that conduction occurred in a reasonably straight line past the electrode poles (and it may not have), conduction velocity would have been approximately 0.04 m/sec. In other experiments on healed infarct preparations, activation time in the vicinity of the electrodes with which fractionated activity was recorded was also similar to the total duration of the electrogram and therefore ranged from 10 to 70 msec (apparent conduction velocities of 0.05 to 0.01 m/sec). It is also possible that some of the fractionated activity might be accounted for by slow or late activation of myocardial fibers that are too deep from the endocardial surface to be impaled with the microelectrode. Activation may be three-dimensional rather than the two-dimensional activation shown on the map.

Is the slow activation of regions where fractionated electrograms were recorded the primary cause of the fractionation? If it is, it would seem that slowing activation to a similar extent in regions where electrograms have a normal configuration should cause fractionation. We slowed conduction in these regions in both normal and 5-day-old infarct preparations by increasing the K^+ concentration to 16 mM, which caused inexcitability, and then by restoring very slow conduction by adding 1 μg/ml epinephrine to the superfusate.[30, 31] When this was done there was a marked decrease in electrogram amplitude, a slowing of its rate of depolarization, and an increase in its duration as shown in figure 6, *A* to *C*. At the high amplification used to display the electrogram, a second component was evident (figure 6, *C*), which always coincided with the repolarization phase of the action potential (figure 6, *1*, *2*, and *3*) and was probably caused by repolarization. Similar double-component electrograms were recorded at all sites on the preparation where slow response action potentials were recorded. The upstroke of the action potential recorded near an extracellular electrode always coincided with the first electrogram component and repolarization always coincided with the second component, even when the microelectrode was moved to different sites around the extracellular recording electrode (see figure 6, *1*, *2*, and *3*).

In none of these experiments in which slow conduction (conduction velocities less than 0.05 m/sec) was caused by high K^+ concentration and epinephrine did multicomponent fractionated electrograms occur. Therefore, slow conduction (alone) is not the cause of fractionated activity, although it does increase the total duration of the electrogram. We also elevated K^+ concentration in experiments in which fractionated electrograms were recorded from healed infarcts. When the K^+ concentration in the superfusate reached 12 to 14 mM, the resting potential and upstroke velocities of the fibers in the vicinity of the fractionated electrograms were significantly depressed and activation time of these regions prolonged. The total duration of the fractionated electrogram increased, its amplitude diminished, and the rate of change of the voltage of the individual spikes comprising the electrogram diminished. However, either the number of components comprising the fractionated electrogram did not change (figure 7) or actually decreased. These results suggest further that the activation time and the action potential characteristics are not the main determinants of the fractionated nature of these electrograms.

Instead of simply slow activation, fractionated electrograms might be caused by slow activation in combination with inhomogeneities in activation around the recording electrode.[28] Such inhomogeneities on a "micro" level would not be apparent in activation maps like the one shown in figure 4. To obtain more detailed information on characteristics of activation in the vicinity of the extracellular bipolar electrode we simultaneously recorded extracellular waveforms with glass capillary electrodes with tip diameters of about 1 to 5 μm. The small tip size enabled us to record extracellular activity from individual muscle fibers[25, 32] at numerous sites within the 1 mm distance between the bipoles.

Recordings are shown in figure 8 for a representative experiment in which the fractionated electrogram had three discrete components separated by short isoelectric segments. Within a 1 mm circumference around the positive electrode pole, a single biphasic deflection was recorded by the extracellular microelectrode. This unipolar electrogram coincided in time with the initial deflection of the fractionated electrogram (figure 8, *A*). As the microelectrode was moved in steps of approximately 0.1 mm toward the negative pole, the amplitude of the waveform coinciding with the first fractionated component decreased and an extracellular potential coincident with the second deflection of the fractionated electrogram appeared (figure 8, *B*). This waveform became larger as the microelectrode was moved to another site (figure 8, *C*). Similarly, the amplitude of this waveform decreased as the extracellular electrode was moved to another site and a deflection coinciding with the third component of the fractionated electrogram appeared (figure 8, *D*) and increased in amplitude (figure 8, *E*) until only this deflection was found (figure 8, *F*). It is apparent from this experiment that an extracellular signal resulting from activation could not be recorded in the vicinity of the bipolar electrode during segments between the major components of the fractionated electrogram. The results of other experiments of this kind are similar.

Spach et al.[32] have shown that a uniform biphasic waveform such as those recorded with the extracellular microelectrode is characteristic of action potentials propagating at uniform velocity in a functionally single strand or bundle of cardiac muscle. Interpreted the same way, the results of the experiment shown in figure 8 indicate the presence of three functional strands or bundles of cardiac muscle, each giving rise to a biphasic waveform. The summation of the extracellular waveforms from each of these strands causes the fractionated electrogram recorded with the bipolar electrode.[25] Furthermore, the results of this experiment show that activation in the area where the fractionated

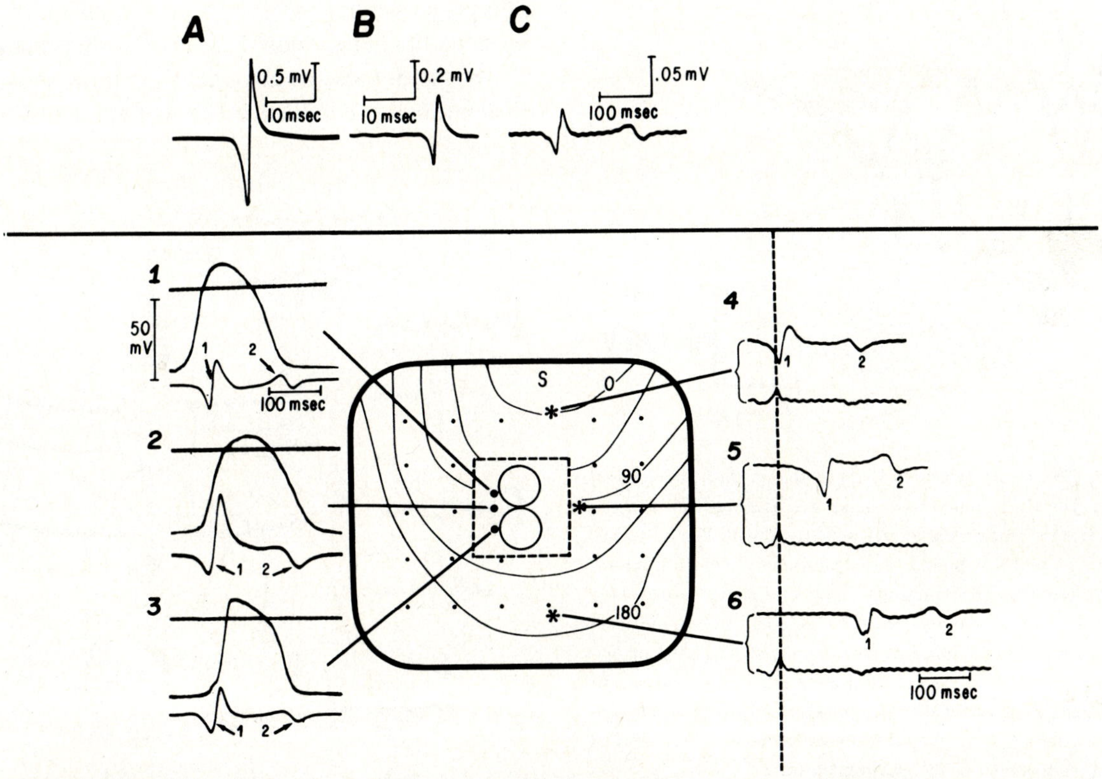

FIGURE 6. Electrograms and action potentials recorded from a normal preparation superfused with high K^+ concentration Tyrode's solution containing epinephrine. At the top, panel *A* shows the control electrogram in normal Tyrode's solution, panel *B* shows the electrogram as the elevated K^+ solution entered the chamber, and panel *C* shows the electrogram in the high-K^+, catecholamine-containing solution. Note the two components to this electrogram. At the bottom center is shown a diagram of the preparation and the activation map in the high-K^+, catecholamine solution. The dots and asterisks indicate sites at which extracellular electrograms were recorded with a roving electrode. They are 1 mm apart. Representative electrograms, recorded with this probe during mapping, are in the top trace of panels *4*, *5*, and *6*. They all have two components (labeled 1 and 2). The electrogram in the bottom trace in each panel was recorded by a reference electrode near the stimulus (S). At the left, in the top traces of panels *1*, *2*, and *3*, action potentials recorded in the vicinity of an extracellular bipolar electrode (indicated by circles) are shown. The bottom trace shows the electrogram. The depolarization phase of the action potential corresponds to the first electrogram component, and repolarization corresponds to the second component. Upstrokes coincident with the second component were not seen (see figures 5 and 10).

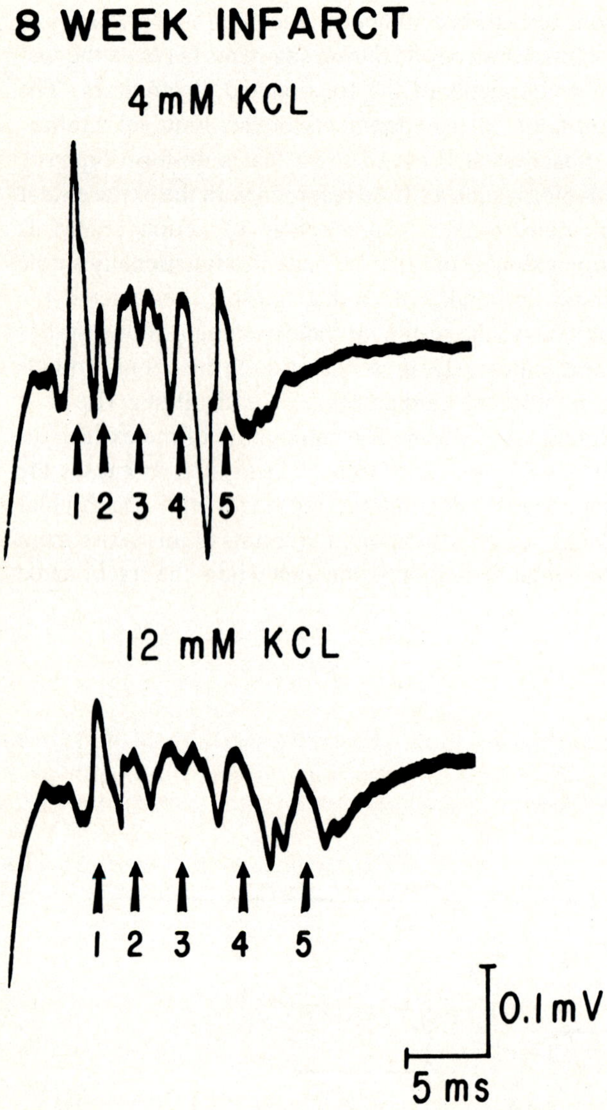

FIGURE 7. Effects of elevated K^+ concentration on a fractionated electrogram. The electrogram shown in the top panel was recorded in a preparation from a 2-month-old infarct, superfused with Tyrode's solution containing 4 mM K^+. Some of the components of the electrogram, indicated by the arrows, are numbered. The electrogram recorded at the same site is shown in the bottom panel during superfusion of the preparation with Tyrode's solution containing 12 mM K. The elevated K^+ concentration depressed the transmembrane potentials and slowed conduction. The amplitude of the electrogram decreased and the total duration increased but the same fractionated components can be identified (arrows and numbers below the electrogram trace).

electrogram was recorded occurred in steps or jumps, progressing from the 40 to 55 msec isochrones. No rapid biphasic deflections were detected at 42 to 46 msec or at 49 to 53 msec. In contrast, when similar experiments were done with extracellular microelectrodes during slow conduction caused by high K^+ concentration and catecholamines, there was a smooth propagation of the waveform; upstrokes of biphasic extracellular electrograms recorded with the microelectrode occurred at all times throughout the duration of the broad bipolar electrogram and there were no time gaps without electrogram upstrokes.

Propagation with the characteristics shown in figure 8 might occur for a number of different reasons, several of which are diagrammed in figure 9. The model shown in panel *A* assumes circuitous conduction (indicated by the arrows) in the vicinity of the bipolar electrode. Conduction velocity in each of three functionally separate strands of muscle is normal (action potentials are normal), yet activation time in the region of the bipolar electrode would appear slow because of the circuitous pathway of propagation. Isoelectric intervals occur during the time the impulse is out of the recording field of the bipolar electrode; components of the fractionated electrogram occur when the impulse returns in one of the muscle strands. (The term "functional strand" is not meant to indicate the actual number of muscle fibers. A functional strand might be composed of a single fiber or a number of closely coupled fibers in which there is uniform propagation.)

The model shown in panel *B* assumes exaggerated discontinuous conduction[33, 34] with large pauses be-

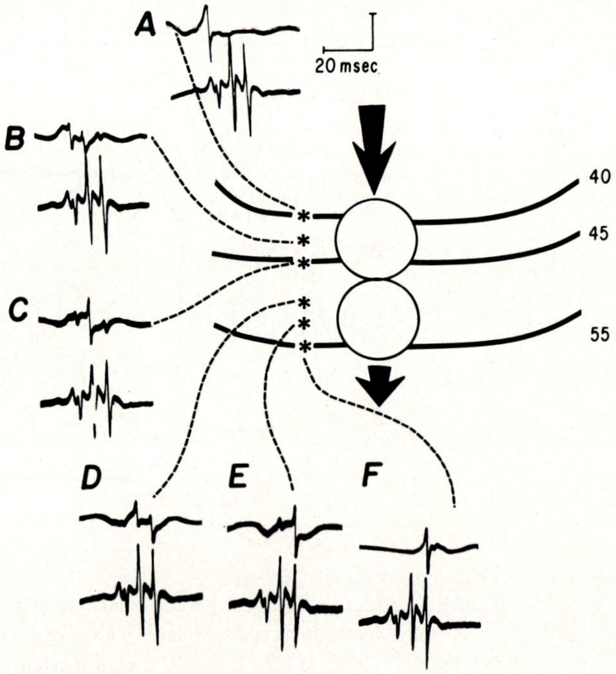

FIGURE 8. In each panel the top trace is the unipolar electrogram recorded with an extracellular microelectrode and the bottom trace is the fractionated electrogram recorded with the bipolar electrode (indicated by the large circles). The dashed lines and the asterisks show the sites where the unipolar electrograms were recorded, relative to the poles of the bipolar electrode. The large black arrows indicate the direction of impulse propagation and the black lines are isochrones showing activation times. The voltage calibration above is 0.2 mV for the bipolar recording and 10 μV for the unipolar recording.

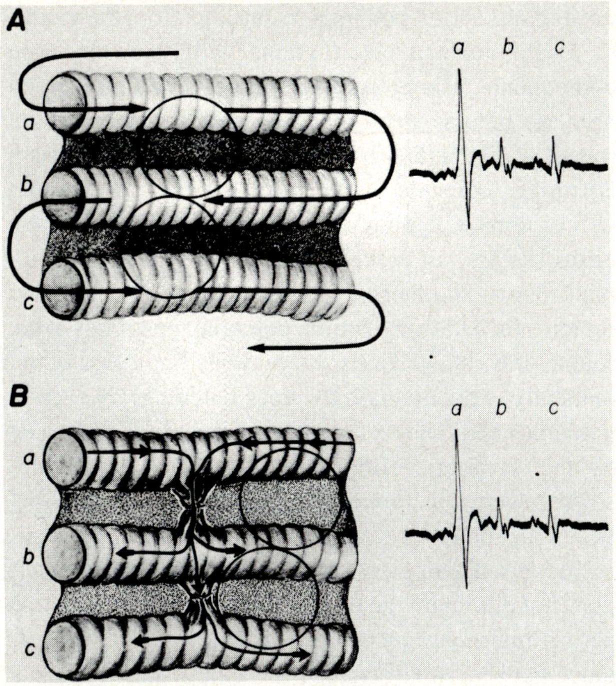

FIGURE 9. Two models that might explain the occurrence of the fractionated electrograms. In *A*, three cardiac fibers or bundles are indicated by the cylindrical structures. These fibers are separated by connective tissue as shown by the results of the anatomic studies and are not interconnected in the region shown by the diagram. However, interconnections do occur at a distant site. The large circles represent the location of the bipoles and the dark arrows show impulse propagation. In *B*, the three cardiac fibers are connected and impulse propagation occurs in a relatively straight line through these connections as indicated by the arrows. If it is assumed that the resistance at the connections is high, there might be a delay in conduction from one fiber to another. The model does not explain the different amplitudes of the electrogram components that may result from different diameters of the bundles or different distances of each bundle from the recording electrodes.

tween activation of each functional muscle strand; unlike the model in panel *A*, the impulse is present at all times in the vicinity of the bipolar electrode. This might occur if the resistance at intercellular contacts (intercalated discs) between myocardial fibers is high, causing slow impulse transmission across high-resistance junctions or barriers.[33–37] Other possible causes for such exaggerated discontinuous conduction include (1) localized increases in other components of intracellular (cytoplasmic) resistance, (2) abrupt changes in cell size or surface-to-volume ratios, (3) marked differences in the number of cells connected across the high-resistance barrier, (4) localized increases in extracellular resistance, or (5) abrupt cell branching.[33–37]

If abrupt increases in intercellular coupling resistance as shown in the second model (figure 9, *B*) accurately explain the multicomponent nature of the fractionated electrograms, we might expect to observe electrotonic prepotentials occurring before the upstrokes of action potentials in regions where fractionated electrograms are recorded.[36, 38–40] We did observe such prepotentials before the upstrokes of action potentials recorded in some areas where "double" potentials occurred. Examples are shown in figures 5 and 10. In the experiment illustrated in figure 10, *D* and *E*, action potentials with upstrokes coinciding either with the first or second component of the "double" potential were recorded in well-defined areas indicated on the diagram. No upstrokes occurred in the segment between the two electrogram components. The upstrokes coinciding with the second electrogram component were preceded by a low-amplitude prepotential (indicated by the open arrow with asterisks in figure 10, *E*), which began during the first electrogram component and spanned the isoelectric segment.

The action potential recordings shown in figure 5 are

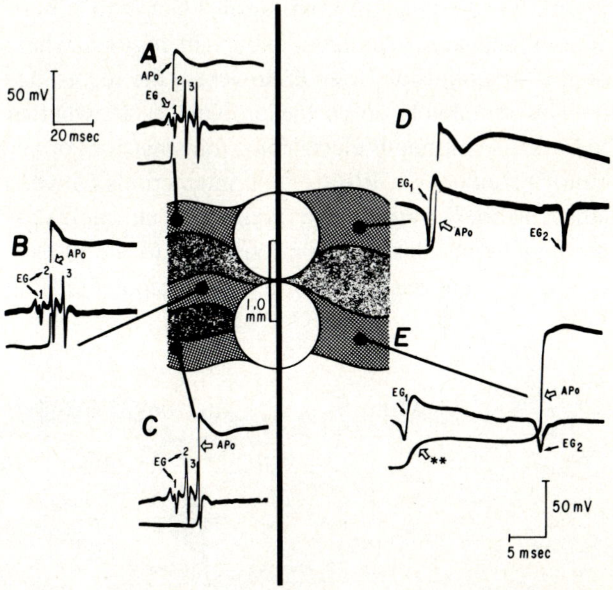

FIGURE 10. Action potentials at sites where fractionated electrograms were recorded in two different experiments, one shown in the left panels (*A* to *C*) and the other shown in the right panels (*D* and *E*). The large circles in the middle of the figure indicate the bipoles of the electrode. The electrograms in panels *A*, *B*, and *C* have three components (EG 1, 2, and 3). The upstrokes of the action potentials are indicated by AP_0. Upstrokes were found corresponding to EG 1 *(A)*, EG 2 *(B)*, and EG 3 *(C)*, but no upstrokes occurred in the segments between components. These action potentials were recorded in three areas indicated by the cross-hatching. No action potentials could be recorded from the stippled region. The electrograms in panels *D* and *E* have two components (EG_1 and EG_2). The action potential upstrokes are indicated by AP_0. Action potential upstrokes coincided either with the first component *(D)* or the second component *(E)* but never occurred in the isoelectric segment between components. Panel *E* also shows the electrotonic prepotential (indicated by asterisks) occurring before the action potential upstroke. Regions where action potentials could not be recorded were also found in this experiment (indicated schematically by shaded area).

more complex. Again, upstrokes were found that coincided either with the first or second electrogram component but not in the isoelectric segment between components. The action potentials with upstrokes occurring during the first electrogram deflection are shown in panels *A* and *B*. Also evident in these recordings are the probable electrotonic effects of distant activation on action potential repolarization: there is an exaggerated repolarization phase (unfilled arrows) before the plateau that coincides with the second electrogram deflection. As the microelectrode was moved toward sites *C* and *D*, two component upstrokes were seen, with each component coinciding with one of the electrogram deflections. At sites *E* and *F* there were only low-amplitude prepotentials before the upstrokes that coincided with the second electrogram deflection. At another site nearby *(G)*, action potentials not preceded by electrotonic potentials were found.

It is apparent from the recordings shown in both figures 5 and 10 that there are strong electrotonic interactions between myocardial fibers in regions where double potentials are found. However, the recordings do not completely solve the problem as to whether there is discontinuous electrotonic transmission, or circuitous conduction. Electrotonic interactions between adjacent fibers might occur even when an impulse is not conducting directly from one fiber to the other.

We did not observe electrotonic prepotentials in most of our action potential recordings from the vicinity of fractionated electrograms with three or more components. Upstrokes of action potentials recorded near the bipolar electrode from the experiment illustrated in figure 8 are shown in figure 10, *A* to *C*. Upstrokes coincided with either the first *(A)*, second *(B)*, or third *(C)* component of the electrogram but the upstrokes are not preceded by prepotentials. This applies also to 20 other action potentials recorded in this region. In addition, action potential upstrokes were found only in well-defined regions (indicated schematically in the diagram by cross-hatching). No action potentials could be recorded in other regions (indicated by the shading). Furthermore, action potential upstrokes were not found to occur during the time between the major three components of the electrogram.

The absence of electrotonic prepotentials, however, does not eliminate the possibility that slow conduction across high-resistance barriers occurred. High-resistance barriers might change the foot of the action potential upstroke without causing the marked prepotential shown in figures 5 and 10.[33, 36] We did not perform the detailed analysis of the foot that would be necessary to determine whether it had been altered.

Anatomic basis for fractionated electrograms. There were marked differences between the microanatomy of regions where normally shaped electrograms were recorded and regions where fractionated electrograms

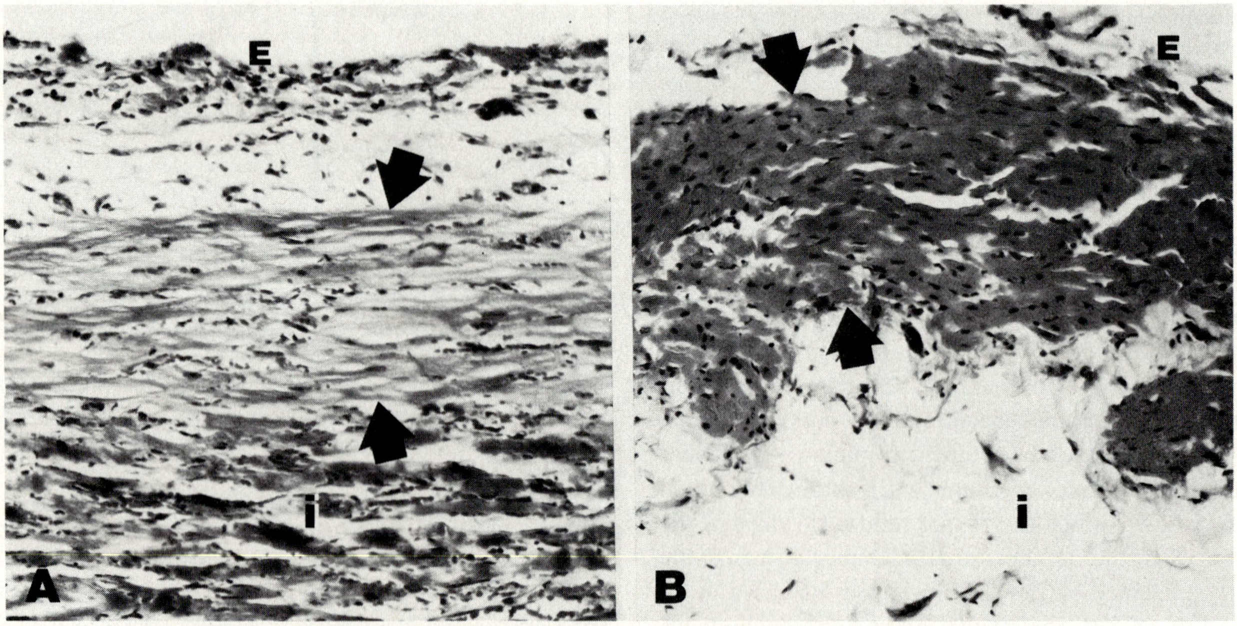

FIGURE 11. Histologic appearance of regions where electrograms without fractionation were recorded in a 5-day-old infarct preparation *(A)* and in a 16-month-old infarct preparation *(B)*. Just beneath the epicardium (E), the surviving muscle fibers are indicated by the arrows. Beneath this histologically normal muscle is the infarct (i). At 5 days the infarct consists of necrotic muscle fibers, whereas at 16 months the infarct zone in this field is composed largely of fat. (Hematoxylin-phloxine-saffron; *A* and *B* × 150.)

were recorded in the infarct preparations. These differences may explain the occurrence of slow, inhomogeneous conduction and fractionated extracellular waveforms. Figure 11, *A*, shows the histologic appearance of the 5-day-old infarct preparation from which the normally shaped electrogram in figure 4 *(left)* was recorded. These histologic features are representative of areas in 5-day-old infarcts where smooth, biphasic electrograms were found. In these regions a thin rim of five to 30 intact ventricular muscle fibers survived the coronary occlusion and overlay the infarct (a mean value of 12 fibers in figure 11 determined from serial sections). These muscle fibers had a normal appearance and were characterized by intact cell membranes, myofibrils exhibiting cross-striations and ovoid nuclei with evenly dispersed chromatin. The muscle fibers were arranged parallel to each other, in closely packed fascicles, separated by edema and normal amounts of connective tissue. The separation of the muscle fibers is indicated by the results of the morphometric analysis. The ratio of muscular to nonmuscular elements (M/NM) at electrogram recording sites in *noninfarcted* subepicardium was 15.9 ± 2 and 12.9 ± 1.9 in the two experiments in which it was determined (average 14.4, which is equivalent to 93.5% muscular tissue and 6.5% nonmuscular tissue). In the experiment illustrated in figure 11, *A*, the M/NM ratio was 6.4 ± 0.8 or 13.5% nonmuscular tissue. The mean value for the four experiments on 5-day-old infarcts that were analyzed was 4.21 ± 1.62 (19.2% nonmuscular tissue). The increase in the nonmuscular component of the epicardial border zone was mainly caused by the edema.

In the 2- to 16-month-old infarcts where normally shaped electrograms such as the ones shown in figure 1 (*E* and *F*) were recorded, closely packed, parallel-oriented subepicardial muscle fibers were also found overlying the fibrotic, healed region (figure 11, *B*). In these areas, there were at least 10 surviving cell layers and sometimes as many as 100.

In figure 11, *B*, showing the site at which the electrogram in figure 1, *E*, was recorded, there are 14 to 18 layers of muscle cells determined from serial sections. The M/NM ratio was 4.56 ± 1.01 in this experiment; nonmuscular tissue composed 17.9% of the epicardial border zone. This is similar to the results of the analysis of the 5-day-old infarcts. The fibrous tissue from the healed infarct did not penetrate into the subepicardial aspect of this rim of muscle.

In contrast, in regions where fractionated electrograms were recorded, large amounts of fibrous tissue from the adjacent healed infarct had invaded the surviving subepicardial muscle layers (figure 12). This expansive growth of fibrous tissue separated the surviving muscle fibers from each other along their length to such an extent that often side-to-side contacts between bundles could not be seen. Moreover, the myocardial fibers were no longer arranged in parallel to one another. In the six experiments in which morphometric analysis was done, the M/NM ratio was 1.35 ± 0.71 (42.6% nonmuscular tissue in the epicardial border zone, significantly different from 5-day-old infarcts ($p < .05$).

An exact correlation between histologic and electrophysiologic results was accomplished from the serial sections of regions where electrograms were recorded. For example, from the data presented in figure 8 it was postulated that there were three functional strands of muscle giving rise to the fractionated electrogram. Figure 12, *A* and *B*, shows the histologic appearance of the area under the bipolar electrode in that experiment. Between three and 10 muscle fibers were found in each of the 120 serial sections that were examined. This epicardial border zone was 41% nonmuscular tissue. In all of the regions analyzed at which multiple component fractionated electrograms were found, the number of individual muscle fibers was usually greater than the number of electrogram components. However, as we indicated before, a functional strand might contain more than one fiber and the number of functional strands could not be determined by the anatomic study. Figure 12, *C*, shows the histologic appearance of the region where the "double" potential of figure 10, *D* and *E*, was recorded. In fact, only two muscle fibers were found throughout the serial sections. However, six to eight muscle fibers were found in the serial sections of another experiment in which double potentials were recorded.

Discussion

Importance of fractionated electrograms. Fractionated electrograms were first recorded with bipolar electrodes from the canine heart during experimental studies on acute ischemia and on healed myocardial infarcts.[28, 41–44] Similar electrograms have also been recorded from patients with ischemic heart disease with catheter electrodes and intraoperative probes, during both sinus rhythm and ventricular tachycardia.[1–11] Fractionated electrograms, recorded during sinus rhythm, have been found to be more numerous in the border zones of aneurysms in patients with healed infarcts and a history of tachycardias than in patients with similar cardiac pathologic status but without tachycardia.[6] In addition, the fractionated electrograms in patients with tachycardias had longer durations.[6] The sites from which fractionated electrograms are recorded during sinus rhythm may therefore delineate regions where reentry occurs, causing tachycardia.[6–8] Fractionated electrograms, however, might also occur in regions other than those in which tachycardia originates.[9, 11, 14, 45]

Fractionated electrograms may not always correlate

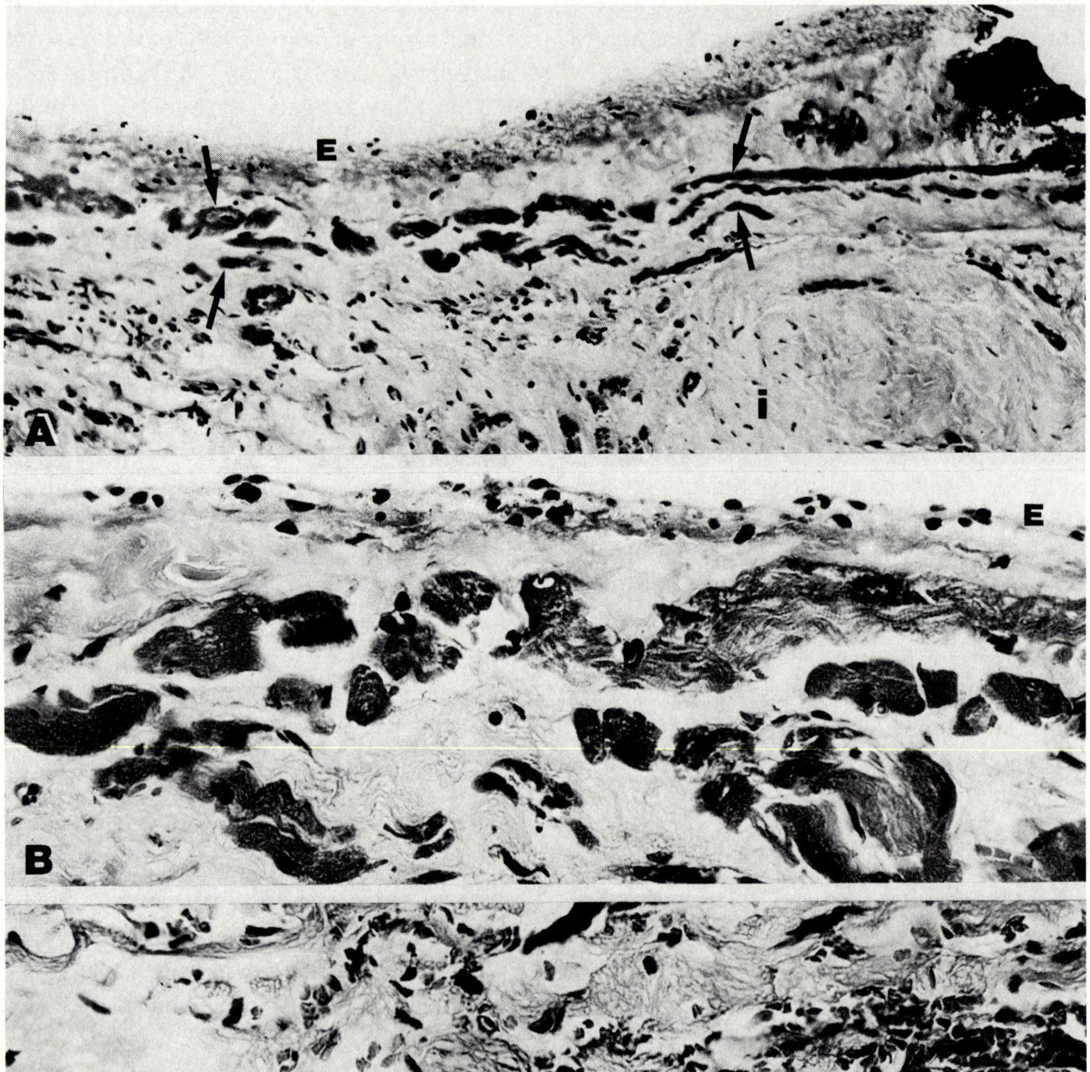

FIGURE 12. Surviving muscle fibers in healed infarcts from which fractionated electrograms were recorded. Beneath the epicardium (E) a few layers of viable muscle, indicated by the arrows, remain at 16 months *(A)*. Directly subjacent is the healed infarct (i). Black ink at the upper right marks the position of the microelectrode used to record extracellular potentials in figure 8. At high magnification *(B)* the entrapped muscle fibers can be readily seen to be separated and distorted by connective tissue. In panel *C*, two isolated muscle fibers, in a different preparation, course between the thickened epicardium and the fat of the subjacent healed infarct. (Hematoxylin-phloxine-saffron; original magnification *A* ×150, *B* × 350, *C* ×400.)

with the occurrence of arrhythmias in canine preparations of ventricular tachycardia. After complete occlusion of the left anterior descending coronary artery, ventricular tachycardia is often inducible during the first week (at a time fractionated electrograms were not usually found in the isolated preparations) but may become more difficult to induce later on (when fractionated electrograms were often found in isolated preparations).[23, 46] We do not have any data explaining this discrepancy. One possibility is that during infarct healing in the canine heart, the area of infarction shrinks markedly. If reentrant tachycardia at 3 to 5 days in this canine preparation requires relatively large circuits,[47, 48] the infarcted area after healing may be too small for reentry despite the persistent slow conduction.

Characteristics of fractionated electrograms. The electrograms recorded in our experiments are not entirely comparable to those in the clinical studies. The bipolar electrograms that we recorded from normal muscle had durations of 5 msec or less and amplitudes of 2 to 4 mV, whereas fractionated electrograms had prolonged durations of 10 to 70 msec and reduced amplitudes that were often less than 1 mV. The durations of both normal and fractionated electrograms were shorter than those of electrograms recorded with a catheter electrode, recently reported by Cassidy et al.[11, 49] (mean duration of 54 msec for normal electrograms and durations of more than 133 msec for fractionated electrograms) or the duration of electrograms recorded intraoperatively by Weiner et al.[6] (mean duration of fractionated electrograms was 97 ± 17 msec). These differences in the absolute values of normal and abnormal electrogram durations may be related to the size of the recording electrodes and the distance between poles. The catheter electrodes used in the studies of Cassidy et al.[11, 49] had a 10 mm distance between bipoles, whereas the electrodes themselves consisted of relatively wide rings. They are therefore expected to record electrical activity from a larger area than our electrodes, which had tip diameters of 0.3 mm and interelectrode-pole distances of 0.5 to 1.0 mm. The bipolar electrodes generally used for intraoperative mapping are also larger than the ones we used.[6] Our data are comparable to the clinical data if electrogram characteristics are expressed as the ratio of amplitude to duration, as suggested by Cassidy et al.[11] Because of the reduced amplitudes and increased durations, fractionated electrograms have significantly decreased ratios compared with normal in both the clinical studies and our experimental study.

Electrophysiologic and anatomic causes of fractionated electrograms. Fractionated electrograms became more apparent as the infarcts healed. Healing was associated with a return in resting potential and action potential characteristics to normal. A similar improvement in action potentials with infarct healing has also been shown in the studies of Myerburg et al.[50] These data show that fractionated electrograms in the healed infarcts are not caused by abnormal or depressed action potentials (although they might be caused by depressed transmembrane potentials in the instances where fractionation has been recorded during acute ischemia).[28, 44] Despite the normal transmembrane potentials in the healed infarcts, activation in the vicinity of the extracellular recording electrodes was much slower than that in the subacute (5-day-old) infarcts; it sometimes took as long as 70 msec for the wavefront to pass by the electrode. We were also sometimes able to show marked inhomogeneities in activation with closely adjacent areas around the electrode activated at very different times. Different components of the fractionated electrograms coincided with activation of the different adjacent regions. It is therefore apparent that the slow and inhomogeneous conduction and the summation of extracellular currents occurring at disparate times cause fractionation. This possibility had been proposed in earlier studies demonstrating fractionated electrograms.[28]

Why is conduction slow and inhomogeneous in healed infarcts when transmembrane action potentials are normal? The answer to this question may be found in the structural changes that occur during infarct healing. Connective tissue from the necrotic region invades the bordering (subepicardial) areas where there is surviving muscle. These muscle fibers become widely separated and their orientation distorted. These structural changes might lead to an increase in the effective axial resistance, a term used by Spach et al.[33] to describe the resistance to current flow in the direction of propagation. The effective axial resistance depends on the intracellular and extracellular resistivities, the size and shape of the cells, cellular packing, and the resistance, extent, and distribution of cell-to-cell couplings.[33] Distortion of the cells by the connective tissue with a resulting decrease in intercellular connections might increase resistance to current flow and thereby slow conduction.[34]

A reduced space constant has been found in regions of chronically infarcted canine myocardium by Spear et al.[51] and supports this suggestion. It is possible that slow electrotonic transmission across high-resistance or inexcitable gaps sometimes caused the marked conduction delays. Models of this kind of propagation have been studied by Wennemark et al.,[52] who used direct current to cause the area of conduction block, and by Antzelevitch et al.[39] and Jalife et al.,[40] who used a sucrose gap. In our study, intervals between deflections comprising the fractionated electrograms ranged from 5 to 20 msec, similar to the delays that can be caused by either a high intracellular resistance[53] or electrotonic transmission across inexcitable areas.[52] However, we never observed delays on the order of 100 or 200 msec that sometimes occurred in the sucrose gap experiments.[40]

Action potentials in regions where we recorded double potentials sometimes showed prepotentials before the upstroke, similar to the prepotentials recorded from regions just distal to an area of block in other experiments in which slow, electrotonic transmission has been demonstrated.[38–40, 52] On occasion we also saw two distinct components during the depolarization phase of the action potential in these regions (figure 5, *A* to *D*), previously shown during electrotonic transmission by Wennemark et al.[52] There is also the possibility that a change in extracellular resistance related to the increased connective tissue alters current flow and conduction velocity. Additional experiments are required to determine whether effective axial resistance is increased or whether electrotonic transmission across inexcitable gaps is occurring in the healed infarcts. The slowed and inhomogeneous activation we observed might also be caused by conduction at normal velocities over circuitous pathways caused by the structural changes (diagrammed in figure 9).

Relevance of experimental data to clinical observations. The pathologic anatomy of endocardial regions where fractionated electrograms are recorded in humans is very similar to that of the epicardial regions of healed infarcts that we studied. Bundles of muscle fibers are widely separated during infarct healing by the ingrowth of large amounts of connective tissue.[54] This anatomic phenomenon and the action potential characteristics we found in our experimental study may explain some of the features of fractionated electrograms. First, fractionated electrograms are sometimes comprised of rapid spikes (no quantification of rapidity is available) called "high frequency" components,[11] although they may also consist of slowly rising deflections. Electrograms with rapid components would not be expected if action potential upstrokes were depressed, since slow upstrokes cause slow rates of extracellular voltage change.[32] On the other hand, rapid spikes might be generated by action potentials with rapid upstrokes. Second, fractionated electrograms have very low amplitudes. Our data suggest that such low amplitudes are not caused by a reduction in the rate of rise or amplitude of the action potential[32] but may be a result of the sparsity of viable muscle fibers surviving in the ischemic region. This would be expected to decrease the density of extracellular current. Low-amplitude electrograms may also be caused by propagation in nonuniformly anisotropic tissue.[34] Third, the very nature of fractionated electrograms — asynchronous or repetitive spikes — appears to be caused by asynchronous excitation of different poorly interconnected muscle bundles or by delay in conduction from one region of a fiber to another region of the same fiber across high-resistance intercellular connections. If, in fact, these areas of fractionated electrograms delineate reentrant circuits in healed infarcts, the role of slow conduction caused by changes in passive properties of cardiac fibers must be given consideration as a cause of reentrant tachycardia.

References

1. Josephson ME, Horowitz LN, Farshidi A, Spear JF, Kastor JA, Moore EN: Recurrent sustained ventricular tachycardia. II. Endocardial mapping. Circulation **57:** 440, 1978
2. Josephson ME, Horowitz LN, Farshidi A: Continuous local electrical activity: a mechanism of recurrent ventricular tachycardia. Circulation **57:** 659, 1978
3. Horowitz LN, Josephson ME, Harken AH: Epicardial and endocardial activation during sustained ventricular tachycardia in man. Circulation **61:** 1227, 1980
4. Waldo AL, Arciniegas JG, Klein H: Surgical treatment of life threatening ventricular arrhythmias: the role of intraoperative mapping and consideration of the presently available surgical techniques. Prog Cardiovasc Dis **23:** 247, 1981
5. Gallagher JJ, Kasell JH, Cox JL, Smith WM, Ideker RE, Smith WM: Techniques of intraoperative electrophysiologic mapping. Am J Cardiol **49:** 221, 1982
6. Weiner I, Mindich B, Pitchon R: Determinants of ventricular tachycardia in patients with ventricular aneurysms: results of intraoperative epicardial and endocardial mapping. Circulation **65:** 856, 1982
7. Klein H, Karp RB, Kouchoukos NT, Zorn GL, James TN, Waldo AL: Intraoperative electrophysiologic mapping of the ventricles during sinus rhythm in patients with a previous myocardial infarction: identification of the electrophysiologic substrate of ventricular arrhythmias. Circulation **66:** 847, 1982
8. Josephson ME, Horowitz LN, Spielman SR, Waxman HL, Greenspan AM: Role of catheter mapping in the preoperative evaluation of ventricular tachycardia. Am J Cardiol **49:** 207, 1982
9. Kienzle MG, Falcone RA, Kempf FC, Miller JM, Harken AH, Josephson ME: Intraoperative endocardial mapping: relation of fractionated electrograms in sinus rhythm to endocardial activation in ventricular tachycardia — surgical implications. J Am Coll Cardiol **1:** 582, 1983
10. Weiner I, Mindich B, Pitchon R: Fragmented endocardial electrical activity in patients with ventricular tachycardia: a new guide to surgical therapy. Am Heart J **107:** 86, 1984
11. Cassidy DM, Vassallo JA, Buxton AE, Doherty JU, Marchlinski FE, Josephson ME: The value of catheter mapping during sinus rhythm to localize site of origin of ventricular tachycardia. Circulation **69:** 1103, 1984
12. Fontaine G, Guiraudon G, Frank R: Double epicardial potentials in idiopathic ventricular tachycardia. Circulation **54**(suppl II): II-78, 1976
13. Ideker RE, Lofland GK, Bardy GH, Smith WM, Worley SJ, Wallace AG, Cox JL, Gallagher JJ: Late fractionated potentials and continuous electrical activity caused by electrode motion. PACE **6:** 908, 1983

14. Waxman HL, Sung RJ: Significance of fragmented ventricular electrogram observed using intracardiac recording techniques in man. Circulation **62:** 1349, 1980
15. Gardner PI, Ursell PC, Fenoglio JJ, Wit AL: Anatomical and electrophysiological basis for electrograms showing fractionated activity. Circulation **66**(suppl II): II-78, 1982
16. Wit AL, Josephson ME: Fractionated electrograms and continuous electrical activity: fact or artifact. *In* Zipes DP, Jalife J, editors: Cardiac electrophysiology and arrhythmias. New York, 1985, Grune & Stratton, p 343
17. Harris AS: Delayed development of ventricular ectopic rhythm following experimental coronary occlusion. Circulation **1:** 1318, 1950
18. Friedman PL, Stewart JR, Fenoglio JJ Jr, Wit AL: Survival of subendocardial Purkinje fibers after extensive myocardial infarction in dogs: in vitro and in vivo correlations. Circ Res **33:** 597, 1973
19. Ursell PC, Gardner PI, Albala A, Fenoglio JJ Jr, Wit AL: Structural and electrophysiological changes in the epicardial border zone of canine infarcts during infarct healing. Circ Res **56:** 436, 1985
20. Friedman PL, Fenoglio JJ Jr, Wit AL: Time course for reversal of electrophysiological and ultrastructural abnormalities in subendocardial Purkinje fibers surviving extensive myocardial infarction in dogs. Circ Res **36:** 127, 1975
21. Weibel ER: Stereological methods, vol 1. London, 1979, Academic Press, p 101
22. Eisenberg BR, Kuda AM, Peter JB: Stereological analysis of mammalian skeletal muscle. I. Soleus muscle of the adult guinea pig. J Cell Biol **60:** 732, 1974
23. El-Sherif N, Scherlag BJ, Lazzara R, Hope RR: Reentrant arrhythmias in the late myocardial infarction period. I. Conduction characteristics in the infarct zone. Circulation **55:** 686, 1977
24. Gardner PI, Ursell PC, Pham TD, Fenoglio JJ Jr, Wit AL: Experimental chronic ventricular tachycardia: anatomic and electrophysiologic substrates. *In* Josephson ME, Wellens HJJ, editors: Tachycardias: mechanisms, diagnosis and treatment. Philadelphia, 1984, Lea and Febiger, p 29
25. Spach MS, Barr RC, Johnson EA, Kootsey JM: Cardiac extracellular potentials: analysis of complex wave forms about the Purkinje networks in dogs. Circ Res **33:** 465, 1973
26. Lazzara R, Scherlag BJ: Role of the slow current in the generation of arrhythmias in ischemic myocardium. *In* Zipes DP, Bailey JC, Elharrar V, editors: The slow inward current and cardiac arrhythmia. The Hague, 1980, Martinus Nijhoff, p 399
27. Spear JF, Michelson EL, Moore EN: Cellular electrophysiologic characteristics of chronically infarcted myocardium in dogs susceptible to sustained ventricular tachyarrhythmias. J Am Coll Cardiol **1:** 1099, 1983
28. Boineau JP, Cox JL: Slow ventricular activation in acute myocardial infarction: a source of reentrant premature ventricular contractions. Circulation **43:** 702, 1973
29. Cranefield PF, Wit AL, Hoffman BF: Conduction of the cardiac impulse. III. Characteristics of very slow conduction. J Gen Physiol **59:** 227, 1972
30. Carmeliet E, Vereecke J: Adrenaline and the plateau phase of the cardiac action potential: importance of Ca, Na and K conductance. Pfluegers Arch **313:** 300, 1972
31. Wit AL, Hoffman BF, Cranefield PF: Slow conduction and reentry in the ventricular conducting system. I. Return extrasystole in canine Purkinje fibers. Circ Res **30:** 1, 1972
32. Spach MS, Barr RC, Serwer GA, Kootsey JM, Johnson EA: Extracellular potentials related to intracellular action potentials in the dog Purkinje system. Circ Res **30:** 505, 1972
33. Spach MS, Miller WT, Geselowitz DB, Barr RC, Kootsey JM, Johnson EA: The discontinuous nature of propagation in normal canine cardiac muscle: evidence for recurrent discontinuities of intracellular resistance that affect the membrane currents. Circ Res **48:** 39, 1981
34. Spach MS, Miller WT, Dolber P, Kootsey JM, Sommer JR, Mosher CE Jr: The functional role of structural complexities in the propagation of depolarization in the atrium of the dog: cardiac conduction disturbances due to discontinuous effective axial resistivity. Circ Res **50:** 175, 1982
35. Heppner DB, Plonsey R: Simulation of electrical interaction of cardiac cells. Biophys J **10:** 1057, 1970
36. Joyner RW: Effects of the discrete pattern of electrical coupling on propagation through an electrical syncytium. Circ Res **50:** 192, 1982
37. Joyner RW, Veenstra R, Rawling D, Chorro A: Propagation through electrically coupled cells: effects of a resistive barrier. Biophys J **45:** 1017, 1984
38. Bandura JP: The role of electrotonus in slow potential development and conduction in canine Purkinje tissue. *In* Zipes DP, Bailey JC, Elharrar V, editors: The slow inward current and cardiac arrhythmia. The Hague, 1980, Martinus Nijhoff, p 327
39. Antzelevitch C, Jalife J, Moe GK: Characteristics of reflection as a mechanism of reentrant arrhythmias and its relationship to parasystole. Circulation **61:** 182, 1980
40. Jalife J, Moe GK: Excitation, conduction and reflection of impulses in isolated bovine and canine cardiac Purkinje fibers. Circ Res **49:** 233, 1981
41. Durrer D, Formijne P, van Dam RTH, Buller J, van Lier AAW, Meijler FL: Electrocardiogram in normal and some abnormal conditions: in revived human fetal heart and in acute and chronic coronary occlusion. Am Heart J **61:** 303, 1961
42. Durrer D, van Lier AAW, Buller J: Epicardial and intramural excitation in chronic myocardial infarction. Am Heart J **68:** 765, 1964
43. Daniel TM, Boineau JP, Sabiston DC: Comparison of human ventricular activation with a canine model in chronic myocardial infarction. Circulation **44:** 74, 1971
44. Waldo AL, Kaiser GA: A study of ventricular arrhythmias associated with acute myocardial infarction in the canine heart. Circulation **42:** 1222, 1973
45. Brugada P, Abdollah H, Wellens HJJ: Significance of continuous electrical activity during ventricular tachycardia. Circulation **68**(suppl III): III-422, 1983 (abst)
46. Karagueuzian HS, Fenoglio JJ Jr, Weiss MB, Wit AL: Protracted ventricular tachycardia induced by premature stimulation of the canine heart after coronary artery occlusion and reperfusion. Circ Res **44:** 833, 1979
47. El-Sherif N, Smith A, Evans K: Canine ventricular arrhythmias in the late myocardial infarction period: epicardial mapping of reentrant circuits. Circ Res **49:** 255, 1981
48. Wit AL, Allessie MA, Bonke FIM, Lammers W, Smeets J, Fenoglio JJ Jr: Electrophysiologic mapping to determine the mechanism of experimental ventricular tachycardia initiated by premature impulses. Am J Cardiol **49:** 166, 1982
49. Cassidy DM, Vassallo JA, Marchlinski FE, Buxton AE, Untereker WJ, Josephson ME: Endocardial mapping in humans in sinus rhythm with normal left ventricles: activation patterns and characteristics of electrograms. Circulation **70:** 37, 1984
50. Myerburg RJ, Gelband H, Nilsson K, Sung RJ, Thurer RJ, Morales AR, Bassett AL: Long term electrophysiologic abnormalities resulting from experimental myocardial infarction in cats. Circ Res **41:** 73, 1977
51. Spear JF, Michelson EL, Moore EN: Reduced space constant in slowly conducting regions of chronically infarcted canine myocardium. Circ Res **53:** 176, 1983
52. Wennemark JR, Ruesta VJ, Brody DA: Microelectrode study of delayed conduction in the canine right bundle branch. Circ Res **23:** 753, 1968
53. Lieberman M, Kootsey JM, Johnson EA, Sawanobori T: Slow conduction in cardiac muscle: a biophysical model. Biophys J **13:** 37, 1973
54. Fenoglio JJ Jr, Pham TD, Harken AH, Horowitz LN, Josephson ME, Wit AL: Recurrent sustained ventricular tachycardia: structure and ultrastructure of subendocardial regions where tachycardia originates. Circulation **68:** 518, 1983

Catheter-mediated electrical ablation of the posterior septum via the coronary sinus: electrophysiologic and histologic observations in dogs

FERNANDO COLTORTI, M.D., GUST H. BARDY, M.D., DENNIS REICHENBACH, M.D., H. LEON GREENE, M.D., ROBERT THOMAS, B.A., DONALD G. BREAZEALE, CLIF ALFERNESS, B.S.E.E., AND TOM D. IVEY, M.D.

ABSTRACT In a series of 12 dogs, the electrophysiologic and histologic effects of a single damped sine-wave shock delivered via standard electrocatheters to the region of the coronary sinus orifice were investigated. Six dogs received 200 J and six received 360 J of stored energy. The shock was delivered to two consecutive proximal poles of a standard quadripolar catheter positioned at the coronary sinus orifice and connected to the positive output (anode) of a defibrillator. A disc electrode positioned on the anterior chest wall served as the cathode (negative pole). During the shock, voltage and current were recorded. Electrophysiologic testing was done before and 4 weeks after the shock. At 4 weeks, animals were killed and serial sections of the atrioventricular groove and conduction system were performed. No significant long-term change in atrioventricular conduction, spontaneous or induced atrial or ventricular arrhythmias was observed. However, transient atrioventricular block was seen in five and idioventricular rhythms in six animals in the short term. No persistent electrocardiographic changes were observed, and no sudden deaths occurred. Microscopically, transmural injury at the anulus proper or basilar ventricular epicardium was inconstant and infrequent. However, transmural atrial injury at the level of the coronary sinus was produced over a 10 ± 5 mm length with the 200 J shock and a 21 ± 6 mm length with the 360 J shock. Neither coronary artery injury nor damage to the conduction system was seen and cardiac tamponade did not occur. However, localized intramural atrial rupture of the coronary sinus wall (on the endocardial aspect only) was observed in each dog, consistent with barotrauma. With the present technique, atrial injury potentially capable of blocking the effects of accessory pathway conduction could be produced without other electrophysiologic alterations or complications. Injury to the anulus proper (and therefore to any accessory pathway per se) is probably unlikely. Barotrauma may play a significant role in the type of injury observed in this study.
***Circulation* 72, No. 3, 612–622, 1985.**

DELIVERY of an electrical shock from a defibrillator to the conduction system through an intracardiac catheter has been used to interrupt the atrioventricular (AV) node/His bundle in experimental preparations as well as in human beings.[1-11] In the first clinical report of the use of such a technique to ablate the AV node/His bundle,[3] a patient was described in whom preexcitation caused by a posterior septal accessory AV connection permanently disappeared after the procedure. Efforts to adapt this technique for intentional interruption of accessory AV connections have followed with variable success.[12-18] Reasons for success or failure of the technique may be manifold and more investigation into individual aspects of the technique is required before it becomes more predictable.

Brodman and Fisher[19] have studied the effects of electrical shocks delivered to various segments of the coronary sinus of dogs via electrode catheters. In their studies, an open-chest preparation was used in which multiple shocks were delivered between two poles of a bipolar electrode catheter. This resulted in fibrosis along the coronary sulcus, potentially capable of interrupting accessory AV connections. Although the study suggested the feasibility of the technique, several questions remained unanswered.

One factor that may affect outcome of catheter-mediated ablation is the changing relationship of atrium,

From the Departments of Medicine, Pathology, and Surgery, Harborview Medical Center, University of Washington, Seattle

Supported in part by the American Heart Association and the Seattle Emergency Medical Services Foundation. Dr. Coltorti is a recipient of a fellowship grant from the Ministero della Pubblica Istruzione, Italy.

Address for correspondence: Gust H. Bardy, M.D., Harborview Medical Center, 325 9th Ave., Seattle, WA 98104.

Received April 22, 1985; revision accepted June 6, 1985.

ventricle, and coronary sinus along the course of the AV groove. An intervention at the os of the coronary sinus may not have the same implications for that applied more distally when the coronary sinus "descends" onto the ventricle. Catheter-mediated ablation interventions should therefore be assessed at a specific anatomic location for gleaning the most information for a particular technique. Another variable is the amount of tissue injury created per shock. Multiple shocks per catheter as done by Brodman and Fisher do not allow for investigation of the effects of energy, voltage, and current on tissue injury. Furthermore, because standard pacing and recording catheters can change dielectric properties after a single shock, and therefore change patterns of current flow,[20] the ability to interpret the effect of several shocks through the same catheter becomes more difficult. In the present study, the intervention was limited to a single damped sine-wave shock delivered at a single site via standard electrocatheters.

Methods

Twelve dogs weighing between 23 and 28 kg were anesthetized with sodium pentobarbital (30 mg/kg), intubated with cuffed endotracheal tubing, and ventilated with a Palmer constant volume ventilator pump adjusted to provide a tidal volume of 20 cc/kg at a rate of 20 breaths/min. Additional pentobarbital was given as needed to maintain anesthesia for the duration of the study. No measurements were made for at least 10 min after additional doses of pentobarbital. Electrodes were placed on the four limbs and on the chest for electrocardiographic monitoring.

With sterile technique and fluoroscopic guidance, one standard quadripolar electrode catheter (No. 6F, USCI, Billerica, MA) with 1 cm interelectrode distance was inserted via a right external jugular vein cut-down and positioned in the high right atrium to record an atrial electrogram (proximal two poles) and to pace the atrium (distal two poles). Another standard quadripolar electrode catheter ("shocking" catheter, No. 6F, USCI) with 1 cm interelectrode distance was inserted via the same vein and positioned in the coronary sinus. Only new catheters were used in the coronary sinus position. In addition, before the shock, the coronary sinus catheter had been inspected and tested for electrical continuity to each electrode. For His bundle recording purposes, a No. 6F USCI quadripolar catheter was inserted via a right femoral vein cut-down and advanced across the tricuspid valve. A fluid-filled polyethylene catheter was inserted via a right femoral artery cut-down to the midabdominal level of the aorta and connected to a Statham (Model P23Db) transducer for arterial pressure monitoring. Fluids were maintained with an intravenous infusion of Ringer's lactate at a rate of 10 ml/kg/hr.

Surface leads I, II, and V_1, intracardiac electrograms and arterial pressure were amplified and displayed on a multichannel oscilloscope (Electronics for Medicine, Model VR 12). A filter setting of 30 to 500 Hz and 1 to 500 Hz was used for bipolar and unipolar signals, respectively. Recordings were printed on-line with the use of an eight-channel Siemens-Elema Mingograf (Model 803) ink jet recorder at paper speeds of 50 to 250 mm/sec. Selected portions were recorded with an Electronics for Medicine optical recorder at paper speeds of 50 to 100 mm/sec. Electrical stimulation of the heart was accomplished with a programmable stimulator (Bloom and Associates, Ltd.) that delivered constant-current rectangular pulses of 1 msec duration at twice the diastolic threshold.

Electrophysiologic studies. Before the stimulation studies, a control 12-lead electrocardiogram and baseline PA, AH, and HV intervals were obtained. Decremental pacing of the right atrium was performed to ascertain the cycle length at which block occurred in the AV node. Stimulation was ended at a point when atrial fibrillation was observed. After conversion to normal sinus rhythm (spontaneous in all dogs), programmed atrial stimulation with the extrastimulus technique was performed to determine the effective and functional refractory periods of the atrium and AV node and to assess the inducibility of atrial arrhythmias. A maximum of two atrial extrastimuli was used for arrhythmia induction.

On completion of the atrial stimulation protocol, the right atrial catheter was moved to the right ventricular apex and the His bundle catheter to the right ventricular outflow tract. Decremental pacing was performed from both sites at cycle lengths down to 200 msec to assess the inducibility of ventricular arrhythmias. Then, programmed stimulation with one extrastimulus was performed at two basic cycle lengths (500 and 400 msec) from the right ventricular apex and right ventricular outflow tract. If no sustained ventricular arrhythmia was induced with this technique, a second extrastimulus was added to the sequence. If a sustained ventricular arrhythmia was not initiated with double extrastimuli, burst pacing with an eight-beat train of stimuli was performed from both sites, starting at a cycle length of 360 msec and ending at a cycle length of 250 msec by 10 msec steps.

At the end of stimulation studies the right ventricular outflow tract catheter was withdrawn, the right ventricular apical catheter was left in place, and the coronary sinus catheter was positioned with the proximal pole at the orifice of the coronary sinus. Position of the catheter in the coronary sinus was confirmed by the following four criteria: (1) characteristic fluoroscopic appearance in the anteroposterior and lateral views, (2) the presence of negative paced P waves in leads II, III, and aVF, (3) the presence of local bipolar electrograms showing an atrial and a ventricular deflection, with the atrial signal falling between the midportion and the end of the P wave, and (4) the unipolar electrogram from the proximal pole showed a loss of the rapid component of the atrial electrogram indicative of an endocavitary potential.

When it was felt that the more proximal of the two shocking electrodes was at the os of the coronary sinus (usually pole 4, except when only three poles could be inserted into the coronary sinus, then pole 3), a single synchronous damped sinusoidal pulse of 200 or 360 J stored energy was delivered to two consecutive poles of the coronary sinus catheter connected to the positive output (anode) of a Physio-Control Life Pak 6a defibrillator. A disc electrode 3.5 cm in diameter (Medtronic Model 6983) was connected to the negative output (cathode) of the defibrillator and positioned on the anterior chest wall opposite the anode as determined by fluoroscopy. A conductive gel (DEFIB-PADS, Medical Products Division, 3-M Co.) was interfaced between the skin and the cathodal electrode. During delivery of the shock, firm pressure was applied to the disc electrode. The two proximal poles (3 and 4) of the coronary sinus catheter were used as the anode in nine dogs, while poles 2 and 3 were used in the remaining three. Poles not used for delivery of shocks and all four electrodes of the right ventricular catheter were disconnected to prevent ground loops and unwanted current pathways. Right ventricular pacing was performed with a temporary external pulse generator when temporary AV block occurred. During the shock, surface leads II, III, and aVF were displayed simultaneously with arterial pressure.

Voltage and current measurements. The waveforms of the voltage across and the current through the electrodes were displayed on an oscilloscope (Tektronix Model 5111A), equipped with a camera for photographic recording. The voltage was recorded in a differential manner by means of a voltage divider with a 1000:1 input to output ratio (Warren Heggen, University Scientific Instruments) interfaced between the defibrillator and a Tektronix 5A14N vertical amplifier. The current was recorded by a Tektronix A6303 current probe that was connected to a Tektronix AM503 current probe amplifier. The current probe was positioned around the cable connecting the positive output of the defibrillator to the two "shocking" poles of the coronary sinus electrode catheter. A second, confirmatory reading of the peak current was obtained by a custom circuit which automatically displayed the peak current on the defibrillator (built by Physio-Control). This adjunct to the displayed current waveform confirmed the absence of current leakage outside the catheter. The experimental schema is shown in figure 1.

Follow-up. After the shock, the dogs were monitored for 2 hr, after which a 12-lead electrocardiogram was obtained. Serial 12-lead electrocardiograms were recorded again at 24 hr, 2 week, and 4 week intervals. On each occasion signs of tricuspid insufficiency, pericardial tamponade, and heart failure were sought on physical examination. Four weeks after the shock, repeat electrophysiologic studies were performed as described earlier. Cannulation of the coronary sinus was attempted in all dogs. At the end of the study, the animals were killed and the hearts were removed and fixed in 10% formalin.

Morphologic studies. After gross inspection for structural damage, each heart was sectioned transversely in 0.5 cm slices from the apex to 2 cm from the AV groove, and each slice was examined grossly. The principal areas of interest (i.e., AV groove and AV conduction system) were removed for more detailed examination in two tissue blocks. One block included the AV node/His bundle and the main fascicles. The other block included the AV junction perpendicular to the anulus spanning 4.5 cm from the coronary sinus orifice and including a 2 cm rim of atrial and a 2 cm rim of ventricular myocardium above and below the AV groove. Each block was embedded in paraffin and sectioned serially. At 1 mm intervals, slides were prepared. A section at each interval was stained with Gomori's trichrome. Verhoeff–Van Gieson stains for visualization of elastic tissue injury were performed on selected sections at points of maximum injury.

Statistics. Results are expressed as mean ± SD. Differences in measures of electrophysiologic parameters before and after the shock were tested by a paired t test. Mean differences of the measurement of transmural atrial injury between the 200 and 360 J groups were tested by a two-sample t test with pooled variance estimate. Statistical significance was assumed at $p < .05$.

Results

The recovery from the procedure was uneventful in all dogs. No signs of hemodynamic compromise consistent with pericardial tamponade, tricuspid insufficiency, or congestive heart failure were observed. No dog died suddenly during the 4 week follow-up period.

Electrocardiographic findings. Immediately after the synchronized shock, all dogs showed nonsustained, self-terminating episodes of ventricular tachycardia. Upon termination of ventricular tachycardia, third-degree AV block was observed in five dogs (dogs 2, 3, 8, 10, and 12). Complete AV block resolved within 15 min in all but one dog (dog 8), in which it lasted up to 45 min. This animal was the only one to require temporary ventricular pacing because of an extremely slow idioventricular escape rhythm. At the end of the 2 hr monitoring period, normal resting AV conduction had resumed in all dogs.

Other short-term electrocardiographic changes included transient PR and ST segment elevation in all dogs, especially evident in the inferior leads. However, at the 2 hr observation period the 12-lead electrocardiogram did not show any change from the control electrocardiogram.

An idioventricular rhythm competing with sinus rhythm was noted at the 24 hr interval in six animals (dogs 4, 5, 8, 10, 11, and 12). This rhythm showed

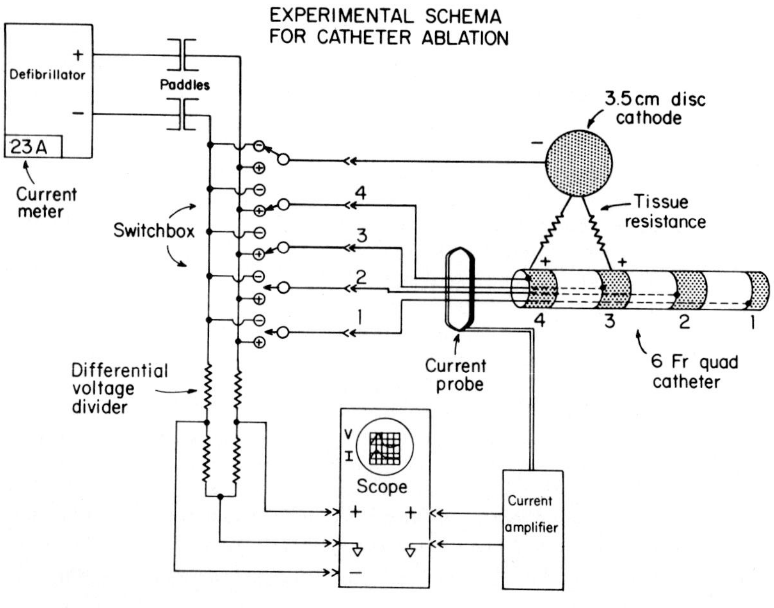

FIGURE 1. Schema for catheter-mediated electrical ablation with a defibrillator and a standard electrode catheter. The proximal pole of the electrode catheter was positioned at the coronary sinus orifice. A damped sine-wave shock was delivered to the two consecutive proximal electrodes (3 and 4) by means of a switch box. These two electrodes, coupled together, served as the anode (positive pole), while a 3.5 cm disc electrode served as the cathode (negative pole). Connections to record current (I) and voltage (V) waveforms are illustrated. A current-sensing transformer built into the Physio-Control defibrillator served as an adjunct to the displayed current waveform confirming the absence of current leakage outside the catheter.

periods of acceleration and deceleration, with a QRS morphology of right bundle branch block and left axis deviation, consistent with an automatic focus located along the posterior base of the left ventricle.

Later serial 12-lead electrocardiograms and monitoring strips were unremarkable for changes suggestive of ischemia or conduction defects. No arrhythmic episode was detected after the first 3 days after the shock and no sudden deaths occurred.

Electrophysiologic findings. Results are summarized in table 1. Evaluation of PA, AH, and HV intervals 1 month after the shock did not show any significant change from baseline values as a group or in any individual dogs. Decremental atrial pacing studies showed that the longest atrial paced cycle length that produced Wenckebach periodicity in the AV node had not changed significantly. Analysis of the programmed premature atrial stimulation data before and after the procedure failed to show any significant differences in the effective and functional refractory periods of the atrium and the AV node. Ease of induction of atrial fibrillation and duration of the induced arrhythmia remained unchanged in all dogs but one (dog 10, table 1), in which external cardioversion was required to terminate the atrial fibrillation upon 4 week follow-up study.

Differences in the ease of induction of ventricular arrhythmias were not observed. Ventricular fibrillation had been induced with double extrastimuli in the baseline preshock study in two dogs (dogs 1 and 6, table 1). Neither animal had inducible ventricular arrhythmias at the 4 week follow-up study. One dog (dog 5, table 1) had ventricular fibrillation induced with double extrastimuli from the right ventricular outflow tract 4 weeks after the shock. No sustained ventricular tachycardia was induced in any dog before or after the shock.

Gross anatomic and histologic findings. Gross inspection of the epicardial aspect of the heart failed to show any sign of healed rupture of the coronary sinus wall. Furthermore there was no pericardial reaction to suggest previous inflammation or hemorrhagic effusion. Examination of the endocardial aspect of the right atrium showed no evidence of damage to the tricuspid valve or to the AV node area.

Scarring was grossly evident around the mouth of the coronary sinus in nine dogs, with narrowing of the coronary sinus orifice in six dogs and complete occlusion in three dogs. In three animals the coronary sinus orifice appeared entirely normal. A brownish discoloration caused by hemosiderin deposits was found occasionally on the endocardium of the posterior left atrium, up to 1 cm above the level of the anulus fibrosus. Gross damage to the circumflex coronary artery was not found in any dog. No congestion or gross changes in the left ventricle secondary to coronary sinus thrombosis were seen.

Histologic findings are summarized in table 2. Sections of the AV node, His bundle, and proximal bundle branches did not reveal any damage in any dog. Coronary sinus injury, however, was present in all animals. Maximum length of coronary sinus injury was 18 ± 6 mm in the 200 J group and 23 ± 4 mm in the 360 J group. Injury consisted of circumferential fibrosis in all dogs and was associated with loss of coronary sinus intimal muscle. Furthermore, the *lumen* of the coronary sinus showed varying degrees of stenosis to complete occlusion, consistent with organization of thrombus (figure 2). Finally, although no gross rupture of the coronary sinus was seen in any dog, a constant histologic finding was rupture of the internal elastica of the coronary sinus with displacement of tissue toward the atrial wall on its endocardial aspect as if segments of the coronary sinus had been forcefully disrupted as a result of barotrauma (figure 3). No such injury was observed along the epicardial aspect of the coronary sinus.

In the left atrial wall, fibrous replacement of atrial myocardium extended for a maximum length of 18 ± 5 mm in the 200 J group and 26 ± 4 mm in the 360 J group, reaching a height of 8 ± 3 mm and 11 ± 2 mm for the 200 and 360 J shocks, respectively. Atrial injury was transmural for a length of 10 ± 5 mm in the 200 J group and 21 ± 6 mm in the 360 J group ($p < .01$). However, transmural fibrosis near the anulus of the mitral valve was inconstant and scanty (figures 2 and 4).

Maximum length of muscle loss and fibrous replacement in the left ventricle paralleled that of the left atrium, being 15 ± 5 mm long in the 200 J group and 19 ± 5 mm long in the 360 J group. However, the depth of involvement of the left ventricular wall was never greater than 5 mm. Additionally, injury width was at most 5 mm at the point of maximum left ventricular injury, except in one dog (dog 12, table 2). Transmural ventricular injury was present only in this one dog and was limited to a length of 3 mm.

Microscopic findings confirmed the absence of injury to the circumflex coronary artery (figures 2 and 4). An occasional finding was the presence of a foreign body reaction with giant cell formation in the areas of maximum injury associated with platinum deposition in the tissue (documented by spectroscopy) (figure 5). This is likely the result of erosion of the electrode after the passage of current.

TABLE 1
Electrophysiologic findings before and after shock[A]

Dog No.	PA b	PA a	AH b	AH a	HV b	HV a	RA DEC P (Wenckebach) b	RA DEC P (Wenckebach) a	AVN ERP b	AVN ERP a
1	30	30	65	62	35	30	250	260	160	240
2	28	38	55	45	34	28	260	260	240	240
3	38	40	75	72	35	30	220	240	220	220
4	25	30	60	45	38	36	210	200	170	190
5	30	22	120	74	40	35	410	200	300	160
6	38	38	58	60	32	35	250	270	260	250
Mean	32	33	72	60	36	32	267	238	225	217
±SD	±5	±7	±24	±13	±3	±3	±73	±31	±54	±35
	p = NS		p = NS		p = NS		p = NS		p = NS	
7	37	42	42	40	38	38	210	220	140	140
8	32	32	50	53	38	38	210	200	140	180
9	46	46	35	38	32	35	190	200	160	170
10	30	25	55	65	32	35	250	250	240	210
11	43	38	52	58	45	43	240	340	250	260
12	42	44	48	48	35	33	240	210	150	150
Mean	38	38	47	50	37	37	223	237	180	185
±SD	±6	±8	±7	±10	±5	±4	±23	±54	±51	±44
	p = NS		p = NS		p = NS		p = NS		p = NS	

Data expressed as milliseconds.

a = after; AF = atrial fibrillation; AH = atrio-Hisian interval; AVN = atrioventricular node; b = before; DEC P = decremental pacing; ERP = effective refractory period; FRP = functional refractory period; HV = His-ventricular interval; NSu = nonsustained; PA = surface P wave to local AVN atrial electrogram interval; RA = right atrium; Su = sustained; VAR = ventricular arrhythmias; VF = ventricular fibrillation.

[A]Dogs 1 to 6 received 200 J shocks, and dogs 7 to 12 received 360 J shocks.

Voltage and current during energy delivery. Delivery of 200 J stored energy resulted in a peak current of 18 ± 2 A and a peak voltage of 3300 ± 100 V. At a 360 J setting, peak current and voltage were 29 ± 3 A and 4150 ± 152 V. Values for peak current as calculated on the oscilloscope screen were always in agreement with readings obtained on the defibrillator display, which therefore excluded any leakage of current outside the catheter.

Current and voltage waveforms were never smooth, like their counterpart obtained with 50 Ω dummy load. They showed a different time course of voltage and current, consistent with a nonlinear resistance or complex impedance during delivery of the shock.[21] An example of current and voltage waveforms recorded during delivery of a 200 J shock is shown in figure 6.

Discussion

Catheter-mediated electrical ablation techniques are receiving increasing attention for a variety of both supraventricular and ventricular arrhythmias.[1–18, 22, 23] This technique has almost supplanted surgery for arrhythmias requiring AV node/His bundle interruption. The relative safety and effectiveness in producing AV block by catheter technique has suggested the possibility that accessory AV pathways also could be ablated without the use of open heart surgery.

The experimental work of Brodman and Fisher[19] supported the feasibility of a catheter technique to ablate left-sided bypass tracts. However, subsequent application of transvenous catheter-mediated electrical ablation procedures to patients with left-sided or posterior septal accessory connections has yielded failures and complications that demand reassessment of the validity and utility of this technique.[16] It is clear from preliminary work that success of the technique is variable[12–18] and less constant than that observed with surgical approaches.[24, 25] More work is necessary to refine the procedure before it can approach AV node/His bundle interruption in safety and efficacy.

In this study, we focused on the electrophysiologic and anatomic effects of delivery of a single electrical shock to the posterior septum via the coronary sinus. Surgical experience with posterior septal accessory pathways has revealed the complexity of the approach necessary to divide them, especially if one is to avoid the AV node/His bundle in the dissection.[24, 25] The approach to the posterior septal region with external cryoablative procedures[26] may avoid the problem of AV block, although experience with this approach re-

TABLE 1
(Continued)

AVN FRP		RA ERP		RA FRP		AF		VAR	
b	a	b	a	b	a	b	a	b	a
300	320	110	160	190	180	NSu	NSu	VF	No
340	340	150	150	180	180	NSu	NSu	No	No
320	310	120	110	160	170	NSu	NSu	No	No
270	270	170	150	190	160	NSu	NSu	No	No
400	270	140	140	180	180	NSu	NSu	No	VF
340	320	150	120	180	190	Su	Su	VF	No
328	305	140	138	180	177				
±44	±29	±22	±19	±11	±10				
p = NS		p = NS		p = NS					
270	280	140	140	170	190	Su	Su	No	No
260	250	140	150	190	180	NSu	NSu	No	No
260	270	160	160	190	190	NSu	NSu	No	No
340	330	150	120	180	140	NSu	Su	No	No
310	340	180	150	220	200	NSu	NSu	No	No
270	225	130	150	180	180	Su	Su	No	No
285	283	150	145	188	180				
±33	±45	±18	±14	±21	±21				
p = NS		p = NS		p = NS					

mains limited and it still requires a sternotomy. Therefore we addressed the specific question of whether a catheter technique can result in damage potentially able to prevent conduction through such posterior septal pathways without affecting the anatomy and the functional characteristics of the normal AV conduction system. We also desired to garner information on the mechanism of catheter-induced electrical injury.

The choice of the present technique was dictated by the following theoretical considerations. If any vectorial component related to delivery of electrical energy is involved in producing the desirable effects, then the current flow should be able to traverse the target area, resulting in adequate current density at that point. Positioning of the cathode on the anterior chest wall opposite to the anode should allow adequate current density

TABLE 2
Anatomic changes after the shock[A]

Dog No.	Coronary sinus injury			Atrial injury			Left ventricular injury			Conduction system injury	Left circumflex arterial injury
	Gross rupture	Elastic rupture	Length (mm)	Max. length (mm)	Length of transmural injury (mm)	Height (mm)	Length (mm)	Width (mm)	Depth (mm)		
1	No	Yes	24	17	7	6	22	4	3	No	No
2	No	Yes	18	16	9	12	13	5	5	No	No
3	No	Yes	7	10	8	6	7	4	2	No	No
4	No	Yes	19	23	20	10	16	3	3	No	No
5	No	Yes	17	18	6	5	18	5	3	No	No
6	No	Yes	23	23	7	9	12	4	1	No	No
Mean ± SD			18±6	18±5	10±5	8±3	15±5	4±1	3±1		
7	No	Yes	22	20	16	11	15	3	1	No	No
8	No	Yes	23	32	22	12	20	4	3	No	No
9	No	Yes	15	24	15	10	14	5	2	No	No
10	No	Yes	24	26	20	14	18	4	2	No	No
11	No	Yes	24	29	30	8	17	4	1	No	No
12	No	Yes	27	26	24	8	27	13	5	No	No
Mean ± SD			23±4	26±4	21±6	11±2	19±5	6±4	2±2		

[A]Dogs 1 to 6 received 200 J shocks, and dogs 7 to 12 received 360 J shocks.

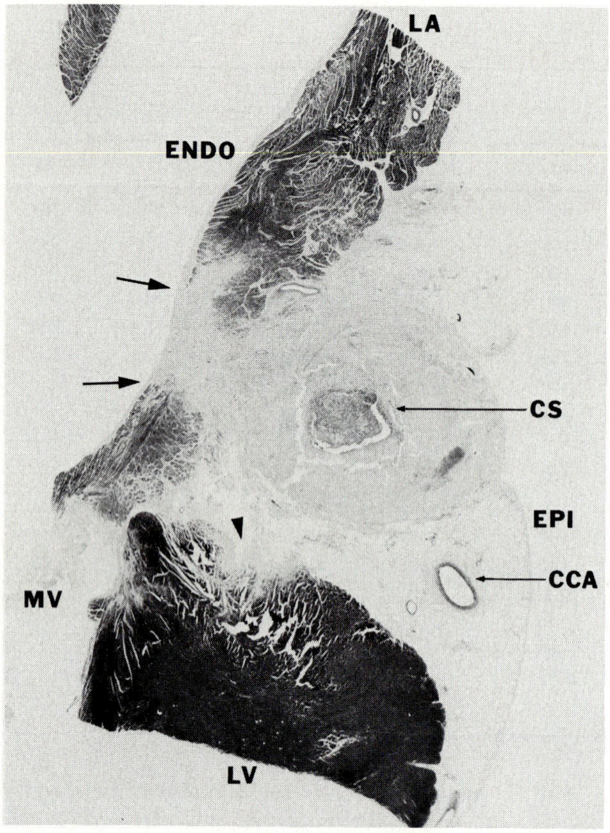

FIGURE 2. Photomicrograph of a cross section of the left atrioventricular groove at the site of maximum injury in dog 7 (360 J). This section is taken 8 mm within the coronary sinus orifice. The coronary sinus lumen is occluded by an organized thrombus. The coronary sinus wall shows loss of muscle and replacement by circumferential fibrosis. Transmural fibrosis of the atrial wall is present (arrows). There is no fibrosis immediately above the anulus fibrosus. The left ventricular wall shows a very limited area of muscle loss and fibrous replacement (arrowhead). The circumflex coronary artery is patent and no wall abnormalities are present. (Gomori's trichrome; original magnification ×5.7.) arrows = site of myocardial fibrosis; CCA = circumflex coronary artery; CS = coronary sinus; ENDO = endocardium; EPI = epicardium; LA = left atrium; LV = left ventricle; MV = mitral valve.

to flow across the area where damage is desirable. Another consideration relates to electrically induced myocardial damage. Cardiac defibrillation studies[27–29] have shown that the use of very small paddles results in high transthoracic resistance, with a reduced total current flow. On the other hand, intracardiac current increases with larger paddles, although the distribution of this current covers a larger cross-sectional area. Therefore the use of smaller paddles should result in less transthoracic current flow, with points of higher current density, which can be useful in producing the desired damage. Additionally, because of the variability of locations of the accessory connections from endocardium to epicardium, an ideal injury should cover the entire thickness of the atrial wall near the anulus. Based on these considerations, we used high-energy shocks and a small (3.5 cm) paddle positioned on the anterior chest wall, opposite the coronary sinus catheter.

The decision to couple together two consecutive poles of the coronary sinus catheter as the anode was based on the consideration that accessory pathways may cover, morphologically or functionally, a zone of myocardium larger than simply the punctate site, which might be expected from catheter mapping. Early surgical experience with posterior septal and left-sided accessory pathways, seems to confirm the impression that accessory AV fibers are often not discrete and can occur over several centimeters.[25, 30, 31] As a consequence, an injury able to prevent accessory pathway conduction ideally should involve a wider area of the atrioventricular sulcus or atrial wall above the anulus fibrosus other than the precise area of earliest activation. Furthermore, the decision to use a pair of electrodes as the anode was taken in view of previous experience indicating that standard catheters may not tolerate high-energy shocks, which can result in failure of the internal wire or the insulation,[20, 32] with subsequent delivery of the shock to poles other than the ones intended.[20] Coupling of two electrodes of equal resistance in parallel would cause total current flow to divide in half through either of them, possibly preventing at least failure of the internal wire. On the other hand, separate shocks of less energy on either pole might not obtain the same result, the first shock possibly weakening the dielectric strength of the catheter.[20]

It is important to emphasize, with respect to ablation techniques, that accessory AV pathways usually skirt the anulus fibrosus in close approximation to it.[33] However, our results show that delivery of high-energy shocks in proximity to the coronary sinus orifice principally produces damage to the wall of the coronary sinus and to left atrial myocardium above the AV groove but not to the anulus proper. Nevertheless, an area of delay could be created so that the accessory connection would become functionally silent. This kind of injury may be all that is necessary or indeed safely possible from a clinical perspective. In our series of dogs, even at high energies, inconsistent injury was produced at the anulus fibrosus. This is consistent with anatomic observations in dogs and in man that the coronary sinus occupies a relatively high position in the pyramidal space with respect to the anulus.

Risk of permanent AV block associated with the surgical approach of posterior septal accessory pathways is a well-known possibility.[25] With the use of the technique described in this study, no functional or

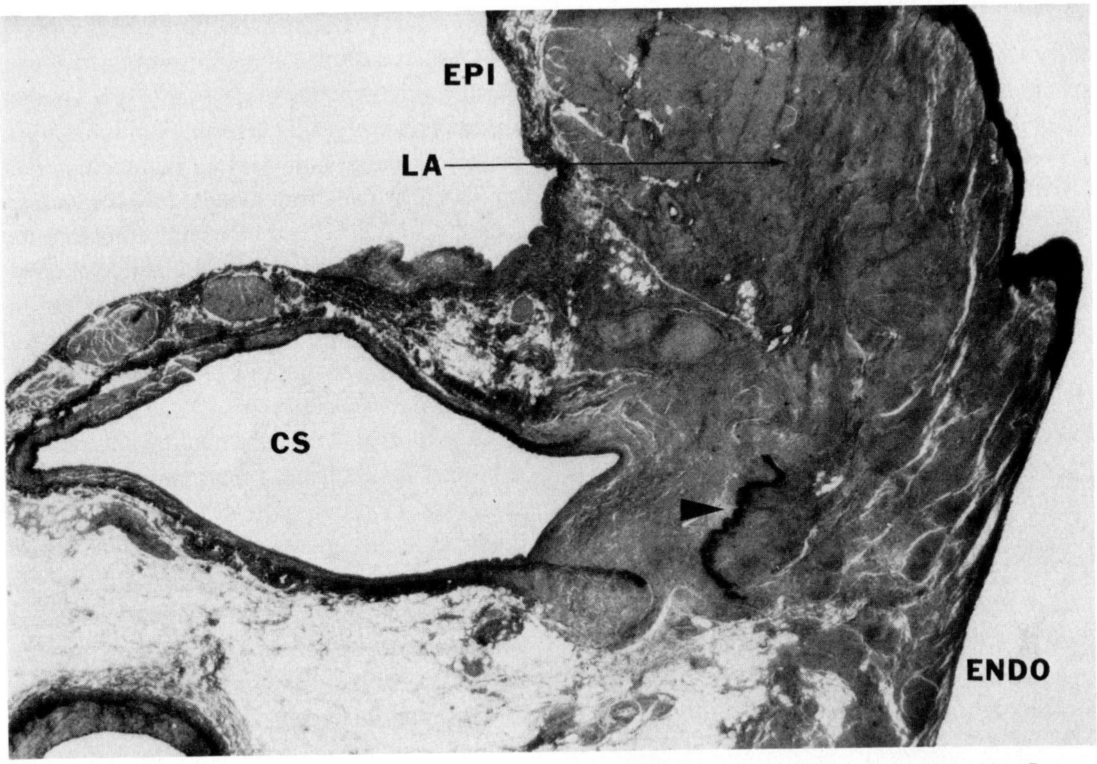

FIGURE 3. Cross section of the left coronary sulcus, taken from dog 4 (200 J) 16 mm within the coronary sinus orifice. Rupture of the internal elastica of the coronary sinus is observed on the endocardial aspect, with a detached part of the elastica itself displaced toward the atrial wall (arrowhead). The integrity of the elastic membrane in the rest of the coronary sinus wall is maintained. The appearance of membrane rupture suggests a barotraumatic mechanism. See text for discussion. (Verhoeff–Van Gieson; original magnification ×26.) arrowhead = disrupted elastic membrane; abbreviations as in figure 2.

morphologic damage was produced to the conduction system. Impairment of AV conduction was observed only transiently in our series of dogs, probably as a consequence of the barotrauma associated with the electrical shock. Furthermore, the arrhythmogenic potential of this particular technique appears to be minimal, as judged from the results of atrial and ventricular stimulation studies and from the long-term absence of spontaneous arrhythmias. The episodes of induced ventricular fibrillation in the preshock studies are of uncertain significance and probably reflect hypersensitivity of dogs to ventricular programmed electrical stimulation. The failure to demonstrate any cardiac abnormalities in these dogs other than that induced after the shock suggests that inducible ventricular fibrillation was a false-positive event. The one dog that had ventricular fibrillation induced after the shock was similar to the other two dogs in that no ventricular abnormality was found except for a region at the shock site corresponding to a 0.27 cm^3 volume of damaged muscle. Although not proved, it is unlikely that this ventricular injury resulted in inducible ventricular fibrillation.

Preservation of normal anatomy of the left circumflex coronary artery was observed in this study, confirming previously reported findings.[19] However, the anatomic relationship of the coronary sinus orifice to the circumflex coronary artery is optimal at the posterior septum. Coronary arterial injury at this location is less likely (assuming no significant right coronary artery extension branch). In the lateral AV groove, on the other hand, such a technique may be more likely to cause coronary arterial injury.

No evidence of gross rupture of the coronary sinus was found in any of our dogs, even when energies as high as 360 J were used. This could have resulted from the use of two electrodes coupled together as the anode, which avoided concentration of electrical energy to a very small area and in essence divided the energy between two electrodes. An interesting finding, however, was the presence of intramural rupture of the coronary sinus in all animals. The morphologic features of this damage would be rather difficult to explain on the basis of a pure electrical or thermal injury. The observation that parts of the internal elastic membrane of the coronary sinus were displaced literally

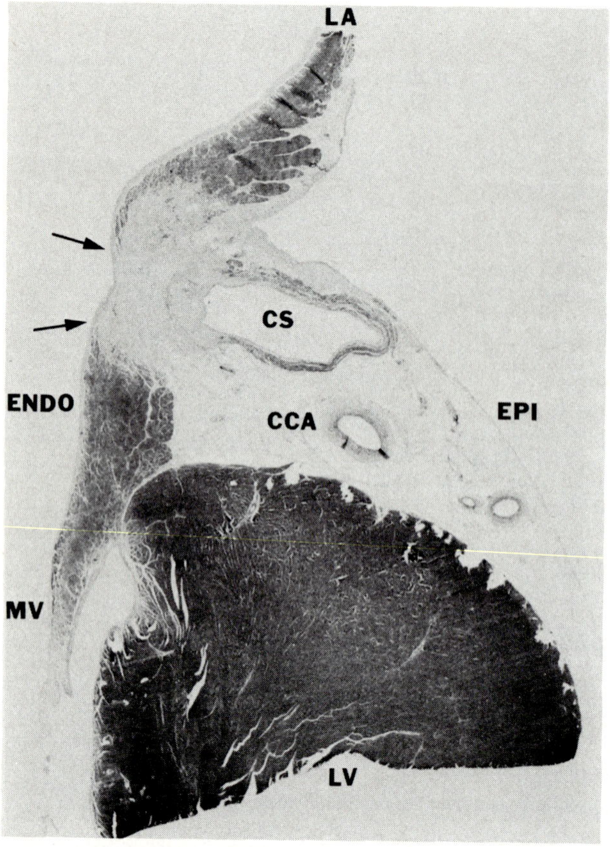

FIGURE 4. Cross section of the left atrioventricular groove, taken 18 mm within the coronary sinus orifice. This dog (No. 4) received 200 J. The left ventricular wall and the coronary artery do not show any damage. Coronary sinus injury is limited. However, transmural atrial fibrosis is present in the atrial wall facing the endocardial aspect of coronary sinus (arrows). Note undamaged atrial muscle just above the mitral valve. This injury could still leave a bypass tract anatomically intact. Conceivably, however, such a boundary of transmural fibrotic tissue could prevent depolarization wavefronts from entering or exiting the accessory pathway. See text for discussion. (Gomori's trichrome; original magnification ×8.7.) Abbreviations as in figure 2.

into the atrial wall would suggest that the pressure increase associated with the electrical discharge was of such a magnitude as to create damage by means of barotrauma. In support of this mechanism, one would expect that close contact between the electrodes of a No. 6F catheter and the coronary sinus wall at the moment of the shock is unlikely to occur because of a disproportion between their respective sizes. This would prevent current directly from contacting the coronary sinus wall, allowing, on the contrary, for some current to be dissipated in the blood. This would result in electrolysis of the blood with plasma (ionic gas) formation.[34, 35] Arcing of the current through the plasma would lead to a shock wave and the barotrauma that gives rise to rupture of the coronary sinus elastica. Coronary sinus rupture with tamponade therefore would be dependent on the degree of barotrauma, with higher energy shocks or multiple shocks more likely to lead to gross coronary sinus rupture. Conceivably, rupture might occur more easily in a small coronary sinus. Therefore adequate angiographic visualization of the coronary sinus should be recommended in potential candidates for catheter-mediated shocks in this locale. Caution should be exercised before proceeding with currently available catheter techniques in children, in patients with a small coronary sinus, and in the more lateral portion of the coronary sinus where the vessel tapers considerably as it becomes the great cardiac vein.

That internal elastic membrane rupture into the atrial wall can result from a barotraumatic mechanism is supported by previous work in underwater pulse technology.[34] Experiments in vitro conducted to assess the reliability of electrode catheters to be used for electrical ablation[32, 35] suggest that high pressures could be generated during delivery of high-energy endocavitary shocks. To which extent arcing through ionic gases formed from electrolysis by high-energy shocks may be one mechanism responsible for barotrauma is unknown.

The role barotrauma has in producing the desired damage rather than creating complications remains to be established. Certainly, barotrauma by itself cannot explain other features of the injury. That discharge of transthoracic or epicardial shocks can result in myocardial injury is a well-known fact.[27, 28, 36, 37] Myocyte necrosis with contraction bands, mineralization of necrotic tissue with subsequent macrophage infiltration, and later fibrosis have all been described in the setting of myocardial electrical injury induced by extracardiac countershocks.[36, 38, 39] Similar findings have been reported recently in canine studies, where the effects of intracardiac shocks delivered through endocardial catheter electrodes were evaluated.[40, 41] Our study design did not allow us to evaluate sequential ultrastructural changes of this kind, even though the observation in our study of areas of macrophage infiltration with giant cell formation is in keeping with the results of those studies[40, 41] and with previous observations made in dogs undergoing transvenous ablation of the AV node.[4] However, all these changes could merely represent a pattern of response of the myocardial cell to injury[42] rather than being specific for an electrical type of injury. Therefore such changes seem insufficient to clarify the mechanism by which endocavitary shocks produce their effects.

With the use of this technique, transmural atrial injury potentially capable of preventing accessory pathway conduction in the posterior septum was con-

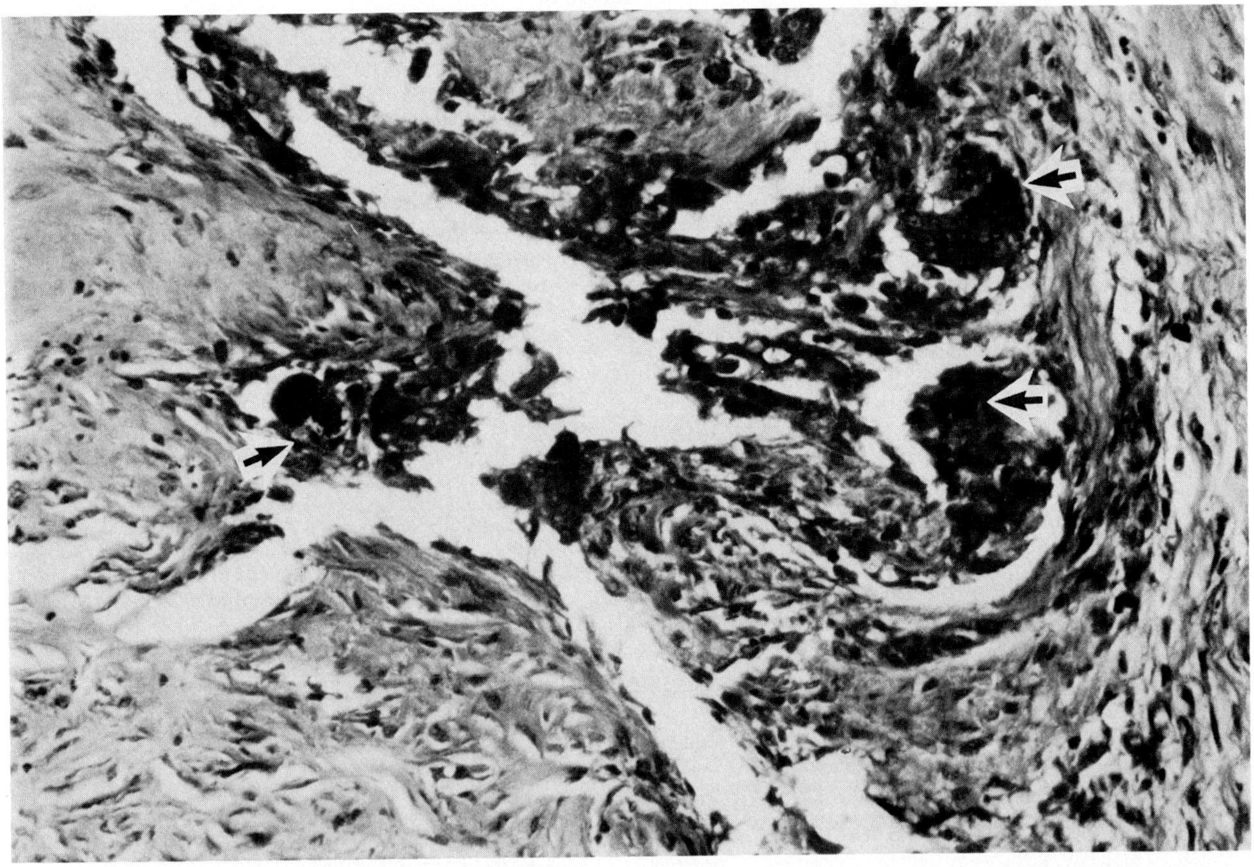

FIGURE 5. High-power photomicrograph from the area of maximum injury in dog 10. A foreign body reaction with giant cell formation is present in the coronary sinus associated with platinum deposition in the tissue (arrows). See text for discussion. (Gomori's trichrome; ×300.)

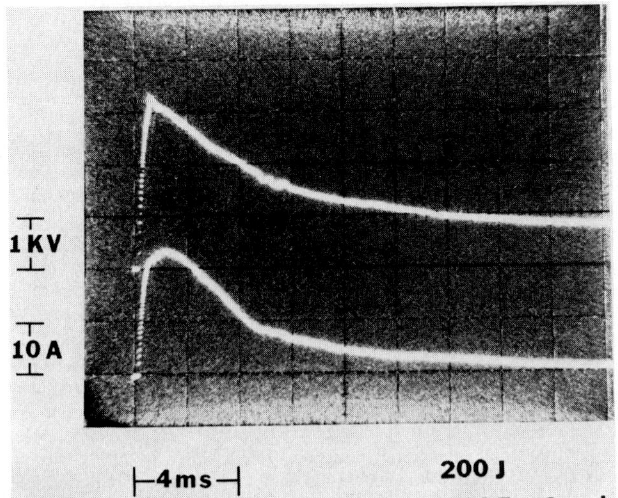

FIGURE 6. Current and voltage waveforms recorded during delivery of 200 J in dog 4. The shock resulted in a peak voltage of 3300 V (top) and a peak current of 23 A (bottom). Note that current and voltage show a different time course, consistent with a nonlinear resistance during delivery of the shock.

sistently produced with a single shock. No AV block, electrophysiologic alterations, pericardial tamponade, or other complications were seen. Atrial intramural rupture of the coronary sinus was observed in each dog, the histologic features of which are suggestive at least in part of a barotraumatic mechanism. The evidence of barotrauma brings into question the controllability of the technique. Changes in the procedure will therefore be necessary for safe application. Successful catheter modification via the coronary sinus of tachycardias using posterior septal accessory pathways may depend on the ability of transmural atrial injury above the anulus proper to effectively block depolarization wavefronts from entering or exiting the accessory pathway, which is likely to persist after the shock.

We thank Lillian T. Kato for typing the manuscript, and Dan Yerkovich and Andrew Luedtke, B.S.E.E, for their help and advice during the course of this study.

References

1. Gonzalez R, Scheinman M, Margaretten W, Rubinstein M: Closed-chest electrode-catheter technique for His bundle ablation in dogs. Am J Physiol **241:** H283, 1981
2. Gonzalez R, Scheinman M, Bharati S, Lev M: Closed chest permanent atrioventricular block in dogs. Am Heart J **105:** 461, 1983
3. Gallagher JJ, Svenson RH, Kasell JH, German LD, Bardy GH, Broughton A, Critelli G: Catheter technique for closed-chest ablation of the atrioventricular conduction system: A therapeutic alternative for the treatment of refractory supraventricular tachycardia. N Engl J Med **306:** 194, 1982

4. Bardy GH, Ideker RE, Kasell J, Worley SJ, Smith WM, German LD, Gallagher JJ: Transvenous ablation of the atrioventricular conduction system in dogs: electrophysiologic and histologic observations. Am J Cardiol **51:** 1775, 1983
5. Scheinman MM, Morady F, Hess DS, Gonzalez R: Catheter-induced ablation of the atrioventricular junction to control refractory supraventricular arrhythmias. JAMA **248:** 851, 1982
6. Critelli G, Perticone F, Coltorti F, Monda V, Gallagher JJ: Closed chest modification of atrioventricular conduction system in man for treatment of refractory supraventricular tachycardia. Br Heart J **49:** 544, 1983
7. Wood DL, Hammill SC, Holmes DR Jr, Osborn MJ, Gersh BJ: Catheter ablation of the atrioventricular conduction system in patients with supraventricular tachycardia. Mayo Clin Proc **58:** 791, 1983
8. Gillette PC, Garson A Jr, Porter CJ, Ott D, McVey P, Zimner A, Blair H: Junctional automatic ectopic tachycardia: new proposed treatment by transcatheter His bundle ablation. Am Heart J **106:** 619, 1983
9. Nathan AW, Bennett DH, Ward DE, Bexton RS, Camm AJ: Catheter ablation of atrioventricular conduction. Lancet **1:** 1280, 1984
10. Scheinman M, Evans-Bell T: Catheter ablation of the atrioventricular junction: a report of the percutaneous mapping and ablation registry. Circulation **70:** 1024, 1984
11. Bhandari A, Morady F, Shen EN, Schwartz AB, Botvinick E, Scheinman MM: Catheter-induced His bundle ablation in a patient with reentrant tachycardia associated with a nodoventricular tract. J Am Coll Cardiol **4:** 611, 1984
12. Weber H, Schmitz L: Catheter technique for closed-chest ablation of an accessory pathway. N Engl J Med **308:** 653, 1983
13. Jackman WM, Friday KJ, Scherlag BJ, Dehning MM, Schechter E, Reynolds DW, Olson EG, Berbari EJ, Harrison LA, Lazzara R: Direct endocardial recording from an accessory pathway: localization of the site of block, effect of antiarrhythmic drugs, and attempt at nonsurgical ablation. Circulation **68:** 906, 1983
14. Critelli G, Monda V, Perticone F, Coltorti F, Scherillo M, Condorelli M: Closed chest ablation of accessory pathways: experimental model and successful application in a patient with incessant supraventricular tachycardia. G Ital Cardiol **14**(I): 181, 1984
15. Morady F, Scheinman MM: Transvenous catheter ablation of a postero-septal accessory pathway in a patient with the Wolff-Parkinson-White syndrome. N Engl J Med **310:** 705, 1984
16. Fisher JD, Brodman R, Kim SG, Matos JA, Brodman E, Wallerson D, Waspe LE: Attempted nonsurgical electrical ablation of accessory pathways via the coronary sinus in the Wolff-Parkinson-White syndrome. J Am Coll Cardiol **4:** 685, 1984
17. Bardy GH, Poole JE, Coltorti F, Ivey TD, Block TA, Greene HL: Catheter ablation of a concealed postero-septal accessory pathway. Am J Cardiol **54:** 1366, 1984
18. Ward DE, Camm JA: Treatment of tachycardias associated with the Wolff-Parkinson-White syndrome by transvenous electrical ablation of accessory pathways. Br Heart J **53:** 64, 1985
19. Brodman R, Fisher JD: Evaluation of a catheter technique for ablation of accessory pathways near the coronary sinus using a canine model. Circulation **67:** 923, 1983
20. Bardy GH, Coltorti F, Ivey TD, Yerkovich D, Greene HL: Effect of damped sine-wave shocks on catheter dielectric strength. Am J Cardiol (in press, vol 56, 1985)
21. Trantham JL, Gallagher JJ, German LD, Broughton A, Guarnieri T, Kasell J: Effects of energy delivery via a His bundle catheter during closed-chest ablation of the atrioventricular conduction system. J Clin Invest **72:** 1563, 1983
22. Hartzler GO: Electrode catheter ablation of refractory focal ventricular tachycardia. J Am Coll Cardiol **2:** 1107, 1983
23. Josephson ME: Catheter ablation of arrhythmias. Ann Intern Med **101:** 234, 1984
24. Sealy WC, Gallagher JJ: The surgical approach to the septal area of the heart based on experiences with 45 patients with Kent bundles. J Thorac Cardiovasc Surg **79:** 542, 1980
25. Gallagher JJ, Sealy WC, Cox JL, German LD, Kasell JH, Bardy GH, Packer DL: Results of surgery for preexcitation caused by accessory atrioventricular pathways in 267 consecutive cases. *In* Josephson ME, Wellens HJJ, editors: Tachycardias: mechanisms, diagnosis, treatment. Philadelphia, 1984, Lea & Febiger, p 259
26. Guiraudon GM, Klein GJ, Sharma AD, Jones DL: Ablation of posterior septal atrioventricular accessory pathways in the Wolff-Parkinson-White syndrome using the closed heart technique. J Am Coll Cardiol **5:** 410, 1985 (abst)
27. Dahl CF, Ewy GA, Warner ED, Thomas ED: Myocardial necrosis from direct current discharge: effect of paddle electrode size and time interval between discharges. Circulation **50:** 956, 1974
28. Doherty PW, McLaughin PR, Billingham M, Kernoff R, Goris ML, Harrison DC: Cardiac damage produced by direct current countershocks applied to the heart. Am J Cardiol **43:** 225, 1979
29. Hoyt R, Grayzel J, Kerber RE: Determinants of intracardiac current in defibrillation: experimental studies in dogs. Circulation **64:** 818, 1981
30. Sealy WC, Gallagher JJ, Wallace AG: The surgical treatment of Wolff-Parkinson-White syndrome: evolution of improved methods for identification and interruption of the Kent bundle. Ann Thorac Surg **22:** 443, 1976
31. Gallagher JJ, Sealy WC, Kasell J: Intraoperative mapping studies in the Wolff-Parkinson-White syndrome. PACE **2:** 523, 1979
32. Fisher JD, Brodman R, Johnston DR, Waspe LE, Kim SG, Matos JA, Scavin G: Nonsurgical electrical ablation of tachycardias: importance of prior in vitro testing of catheters. PACE **7:** 74, 1984
33. Davies MJ, Anderson RH, Becker AE: The conduction system of the heart. London, 1983, Butterworths, p 186
34. Früngel FBA: High speed pulse technology. New York, 1965, Academic Press, vol I, p 476
35. Bardy GH, Coltorti F, Ivey TD, Alferness C, Greene HL: Some factors affecting bubble formation during catheter ablation. PACE **8:** 311, 1985 (abst)
36. Anderson HN, Reichenbach D, Steinmetz GP, Merendino KA: An evaluation and comparison of effects of alternating and direct current electrical discharges on canine hearts. Ann Surg **160:** 251, 1964
37. Ewy GA, Taren D, Bangert J, McClung S, Hellman DA: Comparison of myocardial damage from defibrillator discharges at various dosages. Med Instrum **14:** 9, 1980
38. Van Vleet JF, Tacker WA Jr, Geddes LA, Ferrans VJ: Sequential cardiac morphologic alterations induced in dogs by single transthoracic damped sinusoidal waveform defibrillator shocks. Am J Vet Res **39:** 271, 1978
39. Van Vleet JF, Tacker WA Jr, Geddes LA, Ferrans VJ: Sequential ultrastructural alterations in ventricular myocardium of dogs given large single transthoracic damped sinusoidal waveform defibrillator shocks. Am J Vet Res **41:** 493, 1980
40. Barker-Voelz MA, Van Vleet JF, Tacker WA Jr, Bourland JD, Geddes LA, Schollmeyer MP: Alterations induced by a single defibrillating shock applied through a chronically implanted catheter electrode. J Electrocardiol **16:** 167, 1983
41. Lerman BB, Weiss JL, Bulkley BH, Becker LC, Weisfeldt ML: Myocardial injury and induction of arrhythmia by direct current shock delivered via endocardial catheters in dogs. Circulation **69:** 1006, 1984
42. Reichenbach D, Benditt EP: Myofibrillar degeneration: a response of the myocardial cell to injury. Arch Pathol Lab Med **85:** 189, 1968

Interruption of sympathetic and vagal-mediated afferent responses by transmural myocardial infarction

MICHAEL J. BARBER, PH.D., M.D., THOMAS M. MUELLER, M.D., BECKY G. DAVIES, ROBERT M. GILL, B.S., AND DOUGLAS P. ZIPES, M.D.

ABSTRACT We have demonstrated previously that sympathetic and vagal afferents travel in an apical-to-basal course in the heart, and can be stimulated selectively with epicardial applications of bradykinin and nicotine, respectively. In this study we tested the hypothesis that transmural myocardial infarction interrupts sympathetic and vagal afferent fibers traveling through the infarction and produces regions of afferent denervation in areas apical to the infarction. In open-chest, chloralose-anesthetized dogs, transmural myocardial infarction was created by embolizing a diagonal branch of the left anterior descending coronary artery with a vinyl latex solution that was injected directly into the artery and hardened rapidly. The transmural nature of the infarction was verified by the nitro blue tetrazolium staining technique for dehydrogenase enzymes. Epicardial applications of bradykinin (5 μg) and nicotine (50 μg) were used to stimulate chemically sensitive sympathetic and vagal afferent nerve endings, respectively. Twenty-nine dogs were studied before and 90 min after creation of transmural myocardial infarction. In 20 dogs, epicardial bradykinin applied before production of transmural myocardial infarction produced a maximal pressor response of 13 $\pm$ 3 mm Hg 40 sec after application ($p < .01$ vs preapplication values), while topical nicotine produced a maximal depressor response of 14 $\pm$ 2 mm Hg ($p < .01$ vs preapplication values) 20 sec after application at all sites tested. Ninety minutes after production of transmural myocardial infarction, epicardial sites basal to the infarction continued to respond normally to both drugs, while sites within the area of infarction and apical to the area (noninfarcted myocardium) no longer showed a pressor response to topical bradykinin or a depressor response to topical nicotine. Nerve interruptions in 12 dogs demonstrated that the sympathetic afferent responses elicited by bradykinin were eliminated with bilateral stellectomy, while vagal afferent responses elicited by nicotine were interrupted by transection of the cervical vagi. In 10 dogs, more extensive epicardial mapping of responses to the two drugs revealed that sites were not always afferently denervated in a homogeneous manner. Several sites medial and apical to the transmural myocardial infarction continued to show pressor responses to bradykinin, but were unresponsive to topical nicotine. We conclude that transmural myocardial infarction produces areas of both sympathetic and vagal afferent denervation in infarcted and in noninfarcted myocardium apical to the region of infarction. This afferent denervation is not homogeneous in all areas.
Circulation 72, No. 3, 623–631, 1985.

AFFERENT NERVE FIBERS have endings in the left ventricular wall. Some afferent fibers travel with sympathetic nerves and may be chemically sensitive, mechanosensitive, or both.[1] These sympathetic afferent fibers mediate a pressor and a pseudoaffective response in animals that can be elicited by epicardial[2–4] or intracoronary[2, 4, 5] administration of bradykinin and by other chemical agents. Sympathetic afferents also apparently mediate the sensation of cardiac pain in man.[6, 7] Other afferent fibers travel with the vagus nerves and can be activated by stretch, by epicardial[2, 8, 9] or intracoronary[2, 9] administration of nicotine, and by other chemical agents. These nerves are known to mediate depressor responses produced by ischemia or stretch of the left ventricular myocardium.[1, 10, 11]

We have demonstrated previously that epicardial application of phenol on the anterior and posterior free

From the Krannert Institute of Cardiology, the Department of Medicine and Pharmacology, Indiana University School of Medicine, Veterans Administration Medical Center, Indianapolis.

Supported in part by the Herman C. Krannert Fund, by grants HL-06308 and HL-07182 from the National Heart, Lung, and Blood Institute of the National Institutes of Health, Bethesda, by the American Heart Association, Indiana Affiliate, and by Veterans Administration, Merit Review Funding.

Address for correspondence: Douglas P. Zipes, M.D., Krannert Institute of Cardiology, 1001 W. 10th St., Indianapolis, IN 46202.

Received Jan. 25, 1985; revision accepted June 6, 1985.

wall of the left ventricle distant from the atrioventricular groove interrupts sympathetic, but not vagal afferent, nerves innervating the myocardium, suggesting that sympathetic afferent nerves travel in the subepicardium, but that vagal afferent nerves travel deeper, possibly in the subendocardium.[2] We also have shown that acute and chronic transmural myocardial infarction interrupts sympathetic and vagal efferent transmission to viable, noninfarcted myocardium apical to the infarction, probably by damaging nerves traversing the infarction in a basal-to-apical direction.[12, 13] Little is known, however, of the effects of transmural myocardial infarction on transmission of afferent sympathetic and vagal fibers, the nerve endings of which can be activated by epicardial application of bradykinin and nicotine, respectively. The purpose of this study was to determine if localized transmural myocardial infarction disrupts afferently mediated sympathetic and vagal neural responses elicited apically to the infarction by interrupting afferent fibers traveling in an apical-to-basal direction through the area of infarction.

Methods

We produced transmural myocardial infarction by intracoronary injection of a vinyl latex solution that hardened rapidly[12, 14] to eliminate the influence of collateral circulation found in the canine heart, and to ensure the production of a transmural infarction of the type that has been created with the coronary artery embolization technique.[12, 14, 15]

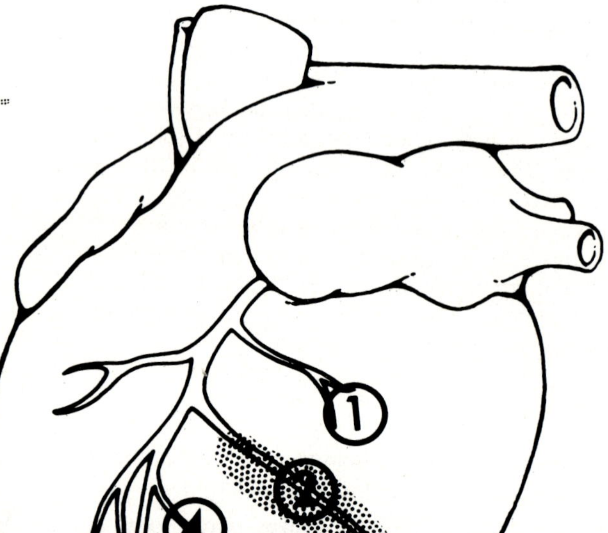

FIGURE 1. Schematic representation of heart showing epicardial sites of drug application (circles labeled 1 through 6) and the region of transmural myocardial infarction (stippling).

Animal preparation. Twenty-nine mongrel dogs of both sexes weighing 14 to 26 kg were anesthetized with α-chloralose (100 mg/kg iv); additional amounts (about 10 mg/kg/hr) were added as needed to maintain a level of light surgical anesthesia. Respiration was controlled with a cuffed endotracheal tube connected to a volume-cycled respirator (Harvard model 607). A left thoracotomy was performed in each dog through the fifth intercostal space, and the heart was supported by suturing the margins of the opened pericardium to the edges of the surgical wound. The cervical vagi were isolated bilaterally in the neck, and the stellate ganglia were isolated in the chest for later surgical interruption. A fluid-filled cannula placed in a femoral artery was used to monitor arterial pressure, and a jugular venous catheter was used to administer drugs. Arterial blood gases and arterial pH were monitored throughout the experiment at intervals not exceeding 30 min, and sodium bicarbonate was infused intravenously or the tidal volume or the respiratory rate was changed to maintain the values for these parameters in the normal range. Arterial pressure and the electrocardiogram were recorded throughout the experiment on a physiologic recorder.

Five to seven millimeters of the first or second diagonal branch of the left anterior descending coronary artery (LAD) was isolated, and two silk ligatures were placed loosely underneath the vessel for use in later cannulation of the artery. Because isolation of the artery itself might disrupt afferent nerve fibers traveling in the adventitia of the artery, control heart rate and blood pressure responses to topical application of bradykinin and nicotine were performed after the dissection (control recordings). This ensured that all areas tested were not afferently denervated by the isolation procedure. All sites tested in this study produced appropriate responses to bradykinin and nicotine after isolation of the coronary artery.[2]

After these manipulations, a banjo thermistor was secured to the epicardial surface of the left ventricular free wall, and epicardial temperature was monitored. Rectal temperature also was monitored, and a heating blanket and thermal lamp were used to keep both epicardial and core temperature within a range of 37° to 39° C. A clear plastic film that covered the wound also aided in maintaining epicardial temperature.

Protocols. In all of the experiments, bradykinin was used to stimulate sympathetic afferent nerve endings[2, 3, 16] and nicotine was used to stimulate vagal afferent nerve endings.[2, 9] Bradykinin triacetate (Sigma) and nicotine (Sigma) were dissolved in normal saline. A 0.5 cm square of surgical gauze moistened with saline was placed on the epicardium several minutes before application of either drug. The gauze was used to prevent the spread of drug outside the area of the epicardium to be tested. Bradykinin (5 μg in 0.20 ml saline solution) or nicotine (50 μg in 0.20 ml saline solution) was dripped onto the gauze sponge. Both nicotine and bradykinin solutions were kept at temperatures between 36.5° and 38° C.[2] At least 10 min was allowed between drug applications. No data were collected in the 15 min period after administration of anesthetic.

To test the effects of transmural myocardial infarction on the afferent innervation of the anterior left ventricle (figure 1), sites above (basal to; site 1), within (site 2), and below (apical to; site 3) the region of coronary artery distribution were tested with topical applications of bradykinin and nicotine before and 90 min after embolization of the coronary artery. Control heart rate and blood pressure responses to the drugs were recorded, and then the isolated coronary artery was cannulated with a PE-50 catheter filled with vinyl latex solution. The cannula was secured in the artery by the silk ligatures, and 0.3 to 0.5 ml of vinyl latex solution (Carolina Biological Supply) was injected rapidly into the artery through the catheter to embolize the vasculature.[2, 14] The catheter was removed and the preparation was allowed to stabilize for 90 min. Responses to drugs were measured 90 min after embolization. In 10 dogs, more extensive mapping was done after multiple drug applications at additional sites (figure 1, sites 4, 5, 6) on the anterior surface of the left ventricle before and 90 min after creation of the transmural myocardial infarction.

In 12 dogs, surgical interruption of sympathetic and vagal afferents was performed to examine afferent pathways mediating pressor responses to bradykinin and depressor responses to nicotine. In half of the dogs (n = 6), the cervical vagal trunks were cut and epicardial sites (figure 1, sites 4, 5) that had demonstrated continued responses to both bradykinin and nicotine after infarction were retested. After these measurements, bilateral stellectomy was performed to interrupt sympathetic afferent pathways and the responses to the drugs tested. In the remaining dogs (n = 6), the order of performance of bilateral stellectomy and vagotomy was reversed.

The relationship of each site tested to the infarcted region was confirmed by the nitro blue tetrazolium staining technique for dehydrogenase enzymes.[12, 17] Four to six hours after embolization, the ventricles were fibrillated and the heart was excised, with wire markers positioned to define the epicardial sites of drug applications. The left ventricle was separated from the rest of the heart and cut in a breadloaf fashion from base to apex. Tissue slices were rinsed in cold tap water and placed in a solution of distilled water (288 ml), phoshate buffer (32 ml, pH 7.4), and nitro blue tetrazolium (100 mg, Sigma) at 37° C for 7 to 12 min.[12, 17, 18] With this method, we verified the location of all sites of drug application in relation to the area of infarction, as well as the transmural nature of the infarction. Data presented in this report were obtained from sites verified to be located above (basal to), within, and below (apical to) the region of latex distribution and transmural myocardial infarction.

Statistics. The responses to nicotine and bradykinin applied topically to the anterior wall of the left ventricle were compared with responses obtained 90 min after creation of transmural myocardial infarction with the use of an analysis of variance and an analysis of variance for repeated measures.[19] Except as stated otherwise, data are reported as mean ± SEM. Statistical significance was achieved when a p value of $<.05$ was obtained.

Results

Twenty-nine dogs were initially entered into the protocol. Of these, 16 demonstrated both a pressor response to topical applications of bradykinin and a depressor response to topical applications of nicotine. All 16 dogs also demonstrated a decrease in heart rate in response to the topical applications of nicotine at all sites tested on the anterior left ventricle. Four of 29 dogs responded to topical bradykinin only, and four animals responded to topical nicotine only. Despite careful control of the level of anesthesia, temperature of the drug solution, epicardial and core temperature of the dogs, blood gases, and the time between drug applications, all of which influence the response to drugs,[2] five dogs did not respond to nicotine or bradykinin. Data from these five dogs were excluded from the study. All 24 animals reported in this study had transmural myocardial infarction confirmed by nitro blue tetrazolium staining and in all, verification of test sites basal, within, or apical to the site of infarction was obtained at autopsy.

Blood pressure responses to bradykinin and nicotine. In the 20 dogs that demonstrated pressor responses to bradykinin before transmural myocardial infarction (control), application of bradykinin to sites basal, within, and apical to the area of potential infarction all produced a significant pressor response ($p < .05$) to the drug (figure 2). This response was maximal approximately 40 sec after application of the drug and

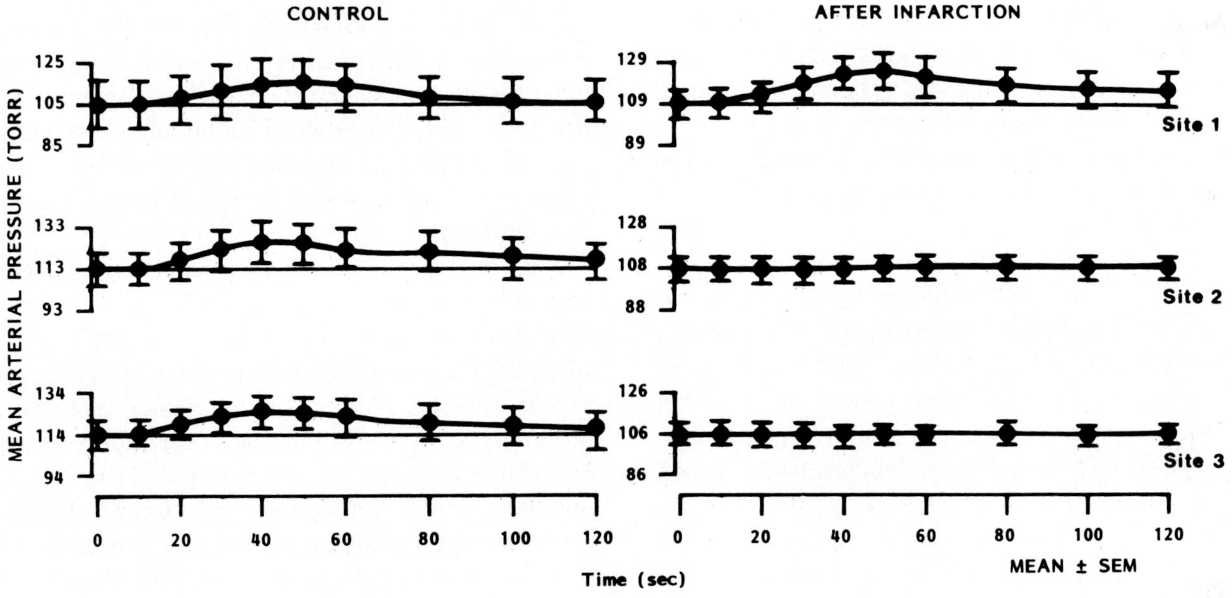

FIGURE 2. Responses of mean arterial pressure to epicardial applications of bradykinin at sites 1, 2, and 3 (see figure 1) in 20 dogs before (control) and 90 min after creation of transmural myocardial infarction. Data are expressed as mean ± SEM.

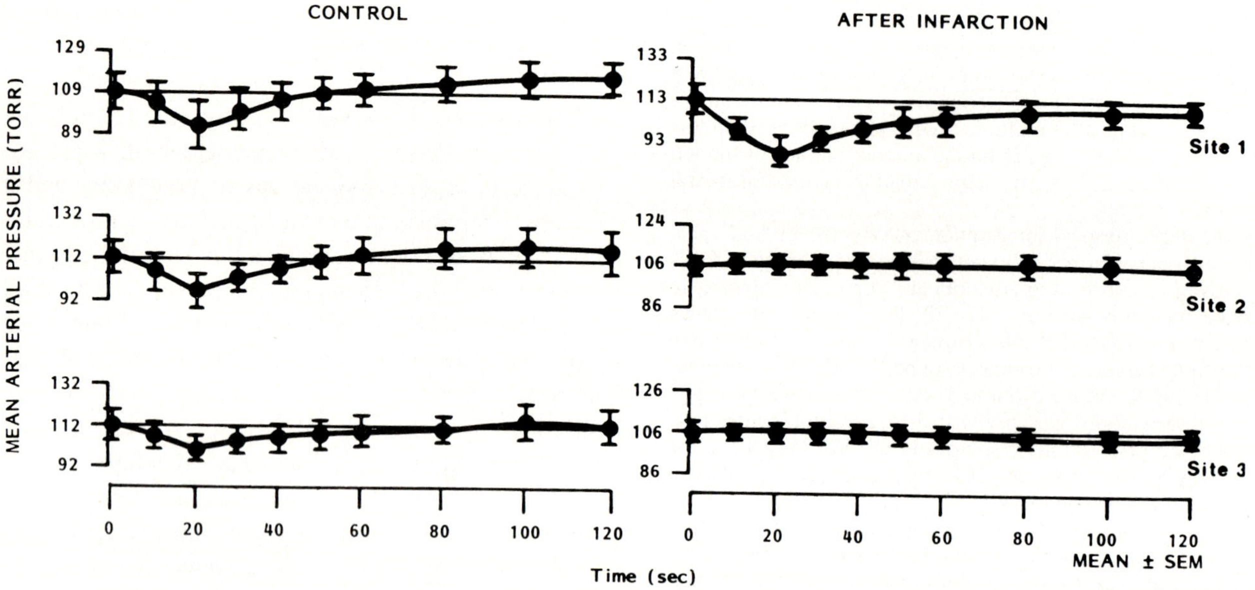

FIGURE 3. Responses of mean arterial pressure to epicardial applications of nicotine at sites 1, 2, and 3 (see figure 1) in 20 dogs before (control) and 90 min after creation of transmural myocardial infarction. Data are expressed as mean ± SEM.

returned to baseline within 120 sec. Ninety minutes after transmural myocardial infarction, sites above (basal to) the site of infarction continued to demonstrate a significant response ($p < .05$) to topical bradykinin, while sites within and below (apical to) the infarction demonstrated no significant change ($p > .10$) in mean arterial pressure when bradykinin was applied topically (figure 2).

In 20 dogs before creation of transmural myocardial infarction, nicotine produced a significant depressor response ($p < .05$) that was maximal approximately 20 sec after application of the drug (figure 3). The response returned to baseline within 60 sec. Ninety minutes after transmural myocardial infarction, sites above (basal to) the infarction continued to demonstrate a significant depressor response ($p < .01$) to topical nicotine, while sites within and below (apical to) the infarction were unresponsive ($p > .10$) to the drug (figure 3).

Heart rate responses to bradykinin and nicotine. Figure 4 illustrates the heart rate data for topical applications of nicotine and bradykinin before and 90 min after transmural myocardial infarction. Throughout all experiments, topical bradykinin (figure 4, *right*) did not significantly affect heart rate ($p > .10$). Topical nicotine before infarction caused significant bradycardia (10 to 20 beats/min) at all sites ($p < .01$). This response was maximal 20 sec after application, and returned rapidly to control without subsequent tachycardia. After creation of transmural myocardial infarction, topical application of nicotine to sites above the infarction continued to elicit significant bradycardia ($p < .01$) 20 sec after application, while nicotine applied to sites within or below (apical to) the infarction had no significant effect on heart rate ($p > .10$).

Mapping of the anterior left ventricular free wall. In 10 dogs with pressor responses to bradykinin and depressor responses to nicotine at all six sites tested before transmural myocardial infarction (figure 1) and in regions above the area of infarction afterward, we mapped the responses to the drugs after infarction.

Figure 5 illustrates the mean data for the 10 dogs used in this portion of the study. Sites above (site 1) and lateral to (site 5) the infarction continued to respond significantly to both drugs ($p < .05$), but those within (site 2) and apical (sites 3 and 6) to the infarction no longer responded to topical bradykinin or nicotine ($p > .10$). Sites medial to the infarction had no significant depressor response to nicotine ($p > .10$), but a significant response to topical bradykinin was maintained ($p < .05$).

Nerve interruptions. In 12 dogs that had sites responsive to both nicotine and bradykinin, nerve interruptions were performed to test the neural pathways responsible for mediating the response to each drug. As shown in tables 1A and 1B, transection of the vagi bilaterally in six dogs eliminated depressor responses to nicotine while the pressor responses of bradykinin remained intact. Subsequent stellectomy bilaterally eradicated the remaining pressor response to bradykinin in these animals. In six other dogs, the order of nerve transections was reversed. Bilateral stellectomy eliminated pressor responses to bradykinin, but did not significantly affect nicotine-induced depressor re-

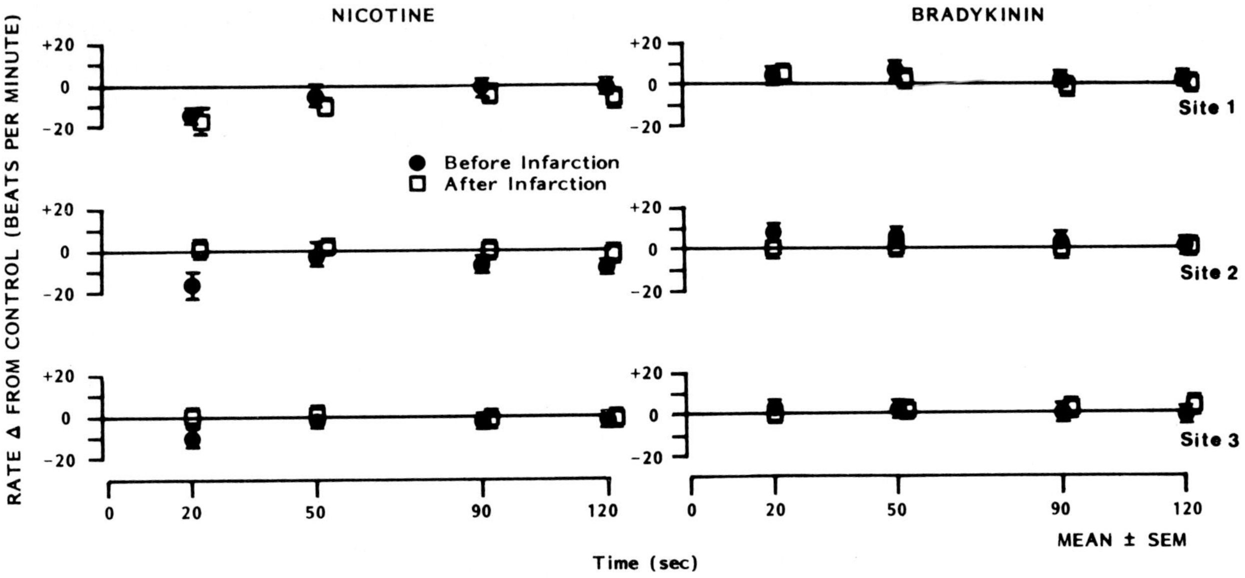

FIGURE 4. Heart rate responses to epicardial applications of nicotine (*left*) and bradykinin (*right*) at sites 1, 2, and 3 (see figure 1) before (filled circles) and 90 min after (open squares) creation of transmural myocardial infarction. Data are expressed as mean ± SEM.

sponses. Subsequent vagotomy prevented the remaining depressor responses to nicotine.

Discussion

The results of this study indicate that a 90 min coronary arterial occlusion produced by the injection of rapidly hardening latex into a diagonal branch of the LAD eliminates afferently mediated blood pressure and heart rate responses to bradykinin and nicotine applied apical to the infarction. Responses were lost at sites over the infarction and in areas of viable, noninfarcted myocardium located apical to the infarction, probably by interruption of afferent nerves passing through the infarction. This interruption of afferent

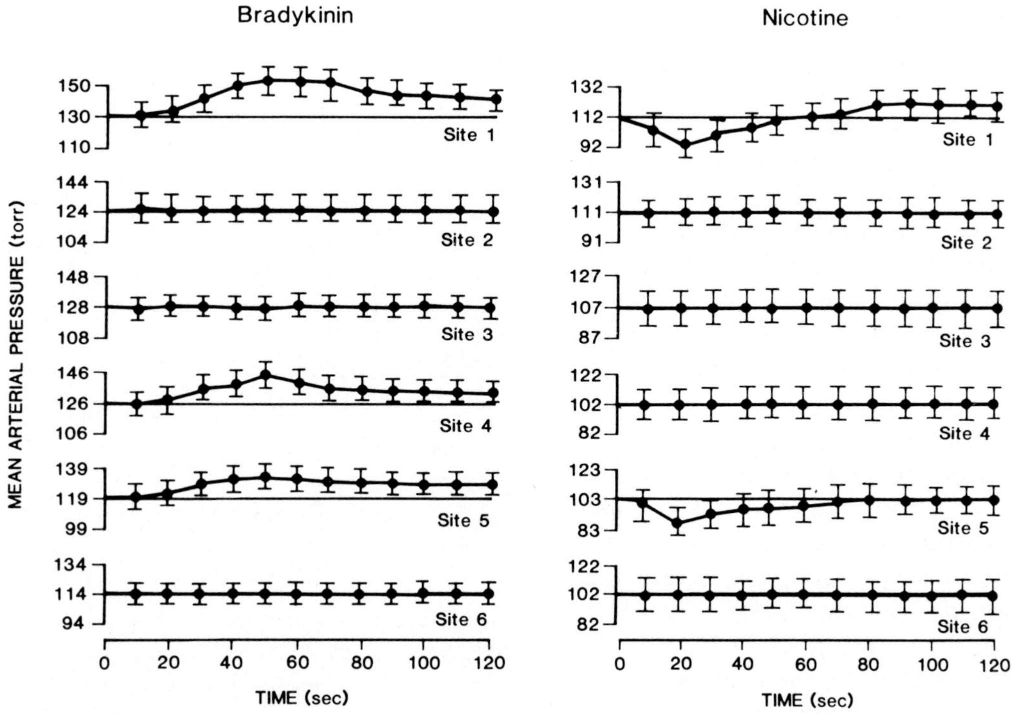

FIGURE 5. Responses of mean arterial pressure in 10 mapping experiments to epicardial applications of bradykinin (*left*) and nicotine (*right*) at the six sites shown in figure 1. Data are expressed as mean ± SEM, and were obtained 90 min after creation of transmural myocardial infarction.

TABLE 1A
Nerve interruption experiments: vagotomy followed by stellectomy (n = 6)

Dog No.	Control	Vagotomy	Stellectomy
Nicotine			
1	−13	−1	−1
2	−8	0	−1
3	−15	0	0
4	−6	1	0
5	−9	−1	1
6	−14	0	0
Mean ± SEM	−11 ± 2	0 ± 1	0 ± 1
	Control vs Vagotomy: .01	Vagotomy vs Stellectomy: NS	
	Control vs Stellectomy: .01		
Bradykinin			
1	8	10	0
2	15	15	1
3	11	10	0
4	17	19	2
5	5	9	1
6	6	7	0
Mean ± SEM	10 ± 2	12 ± 2	1 ± 1
	Control vs Vagotomy: NS	Vagotomy vs Stellectomy: .01	
	Control vs Stellectomy: .01		

All data represent maximal changes in mean arterial pressure (mm Hg) from predrug values.

transmission was selective at one site examined in this study and resulted in vagal, but not sympathetic, afferent interruption. At site 4 (figure 1), the vagal afferents that were activated by nicotine apparently passed through the region of infarction while coursing toward the base of the heart and therefore were interrupted. The sympathetic afferents that were activated by bradykinin at this site probably bypassed the region of infarction in their pathway to the base of the left ventricle.

Course of the nerves in the left ventricular wall. Histologic studies suggest that sympathetic efferent nerves travel over the epicardium, penetrating the myocardium to innervate the endocardium.[20] Parasympathetic efferent fibers appear to reach the left ventricular myocardium via the interventricular septum and travel deeper within the myocardium.[20]

Removing strips of epicardium or painting phenol on the surface of the left ventricle abolishes the contractile effects that occur during stimulation of the stellate ganglia in localized epicardial regions apical to the epicardiectomy or application of phenol.[21–23] Painting a circle of phenol around a multipolar electrode abolishes shortening of the effective refractory period induced by stimulation of sympathetic efferent nerves at both subendocardial and subepicardial poles of the electrode without affecting the increase in effective refractory period duration produced by vagal nerve stimulation.[24] Circles or arcs of phenol positioned close (within 1 to 2 cm) to or at the atrioventricular groove interrupt vagally induced lengthening of effective refractory period,[25] suggesting that the vagal nerves run deep in the myocardium, perhaps in the subendocardium, but ascend as they approach (within 1 to 2 cm) the atrioventricular groove to course in the subepicardium. Consistent with this concept is the demonstration that a 2 to 3 mm deep encircling endocardial incision abolishes vagally induced lengthening of the effective refractory period at endocardial and epicardial sites located apical to the encircling endocardial incision.[26] Elimination of this vagally mediated response may be due to the interruption of vagal efferent fibers coursing along the subendocardium in a basal-to-apical direction.

From the above data it appears that, in dogs, sympathetic efferent nerves travel from base to apex on the surface of the left ventricle, branching off to penetrate the myocardium and innervate the subendocardial portions of the left ventricular wall. Sympathetic efferent transmission can be interrupted by surgical epicardiectomy, superficial sclerosis produced by phenol, or transmural myocardial infarction. Vagal efferent fibers cross the atrioventricular groove in the subepicardium, then appear to travel at deeper levels in the left ventric-

TABLE 1B
Nerve interruption experiments: stellectomy followed by vagotomy (n = 6)

Dog No.	Control	Stellectomy	Vagotomy
Nicotine			
7	−23	−20	−2
8	−7	−10	0
9	−10	−5	0
10	−10	−11	−2
11	−9	−11	1
12	−11	−11	0
Mean ± SEM	−12 ± 2	−11 ± 2	−1 ± 1
	Control vs Stellectomy: NS	Stellectomy vs Vagotomy: .01	
	Control vs Vagotomy: .01		
Bradykinin			
7	15	2	1
8	7	0	2
9	13	0	0
10	24	3	2
11	12	0	0
12	4	0	0
Mean ± SEM	13 ± 3	1 ± 1	1 ± 1
	Control vs Stellectomy: .01	Stellectomy vs Vagotomy: NS	
	Control vs Vagotomy: .01		

All data represent maximal changes in mean arterial pressure (mm Hg) from predrug values.

ular wall (possibly in the subendocardium), and probably penetrate upward to innervate the epicardium. These vagal fibers are interrupted by transmural myocardial infarction, encircling endocardial incision, or the application of phenol to the atrioventricular groove.

Little is known about the left ventricular course of afferent fibers that ultimately travel with the sympathetic or vagal nerves. Harken et al.[6] used phenol on the surface of the heart to produce afferent denervation of the myocardium to treat intractable angina in patients. The sensation of myocardial pain is mediated by afferents traveling with the sympathetic fibers,[27–29] so the assumption was made that phenol produced sympathetic afferent denervation. Mechanosensitive vagal afferents were studied by Thoren[30] in cats. Using electrical stimulation of the fibers, he demonstrated that the nerves transmitting from mechanosensitive endings travel in a general apex-to-base fashion. On the anterior wall of the left ventricle, their course generally is toward the left main coronary artery. On the posterolateral wall of the left ventricle, the fibers sweep basally toward the posterior portion of the atrioventricular groove. Thoren did not comment on the depth of the vagal afferents within the myocardium.

Barber et al.,[2] using epicardial applications of phenol, demonstrated that sympathetic afferents apical to phenol-treated myocardium no longer responded to chemical stimulation, while phenol did not interrupt vagal afferent transmission unless it was painted on the ventricular surface in the atrioventricular groove. They concluded that sympathetic afferents, like their efferent counterparts, travel in the subepicardium while vagal afferents travel a deeper, perhaps subendocardial course. Both vagal and sympathetic afferent fibers cross the atrioventricular groove in the epicardium.

Methodologic consideration. The interpretation of data from these experiments depends on the assumption that bradykinin and nicotine selectively activate sympathetic and vagal afferents, respectively. Several lines of evidence suggest that the topical application of these substances may be used for this purpose. First, bilateral stellectomy eliminated the pressor effect of bradykinin while sectioning the cervical vagi did not. Vagotomy, but not stellectomy, abolished the depressor effect of nicotine. Second, the responses to nicotine and bradykinin are affected in different ways by painting phenol on the surface of the heart,[2] suggesting that the reflexes elicited by the two drugs required separate pathways.

The use of topical nicotine and bradykinin as activators of specific reflexes that could be tested after experimental interventions undoubtedly was aided by excluding data from dogs that did not respond to epicardial nicotine with a depressor response and/or to epicardial bradykinin with a pressor response. Several investigators have demonstrated that the responses to these substances can vary from animal to animal and with different doses of the drugs.[4, 8, 9, 16] We attempted to minimize the variability among animals by carefully controlling level of anesthetic, body temperature, drug temperature, time between drug applications, blood gases, and the manner of drug application.[2] Five of 29 dogs were excluded from the study because they did not demonstrate either a depressor response to nicotine or a pressor response to bradykinin under control (pretransmural myocardial infarction) conditions. A single dose of each drug was used throughout the experiments, so no attempt was made to demonstrate a dose-response relationship in these animals. Thus, under these restricted experimental conditions, the two drugs appeared to serve as selective activators of epicardial reflexes requiring afferent fibers and traveling different limbs of the cardiac autonomic nerves.

In addition to the ability to selectively activate sympathetic or vagal afferent fibers, epicardial application of nicotine or bradykinin on small pieces of gauze provided the advantage of more precise localization of the stimulus. This was important for the purposes of mapping, and it avoided the obvious difficulties attendant to intrapericardial[9] or intravascular[2] administration of drugs. The disadvantage of this method was that only the pathways of afferent nerves subserving receptors on the epicardial surface where the drug was applied could be studied.

The effectiveness of vinyl latex[12, 14] in interrupting collateral blood flow to the ventricles of the canine heart has been demonstrated. One of the goals of the present study was to produce a localized transmural myocardial infarction in the region of a diagonal branch of the LAD that would involve both the endocardial and epicardial layers, where it has been postulated that the afferent nerve fibers course. Euler et al.[14] showed that embolization of coronary arteries effectively and reproducibly resulted in transmural myocardial infarction within the distribution of the artery. Histochemical and histologic analyses of the infarcts studied in our own laboratory[12] demonstrated similar findings. Coronary artery embolization created an infarction that was transmural, yet localized enough so as not to severely compromise left ventricular function. In contrast to these results, preliminary data from our laboratory[31] suggest that coronary artery ligation, which creates a primarily subendocardial infarction with epicardial sparing, does not eliminate the afferent sympathetic response to bradykinin applied over or apical to the infarcted area.

Isolation of a coronary artery and placement of a nonconstricting ring produces degeneration of perivascular adrenergic nerves within 14 days as a result of the surgical procedure and subsequent fibrosis.[32] Vagal denervation would not be expected because of the intramural or subendocardial pathways traveled by the vagus in the ventricle.[2, 26] We have shown repeatedly that a careful, limited dissection that exposes the diagonal branch of the LAD or nonocclusive cannulation of the vessel does not acutely interrupt afferent sympathetic responses to bradykinin[2] or efferently induced shortening of the effective refractory period during stimulation of the stellate ganglia.[12] Such limited dissection must not interrupt all of the perivascular adrenergic nerves. Not all of the sympathetic innervation travels with the coronary artery, since some nerves probably "branch out" to travel over the epicardium[2] and thus are not interrupted by coronary dissection. Most recently we have shown that even an acute nontransmural coronary artery occlusion that produces a viable epicardial layer of myocardium does not interrupt the response to bradykinin in most dogs.[31] Therefore, it would appear likely that transmural myocardial infarction, and not the surgical dissection, was responsible for the results observed in this study.

Implications of the study. The major finding of this study is that transmural myocardial infarction can interrupt afferent neural innervation and thus afferently denervate viable, noninfarcted myocardium apical to the site of infarction. These data, coupled with previously reported evidence from our laboratory,[12, 13] demonstrate that transmural myocardial infarction can interrupt both the afferent and efferent limbs of the autonomic nervous system, innervating the myocardium apical to the transmural myocardial infarction. These areas of denervation may modify reflexes that modulate blood pressure, myocardial and smooth muscle contractility, heart rate, and cardiac electrophysiological properties in a variety of situations. Additionally, creation of autonomic imbalance may be conducive to development of arrhythmias.[33]

It is quite clear, however, that ischemia can also activate sympathetic and vagal reflexes.[34] It is not known from which site or sites activation of afferent reflexes arises and the relationship between such activation and the interruption of afferent reflexes noted here is not clear.

We thank Naomi Fineberg, Ph.D., for statistical analysis of the data and Cindy Rasmussen for typing the manuscript.

References

1. Coleridge JCG, Coleridge HM: Chemoreflex regulation of the heart. *In* Berne RM, editor: The handbook of physiology — section 2. The cardiovascular system. Bethesda, 1979, American Physiological Society, vol I, p 653
2. Barber MJ, Mueller TM, Davies BG, Zipes BP: Phenol topically applied to left ventricular epicardium interrupts sympathetic but not vagal afferents. Circ Res **55:** 532, 1984
3. Staszewska-Barczak J, Ferreira SH, Vane JR: An excitatory nociceptive cardiac reflex elicited by bradykinin and potentiated by prostaglandins and myocardial ischemia. Cardiovasc Res **10:** 314, 1976
4. Uchida Y, Murao S: Bradykinin-induced excitation of afferent cardiac sympathetic nerve fibers. Jpn Heart J **15:** 84, 1974
5. Kaufman MP, Baker DA, Coleridge HM, Coleridge CG: Stimulation by bradykinin of afferent vagal C-fibers with chemosensitive endings in the heart and aorta of the dog. Circ Res **46:** 476, 1980
6. Harken DE, Black H, Dickson JF, Wilson HE: Deepicardialization: a simple, effective surgical treatment for angina pectoris. Circulation **12:** 955, 1955
7. Lindgren I, Olivecrona H: Surgical treatment of angina pectoris. J Neurosurg **4:** 19, 1947
8. Kulaev BS: Characteristics of afferent impulses evoked in cardiac nerves by chemical stimulation of epicardial receptors. Fed Proc 22 (translational suppl): 749, 1963
9. Sleight P: A cardiovascular depressor reflex from the epicardium of the left ventricle in the dog. J Physiol (London) **173:** 343, 1964
10. Coleridge HM, Coleridge JCG, Kidd C: Cardiac receptors in the dog with particular reference to two types of afferent ending in the ventricular wall. J Physiol (London) **174:** 323, 1964
11. Paintal AS: Vagal sensory receptors and their reflex effects. Physiol Rev **53:** 159, 1979
12. Barber MJ, Mueller TM, Henry DP, Felton SY, Zipes DP: Transmural myocardial infarction in the dog produces sympathectomy in noninfarcted myocardium. Circulation **67:** 787, 1983
13. Browne KF, Gill R, Barber MJ, Zipes DP: Vagal denervation of normal endocardium and epicardium apical to transmural infarction. Circulation **68**(suppl III): 247, 1983 (abst)
14. Euler DE, Prood CE, Spear JF, Moore EN: The interruption of collateral blood flow to the ischemic canine myocardium by embolization of a coronary artery with latex: effects on conduction delay and ventricular arrhythmia. Circ Res **49:** 97, 1981
15. Eaton LW, Bulkey BH: Expansion of acute myocardial infarction: its relationship to infarct morphology in a canine model. Circ Res **49:** 80, 1981
16. Felder RB, Thames MD: Responses to activation of cardiac sympathetic afferents with epicardial bradykinin. Am J Physiol **242:** H148, 1982
17. Shatney CH, MacCarter DJ, Lillehei RC: Effects of allopurinol, propranolol and methylmednisolone on infarct size in experimental myocardial infarction. Am J Cardiol **37:** 572, 1976
18. Jones CE, DeVous MD, Thomas JX, DuPont E: The effect of chronic cardiac denervation on infarct size following acute coronary occlusion. Am Heart J **95:** 738, 1978
19. Snedecor GW, Cochran WG: Statistical methods. Ames, IO, 1971, The Iowa State University Press
20. Hirsch EF: The innervation of the vertebrate heart. Springfield, IL, 1970, Charles C Thomas, p 64
21. Geis WP, Kaye MP: Distribution of sympathetic fibers in the left ventricular epicardial plexus of the dog. Circ Res **23:** 165, 1968
22. Randall WC, Szentivanyi M, Pace JB, Wechsler JS, Kaye MP: Patterns of sympathetic nerve projections onto the canine heart. Circ Res **22:** 315, 1968
23. Szentivanyi M, Pace JB, Wechsler JS, Randall WC: Localized myocardial responses to stimulation of cardiac sympathetic nerves. Clin Res **21:** 691, 1967
24. Martins JB, Zipes DP: Epicardial phenol interrupts refractory period responses to sympathetic but not vagal stimulation in canine left ventricular epicardium and endocardium. Circ Res **47:** 33, 1980
25. Takahashi N, Barber MJ, Zipes DP: Efferent vagal innervation of the canine ventricle. Am J Physiol **248:** H89–H97, 1985
26. Chilson DA, Peigh P, Mahomed Y, Zipes DP: Encircling endocardial incision interrupts efferent vagal-induced prolongation of en-

docardial and epicardial refractoriness in the dog. J Am Coll Cardiol **5:** 290, 1985
27. Nishi K, Sakanashi M, Takenaka F: Activation of afferent cardiac sympathetic nerve fibers of the cat by pain producing substances and by noxious heat. Pfluegers Arch **372:** 53, 1977
28. Uchida Y, Murao S: Excitation of afferent cardiac sympathetic nerve fibers during coronary occlusion. Am J Physiol **226:** 1094, 1974
29. White JC: Cardiac pain. Circulation **16:** 644, 1957
30. Thoren P: Characteristics of left ventricular receptors with nonmedullated vagal afferents. Circ Res **40:** 415, 1977
31. Skale BT, Barber MJ, Zipes DP: Time course of the vasopressor response to topical bradykinin during acute myocardial infarction. J Am Coll Cardiol **5:** 439, 1985
32. Dolezel S, Gerova M, Hartmannova B, Dostal M, Janeckova H, Vasku J: Cardiac adrenergic innervation after instrumentation of the coronary artery in the dog. Am J Physiol **246:** H459, 1984
33. Randall WC, Thomas JX, Euler DE, Kozanski GJ: Cardiac dysrhythmias associated with autonomic nervous system imbalance in the conscious dog. *In* Neural mechanisms of cardiac dysrhythmias. New York, 1978, Raven Press, p 123
34. Mark AL: The Bezold-Jarisch reflex revisited: clinical implications of inhibitory reflexes originating in the heart. J Am Coll Cardiol **1:** 90, 1983

Left ventricular ejection fraction after acute coronary occlusion in conscious dogs: relation to the extent and site of myocardial infarction

RICKY M. SCHNEIDER, M.D., ALAN CHU, M.D., MAKOTO AKAISHI, M.D., WILLIAM S. WEINTRAUB, M.D., KENNETH G. MORRIS, M.D., AND FREDERICK R. COBB, M.D.

ABSTRACT The change in left ventricular radionuclide ejection fraction after acute occlusion of the left anterior descending (LAD) or circumflex (LC) coronary artery was compared with the ultimate histologic extent of myocardial infarction in conscious dogs. The acute change in ejection fraction correlated with size of infarction in 14 dogs with occlusions of the LAD coronary artery ($r = .89$, $y = 1.12x + 14.2$) and in 27 dogs with occlusions of the LC coronary artery ($r = .71$, $y = 0.73x + 7.9$); the slope of the regression equation was greater ($p < .05$) for those with LAD than for those with LC occlusions. Multivariate analysis revealed no independent contribution of left ventricular weight, the subendocardial extent of infarction, or change in heart rate to the acute change in ejection fraction. These data indicate that the decrease in ejection fraction after coronary occlusion is determined primarily by the size of the ischemic area, which also determines size of infarction. In dogs instrumented over a long term, infarcts in the LAD myocardial distribution result in greater decreases in ejection fraction than infarcts of comparable size in the LC distribution.
Circulation 72, No. 3, 632–638, 1985.

RESULTS OF A VARIETY of clinical studies support the concept that left ventricular ejection fraction is a measure of ventricular performance that is related to the extent of myocardial infarction.[1–5] In conscious dogs linear relationships exist between changes in global and regional ejection fraction measured by radionuclide angiography after acute coronary occlusion and the extent of myocardium with reduced regional blood flow.[6, 7] Regional myocardial blood flow after coronary occlusion correlates inversely with the extent of histologic necrosis.[8, 9] Thus, the acute change in ejection fraction would also be expected to correlate with ultimate infarct size.

Previous studies that have examined relationships between measurements of left ventricular performance and extent of infarction [1–5] did not consider the influence of anatomic variables such as the location of the infarct and its size relative to the left ventricular weight. The goal of the present study was to assess the relationship between acute changes in ejection fraction after coronary occlusion and direct measurements of the extent of infarction. Studies were performed in awake animals instrumented over the long term to avoid the confounding effects of anesthesia and surgery.

From the Department of Medicine, Division of Cardiology, Duke University Medical Center and the Veterans Administration Medical Center, Durham, and the Mid-Atlantic Heart and Vascular Institute, Department of Medicine, Division of Cardiology, Presbyterian–University of Pennsylvania Medical Center, Philadelphia.

Supported by National Research Services Award grant HL07101 and Research grant HL18537 from the National Institutes of Health, Bethesda, by the Medical Research Service of the Veterans Administration Medical Center, Durham, and by a grant from the Mabel Pew Myrin Trust.

Address for correspondence: Ricky M. Schneider, M.D., Mid-Atlantic Heart and Vascular Institute, Division of Cardiology, Presbyterian–University of Pennsylvania Medical Center, 51 N. 39th St., Philadelphia, PA 19104.

Received June 8, 1984; revision accepted May 23, 1985.

Methods

Experimental animals. Forty-one dogs weighing 20 to 30 kg underwent permanent proximal occlusion of either the left anterior descending (LAD) (14 dogs) or the left circumflex (LC) (27 dogs) coronary artery. They were then maintained for at least 3 days before being killed to permit histologic assessment of infarct size, which was compared with acute changes in radionuclide global and regional ejection fraction.

Surgical preparations. Dogs were anesthetized with sodium thiamylal (30 to 40 mg/kg body weight) and underwent left lateral thoracotomy. Either the LAD or the LC coronary artery was freed by blunt dissection to permit placement of adjustable occluders. Polyethylene loop, snare-type occluders were placed loosely around the vessel and secured to the epicardium. A pacing electrode was sutured to the right atrial appendage. All dogs were allowed to recover for 7 to 14 days before being studied.

Experimental protocols. Snares and electrodes were exteriorized from subcutaneous pouches immediately before each study or 1 day earlier. Morphine sulfate, 5 to 10 mg, was injected intravenously before control studies to provide mild sedation and to minimize discomfort resulting from coronary artery occlusion. Dogs were studied awake while lying loosely restrained on their right sides.

Control hemodynamic measurements were made, and radionuclide angiography was performed in duplicate. The snare was then tightened to occlude the artery permanently. Duplicate radionuclide angiograms were acquired 30 to 60 min after occlusion. In the majority of experiments, to provide a regular cardiac rhythm, rather than the sinus arrhythmia of the conscious dog, the heart was paced from the right atrial appendage at a rate that slightly exceeded the sinus rate at rest; when occlusion resulted in a sinus rate greater than approximately 120 beats/min, pacing was not performed.

Radionuclide angiography. Multigated equilibrium radionuclide angiography was performed after labeling of red blood cells with ^{99m}Tc in vivo. Care was taken to ensure that camera position relative to the thorax remained constant between data acquisitions. Weighted support pads were used to stabilize the chest position.

Global left ventricular ejection fraction was measured in the anterior or ventral projection with slight caudal tilt, a position which provides optimal left ventricular separation from the right ventricle and left atrium.[6, 10] Global ejection fraction measured in this projection by radionuclide angiography correlates closely with that obtained simultaneously with use of ultrasonic dimension crystals over a wide range of ventricular function.[10] Regional ejection fraction was determined in both the anterior and 60 degree left anterior oblique projections with the use of a computer program that divided the left ventricle into quadrants with a nongeometric or count-based center (figure 1).[6] After both LAD and LC coronary artery occlusions, the magnitude of change in regional ejection fraction is significantly greater than the magnitude of change in global ejection fraction, although the quadrants analyzed do not assess left ventricular function in anatomically or physiologically discrete myocardial zones.[6] The mean difference (±SD) between duplicate measurements of global ejection fraction in conscious dogs is 0.02 ± 0.02; the mean difference between global ejection fraction determined by different observers is 0.01 ± 0.01.[6] The mean difference between duplicate measurements of regional ejection fraction ranges from 0.03 ± 0.02 to 0.04 ± 0.04; the mean interobserver variability in these values is 0.02 ± 0.02 to 0.05 ± 0.04.[6]

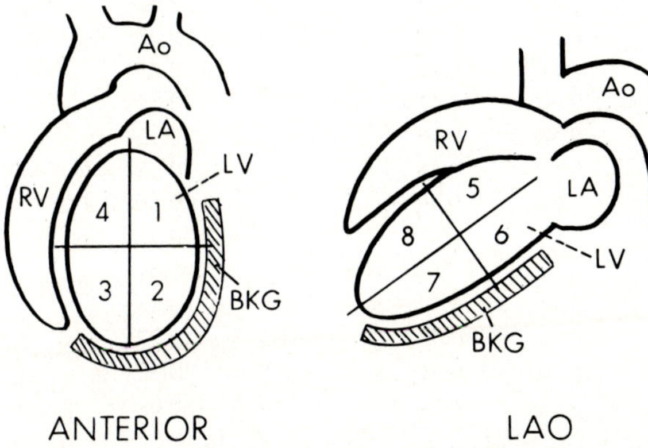

FIGURE 1. Regions assigned by the computer for the determination of regional ejection fractions. Regions 1 to 4 were assigned in the anterior projection and regions 5 to 8 were assigned in the 60 degree left anterior oblique (LAO) projection. The background (BKG) area assigned in each projection for global and regional analysis is indicated. AO = aortic arch: LA = left atrium; LV = left ventricle; RV = right ventricle.

Quantitation of infarction. Dogs were killed a minimum of 3 days after coronary occlusion to allow sharp separation of infarcted and noninfarcted myocardium by routine histologic techniques.[8, 9] The hearts were excised and placed in buffered formalin for 3 days to permit fixation. The left ventricle was sliced into four transverse rings from base to apex. The basal and apical rings were cut into four circumferential regions: anterior, septal, posterior, and lateral. The two middle rings were cut into six circumferential regions: anterior, septal, posterior, posterior papillary muscle, lateral, and anterior papillary muscle. Each circumferential region was cut into four transmural samples from subepicardium to subendocardium, each weighing 1 to 2 g. The tissue samples were weighed, embedded in paraffin, sectioned at two different depths, and stained with hematoxylin and eosin.[8, 9] The samples were arranged so that each histologic section demonstrated the transmural distribution of infarction in the region. Infarcted myocardium was sharply distinguished from intact myocardium and was characterized by complete or partial cellular dissolution, inflammatory cell infiltration, and loss of normal cell architecture. Sketches of the histologic extent of infarcted and of uninvolved myocardium in each tissue sample were then quantitated by planimetry with a graph pen ultrasonic digitizer and computer interface.[8, 9] Total weight of the infarcted tissue was calculated as the sum of weights of infarcted tissue in each individual sample. The weight of infarcted tissue in the subendocardial half of the myocardial wall was determined. Infarct weight was expressed as a percentage of left ventricular weight.

Data analysis. The average of duplicate measurements of global and regional ejection fraction was used in the analysis. The left ventricular region manifesting the maximum change in regional ejection fraction after acute coronary occlusion was identified for each dog.[6] The absolute acute decrease in ejection fraction was divided by the control value, and expressed as a percent of control. Similarly, the acute change in heart rate was calculated as a percent decrease from control.

One-way analysis of variance was used to determine differences between dogs with LAD and those with LC coronary artery occlusions with respect to multiple anatomic and physiologic variables. Linear regression analysis was performed to examine the relationship between the change in global ejection fraction and the percent of the left ventricle that was infarcted. Multiple linear regression analysis was used to evaluate the relative influence of the extent of infarction, the subendocardial extent of infarction, the left ventricular weight, and the change in heart rate in determining global ejection fraction. The criterion Mallows' C_p[11] was applied to all possible subsets regression[12] to select the "best" subset of variables correlating with the change in global ejection fraction. The statistical importance of an individual variable is expressed by its contribution to the r value squared.

Results

Table 1 presents mean left ventricular weights, histologic infarct sizes, and heart rate and radionuclide angiographic data for dogs subjected to LAD or LC coronary artery occlusions. Mean left ventricular weight and percent of left ventricle infarcted did not differ between groups. Mean heart rate was greater at control and after occlusion in the LAD group, but

TABLE 1
Infarct size and ejection fraction

Dog No.	Weight of LV (g)	% LV Infarcted	Heart rate (bpm) Control	Heart rate (bpm) Occlusion	Global EF Control	Global EF Occlusion	Regional EF[A] Control	Regional EF[A] Occlusion
LAD artery occlusion								
1	61.0	0.1	106	112	0.43	0.42	0.57	0.47
2	85.0	0	124	125	0.40	0.37	0.38	0.32
3	86.4	1.4	144	132	0.45	0.43	0.43	0.39
4	85.5	11.6	116	134	0.50	0.26	0.47	0.20
5	97.5	26.9	100	152	0.48	0.23	0.60	0.20
6	139.3	8.0	70	106	0.38	0.29	0.57	0.39
7	112.5	8.0	86	102	0.43	0.33	0.61	0.39
8	82.2	51.7	141	163	0.60	0.22	0.61	0.16
9	113.3	37.0	98	110	0.47	0.23	0.37	0.11
10	98.6	33.0	102	116	0.51	0.25	0.39	0.13
11	120.4	27.8	96	142	0.60	0.32	0.43	0.11
12	88.6	9.5	103	118	0.46	0.30	0.39	0.29
13	86.5	13.3	85	107	0.47	0.34	0.41	0.22
14	134.3	21.4	111	120	0.46	0.26	0.36	0.19
Mean	99.4	17.8	106	124	0.47	0.30	0.47	0.26
SD	21.9	15.6	21	18	0.06	0.07	0.10	0.12
LC artery occlusion								
15	104.5	15.1	75	100	0.51	0.37	0.52	0.32
16	78.0	1.6	60	68	0.57	0.54	0.70	0.55
17	98.5	29.8	100	150	0.59	0.33	0.78	0.37
18	100.3	2.8	60	60	0.46	0.43	0.62	0.49
19	98.0	2.5	67	60	0.63	0.63	0.61	0.58
20	72.5	9.8	108	128	0.56	0.46	0.73	0.46
21	128.0	20.8	60	65	0.52	0.41	0.74	0.41
22	89.5	9.6	60	126	0.58	0.46	0.65	0.37
23	138.0	3.2	77	75	0.51	0.47	0.67	0.53
24	79.5	15.7	72	130	0.56	0.46	0.70	0.46
25	76.0	26.4	70	120	0.66	0.34	0.81	0.35
26	98.4	27.2	60	90	0.55	0.40	0.68	0.36
27	145.2	39.3	65	115	0.57	0.43	0.74	0.46
28	170.7	33.4	75	100	0.61	0.45	0.75	0.46
29	157.5	18.3	75	75	0.55	0.36	0.66	0.30
30	207.0	36.9	75	80	0.59	0.44	0.73	0.45
31	85.0	1.9	75	84	0.56	0.54	0.54	0.42
32	108.0	26.1	78	160	0.57	0.40	0.53	0.38
33	87.5	1.4	95	100	0.51	0.40	0.56	0.49
34	98.8	29.1	79	115	0.60	0.41	0.64	0.32
35	132.3	36.9	67	94	0.51	0.40	0.59	0.33
36	107.5	26.9	96	132	0.60	0.43	0.76	0.45
37	85.2	28.1	127	140	0.53	0.40	0.62	0.36
38	78.1	26.9	82	130	0.66	0.49	0.71	0.42
39	93.3	17.0	114	128	0.66	0.54	0.63	0.41
40	79.0	4.2	99	108	0.44	0.49	0.56	0.55
41	93.3	17.7	94	106	0.47	0.42	0.33	0.22
Mean	107.0	18.8	80	105	0.56	0.44	0.65	0.42
SD	32.7	12.4	18	28	0.06	0.07	0.10	0.09
p value	.38	.84	.11		.03		.13	

EF = ejection fraction; LV = left ventricle.

[A]Region demonstrating the maximum acute decrease in EF following coronary occlusion.

p values reflect results of analysis of variance comparing LAD occlusions to LC occlusions. For heart rate, global EF and regional EF, percent change from control to occlusion was compared in the two groups.

increased to a similar extent (p = .11) in both groups. Mean global and regional ejection fractions were lower in the control state and after occlusion in the LAD group. Percent change in global ejection fraction was greater (p = .03) in dogs with LAD coronary artery occlusion than in those with occlusion of the LC artery (34.2 ± 19.7 vs 20.7 ± 13.1, mean ± SD). Changes in regional ejection fraction were greater than those in global ejection fraction after both LAD and LC artery occlusions; however, the percent change in regional ejection fraction did not differ significantly (p = .13) between groups (45.6 ± 23.1 vs 34.9 ± 14.2).

In figure 2 the percent change in global ejection fraction measured within 1 hr after occlusion of the LAD or LC coronary artery is plotted against the percent of the left ventricle that ultimately infarcted. After LAD artery occlusion, histologic infarct size ranged from 0 to 51.7% of the left ventricular weight and correlated linearly (r = .89) with percent change in global ejection fraction (y = 1.12x + 14.2). After occlusion of the LC artery, infarct size ranged from 1.4% to 36.9% of the left ventricular weight and correlated modestly (r = .71) with change in ejection fraction (y = 0.73x + 7.9). The slope of this relationship was significantly greater (p < .05) for dogs with LAD (1.12) than for those with LC (0.73) artery occlusions, indicating that for comparable ultimate infarct size, acute LAD artery occlusion decreased global ejection fraction to a greater degree than did acute LC artery occlusion. In addition, y axis intercepts were significantly greater than 0 after occlusion of both the LAD (p < .003) and LC (p < .02) arteries, suggesting that after acute coronary occlusion, the reduction in global ejection fraction was influenced by dysfunction in myocardium that did not become irreversibly injured.

Multivariate analysis revealed that the left ventricular weight and the subendocardial extent of infarction did not independently influence the change in ejection fraction after coronary occlusion. After occlusion of the LC, but not after that of the LAD, there was a modest inverse correlation between the change in heart rate and the change in global ejection fraction (r = −.49): that is, increases in heart rate were associated with decreases in ejection fraction. Neither the control value for global ejection fraction, regional ejection fraction, nor heart rate influenced the change in global ejection fraction after coronary occlusion in either group. Thus, although there were baseline differences between the LAD and LC groups with respect to heart rate and global ejection fraction (table 1), these variables were not independently predictive of the change in ejection fraction after occlusion.

Discussion

The major new findings of the present study are that (1) the acute reduction in global ejection fraction that follows coronary artery occlusion is directly related to the extent of final myocardial infarction, and (2) infarction occurring in the LAD as compared with the LC region of the dog left ventricle results in dispropor-

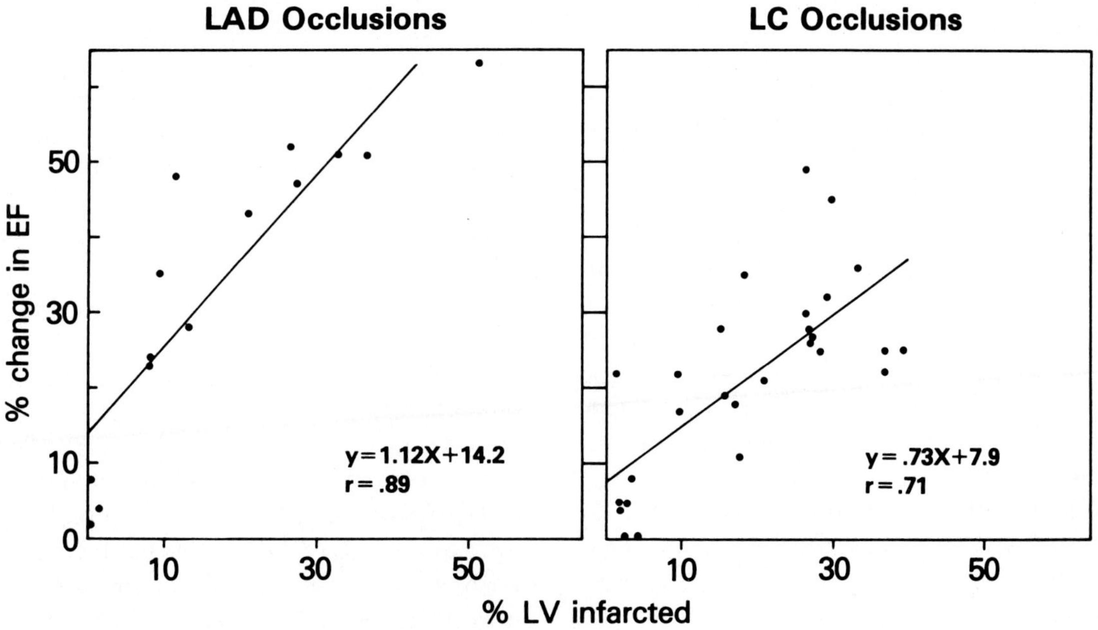

FIGURE 2. Relationships between percent change in global ejection fraction and percent of the left ventricle that infarcted after LAD (*left*) and LC (*right*) artery occlusions. The slope was significantly greater (p < .05) for the LAD than for the LC group. The y intercepts were significantly greater than 0 for both LAD (p < .003) and LC (p < .02) artery occlusions.

tionately greater reduction in global left ventricular function as measured by the radionuclide angiographic technique.

Occlusion of the LAD or LC artery produced a wide range of infarct sizes. The variability resulted in part from the modification of the site of occlusion and in part from inherent variability in the extent of ischemia and subsequent infarction resulting from proximal coronary occlusion in conscious dogs.[8, 9] The entire left ventricle was sectioned into 1 to 2 g samples for direct histologic quantitation of size of infarction. In previous studies of acute coronary occlusion[6, 7] we used similar techniques for tissue sectioning, but analyzed regional myocardial blood flow rather than histologic infarction. In the earlier experiments the size of the ischemic zone was estimated as the percent of the left ventricular weight in which myocardial blood flow was reduced more than 25% from normal zone flow. The acute change in global ejection fraction correlated with size of the ischemic zone in 13 dogs with LAD artery occlusions ($r = .84$, $y = 0.96x + 1.7$) and in 13 dogs with occlusions of the LC artery ($r = .75$, $y = 0.53x + 2.0$).[6, 7]

It is of interest that the slopes of the relationships between decrease in ejection fraction and infarct size tended to be greater than the slopes of the relationships between decrease in ejection fraction and extent of ischemia for both LAD (1.12 vs 0.96) and LC artery occlusions (0.73 vs 0.53). The y axis (change in ejection fraction) intercepts were greater than 0 for the relationships of infarct size to change in ejection fraction, whereas the y intercepts were close to 0 for the relationships of the extent of ischemia to change in ejection fraction. These data indicate that the global ejection fraction is sensitive to mild reductions in regional blood flow; consequently, acute reductions in global ejection fraction are influenced both by the amount of myocardium that infarcts and by the amount that does not infarct after permanent coronary occlusion. It is not surprising that both the extent of acute ischemia after coronary occlusion and the extent of subsequent infarction are directly related to the changes in global ejection fraction, since several studies have demonstrated direct relationships between myocardial ischemia and infarction.[8, 9]

Multivariate analysis demonstrated no consistent relationships between left ventricular weight, the subendocardial extent of infarction, or the change in heart rate and acute changes in global ejection fraction. In our previous examination[6, 7] of the relationship between the size of the ischemic zone and the change in ejection fraction, a more extensive analysis was performed to assess the influence of acute changes in heart rate, aortic blood pressure, and the left ventricular end-diastolic count rate, a radionuclide index of relative left ventricular volume. None of these variables correlated independently with the change in ejection fraction. However, it should be noted that neither the present protocol nor the previous one[6, 7] was designed to assess long-term effects of loading conditions or effects of deliberately altering loading conditions on changes in global ejection fraction. It is likely that certain of these and other unanalyzed variables contributed to the significant scatter in the linear correlations.

A significant finding of this study was that for similar degrees of left ventricular infarction, occlusion of the LAD artery produced greater decreases in global ejection fraction than did occlusion of the LC artery. It is of interest that the decreases in regional ejection fraction after the two occlusions were not significantly different, suggesting that the disproportionate effects of LAD vs LC regional ischemia on left ventricular function were more apparent at a global than at a regional level. Our previous work[6] has indicated a modest linear relationship between acute decreases in regional ejection fraction and size of the ischemic zone after occlusion of both the LAD and LC. This makes it unlikely that the radionuclide angiographic technique preferentially evaluated regional function in dogs that had LAD vs LC artery occlusions in the present study. The present findings with regard to global function are consistent with observations made in experiments in which size of the ischemic zone rather than size of infarction was estimated.[6, 7] In the earlier study the slope of the relationship between the change in global ejection fraction and size of the ischemic zone was also greater for LAD than for LC artery occlusions (0.96 vs 0.53; $p < .01$). While global ejection fraction decreased to a greater extent after LAD than after LC artery occlusions (27.7% vs 13.4%; $p = .004$), regional ejection fraction decreased to a similar extent in the two groups.[6, 7]

The mechanisms or factors responsible for the disproportionate effects of LAD vs LC artery occlusion on global function are not clear. The anatomic distributions of infarction or ischemia were different with occlusion of the LAD artery than with that of the LC, and consequently may have influenced global ejection fraction in different ways. Occlusion of the LAD coronary artery induced infarction of the anterior-apical region, with variable extension toward the base, whereas occlusion of the LC artery induced infarction of the inferior-basal region, with variable extension toward the apex. Larger LAD artery infarcts tended to involve more of the anterior and lateral walls and extended toward the base, whereas larger LC artery infarcts tended to extend more medially and laterally than toward the apex. It has not been determined in studies in the dog to what extent LAD as compared with LC artery occlusions preferentially affect minor- or major-axis shortening, although as noted above the larger infarct regions with LAD artery occlusion may be expected to involve shortening in both the major and minor axes. Previous investigations have indicated that myocardial segment shortening in the dog is greater at the apex than at the base of the left ventricle,[13] and infarction of a left ventricular region that shortens to a greater degree than the remainder of the ventricle may be expected to alter global function disproportionately. On the other hand, shortening of the left ventricular minor axis contributes approximately 87% to generation of the stroke volume.[14]

Studies have suggested that hypofunction may extend for a variable distance outside the ischemic zone, possibly as a result of tethering.[15] It is not known whether the adjacent hypofunctional nonischemic region influences global function or whether the hypofunctional nonischemic region is larger after LAD than after LC artery occlusion. Global left ventricular contraction represents the sum of shortening in the nonischemic and ischemic regions. Although the present studies indicate that hyperfunction in the nonischemic region rarely compensates completely for acute ischemic region hypofunction, in certain studies it has been observed that there is less hypercontraction in nonischemic myocardium remote from the ischemic region after LAD than after LC occlusion in the dog.[16, 17] Such a regional difference would contribute to disproportionate effects of LAD and LC artery occlusion on global ejection fraction.

Finally, in phantom heart studies performed to simulate results of radionuclide angiography during regional left ventricular dysfunction, there was greater attenuation of counts from hypofunctional regions that were distant from the detector and consequently true volume changes from simulated posterior and anterior hypokinesis were underestimated and overestimated, respectively.[18] This theoretical problem, however, had only a minor effect on measurements of ejection fraction in experiments in conscious dogs.[19] It is of interest that in several clinical studies it has been observed that anterior infarction causes greater decreases in left ventricular function than does inferior infarction,[20, 21] but it is not clear from these studies whether the differential effects on global function resulted from different sizes of infarction or different physiologic effects of infarcts of comparable size.[5, 22]

This study demonstrates a major influence of the extent of acute infarction on changes in left ventricular ejection fraction and relatively minor influences of other parameters. The results presented are consistent with those of an earlier experiment[6, 7] in which the size of the ischemic zone was correlated with acute changes in ejection fraction. In both studies anterior ischemia produced greater reduction in global ejection fraction than did inferior ischemia of a similar extent. Although the precise mechanisms responsible for this disproportionate effect have not been determined, the observation is pertinent to the angiographic evaluation of global function in the setting of acute infarction.

We are grateful to Joseph C. Greenfield, Jr., M.D., and Richard H. Helfant, M.D., for support, to Cynthia Silvaggi Baker, R.N., and James A. Stanfield, N.M.T., for assistance in performing the radionuclide studies, to Marjorie Grubb and Robert Murdock, Jr. for technical support, to Kirby Cooper and Eric Fields for surgical preparations, to Michael Taylor and staff for animal care, and to Kathy Tuppeny for secretarial assistance.

References

1. Baltaxe HA, Alonso DR, Lee JG, Prat J, Husted JW, Stakes JW III: Impaired left ventricular contractility in ischemic heart disease: angiographic and histopathologic correlations. Radiology **113:** 581, 1974
2. Ideker RE, Behar VS, Wagner GS, Starr JW, Starmer CF, Lee KL, Hackel DB: Evaluation of asynergy as an indicator of myocardial fibrosis. Circulation **57:** 715, 1978
3. Kostuk WJ, Ehsani AA, Karliner JS, Ashburn WL, Peterson KL, Ross J Jr, Sobel BE: Left ventricular performance after myocardial infarction assessed by radioisotope angiocardiography. Circulation **47:** 242, 1973
4. Rigo P, Murray M, Strauss HW, Taylor D, Kelly D, Weisfeldt M, Pitt B: Left ventricular function in acute myocardial infarction evaluated by gated scintiphotography. Circulation **50:** 678, 1974
5. Hori M, Inoue M, Fukui S, Shimazu T, Mishima M, Ohgitani N, Minamino T, Abe H: Correlation of ejection fraction and infarct size estimated from the total CK released in patients with acute myocardial infarction. Br Heart J **41:** 433, 1979
6. Schneider RM, Roberts KB, Morris KG, Stanfield JA, Cobb FR: Relation between radionuclide angiographic regional ejection fraction and left ventricular regional ischemia in awake dogs. Am J Cardiol **53:** 294, 1984
7. Schneider RM, Roberts KB, Morris KG, Cobb FR: Relationship between left ventricular function and myocardial perfusion during acute left anterior descending or circumflex occlusions in awake dogs. Clin Res **31:** 217A, 1983 (abst)
8. Rivas F, Cobb FR, Bache RJ, Greenfield JC Jr: Relationship between blood flow to ischemic regions and extent of myocardial infarction: Serial measurement of blood flow to ischemic regions in dogs. Circ Res **38:** 439, 1976
9. Irvin RG, Cobb FR: Relationship between epicardial ST-segment elevation, regional myocardial blood flow, and extent of myocardial infarction in awake dogs. Circulation **55:** 825, 1977
10. Swain JL, Morris KG, Bruno FP, Cobb FR: Comparison of multigated radionuclide angiography with ultrasonic sonomicrometry over a wide range of ventricular function in the conscious dog. Am J Cardiol **46:** 976, 1980
11. Daniel C, Wood FS: Fitting equations to data. Wiley, New York, 1971, John Wiley & Sons, p 86
12. Frane JW: All possible subsets regression. *In* Dixon WJ, editor:

BMDP statistical software. Los Angeles, 1981, University of Calif Press, p 264
13. LeWinter MM, Kent RS, Krowner JM, Carew TE, Covell JW: Regional differences in myocardial performance in the left ventricle of the dog. Circ Res **37:** 191, 1975
14. Rankin JS, McHale PA, Arentzen CF, Ling O, Greenfield JC Jr, Anderson RW: The three-dimensional dynamic geometry of the left ventricle in the conscious dog. Circ Res **39:** 304, 1976
15. Sakai K, Watanobe K, Millard RW: The extent of hypokinetic function surrounding focal transmural ischemia. Circulation **68**(suppl III): III-194, 1983 (abst)
16. Heyndrickx GR, Millard RW, McRitchie RJ, Maroko PR, Vatner SF: Regional myocardial functional and electrophysical alterations after brief coronary artery occlusion in conscious dogs. J Clin Invest **56:** 978, 1975
17. Theroux P, Ross J Jr, Franklin D, Covell JW, Bloor CM, Sasayawa S: Regional myocardial function and dimensions early and late after myocardial infarction in the unanesthetized dog. Circ Res **40:** 158, 1977
18. Schneider RM, Jaszczak RJ, Coleman RE, Cobb FR: Disproportionate effects of regional hypokinesis on radionuclide ejection fraction: Compensation using attenuation-corrected ventricular volumes. J Nucl Med **25:** 747, 1984
19. Schneider RM, Jaszczak RJ, Coleman RE, Cobb FR: Differential effects of anterior versus inferior ischemia on global radionuclide ejection fraction: effects of photon attenuation. Circulation **68**(suppl III): III-207, 1983
20. Russell RO Jr, Hunt D, Rackley CE: Left ventricular hemodynamics in anterior and inferior myocrdial infarction. Am J Cardiol **32:** 8, 1973
21. Hamby RI, Hoffman I, Hilsenrath J, Aintablian A, Shanies S, Padmanabhan VS: Clinical, hemodynamic and angiograpic aspects of inferior and anterior myocardial infarctions in patients with angina pectoris. Am J Cardiol **34:** 513, 1974
22. Miller RR, Olson HG, Vismara LA, Bogren HG, Amsterdam EA, Mason DT: Pump dysfunction after myocardial infarction: importance of location, extent and pattern of abnormal left ventricular segmental contraction. Am J Cardiol **37:** 340, 1976

Patterns of myoglobin release after reperfusion of injured myocardium

AVERY K. ELLIS, M.D., PH.D., THOMAS LITTLE, M.D., A. R. ZAKI MASUD, M.D., AND FRANCIS J. KLOCKE, M.D.

ABSTRACT Myoglobin is an intracardiac protein that is released into the blood after myocardial injury and is then cleared rapidly by the kidneys. This study was undertaken to determine whether successful reperfusion of damaged myocardium could be assessed by examination of blood myoglobin concentration-time patterns. After release of a 2 hr occlusion of the mid left anterior descending coronary artery in 11 dogs that had been instrumented over the long term, immunoreactive arterial plasma concentration of myoglobin, [Mb], rose rapidly to a peak within 25 ± 2(SEM) min (range 20 to 40). Individual peaks were three to 165 times the myoglobin levels immediately before release of the occlusion. Myoglobin was cleared rapidly from plasma, falling to one-half its peak level 38 ± 3 min after the peak. Similarly well-defined peaks in [Mb] were evident in plasma from the great cardiac vein (GCV), with a mean time to peak of 16 ± 2 min and a magnitude of two to 177 times prerelease values. In contrast, arterial and GCV creatine kinase activity-time curves showed less defined peaks and they occurred later and with more variability (60 to 330 min after reperfusion). In nine patients with acute infarction, successful coronary artery reopening was also accompanied by a sharp four- to sixteenfold rise in plasma [Mb] within 1 to 2 hr. Elevations in plasma creatine kinase were slower and more prolonged, peaking at 2 to 18 hr. The sharp, early peaks in [Mb] after successful reperfusion were in contrast to the case in one patient in whom reperfusion was not successful and in whom there was only a gradual increase in [Mb]. T_{25-100}, defined as the time required for [Mb] to rise from 25% to 100% of peak, averaged 48 ± 9 min for the nine patients undergoing successful reperfusion. In contrast, T_{25-100} in published series of patients with acute infarction in whom reperfusion was not attempted averaged 5 to 6 hr. In summary, reperfusion of injured myocardium results in a rapid release of myoglobin into the blood in both experimental animals and man. An early peak in the myoglobin concentration-time curve appears to be an additional useful indicator of reopening of the vessel when reperfusion is undertaken and a coronary arteriogram is not available.

Circulation 72, No. 3, 639–647, 1985.

IT IS NOW generally agreed that most transmural myocardial infarctions are associated with fresh thrombi superimposed on atherosclerotic lesions of varying severity.[1] Although the thrombi can often be dissolved with lytic agents, it is frequently difficult to assess whether or not reperfusion has occurred if an immediate coronary arteriographic examination is not performed. Some authors have attempted to use the rate of rise, peak magnitude, and/or time to peak creatine kinase (CK) elevation after reperfusion, but there remains substantial overlap in these parameter values in patients undergoing successful and those undergoing unsuccessful reperfusion.[2–6] Myoglobin is a cardiac protein the levels of which are frequently elevated in plasma of patients with acute infarction and these elevated levels are often apparent before CK is detected.[7] Myoglobin is known to be cleared from the plasma with a half-life of disappearance of less than 10 min.[8] Because of this early appearance and unusually rapid clearance, blood myoglobin concentration-time patterns may provide a useful marker of entry of protein into the vascular space in situations such as myocardial reperfusion.

The present study was undertaken to determine whether successful reperfusion of damaged myocardium could be appreciated by examination of blood myoglobin concentration-time patterns. The problem

From the Departments of Medicine and Physiology, State University of New York at Buffalo School of Medicine, Veterans Administration Medical Center, and Erie County Medical Center, Buffalo.

Supported by a grant from the National Heart, Lung, and Blood Institute (HLB-15194) and by a Research Development Award from the State University of New York at Buffalo.

Address for correspondence: Avery K. Ellis, M.D., CC-172 SUNY Clinical Center, 462 Grider St., Buffalo, NY 14215.

Received March 12, 1985; revision accepted June 13, 1985.

was initially addressed by measuring myoglobin entry into and disappearance from plasma after a period of acute myocardial injury in dogs. The protocol was intended to simulate the procedure for lysis of intracoronary thrombi now being performed clinically. Subsequently, patients undergoing reperfusion with intracoronary streptokinase, percutaneous transluminal coronary angiography (PTCA), and intravenous streptokinase were also studied.

Methods

Fourteen mongrel dogs weighing 15 to 26 kg were anesthetized with sodium pentobarbital and ventilated with a Harvard positive-pressure respirator. Under sterile conditions, a left thoracotomy was performed in each, and one or two pneumatic occluders were placed on the left anterior descending coronary artery (LAD) just distal to the first or second diagonal branch. Electrodes were sewn onto the epicardium in the distributions of the LAD and the undisturbed left circumflex coronary artery (LC). A catheter was placed in the descending aorta for measurement of arterial pressure and subsequent withdrawal of blood samples for determination of systemic arterial myoglobin and CK levels. All animals were allowed to recover for at least 7 days so that elevated myoglobin and CK levels secondary to skeletal muscle damage could return to baseline.

On the day of the short-term study, each animal was anesthetized with thiamylal sodium and halothane, and a cutdown was performed on the external jugular vein. A catheter was placed in the coronary sinus under fluoroscopic control and advanced into the great cardiac vein (GCV), thereby allowing selective sampling from the area of injury in the LAD. Aortic pressure was measured throughout the experimental period, as were lead II of the standard electrocardiogram and the LAD and the LC surface electrograms. After the administration of 1000 units iv heparin, three sets of control arterial and GCV samples for determination of myoglobin concentration, [Mb], and CK activity were obtained. Intravenous lidocaine (25 mg) was administered, and the LAD occluder(s) was inflated for a 2 hr period. One animal developed ventricular fibrillation during the period of occlusion and was not studied further. In two animals the occluders were not inflated. In nine of the remaining 11 animals, the LAD surface electrogram showed ST segment shifts, loss of R wave voltage, and/or widening of the QRS during LAD occlusion.

Arterial and coronary venous samples for determination of myoglobin and CK levels were obtained at 30 min intervals during the 2 hr period of occlusion. At the end of the period, an additional 25 mg of lidocaine was administered intravenously and the occluder(s) was released. Simultaneous arterial and coronary venous samples were then drawn at 1 min intervals for 3 min, at 2 min intervals for 12 min, at 5 min intervals for 25 min, at 10 min intervals for 20 min, and then at 20 min intervals until the completion of the study. In seven animals, sampling was continued for 4 hr after release of the occluder(s); in four other animals, it was continued for 11 hr.

Standard radioimmunoassay[8] and enzymatic[9] methods were used to determine [Mb] and CK activity in each sample. Myoglobin concentration-time curves and CK activity-time curves were analyzed in terms of peak values and time to peak levels. In addition, the half-life of disappearance of arterial myoglobin was determined from the initial portion of the washout phase of the arterial myoglobin concentration-time curve. All values are reported as mean ± SEM unless otherwise stated.

Clinical studies. Ten patients with typical clinical and electrocardiographic evidence of acute myocardial infarction of less than 6 hr duration were studied after giving informed consent. In seven patients, angiography was performed immediately. The artery supplying the area of infarction was totally occluded in four patients, and was estimated to be 99% narrowed in the remainder. Reperfusion was achieved in six patients after administration of intracoronary streptokinase and/or PTCA and was documented by angiography. Neither measure resulted in reperfusion in the seventh patient. Three additional patients were each treated with 1,000,000 units of intravenous streptokinase, which was infused over ~30 min. Each experienced resolution of chest discomfort and ST elevation within 90 min of completion of the infusion. The vessel supplying the area of acute infarction was subsequently demonstrated to be patent at angiography performed 1, 4, and 22 days later.

Venous blood samples for determination of myoglobin levels and CK activity were obtained over an interval of 5 to 60 min before and for at least 3 hr after the reperfusion procedure. Plasma [Mb] was determined with a radioimmunoassay kit developed for human plasma (NMS Pharmaceuticals, Inc., Newport Beach, CA). Plasma CK activity was determined with a commercial kit (SIGMA 45-UV) based on the hexokinase/glucose-6-phosphate dehydrogenase enzyme coupled system.

Results

Animal studies. Myoglobin concentration-time curves were analyzed for the 11 animals completing the occlusion protocol. Although only nine animals showed surface electrographic changes during occlusion, all 11 had clear-cut elevations in myoglobin and CK levels. Hemodynamic parameters remained constant throughout the experimental period in all 11 animals (table 1).

Figure 1 illustrates typical arterial myoglobin and CK concentration-time curves from one animal. [Mb] rose rapidly within a minute of release of occlusion, peaking at 7262 ng/ml 30 min later. The rapid clearance of myoglobin is evident from the disappearance phase of the concentration-time curve, with the concentration falling to one-half of its peak value ~30 min after the peak. The CK activity-time curve also showed a marked increase in enzyme activity after release of occlusion, but the rate of rise was slower and the peak value of 4181 IU/liter occurred ~2 hr after release.

In the two animals in which no electrocardiographic changes were present during LAD occlusion, the asso-

TABLE 1
Summary of hemodynamic data

	Heart rate (bpm)	Mean aortic pressure (mm Hg)
Control	108±9.4	118±5.5
Early occlusion	121±10.6	129±5.5
End-occlusion	112±9.1	132±5.1
After release of occlusion	114±10.6	129±4.2
End of study	116±9.0	125±3.1

All values are expressed as mean ± SEM.

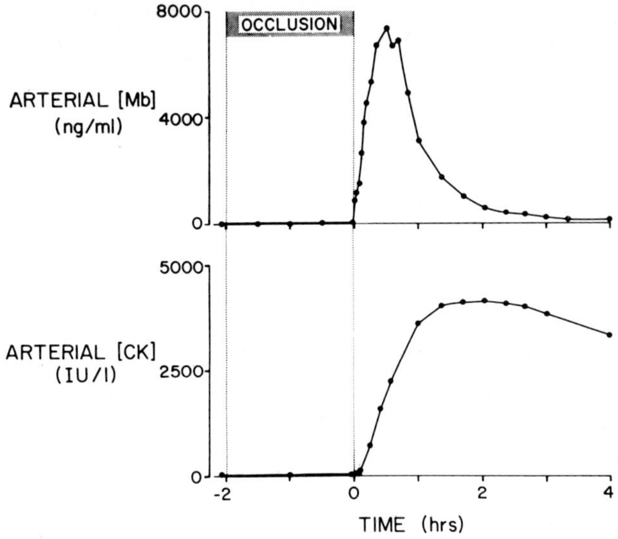

FIGURE 1. Myoglobin concentration-time curve (*top*) and CK activity-time curve (*bottom*) from one animal (dog 9, tables 2 and 3) before, during, and after release of a 2 hr occlusion of the mid LAD occlusion. See text for details.

ciated myoglobin and CK peak levels were smaller than in the other animals (dogs 6 and 8, tables 2 and 3; figure 2). The small peaks and absence of electrocardiographic changes suggest that only small zones of injury were produced by LAD occlusion (possibly because of preexisting collateral vessels in the canine species).

Figure 3 summarizes arterial myoglobin and CK kinetics for all 11 animals. Peak [Mb] occurred between 20 and 40 min after release of occlusion, with an average time to peak of 25 ± 2 min. This is in contrast to the consistently later peaks for CK, which occurred between 1 and 5½ hr after release of occlusion. An additional finding of interest was that [Mb] fell by 50% of its peak value at an average of 63 ± 4 min after reperfusion, that is, 38 min after its peak.

Figure 4 illustrates transcoronary venous-arterial differences for myoglobin and CK in one animal. At the end of the 2 hr occlusion of the LAD, GCV [Mb] was slightly but distinctly elevated, indicating release of the protein into coronary venous blood during the ischemic period. After release of occlusion, there was a rapid rise in both arterial and GCV [Mb], the former peaking at 3724 ng/ml, and the latter peaking fivefold higher, at 17,502 ng/ml. An additional feature of the myoglobin concentration-time curves illustrated in figure 4 was the persistent coronary venous-arterial concentration difference of ~100 ng/ml. Similar persistent coronary venous-arterial concentration differences were present in all 11 animals and averaged 153 ± 33 ng/ml 3 hr after release of occlusion.

Figure 4 also illustrates simultaneous GCV and arterial CK activity as a function of time. During the ischemic period, there was a slight rise in arterial and coronary venous CK activities; a rapid rise in both followed release of occlusion. In contrast to the myoglobin concentration-time curves, there was no clear persistent GCV-arterial concentration difference. Three hours after release of occlusion, mean GCV-arterial CK differences for all 11 animals averaged 32 ± 27 IU/liter (which is not statistically different from zero).

For the two animals in which the occluders were not

TABLE 2
Arterial and GCV myoglobin data in 11 animals subjected to a 2 hr occlusion of the LAD

	Arterial					GCV			
Dog No	Baseline (ng/ml)	End-occlusion (ng/ml)	Peak (ng/ml)	Time to peak (min)	t½ (min)	Baseline (ng/ml)	End-occlusion (ng/ml)	Peak (ng/ml)	Time to peak (min)
1	8	21	612	23	47	8	67	3,227	13
2	15	15	818	30	47	15	63	4,070	26
5	15	170	7,500	25	35	15	720	22,650	12
6	8	15	41	30	50	8	57	136	20
7	15	26	654	20	41	15	63	4,200	15
8	15	15	99	20	32	15	53	632	15
9	15	44	7,262	30	31	15	174	30,830	15
10	17	47	2,680	20	25	18	113	10,398	7
11	18	39	2,129	20	31	20	60	6,935	13
12	71	48	3,724	20	24	79	279	17,502	13
13	27	17	423	40	51	25	75	1,850	30
Mean	20	42	2,538	25	38	21	157	9,311	16
SEM	5	13	826	2	3	6	60	3,046	2

t½ = half-life.

TABLE 3
Arterial and GCV CK data in 11 animals subjected to a 2 hr occlusion of the LAD

	Arterial				GCV			
Dog No	Baseline (IU/l)	End-occlusion (IU/l)	Peak (IU/l)	Time to peak (min)	Baseline (IU/l)	End-occlusion (IU/l)	Peak (IU/l)	Time to peak (min)
1	24	34	500	181	19	35	675	181
2	21	21	743	202	21	28	803	242
5	13	41	4,312	111	14	62	4,870	60
6	12	15	44	140	11	14	54	180
7	21	30	586	120	20	33	672	80
8	16	17	118	330	16	17	118	330
9	20	38	4,181	122	17	55	4,322	102
10	14	24	1,672	60	12	27	1,786	60
11	22	18	1,226	100	20	20	1,310	60
12	54	86	1,881	80	54	100	1,925	80
13	55	54	242	200	56	51	268	200
Mean	25	37	1,409	150	23	40	1,527	143
SEM	5	8	460	23	5	8	495	27

inflated, both myoglobin and CK values remained at control levels (with [Mb] < 42 ng/ml and CK level < 43 IU/liter) throughout the experimental period.

Clinical studies. Figure 5 contrasts myoglobin and CK curves from one patient who underwent successful reperfusion with PTCA with those from the one patient in whom immediate reperfusion was unsuccessful. Rapid increases in myoglobin levels after reperfusion were apparent in each of the six patients in whom intracoronary streptokinase and/or PTCA was successful (figure 6). Peak myoglobin values (1130 to 7200 ng/ml) occurred 49 ± 8 min after the onset of reperfusion and represented a four- to 16-fold increment above the levels observed immediately before reperfusion. CK levels, which rose five- to 42-fold, peaked noticeably later at 11 ± 2 hr after reperfusion.

Data from the patients who received intravenous streptokinase are summarized in figure 7. In each case

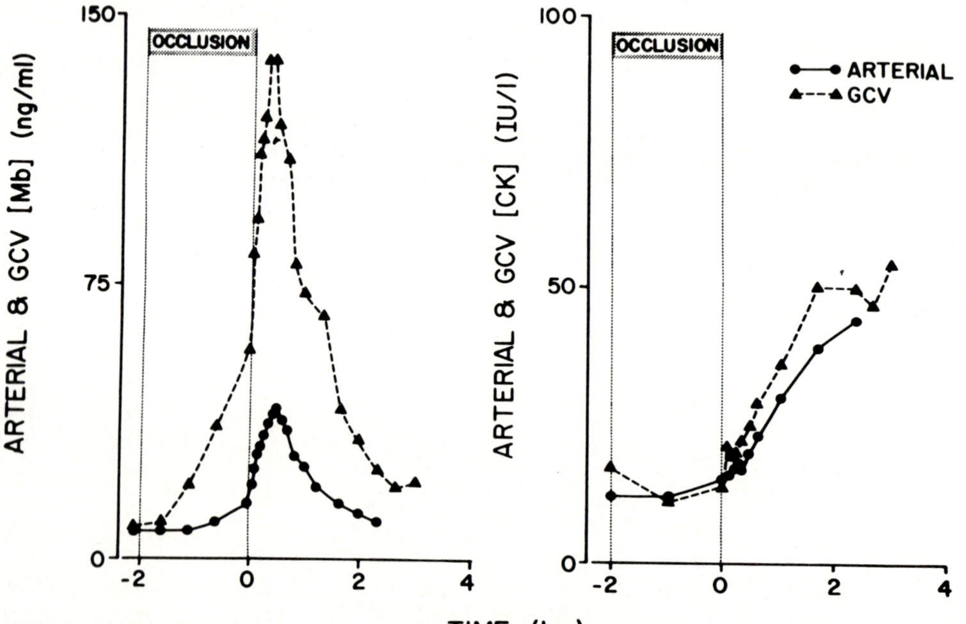

FIGURE 2. Simultaneous arterial and GCV myoglobin (*left*) and CK (*right*) concentration-time curves from an animal that showed no electrocardiographic changes during the LAD occlusion (dog 6, tables 2 and 3). Although peak [Mb] is low, an abnormal pattern is clearly evident. A persistent GCV-arterial [Mb] gradient is present, confirming the release of myoglobin from the myocardium. Although a rise in CK activity is also noted, a clear peak is not evident during the period of observation.

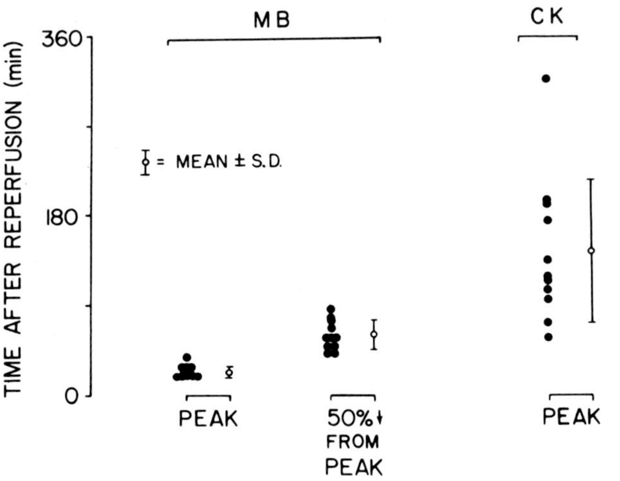

FIGURE 3. Time-to-peak [Mb] (*left*) and CK activity (*right*) after release of occlusion in all 11 animals. In contrast to the CK peaks, peak [Mb] occurred 25 ± 2 min after release of occlusion and then fell to one-half peak value 38 ± 3 min later (*middle*).

there was an abrupt six- to 14-fold rise in [Mb], with peaks occurring 95 to 105 min after completion of the streptokinase infusion. CK activities also rose 23- to 53-fold, with peak levels occurring between 4 and 14 hr after completion of the infusion.

Thus, clinical reperfusion was consistently accompanied by a rapid rise in systemic venous [Mb], with the peak concentration occurring less than 2 hr after therapy. Substantial elevations in CK also occurred with reperfusion, but peak values occurred several hours later.

Discussion

This study demonstrates that myoglobin, a protein that is present in both skeletal and cardiac muscle, is rapidly released into the coronary venous effluent after successful reperfusion of injured myocardium. In all 11 animals successfully undergoing coronary artery occlusion and reperfusion, blood [Mb] increased rapidly after reopening of the vessel, with systemic arterial peaks occurring at 20 to 40 min. These early arterial peaks were followed by a rapid washout of the protein, with half-times of disappearance of 38 ± 3 min. The early peaks in [Mb] contrast with myoglobin concentration-time patterns in animals that sustained myocardial injury but did not undergo reperfusion. In these dogs peak [Mb] occurred at 4 to 7 hr after onset of occlusion.[10, 11] The early peaks and rapid washout of myoglobin also contrast with the patterns of CK activity. Although CK also entered the blood stream rapidly after successful reperfusion of injured myocardium, systemic peaks of this substance occurred significantly later and with greater variability than those of myoglobin, at 1 to 5½ hr after reperfusion.

Similar findings were present in the nine patients who underwent successful coronary reperfusion for acute myocardial infarction produced by arterial occlusions of 99% to 100%. In each case, plasma [Mb] rose rapidly after successful vessel reopening, and each peak level was followed by rapid plasma washout. These findings contrast with the simultaneous CK activity-time curves, which showed a discernible rise

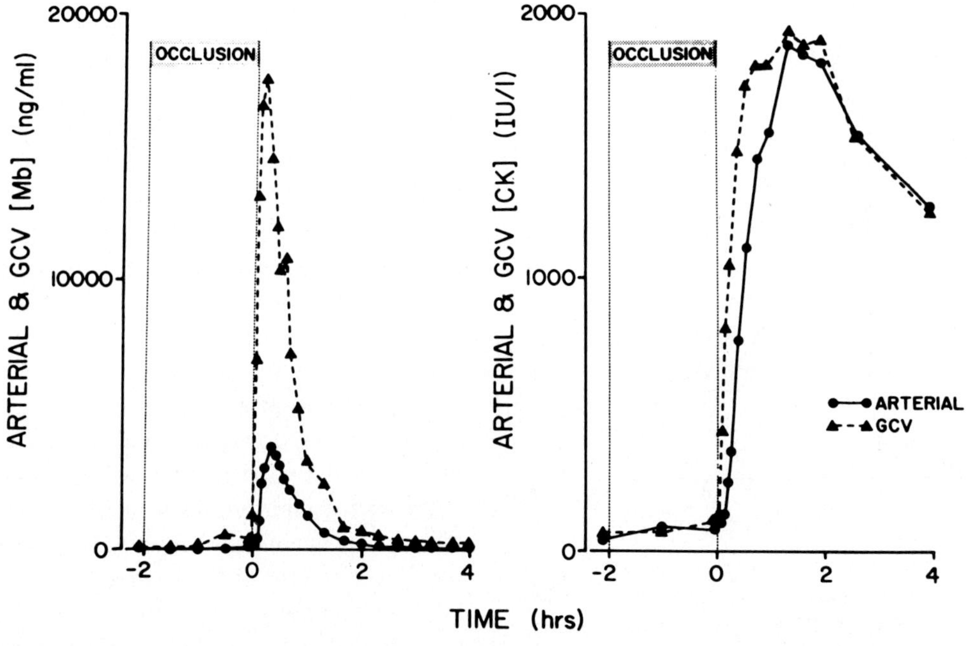

FIGURE 4. Simultaneous arterial and GCV myoglobin concentration-time curves (*left*) and CK activity-time curves (*right*) from one animal (dog 12, tables 2 and 3). See text for details.

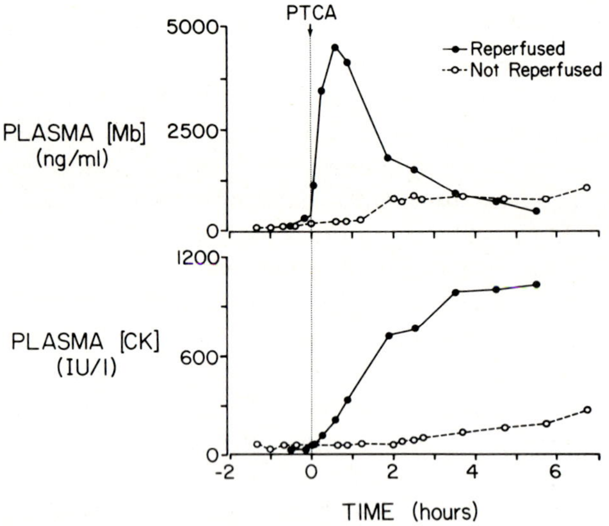

FIGURE 5. Systemic plasma myoglobin concentration-time curves and CK activity-time curves for two patients undergoing thrombolytic therapy for acute myocardial infarction. In the patient in whom reperfusion was successful, plasma [Mb] rose rapidly after PTCA, peaking at 32 min. CK activity also showed a prominent rise but did not reach its peak of 2360 IU/liter until 18 hr. In the patient in whom reperfusion was not successful, plasma [Mb] rose slowly over 7 hr, achieving a maximum level of 1030 ng/ml.

after reperfusion, but peaked at 2 to 18 hr rather than at 1 to 2 hr. Thus, myoglobin is rapidly released into the systemic circulation and is then rapidly cleared, making its early peak more apparent than that of CK after successful coronary arterial reperfusion. With the use of currently available rapid assays, myoglobin levels can be determined within a few hours after a sample is obtained.

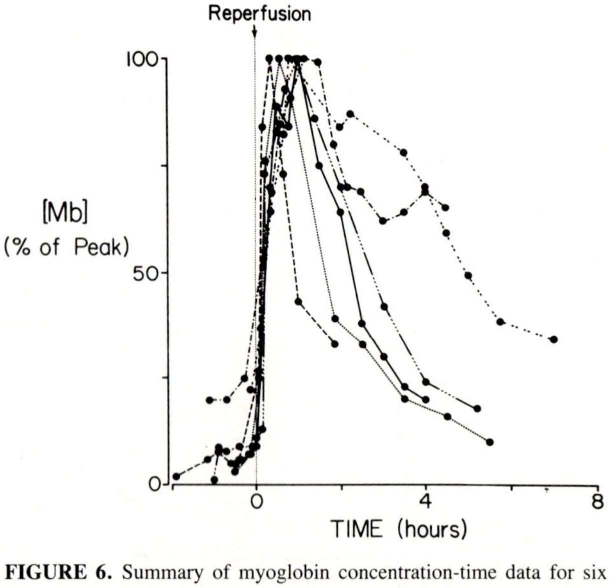

FIGURE 6. Summary of myoglobin concentration-time data for six patients undergoing successful reperfusion with intracoronary streptokinase and/or PTCA. Time of reperfusion is designated time 0. Plasma [Mb] is plotted on the vertical axis as percent of peak myoglobin concentration. See text for details.

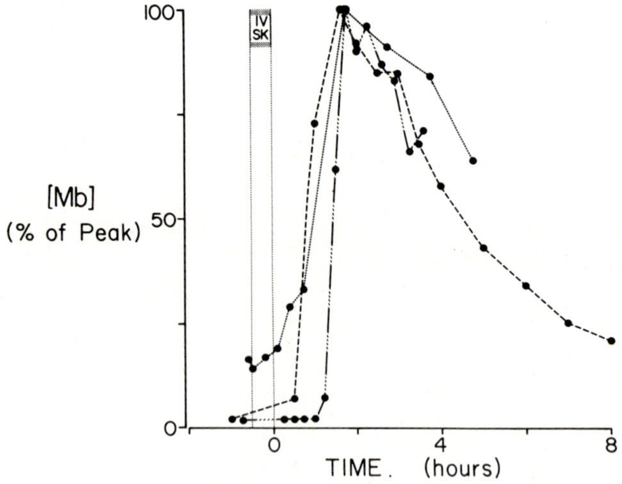

FIGURE 7. Summary of myoglobin concentration-time data for three patients in whom reperfusion with intravenous streptokinase was thought to be successful. Data are plotted as in figure 6. Completion of streptokinase is noted as time 0. See text for details.

The relatively rapid disappearance of myoglobin from plasma has been documented in earlier studies.[8] After intravenous administration of ^{125}I-radiolabeled myoglobin to normal dogs, arterial immunoreactive [Mb] decreased monoexponentially over a two-decade range, with a half-time of disappearance of 8.9 $\pm$ 1.5(SD) min. This half-time after bolus administration contrasts with the half-time of disappearance of 38 $\pm$ 3 min found in the dogs included in the present study. Although a decrease in renal perfusion could theoretically have contributed to the difference,[8] there is no reason to expect an important decrease in renal flow in the face of continuing normal hemodynamics (table 1). A more likely explanation is that there is continuing protein release into the vascular space from damaged myocardium during the first few hours after reperfusion. As discussed above and illustrated in figure 4, coronary venous-arterial myoglobin concentration differences persisted throughout the experimental period in all 11 animals that underwent reperfusion. It is also of interest that myoglobin levels peaked 20 to 40 min after vessel reopening (figure 3) rather than at 1 to 2 min as noted when myoglobin was injected as a bolus.[8] Because coronary flow was not measured in the present study, we are unable to quantitate the magnitude of this continuing protein release.

Mechanisms for continuing myoglobin release remain speculative at this point. Although large-vessel reopening occurs within a relatively short period of time, it is probable that reperfusion at the microcirculatory level is uneven and variable over time. In this situation, myoglobin might be released from different areas within the occluded segment at different times, depending on when microvascular reperfusion actually occurs. A number of studies that have examined experimental ischemia and reperfusion indicate that there can be considerable tissue injury associated with restoration of blood flow to an injured or infarcted area. This additional injury could also produce ongoing myoglobin release. Cobb et al.[12] examined effects of acute cellular injury on coronary flow in a region subjected to a 2 hr occlusion by injecting radiolabeled microspheres at varying times after reestablishment of flow. In the period immediately after reperfusion, a hyperemic response was evident in all areas of ischemic tissue, but was considerably attenuated in the endocardium (which was presumably the area of most severe tissue necrosis and cell swelling). Four hours after the onset of reperfusion, subepicardial flow had returned toward baseline, while subendocardial flow was only 10% to 20% of its preocclusion level.

These findings indicate that prolonged ischemia may initiate tissue reponses that bring about further reductions in flow as reperfusion occurs. Frame et al.[13] examined myocardial reperfusion injury by studying cardiac cell membrane integrity with radiolabeled fragments of anticardiac myosin antibody. In eight animals, serial injections of antibody fragment were made after the onset of reperfusion that followed a 1 hr period of arterial occlusion. In each animal, antibody binding after 45 min of reperfusion was increased beyond that observed immediately after reperfusion, suggesting ongoing and increasing damage to the cell membrane. These studies raise the possibility that reperfusion injury contributes to the observed continuing release of myoglobin after reperfusion.

In the present study we were unable to address the issue of whether reperfusion injury was confined to tissue already destined to become necrotic before reperfusion. The basis for the absence of a continuing difference in GCV-arterial CK activity in contrast to the case for myoglobin in the present study is also unclear at this time. Because arterial levels of CK remain elevated so much longer than those of myoglobin, small GCV-arterial differences may have been difficult to discern analytically. CK released after the initial phase of reperfusion could, theoretically, have been inactivated in situ before its release, although a recent preliminary report by Sato et al.[14] presents evidence against this.[14] Alternatively, CK could have entered the systemic circulation via lymph rather than coronary venous blood. Possibilities such as these will need to be addressed in future studies of the basis of persistent GCV-arterial myoglobin differences.

Our initial patient data confirm the findings in dogs. In the nine patients who underwent successful reperfusion, a sharp myoglobin peak occurred less than 2 hr after reopening of the vessel. This was in contrast to the findings in the patient in whom reperfusion was not successful. In this patient there was only a gradual increase in myoglobin concentration, with no clear peak, and the pattern of myoglobin release was similar to that observed in other studies of patients with acute myocardial infarction in whom reperfusion was not attempted. In this setting peak [Mb] typically occurs within 4 to 12 hr after admission to the coronary care unit, or 6 to 12 hr after onset of symptoms.[15–19] A recent preliminary study that examined patterns of myoglobin release during acute myocardial infarction confirmed the presence of an early peak in [Mb] with successful coronary arterial reperfusion and contrasted this with the later peaks noted in patients who received standard medical therapy.[20]

In addition to the early peaks in [Mb] seen with successful reperfusion, a second, and perhaps practically more important, feature is the consistently rapid rate of rise in [Mb] immediately after reperfusion. The time required for [Mb] to increase from 25% to 100% of its peak value (T_{25-100}) was calculated for all patients studied (figure 8). The nine patients who underwent successful reperfusion, whether by intracoronary streptokinase, intravenous streptokinase, or PTCA, had an average T_{25-100} of 48 ± 27(SD) min. This value is similar in magnitude to that obtained in the 11 animals in the present study, in which T_{25-100} averaged 23 ± 10(SD) min. The T_{25-100} values for patients in whom reperfusion was successful contrast with that in the patient in whom it was unsuccessful (T_{25-100} = 5.7 hr) and with those derived from previous studies in which

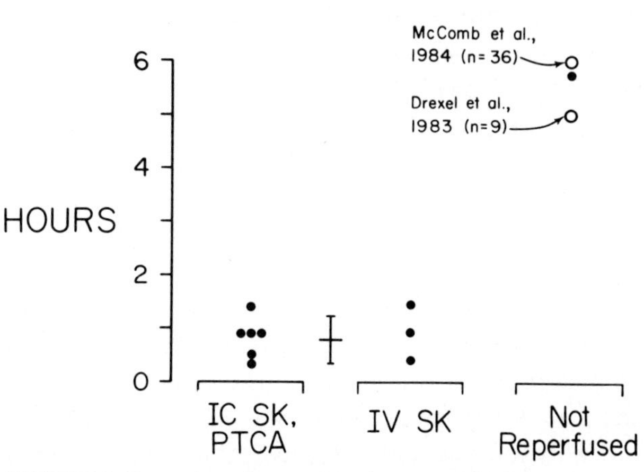

FIGURE 8. T_{25-100} in patients undergoing successful (*left* and *middle*) and the one patient undergoing unsuccessful reperfusion (*right*). The consistently low values of T_{25-100} in the former group of patients contrast with that in the latter patient and with the values in medically treated patients in other series in which reperfusion was not attempted (open circles).

detailed myoglobin concentration-time curves were obtained during myocardial infarctions unassociated with attempts at reperfusion.[18, 19] These differences in T_{25-100} values suggest that this index can distinguish between the two patient groups without overlap.

As noted previously by several laboratories, skeletal muscle and cardiac myoglobin are inseparable by currently available radioimmunoassays. Thus, similar to the situation with measurements of total CK, plasma myoglobin can be elevated independently of cardiac damage when skeletal muscle is injured. We are not aware, however, of peaks related to damage of skeletal muscle that are as rapid and prominent as those produced by reperfusion.

A prominent elevation in CK activity has been reported to be associated with successful coronary arterial reperfusion in patients receiving thrombolytic agents for acute myocardial infarction.[21] Vatner et al.[22] found a more rapid appearance of CK and an earlier time to peak in dogs undergoing reperfusion at 1 and 3 hr after coronary artery occlusion (time to peak CK activity = 4.2 ± 0.4 and 6.8 ± 0.5 hr, respectively) than in similar animals that did not undergo reperfusion (time to peak = 11.4 ± 0.5 hr). Similar results have been noted in patients treated with thrombolytic agents.[2–6] Successful reperfusion in these studies has generally been associated with peaks in CK activity at average times of 13 to 16 hr (vs 20 to 26 hr for patients not undergoing successful reperfusion). However, the large coefficients of variation of 20% to 50% indicate considerable variability and overlap in these values among individual patients in the two groups. Recently it has been noted that individual CK isoenzymes comprise three isoforms based on differences in isoelectric point.[23, 24] Current reports suggest that isoform proportions can be used to separate cases of successful vs unsuccessful reperfusion in the first few hours after lytic therapy.[23]

In summary, reperfusion of injured myocardium results in a rapid release of myoglobin into the blood stream. In both animals and humans undergoing reperfusion, a sharp peak in [Mb] occurs within 1 to 2 hr of vessel reopening. We conclude that myoglobin concentration-time curves are a relatively direct marker of protein entry into the blood stream after reperfusion, and that the myoglobin peaks associated with reperfusion offer a useful additional indicator of reopening of the vessel when revascularization is undertaken and a coronary arteriogram is not available.

We acknowledge the technical assistance of Mary Ahl, Kathleen Harris, Amy Johnson, Richard Kohlmeier, and Kathleen Sayadoff, and the secretarial assistance of Kyle Doran.

References

1. DeWood MA, Spores J, Notske R, Mouser LT, Burroughs R, Golden MS, Land HT: Prevalence of total coronary occlusion during the early hours of transmural myocardial infarction. N Engl J Med **303:** 897, 1980
2. Mathey DG, Kuck K-H, Tilsner V, Krebber H-J, Bleifeld W: Nonsurgical coronary artery recanalization in acute transmural myocardial infarction. Circulation **63:** 489, 1981
3. Schwarz F, Schuler G, Katus H, Mehmel HC, von Olshausen K, Hofmann M, Herrmann H-J, Kübler W: Intracoronary thrombolysis in acute myocardial infarction: correlations among serum enzyme, scintigraphic and hemodynamic findings. Am J Cardiol **50:** 32, 1982
4. Khaja F, Walton JA, Brymer JF, Lo E, Osterberger L, O'Neill WW, Colfer HT, Weiss R, Lee T, Kurian T, Goldberg AD, Pitt B, Goldstein S: Intracoronary fibrinolytic therapy in acute myocardial infarction. N Engl J Med **308:** 1305, 1983
5. Anderson JL, Marshall HW, Bray BE, Lutz JR, Frederick PR, Yanowitz FG, Datz FL, Klausner SC, Hagan AD: A randomized trial of intracoronary streptokinase in the treatment of acute myocardial infarction. N Engl J Med **308:** 1312, 1983
6. Rentrop KP, Feit F, Blanke H, Stecy P, Schneider R, Rey M, Horowitz S, Goldman M, Karsch K, Meilman H, Cohen M, Siegel S, Sanger J, Slater J, Gorlin R, Fox A, Fagerstrom R, Calhoun WF: Effects of intracoronary streptokinase and intracoronary nitroglycerin infusion on coronary angiographic patterns and mortality in patients with acute myocardial infarction. N Engl J Med **311:** 1457, 1984
7. Stone MJ, Waterman MR, Harimoto D, Murray G, Willson N, Platt MR, Blomqvist G, Willerson JT: Serum myoglobin level as a diagnostic test in patients with acute myocardial infarction. Br Heart J **39:** 375, 1977
8. Klocke FJ, Copley DP, Krawczyk JA, Reichlin M: Rapid renal clearance of immunoreactive canine plasma myoglobin. Circulation **65:** 1522, 1982
9. The Committee on Enzymes of the Scandinavian Society for Clinical Chemistry and Clinical Physiology: Recommended method for the determination of creatine kinase in blood modified by the inclusion of EDTA. Scand J Clin Lab Invest **39:** 1, 1979
10. Lwebuga-Mukasa JS, Libby P, Bloor CM, Maroko PR: The evaluation of serum myoglobin following experimental coronary occlusion. Circulation **48** (suppl IV): IV-129, 1973 (abst)
11. Willerson JT, Poliner L, Buja LM, Waterman MR, Gomez-Sanchez CE, Templeton GH, Stone MJ: Myoglobinemia as a clue to the presence of acute myocardial infarction. Clin Res **24:** 422A, 1976 (abst)
12. Cobb FR, Bache RJ, Rivas R, Greenfield JC: Local effects of acute cellular injury on regional myocardial blood flow. J Clin Invest **57:** 1359, 1976
13. Frame LH, Lopez JA, Khaw BA, Falton JT, Haber E, Powell WJ: Early membrane damage during coronary reperfusion in dogs. J Clin Invest **72:** 535, 1983
14. Sato Y, Degawa T, Isojima K, Y-Rit J, Fishbein MC, Karshmer DL, Shell WE, Ganz W: Following early reperfusion, all the creatine kinase depleted from the necrotic myocardium appears in the blood. J Am Coll Cardiol **3:** 522, 1984 (abst)
15. Stone MJ, Willerson JT, Gomez-Sanchez CE, Waterman MR: Radioimmunoassay of myoglobin in human serum. Results in patients with acute myocardial infarction. J Clin Invest **56:** 1334, 1975
16. Reichlin M, Visco JP, Klocke FJ: Radioimmunoassay for human myoglobin. Initial experience in patients with coronary heart disease. Circulation **57:** 52, 1978
17. Varki AP, Roby DS, Watts H, Zatuchni J: Serum myoglobin in acute myocardial infarction: a clinical study and review of the literature. Am Heart J **96:** 680, 1978
18. Drexel H, Dworzak E, Kirchmair W, Milz MM, Puschendorf B, Dienstl F: Myoglobinemia in the early phase of acute myocardial infarction. Am Heart J **105:** 642, 1983
19. McComb J, McMaster EA, MacKenzie G, Adgey AAJ: Myoglobin and creatine kinase in acute myocardial infarction. Br Heart J **51:** 189, 1984
20. Kaiser HF, Helmling E, Glunz H-G: Serum myoglobin in acute revascularization by systemic streptokinase: fast diagnosis of acute

myocardial infarction and control of the efficiency of coronary thrombolysis by a new myoglobin latex test. Circulation **70** (suppl II): II-153, 1984 (abst)
21. Ganz W, Geft I, Shah PK, Lew AS, Rodriguez L, Weiss T, Maddahi J, Berman DS, Charuzi Y, Swan HJC: Intravenous streptokinase in evolving acute myocardial infarction. Am J Cardiol **53:** 1209, 1984
22. Vatner SF, Baig H, Manders WT, Maroko PR: Effects of coronary artery reperfusion on myocardial infarct size calculated from creatine kinase. J Clin Invest **61:** 1048, 1978
23. Puleo P, Perryman MB, Roberts R: Non-invasive detection of reperfusion after thrombolytic therapy based on CK isoform analysis. Circulation **70** (suppl II): II-330, 1984 (abst)
24. Hashimoto H, Abendschein DR, Strauss AW, Sobel BE: Early detection of myocardial infarction in conscious dogs by analysis of plasma MM creatine kinase isoforms. Circulation **71:** 363, 1985

The superiority of maximum fiber elastance over maximum stress-volume ratio as an index of contractile state

THOMAS WISENBAUGH, M.D., GEORGE YU, M.S.M.E., AND JOYCE EVANS, M.S.

ABSTRACT The end-systolic pressure-volume relationship has been used as a load-independent measure of ventricular pump performance. Since comparisons of load between ventricles of different size and thickness may be more accurately made with measurements of wall stress than with those of pressure, the end-systolic stress-volume relationship at one or more levels of end-systolic stress has been used to estimate contractile function in hypertrophied ventricles. Linear regression of end-systolic stress against end-systolic volume for differently loaded beats has a slope termed maximum fiber elastance (fiber Emax) and a volume intercept termed Vo; the maximum stress-volume ratio (MSVR) for a single beat is an approximation of fiber Emax but assumes Vo = 0. However, the influence of preload, afterload, and inotropic state on these indexes has not been examined. We therefore studied the stress-volume relationship in seven open-chest dogs instrumented with ultrasonic crystals and micromanometers. Postextrasystolic potentiation (PESP) increased both the MSVR (5.7 ± 1.83 vs 4.85 ± 1.43 at control, $p < .05$) and fiber Emax (13.93 ± 3.24 vs 9.24 ± 2.15 at control; $p < .05$). Augmentation of preload by infusion of dextran, with the use of nitroprusside to maintain afterload relatively constant, did not significantly influence either the MSVR or fiber Emax. Vo was not significantly influenced by PESP, but was shifted to higher values by augmentation of preload (17.5 ± 14.8 vs 13.9 ± 11.1 ml at control; $p < .05$). Augmentation of afterload by aortic constriction was used to derive fiber Emax, and produced an increase in MSVR directly proportional to the increase in wall stress (6.03 ± 1.39 with end-systolic stress augmented by 93% vs 4.85 ± 1.43 at control; $p < .05$). Thus, MSVR is a less reliable index of inotropic state than fiber Emax since it is afterload dependent.
Circulation 72, No. 3, 648–653, 1985.

THE END-SYSTOLIC pressure-volume relationship has been used as a preload-independent measure of ventricular pump performance.[1-3] Since the load on myocardial fibers comprising the ventricle depends not only on intraventricular pressure, but also on wall thickness and chamber dimensions, it has been proposed that in hypertrophied ventricles stress is a better measure of load than is pressure.[4, 5] Several investigators have therefore used either the end-systolic stress-volume relationship for differently loaded beats[6] or the end-systolic stress-volume ratio from a single beat[7-9] to estimate contractile function in chronically overloaded ventricles. However, existing data are not sufficient to clearly define the sensitivity of either the stress-volume ratio or the slope of the stress-volume relationship at end-systole to changes in contractile state. We therefore examined the effects of postextrasystolic potentiation (PESP) of inotropic state and of altered ventricular volume and load on the maximum stress-volume ratio (MSVR) and the slope of the end-systolic stress-volume relationship (fiber Emax) in open-chest dogs instrumented with sonomicrometer crystals and micromanometer-tip pressure transducers.

Methods

Animal studies were conducted in accordance with the guidelines of the American Physiologic Society. Adult mongrel dogs anesthetized with 1 mg/kg im morphine, 350 mg/kg iv urethane, and 45 mg/kg iv α-chloralose were ventilated on a respirator through an endotracheal tube. Through a left lateral thoracotomy, the pericardium was opened and two orthogonal pairs of 5 MHz piezoelectrical crystals 5 mm in diameter were sutured at the major and minor axes, as previously described.[6] A snare was placed around the descending thoracic aorta. Through branches of the femoral artery, No. 7F micromanometer-tip catheters were introduced into the left ventricle and proximal aorta. A large-bore cannula was inserted into the inferior vena cava through a femoral vein. Bipolar epicardial electrodes were su-

From the Veterans Administration and University of Kentucky Medical Centers, Lexington.

Supported by a grant from the American Heart Association, Kentucky Affiliate.

Address for correspondence: Thomas Wisenbaugh, M.D., Cardiology Division, Room MN670, University of Kentucky Medical Center, 800 Rose St., Lexington, KY 40536.

Received March 8, 1985; revision accepted May 23, 1985.

tured to both the left atrium and left ventricle. Autonomic blockade was produced with 0.1 mg/kg atropine and 2 mg/kg iv propanolol; adequacy of β-blockade was assessed by determining the dose of isoproterenol required to produce a 25% increase in heart rate both before and after administration of propranolol. Heart rate was maintained just above intrinsic rate (120 to 150 beats/min) by atrial pacing. Left ventricular dimensions were measured with a sonomicrometer (Triton Industries) and recorded on a strip-chart recorder and on 16-channel magnetic tape simultaneously with aortic pressure, left ventricular pressure, left ventricular dP/dT, and the electrocardiogram. Measurements were made at four to five different levels of aortic pressure, each produced by tightening the snare during an 8 to 10 sec interruption of ventilation.

PESP was produced by premature ventricular stimuli delivered at a coupling interval of 200 msec by a programmable pacer (Medtronics) every eighth beat at each level of pressure. Myocardial length (or preload), measured as left ventricular end-diastolic dimensions, was increased by rapid infusion of 250 ml dextran. Intravenous nitroprusside was used to maintain constant aortic pressure. Measurements were again made at this and three to four higher levels of aortic pressure produced by tightening the aortic snare. Each experiment was terminated by inducing fibrillation of the heart, which was then removed. The left ventricle, including the septum, was weighed after it was separated from the right ventricle and atria. Data were digitized at 5 msec intervals and transferred to floppy disks with an analog-to-digital converter (Data Acquisition Systems) and microcomputer (IBM PC). Beats just before and after the programmed premature stimulus at each level of varied loading were chosen for analysis.

Ventricular volume was calculated with the equation of Rankin et al.[10] as follows:

$$Vi = (Pi/6)(a - 1.1h)(b - 2h)^2 \quad (1)$$

where Vi is the dynamic internal volume of a prolate ellipsoidal shell in which b is the external diameter of the minor axis, a is the external diameter of the major axis, and h is the equatorial wall thickness.

The external shell volume (Ve) was calculated from the equation

$$Ve = (Pi/6)(ab^2) \quad (2)$$

Since the myocardial volume (Vm = Ve − Vi) can be computed from the measured postmortem mass of the left ventricle and the specific gravity of the myocardium (1.06 g/cm^3), wall thickness can be determined from simultaneous solution of equations 1 and 2. This is done by computer iteration with the Newton Raphson method.[11] Briefly, iteration of the three following computations is performed until convergence on the solution for h:

$$g(h) = 1.1h^3 - (a + 1.1b)h^2 + (ab + 1.1b/4)h - 3Vm/2Pi \quad (3)$$

$$g'(h) = 3.3h^2 - 2(a + 1.1b)h + (ab + 1.1b/4)h \quad (4)$$

$$h = 1h - g(h)/g'(h) \quad (5)$$

where g(h) is a function of h, g′(h) is the first derivative of the function, and 1h represents the value of h from the preceding iteration. This is the method used by Hugenholz et al.[12] for computing dynamic thickness from left ventriculograms in humans. Mean circumferential wall stress is then computed at 5 msec intervals throughout the cardiac cycle with Mirsky's equation for a thick wall ellipse[4] as follows:

$$S = 1.33(Pb/2h)(1 - b^2/(2a^2) - h/b) \quad (6)$$

The end-systolic stress-volume relationship was derived from each series of stress-volume loops with the iterative method of Kono et al.[13] that first locates the end-systolic stress-volume coordinate on each loop and then performs a linear regression on these points. Since we used stress rather than pressure as a measure of afterload in this study, we have referred to the slope of this relationship as fiber Emax to differentiate this quantity from chamber Emax, as used by Sagawa and his colleagues.[1,2] The MSVR within each loop, which assumes an intercept of Vo = 0, was also determined by the computer, which then plotted each loop. Comparisons of MSVR for single beats were made under control conditions, both for a regular atrial and a potentiated beat, with afterload (end-systolic stress) augmented by approximately 100% of control, and with preload augmented while afterload was held constant.

Statistical analysis. Analysis of covariance was used to establish whether or not significant differences in the Emax were produced in each dog by PESP (SYSTAT, Inc.). Comparisons of values for fiber Emax and other parameters under different states were made by analysis of variance for repeated measures and the multiple-comparison test of Dunnett.

Results

The morphologic and baseline hemodynamic characteristics of the dogs are listed in table 1. The hemodynamic responses to PESP, volume loading, and pressure loading are shown in table 2.

Fiber Emax was significantly increased by PESP in each dog, with a mean increase of 51% for the group ($p < .05$). Fiber Emax was not significantly altered by augmentation of preload with infusion of dextran-nitroprusside. The volume intercept, Vo, was not altered by inotropic stimulation with PESP, but was shifted to a larger value by dextran-nitroprusside. An example of the influence of PESP on fiber Emax and Vo is illustrated in figure 1, and the data are summarized in table 3.

TABLE 1
Morphologic and hemodynamic data

Dog	Body weight (kg)	LV weight (g)	HR (bpm)	LVSP (mm Hg)	LVEDP (mm Hg)
437	22.5	107	150	106	7
344	22.4	82	160	108	5
438	17.5	64	150	103	6
567	20.5	82	150	78	8
608	20.5	103	120	135	8
614	20.0	73	150	110	8
663	24.5	106	130	153	8
Mean	21.1	90	144	113	7
SD	±2.2	±18	±14	±24	±1

LV = left ventricular; HR = heart rate; LVSP = LV systolic pressure; LVEDP = LV end-diastolic pressure.

TABLE 2
Hemodynamic response to intervention (mean ± SD)

	Control	PESP	Volume loading	Pressure loading
LVSP	113±24	135±30[A]	113±25	160±38[A]
LVEDP	7±1	9±3	9±2	10±3
Maximum dP/dt	1874±560	3182±909[A]	2396±470[A]	2083±458

Hemodynamic conditions listed in the pressure loading column are those under which MSVR volume ratio was analyzed. Abbreviations and units are as in table 1.
[A]Significant ($p < .05$) difference from control by ANOVA.

PESP produced a modest but significant increase (19%) in the MSVR ratio for single beats under control conditions, as illustrated in figure 2, *left*. The relatively pure increase in preload produced by infusion of dextran-nitroprusside was sufficient to produce a 30% increase in mean end-diastolic volume, but did not significantly alter MSVR. This is illustrated in figure 2, *center*. However, a mean increase of 93% in end-systolic stress produced by aortic constriction resulted in a 24% increase in the MSVR, as illustrated in figure 2, *right*. Thus, the single-beat MSVR was sensitive to the inotropic stimulation produced by PESP and insensitive to changes in preload; however, the MSVR varied directly with increases in afterload. The data are summarized in figures 3 and 4.

Discussion

The two principal findings of this study are (1) the MSVR obtained from a single ventricular beat is an

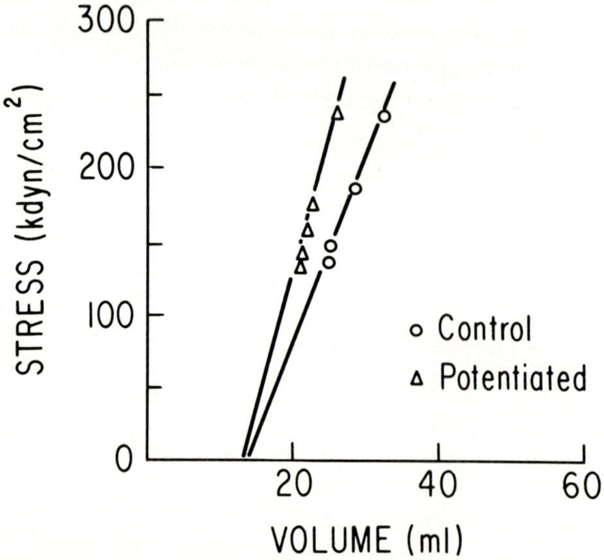

FIGURE 1. End-systolic stress-volume relationships generated under different loading conditions for control and potential beats. The slope, termed fiber Emax, was increased by PESP of inotropic state while the volume intercept, Vo, was unaltered.

TABLE 3
Fiber Emax and Vo (mean ± SD) for control (C), potentiated (PESP), and volume-loaded beats

	Control	PESP	Volume
Fiber Emax	9.24±2.15	13.93±3.24[A]	11.24±4.63
Vo	13.9±11.1	14.1±12.3	17.5±14.8[A]

[A]Significant ($p < .05$) difference from control by ANOVA.

index of inotropic state that is insensitive to changes in myocardial length but is sensitive to changes in afterload, and (2) when examined over a range of end-systolic loads, inotropic stimulation increases fiber Emax without altering the extrapolated Vo.

Estimation of contractile function in chronically overloaded ventricles has been difficult because of the unavailability of a load-independent index of contractile function. Hemodynamic parameters measured during the preejection phase of contraction, such as the maximum left ventricular dP/dt, are sensitive to alterations in preload. Ejection-phase parameters such as ejection fraction and velocity of circumferential fiber shortening (Vcf) are sensitive to alterations in afterload.[14, 15] Emax, based on the relationship between pressure and volume at end-systole, has recently gained acceptance as an index that is sensitive to inotropic state and relatively insensitive to loading conditions.[1–3]

Ventricular afterload can be well characterized by impedence spectra[16] that relate instantaneous pressure to instantaneous flow. Impedence, however, does not take into account the interrelationship between ventricular wall thickness, chamber dimensions, and pressure that may affect load at the myocardial fiber level.[4] Thus, end-systolic or other indexes of contractile state derived with the use of pressure as a measure of afterload may be normal or higher than normal in hypertrophied ventricles when contractile performance per unit mass of myocardium is actually depressed.[17] For this reason, stress-volume relationships are preferred to pressure-volume relationships for use in the comparison of contractile state between ventricles having different thickness-dimension ratios.

Although the end-systolic pressure-volume relationship has been evaluated extensively, there are few reports regarding the influence of inotropic changes on the end-systolic stress-volume relationship. Positive inotropic interventions generally produce an increase in slope but no change in the Vo when pressure is used as a measure of end-systolic load. However, when stress has been used as a measure of load, an increase in Vo with no significant change[6] or even an increase[18]

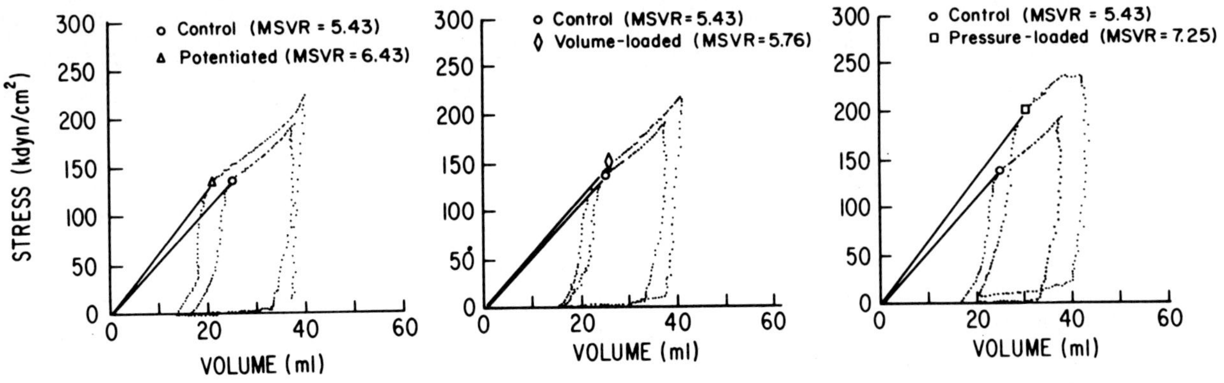

FIGURE 2. MSVR was increased by PESP (*left*), but was also sensitive to increased afterload (*right*). Augmentation of preload, with afterload held constant, did not alter MSVR (*center*).

in slope has been noted in ventricles in which there is chronic overload hypertrophy, suggesting a shift in the stress-volume relationship to larger volumes with depression of the inotropic state. Borow et al.[19] have likewise shown a parallel shift in the end-systolic stress-dimension relationship, with a decrease in end-systolic diameter, for any stress, after short-term inotropic intervention in humans. Weber et al.[20] demonstrated alteration of the slope of the force-length relationship in the isolated dog heart with an indeterminate change in the length intercept. The present data indicate that the stress-volume relationship responds to inotropic stimulation, as does the pressure-volume[1–3] relationship, with an increase in fiber Emax and no significant change in Vo.

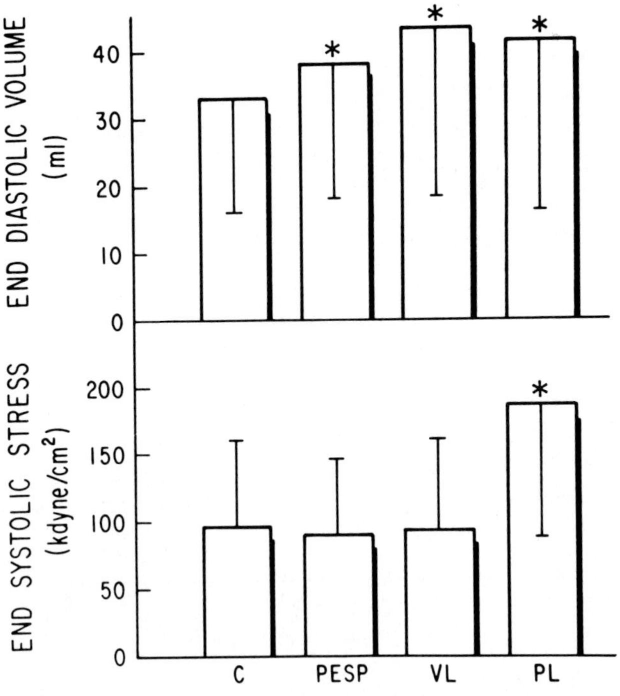

FIGURE 3. Preload was measured as end-diastolic volume (*top*) and afterload was measured as end-systolic stress (*bottom*). $^*p < .05$.

The significance of the increase in Vo that occurred after infusion of dextran-nitroprusside in our study is uncertain, but may be related to the inverse correlation of Vo with resistance noted by Maughan et al.,[21] who studied pressure-volume relationships in excised canine ventricles connected to a servopump system. These investigators observed deficits in pressure for any given end-systolic volume (i.e., a parallel shift to the right) for beats with large end-diastolic volumes and low resistances compared with those with smaller end-diastolic volumes at higher resistances. The viscoelastic property of muscle, termed creep, may possibly account for such parallel shifts at a constant inotropic state in their study[21] and in ours.

Determination of Emax requires repeated measurements of end-systolic ventricular volume over a wide range of systolic pressures. This is difficult in patients in whom hemodynamics are already abnormal, particularly those with critical aortic stenosis.[22] Some investigators have therefore used either ventricular pressure or wall stress and ventricular volume at end-systole under basal conditions as a practical alternative

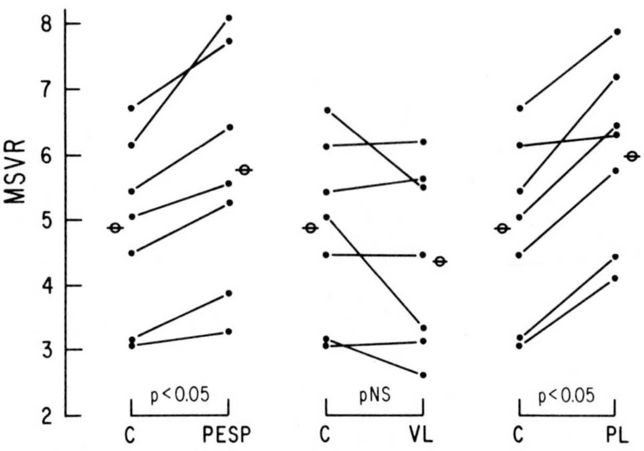

FIGURE 4. MSVR was increased by PESP and pressure loading (PL), but not by volume loading (VL).

to measuring Emax in disease states associated with abnormal ventricular size and loading conditions.[7–9] The ratios of pressure to volume[23] or stress to volume[24] at end-systole have been presumed, but not proven, to be sensitive to contractile state and independent of preload and afterload. Others[25] have used the slope of the relationship of stress to volume during late systole for a single beat to estimate contractile state, but this relationship is affected by afterload.[26] The results of our animal studies demonstrate that, although MSVR is unaltered by short-term changes in preload and is sensitive to short-term inotropic interventions, this ratio also changes in direct proportion to short-term changes in afterload. This is illustrated in figure 5, which also illustrates that the magnitude by which MSVR underestimates fiber Emax depends both on the value of afterload and the magnitude of Vo, since MSVR assumes Vo to be zero.

Thus, a reduced MSVR could be the result of either a depressed inotropic state or reduced afterload. For example, in patients with conditions such as acute mitral regurgitation, MSVR could be depressed as a result of reduced afterload despite the presence of a normal inotropic state. Conversely, increased afterload in patients with decompensated aortic stenosis or regurgitation could partially mask the effects of impaired inotropic state on the MSVR ratio. However, because the computation of ventricular stress provides a means to normalize for abnormal wall thickness and chamber dimensions, this preload-independent index may more accurately assess contractile state in subjects with chronically overloaded ventricles than do traditional indexes of contractility, providing that afterload is not significantly altered from normal.

Limitations of the study. A potential pitfall in the use of the stress-volume relationship to estimate contractile function is related to selection of the time in the cardiac cycle during which it is measured. Several definitions of end-systole have been proposed. The time at which ventricular volume reaches a minimum has been traditionally used; however, Sagawa[1] and Maughan et al.[27] have noted that coincidence of end-ejection, as indicated by minimum ventricular volume or dicrotic notch, with maximal elastance is circumstantial. These investigators have recently derived Emax using the point in each cardiac cycle at which the pressure-volume ratio reaches maximum[21] as an alternative to searching pressure-volume regression lines at frequent intervals during the cardiac cycle for the maximum value.[1] Computer analysis of stress-volume loops in our dogs usually showed that this point in each cardiac cycle very nearly coincided in time with the time of fiber Emax for the series of loops. However, in a few animals it was noted that, when impedence to ejection was markedly reduced by nitroprusside, the MSVR for the loops with the lowest load occurred more near the onset of ejection than the end of ejection. As can be seen in figure 5, the rapid decrease in stress during ejection produced by nitroprusside caused the stress-volume ratio to be slightly greater at a time earlier in the loop than at the time of Emax or end-ejection. In this situation, the stress-volume ratio at end-ejection[8] would be lower, and underestimate fiber Emax by a greater amount, than would MSVR.

Pure alterations in myocardial length, which has been termed preload, are difficult to produce in situ because of the alterations in stroke volume and load (or afterload) that result. We attempted to minimize increases in afterload that accompany increases in preload by using nitroprusside so that the influence of a

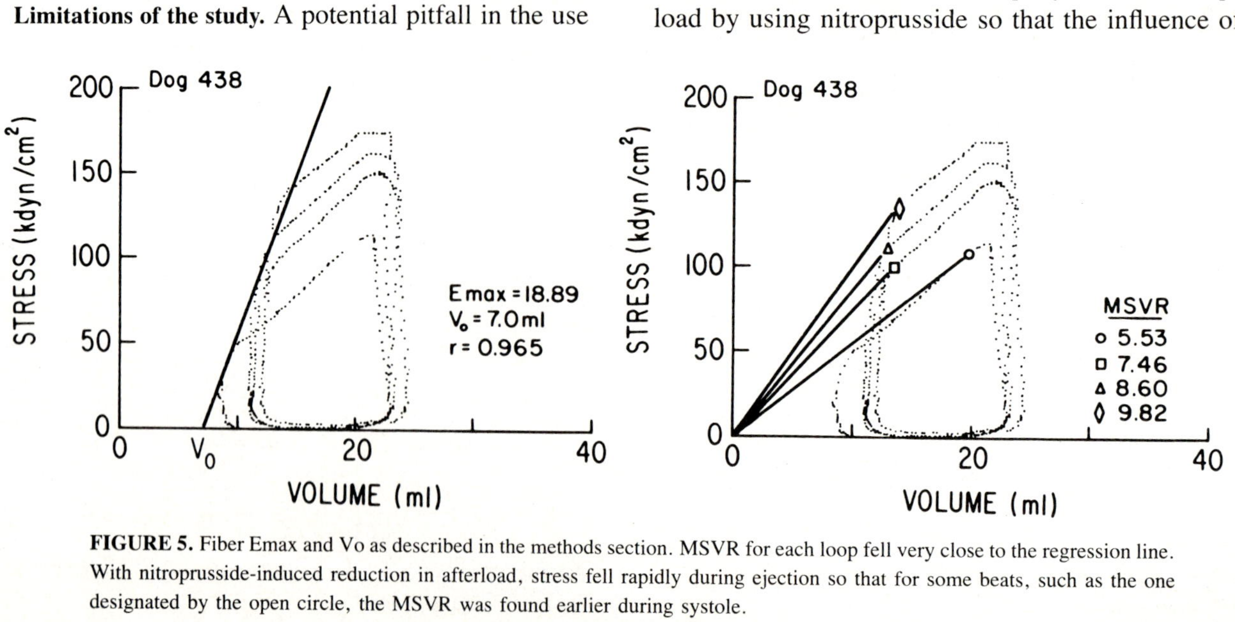

FIGURE 5. Fiber Emax and Vo as described in the methods section. MSVR for each loop fell very close to the regression line. With nitroprusside-induced reduction in afterload, stress fell rapidly during ejection so that for some beats, such as the one designated by the open circle, the MSVR was found earlier during systole.

relatively pure length alteration on MSVR could be examined. Likewise, an increase in afterload results in an increase in end-diastolic length if preload reserve[28] has not already been exhausted. Thus, we were unable to produce pure alterations in afterload, but since relatively pure changes in preload had no significant effect on MSVR, it can be assumed that the increase in MSVR with aortic constriction was a result of augmented afterload.

A variety of methods have been used for measuring ventricular volume. Isolated heart preparations[1–3] probably allow the most accurate determination of ventricular volume. Area-length methods of analysis of radiographic images and minor-axis measurements from M mode echocardiograms have been used extensively in humans. Although the technique based on sonomicrometric measurement of left ventricular major and minor axes used in the present study has been recently validated,[10, 29] the computation of volume with an elliptical model is probably less accurate than methods in which the excised heart is used, since the latter does not require such geometric assumptions. However, ultrasonic techniques have the advantage of allowing continuous measurements of cardiac dimensions in situ without the undesirable effects of contrast agents.

In summary, the MSVR measured from a single ventricular beat is sensitive to the inotropic state and is insensitive to preload; however, the sensitivity of this index to afterload limits its usefulness as a practical index of contractile function. The slope of the end-systolic stress-volume relationship, or fiber Emax, which is increased by inotropic stimulation, accounts for varied afterload over multiple beats, and is therefore a more reliable measure of contractile function than the MSVR when myocardial load is abnormal.

The secretarial assistance of Lynne Cornish is gratefully acknowledged, as are the thoughtful comments of Dr. Blase Carabello during preparation of the manuscript.

References

1. Sagawa K: The end-systolic pressure-volume relation of the ventricle: definition, modifications and clinical use. Am J Cardiol **40:** 748, 1977 (editorial)
2. Sagawa K, Suga H, Shoukas AA, Bakalar KM: End-systolic pressure/volume ratio: a new index of ventricular contractility. Circulation **63:** 1223, 1981
3. Suga H, Sagawa K, Shoukas A: Load independence of the instantaneous pressure-volume ratio of the canine left ventricle and effects of epinephrine and heart rate on the ratio. Circ Res **32:** 314, 1973
4. Mirsky I: Left ventricular stresses in the intact human heart. Biophys J **9:** 189, 1969
5. Hood WP, Rackley CE, Rolett EL: Wall stress in the normal and hypertrophied human left ventricle. Am J Cardiol **22:** 550, 1968
6. Wisenbaugh T, Allen P, Cooper G, Holzgrefe H, Beller G, Carabello B: Contractile function, myosin ATPase activity and isoenzymes in the hyprtrophied pig left ventricle after a chronic progressive pressure overload. Circ Res **53:** 332, 1983
7. Carabello BA, Spann JF: The uses and limitations of end-systolic indexes of left ventricular function. Circulation **69:** 1058, 1984
8. Carabello BA, Nolan SP, McGuire LB: Assessment of preoperative left ventricular function in patients with mitral regurgitation: value of the end-systolic wall stress-end-systolic volume ratio. Circulation **64:** 1212, 1981
9. Osbakken M, Bove AA, Spann JF: Left ventricular function in chronic aortic regurgitation with reference to end-systolic pressure, volume and stress relations. Am J Cardiol **47:** 193, 1981
10. Rankin JS, McHale PA, Arentzen CE, Ling D, Greenfield JC, Anderson RW: The three-dimensional dynamic geometry of the left ventricle in the conscious dog. Circ Res **39:** 306, 1976
11. Miller AR: Pascal programs for scientists and engineers. Berkeley, CA, 1981, Sybex
12. Hugenholtz PG, Kaplan E, Hull E: Determination of left ventricular wall thickness by angiocardiography. Am Heart J **78:** 513, 1969
13. Kono A, Maughan WL, Sunagawa K, Hamilton K, Sagawa K, Weisfeldt ML: The use of left ventricular end-ejection pressure and peak pressure in the estimation of the end-systolic pressure-volume relationship. Circulation **70:** 1057, 1984
14. Mahler F, Ross J, O'Rourke RA, Covell JW: Effects of changes in preload, afterload and inotropic state on ejection and isovolumic phase measures of contractility in the conscious dog. Am J Cardiol **35:** 626, 1975
15. Quinones MA, Gaasch WH, Alexander JK: Influence of acute changes in preload, afterload, contractile state and heart rate on ejection and isovolumic indices of myocardial contractility in man. Circulation **53:** 293, 1976
16. Milnor WR: Arterial impedance as ventricular afterload. Circ Res **36:** 565, 1975
17. Huber D, Grimm J, Koch R, Krayenbuehl HP: Determinants of ejection performance in aortic stenosis. Circulation **64:** 126, 1981
18. Reichek N, Laskey W, Fink L, Sutton MSJ, Unterecker W, Hirshfeld: Relationships of left ventricular end-systolic mechanics to ejection fraction. J Am Coll Cardiol **1:** 664, 1983 (abst)
19. Borow KM, Green LH, Grossman W, Braunwald E: Left ventricular end-systolic stress-shortening and stress-length relations in humans. Am J Cardiol **50:** 1301, 1982
20. Weber KT, Janicki JS, Hefner LL: Left ventricular force-length relations of isovolumic and ejecting contractions. Am J Physiol **231:** 337, 1976
21. Maughan WL, Sunagawa D, Burkhoff D, Sagawa K: Effect of arterial impedance changes on the end-systolic pressure-volume relation. Circ Res **54:** 595, 1984
22. Mehmel HC, Schwarz F, Ruffmann K, Manthey J, von Olshausen K, Kubler W: End-systolic pressure-volume and end-systolic stress-volume relationships in patients with aortic stenosis and with normal valvular function. Basic Res Cardiol **78:** 338, 1983
23. Ramanathan KB, Knowles J, Connor MJ, Tribble R, Kroetz FW, Sullivan JM, Mirvis DM: Natural history of chronic mitral insufficiency: relation of peak systolic pressure/end-systolic volume ratio to morbidity and mortality. J Am Coll Cardiol **3:** 1412, 1984
24. Gash AK, Carabello BA, Cepin D, Spann JF: Left ventricular ejection performance and systolic muscle function in patients with mitral stenosis. Circulation **67:** 148, 1983
25. Pouleur H, Rosseau MF, van Eyll C, Mechelen HV, Brasseur LA, Charlier AA: Assessment of left ventricular contractility from late systolic stress-volume relations. Circulation **65:** 1204, 1982
26. Colan SD, Borow KM, Gamble WJ, Sanders SP: Effects of enhanced afterload (methoxamine) and contractile state (dobutamine) on left ventricular late-systolic wall stress-dimension relation. Am J Cardiol **52:** 1304, 1983
27. Maughan WL, Shoukas AA, Sagawa K, Weisfeldt ML: Instantaneous pressure-volume relationship of the canine right ventricle. Circ Res **44:** 309, 1979
28. Ross J: Afterload mismatch and preload reserve: a conceptual framework for the analysis of ventricular function. Prog Cardiovasc Dis **18:** 255, 1976
29. Sodums MT, Badke FR, Starling MR, Little WC, O'Rourke RA: Evaluation of left ventricular contractile performance utilizing end-systolic pressure-volume relationships in conscious dogs. Circ Res **54:** 731, 1984

Effect of heart rate on the canine end-systolic pressure-volume relationship

W. LOWELL MAUGHAN, M.D., KENJI SUNAGAWA, M.D., DANIEL BURKHOFF, WILLARD L. GRAVES, JR., PH.D., WILLIAM C. HUNTER, PH.D., AND KIICHI SAGAWA, M.D.

ABSTRACT Although the rate dependence of isolated muscle contractility is well known, the ventricular end-systolic pressure-volume relationship (ESPVR) has been reported to be insensitive to heart rate. To resolve this contradiction, we used an isolated, ejecting canine heart preparation perfused at a constant coronary arterial pressure. Heart rate was changed from 60 to 200 beats/min in steps of 20 beats/min. At least 10 pressure-volume loops under different filling pressures were obtained at each heart rate in each of six hearts. Over a heart rate range from 60 to 120 beats/min, the slope of the ESPVR (E_{es}) increased significantly from 3.5 ± 0.4 (SE) to 5.3 ± 0.6 mm Hg/ml. In the range between 120 and 180 beats/min there was little change in E_{es} (5.3 ± 0.6 to 5.4 ± 0.6 mm Hg/ml), but at 200 beats/min E_{es} increased slightly to 5.7 ± 0.5 mm Hg/ml. The volume axis intercept (V_0) of the ESPVR changed little over the range of heart rate from 60 to 160 beats/min (10.2 ± 2 ml to 9.4 ± 1.3 ml) but increased to 15.2 ± 1.2 ml at a rate of 200 beats/min. The change in ESPVR with increase in heart rate from 60 to 120 beats/min (i.e., increase in E_{es} without change in V_0) is the same as those seen with a positive inotropic intervention with calcium or cathecholamines, whereas the V_0 changes over the range from 160 to 200 beats/min is similar to those seen with regional ischemia. The insensitivity of ESPVR in the midrange may be the result of a balance of positive and negative influences on ventricular contraction or a restricted range for the increase in inotropic state with higher rate.
Circulation 72, No. 3, 654–659, 1985.

PHYSIOLOGISTS have long been aware that frequency of contraction influences the contractile state of myocardium. The earliest description of this phenomenon has been credited to Bowditch[1]; many investigators have since shown that in isolated muscle preparations[2–4] and in isovolumically contracting hearts,[5–7] peak systolic tension or pressure is increased as the frequency of contraction increases.

However, several investigators have questioned the importance of the frequency effect on contractility in vivo.[8–14] For example, Kavaler et al.[9] showed that the effect was far less marked or absent in unexcised canine papillary muscles beating in situ. Suga et al.[14] showed that changing heart rate over the midrange caused very little change in the end-systolic pressure-volume relationship (ESPVR).

The purpose of this investigation was to reinvestigate in excised, ejecting canine hearts the effects of extensive change in heart rate on the ESPVR under strictly controlled ejecting conditions, free of reflex stimulation, and over a wider range of heart rates than previously tested.

From the Department of Medicine, Cardiology Division and Division of Biomedical Engineering, Johns Hopkins University, Baltimore.

Supported by USPHS grant HL 14903 and Ischemic Heart Disease (SCOR) grant HL 17655.

Address for correspondence: W. Lowell Maughan, M.D., Cardiology Division, The Johns Hopkins Hospital, Carnegie Bldg. 592, 600 North Wolfe St., Baltimore, MD 21205.

Received July 31, 1984; revision accepted June 6, 1985.

Methods

Surgical preparation. The supported isolated canine heart preparation used in this study has been previously described.[8] Briefly, we used two dogs (20 to 25 kg) per experiment. Both dogs were anesthetized with sodium pentobarbital (25 mg/kg iv bolus) and placed on respirators. One dog supplied oxygenated blood to the heart excised from the second dog as shown in figure 1.

Arterial blood from the femoral arteries of the support animal passed first through a heat exchanger (water bath at 38° C) and a peristaltic pump, then through a "depulsator and debubbling chamber" to the aortic root of the isolated heart. After passing through the coronary vessels, the venous blood was collected and returned to the support dog via the femoral veins. The support dog's arterial pressure was continuously monitored by a pressure transducer (Statham P23Db) via a catheter in the carotid artery. An oxygenator placed in parallel with the support dog (figure 1) was used during the isolation of the donor dog heart and if the support dog became hypotensive during the experiment.

Coronary perfusion pressure was monitored with a catheter in the aortic arch and maintained at a constant level between 80 and 100 mm Hg. Vents were placed in the apices of the right and

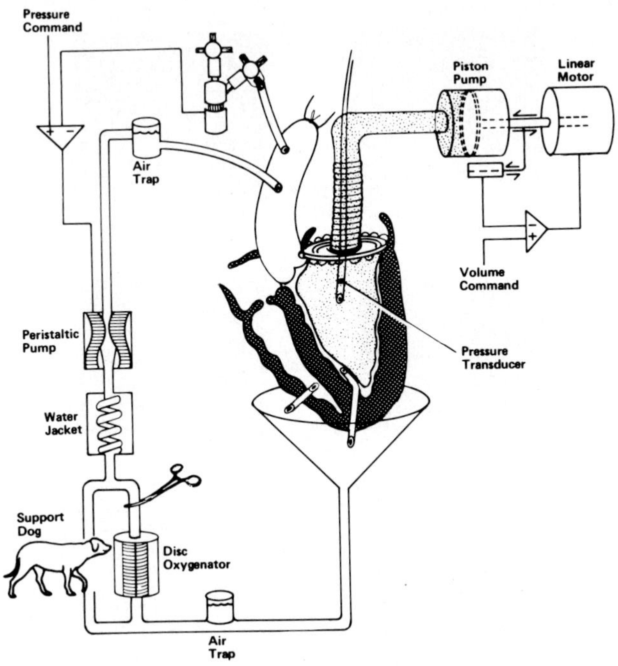

FIGURE 1. Schematic diagram of the isolated canine heart preparation. Coronary perfusion is maintained constant with blood from an oxygenator or second support animal. The left ventricle contains a balloon. Ejection and filling of the left ventricle is controlled by a servomotor with a computer-generated volume-command signal.

left ventricles. The left atrium was opened and the chordae tendineae were severed. A metal ring was sutured to the mitral anulus. A water-filled latex balloon connected to a servocontrolled piston pump[15] was placed within the left ventricle through the metal ring. When the surgical preparation was complete, suction was applied through the left ventricular vent so that the balloon and the left ventricle had very nearly the same volume.

The intrinsic heart rate of the isolated heart tended to be between 100 and 120 beats/min. To obtain lower heart rates it was usually necessary to block the atrioventricular (AV) conduction by damaging the AV node with a suture and to pace the heart from the ventricle at the desired low rates.

Servopump hardware. The right side of figure 1 shows a schematic representation of the ventricular volume control pump system. Details of its design and performance have been previously reported.[15, 16] Briefly, a linear motor (Ling Electronics, Model 411) controlled the piston position of a rolling-diaphragm cylinder (Bellofram SS-4-F-SM). The latex balloon was secured to a tube connected to the outflow tract of the Bellowfram cylinder. The cylinder, connecting tube, and the balloon were all filled with water. A linear displacement transducer (Trans-Tek model 244-000) sensed the position of the piston, producing a signal proportional to the balloon volume. The signal was used in a negative feedback loop for comparison with a volume-command signal from a computer (see below), which represented the desired instantaneous left ventricular volume. The error signal resulting from this comparison was supplied to a power amplifier (Crown DC-300), which in turn drove the linear motor to minimize the difference between the desired and actual left ventricular volume.

Impedance loading system. The ventricular volume-command signal for the volume control servosystem is generated by the interaction between left ventricular pressure signal and a specially designed hybrid computer.[16] The left ventricular pressure, measured by a Konigsburg pressure transducer (P-21) placed inside the balloon, served as the input to an analog computer programmed to solve differential equations that describe both the ventricular preloading and afterloading circuit. The characteristics of this system have been previously described.[16] It allows the ventricle to fill from a fixed pressure source through a preloading system and eject into an afterloading system with precisely controlled afterload resistance, compliance, and characteristic impedance.

Coronary perfusion pressure and left ventricular volume and pressure were recorded simultaneously on a strip chart. Pressure-volume loops were recorded on a storage oscilloscope (Techtronix, Model 5111) and photographed.

Protocol. Left ventricular diastolic pressure was set to produce a peak systolic pressure between 100 and 120 mm Hg at a control coronary perfusion pressure of 80 mm Hg against a control set of arterial impedance parameters (resistance = 3.0 mm Hg-sec/ml, compliance = 0.4 ml/mm Hg, characteristic impedance = 0.2 mm Hg-sec/ml) and at a heart rate of 120 beats/min. The filling pressure, controlled by the computer, was then lowered over 10 sec until the peak systolic pressure became less than 20 mm Hg. The filling pressure was then returned to its initial value.

This was repeated for heart rates of 60, 80, 100, 120, 140, 160, 180, and 200 beats/min. At each heart rate we waited until steady state was reached before recording data. The sequence of the heart rates was varied from heart to heart, and the initial condition was recreated at the end of the sequence to determine whether the contractile state of the preparation changed during the experiment. When a clear change was recognized, the data from the heart was discarded.

Data analysis. The Polaroid pictures of the oscilloscope tracing of pressure-volume loops were used to measure the slope and volume axis parameters of the ESPVR. The ESPVR was traced, the tracing calibrated, and the slope and intercept determined from the tracing.

$(dP/dt)_{max}$ was determined by numerical differentiation of the digitized pressure recording (LSI 11/34 16 bit minicomputer). The $(dP/dt)_{max}$ for corresponding volumes at each heart rate was determined by interpolation with a linear least-squares regression of $(dP/dt)_{max}$ on end-diastolic volume.

Statistical analysis. For each heart, linear regression was applied to the slope vs heart rate relationship and the intercept vs heart rate relationship of the ESPVR over the heart rate ranges from 60 to 120, 120 to 160, and 160 to 200 beats/min. An analysis of variance was applied to compare the slopes of the linear regression over these three ranges. Significance was defined at the $p < .01$ level.

An analysis of variance and covariance with repeated measures (BMDP statistical package) was used for comparison of $(dP/dt)_{max}$.

Results

Figure 2 shows an example of the data from a single heart. The eight panels in the top and middle rows present pressure-volume tracings recorded on the oscilloscope for heart rates from 60 to 200 beats/min. The bottom three panels show the superimposed ESPVR lines for the three heart rate ranges of 60 to 120, 120 to 160, and 160 to 200 beats/min. Notice that in the range from 60 to 120 beats/min there is a progressive increase in the slope of the ESPVR (E_{es}) with increase in heart rate but little change in the volume

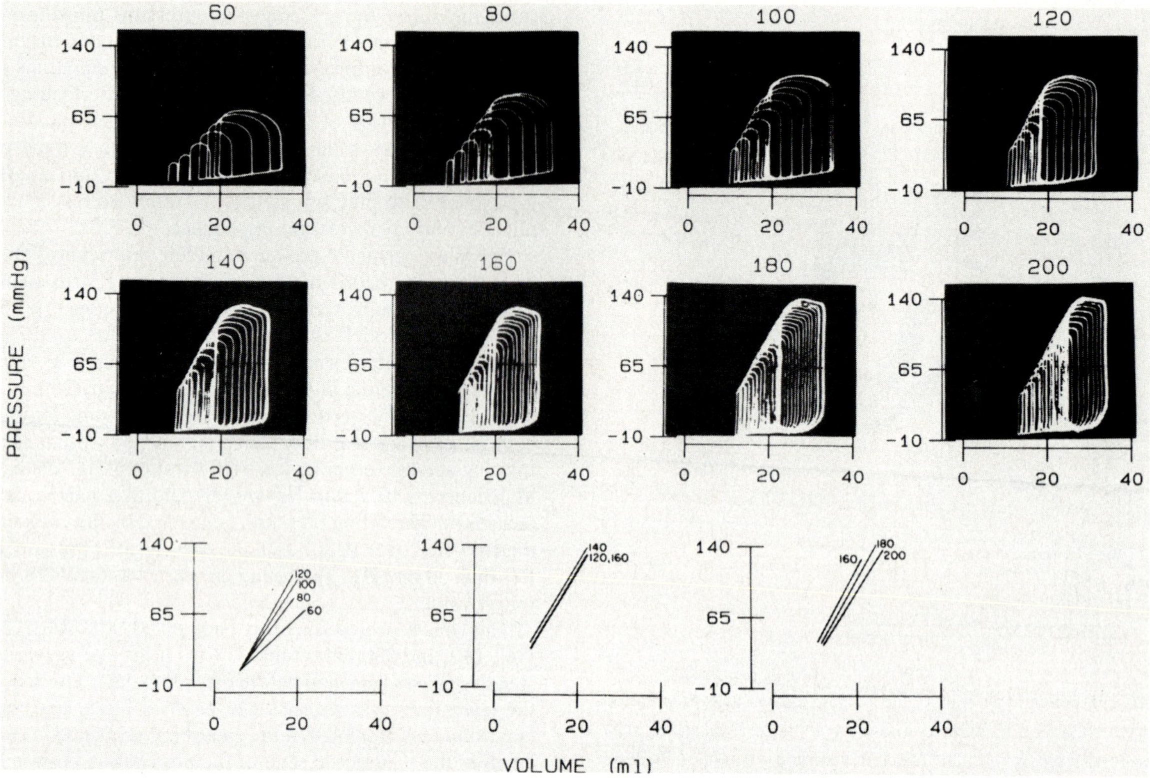

FIGURE 2. Effect of heart rate on ESPVR. An example from one heart. Each of the eight top panels is a photograph of the pressure-volume loops recorded on a storage oscilloscope as filling pressure is lowered over 10 sec. The bottom three panels are tracings of the ESPVR from the top panels over the heart rate ranges 60 to 120, 120 to 160, and 160 to 200 beats/min.

axis intercept (V_0). In the heart rate range from 120 to 180 beats/min there is little change in either the slope or the intercept of the ESPVR line. Over the heart rate range above 180 beats/min there is a progressive, almost parallel rightward shift of the ESPVR.

Figure 3 shows the pooled data from six hearts. The top panel shows the slope of the ESPVR (E_{es}) and the bottom panel shows its volume axis intercept (V_0) over the entire heart rate range. The small bars are standard error of the mean. Over the range from 60 to 120 beats/min E_{es} increased significantly with heart rate (3.5 ± 0.4 to 5.3 ± 0.6 mm Hg/ml; $p < .0001$, $n = 6$); from 120 to 160 beats/min there was no further increase in E_{es} (5.2 ± 0.6 mm Hg/ml; p = NS, $n = 6$); and at 200 beats/min there was a slight further increase in E_{es} (5.7 ± 0.5 mm Hg/ml; $p < .01$, $n = 6$). V_0 was decreased slightly over the heart rate range of 60 to 120 beats/min (10.1 ± 2.0 to 9.2 ± 1.5 ml; $p < .01$, $n = 6$), changed very little over the range 120 to 160 beats/min (9.4 ± 1.3 ml; p = NS, $n = 6$), and increased to 15.2 ± 1.2 ml at a heart rate of 200 beats/min.

The influence of heart rate on the time to end-systole (T_{es}) is shown in figure 4. There was a significant shortening of T_{es} from 237 ± 26.4 (SD) msec at the heart rate of 60 beats/min to 140 ± 20.5 msec at 200

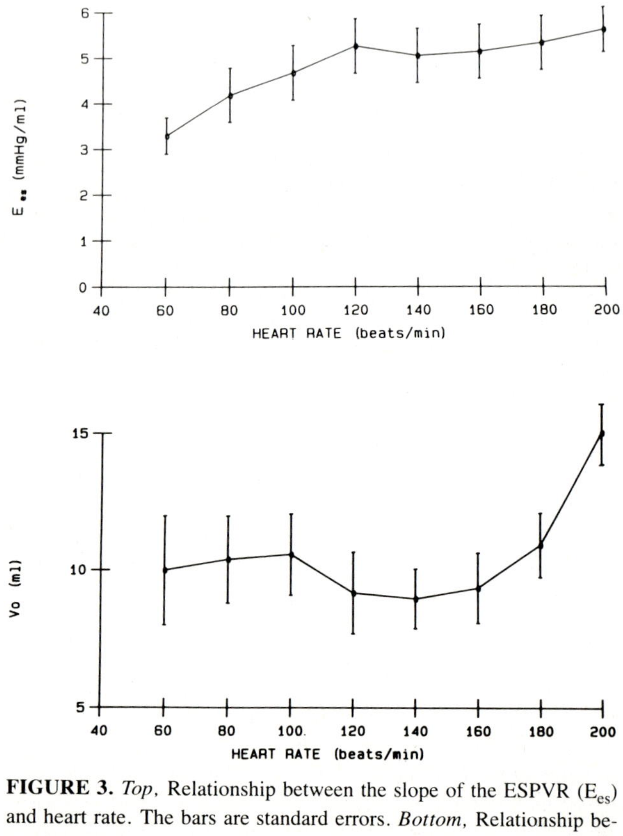

FIGURE 3. *Top*, Relationship between the slope of the ESPVR (E_{es}) and heart rate. The bars are standard errors. *Bottom*, Relationship between the volume intercept (V_0) and heart rate.

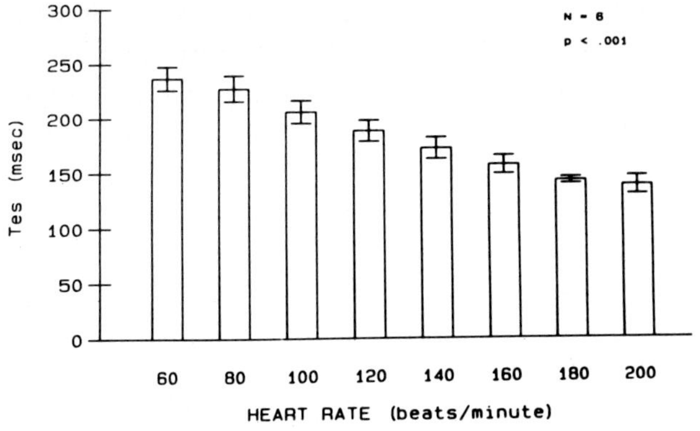

FIGURE 4. The influence of heart rate on the time to end-systole (T_{es}).

beats/min. T_{es} is defined as the time from end-diastole (detected by a threshold rise in dP/dt) to the time at which the pressure-volume loops reached the point that was used for drawing the ESPVR line of an individual beat.

Figure 5 shows the $(dP/dt)_{max}$/heart rate relationship. There was a statistically significant increase in $(dP/dt)_{max}$ over the heart rate range of 60 to 120 beats/min (1192 ± 309 to 1850 ± 368 mm Hg/sec; $p < .001$, $n = 6$). Over the heart rate range 120 to 160 beats/min there was a variable upward trend that was not significant, and from 160 to 200 beats/min there was a downward trend that was not statistically significant (2163 ± 432 to 2011 ± 380 mm Hg/sec; p = NS, $n = 6$).

Discussion

We have shown that in the isolated canine left ventricle, the influence of heart rate on the ESPVR depends on the range over which heart rate varied. Within the range between 60 to 120 beats/min there was a steady increase in E_{es} with insignificant variations in V_0. In the middle range (120 to 180 beats/min) there was very little change in either E_{es} or V_0 of the ESPVR, and over the range above 180 beats/min there was a rightward shift of the relationship with increase in heart rate.

The influence of heart rate on cardiac contractility has been extensively studied and reviewed.[17] A significant influence has been shown in isolated muscle strips,[2–4] isolated hearts,[5–7] intact anesthetized animals,[18, 20] and conscious animals.[19, 20] Species differences have been shown,[3] as well as differences with the presence or absence of anesthesia.[20] In this study we confined our interest to the influence of heart rate on the pumping function of the left ventricle.

Mitchell et al.[12] studied the effect of heart rate on areflexic canine hearts under right heart bypass with controlled aortic pressure and cardiac output. They demonstrated that over the range from 60 to 180 beats/min, the mean rate of pressure rise increased, stroke power increased, and dP/dt increased. However, stroke work remained nearly constant over the entire range.

Lendrum et al.[6] studied the effect of heart rate in isovolumically contracting dog hearts. In their preparation the heart remained in situ, and heart rate was not controlled but changed spontaneously. Monroe and French[7] used an isolated heart compressing air. They reported one heart in which heart rate was changed from 30 to 254 beats/min in four steps. An increase in the slope of the ESPVR was seen with each step of increase in heart rate. In contrast, Suga et al.,[8] using an isolated ejecting canine heart, found that the slope of the ESPVR increased only slightly and inconsistently among different hearts. They reported an increase of 0.54 ± 0.84 mm Hg/ml per 100 beats/min increase in paced heart rate. These studies all suggest that there is a shift to the left of the ESPVR with increasing heart rate but have not convincingly demonstrated the quantitative difference in these shifts over different heart rate ranges.

Our study has the advantage of using an isolated heart, free of the influence of reflex and external factors, ejecting at physiologic preload, and under precisely controlled afterload impedance. These factors, along with precise volume measurements, allowed us to measure ventricular chamber function accurately. In addition, we controlled coronary perfusion pressure precisely, removing another confounding variable.

The mechanism of the frequency range–dependent difference in the effect of heart rate is not revealed from our data. It has been previously suggested that activation has both a positive and a negative inotropic effect.[17] Both effects are most probably mediated through alteration in calcium release and sequestration.

There is evidence that the positive inotropic effect results from increased calcium availability related to

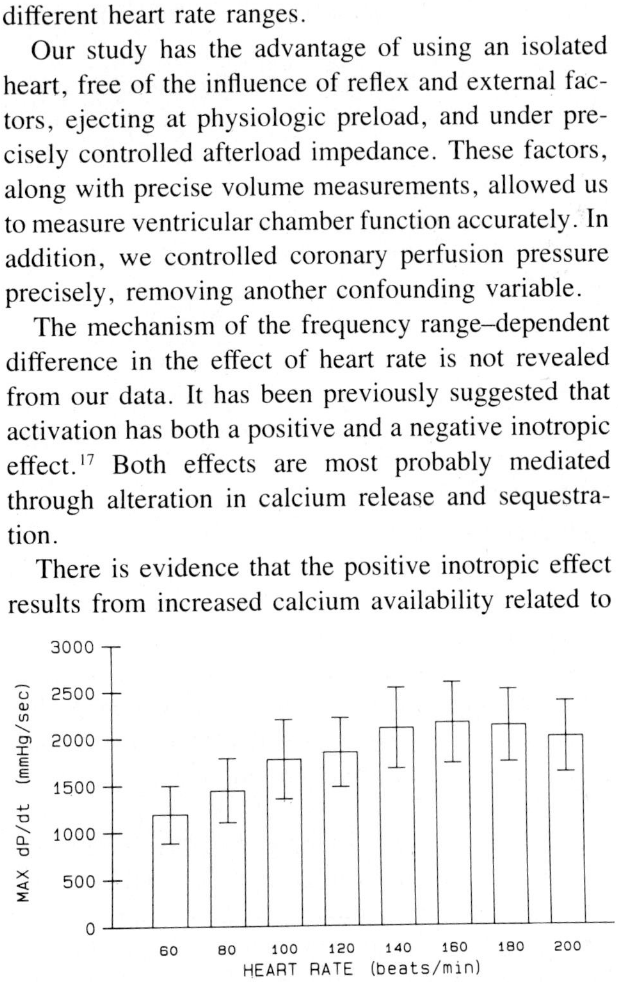

FIGURE 5. The influence of heart rate on $(dP/dt)_{max}$.

accumulation of the calcium entering the cell with each beat.[3] The negative inotropic effect may relate to the finite time required for "mechanical restitution." For a given time constant of mechanical restitution, a shorter duration of electrical diastole allows only a smaller fraction of the "potential" contractile strength to become available on excitation of the ventricle.[21] These factors, together with other factors such as limited coronary reserve, and metabolic limitations probably contribute to the different heart rate responses over different frequency ranges.

Increased heart rate shortened the duration of the T_{es} over the entire range of heart rates studied (figure 4). The disparity between the influence of heart rate on the time course of contraction and the maximum chamber stiffness is particularly apparent in the midrange (120 to 160 beats/min), where no change in the ESPVR and yet significant decrease in T_{es} occurred. This is consistent with the findings of Suga et al.,[14] who reported a significantly shortened T_{es} but no substantial effect of E_{max}. It is also consistent with the findings of Mitchell et al.,[12] who showed that increased dP/dt with increased heart rate was not associated with increased stroke work.

Our data for dP/dt showed a trend similar to that shown in the ESPVR data. That is, over the lower heart rate range there was a significant increase in dP/dt with heart rate, in the middle range there was no significant influence of heart rate on dP/dt, and in the high range there was a trend toward decreasing dP/dt (although not statistically significant). It should be noted that $(dP/dt)_{max}$ has a strong dependence on preload. Preload is altered by heart rate changes, so a valid comparison of dP/dt and heart rate cannot be made without correcting for this load dependence as was done in our analysis.

The shift of the ESPVR in a nearly parallel manner with heart rate increase above 180 beats/min is very similar to the change previously shown in regional ischemia.[22] We have no evidence, however, that regional ischemia was present, nor is there an a priori reason to believe so. An alternative explanation would be that the shape of the heart has changed at the higher heart rate, leading to the ESPVR shift. Further studies are needed to elucidate the mechanism of these changes.

The ESPVR is being used as an index of left ventricular pump function in patients. Several pressure-volume loops under different loading conditions are presently required for measurement of the ESPVR. Because heart rate may change unintentionally during the load manipulation, the present information on the significant influence of change in heart rate itself in the physiologic (low) range on the ESPVR becomes of importance. Unless it is clear that a patient is undergoing evaluation in a range where the ESPVR is insensitive to changes in heart rate, it will be best to ensure, by pacing if necessary, that the heart rate does not vary during the measurement of ESPVR. If extrapolation of the present results to humans is allowed, any significant change in heart rate should be strictly avoided in the low range.

The sensitivity of the ESPVR to heart rate may be useful as an index of the metabolic state of cardiac muscle, since changes in the balance between oxygen demand and calcium delivery will probably lead to changes in the response of the ESPVR to heart rate. Differences between responses of patients with and without regional ischemia have already been demonstrated.[23] Thus the difference in the response of ESPVR to changes in heart rate have the potential to add diagnostic information in patients.

The tightly controlled conditions in this study are the major limitation for extrapolating the results of this study to intact animals or patients. Many of the controlled factors (reflex activity, changing hormonal background, changing coronary perfusion pressure) could significantly modify the response of cardiac performance to changes in heart rate.

Further studies are needed to quantify these changes in patients and to determine the influence of disease states on the sensitivity of ESPVR to heart rate.

References

1. Bowditch HP: Uber die Eigenthumlichkeiten der Reizbarkeit, welche die Muskelfasern des Herzens zeigen. Arb Physiol Anstalt zu Leipzig **6:** 139, 1871
2. Abbott BC, Mommaerts WFHM: A study of inotropic mechanisms in the papillary muscle preparation. J Gen Physiol **42:** 533, 1959
3. Blinks JR, Koch-Weser J: Analysis of the effects of changes in rate and rhythm upon myocardial contractility. J Pharmacol Exp Ther **134:** 373, 1961
4. Sonnenblick EH: Force-velocity relations in mammalian heart muscle. Am J Physiol **202:** 931, 1962
5. Rosenblueth A, Alanis J, Rubio R: Some properties of the mammalian ventricular muscle. Arch Int Physiol **67:** 276, 1959
6. Lendrum B, Feinberg H, Boyd E, Katz LN: Rhythm effects on contractility of the beating isovolumic left ventricle. Am J Physiol **199:** 1115, 1960
7. Monroe RG, French GN: Left ventricular pressure-volume relationships and myocardial oxygen consumption in the isolated heart. Circ Res **9:** 362, 1961
8. Suga H, Sagawa K: Instantaneous pressure-volume relationships and their ratio in the excised, supported canine left ventricle. Circ Res **35:** 117, 1974
9. Kavaler F, Norris RS, Lee RJ, Fisher VJ: Frequency-force behavior of in situ ventricular myocardium in the dog. Circ Res **28:** 533, 1971
10. Boerth RC, Covell JW, Pool PE, Ross J Jr: Increased myocardial oxygen consumption and contractile state associated with increased heart rate in dogs. Circ Res **24:** 725, 1969

11. Covell JW, Ross J Jr, Taylor RR, Sonnenblick EH, Braunwald E: Effects of increasing frequency of contraction on the force-velocity relation of left ventricle. Cardiovasc Res **1:** 2, 1967
12. Mitchell JH, Wallace AG, Skinner NS: Intrinsic effects of heart rate on left ventricular performance. Am J Physiol **205:** 41, 1963
13. Noble MIM, Wyler J, Milne ENC, Trenchard D, Guz A: Effect of changes in heart rate on left ventricular performance in conscious dogs. Circ Res **24:** 285, 1969
14. Suga H, Sagawa K, Shoukas AA: Load independence of the instantaneous pressure-volume ratio of the canine left ventricle and effects of epinephrine and heart rate on the ratio. Circ Res **32:** 314, 1973
15. Suga H, Sagawa K: End-diastolic and end-systolic ventricular volume clamper for isolated canine heart. Am J Physiol **233:** H718, 1977
16. Sunagawa K, Burkhoff D, Lim K, Sagawa K: Impedance loading servo pump system for excised canine ventricle. Am J Physiol **243:** H346, 1982
17. Koch-Weser J, Blinks JR: The influence of the interval between beats on myocardial contractility. Pharmacol Rev **15:** 601, 1963
18. Sugimoto T, Sagawa K, Guyton AC: Effects of tachycardia on cardiac output during normal and increased venous return. Am J Physiol **211:** 288, 1966
19. Vatner SF, Franklin D, Higgins CB, Patrick T, Braunwald E: Left ventricular response to severe exertion in untethered dogs. J Clin Invest **51:** 3052, 1972
20. Higgins CB, Vatner SF, Franklin D, Braunwald E: Extent of regulation of the heart's contractile state in the conscious dog. J Clin Invest **52:** 1187, 1973
21. Burkhoff D, Yue DT, Franz MR, Hunter WC, Sagawa K: Mechanical restitution of isolated perfused canine left ventricles. Am J Physiol **246:** H8, 1984
22. Sunagawa K, Maughan WL, Sagawa K: Effect of regional ischemia on the left ventricular end-systolic pressure-volume relationship of isolated canine hearts. Circ Res **52:** 170, 1983
23. Aroesty J, McKay R, Heller G, Royal H, Grossman W: Left ventricular pressure-volume relations during pacing-induced ischemia. Circulation **68**(suppl III): III-103, 1983

A potential method of correcting intracavitary left ventricular filling pressures for the effects of positive end-expiratory airway pressure

ROY V. DITCHEY, M.D., JOANN LINDENFELD, M.D., E. WAYNE GROGAN, M.D., AND GARY O. ZERBE, PH.D.

ABSTRACT Based on the observation that positive end-expiratory airway pressure (PEEP) causes comparable increments in intrapericardial and right-sided intracardiac pressures, we hypothesized that intracavitary left ventricular filling pressures measured in the presence of PEEP can be corrected for increased intrathoracic pressure by subtracting the effects of PEEP on intracavitary right ventricular filling pressures. Ventricular function curves (aortic blood flow vs intracavitary left ventricular end-diastolic pressure [LVEDP]) were generated with and without 15 cm of water of PEEP in eight dogs. All curves were shifted to the right by PEEP (i.e., intracavitary LVEDP was higher for any submaximal level of aortic blood flow). However, when pressures measured in the presence of PEEP were "corrected" by subtracting the corresponding increment in intracavitary right ventricular end-diastolic pressure caused by PEEP at each level of ventricular filling, control and corrected PEEP data points appeared to fall on the same curve in five dogs, and differed only slightly in three dogs. Mean control and corrected PEEP curves derived by averaging polynomial regression coefficients for each condition differed significantly from uncorrected PEEP curves ($p < .05$), but not from each other. Analogous curves based on mean left atrial pressure were corrected equally well by subtracting the effects of PEEP on mean right atrial pressure. We conclude that the increments in intracavitary right heart filling pressures caused by PEEP can be used to correct intracavitary left heart filling pressures for the effects of PEEP on intrathoracic pressure.
Circulation 72, No. 3, 660–667, 1985.

POSITIVE end-expiratory airway pressure (PEEP) complicates hemodynamic monitoring in critically ill patients by increasing intrathoracic pressure. This effect alters the usual relationship between intravascular filling pressures and cardiac output, and invalidates standard guidelines[1, 2] for optimizing left ventricular preload in patients in low-output states. This is because left ventricular filling and stroke volume are functions of transmural, rather than intracavitary left ventricular end-diastolic pressure (LVEDP).[3] As a result, the increment in pressure around the left ventricle caused by PEEP effectively shifts ventricular function curves based on intracavitary pressures to the right (i.e., ventricular volume and cardiac output are lower for any measured pressure).[4] To remain useful as indexes of left ventricular preload in this setting, intracavitary filling pressures must be corrected for the effects of PEEP on intrathoracic pressure.

We recently found that PEEP causes changes in intracavitary right ventricular end-diastolic pressure (RVEDP) that are similar to changes in mean intrapericardial pressure over a wide range of ventricular filling conditions.[5] Based on this observation, and the knowledge that right ventricular pressure constitutes part of the effective pressure around the left ventricle,[3] we hypothesized that intracavitary left ventricular filling pressures measured in the presence of PEEP can be corrected for increased intrathoracic pressure by subtracting the effects of PEEP on right-sided intracardiac pressures. To test this hypothesis, we generated ventricular function curves with and without 15 cm of water of PEEP in anesthetized dogs. Curves based on intracavitary LVEDP and mean left atrial pressure were "corrected" by subtracting the effects of PEEP on intracavitary RVEDP and mean right atrial pressure, respectively, at each level of ventricular filling.

From the Cardiology Division, University of Colorado Health Sciences Center, Denver.
Supported in part by the Ravin-Goodstein Fund.
Address for correspondence: Roy V. Ditchey, M.D., Cardiology Division, Box 130, University of Colorado Health Sciences Center, 4200 East Ninth Ave., Denver, CO 80262.
Received March 27, 1984; revision accepted May 30, 1985.

Methods

Studies were performed in eight mongrel dogs weighing 22.3 to 32.0 kg. A preliminary left lateral thoracotomy was performed to allow instrumentation. At the time of surgery, a small (approximately 5 cm) incision was made in the superior, left lateral portion of the pericardium, through which an electromagnetic flow probe was placed around the proximal portion of the ascending aorta. In addition, a fluid-filled catheter was placed in the left atrium through the atrial appendage, and a balloon-type pressure manometer was positioned over the lateral surface of the left ventricle within the pericardial space. Each balloon was hand-constructed according to previously described methods,[5, 6] and consisted of condom rubber cemented to both sides of a thin ring of silicone rubber sheeting with an inner chamber containing a silicone rubber tube with multiple sideholes. These balloon manometers were specifically designed for the measurement of pressure between two contiguous surfaces.[7] The pressure-volume characteristics of each balloon were determined before its insertion, and the internal volume necessary to maintain zero pressure was recorded. In addition, a linear pressure response over the range of pressures encountered in each study was confirmed for each balloon in vitro. The balloon rim was attached to the parietal pericardium at one or two points to prevent migration, after which the pericardial incision was closed, and the flow probe electrodes, left atrial catheter, and balloon connecting tubing were exteriorized through small incisions in the lateral chest wall. The chest then was closed in layers, and the dogs were allowed to recover for several days.

On the day of study, the dogs were anesthetized with intravenous morphine (2 mg/kg) and α-chloralose (100 mg/kg), intubated, and mechanically ventilated with 100% oxygen. Fluid-filled catheters were introduced through a femoral artery and femoral and external jugular veins and positioned in the left ventricle, right ventricle, and right atrium, respectively. Catheter positions were confirmed by fluoroscopy and appropriate pressure recordings in all cases. In addition, a transvenous pacing wire and a large-bore catheter for fluid administration were introduced through separate veins and positioned in the right atrium and inferior vena cava, respectively. Propranolol (1 mg/kg) was administered intravenously, after which atrial pacing was instituted at a rate of approximately 10 to 20 beats/min above each animal's intrinsic heart rate. This was done in an attempt to prevent spontaneous or volume-related changes in cardiac sympathetic stimulation and heart rate that might influence the shape of the ventricular function curves generated during each study. Four dogs were given 0.4 mg iv atropine to eliminate Mobitz I atrioventricular block. The right and left atrial and ventricular catheters were connected to Gould P23Db pressure transducers with zero reference set at the midheart level (determined by fluoroscopy). The intrapericardial balloon was connected to a fifth Gould transducer set at the same level and then filled with the volume of air previously shown to maintain zero pressure in the absence of deformation in vitro. The ascending aortic flow probe was connected to a Zepeda SWF-4 square-wave electromagnetic flowmeter and pressures and aortic flow signals were recorded along with a limb-lead electrocardiogram on a Beckman R611 eight-channel recorder. Measurements were made with respiration suspended for several seconds at end-expiration, at a time when pressures and aortic blood flow were stable. Pressures were checked frequently throughout each study for baseline drift, and the end-diastolic flow signal recorded under each set of study conditions was assumed to represent zero flow. Flow probe calibrations were performed in vitro.

To compare the effects of PEEP on intrapericardial and intracardiac pressures, intrapericardial and right and left atrial and ventricular pressures were recorded as airway pressure was increased from 0 to 20 cm of water in 2 cm of water increments by placing the expiratory hose of the ventilator under water. Paired ventricular function curves were then generated by recording pressures and aortic flow signals both with and without 15 cm of water of PEEP under baseline filling conditions, and again after each increment in blood volume as volume was expanded by administering 10% dextran in 100 ml aliquots. This procedure was continued until ascending aortic blood flow (a close approximation of cardiac output) appeared to reach a plateau. Intrapericardial and intracardiac pressures were then recorded again as airway pressure was increased from 0 to 20 cm of water in 2 cm of water increments to determine whether the relative effects of PEEP on intrapericardial and right and left atrial and ventricular pressures were altered by volume loading. At the end of each study, the dog was killed by administration of intravenous potassium chloride, and the ascending aortic blood flow signal was recorded under conditions of circulatory arrest. This signal closely approximated the end-diastolic reference points recorded immediately before the animal was killed in each case.

Ventricular function curves were generated from measurements made with and without 15 cm of water of PEEP by separately plotting ascending aortic blood flow as a function of either intracavitary LVEDP or mean left atrial pressure. Left-sided intracardiac pressures measured in the presence of PEEP were "corrected" by subtracting the increment in the analogous right heart pressure caused by PEEP at each respective level of ventricular filling. Intracavitary LVEDP was corrected by subtracting the increment in intracavitary RVEDP, and mean left atrial pressure was corrected by subtracting the increment in mean right atrial pressure.

Data from each control and uncorrected and corrected PEEP curve were fit to second-order polynomial equations by standard regression techniques. Ascending aortic blood flow (Q_A) was considered a function of left ventricular filling pressure (P) according to the relationship

$$Q_A = a + b_1 P + b_2 P^2$$

where a is the value of Q_A at zero pressure, b_1 and b_2 are regression coefficients that describe the shape of the Q_A vs P curve, and P is either intracavitary LVEDP or mean left atrial pressure. This model was chosen when higher order polynomial regressions demonstrated that mean coefficients corresponding to third- and fourth-order terms did not differ significantly from zero.[8] Mean curves for each condition were derived by averaging regression coefficients.

The differences between control, uncorrected, and corrected PEEP curves were tested statistically by multivariate analysis of regression coefficients using the Bonferroni inequality for multiple simultaneous comparisons.[8]

Results

The effects of incremental increases in end-expiratory airway pressure on intrapericardial and right- and left-sided intracardiac filling pressures are compared in figures 1 and 2. PEEP caused increments in intracavitary RVEDP and mean right atrial pressure that were nearly identical to changes in intrapericardial pressure under baseline filling conditions, and that were similar to (although slightly less than) changes in intrapericardial pressure after volume loading. PEEP caused changes in intracavitary LVEDP and mean left atrial pressure that were similar to (although slightly

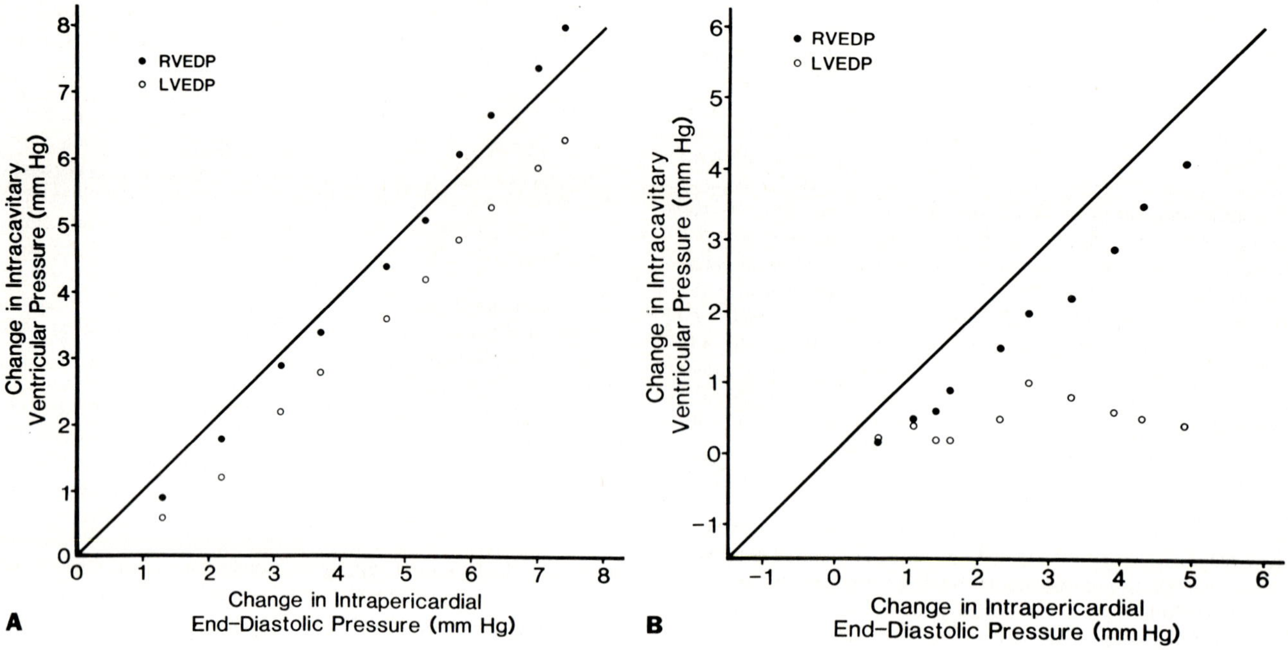

FIGURE 1. Relative effects of PEEP on intrapericardial and intracavitary RVEDP and LVEDP before (*A*) and after (*B*) volume loading. Data points represent average changes from baseline values in eight dogs as end-expiratory airway pressure was increased from 0 to 20 cm of water in 2 cm of water increments. The solid line represents the line of identity. Intracavitary LVEDP in the absence of PEEP averaged 0.6 ± 0.4 and 19.1 ± 1.6 mm Hg before and after volume loading, respectively.

less than) the increments in intrapericardial pressure under baseline filling conditions, but which bore no relationship in either magnitude or direction to the changes in intrapericardial pressure after volume loading.

Ventricular function curves based on intracavitary left heart filling pressures were shifted to the right by PEEP (i.e., pressures were higher for any submaximal level of ascending aortic blood flow) in all eight dogs. This was true whether curves were based on intracavi-

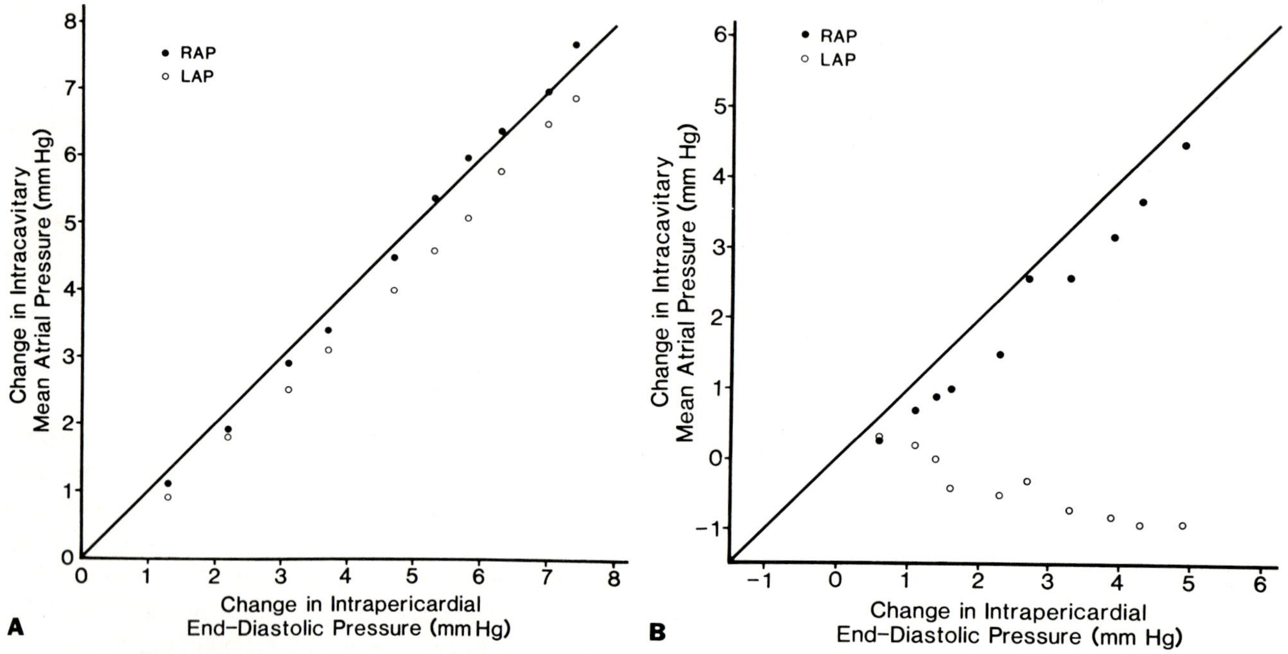

FIGURE 2. Relative effects of PEEP on intrapericardial and intracavitary mean right (RAP) and left (LAP) atrial pressures before (*A*) and after (*B*) volume loading. Data points represent average changes from baseline values in eight dogs as end-expiratory airway pressure was increased from 0 to 20 cm of water in 2 cm of water increments. The solid line represents the line of identity. Mean LAP in the absence of PEEP averaged 0.6 ± 0.5 and 20.3 ± 1.6 mm Hg before and after volume loading, respectively.

tary LVEDP or mean left atrial pressure. Correction by subtracting the increment in intracavitary RVEDP or mean right atrial pressure caused by PEEP from the corresponding left-sided intracardiac pressure shifted these curves back toward control in each case (two examples are shown in figure 3). In five dogs, control and corrected PEEP data points appeared to fall on the same curve; the corrected PEEP curves fell slightly to the right of the control curves in two dogs and slightly to the left of the control curves in one dog. Individual

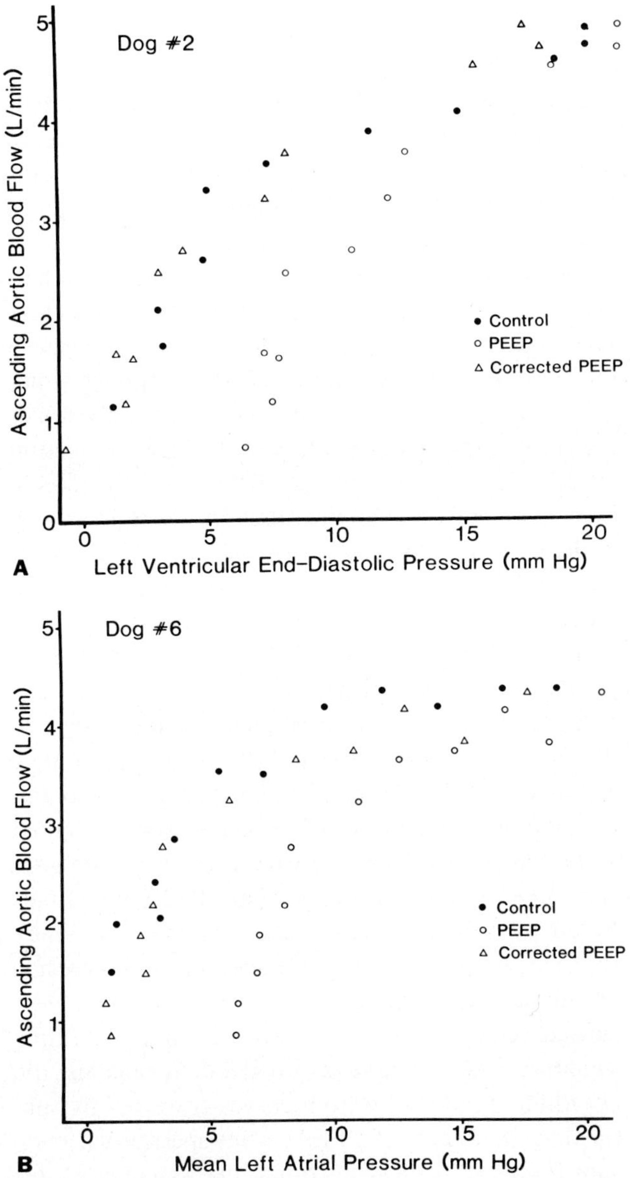

FIGURE 3. Individual ventricular function curves based on intracavitary LVEDP (*A*) and mean left atrial pressure (*B*) obtained in two separate studies. Each intracavitary left heart pressure measured in the presence of PEEP was corrected by subtracting the corresponding increment in right heart pressure (RVEDP or mean right atrial pressure) caused by PEEP at each level of ventricular filling. Control and corrected PEEP data points appear to fall on the same curve in both *A* and *B*.

control, uncorrected, and corrected PEEP curves were well described by second-order polynomial equations ($r = .84$ to $.99$). Mean regression coefficients for control and corrected PEEP curves differed significantly from coefficients for uncorrected PEEP curves ($p < .05$), but not from each other (table 1 and figure 4). This was true whether curves were based on intracavitary LVEDP or mean left atrial pressure. For the purpose of comparison, a second set of corrected curves was generated by subtracting the corresponding increment in intrapericardial pressure from each intracavitary LVEDP and mean left atrial pressure measured in the presence of PEEP. Curves corrected in this manner were also well described by second-order polynomial equations ($r = .93$ to $.99$), and did not differ significantly from either control curves or curves corrected by subtracting the effects of PEEP on intracavitary right heart filling pressures (figure 5).

Discussion

Intracavitary LVEDP and its correlates, mean left atrial and pulmonary arterial wedge pressures, are useful indexes of left ventricular preload when measured in the presence of atmospheric airway pressure.[1, 2] This has proven to be the case[1, 2, 9–13] even though the relationship between these pressures and ventricular filling in any individual patient is influenced to an unknown extent by the compliance of the cardiac chambers and the effective pressure acting on the outer surfaces of the left ventricle. However, standard guidelines for interpreting these pressures are based on studies performed in the presence of atmospheric airway pressure,[1, 2] and are not valid in the presence of PEEP, when the usual relationship between intracavitary pressure and volume is altered by an increase in intrathoracic pressure. Accurate interpretation of intravascular filling pressures must take into account any baseline change in pressure around the left ventricle.

Changes in left-sided intracardiac pressures are not indicative of the effects of PEEP on this external pressure for several reasons. First, although PEEP consistently increases intrathoracic pressure, it decreases left ventricular volume and, under most circumstances, transmural LVEDP.[5, 14, 15] Since, by definition, changes in intracavitary LVEDP must equal the sum of changes in transmural and external pressures ($\Delta \text{LVEDP}_{\text{intracavitary}} = \Delta \text{LVEDP}_{\text{transmural}} + \Delta$ external pressure), net changes in intracavitary pressure are determined by the combined (and opposite) effects of PEEP on intrathoracic pressure and ventricular volume. Furthermore, the magnitude and direction of these changes depend not only on the level of PEEP, but also

TABLE 1
Polynomial regression coefficients (mean ± SEM)

	A			B		
	a	b_1	b_2	a	b_1	b_2
Control	1878±234	309±48	−8.696±1.997	1965±265	301±43	−8.214±1.619
PEEP	−856±564	559±88	−14.621±3.027	−1417±704	600±96	−14.958±2.759
Corrected PEEP	1743±185	336±42	−10.076±1.604	1596±249	372±50	−11.503±1.977

Regression coefficients are for the model: ascending aortic blood flow $= a + b_1P + b_2P^2$, where P = either intracavitary LVEDP or mean left atrial pressure. Data for corrected PEEP curves were derived by subtracting the effects of PEEP on intracavitary right heart filling pressures (see text for explanation). Control and corrected PEEP coefficients differed significantly ($p < .05$) from uncorrected PEEP coefficients, but not from each other. This was true whether curves were based on intracavitary LVEDP (A) or mean left atrial pressure (B).

on the ventricular filling conditions under which PEEP is applied.[5] When baseline ventricular volume is small, PEEP causes pressure around the left ventricle to rise more than transmural pressure falls, and left-sided intracardiac pressures increase.[5] However, with larger initial volumes, comparable reductions in filling due to PEEP cause greater decrements in transmural LVEDP, due to the nonlinear relationship between left ventricular transmural pressure and volume.[3] As a result, transmural pressure falls as much or more than external pressure rises, and intracavitary pressure either remains the same or decreases.[5] This influence of baseline filling conditions on the response of left-sided intracardiac pressues to PEEP is illustrated in figures 1 and 2. When PEEP was applied in the presence of relatively low initial intravascular pressures, both intracavitary LVEDP and mean left atrial pressure increased (although slightly less than intrapericardial pressure). However, after volume loading, changes in left-sided intracardiac pressures bore no consistent relationship to changes in intrapericardial pressure, and often differed in both magnitude and direction.

In contrast, the effects of PEEP on right-sided intracardiac pressures closely approximate changes in intrapericardial pressure regardless of the filling conditions under which PEEP is applied.[5] This is partly because PEEP has opposing effects on right ventricular volume. By increasing intrathoracic pressure, PEEP decreases the driving force for blood return to the thorax,[16] and reduces diastolic right ventricular filling; but, by increasing pulmonary vascular resistance,[15, 17] PEEP increases the systolic load faced by the right ventricle[15] and impedes right ventricular ejection. We have found that PEEP typically increases right-sided intracardiac pressures as much (figures 1 and 2) or slightly more[5] than intrapericardial pressure when baseline filling pressures are low, and by the same amount or slightly less than intrapericardial pressure after volume loading. This suggests that right ventricular volume potentially can either increase or decrease in response to PEEP, depending on the filling conditions present when PEEP is applied. It also suggests that volume loading, by decreasing the effects of PEEP on pulmonary vascular resistance,[17] can shift the balance between the effects of PEEP on right ventricular volume toward decreased filling. However, because the right ventricle is a thin-walled, compliant structure, volume changes that do occur have only minor effects on transmural RVEDP.[5, 15] Since changes in intracavitary pressure must equal the sum of changes in transmural and external pressures for the right as well as the left ventricle, a relatively unchanged transmural pressure predicts that intrapericardial and right-sided intracardiac pressures will increase by similar amounts ($\Delta\ RVEDP_{intracavitary} = \Delta\ RVEDP_{transmural} + \Delta$ external pressure $\cong \Delta$ external pressure).

In the present study, correction for the effects of PEEP on right-sided intracardiac pressures accurately restored the baseline relationships between intracavitary left ventricular filling pressures and ascending aortic blood flow. This was true whether performance curves were based on intracavitary LVEDP and corrected by subtracting the increment in intracavitary RVEDP, or on mean left atrial pressure and corrected by subtracting the increment in mean right atrial pressure caused by PEEP at each level of ventricular filling (figures 3 and 4). Curves corrected in this manner did not differ significantly from curves corrected by subtracting the effects of PEEP on intrapericardial pressure (figure 5). We believe that the accuracy of this correction is partly due to the fact that intracavitary RVEDP *is* part of the effective pressure around the left ventricle, acting across the interventricular septum.[3] This compensates intrinsically for any differences between the effects of PEEP on intrapericardial and right-sided intracardiac pressures. The correlation between

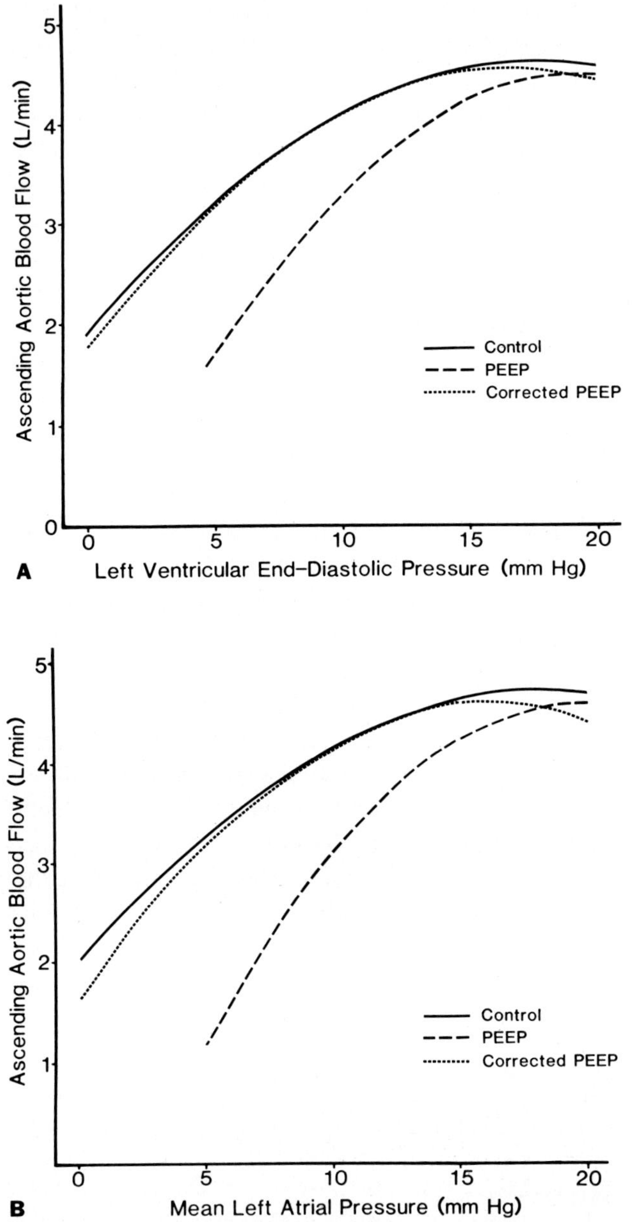

FIGURE 4. Mean ventricular function curves derived by averaging polynomial regression coefficients from eight dogs. Each intracavitary left heart pressure measured in the presence of PEEP was corrected by subtracting the corresponding increment in right heart pressure (RVEDP or mean right atrial pressure) caused by PEEP at each level of ventricular filling. Control and corrected PEEP curves differed significantly from uncorrected PEEP curves ($p < .05$), but not from each other. This was true whether curves were based on intracavitary LVEDP (*A*) or mean left atrial pressure (*B*).

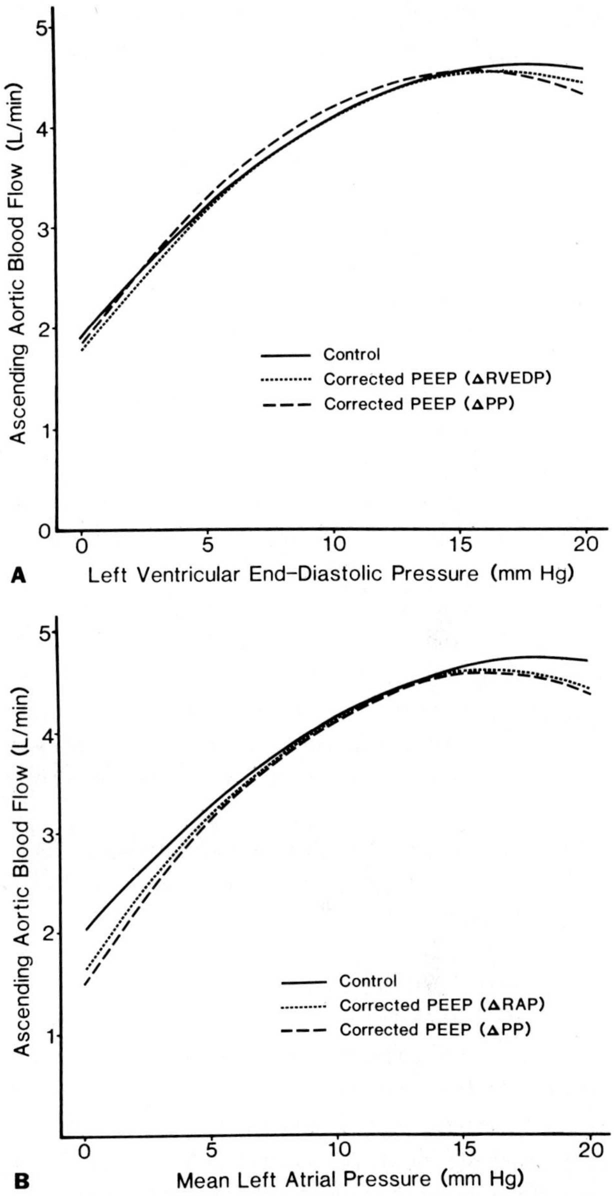

FIGURE 5. A comparison of ventricular function curves corrected by subtracting the effects of PEEP on intrapericardial and intracavitary right heart filling pressures. Mean curves for each condition were derived by averaging polynomial regression coefficients from eight dogs. Each intracavitary LVEDP measured in the presence of PEEP was corrected by subtracting the corresponding increment in either RVEDP (Δ RVEDP) or intrapericardial pressure (Δ PP) caused by PEEP at each level of ventricular filling. Mean left atrial pressures were corrected by subtracting the corresponding increments in either mean right atrial pressure (Δ RAP) or Δ PP. Curves corrected by the two methods did not differ significantly from each other or from control curves. This was true whether curves were based on intracavitary LVEDP (*A*) or mean left atrial pressure (*B*).

control and corrected PEEP curves at high filling pressures also may have been aided by the shape of the normal function curve (i.e., slight undercorrection for a change in external pressure would not be appreciable when operating on a relatively flat portion of the curve). However, from a practical standpoint, it is important only that corrected pressures ultimately have the same relationship to ventricular performance as pressures measured in the absence of PEEP.

Although these findings suggest that the rightward displacement of ventricular function curves caused by PEEP results primarily (if not entirely) from an increase in external pressure, we did not attempt to assess changes in other determinants of ventricular performance. As a result, we can only assume that the effects of PEEP on variables other than transmural pressure[6, 18–20] either offset each other, or were relatively unimportant under the present study conditions. In practice, upward or downward displacement of the relationship between ventricular filling and stroke volume due to a change in either afterload or inotropic state[20] would not negate the usefulness of a corrected filling pressure in evaluating left ventricular preload. However, a change in left ventricular compliance[6, 18, 19] would be directly relevant, and might, under some circumstances, prevent complete correction of intracavitary filling pressures. The extent to which PEEP alters left ventricular compliance, the responsible mechanisms, and whether changes in compliance depend on the intravascular volume present when PEEP is applied have not been clearly established. However, it is tempting to speculate that correction for changes in right-sided intracardiac pressures might compensate partially for any decrease in compliance mediated through changes in right ventricular volume and septal configuration.

In summary, we found that intracavitary left ventricular filling pressures measured in the presence of PEEP and corrected by subtracting the effects of PEEP on right-sided intracardiac pressures have approximately the same relationship to ventricular performance as intracavitary pressures measured under baseline conditions. It seems reasonable to suggest, therefore, that pressures corrected in this manner can be interpreted in accordance with the same guidelines[1, 2] applied to pressures measured in the presence of atmospheric airway pressure. This potentially represents an attractive alternative to esophageal manometry (which is the only practical method of estimating changes in intrathoracic pressure in most clinical settings). Right-sided intracardiac pressures can be measured easily, while esophageal recordings require additional instrumentation and may not accurately reflect changes in pressure around the left ventricle in the presence of PEEP.[21] In practice, our proposal could be implemented with standard, double-lumen catheters for measuring pulmonary arterial wedge and central venous pressures. It would be necessary to ensure that the tip of the catheter was positioned in a dependent portion of the lung to avoid potential discrepancies between wedge and left atrial pressures in the presence of PEEP.[22, 23] Wedge pressures could then be corrected by simply subtracting the difference between central venous pressures recorded with and without positive airway pressure at any given level of filling. Although the appropriate correction factor would need to be determined whenever airway pressure or ventricular filling conditions were altered significantly, we believe that careful application of these techniques would strengthen the relationship between wedge pressures and ventricular performance in this setting.

However, it is important to recognize the limitations of the present study. Our conclusions are based on a comparison of pressure-flow relationships derived under steady-state conditions with and without 15 cm of water of PEEP in dogs. We purposefully suspended respiration for several seconds at end-expiration to allow a relatively pure comparison of pressures and flows in the presence and absence of positive airway pressure. We have not yet validated this method of correction at other levels of PEEP, during cyclic positive pressure ventilation (with or without PEEP) over the range of ventilatory patterns that might be encountered clinically, or in human subjects. Furthermore, the similarity between the effects of PEEP on intrapericardial and right-sided intracardiac pressures is largely a chance occurrence, and depends on the combined effects of several factors that could vary independently in the clinical setting. It remains to be determined whether the method of correction proposed in this study is equally valid in the presence of diseases that alter either right ventricular compliance or the effects of PEEP on intrathoracic pressure and pulmonary vascular resistance.

We would like to express our appreciation to Stephen Bell and Holly Coller for their expert technical assistance, and to Jeanne Boschi and Glenda Murphy for typing the manuscript.

References

1. Russell RO, Rackley CE, Pombo J, Hunt D, Potanin C, Dodge HT: Effects of increasing left ventricular filling pressure in patients with acute myocardial infarction. J Clin Invest **49:** 1539, 1970
2. Crexells C, Chatterjee K, Forrester JS, Dikshit K, Swan HJC: Optimal level of filling pressure in the left side of the heart in acute myocardial infarction. N Engl J Med **289:** 1263, 1973
3. Mirsky I, Rankin JS: The effects of geometry, elasticity, and external pressures on the diastolic pressure-volume and stiffness-stress relations. How important is the pericardium? Circ Res **44:** 601, 1979
4. Marini JJ, Culver BH, Butler J: Effect of positive end-expiratory pressure on canine ventricular function curves. J Appl Physiol **51:** 1367, 1981
5. Ditchey RV: Volume-dependent effects of positive airway pressure on intracavitary left ventricular end-diastolic pressure. Circulation **69:** 815, 1984
6. Haynes JB, Carson SD, Whitney WP, Zerbe GO, Hyers TM, Steele P: Positive end-expiratory pressure shifts left ventricular diastolic pressure-area curves. J Appl Physiol **48:** 670, 1980
7. McMahon SM, Permutt S, Proctor DF: A model to evaluate pleural surface pressure measuring devices. J Appl Physiol **27:** 886, 1969
8. Grizzle JE, Allen DM: Analysis of growth and dose response curves. Biometrics **25:** 357, 1969

9. Forrester JS, Diamond G, Chatterjee K, Swan HJC: Medical therapy of acute myocardial infarction by application of hemodynamic subsets. N Engl J Med **295:** 1356; 1404, 1976
10. Weber KT, Janicki JS, Russell RO, Rackley CE: Identification of high risk subsets of acute myocardial infarction derived from the myocardial infarction research units cooperative study data bank. Am J Cardiol **41:** 197, 1978
11. Rackley CE, Russell RO, Mantle JA, Moraski RE: Cardiogenic shock: recognition and management, Cardiovasc Clin **7:** 251, 1975
12. Greene HL, Kelly DT, Taylor DR, Pitt B: Hemodynamic effects of plasma volume expansion and prognostic implications in acute myocardial infarction. Circulation **49:** 106, 1974
13. Raphael LD, Mantle JA, Moraski RE, Rogers WJ, Russell RO, Rackley CE: Quantitative assessment of ventricular performance in unstable ischemic heart disease by dextran function curves. Circulation **55:** 858, 1977
14. Fewell JE, Abendschein DR, Carlson CJ, Murray JF, Rapaport E: Continuous positive-pressure ventilation decreases right and left ventricular end-diastolic volumes in the dog. Circ Res **46:** 125, 1980
15. Rankin JS, Olsen CO, Arentzen CE, Tyson GS, Maier G, Smith PK, Hammon JW, Davis JW, McHale PA, Anderson RW, Sabiston DC: The effects of airway pressure on cardiac function in intact dogs and man. Circulation **66:** 108, 1982
16. Guyton AC, Jones CE, Coleman TG: Circulatory physiology: cardiac output and its regulation. Philadelphia, 1973, WB Saunders Company, p 430
17. Zarins CK, Virgilio RW, Smith DE, Peters RM: The effect of vascular volume on positive end-expiratory pressure-induced cardiac output depression and wedge-left atrial pressure discrepancy. J Surg Res **23:** 348, 1977
18. Scharf SM, Brown R, Saunders N, Green LH, Ingram RH: Changes in canine left ventricular size and configuration with positive end-expiratory pressure. Circ Res **44:** 672, 1979
19. Jardin F, Farcot J, Boisante L, Curien N, Margairaz A, Bourdarias J: Influence of positive end-expiratory pressure on left ventricular performance. N Engl J Med **304:** 387, 1981
20. Grindlinger GA, Manny J, Justice R, Dunham B, Shepro D, Hechtman HB: Presence of negative inotropic agents in canine plasma during positive end-expiratory pressure. Circ Res **45:** 460, 1979
21. Culver B, Marini J, Butler J: Lung volume and pleural pressure effects on ventricular function. J Appl Physiol **50:** 630, 1981
22. Tooker J, Huseby J, Butler J: The effect of Swan-Ganz catheter height on the wedge-pressure-left atrial pressure relationship in edema during positive pressure ventilation. Am Rev Respir Dis **117:** 721, 1978
23. Shasby DM, Dauber IM, Pfister S, Anderson JT, Carson SB, Manart F, Hyers TM: Swan-Ganz catheter location and left atrial pressure determine the accuracy of the wedge pressure when positive end-expiratory pressure is used. Chest **80:** 666, 1981

Diminished stroke volume during inspiration: a reverse thoracic pump

CRAIG O. OLSEN, M.D., GEORGE S. TYSON, M.D., GEORGE W. MAIER, M.D., JAMES W. DAVIS, M.S., AND J. SCOTT RANKIN, M.D.

ABSTRACT In 12 conscious dogs, a three-dimensional array of pulse-transit ultrasonic transducers was used to measure left ventricular anterior-posterior minor, septal–free wall minor, and basal-apical major diameters. Matched micromanometers measured left ventricular, right ventricular, and intrapleural pressures. Electromagnetic ascending aortic blood flow and right ventricular transverse diameter were measured in five of the dogs. A major cause of the inspiratory decline in stroke volume in this preparation appeared to be reflex tachycardia and autonomic changes associated with inspiration. However, when heart rate was controlled by atrial pacing or pharmacologic autonomic attenuation (propranolol and atropine), stroke volume still decreased around 10%, with an inspiratory decrease in pleural pressure of 10 mm Hg. Based on the measurements of ventricular dimension, venous return to the right ventricle appeared to be augmented significantly during inspiration and the transient increase in right ventricular volume was associated with leftward interventricular septal shifting and altered diastolic left ventricular geometry. However, left ventricular end-diastolic volume was changed minimally, implying that alterations in preload were not important. Moreover, transmural left ventricular ejection pressure, calculated as intracavitary minus pleural pressure, was not significantly changed, and it seemed that neither pressure nor geometric components of afterload were altered significantly by inspiration. The inspiratory fall in left ventricular stroke volume correlated best with the decline in intracavitary left ventricular ejection pressure referenced to atmospheric pressure. It is hypothesized that during ejection, left ventricular pressure referenced to atmospheric pressure is the hydraulic force effecting stroke volume and that the decline in this effective left ventricular ejection pressure is responsible for the inspiratory fall in stroke volume through a reverse thoracic pump mechanism.
Circulation 72, No. 3, 668–679, 1985.

THE EFFECTS of respiratory movement on cardiovascular function are numerous and have been the subject of several extensive monographs.[1–3] Systematic investigation into these effects dates back to 1751 when Albrecht von Haller noted an inspiratory augmentation in venous return to the right ventricle of the dog and cat.[3] Eighteen years earlier Stephen Hales reported his famous series of experiments in the horse and may have been the first to record the inspiratory fall in arterial blood pressure.[4] Although Hales did not make the association between inspiration and the periodic fall in the oscillatory pulse pressure of the carotid artery, numerous subsequent investigators have confirmed this phenomenon and have documented an inspiratory decline in left ventricular stroke volume in both experimental animals[5–11] and man.[12–14]

Several hypotheses have been advanced to explain the inspiratory fall in left ventricular stroke volume, including (1) delayed pulmonary venous transit time,[7, 15, 16] (2) increased pulmonary venous capacitance and diminished left ventricular filling,[17] (3) reduction in left ventricular preload due to leftward interventricular septal shifting,[18, 19] (4) increased left ventricular afterload from altered geometry due to leftward interventricular septal shifting,[8] and (5) increased inspiratory left ventricular transmural pressure, which augments afterload.[6, 9, 20] The present studies were undertaken to investigate the relative importance of these phenomena during spontaneous respiration in a conscious canine preparation.

From the Departments of Surgery and Physiology, Duke University Medical Center, Durham.

This work was supported by NIH grants 2RO1 H109315-17 and RO1 H129436-01, and by research grants from the Whitaker Foundation and the North Carolina Heart Association.

Address for correspondence: Craig O. Olsen, M.D., Box 3492, Duke University Medical Center, Durham, NC 27710.

Received April 26, 1985; revision accepted June 20, 1985.

Dr. Rankin is a recipient of the John A. Hartford Foundation Fellowship.

Methods

Instrumentation and acquisition of data. Twelve healthy adult mongrel dogs (20 to 32 kg) underwent surgical preparation for subsequent studies in the conscious state. The method of implantation of instrumentation has been described previously.[21] Briefly, in all dogs an array of pulse-transit ultrasonic dimension transducers was used to measure three orthogonal left ventricular dimensions: the anterior-posterior minor, septal–free wall minor, and basal-apical major diameters. All transducers, except the one in the septal position, which was positioned near the right ventricular subendocardial surface, were placed epicardially. Silicone rubber introducers were implanted in the right ventricle, left atrium, and intrapleural space of each dog, as were bipolar atrial pacing electrodes. In five dogs, right ventricular septal–free wall transverse diameter and electromagnetic ascending aortic blood flow were measured as well (figure 1, *top left*).

Seven to 14 days after recovery from the implantation procedure, each dog was studied in the conscious state while resting quietly on its right side. The dimension transducers were coupled directly to a custom-designed sonomicrometer.[21] Prewarmed matched micromanometers (PC-350, Millar Instruments, Houston) were passed via the introducers into the mid left and right ventricles and pleural space. Airtight introducer connectors prevented ventricular hemorrhage and pneumothorax. The aortic flow probes were coupled to a sine-wave flowmeter (Statham, M4001, Los Angeles). The performance characteristics of these instruments have been described previously.[22–25]

Cardiac dimensions, pressures, and aortic blood flow were recorded on magnetic tape for subsequent digital analysis. Data were recorded in each experiment during normal spontaneous respiration and deep spontaneous respiration against inspiratory inflow resistance through a gauze sponge. Heart rate was controlled by atrial pacing at 10 min^{-1} higher than the fastest heart rate observed during the respiratory cycle. In six dogs, after completion of initial studies, the autonomic nervous system was pharmacologically attenuated with intravenous propranolol (1 mg kg^{-1}) and atropine (2 mg). Data were collected again during normal and deep spontaneous respirations.

At the conclusion of all studies, the animals were killed, their hearts were excised, and the volume of the left ventricular muscle mass was calculated as the average of three volume displacements of water in a graduated cylinder.

Data analysis. The recorded analog data were filtered once at 50 Hz and digitized at 200 Hz for analysis. Left ventricular transmural pressure was calculated as left ventricular intracavitary pressure minus simultaneous intrapleural pressure. Right ventricular transmural pressure was determined similarly, and interventricular transseptal pressure was computed as left ventricular intracavitary pressure minus right ventricular intracavitary pressure. The first derivative of left ventricular transmural pressure (dP/dt) was calculated from the digitized ventricular pressure waveform with use of a five-point polyorthogonal approximation.[25]

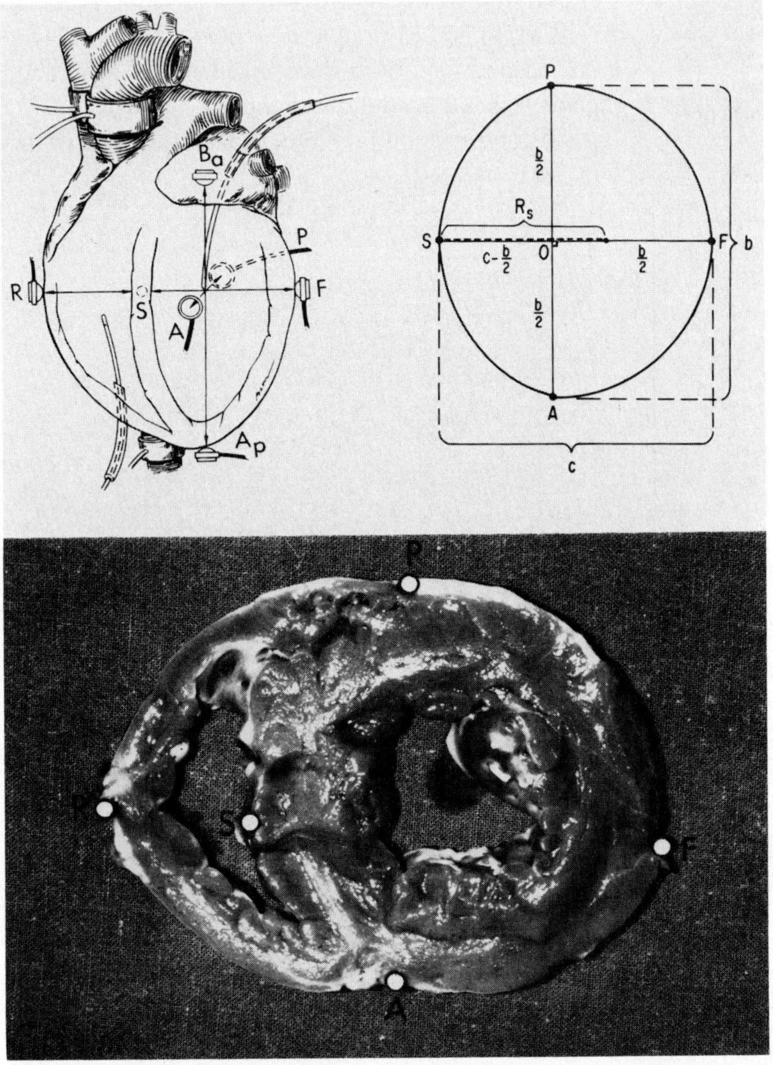

FIGURE 1. *Top left,* Preparation used to assess the three-dimensional geometry of the left ventricle. The anterior-posterior minor (A to P), septal–free wall minor (S to F), and basal-apical (Ba to Ap) major diameters were measured in the conscious dog and fit to a double hemiellipsoidal model. Biventricular and pleural pressures were measured with micromanometers passed through implanted silicone rubber tubes. In five preparations right ventricular transverse diameters (S to R) and ascending aortic blood flow were measured as well. *Top right,* Model of left ventricular latitudinal plane geometry of the left ventricular double hemiellipsoidal model to which dimensions were fitted. A, S, P, and F correspond, respectively, to the placement positions of the anterior, septal, posterior, and lateral free wall dimension transducers. b = external anterior-posterior minor diameter; c = septal–free wall minor diameter; R_S = left ventricular septal radius of curvature in the latitudinal plane. *Bottom,* Postmortem transverse section of myocardium from one dog demonstrating the actual position of the four epicardial and one endocardial dimension transducers. A = anterior; S = septal; P = posterior; F = left ventricular lateral free wall; R = right ventricular free wall.

Measurements of left ventricular dimension were modeled by a double hemiellipsoidal geometry as described previously.[21] External left ventricular volume was calculated as the sum of the two ellipsoidal segments inscribed by ASPA and AFPA from figure 1, *top right.* Calculation of external left ventricular volume yielded results mathematically equivalent to the formula for a general ellipsoid, $(\pi/6)$ a b c, where a is the major diameter, b is the anterior-posterior minor diameter, and c is the septal–free wall minor diameter. Postmortem left ventricular wall volume was subtracted from external left ventricular volume to yield intracavitary left ventricular chamber volume. Aortic blood flow was either measured or derived from the inverted first derivative of left ventricular chamber volume $(-dV_I/dt)$. Geometric deformation of the left ventricle was determined including the latitudinal septal and free wall radii of curvature, as well as septal displacement, and regional left ventricular septal and free wall tensions were calculated according to the Laplace relationship, as described previously.[21]

Comparisons were made between end-diastolic dimensions, chamber volume, regional wall tensions, and measured and calculated pressures at end-expiration and peak inspiration for both normal and deep respirations by an analysis of variance. Similar comparisons were made for end-ejection dimension and volume data from the same cardiac cycles during which end-diastolic data were obtained. In an analogous fashion, peak ejection pressure, aortic blood flow, and calculated tension data were compared at end-expiration and peak inspiration. Linear regression analysis was used to determine the relationship between left ventricular pressures, intrapleural pressures, left ventricular end-diastolic volume, peak aortic blood flow, and left ventricular stroke volumes throughout the respiratory cycle. Unless otherwise specified, all reported data were obtained during control of heart rate by atrial pacing.

Results

Representative analog dimension, pressure, and flow data obtained during three deep inspirations without atrial pacing are illustrated in figure 2. A marked inspiratory increase in heart rate was evident. During inspiration, the fall in intrapleural pressure produced a similar decrease in right and left ventricular intracavitary pressures. Stroke shortening decreased in all three left ventricular dimensions. The end-diastolic diameters and volume changed in a variable fashion because of rate-dependent changes in ventricular filling. This resulted in a progressive and significant inspiratory fall in peak aortic blood flow and stroke volume as inspiration progressed (figure 2).

Atrial pacing (figure 3) and autonomic blockade (figure 4) ablated the respiratory variation in heart rate. End-diastolic diameters and volume changed minimally, but peak aortic blood flow and stroke volume continued to decline during inspiration. During normal spontaneous respiration, intrapleural pressure decreased from an average of -1.6 ± 0.7 mm Hg (mean $\pm$ SEM) at end-expiration to -6.1 ± 0.7 mm Hg at peak inspiration. With deep spontaneous respiration against inspiratory inflow resistance through a gauze sponge, intrapleural pressure decreased from an aver-

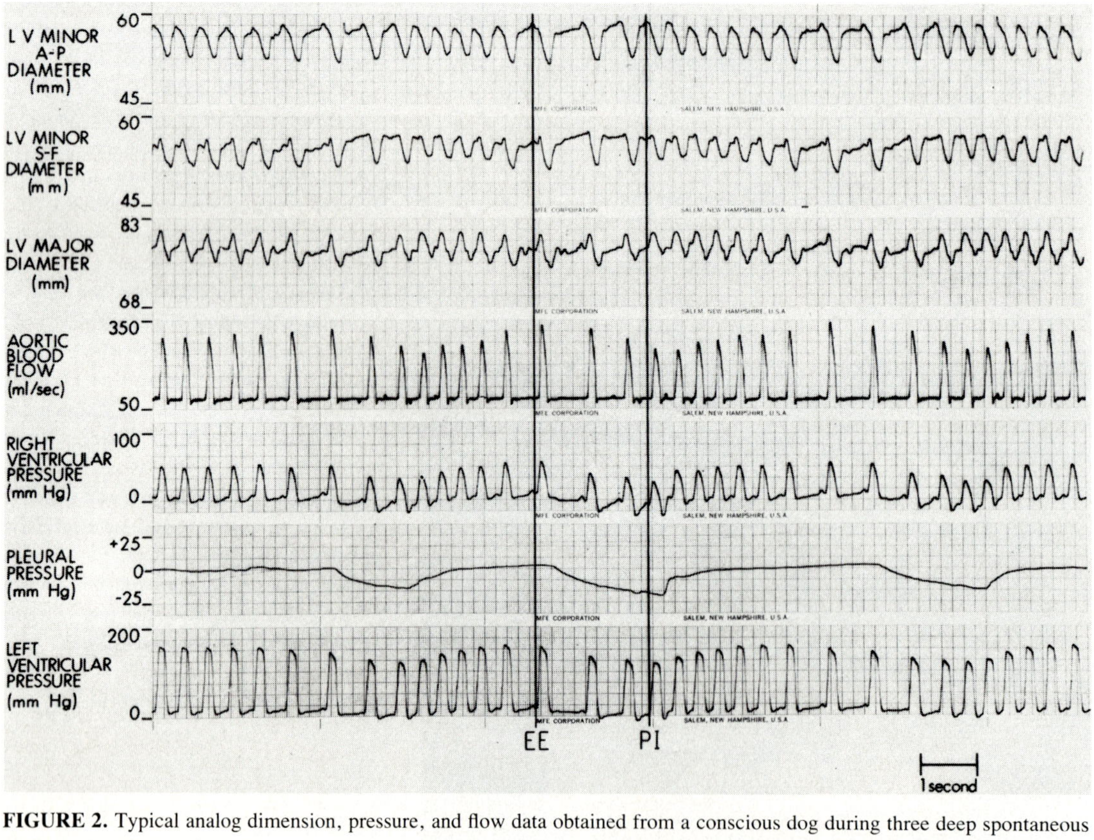

FIGURE 2. Typical analog dimension, pressure, and flow data obtained from a conscious dog during three deep spontaneous respirations without atrial pacing and demonstrating the marked respiratory variation in heart rate. EE = end-diastole at end-expiration; PI = end-diastole at peak inspiration.

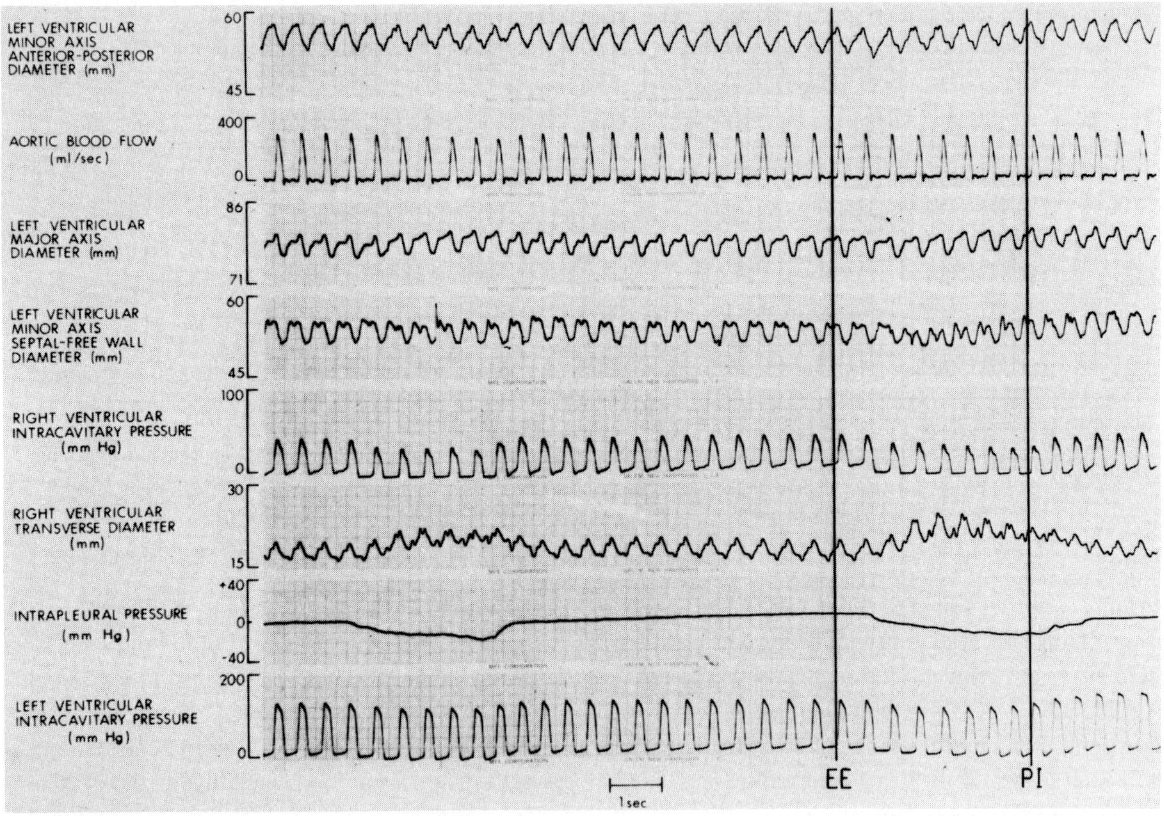

FIGURE 3. Typical analog dimension, pressure, and flow data obtained from a conscious dog during two deep spontaneous respirations with heart rate controlled by atrial pacing. EE and PI are as in figure 2.

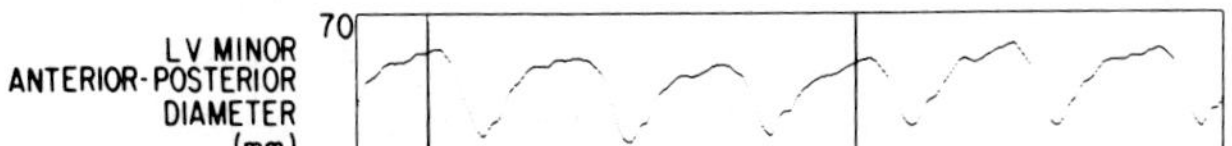

FIGURE 4. Representative digital dimension and pressure data obtained from a conscious dog during a deep spontaneous respiration in which heart rate was controlled by pharmacologic autonomic blockade with propranolol and atropine. EE and PI are as in figure 2.

age of 0.0 ± 0.5 mm Hg at end-expiration to −11.7 ± 0.9 mm Hg at peak inspiration. During inspiration, left ventricular intracavitary end-diastolic and peak ejection pressures decreased by amounts similar to the changes in peak inspiratory intrapleural pressure ($p < .01$), while the corresponding right ventricular intracavitary pressures only decreased by approximately one-half that amount ($p < .01$; table 1). The resulting left ventricular transmural end-diastolic pressure increased slightly ($p < .05$) and peak ejection pressure remained essentially constant ($p > .3$) throughout the respiratory cycle, while right ventricular transmural pressures increased and transseptal pressures decreased during inspiration ($p < .01$; table 1).

The inspiratory fall in end-diastolic transseptal pressure resulted in leftward interventricular septal shifting that reduced the left ventricular end-diastolic septal displacement during deep spontaneous inspirations, a time when left ventricular anterior-posterior minor and major diameters increased slightly (table 2). Thus, left ventricular end-diastolic volume remained essentially constant during the respiratory cycle when heart rate was controlled by atrial pacing ($p > .06$; figure 5), increasing slightly in three dogs, remaining unchanged

TABLE 1
Mean end-diastolic and peak ejection hemodynamic data obtained during spontaneous deep respirations

	PLP (mm Hg)	RVP (mm Hg)	LVP (mm Hg)	RVTMP (mm Hg)	LVTMP (mm Hg)	TSP (mm Hg)
End-diastole						
EE	0.0±0.5	5.9±1.1	10.0±1.1	4.4±1.0	11.8±0.8	7.1±1.0
PI	−11.7±0.9	−0.7±1.6	−0.1±1.2	9.5±1.2	13.4±0.9	3.7±1.0
	B	B	B	B	A	B
Peak ejection						
EE	−1.0±0.6	36.9±3.1	127.8±2.2	36.4±1.8	130.0±4.8	88.2±5.0
PI	−12.6±1.0	31.9±2.4	115.7±4.2	43.1±2.0	129.9±4.6	82.3±3.9
	B	B	B	B		B

Data are presented as mean ± SEM for all 12 experiments.

PLP = intrapleural pressure; RVP = right ventricular intracavitary pressure; LVP = left ventricular intracavitary pressure; RVTMP = right ventricular transmural pressure; LVTMP = left ventricular transmural pressure; TSP = transseptal pressure; EE = end-expiration; PI = peak inspiration.

$^{A}p < .05$; $^{B}p < .01$ by multivariate analysis.

in two dogs, and decreasing slightly in the rest. The pattern of change in each individual dog varied from inspiration to inspiration about a narrow physiologically insignificant range. The end-ejection volume increased slightly on a more consistent basis from dog to dog with each inspiration. Stroke shortening (figures 3 and 4), peak aortic blood flow (figure 3), and stroke volume ($p < .05$; figure 5), however, still fell during inspiration.

Diastolic left ventricular shape was significantly altered during inspiration, with most of the change resulting from leftward displacement of the interventricular septum. The altered left ventricular diastolic geometry during inspiration was indicated by the de-

TABLE 2
Mean end-diastolic and end-ejection dimension data obtained during spontaneous deep respirations

	a (cm)	b (cm)	d (cm)	RVD (cm)
End-diastole				
EE	7.63±0.20	6.32±0.21	2.35±0.11	3.00±0.29
PI	7.65±0.20	6.33±0.20	2.27±0.11	3.25±0.30
%Δ	0.2±0.3	0.1±0.4	−5.4±0.9	9.0±1.3
			A	B
End-ejection				
EE	7.50±0.19	5.91±0.19	2.13±0.13	2.83±0.35
PI	7.52±0.20	5.93±0.19	2.10±0.13	2.96±0.32
%Δ	0.3±0.2	0.2±0.2	−0.9±0.8	5.5±1.9
				B

Data are presented as mean ± SEM for all 12 experiments.

a = basal-apical left ventricular major diameter; b = anterior-posterior left ventricular minor diameter; d = left ventricular septal displacement (segment OS from figure 1); RVD = right ventricular transverse diameter (observations from five experiments); %Δ = percent change determined as (PI − EE)/EE × 100%; other abbreviations and notes are as in table 1.

crease in left ventricular septal displacement (table 2). This resulted in an increased septal radius of curvature during inspiration, as shown in figure 6. Peak developed septal tension, however, decreased during inspiration ($p < .05$; table 3), while peak developed free wall tension remained unchanged ($p > .3$; table 3).

Calculated peak aortic blood flow decreased by an average of 9% during inspiration ($p < .01$; table 3) and measured aortic blood flow showed similar changes (table 3). The inspiratory fall in measured peak ascending aortic blood flow (figure 7, *A*) and left ventricular stroke volume (figure 7, *B*) in the five aortic flow studies correlated with the fall in mean left ventricular intracavitary ejection pressure ($p < .001$) and did not correlate with peak left ventricular transmural pressure or with left ventricular end-diastolic volume during the respiratory cycle ($p > .1$). Inspiratory correlations were observed between intrapleural pressure and left ventricular intracavitary pressure during diastole and systole (figure 7, *C* and *D;* $p < .001$).

The pattern and direction of the changes in dimension, pressure, and flow observed during normal spontaneous respirations were qualitatively similar to those recorded during deep spontaneous respiration. The magnitude of peak inspiratory change during deep respiration was proportionally greater than that observed during normal spontaneous respiration ($p < .01$ by analysis of variance). Similarly, the results obtained during autonomic attenuation with propranolol and atropine were no different than those obtained during atrial pacing.

Discussion

The model of left ventricular geometry we used requires certain assumptions about cardiac shape in order

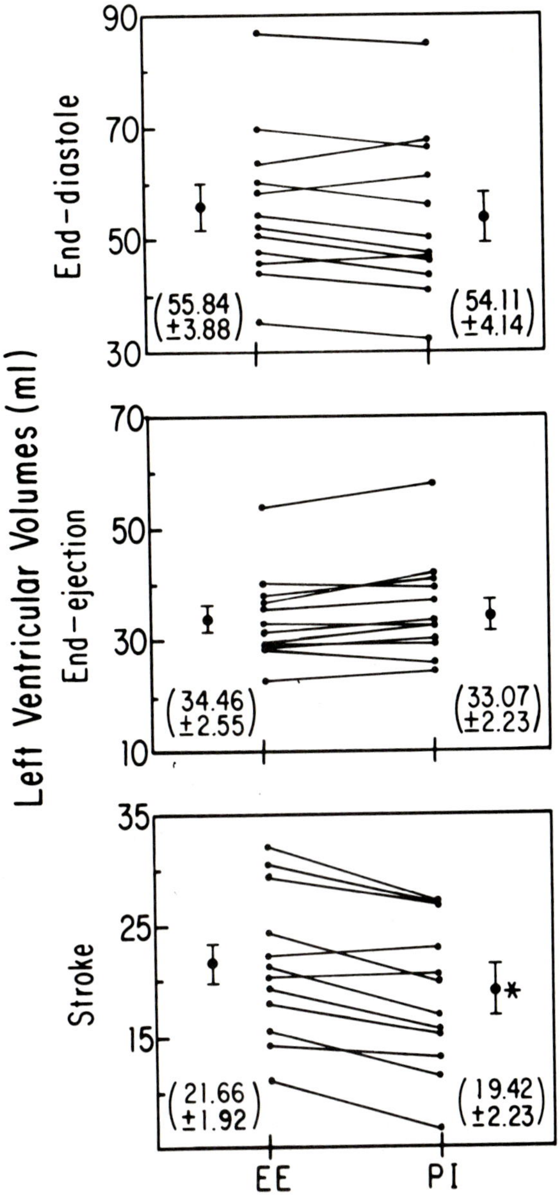

FIGURE 5. *Top,* Left ventricular end-diastolic volumes recorded during the 12 experiments at end-expiration (EE) and peak inspiration (PI). The order of individual studies from top to bottom at EE is: 9, 1, 2, 11, 6, 5, 4, 3, 10, 8, 12, 7. Means ± SEM are shown in parentheses; p > .06. *Middle,* Left ventricular end-ejection volumes for all 12 experiments at EE and PI. The order of individual studies from top to bottom at EE is: 9, 1, 6, 7, 5, 11, 8, 4, 12, 3, 10, 7 (p > .35). *Bottom,* Left ventricular stroke volume recorded during the 12 experiments at EE and PI. The order of individual studies from top to bottom at EE is: 9, 2, 1, 11, 4, 3, 6, 5, 10, 12, 8, 7 (p < .05).

that conclusions about volume changes can be derived. While it is difficult to validate these assumptions, the volume data we obtained by this technique correlate well with those obtained by two other independent methods, namely intraventricular balloon and electromagnetic determination of ascending aortic blood flow (see Appendix). The three principal left ventricular diameters measured in the current study, upon which assumptions about left ventricular shape were based, corresponded closely to the three principal axes (directions) of deformation derived from the eigenvector analysis of left ventricular geometry in an intact dog preparation by Walley et al.[26] The deformations in these principal axes were similar in magnitude and direction to those observed in the present model.[21]

The interventricular septum was shifted leftward during diastole by the inspiratory augmentation in venous return to the right ventricle (table 2). This resulted in an altered left ventricular geometry that reduced chamber compliance, as demonstrated by the upward shift of the normalized pressure-volume curve in figure 8. This observation was consistent from dog to dog and from inspiration to inspiration in each dog. Detailed discussions of this methodology and the normalization procedures have been published previously.[21, 23–25] The reduction in left ventricular chamber compliance that occurs during direct ventricular interactions has been demonstrated previously,[21] and indicates one effect of

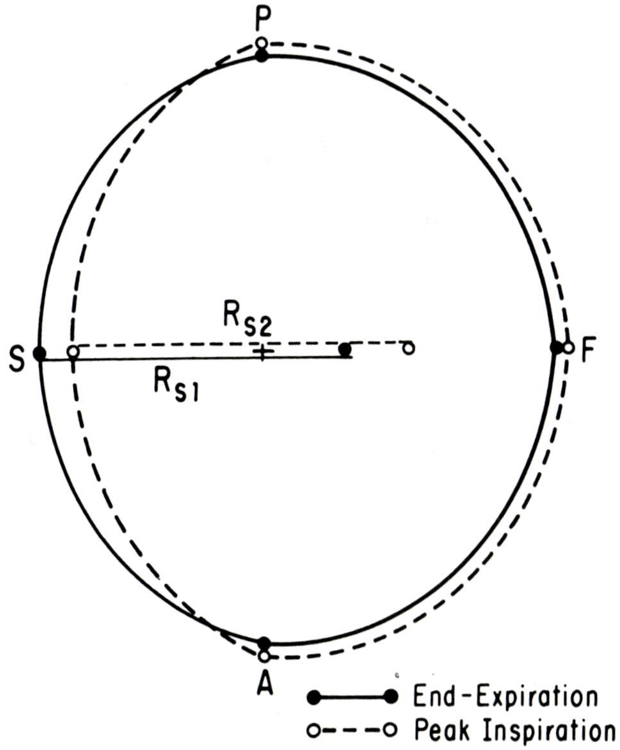

FIGURE 6. Model of the left ventricle latitudinal plane representing change in the average end-diastolic shape during the respiratory cycle over all 12 experiments. During peak deep inspiration (open circles and broken line) the interventricular septum was shifted toward the left ventricle, indicating direct ventricular interaction. A, S, P, and F represent the anterior, septal, posterior, and lateral free walls, respectively. The end-diastolic latitudinal septal radius of curvature was greater during inspiration (R_{S2} = 4.41 cm ± 0.49 cm) than during end-expiration (R_{S1} = 4.25 cm ± 0.49 cm; p < .05).

TABLE 3
Mean ejection data obtained during spontaneous deep respirations

	Ȧo max (ml sec⁻¹)	$\dot{V}_I$ max (ml sec^{-1})	T_S max (mm Hg cm)	T_F max (mm Hg cm)	Ṗ max (mm Hg sec^{-1})
EE	334.8 ± 60.7	313.9 ± 15.8	349.0 ± 22.4	401.4 ± 14.4	2429 ± 89
PI	306.1 ± 55.6	285.2 ± 14.2	325.1 ± 21.2	397.4 ± 13.5	2249 ± 116
%Δ	−8.4 ± 1.0 B	−9.0 ± 1.1 B	−6.7 ± 1.5 A	−0.8 ± 1.1	−6.5 ± 2.0

Data are presented as mean ± SEM for all 12 experiments.
Ȧo max = peak measured ascending aortic blood flow (observations from five experiments); $\dot{V}_I$ max ± peak calculated aortic blood flow; T_S max = peak left ventricular transseptal tension; T_F max = peak left ventricular free wall tension; Ṗ max = peak positive left ventricular transmural dP/dt; other abbreviations and notes are as in tables 1 and 2.

respiration on cardiac function. Figure 8 also attests to the need for accurate measurement of pleural pressure in the assessment of ventricular function, as well as the need for differentiation of end-expiratory from peak inspiratory cardiac cycles in the analysis of diastolic properties.

The accurate measurement of pleural pressure was critical in this study. Pleural pressure should be measured on the surface of the heart at approximately the same vertical level as the intracavitary manometer. The placement of the pleural micromanometer within a large-bore silicone rubber tube with multiple side holes protected the manometer face from motion artifacts but still allowed free communication with the potential space of the pleural cavity. In this manner, reproducible and accurate measurements were made of the pleural pressure affecting cardiac function. Because of the gravitational gradients throughout the chest, measurement of esophageal or peripheral pleural pressure may yield inaccurate results.[27] The use of balloon or fluid-filled catheters may increase the magnitude of impact artifacts and baseline pressure shifts.[20, 28]

In the present studies, the pericardium was left widely open to avoid the potential restrictive effects of scarring or reapproximation of surgically manipulated pericardium. At postmortem examination, the pericardium remained widely open and nonadherent to the right or left ventricles. The effect of an intact pericardium on the results of the present study probably would have been minimal since there were no large changes in ventricular volumes. Moreover, changes in intrapericardial pressure during respiration closely parallel intrapleural pressure changes in the conscious dog.[27, 29] Opening the pericardium in an intact, closed-

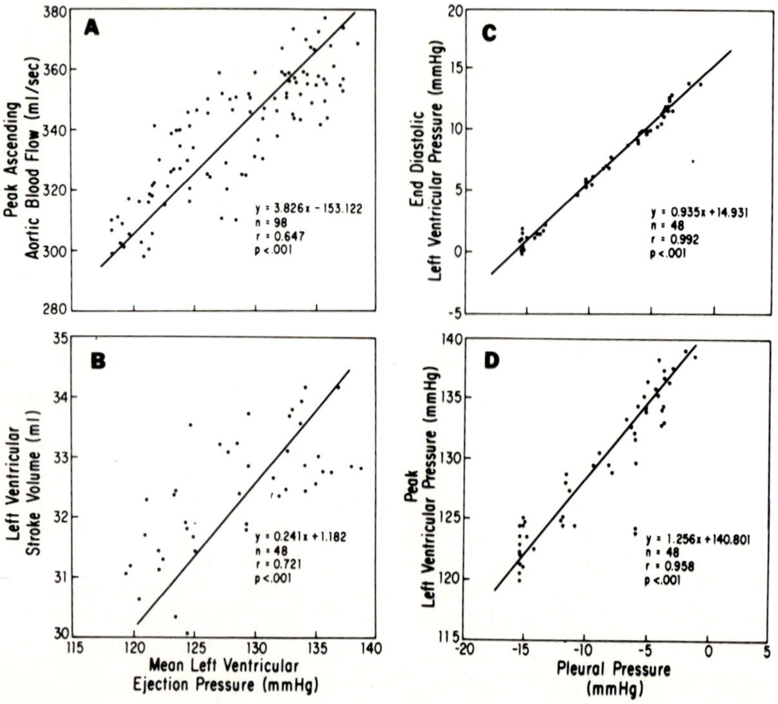

FIGURE 7. *A*, Representative relationship between mean left ventricular intracavitary ejection pressure and peak ascending aortic blood flow during deep spontaneous respirations in one experiment. Linear regression coefficients for the five experiments in which ascending aortic blood flow was measured were m = 8.045 ± 3.860 and b = −772.220 ± 485.785 (r ≥ .503, p < .005). *B*, Relationship between mean left ventricular intracavitary ejection pressure and left ventricular stroke volume measured from ascending aortic blood flow during the same deep spontaneous respirations as in *A*. For all five experiments m = 0.302 ± 0.089 and b = −18.249 ± 10.950 (r ≥ .560, p < .01). *C*, Representative end-diastolic relationship between left ventricular intracavitary pressure and simultaneous intrapleural pressure during the same deep spontaneous respirations as in *A*. For all five experiments m = 0.922 ± 0.084 and b = 12.593 ± 2.438 (r ≥ .835, p < .001). *D*, Same relationship as in *A* except during ejection. For all five experiments m = 1.370 ± 0.230 and b = 142.067 ± 5.733 (r ≥ .835, p < .001).

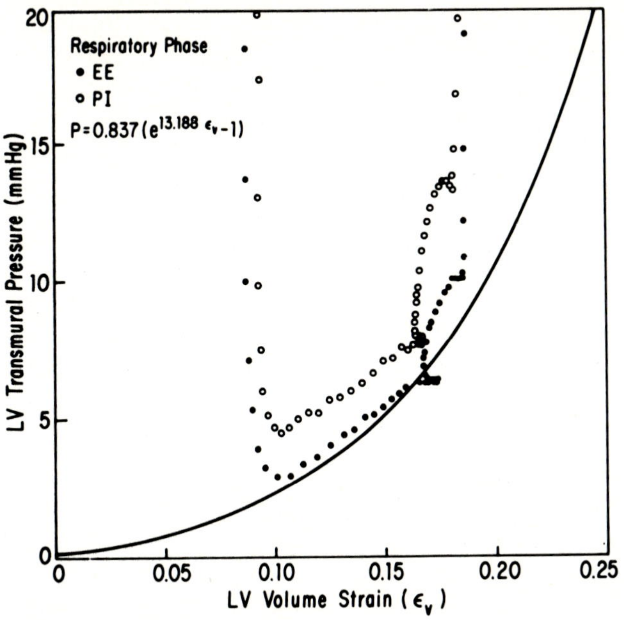

FIGURE 8. The effects of respiration on the normalized left ventricular diastolic pressure-volume relationship in one experiment. The solid curve was obtained by fitting all end-diastolic end-expiration data during a transient vena caval occlusion to the exponential function $P = \alpha (e^{\beta\varepsilon} - 1)$, where α and β are nonlinear coefficients describing the curve and were 0.837 and 13.188, respectively. Superimposed on this curve are data digitized at 200 Hz from two separate cardiac cycles: one from end-expiration (EE, closed circles) and one from peak inspiration (PI, open circles). Peak inspiratory intrapleural pressure was −12.7 mm Hg.

chest canine preparation had no effect on right and left ventricular pressures, left ventricular volumes, or ejection fraction, suggesting that at normal end-diastolic volumes and pressures, the pericardium has minimal influence on ventricular function.[26] An intact pericardium may augment inspiratory leftward septal shifting via the direct ventricular interaction that results from increased right ventricular end-diastolic volumes. However, it is doubtful that such direct ventricular interaction significantly impairs left ventricular function or contributes to the inspiratory fall in left ventricular stroke volume.[19] In a series of unpublished studies from this laboratory in which the pericardium remained intact, the inspiratory changes in the principal measured diameter were similar in direction and magnitude to those observed in the present study.[29]

The marked respiratory variation in heart rate observed during deep, and to a lesser extend during normal respiration, resulted in rather large fluctuations in beat-to-beat left ventricular end-diastolic volume. Several mechanisms have been proposed for this.[30–32] Both atrial pacing and pharmacologic autonomic attenuation with propranolol and atropine effectively ablated the respiratory change in heart rate and neither resulted in a significant change in left ventricular end-diastolic volumes (in some dogs volume increased slightly while in others it decreased minimally). Similar results have recently been observed on radionuclide ventriculograms from healthy human subjects during deep inspirations against resistance.[33]

The inspiratory decrease in left ventricular end-diastolic volume has been thought to result from increased pooling of blood in the lungs[17] or delayed pulmonary transit time of blood.[7, 34] Both would cause a decrease in left ventricular end-diastolic volume (preload) and account for the subsequent fall in left ventricular stroke shortening and peak aortic blood flow that is so apparent in figure 3. Increases in heart rate alone can cause a fall in left ventricular end-diastolic and stroke volumes.[22, 30] However, when heart rate was kept constant by atrial pacing or by pharmacologic autonomic attenuation, as demonstrated in figures 3 and 4, the left ventricular end-diastolic volume remained relatively unchanged, suggesting that under these conditions, increased venous pooling in the lungs or delayed pulmonary transit time was insufficient to prevent adequate left ventricular filling and played only a minor physiologic role.

In addition, leftward shifting of the interventricular septum did not seem to significantly inhibit left ventricular filling when heart rate was kept constant. This is graphically apparent in figure 3. During the prolonged second inspiration, the interventricular septum initially was shifted leftward (reduced minor-axis septal–free wall diameter), with augmented venous return to the right ventricle (increased right ventricular transverse diameter). As inspiration progressed, augmented venous return became less apparent and the septum shifted back to the right, presumably as left ventricular end-diastolic volume increased due to delayed return of the increased pulmonary pooling of blood. Aortic blood flow, however, continued to decrease apparently independent of these events. Similar changes in left ventricular end-diastolic volume and aortic blood flow were observed in several dogs during prolonged deep inspirations.

Another proposed hypothesis has been that leftward shifting of the interventricular septum during inspiration alters ventricular geometry and increases the geometric component of left ventricular afterload.[18, 19] Flattening of the interventricular septum might increase the septal radius of curvature, augment septal wall tension, and impede left ventricular stroke volume during ejection. Although the present studies demonstrated an inspiratory leftward shifting of the septum with altered diastolic geometry that persisted into systole, the increase in septal radius of curvature was small and was outweighed by the larger fall in the transseptal pressure gradient (table 1). Thus, left ventricular septal wall tension actually decreased during inspiration (table 3), and the augmentation in the geometric component of left ventricular afterload from septal shifting did not occur.

Yet another proposed hypothesis is that the inspiratory decline in pleural pressure increased left ventricular transmural pressure (left ventricular intracavitary pressure minus pleural pressure), causing a fall in stroke volume.[6, 9, 12, 20, 34–36] Intracavitary left ventricular ejection pressure decreased by an amount similar to that by which pleural pressure is decreased during inspiration such that left ventricular transmural ejection pressure remained unchanged (table 1). Thus, augmentation of the intraventricular pressure component of left ventricular afterload did not appear to account for the inspiratory fall in left ventricular stroke volume. Similar observations have been made by others.[37]

From the present data, an alternative explanation is proposed for the inspiratory fall in left ventricular stroke volume. The correlations between peak aortic blood flow, left ventricular stroke volume, and mean intracavitary left ventricular ejection pressure (figure 7, *A* and *B*) has led us to the hypothesis that the intracavitary left ventricular pressure referenced to atmospheric pressure is actually the effective ejection pressure of the left ventricle and that the inspiratory decrease in this pressure accounts for the fall in stroke volume. During diastole, the heart is the chamber at the end of the blood flow and pleural pressure is the appropriate external pressure. However, during ejection, when the aortic valve is open and the left ventricle is in continuity with the systemic arterial system, the peripheral vasculature is at the end of the blood flow and atmospheric pressure is the appropriate external pressure. During inspiration, the hydraulic force effecting ejection (intracavitary left ventricular pressure) is decreased by an amount equal to the decline in intrapleural pressure, and left ventricular stroke volume falls as a result of the decrease in this effective left ventricular ejection pressure.

Intrathoracic aortic pressure referenced to atmospheric pressure is reported to fall during inspiration,[6, 12, 20] but to a lesser degree than the inspiratory reduction in intracavitary left ventricular pressure. This is reported to increase left ventricular afterload and decrease stroke volume. In unpublished observations from this laboratory simultaneously measured high-fidelity left ventricular, ascending and descending thoracic aortic, and abdominal aortic pressures were all observed to fall by a similar amount equal to the inspiratory decline in pleural pressure during normal and deep inspiration. Thus, the transmural pressures referenced to pleural pressure at these four simultaneous points of measurement along the central and systemic vascular system did not rise during inspiration, but instead remained essentially unchanged. An increase in left ventricular or transthoracic aortic afterload that might account for the inspiratory fall in stroke volume was not apparent in these studies, or in others.[37] The impedance in effective left ventricular ejection pressure induced by the inspiratory decline in pleural pressure had an effect on left ventricular stroke volume similar to that of an increase in left ventricular afterload, but it apparently occurred by a different mechanism since no measurable increase in transmural left ventricular or transthoracic aortic afterload could be demonstrated. It is therefore more appropriate to refer to the inspiratory effect of pleural pressure on left ventricular function as an impedance of the effective ejection pressure rather than an increase in left ventricular afterload in terms of systolic wall stress.[33]

Right ventricular ejection is not effected during inspiration by the same mechanism that effects left ventricular ejection. During right ventricular ejection, when the pulmonary valve is open, the right ventricle is in continuity with the pulmonary circulation and the left atrium, all of which are subjected to the same inspiratory fall in intrapleural pressure. Thus, pleural pressure is the appropriate external pressure for the right ventricle during ejection and during diastole. Accordingly, during inspiration, the hydraulic force effecting ejection from the right ventricle is not decreased relative to its appropriate external pressure and right ventricular stroke volume would not be expected to fall on the basis of a decreased effective ejection pressure. In fact, the effective ejection pressure of the right ventricle (right ventricular transmural pressure) was increased during inspiration (table 1) as a result of increased venous return (preload), and right ventricular stroke volume was augmented. Right ventricular cavitary volume was not assessed directly in the current study, although increases in the end-diastolic transverse diameter during inspiration (table 2) were believed to represent increased right ventricular end-diastolic volume and were found to correlate linearly with postmortem right ventricular intracavitary balloon volumes (see Appendix). Similar results have been reported by others.[19]

Clinically, an exaggeration of the normal inspiratory decline in left ventricular stroke volume may result in pulsus paradoxus, the absence of a peripheral pulse despite the presence of a cardiac contraction.[38]

Conditions that accentuate the swings in pleural pressure (such as asthma, pulmonary embolism, or pulmonary edema), and conditions that increase the interactive coupling between the right and left ventricles (such as cardiac tamponade or acute right heart failure) may result in either pulsus paradoxus or an increased widening of the inspiratory fall in peak systemic blood pressure. Conversely, the marked increases in the pleural pressure that occur with coughing may produce reversed pulsus paradoxus, the presence of a peripheral pulse in the absence of a cardiac contraction.[39, 40] Conditions that elevate the intrathoracic pressure, such as positive pressure ventilation, Valsalva maneuver, or coughing, augment left ventricular stroke volume as well as forward flow of blood from the thoracic aorta via a thoracic pump mechanism.[40] Factors elevating pleural pressure augment left ventricular pressure and favor left ventricular ejection, while conditions reducing pleural pressure lower the effective left ventricular ejection pressure and impede left ventricular stroke volume. In this regard, deep inspiration may be referred to as a reverse thoracic pump mechanism.

Thus, a hypothesis is proposed that is consistent with, as well as an extension of, the thoracic pump mechanism to explain the long-observed differential effects of inspiration on right and left ventricular stroke volumes. Conceptually, this hypothesis provides a more accurate explanation of cardiorespiratory interaction during inspiration than has previously been offered. Other mechanisms, such as altered preload or afterload, appear to contribute only secondarily, if at all, to the inspiratory fall in left ventricular stroke volume. The principal factor diminishing left ventricular stroke volume during inspiration is the inspiratory fall in the effective intracavitary ejection pressure of the left ventricle.

Appendix

The modified ellipsoid used in the current studies to model left ventricular shape and volume represents the concatenation of two ellipsoidal segments and has been discussed in detail previously.[21] The current model accurately predicted left ventricular stroke volume over a wide range of left ventricular volumes and under various conditions of ventricular interaction with both high and low right ventricular volumes. The stroke volumes and flows calculated from the dimension measurements as $-dV_I/dt$ correlated very well over a wide range of physiologic volumes, with minimal variability when compared with the stroke volumes and flows measured by an ascending aortic electromagnetic flow probe.[21]

The dimension transducers were positioned at approximately 90 degree points around the latitudinal and longitudinal circumferences of the left ventricle. The true three-dimensional position of each transducer was determined in separate validation studies by measurement with the linear chords from all possible paired combinations of the septal and epicardial crystals. The results of one such experiment are shown in figure 9, where the true three-dimensional position of each transducer determined by the chord measurements was compared with the assumed position of these transducers based on the double hemiellipsoidal model (figure 1). The difference in volume calculated from the assumed model and that computed from the actual position based on a three-point derivation of an ellipsoidal segment was minimal (0.9 to 1.8 ml) and accounted for less than a 3% difference in corresponding calculated chamber volumes.

In four studies, in which the hearts were excised with the ultrasonic dimension transducers still in place and before determination of left ventricular wall volume displacement, both atria, the tricuspid and mitral valves, and chordae tendineae were removed. The semilunar valve orifices were individually sutured closed, compliant balloons attached to Lucite disks were introduced into each ventricle, and the sewing rings of the disks were sutured to the anuli of the tricuspid and mitral valves. The excised heart was then suspended in a water bath and left ventricular balloon volumes were varied over a wide range at various right ventricular balloon volumes while recording left and right ventricular ultrasonic dimensions. At various levels of right ventricular balloon volume ranging from 0 to 60 ml, the correlation between the absolute measured and calculated left ventricular chamber volumes was excellent, and the line of regression was very near the line of identity, despite marked differences in relative septal position (figure 10, *A*). In a similar fashion, right ventricular transverse diameter was linearly related to right ventricular cavitary balloon volume (figure 10, *B*).

These data, coupled with those published previously,[21] indicate the validity of the current model in accurately assessing left ventricular volume and geometry.

We are grateful to Mr. James Bradsher and his staff for technical assistance, to Ms. Sandra Justice for preparing the manuscript, and to the Duke Audiovisual Department for the illustration.

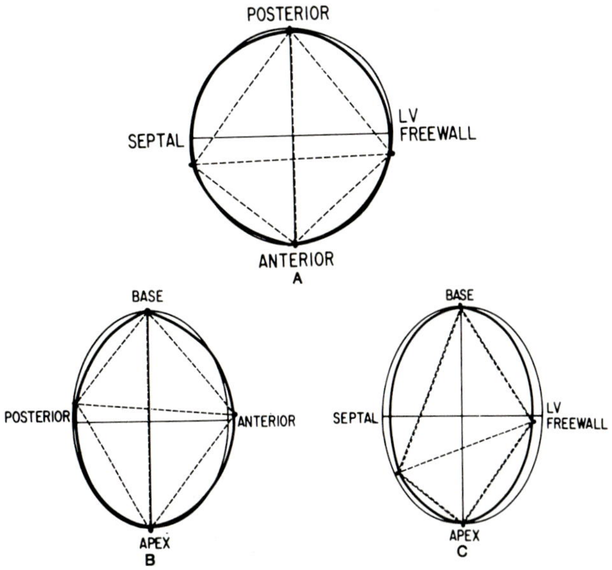

FIGURE 9. Comparison of left ventricular geometry derived from the position of the dimension transducers assumed by the model (thin solid lines) with geometry obtained from the actual position of the dimension transducers calculated from the chord measurements (broken and heavy solid lines). *A*, Latitudinal plane; *B*, longitudinal plane through the anterior and posterior transducers; *C*, longitudinal plane through the septal and free wall transducers. The difference in the actual and assumed volumes calculated by the two methods was less than 3%.

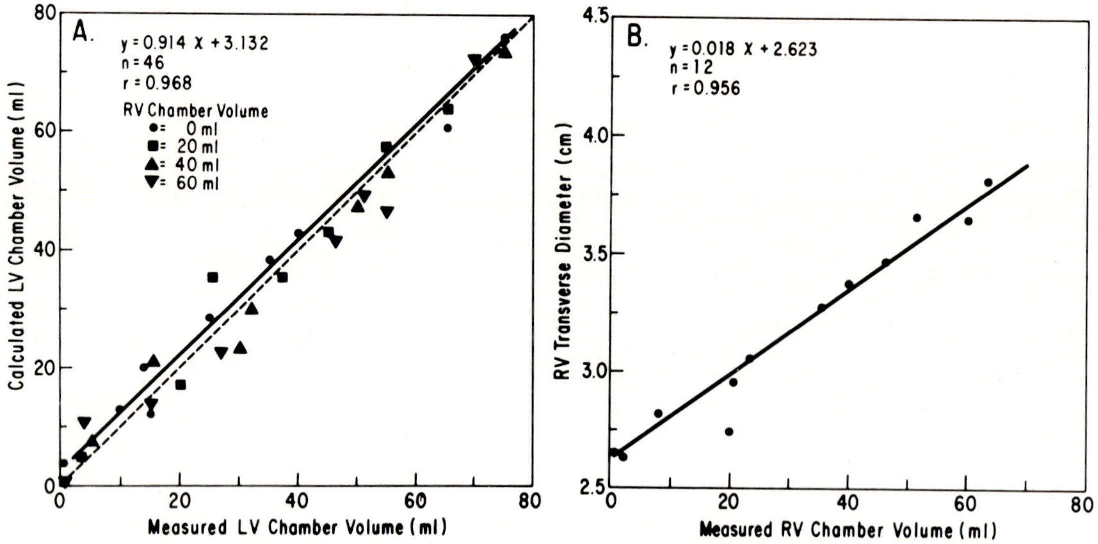

FIGURE 10. *A*, Calculated chamber volume vs measured left ventricular intracavitary balloon volume from four postmortem studies at various levels of right ventricular volume. LV = left ventricle; RV = right ventricle. *B*, Correlation between right ventricular transverse diameter and right ventricular intracavitary balloon volume from one postmortem study.

References

1. Breecher GA: The respiratory pump. *In* Venous return. New York, 1956, Grune and Stratton, pp 71–90
2. Charlier AA: Beat to beat hemodynamic effects of lung inflation and normal respiration in anaesthetized and conscious dogs. Brussels, 1967, Editions Arscia, pp 75–94
3. Franklin KJ: Respiration and the venous return in mammals; the "vis a fronte." *In* A monograph on veins. Springfield, IL, 1937, Charles C Thomas, ch 19, pp 236–267
4. Hales S: I. An account of some hydraulick and hydrostatical experiments made on the blood and blood-vessels of animals. *In* Statistical essays: containing haemastaticles. London, 1773, Innys, Manby, and Woodward, pp 1–3
5. Bugge-Asperheim B, Kill F: Cardiac response to increased aortic pressure. Changes in output and left ventricular pressure pattern at various levels of inotropy. Scand J Clin Lab Invest **24:** 345, 1969
6. Charlier AA, Jaumin PM, Pouleur H: Circulatory effects of deep inspirations, blocked expirations and positive pressure inflations at equal transpulmonary pressures in conscious dogs. J Physiol **241:** 589, 1974
7. Franklin DL, Van Critters RL, Rushmer RF: Balance between right and left ventricular output. Circ Res **10:** 17, 1962
8. Hoffman JIE, Guz A, Charlier AA, Wicken DEL: Stroke volume in conscious dogs; effects of respiration, posture, and vascular occlusion. J Appl Physiol **20:** 865, 1965
9. Schrijen F, Ehrlich W, Permutt S: Cardiovascular changes in conscious dogs during spontaneous deep breaths. Pfluegers Arch **355:** 205, 1975
10. Shabetai R, Fowler NO, Gueron M: The effects of respiration on aortic pressure and flow. Am Heart J **65:** 525, 1963
11. Shuler RH, Ensor C, Gunning RE, Moss WG, Johnson V: The differential effects of respiration on the left and right ventricles. Am J Physiol **137:** 620, 1942
12. Buda AJ, Pinsky MR, Ingels NB Jr, Daughters GT II, Stinson EB, Alderman EL: Effect of intrathoracic pressure on left ventricular performance. N Engl J Med **301:** 453, 1979
13. Goldblatt A, Harrison DC, Glick G, Braunwald E: Studies on cardiac dimensions in intact, unanesthetized man. II. Effects of respiration. Circ Res **8:** 448, 1963
14. Ruskin J, Bache RJ, Rembert JC, Greenfield JC: Pressure-flow studies in man: Effect of respiration on left ventricular stroke volume. Circ Res **48:** 79, 1973
15. Morgan BC, Abel FL, Mullins GL, Guntheroth WG: Flow patterns in cavae, pulmonary artery, pulmonary vein, and aorta in intact dogs. Am J Physiol **210:** 903, 1966
16. Morkin E, Collins JA, Goldman HS, Fishman AP: Pattern of blood flow in the pulmonary veins of the dog. J Appl Physiol **20:** 1118, 1965
17. Macklin CC: Evidences of increases in the capacity of the pulmonary arteries and veins of dogs, cats, and rabbits during inflation of the freshly excised lung. Rev Can Biol **5:** 199, 1946
18. Brinker JA, Weiss JL, Lappe' DL, Rabson JL, Summer WR, Permutt S, Weisfeldt ML: Leftward septal displacement during right ventricular loading in man. Circulation **61:** 626, 1980
19. Santamore WP, Lynch PR, Meier G, Heckman J, Bove AA: Myocardial interaction between the ventricles. J Appl Physiol **41:** 362, 1976
20. Summer WR, Permutt S, Sagawa K, Shoukas AA, Bromberger-Barvea B: Effects of spontaneous respiration on canine left ventricular function. Circ Res **45:** 719, 1979
21. Olsen CO, Tyson GS, Maier GW, Spratt JA, Davis JW, Rankin JS: Dynamic ventricular interaction in the conscious dog. Circ Res **52:** 85, 1983
22. Arentzen CE, Rankin JS, Anderson PAW, Feezor MD, Anderson RW: Force-frequency characteristics of the left ventricle in the conscious dog. Circ Res **42:** 64, 1978
23. Olsen CO, Rankin JS, Arentzen CE, Ring WS, McHale PA, Anderson RW: The deformational characteristics of the left ventricle in the conscious dog. Circ Res **49:** 843, 1981
24. Rankin JS, Arentzen CE, McHale PA, Ling D, Anderson RW: Viscoelastic properties of the diastolic left ventricle in the conscious dog. Circ Res **41:** 37, 1977
25. Rankin JS, McHale PA, Arentzen CE, Ling D, Greenfield JC, Anderson RW: The three-dimensional dynamic geometry of the left ventricle in the conscious dog. Circ Res **39:** 304, 1976
26. Walley KR, Grover M, Raff GL, Benge JW, Hannaford B, Glantz SA: Left ventricular dynamic geometry in the intact and open chest dog. Circ Res **50:** 573, 1982
27. Kenner HM, Wood EH: Intrapericardial, intrapleural, and intracardiac pressures during acute heart failure in dogs studied without thoracotomy. Circ Res **19:** 1071, 1966
28. Rankin JS, Olsen CO, Arentzen CE, Tyson GS, Maier G, Smith PK, Hammon JW, Davis JW, McHale PA, Anderson RW, Sabiston DC Jr: The effects of airway pressure on cardiac function in intact dogs and man. Circulation **66:** 108, 1982
29. Tyson GS Jr, Maier GW, Olsen CO, Davis JW, Rankin JS: Pericardial influences on ventricular filling in the conscious dog: An analysis based on pericardial pressures. Circ Res **54:** 173, 1984
30. Bristlow JO, Ferguson RE, Mintz F, Rapaport E: The influence of heart rate on left ventricular volume in dogs. J Clin Invest **42:** 649, 1963
31. Bainbridge FA: The influence of venous filling upon the rate of the heart. J Physiol **50:** 65, 1915

32. Vatner SF, Boettcher DH, Heyndrickx GR, McRitchie RJ: Reduced baroreflex sensitivity with volume loading in conscious dogs. Circ Res **37:** 236, 1975
33. Karam M, Wise RA, Natarajan TK, Permutt S, Wagner HN: Mechanism of decreased left ventricular stroke volume during inspiration in man. Circulation **69:** 866, 1984
34. Robotham JL, Lixfeld W, Holland L, MacGregor D, Bryan AC, Rabson J: Effects of respiration on cardiac performance. J Appl Physiol **44:** 703, 1978
35. Robotham JL, Mitzner W: A model of the effects of respiration on left ventricular performance. J Appl Physiol **46:** 411, 1979
36. Robotham JL, Rabson J, Permutt S, Bromberger-Barnea B: Left ventricular hemodynamics during respiration. J Appl Physiol **47:** 1295, 1979
37. Scharf SM, Brown R, Saunders N, Green LH: Effects of normal and loaded spontaneous inspiration on cardiovascular function. J Appl Physiol **47:** 580, 1979
38. Kussmaul A: Ueber schwielige Mediastino-Pericarditis und den paradoxen Puls. Berl Klin Wochenshr **10:** 433; 445; 461; 1873
39. Sharpey-Schafer EP: Effect of respiratory acts on the circulation. *In* Fenn WD, Rahn H, editors: Handbook of physiology, vol II, section 3. 1965, Washington, D.C., American Physiological Society, ch 52, pp 1875–1886
40. Niemann JT, Rosborough J, Hansknecht M, Brown D, Criley JM: Cough-CPR: Documention of systemic perfusion in man and in an experimental model: a "window" to the mechanism of blood flow in external CPR. Crit Care Med **8:** 141, 1980

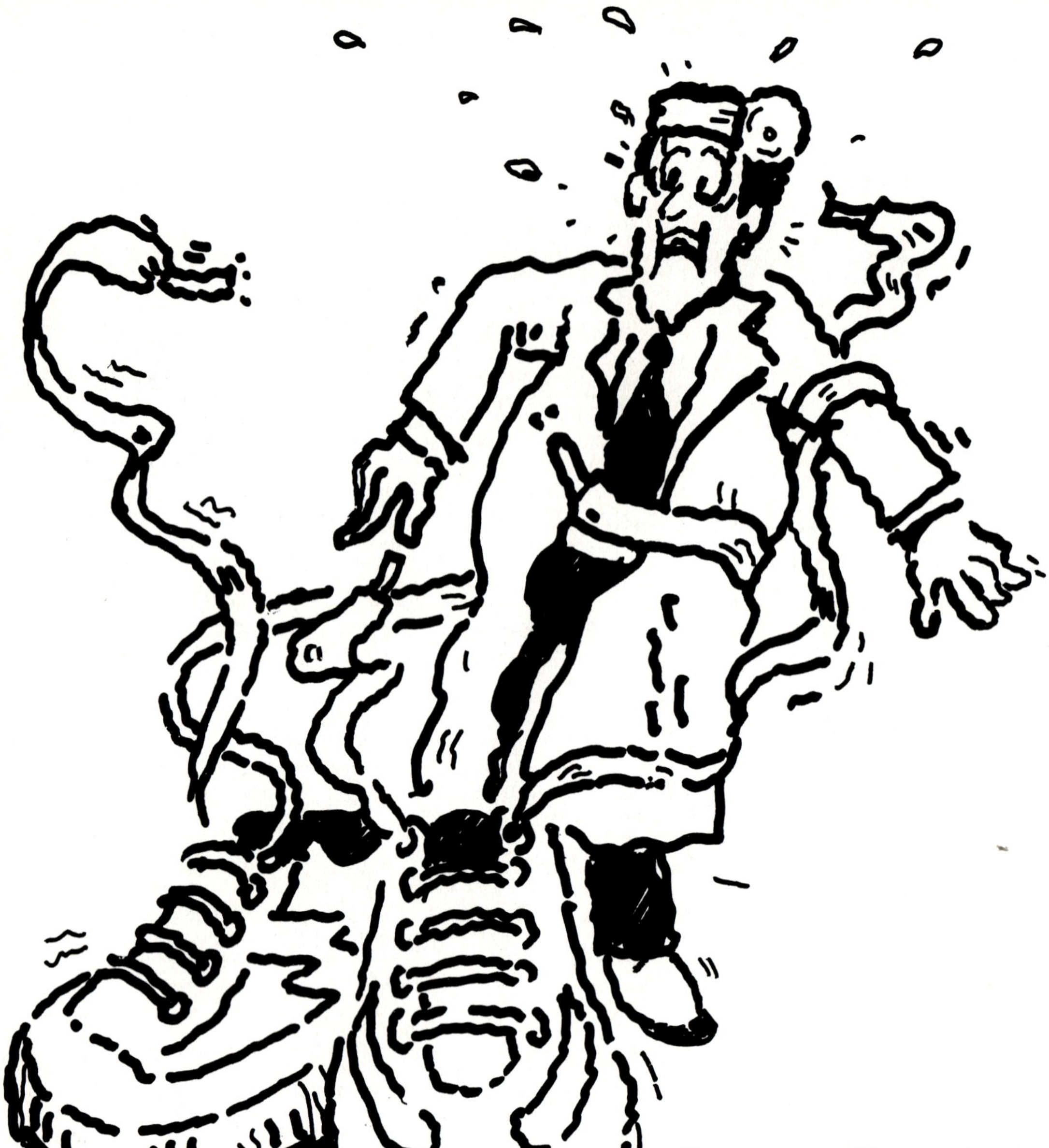

Circulation

VOL 72 NO 4
OCTOBER 1985

An Official Journal of the American Heart Association, Inc.®

FEATURES

Sudden unexpected death in patients with congestive heart failure: a second frontier

MILTON PACKER, M.D.

FOR THE LAST 200 years the management of patients with congestive heart failure has focused on the alleviation of symptoms of the disease that greatly limit the lifestyle of these individuals. For the last 30 years we have concentrated on elucidating the pathophysiologic mechanisms that underlie the hemodynamic abnormalities of the heart failure state and, consequently, we have been enormously successful in developing a variety of potent inotropic, diuretic, and vasodilator drugs that can produce clinical improvement in the vast majority of patients. In our enthusiasm to make our patients feel better, however, we have ignored the fact that the mortality of patients with congestive heart failure remains extremely high, and that no therapeutic intervention has yet been shown to improve long-term *survival*. We should not be surprised that our patients are dying from progression of their underlying heart disease, since the hemodynamic interventions available to us at the present time only incompletely alleviate the markedly abnormal loading conditions in the heart that likely contribute to the progression to terminal right and left ventricular dysfunction. What is surprising, however, is that many of our patients are dying suddenly, unexpectedly, without any evidence of hemodynamic or functional deterioration. As we continue to advance in our ability to pharmacologically improve pump performance, it is likely that sudden unexpected death will soon become the most frequent means of demise in patients with congestive heart failure.

The problem of sudden unexpected death in patients with congestive heart failure. We define sudden unexpected death as death from circulatory failure within 1 hour of onset of symptoms in a patient with advanced left ventricular dysfunction whose heart failure symptoms have remained stable or improved over the previous 2 to 4 weeks and in whom another cause for circulatory collapse cannot be identified clinically. We are thereby excluding patients whose death (albeit sudden) is the terminal event in a progressively worsening clinical picture, characterized by repeated hospitalizations for treatment and progressively shorter periods of clinical stability. We are also excluding the 10% to 15% of patients whose deaths follow the typical symptomatic presentation of an acute myocardial infarction or pulmonary embolism. So defined, sudden unexpected death comprises 35% to 45% of all deaths of patients with congestive heart failure and is equal in frequency to that of deaths secondary to progressive ventricular dysfunction (table 1). Available evidence suggests that the incidence of sudden unexpected death has not changed significantly over the last 10 to 15 years, is not related to the etiology or severity of congestive heart failure, and has not been altered by the advent of direct-acting vasodilator drugs.

Sudden unexpected death in patients with congestive heart failure is most likely the result of a terminal ventricular tachyarrhythmia, either ventricular tachycardia or ventricular fibrillation. Studies using 24 hour ambulatory monitoring indicate that 60% to 90% of patients with congestive heart failure have frequent or complex ventricular ectopy, and that 40% to 60% have nonsustained ventricular tachycardia (table 2). The presence of ventricular arrhythmias and left ventricular dysfunction appear to act *synergically* to determine the subsequent occurrence of sudden death. Hence, it is not surprising that the frequency of sudden unexpected death is greater in patients with congestive heart failure than in any other definable subset of patients in cardiovascular medicine. This risk of sudden death for patients with heart failure is substantially higher than that for patients during the first year after an acute myocar-

From the Division of Cardiology, Department of Medicine, Mount Sinai School of Medicine of The City University of New York, New York.

Address for correspondence: Milton Packer, M.D., Division of Cardiology, Mount Sinai Medical Center, 1 Gustave Levy Place, New York, NY 10029.

Dr. Packer is the recipient of a Research Career Development Award (K04-HL-01229) from the National Heart, Lung, and Blood Institute, Bethesda.

TABLE 1
Frequency of sudden death in patients with congestive heart failure (studies ranked according to increasing severity of heart failure)

References	No. of patients	Cause of CHF	NYHA class	1 year mortality (%)	% SUD of total deaths
Califf et al.[A]	236	CHD	I,II,III,IV	37	41
Franciosa et al.[B]	182	CHD/PMD	II,III,IV	34	45
Burggraf and Parker[C]	28	CHD	II,III,IV	39	33
Massie et al.[D]	59	CHD/PMD	III,IV	37	34
Wilson et al.[E]	77	CHD/PMD	III,IV	48	38
Cohn et al.[F]	106	CHD/PMD	III, IV	50	47
Lee and Packer[G]	203	CHD/PMD	IV	58	39

Despite increasing severity of congestive heart failure as depicted by progressively more limited functional class and greater 1 year mortality, the percentage of patients who died suddenly was similar among the seven studies and was not related to the cause of heart failure. Studies that did not evaluate patients consecutively or used a definition of sudden unexpected death that differed from that used in the text are excluded from this table.

CHD = coronary heart disease; PMD = primary myocardial disease; NYHA class = New York Heart Association functional class; SUD = sudden unexpected death.

References: [A]*In* Braunwald E et al., editors: Congestive heart failure: current research and clinical applications. 1982, New York, Grune & Stratton, p 31. [B]Am J Cardiol **51:** 831, 1983. [C]Circulation **51:** 146, 1975. [D]Circulation **63:** 269, 1981. [E]J Am Coll Cardiol **2:** 403, 1983. [F]N Engl J Med **311:** 819, 1984. [G]Circulation **70**(suppl II): II-113, 1984.

dial infarction, who have been traditionally viewed by cardiologists as being at greatest risk of unexpected circulatory collapse and have consequently become the focus of major rehabilitative and public health programs aimed at preventing the occurrence of fatal arrhythmias.

Predisposing factors to sudden unexpected death in congestive heart failure. What factors underlie the occurrence of malignant ventricular arrhythmias in patients with congestive heart failure? Although previous reports have validly emphasized the importance of structural and hemodynamic factors (such as myocardial fibrosis and ventricular wall stress) in predisposing to the reentry phenomena that are critical to the development of ventricular ectopic rhythms, recent evidence points to three potentially *reversible* arrhythmogenic factors in patients with congestive heart failure: (1) electrolyte deficits, (2) activation of neurohormonal mechanisms, and (3) drug therapy for heart failure (table 3).

Electrolyte depletion. Patients with congestive heart failure have marked deficits of total body and intracellular potassium, which may or may not be reflected by a measurable decrease in serum potassium concentration. The administration of diuretic drugs may further deplete body stores of potassium (as well as magnesium) by promoting the renal excretion of these predominantly intracellular cations, an effect potentiated by coexistent hyperaldosteronism and metabolic alkalosis. Furthermore, the high levels of circulating catecholamines in patients with heart failure may enhance the movement of potassium into cells by a β_2-receptor–mediated mechanism, thereby exacerbating the hypokalemic state and potentiating its arrhythmogenic effects.[1] Recent studies indicate that malignant ventricular ectopic rhythms in some patients with congestive heart failure may be *entirely* the result of potassium and magnesium depletion; short- and long-term electrolyte repletion may abolish these arrhythmias and prevent the recurrence of sudden death without long-term antiarrhythmic drug therapy.[2, 3] As might be expected, potassium and magnesium deficits commonly coexist. Under such circumstances, repletion of magnesium appears to be critical to the success of treatment; therapy with potassium salts alone may fail to restore normal serum levels of potassium or normal sinus rhythm, whereas magnesium administration corrects not only the hypomagnesemia and the hypokalemia but abolishes the accompanying tachyarrhythmias as well.[3]

Activation of neurohormonal mechanisms. The sympathetic nervous system and the renin-angiotensin system are activated in patients with congestive heart failure in an attempt to preserve circulatory homeostasis as cardiac output falls and serve to mediate the systemic vasoconstriction and salt and water retention that characterize patients with this disorder. These systems may be further activated by treatment with diuretic drugs, direct-acting vasodilators, or by the administration of potent inotropic agents. Circulating levels of catecholamines may be directly arrhythmogenic or may contribute to and potentiate the arrhythmogenic effects of hypokale-

TABLE 2
Relationship of ventricular ectopic activity to subsequent occurrence of sudden unexpected death in patients with congestive heart failure (studies ranked according to increasing mortality rates)

	No. of patients	Mortality (%)/ average follow-up (mo)	% patients with VT	Relation of VT to total mortality	Relation of VT to SUD
Huang et al.[A]	35	11/34	60	No	No
Costanzo-Nordin et al.[B]	55	16/?	40	No	No
Meinertz et al.[C]	74	26/11	49	Yes	Yes
Unverferth et al.[D]	69	35/12	41	Yes	—
Holmes et al.[E]	31	45/14	39	Yes	No
Wilson et al.[F]	77	65/12	51	Yes	No

In the first two studies the event rates were too low (< 20%) to show that ventricular arrhythmias were of prognostic significance. In three of the four remaining studies, the occurrence of ventricular tachycardia (≥3 beats) predicted total mortality but not sudden death, suggesting that such malignant ventricular ectopy reflected the severity of hemodynamic and functional abnormalities and was not an independent risk factor. The study by Meinertz et al.[C] showed a relationship between sudden unexpected death and the frequency (but not the occurrence) of ventricular tachycardia, but the extremely high arrhythmia rate (≥ 20 episodes of ventricular tachycardia per 24 hr) proposed by these authors for the identification of high-risk patients is rarely observed in patients with congestive heart failure.

SUD = sudden unexpected death. VT = ventricular tachycardia.

References: [A]Am J Cardiol **51:** 507, 1983. [B]J Am Coll Cardiol **3:** 594, 1984. [C]Am J Cardiol **53:** 902, 1984. [D]Am J Cardiol **54:** 147, 1984. [E]Am J Cardiol **55:** 146, 1985. [F]J Am Coll Cardiol **2:** 403, 1983.

mia.[1] Angiotensin II may exacerbate ventricular arrhythmias by promoting the renal losses of potassium and magnesium by the stimulation of aldosterone synthesis or by potentiating the central and peripheral effects of the sympathetic nervous system. Hence, both neurohormonal systems not only worsen ventricular loading conditions by systemic vasoconstriction, but may provoke life-threatening tachyarrhythmias by their direct and indirect actions on ventricular irritability. These combined effects may explain why plasma catecholamines and plasma renin activity are the most powerful predictors of long-term survival in patients with congestive heart failure.[4, 5]

The most compelling evidence that neurohormonal activation may play a critical role in the pathogenesis of sudden unexpected death in patients with congestive heart failure derives from studies of long-term treatment with neurohormonal antagonists. In a double-blind crossover trial in which captopril was compared with placebo therapy in 14 patients with severe chronic heart failure,[6] converting-enzyme inhibition not only ameliorated the symptoms of heart failure and prolonged exercise tolerance but also reduced the frequency of ventricular premature complexes and the number of episodes of nonsustained ventricular tachycardia during ambulatory monitoring. These antiarrhythmic effects were accompanied by both a reduction in circulating levels of angiotensin II and catecholamines and by an increase in serum and total body potassium. The ability of captopril to promote cation repletion and reduce circulating levels of potentially arrhythmogenic neurohormones may help explain the reduction in overall mortality seen in retrospective analysis of data from patients with heart failure treated with converting-enzyme inhibitors.[5, 7] Alternatively, direct antagonism of the proarrhythmic effects of catecholamines may be achieved by the administration of β-adrenergic–blocking agents. Recent data from the Beta-Blocker Heart Attack Trial (BHAT) indicate that treatment with β-blockers substantially reduces the incidence of sudden death in patients following an acute myocardial infarction that was complicated by congestive heart failure,[8] presumably through an antiarrhythmic mechanism. These observations support the findings of uncontrolled studies that long-term low-dose β-blockade may reduce mortality in patients with a congestive cardiomyopathy.[9]

Therapy with drugs used to treat heart failure. Most of the drugs used to improve cardiac performance and clinical symptoms in patients with congestive heart failure can exacerbate ventricular tachyarrhythmias. Of all the available treatment modalities, diuretic drugs may prove to be the most arrhythmogenic. These agents activate both the sympathetic nervous and renin-angiotensin systems and promote the renal loss of potassium and magnesium, the serum levels of which may be further reduced by the concomitant elevation of circulating catecholamines and aldosterone. All of these factors, acting alone or in concert, may contribute sub-

TABLE 3
Factors predisposing to ventricular arrhythmias in patients with heart failure

- Structural factors
- Hemodynamic factors
- Electrolyte depletion
  - Potassium
  - Magnesium
- Neurohormonal mechanisms
  - Sympathetic nervous system
  - Renin-angiotensin system
- Heart failure therapy
  - Inotropic drugs
  - Diuretic agents
  - ? Direct-acting vasodilators

stantially to the frequency and complexity of malignant ventricular rhythms in patients with congestive heart failure. A similar provocation of arrhythmic events has been postulated to occur during the administration of diuretics in hypertensive patients and may explain the failure of diuretic therapy to reduce overall cardiovascular mortality in these patients in large-scale trials.[10]

Most disturbing is the arrhythmogenic potential of inotropic therapy in patients with congestive heart failure. A long-sought but incompletely realized goal of clinical cardiovascular pharmacologists has been the development of a drug for the treatment of left ventricular dysfunction that increases cardiac contractility without increasing cardiac irritability; unfortunately, most agents that have been developed to date have a narrow toxic-therapeutic ratio. Digitalis may produce serious ventricular tachyarrhythmias not only when its circulating levels are elevated, but also in therapeutic concentrations should potassium stores be depleted. Such malignant arrhythmias may contribute to the increased cardiovascular mortality noted in patients with heart failure and complex ventricular ectopy who receive long-term digitalis therapy after an acute myocardial infarction.[11] Recently developed potent inotropic agents enhance cardiac contractility by increasing intramyocellular levels of cyclic AMP, either by promoting its synthesis (catecholamines) or by retarding its degradation (phosphodiesterase inhibition); both mechanisms are potentially arrhythmogenic. Although intravenously administered catecholamines can increase ventricular ectopy in patients with congestive heart failure, neither dopamine nor dobutamine appear to have increased the risk for sudden death, since these drugs are not generally administered over a long term. Unfortunately, orally active phosphodiesterase inhibitors (such as amrinone, milrinone, and enoximone) are being developed for long-term use and appear to have a similar arrhythmogenic potential, which may explain the high frequency of sudden death in patients with heart failure treated with these agents.[12] Whether the proarrhythmic effects of digitalis and phosphodiesterase inhibitors can be antagonized by concomitant treatment with converting-enzyme inhibitors, β-blockers, or antiarrhythmic agents remains to be seen.

Prevention of sudden unexpected death in patients with congestive heart failure. In attempting to design a therapeutic approach to the prevention of sudden unexpected death in patients with congestive heart failure, two central questions need to be considered: (1) Which patients with congestive heart failure are at high risk of sudden death and should receive prophylactic therapy? (2) Are conventional antiarrhythmic drugs successful in preventing sudden death in these patients?

Identification of patients with heart failure at high risk of sudden death. There is general agreement that patients with *symptomatic* ventricular tachycardia or fibrillation should be treated to prevent future sudden cardiac death, but only a small fraction of patients with congestive heart failure who will die suddenly will experience premonitory symptoms. The clinical picture in most individuals is so dominated by dyspnea and fatigue that sudden death is usually the first manifestation of a clinically important arrhythmia problem. Unfortunately, there remains no clear means of identifying patients who are likely to die suddenly before the terminal event occurs. Some investigators have suggested that the finding of complex ventricular rhythm disturbances (especially nonsustained ventricular tachycardia) on ambulatory electrocardiographic monitoring predicts future fatal arrhythmias, but such malignant ventricular ectopy is usually a reflection of the severity of hemodynamic and functional abnormalities and therefore predicts *total* mortality rather than the occurrence of sudden unexpected death (table 2). Other observers have proposed that the finding of sustained ventricular tachycardia during programmed ventricular stimulation can identify a high-risk patient population, but the arrhythmias in patients with cardiomyopathies may be particularly resistant to electrical provocation,[13] and ventricular tachyarrhythmias may be induced in many patients who are not at risk of future events. Still other investigators have suggested that the finding of late diastolic potentials on signal-averaged electrocardiograms can distinguish those patients with heart failure predisposed to potentially lethal arrhythmias[14]; these findings need to be confirmed, but such abnormalities may prove to be more closely related to the severity of ventricular dysfunction than to ventricular irritability. I believe that there is as yet no validated means of identifying patients with congestive heart failure who are at high risk of sudden unexpected death. Furthermore, because the frequency of sudden death in the overall heart failure population is substantial (20% annual event rate), I view *all* patients with congestive heart failure as being at high risk and would suggest that *all* such patients are candidates for long-term prophylactic treatment, were an effective and well-tolerated therapeutic approach available.

Efficacy of conventional antiarrhythmic drugs in preventing sudden death. Presently available antiarrhythmic agents are seriously flawed in their ability to suppress ventricular tachyarrhythmias in patients with congestive heart failure. Although pharmacologic approaches to the treatment of ventricular ectopy are generally successful in patients with normal ventricular function, the efficacy of antiarrhythmic drugs markedly diminishes as left ventricular ejection fraction declines, such that only a small fraction of patients with heart failure and an ejection fraction less than 30% are responsive to antiarrhythmic drug therapy[15]; the efficacy of these agents may be further reduced in patients with coexistent electrolyte deficiencies. Even the modest response in some patients can be outweighed by the proarrhythmic effects of these drugs in others. Furthermore, many antiarrhythmic agents have potent negative inotropic effects that may exacerbate the heart failure state (especially disopyramide) or interfere with the inotropic actions of digitalis (quinidine). These observations may explain why no antiarrhythmic drug has yet been shown to prevent sudden death in patients with congestive heart failure.

The most successful approaches to the control of arrhythmias in the future for patients with congestive heart failure may be endomyocardial resection of the reentry pathway (guided by electrophysiologic mapping) or the use of an automatic implantable defibrillator.[15] Although use of such aggressive and expensive therapies can be rationalized for the patient with *symptomatic* ventricular tachyarrhythmias, they are not practical solutions to the problem of sudden death for most patients with heart failure.

In conclusion, with the advent of potent inotropic and vasodilator agents that can improve pump performance, sudden unexpected death from ventricular tachyarrhythmias may soon become the most common cause of death in patients with congestive heart failure. Recent evidence indicates that complex ventricular ectopy is nearly universally present in these patients and may be exacerbated by conventional heart failure therapy (digitalis and diuretics) that may lead to electrolyte deficits and activate neurohormonal mechanisms. On the other hand, therapeutic interventions that preserve intracellular cations or reduce circulating levels of vasopressor hormones (converting-enzyme inhibitors or β-blockers) may suppress ventricular ectopic activity and prevent sudden death. The empiric use of conventional antiarrhythmic drugs has generally proved to be an ineffective and potentially dangerous approach to control of arrhythmias in these individuals.

Our attention is slowly shifting from not only making patients with heart failure feel better (the first frontier) but also making patients with heart failure live longer (the second frontier). In doing so, it is imperative that we begin to understand why patients with heart failure die. What factors mediate the progression of left ventricular dysfunction in these patients and what factors predispose to the development of fatal ventricular arrhythmias? Until such information is forthcoming, present evidence suggests that electrolyte deficits and neurohormonal forces may be the most important *treatable* mechanisms of sudden death in patients with congestive heart failure. Prospective large-scale clinical trials are in order to evaluate if converting-enzyme inhibition or β-blockade can really prolong life in these severely ill patients.

References

1. Brown MJ, Brown DC, Murphy MB: Hypokalemia from beta$_2$-receptor stimulation by circulating epinephrine. N Engl J Med **309:** 1414, 1983
2. Bertuso JR, Flaker GC, Ruder MA, Alpert MA: Do patients with cardiac arrest and hypokalemia require antiarrhythmic drug therapy? Circulation **70:**(suppl II): II-443, 1984 (abst)
3. Chadda K, Ballas M, Bodenheimer MM: Efficacy of magnesium replacement in patients with hypomagnesemia and cardiac arrhythmia. Circulation **70:**(suppl II): II-444, 1984 (abst)
4. Cohn JN, Levine TB, Olivari MT, Garberg V, Lura D, Francis GS, Simon AB, Rector T: Plasma norepinephrine as a guide to prognosis in patients with chronic congestive heart failure. N Engl J Med **311:** 819, 1984
5. Lee WH, Packer M: Prognostic value of serum sodium concentration in severe heart failure and its modification by converting-enzyme inhibition. Circulation **70**(suppl II): II-113, 1984 (abst)
6. Cleland JGF, Dargie HJ, Hodsman GP, Ball SG, Robertson JIS, Morton JJ, East BW, Robertson I, Murray GD, Gillen G: Captopril in heart failure. A double-blind controlled trial. Br Heart J **52:** 530, 1984
7. Furberg C, Yusuf S: Effect of vasodilators on survival in chronic congestive heart failure. Am J Cardiol **55:** 1110, 1985
8. Furberg CD, Morton-Hawkins C, Lichtstein E for the Beta-blocker Heart Attack Trial Study Group: Effect of propranolol in postinfarction patients with mechanical or electrical complications. Circulation **69:** 761, 1984
9. Swedberg K, Hjalmarson A, Waagstein F, Wallentin I: Prolongation of survival in congestive cardiomyopathy by beta-receptor blockade. Lancet **1:** 1374, 1979
10. Hollifield JW: Potassium and magnesium abnormalities: diuretics and arrhythmias in hypertension. Am J Med **77**(5A): 28, 1984
11. Bigger JT Jr, Fleiss JL, Rolnitzky LM, Merab JP, Ferrick KJ: Effect of digitalis treatment on survival after myocardial infarction. Am J Cardiol **55:** 623, 1985
12. Packer M, Medina N, Yushak M: Hemodynamic and clinical limitations of long-term inotropic therapy with amrinone in patients with severe chronic heart failure. Circulation **70:** 1038, 1984
13. Naccarelli GV, Prystowsky EN, Jackman WM, Heger JJ, Rahilly GT, Zipes DP: Role of electrophysiologic testing in managing patients who have ventricular tachycardia unrelated to coronary artery disease. Am J Cardiol **50:** 165, 1982
14. Poll DS, Marchlinski FE, Falcone RA, Simson MB: Abnormal signal averaged ECG in nonischemic congestive cardiomyopathy: relationship to sustained ventricular tachyarrhythmias. Circulation **70**(suppl II): II-253, 1984 (abst)
15. Poll DS, Marchlinski FE, Buxton AE, Doherty JU, Waxman HL, Josephson ME: Sustained ventricular tachycardia in patients with idiopathic dilated cardiomyopathy: electrophysiologic testing and lack of response to antiarrhythmic drug therapy. Circulation **70:** 451, 1984

PERSPECTIVE

Cholesterol and cardiovascular disease: no longer whether, but rather when, in whom, and how?

ROBERT I. LEVY, M.D.

IN JANUARY of 1984, the results of the decade-long Lipid Research Clinics (LRC) Coronary Primary Prevention Trial were reported.[1, 2] The results received widespread attention through the news media and have been much discussed and sometimes hotly debated. It is the intention of this article to briefly review this study and some of the findings that led to its initiation in order to detail where we are now and to suggest future directions in research and patient care.

For several decades evidence has been accumulating to indicate that there is a causal relationship between high cholesterol levels in blood and coronary atherosclerosis. The evidence for the cholesterol/atherogenesis connection includes results of direct morphologic studies of the atherosclerotic plaque itself (which by definition contains cholesterol), as well as results of studies in animals (including nonhuman primates in which plaque regression has been demonstrated with cholesterol lowering), and data from metabolic, genetic, and prospective and retrospective epidemiologic studies in man.[3-5]

Despite all of this evidence, some have questioned the cholesterol/atherogenesis connection because it has not been demonstrated directly in man that lowering plasma cholesterol (low-density lipoprotein or LDL) levels reduces progression of atherosclerotic plaque or incidence of heart attack and death from cardiac causes. These individuals point out that epidemiologic findings may represent circumstantial associations and that studies in animals may not necessarily be relevant and demand direct clinical trial evidence in man.

Review of results of all the clinical trials performed before the LRC Coronary Primary Prevention Trial and the NHLBI Type II Intervention Study in aggregate reveals suggestive but not definitive evidence of the value of lowering cholesterol levels. What appeared to be lacking from the design of most of the trials was an appreciation of the logistic (the study power and sample size) requirements essential for a trial designed to test the effects of lowering cholesterol levels on the progression of coronary artery disease.

Many of the clinical trials performed in the past lacked important features. The failure to completely randomize often meant that there was not a comparable control group to compare with the treatment group. The lack of a double-blind design made it difficult to interpret even the most objective of end points. Many of the trials suffered from lack of adequate numbers of participants or adequate follow-up time. In still others adherence of study subjects to diet or other regimens was not documented, resulting in an inadequate cholesterol differential. Finally, when drugs that lower lipid levels are given to subjects, an awareness of the potential side effects of the drugs is necessary. All these factors were reviewed by the National Heart, Lung, and Blood Institute's Atherosclerosis Task Force,[6] which in 1972 recommended (in good part because of logistics) against a national diet-heart trial and for several of the more defined studies that have recently been concluded.

The LRC Coronary Primary Prevention Trial. The LRC Coronary Primary Prevention Trial was a randomized, multicenter, placebo-controlled double-blind study.[1, 2] It enrolled a large number of patients (3806) and was designed to follow them all for a minimum of 7 years to a primary end point of heart attack or cardiac death. It was carried out scrupulously in 12 lipid research clinics, 11 in the United States and one in Canada. The participants were all men (to increase the likelihood of events) between the ages of 35 and 59 years with cholesterol levels above 265 mg% (the 95th percentile for the United States). Volunteers were eligible only if they had no evidence of coronary artery disease on examination or by history and had elevated cholesterol levels. Excluded from the trial were subjects taking lipid-lowering drugs or with hypertension or another disease likely to limit their life expectancy.

Subjects were seen monthly, at first in part to eliminate the faint of heart, and were placed on a modest

From the Office of the Vice President for Health Sciences, Columbia University, New York.

Address for correspondence: Robert I. Levy, M.D., Office of the Vice President for Health Sciences, Columbia University, 630 West 168th St., New York, NY 10032.

modified fat diet designed not so much to lower cholesterol as to offer something to all volunteers entering the trial. (In fact, the power of the study would have been greater and the sample size requirement less if one group received no treatment to lower cholesterol levels and in the other group cholesterol level was lowered by a fixed percentage.) The diet was a modified low-fat, low-cholesterol diet (much less stringent than the current American Heart Association dietary recommendation)[7] containing about 400 mg of cholesterol and a P/S ratio of about 0.8. It was designed to achieve approximately a 3% to 4% reduction in cholesterol.

After five clinic visits the volunteers were randomly assigned to one of two equal groups. The randomization procedure created two comparable groups, identical at the start of the study with respect to clinical characteristics and with a mean age of 47 years and a mean cholesterol level of 291 mg%. The groups were still identical 7 years later except that one had a considerably lower cholesterol level. The lipid-lowering drug cholestyramine was selected for study because it is a known effective LDL-lowering agent that is not absorbed, i.e., it is nonsystemic and does not have the potential systemic effects seen with agents like clofibrate.[8] It was also chosen because a placebo form was known to be available.

The remarkable feature of the LRC Coronary Primary Prevention Trial, in addition to its magnitude (3086 men enrolled, 193,000 clinic visits, 1,055,000 clinic data forms, 341,000 blood tests and 72,000 electrocardiograms) and cost (over $150 million), was the fact that complete follow-up was achieved at the end of the study so that the vital status of all 3806 patients randomized into the trial was known.

With use of intention-to-treat analysis and thereby including both those patients who took cholestyramine regularly and those who took none during most of the trial, it was found that the average 8% differential in cholesterol and 11% differential in LDL between the placebo and treatment group over the 7 years of the study was associated with a statistically significant 19% reduction in occurrence of the primary end point of definite heart attack or cardiac death. This consisted of a 24% reduction in definite cardiac death and a 19% reduction in definite heart attack.

In the group of men randomly assigned to receive cholestyramine the wide range in degree of compliance to the prescribed drug regimen produced a wide differential in cholesterol reductions and thereby created a study within a study. Analysis of these data demonstrated that as compliance increased, reduction in cholesterol level increased, as did the reduction in incidence of definite heart attack and cardiac death. With multivariate analyses it was demonstrated that reduction in cholesterol level and not packet ingestion per se explained the observed reduction in risk. In fact, statistical analysis allowed the development of a linear regression model in which a 25% lowering of cholesterol level, achievable with a full dose of medicine, was associated with a 50% reduction in risk. It is this finding that is responsible for the popularized observation that for every 1% reduction in cholesterol, there was a 2% reduction in incidence of heart attack and cardiac death.

What was perhaps most impressive about the findings of the LRC Coronary Primary Prevention Trial was their consistency. All the cardiovascular events that were recorded, from the definitive end point of heart attack or death from cardiac causes to other "softer" end points, indicated a benefit of treatment (table 1). For example, subjects underwent stress exercise testing every 6 months during the study. Results were positive in 260 of the patients on cholestyramine and in 345 of the patients on placebo, which indicates a reduction in risk of some 25% (p = < .001) for the patients receiving the drug. In the placebo group 287 patients developed angina, compared with 235 patients in the cholestyramine group, a reduction of 20%. In

TABLE 1

Cardiovascular end points in the LRC Coronary Primary Prevention Trial[A]

	Placebo group[B]		Treatment group[B]		% reduction in risk
	No.	%	No.	%	
Definite CHD death[C] and/or definite nonfatal MI	187	9.8	155	8.1	19
Definite CHD death	38	2.0	30	1.6	24
Definite nonfatal MI	158	8.3	130	6.8	19
Positive exercise test	345	19.8	260	14.9	25
Angina (Rose questionnaire)	287	15.1	235	12.4	20
Coronary bypass surgery	112	5.9	93	4.9	21
Congestive heart failure	11	0.6	8	0.4	28
Intraoperative MI	7	0.4	5	0.3	29
Resuscitated coronary collapse	5	0.3	3	0.2	40

MI = myocardial infarction; CHD = coronary heart disease.

[A]Reference 1.

[B]Total placebo group = 1,900; total treatment group (cholestyramine) = 1906.

[C]Primary end point.

the cholestyramine group, 93 patients required coronary bypass surgery vs 112 in the placebo group. Although much smaller in number, there were similar reductions in the development of congestive heart failure, intermittent claudication, and resuscitated coronary arrest in the drug-treated group.

In 1976, in the *Annals of Internal Medicine,*[9] those who supported the lipid hypothesis were challenged in an article entitled "Whether Rather Than How." It was suggested that it was not enough to demonstrate a curvilinear relationship between cholesterol and heart disease in prospective studies like the Framingham Study but rather that it was necessary to demonstrate that if cholesterol level was lowered the risk of heart disease was indeed reduced. This is what the LRC Coronary Primary Prevention Trial has done.

In addition to the results of the LRC Coronary Primary Prevention Trial, recent secondary prevention trials have further supported the value of lowering cholesterol level. In the NHLBIs Type II Coronary Intervention Trial,[9, 10] a design similar to that of the LRC Coronary Primary Prevention Trial was used in hypercholesterolemic patients with existing coronary disease. Change in coronary artery lesions at 0 and 5 years, as demonstrated by comparative angiography, was the end point. It was demonstrated that lowering cholesterol levels was associated with a decrease in progression of atherosclerotic plaque and that this change in progression was related to both a fall in LDL and an increase in high-density lipoprotein (HDL).

Considering all available evidence, we have in fact fulfilled what might be thought of as Koch's postulates for cholesterol and atherosclerosis. Not only have we determined that there is cholesterol in all atherosclerotic plaques and that when the blood levels of cholesterol increase, plaques and the clinical sequelae of plaque progression increase, but we can also demonstrate that when cholesterol levels are lowered the development of plaque and its sequelae, heart attack and cardiac death, decrease.

Extrapolating the evidence. The results of LRC Coronary Primary Prevention Trial are quite clear. What is not so clear is how far these basic findings can be generalized. Some would choose not to extrapolate at all and suggest that the findings are applicable to middle-aged men with cholesterol levels over 265 mg% who take bile acids sequestrants only. That would be a still sizeable number of individuals, some 1 to 2 million in the American population. There is little reason, however, to limit the extrapolation so narrowly. The age group from 35 to 59 years old in this study was chosen arbitrarily. There is no reason to think that lowering of cholesterol levels would not be beneficial in individuals below age 35 or above age 59. Similarly, women were excluded from this study because as a group they do not suffer many cardiac events between ages 35 and 59. However, since in women cholesterol is a major risk factor and coronary artery disease is still the major cause of death, there is every reason to believe that the study results can and should be extrapolated to women. Furthermore, since there is no magic cutoff point above which cholesterol is dangerous, but rather a graded risk relationship at least down to a cholesterol level of 180 mg%, there is every reason to think that the members of the population in the top four quintiles with respect to cholesterol level would benefit from its reduction. Selected reference values for total and lipoprotein cholesterol obtained in the LRC North American Prevalence Study are presented in table 2. If results are extrapolated to women, a wider age range, and to those in the top quintile of cholesterol level, about 40 to 50 million Americans could be considered at risk, a population as large as those now considered at risk of hypertension. With regard to hypertension, since the start of the National High Blood Pressure Education Program in 1972[11] the public health impact of focusing health care professional and public attention has been impressive.

Although more controversial, there are others, like the members of the panel for the recent NIH Consensus Development Conference on lowering of cholesterol,[12] who after reviewing all available evidence extrapolate the potential benefits of lowering cholesterol even further and recommend low-cholesterol diets for the entire American population (except for children under the age of 2). Dietary reduction of plasma cholesterol is safe and cheap and the mechanism by which cholestyramine lowers cholesterol (recently shown to be by increasing hepatic LDL-receptor activity) appears to be similar to the mechanism by which low-fat, low-cholesterol diets do the same. The 10% to 15% lowering of cholesterol level that is possible in the average American with the American Heart Association's prudent phase I diet[7] could have an enormous impact on cardiovascular morbidity and mortality in the United States.

Questions to be answered. Today it is no longer a question of whether to treat those with high cholesterol levels, but rather when, whom, and how to treat? As with any clinical trial, the LRC Coronary Primary Prevention Trial has resulted in many new questions requiring further research. For one, is reduction of LDL by any means beneficial? The LRC Coronary Primary Prevention Trial has demonstrated the benefit of low-

TABLE 2
Selected reference values for plasma cholesterol and lipoprotein cholesterol (mg/dl)[A]

	Plasma cholesterol					LDL cholesterol				HDL cholesterol			
Age (yr)	5	50	75	90	95	5	50	75	95	5	10	50	95
Men													
5–19	115	155	170	185	200	65	95	105	130	35[B]	40[B]	55[B]	75[B]
20–24	125	165	185	205	220	65	105	120	145	30	30	45	65
25–29	135	180	200	225	245	70	115	140	165	30	30	45	65
30–34	140	190	215	240	255	80	125	145	185	30	30	45	60
35–39	145	200	225	250	270	80	135	155	190	30	30	45	60
40–44	150	205	230	250	270	85	135	155	185	25	30	45	65
45–69	160	215	235	260	275	90	145	165	205	30	30	50	70
70+	150	205	230	250	270	90	145	165	185	30	35	50	75
Women													
5–19	120	160	175	190	200	65	100	110	140	35	40	55	70
20–24	125	170	190	215	230	55	105	120	160	35	35	55	80
25–34	130	175	195	220	235	70	110	125	160	35	40	55	80
35–39	140	185	205	230	245	75	120	140	170	35	40	55	80
40–44	145	195	215	235	255	75	125	145	175	35	40	60	90
45–49	150	205	225	250	270	80	130	150	185	35	40	60	85
50–54	165	220	240	265	285	90	140	160	200	35	40	60	90
55+	170	230	250	295	295	95	150	170	215	35	40	60	95

[A]From the LRC Program–North American Prevalence Study.[13, 14]
[B]For HDL values for men age 15 to 19 use values for age group 20 to 24.

ering cholesterol levels with the drug cholestyramine. Since the mechanism is similar, others have suggested that diet should work equally well. What about other lipid-lowering drugs? Should we not be suspicious and cautious in extrapolating the results with cholestyramine to other lipid-lowering agents since findings of both the European Primary Prevention Trial and the Coronary Drug Project indicate that some of these drugs may have serious adverse side effects?[8] Furthermore, in the LRC Coronary Primary Prevention Trial and in the NHLBI Type II Intervention Trial a benefit from reduction of LDL and from an increase in HDL was observed.[12a] An independent benefit seemed to be apparent with small increments in HDL. Should we therefore now be focusing on HDL as well? Is elevation of HDL levels by any means beneficial? Should we be attempting to raise HDL by nonpharmacologic methods like exercise and weight reduction? And what about pharmacologic approaches to raising the HDL level? There are several drugs available for this purpose. Would they be of benefit in preventing heart disease?

In the LRC Coronary Primary Prevention Trial, the major criteria for entry as well as for monitoring and follow-up was total and LDL cholesterol. In the future, should our design to treat and follow-up patients be based on the total cholesterol level or should we be focusing on lipoprotein cholesterol levels? There is much evidence to suggest that treating specific lipoprotein excesses with specific diets and drugs is more effective and that by defining the lipoprotein excess we can provide a more specific and effective regimen for lipid lowering. In the future, will the measurement of lipoprotein apoprotein levels give us a more useful index by which to guide treatment and follow-up than total or lipoprotein cholesterol levels? Immunoassay techniques for the lipoprotein apoproteins are now being developed and tested. It has been suggested that measurement of apoprotein levels may provide more specific and sensitive coronary artery risk information. Evidence is accumulating that measurement of both apoprotein B and apoprotein A_I gives useful and predictive information with regard to coronary heart disease risk.

In the public health arena the potential benefit of lowering cholesterol levels is so great that we must explore the optimal methods of enhancing changes in these levels. Among the health care issues raised are questions such as: How can we reduce the cost of lipid-lowering drugs? The only drugs now shown to be beneficial, the bile acid sequestrants, are expensive, costing patients well over a $100.00 a month. Will the fact that lower cholesterol levels have now been shown to be beneficial lead to increased activity in industry and to the development of more palatable and less costly lipid-lowering drugs? And how can we ensure patient adherence to diet and drug therapy? Even the modest diet changes that are required to reduce the amount of saturated fat and cholesterol in a cholesterol-lowering diet require some degree of motivation and adherence by patients. Habits of a lifetime are difficult to change. We must both educate and motivate our patients. How can we maximize this? And, what are the implications for the meat, dairy, and other food industries? Already a number of food manufacturers are preparing foods lower in saturated fat and cholesterol. The potential in this area is enormous, as is the need to educate Americans on the reading of food labels and the nature of dietary fat and cholesterol.

Finally, a major health care issue that has been the subject of some debate deals with the value of intervention in high-risk subjects vs a mass population approach. Some argue that we should be screening the population at large and treating those with the highest levels of cholesterol. Others argue that it would be much more cost effective to seek to lower the cholesterol level in everyone through diet, thereby reducing the cholesterol-attributable risk in the entire population. As with this issue in hypertension (as well as other risk factor interventions), the answer does not appear to be either/or — the answer is both. There is a clear benefit to identifying and treating individuals at high risk in the population and there is a clear benefit with respect to cost efficiency in seeking to lower the average American cholesterol level through a mass population approach.

When, whom, and how to treat. In terms of when to treat, it would appear that since atherosclerosis begins in the first two decades of life, and is episodically progressive over time, there would be little reason to delay cholesterol reduction. This is especially true if the method is diet, the use of which can be considered safe after age 2 and still appropriate and effective beyond age 65.

The NIH Consensus statement[12] on lowering blood cholesterol recommends that all adults with "high risk blood cholesterol levels" (values above the 90th percentile) be treated intensively by diet and, if the response is inadequate, with appropriate drugs. The statement further recommends that those with "moderate risk blood cholesterol levels" (values between the 75th and 90th percentiles) be treated intensively by dietary means and states that only a small proportion should require drug treatment. Their recommended cholesterol values for defining men and women at "moderate and high risk" requiring treatment are presented in table 3. Some experts recommend a more conservative approach while still others would be even more aggressive.

TABLE 3
Cholesterol values indicating men and women at high risk[A]

Age (yr)	Moderate risk (level in mg/dl)	High risk (level in mg/dl)
20–29	> 200	> 220
30–39	> 220	> 240
40 and over	> 240	> 260

[A]From the NIH Consensus Development Statement on Lowering Blood Cholesterol.[12]

I have used an approach relatively consistent with the NIH recommendations: All individuals (men and women) with cholesterol levels of over 200 mg% should be considered candidates for dietary treatment; treatment is especially indicated for individuals with other risk factors, such as previous coronary artery bypass surgery or diabetes, end-stage renal disease, or other disorders known to be associated with accelerated atherosclerosis.

Every patient should know what his or her plasma cholesterol level is. Any level of cholesterol of 200 mg% or higher (or 175 mg% or higher in children) should be revealed to the patient (or parent) and, if it is due to LDL excess, a diet should be suggested. A cholesterol-lowering diet should certainly be prescribed for any adult patient whose cholesterol level, due to LDL excess, is over 230 mg%. Those patients with other risk factors for coronary heart disease, or with cholesterol levels above 260 mg%, in whom cholesterol level does not fall below 230 mg% with dietary therapy (and the elevation is due to an increase in LDL) should be considered for drug therapy.

In terms of how to treat, it is important to establish a baseline and obtain several measurements so that it can be determined that the patient in truth has an elevated cholesterol level. Secondary causes should be ruled out. The first intervention tried should always be diet. In some patients an improper diet or sensitivity to dietary fat may be the cause of the hypercholesterolemia. In others, diet will help lower the cholesterol enough so that less drug therapy will be necessary, thus lowering costs and the incidence of drug-induced side effects. When deciding upon a treatment strategy, it is important, when possible, to change one factor at a time. If it is known that the patient has complied with therapy, an ineffective regimen should not be continued beyond 8 weeks. When a drug is used, it should be one appropriate for the type of lipoprotein excess the patient has and blood samples should be obtained from the patient regularly. The latter will avoid the possibility of missing inapparent side effects and serve to motivate the patient.

In conclusion, we have now entered into a new era. The question is no longer whether or not lowering cholesterol is beneficial. The questions now, and that have been discussed herein, include when, whom, and how to treat. These are questions that will be debated for a period of time, but practicing physicians today, especially those treating middle-aged Americans at risk for coronary disease, can for the first time do more than say that a high cholesterol level is a risk factor. If a patient is found to have an elevated cholesterol level, a cholesterol-lowering regimen can be prescribed with the knowledge that the patient will likely live longer and better as a result.

References

1. Lipid Research Clinics Program: The Lipid Research Clinics Coronary Primary Prevention Trial Results. I. Reduction in incidence of coronary heart disease. JAMA **251:** 351, 1984
2. Lipid Research Clinics Program: The Lipid Research Clinics Coronary Prevention Trial Results. II. The relationship of reduction in incidence of coronary heart disease to cholesterol lowering. JAMA **251:** 365, 1984
3. Wissler RW: Principles of the pathogenesis of atherosclerosis. *In* Braunwald E, editor: Heart disease. Philadelphia, 1984, W.B. Saunders Co., p 1183
4. Levy RI, Feinleib M: Risk factors for coronary artery disease and their management. *In* Braunwald E, editor: Heart disease. Philadelphia, 1984, W.B. Saunders, Co., p 1205
5. Inter-Society Commission for Heart Disease Resources-Atherosclerosis Study Group (Kannel WB, Chairman): Optimal resources for primary prevention of atherosclerotic diseases. Circulation **70:** 157A, 1984
6. Arteriosclerosis: a report by the National Heart, Lung, and Blood Institute Task Force on arteriosclerosis. Washington, D.C., 1971, Department of Health, Education, and Welfare publication (NIH) 72-137
7. American Heart Association Special Report: Recommendations for the treatment of hyperlipidemia in adults. A joint statement of the Nutrition Committee and the Council on Arteriosclerosis of the American Heart Association. Arteriosclerosis **4:** 445A, 1984
8. Committee of Principle Investigators: WHO cooperative trial on primary prevention of ischemic heart disease with clofibrate to lower serum cholesterol: final mortality follow-up. Lancet **2:** 600, 1984
9. Ahrens EH: The management of hyperlipidemia — whether, rather than how. Ann Intern Med **85:** 87, 1976
10. Brensike JF, Levy RI, Kelsey SF, et al: Effects of therapy with cholestyramine on progression of coronary arteriosclerosis: results of the NHLBI Type II Coronary Intervention Study. Circulation **69:** 313, 1984
11. Levy RI: The National Heart, Lung, and Blood Institute overview 1980. The Director's report on the NHLBI Advisory Council. Circulation **65:** 217, 1982
12. National Institutes of Health Consensus Development Conference Statement: Lowering blood cholesterol. JAMA **253:** 2080, 1985

12a. Levy RI, Brensike JF, Epstein S, Kelsey SF, Passamani ER, Richardson JM, Loh IK, Stone NJ, Aldrich RF, Battagiini JW, Moriarty DJ, Fisher ML, Friedman L, Friedwald W, Detre KM: Influence of changes in lipid values induced by cholestyramine and diet on progression of coronary artery disease: results of the NHLBI Type II Coronary Intervention Study. Circulation **69:** 325, 1984

13. U.S. Department of Health and Human Services: The Lipid Research Clinics Population Studies data book, vol I (The Prevalence Study). Bethesda, 1980, NIH Publication No. 80-1257
14. Rifkind BM, Segal P: Lipid Research Clinics Program reference values for hyperlipidemia and hypolipidemia. JAMA **250:** 1869, 1983

EDITORIAL

Comprehensive health care and noncardiovascular mortality: an unlikely explanation of the findings from the Hypertension Detection and Follow-up Program

SIEGFRIED HEYDEN, M.D., KENNETH SCHNEIDER, M.D., AND J. G. FODOR, M.D.

THE HYPERTENSION Detection and Follow-up Program (HDFP) showed a significant reduction in both cardiovascular and noncardiovascular death rates in patients receiving stepped care. Over the past three years, several reports[1, 2] have suggested that the results of treatment reported in the HDFP were due to comprehensive medical care of hypertensive patients in a stepped care treatment group rather than to a specific hypotensive effect of drug therapy. Also, the clinical significance of the 19% reduction in cardiovascular mortality in patients under stepped care in comparison with those receiving referred care is questionable, because noncardiovascular mortality was reduced by 14% in the former group.

In any hypertension intervention study in which the group on active therapy is seen more frequently than the control group, it is legitimate to ask whether the final benefits result from specific antihypertensive medication and effective blood pressure control or from general contact and comprehensive health care. Because of the implications for management of hypertensive patients it is deemed necessary to advance explanations for reduced noncardiovascular mortality among those that are successfully treated. A decrease in cardiovascular mortality might be expected to be responsible for an increase in mortality from cancer and other important causes of death over a long follow-up time because of competing risk. Therefore, if anything, the noncardiovascular mortality might have been expected to rise rather than fall in response to a decrease of cardiovascular mortality.

Evidence for effective control of "mild" hypertension in lowering noncardiovascular death rate. The number of noncardiovascular deaths by cause for the five years of the HDFP experience are summarized in table 1. In all except three categories, violent deaths and renal and infectious disease, there were fewer deaths in the total stepped care than in the referred care group. Stratum I patients (diastolic blood pressure 90 to 104 mm Hg) accounted for the majority of this difference. For those in strata II (diastolic blood pressure 105 to 114 mm Hg) and III (diastolic blood pressure ≥115 mm Hg) differences were small between stepped care and referred care groups with respect to numbers of both cardiovascular and noncardiovascular deaths.[3]

The greatest reduction in all-cause mortality occurred in the subgroup of stratum I patients with baseline diastolic blood pressure levels of 90 to 94 mm Hg who were free of target organ damage (table 2). They had no evidence of coronary heart disease, stroke, electrocardiographic abnormalities, intermittent claudication, or elevated creatinine levels and were not on blood pressure medication at the initiation of the trial.[4] At that time (1973 to 1974), many physicians would have considered this group to be "healthy" and their diastolic blood pressures would not have mandated any antihypertensive therapy. Yet after five years of HDFP protocol therapy, there was a reduction in deaths in the stepped care group of 34%. Mortality per 1000 from stroke, myocardial infarction, all cardiovascular diseases, and all noncardiovascular diseases in the stepped care group was 6.9, 3.2, 2.9, and 2.7, respectively, lower than in the referred care group. However, there was only a 7.9% reduction in mortality in the stratum I patients in the stepped care compared with the referred care group when target organ damage was present at baseline. This suggests that elevated blood pressure is most successfully treated before the development of target organ damage.

The percentage of patients with diastolic blood pressure of 90 to 104 mm Hg on drug treatment in the stepped care group was 75% at year 2 and remained at

From the Departments of Community and Family Medicine and Pathology, Duke University Medical Center, Durham, and the Department of Community Medicine, University of Newfoundland, St. John's.

Address for correspondence: Kenneth Schneider, M.D., Duke University Medical Center, Department of Pathology, Box 3712, Durham, NC 27710.

TABLE 1
Number of noncardiovascular deaths by cause, stepped care (SC), and referred care (RC) participants, and total and stratum 1 patients (DBP 90 to 104 mm Hg) in HDFP

	Total		Stratum 1 (DBP 90 to 104 mm Hg)	
Cause of death (ICDA codes)[A]	SC	RC	SC	RC
All noncardiovascular diseases	154	179	109	126
Renal disease (580–599)	15	10	7	5
Diabetes mellitus (250)	5	10	4	8
Neoplastic diseases (140–239)	61	74	45	57
Breast cancer (174)	(2)	(5)	(2)	(4)
Gastrointestinal diseases (530–537)	11	20	9	15
Respiratory diseases (460–519)	13	17	9	10
Infectious diseases (000–136)	6	3	4	2
Accidents, suicides, and homicides (800–999)	26	25	20	17
Other diseases	17	20	11	12

DBP = diastolic blood pressure.
[A]From death certificates of HDFP patients (ICDA code is International Classification of Diseases Adapted code).

that level over the next 3 years. In the referred care group only 54% of patients were on drug treatment at year 5. Actively treated patients in the stepped care group with the mildest hypertension (diastolic blood pressure of 90 to 94 mm Hg), by protocol, were under a strict medical treatment regimen with the goal of reducing diastolic blood pressure by 10 mm Hg or reaching 80 to 84 mm Hg. The reduction in pressure in this group was from 92 mm Hg at baseline to 82 mm Hg at year 5 in patients receiving stepped care, while in those receiving referred care it was reduced from 92 mm Hg at baseline to 87 mm Hg at year 5.

No comprehensive preventive medical care beyond blood pressure control was either given or necessary in the HDFP stepped care patients who were essentially "healthy" (those with diastolic blood pressure of 90 to 94 mm Hg and free of target organ damage; table 2). A small subgroup of patients with blood pressures in the same range at baseline but with manifestations of target organ damage and on antihypertensive drug therapy when enrolled in the study might have undergone some additional diagnostic tests and received other therapy. However, the resulting nonsignificant 7.9% lower all-cause mortality rate in the stepped care compared with the referred care group argues against any beneficial effect of a more comprehensive medical regimen after target organ damage has occurred (table 2).

Level of comprehensive health care for stepped care patients. A Department of Health and Human Services publication of working papers for an NHLBI conference on implications of the Hypertension Detection and Follow-up Program (No. 83-2116, 1982) presents the evidence for the close comparability between stepped and referred care in many respects, but not with regard to antihypertensive therapy. A "general medical care" effect on the outcome of 5 years of treatment in patients receiving stepped care should have been reflected in other than strictly hypertension-related findings, i.e., in greater smoking cessation, cholesterol reduction, and weight control. However, in none of these parameters was a preventive medical care effect detectable in the stepped care over the referred care group. Percentage of smokers decreased to 34% in both groups, cholesterol levels declined to 220 mg/dl in both, and average weights remained unchanged.

Employment and retirement rates were virtually identical (table 3) in the two groups and neither annual hospitalization rates nor disability days per year varied significantly. The slightly less likelihood of disability in patients receiving stepped care could have resulted from the lower incidence of the cardiovascular complications of hypertension in that group. This idea is supported by the reported frequency of various illnesses occurring in the past year. A higher incidence of gout at year 5 in the stepped care group was found and would be expected with the more intensive diuretic therapy these patients received. The lower incidence of myocardial infarction, previously unrecorded in hypertension research, was confirmed by a recent report of reduced incidence of fatal coronary heart disease, nonfatal myocardial infarcts, and angina pectoris in patients receiving stepped care.[5] Reported incidence of cancer, diabetes, kidney stones, ulcers, and liver disease were identical in the two groups.

The report also contains a section on the participants' understanding of the problems of high blood pressure, which again reveals similar responses, with 97% of patients in both groups agreeing that individ-

TABLE 2
Results of 5 years of treatment in HDFP stratum I patients in relation to baseline target organ damage

Target organ damage at baseline	SC		RC		% Reduction in deaths in SC group
	n	No. of deaths	n	No. of deaths	
No	1022	36	1023	54	34
Yes	173	30	175	33	7.9

SC = stepped care; RC = referred care.

TABLE 3
Employment status, annual hospitalization rates, and disability (%) at baseline and at 5 year follow-up in stepped care (SC) and referred care (RC) groups[A]

	Baseline		Year 5	
	SC	RC	SC	RC
Employed	64	65	56	56
Not employed	36	35	44	44
Retired (nonmedical)	16	16	25	29
Annual hospitalization rate	13	12	12	15
Hospitalized more than one time	3	3	3	3
Disabled (more than 7 days/year)	21	21	19	21

[A]U.S. Department of Health and Human Services, Public Health Service: Implications of the Hypertension Detection and Follow-up Program. N.I.H. publication No. 83-2116, 1982.

uals with hypertension should see a doctor regularly, and 93% in both groups believing that the long-range benefits of medication for high blood pressure include a lesser chance of developing a heart attack. As far as self-perception of health is concerned, 19% of those in the referred care and 20% of those in the stepped care group evaluated their health as "excellent," 45% and 46%, respectively, reported it as "good," 27% and 26% said it was "fair," and only 9% and 7% reported it was "poor."

The report concludes that the improved cardiovascular status resulting from better control of hypertension in patients receiving stepped care may have indirectly caused a decrease in noncardiovascular deaths.

Complications refractory to comprehensive medical care. Development of left ventricular hypertrophy (LVH) in patients with normal electrocardiograms at baseline was 37.5% greater in the referred care than in the stepped care group. Among patients with an increase in R wave amplitude at baseline, at 5 years there was a 66.7% greater occurrence of LVH with ST-T segment changes in the referred care compared with the stepped care group.[6]

In those patients with electrocardiographic evidence of tall R waves or LVH at baseline, the rate of regression toward normal was 54.3% in the stepped care and 42.9% in the referred care group ($p < .01$). Reversal of enlarged cardiac silhouette on chest x-rays was noted in 47% of those in the stepped care and in 38% of those in the referred care group ($p < .01$). It appears unlikely that this regression of highly abnormal electrocardiographic and chest x-ray findings in a significantly larger number of patients receiving stepped care could have occurred with an improved general health care program. It is equally unlikely that a comprehensive medical care system could effect a 45% reduction in death from stroke and, among patients free of target organ damage at entry, a 25% decrease in incidence of fatal coronary heart disease and nonfatal myocardial infarction in the stepped care compared with the referred care group.

Noncardiovascular mortality in hypertension intervention trials. In contrast to other interventional studies, HDFP patients were unselected with respect to comorbidity and hypertension-related or unrelated risk factors at baseline. Trials such as those undertaken by the United States Public Health Service (USPHS) Hospitals,[7] and the Australian Mild Hypertension[8] and the Oslo studies,[9] excluded mildly (90 to 94 mm Hg) hypertensive individuals or did not compare those with and without baseline target organ damage. Therefore, they did not yield information on these subgroups, which were studied in detail in HDFP. All three studies failed to show any reduction in noncardiovascular mortality in patients under active treatment. It is relevant to note that the overall mortality was unusually low in these three studies: Two of 193 patients under active therapy (1%) and four of 196 placebo-treated patients (2%) in the USPHS Hospitals Study died.[7] There were nine fatal events from all causes in 1721 Australian patients in the active treatment group and 19 fatal events among 1706 patients in the placebo group. In the Oslo Study[9] total deaths numbered 10 of 406 patients under active treatment and nine of 379 patients receiving no treatment. In comparison with these very low numbers, HDFP reported a total of 349 deaths in the stepped care and 419 deaths in the referred care group, corresponding to a 6.4% and 7.7% mortality, respectively ($p < .01$).

The Gothenburg Study[10] recruited hypertensive patients without any regard to coexisting risk factors and morbidity. The authors found that the lower mortality from cardiovascular causes in the treatment group was not compensated for by an increased mortality from other causes. They recognized a tendency to lower mortality from noncardiovascular causes, and concluded that if this tendency were to be found in a larger series, it could be due to some overall effect of antihypertensive treatment. The lower noncardiovascular mortality in the treatment group was similar to that found in the HDFP (2.8% in the stepped care and 3.3% in the referred care group).

Lack of effect of comprehensive care on blood pressure control. In describing the placebo group of the USPHS Hospital Study,[8] the authors emphasized that these patients received placebo in a very positive health care setting, including regular systematized follow-up within a system that provided comprehensive medical care. This care did not produce a fall in the mean diastolic blood pressure.

Noncardiovascular mortality in two epidemiologic studies. In two prospective epidemiologic studies, the Evans County and the Framingham cohorts, a modest positive association between hypertension and risk of dying from noncardiovascular causes was demonstrated for the era before antihypertensive drug therapy became widely accepted. For the purpose of this article, we have carried out analyses of the Evans County cohort, which disclosed excess noncardiovascular mortality in hypertensive individuals as compared with normotensive subjects as ascertained in a community-based survey begun in 1960 and continued to 1980. The ratio of age-adjusted noncardiovascular mortality of men with hypertension compared with that of nonhypertensive men was 1.06 in lower social class white men, 1.34 in high social status white men (neither of these statistically significantly different from 1), and 1.73 in the black men ($p < .05$).

Among men in the Framingham study population who were 45 to 74 years old, the age-adjusted noncardiovascular death rate was 1.2 times higher in hypertensive compared with normotensive individuals between 1955 and 1973 (72.2 per 10,000 men vs 59.4 per 10,000 men). Among women in this study group, all-cause mortality rates in hypertensive and normotensive individuals were 50% lower than in men and noncardiovascular death rates were similar in normotensive and hypertensive women.[11]

Discussion. The design of the HDFP was thought to be flawed because patients who receive comprehensive medical care have lower mortality than those who get less intense care.[1, 2]

It is impossible to completely differentiate between the impact of general medical care for hypertensive patients and that of stepwise antihypertensive care in the HDFP. The counter argument can be summarized as follows: Noncardiovascular mortality decreased significantly in the stepped care group, which is proof of a comprehensive medical care effect; therefore, the HDFP results with respect to reduced cardiovascular mortality are not due to antihypertensive medication per se. This ignores the data that show hypertension to have a deleterious effect on noncardiovascular mortality.

When data from five recently completed hypertension intervention trials were reviewed, it became evident that strict exclusion criteria for three of the studies prevented the admission of hypertensive patients with target organ damage. Among 2320 patients randomly assigned to the active treatment groups only 21 deaths occurred; among 2281 patients randomly assigned to the control groups only 32 deaths were recorded. It would be unreasonable to expect noncardiovascular mortality to show any significant difference between the two treatment groups when the total number of deaths was so low (53 or 1.2%), probably as a result of the strict exclusion criteria, in all three studies.

Neither the Australian nor the Oslo study followed patients with diastolic blood pressures below 95 mm Hg. In the USPHS study, baseline mean diastolic blood pressure was 99 mm Hg, with the mode in the range of 90 to 95 mm Hg. The total number of deaths in this study of 389 hypertensives was small: only four deaths occurred in the placebo group and only two in the actively treated group. The HDFP experience, with its 2045 hypertensive subjects with diastolic blood pressures in the range of 90 to 94 mm Hg, showed a 34% decrease in total mortality.

It is not surprising to clinicians that patients with uncontrolled hypertension, when randomly assigned to a control group of an intervention trial, would suffer from increased noncardiovascular complications, particularly if these patients have a variety of coexisting risk conditions and morbidity at baseline. If untreated hypertension diminishes cardiac reserve, then these patients are at higher risk of death when faced with life-threatening consequences of various noncardiac diseases.

A test of total health care exclusive of blood pressure control was carried out in the 7 year study of the USPHS Hospitals.[7] As expected, blood pressure was not reduced, but in fact rose to an unacceptably high level in 24 of 196 control patients.

It is interesting to consider how noncardiovascular diseases affected hypertensive patients before effective means of treating large numbers of patients became available. Data from the Framingham Study indicated that death rate from noncardiovascular causes among white male hypertensive patients in the first 18 years (1955 to 1973) was higher than in age-matched normotensive men; this was in addition to the well-known increased mortality from cardiovascular disease among hypertensive men (cardiovascular deaths per 10,000 159.9 vs 58.0 in normotensive men).[11] Complementary to these observations are the slightly higher than expected noncardiovascular mortality rates among hypertensive white men and the significantly higher noncardiovascular mortality rates among black men with hypertension in comparison with normotensive men in Evans County between 1960 and 1980.

There can be little doubt that the reduction in cardiovascular events achieved by the stepped care program of the HDFP, including reductions in stroke, LVH, radiographic evidence of cardiomegaly, fatal and nonfatal myocardial infarction, and angina pectoris, were attributable primarily to control of blood pressure, possibly with some additional contribution of comprehensive medical care. The reduction in rates of noncardiovascular death may be due to a similar mechanism: improvement of cardiac reserve in patients compromised by other major disease entities.

We acknowledge the contribution by Dr. Henry Blackburn, Professor of Epidemiology, University of Minnesota, for encouragement in conceiving this article and his very helpful suggestions in the formulation of the manuscript.

Addendum

In a cohort of California men and women from 60 to 79 years old, Khaw and Barrett-Connor (Am J Epidemiol **120:** 550, 1984) reported that systolic blood pressure was a significant independent predictor of cancer mortality in men. In women there was a similar but not statistically significant trend. They raise the possibility that hypertension might decrease cancer survival. "In fact, the positive relationship between systolic blood pressure and cancer may suggest some benefit" from antihypertensive treatment.

References

1. Freis ED: Sounding Board: Should mild hypertension be treated? N Engl J Med **307:** 306, 1982
2. McAlister, NH: Should we treat "mild" hypertension? JAMA **249:** 379, 1983
3. Hypertension Detection and Follow-up Program Cooperative Group: Five-year findings of the Hypertension Detection and Follow-up Program. I. Reduction in mortality of persons with high blood pressure, including mild hypertension. II. Mortality by race-sex and age. JAMA **242:** 2562, 2572, 1979
4. Hypertension Detection and Follow-up Program Cooperative Group: The effect of treatment on mortality in "mild" hypertension. Results of the Hypertension Detection and Follow-up Program. N Engl J Med **307:** 976, 1982
5. Hypertension Detection and Follow-up Program Cooperative Group: Effect of stepped care treatment on the incidence of myocardial infarction and angina pectoris. Hypertension 6(suppl I): I-198, 1984
6. Hypertension Detection and Follow-up Program Cooperative Group: Five-year findings of the Hypertension Detection and Follow-up Program. Prevention and reversal of left ventricular hypertrophy with antihypertensive drug therapy. Circulation **64**(suppl IV): IV-1235, 1981; Hypertension **7:** 105, 1985
7. Smith WM: Treatment of mild hypertension results of a ten-year intervention trial. U.S. Public Health Service Hospitals Cooperative Study Group. Circ Res **40**(suppl I): I-98, 1977
8. Management Committee: The Australian therapeutic trial in mild hypertension. Lancet **1:** 1262, 1980
9. Helgeland A: Treatment of mild hypertension: A five year controlled drug trial. The Oslo Study. Am J Med **69:** 725, 1980
10. Berglund G, Sannerstedt R, Andersson O, Wedel H, Wilhelmsen L, Hansson L, Sievertsson R, Wikstrand J: Coronary heart disease after treatment of hypertension. Lancet **1:** 1, 1978
11. Kannel WB, Gordon T: The Framingham Study. Washington, D.C., 1974, U.S. Government Printing Office. DHEW Publication No. 599

PLATELETS AND VASCULAR OCCLUSION: PLATELET-DERIVED MEDIATORS

Part I

The potential contribution of platelets to atherogenesis, thrombogenesis, and vasospasm has prompted considerable interest in their role in syndromes of vascular occlusion. Recently identified, novel platelet-derived products and pharmacologic probes have helped to illuminate these areas. Accordingly, key advances in cell biology, biochemistry, and pharmacology of platelet–vessel wall interactions will be considered in this and forthcoming issues of *Circulation* in groups of papers based on presentations at a recent symposium entitled "Platelet inhibition and vascular occlusion in man" held in London, England, in August 1984. To provide our readers with an in-depth presentation of the basic science and clinical implications of platelet biology, the material is being published as a featured symposium. Selection of reviewers and editorial decisions for the manuscripts from the symposium were made with the help of Drs. Garret A. FitzGerald, Nashville, Tennessee, and Carlo Patrono, Rome, Italy, chairmen of the meeting.

Part II, "Pharmacology of platelet inhibition," will appear in the December 1985 issue of *Circulation*.

Inhibition of platelet function in thrombosis

AARON J. MARCUS, M.D., LENORE B. SAFIER, M.S., HARRIS L. ULLMAN, M.S., M. JOHAN BROEKMAN, Ph.D., NAZIBA ISLAM, M.S., THOMAS D. OGLESBY, Ph.D., ROBERT R. GORMAN, Ph.D., AND JEAN W. WARD, B.S.

ABSTRACT Accumulating experimental and clinical evidence indicates that a time for reappraisal of therapeutic modalities designed to inhibit the eicosanoid pathway as it may affect vascular disease may be approaching. Pharmacologic agents originally used were chosen because they were capable of suppressing platelet functions such as aggregation, release, and adhesion. The goals of clinical trials were to evaluate medications that would prevent or reduce platelet accumulation in critically located blood vessels of the heart, brain, and extremities and on vascular prostheses. Evaluation of results of therapeutic trials has been difficult and this is superimposed on less-than-complete knowledge of the basic pharmacology of the drugs that have been used. Participation of neutrophils and possibly macrophages in the thrombotic process is now well recognized on morphologic grounds. Because different cell types such as platelets, neutrophils, and endothelial cells have been shown to interact biochemically by sharing precursors and intermediates of the eicosanoid pathway, the pharmacologic approach to inhibition of vascular diseases may require reevaluation. Neutrophils appear to lack a cyclooxygenase pathway but serve as a source of the lipoxygenase product leukotriene B_4 (LTB_4). Actions of LTB_4 include neutrophil aggregation, adhesion of neutrophils to endothelial cells, chemotaxis, chemokinesis, and plasma exudation. We have demonstrated in vitro that released free arachidonic acid from aspirin-treated platelets can serve as a source of neutrophil LTB_4. Leukotrienes C_4, D_4, and E_4 are agonists for various functions of vascular endothelium and smooth muscle. Most pharmacologic agents used in the treatment of vascular diseases inhibit the cyclooxygenase pathway. A possible contribution of leukotrienes and hydroxy fatty acids to vascular diseases may need to be considered in the development of new pharmacologic agents for the prophylaxis and treatment of thrombosis.
Circulation 72, No. 4, 698–701, 1985.

THROMBI forming in arteries are similar to hemostatic platelet plugs in that they are produced in response to injury of vascular surfaces. Morphologically these thrombi consist of platelets that have adhered initially to the subendothelium and then to each other. The thrombus also contains a mixture of neutrophils, macrophages, fibrin, and erythrocytes, especially in the distal portion.[1] Currently, it is thought that increased platelet-vessel and platelet-platelet interactions are critical factors in the development of arterial and venous thrombi as well as in the pathogenesis of thromboembolic phenomena.[2] If we assume that the foregoing hypotheses are correct, then aspirin, which induces a functional platelet defect demonstrable as prolongation of the bleeding time, should be useful for prevention of thromboembolic events. Aspirin acetylates platelet proteins, especially the arachidonic acid cyclooxygenase. This results in complete inhibition of TXA_2, HHT, and malondialdehyde formation.* However, platelet arachidonic acid release and lipoxygenase activity are not affected by aspirin. Thus, the lipoxygenase product 12-HETE continues to be synthesized in stimulated platelets from donors who have ingested aspirin. Although 12-HETE has no demonstrable effect on platelet function, it can be shown to interact biochemically with neutrophils in vitro.[3, 4] Furthermore, if a combined suspension of platelets and neutrophils is stimulated with the nonspecific agonist ionophore A23187, released arachidonate from aspirin-treated platelets can be converted to LTB_4 by the

From the Departments of Medicine, Divisions of Hematology/Oncology, New York Veterans Administration Medical Center and Cornell University Medical College, New York, NY, and Department of Experimental Sciences, The Upjohn Co., Kalamazoo, MI.

Supported by grants from the Veterans Administration, National Institutes of Health (HL 18828-09 SCOR, HL 29034, and RR 05396), the New York Heart Association, and the Edward Gruenstein Fund.

Address for correspondence: Aaron J. Marcus, M.D., Hematology/Oncology, 13 W, NYVA Medical Center, 408 First Ave., New York, NY 10010.

*The following abbreviations are used throughout this article: TXA_2, thromboxane A_2; HHT, 12S-hydroxy-5,8,10-heptadecatrienoic acid; LTB_4 (leukotriene B_4), 5S, 12R-dihydroxy-6-*cis*, 8,10-*trans*, 14-*cis*-eicosatetraenoic acid; 5,12-DiHETE, 5S, 12S-dihydroxy-6-*trans*, 8-*cis*, 10-*trans*, 14-*cis*-eicosatetraenoic acid; 5-HETE, 5S-hydroxy-6-*trans*, 8,11,14-*cis*-eicosatetraenoic acid; THETE, trihydroxyeicosatetraenoic acids; 12-HETE, 12S-hydroxy-5, 8-*cis*, 10-*trans*, 14-*cis*-eicosatetraenoic acid; 12,20-DiHETE, 12S, 20-dihydroxyeicosatetraenoic acid; TLC, thin-layer radiochromatography; HPLC, high-performance liquid chromatography.

neutrophil.[4] Thus eicosanoid metabolism in platelets is only partially inactivated after administration of aspirin and products that can react with other cells in the microenvironment are still biosynthesized.

In this review we will summarize recent studies in our laboratory involving platelets and neutrophils from untreated donors and those who had previously ingested aspirin. The results further extend our previous observations that the eicosanoid pathway is particularly amenable to metabolic interchange of biochemical products generated by different cell types.[3–5]

Methods

All experiments were carried out on freshly prepared platelet and neutrophil suspensions. In recent studies[3] both cell types originated from the same donor. When indicated, 650 mg aspirin was ingested 1 to 3 hr before venipuncture. Cell preparations and radioisotope labeling, experimental procedures, lipid extractions, and separations were carried out as previously described.[3, 4, 6]

Results and discussion

Ionophore stimulation of [^{3}H] arachidonate–labeled platelets and unlabeled neutrophils. To ascertain whether precursors originating from platelets can contribute to synthesis of eicosanoids produced by neutrophils, cell suspensions containing radiolabeled platelets and unlabeled neutrophils were stimulated with ionophore A23187.[4] Radioactive metabolites not synthesized by platelets alone were identified by TLC. Among these was LTB_4, the importance of which has already been mentioned. Also detected were 5,12-DiHETE, 5-HETE, and possibly THETE. Production of these radioactive eicosanoids by labeled platelet–unlabeled neutrophil suspensions was not spontaneous but required ionophore stimulation of both cell types. It was of interest that the metabolic interchange observed was of sufficient magnitude to permit actual visualization of LTB_4 and 5,12-DiHETE on stained thin-layer plates.

Radioactive lipid extracts were analyzed by HPLC in addition to TLC. A radioactive HPLC peak comigrated with synthetic LTB_4. This material demonstrated an ultraviolet spectrum similar to that of LTB_4 and also promoted neutrophil aggregation. When material from this peak was studied by TLC, it was found to contain both LTB_4 and 5,12-DiHETE.

As already mentioned, platelets were the sole source of radioactivity in these studies. Thus the radioactive LTB_4, 5,12-DiHETE, and 5-HETE detected originated from platelet precursors after ionophore stimulation. This was the first direct demonstration of a platelet contribution to formation of neutrophil eicosanoids such as leukotrienes and hydroxy acids.

Possible pathways in the formation of labeled neutrophil eicosanoids from platelet precursors as induced by ionophore stimulation. In the above experiments, platelets from donors who had ingested aspirin were used. Thus three platelet precursors were available for neutrophil metabolism: free arachidonic acid, 12-HPETE, and 12-HETE. Neutrophils were stimulated with ionophore A23187 in the presence of either [^{14}C] arachidonate or [^{3}H] 12-HETE. Results of these experiments indicated that platelet-derived 12-HETE served as precursor of 5,12-DiHETE synthesized by ionophore-stimulated neutrophils and that platelet-derived arachidonate was the precursor of LTB_4 and 5-HETE produced by neutrophils in which the 5-lipoxygenase enzyme had been activated by ionophore.

The identity of 5,12-DiHETE was further confirmed when unlabeled platelets were stimulated with ionophore in the presence of [^{3}H] 5-HETE. A radioactive TLC peak comigrated in two solvent systems with an authentic 5,12-DiHETE standard as well as with 5,12-DiHETE derived from incubation of neutrophils with [^{3}H] 12-HETE and ionophore. Thus 5,12-DiHETE can be formed by dual pathways in a stimulated, combined platelet-neutrophil system. It should be noted that despite formation of 5,12-DiHETE by platelets from 5-HETE, no detectable trihydroxy acids (THETE), products of omega oxidation, were produced in the absence of neutrophils.[4]

Experiments involving unstimulated neutrophils and platelets activated by agonists known to occur in vivo. The studies to be described here are in contrast to those reported above, in which cells were stimulated by ionophore simultaneously. Thrombin or collagen do not initiate eicosanoid metabolism in neutrophils, but they do so in platelets. Addition of thrombin or collagen to cell suspensions containing [^{3}H] arachidonate–labeled platelets and unlabeled neutrophils resulted in an eicosanoid pattern that differed markedly from that observed after exposure to ionophore. A labeled compound subsequently identified as 12,20-DiHETE, which could not be synthesized by platelets or neutrophils alone, was produced. The Rf value of this product by radio-TLC was incompatible with any previously identified neutrophil or platelet eicosanoid. The new compound could also be produced by addition of 5.7 μM [^{14}C] arachidonate, a concentration that was nonstimulatory for neutrophils but did activate platelets, to unlabeled platelet-neutrophil mixtures.

Results of subsequent experiments indicated that 12-HETE, the major product of the platelet lipoxygenase pathway, was involved in production of the new eicosanoid. Combined suspensions of [^{3}H] arachidonate-labeled platelets and unlabeled neutrophils were prepared from donors who had ingested aspirin before the experiment. Such platelets, when stimulated by thrombin in the absence of neutrophils, produced 12-HETE only. When the labeled platelet–unlabeled neutrophil suspension was exposed to thrombin, there was a 70% decrease in 12-HETE and the new eicosanoid was present. These results are summarized in table 1. Also demonstrated in table 1 is the relative lack of production of the new eicosanoid in the setting of ionophore stimulation. Instead, ionophore exposure resulted in synthesis of 5,12-DiHETE, the 12-HETE metabolite described above.[4]

It was possible to demonstrate directly that platelet 12-HETE was indeed the precursor of the new eicosanoid. This was done by adding [^{3}H] 12-HETE (9.4 pmol/ml) to unlabeled neutrophil suspensions. The radioactive product observed had an Rf value identical to that previously obtained with thrombin- or collagen-stimulated combined cell suspensions.

HPLC experiments. The observations made by TLC were confirmed and extended by reversed-phase HPLC. Thrombin-stimulated platelets in the presence of neutrophils generated a reversed-phase HPLC peak that was identical to that eluted when purified 12-HETE was added to neutrophils in the absence of platelets. No peak was eluted at this retention time (10.75 min) when platelets alone or neutrophils alone were exposed to thrombin.

Production of the new eicosanoid by neutrophils from purified platelet 12-HETE increased with both time and cell quantity. As in previous experiments, addition of ionophore to neutrophils in the presence of 12-HETE resulted in a decrease in production of the new metabolite by 95%. Inhibition was also observed with 5,8,11,14-eicosatetraynoic acid. Additional experiments demonstrated that the new eicosanoid was not cell-associated after its production, 100% of the product was recovered in the supernatant after a 5 min incubation period. The ultraviolet absorption spectrum of the isolated product after esterification and straight-phase HPLC demonstrated an absorption maximum at 235 nm. This did not differ significantly from that of the parent compound (12-HETE).

Gas chromatography–mass spectrometric analyses. The purified esterified product obtained by straight-phase HPLC was converted to the trimethylsilyl ether and analyzed by gas chromatography–mass spectrometry. The derived product eluted from an SE-30 column with an equivalent chain length value of C-24.6. The mass spectrometric studies suggested that the new compound was a dihydroxy derivative of arachidonic acid. After hydrogenation, the mass spectrum of the material was consistent with the assumption that the compound retained a hydroxyl group at C-12 and had an additional hydroxyl group between C-12 and C-20. Additional procedures were carried out to confirm the C-20 position of the omega hydroxyl. The compound was subjected to catalytic hydrogenation, Jones oxidation, and methylation. This was followed by gas chromatography–mass spectrometry. The spectrum proved conclusively that the structure of the new metabolite was (12S)-12,20-dihydroxy-5,8,10,14-eicosatetraenoic acid. The same compound has recently been described by Wong et al.[7] after incubation of arachidonic acid or 12-HETE with suspensions of neutrophils that also contained platelets. These authors also concluded that 12-HETE formed by platelets was further metabolized by omega-hydroxylation in leukocytes.[7]

We have therefore shown that platelet 12-HETE can be further metabolized by neutrophils to two different products: 5S,12S-DiHETE in the case of activated neutrophils and 12,20-DiHETE when neutrophils are not stimulated. Platelet 12-HETE cannot directly give rise to leukotriene A_4; however, Maclouf et al.[8] have suggested that platelet-derived 12-HPETE can activate the neutrophil 5-lipoxygenase pathway.

Eicosanoids in thrombotic diseases. It is now becoming appreciated that the proinflammatory eicosanoids that

TABLE 1
Metabolism of platelet 12-HETE by neutrophils after ingestion of aspirin

Incubation mixture	12S, 20-DiHETE	5S, 12S-DiHETE	12-HETE
Platelets, buffer	40	34	147
Platelets, thrombin	81	54	13897
Platelets, neutrophils, thrombin	4645	86	4129
Platelets, neutrophils, ionophore	312	3034	5876

Numbers indicate disintegrations per minute (dpm), corrected to 100% recovery from TLC plates and to 1×10^5 dpm spotted. [^{3}H] Arachidonate-labeled platelets (3×10^8) were incubated with neutrophils (3×10^7) and then with either thrombin (5 units/ml) or 1 μM ionophore. Five minutes later, lipids were extracted, separated by TLC along with authentic standards, stained with iodine, and scanned. Identified areas were scraped and quantified by scintillation counting.[3]

are produced via the lipoxygenase pathway exert important effects (at least in experimental systems) in the microcirculation. This includes an increase in permeability of postcapillary venules, adhesion of neutrophils to endothelial cells, and leukocyte extravasation. As in the studies reported here, these reactions are not inhibited by aspirin or nonsteroidal anti-inflammatory agents. Because steroids may act on phospholipases and inhibit arachidonic acid release, they may function as inhibitors of leukotriene biosynthesis. Leukotrienes, which seem to act on vascular endothelium and smooth muscle, may play a role in occlusive vascular diseases, which remains to be elucidated.

Current concepts of the role and possible contributions of thromboxane and prostacyclin to thrombotic disease may require additional elaboration to accommodate contributions of lipoxygenase products. In addition, cell-cell interactions may take place between different cell types in the vascular microenvironment. While these new developments and experimental approaches are in progress, we still recommend the use of aspirin (325 mg) daily as well as dipyridamole (about 75 mg) three times daily for patients at risk for thrombotic disease. This includes the cerebral, coronary, or peripheral circulation. This approach has also been shown to be fruitful for the maintenance of coronary bypass graft patency. It should be stressed that these recommendations are empirical and have as their basis an indication of positive experience in recent clinical trials.[2] However, as already mentioned, we are approaching a time for reevaluation and reassessment of the role of the entire eicosanoid pathway in vascular diseases.[9]

References

1. Marcus AJ: Recent progress in the role of platelets in occlusive vascular disease. Stroke **14:** 475, 1983
2. Marcus AJ: Editorial retrospective: aspirin as an antithrombotic medication. N Engl J Med **309:** 1515, 1983
3. Marcus AJ, Safier LB, Ullman HL, Broekman MJ, Islam N, Oglesby TD, Gorman RR: 12 S, 20-Dihydroxyicosatetraenoic acid: a new icosanoid synthesized by neutrophils from 12S-hydroxyicosatetraenoic acid produced by thrombin- or collagen-stimulated platelets. Proc Natl Acad Sci USA **81:** 903, 1984
4. Marcus AJ, Broekman MJ, Safier LB, Ullman HL, Islam N, Serhan CN, Rutherford LE, Korchak HM, Weissmann G: Formation of leukotrienes and other hydroxy acids during platelet-neutrophil interactions *in vitro*. Biochem Biophys Res Commun **109:** 130, 1982
5. Marcus AJ, Weksler BB, Jaffe EA, Broekman MJ: Synthesis of prostacyclin from platelet-derived endoperoxide by cultured human endothelial cells. J Clin Invest **66:** 979, 1980
6. Marcus AJ: Platelet arachidonic acid metabolism. *In* Harker LA, Zimmerman TS, editors: Measurements of platelet function. New York, 1983, Churchill Livingstone, p 126
7. Wong PY-K, Westlund P, Hamberg M, Granstrom E, Chao PH-W, Samuelsson B: ω-Hydroxylation of 12-L-hydroxy-5,8,10,14-eicosatetraenoic acid in human polymorphonuclear leukocytes. J Biol Chem **259:** 2683, 1984
8. Maclouf J, Fruteau de Laclos B, Borgeat P: Stimulation of leukotriene biosynthesis in human blood leukocytes by platelet-derived 12-hydroperoxy-icosatetraenoic acid. Proc Natl Acad Sci USA **79:** 6042, 1982
9. Marcus AJ: The eicosanoids in biology and medicine. J Lipid Res **25:** 1511, 1984

A review of possible roles of the platelet 12-lipoxygenase

ALAN R. BRASH, PH.D.

THE 12-LIPOXYGENASE ENZYME of platelets was the first lipoxygenase to be discovered in animal tissue,[1] yet its physiologic significance remains far from clear. The enzyme catalyzes the reaction of arachidonic acid with molecular oxygen to form 12(*S*)-hydroperoxy-eicosatetraenoic acid (12-HPETE); under most conditions the majority of the hydroperoxide is reduced to the hydroxy form (12-HETE) and released from the cell. What is the function of this very simple transformation? At present we have no definitive answer. The pathways of arachidonic acid metabolism that are understood lead to the formation of potent biological mediators such as the prostaglandins and leukotrienes. However, there is no obvious analogy to these mediators in the 12-lipoxygenase pathway. For this reason, even the most elementary consequences of the platelet 12-lipoxygenase reaction are included in the following list of possible functions of the pathway:

(1) Reaction forms 12-HPETE or 12-HETE as a specific mediator?

(2) Reaction consumes molecular oxygen.

(3) Reaction consumes free arachidonic acid.

(4) Reaction forms a hydroperoxide.

(5) Specific mediators are formed from 12-HPETE (or 15-HPETE)?

(6) Involvement in cell-cell interactions?

Figure 1 illustrates the overall reaction in its most elementary form. Lipoxygenases react the polyunsaturated lipid substrate (LH in figure 1) with molecular oxygen to form a lipid hydroperoxide (L-OOH). The cyclooxygenase reaction involves two steps of lipoxygenase-like oxygenation. For comparison, figure 1 also shows the simple equation for p-450. This enzyme complex can be regarded both as a monooxygenase (formation of L-OH) and as a mixed-function oxidase (multiple cosubstrates are used in the reduction of molecular oxygen to water). Note that a reducing cofactor is required by p-450 but not by the lipoxygenase or cyclooxygenase.

In the following review of the 12-lipoxygenase, the possible physiologic functions are considered by reference to six consequences of the simple reaction:

$$LH + O_2 \rightarrow L\text{-}OOH$$

Reaction forms 12-HPETE or 12-HETE as a specific mediator? This section is a review of the evidence that 12(*S*)-HPETE or 12(*S*)-HETE functions as a specific biological agonist acting via specific receptors. (The possible importance of the hydroperoxide group of 12-HPETE will be considered later.) Certainly, it can be argued that specific receptors for such simple structures could exist. For example, specific radioimmunoassays have been developed for 12-HETE.[2] However, there is very little evidence to support the notion that the primary products of the 12-lipoxygenase pathway are specific agonists. Furthermore, there is no convincing precedent for this with related structural analogs such as the other HPETEs. Notably, submicromolar concentrations of 12-H(P)ETE are inactive in eliciting contraction or relaxation of smooth muscle. In contrast, the prostaglandins and leukotrienes each exhibit a distinct profile of myotropic activity in the nanomolar range. Although the very first report of chemotactic activity for leukocytes among the eicosanoids concerned 12-HETE,[3] and 12-HPETE was later found to be more active,[4] both products are now recognized as extremely weak agonists compared with LTB_4.[5] More recently, a series of studies by Nakao et al.[6] have suggested that 12-HETE induces migration of aortic smooth muscle cells at the astoundingly low concentration of 10^{-15} M. An unresolved question concerning these experiments is the fact that all incubations contained 5% to 10% fetal calf serum. Because bovine platelets synthesize 12-HETE,[7] the serum potentially could contain roughly 10^6 times more 12-HETE than is subsequently added to induce chemotaxis of the smooth muscle cells. However, if these findings are confirmed, they stand as an important exception to the current impression that 12-HETE is a biologically inactive compound.

From the Division of Clinical Pharmacology, Department of Pharmacology, Vanderbilt University School of Medicine, Nashville, TN.

Supported by NIH grant GM 15431.

Address for correspondence: Alan R. Brash, Ph.D., Division of Clinical Pharmacology, Department of Pharmacology, Vanderbilt University School of Medicine, Nashville, TN 37232.

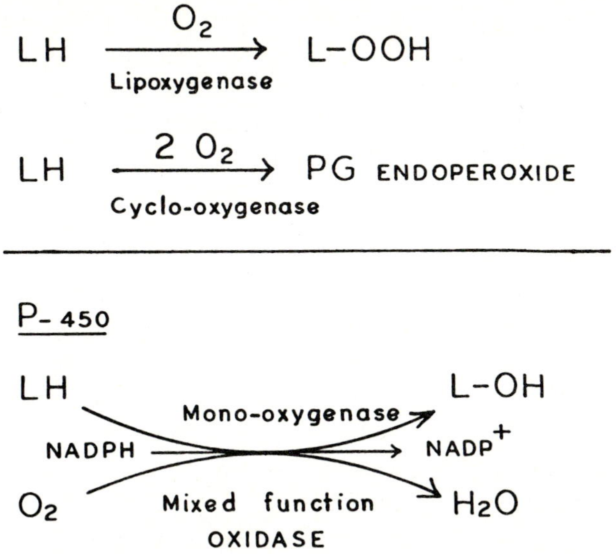

FIGURE 1. Oxygenation of lipid substrates (LH) by lipoxygenase, cyclooxygenase, and p-450.

Several studies have pursued the possibilities for specific interaction of 12-HETE on platelet function. Invariably, micromolar concentrations are required to elicit any effect, and this is a higher concentration than is likely to be achieved in vivo. Potentially, studies with 12-lipoxygenase inhibitors hold the key to understanding the role of the pathway. However, it has yet to be demonstrated that the available 12-lipoxygenase inhibitors are suitable for tests of cellular function. This problem is exemplified by the series of acetylenic analogs of arachidonic acid. The most widely used member of this series, 5,8,11,14-eicosatetraynoic acid (ETYA), is both a lipoxygenase and cyclooxygenase inhibitor, and it has been used to test platelet function in several studies.[7–9] Although ETYA will inhibit both these enzymes, there are analogs with selective lipoxygenase or cyclooxygenase inhibitory[10, 11] activities and therefore this problem can be circumvented. However, there are yet other analogs that inhibit neither enzyme, and these analogs are equipotent with the enzyme inhibitors in modifying indexes of platelet[12] and leukocyte function.[13] It remains to be seen whether this same problem will arise with the more recently developed 12-lipoxygenase inhibitors such as the flavonoids related to esculetin.[14]

Currently, the balance of evidence weighs heavily against 12-H(P)ETE acting as a specific agonist acting via specific receptors. There is no evidence for specific modification of the aggregation, adhesion, or secretory functions of platelets. This must be considered as one of the least likely functions of the platelet 12-lipoxygenase.

Reaction consumes molecular oxygen. Several years ago this was considered as a possible function of the lipoxygenases commonly found in plants,[15] although little evidence has been presented to substantiate the possibility. With regard to the 12-lipoxygenase of platelets, it is relevant to point out the potentially high capacity to oxygenate arachidonic acid and hence the corresponding capacity to deplete cellular levels of oxygen. In a well-stirred system such as the circulating blood or in platelet-rich plasma in vitro it is inconceivable that a significant depletion of oxygen could be attained. The only realistic possibility for oxygen depletion is within a mass of clumped platelets. For example, within a platelet plug on a blood vessel wall, the activity of the 12-lipoxygenase might render the system anaerobic.

Several articles have drawn attention to the fact that the 12-lipoxygenase is slow to be activated in the intact platelet[16, 17] and it remains active well beyond the time required to aggregate the cells.[2, 8] This is in contrast to the cyclooxygenase, which is inactivated after a short burst of activity. Although it may appear unlikely that depletion of oxygen is the physiologic function of the platelet 12-lipoxygenase, this possibility should not be rejected out of hand. Clearly, the activation and aggregation of platelets is followed by gross structural and metabolic changes within the cell. There are no data one way or the other to indicate whether forced depletion of oxygen by lipoxygenase activity could contribute to these changes. Nevertheless, if there is significant enzymatic activity in a closed system such as a clump of aggregated cells, then it may well be worth calculating the rate of oxygen depletion by the lipoxygenase and the rate of replenishment by diffusion from the surrounding fluids.

Reaction consumes arachidonic acid. Potentially, arachidonic acid is a far more potent mediator than 12-HETE. By conversion to prostaglandins, thromboxane A_2, and leukotrienes it forms highly active agonists. In contrast, no highly active metabolites of 12-H(P)ETE have been described. Therefore, there emerges the very real possibility that the function of the 12-lipoxygenase pathway is to inactivate free arachidonic acid and thus prevent the generation of biologically active products.

There is another potentially significant consequence of the metabolism of arachidonic acid to 12-H(P)ETE. In the unactivated platelet, the cell membranes are relatively rich in esterified arachidonic acid. During cell activation the structure of the cell membrane is altered to permit change in shape, adhesion, and secretion. The 12-lipoxygenase eliminates free arachidonic acid, and as stated earlier it continues to function well after the immediate events of platelet activation. Therefore it is quite possible that the 12-lipoxygenase could act to eliminate arachidonic acid and hence, either facilitate structural changes that accompany the adhesion and secretory process and/or prevent the reversal of structural changes in the membrane.

The idea that the platelet lipoxygenase functions as a metabolic sink for free arachidonic acid may not be very exciting, but it remains a very real possibility that is in accord with our current understanding of arachidonic acid metabolism and the events that accompany platelet activation.

Reaction forms a hydroperoxide: effects on cellular metabolism. The platelet 12-lipoxygenase forms 12-HPETE, but under most experimental conditions it is the hydroxy analog 12-HETE that is released from the cells. Reduction of the hydroperoxide involves a sequence of redox reactions, and ultimately the reducing equivalents are generated at the expense of glucose. As the hydroperoxide is reduced, glutathione is oxidized and then replenished with equivalents from NADPH, which is itself regenerated via the hexose monophosphate shunt. It is therefore apparent that the formation of a hydroperoxide per se could influence cellular metabolism in the platelet and thus modulate cellular function. Notably, lipoxygenases generate hydroperoxides in a reaction that needs no cofactors; in contrast, cellular formation of hydrogen peroxide requires the reduction of molecular oxygen at the expense of NAD(P)H.

The quantitative relationship between 12-HPETE formation, hydroperoxide reduction, and platelet redox balance was examined by Bryant et al.[18] They found that the synthesis and subsequent reduction of 3 to 10 nmol (1 to 3 μg) of 12-HPETE by 3×10^8 platelets required the consumption of 10 times more reduced glutathione (GSH) than was present in the resting cell. In other words, a very rapid regeneration of GSH is required to enable the cells to deal with this amount of hydroperoxide.

Could a temporary depletion of GSH exert (indirect) effects on cellular function? Bosia et al.[19] have shown that chemical agents that deplete cellular GSH cause inhibition of platelet aggregation and secretion. Cross-binding of disulfide proteins was also shown to accompany GSH depletion and this may be related to the antiaggregatory effects.[19] If these findings have any relevance to the formation of 12-HPETE in platelets, then 12-HPETE and other lipid hydroperoxides should inhibit aggregation and secretion. In fact there are conflicting reports in the literature. There is some evidence to suggest that an intact 12-lipoxygenase pathway is required for the normal process of platelet aggregation in the rat[8] and in man.[9] This idea is supported by reports that 12-HPETE can enhance cyclooxygenase metabolism.[16, 20] In contrast, Aharony et al.[21] and Vericel and Lagarde[22] found that 12-HPETE and 15-HPETE exerted an antiaggregatory and antisecretory effect on human platelets with median inhibitory concentrations in the range of 2 to 6 μM; these effects are compatible with the concept of GSH depletion by hydroperoxide, leading to an inhibitory effect on platelet function. However, the hydroxy analogs (12-HETE and 15-HETE) also exhibited significant activity (median inhibitory concentration 10 μM[21]), and therefore GSH depletion can only be a partial explanation of these findings.

The important question in terms of a cellular control mechanism is whether 12-lipoxygenase activity could significantly deplete cellular GSH under physiologic conditions. This must remain doubtful. There is every indication that platelets are very well equipped to eliminate peroxide; one important index of this is the fact that it is very difficult to isolate the hydroperoxide 12-HPETE from platelet suspensions. Extreme circumstances are required before the cellular redox balance is seriously disturbed. These extreme circumstances might include (1) absence of glucose in the medium, (2) dietary deficiency of selenium,[23] (3) the rapid formation of large amounts of 12-HPETE from an exogenous source of arachidonic acid, or (4) the possible contribution of unknown factors that might strain the GSH regeneration system. These conditions have to be contrived intentionally in the laboratory and it seems unlikely they would arise in vivo. The balance of evidence does not favor the concept that generation of a hydroperoxide per se is the function of the platelet 12-lipoxygenase.

Specific mediators are formed from 12-HPETE (or 15-HPETE)? Arachidonic acid can be converted to endoperoxides, epoxides, and diH(P)ETEs under the influence of the platelet 12-lipoxygenase. However, there is no evidence that any of these products have biological activity. Furthermore, the compounds are formed in extremely low yield. In fact, they have been demonstrated to be formed only under very contrived conditions in vitro. Their mechanisms of biosynthesis can be categorized as: (1) Nonenzymatic decomposition of 12-HPETE; this gives epoxy-hydroxy and trihydroxy products.[24–26] There is evidence that the epoxy-hydroxy compounds are formed via an unstable endoperoxide reaction intermediate.[27] (2) Formation of 15(*S*)-HPETE and further conversion to 15-series leukotrienes. There is evidence that these reactions are enzymatic and that the 12-lipoxygenase may be the enzyme responsible for the transformation.[28] It has also been shown that bradykinin is a specific stimulus for the synthesis of these products in human platelets.[29]

Formation of the first group of products, the nonenzymatic breakdown products of 12-HPETE, depends on accumulation of the hydroperoxide in the cells. Selenium deficiency (glutathione peroxidose deficiency) is one extreme circumstance known to promote this condition. The demonstration of product formation has also always depended on addition of exogenous arachidonic acid. This is necessary to increase the yield of 12-HPETE and thus to overcome the very efficient mechanisms for reduction to 12-HETE within the cell. The nonenzymatic breakdown products are not formed from 12-HETE.

The second group of products, the 15-series dihydroxy leukotrienes, also require the addition of exogenous substrate to form detectable amounts of the compounds. The yields from exogenous arachidonic acid are very low; addition of 15-HPETE improves the yield,[28] but this is a very artificial condition. The preliminary report that bradykinin stimulates biosynthesis of these products certainly deserves further attention. However, our current state of knowledge tends to suggest that all the products considered in this section are no more than biochemical artifacts formed under extreme conditions in vitro.

Involvement in cell-cell interactions

Inactivation of prostaglandin (PG)I_2 synthase. Prostacyclin synthesis is very sensitive to inhibition by fatty acid hydroperoxides.[30] Consequently it has been suggested that the 12-lipoxygenase activity of platelets could result in inhibition of PGI_2 synthesis in the vascular endothelium. However, there are at least two major problems with this simple hypothesis. First, an exogenous source of arachidonic acid is needed to generate large amounts of 12-HPETE. Second, it is questionable whether the hydroperoxide 12-HPETE can escape from the platelet without being reduced to 12-HETE. This particular point was studied by Turk et al.[31] Indomethacin-treated platelets were stirred together with aortic microsomes. In effect, the PGI_2 synthase activity of the microsomes served as an assay for the escape of platelet-derived 12-HPETE into the extracellular medium. It was found that the synthesis of PGI_2 from PGH_2 was not compromised by prior stimulation of the 12-lipoxygenase pathway in intact platelets. Thus it could be inferred from these results and the appropriate controls that 12-HPETE was reduced to 12-HETE before its release into the medium.

Novel eicosanoid products derived via platelet-leukocyte interactions. The consecutive actions of oxygenases in separate cell types can lead to the formation of novel products. This aspect of cell interactions is the subject of another contribution to this symposium[32] and is reviewed very briefly here. The first of the double oxygenation products to be identified, 5(*S*),12(*S*)-DiHETE, was originally detected as a product of porcine leukocytes.[33] White cells of this species contain both 5-lipoxygenase and 12-lipoxygenase activities. Subsequently, the formation of 5(*S*) 12(*S*)-DiHETE was studied in mixtures of human platelets and leukocytes.[34, 35] More recently, the ω-oxidation metabolite of 12-HETE, namely 12,20-DiHETE, was detected in platelet-leukocyte mixtures.[36, 37] As yet, these products have not been shown to exhibit marked biological activity.

Platelet lipoxygenase products and vascular relaxation. We have investigated the biological activity of lipoxygenase-derived products in causing relaxation of vascular smooth muscle. It seemed possible that a 12-lipoxygenase or 15-lipoxygenase product could account for the biological activity known as "endothelial cell derived relaxing factor," EDRF.[38] We have taken two approaches to testing the ability of lipoxygenase products to relax arterial smooth muscle. First, we have tested the biological activity of authentic standards. These included 14,15-LTA_4 and its derivatives, which were prepared in our laboratory. In this way we were able to discount the involvement of all the prostaglandins and leukotrienes. The 15-lipoxygenase products tested included 14,15-LTA_4,14,15-LTC_4, 14,15-DiHETE, 8,15-DiH(P)ETES, and 5,15-DiHPETE. None were active in concentrations up to 5 μM.*

Our second approach was to encourage the generation of unstable lipoxygenase products and by-products in situ in the bioassay tissue bath. This was accomplished with hemoglobin to catalyze the autoxidation of authentic HPETEs added to the buffer. Hemoglobin is well known to promote the autoxidative breakdown of HPETEs to hydroxy, epoxy, and peroxy derivatives.[39] In this way unstable products can be formed in the tissue bath and their biological activity measured. However, the results proved to be negative. As shown in figure 2 (*top*), addition of 15-HPETE (5 μM) and then hemoglobin (50 μg/ml) to a ring of rabbit aorta precontracted with 10^{-7} M norepinephrine led to an immediate relaxation. This relaxation is an artifact caused by the autoxidative destruction of the norepinephrine; however, this does indicate that the expected autoxidation takes place when 15-HPETE

*Murray JJ, Brash AR: Unpublished observations.

and hemoglobin are mixed together in the buffer. When a stable agonist was used to precontract the rabbit aorta ($PGF_{2\alpha}$, 10^{-5} M), it can be seen that the autoxidation catalyzed by the mixture of 15-HPETE and hemoglobin had no effect on the tone of the vascular smooth muscle (figure 2, bottom). Subsequent addition of acetylcholine (10^{-6} M) effected a pronounced relaxation typical of the endothelial cell–dependent response.

Further work is in progress on the possible involvement of lipoxygenase products in the endothelial cell–dependent relaxation of blood vessels. This topic is also addressed by Vanhoutte and Houston.[40]

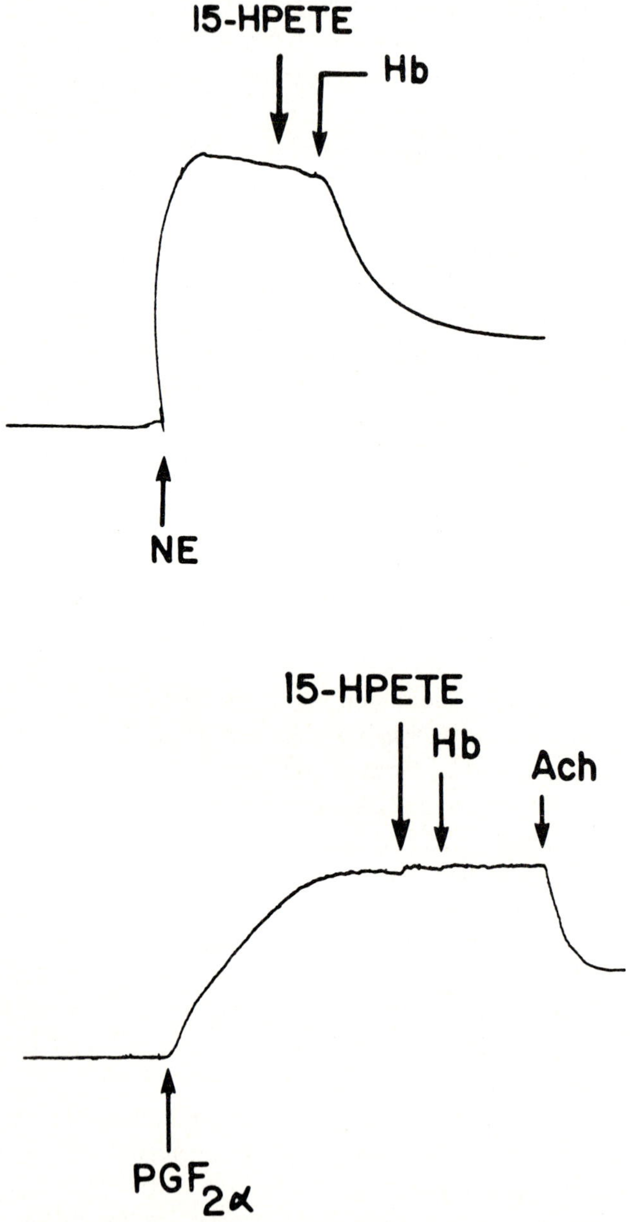

FIGURE 2. Effect of autoxidized 15-HPETE on vascular tone. *Top*, Rabbit aorta precontracted with 10^{-7} M norepinephrine then treated with 5 μM 15-HPETE and 50 μg/ml hemoglobin. *Bottom*, Precontraction with 10^{-5} M $PGF_{2\alpha}$, treatment with same concentrations 15-HPETE and hemoglobin and then 10^{-6} M acetylcholine.

Conclusion. The problem of assigning a physiologic role to the platelet 12-lipoxygenase is somewhat similar to the unsolved question of the role of lipoxygenases in plants. In the case of the plant lipoxygenases, the main substrate is linoleic acid, the simplest member of the series of polyunsaturated fatty acids. The plant enzymes convert linoleic acid either to its 9-hydroperoxy or 13-hydroperoxy derivative. Because linoleic acid has only two double bonds, there is no possibility for its further metabolism to prostaglandin or leukotriene-like structures. Thus, in plant tissues and in platelets, both rich in lipoxygenase activity, polyunsaturated fatty acid is converted to a simple hydroperoxy derivative. In neither case does it appear that the objective is to form biological mediators analogous to the prostaglandins and leukotrienes.

Six potential consequences of platelet 12-lipoxygenase activity have been considered in this review. Undoubtedly some of these are farfetched. Nevertheless it is worth adding up the evidence for and against before rejecting the hypothesis. It does seem improbable that 12-HPETE or any of its minor dihydroxy or other derivatives acts as a specific mediator or agonist. Furthermore, the concept that lipoxygenase activity could deplete cellular oxygen or cellular gluthathione demands that there is an exceptionally high turnover of the enzyme. In fact, it is difficult to make a convincing case that the 12-lipoxygenase of platelets is involved in the rapid series of events that results in adhesion, aggregation, and secretion of the granular contents of the cell. Rather, the evidence points to the fact that the 12-lipoxygenase continues to turnover well after the cells are fully aggregated. This may be related to some aspect of cell-cell interaction, or possibly it marks the metabolism of the potent biological mediator arachidonic acid to the relatively innocuous product 12-H(P)ETE.

References

1. Hamberg M, Samuelsson B: Prostaglandin endoperoxides: novel transformations of arachidonic acid in human platelets. Proc Natl Acad Sci USA **721:** 3400, 1974
2. Hwang DH: Characteristics of the formation of the platelet lipoxygenase product from endogenous arachidonic acid. Lipids **17:** 845, 1982
3. Goetzl EJ, Woods JM, Gorman RR: Stimulation of human eosinophil and neutrophil polymorphonuclear leukocyte chemotaxis and random migration by 12-L-hydroxy-5,8,10,14-eicosatetraenoic acid. J Clin Invest **59:** 179, 1977
4. Goetzl EJ, Hill HR, Gorman RR: Unique aspects of the modulation of human neutrophil function by 12-L-hydroperoxy-5,8,10,14-eicosatetraenoic acid. Prostaglandins **19:** 71, 1980
5. Ford-Hutchinson AW, Bray MA, Doig MV, Shipley ME, Smith MJH: Leukotriene B_4, a potent chemokinetic and aggregating sub-

stance released from polymorphonuclear leukocytes. Nature (London) **286:** 264, 1980
6. Nakao J, Ito H, Koshihara Y, Murota S: Age-related increase in the migration of aortic smooth muscle cells induced by 12-L-hydroxy-5,8,10,14-eicosatetraenoic acid. Atherosclerosis **51:** 179, 1984
7. Nugteren DH: Arachidonate lipoxygenase in blood platelets. Biochim Biophys Acta **380:** 299, 1975
8. Dutilh CE, Haddeman E, Jouvenaz GH, ten Hoor F, Nugteren DH: Study of the two pathways for arachidonate oxygenation in blood platelets. Lipids **14:** 241, 1979
9. Dutilh CE, Haddeman E, Don JA, ten Hoor F: The role of arachidonate lipoxygenase and fatty acids during irreversible blood aggregation in vitro. Prostaglandins Med **6:** 111, 1981
10. Wilhelm TE, Sankarappa SK, VanRollins M, Sprecher H: Selective inhibitors of platelet lipoxygenase: 4,7,10,13-icosatetraynoic acid and 5,8,11,14-henicosatetraynoic acid. Prostaglandins **21:** 323, 1981
11. Sun FF, McGuire JC, Morton DR, Pike JE, Sprecher H, Kunau WH: Inhibition of platelet arachidonic acid 12-lipoxygenase by acetylenic acid compounds. Prostaglandins **21:** 333, 1981
12. Sams AR, Sprecher H, Sankarappa SK, Needleman P: Selective inhibitors of platelet arachidonic acid metabolism: aggregation independent of lipoxygenase. Adv Prostaglandin Thromboxane Leuk Res **9:** 19, 1982
13. Smith RJ, Sun FF, Iden SS, Bowman BJ, Sprecher H, McGuire JC: An evaluation of the relationship between arachidonic acid lipoxygenation and human neutrophil degranulation. Clin Immunol Immunopathol **20:** 157, 1981
14. Seyika K, Okuda H, Arichi S: Selective inhibition of platelet lipoxygenase by esculetin. Biochim Biophys Acta **713:** 68, 1982
15. Garssen GJ, Vliegenthart JFG, Boldingh J: An anaerobic reaction between lipoxygenase, linoleic acid and its hydroperoxides. Biochem J **122:** 327, 1971
16. Hamberg M, Hamberg G: On the mechanism of oxygenation of arachidonic acid by human platelet lipoxygenase. Biochem Biophys Res Commun **95:** 1090, 1980
17. Schafer AI, Turner NA, Handin RI: Platelet lipoxygenase-dependent oxygen burst: evidence for differential activation of lipoxygenase in intact and disrupted human platelets. Biochim Biophys Acta **712:** 535, 1982
18. Bryant RW, Simon TC, Bailey JM: Role of glutathione peroxidase and hexose monophosphate shunt in the platelet lipoxygenase pathway. J Biol Chem **257:** 14937, 1982
19. Bosia A, Spangenberg P, Losche W, Arese P, Till V: The role of the GSH-disulfide status in the reversible and irreversible aggregation of human platelets. Thromb Res **30:** 137, 1983
20. Morita I, Takahashi R, Saito Y, Murota S: Stimulation of eicosapentaenoic acid metabolism in washed human platelets by 12-hydroperoxyeicosatetraenoic acid. J Biol Chem **258:** 10197, 1983
21. Ahorony D, Smith JB, Silver MJ: Regulation of arachidonate-induced platelet aggregation by the lipoxygenase product, 12-hydroperoxyeicosatetraenoic acid. Biochim Biophys Acta **718:** 193, 1982
22. Vericel E, Lagarde M: 15-Hydroperoxyeicosatetraenoic acid inhibits human platelet aggregation. Lipids **15:** 472, 1980
23. Bryant RW, Bailey JM: Altered lipoxygenase metabolism and decreased glutathione peroxidase activity in platelets from selenium-deficient rats. Biochem Biophys Res Commun **92:** 268, 1980
24. Falardeau P, Hamberg M, Samuelsson B: Metabolism of 8,11,14-eicosatrienoic acid in human platelets. Biochim Biophys Acta **441:** 193, 1976
25. Jones RL, Kerry PJ, Poyser NL, Walker IC, Wilson NH: The identification of trihydroxy-eicosatrienoic acids as products from the incubation of arachidonic acid with washed blood platelets. Prostaglandins **16:** 583, 1978
26. Bryant RW, Bailey JM: Isolation of a new lipoxygenase metabolite of arachidonic acid, 8,11,12-trihydroxy-5,9,14-eicosatrienoic acid from human platelets. Prostaglandins **17:** 9, 1979
27. Pace-Asciak CR, Granström E, Samuelsson B: Arachidonic acid epoxides: isolation and structure of two hydroxy epoxide intermediates in the formation of 8,11,12- and 10,11,12-trihydroxy-eicosatrienoic acids. J Biol Chem **258:** 6835, 1983
28. Maas RL, Brash AR: Evidence for a lipoxygenase mechanism in the biosynthesis of epoxide and dihydroxy leukotrienes from 15(S)-hydroperoxyeicosatetraenoic acid by human platelets and porcine leukocytes. Proc Natl Acad Sci USA **80:** 2884, 1983
29. Wong PY-K, Westlund P, Granström E, Harnberg M, Chao PH-W, Samuelsson B: Effects of bradykinin on the metabolism of arachidonic acid in human platelets and leukocytes: formation of 14,15-DiHETE and 12,20-DiHETE. Thromb Haemost **50:** 129, 1983
30. Gryglewski RJ, Bunting S, Moncada S, Flower RJ, Vane JR: Arterial walls are protected against deposition of platelet thrombi by a substance (prostaglandin X) which they make from prostaglandin endoperoxides. Prostaglandins **12:** 685, 1976
31. Turk J, Wyche A, Needleman P: Inactivation of vascular prostacyclin synthetase by platelet lipoxygenase products. Biochem Biophys Res Commun **95:** 1628, 1980
32. Marcus AJ, Safier LB, Ullman HL, Broekman MJ, Islam N, Oglesby TD, Gorman RR, Ward JW: Inhibition of platelet function in thrombosis. Circulation **72:** 698, 1985
33. Borgeat P, Picard S, Vallerand P, Sirois P: Transformation of arachidonic acid in leukocytes: isolation and structural analysis of a novel dihydroxy derivative. Prostaglandins Med **6:** 557, 1981
34. Borgeat P, Fruteau deLaclos B, Picard S, Drapeau J, Vallerand P, Corey EJ: Studies on the mechanism of formation of the 5S,12S-dihydroxy-6,8,10,14 (E,Z,E,Z)-icosatetraenoic acid in leukocytes. Prostaglandins **23:** 713, 1982
35. Marcus AJ, Broekman MJ, Safier LB, Ullman HL, Islam N: Formation of leukotrienes and other hydroxy acids during platelet-neutrophil interactions in vitro. Biochem Biophys Res Commun **109:** 130, 1982
36. Marcus AJ, Safier LB, Ullman HL, Broekman MJ, Islam N, Oglesby TD, Gorman RR: 12S,20-Dihydroxyicosatetraenoic acid: a new icosanoid synthesized by neutrophils from 12S-hydroxyicosatetraenoic acid produced by thrombin- or collagen-stimulated platelets. Proc Natl Acad Sci USA **81:** 903, 1984
37. Wong PY-K, Westlund P, Hamberg M, Granstrom E, Chao PH-W, Samuelsson B: ω-Hydroxylation of 12L-hydroxy-5,8,10,14-eicosatetraenoic acid in human polymorphonuclear leukocytes. J Biol Chem **259:** 2683, 1984
38. Furchgott RF, Zawadzki JV: The obligatory role of endothelial cells in the relaxation of arterial smooth muscle by acetylcholine. Nature **288:** 373, 1979
39. Hamberg M: Decomposition of unsaturated fatty acid hydroperoxides by hemoglobin: structures of major products of 13L-hydroperoxy-9,11-octadecadienoic acid. Lipids **10:** 87, 1975
40. Vanhoutte PM, Houston DS: Platelets, endothelium, and vasospasm. Circulation **72:** 728, 1985

Evidence for 15-HETE synthesis by human umbilical vein endothelial cells

ROBERT R. GORMAN, PH.D., THOMAS D. OGLESBY, PH.D., GORDON L. BUNDY, PH.D., AND NANCY K. HOPKINS, B.S.

ABSTRACT Incubation of cultured human umbilical vein endothelial cells with [1-^{14}C]-arachidonic acid, followed by RP-HPLC analysis, resulted in the appearance of two principal radioactive products besides 6-keto-$PGF_{1\alpha}$. The first peak was HHT, a hydrolysis product of the prostaglandin endoperoxide. The second peak was esterified, converted to the trimethylsilyl ether derivative, and analyzed by GC/MS and was shown to be the lipoxygenase product 15-HETE. Stimulation of endothelial cells with thrombin enhanced 15-HETE synthesis from arachidonate. Subsequent experiments showed that 5-HETE and 12-HETE were also synthesized by endothelial cells, but no evidence of leukotriene synthesis was found. Incubation of the 15-HETE precursor 15-HPETE with endothelial cells resulted in the formation of four distinct ultraviolet light–absorbing peaks. Ultraviolet and GC/MS analysis showed these peaks to be 8,15-diHETEs that differed only in their hydroxyl configuration and *cis-trans* double-bond geometry. Formation of 8,15-diHETE molecules suggests the prior formation of the unstable epoxide molecule 14,15-LTA_4 or an attack at C-10 of 15-HPETE by an enzyme with mechanistic features in common with a 12-lipoxygenase. The observation that endothelial cells can synthesize both 15-HETE and 8,15-diHETE molecules suggests that this cell type contains both a 15-lipoxygenase and a system that can synthesize 14,15-LTA_4.
Circulation 72, No. 4, 708–712, 1985.

PGI_2* is the principal prostaglandin biosynthesized by cultured human umbilical vein endothelial cells in response to thrombin, histamine, A-23187, trypsin, and ATP.[1-5] Recently, LTC_4 and LTD_4 were shown to stimulate PGI_2 biosynthesis in human endothelial cells, and agonist-specific desensitization to LTC_4 was also observed.[6, 7] Although leukotrienes are known to stimulate prostaglandin biosynthesis in endothelial cells, no physical evidence of arachidonate lipoxygenation by endothelial cells has appeared. In this report we present evidence that human umbilical vein endothelial cells do contain a 15-lipoxygenase.

From the Cell Biology and Lipid Research Departments, The Upjohn Company, Kalamazoo, MI.

Address for correspondence: R. R. Gorman, Ph.D., Cell Biology Department, The Upjohn Co., Kalamazoo, MI 49008.

*Abbreviations used are as follows: PGI_2, prostaglandin I_2; LTC_4, 5(*S*)-hydroxy,6(*R*)-*S*-glutathionyl-7-9-*trans*-11,14-*cis*-eicosatetraenoic acid; LTD_4, 5(*S*)-hydroxy, 6(*R*)-*S*-cysteinylglycine-7,9-*trans*-11, 14-*cis*-eicosatetraenoic acid; LTB_4, [5(*S*),6*Z*,8*E*,10*E*,12(*R*),14*Z*]-5, 12-dihydroxyeicosa-6,8,10,14-tetraenoic acid; 12-HETE, 12(*S*)-hydroxy-5,8,10,14-eicosatetraenoic acid; 5-HETE, 5(*S*)-hydroxy-5,8,10, 14-eicosatetraenoic acid; 15-HETE, 15(*S*)-hydroxy-5,8,11-*cis*-13-*trans*-eicosatetraenoic acid; 15-HPETE, 15(*S*)-hydroperoxy-5,8,11-*cis*-13-*trans*-eicosatetraenoic acid; 8,15-diHETE, 8,15(*S*)-dihydroxy-5, 8,11,13-eicosatetraenoic acid; 14,15-LTA_4, 14(*S*), 15(*S*)-*trans*-oxido-5,8-*Z*-10,12-*E*-eicosatetraenoic acid; NDGA, nordihydroguaiaretic acid; HHT, 12-L-hydroxy-5,8,10-heptadecatrienoic acid; RP-HPLC and HPLC, reversed-phase and straight-phase high-pressure liquid chromatography; GC/MS, gas chromatography–mass spectrometry.

Experimental procedures

Materials. Arachidonic acid was obtained from Nu-Chek Prep Inc. (Elysian, MN) and [1-^{14}C]-arachidonic acid (specific activity, 53 mCi/mmol) and [^{3}H]-arachidonic acid (87 Ci/mmol) were obtained from New England Nuclear (Boston). The radiolabeled arachidonate was diluted to give a final specific activity of 4.6 mCi/mmol and the mixture was purified by HPLC the day it was used, as described below. 15-HPETE and [1-^{14}C]-15-HPETE were biosynthesized from arachidonate via soybean lipoxidase (Sigma Chemical Co., St. Louis) according to the methods of Van Os et al.[8] 14,15-LTA_4 was kindly provided by F. A. Fitzpatrick, The Upjohn Co. (Kalamazoo, MI). NDGA, bovine serum albumin, and aspirin were from Sigma Chemical Co., St. Louis.

Medium 199 with Earle's salts was purchased from Flow Laboratories, (McLean, VA). L-Glutamine and HEPES buffer were purchased from Microbiological Associates, Walkersville, MD.

Culture of endothelial cells. Endothelial cells were derived from human umbilical cord veins as described by Jaffe et al.[9] Cells were exposed to an atmosphere of 95% air and 5% CO_2 and were fed twice a week until they were subcultured. Confluency was usually reached in 4 to 5 days.

Incubation of endothelial cells with arachidonic acid or 15-HPETE. Before the incubation of cells with arachidonate or 15-HPETE, the confluent monolayers were harvested from the culture flasks by a 5 min incubation with a 1:1 mixture of 0.2% collagenase: 0.5% bovine serum albumin, 0.02% EDTA. After washing, the cells were resuspended in cord buffer (137 mM NaCl, 4 mM KCl, 10 mM HEPES, pH 7.5, and 11 mM glucose) to a concentration of 1 to 3 × 10^6 cells/ml, and allowed to equilibrate at 37° C for 10 min.

Reactions were initiated by transferring 10 ml of cells to a silanized vessel containing the desired amount of 15-HPETE or arachidonic acid. Incubations were carried out at 37° C with stirring.

The reactions were terminated by the addition of two volumes of cold acetone. The precipitate was removed by centrifugation and the acetone was removed in vacuo. The residual aqueous phase was acidified to pH 4.0 with 1N H_3PO_4 and applied to a C_{18} Sep-Pak column (Waters Associates, Milford, MA). Hydroxylated fatty acids were eluted with ethyl acetate according to the method of Powell.[10]

Analysis of incubation products by HPLC. Monohydroxy fatty acids were separated on a 5 μm 10 mm × 250 mm Ultrasphere-ODS column at 3.5 ml/min isocratically with methanol/water/glacial acetic acid (80:20:0.01) and *p*-hydroxyheptyl benzoate was used as an internal standard with ultraviolet detection at 235 nm. The system resolved 15-HETE, 12-HETE, and 5-HETE (retention times = 14, 16.2, and 19 min, respectively). Radioactivity in the peaks was detected with a Flo-One HS radioactive flow detector (after ultraviolet detection) and Flo Scint II scintillant (Radiomatic Instruments and Chemical Co., Inc., Tampa, FL).

Dihydroxy fatty acids synthesized from 15-HPETE were separated as above except that the mobile phase was methanol/water/glacial acetic acid (73.75:26.25:.01) and detection was at 270 nm.

Purification of reverse-phase peaks by HPLC. Monohydroxy and dihydroxy fatty acids collected from RP-HPLC were methylated with etheral diazomethane and the resulting methyl esters were dissolved in hexane with sonication. Purification of dihydroxy and monohydroxy fatty acids was achieved on a Bakerbond chiral column (4.6 mm × 25 cm) (J. T. Baker Research Products, Phillipsburg, NJ). Monohydroxy fatty acids were eluted isocratically in hexane/2-propanol (98:2) at a flow rate of 1.5 ml/min with ultraviolet detection at 235 nm. Dihydroxy fatty acids were isocratically eluted at 2.0 ml/min with hexane/2-propanol (96:4), with ultraviolet detection at 270 nm.

GC/MS of purified products. The purified methyl esters of the monohydroxy and dihydroxy fatty acids were derivatized with bis-(trimethylsilyl) trifluoroacetamide/1% trimethyl-chlorosilane (Pierce Chemical Company, Rockford, IL) and analyzed by GC/MS, as previously described.[11]

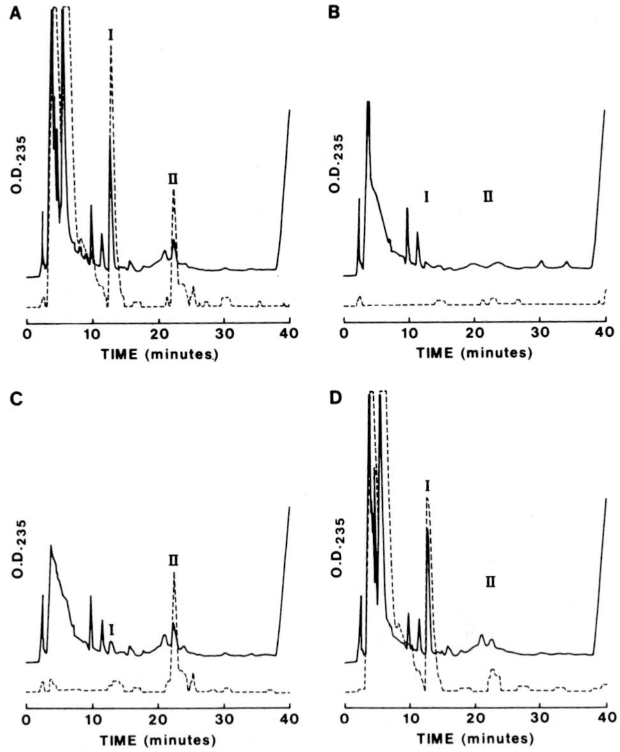

FIGURE 1. RP-HPLC chromatogram of [1-^{14}C]-arachidonic acid metabolism by endothelial cells. *A*, Endothelial cells (30 × 10^6) were incubated for 10 min at 37° C with 50 μM [1-^{14}C]-arachidonic acid. After extraction, the radioactive products were analyzed by RP-HPLC as described in the methods. *B*, Same as in *A* except the cells were boiled 10 min before the addition of arachidonate. *C*, Same as in *A* except the cells were incubated with 1 mM aspirin for 30 min before the addition of arachidonate. *D*, Same as in *A* except cells were incubated for 10 min with 30 μM NDGA before the addition of arachidonate. Solid line denotes ultraviolet detection at 235 nm, and dotted line indicates radioactivity.

Results

Incubation of human endothelial cells (30 × 10^6) with 50 μM [1-^{14}C]-arachidonic acid for 10 min at 37° C results in the formation of two major radioactive ultraviolet light–absorbing peaks on RP-HPLC (figure 1). Radioactive peaks were also evident at the origin, but were identified as PGE_2 and 6-keto-$PGF_{1\alpha}$, known products of arachidonate metabolism in endothelial cells.[1-3] Peak I is also known from previous work to be the PGH_2 hydrolysis product HHT. Peak II is a new product with a retention time of 20.5 min that chromatographs in the monohydroxy arachidonate region (figure 1, *A*). Boiling the endothelial cells for 10 min completely inhibited the synthesis of both peaks I and II (figure 1, *B*). Preincubation of the endothelial cells with 1 mM aspirin, a cyclooxygenase inhibitor, inhibited peak I formation, but did not significantly influence peak II synthesis (figure 1, *C*). Incubation with the lipoxygenase inhibitor NDGA at a concentration of 30 μM inhibited peak II formation approximately 85%, and inhibited peak I synthesis about 30% (figure 1, *D*).

To determine the structural identity of peak II, the molecule was esterified with diazomethane, derivitized to the trimethylsilyl ether, and analyzed by GC/MS.[11] The methyl ester, trimethylsilyl ether derivative of peak II gave prominent ions at 225 (base peak), 316 (M^+-90), 335 (M^+-71), 375 (M^+-31), 391 (M^+-15), and the molecular ion at 406. This mass spectrum is identical to the published mass spectrum of the methyl ester, trimethylsilyl ether derivative of 15-HETE.[12]

Incubation of [1-^{14}C]-arachidonic acid with endothelial cells for extended periods of time (60 min) revealed increased 15-HETE synthesis and the presence of additional radioactive products in addition to 15-HETE (figure 2, *A*). Peak I was HHT, peak II was 15-HETE, and the new peaks III and IV cochromato-

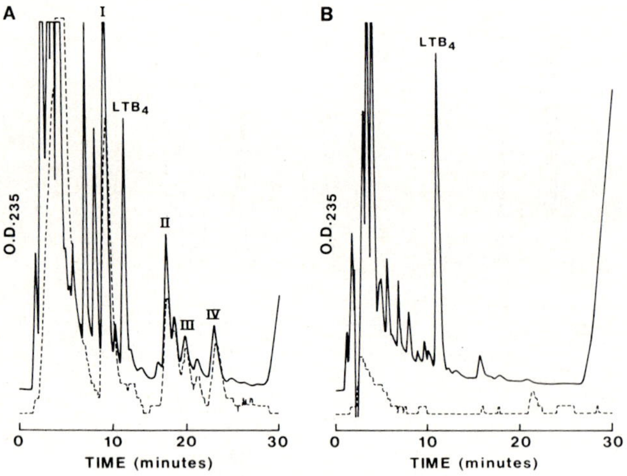

FIGURE 2. Extended incubation of [1-^{14}C]-arachidonic acid with endothelial cells. *A*, Endothelial cells (30 × 10^6) were incubated at 37° C with 50 μM [1-^{14}C]-arachidonate for 60 min. After extraction, the radioactive products were analyzed by RP-HPLC coupled with radioactive flow detection. *B*, Same as in *A* except the cells were boiled for 10 min before the addition of arachidonate. Solid line denotes ultraviolet detection at 235 nm, and dotted line indicates radioactivity. The LTB_4 peak is an internal standard.

graphed with 12-HETE and 5-HETE standards, respectively. NDGA (30 μM) completely inhibited the synthesis of peaks, II, III, and IV (data not shown). The LTB_4 peak was an exogenously added internal standard. There was no evidence of hydroxy fatty acid synthesis after incubation of heat-inactivated endothelial cells with [1-^{14}C]-arachidonic acid for 60 min (figure 2, *B*).

15-HETE synthesis from arachidonate was enhanced by thrombin stimulation. When endothelial cells are incubated with a combination of 50 μM arachidonate and 2 units of thrombin per 10^6 cells, 15-HETE synthesis is increased to 189% of the control arachidonate response (figure 3). A-23187 also enhances the arachidonate response (data not shown).

Since endothelial cells synthesize 15-HETE (by way of a 15-hydroperoxy arachidonate intermediate), we evaluated 15-HPETE metabolism in endothelial cells. Incubation of 15 × 10^6 endothelial (1.5 × 10^6/ml) cells with 30 μM 15-HPETE for 15 min at 37° C resulted in the formation of four major ultraviolet light–absorbing peaks on the RP-HPLC (figure 4, *A*). Peaks I, II, III, and IV were found to have RP-HPLC retention times (14.5 to 21.0 min) analogous to those of dihydroxy arachidonate molecules. Incubation of endothelial cells at 100° C for 10 min completely inhibited the formation of peaks I to IV (figure 4, *B*). Ultraviolet spectrophotometry revealed that each peak had a conjugated triene structure with identical ultra violet maxima at 258, 268, and 279 nm, and esterifica-

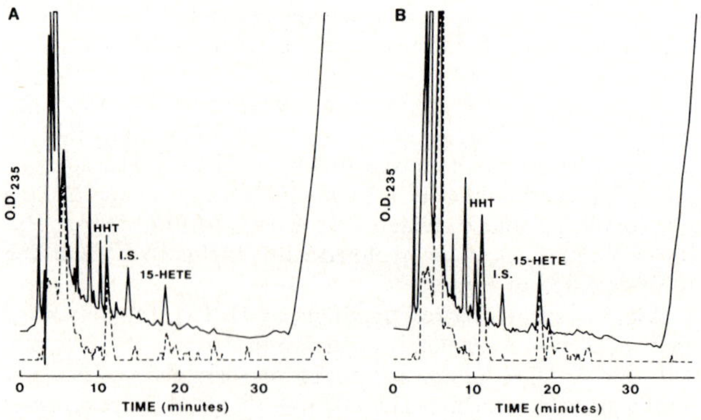

FIGURE 3. Stimulation of 15-HETE synthesis by thrombin. *A*, Endothelial cells (15 × 10^6) were exposed to 50 μM arachidonate for 10 min at 37° C. *B*, Same as in *A* except 2 units of thrombin were added per 10^6 cells. After extraction the metabolites were analyzed by RP-HPLC with radioactivity and ultraviolet detection.

tion and derivitization of the four unknown peaks followed by GC/MS showed that the four molecules had C numbers of 24.6 to 25.2 min and gave essentially identical mass spectra. The prominent ions were observed at 129 (M^+-365), 173 (M^+-321), 217 (M^+-277), 263 (M^+-231), 353 (M^+-141), 463 (M^+-31), 479 (M^+-15), and the molecular ion at 494. These spectra are identical to the published mass spectrum of the same derivative of 8,15-diHETE.[13, 14] We were not able to detect 8,15-diHETE formation from arachidonate. Presumably the amounts made were below our detection limits.

The formation of 8,15-diHETE from 15-HPETE suggests that endothelial cells may synthesize 14,15-LTA_4 from 15-HPETE.[13, 14] However, these data do

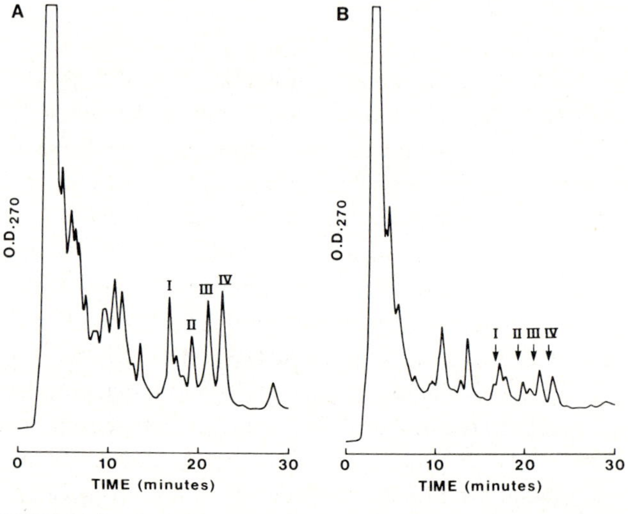

FIGURE 4. RP-HPLC chromatogram of 15-HPETE metabolism by endothelial cells. *A*, Endothelial cells (15 × 10^6) were incubated for 15 min at 37° C with 30 μM 15-HPETE. After extraction, the metabolites were analyzed by RP-HPLC with ultraviolet detection at 270 nm. *B*, Same as in *A* except cells were boiled for 10 min before the addition of 15-HPETE.

not indicate if the conversion of 14,15-LTA_4 to the 8,15-diHETE molecules is actually an enzymatic process. To assess this, we incubated 10 μM 14,15-LTA_4 with 15 $\times$ 10^6 endothtelial cells for 10 min at 37° C. RP-HPLC analysis showed that 14,15-LTA_4 in the presence of endothelial cells primarily formed peaks I and III of the 8,15-diHETE series, with very small amounts of peaks II and IV (figure 5). However, incubation of 14,15-LTA_4 with heat-inactivated endothelial cells resulted in essentially the same profile, with large peaks for I and III, and small peaks for II and IV (figure 5). This is very different from the chromatogram obtained with 15-HPETE and endothelial cells, on which nearly equal amounts of peaks, I, III, and IV were observed with a somewhat smaller peak II (figure 4, *A*). These data suggest that the 8,15-diHETE peaks II and IV are enzymatically formed from endogenously produced 14,15-LTA_4, but that exogenously added 14,15-LTA_4 is nonenzymatically hydrolyzed before it can be metabolized by the endothelial cell.

Discussion

Several laboratories have shown that human umbilical vein endothelial cells actively metabolize arachi-

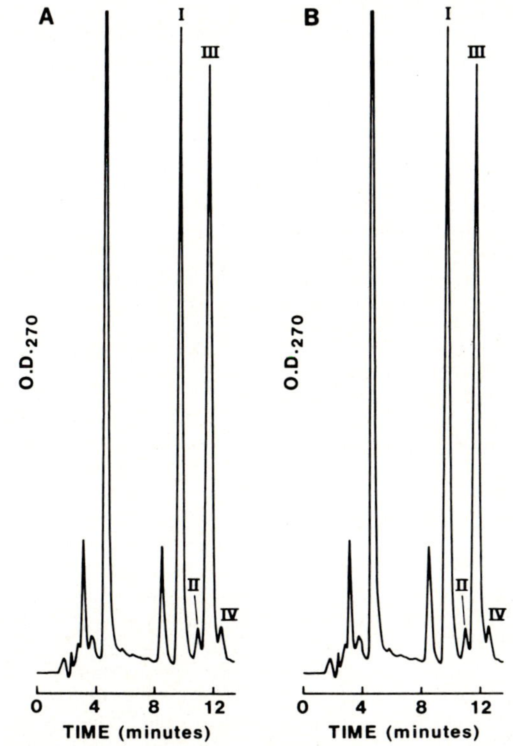

FIGURE 5. 14,15-LTA_4 metabolism by human endothelial cells. *A*, Human endothelial cells (15 $\times$ 10^6) were incubated at 37° C for 10 min with 10 μM 14,15-LTA_4. The products of the incubation were analyzed by RP-HPLC with ultraviolet detection at 270 nm. *B*, Same as in *A* except cells were boiled for 10 min before the addition of 14,15-LTA_4. Peaks I to IV correspond to the four 8,15 diHETE molecules observed in figure 4.

donic acid to form PGE_2 and PGI_2.[3,4] Endogenous arachidonate is released from endothelial cell phospholipids by phospholipase activity[15] and converted into eicosanoids after stimulation by various methods.[1-7] The prostaglandins can then either escape and inhibit platelet or neutrophil aggregation and adhesion, or inhibit their own synthesis in endothelial cells by feedback.[16-19] Although the cyclooxygenase pathway in endothelial cells is well characterized, we were interested in the possibility that endothelial cells might have both a cyclooxygenase and lipoxygenase system.

Incubation of human umbilical vein endothelial cells with [1-^{14}C]-arachidonic acid followed by extraction and appropriate RP-HPLC showed two prominent radioactive peaks with ultraviolet light absorbance at 235 nm. Peak I was identified as the cyclooxygenase product HHT, while peak II eluted in the monohydroxy arachidonate region. GC/MS analysis of peak II indicated that the unknown compound was 15-HETE. The precursor of 15-HETE biosynthesis is 15-HPETE. Incubation of 15-HPETE with endothelial cells results in the formation of four isomers of 8,15-diHETE with essentially identical mass spectra. The ultraviolet absorbance patterns of the four 8,15-diHETE molecules are also identical and reveal a conjugated triene system with absorption maxima at 258, 268, and 279 nm. Compounds I and III have retention times on RP-HPLC and ultraviolet spectra that are identical to those of diastereomeric (8*R*,15*S*)- and (8*S*,15*S*)-dihydroxy acids formed from the hydrolysis of synthetic 14,15 LTA_4. These compounds were detected by Maas et al.[13] in incubations of 15-HPETE with porcine leukocytes, and are thought to be formed by the incorporation of oxygen from water at C-8. Peak I was identified as (8*R*,15*S*)-dihydroxy-5-*cis*-9,11,13-*trans*-eicosatetraenoic acid, and peak III as (8*S*,15*S*)-dihydroxy-5-*cis*-9,11,13-*trans*-eicosatetraenoic acid.[13] These hydrolysis products correspond to the 5,12-dihydroxy acids formed nonenzymatically from LTA_4 via acid-catalyzed formation of a carbonium ion.[20] The mechanism of formation of compounds II and IV is not clear. Originally, an attack on the 14,15-LTA_4 epoxide by either hydroxyl radical or superoxide anion by direct nucleophilic attack or by electron transfer was proposed.[14]

More recently, a reaction scheme was proposed that has many mechanistic features in common with the 12-lipoxygenase.[21] The mechanism involves the removal of the pro(S) hydrogen at C-10, and migration of the radical to C-14. This radical centers on C-14, then reacts with the carbon-bound hydroperoxy oxygen with homolytic cleavage of the oxygen-oxygen bond to form 14,15-LTA_4. In addition, according to this hypothesis, migration of a radical centered on C-10 in the opposite direction gives antarafacial addition of oxygen at C-8, leading to the formation of compounds II and IV.[21] Since we have indirect evidence by HPLC of 12-HETE formation, a similar mechanism in endothelial cells is possible. It is believed that compound II is (8*S*,15*S*)-dihydroxy-5-*cis*-9-*trans*-11-*cis*-13-*trans*-eicosatetraenoic acid, and compound IV is (8*R*,15*S*)-dihydroxy-5-*cis*-9-*trans*-11-*cis*-13-*trans*-eicosatetraenoic acid.[13] Although the absolute stereochemistry of the 8,15-diHETE molecules produced by endothelial cells is not known, our data suggest that 14,15-LTA_4 is produced from 15-HPETE, and that two enzymatic (II, IV) and two nonenzymatic peaks (I, III) are synthesized from 15-HPETE by human endothelial cells. At the present time we do not know if these molecules are produced by a single enzyme or a sequence of enzymes. It is possible that 14,15-LTA_4 could be formed by interaction with hemoproteins (Cyt P-450, Cyt c) instead of by a specific 14,15-LTA_4 synthase.[22, 23] However, the high concentrations of these proteins that would be required to catalyze 14,15-LTA_4 synthesis from 15-HPETE make this an unlikely alternative.

The presence of 11-, 12-, and 15-OH arachidonate derivatives in vascular smooth muscle cells is well documented, and a recent report showed that 12-HETE was chemotactic for smooth muscle cells.[24] With both smooth muscle and endothelial cells displaying hydroxy fatty acid metabolism, the interesting possibility of transcellular metabolism between these two vascular cells as well as circulating cells cannot be ignored. Although the physiologic significance of 15-HETE and 8,15-diHETE in endothelial cells is not known, the presence of these molecules in our experiments suggests that the involvement of 15-lipoxygenase products in neutrophil-endothelial cell and platelet-endothelial cell interactions warrants further study.

References

1. Weksler BB, Marcus AJ, Jaffe EA: Synthesis of prostaglandin I_2 (prostacyclin) by cultured human and bovine endothelial cells. Proc Natl Acad Sci USA **74:** 3922, 1977
2. Marcus AJ, Weksler BB, Jaffe EA: Enzymatic conversion of prostaglandin endoperoxide H_2 and arachidonic acid to prostacyclin by cultured human endothelial cells. J Biol Chem **253:** 7138, 1978
3. Weksler BB, Ley CW, Jaffe EA: Stimulation of endothelial cell prostacyclin production by thrombin, trypsin, and the Ionophore A-23187. J Clin Invest **62:** 923, 1978
4. Baenziger NL, Force LE, Becherer PR: Histamine stimulates prostacyclin synthesis in cultured human umbilical vein endothelial cells. Biochem Biophys Res Commun **92:** 1435, 1980
5. Pearson JD, Slakey LL, Gordon JL: Stimulation of prostaglandin production through purinoreceptors on cultured porcine endothelial cells. Biochem J **214:** 273, 1983
6. Cramer EB, Pologe L, Pawlowski NA, Cohn ZA, Scott WA: Leukotriene C promotes prostacyclin synthesis by human endothelial cells. Proc Natl Acad Sci USA **80:** 4109, 1983
7. Benjamin CW, Hopkins NK, Oglesby TD, Gorman RR: Agonist specific desensitization of leukotriene C_4–stimulated PGI_2 biosynthesis in human endothelial cells. Biochem Biophys Res Commun **117:** 780, 1983
8. Van Os CPA, Geertruida PM, Rijke S, Halbeck HV, Verhagen J, Vliegenthart JFG: Double dioxygenation of arachidonic acid by soybean lipoxygenase-1. Biochim Biophys Acta **663:** 177, 1981
9. Jaffe EA, Nachman RL, Becker CG, Minick CR: Synthesis of antihemophilic factor antigen by cultured human endothelial cells. J Clin Invest **52:** 2745, 1973
10. Powell WE: Rapid extraction of oxygenated metabolites of arachidonic acid from biological samples using octadecylsilyl silica. Prostaglandins **20:** 947, 1980
11. Sun FF, Stafford JE: Metabolism of prostaglandin $F_{2\alpha}$ in rhesus monkey. Biochim Biophys Acta **369:** 95, 1974
12. Turk J, Maas RL, Brash AR, Roberts LJ, Oates JA: Arachidonic acid 15-lipoxygenase products from human eosinophils. J Biol Chem **257:** 7068, 1982
13. Maas RL, Brash AR, Oates JA: A second pathway of leukotriene biosynthesis in porcine leukocytes. Proc Natl Acad Sci USA **78:** 5523, 1981
14. Lundberg U, Radmark O, Malmsten C, Samuelsson B: Transformation of 15-hydroperoxy-5,9,11,13-eicosatetraenoic acid into novel leukotrienes. FEBS Letters **126:** 127, 1981
15. Hong SL: Effect of bradykinin and thrombin on prostacyclin synthesis in endothelial cells from calf and pig aorta and human umbilical cord vein. Thromb Res **18:** 787, 1980
16. Marcus AJ, Weksler BB, Jaffe EA, Broekman MJ: Synthesis of prostacyclin from platelet-derived endoperoxide by cultured human endothelial cells. J Clin Invest **66:** 979, 1980
17. Pearson JD, Carleton JS, Beesley JE, Hutchings A, Gordon JL: Granulocyte adhesion to endothelium in culture. J Cell Sci **38:** 225, 1979
18. Czervionke RL, Hoak JC, Fry GL: Effect of aspirin on thrombin-induced adherence of platelets to cultured cells from the blood vessel wall. J Clin Invest **62:** 847, 1978
19. Hopkins NK, Gorman RR: Regulation of endothelial cell cyclic nucleotide metabolism by prostacyclin. J Clin Invest **67:** 540, 1981
20. Hansson G, Lindgren JA, Dahlen SE, Hedqvist P, Samuelsson B: Identification and biological activity of novel ω-oxidized metabolites of leukotriene B_4 from human leukocytes. FEBS Letters **130:** 107, 1981
21. Mass RL, Brash AR: Evidence for a lipoxygenase mechanism in the biosynthesis of epoxide and dihydroxy leukotrienes from 15(S)-hydroperoxyeicosatetraenoic acid by human platelets and porcine leukocytes. Proc Natl Acad Sci USA **80:** 2884, 1983
22. Sok DE, Chung T, Sih CJ: Mechanisms of leukotriene formation: hemoglobin-catalyzed transformation of 15-HPETE to 8,15-DiHETE and 14,15-DiHETE isomers. Biochem Biophys Res Commun **110:** 273, 1983
23. Radmark O, Shimizu T, Fitzpatrick FA, Samuelsson B: Hemoprotein catalysis of leukotriene formation. Biochim Biophys Acta **792:** 324, 1984
24. Nakao J, Ito H, Ooyama T, Chang WC, Murota S: Calcium-dependency of aortic smooth muscle cell migration by 12-L-hydroxy-5,8,10,14 eicosatetraenoic acid. Atherosclerosis **46:** 309, 1983

A role for PAF-acether (platelet-activating factor) in platelet-dependent vascular diseases?

J. BENVENISTE AND M. CHIGNARD

ABSTRACT Platelets — isolated or in conjunction with leukocytes — interact with vessel walls in many experimental and human diseases. Several mediators are held responsible for platelet activation and interaction with leukocytes, among which PAF-acether (platelet-activating factor) is a prime candidate. This phospholipid mediator is released by most inflammatory cells, including neutrophils, by isolated organs such as kidney and heart, is a potent platelet and neutrophil agonist, and exerts major vasoactive properties. Its biosynthesis involves a two-step enzymatic process yielding the active molecule from the membrane alkyl-ether choline-containing phospholipids. The first step implicates a phospholipase A_2 that hydrolyzes a long-chain fatty acid (which can be arachidonic acid) from membrane phospholipids, leaving the intermediate compound lyso PAF-acether, a PAF-acether precursor that is acetylated by an acetyltransferase in a second step. It can also result from deacetylation of PAF-acether by an acetylhydrolase. PAF-acether release might explain the intervention of platelets in diseases such as glomerulonephritis and allergic vasculitis, in which the involvement of neutrophils and platelets is frequently noted. The end result of these complex sets of cell-to-cell interactions is the release of most known inflammatory mediators, influencing vascular permeability, cell infiltration, and smooth muscle contraction. Nevertheless, direct evidence for the implication of these rather well-defined cellular and molecular interactions in human pathologic states remains to be obtained.
Circulation 72, No. 4, 713–717, 1985.

THE INVOLVEMENT of platelets is a common feature in various human or experimental vascular diseases. Indeed, activated platelets release coagulation and growth factors, enzymes, vasoactive amines, lipid mediators, and basic proteins, all endowed with properties that can result in vessel wall injury. In thrombi, neutrophil-platelet interaction is often seen, for which several mediators are held responsible because they are released from neutrophils and are potent inducers of platelet aggregation and release. One of them, PAF-acether (platelet-activating factor), is a phospholipid that is synthesized by various cell types and organs. Therefore platelets can be instrumental in physiologic and pathologic phenomena, not only via the known pathways of hemostasis and coagulation but also as a result of their interaction with, for example, stimulated leukocytes.

A phospholipid mediator of platelet activation. In 1971, it was recognized that antigen-induced degranulation of immunoglobulin E (IgE)-sensitized basophils provoked the release in the extracellular medium of a soluble mediator, which was named platelet-activating factor (PAF).[1] We subsequently demonstrated its presence in human leukocytes and its ability to activate human platelets. Later, its physicochemical characteristics, including its phospholipid nature and the backbone of its molecular structure, were discovered, and we thereby proposed the recognition of a new class of phospholipid mediator.[2] Finally, its structure was elucidated and its full synthesis achieved.[3–5] PAF (1-0-alkyl-2-0-acetyl-*sn*-glyceryl-3-phosphorylcholine) is now termed "PAF-acether" to emphasize the structural features necessary for biological activity (figure 1).

Synthetic PAF-acether with C_{18} or C_{16} chains at position 1 have an equipotent activity in inducing platelet aggregation and desensitization or granule enzyme release from neutrophils.[6] By contrast, some structural features are mandatory for PAF-acether activity, such as an ether-linkage at position 1, the presence and the steric position of the short 2-acyl chain, and the presence of the choline head group.[4, 7, 8–11] These data are in favor of a specific platelet receptor for PAF-acether. Indeed, recent studies show PAF-acether–specific platelet binding sites.

PAF-acether aggregates rabbit and human platelets at a concentration of 1×10^{-9}M to 10^{-11}M. Circulating basophils are a source for PAF-acether in the rabbit[1] but probably not in man.[12, 13] Release of PAF-acether in the presence of the ionophore A 23187 or phagocytotic particles was observed from murine mac-

From the Institut National de la Santé et de la Recherche Médicale, INSERM U 200, Clamart, France.

Address for correspondence: J. Benveniste, INSERM U 200, 32 rue des Carnets, 92140 Clamart, France.

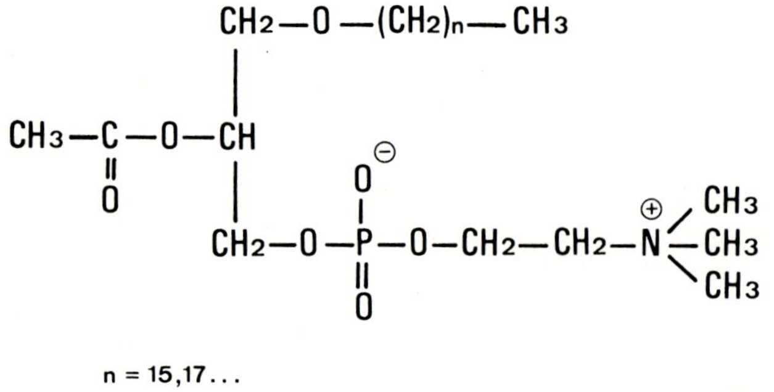

FIGURE 1. Structure of PAF-acether.

rophages but not from mastocytes.[14] PAF-acether is also released by the platelets themselves, therefore providing a molecular basis for the suggested third way of platelet aggregation.[15] PAF-acether has been recovered from rat, rabbit, and human alveolar macrophages,[16] human blood monocytes, and neutrophils, whereas 100% pure lymphocyte preparations failed to release the mediator.[17, 18] Therefore, PAF-acether, once described as a mediator of immediate hypersensitivity, is in fact formed by several cells, mostly proinflammatory ones, under various immune and nonimmune stimuli. Release in vivo in the vasculature of PAF-acether from IgE-sensitized basophils has been documented, and platelets returning to the circulation, after PAF-acether–induced thrombocytopenia, are specifically desensitized to PAF-acether.[19] First reports on the presence of PAF-acether in human blood in allergic and renal diseases are appearing.[20, 21] These results indicate that leukocyte-platelet interaction via the release of PAF-acether might take place in vivo.

Assay and characterization of PAF-acether. PAF-acether is quantified by aggregation of (or radiolabeled serotonin release from) washed rabbit platelets. Platelets are made refractory to adenosine-5′-diphosphate (ADP) and to arachidonic acid (AA). Using this very sensitive platelet bioassay (aggregation), one can detect as low as 5 pg of PAF-acether. The concentrations of PAF-acether are calculated over a standard curve established from aggregations of the rabbit washed platelets triggered by increasing concentrations of synthetic PAF-acether.

Besides aggregation of AA- and ADP-insensitive platelets, criteria for PAF-acether identification are (1) elution pattern identical to that of synthetic PAF-acether on silicic acid thin-layer or high-pressure liquid chromatography,[22] (2) inactivation by phospholipases A_2, C, and D and insensitivity to lipase from *Rhizopus arrhizus*,[2] and (3) absence of aggregation of PAF-acether–desensitized platelets.[6]

PAF-acether formation in platelets. It has been known since 1977 that when the two pathways of platelet aggregation (AA- and ADP-dependent) are inoperative, aggregations can still be launched by the calcium ionophore or thrombin, thus calling for the existence of more than two pathways. We indeed observed PAF-acether formation by rabbit and human washed platelets challenged by ionophore A 23187.[15] It was shown that this formation occurred even in the presence of inhibitors of the ADP and AA pathways. Later on we demonstrated that this synthesis was also triggered by thrombin and collagen but not by ADP, AA, or PAF-acether itself.[23] Other authors have reported on the formation of PAF-acether by calcium ionophore-stimulated rabbit or human platelets.[24]

PAF-acether biosynthesis. Involvement of a phospholipase A_2 (PLA_2) in PAF-acether formation was quickly suspected, mainly because all platelet agonists that trigger PAF-acether formation are potent PLA_2 activators. Accordingly, all tested PLA_2 inhibitors (EDTA, EGTA, bromophenacyl bromide, dibutyryl cyclic AMP, and compound 874CB) totally suppressed PAF-acether formation from washed rabbit platelets challenged either by the calcium ionophore A 23187 or by thrombin.[25] Although these different inhibitors are not specific for PLA_2, the fact that they are all active in spite of their different chemical structures allows one to conclude that PLA_2 is most probably involved in PAF-acether formation. The result of PLA_2 action on ether-linked choline-containing phospholipids, lyso PAF-acether, has no platelet aggregating properties, but after acetylation it is transformed into a compound with biological activity and chromatographic behavior indistinguishable from that of native PAF-acether. Lyso PAF-acether is formed upon calcium ionophore A 23187- or thrombin-induced rabbit platelet activation. Interestingly, the use of PLA_2 inhibitors mentioned above also led to the total suppression of lyso PAF-acether formation.[25] Furthermore, an enzyme capable of transferring an acetyl group on position 2 of the lyso PAF-acether has been demonstrated in spleen, leukocytes, and murine macrophages.[26, 27] It is indeed present in rabbit and human platelets because incubation of platelet lysates with synthetic lyso PAF-acether and acetyl–coenzyme A led to the formation of PAF-acether. This acetyltransferase activity was increased when platelets were activated by thrombin before lysis, reached a maximum between 1 and 2 min after thrombin stimulation, and returned to near its basal level within 5 min. The peak of activity preceded the plateau of PAF-acether formation.

The simultaneous release of PAF-acether and arachidonate metabolite from platelets. The probable precursor for lyso PAF-acether and PAF-acether synthesis is an ether-linked glycerylphosphorylcholine (GPC), i.e., a phosphatidylcholine with an ether bond in position 1 of the glycerol. When platelet phospholipid extracts were subjected to alkaline hydrolysis followed by chemical acetylation, the potential precursor was successively transformed into lyso PAF-acether and PAF-acether. Rabbit platelets (5×10^8) contained 2 to 3 nmol (i.e., 8 to 10 nmol considering a yield of 25%) of ether-linked GPC. Upon thrombin stimulation, around 0.3 nmol lyso PAF-acether and 5 pmol PAF-acether were formed (10% and less than 0.2%, respectively, of the total ether-linked GPC).[28] In platelets, the ether-linked GPC represented 11%,[29] 18%,[30] and 17%[31] of total GPC.

The reaction leading to lyso PAF-acether via PLA_2 also triggers the freeing of fatty acid. This fatty acid linked to the glycerol backbone in position 2 could be AA, the mediator of the second pathway of platelet activation. Indeed, in rabbit platelets, alkylacyl GPC contains AA in a higher amount than diacyl GPC.[29] Comparable differences were noted with human platelets, 44% and 23% for alkylacyl and diacyl GPC, respectively.[30] This AA can be mobilized upon platelet activation.[28] Similar results have been obtained in macrophages and neutrophils.

These data indicate that from the very same molecule, two mediators of platelet activation can be formed: thromboxane A_2 and PAF-acether. Thus PLA_2 appears to be a key enzyme for platelet activation.

Mechanisms of leukocyte-platelet interactions. Several mechanisms implicating various cell types with proinflammatory functions may explain the platelet-dependent amplification of vascular permeability and inflammatory lesions. Degranulation of basophils sensitized by IgE antibodies triggers activation of platelets, which leads to immune complex deposition in acute serum sickness in rabbits, a disease that involves mainly renal and peripheral small arteries.

The well-known interactions of neutrophils with platelets in various experimental preparations and in human pathologic states (reviewed in ref. 32) was poorly understood until it was found that activated neutrophils release thromboxane A_2 and PAF-acether.[10, 17, 18, 33, 34] Moreover, since 1981 many studies have emphasized the role of PAF-acether as a neutrophil-activating agonist. Since the initial descriptions,[9, 35] most of the neutrophil functions have been shown to be triggered by PAF-acether (e.g., aggregation, adherence, degranulation, chemotaxis and chemokinesis, release of superoxide anions and leukotriene B_4, and increase in C_3 receptor expression). Thus practically all known mechanisms of neutrophil activation can in turn bring platelets into the inflammatory site.

Another example of leukocyte-platelet interaction can be found in the onset of bronchoconstriction in the guinea pig, baboon, and man. Alveolar macrophages release PAF-acether when stimulated by a variety of agents such as zymosan particles, bacteria, immune complexes, and, in hyperimmunized animals, the specific antigen.[16] PAF-acether injected either intravenously or administered intratracheally is capable of inducing a potent bronchoconstriction that appears to be temporally related to a decrease in the number of blood platelets and neutrophils and to cell deposition in lung capillaries. These observations have been made in the guinea pig, the rabbit, the baboon, and man. Therefore mediators released from alveolar macrophages upon antigenic or nonantigenic (phagocytosis) stimulation induce platelet and neutrophil aggregation within the lung vessels. This process triggers bronchoconstriction via unknown pathways. Recently, ultrastructural evidence for the presence of aggregated platelets in the extravascular space, close to the lung smooth muscle, has been obtained after intravenous administration of PAF-acether to guinea pigs. This cascade of events, successively implicating lung macrophages, platelets, capillaries, and bronchi, offers an alternative explanation for unexplained bronchospasm in human pathologic states.

Direct vascular effects of PAF-acether. When PAF-acether was administered intradermally to the rat or to humans it induced edema and in the latter case hyperalgesia.[36-39] This effect appears to be independent of platelets and neutrophil activation.[37, 39] Recently, a dual response — early and late — was reported in human skin.[36]

Intravenous injection of PAF-acether in rabbits, guinea pigs, baboons, and rats triggered hypotension. The phospholipid seems to be the same molecule as the antihypertensive polar renomedullary lipid described 25 years ago.[40] In dogs PAF-acether induces an acute circulatory collapse.[41] In all species the hypotensive effect is independent of platelet aggregation, this being particularly clear in the rat.

The only vascular response in vitro to PAF-acether stimulation that has been observed is in the rat portal vein preparation.[42] There is no effect on isolated vascular muscle preparations.[43] However, vessels respond to PAF-acether when present in an intact organ such as the heart. Injection of PAF-acether in isolated guinea pig heart Langendorff preparations triggers dramatic impairment in the mechanical performance of the heart and decrease in flow rate. These data would suggest an effect on the coronary circulation in the perfused organ.[44] Nevertheless, we have been unable to show any direct effect in isolated canine coronary arteries (R. Santamaria, unpublished observations). Several authors have pointed out the platelet-independent effect of PAF-acether. Platelet depletion abolished the lung mechanical changes but not ventilatory and circulatory alterations provoked by intravenous injection of PAF-acether.[45] Furthermore, the phospholipid raised airway and vascular pressure and induced edema in guinea pig lungs perfused with platelet-free solution.[46] However, most of the effects in vitro and those obtained after platelet depletion must be examined in caution, since the experimental conditions are far from being physiologic. Moreover, high doses of PAF-acether are used in most of these experiments. Therefore, even if these experiments are useful to define the potential role of PAF-acether and to unveil some of the involved mechanisms, they do not necessarily reflect its mode of action in physiology and pathology in experimental animals and in man.

Conclusion. Activation of platelets and neutrophils in the vascular bed is a common feature in vascular diseases. Because PAF-acether is formed by and acts on platelets and neutrophils, it may represent one of the critical links in cell-to-cell interactions, thus providing the cellular and molecular basis for potent amplifying injurious mechanisms. It also appears to have direct effect on the vasculature. However, only the development of new drugs capable of interacting specifically with the biosynthetic pathways or sites of action of the various potential mediators so far described will bring about the elucidation of their precise role in various pathologic situations.

References

1. Benveniste J, Henson PM, Cochrane CG: Leukocyte-dependent histamine release from rabbit platelets: the role of IgE, basophils and a platelet-activating factor. J Exp Med **136:** 1356, 1972
2. Benveniste J, Le Couedic JP, Polonsky J, Tencé M: Structural analysis of purified platelet-activating factor by lipases. Nature **269:** 170, 1977
3. Benveniste J, Tencé M, Varenne P, Bidault J, Boullet C, Polonsky J: Semi-synthèse et structure proposée du facteur activant les plaquettes (PAF): PAF-acéther, un alkyl éther analogue de la phosphatidylcholine. CR Acad Sci Paris **289D:** 1037, 1979
4. Demopoulos CA, Pinckard RN, Hanahan DJ: Platelet-activating factor: Evidence for 1-0-alkyl-2-acetyl-sn-glyceryl-3-phosphorylcholine as the active component (a new class of lipid chemical mediators). J Biol Chem **254:** 9355, 1979
5. Godfroid JJ, Heymans F, Michel E, Redeuilh HC, Steiner E, Benveniste J: Platelet-activating factor (PAF-acether): total synthesis of 1-0-octadecyl 2-0-acetyl sn-glycero-3-phosphorylcholine. FEBS Lett **116:** 161, 1980
6. Smith RJ, Bowman BJ, Iden SS: Characteristics of 1-0-hexadecyl- and 1-0-octadecyl-2-0-acetyl-sn-glyceryl-3-phosphorylcholine– stimulated granule enzyme release from human neutrophils. Clin Immunol Immunopathol **28:** 13, 1983
7. Lalau Keraly C, Coëffier E, Tencé E, Borrel MC, Benveniste J: Specific desensitization of rabbit platelets by platelet-activating factor (PAF-acether) and derivatives. Br J Haematol **51:** 313, 1982
8. Tencé M, Coëffier E, Heymans F, Polonsky J, Godfroid JJ, Benveniste J: Structural analogs of platelet-activating factor (PAF-acether). Biochimie **63:** 723, 1981
9. O'Flaherty JT, Wykle RL, Miller CH, Lewis JC, Waite M, Bass DA, McCall CC, DeChatelet LR: 1-0-alkyl-sn-glyceryl-3-phosphorylcholines: a novel class of neutrophil stimulants. Am J Pathol **103:** 70, 1981
10. Wykle RL, Miller C, Lewis JC, Schmitt JD, Smith JA, Surles JR, Piantadosi C, O'Flaherty JT: Stereospecific activity of 1-0-alkyl-2-0-acetyl-sn-glyceryl-3-phosphorylcholine and comparison of analogs in the degranulation of platelets and neutrophils. Biochem Biophys Res Commun **100:** 1651, 1981
11. Satouchi K, Pinckard RN, McManus LM, Hanahan DJ: Modification of the polar head group of acetyl-sn-glyceryl-ether-phosphorylcholine and subsequent effects upon platelet activation. J Biol Chem **256:** 4425, 1982
12. Betz SJ, Lotner GZ, Henson PM: Generation and release of platelet-activating factor (PAF) from enriched preparations of rabbit basophils: failure of human basophils to release PAF. J Immunol **125:** 2749, 1980
13. Sanchez-Crespo M, Alonso F, Egido J: Platelet-activating factor in anaphylaxis and phagocytosis. I. Release from human peripheral polymorphonuclears and monocytes during the stimulation by ionophore A 23187 and phagocytosis but not from degranulating basophils. Immunology **40:** 645, 1980
14. Mencia-Huerta JM, Benveniste J: Platelet-activating factor and macrophages. I. Evidence for the release from rat and mouse peritoneal macrophages and not from mastocytes. Eur J Immunol **9:** 409, 1979
15. Chignard M, LeCouedic JP, Tencé M, Vargaftig BB, Benveniste J: The role of platelet-activating factor in platelet aggregation. Nature **279:** 799, 1979
16. Arnoux B, Duval D, Benveniste J: Release of platelet-activating factor (PAF-acether) from alveolar macrophages by the calcium ionophore A 23187 and phagocytosis. Eur J Clin Invest **10:** 437, 1980
17. Jouvin-Marche JE, Ninio E, Beaurain G, Tencé M, Niaudet P, Benveniste J: Biosynthesis of paf-acether (platelet-activating factor). VII. Precursors of paf-acether and acetyltransferase activity in human leukocytes. J Immunol **133:** 892, 1984
18. Lotner GZ, Lynch JM, Betz SJ, Henson PM: Human neutrophil-derived platelet-activating factor. J Immunol **124:** 676, 1980
19. Henson PM, Pinckard RN: Basophil-dervied platelet-activating factor (PAF) as an in vivo mediator of acute allergic reactions: demonstration of specific desensitization of platelets to PAF during IgE-induced anaphylaxis in the rabbit. J Immunol **119:** 2179, 1977
20. Grandel KE, Eisenstadt TC, Wanderer AA, Wasserman SI, Farr RS: A platelet-activating factor-like lipid in the plasma of patients during the induction of acquired cold urticaria. Fed Proc **43:** 1925, 1984 (abst)
21. Caramelo C, Fernandez-Gallardo S, Marin-Cao D, Inarrea P, Santos JC, Lopez-Novoa JM, Sanchez-Crespo M: Presence of platelet-activating factor in blood from humans and experimental animals: its absence in anephric individuals. Biochem Biophys Res Commun **120:** 789, 1984
22. Tencé M, Polonsky J, Le Couedic JP, Benveniste J: Release, purification, and characterization of platelet-activating factor (PAF). Biochimie **62:** 251, 1980
23. Chignard M, Le Couedic JP, Vargafting BB, Benveniste J: Platelet-activating factor (PAF-acether) secretion from platelets: effect of aggregating agents. Br J Haematol **46:** 455, 1980
24. Alam I, Smith JB, Silver MJ: Human and rabbit platelets form platelet-activating factor in response to calcium ionophore. Thomb Res **30:** 71, 1983
25. Benveniste J, Chignard M, Le Couedic JP, Vargafting BB: Biosynthesis of platelet-activating factor (PAF-acether). II. Involvement of phospholipase A_2 in the formation of PAF-acether and lyso-PAF-acether from rabbit platelets. Thomb Res **25:** 375, 1982
26. Wykle RL, Malone B, Snyder F: Enzymatic synthesis of 1-alkyl-2-acetyl-sn-glycero-3-phosphocholine, a hypotensive and platelet-aggregating lipid. J Biol Chem **255:** 10256, 1980
27. Ninio E, Mencia-Huerta JM, Heymans F, Benveniste J: Biosynthe-

sis of platelet-activating factor. I. Evidence for an acetyltransferase activity in murine macrophages. Biochm Biophys Acta **710:** 23, 1982
28. Chignard M, Le Couedic JP, Coëffier E, Benveniste J: Paf-acether formation and arachidonic acid freeing from platelet ether-linked glyceryl-phosphorylcholine. Biochem Biophys Res Commun **124:** 637, 1984
29. Sugiura T, Soga N, Nitta H, Waku K: Occurrence of alkyl ether phospholipids in rabbit platelets: composition and fatty chain profiles. J Biochem **94:** 1719, 1983
30. Mueller HW, Purdon AD, Smith JB, Wykle RL: 1-0-alkyl-linked phosphoglycerides of human platelets: distribution of arachidonate and other acyl residues in the ether-linked and diacyl species. Lipids **18:** 814, 1983
31. Tencé M, Jouvin-Marche E, Bessou G, Record M, Benveniste J: Ether-phospholipid composition in neutrophils and platelets. Thromb Res (in press, 1985)
32. Henson PM: Platelet-activating factor (PAF) as a mediator of neutrophil-platelet interactions in inflammation. *In* Russio-Marie F, Vargaftig BB, Benveniste J, editors: Pharmacology of inflammation and allergy: lipids and cells. Paris, 1981, Editions INSERM, vol 100, p 63
33. Higgs GA, Bunting S, Moncada S, Vane JR: Polymorphonuclear leukocytes produce thromboxane A_2-like activity during phagocytosis. Prostaglandins **12:** 749, 1976
34. Camussi G, Aglietta M, Coda R, Bussolino F, Piacibello W, Tetta C: Release of platelet-activating factor (PAF) and histamine. II. The cellular origin of human PAF: monocytes, polymorphonuclear neutrophils and basopils. Immunology **42:** 191, 1981
35. Camussi G, Tetta C, Bussolino F, Caligaris-Cappio F, Coda R, Masera C, Segoloni G: Mediators of immune complex-induced aggregation of polymorphonuclear neutrophils. II. Platelet-activating factor as the effector substance of immune induced aggregation. Int Arch Allergy Appl Immunol **64:** 25, 1981
36. Archer CB, Page CP, Paul W, Morley J, McDonald DM: Inflammatory charcteristics of platelet-activating factor (PAF-acether) in human skin. Br J Dermatol **110:** 45, 1984
37. Björk J, Smedegard G: Acute microvascular effects of paf-acether, as studied by intravital microscopy. Eur J Pharmacol **96:** 87, 1983
38. Humphrey DM, McManus LM, Satouchi K, Hanahan DJ, Pinckard RN: Vasoactive properties of acetyl-glyceryl-ether-phosphorylcholine analogues. Lab Invest **46:** 422, 1982
39. Pirotzky E, Page CP, Roubin R, Pfister A, Paul W, Bonnet J, Benveniste J: Paf-acether-induced plasma exudation in rat skin is independent of platelets and neutrophils. Microcirc Endothel Lymph **1:** 107, 1984
40. Blank ML, Snyder F, Byers LW, Brooks B, Muirhead EE: Antihypertensive activity of an alkyl ether analog of phosphatidylcholine. Biochem Biophys Res Commun **90:** 1194, 1979
41. Bessin P, Bnnet J, Apffel D, Soulard C, Desgroux L, Pelas I, Benveniste J: Acute circulatory collapse caused by platelet-activating factor (paf-acether) in dogs. Eur J Pharmacol **86:** 403, 1983
42. Santamaria R, Pourrias B, Benveniste J: Effet du paf-acéther sur la veine porte de rat. J Pharmacol (Paris) **14**(suppl): 83, 1983 (abst)
43. Cerrina J, Raffestin B, Labat C, Boullet C, Bayol A, Gateau O, Brink C: Effects of paf-acether on isolated muscle preparations from the rat, guinea pig and human lung. *In* Benveniste J, Arnoux B, editors: Platelet-activating factor and structurally-related ether lipids. Amsterdam, 1983, Elsevier Science Publishers, p 205
44. Benveniste J, Boullet C, Brink C, Labat C: The actions of paf-acether (platelet-activating factor) on guinea-pig-isolated heart preparations. Br J Pharmacol **80:** 81, 1983
45. Halonen M, Palmen JD, Lohman IC, McManus LM, Pinckard N: Differential effects of platelet depletion on the physiologic alteration of IgE anaphylaxis and acetyl glyceryl ether phosphoryl choline infusion in the rabbit. Am Rev Respir Div **124:** 416, 1981
46. Hamasaki Y, Mojarad M, Saga T, Tai HH, Said SI: Platelet-activating factor raises airway and vascular pressures and induces edema in lungs perfused with platelet-free solution. Am Rev Respir Dis **120:** 742, 1984

Production of platelet-activating factor by human vascular endothelial cells: evidence for a requirement for specific agonists and modulation by prostacyclin

GUY A. ZIMMERMAN, M.D., THOMAS M. MCINTYRE, PH.D., AND STEPHEN M. PRESCOTT, M.D.

ABSTRACT Primary cultures of confluent endothelial cells derived from human umbilical veins produce platelet-activating factor (PAF) (1-alkyl-2-acetyl-*sn*-glycero-3-phosphocholine) when stimulated with appropriate agonists. Highly purified human thrombin and calcium ionophore A23187 stimulate the incorporation of [^{3}H] acetate into a lipid product that has been identified as PAF by its behavior in thin-layer chromatographic and high-performance liquid chromatographic systems, the presence of characteristic biologic activity, and appropriate response to phospholipases. A number of other humoral mediators, examined because they directly influence the activity of vascular cells or because they may mediate endothelial injury, do not stimulate PAF production by endothelial cells. This indicates that the synthesis of PAF by cultured human endothelial cells is a response to specific agonists and is not an unregulated event that occurs as a result of nonspecific cellular perturbation. The PAF produced by thrombin-treated endothelial cells is a potent stimulus for platelet activation, as assayed by the aggregation of human platelets in autologous plasma. The production of PAF by endothelial monolayers is attenuated by prostacyclin, another product of stimulated endothelial cells. Conversely, PAF production is enhanced by treatment of the endothelial cells with indomethacin, an inhibitor of prostacyclin synthesis from arachidonic acid, indicating that endogenously generated prostacyclin may modulate PAF synthesis. The potential to synthesize PAF, a unique lipid autocoid that stimulates the activation of both platelets and polymorphonuclear leukocytes, suggests that endothelial cells can directly influence the activity of these circulating effector cells. This biologic potential may be important in the interaction of the endothelium with circulating blood cells in physiologic conditions and in syndromes of vascular injury.
***Circulation* 72, No. 4, 718–727, 1985.**

PLATELET-ACTIVATING FACTOR (PAF), originally described as an albumin-bound material produced by rabbit basophils that stimulated the release of histamine from autologous platelets,[1] is a mediator that may be important in the pathogenesis of a variety of immunologic and inflammatory syndromes (reviewed in refs. 2 and 3). The biochemical and biologic qualities of the factor have been further characterized,[2–4] and its chemical identity has been shown to be 1-alkyl-2-acetyl-*sn*-glycero-3-phosphocholine[3, 5, 6] (figure 1). PAF activates leukocytes, platelets, and other effector cells isolated from experimental animals[2, 3] and causes a syndrome with features suggestive of anaphylactic shock when injected into rabbits or baboons.[3] A mediator with biochemical properties and biologic activity characteristic of PAF is produced by macrophages, monocytes, polymorphonuclear leukocytes (PMNs), and platelets isolated from experimental animals[2, 3] in addition to basophils.[1] Several human cell types that are active in immunologic and inflammatory responses have been reported to synthesize PAF, including circulating monocytes,[7–9] alveolar macrophages,[10] PMNs,[7, 11, 12] and platelets.[13] Clark et al.[7] reported that PAF synthesized by stimulated human monocytes and PMNs is indistinguishable from PAF released from rabbit basophils. These observations have suggested that PAF is an autocoid that may mediate inflammatory events in humans, including some syndromes of inflammatory vascular injury.[14, 15] PAF causes vasoconstriction followed by inflammation and edema when injected into the skin of normal subjects,[3] consistent with this hypothesis. Furthermore, PAF is a potent

From the Nora Eccles Harrison Cardiovascular Research and Training Institute and the Department of Internal Medicine, University of Utah School of Medicine, Salt Lake City.

Supported by awards from the Nora Eccles Treadwell Foundation and the Richard A. and Nora Eccles Harrison Fund for Cardiovascular Research, and a grant from the American Heart Association (Montana Affiliate). Dr. Zimmerman was the recipient of a Public Health Service Clinical Investigator Award (HL00696) from the National Heart, Lung, and Blood Institute when this work was done.

Address for correspondence: Guy A. Zimmerman, M.D., Nora Eccles Harrison CVRTI, Bldg. 100, University of Utah, Salt Lake City, UT 84112.

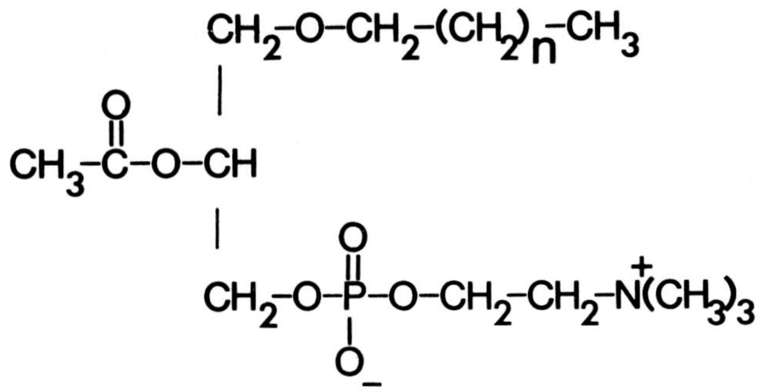

PLATELET-ACTIVATING FACTOR

FIGURE 1. The structure of PAF.

stimulus for the activation of human PMNs[14, 16–20] and platelets[21] in vitro.

In previous studies we found that human endothelial cells produce PAF when stimulated with thrombin, demonstrating an additional cellular source of this mediator.[22] The polar lipid product was identified as PAF by its migration with authentic PAF in two chromatographic systems, incorporation of tritiated precursors of PAF into the molecule, the ability of the lipid to stimulate PMN aggregation, a biologic activity characteristic of PAF,[14, 17–20] and the loss of labeled acetate and biologic activity when the material was treated with phospholipase A_2.[3, 4] Camussi et al.[23] independently reported that human endothelial cells synthesize PAF.

The production of PAF by vascular endothelial cells may mediate some of the responses of the endothelium to inflammation and injury and could potentially explain the increased adherence of leukocytes and platelets to the vascular surface under such conditions. Therefore we have further characterized the production of the lipid by stimulated endothelial cells. We report here: (1) that the synthesis of PAF by cultured human endothelium requires stimulation by specific agonists, (2) that PAF production is minimally altered by preincubation of endothelial cells with acetate, (3) that a variety of potential agonists that have vasoactive or proinflammatory properties do not stimulate its accumulation, (4) that the production of PAF by stimulated endothelial cells is enhanced by inhibition of cyclooxygenase and inhibited by treatment of the monolayers with prostacyclin (PGI_2), and (5) that the endothelial cell–derived lipid can activate human platelets. These findings are correlated with our previous observations on the synthesis of PAF by human endothelium.

Methods

Materials. The sodium salt of [^{3}H] acetic acid (2.8 Ci/mmol) was purchased from New England Nuclear. Lipid standards and unlabeled PAF were from Avanti Polar Lipids, Inc. Highly purified human thrombin and coagulation factor X_a, PGI_2, and cyanobacterial peptide[24] were the generous gifts of George Broze (Washington University, St. Louis), John Pike (Upjohn Diagnostics, Inc., Kalamazoo, MI), and Harold W. Siegelman (Brookhaven National Laboratory, Upton, NY), respectively. The biologic activity of thrombin was demonstrated by its ability to cause platelet aggregation and to stimulate the release of ^{14}C-serotonin from isolated, prelabeled platelets. All other reagents were purchased from Sigma Chemical Co. except as noted and were of the highest grade available.

Human umbilical vein endothelial cell culture. Endothelial cells were isolated from umbilical veins and cultured in modified medium 199 with 20% pooled human serum as described.[22, 25] The production of PAF by the endothelial monolayers was studied after they became completely confluent,[25] which usually occurred 4 to 9 days after their isolation and inoculation onto 35 mm gelatinized Petri dishes. The identity of endothelial cells grown in this fashion was verified by morphologic appearance,[26] the presence of human factor VIII antigen,[26] and the production of PGI_2 in response to thrombin,[27] bradykinin,[28] and histamine.[29] Contamination by cells that did not have morphologic characteristics absolutely typical of confluent endothelial cells was determined by phase-contrast microscopy to be 0.2% or less in all monolayers used. Only primary cultures were studied.

Incorporation of [^{3}H] acetate into [^{3}H] PAF. PAF synthesis in response to agonist stimulation was assayed with a minor modification of our previously described technique.[22] The reaction was initiated by replacing the growth medium with 1 ml of Hanks' buffered salt solution containing 10 mM HEPES (N-2-hydroxyethyl-piperazine-N′-2-ethylsulfonic acid) buffer (pH 7.4), 25 μCi of carrier-free [^{3}H] acetate, and the appropriate agonist (thrombin, calcium ionophore A23187, etc.) or control solution. In some experiments the monolayers were preincubated for various times (0 to 25 min) at 37° C with [^{3}H] acetate and the reaction was initiated by exchanging the preincubation medium for medium containing labeled acetate with or without the agonist. The monolayers were incubated for 5 or 10 min at 25° C or the indicated temperature; experiments done at 37° used a variable-powered, constant-temperature heating platform.

In experiments to test the effect of indomethacin, the indomethacin was first dissolved in dimethylsulfoxide and diluted to the final concentration (25 μM) in Hanks' balanced salt solution. The final concentration of dimethylsulfoxide was 0.1% or less in each experiment and was included in the control buffer. The endothelial monolayers were preincubated with indomethacin or control solution for 15 min before addition of the agonist. In experiments with prostacyclin, it was dissolved in 50 mM Tris buffer (pH 9.5) and diluted to a final concentration of 2 mM immediately before addition to the endothelial cell monolayer, and was incubated with the monolayers for 2 to 10 min before addition of the agonist. Pharmacologic concentrations of PGI_2 were used because the amount of active prostaglandin that entered the cells was unknown and because we did not use drugs that may potentiate the effects of PGI_2, such as isobutylmethylxanthine.

After incubation of the endothelial cell monolayers with labeled acetate under the specific conditions described, the reaction was stopped by adding 50 mM acetic acid in methanol. The cells were then scraped from the plate and it was washed twice with 1 ml methanol. The cell fraction and the methanol washes were pooled, and 7 nmol labeled carrier PAF and 1.25 ml of chloroform were added. The resulting monophase was split with chloroform and 0.1M sodium acetate and the lower phase was washed three times with preequilibrated upper phase. The lower phase was dried under N_2, and the lipids were resuspended in a known volume of chloroform/methanol (9:1). A portion was used to determine the total radioactivity and the lipids in the remainder were separated by thin layer chromatography (TLC) as described.[22] Areas containing PAF were scraped from the plate and the radioactivity was determined by scintillation spectrophotometry. Duplicate assays showed that the mean variation of PAF production by monolayers from the same isolate studied on the same day was ±5%.

High-performance liquid chromatography (HPLC) of fractions containing PAF. In some experiments the extracts from endothelial monolayers were chromatographed on TLC plates, and the areas migrating with authentic PAF were scraped into a centrifuge tube. The lipids were eluted with chloroform/methanol (2:1, vol/vol) and then methanol. The lipids in this extract were then separated by HPLC as described.[22]

Recovery of platelet-activating activity from thrombin-stimulated endothelial cells. Six dishes of endothelial cells were stimulated with thrombin (2 U/ml) for 5 min and extracted as previously outlined, with the exception that carrier PAF was not included. The lipids in the extract were separated by HPLC, 0.5 ml volumes of the effluent were collected, dried under nitrogen, and redissolved in 75 μl of 0.15M NaCl containing 1 mg/ml fatty acid–free bovine serum albumin. In addition, 5 nmol of authentic PAF was applied to the HPLC and fractions were collected and processed in the same way, except that the lipid in each fraction was redissolved in 0.5 ml of NaCl containing fatty acid–free bovine serum albumin.

The recovery of bioactivity was assayed by analyzing each fraction for the ability to stimulate the aggregation of cytochalasin B–treated human granulocytes as described.[22] The HPLC fractions containing this activity were found to elute at the same time as those containing authentic PAF,[22] which also retained proaggregatory activity for neutrophils (not shown).

Aliquots of the fractions that contained neutrophil proaggregatory activity were then pooled and evaluated for their ability to stimulate human platelet aggregation[21] by means of a modification of a published method.[30] Venous blood from a normal man who had taken no drugs for 14 days was drawn with a "two syringe" technique and anticoagulated with 1 volume of 3.8% sodium citrate to 9 volumes of blood. Platelet-rich plasma was removed with a plastic transfer pipet after centrifugation at 250 *g* for 10 min at room temperature and kept at 37° C in an atmosphere of 5% CO_2 until use. Platelet-poor plasma was prepared by centrifuging the remaining blood at 750 *g* for 20 min; the platelet-poor plasma was then handled in the same way as the platelet-rich plasma. Platelet aggregometry was carried out in a Payton Model DB 2 channel aggregometer. Aliquots (0.45 ml) of the platelet-rich plasma were stirred at 900 rpm at 37° C for 2 min, 50 μl of sample (extract from endothelial cells or authentic PAF retrieved from HPLC, authentic PAF not subjected to HPLC, or control buffer) was added, and the resulting aggregation wave was recorded for 5 min. Light transmission was set at 0% with platelet-rich plasma and 100% with platelet-poor plasma, with 100% transmission causing a pen deflection of 21.5 cm on the recorder.

Results

PAF production by human endothelial cells occurs in response to agonist stimulation. Human thrombin reproducibly stimulated confluent endothelial monolayers to produce PAF. In experiments with primary endothelial cell cultures from 21 different isolates, thrombin caused a 15-fold increase in the incorporation of [^{3}H] acetate into the polar lipid migrating with authentic PAF when compared with monolayers treated with buffer (figure 2). The amount of [^{3}H] acetate that accumulated in the PAF fractions in these experiments was similar to the incorporation in studies with six other endothelial isolates that we previously reported.[22] Endothelial monolayers treated for 5 min with 1 or 2 U/ml thrombin did not contract[31] nor was there morphologic evidence of injury under the conditions of these experiments; they excluded trypan blue, and maintained unchanged monolayer morphology for up to 72 hr after treatment with thrombin (2 U/ml for 5 to 30 min). Calcium ionophore A23187 also stimulated endo-

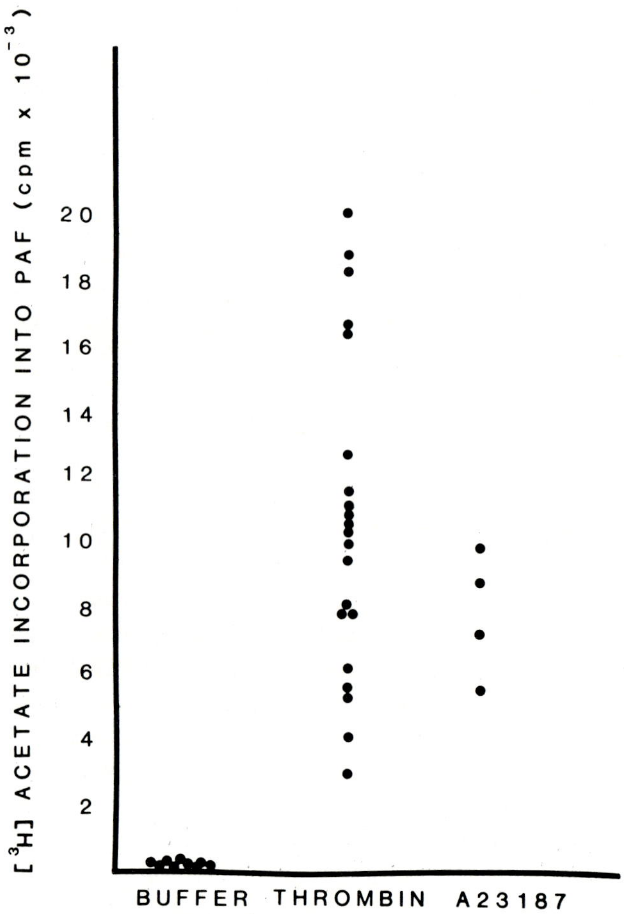

FIGURE 2. Thrombin and calcium ionophore A23187 stimulate the production of PAF by cultured human endothelial cells. Primary monolayers of confluent umbilical vein endothelial cells were stimulated with human thrombin (2 U/ml) or ionophore A23187 (5 μM) in the presence of [^{3}H] acetate, the incubation was continued for 5 or 10 min at 25° C, and the lipid products were extracted and analyzed by TLC as described in Methods. The results of experiments with 21 different endothelial cultures are shown. Thrombin and ionophore reproducibly stimulated the incorporation of labeled acetate into PAF, whereas little acetate was incorporated when the cells were treated with buffer in place of one of these agonists (mean counts per minute: buffer, 210 ± 96 [n = 17]; thrombin, 10,796 ± 4873 [n = 21]; ionophore A23187, 7894 ± 1869 [n =4]).

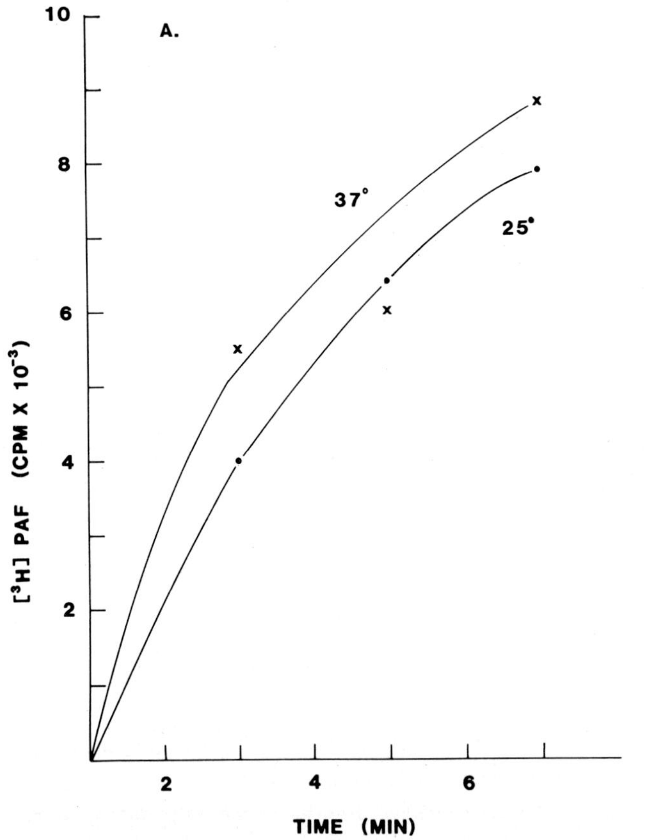

FIGURE 3A. Effect of temperature and prelabeling on the incorporation of [^{3}H] acetate into PAF by stimulated endothelial cells. Duplicate monolayers of endothelial cells from the same culture were stimulated for various times at 25° or 37° C as described in Methods and figure 2. There was a small increase in [^{3}H] acetate incorporation into PAF in monolayers incubated at 37° C compared with those incubated at 25° C.

thelial cells to produce PAF; the magnitude of the stimulation was similar to that in response to thrombin (figure 2).

In an experiment to determine the daily variability of the response, confluent endothelial monolayers from the same culture were stimulated with thrombin and ionophore A23187 on successive days. The response to thrombin was 24% greater, and that to A23187 was 16% greater, on the second day as compared with the first, whereas the variation in duplicate monolayers assayed on the same day was 5% or less (Methods). We have previously shown that the cell number in endothelial cell monolayers does not change significantly over a period of several days after the cultures become tightly confluent,[32] as have others.[26, 33] These data suggest that a small increase in PAF synthetic capacity may occur with time in confluent monolayers.

The incorporation of [^{3}H] acetate into PAF was enhanced when the incubations were done at 37° C rather than 25° C (figure 3A), but the incremental increase at each time point was relatively small. For this reason all other experiments were done at 25°. Preincubation of endothelial monolayers with [^{3}H] acetate for up to 25 min before stimulation did not increase the incorporation of the label into PAF over that achieved when the acetate and the agonist were added simulaneously (figure 3B). This result indicates that exogenous acetate is rapidly assimilated into the cellular pool that is available for PAF synthesis, presumably as acetyl coenzyme A, and suggests that the intracellular distribution of acetate is uniform rather than compartmental.

Enhanced synthesis of PAF by stimulated endothelial cells requires specific agonists. We evaluated a variety of humoral mediators that are known to act directly on vascular endothelial cells, or are postulated to directly modify the biological or biochemical activity of these cells, for their ability to stimulate PAF production. Table 1 lists a group of these mediators that did not

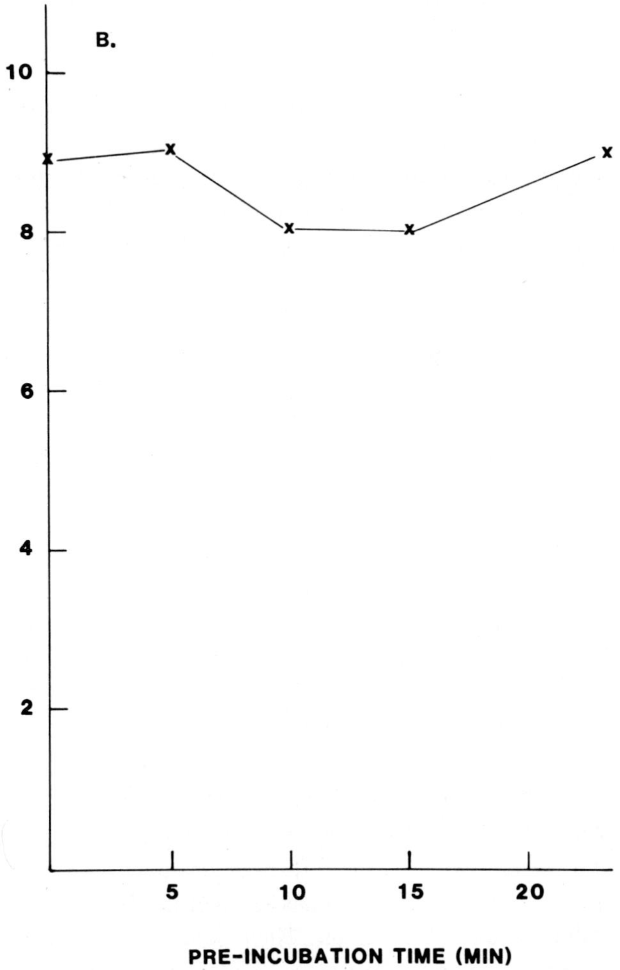

FIGURE 3B. Monolayers of endothelial cells from the same culture were preincubated with [^{3}H] acetate for the times shown and then stimulated for 5 min as described. The incorporation of [^{3}H] acetate into PAF was not significantly altered by preincubation of the endothelial cells with the labeled compound when compared with addition of the acetate and the agonist simultaneously (0 preincubation time).

TABLE 1

Potential mediators of vascular effects that did not induce the synthesis of PAF by cultured endothelial cells[A]

Endotoxin (10 μg/ml)[B]	Serotonin (1 μM)
Angiotensin II (1 μg/ml)	Epinephrine (1 μM)
Zymosan-activated plasma (10%)[C]	Collagen (100 μg/ml)
n-Formylmethionyl-leucyl-phenylalanine (1 μM)	Coagulation factor X_a (2 μg/ml)
Concanavalin A (1 μg/ml)	Vasoactive intestinal peptide (3 μg/ml)
Acetylcholine (10 μM)	Insulin (25 mM)
Substance P (1 μM)	Gastrin (3 μg/ml)
Homocysteine (100 μM)	Trypsin (0.0025%)[E]
Fibrinogen (10 μg/ml)	Phorbol myristate acetate (1 μM)
Fibrin and fibrin peptides[D]	Cyanobacterial peptide (0.1 μg/ml)
Urokinase (250 U/ml)	Streptokinase (250 U/ml)

[A]These compounds were tested in the standard assay, which measures the incorporation of [^{3}H] acetate into PAF (Methods and figure 2), at the concentrations shown in parentheses. In each experiment positive controls of thrombin (2 U/ml) or the calcium ionophore A23187 (5 μM) were included and gave values of 10,000 to 20,000 cpm of [^{3}H] acetate incorporation into PAF. The compounds listed did not result in incorporation over control (buffer-only) incubations.

[B]Lipopolysaccharide from *Escherichia coli* serotype 055:B5.

[C]Used as a source of C5a desarg and prepared as described.[32]

[D]Human fibrinogen (10 μg) was treated with 0.20 U thrombin in 0.1 ml of buffer for 120 min at 37° C and chilled, and an aliquot of the fluid phase (1:1000 dilution) was added with labeled acetate to the endothelial cell monolayer.

[E]A 10-fold higher concentration gave a small increase over background (<10% of the thrombin response).

enhance PAF production. These findings indicate that the synthesis of PAF by human endothelial cells in response to thrombin (figure 2) is not a response that occurs when the cells are perturbed in a nonspecific fashion. Furthermore, the results are important because several of the humoral mediators that we tested (table 1) also enhance the adherence of inflammatory cells to endothelium,[32, 34–36] an interaction that could be explained by production of PAF by the endothelial cells.[22] We have previously shown that PAF itself does not stimulate endothelial cells to make additional PAF.[22]

PAF synthesized by endothelial cells activates human platelets. Endothelial monolayers were stimulated with thrombin (2 U/ml) and extracted, and the pooled extract was separated by HPLC. Fractions of the effluent that migrated with authentic PAF were tested for their ability to aggregate human PMNs, as described,[22] and were found to potently induce aggregation of the isolated leukocytes (Methods). Aliquots of the endothelial cell fractions that contained PMN proaggregatory activity were tested for their ability to stimulate platelet aggregation, along with fractions that contained authentic PAF that had been passed over the HPLC column in an identical manner. The results of this experiment are shown in figure 4A and document that the lipid product from thrombin-stimulated endothelial cells causes the aggregation of human platelets. The concentration curve for authentic PAF indicated a threshold between 10^{-9}M and 10^{-8}M (figure 4B), suggesting that the amounts of PAF synthesized by human endothelial cells[22] could potentially result in the activation of platelets in plasma or blood.

Effect of treatment of endothelial cells with indomethacin and prostacyclin on the synthesis of PAF. When endothelial monolayers were incubated with the cyclooxygenase inhibitor indomethacin before stimulation, the synthesis of PAF was enhanced (table 2). The magnitude of the increased response was highly variable, although the qualitative response itself was consistent. The increase that followed indomethacin occurred after stimulation with different agonists[22a] and at submaximal as well as maximal responses. Indomethacin pretreatment reduced the release of PGI_2 from stimulated endothelial cells by 90% or greater (not shown). These experiments suggested that PGI_2, the major cyclooxygenase product of stimulated human macrovascular endothelium,[27, 37] inhibits the production of PAF. Consistent with this hypothesis, we found that the addition of exogenous PGI_2 caused a small, but reproducible, attenuation of PAF accumulation in stimulated endothelial cells (table 2).

Discussion

In previous studies, we found that primary cultures of human umbilical vein endothelial cells synthesize PAF when stimulated with thrombin.[22] Thrombin treatment of cultured umbilical vein endothelial cells caused a dose-related increase in incorporation of tritiated acetate into a polar lipid that migrated with authentic PAF when the lipid products were separated by TLC; the concentrations of thrombin that stimulated

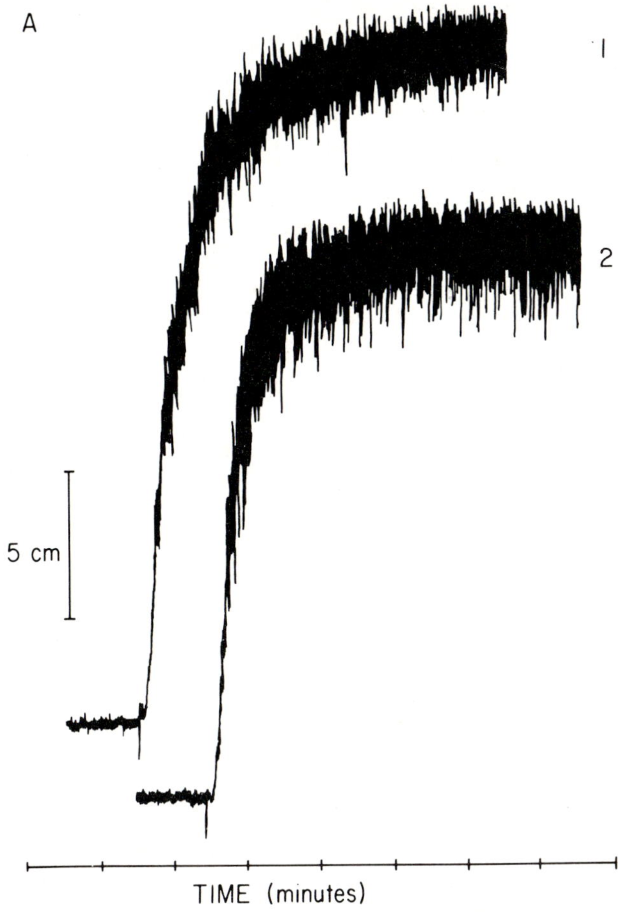

FIGURE 4A. PAF recovered from thrombin-treated endothelial cells stimulates human platelet aggregation. Endothelial monolayers were treated with thrombin (2 U/ml) for 5 min at 37° C, the lipids were extracted and separated by HPLC, and the fractions migrating at the same time as authentic PAF were collected (Methods). An aliquot from combined portions of these fractions stimulated the aggregation of human platelets in platelet-rich plasma (curve 1). An aliquot from fractions containing authentic PAF that has been processed in the same way as the endothelial cell extracts also stimulated platelet aggregation (curve 2). The aggregation waves were traced directly from the original strip-chart recordings.

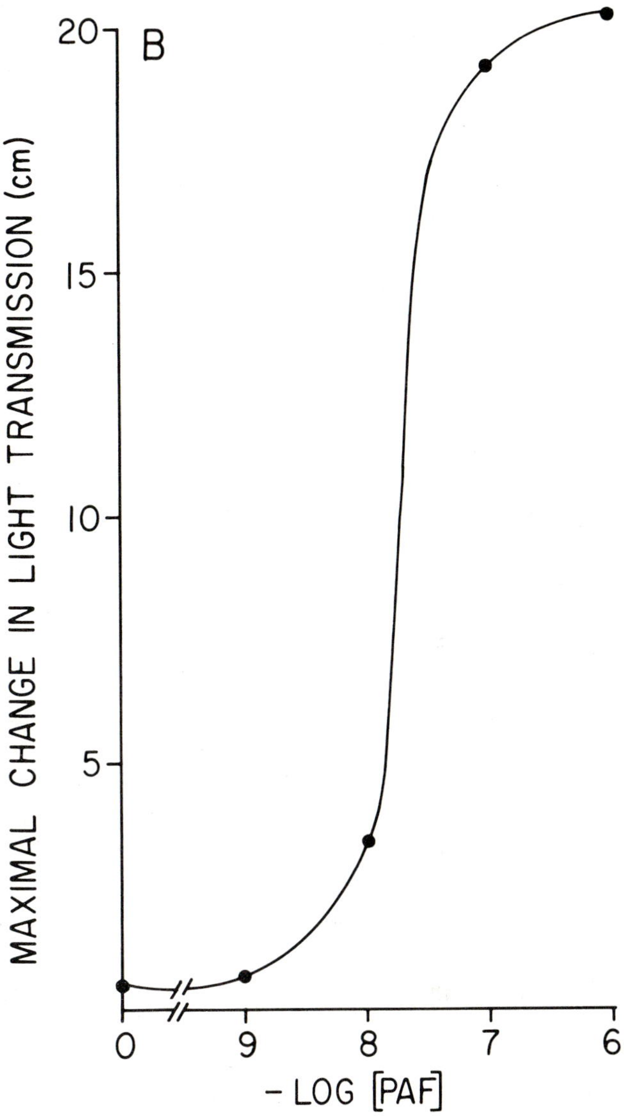

FIGURE 4B. Authentic PAF (that had not been subjected to HPLC) caused a concentration-dependent increase in platelet aggregation. The aggregation wave stimulated by 10^{-8}M PAF reversed and returned to baseline spontaneously; aggregation curves stimulated by higher concentrations of PAF did not reverse during the 5 min recording period.

production of the lipid were similar to those that stimulate other endothelial cell responses, such as PGI_2 release. The accumulation of the product was maximal 5 min after treatment of the endothelial monolayers with thrombin, did not occur when the thrombin was inactivated, and required divalent cations. When the [^{3}H] acetate-containing lipid was eluted from the thin-layer chromatogram and treated with phospholipase A_2, greater than 90% of the radiolabel was lost from the molecule, confirming that the [^{3}H] acetate was located at the *sn*-2 position of the glycerol chain.

The radiolabeled polar lipid produced by thrombin-stimulated endothelial cells also eluted with authentic [^{3}H] PAF when extracts were analyzed by HPLC. Fractions of the lipid extract from thrombin-stimulated cells that eluted at the same time as authentic PAF caused the aggregation of isolated human PMNs. The ability of the lipid to activate the PMNs, as measured

TABLE 2
Effect of pretreatment of endothelial cells with indomethacin or exogenous PGI_2 on agonist-stimulated production of PAF

Pretreatment	% Response compared with buffer pretreatment
Indomethacin (n = 14)	185 ± 102 ($p < .01$)[A]
PGI_2 (n = 9)	78 ± 15 ($p < .01$)

[A]The results were analyzed for statistical significance with a two-tailed, unpaired Student's t test.

by aggregation, was lost when the fractions were incubated with phospholipase A_2 but not when they were incubated with buffer. Thus the polar lipid produced by human endothelial cells in response to thrombin was characterized as PAF by its migration in two chromatographic systems, the presence of biological activity characteristic of PAF,[14, 19] and loss of the biologic activity and radiolabeled acetate when treated with phospholipase A_2.[3, 4] Under the conditions of these experiments the PAF remained associated with the endothelial cells and was not released into the overlying buffer. Additionally, we found that stimulated human endothelial cells can convert 1-[^{3}H]alkyl-*sn*-glycero-3-phosphocholine to [^{3}H]alkyl-2-acyl-GPC and to [^{3}H] PAF, indicating that the cells have the appropriate enzymes to acylate the labeled alkyl lipid to a potential precursor molecule (1-alkyl-2-acyl-GPC)[22] or to PAF itself.

The experiments reported here confirm that thrombin reproducibly stimulates primary cultures of human endothelium to incorporate labeled acetate into the lipid product and that calcium ionophore A23187 can also act as an agonist (figure 2). Thrombin and ionophore A23187 stimulate other biochemical activities of human endothelial cells, including the release of arachidonate and the synthesis of PGI_2.[27] Although thrombin was a potent agonist for PAF production by the endothelial cells (figure 2), a number of other humoral agents did not stimulate PAF accumulation (table 1). Each of these agents was studied because it has been reported to enhance the adherence of platelets or PMNs to endothelium or to mediate endothelial injury, is locally generated during thrombosis, or directly stimulates a biologic response of endothelial cells, and thus was a potential agonist for PAF production. The fact that these agents did not stimulate PAF accumulation under the conditions of these experiments indicates that the production of PAF by endothelial monolayers is a regulated event that requires the action of specific agonists. This conclusion is also supported by additional observations from our laboratories that demonstrate that histamine, bradykinin, and ATP are agonists for PAF synthesis by human endothelial cells and that they appear to stimulate PAF production by interacting with specific receptors.[22a]

Camussi et al.[23] have reported that umbilical vein endothelial cells synthesize and release PAF in response to ionophore A23187, rabbit antihuman factor VIII, angiotensin II, and vasopressin. Their studies differ from our findings in that they did not observe PAF synthesis in response to thrombin (in the absence of indomethacin; see below) unless the endothelial cells were repetitively stimulated with the agonist, and they reported that PAF is released from stimulated endothelial monolayers whereas we have found it to remain cell associated.[22] The first discrepancy may be explained, in part, by differences in the time of incubation of endothelial cells with thrombin, since we have found that the maximal accumulation of PAF in response to thrombin occurs at 5 to 10 min after stimulation[22] and Camussi et al.[23] assayed supernates from endothelial monolayers after 45 min of stimulation with thrombin. The explanation for different findings with regard to release of PAF from the endothelial monolayers is unclear at this time. Camussi et al.[38] have also reported that PAF is released from rabbit aortic endothelial cells injured by treatment with antibody directed against angiotensin-converting enzyme, a plasma membrane component of endothelium. In our experiments, endothelial cells maintained normal morphology and monolayer architecture after stimulation with thrombin, suggesting that there was no significant injury.

Figures 4A and 4B illustrate that the lipid isolated from thrombin-stimulated human endothelial cells is a potent activator of human platelets. The phospholipid product in the fractions containing this biologic activity migrated with authentic PAF in the HPLC separation and also stimulated the aggregation of human granulocytes (Results and ref. 22). The ability to activate both PMNs and platelets directly is an unusual biologic property of PAF[2, 3, 13, 14, 16–21] that is shared with no other phospholipids yet identified. Thus the presence of this bioactivity is further evidence that the lipid product from thrombin-stimulated endothelial cells is PAF. Furthermore, the ability of thrombin-stimulated endothelial cells to produce a mediator that activates platelets may contribute to the accumulation of thrombocytes on the endothelial surface in response to procoagulants[39, 40] or when the endothelium is injured.[41] Thus the production of PAF by endothelium may be one mechanism by which thromboresistance is lost under these conditions.[22]

Indomethacin, an inhibitor of cyclooxygenase and of the production of PGI_2 and other metabolites of arachidonic acid via the cyclooxygenase pathway,[27] enhanced the accumulation of PAF by endothelial monolayers (table 2). This finding suggests an interaction between arachidonic acid metabolism and PAF production in endothelial cells. The experiments in which exogenous PGI_2 suppressed PAF production (table 2) support this possibility. Camussi et al.[23] also reported that exogenous PGI_2 inhibited PAF release by stimulated endothelial cells and that indomethacin had a variable effect on PAF release. Although pharmacologic concentrations of prostacyclin were used (Methods), the findings in table 2 additionally suggest that endogenously generated PGI_2 may influence the synthesis or degradation of PAF. Modulation of synthesis seems more likely, since an equivalent effect of indomethacin was seen at a variety of concentrations of agonist (i.e., the concentration-response curve was shifted upward). PGI_2 inhibits arachidonate release and increases intracellular cyclic AMP in the presence of the phosphodiesterase inhibitor isobutylmethylxanthine in cultured endothelium,[42, 43] indicating that endogenous PGI_2 can influence biochemical events in vascular cells.[43] The data in table 2 suggest that the inhibition of endothelial cell prostacyclin synthesis with indomethacin, or other cyclooxygenase blockers, will enhance PAF accumulation in response to stimulation with appropriate agonists, such as thrombin. Because PAF stimulates enhanced platelet adhesiveness (ref. 21 and figure 4), increased PAF synthesis may favor platelet adherence to the endothelial surface. Czervionke et al.[40] have observed augmented platelet adherence to aspirin-treated endothelial monolayers that were stimulated with thrombin, an effect that they attributed to decreased PGI_2 release and a resultant abrogation of the direct inhibitory effect of PGI_2[27, 45] on the platelets. Our studies suggest that increased PAF production is an alternative mechanism for the enhanced platelet adherence under these conditions.

In additional studies we have found that several agonists that stimulate PGI_2 release by endothelial cells (thrombin, bradykinin, histamine, ATP) also stimulate PAF synthesis, although the durations of production of the two autocoids are quite different.[22a] These observations suggest that a common phospholipid precursor may provide arachidonate and 1-alkyl-*sn*-glycero-3-phosphocholine for metabolism to PGI_2 and PAF, respectively; 1-alkyl-2-arachidonoyl-*sn*-glycero-3-phosphocholine has been reported to provide both arachidonate and 1-alkyl-GPC for subsequent metabolism in stimulated neutrophils.[44]

The observations that we have described indicate that the production of PAF can be added to the list of biosynthetic potentials of the human vascular endothelial cell.[46] The ability of PAF to activate platelets and neutrophils suggests that this biosynthetic capability may be important in the interaction of endothelium with circulating blood cells and perhaps with other adjacent cells as well. The ability of stimulated endothelial cells to produce PAF, a platelet activator, and PGI_2, a potent inhibitor of platelet activity,[27, 45] indicates the potential for the endothelium to regulate the interaction between the two cells directly (figure 5). This may be important in vascular homeostasis, since platelets are required to maintain endothelial integrity.[22] The production of the two autocoids may similarly affect the interaction of polymorphonuclear leukocytes and endothelial cells.[22, 25] The potential to produce PAF also suggests, however, that this response of stimulated endothelial cells may contribute to pathologic thrombosis and vascular injury. Products released from activated platelets[36, 47] and granulocytes[34, 36, 48–50] can directly injure endothelium, and both of these effector cells adhere to sites of vascular damage under the appropriate conditions.[34, 39, 41, 51, 52] The unregulated production of PAF by endothelial cells, or an uncontrolled response of the PMNs and platelets to this inflammatory mediator, may thus influence the local activation of the blood cells and pro-

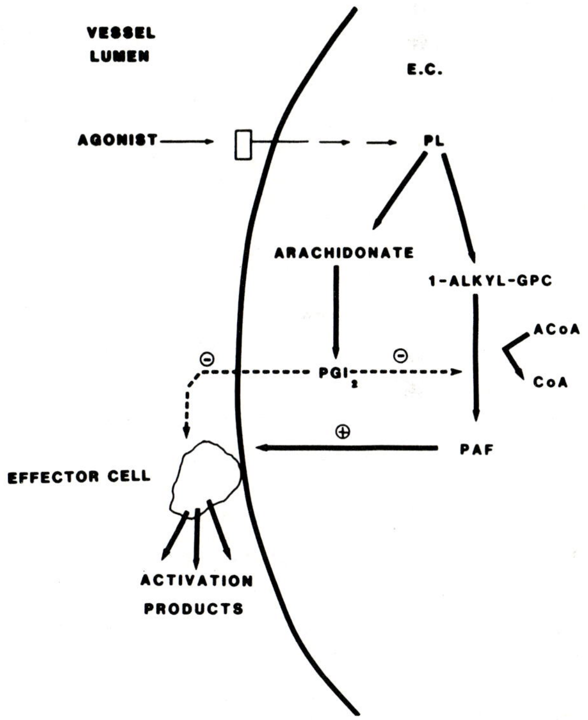

FIGURE 5. A proposed schema for the role of lipid metabolites of endothelial cells in regulating interactions with circulating blood cells. In response to appropriate agonist stimulation (thrombin, others), arachidonic acid (AA) and 1-alkyl-GPC are released from membrane phospholipids (PL) and are metabolized to PGI_2 and PAF, respectively. 1-alkyl-GPC is converted to PAF after addition of acetate at the *sn*-2 position, a reaction catalyzed by an acetyltransferase, with acetyl coenzyme A (ACoA) as the acetyl donor. PAF may then promote the adherence and activation of circulating effector cells, such as platelets or PMNs. PGI_2 is synthesized from AA via subsequent steps catalzyed by cyclooxygenase and prostacyclin synthetase; it is a potent inhibitor of platelet activation stimulated by PAF[21] and other agonists and may modulate some PMN responses as well. In addition, PGI_2 may modulate the synthesis of PAF from 1-alkyl-GPC by inhibiting its release from phospholipid precursors (as with arachidonate; ref. 42) or by other mechanisms.

mote the initiation or amplification of vascular injury. Although there is currently no direct evidence for the participation of PAF in human vascular disease, the observations that it causes pulmonary hypertension and edema,[15] coronary vasoconstriction,[53] and increased dermal capillary permeability[54] in animal preparations support this possibility.

We thank George Broze, John Pike, and Harold Siegelman for the generous gift of biologic materials, Donelle Benson, Alexandra McGee, and Anthony Seeger for technical assistance, the staff of the LDS Hospital Labor and Delivery Service for their valuable help in the collection of umbilical vein samples, and the electronics core facility of the Nora Eccles Harrison CVRTI for construction of the variable-power heating plate. We also appreciate the skillful assistance of Carol Evans and Jerri Duncan-Goff in the preparation of the figures and manuscript.

References

1. Benveniste J, Henson PM, Cochrane CG: Leukocyte-dependent histamine release from rabbit platelets: the role of IgE, basophils, and a platelet-activating factor. J Exp Med **136:** 1356, 1972
2. Benveniste J, Vargaftig BB: Platelet-activating factor: an ether lipid with biological activity. *In* Mangold HK, Paltauf F, editors: Ether lipids: biochemical and biomedical aspects. New York, 1983, Academic Press, Inc., p 355
3. Pinckard RN, McManus LM, Hanahan DJ: Chemistry and biology of acetyl glyceryl ether phosphorylcholine (platelet-activating factor). *In* Weissman G, editor: Advances in inflammation research, vol 4. New York, 1982, Raven Press, p 147
4. Benveniste J, Le Couedic JP, Polonsky J, Tence M: Structural analysis of purified platelet-activating factor by lipases. Nature **269:** 170, 1977
5. Demopoulos CA, Pinckard RN, Hanahan DJ: Platelet activating factor: evidence for 1-0-alkyl-2-acetyl-*sn*-glyceryl-3-phosphorylcholine as the active component (a new class of lipid chemical mediators). J Biol Chem **254:** 9355, 1979
6. Hanahan DJ, Demopoulos CA, Liehr J, Pinckard RN: Identification of platelet activating factor isolated from rabbit basophils as acetyl glyceryl ether phosphorylcholine. J Biol Chem **255:** 5514, 1980
7. Clark PO, Hanahan DJ, Pinckard RN: Physical and chemical properties of platelet-activating factor obtained from human neutrophils and monocytes and rabbit neutrophils and basophils. Biochim Biophys Acta **628:** 69, 1980
8. Sanchez-Crespo M, Alonso F, Egido J: Platelet-activating factor in anaphylaxis and phagocytosis. I. Release from human peripheral polymorphonuclears and monocytes during the stimulation by ionophore A23187 and phagocytosis but not from degranulating basophils. Immunology **40:** 645, 1980
9. Camussi G, Aglietta M, Coda R, Bussolino F, Piacibello W, Tetta C: Release of platelet-activating factor (PAF) and histamines. II. The cellular origin of human PAF: monocytes, polymorphonuclear neutrophils and basophils. Immunology **42:** 191, 1981
10. Arnoux B, Duval D, Benveniste J: Release of platelet-activating factor (PAF-acether) from alveolar macrophages by the calcium ionophore A23187 and phagocytosis. Eur J Clin Invest **10:** 437, 1980
11. Lotner GZ, Lynch JM, Betz SJ, Henson PM: Human neutrophil-derived platelet activating factor. J Immunol **124:** 676, 1980
12. Betz SJ, Henson PM: Production and release of platelet-activating factor (PAF): dissociation from degranulation and superoxide production of the human neutrophil. J Immunol **125:** 2756, 1980
13. Chignard M, Le Couedic JP, Tence M, Vargaftig BB, Benveniste J: The role of platelet-activating factor in platelet aggregation. Nature **279:** 799, 1979
14. O'Flaherty JT, Wykle RL, Miller CH, Lewis JC, Waite M, Bass DA, McCall CE, DeChatelet LR: 1-0-alkyl-*sn*-glyceryl-3-phosphorylcholines: a novel class of neutrophil stimulants. Am J Pathol **103:** 70, 1981
15. Heffner JE, Shoemaker SA, Canham EM, Patel M, McMurtry IF, Morris HG, Repine JE: Acetyl glyceryl ether phosphorylcholine-stimulated human platelets cause pulmonary hypertension and edema in isolated rabbit lungs: role of thromboxane A_2. J Clin Invest **71:** 351, 1983
16. Goetzl EJ, Derian CK, Tauber AI, Valone FH: Novel effects of 1-0-hexadecyl-2-acyl-*sn*-glycero-3-phosphorylcholine mediators on human leukocyte function: delineation of the specific roles of the acyl substituents. Biochem Biophys Res Commun **94:** 881, 1980
17. O'Flaherty JT, Wykle RL, Lees CJ, Shewmake T, McCall CE, Thomas MJ: Neutrophil-degranulating action of 5,12-dihydroxy-6,8,10,14-eicosatetraenoic acid and 1-0-alkyl-2-0-acetyl-*sn*-glycero-3-phosphocholine: comparison with other degranulating agents. Am J Pathol **105:** 264, 1981
18. O'Flaherty JT, Lees CJ, Miller CH, McCall CE, Lewis JC, Love SH, Wykle RL: Selective desensitization of neutrophils: further studies with 1-0-alkyl-*sn*-glycero-3-phosphocholine analogues. J Immunol **127:** 731, 1981
19. Shaw JO, Pinckard RN, Ferrigni KS, McManus LM, Hanahan DJ: Activation of human neutrophils with 1-0-hexadecyl/octadecyl-2-acetyl-*sn*-glyceryl-3-phosphorylcholine (platelet activating factor). J Immunol **127:** 1250, 1981
20. Lin AH, Morton DR, Gorman RR: Acetyl glyceryl ether phosphorylcholine stimulates leukotriene B_4 synthesis in human polymorphonuclear leukocytes. J Clin Invest **70:** 1058, 1982
21. McManus LM, Hanahan DJ, Pinckard RN: Human platelet stimulation by acetyl glyceryl ether phosphorylcholine. J Clin Invest **67:** 903, 1981
22. Prescott SM, Zimmerman GA, McIntyre TM: Human endothelial cells in culture produce platelet-activating factor (1-alkyl-2-acetyl-*sn*-glycero-3-phosphocholine) when stimulated with thrombin. Proc Natl Acad Sci USA **81:** 3534, 1984

22a. McIntyre TM, Zimmerman GA, Satoh K, Prescott SM: Cultured endothelial cells synthesize both platelet-activating factor and prostacyclin in response to histamine, bradykinin, and ATP. J Clin Invest vol 76, July 1985

23. Camussi G, Aglietta M, Malavasi F, Tetta C, Piacibello W, Sanavio F, Bussolino F: The release of platelet-activating factor from human endothelial cells in culture. J Immunol **131:** 2397, 1983
24. Slatkin DN, Stoner RD, Adams WH, Kycia JH, Siegelman HW: Atypical pulmonary thrombosis caused by a toxic cyanobacterial peptide. Science **220:** 1383, 1983
25. Zimmerman GA, Wiseman GA, Hill HR: Human endothelial cells modulate granulocyte adherence and chemotaxis. J Immunol **134:** 1866, 1985
26. Jaffe EA, Nachman RL, Becker CG, Minick CR: Culture of human endothelial cells derived from umbilical veins: identification by morphologic and immunologic criteria. J Clin Invest **52:** 2745, 1973
27. Weksler BB, Ley CW, Jaffe EA: Stimulation of endothelial cell prostacyclin production by thrombin, trypsin, and the ionophore A23187. J Clin Invest **62:** 923, 1978
28. Hong SL: Effect of bradykinin and thrombin on prostacyclin synthesis in endothelial cells from calf and pig aorta and human umbilical cord vein. Thromb Res **18:** 787, 1980
29. Baenziger NL, Fogerty FJ, Mertz LF, Chernuta LF: Regulation of histamine-mediated prostacyclin synthesis in cultured human vascular endothelial cells. Cell **24:** 915, 1981
30. Weksler BB, Gillick M, Pink J: Effect of propranolol on platelet function. Blood **49:** 185, 1977
31. Laposata M, Dovnarsky DK, Shin HS: Thrombin-induced gap formation in confluent endothelial cell monolayers in vitro. Blood **62:** 549, 1983
32. Zimmerman GA, Hill HR: Inflammatory mediators stimulate granulocyte adherence to cultured human endothelial cells. Thromb Res **35:** 203, 1984
33. Eldor A, Vlodavsky I, Hy-Am E, Atzmon R, Weksler BB, Raz A, Fuks Z: Cultured endothelial cells increase their capacity to synthesize prostacyclin following the formation of a contact inhibited cell monolayer. J Cell Physiol **114:** 179, 1983
34. Yamada O, Moldow CF, Sacks T, Craddock PR, Boogaerts MA, Jacob HS: Deleterious effects of endotoxin on cultured endothelial cells: an in vitro model of vascular injury. Inflammation **5:** 115, 1981
35. Hoover RL, Briggs RT, Karnovsky MJ: The adhesive interaction

between polymorphonuclear leukocytes and endothelial cells in vitro. Cell **14:** 423, 1978
36. Boogaerts MA, Yamada O, Jacob HS, Moldow CF: Enhancement of granulocyte-endothelial cell adherence and granulocyte-induced cytotoxicity by platelet release products. Proc Natl Acad Sci USA **79:** 7019, 1982
37. Johnson AR: Human pulmonary endothelial cells in culture: activities of cells from arteries and cells from veins. J Clin Invest **65:** 841, 1980
38. Camussi G, Pawlowski I, Bussolino F, Caldwell PRB, Brentjens J, Andres G: Release of platelet activating factor in rabbits with antibody-mediated injury of the lung: the role of leukocytes and of pulmonary endothelial cells. J Immunol **131:** 1802, 1983
39. Chen S, Barmatoski S, Barnhart MI: Effect of thrombin on platelet-vessel wall interactions. Scanning Electron Microscopy **3:** 783, 1979
40. Czervionke RL, Hoak JC, Fry GL: Effect of aspirin on thrombin-induced adherence of platelets to cultured cells from the blood vessel wall. J Clin Invest **62:** 847, 1978
41. Buchanan MR, Dejana E, Gent M, Mustard JF, Hirsch J: Enhanced platelet accumulation onto injured carotid arteries in rabbits after aspirin treatment. J Clin Invest **67:** 503, 1981
42. Adler B, Gimbrone MA, Schafer AI, Handin RI. Prostacyclin and β-adrenergic catecholamines inhibit arachidonate release and PGI_2 synthesis by vascular endothelium. Blood **58:** 514, 1981
43. Hopkins NK, Gorman RR: Regulation of endothelial cell cyclic nucleotide metabolism by prostacyclin. J Clin Invest **67:** 540, 1981
44. Swendsen CL, Ellis JM, Chilton FH III, O'Flaherty JT, Wykle RL: 1-0-alkyl-2-acyl-*sn*-glycero-3-phosphocholine: a novel source of arachidonic acid in neutrophils stimulated by the calcium ionophore A23187. Biochem Biophys Res Commun **113:** 72, 1983
45. Majerus PW: Arachidonate metabolism in vascular disorders. J Clin Invest **72:** 1521, 1983
46. Nossel HL, Vogel HJ: Pathobiology of the endothelial cell. New York, 1982, Academic Press, pp 1–486
47. Nachman RL, Weksler B, Ferris B: Characterization of human platelet vascular permeability-enhancing activity. J Clin Invest **51:** 549, 1972
48. Sacks T, Moldow CF, Craddock PR, Bowers TK, Jacob HS: Oxygen radicals mediate endothelial cell damage by complement-stimulated granulocytes. J Clin Invest **61:** 1161, 1978
49. Weiss SJ, Young J, LoBuglio AF, Slivka A, Nimeh NF: Role of hydrogen peroxide in neutrophil-mediated destruction of cultured endothelial cells. J Clin Invest **68:** 714, 1981
50. Harlan JM, Killen PD, Harker LA, Striker GE: Neutrophil-mediated endothelial injury in vitro: mechanisms of cell detachment. J Clin Invest **68:** 1394, 1981
51. Stewart GJ, Ritchie WGM, Lynch PR: Venous endothelial damage produced by massive sticking and emigration of leukocytes. Am J Pathol **74:** 507, 1974
52. MacGregor RR, Friedman HM, Macarak EJ, Kefalides NA: Virus infection of endothelial cells increases granulocyte adherence. J Clin Invest **65:** 1469, 1980
53. Feuerstein G, Boyd LM, Ezra D, Goldstein RE: Effect of platelet-activating factor on coronary circulation of the domestic pig. Am J Physiol **246:** H466, 1984
54. Humphrey DM, McManus LM, Satouchi K, Hanahan DJ, Pinckard RN: Vasoactive properties of acetyl glyceryl ether phosphorylcholine and analogues. Lab Invest **46:** 422, 1982

Platelets, endothelium, and vasospasm

P. M. VANHOUTTE, M.D., AND D. S. HOUSTON, M.D.

THE VASCULAR ENDOTHELIUM synthesizes prostacyclin, a potent antiaggregatory substance with vasodilator properties. It also activates (e.g., angiotensin I) or inactivates (e.g., bradykinin, serotonin) a number of vasoactive substances present in the blood (figure 1). Thus, it is far from being a passive diffusion barrier, but it can actively alter the amounts of vasoactive substances reaching the deeper layers of the blood vessel wall. In addition, endothelial cells can modulate powerfully the responsiveness of the vascular smooth muscle of the tunica media. Indeed, Furchgott and Zawadzki[1] first noted that rings of rabbit aorta, contracted with norepinephrine, would relax upon exposure to acetylcholine if they were handled carefully to preserve the endothelial layer; if the endothelium was simply mechanically rubbed off, no relaxation was seen. Similar findings have been obtained in a host of other blood vessels, including coronary arteries (figure 2), and with a variety of agents (figure 3).[2-6] The prototypic response to acetylcholine probably is only a pharmacologic curiosity since endothelial cells are not innervated by cholinergic neurones, and any acetylcholine that would reach the blood would be degraded at once by circulating cholinesterases. However, the finding that a number of other substances present in the blood under normal or pathologic conditions can cause potent endothelium-dependent responses implies that such responses may play a role in health and disease. This article briefly discusses this possibility in regard to the interaction between platelets and endothelial cells (see references 7 and 8).

Contractile responses to aggregating platelets. Cohen et al.[9, 10] observed that isolated rings of canine coronary artery contract if autologous platelets aggregate in the organ chamber in which the rings are suspended. Such contractions are markedly enhanced if the endothelium is removed (figure 4). If the rings are first contracted with prostaglandin $F_{2\alpha}$, a definite relaxation to aggregating platelets is observed in rings with endothelium, but only further contraction is observed in denuded rings (figure 5). In segments of canine coronary artery perfused with physiologic salt solution, relaxation in response to platelets is observed only if the platelets are added intraluminally and if the segment still contains endothelial cells. If the platelets aggregate intraluminally after removal of the endothelium, or are added to the bath surrounding the outside of the blood vessel, strong contractions ensue (figure 6).[11] Thus, aggregating platelets release sustances that trigger potent endothelium-dependent inhibitory responses of the smooth muscle in the media. Of the other canine blood vessels studied (femoral artery, femoral vein, and saphenous vein,[12] pulmonary artery,[13] saphenous artery[14]), only the coronary artery displays a sustained or consistent relaxation response to platelets aggregating in the organ chamber (figure 7).

Mediators of the endothelium-dependent responses to platelets

Serotonin. Almost all of the serotonin (5-hydroxytryptamine) in the blood is contained in the platelets,[15] which release the monoamine when they aggregate. Concentrations of exogenous serotonin comparable to those released from aggregated platelets cause contractions of isolated canine coronary arteries.[9, 10] Serotonin-induced contractions of the coronary artery of the dog are enhanced in vitro and in vivo by removal of the endothelium.[9, 10, 16] In isolated coronary arteries contracted with prostaglandin $F_{2\alpha}$, serotonin can cause endothelium-dependent relaxation, albeit not as profound as that induced by acetylcholine.[9, 10, 17] The contraction of the canine coronary artery caused by serotonin is antagonized by ketanserin,[18, 19] suggesting that it is mediated by S_2-serotonergic receptors on the smooth muscle. By contrast, the endothelium-dependent relaxation in response to serotonin is not affected by ketanserin, but is abolished by methiothepin, suggesting the involvement of S_1-serotonergic receptors (figure 8).[20]

S_2-Serotonergic antagonists reduce the contractions evoked by aggregating platelets.[9] Thus, it seems likely that serotonin released from the platelets contributes to the contractile response of the coronary artery. However, endothelium-dependent responses to aggregating platelets persist in the presence of concentrations of

From the Department of Physiology and Biophysics, Mayo Clinic and Mayo Foundation, Rochester, MN 55905.

Address for correspondence: P. M. Vanhoutte, M.D., Department of Physiology and Biophysics, Mayo Clinic and Mayo Foundation, Rochester, MN 55905.

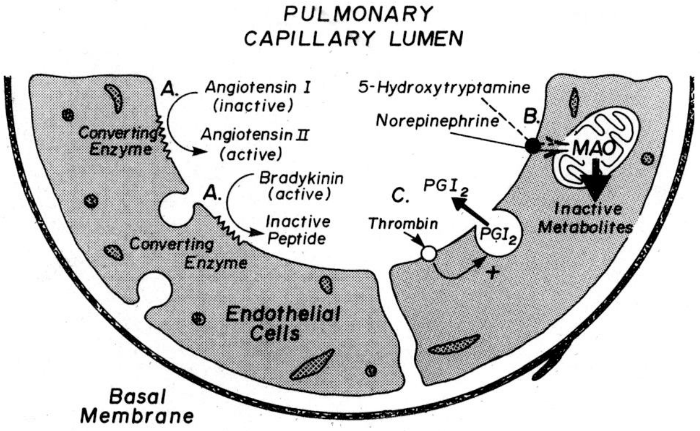

FIGURE 1. The handling of vasoactive substances by endothelial cells. *A*, Substances such as angiotensin I and bradykinin are converted by enzymes on the endothelial surface, with the resulting formation of active and inactive substances, respectively. *B*, Substances such as norepinephrine and serotonin are actively taken up (o) and degraded enzymatically by monoamine oxidase (MAO). *C*, Prostacyclin (PGI_2), a potent vasodilator, is produced by endothelial cells in response to a number of stimuli, including thrombin. (Modified from Shepherd JT, Vanhoutte PM: The human cardiovascular system. Facts and concepts. New York, 1979, Raven Press.)

methiothepin, preventing responses to serotonin (figure 5).[20] Thus, it is unlikely that serotonin is solely responsible for platelet-induced endothelium-dependent relaxation in response to aggregating platelets.

Thromboxane. Thromboxane A_2 is produced by activated and aggregating platelets. It further stimulates platelet activation, and causes contraction of coronary smooth muscle.[21] There are no reports of endothelium-dependent relaxation induced by thromboxane A_2. The

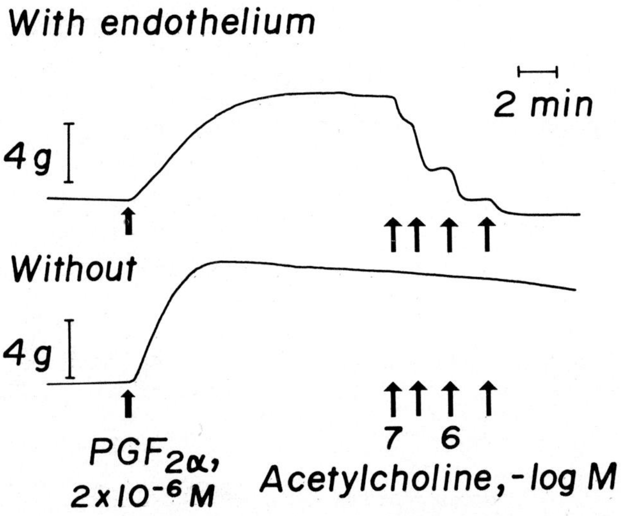

FIGURE 2. Tracing of isometric tension recording of isolated rings of canine coronary artery. Prostaglandin $F_{2\alpha}$ ($PGF_{2\alpha}$) added to the organ bath causes a contraction. In rings that have been denuded of endothelium, cumulative addition of acetylcholine causes no change in tension, whereas in rings with intact endothelium, concentration-dependent relaxation results. (Reprinted, with permission, from Shepherd and Vanhoutte.[44])

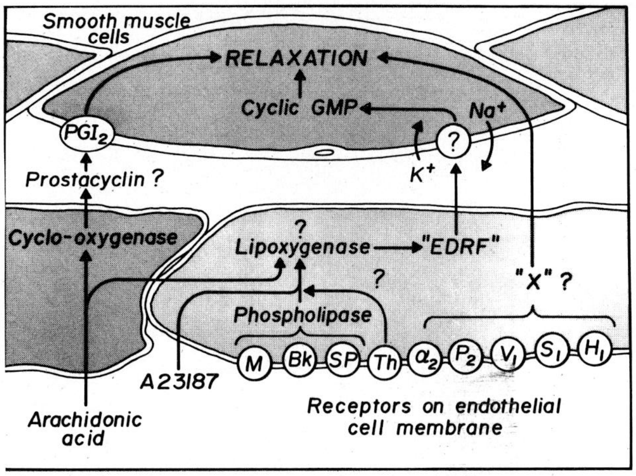

FIGURE 3. Postulated mechanisms of endothelially mediated relaxation of vascular smooth muscle. A host of substances can induce endothelially mediated relaxation (see text). More than one endothelium-derived relaxing factor (EDRF) may be produced, or the formation of the same factor may result from a number of mechanisms. The action of EDRF(s) on the smooth muscle cell appears to involve stimulation of the membrane Na^+/K^+ pump, and to be mediated by increases in cyclic GMP in the smooth muscle cell. M = muscarinic receptor; BK = bradykinin receptor; SP = substance P receptor; Th = thrombin receptor; α_2 = α_2-adrenoceptor; P_2 = P_2 purinergic receptor; V_1 = V_1-vasopressinergic receptor; PGI_2 = prostacyclin receptor; S_1 = S_1-serotonergic receptor; H_1 = H_1-histaminergic receptor; X = unknown intermediate; A23187 = calcium ionophore.

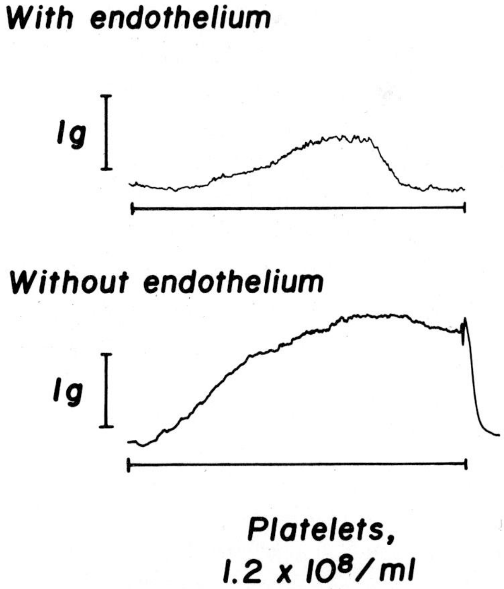

FIGURE 4. Traces of isometric tension recording of isolated rings of canine coronary with and without endothelium. Platelets added to the organ chamber promptly aggregate and evoke contraction (the time of exposure to platelets shown is approximately 20 min). The contractions produced in rings with intact endothelium are smaller and more transient than those in rings form which the endothelium has been removed, indicating that platelets not only directly stimulate smooth muscle contraction, but also initiate an endothelially mediated inhibition. (Data from Cohen RA, Shepherd JT, Vanhoutte PM: Inhibitory role of the endothelium in the response of isolated coronary arteries to platelets. Science **221:** 273, 1983.)

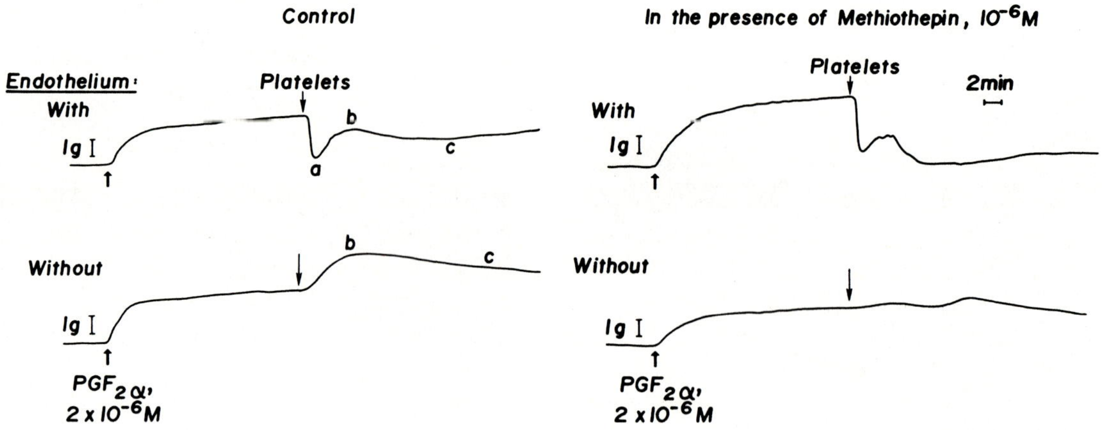

FIGURE 5. *Left,* If rings of canine coronary artery with and without endothelium are first contracted with prostaglandin $F_{2\alpha}$ ($PGF_{2\alpha}$), addition of platelets (6.1 $\times$ 10^7/ml) causes relaxation in rings with endothelium, but only further contraction in rings without endothelium. This highlights the potent, endothelium-mediated relaxing effect of platelets. A similar relaxation can be seen if the rings are contracted with norepinephrine instead of $PGF_{2\alpha}$. *Right,* Methiothepin, in a concentration that abolishes endothelially mediated relaxation in response to serotonin, does not affect the endothelium-dependent relaxation in response to aggregating platelets. (Reprinted, with permission, from Houston et al.[20])

thromboxane synthetase inhibitor dazoxiben reduces the ischemic response to atrial pacing in subjects with coronary artery disease,[22] suggesting that thromboxane A_2 may contribute to constriction of coronary vessels even in the absence of overt spasm. Thromboxane B_2 can be measured in the fluid from organ chambers where the interaction between aggregating platelets and isolated blood vessels are studied.[10, 13] However, inhibitors of cyclooxygenase do not alter the response of coronary arteries to aggregating platelets.[9, 20] Thus, it seems unlikely that thromboxane A_2 contributes to the endothelium-dependent response to the latter.

Adenine nucleotides. ADP and ATP are contained in large quantities in the dense granules of platelets and are released during aggregation. Both compounds cause similar endothelium-dependent relaxation in a

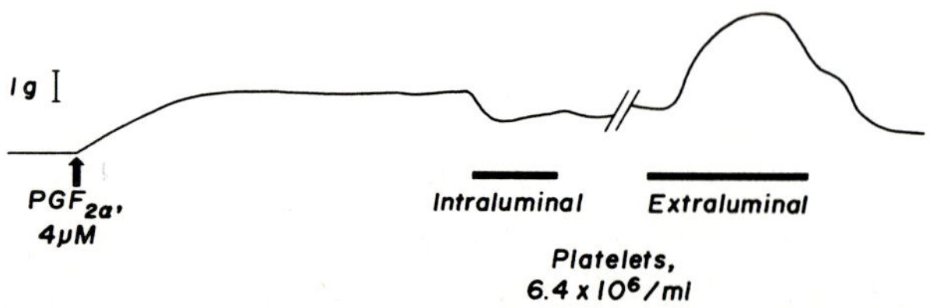

FIGURE 6. Further evidence of the obligatory role of endothelial cells in the relaxation of a canine coronary artery induced by platelets. A segment of canine coronary artery was perfused with physiologic saline solution; hooks in the vessel wall allowed the recording of wall tension (equivalent to tension measurement in the ring preparation). The vessel was constricted with prostaglandin $F_{2\alpha}$ ($PGF_{2\alpha}$). If only the luminal surface is exposed to aggregating platelets by their addition to the perfusate, a relaxation occurs; if, however, the platelets are added to the organ bath surrounding the outside of the vessel, only further contraction occurs. (Reprinted, with permission, from Cohen et al.[11])

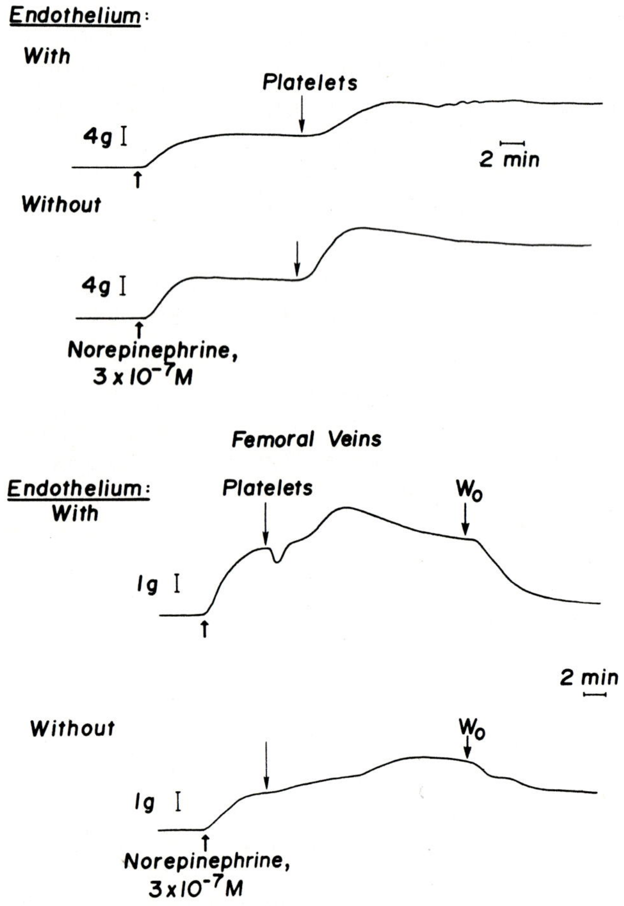

FIGURE 7. Responses of canine femoral arteries and femoral veins with and without endothelium to aggregating platelets. Vessels were contracted with norepinephrine before addition of platelets. Although small transient or occasional periods of relaxation in response to platelets may be observed in these vessels, the sustained major relaxation seen in the coronary artery does not occur. (Data from Houston et al.[12])

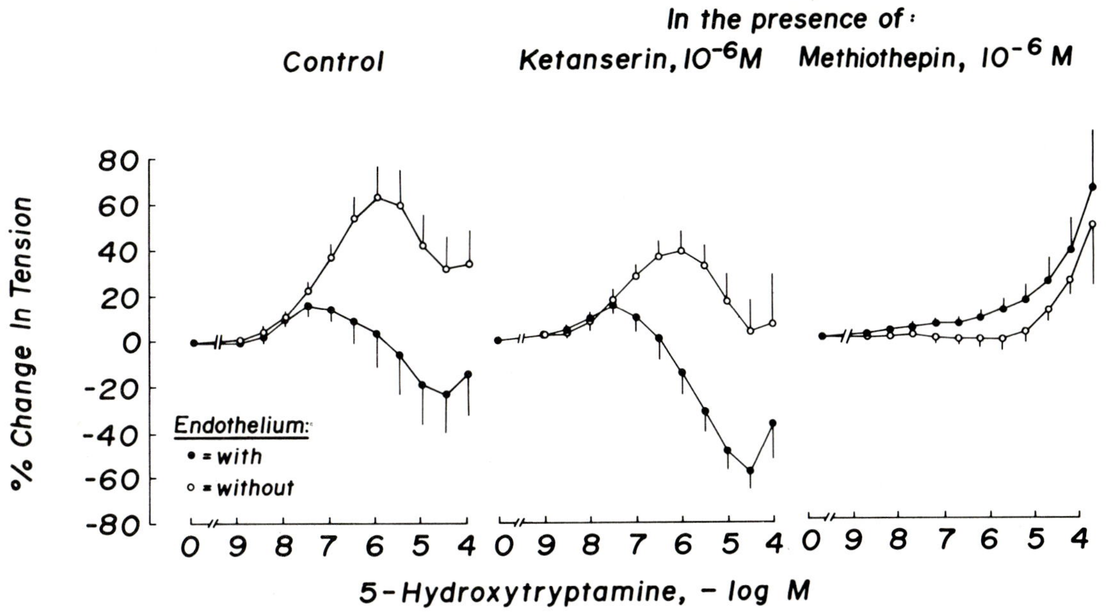

FIGURE 8. Concentration/effect relationships of canine coronary artery, with and without endothelium, contracted with prostaglandin $F_{2\alpha}$ (2×10^{-6}M) to cumulative addition of serotonin. In rings with endothelium, lower concentrations of serotonin (up to 10^{-7}) produce a slight contraction; higher concentrations cause relaxation. In rings without endothelium a much stronger contraction is observed. The difference between the curves reflects the inhibitory effect of the endothelium stimulated by serotonin. Ketanserin, a selective S_2-serotonergic antagonist, reduces the contractile effect of serotonin and shifts both curves downward. Methiothepin, an S_1-serotonergic antagonist, abolishes the endothelium-dependent inhibitory effect. (Reprinted, with permission, from Houston et al.[20])

number of isolated arteries, including the canine coronary artery.[20, 23, 24] The endothelium-dependent relaxation in response to platelets is almost abolished by apyrase (an enzyme that hydrolyzes ATP and ADP to AMP and inhibits the endothelium-dependent relaxations induced by adenine nucleotides) (figure 9).[20] If endothelial receptors are saturated with ADP, the platelets cause contraction only, even though acetylcholine is still capable of causing relaxation (figure 9). Thus, the endothelium-dependent relaxation of isolated coronary arteries in response to aggregating platelets is due mainly to the release of ADP and ATP.

Platelet-activating factor. Platelet-activating factor is a phospholipid released by leukocytes, mast cells, and platelets.[25] Is is a potent aggregating agent at concentrations as low as 10^{-12}M in some species. In a number of animals, including the rat in which it does not activate platelets, platelet-activating factor causes profound hypotension.[26-28] Both the platelet-stimulating and hypotensive effects of platelet-activating factor are antagonized by compound CV-3988.[29] The precursor, 2-lyso-platelet–activating factor, is inactive.[30] In the isolated aorta of the rat, platelet-activating factor causes relaxation that is abolished by removal of the endothelium.[26, 31]

In canine coronary and femoral arteries, relaxation induced by platelet-activating factor is observed only

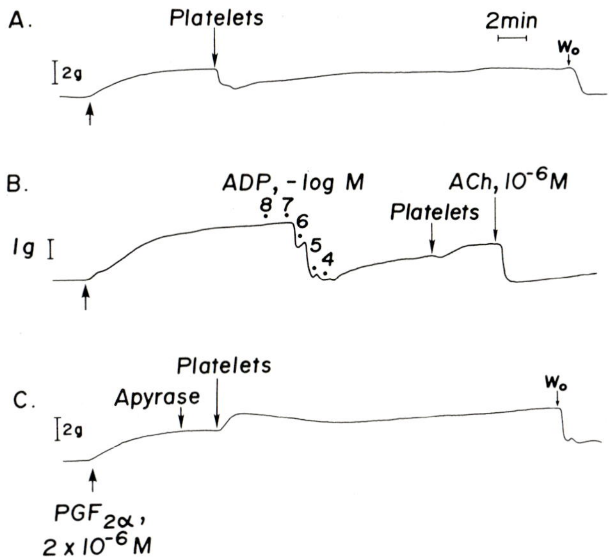

FIGURE 9. Evidence that adenine nucleotides play a major role in the endothelial-dependent relaxation of canine coronary arteries induced by aggregating platelets. Rings with intact endothelium that contracted with prostaglandin $F_{2\alpha}$ ($PGF_{2\alpha}$) show a typical relaxation response to platelets (*A*); this relaxation is abolished and contraction is seen if apyrase (an enzyme that degrades ATP and ADP) is present in the bath (0.67 units/ml) (*C*). Canine coronary rings with intact endothelium and contracted with prostaglandin $F_{2\alpha}$ ($PGF_{2\alpha}$) relax on exposure to cumulative concentrations of ADP; with the purinergic receptors saturated, aggregating platelets can no longer induce relaxation, although the endothelium-dependent response to acetylcholine (ACh) persists (*B*). W_o = washout. (Modified from ref. 20.)

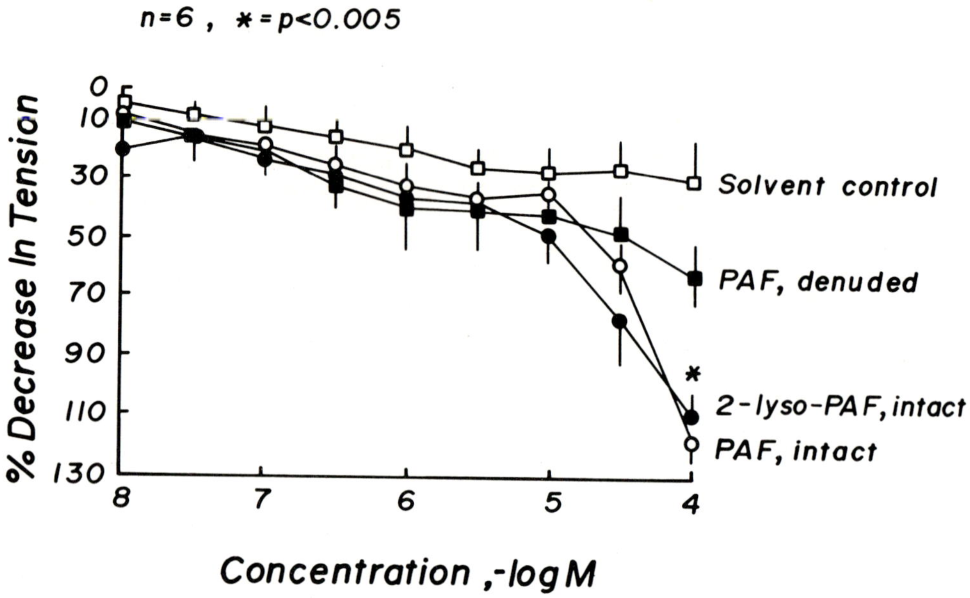

FIGURE 10. Concentration-effect curves in canine coronary artery, with and without endothelium, contracted with prostaglandin $F_{2\alpha}$ ($PGF_{2\alpha}$; 2×10^{-6}M) in response to cumulative additions of platelet-activating factor (PAF) and its 2-lyso derivative (2-lyso-PAF) and the ethanol solvent used. Changes in tension are expressed as percent of contraction obtained with $PGF_{2\alpha}$. Relaxation induced by PAF and 2-lyso-PAF occurs in rings with intact endothelium above 10^{-5}M; this effect is endothelium dependent (*$p < .005$ comparing responses of intact and denuded vessels to 10^{-4}M PAF) (*top*). The lack of a difference between responses to PAF and 2-lyso-PAF suggests that this relaxation is not a specific, receptor-mediated effect of PAF. Further evidence in support of this interpretation is the lack of effect of the PAF antagonist CV-3988 on the endothelium-dependent response to high concentrations of PAF (*bottom*). The lack of effect of indomethacin on this response (*bottom*) shows that production of prostacyclin by the endothelium is not responsible for the relaxation induced by PAF.

at high concentrations (figure 10). This relaxation is endothelium dependent, but it persists in the presence of CV-3988; 2-lyso-platelet–activating factor causes relaxation similar to that caused by platelet-activating factor. It seems unlikely, therefore, that endothelium-dependent relaxation is due to the interaction of platelet-activating factor with a receptor similar to those mediating platelet activation and hypotension. At the high concentrations required to observe it, a direct membrane effect of these lipids analogous to that observed with arachidonic and oleic acid[32] is a more likely explanation. The synthesis of prostacyclin is not involved, since incubation of the blood vessels with the inhibitor of cyclooxygenase indomethacin does not block the response (figure 10). Unless very high local concentrations of platelet-activating factor (and 2-lyso-platelet–activating factor, which is also contained in platelets)[33] are achieved at the sites of platelet aggregation, it is unlikely that these substances contribute directly to platelet-induced relaxation.

Vasopressin. Human platelets contain vasopressin,[34] which evokes endothelium-dependent relaxation of canine coronary and cerebral arteries.[35] This relaxation is blocked by the V_1-vasopressinergic antagonist $d(CH_2)_5Tyr(Me)AVP$. However, the antagonist does not affect endothelium-dependent relaxation in response to platelets.*

Potential role in health and disease. It is a giant leap from studies in organ chambers with artificial solution and containing healthy canine tissue to a diseased coronary artery on a pumping human heart, so that inferences about human pathology must necessarily be tentative. Nonetheless, one cannot but speculate that these observations in isolated canine blood vessels may be key to the understanding of coronary arterial spasm. It is appealing to propose that the body has evolved a particularly effective defense against thrombosis in a critical vascular bed with little collateral blood supply, namely the myocardium. Thus, one can imagine that if, for any reason, platelets began to aggregate in a normal coronary artery with an intact endothelium, the response of the smooth muscle of the blood vessel to the substances released from the platelets would be relaxation. This would be reinforced if the platelet aggregation were to set the coagulation cascade in motion, which would cause the formation of thrombin. Indeed, in peripheral, cerebral, and coronary arteries, thrombin causes endothelium-dependent

*Houston DS, Vanhoutte PM: Unpublished observation.

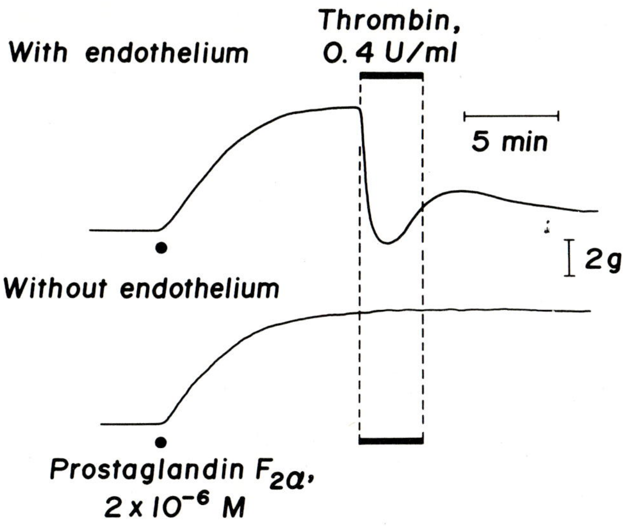

FIGURE 11. Isometric tension recording of porcine coronary artery, with and without endothelium, contracted with prostaglandin $PGF_{2\alpha}$. Thrombin produces relaxation that is entirely dependent on the presence of endothelium. A similar endothelium-dependent relaxation is seen in the canine coronary artery. (Reprinted, with permission, from Shepherd and Vanhoutte.[44])

relaxation, which overcomes the direct constrictor effect that it has on smooth muscle (figure 11).[23, 24, 35–37] The endothelium-dependent relaxation to thrombin is abolished but the direct contractile effect is augmented by hypoxia.[36, 37] An endothelium-dependent dilatation triggered by the platelet products (and thrombin) would tend to flush away the beginning aggregate before it could occlude the vessel (figure 12). If, on the other hand, the endothelium were absent, damaged, or for some reason failed to function properly, the response of the vessel to platelet products and thrombin would be contraction, as observed in the rings denuded of endothelium in vitro (figure 12). Such contraction would further reduce the luminal area and increase the obstruction to blood flow.[38] Clinical coronary arterial spasm may be just such a contraction.

A potential pivotal role of the endothelium becomes apparent when one recalls that disruption of the endothelium by an atheromatous plaque is a ubiquitous feature of coronary disease, and that such plaques and partial obstructions can initiate platelet activation. It has been demonstrated that patients with classic and Prinzmetal's angina have increased coronary sinus levels of thromboxane B_2 (the metabolite of the potent vasoconstrictor prostanoid produced by activated platelets, thromboxane A_2) during atrial pacing, whereas normal subjects do not,[39, 40] indicating that platelet activation does occur in the diseased coronary circulation. Besides triggering relaxation of the smooth muscle of the tunica media, an intact endothelium could combat platelet-induced spasm in a number of other ways, including (1) by acting as a diffusion barrier preventing vasoconstrictor substances from reaching the smooth muscle cells, (2) by metabolizing vasoactive platelet products such as serotonin and catecholamines with

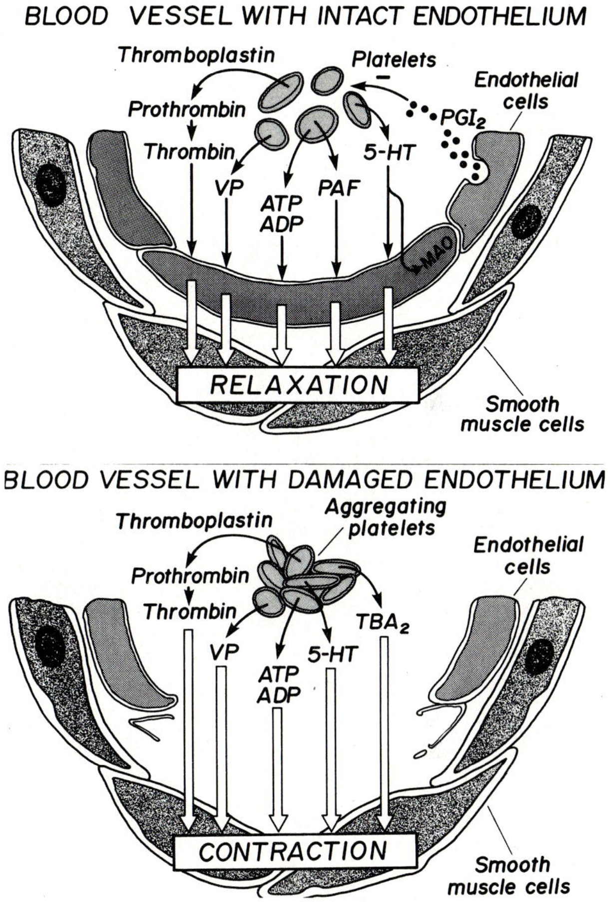

FIGURE 12. Schematic representation of the role of endothelial cells in the prevention of vasospasm. Aggregating platelets release adenine nucleotides (ATP and ADP), serotonin (5-HT), thromboxane A_2 (TBA_2), platelet-activating factor (PAF), and vasopressin (VP), and initiate the coagulation cascade with production of thrombin. *Top*, The presence of an intact endothelium prevents platelet aggregation through production of the platelet inhibitor, prostacyclin (PGI_2); PGI_2 is also a vasodilator. Serotonin is taken up by endothelial cells and degraded by monoamine oxidase (MAO). PAF (in high concentrations), 5-HT, VP, adenine nucleotides, and thrombin can all stimulate the endothelial production of a relaxing factor or factors that have an inhibitory effect on smooth muscle. Relaxation and vasodilatation would tend to flush away any developing aggregate or thrombus. Finally, an intact endothelium and basement membrane probably serve as a diffusion barrier to prevent the above-mentioned substances from reaching the smooth muscle layers of the media. *Bottom*, Platelet aggregation is enhanced by contact with collagen in the exposed vessel wall. Depending on the blood vessel, the thrombin, VP, 5-HT, adenine nucleotides, and thromboxane produced all directly activate vascular smooth muscle. These effects would be unopposed if the endothelium were damaged or dysfunctional. Vasospasm may thus result in areas of endothelial abnormality.

monoamine oxidase (figure 1), and (3) by producing the vasodilator and platelet inhibitor prostacyclin in response to (and even out of) substances released from platelets.[41, 42]

We would like to thank Mrs. Janet Beckman for typing the manuscript and Mr. Robert Lorenz for preparation of the illustrations.

References

1. Furchgott RF, Zawadzki JV: The obligatory role of endothelial cells in the relaxation of arterial smooth muscle by acetylcholine. Nature **286:** 373, 1980
2. Furchgott RF, Zawadzki JV, Cherry PD: Role of endothelium in the vasodilator response to acetylcholine. *In* Vanhoutte PM, Leusen I, editors: Vasodilatation. New York, 1981, Raven Press, pp 49–66
3. De Mey JG, Vanhoutte PM: Heterogeneous behavior of the canine arterial and venous wall: importance of the endothelium. Circ Res **51:** 439, 1982
4. Furchgott RF: Role of the endothelium in responses of vascular smooth muscle. Circ Res **53:** 557, 1983
5. Furchgott RF: The role of endothelium in the responses of vascular smooth muscle to drugs. Ann Rev Pharmacol Toxicol **24:** 175, 1984
6. Vanhoutte PM, Rimele TJ: Role of the endothelium in the control of vascular smooth muscle function. J Physiol (Paris) **78:** 681, 1983
7. Vanhoutte PM, Cohen RA: The elusory role of serotonin in vascular function and disease. Biochem Pharmacol **32:** 3671, 1983
8. Cohen RA, Shepherd JT, Vanhoutte PM: Vasodilatation mediated by the coronary endothelium in response to aggregating platelets. *In* Vanhoutte PM, Vatner SF, editors: Vasodilator mechanisms. Basel, 1985, Karger, pp 35–42
9. Cohen RA, Shepherd JT, Vanhoutte PM: Inhibitory role of the endothelium in the response of isolated coronary arteries to platelets. Science **221:** 273, 1983
10. Cohen RA, Shepherd JT, Vanhoutte PM: 5-Hydroxytryptamine can mediate endothelium-dependent relaxation of coronary arteries. Am J Physiol **245:** H-1077, 1983
11. Cohen RA, Shepherd JT, Vanhoutte PM: Endothelium and asymmetrical responses of the coronary arterial wall. Am J Physiol **247:** H403, 1984
12. Houston DS, Shepherd JT, Vanhoutte PM: Platelets cause endothelium-dependent relaxations in some but not all isolated canine vessels. Fed Proc **43:** 1084, 1984
13. McGoon MD, Vanhoutte PM: Aggregating platelets contract isolated canine pulmonary arteries by releasing 5-hydroxytryptamine. J Clin Invest **74:** 828, 1984
14. Lindblad LE, Shepherd JT, Vanhoutte PM: Cooling augments platelet-induced contraction of peripheral arteries of the dog. Proc Soc Exp Biol Med **176:** 119, 1984
15. Crawford NV: Systemic venous platelet-bound and plasma free serotonin levels in non-carcinoid malignancy. Clin Chim Acta **12:** 274, 1965
16. Bove AA, Dewey JD: Effects of serotonin and histamine on proximal and distal coronary vasculature in dogs: comparison with alpha-adrenergic stimulation. Am J Cardiol **52:** 1333, 1983
17. Cocks TM, Angus JA: Endothelium-dependent relaxation of coronary arteries by noradrenaline and serotonin. Nature **305:** 627, 1983
18. Van Nueten JM, Janssen PAJ, Van Beek J, Xhonneux R, Verbeuren TJ, Vanhoutte PM: Vascular effects of ketanserin (R41468), a novel antagonist of 5-HT_2 serotonergic receptors. J Pharmacol Exp Ther **218:** 217, 1981
19. Brazenor RM, Angus JA: Actions of serotonin antagonists on dog coronary artery. Eur J Pharmacol **81:** 569, 1982
20. Houston DS, Shepherd JT, Vanhoutte PM: Adenine nucleotides, serotonin and endothelium-dependent relaxations to platelets. Am J Physiol **248:** H389, 1985
21. Ellis EF, Oelz O, Roberts LJIII, Payne NA, Sweetman BJ, Nies AL, Oates JA: Coronary arterial smooth muscle contraction by a substance released from platelets: evidence that it is thromboxane A_2. Science **193:** 1135, 1976
22. Thaulow E, Dale J, Myhre E: Effects of a selective thromboxane synthetase inhibitor, Dazoxiben, and of acetylsalicylic acid on myocardial ischemia in patients with coronary artery disease. Am J Cardiol **53:** 1255, 1984
23. De Mey JG, Vanhoutte PM: Role of the intima in cholinergic and purinergic relaxation of isolated canine femoral arteries. J Physiol (London) **316:** 347, 1981
24. De Mey JG, Claeys M, Vanhoutte PM: Endothelium-dependent inhibitory effects of acetylcholine, adenosine triphosphate, thrombin and arachidonic acid in the canine femoral artery. J Pharmacol Exp Ther **222:** 166, 1982
25. Vargaftig BB, Benveniste J: Platelet-activating factor today. Trans Pharmacol Sci **4:** 341, 1983
26. Kamitani T, Katamoto M, Tasumi M, Katsuta K, Ono T, Kikuchi H, Kumada S: Mechanism(s) of the hypotensive effect of synthetic 1-0-octadecyl-2-0-acetyl-glycero-3-phosphocholine. Eur J Pharmacol **98:** 357, 1984
27. Caillard CG, Mondot S, Zundel JL, Julou L: Hypotensive activity of PAF-acether in rats. Agents Actions **12:** 725, 1972
28. Lai FM, Shepherd CA, Cervoni P, Wissner A: Hypotensive and vasodilatory activity of (+ −) 1-0-octadecyl-2-acetyl glyceryl-3-phosphorylcholine in the normotensive rat. Life Sci **32:** 1159, 1983
29. Terashita Z, Tsushima S, Yoshioka Y, Nomura H, Inada Y, Nishikawa K: CV-3988: a specific antagonist of platelet activating factor (PAF). Life Sci **32:** 1975, 1983
30. Blank ML, Cress DA, Lee T-C, Malone B, Surles JR, Piantadosi C, Hajdu J, Snyder F: Structural features of platelet activating factor (1-alkyl-2-acetyl-*sn*-glycero-3-phosphocholine) required for hypotensive and platelet serotonin responses. Res Commun Chem Pathol Pharmacol **38:** 3, 1982
31. Cervoni P, Herzlinger HE, Lai FM, Tanikella TE: Aortic vascular and atrial responses to (+ −)-1-0-octadecyl-2-acetyl-glyceryl-3-phosphorylcholine. Br J Pharmacol **79:** 667, 1983
32. Cherry PD, Furchgott RF, Zawadzki JV: The endothelium-dependent relaxation of vascular smooth muscle by fatty acids. Fed Proc **42:** 619, 1983
33. Benveniste J: Platelet-activating factor (PAF-acether): present status. Agents Actions **11:** 542, 1981
34. Preibisz JJ, Sealey JE, Laragh JH, Cody RJ, Weksler BB: Plasma and platelet vasopressin in essential hypertension and congestive heart failure. Hypertension **5**(suppl I): I-129, 1983
35. Katusic ZS, Shepherd JT, Vanhoutte PM: Vasopressin causes endothelium-dependent relaxations of the canine basilar artery. Circ Res **55:** 575, 1984
36. De Mey JG, Vanhoutte PM: Anoxia and endothelium dependent reactivity of the canine femoral artery. J Physiol **335:** 65, 1983
37. Ku DD: Coronary vascular reactivity after acute myocardial ischemia. Science **218:** 576, 1982
38. Gertz SD, Uretsky G, Wainberg RS, Navot N, Gotsman M: Endothelial cell damage and thrombus formation after partial arterial constriction: relevance to the role of coronary artery spasm in the pathogenesis of myocardial infarction. Circulation **63:** 476, 1981
39. Cortellaro M, Boschetti C, Antoniazzi V, Moreo G, Repetto S, Verna E, Boscarini M, Limido A, Binaghi G, Polli EE: Transcoronary platelet thromboxane A_2 formation without platelet trapping in patients with coronary stenosis — effect of sulphinpyrazone treatment. Thromb Haemostas **50:** 857, 1983
40. Tada M, Kuzuya T, Inoue M, Kodama K, Mishima M, Yamada M, Inui M, Abe H: Elevation of thromboxane B2 levels in patients with classic and variant angina pectoris. Circulation **64:** 1107, 1981
41. Marcus AJ, Weksler BB, Jaffe EA, Broekman MJ: Synthesis of prostacyclin from platelet-derived endoperoxides by cultured human endothelial cells. J Clin Invest **66:** 979, 1980
42. Shafer AI, Crawford DD, Gimbrone MA: Unidirectional transfer of prostaglandin endoperoxides between platelets and endothelial cells. J Clin Invest **73:** 1105, 1984
43. Shepherd JT, Vanhoutte PM: The human cardiovascular system. Facts and concepts. New York, 1979, Raven Press, pp 1–351
44. Shepherd JT, Vanhoutte PM: Spasm of the coronary arteries: causes and consequences (the scientist's viewpoint). Mayo Clin Proc **60:** 33, 1985

Locally acting growth factors for vascular smooth muscle cells: endogenous synthesis and release from platelets

DANIEL F. BOWEN-POPE, PH.D., RUSSELL ROSS, PH.D., AND RONALD A. SEIFERT, PH.D.

ABSTRACT Release of platelet-derived growth factor (PDGF) from platelets has been postulated to stimulate at least some of the cell proliferation seen at sites of tissue damage, both beneficially (wound healing) and perniciously (during formation of atherosclerotic lesions). Two other growth factors have been localized to the platelet: epidermal growth factor and transforming growth factor. These factors may function synergistically with PDGF in promoting smooth muscle cell proliferation in the injured vessel wall. PDGF-like molecules (PDGF-c) that bind to the PDGF receptor and are at least partially recognized by antiserum against PDGF may also be synthesized by vessel wall cells themselves under certain circumstances. Arterial endothelial cells secrete several mitogens, one of which is a PDGF-c. Release is greatly stimulated by exposure of the cells to physiologic concentrations of thrombin. Also, aortic smooth muscle cells from 2-week-old rats secrete mitogenic levels of PDGF-c. In this case, PDGF-c accounts for all the mitogenic activity in conditioned medium (when assayed on 3T3 cells). Smooth muscle cells obtained from adult rat aortae secrete 150-fold less PDGF-c. In a third example, when adult rat carotid arteries are damaged with a balloon catheter, smooth muscle cells migrate into the intima of the artery and proliferate. By 2 weeks, the number of smooth muscle cells in the artery has doubled. When these intimal smooth muscle cells are cultured, they are found to secrete PDGF-c. These findings suggest that activation of endogenous synthesis of PDGF-c may contribute to the smooth muscle cell proliferation seen in response to vascular injury.
Circulation 72, No. 4, 735–740, 1985.

IT IS NOW recognized that smooth muscle cell proliferation plays an important role in the formation of the proliferative lesions of atherosclerosis.[1–5] The involvement of platelet-derived growth factor (PDGF) in this process was suggested by an observation made by Russell Ross and his collaborators in the early 1970s that cultured arterial smooth muscle cells grew poorly in plasma-derived serum and that addition of platelet extract greatly increased the growth rate.[6] Ross and his collaborators proposed that platelets contained a growth factor, now called platelet-derived growth factor or PDGF, which might contribute to the proliferation of vascular smooth muscle cells that occurs beneficially at sites of wound healing and perniciously during the process of formation of atherosclerotic lesions.[7]

PDGF-like molecules (PDGF-c) from platelets. In normal blood, all PDGF seems to be sequestered within the platelets — none can be detected in the plasma.[8, 9] At sites of platelet adhesion and/or activation, platelets release the contents of their alpha granules.[10] The PDGF that is released is predicted to bind to, and activate, nearby smooth muscle cells.[7] This model provides a mechanism for the topical administration of growth factors to sites at which they are necessary for promoting tissue regeneration. Discoveries in the last few years, however, suggest both narrower and wider views of the role of PDGF in vascular biology: wider in that they suggest PDGF may be provided at sites of vascular trauma by mechanisms in addition to platelet-degranulation, and narrower in that they suggest PDGF is not the only important polypeptide growth factor present in platelets.

It was difficult to study PDGF critically when it could be identified only as a growth-promoting substance from platelets. However, PDGF has now been purified in several laboratories,[11–14] it has been partially sequenced,[15–17] and antisera have been raised against it.[9, 18–20] It is known to be a protein of approximately 30,000 daltons with a basic isoelectric point and considerable hydrophobicity.[21, 22] With availability of pure PDGF, the molecule could be radioiodinated and the

From the Department of Pathology, SM-30, University of Washington School of Medicine, Seattle.

Supported in part by grants from NIH (HL-18645) and R. J. Reynolds Industries, Inc.

Address for correspondence: Daniel F. Bowen-Pope, Ph.D., Department of Pathology, SM-30, University of Washington School of Medicine, Seattle, WA 98195.

properties of its cell-surface receptor could be determined. The binding of radioiodinated PDGF to PDGF-responsive cells has proven to be a useful method for determination of which cells are likely to be responsive to PDGF and has also allowed us to develop a sensitive radioreceptor assay for specifically detecting PDGF-c in test samples.[23, 24] We have found that PDGF-responsive cells show very high affinity binding of ^{125}I-PDGF (figure 1).[23, 25–27] This binding site does not cross react with any other growth factor or protein tested except at much higher concentrations.[28] The number of binding sites varies within rather broad limits. In general, we find that connective tissue cells, including vascular smooth muscle cells, express PDGF receptors, while epithelial, skeletal muscle, and nerve cells do not.[28] Cells from species as evolutionarily distant from humans as fish and rodents still bind ^{125}I-human PDGF with comparable affinity (figure 1). This high degree of conservation is consistent with the possibility that PDGF and its receptor serve some important role in vertebrate physiology. The techniques we have developed for determining expression of PDGF receptors and for measuring levels of PDGF-c have allowed us to extend the original hypothesis about the involvement of PDGF and PDGF-c molecules in vascular physiology.

PDGF-c from endothelial cells. Cultured endothelial cells have been reported to release growth-promoting activity into culture medium.[29–31] We have used the PDGF radioreceptor assay to demonstrate that at least one of the mitogens made by cultured endothelial cells is PDGF-like, in that it binds to the PDGF receptor and is recognized by an antiserum prepared in goats immunized with pure PDGF.[32] Comparisons between potency of endothelial cell conditioned medium in competing for PDGF binding to test cells and in stimulating ^{3}H-thymidine corporation to test cells suggest that the PDGF-c represents less than 25% of the total growth-promoting activity produced by endothelial cells.[32, 33] This is supported by the observation that the antibody against PDGF, which completely neutralizes the PDGF binding competitor, only neutralizes about 25% of the growth-promoting activity of endothelial cell conditioned medium.

Both rapidly growing and quiescent cultured endothelial cells secrete PDGF-c constitutively, but the rate of release can be varied somewhat by specific conditions. Both tumor promoters and endotoxin can stimulate the rate of release about twofold.[34] This increased rate of release seems to be associated with the injurious effects of these agents on the endothelial cells. We have also found[34a] that release of PDGF-c by cultured human and bovine endothelial cells can be stimulated at least threefold by physiologic concentrations of thrombin. This increased release is not associated with any change in the intracellular levels of PDGF-c, suggesting that thrombin is not stimulating release of preformed active PDGF. The effect of thrombin may be on the rate of synthesis of PDGF-c by endothelial cells or on the rate of processing of an inactive PDGF processor to a secreted active PDGF-c. The above findings with endothelial cells suggest that the original

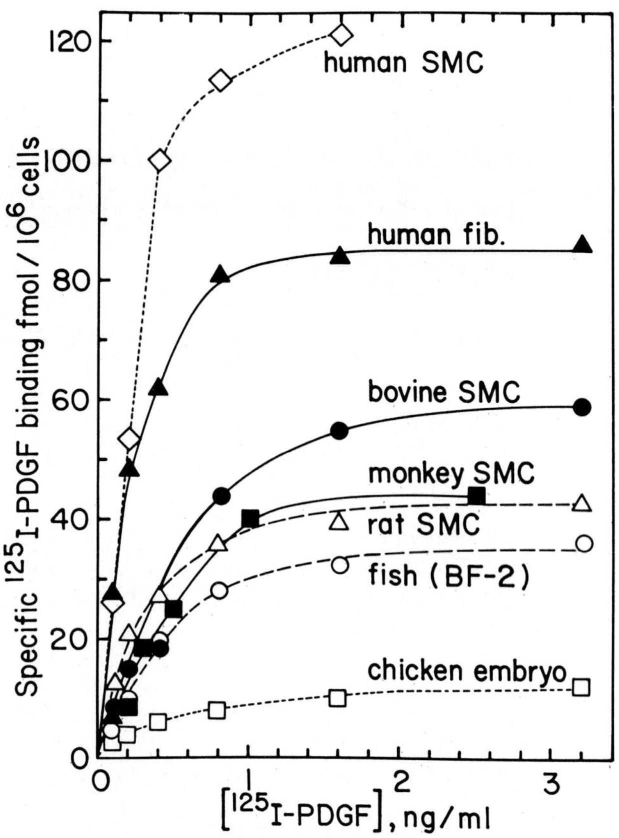

FIGURE 1. Specific binding of ^{125}I-PDGF to cultured cells from different species. Monolayer cultures of each cell type were prepared in 24-well culture trays. When the cutlures were confluent, the medium was replaced with culture medium containing 2% plasma-derived serum or 2% calf whole blood serum from which the PDGF had been removed by cation exchange chromatography.[56] After 2 days, the cultures were rinsed once with ice-cold saline, then incubated for 4 hr at 4° C with gentle oscillation in 1 ml of medium containing 0.25% bovine serum albumin and the concentration of ^{125}I-PDGF shown on the abscissa, or with ^{125}I-PDGF plus a 100-fold excess of unlabeled PDGF to determine nonspecific binding (always less than 15% of total binding), or with medium alone to determine cell number by electronic particle counting. The cell types examined were as follows: open diamond, adult human aortic smooth muscle; solid triangle, adult human foreskin fibroblasts; solid circle, bovine aortic smooth muscle; solid square, adult monkey (*Macaca nemestrina*) aortic smooth muscle; open triangle, adult rat aortic smooth muscle; open circle, Blue-gill fry fish cell line BF-2 (American Type Culture Collection); open square, secondary cultures of chicken embryo cells. (Reprinted, with permission, from Bowen-Pope et al.[28]).

hypothesis of the involvement of PDGF in response to injury might be extended to include the possibility that endothelial cells produce PDGF-c in the vicinity of an injury, possibly stimulated by the local formation of thrombin from prothrombin. This endothelial cell–derived PDGF-c could then serve to augment the PDGF that is provided by platelets.

PDGF-c from smooth muscle cells. A second vascular cell that can make a PDGF-c under certain conditions is the smooth muscle cell itself. We have recently reported[35] that aortic smooth muscle cells cultured from the aortae of 2-week-old rats secrete substantial levels of PDGF-c, while smooth muscle cells from adult rats do not. This PDGF-c is recognized by goat anti-PDGF antiserum. We have used antibody neutralization to show that this PDGF-c is mitogenic for mouse 3T3 cells and is, in fact, the only such mitogen secreted by pup rat smooth muscle cells. This situation is quite different from that found with cultured endothelial cells and with blood platelets. In those cases the PDGF-c component accounts for only a portion of the total mitogenic activity. Since smooth muscle cells respond mitogenically to PDGF-c, the PDGF-c produced by pup rat smooth muscle cells may be an example of what Sporn and Todaro have called an "autocrine hormone," a hormone that stimulates the cells that produce it.[36] Autocrine production of PDGF-c by aortic smooth muscle cells may contribute toward stimulating the more rapid proliferation of these cells and the synthesis of connective tissue components that occurs during the period of growth of the young rat.[37, 38]

We have recently reported[39] that production of a PDGF-c by adult rat smooth muscle cells might also be activated under conditions associated with wounding. In these studies, the carotid artery was deendothelialized with a balloon catheter. Two weeks after this injury, extensive proliferation of smooth muscle cells in the intima of the artery had occurred.[40] At this point the intima was dissected away from the media and cultured. When the PDGF-related phenotype of the intimal smooth muscle cells was compared with that of smooth muscle cells from uninjured media, it was found that the number of PDGF receptors, expressed by the intimal smooth muscle cells, was only 50% as high as the level of PDGF receptors expressed by cells from the uninjured media. In addition, cells from the intima produced 10-fold higher levels of a PDGF than did smooth muscle cells from the uninjured media. As is the case for the pup and adult rat smooth muscle cells (which maintain the differences in PDGF-related phenotype for at least 18 subcultures in vitro) the differences between intimal and medial smooth muscle cells seem to be at least partially stable in culture since the differences between medial and neointimal smooth cells were observed when cells that had been cultured in vitro for at least 3 weeks were used. These findings suggest that production of PDGF-c by smooth muscle cells might be activated in response to wounding and might supplement the PDGF derived from attached degranulated platelets and from activated endothelial cells in contributing toward the extensive and prolonged proliferation of smooth muscle cells in the intima of the wounded vessel. The relative importance of these three sources of PDGF in stimulating smooth muscle cell proliferation is not yet known and may depend on the type of injury and on the time after injury.

Other growth factors from platelets. Platelets also contain other growth factors that may also play roles in stimulating proliferation of vascular smooth muscle cells. With the use of antiserum against PDGF, it has been demonstrated that PDGF accounts for only about 50% of the growth-promoting activity present in human platelets, at least when assayed with attached cultured cells.[19, *] Two additional growth factors, or types of growth factor, are now known to be present in significant concentrations in human platelets: an epidermal growth factor (EGF)–like mitogen and a transforming growth factor (TGF). Despite its name, EGF is a potent mitogen for many connective tissue cell types, including smooth muscle cells.[41] EGF was first discovered because of its presence in huge quantities within the mouse salivary glands.[42] Although EGF is now one of the best-characterized growth factors, and has served as a model for many of the biochemical and cell biological studies performed with PDGF, its source and physiologic roles in humans are far from clear. It is not, for example, present in high concentrations in the human salivary gland. Even in the mouse, the relationship between the high concentrations in salivary glands and the concentrations seen in other tissues is far from clear since surgical removal of the salivary gland does not alter levels of EGF in other tissues and in blood.[43] While investigating interactions between the receptors for PDGF and for EGF, we made measurements of EGF levels in blood, distinguishing what was in platelets from what was in plasma. We found that all EGF detectable in blood appeared to be present within the platelets.[44] Oka and Orth[45] made a similar observation and concluded that platelets are the major repository of EGF in man.

*Bowen-Pope DF, et al: Unpublished observation.

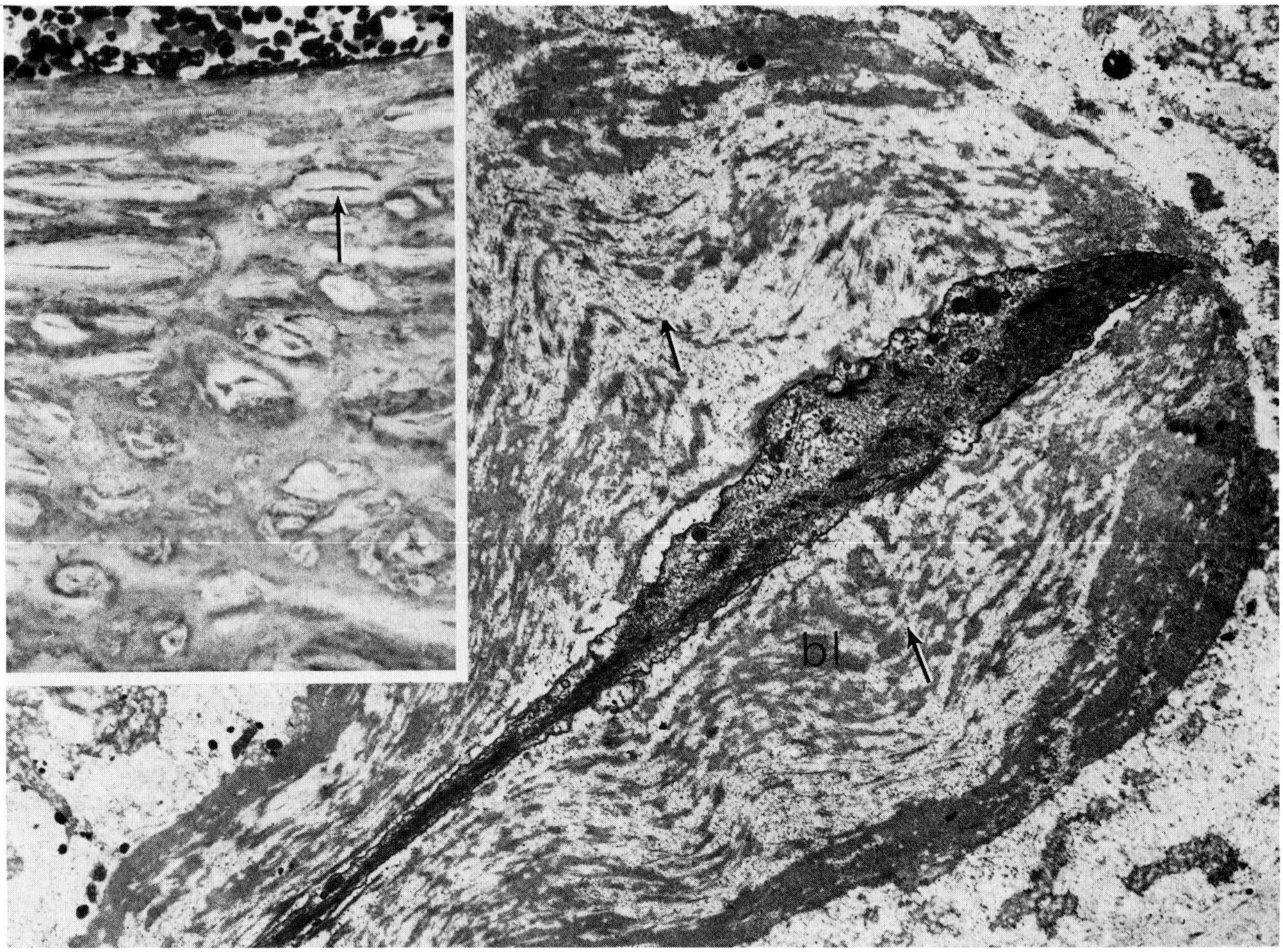

FIGURE 2. Electron micrograph of a cell within the fibrous cap of an advanced atherosclerotic lesion of a human superficial femoral artery. The cell is surrounded by concentric layers of amorphous material resembling basal lamina (bl). Small dark-staining ruthenium red granules (arrows) are interspersed among the basal lamina-like material (bl) (× 10,500). *Inset,* A light micrograph of a fibrous cap showing the distribution of cells similar to that in the electron micrograph. One such cell is indicated by the arrow (× 170). (Adapted from Ross et al.[5]).

The third growth factor is a so-called transforming growth factor. TGFs are operationally defined as substances that promote the growth in suspension of cultured cells that otherwise require attachment to a substratum.[46] Ability to grow in soft agar is one of the characteristics of oncogenically transformed cells that most reliably distinguishes them from their nontransformed counterparts.[47] Class alpha TGFs were first found to be secreted by cultured transformed cells. They resemble EGF in that they bind to the EGF receptor[48] and are related to them in amino acid sequence.[49] Class beta TGFs do not bind to the EGF receptor and depend on the presence of EGF in order to display optimal ability to promote growth in soft agar.[50, 51] Surprisingly, the normal tissue richest in class beta TGFs seems to be the blood platelets.[52, 53] Assoian et al.[54] have provided evidence that the TGF-beta in platelets may be strongly supported in its activity by EGF and PDGF together, so that a platelet contains a complete set of the three growth factors needed to support optimal growth in soft agar: PDGF, EGF, and TGF-beta.

It is intriguing to speculate on why normal platelets contain factors that are associated with the production of the transformed phenotype. One possibility is that the environment of a smooth muscle cell in a damaged artery, and possibly in a normal artery as well, is not identical to that of an attached cell in monolayer culture and that it shares some characteristics with suspension in soft agar. Figure 2 is a transmission electron micrograph of the fibrous cap of a human atherosclerotic lesion. It illustrates the fact that smooth muscle cells in vivo are suspended within a complex extracellular matrix.[5] It is possible that the normal function of the so-called TGFs is to stimulate the proliferation of just such cells in vivo and that certain oncogenic viruses have acquired the ability to activate the gene for this growth factor.[54, 55]

In summary, we would like to suggest that any model for describing the involvement of growth factors in the response of a vessel to injury should consider at least three factors: (1) that the cells adjacent to, or involved in, the damaged area may themselves synthesize mitogens to which they or their neighbors can respond, (2) that the blood platelets contain a variety of different growth factors, each of which may be able to stimulate growth under different conditions and/or may be able to act synergistically with other growth factors present in the platelet or in the wound environment, and (3) that the physiologic state, or local environment of a cell in vivo, may determine how cells will respond to different growth factors. Proliferation of cells in a wound may require factors that have been studied because of the association with oncogenic transformation, but that are encoded by cellular genes and presumably have functions in normal physiologic processes. Recent advances in our ability to specifically detect and measure growth factors that may be involved in these processes should allow us to test possibilities.

We would like to thank Mara Berkley for typing the manuscript.

References

1. Stary HC: Kinetics of cellular proliferation in experimental atherosclerosis. Arch Pathol **89:** 173, 1970
2. Stemerman MB, Ross R: Experimental arteriosclerosis. I. Fibrous plaque formation in primates, an electron microscopic study. J Exp Med **136:** 769, 1972
3. Fowler S: Characterization of cell populations from aortas of Rhesus monkeys with experimental atherosclerosis. Circ Res **46:** 520, 1980
4. Thomas WA, Kim DN: Atherosclerosis as a hyperplastic and/or neoplastic disease. Lab Invest **48:** 245, 1983
5. Ross R, Wight TN, Strandness E, Thiele B: Human atherosclerosis: I. Cell constitution and characteristics of advanced lesions of the superficial femoral artery. Am J Pathol **114:** 79, 1984
6. Ross R, Glomset JA, Kariya B, Harker L: Platelet-dependent serum factor that stimulates the proliferation of arterial smooth muscle cells in vitro. Proc Natl Acad Sci USA **71:** 1207, 1974
7. Ross R, Glomset JA: The pathogenesis of atherosclerosis. N Engl J Med **295:** 369; 420, 1976
8. Bowen-Pope DF, Malpass TW, Foster DM, Ross R: Platelet-derived growth factor in vivo: levels, activity and rate of clearance. Blood **64:** 458, 1984
9. Huang JS, Huang SS, Deuel TF: Human platelet-derived growth factor: radioimmunoassay and discovery of specific plasma-binding protein. J Cell Biol **97:** 383, 1983
10. Baumgartner HR, Muggli R: Adhesion and aggregation: morphological demonstration and quantitation in vivo and in vitro. *In* Gordon JI, editor: Platelets in biology. Amsterdam, 1976, Elsevier/North Holland Biomedical Press, pp 32–60
11. Heldin C-H, Wasteson A, Westermark B: Platelet-derived growth factor: purification and partial characterization. Proc Natl Acad Sci USA **76:** 3722, 1979
12. Antoniades HN, Scher CD, Stiles CD: Purification of human platelet-derived growth factor. Proc Natl Acad Sci USA **76:** 1809, 1979
13. Deuel TF, Huang JS, Proffitt RT, Baenziger JU, Chang D, Kennedy BB: Human platelet-derived growth factor — purification and resolution into two active protein fractions. J Biol Chem **256:** 8896, 1981
14. Raines E, Ross R: Platelet-derived growth factor. I. High yield purification and evidence for multiple forms. J Biol Chem **257:** 5154, 1982
15. Antoniades HN, Hunkapiller MW: Human platelet-derived growth factor (PDGF): amino-terminal amino acid sequence. Science **220:** 963, 1983
16. Waterfield MD, Scrace GT, Whittle N, Stroobant P, Johnsson A, Wasteson A, Westermark B, Heldin C-H, Huang JS, Deuel TF: Platelet derived growth factor is structurally related to the putative transforming protein $p28^{sis}$ of simian sarcoma virus. Nature **304:** 35, 1983
17. Johnsson A, Heldin C-H, Wasteson A, Westermark B, Deuel TF, Huang JS, Seeburg PH, Gray A, Ullrich A, Scrace G, Stroobant P, Waterfield MD: The c-sis gene encodes a precursor of the B chain of platelet derived growth factor. EMBO J **3:** 921, 1984
18. Antoniades HN, Scher CD: Radioimmunoassay of a human serum growth factor for Balb/c 3T3 cells: derivation from platelets. Proc Natl Acad Sci USA **74:** 1973, 1977
19. Heldin C-H, Westermark B, Wasteson A: Demonstration of an antibody platelet derived growth factor. Exp Cell Res **136:** 255, 1981
20. Bowen-Pope DF, Vogel A, Ross R: Production of platelet-derived growth factor-like molecules and reduced expression of platelet-derived growth factor receptors accompanies transformation by a wide spectrum of agents. Proc Natl Acad Sci USA **81:** 2396, 1984
21. Stiles CD: The molecular biology of platelet-derived growth factor. Cell **33:** 653, 1983
22. Bowen-Pope DF, Ross R: Platelet-derived growth factor. *In* Daughaday WH, editor: Clinics in metabolism and endocrinology: tissue growth factors. London, 1984, WB Saunders Co., Ltd., pp 191–205
23. Bowen-Pope DF, Ross R: Platelet-derived growth factor. II: Specific binding to cultured cells. J Biol Chem **257:** 5161, 1982
24. Bowen-Pope DF, Ross R: Methods for studying the PDGF receptor. *In* O'Malley BW, Birnbaumer L, editors: Methods in enzymology. Peptide hormones. New York, 1985, Academic Press, pp 69–100
25. Heldin C-H, Westermark B, Wasteson A: Specific receptors for platelet-derived growth factor on cells derived from connective tissue and glia. Proc Natl Acad Sci USA **78:** 3664, 1981
26. Huang JS, Huang SS, Kennedy B, Deuel TF: Platelet-derived growth factor: specific binding to target cells. J Biol Chem **257:** 8130, 1982
27. Williams LT, Tremble P, Antoniades HN: Platelet-derived growth factor binds specifically to receptors on vascular smooth muscle cells and the binding become nondissociable. Proc Natl Acad Sci USA **79:** 5867, 1982
28. Bowen-Pope DF, Seifert RA, Ross R: The platelet-derived growth factor receptor. *In* Boynton AL, Leffert HL, editors: Cell proliferation: recent advances. New York, Academic Press (in press)
29. Gajdusek C, DiCorleto P, Ross R, Schwartz SM: An endothelial cell-derived growth factor. J Cell Biol **85:** 467, 1980
30. Wang C-H, Largis EE, Schaffer SA: The effects of endothelial cell-conditioned media on the proliferation of aortic smooth muscle cells and 3T3 cells in culture. Artery **9:** 358, 1981
31. DiCorleto PE, Gajdusek CM, Schwartz SM, Ross R: Biochemical properties of the endothelium-derived growth factor: comparison to other growth factors. J Cell Physiol **114:** 339, 1983
32. DiCorleto PE, Bowen-Pope DF: Cultured endothelial cells produce a platelet-derived growth factor-like protein. Proc Natl Acad Sci USA **80:** 1919–1923, 1983
33. DiCorleto PE: Cultured endothelial cells produce multiple growth factors for connective tissue cells. Exp Cell Res (in press)
34. Fox PL, DiCorleto PE: Regulation of production of a platelet-derived growth factor-like protein by cultured bovine aortic endothelial cells. J Cell Physiol (in press)

34a. Harlan JM, Bowen-Pope DF, Thompson PJ, Ross R: Alpha-thrombin induces secretion of PDGF-like molecules from cultured human endothelial cells. Clin Res **33:** 342a, 1985

35. Seifert RS, Schwartz SM, Bowen-Pope DF: Developmentally regulated production of platelet-derived growth factor-like molecules. Nature **311:** 669, 1984

36. Sporn MB, Todaro GJ: Autocrine secretion and malignant transformation of cells. N Engl J Med **303:** 878, 1980
37. Bucher B, Travo P, Laurent P, Stoclet JC: Use of vascular smooth-muscle single cell suspensions for rapid cell number determination in rat thoracic aorta media layer. Cell Biol Int Rep **6:** 113, 1982
38. Gerrity RG, Cliff WJ: The aortic tunica media of the developing rat. I. Quantitative stereologic and biochemical analysis. Lab Invest **32:** 585, 1975
39. Walker LN, Bowen-Pope DF, Reidy MA: Secretion of platelet-derived growth factor (PDGF)-like activity by arterial smooth muscle cells is induced as a response to injury. J Cell Biol **99:** 416a, 1984 (abst)
40. Clowes AW, Reidy MA, Clowes MM: Kinetics of cellular proliferation after arterial injury. I. Smooth muscle growth in the absence of endothelium. Lab Invest **49:** 327, 1983
41. Adamson ED, Rees AR: Epidermal growth factor receptors. Mol Cell Biochem **34:** 129, 1981
42. Savage CR, Cohen SJ: Epidermal growth factor and a new derivative. Rapid isolation procedures and biological and chemical characterization. J Biol Chem **247:** 7609, 1972
43. Byyny RL, Orth DN, Cohen S, Doyne ES: Epidermal growth factors: effects of androgens and adrenergic agents. Endocrinology **95:** 776, 1974
44. Bowen-Pope DF, Ross R: Is epidermal growth factor present in human blood? Alteration of EGF binding specificity in the radioreceptor assay. Biochem Biophys Res Commun **114:** 1036, 1983
45. Oka Y, Orth DN: Human plasma epidermal growth factor/beta-urogastrone is associated with blood platelets. J Clin Invest **72:** 249, 1983
46. Sporn MB, Newton DL, Roberts AB, DeLarco JE, Todaro GJ: Retinoids and suppression of the effects of polypeptide transforming factors — a new molecular approach to chemoprevention of cancer. *In* Satorelli AC, Lazo JS, Bertino JR, editors: Molecular actions and targets for cancer chemotherapeutic. New York, 1981, Academic Press, pp 541–554
47. Macpherson I, Montagnier L: Agar suspension culture for the selective assay of cells transformed by polyoma virus. Virology **23:** 291, 1968
48. Todaro GJ, DeLarco JE, Cohen S: Transformation by murine and feline sarcoma viruses specifically blocks binding of epidermal growth factor to cells. Nature **264:** 26, 1976
49. Marquardt H, Hunkapillar MW, Hood LE, Twardzik DR, DeLarco JE, Stephenson JR, Todaro GJ: Transforming growth factors produced by retrovirus-transformed rodent fibroblasts and human melanoma cells: amino acid sequence homology with epidermal growth factor. Proc Natl Acad Sci USA **80:** 4684, 1983
50. Roberts AB, Anzano MA, Lamb LC, Smith JM, Frolik CA, Marquardt H, Todaro GJ, Sporn MB: Isolation from murine sarcoma cells of novel transforming growth factors potentiated by EGF. Nature **295:** 417, 1982
51. Roberts AB, Anzano MA, Lamb LC, Smith JM, Sporn MD: New class of transforming growth factors potentiated by epidermal growth factor: isolation from non-neoplastic tissues. Proc Natl Acad Sci USA **78:** 5339, 1981
52. Childs CB, Proper JA, Tucker RF, Moses HL: Serum contains a platelet-derived transforming growth factor. Proc Natl Acad Sci USA **79:** 5312, 1982
53. Assoian RK, Komoriya A, Meyers CA, Miller DM, Sporn MB: Transforming growth factor-beta in human platelets. Identification of a major storage site, purification, and characterization. J Biol Chem **258:** 7155, 1983
54. Assoian RK, Grotendorst GR, Miller DM, Sporn MB: Cellular transformation by coordinated action of three peptide growth factors from human platelets. Nature **309:** 804, 1984
55. Bowen-Pope DF: The growth factor-platelet–transformation connection. *In* Browder L, editor: Developmental biology. The cell surface in development and cancer. Plenum Press (in press)
56. Vogel A, Raines E, Kariya B, Rivest MJ, Ross R: Coordinate control of 3T3 cell proliferation by platelet-derived growth factor and plasma components. Proc Natl Acad Sci USA **75:** 2810, 1978

Adenosine diphosphate as a mediator of platelet aggregation in vivo: an editorial view

G. V. R. Born

Platelets in hemostasis

When blood vessels are injured so that they bleed, circulating platelets adhere to the damaged vessel walls and aggregate, so diminishing or arresting the hemorrhage. This interaction between platelets and vessel walls therefore has an easily demonstrable physiologic function. There is much clinical and experimental evidence that a deficiency or defect in circulating platelets is associated with "spontaneous" hemorrhages from small vessels. This suggests that platelets are somehow essential for the functional integrity of these vessels, but if there is such a mechanism it has yet to be established.

Platelets in atherogenesis

The old thrombogenic hypothesis of atherosclerosis[1, 2] has recently reappeared in modern costume as claims that platelets contribute to atherogenesis in three ways: first, through damaging arterial endothelial cells by releasing injurious agents, presumably where circulating platelets adhere[3]; second, through the release in such situations of a factor responsible for smooth muscle proliferation in the arterial wall[4]; and third, through the formation of persistent mural thrombi, which are organized into intimal thickenings. Such evidence as there is for these propositions fails to establish any of them as relevant to atherosclerosis in animals or human beings.[5] Underlying all three claims is the assumption that some normal circulating platelets settle on arterial walls long enough to release some of their contents. There is no observational basis for this assumption in normal arteries, although quantitative observations should now be possible with modern imaging techniques.

Because the assumption is essential for the various claims referred to above, we have begun an investigation designed to quantify the adhesion of circulating platelets in different types of blood vessel.[6] So far, the observations have been mainly on small veins. However, some observations were made also on small arteries for comparison. The venous vessels were chosen for quantification in preference to arteries because the comparative slowness of blood flow made it easier to develop and control the new methods required.

The results showed that the injection of hamster platelets, made fluorescent by labeling in vitro with fluorescein isothiocyanate, into the circulation of other hamsters makes it possible to quantify the flowing and sticking of platelets in vivo. The experiments provide evidence that there is very little tendency for circulating platelets to stick to the walls of small veins and arterioles, even under conditions in which the adhesion propensities of both platelets and vessel walls might be expected to be increased by preparative manipulations. In venules such sticking as there was affected only a very small proportion of circulating platelets and those only for very short periods. In arterioles, sticking appeared to increase somewhat under conditions in which the blood flow could be assumed to be nonlaminar. If the sticking behavior of platelets is at all similar in larger arteries, it seems unlikely that it would permit the release of platelet constituents capable of affecting the arterial walls, except just possibly under hemodynamic conditions such as occur at branches or other major unevennesses in the walls; but platelets are not normally found even there.

It is assumed further that arterial endothelium is continuously subject to "damage" or "injury" of some kind as a precondition for the adherence of platelets. There is no convincing evidence for this generalization, especially not in human beings. The first lesions of atherosclerosis, the fatty streaks, commonly begin during childhood or adolescence. It seems most improbable that these could be caused by any conceivable "injury." Specifically, the common assertion that damage is produced by shear stresses in the high-pressure blood system is inherently improbable because of

From the Department of Pharmacology, King's College, London.
Supported by the British Heart Foundation, the Minna-James-Heineman Foundation of Hanover, and the Fritz Thyssen Foundation of Cologne.
Address for correspondence: G. V. R. Born, Department of Pharmacology, King's College, Strand, London WC2R 2LS, United Kingdom.

functional adaptations in the course of evolution. The only finding that could conceivably apply to human arteries is that guinea pig aorta has a higher replacement rate of endothelium around the openings of branches than elsewhere.[7] This is most simply explained by assuming that endothelial turnover depends, *inter alia,* on hemodynamic effects of nonlaminar blood flow over such areas. But this should be thought of more correctly as a quasiphysiologic effect and, even there, platelets are rarely if ever seen adhering to the walls. The turnover rate of endothelium is increased in experimental hypertension.[8] This is compatible with hypertension as a "risk factor" for coronary heart disease. It seems more likely that this is caused by an accelerating effect of interendothelial gaps on plasma lipoprotein accumulation[9, 10] than to an increase in the indiscriminate or even selective deposition of platelets on arterial walls.

Platelets in thrombogenesis

There is conclusive evidence that occlusive thrombi in arteries damaged by atherosclerosis contain platelets as a major, if not the main, component.[11] The formation of platelet thrombi appears so similar to that of hemostatic plugs of platelets that analysis of the mechanism of the latter is likely to provide an understanding of the former. This article poses questions about how the thrombogenic mechanism depends on the hemodynamic and chemical environment in which platelets aggregate on acutely damaged vessel walls.

Both the gross and the histologic appearance of arterial thrombi establish that their central mass consists mainly of aggregated platelets. What, therefore, is the mechanism responsible for rapid and extensive platelet aggregation in an artery as an apparently random event in time?[12] Close serial sectioning of obstructed coronary arteries has established that the platelet thrombus responsible is invariably associated with recent hemorrhage into an underlying atherosclerotic plaque.[11, 13] The hemorrhages occur through fissures or fractures in the plaque, and the sudden appearance of such a fissure or fracture may well be the random, individually unpredictable event affecting coronary arteries that has to be assumed to occur to account for the clinical onset of acute coronary thrombosis.[12]

How does hemorrhage into a ruptured plaque start off platelet thrombogenesis? This can be regarded as part of the general question of how platelets are caused to aggregate through hemorrhage, and most effectively through hemorrhage from arteries. Until recently this question was commonly answered by assuming that the process depends on the adhesion of platelets to collagen, which is exposed where damaged vessel walls are denuded of endothelium. Adhering platelets then release other agents, including thromboxane A_2 and ADP, which in turn are responsible for the adhesion of more platelets as growing aggregates. This explanation is unlikely to be correct for the following reasons. First, hemostatic and thrombotic aggregates of platelets grow without delay and very rapidly. For example, when an arteriole 200 μm in diameter is cut laterally, the rate of accession of platelets to the hemostatic plug is of the order of 10^4/sec.[14] In contrast, although the adhesion of platelets to collagen itself is almost instantaneous, the subsequent aggregation of platelets, even under optimal conditions for their reactivity, begins only after a delay or lag period of several seconds.[15] Second, platelets tend to aggregate as mural thrombi when anticoagulated blood flows through the plastic vessels of artificial organs such as oxygenators or dialyzers[16] that contain no collagen or anything else capable of activating platelets similarly. This implies that there are conditions under which platelets are activated in the blood by something other than collagen or other constituents of the walls of living vessels.

The plaque on which a thrombus grows has usually narrowed the arterial lumen. At constant blood pressure the flow of blood is faster through the constriction than elsewhere in the artery. Therefore high flow and wall shear rates do not prevent the aggregation of platelets as thrombi.[17] Indeed, the question arises of whether the activation of platelets that precedes their aggregation depends in some way on such abnormal hemodynamic conditions.

The effectiveness of platelet aggregation in plugging a leak is at least as effective in arterioles as in venules. Because the hemodynamic situation should be more unfavorable to the formation of aggregates in arterioles than in venules, an explanation of arteriolar hemostasis is likely to account in principle also for that in venules. For that reason, the following considerations are limited to arterioles.

When an arteriole is cut, platelets are seen to adhere with great rapidity to the damaged vessel wall, while the red cells continue to rush by. This high flow velocity in relation to the small size of the vessels implies the presence in the fluid of strong mechanical forces acting normally and tangentially on and near the vessel walls. The cut causes peripheral resistance to the flow to diminish suddenly, and if the inflow pressure remains constant the mean flow velocity increases. Thus the fluid-mechanical forces on platelets adhering and aggregating on the vessel wall becomes greater still. With increasing size the platelet aggregates tend to constrict the cut, causing a further, although usually temporary, increase in flow velocity.

The blood-flow velocities that would be experienced by platelets closest to the vessel wall, and therefore with the highest probability of colliding with the sites of damage, can be calculated. Human platelets have a major diameter of about 1.5 μm. In an arteriole of medium size, the flow velocity of plasma and of any cells in it at a distance of 1 μm from the wall is of the order of 10 to 100 μm/msec. Therefore a platelet flowing within a distance no greater than its own diameter would pass an injury site 100 μm long in at most 10 msec. In the absence of other influences, this would seem to be the time available for such a platelet to adhere to the damaged wall.

The time just calculated as available to circulating platelet "at risk" for adhering to a wall lesion has to be compared with what is known about the time required for platelets to be activated into a condition in which their collision with such a lesion would very probably result in adhesion.[14] That a process of activation is an essential prerequisite for adhesion and aggregation is implied by the nonreactivity of normal circulating platelets. Presumably, activation consists of a sequence of physical and biochemical events analogous to the activation of muscle.[18] The sequence is still being worked out, but several similarities with muscle are already established. Thus it is known that in platelets an early event is an increased influx of sodium unaccompanied by an equivalent amount of chloride[19] and that activation is associated with an increase of free calcium in platelets.[20, 21]

Because activation is indicated by adhesiveness, the change must involve one or more constituents of the outer surface of platelets. There is evidence that the essence is the exposure of surface receptors for fibrinogen, which has long been known to be an essential and specific plama cofactor for platelet aggregation.[22, 23] The activation time of platelets may then be defined as the interval between the encounter of platelets with an activating agent such as ADP and their ability to react with plasma fibrinogen.

That circulating platelets can be activated to adhere in much less time than that required by their gross changes in shape, i.e., $t\frac{1}{2}$ = 1 to 2 sec at 37° C,[24] is indicated by direct experimental observations. An arteriole can be irradiated by a laser in such a way that damage is limited to a few square micrometers of endothelium.[25] The site of damage is covered almost immediately with platelets that must have been activated in small fractions of a second.

Very similar events follow the application of the activating agent ADP by microiontophoresis to the outside of an arteriole or venule under conditions in which appropriate controls indicate that there is no evidence at all of damage to the endothelial layer.[26] Platelet aggregates grow in the vessel exactly opposite the tip of the micropipette, while the blood continues to flow rapidly and without noticeable disturbance over the site. This is explained most simply by assuming that sufficient ADP diffuses between the endothelial cells into the blood to reach platelets passing close to the wall and that this ADP activates them very rapidly indeed.

An extension of this technique has provided a basis for calculating an average activation time for circulating platelets. It was found that the size of platelet aggregates produced by the iontophoretic application of ADP increases exponentially. The rate constant of this increase depended on the mean blood flow velocity, determined in the same vessels at the same time.[26] The shape of the experimentally determined curve was simulated closely by a theoretical curve[27] that was derived on the single assumption that platelets require an activation time of about 100 to 200 msec. This time is still one to two orders of magnitude greater than that indicated by the earlier theoretical considerations, so either this experimental derivation overestimates the true activation time or the earlier considerations failed to take something into account that would allow flowing platelets more than a few milliseconds for activation. For example, more time would be available if the blood flow near the vessel wall were nonlaminar, so that platelets caught up in vortices, however small, might be exposed to localized activating conditions for longer than they would otherwise be. When branching vessels of the microcirculation are observed microscopically, platelets can often be seen trapped in vortices for variable times of up to several seconds. Such delays may occur in the immediate vicinity of major vessel wall lesions, whether caused by disease such as the sudden rupture of an atheromatous plaque[11, 28] or by traumatic injury such as a puncture or transection. However, there is no evidence of even the smallest disturbances in the flow of blood in a normal vessel in which platelets are caused to adhere by iontophoretically applied ADP. Moreover, it seems most unlikely that any endothelial unevenness produced by laser injury would give rise to flow disturbances large enough to delay the passage of platelets.

The chemical environment of platelets aggregating in vivo has been in doubt until recently. Platelets are activated by various chemical agents in vitro, and it is uncertain which if any of these are responsible for the hemostatic aggregation of platelets in living blood vessels. Recent evidence[29] suggests that ADP is involved in activating platelets in vivo. Novel techniques were developed for the reproducible determination of bleeding times from small arteries of rats and rabbits in the territory supplied by the superior mesenteric artery. One of its main branches was cannulated and infusions were made into the mesenteric circulation of one or other of two enzyme systems that are specific for removing ADP. The reactions catalyzed by these enzymes are as follows:

$$\text{ADP} + \text{creatine phosphate} \underset{}{\overset{\text{creatine phosphokinase}}{\rightleftarrows}} \text{ATP} + \text{creatine}$$

$$\text{ADP} + \text{phosphoenolpyruvate} \underset{}{\overset{\text{Pyruvate kinase}}{\rightleftarrows}} \text{ATP} + \text{pyruvate}$$

For both reactions, the equilibrium at physiologic pH is far to the right. In both species these infusions increased the bleeding times very significantly. This suggests that the observed increases in bleeding time are caused by removal from the blood plasma of ADP, the presence of which makes a major contribution to the activation and hemostatic aggregation of arriving platelets. This conclusion is supported by control experiments in which creatine phosphate was infused alone, without creatine phosphokinase. We have shown this enzyme to be present in blood plasma of both rats and rabbits, in concentrations somewhat higher than in human plasma.[30] Completion of the ADP-removing system by the naturally occurring plasma enzymes could therefore account for the observed increases in bleeding time in these control experiments. In each experiment, control bleeding times were measured before and after infusions of the enzyme systems. Changes in general factors that could be expected to influence bleeding time values, namely the moderate decreases in blood pressure, blood platelet concentration, and hematocrit that were observed, were thereby taken into account. There is other evidence[31] that the bleeding time is not affected by moderate decreases in blood platelet concentrations, i.e., as long as they remain above about 5×10^7 platelets/ml.

One reservation about the conclusion arises out of the presence of nucleotide-dephosphorylating enzymes in normal blood, both in plasma[32] and as ectoenzymes on the surfaces of different types of circulating cells.[33, 34] These enzymes hydrolyze the γ-phosphate of ATP several times more rapidly than β-phosphate of ADP. Both of the infused enzyme systems convert ADP to ATP, which the dephosphorylating enzymes presumably reconvert into ADP. It must be assumed, therefore, that the overall balance between the reaction rates in both directions is sufficient to diminish the concentration of ADP.

Another reservation comes from recent observations showing that creatine phosphate plus creatine phosphokinase inhibits platelet aggregation induced by the stable thromboxane analogue U46619[35] under conditions in which the concomitant presence of ADP is unlikely.[36] More evidence in support of an essential role of ADP in platelet hemostasis will therefore depend on substituting for the above enzyme systems one, such as apyrase, which only dephosphorylates ADP to AMP. Apyrase has already been shown to increase the bleeding time from transected vessels in isolated rabbit mesenteries[31] and from punctures or cuts into artificial vessels.[37] Apyrase also prevents the activation of platelets during their preparation.[38] All this is in vitro or ex vivo evidence for the dependence of the hemostatic aggregation of platelets on free ADP in the blood. The results reported here are the first to provide similar evidence in vivo, as far as the primary physiologic function of platelets is concerned. Intravascular coagulation associated with the generalized Schwartzman phenomenon in rabbits can be prevented by the infusion of creatine phosphate with creatine phosphokinase,[39] but that is under pathologic conditions in which damaged vascular or blood cells, possibly including platelets, can be expected to release ADP among other agents into the circulating blood.[40]

Our observations increase current interest in the following questions. First, is it possible to demonstrate plasma ADP directly in blood at sites of hemostasis or thrombosis at concentrations required to activate platelets? Second, what is the cellular source (or sources) of the ADP? And third, how does this evidence affect therapeutic possibilities for the prevention or reversal of intravascular, particularly arterial, thrombosis?

It has recently become possible to provide more direct evidence for the presence of ADP in blood emerging from vascular injuries in experimental animals and human subjects.[41, 42]

A new technique was developed for the measurement of extracellular free ATP in very small samples of whole blood with the luciferin-luciferase enzyme system. The method had a very low background corresponding to approximately 10^{-16} moles of ATP. ATP was measured in blood as it emerged during hemostasis after precise puncture of rat and rabbit arteries and after standardized incisions of human skin by the Simplate device.

The initial concentration of free ATP in blood emerging 2 to 4 sec after vascular injury was about 2×10^{-7}M in rats and rabbits and about 2×10^{-6}M in humans. The free ATP concentration increased to about 10^{-5}M 3 to 5 min after injury, and these increases could be prevented by heparin (20 U/ml).

The source of the initial free ATP was identified as damaged cells in the injured vessel walls. It could be inferred that sufficient ADP, both released as such with ATP and generated by the rapid enzymic dephosphorylation of ATP, is present at the site of injury to initiate the hemostatic aggregation of platelets. The results confirm a long-standing proposition[43] that at sites of vascular injury, enough ADP is rapidly released from damaged cells into the blood to account for the hemostatic aggregation of platelets.

Whatever the source of hemostatic ADP, its demonstration suggests novel therapeutic possibilities in the prevention of arterial thrombosis when it is initiated by platelet aggregation.[12] One such possibility would turn on the feasibility of infusing enzyme systems that remove free ADP from the blood. In spite of immunologic and other problems, it is conceivable that one or other enzyme with this specificity and a sufficiently long half-life in blood could be investigated for this purpose in appropriate clinical conditions. Furthermore, on the basis of our demonstration that bleeding times were increased also by infusing substrates only, with the implication that the systems are completed by the endogenous plasma enzymes, it is conceivable that therapeutic removal of ADP can be achieved by administering creatine phosphate or phosphoenolpyruvate in a way that provides adequate concentrations in the circulating blood.

References

1. von Rokitansky: Handbuch der pathologischen Anatomie. Vienna, 1941–1946, Braumüller and Seidel
2. Duguid JB: Pathogenesis of atherosclerosis. Lancet **2:** 925, 1949
3. Mustard JF, Moore S, Packham MA, Kinlough Rathbone RL: Platelets, thrombosis and atherosclerosis. Proc Biochem Pharmacol **13:** 312, 1977
4. Ross R, Glomset JA: Atherosclerosis and the arterial smooth muscle cell: proliferation of smooth muscle is a key event in the genesis of the lesions of atherosclerosis. Science **180:** 1332, 1973
5. Walton KW: Pathogenetic mechanisms in atherosclerosis. Am J Cardiol **35:** 542, 1975
6. Kortenhaus H, Schroer H, Born GVR: Quantification of the adhesion of platelets in hamster venules *in vivo*. Proc R Soc Lond B **215:** 135, 1982
7. Payling-Wright HP, Born GVR: Possible effect of blood flow on the turnover rate of vascular endothelial cells. *In* Hartert HH, Copley AL, editors: Theoretical and clinical haemorheology. Berlin, 1971, Springer-Verlag, pp 220–226
8. Payling-Wright HP: Mitosis patterns in aortic endothelium. Atherosclerosis **15:** 93, 1972
9. Stehbens WE: Endothelial cell mitosis and permeability. J Exp Physiol **50:** 90, 1965
10. Caro CG: Mechanical factors in atherogenesis. *In* Cardiovascular flow dynamics and measurement. Baltimore, 1977, University Park Press
11. Davies MJ, Thomas T: The pathological basis and microanatomy of occlusive thrombus formation in human coronary arteries. Philos Trans R Soc Lond B **294:** 225, 1981
12. Born GVR: Arterial thrombosis and its prevention. *In* Hayase S, Murao S, editors: Proceedings of VIIIth World Congress of Cardiology. Amsterdam, 1979, Excerpta Medica, pp 81–91
13. Friedman H: Pathogenesis of coronary thrombosis, intramural and intraluminal haemorrhage. *In* Halonen LA, editor: Thrombosis and coronary heart disease. Basel, 1970, Karger, vol 4:3
14. Born GVR, Richardson PD: Activation time of blood platelets. J Membrane Biol **57:** 87, 1980
15. Wilner GD, Nossel HL, LeRoy ED: Aggregation of platelets by collagen. J Clin Invest **47:** 2616, 1969
16. Richardson PD, Galetti P, Born GVR: Regional administration of drugs to control thrombosis in artificial organs. Trans Am Soc Artif Intern Organs **22:** 22, 1976
17. Born GVR: Fluid-mechanical and biochemical interactions in haemostasis. Br Med Bull **33:** 193, 1977
18. Pringle JWS: Stretch activation of muscle: function and mechanism. The Croomian Lecture 1977, The Royal Society
19. Feinberg H, Sandler WC, Scorer M, LeBreton GC, Grossman B, Born GVR: Movement of sodium into human platelets induced by ADP. Biochim Biophys Acta **470:** 317, 1977
20. Kaser-Glanzmann R, Jakabova M, George JN, Luscher EF: Stimulation of calcium uptake in platelet membrane vesicles by adenosine 3′, 5′-cyclic monophosphate and protein kinase. Biochim Biophys Acta **466:** 429, 1977
21. Le Breton CG, Sandler WC, Feinberg H: The effect of D_2O and chlortetracyclin on ADP-induced platelet shape change and aggregation. Thromb Res **8:** 477, 1976
22. Born GVR, Cross MJ: Effects of inorganic ions and of plasma proteins on the aggregation of blood platelets by adenosine diphosphate. J Physiol (Lond) **170:** 394, 1964
23. Cross MJ: Effect of fibrinogen on the aggregation of platelets by adenosine diphosphate. Thromb Diath Haemorrh **12:** 524, 1964
24. Born GVR: Observations on the change in shape of blood platelets brought about by adenosine diphosphate. J Physiol **209:** 487, 1970
25. Arfors KE, Cockburn JS, Gross JF: Measurement of growth rate of lase-induced intravascular platelet aggregation, and the influence of blood flow velocity. Microvasc Res **11:** 79, 1976
26. Begent NA, Born GVR: Growth rate *in vivo* of platelet thrombi produced by iontophoresis of ADP, as a function of mean blood flow velocity. Nature **227:** 926, 1970
27. Richardson PD: Effect of blood flow velocity on growth rate of platelet thrombi. Nature **245:** 103, 1973
28. Constantinides P: Plaque fissures in human coronary thrombosis. J Atherosclerosis Res **6:** 1, 1966
29. Zawilska KM, Born GVR, Begent NA: Effect of ADP-utilizing enzymes on the arterial bleeding time in rats and rabbits. Br J Haematol **50:** 317, 1982
30. Forster G, Bernt E, Bergmeyer HV: Creatine kinase. *In* Bergmeyer HV, editor: Methods of enzymatic analysis. New York, 1974, Academic Press, Inc., vol 2, pp 784–797
31. Bergqvist D, Arfors KE: Influence of platelet count on haemostatic plug formation and plug stability: an experimental study in rabbits with graded thrombocytopenia. Thromb Diath Haemorrh **30:** 586, 1973
32. Haslam RJ, Mills DCB: The adenylate kinase of human plasma, erythrocytes and platelets in relation to degradation of adenosine diphosphate in plasma. Biochem J **103:** 773, 1967
33. De-Pierre JW, Karnovsky ML: Plasma membranes of mammalian cells: a review of methods for their characterisation and isolation. J Cell Biol **56:** 275, 1973
34. Manery JF, Dryden EE: Ecto-enzymes concerned with nucleotide metabolism. *In* Baer HP, Drummond GI, editors: Physiological and regulatory functions of adenosine and adenine nucleotides. New York, 1979, Raven Press, pp 323–339
35. Nunn B, Chamberlain PD: Further evidence against the validity of using an ADP-removing enzyme system (CP/CPK) for demonstrating the role of secreted ADP in platelet activation. Thromb Res **30:** 19, 1983
36. Huang EM, Detweiler TC: Reassessment of the evidence for the role of secreted ADP in biphasic platelet aggregation. J Lab Clin Med **95:** 59, 1980
37. Born GVR, Bergqvist D, Arfors KE: Evidence for inhibition of platelet activation in blood by drug effect on erythrocytes. Nature **259:** 233, 1976
38. Mustard JF, Perry DW, Ardlie NG, Packham MA: Preparation of

suspension of washed platelets from humans. Br J Haematol **22:** 193, 1972
39. Zawilska K, Izrael V, Chelloul N, Caen J: Prevention de la coagulation intravasculaire disseminee au course du Phenamenene de Schwartzmann generalise chez le lapin par un system enzymatique consommant l'ADP plasmatique. Actualitees Hematologiques **9:** 269, 1975
40. Born GVR, Gorog P, Kratzer MAA: Aggregation of platelets in damaged vessels. Philos Trans R Soc Lond B **294:** 241, 1981
41. Kratzer MAA, Born GVR: Free ATP in blood during haemorrhage. Thromb Haemost **46:** 393, 1981
42. Born GVR Kratzer MAA: Source and quantification of extracellular adenosine triphosphate during haemostasis in rats, rabbits and man. J Physiol (Lond) **354:** 419, 1984
43. Born GVR: Aggregation of blood platelets by adenosine diphosphate and its reversal. Nature **194:** 927, 1962

Melvin Paul Judkins (1922–1985)

Melvin Paul Judkins died on January 28, 1985, after a day of strenuous exertion on behalf of his father-in-law, who preceded him in death by a few hours. Dr. Judkins' freely bestowed gifts reflected dedicated excellence — as with his exquisite method for in vivo visualization of the coronary circulation, which is today the one most used throughout the world. It brought the "greats" and the "nameless foot soldiers" in cardiology and radiology to his laboratories — a tacit tribute to his preeminence in both fields. He also shared in the development of transluminal angioplasty, which today has ever-increasing coronary application. He has literally entered the lives of thousands upon thousands, with an immensely beneficial impact. Dr. Judkins was a giant in modern cardiovascular diagnosis, a creative genius, a master teacher, and a tireless worker. He was folksy, artfully humorous, intensely practical, and a marvel in making the complex simple. In all labors, his wife, Eileen, fully shared round the clock.

From 1970 to 1978, Dr. Judkins was Professor and Chairman of the Department of Radiation Sciences at his alma mater, The Loma Linda University School of Medicine. In two decades he authored more than 150 major scientific papers, books, chapters, and exhibits. He presided over The Society for Cardiac Angiography et al., and led or served numerous national and international committees. He also served on the editorial boards of *The American Journal of Cardiology* and *Applied Radiology* and as editorial consultant to *Chest, Circulation, Radiology,* and *Cardiovascular and Interventional Radiology.*

To his many admirers, Mel was a towering, yet simply based gentle man who left us much too soon. Robert Frost's verse speaks for him in a way that even his modesty might permit him to accept: "Two roads diverged in a wood, and I — I took the one less traveled by, and that has made all the difference."

Winston A. Mitchell, M.D.
Howard Memorial Hospital
Willets, CA

The effects of sublingually administered nitroglycerin on forearm vascular resistance in patients with heart failure and in normal subjects

TSUTOMU IMAIZUMI, M.D., AKIRA TAKESHITA, M.D., TOSHIAKI ASHIHARA, M.D., AND MOTOOMI NAKAMURA, M.D.

ABSTRACT This study examined the effects of sublingually administered nitroglycerin on forearm resistance vessels in normal subjects (n = 9) and in patients with congestive heart failure (n = 8). Forearm blood flow was measured with a strain-gauge plethysmograph and forearm vascular resistance was calculated. To assess the magnitude of reflex forearm vasoconstriction triggered by decreased central venous pressure after sublingual nitroglycerin, lower body negative pressure (LBNP) was applied to produce a comparable decrease in central venous pressure to that after nitroglycerin. The change in forearm vascular resistance during LBNP was compared with that after nitroglycerin. In normal subjects, LBNP increased but nitroglycerin did not change forearm vascular resistance. In patients with congestive heart failure neither nitroglycerin nor LBNP changed forearm vascular resistance. The direct vasodilator effect of nitroglycerin on forearm resistance vessels assessed by the difference between the change in forearm vascular resistance produced by nitroglycerin and that during LBNP tended to be less in patients with congestive heart failure than in normal subjects, which might have resulted from decreased vasodilator capacity of resistance vessels in patients with congestive heart failure. Changes in forearm vascular resistance with a cold pressor test were not different between normal subjects and patients with congestive heart failure. These data suggest that in normal subjects, nitroglycerin does not alter forearm vascular resistance because its dilator effect is offset by reflex vasoconstriction. In patients with congestive heart failure, reflex vasoconstriction is impaired but the direct vasodilator effect of nitroglycerin also tends to be reduced, so that as a net effect forearm vascular resistance is not altered.
Circulation 72, No. 4, 747–752, 1985.

NITROGLYCERIN is used in unloading therapy for patients with congestive heart failure.[1] It is predominantly considered a venodilator drug because, like other nitrates, it does not alter total vascular resistance when it is administered systemically.[2,3] However, nitroglycerin exerts marked vasodilatation when it is injected locally into an artery.[4] It is believed that the direct vasodilator effect of nitroglycerin may be offset by reflex vasoconstriction triggered by a reduction in preload.[5,6]

Reflex vasoconstriction in forearm resistance vessels that occurs with systemically administered nitroglycerin in response to a reduction in preload may be assessed by examining the forearm vascular response to lower body negative pressure (LBNP), which is adjusted to produce a comparable decrease in central venous pressure to that with nitroglycerin. Thus, by comparing the change in forearm vascular resistance produced by nitroglycerin with that during LBNP, one may assess the direct vasodilator effect of nitroglycerin on forearm resistance vessels.

In this study, we assessed the direct vasodilator as well as indirect reflex vasoconstrictor effect of nitroglycerin administered sublingually on forearm resistance vessels in patients with congestive heart failure and normal subjects. There are several reasons for this study. First, it is important to demonstrate that sublingually administered nitroglycerin is not a selective venodilator but dilates the arteries as well as the veins. The arterial dilator effect of nitroglycerin, which may be offset normally by reflex vasoconstriction, may manifest when baroreflex function is impaired. Results of a recent study suggest that reflex forearm vasocon-

From the Research Institute of Angiocardiology and Cardiovascular Clinic, Kyushu University, Fukuoka, Japan.

Address for correspondence: Akira Takeshita, M.D., Research Institute of Angiocardiology and Cardiovascular Clinic, Faculty of Medicine, Kyushu University, 3-1-1 Maidashi, Higashi-ku, Fukuoka 812, Japan.

Received Nov. 5, 1984; revision accepted May 23, 1985.

striction in response to a decrease in central venous pressure is impaired in patients with congestive heart failure.[7] Thus the effects of nitroglycerin on forearm resistance vessels in patients with congestive heart failure might be different from those in normal subjects because offsetting indirect reflex vasoconstriction may be impaired. Second, it is important to know the effect of nitroglycerin on muscle blood flow because exercise capacity may depend on muscle blood flow.[8, 9] Failure to alter total vascular resistance by systemically administered nitroglycerin does not necessarily mean that regional vascular resistance is not altered. Although total vascular resistance is not changed by nitroglycerin,[2, 3] it is conceivable that blood flow to muscles may be altered by the drug. Data in animals suggest that the effect of nitroglycerin on vascular resistance may be different between skeletal muscle and other organs.[3]

Methods

Subjects. Nine normal subjects (eight men, one woman) and eight patients with congestive heart failure (seven men, one woman) were studied. Ages of normal subjects ranged from 30 to 65 years (mean 42 ± 4) and those of patients with congestive heart failure ranged from 33 to 55 years (mean 43 ± 3 years). Ages of these two groups were not different. Normal subjects were free of any cardiovascular disease by history, physical examination, and electrocardiographic studies. All patients with congestive heart failure had clinical, roentgenographic, and hemodynamic evidence of congestive heart failure. Five patients had rheumatic heart disease, two had congestive cardiomyopathy, and one had ischemic heart disease. All of these patients were in NYHA functional class III or higher. All patients had cardiomegaly on chest roentgenogram. Five patients underwent cardiac catheterization within 3 weeks after the study, which showed the elevated mean pulmonary capillary wedge or pulmonary diastolic pressure (average 31 ± 4 mm Hg). Five patients were on a maintenance dosage of digoxin when the study was done. Five patients were taking furosemide and one prazosin. None were on nitrates. Informed written consent was obtained from all subjects.

Measurement of forearm blood flow. The study was done with the subjects in the supine position and in the postabsorptive state. Forearm blood flow was measured with a mercury-in-Silastic strain-gauge plethysmograph with a venous occlusion technique as previously described.[10] The strain gauge was placed approximately 5 cm below the antecubital crease. Forearm blood flow (ml/min/100 ml of forearm) was calculated from the rate of increase in forearm volume while venous return from the forearm was prevented by inflating the cuff at the upper arm. The pressure in the venous occlusion or congesting cuff was 40 mm Hg. Circulation to the hand was arrested by inflating a cuff around the wrist. The wrist cuff was inflated before the determination of forearm blood flow and continuously throughout the measurements. Blood pressure was measured with a sphygmomanometer in the other arm. Forearm vascular resistance was calculated by dividing the difference in the mean blood pressure (mm Hg) and central venous pressure (mm Hg) by the forearm blood flow. These values are expressed as units throughout this report. Mean blood pressure was calculated by adding one-third of the pulse pressure to the diastolic pressure. An average of five to eight flow measurements made at 15 sec intervals was used for later analysis.

LBNP. The lower half of the subject's body below the iliac crest was enclosed in a box sealed and connected to a vacuum. To examine reflex forearm vasoconstriction, the pressure inside the box was lowered below the atmospheric pressure, which decreased venous return and caused reflex forearm vasoconstriction. A catheter was inserted into an antecubital vein, which was advanced into the superior vena cava; central venous pressure was measured with a pressure transducer (Toyo Baldwin, TM1).

Cold pressor test. Ice was placed on the subject's forehead for 45 sec and forearm blood flow was measured throughout. Blood pressure was measured before and at the end of the cold pressor test. Forearm vascular resistance at the termination of cold stimulus was compared with that at control.

Protocols. After stable blood pressure and central venous pressure were obtained, forearm blood flow at control was measured. The subjects were then given one tablet of sublingual nitroglycerin (0.3 mg). Forearm blood flow was recorded at every 15 sec, central venous pressure was recorded continuously, and blood pressure was measured every 30 sec until a stable and maximal reduction in central venous pressure was obtained, which took about 5 min. After administration of nitroglycerin we waited for at least 60 min, by which time central venous pressure and blood pressure returned to the control values. LBNP was then applied to produce a comparable reduction in central venous pressure to that observed after sublingual nitroglycerin. LBNP was continued for the same duration as that required to reach the maximal reduction in central venous pressure after nitroglycerin.

Statistical analysis. Statistical analysis was done with paired and unpaired t tests; $p < .05$ was considered significantly different. All values were expressed as mean ± SEM.

Results

Basal hemodynamic values are shown in table 1. Heart rate was faster ($p < .01$) and central venous pressure was higher ($p < .001$) in patients with congestive heart failure than in normal subjects. Neither resting forearm blood flow nor forearm vascular resistance was different between patients with congestive heart failure and normal subjects.

Representative recordings of forearm blood flow in response to nitroglycerin and LBNP in a normal subject are illustrated in figure 1. Nitroglycerin produced no significant changes in forearm blood flow or forearm vascular resistance, whereas LBNP with a comparable reduction in central venous pressure to that after nitroglycerin decreased forearm blood flow and increased forearm vascular resistance.

Responses to nitroglycerin and LBNP are summarized in table 2. In normal subjects, nitroglycerin decreased central venous pressure ($p < .01$) but did not alter blood pressure, forearm blood flow, or forearm vascular resistance. LBNP decreased central venous pressure ($p < .01$) to an extent that was not different from that with nitroglycerin. However, LBNP decreased forearm blood flow ($p < .01$) and increased forearm vascular resistance ($p < .0025$).

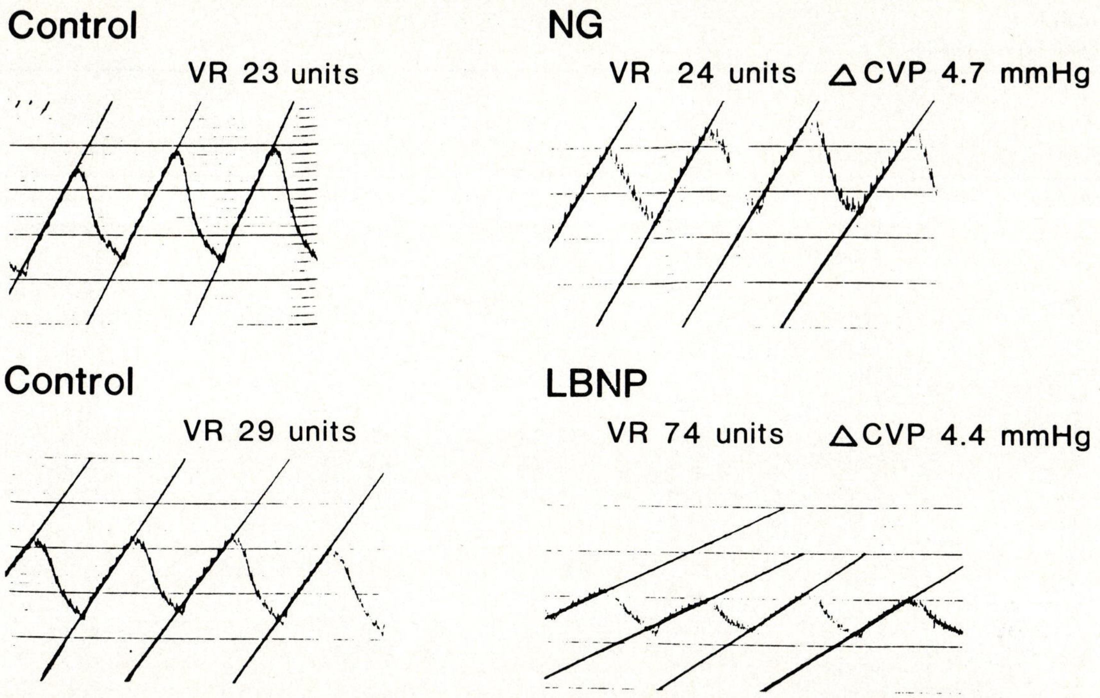

FIGURE 1. Representative recordings of forearm blood flow in a normal subject. With a comparative reduction in central venous pressure (CVP), LBNP increased forearm vascular resistance (VR), whereas nitroglycerin did not change vascular resistance.

In patients with congestive heart failure nitroglycerin decreased central venous pressure ($p < .001$). This reduction in central venous pressure with nitroglycerin was larger than that in normal subjects ($p < .025$). Nitroglycerin did not change forearm blood flow or forearm vascular resistance. LBNP decreased central venous pressure ($p < .01$) to an extent that was not different from that with nitroglycerin. LBNP did not change forearm blood flow or forearm vascular resistance.

Responses to the cold pressor test are given in table 3. Cold stimuli increased mean blood pressure ($p < .001$ for both groups) and forearm vascular resistance in normal subjects as well as in patients with congestive heart failure ($p < .05$ for normal subjects and $p < .025$ for patients with congestive heart failure). However, the increase in mean blood pressure as well as in forearm vascular resistance in response to the cold pressor test was not different between two groups.

Discussion

The effects of nitroglycerin on resistance vessels are likely to result from an interaction between the direct vasodilator effect and indirect reflex vasoconstriction triggered by the reduction in central venous pressure. In this study we assumed that the magnitude of reflex vasoconstriction that should have occurred after sublingual administration of nitroglycerin might be assessed by measuring reflex vasoconstriction during LBNP when LBNP was adjusted to produce a comparable reduction in central venous pressure to that observed after nitroglycerin. This assumption is valid only when the gain of the vasoconstrictor reflex is not altered by nitroglycerin. However, results of a previous study from our laboratory indicated that the relationship between central venous pressure and forearm vascular resistance during LBNP is not altered by nitroglycerin.[11] We should also consider the possibility that the magnitude of an adaptation of the baroreflex during persistent stimulation might have been different between nitroglycerin and LBNP. If so, the assumption may not be reasonable. The development of an adaptation is time-dependent.[12] However, in this study we examined forearm vascular responses to nitroglycerin and to LBNP at a similar time interval. It has not been shown that nitroglycerin alters the rate or magnitude of an adaptation of the reflex mechanisms. Thus it is unlikely that the magnitude of an adaptation of the reflex mechanisms was different between nitroglycerin and LBNP. On the basis of these considerations, we assumed that the direct vasodilator effect of nitroglycerin on forearm resistance vessels might be approximated by obtaining the difference between the change in forearm vascular resistance during LBNP and that with nitroglycerin.

The results of this study indicate that in normal

TABLE 1
Basal hemodynamics

Subject	BP (mm Hg)	MBP (mm Hg)	HR (bpm)	CVP (mm Hg)	FoBF (ml/min 100 ml)	FoVR (units)
Normal						
1	104/67	79	69	4.8	4.2	19.7
2	128/80	96	61	4.6	3.7	24.7
3	121/71	88	34	2.0	3.4	25.3
4	116/80	92	—	2.9	4.1	21.7
5	109/73	85	59	2.0	2.9	28.6
6	110/79	88	61	2.0	3.5	24.6
7	131/65	87	59	2.0	3.0	28.3
8	110/73	85	55	4.8	3.2	25.6
9	108/57	74	62	2.6	3.2	22.3
Mean	115/79	86	58	3.1	3.5	24.3
SE	3/3	2	3	0.4	0.1	1.1
CHF						
1	98/77	81	82	7.0	2.9	25.5
2	120/77	92	80	10.2	2.5	32.7
3	157/98	118	78	5.4	4.2	26.8
4	102/73	83	67	15.7	4.1	16.4
5	113/60	78	58	6.9	2.1	33.9
6	123/100	108	114	18.9	2.5	35.6
7	135/72	93	100	8.0	4.7	18.1
8	117/67	84	—	19.0	2.4	27.1
Mean	121/78	92	83	11.4	3.2	27.0
SE	6/5	13	7	1.9	0.3	2.5
p value (CHF vs normal)	NS	NS	<.01	<0.0001	NS	NS

BP = blood pressure; MBP = mean blood pressure; HR = heart rate; CVP = central venous pressure; FoBF = forearm blood flow; FoVR = forearm vascular resistance (calculated by dividing the difference in MBP and CVP by FoBF); CHF = congestive heart failure.

subjects, nitroglycerin did not alter but LBNP increased forearm vascular resistance with a comparable reduction in central venous pressure. Changes in forearm vascular resistance during LBNP were significantly greater ($p < .05$) than those with nitroglycerin (table 2), suggesting that nitroglycerin exerted the direct vasodilator effect on forearm resistance vessels. These results suggest that nitroglycerin did not alter forearm vascular resistance in normal subjects because its potent direct vasodilator effect on forearm resistance vessels was offset by reflex vasoconstriction triggered by the reduction in central venous pressure. In patients with congestive heart failure, neither nitroglycerin nor LBNP alftered forearm vascular resistance. Thus the mechanisms by which nitroglycerin did not alter forearm vascular resistance appear to be different between normal subjects and patients with congestive heart failure.

An attenuation of vasoconstrictor response to a decrease in central venous pressure has been reported previously in patients with congestive heart failure.[7] Failure to respond to LBNP in patients with congestive heart failure was not caused by the inability for forearm resistance vessels to respond to vasoconstrictor stimuli, since the vasoconstrictor response to the cold pressor test was not altered (table 3). Abnormal responses to LBNP in patients with congestive heart failure were probably related to an impairment of arterial and/or cardiopulmonary baroreflexes.[7] Five of eight patients with congestive heart failure were taking digitalis when the study was done. However, impaired reflex forearm vasoconstriction was probably not caused by digitalis because digitalis has been shown to augment but not attenuate the gain of baroreflex control of forearm resistance vessels in response to LBNP.[7, 13]

The direct vasodilator effect of nitroglycerin on forearm resistance vessels assessed by the difference between changes in forearm vascular resistance during LBNP and those with nitroglycerin tended to be smaller ($p < .1$) in patients with congestive heart failure than in normal subjects. Decreased vasodilator capac-

TABLE 2
Responses to nitroglycerin and LBNP

Subject	NG ΔMBP (mm Hg)	NG ΔCVP (mm Hg)	NG ΔFoBF (ml/min) 100 ml)	NG ΔFoVR (units)	LBNP ΔMBP (mm Hg)	LBNP ΔCVP (mm Hg)	LBNP ΔFoBF (ml/min 100 ml)	LBNP ΔFoVR (units)	Difference between ΔFoVR (LBNP) and ΔFoVR (NG) (units)
Normal									
1	−15	−2.6	−1.4	+4.4	−15	−3.2	−1.2	+3.1	−1.3
2	−4	−3.0	−0.1	−0.4	+6	−2.0	−1.5	+20.5	+20.1
3	−7	−1.4	−0.7	+4.5	−1	−1.4	−0.6	+5.6	+1.1
4	+5	−3.6	+1.5	−4.3	+8	−2.9	−2.5	+40.8	+45.1
5	0	−2.1	+0.5	−3.6	+2	−2.2	−0.5	+7.7	+11.3
6	−1	−2.4	−1.1	+11.8	−4	−2.6	−0.8	+6.7	−5.1
7	0	−2.4	−0.3	+4.5	−1	−4.4	−1.4	+27.0	+22.5
8	−2	−2.8	+0.2	−1.8	+3	−4.8	−2.0	+47.7	+49.5
9	−1	−3.8	+0.9	−4.2	−1	−5.4	−1.0	+12.2	+16.4
Mean	−3	−2.7	−0.3	+1.3	−0.3	−3.2	−1.3	+19.0	+17.7
SE	2	±0.2	0.3	1.8	2.1	0.4	0.2	5.4	6.4
p value (vs control)	NS	<.01	NS	NS	NS	<.01	<.01	<.025	<.05
CHF									
1	0	−4.4	+1.0	−5.4	−2	−3.3	−0.8	+10.4	+15.8
2	−3	−3.0	−0.4	+6.3	−5	−3.0	−0.7	+11.6	+5.3
3	−4	−2.5	0	−0.3	+5	−2.8	−0.5	+5.7	+6.0
4	−1	−3.5	+0.4	−0.9	0	−5.1	+0.2	+0.4	+1.3
5	−12	−4.1	+0.2	−6.3	+3	−2.0	0	+2.3	+8.4
6	−2	−4.2	+0.8	−8.1	0	−4.5	+0.7	−6.3	+1.8
7	0	−4.0	+0.3	−0.3	−2	−4.0	−0.6	+3.1	+3.4
8	−2	−3.0	+0.2	−1.7	−1	−3.0	−0.3	+4.8	+6.5
Mean	−3	−3.6	0.3	−2.1	0	−3.5	−0.3	+4.0	+6.1
SE	1	0.2	0.1	1.6	1	0.3	0.2	2.0	1.6
p value (vs control)	<.05	<.025	NS	NS	NS	<.01	NS	NS	<.01

NG = nitroglycerin; other abbreviations as in table 1.

ity of resistance vessels has been shown in animals[14] as well as in patients with congestive heart failure.[8] It has been shown that impaired vasodilator capacity of resistance vessels is caused by the increase in sodium content of the vessels and interstitial edema.[8] Thus, in patients with congestive heart failure, reflex vasoconstriction was impaired but the direct vasodilator effect of nitroglycerin also tended to be reduced, so that as a net effect forearm vascular resistance was not altered.

It is important to know whether vasodilator drugs increase blood flow to muscle in patients with congestive heart failure, since exercise capacity may depend on muscle blood flow.[8] It is not possible to predict the effect of nitroglycerin on regional vascular beds from its effect on total vascular resistance. Flaim et al.[15] have shown in an animal study that nitroglycerin has no significant effect on blood flow or vascular resistance in skeletal muscle in heart failure. The results of this study indicate that sublingually administered nitroglycerin in patients with congestive heart failure did not alter blood flow or vascular resistance in the forearm.

Because forearm blood flow is composed of both muscle and skin blood flow,[16-19] we cannot determine the changes in blood flow in muscle from changes in forearm blood flow. However, previous studies have suggested that responses to nitroglycerin at rest are not markedly different between muscle and skin in normal subjects as well as in patients with heart failure.[4, 15] Thus we believe that proportional changes in muscle blood flow in response to nitroglycerin may be similar to those in forearm blood flow.

In summary, nitroglycerin did not alter forearm vascular resistance either in normal subjects or in patients with congestive heart failure. In normal subjects the direct vasodilator effect of nitroglycerin on forearm

TABLE 3
Responses to the cold pressor test

Subject	ΔMBP (mm Hg)	ΔFoBF (ml/min 100 ml)	ΔFoVR (units)
Normal			
1	+8	−1	+11.6
2	+11	0	+2.0
3	+9	−0.1	+6.0
4	+10	−1.1	+21.1
5	+7	−0.1	+5.0
Mean	+9	+0.5	+9.1
SE	0.6	0.2	3.0
p value	<.001	NS	<.05
CHF			
1	+8	−0.4	+10.3
2	+5	−0.7	+17.0
3	+8	−0.3	+5.5
4	+8	−1.1	+5.6
5	+4	−0.8	+32.0
6	+3	−1.1	+9.1
7	+3	−0.8	+10.0
Mean	+6	−0.7	+12.8
SE	1.0	0.1	3.5
p value	<.001	<.001	<.025

resistance vessels appeared to be offset by indirect reflex vasoconstriction triggered by the decrease in central venous pressure. In patients with congestive heart failure, indirect reflex vasoconstriction was impaired but the direct vasodilator effect of nitroglycerin also tended to be reduced, so that as a net effect forearm vascular resistance was not altered.

We appreciate technical and secretarial assistance of Tomoko Hirokawa.

References

1. Massie BM, Chatterjce K, Parmley WW: Vasodilator therapy for acute and chronic heart failure. *In* Yu PN, Goodwin JF, editors: Progress in cardiology. Philadelphia, 1979, Lea & Febiger, pp 197–234
2. Mookherjee S, Fuleihan D, Warner RA, Vardan S, Obeid A: Effect of sublingual nitroglycerin on resting pulmonary gas exchange and hemodynamics in man. Circulation **57:** 106, 1978
3. Flaim SF: Peripheral vascular effects of nitroglycerin in a conscious rat model of heart failure. Am J Physiol **243:** H934, 1982
4. Needleman P, Johnson EM Jr: Vasodilators and the treatment of angina. *In* Gilman AG, Goodman LS, Gilman A, editors: The pharmacological basis of therapeutics, New York, 1980, Macmillan, Inc., pp 819–833
5. Abrams J: Nitroglycerin and long-acting nitrates. N Engl J Med **302:** 1234, 1980
6. Petrovich LJ, Smith GB, Quinones MA, Adyanthaya AV, Alexander JK: Hemodynamic effects of nitroglycerin vs pure preload reduction: masked arteriolar dilatory effect. Circulation **58**(suppl II): II-223, 1978
7. Ferguson DW, Abboud FM, Mark AL: Selective impairment of baroreflex-mediated vasoconstrictor response in patients with ventricular dysfunction. Circulation **69:** 451, 1984
8. Zelis R, Longhurst J: The circulation in congestive heart failure. *In* Zelis R, editor: The peripheral circulations, New York, 1975, Grune & Stratton, p 283
9. Zelis R, Flaim SF: The circulation in congestive heart failure. Mod Concepts Cardiovasc Dis **51:** 79, 1982
10. Takeshita A, Imaizumi T, Ashihara T, Yamamoto K, Hoka S, Nakamura M: Limited maximal vasodilator capacity of forearm resistance vessels in normotensive young men with a familial predisposition to hypertension. Circ Res **50:** 671, 1982
11. Noguchi K, Takeshita A, Ashihara T, Yamamoto K, Nakamura M: Effects of trapidil on forearm veins and arteries in man. J Cardiovasc. Pharmacol **5:** 768, 1983
12. Richter DW, Keck W, Seller H: The course of inhibition of sympathetic activity during various patterns of carotid sinus nerve stimulation. Pfluegers Arch **317:** 110, 1970
13. Imamura T, Takeshita A, Ashihara T, Yamamoto K, Hoka S, Nakamura M: Digitalis augments cardiopulmonary baroreflex control of forearm vascular resistance in man. Circulation **71:** 11, 1985
14. Zelis R, Lee G, Mason DT: Influence of experimental edema or metabolically determined blood flow. Circ Res **34:** 482, 1974
15. Flaim SF, Weitzel RL, Zelis R: Mechanism of action of nitroglycerin during exercise in a rat model of heart failure: improvement of blood flow to the renal, splanchnic and cutaneous beds. Circ Res **49:** 458, 1981
16. Zelis R, Mason DT, Braunwald E: Partition of blood flow to the cutaneous and muscular beds of the forearm at rest and during leg exercise in normal subjects and in patients with heart failure. Circ Res **24:** 799, 1969
17. Beiser CD, Zelis R, Epstein SE, Mason DT, Braunwald E: The role of skin and muscle resistance vessels in reflexes mediated by the baroreceptor system. J Clin Invest **49:** 225, 1970
18. Rowell L, Wyss C, Brengelmann GL: Sustained human skin and muscle vasoconstriction with reduced baroreceptor activity. J Appl Physiol **34:** 639, 1973
19. Johnson JM, Niederberger M, Rowell LB, Eisman MM, Brengelmann GL: Competition between cutaneous vasodilator and vasoconstrictor reflexes in man. J Appl Physiol **35:** 798, 1973

Death and other time-related events after valve replacement

EUGENE H. BLACKSTONE, M.D., AND JOHN W. KIRKLIN, M.D.

ABSTRACT A total of 1533 patients received primary aortic and/or mitral valve replacement, with or without tricuspid valve surgery or other associated cardiac procedures, from January 1, 1975, to July 1, 1979. Actuarial survival at 5 years was 74%. The hazard function (instantaneous risk) of death was highest immediately after operation. Among the incremental risk factors for premature death from any cause were preoperative NYHA class, any valve lesion other than aortic stenosis, aortic cross-clamp time, and combined aortic and mitral valve replacement. Ten modes of death were identified, each with its unique hazard function and risk factors. The commonest mode was cardiac failure. Sudden death was the next commonest, and the early phase of its hazard function peaked about 3 weeks after operation. Seventy-five patients (6.7% of the 1533) had 103 valve *reoperations* in the follow-up period. Actuarial survival after reoperation was less than that after the primary operation; whether the reoperation was the first, second, or third was a risk factor. Actuarial freedom from prosthetic valve endocarditis (PVE) was 97% at 1 year, and that of periprosthetic leakage without evident infection was 98.8%; the hazard function for the event PVE had an early phase peaking at about 6 weeks and a constant low phase throughout, whereas that of periprosthetic leakage had a single early peaking phase. After reoperations, the actuarial freedom from PVE and periprosthetic leakage was less than that after the original operation. The risk factors for the development of periprosthetic leakage without evident infection were similar but not identical to those for PVE. Among patients receiving a bioprosthesis, 91% were free of bioprosthetic degeneration 5 years after operation. The hazard function was single and continuously rising, and young age and female gender were risk factors. Actuarial freedom from acute prosthetic thrombosis was 97.9% at 5 years. The single hazard function for this event peaked at 10 months. The risk of thrombosis was higher in female patients. The uses of this integrated study, and the inferences from it, are described.
Circulation 72, No. 4, 753–767, 1985.

THE REPLACEMENT of diseased cardiac valves is an accepted form of treatment for many patients with valvular heart disease. The in-hospital mortality for most of these operations is now low but does not approach zero, and premature death and other unfavorable events continue to complicate the subsequent course of patients undergoing them. In-hospital and later death, as well as other events, have usually been addressed separately and as isolated complications, and the nature of their time-relatedness has been assumed.

We performed an integrated study of most of the time-related events that occur after valve replacement, dated from the time of operation and without the artificiality of separating them into those occurring in hospital and those occurring later. Methods specifically developed for the study of time-related events and their risk factors were used. The results can be used to develop inferences as to the current reasons for surgical failures and methods for neutralizing them and to evaluate results from different experiences.

Materials and methods

The study group consists of all patients undergoing primary cardiac valve replacement, with or without an associated cardiac procedure, between January 1, 1975, and July 1, 1979. Among the 1533 patients, 842 had aortic valve replacement, 478 had mitral valve replacement, and 213 had combined mitral and aortic valve replacement. Patients receiving valve replacement for mitral incompetence on the basis of ischemic heart disease were included. Patients who previously had replacement of a different valve or who underwent valve replacement in infancy or childhood (age less than 20 years) as part of the treatment for a congenital cardiac malformation were excluded. A few children receiving replacement for rheumatic valve disease were included. Associated surgical procedures included

From the Division of Cardiothoracic Surgery, Department of Surgery, University of Alabama at Birmingham School of Medicine and Medical Center, and the Birmingham Veterans Administration Hospital.

Address for correspondence: John W. Kirklin, M.D., Department of Surgery, University of Alabama at Birmingham, University Station, Birmingham, AL 35294.

Received March 6, 1985; revision accepted July 11, 1985.

coronary artery bypass grafting (n = 412 patients), resection of left ventricular aneurysm (n = 13), resection of ascending aortic aneurysm (n = 82), tricuspid annuloplasty (n = 73), tricuspid replacement (n = 6), resection of subaortic stenosis (n = 13), repair of atrial septal defect (n = 6), and others (n = 6). Median age of the 1533 patients was 57 years (range 8 to 85 years); 70% were between 41 and 69 years of age and 95% were between 22 and 76 years.

The time-related events studied were death (considered to be premature in the context of a 5 year follow-up and an observed median survival of 8.6 years for male persons and 11.2 years for female persons aged 75 to 80 years in the 1976 U.S. Life Table), mode of death, reoperation on the valve originally replaced, and the valve complications of prosthetic valve endocarditis (PVE), periprosthetic leakage without evidence of PVE, bioprosthetic degeneration, and acute prosthetic thrombosis.

Information concerning early, in-hospital events was obtained from review of individual hospital charts and that concerning events occurring after hospital dismissal was obtained from personal evaluation of the patient at return visits and from replies to letters sent to the patients and their physicians. If the returned information was incomplete, it was completed by telephone calls to the patients and their physicians. The follow-up interval ended in January 1981 for patients with mitral valve replacement, in June 1981 for those with aortic valve replacement, and in November 1981 for those with combined aortic and mitral valve replacement. Only one of the 1533 patients was untraceable. The median follow-up period was 43 months.

The operations were done with simple hypothermic ischemic cardiac arrest until 1977 and with cold cardioplegic cardiac arrest thereafter.[1] The Bjork-Shiley valve was the most commonly used mechanical prosthesis, with three patients receiving a Starr-Edwards prosthesis in the mitral position and two in the aortic position and one patient receiving a Lillehei-Kaster prosthesis in the aortic position. Both the Hancock (n = 241) and Carpentier-Edwards (n = 235) bioprostheses (porcine heterografts) were used; in addition, three patients received a porcine heterograft of unspecified type, and one patient received an aortic homograft for aortic valve replacement. Interrupted simple sutures of Dacron were most frequently used in suturing the prosthetic device in place, but interrupted pledgetted mattress sutures and, in the mitral position, continuous polypropylene sutures were used in many patients. Patients receiving Bjork-Shiley or other mechanical prostheses systematically received warfarin, beginning 48 hr after operation and to continue throughout life. Patients receiving bioprostheses usually were not given warfarin, even early after surgery. Prophylactic antibiotic treatment was given for 4 to 6 days early after surgery and was advised for later dental extractions, operations, and injuries but the details of compliance are not known. In most reoperations, the original prosthetic device was replaced. Repair rather than re-replacement was done in one of the 42 operations for PVE and in 12 of the 37 for periprosthetic leakage without evident infection; thrombectomy rather than replacement was done in three of the 11 reoperations for acute thrombosis.

Among the 1533 patients, 67 (4.4%) died in the hospital after the operation; 271 patients (17.7%) died later. Also, 75 patients (4.9%) underwent 103 reoperations on the valves that had been replaced. Fifty-eight patients (3.8%) developed 65 episodes of PVE, and 31 (2.0%) developed 39 episodes of periprosthetic leakage without evident infection. Thirteen (2.9% of 446 patients receiving a bioprosthesis) developed bioprosthetic degeneration, and 19 (1.8% of the 1084 patients receiving a Bjork-Shiley prosthesis) developed acute thrombotic occlusion (one patient with a bioprosthesis developed this complication).

No attempt was made to separate the events into those occurring in-hospital (or within 30 days of operation) and those occurring later because of the artificiality imposed by such a strategy. Instead, all events were dated to the conclusion of cardiopulmonary bypass (no deaths occurred between the time patients were taken to the operating room and the start of cardiopulmonary bypass), which for convenience is referred to as the time of operation. The identification and classification of events, including modes of death, were done by the investigators after repeated detailed review of in-hospital and follow-up documents, some from hospitals elsewhere, and after personal telephone calls to patients, their families, and their physicians.

The mode of death (the category, syndrome, or pattern describing the subsystem failure or event that appeared to be associated with the death) was determined for each of the 298 patients who died after the original operation without reoperation; the 40 patients dying after reoperation were not included. Ten categories emerged: death with cardiac failure (acute, subacute, or chronic), sudden death (defined according to the Framingham study criteria of unexpected death without evidence of arrhythmia, occurring within an hour of the onset of symptoms[2]), arrhythmic death (deaths, usually sudden, with documented life-threatening ventricular arrhythmias in close proximity to the death), death with documented uncontrolled and symptomatic infection (mediastinitis, blood stream or prosthetic infection), other cardiac deaths (delayed cardiac tamponade, death after a subsequent unrelated cardiac operation), death with postoperative hemorrhage, neurologic death, death with cancer, death with trauma, and death with other specific but miscellaneous modes (hepatitis, late acute or subacute pulmonary insufficiency, long-term drug and/or alcohol abuse, chronic renal failure, cirrhosis of the liver, diverticulitis with complications, systemic lupus erythematosus, massive hemoptysis of undetermined etiology, and after unrelated noncardiac surgery). There were no more than four patients in any one category of the miscellaneous modes. Assignment of mode of death was made independently by the two authors and was virtually self-evident and agreed upon in 271 patients. In 27 patients, the mode of death was either not agreed upon or undiscernible, and therefore no mode was assigned.

Reoperations refer to any subsequent operation on a prosthetic valve inserted at the original operation. Ten of the 75 first reoperations were performed in other institutions. The definitions of PVE with or without periprosthetic leakage used by Ivert et al.[3] and that of periprosthetic leakage without evidence of PVE used by Dhasmana et al.[4] were used, and these complications were included whether or not they led to reoperation. Bioprosthetic degeneration was considered as an event only when it became severe enough to cause reoperation or death (no instances of the latter occurred). Acute prosthetic thrombosis was considered as an event only under the same circumstances (11 required reoperation and nine caused death without reoperation).

A time-relatedness analysis was made for each event, starting with an actuarial analysis (Kaplan-Meier method[5]) as a method of presenting the data in as direct a manner as possible. The degree of uncertainty in each actuarial analysis is expressed by the 70% confidence limits (CL) (corresponding to 1 SD). In some instances the actuarial analyses have been stratified, and the possibility was tested that differences between the stratified elements are due to chance.[6] A parametric method was used to generate the hazard function, or the instantaneous risk of an event occurring in individuals not yet experiencing the event.[7] The details of the method, the equations, and the shaping parameter estimates and risk factor coefficients for the hazard functions of each event are contained in appendixes 1 and 2. These may be used to recalculate the various nomograms and may be compared with estimates made from a different data set. The hazard function is expressed as incidence of the event per month (an arbitrarily selected unit of time). The hazard function analysis determines whether or not the risk is a constant one with time or whether it is in one or several phases. When there is more than one phase in the hazard function, the hazard function(s) that change(s) with time is (are) added to any constant hazard function that is present. Thus, when an early declining phase of increased risk and a constant phase are both present, the hazard function during the postoperative interval in which the early phase is present is the sum of both the early and constant hazard functions. The 70% confidence limits around the hazard function are presented to facilitate estimating the likelihood that differences are not due to chance. For some analyses, the parametric survivorship function has been used to calculate the probability of an event occurring within any time period. The survival and hazard functions are presented along with those of an age-race-sex–matched U.S. population, taken from the 1976 life tables.

Incremental risk factors (variables, either dichotomous or continuously variable, that are associated with increased risk in risk-containing situations[8]) have been determined simultaneously for each phase of a hazard function by a multivariate step-wise elimination procedure, thus generating equations from which nomograms can be plotted and stratified.[7] Variables were excluded when the p value for their association with an event was $\geq .1$. Risk factors for a constant phase pertain *throughout* the postoperative period, and in the case of more than one phase those for the changing (decreasing or increasing with time) early or late phase pertain only during the time of changing hazard function. The equations and coefficients of the parametric hazard and survivorship functions, and those of the multivariate equations are given in appendix 2.

The possible risk factors (dichotomous unless otherwise stated) analyzed for each time-related event, including the modes of death, after the original operation were age (years) at the time of operation; gender (male or female); race (white or black, in this study); pure incompetence vs pure stenosis vs mixed lesion at each valve; in the case of mitral incompetence, ischemic vs nonischemic origin; NYHA functional class (I through V, V indicating a state of shock requiring emergency operation); atrial fibrillation; native valve endocarditis; date of operation (years since January 1, 1975); cardiopulmonary bypass time (minutes); cardioplegia; in the case of cardioplegia, aortic cross-clamp (cardiac ischemic) time (minutes); valve replacement location (aortic, mitral, or both); tricuspid repair or replacement; concomitant coronary artery bypass grafting, resection of ascending aortic aneurysm, or other associated procedure; valve replacement device (mechanical vs bioprosthesis); and size of valve replacement device. Continuous variables were tested in the model both in their original units and in transformations to logarithmic and squared units, and that which fit the data best was selected. In addition, the potential interactions were examined between age and the valve replaced; NYHA functional class and valve replaced; and cardiac ischemic time (in the cardioplegic group) and NYHA functional class. Reoperation was not considered as a possible risk factor for death after the original valve operation because it too is an event after valve replacement.

In the case of events following one or more reoperations on the original valve replacement device, the risk factor analysis specific to each reoperation (i.e., the first reoperation, the second reoperation, etc.) included the same variables, except that "native valve endocarditis" was replaced by "prosthetic valve endocarditis." In addition, the reoperation number (first, second, third, or fourth reoperation) was entered as a possible risk factor, as was the indication for the reoperation (PVE, periprosthetic leakage in the absence of any evidence for PVE, bioprosthetic degeneration, and acute prosthetic thrombosis), and the procedure used at reoperation (replacement vs repair).

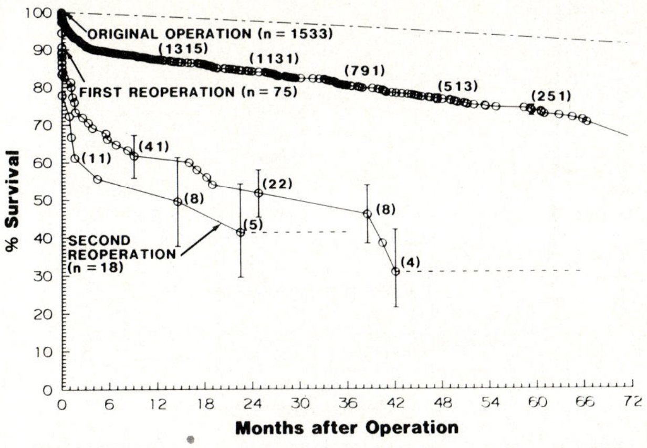

FIGURE 1. Actuarial survival after primary (original) valve replacement (1975 to July 1979; n = 1533, 338 deaths). In this and subsequent actuarial depictions, each individual event (death in this instance) is represented by a circle; the bars enclose the 70% confidence limits ($\pm$ 1 SD) of the actuarial point estimate. The numbers in parentheses indicate the number of patients traced at that time. The top line (— - —) represents data for an age-race-sex–matched general population. Time 0 is the conclusion of cardiopulmonary bypass. The next line pertains to the primary valve replacement operation, the next lower to the first reoperation (36 deaths), and the lowest to the second reoperation (10 deaths). $p < .0001$ for the actuarial difference between original operation and first reoperation; $p < .5$ for the difference between first and second reoperation. Actuarial survival after the third reoperation (n = 8, four deaths) was 75% (CL 57% to 87%) at 24 hr after surgery, the same at 2 weeks, 56% (CL 36% to 74%) at 1 year, and 38% at 2 years (CL 20% to 60%); after the fourth reoperation (n = 2), one of the patients died 1 hr after surgery and the other died 10 months later.

For events other than death following a given operation, the patient was censored at the time of another operation, if one occurred. In the case of the event death, no censoring was done at the time of any reoperation except in the analyses of modes of death.

Results

Premature death

Original valve replacement operation. Actuarial survival after the original valve replacement operation was 98.5% at 24 hr (CL 98.2% to 98.8%), 96.3% at 2 weeks (CL 95.8% to 96.8%), 87.3% at 1 year (CL 86.4% to 88.1%), and 73.6% at 5 years (CL 72.2% to 75.0%) (figure 1). The hazard function or instantaneous risk of death was highest immediately after operation, fell rapidly during the first postoperative month, and became a constant lower hazard phase by about 3 months after operation (figure 2).

Older age was an incremental risk factor for premature death in both the early phase ($p = .01$) and the constant phase ($p = .02$); the age effect is not very strong, however, since 5 year survival predicted from the multivariate equation (see appendixes 1 and 2) for aortic valve replacement during 60 min of aortic cross-

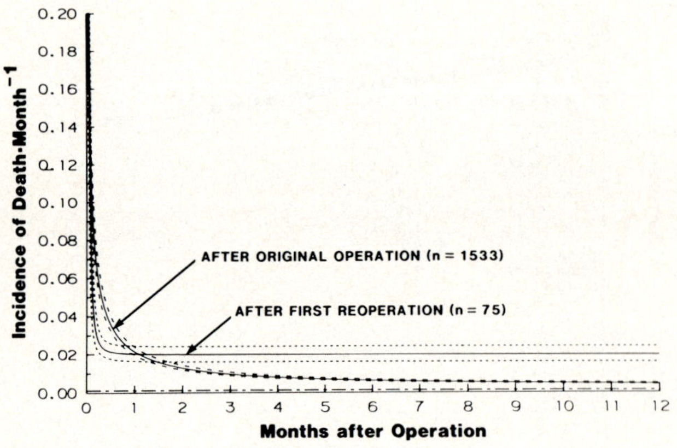

FIGURE 2. Hazard function for death in the first 12 months after the primary valve replacement (n = 1533) and after the first reoperation (n = 75). The instantaneous risk of death is along the vertical axis, and the time after operation is along the horizontal axis. In this and subsequent hazard function depictions, the dashed lines enclose the 70% confidence limits (± 1 SD), and the hazard function of a matched population is shown (— - —). In both hazard functions there is an early phase of rapidly falling risk and a constant phase that extends throughout the follow-up period.

clamping with cold cardioplegia is 80% (CL 78% to 81%) for a 60-year-old man, whereas it is 75% (CL 72% to 77%) for a 75-year-old man. Black race was a risk factor in the constant phase ($p < .0001$). Only isolated aortic stenosis among the various valve lesions did not increase the risk of death in any phase. Aortic incompetence was a risk factor in the early phase ($p = .003$), as was mitral stenosis and/or incompetence ($p < .0001$). Ischemic mitral incompetence, with or without concomitant coronary artery bypass grafting, was a powerful risk factor in the constant phase ($p = .003$). Preoperative functional status (NYHA class) was a risk factor for premature death only in the early phase ($p < .0001$). Among the surgical variables, longer aortic cross-clamp time was a risk factor in the early phase ($p < .0001$), as was combined aortic and mitral valve replacement ($p < .0001$).

According to the parametric time-related risk factor analysis (see appendix 2), the predicted 2 week, 1 year, and 5 year survival of a patient 60 years of age undergoing isolated valve replacement for aortic stenosis is 99%, 94%, and 78%, respectively (table 1). The predicted 5 year survival is lower when (1) aortic valve replacement is combined with mitral valve replacement, (2) the aortic lesion is incompetence rather than stenosis, (3) the operation is isolated mitral valve replacement for stenosis or incompetence, and especially (4) the operation is for ischemic mitral incompetence (table 1). When the operation is aortic valve replacement for aortic stenosis and the conditions were the same as in table 1, the predicted 5 year survival, including in-hospital deaths, for patients in NYHA classes II, III, IV, and V before surgery is 82%, 80%, 75%, and 63%, respectively.

Reoperation after valve replacement. The actuarial survival after reoperation on the prosthetic valve previously inserted was 31% (CL 21% to 43%) at 3½ years (figure 1), considerably lower than that after the original valve replacement operation. The hazard function for death was different after reoperation in that the early phase was initially higher but dropped

TABLE 1
Parametrically predicted survival after isolated primary valve replacement according to the valve lesion[A]

	Predicted survival					
	2 wk		1 yr		5 yr	
Valve lesions	%	CL (%)	%	CL (%)	%	CL (%)
Aortic stenosis	98.7	98.3–99.0	93.5	92.7–94.3	79.7	78.1–81.3
Aortic stenosis and mitral stenosis and/or incompetence	97.5	96.5–98.2	90.6	88.6–92.3	76.6	74.4–78.8
Aortic incompetence	97.2	96.3–97.9	89.9	88.0–91.6	75.9	73.7–78.0
Aortic incompetence and mitral stenosis or incompetence	94.5	92.6–95.9	83.8	80.0–86.9	69.5	65.7–73.1
Mitral stenosis and/or incompetence	95.7	94.7–86.5	86.4	84.4–88.3	72.3	70.0–74.5
Ischemic mitral incompetence	95.3	94.3–96.1	78.4	73.3–82.7	44	32–57
Total group (n = 1533)	95.8	95.3–96.2	87.2	86.3–87.9	73.9	72.7–75.2

CL = 70% confidence limits.

[A]Obtained by solution of the multivariate equation (see appendixes 1 and 2) for death in all modes. In solving for the predicted survivals for the individual valve lesions, NYHA functional class was set at III, age at 60 years, 15% of the patients black, and the aortic cross-clamp time (with cardioplegia) 60 min. Actuarial survival for the total group (n = 1533) for 5 years was 73.6% (CL 72.2% to 75.0%).

more rapidly, essentially to disappear at about 2 weeks; the hazard function after this was a constant phase that was higher than that after primary valve replacement (figure 2).

There were fewer incremental risk factors for premature death after valve reoperations than after the original valve replacement operation. No demographic variables appeared. The number of the reoperation was a risk factor, the risk of death in the early phase increasing with each subequent reoperation (p = .04). Among the valve lesions, only mitral valve disease (stenosis and/or incompetence) increased the risk, and that was in the constant phase (p = .0005). Higher NYHA functional class was a risk factor in the early phase (p = .04). Among the surgical variables, only use of a mechanical prosthesis (rather than a bioprosthesis or repair) was a risk factor, and then in the constant phase (p = .04).

According to the time-related risk factor analysis (see appendix 2), for a patient in NYHA class I the predicted 2 week survival after the original operation and that after the first reoperation are 99.7% (CL 99.6% to 99.8%) and 98.9% (CL 97.9% to 99.4%), respectively, and those for 5 years are 82% (CL 81% to 84%) and 46% (CL 35% to 58%), respectively. With more advanced preoperative disability and/or repeated reoperations, both early and late predicted survival are lower (table 2).

Modes of death. Ten modes of death after the original valve replacement operation were identified (table 3). The hazard functions for the various modes were highly variable (figure 3).

Cardiac failure. The commonest mode of death was cardiac failure (acute in 38 patients, subacute in 34, and chronic in 29). The median interval between operation and death was 3 days, 2.7 weeks, and 25 months, respectively, for the three subgroups. The instantaneous risk (hazard function) of death with cardiac failure in the early phase was highest immediately after operation and became a lower constant phase about 6 months after surgery.

The incremental risk factors for death with cardiac

TABLE 2

Parametrically predicted 2 week and 5 year survival after aortic valve replacement for aortic stenosis: primary operation vs reoperation and preoperative NYHA functional class[A]

	Survival							
	Primary operation		Reoperation 1		Reoperation 2		Reoperation 3	
NYHA class	%	CL (%)	%	CL (%)	%	CL (%)	%	CL (%)
I								
2 wk	99.7	99.6–99.8	98.9	97.9–99.4	—[B]	—	—	—
5 yr	82.3	80.6–83.9	46	35–58	—	—	—	—
II								
2 wk	99.5	99.3–99.6	97.9	95.8–99.0	96.3	92.4–98.2	—	—
5 yr	81.6	80.0–83.2	46	34–58	45	34–57	—	—
III								
2 wk	98.7	98.3–99.0	95.1	91.5–97.3	90.6	85.1–94.2	82	71–90
5 yr	79.7	78.1–81.3	44	34–56	42	32–54	38	28–50
IV								
2 wk	96.6	95.5–97.5	88	83–91	77	71–82	61	47–74
5 yr	74.6	72.0–77.0	41	31–52	36	27–46	28	20–39
V								
2 wk	91	88–94	71	62–78	53	42–64	35	21–52
5 yr	63	56–69	33	25–43	25	17–34	16	9–27
Mean NYHA class	2.9(±0.71 SD) (n = 1533)		3.7(±1.22 SD) (n = 75)		3.4(±1.29 SD) (n = 18)		3.6(±0.92 SD) (n = 8)	

CL = 70% confidence limits.

[A]The digital nomogram is a solution of the multivariate equation for death after the original valve replacement or valve re-replacement (see appendixes 1 and 2). In the solution of the equation, age was set at 60 years, mechanical prosthesis–yes, cardioplegia–yes, cross-clamp time 60 min, and 15% of the patients black.

[B]In the categories where no survival estimate is given, there were no examples in the data set and the estimate would be an extrapolation of the experience.

TABLE 3

Mode of death after the original valve replacement operation[A]

Symbol[B]	Modes of death	n
A	Cardiac failure	101
B	Sudden	62
C	Neurologic	27
D	Cancer	24
E	Hemorrhage	11
F	Infection	9
G	Arrhythmias	7
H	Other cardiac modes	7
I	Trauma	6
J	Miscellaneous	17
	Total	271

[A]In 27 additional patients a mode of death could not be agreed upon; their hazard function is depicted as *K* in figure 3. Seventy-five patients had reoperations, of whom 40 died after the first or subsequent operations and are not included in this analysis.

[B]Symbols used in figure 3.

failure were similar to those for all deaths (table 4). Longer aortic cross-clamp time and increased preoperative functional disability only slightly increased predicted 2 week mortality after valve replacement for aortic stenosis, but both were associated with an evident increase in risk when the operation was for aortic incompetence, mitral valve disease, and particularly when it was a double valve replacement for aortic incompetence and mitral valve disease (figure 4).

Sudden death. Sudden death (62 events) was the next commonest mode of death (see table 3). Its hazard function peaked at about 3 weeks after operation and fell to become constant by about 8 months after surgery (see figure 3). The risk factors for sudden death included three variables (aortic incompetence, mitral valve stenosis and/or incompetence, and NYHA functional class), which were also risk factors for death with cardiac failure (table 5). Fifteen of the patients with sudden death had autopsy examination. In eight the prosthetic valve and the periprosthetic area appeared normal and no explanation was found for the death. Unexpectedly, there was extensive dehiscence of the valve in two patients, PVE with dehiscence in two, thrombosis of a Carpentier-Edwards bioprosthesis in one, and massive pulmonary embolization in two.

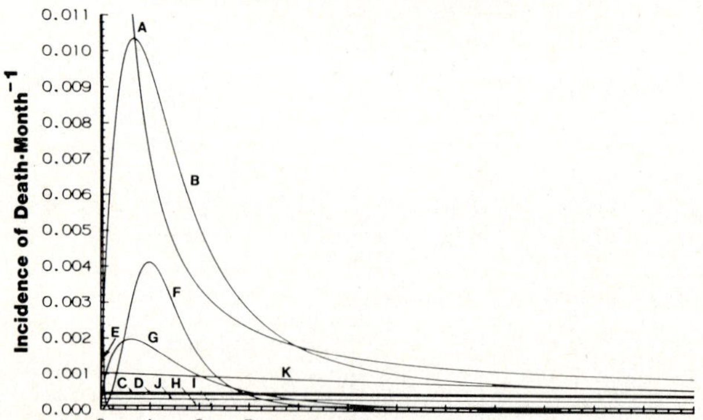

FIGURE 3. Nomogram of the hazard function of each mode of death after the original valve replacement. (See table 3 for meaning of symbols.) An age-sex-race–matched general population has an incidence of deaths/month of 0.001 across a 5 year period.

TABLE 4

Incremental risk factors for death with cardiac failure after original valve replacement operation (January 1975–July 1979; n = 1533, 101 events)

	Time of influence (phase)	
Incremental risk factor	Throughout and constant (p value)	Early and decreasing (p value)
Demographic variable		
(Older) age (yr) at operation	>.1	.002
Black race	.004	>.1
Valve lesion		
Aortic incompetence	>.1	.003
Mitral valve stenosis and/or incompetence	>.1	<.0001
Ischemic mitral incompetence	<.0001	>.1
(Higher) NYHA functional class	>.1	<.0001
Surgical variables		
Aortic cross-clamp time (min) in cardioplegic group	>.1	.008
Tricuspid procedure	>.1	.008
Coronary artery bypass grafting	>.1	.008

In this and subsequent tables, p > .1 excludes the variable as a risk factor in that phase.

Neurologic. The hazard function for neurologic death (27 events) was constant and low across the time of this study (see figure 3). Older age at operation (p = .008) was the only risk factor. Autopsy was performed in four of the 27 patients and in all four there was evident intracranial disease (cerebral embolus in one, cerebral thrombosis in the bulbar area in one, multiple areas of cerebral hemorrhage in one, and diffuse brain necrosis in one. In addition, seven other patients with a neurologic mode of death had evidence of intracranial hemorrhage at the time of intracranial surgery or study by computed tomography.

Other modes of death. The hazard function for death with cancer was constant across time (see figure 3); only older age at operation (p = .07) was a risk factor. The hazard function of death with hemorrhage had a single phase and was highest immediately after operation and declined rapidly to essentially disappear after

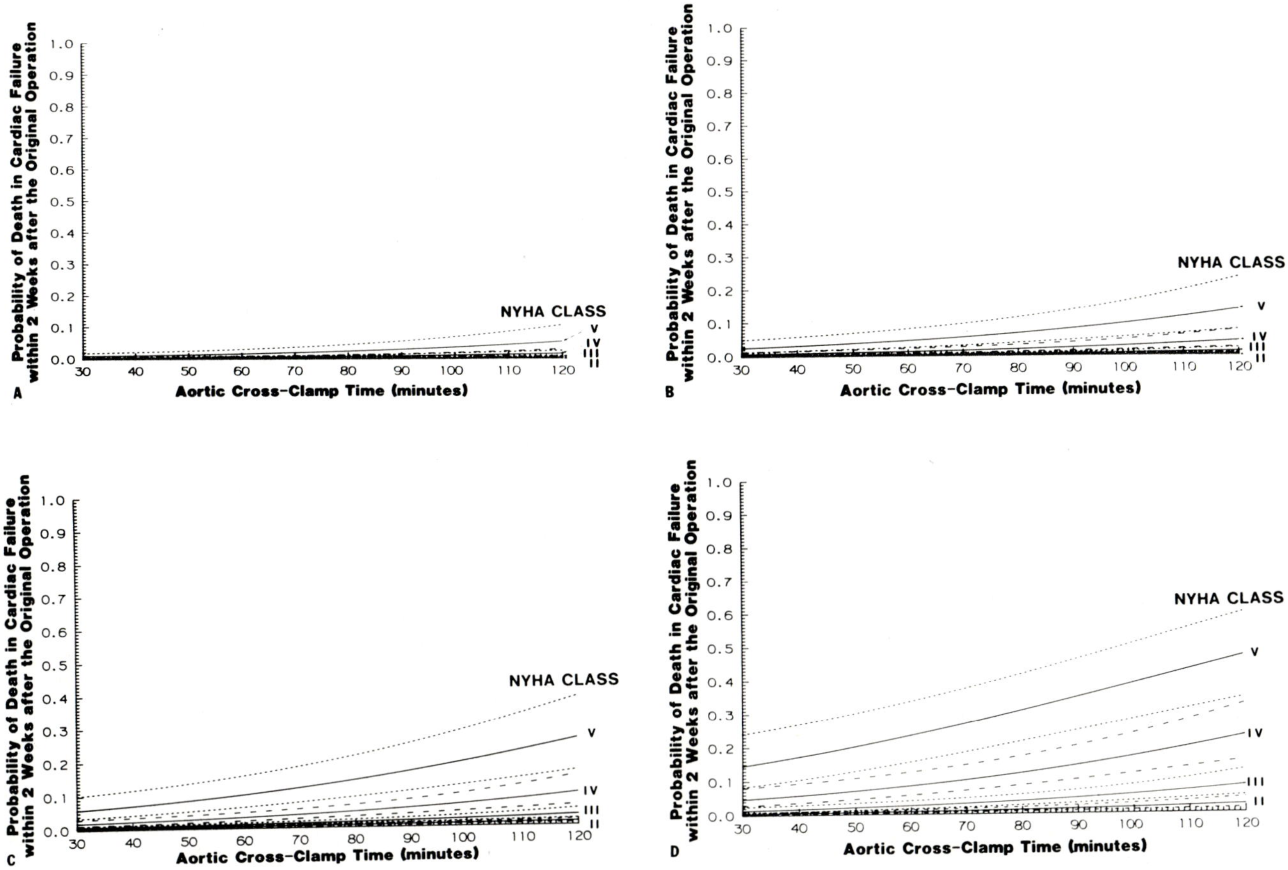

FIGURE 4. Nomograms of probability of cardiac death within 2 weeks of a valve replacement operation, according to the length of the aortic cross-clamp time during cold cardioplegia, preoperative NYHA class, and the valve lesion. The nomograms are solutions of the multivariate equations (see appendixes 1 and 2), with the other entries being age of 60 years, 15% of the patients black, no coronary artery bypass grafting, and no tricuspid valve procedure. *A*, Aortic valve replacement for aortic stenosis. *B*, Aortic valve replacement for aortic incompetence. *C*, Mitral valve replacement for stenosis and/or incompetence, isolated or combined with aortic valve replacement for aortic stenosis. *D*, Double valve replacement for aortic incompetence and mitral stenosis and/or incompetence.

3 to 4 days. The incremental risk factors were higher NYHA functional class (p = .008), older age (p = .04), and duration of aortic cross-clamp time (p = .02). Among the nine patients dying with infection, only one, who died with septic shock and severe hyperthermia, had PVE. In seven patients extensive mediastinitis was the primary focus of infection. The ninth patient, a diabetic, had septic shock and fungal and bacterial infections of the blood stream and fungal native valve endocarditis before surgery; the patient died early after valve replacement and at autopsy had fungus (*Candida*) infection of many organs. The hazard function for death with arrhythmia (seven events) peaked at about 2 weeks after surgery and fell to a very low level within 6 months after operation. In only one of the patients (aortic valve replacement and coronary artery bypass grafting) with this mode of death was autopsy done; the grafts were open, the valve replacement area was normal, and no myocardial necrosis was found. The patient had documented ventricular tachyarrhythmia before death.

Reoperation. The actuarial incidence of reoperation after the original valve replacement was 2.5% (CL 2.2% to 3.0%) within 6 months, 4.3% (CL 3.8% to 4.8%) within 2 years, and 6.7% (CL 5.9% to 7.7%) within 5 years (figure 5). The hazard function for reoperation after the original operation had an early peak at about 3 months after operation, a rather rapid fall to a low and constant hazard function, and a rising third phase of hazard function beginning at about 3 years after surgery. The shape of the hazard function was different for mechanical valves and bioprostheses, with the late rise in hazard function characterizing only the latter (figure 6).

Thirty-four (45%; CL 39% to 52%) of 75 patients undergoing a first reoperation had PVE, in contrast to the original valve replacement operation in which 67 (4.4%; CL 3.8% to 5.0%) of the 1533 patients had

TABLE 5

Incremental risk factors for sudden death after original valve replacement operation (n = 1533, 62 events)

Incremental risk factor	Time of influence (phase): Throughout and constant (p value)	Time of influence (phase): Early and decreasing (p value)
Demographic variable		
Male gender	.02	>.1
Valve lesions		
Aortic incompetence	>.1	.08
Mitral valve stenosis and/or incompetence	>.1	.04
(Higher) NYHA functional class	>.1	.04
Surgical variables		
Use of bioprosthesis	.07	>.1

native valve endocarditis. Five (28%; CL 16% to 43%) of 18 patients undergoing a second reoperation had valve infection, as did three (38%; CL 17% to 62%) of eight patients undergoing the third reoperation. Other indications for the first reoperation were periprosthetic leakage without evident PVE (n = 17), bioprosthetic degeneration (n = 13), and thrombosis of a Bjork-Shiley prosthesis (n = 11). Periprosthetic leakage without evident PVE (in 13 of 18 patients undergoing a second reoperation, five of eight undergoing a third, and two of two undergoing a fourth) and PVE were the only indications for the second and subsequent reoperations.

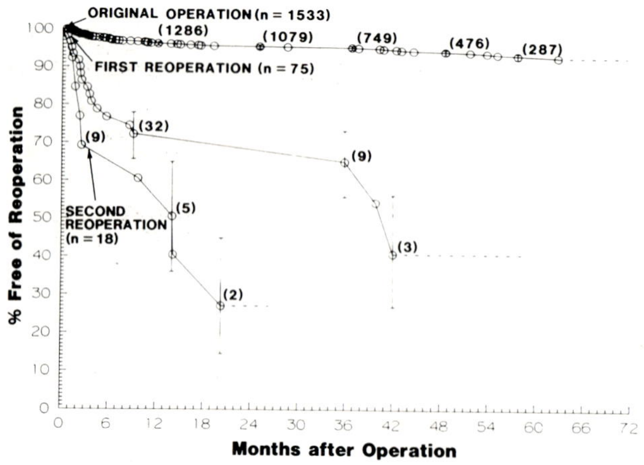

FIGURE 5. Actuarial freedom from reoperation after the primary valve operation (n = 1533, 75 events) and after the first reoperation (18 events) and the second reoperation (eight events). The actuarial freedom from reoperation after the third reoperation (n = 8, two events) is 83% (CL 63% to 94%) at 6 months and 56% (CL 31% to 78%) at 2 years (not shown). After the fourth reoperation (n = 2) there were no further reoperations (not shown). $p < .0001$ for the difference between the original operation and the first reoperation; $p = .12$ for difference between the first and second reoperation.

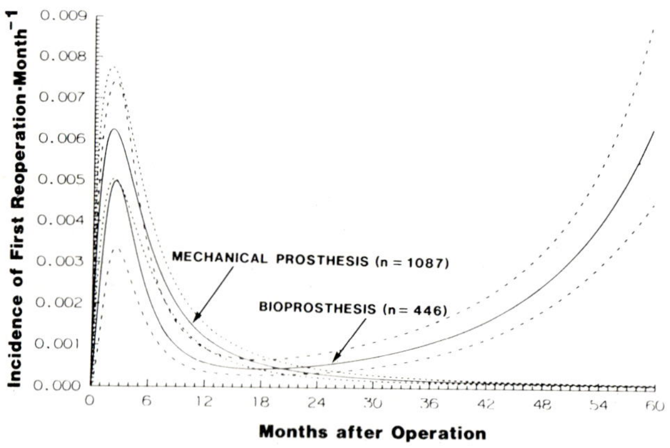

FIGURE 6. Nomogram of the hazard function for reoperation for mechanical prostheses and bioprostheses, determined by separate analyses. In the hazard function for mechanical prostheses there is an early peaking phase and a constant phase; in that for bioprostheses there is an early peaking phase and a second rising late phase.

Although reoperation was not considered as a possible risk factor for death after the original operation, its occurrence in a patient increased the subsequent risk of death (see figure 1). If considered an additional "mode of death," it would be the third most common (table 3).

PVE. The actuarial freedom from PVE after the original valve replacement operation was 97.0% (CL 96.5% to 97.4%) at 1 year and 95.6% (CL 95.0% to 96.2%) at 5 years after the original operation; it was lower after reoperations (figure 7). The hazard function for PVE peaked at 6 weeks after the original operation and then declined to a lower constant hazard function by about 6 months after surgery (figure 8). The early peak of the single hazard function after reoperations was higher than that after the original operation. The incremenetal risk factors were different for

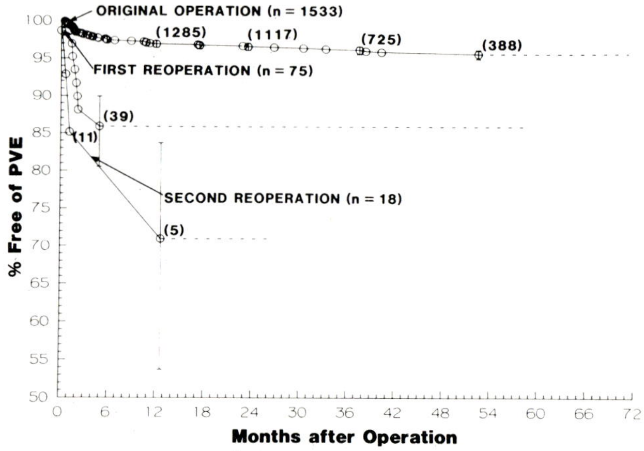

FIGURE 7. Actuarial freedom from PVE after the original valve replacement (54 events) and after reoperations. Note the expanded vertical axis. $p < .0001$ for difference between original operation and first reoperation (eight events); $p = .4$ for the difference between first and second reoperation (three events). PVE was not identified after the third or fourth reoperation.

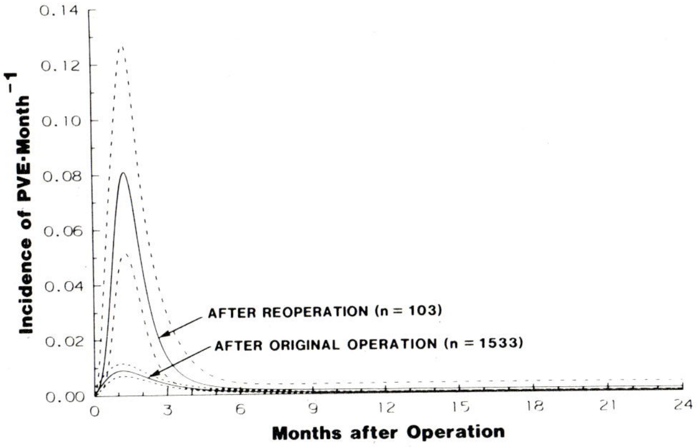

FIGURE 8. Nomogram of the hazard function for PVE after the original valve replacement and after any reoperation (n = 103 in 75 patients). In both hazard functions there is an early peaking phase and a constant phase.

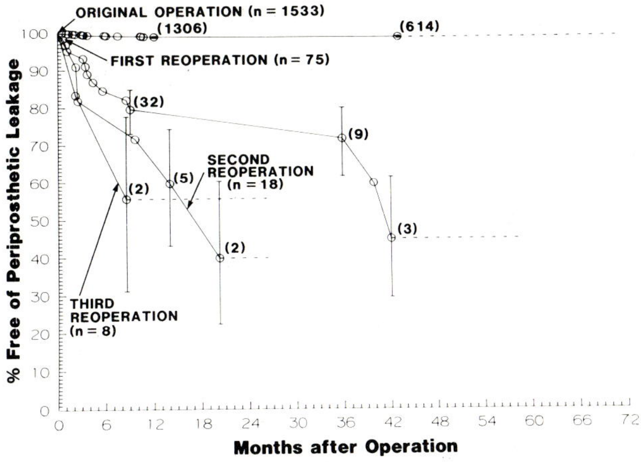

FIGURE 9. Actuarial freedom from periprosthetic leakage without evident infection after the original valve replacement (19 events) and after the first (n = 75, 13 events), second (n = 18, five events), and third (n = 8, two events) reoperations. Periprosthetic leakage did not develop in either of the two patients undergoing a fourth reoperation.

PVE after the original operation compared with that after reoperations (table 6).

Periprosthetic leakage. Actuarial freedom from periprosthetic leakage without evident infection after the original valve replacement operation was 98.8% (CL 98.4% to 99.0%) at 1 year and 98.5% (CL 98.2% to 98.8%) at 5 years. Freedom from periprosthetic leakage was lower after reoperations (figure 9). The single phase hazard function for leakage after the original valve replacement operation peaked at about 2 months after operation and steadily declined thereafter; that after the re-replacement operations was high initially and declined slowly (figure 10). The incremental risk factors for periprosthetic leakage without evident infection after the original valve replacement (table 7) resembled but were not the same as those for PVE (see table 6). Among the 12 patients undergoing suture-repair of periprosthetic leakage without evident infection, only one redeveloped periprosthetic leakage without evident infection; two others subsequently had evident PVE.

The similarities between the two events, PVE and periprosthetic leakage without evident infection, are indicated by the similarity of their risk factors and by the similarity but not identity of their hazard functions (see figures 9 and 10). Also, the hazard function for periprosthetic leakage without evident infection was constant with time after reoperation for periprosthetic leakage, whereas it had a peak at 3 months after reoperation for PVE (figure 11, *A*). The hazard functions for PVE after reoperation for periprosthetic leakage without evident infection and after reoperation for PVE

TABLE 6
Incremental risk factors for PVE after the original valve replacement operation (n = 1533, 54 events) and after reoperation (n = 103 reoperations in 75 patients, 11 events)

	Operation		
	Original valve replacement		Reoperation–single phase (p value)
Incremental risk factors	Constant phase (p value)	Early phase (p value)	
Demographic variables			
Male gender	>.1	.01	.03
Black race	.01	.02	>.1
Endocarditis	>.1	<.0001	>.1
Surgical variables			
Mechanical prosthesis	>.1	.004	>.1
Mitral replacement at original operation	>.1	>.1	.05

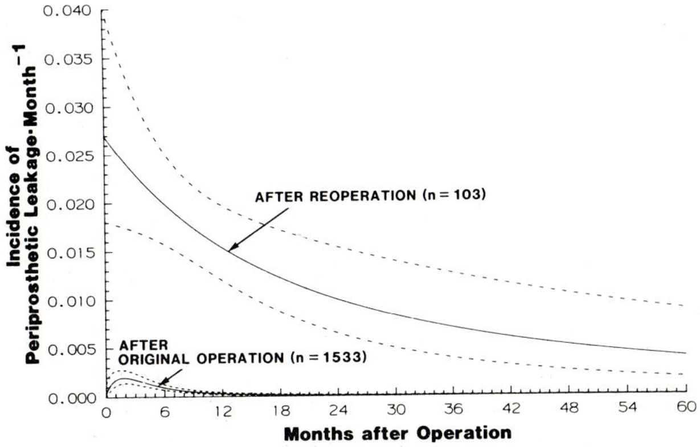

FIGURE 10. Nomogram of the hazard function for periprosthetic leakage without evident infection after the original valve replacement and after any reoperation, determined by separate analyses. In both hazard functions there is only a single phase.

TABLE 7
Incremental risk factors for periprosthetic leakage without evident infection after the original valve replacement operation (n = 1533, 19 events) and after reoperation (n = 103, 20 events)

Incremental risk factors	Operation: Original valve replacement operation–single phase (p value)	Reoperation–single phase (p value)
Demographic variables		
(Younger) age at operation	.02	.1
Male gender	.05	>.1
Black race	.05	.01
Endocarditis	.08	>.1
Surgical variables		
Mitral valve replacement (isolated or combined)	.004	>.1
Valve replacement rather than repair	NA	.08

NA = not applicable.

both peaked at about 6 weeks after surgery and gradually declined toward zero thereafter (figure 11, *B*).

Bioprosthetic degeneration. Actuarial freedom from bioprosthetic degeneration in patients receiving a porcine heterograft fell to 91% (CL 88% to 93%) by 5 years. The hazard function had a single rising phase (figure 12). Young age at the time of insertion of the bioprosthesis ($p < .0001$) and female gender ($p = .02$) were the risk factors for bioprosthetic degeneration. The predicted probability of important bioprosthetic degeneration within 5 years in persons aged 30 years at the time of insertion is 23% for women and 6% for men (figure 13).

Acute prosthetic thrombosis. Actuarial freedom from thrombosis after the original valve replacement was 97.9% (CL 97.4% to 98.4%) at 36 months among patients receiving the Bjork-Shiley prosthesis. The hazard function for acute thrombosis of Bjork-Shiley prostheses peaked at 10 months and declined nearly to zero by 6 years (figure 14). The single risk factor was female gender ($p = .0006$). There was no recurrence of the acute thrombosis in the three patients in whom simple thrombectomy, rather than valve replacement, was done.

Discussion

Special features of the study. The proportion of traced patients in this study is high (99.9%) and the follow-up sufficiently thorough that undetected events are unlikely. The concept of modes, or syndromes, of death (see definition under Materials and methods) has been used to avoid assignment of the cause of death, always a controversial matter. Assignment of a mode of death is not dependent on autopsy data, which are frequently missing, and generally not controversial (see Materials and methods) as compared with "cause of death." Knowledge of the frequency and time-relatedness of the various modes of death, and of their specific risk factors, provides insight into the potential improvements that are most likely to reduce the overall inci-

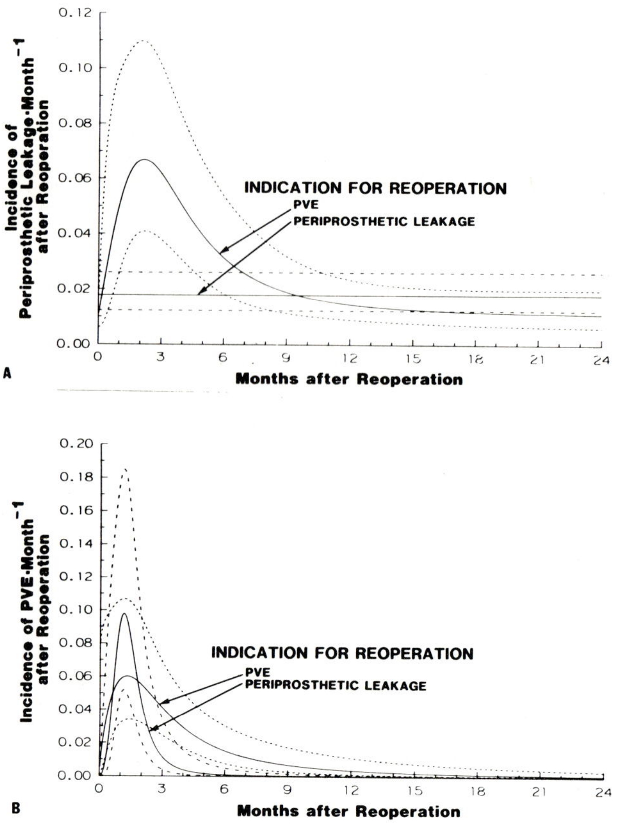

FIGURE 11. Nomograms of the hazard function for periprosthetic leakage without evident infection (*A*) (n = 37) and PVE (*B*) (n = 42) after the primary valve replacement operation, determined separately for patients stratified according to two of the indications for reoperation.

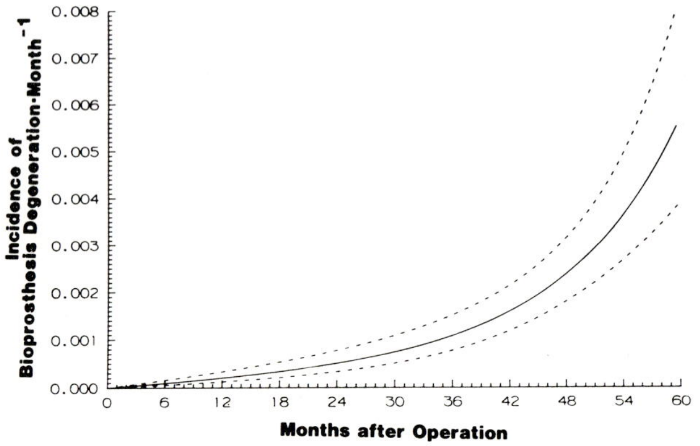

FIGURE 12. Hazard function for bioprosthetic degeneration after the original valve replacement (n = 446). There is only a single phase.

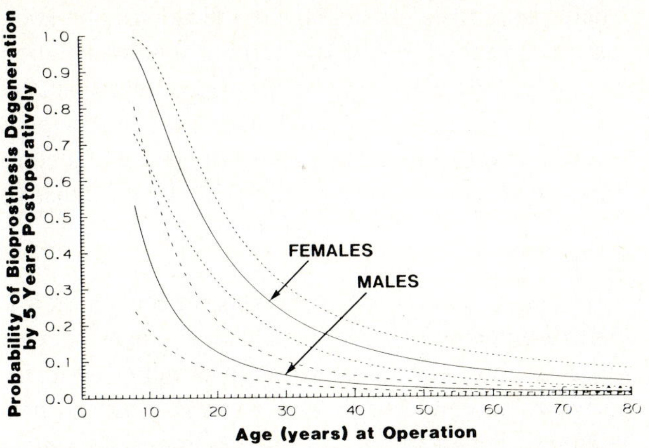

FIGURE 13. Nomogram of the estimated probability of bioprosthetic degeneration within 5 years of insertion, according to the patient's sex and age at insertion.

dence of premature death in patients who have undergone valve replacement. The variability of the autopsy findings within one mode of death, however, indicates the need for caution in using this information.

The relative frequency with which events, including death, occur in the first few months after hospital dismissal makes it evident that the artificiality of emphasizing in-hospital deaths underestimates the incidence of early events. This has been avoided in this study by the use of a method that identifies differing risks across time by decomposing them into hazard phases, with their unique incremental risk factors.

Two important events have not been addressed by this study. One is thromboembolism and the other warfarin-related hemorrhage. There is a considerable degree of uncertainty in attributing death to either of these, but no doubt they have been the causes of some sudden and neurologic deaths.

A limitation of this study is that no prophylactic valve reoperations have been performed in these patients. In all likelihood, there is an overall lower incidence of death and other time-related untoward events after prophylactic valve reoperations than after those done for the indications present in this group of patients. However, the multivariate equation derived from the data in this study (see appendixes 1 and 2) can be used to estimate the probability of death (and other time-related events) in a specific patient after a valve reoperation done prophylactically and in anticipation of failure of a prosthetic valve. The NYHA functional class can be set for that patient, and in the case of most prophylactic operations is I or II. The aortic cross-clamp time can be predicted with reasonable certainty by the surgeon. The other variables in the multivariate equation can also be set specifically for the patient at hand. Thereby the predicted 2 week or 5 year survival can be determined for the patient (as was done in table 2), and these can be compared with those of no reoperation.

The early and late survival probabilities of individual patients being considered for an original valve operation can also be estimated from the multivariate equations in a similar manner. These can be compared with the probability of survival with nonsurgical treatment, as an aid in making the decision about valve replacement.

The data and methodology can also be used to make valid comparisons with experiences in a different era in the same institution or in different institutions, a process that otherwise can be difficult because of potential differences in the age, functional status, and valve lesions of the patients (see appendix 3). Such comparisons can be useful in assessing progress, evaluating the quality of programs, and identifying means of improving results.

Premature death and its modes. The overall 5 year actuarial survival of about 75% is similar to that in previous reports.[9–13] The inadequacy of using hospital survival figures as criteria of the early risks and result of a valve replacement operation is evident from the fact that the early phase of higher risk does not end with hospital dismissal or on postoperative day 30, but rather does not merge with a constant risk phase until about 3 months after operation.

It may be inferred from the data that improvement in survival after valve replacement operations could be achieved by reducing the incidence of deaths with cardiac failure and those that occur suddenly. The risk factors for these two most common modes of death suggest that they are associated with preoperatively important left ventricular secondary cardiomyopathy and dysfunction. The deaths in these modes that occur in the very early days after operation might be reduced

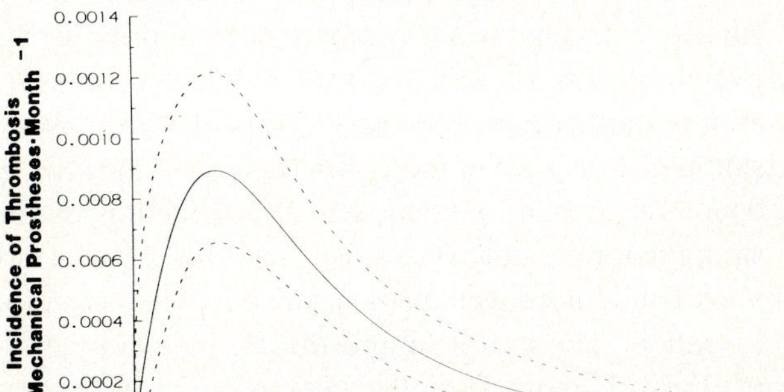

FIGURE 14. Nomogram of the hazard function for acute thrombosis of a Bjork-Shiley prosthesis after insertion at the original operation (n = 1084), 19 events). There is only a single phase in the hazard function.

by better myocardial protection and a more efficient surgical technique with its shorter cross-clamp time (see figure 4). The deaths occurring later in the early phase and in the constant phase are unlikely to be improved by these measures and may be inevitable once the existing degree of ventricular disease has developed. Therefore, in the ongoing management of patients with valvular heart disease, the competing risks of continuation of the natural evolution of the ventricular disease (which appears to be particularly disadvantageous in the case of aortic incompetence and mitral valve disease) and those of prompt valve replacement must be repeatedly reconsidered. The adverse effect of ischemic mitral incompetence on late survival, also observed by Kay et al.,[14] is no doubt related to its association with important ischemic cardiomyopathy, and once developed this probably has an immutable detrimental effect on late survival. Therefore its prevention is also to be stressed.

Although the event reoperation followed by death was not considered as a mode of death in a formal way (see table 3), it does account for 40 deaths (the third most common "mode") among the original 1533 patients and does have an early phase of high risk after operation (see figure 2). Favorably influencing the risk factors for the indications for reoperation (PVE, periprosthetic leakage without evident infection, valve thrombosis, and bioprosthetic degeneration) would reduce the overall risk of premature death after valve replacement. PVE, usually with periprosthetic leakage, is often difficult to distinguish from periprosthetic leakage through evident infection. The similarities between the risk factors for PVE and those for periprosthetic leakage without evident infection, and the similarities between the hazard functions of these two events, suggest that some of the latter may in fact be instances of PVE. A precise surgical technique, scrupulous attention to the details of asepsis, and effective antibiotic prophylaxis are important in improving the overall results of primary valve replacement operations. Furthermore, the hairy chests of men may result in the presence of more skin bacteria at the time of operation than in women, and the reduction of the strength of male gender as a risk factor for these events may require improved methods of skin preparation for operation. The use of bioprostheses, including cryopreserved homografts in the aortic position, whenever there is native valve endocarditis or PVE could be expected to minimize these complications and thus the need for reoperation.[3, 15]

Because the increase in risk of premature death after valve replacement that is associated with older age is small, patients should not be advised against operation just because they are elderly. Neither should operation be advised prematurely, on the basis of advancing years. The association of black race with an increased hazard of premature death in the early phase of a number of modes may be related to the higher incidence of hypertension and left ventricular hypertrophy in blacks.

The study does not provide support for the preference of bioprostheses over mechanical valves, or vice versa, except when the operation is being done for native valve endocarditis (see above). Although bioprosthetic degeneration, a slow process in older male patients (see figure 13), may require reoperation, the risk of this is low when done while the patient's functional status is good (see table 2). The relative rapidity of bioprosthetic degeneration in persons less than about 45 years old, and especially in women, cautions against the use of bioprostheses in such individuals.

Reoperation. There is a tendency to consider valve reoperation after an original valve replacement operation as a benign event, but this is not supported by this study. An increasing risk of complications after multiple valve reoperations has also been reported by Sandza et al.[17] This and the increased risks of death, reoperation, PVE, and periprosthetic leakage without evident infection after valve reoperations make it apparent that every effort should be made to make the first operation a lasting one.

PVE. Although PVE occurs uncommonly after an original valve replacement operation, it is a serious complication with a mortality of 63% in the patients in this series[3] and a similar mortality in the experience of others.[18, 19] Its early peaking hazard phase is probably caused by organisms present in the patient's valve area or introduced there at the time of operation, whereas its constant phase is probably related to transient bacteremias during which organisms lodge in the valve area.[3] It is likely that the contention of Miller et al.[18] that the hazard of this event across time is constant resulted from their failure to decompose in detail the early period after operation.

Periprosthetic leakage without evident infection. In view of the data in this study, when the leakage is mild, nothing should be done surgically because the reoperation in this setting carries the same risks of untoward postoperative events as do other reoperations. When reoperation is indicated and there is no suggestion that PVE is present, the data support the use of repair of the leakage whenever possible, rather than rereplacement.

Bioprosthetic degeneration. The particular tendency of

young patients to develop degeneration of porcine bioprostheses, previously reported by Magilligan et al.,[20] Dunn,[21] Geha et al.,[22] Williams et al.,[23] and others is again emphasized by this study. The association of female gender with an increased risk of bioprosthetic degeneration has not been noted previously. The inference from these analyses is that currently available porcine bioprostheses should not be used, with rare exceptions, in women less than about 55 years of age and in men less than about 45 years of age.

Acute valve thrombosis. The early and transiently peaking hazard function of this low-frequency event in addition to the untoward events that tend to follow valve re-replacement suggest the advisability of declotting the prosthetic valve, rather than replacing it, whenever possible. This very important complication is not limited to the Bjork-Shiley valve, which was the type of mechanical device used nearly exclusively in the patients in this study, but was experienced by one patient in this series with a bioprosthesis, has been seen by us in one patient with a St. Jude Medical valve, and is reported by Miller et al.[18] as occurring in patients receiving the Starr-Edwards Silastic ball valve mitral prosthesis.

We appreciate the cooperation of our surgical colleagues, Drs. R. B. Karp, N. T. Kouchoukos, A. D. Pacifico, G. L. Zorn, and J. K. Kirklin, for permitting us to include patients operated on by them in this study and for assisting us in the interpretation of the data. Drs. Joseph Defauw, Janardan Dhasmana, Torjborn Ivert, Richard A. Reynolds, Ismail Sallam, Steven Westaby, and Frederick Wideman, as well as Robert Brown, Kathy Peterson, and Phyllis Smith, assisted in obtaining the follow-up data. Sandy O'Brien assisted in the preparation of the graphics. Drs. David Naftel and Malcolm Turner, Department of Biostatistics and Biomathematics, collaborated with us in the statistical work. Nancy Ferguson and Debbie Nuby contributed greatly in the formation of the tables and the typing and editing of the manuscript.

References

1. Conti VR, Bertranou EG, Blackstone EH, Kirklin JW, Digerness SB: Cold cardioplegia versus hypothermia for myocardial protection: randomized clinical study. J Thorac Cardiovasc Surg **76:** 577, 1978
2. Kannel WB, Gordon T: Cardiovascular diseases and death following myocardial infarction and angina pectoris: Framingham Study, 20-year follow-up. *In* The Framingham Study: an epidemiological investigation of cardiovascular diseases. Section 32, Bethesda, 1977, U. S. Department of Health, Education, and Welfare, Public Health Service, National Institutes of Health
3. Ivert TSA, Dismukes WE, Cobbs CG, Blackstone EH, Kirklin JW, Bergdahl LAL: Prosthetic valve endocarditis. Circulation **69:** 223, 1984
4. Dhasmana JP, Blackstone EH, Kirklin JW, Kouchoukos NT: Factors associated with periprosthetic leakage following primary mitral valve replacement: with special consideration of the suture technique. Ann Thorac Surg **35:** 170, 1983
5. Kaplan EL, Meier P: Nonparametric estimation from incomplete observations. J Am Stat Assoc **53:** 457, 1958
6. Gehan EA: A generalized Wilcoxon test for comparing arbitrarily singly-censored samples. Biometrika **52:** 203, 1965
7. Blackstone EH, Naftel DC, Turner ME Jr: The decomposition of time-varying hazard into phases, each incorporating a separate stream of concomitant information. J Am Stat Assoc (in press)
8. Kirklin JW: A letter to Helen. J Thorac Cardiovasc Surg **78:** 643, 1979
9. Barnhorst DA, Oxman HA, Connolly DC, Pluth JR, Danielson GK, Wallace RB, McGoon DC: Long-term follow-up of isolated replacement of the aortic or mitral valve with the Starr-Edwards prosthesis. Am J Cardiol **35:** 228, 1975
10. Karp RB, Cyrus RJ, Blackstone EH, Kirklin JW, Kouchoukos NT, Pacifico AD: The Bjork-Shiley valve: intermediate-term follow-up. J Thorac Cardiovasc Surg **8:** 602, 1981
11. Tepley JF, Grunkemeier GL, Sutherland HD, Lambert LE, Johnson VA, Starr A: The ultimate prognosis after valve replacement: an assessment at twenty years. Ann Thorac Surg **32:** 111, 1981
12. Cheung D, Flemma RJ, Mullen DC, Lepley D Jr, Anderson AJ, Weirauch E: Ten-year follow-up in aortic valve replacement using the Bjork-Shiley prosthesis. Ann Thorac Surg **32:** 138, 1981
13. Macmanus Q, Grunkemeier GL, Lambert LE, Starr A: Non-cloth-covered caged-ball prostheses: the second decade. J Thorac Cardiovasc Surg **76:** 788, 1978
14. Kay PH, Nunley DL, Grunkemeier GL, Pinson CW, Starr A: Late results of combined mitral valve replacement and coronary bypass surgery. J Am Coll Cardiol **5:** 29, 1985
15. Kirklin JW, Barratt-Boyes BG: Aortic valve disease. *In* Cardiac surgery. New York, 1985, John Wiley and Sons, ch 12, p 409
16. Miller DC, Oyer PE, Stinson EB, Reitz BA, Jamieson SW, Baumgartner WA, Mitchell RS, Shumway NE: Ten to fifteen year reassessment of the performance characteristics of the Starr-Edwards Model 6120 mitral valve prosthesis. (Discussion) J Thorac Cardiovasc Surg **85:** 19, 1983
17. Sandza JG Jr, Clark RE, Ferguson TB, Connors JP, Weldon CS: Replacement of prosthetic heart valves: a fifteen-year experience. J Thorac Cardiovasc Surg **74:** 864, 1977
18. Miller DC, Oyer PE, Stinson EB, Reitz BA, Jamieson SW, Baumgartner WA, Mitchell RS, Shumway NE: Ten to fifteen year reassessment of the performance characteristics of the Starr-Edwards Model 6120 mitral valve prosthesis. J Thorac Cardiovasc Surg **85:** 1, 1983
19. Miller DC, Oyer PE, Mitchell RS, Stinson EB, Jamieson SW, Baldwin JC, Shumway NE: Performance characteristics of the Starr-Edwards Model 1260 aortic valve prosthesis beyond ten years. J Thorac Cardiovasc Surg **88:** 193, 1984
20. Magilligan DJ Jr, Lewis JW Jr, Jara FM, Lee MW, Alam M, Riddle JM, Stein PD: Spontaneous degeneration of porcine bioprosthetic valves. Ann Thorac Surg **30:** 259, 1980
21. Dunn JM: Porcine valve durability in children. Ann Thorac Surg **32:** 357, 1981
22. Geha AS, Laks H, Stansel HC, Cornhill JF, Kilman JW, Buckley MJ, Roberts WC: Late failure of procine valve heterografts in children. J Thorac Cardiovasc Surg **78:** 351, 1979
23. Williams JB, Karp RB, Kirklin JW, Kouchoukos NT, Pacifico AD, Zorn GL Jr, Blackstone EH, Brown RN, Piantadosi S, Bradley EL: Consideration in selection and management of patients undergoing valve replacement with gluteraldehyde-fixed porcine bioprostheses. Ann Thorac Surg **30:** 247, 1980

Appendix 1

Identification of the structure and risk factors of the time-related distribution of events

The parametric method is conceptualized in the cumulative hazard domain $\Lambda(t)$. Cumulative hazard is related to the survivorship function S(t) by the expression:

$$S(t) = \exp\left[-\Lambda(t)\right] \quad (1)$$

and to the hazard function $\lambda(t)$ by its first derivative with respect to time (exp is the base of the natural logarithms). The system considers up to three additive phases of hazard:

$$\Lambda(t) = \mu_1 G_1(t) + \mu_2 G_2(t) + \mu_3 G_3(t) \quad (2)$$

The μ's are scaling parameters and G's are shaping parameters.

$$G_1(t) = \left[1 - \frac{m}{|m|}\left(\frac{m+|m|}{2|m|} + \frac{\alpha t}{|m|v}\right)^{-v}\right]^{m} \quad (3)$$

represents early, decreasing risk (or a risk that rises transiently then declines). Based on the data in this study, its parameters and forumula were simplified to:

$$G_1(t) = 1 / \left[1 + (\rho / t)^v\right],\ g_1(t) = G_1(v / t) / \left[1 + (\rho / t)^v\right] \quad (4)$$

where $g_1(t)$ is the representation of $G_1(t)$ in the hazard domain, ρ represents the half-time for early cumulative hazard, and v determines the shape of the hazard function in the vicinity of time zero.

$$G_2(t) = t,\ g_2(t) = 1 \quad (5)$$

represents a constant hazard phase that is present throughout the experience.

$$G_3(t) = \left[\exp(t / \delta)^{\gamma} - 1\right]^{\eta} \quad (6)$$

represents the increasing late phase of hazard. In this study, $\gamma = 2$ and $\eta = 1$ throughout, so only δ has been estimated, which corresponds to the time at which the hazard function begins to rise steeply. With these simplifications:

$$g_3(t) = 2t\left[\exp(t / \delta)^2\right] / \delta^2 \quad (7)$$

The scaling parameters were made parametric functions of concomitant information (possible risk factors):

$$\mu_1 = \ln\left[1 + \exp(\underset{\sim}{\beta}{}_1' \underset{\sim}{\times}{}_1)\right] \quad (8)$$

where ln is the natural logarithm and

$$\underset{\sim}{\beta}{}_1' \underset{\sim}{\times}{}_1 = \beta_0 + \beta_1 \times_1 + \beta_2 \times_2 + \ldots \beta_k \times_k \quad (9)$$

that is, a linear regression model. Equation 8 is the logistic equation, expressed in cumulative hazard. The parametric scaling function for the constant and increasing hazard phases are log-linear (proportional hazards) regression models:

$$\mu_2 = \exp(\underset{\sim}{\beta}{}_2' \underset{\sim}{\times}{}_2) \quad (10)$$

and

$$\mu_3 = \exp(\underset{\sim}{\beta}{}_3' \underset{\sim}{\times}{}_3) \quad (11)$$

All parameters and regression coefficients were estimated simultaneously by the method of maximum likelihood. Structural parsimony of the model was determined by the likelihood ratio test. Asymptotic p values for regression coefficients were based on the ratio of each coefficient to its standard deviation, and confidence limits for estimated functions were determined by the method of statistical differentials.

Appendix 2

Parameter estimates and regression coefficients

For each event analyzed, shaping parameter estimates and intercepts are given for the parametric estimates of events across time (hazard function and survivorship function); these plus regression coefficients are given from the multivariate analysis of the event. These are organized according to their time of influence on the hazard function: throughout and constant, early and decreasing, and late and increasing. For dichotomous variables, the presence of the stated factor takes on the value of 1, its absence 0; thus its coefficient is used when the factor is present and not used when it is absent. In the text, an average value for a dichotomous variable is used occasionally; in this case, that value is multiplied by the listed coefficient. For continuous variables, the units of the variable are multiplied by the coefficient in the equation.

(1) Death
Parametric estimate. Constant phase: intercept −5.816. Early phase: $\rho = 2.515$, $v = 0.5333$, intercept −1.852.
Parametric multivariate estimates. Constant phase: intercept −6.802, age 0.01531, black race 0.8899, ischemic mitral incompetence 1.271. Early phase: $\rho = 3.333$, $v = 0.5209$, intercept −7.714, age 0.2493, aortic incompetence 0.8924, mitral valve stenosis and/or incompetence × NYHA functional class (interaction term) 0.4602, NYHA functional class 1.100, cardioplegia −1.901, aortic cross-clamp time if cardioplegia was used 0.0284, combined mitral and aortic valve replacement 1.601, combined mitral and aortic valve replacement × aortic cross-clamp time (with cardioplegia) −0.01384.

(2) Death after first reoperation
Parametric estimate. Constant phase: intercept −4.214. Early phase: $\rho = 0.001882$, $v = 1.958$, intercept −1.763.

(3) Death after all reoperations
Parametric estimate. Constant phase: intercept −3.862. Early phase: $\rho = 0.003302$, $v = 1$, intercept −1.483.
Parametric multivariate estimates. Constant phase: intercept −5.516, mitral valve stenosis and/or insufficiency at original operation 1.342, mechanical prosthesis 1.154. Early phase: intercept −7.133, reoperation number 0.7679, NYHA functional class 1.093.

(4) Death with cardiac failure
Parametric estimate. Constant phase: intercept −7.291. Early phase: $\rho = 0.3770$, $v = 0.5954$, intercept −3.052.
Parametric multivariate estimates. Constant phase: intercept −7.464, black race 1.085, ischemic mitral incompetence 2.322. Early phase: $\rho = 0.3718$, $v = 0.6023$, intercept −11.71, age 0.04575, aortic incompetence 1.100, mitral valve stenosis and/or incompetence 1.946, NYHA functional class 1.290, cardioplegia −2.235, aortic cross-clamp time if cardioplegia was used 0.02101, tricuspid procedure 1.116, coronary artery bypass grafting 0.9684.

(5) Sudden death
Parametric esimate. Constant phase: intercept −7.531. Early phase: $\rho = 1.434$, $v = 1.736$, intercept −3.772.
Parametric multivariate estimates. Constant phase: intercept −8.913, males 1.453, use of bioprosthesis 0.7277. Early phase: $\rho = 1.488$, $v = 1.986$, intercept −6.505, aortic incompetence 0.7533, mitral valve stenosis and/or incompetence 0.9012, NYHA functional class 0.6577.

(6) Neurologic death
Parametric estimate. Constant phase: intercept −7.630.
Parametric multivariate estimates. Constant phase: intercept −10.85, age 0.05478.

(7) Death with cancer
Parametric estimate. Constant phase: intercept −7.748.
Parametric multivariate estimates. Constant phase: intercept −10.20, age 0.04231.

(8) Death with hemorrhage
Parametric estimate. Early phase: ρ = 0.004278, ν = 1.650, intercept −4.925.
Parametric multivariate estimates. Early phase: ρ = 0.004333, ν = 1.648, intercept −13.07, age 0.0651, NYHA functional class 1.082, aortic cross-clamp time if cardioplegia was used 0.01644.

(9) Death with infection
Parametric estimate. Early phase: ρ = 1.249, ν = 2.900, intercept −5.066.

(10) Death with arrhythmias
Parametric estimate. Early phase: ρ = 1.538, ν = 1.585, intercept −5.300.

(11) Death in other cardiac modes
Parametric estimate. Constant phase: intercept −8.980.

(12) Death with trauma
Parametric estimate. Constant phase: intercept −9.134.

(13) Death in miscellaneous modes
Parametric estimate. Constant phase: intercept −8.093.

(14) Death with uncertain modes
Parametric estimate. Early phase: ρ = 39.62, ν = 1, intercept −3.173.

(15) Reoperation
Parametric estimate. Early phase: ρ = 4.522, ν = 1.724, intercept −3.107. Increasing phase: δ = 55.18, intercept −4.525.

(16) Reoperation for mechanical prostheses
Parametric estimate. Constant phase: intercept −9.520. Early phase: ρ = 5.097, ν = 1.594, intercept −2.938.

(17) Reoperation for bioprostheses
Parametric estimate. Early phase: ρ = 3.847, ν = 2.090, intercept −3.536. Increasing phase: δ = 42.42, intercept −4.358.

(18) PVE after original operation
Parametric estimate. Constant phase: intercept −8.028. Early phase: ρ = 1.956, ν = 2.056, intercept −3.648.
Parametric multivariate estimates. Constant phase: intercept −8.330, black race 1.514. Early phase: ρ = 2.104, ν = 2.073, intercept −7.098, males 1.210, black race 1.169, native valve endocarditis 2.364, mechanical prosthesis 1.816.

(19) PVE after all reoperations
Parametric estimate. Early phase: ρ = 1.940, ν = 2.183, intercept −1.723.
Parametric multivariate estimates. Early phase: ρ = 2.049, ν = 2.158, intercept −4.282, males 2.490, mitral valve replacement at original operation 1.457.

(20) Periprosthetic leakage after original operation
Parametric estimate. Early phase: ρ = 4.416, ν = 1.613, intercept −4.239.
Parametric multivariate estimates. Early phase: 4.681, ν = 1.595, intercept −4.520, age −0.03727, males 1.076, black race 1.033, native valve endocarditis 1.128, mitral valve replacement (isolated or combined) 1.700.

(21) Periprosthetic leakage after all reoperations
Parametric estimate. Early phase: ρ = 36.93, ν = 1, intercept 0.5335.
Parametric multivariate estimates. Constant phase: intercept −5.567, age −0.02448, black race 1.383, valve replacement rather than repair 1.804.

(22) PVE after reoperation when PVE was indication for reoperation
Parametric estimate. Early phase: ρ = 3.000, ν = 1.661, intercept −1.071.

(23) Periprosthetic leakage after reoperation when PVE was indication for reoperation
Parametric estimate. Constant phase: intercept −4.562. Early phase: ρ = 3.645, ν = 2.025, intercept −0.9921.

(24) PVE after reoperation when periprosthetic leakage was indication for reoperation
Parametric estimate. Early phase: ρ = 1.379, ν = 3.257, intercept −1.816.

(25) Periprosthetic leakage when periprosthetic leakage was indication for reoperation
Parametric estimate. Constant phase: intercept −4.027.

(26) Bioprosthetic degeneration
Parametric estimate. Increasing phase: δ = 45.22, intercept −4.127.
Parametric multivariate estimates. Increasing phase: δ = 39.52, intercept 1.459, age (natural logarithm) −1.893, females 1.443.

(27) Acute prosthetic thrombosis
Parametric estimate. Early phase: ρ = 18.33, ν = 1.817, intercept −3.632.
Parametric multivariate estimates. Early phase: ρ = 18.94, ν = 1.799, intercept −4.165, females (if mitral valve replacement) 1.611.

Appendix 3

Comparison of differing experiences

A rigorous comparison of the results of different experiences requires the actual combination of the data sets; this is usually not feasible. Alternatively, the same multivariate analysis model can be fitted to differing experiences and the shaping and risk factor coefficients compared; this is also often not feasible. The approach most often possible is the application of the model from one study, such as that presented in appendixes 1 and 2, to the new experience in each of two ways. First, from the multivariate equation the expected incidence of an event (cumulative hazard function) can be calculated for each patient, with his specific incremental risk factors and his duration of follow-up. The summation of these individual cumulative hazard incidences totals the number of events *expected* in the total patient group. A chi-square test of the difference between the number of *observed* and expected events is then performed to determine whether that difference is greater than that expected by chance. This method gives an overall comparison of experiences.

Second, parametric survivorship functions, representing freedom from the event of interest, can be generated for each patient from the multivariate analysis. The average of these curves, with its confidence limit (a reasonable approximation to the expected curve for the given prevalence of risk factors) is compared with the observed actuarial estimate for the second group with its confidence limits.

Noninvasively diagnosed peripheral arterial disease as a predictor of mortality: results from a prospective study

MICHAEL H. CRIQUI, M.D., M.P.H., STEVEN S. COUGHLIN, M.P.H., AND ARNOST FRONEK, M.D., PH.D.

ABSTRACT Intermittent claudication has been reported in previous studies to approximately double the risk of subsequent mortality. However, a history of claudication is often present in the absence of significant peripheral arterial disease (PAD) and absent in the presence of PAD. For this reason we evaluated the association between large-vessel and small-vessel PAD, measured by highly reliable and valid noninvasive tests, and mortality in 567 older subjects from a defined population followed-up for an average of 4 years. Large-vessel PAD was strongly and significantly predictive of all-cause mortality in both men and women with a relative risk of 4 to 5, and this finding was independent of other cardiovascular disease risk factors in multivariable analysis. In addition, this finding persisted after exclusion of subjects with extant cardiovascular disease at baseline. The associations of both claudication and abnormal peripheral pulses with mortality were weaker than the large-vessel PAD association. Isolated small-vessel PAD was unrelated to subsequent mortality. These findings suggest older subjects of both sexes at a high risk of impending mortality can be identified through noninvasive testing for large-vessel PAD.
Circulation 72, No. 4, 768–773, 1985.

IT IS well recognized that the atherosclerotic process is frequently generalized, affecting vessels in various parts of the body. Previous reports have noted the strong association between coronary heart disease and peripheral arterial disease (PAD) and the similarity of risk factors, particularly cigarette smoking and diabetes, for both diseases.[1, 2] Concordant with these observations, the symptomatic expression of PAD, intermittent claudication, has been noted to be predictive of mortality in previous studies, with an approximate doubling of risk.[1, 3, 4] However, after adjustment for risk factors and signs and symptoms of coexisting coronary heart disease, this risk tends to be reduced, suggesting claudication may not be an *independent* marker for mortality.[3]

It is evident that considerable "noise" is present in such analyses, since in population studies, many subjects who report typical symptoms of claudication may not have PAD and many subjects with PAD have atypical or no symptoms.[5–7] In a population-based study of older subjects, we used highly reliable and accurate noninvasive techniques to measure PAD, and here report the mortality experience of subjects with and without noninvasively measured PAD after 4 years of follow-up. We also analyzed the prognostic significance of claudication and pulse palpation for mortality as compared with noninvasive testing.

From the Departments of Community and Family Medicine, and Surgery and Bioengineering, University of California, San Diego, and the Graduate School of Public Health, San Diego State University.

Supported by NIH grant HL 22255. Dr. Criqui is a recipient of a Research Career Development Award (HL 00946) from the NHLBI.

Addres for correspondence: Michael H. Criqui, M.D., M.P.H., Division of Epidemiology, Department of Community and Family Medicine, M-007, University of California, San Diego, La Jolla, CA 92093.

Received April 8, 1985; revision accepted July 18, 1985.

Methods

All 624 subjects were residents of a geographically defined community initially studied under a Lipid Research Clinics (LRC) protocol that involved two evaluations, visit 1 and visit 2.[8] At visit 2, about half of the subjects were from a random sample of the LRC visit 1 cohort and the others were selected from the visit 1 cohort for hyperlipidemia, defined as being at or above age- and sex-specific 90th percentiles for cholesterol or 95th percentiles for triglycerides or taking lipid-lowering medications. The PAD study involved a subset of visit 2 subjects, and the PAD subjects were comparable to visit 2 subjects with regard to age, sex, and the proportion with hyperlipidemia (47.9%). Subjects were from a predominantly white, upper-middle-class community in southern California, and informed consent was obtained after the procedures had been fully explained.

Fifty-seven subjects (9.1%) were excluded from these analyses because of missing data or unreliable noninvasive testing results. Two hundred and fifty-seven men and 310 women ranging in age from 38 to 82 years with an average age of 66 years remained.

Criteria for PAD measurements

Intermittent claudication. Claudication was assessed by the standard Rose Questionnaire developed at the London School of Hygiene and Tropical Medicine.[9] Claudication was defined by the Rose criteria: exercise calf pain not present at rest relieved within 10 min only by rest. We also defined as "possible" claudication, exercise calf pain not present at rest but otherwise not fully concordant with the Rose criteria. The remaining subjects, including subjects with leg pain at rest and subjects with exercise pain not including the calf, were categorized as not having claudication.

Pulse palpation. On 508 (89.6%) of the subjects, a single examiner performed a standardized bilateral palpation of the femoral, posterior tibial, and dorsalis pedis arteries with pulses subjectively graded from 0 to 4, and auscultation of the groin for femoral bruits. Pulses lower than grade 3 or audible bruits were considered abnormal. This examination was done before noninvasive testing, and the examiner was unaware of the subject's responses to the claudication questionnaire.

Noninvasive testing. Four different noninvasive measurements of limb perfusion in the lower extremities were made: segmental blood pressure, flow velocity, postocclusive reactive hyperemia, and pulse reappearance half-time.

SEGMENTAL BLOOD PRESSURE. The ratio of arm systolic blood pressure to pressure at five different levels of the lower extremity (upper thigh, above knee, below knee, above ankle, and toe) were recorded by the sphygmomanometric technique and a mercury-in-Silastic gauge attached to the toe.[10–12]

FLOW VELOCITY. The Doppler effect produced by back-scattered ultrasound from red blood cells in motion was used to measure flow velocity in the femoral and posterior tibial arteries.[13]

POSTOCCLUSIVE REACTIVE HYPEREMIA. The phenomenon was used to mimic exercise blood flow requirements. Arterial flow was halted by inflating a cuff below the knee to a suprasystolic value for 4 min. Upon release of the cuff, the Doppler flow velocity response (reactive hyperemia) was recorded from the femoral artery. The percentage increase above baseline as well as the time for the response to return to 50% of peak were recorded.[14]

PULSE REAPPEARANCE HALF-TIME. Simultaneously with the postocclusive reactive hyperemia test, the pulse reappearance half-time, or time it took after releasing the cuff for the pulse amplitude to reach one-half the baseline value, was recorded.[15]

Large-vessel PAD. Large-vessel PAD was defined as either an abnormal segment–to–arm blood pressure ratio ($LV_{BP}+$) or an abnormal large-vessel flow velocity ($LV_{FV}+$).

$LV_{BP}+$ was defined as

(both an above ankle and below knee ratio $\leq$ 0.8)

or

(an above ankle *or* below knee ratio $\leq$ 0.8, *and* [a toe ratio $\leq$ 0.7 *or* an above knee ratio $\leq$ 0.8 *or* an upper thigh ratio $\leq$ 0.8])

$LV_{FV}+$ was defined as *either* a

(femoral peak forward flow of $\leq$ 20 cm/sec)

and

(a femoral pulse decay of $\geq$ 260 msec *or* a femoral deceleration of $\leq$ 100 cm/sec^2)

or

(a posterior tibial peak forward flow of $\leq$ 10 cm/sec)

and

(a posterior tibial pulse decay of $\geq$ 220 msec *or* a posterior tibial deceleration of $\leq$ 70 cm/sec^2)

Although these tests measure dynamic aspects of perfusion rather than the degree of anatomic obstruction, they have been demonstrated to have a very high correlation with moderate or greater large-vessel PAD determined angiographically.[10–13]

Small-vessel PAD. Small-vessel PAD was defined by an isolated toe pressure abnormality or a pulse reappearance half-time abnormality or a combination of abnormalities in pulse reappearance half-time, postocclusive reactive hyperemia, and time for hyperemic response to fall to 50% of peak. Specifically, the presence of small-vessel PAD was defined as

(a toe ratio $\leq$0.7 with the above ankle ratio *and* the below knee ratio normal)

or

(a pulse reappearance half-time $\geq$20 sec)

or

(a pulse reappearance half-time $\geq$15 sec *and* a postocclusive reactive hyperemia $\leq$75% *and* time for hyperemic response to fall to 50% of peak $\geq$40 sec)

The cutpoints chosen represent extreme values from previous studies of normal control subjects.[14, 15] Because small-vessel PAD cannot be reliably assessed angiographically, anatomic correlation of these tests is impractical.

Surgery for PAD. Subjects were asked whether they had ever had surgery for poor circulation to the extremities, other than for varicose veins, and the nature and location of the surgery. Subjects with documented surgery for PAD underwent the noninvasive testing along with other subjects. For this analysis, surgical subjects were arbitrarily considered to have had large-vessel PAD.

Covariates. Age at last birthday and past and current cigarette smoking were determined by questionnaire. Pack-years was chosen as the smoking variable, rather than current smoking, because of both the low prevalence of current smokers in this older population and the possibility of selective cessation of smoking in ill individuals. A past history of angina, myocardial infarction, or stroke were also determined by questionnaire.

Blood pressure was measured in the sitting position with a random zero sphygmomanometer.[16] High-density (HDL), low-density (LDL), and very low–density (VLDL) lipoprotein cholesterol levels were measured by standardized LRC Program methods.[17]

Dependent variables. The dependent variable was all-cause mortality during an average follow-up time of approximately 4 years. The study population is surveyed routinely on an annual basis as part of an ongoing LRC follow-up study, and reported deaths are confirmed by obtaining death certificates. The underlying cause of death on each death certificate was determined, but the small number of deaths (30) precluded cause-specific multivariable analyses.

Statistical analysis. Sex-specific, unadjusted death rates by claudication, pulse palpation, and PAD categories, as well as simple relative risks, were calculated. Two categories of PAD were evaluated: large-vessel PAD, with or without concomitant small-vessel PAD, and isolated small-vessel PAD, both compared with subjects free of any PAD. The category of *isolated* small-vessel PAD was defined because of the possibility that small-vessel PAD accompanying large-vessel PAD might reflect, to some degree, reduced small-vessel flow as a result of proximal stenoses in larger vessels. Adjustment for covariates, including age, was performed with the Cox proportional hazards model, which calculates the statistical significance for each variable in the model and which also adjusts for differences in follow-up time for deceased subjects.[18] Subjects with isolated small-vessel PAD were excluded from Cox models evaluating the risk of large-vessel PAD and subjects with large-vessel PAD were excluded from Cox models evaluating the risk of isolated small-vessel PAD.

Results

Table 1 shows the sex-specific and combined crude mortality rates in subjects with large-vessel PAD or isolated small-vessel PAD vs subjects with normal results of noninvasive testing. Sixty-nine of 567 subjects (12.2%) had large-vessel PAD, and an additional 90 (15.9%) had isolated small-vessel PAD. The overall death rate was 30 of 567 (5.3%). However, 14 of the 69 subjects with large-vessel PAD (20.3%), died in the follow-up period compared with five of the 90 subjects with isolated small-vessel PAD (5.6%) and 11 of the 408 (2.7%) subjects without PAD, giving crude relative risks of mortality of 7.5 for large-vessel PAD and 2.1 for isolated small-vessel PAD. Although death rates were lower overall in women (3.2% vs 7.8% in men), the *relative* risk for large-vessel PAD for death was, if anything, greater in women (8.2 vs 6.8 in men).

Table 2 shows that the preponderance of deaths were cardiovascular in the groups with large-vessel PAD and isolated small-vessel PAD, whereas among subjects with normal findings the majority of deaths were from cancer. The numbers of deaths were too small for reliable inference concerning cause-specific mortality. However, the crude relative risk of large-vessel PAD for cardiovascular death (11.8), was much greater than the relative risk for cancer (4.2).

Table 3 presents relative risks for Rose claudication, Rose or possible claudication, and abnormal pulse examination (defined as a femoral bruit or a diminished or absent femoral or posterior tibial pulse). For all subjects the relative risk for Rose claudication was 1.9, which improved to 3.7 when possible claudication was added. The relative risk for abnormal pulse examination was similar at 3.4. However, each of these values were less than half the relative risk for noninvasively measured large-vessel PAD.

To distinguish the extent to which the large-vessel PAD mortality association was confounded by, alternatively, age and sex, the traditional cardiovascular disease risk factors, or extant cardiovascular disease at baseline, three sets of Cox models were run.

Table 4 shows the first set of Cox model results with only age, sex, and large-vessel PAD entered as predictor variables. A decade of aging independently increased the risk of death about 69% and men were at about twice the risk of women. Both results were of borderline statistical significance. However, large-vessel PAD was powerfully and independently predictive of mortality, with a relative risk of 5.23 (95% confidence interval = 2.28 to 12.02, $p = .0001$). A Cox model with isolated small-vessel PAD, age, and sex entered as predictor variables (not shown) revealed no independent statistically significant association of isolated small-vessel PAD with mortality.

The left-hand column in table 5 shows for all subjects, the statistical significance for large-vessel PAD and for each of the covariates in the second set of Cox models. After controlling for HDL, LDL, VLDL, systolic blood pressure, and pack-years of cigarette smoking in addition to age and sex, the association between large-vessel PAD and mortality decreased only slightly, with a relative risk of 4.23 (95% confidence interval = 1.80 to 9.97, $p = .001$), indicating little

TABLE 1
Mortality rates and relative risks in men and women with large-vessel PAD or isolated small-vessel PAD compared with normal subjects

	LV-PAD	Isolated SV-PAD	Normal	Total	Relative risk: LV-PAD/ normal	Relative risk: Isolated SV-PAD/ normal
Men (n)	35	39	183	257		
Deaths (n)	9	4	7	20		
% Deaths	25.7	10.3	3.8	7.8	6.8	2.7
Women (n)	34	51	225	310		
Deaths (n)	5	1	4	10		
% Deaths	14.7	2.0	1.8	3.2	8.2	1.1
All subjects (n)	69	90	408	567		
Deaths (n)	14	5	11	30		
% Deaths	20.3	5.6	2.7	5.3	7.5	2.1

LV-PAD = large-vessel PAD; SV-PAD = small-vessel PAD.

TABLE 2

Distribution of deaths in subjects with large-vessel PAD, isolated small-vessel PAD, and normal findings, and relative risks of large-vessel PAD for cardiovascular and cancer mortality

	LV-PAD (n = 69, deaths = 14)	Isolated SV-PAD (n = 90, deaths = 5)	Normal (n = 408, deaths = 11)	Relative risk (LV-PAD/ normal)
Cardiovascular	8	5	4	11.8[A]
Cancer	5	0	7	4.2[B]
Other	1	0	0	—

[A](8/69)/(4/408) = 11.8.
[B](5/69)/(7/408) = 4.2.

confounding of the large-vessel PAD–mortality association by these additional covariates. The only other variable significantly associated with mortality in this model was VLDL cholesterol (p = .02), although age, cigarette smoking, and HDL cholesterol all showed p values close to statistical significance.

The right-hand column in table 5 shows the third set of Cox results, which excluded the 61 subjects with a history of angina, myocardial infarction, or stroke at baseline. There were 20 deaths in the 415 subjects without a previous history of angina, myocardial infarction, or stroke. In this group, the relative risk of large-vessel PAD was 4.51 (95% confidence interval = 1.74 to 11.69, p = .002), which, if anything, was somewhat higher than that for the entire group. The p values for the covariates were slightly higher than those for the data for all subjects, probably because of the smaller sample size. An exception was pack-years of cigarettes, which became significant (p = .02) in this analysis. Comparable Cox models for isolated small-vessel PAD, both with and without baseline cardiovascular disease exclusions, showed no significant associations of small-vessel PAD with mortality.

TABLE 3

Relative risks of mortality in men and women with Rose claudication, Rose or possible claudication, or abnormal pulse examination compared with other subjects

	Rose claudication	Rose or possible claudication	Abnormal pulse examination[A]
Men	2.7	4.0	2.8
Women	B	1.9	5.4
All subjects	1.9	3.7	3.4

[A]Abnormal femoral pulse or bruit or abnormal posterior tibial pulse.
[B]No deaths occurred among the six women with Rose claudication.

TABLE 4

Relative risks of mortality derived from the Cox model for age, sex, and large-vessel PAD[A]

	Relative risk	p value
Age (10 years)	1.69	.05
Male vs female	1.99	.09
Large-vessel PAD	5.23[B]	.0001

[A]Subjects with isolated small-vessel PAD excluded.
[B]95% confidence interval = 2.28 to 12.02.

Discussion

Previous reports have documented that intermittent claudication is a risk factor for mortality,[1, 3, 4] although the independence of this finding has been less certain.[3] We hypothesized that if PAD is a marker for subsequent mortality, a much more accurate assessment of PAD should provide a more accurate, and larger, estimate of risk, because misclassification bias would be greatly reduced.[19] We have described the prognostic significance in a defined population of accurately assessed large-vessel PAD for mortality and our results have suggested a greater than fourfold excess risk for subjects with large-vessel PAD, independent of other cardiovascular risk factors or disease at baseline.

By contrast, isolated small-vessel PAD was not significantly related to mortality in multivariable analysis. We have recently reported that isolated small-ves-

TABLE 5

Statistical significance in Cox model of large-vessel PAD and all covariates in all subjects and in subjects free of cardiovascular disease at baseline

	p values	
	All subjects (n = 476, deaths = 25)[A]	Excluding subjects with history of angina, MI, or stroke at baseline (n = 415, deaths = 20)[A]
Large vessel PAD	.001 (RR = 4.23[B])	.002 (RR = 4.51[C])
Age	.07	.15
Sex	.36	.44
HDL	.06	.09
LDL	.35	.82
VLDL	.02	.03
Systolic BP	.36	.61
Smoking (pack-years)	.06	.02

MI = myocardial infarction; RR = relative risk; BP = blood pressure.
[A]Subjects with isolated small-vessel PAD excluded.
[B]95% confidence interval = 1.80 to 9.97.
[C]95% confidence interval = 1.74 to 11.69.

sel PAD is also unrelated to claudication, abnormal pulses, sex, hyperlipidemia, or age after age 60.[5,6]

The risk associated with large-vessel PAD was clearly higher than that for less accurate determinations of large-vessel PAD by claudication or abnormal pulses (table 1 vs table 3). We had expected that PAD would be predictive of higher mortality mainly from atherosclerotic disease. The data in table 2 support this idea, although there was some excess of cancer deaths in the group with large-vessel PAD, perhaps reflecting the powerful effect of smoking on both cardiovascular disease and cancer and/or possibly poorer general health and survival in subjects with large-vessel PAD. Overall, the numbers were too small to draw firm conclusions.

Before our multivariable analysis, we were aware of the well known associations between cigarette smoking and both large-vessel PAD and mortality, and we considered the possibility that large-vessel PAD was simply a marker for cigarette smoking. Thus we were particularly interested in the multivariable analysis to note that the large-vessel PAD–mortality association was largely independent of cigarette smoking, even though cigarette smoking was itself independently associated with mortality. The only other statistically significant result was a positive association for VLDL cholesterol, which was contrary to our expectation since VLDL is essentially a surrogate for triglycerides, which is not thought to be an independent risk factor of cardiovascular disease.[20] However, this issue remains controversial, and in our population VLDL was a more important risk factor than LDL for all-cause mortality.

In a previous study from Finland, only a small part of the association between claudication and mortality was attributable to risk factors of cardiovascular disease,[3] and our study had a similar result for the large-vessel PAD association with mortality. It thus appears as though the increased specificity in measuring extant atherosclerosis, albeit in the lower extremities, leads to a better prediction of mortality even with simultaneous consideration of multiple risk factors of cardiovascular disease.

In the Finnish study, adjusting for signs and symptoms of coronary heart disease eliminated the independent effects of claudication on mortality, whereas in our study, after exclusion of subjects with angina, myocardial infarction, or stroke at baseline, the relative risk for large-vessel PAD was, if anything, higher. Thus, in our population the prognostic significance of large-vessel PAD for mortality was independent of both risk factors of and extant cardiovascular disease. A recent Swedish study of patients with claudication used venous occlusion plethysmography to diagnose PAD. Patients with positive plethysmographic results had a 2.2 to 4.9 times greater 10 year mortality rate, depending on age, with younger patients having a greater relative risk.[21] The increased mortality risk was mainly caused by myocardial infarction. However, the data were not adjusted for other cardiovascular risk factors or disease at baseline.

The relative risk of 4 to 5 of large-vessel PAD for mortality is similar to recent reports of the relative risk of an ischemic exercise electrocardiography test for coronary heart disease morbidity[22] or coronary heart disease and cardiovascular disease mortality.[23] It should be noted that, unlike exercise electrocardiography, these noninvasive PAD tests require no exertion and are essentially without risk.

In conclusion, the prognostic significance of large-vessel PAD in our population was largely independent of risk factors of cardiovascular disease, and independent of extant cardiovascular disease at baseline. These results suggest that men and women at high risk of impending mortality might be identifiable by noninvasive PAD testing, and thus such testing may alert us to patients who require additional evaluation or who might benefit from additional intervention. We would caution that these results, although highly statistically significant, are based on only 30 deaths. Our follow-up of this population is continuing.

References

1. Peabody CN, Kannel WB, McNamara PM: Intermittent claudication: surgical significance. Arch Surg **109:** 693, 1974
2. Friedman SA, Pandya M, Greif E: Peripheral arterial occlusion in patients with acute coronary heart disease. Am Heart J **86:** 415, 1973
3. Reunanen A, Takkunen H, Aromaa A: Prevalence of intermittent claudication and its effect on mortality. Acta Med Scand **211:** 249, 1982
4. Hughson WG, Mann JI, Tibbs DJ, Woods HF, Walton I: Intermittent claudication: factors determining outcome. Br Med J **1:** 1377, 1978
5. Criqui MH, Fronek A, Barrett-Connor E, Klauber MR, Gabriel S, Goodman D: The prevalence of peripheral arterial disease in a defined population. Circulation **71:** 510, 1985
6. Criqui MH, Fronek A, Klauber MR, Barrett-Connor E, Gabriel S: The sensitivity, specificity, and predictive value of traditional clinical evaluation of peripheral arterial disease: results from noninvasive testing in a defined population. Circulation **71:** 516, 1985
7. Marinelli MR, Beach KW, Glass MJ, Primozich JF, Strandness DE: Non-invasive testing vs. clinical evaluation of arterial disease: a prospective study. JAMA **241:** 2031, 1979
8. The Lipid Research Clinics Program Prevalence Study, Epidemiology Committee: Plasma lipid distributions in selected North American populations. Circulation **60:** 427, 1979
9. Rose GA, Blackburn H: Cardiovascular survey methods. Geneva, 1968, World Health Organization
10. Fronek A, Johansen KH, Dilley RB, Bernstein EF: Non-invasive physiologic tests in the diagnosis and characterization of peripheral arterial occlusive disease. Am J Surg **126:** 205, 1973

11. Winsor T: Influence of arterial disease on the systolic blood pressure gradients of the extremity. Am J Med Sci **220:** 117, 1950
12. Strandness DE Jr: Peripheral arterial disease: A physiologic approach. Boston, 1979, Little Brown and Co.
13. Fronek A, Coel M, Bernstein EF: Quantitative ultrasonographic studies of lower extremity flow velocities in health and disease. Circulation **53:** 957, 1976
14. Fronek A, Johansen KH, Dilley RB, Bernstein EF: Ultrasonographically monitored post-occlusive reactive hyperemia in the diagnosis of peripheral arterial occlusive disease. Circulation **48:** 149, 1973
15. Fronek A, Coel M, Bernstein EF: The pulse reappearance time — an index of over-all blood flow impairment in the ischemic extremity. Surgery **81:** 376, 1977
16. Labarthe DR, Hawkins CM, Remington RD: Evaluation of performance of selected devices for measuring blood pressure. Am J Cardiol **32:** 546, 1973
17. National Heart and Lung Institute, National Institutes of Health. Manual of laboratory operations, Lipid Research Clinics Program. Vol 1: Lipid and lipoproteins analysis. Washington, DC, 1975, DHEW Publication No. (NIH) 75-628
18. Cox DR: Regression models and life tables (with discussion). J R Stat Soc B **34:** 187, 1972
19. Copeland KT, Checkoway H, McMichael AJ: Bias due to misclassification in the estimation of the relative risk. Am J Epidemiol **105:** 488, 1977
20. Hulley SB, Rosenman RH, Bawol RD, Brand RJ: Epidemiology as a guide to clinical decisions: the association between triglyceride and coronary heart disease. N Engl J Med **302:** 1383, 1980
21. Kallero KS: Mortality and morbidity in patients with intermittent claudication as defined by venous occlusion plethysmography: a ten-year follow-up study. J Chron Dis **34:** 455, 1981
22. Giagnoni E, Secchi MB, Wu SC, Morabito A, Oltrona L, Mancarella S, Volpin N, Fossa L, Bettazzi L, Arangio G, Sachero A, Folli G: Prognostic value of exercise EKG testing in asymptomatic normotensive subjects: a prospective matched study. N Engl J Med **309:** 1085, 1983
23. Ekelund LG, Karon JM, Gordon DJ, Probstfield JL, Rubenstein C, Shetfield LT: Predictive value of the exercise tolerance test for coronary heart disease mortality in men: the Lipid Research Clinics Follow-up Study. Presented at the 24th Annual Conference on Cardiovascular Disease Epidemiology, Tampa, FL, March 1984

Prognostic significance and natural history of left ventricular thrombi in patients with acute anterior myocardial infarction: a two-dimensional echocardiographic study

PAOLO SPIRITO, M.D., PAOLO BELLOTTI, M.D., FRANCESCO CHIARELLA, M.D., STEFANO DOMENICUCCI, M.D., ANGELA SEMENTA, M.D., AND CARLO VECCHIO, M.D.

ABSTRACT Fifty-eight patients with transmural anterior myocardial infarction were prospectively studied with serial two-dimensional echocardiography to determine the clinical implications and prognostic significance of detection of left ventricular thrombus during acute myocardial infarction, the incidence of systemic embolization, and the possible occurrence of spontaneous regression of left ventricular thrombi. Patients were not treated with anticoagulants or platelet inhibitors during the acute phase of infarction or during follow-up. Two-dimensional echocardiograms were obtained within 24 hr of myocardial infarction, every 24 hr until day 5, every 48 hr until day 15, and every month for a follow-up of 2 to 11 months (mean 7), in the surviving patients; a total of 774 echocardiograms were obtained. Left ventricular thrombi were identified in 24 (41%) of the 58 study patients, and developed within 48 hr of infarction in 11 of these patients. Ten (91%) of the 11 patients with early thrombus formation died during hospitalization or during follow-up, while only two (15%) of the 13 who developed a thrombus after 48 hr of infarction died ($p < .005$). Incidence of Killip class III or IV, total lactic dehydrogenase values, and extent of wall motion abnormalities were significantly higher in patients who developed a thrombus within 48 hr of infarction than in patients without thrombus. On the other hand, in patients who developed a thrombus after 48 hr of infarction, these parameters were not significantly different from those in patients who did not develop a thrombus. Spontaneous regression of thrombi was documented in three (20%) of the 15 patients who survived the acute phase of myocardial infarction. The incidence of clinically evident systemic embolic events was low: one of the 24 patients with left ventricular thrombus experienced transient ischemic attacks, and no embolic events were detected in patients without thrombus. We conclude that development of left ventricular thrombi within 2 days of acute anterior myocardial infarction occurs in patients with the most extensive infarcts and is predictive of high mortality. Our data also demonstrate that spontaneous regression of thrombi may occur. Finally, in our study patients, none of whom were treated with anticoagulants or platelet inhibitors, the incidence of clinically evident systemic embolic events was low.
Circulation 72, No. 4, 774–780, 1985.

TWO-DIMENSIONAL ECHOCARDIOGRAPHY has recently demonstrated that left ventricular thrombi are common in patients with acute anterior myocardial infarction.[1-5] However, the clinical implications and prognostic significance of detection of thrombi during acute myocardial infarction, the incidence of systemic embolization, and the possible occurrence of spontaneous regression of left ventricular thrombus have not yet been investigated in prospective studies conducted in a large population of patients not treated with anticoagulants. Therefore, it is not known if the detection of left ventricular thrombi during acute anterior myocardial infarction should alter the course of treatment. To address these questions, we obtained serial two-dimensional echocardiograms, at short intervals, in the acute phase and during the months after anterior myocardial infarction in a consecutive series of patients who were not treated with anticoagulants or platelet inhibitors.

From the Divisione di Cardiologia and Servizio di Anatomia ed Istologia Patologica, Ente Ospedaliero Ospedali Galliera, Genoa, Italy.

Address for correspondence: Dr. Paolo Spirito, Divisione di Cardiologia, Ente Ospedaliero, Ospedali Galliera, Via Volta 8, 16128 Genoa, Italy.

Received Dec. 31, 1984; revision accepted May 30, 1985.

Methods

Selection and characterization of patients. Fifty-nine consecutive patients admitted to the coronary care unit of the Ente Ospedaliero Ospedali Galliera within 24 hr of transmural anterior myocardial infarction and who had no evidence of prior anterior myocardial infarction entered the study. A satisfactory visualization of the left ventricular cavity in the echocardiographic apical views could not be obtained in one patient, who was excluded from further study. The remaining 58 patients comprise our study population.

The patients ranged in age from 35 to 87 years (mean 63); 44 (76%) were men. The diagnosis of acute anterior myocardial infarction was documented in each patient by a typical history of chest pain, serial electrocardiographic changes, and serial elevation of serum enzymes. The electrocardiographic criterion for diagnosis of transmural infarction was the appearance of Q waves of greater than 0.04 sec in the anterior precordial leads. Total creatine kinase (CK) and CK-MB activity was measured on admission, at 12 hr after the onset of symptoms, and then every 4 hr for the next 16 hr. Total lactic dehydrogenase (LDH) activity was measured on admission, and daily for the first 3 hospital days. By clinical criteria, each study patient was assigned to the highest (most severe) Killip class[6] he reached during hospitalization. In patients who developed left ventricular thrombi, Killip class was also assessed at the time of the first echocardiographic detection of thrombus. Four patients had electrocardiographic documentation of a prior inferior infarction in addition to the acute anterior infarct. By design, no study patient was treated with anticoagulants or platelet inhibitors in the acute phase of infarction or during the follow-up period.

Two-dimensional echocardiography. An Advanced Technology Laboratory (ATL) Mark 300 mechanical sector scanner with a 3 MHz transducer was used to perform the echocardiographic studies. Two-dimensional echocardiographic images were recorded on a Panasonic NW-8200 videotape. A Sony U-matic videotape VO-5800 PS was used to review the studies in slow-motion and real-time modes. In each patient, two-dimensional echocardiograms were obtained within 24 hr of acute infarction, every 24 hr until day 5, every 48 hr until day 15, and every month for a follow-up of 2 to 11 months (mean 7) in the surviving patients. A total of 774 two-dimensional echocardiograms were obtained in the 58 study patients.

Images were obtained in the parasternal long- and short-axis and apical two- and four-chamber views with the use of standard transducer positions. In most studies, images were also obtained from the apical short-axis view and from sector orientations intermediate between the two- and four-chamber views. Routinely, while recording from the apical views, depth was adjusted to examine the left ventricular apex more thoroughly. Multiple gain and reject settings were also used to improve definition of the epicardium, endocardium, and margins of the thrombus.

Left ventricular thrombus was diagnosed when an echodense mass with defined margins was visualized contiguous to the endocardial surface, and it was clearly identifiable throughout the cardiac cycle.[1, 7, 8] Multiple sector orientations from the apical windows were used to differentiate left ventricular thrombi from muscle trabeculations, chordal structures, and false masses that may result from oblique angulation of the ultrasound beam through the left ventricular wall.[7] Agreement of two observers who were blinded to each other's interpretation was required before an echocardiogram was considered positive for left ventricular thrombus. To minimize false-positive diagnoses, studies in which there was observer disagreement that persisted after joint review of the study were considered negative for thrombus.[9] However, our protocol provided for serial two-dimensional echocardiograms obtained at short intervals in each patient, and the comparison of sequential echocardiograms was helpful in reducing the number of equivocal studies. Echocardiograms were considered equivocal, and therefore negative for left ventricular thrombus in only two of the 58 study patients.

The serial echocardiograms obtained in each patient were also analyzed with regard to shape of the left ventricular thrombus, and thrombi were classified either as mural, when they were flat and parallel to the endocardial surface, or protruding, when they were spherical and projected into the left ventricular cavity.[7]

Left ventricular wall motion analysis. Left ventricular wall motion was assessed from the combined analysis of the echocardiographic apical two- and four-chamber views. In these two-dimensional planes, the left ventricle was divided into nine segments that identified the left ventricular apex, the basal and midventricular regions of the interventricular septum, and the posterolateral, inferior, and lateral free walls.[10, 11] Wall motion in each segment was classified as normal, hypokinetic, akinetic, dyskinetic, or hyperkinetic on the basis of a visual assessment of left ventricular wall movement during systole. A wall motion index was calculated according to the method of Gibson et al.,[11] in which a numerical score is assigned to each segment on the basis of the severity of the wall motion abnormalities as follows: normal, 0; hypokinetic, +1; akinetic, +2; dyskinetic, +3; and hyperkinetic, −1. A left ventricular wall motion index was then calculated by adding the scores from each segment and dividing by the number of segments analyzed. In each patient, left ventricular wall motion was assessed twice, from the echocardiogram recorded on day 1 of infarction and from the echocardiogram obtained 30 days after infarction. In patients who died within 30 days of suffering myocardial infarction, the second assessment of wall motion was made from the last echocardiogram recorded before death. In the 58 study patients, a total of 116 echocardiograms were analyzed to calculate wall motion index. Of the 1044 possible left ventricular segments, 960 (92%) were considered adequate for analysis.

Statistical analysis. Continuous data were expressed as mean ± SD. Differences between two means were analyzed by the unpaired or paired Student's t test, as appropriate. Differences between three means were tested by the one-way analysis of variance. Differences between proportions were analyzed by the chi-square test.

Results

Incidence of left ventricular thrombi and prognosis. Left ventricular thrombi were identified in 24 (41%) of the 58 study patients, and were either confined to the left ventricular apex, or extended from the apex over the interventricular septum. The thrombus was protruding in 14 (58%) of the patients, and mural in 10 (42%). In none of the patients did the thrombus show vigorous mobility within the left ventricular cavity during the cardiac cycle. In each patient, left ventricular thrombus was associated with adjacent wall motion abnormalities. Incidence of Killip class III or IV, peak total LDH values, extent of wall motion abnormalities, and mortality were significantly higher in patients who developed thrombi than in patients who did not (table 1).

However, during the course of the study a relationship became evident within the group of patients with thrombi between time of development of thrombus and clinical outcome. Ten (91%) of the 11 patients who developed thrombi within 48 hr of acute infarction died during hospitalization (eight patients), or during fol-

TABLE 1

Clinical data and wall motion index in patients with and without left ventricular thrombus (LVT) after acute myocardial infarction

	Age (years)	Sex (No. of men)	CK (IU/l)	MB (IU/l)	LDH (IU/l)	Killip class III or IV (No. of patients)	Wall motion index[A] Day 1	Wall motion index[A] Day 30	Mortality (No. of patients)
Patients with LVT (n = 24)	63±12	21 (88%)	2410±832	275±91	1902±639	10 (42%)	0.46±0.23	0.67±0.34	12 (50%)
Patients without LVT (n = 34)	64±13	23 (68%)	1935±886	232±146	1440±582[D]	4 (12%)[C]	0.31±0.26[B]	0.35±0.26[D]	4 (12%)[D]

[A]Wall motion index was calculated from the echocardiograms obtained on day 1 and on day 30 of myocardial infarction (or from the last echocardiogram recorded before death in patients who died within 30 days of infarction).

[B]$p < .05$ compared with patients with LVT; [C]$p < .025$ compared with patients with LVT; [D]$p < .01$ compared with patients with LVT.

low-up (two patients), while only two (15%) of the 13 who developed thrombi after 48 hr of acute infarction died ($p < .005$). We therefore decided to further analyze our clinical and echocardiographic findings in these two subgroups of patients (the group with early and that with late development of thrombus). Data from these two patient subgroups were also compared with those obtained in patients who did not develop left ventricular thrombi.

Peak CK and CK-MB values did not differ significantly among the three study groups. Peak total LDH values were significantly higher in patients who developed a thrombus early during myocardial infarction than in patients who did not develop a thrombus, while in patients with late-developing thrombus this variable did not differ significantly from that in the other two groups (table 2). Incidence of Killip classes III or IV and mortality were also significantly higher in patients with early-developing thrombi than in patients without thrombi, while in patients who developed thrombi late, these variables did not differ significantly from those in patients without thrombi (table 2; figures 1 and 2).

Wall motion indexes calculated from the echocardiograms obtained on day 1 and day 30 of infarction (or from the last echocardiogram obtained before death in patients who died within 30 days of infarction) were significantly higher (indicating more extensive wall motion abnormalities) in patients who developed a thrombus early than in patients without thrombus (table 3). In patients with late thrombus formation, wall motion index obtained on day 1 of infarction was not significantly different from that in the other two groups; wall motion index obtained on day 30 was significantly lower than that in patients with early-developing thrombi, but higher than that in patients without thrombi.

In addition, wall motion indexes obtained at these two times during the course of infarction were compared within each group of patients. In patients who developed an early thrombus, left ventricular wall motion was significantly more compromised at the time of its second assessment than at the first assessment, while in patients who developed a thrombus late and in patients without thrombi, wall motion indexes did not differ significantly at the first and second assessments (table 3).

We also analyzed the relationship between patient clinical condition (Killip class) at the time when a thrombus was first detected and subsequent patient clinical course. Of the 11 patients who developed

TABLE 2

Clinical data on patients with left ventricular thrombus (LVT) within 48 hr of acute myocardial infarction (AMI), with LVT after 48 hr of AMI, and without LVT

	Age (years)	Sex (No. of men)	Killip class III or IV (No. of patients)	CK (IU/l)	MB (IU/l)	LDH (IU/l)	Mortality (No. of patients)
LVT within 48 hr of AMI (n = 11)	66±8	9 (82%)	7 (64%)	2448±920	281±114	2087±667	10 (91%)
LVT after 48 hr of AMI (n = 13)	59±13	12 (92%)	3 (23%)	2368±772	268±64	1695±555	2 (15%)[A]
No LVT (n = 34)	64±13	23 (68%)	4 (12%)[A]	1935±886	232±146	1440±582[B]	4 (12%)[B]

[A]$p < .005$ compared with patients with LVT within 48 hr of AMI; [B]$p < .001$ compared with patients with LVT within 48 hr of AMI.

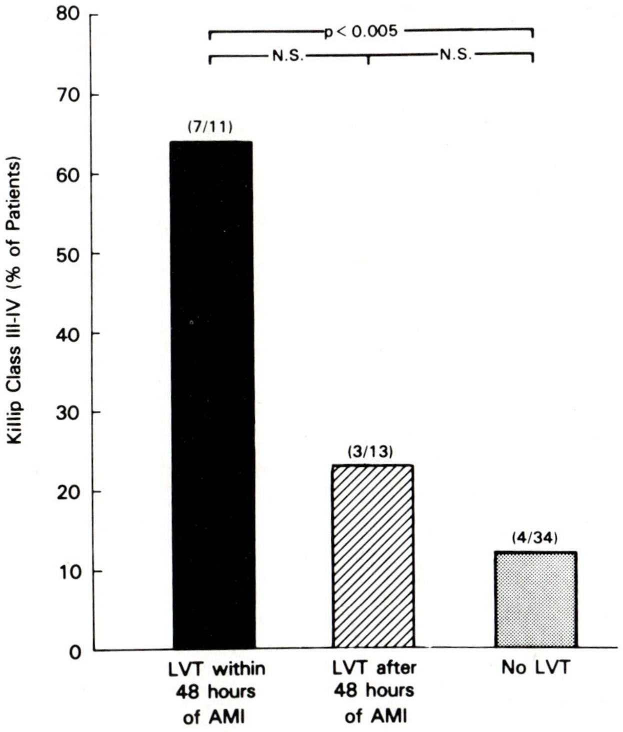

FIGURE 1. Patients who developed left ventricular thrombus (LVT) within 48 hr of acute myocardial infarction (AMI), those who developed LVT after 48 hr of AMI, and patients without LVT are compared with regard to incidence of Killip class III or IV.

thrombi early after infarction, four were in Killip class I or II at the time of first detection of the thrombus. Three of these patients died suddenly and unexpectedly during hospitalization. Autopsy demonstrated cardiac rupture and extensive myocardial necrosis in each patient. The remaining seven patients with early-de-

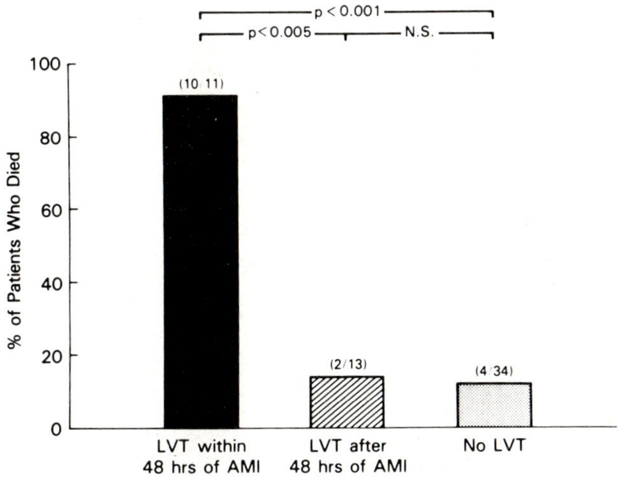

FIGURE 2. Patients who developed left ventricular thrombus (LVT) within 48 hr of acute myocardial infarction (AMI), those who developed LVT after 48 hr of AMI, and patients without LVT are compared with regard to mortality.

TABLE 3
Wall motion index on day 1 and day 30[A] of myocardial infarction (MI) in patients with early left ventricular thrombus (LVT), in patients with late-developing LVT, and in patients without LVT

	Wall motion index on day 1 of MI	Wall motion index on day 30 of MI
LVT within 48 hr of MI (n = 11)	0.50±0.21	0.82±0.25
LVT after 48 hr of MI (n = 13)	0.42±0.25	0.55±0.14[B]
No LVT (n = 34)	0.31±0.26[B]	0.35±0.26[C,D]

[A]In patients who died within 30 days of MI, wall motion index was calculated from the last echocardiogram recorded before death.
[B]p < .04 compared with patients with early LVT; [C]p < .001 compared with patients with early LVT; [D]p < .05 compared with patients with late LVT.

veloping thrombi were in Killip class III or IV when the thrombus was first identified. These patients died during hospitalization (five patients) or during follow-up (two patients). Each of the 13 patients who developed thrombus late were in Killip class I or II at the time of first detection. Three of these patients progressed to class III or IV during hospitalization, and two of these three patients died (one of cardiogenic shock on day 5, the other of reinfarction 3 months after the initial infarction).

Causes of death. Sixteen study patients died and the causes of death are summarized in table 4. In the group of patients who developed a thrombus within 48 hr of infarction, cardiogenic shock (five patients) and cardiac rupture (three patients) were the most common causes of death. Reinfarction during follow-up was the cause of death in three of the six patients who died among the patients who either developed a thrombus late, or did not develop one at all. The remaining three

TABLE 4
Causes of death in 16 study patients

	LVT within 48 hr of AMI (No. of patients)	LVT after 48 hr of AMI (No. of patients)	No LVT (No. of patients)
Cardiogenic shock	5	1	2
Reinfarction	1	1	2
Cardiac rupture	3	0	0
Unexplained sudden death[A]	1	0	0

AMI = acute myocardial infarction; LVT = ventricular thrombus.
[A]This patient had recurrent nonsustained ventricular tachycardia, was treated with amiodarone, and died during sleep at home 3 months after myocardial infarction.

patients in this group died of cardiogenic shock (two died within 24 hr of acute infarction and the third died on day 5).

Autopsy. Autopsies were performed in 13 of the 16 study patients who died. In 12 of the 13 patients, autopsy findings confirmed the echocardiographic interpretation (positive for left ventricular thrombus in nine patients and negative in three). In one patient, autopsy identified a thrombus that had not been detected by echocardiography.

In each patient, the location of the thrombus within the left ventricular cavity as verified at autopsy was in agreement with that predicted by echocardiography.

Spontaneous regression of left ventricular thrombi. Spontaneous regression of thrombus could be demonstrated in three (20%) of the 15 patients who survived the acute phase of myocardial infarction (figure 3). In these three patients, the regression was documented on the echocardiograms obtained on days 12, 26, and 257 after the thrombus was first identified. The thrombus was located at the left ventricular apex in the first two patients, and extended from the apex over the interventricular septum in the third patient (figure 3, *B*). The left ventricular wall adjacent to the thrombus was akinetic or dyskinetic in each of the three patients and remained so after the thrombus resolved. Of note is the fact that, in the patient in whom regression of thrombus was documented 257 days after its first detection, a large left ventricular aneurysm developed early after infarction, but it did not prevent the subsequent spontaneous regression of thrombus (figure 3, *C*).

Systemic embolic events. Clinically apparent systemic embolic events occurred in only one patient with a left ventricular thrombus who had two transient ischemic attacks on days 9 and 11 after infarction. No changes in size of thrombus were detected on the echocardiograms obtained during the days after transient ischemic attacks. The patient died of reinfarction 3 months after his first infarction. No systemic embolic events occurred in the group of patients without thrombus. Therefore, the total incidence of embolic events in our study population was 2%.

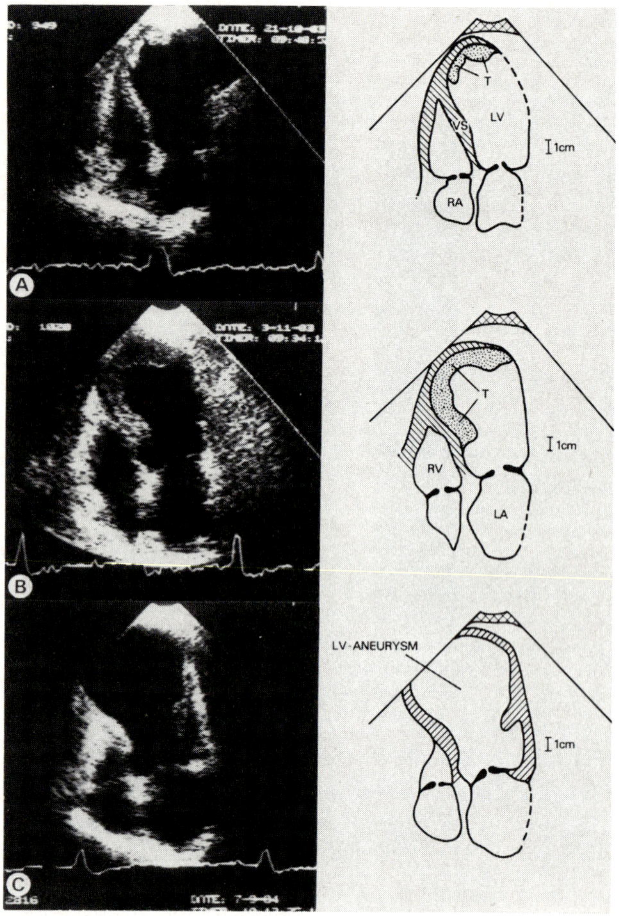

FIGURE 3. Stop-frame images of two-dimensional echocardiograms obtained at end-diastole in the same patient during hospitalization (*A*) and during follow-up (*B* and *C*). Each stop frame is accompanied by a schematic illustration. *A*, Sixteen days after myocardial infarction, a relatively small, lobulated thrombus is visualized at the left ventricular apex. *B*, Thirty days after infarction, the thrombus is greatly increased in size, and it now extends from the apex over the interventricular septum. *C*, Nine months (257 days) after infarction, no thrombus is visualized, and a large left ventricular aneurysm is present. LA = left atrium; LV = left ventricle; VS = interventricular septum; RA = right atrium; RV = right ventricle; T = thrombus.

Discussion

Incidence and prognostic significance of detection of thrombi. Previous two-dimensional echocardiographic studies have shown that the incidence of left ventricular thrombus is high in patients with acute anterior myocardial infarction (30% to 43% of the patients).[1-5, 12] In the present investigation, thrombi were detected in about 40% of the study patients. Wall motion abnormalities were more extensive, and peak total LDH, incidence of Killip class III or IV, and mortality were significantly higher in patients who developed compared with patients who did not develop thrombi. However, the high number of serial echocardiograms obtained in our study patients early during infarction has allowed the identification of a relationship between time of development of thrombus and clinical outcome. More than 90% of the patients who developed thrombi within 2 days of acute anterior infarction died during hospitalization or follow-up. Cardiogenic shock and cardiac rupture, both indicative of extensive myocardial necrosis,[13-15] were the most common causes of death in these patients. On the other hand, only 15% of the patients who developed thrombi more than 2 days after acute infarction died, and their mortality rate was not different from that of patients who did not develop thrombi. Furthermore, the analysis of clinical variables and left ventricular contractility in these patient subgroups substantiated the conclusion that the time of development of thrombus after acute myocardial infarction identifies subsets of patients with different clinical profiles and outcome. For example, in the group of patients who developed a thrombus early, incidence of Killip class III or IV, peak total LDH, and extent of wall motion abnormalities were significantly higher compared with those in patients who did not develop a thrombus. On the other hand, patients who developed a thrombus late did not differ significantly from patients without thrombi with regard to Killip class, enzyme values, and left ventricular wall motion (assessed in the acute phase of infarction). These findings demonstrate that development of left ventricular thrombus within 48 hr of myocardial infarction occurs in patients with the most extensive infarcts and is associated with particularly high mortality.

Although the majority of patients with acute myocardial infarction and large infarcts usually present with or progress to Killip class III or IV, about 15% of patients with extensive myocardial damage and high pulmonary pressures are not identified on the basis of clinical evaluation, but only by means of invasive hemodynamic measurements.[16] Four of our study patients who developed left ventricular thrombus within 48 hr of myocardial infarction had been assigned by clinical criteria to Killip class I or II at the time of admission. Of note is the fact that three of these four patients died suddenly and unexpectedly during hospitalization. Autopsy demonstrated cardiac rupture and extensive myocardial necrosis in each of these three patients. This finding would suggest that echocardiographic detection of early formation of thrombus during acute anterior infarction may identify a subset of patients whose poor prognosis would not be predicted on the basis of their clinical presentation.

Spontaneous regression of thrombus. Spontaneous regression of left ventricular thrombus in patients with myocardial infarction who are not treated with anticoagulants has been previously reported in three patients.[5, 17] In our study, thrombus resolved in three of the 15 patients (20%) who survived the acute phase of infarction. The period of time between formation of the thrombus and its spontaneous regression was greatly variable in these three patients, ranging from a minimum of 12 days to a maximum of 9 months. The left ventricular segments contiguous to the thrombus were akinetic or dyskinetic in each patient and remained so after the thrombus resolved. Regression of thrombus was not associated with clinically evident embolic events in any of the three patients. During follow-up, one of these patients developed a large left ventricular aneurysm associated with poor global left ventricular contractility and, interestingly, the presence of this large aneurysm did not prevent subsequent spontaneous regression of thrombus (figure 3).

Incidence of systemic embolic events. The incidence of clinically apparent systemic embolic events in patients with myocardial infarction and echocardiographic documentation of left ventricular thrombus is controversial, and the available data are from small numbers of patients, the majority of whom were treated with anticoagulants. Asinger et al.[1] reported no evidence of systemic embolization during a mean follow-up of 9 months in nine patients with anterior myocardial infarction and left ventricular thrombus, seven of whom were treated with anticoagulants. In a preliminary study, Kothari et al.[12] reported one embolic event in 11 patients who received anticoagulants and one embolic event in eight patients not treated with anticoagulants; no data on follow-up were provided. In contrast, Keating et al.[3] reported embolic events in six of seven patients who were not treated with anticoagulants (mean follow-up 1 month) and no embolic events in nine patients on anticoagulants (mean follow-up 11 months). More recently, Weinreich et al.[5] reported systemic embolization in seven of 18 patients who did not receive anticoagulants and in none of 25 patients treated with anticoagulants (minimum follow-up 6 months).

None of our 58 study patients was treated with anticoagulants or platelet inhibitors during the acute phase of infarction or follow-up. The incidence of clinically apparent systemic embolic events was low, with only one patient with left ventricular thrombus having transient ischemic attacks. No embolic events occurred in the remaining patients with or without thrombus during a mean follow-up of 7 months. Therefore, in our study population the total incidence of clinically apparent systemic embolic events was 2%. While this incidence is in agreement with the 0.6% to 6.4% reported in several large series of patients with myocardial infarction,[18-20] it contrasts with the substantially higher incidence of systemic embolization identified by Keating et al.,[3] and Weinreich et al.[5] in study populations similar to ours. We do not have a definite explanation for these conflicting findings. Our study patients were a consecutive series, and no patient was treated with either anticoagulants or platelet inhibitors; therefore, our results should not be importantly affected by selection factors. Several investigators have described the vigorous mobility of left ventricular thrombi within the left ventricular cavity as an echocardiographic feature associated with embolization.[21–24] None of the thrombi identified in our study patients showed vigorous mobility during the cardiac cycle. This morphologic feature could explain, in part, the relatively low incidence of embolic events in our population. However, larger prospective studies are needed to define the clinical and echocardiographic profile of patients with myocardial infarction and left ventricular thrombus who are potentially at higher risk of systemic embolization and who may benefit from treatment with anticoagulants.

In conclusion, our findings indicate that development of left ventricular thrombus within 2 days of acute anterior myocardial infarction occurs in patients with the most extensive infarcts and is predictive of high mortality. Our study also demonstrates that spontaneous regression of thrombus may occur in patients with myocardial infarction, despite the persistence of severe wall motion abnormalities. Finally, in our study patients with left ventricular thrombi, none of whom were treated with anticoagulants or platelet inhibitors, the incidence of clinically apparent systemic embolic events was low.

References

1. Asinger RW, Mikell FL, Elsperger J, Hodges M: Incidence of left ventricular thrombosis after acute transmural myocardial infarction. N Engl J Med **305:** 297, 1981
2. Friedman MJ, Carlson K, Marcus FI, Woolfenden JM: Clinical correlations in patients with acute myocardial infarction and left ventricular thrombus detected by two-dimensional echocardiography. Am J Med **72:** 894, 1982
3. Keating EC, Gross SA, Schlamowitz RA, Glassman J, Mazur JH, Pitt WA, Miller D: Mural thrombi in myocardial infarctions. Prospective evaluation by two-dimensional echocardiography. Am J Med **74:** 989, 1983
4. Visser CA, Kan G, Lie KI, Durrer D: Left ventricular thrombus following acute myocardial infarction: a prospective serial echocardiographic study of 96 patients. Eur J Cardiol **4:** 333, 1983
5. Weinreich DJ, Burke JF, Pauletto FJ: Left ventricular mural thrombi complicating acute myocardial infarction. Long-term follow-up with serial echocardiography. Ann Intern Med **100:** 789, 1984
6. Killip T, Kimball JT: Treatment of myocardial infarction in a coronary care unit. A two year experience with 250 patients. Am J Cardiol **20:** 457, 1967
7. Asinger RW, Mikell FL, Sharma B, Hodges M: Observations on detecting left ventricular thrombus with two-dimensional echocardiography: emphasis on avoidance of false positive diagnoses. Am J Cardiol **47:** 145, 1981
8. Mikell FL, Asinger RW, Elsperger JK, Anderson RW, Hodges M: Regional stasis of blood in the dysfunctional left ventricle: echocardiographic detection and differentiation from early thrombosis. Circulation **66:** 755, 1982
9. Stratton JR, Lighty GW Jr, Pearlman AS, Ritchie JL: Detection of left ventricular thrombus by two-dimensional echocardiography: sensitivity, specificity, and causes of uncertainty. Circulation **66:** 156, 1982
10. Heger JJ, Weyman AE, Wann SL, Rogers EW, Dillon JC, Feigenbaum H: Cross-sectional echocardiographic analysis of the extent of left ventricular asynergy in acute myocardial infarction. Circulation **61:** 1113, 1980
11. Gibson RS, Bishop HL, Stamm RB, Crampton RS, Beller GA, Martin RP: Value of early two-dimensional echocardiography in patients with acute myocardial infarction. Am J Cardiol **49:** 1110, 1982
12. Kothari AJ, Paczkowski K, Baker KM, Schreck SC, Butcher RJ, Kline DM, Menapace FJ: Ventricular thrombi in acute myocardial infarction: incidence, complications, and effects of anticoagulation. J Am Coll Cardiol **3:** 601, 1984 (abst)
13. Page DL, Caulfield JB, Kastor JA, DeSanctis RW, Sanders CA: Myocardial changes associated with cardiogenic shock. N Engl J Med **285:** 133, 1971
14. Gutovitz AL, Sobel BE, Roberts R: Progressive nature of myocardial injury in selected patients with cardiogenic shock. Am J Cardiol **41:** 469, 1978
15. London RE, London SB: Rupture of the heart. A critical analysis of 47 consecutive autopsy cases. Circulation **31:** 202, 1965
16. Forrester JS, Diamond G, Swan HJC: Bedside diagnosis of latent cardiac complications in acutely ill patients. JAMA **30:** 338, 1972
17. Tramarin R, Pozzoli M, Febo O, Opasich C, Cobelli F, Specchia G: Echocardiographic assessment of therapy efficacy in left ventricular thrombosis post myocardial infarction. Circulation **68** (suppl III): III-331, 1983 (abst)
18. Wright IS, Marple CD, Beck DF: Report of the committee for the evaluation of anticoagulants in the treatment of coronary thrombosis with myocardial infarction. Am Heart J **36:** 801, 1948
19. Hilden T, Raaschov F, Iversen K, Schwartz M: Anticoagulants in acute myocardial infarction. Lancet **2:** 327, 1961
20. Veterans Administration Hospital Investigators: Anticoagulants in acute myocardial infarction. results of a cooperative clinical trial. JAMA **225:** 724, 1973
21. DeMaria AN, Bommer W, Neumann A, Grehl T, Weinart L, DeNardo S, Amsterdam EA, Mason DT: Left ventricular thrombi identified by cross-sectional echocardiography. Ann Intern Med **90:** 14, 1979
22. Nagvi N, Popp RL, Coltart DJ: Diagnosis of left ventricular thrombosis by two-dimensional echocardiography. Eur J Cardiol **11:** 235, 1980
23. Visser CA, Kan G, Meltzer RS, Roelandt J, Durrer D: Two-dimensional echocardiographic features of left ventricular thrombi causing peripheral embolization. Circulation **68**(suppl III): III-111, 1983 (abst)
24. Haugland MJ, Asinger RW, Mikell FL, Elsperger J, Hodges M: Embolic potential of left ventricular thrombi detected by two-dimensional echocardiography. Circulation **70:** 588, 1984

Non–Q wave perioperative myocardial infarction: assessment of the incidence and severity of regional dysfunction with quantitative two-dimensional echocardiography

THOMAS FORCE, M.D., ANDREW J. KEMPER, M.D., PETER BLOOMFIELD, M.B., DONALD E. TOW, M.D., SHUKRI F. KHURI, M.D., MIGUEL JOSA, M.D., AND ALFRED F. PARISI, M.D.

ABSTRACT Since the widespread use of hypothermic potassium cardioplegia began, marked reductions in perioperative mortality and the rate of Q wave–associated myocardial infarctions have been noted. No study to date has evaluated whether there has been an equally dramatic improvement in the incidence of postoperative myocardial infarctions unassociated with Q wave development. We used a previously validated quantitative two-dimensional echocardiographic analytic algorithm to determine the incidence and severity of regional wall motion abnormalities (RWMAs) and first-pass radionuclide ventriculography to assess deterioration in global left ventricular function in the four following groups of patients (total n = 65): (1) those with peak postoperative creatine kinase (CK)–MB levels equal to or less than the mean value for patients undergoing coronary artery bypass surgery at our institution (n = 10), (2) those with CK-MB levels between the mean and 1 SD above the mean (n = 10), (3) those with peak CK-MB levels higher than 1 SD above the mean (n = 25), and (4) those with new pathologic Q waves on the postoperative electrocardiogram (n = 20). All patients had electrocardiograms without pathologic Q waves and normal wall motion and ejection fraction by contrast ventriculography before surgery. The incidence of postoperative RWMA by two-dimensional echocardiography for groups 1 through 4 was 0%, 20%, 55%, and 89%, respectively. Percent of abnormal left ventricular segments, wall motion scores, and the deterioration in left ventricular ejection fraction as assessed by radionuclide ventriculography were similar for patients with new RWMAs whether or not new Q waves developed (p = NS for all). In summary, although the incidence of both Q wave and non–Q wave perioperative myocardial infarctions appears to have declined significantly with the use of cold potassium cardioplegia, the incidence of non–Q wave infarction remains high and in this study was calculated to be three times greater than the 4.5% incidence of Q wave infarction. Furthermore, the impact of these non–Q wave myocardial infarctions on left ventricular function is significant and equal to that of Q wave infarctions. Future evaluations of methods of myocardial preservation should include analyses of regional left ventricular function designed to identify these patients.
Circulation 72, No. 4, 781–789, 1985.

MYOCARDIAL PRESERVATION with hypothermic potassium cardioplegia (cold cardioplegia) has been a major factor in the decline in perioperative mortality and Q wave myocardial infarction seen since the advent of coronary artery bypass surgery (CABG).[1] However, there may be a risk of significantly underestimating remaining problems with respect to preservation if mortality or statistics on Q wave infarction alone are examined.[2–4] In a study done before cold cardioplegia was used, Bulkley and Hutchins[5] reported that over 80% of patients with perioperative myocardial infarction did not develop pathologic Q waves on the electrocardiogram, even when transmural necrosis was seen at postmortem examination. Similarly, contrast ventriculographic studies done before cold cardioplegia was used showed new postoperative regional wall motion abnormalities (RWMAs) in 2.3 to 5.5 times as

From the Departments of Medicine (Cardiology) and Surgery, Brockton-West Roxbury Veterans Administration Medical Center; Brigham and Women's Hospital; and Harvard Medical School, Boston.

Supported by the Medical Research Service of the Veterans Administration and the David Littmann Memorial Foundation (Dr. Force).

Received Jan. 30, 1985; revision accepted June 27, 1985.

Address for correspondence: Thomas Force, M.D., Veterans Administration Medical Center, 1400 VFW Parkway, West Roxbury, MA 02132.

many patients as those developing pathologic Q waves.[6–8]

Similar studies have not been performed since the use of cold cardioplegia has become widespread. Thus, although cardioplegia has dramatically reduced the incidence of Q wave myocardial infarction, the effect it has had on the incidence of deterioration in regional function due to non–Q wave myocardial infarction is not known. Furthermore, neither the extent of these regional abnormalities nor their effects on global left ventricular function have been examined adequately. This may be due to the lack of adequate noninvasive methods of regional wall motion analysis. In the perioperative period, current methods have been unable to differentiate the normal apparent septal hypokinesis seen in most patients undergoing uncomplicated CABG from that due to infarction.[9–17] In a prior study we evaluated a quantitative two-dimensional echocardiographic analytic algorithm for wall motion using a floating-axis system and found it to be a reliable method for analyzing regional left ventricular function, including that of the interventricular septum.[18] Subsequently we found it to be accurate at differentiating patients with perioperative Q wave myocardial infarction from patients undergoing uncomplicated CABG.[19] Sensitivity of the method was 88% and specificity was 80%. In the present study, we applied this system of analysis to 65 patients undergoing CABG to determine the incidence of perioperative RWMAs unassociated with new Q waves on the electrocardiogram. We also compared the effects of these RWMAs on regional and global left ventricular function with those in a group of patients with Q wave–associated perioperative myocardial infarction.

Methods

Patient selection. Only patients with no documented history of a prior myocardial infarction who were scheduled for CABG surgery were considered eligible for study. Patients undergoing concomitant valve replacement or aneurysmectomy were excluded. The electrocardiograms of all subjects were reviewed and patients with preexisting pathologic Q waves (>0.04 sec in duration) were excluded. The preoperative contrast ventriculograms (done no more than 3 months before surgery) were reviewed and only patients with normal regional wall motion, by the consensus of three observers, and global ejection fraction greater than or equal to 55% were considered eligible. After CABG, all perioperative electrocardiograms were reviewed and patients who survived for 24 hr after surgery and who did not develop new pathologic Q waves were divided into three groups based on the peak creatine kinase (CK)–MB isoenzyme level. We had previously determined the mean and SD of peak CK-MB at our hospital to be 92 ± 49 IU/liter by reviewing the data on a consecutive series of 106 patients who underwent CABG without developing new Q waves. Group 1 was defined as those patients with peak CK-MB between 0 and 92 IU/liter. The peak value for group 2 patients was between 93 and 141 IU/liter and that for group 3 patients was greater than 141 IU/liter. The final group studied, group 4, was composed of those patients who developed new pathologic Q waves in the perioperative period.

Before the commencement of the study we established goals with regard to the number of patients from each group that would be included in the study because we wished to avoid studying large numbers of patients with high probabilities of having normal postoperative wall motion. Accordingly, based on data from our prior studies,[18, 19] our goal was to include 10 patients from group 1, 10 patients from group 2, 25 patients from group 3, and 20 patients from group 4.

Surgical technique. All patients underwent cardiopulmonary bypass at a systemic temperature of 25° C. The left ventricle was vented through the right superior pulmonary vein. Distal bypass graft anastomoses were performed during one period of aortic cross-clamping. Myocardial preservation was achieved with cold (4° C) potassium crystalloid cardioplegia administered through the aortic root and through the free ends of the grafts immediately after the distal anastomoses were completed. Topical hypothermia was produced with iced saline slush. Myocardial temperature was continuously monitored in the interventricular septum anteriorly in all patients and was maintained below 15° C throughout the period of aortic cross-clamping. The proximal anastomoses were performed with an aortic side-biting clamp while the patient was being rewarmed. In all patients segments of reversed saphenous vein were used exclusively. The pericardium was left open after surgery in each case.

Determination of cardiac enzyme levels. Total serum CK activity was determined by a modification of the method of Rosalki.[20] Total CK-MB levels were determined by a modification of the method of Somer and Konttinen,[21] as described by Wlodarski et al.[22] Blood samples were drawn immediately, 8, and 24 hr after surgery. Occasionally some patients had additional samples drawn at the discretion of their physicians.

Two-dimensional echocardiographic studies. The methods of image acquisition and quantitative analysis have been previously described in detail,[18, 19] and are reiterated briefly.

Image acquisition techniques. Two-dimensional echocardiographic studies were performed by a technician, blinded to the purpose of the study and the clinical status of the patient, with a commercially available Hewlett-Packard phased-array sector scanner (Model 77020A) with 2.5 and 3.5 MHz transducers or an ATL-ADR (Advanced Technology Labs, Inc.) 90 degree mechanical sector scanner and recorded on videotape (Sony Betamax). To allow recovery of function in regions rendered ischemic during surgery the studies were performed as late as possible in the hospital course.

Endocardial tracings were made on a transparent overlay placed on a video monitor screen. All tracing was performed without knowledge of group assignment, clinical status of the patient, CK-MB level, or electrocardiographic or radionuclide ventriculographic data.

Quantitative image analysis. Quantitative analysis of regional wall motion was made from the apical four-chamber and two-chamber (with aorta) views as described by Feigenbaum.[23] The method of floating-axis analysis with an Irex Cardio 80 computer has been previously described.[18, 19] The long axis of the left ventricle is defined by internal points of reference for each diastolic and systolic image. The long axis is identified from the midpoint of the apex to the midpoint of the mitral valve for the apical four-chamber view and from the apex to the junction of the mitral and aortic valve in the apical two-chamber view. The midpoint of the long axis for each end-diastolic and end-systolic image is determined by the computer. The end-systolic image is transposed so that the long axes and midpoints of each image are exactly superimposed. From the midpoint of the long axis 24 radii are drawn to the systolic and diastolic outlines of the left ventricle. The percentage change in area (area shrinkage) for each segment is then calculated from the formula (end-diastolic area − end-systolic area)/end-distolic area × 100%.

For the apical four-chamber view the following segments were defined[18, 19]: basal septal, apical septal, apical, apical lateral, and basal lateral. The apical two-chamber view was similarly divided into anterobasal, anteroapical, apical, inferoapical, and inferobasal segments. The mean percent area shrinkage was determined for each region. Hypokinesis was defined as mean percent area shrinkage more than 2 SDs below the mean value for a group of normal subjects studied previously.[19]

A wall motion score was generated for each patient, based on the number of regions involved and the severity of the abnormality, with a modification of the method of Heger et al.[24] Akinesis was defined as mean percent area shrinkage for a segment of between −10% (that is, 10% systolic expansion of the area) and +10%, and was given a score of 2. Dyskinesis was defined as systolic expansion of the area of more than 10% and was given a score of 3. Hypokinesis was a mean percent area shrinkage of between +10% and 2 SDs below the normal mean[19] and was assigned a score of 1. Normal area shrinkage was scored as 0. Total score was derived by multiplying the number of dyskinetic segments by 3, akinetic segments by 2, and hypokinetic segments by 1 and adding the total. The score for the apical segment was derived by taking the mean of the score in apical four- and two-chamber views. Because normal apical endocardial motion can be minimal[19, 25] and we wanted to minimize false-positive results, isolated apical hypokinesis was not considered abnormal.[26] Isolated apical akinesis or dyskinesis and apical hypokinesis in association with other regional abnormalities were considered abnormal and were scored accordingly.

To assess the probability that our patient selection criteria might have failed to exclude some patients with abnormal preoperative two-dimensional echocardiograms, we applied this echocardiographic analysis system to 15 eligible patients before CABG. Eleven (73%) had complete studies. Of these, two (18%) had a regional abnormality by quantitative two-dimensional echocardiography (a specificity of 82%). In both of these, the abnormality was mild hypokinesis involving only one segment (wall motion score = 1).

Radionuclide ventriculography. First-pass radionuclide ventriculography was performed during the week before surgery and again 10 to 14 days after surgery. Details of the technique have been published previously.[27] Briefly, a bolus of 15 mCi of ^{99m}Tc pertechnetate was injected into a large-bore intravenous catheter placed in an antecubital vein. A multicrystal scintillation camera in the 30 degree left anterior oblique position with 20 degrees of caudal tilt was interfaced with a computer that acquired data at 40 frames/sec. The left ventricular region of interest was defined manually and a time-activity curve was generated for the left ventricle with use of a computer algorithm. Ejection fraction was determined by averaging the counts of 5 to 8 consecutive beats. Ejection fraction determined by this technique is highly reproducible ($y = 3.4 + 0.92x$, where y is the first determination and x is the second; $r = .97$).[27] Measurements of left ventricular ejection fraction in our hospital are significantly correlated with contrast cineangiography ($r = .88$, SEE = 0.07).[28] However, ejection fractions determined by radionuclide ventriculography are consistently lower than those derived from contrast cineangiograms. The regression equation is $y = 1.16x + 3.6$, where y is the contrast angiographic value and x is the ventriculographic value.[29] Thus, a radionuclide ventriculographic ejection fraction of 44% is equivalent to a contrast angiographic ejection fraction of 55%, the lower limit of normal in our laboratory.

Adequacy of revascularization. Adequacy of revascularization was assessed grossly by dividing the coronary circulation into three arterial distributions — the anterior (left anterior decending artery and diagonal branches), the lateral (circumflex artery and marginal branches), and the inferior (posterior descending artery and left ventricular extension branches). Maximal number of coronary arteries that could be diseased was thus three. For the purpose of this study, if a graft were placed to a region, that region was considered adequately revascularized even if a branch of the major vessel were diseased and did not receive a graft.

Statistical analyses. Differences between groups with respect to the frequency of an event were determined by the multiple chi-square analysis. Presence of significant differences between multiple groups was determined by analysis of variance and the modification of Tukey's method for unequal sample sizes. When comparisons involved only two groups, significance was determined by the t test for independent means.

Variability. Variability in the process of identifying the long axis of the ventricle was examined previously.[18] When two observers identified the long axis of the same diastolic and systolic endocardial outline, the interobserver difference in mean percent area shrinkage was 4% and 3% for the septum and lateral walls, respectively. Variability in our method of tracing endocardial outlines has also been examined.[19, 30] Correlation coefficients for mean percent area shrinkage ranged from .88 to .97 for various regions of the ventricle and SEEs were less than 6% (intraobserver) and 9% (interobserver). These analyses were not repeated.

Results

Patient population. Preoperative characteristics of the four groups were similar. Ejection fraction by contrast angiography (69 ± 5%, 63 ± 8%, 68 ± 6%, 67 ± 8% for groups 1 through 4, respectively) and mean number of vessels diseased (2.5 ± 0.7, 2.9 ± 0.4, 2.7 ± 0.7, 2.7 ± 0.6 for groups 1 through 4) were not significantly different. The patients in groups 1 through 3 were enrolled over a 16 month period and those in group 4 were enrolled over a 34 month period. Eighty patients (58% of all eligible patients) had a peak CK-MB of 92 IU/liter or less. Ten of these were randomly chosen for entry into the study. Thirty-two patients (23% of all eligible patients) had a peak CK-MB of 93 to 141 IU/liter and 10 of these were also selected. All 20 of the patients from groups 1 and 2 survived to undergo two-dimensional echocardiographic examination. All 25 group 3 patients (18% of all eligible patients) were entered into the study, but two were transferred to another institution and one died before undergoing two-dimensional echocardiographic examination. Thus, 22 or 88% of all eligible group 3 patients were studied. All eligible group 4 patients were entered into the study; one died and the remaining 19 (95%) underwent two-dimensional echocardiographic examination. The overall incidence of Q wave perioperative myocardial infarction during the 16 month period was 4.5%. The new Q waves were located in anterior leads in eight patients, the inferior leads in seven, the lateral leads in one, the inferior and lateral leads in two, and the anterior and inferior leads in two.

Complete two-dimensional echocardiographic examinations technically adequate for quantitative analysis were obtained for 79% of patients with new Q waves and 83% of those without new Q waves on the electrocardiogram. Studies in patients in group 1 were performed 12.2 ± 3.7 days after surgery, those in group 2 were performed at 12 ± 5.9 days, those in group 3 at 13.6 ± 6.8 days, and those in group 4 at 13.5 ± 4.8 days (p = NS). A large pericardial effusion was present on the initial study in one group 3 patient, but since the effusion had partially resolved to moderate size by the time of the follow-up study, data from the patient were included in the analysis. Seventy-four percent of patients who developed new Q waves on the electrocardiogram and 86% of patients without new Q waves underwent preoperative and postoperative radionuclide ventriculographic examinations.

Incidence of RWMAs. RWMAs were detected in none of the group 1 patients, two (20%) of the group 2 patients, 12 (55%) of the group 3 patients, and 17 (89%) of the group 4 patients ($p < .01$ for groups 3 and 4 vs group 1; $p < .01$ for group 4 vs group 2; no other comparisons showed a statistically significant difference). The increasing risk of a RWMA with increasing peak CK-MB can also be seen by comparing peak CK-MB values in those with vs those without such regional abnormalities (229 ± 128 vs 143 ± 149 IU/liter, respectively, $p < .01$).

Severity of RWMAs. Those patients in groups 2 and 3 with new RWMAs were compared with those in group 4 with new RWMAs to determine the relative severity of systolic dysfunction. These data are presented in table 1 and in figures 1 and 2. There were no significant differences in extent or severity of regional involvement (assessed as number of abnormal regions

TABLE 1
Summary of regional function data

	% of abnormal regions per patient	Mean wall motion score	Mean score per abnormal segment
Non–Q wave infarction (n = 14)	43±25	6.2±4.1	1.6±0.8
Q wave infarction (n = 17)	46±22	5.8±4.0	1.5±0.7

p = NS for all comparisons between Q wave and non–Q wave groups.

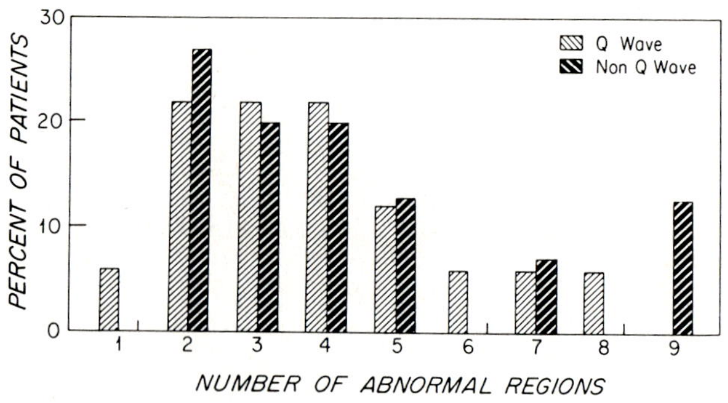

FIGURE 1. Frequency distribution of the number of abnormal regions per patient in Q wave and non–Q wave myocardial infarction groups.

per patient [figure 1], wall motion score [figure 2], or mean score per abnormal segment [table 1]), in patients with non–Q wave and those with Q wave infarction. Absolute mean percent area shrinkage for Q wave and non–Q wave groups was compared on a segment-by-segment basis. Again, no significant differences were found.

Global left ventricular function. Changes in global left ventricular function were assessed by changes in ejection fraction from before to after surgery by radionuclide ventriculography. Before surgery the mean ejection fractions for the four groups were not significantly different and ranged from 50 ± 6.5% for group 1 to 53.5 ± 7.5% for group 3. All values were equal to or greater than 44%. Figure 3 is a plot of the change in ejection fraction in (1) patients without new Q waves and normal regional wall motion after surgery, (2) patients without new Q waves but with abnormal regional wall motion, and (3) patients with new Q waves and abnormal regional wall motion. Mean deterioration in ejection fraction for the patients without new Q waves but with a regional abnormality (8.9 ± 10%) was not significantly different from that in the Q wave group (6.7 ± 10.7%). Both of these values are signifi-

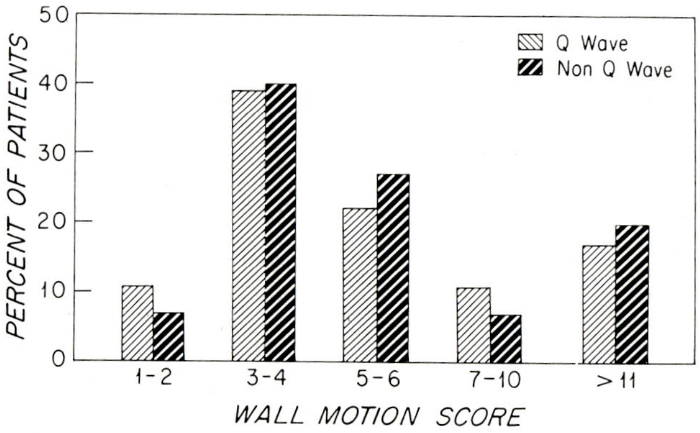

FIGURE 2. Frequency distribution of the wall motion scores in Q wave and non-Q wave myocardial infarction groups.

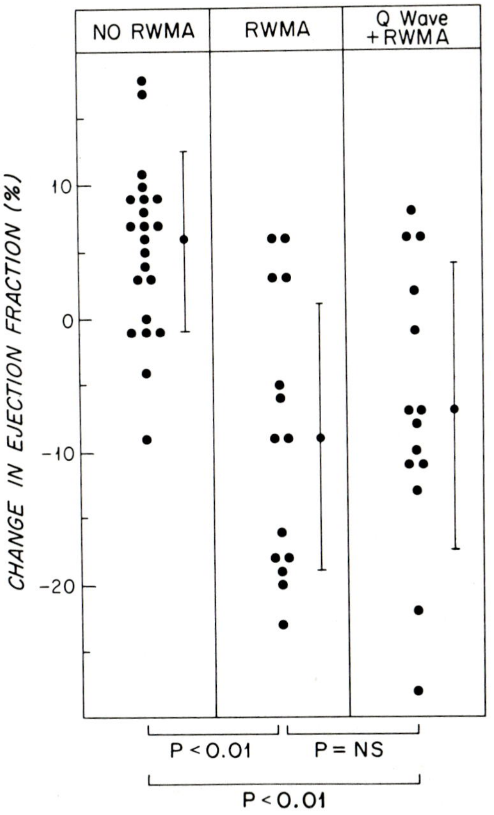

FIGURE 3. Change in radionuclide ventriculographic ejection fraction from preoperative to postoperative study. No RWMA = patients with normal postoperative regional wall motion; RWMA = patients with new postoperative RWMAs but without new Q waves; Q wave + RWMA = patients from group 4 (Q waves on postoperative electrocardiograms) with new RWMAs.

cantly different from the results for the patients who did not develop Q waves or a regional abnormality. This group increased their ejection fraction by 5.7 ± 6.7% ($p < .001$).

Clinical correlates of non–Q wave myocardial infarction. Unstable angina (i.e., uncontrolled angina at rest requiring surgery within 7 days) was a significant predictor of subsequent development of a wall motion abnormality. Seventy-one percent of the patients with unstable angina developed a wall motion abnormality vs 29% of those with stable angina ($p < .05$). Neither extent of coronary disease nor preoperative ejection fraction were predictive of RWMA.

Operative variables examined were aortic cross-clamp time (as an index of ischemic time) and adequacy of revascularization. Longer cross-clamp time was not required in those patient groups with higher peak CK-MB levels or in those who developed wall motion abnormalities (normal wall motion, 47 ± 14 min; abnormal wall motion, 51 ± 20 min). Similarly, inadequate revascularization was not more common in the groups with higher peak CK-MB. However, in those patients with the highest levels of CK-MB (group 3), inadequate revascularization tended to predict the development of wall motion abnormalities. Eighty-three percent of inadequately revascularized group 3 patients developed a regional abnormality vs 41% of adequately revascularized patients. The trend failed to reach statistical significance.

Discussion

Experimental observations in animals have shown that the use of hypothermia and potassium cardioplegia can effectively preserve regional and global ventricular function as well as myocardial ultrastructure during prolonged periods of anoxia.[31–33] Similar data exist for patient studies,[2, 34, 35] but the Coronary Artery Surgery Study has provided the strongest evidence that hypothermic cardioplegia is beneficial. Berger et al.[1] reported reductions in operative mortality of nearly 5% over normothermic intermittent ischemic arrest. Also, rates of Q wave infarction were reduced by half when compared with normothermia or hypothermia alone. Although this data is certainly encouraging, several workers in the field have expressed the concern that statistics on survival and Q wave myocardial infarction alone may be too insensitive to properly evaluate the adequacy of current preservation techniques.[2–4]

Support for this viewpoint comes from the study of Bulkley and Hutchins, which was done before cold cardioplegia was used.[5] In their postmortem study of patients who died within 1 month of cardiac surgery, they found operative myocardial injury of some degree in 83% of patients and regional transmural necrosis in 38%. In only 14% of the patients with transmural necrosis was the injury detected by Q waves on the electrocardiogram. Further support comes from studies in which ^{99m}Tc pyrophosphate was used for imaging of myocardial infarction.[36–41] Although done before the advent of cold cardioplegia and not specifically addressing the problem of non–Q wave myocardial infarction, most of these studies have reported an incidence of positive ^{99m}Tc pyrophosphate scans without associated Q waves on the electrocardiogram at least as great as the incidence of positive scans with new Q waves on the electrocardiogram. Gray et al.[40] and Platt et al.[37] found incidences of positive scans without new Q waves that were 1.5 and 2 times the incidence of positive scans with new Q waves. Given the limited sensitivity of planar imaging for detecting non–Q wave myocardial infarction,[42–44] the true relative incidence may be significantly higher. Indeed, the three contrast ventriculographic studies (again, done before cold cardioplegia was used) that examined this question[6-8] found that the incidence of deterioration in wall motion without associated Q waves on the electrocardiogram was 2.3 to 5.5 times greater than the 6.2% to 15% incidence of Q wave myocardial infarction.

In summary, use of hypothermic cardioplegia has dramatically reduced the incidence of Q wave infarction. However, contrast ventriculographic studies with adequate numbers of patients analogous to the ones referenced above have not been done since the use of cold cardioplegia has become widespread. Thus, it is not clear whether the newer preservation technique has similarly reduced the occurrence of left ventricular regional dysfunction unassociated with Q waves on the electrocardiogram, which seemingly is a more common outcome of inadequate preservation than is Q wave infarction.

There are several reasons for this lack of data. Since suboptimal preservation presumably occurs infrequently, prohibitively large numbers of consecutive (unselected) patients would need to undergo contrast ventriculography — a procedure that investigators are hesitant to do and patients are equally hesitant to undergo in the perioperative period — to collect a series of adequate size to draw meaningful conclusions. Thus, Raabe et al.[45] studied 50 consecutive patients but found only eight with RWMAs. Although noninvasive techniques would be ideal, regional wall motion analysis with radionuclide ventriculography has been limited by its inherent fixed external-frame-of-reference system, which cannot correct for the exaggerated anteromedial systolic translation of the postoperative heart.[9, 11-17] Consequently there is false enhancement of lateral wall motion and false hypokinesis of septal segments, as noted in comparison with systolic thickening data.[18]

We used a quantitative two-dimensional echocardiographic analysis system that has been evaluated in two previous reports.[18, 19] This method used an internal frame of reference or floating-axis system that corrected for the exaggerated postoperative systolic translation of the heart. Thus, regional endocardial motion closely reflected regional systolic function as measured by systolic thickening analysis.[18] With two-dimensional echocardiographic floating-axis analysis, we detected RWMAs in 88% of patients who underwent CABG and developed new pathologic Q waves on postoperative electrocardiograms.[19] Specificity was 80% and was increased to 90% without a decrease in sensitivity when isolated apical hypokinesis was considered normal, as suggested by the data of Sheehan et al.[25] and Schnittger et al.[26]

In the present study we again detected RWMAs in a high percentage of patients (89%) with new pathologic Q waves. In the patients without Q waves, the risk of developing a new wall motion abnormality increased with higher peak CK-MB values. To extrapolate an overall incidence of new RWMAs unassociated with new Q waves, the percentage of all CABG patients falling into each group during the 16 month period of the study can be multiplied by the observed incidences of wall motion abnormalities within each group. Thus, the expected incidence of RWMAs without new Q waves would be 14.4% (with a standard error of 3.5%) of 3.2 times the incidence of Q wave myocardial infarction. This relative incidence is similar to that reported in the contrast ventriculographic studies done before the advent of cold cardioplegia,[6-8] although absolute incidence is markedly lower. Thus, improved methods of preservation appear to have reduced the occurrence of non–Q wave myocardial infarction in parallel with the reduction in Q wave infarction so that absolute incidence has dropped significantly but relative incidence remains high. These data confirm the suspicions of Conti et al.[2] and others[3, 4] that a measure more sensitive than ones employed previously must be used to evaluate new methods of preservation.

To ensure that the observed incidence of non–Q wave infarction was not due to minor amounts of hypokinesis, we examined the effects of the non–Q wave myocardial infarction on regional and global ventricular function. Previous studies examining this question have been limited by the use of highly nonspecific electrocardiographic criteria for patient selection,[46, 47] qualitative assessment of contrast ventriculograms,[46] nonblinded reviewers,[47] study patients with unusual distributions of location of infarction,[47] and small study populations.[48] In general, however, results of these studies have suggested that the effects on left ventricular function of both non–Q wave and Q wave infarctions are minimal. Our results differ significantly. We found that not only are the effects on regional and global left ventricular function similar, but also that they are important in the majority of patients. We detected no difference between Q wave and non–Q wave infarction groups with respect to any parameter of regional or global function, and the ejection fraction of 43% in patients with new wall motion abnormalities deteriorated by at least 10%. Given that in patients with no evidence of myocardial infarction ejection fractions increased by a mean of 6%, this is a significant decline.

Limitations. The first potential question is whether our results can be generalized to patients being treated at other institutions. Several factors argue that they can. First, the graft patency rates (80% at 1 year) for series of patients at our institution[49, 50] are equivalent to those reported by others.[51–54] Second, the perioperative rate of Q wave infarction during the time of our study of 4.5% is similar to the overall rate of 3.8%[1] and the rate of 6.4% for the randomized subgroup in the Coronary Artery Surgery Study.[55] Since results with respect to these two easily identifiable outcomes of operative therapy are comparable to those at other institutions, there is no reason to suspect that marked variances in other aspects of operative and postoperative care exist.

The second limitation of our study is the lack of preoperative two-dimensional echocardiograms on our patients. Thus, the possibility that patients with preexistent wall motion abnormalities were entered into the study is raised. Given the stringent entrance criteria of no pathologic Q waves on the electrocardiogram and normal wall motion and ejection fraction by contrast ventriculography, we believe this is unlikely. To confirm this we analyzed two-dimensional echocardiograms from 15 preoperative patients who met our entrance criteria. Although 18% had a regional abnormality as assessed by quantitative two-dimensional echocardiography, the abnormalities were minimal (mild hypokinesis of one segment). Thus, it seems unlikely that many patients with preexisting significant RWMAs would have been studied.

Finally, our results may have been affected by the timing of the echocardiographic examinations, which were performed a mean of 13 days after surgery. Regional and global left ventricular function may not necessarily be stable over time in this patient population. Quantitative data on the evolution of regional contraction abnormalities in man after acute myocardial infarction are very limited. It is clear that global left ventricular function may change significantly in individual patients during the first year after nonoperative acute infarction.[56–60] For these patients as a group, however, ejection fraction changes very little during this time.[56–60] Postoperative changes in ventricular function do occur over time and may be related to perioperative alterations in preload and afterload,[61] diastolic compliance,[62] sympathetic nervous system activity,[63, 64] and potentially to the resolution of intraoperative or preoperative ischemia.[65] Global ejection fraction decreases very early after CABG, but then improves to near preoperative levels by the first postoperative week.[66, 67] Minimal further improvement may occur over the next year.[61] Thus, a greater incidence and severity of RWMAs might have been observed if studies had been performed during the very early postoperative period. Extrapolation from data on nonoperative acute infarction suggests that it is unlikely that any substantial improvement in wall motion would have been observed if studies had been performed at late follow-up.

In conclusion, hypothermic potassium cardioplegia has certainly reduced the incidence of perioperative Q wave myocardial infarction, and appears to have reduced the incidence of RWMAs without associated Q waves on the electrocardiogram (non–Q wave infarction) to a similar degree. However, non–Q wave infarction remains roughly three times more common than Q wave infarction, and half of the patients with non–Q wave infarcts will have a significant deterioration in ventricular function. Our findings indicate that evaluations of newer techniques of myocardial preservation should include a method that allows prospective quantitative analysis of regional left ventricular function.

We thank Dr. Peter Kowey for his review of this manuscript, Carol Cohen, Michelle Gilfoil, and Lori Perkins for their technical assistance, and Donna Kantarges and Clare Smith for their help in the preparation of this manuscript.

References

1. Berger RL, Davis KB, Kaiser GC, Foster ED, Hammond GL, Tong TGL, Kennedy JW, Sheffield T, Ringqvist I, Wiens RD, Chaitman BR, Mock M: Preservation of the myocardium during coronary artery bypass grafting. Circulation **64** (suppl II): II-61, 1981
2. Conti VR, Bertranon EG, Blackstone EH, Kirklin JW, Digerness SB: Cold cardioplegia versus hypothermia for myocardial protection. J Thorac Cardiovasc Surg **76:** 577, 1978
3. Singh AK, Farrugia R, Teplitz C, Karlson K: Electrolyte versus blood cardioplegia: randomized clinical and myocardial ultrastructural study. Ann Thorac Surg **33:** 218, 1981
4. Stiles QR, Kirklin JW: Myocardial preservation symposium. J Thorac Cardiovasc Surg **82:** 870, 1981
5. Bulkley BH, Hutchins GM: Myocardial consequences of coronary artery bypass graft surgery. The paradox of necrosis in areas of revascularization. Circulation **56:** 906, 1977
6. Lim JS, Proudfit WL, Sheldon WC, Alosilla C, Phillips DF, Loop FD: Perioperative myocardial infarction related to coronary bypass surgery. Am Heart J **96:** 463, 1978
7. Achuff SC, Griffith LSC, Conti CR, Humphries JO, Brawley RK, Gott VL, Ross RS: The "angina-producing" myocardial segment: an approach to the interpretation of results of coronary bypass surgery. Am J Cardiol **36:** 723, 1975
8. Warren SG, Wagner GS, Bethea CF, Roe CR, Oldham HN, Kong Y: Diagnostic and prognostic significance of electrocardiographic and CPK isoenzyme changes following coronary bypass surgery: correlation with findings at one year. Am Heart J **93:** 189, 1977
9. Dinsmore RE, Pohost GM: Abnormal interventricular septal motion following cardiac surgery: clinical, surgical, echocardiographic and radionuclide correlates. Am Heart J **97:** 27, 1979
10. Rubenson DS, Tucker CR, London E, Miller DC, Stinson EB, Popp RL: Two-dimensional echocardiographic analysis of segmental left ventricular wall motion before and after coronary artery bypass surgery. Circulation **66:** 1025, 1982
11. Righetti A, Crawford MH, O'Rourke RA, Schelbert H, Daily PO, Ross J Jr: Interventricular septal motion and left ventricular function after coronary bypass surgery. Am J Cardiol **39:** 372, 1977
12. Rozanski A, Berman DS, Gray R, Levy R, Raymond M, Maddahi J, Pantaleo N, Waxman AD, Swan MJC, Matloff J: Use of thal-

lium-201 redistribution scintigraphy in the preoperative differentiation of reversible and nonreversible myocardial asynergy. Circulation **64:** 936, 1981
13. Rozanski A, Berman D, Gray R, Diamond G, Raymond M, Prause J, Maddahi J, Swan HJC, Matloff J: Preoperative prediction of reversible myocardial asynergy by postexercise radionuclide ventriculography. N Engl J Med **307:** 212, 1982
14. Lindsay J Jr, Nolan NG, Kotlyarov EV, Goldstein SA, Bacos JM: Radionuclide evaluation of the interventricular septum following coronary artery bypass surgery. Radiology **142:** 489, 1982
15. Murphy JH, Okada RD, Boucher CA, Strauss HW, Pohost GM, Daggett WA: Relationship between septal perfusion and abnormal septal motion after coronary artery bypass surgery. Am J Cardiol **49:** 919, 1982
16. Phillips HR, Carter JE, Okada RD, Levine FH, Boucher CA, Osbakken M, Lappas D, Buckley MJ, Pohost GM: Serial changes in left ventricular ejection fraction in the early hours after aortocoronary bypass grafting. Chest **83:** 28, 1983
17. Rakowski H, Gilbert BW, Phaneuf DC, Schreiber J, Crobac M, Koilpillai C, Weisel RD: Late improvement in septal and left ventricular wall motion following aorto-coronary bypass surgery. J Am Coll Cardiol **1:** 619, 1983 (abst)
18. Force T, Bloomfield P, O'Boyle JE, Pietro DA, Dunlap RW, Khuri SF, Parisi AF: Quantitative two-dimensional echocardiographic analysis of motion and thickening of the interventricular septum after cardiac surgery. Circulation **68:** 1013, 1983
19. Force T, Bloomfield P, O'Boyle JE, Khuri SF, Josa M, Parisi AF: Quantitative two-dimensional echocardiographic analysis of regional wall motion in patients with perioperative myocardial infarction. Circulation **70:** 233, 1984
20. Rosalki SB: An improved procedure for serum creatine phosphokinase determination. J Lab Clin Med **69:** 696, 1967
21. Somer H, Konttinen A: A method allowing the quantitation of serum creatine kinase isoenzymes. Clin Chim Acta **36:** 531, 1972
22. Wlodarski FM, Howard PL, Trainer TD: Creatine phosphokinase isoenzymes: a comparison of a kinetic and an electrophoretic method in the diagnosis of myocardial infarction. Clin Chim Acta **76:** 171, 1977
23. Feigenbaum H: Echocardiography. Philadelphia, 1981, Lea and Febiger
24. Heger JJ, Weyman AE, Wann LS, Rogers EW, Dillon JC, Feigenbaum H: Cross-sectional echocardiographic analysis of the extent of left ventricular asynergy in acute myocardial infarction. Circulation **61:** 1113, 1980
25. Sheehan FH, Stewart AK, Dodge HT, Mitten S, Bolson EL, Brown BG: Variability in the measurement of regional left ventricular wall motion from contrast angiograms. Circulation **68:** 550, 1983
26. Schnittger I, Fitzgerald PJ, Gordon EP, Alderman EL, Popp RL: Computerized quantitative analysis of left ventricular wall motion by two-dimensional echocardiography. Circulation **70:** 242, 1984
27. Scharf SM, Brown R, Tow DE, Parisi AF: Cardiac effects of increased lung volume and decreased pleural pressure in man. J Appl Physiol **47:** 257, 1979
28. Folland ED, Parisi AF, Moynihan PF, Jones DR, Feldman CL, Tow DE: Assessment of left ventricular ejection fraction and volumes by real-time, two dimensional echocardiography. Circulation **60:** 760, 1979
29. Tow DE, Parisi AF, Folland ED, Sasahara AA: Proceedings of II International Congress of World Federation of Nuclear Medicine and Biology. September 17–21, 1978, Washington, D.C., p 99
30. Moynihan PF, Parisi AF, Feldman CL: Quantitative detection of regional left ventricular contraction abnormalities by two-dimensional echocardiography. Circulation **63:** 752, 1981
31. Hearse DJ, Stewart DA, Braimbridge MV: Hypothermic arrest and potassium arrest. Metabolic and myocardial protection during elective cardiac arrest. Circ Res **36:** 481, 1975
32. Schaff HV, Dombroff R, Flaherty JT, Bulkley BH, Hutchins GM, Goldman RA, Gott VL: Effect of potassium cardioplegia on myocardial ischemia and post arrest ventricular function. Circulation **58:** 240, 1978
33. Engelman RM, Levitsky S, O'Donoghue MJ, Anvil J: Cardioplegia and myocardial preservation during cardiopulmonary bypass. Circulation **58** (suppl I): I-107, 1978
34. Weisel RD, Lipton IH, Lyall RM, Baird RJ: Cardiac metabolism and performance following cold potassium cardioplegia. Circulation **58** (suppl I): I-217, 1978
35. Fischer VW, Barner HB: Ultrastructural integrity of human ventricular myocardium following cardioplegic arrest. Ann Thorac Surg **27:** 49, 1979
36. Klausner SC, Botvinick EH, Shames D, Ullyot DJ, Fishman NH, Roe BB, Ebert PA, Chatterjee K, Parmley WW: The application of radionuclide infarct scintigraphy to diagnose perioperative myocardial infarction following revascularization. Circulation **56:** 173, 1977
37. Platt MR, Mills LJ, Parkey RW, Willerson JT, Bante FJ, Shapiro W, Sugg WL: Perioperative myocardial infarction diagnosed by technetium-99m stannous pyrophosphate myocardial scintigrams. Circulation **54** (suppl III): III-24, 1976
38. Righetti A, Crawford MH, O'Rourke RA, Hardarson T, Schelbent H, Daily PO, DeLuca M, Ashburn W, Ross J Jr: Detection of perioperative myocardial damage after coronary artery bypass graft surgery. Circulation **55:** 173, 1977
39. Burdine JA, DePuey EG, Mathur VS, Hall RJ: Scintigraphic, electrocardiographic, and enzymatic diagnosis of perioperative myocardial infarction in patients undergoing myocardial revascularization. J Nucl Med **20:** 711, 1979
40. Gray RJ, Matloff JM, Conklin CM, Gary W, Charuzi Y, Wolfstein R, Swan HJC: Perioperative myocardial infarction: late clinical course after coronary artery bypass surgery. Circulation **66:** 1185, 1982
41. Fennel WH, Chua KG, Cohen L, Morgan J, Karunaratne HB, Resnekov L, Al-Sadir J, Lin C-Y, Lamberti JJ, Anagnostopoulos CE: Detection, prediction, and significance of perioperative myocardial infarction following aorta-coronary bypass. J Thorac Cardiovasc Surg **78:** 244, 1979
42. Walsh WF, Karunaratne HB, Resnekov L, Fill HR, Harber PV: Assessment of diagnostic value of technetium-99m pyrophosphate myocardial scintigraphy in 80 patients with possible acute myocardial infarction. Br Heart J **39:** 974, 1977
43. Massie BM, Botvinick EH, Werner JA, Chatterjee K, Parmley WW: Myocardial scintigraphy with technetium-99m stannous pyrophosphate: An insensitive test for nontransmural myocardial infarction. Am J Cardiol **43:** 186, 1979
44. Corbett JR, Lewis M, Willerson JT, Nicol PH, Huxley RL, Simon T, Rude RE, Henderson E, Parkey R, Rellas JS, Buja LM, Sokolov JJ, Lewis SE: ^{99m}Tc-Pyrophosphate imaging in patients with acute myocardial infarction: comparison of planar imaging with single-photon tomography with and without blood pool overlay. Circulation **69:** 1120, 1984
45. Raabe DS Jr, Morise A, Sbarbaro JA, Gundel WD: Diagnostic criteria for acute myocardial infarction in patients undergoing coronary artery bypass surgery. Circulation **62:** 869, 1980
46. Codd JE, Wiens RD, Kaiser GC, Barner HB, Tyras DH, Mudd JG, Willman VL: Late sequelae of perioperative myocardial infarction. Ann Thorac Surg **26:** 208, 1978
47. Burton JR, Fitzgibbon GM, Keon WJ, Leach AJ: Perioperative myocardial infarction complicating coronary bypass. Clinical and angiographic correlations and prognosis. J Thorac Cardiovasc Surg **82:** 758, 1981
48. Roberts AJ, Spies SM, Lichtenthal PR, Moran JM, Sanders JH, Michaelis LL: Changes in left ventricular performance related to perioperative myocardial infarction in coronary artery bypass graft surgery. Ann Thorac Surg **35:** 516, 1983
49. Sharma GVRK, Khuri SF, Folland ED, Barsamian EM, Parisi AF: Prognosis for aortocoronary graft patency: a comparison of preoperative and intraoperative assessments. J Thorac Cardiovasc Surg **85:** 570, 1983
50. Sharma GVRK, Khuri SF, Josa M, Folland ED, Parisi AF: The effect of antiplatelet therapy on saphenous vein coronary artery bypass graft patency. Circulation **68** (suppl II): II-218, 1983
51. McEnany MT, Salzman EW, Mundth ED, DeSanctis RW, Harthorne JW, Weintraub RM, Gates S, Austen WG: The effect of antithrombotic therapy on patency rates of saphenous vein coronary artery bypass grafts. J Thorac Cardiovasc Surg **83:** 81, 1982
52. Pantely GS, Goodnight SH Jr, Rahimtoola SH, Harlan BJ, DeMots H, Calvin L, Rösch J: Failure of antiplatelet and anticoagulant therapy to improve patency of grafts after coronary-artery bypass. N Engl J Med **301:** 962, 1977
53. Cheseboro JH, Clements IP, Fuster V, Elveback LR, Smith HC,

Bardsley WT, Frye RL, Holmes DR Jr, Vlietstra RE, Pluth JR, Wallace RB, Puga FJ, Orszulak TA, Pichler JM, Schaff HV, Danielson GK: A platelet inhibitor drug trial in coronary artery bypass operations. N Engl J Med **307:** 73, 1982
54. Kouchoukos N, Karp RB, Oberman A, Russel RO Jr, Alison HW, Holt JH Jr: Longterm patency of saphenous veins for coronary bypass grafting. Circulation **58** (suppl I): I-96, 1978
55. CASS Principal Investigators and their associates: Coronary artery surgery study (CASS): a randomized trial of coronary artery bypass surgery. Survival data. Circulation **68:** 939, 1983
56. Wackers FJ, Berger HJ, Weinberg MA, Zaret BL: Spontaneous changes in left ventricular function over the first 24 hours of acute myocardial infarction: implications for evaluating early therapeutic interventions. Circulation **66:** 748, 1982
57. Schelbert HR, Henning H, Ashburn WL, Verba JW, Karliner JS, O'Rourke RA: Serial measurements of left ventricular ejection fraction by radionuclide angiography early and late after myocardial infarction. Am J Cardiol **38:** 407, 1976
58. Reduto LA, Berger HJ, Cohen LS, Gottschalk A, Zaret BL: Sequential radionuclide assessment of left and right ventricular performance after acute transmural myocardial infarction. Ann Intern Med **89:** 441, 1978
59. Borer JS, Rosing DR, Miller RH, Stark RM, Kent KM, Bacharach SL, Green MV, Lake CR, Cohen H, Holmes D, Donohue D, Baker W, Epstein SE: Natural history of left ventricular function during 1 year after acute myocardial infarction: comparison with clinical electrocardiographic and biochemical determinations. Am J Cardiol **46:** 1, 1980
60. Ramanathan K, Bodenheimer MM, Banka VS, Helfant RH: Natural history of contractile abnormalities after acute myocardial infarction in man: severity and response to nitroglycerin as a function of time. Circulation **63:** 731, 1981
61. Mintz LJ, Ingels NB, Daughters GT, Stinson EB, Alderman EL: Sequential studies of left ventricular function and wall motion after coronary arterial bypass surgery. Am J Cardiol **45:** 210, 1980
62. Levine FH, Copeland JG, Melvin DB, Stinson EB: Extended evaluation of anoxia on ventricular performance and compliance. Circulation **46** (suppl II): II-182, 1972 (abst)
63. Boudoulas H, Lewis RP, Vasko JS, Karayannacos PE, Beaver BM: Left ventricular function and adrenergic hyperactivity before and after saphenous vein bypass. Circulation **53:** 802, 1976
64. Hammermeister KE, Kennedy JW: Myocardial revascularization and ventricular performance. Circulation **48:** 450, 1973
65. Chatterjee K, Swan HJC, Parmley WW, Sustaita H, Marcus H, Matloff J: Depression of left ventricular function due to acute myocardial ischemia and its reversal after aortocoronary saphenous vein bypass. N Engl J Med **286:** 1117, 1972
66. Roberts AJ, Spies SM, Sanders JH, Moran JM, Wilkinson CJ, Lichtenthal PR, White RL, Michaelis LL: Serial assessment of left ventricular performance following coronary artery bypass grafting. J Thorac Cardiovasc Surg **81:** 69, 1981
67. Reduto LA, Lawrie GM, Reid JW, Whissenand HH, Noon GP, Kanon D, De Bakey ME, Miller RR: Sequential postoperative assessment of left ventricular performance with gated cardiac blood pool imaging following aortocoronary bypass surgery. Am Heart J **101:** 59, 1981

Subendocardial infarction in retrospect: pathologic, cardiographic, and ancillary features

HAROLD D. LEVINE, M.D.

ABSTRACT Fifty-three patients with subendocardial infarction (SEMI) were studied at autopsy; all were elderly and the group was equally divided by sex. About half had more than one SEMI; the recurrences or extensions often involved superjacent, but not infrequently adjacent, areas. Six showed fibrinous pericarditis. This larger study showed more widespread and severe coronary narrowing than an earlier report. Six patients had thrombi in the right coronary artery. Six showed electrocardiographic evidence of concomitant anteroseptal and inferior (Roesler-Dressler) infarction, and 12 had intraventricular block generally preceding higher-grade block or arrhythmias. At some time during their terminal hospitalization, 27 patients, or half, developed distinctive protracted RS-T depression or T wave inversion. Twenty-four of the SEMIs were diagnosed on accepted criteria as transmural infarct; that diagnosis was sustained in only four. Thus neither the presence of changes in RS-T segment or T wave nor the absence of QRS changes are mandatory for the diagnosis of SEMI; this invalidates the common assumption that the diagnosis is not justified unless these conditions are met.
Circulation 72, No. 4, 790–800, 1985.

ON THE PRESUMPTION that it is uncommon[1, 2] relatively benign,[3, 4] and represented in the electrocardiogram (ECG) only by changes in ventricular repolarization, subendocardial infarction (SEMI) was at first regarded as quite distinct from "garden variety" transmural infarction. Recent consensus, by contrast, has recognized SEMI as more common,[5–9] more serious in impact,[10–13] tending to recur or extend,[5, 9, 14–17] and associated with changes in depolarization.[5, 9, 18–22] By and large the diagnosis has been clinical and electrocardiographic and based on (1) a history of prolonged chest pain or compression, (2) the observation of a diagnostic rise in the peak level of enzymes in the blood, (3) the new development of widespread depression of RS-T segments (figure 1) or inversion of T waves (figure 2) lasting at least 48 hr, and (4) the absence of changes in the QRS complex. It has been assumed that satisfaction of these criteria establishes the diagnosis with the implication that, if the criteria are not met, the diagnosis is not justified.

Pathologic substantiation of the diagnosis has, to no small extent, been scanty or lacking. Confusion has been compounded by (1) inconsistent definition of the necessary extent of infarction, (2) the introduction of a less restrictive term, "non-transmural" myocardial infarction, which by some authorities is and by others is not used interchangeably with SEMI, (3) the more recent designations "Q wave" vs "non–Q wave" infarctions, and (4) the introduction into chemical parlance of such terms as "acute coronary insufficiency," "unstable angina pectoris," "rule out myocardial infarction," "acute mild" or "acute atypical infarction," and even the label SEMI itself, used with similar imprecision. Out of this overwhelming confusion and ambiguity emerges a compelling need for a wholesale reassessment of the entire subject, the point of departure being anatomic and the sole requirement for the diagnosis being the demonstration of bona fide SEMI at postmortem examination. Although subject to the distortion inherent in all retrospective studies, this offers the dividend of an incontestable verification of SEMI in every patient included.

Materials and methods

The clinical charts of 53 patients treated at Brigham and Women's Hospital were reviewed and correlated with the autopsy findings of the same patients. Twenty-one of these were consecutive patients from a personal consultation practice (in this sense "selected"), and 32 were culled at random from autopsy records as they became available (thus "unselected"). All had indubitable (acute, healing, or healed) SEMIs and were accumulated over the years following an earlier publication from this hospital.[23] Unless an anatomically distinct SEMI ex-

From the Department of Medicine, Brigham and Women's Hospital and Harvard Medical School, Boston.

Address for correspondence: Harold D. Levine, M.D., Deaconess Medical Office Bldg., 110 Francis St., Boston, MA 02215.

Received Feb. 11, 1985; revision accepted June 27, 1985.

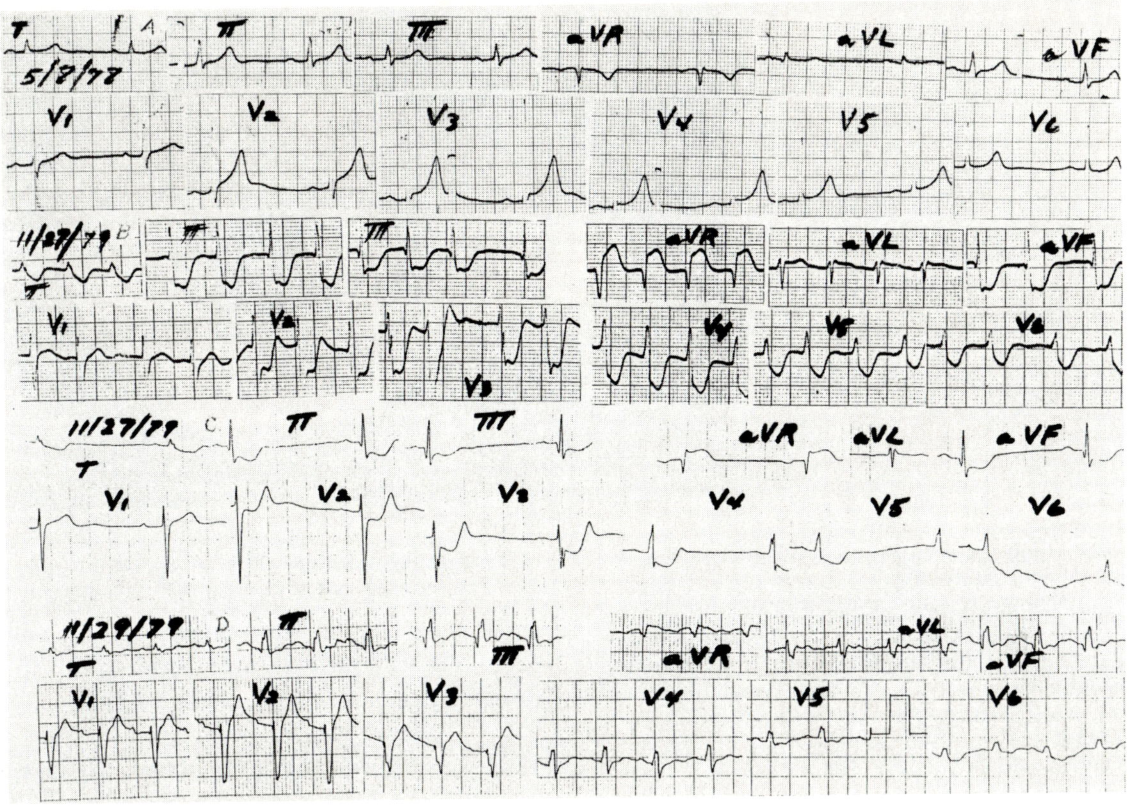

FIGURE 1. Extreme RS-T shifts in an 81-year-old patient with acute SEMI (same patient as in figure 3). *A*, Tracings in 1978 showing normal sinus bradycardia (rate 50 beats/min) and tall R wave in V_1 suggesting old posterobasal infarct. *B*, Tracings recorded on admission for acute chest pain showing atrial fibrillation, inconspicuous Q waves in leads II, III, and aVF, RS-T depression in leads II, III, aVF, and V_2 to V_6 with RS-T elevation in lead aVR. *C*, Tracings late that evening showing return to sinus bradycardia (rate 47 beats/min, sick sinus syndrome?) and persistent but less pronounced RS-T shifts. *D*, Preterminal tracings 2 days later showing sinus tachycardia (110 beats/min), more prominent Q waves in leads II, III, and aVF, and left bundle branch block.

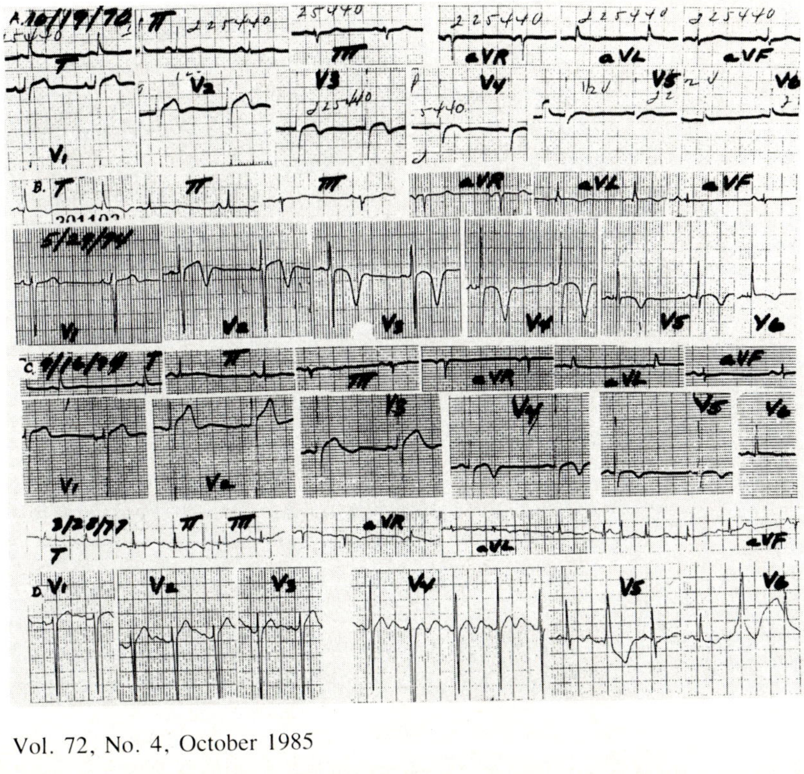

FIGURE 2. T wave inversions during and after acute SEMIs. *A*, Tracings from 87-year-old man during initial hospitalization in 1970 for protracted chest pain and marked enzyme elevations, showing "localized" T wave inversion. *B*, Tracings on rehospitalization in 1974 for syncope and sustained interscapular pain with marked rise in creatine kinase level, showing sharp T wave inversion in leads V_2 to V_6, most pronounced in V_3 and V_4. *C*, Tracings 4 months later showing partial recession of T wave changes. *D*, ECG in terminal admission 2½ years later for lung abscess, showing left ventricular hypertrophy, prominent U waves, and atrial and ventricular premature beats. Postmortem examination showed lung abscess, atherosclerosis of surface coronary arteries, marked involvment of medium-sized arteries, two distinct subendocardial scars, but no acute infarct. Same patient as in figure 4.

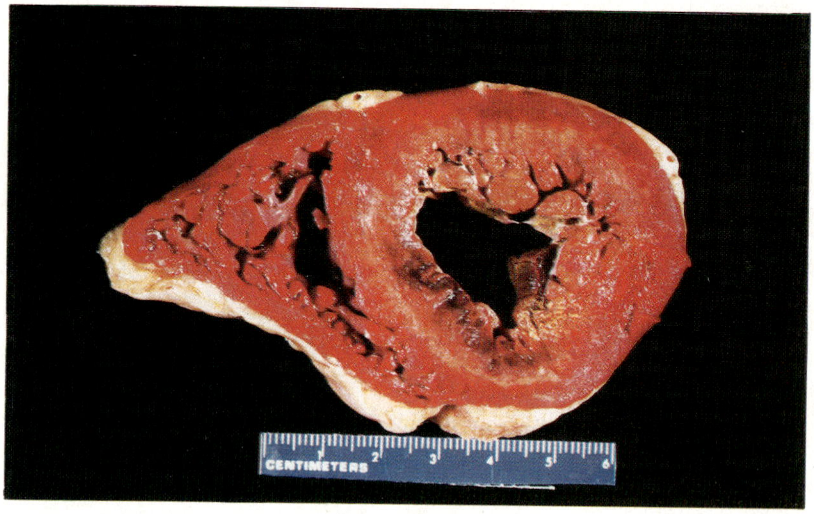

FIGURE 3. Acute circumferential SEMI, stained with triphenyl tetrazolium chloride, which extended from atrioventricular ring to apex and involved two-thirds of left ventricular thickness. Same patient as in figure 1.

isted elsewhere in the same heart, patients with transmural infarction per se were empirically excluded.

Topographically SEMIs were classified as either circumferential (figures 3 and 4), including in at least one plane its entire circumference, or segmental and involving only a portion of the ventricular subendocardium. The age of an infarct was judged as acute ("subacute" cases were empirically combined with "acute") or healed.

From coronary cineangiography in the living patient (40 patients) or from postmortem angiography (the latter by preference if both were done), estimates were made of the degree of stenosis of the left main (LM), its anterior descending branch (LAD), its circumflex branch (LCX), and the right (RCA) coronary arteries.

Measurements of the actual volume of infarcted muscle were not attempted. On the assumption that the accession of certain enzymes into the blood serum during a suspected acute episode reflects the volume of damaged tissue,[24–26] the clinical records of all 41 patients with acute SEMI were scrutinized for peak enzyme levels attained during their terminal illness, thus providing an estimate of infarct volume.*

Because earlier and scantier experiences[23] suggested that certain extracoronary factors play an important role in diminishing coronary blood flow, an attempt was made to reassess the role of such accessory conditions tending to curtail global coronary flow (shock, other "low flow" states, those diminishing the oxygen capacity of the blood, and those increasing the left ventricular end-diastolic blood pressure).

Finally, attention was directed to electrocardiographic changes, principally those observed at the onset of, or developing during, the terminal hospitalization of these 53 patients.

Results

Study population. In the 36 patients in whom it could be estimated, the time from first SEMI to death ranged from 3 days to 15 years (mean 10 months, average 2.3 years). There were 27 men and 26 women, the men averaging 69.1 years and the women 69.8 years at death.

Topography, age, and extent of SEMI. Almost half of the SEMIs were multiple. Of the 53 patients, 16 had single acute SEMIs (nine segmental, seven circumferential) (figures 3 and 4) and 13 had single old SEMIs (eight segmental, five circumferential). In 25 patients acute SEMI was associated with at least one healed SEMI considered to be separate from the acute infarct (figure 5); in 11 of the 25 there was more than one associated old SEMI. In a few of them repetitive SEMI had been recognized clinically (figure 6). In eight patients of the entire group the existence of old transmural infarction was also substantiated pathologically.

Most of the SEMIs were quite sharply layered (figure 3), many were irregular and mottled, a few were the obvious end-stage of a conglomeration of serial infarctions (figure 7), and one or two consisted of aggregations of similar but discrete punctate necroses. Although a deliberate numerical estimate of infarct depth was not attempted, general statements and color photographs indicated that most involved the inner third of the ventricular wall; in three it extended beyond two-thirds of the thickness of the ventricular wall. None extended to the epicardium.

Coronary artery stenosis in SEMI. The degree of stenosis of the LAD, measured in 30 patients, ranged from 50% to 100% (mean 90%, average 84.1%). Narrowing of the LCX, measured in 29, ranged from 40% to 100% (mean 85%, average 80%), and that of the RCA, measured in 38, ranged from 30% to 100% (mean 95%, average 90.1%), the latter including seven in whom the occlusion was total and partly or completely thrombotic (figures 4 and 11).

Papillary muscle dysfunction. Papillary muscle necrosis or fibrosis, generally of striking degree, was found in eight of the 53 patients. In all a well-marked systolic murmur had been heard before, or first developed dur-

*Normal enzyme range at this laboratory (IU/liter): creatine kinase 50 to 60 (women), 50 to 180 (men); muscle band fraction of creatine kinase, < 2.2% of total creatine kinase; lactate dehydrogenase 88 to 196; and aspartate aminotransferase 22 to 47.

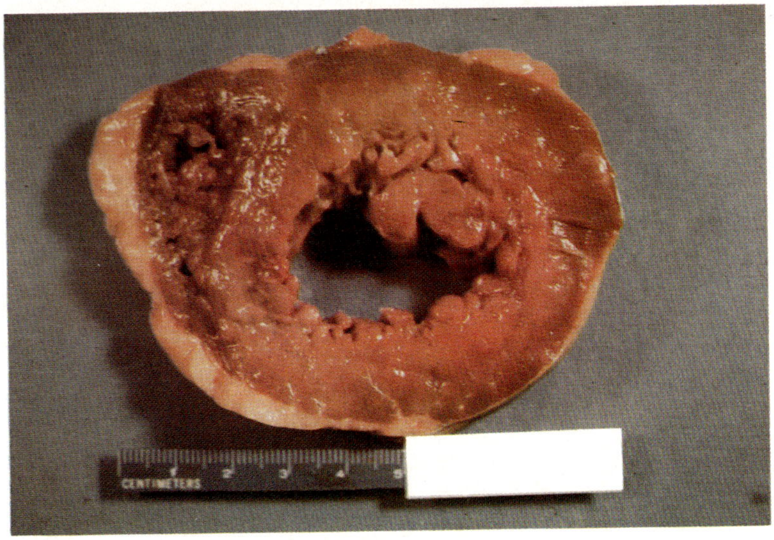

FIGURE 4. Acute circumferential SEMI, pale brown, in unstained transverse section. The patient, 62 years old, was allegedly well until 1 month before fatal cardiogenic shock. There was complete, partly thrombotic occlusion of the right coronary artery, segmental narrowing of the left main, left anterior descending and left circumflex arteries, and, in a contiguous section not shown here, old endocardial thickening of lateral wall of the left ventricle summarized as "extensive SEMI of left ventricle of different ages." Microsopic results showed focal acute pericarditis and perivascular round cell infiltration in the pericardium. Same patient as in figure 2.

ing, the terminal hospitalization. In one patient the diagnosis was first suspected by the detection of this syndrome and the reflection that the papillary muscle may be considered an extension of the subendocardial laminae of the ventricular wall.

Pericarditis in SEMI. Paradoxically, six patients had clinical and pathologic evidence of acute pericarditis. In four a friction rub had been heard. Fibrinous pericarditis was found in all six but in none did the infarct extend to the epicardium. In one, perivascular round cell infiltration was demonstrated in the pericardium. Rheumatoid arthritis or uremia may have been implicated in three but in the remaining three there was no explanation for the pericarditis other than SEMI.

Mural thrombosis. Left ventricular thrombi adjacent to SEMI were detected in only three patients, one with disseminated intravascular coagulation.

Accessory noncoronary factors. Search for factors ancillary to coronary arterial narrowing and adversely affecting myocardial oxygenation disclosed, in a substantial proportion of these patients, the six entities detailed in table 1 (see also figures 6 to 8).

Cardiographic features. Serial electrocardiographic tracings were available in 51 of the 53 patients. From the appearance of the tracings recorded initially in the terminal hospitalization, patients were divided empirically into five groups: (1) nine patients showing widespread depression of the RS-T segments persistent over at least 2 days, (2) seven patients showing widespread inversion of T waves also lasting at least 2 days, (3) 12 patients showing conduction disturbances

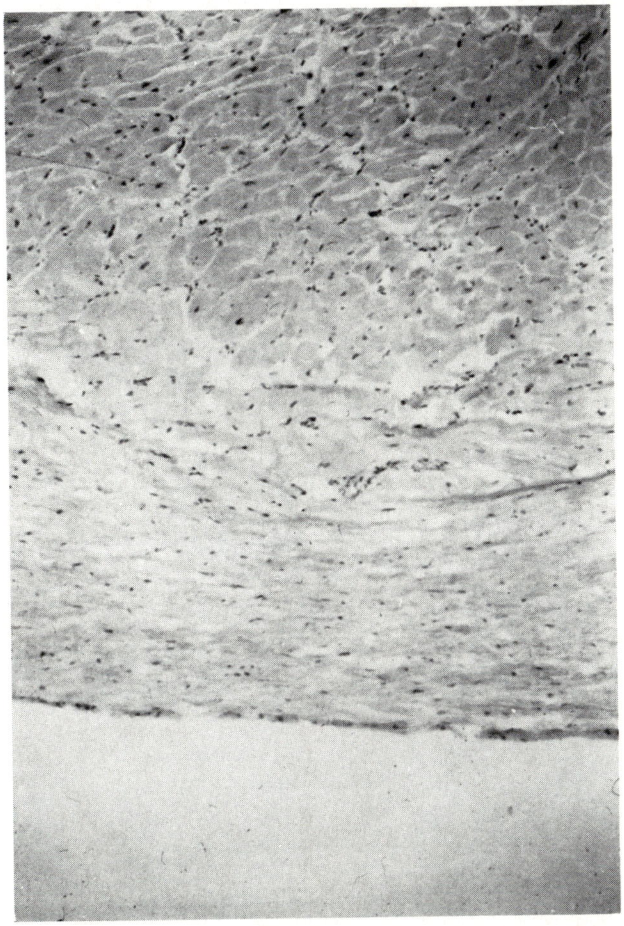

FIGURE 5. Histologic old and fresh SEMI in 59-year-old man with angina since 1962, a series of acute myocardial infarcts since 1968, and emergency triple bypass surgery with right coronary artery thromboendarterectomy in 1972. ECG showed right bundle branch block and probable old posterobasal infarct (tall R and R^1 in lead V_1). The patient died of high-grade atrioventricular block and ventricular fibrillation in 1983. Autopsy (gross) showed old inferior segmental and fresh circumferential SEMI involving basalar two-thirds of left ventricle and papillary muscles. Microscopy shows thick band of subendocardial fibrosis (below) subtending fresh coagulation necrosis of superjacent "new" subendocardium (above).

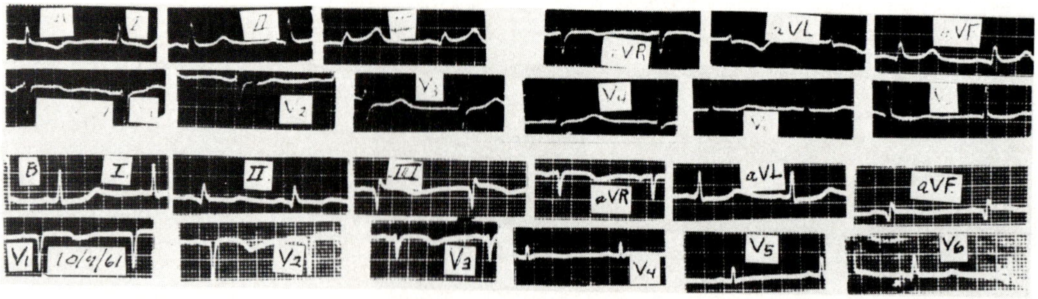

FIGURE 6. Dynamic change of concurrent anterior and inferior (Roesler-Dressler) infarction recorded on 2 consecutive days in 1961 in a woman, then age 61, with angina pectoris and myxoedema of 10 years' duration. Subsequent acute infarcts occurred in 1962, 1966, 1968, 1975, and 1976, the latter two diagnosed clinically as subendocardial. "Cardiac scan" in 1977 was compatible with SEMI.

(atrioventricular, intraventricular or fascicular block, and/or ventricular arrhythmias, (4) five patients regarded on the basis of currently and commonly employed criteria, including Q waves of significant duration, as having acute myocardial infarction, and (5) 19 patients regarded as having old myocardial infarction by similar criteria. Although serial tracings commonly continued to show the usual changes within each of these categories, many were unstable and evolved, as demonstrated in table 2, superimposed changes characteristic of one or more of the other groups.

Discussion

Pathologic aspects. For a population with coronary artery disease, this group was disproportionately elderly and female. That the degree of coronary narrowing in this expanded experience with SEMI exceeds that in the original handful of patients[23] may be due simply to the selection bias of an aging population, but it poses the question of whether the elderly patient, and par-

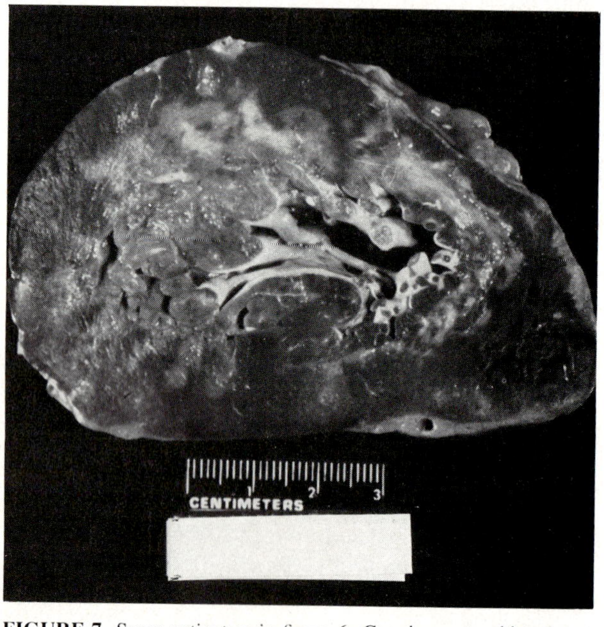

FIGURE 7. Same patient as in figure 6. Conglomerate old and acute SEMIs. The left main coronary artery was the site of an aneurysm extending to proximal left circumflex and left anterior descending arteries. The right coronary artery was totally occluded. All but one of the grafts had become occluded.

TABLE 1

Factors ancillary to coronary narrowing affecting myocardial oxygenation

General condition	n	Subgroups	n
Massive blood loss or shock (or both) after surgical or diagnostic procedures	5	Massive hemorrhage in ruptured AA	2
		Refused transfusion	2
		Hypotension after cardiac catheterization	1
Myxoedema (figures 6 and 7	4	Severe angina prevented optimal control of hypothyroidism	4
Acute pulmonary embolism (figure 8)	8	Additional old SEMIs	7
		Multiple PEs	6
		SEMI preceded PE	5
		PE preceded SEMI	2
		Sequence uncertain	1
Respiratory collapse from other causes	2	Acute recurrent pneumothorax	1
		Severe cervical arthritis with acute spinal cord compression	1
Aortic valve disease	4	Significant aortic stenosis	2
		Significant aortic regurgitation	2
Abnormalities of blood	6	Blood dyscrasias	5
		Pernicious anemia	1
		DiGuglielmo's leukemia	1
		Sickle cell anemia	1
		DIC	2
		Unusual chronic carbon monoxide exposure	1

AA = aortic aneurysm; PE = pulmonary embolism; DIC = disseminated intravascular coagulation.

TABLE 2
Static and dynamic electrocardiographic features of SEMI

ECG on admission	n	Early developments → Later developments	n	Pathologic highlights
Protracted RS-T depression	9	IVB	2	Old TMI, acute anterior SEMI (fig. 11)
		Supraventricular tachycardia	1	
		Complete AVB	1	
		No further ECG changes	5	
Protracted and widespread T wave inversion	7	Superimposed RS-T depression	1	
		Persistent T wave inversion		
		3 yr → VF →	1	Diffuse disease of middle-sized coronary arteries, no acute infarct
			1	Acute segmental anteroseptal and lateral SEMI
		No further ECG changes	4	
IVB				
LBBH	4	Higher grade IVB (figs. 9, 10)	6	
RBBB	6	Less pronounced IVB		
LAH	2	VF	3	
		Increasing AVB → acute anterolateral MI	1	
		acute inferior MI	1	Old inferior TMI and acute circumferential SEMI
Acute TMI	5	IVB	2	(None of this group showed TMI)
Anterolateral		Increasing AVB (fig. 12)	2	
Inferior				
RD infarct		RS-T elevation in inferior and anteroseptal areas	1	Old segmental SEMI and acute circumferential SEMI
Old TMI	19	RS-T depression in precordial leads	5	
		Pronounced T wave inversion	3	(Only 4 of this group showed TMI)
		Bifascicular block with prolonged PR interval	1	
		PVT → VF →	1	
		Acute inferior MI	1	Acute circumferential SEMI and old MI
		No further ECG changes	8	

IVB = intraventricular block; AVB = atrioventricular block; LBBB = left bundle branch block; RBBB = right bundle branch block; LAH = left anterior hemiblock; TMI = transmural myocardial infarct; RD infarct = Roesler-Dressler infarct (ref. 27); PVT = paroxysmal ventricular tachycardia; VF = ventricular fibrillation.

ticularly the elderly woman, is prone to infarction at the subendocardial level.

Multiple infarctions and early recurrence. From being subendocardial at their inception, myocardial infarcts, later in the same or in a subsequent acute episode, allegedly exhibit "transmural breakthrough."[14, 28] Juxtaposition of scarred with freshly infarcted myocardium, as shown in figure 5, suggests rather that these were successive infarcts of different ages. The argument for successive infarction was supported in the present study by a frequent history of parallel and corroborative discrete repetitive clinical, enzymatic, and electrocardiographic episodes. From the multiplicity and the diverse location of SEMIs reported here, the contention seems valid that the conditions that led to the original SEMI may cause other areas, and not necessarily the superjacent subepicardium — the "new subendocardium" so to speak — to emerge as susceptible to infarction. This may explain Erhardt's report[9] that in 88% of his patients with terminal SEMI who had had previous infarcts, the earlier infarcts were also subendocardial, and the impression of Marmor et al.[17] that each wave of necrosis may involve the same or a nearby site of coronary obstruction.

Infarct size in SEMI. The phenomenally high enzyme levels in patients with acute SEMI were quite unexpected. If peak enzyme level is correlated with the volume of infarcted muscle, these results suggest that SEMIs are large. Although thin compared with transmural infarctions SEMIs are more extensive and may wrap around a substantial portion, if not all, of the subendocardial circumference. Except in the study of

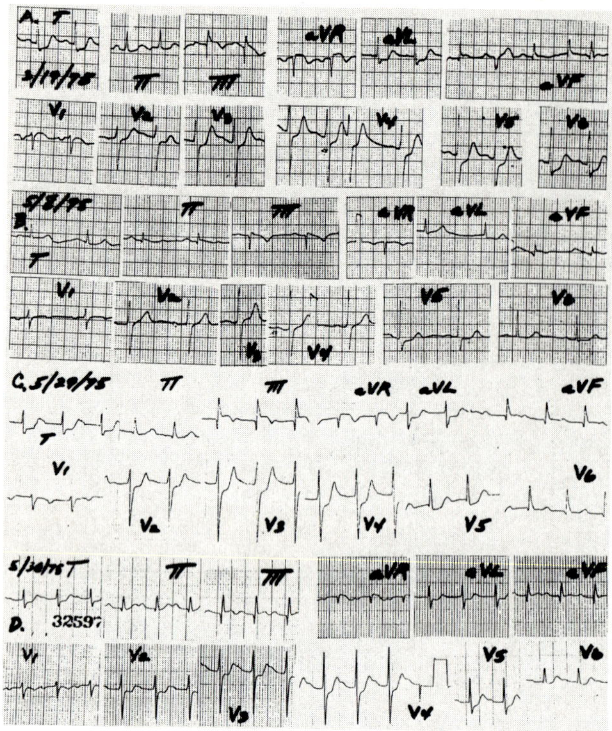

FIGURE 8. RS-T shifts attributable to SEMI and/or acute cor pulmonale, QRS changes attributed to transmural infarction. *A*, On admission, an 85-year-old woman with dyspnea and chest pain showed Q waves in leads III and aVF, depressed RS-T segment in leads I, aVL, and V_3 to V_6, elevated RS-T segment in aVR, and atrial and ventricular premature beats and was diagnosed as having acute inferior transmural infarction. *B*, Tracings on readmission 6 weeks later for recurrent pain showing persistent Q waves in leads II, III, and aVF but much less pronounced RS-T shifts. *C*, Tracings after severe recurrence showed first-degree atrioventricular block and pronounced RS-T depression ("staircase ascent") in leads I, aVL, and midprecordial leads and elevated RS-T in aVR. The patient then developed transient complete atrioventricular block and paroxysms of atrial flutter and fibrillation (not shown). Pulmonary embolism was suspected but rated unlikely by lung scan. *D*, Terminal tracings showing persistent but less pronounced RS-T shifts, persistent P-R delay. Both acute pulmonary embolism and acute SEMI were found at postmortem examination.

Erhardt,[9] precise anatomic measurements have not been made of the volume of tissue that is infarcted in SEMI. Such studies in the future might well show that the breadth of these infarcts much more than compensates for their relative lack of depth.

Pericarditis in acute SEMI. Hutter et al.[16] found pericarditis to be as frequent in nontransmural as in transmural infarctions. The finding of pericarditis in their study and in the present report is difficult to explain. The pericarditis of acute myocardial infarction is commonly considered to be caused by direct extension of infarction to pericardium and the detection of a friction rub decisive evidence for cross-the-wall infarction. Acute pericarditis may be the sole or predominant manifestation of Dressler's postinfarction syndrome, which is commonly regarded as an autoimmune process. Many patients with pericarditis as a feature of that

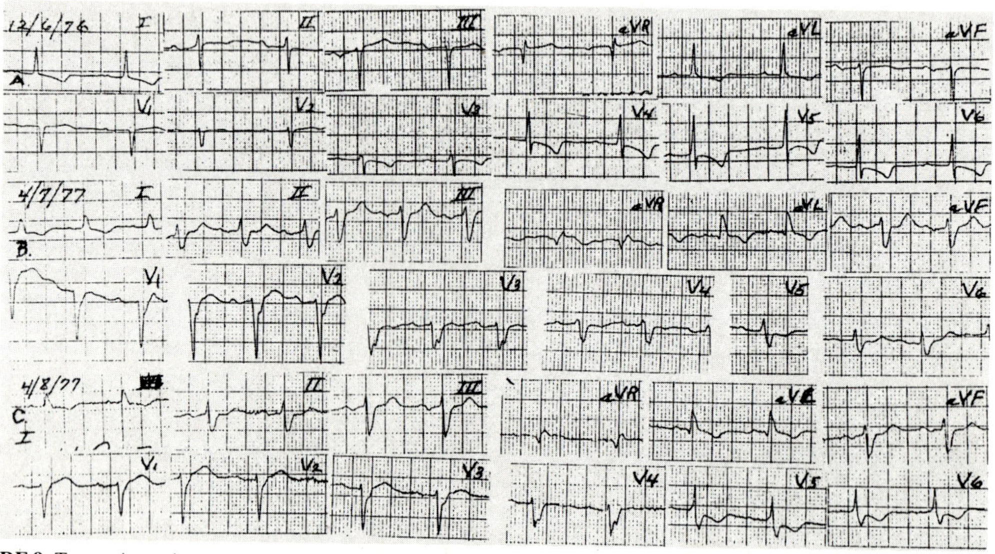

FIGURE 9. T wave inversion and advancing conduction disturbances in a 91-year-old woman with acute myocardial infarction 1 year before SEMI. *A*, Tracings in initial hospitalization for painless congestive failure showing left anterior hemiblock and first-degree atrioventricular block with "poor R wave progression." QRS complex was not prolonged. Peak creatine kinase level was 1224 IU/liter. *B*, Initial tracings in terminal admission 4 months later for severe dyspnea and chest pain, showing either intraventricular (possibly right bundle branch block with rightward and superior terminal forces) or "peri-infarction block" with left axis deviation of terminal 0.04 sec vector. Creatine kinase, 1500 IU/liter; MB fraction increased. *C*, Preterminal tracings the next day. The PR interval and QRS complex were still prolonged. RS-T depression and T wave inversion were more prominent in leads V_5 and V_6. Autopsy showed old healed circumferential and acute posterior segmental SEMI.

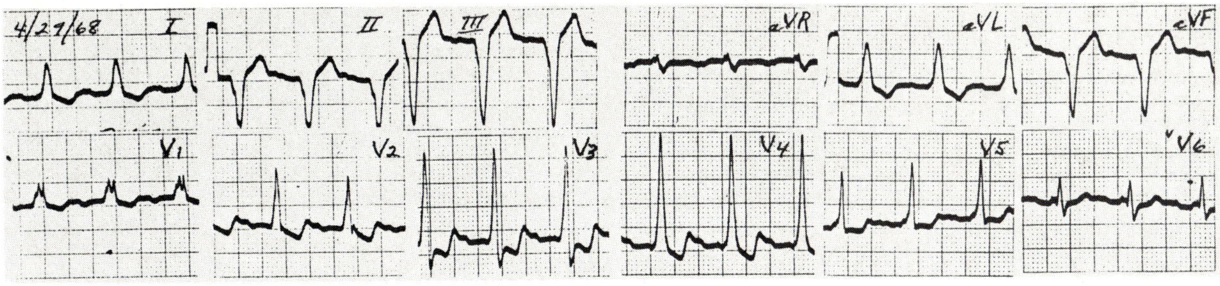

FIGURE 10. SEMI associated with bifascicular and possibly trifascicular block (right bundle branch block, left anterior hemiblock, and prolonged PR interval, best seen in lead V_2, the latter compatible with delayed conduction in atrioventricular conduction system or in posterior fascicle of left bundle branch). Alternative or additional anomalous atrioventricular excitation not excluded. This 84-year-old patient with tertiary lues and healed tuberculosis had periodic complete atrioventricular block in terminal admission. Autopsy showed healed posterolateral and apical SEMI, in some areas only recently healed.

syndrome, blossoming sometime after an acute infarction, have in retrospect manifested that very same complication during their initial acute infarction. If the recurrence is autoimmune in nature, the same might be assumed for the original bout of pericarditis, a possibility considered but rejected by Hutter et al.[16]

If this argument is valid, these patients could appropriately be considered to have an accelerated or "syninfarction" autoimmune pericarditis. In other words, the concomitance of pericarditis with infarction need not signal extension of infarct to pericardium. Unfortunately, although potentially pertinent, serologic or im-

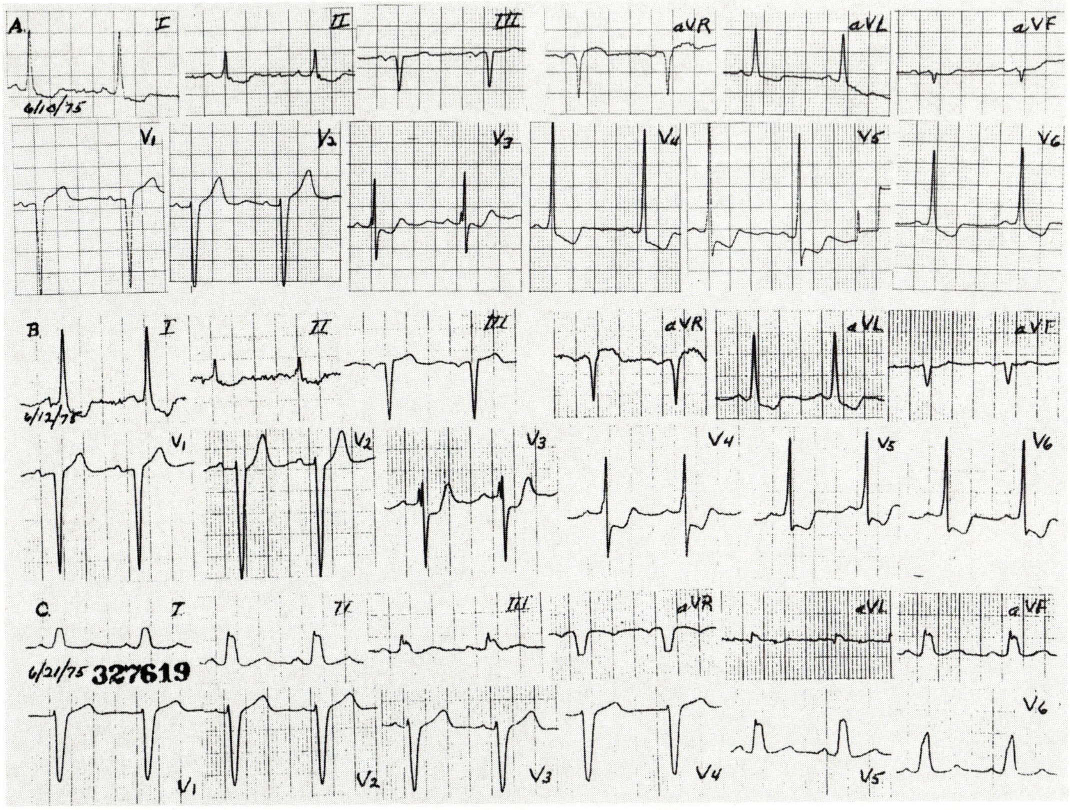

FIGURE 11. Left bundle branch block developing in patient with old inferior transmural infarct and fresh segmental SEMI. Serial tracings in terminal admission of 75-year-old hypertensive woman with previous angina pectoris. *A*, tracings showing the R wave voltage and RS-T shifts of left ventricular hypertrophy. *B*, Tracings 2 days later suggesting old transmural infarction, still lacking left precordial Q waves but now with deeper and straighter RS-T depression in leads V_4 to V_6, a change that persisted for several days and measured 5 to 6 mm the day before death. *C*, Preterminal tracings showing complete left bundle branch block. Postmortem examination showed old inferior wall scar and acute "almost transmural" segmental anterior wall infarct. The left main coronary artery was more than 90% occluded, and the right coronary artery was the site of acute thrombus producing 90% stenosis of its lumen. Aortic stenosis was also present.

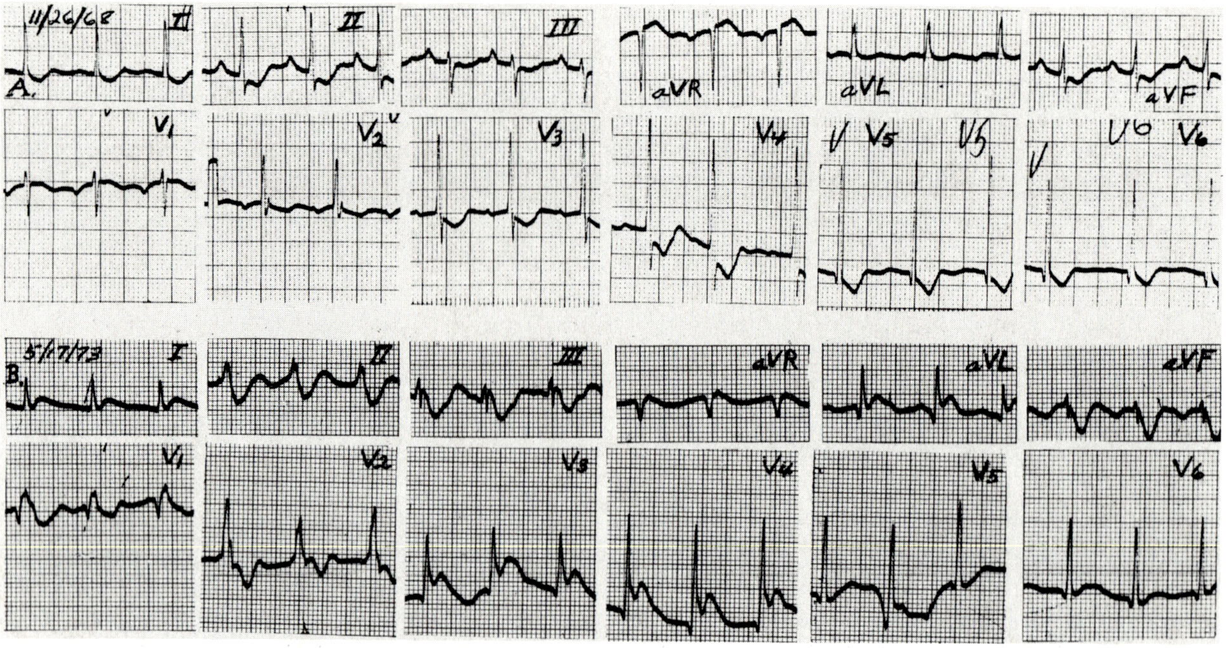

FIGURE 12. Acute SEMI with development of right bundle branch block and simulated transmural anterior wall infarct in 77-year-old patient who had undergone mitral valvuloplasty by 15 years before. *A*, Tracings recorded in asymptomatic interval showing left ventricular hypertrophy (leads V_5 and V_6 half-standardized). *B*, Preterminal tracings showing development of right bundle branch block and of prolonged PR interval with elevated RS-T and new Q waves in leads V_3 and V_4 (leads V_4 to V_6 half-standardized). Autopsy showed acute segmental SEMI involving anterior and posteroseptal areas, papillary muscles, and left atrium and sparing lateral subendocardium. There was 95% stenosis of the left anterior descending artery and no transmural infarction was evident.

munologic data were not obtained in these patients.

Cardiographic aspects. At the onset of their terminal illness, nine patients showed protracted RS-T segment depression and seven had protracted and widespread T wave inversion. An additional 11 (e.g., figures 9 and 11) developed such changes during that hospitalization. Thus 27 showed changes in repolarization. Clearly, if we depend on RS-T or T wave changes for the diagnosis, it would have been missed in about half of these 53 patients. Furthermore, in none of the five patients diagnosed on the basis of QRS and T wave changes as having acute transmural infarction and in only four of 19 diagnosed on the basis of QRS changes as having old transmural infarction was coexistent transmural infarction substantiated at postmortem examination. These observations support the growing protest that in SEMI,[2, 5, 19–22, 29–39] the ECG may indeed show changes in, or even restricted to, the QRS complex and that it is erroneous to exclude that diagnosis if significant Q waves are recorded. Possibly pertinent are the observations of Wilson et al.[40] that QS complexes may be recorded at an epicardial electrode overlying the transmural core of a full-thickness wedge-shaped infarct and QR complexes at the flanking epicardial surface tapping intact subepicardium overlying the subendocardial extension of such an infarct.[31]

Are there other possible electrocardiographic clues to the diagnosis? The cluster of six patients developing changes attributable to concurrent inferior and anteroseptal infarction (Roesler-Dressler infarcts, figure 6) is noteworthy. Although Roesler and Dressler implied that these infarcts are primarily septal and that the anterior and inferior "transmural" portions are an extension of, and part and parcel of, the septal infarct, this electrocardiographic configuration may serve as a clue to a subendocardial location on the empiric ground of the present experience alone.

It is difficult to explain this type of infarct on the basis of current electrocardiographic teaching. One possibility is that the changes may be artifactual and the result a much faster spread of the activating impulse along the endocardium than its centrifugal conduction through working myocardium. Activation at the endocardial aspect of the anterior and posterior walls might then be only slightly out of phase and, assuming the direction of anterior activation to be about 180 degrees from that of posterior activation, the "anterior" and "inferior" R waves could in effect cancel each other, inducing QRS changes suggesting coexistent transmural infarction at both poles. Nor is the development of advancing intraventricular or atrioventricular block or of ectopic ventricular rhythms, as observed in this study, distinctive of SEMI, attesting the subendocardial substructure of all myocardial infarcts. Perhaps the best that can be anticipated would be a differentiation between SEMI and transmural infarction based on statistical probability. The concepts underlying "peri-infarction block" and the "hemiblocks," proposed and developed during the past generation, must have a profound potential bearing on this diagnosis. During their terminal illness and before going on to higher-grade block or arrhythmias, 12 of these 53 patients developed either peri-infarction block (figure 9) or hemiblock (figure 10). Although Grant[41] and Rosenbaum et al.[42] attributed these changes to conduction disturbances in the bundle branches, the latter emphasized that necrosis of heart muscle per se at or near the subendocardium may induce more profound electrocardiographic changes than similar damage near the epicardium. Certainly these "Roesler-Dressler" infarcts, as well as peri-infarction blocks and hemiblocks, deserve further study as possible indicators of SEMI.

The "head start" intrinsic to its gradual partial depolarization before end-diastole presumably explains the normal domination of Purkinje tissue over the cardiac rhythm.[43] The frequency of block and ectopy in patients with SEMI may be explained by (1) the fact that electrical activation, which proceeds outward from endocardium to epicardium, is at the mercy of blood flow, which proceeds inward from epicardium to endocardium, and (2) the concentration of the major trunks of the atrioventricular conduction system at the crest of the interventricular conduction system and the rich subendocardial distribution of the Purkinje network. The resultant propensity to ectopy may be enhanced by electrochemical changes at the margins of infarcted tissue and perhaps by a tactile vulnerability analogous to the induction of premature ventricular beats on simple contact of catheter tip with ventricular endocardium.[44]

These findings may be discounted because this is a retrospective study, but they cannot be ignored. The court of final appeal remains the postmortem examination. A prospective approach is not disparaged; rather a modification in guidelines and in the direction of future studies, prospective or retrospective, is encouraged, including more frequent ventriculographic studies, data bearing upon an autoimmune state, a forthright statement of how many patients underwent autopsy, precise measurement of depth and volume of infarcted muscle, and explicit determination of whether, and over how large an area, the process of infarction actually reached the epicardium.

I am happy to express my sincerest gratitude to the late Dr. Monroe J. Schlesinger, who encouraged my continued interest in SEMI; to many colleagues at the Brigham and Women's Hospital, including Drs. Thomas W. Smith, Eugene Braunwald, Peter L. Friedman, Fred Schoen, Ramzi S. Cotran, and B. Leonard Holman, for their invaluable criticism of the manuscript; and through correspondence to Dr. Thomas E. Lowe of Toorak, Australia (regarding muscle bundles), Dr. Jesse E. Edwards of St. Paul (regarding semantics), Dr. Tom Raffin of Stanford, and Dr. Goodwill M. Stewart (who referred many of these patients to me in consultation). My heartfelt thanks also go to Mrs. Beatrice Scheff for invaluable secretarial assistance and to Barbara for a half century of constant support and forebearance.

References

1. Barnes AR, Ball RG: The incidence and situation of myocardial infarction in one thousand consecutive post-mortem examinations. Am J Med Sci **183:** 215, 1932
2. Savage RM, Wagner GS, Ideker RE, Podolsky SA, Hackel DB: Correlation of post-mortem anatomic findings with electrocardiographic changes in patients with typical anterior and posterior infarcts. Circulation **55:** 279, 1977
3. Alzamora-Castro V: Contribution al conocimiento del significado de las modificaciones del segmento ST: angina pectoris e infartos-subendocardicos. Arch Inst Cardiol Mexico **17:** 870, 1947
4. Friedberg CK: Symposium: Myocardial infarction 1972. Part I. Introduction. Circulation **45:** 179, 1972
5. Yu PNG, Stewart JM: Subendocardial myocardial infarction with special reference to the electrocardiographic changes. Am Heart J **39:** 862, 1950
6. Rosenberg BA, Malach M: Acute myocardial infarction in a city hospital: follow-up study of 131 survivors. Am J Cardiol **8:** 799, 1961
7. Lown B, Vassaux C, Hood WB Jr, Fakhro AM, Kaplinsky E, Roberge G: Unresolved problems in coronary care. Am J Cardiol **20:** 494, 1967
8. Stimmel B, Katz AM, Donoso E: Q wave development in acute subendocardial infarction. Arch Intern Med **131:** 676, 1973
9. Erhardt LR: Clinical and pathological observations in different types of acute myocardial infarction. Acta Med Scand [Suppl] **560:** 7, 1974
10. Madias JE, Gorlin R: The myth of acute "mild" myocardial infarction. Ann Intern Med **86:** 347, 1977
11. Cannom DS, Levy W, Cohen LS: The short- and long-term prognosis of patients with transmural and non-transmural myocardial infarction. Am J Med **61:** 452, 1978
12. Levy W, Cannom DS, Cohen LS: The non-transmural myocardial infarction in perspective. Cardiovasc Rev Rep **21:** 1285, 1981
13. Hollander G, Herschel O, Greengart A, Shani J, Lichstein E: High mortality early reinfarction with first non-transmural myocardial infarction. Am Heart J **108:** 1412, 1984
14. Kossowsky WA, Mohr BD, Rafii S, Lyon AF: Superimposition of transmural infarction following acute subendocardial infarction. How frequent? Chest **69:** 758, 1976
15. Madigan NP, Rutherford BD, Frye RL: The clinical course, early prognosis and coronary anatomy of subendocardial infarction. Am J Med **60:** 634, 1976
16. Hutter AM Jr, DeSanctis RW, Flynn T, Yeatman LA: Non-transmural myocardial infarction; a comparison of hospital and late clinical course with that of matched patients with transmural anterior and transmural inferior myocardial infarction. Am J Cardiol **48:** 595, 1981
17. Marmor A, Sobel BE, Roberts R: Factors presaging early recurrent myocardial infarction ("extension"). Am J Cardiol **48:** 603, 1981
18. Krone RJ, Friedman E, Thanavaro S, Miller JP, Kleiger RE, Oliver GC: Long term prognosis after first Q wave (transmural) or non-Q-wave (non-transmural) myocardial infarction: analysis of 593 patients. Am J Cardiol **52:** 234, 1983
19. Myers GB, Sears CH, Hiratzka T: Correlation of electrocardiographic and pathologic findings in ring-like subendocardial infarction of the left ventricle. Am J Med Sci **222:** 417, 1951

20. Cook RW, Edwards JE, Pruitt RD: Electrocardiographic changes in acute subendocardial infarction. I. Large subendocardial and large non-transmural infarcts. Circulation **18:** 603, 1958
21. Raunio H, Rissanen V, Ramppanen T, Jokinen T, Rehnberg S, Helin M, Pyorale K: Changes in the QRS complex and ST segment in transmural and subendocardial myocardial infarctions: a clinicopathologic study. Am Heart J **98:** 176, 1979
22. Abbott JA, Scheinman MM: Non-diagnostic electrocardiogram in patients with acute myocardial infarction. Am J Med **55:** 608, 1973
23. Levine HD, Ford RV: Subendocardial infarction: report of six cases and critical survey of the literature. Circulation **1:** 246, 1950
24. Sobel BE, Bresnahan GE, Shell WE, Yoder RD: Estimation of infarct size in man and its relation to prognosis. Circulation **46:** 640, 1972
25. Mathey D, Bleifeld W, Hanrath P, Effert S: Attempt to quantitate relation between cardiac function and infarct size in acute myocardial infarction Br Heart J **36:** 271, 1974
26. Reimer KA, Hackel DB, Ideker RE, Mikat EM, Hartwell TD, Parker CB, Braunwald EB, Gold HK, Raabe DS, Rude RE, Sobel BE, Stone PH, Roberts R, and the MILIS Study Group: Comparison of enzymatic and anatomic estimates of myocardial infarct size in man. Clin Res **31:** 214A, 1983
27. Roesler H, Dressler W: An electrocardiographic pattern of infarction of the internventricular septum extending from the anterior to the posterior aspect of the heart. Am Heart J **34:** 817, 1947
28. Eliot RS, Holsinger JW: A unified concept of the pathophysiology of myocardial infarction and sudden death. Chest **62:** 469, 1972
29. Georas CS, Dahlquist E, Cutts FB: Subendocardial infarction: correlation of clinical, electrocardiographic and pathologic data in 17 cases. Arch Intern Med **111:** 488, 1963
30. Kleinfeld M, Magin J, Stein E: The effect of tetraethylpyrophosphate (TEPP) on the transmembrane potentials of pacemaker and non-pacemaker fibers of isolated rabbit atrium. Circ Res **8:** 240, 1960
31. Madias JE, Chahine RA, Gorlin R, Blacklow DJ: A comparison of transmural and non-transmural acute myocardial infarction. Circulation **49:** 498, 1974
32. Coll S, Castaner A, Sanz G, Roig E, Magrina J, Navarro-Lopez F, Betriu A: Prevalence and prognosis after a first nontransmural myocardial infarction. Am J Cardiol **51:** 1584, 1983
33. Wilkinson RS Jr, Schaefer JA, Abildskov JA: Electrocardiographic and pathologic features of myocardial infarction in man. Am J Cardiol **11:** 24, 1963
34. Boineau JP, Blumenschein SD, Spaach MS, Sabiston DC: Relationship between ventricular depolarization and electrocardiogram in myocardial infarction. J Electrocardiol **1:** 233, 1968
35. Abbott JA, Scheinman MM: Nondiagnostic electrocardiogram in patients with acute myocardial infarction. Am J Med **55:** 608, 1973
36. Schamroth L: The electrocardiology of coronary artery disease. Oxford, 1975, Blackwell Scientific Publications
37. Helfant L: Q-waves in coronary heart disease: newer understanding of their clinical implications. Am J Cardiol **38:** 622, 1976 (editorial)
38. Sullivan W, Vlodaver Z, Tuna N, Long L, Edwards JE: Correlation of electrocardiographic and pathological findings in healed myocardial infarction. Am J Cardiol **42:** 724, 1978
39. Phibbs B: "Transmural" versus "non-transmuarl" myocardial "infarction: an electrocardiographic myth. J Am Coll Cardiol **1:** 561, 1983
40. Wilson FN, Johnston FD, Hill IGW, Grout GC: The electrocardiogram in the later stages of experimental myocardial infarction. Trans Assoc Am Phys **48:** 154, 1933
41. Grant RP: Peri-infarction block. Prog Cardiovasc Dis **2:** 237, 1959
42. Rosenbaum MB, Elizari MV, Lazzari JO: The hemiblocks. Tampa Tracings. Oldsmar, FL, 1970, pp 4–7
43. Scheinman MM, Abbott JA: Clinical significance of transmural versus non-transmural electrocardiographic changes in patients with acute myocardial infarction. Am J Med **55:** 602, 1973
44. Levine HD, Hellems HK, Dexter L, Tucker AS: Studies in intracardiac electrography in man. II. The potential variations in the right ventricle. Am Heart J **37:** 64, 1949

Detection of local abnormalities in ventricular activation sequence by body surface isochrone mapping in patients with previous myocardial infarction

KOZUE IKEDA, M.D., ISAO KUBOTA, M.D., AKIRA IGARASHI, M.D., MICHIYASU YAMAKI, M.D., KAI TSUIKI, M.D., AND SHOJI YASUI, M.D.

ABSTRACT Body surface isochrone mapping was performed in 36 normal subjects and in 85 patients with previous myocardial infarction. Eighty-seven unipolar electrocardiograms distributed over the anterior chest and the back were recorded simultaneously. For each lead, activation time was measured as the time from the onset of QRS to the peak of the R wave. The lead points where R waves were not observed were designated the "no R wave area" (NR area). Isochrone maps of normal subjects had a consistent pattern, with isochrone lines extending from the right upper anterior chest to the left anterior chest and then to the back. NR area was small and was located only on the right upper chest or the upper back. On the isochrone maps of patients with myocardial infarction, abnormal findings were observed; NR area was found in 26 of 28 patients with anterior infarction on the upper to middle anterior chest, in 13 of 22 patients with inferior infarction on the lower chest, and in 24 of 25 patients with anterior and inferior infarction on the upper to lower anterior chest. Activation time was delayed near the NR area (peri–NR area delay) in 37 patients. In patients with apical infarction, an islandlike zone of delayed activation was typically found on the left precordium. These abnormal patterns are considered to indicate local abnormalities in the activation of infarcted myocardium; the NR area indicates dead unexcitable scar, and the peri–NR area delay and islandlike zone of delayed activation indicate partially infarcted myocardium of slow activation. Patients with NR area had greater degree of left ventricular asynergy and lower ejection fraction than those without. Patients with peri–NR area delay had higher incidence of ventricular arrhythmia than those without. Body surface isochrone mapping provides new evidence of myocardial infarction that is not available by the conventional analysis of the electrocardiogram.
Circulation 72, No. 4, 801–809, 1985.

BODY SURFACE potential mapping has been used increasingly for the diagnosis of myocardial infarction.[1–7] In the analysis of mapping data, the most conventionally used technique is the instant-by-instant observation of the isopotential maps. Isopotential display has the advantage of presenting simultaneous comparisons of potential at many body surface sites and can demonstrate abnormal potential distribution in patients with myocardial infarction who had no classical diagnostic Q wave in standard 12-lead electrocardiograms (ECGs).[3, 7] However, detection of subtle disorders in the activation sequence may not always be easy in isopotential mapping because it is very time consuming to analyze many isopotential maps of various times. Comparison of time factors such as local activation time between different leads is difficult in the isopotential map display.

Flowers et al.[1, 2] analyzed isopotential maps of anterior and inferoposterior myocardial infarction by departure map technique and found areas of abnormal positivity at the mid and late QRS period. They proposed that the mid and late activation changes detected by the departure map were related to ischemically induced alterations in the temporal sequence of ventricular activation. In this study we attempted to detect the local abnormalities in ventricular activation sequence directly by body surface isochrone mapping.

The isochrone map is a display of the distribution of ventricular activation time, and many investigators

From the First Department of Internal Medicine, Yamagata University School of Medicine, Yamagata, Japan.

Address for correspondence: Kozue Ikeda, M.D., The First Department of Internal Medicine, Yamagata University School of Medicine, Zao-Iida, Yamagata 990-23, Japan.

Received Feb. 28, 1985; revision accepted June 20, 1985.

have performed epicardial isochrone mapping in patients with Wolff-Parkinson-White syndrome,[8] bundle branch block,[9] and ventricular tachyarrhythmias.[10–12] However, few have performed body surface isochrone mapping to detect abnormalities in the ventricular activation sequence.[13] We made body surface isochrone maps of patients with myocardial infarction and tried to detect local abnormalities in ventricular activation, which are hard to detect on standard 12-lead ECGs and isopotential map displays. Information about the local ventricular activation sequence may help to determine the extent and severity of ischemic damage and to predict the occurrence of ventricular arrhythmias after infarction.

Materials and methods

Subjects. From 614 consecutive patients who underwent left ventriculography and selective coronary arteriography in Yamagata University Hospital from August 1979 to July 1984, 85 satisfying all of the following criteria were selected for this study: (1) a clinical diagnosis of myocardial infarction established by typical chest pain and serum enzyme changes; (2) asynergic site proved by left ventriculography; in this study, asynergy implies akinesis or dyskinesis according to the reporting system of the American Heart Association[14]; (3) significant stenosis of 70% or more in at least one major coronary artery; (4) no other heart disease such as congenital heart disease, myocardial disease, or valvular heart disease; and (5) no conduction disturbance such as right bundle branch block, left bundle branch block, or Wolff-Parkinson-White syndrome. The QRS duration was less than 0.12 sec.

The patient group consisted of 73 men and 12 women 35 to 69 years of age (mean 55). The time from the onset of the myocardial infarction to the cardiac catheterization ranged from 2 to 11 months (mean 5.1).

Thirty-six clinically normal subjects were also studied (the normal group). They were all men, 22 to 51 years of age (mean 33). All had normal physical and electrocardiographic findings. None of them had a history of heart disease or hypertension.

Informed consent was given by all subjects before the study commenced.

Left ventriculography and coronary arteriography. Biplane left ventriculograms in the 30 degree right anterior oblique and 60 degree left anterior oblique projections were recorded on 35 mm film taken at 50 frames/sec with the Toshiba 9 inch image amplifier system (Angiorex/U-arm). The left ventricle was opacified with contrast medium (meglumine diatrizoate) injected into the left ventricle at a rate of 13 ml/sec for 3 sec. The left ventricular ejection fraction was calculated from biplane left ventriculograms according to the area-length method of Dodge et al.,[15] with the use of Siemens cardiac catheterization SICOR system.[16] Left ventricular wall motion was evaluated qualitatively by three or more observers who had no knowledge of mapping data, according to the reporting system of the American Heart Association.[14] Regional wall motion was graded as follows: normal = 0, hypokinesis = 1, akinesis = 2, and dyskinesis = 3. These scores were given separately to the seven segments (anterobasal, anterolateral, apical, diaphragmatic, posterobasal, septal, and posterolateral) of the left ventricular wall. The asynergy index was determined by adding the seven scores.

In this study, segments of akinesis or dyskinesis were referred to as the asynergic sites. Asynergy of the anterobasal, anterolateral, and/or septal segments with or without apical asynergy was referred to as anterior asynergy. Asynergy of the diaphragmatic, posterobasal, and/or posterolateral segments with or without apical asynergy was referred to as inferior asynergy. Asynergy of only the apical segment was referred to as apical asynergy.

Selective coronary arteriographic studies were carried out in multiple projections according to the Judkins technique. Coronary arterial narrowing of 70% or more in the luminal diameter was considered significant.

Body surface mapping

Map recording. Body surface mapping was performed with a body surface potential mapping system, HPM-5100S unit (Chunichi Denshi Co.) within a week before the cardiac catheterization. Because the procedure for data sampling and processing has been described in detail elsewhere,[17] it will be reviewed here only briefly. Eighty-seven body surface leads were arranged in a latticelike pattern (13 × 7 matrix) except for four lead points in the midaxillary lines and covered the entire thoracic surface (59 leads on the anterior chest and 28 leads on the back). ECGs from these 87 unipolar leads with Wilson's central terminal as reference, standard 12-lead ECGs, and the Frank X, Y, Z ECGs were sampled simultaneously. The stored signals of each ECG were then displayed on a graphic terminal (Tektronix 4006-1). If noise was detected in any of the signals, data sampling was repeated. The flat portion of the PQ segment was chosen for the baseline. After the baseline adjustment, the data were recorded in a magnetic cassette tape in a digital format. This system had a resolution of 10 μV, in the dynamic range ± 5 mV, with a sampling rate of 1000 samples/sec/channel. The data sampling was done at the resting expiratory level and in the supine position.

Data analysis. The map data were processed off-line on a minicomputer (Texas Instrument 980-B) by means of the program for isochronal map analysis developed at our institution. For this study, the onset of QRS was determined from superimposed Frank X, Y, Z leads and the spatial magnitude and was called "zero time." For each lead, the duration from zero time to the time of the peak of the R wave was measured and was designated "activation time." When two R waves were present in a lead, the greater R wave was chosen for the measurement. When the R wave was absent in a lead, the area where the lead points were located was called the "no R-wave area" (NR area). The body surface distribution of the activation times was displayed as an isochrone map. On the display of isochrone maps, the rectangular area represented the torso surface, with the left half reflecting the anterior chest and the right half the back. Thus both the right and left edges represented the right midaxillary line. Each contour line connected points of equal activation time. The interval of isochrone lines was 5 msec. NR areas were indicated by crosses.

Examinations for ventricular arrhythmia. Holter monitoring was done in 25 patients and treadmill exercise testing was done in all 85 patients within a week before or after the cardiac catheterization. Twenty-four hour ambulatory ECGs of modified leads V_1 and V_5 were recorded by a Holter recorder (Avionics model 445B). All recordings were analyzed by a computer-assisted system (Avionics Cardioscanner) as to the presence of ventricular premature contractions (VPCs). Submaximal treadmill exercise was performed according to Bruce's protocol.[18] The ECG of lead CM5 was continuously monitored before, during, and at least 10 min after the exercise.

All patients were followed for 6 months to 5 years (mean 3.1 years) after the onset of myocardial infarction as to the occurrence of ventricular tachycardia.

Statistical analysis. Group mean data were expressed as mean ± SD. Statistical difference was examined by the unpaired t test or the chi-square test; $p < .05$ was considered significant.

Results

Isochrone maps of normal subjects. Figure 1 represents isochrone maps of normal subjects. Figure 1, *A*, is an isochrone map from a 44-year-old man. On this map, activation time was shortest on the right upper anterior chest. Isochrone lines extended from the right upper anterior chest to the left anterior chest in the leftward and downward direction. After they reached the left lateral chest, isochrone lines propagated to the back in a rightward and upward direction. The activation time was longest on the upper back.

Figure 1, *B*, is another example of normal isochrone map obtained from a 26-year-old man. Although there were slight interindividual differences, the total distribution pattern of the isochrone map was almost the same as that in the first case. Activation time was shortest on the right upper anterior chest. Isochrone lines spread from the right upper chest over the left anterior chest and finally to the back. Small NR areas were found on the upper back (only two lead points).

As shown in figure 1, isochrone maps of normal subjects had a consistent distribution pattern, extending from the right upper anterior chest toward the left anterior chest and then to the back. At the fifth intercostal level (row 4, indicated by arrows), the 30 msec isochrone line crossed near the anterior median line, the 40 msec isochrone line passed nearby the left axillary line, and the 50 msec isochrone line crossed near the posterior median line. The difference between the activation times of neighboring lead points did not exceed 20 msec except on the right axillary zone and upper back. NR area was found in 24 of the 36 normal subjects on the upper right anterior chest or on the upper back. All these NR areas were small (three lead points in four subjects, two lead points in seven, and one lead point in 13). NR area did not exist on the right lower anterior chest, central sternal region, left anterior or left lateral chest, or lower back.

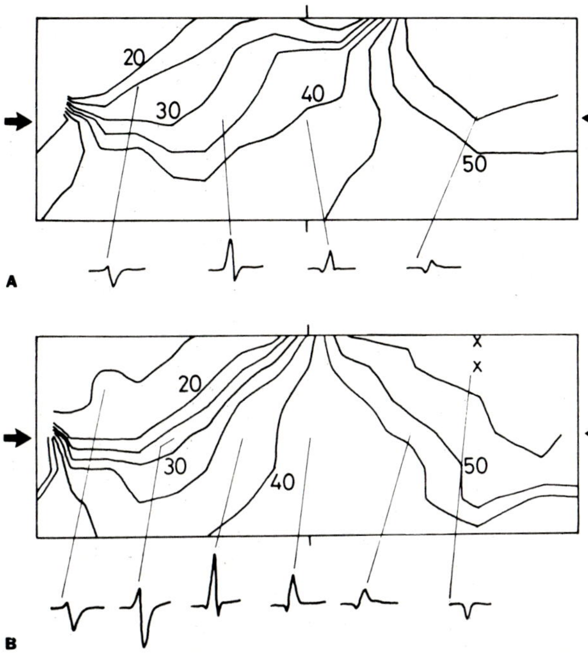

FIGURE 1. Isochrone maps from normal subjects. *A*, Isochrone map from a 44-year-old man. The rectangular area represents the torso surface, with the left half reflecting the anterior chest and the right half the back. Each contour line connects the points of equal activation time at 5 msec intervals. The numerals indicate the activation time. ECGs of the QRS period from some lead points are also illustrated. Arrows indicate the level of fifth intercostal space. *B*, Isochrone map from a 26-year-old man. Crosses indicate the NR area. See text for details.

Isochrone maps in patients with myocardial infarction. The patients were divided into four groups according to the asynergic site of the left ventricle: group 1 (anterior asynergy group), 28 patients; group 2 (inferior asynergy group), 22 patients; group 3 (anterior and inferior asynergy group), 25 patients; group 4 (apical asynergy group), 10 patients.

Group 1 (anterior asynergy group). Group 1 consisted of 28 patients, 25 men and three women 41 to 67 years of age.

Figure 2 shows the isochrone map obtained from a patient in group 1. The left ventricular asynergic site was located in the anterolateral and apical segments (both were dyskinetic). On the isochrone map, NR area lay over the upper right anterior chest and central sternal regions. The earliest isochrone line appeared on the left upper lateral chest at 40 msec from the onset of QRS. Isochrone lines extended from the left upper anterior chest to the left lateral chest and then to the back. On the middle right to lower anterior chest, isochrone lines propagated from the lower chest toward the NR area, in the opposite direction from the normal isochrone maps. Isochrone lines crowded on the lower portion of the right anterior chest. On the lower side of the NR area, activation time was much delayed (70 to 80 msec); this phenomenon was referred to as "peri–NR area delay." Peri–NR area delay was judged to be present when a zone of three or more leads of delayed activation was found near the NR area; delayed activation was considered significant when the activation time was obviously outside what was found in normal subjects for that torso area with coexistent increased density of isochrone lines. Contrary, on the left side of the NR area, isochrone lines were suddenly interrupted and peri–NR area delay was not observed on the isochrone map.

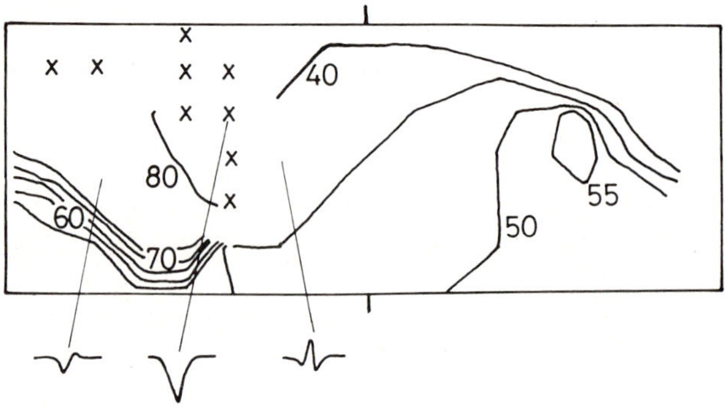

FIGURE 2. Isochrone maps from a patient in group 1 (anterior asynergy). An NR area was located on the upper to middle anterior chest. Peri–NR area delay was observed on the right anterior chest.

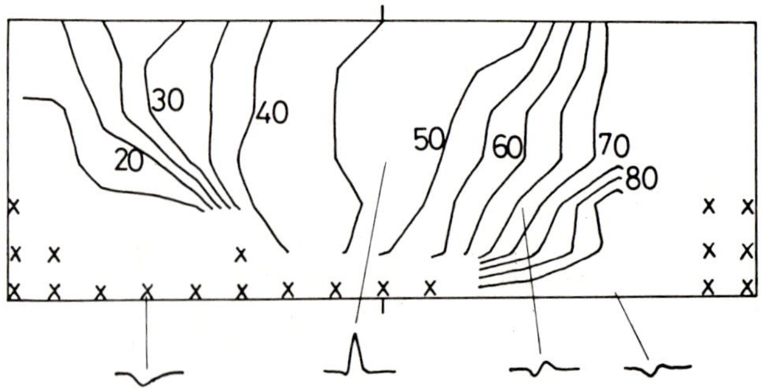

FIGURE 4. Isochrone map from a patient in group 2 (inferior asynergy). An NR area was located on the lower chest. Peri–NR area delay was observed on the back.

Figure 3 represents an isochrone map of another patient in group 1. The asynergic site was anterolateral segment (akinesis). NR area was found on the upper anterior chest. Activation times on the left upper chest were slightly longer than those on the left middle anterior chest. Isochrone lines propagated on the left anterior chest in the upward direction and finally toward the NR area, as if they moved around the NR area. We thought that slight peri–NR area delay was present in this case.

In 26 of the 28 patients (93%) of group 1, NR area was found on the upper to middle anterior chest. The mean size of NR area in these 26 patients was 11.6 ± 3.0 leads. Peri–NR area delay was found in 10 patients (36%).

Group 2 (inferior asynergy group). This group consisted of 22 patients, 20 men and two women 40 to 69 years of age.

Figure 4 is an isochrone map of a patient in group 2. The asynergic site was located in the apical, diaphragmatic, and posterobasal segments (akinesis, akinesis, and dyskinesis, respectively). NR area was located widely on the lower chest. Isochrone lines were converged on the inferior chest near the NR area. Activation time was much delayed on the back (over 70 msec), especially in the inferior portion. Peri–NR area delay was judged to be present on the back in this case.

Of the 22 patients in group 2, 13 patients (59%) had NR area on the lower chest. The mean size of NR area was 11.5 ± 3.2 leads. Peri–NR area delay was observed in 11 patients (50%).

Group 3 (anterior and inferior asynergy group). Group 3 consisted of 25 patients, 18 men and seven women 35 to 69 years of age.

Figure 5 represents an isochrone map of a patient in group 3. The asynergic site was located in the anterolateral, apical, and diaphragmatic segments (akinesis, dyskinesis, and dyskinesis, respectively). A large NR area lay over almost the entire anterior chest except for the left lateral portion. Isochrone lines extended from the left upper chest to the back. But on the lower portion of the left lateral chest, a zone of delayed activation time was present. This was also determined to be peri–NR area delay.

Figure 6 is another isochrone map of a patient in group 3. The asynergic site was located in the anterolateral, apical, and diaphragmatic segments (all dyskinesis). NR area was located on the upper portion of the anterior chest. Activation time was earliest in the

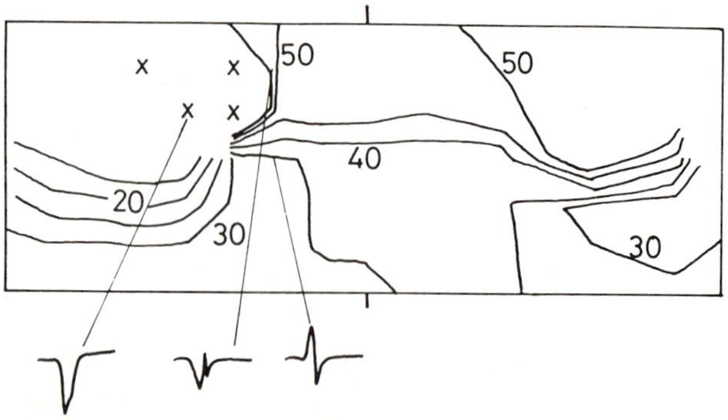

FIGURE 3. Isochrone map from a patient in group 1. The NR area is smaller than that in figure 2. A slight peri–NR area delay was found on the left upper anterior chest.

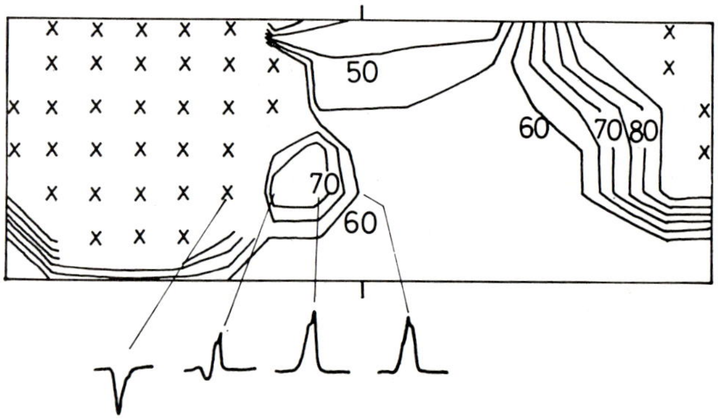

FIGURE 5. Isochrone map from a patient in group 3 (anterior and inferior asynergy). A large NR area was located on the anterior chest. Peri–NR area delay was observed on the left lateral chest.

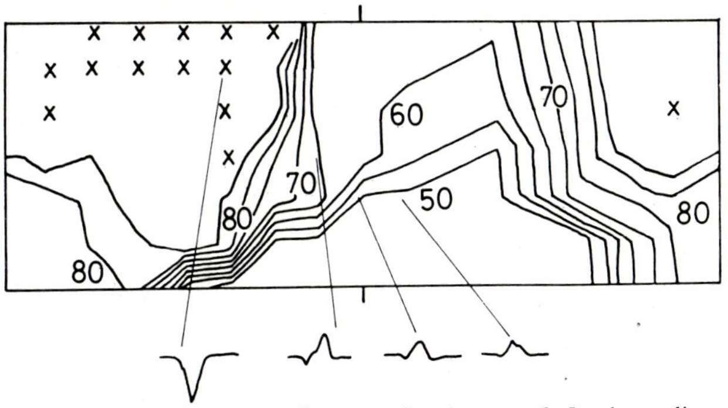

FIGURE 6. Isochrone map from a patient in group 3. Isochrone lines propagated from the left lower chest toward the NR area in an upward and rightward direction. This pattern was considered to be an extreme example of peri–NR area delay.

left-lateral inferior chest and the lower back. Isochrone lines extended from inferior to superior toward the NR area. On the left anterior chest, activation time was much delayed beside the NR area. In this case, the area of the peri–NR area delay was extremely wide and occupied almost all the anterior chest except for the NR area.

NR areas were found in 24 of 25 patients (96%) in group 3 and extended over the upper to lower right and left anterior chest. The group mean size of NR area was 21.0 ± 3.3 leads and significantly greater than those in groups 1 and 2 ($p < .01$, $p < .01$). Peri–NR area delay was found in 16 patients (64%).

Group 4 (apical asynergy group). Group 4 consisted of 10 patients, all men, 45 to 66 years of age.

Figure 7A represents an isochrone map of a patient in group 4. The asynergic site was located in the apical segment. A small NR area was found on the right anterior chest, but on the left anterior chest no NR area was present. Isochrone lines crowded on the left anterior chest and formed an islandlike zone of delayed activation time (indicated by an arrow). As was shown in figure 7B standard 12-lead ECGs failed to detect this abnormal activation pattern.

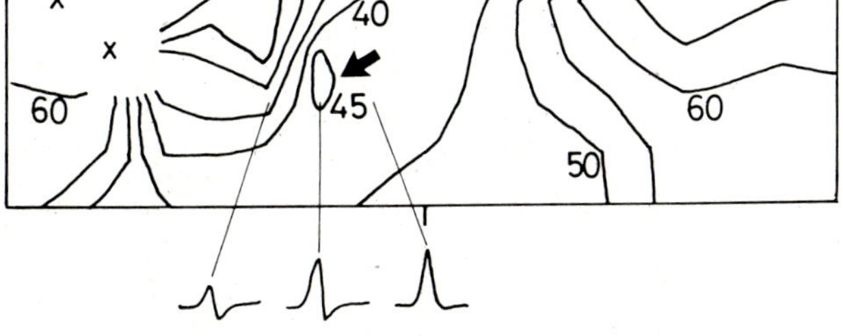

FIGURE 7A. Isochrone map from a patient in group 4 (apical asynergy). Isochrone lines crowded on the left anterior chest and formed an islandlike zone of delayed activation (indicated by an arrow).

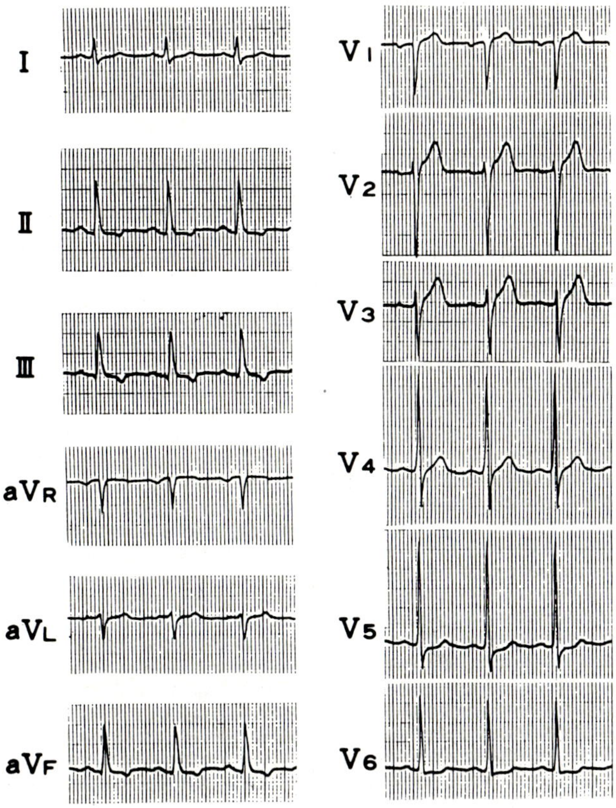

FIGURE 7B. Standard 12-lead ECG from the same patient as in figure 7A.

Out of the 10 patients in group 4, four (40%) had NR areas on the anterior chest. The mean size of the NR area in the four patients was 7.0 ± 2.0 leads, significantly smaller than those in groups 1, 2, and 3 ($p < .05$, $p < .05$, and $p < .01$, respectively). Peri–NR area delay was not observed in any case. Crowds of isochrone lines were considered significant when activation time was delayed by over 20 msec between neighboring leads except on the right axillary zone and upper back. Isochrone lines crowded on the left anterior chest in nine patients and formed an island of delayed activation as in figures 7A and 7B in five patients.

Table 1 summarizes the abnormal findings on the body surface isochrone maps in patients with myocardial infarction (NR area, peri–NR area delay, crowd of isochrone lines, and islandlike zone of delayed activation). Islandlike zones of delayed activation were found in nine patients, all of whom had asynergy in the apical segment. Of the 85 patients, 83 (98%) had abnormal patterns on isochrone maps.

Correlation of the isochrone map findings with asynergy index, ejection fraction, and incidence of ventricular arrhythmias. Patients were divided into three sets of subgroups according to the findings of the isochrone

TABLE 1
Abnormal findings on the isochrone maps

Group	n	NR area	Peri–NR area delay	Crowd of isochrone lines	Islandlike zone	One or more abnormalities[A]
1	28	26 (93)	10 (36)	11 (39)	1 (4)	28 (100)
2	22	13 (59)	11 (50)	9 (41)	0 (0)	20 (91)
3	25	24 (96)	16 (64)	17 (68)	3 (12)	25 (100)
4	10	4 (40)	0 (0)	9 (90)	5 (50)	10 (100)
total	85	67 (79)	37 (44)	46 (54)	9 (11)	83 (98)

Numbers in parentheses are percentages of the group.
[A]Number of patients who had at least one of the abnormal findings.

maps: those with and without NR area, those with and without peri–NR area delay, and those with and without crowds of isochrone lines. Between each subgroup, asynergy index, left ventricular ejection fraction, and the incidence of VPCs were compared (table 2).

The group with NR area had a higher asynergy index ($p < .01$) and lower ejection fraction ($p < .01$) than the group without NR area. The group with peri–NR area delay had a higher asynergy index ($p < .01$) and lower ejection fraction ($p < .01$) than the group without peri–NR area delay. However, a significant difference was not found in asynergy index or ejection fraction between the groups with and without crowds of isochrone lines.

The incidence of VPCs was significantly higher in the group with peri–NR area delay than in the group without ($p < .05$). It also tended to be higher in the group with crowds of isochrone lines than in the group without, but the difference was not significant. There was no significant difference in the incidence of VPCs between the groups with and without NR area.

During the follow-up period, episodes of ventricular tachycardia were found in three patients in group 3 (anterior-inferior asynergy). All of them had peri–NR area delay.

Discussion

The purpose of this study was to detect local abnormalities in ventricular activation sequence in patients with previous myocardial infarction by body surface isochrone mapping.

Interpretations of the body surface isochrone maps. From the results of this study, body surface isochrone maps of normal subjects showed a consistent pattern in which isochrone lines propagated from the right upper anterior to left lateral chest and finally to the back. The leftward extension of the isochrone lines is considered to reflect the ventricular excitation from the septum to the left ventricular free wall. We could not separate the excitation of the right ventricle by this analysis. Thus we focused our attention on the relationship between the left ventricular asynergic site and the distribution pattern of the isochrone lines in patients with previous myocardial infarction.

The results in patients revealed that the NR area was usually located on the upper to middle anterior chest in group 1 (anterior asynergy), on the lower anterior chest and the back in group 2 (inferior asynergy), and on the upper to lower anterior chest in group 3 (anterior and inferior asynergy). NR area was found in 93% of group 1, 59% of group 2, and 96% of group 3 patients. Sometimes activation time was very delayed near the

TABLE 2
Correlation of the isochrone map findings with the findings of left ventriculography and the incidence of VPCs

	NR area		Peri–NR area delay		Crowd of isochrone lines	
	+	–	+	–	+	–
AI	7.1±3.3[B]	4.8±2.3	8.6±3.0[B]	5.1±2.5	6.9±3.4	6.3±3.0
EF (%)	47.0±12.8[B]	56.0±11.5	43.7±12.3[B]	53.0±12.2	49.8±12.3	48.1±13.9
VPC (%)[C]	36	33	49[A]	25	39	31

AI = asynergy index; EF = left ventricular ejection fraction.
[A]$p < .05$; [B]$p < .01$ compared with the negative subgroup.
[C]Incidence of VPCs during Holter monitoring or treadmill test.

NR area (peri–NR area delay). This delay was most frequently found in patients with larger infarction, as in group 3 (67%). On the other hand, in cases of small infarction of the apical segment (group 4), NR area was less frequent (40%). But a crowd of isochrone lines frequently existed on the left anterior chest (nine of 10, 90%). In typical cases, local delay of the activation time was indicated by an island of isochrone lines on the left precordial region. As shown in table 2, patients with NR area had a greater asynergy index and lower ejection fraction than those without. Furthermore, patients with peri–NR area delay had a greater asynergy index and lower ejection fraction.

We propose the following interpretations for these findings: the NR area indicates the central portion of a large infarction, which was almost unexcitable scar; the peri–NR area delay, crowds of isochrone lines, and islandlike zones of delayed activation indicate the area of partial or small infarction, where excitation propagated slowly through the surviving myocardial cell. These hypotheses agree closely with the results of Durrer et al.[19] on epicardial and intramural ECGs in experimental chronic myocardial infarction. They concluded that QS complexes on epicardium were present only where the infarction was transmural. Where living intrainfarction muscle fibers were present, excitatory waves followed circuitous routes and the mean conduction velocity was reduced.

Local delay of activation has been considered to have a close relationship with ventricular arrhythmias.[11, 20] Patients with peri–NR area delay had a higher incidence of VPCs than those without. All the patients with episodes of ventricular tachycardia had peri–NR area delay. Although these results are preliminary, they suggest that peri–NR area delay will be an aid in identifying high-risk patients with ventricular tachyarrhythmias.

When NR area is not associated with peri–NR area delay, the excitation may be suddenly interrupted beside the infarcted area or may be delayed in a very small site near the infarcted area, undetectable by the body surface isochrone map. Further study must be conducted to address this problem.

Influences of the time after infarction on the isochrone maps. QRS waveforms sometimes change, especially in the acute phase of myocardial infarction, as well as the extent of asynergy of ventricular wall. Figure 8 represents isochrone maps of a patient who underwent left ventriculography twice. The first left ventriculographic study was performed 4 weeks after the onset of myocardial infarction. Anterolateral and apical segments were dyskinetic and ejection fraction was 46%.

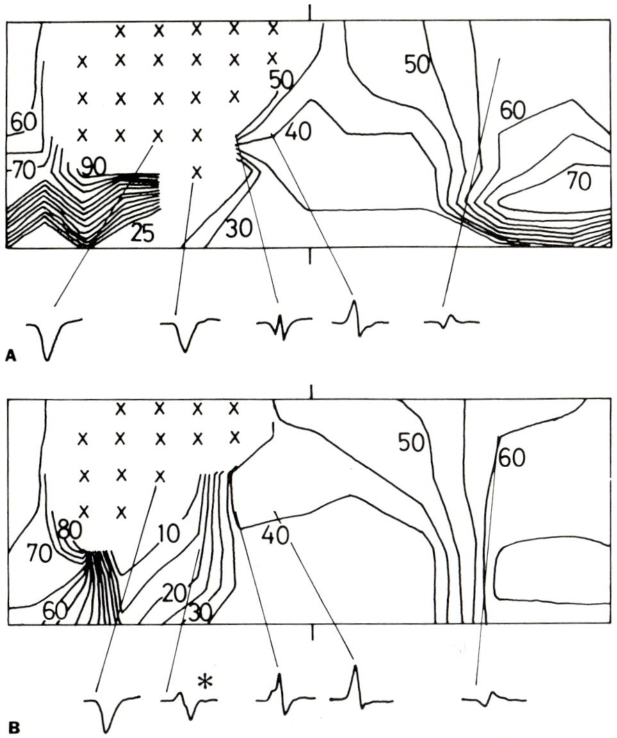

FIGURE 8. Isochrone maps from a patient in group 1 recorded at 4 weeks (*A*) and 7 months (*B*) after the infarction. In *B*, the size of NR area becomes smaller than in *A*. Several leads on the left and lower part of the NR area in *A* showed the development of R waves (*B*, indicated by asterisk), indicating a zone of slow conduction.

Figure 8, *A*, is the isochrone map at that time. NR area was located on the upper to middle anterior chest. Isochrone lines appeared on the lower anterior chest at 25 msec and propagated leftward and upward. On the left lateral chest, activation time was later near the NR area and peri–NR area delay was judged to be present. On the right lower chest, isochrone lines crowded and slowly propagated toward the NR area.

Six months later, the patient underwent a second left ventriculographic study. Asynergy of anterolateral and apical segments was reduced to akinesis and ejection fraction increased to 61%. Figure 8, *B*, is the isochrone map at the second left ventriculographic examination 7 months after the onset of infarction. NR area decreased in size, especially on the left anterior chest, and was replaced by a zone of slow conduction (indicated by an asterisk) and a crowd of isochrone lines. On the right anterior chest the distribution pattern of isochrone lines was not much different from the first time.

We thought that the NR area detected at the first study included the electrically silent myocardium with reversible damage as well as the dead unexcitable myocardium. We supposed that during the interval between the two recordings, reversibly damaged myocardium had recovered and the irreversibly damaged area still existed. At the second ventriculographic study, we thought that the NR area indicated the infarcted scar and the crowd of isochrone lines indicated the partially infarcted slow conduction area.

To avoid the influence of short-term reversible change on the isochrone maps, we analyzed the ECGs at the early chronic phase of myocardial infarction (2 to 11 months) in this study. However, comparison of isochrone map patterns at the acute and chronic phases may be used to evaluate the balance of reversible and irreversible damage in the infarcted myocardium.

Limitations of body surface isochrone maps. Isochrone maps have been made from epicardial bipolar ECGs. In this study, we tried to construct isochrone maps from body surface unipolar ECGs. Designation of the activation time on the body surface unipolar ECGs is a problem,[13] and we chose the peak of the R wave because it has been conventionally used to measure the ventricular activation time in clinical electrocardiology.[21] On the precordial ECG, the deflection from the peak of the R wave to the termination of the R wave or to the nadir of the S wave is called "intrinsicoid deflection," which is assumed to occur when the depolarization force reaches the myocardium beneath it. The peak of the R wave is the onset of the intrinsicoid deflection and is considered to represent the arrival of the depolarization force at the myocardial surface under the precordial lead.

Therefore the existence of the QS complex implies that the activation is proceeding away from the recording site and does not necessarily mean that the area is not activated. In fact, the NR area is sometimes seen in normal subjects on the right upper anterior chest and upper back, where the ECG leads are supposed to face the endocardial surface. But when the NR area is located on the other part of the torso surface of a patient with myocardial infarction, it may be reasonable to assume that the area reflects the inactive myocardium damaged by the infarction.

The potential on the epicardial surface is transmitted through the lungs, muscle layer, and skin to the body surface. The body surface potential at a point is mainly determined by the epicardial potentials beneath it, although it is also affected by potentials of the other part of the epicardium to some extent. The activation time measured in this study may be somewhat different from the local activation time of the corresponding point of the epicardial surface. However, the results of this study indicated that body surface isochrone maps reflected the normal left ventricular activation sequence from septum to the free wall and depicted abnormalities corresponded well with the asynergic site in patients with myocardial infarction. Thus we believe that body surface isochrone maps can be used clinically to determine the activation sequence of the myocardium.

Clinical implications. Peri–NR area delay and the island of delayed activation or the crowd of isochrone lines are not easily detected by the conventional analysis of ECGs. The island of delayed activation on the precordium was characteristic of apical infarction. It has been difficult to diagnose the infarction of the apical segment by the ECG. Thus body surface isochrone mapping will be a useful analytic method for apical infarction.

Patients with peri–NR area delay had a higher incidence of VPCs than those without. All the patients with episodes of ventricular tachycardia had peri–NR area delay. Local delay of activation indicated by the body surface isochrone map may be used to predict the occurrence of serious ventricular arrhythmias. Furthermore, as mentioned above, isochrone mapping may aid in evaluating the balance of reversible and irreversible damage in the infarcted myocardium. Further study will be carried out to address these points.

Although body surface isochrone mapping has several limitations, it is able to represent local abnormalities in ventricular activation sequence. Information from the body surface isochrone maps will provide new evidence for the occurrence of myocardial infarction.

References

1. Flowers NC, Horan LG, Sohi GS, Hand RC, Johnson JC: New evidence for inferoposterior myocardial infarction on surface potential maps. Am J Cardiol **38:** 576, 1976
2. Flowers NC, Horan LG, Johnson JC: Anterior infarctional changes occurring during mild and late ventricular activation detectable by surface mapping techniques. Circulation **54:** 901, 1976
3. Vincent GM, Abildskov JA, Burgess MJ, Millar K, Lux RL, Wyatt RF: Diagnosis of old inferior myocardial infarction by body surface isopotential mapping. Am J Cardiol **39:** 510, 1977
4. Ohta T, Kinoshita A, Ohsugi J, Isomura S, Takatsu F, Ishikawa H, Toyama J, Nagaya T, Yamada K: Correlation between body surface isopotential maps and left ventriculograms in patients with old inferoposterior myocardial infarction. Am Heart J **104:** 1262, 1982
5. Montague TJ, Smith ER, Spencer CA, Johnstone DE, Lalonde LD, Bessoudo RM, Gardner MJ, Anderson RN, Horacek BM: Body surface electrocardiographic mapping in inferior myocardial infarction: manifestation of left and right ventricular involvement. Circulation **67:** 665, 1983
6. Tonooka I, Kubota I, Watanabe Y, Tsuiki K, Yasui S: Isointegral analysis of body surface maps for the assessment of location and size of myocardial infarction. Am J Cardiol **52:** 1174, 1983
7. Hirai M, Ohta T, Kinoshita A, Toyama J, Nagaya T, Yamada K: Body surface isopotential maps in old anterior myocardial infarction undetectable by 12-lead electrocardiograms. Am Heart J **108:** 975, 1984
8. Gallagher JJ, Kasell J, Sealy WC, Pritchett ELC, Wallace AG: Epicardial mapping in the Wolff-Parkinson-White syndrome. Circulation **57:** 854, 1978
9. Wyndham CRC, Smith T, Meeran MK, Mammana R, Levitsky S,

Rosen KM: Epicardial activation in patients with left bundle branch block. Circulation **61:** 696, 1980
10. Klein GJ, Ideker RE, Smith WM, Harrison LA, Kasell JK, Wallace AG, Gallagher JJ: Epicardial mapping of the onset of ventricular tachycardia initiated by programmed stimulation in the canine heart with chronic infarction. Circulation **60:** 1375, 1979
11. Richards DA, Blake GJ, Spear JF, Moore EN: Electrophysiologic substrate for ventricular tachycardia: correlation of properties in vivo and in vitro. Circulation **69:** 369, 1984
12. Bardy GH, Ungerleider RM, Smith WM, Ideker RE: A mechanism of Torsades de Pointes in a canine model. Circulation **67:** 52, 1983
13. Okajima M, Doniwa K, Ishikawa T, Niimi N, Koike Y: On body surface VAT "isochrone" maps generated by computer using simulated excitation sequences in ventricular model. Proceedings of Computers in Cardiology, October 1980, Williamsburg, VA, 1981, p 187
14. Austen WG, Edwards JE, Frye RL, Gensini GG, Gott VL, Griffith LSC, McGoon DC, Murphy ML, Roe BB: A reporting system on patients evaluated for coronary artery disease. Report of the Ad Hoc Committee for grading of coronary artery disease, Council on Cardiovascular Surgery, American Heart Association. Circulation **51:** 5, 1975 (News from the AHA)
15. Dodge HT, Sandler H, Ballew DW, Lord DJ: The use of biplane angiocardiography for the measurement of left ventricular volume in man. Am Heart J **60:** 762, 1960
16. Mannebach H, Fassbender D, Trieb G, Gleichmann U: AVD: A new system for the computer-aided analysis of ventricular wall motion abnormalities. Initial experience. Elektromedica **3:** 85, 1982
17. Watanabe T, Toyama J, Toyoshima H, Oguri H, Ohno M, Ohta T, Okajima M, Naito Y, Yamada K: A practical microcomputer-based mapping system for body surface, precordium, and epicardium. Comput Biomed Res **14:** 341, 1981
18. Bruce RA: Exercise testing of patients with coronary artery disease: principles and normal standard for evaluation. Ann Clin Res **3:** 323, 1971
19. Durrer D, Van Lier AAW, Buller J: Epicardial and intramural excitation in chronic myocardial infarction. Am Heart J **68:** 765, 1964
20. Josephson ME, Horowitz LN, Farshidi A: Continuous local electrical activity: a mechanism for recurrent ventricular activity. Circulation **57:** 659, 1978
21. Lipman BS, Dunn M, Massie E: Clinical electrocardiography, ed 7. Chicago, 1984, Year Book Medical Publishers, Inc., pp 42–54

Erratum

In an article by Eichler et al. that was published in the April 1985 issue of Circulation (**71:** 779, 1985), a sentence in the Abstract appeared incorrectly. The sentence should have read: "The hemodynamic effects of this drug (1 mg/kg followed by 25 μg/kg/min over 36 hr) were studied, in 30 patients randomly assigned to a tiapamil or control group within 12 hr of the onset of acute myocardial infarction, by Swan-Ganz catheterization and gated blood pool scans."

Noninvasive estimation of valve area in patients with aortic stenosis by Doppler ultrasound and two-dimensional echocardiography

TERJE SKJAERPE, M.D., LARS HEGRENAES, M.D., AND LIV HATLE, M.D.

ABSTRACT In 30 patients with aortic stenosis, 14 of whom also had significant aortic regurgitation, the velocities in the stenotic jet (V′) and below the valve (V) were recorded by Doppler ultrasound. With two-dimensional echocardiography, two subvalvular areas (A) were calculated from leading-to-leading edge ("large") and trailing-to-leading edge ("inner") diameter measurements. The aortic valve area was calculated by the equation of continuity (A′ = A × peak V/peak V′) and by calculating stroke volume below the valve [A × integral of V(t)] and dividing by the integral of V′(t) (= A″). Based on cardiac output estimations from single-plane angiographic images, Gorlin's formula was used to calculate invasive valve areas. In patients with no or mild aortic regurgitation a second invasive estimate was based on cardiac output measured by the Fick method. The best correlation was found when A′ (with "large" diameter) was compared with invasive results based on cardiac output measured by the Fick method (r = .89, SEE ± 0.12, n = 16); the worst was found when A″ (with "large" diameter) was compared with invasive results based on cardiac output measurements by single-plane angiography (r = .80, SEE ± 0.20, n = 30). The results indicate that valve area in patients with aortic stenosis can be reliably estimated noninvasively, even in those with significant aortic regurgitation.
Circulation 72, No. 4, 810–818, 1985.

BECAUSE the pressure drop across a stenotic valve depends both on the effective valve area and the flow across the valve, the information it offers about the severity of the obstruction is not complete. The quantitation of valvular stenosis therefore includes an estimation of the valve area.

Ideally a method for the estimation of a valve area should be independent of valve insufficiency, of diseases of other valves, and of ventricular performance. If the valve area varies during the antegrade flow period, the method should give an estimate of the effective area. The method should also be noninvasive to allow frequent follow-up of the patient. So far the various methods described to estimate the valve area in patients with aortic stenosis only partly fulfill these criteria, either because the methods are invasive or semi-invasive,[1, 2] or because they rely on the absence of significant aortic regurgitation[1-3] or mitral regurgitation.[4]

From the Section of Cardiology, Department of Medicine, University Hospital, Trondheim, Norway.
Supported by the Norwegian Research Council for Science and the Humanities and by the Norweigna Council on Cardiovascular Diseases.
Address for correspondence: Terje Skjaerpe, M.D., Section of Cardiology, Department of Medicine, University Hospital, 7000 Trondheim, Norway.
Received Feb. 15, 1985; revision accepted June 6, 1985.

In this work we evaluated a completely noninvasive method designed to be accurate despite any coexisting regurgitation.

Methods

Theoretical considerations. When there is an obstruction in a flow channel, the product of flow area and flow velocity will be constant at the obstructed and the nonobstructed part of the flow channel, according to the equation of continuity:

$$A \times V = A' \times V' \qquad (1)$$

where V and A are the spatial mean velocity and the area proximal to the obstruction, and V′ and A′ are the spatial mean velocity and the area at the obstruction. If V, A, and V′ are known, the stenotic area can be calculated by rearranging equation 1 as follows:

$$A' = A \times V/V' \qquad (2)$$

This equation is valid both in time-steady flow and at each moment during pulsatile flow, provided that the velocity profile does not change from A to A′. It is also assumed that A is constant. If A′ is elastic and varies because of the changing pressure drop across the obstruction during pulsatile flow, the size of the valve area calculated by equation 2 will depend on when V and V′ are recorded. If peak V and V′ are recorded, it can probably be assumed that the maximal A′ is calculated, since the pressure drop is highest at this moment, forcing the valve to open maximally.

There are two ways of calculating mean A′. One is to estimate the area at frequent intervals during one flow period and calculate a temporal mean area (mean A′). Equation 2 must then be modified to:

$$\text{Mean } A' = A \times \text{int}(V(t)/V'(t))/t \quad (3)$$

where int(V(t)/V′(t)) is V/V′ integrated over one cycle and t is the time of one flow period (see Appendix for how equation 3 is developed). This equation involves the laborious procedure of measuring V and V′ at frequent corresponding intervals on two velocity curves and integrating the quotients.

The other way is to calculate an effective area of A′ (A″) by estimating volume flow through A and A′, which must be equal:

$$A \times \text{int}V(t) = A'' \times \text{int}V'(t) \quad (4)$$

where intV(t) and intV′(t) are the integrals of the velocity curves recorded at A and A′. The effective valve area is obtained by rearranging equation 4 into:

$$A'' = A \times \text{int}V(t)/\text{int}V'(t) \quad (5)$$

The effective valve area is equivalent to a constant area that lets the same volume of flow pass through it when the pressure drop and the duration of flow are identical. The integrals of the velocity curves are easily obtained with a computer and a digitizing tablet or with a mechanical planimeter. The left side of equation 4, when applied to the left ventricular outflow tract (LVOT), defines the stroke volume of the heart, which is an important advantage.

When the velocities proximal to the obstruction are recorded, it must be realized that they are influenced by the obstruction. According to fluid mechanics, dead water zones are formed around a central, tapering core of flow with increasing velocities (figure 1). Because of the corresponding peaking of the velocity profile, recordings representative of the cross-sectional mean velocity should be made proximal to this level. In our experience, the increase in velocities in the LVOT, caused by the valvular stenosis, starts about 0.5 to 1.5 cm proximal to the valve. This is in agreement with the results of another report.[5] Recent experience has shown that the velocity curve of the jet in aortic stenosis can be recorded in almost all patients[5a] and that cardiac output can be measured with echocardiography and Doppler ultrasound by recording the diameter and the velocities in the upper LVOT in patients with normal aortic valves.[6, 7] This was the background for the present attempt to apply equations 2 and 5 to estimate the valve area in patients with aortic stenosis.

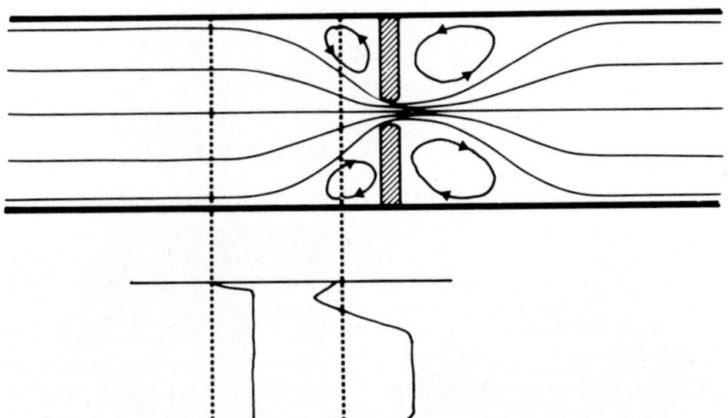

FIGURE 1. When there is an obstruction of a flow channel, an increase in velocities proximal to the obstruction (level B) will be observed. If, as in the LVOT, the flow proximal to the obstruction is accelerated, the velocity profile at level A is flattened. Velocities representing the spatial mean velocity should therefore be recorded at this level.

Patients. Thirty-six consecutive patients were studied. Informed consent was obtained from all. Six were excluded, four because the cardiac output or the pressure drop was not obtained as a result of problems experienced during catheterization, and two because they had significant aortic and mitral regurgitation, precluding calculation of valve area from Gorlin's formula. None were excluded because of failure in obtaining the echocardiographic and Doppler measurements. Of the remaining 30 patients, 10 were women and 20 were men, ranging in age from 38 to 76 years (mean 63.1).

Twenty-one patients were examined with echocardiography/Doppler within 2 days of the catheterization, and three within 4 days. Six patients were examined just before replacement of the valve, and the interval from the time of catheterization ranged from 27 to 87 days (mean 60). None had clinical signs indicating increasing severity of the aortic stenosis during this period.

By angiographic criteria for regurgitation,[8] nine patients had mild (+) aortic regurgitation, nine had moderate (+ +), two had moderate to severe (+ + +), and three had severe (+ + + +). Eight patients had mild (+) mitral regurgitation. Three patients had atrial fibrillation.

Diameter measurements. For the subvalvular diameter measurements we used an Irex III B (Irex Corp.) 3.5 MHz phased-array or an ATL mark III (Advanced Technology Laboratories) 3 MHz mechanical sector scanner. The LVOT and the aortic root were visualized in the parasternal long-axis view, using the intercostal space from which the clearest image of these structures was obtained (figure 2).

At least five copies of the two-dimensional image were recorded. The transducer was repositioned between each recording. The diameter was measured preferably in systole, but sometimes measurements were made in late diastole because the upper part of the LVOT was clearly visualized only in this part of the cardiac cycle. Despite careful adjustment of gain, the presence of calcium deposits in the wall of the LVOT might cause some blooming of the echoes. Therefore, on each image two diameters were measured, one "large," obtained from leading edge measurements, and one "inner" diameter measured from the trailing edge of the anterior echo to the leading edge of the posterior echo. Because the leading edge of the anterior echo was often difficult to define due to the calcium deposits, the "large" diameter was not allowed to exceed the "inner" diameter by more than 2 mm. If the diameters measured on different recordings varied in size, the largest obtained in at least two

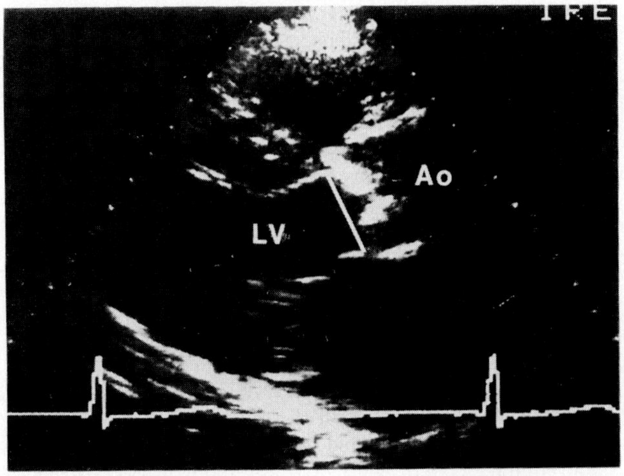

FIGURE 2. The diameter is measured just below the aortic valve to avoid any influence of the systolic thickening of the septum and movement of the anterior mitral valve leaflet. LV = left ventricle; Ao = aorta.

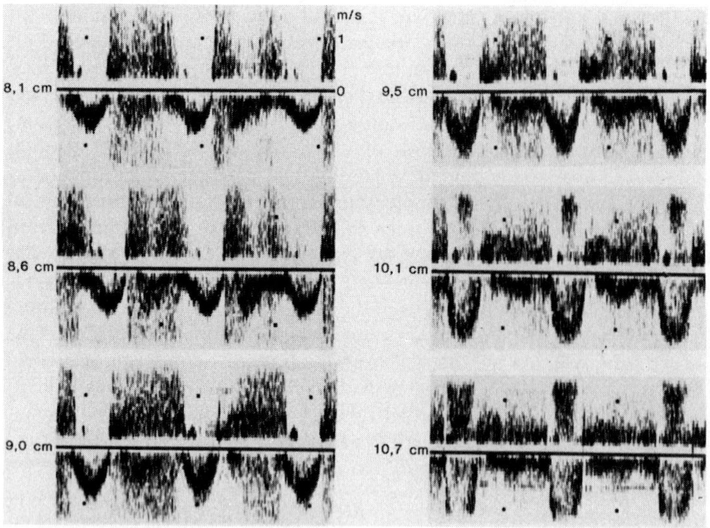

FIGURE 3. Velocities recorded with pulsed Doppler in the distal part of the LVOT. The aortic valve is located at about 10.7 cm from the transducer (the level showing maximal aliasing of the velocities). In this patient, steeply increasing velocities were recorded from 9.5 cm. The velocities recorded at 9.0 cm were therefore chosen as representing the spatial mean.

recordings was chosen for the subsequent calculations. The cross-sectional area was calculated by assuming a circular shape of the distal part of the LVOT.

Velocity recordings. The velocity recordings were obtained with the Irex III B, which includes a 2 MHz Doppler instrument (Pedof, Vingmed), allowing pulsed- or continuous-wave Doppler measurements to be made simultaneously with imaging. Velocity recordings with a separate, optimized Doppler transducer were also possible.

The subvalvular velocities were recorded from the apex with pulsed-wave Doppler. The image and the audio signal were used to align the ultrasound beam to the direction of flow. The positioning of the sample volume was made as follows: When the sample volume was moved out of the LVOT, gradually increasing velocities were recorded until a much steeper rise occurred 0.5 to 1.5 cm proximal to the valve (figure 3). The corresponding increase in pitch of the audio signal was easily heard. The sample volume was placed just proximal to this level.

The velocities in the stenotic jet were recorded with continuous-wave Doppler. A meticulous search for the highest velocities was made by recording from the apex, along the right sternal border, from the suprasternal notch, and sometimes also from the right and left supraclavicular regions. The separate Doppler transducer was used because the combined echocardiographic/Doppler transducer — even in Doppler-only mode — may fail to display the highest velocities because of suboptimal sensitivity. Typical recordings from the LVOT and the stenotic jet are shown in figure 4.

The peak and the mean pressure drops were calculated as described by Hegrenaes and Hatle.[5a] Integration of the velocity curves was made with a digitizing tablet and a computer (Cardio 80, Kontron AG) or with a mechanical planimeter (Cora senior, G. Coradi AG). The subvalvular integrals and peak velocities were averaged over 5 beats in sinus rhythm and over 10 beats in atrial fibrillation. In some patients it was difficult to obtain optimal velocity recordings from the stenotic jet in more than a few beats, and the integrals and peak velocities of the recordings from the jet were averaged over only 3 beats. Beats giving the largest integrals were selected, provided that the heart rate was stable. In three patients with atrial fibrillation it was possible to average the integral over 10 consecutive beats. The opening and closing of the aortic valve was identified to ensure that diastolic velocities were not included.

The valve area was calculated from both equations 2 and 5. Two estimates were obtained from each equation by the two diameters measured echocardiographically.

The subvalvular integral was multiplied with the cross-sectional area of the LVOT and the heart rate to give an estimate of total cardiac output (effective cardiac output + regurgitant volume).

In eight patients the velocities in the LVOT were recorded at multiple levels, and the differences in integral size and peak velocity from one level to the next were calculated.

Catheterization. The patients received a mild sedative 1 hr before catheterization; otherwise there was no change in medication between the noninvasive and invasive measurements.

The pressures were recorded with a fluid-filled No. 7F pigtail catheter connected to an Elema 746 pressure transducer. The pressure difference was calculated by superimposing pressure recordings obtained by pullback of the catheter from the left ventricle to the ascending aorta. Beats with comparable RR

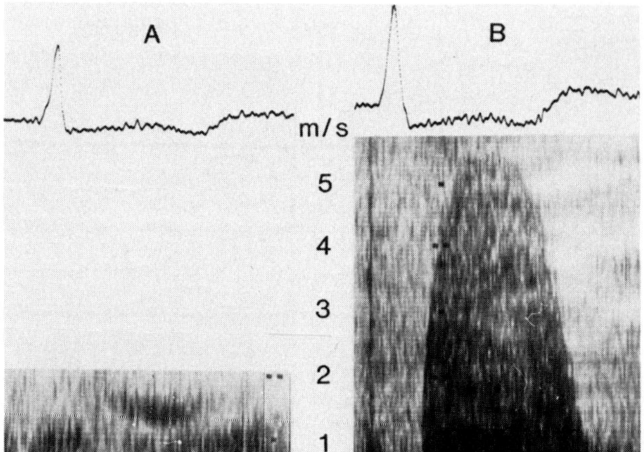

FIGURE 4. Representative subvalvular (*A*) and valvular (*B*) velocity recordings. The paper was run at a speed of 100 mm/sec to increase the accuracy when the curves were integrated.

TABLE 1
Catheterization data[A]

	Pressure drop (mm Hg)		Cardiac output (l/min)		Aortic valve area (cm^2)	
Patients	Peak	Mean	F	A	G/F	G/A
All (n = 30)	89±31	62±22	5.5±1.9	6.5±2.5		0.92±0.47
With no or mild AI (n = 16)	90±35	64±24	5.4±1.6	5.5±1.4	0.74±0.33	0.74±0.22
With > mild AI (n = 14)	88±29	60±20	5.6±2.3	7.7±3.0		1.14±0.58
Doppler < 4 days from cath. (n = 24)	91±32	64±23	5.7±2.0	6.7±2.7		0.95±0.52
Doppler > 4 days from cath. (n = 6)	84±32	54±16	4.8±1.4	5.9±1.3		0.82±0.13

F = Fick method; A = single-plane angiography; G = Gorlin's formula; AI = aortic regurgitation.
[A]In groups including patients with more than mild aortic regurgitation, only the valve areas for which the calculations are based on single-plane angiographic estimates of flow are shown. Values presented as mean ± 1 SD.

intervals were used for assessing the peak and mean pressure drops. In the presence of premature beats the following 2 sinus beats were disregarded. The peak pressure drop was obtained as an average of the largest instantaneous pressure drop from 3 representative beats. In the same beats the area between the ventricle and the aortic pressure curves in systole were planimetered to give the mean pressure drop. In atrial fibrillation, beats with a preceding RR interval representative of the mean heart rate were chosen. Cardiac output was measured by the direct Fick method.[9] The oxygen content in air and blood was measured with an OM-11 (Beckman Instruments Inc.) and an OSM 2 (Radiometer, Copenhagen), respectively. Because effective cardiac output will underestimate flow across the valve in patients with aortic regurgitation, total cardiac output was also calculated from single-plane angiographic images by a modification[10] of the Dodge-Sandlers method. Aortic valve area was calculated with Gorlin's formula.[1]

Results

There were no statistically significant differences in heart rate ($p > .05$) and systolic and diastolic blood pressure ($p > .1$ and $p > .5$) between the noninvasive and invasive examinations.

The invasive results are presented in table 1 and the noninvasive results in table 2. The "large" diameter was 2.2 ± 0.3 cm and the "inner" diameter was 2.0 ± 0.3 cm (mean ± SD). In patients with no or mild aortic regurgitation two invasive estimates of the valve area were calculated, one with cardiac output measured by single-plane angiographic images and one with measurements obtained by the Fick method, assuming that the regurgitant volume in patients with mild aortic regurgitation is within the error of the Fick method. This is supported by the findings in figure 5, where cardiac output measurements by the two methods are compared. There is no tendency for the Fick method to underestimate flow across the valve in patients with mild aortic regurgitation when compared with single-plane angiographic measurements. The same assumption was made about the regurgitant volume in patients with mild mitral regurgitation when total cardiac output was quantitated from single-plane angiographic images.

Table 3 shows the correlations obtained when measurements of pressure drops, cardiac output, and valve areas were compared. The rather poor correlation between noninvasive and invasive measurements of flow might be explained by the time interval of 1 to 3 months between the two measurements in some patients. Therefore, noninvasive measurements of cardiac output were also compared with invasive measurements (Fick) in a subgroup of patients (patients with no or mild aortic regurgitation, examined with echocardiography/Doppler within 4 days of catheterization).

TABLE 2
Noninvasive results[A]

	Pressure drop (mm Hg)		Cardiac output (l/min)		Aortic valve area (cm^2)			
Patients	Peak	Mean	D/El	D/Ei	A''/El	A''/Ei	A'/El	A'Ei
All	92±32	61±23	5.9±1.8	5.0±1.6	0.82±0.35	0.70±0.29	0.92±0.42	0.78±0.36
With no or mild AI	92±35	64±25	4.9±1.3	4.3±1.1	0.71±0.26	0.61±0.22	0.77±0.27	0.66±0.22
With > mild AI	92±30	58±20	7.0±1.7	5.9±1.7	0.95±0.39	0.80±0.33	1.10±0.50	0.93±0.44
Doppler < 4 days from cath.	93±33	62±24	5.9±1.9	5.0±1.7	0.83±0.38	0.71±0.32	0.94±0.47	0.79±0.40
Doppler > 4 days from cath.	88±30	58±21	5.7±1.5	5.0±1.4	0.76±0.10	0.67±0.11	0.86±0.07	0.76±0.07

D/El = Doppler/echo measurements, "large" diameter used; D/Ei = Doppler/echo, "inner" diameter used; A'' = valve area calculated by equation 5, "large" (El) and "inner" (Ei) diameter; A' = valve area calculated by equation 2, same diameters.
[A]Values presented as mean ± 1 SD.

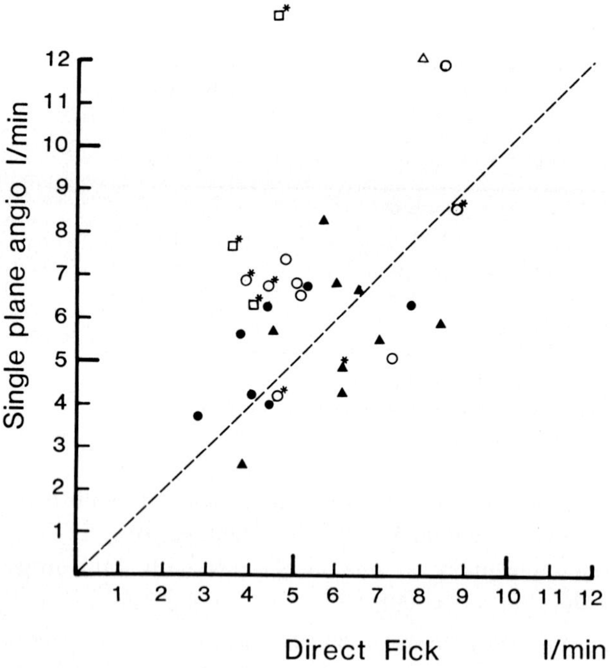

FIGURE 5. Effective cardiac output measurements obtained by the Fick method compared with total cardiac output measurements from single-plane angiographic images. Symbols represent patients with the following degrees of aortic regurgitation: ● = no aortic regurgitation; ▲ = mild; ○ = moderate; △ = moderate to severe; □ = severe. Data points marked with an asterisk represent patients who also had mild mitral regurgitation.

TABLE 3
Comparison of pressure drops, cardiac output, and valve areas

	Correlations				
Comparisons	r value	p value	Regression equation	SEE	No. of patients
Pressure drops					
Peak	.93	<.001	y=0.94x+7.60	11.75	30
Mean	.92	<.001	y=0.95x+2.48	9.23	30
Cardiac output					
D/El-A	.70	<.001	y=0.52x+2.53	1.29	30
D/Ei-A	.71	<.001	y=0.46x+1.99	1.13	30
D/El-F	.46	<.1	y=0.37x+2.93	1.12	16
D/Ei-F	.45	<.1	y=0.32x+2.52	0.99	16
A-F	.49	<.1	y=0.34x+3.89	1.39	16
D/El-F^	.71	<.01	y=0.54x+1.76	0.88	12
D/Ei-F^	.69	<.02	y=0.47x+1.44	0.76	12
Valve area					
A''/El-G/A	.80	<.001	y=0.59x+0.27	0.20	30
A''/Ei-G/A	.82	<.001	y=0.51x+0.23	0.17	30
A'/El-G/A	.87	<.001	y=0.79x+0.20	0.21	30
A'/Ei-G/A	.87	<.001	y=0.68x+0.16	0.17	30
A''/El-G/F	.87	<.001	y=0.70x+0.18	0.13	16
A''/Ei-G/F	.86	<.001	y=0.59x+0.17	0.11	16
A'/El-G/F	.89	<.001	y=0.74x+0.21	0.12	16
A'/Ei-G/F	.89	<.001	y=0.62x+0.20	0.10	16
G/A-G/F	.73	<.01	y=0.49x+0.37	0.15	16

Abbreviations as in tables 1 and 2.
^Subgroup: patients with no or mild aortic regurgitation examined with echo/Doppler within 4 days of catheterization.

Figures 6 to 9 graphically present comparisons between noninvasive and invasive estimates of valve areas. The noninvasive areas were calculated with the "large" diameter. There is tendency for the larger valve areas to be underestimated, especially when calculated by equation 5. When the "inner" diameter was used, this tendency was more pronounced, affecting also smaller valve areas (table 3).

The valve areas calculated from equations 2 and 5 are compared in figure 10. The largest difference between the estimates in one patient was 37% (0.41 cm^2).

In five patients a second diameter measurement was made on another occasion. In two the diameter was identical to the first measurement, in two there was a difference of 1 mm, and in one there was a difference of 2 mm.

In the eight patients in whom the velocities were recorded at several levels in the LVOT, it was decided which was the last level to show only a gradual increase in velocities and which was the first level to definitely indicate the steeper rise. Peak velocities and velocity integrals were measured from recordings made at these two levels. Differences in peak velocity and integral size in paired recordings ranged from 5% to 14% (mean 9%).

Discussion

The obvious difficulty in evaluating a new method for estimating valve areas is the problem of what to compare it with. Even in the absence of aortic regurgitation, Gorlin's formula may produce errors of up to 20% to 40% by including an empirical constant, the discharge coefficient.[11] Additional errors may be introduced by incorrect measurements of cardiac output and pressure drop. Besides, in the presence of aortic regurgitation, the valve area will be underestimated. It is possible to substitute effective cardiac output in the formula with total cardiac output calculated from single-plane angiographic images, except when there is significant mitral regurgitation. However, cardiac output measurements with this method may be less accurate in hypertrophic than in nonhypertrophic ventricles because of the influence of the larger papillary muscles. This may explain the poor correlation between invasive measurements of cardiac output and of valve area in these patients (table 3) and also the larger standard error of the estimate in figures 8 and 9. Considering these limitations, the correlations obtained in figures 6 to 9 indicate that the present method is

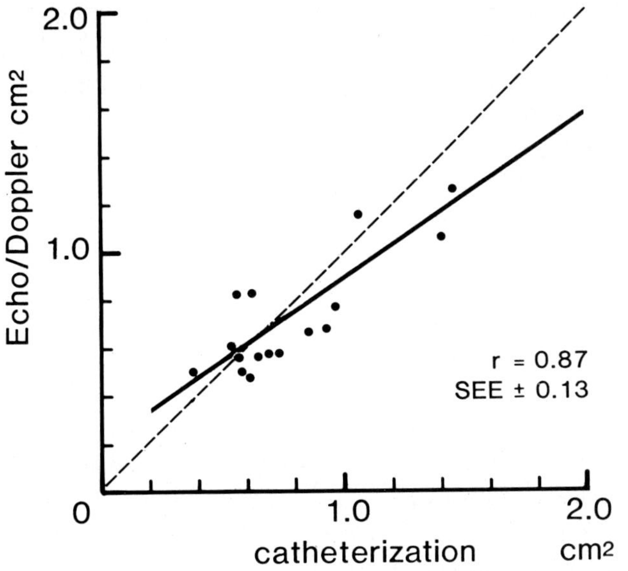

FIGURE 6. Aortic valve area in patients with no or mild aortic regurgitation. Cardiac output (Gorlin's formula) was measured by the Fick method. The noninvasive results are based on integration of the velocity curves (equation 5) and the "large" subvalvular diameter.

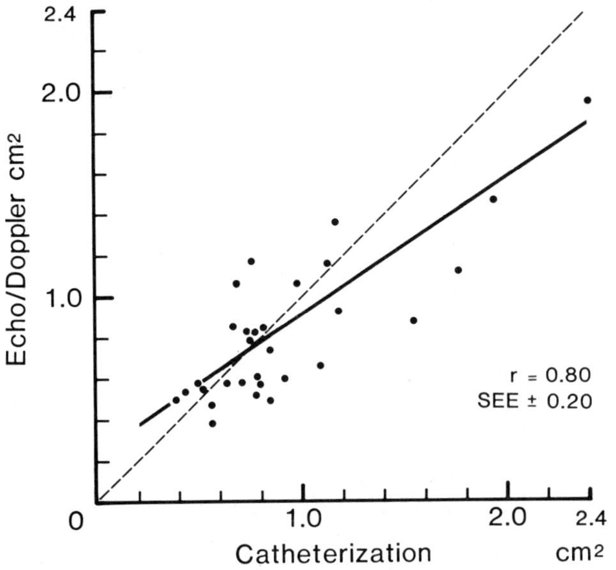

FIGURE 8. Aortic valve area in all patients. Cardiac output (Gorlin's formula) was measured by single-plane angiography. The noninvasive measurements are based on integration of the velocity curves (equation 5) and the "large" subvalvular diameter.

reasonably accurate for estimating the aortic valve area.

Figure 10 shows that valve areas calculated by equation 2 are equal to or larger than those calculated from equation 5. The assumption that equation 2 calculates a maximal area and equation 5 an effective area is thus supported. This difference seems to be less marked when the valve area is small, possibly indicating that those valves are more calcified and less elastic. The difference cannot be explained by the peak velocity in the stenotic jet being less well recorded than the rest of the velocity curve, since both the peak and mean pressure drops calculated from the velocity recordings correlated well with the corresponding invasive measurements (table 3).

Valve areas calculated from equation 2 correlated better with invasive results (figures 7 and 9) than did the valve areas calculated from equation 5 (figures 6 and 8). Especially the larger areas seemed to be underestimated by equation 5. The reason for this is difficult

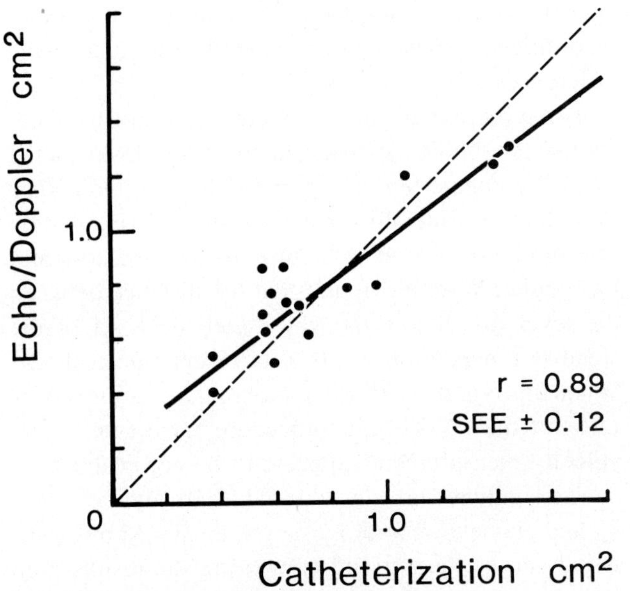

FIGURE 7. Same as in figure 6, except that the noninvasive results are based on peak velocity measurements (equation 2).

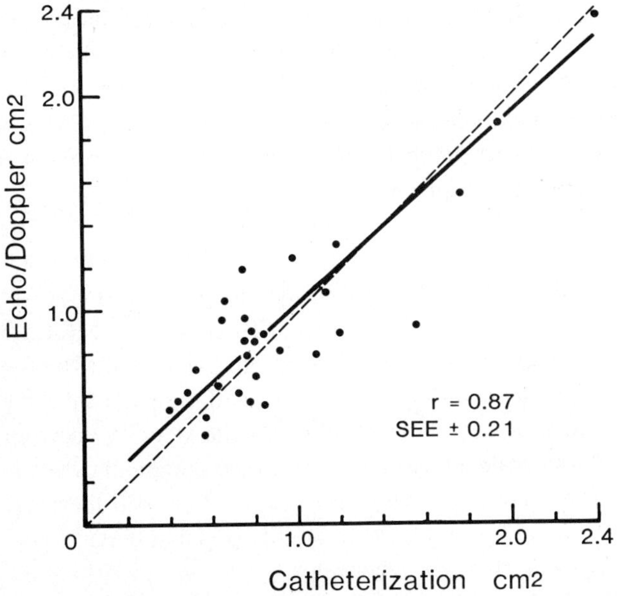

FIGURE 9. Same as in figure 8, except that the noninvasive results are based on peak velocity measurements (equation 2).

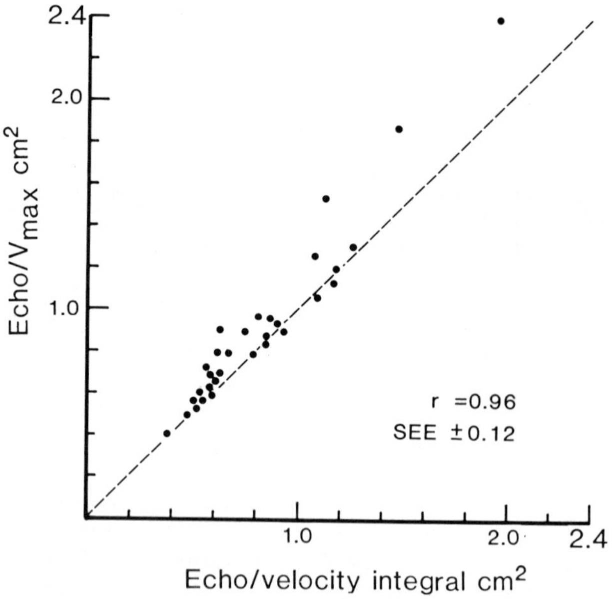

FIGURE 10. Aortic valve area calculated from equation 2 (vertical axis) and equation 5 (horizontal axis). The "large" diameter was used in both equations.

to ascertain because there were few patients with large valve areas in this series and because the measurements were not done simultaneously. However, according to Rodrigo,[11] the discharge coefficient in Gorlin's formula can only be assumed to be constant when the valve area is small compared with the area proximal to the valve. Larger valve areas will be overestimated. One therefore cannot exclude that the larger valve areas in figures 6 and 8 are overestimated by Gorlin's formula rather than underestimated by equation 5. Thus in figures 7 and 9 the overestimation of effective valve area made by equation 2 may seem to be balanced by an overestimation of similar magnitude by assuming the discharge coefficient in Gorlin's formula to be constant, accidentally causing the two methods to correlate well. The tendency for Gorlin's formula to overestimate large valve areas was also shown by Warth et al.[2]

Reliability of velocity and diameter measurements. The reliability of the estimates of the right sides of equations 2 and 5 is best established for V′ and intV′(t). In accordance with the results of Hegrenaes and Hatle,[5a] the peak and mean pressure drops calculated from the velocity recordings correlated well with the invasive results (table 3), indicating that the velocity curve of the stenotic jet was adequately recorded in all patients. The accuracy of valve area estimations will therefore largely depend on the reliability of subvalvular velocity and diameter recordings.

Ihlen et al.[12] and Gussenhoven et al.[13] found the reproducibility of subvalvular diameter measurements to be good in patients with noncalcified aortic valves. In the case of calcific aortic stenosis, the accuracy is probably less good. Cohen et al.[14] measured the subvalvular diameter to predict the prosthetic valve size in adult patients with aortic stenosis. Errors up to 2 mm were made. This is similar to the difference in diameters on repeated measurements that we found in five patients and indicates that an error of about 10% to 20% in the assessment of subvalvular area has to be expected in some patients.

In some patients the diameter was measured in late diastole because the upper LVOT was poorly visualized in systole. In the case of different diameters in systole and diastole, the systolic value should probably be used. However, there is reason to believe that this diameter does not change much during the cardiac cycle.[12]

Assessment of the reliability of the subvalvular velocity recordings is difficult. In some patients stable velocities were recorded over a distance of 1 to 2 cm in the upper LVOT, making the decision on which velocities to use easy. In general, however, the velocities increased gradually until the more rapid increase 0.5 to 1.5 cm proximal to the valve. Even if this rapid increase could occur quite suddenly, there was necessarily a range of velocities from which the correct one was difficult to choose. In figure 3 this range is represented by the velocities recorded at 9.0 and 9.5 cm. These recordings are from a patient in whom the change from gradually to steeply increasing velocities was less marked than usual. The resulting differences in maximal velocity and integral size, about 14%, therefore probably represent the upper limit of the error in calculated valve area, introduced by subvalvular velocity recordings. In seven other patients this range gave differences of 12% or less.

It may be argued that diameter and velocity measurements should be made at the same level in the LVOT (compare figures 2 and 3). Because the LVOT may show considerable axial movement during systole (we have noticed up to 1 cm), this is not possible. Pasipoularides et al.[5] found that the distance between the level just below the valve and the level of the stenosis ranged from 0.26 to 0.95 cm (mean 0.52). When this is added to the distance of the systolic movement of the LVOT, our procedure for diameter and velocity measurements appears to be acceptable.

The combined error produced by subvalvular velocity and diameter recordings can be evaluated by calculating cardiac output and comparing the results with invasive measurements (table 3). The poor correlation obtained is probably partly explained by the fact that the measurements were done simultaneously, partly by the inaccuracy of subvalvular velocity and diameter measurements as discussed above, but also by the inaccuracies of the invasive methods (table 3). Nevertheless, the standard error of the estimate as obtained in the subgroup of patients is not very different from that reported in other studies in which the noninvasive and invasive measurements of cardiac output were made simultaneously.[12, 15–18] In the same group of patients the largest underestimation of cardiac output occurring when the "inner" diameter was used was 49%, compared with 38% when the "large" diameter was used. This may indicate that the "large" diameter is to be preferred for calculations of volume flow and valve area, but again, due to the fact that measurements were not made simultaneously, it is difficult to make any final evaluation of the problem.

The reasons why noninvasive measurements of pressure drops correlated better with the invasive results than did the measurements of cardiac output are probably that both the invasive and noninvasive methods are more accurate in assessing pressure drops than volume flow and that variations in flow will produce comparatively smaller variations in pressure drop because the ejection time also varies. Variations in heart rate will also influence cardiac output and pressure drop differently.

If the errors in diameter and velocity measurements are added, they may be of the same magnitude as the difference between the valve areas estimated from equation 2 and 5. The simplicity of equation 2 probably justifies its use in the clinical routine. If the estimated area is borderline regarding the decision of how to treat the patient, it might be helpful to calculate the area from equation 5 as well.

Our results show that this method can also be used when there is significant aortic regurgitation, which was present in 14 patients. Even though it was not present in this series, significant mitral regurgitation should not invalidate the method. Thus the limitations of other methods[1–4] are eliminated. No empirical constant is used, reducing errors caused by individual variations. The approximation made by Kosturakis et al.[3] by assuming the temporal mean velocity in the stenotic jet to be 0.88 × peak velocity is also avoided. According to our observations, the quotient Vmean/Vpeak can range from 0.69 to 0.87. By assuming a fixed quotient, the method will tend to average the results. On the other hand, the error made may not be important compared with other errors inherent in any method used to estimate valve areas.

The left and right sides of equation 4 describe the stroke volume at two levels that are in series and closely located. Hemodynamic changes should therefore affect both sides of the equation similarly, making the method independent of left ventricular performance.

Fujii et al.[19] have simultaneously and independently of our study used equation 2 to calculate the valve area in aortic stenosis and have derived similar results.

There may be some practical problems in using equations 2 and 5. Especially in patients with emphysema, in whom the subvalvular diameter can be very difficult to measure, the results should be accepted with some reservation. Caution should also be exercised when calcifications are seen to protrude into the LVOT. This was seen in two patients in the present series. We attempted to solve the problem by placing the sample volume just proximal to the calcification. Thereby the increase in velocity, secondary to the decrease in cross-sectional area caused by the calcifications, was avoided. The calculation of the subvalvular area was made as described earlier, disregarding the calcifications. This apparently was successful, since the noninvasive estimates of valve area were quite close to the invasive results (invasive results, based on Fick method, 0.59 and 0.86 cm^2; noninvasive results with the "large" diameter, 0.50 and 0.66 cm^2 [equation 5], 0.56 and 0.79 cm^2 [equation 2]).

If subvalvular obstruction caused by septal hypertrophy is present, the subvalvular velocity profile may be unpredictable and calculated valve area should be looked upon only as a rough estimate. Significant subvalvular obstruction was not seen in any patient in this study. In fact, problems were more frequently encountered when collecting the invasive than the noninvasive data, emphasizing the usefulness of the noninvasive method.

Appendix

If the stenotic area (A′) of a flow channel varies because of the changing pressure drop across the obstruction during pulsatile flow, the equation of continuity can be developed to calculate the temporal mean of A′.

The equation of continuity is valid at any moment during pulsatile flow:

$$A \times k(prof) \times V = A' \times k(prof)' \times V'$$

A and V are the area and maximal velocity proximal to the obstruction, and V′ is the maximal velocity at the obstruction; k(prof) is a constant describing the velocity profile [k(prof) = 1 if the profile is flat, k(prof) = ½ if the profile is parabolic]. If k(prof) = k(prof)′, the equation can be reduced and rearranged to:

$$A'/A = V/V'$$

Both sides are then integrated over one flow period:

$$int(A'/A) = int(V/V')$$

If A is constant:

$$\text{int}(A') = A \times \text{int}(V/V')$$

Temporal mean of A′ = int(A′)/t, where t is the duration of one flow period:

$$\text{mean } A' = A \times \text{int}(V/V')/t$$

References

1. Gorlin R, Gorlin SG: Hydraulic formula for calculation of the area of the stenotic mitral valve, other cardiac valves, and central circulatory shunts. I. Am Heart J **41:** 1, 1951
2. Warth DC, Stewart WJ, Block PC, Weyman AE: A new method to calculate aortic valve area without left heart catheterization. Circulation **70:** 978, 1984
3. Kosturakis D, Allen HD, Goldberg SJ, Sahn DJ, Valdes-Cruz LM: Noninvasive quantification of stenotic semilunar valve areas by Doppler echocardiography. J Am Coll Cardiol **3:** 1256, 1984
4. Seitz WS, Kashani IA: Noninvasive determination of the aortic valve area in stenosis: hydraulic orifice formula for application to echocardiography and correlation with catheterization. Eur Heart J **4:** 31, 1983
5. Pasipoularides A, Murgo JP, Bird JJ, Craig WE: Fluid dynamics of aortic stenosis: mechanisms for the presence of subvalvular pressure gradients. Am J Physiol **246:** H542, 1984

5a. Hegrenaes H, Hatle L: Aortic stenosis in adults: noninvasive estimation of pressure drop with Doppler. Br Heart J (in press)

6. Hatle L, Angelsen B: Doppler ultrasound in cardiology, ed 2. Philadelphia, 1985, Lea & Febiger, p 306
7. Lewis JF, Kuo LC, Nelson JG, Limacher MC, Quinones MA: Pulsed Doppler echocardiographic determination of stroke volume and cardiac output: clinical validation of two new methods using the apical window. Circulation **70:** 425, 1984
8. Croft CH, Lipscomb K, Mathis K, Firth BG, Nicod P, Tilton G, Winniford MD, Hillis LD: Limitations of qualitative angiographic grading in aortic or mitral regurgitation. Am J Cardiol **53:** 1593, 1984
9. Yang SS, Bentivoglio LG, Maranhao V, Goldberg H: From catheterization data to hemodynamic parameters, ed 2. Philadelphia, 1978, F. A. Davies, p 56
10. Wynne J, Green LH, Mann T, Levin D, Grossman W: Estimation of left ventricular volume in man from biplane cineangiograms filmed in oblique projections. Am J Cardiol **41:** 726, 1978
11. Rodrigo FA: Estimation of valve area and "valvular resistance": a critical study of the physical basis of the methods employed. Am Heart J **45:** 1, 1953
12. Ihlen H, Amlie JP, Dale J, Forfang K, Nitter-Hauge S, Otterstad JE, Simonsen S, Myhre E: Determination of cardiac output by Doppler echocardiography. Br Heart J **51:** 54, 1984
13. Gussenhoven WJ, Van Leenen BF, Kuis W, De Villeneuve VH, Bom N, Van Meurs-Van Woezik H: Comparison of internal diameter of great arteries in congenital heart disease. Br Heart J **49:** 45, 1983
14. Cohen JL, Austin SM, Kim CS, Christakos ME, Hussain SM: Two-dimensional echocardiographic preoperative prediction of prosthetic aortic valve size. Am Heart J **107:** 108, 1984
15. Goldberg SJ, Sahn DJ, Allen HD, Valdes-Cruz LM, Hoenecke H, Carnahan Y: Evaluation of pulmonary and systemic blood flow by 2-dimensional Doppler echocardiography using fast Fourier transform spectral analysis. Am J Cardiol **50:** 1394, 1982
16. Sanders SP, Yeager S, Williams RG: Measurements of systemic and pulmonary blood flow and QP/QS ratio using Doppler and two-dimensional echocardiography. Am J Cardiol **51:** 952, 1983
17. Loeppky JA, Hoekenga DE, Greene ER, Luft UC: Comparison of noninvasive pulsed Doppler and Fick measurements of stroke volume in cardiac patients. Am Heart J **107:** 33, 1984
18. Huntsman LL, Stewart DK, Barnes SR, Franklin SB, Colocousis JS, Hessel EA: Noninvasive Doppler determination of cardiac output in man: clinical validation. Circulation **67:** 593, 1983
19. Fujii K, Kitabatake A, Asao M, Tanouchi J, Ishihara K, Morita T, Masuyama T, Ito H, Hori M, Inoue M, Abe H: Noninvasive evaluation of valvular stenosis by a quantitative Doppler technique. J Cardiovasc Ultrasonogr **3:** 201, 1984

Assessment and follow-up of patients with aortic regurgitation by an updated Doppler echocardiographic measurement of the regurgitant fraction in the aortic arch

THIERRY TOUCHE, M.D., RICHARD PRASQUIER, M.D., ALAIN NITENBERG, M.D., DOMINIQUE DE ZUTTERE, M.D., AND RENÉ GOURGON, M.D.

ABSTRACT The purpose of this study was to determine the value and limitations of an updated Doppler echocardiographic measurement of the aortic regurgitant fraction derived from the comparison of forward and reverse flows in the aortic arch. The method was based on the improvements in sampling and displaying Doppler frequencies and blood velocities provided by pulsed-emission, two-dimensional location, and spectral analysis and on an account for variations of aortic diameter through an M mode record of the aortic arch. Relevant statistical comparisons were performed between simultaneous noninvasive and invasive determinations of the regurgitant fraction in a group of 30 patients with aortic regurgitation (group I) and between simultaneous noninvasive and invasive measurements of variations of the regurgitant fraction induced by atrial pacing or vasodilator administration in 12 patients of this group. The two basal determinations were closely correlated (r = .90). The invasive regurgitant fraction ranged from 0% to 80%. The standard error of the Doppler estimate was 8.8% in group I as a whole and was only 6% in a subgroup of 20 patients with a high systolic aortic flow pattern, defined as both peak velocity above 0.8 m/sec and duration of systolic flow above 0.24 sec. This pattern was present in almost all (19/22) patients in whom the aortic regurgitation was more than moderate by invasive criterion (regurgitant fraction above 40%). The standard error of the Doppler estimate of variations of the regurgitant fraction was only 6.6%. Among 100 additional patients with aortic regurgitation (group II), only 12 had no pandiastolic reverse flow in the arch, and their regurgitation was always mild at aortographic examination. Among 100 patients without aortic regurgitation (group III) four had a pandiastolic reverse flow in the arch and each had a left-to-right shunt issued from the aorta at the invasive study. The false-negative and false-positive diagnoses of aortic regurgitation on aortic arch records were all corrected by the Doppler sampling beneath the aortic valve. Provided that left ventricular sampling confirms the regurgitation and that aortic sampling displays the high systolic flow pattern, the Doppler measurement of the regurgitant fraction in the aortic arch is remarkably suited to the assessment and follow-up of patients with aortic regurgitation.
Circulation 72, No. 4, 819–824, 1985.

ECHOCARDIOGRAPHIC measurements of left ventricular dimensions contribute to the assessment and follow-up of patients with aortic regurgitation,[1, 2] although their prognostic value is still controversial.[3] Noninvasive quantitation of the magnitude of the regurgitation would improve the assessment of these patients and could provide important additional data regarding the prognosis. Boughner[4] in 1975 measured the aortic regurgitant fraction in the aortic arch by means of a continuous-wave Doppler instrument, but the measurement was difficult and even impossible in some patients because of interference with venous flows present along the ultrasonic beam. Since the introduction of pulsed-wave Doppler, which provides range resolution along the beam and can be performed under two-dimensional location, numerous indexes have been proposed based either on flow comparisons in the aorta[5–7] or on mappings of the regurgitant jet in the left ventricle.[8–10] However, these new indexes were

From Services d'Explorations Fonctionnelles et de Cardiologie, Hôpital Bichat, and Unité de Recherche INSERM 251, Faculté Xavier Bichat, Paris, France.
Supported in part by grants from CNAMTS and Fédération de Cardiologie.
Address for correspondence: Thierry Touche, M.D., Service d'Explorations Fonctionnelles, Hôpital Bichat, 46 rue Henri Huchard, 75018 Paris, France.
Received July 20, 1984; revision accepted June 13, 1985.
Presented in part at the 56th Scientific Sessions of the American Heart Association, November 1983, Anaheim, CA.

compared with three- or four-point aortographic gradings, which have their own serious limitations.[11, 12] Furthermore, this semiquantitative reference did not permit comprehensive statistical assessment (including SEE) of the quantitative Doppler indexes. The aim of our study was threefold: (1) to assess an improved Doppler method of measurement of the aortic regurgitant fraction in the aortic arch, (2) to test the value of the method for the measurement of variations of the regurgitant fraction, and (3) to assess the sensitivity and specificity of Doppler aortic arch records obtained in large additional groups of patients with or without aortic regurgitation.

Methods

Patients. Group I included 30 patients with aortic regurgitation who underwent a simultaneous invasive and noninvasive measurement of the aortic regurgitant fraction. Twelve patients were then restudied under atrial pacing or while on vasodilators. Patients with left ventricular asynergy, tricuspid regurgitation, arrhythmias, mitral regurgitation, or ventricular septal defect were excluded because these abnormalities would have hampered the invasive determinations of left ventricular volumes, cardiac output, and/or aortic regurgitant fraction. The ages, etiologies and associated lesions are listed in table 1.

Group II included 100 patients with aortic regurgitation confirmed by aortography and/or surgery, and group III included 100 patients with valvular, congenital, or ischemic heart disease diagnosed by left and right heart catheterization and unassociated with aortic regurgitation. These additional groups were studied to review the timing, magnitude, sensitivity, and specificity of the diastolic flow values that can be recorded by pulsed Doppler in the aortic arch.

Invasive determination of the regurgitant fraction. Cardiac output was averaged from three thermodilution determinations with the Swan-Ganz catheter. Effective stroke volume was calculated as cardiac output divided by heart rate. Total stroke volume was the difference between end-diastolic and end-systolic volumes determined from a 30 degree right anterior oblique cineangiogram with the area-length method and a correction formula.[13] Angiography was performed immediately after the thermodilution cardiac output measurement. The regurgitant

TABLE 1
Patients and individual results (group I)

Patient No.	Sex/Age (yr)	Etiology	Associated lesions	Invasive RF (%)	TVI ratio (%)	HSF	CSA ratio (%)	Doppler RF (%)
1	M/58	AA	—	21	38	−	100	38
2	M/29	UE	—	66	80	+	81	65
3	M/55	AA	—	45	40	+	98	39
4	M/28	RHD	—	50	49	+	87	43
5	F/40	RHD	MS	15	38	−	79	30
6	M/22	RHD	—	50	77	−	83	64
7	F/31	RHD	MS	TF	35	+	90	31
8	M/20	VP	—	40	26	+	87	23
9	M/23	VP	—	53	51	+	100	51
10	M/19	AP+BE	—	80	87	+	85	74
11	M/61	UE	—	65	58	+	97	56
12	M/41	UE	—	64	62	+	100	62
13	M/56	AA	—	68	65	+	100	65
14	F/40	RHD	MS	0	0	−	100	0
15	M/16	RHD	—	56	70	+	84	59
16	F/31	RHD	MS	64	97	+	75	73
17	M/75	AA	—	63	71	+	94	67
18	M/29	BE	—	76	78	+	91	71
19	M/21	RHD	—	53	64	+	82	52
20	M/61	UE	—	41	56	−	89	50
21	M/60	BE	—	79	79	+	88	70
22	M/42	RHD	—	47	47	+	85	40
23	F/58	UE	—	59	49	−	100	49
24	F/61	UE	AS	19	0	−	100	0
25	M/63	UE	AS	16	TF	TF	TF	TF
26	M/26	RHD	—	42	45	+	88	40
27	M/25	RHD	—	69	85	+	78	66
28	M/52	AA	—	77	87	+	90	78
29	M/32	RHD	MS	33	35	−	93	33
30	F/59	AP	—	59	48	+	97	47

RF = regurgitant fraction; HSF = high systolic flow; CSA = cross-sectional area; AA = aortic aneurysm; UE = undetermined etiology; RHD = rheumatic heart disease; VP = aortic valvuloplasty; AP = aortic prosthesis; BE = bacterial endocarditis; MS = mitral stenosis; AS = severe aortic stenosis; TF = technical failure.

fraction was calculated as: (total stroke volume − effective stroke volume)/total stroke volume. In a concomitant series of 35 consecutive patients without valvular regurgitation or left ventricular segmental wall abnormalities, the technique provided stroke volume values very close to those obtained by the thermodilution measurement (thermodilution stroke volumes: 32 to 118 ml, r = .93, angiographic stroke volume = 0.91 × thermodilution stroke volume + 8.8 ml, SEE = 6.3 ml).

Ultrasound examination. The aortic arch was examined from the suprasternal notch with a 3 MHz probe for mechanical two-dimensional imaging, M mode, and pulsed Doppler with spectral analysis. Two-dimensional imaging of the bend between horizontal and descending segments of the arch (aortic isthmus, figure 1, *A*) allowed selection of a sampling depth at which the Doppler beam paralleled the axis of the vessel (zero intercept angle). At this sampling site Doppler frequencies were maximal for both forward and reverse flows and the corresponding blood velocities could be calculated by a constant conversion factor (figure 1). Whenever necessary to optimize the Doppler signal-to-noise ratio, the operator switched to a small nonimaging 3 MHz Doppler transducer, a short additional time being necessary to locate the aortic flow at the predetermined depth. Doppler filters were adjusted to minimal values (100 or 200 Hz) and gains were reduced to obtain a contrasted but uninterrupted display of the modal Doppler frequencies (darkest shades of the gray scale display of the Doppler spectrum) (figure 1, *B*).

In group I the Doppler record was obtained simultaneously with the cardiac output measurement. An M mode record of the aortic arch diameter was performed under two-dimensional guidance of the long-axis view of the horizontal segment of the arch so that arterial branchings were avoided (figure 2, *A*). The operators analyzing the Doppler and M mode records were unaware of angiographic results and invasive data processing.

Ultrasound data analysis

Group I. The envelopes of the modal Doppler frequencies were traced. In seven patients increased systolic velocities were associated with frequency aliasing (figure 1, *B*) at the selected sampling depths (7 to 9 cm), and this was corrected before the tracing by a translation of the aliased portion of the curve (figure 1, *C*). Systolic and diastolic envelopes were planimetered (figure 1, *D*). The ratio of diastolic to systolic areas was calculated to give the time-velocity integral (TVI) ratio (%). In two patients of group I the aortic regurgitation was not associated to the typical pandiastolic reverse flow, and only low amplitude diastolic flows were observed, with a reverse component limited to early diastole. In these cases the TVI ratio was considered to be 0%. In the rest of group I the TVI ratios were averaged on five consecutive, technically adequate cycles; the mean and maximal differences between the TVI ratios determined by two independent operators were 4% and 8%. Peak systolic velocity and duration of systolic flow were measured. Whenever their respective values were both over 0.8 m/sec and 0.24 sec, respectively, the patients were included in a high systolic flow subgroup.

The regurgitant fraction was the ratio of diastolic to systolic flow in the arch. Each flow was the product of the corresponding TVI times a corresponding aortic cross-sectional area. Therefore the regurgitant fraction was the ratio of diastolic to systolic TVI times the ratio of diastolic to systolic cross-sectional area. Each aortic cross-sectional area was equal to the square of an aortic diameter times $\pi/4$. Therefore the diastolic to systolic area ratio was equal to the square of a diastolic to systolic diameter ratio (figure 2, *B*). Whenever significant, the aortic diameter variations (figure 2, *A*) included a rapid early systolic increase, a midsystolic plateau at a maximal diameter value, a dicrotic notch, and a progressive decrease to an end-diastolic minimal value. In calculations of the diameter ratio, the systolic value was the maximal diameter and the diastolic value was the average of maximal and minimal diameters (figure 2, *C*). In group I as a whole these systolic and diastolic values were compared with the true mean systolic and mean diastolic diameters, calculated by dividing the planimetered M mode aortic systolic and diastolic areas by the duration of systole and diastole, respectively (figure 2, *D*). The simplified values slightly overestimated the mean systolic diameter (averaged difference

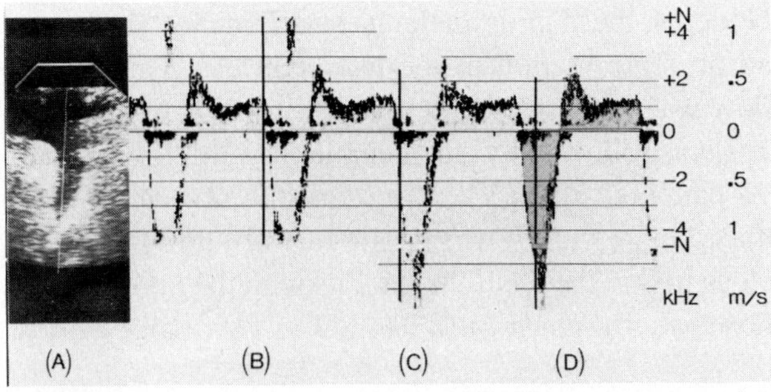

FIGURE 1. Pulsed Doppler record of the aortic arch in aortic regurgitation. *A*, Two-dimensional selection of a sampling site providing a zero intercept angle with aortic flows. This is obtained within the bend between the horizontal and descending segments of the arch. *B*, Spectral display of Doppler frequencies; the signal of the systolic flow (directed away from the transducer) is displayed with negative values, the signal of the diastolic flow (directed toward the transducer) with positive values. *C*, Correction of frequency aliasing by a translation of the aliased portion of the curve. *D*, Tracing and planimetry of the envelopes of the modal Doppler frequencies in systole and diastole. The conversion factor from Doppler frequencies (kHz) to blood velocities (m/sec) is 0.246. +N and −N are the Nyquist limits (maximal measurable frequencies at the selected maximal sampling depth).

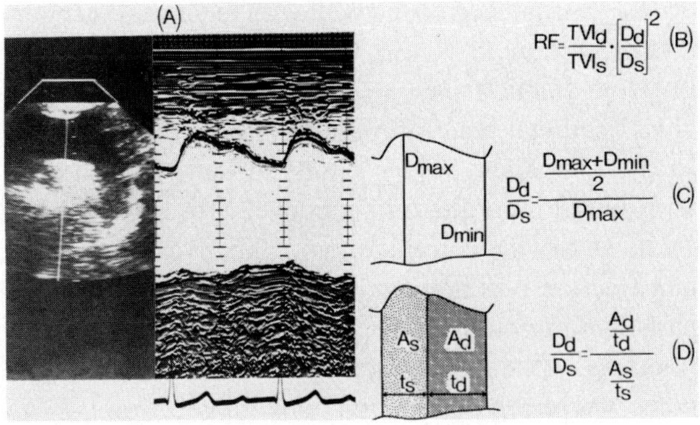

FIGURE 2. Account for variations of aortic diameter in the calculation of the aortic regurgitant fraction. *A*, M mode record of the aortic arch under two-dimensional location. *B*, The regurgitant fraction (RF) is equal to a diastolic (d) to systolic (s) time-velocity integral (TVI) ratio, times a squared diastolic to systolic diameter (D) ratio. *C*, Simplified determination of the diameter ratio: the systolic diameter is the maximal diameter (D_{max}) and the diastolic diameter is the mean of maximal and minimal (D_{min}) diameters. *D*, Determination of the ratio of the true mean diastolic diameter to the true mean systolic diameter. Mean diameters were obtained by dividing planimetered M mode aortic systolic and diastolic areas (A) by the duration (t) of systole and diastole, respectively. The subsequent diameter ratio was not significantly different from the diameter ratio obtained by the simplified determination (see in text).

0.8 mm, paired t = 5.4, $p < .01$) and the mean diastolic diameter (averaged difference 0.6 mm, paired t = 4.5, $p < .01$), but the difference in diameter ratios was insignificant (paired t = 1.4).

Groups II and III. In group II (patients with aortic regurgitation) we studied the frequency of absence of a pandiastolic reverse flow in the arch. In the corresponding subgroup of patients we reviewed the results of the aortographic grading and of the Doppler diagnosis of the aortic regurgitation by left ventricular sampling. In group III (patients without aortic regurgitation) we studied the frequency of presence of a pandiastolic reverse flow in the arch. In the corresponding subgroup we reviewed the diagnosis provided by the invasive study and the results of the Doppler search of an aortic regurgitant jet in the left ventricle. In the remaining group III patients some reverse flow was found in the arch in the early diastole, frequently followed by a middiastolic forward flow. In these patients the relative magnitude of the net diastolic flow was evaluated on a representative cycle by calculating a TVI ratio, equal to: (diastolic reverse flow − diastolic forward flow)/systolic forward flow. As in group I, a subgroup of patients with the high systolic flow pattern was constituted.

Results

The individual results in group I at the basal state are presented in table 1. Two patients were discarded from the statistical comparison, one because of ventricular premature beats during angiography and the other because of lack of adequate Doppler signal in the aortic arch. The invasive regurgitant fraction ranged from 0% to 80%. The patient with an invasive regurgitant fraction equal to zero had a total stroke volume that did not exceed the effective stroke volume, with minimal regurgitation on aortography. TVI ratios ranged from 0% to 97% and correlated well with the invasive regurgitant fraction: r = .86, TVI ratio (%) = 1.05 × invasive fraction (%) + 2%, SEE = 12.4%. The cross-sectional area ratio ranged from 75% to 100%, with the smallest values observed in young patients with severe regurgitation (patients 2, 16, and 27, table 1); however, the correlation with the invasive regurgitant fraction was not significant (r = .22). The comparison between invasive and noninvasive regurgitant fractions at the basal state is shown in figure 3, *left*: noninvasive regurgitant fractions ranged from 0% to 78%, with r = .90, noninvasive fraction (%) = 0.92 invasive fraction (%) + 3%, and SEE = 8.8%. The high systolic flow pattern was present in 20/28 (71%) patients. In this subgroup the agreement between the two determinations was excellent: r = .92, SEE = 6%. The high systolic flow pattern was found in 19 of the 22 patients with invasive regurgitant fractions above 40%.

The comparison between the induced variations of the regurgitant fraction is presented in figure 3, *right*. Variations of the invasive regurgitant fraction (second value − basal value) ranged from −24% to +11%, with increases in only two patients (in one electrocardiographic signs of myocardial ischemia appeared during atrial pacing and in the other vasodilator dose and delay after the first angiographic study may have been insufficient). The variations of the noninvasive fraction always occurred in the same direction (r = .82, and SEE = 6.6%).

In group II the aortic regurgitation was associated with a pandiastolic reverse flow in the arch in 88 of 100 patients and with a reverse flow limited to early diastole in 12 of 100 patients. The review of the 12 corresponding case reports indicated that the regurgitation had been diagnosed by Doppler examination of the left ventricular outflow tract in each case and that it had always been graded 1/4 on aortographic examination.

In group III a pandiastolic reverse flow was recorded in the absence of aortic regurgitation in four of 100 patients: one rupture of the sinus of Valsalva in the right atrium, one abnormal coronary artery with aortopulmonary shunt, and two patent ductus arteriosus. None of these four patients had Doppler signals of aortic regurgitation in the left ventricle. The reverse flow was limited to early diastole in 96 of 100 patients and was followed by a detectable forward flow in 50 of 96 patients. The TVI ratio (diastolic reverse flow − diastolic forward flow/systolic forward flow) was very close to 0 in the 43 of 96 patients with the high systolic flow pattern (mean = 0.5%, SD = 8%, range −16%

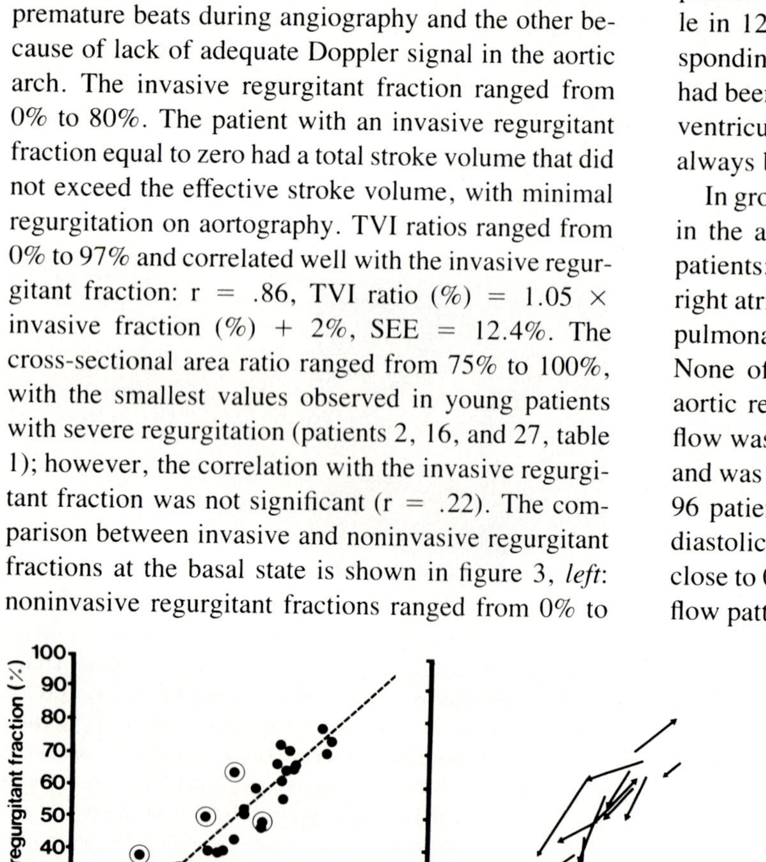

FIGURE 3. Comparison between invasive and noninvasive measurements of the aortic regurgitant fraction. *Left*, Basal results in patients fulfilling (●) and not fulfilling (⊙) the high systolic flow pattern. *Right*, Induced variations of the regurgitant fraction. See statistical results in the text.

to +15%). On the contrary, among the 53 of 96 patients without this pattern, positive or negative net diastolic flows of high relative magnitude were frequently encountered (mean TVI ratio = 8%, SD = 19%, range −27% to +48%).

Discussion

A number of Doppler methods have been proposed for the assessment of aortic regurgitation.[4–10, 14–16] As for other types of valvular regurgitation, the Doppler methods can be divided in two groups: (1) mappings of the regurgitant jet, by pulsed Doppler under two-dimensional location[8–10] or recently by two-dimensional color-coded pulsed Doppler, measuring the length of the jet,[8, 14] its areas on long- and short-axis views of the left ventricle[10] or on a short-axis view just beneath the aortic orifice[9]; (2) flow comparisons between increased forward flow through the aortic valve and normal or low forward flow through another cardiac sampling site[15] or more frequently between forward and reverse flows at the same site, either the ascending aorta[5, 6, 16] or the aortic arch.[4, 5, 7] In the search of an optimal Doppler approach to the assessment of aortic regurgitation, the discussion will focus on the specific advantages of our proposed method.

Technical features. The choice of the aortic arch for the Doppler measurement of the aortic regurgitant fraction has already been reported by Boughner.[4] In our study, pulsed emission provided range resolution along the beam, allowing discrimination between the low diastolic aortic velocities associated with the aortic regurgitation and the low diastolic velocities present in carotid arteries and innominate[4] or jugular veins. Two-dimensional location permitted us to select a standardized sampling site (the aortic isthmus) where the Doppler beam paralleled the aortic flow. Unlike other techniques of Doppler signal processing, spectral analysis allowed identification and correction of frequency aliasing, inadequate filtering, and excessive noise in the instrument. The account for variations of aortic diameter and section, by multiplying the TVI ratio by a cross-sectional area ratio, improved the correlation coefficient, standard error of the estimate, and slope. This correction was essential in young patients with severe regurgitation. Conversely, it could have been neglected when the area ratio was above 90% (15 patients, 13 with regurgitant fractions below 40% and/or ages over 50, table 1). Area ratios above 90% can be predicted when the ratio of minimal to maximal aortic diameter exceeds 90%.

The aortic isthmus had several potential technical advantages over other sampling sites. The ascending aorta[5, 6, 16] has large movements during the heart cycle and a nonuniform distribution of blood velocities.[15] In this study, aortic arch records displayed narrow spectra in both systole and diastole and were not clearly modified during attempts to vary the sampling position within the selected aortic section. This suggested a laminar flow and a reasonably flat velocity profile at that site, which was also supported by experimental data.[17] Sampling the regurgitant flow in the left ventricle permits various evaluations of the dimensions of the regurgitant jet, which have been correlated to angiographic gradings.[8–10] This approach is aided by two-dimensional color-coded pulsed Doppler.[13] However, the estimated size of the flow disturbance varies with the sensitivity of the instrument in a given patient and does not account for the duration of regurgitation and for its changes within diastole. Flow comparisons with two different sampling sites[14] instead of one may be affected more markedly by the potential errors in the determinations of dimensions and incident angles.

Sources of error. Diastolic flows were constantly observed in the aortic isthmus, even in patients without aortic regurgitation (group III). In this group of patients the typical pattern was an early diastolic reverse flow followed by a middiastolic forward flow, as on the record of a normal subject compared to six records of the study in figure 4. The relative magnitude of the net diastolic flow was negligible in a subgroup of these patients fulfilling a high systolic flow pattern. In patients with aortic regurgitation (group I) and with the same high systolic flow criteria, an excellent agreement between invasive and noninvasive measurements of the aortic regurgitant fraction was observed. This subgroup included almost all patients with more than moderate aortic regurgitation. Conversely, when the high systolic flow pattern was not observed, the relative magnitude of diastolic flows in the absence of aortic regurgitation (group III) could be considerable in particular patients. Therefore calculation of the regurgitant fraction should not be performed in patients

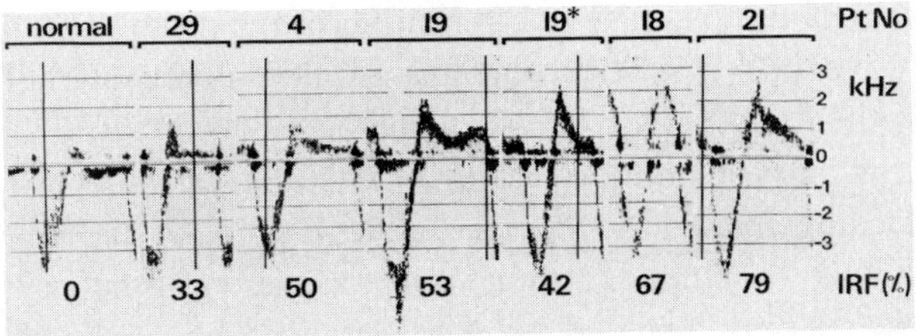

FIGURE 4. Pulsed Doppler records of the aortic arch in a normal subject and in five patients with aortic regurgitation. The five patients belong to group I (see table 1 for additional data). Example of duplication of the record under atrial pacing (patient 19*). IRF = invasive regurgitant fraction.

with aortic regurgitation and no high systolic flow. In these patients other criteria should be used to assess the regurgitation. For instance, lack of any end-diastolic reverse flow was observed in our group II patients only in association with mild regurgitation (angiographic grade 1/4). In another study using aortic arch sampling,[7] an end-diastolic plateau of low amplitude with respect to the peak systolic amplitude corresponded to mild or moderate regurgitation. A regurgitant jet localized in the most distal left ventricular outflow tract also suggests a mild regurgitation.[8] In our series left ventricular sampling was also useful to correct the false diagnosis of aortic regurgitation suggested by aortic arch records in the presence of shunts issued from the aorta.

Validation of the method. The comparison of simultaneous invasive and noninvasive assessments obviated the variability of the regurgitation with physiologic conditions.[18] The two determinations of the same quantitative physiologic index provided optimal data for a relevant statistical comparison. Semiquantitative and subjective aortographic gradings have been used as standards to validate new quantitative indexes for assessing aortic regurgitation.[5–7, 9, 10] These comparisons are hampered by the limited quantitative information provided by three-point gradings, or by the important overlaps between four or five grades.[11, 12] We recognize that the invasive measurement of the aortic regurgitant fraction has its limitations, although a reasonable agreement was obtained between thermodilution and angiographic stroke volumes in our abovementioned series of 35 patients without regurgitation. Notwithstanding the difficulties in the search of a "gold standard," the excellent agreement with the best available clinical measurement of the regurgitant fraction fully justifies the clinical use of the Doppler method.

Utility of the method. The Doppler measurement of the regurgitant fraction may be used to obviate particular limitations of the invasive measurement, such as associated mitral regurgitation or beat-to-beat changes present during arrhythmias. Furthermore, it should improve the routine assessment and follow-up of patients with aortic regurgitation, which remains a difficult clinical problem despite the contribution of the echocardiographic assessment of left ventricular dimensions.[1–3] The major reason why the severity of the leak has not been included in the follow-up of these patients thus far was that no accurate and repeatable noninvasive measurement was available. Such a measurement is provided by the aortic regurgitant fraction calculated in the aortic arch by the present Doppler techniques.

We thank N. Laffay, M.D., and S. Zouiouèche, M.D., who performed a part of the invasive studies, and B. Diebold, M.D., who discussed the manuscript.

References

1. Henry WL, Bonow RO, Borer JS, Ware JH, Kent KM, Redwood DR, McIntosh CL, Morrow AG, Epstein SE: Observations on the optimum time for operative intervention for aortic regurgitation. I. Evaluation of the results of aortic valve replacement in symptomatic patients. Circulation **61:** 471, 1980
2. Henry WL, Bonow RO, Rosing DR, Epstein SE: Observations on the optimum time for operative intervention for aortic regurgitation. II. Serial echocardiographic evaluation of asymptomatic patients. Circulation **61:** 484, 1980
3. Fioretti P, Roelandt J, Bos RJ, Meltzer RS, van Hoogenhuijze D, Serruys PW, Nauta J, Hugenholtz PG: Echocardiography in chronic aortic insufficiency. Is valve replacement too late when left ventricular end-systolic dimension reaches 55 mm? Circulation **67:** 216, 1983
4. Boughner DR: Assessment of aortic insufficiency by transcutaneous Doppler ultrasound. Circulation **52:** 874, 1975
5. Veyrat C, Cholot N, Abitbol G, Kalmanson D: Non-invasive diagnosis and assessment of aortic valve disease and evaluation of aortic prosthesis function using echo pulsed Doppler velocimetry. Br Heart J **43:** 393, 1980
6. Quinones MA, Young JB, Waggoner AD, Ostojic MC, Ribeiro LGT, Miller RR: Assessment of pulsed Doppler echocardiography in detection and quantification of aortic and mitral regurgitation. Br Heart J **44:** 612, 1980
7. Diebold B, Peronneau P, Blanchard D, Colonna G, Guermonprez JL, Forman J, Sellier P, Maurice P: Non-invasive quantification of aortic regurgitation by Doppler echocardiography. Br Heart J **49:** 167, 1983
8. Ciobanu M, Abbasi A, Allen M, Hermer A, Spellberg R: Pulsed Doppler echocardiography in the diagnosis and estimation of severity of aortic insufficiency. Am J Cardiol **49:** 330, 1982
9. Veyrat C, Lessana A, Abitbol G, Ameur A, Benaim R, Kalmanson D: New indexes for assessing aortic regurgitation with two-dimensional echocardiographic measurement of the regurgitant aortic valvular area. Circulation **68:** 998, 1983
10. Veyrat C, Ameur A, Gourtchiglouian C, Lessana A, Abitbol G, Kalmanson D: Calculation of pulsed Doppler left ventricular outflow tract regurgitant index for grading the severity of aortic regurgitation. Am Heart J **108:** 507, 1984
11. Hunt D, Baxley WA, Kennedy JW, Judge TP, Williams JE, Dodge HT: Quantitative evaluation of cineaortography in the assessment of aortic regurgitation. Am J Cardiol **31:** 696, 1973
12. Croft CH, Lipscomb K, Mathis K, Firth BG, Nicod P, Tilton G, Winniford MD, Hillis LD: Limitations of qualitative angiographic grading in aortic or mitral regurgitation. Am J Cardiol **53:** 1593, 1984
13. Dodge HT, Sandler H, Baxley WA, Hawley RR: Usefulness and limitations of radiographic methods for determining left ventricular volume. Am J Cardiol **18:** 10, 1966
14. Sahn DJ, Valdes-Cruz L, Scagnelli S, Tomizuka F, Elias W, Covell J: Two dimensional Doppler color flow mapping for spatial localization and quantitation of aortic insufficiency: validation of a new diagnostic modality using an open chest animal model. Circulation **70**(suppl II): II-38, 1984 (abst)
15. Kitabatake A, Ito K, Asao M, Tanouchi J, Ishibara K, Morita T, Fujii K, Tada M, Inoue M, Abe H, Yoshima H: A new approach to estimate aortic regurgitant fraction by duplex Doppler echocardiography. Circulation **70**(suppl II): II-398, 1984 (abst)
16. Jenni R, Vieli A, Anliker M, Krayenbuehl HP: Quantitation of aortic regurgitation using 16-gate Doppler 2-D echo. Circulation **70** (suppl II): II-246, 1984 (abst)
17. Schultz DL: Pressure and flow in large arteries. *In* Bergel DH, editor: Cardiovascular fluid dynamics. London, 1972, Academic Press, Inc., p 287
18. Brawley RK, Morrow AG: Direct determinations of aortic blood flow in patients with aortic regurgitation: effects of alterations in heart rate, increased ventricular preload or afterload, and isoproterenol. Circulation **35:** 32, 1967

Fetal atrioventricular valve insufficiency associated with nonimmune hydrops: a two-dimensional echocardiographic and pulsed Doppler ultrasound study

NORMAN H. SILVERMAN, M.D., CHARLES S. KLEINMAN, M.D., ABRAHAM M. RUDOLPH, M.D., JOSHUA A. COPEL, M.D., ELLEN M. WEINSTEIN, M.D., MARLENE A. ENDERLEIN, B.S., AND MITCHELL GOLBUS, M.D.

ABSTRACT Of 466 fetuses who underwent cardiac ultrasound examination with cross-sectional and M mode echocardiography and pulsed Doppler ultrasound and in whom we were able to follow the natural history, 12 were found to have atrioventricular valve insufficiency and nonimmune hydrops. Eleven fetuses (all of whom had structural heart disease) died either in utero or during the early postnatal period. In the one surviving hydropic fetus with supraventricular tachyarrhythmia and atrioventricular valve regurgitation but without structural heart disease, all the abnormalities disappeared on treatment with digoxin and verapamil. Seven fetuses who had atrioventricular valve insufficiency but did not develop nonimmune hydrops all survived pregnancy and the early neonatal period. The syndrome of atrioventricular valve insufficiency, nonimmune hydrops, and structural heart disease has a poor prognosis. The hydrops in this instance reflects fetal cardiac failure related to venous hypertension and low colloid oncotic pressure.
Circulation 72, No. 4, 825–832, 1985.

ADVANCES in ultrasound technology have made it possible to examine human fetal cardiac development and function in utero[1-13] and have even permitted the study of early embryogenesis in experimental animals.[14] Structural and functional heart disease in utero has been examined by a number of investigators applying M mode and cross-sectional echocardiographic imaging techniques to the examination of the human fetus during the second and third trimesters of pregnancy.[1-13] This information has been used to counsel prospective parents and, in several instances, to formulate management for the remainder of pregnancy, during delivery, and in the neonatal period.[15-23]

Recently several workers have applied range-gated pulsed Doppler ultrasound to quantitate fetal descending aortic and/or umbilical blood flow by measuring mean flow velocity and cross-sectional vessel area.[11, 12, 24-28] This method has also been used to provide qualitative information about intracardiac blood flow.[11, 12, 24, 25, 28]

We used the combination of cross-sectional echocardiography and pulsed Doppler ultrasound to evaluate 466 fetuses referred to our centers for evaluation of the presence of congenital heart disease. We detected atrioventricular valve insufficiency in 23 of these 466 fetuses in the second and third trimesters of pregnancy. Of these fetuses, 16 had associated nonimmune hydrops. Four of the pregnancies were terminated. Eleven of the 12 fetuses with structural heart disease either died in utero or within the first week after birth. Seven fetuses with atrioventricular valve insufficiency and structural heart disease but without nonimmune hydrops survived pregnancy and the neonatal period.

Methods

Four hundred sixty-six fetuses, ranging from 16 to 40 weeks gestational age, whose mothers had been referred to the fetal echocardiographic laboratories of the University of California San Francisco Medical Center or the Yale University School of Medicine underwent cross-sectional and M mode echocardiographic studies as described in previous reports, with either

From the Departments of Pediatrics and Obstetrics, Gynecology, and Reproductive Sciences, and the Cardiovascular Research Institute, University of California, San Francisco, and the Departments of Pediatrics, Genetics, and Obstetrics and Gynecology, Yale University School of Medicine, New Haven, CT.

Supported in part by a grant from the March of Dimes Birth Defects Foundation.

Address for correspondence: Norman H. Silverman, M.D., M342A, University of California, San Francisco, San Francisco, CA 94143.

Received Dec. 11, 1984; revision accepted June 27, 1985.

Presented in part at the Society of Pediatric Research Meeting, May 1984, San Francisco.

Advanced Technologies Laboratories MK-500 or MK-600 ultrasonographs.[4, 7, 9, 10, 15, 29]

The two-dimensional equipment was interfaced with 3.5 or 5 MHz transducers. Range-gated pulsed Doppler examination was guided from the cross-sectional image where the Doppler carrier frequency was 3.0 or 5 MHz. The sample volume was always kept to minimum size, 1.5 mm in axial direction, and could be placed at any position within the 90 degree sector arc up to a depth of 16 cm. The direction of flow was depicted on the videomonitor as a "positive" deflection when flow was toward the transducer, whereas flow away from the transducer face was depicted as a "negative" deflection with respect to the baseline. The Doppler frequency shift was analyzed by fast Fourier transform algorithm with the intensities of the spectral frequencies depicted in shades of gray. Doppler interrogation was usually performed at 5 to 14 cm distance from the transducer. Atrioventricular valve insufficiency was recognized by the audio output and from the characteristics of the spectral output with reference to the systolic portion of the visible atrioventricular valve motion on the simultaneous M mode display. In the normal heart this period was quiet in systole but showed either disturbed flow consistent with the direction of tricuspid insufficiency or marked systolic aliasing (figure 1). The type of signal displayed depended to some extent on the distance from the transducer. We attempted to obtain flow signals by placing the sample volume as parallel as possible to the direction of blood flow.

In all 466 fetuses we examined, atria, ventricles, and great arteries and veins were defined in each study. Characteristic flow signals were defined in each location.[26] Doppler, M mode signals, and cross-sectional images were recorded on videotape. The Doppler signals were also recorded on paper at speeds of 75 mm/sec for a permanent record with a Tektronix page printer.

Tricuspid or atrioventricular valve insufficiency was assessed as mild, moderate, or marked based on multiple serial positioning of the sample volume in the atria to define how localized the regurgitant jet was and how far from the valve this jet could be recorded.

Results

Among the 466 fetuses we studied, using a combined two-dimensional echocardiographic/Doppler approach, we found 16 fetuses with a combination of atrioventricular valve insufficiency and nonimmune hydrops. Four pregnancies were terminated and therefore excluded from this report. This report is concerned with the 12 remaining fetuses and their natural history. The relevant history, findings, and outcome are summarized in table 1. In addition there were seven fetuses with atrioventricular valve insufficiency without associated hydrops whose data are displayed in table 2. Although the pathologic spectrum is similar to that in table 1, there was no associated nonimmune hydrops and most of the infants survived the first week of life. There were an additional 26 fetuses with nonimmune hydrops in whom there was no atrioventricular valve insufficiency. Results from many of these fetuses have been reported previously.[10,30]

Of the 12 instances of atrioventricular valve insufficiency associated with nonimmune hydrops, 11 with structural heart disease died either in utero or shortly

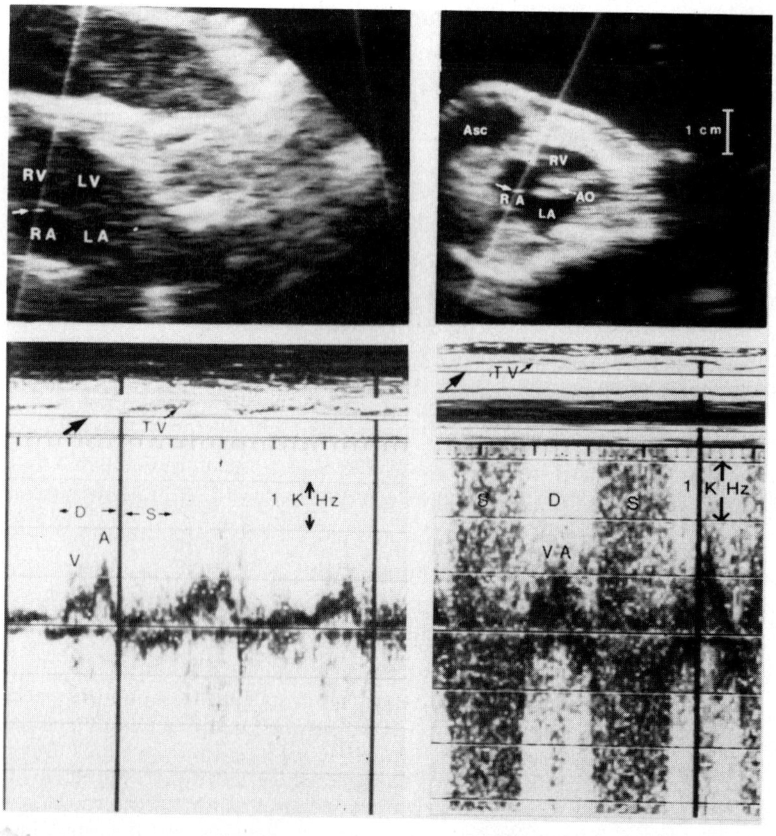

FIGURE 1. *Top panels,* Cross-sectional echocardiographic images showing the Doppler cursor and sample volume within the atria (small arrows). *Bottom panels,* M mode tracing with the sample volume (large arrow) located behind the echo of the tricuspid valve (TV) (small arrow). Below the M mode recordings the spectral Doppler output is shown. The scale marker is 1 kHz per division. Flow above the central baseline represents flow toward the transducer, flow below the baseline represents flow away from the transducer. *Left,* The top frame is an apical four-chamber view of a normal 20 week fetus with the Doppler cursor directed through the right heart and the sample volume placed behind the tricuspid valve within the right atrium (RA). In the bottom panel, the characteristic pattern with forward flow in diastole (D). The A peak from atrial contraction is higher than the V peak of venous filling. In systole (S), there is no flow signal. *Right,* Image from fetus 3, short-axis plane through the right heart. The sample volume is proximal to the tricuspid valve in the right atrium (RA). AO = aorta; Asc = ascites; LA = left atrium; RV = right ventricle. A 1 cm marker is shown. At bottom right, the systolic portion of the image (S) shows marked flow disturbance with aliasing (the dominant negative direction away from the right ventricle and the transducer). The diastolic V and A points are present but less clearly separated than in the normal patient.

TABLE 1
Presentation and outcome of fetuses with atrioventricular valve insufficiency and nonimmune hydrops

Fetus No.	Weeks gest.	Presenting problem	Findings	Outcome
1	20	Lithium ingestion	20 wk: tricuspid insufficiency and questionable valve displacement; 24 wk: definite displacement of tricuspid valve characteristic of Ebstein's anomaly; 34 wk: hydrops	Vaginal delivery, born cyanotic, maintained on PGE_1, presented with low blood pressure, died at 30 hr, autopsy confirmed diagnosis of Ebstein's anomaly
2	36	Arrhythmia	Complex bradyarrhythmia, AV canal defect, AV valve insufficiency, interrupted IVC, polysplenia, hydrops	Vaginal delivery, presented with low blood pressure and cardiac failure, died at 20 hr, autopsy confirmed diagnosis
3	20	Twin pregnancy with hydropic twin	Tricuspid valve insufficiency, no recordable pulmonary valve, small main pulmonary artery segment, 1 twin hydropic, 1 normal	Twin died and pregnancy aborted spontaneously, autopsy refused
4	35	Hydropic fetus	Aortic atresia, diminutive left ventricle and mitral valve, tricuspid insufficiency, hydrops	Vaginal delivery, died within 20 hr, autopsy confirmed diagnosis
5	34	Lithium treatment for depression, hydrops noted 24 wk gestation	Ebstein's anomaly noted on echo and tricuspid insufficiency by Doppler exam	Died on second day of life, autopsy confirmed diagnosis
6	38	Polyhydramnios and hydrops	Right atrial and right ventricular dilatation, pulmonary outflow not clearly seen, tricuspid insufficiency	Died at 4 hr, autopsy confirmed dysplastic pulmonary valve
7	29	Polyhydramnios, sustained tachycardia (240/min)	Normal cardiac anatomy, hydrops, mother given digitalis, verapamil, and eventually furosemide	Hydrothorax and ascites, resolved 14 days after treatment, born at 38 wk gestation
8	26	Fetal hydrops, bradycardia, Sjogren's syndrome, arthritis, ANA positive to 1:160	Complete heart block with ventricular rate of 55/min, hydrops, AV valve insufficiency	Spontaneous abortion at 30 wk, at postmortem tricuspid valve thickened and right ventricle hypertrophied
9	23	Nonimmune hydrops at 23 wk gestation	AV canal defect, mild AV valve insufficiency, pulmonary atresia, asplenia	Died on first day of life, could not be resuscitated, postmortem refused
10	25	Ascites, pericardial effusion; mother has Ebstein's anomaly at 24 weeks	Ebstein's anomaly, same degree as maternal disorder, nonimmune hydrops, moderate AV valve insufficiency	Born with hydrops, severe tricuspid valve insufficiency after birth with right-to-left atrial shunt, died at 5 days
11	29	Bradycardia (45–50/min)	Ambiguous atrial situs, AV canal defect, double-outlet right ventricle and pulmonic stenosis, mild atrioventricular valve insufficiency by Doppler exam	Maintained on terbutaline to prevent premature labor, heart rate increased to 70/min, AV valve regurgitation increased, nonimmune hydrops developed, baby died on first day of life, autopsy confirmed right isomerism and other in utero findings
12	31	Maternal polyhydramnios and nonimmune fetal hydrops	AV canal defect and AV valve insufficiency	Amniocentesis showed trisomy 21, baby delivered at term, died on first day of life

ANA = antinuclear antibody; AV = atrioventricular; IVC = inferior vena cava.

after delivery. The sole survivor was a 29 week fetus with sustained supraventricular tachycardia whose tachyarrhythmia, atrioventricular valve regurgitation, and hydrops fetalis resolved in utero after transplacental therapy with digoxin and verapamil.

Our first fetus discovered to have atrioventricular valve insufficiency was a 20 week product of a 42-year-old gravida IV para III who had received high-dosage lithium for depression during the first trimester. The examination showed an enlarged right atrium and probable displacement of the tricuspid valve. Doppler insonation of the right atrium from a four-chamber view showed marked tricuspid insufficiency. The diagnosis of Ebstein's anomaly was suspected (figure 2). At 24 weeks gestation the degree of tricuspid insufficiency appeared qualitatively unchanged but there had been further enlargement of the right atrium and the umbilical vein, possibly reflecting venous hy-

TABLE 2
Presentation and outcome of fetuses with atrioventricular valve insufficiency and without nonimmune hydrops

Fetus No.	Weeks gest.	Presenting problem	Findings	Outcome
1	34	Severe growth retardation	Pulmonary insufficiency, tricuspid insufficiency	Cesarean section undertaken, severe growth retardation with birth weight 1250 g, postnatal echocardiogram confirmed pulmonary and tricuspid insufficiency, infant alive and well
2	34	Bradycardia (85/min)	Right isomerism, AV canal defect, double-outlet right ventricle and pulmonary stenosis, AV valve insufficiency	Prenatal findings confirmed after birth, Blalock-Taussig shunt performed, patient alive at 2 mo of age
3	38	Intermittent bradycardia to 50/min, anti-Rho antibody positive	Complete heart block at echocardiography, mild AV valve insufficiency	Epicardial pacemaker inserted, baby doing well
4	26	Bradycardia to 60/min, mother had hepatitis during pregnancy	Complete heart block with AV valve insufficiency	No problem with heart block since delivery
5	34	Dermatomyositis, bradycardia	Complete heart block and mild AV valve insufficiency	Situs inversus, baby born with dextrocardia, catheterization showed small atrial septal defect and patent ductus arteriosus, asymptomatic at 6 mo
6	32	Bradycardia	Isolated levocardia, atrial isomerism, complete AV canal defect, severe subpulmonary stenosis, mild AV valve insufficiency, sinus bradycardia	Delivery at 36 wk gestation, cardiac catheterization showed right isomerism and mild AV valve regurgitation, child alive after Blalock-Taussig shunt
7	32	General ultrasound exam showed duodenal atresia	Complete AV canal defect with mild AV valve insufficiency, chromosome analysis showed normal complement	Small for dates, operation to bypass duodenal atresia, echocardiography after birth confirmed in utero findings

AV = atrioventricular.

pertension. The tricuspid valve showed obvious displacement of its septal leaflet. Examination at 35 weeks gestation showed fetal hydrops in addition to the atrioventricular valve insufficiency. Analysis of the amniotic fluid showed fetal pulmonary maturity. Labor was induced and the infant delivered. She was cyanotic (Pa_{O_2} 34 mm Hg) and had marked hydrops and poor peripheral perfusion, with an arterial blood pressure of only 40/20 mm Hg. Postnatal echocardiographic and Doppler examination confirmed the prenatal findings. Contrast echocardiography showed marked right-to-left atrial shunting.

Despite administration of prostaglandin E_1, isoproterenol, and dopamine, the baby died 30 hr after delivery. Autopsy confirmed the diagnosis of Ebstein's anomaly.

The second fetus we encountered was the product of a gravida II para I referred for evaluation of a fetal cardiac arrhythmia at 35 weeks gestation. The fetus was noted to be hydropic with atrioventricular valve insufficiency on Doppler examination and complex congenital heart disease consisting of an atrioventricular canal defect associated with left atrial isomerism (figure 3). Labor was induced and delivery was uneventful. Neonatal ultrasound examination confirmed the prenatal diagnosis of atrioventricular valve insufficiency. The blood pressure was low and could not be maintained despite infusion of isoproterenol and dopamine. The infant died 32 hr after birth and autopsy confirmed the findings.

The next case involved a 23 week monoamniotic twin pregnancy. Nonimmune hydrops was noted during an obstetric ultrasound examination and the patient was referred for cardiac ultrasound study, which showed the presence of pulmonary atresia. The right ventricle and right atrium appeared enlarged in the four-chamber view (figure 4). Doppler insonation of the main pulmonary artery showed no forward flow into the pulmonary artery. There was no observable pulmonary valve motion. Pulsed Doppler insonation of the right atrium showed marked tricuspid insufficiency (figure 1, *right*). The other twin was morphologically normal. The pregnancy terminated spontaneously 4 weeks later. Both fetuses were stillborn and severely macerated. Postmortem examination was refused.

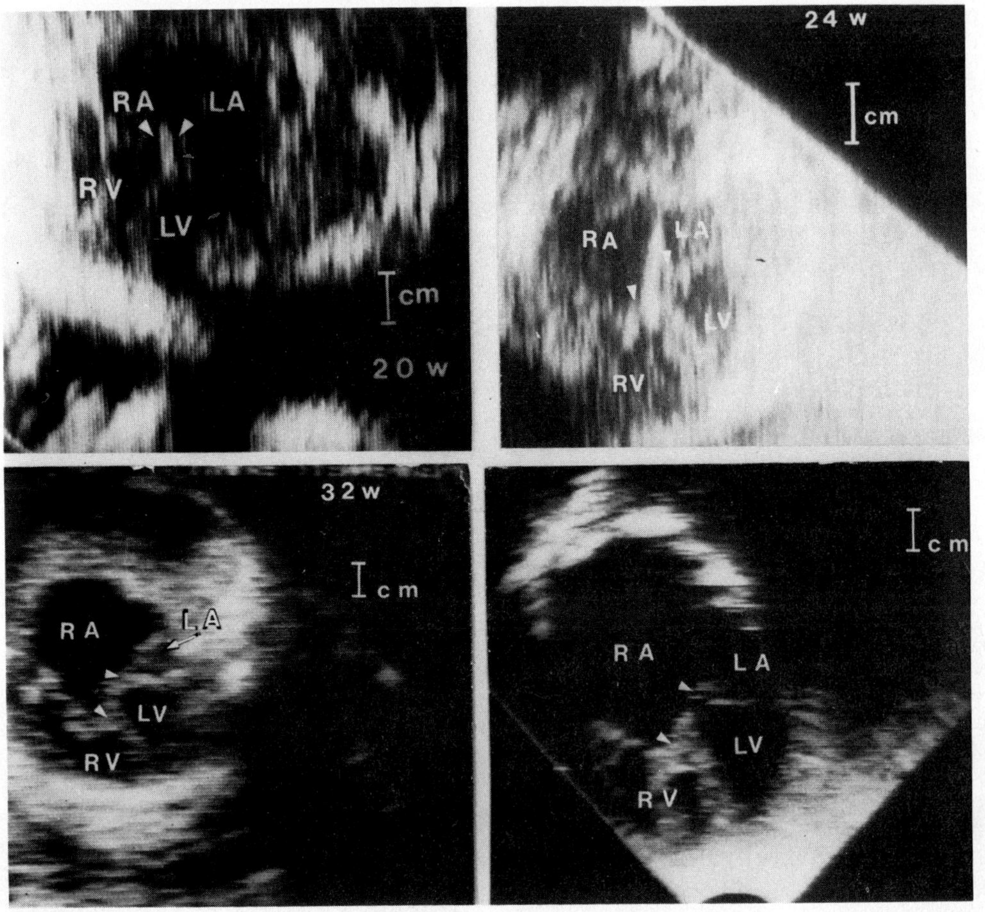

FIGURE 2. Four frames in equivalent orientation, four-chamber plane, from fetus 1 with Ebstein's anomaly, showing the findings at 20 weeks (*top left*), 24 weeks (*top right*), 32 weeks (*bottom left*), and after birth at 35 weeks (*bottom right*). The four chambers identified are the right atrium (RA), right ventricle (RV), left atrium (LA), and left ventricle (LV). The arrows indicate the septal insertion of the tricuspid and mitral valves. At 20 weeks the heart appears structurally normal (although other views suggested right atrial enlargement). At 24 weeks right atrial enlargement and tricuspid displacement are apparent. At 32 weeks the tricuspid displacement is marked, the right atrial enlargement has progressed, and pleural effusions are noted. After birth there is a similar pattern to that at 32 weeks. A large right-sided pericardial effusion can be seen.

The fourth fetus was examined at 32 weeks of gestation and was found to have nonimmune hydrops with marked ascites and pericardial effusion. Fetal echocardiography confirmed the presence of aortic atresia, a minute ascending aorta, and a diminutive mitral valve and left ventricle (figure 5). Doppler flow study showed marked systolic flow disturbance within the enlarged right atrium with aliasing indicating tricuspid insufficiency. The jet could be recorded only toward the lateral atrial wall, suggesting that the insufficiency was mild. The baby died within 6 hr of delivery. The autopsy findings confirmed the sonographic observations in utero. Data pertaining to the other fetuses in this study are summarized in tables 1 and 2.

Discussion

These cases demonstrate the ability of range-gated pulsed Doppler echocardiography to detect flow disturbances in fetuses with cardiovascular compromise related to abnormalities either of cardiac structure or of rhythm.

Hydrops fetalis was present in all 12 fetuses who demonstrated atrioventricular valve regurgitation. The 11 fetuses with structural heart disease died in utero or during the first few days of life.

We encountered an additional seven fetuses who had atrioventricular valve insufficiency without nonimmune hydrops. The prognosis appears somewhat better than that of the group in whom there was atrioventricular valve insufficiency and nonimmune hydrops (table 2). Although the prognosis of nonimmune hydrops in general is poor, 82% mortality,[30] our series suggests that nonimmune hydrops associated with atrioventricular valve insufficiency makes the prognosis even poorer.

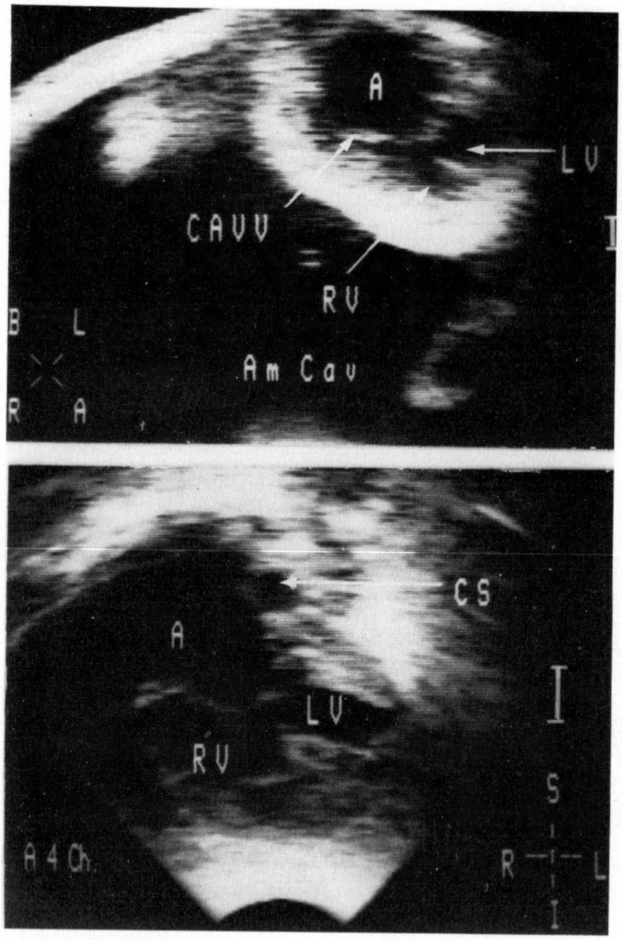

FIGURE 3. Four-chamber view taken from the examination in utero (*top*) and after birth (*bottom*). The top panel shows the single large common atrium (A) and the common atrioventricular valve (CAVV). The left ventricle (LV) and right ventricle (RV) are separated by the ventricular septum and a large ventricular septal defect. There is polyhydramnios filling the amniotic cavity (Am Cav). A 1 cm scale marker is shown. A = apex; B = base; L = left; R = right. The bottom panel shows the same intracardiac anatomy after birth except a large coronary sinus (CS) can be seen. I = inferior; L = left; R = right; S = superior.

The high incidence of cardiac pathology in the presence of nonimmune fetal hydrops has been recognized,[9, 30] suggesting that hydrops fetalis represents end-stage fetal cardiac decompensation in some cases.

It has been assumed that hydrops is the result of fetal systemic venous hypertension. The response of the fetal circulation to obstructive lesions such as hypoplastic left heart syndrome with aortic atresia or pulmonary atresia is to redistribute flow, thereby bypassing the obstruction. Thus cardiac failure and fetal hydrops appear to be uncommon findings in the presence of valvular stenotic lesions at birth. However, atrioventricular valve insufficiency is associated with a mandatory increased volume load on the heart. The fetal heart has only a limited ability to increase its output in response to an increase in ventricular filling pressure. Several studies in fetal lambs have shown that the ventricular output is near the peak at ventricular end-diastolic pressures that are present in the normal resting state; any further increase in preload has a limited effect on stroke volume.[31–33] This could be the result of either myocardial immaturity with limited inotropic reserves or reduced compliance of the fetal ventricles.[34] Because the foramen ovale provides a large communication between the left atrium and systemic veins, the volume loading causes systemic venous hypertension regardless of whether there is insufficiency of a mitral, a tricuspid, or a common atrioventricular valve.

The elevated systemic venous hypertension coupled with low colloid osmotic pressure during fetal life

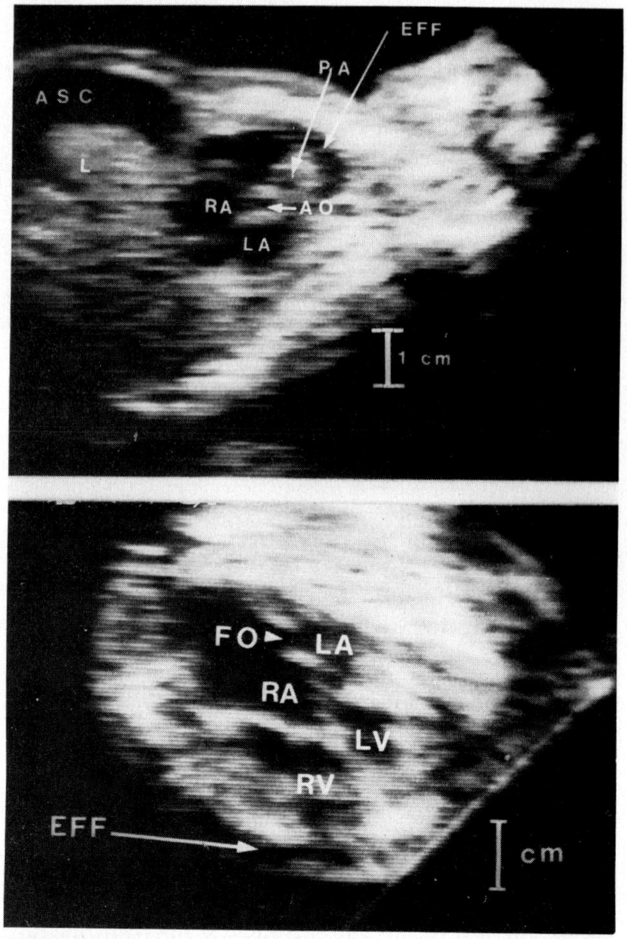

FIGURE 4. *Top,* Longitudinal view through one twin fetus at 23 weeks showing the finding of hydrops with skin edema, ascites (Asc), and pericardial effusion (EFF). The heart orientation is in a plane equivalent to a short-axis plane showing a large right atrium (RA), smaller left atrium (LA), aorta (AO), and pulmonary artery (PA). The pulmonary valve leaflets did not open and there was no recordable Doppler signal within the pulmonary artery. L = liver. A 1 cm marker is shown. *Bottom,* A four-chamber plane with the enlarged right atrium (RA) and right ventricle (RV). The fossa ovalis (FO) is patent (arrow) and the smaller left atrium (LA) and left ventricle (LV) are seen.

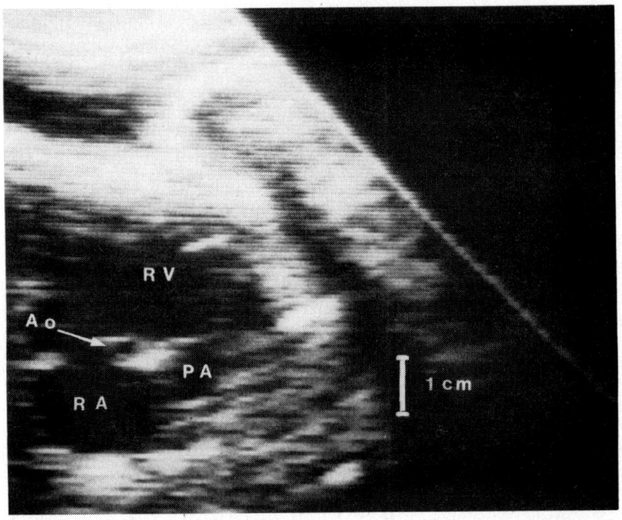

FIGURE 5. Short-axis projection in fetus 4 shows a minute aortic root (Ao) and large right atrium (RA). Right ventricle (RV) and pulmonary artery (PA). A 1 cm marker shows the aorta to be no larger than 4 mm. RV = right ventricle; PA = pulmonary artery.

leads to the presence of edema and hydrops in the fetus. The physiologic low serum albumin level may be further aggravated by decreased hepatic albumin formation in the presence of retrograde inferior vena caval flow and loss of albumin into the extravascular space. The venous pressure could not be measured in our fetuses, but the atrium receiving regurgitant flow was usually large and the umbilical vein dilated when compared with the umbilical artery cross-sectional area.

Pulsed Doppler ultrasound has provided the means to ascertain the presence of atrioventricular or semilunar valve regurgitation and would seem to confirm the postulate that the severity of the venous hypertension load attending such valve dysfunction may be the factor that distinguishes the hydropic fetus from the nonhydropic fetus with the same underlying cardiac lesion. We have been able to follow the natural history of seven other fetuses with similar lesions and atrioventricular valve insufficiency without nonimmune hydrops, all of whom have survived through pregnancy and the early neonatal period (table 2). The atrioventricular valve insufficiency appears to have been less severe by the limited methods we were able to use to define severity.

The difference in the clinical manifestations of the fetuses with atrioventricular valve insufficiency could be related to the severity of the lesion. However, it could also be the result of the duration of the insufficiency, as well as changes in the degree of insufficiency associated with growth. This is exemplified in fetuses 1 and 11, in whom atrioventricular valve insufficiency was noted before hydrops was observed. The increasing severity of the hemodynamic disturbance could well be related to increase in heart size with increasing valvular insufficiency occurring in association with increased size of the valve anulus caused by growth and dilatation.

A relatively small subgroup of patients with congenital heart disease develop hydrops fetalis (i.e., absent pulmonary valve syndrome, Ebstein's malformation of the tricuspid valve, as well as atrial isomerism with atrioventricular canal defects) largely secondary to atrioventricular or semilunar valve insufficiency rather than systolic pump failure.

The findings in our patients suggest that early identification of atrioventricular valve regurgitation in utero may, in selected cases, identify the fetus with structural or functional cardiac impairment who may be at risk for the development of hydrops fetalis. In such cases, prompt transplacental medication or early delivery may be considered.

The detection of atrioventricular valve insufficiency may be used to direct efforts at in utero therapy of arrhythmias and may be used to formulate plans for delivery of the affected fetus and, in the future, may be useful for identifying fetuses who may be candidates for cardiac surgery in utero. The detection of tricuspid insufficiency in aortic atresia, which occurred in one fetus in this series, may suggest that palliative surgery would not make these infants appropriate candidates for a subsequent Fontan operation.[35]

Although it is possible to criticize this study on the basis of not assessing interobserver and intraobserver error, we kept the exposure of the fetuses to ultrasound to a minimum in accordance with recent recommendations.[36]

These studies suggest that the detection of atrioventricular valve insufficiency provides practical information of value for managing the high-risk pregnancy. The combined ultrasound technique augments our understanding of the pathophysiologic nature of the human fetus affected with congenital heart disease.

We thank Ms. Martha Prince for preparation of the manuscript and photographic material, Ms. Mary Helen Briscoe for the artwork, Mr. Rick Soloway for the photography, and Mrs. Heather Silverman for editorial assistance.

References

1. Sahn DJ, Lange LW, Allen HD, Goldberg SJ, Anderson C, Giles H, Haber K: Quantitative real-time cross-sectional echocardiography in the developing normal human fetus and newborn. Circulation **62:** 588, 1980
2. Lange LW, Sahn DJ, Allen HD, Goldberg SJ, Anderson C, Giles H: Quantitative real-time cross-sectional echocardiographic imag-

ing of the human fetus during the second half of pregnancy. Circulation **62:** 799, 1980
3. Allan LD, Tynan MJ, Campbell S, Wilkinson JL, Anderson RH: Echocardiographic and anatomical correlates in the fetus. Br Heart J **44:** 444, 1980
4. Kleinman CS, Hobbins JC, Jaffe CC, Lynch DC, Talner NS: Echocardiographic studies of the human fetus: prenatal diagnosis of congenital heart disease and cardiac dysrhythmias. Pediatrics **65:** 1059, 1980
5. Allan LD, Tynan M, Campbell S, Anderson RH: Identification of congenital cardiac malformations by echocardiography in midtrimester fetus. Br Heart J **46:** 358, 1981
6. Allan LD, Tynan MJ, Campbell S, Anderson RH: Normal fetal cardiac anatomy — a basis for the echocardiographic detection of abnormalities. Prenatal Diagn **1:** 131, 1981
7. DeVore GR, Donnerstein RL, Kleinman CS, Platt LD, Hobbins JC: Fetal echocardiography. I. Normal anatomy as determined by real-time–directed M-mode ultrasound. Am J Obstet Gynecol **144:** 249, 1982
8. Allan LD, Joseph MC, Boyd EG, Campbell S, Tynan M: M-mode echocardiography in the developing human fetus. Br Heart J **47:** 573, 1982
9. Kleinman CS, Donnerstein RL, DeVore GR, Jaffe CC, Lynch DC, Berkowitz RL, Talner NS, Hobbins JC: Fetal echocardiography for evaluation of in utero congestive heart failure. N Engl J Med **306:** 568, 1982
10. Kleinman CS, Donnerstein RL, Jaffe CC, DeVore GR, Weinstein EM, Lynch DC, Talner NS, Berkowitz RL, Hobbins JC: Fetal echocardiography. A tool for evaluation of in utero cardiac arrhythmias and monitoring of in utero therapy: analysis of 71 patients. Am J Cardiol **51:** 237, 1983
11. Wladimiroff JW, McGhie J, Vosters R: Fetal cardiac activity. *In* Rijsterborgh H, editor: Echocardiology. The Hague, 1981, Martinus Nijhoff Publishers, p 417
12. Eik-Nes SH, Brubakk AO, Ulstein MK: Measurement of human fetal blood flow. Br Med J **280:** 283, 1980
13. Redel DA, Hansmann M: Fetal obstruction of the foramen ovale detected by two-dimensional Doppler echocardiography. *In* Rijsterborgh H, editor: Echocardiology. The Hague, 1981, Martinus Nijhoff Publishers, p 425
14. Loeber C, Goldberg SJ, Hendrix MJC, Sahn DJ: Dynamic mammalian cardiogenesis investigated by high-resolution ultrasound in guinea pigs. Circulation **68:** 841, 1983
15. Silverman NH, Snider AR, Golbus MS, Stanger P: Perspectives in fetal echocardiography. *In* Dellenbach P, editor: Ler symposium international d'echocardiologie foetale. Strasbourg, 1982, Milupa Dietique, p 95
16. Redel DA, Hansmann M: Prenatal diagnosis and treatment of heart disease. *In* Dellenbach P, editor: Ler symposium international d'echocardiologie foetale. Strasbourg, 1982, Milupa Dietique, p 127
17. Hansmann M, Redel DA: Prenatal symptoms and clinical management of heart disease. *In* Dellenbach P, editor: Ler symposium international d'echocardiologie foetale. Strasbourg, 1982, Milupa Dietique, p 137
18. Nesser HJ, Redel DA, Salzer HR: Echocardiography in utero of tricuspid atresia. *In* Dellenbach P, editor: Ler symposium international d'echocardiologie foetale. Strasbourg, 1982, Milupa Dietique, p 248
19. DeGeeter B, Nisand I, Kohler A, Durand JL, Dellenbach P, Kieny R: Etude du coeur foetale en routine. *In* Dellenbach P, editor: Ler symposium international d'echocardiologie foetale. Strasbourg, 1982, Milupa Dietique, p 87
20. Leslie J, Shen SC, Srauss L: Hypertrophic cardiomyopathy in a midtrimester fetus born to a diabetic mother. J Pediatr **100:** 631, 1982
21. Sahn DJ, Shenker L, Reed KL, Valdes-Cruz LM, Sobonya R, Anderson C: Prenatal ultrasound diagnosis of hypoplastic left heart syndrome in utero associated with hydrops fetalis. Am Heart J **104:** 1368, 1982
22. Sharf M, Abinader EG, Shapiro I, Rosenfeld T, Eibschitz I: Prenatal echocardiographic diagnosis of Ebstein's anomaly with pulmonary atresia. Am J Obstet Gynecol **147:** 300, 1983
23. Silverman NH, Enderlein MA, Golbus MS: Ultrasonic recognition of aortic valve atresia in utero. Am J Cardiol **5:** 20s, 1985
24. Berman WJ, editor: Pulsed Doppler ultrasound in clinical pediatrics. Mount Kisco, NY, 1983, Futura Publishing Co.
25. Kurjak A, Rajhvajn B Jr: Ultrasonic measurements of umbilical blood flow in normal and complicated pregnancies. J Perinat Med **10:** 3, 1982
26. Maulik D, Nanda NC, Saini VD: Fetal Doppler echocardiography: methods and characterization of normal and abnormal hemodynamics. Am J Cardiol **53:** 572, 1984
27. Hata T, Hata K, Kitao M: Fetal intracardiac blood-flow patterns assessed by pulsed Doppler and B-mode ultrasound. J Cardiovasc Ultrasonogr **3:** 101, 1984
28. Tonge HM, Struijk PC, Wladimiroff JW: Blood flow measurements in the fetal descending aorta: technique and clinics. Clin Cardiol **7:** 323, 1984
29. Silverman NH, Golbus MS: Echocardiographic techniques for assessing normal and abnormal fetal cardiac anatomy. J Am Coll Cardiol **5:** S20, 1985
30. Mahoney BS, Filly RA, Callen PW, Chinn DH, Golbus MS: Severe nonimmune hydrops fetalis: sonographic evaluation. Radiology **151:** 757, 1984
31. Heymann MA, Rudolph AM: Effects of increasing preload on right ventricular output in fetal lambs in utero. Circulation **48**(suppl IV): IV-37, 1983
32. Gilbert RD: Effects of afterload and baroreceptors on cardiac function in fetal sheep. J Dev Physiol **4:** 299, 1982
33. Thornburg KL, Morton MJ: Filling and arterial pressures as determinants of RV stroke volume in the sheep fetus. Am J Physiol **244:** H656, 1983
34. Friedman WF, Lesch M, Sonnenblick EH Intrinsic physiologic properties of the developing heart in neonatal heart disease. New York, 1972, Grune & Stratton, p 27
35. Lang P, Norwood WI: Hemodynamic assessment after palliative surgery for hypoplastic left heart syndrome. Circulation **68:** 104, 1983
36. Diagnostic ultrasound imaging in pregnancy. U.S. Dept. of Health & Human Services. Public Health Service and National Institutes of Health. N.I.H. Publication No. 84-667. U.S. Government Printing Office, Washington, DC, pp 21–56

Comparative long-term effects of coronary artery bypass graft surgery and percutaneous transluminal coronary angioplasty on regional coronary flow reserve

ERIC R. BATES, M.D., FRED M. AUERON, M.D., VICTOR LEGRAND, M.D., MICHAEL T. LEFREE, B.S., G. B. JOHN MANCINI, M.D., JOHN M. HODGSON, M.D., AND ROBERT A. VOGEL, M.D.

ABSTRACT To evaluate the relative long-term improvement in coronary artery hemodynamics after revascularization by coronary artery bypass graft surgery (CABG) or percutaneous transluminal coronary angioplasty (PTCA), regional coronary flow reserve (CFR) was measured, by digital computer analysis of 35 mm cine film, in 50 men undergoing cardiac catheterization. CFR (mean ± SEM) in 12 atherosclerotic arteries before revascularization was 1.02 ± 0.05. Mean CFR in 29 normal arteries of men with normal coronary arteriograms was significantly higher (2.59 ± 0.11) than that in 16 atherosclerotic arteries of patients revascularized by CABG (2.02 ± 0.17, $p < .01$) or in 14 atherosclerotic arteries of those revascularized by PTCA (1.97 ± 0.12, $p < .01$). No difference in CFR between the CABG and PTCA groups was found and variables known to influence CFR were similar between groups. Equivalent and significant long-term improvement in coronary artery hemodynamics is provided by CABG or PTCA. We postulate that the difference in CFR in the men with normal arteries and those who underwent revascularization was related to the effects of the general atherosclerotic process, which remain despite successful treatment by these techniques.
Circulation 72, No. 4, 833–839, 1985.

MYOCARDIAL REVASCULARIZATION can now be accomplished by either coronary artery bypass graft surgery (CABG) or percutaneous transluminal coronary angioplasty (PTCA).[1–4] Although symptomatic, metabolic, hemodynamic, and functional improvement has been demonstrated with each technique,[5–15] little data exist comparing the two.[16, 17] One difficulty in undertaking comparative studies resides in the clinical disparities in groups of patients undergoing these procedures. While patients who undergo CABG are more likely to have chronic symptoms, a history of myocardial infarction, and multivessel disease, those treated by PTCA characteristically have recent onset of symptoms, normal ventricular function, and single-vessel disease. More importantly, the lack of a generally available clinical test sensitive enough to evaluate subtle regional differences in coronary blood flow or myocardial function due to either technique has inhibited investigation.

The coronary reactive hyperemic response is an important, reproducible physiologic parameter.[18, 19] It can be measured by determining the ratio of maximal coronary blood flow to resting flow. Increasingly significant obstructive coronary artery disease progressively exhausts this coronary flow reserve (CFR) by reducing peak flow.[20, 21] Three techniques have recently been developed that allow the measurement of regional CFR in man. The first uses a pulsed Doppler coronary artery catheter, which can measure proximal coronary flow velocity in the catheterization laboratory.[22] The second uses a Doppler velocity probe, which can be applied directly to selected epicardial coronary arteries at the time of open heart surgery to measure the reactive hyperemic response to transient arterial occlusion.[23] The third is a digital radiographic technique performed during routine cardiac catheterization that measures the myocardial reactive hyperemic response to intracoronary injection of contrast medium.[24, 25]

The present study, in which we used the third tech-

From the Division of Cardiology, Veterans Administration Medical Center, Ann Arbor.

Supported in part by grants from the Veterans Administration, the Merck Fellowship Foundation of the American College of Cardiology, and the Michigan Heart Association.

Address for correspondence: Eric R. Bates, M.D., Division of Cardiology, Veterans Administration Medical Center, Ann Arbor, MI 48105.

Received Feb. 7, 1985; revision accepted June 20, 1985

nique, was designed to evaluate the relative improvement in long-term regional CFR after myocardial revascularization by CABG or PTCA.

Methods

Patient population. The patient population consisted of 50 men undergoing coronary arteriography. These patients were divided into four groups for analysis. Group I was composed of 10 patients with symptomatic coronary artery disease (a total of 12 diseased arteries) who subsequently underwent revascularization by CABG or PTCA. Eleven patients with 16 arteries previously treated by CABG formed group II, and 13 patients with 14 arteries previously treated by PTCA formed group III; these patients were studied to evaluate postrevascularization vessel patency. In group II patients all grafts were patent and nonstenotic, and in those in group III there was a residual translesional pressure gradient of 20 mm Hg or less at the time of angioplasty and no angiographic evidence of restenosis at follow-up. Twenty-nine arteries in 16 patients with atypical chest pain and normal coronary arteriograms formed group IV and served as the normal control group. Patients were excluded if they had valvular heart disease, electrocardiographic evidence of left ventricular hypertrophy, more than mild hypokinesis documented on the contrast ventriculogram, or angiographically visible coronary collateral vessels. Data from 15% of arterial distributions were excluded from analysis because of use of an inadequate contrast injection technique, motion artifact, poor visualization of the perfusion bed, or failure of the angiographer to acquire arteriographic data suitable for digital processing.

Prescribed medication regimens were not followed the morning of the cardiac catheterization. Patients were premedicated with 10 mg diazepam and 50 mg diphenhydramine. This study was approved by the institutional committees on human research and informed consent was obtained from each patient.

Arteriographic technique. To obtain images for digital processing, the following arteriographic technique was used. Standard left ventriculography and multiple-view selective coronary arteriography were performed by the Judkins technique. Arteriography for subsequent functional image digital processing was obtained in the left anterior oblique projection on 35 mm cine film. Fixed parameter (kV, mA, and pulse width) cineradiography at 30 frames/sec was used. Patients were required to cease respiration and remain motionless during filming. Vein grafts and coronary arteries were opacified by a fixed dose of 5 to 8 ml of sodium meglumine diatrizoate (Renografin-76) injected by an electrocardiographically triggered power injector gated to the R wave of the electrocardiogram. Reflux of contrast medium into the aorta was considered proof that a maximal bolus of contrast was delivered to the artery and that the catheter was not impeding coronary blood flow. Baseline studies were performed at least 3 min after the previous injection of contrast. Studies under hyperemic conditions were performed 10 sec after intracoronary injection of an identical dose of contrast medium. Cineradiography was initiated at least one full cardiac cycle before injection of contrast. A density step wedge was imaged and checked densitometrically after film processing to ensure that the film gray scale was kept constant on a day-to-day basis.

Digital processing of the functional image. Digital image processing was performed by a technique similar to that previously described.[24-27] Three general operations were required: digitization, mask-mode substraction, and functional image generation. Arteriograms were displayed on a cine film projector (Vanguard Corporation, XR-35) equipped with a primary beam splitter coupled to a fixed-gain video camera and a video analog-to-digital converter. Five to seven end-diastolic frames from consecutive cardiac cycles were chosen, with use of the criterion of closest duplication of arterial position, beginning with the end-diastolic frame just before injection of contrast medium. These frames were digitized into 512 × 512 × 8-bit matrixes. Video-amplified gain and projector light levels were adjusted to provide a linear correspondence between contrast x-ray absorption and digital scale. The digital images were stored in the disk memory of a digital radiographic computer (DPS-4100C, ADAC Labs, Edenvale, CA) for subsequent processing.

Image enhancement was performed by standard mask-mode subtraction with use of the end-diastolic frame before injection of contrast as the mask. A single contrast intensity and appearance time–modulated functional image was then generated from each set of enhanced frames (figure 1).[25] The intensity value of each pixel corresponded to the maximum contrast density reached during each acquisition, while the appearance time of contrast in the pixel was color modulated, with a different color assigned to each postinjection cardiac cycle (red for the first cycle, yellow for the second, etc.). Only pixels with an intensity above a preset threshold appeared on the final functional image. This threshold was manually set at a level that excluded most of the background noise intensity. Acquisition and processing were identical for each pair of basal and hyperemic images so that each set was technically comparable.

Analysis of functional images. Mean myocardial contrast density and appearance were determined by a computer program that averaged pixel values in a region of interest defined by the operator in the basal images and in the same area of the hyperemic images (figure 1). Large epicardial coronary arteries and areas that overlapped with the aortic root, diaphragm, or coronary sinus were excluded from analysis. Since contrast density is directly related to the volume of distribution in the myocardium and flow is inversely related to myocardial contrast appearance time, digital estimation of coronary blood flow was calculated as

$$Q \propto \text{volume/time} \propto CD/AT$$

where Q = mean regional cornary flow; CD = mean maximal contrast density; and AT = mean contrast appearance time. CFR, the ratio of hyperemic (H) flow to basal (B) flow, corrected for heart rate (HR), was calculated as

$$CFR = Q_H/Q_B = CD_H/CD_B \times AT_B/AT_H \times HR_H/HR_B$$

Studies in dogs have demonstrated an excellent correlation between CFR measured by electromagnetic flow probe and the ratio CD/AT measured by digital subtraction angiography ($r = .92$). The digital measurements were accurate (regression slope = .90), reproducible (±13%), and had low interobserver ($r = .99$) and intraobserver ($r = .98$) variability.[25]

Data analysis. Data are expressed as mean ± SEM. Statistical comparisons between groups were obtained with the two-tailed, unpaired t test. Significant differences were assumed when confidence limits exceeded 95% ($p < .05$).

Results

Clinical characteristics. The clinical characteristics of the patients groups are listed in table 1. Nine of 11 patients in group II (CABG) had triple-vessel disease, while nine of 13 patients in group III (PTCA) had single-vessel disease. Forty-two of the 48 diseased arteries in group II and III patients were successfully revascularized. Two patients each in groups II and III

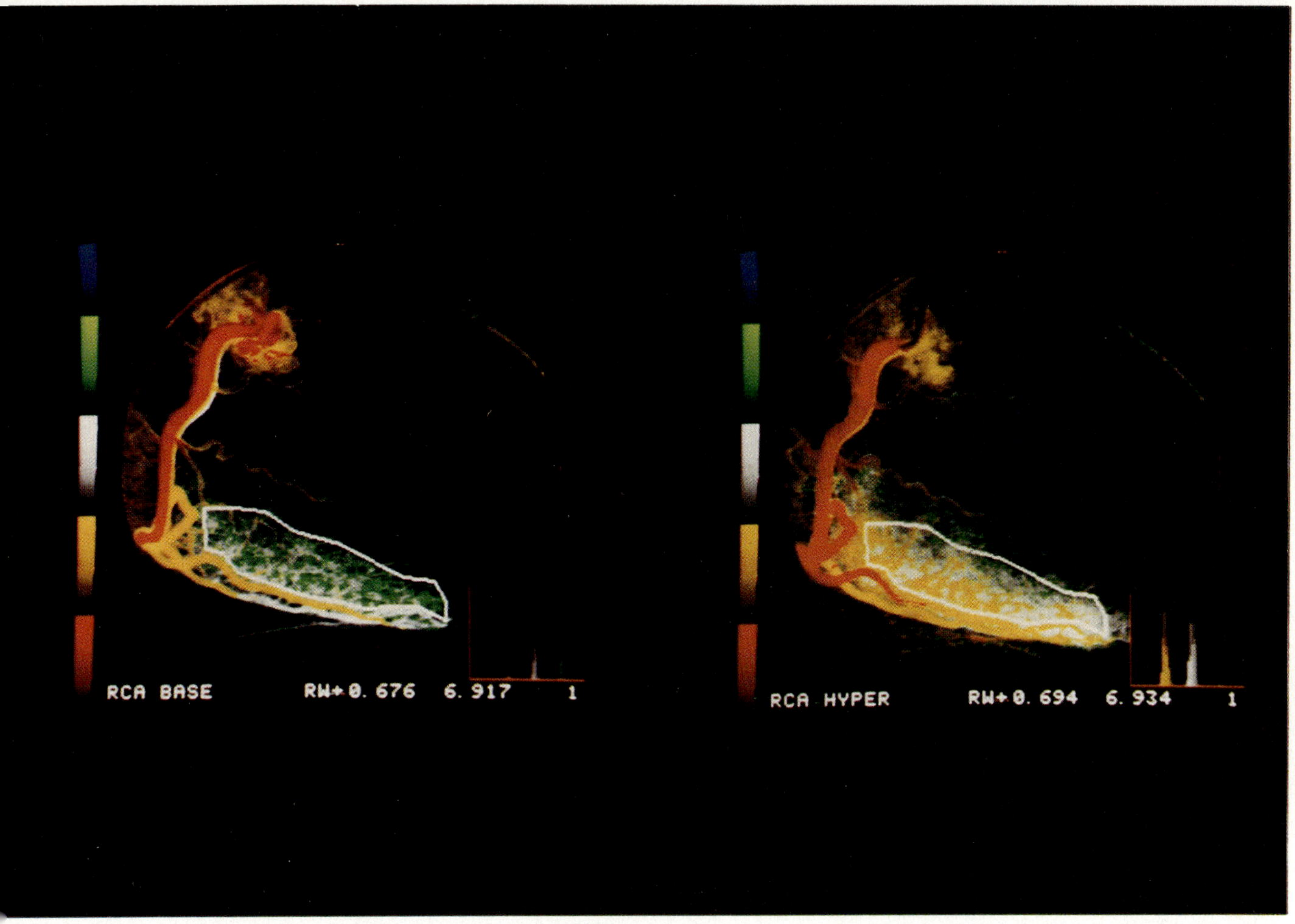

FIGURE 1. Contrast medium appearance pictures of a normal right coronary artery in the right anterior oblique projections at baseline (*left*) and under hyperemic (*right*) conditions. CFR was calculated to be 2.49 in the region of interest.

still had exertional chest pain; the others were pain free. The hemoglobin averaged 14.9 ± 0.7 g/dl in group II and 15.0 ± 0.3 g/dl in group III and the interval between revascularization and catheterization in these two groups was 15.4 ± 2.0 and 32.6 ± 4.2 weeks, respectively.

Cardiac catheterization. Data obtained at cardiac catheterization for the four patient groups are listed in table 2. There were no significant differences in heart rate, mean aortic pressure, or pressure-rate product between groups. Although group III patients had a significantly lower left ventricular ejection fraction than the men with normal arteries (group IV) ($p < .01$), the value was not statistically different from that in group II, and was well within normal physiologic limits. No difference in left ventricular end-diastolic pressures existed. Percent luminal stenosis of arteries was 80 ± 4% in group I and 17 ± 3% in group III.

CFR. Individual values for CFR for each group are plotted in figure 2. CFR in five patients who subsequently underwent CABG and in five patients who subsequently underwent PTCA are grouped together in group I because they were equivalent (1.10 ± 0.05 vs 0.95 ± 0.06). Mean values for CFR for groups I, II, III, and IV were 1.02 ± 0.05, 2.02 ± 0.17, 1.97 ± 0.12, and 2.59 ± 0.11, respectively. While CFR in patients with atherosclerotic arteries revascularized by CABG or PTCA was significantly higher than in those with arteries not revascularized ($p < .0001$), it was significantly lower than CFR in men with normal arteries ($p < .01$). No difference in CFR in groups II and III was found.

Discussion

Autoregulatory changes maintain basal coronary blood flow in arteries with flow-limiting stenoses by decreasing distal coronary resistance, but this limits potential further increases in flow. In arteries with high-grade stenoses suitable for revascularization by CABG or PTCA, CFR is exhausted. An improvement

TABLE 1
Characteristics of the 50 study patients

	Group I (n = 10)	Group II (n = 11)	Group III (n = 13)	Group IV (n = 16)
Age (yr)[A]	56±3	57±2	55±3	48±2
No. of diseased vessels	19	31	17	0
No. of vessels revascularized	18	27	15	0
No. of vessels studied	12	16	14	29
LAD	7	5	6	9
Diagonal branch	0	3	0	0
Left circumflex	2	6	2	8
RCA	3	2	6	12
Medications before testing				
Nitrates	10	3	3	10
β-blockers	2	9	0	11
Ca^{++}-blockers	6	2	9	3

LAD = left anterior descending artery; RCA = right coronary artery.
[A]Mean ± SEM.

in individual arterial CFR several months after CABG and immediately after PTCA, as measured by coronary radiography, has been demonstrated previously.[26, 27] We have since modified our image analysis algorithm and use contrast density information to reflect regional vascular volume and the CD/AT ratio to more accurately estimate coronary blood flow.[25] While the CFR values found for vessels without severe obstruction are higher when CD/AT ratios than when AT ratios are used,[24–27] findings with both methods indicate that CFR is absent in vessels with high-grade stenoses suitable for revascularization. In this report, the long-term effects of revascularization as determined by these two techniques were compared with this refined image algorithm. Equivalent and significant long-term improvements in regional CFR were found in arteries revascularized by either CABG or PTCA. Additionally, even though revascularization was quite successful in each artery, normal CFR was not restored.

Clinical implications. CABG has been the most popular means of restoring regional myocardial blood flow to perfusion beds distal to coronary stenoses for 15 years. More recently, PTCA has emerged as an alternative revascularization treatment for single-vessel obstructive coronary artery disease. It has clearly been demonstrated that successful revascularization by CABG or PTCA produces symptomatic, metabolic, hemodynamic, and functional improvement.[5–15] The current investigation is the first to suggest that equivalent improvement in individual coronary artery hemodynamics is achieved by the two techniques and further justifies the use of revascularization by CABG or PTCA in properly selected patients.

Theoretical implications. The failure of successful revascularization to restore normal CFR to atherosclerotic coronary arteries is probably the most interesting finding of this study and one for which an explanation is not readily apparent. The patients in each group had equivalent basal oxygen demands, as estimated by pressure-rate product, and normal global left ventricular function. Patients with severe regional wall motion abnormalities, collateral blood flow, or left ventricular hypertrophy were excluded because these factors can have an effect on CFR independent of that of coronary

TABLE 2
Cardiac catheterization data

	Group I (n = 10)	Group II (n = 11)	Group III (n = 13)	Group IV (n = 16)
Heart rate (beats/min)	75±2	75±3	74±3	71±3
Mean aortic pressure (mm Hg)	92±3	95±4	97±3	93±3
Pressure-rate product ($\times 10^{-2}$)	99±4	96±5	98±5	90±6
Left ventricular ejection fraction (%)	65±4	67±3	59±3[A]	73±3
Left ventricular end-diastolic pressure (mm Hg)	13±2	10±2	14±2	13±1

Data expressed as mean ± SEM.
[A]$p < .01$, as compared with the control group (group IV).

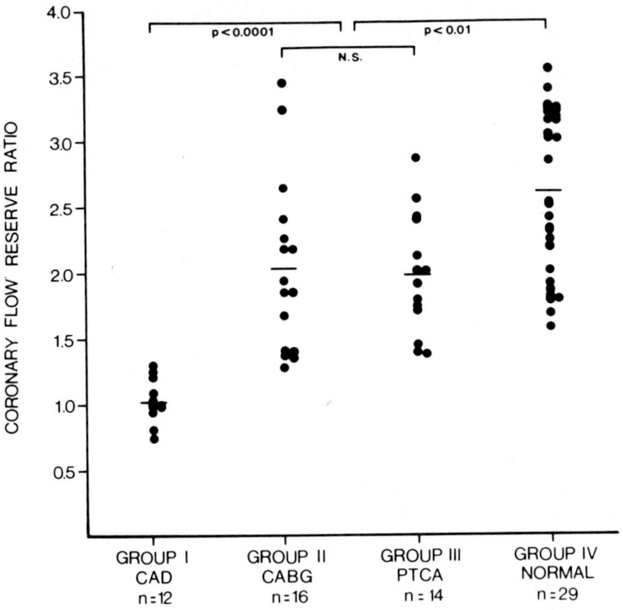

FIGURE 2. Long-term CFR values for the patient groups as determined by digital coronary radiography. CAD = coronary artery disease.

stenoses.[28–31] By using contrast medium as a direct vasodilator stimulus, rather than depending on the ischemic stimulation of vessel occlusion often used in the operating room, we avoided measurement of any influence dual blood supply may have had on determinations of graft CFR. Also, the arteries subjected to PTCA had very mild residual luminal stenoses and would thus not be expected to be associated with limitations of peak coronary blood flow.[20, 21] In the early postrevascularization period patients were receiving antianginal medications prescribed by their referring physicians for prophylactic reasons, not because of persistent ischemia; none received antianginal medications on the day of the catheterization.

It is unlikely that use of a saphenous vein graft as the proximal conduit for coronary blood flow influences coronary artery hemodynamics. No change in timing of the resting pulse wave, pressure contour, or distal blood flow was found by Kakos et al.[32] in bypassed normal canine coronary arteries. Others have shown graft CFR to be normal in the canine model.[33] Likewise, Brandt et al.[34] have demonstrated restoration of normal CFR by CABG in a nonatherosclerotic human right coronary artery originating from the left sinus of Valsalva.

It is postulated that the difference in CFR in men with normal arteries and those who underwent revascularization is related to the atherosclerotic disease process. First, although obstructive coronary artery disease, as defined by the coronary arteriogram, is often detected as discrete proximal luminal stenoses treatable by CABG or PTCA, anatomic descriptions have repeatedly demonstrated the diffuse nature of atherosclerotic plaque in diseased epicardial coronary arteries.[35–37] Secondly, local vasomotor reactivity may not be normal in atherosclerotic arteries. Neovascularization in the region of atherosclerotic plaque has been visualized by cinematography after silicone polymer injections into the arteries of isolated human hearts.[38] These transmural vascular networks potentially provide higher concentrations of vasoconstrictor substances and the proliferation of autonomic nerve terminals known to accompany neovascularization may enhance local catecholamine levels.[38] Also, endothelial damage due to mechanical injury or atherogenesis has been shown to inhibit arterial smooth muscle relaxation.[39, 40] Finally, vascular reactivity at the arteriolar level may be affected by the atherosclerotic disease process through intimal thickening and fibrosis,[41] altered α-adrenergic tone,[42] or chronic microembolization of platelet aggregates.[43]

The effect of experimental atherosclerosis on CFR has been studied in the cynomolgus monkey.[44] After an atherogenic diet was given to induce lesions producing an average of 60% luminal stenosis, a normal diet was given for a regression period of 18 months. While the degree of stenosis was reduced to 25%, intimal fibrosis was increased and CFR was only partially restored. The authors concluded that intimal fibrosis substantially limited arterial hemodynamic improvement.

Study limitations. The limitations of the digital radiographic technique we used have been previously summarized and include those related to specific hardware requirements, motion artifact, use of contrast medium as the hyperemic stimulus, and the mathematic assumptions necessary for calculation of blood flow.[24–27, 45] Despite these difficulties, a good correlation between electromagnetic flowmeter and digital radiographic determinations of relative regional CFR has been demonstrated.[25] Also of concern is the fact that about a quarter of the normal CFR values were less than 2. We have recently shown that patients with chest pain, normal coronary arteriograms, and low regional CFR frequently have associated regional abnormalities on radionuclide exercise tests.[46] These patients probably have ischemic heart disease without epicardial coronary stenoses.[47, 48] Since this normal group was defined only by the arteriogram, without radionuclide exercise test data, it is likely that the difference in CFR in the group with normal arteries and the group undergoing revascularization is larger than stated.[49] The wide range of CFR values found in each patient group probably reflects the multiplicity of factors that can influence arterial CFR.[49, 50]

In summary, revascularization by CABG or PTCA restores equivalent CFR to individual coronary arteries. Although normal CFR is not achieved, this improvement in coronary arterial hemodynamics is sufficient to reverse clinically detectable myocardial ischemia. The difference in CFR in normal and revascularized arteries requires further evaluation. Confirmation that physiologic perturbations accompany the previously documented anatomic changes caused by the presence of coronary atherosclerosis, despite successful revascularization of angiographically visible proximal stenoses, would be of importance in understanding the pathophysiology of obstructive coronary disease.

We are indebted to Mr. Glenn Beauman for technical assistance and to Ms. Diane Bauer for assistance in preparing the manuscript.

References

1. Favaloro RG: Saphenous vein graft in the surgical treatment of coronary artery disease. Operative technique. J Thorac Cardiovasc Surg **59:** 178, 1969
2. Favaloro RG: Direct myocardial revascularization: A ten year journey. Myths and realities. Louis F. Bishop Lecture. Am J Cardiol **43:** 109, 1979
3. Gruentzig AR, Senning A, Siegenthaler WE: Nonoperative dilatation of coronary artery stenosis: Percutaneous transluminal coronary angioplasty. N Engl J Med **301:** 61, 1979
4. Gruentzig AR: Percutaneous transluminal coronary angioplasty: six years' experience. Am Heart J **107:** 818, 1984
5. Peduzzi P, Hultgren HN: Effect of medical vs surgical treatment on symptoms in stable angina pectoris. The Veterans Administration Cooperative Study of Surgery for Coronary Arterial Occlusive Disease. Circulation **60:** 888, 1979
6. Kent KM, Bentivoglio LG, Block PC, Cowley MJ, Dorros G, Gosselin AJ, Gruentzig A, Myler RK, Stertzer SH, Williams DO, Fisher L, Gillespie MJ, Detre K, Kelsey S, Mullin SM, Mock MD: Percutaneous transluminal coronary angioplasty: report from the Registry of the National Heart, Lung, and Blood Institute. Am J Cardiol **49:** 2011, 1982
7. Kloster FE, Kremkau EL, Ritzmann LW, Rahimtoola SH, Rosch J, Kanarek PH: Coronary bypass for stable angina: a prospective randomized study. N Engl J Med **300:** 149, 1979
8. Williams DO, Riley RS, Singh AK, Most AS: Restoration of normal coronary hemodynamics and myocardial metabolism after percutaneous transluminal coronary angioplasty. Circulation **62:** 653, 1980
9. Barry WH, Pfeiffer JF, Lipton MJ, Tilkian AG, Hultgren HN: Effects of coronary artery bypass grafting on resting and exercise hemodynamics in patients with stable angina pectoris: a prospective randomized study. Am J Cardiol **37:** 823, 1976
10. Rothman MT, Baim DS, Simpson JB, Harrison DC: Coronary hemodynamics during percutaneous transluminal coronary angioplasty. Am J Cardiol **49:** 1615, 1982
11. Rahimtoola SH: Postoperative exercise response in the evaluation of the physiologic status after coronary bypass surgery. Circulation **65**(suppl II): II-106, 1982
12. Ritchie JL, Narahara KA, Trobaugh GB, Williams DL, Hamilton GW: Thallium-201 myocardial imaging before and after coronary revascularization. Assessment of regional myocardial blood flow and graft patency. Circulation **56:** 830, 1977
13. Scholl JM, Chaitman BR, David PR, Dupras G, Brevers G, Val PG, Crepeau J, Lesperance J, Bourassa MG: Exercise electrocardiography and myocardial scintigraphy in the serial evaluation of the results of percutaneous transluminal coronary angioplasty. Circulation **66:** 380, 1982
14. Kent KM, Borer JS, Green MV, Bachrach SL, McIntosh CL, Conkle DM, Epstein SE: Effects of coronary artery bypass on global and regional left ventricular function during exercise. N Engl J Med **298:** 1434, 1978
15. Kent KM, Bonow RO, Rosing DR, Ewels CJ, Lipson LC, McIntosh CL, Bachrach S, Green M, Epstein SE: Improved myocardial function during exercise after successful percutaneous transluminal coronary angioplasty. N Engl J Med **306:** 441, 1982
16. Williams D, Singh A, Most A: Sustained efficacy of coronary angioplasty documented by stress testing at one year. J Am Coll Cardiol **1:** 644, 1983 (abst)
17. Meier B, Gruentzig AR, Siegenthaler WE, Schlumpf M: Long-term exercise performance after percutaneous transluminal coronary angioplasty and coronary artery bypass grafting. Circulation **68:** 796, 1983
18. Coffman JD, Gregg DE: Reactive hyperemia characteristics of the myocardium. Am J Physiol **199:** 1143, 1960
19. Olsson RA, Gregg DE: Myocardial reactive hyperemia in the unanesthetized dog. Am J Physiol **208:** 224, 1965
20. Gould KL, Lipscomb K, Hamilton GW: Physiologic basis for assessing critical coronary stenosis: instantaneous flow response and regional distribution during coronary hyperemia as measure of coronary flow reserve. Am J Cardiol **33:** 87, 1974
21. Gould KL, Lipscomb K: Effects of coronary stenoses on coronary flow reserve and resistance. Am J Cardiol **34:** 48, 1974
22. Cole JS, Hartley CJ: The pulsed Doppler coronary artery catheter. Preliminary report of a new technique for measuring rapid changes in coronary flow velocity in man. Circulation **56:** 18, 1977
23. Marcus M, Wright C, Doty D, Eastham C, Laughlin D, Krumm P, Fastenow C, Brody M: Measurements of coronary velocity and reactive hyperemia in the coronary circulation of humans. Circ Res **49:** 877, 1981
24. Vogel RA, LeFree MT, Bates ER, O'Neill WW, Foster RK, Kirlin PC, Smith D, Pitt B: Application of digital techniques to selective coronary arteriography: Use of myocardial contrast appearance time to measure coronary flow reserve. Am Heart J **107:** 153, 1984
25. Hodgson JMcB, LeGrand V, Bates ER, Mancini GBJ, Aueron FM, O'Neill WW, Simon SB, Beauman GJ, LeFree MT, Vogel RA: Validation in dogs of a rapid angiographic technique to measure relative coronary blood flow during routine cardiac catheterization. Am J Cardiol **55:** 188, 1985
26. O'Neill WW, Walton JA, Bates ER, Colfer HT, Aueron FM, LeFree MT, Pitt B, Vogel RA: Criteria for successful coronary angioplasty, as assessed by alterations in coronary vasodilator reserve. J Am Coll Cardiol **3:** 1382, 1984
27. Bates ER, Vogel RA, LeFree MT, Kirlin PC, O'Neill WW, Pitt B: The chronic coronary flow reserve provided by saphenous vein bypass grafts as determined by digital coronary radiography. Am Heart J **108:** 462, 1984
28. Pichard AD, Gorlin R, Smith H, Ambrose J, Meller J: Coronary flow studies in patients with left ventricular hypertrophy of the hypertensive type. Evidence for an impaired coronary vascular reserve. Am J Cardiol **47:** 547, 1981
29. Marcus ML, Doty DB, Hiratzka LF, Wright CB, Eastham CL: Decreased coronary reserve: A mechanism for angina pectoris in patients with aortic stenosis and normal coronary arteries. N Engl J Med **307:** 1362, 1982
30. Pichard AD, Smith H, Holt J, Meller J, Gorlin R: Coronary vascular reserve in left ventricular hypertrophy secondary to chronic aortic regurgitation. Am J Cardiol **51:** 315, 1983
31. White CW, Wright CB, Doty DB, Hiratzka LF, Eastham CL, Harrison DG, Marcus ML: Does visual interpretation of the coronary arteriogram predict the physiologic importance of a coronary stenosis? N Engl J Med **310:** 819, 1984
32. Kakos GS, Oldham HN, Dixon SH, Davis RW, Haggen P-O, Sabiston DC: Coronary artery hemodynamics after aorto-coronary artery vein bypass. J Thorac Cardiovasc Surg **63:** 849, 1972
33. Folts JD, Kahn DR, Bittar N, Rowe GG: Effects of partial obstruction on phasic flow in aortocoronary grafts. Circulation **51/52** (suppl I): I-148, 1975
34. Brandt B, Martins JB, Marcus ML: Anomolous origin of the right coronary artery from the left sinus of Valsalva. N Engl J Med **309:** 596, 1982

35. Arnett EN, Isner JM, Redwood DR, Kent KM, Baker WP, Ackerstein H, Roberts WC: Coronary artery narrowing in coronary heart disease: comparison of cineangiographic and necropsy findings. Ann Intern Med **91:** 350, 1979
36. Roberts WC, Jones AA: Quantitation of coronary arterial narrowing at necropsy in sudden coronary death: analysis of 31 patients and comparison with 25 control subjects. Am J Cardiol **44:** 39, 1978
37. Roberts WC, Jones AA: Quantification of coronary arterial narrowing at necropsy in acute transmural myocardial infarction: analysis and comparison of findings in 27 patients and 22 controls. Circulation **61:** 786, 1980
38. Barger AC, Beeuwkes R, Lainey LL, Silverman KJ: Hypothesis: vasa vasorum and neovascularization of human coronary arteries. A possible role in the pathophysiology of atherosclerosis. N Engl J Med **310:** 175, 1984
39. Furchgott RF, Zawadzki JV: The obligatory role of endothelial cells in the relaxation of arterial smooth muscle by acetylcholine. Nature **288:** 373, 1980
40. Habib JB, Wells SL, Williams CL, Henry PD: Atherosclerosis impairs endothelium-dependent arterial relaxation. Circulation **70** (suppl II): II-123, 1984 (abst)
41. Saphir O, Ohringer L, Wong R: Changes in the intramuscular coronary branches in coronary arteriosclerosis. Arch Pathol **62:** 159, 1956
42. Cannnon RO, Watson RM, Rosing DR, Epstein SE: Angina caused by reduced vasodilator reserve of the small coronary arteries. J Am Coll Cardiol **1:** 1359, 1983
43. Folts JD, Crowell EB, Rowe GG: Platelet aggregation in partially obstructed vessels and its elimination with aspirin. Circulation **54:** 365, 1976
44. Armstrong ML, Heistad DD, Marcus ML, Piegors DJ, Aboud FM: Hemodynamic sequelae of regression of experimental atherosclerosis. J Clin Invest **71:** 104, 1983
45. Vogel RA: The radiographic assessment of coronary blood flow parameters. Circulation **72:** ?, 1985
46. LeGrand V, Hodgson JMcB, Bates ER, Aueron FM, Mancini GBJ, Smith JS, Vogel RA: Abnormal coronary flow reserve and abnormal radionuclide exercise tests in patients with normal coronary angiograms. J Am Coll Cardiol **5:** 531, 1985 (abst)
47. Opherk D, Zebe H, Weihe E, Mall G, Durr C, Gravert B, Mehmel HC, Schwarz F, Kubler W: Reduced coronary dilatory capacity and ultrastructure changes of the myocardium in patients with angina pectoris but normal coronary arteriograms. Circulation **63:** 817, 1981
48. Berger HJ, Sands MJ, Davies RA, Wackers FJ, Alexander J, Lachman AS, Williams BW, Zaret BL: Exercise left ventricular performance in patients with chest pain, ischemic-appearing exercise electrocardiograms, and angiographically normal coronary arteries. Ann Intern Med **94:** 186, 1981
49. Rozanski A, Diamond GA, Forrester JS, Berman DS, Morris D, Swan HJC: Alternative referent standards for cardiac normality. Implications for diagnostic testing. Ann Intern Med **101:** 164, 1984
50. Hoffman JIE: Maximal coronary flow and the concept of vascular reserve. Circulation **70:** 153, 1984

Senning repair for transposition of the great arteries in the first week of life

G. PAUL MATHERNE, M.D., JERRY D. RAZOOK, M.D., WEBB M. THOMPSON, JR., M.D., MARY M. LANE, M.P.H., CYNTHIA K. MURRAY, M.P.H., AND RONALD C. ELKINS, M.D.

ABSTRACT Infants with D-loop transposition of the great arteries (D-TGA) may have unacceptable results after balloon septostomy while awaiting surgery. It has been our policy to repair defects in infants with D-TGA and intact ventricular septum or small ventricular septal defect at the time of diagnosis. We report our experience with the Senning operation in 18 newborns less than 1 week of age. The mean age at operation was 3 days (range 12 hr to 7 days) and the mean weight was 3.5 kg (range 2.8 to 4.8). There were two early postoperative deaths (11%) and one late death (5%). Early mortality was associated with preoperative acidosis and congestive heart failure. Late mortality was associated with severe left ventricular outflow tract obstruction (LVOTO). The 15 long-term survivors have been followed for an average of 27 months and 11 of the 16 perioperative survivors have undergone postoperative catheterizations. There was no evidence of systemic or pulmonary venous obstruction. One patient developed LVOTO that led to his death. Two patients had residual atrial shunts. Electrocardiograms revealed no major arrhythmias. All patients are clinically asymptomatic. Good hemodynamic, electrocardiographic, and clinical results can be obtained with correction of D-TGA in the first week of life.
Circulation 72, No. 4, 840–845, 1985.

MANAGEMENT OF D-loop transposition of the great arteries (D-TGA) has undergone dramatic change in the past 35 years. The development of the Blalock-Hanlon,[1, 2] Mustard,[3] Senning,[4, 5] and Jatene[6] procedures, along with Rashkind balloon septostomy,[7] has led to significant decreases in mortality and morbidity.

Recently, interest has been focused on the correct age for repair. The trend has been toward earlier correction to avoid morbidity and mortality.[8–17] The long-term results of early repair are comparable to those of later repair without the risks associated with uncorrected D-TGA.[11, 16, 17]

While palliation is achieved in many infants with D-TGA with balloon septostomy, significant complications can occur while these infants are awaiting surgery. Gutgesell et al.[18] have reported a 22% incidence of death, cerebrovascular accident, or obstructive pulmonary vascular disease in infants with palliated D-TGA awaiting surgery.[18] Because of this unacceptable morbidity and mortality, it has been the policy at our institution to repair defects in all infants with D-TGA at the time of diagnosis. We report the results of 18 infants with D-TGA corrected with the Senning procedure during the first week of life.

Methods

Patients. From April 1979 through January 1984, 18 infants 1 week or less old underwent Senning repair for D-TGA. The patient population was derived from records of the Departments of Pediatric Cardiology and Thoracic Surgery. Infants with a patent ductus arteriosus (PDA) or small ventricular septal defect (VSD) without adequate mixing were included. Initial evaluation included cardiac catheterization at our institution in 13 and at a referring hospital in five.

Surgical procedure. A modified Senning operation was performed in all 18 infants. The atrial patch was augmented with knitted Dacron in 11 patients and enlargement of the new pulmonary venous atrium with a pericardial patch was necessary in one patient. All PDAs were ligated and three patients had suture closure of a VSD. Hypothermic circulatory arrest was used in all patients (18° C in 17 and 20° C in 1). The mean period of circulatory arrest was 57 min (range 47 to 77).

Follow-up. Clinical history, physical examination, and growth parameters were reviewed along with chest roentgenograms and electrocardiograms. Postoperative cardiac catheterization was performed in 11 patients. Measurement for left ventricular outflow tract obstruction (LVOTO) was performed if clinically indicated by elevated left ventricular pressures or by the presence of a murmur suggestive of LVOTO. Pulmonary venous pressures were measured if indicated by clinical evidence of obstruction. Systemic venous obstruction was determined by measuring the gradient between the mean superior vena caval or inferior vena caval pressure and the mean system-

From the Departments of Pediatrics, Pediatric Cardiology, and Surgery, University of Oklahoma Health Sciences Center, Oklahoma City.
Address for correspondence: Ronald C. Elkins, M.D., Section of Thoracic Surgery, PO Box 26307, Oklahoma City, OK 73126.
Received April 29, 1985; revision accepted July 5, 1985.

ic venous atrial pressure. Intracardiac shunts were determined by oximetry data.

Survival analysis. Survival was analyzed by the Kaplan-Meyer method for actuarial survival.[19]

Results

Patient profile. Eighteen neonates with D-TGA underwent Senning repair between April 1979 and January 1984 (table 1). This group comprised all but five newborns with D-TGA seen at our institution during that period; one infant was excluded because repair was delayed until 2 months of age and four infants were excluded because they had VSDs. Six of the patients had no associated cardiac defects, five had associated PDA, four had an associated VSD, and three patients had both PDA and a VSD. LVOTO was not seen preoperatively. All of the patients with VSDs had small defects without adequate mixing. The age range at operation was 12 hr to 7 days (mean 3 days), and the weight range was 2.8 to 4.8 kg (mean 3.5). Sixteen patients had undergone Rashkind balloon septostomy before operation.

Preoperative and postoperative profile. Preoperative complications consisted mainly of hypoxemia and congestive heart failure. Seven patients underwent a trial of prostaglandin E_1 for persistent hypoxemia, and three of the patients received digoxin for congestive heart failure. Three patients underwent repeat Rashkind septostomy because of persistent hypoxia. Other preoperative complications were transient supraventricular tachycardia during catheterization in one patient and a blood culture positive for *Staphylococcus aureus* in one patient.

After surgical repair, all of the patients were weaned from cardiopulmonary bypass. Seven patients had transient postoperative complications that resolved without sequelae, while two patients had complications that led to their deaths. Transient complications included junctional rhythm in four, supraventricular tachycardia in one, ventricular fibrillation in one, cardiac arrest in one, and seizures in one patient. Two patients with transient junctional rhythms developed passive arrhythmias on follow-up; one of these patients had first-degree atrioventricular block and the other had ectopic atrial pacemaker and occasional junctional beats. Fatal complications included ventricular failure in one patient and severe ischemic central nervous system damage in one patient. No patient demonstrated evidence of systemic or pulmonary venous obstruction postoperatively. However, one patient who died had evidence of systemic venous obstruction and required augmentation of the systemic atrium during weaning from bypass. No patient underwent reoperation for systemic or pulmonary venous obstruction.

Among the 16 perioperative survivors the duration of ventilator support ranged from ½ to 7 days (mean 1.5). The duration of hospitalization was from 7 to 21 days (mean 11).

Mortality. The overall mortality was 17% (3/18; table 2). Two patients died during the perioperative period (perioperative mortality 11%) and one patient died at 33 months of age.

The two patients that died during the perioperative period had very complicated preoperative courses. Both patients developed severe acidosis and hypoxia that required urgent surgical correction. One patient whose pH was less than 7.03 for 5 hr before surgery developed severe neurologic dysfunction shortly after surgery. He died on the tenth postoperative day without neurologic recovery. The second patient was responsive only to deep pain with nonreactive pupils upon arrival at our institution. The emergency surgical procedure was complicated by obstruction of the superior and inferior venae cavae when the patient was first weaned from cardiopulmonary bypass, which required augmentation of the systemic atrium. The patient was weaned from bypass the second time, but died a short time later from continued hypotension and poor ventricular function. Autopsy in both infants revealed good surgical repair without evidence of systemic or pulmonary venous obstruction.

The patient who died late after surgery was found to have LVOTO and a residual VSD on postoperative catheterization at 12 months of age. At the initial catheterization he was thought to have a small 3 to 4 mm supracristal VSD, but LVOTO was not found. At 27 months of age, he underwent patch closure of the VSD, pulmonary commissurotomy, and infundibular resection. Postoperative catheterization revealed residual severe LVOTO. At 33 months of age, he under-

TABLE 1
Patient characteristics

No. of patients	18
Ratio of male/female patients	15/3
Age at operation (days)	
Mean (SEM)	3.0 (0.5)
Range	0.5–7.3
Weight at operation (kg)	
Mean (SEM)	3.5 (0.1)
Range	2.8–4.2
Associated defects	
PDA	5
VSD	4
PDA VSD	3
Rashkinds	16

TABLE 2
Findings at follow-up

Perioperative survivors	16/18 (89%)
Long-term survivors	15/18 (83%)
Length of follow-up (months)	
Mean (SEM)	27.0 (4.2)
Range	9–64
Postoperative catheterization	11/16 (69%)
Age at 1st postop. cath. (months)	
Mean (SEM)	14.6 (1.8)
Range	4–26
Pressures at postop. catheterization (mm Hg)	
Mean SVC (SEM)	6.7 (0.8)
Mean SA (SEM)	5.3 (0.6)
Mean SVC-SA gradient (SEM)	1.0 (0.3)
Mean LV	30.4 (2.8)
Electrocardiography (n)	
Sinus rhythm	11
SR primary AV block	1
Junctional rhythm	1
Ectopic pacemaker	1
Sinus bradycardia	1
Chest roentgenography (n)	
Normal	12
Increased pulmonary vasculature	1
Increased pulmonary vasculature and enlarged heart	2

SVC = superior vena caval; SA = sinoatrial; LV = left ventricular.

went repeat infundibular resection, but some LVOTO persisted and he died after surgery from ventricular failure. Autopsy revealed evidence of the previous surgical procedures along with a stenotic pulmonic valve and biventricular hypertrophy. There was no evidence of systemic or pulmonary venous obstruction.

General clinical follow-up. The 15 long-term survivors have been followed from 9 to 64 months (mean 27; table 2). All patients were asymptomatic and doing well without limitations of activity and with grossly normal development. Two patients have weights lower than the 5th percentile for their ages, but the remaining patients are growing normally.

Chest roentgenography. Chest roentgenograms showed no evidence of pulmonary venous congestion in any patient. Twelve patients had normal cardiac silhouettes and normal pulmonary vascular markings. Two patients with a residual atrial shunt had evidence of increased pulmonary vascularity; one of these had mild cardiomegaly. One other patient had mild cardiomegaly with prominent pulmonary vascular markings.

Electrocardiography. No major arrhythmias were detected in any patient. Sinus rhythm was present in 11 patients, as determined from the follow-up electrocardiogram. Five patients had passive arrhythmias, including first-degree atrioventricular block, junctional rhythm, ectopic atrial pacemaker with occasional junctional beats, and sinus bradycardia with occasional junctional beats.

The patient with the sinus bradycardia had a possible episode of supraventricular tachycardia at another hospital, but the episode was not documented and has not recurred.

Cardiac catheterization. Postoperative cardiac catheterization was performed in 69% (11/16) of the patients who survived the perioperative period. The mean age at catheterization was 14.5 months (range 4 to 26). No patient demonstrated evidence of pulmonary or systemic venous obstruction. The superior vena caval–to–systemic venous atrial gradient ranged from 0 to 2.5 mm Hg. We were unable to enter the inferior vena cava from the femoral vein in two patients, but neither showed angiographic or hemodynamic evidence of systemic venous obstruction. All patients had evidence of good systemic and pulmonary ventricular function. Two patients had evidence of residual atrial shunts. One of the patients with a residual atrial shunt had evidence of mild LVOTO (23 mm Hg gradient) that was thought to be secondary to flow. One patient had severe LVOTO, with an 85 mm Hg gradient. One patient showed evidence of mitral incompetence that was thought to be catheter induced.

Survival analysis. Survival was analyzed with the Kaplan-Meyer method for actuarial survival for small samples.[19] The resulting estimated cumulative patient survival curve for the 18 patients is shown in figure 1. The estimated 2 year survival rate is 89%, with nine patients so far having survived 2 years.

Discussion

The infant with D-TGA after septostomy is at risk for many complications, including recurrent hypoxia,[20] cerebrovascular accidents,[18, 21, 22] pulmonary

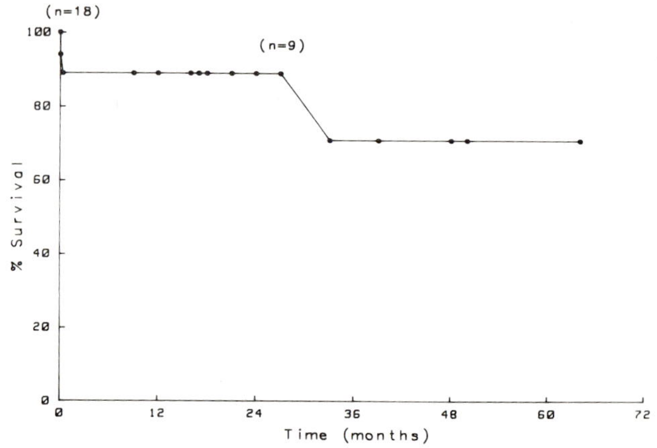

FIGURE 1. Cumulative patient survival computed by the Kaplan-Meyer method.

hypertension,[23, 24] growth retardation,[25] and death. Mortality for infants after septostomy and before correction varies from 12% to 28%.[18, 20, 26–30] The high mortality for infants awaiting repair has led to earlier repair,[8–17] but the optimal age has remained controversial.

Our data show that the Senning procedure can be performed in the first week of life with excellent results. The perioperative mortality of 11% (2/18) is comparable to that in other series in infants[14, 16, 17] and in older patients.[5, 11, 31–34] The two patients who died in the perioperative period were both moribund at the time of surgery because of complicated preoperative courses. The patient who died late after surgery developed intractable LVOTO and expired after the second surgical procedure to relieve the obstruction. It is encouraging that no deaths were associated with complications related to the Senning procedure; all were associated with preoperative condition or additional cardiac anomalies.

Few studies have taken into account preoperative morbidity and mortality along with perioperative mortality in the analysis of final outcome of treatment of D-TGA. Among infants with uncomplicated D-TGA who were treated with septostomy, Gutgesell et al.[18] reported 8% mortality during the first month of life. Among the 1 month survivors they reported an additional 14% incidence of death or major complication in infants awaiting surgical correction. Their estimated 2 year survival for patients with uncomplicated and complicated (significant VSD and LVOTO) D-TGA was 70%. Our survival rate of 90% at 2 years compares favorably. Although the study by Gutgesell et al.[18] included patients with complicated D-TGA and included patients who had undergone the Mustard procedure, it highlights the significant morbidity and mortality that occur in infants with D-TGA after septostomy and before surgical correction.

Postoperative complications in survivors were transient without sequelae. No patient with postoperative rhythm disturbances showed evidence of significant arrhythmias on long-term follow-up. There were no long-term neurologic sequelae in the patients who experienced cardiopulmonary arrest or seizures. While the incidence of postoperative complications was disquieting, the long-term morbidity and mortality was not affected.

The long-term complications of the Senning procedure include pulmonary[11, 17, 32, 34] and systemic venous obstruction,[11, 17, 32] arrhythmias,[5, 14, 17, 31, 33] and residual atrial shunts.[5, 11, 17] The incidence of these complications with the Senning procedure is lower than with the Mustard operation, but they remain a significant problem. Some authors[8, 35] have suggested that complications occur more frequently with the Mustard operation in young patients, but this has not been found with the Senning procedure.[11]

Systemic venous obstruction was not found in the patients in our series. This compares favorably with the reported incidence of up to 5% in infants[17] and up to 10% in older patients.[11] Although the length of follow-up is limited (mean 27 months), our results are encouraging. Pulmonary venous obstruction was also not found in our patients. Others have reported incidences of up to 16% in infants[17] and 10% in older patients.[11]

The incidence of residual atrial shunts was 11% (2/18) in this series. Neither of the patients with a shunt is symptomatic, although one weighs less than the 5th percentile weight for his age. It is planned that both patients will have elective repair in the future. Development of atrial shunts has been reported after the Senning procedure, with an incidence up to 15% in older patients[5] and an incidence of up to 12.5% in infants.[11] Whether this complication is related to age and size or some other factor is not known, but it has not been a significant cause of morbidity and mortality.

The incidence of LVOTO was 11% (2/18). In one patient it was severe and led to death and in the other patient it was mild and believed to be secondary to flow from an atrial shunt. In other series, LVOTO has been reported to occur in up to 59% of the patients, with severe LVOTO in 8%.[11, 17]

The incidence of passive arrhythmias was 25% in our series and no active arrhythmias were noted. No morbidity or mortality was related to arrhythmia. Other series have reported transient junctional rhythm postoperatively[5, 14, 17, 31, 32] and on follow-up.[5, 17] The presence of active arrhythmias that require pacemaker implantation have also been reported after the Senning procedure.[11, 14] Whether or not passive arrhythmia will change to active ones is not known, but these patients will require close follow-up.

No patient in this series showed evidence of cardiorespiratory compromise. They were all reported to be in general good health with grossly normal development. Two patients did have weights lower than the 5th percentile for their ages. One patient had an atrial septal defect on postoperative catheterization that may have been the cause of growth failure. The other patient had a normal postoperative study and there was no identifiable cause for his low weight.

This report and others[36] have demonstrated the ability to surgically correct the heart defects of children with uncomplicated D-TGA during the first week of life and the operative mortality in this and the other studies was similar. The decision of whether to use the Jatene arterial switch procedure or to perform a Senning procedure should be based on the child's anatomy and the surgeons experience. The Senning procedure is not as technically demanding as the Jatene and may not result in as many late operative complications. The incidence of late anastomotic stricture at the coronary artery anatomosis or the arterial, pulmonary, or aortic anastomosis is not known, particularly in children who undergo the Jatene procedure as neonates. The incidence of late operative complications in this series of patients is gratifyingly low, but the incidence of late sequelae due to the right ventricle and the tricuspid valve being subjected to systemic pressures indicate the necessity for continued long-term follow-up.

Correcting heart defects in infants with D-TGA during the first week of life offers several advantages over later repair. With early repair the significant morbidity and mortality associated with palliation in infants with D-TGA[18, 20–30] can be avoided, thereby improving the overall mortality and morbidity of infants with D-TGA. Early repair also has the advantage of decreasing the duration of cyanosis, which has been associated with poor somatic growth[37, 38] and decreased cognitive and gross motor development[39, 40] and has been postulated to be associated with late right ventricular dysfunction.[33, 41] While the period of follow-up in this study was short (mean 27 months) and the number of patients was small (n = 18), the results presented are convincing evidence in favor of early elective repair of infants with D-TGA.

We gratefully acknowledge the willingness of Drs. Charles L. Cooper and Michael J. Hirschklau of St. Francis Hospital in Tulsa to allow us to include their patients in this report.

References

1. Blalock A, Hanlon CR: Interatrial septal defect — its experimental production under direct vision without interruption of the circulation. Surg Gynecol Obstet **87:** 183, 1948
2. Blalock A, Hanlon CR: The surgical treatment of complete transposition of the aorta and the pulmonary artery. Surg Gynecol Obstet **90:** 1, 1950
3. Mustard WT: Successful two stage correction of transposition of the great vessels. Surgery **55:** 469, 1964
4. Senning A: Surgical correction of transposition of the great vessels. Surgery **45:** 966, 1959
5. Quaegebeur JM, Rohmer J, Brom AG: Revival of the Senning operation in the treatment of transposition of the great arteries. Thorax **32:** 517, 1977
6. Jatene AD, Fontes VF, Paulista PP, Souza LCB, Neger F, Galantier M, Sousa JEMR: Anatomic correction of transposition of the great vessels. J Thorac Cardiovasc Surg **72:** 364, 1976
7. Rashkind WJ, Miller WW: Creation of an atrial septal defect without thoracotomy — a palliative approach to transposition of the great arteries. JAMA **196:** 991, 1966
8. Stark J, deLeval MR, Waterston DJ, Graham GR, Bonham-Carter RE: Corrective surgery of transposition of the great arteries in the first year of life. J Thorac Cardiovasc Surg **67:** 673, 1974
9. Egloff LP, Freed MD, Dick M, Norwood WI, Castaneda AR: Early and late results with Mustard operation in infancy. Ann Thorac Surg **26:** 474, 1978
10. Turley K, Ebert PA: Total correction of transposition of the great arteries. J Thorac Cardiovasc Surg **76:** 312, 1978
11. Marx GR, Hougen TJ, Norwood WI, Fyler DC, Castaneda AR, Nadas AS: Transposition of the great arteries with intact ventricular septum: results of Mustard and Senning operations in 123 consecutive patients. J Am Coll Cardiol **1:** 476, 1983
12. Kawabori I, Guntheroth WG, Morgan BC, Mohri H, Dillard DH: Surgical correction in infancy to reduce mortality in transposition of the great arteries. Pediatrics **60:** 83, 1977
13. Bailey LL, Jacobson JG, Merritt WH, Doroshaw RW, Petry EL: Mustard operation in the first month of life. Am J Cardiol **49:** 766, 1982
14. Fortune RL, Paquet M, Collins-Nakai RL, Duncan NF: Intracardiac repair of dextro-transposition of the great arteries in the newborn period. Early and late results. J Thorac Cardiovasc Surg **85:** 371, 1983
15. Idriss FS, Paul MH, Deleon SY, Muster AJ, Nikaidoh H, Tin N: Mustard operation for transposition of the great arteries in the first three months of life. Am J Cardiol **43:** 346, 1979 (abst)
16. Mahony L, Turley K, Ebert P, Heymann MA: Long-term results after atrial repair of transposition of the great arteries in early infancy. Circulation **66:** 253, 1982
17. DeLeon VH, Hougen TJ, Norwood WI, Lang P, Marx GR, Castaneda A: Results of the Senning operation for transposition of the great arteries with intact ventricular septum in neonates. Circulation **70**(suppl I): I-21, 1984
18. Gutgesell HP, Garson A, McNamara DG: Prognosis for the newborn with transposition of the great arteries. Am J Cardiol **44:** 96, 1979
19. Lee ET: Statistical methods for survival data analysis. Belmont, CA, 1980, Lifetime Learning Publications, p 76
20. Henny CG, Goldring D, Hartman AF, Weldon CS, Straus AW: Treatment of D-Transposition of the great arteries: management of hypoxemia after balloon atrial septostomy. Am J Cardiol **47:** 299, 1981
21. Tynan M: Survival of infants with transposition of great arteries after balloon atrial septostomy. Lancet **1:** 621, 1971
22. Parsons CG, Astley R, Burrows FGO, Singh SP: Transposition of the great arteries. A study of 65 infants followed 1 to 4 years after balloon septostomy. Br Heart J **33:** 725, 1971
23. Newfeld EA, Paul MH, Muster AJ, Idriss FS: Pulmonary vascular disease in transposition of the great vessels and intact ventricular septum. Circulation **59:** 525, 1979
24. Clarkson PM, Neutze JM, Wardill JC, Barratt-Boyes BG: The pulmonary vascular bed in patients with complete transposition of the great arteries. Circulation **53:** 539, 1976
25. Levy RJ, Rosenthal A, Castaneda AR, Nadas AS: Growth after surgical repair for simple D-Transposition of the great arteries. Ann Thorac Surg **25:** 225, 1978
26. Rashkind WJ, Miller WW: Transposition of the great arteries. Results of palliation by balloon atrioseptostomy in thirty-one infants. Circulation **38:** 453, 1968
27. Clarkson PM, Barratt-Boyes BG, Neutze JM, Lowes JB: Results over a ten year period of palliation followed by corrective surgery for complete transposition of the great arteries. Circulation **45:** 1251, 1972
28. Kidd BSL: The fate of children with transposition of the great arteries following balloon atrial septostomy. *In* Kidd BSL, Rowe RD, editors: The children with congenital heart disease after surgery. New York, 1976, Futura, p 153
29. Gutgesell HP, McNamara DG: Transposition of the great arteries: results of treatment with early palliation and late intracardiac repair. Circulation **51:** 32, 1975
30. Neches WH, Mullins CE, McNamara DG: The infant with transposition of the great arteries. II. Results of balloon atrial septostomy. Am Heart J **84:** 603, 1972
31. Parenzan L, Locatelli G, Alfieri O, Villani M, Invernizzi G, Pacifico AD: The Senning operation for transposition of the great arteries. J Thorac Cardiovasc Surg **76:** 305, 1978
32. Otero Coto E, Norwood WI, Lang P, Castaneda AR: Modified

Senning operation for treatment of transposition of the great arteries. J Thorac Cardiovasc Surg **78:** 721, 1979

33. Bender HW Jr, Graham TP Jr, Boucek RJ, Walker WE, Boerth RG: Comparative operative results of the Senning and Mustard procedures for transposition of the great arteries. Circulation **62**(suppl I): I-197, 1980
34. Alvarez Diaz F, Cabo Salvador J, Rivas J, Alvarado F, Cordovilla Zurdo G: Technical advances in the Senning operation. Thorac Cardiovasc Surg **31:** 105, 1983
35. Clarkson PM, Neutze JM, Barratt-Boyes BG, Brandt PWT: Late postoperative hemodynamic results and cineangiographic findings after mustard atrial baffle repair of transposition of the great arteries. Circulation **53:** 525, 1976
36. Castaneda AR, Norwood WI, Jonas RA, Colon SD, Sanders SP, Lang P: Transposition of the great arteries and intact ventricular septum: anatomical repair in neonate. Ann Thorac Surg **38:** 438, 1984
37. Feldt RH, Strickler GS, Weidman WH: Growth of children with congenital heart disease. Am J Dis Child **117:** 573, 1969
38. Linde LM, Dunn OJ, Schireson R, Rasof B: Growth in children with congenital heart disease. J Pediatr **70:** 413, 1967
39. Newburger JW, Silbert AR, Buckley LP, Fyler DC: Cognitive function and age at repair of transposition of the great arteries in children. N Engl J Med **310:** 1495, 1984
40. Newburger JW, Tucker AD, Silbert AR, Fyler DC: Motor function and timing of surgery in transposition of the great arteries, intact ventricular septum. Pediatr Cardiol **4:** 317, 1983 (abst)
41. Graham TP Jr, Atwood GF, Boucek RJ Jr, Boerth RC, Bender HW: Abnormalities of right ventricular function following Mustard's operation for transposition of the great arteries. Circulation **52:** 678, 1975

Comparative systemic and renal effects of dopamine and angiotensin-converting enzyme inhibition with enalaprilat in patients with heart failure

CAROL S. MASKIN, M.D., STEVEN OCKEN, M.D., BRIAN CHADWICK, R.N., AND THIERRY H. LEJEMTEL, M.D.

ABSTRACT Renal and systemic hemodynamics were measured during titration of dopamine and serially after intravenous administration of enalaprilat in nine patients with chronic severe congestive heart failure. During titration of dopamine, renal blood flow increased by 99%, from 304 ± 120 to 604 ± 234 ml/min ($p < .01$) at a dose of dopamine of 2.1 μg/kg/min, which produced only a 21% increase in cardiac index, from 1.96 ± 0.36 to 2.38 ± 0.35 liters/min/m^2 ($p < .05$). Cardiac index was increased maximally at a dose of 4.0 μg/kg/min dopamine; however, renal blood flow was not further augmented. In contrast, after intravenous administration of enalaprilat, peak improvement of renal blood flow and cardiac index occurred concomitantly. Renal blood flow increased by 35%, from 316 ± 97 to 427 ± 107 ml/min ($p < .05$), and cardiac index increased by 18%, from 1.99 ± 0.40 to 2.35 ± 0.40 liters/min/m^2 ($p < .05$). At similar increases in cardiac index, dopamine produced a greater increase in renal blood flow than enalaprilat: 604 ± 234 vs 427 ± 107 ml/min ($p < .05$). Mean systemic arterial pressure, however, was greater with dopamine than with enalaprilat (78.1 ± 16.7 vs 70.2 ± 17.2 mm Hg; $p < .05$) at peak effect. Thus, although both drugs appear to be potent renal vasodilators in patients with severe congestive heart failure, dopamine may be more effective in augmenting renal blood flow.
Circulation 72, No. 4, 846–852, 1985.

IN PATIENTS with severe congestive heart failure, blood flow to the kidneys is reduced.[1] Although it is unclear whether this reduction in renal blood flow is proportionate to the fall in cardiac output,[2,3] drugs that increase cardiac performance as well as specifically dilate the renal vasculature are of particular interest in the treatment of this entity.

Both inhibition of the angiotensin II–converting enzyme[4] and stimulation of dopaminergic receptors[5] have been shown to selectively increase renal blood flow in patients with congestive heart failure. Because both pharmacologic interventions are now available[6–8] or are under investigation for long-term use in patients with congestive heart failure, it is of interest to compare their relative effects on systemic and renal hemodynamics. Accordingly, this study was undertaken to evaluate the effects of ascending doses of dopamine on cardiac output and renal blood flow in patients with congestive heart failure and to compare these effects with those of intravenously administered enalaprilat, an angiotensin-converting enzyme inhibitor presently under investigation.

From the Division of Cardiology, Department of Medicine, The Albert Einstein College of Medicine, Bronx, NY.

Address for correspondence: Thierry H. LeJemtel, Division of Cardiology, Albert Einstein College of Medicine, 1300 Morris Park Ave., Bronx, NY 10461.

Received March 5, 1985; revision accepted June 27, 1985.

Methods

Patients. Eight men and one woman with severe congestive heart failure, consistent with functional class III or IV according to the New York Heart Association, were studied (average age 59 years, range 34 to 71). The etiology of heart failure was coronary artery disease in five patients and an idiopathic cardiomyopathy in four. Left ventricular ejection fraction was less than 20% in all patients. Eight patients were in sinus rhythm, and one patient was in atrial fibrillation. All were markedly limited in physical activity by fatigue and/or dyspnea, and the average maximum oxygen uptake during graded treadmill exercise was 11.5 ± 2.0 ml/kg/min. No patient had sustained a myocardial infarction within 1 month of the study. Patients were on optimal and stable doses of furosemide and digoxin for 2 weeks, and the mean digoxin level immediately before the study was 1.2 ng/ml. Creatinine clearance, determined during a 24 hr urine collection the day before the study, averaged 72 ± 10.5 ml/min.

Patients were admitted to the coronary care unit and maintained on a 2 g/day sodium diet for at least 3 days before the study. Daily doses of digoxin and furosemide were maintained throughout the study and administered at night. The nature, potential benefits, and possible risks of the study were fully explained to the patients, who gave their written consent.

Hemodynamics. On the day of study, right heart catheterization was performed in all patients by means of a triple-lumen, flow-directed, balloon-tipped catheter (Edwards Laboratories). An intra-arterial catheter was inserted percutaneously into a radial artery for measurement of systemic arterial pressure. Systemic arterial, right atrial, pulmonary arterial, and pulmonary capillary wedge pressures were determined with Gould Statham P23ID transducers and recorded on an Electronics for Medicine photographic recorder. Cardiac output was determined in triplicate (less than 10% variation) by the thermodiluton technique, with iced 5% dextrose and a bedside computer (Model 9250A). Heart rate was recorded continuously from two bedside electrocardiographic monitoring devices.

Renal blood flow was determined as the left renal venous blood flow by the continuous thermodilution technique[9–11] with a No. 7F dual thermistor catheter (Webster Laboratories). The catheter is preformed with a curved terminal bend as previously described,[12, 13] to facilitate introduction and stable positioning in the renal vein. The injection orifice is located 15 mm proximal to the distal end and on the concavity of the bend to prevent vascular wall contact, with the opening obliquely oriented at 30 to 40 degrees against the blood stream to increase turbulence and to ensure optimal indicator/blood admixture. The external "dilution" thermistor is located 10 mm proximal to the injection orifice, and the second "indicator" thermistor is within the catheter just proximal to the orifice. The catheter was introduced into the femoral vein via the Seldinger technique and guided into the left renal vein under fluoroscopy. Optimal positioning within the renal vein and the absence of accessory veins were confirmed by injection of meglumine diatrizoate through the catheter. The position was confirmed by determination of the oxygen saturation of venous blood withdrawn from the catheter, which was greater than 85% in all cases. Determination of oxygen saturation of blood withdrawn from the catheter was repeated frequently during the study. At the end of the study, the position of the catheter was reconfirmed under fluoroscopy.

For each determination of blood flow, room temperature 5% dextrose was infused through the catheter by a Harvard pump (Model 921) at a constant rate of 50 ml/min until the resistance deflections of both thermistors consequent to the thermal dilution temperature changes were stable. Each renal blood flow was measured at least five times, and three measurements within 10% were averaged. A standard three-channel thermodilution Wheatstone Bridge (Webster Laboratories) was used to convert the resistance changes into calibrated voltages, which were recorded on photographic paper. Blood flow was then calculated from the formula derived by Ganz et al.[9]:

$$F_B = F_I \times 1.08\ (\Delta T_I/\Delta T_B) - 1$$

where F = flow (ml/min); B = blood; I = indicator; T = temperature (°C). A previously validated modification of this formula, derived to correct for thermotransport within the Webster catheter at blood flow rates ranging from 300 to 1500 ml/min,[14] was used:

$$F_{B\text{-corr}} = (F_{B\text{-uncorr}} \times 1.427) - 130$$

Such correction was made in the calculation of renal blood flow in patients 1, 2, 3, 5, 7, and 8.

The following parameters were determined: cardiac index (liters/min/m^2) = cardiac output/body surface area; stroke volume index (ml/m^2) = cardiac index × 1000/heart rate; systemic vascular resistance (dyne-sec-cm^{-5}) = 80 × (mean systemic arterial pressure − right atrial pressure)/cardiac output; renal vascular resistance (dyne-sec-cm^{-5} × 10^3) = 80 (mean systemic arterial pressure − right atrial pressure)/renal blood flow.

Hemodynamic parameters were determined during the first control period before infusion of dopamine, at each dose (μg/kg/min) during the dopamine titration, during the second control period before administration of enalaprilat by intravenous bolus, and thereafter at intervals of 30, 60, 90, and 120 min after the administration of enalaprilat.

Plasma renin activity. Blood samples were withdrawn for determinations of plasma renin activity in all patients during the control periods before infusion of dopamine and before administration of enalaprilat, at the dose rate resulting in peak augmentation of renal blood flow during infusion of dopamine, and at the time of maximum increase in renal blood flow after the intravenous bolus of enalaprilat. Before each control period, patients assumed the supine position for 30 to 60 min and remained supine during the dopamine titration and for 2 hr after administration of enalaprilat. Mixed venous blood was withdrawn from the indwelling thermodilution catheter into chilled collection tubes containing ethylenediaminetetraacetate. Specimens were immediately centrifuged and the plasma was removed and maintained at 4°C. Plasma renin activity (ng/ml/hr) was measured by radioimmunoassay of generated angiotensin I by use of a commercially available kit (Immutrope ER, Squibb & Sons, Princeton, NJ).

Drug administration

Dopamine. After baseline determinations and while the patient was in the fasting state, dopamine was infused at an initial dose of 1 μg/kg/min and increased every 10 min by 1 μg/kg/min until a maximal cardiac output was reached or undesirable side effects were elicited. Adverse effects were defined as a 10% increase in heart rate or systolic arterial pressure above control values or as precipitation of recurrent episodes of nonsustained ventricular tachycardia. Measurements were repeated after 5 min at each rate of infusion.

Enalaprilat. Three hours after administration of dopamine and after return of systemic and renal hemodynamics to baseline values, enalaprilat was administered to all patients as a single intravenous bolus at a dose of 2.5 mg in four patients, 10 mg in three, and 5 mg in the remaining two. A dose-ranging study in these patients demonstrated similar peak hemodynamic responses to doses ranging from 2.5 to 10 mg. Measurements were repeated at 30, 60, 90, and 120 min after intravenous bolus of enalaprilat.

Statistical analysis. The results are expressed as mean ± SD and were considered significant at $p < .05$. Statistical significance for effects of titration of dopamine and duration of effects of enalaprilat are based on the results of analysis of variance techniques. Comparison of the systemic and renal hemodynamic effects of dopamine and enalaprilat were made using a two-factor repeated measures analysis of variance.

Results

Hemodynamic results. During infusion of dopamine at increasing rates, renal blood flow and cardiac index did not rise in parallel (figure 1). In eight of the nine patients, renal blood flow increased maximally at an infusion rate of 2 μg/kg/min, whereas in one patient this occurred at an infusion rate of 3 μg/kg/min. Thus, at an average infusion rate of 2.1 μg/kg/min, renal blood flow increased from 304 ± 120 ml at control to a peak of 604 ± 234 ml/min ($p < .01$), and cardiac index increased from 1.96 ± 0.36 to 2.38 ± 0.35

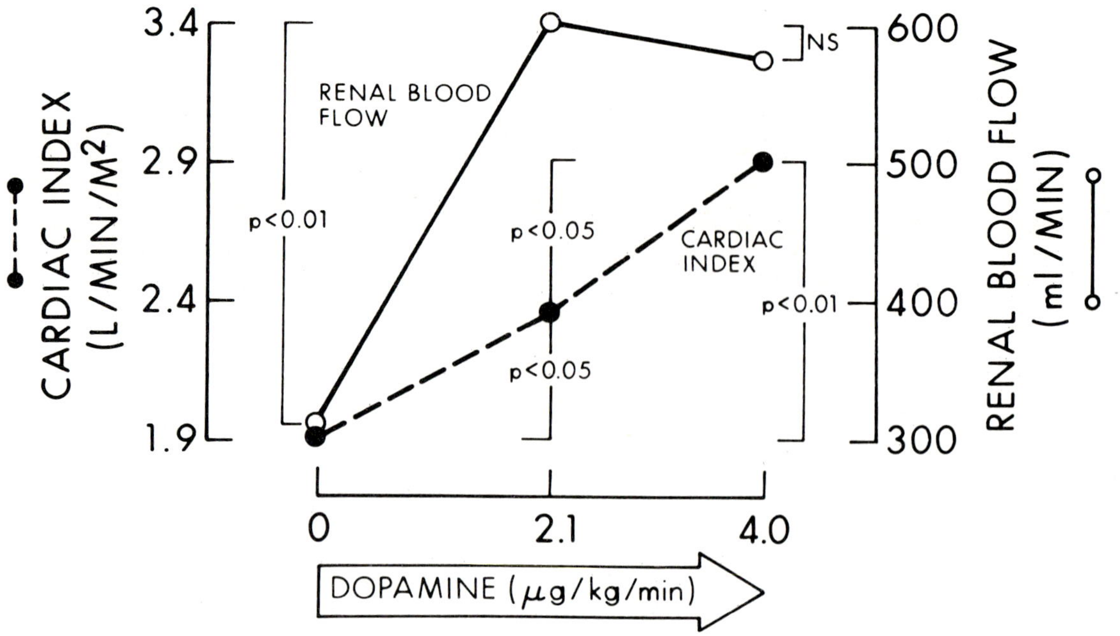

FIGURE 1. Changes in cardiac index and renal blood flow in response to ascending doses of dopamine.

liters/min/m^2 ($p < .05$). The ratio of renal blood flow to cardiac output, which was 17 ± 7% during the control period, increased to 27 ± 8%. Concomitantly, systemic and renal vascular resistances fell from 1682 ± 524 to 1348 ± 324 dyne-sec-cm^{-5} ($p < .05$) and from 20.5 ± 5.4 to 11.0 ± 2.9 dyne-sec-cm^{-5} × 10^3 ($p < .05$), respectively.

A maximum increase in cardiac index was obtained in seven patients at a rate of infusion averaging 4 μg/kg/min (range 3 to 5). In the remaining two patients, ventricular arrhythmias limited the maximum rate of infusion to 4 μg/kg/min. Thus, at a mean infusion rate of 4.0 μg/kg/min, cardiac index increased further from 2.38 ± 0.35 to a peak of 2.87 ± 0.46 liters/min/m^2 ($p < .05$), whereas renal blood flow had not changed significantly, 604 ± 234 vs 572 ± 222 ml/min. The peak increase in cardiac index was accompanied by a further reduction in systemic vascular resistance from 1384 ± 322 to 1114 ± 271 dyne-sec-cm^{-5} ($p < .01$). Renal vascular resistance was unchanged, 11.0 ± 2.9 vs 11.6 ± 2.6 dyne-sec-cm^{-5} × 10^3. At maximum increase in cardiac index, the changes in mean systemic arterial and pulmonary capillary wedge pressures were not significant when compared with control values, 81.8 ± 17.1 vs 80.2 ± 15.9 mm Hg and 22.8 ± 5.8 vs 20.9 ± 6.3 mm Hg, respectively. Similarly, heart rate did not change significantly.

After intravenous administration of enalaprilat, left ventricular performance improved in all patients (table 1). The maximal increase in cardiac index and renal blood flow and the maximal decrease in mean systemic arterial pressure occurred simultaneously 30 min after administration of enalaprilat (figure 2). At that point, cardiac index had increased from 1.99 ± 0.40 to 2.35 ± 0.40 liters/min/m^2 ($p < .05$) and renal blood flow from 316 ± 97 to 427 ± 108 ml/min ($p < .01$), whereas mean systemic arterial pressure had decreased from 79.1 ± 15.4 to 70.2 ± 17.2 mm Hg ($p < .01$). Changes in other parameters are detailed in table 1. The ratio of renal blood flow to cardiac output increased from 18 ± 5% at control to a peak of 23 ± 7% ($p < .05$). Renal blood flow increased in every patient, notwithstanding reduction in mean systemic arterial pressure by as great as 20 mm Hg or to as low as 46 mm Hg. At 60 min after the intravenous bolus of enalaprilat, mean systemic arterial pressure, renal blood flow, and systemic vascular resistance were still significantly different from baseline values. The other parameters were not, although they had not returned to baseline values at 60 min.

Both dopamine and enalaprilat produced relatively greater increases in renal blood flow than cardiac index. However, with dopamine, the peak renal blood flow was significantly greater than that attained with enalaprilat, 604 ± 254 vs 427 ± 107 ml/min ($p < .05$), whereas the cardiac index values measured concomitantly were similar with both drugs, 2.38 ± 0.35 vs 2.35 ± 0.40 liters/min/m^2 (figure 3). Mean systemic arterial pressure was significantly lower with enalaprilat than with dopamine, 70.2 ± 17.2 vs 78.1 ± 16.7 mm Hg ($p < .05$). Systemic vascular resistance

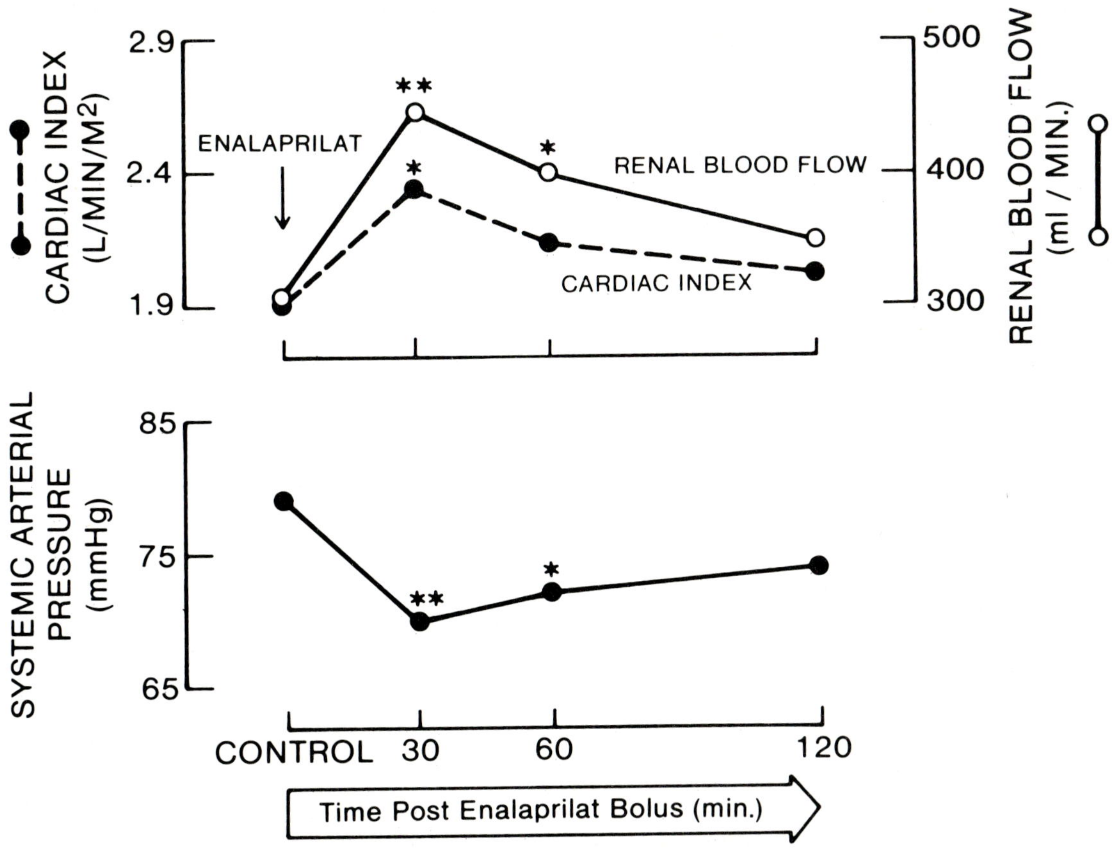

FIGURE 2. Cardiac index, renal blood flow, and mean systemic arterial pressure during the control period and at 30, 60, and 120 min after intravenous bolus of enalaprilat. $*p < .05$; $**p < .01$.

was also lower but not significantly, 1235 ± 414 vs 1348 ± 324 dyne-sec-cm^{-5}.

Plasma renin activity. After the intravenous bolus of enalaprilat, plasma renin activity measured at peak increase in renal blood flow rose from 3.5 ± 0.5 to 10.6 ± 1.1 ng/ml/hr ($p < .05$). During infusion of dopamine, plasma renin activity did not change significantly when compared with control values, 3.8 ± 0.4 vs 3.5 ± 0.8 ng/ml/hr.

Discussion

In this study, renal blood flow was determined by local thermodilution technique during titration of dopamine and serially after intravenous administration of enalaprilat in patients with chronic severe congestive heart failure, with concomitant assessment of systemic hemodynamic parameters. During titration of dopamine, improvement of renal blood flow was greater than that achieved with enalaprilat and was found to peak at a low dose before maximal augmentation of cardiac performance. In contrast, peak increase in renal blood flow and cardiac output subsequent to administration of enalaprilat occurred concurrently.

In instrumented dogs, dopamine selectively increases renal blood flow predominantly by dilating the renal vasculature rather than by enhancing cardiac performance.[15] Similarly, Hollenberg et al.,[16] using the xenon washout technique, demonstrated in normal subjects that renal blood flow was optimized by a dose of 3 μg/kg/min dopamine. In hypertensive patients, Breckenridge et al.[17] showed an improvement in the renal fraction of the cardiac output in response to dopamine in doses of 1 to 2 μg/kg/min. In patients with congestive heart failure, McDonald et al.[5] found an increase in renal blood flow at an average dose of 2.6 μg/kg/min dopamine (range 1.3 to 3.6).

Rosenblum et al.,[18] using the para-aminohippurate clearance method, observed similar improvements in renal blood flow as well as the renal fraction of cardiac output in patients with heart failure in response to dopamine doses ranging in individuals from 2.1 to 5.8 μg/kg/min. However, the dose-response relationships for the renal and systemic hemodynamic effects of dopamine were not characterized in these two previous studies.

Indeed, the para-aminohippurate clearance method previously used to determine renal blood flow, did not provide for the instantaneous and repetitive measurements needed to establish a dose-response curve.[19] In contrast, measurement of renal blood flow by local

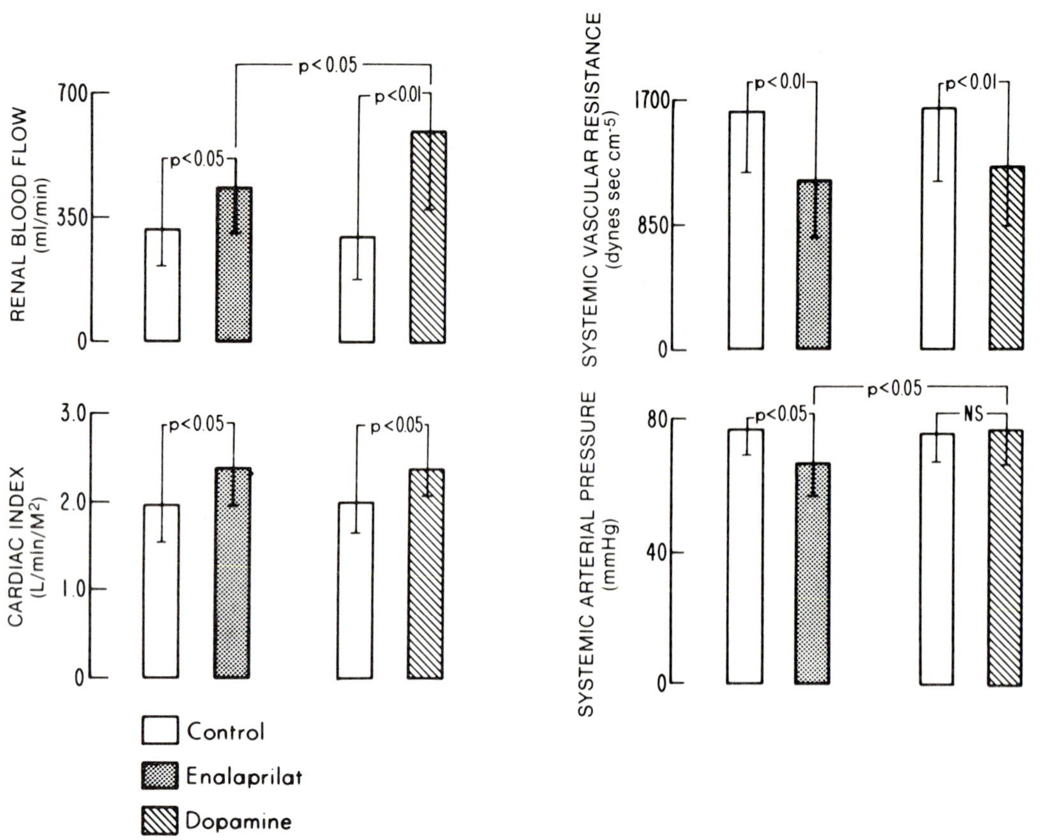

FIGURE 3. Cardiac index, mean systemic arterial pressure, and systemic vascular resistance during the control period and at peak increase in renal blood flow after intravenous bolus of enalaprilat and during infusion of dopamine.

thermodilution technique is more appropriate for such an analysis by allowing temporal correlations with systemic hemodynamic parameters.

In this study, the maximum increase in renal blood flow averaged 99% and was attained at a dopamine dose of 2.1 μg/kg/min, which produced only a 21% increase in cardiac output. Such selective improvement in renal perfusion is consistent with specific renal vasodilatation, mediated via stimulation of postsynaptic dopaminergic receptors. In addition, stimulation of presynaptic dopaminergic receptors with adrenergic-inhibiting activity may have facilitated renal vasodilatation in patients with severe heart failure in whom heightened sympathetic activity contributes to elevated renal vascular resistance.[20] At peak increase in cardiac output, which occurred at an average dopamine dose of 4 μg/kg/min, renal blood flow had not increased further. In fact, it had even decreased in some patients who experienced a concomitant increase in systemic arterial pressure. Indeed, with higher doses of dopamine, further improvement in renal blood flow may have been effectively countered by concurrent dopamine-mediated stimulation of renal vascular α-adrenergic receptors. In fact, studies by McNay et al.[15] have demonstrated that the renal vasoconstrictor effects of dopamine can be completely eliminated in dogs by pretreatment with the α-adrenergic blocking agent phenoxybenzamine.

Intravenous administration of enalaprilat improved cardiac performance in all patients, whereas systemic arterial pressure and vascular resistance were significantly reduced. Renal blood flow was improved substantially by enalaprilat. However, in contrast to the response to dopamine, peak augmentation of renal blood flow and cardiac output were concurrent, thereby suggesting similar mechanisms for both systemic and regional circulatory effects. The selective improvement in renal blood flow observed after administration of enalaprilat is consistent with a major role of angiotensin II in mediating renal vasoconstriction and thereby reduced renal blood flow in patients with severe heart failure. The rise in plasma renin activity noted at peak hemodynamic effect attests to the inhibition of the angiotensin-converting enzyme by enalaprilat. Whether inhibition of bradykinin degradation or enhanced prostaglandin production also contribute to the systemic hemodynamic effects of enalaprilat is still unclear. Nonetheless, these mechanisms do not appear to be important mediators of renal vasodilatation.[21]

Our findings with enalaprilat were consistent with

the short-term effects of the angiotensin-converting enzyme inhibitor captopril on renal hemodynamics reported by Creager et al.[22]; however, they differ from the experience of Powers et al.[23] In the latter study, despite short-term improvement in systemic hemodynamics, renal flow, determined by para-aminohippurate clearance, did not change during the first few days of therapy with captopril. Of importance, the reduction

TABLE 1
Short-term regional and systemic hemodynamic effects of enalaprilat

Patient	Dose (mg)	T (min)	CI (l/min/m²)	HR (beats/min)	SAP (mm Hg)	PCWP (mm Hg)	SVR (dyne-sec-cm⁻⁵)	RBF (ml/min)	RVR (dyne-sec-cm⁻⁵ × 10³)
1	2.5	0	2.40	96	100	20	1729	438	17.3
		30	2.84	92	80	12	1199	465	13.4
		60	2.87	86	90	18	1276	502	13.4
		120	2.44	92	95	22	1555	452	19.2
2	5.0	0	1.73	110	77	34	1764	309	17.3
		30	2.12	106	70	30	1332	373	13.1
		60	2.03	108	70	30	1572	337	14.2
		120	2.05	114	80	37	1368	277	20.2
3	2.5	0	2.42	89	80	22	1213	412	15.5
		30	2.56	86	70	12	1004	522	10.7
		60	2.54	85	70	18	1071	533	9.4
		120	2.40	83	72	16	1101	445	12.9
4	2.5	0	1.57	95	68	22	1551	225	21.0
		30	1.80	78	58	15	1145	320	12.5
		60	1.67	78	58	18	1214	318	12.3
		120	1.56	83	59	15	1351	292	14.0
5	5.0	0	1.55	128	100	26	2230	409	16.4
		30	1.90	124	100	26	1821	605	11.1
		60	2.12	118	95	20	1674	685	10.0
		120	1.91	118	95	20	1944	534	12.9
6	2.5	0	2.20	100	59	20	1044	170	23.5
		30	2.57	98	51	14	768	280	12.3
		60	1.85	100	59	20	1164	209	19.5
		120	2.04	94	58	19	1056	165	25.2
7	10.0	0	2.37	72	78	16	1494	365	16.2
		30	2.84	68	70	10	1149	505	10.8
		60	2.75	67	71	15	1186	469	11.1
		120	2.36	71	70	15	1191	405	13.6
8	10.0	0	2.18	79	60	23	1264	305	15.7
		30	2.71	75	46	2	754	434	4.9
		60	2.44	74	47	12	855	349	10.8
		120	2.04	74	53	7	1155	327	13.0
9	10.0	0	1.45	100	90	29	2568	215	30.0
		30	1.85	106	87	23	1941	336	19.4
		60	1.47	104	89	28	2080	207	30.5
		120	1.68	102	85	20	2080	286	21.3
Mean		0	1.99	96.6	79.1	23.6	1651	316	19.2
±SD			0.40	16.4	15.4	5.4	492	97	4.9
Mean		30	2.35	92.6	70.2	16.0	1235	427	12.0
±SD			0.43	17.8	17.2	8.8	414	108	3.8
p value			<.05		<.01	<.05	<.01	<.01	<.01
Mean		60	2.19	91.1	72.1	19.9	1375	401	14.6
±SD			0.49	17.1	16.4	5.8	375	158	6.7
p value					<.05		<.05	<.05	<.05
Mean		120	2.05	92.3	74.1	19.0	1422	354	16.9
±SD			0.31	16.5	15.7	8.1	369	114	4.6

T = time; CI = cardiac index; HR = heart rate; SAP = mean systemic arterial pressure; PCWP = pulmonary capillary wedge pressure; SVR = systemic vascular resistance; RBF = renal blood flow; RVR = renal vascular resistance.

in systemic arterial pressure noted by Powers et al.[23] was more profound than that observed by other investigators[4, 22, 24] and a significant correlation was present between changes in systemic arterial pressure and renal blood flow. In particular, renal blood flow decreased when mean systemic arterial pressure fell below 60 mm Hg, which may endanger renal autoregulation.[25] Differences in patient population, severity and chronicity of the disease, and sodium intake may also partially explain the disparate results.[26, 27]

Although dopamine and enalaprilat increased cardiac output similarly, the improvement in renal blood flow was less marked with enalaprilat than with dopamine. Because renal perfusion pressure was lower during administration of enalaprilat, comparison of the direct renal vasodilator activity of the two drugs was not attempted. Nevertheless, because the increase in renal blood flow produced by dopamine is not associated with a fall in systemic arterial pressure, loss of renal autoregulation is unlikely to occur. In contrast, the renal response to angiotensin-converting enzyme inhibition may not always be beneficial, since renal autoregulation may be lost because of an excessive decrease in systemic arterial pressure. Accordingly, the development of new, orally active, dopamine-like agents, or the administration of oral levodopa,[28] appears to be of great promise in the treatment of chronic congestive heart failure. However, although both dopamine and enalaprilat were shown to increase renal blood flow, the concomitant effects on renal glomerular filtration and urinary sodium excretion were not evaluated. Accordingly, further studies are needed to determine whether the improvement in renal blood flow observed with dopamine and enalaprilat is associated with changes in renal function.

References

1. Merril AJ: Edema and decreased renal blood flow in patients with chronic congestive heart failure: evidence of "forward failure" as the primary cause of edema. J Clin Invest **49:** 389, 1945
2. Wade OL, Bishop JM: Cardiac output and regional blood flow. Oxford, 1962, Blackwell Scientific Publishers, p 134
3. Leithe ME, Margorien RD, Hermiller JB, Unverferth DV, Leier CV: Relationship between central hemodynamics and regional blood flow in normal subjects and in patients with congestive heart failure. Circulation **69:** 57, 1984
4. Faxon DP, Creager MA, Halperin JL, Gavras H, Coffman JD, Ryan TJ: Central and peripheal hemodynamic effects of angiotensin inhibition in patients with refractory congestive heart failure. Circulation **61:** 925, 1980
5. McDonald RH, Goldberg LI, McNay J, Tuttle EP: Effects of dopamine in man: augmentation of sodium excretion, glomerular filtration rate and renal plasma flow. J Clin Invest **43:** 116, 1964
6. Captopril Multicenter Research Group: A placebo-controlled trial of captopril in refractory chronic congestive heart failure. J Am Coll Cardiol **2:** 755, 1983
7. Ventura HO, Messerli FH, Frohlich ED, Kobrin I, Oigman W, Dunn FG, Carey RM: Immediate hemodynamic effects of a dopamine-receptor agonist (fenoldopam) in patients with essential hypertension. Circulation **69:** 1142, 1984
8. Stefoni S, Docci D, Vangelista A, Mosconi G, Coli C, Prandini R: Long-term treatment of chronic renal insufficiency with ibopamine (SB 7505), a new orally active dopamine-related drug. Clin Nephrol **18:** 168, 1982
9. Ganz W, Tamura K, Marcus HS, Donoso R, Yoshida S, Swan HJC: Measurement of coronary sinus blood flow by continuous thermodilution in man. Circulation **44:** 181, 1971
10. Warembourg H, Ketellers JY, LeKieffre J, Bertrand M, Houdas Y, Carre A: La mesure du debit sanguin renal par la methode de thermodilution. Arch Mal Coeur **65:** 218, 1972
11. Warembourg H, LeKieffre J, Ketellers JY, Bertrand ME, Houdas Y, Carre E: Etude du debit veineux renal par la methode de thermodilution au cours des hypertensions arterielles secondaires. Arch Mal Coeur **67:** 701, 1974
12. Sato Y, Matsuzawa H, Eguchi S: Comparative study of effects of adrenaline, dobutamine and dopamine on systemic hemodynamics and renal blood flow in patients following open heart surgery. Jpn Circ J **46:** 1059, 1982
13. Hornych A, Brod J, Sclechta V: The measurement of the renal venous outflow in man by the local thermodilution method. Nephron **8:** 17, 1971
14. Haggmark S, Biber B, Sjodin J, Winso O, Gustavsson B, Reiz S: The continuous thermodilution method for measuring high blood flows. Scand J Clin Lab Invest **42:** 315, 1982
15. McNay JL, McDonald RH, Goldberg LI: Direct renal vasodilatation produced by dopamine in the dog. Circ Res **16:** 510, 1965
16. Hollenberg NK, Adams DF, Mendell P, Abrams HL, Merrill JP: Renal vascular response to dopamine: haemodynamic and angiographic observations in normal man. Clin Sci Molec Med **45:** 733, 1973
17. Breckenridge A, Orme A, Dollery CT: The effect of dopamine on renal blood flow in man. Eur J Clin Pharmacol **3:** 131, 1971
18. Rosenblum R, Razzak A, Lawson D: Dopamine in man: cardiorenal hemodynamics in normotensive patients with heart disease. J Pharmacol Exp Ther **183:** 256, 1972
19. Silkans JL, Jeck D, Eron J, Edelman CM, Chervu LR, Blaufox MD, Spitzer A: Simultaneous measurement of glomerular filtration rate and renal plasma flow using plasma disappearance curves. J Pediatr **83:** 749, 1973
20. Cannon PJ: The kidney in heart failure. N Engl J Med **296:** 26, 1977
21. Hollenberg NK: Renal response to angiotensin-converting enzyme inhibition. Am J Cardiol **49:** 1425, 1982
22. Creager MA, Halperin JL, Bernard DB, Faxon DP, Melidessian CD, Gavras H, Ryan TJ: Acute regional circulatory and renal hemodynamic effects of converting enzyme inhibition in patients with congestive heart failure. Circulation **64:** 483, 1981
23. Powers ER, Bannerman KS, Stone J, Reison DS, Escala EL, Kalisher A, Weiss MB, Sciacca RL, Cannon PJ: The effect of captopril on renal coronary and systemic hemodynamics in patients with severe congestive heart failure. Am Heart J **104:** 1203, 1982
24. Dzau VJ, Colluci WS, Williams GH, Curfman G, Meggs L, Hollenberg NK: Sustained effectiveness of converting enzyme inhibition in patients with severe heart failure. N Engl J Med **302:** 1373, 1980
25. Blythe WB: Captopril and renal autoregulation. N Engl J Med **308:** 390, 1983
27. Dzau VJ, Colucci WS, Hollenberg NK, Williams GH: Relation of the renin-angiotensin-aldosterone system to clinical state in congestive heart failure. Circulation **63:** 645, 1981
27. Hollenberg NK, Salomon HS, Adams DF, Abrams HL, Merrill JP: Renal vascular responses to angiotensin and norepinephrine in normal man. Circ Res **31:** 750, 1972
28. Rajfer SI, Anton AH, Rossen JD, Goldberg LI: Beneficial hemodynamic effects of oral levodopa in heart failure. N Engl J Med **310:** 1357, 1984

Verapamil-induced improvement in left ventricular diastolic filling and increased exercise tolerance in patients with hypertrophic cardiomyopathy: short- and long-term effects

ROBERT O. BONOW, M.D., VASKEN DILSIZIAN, M.D., DOUGLAS R. ROSING, M.D., BARRY J. MARON, M.D., STEPHEN L. BACHARACH, PH.D., AND MICHAEL V. GREEN, M.S.

ABSTRACT Verapamil improves exercise tolerance and decreases symptoms in many patients with hypertrophic cardiomyopathy. The mechanisms responsible for these effects are not completely understood, although previous studies indicate that verapamil enhances left ventricular relaxation and diastolic filling in such patients. To investigate the association between changes in left ventricular filling and exercise tolerance after verapamil, we studied 55 patients with hypertrophic cardiomyopathy by radionuclide angiography and graded treadmill testing before and after 1 to 4 weeks of therapy with orally administered verapamil, 320 to 640 mg/d. The verapamil-induced increase in peak left ventricular filling rate at rest (from 3.1 ± 1.3 to 3.7 ± 1.3 end-diastolic volumes/sec; $p < .001$) was associated with an increase in exercise tolerance (from 5.9 ± 3.6 to 8.7 ± 4.7 min; $p < .001$); exercise capacity increased in 34 of 43 patients (79%) manifesting an increase in peak filling rate but only one of 12 patients (8%) with unchanged or decreased peak filling rate ($p < .001$). This initial trend persisted in 25 patients studied after 1 year of therapy; 11 of 16 patients (69%) with a persistent increase in peak filling rate had persistent improvement in exercise tolerance relative to preverapamil values, compared with only one of nine patients (11%) in whom peak filling rate was unchanged or decreased relative to preverapamil levels ($p < .02$). Verapamil withdrawal after 1 to 2 years in 24 patients resulted in reduction in peak filling rate ($p < .001$) and was associated with deterioration in exercise tolerance in 17 patients (71%). Hence, verapamil-induced changes in left ventricular peak filling rate were associated significantly with objective symptomatic improvement. These data support the concept that enhanced left ventricular diastolic filling is an important mechanism contributing to the clinical improvement experienced by many patients with hypertrophic cardiomyopathy during therapy with verapamil.
Circulation 72, No. 4, 853–864, 1985.

IMPAIRED RELAXATION and diastolic filling of the left ventricle contribute importantly to the spectrum of symptoms experienced by patients with hypertrophic cardiomyopathy. Several studies of hypertrophic cardiomyopathy indicate that verapamil, administered intravenously or orally, improves indexes of left ventricular relaxation and diastolic filling.[1–4] Verapamil also reduces symptoms and increases exercise tolerance in many patients with this disease.[5–9] However, the relationship between enhanced left ventricular diastolic filling resulting from verapamil and improved exercise tolerance has not been demonstrated conclusively.

From the Cardiology Branch, National Heart, Lung, and Blood Institute, National Institutes of Health, Bethesda, MD.
Address for correspondence: Robert O. Bonow, M.D., Bldg. 10, Room 7B15, National Institutes of Health, Bethesda, MD 20205.
Received March 5, 1985; revision accepted July 5, 1985.

In this study, we investigated the association between improved left ventricular diastolic filling and improved exercise capacity induced by therapy with orally administered verapamil, both short- and long-term, in patients with hypertrophic cardiomyopathy. Left ventricular diastolic filling characteristics were assessed by radionuclide angiography, and exercise tolerance was measured objectively by graded treadmill exercise testing. To evaluate further the interrelationship between left ventricular diastolic filling and exercise capacity and the reversible effects of verapamil, we also studied the effects of verapamil withdrawal after long-term therapy in a subgroup of patients.

Methods

Patient selection. We studied the effects of verapamil administered orally in a total of 70 patients with hypertrophic cardiomyopathy by radionuclide angiography and graded treadmill testing. Patients ranged in age from 14 to 69 years (mean 47). There were 37 men and 33 women. All had echocardiographic confirmation of a hypertrophied, nondilated left ventricle in the absence of another cardiac or systemic disease capable of producing myocardial hypertrophy.[10, 11] Disproportionate septal thickening was present in 67 patients (96%). Cardiac catheterization in 68 patients demonstrated obstruction of the left ventricular outflow tract at rest (gradient of ≥30 mm Hg) in 25 patients (37%), a provocable outflow gradient during Valsalva maneuver, amyl nitrite inhalation, or intravenous infusion of isoproterenol in 27 patients (40%), and no rest or provocable gradient in 16 patients (23%). The two patients not catheterized manifested marked systolic anterior motion of the anterior mitral valve on M mode echocardiography, compatible with the presence of a resting outflow gradient. All patients were limited by moderate-to-severe symptoms of angina, exertional dyspnea, orthopnea, or paroxysmal nocturnal dyspnea (New York Heart Association functional class III to IV). All patients were in normal sinus rhythm.

Short-term administration of verapamil. Fifty-five of the 70 patients were studied before and after short-term therapy with verapamil of 5 to 25 days (mean 9). In 28 patients verapamil was administered in a randomized, double-blind, crossover manner at least 48 hr after cessation of all cardiac drugs. Verapamil (80 mg) or placebo were given every 6 hr. After nine low-dose capsules of the drug, high-dose capsules (120 mg) were administered every 6 to 8 hr for 48 hr and radionuclide angiography and graded exercise testing were performed. Two patients were studied during low-dose verapamil, since heart rate or blood pressure effects prevented high-dose administration. Fifteen of the 28 patients received placebo before verapamil, and the other 13 received verapamil before placebo. Results obtained during the placebo phase were considered "control" data for subsequent comparison with the effects of verapamil.

In the other 27 patients, verapamil was administered in an unblinded manner. Control studies were performed after cardiac medications were withdrawn for at least 48 hr. Verapamil was then administered orally, beginning at a dose of 240 or 320 mg/d. The dose was increased gradually every 36 to 48 hr as possible to a dose of 480 to 640 mg/d. The final dosage was determined by the clinical response of each patient and was limited in some patients because of atrioventricular dissociation, Mobitz I second-degree atrioventricular block, or systemic hypotension. Radionuclide angiography and graded treadmill testing were repeated after each patient received what was considered the optimal dose for at least 36 hr.

For the 55 patients undergoing short-term studies, the final daily verapamil dose was 240 mg in two patients, 320 mg in 14 patients, 360 mg in 16 patients, 480 mg in 22 patients, and 640 mg in one patient. Radionuclide angiography and exercise testing were performed within 1 week of verapamil initiation in 40 patients and within 8 to 25 days in the other 15 patients.

Long-term administration of verapamil. Twenty-five of the 70 patients were studied before and after long-term therapy of 1 to 2 years (mean 15 months). Drug dosage ranged from 320 to 640 mg/d. Eighteen of these patients were also included in the short-term study, so that serial control, short-term verapamil, and long-term verapamil data were obtained in these 18 patients. In 11 of these 18 patients, drug dosage was the same during the short- and long-term studies. In one patient the dose of verapamil was decreased from 480 to 320 mg/d between 1 week and 1 year; in the other six, increases in dosage were made during the course of the 1 to 2 year period because of persistent or progressive symptoms, from a median dose of 320 to 480 mg/d.

Verapamil withdrawal. We also studied the effects of verapamil withdrawal on left ventricular function and exercise performance in 24 patients after long-term verapamil therapy was complete. Sixteen of these patients were among the 25 patients in the long-term verapamil study, and the other eight patients were studied after long-term therapy but did not undergo initial control testing before verapamil treatment was begun. In these 24 patients, verapamil was discontinued after the long-term radionuclide angiographic and exercise tests were completed. The studies were then repeated 48 to 96 hr (mean 64) after verapamil was discontinued.

Gated equilibrium blood pool cardiac scintigraphy. Radionuclide angiography was performed at rest with red blood cells labeled in vivo with 15 to 20 mCi of technetium-99m. Imaging was performed with patients in the supine position by means of a conventional Anger camera equipped with a high-sensitivity, parallel-hole collimator oriented in a modified left anterior oblique position to isolate the left ventricle from other cardiac structures. The cardiac image sequence spanning the average cardiac cycle was constructed from several hundred cardiac cycles by computer-based electrocardiographic gating, using list-mode data acquisition (framing rate up to 100 images/sec) with exclusion of extrasystolic and postextrasystolic cardiac cycles and combined forward and reverse gating from the R wave.[12] High temporal resolution left ventricular time-activity curves, representing a measure of relative left ventricular volume changes with time throughout the average cardiac cycle, were generated from the cardiac image sequence with use of fixed left ventricular and background regions of interest.[2, 12]

Left ventricular ejection fraction was determined automatically by computer analysis of the time-activity curve. The peak rates of left ventricular ejection and rapid diastole filling were computed by fitting third-order polynomial functions to the systolic ejection phase and the rapid filling phase of the time-activity curve, with use of a least-squares technique.[2, 3, 13] Peak ejection and filling rates were computed in counts per second, normalized for the number of counts at end-diastole and expressed as relative end-diastolic volumes per second (EDV/sec). Time to peak filling rate was computed as the time difference between end-systole (nadir of the time-activity curve) and the time corresponding to peak rate of filling. The reproducibility limits of these measurements in patients with hypertrophic cardiomyopathy have been reported previously.[2, 3] A change in peak filling rate of 0.4 EDV/sec (±2 SDs) or greater was considered to be a significant change from baseline values.

In 34 patients studied during short-term administration of verapamil, we also performed radionuclide angiography during maximum supine exercise both before and after verapamil, with a bicycle ergometer and a restraining harness to minimize patient motion under the camera. Exercise loads were increased by 25 W every 2 min until the development of angina or limiting fatigue or dyspnea. Heart rate and blood pressure were monitored during exercise. Imaging was begun shortly after the onset of exercise, but only that portion of the data series that occurred during maximal exercise, encompassing approximately the last 2 to 3 min of exercise, was selected for analysis.

Graded treadmill exercise testing. Two different graded treadmill protocols, requiring different intensities of exercise, were used in this study to evaluate exercise capacity.[6, 7] The selection of the specific protocol used for each patient was a clinical decision based on age, sex, severity of symptoms, and expected exercise tolerance, with the goal that a symptomatic end point would be reached within 2.5 to 12.5 min of exercise. In the protocol requiring less intense exercise (protocol I), the treadmill was driven at a constant speed of 2.2 mph at a inclination of 0%. Every 2.5 min the inclination was increased by 2.5% until a maximum of 22.5 min elapsed. The maximum workload at this final stage was 2.2 mph at 20% incline. In the more intense exercise protocol (protocol II), the treadmill was driven initially at 1.9 mph at an inclination of 10%. Every 2.5 min the treadmill speed and inclination were increased by 0.4 mph and 2%, respectively. After 15 min the inclination was held constant at 20% and the speed was increased 0.8 mph every 2.5 min. Exercise tolerance was assessed by protocol II in 59 of the 70 patients and protocol I in the other 11 patients. Subsequent exercise tests in the same patient were always performed with the same exercise protocol used in the initial study. In either protocol, exercise was terminated when the patient complained of angina, lightheadness, or limiting fatigue or dyspnea. No patient was forced to discontinue exercise because of the development of ventricular tachycardia.

To determine the reproducibility of exercise testing in patients with hypertrophic cardiomyopathy, exercise tolerance in 19 patients was studied twice during administration of placebo, at least 48 hr apart.[7] The standard deviation of the mean difference (−11 sec) in exercise capacity between the two tests was 50 sec. Hence, a change in exercise capacity greater than 2 SDs (±100 sec) was considered a significant change compared with baseline values.

Echocardiography. M mode echocardiograms were obtained with a 2.25 MHz, 1.25 cm diameter, unfocused Aerotech transducer and a Hoffrel 101 ultrasound receiver interfaced with a Honeywell 1856 strip-chart recorder or an Irex System II ultrasound unit with either a 2.25 or 3.5 MHz transducer (1.3 cm diameter). Ventricular septal and posterior left ventricular free wall thicknesses were measured before atrial systole with the ultrasound beam directed through the distal margins of the mitral leaflets.[14]

Systolic anterior motion of the mitral valve was assessed with a semiquantitative grading system that was modified from that of Gilbert et al.[15] Systolic anterior motion was defined as minimal if the minimum mitral-septal distance exceeded 10 mm, mild if this distance was 10 mm or less but there was no mitral-septal contact, moderate if there was only brief mitral septal contact (less than 30% of echocardiographic ventricular systole), and severe if there was prolonged (30% or more of echocardiographic systole) mitral-septal contact. These studies were interpreted by an experienced observer who was unaware of the results of radionuclide angiographic and exercise testing. Serial echocardiographic studies corresponding temporally to the serial radionuclide angiographic and graded exercise tests were obtained in 47 of the 62 patients studied before and after verapamil.

Statistical methods. The effects of verapamil on indexes of left ventricular function and exercise tolerance were analyzed with the paired t test. Serial studies obtained in patients under control conditions, during short-term therapy with verapamil, and during long-term therapy with verapamil were evaluated by analysis of variance of repeated measures. The relationship between changes in left ventricular diastolic filling and changes in exercise tolerance were assessed by linear regression analysis, chi-square analysis, and analysis of variance.

Results

Effects of short-term therapy with verapamil. During short-term administration of verapamil (table 1), indexes of left ventricular systolic function were unchanged compared with control values. However, as previously reported,[2] indexes of left ventricular diastolic filling at rest significantly improved: peak filling rate increased and time to peak filling decreased, despite the reduction in heart rate (which would be expected to reduce peak filling rate and prolong time to peak filling rate). Peak filling rate increased (figure 1) from 3.1 ± 1.3 EDV/sec (mean ± SD) under control conditions to 3.7 ± 1.3 EDV/sec with verapamil ($p < .001$). Forty-three of the 55 patients manifested an increase in resting peak filling rate of 0.4 EDV/sec or greater, a change considered meaningfully greater than the control value.

TABLE 1
Effects of short-term administration of verapamil (55 patients)

	Control	Verapamil	p value
Heart rate at rest (beats/min)	75±16	68±10	< .001
LV systolic function (rest)			
LV ejection fraction (%)	73±13	72±13	NS
Peak LV ejection rate (EDV/sec)	3.7±0.8	3.6±0.8	NS
Time to end-systole (msec)	360±46	365±34	NS
LV diastolic filling (rest)			
Peak LV filling rate (EDV/sec)	3.1±1.3	3.7±1.3	< .001
Time to peak LV filling rate (msec)	184±46	161±30	< .001
Exercise capacity (min)	5.9±3.6	8.7±4.7	< .001

Data are mean ± SD.
LV = left ventricular.

Verapamil increased exercise capacity significantly (figure 1) from 5.9 ± 3.6 min under control conditions to 8.7 ± 4.7 min ($p < .001$). Exercise time increased by greater than 100 sec in 35 patients (64%). The magnitude of the change in exercise tolerance was associated with the change in peak filling rate. Exercise capacity improved significantly in the 43 patients manifesting an increase in peak filling rate after verapamil (figure 2), from 6.1 ± 3.8 to 9.6 ± 4.7 min ($p < .001$). However, in the 12 patients in whom peak filling rate was unchanged or decreased after verapamil, exercise capacity was not substantially altered (from 5.2 ± 2.7 to 5.7 ± 3.2 min; p = NS). Representative left ventricular time-activity curves are shown in figure 3 for a patient in whom improved left ventricular diastolic filling with verapamil was associated with increased exercise tolerance and for a patient in whom neither diastolic filling nor exercise tolerance increased with verapamil.

In the subset of 28 patients who received verapamil in a randomized, double-blind fashion, the results of short-term administration of verapamil were similar to those of the total group. Verapamil increased both resting peak filling rate (from 3.1 ± 1.2 to 3.8 ± 1.3 EDV/sec; $p < .005$) and exercise tolerance (from 5.3

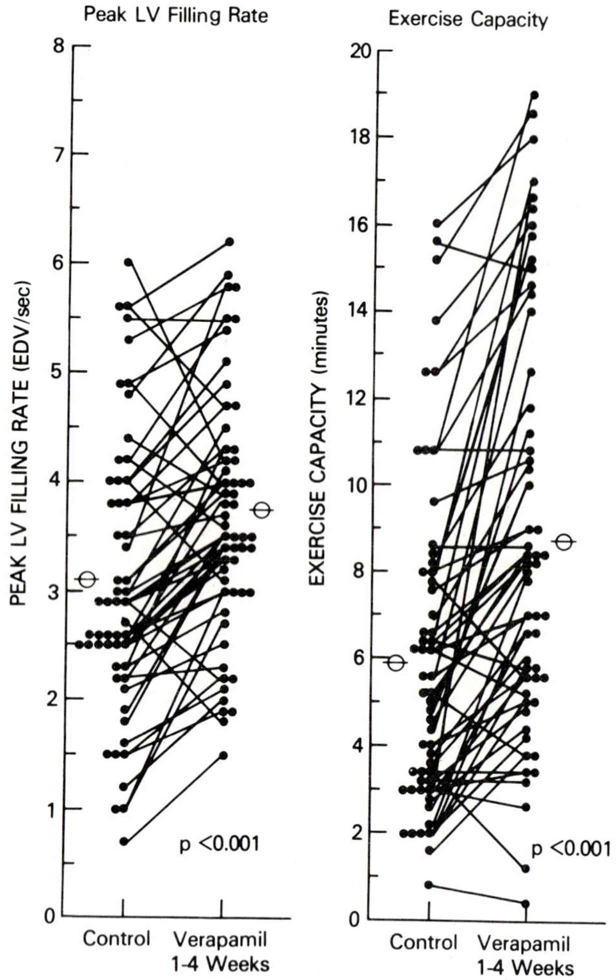

FIGURE 1. Effects of short-term therapy with verapamil (1 to 4 weeks) on peak left ventricular (LV) filling rate at rest and on exercise capacity. Open circles with lines indicate mean values.

± 3.1 to 8.5 ± 4.3 min; $p < .001$). Exercise time was greater with verapamil than with placebo in 12 of 15 patients who received verapamil after placebo and in 10 of 13 patients who received verapamil before placebo. Hence the improvement in exercise time by verapamil could not be attributed purely to a training effect. In the 21 patients in whom peak filling rate increased after verapamil, exercise tolerance increased significantly (from 5.4 ± 3.4 to 9.4 ± 4.5 min; $p < .001$), whereas exercise time was not altered (from 5.1 ± 2.2 to 5.7 ± 2.3 min) in the seven patients in whom peak filling rate was decreased or unchanged after verapamil.

Similar data were obtained in the 34 patients who were studied by radionuclide angiography during exercise before and after short-term therapy with verapamil. Verapamil did not alter ejection fraction during exercise (from 71 ± 9% to 71 ± 9%) but significantly decreased exercise heart rate (from 123 ± 13 to 113 ± 2 beats/min; $p < .001$). Despite the significant decrease in heart rate, there was a significant increase in peak filling rate (from 6.4 ± 1.8 to 7.1 ± 1.9 EDV/sec; $p < .02$) and a decrease in time to peak filling rate (from 130 ± 40 to 113 ± 30 msec; $p < .005$). As in the data obtained at rest, there was a significant association between increased peak filling rate during exercise and exercise tolerance. Fifteen of 18 patients with an increase in exercise peak filling rate manifested an increase in exercise tolerance compared with only seven of 16 patients in whom exercise peak filling rate was unchanged or decreased ($p < .02$ by chi-square analysis). An example of improved left ventricular filling at rest and during exercise after verapamil is presented in figure 4.

Effects of long-term therapy with verapamil. Serial data obtained in the 18 patients studied before and after both short- and long-term administration of verapamil demonstrated that the initial increase in resting peak filling rate during short-term therapy declined in most patients over the course of 1 to 2 years (figure 5), so

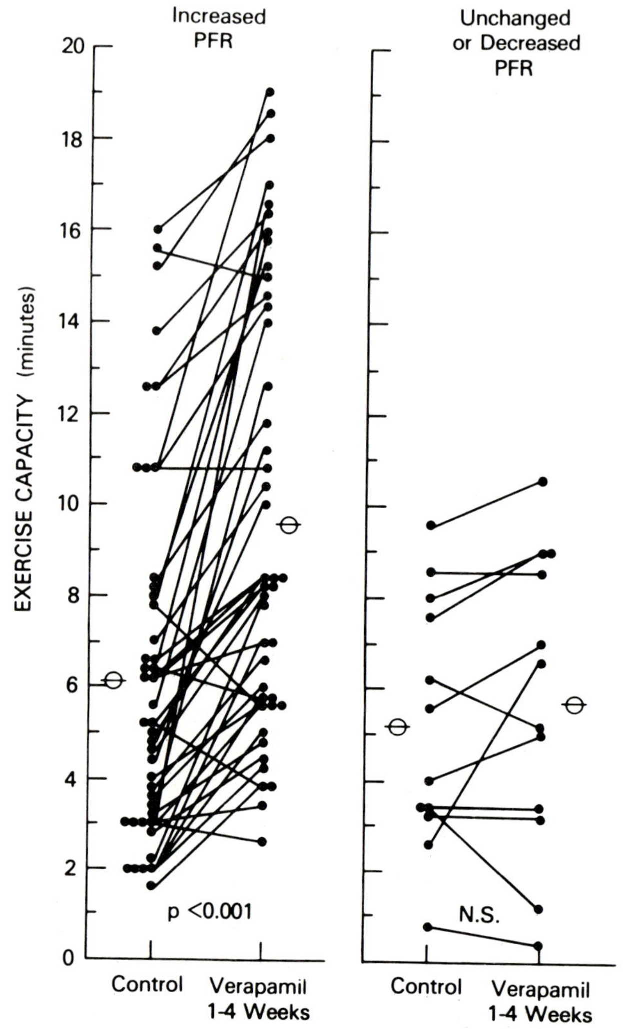

FIGURE 2. Effects of short-term therapy with verapamil on exercise capacity. PFR = peak filling rate.

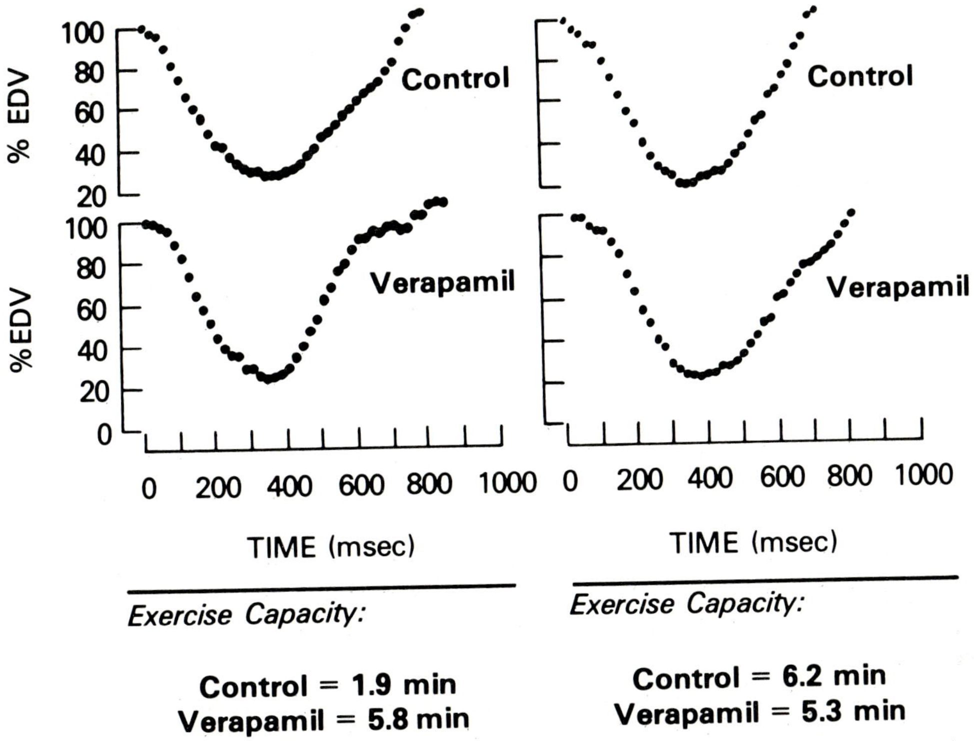

FIGURE 3. Left ventricular time-activity curves obtained at rest from two patients before (control) and after 1 week of orally administered verapamil. Each point represents 20 msec. *Left,* Improved peak filling rate after verapamil (from 1.9 to 3.4 EDV/sec) is associated with increased exercise capacity from 1.9 to 5.8 min. *Right,* Lack of increase in peak filling rate by verapamil (from 2.9 to 2.2 EDV/sec) is associated with no improvement in exercise tolerance.

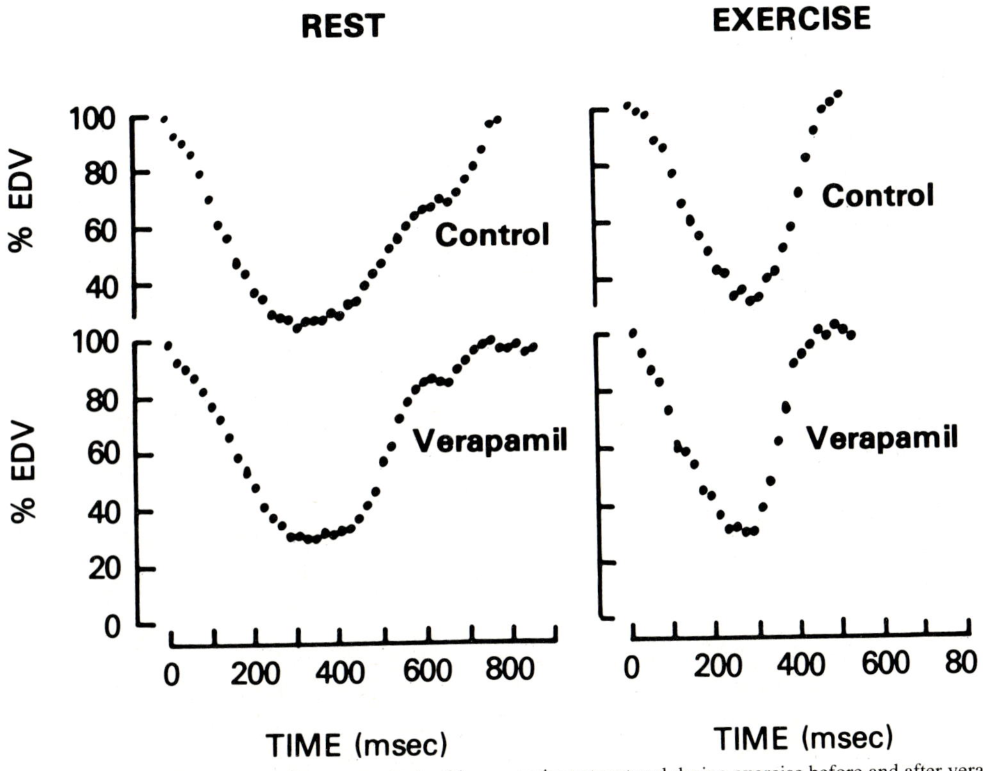

FIGURE 4. Left ventricular time-activity curves obtained in one patient at rest and during exercise before and after verapamil. Despite increases in cardiac cycle length, verapamil increases peak filling rate both at rest (from 2.5 to 4.0 EDV/sec) and during exercise (from 5.7 to 7.1 EDV/sec) and is associated with a decrease in time to peak filling rate at rest (from 184 to 149 msec) and exercise (from 123 to 75 msec). Verapamil augmented exercise tolerance in this patient from 3.0 to 5.6 min.

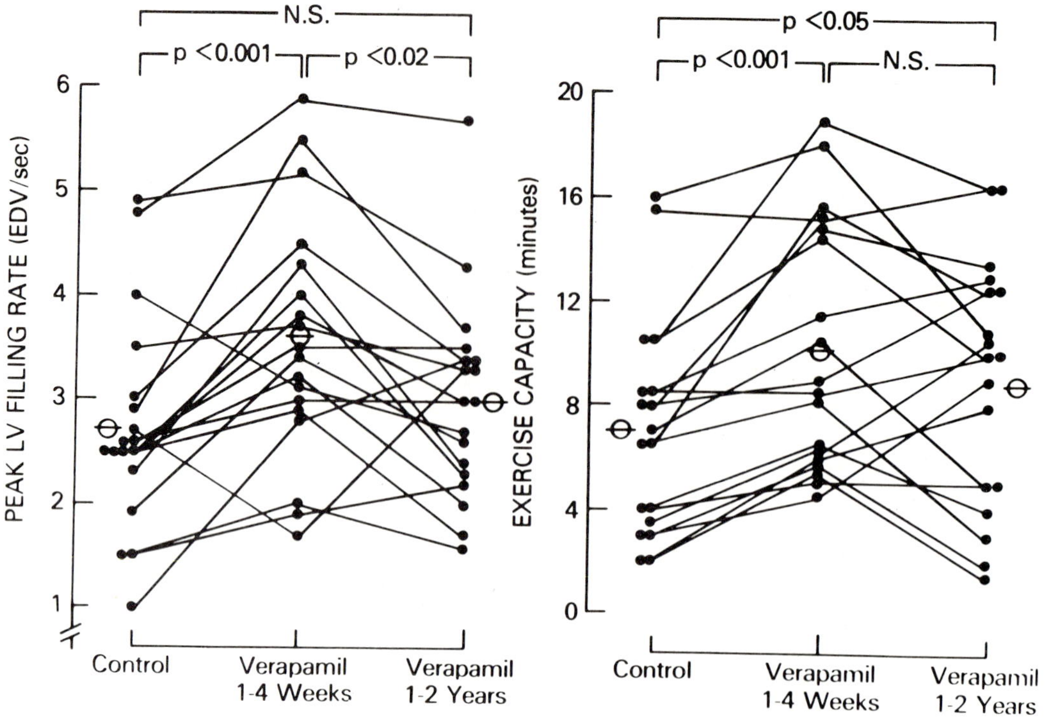

FIGURE 5. Serial changes in peak left ventricular (LV) filling rate at rest and in exercise capacity during both short- and long-term administration of verapamil.

that the mean value was significantly lower at 1 to 2 years than that measured at 1 to 4 weeks and was not significantly changed from the initial control value. Nonetheless, 10 patients (56%) still exhibited an increase in peak filling rate of 0.4 EDV/sec compared with control values. In similar fashion, exercise capacity, which increased in the majority of patients during short-term therapy, was only slightly greater than control values at 1 to 2 years of therapy. Nonetheless, exercise capacity at 1 to 2 years of therapy remained significantly greater than control and in nine patients (50%) was greater than 100 sec compared with control values.

Similar long-term results were evident when all 25 patients studied before and after long-term treatment were considered (table 2). Left ventricular systolic function was not altered by long-term therapy with verapamil. As with the short-term effects, however, resting peak filling rate was significantly greater than control values, and 16 patients (64%) had a persistent increase in peak filling rate of greater than 0.4 EDV/sec. Exercise capacity after long-term drug administration remained significantly longer than control values; 12 patients (48%) manifested an increased exercise capacity of greater than 100 sec compared with control.

These long-term effects of verapamil on exercise capacity were associated significantly with the drug's long-term effects on left ventricular diastolic filling. Verapamil-induced changes in exercise tolerance after 1 to 2 years of therapy are presented in figure 6 for all 25 patients studied before and after long-term treatment with verapamil. The 16 patients with a persistent increase in resting peak filling rate after 1 to 2 years of therapy manifested a significant increase in exercise tolerance over this period, from 6.8 ± 3.8 to 10.8 ± 3.9 min ($p < .001$). In contrast, in the nine patients with no change or a decrease in peak filling rate com-

TABLE 2
Effects of long-term administration of verapamil (25 patients)

	Control	Verapamil	p value
Heart rate at rest (beats/min)	79 ± 20	68 ± 11	< .001
LV systolic function (rest)			
LV ejection fraction (%)	71 ± 11	71 ± 11	NS
Peak LV ejection rate (EDV/sec)	3.5 ± 0.8	3.3 ± 0.7	NS
Time to end-systole (msec)	369 ± 52	366 ± 43	NS
LV diastolic filling (rest)			
Peak LV filling rate (EDV/sec)	2.8 ± 1.3	3.2 ± 1.2	< .05
Time to peak LV filling rate (msec)	186 ± 46	181 ± 34	NS
Exercise capacity (min)	7.2 ± 3.9	9.3 ± 4.3	< .02

Data are mean ± SD.
LV = left ventricular.

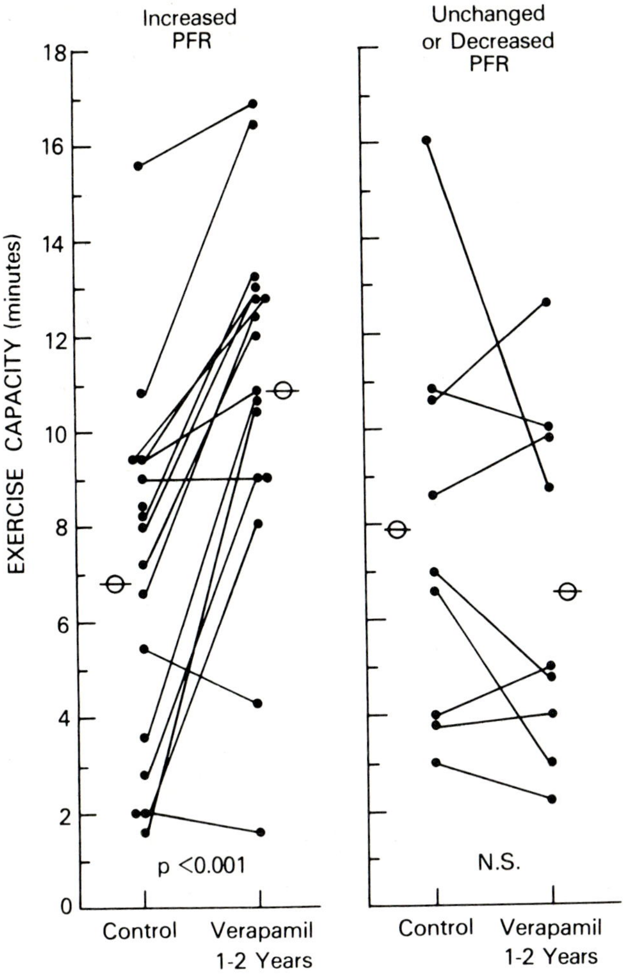

FIGURE 6. Effects of verapamil on exercise capacity during long-term therapy with verapamil (1 to 2 years). PFR = peak filling rate.

pared with initial control values, exercise tolerance at 1 to 2 years was unchanged from control values (from 7.8 ± 4.2 to 6.6 ± 3.6 min; p = NS).

Change in diastolic filling vs change in exercise capacity. The magnitude of the change in exercise capacity during treatment with verapamil and the influence of verapamil-induced changes in left ventricular diastolic filling on exercise tolerance were similar during both short- and long-term studies (figure 7). During both short- and long-term therapy, patients with an increase in resting peak filling rate compared with initial control values manifested a greater increase in exercise capacity than patients in whom peak filling rate was unchanged or decreased. Thirty-four of 43 patients (79%) with a verapamil-induced increase in peak filling rate during short-term therapy had an increase in exercise time greater than 100 sec relative to control values (table 3), compared with only one of 12 patients (8%) in whom peak filling rate was unchanged or decreased during short-term treatment with verapamil. The results were similar during long-term studies: 11 of 16 patients (69%) with a persistent increase in peak filling rate compared with initial control values manifested a persistent improvement in exercise tolerance, compared with only one of nine patients (11%) in whom peak filling rate was unchanged or decreased. By analysis of variance, the magnitude of the increase in peak filling rate was significantly related to the magnitude of change in exercise capacity during both short- and long-term studies (figure 8). Moreover, by linear regression analysis, a weak but significant correlation was observed between change in peak filling rate and change in exercise tolerance during short-term therapy ($r = .38$, $p < .05$); a stronger correlation was observed after long-term therapy ($r = .60$, $p < .01$).

Echocardiographic data. Among the 47 patients with serial echocardiographic data, 22 patients did not manifest significant mitral systolic anterior motion under basal conditions either before or during administration of verapamil. The remaining 25 patients had

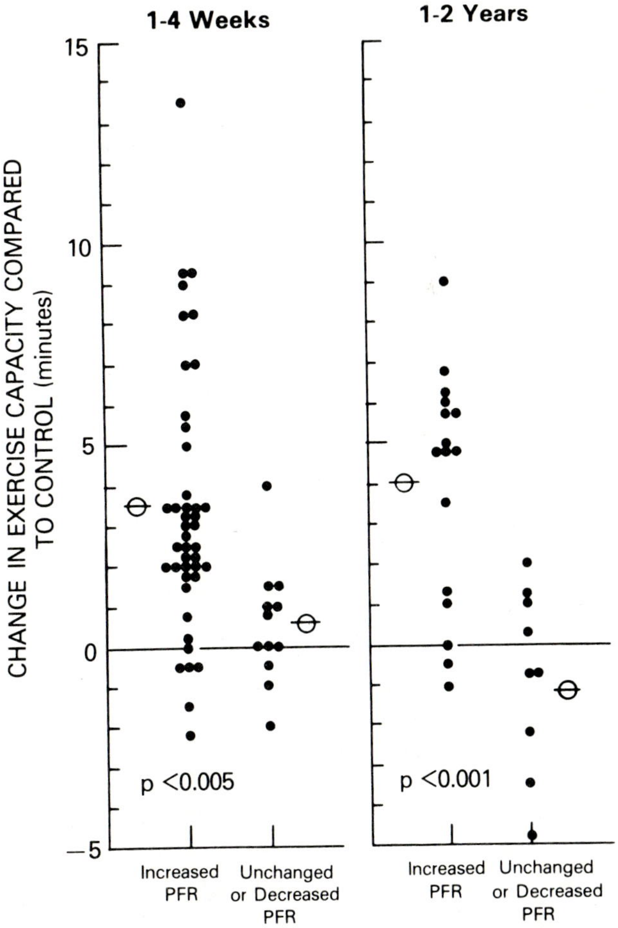

FIGURE 7. Change in exercise capacity compared with control values during short- and long-term therapy with verapamil. The change in exercise capacity is computed as the exercise time with verapamil minus the exercise time under control conditions. Patients are subdivided as in figures 2 and 6. PFR = peak filling rate.

TABLE 3
Verapamil-induced changes in diastolic filling and exercise capacity

	Total No.	Verapamil effect on exercise capacity: Increased[A]	Unchanged or decreased	p value[B]
Short-term verapamil therapy				
Patients with increased PFR[C]	43	34 (79%)	9 (21%)	< .001
Patients with unchanged or decreased PFR	12	1 (8%)	11 (92%)	
Long-term verapamil therapy				
Patients with increased PFR[C]	16	11 (69%)	5 (31%)	< .02
Patients with unchanged or decreased PFR	9	1 (11%)	8 (89%)	

PFR = peak left ventricular filling rate at rest.
[A]Increase defined as greater than 100 sec increase in exercise time compared with control values.
[B]Statistical significance by chi-square analysis.
[C]Increase defined as 0.4 EDV/sec or greater increase in peak filling rate compared with control values.

systolic anterior motion before verapamil (moderate-to-severe in 23 and mild in two). In nine of these 25 patients, administration of verapamil resulted in a substantial reduction in the severity of mitral systolic anterior motion. In each of these nine patients, administration of verapamil resulted in both an increase in resting peak left ventricular filling rate and an improvement in exercise tolerance. Eleven of the other 16 patients with no reduction in severity of systolic anterior motion also manifested an increase in peak filling rate with verapamil. Thus verapamil increased peak filling rate in a total of 20 patients with systolic anterior motion, of whom nine (45%) demonstrated a concomitant reduction in the severity of systolic anterior motion. In comparison, none of the five patients in whom peak filling rate was unchanged or decreased with verapamil had a reduction in severity of systolic anterior motion.

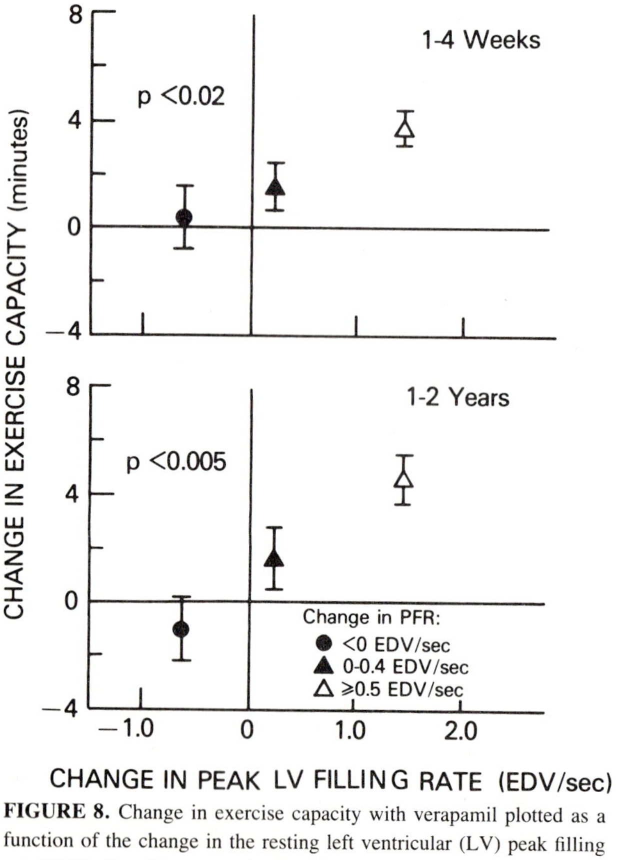

FIGURE 8. Change in exercise capacity with verapamil plotted as a function of the change in the resting left ventricular (LV) peak filling rate (PFR). *Top,* Short-term therapy; *bottom,* long-term therapy. Statistical significance computed by analysis of variance.

Effects of verapamil withdrawal. Left ventricular systolic function was not altered by verapamil withdrawal after long-term therapy (table 4), but left ventricular diastolic filling significantly deteriorated: peak filling rate decreased significantly (figure 9), and time to peak filling rate increased. This was associated with a reduction in exercise capacity in 17 of the 24 patients (71%). However, this change in exercise tolerance for the group (from 8.5 ± 5.0 to 7.5 ± 5.2 min) did not achieve statistical significance.

Discussion

Relaxation and diastolic filling of the hypertrophied left ventricle are impaired in many patients with hypertrophic cardiomyopathy.[1-4, 16-22] Prolonged or incomplete left ventricular relaxation and subsequent reduction in the rate and the extent of rapid filling result in reduced diastolic volume, reduced stroke volume, and altered diastolic pressure-volume relationships.[16, 23-27] On the basis of these common physiologic abnormalities, it has been postulated, and generally accepted, that these abnormalities in left ventricular diastolic function contribute importantly to the clinical manifestations and severity of symptoms in patients with this disease.

The demonstration that verapamil and nifedipine improve indexes of left ventricular relaxation, filling, and diastolic distensibility[1-4, 27-30] suggest that an im-

TABLE 4
Effects of verapamil withdrawal (24 patients)

	Verapamil 1–2 yr	Verapamil withdrawal	p value
Heart rate at rest (beats/min)	64±10	74±12	< .001
LV systolic function (rest)			
LV ejection fraction (%)	72±7	73±6	NS
Peak LV ejection rate (EDV/sec)	3.4±0.6	3.5±0.6	NS
Time to end-systole (msec)	352±32	348±31	NS
LV diastolic filling (rest)			
Peak LV filling rate (EDV/sec)	3.5±1.2	2.9±1.0	< .001
Time to peak LV filling rate (msec)	181±40	195±44	< .02
Exercise capacity (min)	8.5±4.9	7.5±5.2	NS

LV = left ventricular.

portant mechanism for the salutary clinical effects of the calcium channel–blocking agents in patients with hypertrophic cardiomyopathy is enhanced left ventricular diastolic function. The significant relationship in this study between improved rapid diastolic filling during therapy with verapamil and clinical improvement, measured objectively by exercise testing, supports this concept. Our data demonstrate that verapamil-induced improvement in left ventricular diastolic filling in patients with hypertrophic cardiomyopathy is associated with increased exercise capacity during both short- and long-term oral therapy.

In many of the patients in this study, it was not possible to exclude with certainty the possible contribution of a training effect with regard to the apparent improvement in exercise capacity by verapamil. However, several arguments suggest that potential training effects, if present, did not influence the exercise data importantly. First, in the 19 patients who exercised twice during the placebo phase, separated by at least 48 hr, to determine exercise reproducibility, the mean change between the first and second study was −11 sec, with 11 patients manifesting a decrease in exercise time during the second study compared with the first. Second, 28 of the 55 patients studied during short-term therapy with verapamil received the drug in a randomized, double-blind, cross-over fashion, with verapamil administered to 13 patients before placebo. The relative numbers of patients experiencing improved exercise tolerance with verapamil were the same whether verapamil was administered first or second in this protocol. Regarding the significant relationship between exercise tolerance and improved distolic filling after verapamil, patients with increased peak filling rate after verapamil were subject to the same potential training effects on exercise capacity during both short- and long-term therapy with verapamil as those patients in whom peak filling rate did not increase.

Data obtained in the patients who underwent serial studies (figure 5) indicate that the initial increase in peak filling rate after several weeks declined in most patients over the subsequent 1 to 2 years. Exercise capacity also decreased in over half of the patients between short- and long-term studies. This deterioration in left ventricular diastolic filling and exercise capacity during long-term drug administration occurred despite doses of verapamil that were the same or higher than the initial dosage. Hence, these serial data might indicate the development of tachyphylaxis or drug tolerance. However, the results obtained during verapamil withdrawal (table 4, figure 9) demonstrate persistent long-term, reversible verapamil effects. Both diastolic filling and exercise tolerance deteriorated further in the majority of patients when the drug was

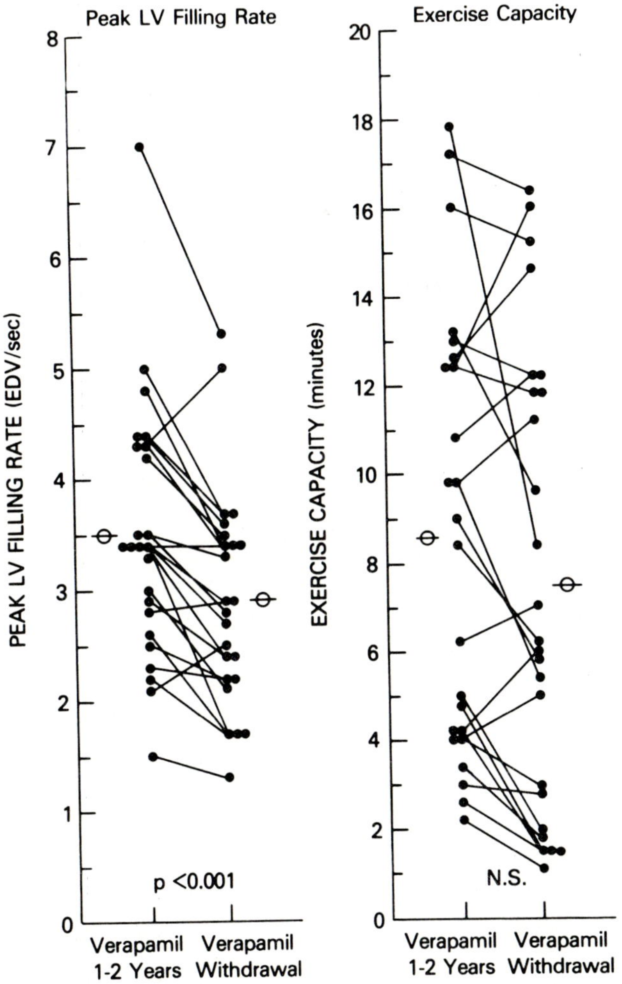

FIGURE 9. Effects of verapamil withdrawal after long-term therapy on peak left ventricular (LV) filling rate (PFR) at rest and on exercise capacity.

discontinued after 1 to 2 years. These findings suggest that disease progression rather than drug tolerance occurred during the course of long-term therapy with verapamil and that verapamil continued to exert a beneficial effect on left ventricular diastolic filling.

Improved left ventricular relaxation and filling by verapamil, reported by several investigators,[1-4] results from the complex interrelationship of several potential drug effects, including altered left ventricular loading conditions, increased coronary blood flow, and reduced ventricular ischemia, in addition to possible direct myocardial effects. Although the actual mechanism or mechanisms responsible for improved left ventricular relaxation and filling by verapamil are difficult to establish, the beneficial clinical effects of improved diastolic function in reducing symptoms and increasing exercise tolerance are more readily explained. Increased rate and extent of rapid diastolic filling after verapamil[1-4] is associated with increased end-diastolic volume and stroke volume, with unchanged or reduced diastolic filling pressures.[5, 8, 9, 27, 31] Thus improved forward stroke volume is achieved while elevated pulmonary venous pressures are reduced (or at least not increased). Moreover, because the magnitude of the left ventricular outflow tract gradient is influenced by left ventricular volume,[32-34] enhanced left ventricular filling and increased ventricular volumes may reduce the outflow gradient, which has been reported after administration of verapamil.[5, 27, 31] This may result in decreased systolic wall tension and reduced oxygen requirements, further alleviating symptoms. Although the echocardiographic data did not demonstrate a consistent verapamil-induced reduction in the degree of systolic anterior motion of the mitral valve (an estimate of the severity of the subaortic gradient), systolic anterior motion was markedly reduced or obliterated in over one-third of those patients manifesting systolic anterior motion before therapy with verapamil.

In this study, we used the peak rate of rapid diastolic filling as an index of left ventricular relaxation and filling. This index cannot be considered a pure measure of diastolic performance, since it may also be influenced by heart rate, left ventricular systolic function, left ventricular volume, and possibly myocardial thickness. There is no evidence that the verapamil-induced increase in peak filling rate we observed in this study resulted from changes in heart rate or systolic function. Changes in peak filling rate are directly related to changes in heart rate. Because the reduction in heart rate by verapamil would by itself be expected to decrease the peak filling rate, the observed increase in peak filling rate by verapamil could not be explained by changes in heart rate. Changes in peak filling rate measured by radinuclide angiography are also directly related to changes in ejection fraction.[35] Oral therapy with verapamil does not alter indexes of left ventricular systolic function in hypertrophic cardiomyopathy,[2, 9] although intravenous administration of verapamil may result in clinically measurable negative inotropic effects.[27]

In the current study, ejection fraction was not changed by short- or long-term oral therapy with verapamil and therefore did not influence peak filling rate measurements importantly. The issue regarding the influence of changes in left ventricular volume on this index of diastolic function is more complex and difficult to resolve. Improved rapid diastolic filling after verapamil may result in increased end-diastolic volume.[5, 9, 27] On the other hand, increased end-diastolic volume could, in itself, influence the measurement of peak filling rate, although this effect might be minimized by normalizing the filling rate value (in counts/sec) by end-diastolic volume (that is, end-diastolic counts), as was done in this study. In our previous experience with verapamil administered intravenously in the catheterization laboratory,[27] the consistent increase in end-diastolic volume after verapamil was not associated uniformly with increased peak filling rate; peak filling rate increased only in those patients with enhanced left ventricular relaxation (reduction in the time constant of left ventricular pressure decline) or in one patient with a marked increase in pulmonary wedge pressure (implicating a greater driving pressure across the mitral valve in early diastole). Thus increases in end-diastolic volume alone may not necessarily alter the peak rate of diastolic filling when this index is normalized for end-diastolic volume. In the current study, we did not measure absolute ventricular volumes (a limitation of the radionuclide method) to investigate the possible relationship between enhanced peak filling rate and changes in end-diastolic volume. Previous experience with M mode echocardiography indicated no change in left ventricular dimensions after orally administered verapamil,[2] which may represent the inability of echocardiographic measurements to estimate volumes adequately in the irregularly shaped left ventricular cavities of patients with hypertrophic cardiomyopathy rather than definite evidence against a verapamil effect on left ventricular volume. Similarly, orally administered verapamil has not altered left ventricular wall thickness by this technique after 1 year of treatment,[7] indicating either lack of a verapamil effect on left ventricular mass or the inability of M mode echocardiography to assess mass accurately because of the inhomogeneous nature of the severity of hypertrophy throughout the left ventricle.[11]

Our data indicate a significant relationship between verapamil-induced changes in peak filling rate at rest and improvement in exercise tolerance. Similar findings were observed regarding changes in peak filling rate during exercise. However, all measurements of filling rate obtained during exercise must be interpreted with great caution because of two factors. First, at higher heart rates there is loss of the diastasis interval, so that the rapid diastolic filling period (a period of ventricular filling influenced by active relaxation) overlaps with atrial systole (during which the ventricle fills passively during atrial contraction). This is shown in figure 4, in which the volume curves at rest have a definite period of diastasis, which is lost during exercise. Hence, the ability to study the rapid diastolic filling period, as a reflection of active relaxation and filling (which might be influenced by calcium-channel blockers or other interventions), is lost during exercise because of the compounding effect of superimposed atrial systole.

Second, the direct relationship between heart rate and peak filling rate is more pronounced during exercise. Under resting conditions, changes in cardiac cycle length are buffered by changes in duration of the diastasis interval. However, during exercise to higher heart rates and loss of the diastasis interval, the buffering effect of diastasis is lost, so that the measurement of peak filling rate is more sensitive to fluctuations in heart rate. This has important implications in the measurement of peak filling rate during exercise in patients before and after verapamil because of the consistent reduction in heart rate during exercise after verapamil. In this regard, during short-term therapy with verapamil, the separation of patients with improved and unimproved exercise tolerance on the basis of an increase or a decrease or no change in peak filling rate during exercise was not as definite as that observed in the peak filling rate data at rest. This may reflect the increasing dependence of peak filling rate on heart rate during exercise, so that potential beneficial effects of verapamil on left ventricular filling are masked by the significant decreases in heart rate. Because of these considerations, we believe that the changes in indexes of left ventricular filling under resting conditions may be more reliable indicators of alterations in diastolic function than those measured during exercise.

In summary, our results demonstrate that the increased rate of left ventricular rapid diastolic filling, as an index of improvement in diastolic function, is closely linked to clinical response to verapamil therapy in patients with hypertrophic cardiomyopathy. Patients with increased rate of diastolic filling are likely to experience an increase in exercise tolerance, whereas patients with no improvement in diastolic filling rate are not. Although the peak filling rate may be altered by factors other than left ventricular relaxation and filling, in the absence of more definitive data demonstrating a causal role of changes in heart rate, systolic function, or left ventricular volume or mass in augmenting this index of diastolic function after verapamil, our findings provide further evidence that impaired relaxation and filling of the hypertrophied left ventricle contribute importantly to the severity of symptoms in patients with this disease. These data also support the concept that enhanced left ventricular diastolic filling is a mechanism leading to the clinical improvement experienced by many patients with hypertrophic cardiomyopathy during long-term therapy with verapamil.

References

1. Hanrath P, Mathey DG, Kremer P, Sonntag F, Bleifeld W: Effect of verapamil on left ventricular isovolumic relaxation time and regional left ventricular filling in hypertrophic cardiomyopathy. Am J Cardiol **45:** 1258, 1980
2. Bonow RO, Rosing DR, Bacharach SL, Green MV, Kent KM, Lipson LC, Maron BJ, Leon MB, Epstein SE: Effects of verapamil on left ventricular systolic function and diastolic filling in patients with hypertrophic cardiomyopathy. Circulation **64:** 787, 1981
3. Bonow RO, Frederick TM, Bacharach SL, Green MV, Goose PW, Maron BJ, Rosing DR: Atrial systole and left ventricular filling in patients with hypertrophic cardiomyopathy: effect of verapamil. Am J Cardiol **51:** 1386, 1983
4. Hess OM, Grimm J, Krayenbuehl HP: Diastolic function in hypertrophic cardiomyopathy: effects of propranolol and verapamil on diastolic stiffness. Eur Heart J **4**(suppl F): 47, 1983
5. Kaltenbach M, Hopf R, Kober G, Bussman WD, Keller M, Paterson Y: Treatment of hypertrophic obstructive cardiomyopathy with verapamil. Br Heart J **42:** 35, 1979
6. Rosing DR, Kent KM, Maron BM, Epstein SE: Verapamil therapy: a new approach to the pharmacologic treatment of hypertrophic cardiomyopathy. II. Effects on exercise capacity and symptomatic status. Circulation **60:** 1208, 1979
7. Rosing DR, Condit JP, Maron BJ, Kent KM, Leon MB, Bonow RO, Lipson LC, Epstein SE: Verapamil therapy: a new approach to the pharmacologic treatment of hypertrophic cardiomyopathy. III. Effect of long-term administration. Am J Cardiol **48:** 545, 1981
8. Hanrath P, Schluter M, Sonntag F, Diemert J, Bleifeld W: Influence of verapamil therapy on left ventricular performance at rest and during exercise in hypertrophic cardiomyopathy. Am J Cardiol **52:** 544, 1983
9. Anderson DM, Raff GL, Ports TA, Brundage BH, Parmley WW, Chatterjee K: Hypertrophic obstructive cardiomyopathy: effects of acute and chronic verapamil treatment on left ventricular systolic and diastolic function. Br Heart J **51:** 523, 1984
10. Maron BJ, Epstein SE: Hypertrophic cardiomyopathy: a discussion of nomenclature. Am J Cardiol **43:** 1242, 1979
11. Maron BJ, Gottdiener JS, Epstein SE: Patterns and significance of distribution of left ventricular hypertrophy in hypertrophic cardiomyopathy: a wide-angle two-dimensional echocardiographic study of 125 patients. Am J Cardiol **48:** 409, 1981
12. Bacharach SL, Green MV, Borer JS: Instrumentation and data processing in cardiovascular nuclear medicine: evaluation of ventricular function. Semin Nucl Med **9:** 257, 1979

13. Bacharach SL, Green MV, Borer JS, Hyde JE, Farkas SP, Johnston GS: Left ventricular peak ejection rate, filling rate, and ejection fraction: frame rate requirements at rest and during exercise. J Nucl Med **20:** 189, 1980
14. Henry WL, Clark CE, Epstein SE: Asymmetric septal hypertrophy (ASH): echocardiographic identification of the pathognomonic anatomic abnormality of IHSS. Circulation **47:** 225, 1973
15. Gilbert BW, Pollick C, Adelman AG, Wigle ED: Hypertrophic cardiomyopathy: subclassification by M-mode echocardiography. Am J Cardiol **45:** 861, 1980
16. Grossman W, McLaurin LP: Diastolic properties of the left ventricle. Ann Intern Med **84:** 316, 1976
17. Sanderson JE, Gibson DG, Brown DJ, Goodwin JF: Left ventricular filling in hypertrophic cardiomyopathy: an angiographic study. Br Heart J **39:** 661, 1977
18. Sanderson JE, Traill TA, St. John Sutton MG, Brown DJ, Gibson DG, Goodwin JF: Left ventricular relaxation and filling in hypertrophic cardiomyopathy: an echocardiographic study. Br Heart J **40:** 596, 1978
19. St. John Sutton MG, Tajik AJ, Gibson DG, Brown CJ, Seward JB, Giuliani ER: Echocardiographic assessment of left ventricular filling and septal and posterior wall dynamics in idiopathic hypertrophic subaortic stenosis. Circulation **57:** 512, 1978
20. Hanrath P, Mathey DG, Siegert R, Bleifeld W: Left ventricular relaxation and filling in different forms of left ventricular hypertrophy: an echocardiographic study. Am J Cardiol **45:** 15, 1980
21. Murgo JP, Craig WE: Relaxation abnormalities in hypertrophic cardiomyopathy. Circulation **62**(suppl III): III-316, 1980 (abst)
22. Alvares RF, Shaver JA, Gamble WH, Goodwin JF: Isovolumic relaxation period in hypertrohic cardiomyopathy. J Am Coll Cardiol **3:** 71, 1984
23. Gotsman MS, Lewis BS: Left ventricular volumes and compliance in hypertrophic cardiomyopathy. Chest **66:** 498, 1974
24. Gaasch WH, Levine HJ, Quinones MA, Alexander JK: Left ventricular compliance: mechanisms and clinical implications. Am J Cardiol **38:** 645, 1976
25. Gaasch WH, Cole JS, Quinones MA, Alexander JK: Dynamic determinants of left ventricular diastolic pressure-volume relations in man. Circulation **51:** 317, 1975
26. Grossman W, Barry WH: Diastolic pressure-volume relations in the diseased heart. Fed Proc **39:** 148, 1980
27. Bonow RO, Ostrow HG, Rosing DR, Cannon RO, Lipson LC, Maron BJ, Kent KM, Bacharach SL, Green MV: Verapamil effects on left ventricular systolic and diastolic function in patients with hypertrophic cardiomyopathy: pressure-volume analysis with a nonimaging scintillation probe. Circulation **68:** 1062, 1983
28. Lorell BH, Paulus WJ, Grossman W, Wynne J, Cohn PF: Modification of abnormal left ventricular diastolic properties by nifedipine in patients with hypertrophic cardiomyopathy. Circulation **65:** 499, 1982
29. Senn M, Hess OM, Krayenbuehl HP: Nifedipin in der Behandlung der hypertrophen, nicht-obstruktiven Kardiomyopathie. Schweiz Med Wochenschr **112:** 1312, 1982
30. Paulus WJ, Lorell BH, Craig WE, Wynne J, Murgo JP, Grossman W: Comparison of the effects of nitroprusside and nifedipine on diastolic properties in patients with hypertrophic cardiomyopathy: altered left ventricular loading or impaired muscle inactivation? J Am Coll Cardiol **2:** 879, 1983
31. Rosing DR, Kent KM, Borer JS, Seides SF, Maron BJ, Epstein SE: Verapamil therapy: a new approach to the pharmacologic treatment of hypertrophic cardiomyopathy. I. Hemodynamic effects. Circulation **60:** 1201, 1979
32. Braunwald E, Oldham HN, Ross J Jr, Linhart JW, Mason DT, Font L: The circulatory response of patients with idiopathic hypertrophic subaortic stenosis to nitroglycerin and to the Valsalva maneuver. Circulation **29:** 422, 1964
33. Braunwald E, Lambrew CT, Rockoff SD, Ross J Jr, Morrow AG: Idiopathic hypertrophic subaortic stenosis. I. A description of the disease based upon an analysis of 64 patients. Circulation **30**(suppl IV): IV-3, 1964
34. Epstein SE, Henry L, Clark CE, Roberts WC, Maron BJ, Ferrans VJ, Redwood DR, Morrow AG: Asymmetric septal hypertrophy. Ann Intern Med **81:** 650, 1974
35. Bonow RO, Leon MB, Rosing DR, Kent KM, Lipson LC, Bacharach LC, Green MV, Epstein SE: Effects of verapamil and propranolol on left ventricular systolic function and diastolic filling in patients with coronary artery disease: radionuclide angiographic studies at rest and during exercise. Circulation **65:** 1337, 1981

Importance of internal controls, statistical methods, and side effects in short-term trials of vasodilators: a study of hydralazine kinetics in patients with aortic regurgitation

CHARLES R. MCKAY, M.D., MICHELE NANA, M.D., DAVID T. KAWANISHI, M.D., URI ELKAYAM, M.D., P. ANTHONY N. CHANDRARATNA, M.D., JOYCE N. WEISS, PH.D., AND SHAHBUDIN H. RAHIMTOOLA, M.D.

ABSTRACT We determined that the spontaneous changes in cardiac output (CO) over 12 hr in 21 patients with chronic severe aortic regurgitation averaged ±8.9% ($p = .03$). We then measured changes in CO over time after administering incremental doses of oral hydralazine (50, 100, 150, and 200 mg) every 12 hr and analyzed these changes by several methods. Changes over time of only +14% were highly significant ($p < .001$) when analyzed by t test, but were not significant by repeated-measures analysis of variance (ANOVA). When changes in CO were compared with internal control values (spontaneous changes over 12 hr), only changes of 20% or more were significant ($p < .05$). Transient "peak effects" markedly overestimated the maximum effects after all doses. We then compared the incremental doses of hydralazine, given either every 8 or every 12 hr, with respect to (1) the hemodynamic changes induced, and (2) the relative incidence of acute side effects. Maximal increases in CO were similar when hydralazine was given every 8 hr (16 patients) and every 12 hr (21 patients), and ranged from +14% after 50 mg to +61% after 200 mg. After the 150 and 200 mg doses, marked sustained increases in CO were present at 8 hr and mild increases in CO were still present at 12 hr. Hydralazine every 8 hr was associated with side effects in 25% to 86% of patients, but when the drug was given every 12 hr it was associated with side effects in only 5% to 19% of patients ($p < .001$). We conclude that (1) there are significant variations in control hemodynamics over time, (2) time-related effects should preferably not be compared with a single pretherapy baseline but instead should be compared, by repeated-measures ANOVA, with a value from a control group, (3) transient peak effects should preferably not be used to analyze time-related hemodynamic changes, (4) oral hydralazine given in 150 to 200 mg doses every 12 hr induces marked increases in CO and moderate sustained effects over 12 hr, with a lower incidence of acute side effects. This regimen would be expected to improve patient compliance and long-term benefits.
***Circulation* 72, No. 4, 865–872, 1985.**

HYDRALAZINE has beneficial hemodynamic effects in patients with congestive heart failure[1, 2] and those with valvular regurgitation.[3–7] Optimal oral doses of hydralazine have usually been determined by increasing the dose every 3 to 6 hr[7–10]; however, in some of these studies maximal effects were seen only after 24 hr[8, 10] and the incidence of side effects was high, ranging from 41% to 50%.[7–9] Moreover, the hemodynamic effects of therapy were evaluated by comparing a single "peak effect" to a single pretherapy baseline value rather than to a value from a control group of patients who were not treated.

The present study was undertaken (1) to determine spontaneous changes in values for various hemodynamic parameters in patients with chronic severe aortic regurgitation who were not receiving hydralazine therapy (control group), (2) to determine whether the conclusions regarding optimal hydralazine doses are different if the drug effects are analyzed by comparison with a single baseline determination, a single peak effect, or the values from a control group (spontaneous

From the Section of Cardiology, Department of Medicine and Division of Biometry, University of Southern California School of Medicine, Los Angeles.

Supported in part by a grant from the American Heart Association — Greater Los Angeles Affiliate.

Address for correspondence: Charles R. McKay, M.D., Section of Cardiology, USC School of Medicine, 2025 Zonal Ave., Los Angeles, CA 90033.

Received Feb. 5, 1985; revision accepted June 27, 1985.

Presented in part at the Annual Scientific Session of the American Heart Association, Anaheim, CA, November 1983.

changes), and (3) to determine the optimal effective level and frequency of dose of oral hydralazine that induces sustained beneficial hemodynamic effects with minimal side effects.

Methods

Patient population. Thirty-seven patients (six women and 31 men) with symptomatic, severe, chronic aortic regurgitation were studied. Their mean age was 48 years (range 21 to 70). All patients reported dyspnea (NYHA functional class II or III); other symptoms included occasional chest pains in three patients and palpitations or dizziness after exertion in five patients. All patients had peripheral and cardiac findings of severe aortic regurgitation, and all had 3+ to 4+ aortic regurgitation demonstrated by aortic root cineangiography. The angiographic left ventricular ejection fraction was 0.55 ± 0.15 (mean ± SD) and ranged from 0.26 to 0.80. Five patients had mild mitral regurgitation and none had mitral stenosis. Four had 30% to 50% stenosis in one coronary artery. In one patient who had undergone mitral valve replacement previously, the prosthetic mitral valve function was demonstrated to be normal by clinical findings, hemodynamic data, and angiography. The cause of the aortic regurgitation was judged to be congenital in four, remote endocarditis in four, presumed rheumatic disease in eight, and idiopathic in 21.

Hemodynamics. Diagnostic cardiac catheterization studies were performed in all patients, after which the right heart balloon flotation catheter used for the diagnostic study was left in place. Patients were monitored for 18 to 24 hr in the intensive cardiac care unit. After this observation period, recordings were made of the following at predetermined intervals: (1) heart rate (HR) and blood pressure, (2) right atrial, pulmonary arterial, and pulmonary arterial wedge (PAW) pressures by use of the Statham P23Db transducer with the zero level at the midchest position, and (3) cardiac output (CO) by the thermodilution method and with use of an average of three determinations. The usual calculations were made for derived hemodynamic parameters.[11]

Spontaneous changes. Spontaneous changes in all hemodynamic parameters were determined, without intervention, in 21 patients with chronic aortic regurgitation. There were 18 men and three women with a mean age of 48 years (range 21 to 62). With the patient resting supine in bed, hemodynamic data were collected at an index time (0 hr) and then 1, 2, 4, 6, 8, 10, and 12 hr later.

The average value for each parameter for each patient was calculated over the 12 hr observation period. The spontaneous change for each patient was then calculated as the coefficient of variation (CV% = standard deviation SD/mean × 100).[12] The average of these coefficients of variation for all 21 patients is reported as the spontaneous change in each parameter. The mean baseline value without intervention was also used to calculate percent changes in each parameter after intervention. Since the coefficient of variation has the same denominator, it can be directly compared with the percent change in each parameter after each dose of hydralazine.

Hydralazine dose schedules. Incremental doses of hydralazine (50, 100, 150, and 200 mg doses) were given to determine dose-response relationships. Because the clinical goal is to maintain a therapeutically significant increase in CO without a return to the control value and without side effects, there was no washout period between doses.

In 16 patients, the doses of hydralazine listed above were given every 8 hr. There were 13 men and three women with a mean age of 52 years (range 23 to 70). Hemodynamic data were collected just before each dose was administered and 1, 2, 4, 6, and 8 hr later. End points that precluded further increases in dose were an increase in CO of 50% or more[6] for 8 hr; adverse effects, including tachycardia of 140/min for more than 1 hr; or symptoms of intolerable palpitations, flushing, or dizziness.

In 21 patients, the same incremental doses were given every 12 hr. There were 18 men and three women with a mean age of 48 years (range 21 to 62). Hemodynamic data were collected just before each dose was administered and 1, 2, 4, 6, 8, 10, and 12 hr later. The same end points were used to preclude further increases in dose.

Statistical analysis. Hemodynamic data were analyzed by one-way repeated-measures analysis of variance (ANOVA) and by the Student-Newman-Keuls multiple-range tests when overall statistical significance was achieved.[13, 14] Single comparisons were performed with Student's t test for paired data. Analyses were performed with the use of the CLINFO system and the SAS statistical package on the IBM 370 system at the University of Southern California. The proportion of patients who experienced side effects on either regimen was compared with the Mantel-Haenszel chi-square statistic.[15] Here death was the side effect and time was dose; this approach seemed best for the analysis of data in a situation in which there was patient attrition.

Results

Group comparison. Baseline characteristics were compared in 21 patients receiving hydralazine every 12 hr and the 16 patients receiving hydralazine every 8 hr. There were no significant differences with respect to age, functional class, Estes left ventricular hypertrophy score on the electrocardiogram, resting left ventricular ejection fraction, or resting CO between these two groups.

Spontaneous changes. Spontaneous changes in CO over 12 hr without intervention are shown in figure 1. Mean COs ranged from 4.9 to 5.4 liters/min ($p = .03$). Spontaneous changes in hemodynamic parameters over 12 hr as measured by the coefficients of variation are listed in table 1. The spontaneous changes in CO (8.9%), mean arterial pressure (6.3%), and HR (7.1%) were relatively small; larger variations were encountered in other parameters, for example, mean PAW (18.4%) and right atrial pressure (37.8%).

Comparison of dose effects. We analyzed changes in CO over 12 hr by the four following methods after administration of incremental doses of hydralazine: (1) by determining changes at single times after each dose by Student's t test for paired data, (2) by determining changes over time by repeated-measures ANOVA and comparing them with a single baseline CO, (3) by determining changes over time by ANOVA and comparing them with internal control values, and (4) by determining peak effect CO retrospectively and applying the paired t test.

Changes at single times by t test. Figures 2 and 3 (*middle* panels) show the mean CO for 21 patients over the 12 hr after the 50 and 100 mg doses of hydralazine were

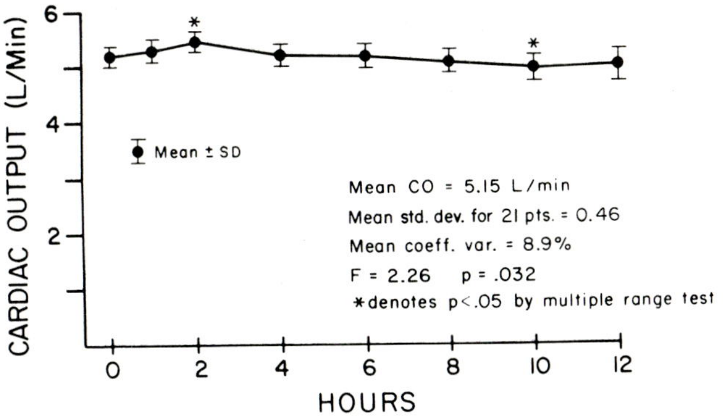

FIGURE 1. Spontaneous changes in CO over 12 hr in 21 patients with chronic severe aortic regurgitation. Changes were statistically significant by repeated-measures ANOVA ($p = .032$). The means for hour 2 and hour 10 were significantly different ($p < .05$) by the Student-Newman-Keuls multiple-range test.

given. Changes in CO at each time are compared with a single baseline determination obtained before the 50 mg dose by paired t test. Probability values, listed at the bottom of each figure, show "significant" changes even for very small increases from baseline.

Changes over time compared with a single baseline value. Changes over time were also analyzed by repeated-measures ANOVA and compared with a single baseline value. Probability values are listed at the bottom of figures 2 and 3. None of these changes were significant after the 50 mg dose ($p < .07$), while changes of +16% above the baseline CO were significant after 100 mg of hydralazine.

Changes compared with internal control values. Changes over time were also compared with internal control values (spontaneous changes) over 12 hr. Probability values are listed at the bottom of figures 2 and 3. No changes were significant after the 50 mg dose, and increases in CO of +20% were significant after 100

TABLE 1
Spontaneous changes in values of hemodynamic parameters over 12 hr in 21 patients with chronic severe aortic regurgitation

Parameter	Mean value	Average coefficient of variation (%)
HR	74 (beats/min)	7.1
CO	5.2 (l/min)	8.9
Stroke volume index	39.8 (ml)	12.0
Mean right atrial pressure	4.5 (mm Hg)	37.8
Mean pulmonary artery pressure	20.9 (mm Hg)	13.2
Mean PAW pressure	12.1 (mm Hg)	18.4
Mean systemic arterial pressure	82.3 (mm Hg)	6.3
Systemic vascular resistance	1250 (dynes-sec-cm^{-5})	11.1
Pulmonary vascular resistance	115 (dynes-sec-cm^{-5})	33.6

mg of the drug. Thus, after low doses of hydralazine, the importance of small-to-moderate changes in CO and the duration of effects were overestimated unless internal controls were incorporated into the analysis.

Changes over time or transient peak effect. Table 2 compares two methods of determining maximal effects of oral hydralazine on CO. Peak effect CO is the maximum CO determined for a patient after each dose, regardless of time after dose. It occurred from 2 to 6 hr after the dose and most often occurred 2 hr after the higher doses. Peak effects were compared with baseline values by paired t test. The mean effects at 2, 4, and 6 hr after each dose were compared with the same baseline values by repeated-measures ANOVA.

For all doses, the peak effect COs were uniformly higher than those obtained over time. After the 50 mg dose, the transient peak effect CO was much higher than any average CO 2 to 6 hr after the dose. This peak effect was statistically significant while none of the changes in CO over time were significant at $p < .05$ (figure 2). After higher doses, the p values for the peak

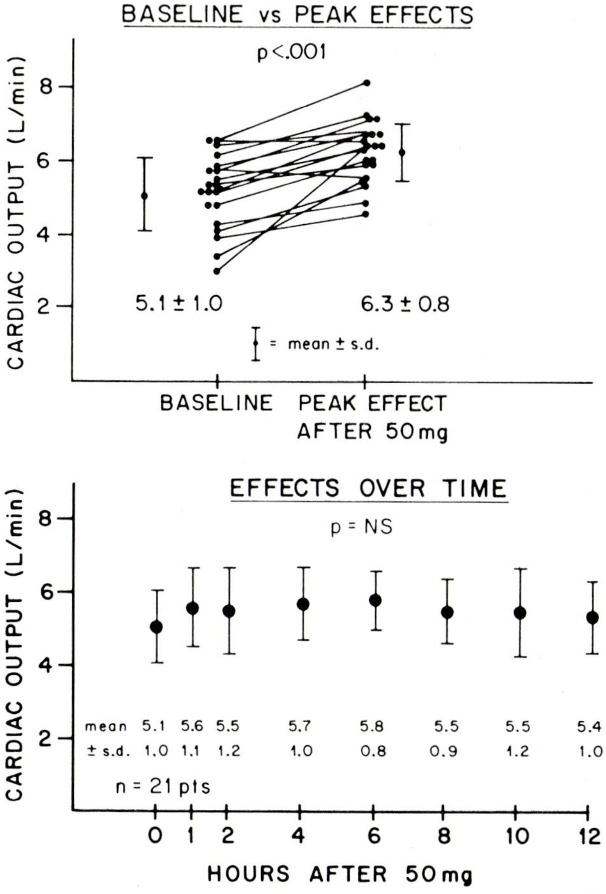

FIGURE 2. Change in CO over 12 hr after 50 mg oral hydralazine in patients with aortic regurgitation. *Top,* Individual baseline and peak effect CO. *Middle,* Mean changes over time. *Bottom,* Analyses of changes over time by t test, ANOVA compared with a single baseline value (B), and ANOVA compared with spontaneous changes (SC).

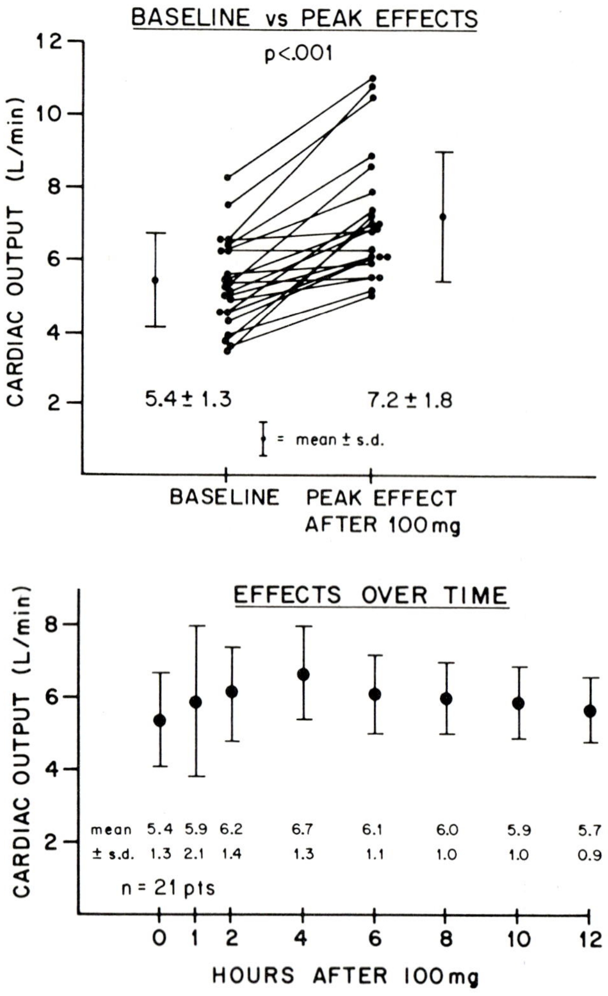

t-test vs. Baseline	-	.02	.01	.001	.001	.001	.002	.005
ANOVA vs. Baseline	-	.05	.01	.001	.01	.05	.05	NS
ANOVA vs. Spontaneous Changes	-	NS	.05	.01	.05	NS	NS	NS

FIGURE 3. Changes in CO over 12 hr after 100 mg oral hydralazine in patients with aortic regurgitation. Panels are as for the 50 mg dose in figure 2.

effect COs were uniformly smaller than those for the COs over time. Thus, retrospectively selecting the peak effect markedly overestimates the maximal response to hydralazine and may lead to a likely erroneous conclusion that the lower doses of hydralazine are "effective."

Dose response

Response to dosing every 8 hr. When hydralazine was given every 8 hr, the maximal changes in CO were seen 2 to 6 hr after each dose (figure 4). The maximal increase after the 50 mg dose was 17% (p = NS). CO increased +32% 2 hr after the 100 mg dose (p < .01), +47% 2 hr after the 150 mg dose (p < .01), and +53% 2 hr after the 200 mg dose (p < .01). However, with doses above 100 mg, CO did not return toward the range of spontaneous changes (baseline ±8.9%) at 8 hr, but remained 27% (p < .05) to 42% (p < .01) above the baseline value.

Changes in values for other hemodynamic parameters at the time of these maximal effects on CO showed that the 53% increase in CO after the 200 mg dose was associated with an increase in HR of 20% (p < .05), an increase in stroke volume index of 36% (p < .01), a decrease in mean arterial pressure of −9% (p = NS), and a decrease in systemic vascular resistance of −49% (p < .01). PAW pressure remained within the range of spontaneous changes.

The magnitude of each response in each individual patient was also evaluated (figure 5). After 50 mg of hydralazine increases in CO of 10% to 29% were seen only on one or two determinations in 57% of patients, increases of 30% to 49% were seen only on one or two determinations in 44% of patients, and increases of 50% or more on one or two occasions or increases of 30% to 49% on three or more determinations were rare. However, after 150 mg of the drug, increases in CO of 50% or more and increases of 30% to 40% on

TABLE 2

Maximal effects of oral hydralazine given every 12 hr on CO: comparison of changes over time and transient peak effect

	50 mg dose		100 mg dose		150 mg dose		200 mg dose	
	CO	p value	CO	p value	CO	p value	CO	p value
Baseline	5.1±1.0	—	5.4±1.3	—	5.7±1.1	—	5.4±1.0	—
Peak effect[A]	6.3±0.8	.001	7.2±1.8	.001	8.2±2.0	.0001	8.4±1.7	.00001
Mean effect at[B]:								
2 hr	5.5±1.2	NS	6.2±1.9	.05	7.4±2.0	.001	7.8±1.6	.001
4 hr	5.7±1.0	NS	6.7±1.3	.01	7.3±1.3	.001	7.5±1.9	.001
6 hr	5.8±0.8	NS	6.1±1.1	.05	7.0±1.3	.01	7.4±1.0	.001

NS = p > .05.

[A]Baseline vs a retrospectively determined peak effect CO evaluated by paired t test.

[B]Baseline vs mean CO 2, 4, and 6 hr after each dose analyzed by repeated-measures ANOVA and Student-Newman-Keuls multiple-range tests.

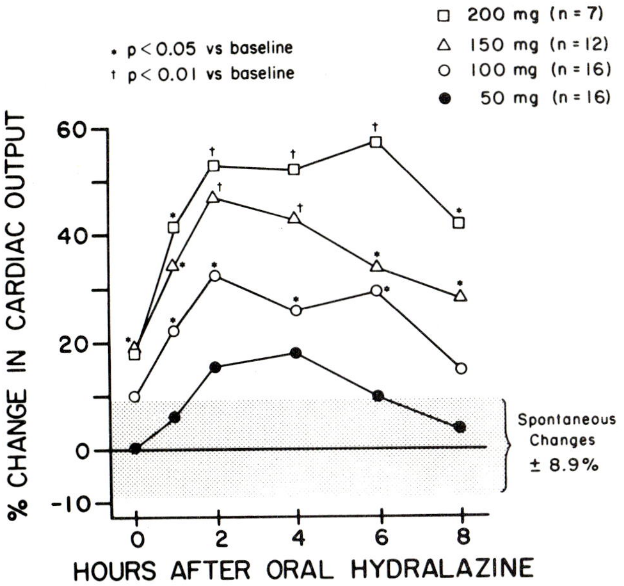

FIGURE 4. Pecent change in CO after incremental doses of oral hydralazine every 8 hr. The stippled area represents the range of spontaneous changes (mean coefficient of variation) without intervention.

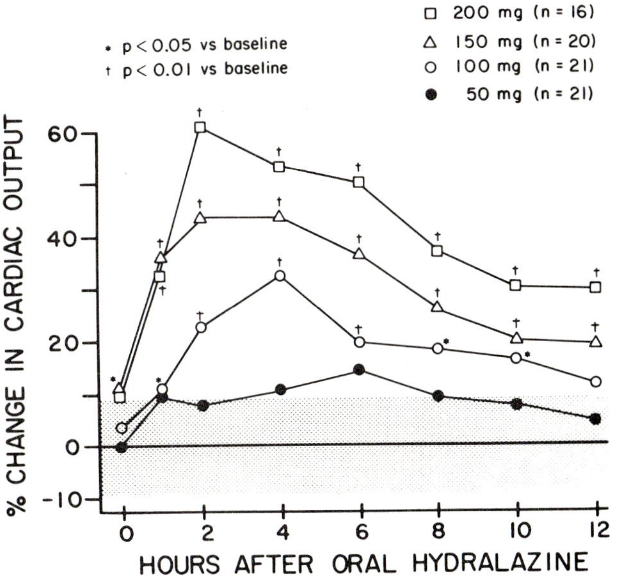

FIGURE 6. Percent change in CO compared with control after incremental doses of hydralazine every 12 hr. The stippled area represents the range of spontaneous changes without intervention.

three or more determinations were seen in approximately one-third of the patients. Increases in CO of 50% or more persisted at 8 hr in 25% of patients after the 150 mg and in 43% of patients after the 200 mg dose.

Response to dosing every 12 hr. When hydralazine was given every 12 hr maximal changes in CO were also seen 2 to 6 hr after each dose and were similar to those seen with the 8 hr schedule (figure 6). The increases in CO after 50 mg ranged from 11% to 14% (p = NS). CO increased +32% 2 hr after the 100 mg dose ($p < .01$), +45% 2 hr after the 150 mg dose ($p < .01$), and +61% 2 hr after the 200 mg dose ($p < .01$). Mild-to-moderate increases in CO persisted at 12 hr. For example, after the 150 mg dose, CO remained 18% ($p < .01$) above the baseline value; after the 200 mg dose, the CO remained 30% ($p < .01$) above baseline.

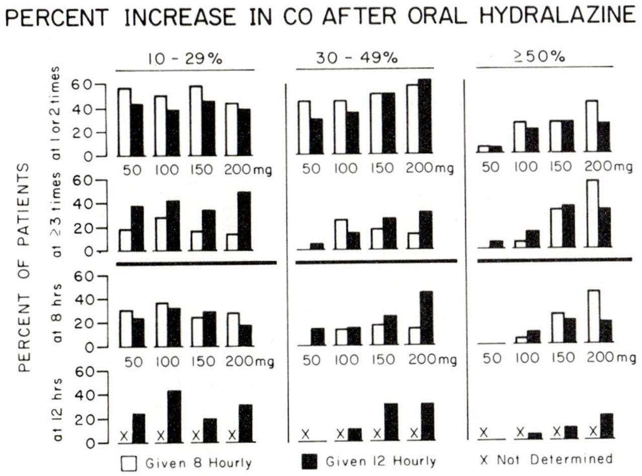

FIGURE 5. Percentage of patients who achieved various levels of increase in CO (10% to 29%, 30% to 49%, and ≥50%) after incremental doses of hydralazine every 8 or 12 hr.

Changes in values for other hemodynamic parameters at the time of these maximal effects on CO showed that the 61% increase in CO after the 200 mg dose was associated with an increase in HR of 24% ($p < .01$), an increase in stroke volume index of +32% ($p < .01$), a decrease in mean arterial pressure of −4% (p = NS), and a decrease in systemic vascular resistance of −33% ($p < .01$). PAW pressure remained within the range of spontaneous changes.

The magnitude of each response in each individual patient was also evaluated (figure 5). Patient responses after the 50 and 100 mg doses given every 12 hr were similar to responses in those given the same doses every 8 hr. After 150 mg, however, increases in CO of 30% to 49% persisted over three or more determinations, or to 8 hr after dosing, in 25% of patients. Increases in CO of 50% or more persisted for three or more determinations, or to 8 hr, in 20% to 38% of patients. After 200 mg of drug increases in CO of 30% to 49% were seen on three or more determinations in 33% of patients and at 8 hr in 44% of patients. Increases in CO of 50% or more that persisted for three or more determinations were seen in 33% of patients. Note that at 12 hr increases in CO of 30% to 49% were seen after both the 150 and 200 mg doses in 30% of patients, but increases of 50% or more were seen in only 10% to 19% of patients.

Side effects. When hydralazine was given every 8 hr,

the incidence of acute side effects with each successive dose increased from 25% at 100 mg to 86% at 200 mg (table 3). Twelve patients experience palpitations, two had dizziness, and one had tachycardia. However, when hydralazine was given every 12 hr, the incidence of acute side effects with each dose ranged from 5% at the 100 mg dose to 19% at the 200 mg dose. Four patients experienced palpitations; four had dizziness. Tachycardia, hypotension, and flushing were not observed. The chi-squared test revealed that the increased incidence of side effects with the 8 hr dosage schedule was significant ($\chi^2 = 10.0$, $p < .001$, table 3).

Discussion

Spontaneous changes in hemodynamic parameters. Our data show that for patients with severe aortic regurgitation, spontaneous changes in various hemodynamic parameters range from 7% to 37% (table 1); moreover, these changes over time can reach statistical significance without intervention (figure 1). Therefore, the magnitude of spontaneous changes should be assessed to determine statistical and clinical importance of hemodynamic changes observed after therapeutic interventions.

Importance of internal controls and statistical methods. Our data demonstrate that changes in CO over time after hydralazine are best analyzed by repeated-measures ANOVA. Moreover, small changes in CO may reach statistical significance, even by ANOVA, when an arbitrary baseline CO is used for comparison (figure 3). We have shown that analyses that compare a single baseline determination and a retrospectively determined peak effect overestimate the statistical and clinical importance of effects of small and moderate doses (table 2). A comparison of changes over time after intervention with internal control values yields better statistical and clinical interpretations of the maximal effects and the duration of effects. Recently, Bailar et al.[16] have emphasized that a study incorporating internal controls will support substantially stronger inferences than a study without internal controls; our present study demonstrates that for hemodynamic studies, internal controls that include spontaneous changes over time are important.

Previous authors, including ourselves and many others not cited, have reported hemodynamically "effective" doses of hydralazine in patients with heart failure[2, 8–10] or valvular regurgitation[3, 4, 6, 7] based on an analysis that did not take spontaneous changes into consideration. It is therefore possible that these studies may have yielded overoptimistic and possibly erroneous conclusions regarding the beneficial effects of certain doses, optimal doses, and dosing schedules of hydralazine. This may also apply to the evaluation of effects of other therapeutic agents. Furthermore, it needs to be emphasized that a statistically significant change in parameter value does not necessarily imply the clinical significance of that change.

Optimal doses of hydralazine in patients with aortic regurgitation

Comparison of dose intervals. Our study demonstrates that higher doses of hydralazine (150 to 200 mg) given every 8 or 12 hr induce significant increases of 40% to 60% in CO in patients with chronic severe aortic regurgitation. These doses may thus induce maximal transient reductions in systemic vascular resistance, regardless of dosing interval. Much higher doses may be needed to induce further changes. These data are consistent with results of previous studies, which show that the peak hemodynamic effect is partially determined by the transient peak plasma level of hydralazine.[17] These high doses, when given every 12 hr, but not when given every 8 hr, were well tolerated without cumulative hemodynamic effects and without a high incidence of acute side effects. The cumulative hemodynamic effects and incidence of side effects after repeated 200 mg doses of hydralazine were not determined in this study.

Over the short term, increases in CO after hydralazine are achieved in patients with aortic regurgitation at the expense of the regurgitant volume.[6, 18] Peak increases in CO of over 50% have been associated with a decrease in regurgitant fraction from 0.64 to 0.48.[6] Thus, only large increases in CO have been associated with significant reductions in regurgitant flow. The effects of lesser increases in CO on reductions in regurgitant fraction are not known. The long-term effects of hydralazine with respect to changes in CO are also unknown and need to be studied.[4, 19] Of interest is the fact that in a previous study, oral doses of hydralazine beginning at 50 mg and increased in small increments

TABLE 3
Hydralazine kinetics: incidence of acute side effects with incremental doses

Oral dose of hydralazine (mg)	Incidence of side effects with dosing: Every 8 hr	Every 12 hr
100	4/16 (25%)	1/21 (5%)
150	5/12 (42%)	4/20 (20%)
200	6/7 (86%)	3/16 (19%)

$\chi^2 = 10.0$; $p < .001$.

every 4 to 6 hr induced transient marked increases in CO in only four of 10 patients with chronic severe aortic regurgitation.[4] In doses of 50 and 100 mg, 5% to 25% of our patients had transient increases in CO; sustained increases in CO were rare. Doses of 150 to 200 mg of hydralazine given every 8 hr induced cumulative effects at 8 hr in 25% to 43% of our patients and the incidence of side effects was 25% to 86%. However, when hydralazine was given in doses of 150 to 200 mg every 12 hr, 30% to 45% of patients had persistent marked increases in CO, only 10% to 19% had cumulative increases at 12 hr, and the incidence of side effects was only 5% to 19%.

The small changes in PAW pressure observed in our patients have been noted previously.[2, 4, 6] Large decreases would not be expected over the short term unless significant mitral regurgitation were present and were concomitantly reduced.[3, 7]

Previous optimization procedures. For patients with valve regurgitation and heart failure, hemodynamic monitoring and frequent increases of dose every 4 to 6 hr, with no washout period, have commonly been used to determine optimal doses of oral hydralazine.[2–10] Some of these protocols have demonstrated further increased effects on CO after 24 hr on the same oral dose[8] and the need to adjust medications over 24 to 72 hr.[8, 9] With usual doses of 300 to 400 mg/day a 21% incidence of early "nonresponders" who had excessive decreases in blood pressure, increases in HR, or adverse symptoms without an increase in stroke volume index has been demonstrated.[3, 10] These studies also noted a high incidence of severe late side effects that precluded further use of hydralazine.[3, 9, 10] On the other hand, some patients may require unusually high doses to achieve beneficial hemodynamic effects.[20] Thus, dose optimization procedures in which dose is increased every 4 or 6 hr may frequently induce acute side effects in individual patients before optimal increases in CO can be achieved with higher doses. Our data suggest that the side effects observed by others may have been due to cumulative biologic effects of the dosing schedules that were used, and could have been reduced by the every-12-hr schedule.

Pharmacokinetics of hydralazine. Pharmacokinetics of hydralazine have been studied previously in patients with systemic hypertension and with congestive heart failure.[21] Small oral doses of about 1 mg/kg in patients with systemic hypertension resulted in decreased mean arterial pressure after 30 min; the peak effect was usually seen at 2 hr, and a sustained effect was seen for 8 to 12 hr. Changes in mean arterial pressure after a single effective dose were similar to changes after five of these low doses when hydralazine was given every 12 hr.[17] Thus, low doses given every 12 hr induce minimal cumulative effects in hypertensive patients. Changes in mean arterial pressure have been related to peak plasma concentrations as determined by a specific assay method.[17] However, sustained arteriolar effects are present at 8 to 12 hr and greatly exceed the plasma half-life of 10 to 15 min.[22]

The major plasma metabolite of hydralazine (hydralazine pyruvic acid hydrazone) has no effect on blood pressure. Direct hydralazine binding to arterial smooth muscle cells, possibly by chelation, appears to be the mechanism of action.[21] Thus, factors that affect first-pass metabolism through the liver will determine bioavailability (peak hydralazine levels) and, therefore, peak biologic effects. Hydralazine bioavailability increases after eating, decreases with hepatic congestion, and increases in patients with a slow-acetylator phenotype. Increased plasma levels after incremental doses are possibly due to saturation of the noninducible n-acetyl transferase system.[22] Thus, acetylator phenotype is a determinant of which patients will experience adverse symptoms. We have demonstrated that increasing maximal effects on CO are seen with incremental oral doses. We have also shown that similar maximal effects are seen after each dose from 50 to 200 mg, whether given every 8 or every 12 hr. Our findings are consistent with the previously demonstrated kinetics of hydralazine in hypertensive patients.

In conclusion, significant spontaneous changes in CO and other hemodynamic parameters occur over 12 hr in patients with severe aortic regurgitation. The statistical and clinical importance of lower doses (50 to 100 mg) of hydralazine are overestimated when single baseline determinations and transient peak effects are used to determine optimal doses. Use of internal controls plus evaluation of time-related effects by repeated-measures ANOVA provide "better" information regarding the effects, optimal dose, and proper dosing intervals for a pharmacologic intervention.

In patients with chronic severe aortic regurgitation, oral hydralazine given in doses of 50 and 100 mg induces transient increases in CO of 50% or more in a small percentage of patients (5% to 25%); however, sustained increases in CO are rare.

In patients with chronic severe aortic regurgitation, oral hydralazine given in doses of 150 to 200 mg induces significant sustained increases in CO, which have previously been demonstrated to be associated with significant decreases in regurgitant flow. Moreover, when these doses are given every 12 hr, they are associated with significantly fewer acute side effects than doses every 8 hr. Therefore, hydralazine may be given in doses of 150 mg or more every 12 hr in these patients. This regimen would be expected to improve patient compliance, and thus long-term benefits. Results of this short-term study should not be considered to indicate benefits of long-term therapy with hydralazine. Studies in progress are intended to provide data on the long-term effects of this drug in patients with chronic aortic regurgitation.[23]

References

1. Judson WE, Hollander W, Wilkins RW: The effects of intravenous Apresoline (hydralazine) on cardiovascular and renal function in patients with and without congestive heart failure. Circulation **13:** 664, 1956
2. Chatterjee K, Parmley WW, Massie B, Greenberg B, Werner J, Klausner S, Norman A: Oral hydralazine therapy for chronic refractory heart failure. Circulation **54:** 879, 1976
3. Greenberg BH, DeMots H, Murphy E, Rahimtoola SH: Arterial dilators in mitral regurgitation: effects on rest and exercise hemodynamics and long-term follow-up. Circulation **65:** 181, 1982
4. Greenberg BH, DeMots H, Murphy E, Rahimtoola SH: Beneficial effects of hydralazine on rest and exercise. Hemodynamics in patients with chronic severe aortic insufficiency. Circulation **62:** 49, 1980
5. Elkayam U, McKay CR, Weber L, Eisenberg D, Rahimtoola SH: Favorable effects of hydralazine on hemodynamic response to isometric exercise and hydralazine in aortic regurgitation patients. Am J Cardiol **53:** 1603, 1984
6. Greenberg BH, DeMots H, Murphy E, Rahimtoola SH: Mechanism for improved cardiac performance with arteriolar dilators in aortic insufficiency. Circulation **63:** 263, 1981
7. Greenberg BH, Massie B, Brundage BH, Botvinick E, Parmley WW, Chatterjee K: Beneficial effects of hydralazine in severe mitral regurgitation. Circulation **58:** 273, 1978
8. Chatterjee K, Ports TA, Brundage BH, Massie B, Holly A, Parmley WW: Oral hydralazine in chronic heart failure: sustained hemodynamic effects. Ann Intern Med **92:** 600, 1980
9. Massie B, Ports T, Chatterjee K, Parmley W, Olstand J, O'Young J, Haughorn F: Long-term vasodilator therapy for heart failure: Clinical response and its relationship to hemodynamic measurements. Circulation **63:** 269, 1981
10. Walsh WF, Greenberg BH: Results of long-term vasodilator therapy in patients with refractory congestive heart failure. Circulation **64:** 499, 1981
11. Elkayam U, Weber L, Torkan B, Berman B, Rahimtoola SH: Acute hemodynamic effects of oral nifedipine in severe chronic congestive heart failure. Am J Cardiol **52:** 1041, 1983
12. Simpson GG, Roe A, Lewontin RC: Quantitative zoology. New York, 1960, Harcourt, Brace & Co., pp 89–95
13. Zar JH: Biostatistical analysis. Englewood Cliffs, NJ, 1974, Prentice-Hall, pp 151–155
14. Glantz SA: A primer of biostatistics. New York, 1981, McGraw-Hill, pp 249–261
15. Breslow NE, Day NE: Statistical methods in cancer research. Lyon, France, 1980, International Agency for Research on Cancer, p 122
16. Bailar JC III, Louis TA, Lavori PW, Polansky M: Statistics in medicine: studies without internal controls. N Engl J Med **311:** 156, 1984
17. Shepherd AM, McNay J, Ludden T, Lin MS, Musgrave G: Plasma concentration and acetylator phenotype determine response to oral hydralazine. Hypertension **3:** 580, 1981
18. Kawanishi DT, McKay CR, Chandraratna PAN, Nanna M, Reid CL, Elkayam U, Siegel M, Rahimtoola SH: Circulatory response to exercise in patients with chronic severe aortic regurgitation. J Am Coll Cardiol **3:** 534, 1984 (abst)
19. Greenberg BH, Rahimtoola SH: Long-term vasodilator therapy in aortic insufficiency: Evidence for regression of left ventricular dilatation and hypertrophy and improvement in systolic pump function. Ann Intern Med **93:** 440, 1980
20. Packer M, Muller J, Medina N, Gorlin R, Herman M: Dose requirements of hydralazine in patients with severe chronic congestive heart failure. Am J Cardiol **45:** 655, 1980
21. Koch-Weser J: Hydralazine drug therapy. N Engl J Med **295:** 320, 1976
22. Ludden TM, McNay JL, Shepherd AM, Lin MS: Clinical pharmacokinetics of hydralazine. Clin Pharmacokinet **7:** 185, 1982
23. McKay CR, Nanna M, Elkayam U, Kawanishi D, Chandraratna PAN, Rahimtoola SH: Long-term vasodilator treatment of chronic aortic regurgitation: preliminary evidence of hemodynamic and functional improvement. Circulation **68**(suppl III): III-300, 1983 (abst)

Use of an ultra short–acting β-blocker in patients with acute myocardial ischemia

JAMES M. KIRSHENBAUM, M.D., ROBERT A. KLONER, M.D., PH.D., ELLIOTT M. ANTMAN, M.D., AND EUGENE BRAUNWALD, M.D.

ABSTRACT Esmolol is a new ultra short–acting (half-life $[t\frac{1}{2}]_\beta$ 9 min) β_1-adrenergic–receptor antagonist reported to have no intrinsic sympathomimetic activity. The safety and efficacy of esmolol in lowering the ventricular rate and rate-pressure product in patients with acute myocardial infarction (n = 5), postmyocardial infarction angina (n = 10), or acute unstable angina (n = 4), and without cardiogenic shock were studied. After a 30 min observation period, esmolol was titrated to a maximum dose of 300 μg/kg/min and infused for up to 420 min. The ventricular rate fell from 92 ± 11 (mean ± SD) to 77 ± 13 beats/min ($p < .01$) and the systolic arterial pressure decreased from 120 ± 13 to 97 ± 11 mm Hg ($p < .01$) during the initial 30 min titration period. There was no significant change during the maintenance phase, and both the ventricular rate and arterial pressure returned rapidly toward baseline values within 30 min of termination of the infusion. The cardiac index fell from 2.8 ± 0.6 to 2.2 ± 0.6 liters/min/m^2 ($p < .01$) during the same period, and also returned to the baseline level 30 min after termination of the infusion. There was no significant change in the pulmonary capillary wedge pressure, respiratory rate, or PR interval. Five patients required termination of infusion because of hypotension and all recovered uneventfully within 30 min of stopping the esmolol. One patient required a brief infusion of dopamine to restore hemodynamic stability. This experience suggests that in the absence of congestive heart failure or shock, esmolol is effective in slowing the heart rate and lowering the arterial pressure and the rate-pressure product in patients with acute myocardial ischemia. Furthermore, the hemodynamic effects are rapidly reversed after termination of infusion. Thus, esmolol may be of value in patients with acute myocardial ischemia in whom rapid titration of β-adrenergic blockade is clinically desirable.
Circulation 72, No. 4, 873–880, 1985.

THE USE OF currently available β-adrenergic–blocking agents in the management of patients with acute myocardial ischemia frequently raises concern about the potential initiation or exacerbation of congestive heart failure, severe sinus bradycardia, advanced degrees of atrioventricular block, or bronchospasm.[1–3] The development of these adverse effects may be unpredictable before starting β-blocker therapy and may result from antagonism of intrinsic sympathetic tone or direct depression of myocardial function and of the specialized automatic and conductive tissues.[2, 4, 5] Furthermore, the relatively long duration of action of standard β-blockers precludes rapid termination of drug effect should adverse reactions develop. This risk may restrict the use of β-blockers in patients with acute myocardial infarction (AMI) or unstable angina, a group particularly likely to benefit from such agents.[6, 7] A recently developed ultra short–acting β-blocker, esmolol, may prove useful in these clinical situations because of its unique kinetic profile.[8]

Esmolol, methyl 3-[4-(2-hydroxy-3-[isopropylamino]propoxy)phenyl] propionate (American Critical Care, McGaw Park, IL), is a cardioselective β_1-adrenergic–receptor antagonist without intrinsic sympathomimetic activity that has an extremely brief duration of action (half-life $[t\frac{1}{2}]_\beta$ = 9 min) because of its rapid metabolic degradation by serum and tissue ester-

From the Samuel A. Levine Cardiac Unit, Cardiovascular Division, Department of Medicine, Brigham and Women's Hospital and Harvard Medical School, Boston.

Supported in part by grant 5T32 HL-07049 from the National Heart, Lung, and Blood Institute, Bethesda; by a grant from the American Critical Care Corporation, McGaw Park, IL; and by funds contributed in part by the Massachusetts Heart Association, Boston. Data Organization and analysis assisted by the CLINFO data management and analysis system at Brigham and Women's Hospital, Boston. Supported by GCRC grant No. M01 RR00888-10 CLR. Dr. Kloner is an Established Investigator of the American Heart Association.

Address for correspondence: Elliot Antman, M.D., Cardiovascular Division, Brigham and Women's Hospital, 75 Francis St., Boston, MA 02115.

Received May 6, 1985; revision accepted July 18, 1985.

Presented at the American Heart Association Scientific Sessions, November 12, 1984, Miami Beach.

ases.[9,10] This short duration of action permits rapid titration during intravenous infusion to desired levels of β-adrenergic blockade. In addition, the rapid disappearance of β-blockade upon termination of infusion may allow ready reversal of side effects should they develop. Initial studies have demonstrated the safety and efficacy of esmolol in reducing the heart rate response to isoproterenol in animals and man, as well as for controlling the ventricular rate in patients with supraventricular tachycardia.[11–14] In experimental studies esmolol has been shown to reduce myocardial ischemic damage.[14] We report here the first experience with esmolol in treating patients with acute ischemia, including those with myocardial infarction or unstable angina.

Methods

There were 19 patients (eight men and 11 women, age 61 ± 11 [mean ± SD] years, range 31 to 80) who entered the study. Five patients were studied between 4 and 24 hr after onset of an AMI, 10 patients were treated because of angina at rest developing more than 24 hr but less than 1 week after AMI, and four patients had received therapy for acute unstable angina but had not suffered a recent infarction. All patients were in sinus rhythm with ventricular rates of more than 75 beats/min before the esmolol infusion, which was carried out in the coronary care unit of Brigham and Women's Hospital.

AMI was diagnosed by a history of typical chest pain lasting 30 min or more, as well as a transient increase in total serum creatine kinase (CK) above the normal range associated with the presence of the myocardial specific isoenzyme CK-MB* (at twice the normal range), and evolutionary ST-T wave and QRS criteria for myocardial infarction, including R wave loss and development of pathologic Q waves. Unstable angina was characterized by ischemic chest pain occurring at rest, accompanied by transient electrocardiographic changes of ST segment elevation or depression or T wave changes. Any such episodes in which electrocardiographic changes and ischemic pain occurred in the absence of serum CK elevation more than 24 hr after AMI were also considered indicative of unstable angina.

Patients were excluded if they had systolic blood pressure less than 90 mm Hg before therapy, PR intervals greater than 0.22 sec or new left or right bundle branch block, a prior history of bronchospasm or severe chronic obstructive pulmonary disease, cardiogenic shock or pulmonary capillary wedge pressure in excess of 22 mm Hg, severely impaired renal or hepatic function, significant cardiac valvular disease, or if they had received any β-blockers for at least two excretory t½s. All patients who participated gave written informed consent, and the study protocol was approved by the Human Subjects Committee of the Brigham and Women's Hospital. After consent was obtained, a 24 hr electrocardiographic monitor was applied; baseline hemodynamics were determined immediately before initiation of the esmolol infusion.

Treatment protocol. A 10 mg/ml solution of esmolol was infused with an IMED model 927 volumetric infusion pump (San Diego, CA) into a peripheral vein in each patient. The drug was administered over a 30 min titration period consisting of six consecutive 5 min infusion periods. Each infusion period consisted of a 500 μg/kg/min loading dose for 1 min followed by 4 min infusions of 50, 100, 150, 200, 250, and 300 μg/kg/min of esmolol. This regimen was followed until either the peak dose of 300 μg/kg/min had been given or systolic pressure less than 90 mm Hg, PR interval greater than 0.22 sec or left or right bundle branch block, bronchospasm, cardiogenic shock, or pulmonary capillary wedge pressure greater than 22 mm Hg developed. If necessary, the dose of esmolol was decreased to restore the systolic arterial pressure towards 90 mm Hg.

The maximal rate of infusion that each patient tolerated was continued during a maintenance period that lasted up to an additional 7 hr, following which the infusion was stopped. Patients were monitored for at least 30 min after termination of the infusion. Heart rate was determined from the electrocardiogram after each 5 min titration period, hourly during the maintenance phase, and every 5 min during the 30 min follow-up period. Blood pressure (measured by the cuff occlusion method), respiratory rate, pulmonary arterial pressure, and the mean pressure in the pulmonary capillary wedge position were similarly monitored. Cardiac output was determined at baseline, after the titration period, at the end of the maintenance period, and 30 min after termination of the infusion by the thermodilution method with an Instrumentation Laboratories (Lexington, MA) model 701 cardiac output computer (mean of three to five measurements) in 13 patients and by the Fick method in two patients. Swan-Ganz catheters were inserted in 15 patients.

In addition the following parameters were calculated:

$$\text{Mean arterial pressure (MAP) (in mm Hg)} = (2 \times \text{diastolic} + \text{systolic pressure})/3$$

$$\text{Total systemic peripheral vascular resistance (in dynes-sec-cm}^{-5}) = (\text{MAP} - \text{RA/CO} \times 80)$$

$$\text{Stroke volume index (in ml/min/m}^2) = \text{CO/(HR} \times \text{body surface area)}$$

$$\text{Double product} = (\text{Systolic BP} \times \text{HR})$$

where RA = right atrial pressure; CO = cardiac output; HR = heart rate; BP = blood pressure. Physical examination and standard laboratory tests (urinalysis; complete blood count and chemistries) were performed before and after the esmolol infusion.

Statistical analysis. Data were analyzed by a repeated-measures analysis of variance. The model included factors for period of drug administration and for patients. Contrasts within main effects were done by Tukey's method, with significance assumed at $p < .05$. Conformity to assumptions required for the model were tested by visual examination of plots of residuals.

Data are presented as mean ± SD.

Results

Data for each of the 19 patients are presented in table 1. Esmolol produced a clinically significant reduction in heart rate within the first 5 min of the titration phase (figure 1, *A*). The mean pretreatment heart rate of 92 ± 11 beats/min (range 77 to 126) decreased to 83 ± 11, 80 ± 11, 77 ± 8, 76 ± 8, 75 ± 8, 74 ± 8 beats/min, respectively, after infusion rates of 50 (n = 19), 100 (n = 19), 150 (n = 18), 200 (n = 15), 250 (n = 15), and 300 (n = 15) μg/kg/min.

Figure 1, *B*, demonstrates the peak effects on ventricular rate at the completion of the titration and main-

*CK-MB determinations were made with a DEAE non-exchange column (Dupont ACA analyzer).

tenance phases, as well as the heart rate 15 and 30 min after termination of the infusion. The peak effect on ventricular response was usually achieved at a dose of 150 μg/kg/min. Sixteen patients (group A) completed the titration phase and advanced to the maintenance phase at doses of 150 to 300 μg/kg/min (figure 2). The maintenance infusion lasted for 360 ± 94 min (range 120 to 420). There was no clinically significant change in heart rate during the maintenance phase. Three patients (group B) entered the titration phase but did not advance to the maintenance phase and are discussed below. Thirty minutes after the esmolol infusion was stopped the mean heart rate returned to within 4% of baseline values in patients in groups A and B.

Hemodynamics. Arterial pressure at baseline in the 19 patients was (systolic/diastolic, mean) 120/72, 88 mm Hg, and fell to 97/63, 75 mm Hg, at the end of the titration period. These decreases averaged 15% (systolic), 19% (diastolic), and 16% (mean) of baseline values. There was no significant change in blood pressure during the maintenance phase and blood pressure returned to 110/69, 83 mm Hg, 30 min after the esmolol infusion was stopped. During recovery, pressures returned to averages of 93% (systolic), 94% (diastolic), and 94% (mean) of baseline levels (figure 3; table 1).

Eight patients were receiving intravenous nitroglycerin at the start of the esmolol infusion because of severe, recurrent angina. Six of the eight required discontinuation of nitroglycerin to maintain systolic pressure at approximately 90 mm Hg. Subsequently, one patient developed transient angina while receiving esmolol and one required parenteral nitroglycerin after esmolol because of recurrent chest pain.

Among the 16 patients in group A, seven were unable to continue therapy at the dose of 300 μg/kg/min during the maintenance phase because systolic blood pressure persistently fell below 90 mm Hg. In five of these seven patients, a reduction in the infusion rate from 300 μg/kg/min to the range of 100 to 200 μg/kg/min permitted maintenance of peak reductions in heart rate with return of systolic blood pressure to approximately 90 mm Hg. However, two patients required termination of the maintenance infusion because of hypotension, even at such low doses. One patient with an inferior AMI developed a sudden recurrent ischemic episode complicated by electrocardiographic changes including heightened ST-T abnormalities, marked hypotension, elevation of pulmonary capillary wedge pressure, and transient mitral regurgitant murmur after tolerating a 3 hr esmolol infusion of 200 μg/kg/min. Her blood pressure and pulmonary capillary wedge pressure recovered in less than 20 min after termination of esmolol and a brief infusion of dopamine. The other patient with an anterior AMI had tolerated the 300 μg/kg/min infusion for 90 min without difficulty when he suddenly developed a profound postprandial vagal episode with nausea, vomiting, and hypotension. All symptoms and signs resolved in less than 30 min after esmolol was discontinued and 25 mg of prochlorperazine was given by the rectal route.

The limiting factor in the three patients (group B) who were unable to enter the maintenance phase was hypotension (systolic blood pressure fell below 90 mm Hg). Of these, two were evolving acute anterior infarctions at the time of the esmolol infusion and one subsequently died 48 hr later from cardiogenic shock. The third patient's systolic blood pressure fell below 90 mm Hg only at the 300 μg/kg/min dose. In each of these three patients blood pressure and heart rate both returned to control levels within 30 min of discontinuation of the esmolol infusion and none suffered any persistent sequelae as a result of transient hypotension. The time course of the recovery of heart rate and systolic pressure in these four patients with significant hypotension is depicted in figure 4.

Pulmonary capillary wedge pressure was not significantly altered during esmolol infusion (table 2).

The stroke volume index varied; both increases and decreases were observed. On average there was a 3% reduction in the stroke volume index at the completion of the titration period. This modest effect on stroke volume combined with the more appreciable reduction in heart rate caused a significant decrease in cardiac output, with an average fall in cardiac index of 21% by the end of the titration period. There was no concurrently clinically significant change in total peripheral resistance. Thus, the fall in arterial pressure was primarily due to the decline in cardiac output. Both the cardiac index and the stroke volume index returned to control levels within 30 min of termination of the esmolol infusion.

In accordance with the fall in both systolic blood pressure and heart rate there was a significant decrease of 33% in the rate-pressure product (table 2). The respiratory rate, pulmonary vascular resistance, and PR interval did not change significantly (table 2).

Side effects. No clinically important blood, urine, or electrocardiographic effects were noted during the esmolol infusion, as determined by comparing preinfusion and postinfusion electrocardiograms and results of blood and urine tests. There were no episodes of symptomatic bronchospasm, atrioventricular conduction delay, or initiation or exacerbation of congestive

TABLE 1
Patient baseline data and responses to esmolol at peak titration and maintenance doses and at 15 and 30 min after end of infusion

Patient No.	Age (yr)/sex	Dx	Esmolol dose (μg/kg/min) Peak titration	Esmolol dose (μg/kg/min) Peak maintenance	Heart rate (beats/min) Baseline	Peak T	Peak M	Recovery 15 min	Recovery 30 min
1	58/M	pMI	300	0	93	74	—	89	93
2	65/F	UA	300	300	102	77	74	90	92
3	63/F	UA	300	200	76	63	60	60	60
4	69/F	pMI	150	100	108	94	90	102	104
5	65/M	AMI	300	50	106	88	92	106	104
6	48/M	pMI	300	200	92	74	84	88	95
7	51/F	pMI	300	300	83	67	68	79	76
8	58/M	pMI	300	300	82	74	79	88	90
9	74/F	pMI	300	300	79	62	67	72	70
10	60/M	pMI	300	150	80	60	66	74	77
11	69/F	AMI	100	0	118	115	—	125	118
12	62/M	UA	300	300	97	79	77	85	91
13	31/M	pMI	300	300	92	82	81	85	85
14	62/M	UA	300	300	84	68	70	77	77
15	47/M	pMI	300	300	85	66	69	75	77
16	80/F	pMI	300	150	99	85	87	98	98
17	71/F	AMI	150	150	95	81	74	88	96
18	55/F	AMI	150	0	87	78	—	86	88
19[A]	63/F	AMI	300	200	89	77	75	(93)	(93)
Mean ± SD	61 ± 11				92 ± 11	77 ± 13[B]	76 ± 9[B]	87 ± 15[C]	88 ± 14[C]

pMI = resting angina occurring 24 hr to 7 days after a myocardial infarction; UA = acute unstable angina; T = titration phase; M = maintenance phase.

[A]The recovery values for patient 19 are not included in the data analysis because the patient received a short dopamine infusion at time of recovery data collection.

[B]$p < .01$ vs baseline; [C]$p < .01$ vs maintenance; [D]$p < .05$ vs maintenance.

heart failure. In neither of the two patients with prior histories of chronic obstructive pulmonary disease was there any exacerbation of wheezing or development of dyspnea. Patients who had a hemodynamically significant drug-induced decline in systolic pressure rapidly responded to either a dose reduction or terminaton of the infusion and in all systolic pressure returned to greater than 90 mm Hg within 15 min of discontinuing the drug. One patient required a brief infusion of dopamine. This clinical course compares favorably with that reported after infusions up to 24 hr in length in normal human volunteers.[12]

Long-term oral β-blockade. All 14 patients in group A who completed the maintenance phase without complications were subsequently started on varying doses of oral β-blockers. At the discretion of their treating physicians, 10 patients were placed on cardioselective β-adrenergic blockers (nine metoprolol, one atenolol) and four received nonselective β-adrenergic blockers (two nadolol, two propranolol). All 14 tolerated the oral drugs without clinically symptomatic adverse reactions during the period of in-hospital follow-up, which lasted up to 10 days. Metoprolol was discontinued at the discretion of the treating physician in one patient because of brief asymptomatic sinus pauses.

Two of the three patients in group B who did not enter the maintenance phase because of drug-induced hypotension eventually tolerated low doses of oral metoprolol after their conditions had stabilized clinically and hemodynamically. Their systolic blood pressures at hospital discharge were 90 to 110 mm Hg. The patient who developed postprandial vagal symptoms during the maintenance infusion phase was subsequently started on 50 mg/day atenolol without difficulty.

Discussion

Symptomatic coronary artery disease as manifested as angina or AMI results from an imbalance between myocardial oxygen supply and demand. By reducing heart rate, arterial pressure, and myocardial contractility, important determinants of myocardial oxygen consumption,[15] β-adrenergic blockers have become a mainstay of therapy of exertional angina pectoris.[16, 17]

TABLE 1
(Continued)

Blood pressure (mm Hg)				
	Peak		Recovery	
Baseline	T	M	15 min	30 min
100/64	87/55	—	94/59	102/66
130/86	110/70	88/62	98/66	100/70
150/100	120/90	88/60	92/64	104/74
128/61	79/53	105/65	120/70	117/65
122/76	104/76	88/74	98/76	94/62
118/—	88/—	96/—	98/—	102/—
115/52	93/43	100/45	96/41	100/42
110/82	108/82	100/65	122/84	130/84
108/80	110/82	92/62	94/64	94/76
138/80	90/70	102/64	118/80	124/78
130/82	90/65	—/—	102/68	128/72
128/72	112/58	110/72	120/83	140/82
100/74	96/70	90/60	95/74	99/78
130/84	98/58	92/74	96/70	102/72
111/53	99/53	104/56	107/54	105/53
109/61	84/53	92/49	109/55	110/55
108/60	96/55	109/65	122/64	124/70
112/84	86/65	—/—	100/58	106/66
129/50	96/44	120/50	(90/65)	(94/65)
120 ± 13	97 ± 11[B]	99 ± 9[B]	105 ± 11	110 ± 14[D]
72 ± 14	63 ± 13[B]	62 ± 9[B]	66 ± 11	69 ± 11

In recent studies β-adrenergic blockers appear to reduce the size of experimental and naturally occurring myocardial infarctions,[6, 18–21] and to reduce mortality and the incidence of reinfarction in patients surviving AMI.[22–24] However, β-blockade was associated with significant adverse reactions in 2% to 7% of patients, and these reactions consisted principally of cardiac failure, bradycardia, hypotension, or atrioventricular block.[5, 25–27] Adverse reactions can occur rapidly and after relatively small doses of drug and can develop with cardioselective β-blockers or those with intrinsic sympathomimetic activity.[25] Therefore, it is often recommended that initial doses of β-adrenergic–receptor antagonists in acutely ischemic patients be administered cautiously and in small amounts.[3] Should adverse effects be noted, the use of inotropic agents may be required, which would complicate the management of these acutely ill patients.

Esmolol is an ultrashort–acting β-blocker that is rapidly degraded by tissue and serum esterases, permitting resolution of β-blockade within minutes of termination of an intravenous infusion. This study was designed to assess the safety and efficacy of esmolol in diminishing the ventricular rate and the rate-pressure product in patients with acute ischemic heart disease.

Esmolol caused a rapid reduction in ventricular rate that, when coupled with the rapid return to the baseline rate after termination of the infusion, is indicative of a clear drug effect. The fall in heart rate was matched by a similar decline in arterial pressure. The maximal

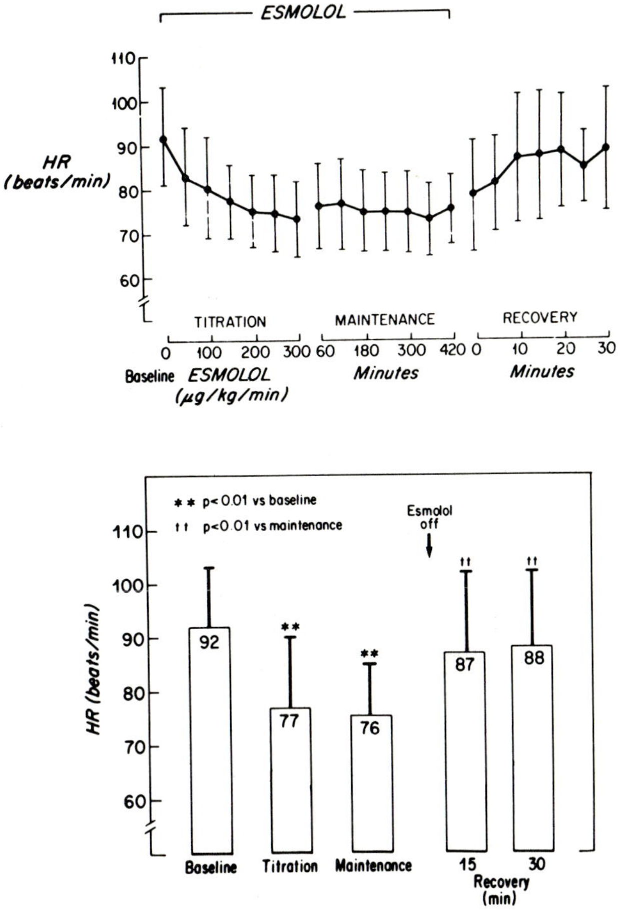

FIGURE 1. *A*, Ventricular response in all 19 patients during the titration, maintenance, and recovery phases. *B*, Ventricular rate (mean ± SD) achieved at peak tolerated titration and maintenance infusions, and peak recovery rates 15 and 30 min after termination of the esmolol infusion.

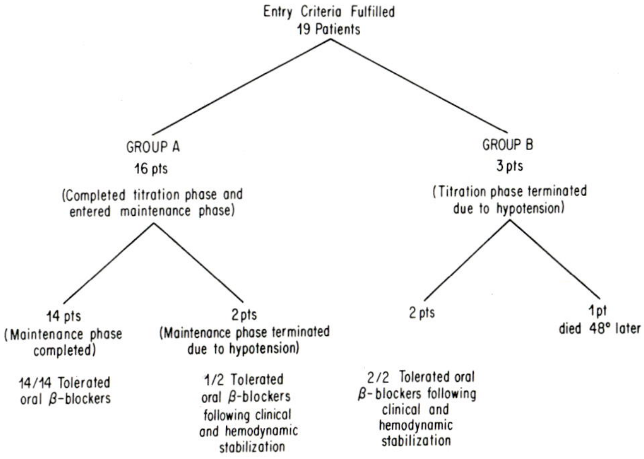

FIGURE 2. Clinical outcome in the 19 patients with fulfilled inclusion criteria and entered the esmolol infusion study.

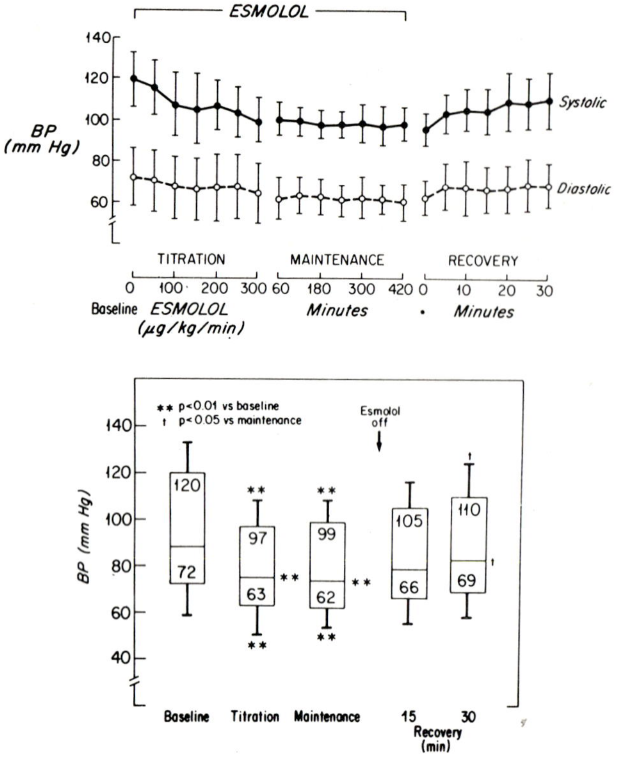

FIGURE 3. *A*, Arterial pressure response in all 19 patients during the titration, maintenance, and recovery phases. *B*, Systolic, diastolic, and mean (± SD) arterial pressure achieved at peak tolerated titration and maintenance infusions, and peak recovery pressures 15 and 30 min after esmolol.

reduction in heart rate occurred at doses below those causing the greatest reductions in blood pressure. Little additional negative chronotropic effect was observed at infusion rates in excess of 150 to 200 µg/kg/min (figure 1).

The magnitude of reduction in heart rate was similar to that obtained by Wirtzfeld et al.,[28] who administered 10 mg metoprolol to patients with AMI and noted a 16% reduction in heart rate. Amsterdam et al.[29] reported a decrease in heart rate from 99 to 81 beats/min after propranolol (0.03 to 0.05 mg/kg) in 10 patients with AMI. Similar findings in heart rate reduction were obtained by Gold et al.[30] Although Mueller et al.[31] reported a smaller decrement (9%) in heart rate after propranolol (0.1 mg/kg), the baseline heart rate in their patients averaged 80 vs 93 beats/min in our patients with acute myocardial ischemia.

The maximal negative chronotropic effect (achieved by infusion rates of 100 to 200 µg/kg/min) was associated with a systolic pressure greater than 90 mm Hg in 17 of 19 patients. The double product (systolic pressure × heart rate) declined by more than 30% in most of our patients without clinically significant hemodynamic compromise. As noted above, systemic hypotension was frequently the dose-limiting factor preventing the incremental augmentation of esmolol infusion rates. This is in contrast with the findings in studies of other β-adrenergic antagonists in patients with AMI in whom only a small effect on systemic arterial pressure was noted.[28–30, 32] This may be explained by recent studies in rabbits that demonstrated a decrease in total peripheral resistance with a subsequent fall in blood pressure during esmolol infusion.[33] While there was a small diminution in systemic resistance in our patients, most other studies have reported a persistent augmentation of peripheral resistance during the administration of the longer-acting β-blockers.[28, 29, 34–36] Whether esmolol in fact has a unique effect on peripheral vascular tone cannot be definitely demonstrated in this small series of patients.

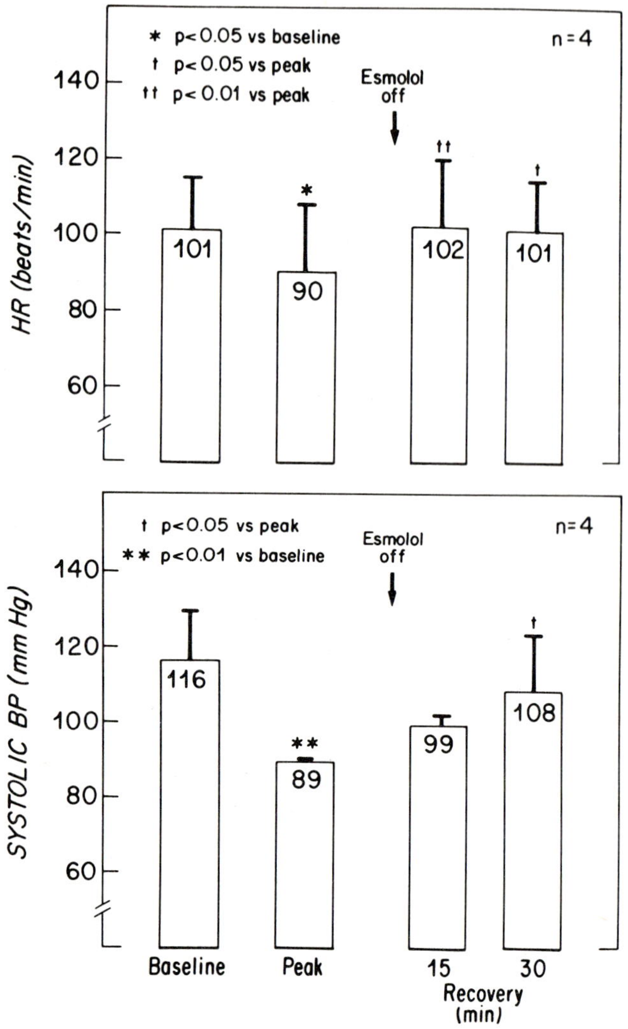

FIGURE 4. *A*, Heart rate response in four patients with hypotensive reactions. The heart rate returned toward baseline 15 min after completion of the esmolol infusion. *B*, Systolic arterial pressure response in four patients with hypotensive reactions. There was complete return to baseline pressure 30 min after infusion termination. One patient (data not shown) required a short course of dopamine to restore hemodynamic stability.

TABLE 2
Summary of patient hemodynamic, pulmonary, and electrical responses to esmolol

	Baseline	Titration	Maintenance	Recovery (30 min p̄ esmolol)
Rate-pressure product ($\times 10^3$)	11 ± 1.8	7.4 ± 1.2[C]	7.5 ± 1.1[C]	9.8 ± 2.3[B]
Cardiac index (l/min/m^2)	2.8 ± 0.6	2.2 ± 0.6[C]	2.6 ± 0.7[D]	2.8 ± 0.6[D]
Mean PCW (mm Hg)	13 ± 5	14 ± 5	14 ± 5	13 ± 5
RR (breaths/min)	19 ± 2	19 ± 2	19 ± 2	19 ± 2
PR interval (sec)	0.17 ± 0.03	0.17 ± 0.03	0.17 ± 0.03	0.17 ± 0.03
SVI (ml/min/m^2)	31 ± 8	30 ± 9	35 ± 10[A]	32 ± 10
TPR (dynes-sec-cm^{-5})	1351 ± 552	1452 ± 460	1162 ± 398	1283 ± 563
PVR (dynes-sec-cm^{-5})	86 ± 61	126 ± 85	101 ± 54	101 ± 66

PCW = mean pulmonary capillary wedge pressure; RR = respiratory rate; SVI = stroke volume index; TPR = total peripheral resistance; PVR = pulmonary vascular resistance.
[A]$p < .05$ vs baseline; [B]$p < .01$ vs maintenance; [C]$p < .01$ vs baseline; [D]$p < .01$ vs titration.

There was no significant change in left ventricular filling pressure during either the titration or maintenance phases of esmolol infusion, except in the one patient who experienced a sudden ischemic episode during the infusion. This is similar to observations made in several prior studies of β-blockers in patients with acute ischemia.[28–30, 34] Even in our seven patients with abnormally elevated pulmonary capillary pressures (≥12 mm Hg), there was no evidence of congestive heart failure or pulmonary edema.

Duration of action. All values for hemodynamic parameters initially influenced by esmolol returned toward baseline within 30 min of terminating the infusion. This is in agreement with prior observations in animals, normal human volunteers, and patients with supraventricular tachycardia.[8–14] Serum and tissue esterases are thought to be the prime mechanism of esmolol's "ultra short" ($t\frac{1}{2}_\beta$ = 9 min) duration of action. The presence of left ventricular dysfunction as manifested by a markedly diminished cardiac output in the setting of adequate filling pressures did not prolong the drug effect. Even in the three patients who were unable to complete the titration phase because of hypotension, the resolution of β-blockade occurred in less than 30 min.

Clinical implications. Esmolol was effective in slowing the heart rate in our patients with AMI or unstable angina without cardiogenic shock. The rapid metabolism of esmolol permitted tighter immediate control over the desired degree of β-blockade than would have been possible with currently available long-acting β-adrenergic–receptor antagonists. The effects of the drug on heart rate and blood pressure were rapidly eliminated on termination of the infusion. In three recent large-scale studies of the value of β-blockade therapy after myocardial infarction a history of bradycardia, hypotension, congestive heart failure, atrioventricular block, or asthma excluded 18% to 28% of otherwise eligible patients.[22–24] These patients may, however, have been the very patients most likely to benefit from such therapy. While use of esmolol in such a subset of patients has yet to be reported, its rapid reversal of action may allow the safe initiation of β-blockade in some of these high-risk patients.

Recent studies suggest that there is a brief period of several hours after acute coronary occlusion during which revascularization may limit eventual size of infarction or reduce mortality.[18, 37, 38] The immediate administration of cardioprotective agents, such as β-adrenergic blockers, calcium-channel blockers, or other drugs, may prolong the critical time period during which reperfusion, whether thrombolytic, mechanical, or surgical, would be beneficial. Lange et al.[14] and Hammerman et al.[39] have demonstrated enhanced salvage of ischemic myocardium in dogs after coronary occlusion when β-adrenergic–receptor blockade was added to reperfusion alone. The rapid offset of action of esmolol may offer important clinical benefits in titrating β-blockade in patients undergoing thrombolytic therapy for AMI. Finally, it will be important to determine whether a beneficial hemodynamic response to a brief infusion of esmolol predicts long-term efficacy and safety with oral β-adrenergic blockers.

We acknowledge the secretarial assistance of Nancy Watterson and Mary Gillan, and the statistical and technical advice of Sharon Hale. We thank the American Critical Care Corporation for supplying esmolol and for the support and advice provided by Atul R. Laddu, M.D., Robert J. Lee, Ph.D., and Lori Blanski, R.N. All patients who participated gave written informed consent, and the study protocol was approved by the Human Subjects Committee of the Brigham and Women's Hospital.

References

1. Frishman W, Silverman R: Clinical pharmacology of the new beta-adrenergic blocking drugs. Part 3. Comparative clinical experience and new therapeutic applications. Am Heart J **98:** 119, 1979
2. Ahlquist RP: Present state of alpha and beta adrenergic drugs III. Beta blocking agents. Am Heart J **93:** 117, 1977
3. McDevitt DG: Adrenoceptor blocking drugs: clinical pharmacology and therapeutic use. Drugs **17:** 267, 1979
4. Nies AS, Shand DG: Clinical pharmacology of propranolol. Circulation **52:** 6, 1975
5. Frishman W, Silverman R, Strom J, Elkayam U, Sonnenblick E: Clinical pharmacology of the new beta-adrenergic blocking drugs. part 4. Adverse effects. Choosing a beta-adrenoceptor blocker. Am Heart J **98:** 256, 1979
6. Braunwald E, Muller JE, Kloner RA, Maroko PR: Role of beta-adrenergic blockade in the therapy of patients with myocardial infarction. Am J Med **74:** 113, 1983
7. Fischl SJ, Herman MV, Gorlin R: The intermediate coronary syndrome. Clinical, angiographic and therapeutic aspects. N Engl J Med **288:** 1193, 1973
8. Zaroslinski J, Borgman RJ, O'Donnell JP, Anderson WG, Erhardt RW, Kam ST, Reynolds RD, Lee RJ, Groczynski JR: Ultra-short acting beta-blockers: A proposal for the treatment of the critically ill patient. Life Sci **31:** 899, 1982
9. Yacobi A, Kartzinel R, Lai CM, Sum CY: Esmolol: A pharmacokinetic profile of a new cardioselective beta-blocking agent. J Pharm Sci **72:** 710, 1983
10. Sum CY, Yacobi A, Kartzinel R, Stampfli H, Davis CS, Lai CM: Kinetics of esmolol, an ultra short–acting beta-blocker, and of its major metabolite. Clin Pharmacol Ther **34:** 427, 1983
11. Gorczynski RJ, Shaffer JE, Lee RJ: Pharmacology of ASL-8052, a novel beta-adrenergic receptor antagonist with an ultrashort duration of action. J Cardiovasc Pharmacol **5:** 668, 1983
12. Angaran D, Fitzpatrick P, Gray R, Hochman J, Kaplan K, Lester R, Schwartz M, Turlapaty P: Antiarrhythmic efficacy and safety of esmolol — an ultra-short acting beta blocker. Clin Res **32:** 48A, 1984
13. Byrd RC, Sung RJ, Marks J, Parmley WW: Safety and efficacy of esmolol (ASL-8052: an ultrashort-acting beta-adrenergic blocking agent) for control of ventricular rate in supraventricular tachycardias. J Am Coll Cardiol **3:** 394, 1984
14. Lange R, Kloner RA, Braunwald E: First ultra-short-acting beta-adrenergic blocking agent: its effect on size and segmental wall dynamics of reperfused myocardial infarcts in dogs. Am J Cardiol **51:** 1759, 1983
15. Boerth RC, Covell JW, Pool PE, Ross J Jr: Increased myocardial oxygen consumption and contractile state associated with increased heart rate in dogs. Circ Res **24:** 725, 1969
16. Wolfson S, Heinle RA, Herman MV, Kemp HG, Sullivan JM, Gorlin R: Propranolol and angina pectoris. Am J Cardiol **18:** 345, 1966
17. Frishman WH: Beta-adrenoceptor antagonists: new drugs and new indications. N Engl J Med **305:** 500, 1981
18. Reimer KA, Rasmussen MM, Jennings RB: Reduction by propranolol of myocardial necrosis after temporary coronary occlusion in dogs. Circ Res **33:** 353, 3973
19. Herlitz J, Elmfeldt D, Hjalmarson A, Holmberg S, Malek I, Nyberg G, Ryden L, Swedberg K, Vedin A, Waagstein F, Waldenstrom A, Waldenstrom J, Wedel H, Wilhelmsen L, Wilhelmsson C: Effect of metoprolol on indirect signs of the size and severity of acute myocardial infarction. Am J Cardiol **51:** 1282, 1983
20. The International Collaborative Study Group: Reduction of infarct size with the early use of timolol in acute myocardial infarction. N Engl J Med **310:** 9, 1984
21. Hjalmarson A, Herlitz J: Limitation of infarct size by beta blockers and its potential role for prognosis. Circulation **67**(suppl II): II-68, 1983
22. Beta-Blocker Heart Attack Trial Research Group. A randomized trial of propranolol in patients with acute myocardial infarction. 1. Mortality results. JAMA **247:** 1707, 1982
23. The Norwegian Multicenter Study Group: Timolol-induced reduction in mortality and reinfarction in patients surviving acute myocardial infarction. N Engl J Med **304:** 801, 1981
24. Hjalmarson A, Herlitz J, Malek I, Ryden L, Vedin A, Waldenstrom A, Wedel H, Elmfeldt D, Holmberg S, Nyberg G, Swedberg K, Waagstein F, Waldenstrom J, Wilhelmsen L: Effect on mortality of metoprolol in acute myocardial infarction. A double-blind randomized trial. Lancet **2:** 823, 1981
25. Greenblatt DJ, Koch-Weser J: Adverse reactions of beta-adrenergic receptor blocking drugs: a report from the Boston Collaborative Drug Surveillance Program. Drugs **7:** 118, 1974
26. Herlitz J, Pennert K, Wedel H, Vedin A, Wilhelmsson C, Wilhelmsen L, Hjalmarson A: Goteborg Metoprolol Trial: Tolerance. Am J Cardiol **53:** 46D, 1984
27. Friedman LM: How do the various beta blockers compare in type, frequency and severity of their adverse effects? Circulation **67** (suppl I): I-89, 1983
28. Wirtzfeld A, Klein G, Delius W, Sack D: Treatment of acute myocardial infarction with metoprolol. Dtsch Med Wochenschr **103:** 566, 1978
29. Amsterdam EA, Hilliard G, Williams DO, Caudill C, Vismara L, Massumi RA, Mason DT: Hemodynamic effects of propranolol in acute myocardial infarction. Circulation **48**(suppl IV): IV-138, 1973
30. Gold HK, Leinbach RC, Maroko PR: Propranolol-induced reduction of signs of ischemic injury during acute myocardial infarction. Am J Cardiol **38:** 689, 1976
31. Mueller HS, Ayres SM, Religa A, Evans RG: Propranolol in the treatment of acute myocardial infarction. Effect on myocardial oxygenation and hemodynamics. Circulation **49:** 1078, 1974
32. Waagstein F, Hjalmarson AC: Double-blind study of the effect of cardioselective beta-blockade on chest pain in acute myocardial infarction. Acta Med Scand **587** (suppl):201, 1975
33. Murthy VS, Hwang-TF, Zagar ME, Vollmer RR, Schmidt DH: Cardiovascular pharmacology of ASL-8052, an ultra-short acting beta blocker. Eur J Pharmacol **94:** 43, 1983
34. Malek I, Waagstein F, Hjalmarson A, Holmberg S, Swedberg K: Hemodynamic effects of the cardioselective beta-blocking agent metoprolol in acute myocardial infarction. A 24-hour catheterization study. Acta Med Scand **204**(suppl): 195, 1978
35. Bay G, Lund-Larsen P, Lorentsen E, Sivertssen E: Hemodynamic effects of propranolol (inderal) in acute myocardial infarction. Br Med J **1:** 141, 1967
36. Taylor SH, Silke B, Lee PS: Intravenous beta-blockade in coronary heart disease. Is cardioselectivity or intrinsic sympathomimetic activity hemodynamically useful? N Engl J Med **306:** 631, 1982
37. Laffel GL, Braunwald E: Thrombolytic therapy: a new strategy for the treatment of acute myocardial infarction. N Engl J Med **311:** 710; 770, 1984
38. Kennedy JW, Ritchie JL, Davis KB, Fritz JK: Western Washington Randomized trial of intracoronary streptokinase in acute myocardial infarction. J Engl J Med **309:** 1477, 1983
39. Hammerman H, Kloner RA, Briggs LL, Braunwald E: Enchangement of salvage of reperfused myocardium by early beta-adrenergic blockade (timolol). J Am Coll Cardiol **3:** 1438, 1984

Exercise thallium-201 scintigraphy in dogs: effects of long-term coronary occlusion and collateral development on early and late scintigraphic images

MICHAEL V. COHEN, M.D., AND RICHARD M. STEINGART, M.D.

ABSTRACT To examine the effects of coronary collateral development on thallium-201 (^{201}Tl) distribution the left circumflex coronary artery was ligated in eight dogs. Three days later these animals ran on a treadmill, and 201-thallous chloride was injected into the right atrium at peak exercise. Scintigraphic scanning was begun within 10 min and continued for 3 hr. Scanning was repeated weekly for 6 weeks. In the last week radioactive microspheres were injected into the left atrium at peak exercise to measure regional myocardial blood flow. The scintigraphically determined disparity between perfusion of the ischemic and normal myocardium was most marked at 3 days after ligation. This difference gradually lessened over the first 4 weeks until there was no difference in ^{201}Tl distribution to normally perfused myocardium and tissue distal to the ligation. Concomitant with the improvement in the scintigrams, exercise hemodynamics also improved over this 4 week period with significant increases in cardiac output and decreases in left atrial pressure. Serial coronary angiographic studies in two animals demonstrated the appearance of collaterals in the initial weeks after coronary occlusion, and by 4 weeks the left circumflex artery distal to the obstruction was completely opacified by collateral flow. The ratio of directly measured exercise blood flow to the left circumflex and normally perfused tissues was 0.89 ± 0.08 at 6 weeks after ligation. Scintigraphic ^{201}Tl redistribution after 3 hr also changed over the weeks after ligation. Three days after ligation washout from the ischemic area was significantly slower than that from the normal myocardium. By 6 weeks loss of ^{201}Tl from the two regions occurred at nearly equal rates. Thus myocardial perfusion and function during exercise after coronary occlusion are dynamic events that change with time. It is likely that coronary collateral development is responsible for these phenomena. Therefore coronary collaterals do have salutary effects in the dog.
Circulation 72, No. 4, 881–891, 1985.

THE FUNCTIONAL SIGNIFICANCE of coronary collaterals has been debated for many years. On the basis of analysis of clinical presentation and myocardial function in patients with coronary artery disease, several investigators have concluded that coronary collaterals are merely markers of the underlying disease.[1–6] However, other clinical studies have concluded that coronary collaterals are indeed able to prevent infarction,[7–10] preserve myocardial function,[11–16] and prolong survival.[17, 18] Perhaps the reasons for these conflicting conclusions rest in the difficulties encountered in designing an appropriate clinical study to answer the question and in the almost impossible task of selecting nearly identical subjects differing only in the presence or absence of collaterals. Because of these problems, animal preparations in which variables can be closely controlled have been used to study the significance of coronary collaterals.

Coronary collaterals in the experimental animal do limit infarction,[19, 20] restore blood flow to ischemic myocardium,[21] preserve myocardial function,[21, 22] and improve survival after coronary occlusion.[23, 24] However, most studies have compared groups of animals with poorly developed coronary collaterals to those with well-developed collaterals.[19, 20, 22–24] These group comparisons suffer from many of the same doubts raised by the clinical studies. Only a few investigators have studied the longitudinal effects of collateral development in the same individual animals.[21] To better examine the sequential functional effects of coronary

From the Division of Cardiology and Departments of Medicine and Nuclear Medicine, Montefiore Medical Center and Albert Einstein College of Medicine, Bronx, NY.

Supported in part by NHLBI grant HL-17809. Dr. Cohen is the recipient of NHLBI Research Career Development Award HL-00281.

Address for correspondence: Michael V. Cohen, M.D., Division of Cardiology, Montefiore Medical Center, 111 East 210th St., Bronx, NY 10467.

Received Sept. 28, 1984; revision accepted July 5, 1985.

Presented in part at the National Meeting of the American Federation for Clinical Research, Washington, DC, May 1982.

collateral development after coronary occlusion, we used exercise thallium-201 (^{201}Tl) scintigraphy in chronically instrumented dogs to make multiple observations in the same animal during a period that is known to encompass dramatic histologic changes in collateral structure. Our results demonstrate the functional counterpart of these anatomic changes and define the ability of coronary collaterals to limit the intensity of stress-induced myocardial ischemia.

Methods

Experimental preparation. Eight mongrel dogs (20 to 30 kg) were anesthetized with sodium pentobarbital (30 mg/kg) and intubated. Through a left thoracotomy, 15-gauge polyethylene catheters were inserted into the left atrial appendage and descending thoracic aorta and secured with purse-string sutures. The left circumflex coronary artery (LCf) was isolated immediately beyond the first major marginal branch. After premedication of the dogs with quinidine gluconate (6 mg/kg im) and lidocaine (40 mg iv) and initiation of a continuous intravenous infusion of lidocaine (1 mg/min), the LCf was totally ligated. Ventricular premature contractions were treated with 20 mg iv bolus injections of lidocaine. The LCf was incised immediately distal to the ligature and an 18-gauge catheter inserted and advanced to a point proximal to the next marginal branch where it was secured. The edges of the pericardium were approximated and the chest was closed in layers. All catheters were brought out through the chest wall and filled with a dilute solution of sodium heparin (1000 U/ml).

Experimental protocol. One or 2 days before any operative intervention a catheter was inserted into a foreleg vein of all animals. The dogs ran on a treadmill at increasing speeds and inclines until heart rate stabilized at approximately 220 beats/min. Two millicuries of 201-thallous chloride was then injected intravenously. The animals ran for an additional minute and after a brief cooldown period were anesthetized with sodium pentobarbital. Scanning commenced 10 min after injection of radioisotope.

Three to 4 days after surgery and occlusion of the LCf, all dogs were able to run on the treadmill and underwent repeat exercise ^{201}Tl scintigraphy. Heart rate and phasic and mean left atrial and aortic pressures were recorded while the dogs were resting quietly. Cardiac output was measured in duplicate by the indicator dilution method. A bolus of indocyanine green was injected into the left atrium while arterial blood was withdrawn by a Harvard constant-withdrawal pump and sampled by a Gilford densitometer (103IR) inserted in the line. After completion of the baseline recordings, the treadmill was started and the speed and incline were slowly increased. Although the goal was to reproduce the heart rate attained during the preoperative exercise study, animals rarely performed as well during this initial postoperative exercise session. Two millicuries of ^{201}Tl was injected after heart rate plateaued, and the animal continued to run 1 min longer. Scanning was begun 10 min after the completion of exercise.

The exercise studies and ^{201}Tl scans were repeated weekly for 6 weeks in all eight dogs every 2 weeks for an additional 6 weeks in three animals. After the initial postoperative scan, all dogs were able to exercise to heart rates of at least 220 beats/min.

Myocardial scintigrams. The dogs were scanned with the right chest on the table. A gamma camera (Picker Nuclear) equipped with an all-purpose collimator was positioned parallel to the left chest and centered approximately 1 inch above the cardiac impulse. Placement of three ^{57}Co markers on the chest wall at specified reference points assisted in centering the heart in the camera field and ensured reproducible orientation in all serial studies. A 15% energy window centered at 77 keV was used to collect ^{201}Tl scintigraphic data. Data were acquired in a 64 × 64 pixel matrix on a PDP 1134 computer (Digital Equipment Corp). Scanning was begun 10 min after ^{201}Tl injection and continued for 36, 5 min frames with the camera-animal relationship held constant. The initial 5 min frame contained a minimum of 450,000 counts, with at least 75,000 counts in the region of the left ventricle. This scintigraphic procedure was duplicated for each of the control and six or seven postligation studies.

Before the exercise studies, 0.1 mCi of ^{201}Tl was injected into the LCf catheter to determine the scintigraphic perfusion territory of the LCf. The animals were then positioned under the gamma camera and a 10 min acquisition was begun. In this way the territories of the LCf (active) and left anterior descending coronary artery (LAD) (inactive) were clearly and reproducibly circumscribed.

All postexercise scans were processed in a blinded fashion. A region of interest was drawn manually around the perimeter of the left ventricle with the operator designating the pixel on the circumference corresponding to the left ventricular apex. The operator also designated a rectangular background region of interest situated four pixels from the edge of the ventricle. A computer algorithm then determined the centroid of the left ventricle and generated 24 radials, at 15 degree increments, from this centroid to pixels on the circumference. By conversion, that point on the circumference opposite the apex was designated radius 1, with numbering proceeding clockwise around the ventricle. Guided by the results of the intracoronary ^{201}Tl injections, which helped to demarcate the perfusion territory of the distal LCf, average counts within radials 3 to 11 (30 to 150 degrees) were designated as LCf activity, whereas counts from radials 14 to 18 (195 to 255 degrees) were designated as LAD activity. Radials 12 and 13 were not included in the analysis because LAD and LCf distributions tend to overlap in this region.

Background subtraction was accomplished with a modification[25] of the bilinear interpolation algorithm first described by Goris et al.[26] Because the gamma camera–animal relationships were not changed over the 3 hr of scanning, these same regions of interest were used to analyze each of the 36 frames with background determined separately for each frame.

For analysis of LAD and LCf count activity within the initial 5 min scan, count data were expressed as a percentage of the highest average radial activity in the heart. For analysis of ^{201}Tl "washout" within the LAD and LCf distributions, data were expressed as a percentage of the average LAD ^{201}Tl activity in the initial 5 min frame from that scan.

Scintigraphic measurement of the LCf/LAD ^{201}Tl activity ratio at 10 to 14 min after exercise provides a measure of the distribution of blood flow at peak exercise.[27] Scintigraphic analysis of subsequent redistribution can be used to distinguish between hypoperfusion of viable myocardium and infarction as a cause of the initial flow disparity.[28]

Coronary angiography. In two animals coronary angiograms were obtained 2 days after coronary occlusion and again 2 and 4 weeks later. Two days after the operative procedure the dogs were reanesthetized with sodium pentobarbital (15 to 20 mg/kg) and transported to the coronary angiographic suite where a femoral cutdown was performed. The animal was placed in a lateral position, with the right chest closest to the image intensifier (Philips). A previously described preformed Kifa catheter[29] was inserted into the femoral artery and advanced with fluoroscopic guidance into the aortic root and then into the ostium of the left coronary artery. Five to 7 ml of contrast agent (meglumine diatrizoate) was injected by hand into the coronary artery, and the image was recorded on 35 mm film at a rate of 50 frames/sec. After completion of the procedure, the Kifa catheter was removed and thrombus was extracted proximal and distal to the arterial incision with a balloon catheter. The vessel was then repaired. Subsequent angiographic procedures were performed by cutting down on the same or contralateral femoral artery after initially anesthetizing the dogs with sodium pentobarbital (30 mg/kg).

Radioactive microspheres. In the sixth week after coronary ligation, myocardial blood flow was measured during exercise with radioactive microspheres before the ^{201}Tl injection. Two to 4×10^6 radioactively labeled 15 μm microspheres suspended in 10 ml of 6% dextran to which 2 drops of polysorbate 80 (Tween 80) had been added to prevent aggregation were agitated in an ultrasonic bath for at least 20 min before injection. With the animal running on the treadmill and after the target heart rate was reached, hemodynamics were recorded and a timed constant-rate withdrawal of arterial blood was begun. Shortly thereafter the microspheres were injected into the left atrium, followed immediately by a bolus of indocyanine green for measurement of cardiac output.

Preparation of myocardial samples. After completion of the longitudinal exercise/scanning protocol, the dogs were anesthetized with sodium pentobarbital (30 mg/kg) and the heart was exposed through a left thoracotomy. Coincident with the left atrial administration of 20 ml of a saturated solution of KCl to arrest the heart, 2 to 3 ml of a concentrated solution of Evans blue dye was injected into the distal LCf to outline its perfusion territory. The heart was extirpated and the atria were trimmed away. After filling of the ventricular chambers with gauze, the heart was frozen and then sliced from apex to base into 0.5 cm thick slices. The left ventricular rings were separated into stained (LCf perfusion territory distal to the ligature) and unstained portions. These pieces were then divided into wedges and each wedge was subdivided into inner (or endocardial) and outer (or epicardial) halves. Isotope activity of all myocardial pieces and reference arterial blood samples was counted in a gamma spectrometer (Nuclear Chicago Model 1185), and the counts per minute and counts per minute per gram were determined by standard computer programs after correction for decay and overlap of isotope energies.

Determination of myocardial blood flow. Myocardial flow (ml/min/g) to each piece was calculated by the reference arterial sample method. Average flow to the entire stained and unstained myocardial regions as well as inner and outer portions of the left ventricular wall were obtained by summing the counts per minute as well as the wet weights of all pieces within the region of interest and then expressing the results as milliliters per minute per gram. Collateral flow is defined as the flow to the stained LCf tissue beyond the ligation.

Statistical analysis. All results are expressed as mean ± SE. The significance of differences in scintigraphic ^{201}Tl ratios within a heart and in regional myocardial blood flows was determined by a paired Student's t test.[30] The significance of changes in hemodynamics, double product, and ^{201}Tl activity over time was determined by an analysis of variance procedure with intergroup comparisons.[30] A p value of $<.05$ was considered significant.

Results

Hemodynamics at rest and during exercise before ligation and during the postligation studies done 3 days to 6 weeks after LCf occlusion are summarized in table 1. Before surgery and LCf occlusion the average heart rate rose from 96 ± 5 beats/min at rest to 229 ± 8 beats/min at a speed of 5.2 ± 0.3 mph and incline of 11.1 ± 0.7%. Three days after coronary occlusion, the maximal exercise heat rate was significantly lower, 204 ± 4 beats/min ($p < .05$). The dogs could run at only 4.0 ± 0.5 mph and 8.4 ± 2.0% grade. The average double product (heart rate × mean blood pressure) of 12,765 ± 1286 mm Hg/min at rest rose to 22,802 ± 1618 mm Hg/min during running ($p < .001$) (figure 1). Cardiac output doubled to 6.1 liters/min, and average left atrial pressure increased from 7.5 to 23.1 mm Hg.

Exercise tolerance and cardiac function subsequently improved. Thus, at week 1 maximal heart rate was

TABLE 1
Hemodynamics at rest and during peak exercise before and after LCF occlusion (mean ± SEM)

	Rest				Exercise			
	HR (bpm)	AoP (mm Hg)	LAP (mm Hg)	CO (l/min)	HR	AoP	LAP	CO
Preligation	96±5	—	—	—	229 ± 8^{B}	—	—	—
Postligation								
3 days	135 ± 7^{E}	96±8	7.5±2.6	2.8±0.3	$204\pm4^{B,D}$	111±9	23.1 ± 4.2^{A}	6.1 ± 0.7^{B}
1 wk	123 ± 8^{D}	95±7	9.6±1.0	3.3±0.3	230 ± 3^{B}	107±9	19.0 ± 4.1^{A}	$8.3\pm0.9^{A,C}$
2 wk	118±8	101±6	11.4±2.8	3.2±0.3	231 ± 4^{B}	107±6	15.1±2.2	$8.0\pm0.8^{B,C}$
3 wk	122 ± 9^{D}	105±7	7.5±2.2	3.3±0.2	228 ± 4^{B}	115±7	11.1 ± 2.0^{C}	$8.1\pm0.7^{B,C}$
4 wk	111±5	103±8	8.1±2.2	3.5±0.3	219 ± 8^{B}	111±8	10.7 ± 2.2^{C}	$8.3\pm0.8^{A,C}$
5 wk	122 ± 6^{D}	107±6	8.5±1.8	3.6±0.3	221 ± 5^{B}	115±9	10.5 ± 2.0^{C}	$8.5\pm0.9^{A,C}$
6 wk	115±9	99±6	8.9±2.4	3.8±0.3	227 ± 6^{B}	109±9	11.2 ± 1.8^{C}	$8.6\pm1.1^{A,C}$

AoP = mean aortic pressure; CO = cardiac output; HR = heart rate; LAP = mean left atrial pressure.
Statistical significance of paired differences between rest and exercise states: $^{A}p < .005$; $^{B}p < .001$.
Statistical significance of differences between first and subsequent postligation studies: $^{C}p < .05$.
Statistical significance of differences between preligation and postligation heart rates: $^{D}p < .05$; $^{E}p < .005$.

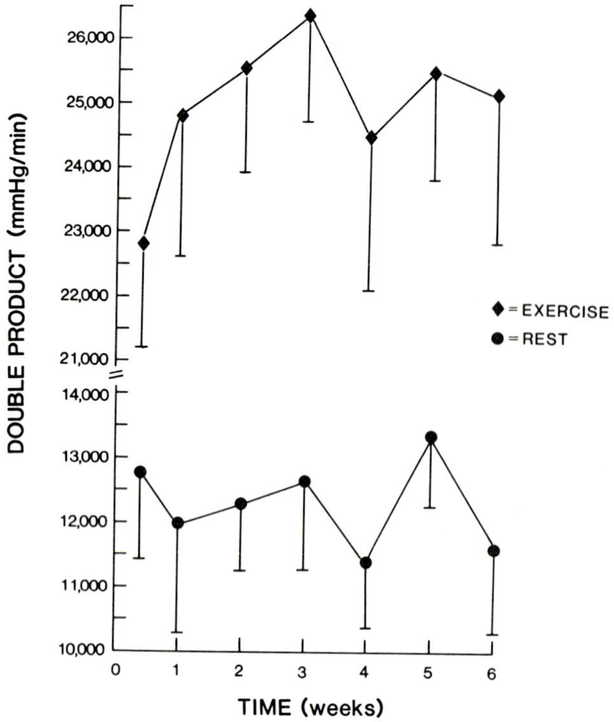

FIGURE 1. Resting and exercise double products after ligation of the LCf. The exercise double product was lowest 3 days after ligation and increased progressively over the next 3 weeks, although the changes were not statistically significant. The rise reflected improving exercise performance. The exercise value was always significantly greater ($p < .001$) than the index at rest. The vertical bars represent 1 SEM.

back to 230 beats/min (table 1) and double product was higher (figure 1). Exercise cardiac output rose to 8.3 liters/min by week 1, significantly greater than the 3 day level ($p < .05$), and thereafter plateaued. Left atrial pressure during peak exercise began to decrease by 1 week after ligation. At 3 weeks peak atrial pressure was only 11.1 mm Hg, significantly lower than at 3 days ($p < .05$). This improvement in cardiac function was accompanied by increasing ability to run for longer periods at faster speeds and steeper inclines. Although exercise double products increased progressively up to 3 weeks after coronary ligation, these changes were not statistically significant. There were no significant differences in double product, exercise tolerance, or hemodynamics between weeks 6 and 12 in the three dogs that continued the protocol.

The myocardium in the perfusion territory of the occluded vessel, or risk area, averaged 22.6 ± 4.6% of the entire left ventricle. Because of likely resorption of necrotic myocardium and possible replacement by fibrous tissue at 6 weeks in these dogs, we believed that infarct size immediately after occlusion could not be determined accurately. Exercise myocardial blood flow to the normal tissue 6 weeks after coronary occlusion was 3.11 ± 0.09 ml/min/g, whereas perfusion to the LCf tissue averaged 2.75 ± 0.34 ml/min/g without appreciable radial flow gradient. Thus the ratio of ischemic to normal blood flow was 0.89 ± 0.08. Transmural flow distribution favored the endocardium in the normally perfused regions (inner/outer left ventricular wall flow ratio 1.12 ± 0.07), whereas mild redistribution of flow toward the epicardium was still apparent in the myocardium beyond the coronary occlusion 6 weeks after LCf ligation (inner/outer left ventricular wall flow ratio 0.94 ± 0.06).

Figure 2 illustrates mean ^{201}Tl radial activity 10 to 14 min after exercise in the scans acquired before and 3 days and 6 weeks after LCf ligation. The data are expressed as a percentage of the highest mean radial activity in a given heart. Before ligation, the circumferential profile plot demonstrated a peak in ^{201}Tl activity within the circumflex distribution. Three days after LCf ligation, activity in the LCf distribution was markedly reduced relative to control, whereas LAD activity was relatively increased. By 6 weeks after LCf occlusion, LCf ^{201}Tl activity in the initial frame was intermediate between that observed before and at 3 days after LCf ligation, whereas LAD activity was unchanged from the 3 day scan. No further changes were noted in weeks 7 to 12.

The ratios of mean LCf/LAD activity (mean ± SE) 10 to 14 min after injection of ^{201}Tl for the preligation scan and the exercise scintigrams done at 3 days and 2, 3, 4, 5, and 6 weeks after LCf ligation are shown in figure 3. Before ligation, LCf and LAD activities were equal. At 3 days after LCf ligation, LCf activity in the initial frame of the 3 hr study was 73.6 ± 6.6% of LAD activity ($p < .02$). During the next 2 weeks, LCf activity remained significantly lower. By 4 weeks LCf activity was 87.4 ± 4.6% of LAD activity (p = NS), and there was no further change in subsequent weeks. The LCf/LAD activity ratios at 3 days and 2 weeks after LCf ligation were significantly lower than the ratio before ligation ($p < .05$). By the third week after ligation and thereafter, the LCf/LAD ratios in the initial frame of the 3 hr studies were no longer significantly different from preligation values. Thus the large exercise scintigraphic defect apparent 3 days after coronary occlusion showed progressive shrinkage in subsequent weeks until perfusion of the identified abnormal region became nearly indistinguishable from that of normal myocardium.

Dynamic changes in the rate of ^{201}Tl loss from the LAD and LCf distributions were observed over the 6 weeks after LCf ligation. Figure 4 illustrates the mean LCf and LAD ^{201}Tl activities for the eight dogs in each

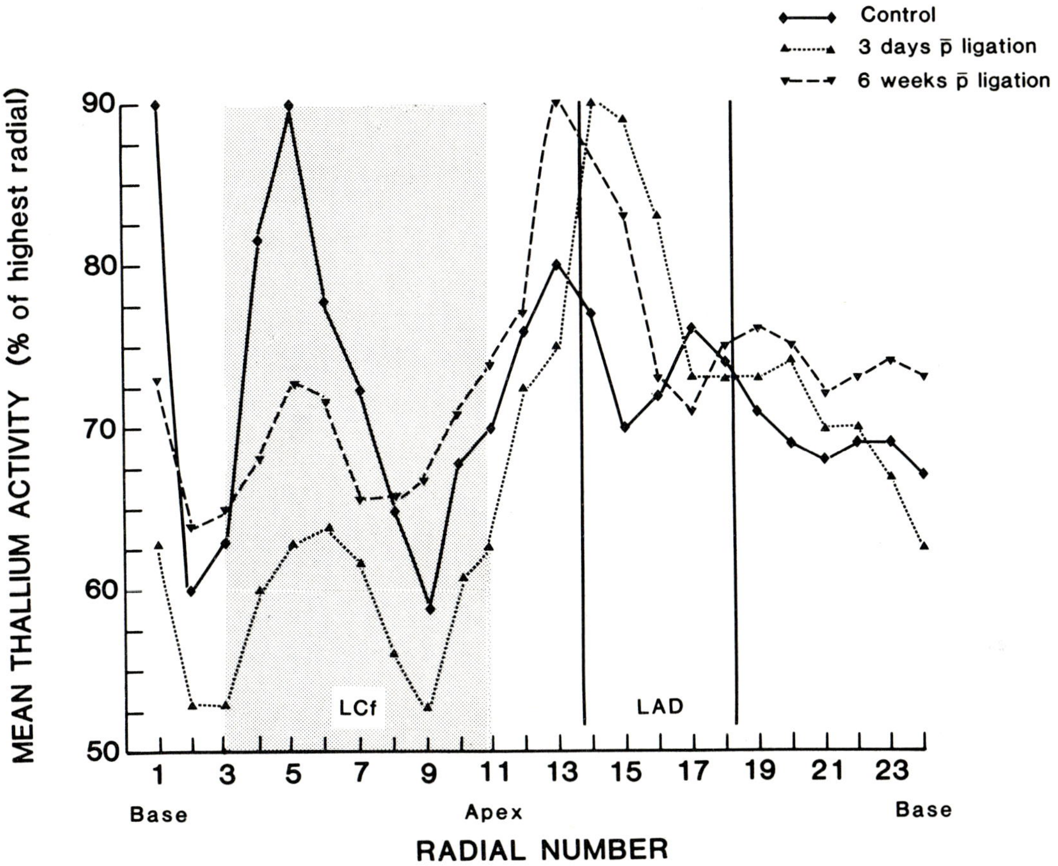

FIGURE 2. Mean scintigraphic myocardial ^{201}Tl activity in each of 24 radials for the six experimental animals 10 to 14 min after injection. Mean radial profiles from before (control) and 3 days and 6 weeks after LCf ligation are shown. Activity in the LCf region is significantly depressed immediately after ligation. Significant recovery is evident by 6 weeks. Activity in the LAD territory is comparable before and after ligation.

of the 36-frame studies acquired before (figure 4, *A*) and at 3 days (figure 4, *B*) and 6 weeks (figure 4, *C*) after LCf ligation. Data from each dog were expressed as a percentage of ^{201}Tl activity in the LAD territory of that dog in the first frame of each 36-frame study. Before LCf ligation, LAD and LCf activities were equivalent immediately after exercise, and the washout rates from the two regions were similar (figure 4, *A*). Three days after LCf ligation, LCf activity was initially lower than LAD activity. The decline in LAD and LCf activities thereafter was dissimilar, so that the washout curves converged over the 3 hr scanning interval (figure 4, *B*). At 6 weeks after LCf ligation, LCf activity was slightly, but not significantly, lower than LAD activity in the first frame of the study (figure 4, *C*). The rates of ^{201}Tl loss from the two distributions were more nearly equal, although there continued to be some convergence of the curves by 2 hr (see below).

Before LCf ligation, the rates of ^{201}Tl loss from the LAD and LCf distributions were equal, averaging 52.5 ± 5.5% and 54.5 ± 5.5% over 3 hr for the LAD and LCf distributions, respectively (figure 5, *A*). Three days after LCf ligation, the loss of ^{201}Tl from the LCf distribution (49.9 ± 6.1%) was significantly slower than that from the LAD distribution (68.5 ± 9.2%) ($p < .025$) (figure 5, *A*). The time-activity curves therefore converged over the 3 hr observation period (figure 4, *B*). During the ensuing 5 study weeks, the rate of ^{201}Tl loss from the LAD distribution remained constant, whereas that from the LCf distribution tended to increase. When the differences in the postligation LAD and LCf washout rates were compared with the preligation values, marked change was noted at 3 days (figure 5, *B*). The difference in LAD and LCf washout rates then gradually disappeared over the ensuing 5 weeks and was no longer significantly different from the preligation value at 6 weeks after LCf ligation.

In two animals coronary collateral development was monitored with serial angiograms. Two days after coronary occlusion there was no opacification of the LCf beyond the site of ligation (figure 6, *A*). Contrast agent remained in the LCf stump distal to the last patent marginal branch for several minutes after disappearance from the other vessels. Two weeks later col-

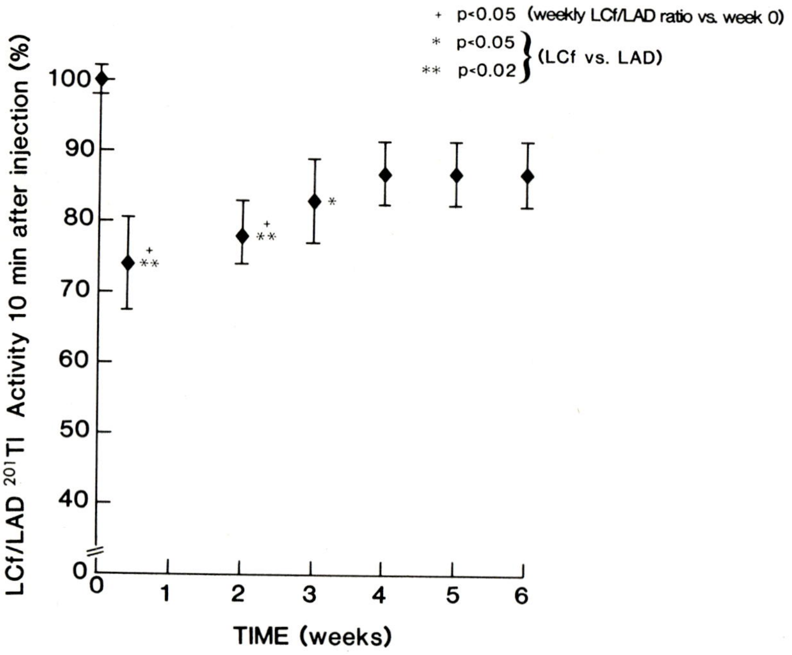

FIGURE 3. Mean ratio of LCf and LAD scintigraphic myocardial ^{201}Tl activities for the 6 dogs 10 to 14 min after injection. The LCf/LAD ratio from the control scan (week 0) and from scans done at 3 days and 2 through 6 weeks after LCf ligation are shown. A marked fall in the ratio is evident immediately after coronary ligation, with subsequent significant increases during the next 3 weeks. After 4 weeks there is little additional change, and the ratios are not different from those measured in week 0. Data are mean ± SEM.

lateral vessels were evident and contrast agent could be seen in the distal LCf, but washout was still delayed. By 4 weeks abundant collateral channels from the proximal LCf, including the sinoatrial node artery and the mid and distal LAD, were present. Furthermore, the entire LCf distal to the ligation was well opacified (figure 6, *B*), and the crux and atrioventricular node arteries could be easily identified. Dye washout from the distal LCf was only slightly slower than that from the LAD. In figure 6 these changes in the angiogram

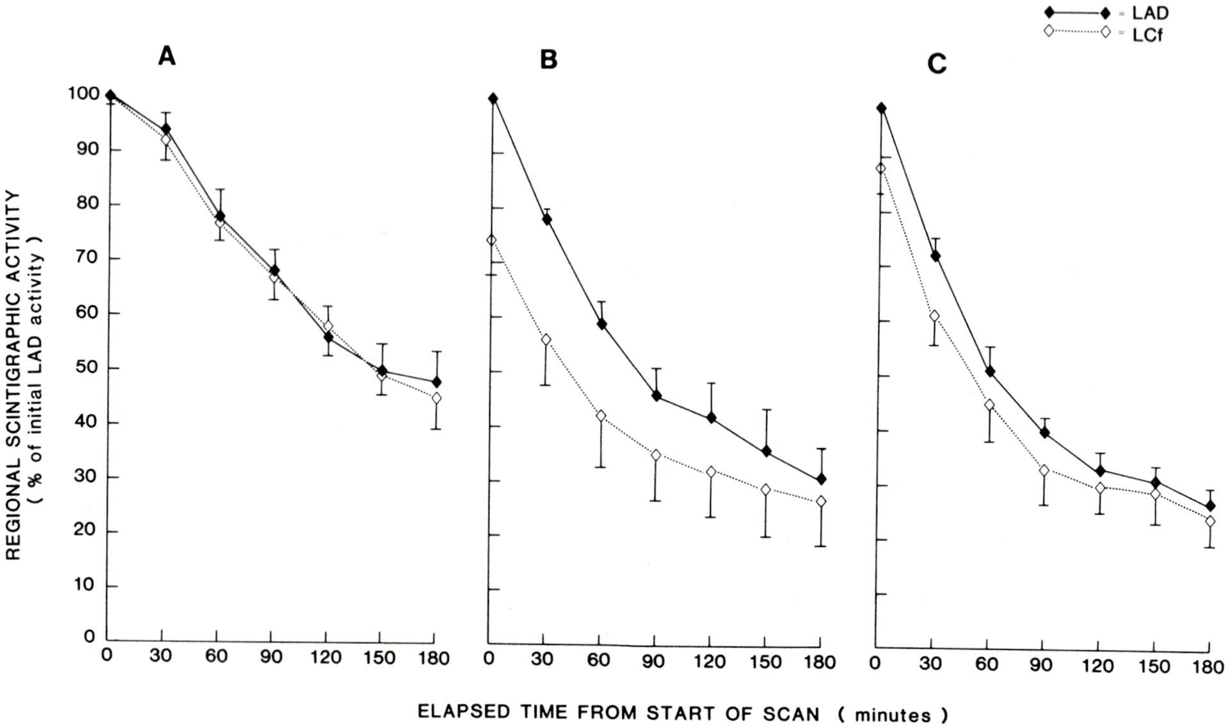

FIGURE 4. LAD and LCf scintigraphic ^{201}Tl activities over the 3 hr scanning interval before (*A*) and 3 days (*B*) and 6 weeks (*C*) after LCf ligation. Before ligation the two washout curves are superimposed. Three days after ligation initial activity in LCf territory is significantly lower than that in LAD myocardium, and LCf washout is considerably slower. Therefore the two washout curves converge by 3 hr. At 6 weeks the initial LAD and LCf activities and subsequent washouts are almost equal. Therefore the two curves are nearly parallel for the 3 hr observation period. Data are mean ± SEM.

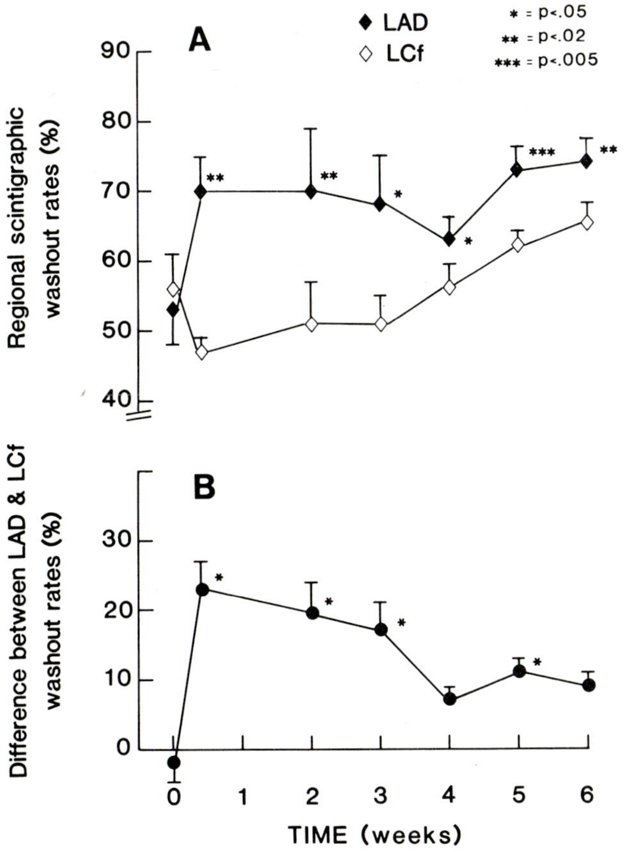

FIGURE 5. *A*, LAD and LCf scintigraphic ^{201}Tl washout rates before (week 0) and after LCf ligation. Statistical comparisons are for LAD vs LCf washout rates. Immediately after LCf ligation, washout in the LAD myocardium is significantly faster, whereas the LCf washout rate tends to fall. Subsequently LCf washout increases back toward normal and the difference between the two washout rates diminishes. *B*, Difference in LAD and LCf washout rates during the control scan and each of the six postligation scans. Statistical comparisons are with the control state (week 0). By 6 weeks the difference is no longer significant. Data are mean ± SEM.

are compared with the changes in the thallium scintigraphic images recorded 1 day after the respective angiograms in the same dog. Three days after coronary occlusion, when few collaterals were apparent, a large scintigraphic defect corresponding to the region of absent or poor myocardial perfusion was obvious (figure 6, *A*). However, by 4 weeks (figure 6, *B*), when coronary collaterals had become abundant and accounted for substantial restoration of flow to the distal LCf perfusion territory, the scintigram was nearly normal.

Discussion

In this study, large, reversible, exercise-induced scintigraphic defects were apparent shortly after coronary occlusion. Exercise in these animals resulted in dramatic increases in left atrial pressure and only modest rises in cardiac output. In subsequent weeks scintigraphic defects shrank, and after 4 weeks there was no statistically significant difference in radioisotope uptake or washout by normal tissue and myocardium in the perfusion territory of the ligated vessel. Hemodynamics and exercise performance also improved in the initial 4 weeks after occlusion. Exercise elicited smaller increases in left atrial pressure and larger rises in stroke volume and cardiac output.

Numerous studies have demonstrated that directly measured myocardial thallium distribution shortly after intravenous injection is proportional to blood flow.[31–33] In particular this has been clearly demonstrated in an exercising canine preparation similar to the one used in this study.[31] Our previous work has extended these conclusions to scintigraphic measurements of myocardial thallium activity.[27] Therefore, increasing LCf/LAD (ischemic/normal) myocardial scintigraphic ^{201}Tl ratios correlate with increasing tissue perfusion of the once ischemic myocardium. At 6 weeks, when scintigraphic defects were nearly absent, myocardial blood flow to muscle in the distribution of the occluded vessel was practically normal even during the stress of exercise. These flow data confirm earlier observations.[21] Persistent small scintigraphic and flow deficits at 6 weeks are probably related to replacement of infarcted tissue by poorly vascularized fibrous tissue and the fundamental inability of coronary collaterals to deliver normal flows during stress.[34–37] Scintigraphic studies up to 12 weeks after coronary occlusion showed no additional improvement.

The most likely explanation for the improvement in exercise scintigraphic images, exercise performance, and hemodynamics in the weeks after coronary occlusion is development of coronary collaterals. The time course of the improvement in the dogs in this study parallels the three-phase collateral transformation demonstrated by Schaper et al.,[38–41] in which a thin-walled 40 μm conduit is eventually converted into a 1 mm thick-walled arteriole. Hence coronary collateral development could account for the gradually increasing perfusion of the ischemic tissue with subsequent lessening of exercise-induced myocardial dysfunction and improvement in hemodynamics. Previous studies[21, 22] have clearly demonstrated a significant correlation between increasing coronary collateral flow and improved hemodynamic performance during exercise. Thus coronary occlusion in exercising dogs with initially low collateral flow caused cardiac failure with a rise in left atrial pressure to nearly 30 mm Hg and a significant decrease in cardiac output.[21] With further collateral development, coronary occlusion in the same running dogs resulted in a much smaller rise in

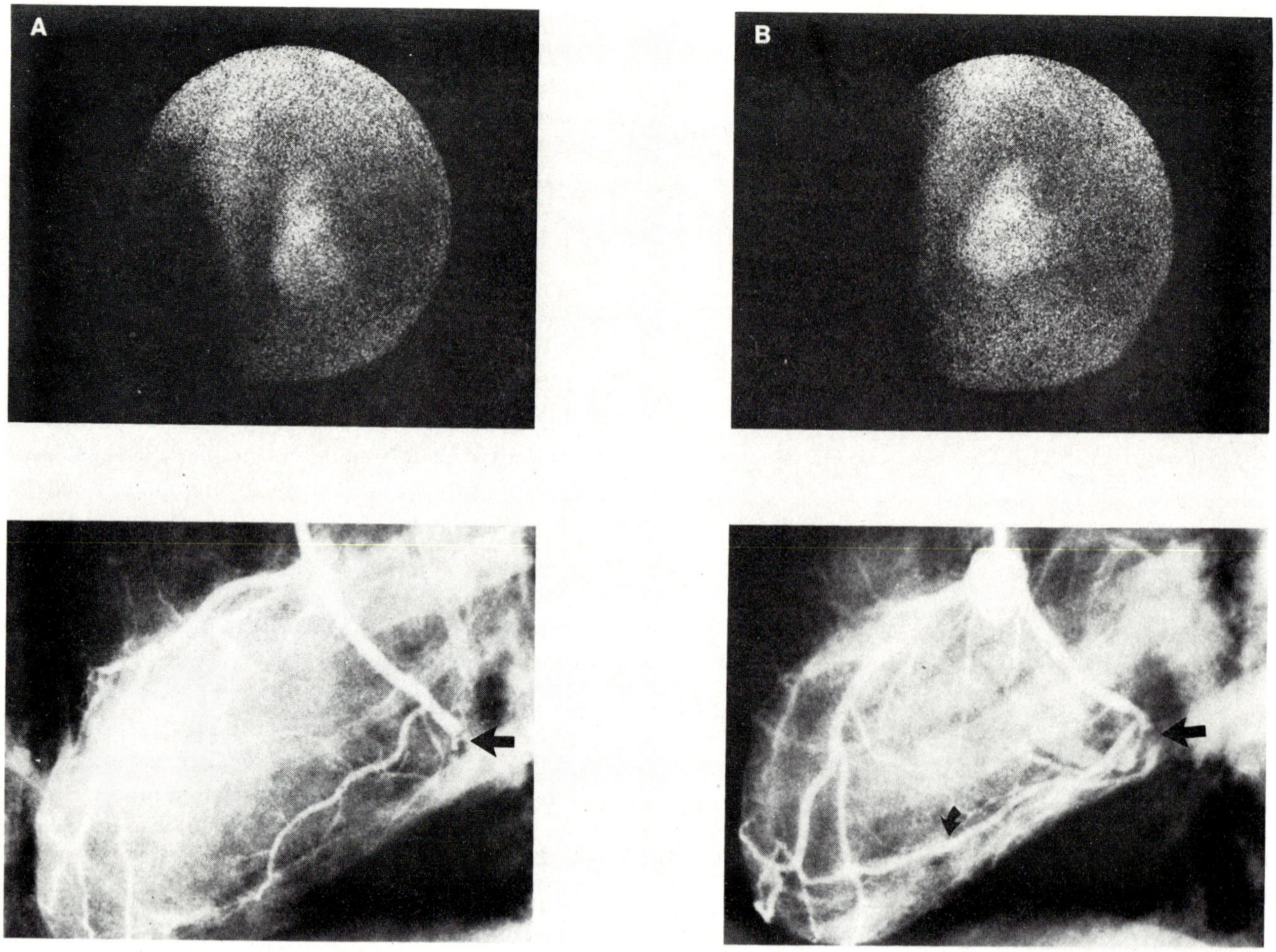

FIGURE 6. *A*, Unretouched Polaroid picture of a ^{201}Tl scintigram taken 10 min after cessation of exercise performed 3 days after coronary occlusion. A frame from a coronary angiogram completed 1 day earlier appears beneath the scintigram. There is a large scintigraphic defect apparent in the distribution of the LCf. The arrow in the angiographic frame indicates the site of LCf ligation. The radiopaque contrast agent injected into the ostium of the left coronary artery flowed only to the point of arterial obstruction. There were no visualized collateral channels and no contrast agent was ever observed in the distal LCf. *B*, Scintigraphic and angiographic frames from studies performed 4 weeks after those presented in *A*. Only a small scintigraphic defect remains, and the improvement after the initial study is obvious. The level of the LCf ligation is again indicated by the straight arrow. But now the entire distal LCf (curved arrow) is normally opacified by numerous intracoronary and intercoronary collateral channels. Because of the slightly different projection, the short marginal artery originating just before the site of ligation in *A* is in part superimposed on the initial segment of the collateralized LCf. Runoff from the distal LCf was only slightly slower than that from normal vessels.

left atrial pressure and a smaller fall in cardiac output, thus documenting the ability of collaterals to preserve myocardial perfusion despite interruption of normal antegrade sources and to attenuate the effects of this interruption on cardiac function. The serial coronary angiographic studies in this investigation further demonstrate that coronary collateral development parallels the improvement in exercise hemodynamics as well as in the exercise thallium scintigrams (figure 6). Furthermore, nearly normal exercise flows in the ischemic region at 6 weeks attest to the ability of coronary collaterals to rapidly restore perfusion of myocardium after coronary occlusion.

Explanations for the serial changes in hemodynamics and scintigraphic images other than increasing collateral blood flow are possible but less likely. Decreased exercise performance in the initial postsurgical study could have been related in part to anesthesia and thoracotomy performed just 3 days earlier. Decreased exercise capacity at this time because of discomfort or the detraining effect of surgery might have limited the rise in cardiac output, although the increase in left atrial pressure would also have been attenuated. Further recovery from the surgical insult might have accounted for better exercise performance and the increased cardiac output in later studies, but left atrial pressure would also have been expected to increase rather than decrease, as seen in the experimental animals. The gradual and significant decline in left atrial pressure during exercise over the initial 3 to 4 weeks of study is more consistent with an improvement in left ventricular function, and the limitation of early performance more likely the result of acute cardiac failure. To support this contention, parallel studies in four dogs similarly instrumented except that the LCf was not ligated revealed that aortic and left atrial pressures, cardiac output, and double product as well as exercise performance did not change significantly from 3 days to 10 to 14 days after surgery, a period during which the most impressive changes in hemodynamics were occurring in the experimental animals described above.

Compensatory hypertrophy of normal myocardium theoretically could result in improvement of global left ventricular function. However, improvement was evident between the first evaluation at 3 days and the second at 7 days after coronary ligation, hardly enough time for significant hypertrophy to occur.

It is also possible that changes in ventricular geometry rather than increasing collateral blood flow over time were responsible for the apparent shrinking of the scintigraphic defect. Gewirtz et al.[42] demonstrated that short-term aortic constriction that doubled left atrial pressure and caused substantial decreases in distal aortic pressure could result in left ventricular dilatation. ^{201}Tl scintigrams obtained during the aortic constrictions showed prominent apical defects, presumably caused by thinning of the tissue. However, in the present experiments imaging was begun 10 min after exercise in anesthetized dogs. Blood pressure in these animals had returned to or had fallen slightly below baseline levels and therefore would not have been responsible for thinned, count-deficient myocardium. Alternatively, a large scintigraphic defect in the initial study might have been caused by bulging of a large LCf scar. But if the diminution of LCf counts was simply caused by bulging of a scar, one would have expected the left ventricular cavity to have dilated and the LCf myocardium to have thinned. As seen in figure 6, left ventricular size was not grossly different at 3 days and 4 weeks after coronary ligation and the count-deficient area in the LCf distribution had normal thickness. Furthermore, the heart size did not change over the 3 hr scanning interval, and the circumferential region of interest closely approximated the ventricular borders. If the LCf distribution were largely scarred, the documented marked redistribution of ^{201}Tl activity over the 3 hr of scanning would not have been observed. Finally, since there was only a small flow deficit at 6 weeks and the amount of infarcted tissue at postmortem examination was small, it is unlikely that changes in compliance of infarcted tissue or contraction of scar would account for improvement of the scintigrams done several weeks after coronary ligation. Nevertheless, a small contribution of these mechanical effects cannot be completely excluded.

If absolute blood flow to the normal myocardium were highest in the initial exercise study after coronary occlusion and then during subsequent weeks were lower, the ischemic/normal ^{201}Tl activity ratio would have appeared to increase even if ischemic myocardial uptake had been unchanged. However, previous studies[21] have demonstrated that normal myocardial flows are lower in the exercising dog shortly after coronary occlusion than in the same animals with long-standing occlusions exercising at similar workloads. Presumably cardiac failure and poor exercise tolerance in the early exercise studies limit the rise in myocardial flow in the noninvolved segments. The flow increases are seen later after long-term coronary occlusion when the limitations are no longer present. These changes in normal tissue flow, if unaccompanied by changes in perfusion of ischemic myocardium, would have produced a fall, rather than the observed increase, in the ischemic/normal activity ratio over 6 weeks and cannot account for the observed improvement in scintigraphic images.

In the routine performance of exercise ^{201}Tl scintigraphy in patients with severe coronary obstructive disease, occasional subjects will have no evidence of scintigraphic defects.[16, 43–46] In fact, several investigators have already concluded that collaterals in man may attenuate or eliminate ^{201}Tl defects[16, 43–47] as well as modify redistribution,[43, 48, 49] although agreement is not universal.[6, 50] Buda et al.[47] did serial ^{201}Tl scintigrams in patients 3 weeks and 3 months after myocardial infarction. Similar to the present observations in dogs, scintigraphic defects were significantly smaller in the follow-up studies despite greater rate-pressure products. They also postulated that increased myocardial perfusion related to collateral development was the most likely explanation. Patients studied by Kondo et al.[49] with collateral vessels were significantly more likely to have complete or partial ^{201}Tl redistribution than patients without anastomotic vessels ($p < .02$). As demonstrated by Khaw et al.[33] in animal preparations, delayed distribution of ^{201}Tl is a function of the distribution of viable myocardium. Therefore the presence of collateral vessels is associated with the maintenance of myocardial viability.

To the extent that collaterals do have these effects on early and late ^{201}Tl distribution, attempts to predict the severity of coronary artery disease from exercise scintigrams[51] are consigned to failure. As demonstrated in this investigation in dogs with the same coronary lesion throughout the study, the magnitude of the ^{201}Tl defect was greatly influenced by the degree of collateral development. Thus it must be recognized that ^{201}Tl scintigrams are likely to be affected by the collateral circulation as well as by the severity of the lesions.

Our results provide evidence that coronary collaterals in an experimental preparation can restore blood flow to ischemic myocardium and improve global cardiac function. These observations further strengthen the contention that coronary collaterals have salutary effects. By diminishing myocardial ischemia, collaterals attenuate initial scintigraphic defects and in turn may alter the pattern of redistribution. These latter observations should not be overlooked when clinical scintigrams are being evaluated.

We wish to acknowledge Ann DeVita, Dominick Moreschi, and Robert Bontemps for technical assistance, Ari Rabinowitz for programming support, and Lori Fields for help in preparing the manuscript.

References

1. Mason DT, Amsterdam EA, Miller RR, Hughes JL III, Bonanno JA, Iben AB, Hurley EJ, Massumi RA, Zelis R: Consideration of the therapeutic roles of pharmacologic agents, collateral circulation and saphenous vein bypass in coronary artery disease. Am J Cardiol **28:** 608, 1971
2. Miller RR, Amsterdam EA, Zelis R, Massumi RA, Mason DT: Determinants and functional significance of the coronary collateral circulation in ischemic heart disease. *In* Russek HI, editor: Cardiovascular disease: new concepts in diagnosis and therapy. Baltimore, 1974, University Park Press, pp 75–83
3. Bartel AG, Behar VS, Peter RH, Orgain ES, Kong Y: Graded exercise stress tests in angiographically documented coronary artery disease. Circulation **49:** 348, 1974
4. Gorlin R: Coronary collaterals. Major Probl Intern Med **11:** 59, 1976
5. Williams DO, Amsterdam EA, Miller RR, Mason DT: The role of the coronary collateral circulation in acute and chronic coronary artery disease. *In* Mason DT, editor: Advances in heart disease. New York, 1977, Grune & Stratton, vol 1, pp 253–67
6. Berger BC, Watson DD, Taylor GJ, Burwell LR, Martin RP, Beller GA: Effect of coronary collateral circulation on regional myocardial perfusion assessed with quantitative thallium-201 scintigraphy. Am J Cardiol **46:** 365, 1980
7. Blumgart HL, Schlesinger MJ, Davis D: Studies on the relation of the clinical manifestations of angina pectoris, coronary thrombosis, and myocardial infarction to the pathologic findings: with particular reference to the significance of the collateral circulation. Am Heart J **19:** 1, 1940
8. Allison RB, Rodriguez FL, Higgins EA Jr, Leddy JP, Abelmann WH, Ellis LB, Robbins SL: Clinicopathologic correlations in coronary atherosclerosis: four hundred thirty patients studied with postmortem coronary angiography. Circulation **27:** 170, 1963
9. Fulton WFM: Anastomotic enlargement and ischaemic myocardial damage. Br Heart J **26:** 1, 1964
10. Baroldi G: Functional morphology of the anastomotic circulation in human cardiac pathology. Methods Achiev Exp Path **5:** 438, 1971
11. Levin DC, Sos TA, Lee JG, Baltaxe HA: Coronary collateral circulation and distal coronary runoff: the key factors in preserving myocardial contractility in patients with coronary artery disease. Am J Roentgenol **119:** 474, 1973
12. Hecht HS, Aroesty JM, Morkin E, LaRaia PJ, Paulin S: Role of the coronary collateral circulation in the preservation of left ventricular function. Radiology **114:** 305, 1975
13. Ensslen R, Schwarz F, Thormann J, Feige A: Die protektive Wirkung von Kollateralen auf die regionale linksventrikulare Funktion bei koronarer Herzkrankheit. Verh Dtsch Ges Kreislaufforsch **42:** 327, 1976
14. Schwarz F: Correlation between the degree of coronary artery obstruction and myocardial dysfunction. *In* Schaper W, editor: The pathophysiology of myocardial perfusion. Amsterdam, 1979, North-Holland Biomedical Press, pp 305–344
15. Sesto M, Schwarz F: Regional myocardial function at rest and after rapid ventricular pacing in patients after myocardial revascularization by coronary bypass graft or by collateral vessels. Am J Cardiol **43:** 920, 1979
16. Kolibash AJ, Bush CA, Wepsic RA, Schroeder DP, Tetalman MR, Lewis RP: Coronary collateral vessels: spectrum of physiologic capabilities with respect to providing rest and stress myocardial perfusion, maintenance of left ventricular function and protection against infarction. Am J Cardiol **50:** 230, 1982
17. Webster JS, Moberg C, Rincon G: Natural history of severe proximal coronary artery disease as documented by coronary cineangiography. Am J Cardiol **33:** 195, 1974
18. Williams DO, Amsterdam EA, Miller RR, Mason DT: Functional significance of coronary collateral vessels in patients with acute myocardial infarction: relation to pump performance, cardiogenic shock and survival. Am J Cardiol **37:** 345, 1976
19. Blumgart HL, Zoll PM, Freedberg AS, Gilligan DR: The experimental production of intercoronary arterial anastomoses and their functional significance. Circulation **1:** 10, 1950
20. Schaper W, Jageneau A, Xhonneux R: The development of collateral circulation in the pig and dog heart. Cardiologia **51:** 321, 1967
21. Cohen MV, Yipintsoi T: Restoration of cardiac function and myocardial flow by collateral development in dogs. Am J Physiol **240:** H811, 1981
22. Cohen MV, Yipintsoi T: Myocardial performance and collateral flow after transient coronary occlusion in exercising dogs. Am J Physiol **237:** H520, 1979
23. Garza DA, White FC, Hall RE, Bloor CM: Effect of coronary collateral development on ventricular fibrillation threshold. Basic Res Cardiol **69:** 371, 1974
24. Meesmann W, Stephan K, Gulker H, Kramer B, Komhard W, Rehwald U, Menken U: Arrhythmias, vulnerability, and focal blocks in the early phase of experimental myocardial infarction in relation to coronary collateral vessels. *In* Kaltenbach M, Lichtlen P, Balcon R, Bussmann W-D, editors: Coronary Heart Disease: 3rd International Symposium Frankfurt. Stuttgart, 1978, Georg Thieme, pp 55–60
25. Watson DD, Campbell NP, Read EK, Gibson RS, Teates CD, Beller GA: Spatial and temporal quantitation of plane thallium myocardial images. J Nucl Med **22:** 577, 1981
26. Goris ML, Daspit SG, McLaughlin P, Kriss JP: Interpolative background subtraction. J Nucl Med **17:** 744, 1976
27. Steingart RM, Cohen MV: 201-Thallium scintigraphic quantitation of regional flow disparity and subsequent redistribution in dogs. J Nucl Med (in press)
28. Schwartz JS, Ponto R, Carlyle P, Forstrom L, Cohn JN: Early redistribution of thallium-201 after temporary ischemia. Circulation **57:** 332, 1978
29. Cohen MV, Eldh P: Experimental myocardial infarction in the closed-chest dog: controlled production of large or small areas of necrosis. Am Heart J **86:** 798, 1973
30. Zar JH: Biostatistical analysis. Englewood Cliffs, NJ, 1974, Prentice-Hall
31. Nielsen AP, Morris KG, Murdock R, Bruno FP, Cobb FR: Linear relationship between the distribution of thallium-201 and blood flow in ischemic and nonischemic myocardium during exercise. Circulation **61:** 797, 1980
32. Chu A, Murdock RH Jr, Cobb FR: Relation between regional distribution of thallium-201 and myocardial blood flow in normal, acutely ischemic, and infarcted myocardium. Am J Cardiol **50:** 1141, 1982

33. Khaw BA, Strauss HW, Pohost GM, Fallon JT, Katus HA, Haber E: Relation of immediate and delayed thallium-201 distribution to localization of iodine-125 antimyosin antibody in acute experimental myocardial infarction. Am J Cardiol **51:** 1428, 1983
34. Schaper W, Flameng W, Winkler B, Wusten B, Turschmann W, Neugebauer G, Carl M, Pasyk S: Quantification of collateral resistance in acute and chronic experimental coronary occlusion in the dog. Circ Res **39:** 371, 1976
35. Scheel KW, Galindez TA, Cook B, Rodriguez RJ, Ingram LA: Changes in coronary and collateral flows and adequacy of perfusion in the dog following one and three months of circumflex occlusion. Circ Res **39:** 654, 1976
36. Scheel KW, Ingram LA, Wilson JL: Effects of exercise on the coronary and collateral vasculature of beagles with and without coronary occlusion. Circ Res **48:** 523, 1981
37. Schaper W: Influence of physical exercise on coronary collateral blood flow in chronic experimental two-vessel occlusion. Circulation **65:** 905, 1982
38. Schaper W, Schaper J, Xhonneux R, Vandesteene R: The morphology of intercoronary anastomoses in chronic coronary artery occlusion. Cardiovasc Res **3:** 315, 1969
39. Schaper W, DeBrabander M, Lewi P: DNA synthesis and mitoses in coronary collateral vessels of the dog. Circ Res **28:** 671, 1971
40. Schaper W: The collateral circulation of the heart. Amsterdam, 1971, North-Holland Publishing Co.
41. Schaper W, Schaper J, Pasyk S: Development of a collateral circulation in chronic experimental coronary occlusion. *In* Lichtlen PR, editor: Coronary angiography and angina pectoris. Stuttgart, 1976, Georg Thieme, pp 325–33
42. Gewirtz H, Grotte GJ, Strauss HW, O'Keefe DD, Akins CW, Daggett WM, Pohost GM: The influence of left ventricular volume and wall motion on myocardial images. Circulation **59:** 1172, 1979
43. Verani MS, Jhingran S, Attar M, Rizk A, Quinones MA, Miller RR: Poststress redistribution of thallium-201 in patients with coronary artery disease, with and without prior myocardial infarction. Am J Cardiol **43:** 1114, 1979
44. Rigo P, Becker LC, Griffith LSC, Alderson PO, Bailey IK, Pitt B, Burow RD, Wagner HN Jr: Influence of coronary collateral vessels on the results of thallium-201 myocardial stress imaging. Am J Cardiol **44:** 452, 1979
45. Wainwright RJ, Maisey MN, Edwards AC, Sowton E: Functional significance of coronary collateral circulation during dynamic exercise evaluated by thallium-201 myocardial scintigraphy. Br Heart J **43:** 47, 1980
46. Eng C, Patterson RE, Horowitz SF, Halgash DA, Pichard AD, Midwall J, Herman MV, Gorlin R: Coronary collateral function during exercise. Circulation **66:** 309, 1982
47. Buda AJ, Dubbin JD, MacDonald IL, Strauss HD, Orr SA, Meindok H: Spontaneous changes in thallium-201 myocardial perfusion imaging after myocardial infarction. Am J Cardiol **50:** 1272, 1982
48. Cooper R, Puri S, Francis CK, Spencer RP: Role of coronary artery disease and collateral circulation in redistribution of thallium-201. Clin Nucl Med **5:** 292, 1980
49. Kondo M, Miyazaki S, Takahashi M, Shimono Y: Assessment of viable myocardium within infarct zone by exercise thallium-201 scintigraphy. Jpn Circ J **48:** 219, 1984
50. Verani MS, Marcus ML, Razzak MA, Ehrhardt JC: Sensitivity and specificity of thallium-201 perfusion scintigrams under exercise in the diagnosis of coronary artery disease. J Nucl Med **19:** 773, 1978
51. Glass EC, Joye JA, Hines HH, DeMaria AN, DeNardo GL, Amsterdam EA, Mason DT: Assessment of the extent of clinical coronary artery disease using Tl-201: a new computerized myocardial imaging approach that correlates with angiographic-defined vessel obstruction. Clin Res **28:** 173A, 1980 (abst)

Effects of synthetic atrial natriuretic peptide on renal function and renin release in acute experimental heart failure

TERRY A. SCRIVEN, B.A., AND JOHN C. BURNETT, JR., M.D.

ABSTRACT Studies were performed in anesthetized control dogs (n = 6) and in dogs (n = 6) with acute low-output heart failure produced by inflation of a balloon in the thoracic inferior vena cava. Studies were designed to determine the effects of synthetic atrial natriuretic peptide on renal function and renin release in this acute high-renin, sodium-retaining preparation. Intrarenal infusion of synthetic atrial natriuretic peptide (0.3 $\mu g \cdot kg^{-1} \cdot min^{-1}$) resulted in decreases in arterial pressure and renal blood flow in both groups. Glomerular filtration rate increased in both low-output (Δ +10.7 ± 3.1 ml/min) and control (Δ +8.7 ± 2.9 ml/min) groups. Fractional lithium excretion, a marker of proximal tubule reabsorption, also increased in both low-output (Δ +12.0 ± 4.6%) and control (Δ +14.3 ± 5.0%) groups. Renin secretory rate decreased in the low-output group from 852.8 ± 183.0 to 149.5 ± 73.7 ng/min and in the control group from 308.5 ± 84.5 to 44.5 ± 27.5 ng/ml. Intrarenal infusion of atrial natriuretic peptide resulted in an attenuated increase in both urinary sodium excretion (Δ +42.3 ± 10.7 vs Δ +201.2 ± 37.9 μeq/min) and fractional excretion of sodium (Δ +0.48 ± 0.13% vs Δ +2.85 ± 0.45%) in the low-output as compared with the control group. Our studies demonstrate that administration of synthetic atrial natriuretic peptide results in an increase in glomerular filtration rate and a decrease in proximal tubule reabsorption, as estimated by lithium excretion, in both control dogs and those with acute low-output heart failure. Furthermore, despite a decrease in arterial pressure, synthetic atrial natriuretic peptide markedly inhibits renin secretion under control conditions and in the high-renin state. Despite similar increases in glomerular filtration rate and decreases in proximal tubule reabsorption and renin release, the natriuretic response to synthetic atrial natriuretic peptide, although present, is markedly attenuated in this preparation of acute experimental heart failure.
Circulation 72, No. 4, 892–897, 1985.

RECENT INVESTIGATIONS have established that mammalian atria possess specific secretory granules that synthesize and release natriuretic and vasoactive peptides that have a fundamental physiologic role in regulation of cardiovascular volume. These peptides have been referred to as atrial natriuretic factor, atrial natriuretic peptides, cardionatrin, atriopeptin, and auriculin.[1-6] Previous studies from our laboratory have reported that intrarenal infusion of synthetic atrial natriuretic peptide results in a marked increase in urine volume and sodium excretion.[7] This marked natriuresis is associated with a significant increase in glomerular filtration rate and a decrease in whole-kidney proximal tubule reabsorption as determined by the clearance of lithium. These studies have also demonstrated that intrarenal administration of synthetic atrial natriuretic peptide results in marked inhibition of renin release despite a sustained decrease in arterial pressure.

Congestive heart failure is a syndrome characterized by sodium retention and activation of the renin-angiotensin system. To date, no studies have definitely investigated the renal hemodynamic and excretory response to atrial natriuretic peptide in a preparation of heart failure. Preliminary studies in dogs with experimental heart failure have reported that intravenous infusion of synthetic atrial natriuretic peptide is associated with a blunted natriuretic response.[8] This blunted natriuretic response occurred despite an increase in creatinine clearance. Recent studies by Chimoskey et al.[9] in hamsters with familial cardiomyopathy and con-

From the Department of Medicine and of Physiology and Biophysics, Mayo Medical School, Rochester, MN.

Supported by the American Heart Association grant-in-aid 83-964 and by the Hearst and Mayo Foundations. Terry A. Scriven was supported by an NIH Medical Student Short-Term Training grant (HL07551).

Address for correspondence: John C. Burnett, Jr., M.D., Division of Cardiovascular Disease, Department of Medicine, Mayo Medical School, Rochester, MN 55905.

Received March 15, 1985; revision accepted June 27, 1985.

gestive heart failure have shown a deficiency in atrial natriuretic peptide activity in these animals.[9] These investigators speculated that the abnormalities in volume regulation accompanying heart failure could in part be mediated by an absence of atrial natriuretic peptide. The present study was therefore designed to test the hypothesis that exogenous administration of atrial natriuretic peptide to dogs with acute low-output heart failure, a preparation that produces the renal and neurohumoral adjustments characteristic of congestive heart failure, would correct defects in renal sodium handling and the renin-angiotensin system.

The present study investigates the effects of synthetic atrial natriuretic peptide on renal function and renin release in the presence and absence of acute low-output heart failure produced by inflation of a balloon in the thoracic inferior vena cava. Specifically, these studies focus on the effect of synthetic atrial natriuretic peptide on renal blood flow, glomerular filtration rate, proximal tubular reabsorption, renin secretion, and arterial pressure in this experimental preparation of heart failure.

Methods

Experiments were performed in two groups of 14 to 25 kg mongrel dogs: a control group and a group in which acute low-output heart failure was induced by balloon inflation. The low-output state was produced by introduction of a Bardex-Foley No. 16F catheter into the thoracic inferior vena cava via the right femoral vein, with subsequent inflation to increase inferior vena caval venous pressure approximately 8 to 10 mm Hg above baseline. The position of the balloon in the thoracic inferior vena cava was confirmed at the termination of the experiment by exploration of the vena cava through a thoracotomy incision. This preparation, extensively used in previous investigations of the pathophysiology of congestive heart failure, produces the systemic hemodynamic and neurohumoral adjustments that characterize this syndrome.[10, 11]

Immediately before the experiment, each dog was anesthetized with pentobarbital (30 mg/kg iv). The femoral artery was catheterized for measurement of mean arterial pressure. Double cannulation of the left femoral vein was performed. One catheter was placed in the thoracic vena cava to measure venous pressure and the second was used for infusion of inulin in isotonic saline at a rate of 1 ml/min to achieve a plasma inulin concentration of 50 mg/dl. In the low-output group, the No. 16F Foley catheter was introduced into the right femoral vein and advanced into the thoracic inferior vena cava, as described above. Isotonic saline was perfused at 10 ml/hr through the catheter to maintain patency and to minimize thrombosis of the catheter tip. A left flank incision was then made and the left kidney was exposed. The ureter was cannulated with polyethylene tubing. The renal vasculature was isolated in situ. An angled 22-gauge needle was introduced into the renal vein for renal venous sampling, which was maintained patent with a 10 ml/hr heparinized saline infusion. A 22-gauge curved needle was placed in the renal artery for infusion of synthetic atrial natriuretic peptide. During non–atrial natriuretic peptide infusion periods of the experiment 1 ml/min isotonic saline was infused through the renal artery needle. Both needles were connected to Sage Instruments syringe pumps (Model 391A). An electromagnetic flow probe (Micron Instruments, Model MC-4025) was placed on the renal artery proximal to the needle and connected to a flowmeter (Micron Instruments, Inc., Model RC1008).

After completion of surgery, the balloon was inflated as described above in the low-output group; no inflation procedure was performed in the control group. The dogs were then allowed to stabilize for approximately 1 hr. During the control period, 15 min clearance was determined twice, followed by the intrarenal infusion of 26-amino acid (8-33) synthetic atrial natriuretic peptide (Peninsula Labs, Belmont, CA) at a rate of 0.3 $\mu g \cdot kg^{-1} \cdot min^{-1}$ for a total of 45 min. Fifteen minutes after initiation of the infusion of synthetic atrial natriuretic peptide, clearance was determined twice. Glomerular filtration rate was determined by the clearance of inulin. Plasma and urine levels of inulin were measured by the anthrone method. Plasma and urine sodium and potassium levels were determined by use of ion-selective electrodes (Beckman E 2A analyzer). Urine and plasma lithium concentrations were measured by flame-emission spectrophotometry (Instruments Lab, Model 357). Whole-kidney proximal tubular reabsorption of sodium was estimated by the lithium-clearance technique. This technique has been shown to be a reliable method for estimating proximal tubular handling of sodium, since lithium is reabsorbed exclusively by the proximal tubule.[12, 13] Thus, the fractional excretion of lithium serves as a measure of whole-kidney fractional delivery of sodium from the proximal tubule. Dogs were given 300 mg of lithium orally the night before each experiment. Samples for determination of plasma renin activity were obtained from arterial and renal vein catheters during each clearance period. Renin secretion rate was calculated from the product of renal plasma flow and the renal-arteriovenous plasma renin activity difference. For clarity of presentation, the renin secretion rate units of nanograms of angiotensin I per hour per minute were simplified to nanograms per minute. Plasma renin activity was measured by radioimmunoassay.[14]

All data on clearance during the control and atrial natriuretic peptide infusion periods were averaged and expressed as mean values ± SE. The data were analyzed with paired and unpaired t tests.

Results

Table 1 and figures 1 to 5 list the renal hemodynamic and excretory function data obtained at baseline and during the intrarenal infusion of synthetic atrial natriuretic peptide in the two groups of dogs.

Hemodynamics. A decrease in mean arterial pressure was observed during intrarenal infusion of synthetic atrial natriuretic peptide in both the control (120 ± 4 to 114 ± 4 mm Hg, $p < .05$) and low-output (113 ± 5 to 107 ± 4 mm Hg, $p < .05$) groups. Renal blood flow also slightly decreased in the control group (157 ± 24 to 146 ± 21 ml/min) and low-output group (143 ± 21 to 137 ± 23 ml/min) during administration of atrial natriuretic peptide; however, these decreases in renal blood flow were not significant. Renal vascular resistance did not change in either group in response to atrial natriuretic peptide. Glomerular filtration rate increased in the control group from 34.0 ± 3.9 to 45.3 ± 3.6 ml/min ($p < .05$) and glomerular filtration rate

TABLE 1

Renal hemodynamic and excretory response to intrarenal infusion of synthetic atrial natriuretic peptide in dogs in the control and acute low-output heart failure groups

	MAP (mm Hg)	IVCP (mm Hg)	RBF (ml/min)	GFR (ml/min)	RVR (mm Hg·ml·min^{-1})	V (ml/min)	$U_{Na}V$ (μeq/min)
Control group (n = 6)							
Baseline	120±4	1.9±0.4	157±24	34.0±3.9	0.88±0.19	0.47±0.15	29.9±7.8
ANP	114±4[A]	1.8±0.4	146±21	45.3±3.6[A]	0.84±0.13	2.49±0.44[C]	231.0±42.5[C]
Acute low-output heart failure group (n = 6)							
Baseline	113±5	10.8±1.2[D]	143±21	23.3±4.4	0.89±0.16	0.11±0.03	10.8±2.3
ANP	107±4[A]	10.8±1.3[D]	137±23	33.9±5.6[A]	0.91±0.17	0.41±0.10[B,D]	46.2±12.3[B,D]

ANP = atrial nartiuretic peptide; MAP = mean arterial pressure; IVCP = inferior vena cava pressure; RBF = renal blood flow; GFR = glomerular filtration rate; RVR = renal vascular resistance; V = urine flow; $U_{Na}V$ = urinary sodium excretion; FE_{Na} = fractional excretion of sodium; FE_{Li} = fractional excretion of lithium; RSR = renin secretory rate.

[A]$p < .05$; [B]$p < .02$; [C]$p < .005$, by paired t test. [D]$p < .05$ by unpaired t test.

similarly increased in the low-output group from 23.3 ± 4.4 to 33.9 ± 5.6 ml/min ($p < .05$).

Excretory function. When compared with the marked diuresis and natriuresis observed in control dogs, a significantly blunted natriuretic and diuretic response to intrarenal infusion of synthetic atrial natriuretic peptide was observed in the dogs with acute low-output heart failure. In control dogs urine flow increased from 0.47 ± 0.15 to 2.49 ± 0.44 ml/min ($p < .005$) and in the low-output group it increased from 0.11 ± 0.03 to 0.41 ± 0.10 ml/min ($p < .05$). Thus, the diuretic response was significantly blunted ($p < .005$) in the dogs in the low-output group (Δ +0.30 ± 0.08 ml/min) as compared with that in dogs in the control group (Δ +2.02 ± 0.37 ml/min).

Sodium excretion increased in the control group (29.9 ± 7.8 to 231.0 ± 42.5 μeq/min, $p < .005$) and in the low-output group (10.8 ± 2.3 to 46.2 ± 12.3 μeq/min, $p < .02$). Fractional excretion of sodium increased in the control dogs (0.57 ± 0.13% to 3.42 ± 0.54%, $p < .005$). A lesser increase in fractional excretion of sodium was observed in the low-output group (0.42 ± 0.16% to 0.90 ± 0.13%, $p < .05$). Thus, the natriuretic response to intrarenal administration of synthetic atrial natriuretic peptide was markedly attenuated ($p < .005$) in the dogs with acute low-output heart failure as compared with that in control dogs. Absolute urinary sodium excretion increased Δ +42.3 ± 10.7 μeq/min in the low-output group, compared with Δ +201.2 ± 37.9 μeq/min in the control group. The change in fractional sodium excretion with infusion of atrial natriuretic peptide was Δ +0.48 ± 0.13% in the low-output group, as compared with Δ +2.85 ± 0.45% in the normal group. Despite the blunted natriuretic response to atrial natriuretic peptide in the low-output group, fractional lithium excretion increased significantly in both the control dogs (29.8 ± 4.1 to 44.1 ± 4.6%, $p < .05$) and those with low-output heart failure (17.7 ± 3.1% to 30.2 ± 4.3%, $p < .05$).

Renin secretory rate was significantly elevated in dogs with acute low-output heart failure as compared with that in normal animals (852.8 ± 183.0 vs 308.5 ± 84.5 ng/min, $p < .05$). Nevertheless, the intrarenal infusion of synthetic atrial natriuretic peptide produced a significant decrease in renin secretory rate in both groups. Administration of synthetic atrial natriuretic peptide resulted in a decrease in renin secretory rate in

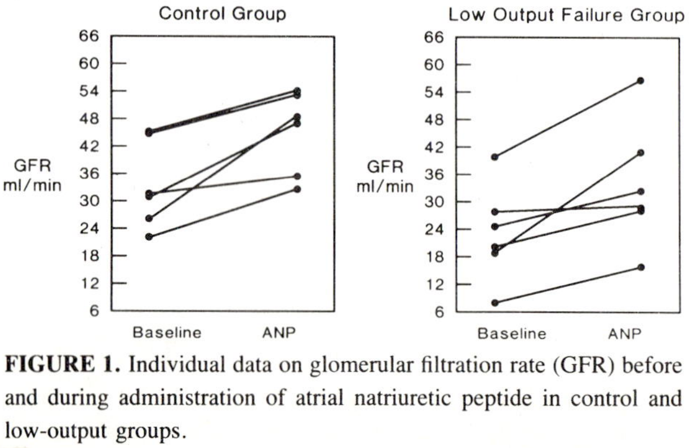

FIGURE 1. Individual data on glomerular filtration rate (GFR) before and during administration of atrial natriuretic peptide in control and low-output groups.

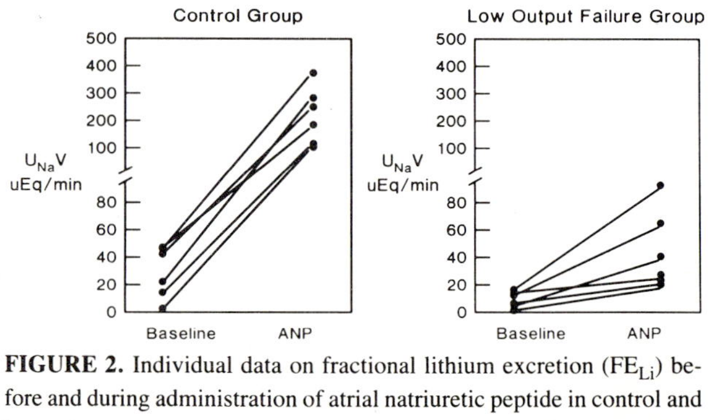

FIGURE 2. Individual data on fractional lithium excretion (FE_{Li}) before and during administration of atrial natriuretic peptide in control and low-output groups.

TABLE 1
(Continued)

FE_{Na} (%)	FE_{Li} (%)	RSR (ng/min)
0.57±0.13	29.8±4.1	308.5±84.5
3.42±0.54[C]	44.1±4.6[A]	44.5±27.5[A]
0.42±0.16	17.7±3.1	852.8±183.0[D]
0.90±0.13[B,D]	30.2±4.3[A]	149.5±73.7[C]

normal dogs from 308.5 ± 84.5 to 44.5 ± 27.5 ng/min ($p < .05$). In the low-output group, intrarenal infusion of atrial natriuretic peptide decreased renin secretory rate from 852.8 ± 183.0 to 149.5 ± 73.7 ng/min ($p < .005$).

Discussion

The intrarenal infusion of synthetic atrial natriuretic peptide in control dogs and those with low-output heart failure resulted in a significant increase in glomerular filtration rate and a decrease in proximal tubule reabsorption as estimated by changes in lithium excretion. Intrarenal administration of the synthetic atrial natriuretic peptide significantly decreased arterial pressure as well as renin secretory rate in both groups. Despite similar alterations in glomerular filtration rate, proximal tubular reabsorption, and renin release in the two groups, the natriuretic and diuretic response to atrial natriuretic peptide was markedly attenuated in animals with acute low-output heart failure as compared with that in control dogs.

Glomerular filtration rate increased in both the control and low-output groups. The observed increase in glomerular filtration rate was consistent with previous reports of effects of synthetic atrial natriuretic peptide in normal dogs.[7, 15] Previous studies have suggested

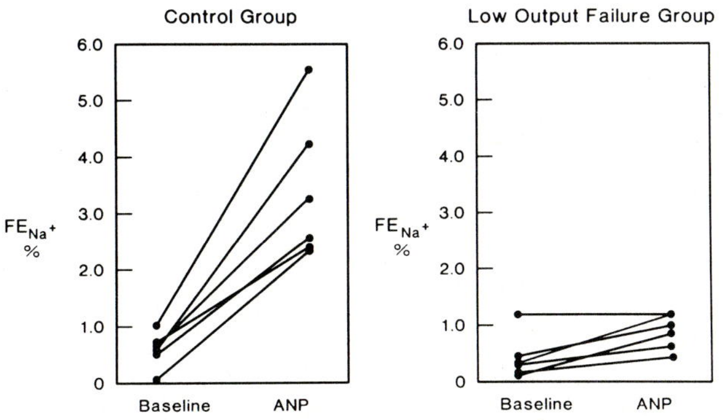

FIGURE 3. Individual data for absolute urinary sodium excretion ($U_{Na}V$) before and during administration of atrial natriuretic peptide in control and low-output groups.

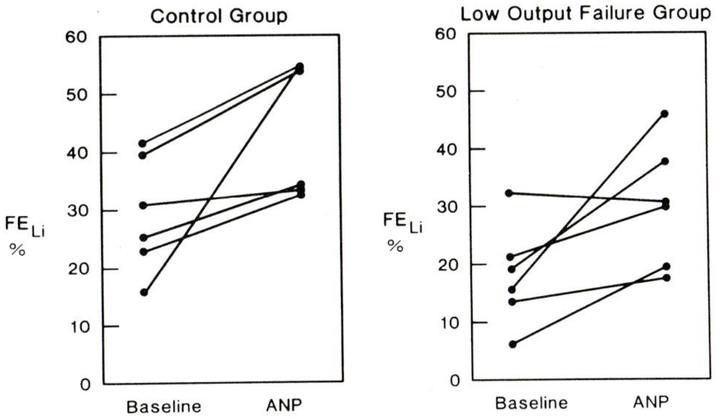

FIGURE 4. Individual data for fractional excretion of sodium (FE_{Na^+}) before and during administration of atrial natriuretic peptide in control and low-output groups.

that the increase in glomerular filtration rate observed with infusion of this substance may be the result of an increase in postglomerular arteriolar resistance or in the coefficient for ultrafiltration.[7, 16]

The present study revealed a significant increase in whole-kidney fractional excretion of lithium with intrarenal infusion of synthetic atrial natriuretic peptide in both groups. Previous studies from our laboratory, as well as others, have reported an action of atrial natriuretic peptide on proximal tubule reabsorption.[7, 17] However, the increased filtered load of lithium accompanying increased glomerular filtration in each group may have contributed to its increased excretion.

Despite a significant increase in glomerular filtration rate and a decrease in proximal tubule reabsorption, the natriuretic response to synthetic natriuretic peptide was markedly attenuated in the low-output group. Such a response is similar to the excretory response to acute volume expansion previously observed in animals with experimental heart failure.[18] These latter studies in dogs with heart failure demonstrated that acute saline volume expansion, a physiologic maneuver recently reported to be associated with increased levels of immunoreactive atrial natriuretic peptide,[19] is characterized by an increase in glomerular filtration

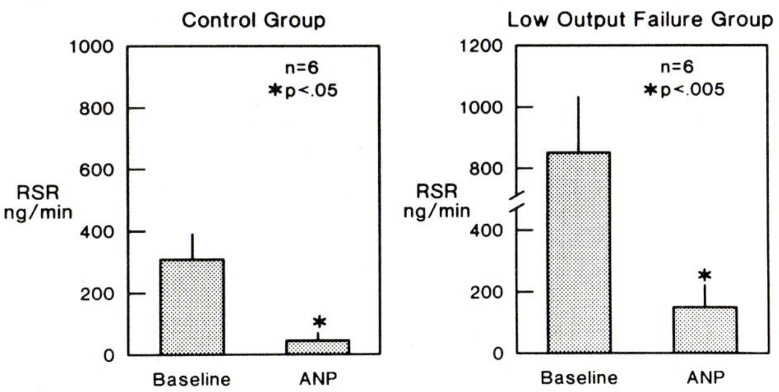

FIGURE 5. Renin secretory rate (RSR) before and during administration of atrial natriuretic peptide in control and low-output groups.

rate and a decrease in proximal tubule reabsorption with a blunted natriuresis. The blunted natriuresis was attributed to enhanced solute reabsorption beyond the proximal tubule, perhaps in part mediated by enhanced circulating levels of aldosterone, which are known to be elevated in models of low-output heart failure,[10, 11] and/or alterations in physical factors, which occur during perturbations in renal perfusion and venous pressures.[20, 21] The present studies further support the hypothesis that the defect in the renal handling of sodium in heart failure may be mediated by factors that act beyond the proximal tubule and are therefore independent of the action of atrial natriuretic peptide on glomerular filtration rate and proximal tubular reabsorption. Thus, the present studies provide further insight into the understanding of heart failure by focusing on the importance of nephron segments beyond the proximal tubule in the pathophysiology of congestive heart failure.

Balloon inflation in the thoracic inferior vena cava resulted in an increase in renin secretion. The mechanism of the increase in renin release during balloon inflation may be multifactorial, with factors including decreased delivery of solute to the macula densa, increased renal nerve activity, and decreased distention of renal baroreceptors.[22] Intrarenal administration of atrial natriuretic peptide nevertheless resulted in a decrease in renin secretory rate in both control dogs and those with low-output heart failure. This observation is consistent with previous reports that atrial natriuretic peptide decreases renin release despite a sustained decrease in arterial pressure.[7, 15] The mechanism by which atrial natriuretic peptide decreases renin secretory rate remains unclear. Previous investigations have reported an inverse relationship between sodium chloride delivery to the macula densa and renin release.[23] Probable enhanced delivery of sodium chloride to the macula densa during intrarenal infusion of atrial natriuretic peptide thus would be expected to signal the juxtaglomerular cells to decrease renin release. Recent studies by Opgenorth et al.[24] support a macula densa mechanism in the mediation of atrial natriuretic peptide–induced inhibition of renin release.[24] However, the possibility of an additional direct suppression of renin release from the juxtaglomerular cells by this peptide cannot be excluded.

In summary, results of the present study demonstrate that the natriuretic response to atrial natriuretic peptide, although present, is markedly attenuated in the acute high-renin, sodium-retaining preparation of heart failure we used. This blunted natriuretic response occurs despite the unique ability of this peptide to increase glomerular filtration rate and decrease proximal tubule reabsorption. Furthermore, atrial natriuretic peptide serves as a potent inhibitor of the renin-angiotensin system in this high-renin state, despite a decrease in arterial pressure.

We thank Denise Heublein for her expert technical assistance, and June M. Hanke and Lori Meyer for secretarial assistance.

References

1. DeBold AJ, Borenstein HB, Veress AT, Sonnenberg H: A rapid and potent natriuretic response to intravenous injection of atrial myocardial extracts in rats. Life Sci **28:** 89, 1981
2. Flynn TG, DeBold ML, DeBold AJ: The amino acid sequence of an atrial peptide with potent diuretic and natriuretic properties. Biochem Biophys Res Commun **117:** 859, 1983
3. Atlas SA, Kleinert HD, Camargo MJ, Januszewicz A, Sealey JE, Laragh JH, Schilling JW, Lewichki JA, Johnson LK, Maack T: Purification, sequencing and synthesis of natriuretic and vasoactive rat atrial peptides. Nature **309:** 717, 1984
4. Currie MG, Geller DM, Cole BR, Boyland JG, Yusheng W, Holmberg SW, Needleman P: Purification and sequence analysis of bioactive atrial peptides (atriopeptins). Science **223:** 67, 1984
5. Misono KS, Fukumi H, Grammer RT, Inagami T: Rat atrial natriuretic factor: complete amino acid sequence and disulfide linkage essential for biological activity. Biochem Biophys Res Commun **119:** 524, 1984
6. Seldah NG, Lazure C, Chretian M, Thibault G, Garcia R, Cantin M, Genest J: Amino acid sequence of homologous rat atrial peptides: natriuretic activity of native and synthetic forms. Proc Natl Acad Sci USA **81:** 2640, 1984
7. Burnett JC Jr, Granger JP, Opgenorth TJ: Effects of synthetic atrial natriuretic factor on renal function and renin release. Am J Physiol **247:** F863, 1984
8. Freeman RH, Davis JO, Vari RC, Sweet WD: The anti-renin/anti-aldosterone actions of synthetic atrial natriuretic factor in conscious dogs with caval constriction and ascites. Proc Am Soc Nephrol 159A, 1984
9. Chimoskey JE, Spielman WS, Brandt MA, Heidemann SR: Cardiac atria of BIO 14.6 hamsters are deficient in natriuretic factor. Science **223:** 820, 1984
10. Davis JO, Pechet MM, Ball WS Jr, Goodkin MJ: Increased aldosterone secretion in dogs with right-sided congestive heart failure and in dogs with thoracic inferior vena cava constriction. J Clin Invest **36:** 689, 1957
11. Watkins L, Burton JA, Haber E, Cant JR, Smith FW, Barger AC: The renin-angiotensin-aldosterone system in congestive failure in conscious dogs. J Clin Invest **57:** 1606, 1976
12. Hayslett JP, Kashgarian M: A micropuncture study of the renal handling of lithium. Pflugers Arch **380:** 159, 1979
13. Thomsen K, Holstein-Rathlow NH, Leyssac PP: Comparison of three measures of proximal tubular reabsorption: lithium clearance, occlusion time, and micropuncture. Am J Physiol **241:** F348, 1981
14. Haber E, Loerner D, Page T, Kleman K, Purnode A: Application of a radioimmunoassay for angiotensin I to the physiologic measurement of plasma renin activity in normal human subjects. J Clin Endocrinol **29:** 1329, 1969
15. Maack T, Marion DH, Camargo MJF, Kleinert HD, Laragh JH, Vaughan ED, Atlas SA: Effects of synthetic atrial natriuretic factor on kidney function and the renin-aldosterone system in the dog. Am J Med **77:** 1069, 1984
16. Camargo MJF, Kleinert HD, Atlas SA, Sealey JE, Laragh JH, Maack T: Ca-dependent hemodynamic and natriuretic effects of atrial extract in isolated rat kidney. Am J Physiol **246:** F447, 1984
17. Dousa TP, Hammond TG, Yusufi ANK, Knox FG: Synthetic atrial natriuretic factor inhibits Na-coupled solute reabsorption in proximal tubules. J Clin Invest **75:** 1983, 1985
18. Schneider EG, Dresser TP, Lynch RE, Knox FG: Sodium reab-

sorption by proximal tubule of dogs with experimental heart failure. Am J Physiol **220:** 952, 1971
19. Lang RE, Luft F, Gauter D, Thoelken G, Unger T: Radioimmunoassay determination and characterization of atrial natriuretic peptide in plasma. Proc Am Soc Nephrol 162A, 1984
20. Hartupee DA, Burnett JC Jr, Mertz JI, Knox FG: Bradykinin-induced vasodilation without natriuresis by control of interstitial pressure. Am J Physiol **243:** F325, 1982
21. Burnett JC Jr, Knox FG: Renal interstitial pressure and sodium excretion during renal vein constriction. Am J Physiol **238:** F279, 1980
22. Davis JO, Freeman RH: Mechanisms regulating renin release. Physiol Rev **56:** 1, 1976
23. Keeton TK, Campbell WB: The pharmacologic alteration of renin release. Pharmacol Rev **31:** 181, 1981
24. Opgenorth TJ, Burnett JC Jr, Granger JP: Mechanism of inhibition of renin secretion by atrial natriuretic peptide. Clin Res **23:** 494A, 1985

Frequency-dependent effects of amitriptyline on ventricular conduction and cardiac rhythm in dogs

STANLEY NATTEL, M.D.

ABSTRACT Although overdoses of tricyclic antidepressant are known to produce both sinus tachycardia and ventricular tachyarrhythmias in man, these have been assumed to occur by independent mechanisms. This study was designed to evaluate the relationship of ventricular activation frequency to the cardiotoxic effects of amitriptyline. When amitriptyline was infused into dogs with formalin-induced atrioventricular (AV) block to evaluate a broad range of pacing frequencies, the drug produced dose-related QRS prolongation that was markedly frequency dependent. Similar frequency-dependent depression of the maximum rate of depolarization ($\dot{V}_{max}$) was noted for canine Purkinje fibers superfused with amitriptyline in vitro. The time constant of recovery from amitriptyline-induced block was dose independent and averaged 228 msec in vivo and 216 msec in vitro. When amitriptyline was infused into dogs with intact AV conduction, sinus tachycardia occurred within 15 min, followed by progressive QRS prolongation and ventricular tachyarrhythmias after an average of 29 min. Slowing of sinus rate by vagal stimulation (seven dogs) or intravenous metoprolol (five dogs) reproducibly reversed the QRS prolongation and ventricular tachyarrhythmias caused by amitriptyline. These studies show that amitriptyline produces frequency-related depression of ventricular conduction in vivo, with a time dependence similar to effects on the maximum rate of depolarization in vitro. Interventions that slow heart rate reverse the adverse effects of amitriptyline on ventricular conduction and cardiac rhythm.
Circulation 72, No. 4, 898–906, 1985.

LOCAL ANESTHETIC drugs have been shown to have important frequency-dependent effects on the maximum rate of depolarization ($\dot{V}_{max}$) and the inward sodium current of mammalian cardiac tissues.[1] These observations have been incorporated into powerful new models of the interaction between antiarrhythmic drugs and cardiac sodium channels.[2, 3] Although these models have important potential clinical implications,[4] there is relatively little information available about the occurrence in vivo and clinical relevance of frequency-dependent drug effects on ventricular conduction.

The tricyclic antidepressants are local anesthetic drugs[5–7] with potentially useful antiarrhythmic effects.[8] Overdoses of tricyclic antidepressants produce slowing of ventricular conduction and tachyarrhythmias.[9–12] The relative role of local anesthetic properties, anticholinergic actions, and blockade of norepinephrine uptake in producing tricyclic-induced ventricular tachyarrhythmias has been debated.[13] We have shown that amitriptyline infusion predictably results in sinus tachycardia at low doses, followed by QRS prolongation and ventricular tachyarrhythmias at higher doses.[14, 15] These findings correspond to clinical observations suggesting that anticholinergic actions of the tricyclics are not directly responsible for ventricular arrhythmogenesis and that ventricular conduction slowing may play an important role in arrhythmia production as originally suggested by Vohra et al.[16]

The possibility that sinus tachycardia caused by tricyclic antidepressant overdose plays a permissive role in slowing of ventricular conduction, and in arrhythmogenesis has not been considered. Observations supporting this idea include the anecdotally described reversal of amitriptyline-induced ventricular arrhythmias and conduction slowing by physostigmine in man[17] and by physostigmine, neostigmine, and practolol in puppies.[18]

This investigation was designed to evaluate the frequency dependence of the effects of amitriptyline on

From the Departments of Pharmacology and Therapeutics and Medicine, McGill University, and the Divisions of Cardiology and Clinical Pharmacology, Montreal General Hospital, Montreal, Quebec.

Supported by operating grants from the Medical Research Council of Canada and the Quebec Heart Foundation. Dr. Nattel is a Medical Research Council Scholar.

Address for correspondence: Stanley Nattel, M.D., Department of Pharmacology and Therapeutics, 3655 Drummond St., Montreal, Quebec H3G 1Y6, Canada.

Received Jan. 28, 1985; revision accepted July 5, 1985.

ventricular conduction in vivo and to relate these frequency-dependent effects to changes in $\dot{V}_{max}$ of canine cardiac Purkinje fibers in vitro and to amitriptyline-induced ventricular arrhythmias in intact dogs. Preliminary results of these studies have been presented in abstract form.[19]

Methods

General. Mongrel dogs of either sex were used for all experiments. For experiments in vivo, dogs were anesthetized with morphine (2 mg/kg im) and alphachloralose (100 mg/kg iv). This form of anesthesia was chosen because it results in baseline cardiovascular variables and effects of amitriptyline similar to those found in the awake, nonsedated dog.[14, 15] Catheters were inserted into the left femoral artery and both femoral veins and kept patent with heparinized saline solution (0.9%). A Statham P23 1D transducer (Statham Medical Instruments, Los Angeles) and electrophysiologic amplifiers and a paper recorder (Grass Instruments Co.) were used to monitor blood pressure, electrocardiographic leads II and aVR, and a right atrial electrogram or stimulus artifacts. All dogs were ventilated via an endotracheal tube at a rate of 10/min with a tidal volume obtained from a nomogram. The control heart rate of these dogs averaged 58 ± 8 beats/min and blood pressure averaged 153 ± 22/100 ± 20 mm Hg.

Tissues for studies in vitro were obtained from dogs anesthetized with sodium pentobarbital (30 mg/kg iv). Free-running false tendons were dissected from either ventricle along with subjacent muscle and attached to the paraffin-coated bottom of a Lucite tissue chamber. The preparation was stimulated with 2 msec square-wave pulses of twice diastolic threshold current via bipolar Teflon-coated platinum electrodes. A digital timing unit and stimulus isolator (Bloom Instruments, Flying Hills, PA) were used to control stimulus delivery. The tissue was superfused with modified Tyrode's solution oxygenated with 95% O_2/5% CO_2 and containing the following consituents: Na^+, 141 mM; HCO_3-; 22 mM; dextrose, 5.5 mM; K^+, 4 mM; Mg^{2+}, 0.5 mM; $H_2PO_4^-$, 0.9 mM; Ca^{2+}, 2mM; and Cl^-, 125 mM. Temperature of the solution was kept at 37° ± 0.2° C by a heating element under negative feedback control from a thermistor in the tissue bath (Hanna Instruments, Philadelphia). Glass microelectrodes filled with 3M KCl solution and with resistances of 8 to 20 megohm were coupled via a Ag-AgCl junction to a microelectrode amplifier (WPI Model KS-700). Transmembrane potential was displayed on a Tektronix 5115 storage oscilloscope and was differentiated electronically (differentiation linear over 20 to 1000 V/sec). Transmembrane potentials were converted into digital form with a 100 kHz analog-to-digital converter (Tecmar, Inc.) and analyzed with an IBM personal computer and custom-made software routines (Bascom Consultants Inc., Montreal, Quebec).

Frequency-dependent effects of amitriptyline on conduction in vivo. A right thoracotomy was performed and complete atrioventricular (AV) block was produced by injection of small quantities (average 0.15 ml) of formalin.[20] A bipolar, Teflon-coated, stainless steel electrode inserted into the right ventricle was used to stimulate the heart with 4 msec square-wave pulses of twice diastolic threshold current. Electrocardiographic recordings were obtained at 100 mm/sec paper speed during sustained stimulation at basic cycle lengths of 300 and 1000 msec and in the presence of premature beats and pauses. Single premature beats were initiated after every eight basic complexes at 1 Hz, and pauses were introduced after 18 basic activations at 2.5 to 3.3 Hz. Effective refractory period, defined as the longest premature coupling interval at which ventricular activation failed, was measured by the extrastimulus technique. Spontaneous escape intervals were measured by temporarily interrupting stimulation after at least 30 sec of continuous pacing at a selected frequency.

Induction of arrhythmia was attempted in some experiments with up to two extrastimuli and burst pacing. Ventricular tachycardia was defined as three or more successive broad QRS complexes at a rate greater than the underlying sinus or paced rate with evidence of AV dissociation.

The effects of amitriptyline were studied by a multiple infusion system developed during preliminary investigations. Stable drug effects were observed for over 20 min during continuous infusions of amitriptyline that had been preceded by 15 min loading infusions at 50% greater rate. Results were obtained during infusion at rates of 0.17, 0.33, and 0.67 mg/kg/min, which paralleled the range over which amitriptyline cardiotoxicity in the dog resembles the drug's toxic effects in man.[14, 15] Plasma amitriptyline concentrations were measured by previously developed high-pressure liquid chromatographic techniques.[14]

Frequency-dependent effects of amitriptyline on $\dot{V}_{max}$ in vitro. After a 1 hr stabilization period, control action potential characteristics were measured at basic cycle lengths of 300 and 1000 msec. Amitriptyline was then added to the superfusate at concentrations of 0.2 or 1 mg/liter, and measurements were repeated after 30 and 60 min. After 1 hr of drug superfusion, the effects of changes in basic stimulation frequency and of premature and delayed activation were evaluated. Premature or delayed action potentials with a take-off potential more than 2 mV different from basic action potentials were not included in analyses of changes in $\dot{V}_{max}$. Results presented are for experiments in which continued impalement of the same cell was maintained during both control and drug superfusion periods. The concentration range selected was based on estimates of the range of free plasma concentrations associated with significant electrophysiologic effects in previous experiments.[14]

The voltage dependence of $\dot{V}_{max}$ was studied by increasing superfusate potassium concentration to 14 mM by the addition of potassium chloride. The resulting $\dot{V}_{max}$ inactivation curves were fitted to an equation based on the observations of Weidmann.[21] Nonlinear curve fitting techniques were used to obtain the transmembrane potential for 50% inactivation of $\dot{V}_{max}$ (V_{50}) and the slope factor (S), which characterize the inactivation curve. Only curves that were reproducible upon potassium washout were used. Results were obtained first under control conditions, then after 1 hr of amitriptyline infusion at one cycle length, and finally during continued amitriptyline infusion at a second basic cycle length. The cycle lengths studied were 1000 and 300 msec (or the shortest cycle length greater than 300 msec at which sustained capture was obtained). Five experiments were performed to study the effects of 0.2 mg/liter amitriptyline and five with 1 mg/liter amitriptyline.

Effects of amitriptyline, vagal stimulation, and metoprolol. Amitriptyline was infused via the right femoral vein of closed-chest, anesthetized dogs at 0.5 mg/kg/min for 30 min followed by 1 mg/kg/min for up to 30 min. When ventricular tachyarrhythmia occurred, the infusion rate was reduced by one-third and the infusion was continued. We have shown that this protocol results in ventricular tachyarrhythmias in most dogs and that the effects of amitriptyline are constant for at least 30 min after the dose reduction.[15] The vagi were isolated from the carotid sheaths in the neck but not decentralized and were stimulated with supramaximal voltage, square-wave bipolar pulses of 0.2 msec duration and 12 Hz frequency. To produce appreciable vagal effects in the presence of amitriptyline, it was necessary to administer an acetylcholinesterase inhibitor. We used a single dose of neostigmine (2.5 mg iv) given 1 min after the reduction in infusion rate. In experiments studying metoprolol, 2.5 mg of metoprolol (approximately 0.15 mg/kg) was administered intravenously 1 min after the onset of ventricular arrhythmia.

Statistical analysis. Group data are presented as mean ± SD. Comparisons between group means were made by two-way analysis of variance with Scheffé's test.[22]

The frequency dependence of drug effects in vitro was determined by calculating an F ratio for interaction effects.[22] Raw data and two-tailed tests were used for all statistical comparisons. A probability of 5% or less was taken to indicate statistical significance. Linear and nonlinear curve fitting was performed by least squares regression.

Results

Frequency-dependent effects of amitriptyline on ventricular conduction in vivo. Infusion of amitriptyline resulted in QRS prolongation that depended on both the frequency of activation and the drug infusion rate (table 1). Overall QRS morphology was not altered by the drug, but the slope of all portions of the QRS was decreased. Measurements of QRS duration were made from corresponding points at the first rapid voltage deflection to the last rapid deflection, with use of the same lead for both control and drug infusion periods. QT intervals at a basic cycle length of 1000 msec were decreased by amitriptyline, but at a basic cycle length of 300 msec large doses of amitriptyline increased the QT interval by increasing the QRS duration. Refractory periods decreased at the smaller infusion rates and increased at the largest infusion rate. Escape intervals varied greatly between dogs and were increased by amitriptyline. In three animals escape intervals were studied at four basic cycle lengths between 300 and 1000 msesc and were increased by the drug at all frequencies.

Amitriptyline-induced QRS prolongation could be eliminated by pauses in the pacing protocol. Figure 1 shows the effect of an 8 sec pause interrupting stimulation at a basic cycle length of 350 msec during infusion of amitriptyline at 0.67 mg/kg/min. Within four complexes after the resumption of stimulation, the QRS returned to prepause values. Over 90% of steady-state change in QRS duration was obtained within 1 sec after a pause in all animals.

To quantitate the time dependence of QRS prolongation in the presence of amitriptyline, the response to variations in diastolic interval was studied. Diastolic interval was altered by introducing a premature stimulus (S_2) after a train of eight basic stimuli (S_1) at 1 Hz. The increase in QRS duration of premature complexes compared with the QRS duration of the last complex of the basic train was a log-linear function of the S_1S_2 coupling interval (figure 2). Similar results were obtained in each experiment by means of either premature stimuli or pauses to vary the S_1S_2 interval. Pauses were introduced after 18 basic complexes at a cycle length of 300 to 350 msec. The time constant of recovery from amitriptyline-induced QRS prolongation was obtained from the relationship between changes in QRS duration and S_1S_2 interval in each experiment.

Changes in QRS duration that were large enough to measure the time constant accurately were observed in all experiments at the two higher infusion rates. The time constants for QRS prolongation averaged 229 ± 34 and 226 ± 7 msec for the 0.33 and 0.67 mg/kg/min infusion rates, respectively.

Frequency-dependent effects of amitriptyline on $\dot{V}_{max}$ in vitro. Amitriptyline decreased action potential duration and $\dot{V}_{max}$ of canine Purkinje fibers. Under control conditions, $\dot{V}_{max}$ was not significantly changed by decreas-

TABLE 1

Changes in electrophysiologic variables produced by infusion of amitriptyline into six dogs with complete AV block

	QRS (msec)		QT (msec)		ERP (msec)		Esc. Int. (sec)		Ami. Conc. (mg/l)	
	BCL 1000	BCL 300	BCL 1000	BCL 300	BCL 1000	BCL 300	BCL 1000	BCL 300	Prestudy	Poststudy
Control	94±13	94±13	288±24	235±17	221±12	179±6	2.5±1.3	6.9±5.6	—	—
Amitriptyline (mg/kg/min)										
0.17	95±12	110±8^B	265±19^C	237±23	197±10^C	173±5	5.9±5.5	9.3±7.8	1.85±0.65	1.86±0.5
0.33	102±13	146±9^D	261±26^C	269±29^C	237±58	222±68	6.8±5.5	8.1±5.7	3.76±1.13	4.15±1.7
0.67^A	107±14^C	186±22^D	270±18^B	308±33^D	319±107^B	317±90^B	9.3±8.1	12.5±3.5	6.60±0.51	6.59±0.3

ERP = effective refractory period; Esc. Int. = pause before spontaneous ventricular escape after interrupting a 30 sec period of pacing; Ami. Conc. = plasma amitriptyline concentration immediately before (prestudy) and after (poststudy) measurement of electrophysiologic variables during a given drug infusion; BCL 1000, BCL 300 = measurements made at a paced basic cycle length of 1000 and 300 msec.

^{A}It was frequently impossible to maintain pacing at a cycle length of 300 msec during the 0.67 mg/kg/min infusion of amitriptyline. Measurements during this infusion were made at the shortest cycle length permitting sustained capture, averaging 350 msec.

Statistical comparisons (vs control at the same cycle length, by analysis of variance with Scheffé's test): $^Bp < .05$; $^Cp < .01$; $^Dp < .001$.

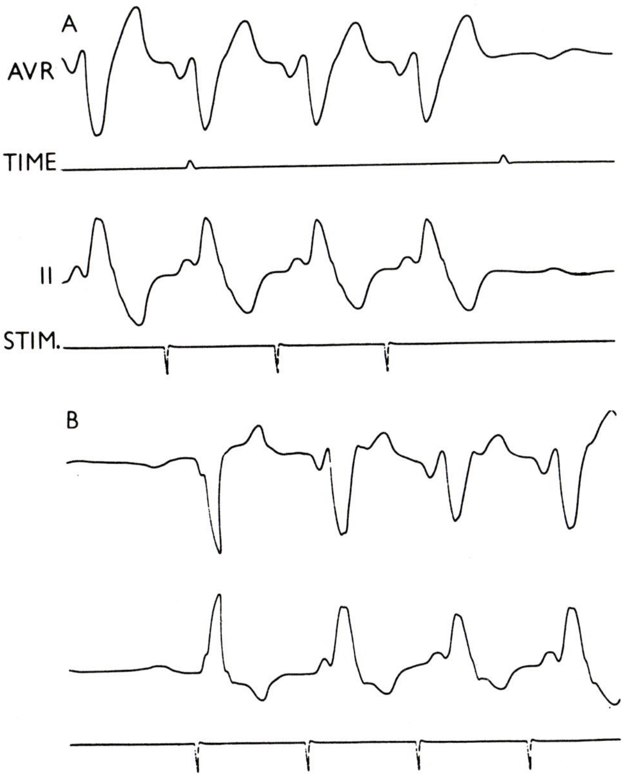

FIGURE 1. Recovery from amitripytline-induced QRS prolongation after a pause. Panels *A* and *B* show electrocardiographic leads aVR and II and stimulus artifacts in a dog with complete AV block during infusion of amitriptyline at 0.67 mg/kg/min. The time marker in panel *A* shows a 1 sec calibration between the two vertical deflections. Continuous pacing at a cycle length of 350 msec was interrupted by an 8 sec pause. Panel *A* shows the last electrograms before the pause, with QRS durations of 0.16 sec. The first QRS after the pause (panel *B*) has a duration of 0.08 sec, equal to the control QRS duration before infusion of amitriptyline. Within four complexes after the resumption of pacing, the QRS duration has returned to 0.16 sec. All tracings were obtained with a curvilinear pen recorder.

ing basic cycle length from 1000 to 300 msec. The electrophysiologic changes resulting from 1 hr of amitriptyline infusion are summarized in tables 2A and 2B. Lower concentrations of amitriptyline (0.2 mg/liter) did not alter $\dot{V}_{max}$ at a basic cycle length of 1000 msec but significantly reduced $\dot{V}_{max}$ at a cycle length of 300 msec. Higher concentrations of amitriptyline reduced $\dot{V}_{max}$ at both cycle lengths but produced greater depression of $\dot{V}_{max}$ as the frequency was increased. Action potential duration was reduced by amitriptyline and this effect was attenuated at higher frequencies.

The effects of amitriptyline on $\dot{V}_{max}$ were found to have marked frequency and voltage dependence. In the presence of amitriptyline, premature stimuli produced reductions in $\dot{V}_{max}$ that were log-linearly related to the premature coupling interval (figure 2). The time constant for recovery from amitriptyline-induced block of $\dot{V}_{max}$ was measured in five fibers exposed to 1 mg/liter of the drug and averaged 216 ± 32 msec. Changes in $\dot{V}_{max}$ resulting from 0.2 mg/liter amitriptyline were much smaller, making accurate quantitation of the time constant at the lower concentration difficult.

Amitriptyline shifted the voltage dependence of $\dot{V}_{max}$ to more negative membrane potentials (figure 3). Decreasing the basic cycle length shifted the curve downward without any further rightward shift on the voltage axis. Nonlinear curve fitting of the experimental data showed that amitriptyline produced a concentration-related change in the voltage dependence of $\dot{V}_{max}$ and that changes in frequency did not alter the voltage dependence of $\dot{V}_{max}$ at a given amitriptyline concentration (table 2B).

Effects of changes in spontaneous rate on amitriptyline-induced conduction slowing and arrhythmia. Amitriptyline was infused into 13 closed-chest dogs with intact AV conduction, and ventricular tachyarrhythmias occurred in 12. Amitriptyline increased sinus rate from 57 ± 12 beats/min (control) to a maximum of 173 ± 37 beats/min after 15 min of infusion. QRS duration was altered more slowly by amitriptyline, increasing from 58 ± 8 msec (control) to 75 ± 18 msec after 15 min of drug infusion and then to a maximum of 127 ± 23 msec immediately before the onset of ventricular tachyarrhythmia after an average of 29 min of infusion.

Neostigmine transiently reversed ventricular tachyarrhythmias in one of seven dogs, without altering the cardiac rhythm among the other six. In all seven dogs, vagal stimulation resulted in complete abolition of ventricular tachycardia, slowing of heart rate, and decreases in QRS duration (figure 4). After vagal stimulation was stopped, heart rate gradually increased to previous values, QRS complexes widened, and ventricular tachycardia recurred. Vagal stimulation was then repeated, resulting in sinus rhythm with narrowed QRS complexes. This sequence could be reproduced repeatedly for 30 min after the initial occurrence of ventricular tachyarrhythmia.

Metoprolol was administered to five dogs with ventricular tachyarrhythmia and restored sinus rhythm at a slower rate in all. Although metoprolol was slightly less effective than vagal stimulation, its effects on RR intervals and QRS duration were qualitatively similar (table 3). Vagal stimulation did not significantly alter blood pressure compared with prearrhythmia values, but metoprolol often produced profound and progressive hypotension, sometimes leading to death.

Spontaneous ventricular tacyarrhythmias did not occur among any dogs with complete AV block. Pro-

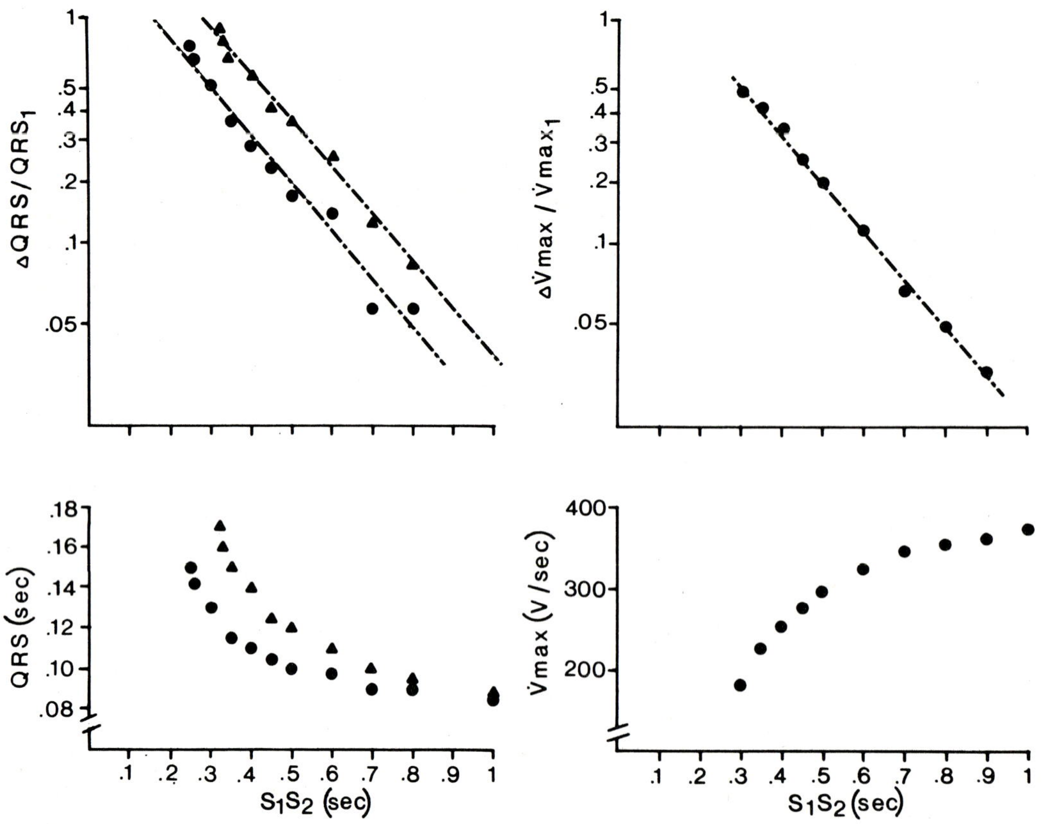

FIGURE 2. Relationship of amitriptyline-induced block to recovery time. *Left,* Relationship between changes in QRS duration and coupling interval during infusion of amitriptyline at 0.33 mg/kg/min (circles) and at 0.67 mg/kg/min (triangles) in a typical experiment in vivo. One premature stimulus with a selected coupling interval was introduced after every eight basic stimuli at a frequency of 1 Hz. The bottom graph shows the relationship between the QRS durations of premature responses and their coupling intervals. The top graph shows the relationship between increases in QRS duration (relative to the QRS of basic complexes) and coupling intervals. The regression lines of best fit to the derived points are shown. The time constants for QRS prolongation were 211 msec (at the slower drug infusion rate) and 217 msec (at the faster infusion rate) in this experiment. *Right,* Relationship between changes in $\dot{V}_{max}$ and coupling interval in a typical experiment in vitro. Before amitriptyline superfusion, the $\dot{V}_{max}$ of a premature action potential was not reduced unless it was elicited during phase 3 of the preceding action potential. After 1 hr of superfusion with amitriptyline at 1 mg/liter, premature stimulation reduced $\dot{V}_{max}$ over a broad range of coupling intervals (bottom graph). One premature stimulus was applied after every eight basic stimuli at a frequency of 1 Hz. The top graph shows the relationship between changes in $\dot{V}_{max}$ of premature action potentials (relative to the $\dot{V}_{max}$ of basic action potentials) and the premature coupling interval as well as the regression line of best fit. The time constant for changes in $\dot{V}_{max}$ was 211 msec in this experiment.

grammed electrical stimulation was applied in seven dogs and reproducibly resulted in ventricular tachyarrhythmias along with marked conduction slowing in six. Ventricular tachyarrhythmias consisted of ventricular tachycardia in five dogs and ventricular fibrillation in one.

Discussion

We have demonstrated that amitriptyline has frequency-dependent effects on ventricular conduction in vivo, with a similar time dependency to the drug's depressant effects on $\dot{V}_{max}$ in vitro. Furthermore, interventions that slow heart rate (including vagal stimulation, metoprolol, and AV block) reverse or prevent both conduction slowing and ventricular tachyarrhythmias caused by infusion of amitriptyline. In contrast to the extensive information about frequency-dependent effect of drugs on cardiac tissue in vitro, little has been published about corresponding effects in vivo. Lidocaine has been shown to produce time-dependent conduction slowing in intact hearts.[23] but the time dependency was not quantified. A major restriction in studying rate-dependent drug effects in vivo is the often-limited range of frequencies that can be evaluated because of interference from supraventricular pacemakers. This problem can be avoided by using animals with complete AV block, as described in this study.

We used $\dot{V}_{max}$ as an index of amitriptyline's effects on cardiac sodium channels in vitro. The limitations of this approach are well recognized.[1, 24] It is nevertheless

TABLE 2A
Effects of amitriptyline on action potential characteristics of canine cardiac Purkinje fibers[A]

	Control		Amitriptyline (0.2 mg/l)			Control		Amitriptyline (1 mg/l)		
	BCL 1000	BCL 300	BCL 1000	BCL 300	P_{intrxn}	BCL 1000	BCL 300	BCL 1000	BCL 350[B]	P_{intrxn}
MAP (mV)	−86±2	−90±2	−85±1	−86±1[C]	NS	−88±4	−90±2	−87±2	−88±2	NS
APA (mV)	128±3	132±2	126±4	123±3[D]	NS	127±5	126±3	120±7[C]	112±9[D]	NS
APD_{50} (msec)	213±30	121±8	116±17[E]	74±15[C]	<.05	171±37	106±8	81±23[E]	75±13[C]	<.01
APD_{90} (msec)	280±23	169±9	211±14[E]	146±8	<.01	266±29	169±10	214±19[E]	169±20	<.01
$\dot{V}_{max}$ (V/sec)	718±104	683±107	681±107	548±116[E]	<.01	695±76	658±124	525±101[E]	380±129[E]	<.05

BCL = basic cycle length; MAP = transmembrane potential at the time of activation; APA = action potential amplitude; APD_{50}, APD_{90} = action potential duration to 50% and 90% of repolarization; P_{intrxn} = statistical significance of the interaction between pacing cycle length and drug effects, by F test for interaction.

[A]Results are from five experiments studying amitriptyline at 0.2 mg/l and 10 experiments at 1 mg/l.

[B]Sustained capture could not always be maintained at a cycle length of 300 msec at this amitriptyline concentration. The shortest possible cycle length over 300 msec was then used, and the average cycle length studied was 350 msec.

Statistical comparisons (vs control at the same basic cycle length): [C]$p < .05$; [D]$p < .01$; [E]$p < .001$.

TABLE 2B
Effects of amitriptyline on the voltage dependence of $\dot{V}_{max}$ in canine cardiac Purkinje fibers

		Amitriptyline (0.2 mg/l)			Amitriptyline (1 mg/l)	
	Control	BCL 1000	BCL 300	Control	BCL 1000	BCL 350
V_{50} (mV)	−66.7±1.4	−71.6±2.2[C]	−72.2±1.9[C]	−70.8±2.1	−78.2±1.3[C]	−78.8±1.2[C]
S	3.90±0.62	3.52±0.47	3.69±0.78	4.09±0.55	2.48±0.27[B]	2.97±0.43[A]

V_{50} = transmembrane potential at which 50% reduction of $\dot{V}_{max}$ was achieved; S = slope factor. Both values were obtained from nonlinear curve fitting of the K^+-depolarized MAP − $\dot{V}_{max}$ relationship to the equation: $(\dot{V}_{max})_t = (\dot{V}_{max})_o/(1 + \exp(V_{50} - MAP)/S)$, where $(\dot{V}_{max})_t$ = $\dot{V}_{max}$ of the test action potential, $(\dot{V}_{max})_o$ = $\dot{V}_{max}$ before K^+ depolarization, and MAP = activation potential of the test action potential. The mean correlation coefficient for the fits obtained was .99. Results were obtained from five experiments at each amitriptyline concentration.

Statistical comparisons (vs control): [A]$p < .05$; [B]$p < .01$; [C]$p < .001$.

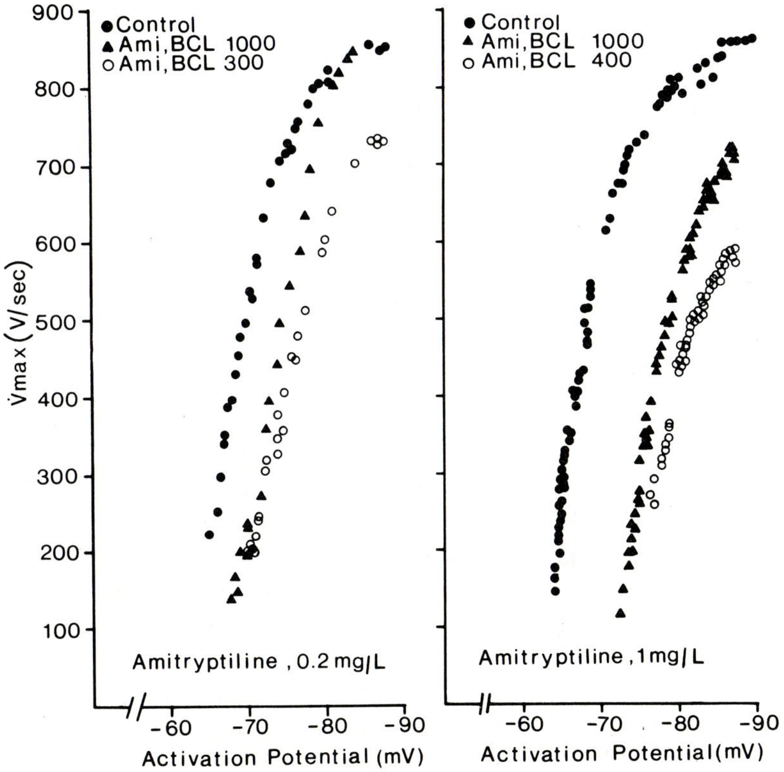

FIGURE 3. Effect of amitriptyline (Ami) on the relationship between $\dot{V}_{max}$ and activation potential. The $\dot{V}_{max}$ of action potentials was measured as a function of transmembrane potential at the onset of activation. Membrane potential was altered by increasing superfusate potassium concentration to 14 mM and then returning to control Tyrode's solution. Under control conditions, changes in frequency did not alter membrane responsiveness. This figure shows the changes in membrane responsiveness in typical experiments after 1 hr of superfusion with 0.2 mg/liter of amitriptyline (*left*) and 1 mg/liter of amitriptyline (*right*). Amitriptyline produced a concentration-dependent rightward shift of the membrane responsiveness curve. Decreasing the cycle length in the presence of amitriptyline resulted in a downward shift of the curve, without changing its voltage dependence. BCL = basic cycle length (msec).

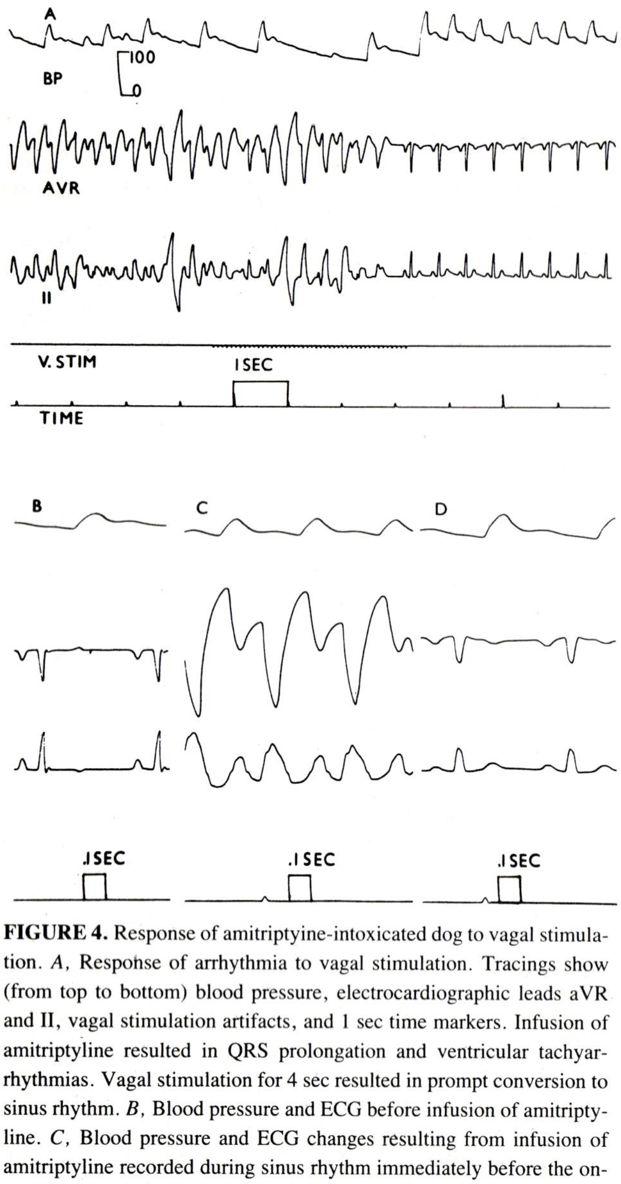

FIGURE 4. Response of amitriptyine-intoxicated dog to vagal stimulation. *A*, Response of arrhythmia to vagal stimulation. Tracings show (from top to bottom) blood pressure, electrocardiographic leads aVR and II, vagal stimulation artifacts, and 1 sec time markers. Infusion of amitriptyline resulted in QRS prolongation and ventricular tachyarrhythmias. Vagal stimulation for 4 sec resulted in prompt conversion to sinus rhythm. *B*, Blood pressure and ECG before infusion of amitriptyline. *C*, Blood pressure and ECG changes resulting from infusion of amitriptyline recorded during sinus rhythm immediately before the onset of ventricular tachycardia. *D*, Reversal of amitriptyine-induced ECG changes resulting from the brief period of vagal stimulation shown in panel *A*. All records were obtained with a curvilinear-motion pen recorder.

a well-characterized and standard method to study the cellular effects of antiarrhythmic drugs. Its advantages include simplicity and the ability to study tissues at physiologic temperatures and with superfusates that mimic the normal extracellular milieu. Much of our current understanding of cellular mechanisms of antiarrhythmic drug action depends on the use of $\dot{V}_{max}$ as an index of maximum sodium permeability,[1] although more direct measurements of sodium current will certainly provide important improvements in the understanding of drug mechanisms.

Considerable work has been done to characterize the biophysical properties that determine the time course of the blocking actions of various drugs.[24–28] Amitriptyline and imipramine have similar chemical structures and molecular weights, but our data suggest a more rapid time course for amitriptyline induced block than has been shown for imipramine in vitro.[25] The differences may be caused by differences in the experimental preparations used or by differences in rate of block, which can occur even with relatively small modifications of drug structure.[26, 27]

The mechanism of frequency-dependent drug effects on cardiac sodium channels is an area of major ongoing investigation. Suggested mechanisms include drug-receptor association and dissociation rates that depend on the state of the sodium channel[2] and access to the sodium channel that depends on the drug's biophysical properties and the state of the channel.[3] Those models predict that the block produced by tertiary amine local anesthetics (like amitriptyline) may be enhanced by depolarization and that recovery from depolarization-induced block is time dependent. The observed shifts in the voltage dependence of $\dot{V}_{max}$ and the frequency dependence of $\dot{V}_{max}$ depression caused by amitriptyline are therefore typical of drug effects described in these models. Furthermore, changes in QRS duration in the presence of amitriptyline in vivo follow a similar pattern and can be explained in terms of the models. With each activation, amitriptyline binds to sodium channels and begins to unbind during diastole. If diastole is sufficiently long, sodium channels become completely unblocked between activations and conduction is unaltered. As heart rate is increased, the diastolic period is shortened and there is insufficient time for complete drug unbinding between beats. The

TABLE 3
Changes in electrocardiographic intervals produced by amitriptyline, and effects of vagal stimulation and metoprolol during continued infusion

		Amitriptyline	
	Control	Prearrhythmia	Vagal stimulation
RR (sec)	1.02±0.36	0.34±0.08^C	0.56±0.14^A
QRS (sec)	0.055±0.005	0.131±0.019^C	0.079±0.019^A
		Amitriptyline	
		Prearrhythmia	After metoprolol
RR	0.95±0.29	0.33±0.05^C	0.49±0.05^B
QRS	0.060±0.009	0.135±0.023^C	0.099±0.016^C

All measurements were made during sinus rhythm, including those immediately before arrhythmia and after conversion to sinus rhythm by vagal stimulation (studied in seven dogs) or metoprolol (in five dogs).

Statistical comparisons (vs corresponding control value, by two-way analysis of variance with Scheffé's test): $^Ap < .05$; $^Bp < .01$; $^Cp < .001$.

presence of persistent drug-associated (blocked) sodium channels reduces maximum sodium current and conduction velocity, resulting in QRS prolongation. Marked QRS prolongation is associated with the appearance of ventricular tachyarrhythmias. Slowing the underlying rate in the presence of amitriptyline allows greater diastolic time for drug unbinding from sodium channels, which reduces the degree of sodium channel block, improves ventricular conduction, and eliminates ventricular arrhythmias.

Amitriptyline slowed conduction with variable effects on refractory periods. At lower concentrations, refractoriness was decreased or unaltered by amitriptyline. At high concentrations, refractory periods were increased, presumably because of interval dependent inactivation of sodium channels.[8, 29] Sinus tachycardia in the presence of amitriptyline would favor reentry by increasing rate-dependent conduction slowing. If the heart rate was sufficiently rapid that ventricular activation occurred during phase 3 of the preceding action potential, further voltage-dependent conduction slowing would result. The establishment of reentry circuits would depend on the balance between changes in conduction and refractoriness caused by amitriptyline. The inducibility of arrhythmia by programmed stimulation in the presence of amitriptyline favors a reentrant type of arrhythmic mechanism. We found no evidence that amitriptyline enhances automaticity, either by measuring escape intervals in this study or by monitoring spontaneous ventricular rate in previous work.[14] The lack of overdrive enhancement of escape intervals is evidence against the possibility that amitriptyline causes ventricular tachyarrhythmias by inducing triggered automaticity.[30]

Reversal of conduction slowing might be expected to abolish the conditions permitting reentrant arrhythmias in the presence of amitriptyline. This could explain the antiarrhythmic effects of vagal stimulation and metoprolol in this study and could account for the beneficial effects of alkalinization (the clinical treatment of choice) on arrhythmias caused by amitriptyline.[15] Increases in pH have been shown to accelerate the recovery of sodium channels blocked by weakly basic local anesthetics,[31, 32] presumably by decreasing protonation of the drug-receptor complex. Amitriptyline has a pK_a of 9.4, implying that its nonionized drug fraction should be sensitive to pH changes over the physiologic range. Increasing the proportion of amitriptyline that is nonionized would presumably facilitate egress of the drug from the sodium channel, possibly accounting for the improvements in conduction and reversal of arrhythmia that have been observed.[15]

Amitriptyline is believed to cause sinus tachycardia by an anticholinergic mechanism.[13, 14] Ventricular tachyarrhythmias are thought to result from conduction slowing caused by amitriptyline's direct actions on sodium channels.[13, 14] The experiments described here suggest that amitriptyline-induced sinus tachycardia and ventricular tachyarrhythmias are not merely coincidental in occurrence but also that sinus tachycardia contributes importantly to ventricular arrhythmogenesis by enhancing the frequency-dependent depressant effects of amitriptyline. This constitutes, to our knowledge, the clearest demonstration to date of a clinically relevant consequence of the frequency-dependent effects of local anesthetic drugs on the heart.

I would like to thank Steven Nuara and Carol Matthews for their excellent technical assistance and Merck-Frosst Pharmaceuticals of Montreal, Canada, for providing purified amitriptyline to standardize the HPLC assay. Dr. Sanfacon of Louis-H. Lafontaine Hospital provided invaluable advice regarding the technique for measurement of amitriptyline concentration.

References

1. Grant AO, Starmer CF, Strauss HC: Antiarrhythmic drug action-blockade of the inward sodium current. Circ Res **5:** 427, 1984
2. Hondeghem LM, Katzung BG: Time and voltage-dependent interactions of antiarrhythmic drugs with cardiac sodium channels. Biochim Biophys Acta **472:** 373, 1977
3. Starmer CF, Grant AO, Strauss HC: Mechanisms of use-dependent block of sodium channels in excitable membranes by local anesthetics. Biophys J **46:** 15, 1984
4. Hondeghem LM, Katzung BG: Antiarrhythmic agents: the modulated receptor mechanism of action of sodium and calcium channel-blocking drugs. Annu Rev Pharmacol Toxicol **24:** 387, 1984
5. Weld FM, Bigger JT: Electrophysiological effects of imipramine on ovine cardiac Purkinje and ventricular muscle fibers. Circ Res **46:** 167, 1980
6. Rawling DA, Fozzard HA: Effects of imipramine on cellular electrophysiological properties of cardiac Purkinje fibers. J Pharmacol Exp Ther **209:** 371, 1979
7. Brennan FJ: Electrophysiologic effects of imipramine and doxepin on normal and depressed cardiac Purkinje fibers. Am J Cardiol **46:** 599, 1980
8. Giardina EV, Bigger JT, Glassman AH, Perel JM, Kantor SJ: The electrophysiologic and antiarrhythmic effects of imipramine hydrochloride at therapeutic plasma concentrations. Circulation **60:** 1045, 1979
9. Sedal L, Korman MG, Williams PO, Mushkin G: Overdose of tricyclic antidepressants: a report of two deaths and a prospective study of 24 patients. Med J Aust **2:** 74, 1972
10. Serafimovski N, Thorball N, Rassmussen I, Lunding M: Tricyclic antidepressive poisoning with special reference to cardiac complications. Acta Anaesth Scand [Suppl] **57:** 55, 1975
11. Thorstrand C: Clinical features in poisoning by tricyclic antidepressants with special reference to the ECG. Acta Med Scand **199:** 337, 1976
12. Biggs JT, Spiker DG, Petit JM, Ziegler VE: Tricyclic antidepressant overdose-incidence of symptoms. JAMA **238:** 135, 1977
13. Marshall JB, Forker AD: Cardiovascular effects of tricyclic antidepressant drugs: therapeutic usage, overdose, and management of complications. Am Heart J **103:** 401, 1982
14. Nattel S, Keable H, Sasyniuk BI: Experimental amitriptyline intoxication: electrophysiologic manifestations and management. J Cardiovasc Pharmacol **6:** 83, 1984
15. Nattel S, Mittleman M: Treatment of ventricular tachyarrhythmias resulting from amitriptyline toxicity in dogs. J Pharmacol Exp Ther **231:** 430, 1984

16. Vohra J, Burrows G, Hunt D, Sloman G: The effect of toxic and therapeutic doses of tricyclic antidepressant drugs on intracardiac conduction. Eur J Cardiol **3:** 219, 1975
17. Tobis J, Das BN: Cardiac complications in amitriptyline poisoning: successful treatment with physostigmine. JAMA **235:** 1974, 1976
18. Brown TCK. Tricyclic antidepressant overdosage: experimental studies on the management of circulatory complications. Clin Toxicol **9:** 255, 1976
19. Nattel S: Frequency-dependent effects of amitriptyline determine arrhythmogenesis. Clin Invest Med **7**(suppl 2): 34, 1984 (abst)
20. Steiner C, Kovalic TW: A simple technique for production of chronic complete heart block in dogs. J Appl Physiol **25:** 631, 1968
21. Weidmann S: The effect of the cardiac membrane potential on the rapid availability of the sodium-carrying system. J Physiol **127:** 213, 1955
22. Sachs L: Applied statistics. New York, 1984, Springer-Verlag
23. Saito S, Chen CM, Buchanan J, Gettes LS, Lynch MR: Steady state and time-dependent slowing of conduction in canine hearts: effects of potassium and lidocaine. Circ Res **42:** 246, 1978
24. Gintant GA, Hoffman BF, Naylor RE: The influence of molecular form of local anesthetic-type antiarrhythmic agents on reduction of the maximum upstroke velocity of canine cardiac Purkinje fibers. Circ Res **52:** 735, 1983
25. Courtney KR: Interval-dependent effects of small antiarrhythmic drugs on excitability of guinea-pig myocardium. J Mol Cell Cardiol **12:** 1273, 1980
26. Ehring G, Hondeghem LM: Antiarrhythmic structure activity relationships in a series of lidocaine and procainamide derivatives. Proc West Pharmacol Soc **24:** 221, 1981
27. Moyer J, Ehring G, Hondegham L: Kinetics of interaction of a series of aprindine derivatives with the cardiac sodium channel. Fed Proc **41:** 1737, 1982 (abst)
28. Campbell TJ: Resting and rate-dependent depression of maximum rate of depolarisation ($\dot{V}_{max}$) in guinea pig ventricular action potentials by mexiletine, disopyramide and encainide. J Cardiovasc Pharmacol **5:** 291, 1983
29. Nattel S, Zeng F-D: Frequency dependent effects of antiarrhythmic drugs on action potential duration and refractoriness. J Pharmacol Exp Ther **229:** 283, 1984
30. Ferrier GR, Saunders JH, Mendez C: A cellular mechanism for the generation of ventricular arrhythmias by acetylstrophanthidin. Circ Res **32:** 600, 1973
31. Grant AO, Strauss LJ, Wallace AG, Strauss H: The influence of pH on the electrophysiological effects of lidocaine in guinea pig ventricular myocardium. Circ Res **47:** 542, 1980
32. Grant AO, Trantham JL, Brown KK, Strauss H: pH-dependent effects of quinidine on the kinetics of dV/dt_{max} in the guinea pig ventricular myocardium. Circ Res **50:** 210, 1982

Delayed effects of early infarct-limiting therapies on healing after myocardial infarction

BODH I. JUGDUTT, M.B., CH.B., M.SC.

With the technical assistance of Marie Riesel and John Henriksen

ABSTRACT The effect of early infarct-limiting therapy on the hydroxypyroline (OHP, a marker of collagen) content and topography of 7-day-old infarcts was studied in 76 conscious dogs (69 ligated; seven sham operated). Two hours after their left anterior descending coronary arteries were occluded, 69 dogs were randomly assigned to receive 6 hr intravenous infusions of saline (controls; n = 29), low-dose nitroglycerin (NG; n = 13), prostacyclin (PGI_2; n = 14), or ibuprofen (IBU; n = 13). Regional OHP (mg/g dry weight) was measured by spectrophotometry, and size of infarction and topography were determined by computerized planimetry. Infarct size was less in the NG, PGI_2, and IBU groups compared with that in the saline group, both when measured as a percent of the arteriographic occluded bed ($p < .001$) and as a percent of the left ventricle ($p < .005$). For each treatment group (1) the level of OHP was higher ($p < .001$) in the region of infarction (saline group, 9.9 ± 0.7 mg/g; NG group, 14.9 ± 1.9 mg/g; PGI_2 group, 12.9 ± 0.9 mg/g; IBU group, 10.6 ± 1.4 mg/g) than in normal zones (4.4 ± 0.2 mg/g), with more ($p < .05$) OHP in border than center regions, and (2) the total OHP in the infarct zone was linearly related to size of infarction as a percent of the left ventricle (r = .89 to .94). However, the slopes of regressions for the NG, PGI_2, and IBU groups were greater ($p < .001$) than the slope for the saline group. Also, levels of OHP in the infarct zone were greater in the NG than in the saline group (14.9 ± 1.9 vs 9.9 ± 0.7 mg/g, $p < .02$). Thinning ratios (average infarct/normal wall thickness) were similar in the sham-operated (1.03 ± 0.02), no infarct (1.03 ± 0.03), saline (0.92 ± 0.02), NG (0.94 ± 0.02), and PGI_2 (0.96 ± 0.01) groups, and were greater ($p \leq .02$) than the ratio in the IBU group (0.80 ± 0.02). Expansion indexes (infarct/noninfarct containing endocardial segment) were similar in the sham-operated (1.02 ± 0.02), no infarct (1.01 ± 0.03), NG (1.07 ± 0.03), and PGI_2 (1.02 ± 0.01) groups and were less ($p < .05$) than those in the saline (1.20 ± 0.03) and IBU (1.26 ± 0.02) groups. Thus, early therapy with NG, PGI_2, or IBU reduced the size of infarction but did not reduce the amount of collagen in the area of infarction by 1 week. Instead, NG appeared to increase collagen content. More importantly, IBU produced more infarct thinning while NG and PGI_2 reduced infarct expansion by 1 week.
Circulation 72, No. 4, 907–914, 1985.

PROGNOSIS in survivors of myocardial infarction might be influenced not only by the size, but also by the collagen content and thickness of the infarct or scar. Although nitroglycerin (NG),[1,2] prostacyclin (PGI_2),[3] and ibuprofen (IBU)[4] therapy instituted in the early stages of infarction have been shown to reduce the size of experimental infarction, their effects on collagen content in the infarct zone and topography during the early phase of healing are not known. Infarct "expansion," or thinning, stretching, and dilatation of the infarct, is common in the first week after infarction and is associated with increased early mortality.[5-8] Early therapy with some anti-inflammatory agents has been shown to lead to thinner scars.[9-12] Specifically, both indomethacin[10] and IBU,[12] given at 15 min and 3 hr after coronary occlusion, cause marked thinning of 6-week-old infarcts in dogs, although indomethacin increases[13] while IBU reduces[4] the size of experimental infarction. More importantly, infarct thinning and expansion after early indometha-

From the Cardiology Division of the Department of Medicine and the Surgical and Medical Research Institute, University of Alberta, Edmonton, Alberta.

Supported in part by grants from the Medical Research Council of Canada. Dr. Jugdutt is recipient of a Senior Clinical Investigator Award from the Canadian Heart Foundation.

Address for correspondence: Dr. B. Jugdutt, 2C243 Walter MacKenzie Health Sciences Center, Division of Cardiology, University of Alberta, Edmonton, Alberta, T6G 2R7, Canada.

Received April 1, 1985; revision accepted June 6, 1985.

Presented in part at the Scientific Sessions of the 57th Annual Meeting of the American Heart Association in Miami Beach, November 1984.

cin therapy were also detected in 7-day-old infarcts.[11]

This study was undertaken to determine if NG, PGI_2, or IBU, given early after coronary occlusion to reduce size of infarction in conscious dogs, would also alter the collagen content and topography of 7-day-old infarcts.

Methods

Ninety-five mongrel dogs weighing 14 to 24 kg were instrumented while under general anesthesia (sodium pentobarbital, 25 to 35 mg/kg iv) through a left lateral thoracotomy, as described previously.[14] Briefly, a plastic occluder snare was placed around the left anterior descending coronary artery just distal to the first diagonal branch. Plastic catheters were placed in the external jugular vein, internal carotid artery, and left atrium. Distal ends of the catheters and snare were tunneled subcutaneously and exteriorized behind the neck. After surgery, penicillin (1 million units) and streptomycin (1 g) were given intramuscularly and the catheters were filled with heparinized saline.

Experiments were done 7 to 10 days later on 91 healthy surviving dogs. On the morning of each study, the dogs were made to stand in a sling for support. Left atrial and aortic pressures (Statham P23 Db) and lead II of the electrocardiogram were recorded continuously on a pen recorder (Gould). After 30 min of baseline recordings, a permanent coronary occlusion was created in each of 84 dogs by pulling the snare and clamping the plastic tube. Five minutes after occlusion, morphine (0.3 to 0.5 mg/kg iv) was given for analgesia and mild sedation, and lidocaine (1 mg/kg iv) was administered to suppress ventricular arrhythmias. Two hours after occlusion, 75 surviving dogs were randomly allocated to the control or one of the three treatment groups. Control dogs (group 1, n = 32) were given intravenous infusions of 200 ml of 0.9% saline over 6 hr. In group 2 (14 dogs), low-dose intravenous infusions of NG (commercially available Nitrostat IV, Parke-Davis) were titrated to reduce mean arterial pressure by 10%, but not below 80 mm Hg. In group 3 (15 dogs), low-dose intravenous infusions of PGI_2 (Upjohn Co.) were titrated as in group 2. In group 4 (14 dogs), low-dose (6.25 mg/kg per hr) intravenous IBU (Upjohn Co.) was given. This dose of IBU is similar to that previously shown to produce myocardial salvage.[4] Infusions in the therapy groups were given for 6 hr in 200 ml 0.9% saline with use of a Harvard pump. Average infusion rates (μg/kg/min) were as follows: NG, 10 (range 3 to 16); PGI_2, 0.5 (range 0.25 to 2.0); IBU, 105. Occlusions were not created in the seven other dogs, but they underwent sham operations and received morphine, lidocaine, and saline in group 1. No further morphine, lidocaine, or other drugs were given during the infusions.

Of the 75 treated dogs, six died between 2 hr and 6 days after occlusion (three from group 1, one from group 2, one from group 3, and one from group 4). At 7 days, hemodynamic recordings were repeated in the 76 surviving dogs (seven sham-operated dogs; 69 ligated and treated) before they were killed. The dogs were then anesthetized (30 mg/kg iv sodium pentobarbital) and their hearts were arrested in diastole with intravenous KCl. The hearts were removed, washed free of blood, and weighed.

Measurement of size of the occluded bed and infarction. Postmortem coronary arteriography was performed on the fresh hearts to define anatomic boundaries of the occluded bed, as described previously.[14] Briefly, simultaneous injections of a barium sulfate–gelatin mass were made under controlled pressure (160 mm Hg) via cannulas placed at the origins of the right, left circumflex, and anterior descending coronary arteries and distal to the ligation. No dyes were incorporated because they were found to interfere with the hydroxyproline (OHP) assays. Injected hearts were packed with gauze to preserve diastolic proportions, and fixed in 10% phosphate-buffered formalin for 48 hr. Hearts were then radiographed in two perpendicular planes. Five equally spaced transverse sections (1 to 1.5 cm thick) were then made from the level of the occlusion to the apex and section radiographs were made.[14] Boundaries of the occluded bed were marked on section radiographs, by consensus of two observers, at the "watersheds" between interdigitating terminal branches of occluded and unoccluded arteries.[14]

The left ventricular transverse sections were weighed after the right ventricle, fatty and valvular tissue, large epicardial vessels, and fibrous connections were removed. Outlines of the ventricular rings and infarcts were then made on plastic overlays and boundaries of the occluded bed were copied from marked section radiographs. The following were calculated by computerized planimetry (HP 9835A computer and HP 9874A digitizer): areas of ventricular rings and cavities; areas of infarct, occluded bed, and noninfarcted myocardium; thicknesses of infarct and ventricular ring along radials at 5 degree angular intervals (figure 1); endocardial lengths of infarcted and noninfarcted segments; circumferences of the rings and infarct; and mass of the infarct and occluded bed for each ring by relating the average areas (top and bottom surfaces) to the weight of the ring.[14] Total infarct and occluded bed masses were then computed for each heart by summing values for each ring. The "thin-

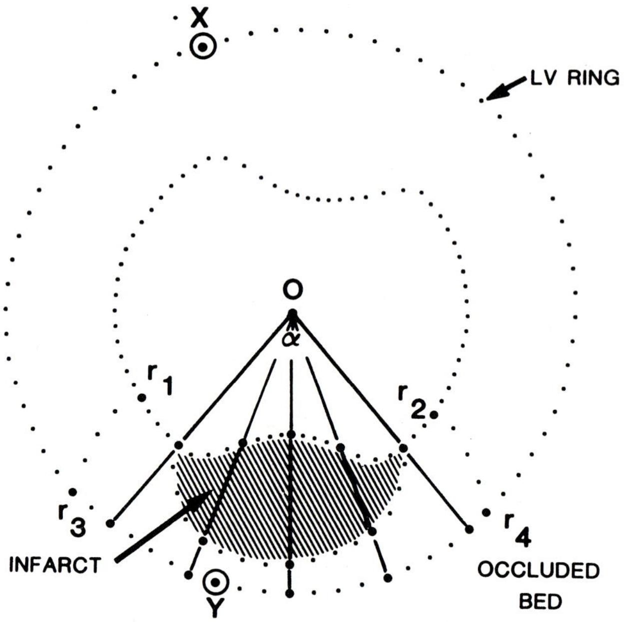

FIGURE 1. Map of the infarct, occluded bed, and left ventricular (LV) section generated by computerized planimetry. Points along inner and outer contours are at 5 degree intervals. The center 0 of the inner contour represents the computed zero moment of inner perimeter. Radii were constructed at intersections of the inner contour with the infarct and extended to the outer contour so that measurements could be made of the angular extent of the infarct (α) and distances along selected radii (α/4 apart) and along circumferences between appropriate pairs of points in the wall (large dots). Between the extreme radials, the average infarct wall thickness was computed. The average normal wall thickness was computed from similar measurements between radials mirrored on the opposite normal wall. Intersections of the boundaries of the occluded bed with the inner and outer contours (r_1-r_4) and the right ventricle with the outer LV contour (X,Y) were also recorded.

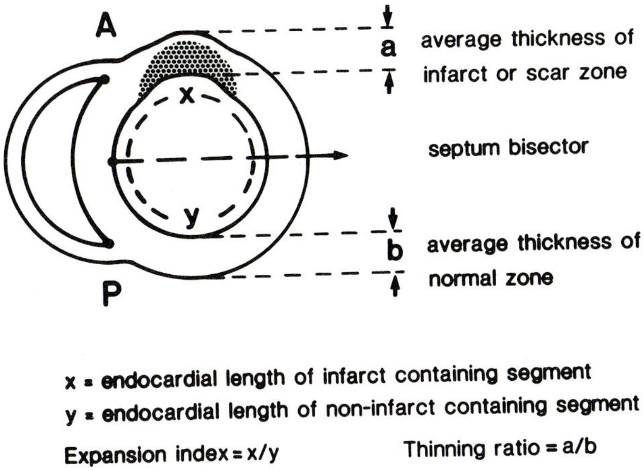

FIGURE 2. Method of calculating expansion index and thinning ratio. A midventricular section with an anterior infarct (stippled area). A line was drawn from the midpoint of the septum between anterior (A) and posterior (P) junctions with the right ventricle, perpendicular to the line through A and P, to meet the free wall. The expansion index was expressed as the ratio of anterior and posterior inner segment lengths (x/y). The thinning ratio was calculated as the ratio of the average infarct to noninfarct wall thickness (a/b).

ning ratio" and "expansion index" were calculated as shown in figure 2, by a modification of the method of Eaton and Bulkley.[7] Similar measurements (except for infarct size, which was absent) were made on hearts from the sham-operated and no-infarct groups.

Determination of total and regional OHP content. Transmural myocardial tissue samples were taken from the central zone of the infarct or occluded bed and center of the nonoccluded bed. Samples were obtained in duplicate from two consecutive transverse rings in the midventricular region between the occlusion site and left ventricular apex. The first set of samples was used for assay of OHP content in the total area of infarction (figure 3, *A*). In the second set, the infarct was cut into center, margin, and border regions (figure 3, *B*). All samples were weighed (50 to 200 mg), freeze-dried to constant dry weight (for 12 hr), reweighed, and hydrolyzed in 6N HCl at 125° C for 3 hr and at 200 psi pressure in an autoclave. Instead of being subjected to neutralization and decoloration, 1 ml aliquots of the acid hydrolysate were evaporated, washed with 1 ml water, and redried in the tubes, as described by Bergman and Loxley.[15] OHP content was measured on a spectrophotometer (Unican SP-1800) by the method of Neuman and Logan[16] as modified by Martin and Axelrod,[17] and expressed in milligrams per gram dry tissue weight.

Histology. Slices from transverse sections through the middle region of the infarcts corresponding to the midventricular ring were used for histologic analysis. Slices were dehydrated, cleared, embedded, cut into 5 μm sections, and mounted on 6 × 4 cm or larger slides. Triplicate sections were stained with hematoxylin-eosin, Mallory's stain, and Masson's trichrome, respectively. Special slides of whole ventricular sections were made for projection, morphometric analysis, and planimetry (40 infarcted hearts). Histologic features of necrosis and healing were graded semiquantitatively (0 = absent; 4 = most marked) as described previously by others.[11, 18, 19]

Statistics. Data at different steps of collection were coded, except for presence or absence of infarction, on outlines for planimetry. The following statistical methods were used: (1) analysis of variance (ANOVA) for significance of differences within and among groups, with Tukey's test for multiple comparisons, (2) linear regression analysis by the least square fit method, and the significance of r values and slopes by ANOVA, (3) 2 × 4 chi-squared test (with ANOVA) to assess the significance of differences in event frequency among treatment groups, and (4) repeated-measures ANOVA for hemodynamic changes. Results are given as mean ± SEM. Statistical significance was assumed at the .05 level.

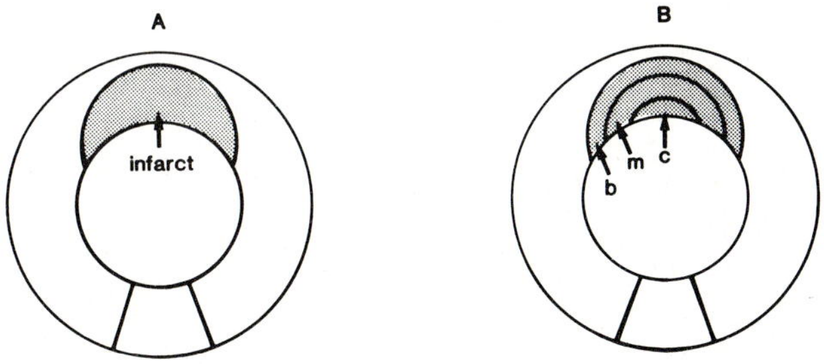

FIGURE 3. Methods of sampling for OHP. *A*, Entire infarct (stippled area) and transmural normal wall samples were taken. *B*, The samples were cut into border (b), margin (m), and center (c) regions.

Results

Of the 84 dogs that were subjected to occlusion of the left anterior descending coronary artery, nine died during the first 2 hr (10%), six died after randomization (three in the saline group [group 1], one in the NG group [group 2], one in the PGI_2 group [group 3], and one in the IBU group [group 4]) between 2 hr and 6 days (7%) after occlusion, and 69 survived 7 days. In all dogs with occlusions, autopsy and postmortem coronary arteriographic examination confirmed complete coronary occlusion, and electrocardiograms showed ST segment elevation in leads I, aVL, and V_4 after occlusion. All seven sham-operated dogs survived the 7 days and had normal electrocardiograms and arteriograms. Results for the 69 dogs with occlusions and the seven sham-operated dogs that were killed at 7 days are presented. Among the four treatment groups the incidence of Q waves (>0.03 sec or 0.2 mV) was similar (20/29 vs 5/13 vs 6/14 vs 5/13), as were the Lown scores for arrhythmia (1.4 vs 0.8 vs 0.9 vs 0.9).

Hemodynamics (table 1). Before occlusion, heart rate, mean arterial pressure, and mean left atrial pressure in all dogs were similar. In all groups, over the first 2 hr after coronary occlusion heart rate (84 ± 1 vs 103 ± 1 beats/min) and mean left atrial pressure (6.9 ± 0.2 vs 13.8 ± 0.5 mm Hg) increased ($p < .001$), but mean arterial pressure did not change (106 ± 1 vs 104 ± 1 mm Hg). In groups 1 and 4, these changes were maintained over the next 6 hr. In groups 2 and 3, decreases ($p < .001$) in the mean arterial pressure averaged 10% and 9%, respectively, and were maintained over the 6 hr infusion. Sustained decreases ($p < .001$) in mean left atrial pressure were also produced during the infusion of NG and PGI_2. At 7 days, there were no differ-

TABLE 1
Hemodynamics in the treatment groups (mean ± SEM)

Group	Timing	Heart rate (beats/min)	Mean arterial pressure (mm/Hg)	Mean left atrial pressure (mm/Hg)
1 (n = 29)	Before occlusion	86±2	107±2	6.6±0.2
	After occlusion			
	First 2 hr	103±2[A]	104±2	14.1±0.7[A]
	Next 6 hr	98±3	101±3	15.2±0.8
2 (n = 13)	Before occlusion	79±3	107±2	7.3±0.5
	After occlusion			
	First 2 hr	103±3[A]	105±2[B]	15.3±1.2[A,B]
	Next 6 hr	100±4	95±2	5.5±0.8
3 (n = 14)	Before occlusion	88±3	108±2	6.4±0.4
	After occlusion			
	First 2 hr	103±3[A]	106±2[B]	13.5±1.1[A,B]
	Next 6 hr	100±3	96±2	7.5±0.4
4 (n = 13)	Before occlusion	78±3	104±2	7.6±0.4
	After occlusion			
	First 2 hr	100±4[A]	101±2	12.9±0.4[A]
	Next 6 hr	102±3	99±3	11.9±0.4

[A]$p < .001$, significance of difference between average value over first 2 hr after occlusion and the preocclusion value.
[B]$p < .001$, significance of difference between average values over the first 2 hr and those over the next 6 hr after occlusion.

ences in resting arterial pressure or heart rate among the four groups, although left atrial pressure remained lower in therapy groups compared with that in the control dogs.

Size of infarction. Data on size of infarction in the 69 dogs with occlusions are summarized in figure 4. Infarct size in groups 2, 3, and 4 was less than in group 1, both when expressed as a percent of the occluded bed ($p < .001$) and as a percent of the left ventricle ($p < .05$). As noted previously, occlusions at a constant anatomic location result in a wide range of sizes of infarcts and occluded beds,[1-4, 13, 14] but there was no difference in mean occluded bed mass or left ventricular mass among the four groups. Size of the occluded bed as a percent of the left ventricle in the four groups was as follows: 31.4 ± 2.7% in group 1, 33.6 ± 3.0% in group 2, 33.1 ± 2.7% in group 3, and 37.1 ± 3.2% in group 4. Also, in each of the four groups, infarct size (as a percent of the left ventricle) was linearly related to the size of the occluded bed (as percent of left ventricle) and 14 dogs with small occluded beds (<20% of left ventricle) had no infarcts (four in group 1, four in group 2, four in group 3, and two in group 4). As has been reported previously,[1-4] the slope of the linear regression in the saline group was greater ($p < .05$) than that in the NG, PGI_2, and IBU groups. The regression equation for group 1 was $y = 0.84x - 4.08$; $r = .93$, $p < .01$, and that for the therapy groups 2, 3, and 4 combined was $y = 0.16x - 0.96$; $r = .66$, $p < .05$. There were no infarcts in the seven sham-operated dogs.

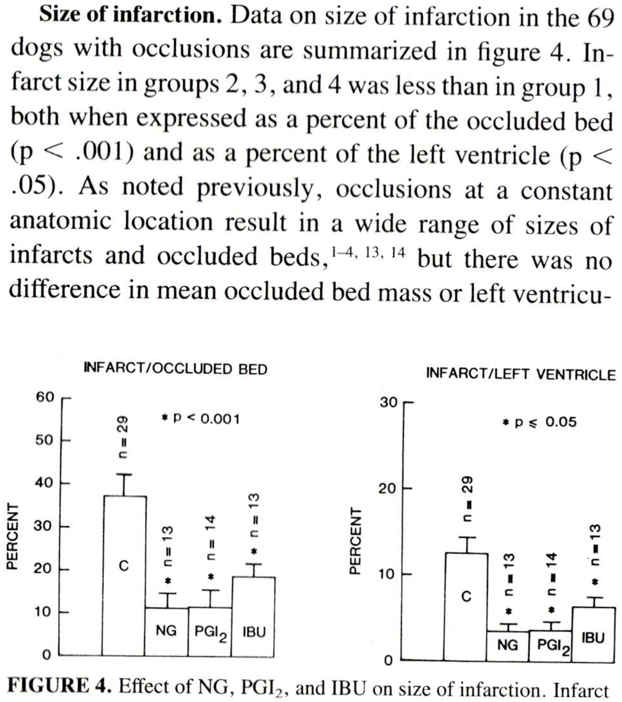

FIGURE 4. Effect of NG, PGI_2, and IBU on size of infarction. Infarct size, both as a percent of the occluded bed (*$p < .001$; *left*) and of the left ventricle (*$p < .05$; *right*), in dogs given NG, PGI_2, and IBU is compared with that in saline controls (C).

Concentrations of OHP. OHP data from hearts of dogs with infarcts in the four treatment groups and from hearts of dogs without infarcts and those that were sham operated are summarized in figure 5. OHP content in central zones of the occluded and nonoccluded beds in hearts without infarcts (5.5 ± 0.4 vs 4.4 ± 0.2 mg/g) and hearts from sham-operated dogs (4.4 ± 0.3 vs 4.4 ± 0.3 mg/g) were similar. However, OHP content in the infarct zone was greater ($p < .001$) than in the corresponding normal zone for each treatment group: 9.9 ± 0.7 vs 4.4 ± 0.2 mg/g in group 1, 14.9 ± 1.9 vs 5.2 ± 0.3 mg/g in group 2, 12.9 ± 0.9 vs 5.3 ± 0.6 mg/g in group 3, and 10.6 ± 1.4 vs 4.2 ± 0.2 mg/g in group 4. Interestingly, OHP content in the infarct zone was higher in group 2 than in group 1 (14.9 ± 1.9 vs 9.9 ± 0.7 mg/g, $p < .02$). Although there was a similar qualitative trend in this value in groups 3 and 4 compared with group 1, these differences were not statistically significant.

Regional differences in OHP content in the infarct zone for the four treatment groups are listed in table 2. A gradient was found, with more ($p < .05$) OHP in the outer border than in inner center regions. Again, more OHP was present in most of the infarct regions in dogs in groups 2 to 4 than in these regions in group 1 dogs. These differences might be a reflection of more rapid collagen deposition in infarcts of dogs in the therapy groups than in those of control dogs.

OHP in the total infarct zone (infarct zone OHP in mg/g multiplied by infarct mass in grams for each left ventricle) was linearly related to the size of infarction (as a percent of left ventricle) in all four treatment groups (table 3). The slopes of linear regression were greater ($p < .001$) for groups 2 (10.81 ± 0.59), 3

TABLE 2

OHP content in the region of infarction (mg/g dry weight) after the various treatments (mean ± SEM)

Group	Infarct center	Infarct margin	Infarct border	Normal zone
1 (n = 25)	6.1±0.3	8.7±0.5	10.8±0.7[A]	4.4±0.2
2 (n = 9)	9.1±0.9[B]	11.3±1.1[C]	15.1±1.9[A,C]	5.2±0.3
3 (n = 10)	8.5±0.6[B]	11.0±0.6[C]	13.2±0.9[A]	5.3±0.6
4 (n = 11)	7.7±0.7[C]	10.7±1.3	11.8±1.5[A]	4.2±0.2

[A]p < .05, significance of difference between infarct border and other infarct regions within a group.

[B]p < .001; [C]p < .02, significance of differences between corresponding regions in the therapy groups and those in the saline group.

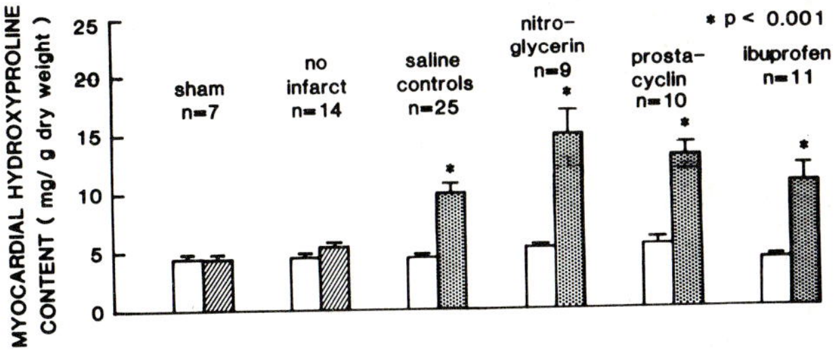

FIGURE 5. Effect of NG, PGI_2, and IBU on myocardial OHP content. *p < .001, for comparison of OHP content in the infarct zones (stippled bars) and with that in corresponding normal center zones of the nonoccluded bed (clear bars), as shown in figure 3, *A*. Hatched bars = normal center zone of the occluded bed in hearts from dogs in sham-operated and no infarct groups.

(6.68 ± 0.26), and 4 (7.00 ± 0.36) and all therapy groups combined (6.83 ± 0.13) than for the control group (4.04 ± 0.09), suggesting greater collagen deposition relative to infarct size in all therapy groups. Similar correlations were found between OHP in the infarct zone (mg/g dry weight) and infarct area (cm^2) for the midventricular ring in each treatment group.

Topographic changes. The main topographic measurements made of midventricular sections in the 76 hearts are summarized in figure 6. The infarcts were predominantly subendocardial, with maximal transmural extent (as percent full wall thickness in rings with the largest infarcts) being greater ($p < .05$) in group 1 than in the treatment groups (80% vs 54% vs 61% vs 69%, respectively). Transmural extent of infarction was not different among therapy groups. Infarct areas (as a percent of the left ventricle) were also greater ($p < .05$) in control dogs than in those receiving treatment, but were similar among therapy groups. However, the thinning ratio (figure 6, *A*) for the group 4 dogs (0.80 ± 0.02) was less ($p < .001$) than in dogs in the sham-operated (1.03 ± 0.03) or the no-infarct group (1.03 ± 0.03), and less ($p < .02$) than in groups 1 (0.92 ± 0.02), 2 (0.94 ± 0.02), or 3 (0.96 ± 0.01).

Also, the expansion index (figure 6, *B*) for group 4 (1.26 ± 0.02) was similar to that in group 1 (1.20 ± 0.03), but greater than that in group 2 (1.07 ± 0.03) or 3 (1.02 ± 0.01), or the sham-operated (1.02 ± 0.02) or no-infarct (1.01 ± 0.03) group. In addition, the left ventricular cavity area and endocardial circumference in groups 4 and 1 were similar and were greater ($p < .05$) than those in groups 2 and 3 and in the sham-operated and no-infarct groups.

There were no statistically significant correlations for infarcted hearts in the four treatment groups between (1) the thinning ratio and collagen content ($r < -.40$) or infarct size ($r < .30$), (2) the expansion index

TABLE 3

Linear regressions between OHP in the total infarct zone and infarct size[A]

Group	n	Equation	Correlation	SEE
1	25	y = 4.04x − 6.47	r = .89, p < .001	20.87
2	9	y = 10.83x + 1.30	r = .92, p < .001	14.84
3	10	y = 6.68x + 15.20	r = .94, p < .001	10.19
4	11	y = 7.00x + 2.66	r = .89, p < .001	22.35
Groups 2, 3, 4	30	y = 6.83x + 12.55	r = .87, p < .001	18.35
All groups (1 to 4)	55	y = 3.52x + 18.31	r = .73, p < .001	27.97

[A]As a percent of the left ventricle.

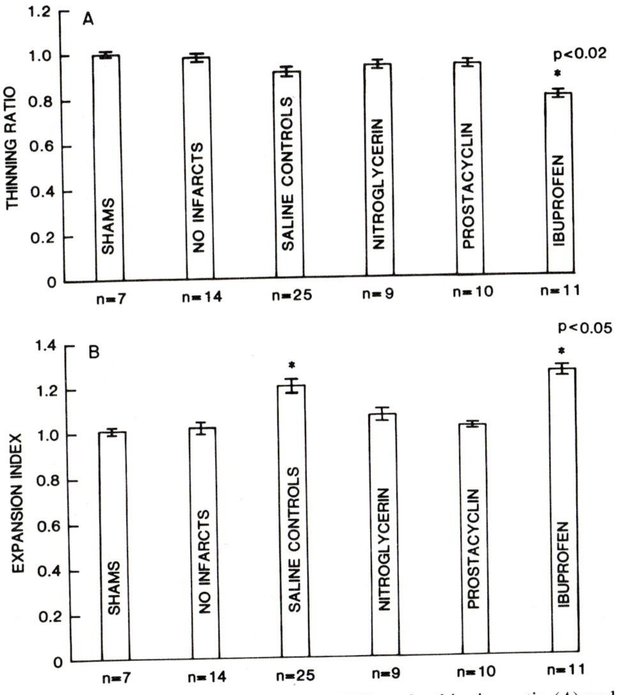

FIGURE 6. Effect of NG, PGI_2, and IBU on the thinning ratio (*A*) and expansion index (*B*). *p < .02 for IBU vs other groups (*A*); *p < .05, for IBU and saline control vs other groups (*B*).

and collagen content (r < .60) or infarct size (r < .56), and (3) the expansion index and thinning ratio (r < −.54).

Histology. Previously reported features of necrosis[18, 19] were observed in the hearts with 7-day-old infarcts. Coagulation necrosis predominated in central regions and fibroblastic and collagenous proliferation were seen at the subepicardial and lateral borders of necrotic muscle. Pigmented mononuclears, phagocytes, macrophages, and capillary neovascularization were prominent. Planimetered visual and histologic values for necrosis were in agreement (visual = 0.96 histologic + 5.7; r = .95, n = 40, p < .001). No differences were found in necrosis, hemorrhage, vascular proliferation, fibroblasts, or collagen content among infarcts in hearts from dogs in the four treatment groups, but there was slightly less (p = .1) edema, neutrophils, and macrophages in the group 4 hearts.

Discussion

In this study, therapy with low-dose NG, PGI_2, or IBU between 2 and 8 hr after occlusion of the left anterior descending coronary artery reduced the size of 7-day-old infarcts in conscious dogs. Compared with saline, the therapies decreased infarct size by more than 50% of the occluded bed (NG 70%, PGI_2 70%, IBU 51%). This is in agreement with previous reports,[1–4] although in those studies, drugs were given (1) over the first 6 hr after left circumflex occlusion and infarcts measured at 2 days,[1, 3, 4] or (2) between 2 and 6 hr after occlusion and size of infarction was measured at 7 days.[2] The early hemodynamic changes during drug treatment in this study were similar to those reported previously.[1–4]

There were two important new findings. First, none of the early infarct-limiting therapies impaired collagen deposition and, in fact, NG increased collagen content in the area of infarction. Thus, in each treatment group (1) OHP content was greater in infarct than normal regions, (2) OHP levels in the infarct zone were directly related to size of infarction, and (3) there was a gradient in OHP level, with a higher content at the infarct border than center. This latter finding is in agreement with the histologic observation, in this study and others,[18, 19] that fibroblast proliferation and collagen deposition proceeds inwards from epicardial and lateral borders of the infarct. Also, the smaller infarcts in the NG group contained more OHP than did those in the saline controls. Although regional data revealed that, compared with that in control hearts, there was more OHP in infarct centers of hearts from all three therapy groups, in the infarct margins of hearts in groups 2 and 3, and in the infarct border of the hearts from group 2, and that the slope of the relationship between OHP content in the region of the infarct and infarct size was steeper for each therapy group, the average OHP content in groups 3 and four was not greater than that in the control group. The fact that significant but different linear correlations between OHP content in the infarct zone and infarct size were found for each treatment group and all groups combined suggests that the greater collagen content in group 2 was not merely a reflection of reduced infarct size.

Second, infarct topography differed among therapy groups. Thus, IBU caused more infarct thinning while NG and PGI_2 reduced infarct expansion. The thinning ratio with IBU was 13% less than with saline, 15% less than that with NG, 17% less than that with PGI_2, and 22% less than that in animals in sham-operated and no infarct groups. Also, the percent increase in expansion index, compared with that in animals undergoing a sham operation or without infarcts, was 24% with IBU, 18% with saline, 5% with NG, and zero with PGI_2.

The main mechanisms for myocardial salvage with low-dose NG, PGI_2, and IBU have been reviewed.[1–4, 20, 21] Briefly, both NG[1, 2] and PGI_2[3] reduce preload and afterload and increase collateral blood flow,[1–3] so that salvage could be attributed to reduced myocardial oxygen demands and increased nutrient supply. Other explanations include (1) NG-mediated release of another vasoactive compound such as prostaglandin E[22] or PGI_2,[23] (2) relief of coronary spasm and a direct action on collaterals by the two drugs, (3) cellular and metabolic effects of PGI_2, such as inhibition of platelet aggregation, disaggregation of clumped platelets, and stabilization of lysosomes in cardiac cells and possibly phagocytic cells.[3, 20, 24] Exogenous PGI_2 might also be beneficial because of reduced synthesis of the endogenous form in damaged endothelium of ischemic regions.[24] In contrast, myocardial salvage with IBU is not associated with altered myocardial oxygen demands or collateral blood flow,[4] suggesting that anti-inflammatory, cellular, and metabolic effects might be important.[21, 25–30] Thus, IBU in low doses, as used clinically, is known to produce weak inhibition of prostaglandin synthesis,[25] to prevent platelet aggregation by inhibiting thromboxane synthesis,[26, 27] to inhibit leukocyte migration[28] and stabilize lysosomal membranes,[29] and to inhibit the ability of stimulated granulocytes to aggregate, generate radical oxygen, or damage the endothelial wall.[30]

The effects of NG and PGI_2 on healing have not been previously studied. It is not known whether the reduced preload and afterload between 2 and 8 hr after occlusion with these two agents contributed to the reduced infarct expansion seen in this study. Since the half-lives of all three agents are short, it is unlikely that the effects observed at 7 days were due to their continued presence after the infusions were stopped. The resting hemodynamics at 7 days suggests that preload might have been persistently lower in all three therapy groups compared with in control dogs, with no difference among the therapy groups. Thus, the delayed effects seen at 7 days were probably due to other differences in the early actions of the drugs. Although early IBU therapy (low dose of 12.5 mg/kg iv, at 15 min and 3 hr) has been reported to cause thinner scars at 6 weeks in dogs,[12] the effect at 1 week was not studied. Also, late IBU therapy (12.5 mg/kg iv every 12 hr, beginning 6 hr after infarction) increased infarct collagen in rats.[31] In this study, only early NG produced a quantitatively significant increase in collagen content in the region of infarction. The possibility that NG could have resulted in persistently open collaterals, thus increasing nutrient influx and causing more rapid collagen deposition, seems unlikely because PGI_2, also a potent coronary vasodilator, would be expected to have a similar effect. Whether NG might have stimulated early collagen synthesis is not known. The effect of the increased collagen content on the mechanical strength of the scar and expansion and thinning is not clear since both NG and PGI_2 reduced expansion. The greater thinning with IBU could have been entirely due to its early anti-inflammatory effects,[4, 21, 28] resulting in less edema and cellular infiltration. Although the larger and more transmural infarcts in control dogs might be expected to expand,[7] expansion of the smaller infarcts in the IBU group is less easily explained unless it is assumed that IBU-induced thinning weakened the infarcts. However, no significant correlations were found among thinning or expansion and collagen content or size of infarction, or between expansion and thinning, suggesting that the relationship among these parameters is complex.

In conclusion, the results suggest that although early therapy with all three drugs reduced size of infarction, IBU produced marked infarct thinning and expansion similar to that in control dogs. NG and PGI_2 did not have this deleterious effect on healing and both reduced infarct expansion. NG also increased infarct collagen. Delayed effects of some early infarct-limiting therapies can thus negate their beneficial effects on size of infarction. The effects of infarct-limiting pharmacologic therapies on healing should therefore be studied before they are applied in man.

I am indebted to Catherine Jugdutt for secretarial assistance and Christine Scott for typing, Moira McCubbin for hydroxyproline assays, Christine Wortman, B.Sc., and Gordon Blinston, Ph.D., for statistics and computing, medical students Brian Hayden and Ralph Sinn for assistance during the summer of 1981, and Roger Amy, M.D. (Department of Pathology) for histopathology.

References

1. Jugdutt BI, Becker LC, Hutchins GM, Bulkley BH, Reid PR, Kallman CH: Effect of intravenous nitroglycerin on collateral blood flow and infarct size in the conscious dog. Circulation **63:** 17, 1981
2. Jugdutt BI: Myocardial salvage by intravenous nitroglycerin in conscious dogs: loss of beneficial effect with marked nitroglycerin-induced hypotension. Circulation **68:** 673, 1983
3. Jugdutt BI, Hutchins GM, Bulkley BH, Becker LC: Dissimilar effects of prostacyclin, prostaglandin E_1 and prostaglandin E_2 on myocardial infarct size after coronary occlusion in conscious dogs. Circ Res **49:** 685, 1981
4. Jugdutt BI, Hutchins GM, Bulkley BH, Becker LC: Salvage of ischemic myocardium by ibuprofen during infarction in the conscious dog. Am J Cardiol **46:** 74, 1980
5. Hutchins GM, Bulkley BH: Infarct expansion versus extension: two different complications of acute myocardial infarction. Am J Cardiol **41:** 1127, 1978
6. Eaton LW, Weiss JL, Bulkley BH, Garrison JB, Weisfeldt ML: Regional cardiac dilatation after acute myocardial infarction. Recognition by two-dimensional echocardiography. N Engl J Med **300:** 57, 1979
7. Eaton LW, Bulkley BH: Expansion of acute myocardial infarction: its relationship to infarct morphology in a canine model. Circ Res **49:** 80, 1981
8. Hochman JC, Bulkley BH: Pathogenesis of left ventricular aneurysms: an experimental study in the rat model. Am J Cardiol **50:** 83, 1982
9. Hammerman H, Kloner RA, Hale S, Schoen FJ, Braunwald E: Dose-dependent effects of short-term methylprednisolone on myocardial infarct extent, scar formation, and ventricular function. Circulation **68:** 446, 1983
10. Hammerman H, Kloner RA, Schoen FJ, Brown EJ Jr, Hale S, Braunwald E: Indomethacin-induced scar thinning following experimental myocardial infarction. Circulation **67:** 1290, 1983
11. Hammerman H, Schoen FJ, Braunwald E, Kloner RA: Drug-induced expansion of the infarct: morphologic and functional correlations. Circulation **69:** 611, 1984
12. Brown EJ, Kloner RA, Schoen FJ, Hammerman H, Hale S, Braunwald E: Scar thinning due to ibuprofen administration following experimental myocardial infarction. Am J Cardiol **51:** 877, 1983
13. Jugdutt BI, Hutchins GM, Bulkley BH, Pitt B, Becker LC: Effect of indomethacin on collateral blood flow and infarct size in the conscious dog. Circulation **59:** 734, 1979
14. Jugdutt BI, Hutchins GM, Bulkley BH, Becker LC: Myocardial infarction in the conscious dog: three-dimensional mapping of infarct, collateral flow and region at risk. Circulation **60:** 1141, 1979
15. Bergman I, Loxley R: Two improved and simplified methods for the spectrophotometric determination of hydroxyproline. Anal Chem **35:** 1961, 1963
16. Neuman RF, Logan MA: The determination of hydroxyproline. J Biol Chem **184:** 299, 1950
17. Martin CJ, Axelrod AE: A modified method for the determination of hydroxyproline. Proc Soc Exp Biol Med **83:** 461, 1953
18. Mallory GK, White PD, Salcedo-Salgar J: The speed of healing of myocardial infarction: a study of the pathologic anatomy in seventy-two cases. Am Heart J **18:** 647, 1939
19. Fishbein MC, Maclean D, Maroko PR: The histopathologic evolution of myocardial infarction. Chest **73:** 843, 1978
20. Jugdutt BI. Prostaglandins in myocardial infarction: with emphasis

on myocardial preservation. Prostaglandins and Medicine **7:** 109, 1981
21. Jugdutt BI, Becker LC: Prostaglandin inhibition and myocardial infarct size. Clin Cardiol **4:** 117, 1981
22. Morcillio E, Reid PR, Dubin N, Chodgaonkar R, Pitt B: Myocardial prostaglandin E release by nitroglycerin and modification by indomethacin. Am J Cardiol **45:** 53, 1980
23. Levin RI, Jaffe EA, Weksler BB, Tack-Goldman K: Nitroglycerin stimulates synthesis of prostacyclin by cultured human endothelial cells. J Clin Invest **67:** 762, 1981
24. Needleman P, Kaley B: Cardiac and coronary prostaglandin synthesis and function. N Engl J Med **298:** 1122, 1978
25. Davies EF, Avery GS: Ibuprofen: a review of its pharmacological properties and therapeutic efficacy in rheumatic disorders. Drugs **2:** 416, 1971
26. Packham MA, Mustard JF: Clinical pharmacology of platelets. Blood **50:** 555, 1977
27. Majerus PW: Why aspirin? Circulation **54:** 357, 1976
28. Brown KA, Collins AJ: Action of non-steroidal, anti-inflammatory drugs on human and rat peripheral leukocyte migration in vitro. Ann Rheum Dis **36:** 239, 1977
29. Lefer AM, Polansky E: Beneficial effects of ibuprofen in acute myocardial ischemia. Cardiology **64:** 265, 1979
30. Hammerschmidt DE, Flynn PJ, Vercellotti GM, Coppo PA, Jacob HS: Synergy among agents inhibiting granulocyte responses to activated complement: a rationale for new therapeutic strategies in shock and myocardial infarction. Clin Res **29:** 334A, 1981
31. Cannon RO, Speir E, Bolli R: Beneficial effects of ibuprofen on collagen after acute myocardial infarction. Circulation **64**(suppl IV): IV-138, 1981 (abst)

Enhancement of recovery of myocardial function by oxygen free–radical scavengers after reversible regional ischemia

MARY LEE MYERS, M.D., ROBERTO BOLLI, M.D., RAYMOND F. LEKICH, M.S., CRAIG J. HARTLEY, PH.D., AND ROBERT ROBERTS, M.D.

ABSTRACT Reperfusion after reversible regional ischemia has been shown to result in delayed recovery of myocardial function, but the mechanism responsible for this phenomenon remains unknown. We explored the potential role of oxygen-free radicals as mediators of postischemic dysfunction in open-chest dogs undergoing a 15 min occlusion of the left anterior descending coronary artery (LAD) followed by 2 hr of reperfusion. Treated animals (n = 19) received an infusion of the oxygen free–radical scavengers superoxide dismutase (SOD; 15,000 U/kg) and catalase (CAT; 55,000 U/kg) for 1 hr starting 15 min before LAD occlusion, while control animals (n = 20) received an equal volume of saline. SOD and CAT produced no discernible effect on heart rate, aortic pressure, or left atrial pressure. Collateral flow to the ischemic zone (radioactive microspheres) was 0.07 ± 0.01 ml/min/g in both groups. The size of the occluded bed as determined by postmortem perfusion was 26.1 ± 1.2% of the left ventricle in the control group and 26.5 ± 0.9% in the treated group. Systolic wall thickening (an index of regional function) was assessed with an epicardial pulsed-Doppler probe. The two groups exhibited comparable systolic thickening under baseline conditions and similar degrees of dyskinesia during ischemia. Nevertheless, recovery of function (expressed as percent of baseline) was considerably greater in the treated dogs, both at 1 hr (43.8 ± 14.3 vs 12.8 ± 11.6) and 2 hr of reperfusion (74.2 ± 8.4 vs 31.6 ± 9.8, $p < .005$). This improved recovery of function obtained with SOD and CAT suggests that oxygen-free radicals play an important role in the genesis of myocardial dysfunction after a brief episode of regional ischemia.
Circulation 72, No. 4, 915–921, 1985.

REPERFUSION after a brief period of experimental coronary artery occlusion results in delayed recovery of regional function despite the absence of myocardial cell necrosis.[1–4] The mechanism underlying this persistent but ultimately reversible dysfunction, or myocardial "stunning,"[5] remains unclear. There is, however, mounting evidence to implicate oxygen-free radicals as mediators of reperfusion injury in various organ systems, including the heart.[6] These byproducts of oxygen metabolism, which include the superoxide anion (O^-_2), hydrogen peroxide (H_2O_2), and the hydroxyl radical ($OH^\cdot$), are highly reactive substances capable of producing marked cellular damage. It has recently been shown that administration of the oxygen free–radical scavengers superoxide dismutase (SOD), a scavenger of the superoxide anion, and catalase (CAT), a scavenger of hydrogen peroxide, results in a significant decrease in infarct size in a canine preparation of 90 min of coronary artery occlusion.[7] Furthermore, free-radical scavengers have been reported to improve global ventricular function after prolonged hypothermic ischemic arrest.[8–10]

Results obtained in such preparations of irreversible ischemic injury, or prolonged global ischemia, cannot necessarily be extrapolated to the setting of a brief episode of regional ischemia. Thus, the role of oxygen-free radicals in the pathogenesis of postischemic dysfunction after transient coronary occlusion remains unknown. Accordingly, the present study was undertaken to determine whether the free-radical scavengers SOD and CAT could enhance recovery of function after reversible regional ischemia in open-chest dogs

From the Experimental Animal Laboratory, Section of Cardiology, Department of Medicine, Baylor College of Medicine, Houston.

Address for correspondence: M. L. Myers, M.D., 375 South St., Victoria Hospital, London, Ontario, Canada N6A 4G5.

Received April 1, 1985; revision accepted July 12, 1985.

This study was carried out during Dr. Myers' tenure as a Fellow of the Medical Research Council of Canada. The results were presented in part at the thirty-fourth meeting of the American College of Cardiology, Anaheim, CA, March, 1985.

undergoing 15 min of coronary artery occlusion followed by 2 hr of reperfusion. This duration of ischemia was selected because it is well established that it does not result in myocardial cell necrosis,[2-4, 11-13] but nevertheless does produce delayed recovery of function.[1-5]

Methods

Instrumentation. Mongrel dogs of both sexes weighing 15 to 29 kg were anesthetized with intravenous 30 mg/kg sodium pentobarbital, intubated, and ventilated with room air via a Harvard ventilator. Ventilatory parameters were adjusted on the basis of arterial blood gas determinations to maintain normal pH and satisfactory oxygenation. A polyethylene catheter was positioned in the aorta via the left common carotid artery. The left pleural cavity was entered through the fifth intercostal space and the pericardium was incised. A polyethylene catheter was placed in the left atrium, and a No. 8F Millar pressure transducer was introduced into the left ventricle via an apical stab wound. The left anterior descending coronary artery (LAD) was isolated and encircled with a snare at a site distal to the first major diagonal branch, so as to produce an ischemic zone encompassing approximately one-quarter of the left ventricle. A Doppler flow velocity probe was placed around the LAD distal to the snare. A Doppler ultrasonic wall thickening probe[14] was sutured to the epicardium overlying the portion of the left ventricle to be rendered ischemic, and a second probe was positioned on the posterior left ventricular wall to serve as a control. Aortic pressure, left ventricular pressure, left ventricular dP/dt, left atrial pressure, LAD blood flow velocity, myocardial thickening, and lead II of the electrocardiogram were recorded simultaneously on an eight-channel Gould-Brush recorder (200 series).

Protocol. After baseline recordings were obtained, animals received either 15,000 U/kg (SOD)* (purified from bovine erythrocytes; activity 3000 U/mg protein) plus 55,000 U/kg CAT* (purified from bovine liver; activity 11,000 Sigma units/mg protein) in normal saline, or an equal volume of saline alone. The infusion was administered directly into the left ventricle via the Millar catheter at 0.6 ml/min starting 15 min before coronary artery occlusion, and continued until 30 min after the onset of reperfusion. The LAD was occluded for 15 min and then reperfused. Restoration of flow was confirmed by noting the immediate reactive hyperemic response detected by the coronary flow velocity probe. No attempt was made to resuscitate animals that developed ventricular fibrillation during ischemia or reperfusion. Hemodynamic and wall thickening data were obtained during ischemia and after 30, 60, and 120 min of reperfusion. At the conclusion of the study, the animals were given heparin (6000 units) followed by a lethal dose of potassium chloride, and the hearts were excised.

Determination of size of the occluded bed. A postmortem dual perfusion technique was used to determine the size of the occluded coronary vascular bed. Cannulae were inserted into the LAD immediately proximal and distal to the site of coronary artery occlusion. The distal LAD bed was perfused with normal saline. The proximal LAD and circumflex arteries were perfused in a retrograde fashion with a 0.5% solution of monastral blue dye while the left coronary ostium was digitally occluded. The two vascular beds were perfused simultaneously for 2 min at equal physiologic pressure (100 mm Hg) to prevent flow across collateral channels. The heart was then cut into 1.0 cm slices in a plane parallel to the atrioventricular groove, and all atrial, valvular, and right ventricular tissue was excised. The slices were incubated in a 1% solution of triphenyl tetrazolium chloride (TTC) for 20 min at 38° C to verify the absence of irreversible injury. This agent stains only viable dehydrogenase-containing myocardium dark red.[15, 16] The portion of the left ventricle supplied by the previously occluded LAD (occluded coronary bed) was identified by the absence of blue dye, and separated from the rest of the left ventricle. Both components were weighed to determine occluded bed size as a percentage of the left ventricle.

Regional myocardial blood flow. Regional myocardial blood flow was determined by the radioactive microsphere technique[17] 10 min after LAD occlusion. Microspheres (15 $\pm$ 3 μm [mean $\pm$ SD] in diameter, Dupont Co.) were obtained as 1 mCi of nuclide suspended in 10 ml of 10% dextran containing Tween 80. After 2 min of vigorous mixing on a vortex agitator, approximately 2 million spheres were suspended in 3 ml of normal saline and injected into the left atrium over 10 sec, following which the catheter was flushed with an additional 10 ml of saline. Beginning 15 sec before and continuing for 2 min after injection, a reference blood sample was withdrawn from the aorta with a Harvard pump at a constant rate of 4.05 ml/min. After postmortem perfusion and TTC staining, four transmural samples (1.0 to 1.5 g) were obtained from both the occluded and nonoccluded beds. To avoid admixture of ischemic and nonischemic tissue, ischemic samples were obtained at least 1 cm inside the margin of the unstained region.[18] Each tissue sample was weighed, and all samples were subsequently counted for 5 min in a gamma counter. Regional myocardial blood flow was calculated by standard methods.[17]

Regional myocardial function. Regional myocardial function was assessed with a pulsed-Doppler epicardial wall thickening probe. Theoretical and experimental validation of this technique has been previously published.[14, 19] In brief, the pulsed-Doppler technique uses a single epicardial transducer to determine systolic myocardial wall displacement by digitally integrating the velocity of myocardial layers passing through the range-gated sample volume. A representative example of the wall thickening tracings obtained with this probe is illustrated in figure 1. The beginning and end of systole were determined from the onset of the upstroke of the left ventricular pressure tracing and peak negative dP/dt, respectively. Systolic thickening fraction was calculated by dividing net systolic thickening by end-diastolic wall thickness as determined by the range gate depth. Net systolic thickening was defined as the maximal systolic increase in wall thickness from the end-diastolic values.[20] When paradoxical wall thinning persisted for 50% or more of systole, the maximal extent of wall thinning was subtracted from wall thickening.[20] Thickening fraction determined by the Doppler method correlates closely with thickening fraction measured with two ultrasonic transit-time crystals.[14, 19] The use of the Doppler probe is advantageous, however, in that the single epicardial transducer eliminates the trauma of intramyocardial crystal insertion that occurs with the transit-time method.

Statistical analysis. All values are reported as mean $\pm$ SEM. Student's unpaired t test was used to compare mean values between control and treated animals, while the paired t test was used to analyze intragroup variation. A p value $< .05$ was considered indicative of statistical significance.

Results

Of the 51 dogs initially instrumented, one (treated group) died of ventricular fibrillation during ischemia, and nine died during reperfusion (four in the control group and five in the treated group). The protocol was discontinued in one dog from each group because coro-

*Sigma Chemical Company, St. Louis.

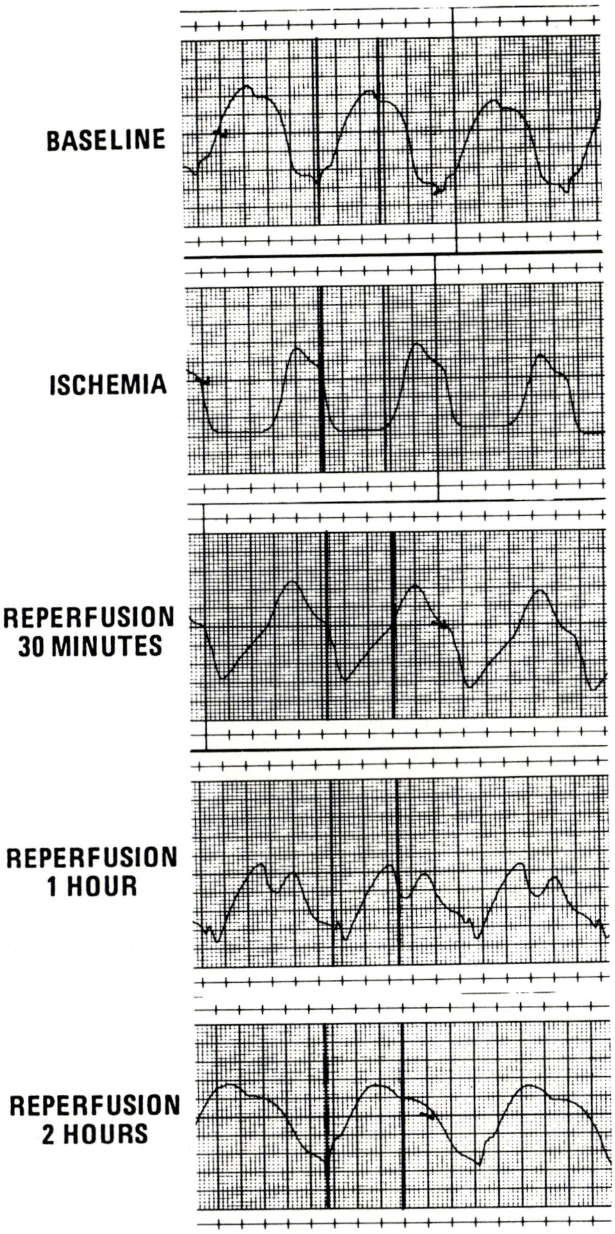

FIGURE 1. Representative wall thickening tracings from one animal. Vertical lines indicate the beginning and end of systole. Systolic wall thickening present under baseline conditions was replaced by paradoxical thinning (dyskinesia) during LAD occlusion. Dyskinesia persisted at 30 min of reperfusion, but active systolic thickening resumed by 1 hr of reperfusion.

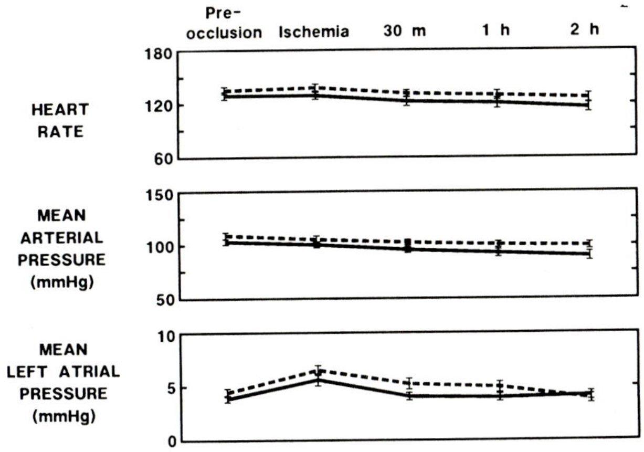

FIGURE 2. Heart rate, mean arterial pressure, and mean left atrial pressure in control (dashed line) and treated (continuous line) groups. There were no significant differences between treated and control groups throughout the study.

nary artery occlusion failed to produce dyskinesia. Analysis of data was thus carried out for 20 control dogs and 19 treated dogs. The presence of TTC staining confirmed the absence of irreversible injury in all animals.

Hemodynamic results are summarized in figure 2. There were no significant differences between the two groups with respect to preocclusion heart rate, mean arterial blood pressure, or mean left atrial pressure. Infusion of SOD and CAT did not appreciably affect these hemodynamic variables (table 1). During coronary occlusion, both groups exhibited a significant ($p < .0001$) increase in left atrial pressure and a significant ($p < .02$) decrease in arterial pressure, with no consistent change in heart rate. No significant hemodynamic differences developed between the groups throughout the course of the study.

The two groups were closely comparable with respect to both size of the occluded bed and coronary collateral blood flow (table 2). Occluded bed size was 26.1 ± 1.2% of the left ventricle (20.2 ± 0.9 g) in the control group and 26.5 ± 0.9% of the left ventricle (23.5 ± 1.4 g) in the treated group. Transmural ischemic zone blood flow was 0.07 ± 0.01 ml/min/g in both groups. Blood flow to the nonischemic zone was also similar: 1.16 ± .09 ml/min/g in control dogs and 0.99 ± 0.09 ml/min/g in the dogs given SOD plus CAT (NS).

Systolic thickening fraction in the control (nonischemic) region remained similar in the two groups throughout the study (table 3). Baseline systolic thickening fraction in the LAD-dependent territory was 32.8 ± 1.8% in the control group and 34.3 ± 1.8% in

TABLE 1
Systemic hemodynamics and regional myocardial function before and 10 min after administration of SOD + CAT

	Baseline	SOD + CAT
Mean arterial pressure (mm Hg)	103±3.4	103±2.8
Heart rate (beats/min)	135±4.4	129±4.2
Mean left atrial pressure (mm Hg)	3.5±0.33	3.8±0.31
Systolic thickening fraction (%) — LAD territory	34.3±1.8	35.2±1.8

Values are mean ± SEM.

TABLE 2
Size of the occluded bed and regional myocardial blood flow

	Occluded bed (g)	Left ventricle (g)	Occluded bed / Left ventricle (%)	Ischemic zone flow (ml/min/g)	Nonischemic zone flow (ml/min/g)
Control (n = 20)	20.2	76.6	26.1	0.07	1.16
	±0.9	±2.5	±1.2	±.01	±.09
SOD + CAT (n = 19)	23.5	86.9	26.5	0.07	0.99
	±1.4	±3.6	±0.9	±.01	±.09

Values are mean ± SEM.

the treated group (NS). There was no significant change in thickening fraction with infusion of SOD and CAT (table 1). The results of serial measurements of systolic thickening expressed as a percentage of baseline are displayed in figure 3. The two groups did not differ with respect to systolic thinning (dyskinesia) during ischemia. Nevertheless, there was improved recovery of function after reperfusion in the animals treated with SOD and CAT. Systolic thickening recovered to 43.8 ± 14.3% of baseline in treated animals vs only 12.8 ± 11.6% in controls after 1 hr of reperfusion ($p = .09$), with further improvement to 74.2 ± 8.4% of baseline in the treated group vs only 31.6 ± 9.8% in the control group after 2 hr of reperfusion ($p < .005$).

Discussion

This study demonstrates that the oxygen free–radical scavengers SOD and CAT significantly enhance recovery of myocardial function after reversible regional ischemia. Regional systolic function after 15 min of coronary artery occlusion and 2 hr of reperfusion recovered to 74% of baseline in the treated group as compared with only 31% in the control group ($p < .005$). SOD and CAT did not produce any hemodynamic changes that might account for this beneficial effect. Furthermore, the two groups were virtually identical with respect to collateral blood flow and size of the occluded bed. These findings provide evidence that toxic oxygen metabolites play an important role in the genesis of regional postischemic myocardial dysfunction. Other studies have suggested a role for oxygen-free radicals in the dysfunction that follows hypothermic global myocardial ischemia,[8–10] as well as in the cellular destruction associated with myocardial infarction.[7] No previous study, however, has implicated free radicals in the delayed recovery of function that occurs after a brief episode of regional ischemia unassociated with myocardial cell necrosis.

The phenomenon of myocardial stunning was first demonstrated by Heyndrickx et al.,[1] who noted persistent depression of regional function after 15 min of coronary artery occlusion and 3 hr of reperfusion. Using the same duration of ischemia, Kloner et al.[3] demonstrated functional recovery of only 12% after 90 min of reperfusion, with improvement to 58% at 3 days. In the present study, recovery of function in the control group was 13% of baseline at 1 hr, with improvement to 32% at 2 hr, and was thus somewhat greater, but nevertheless comparable to that observed by Kloner et al. Although the intramyocardial crystal insertion required in these previous experiments inevitably results in some tissue injury, this factor was virtually eliminated in the present study with the use of the single epicardial Doppler probe.

Despite considerable investigative effort, the cause of persistent dysfunction after a brief episode of ischemia remains unknown. Myocardial ATP concentration decreases rapidly after coronary artery occlusion,[4] and some studies have suggested a parallel between replenishment of ATP and recovery of myocardial

TABLE 3
Nonischemic zone systolic thickening fraction (%)

	Before occlusion	Ischemia	30 min	1 hr	2 hr
Control (n = 20)	23.4	23.7	22.3	22.0	19.6
	±1.3	±1.2	±1.0	±1.0	±0.8
SOD + CAT (n = 19)	24.7	24.6	22.6	23.4	21.9
	±1.7	±1.3	±1.8	±1.6	±1.5

Values are mean ± SEM.

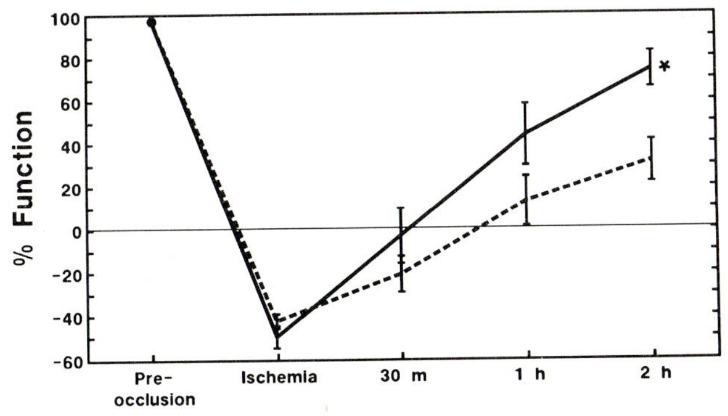

FIGURE 3. Recovery of regional function after 15 min of coronary artery occlusion in control (dashed line) and treated (continuous line) groups. Function is represented as a percentage of baseline systolic thickening fraction. *$p < .005$ vs control group. The p value relative to the 1 hr data was .09.

function.[3, 21] More recent investigations, however, have failed to substantiate this hypothesis.[22–24] Our results suggest an alternative mechanism that may contribute to myocardial stunning: the generation of cytotoxic oxygen-free radicals.

Oxygen-free radicals have been previously identified as mediators of cell injury in a wide range of pathologic processes,[25] including pulmonary oxygen toxicity,[26] radiation injury,[27] and various inflammatory conditions.[28] Increasingly, interest has focused on their role in the setting of ischemia and reperfusion, where injury has been convincingly linked to free-radical production in the small intestine,[29] kidney,[30] and central nervous system.[31] Recent investigations have also implicated oxygen-free radicals in myocardial postischemic injury. Jolly et al.[7] have demonstrated a significant reduction in the size of myocardial infarction with the administration of SOD and CAT in a canine preparation of 90 min of coronary artery occlusion followed by reperfusion. The administration of free-radical scavengers has produced improved recovery of global left ventricular function in isolated heart and cardiopulmonary bypass preparations of prolonged hypothermic global ischemia.[8–10] In addition, Burton[32] has recently reported that treatment with SOD significantly improves contractile performance in an isolated perfused septal preparation subjected to 1 hr of ischemia followed by reperfusion. Our data extend these observations to the dysfunction that occurs after brief regional myocardial ischemia in the intact, normothermic animal, and thus, for the first time, provide evidence that free radicals play a significant role in the setting of transient coronary occlusion.

Many physiologic processes are known to result in production of oxygen-free radicals[33, 34]: enzymatic reactions, electron transport processes within the mitochondria and endoplasmic reticulum, intracellular autoxidation of various compounds, arachidonic acid metabolism, and the activation of phagocytic cells. The source of oxygen-free radicals in tissues subjected to ischemia and reperfusion is not yet clear. Under normal conditions, approximately 2% of the oxygen metabolized within the mitochondria undergoes univalent reduction,[35] a process that results in the production of oxygen-free radicals.[36] Ischemia-induced mitochondrial dysfunction may result in increased utilization of this radical-generating pathway, particularly when the mitochondria are exposed to a sudden increase in oxygen concentration at the time of reperfusion.[37]

The activated neutrophil, which produces superoxide anion, hydrogen peroxide, and the hydroxyl radical,[28] constitutes a potential extracellular source of free radicals. Acute myocardial ischemia results in complement activation with production of C5a, a powerful chemotactic factor.[38] Compelling evidence to support the neutrophil as a mediator of postischemic damage is provided by a recent investigation in which antibody-induced neutrophil depletion resulted in a significant decrease in infarct size.[39] In addition, Rowe et al.[40] have demonstrated that activated leukocytes can disrupt canine sarcoplasmic reticulum calcium transport via an oxygen-free radical mechanism.

Another postulated source of free radicals is the enzyme xanthine oxidase, which, in the presence of oxygen, catalyzes the conversion of hypoxanthine to xanthine with simultaneous generation of superoxide.[41] While one substrate (hypoxanthine) accumulates during ischemia as a result of ATP degradation, the other (molecular oxygen) is provided by reperfusion, which could theoretically result in a burst of superoxide production. Evidence regarding the significance of this mechanism is contradictory. In preliminary reports by Akizuki et al.[42] and Werns et al.,[43] treatment with allopurinol, a xanthine oxidase inhibitor, was associated with a decrease in the size of myocardial infarction. A recent report by Reimer and Jennings,[44] however, showed no decrease in infarct size after administration of allopurinol in a preparation of 40 min of occlusion followed by reperfusion. Although xanthine oxidase appears to play a significant role in the pathogenesis of reperfusion injury in other organs,[41] the activity of this enzyme in the heart is relatively low.[45] It is difficult to reconcile these contrasting results. Nevertheless, the lack of beneficial effect observed by Reimer and Jennings is not in conflict with our findings, since the production of superoxide anion via xanthine oxidase is only one of several potential sources of oxygen-free radicals. Furthermore, we assessed contractile function in a preparation of reversible ischemia, in contrast to Reimer and Jennings, who assessed size of infarction in a preparation of irreversible myocardial cell injury.

Although extrapolation of experimental data to man must be done with caution, the results of this study may have therapeutic implications. There are numerous clinical settings of transient myocardial ischemia in which postischemic dysfunction may occur: unstable or variant angina, cardiac transplantation, open heart surgery with cardioplegic arrest, or acute myocardial infarction with early reperfusion (either spontaneous or induced with thrombolytic therapy). The presence of myocardial stunning in these situations may be associated with significant left ventricular dysfunction and its potential serious sequelae. Our results suggest that enhanced recovery of myocardial function under these varying clinical circumstances may be achieved with the elimination of toxic oxygen radicals.

The expert technical assistance of Terrence Edwards is gratefully acknowledged, as is the secretarial assistance of Lisa Gearinger in the preparation of the manuscript.

References

1. Heyndrickx GR, Millard RW, McRitchie RJ, Maroko PR, Vatner SF: Regional myocardial functional and electrophysiological alterations after brief coronary artery occlusion in conscious dogs. J Clin Invest **56:** 978, 1975
2. Heyndrickx GR, Baig H, Nellens P, Leusen I, Fishbein MC, Vatner SF: Depression of regional blood flow and wall thickening after brief coronary occlusions. Am J Physiol **234:** H653, 1978
3. Kloner RA, DeBoer LW, Darsee JR, Ingwall JS, Hale S, Tumas J, Braunwald E: Prolonged abnormalities of myocardium salvaged by reperfusion. Am J Physiol **241:** H591, 1981
4. Kloner RA, DeBoer LW, Darsee JR, Ingwall JS, Braunwald E: Recovery from prolonged abnormalities of canine myocardium salvaged from ischemic necrosis by coronary reperfusion. Proc Natl Acad Sci USA **78:** 7152, 1981
5. Braunwald E, Kloner RA: The stunned myocardium: prolonged, postischemic ventricular dysfunction. Circulation **66:** 6; 1146, 1982
6. Gardner TJ, Stewart JR, Casale AS, Downey JM, Chambers DE: Reduction of myocardial ischemic injury with oxygen-derived free radical scavengers. Surgery **94:** 423, 1983
7. Jolly S, Kane WJ, Bailie MB, Abrams GD, Lucchesi BR: Canine myocardial reperfusion injury: Its reduction by the combined administration of superoxide dismutase and catalase. Circ Res **54:** 277, 1984
8. Shlafer M, Kane PF, Wiggins VY, Kirsh MM: Possible role for cytotoxic oxygen metabolites in the pathogenesis of cardiac ischemic injury. Circulation **66**(suppl I): I-85, 1982
9. Stewart JR, Blackwell WH, Crute SL, Loughlin V, Greenfield LJ, Hess ML: Inhibition of surgically induced ischemia/reperfusion injury by oxygen free radical scavengers. J Thorac Cardiovasc Surg **86:** 262, 1983
10. Casale AS, Bulkley GB, Bulkley BH, Flaherty JT, Gott VL, Gardner TJ: Oxygen free-radical scavengers protect the arrested, globally ischemic heart upon reperfusion. Surg Forum **34:** 313, 1983
11. Tennant R, Grayzel DM, Sutherland FA, Stringer SW: Studies on experimental coronary occlusion. Chemical and anatomical changes in the myocardium after coronary ligation. Am Heart J **12:** 168, 1936
12. Jennings RB, Sommers HM, Smyth GA, Flack HA, Lim H: Myocardial necrosis induced by temporary occlusion of a coronary artery in the dog. Arch Pathol **70:** 68, 1960
13. Ahmed SA, Williamson JR, Roberts R, Clark RE, Sobel BE: The association of increased plasma MB CPK activity and irreversible ischemic myocardial injury in the dog. Circulation **54:** 187, 1976
14. Hartley CJ, Latson LA, Michael LH, Seidel CL, Lewis RM, Entman ML: Doppler measurement of myocardial thickening with a single epicardial transducer. Am J Physiol **245**(Heart Circ Physiol 14): H1066, 1983
15. Lie JT, Pairolero PC, Holley KE, Titus JL: Macroscopic enzyme-mapping verification of large, homogeneous, experimental myocardial infarcts of predictable size and location of dogs. J Thorac Cardiovasc Surg **69:** 599, 1975
16. Fishbein MC, Meerbaum S, Rit J, Lando V, Kanmatsuse K, Mercier J, Corday E, Ganz W: Early phase acute myocardial infarct size quantification: validation of the triphenyl tetrazolium chloride tissue enzyme staining technique. Am Heart J **101:** 593, 1981
17. Heymann MA, Payne BD, Hoffman JI, Rudolph AM: Blood flow measurements with radionuclide-labeled particles. Prog Cardiovasc Dis **20:** 55, 1977
18. Patterson RE, Kirk ES: Apparent improvement in canine collateral myocardial blood flow during vasodilatation depends on criteria used to identify ischemic myocardium. Circ Res **47:** 108, 1980
19. Zhu WX, Bolli R, Lekich RF, Myers ML, Hartley CJ, Roberts R: Validation of a single nontraumatic epicardial crystal in the measurement of transmural and epicardial wall thickening. Clin Res **33:** 239A, 1985 (abst)
20. Roan P, Scales F, Saffer S, Buja LM, Willerson JT: Functional characterization of left ventricular segmental responses during the initial 24 hours and first week after experimental canine myocardial infarction. J Cli Invest **64:** 1074, 1979
21. Reimer KA, Hill ML, Jennings RB: Prolonged depletion of ATP and of the adenine nucleotide pool due to delayed resynthesis of adenine nucleotide following reversible myocardial ischemic injury in dogs. J Mol Cell Cardiol **13:** 229, 1981
22. Hoffmeister HM, Manser M, Schaper W: Pharmacological accumulation of adenosine during repeated ischemia: preservation of ATP but failure to prevent postischemic dysfunction. Circulation **70:** III-194, 1984 (abst)
23. Neely JR, Grotyhann LW: Role of glycolytic products in damage to ischemic myocardium: Dissociation of adenosine triphosphate levels and recovery of function of reperfused ischemic hearts. Circ Res **55:** 816, 1984
24. Bolli R, Zhu WX, Myers ML, Hartley CJ, Roberts R: Beta-adrenergic stimulation reverses postischemic myocardial dysfunction without producing subsequent functional deterioration. Am J Cardiol (in press)
25. Bulkley GB: The role of oxygen free radicals in human disease processes. Surgery **94:** 407, 1983
26. Frank L, Massaro D: The lung and oxygen toxicity. Arch Intern Med **139:** 347, 1979
27. Menzel DB: Toxicity of ozone, oxygen and radiation. Ann Rev Pharmacol **10:** 379, 1970
28. Fantone JC, Ward PA: Role of oxygen-derived free radicals and metabolites in leukocyte-dependent inflammatory reactions. Am J Pathol **107:** 397, 1982
29. Parks DA, Bulkley GB, Granger DN, Hamilton SR, McCord JM: Ischemic injury in the cat small intestine: Role of superoxide radicals. Gastroenterology **82:** 9, 1982
30. Paller MS, Hoidal JR, Ferris TF: Oxygen free radicals in ischemic acute renal failure in the rat. J Clin Invest **74:** 1156, 1984
31. Demopoulos HB, Flamm ES, Pietronigro DD, Seligman ML: The free radical pathology and the microcirculation in the major central nervous system disorders. Acta Physiol Scand **492**(suppl): 91, 1980
32. Burton K: Superoxide dismutase enhances recovery following myocardial ischemia. Am J Physiol **248:** H637, 1985
33. Fridovich I: The biology of oxygen radicals. Science **201:** 875, 1978
34. Freeman BA, Crapo JD: Biology of disease: free radicals and tissue injury. Lab Invest **47:** 412, 1982
35. McCord JM: The superoxide free radical: its biochemistry and pathophysiology. Surgery **94:** 412, 1983
36. Boveris A: Mitochondrial production of superoxide radical and hydrogen peroxide. Adv Exp Med Biol **78:** 67, 1977
37. Del Maestro R: An approach to free radicals in medicine and biology. Act Physiol Scand **492**(suppl): 153, 1980

38. Pinckard RN, O'Rourke RA, Crawford MH, Grover FS, McManus LM, Ghidoni JJ, Storrs SB, Olson MS: Complement localization and mediation of ischemic injury in baboon myocardium. J Clin Invest **66:** 1050, 1980
39. Romson JL, Hook BG, Kimbel SL, Abrams GD, Schork A, Lucchesi BR: Reduction in the extent of ischemic myocardial injury by neutrophil depletion in the dog. Circulation **67:** 1016, 1983
40. Rowe GT, Manson NH, Coplan M, Hess ML: Hydrogen peroxide and hydroxyl radical mediation of activated leukocyte depression of cardiac sarcoplasmic reticulum. Circ Res **53:** 584, 1983
41. McCord JM: Oxygen-derived free radicals in postischemic tissue injury. N Engl J Med **312:** 159, 1985
42. Akizuki S, Yoshida S, Chambers D, Eddy L, Parmley L, Yellon D, Downey J: Blockage of the O_2^- radical producing enzyme, xanthine oxidase, reduces infarct size in the dog. Fed Proc **43:** 540, 1984 (abst)
43. Werns SW, Shea MJ, Driscoll EM, Mitsos SE, Fantone JC, Pitt B, Lucchesi BR: Effect of xanthine oxidase inhibition on canine myocardial ischemia. Clin Res **33:** 237A, 1985 (abst)
44. Reimer KA, Jennings RB: Failure of the xanthine oxidase inhibitor allopurinol to limit infarct size after ischemia and reperfusion in dogs. Circulation **71:** 1069, 1985
45. Morgan EJ: The distribution of xanthine oxidase. I. Biochem J **20:** 1281, 1926

Effect of serial brief ischemic episodes on extracellular K^+, pH, and activation in the pig

WILLIAM F. FLEET, TIMOTHY A. JOHNSON, CHRIS A. GRAEBNER, AND LEONARD S. GETTES

ABSTRACT This study was performed to determine the reproducibility of the ionic and electrical changes associated with serial ischemic episodes. We used ion-selective and bipolar plunge electrodes to determine the changes in left ventricular extracellular potassium ($[K^+]_e$), extracellular pH (pH_e), and local activation during sequential 10 min occlusions of the left anterior descending coronary artery separated by 50 min of reperfusion in open-chest anesthetized pigs. We found that uniformly during the initial occlusion, and in approximately 50% of animals during the second occlusion, $[K^+]_e$ rose more rapidly but to a lower level than in subsequent occlusions. By the third occlusion the changes in $[K^+]_e$ were reproducible. Extracellular acidosis was greatest in the first occlusion and decreased progressively with each subsequent occlusion. Local activation was characterized by a decrease in spontaneous improvement and increase in block with each successive occlusion. The occurrence of ventricular fibrillation could not be directly attributed to the magnitude of the change in $[K^+]_e$ or pH_e. Moreover, the occurrence of ventricular fibrillation in one occlusion did not necessarily predict its occurrence thereafter. Our results indicate that serial episodes of ischemia are associated with different but predictable changes in ionic and electrical events that may be clinically relevant and that must be appreciated before the results from similar protocols with serial ischemic episodes can be interpreted meaningfully.

Circulation 72, No. 4, 922–932, 1985.

ACUTE MYOCARDIAL ISCHEMIA causes a rapid depletion of energy-rich substrates,[1–3] a rise in the extracellular concentration of K^+ ($[K^+]_e$),[4–9] a fall in extracellular and intracellular pH,[10–13] and slowing of conduction through the ischemic area.[14–18] Acute coronary occlusion of more than 20 min duration causes irreversible cellular injury.[19] Shorter periods of ischemia cause ionic and electrical changes that are rapidly reversed by reperfusion,[6, 4] although mechanical[20–22] and metabolic[23, 24] changes may persist for long periods after reperfusion.

If the ionic and electrical changes induced by brief episodes of ischemia were reproducible or predictable as well as reversible, they could then be used to study the effects of interventions designed to influence the ischemic process. Prior work from our laboratory[6] and from the laboratories of others[7, 8] suggests that the rise in $[K^+]_e$ induced by serial 10 min occlusions may be reproducible. However, these studies were not designed to address this issue specifically and did not measure the associated changes in pH or electrical activity. Changes in myocardial blood flow, ventricular activation, electrocardiographic waveform, and arrhythmias are reproducible when two 5 min periods of ischemia are separated by 40 min of reperfusion[25] but are not reproducible when the occlusions are separated by only 3 min. Occlusions greater than 5 min in duration have not been studied in this manner. Moreover, no studies have tested the reproducibility of the changes in extracellular pH (pH_e) during serial brief episodes of ischemia, nor has the reproducibility of the electrical and ionic changes been studied concomitantly.

We have studied the simultaneous changes in myocardial $[K^+]_e$, pH_e, and local activation, as well as the incidence of ventricular fibrillation, during serial 10 min occlusions of the left anterior descending coronary artery (LAD) in open-chest swine. Our results provide a basis for the interpretation of experiments that use serial ischemic episodes to test the effects of physiologic and pharmacologic interventions and may apply to clinically occurring repetitive episodes of myocardial ischemia in man.

From the Department of Medicine, Division of Cardiology, University of North Carolina at Chapel Hill.
Supported by grant P01 HL27430 from the NHLBI.
Address for correspondence: Leonard S. Gettes, M.D., 349 Burnett Womack Bldg. 229H, Chapel Hill, NC 27514.
Received Jan. 14, 1985; revision accepted July 18, 1985.

Methods

Electrodes. Miniature K^+-sensitive plunge electrodes, modified from designs described earlier,[26] were fashioned from Teflon-coated silver wire 0.005 inch in diameter. The cut end of each wire was chloridized in sodium hypochlorite (NaOCl), covered with a mixture of cellulose acetate and titanium dioxide, soaked in 3 mM KCl solution, and covered with a polyvinyl chloride–based membrane containing the K^+ ionophore valinomycin. The pH-sensitive electrodes[11] were constructed in an analogous manner with the H^+ ionophore p-octadecyloxy m-chlorophenylhydrazone.[27] The response characteristics and time constants of these electrodes in vitro and in vivo were similar to those of previously described designs.[11, 26] Reference electrodes, similarly constructed, lacked only an ion-selective membrane. A K^+-sensitive, pH-sensitive, and common reference electrode were placed into a 20 gauge short-beval needle for insertion into the midmyocardium. Each electrode was bent back on itself just beyond the tip so that the needle could be withdrawn, leaving the electrode embedded in the myocardial tissue. The K^+-sensitive electrodes were calibrated in solutions of 3, 10, and 20 mM KCl before and again after each experiment, and the pH-sensitive electrodes were calibrated in solutions of pH 6 and 8. Data were accepted only from those electrodes that demonstrated a 57 to 61 mV shift per decade change in K^+ or H^+ activity both before and after each experiment.

Millivolt readings from the K^+- and pH-sensitive electrodes were amplified by a high-impedance instrumentation amplifier and serially connected to a low pass filter (1 kHz). The amplified signals from all ion-selective electrodes were sampled every 15 sec by a DEC PDP-11/03 minicomputer during the S-T segment of the cardiac cycle, thus avoiding interference from the electrocardiographic signal. Epicardial temperature was monitored with a Yellow Springs temperature probe sutured onto the left ventricular epicardium. Millivolt readings from ion-selective electrodes were converted to changes in local K^+ and H^+ activity with the Nernst equation and epicardial temperature. Absolute values of myocardial K^+ activity and pH_e were determined by relating the measured changes in these variables to the values of arterial $[K^+]$ and pH obtained just before each occlusion. Changes in pH were referenced to arterial pH because interstitial pH and arterial pH have been shown to differ only minimally despite differences in P_{CO_2}.[12] The results are expressed as millimolar K^+ concentration ($[K^+]$), calculated from K^+ activity with an activity coefficient of 0.746.[28]

Local midmyocardial bipolar ventricular electrograms were recorded by Teflon-coated stainless steel bipolar plunge electrodes.[14] One electrode was placed in the nonischemic area, one or two electrodes were placed along the lateral margin, and two or three electrodes were placed in the center of the ischemic zone. These bipolar electrograms were filtered between 50 and 500 Hz and continuously displayed with a lead I electrocardiogram on the oscilloscope of a Honeywell visicorder. Recordings were made every minute during occlusions at paper speeds of 200 and 400 mm/sec. Local activation was determined from the onset of the QRS complex in the electrocardiogram to the peak of the high-frequency deflection in each local electrogram. Activation delay was determined by subtracting the starting activation time from the activation time at each minute of ischemia. Activation block was said to occur when no high-frequency deflection was discernible.[16]

Experimental protocol. Domestic pigs of either sex weighing 20 to 25 kg were immobilized with ketamine (10 mg/kg) and anethetized with thiamylal sodium (25 mg/kg). Anethesia was then maintained with α-cholralose in polyethylene glycol (mol wt = 400) as needed in doses ranging from 30 to 50 mg/kg/hr. No anesthetic was given within 20 min of an occlusion. The animals were ventilated through an endotracheal tube on a positive-pressure respirator (Harvard Apparatus) with a minute volume and oxygen mixture sufficient to maintain arterial oxygen saturation greater than 95%, arterial P_{CO_2} at 35 to 45 mm Hg, and arterial pH at 7.35 to 7.45. A femoral venous catheter was used to infuse drugs and 0.9% saline solution. Systemic arterial pressure was measured by a Millar pressure transducer placed in the descending aorta via the femoral artery. Arterial blood samples were obtained before each occlusion for determination of pH, P_{CO_2}, and P_{O_2} and for the independent determination of serum $[K^+]$.

After a midsternal thoracotomy, the LAD was dissected distal to the second diagonal branch, and a polyethylene snare was placed around the LAD. Two methods were used to position as many as nine electrode groups along the lateral border and in the center of the ischemic zone (figure 1). In six animals the artery was occluded for 30 sec to demarcate the border of the ischemic zone (group A). During this period, one or two electrodes were placed along the lateral margin. The snare was then released, and the remaining electrodes were inserted. In nine animals (group B) the artery was occluded for 10 min, during which all electrodes were inserted. The integrity of K^+ and pH electrodes

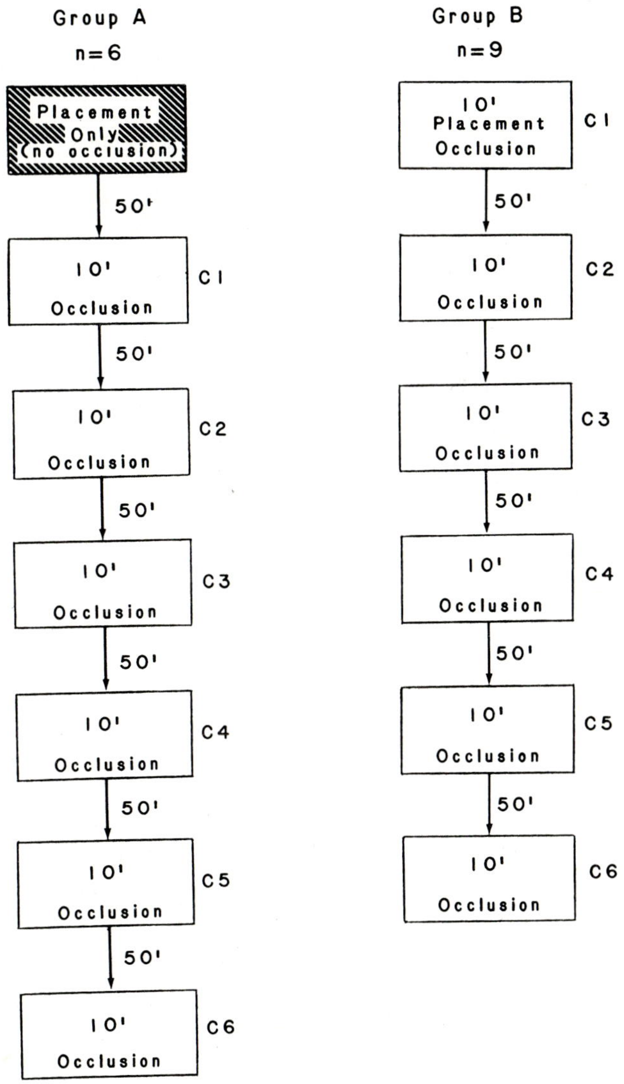

FIGURE 1. Schematic representation of the different protocols used in this study.

in vivo was determined 30 min after placement by the response to a bolus injection of 1.5 meq KCl in 3 ml of normal saline[6] or to 45 sec of respiratory acidosis, respectively. Data were accepted only from electrodes that responded promptly to each KCl bolus or period of acidosis.

A series of five or six occlusions of the LAD was initiated 50 min after placement of the electrodes (see figure 1). Each occlusion was 10 min in duration, and episodes were separated by 50 min of reperfusion. Right atrial pacing was used to maintain a constant heart rate of 90 beats/min in all experiments in which the spontaneous rate was slower than this, or at the rate of the initial occlusion when the spontaneous rate was faster than 90 beats/min. Release of each occlusion was performed slowly over 30 to 60 sec to reduce the incidence of reperfusion arrhythmias. Animals that fibrillated were quickly defibrillated by 10 to 20 W-sec applied directly to the heart. Integrity of electrodes was retested after defibrillation by a second KCl bolus and period of respiratory acidosis. After termination of each experiment, either by spontaneous ventricular fibrillation or by the injection of a large KCl bolus, the hearts were removed and the electrodes were dissected free of myocardial tissue for recalibration. All electrodes included in the study were located in the midmyocardium ($\geq$3 mm from endocardium and epicardium).

Electrodes were categorized as being in the center of the ischemic zone when they were more than 5 mm from the visible cyanotic border and at the margin of the ischemic zone when they were within 5 mm of the border.[29-31] The number of functioning K^+-sensitive electrodes in each experiment varied from four to eight, and the number of functioning pH-sensitive electrodes varied from three to six. To minimize the impact of these differences in the number of working electrodes, when mean values were determined, results from all electrodes in a given location (center or margin) from each animal were pooled to compute mean changes in $[K^+]_e$ and pH_e at each location at each minute of ischemia. Thus each experiment was weighted equally. Statistical evaluation was performed with Student's t test for paired and unpaired data.

The occlusions are identified as C_1 to C_6. In group A the electrodes were inserted without the benefit of a 10 min occlusion and thus C_1 was the first experimental occlusion. In group B the electrodes were inserted during C_1 and the experimental occlusions commenced with C_2 (figure 1).

Results

A total of 15 animals were studied; six were in group A and nine were in group B. Eight animals completed the series of occlusions without an episode of ventricular fibrillation. Of these, four were in group A and four were in group B. Seven animals had at least one episode of ventricular fibrillation. Two of these were in group A and five were in group B (not statistically significant). $[K^+]_e$ was measured in all 15 animals; pH_e was measured in eight, six in group A (two of which fibrillated) and two in group B (both without ventricular fibrillation). The mean heart rates, starting $[K^+]_e$, and starting pH_e for each occlusion are shown in table 1. There were no significant differences between occlusions in these variables.

Extracellular K^+. Figure 2 shows two representative experiments in which the electrodes were placed 50 min before the first occlusion (group A). For each experiment, the changes in $[K^+]_e$ recorded by a single K^+-selective electrode located in the center of the ischemic zone during successive occlusions are superimposed. In the experiment shown in figure 2, *A*, $[K^+]_e$ during C_1 rose slightly more rapidly in the early minutes of ischemia than during C_2. However, $[K^+]_e$ during C_1 reached a plateau after 5 min of ischemia, whereas in C_2 $[K^+]_e$ continued to rise and attained a higher peak. The $[K^+]_e$ changes during C_2 to C_5 were then reproducible. In the experiment shown in figure 2, *B*, the change in $[K^+]_e$ was again more rapid during C_1 than during C_2 and reached a greater peak value in C_2. However, unlike the experiment shown in figure 2, *A*, peak $[K^+]_e$ was slightly greater in C_3 than in C_2. The $[K^+]_e$ change was then reproducible in C_3 to C_6.

Figure 3 shows two representative experiments in which the electrodes were placed during the first occlusion, C_1 (group B). In the experiment shown in figure 3, *A*, the change in $[K^+]_e$ during C_2 (the first experimental occlusion) predicted the $[K^+]_e$ changes during subsequent occlusions. In the experiment shown in figure 3, *B*, the peak $[K^+]_e$ in C_3 was greater than in C_2, but thereafter the changes in $[K^+]_e$ were reproducible. Thus the changes observed in $[K^+]_e$ during C_2 to C_5 were similar in groups A and B.

These experiments are representative of the patterns consistently observed in the center of the ischemic zone. The occurrence of ventricular fibrillation during one occlusion did not affect the reproducibility of subsequent occlusions. In all experiments, release of occlusion caused a return of $[K^+]_e$ to preischemic values within 5 min. The changes in $[K^+]_e$ during C_2 predicted the changes during C_3 to C_5 in 54% of all experiments. In the remaining 46%, reproducibility of $[K^+]_e$

TABLE 1

Mean values (±SEM) of heart rate, $[K^+]_e$, and pH_e just before the start of each of five sequential occlusions (C_1 to C_5)

	C_1	C_2	C_3	C_4	C_5
HR (beats/min)	125±4	121±5	126±6	128±6	125±6
$[K^+]_e$ (mM)	4.1±0.1	4.3±0.2	4.2±0.1	4.3±0.1	4.1±0.15
pH_e	7.39±0.03	7.39±0.01	7.39±0.01	7.40±0.01	7.39±0.11

HR = heart rate.

n = 8 animals. Differences were not statistically significant.

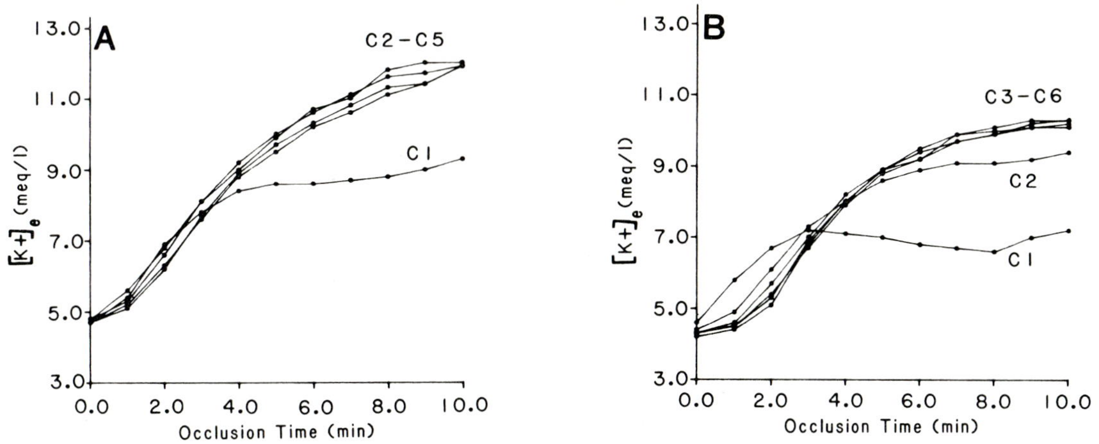

FIGURE 2. $[K^+]_e$ measured by single K^+-selective electrodes in the center of the ischemic zone during two separate experiments (panels *A* and *B*) from group A. In each experiment, $[K^+]_e$ was measured during serial 10 min occlusions of the LAD separated by 50 min of reperfusion.

was not attained until C_3. As previously described,[6] $[K^+]_e$ rose more slowly and to a lower peak value at the margin than in the center. However, the pattern of reproducibility was the same in both regions.

Our results indicate that once two occlusions produce similar changes in $[K^+]_e$, i.e., $C_3 = C_2$ or $C_4 = C_3$, the changes in $[K^+]_e$ during two subsequent occlusions will be similar. This is illustrated in figure 4, which shows the mean value of $[K^+]_e$ at each minute of ischemia during the second of the two matching occlusions (labeled M) and during two subsequent occlusions, M + 1 and M + 2. The changes in $[K^+]_e$ during these three occlusions did not differ significantly either in the center (figure 4, *A*) or at the margin (figure 4, *B*).

Extracellular pH. Occlusion of the LAD caused a fall in pH_e from a preischemic value of 7.39 + 0.02, which began within 30 to 45 sec of occlusion and returned to preischemic values within 6 min of release. The fall in pH_e did not have a plateau phase during C_1. The pattern of change in pH_e recorded by single electrodes in the center (panel *A*) and margin (panel *B*) of the ischemic zone during sequential occlusions differed from that of changes in $[K^+]_e$. This is illustrated in figure 5, which shows the changes in pH_e during five sequential occlusions from a single representative experiment in a group A animal. The figure demonstrates that acidosis was greatest during the initial experimental occlusion (C_1 in this instance) and decreased progressively with each occlusion. The progressive decrease in acidosis with successive occlusions was consistently observed in all experiments in both groups A and B. Figure 6 shows the mean value of pH_e at each minute of ischemia during each of five sequential occlusions. The data in this figure are taken from the four animals in group A that did not fibrillate during any occlusion.

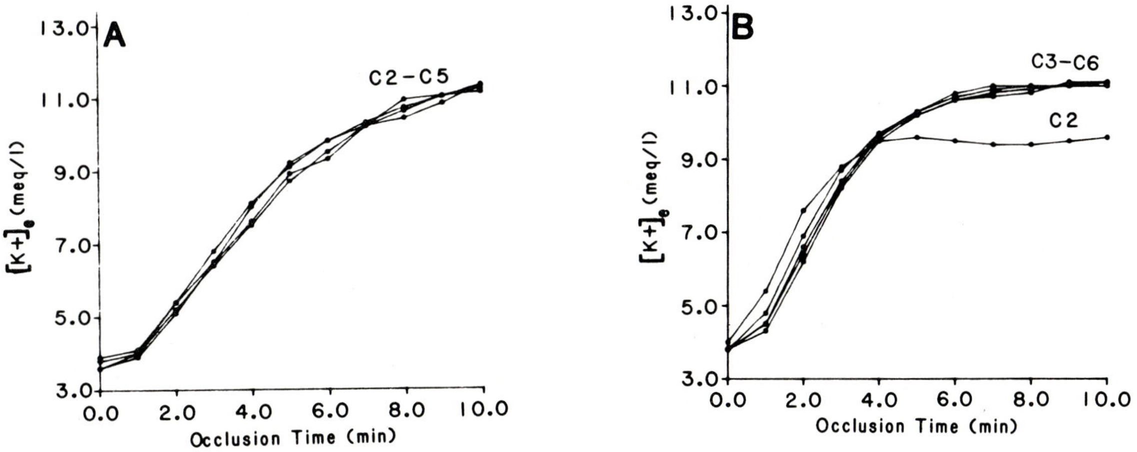

FIGURE 3. $[K^+]_e$ measured by single K^+-selective electrodes in the center of the ischemic zone during two separate experiments (panels *A* and *B*) from group B. In each experiment, $[K^+]_e$ was measured during serial 10 min occlusions of the LAD separated by 50 min of reperfusion.

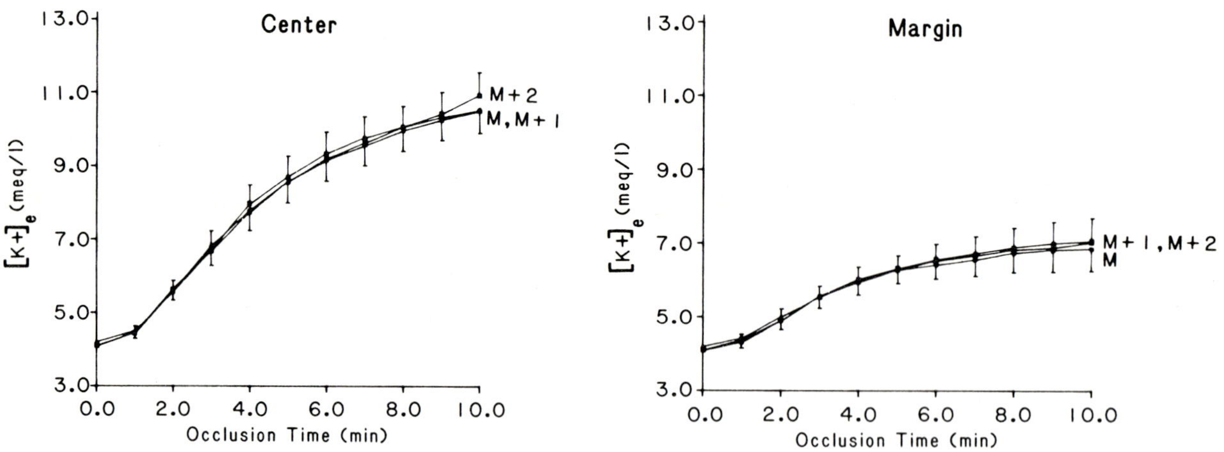

FIGURE 4. Mean values of $[K^+]_e$ in the center (*A*) and at the margin (*B*) of the ischemic zone at each minute of ischemia during M (the second of two occlusions that yielded matching changes in $[K^+]_e$) and during the two subsequent occlusions, M + 1 and M + 2; n = 8 animals without ventricular fibrillation (groups A and B).

Although the changes in pH_e were not reproducible during sequential occlusions, the differences in pH_e from one occlusion to the next were predictable. Figure 7 shows the mean pH_e at each minute of ischemia during the second of two occlusions that yielded matching changes in $[K^+]_e$ (M) and the two subsequent occlusions (M + 1, M + 2). Figure 8 shows that the mean differences in pH_e between M and M + 1 increased throughout the occlusion and were approximately 0.1 pH units at the center and 0.05 pH units at the margin after 10 min of ischemia.

Activation delay. The patterns of the changes in activation delay were assessed in the eight animals that did not have ventricular fibrillation. In this group, a total of 22 electrodes were placed in the center of the ischemic zone. At 13 electrode sites (59%) a discrete activation spike could be identified throughout all occlusions. At the remaining nine sites (41%) activation block occurred in the course of one or more of the occlusions. Figure 9, *A*, showing data from a group A animal, illustrates the characteristic activation pattern at sites with perceived activation during all occlusions. C_1 resulted in an initial delay in activation within 1 min of the occlusion. This was followed by a phase of spontaneous improvement that lasted approximately 3 min. Thereafter local activation again became increasingly delayed. The spontaneous improvement in activation occurred later and was less marked in C_2 and

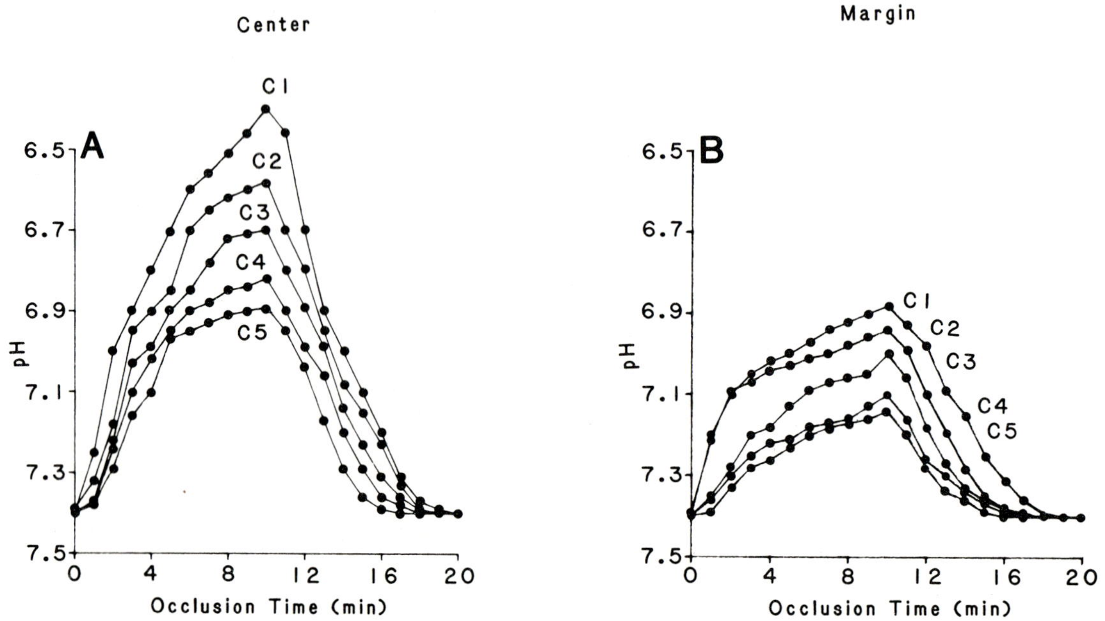

FIGURE 5. pH_e measured by single pH-sensitive electrode in the center of the ischemic zone (*left*) and one electrode at the margin (*right*) in a representative experiment from group A. Values are shown from five sequential occlusions, C_1 to C_5.

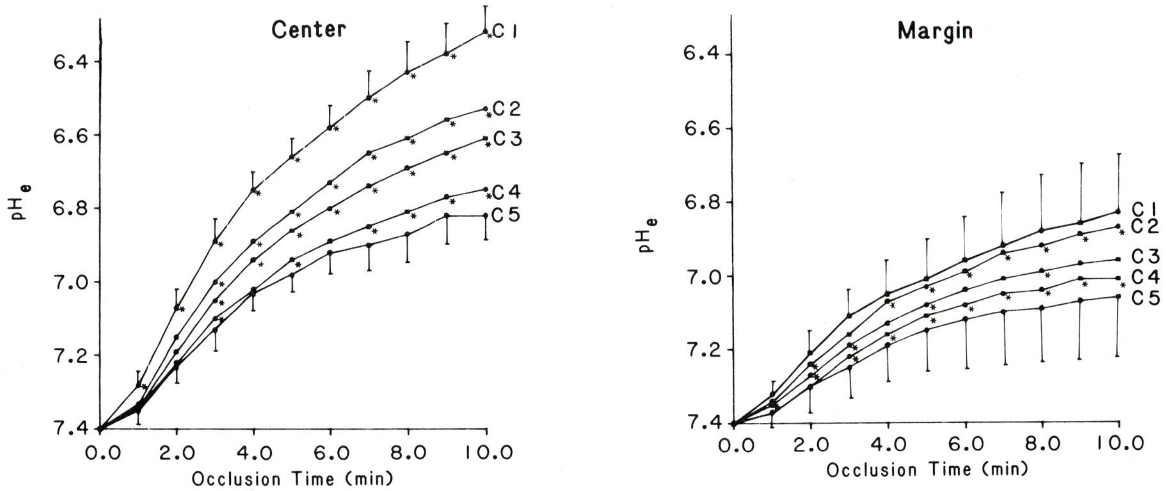

FIGURE 6. Mean pH_e ($\pm$ SEM) in the center and at the margin of the ischemic zone at each minute of ischemia during five successive occlusions (C_1 to C_5). *$p < .05$ compared with the subsequent occlusion; $n = 4$ animals without ventricular fibrillation (group A).

C_3. Spontaneous improvement did not occur at all in C_4 or C_5. Figure 9, *B*, shows the declining incidence of spontaneous improvement in each occlusion at the 13 electrode sites with preserved activation in the eight animals without ventricular fibrillation. The panel demonstrates that spontaneous improvement was never observed after C_3.

Figure 10, *A*, also showing data from a group A animal, illustrates the characteristic pattern observed at the nine electrode sites demonstrating activation block during one or more of the occlusions. During C_1 the changes in activation were similar to that shown in figure 9, *A*. In C_2, activation block occurred after 3 min of ischemia but activation was restored before the end of the occlusion. In C_3 and in all subsequent occlusions, activation block persisted throughout the occlusion. Figure 10, *B*, shows the combined data from the nine electrode sites and illustrates that activation block occurred with increasing frequency with each occlusion. Furthermore, once activation block occurred at a particular location, it was observed in all subsequent occlusions at that location. The time to onset of block was either the same or shorter in each subsequent occlusion.

We often observed both patterns of activation changes (loss of spontaneous improvement and the development of block) in the same heart. Moreover, since only two or three centrally placed electrodes were used in each animal, it is possible that both patterns were present in all hearts. The changes in local activation in the center of the ischemic zone were rapidly reversed by reperfusion. Activation delay was

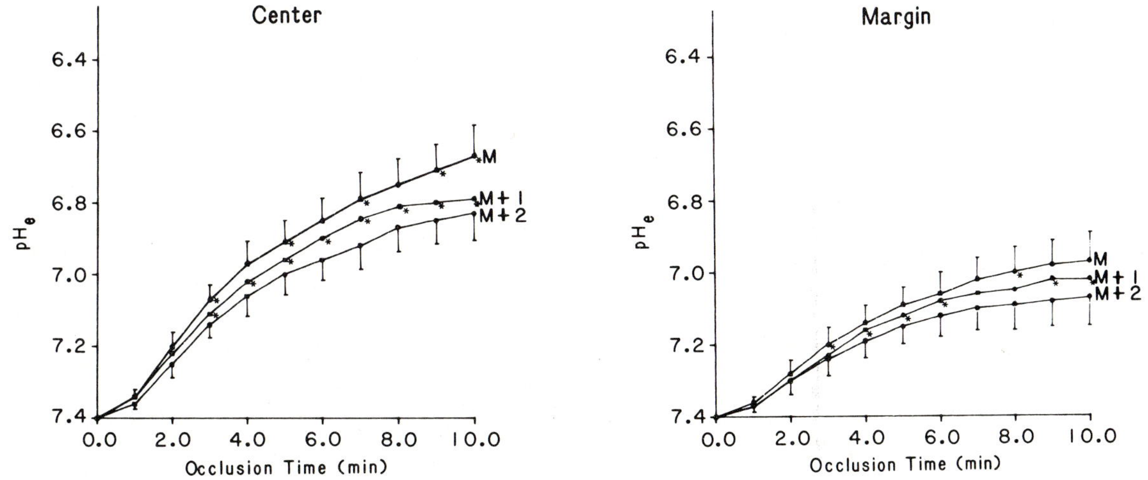

FIGURE 7. Mean pH_e ($\pm$ SEM) in the center and at the margin of the ischemic zone at each minute of occlusion during M (the second of two occlusions that yielded matching changes in $[K^+]_e$) and during the two subsequent occlusions, M + 1 and M + 2. *$p < .05$ compared with the subsequent occlusion; $n = 6$ animals without ventricular fibrillation (groups A and B).

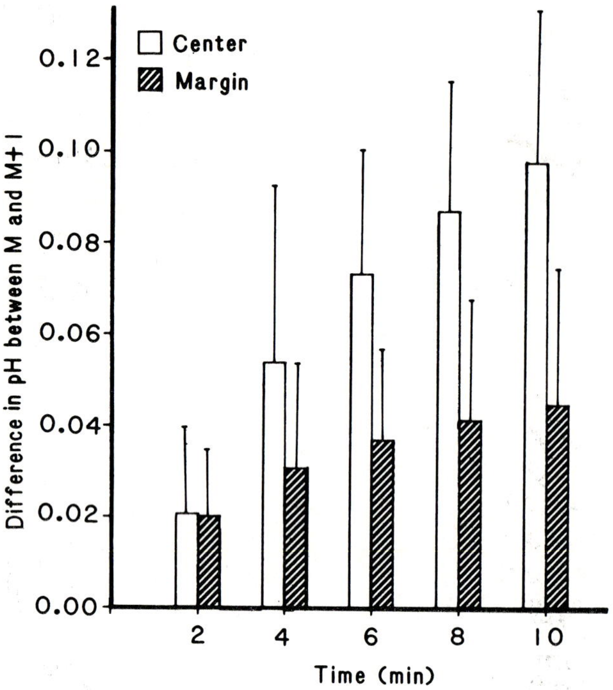

FIGURE 8. Mean differences (± SEM) in pH_e at alternate minutes of ischemia between M and M + 1 at the center and at the margin; n = 6 animals without ventricular fibrillation (groups A and B).

minimal or did not occur at the lateral margin of the ischemic zone. The animals with ventricular fibrillation were excluded from the analysis shown in figures 9 and 10 to keep constant the number of electrodes. Analysis of these animals showed changes in activation similar to those of the animals without ventricular fibrillation.

Ventricular fibrillation. The incidence of ventricular fibrillation in each occlusion is summarized in table 2. Ventricular fibrillation occurred only in later occlusions (C_3 to C_5). Two of the five animals that fibrillated in C_4 did not fibrillate in C_5. Thus, in contrast to the occurrence of conduction block, the occurrence of ventricular fibrillation in a given occlusion did not predict its occurrence in subsequent occlusions.

Among the seven animals with ventricular fibrillation, we compared the values of $[K^+]_e$, pH_e, and activation delay measured just before the onset of ventricular fibrillation to those values at the same time in the immediately preceding occlusion in which ventricular fibrillation did not occur. We were unable to detect a significant difference in $[K^+]_e$ change or activation at the onset of ventricular fibrillation compared with those occurring at the same time in the preceding occlusion in which ventricular fibrillation did not occur. The pH_e values were recorded in only two animals with ventricular fibrillation. In both experiments, pH_e at each electrode was slightly lower (0.05 to 0.10 pH units) in the preceding occlusion without fibrillation than in the occlusion with ventricular fibrillation, as predicted by the data shown in figures 5 to 8.

Discussion

In a series of 10 min coronary artery occlusions separated by 50 min of reperfusion, the following observations were made: (1) Changes in $[K^+]_e$ during the initial occlusion differ from later occlusions, but changes in $[K^+]_e$ eventually become reproducible. (2) Reproducibility of the change in $[K^+]_e$ cannot be assumed until two matching occlusions are obtained. (3) The magnitude of extracellular acidosis decreases with each occlusion. (4) The change in local activation is characterized by a decreasing incidence of spontane-

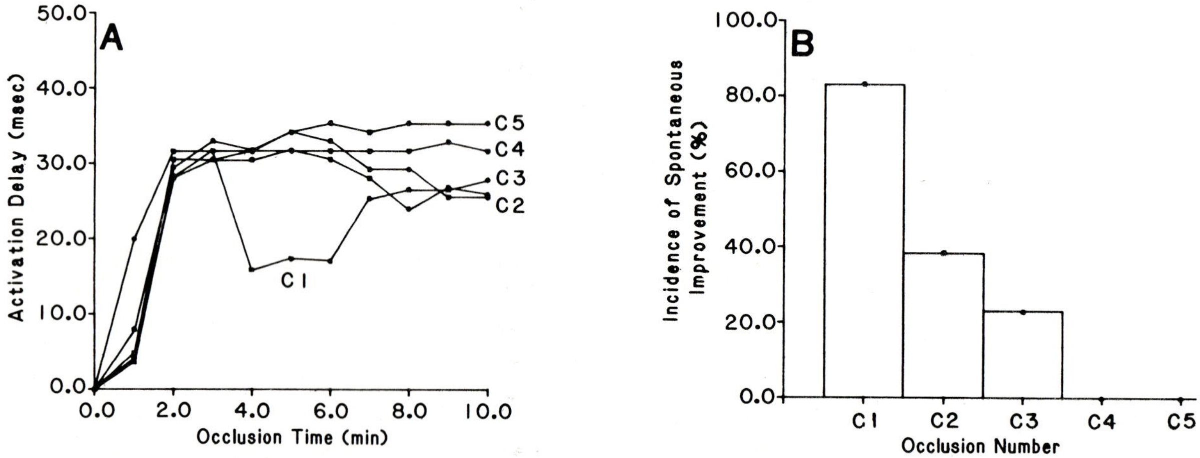

FIGURE 9. *A*, Change in local activation at each minute of ischemia as measured by a bipolar electrode in the center of the ischemic zone during five serial 10 min occlusions of the LAD. *B*, Incidence of spontaneous improvement in activation delay recorded at the electrode sites demonstrating activation spikes throughout each of the five serial occlusions in the eight animals without ventricular fibrillation; n = 6 electrodes in C_1 (group A) and 13 electrodes in C_2 to C_5 (groups A and B).

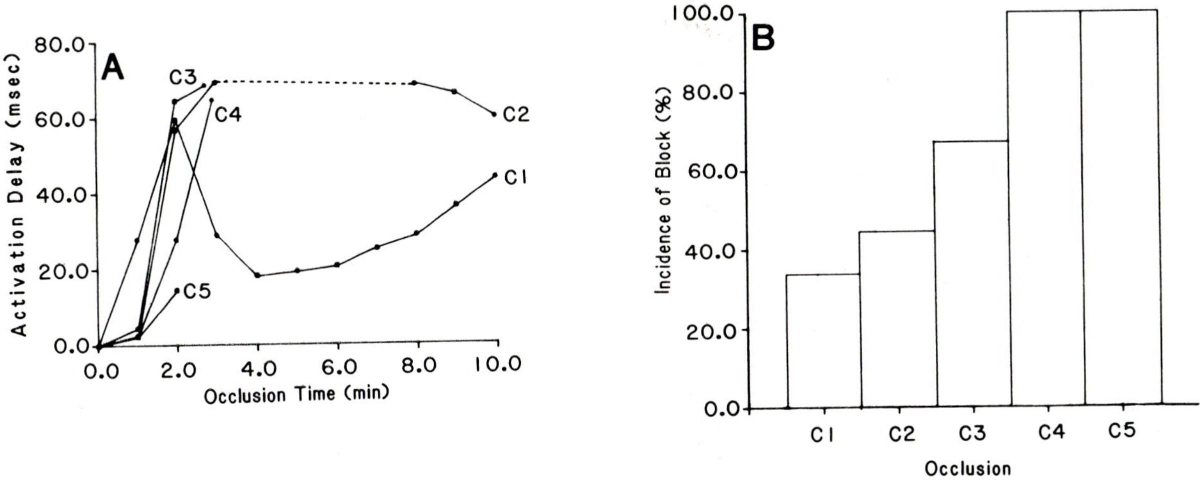

FIGURE 10. *A*, Change in local activation at each minute of ischemia, as recorded by a single bipolar electrode in the center of the ischemic zone, during five serial occlusions of the LAD. In C_2 the local activation spike was not discernible from 4 to 7 min of ischemia, but local activation was then restored by 8 min of ischemia. Activation block occurred during C_3 to C_5 and persisted until release of each occlusion. *B*, Incidence of activation block recorded at the electrode sites at which the activation block occurred during one or more of the serial occlusions of the LAD in the eight animals without ventricular fibrillation; n = 4 electrodes in C_1 (group A) and 9 electrodes in C_2 to C_5 (groups A and B).

ous improvement and an increasing incidence of local activation block. (5) Ventricular fibrillation is more common in later occlusions but is not reproducible. (6) The occurrence of ventricular fibrillation cannot be attributed solely to the magnitude of the $[K^+]_e$ rise or pH_e fall.

The different protocols (groups A and B) were used to determine whether the observed differences between C_1 and C_2 were attributable to the additional 50 min during which electrodes were in situ in the group A animals. Our hypothesis was as follows. If the differences between C_1 and C_2 were caused by time-dependent changes in electrodes and/or myocardial response characteristics, then changes in $[K^+]_e$ during C_2 of group B animals should be identical to changes during C_1 of group A animals, since in each case electrodes were in situ for 50 min before occlusion. Conversely, if differences between C_1 and C_2 were due to effects of the initial 10 min ischemic episode on subsequent changes, then the C_2 occlusions of groups A and B should be similar, since in each case C_2 followed an initial 10 min occlusion. The fact that C_2 in groups A and B were similar indicates that the initial ischemic period was the critical factor responsible for the difference in subsequent occlusion. Additionally, we felt it important to demonstrate the reproducibility of $[K^+]_e$ changes with the group B protocol because the group B protocol offers the advantage of 1 hr less operative time than the group A protocol and permits the more precise placement of the electrodes.

Extracellular pH was measured by ion-selective (H^+) electrodes similar in design and size to the K^+-selective electrodes.[26] These electrodes were used in the final eight animals of the series (six in group A, two in group B). The consistency of the results in these experiments was such that further experiments were not considered necessary.

We recognize that our measurements of local activation are inadequate to permit precise quantitative statements regarding activation time or sequence in the ischemic zone. It was our intent to use our measurements only to determine the reproducibility of the ischemia-induced change in local activation and to establish the qualitative nature of any changes in local activation delay associated with the repetitive occlusions.

The differences in the changes of $[K^+]_e$ and pH_e

TABLE 2
Occurrence of ventricular fibrillation in seven animals during serial 10 min occlusions (C_1 to C_5)

Animal	C_1	C_2	C_3	C_4	C_5
1	–	–	+	+	+
2	–	–	+	+	+
3	–	–	–	+	+
4	–	–	–	+	–
5	–	–	–	+	–
6	–	–	–	–	+
7	–	–	–	–	+

+ = occurrence of ventricular fibrillation.
Note that in animals 4 and 5, ventricular fibrillation occurred during C_4 but did not occur during C_5.

observed in the repetitive occlusions cannot be attributed to changes in the response characteristics of the electrodes because data were used only from electrodes that exhibited similar calibrations before and after each experiment. Other possible confounding influences such as changes in temperature and in K^+-independent direct current potentials have previously been shown to be insignificant.[6] We did not determine whether changes in collateral flow contributed to our results. However, it is unlikely that the development of collateral circulation contributed significantly, since collateral circulation in the pig is minimal.[32] Furthermore, if collaterals were to develop during repetitive occlusions, it is likely that their influences would be more pronounced at the margin than at the center of the ischemic zone. The fact that similar patterns of change in $[K^+]_e$ and pH_e were observed at both locations argues against the possibility that changes in flow contributed substantially to our results.

We also cannot exclude a possible confounding effect of the long duration of our experiments. However, the reproducibility of the change in $[K^+]_e$ in the later occlusions and the equality of epicardial temperature in each occlusion suggest that this factor alone does not explain the progressive changes in pH_e and activation with each occlusion or the development of ventricular fibrillation during the later occlusions.

We have shown that successive periods of brief ischemia produce progressively less acidosis. This phenomenon may be significant in view of the possible role of intracellular acidosis in cellular necrosis[33, 34] and the protective effects of mild acidosis on hypoxic myocardium.[35-37] The progressive decrease in extracellular acidosis with each occlusion may be explained by a decrease in acid production, a decrease in transport of intracellular protons into the extracellular space, and/or an increase in buffering capacity of the intracellular or extracellular compartments. The ischemia-induced H^+ ions are probably derived from glycolytically produced lactic acid and the hydrolysis of ATP.[38, 39] Although our studies do not clarify the mechanism(s), it is possible that depletion of glycogen[22] and/or ATP[24] stores might contribute to our findings.

Our results indicate that the changes in $[K^+]_e$ and pH_e are not closely correlated. This lack of correlation is demonstrated by the following observations: (1) the changes in $[K^+]_e$ reached a plateau during the early minutes of C_1, whereas pH_e continued to fall throughout this occlusion, and (2) maximum $[K^+]_e$ values increased from C_1 to C_3 and then became reproducible in subsequent occlusions while acidosis decreased progressively. A close relationship between K^+ efflux and intracellular acidosis during ischemia has been suggested,[40] and other investigators have correlated the release of K^+ during ischemia with release of lactate and phosphate.[41, 42] Our results do not necessarily suggest a lack of close relationship between K^+ efflux and intracellular acidosis, since we measured only pH_e. The relationship of pH_e to intracellular pH under conditions of ischemia is not known with certainty,[43] and measurements of intracellular pH during ischemia by various techniques have shown differing results.[10, 43]

The diffusion of carbon dioxide, which rises quickly during ischemia,[44] across cell membranes should tend to equalize pH in the intracellular and extracellular compartments,[45, 46] but differences in buffering capacities may cause differences in pH between the two compartments during ischemia despite similar values of P_{CO_2}.

The spontaneous improvement and return of local activation after an initial delay with or without block has been described previously[29, 47-50] and probably correlates with the spontaneous increase in action potential amplitude, recovery in resting membrane potential, decrease in ST and TQ potentials, and recovery of excitability that have been reported by others.[29, 48, 50] The progressively more delayed activation observed in subsequent occlusions might be caused by depletion of factors that favorably affect propagation through acutely ischemic myocardium, such as endogenous catecholamines. Depletion of myocardial catecholamines by brief episodes of ischemia have been reported previously.[5, 51] Catecholamines may improve ventricular conduction during simulated ischemia[52] and during ischemia by affecting resting membrane potential in depressed fibers,[53] by increasing the magnitude of the slow inward current,[54] and possibly by preventing cellular uncoupling.[55] Thus their depletion could lead to the progressive delay in local activation seen in this study. This hypothesis remains to be tested.

We found the incidence of ventricular fibrillation to be greater in the later occlusions. Other investigators have implicated both an increase in $[K^+]_e$[7, 56-58] and a slowing of ventricular activation[15-17, 47] in the genesis of ventricular fibrillation. We were unable to document a difference in $[K^+]_e$ or activation delay at the onset of fibrillation in the occlusions with and without ventricular fibrillation. This suggests that the occurrence of ventricular fibrillation may not be related solely to the magnitude of the change in $[K^+]_e$ or activation.

However, it does not exclude the possibility that ventricular fibrillation is related to more complex and subtle changes in $[K^+]_e$, pH_e, and electrical properties than were measured in this study, such as the inhomogeneity of the ionic and electrical changes and/or the size of the central and marginal ischemic zones.

The implications of our study are twofold. From a clinical perspective, our results suggest that closely spaced episodes of reversible acute transmural ischemia of approximately equal duration, as may occur in patients with coronary vasospasm,[59] may produce dissimilar ionic, metabolic, and electrical changes. Furthermore, these patients may be at risk for development of ventricular fibrillation in later episodes of ischemia, even if the initial episodes are free of arrhythmias.

From a laboratory investigative perspective, our results indicate that studies designed to test the effects of pharmacologic interventions on the ionic and electrical events that characterize acute ischemia must take into consideration the differences in these parameters that occur in repeated ischemic periods. However, such studies can be meaningfully interpreted if it is appreciated that changes in $[K^+]_e$ may not become reproducible until the third occlusion, that changes in pH_e are not reproducible but the differences are predictable, that ventricular activation becomes progressively depressed with successive occlusions, that the presence of ventricular fibrillation in one ischemic episode does not invariably predict its presence in subsequent episodes, and that the occurrence of ventricular fibrillation is not determined solely by the magnitude of the change in $[K^+]_e$, pH_e, or local activation.

References

1. Jennings RB, Hawkins HK, Lowe JE, Hill ML, Klotman S, Reimer RA: Relation between high energy phosphate and lethal injury in myocardial ischemia in the dog. Am J Pathol **92:** 187, 1978
2. Braash W, Gudbjarnason S, Puri PS, Ravens KG, Bing RJ: Early changes in energy metabolism in the myocardium following acute coronary artery occlusion in anesthetized dogs. Circ Res **23:** 429, 1968
3. Dunn RB, Griggs DW: Transmural gradients in ventricular tissue metabolites produced by stopping coronary blood flow in the dog. Circ Res **37:** 438, 1975
4. Wiegand V, Guggi M, Meesmann W, Kessler M, Greitschus F: Extracellular potassium activity change in the canine myocardium after acute coronary occlusion and the influence of beta-blockade. Cardiovasc Res **13:** 297, 1979
5. Hirche HJ, Franz LB, Bissig R, Lang R, Schramm M: Myocardial extracellular K^+ and H^+ increase and noradrenaline release as possible cause of early arrhythmia following acute coronary artery occlusion in pigs. J Mol Cell Cardiol **12:** 579, 1980
6. Hill JL, Gettes LS: Effect of acute coronary artery occlusion on local myocardial extracellular K^+ activity in swine. Circulation **61:** 768, 1980
7. Weiss J, Shine KI: Extracellular potassium accumulation during myocardial ischemic: implications for arrhythmogenesis. J Mol Cell Cardiol **13:** 699, 1981
8. Weiss J, Shine KI: Extracellular K^+ accumulation during myocardial ischemia in isolated rabbit heart. Am J Physiol **242:** H619, 1982
9. Kleber AG: Resting membrane potential, extracellular potassium activity, and intracellular sodium activity during acute global ischemia in isolated perfused guinea pig hearts. Circ Res **52:** 442, 1983
10. Garlick PB, Radda GK, Seely PJ: Studies of acidosis in the ischemic heart by phosphorous nuclear magnetic resonance. Biochem J **184:** 547, 1979
11. Cobbe SM, Poole-Wilson PA: The time of onset and severity of acidosis in myocardial ischemia. J Mol Cell Cardiol **12:** 745, 1980
12. Walters FJM, Wilson GJ, Steward DJ, Domenech RJ, MacGregor DC: Intramyocardial pH as an index of myocardial metabolism during cardiac surgery. J Thoracic Cardiovasc Surg **78:** 319, 1979
13. Cobbe SM, Parker DJ, Poole-Wilson PH: Tissue and coronary venous pH in ischemic canine myocardium. Clin Cardiol **5:** 153, 1982
14. Durrer D, Formijne P, van Dam RT, Buller J, van Lier AAW, Meyler FL: The electrocardiogram in normal and some abnormal conditions. Am Heart J **61:** 303, 1961
15. Waldo AL, Kaiser GA: A study of ventricular arrhythmias associated with acute myocardial infarction in the canine heart. Circulation **47:** 1222, 1973
16. Boineau JP, Cox JL: Slow ventricular activation in acute myocardial infarction. Circulation **48:** 702, 1973
17. Hope RR, Williams DO, El-Sherif N, Lazzara R, Scherlag BJ: The efficacy of antiarrhythmic agents during acute myocardial ischemia and the role of heart rate. Circulation **50:** 507, 1974
18. Williams DO, Scherlag BJ, Hope RR, El-Sherif N, Lazzara R: The pathophysiology of malignant ventricular arrhythmias during acute myocardial ischemia. Circulation **50:** 1163, 1974
19. Jennings RB, Sommers HM, Herdson PB, Kaltenback JP: Ischemic injury of myocardium. Ann NY Acad Sci **156:** 61, 1969
20. Heyndrickx GR, Millard RW, McRitchie LJ, Maroko PR, Vatner SF: Regional myocardial function and electrophysiological alterations after brief coronary artery occlusion in conscious dogs. J Clin Invest **56:** 978, 1975
21. Heyndrickx GR, Baig H, Nellens P, Larsen I, Fishbein MC, Vatner SF: Depression of regional blood flow and wall thickening after brief coronary occlusions. Am J Physiol **234:** H653, 1978
22. Wood JM, Hanley HG, Entman ML, Hartley CJ, Swain JA, Busch U, Chen-Hong C, Lewis RM, Morgan WJ, Schwartz A: Biochemical and morphological correlates of acute experimental myocardial ischemia in the dog. Circ Res **44:** 52, 1979
23. Vial C, Font B, Goldschmidt D, Pearlman AS, Delaye J: Regional myocardial energetics during brief periods of coronary occlusion and reperfusion: comparison with S-T segment changes. Cardiovasc Res **12:** 470, 1978
24. Reimer KA, Hill ML, Jennings RB: Prolonged depletion of ATP and of the adenine nucleotide pool due to delayed resynthesis of adenine nucleotides following reversible myocardial ischemic injury in dogs. J Mol Cell Cardiol **13:** 229, 1981
25. Barber MJ: Effect of the interval between repeated brief coronary artery occlusions on arrhythmia, electrical activity and myocardial blood flow. J Am Coll Cardiol **2:** 699, 1983
26. Hill JL, Gettes LS, Lynch MR, Hebert NC: Flexible valinomycin electrodes for on-line determination of intravascular and myocardial K^+. Am J Physiol **235:** H455, 1978
27. Le Blanc OH, Brown JF, Klebe JF, Niedrach LW, Slusarczuk GMJ, Stoddard WH: Polymer/membrane sensors for continuous intravascular monitoring of blood pH. J Appl Physiol **40:** 644, 1976
28. Meites L: Mean activity coefficients. *In* Handbook of analytic chemistry. New York, 1963, McGraw-Hill Book Co., Inc., pp 8–12
29. Janse MJ, Cinca J, Morena H, Fiolet JWT, Kleber AG, DeVries GP, Becher AE, Durrer D: The "border zone" in myocardial ischemia: an electrophysiologic, metabolic, and histochemical correlation in the pig heart. Circ Res **44:** 576, 1979
30. Brooks H, Al-Sadir J, Schwartz J, Rich B, Harper P, Resnekov L: Biventricular dynamics during quantitated anteroseptal infarction in the porcine heart. Am J Cardiol **36:** 765, 1975
31. Hearse DJ, Opie LH, Katzeff IE, Lubbe WF, Van Der Werff TJ, Peisach M, Boulle G: Characterization of the "border zone" in acute regional ischemia in the dog. Am J Cardiol **40:** 716, 1977
32. Janse MJ, Wilms-Schopman F: Effect of changes in perfusion pressure on the position of the electrophysiologic border zone in acute regional ischemia in isolated perfused dog and pig hearts. Am J Cardiol **50:** 74, 1982

33. Dehaan RL, Field J: Mechanisms of cardiac damage in anoxia. Am J Physiol **197:** 449, 1959
34. Hoffstein S, Weissman G, Fox AC: Lysosomes in myocardial infarction: studies by means of cytochemistry and subcellular fractionation, with observation on the effects of methylprednisone. Circulation **53**(suppl I): I-34, 1976
35. Bing OHL, Brooks WW, Messer JV: Heart muscle viability following hypoxia: protective effect of acidosis. Science **180:** 1296, 1973
36. Greene HL, Weisfeldt ML: Determinants of hypoxic and posthypoxic contracture. Am J Physiol **232:** H526, 1977
37. Lakatta EG, Nayler WG, Poole-Wilson PA: Calcium overload and mechanical function in post-hypoxic myocardium: biphasic effect of pH during hypoxia. Eur J Cardiol **10:** 77, 1979
38. Opie LH: Effects of regional ischemia on metabolism of glucose and fatty acids. Circ Res **38**(suppl I): I-52, 1975
39. Gevers W: Generation of protons by metabolic processes in heart cells. J Mol Cell Cardiol **9:** 867, 1979
40. Boyle PJ, Conway EJ: Potassium accumulation in muscle and associated changes. J Physiol **100:** 1, 1941
41. Case RB: Ion alterations during myocardial ischemia. Cardiology **56:** 245, 1971/1972
42. Mathur PP, Case RB: Phosphate loss during reversible myocardial ischemia. J Mol Cell Cardiol **5:** 375, 1973
43. Poole-Wilson PA: Measurement of myocardial intracellular pH in pathological states. J Mol Cell Cardiol **10:** 511, 1978
44. Case RB, Felix A, Castellana FS: Rate of rise in myocardial pCO_2 during early myocardial ischemia in the dog. Circ Res **45:** 324, 1979
45. Poole-Wilson PA, Cameron IR: Intracellular pH and K^+ of cardiac and skeletal muscle in acidosis and alkalosis. Am J Physiol **229:** 1305, 1975
46. Fenn WO: The carbon dioxide dissociation curve of nerve and muscle. Am J Physiol **85:** 207, 1928
47. Scherlag BJ, El-Sherif N, Hope R, Lazzara R: Characterization and localization of ventricular arrhythmias resulting from myocardial ischemia and infarction. Circ Res **35:** 372, 1974
48. Morena H, Janse MJ, Fiolet JWT, Krieger WJ, Crijans H, Durrer D: Comparison of the effects of regional ischemia, hypoxia, hyperkalemia, and acidosis on intracellular and extracellular potentials and metabolism in the isolated porcine heart. Circ Res **46:** 634, 1980
49. Cinca J, Figueras J, Senador G, Garcia-Moreno E, Salas A, Rius J: Transmural DC electrograms after coronary artery occlusion and latex embolization in pigs. Am J Physiol **246:** H475, 1984
50. Kleber AG, Janse MJ, Van Capelle FJL, Durrer D: Mechanism and time course of S-T and T-Q segment changes during acute regional myocardial ischemia in the pig heart determined by extracellular and intracellular recordings. Circ Res **42:** 603, 1978
51. Hirche HS, Bischoff A, Addicks K, Hartone S, Knopf H, McDonald FM: Acute myocardial ischemia in the anesthetized pig: effects of dextro- and racemic propranolol on myocardial catecholamine release. Fed Proc **43:** 3086, 1984
52. Weiss J, Shine KI: $[K^+]_o$ accumulation and electrophysiological alterations during early myocardial ischemia. Am J Physiol **243:** H318, 1982
53. Hoffman BF, Singer DH: Appraisal of the effects of catecholamines on cardiac electrical activity. Ann NY Acad Sci **139:** 914, 1967
54. Reuter H: Calcium channel modulation by neurotransmitters, enzymes and drugs. Nature **301:** 569, 1983
55. Demello WC: Modulation of junctional permeability. Fed Proc **43:** 2692, 1984
56. Cherbakoff A, Toyama S, Hamilton WF: Relationship between coronary sinus plasma potassium and cardiac arrhythmias. Circ Res **5:** 517, 1957
57. Harris SA, Bisteni A, Russell RA, Brigham JC, Firestone JF: Excitatory factors in ventricular tachycardia resulting from myocardial ischemia: potassium a major excitant. Science **119:** 200, 1954
58. Gettes LS, Hill JL, Saito T, Kagiyama Y: Factors related to vulnerability to arrhythmias in acute myocardial infarction. Am Heart J **103:** 667, 1982
59. Robertson RM, Breining JB, Robertson D: Chronic recurrent variant angina. South Med J **72:** 1297, 1979

Autonomic control of ventricular tachycardia: sympathetic neural influence on spontaneous tachycardia 24 hours after coronary occlusion

JAMES B. MARTINS, M.D.

ABSTRACT This study was performed to determine whether sympathetic nerves influence the rate of ventricular tachycardia occurring spontaneously in dogs 24 hr after occlusion of the anterior descending coronary artery. Seventeen chloralose-anesthetized dogs underwent activation mapping during spontaneous ventricular tachycardia with QRS morphologies similar to those recorded in the conscious state. Bilateral stellate ganglionectomy (n = 8) decreased mean arterial pressure from 71 ± 4 (mean ± SE) to 52 ± 5 mm Hg ($p < .001$) and heart rate from 121 ± 9 to 79 ± 15 beats/min ($p < .025$) by decreasing the number of complexes of ventricular tachycardia from 120 ± 9 to 49 ± 15 per minute ($p < .001$). Subsequent unilateral sympathetic nerve stimulation (n = 4) was shown to accelerate ventricular tachycardia foci originating from the ipsilateral aspect of the infarction. Regional sympathetic denervation (n = 7) was performed by application of phenol to the epicardium surrounding an electrode at the site of origin of at least one morphology of ventricular tachycardia. Mean arterial pressure did not change, but total heart rate decreased from 122 ± 9 to 106 ± 9 beats/min ($p < .01$) and the number of complexes of ventricular tachycardia with a morphology arising from the phenol-treated area fell from 68 ± 12 to 28 ± 9 ($p < .001$). Evidence for regional denervation was documented by prolongation of duration of electrograms and local repolarization times limited to the phenol-treated area. We conclude that sympathetic nerves directly control rate of spontaneous ventricular tachycardia 24 hr after myocardial infarction in the dog.
Circulation 72, No. 4, 933–942, 1985.

SYMPATHETIC neural influences importantly influence electrophysiologic changes in the ventricle during acute myocardial ischemia[1,2] and may modulate the occurrence of ventricular fibrillation.[3,4] Ventricular tachycardias occurring during the course of myocardial ischemia might also be modulated by sympathetic nerves. One such ventricular tachycardia occurs spontaneously 8 hr to 4 days after occlusion of the anterior descending coronary artery in the dog.[5] Recent studies suggest that this ventricular tachycardia originates in surviving subendocardial Purkinje fibers[6–11] due to triggered activity,[12] abnormal automaticity,[6–8,13] or both.[14] While studies in vitro suggest that these arrhythmogenic mechanisms are responsive to catecholamines,[15–18] sympathetic nerves may still not modulate this ventricular tachycardia if the neural transmitter does not reach the cells responsible for the tachycardia. This might occur if denervation produced by ischemia of cardiac nerves[19,20] occurred at the site of origin of the tachycardia. The purpose of the present study was to determine if sympathetic neural influences control the rate of ventricular tachycardia 24 hr after occlusion of the anterior descending coronary artery. Sympathetic neural influences were removed in two ways. Bilateral stellate ganglionectomy was performed, the effects of which could then be reversed by sympathetic nerve stimulation. To exclude hemodynamic effects of stellate ganglionectomy that may modify rate of ventricular tachycardia by changing the stretch of cardiac tissue,[21] irreversible but local sympathectomy limited to a focus of tachycardia was also produced by epicardial application of phenol.[22]

From the Department of Internal Medicine and Cardiovascular Center, University of Iowa, Iowa City, Iowa.

Supported in part by grant HL26567 from the National Heart, Lung, and Blood Institute, Bethesda, and funds from the Veterans Administration, Iowa City, and the American Heart Association, Iowa Affiliate, Des Moines. This work was done during Dr. Martins' tenure as a Clinician-Scientist awardee of the American Heart Association, Dallas.

Address for correspondence: James B. Martins, M.D., Cardiovascular Division, Department of Internal Medicine, University of Iowa Hospitals and Clinics, Iowa City, IA 52242.

Received March 12, 1985; revision accepted July 18, 1985.

Methods

General. Mongrel dogs of both sexes (n = 21) were anesthetized with droperidol (60 mg) and fentanyl (1.2 mg) and pentobarbital sodium (15 mg/kg) and mechanically ventilated. The heart of each was exposed through a left thoracotomy. The proximal left anterior descending coronary artery was bluntly dissected within 1 cm from the tip of the atrial appendage and proximal to the last major diagonal branch. A 21-gauge needle was placed along the artery and a 2-0 silk ligature was tied around the vessel and the needle. The needle was then withdrawn. This procedure resulted in a coronary stenosis that was maintained for 20 min. The vessel was then permanently occluded by another ligature. The ligature was always distal to the first septal perforator, as determined by subsequent necropsy. The chest was closed and the animal was allowed to recover.

Seventeen dogs survived to be studied 24 hr later; the others either developed ventricular fibrillation on occlusion of the coronary artery or were found dead the next day. Each was sedated with 2.3 mg/kg morphine and three surface electrocardiographic recordings were obtained at a paper speed of 25 mm/sec for 1 to 3 min (see below). Each dog was then anesthetized with α-chloralose (100 mg/kg). Thereafter, chloralose was administered by constant infusion at 8 mg/kg/hr to maintain anesthesia. Chloralose was prepared in a 1% solution dissolved in 40% polyethylene glycol (average molecular weight, 200). The trachea was intubated and the animal was ventilated with a volume-cycled respirator with air enriched with oxygen (2 liters/min). Tidal volume was regulated by measurement of arterial P_{CO_2} and 20 meq/hr iv sodium bicarbonate was given to maintain pH in the normal range.

The sternum was split and the pericardium was incised and sutured to the sternal incision to support the heart. A plastic sheet was placed over the sternal incision and a temperature probe was sutured to the pulmonary artery. Temperature was maintained constant at 37.5° C by adjustment of the distance of the operating table lamp to the heart. All animals underwent bilateral vagotomy by ligation and section of the mid cervical vagi. The femoral vein was cannulated to infuse 0.9% NaCl at 200 ml/hr and to administer drugs. The femoral artery was cannulated to record arterial pressure. Mean arterial pressure was measured by electrical filtering.

Electrophysiologic measurements. Surface electrocardiograms were recorded in the conscious and anesthetized state by use of standard surface leads I, aVF, and either V_5R or V_6. The surface morphologic appearance of each QRS complex in V_5R was categorized as either a right or left bundle branch block pattern according to whether the overall QRS deflection was positive or negative, respectively. In addition, the electrical axis in the frontal plane was determined to be in one of four quadrants (left and inferior, left and superior, right and inferior, or right and superior) by the major QRS deflection measured in leads I and aVF (figure 1).

After the chest was opened the sinus node was clamped and temporary overdrive atrial pacing was performed by attaching a bipolar electrode to the atrial appendage. Atrial pacing was performed with a programmable stimulator with constant-current outputs at two times diastolic threshold with pulses of 2 msec duration. Atrial pacing was performed at rates just greater than the rate of ventricular tachycardia (range of atrial pacing rates required was 150 to 200 beats/min) to measure His bundle, Purkinje activity, and QT intervals (see below). Bipolar His bundle recording wires (Teflon-coated stainless steel) were placed in the region of the His bundle via a needle passed through the right ventricular free wall and cavity.[23] Ventricular origin of wide QRS morphologies was documented by absence of His bundle deflections (which were present during overdrive atrial pacing; figure 1). Junctional origin of normal surface QRS morphologies was confirmed by normal HV intervals of that complex. Heart rate was determined by counting individual surface QRS complexes for 2 to 3 min in succession. The number of complexes of ventricular tachycardia of each morphology was also tallied and averaged per minute over the 2 to 3 min sampling period.

Activation mapping[24] was performed during spontaneous ventricular tachycardia observed during recordings made in dogs in the conscious state. Electrograms were filtered from 40 to 500 Hz, amplified, and registered on a storage oscilloscope and on an oscillographic recorder at paper speeds of 200 mm/sec. Bipolar electrograms were recorded from reference Teflon-coated stainless steel wire electrodes in the posterior left ventricular base and the outflow tract of the right ventricle and from a roving epicardial bipolar electrode (2 mm interelectrode distance) placed on the ventricular epicardium at up to 54 predetermined positions. The interval from the onset of the surface QRS to the intrinsicoid deflection on the roving electrogram was measured for each site. In this manner, the earliest epicardial electrical activity during a ventricular tachycardia of a particular morphology was determined. After this, a 16-pole electrode needle with 1 mm interelectrode spacing[25] was placed perpendicular to the epicardium in that site and endocardial and epicardial electrograms were recorded during spontaneous ventricular tachycardia. These positions on the needle were chosen as follows. At each needle site adjacent pairs of electrodes were recorded sequentially during atrial overdrive pacing. The endocardial bipolar electrograms were defined as those indicating the earliest electrical activation of all of that needle's pairs and

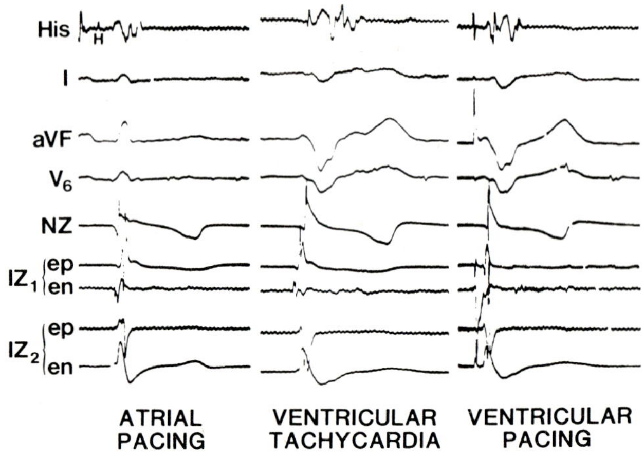

FIGURE 1. Recordings from one animal in our study. From top to bottom recordings are from the His bundle region and surface electrocardiographic recording leads I, aVF, and V_6 and intracardiac bipolar electrograms from the normal zone (NZ) and ischemic zone (IZ) both from epicardium (ep) and endocardium (en). *Left,* Recordings made during atrial pacing demonstrate a normal surface QRS activated via the His bundle (H). Note that endocardial electrogram from IZ_1 demonstrates a Purkinje potential preceding the ventricular muscle potential. *Middle,* Recordings during spontaneous ventricular tachycardia with a surface QRS of right and superior axis and right bundle branch block morphology. Prior activation mapping (not shown) demonstrated that the endocardial site of IZ_1 was the earliest electrical activity during tachycardia; electrical activation in endocardium of IZ_1 precedes activity in IZ_2 (only 1 cm away) and all other surface, intracardiac, and His bundle recordings. *Right,* Further demonstration that the electrode in endocardium of IZ_1 was near the site of origin of ventricular tachycardia of this morphology, since pacing from that electrode reproduced the same morphology as in the spontaneous tachycardia of the *middle* panel.

which frequently contained Purkinje spikes (figure 1).[26] These were usually located 7 to 8 mm in from the outermost epicardial electrode. Epicardial electrograms were taken from the outermost bipolar pair of electrodes and were the latest activated on that needle during atrial pacing rhythm. Additional multipolar electrodes were placed 1 cm from the original electrode position in four quadrants surrounding it. This procedure was repeated until the earliest electrical activity during ventricular tachycardia of a single QRS morphology was found surrounded by electrodes recording later activity (figure 1). This position was the presumed site of origin of ventricular tachycardia of that QRS morphology.

To confirm this position as the origin of a ventricular tachycardia of a particular morphology, pacing from the ventricular multipolar electrode needle was performed to produce the same surface morphology[10] (figure 1). A single electrode adjacent to the bipolar electrode recording earliest activity on each multipolar needle was used for pacing. This single electrode formed the cathode while the anode was a 7 mm^2 stainless steel electrode located in the subcutaneous tissue of the abdomen. Pacing was performed at two times diastolic threshold.

Local bipolar electrograms (1 mm interelectrode spacing) also were recorded for the purposes of measuring local electrophysiologic properties in the following manner. Overdrive atrial pacing was instituted at a rate just faster than that of the spontaneous ventricular tachycardia (range of basic cycle lengths required was 300 to 400 msec). Electrograms were filtered at from 1.2 to 500 Hz. Recordings were made at high gain to measure T waves on each bipolar electrogram at paper speeds of 500 mm/sec. Activation times to epicardium and endocardium were recorded from the His bundle deflection or onset of the surface QRS to the intrinsicoid deflection of each electrogram. Duration of individual electrograms was measured from the first to the last rapid deviation from the isoelectric line.[1] Local repolarization times on each individual bipolar electrogram were recorded from the onset of the local electrogram QRS to the peak or ending of the T wave (figure 2). Data from each electrogram recording between interventions was accepted only if pacing rates between interventions were constant, electrogram activation sequences remained constant, and electrogram morphologies remained unchanged.[27] All dogs in this study met these criteria.

Protocols. After activation mapping and recording of electrograms during atrial overdrive pacing, rates of spontaneous ventricular tachycardia were recorded over 2 to 3 min. Sympathectomy was then performed by one of two methods applied randomly to two groups of dogs. Stellate ganglionectomy was performed in eight dogs by isolation and incision of all proximal rami communicans from both right and left stellate ganglia; the anterior and posterior ansae were intact. In a subgroup of four of the original eight plus two additional animals, stimulation of the individual stellate ganglia was performed by placing bipolar stainless steel electrodes on the anterior ansa subclavii of each ganglion. Stimulation parameters were 4 msec pulses with suprathreshold currents at 1 to 8 Hz.

Regional sympathectomy was performed in seven dogs by application of 88% phenol to the epicardium surrounding an electrode recording the site of origin during a ventricular tachycardia of a particular morphology. The radius of the circle of phenol was 2 to 3 cm, as described previously.[22] Recording of electrograms and spontaneous rates of ventricular tachycardia was performed after epicardial temperature returned to the control level after replacement of the plastic sheet covering the sternal incision and 20 min after sympathectomy.

The dogs were killed with rapid ventricular pacing to produce ventricular fibrillation. The multipolar electrode sites were related to gross white and hemorrhagic areas of infarction.

Statistical analysis. The data are expressed as mean ± SE. The comparisons within groups were performed by Student's t test.[28]

Results

Mapping and gross anatomic data. In the conscious state just before study all 15 dogs from the original two groups had spontaneous ventricular tachycardia of one to five distinct QRS morphologies. One dog had five, one had four, two had three, five had two, and six had only one morphology of ventricular tachycardia. Of

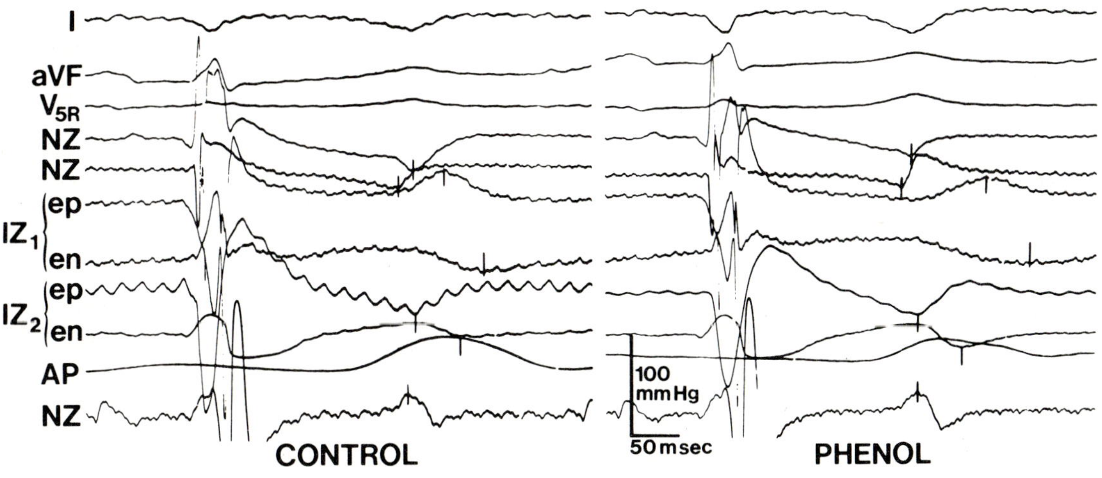

FIGURE 2. Surface and intracardiac bipolar electrograms taken from one dog in this study during overdrive atrial pacing. Tracing are labeled as in figure 1, except for the addition of aortic pressure, which is labeled AP. Intracardiac electrograms were recorded at high gain with filter settings from 1.2 to 500 Hz. Duration of local repolarization is indicated by the vertical bar located on each t wave. After phenol was applied to the epicardium surrounding the electrode in IZ_1, repolarization times in IZ_1 were prolonged compared with their control values as well as with values in other areas after phenol was applied. Aortic pressure did not change after phenol.

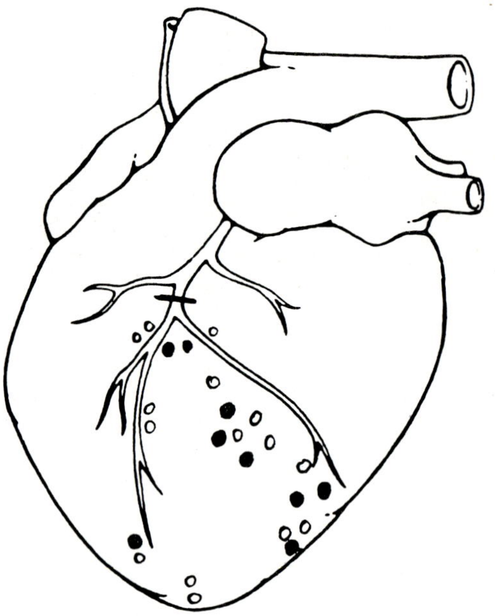

FIGURE 3. Schema of the anterior surface of the canine heart with the anterior descending coronary artery ligated (horizontal bar) just proximal to the last diagonal. The approximate sites of the original 24 ventricular tachycardias of different morphologies are shown by circles. In this report sites of origin along the anterior descending artery are described as arising from the septal, free wall side of the infarct, while sites of origin along the diagonal vessel are described as arising from the lateral aspect of the infarct. Filled circles indicate the sites that were denervated by epicardial application of phenol.

these 31 morphologies observed in the conscious state, 24 were fully mapped. During these tachycardias the sites of origin were always identified by a local endocardial bipolar electrogram that always coincided with or preceded the surface QRS by up to 20 msec (figure 1); no other electrical activity occurred earlier, including that activity on the same needle in the epicardium. The predominant morphology was the rightward and superior axis tachycardia with a right bundle branch block pattern that occurred in 13 dogs. Activation mapping suggested that sites of origin of this tachycardia were near the subendocardium in the border of the anteroseptal infarct ranging over the left lateral, free wall aspect from base to apex (figure 3). The second most common morphology (n = 7) was a right and inferior axis tachycardia with a right bundle branch block pattern; this tachycardia appeared to originate on the endocardium ranging over the septal, free wall side of the infarction (figure 3). Four animals had ventricular tachycardia of a left-axis, left bundle branch block morphology that appeared to originate from the inferior septal, free wall side of the infarction (figure 3). Therefore, the origins of ventricular tachycardia studied occupied all possible sites on the perimeter of the infarction conforming to the left anterior descending perfusion bed.

The rate of ventricular tachycardia before anesthesia averaged 156 ± 6/min, but after anesthesia and during mapping the average rate was 121 ± 7/min ($p < .01$). To examine the stability of this tachycardia, six dogs were observed for 1 hr without intervention under the experimental conditions of constant infusion of chloralose dissolved in polyethylene glycol. Rate of tachycardia did not change (123 ± 15/min at initial control and 122 ± 10/min at late control, $p > .5$). In addition, the ratio of individual morphologies to the overall rate of ventricular tachycardia was also constant. To determine whether polyethylene glycol alone would influence rate of tachycardia, we also administered a constant infusion of polyethylene glycol only to two dogs. In these animals rate of ventricular tachycardia increased by 12 and 24 beats/min 1 hr after control rates of 180 and 128 beats/min, respectively, reflecting the lack of chloralose infusion. Thus, polyethylene glycol alone produced no effect on rate of ventricular tachycardia.

Effects of global cardiac sympathetic denervation. Bilateral stellate ganglionectomy (n = 8) decreased both heart rate (by 35%) and complexes of tachycardia per minute (by 60% table 1); in seven of eight dogs there was a decrease in rate while in one there was an increase. The overall heart rate decreased to a lesser extent than the rate of ventricular tachycardia after stellectomy because of the appearance of frequent junctional complexes. In addition, the shortest cycle length of ventricular tachycardia (in msec) was pro-

TABLE 1
Effects of global cardiac sympathetic denervation

	Control	Stellate ganglio-nectomy	p value
Spontaneous rhythm			
Heart rate (bpm)	121±9	79±15	<.025
VT complexes (per min)[A]	120±9	49±15	<.001
Shortest VT cycle length (msec)	464±49	647±93	<.025
Overdrive pacing			
Mean arterial pressure (mm Hg)	71±4	52±5	<.001
Activation time (msec)			
To normal zone	28±5	29±5	>.09
To ischemic zone	26±4	29±4	<.01
Electrogram duration (msec)			
Normal zone	21±4	20±4	>.2
Ischemic zone	21±3	24±4	<.01
Repolarization time (msec)			
Normal zone	184±6	192±8	<.01
Ischemic zone	189±9	206±11	<.01

[A]Excluding only junctional complexes.

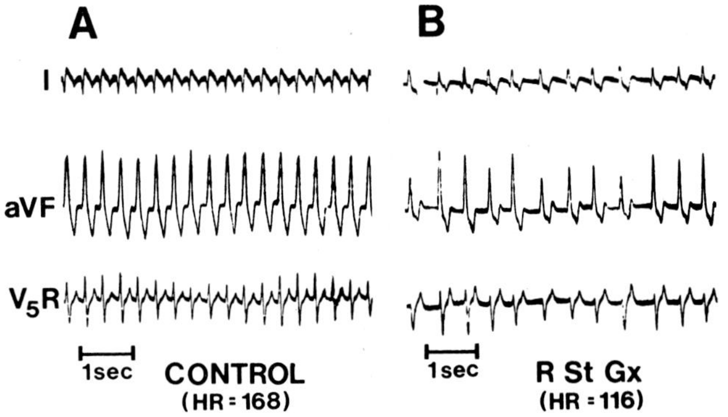

FIGURE 4. Surface electrocardiographic recordings from one animal in our study. *Left,* In the control state, ventricular tachycardia with a right and inferior axis, right bundle branch block morphology was recorded. *Right,* After right stellate ganglionectomy (RSTGX), heart rate slowed. After left stellate ganglionectomy no further slowing occurred (data not shown).

longed by 40%. During continuous recording of bipolar electrograms from sites of origin of tachycardia, there was no evidence of endocardial electrical activity without an associated surface QRS; thus, there was no macro exit block (block from the endocardial origin to the rest of the heart) produced by stellate ganglionectomy. During atrial pacing mean arterial pressure fell by 27% and repolarization time was prolonged in both normal and ischemic zones (by 4% and 9%, respectively; table 1). Activation time and electrogram duration in normal zones did not change with stellate ganglionectomy, but activation time and electrogram duration in ischemic zones were prolonged by 12% and 14%, respectively (table 1).

To exclude the possibility that the results of stellate ganglionectomy were due to deterioration of the preparation, sympathetic nerve stimulation was performed in a subgroup of six animals. During atrial pacing, bilateral sympathetic nerve stimulation shortened duration of bipolar electrograms toward control from 25 $\pm$ 3 to 23 $\pm$ 3 msec in ischemic zones ($p < .025$ compared with data in table 1). Similarly, local repolarization time in ischemic zones was shortened from 211 $\pm$ 8 to 188 $\pm$ 6 msec ($p < .01$). During spontaneous rhythm, sympathetic stimulation produced a junctional tachycardia at a faster rate than the prestellectomy ventricular tachycardia in the first two dogs of the initial eight. Therefore, analysis of tachycardia response to individual right or left sympathetic stimulation was not performed until the last two dogs. The first of these dogs had ventricular tachycardia of a single morphology that slowed with right but not left stellate ganglionectomy (figure 4); stimulation of the right sympathetic nerves alone reproducibly returned tachycardia with an origin on the septal free wall side of the infarct to the prestellectomy rate (figure 5). Three more animals then underwent individual right and left sympathetic nerve simulation to determine whether ventricular tachycardia originating from the septal side of the infarct might accelerate with right sympathetic stimulation and whether ventricular tachycardia from the lateral aspect of the infarct might accelerate with left sympathetic stimulation. Table 2 lists data demonstrating that either right or left sympathetic stimulation could reproducibly accelerate the rate of tachycardia, but that the specific origin of the tachycardia that is accelerated is predicted by its relationship to the infarction. Thus, sympathetic nerve stimulation demonstrated return of electrophysiologic

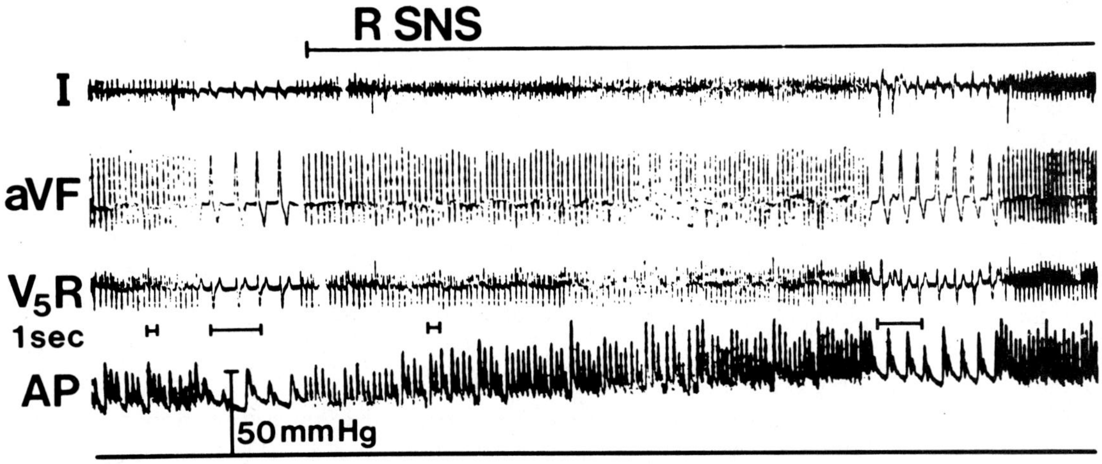

FIGURE 5. Recording from the same animal as in figure 4. Surface electrocardiographic recordings and aortic pressure were recorded simultaneously at two paper speeds indicated by the 1 sec time lines. The horizontal line at the bottom is 0 aortic pressure. On the left hand portion of the tracing ventricular tachycardia after bilateral stellate ganglionectomy is shown. The right hand portion of the figure was recorded during continuous right sympathetic stimulation (RSNS). Sympathetic stimulation produced increases in rate of tachycardia and arterial pressure.

TABLE 2
Effects of right or left sympathetic nerve stimulation on rate of ventricular tachycardia (VT)

Dog No.	Denervation	Right SNS (VT from septal side)	Left SNS (VT from lateral side)
1	130	180	—
2	<30	170	80
3	150	180	220
4	<120	133	170

SNS = sympathetic nerve stimulation.

properties and rate of tachycardia toward the prestellectomy level.

Effects of regional sympathetic denervation. After application of phenol (n = 7 dogs) to the epicardium surrounding an electrode near the site of origin of ventricular tachycardia of at least one morphology, overall heart rate and the number of complexes of tachycardia with that morphology decreased by 13% and 60%, respectively (figure 6, table 3). Six of seven dogs had a decrease in rate of ventricular tachycardia while in one dog rate did not change; in the latter the origin of tachycardia was mapped to the inferior and septal, free wall side of the infarction. In addition, the shortest cycle length also increased. During continuous recording of bipolar electrograms from ventricular tachycardia origins there was no evidence of endocardial electrical activity without an associated surface QRS; thus, there was no evidence of macro exit block (block from endocardial origin to the rest of the heart) produced by

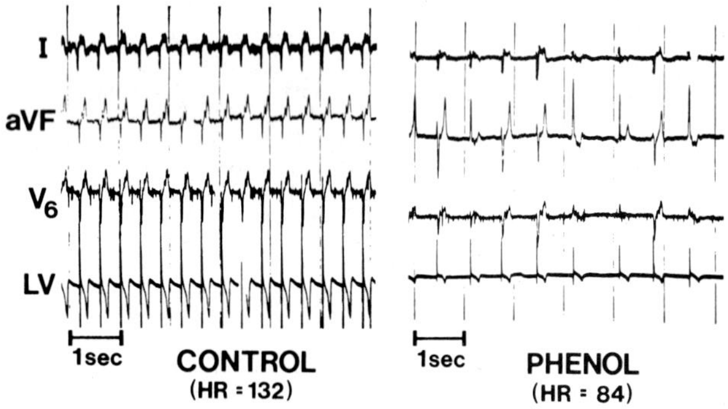

FIGURE 6. Recordings from a dog with regional denervation of the area from which tachycardia originated. Surface electrocardiographic leads were recorded with a bipolar left ventricular electrogram (LV). *Left,* In the control state, a uniform ventricular tachycardia with a rightward and superior axis, right bundle branch block morphology was recorded continuously. *Right,* After phenol was applied around the electrode indicating earliest electrical activity of this morphology of ventricular tachycardia, tachycardia was markedly slowed such that only the first, third, fourth, and seventh complexes reflect the control morphology. Other complexes reflect other foci of ventricular tachycardia or junctional escape complexes. The left ventricular electrogram decreased in size because of the change in amplification.

TABLE 3
Effects of regional cardiac sympathetic denervation

	Control	Phenol application	p value
Spontaneous rhythm			
Heart rate (bpm)	122±9	106±9	<.01
VT complexes (per min)[A]	68±12	28±9	<.001
Shortest VT cycle length (msec)[A]	429±27	505±32	<.01
During overdrive pacing			
Mean arterial pressure (mm Hg)	78±4	80±4	>.4
Activation time (msec)			
To normal zone	36±9	34±9	>.5
To ischemic zone	43±8	43±7	>.5
Electrogram duration (msec)			
Normal zone	17±4	17±4	>.4
Ischemic zone	21±3	24±3	<.06
Repolarization time (msec)			
Normal zone	184±9	186±11	>.4
Ischemic zone	212±14	232±17	<.025

[A]With morphology from treated focus(i), excludes junctional and other ectopic foci.

regional denervation. Similar to stellectomy, duration of electrograms in the ischemic zone was prolonged by 14% and local repolarization time in the phenol-treated area was prolonged by 9% (figure 2, table 3). In contrast to results with stellate ganglionectomy, mean arterial pressure, repolarization time in the normal zone, and activation time to the ischemic zone did not change after application of phenol.

In one dog isoproterenol was infused at 5 μm/min to determine whether the phenol-treated area would respond to a sympathetic agonist. Isoproterenol accelerated other foci of ventricular tachycardia that were not mapped or treated with phenol. This prevented assessment of the effect of isoproterenol on the rate of ventricular tachycardia originating from the phenol-treated site. However, as has been shown in previous experiments,[22] during atrial pacing isoproterenol shortened both duration of bipolar electrograms and local repolarization time in the phenol-treated ischemic zone. In addition, bilateral sympathetic nerve stimulation did not shorten duration of bipolar electrograms or repolarization time limited to the phenol-treated area, confirming the existence of local denervation.[22] Therefore, the electrophysiologic response of the denervated area to isoproterenol was normal during atrial pacing. However, because of acceleration of other foci of ventricular tachycardia, we could not assess the effect of isoproterenol on the tachycardia from the denervated site.

Discussion

This study demonstrates two new observations. First, sympathetic nerves control rate of ventricular tachycardia originating from endocardial Purkinje fibers 24 hr after coronary occlusion in the dog. Second, these effects are mediated because of the direct influence of sympathetic nerves on the focus of the tachycardia and not indirectly through hemodynamic changes.

Methodologic considerations. The origin of the ventricular tachycardia was determined by activation mapping in an effort to find the earliest electrogram activity before the onset of the surface QRS. This method, involving a single roving electrode, is valid for use under conditions of a continuously repetitive tachycardia in which information from many cardiac cycles can be added together, comparing many recordings of the roving electrode, such as in the case of patients with reentrant ventricular tachycardia when intraoperative activation mapping is used to guide antiarrhythmic surgery.[24, 29] The limitation of epicardial activation mapping without heart-lung bypass is that foci of tachycardia arising from the intraventricular septum are difficult to characterize accurately because the interventricular surface is not accessible except by individual plunge electrodes.

In the present study we specifically did not perform extrastimulus pacing protocols such as those used to record refractoriness in an effort to prevent reentry tachycardias. In fact, we believe that the tachycardias studied in our preparation were not reentrant. The evidence for this assertion is based upon previous studies in the same preparation of myocardial ischemia in which both spontaneous and induced tachycardias were studied. Thus, the spontaneous tachycardias were multiformed and comparatively slow and hemodynamically tolerated,[11, 30] had radial activation spread away from a small region (<1 cm),[11] and were not able to be terminated or initiated by pacing.[11, 17, 30]

The phenol denervation technique used in these experiments produces electrophysiologic effects indirectly by interruption of epicardial sympathetic nerves en route to a test electrode. This electrode was placed in an area that displayed the earliest endocardial electrical activity during ventricular tachycardia compared with bipolar electrograms recorded from multipolar plunge electrodes surrounding it by only 1 cm. The phenol was applied in 3 to 5 mm thick line inscribed on a circle with a radius of 2 to 3 cm centered on the test electrode.[22] Since phenol produced necrosis to a depth of only 0.25 mm,[31] we would not expect direct effects on ventricular tachycardia originating in endocardial fibers 2 cm or more away. Indeed, when electrophysiologic measurements were performed in ischemic regions of reserpine-treated dogs, phenol applied as described herein produced no electrophysiologic effect.[1] However, it is theoretically possible that tachycardias originating in the endocardium but exiting via narrow layers of viable epicardium that range from less than 1 to 2 mm in thickness[11, 32] could be directly slowed by epicardial phenol, which produces macro exit block, i.e., block of endocardial wave fronts in epicardium 1 to 2 cm away. In no experiment did we find evidence of macro exit block as might be evidenced by endocardial electrical activity continuing at the presympathectomy rate while tachycardia slowed. Thus, application of phenol to the epicardium as performed in the present experiments did not produce electrophysiologic effects or slowing of ventricular tachycardia by direct actions on ischemic or normal myocardium.

In this study the evidence for regional sympathetic denervation with application of phenol was based on electrophysiologic criteria. This was reasonable considering the following. The electrophysiologic effects of regional sympathetic denervation are well described in normal muscle; refractory period responses to sympathetic nerve stimulation are eliminated where norepinephrine concentrations and catecholamine histofluorescence are also absent.[22] In addition, in the present study phenol produced electrophysiologic effects compatible with those of sympathetic denervation, which have been described previously in ischemic ventricles. In the present study phenol tended to prolong local electrogram durations and local repolarization times were definitely prolonged. These data are compatible with loss of sympathetic nerve influence, which has been shown previously to improve ischemic zone conduction by shortening overdrive cycle lengths, resulting in Wenckebach conduction delay,[33] or by shortening electrogram duration, as in the present study. Also, as shown in this study, sympathetic denervation produced by stellate ganglionectomy prolongs local repolarization times, and we and others have shown[34] that subsequent sympathetic nerve stimulation shortens repolarization time or refractoriness.[34] While these electrophysiologic effects are evidence of sympathetic denervation, they do not necessarily suggest mechanisms by which sympathetic denervation affected the rate of ventricular tachycardia.

While the application of phenol is an effective technique to produce regional sympathetic denervation, its use could be limited by the fact that it cannot be applied to the intraventricular septum. Therefore, phenol applied to the entire epicardial surface could not be expected to produce results comparable to stellate ganglionectomy since morphologies of ventricular tachycardia that arise from septal origins inaccessible to phenol may not be denervated. In addition, one would like to denervate only a portion of the ischemic zone to compare denervated with innervated ischemic responses. However, denervation produced by phenol requires a 2 to 3 cm circle to ensure transmural denervation.[22] Thus, it is difficult to consistently and effectively denervate a small area in order to leave a portion of the ischemic zone innervated (although this occasionally occurs; figure 2). Therefore, comparisons between innervated and denervated ischemic zones in the same heart are difficult with the phenol technique.

Another methodologic consideration is that we produced acute sympathetic denervation. Effects of chronic denervation may have produced different results since it may be more effective in preventing ventricular fibrillation associated with acute ischemia.[35] Chronic denervation applied before coronary occlusion may simply decrease size of infarction[36] such that the same arrhythmias may not be present or significantly altered as a result of the procedure.[37] In addition, supersensitivity resulting from chronic denervation may alter responsiveness to circulating catecholamines.

Effects of sympathetic denervation on ventricular tachycardia. Sympathetic denervation produced by either method in the present study slowed the rate of ventricular tachycardia. The effects of stellate ganglionectomy were reversible in that electrical stimulation of the distal cut end of one or both of the stellate ganglia reversed electrophysiologic changes and returned the rate of tachycardia to the predenervation level. The changes in hemodynamics produced by stellate ganglionectomy may alone modulate the rate of automaticity by the amount of stretch of Purkinje fibers.[21] The results of phenol denervation argue against these hemodynamic mechanisms because there was no change in arterial pressure during atrial overdrive pacing. Therefore, the phenol studies support the role of a direct action of sympathetic efferent nerves acting on a tachycardia focus.

The precise mechanism(s) by which sympathetic denervation modulate(s) rate of ventricular tachycardia is unclear. There may be at least two direct effects of sympathetic nerves on foci of tachycardia. One effect could be direct action on the Purkinje fiber(s) that are abnormally automatic[6, 16] or triggered.[15] Another effect might be modulation of conduction out of the focus of ventricular tachycardia such that micro exit block (≤ 2 mm) of some of the impulses may occur, as has been reported with nifedipine in vitro.[38] In the present study these two mechanisms could not be differentiated. However, the possibility that conduction in the ischemic zone is modulated by sympathetic influences is supported by the present and other studies that have shown that duration of electrograms in the ischemic zone[1] or the cycle length at which conduction delay occurs[33] is modified by sympathetic nerves.

In the present study we found that ventricular tachycardia originating around the entire border of the infarction responded to sympathetic denervation. This border origin of tachycardia helps to explain why the ventricular tachycardia responds to sympathetic denervation, since the center of the infarction is thought to be denervated.[19] Moreover, sympathetic innervation to the anterior ventricles is redundant, coming from both right and left ganglia.[27, 39, 40] This distribution of innervation with superimposed ischemia suggests a possible mechanism by which sympathetic innervation could be maintained in border areas. Ischemic damage could interfere with neural pathways from the left stellate ganglion en route to septal, free wall aspects of the infarction, since they traverse the ischemic zone,[20] while the right neural pathways to septal sites would remain intact. The converse could also be true for right sympathetic denervation, with the left innervation remaining intact to lateral areas of infarction. This hypothesis is suggested by the observation that ventricular tachycardia originating from the septal free wall side of the infarct accelerates during right sympathetic nerve stimulation. The converse also appears to be true (table 2). Thus, it appears that the highly selective[39, 40] cardiac control by sympathetic nerves may be even more selective after myocardial infarction such that sympathetic nerves on one side may only modulate the rate of ventricular tachycardia originating from sites of origin on the ipsilateral aspect of the infarct. Further work on this hypothesis is needed for confirmation.

Possible clinical correlations. We speculate that patients suffering from acute myocardial infarction may have ventricular tachycardia similar to that recorded herein 24 hr after onset of infarction. This tachycardia is not induced or terminated by pacing,[41] appears multiform,[42] and is not necessarily associated with hemodynamic deterioration or subsequent development of ventricular fibrillation.[43] The rhythms in the dog are faster than those reported for humans, but this may result from the prior performance of thoracotomy in the dog, which may increase sympathetic influence and accelerate the tachycardia.

Recent studies in patients[42] suggest that verapamil

may be effective in eliminating these multiform accelerated idioventricular rhythms. This study suggests the possibility that other interventions that impair sympathetic neural activity or block effects of sympathetic neural transmitter may also slow these rhythms.

It is tempting to consider the possibility that local denervation might be applied to the treatment of ventricular tachycardia in general as a therapeutic measure. It must be remembered, however, that reinnervation may occur in previously denervated areas as early as 6 to 9 months after denervation.[44]

I thank Greg Neighbors, Steve Greif, and Michael T. Leonard for technical assistance and Linda Bang for secretarial assistance.

References

1. Martins JB, Mueller TM, Zipes DP: Sympathetic denervation limited to a region of acutely ischemic canine myocardium increases excitability threshold and duration of bipolar electrograms. Am J Cardiol **51:** 1768, 1983
2. Ruffy R, Lovelace DE, Knoebel SB, Zipes DP: Influence of secobarbital and α-chloralose, and of vagal and sympathetic interruption, on left ventricular activation after acute coronary artery occlusion in the dog. Circ Res **48:** 884, 1981
3. Martins JB: Sympathetic influences in myocardial ischemia: possible mechanisms of arrhythmogenesis. Cardiol Clin **1:** 51, 1983
4. Corr PB, Gillis RA: Autonomic neural influences on the dysrhythmias resulting from myocardial infarction. Circ Res **43:** 1, 1978
5. Harris AS: Delayed development of ventricular ectopic rhythms following experimental coronary occlusion. Circulation **1:** 1318, 1950
6. Lazzara R, El-Sherif N, Scherlag BJ: Electrophysiological properties of canine Purkinje cells in one-day-old myocardial infarction. Circ Res **33:** 722, 1973
7. Friedman PL, Stewart JR, Fenoglio JJ, Wit AL: Survival of subendocardial Purkinje fibers after extensive myocardial infarction in dogs: In vitro and in vivo correlations. Circ Res **33:** 597, 1973
8. Friedman PL, Stewart JR, Wit AL: Spontaneous and induced cardiac arrhythmias in subendocardial Purkinje fibers surviving extensive myocardial infarction in dogs. Circ Res **33:** 612, 1973
9. Scherlag BJ, El-Sherif N, Hope R, Lazzara R: Characterization and localization of ventricular arrhythmias resulting from myocardial ischemia and infarction. Circ Res **35:** 372, 1974
10. Horowitz LN, Spear JF, Moore EN: Subendocardial origin of ventricular arrhythmias in 24-hour-old experimental myocardial infarction. Circulation **53:** 56, 1976
11. El-Sherif N, Mehra R, Gough WB, Zeiler RH: Ventricular activation patterns of spontaneous and induced ventricular rhythms in canine one-day-old myocardial infarction: evidence for focal and reentrant mechanisms. Circ Res **51:** 152, 1982
12. El-Sherif N, Gough WB, Zeiler RH, Mehra R: Triggered ventricular rhythms in 1-day-old myocardial infarction in the dog. Circ Res **52:** 566, 1983
13. Marech H, Dangman KH, Danilo P, Rosen MR: An evaluation of automaticity and triggered activity in the canine heart 1 to 4 days after myocardial infarction. Circulation **71:** 1224, 1985
14. Constantin L, Leonard MT, Martins JB: Mechanisms of spontaneous ventricular tachycardia in one day old canine myocardial infarction. Clin Res **32:** 729, 1984 (abst)
15. Wit AL, Fenoglio JJ, Wagner BM, Bassett AL: Electrophysiological properties of cardiac muscle in the anterior mitral valve leaflet and the adjacent atrium in the dog. Circ Res **32:** 731, 1973
16. Pappano AJ, Carmeliet EE: Epinephrine and the pacemaking mechanisms at plateau potentials in sheep cardiac Purkinje fibers. Pfluegers Arch **382:** 17, 1979
17. Davis J, Glassman R, Wit AL: Method for evaluating the effects of antiarrhythmic drugs on ventricular tachycardias with different electrophysiologic characteristics and different mechanisms in the infarcted canine heart. Am J Cardiol **49:** 1176, 1982
18. Constantin L, Martins JB: Beta adrenergic influences in the ischemic zone control rate of spontaneous ventricular tachycardia occurring 24 hours after experimental coronary occlusion. Fed Proc **43:** 1009, 1984 (abst)
19. Mathes P, Gudjarnason S: Changes in norepinephrine stores in the canine heart following experimental myocardial infarction. Am Heart J **81:** 211, 1971
20. Barber MJ, Mueller TM, Henry DP, Felten SY, Zipes DP: Transmural myocardial infarction in the dog produces sympathectomy in noninfarcted myocardium. Circulation **67:** 787, 1983
21. Singer DH, Lazarra R, Hoffman BF: Inter-relationships between automaticity and conduction in Purkinje fibers. Circ Res **21:** 537, 1967
22. Martins JB, Zipes DP: Epicardial phenol interrupts refractory period responses to sympathetic but not vagal stimulation in canine left ventricular epicardium and endocardium. Circ Res **47:** 33, 1980
23. Scherlag BJ, Kosowsky BD, Damato AN: A technique for ventricular pacing from the His bundle of the intact heart. J Appl Physiol **22:** 584, 1967
24. Horowitz LN, Josephson ME, Harken AH: Epicardial and endocardial activation during sustained ventricular tachycardia in man. Circulation **61:** 1227, 1980
25. Kasell J, Gallagher JJ: Construction of a multipolar needle electrode for activation study of the heart. Am J Physiol **233:** H312, 1977
26. Martins JB, Zipes DP: Effects of sympathetic and vagal nerves on recovery properties of the endocardium and epicardium of the canine left ventricle. Circ Res **46:** 100, 1980
27. Martins JB, Zipes DP, Lund DD: Distribution of local repolarization changes produced by efferent vagal stimulation in the canine ventricles. J Am Coll Cardiol **2:** 1191, 1983
28. Steel RGD, Torrie JH: Principles and procedures of statistics. New York, 1960, McGraw-Hill, pp 99–156
29. Miller JM, Kienzle MG, Harken AH, Josephson ME: Morphologically distinct sustained ventricular tachycardias in coronary artery disease: significance and surgical results. J Am Coll Cardiol **4:** 1073, 1984
30. Scherlag BJ, Kabell G, Brachmann J, Harrison L, Lazzara R: Mechanisms of spontaneous and induced ventricular arrhythmias in the 24 hour infarcted dog heart. Am J Cardiol **51:** 207, 1983
31. Kaye MP, Brynjolfsson GG, Geis WP: Chemical epicardiectomy. Cardiologia **53:** 139, 1968
32. Wit AL, Allessie MA, Bonke FIM, Lammers W, Smeets J, Fenoglio JJ: Electrophysiologic mapping to determine the mechanism of experimental ventricular tachycardia initiated by premature impulses. Am J Cardiol **49:** 166, 1982
33. El-Sherif N: Reentrant ventricular arrhythmias in the late myocardial infarction period 6. Effect of the autonomic system. Circulation **58:** 103, 1978
34. Gaide MS, Myerburg RJ, Kozlovskis PL, Bassett AL: Elevated sympathetic response of epicardium proximal to healed myocardial infarction. Am J Physiol **245:** H646, 1983
35. Ebert PA, Vanderbeek RB, Allgood RJ, Sabiston DC: Effect of chronic cardiac denervation on arrhythmias after coronary artery ligation. Cardiovasc Res **4:** 141, 1970
36. Jones CE, Beck LY, DuPont E, Barnes GE: Effects of coronary ligation on the chronically sympathectomized dog ventricle. Am J Physiol **4:** H429, 1978
37. Harris AS, Estandia A, Tillotson RF: Ventricular ectopic rhythms and ventricular fibrillation following cardiac sympathectomy and coronary occlusion. Am J Physiol **165:** 505, 1951
38. Gough WB, Zeiler RH, El-Sherif N: Effects of nifedipine on triggered activity in 1-day-old myocardial infarction in dogs. Am J Cardiol **53:** 303, 1984
39. Yanowitz F, Preston JB, Abildskov JA: Functional distribution of right and left stellate innervation of the ventricles. Circ Res **18:** 416, 1966
40. Randall WC, Szentivanyi M, Pace JB, Wechsler JS, Kaye MP: Patterns of sympathetic nerve projection into the canine heart. Circ Res **22:** 315, 1968
41. Wellens HJJ, Lie KI, Durrer D: Further observations on ventricular tachycardia as studied by electrical stimulation off the heart: chron-

ic recurrent ventricular tachycardia and ventricular tachycardia during acute myocardial infarction. Circulation **49:** 647, 1974
42. Sclarovsky S, Strasberg B, Fuchs J, Lewin RF, Arditi A, Klainman E, Kracoff OH, Agmon J: Multiform accelerated idioventricular rhythm in acute myocardial infarction: electrocardiographic characteristics and response to verapamil. Am J Cardiol **52:** 43, 1983
43. Bigger JT Jr, Dresdale RJ, Heissenbuttel RH, Weld FM, Wit AL: Ventricular arrhythmias in ischemic heart disease: mechanism, prevalence, significance and management. Prog Cardiovasc Dis **19:** 255, 1977
44. Kaye MP, Randall WC, Hageman GR, Geis WP, Priola DV: Chronology and mode of reinnervation of the surgically denervated canine heart: functional and chemical correlates. Am J Physiol **233:** H431, 1977

Circulation

VOL 72 NO 5
NOVEMBER 1985

An Official Journal of the American Heart Association, Inc.®

FEATURES

Atherogenic lipoproteins and coronary artery disease: concepts derived from recent advances in cellular and molecular biology

ROBERT W. MAHLEY, M.D., PH.D.

RECENT ADVANCES have contributed to our understanding of lipoproteins, their metabolism, and their involvement in atherogenesis (for review see refs. 1 to 6). In this review, attention will be focused on specific types of lipoproteins and the mechanisms whereby they may be either atherogenic or antiatherogenic. Human genetic diseases of lipid metabolism and diet-induced changes in lipoproteins have provided unique insights.

Atherosclerotic lesions, as they occur in man or as induced by high-fat, high-cholesterol diets in experimental animals, share many common properties. Narrowing of the vessel lumen is characterized by the deposition of cholesterol in and around cells of the arterial wall in association with cellular proliferation and fibrosis. The cholesterol that accumulates in the arterial wall is derived from plasma lipoproteins; therefore, to understand the mechanisms involved in atherogenesis, it is important to identify the specific lipoproteins responsible for the delivery of cholesterol to the cells and to identify the cell type responsible for the accumulation of the cholesterol. Lipid transport into and out of the vessel wall appears to be a constant and dynamic process. Disease of clinical significance develops when influx and deposition of cholesterol exceeds egress of cholesterol from the arterial wall. The hyperlipidemia that develops in the genetic diseases to be discussed, or that develops with the consumption of high levels of fat and cholesterol, accelerates the lipid deposition and upsets the balance between influx and egress.

Plasma lipoproteins and their metabolism. A brief consideration of the normally occurring major plasma lipoproteins and their metabolism[4] is essential for understanding the role of specific lipoproteins in atherogenesis. Chylomicrons are synthesized by the intestine to transport dietary triglyceride and cholesterol. As they circulate in the plasma compartment, the triglycerides are hydrolyzed by the action of lipoprotein lipase, resulting in the production of cholesterol-enriched chylomicron remnants. The chylomicron remnants are rapidly cleared from the plasma by the liver (figure 1, step 1), and their cholesterol converted to bile acids and excreted or used in membrane and hepatic lipoprotein biosynthesis. Very low–density lipoproteins (VLDLs) are triglyceride-rich particles synthesized by the liver. As the VLDLs circulate, they are acted upon by lipases, which liberates the fatty acids for use as an energy source in various tissues, and are converted to intermediate-density lipoproteins (IDLs). The IDLs are either removed from plasma by the liver (figure 1, step 2) or are converted to low-density lipoproteins (LDLs) by further action of the lipases (figure 1, step 3). By virtue of the removal of triglyceride from the VLDLs, the IDLs and LDLs become enriched in cholesterol. The LDLs are the end product of VLDL catabolism and are the major cholesterol-transporting lipoproteins in the plasma. They are catabolized by both the liver and extrahepatic tissues (figure 1, step 4). High-density lipoproteins (HDLs) are derived from several sources and appear to play a dynamic role in acquiring and redistributing cholesterol among cells (see figure 2, to be discussed below).

Each of the lipoproteins possess one or more protein constituents called apolipoproteins. An important function of certain apolipoproteins is to mediate the binding of the lipoproteins to specific receptors on the surface of cells. Receptor-mediated uptake of lipoproteins by cells is the mechanism by which lipoproteins

From the Gladstone Foundation Laboratories for Cardiovascular Disease, Cardiovascular Research Institute, Departments of Pathology and Medicine, University of California, San Francisco.

Address for correspondence: Robert W. Mahley, M.D., Ph.D., Gladstone Foundation Laboratories, P.O. Box 40608, San Francisco, CA 94140.

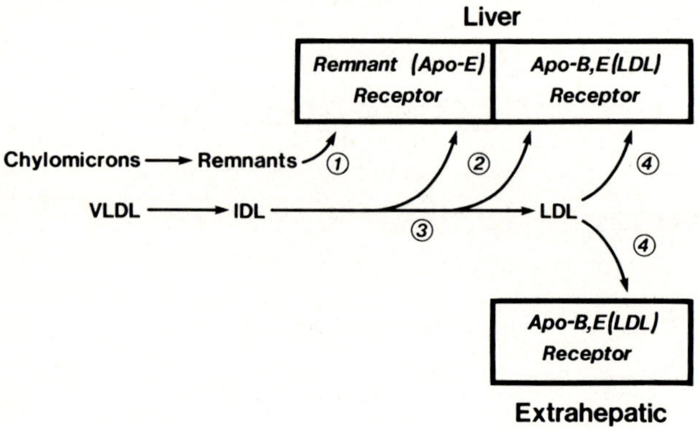

FIGURE 1. General scheme of lipoprotein metabolism.

are cleared from the plasma and catabolized by the cells.[2,4] The two apolipoproteins that have been shown to mediate binding to the lipoprotein receptors are apolipoprotein E (apo-E) and apolipoprotein B (apo-B). Apo-E is the protein determinant responsible for receptor-mediated uptake of chylomicron remnants and a subclass of HDL, the HDL-with apo-E. Apo-B is responsible for mediating receptor binding of LDL. Either apo-B or apo-E appears to be involved in mediating uptake of IDL.

Two distinct cell surface receptors are involved in lipoprotein metabolism (figure 1). The apo-B,E(LDL) receptor, as originally described by Goldstein, Brown, and associates,[1,7] interacts with either apo-B– or apo-E–containing lipoproteins.[2] They are present within the liver and most extrahepatic tissues. A second receptor that appears to be unique to the liver is referred to as the chylomicron remnant receptor (a receptor postulated to be the apo-E receptor).[2] This receptor interacts with apo-E–containing lipoproteins but not with apo-B–containing LDL.

Atherogenic and antiatherogenic lipoproteins. Two genetic diseases of lipoprotein metabolism (type III hyperlipoproteinemia and familial hypercholesterolemia) are associated with accelerated atherosclerosis. Although these relatively uncommon disorders are not responsible for large numbers of patients with coronary artery disease, they provide key insights into the role of specific lipoproteins in atherogenesis. The importance of understanding these disorders lies in the close parallels between the lipoproteins seen in these genetic disorders and those induced by the consumption of diets high in saturated fat and cholesterol. Changes in lipoproteins induced by diet are a major factor responsible for the widespread hypercholesterolemia seen in the U.S. population and the associated high incidence of coronary artery disease.

Type III hyperlipoproteinemia. Type III hyperlipoproteinemia is associated with hypertriglyceridemia and hypercholesterolemia that is characterized by the accumulation in the plasma of cholesterol-rich remnants of chylomicrons and VLDLs or IDLs, which are referred to collectively as β-VLDLs. Patients with type III hyperlipoproteinemia develop accelerated atherosclerosis involving both coronary and peripheral arteries. In considering the potentially atherogenic lipoproteins seen in this disorder, it is important to note that patients with type III hyperlipoproteinemia usually have low levels of LDL and HDL and that the hyperlipidemia is associated exclusively with an elevation in the level of β-VLDL. The underlying genetic defect responsible for the lipoprotein abnormalities is the synthesis of an abnormal form of apo-E, i.e., a form that does not bind normally to either the apo-B,E(LDL) or remnant (apo-E) lipoprotein receptors. A brief description of apo-E and its role in lipoprotein metabolism illustrates how this defect interferes with the catabolism of specific lipoproteins and how these lipoproteins contribute to the development of accelerated atherosclerosis (for a complete discussion of type III hyperlipoproteinemia and how other genetic, environmental, and hormonal factors modulate expression of the disease, see refs. 8 and 9).

The molecular defect in type III hyperlipoproteinemia is caused by the inheritance of genes coding for dysfunctional forms of apo-E. As has been described for other proteins, e.g., hemoglobin, there are multiple alleles in the population that code for apo-E isoforms that differ in protein structure by single amino acid substitutions. The most common isoform of apo-E

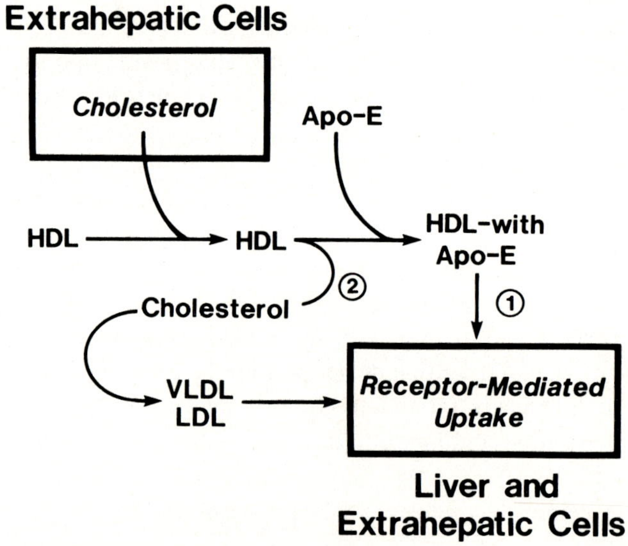

FIGURE 2. Role of HDL in acquiring cholesterol from cells containing excess cholesterol and redistributing the cholesterol to cells requiring it for steroid hormone production and membrane biosynthesis [extrahepatic cells, e.g., adrenal, testis, etc., with apo-B,E(LDL) receptors] or to the liver for elimination from the body.

seen in the population is apo-E3 (approximately 60% of the population is homozygous for apo-E3). Type III hyperlipoproteinemia is most often associated with apo-E2 homozygosity. Four variant isoforms of apo-E have been identified in studies of a number of patients with type III hyperlipoproteinemia.[2,4,8,9] These variant forms of apo-E exhibit defective binding to lipoprotein receptors, which accounts for the delayed clearance and increased concentration of apo-E–containing, cholesterol-rich lipoproteins in type III patients. The amino acid substitutions that affect receptor binding occur in the midportion of the apo-E molecule and involve substitutions of neutral amino acids for the normally occurring lysine or arginine residues (table 1). It has now been established that the region of the apo-E molecule responsible for mediating apo-B,E(LDL) and remnant (apo-E) receptor binding involves basic amino acids (arginine and lysine) in the vicinity of residues 140 to 160.[2,4,9] The description of this ligand binding domain of apo-E has helped to identify the postulated multiple binding sites on the apo-B,E(LDL) receptor, a region enriched in the acidic amino acids glutamic and aspartic acids.[10]

The abnormal apo-E, defective in its ability to bind to the lipoprotein receptors, disrupts the normal metabolism of chylomicrons and VLDLs (the β-VLDLs) (figure 1, steps 1 and 2). The impaired receptor-mediated uptake of these lipoproteins results in their accumulation in the plasma. In addition, the presence of the abnormal form of apo-E interferes with the normal formation of LDL from β-VLDL and IDL in type III patients (figure 1, step 3). This could contribute to the low level of LDL seen in patients with type III hyperlipoproteinemia and could contribute further to the accumulation of β-VLDL in the plasma.[4,8,9] The cholesterol-rich remnants of chylomicrons and VLDL (the β-VLDLs) that accumulate must now be cleared from the plasma by an alternative pathway. The alternate route may well be through macrophages (scavenger cells), including macrophages of the arterial wall that participate in foam cell production in atherosclerotic lesions.

TABLE 1
Human apo-E variants and their receptor binding activities

Substitutions[A]	Receptor binding activity relative to apo-E3[B] (%)
$Arg_{158} \rightarrow Cys$	<2
$Arg_{145} \rightarrow Cys$	45
$Lys_{146} \rightarrow Gln$	40
$Cys_{112} \rightarrow Arg$, $Arg_{142} \rightarrow Cys$	<20

Arg = arginine; Cys = cysteine; Lys = lysine; Gln = glutamine.

[A]The designation of the variants, as listed, refers to the site(s) where their structures vary from that of "normal" apo-E3. For example, the notation $Arg_{158} \rightarrow Cys$ indicates that cysteine is substituted for the normally occurring arginine at residue 158.

[B]Apo-E3 binding activity is set at 100%. The binding activities of the variants associated with type III hyperlipoproteinemia are expressed as a percentage of the "normal" apo-E3 binding to both apo-B,E(LDL) and remnant (apo-E) receptors.

Several lines of evidence implicate β-VLDLs in atherogenesis and suggest that macrophages are involved in the process (for review see refs. 2, 3, 5, 6, and 9). Macrophages possess a receptor that interacts specifically with β-VLDL. Both chylomicron and VLDL remnants bind to this receptor and cause massive cholesteryl ester accumulation in the cultured macrophages. In addition, it has been shown that foam cells within the arterial wall possess receptors for β-VLDL.[11]

In further support of the postulate that β-VLDL may be atherogenic, animals fed diets high in fat and cholesterol have markedly elevated levels of β-VLDL (chylomicron and VLDL remnants) in their plasma and develop accelerated atherosclerosis.[2,5,6] These diet-induced β-VLDLs also cause cholesteryl ester accumulation in macrophages. Furthermore, lipoproteins resembling β-VLDLs are seen in the plasma of humans after consumption of a single high-fat, high-cholesterol meal, and it is reasonable to speculate that these transiently present lipoproteins may contribute to the atherogenic risk seen in populations consuming such diets.[5] Dietary intervention could be expected to alter the production of these potentially atherogenic lipoproteins.

Unlike type III hyperlipoproteinemia, in which the accumulation of β-VLDL is caused by the presence of the receptor-defective apo-E, the β-VLDL accumulation seen after fat and cholesterol feeding appears to be secondary to the down-regulation of expression of apo-B,E(LDL) receptors.[2,12] Cholesterol feeding decreases the number of apo-B,E(LDL) receptors in the liver, whereas cholesterol feeding does not decrease the expression of remnant (apo-E) receptors.[2] Presumably, lipoprotein overproduction induced by the dietary fat and cholesterol, in association with a decrease in apo-B,E(LDL) receptors, exceeds the ability of the remnant receptors to clear the excess particles from the plasma, and both the chylomicron and VLDL remnants accumulate. Thus, either an impaired ability of apo-E–containing lipoproteins to interact with the receptors, as seen in type III hyperlipoproteinemia, or a decreased expression of the apo-B,E(LDL) receptor, as seen in fat and cholesterol feeding in animals, results in accumulation of remnant lipoproteins. Both conditions are associated with accelerated atherosclerosis.

A comparison of the changes in HDL in both type III hyperlipoproteinemia and with fat and cholesterol feeding in animals suggests how these lipoproteins may function as protective or antiatherogenic lipoproteins (for review see refs. 2, 5, 6, and 9). The changes include a reduction in the typical HDL, i.e., HDL-without apo-E, and an increase in HDL-with apo-E (HDL_1 or HDL_c). These changes appear to reflect the role of HDL in the process referred to as reverse cholesterol transport. Cholesterol deposited in extrahepatic tissues, including cells of the arterial wall, may be acquired by HDL, especially HDL-without apo-E (figure 2). The cholesterol appears to be esterified in the plasma, resulting in an increase in the size of the HDL particles and the acquisition of apo-E. Because apo-E is synthesized by various cells, including macrophages,[4] it is available within the interstitial fluid to become associated with the cholesterol-enriched HDL, i.e., HDL-with apo-E. The presence of the apo-E on these lipoproteins can now target the HDL-with apo-E to cells with either the apo-B,E(LDL) or remnant (apo-E) receptors (figure 2, step 1). Alternatively, it has been postulated that the cholesterol in HDL can be transferred to other lipoproteins (e.g., VLDL or LDL) that are then taken up by receptor-mediated endocytosis (figure 2, step 2). By either process, the HDL can participate in the redistribution of cholesterol from cholesterol-loaded cells to cells requiring cholesterol or to the liver for elimination of cholesterol from the body.

The decreased level of HDL-without apo-E in type III patients (or with fat and cholesterol feeding) could reflect the use of these particles as precursors in the formation of the cholesterol-loaded, HDL-with apo-E. The association of low levels of HDL with an increased risk of coronary artery disease may well be caused by the lack of sufficient quantities of HDL necessary to facilitate the egress of cholesterol from cells of the arterial wall in the face of large quantities of lipoproteins (e.g., β-VLDL), resulting in the deposition of cholesterol within these cells. Studies in vivo and in vitro have shown that high levels of HDL prevent the development of atherosclerosis in dogs and prevent accumulation of cholesteryl ester in macrophages, even when high levels of remnant lipoproteins (β-VLDL) are present.[13]

Familial hypercholesterolemia. The role of LDLs in the development of accelerated atherosclerosis is dramatically illustrated by studies of patients with familial hypercholesterolemia. As demonstrated by the classic studies of Goldstein and Brown (for review see refs. 2, 7, 12, and 14), patients with this disorder lack or have defective apo-B,E(LDL) receptors (figure 1, step 4; defective receptors prevent normal LDL and IDL uptake and catabolism). Patients homozygous for this disorder often die in the second decade of life from coronary artery disease. It should be kept in mind that these subjects also have abnormally high levels of IDL, resembling VLDL remnants, that could be contributing to the atherogenic process through the mechanisms discussed above.

Not only do LDLs accumulate in the plasma of individuals with familial hypercholesterolemia but also in the plasma of animals fed diets high in fat and cholesterol.[5,6] The increase in plasma LDLs in the various animal preparations is very likely secondary to the down-regulation in expression of the apo-B,E(LDL) receptors. The decrease in the number of these receptors would be expected to decrease LDL catabolism and to result in an increase of the plasma concentration. This may well be the mechanism whereby the consumption of high-fat, high-cholesterol diets by humans results in elevated plasma cholesterol levels and predisposes man to an increased risk of developing coronary artery disease.

However, the precise mechanism whereby LDLs are atherogenic is not entirely clear (for review see refs. 3, 5, 6, 12, and 15). High levels of LDLs may in fact lead to endothelial damage (including the possibility of subtle derangement in endothelial cell metabolism) and to an increased flux of LDLs into the arterial wall. The LDLs do accumulate in the arterial wall in association with atherosclerotic lesions, and these lesions are associated with cholesterol accumulation in smooth muscle cells and macrophages. However, at the present time it is difficult to explain how the smooth muscle cells could acquire excess cholesterol, since, at least in tissue culture, the apo-B,E(LDL) receptors are efficiently down-regulated by delivery of cholesterol to these cells and will not accumulate excess cholesterol. Furthermore, based on studies in vitro, macrophages do not accumulate massive amounts of cholesteryl ester after incubation with even high concentrations of normal LDL.

An intriguing hypothesis has been put forth that suggests how macrophages may become loaded with cholesterol in response to high levels of LDL. It has been shown that chemically modified LDL can be recognized by unique receptors on macrophages (referred to as the acetyl LDL receptor or the receptor for chemically modified LDL) (for review see refs. 2, 3, 5, and 15). In the laboratory, LDL modified by acetylation, acetoacetylation, oxidation, or malondialdehyde modification can be recognized by this receptor and can cause massive accumulation of cholesteryl ester within the macrophages. Such modifications of LDLs could occur in the plasma as the lipoproteins circulate or in the arterial wall as they perfuse through the tissue. In addition, LDL complexed to glycosaminoglycans, such as dextran sulfate, can also be recognized and taken up by macrophages, causing cholesterol accumulation. However, despite the attractiveness of these postulated mechanisms, more data are needed to establish their importance in the pathogenesis of atherosclerosis.

Conclusions. Accelerated atherosclerosis occurs in patients with type III hyperlipoproteinemia and familial hypercholesterolemia. The genetic defects in these disorders focus attention on specific types of lipoproteins as being responsible for the development of accelerated coronary artery disease. The accumulation of chylomicron remnants of intestinal origin and of VLDL or IDL remnants of hepatic origin appears to correlate with coronary disease seen in patients with type III hyperlipoproteinemia. The presence of abnormal apo-E prevents normal receptor-mediated catabolism of these lipoproteins. The type III hyperlipoproteinemic patients also have changes in their HDL that suggest how these lipoproteins participate in the process of reverse cholesterol transport and function as antiatherogenic lipoproteins. Patients with familial hypercholesterolemia have an elevation of plasma LDL (and to a lesser extent an increase in IDL), which is secondary to defective apo-B,E(LDL) receptors that impair normal catabolism. Animals fed diets high in fat and cholesterol have an accumulation of β-VLDL remnants, IDL, and LDL resembling the lipoproteins in patients with both genetic defects.

Attention has been focused on macrophages as playing a key role in atherogenesis and as being at least one of the progenitors of foam cells in arterial lesions. Many studies have highlighted the importance of macrophages, which are presumably derived from circulating monocytes that enter the arterial wall. Such cells within the arterial wall express receptors for both β-VLDL (chylomicron and VLDL remnants) and chemically modified LDL. Thus, in the presence of specific lipoproteins, macrophages are converted to cells with the appearance of foam cells. The precise stimulus that causes monocyte-macrophages to enter specific regions of the arterial wall remains to be determined. They may be responding to the trapping of the abnormal lipoproteins in the matrix of the arterial wall or alterations in endothelial cells. Initially they may be part of a protective, reparative process. However, pathologic changes could result when these cells become excessively overloaded with cholesterol. Certainly in advanced atherosclerotic lesions, cell death and necrosis represent part of the complexity of the lesion and lead to the deposition of extracellular cholesterol and the destruction of the normal architecture of the arterial wall.

This discussion provides insights into the mechanisms whereby the consumption of diets high in saturated fat and cholesterol could predispose humans to an increased risk of coronary artery disease. Such diets could stimulate the production of chylomicron and VLDL remnants and could lead to impaired catabolism of the remnant lipoproteins and LDL by suppression of apo-B,E(LDL) receptors. An NIH Consensus Panel, which reviewed all available data, has reported recently that the plasma cholesterol levels of our population are excessively high by comparison to certain other peoples of the world, that these high levels correlate with our increased incidence of coronary artery disease, and that a reduction of plasma cholesterol levels by diet modification (consumption of a prudent, low-fat, low-cholesterol diet) should be a goal for our entire population.[16] Consideration of the available studies — epidemiologic studies, clinical trials, animal preparations, and metabolic ward studies, including data discussed in this review — support these conclusions. A beneficial effect on the incidence of coronary artery disease can be expected by the population-wide adoption of a prudent, low-fat and low-cholesterol diet.

I greatly appreciate the excellent assistance of Sylvia Richmond, Barbara Allen, and Sally Gullatt Seehafer in the preparation of this manuscript. In addition, I thank James X. Warger and Norma Jean Gargasz for preparation of the illustrations.

References

1. Havel RJ, Goldstein JL, Brown MS: Lipoproteins and lipid transport. *In* Bondy PK, Rosenberg LE, editors: Metabolic control of disease. Philadelphia, 1980, W. B. Saunders, p 393
2. Mahley RW, Innerarity TL: Lipoprotein receptors and cholesterol homeostasis. Biochim Biophys Acta **737:** 197, 1983
3. Brown MS, Goldstein JL: Lipoprotein metabolism in the macrophage: implications for cholesterol deposition in atherosclerosis. Annu Rev Biochem **52:** 223, 1983
4. Mahley RW, Innerarity TL, Rall SC Jr, Weisgraber KH: Plasma lipoproteins: apolipoprotein structure and function. J Lipid Res **25:** 1277, 1984
5. Mahley RW: Development of accelerated atherosclerosis: concepts derived from cell biology and animal model studies. Arch Pathol Lab Med **107:** 393, 1983
6. Mahley RW: Atherogenic hyperlipoproteinemia: the cellular and molecular biology of plasma lipoproteins altered by dietary fat and cholesterol. Med Clin North Am **66:** 375, 1982
7. Goldstein JL, Brown MS: The LDL receptor defect in familial hypercholesterolemia: implications for pathogenesis and therapy. Med Clin North Am **66:** 335, 1982

8. Mahley RW, Angelin B: Type III hyperlipoproteinemia: recent insights into the genetic defect of familial dysbetalipoproteinemia. Adv Intern Med **29:** 385, 1984
9. Mahley RW, Innerarity TL, Rall SC Jr, Weisgraber KH: Lipoproteins of special significance in atherosclerosis: insights provided by studies of type III hyperlipoproteinemia. Ann NY Acad Sci **454:** 209, 1985
10. Yamamoto T, Davis CG, Brown MS, Schneider WJ, Casey ML, Goldstein JL, Russell DW: The human LDL receptor: a cysteine-rich protein with multiple Alu sequences in its mRNA. Cell **39:** 27, 1984
11. Pitas RE, Innerarity TL, Mahley RW: Foam cells in explants of atherosclerotic rabbit aortas have receptors for β-very low density lipoproteins and modified low density lipoproteins. Arteriosclerosis **3:** 2, 1983
12. Brown MS, Goldstein JL: How LDL receptors influence cholesterol and atherosclerosis. Sci Am **251:** 58, 1984
13. Innerarity TL, Pitas RE, Mahley RW: Modulating effects of canine high density lipoproteins on cholesteryl ester synthesis induced by β-very low density lipoproteins in macrophages: possible *in vitro* correlates with atherosclerosis. Arteriosclerosis **2:** 114, 1982
14. Goldstein JL, Brown MS: Familial hypercholesterolemia. *In* Stanbury JB, Wyngaarden JB, Frederickson DS, Goldstein JL, Brown MS, editors: The metabolic basis of inherited disease. New York, 1983, McGraw-Hill Book Co., Inc., p 672
15. Steinberg D: Lipoproteins and atherosclerosis: a look back and a look ahead. Arteriosclerosis **3:** 283, 1983
16. Consensus Conference (Office of Medical Applications of Research, National Institutes of Health): Lowering blood cholesterol to prevent heart disease. JAMA **253:** 2080, 1985

EDITORIAL

A consideration of antiarrhythmic therapy

DOUGLAS P. ZIPES, M.D.

THE PURPOSE of this article is to place into perspective newer avenues of antiarrhythmic therapy, including drugs and nonpharmacologic approaches.

Antiarrhythmic drugs

Types. A variety of antiarrhythmic drugs are available, both conventional and investigational. They can be divided into groups: those that exert blocking actions predominantly on sodium, potassium, or calcium channels, and those that block β-adrenergic receptors. Exensive subclassification[1] of these drugs does not seem to be useful, primarily because it does not help in choosing effective drug therapy for a given patient. The classifications are also limited because they are based on the electrophysiologic effects exerted by an arbitrary concentration of the drug, generally on normal Purkinje fibers, often not even in arrhythmic preparations. The effects of these drugs depend on tissue type, species, the degree of acute or chronic damage, heart rate, membrane potential, the ionic composition of the extracellular milieu, and other factors. Thus, for example, lidocaine exerts little effect on a normal Purkinje fiber action potential upstroke at a pacing cycle length of 1000 msec but can profoundly depress it when the cell becomes depolarized and discharges at a rapid rate, such as might occur during ischemia-induced tachycardia. Many drugs exhibit actions that belong in multiple categories or operate indirectly, such as by altering hemodynamics, myocardial metabolism, or autonomic transmission. Some drugs have active metabolites that exert effects different from the parent compound. Not all drugs in the same class have identical effects, while some drugs in different classes have similar actions.

From the Krannert Institute of Cardiology, Department of Medicine, Indiana University School of Medicine, and the Richard L. Roudebush Veterans Administration Medical Center, Indianapolis.

Supported in part by the Herman C. Krannert Fund, by grants HL-06308 and HL-07182 from the National Heart, Lung, and Blood Institute, by the American Heart Association, Indiana Affiliate, and by the Veterans Administration.

Address for correspondence: Douglas P. Zipes, M.D., Krannert Institute of Cardiology, 1001 W. 10th St., Indianapolis, IN 46202.

Supraventricular tachycardia

Choice of drugs for supraventricular tachycardias

General. Antiarrhythmic therapy, like antibiotic therapy, must be individualized, but unlike choosing a specific antimicrobial drug by testing its efficacy against the specific offending organism cultured from the patient, the appropriate and selective antiarrhythmic agent must be determined empirically. The need for such empiricism in treating many patients with supraventricular tachycardias such as atrioventricular nodal (AVN) reentry and tachycardias associated with an accessory pathway (AV reentry) has been modified dramatically over the past decade or more, in part because of results from invasive electrophysiologic studies that test the patient's response to a drug (table 1). These studies have made it possible to deduce the pathways involved in the presumed reentrant mechanism and to determine their electrophysiologic properties.[2] The effects on these pathways of drugs with known and different mechanisms of action have been determined and these drugs can be anticipated to exert predictable effects because the pathways respond, for the most part, in a predictably normal electrophysiologic manner. This predictability is a key factor in choosing therapy. Moreover, when a drug terminates AV or AVN reentry, the mechanism by which this has occurred, e.g., the production of block in one of the reentry pathways, can be elucidated. Since the mechanism responsible for initiating and maintaining the tachycardia is often fairly constant from one episode to another, predictable responses to long-term therapy can be anticipated. Also, the electrophysiologic information obtained from invasive studies has permitted more accurate diagnosis of the supraventricular tachycardia by scalar electrocardiography and that information, coupled with data on predictable drug actions, permit drug selection that can be anticipated to exert a high degree of efficacy.

Thus, for example, in a patient with the usual AV reentry (presumptively diagnosed electrocardiographically by a delta wave during sinus rhythm and regular tachycardia with a normal QRS complex at about

TABLE 1
Tachyarrhythmias

	Supraventricular^	Ventricular
Pathways elucidated	Yes	No
EP properties of pathways known	Yes	No
Pathways electrophysiologically normal and/or drug response predictable	Yes	No
Mechanism of tachyarrhythmia constant	Usually	Sometimes
Accurate therapeutic decision from scalar ECG	Often	Seldom

EP = electrophysiologic; ECG = electrocardiogram.
^AVN reentry or reentry associated with an accessory pathway.

200/min with a retrograde P wave in the ST segment), the reentrant loop can be surmised with a high degree of probability and specific drugs can be selected to exert a major depressant effect on the slow calcium channel–dependent AVN tissue used for anterograde conduction while other drugs can be chosen to affect the fast sodium channel–dependent tissue of the usual AV accessory pathway used retrogradely. The pathways in AVN reentry can be deduced in a similar fashion. The major unknown is whether the quantitative effects, not the qualitative effects, are appropriate to abolish the reentry loop or slow the ventricular rate if atrial fibrillation results. Founded firmly on the knowledge derived from these invasive electrophysiologic and electropharmacologic studies, a more focused therapeutic plan with a high likelihood of success can be outlined for most patients with these tachycardias. In essence, a tight-fitting match can be created between the mechanism of the tachycardia and the prescribed therapy. Given these considerations, what are the available choices?

Immediate termination. For the immediate termination of AV and AVN reentry, after simple vagal maneuvers have been tried, intravenous verapamil is the drug of choice because of its ability to slow conduction and prolong refractoriness in the AV node. Should atrial fibrillation supervene in the patient with the Wolff-Parkinson-White syndrome, the ventricular response over the accessory pathway may increase after intravenous (generally not after oral) verapamil. In that situation or for the patient presenting initially with atrial fibrillation and conduction over an accessory pathway, a drug that prolongs the refractory period of the accessory pathway (e.g., procainamide) should be used or application of electrical direct-current cardioversion considered, depending on the clinical situation. In some instances the drug that successfully terminates AV or AVN reentry can then be used for long-term oral therapy to prevent recurrences, considering the response to the acute episode akin to an electrophysiologic evaluation.

Long-term oral therapy. For long-term oral therapy to prevent recurrences of AV or AVN reentry, drugs that affect the AV node, such as digitalis, β-adrenergic–receptor blockers, or slow-channel blockers like verapamil or diltiazem, can be tried alone or in combination with drugs such as procainamide, quinidine, or disopyramide that affect the accessory pathway in AV reentry or the retrogradely conducting pathway in the usual variety of AVN reentry. Digitalis is contraindicated as single therapy in patients with Wolff-Parkinson-White syndrome and atrial fibrillation because it may increase the ventricular response.

Of the newer agents, amiodarone is particularly effective for patients with AV or AVN reentry. Although its side effects are many, for the most part they appear to be dose-related and, if lower doses are successful, as they seem to be for many patients with supraventricular tachycardias, side effects can be minimized. Amiodarone depresses conduction and prolongs refractoriness in both the AV node and accessory pathway, a particularly advantageous feature should atrial fibrillation occur. Encainide, flecainide, and propafenone, quite different from amiodarone with respect to electrophysiologic properties, similarly affect both the AV node and the accessory pathway to suppress both AV and AVN reentry and to decrease the ventricular response during atrial fibrillation. In general, side effects with these latter three drugs are quite tolerable, so it is logical to try therapy with them before amiodarone.

Thus, amiodarone, flecainide, encainide, or propafenone, alone or in combination with drugs that affect the AV node, would be the drugs of choice from the selection of newer agents to treat AV or AVN reentry that recurs despite treatment with conventional drugs. Efficacy is probably distributed fairly evenly among them.

In some patients who are dependent hemodynamically on atrial systole, such as those with hypertrophic cardiomyopathy, recurrent atrial flutter, or fibrillation can be a very troublesome and symptomatic arrhythmia. We have found amiodarone to be very effective in these patients, infrequently restoring sinus rhythm if atrial flutter or atrial fibrillation is present, but maintaining it after electrical reversion in the majority of patients. Often very low doses, e.g., 200 mg/day or on alternate days, are sufficient and side effects are minimal in this dose range.

Sinus nodal reentry less frequently presents a clinical problem due in part to slower rates of tachycardia, and probably should be treated initially with drugs that affect the sinus node, such as digitalis or β- and slow-channel blockers. For other atrial tachycardias, slowing the ventricular response is often the therapeutic end point and the choice of drug or drugs that will be used to suppress the tachycardia itself is made empirically.

Choice of nonpharmacologic therapy for supraventricular tachycardias. Electrical devices that automatically or when activated by the patient or physician deliver competitive stimuli to the atrium or (less commonly) to the ventricle may be useful in selected patients with AV and AVN reentry. Rapid atrial pacing, or stimuli timed to a portion of the cardiac cycle, terminate virtually 100% of these two types of tachycardia. However, because pharmacologic management is usually successful, such approaches generally are reserved for the patient with recurrent tachycardia despite multiple drug trials or who is intolerant of drug management. A potential problem with these devices is that competitive atrial pacing may initiate atrial flutter or atrial fibrillation that may, particularly in the patient with an anterogradely conducting accessory pathway with a short refractory period, precipitate very rapid ventricular rates. However, an electrical device for the carefully screened and evaluated patient with AV or AVN reentry, often combined with drugs, can be a very successful and acceptable form of therapy.

On occasion, pacemakers can be used to prevent the onset of a variety of supraventricular tachycardias by pacing at rapid rates, at normal rates when the onset of tachycardia is related to bradycardia, or at short AV intervals to prevent retrograde invasion of an accessory pathway or reentry in the AV node.

Surgery to interrupt an accessory pathway[3] should be considered for the patients with recurrent symptomatic tachycardia despite multiple drug trials, those with life-threatening tachycardia such as atrial fibrillation precipitating ventricular fibrillation, or for those whose consignment at a young age to a lifetime of pill consumption is unacceptable. Surgery for atrial flutter, AVN reentry, and some unusual forms of supraventricular tachycardia is still in the investigational stage, as is electrical ablation with catheter-delivered energy. These are areas to watch closely for future developments.

Ventricular tachycardia and ventricular fibrillation

Choice of drugs for ventricular tachyarrhythmias

General. Selecting therapy for the patient with ventricular tachyarrhythmias cannot be approached as logically and predictably as can treatment for supraventricular tachycardias (table 1). Individual pathways involved in the tachycardia cannot be studied, for the most part because the area of reentry, if that is the responsible mechanism, occurs in a small portion of the ventricle, precluding accurate electrophysiologic assessment with relatively gross extracellular stimulating and recording techniques. The right ventricle, generally remote from the origin of the ventricular tachycardia, is often the site of recording and stimulating and cannot be expected to provide electrophysiologic data relevant to a reentry loop or an automatic focus originating in the left ventricle. Even if the left ventricle is explored, the electrophysiologic properties of the microreentrant pathways cannot be discerned with the present tools. However, data from a variety of studies suggest that, if these pathways could be studied electrophysiologically, they probably would be very complex, including both normal and diseased tissue. In some cells, propagation or automaticity may be dependent on slow-channel activity and in others, it may depend on the fast sodium channel. Because the damaged area is so complex, in sharp contrast to the predictable response in many patients with supraventricular tachycardias, its response to antiarrhythmic agents with mechanisms of action based on data obtained in vitro in normal tissues cannot be predicted accurately.

Damaged ventricular myocardial and Purkinje tissue generally depolarize when injured, at least initially, and probably cell groups with several levels of maximum diastolic membrane potential exist, influenced by the nature and degree of damage, healing, and interposed scar tissue matrixes. In addition, alterations of the autonomic nervous system,[4] heterogeneous blood flow patterns creating heterogeneous tissue concentrations of drugs, modulation of drug effects by active and inactive channel states, diastolic membrane potential and heart rate,[5] varying drug kinetics due to genetic and other factors that influence the serum concentration of the parent compound and active metabolites, hemodynamic events, and other confounding variables may affect the cellular response to the drug and consequently the drug's efficacy or toxicity. Although a predictable drug response can be anticipated in a few patients with unique types of ventricular tachycardia, it is not surprising that a focused therapeutic attack with a predictably high degree of success is difficult to anticipate for a specific patient with a ventricular tachyarrhythmia. Even the ideal end point with which to judge the therapeutic response, such as the suppression of spontaneous ventricular ectopic activity or response to programmed electrical stimulation, still has not been unquestionably determined.

Mechanisms. Most times we do not know why a drug terminates or prevents recurrence of a ventricular arrhythmia. Measurements of parameters such as refractoriness, excitability, and conduction are very useful in the characterization of the drug, but may not necessarily relate to the mechanism by which the drug is antiarrhythmic. Experimental studies usually establish the properties of antiarrhythmic agents rather than their antiarrhythmic properties. For example, a drug like amiodarone may suppress arrhythmias by exerting direct electrophysiologic actions on ventricular muscle and specialized conducting tissue that include prolongation of refractoriness and slowing of conduction velocity, or may act indirectly by slowing the heart rate, reducing ischemia, improving myocardial blood flow, or blocking α- or β-adrenergic receptors or the conversion of T_4 to T_3, reducing platelet adhesiveness or other factors. Very probably, in a general sense, antiarrhythmic drugs "isolate" the arrhythmogenic area by selectively making "sick cells sicker" and in some way uncoupling them electrically from the rest of the ventricle. It would not be at all surprising to find in damaged ventricles islands of "arrhythmic activity" that do not propagate to neighboring myocardium and thus do not produce clinically evident/manifest arrhythmias.

In contrast to many supraventricular tachycardias, it is seldom feasible to deduce the mechanism of a clinically occurring ventricular tachycardia from its response to a drug, given our present state of knowledge. Most drug actions are too nonspecific. For example, suppression of a ventricular tachycardia by verapamil may lead to the conclusion that the slow calcium current plays an important role in the mechanism of the tachycardia. However, the clinically used drug is a racemic mixture of two isomers, one of which exerts a slight but definite effect on the fast sodium channel. Also, among several other actions that may affect the arrhythmia, verapamil influences myocardial blood flow and produces reflex sympathetic stimulation while also producing α-blockade, all factors that could alter arrhythmogenicity independently from slow-channel suppression. Conversely, if lidocaine terminates an arrhythmia, it may be concluded that the slow inward current played no important role in the arrhythmic mechanism. However, lidocaine could eliminate an arrhythmia originating in a calcium channel–dependent automatic focus by blocking conduction in fast sodium channel–dependent tissue exiting from the focus rather than by actually suppressing the slow calcium channel–dependent automatic focus.[6] The clinical result still would be suppression of the tachycardia. Indeed, except for reciprocating tachycardias associated with an accessory pathway in patients with the Wolff-Parkinson-White syndrome,[2] for which virtually all evidence supports a reentrant mechanism, the electrophysiologic mechanisms responsible for other tachycardias remain speculative and there exist no pharmacologic, electrical, or surgical approaches so specific as to establish unquestionably the responsible electrophysiologic mechanism.

Variability. These factors make rational antiarrhythmic choices difficult for treating ventricular tachyarrhythmias. Also, in contrast to the fairly consistently recurring mechanisms in supraventricular tachycardias, the electrophysiologic mechanisms responsible for ventricular tachyarrhythmias may vary. For example, in the same patient, ventricular tachycardia may result from stable prior anatomic injury, e.g., ventricular scar or aneurysm, from acute myocardial ischemia, or from reperfusion that terminates acute ischemia. Each of these three causes may occur in the same patient, and probably will have unique electrophysiologic mechanisms and react differently to the same antiarrhythmic drugs. Ventricular fibrillation may respond to the same antiarrhythmic agent in still another fashion. Altered disease states may add to intrapatient variability of response. Thus, the anatomic-electrophysiologic status of a patient 2 weeks after a myocardial infarction probably is not the same as it is 6 months later. Therefore, it may be unreasonable to think that any single antiarrhythmic drug, e.g., quinidine, will be uniformly effective in reducing the incidence of sudden death in large numbers of patients in groups that are considered to be homogeneous but that actually are heterogeneous, such as patients who have had a myocardial infarction. The marked variability between patients, and potentially in the same patient, precludes determination of a consistent response to a single drug, and its seems unrealistic to rely on the effectiveness of one agent to suppress all the possible arrhythmogenic mechanisms in a given patient.

Ideal drug. We do not now have, and it is not likely that we will have in the near future, that elusive Holy Grail of antiarrhythmic therapy: the single antiarrhythmic agent with minimal side effects and ideal kinetics that is uniformly and predictably effective in preventing recurrence of ventricular tachyarrhythmia in a large percentage of patients with life-threatening arrhythmias. Unless an arrhythmia results from a common cause, e.g., ischemia, that can be prevented uniformly and in a predictable fashion with a closely related group of drugs like β-adrenergic–receptor blockers, it is not likely that one drug will be effective "across the board." Each of the new (and old) drugs successfully suppresses electrically induced arrhythmias in approximately the same percentage of patients (about 20% to 30% of those referred for treatment of drug-resistant ventricular arrhythmias). Drugs suppress a higher percentage of spontaneously occurring ventricular arrhythmias. While one drug may be effective in one patient and not in another, it is not certain that any one of them is clearly more efficacious overall than the others. Amiodarone may be an exception. However, since only one drug chosen from a wide selection may be effective in a given patient, and since the drugs produce different side effects and patient tolerance differs, the availability of a wide variety from which to choose may be justified.

Comparison. It should be stressed that for several reasons it is very difficult to compare antiarrhythmic drug efficacy quantitatively, i.e., drug A is superior to drug B because it is effective in 25% more patients or more arrhythmias. Studies in patients with serious and symptomatic recurrent ventricular tachyarrhythmias generally are flawed, most often because the serious nature of the tachyarrhythmia precludes the use of scientifically rigorous principles that require placebo-controlled, blinded, prospective, and randomized trials. In addition, varying therapeutic end points (e.g., suppression of ambient arrhythmia present on long-term electrocardiographic recordings vs response to programmed electrical stimulation [with varying protocols]), and varying populations of patients (e.g., treated groups "top heavy" with patients having class 4 congestive heart failure and sustained ventricular tachycardia vs groups laden with patients having nonsustained ventricular tachycardia and no structural heart disease) are two of the many problems making comparative assessments difficult. Accurate tabulation of the prevention of symptomatic recurrences of ventricular tachycardia and ventricular fibrillation is extremely difficult to obtain and most often control data based on past history, natural history, or comparison between responders and nonresponders is used. Such data have inherent inaccuracies, magnified by the variable recurrence rate of most arrhythmias. Finally, patients referred to a medical center for treatment, who generally comprise the study groups in most of the published articles, are a selected group that may not represent the usual patient population seen in clinical practice.

Immediate termination. Given this lengthy list of qualifications, what are the antiarrhythmic drug choices for patients with recurrent ventricular tachyarrhythmias not responsive to conventional antiarrhythmic drugs?

A variety of investigational drugs have been used intravenously for immediate termination of ventricular tachycardia. However, none of them show clear superiority over conventional choices, although some have been successful in selected patients after conventional drugs have failed. Therefore, after a trial of lidocaine, and then perhaps intravenous procainamide and/or bretylium, electrical cardioversion would be recommended. If the arrhythmia recurs despite use of these drugs, we would probably then use intravenous amiodarone. For the patient with hemodynamic deterioration, direct-current cardioversion/defibrillation is certainly indicated.

Long-term oral therapy. Because of the fairly equal distribution of efficacy among most of the drugs, and the inability to predict beforehand that a particular patient will respond to a particular drug, generally the side effect profiles of the drugs most influence the initial choice of long-term oral therapy, a fact that is indicative of the general state of antiarrhythmic drug selection. Therefore, despite the apparently greater efficacy of amiodarone, it is often selected after other investigational drugs have been tried. Initial choices include propafenone or flecainide, in no particular order. Perhaps mexiletine would be tried next. Insufficient data exist regarding ethmozine, encainide, cibenzoline bepridil, and sotalol to place them in reasonable categories of effectiveness as yet.

Drugs in combination may be effective and also permit the use of lower doses of each drug, which may reduce side effects. Although suggestions for specific combinations have been offered, e.g., use of drugs with different electrophysiologic actions, no combination has emerged that is clearly superior to others and we generally opt for an empirical approach not unlike that used for the selection of single agents. It should be remembered that the drugs chosen may be synergistic, antagonistic, or noninteractive. Drugs that have each achieved partial suppression of the arrhythmia may be combined. From a practical standpoint, when we reach the point at which multiple drug therapy should be considered, the patient often is receiving amiodarone as the last attempt at single-agent therapy, and rather than wait weeks or months for its elimination, other agents are added to the amiodarone regimen. It is probably a good rule to reduce doses of both drugs when combinations, particularly with amiodarone, are used.

The above recommendations are applicable to patients with recurrent symptomatic ventricular tachyarrhythmias. However, it is very important to remember that ventricular tachyarrhythmias probably result from diverse electrophysiologic mechanisms and these guidelines may not necessarily apply to arrhythmias resulting directly from ischemia, either at its onset or termination. Since we have scanty clinical information about which ventricular arrhythmias result solely from an anatomic obstacle, e.g., ventricular scar or aneurysm, and which are related to an ischemic event, or a combination of the two, hard and fast rules cannot be advanced. Experimental animal data, however, suggest that arrhythmias related to the onset or termination of ischemia are better treated by anti-ischemic and antisympathetic approaches than with local anesthetic–type drugs. In this regard, the only agents demonstrated to reduce mortality after myocardial infarction are β-adrenergic–receptor blockers, not local anesthetics. Slow-channel blockers and local anesthetics are presently being evaluated in this postinfarction setting.

Choice of nonpharmacologic therapy for ventricular tachyarrhythmias

Surgery. Should drug therapy prove ineffective or not well tolerated, surgery[7, 8] or electrical devices[9, 10] may be considered alone or in combination. The surgical candidate generally is a patient who has recurrent life-threatening ventricular tachycardia that can be mapped preoperatively and/or intraoperatively, a reasonably localized ventricular lesion such as an aneurysm, and sufficient myocardial reserve to withstand the stress of surgery. Coronary bypass surgery alone may be indicated only if ischemia is definitely established as the cause of the arrhythmia. Therapy with an electrical device can be combined with surgery in that leads for an implantable cardioverter/defibrillator can be sewn in place at the time of ablative surgery. Determination of the antiarrhythmic efficacy of electrical and chemical ablation techniques awaits documentation from further experience.

Electrical devices. An implantable cardioverter-defibrillator[9, 10] may be considered for the patient who has recurrent life-threatening ventricular tachyarrhythmia and may not be a surgical candidate because he cannot tolerate the surgery or has ventricular tachyarrhythmia that cannot be mapped or resected or progresses rapidly to ventricular fibrillation. One advantage of electrical cardioversion or defibrillation is that it successfully terminates the ventricular tachyarrhythmia in a very high percentage of patients with life-threatening ventricular arrhythmias independent of the cause of the heart disease, heart rate changes, hemodynamic status, levels of autonomic tone, pharmacokinetic influences, and all of the other variables mentioned earlier. In 1980 Mirowski et al.[9] demonstrated the usefulness of an implantable device in patients with ventricular fibrillation, and more recently we[10] presented data on an implantable pacemaker-cardioverter for patients with ventricular tachycardia. Next-generation devices of this type will be capable of delivering competitive pacing stimuli, synchronous cardioversion, or defibrillation shocks automatically in a programmable, escalating fashion, depending on the spontaneous cardiac rhythm. They also may have recording capabilities so that a record of the rhythm disturbance and device performance may be obtained.

Such electrical therapy has the drawback of not preventing a tachyarrhythmia from occurring, even though it promptly terminates it after the onset. Although efforts to use electrical therapy to prevent arrhythmias are being explored, in reality such antitachycardia devices probably will be used in conjunction with antiarrhythmic drug therapy to decrease recurrence of arrhythmias and minimize the number of times a patient may need to be shocked electrically. Having an implantable pacemaker-cardioverter-defibrillator available may permit some leeway in drug selection in the event that the drug fails to prevent recurrence of arrhythmia or is arrhythmogenic. One can envision giving a drug in lower doses that are well tolerated to prevent nine of 10 episodes of ventricular fibrillation, with the device terminating what would have been the tenth episode. In addition, such devices could permit, for the first time, the ethical study of control or placebo-treated groups of patients who have had recurrent ventricular tachycardia or ventricular fibrillation in order to evaluate drug efficacy according to more scientifically acceptable methods. Recording capabilities will document accurately the rhythm disturbance to provide proof of the arrhythmic event.

At present, the use of such devices is restricted, appropriately, to limited patient populations. Further progress in accurate and reliable identification of tachycardias is required before recommending more widespread application of such electrical approaches. Although more expensive than ordinary pacemakers, these devices probably will become cost-effective by enabling rapid patient discharge from the hospital and reducing the need for frequent readmission of patients with recurrent ventricular tachycardia and fibrillation. Electrophysiologic studies to test the efficacy of drugs and the electrical device can be performed noninvasively with the pacemaker-cardioverter in an outpatient setting.[10] Most importantly, however, the defibrillator[9] appears to reduce the incidence of sudden death in a heterogeneous population of patients with coronary artery disease, cardiomyopathy, long QT syndrome, and other problems. Reduction in defibrillation threshold may make possible transvenous implantation of defibrillators. As this mode of therapy becomes perfected, with accurate identification of tachycardias and safe, effective administration of therapy, application may even reach the point of prophylactic implantation in high-risk populations before a potentially lethal arrhythmia occurs. Further investigation into the effects of drugs on the efficacy of these devices is necessary.

Selection of candidates for therapy

One must consider carefully which patients with ventricular arrhythmias should be treated, particularly in view of the proarrhythmic effects of these agents. Initially, attempts should be made to uncover easily treatable causes of arrhythmias, such as hypokalemia. No data exist to support treating patients with asymptomatic premature ventricular complexes (PVCs). Thus, suppression of spontaneous PVCs rather than suppression of recurrences of sustained or nonsustained ventricular tachycardia or ventricular fibrillation may not be relevant in defining a drug's therapeutic potency. In fact, it is difficult to understand the recent infatuation with so-called PVC killers (a repugnant and very unscientific term) unless these drugs also suppress ventricular tachycardia and fibrillation. Suppression of PVCs and of ventricular tachycardia or fibrillation may have different "thresholds." That is, different drugs or different concentrations of the same drug may suppress PVCs and not tachycardia or vice versa, possibly because the electrophysiologic mechanism responsible for the PVC may be different from that responsible for the ventricular tachycardia.[11]

We would consider for therapy those patients with structural heart disease who have asymptomatic or symptomatic sustained or nonsustained ventricular tachycardia and those without structural heart disease who have symptomatic sustained or nonsustained ventricular tachycardia. Patients resuscitated from ventricular fibrillation not associated with an acute myocardial infarction should also be treated. While convincing objective data to support this approach do not exist in all groups of patients, this seems to strike a reasonable balance between the risks of therapy and the risks of the arrhythmia. Close monitoring of the patient's response is necessary to avoid drug-induced arrhythmogenic responses. Future studies may demonstrate that so-called idiosyncratic drug reactions may be explained by patients with genetically determined unusual metabolic pathways that result in production of arrhythmogenic metabolites.

Future considerations

There can be no doubt that in vitro and in vivo electrophysiologic studies in animals and humans have advanced our knowledge of the mechanisms of arrhythmogenesis and of drug action and that such studies must continue. However, advances in understanding actions of antiarrhythmic agents that have directly benefited the patient with ventricular arrhythmia have been slow and, except for producing a wider choice of drugs, we have progressed little clinically over the past 25 years. Most of these new drugs, however, are simply another iteration of existing drugs, with slightly different efficacy or side effect profiles. Progress must come from knowledge of the autonomic, metabolic, or cellular changes associated with the genesis of cardiac arrhythmias to provide insight into therapy that actually corrects basic defects rather than simply suppresses them. New diagnostic procedures such as the use of nuclear magnetic resonance, positron-emission tomography, NAD-NADH fluorescence, or voltage-sensitive dyes may not only provide insight into arrhythmogenic mechanisms, or at least the abnormal environment in which arrhythmias arise, but may help differentiate subpopulations of patients that may respond predictably to one or another antiarrhythmic drug. One can envision development of site-specific antiarrhythmic agents that could be directed to designated areas of the myocardium identified by such imaging techniques. While conventional invasive electrophysiologic studies are essential to categorize the usual electrophysiologic effects of a drug on specialized conducting tissue and muscle and may be useful in rapidly assessing drug efficacy, it is difficult to see how such studies, in their present form, will be able to provide further insight into mechanisms of drug action or deliver us from the need for empirical drug selection. Major criticisms of almost all of these studies involve their lack of adequate controls, small numbers of patients, and short-term follow-up.

In 1914, Wenckebach noted empirically that two patients with paroxysmal atrial fibrillation who were treated prophylactically for malaria with an extract of cinchona bark (quinine) frequently reverted to sinus rhythm. While we have made enormous strides over the intervening 70 years, pharmocologic control of arrhythmia still remains predicated on an individual, patient-by-patient, pharmacologic experiment, determined by trial and error, and tempered by good clinical judgment, whether one uses criteria obtained from noninvasive or invasive studies.

References

1. Vaughn Williams EM: A classification of antiarrhythmic actions reassessed after a decade of new drugs. J Clin Pharmacol **24:** 129, 1984
2. Durrer D, Schoo L, Schuilenberg RM, Wellens HJJ: The role of

premature beats in the initiation and termination of supraventricular tachycardia in the Wolff-Parkinson-White syndrome. Circulation **36:** 644, 1967
3. Cobb FR, Blmenschein SD, Sealy WC, Boineau JP, Wagner GS, Wallace AG: Successful surgical interruption of the bundle of Kent in a patient with Wolff-Parkinson-White syndrome. Circulation **38:** 1018, 1968
4. Barber MJ, Mueller TM, Henry D, Felten SY, Zipes DP: Transmural myocardial infarction in the dog produces sympathectomy in noninfarcted myocardium. Circulation **67:** 787, 1983
5. Hondeghem L, Katzung BG: Test of a model of antiarrhythmic drug action. Effects of quinidine and lidocaine in myocardial conduction. Circulation **61:** 1217, 1980
6. Evans JJ, Gilmour RF Jr, Zipes DP: The effects of lidocaine and quinidine on impulse propagation across the canine Purkinje-muscle junction during combined hyperkalemia, hypoxia and acidosis. Circ Res **55:** 185, 1984
7. Guiraudon G, Fontaine G, Frank R, Escande G, Etievent P, Cabrol C: Encircling endocardial ventriculotomy: a new surgical treatment for life-threatening ventricular tachycardias resistant to medical treatment following myocardial infarction. Ann Thorac Surg **26:** 438, 1978
8. Josephson ME, Harken AH, Horowitz LN: Endocardial excision. A new surgical technique for the treatment of recurrent ventricular tachycardia. Circulation **60:** 1430, 1979
9. Mirowski M: The automatic implantable cardioverter-defibrillator. J Am Coll Cardiol **6:** 461, 1985
10. Zipes DP, Heger JJ, Miles WM, Mahomed Y, Brown JW, Spielman SR, Prystowsky EN: Early experience with the implantable cardioverter. N Engl J Med **311:** 485, 1984
11. Myerburg RJ, Kessler KM, Kiem I, Pefkaros KC, Conde CA, Cooper D, Castellanos A: Relationship between plasma levels of procainamide, suppression of premature ventricular complexes, and prevention of recurrent ventricular tachycardia. Circulation **64:** 280, 1981

Increased lung vasoreactivity in children from Leadville, Colorado, after recovery from high-altitude pulmonary edema

JAMES W. FASULES, M.D., JAMES W. WIGGINS, M.D., AND ROBERT R. WOLFE, M.D.

ABSTRACT Cardiac catheterization was performed on seven children after recovery from high-altitude pulmonary edema. All were life-long residents at elevations above 10,000 feet. Three of the seven had developed pulmonary edema without antecedent travel to low altitude but had an upper respiratory infection. Response of pulmonary arterial pressure to 16% inspired oxygen in all seven was compared with that in six well children who resided at a similar altitude and had no history of high-altitude pulmonary edema. With hypoxia the susceptible patients had a greater mean pulmonary arterial pressure (56.3 ± 23.8) than the nonsusceptible children (18.8 ± 3.9, $p < .05$). Comparison with historical hemodynamic responses in children at high altitudes showed a similar greater mean pulmonary arterial pressure in the susceptible children. Thus, in children from high altitudes, increased pulmonary vasoreactivity to hypoxia may play a role in the pathogenesis of high-altitude pulmonary edema. The development of pulmonary edema in high-altitude residents with upper respiratory infections and no antecedent low-altitude journey is consistent with the presence of other factors such as inflammation, which may play a role in the pathogenesis of the edema. The finding of right ventricular hypertrophy on an electrocardiogram in children from high altitudes may be predictive of their susceptibility to high-altitude pulmonary edema.
Circulation 72, No. 5, 957–962, 1985.

HIGH-ALTITUDE PULMONARY EDEMA in Colorado residents of areas of high altitude occurs predominantly in children.[1, 2] Characteristically the children develop pulmonary edema on return to high altitude after a visit to low altitude. Some children have repeated episodes of high-altitude pulmonary edema, suggesting that they are particularly susceptible. However, the mechanisms of the edema are unknown.

It is known that during the acute episode both children and adults have acutely elevated pulmonary arterial pressure, suggesting that pulmonary hypertension may be a factor in the pathogenesis of the edema.[3] Increased pulmonary vasoconstriction to acute hypoxia has been found at low altitude in some adults after recovery from high-altitude pulmonary edema.[4, 5] Increased pulmonary vasoreactivity could contribute to excessive pulmonary hypertension in susceptible subjects ascending to high altitude. We can find only two reported instances in which hypoxic pulmonary vasoreactivity was measured in children who had recovered from high-altitude pulmonary edema, and both appeared to have large increases in pulmonary arterial pressure during the hypoxic challenge.[3] However, at cardiac characterization in one of the two children 1 year later, the hyperresponsiveness was decreased.

We hypothesized that increased vasoconstriction in response to hypoxia plays a role in the pathogenesis of high-altitude pulmonary edema in children who reside at high altitudes. If so, children living at high elevations who have a history of high-altitude pulmonary edema should have larger hypoxic pulmonary pressor responses than do children without such history. To address this question we measured pulmonary vascular responses to acute hypoxia in children from high-altitude areas who were referred to us for heart catheterization between 1978 and 1984. The seven children without other heart and lung disease who had a history of prior high-altitude pulmonary edema and the six normal, or near-normal, children without such history constitute the basis of this report. The measurements of

From the Department of Pediatrics and the Cardiovascular Pulmonary Research Laboratory, University of Colorado School of Medicine, Denver.

Supported by NIH grants HL 14985 and HL 07171.

Address for correspondence: J. W. Fasules, M.D., Pediatric Cardiology, University of Colorado Health Sciences Center, 4200 East Ninth Ave., C220, Denver, CO 80262.

Received Feb. 15, 1985; revision accepted July 25, 1985.

pulmonary vascular reactivity in susceptible children could increase our understanding of pathophysiologic mechanisms of high-altitude pulmonary edema.

Methods

Our definition of high-altitude pulmonary edema included (1) respiratory illness, (2) chest roentgenographic infiltrates consistent with pulmonary edema, and (3) response to oxygen therapy with rapid relief of symptoms and clearing of infiltrates. No children with heart disease were included in the study.

Patients. Patient 1 (E. H) was a 10-year-old boy who developed nausea, cyanosis, pallor, lethargy, tachypnea, and a nonproductive cough within 12 hr of return from sea level to his home at 3060 m elevation in Colorado. On admission to the hospital in Salida (2150 m), blood pressure was 100/78 mm Hg and rales were heard over both lung fields. He was treated with furosemide and oxygen with rapid relief of symptoms. A similar episode occurred at age 11 years after his return home from a trip to sea level. He was again treated with oxygen and furosemide with rapid improvement. He continued to reside at 3060 m until cardiac catheterization was performed in Denver (1600 m) 1 year later.

Patient 2 (D. F.) was an 8-year-old girl who developed cough, headache, emesis, and lethargy within 24 hr of return to Leadville (3100 m) from a trip to a lower altitude. She was admitted to the hospital in Leadville where her symptoms improved rapidly with oxygen and furosemide. Two days later the chest roentgenogram was normal. However, within 12 hr of discharge she was readmitted to the hospital because of recurrent symptoms and radiographic infiltrates. She rapidly improved with administration of oxygen. The patient remained in Leadville until cardiac catheterization was performed in Denver 10 days later.

Patient 3 (A. M.), a 4-year-old boy of Leadville, developed coryza, cough, and fever for 3 days and lethargy for 1 day while at home in Leadville. Examination revealed cyanosis, dehydration, lethargy, and fever. The arterial blood oxygen tension was 25 mm Hg. He was treated with oxygen, penicillin, and intravenous fluids and was evacuated to Denver where, on arrival, he was much improved. After remaining in Denver for 10 days he underwent cardiac catheterization there.

Patient 4 (S. S.), a 6-year-old girl of Leadville, had coryza and fever that continued for 2 weeks despite treatment with amoxicillin. Her admission to the hospital in Leadville was preceded by nausea, emesis, cough, dyspnea, and cyanosis over the previous 24 hr. Examination showed a cardiac gallop rhythm and bilateral pulmonary rales. Her arterial oxygen tension was 30 mm Hg. Treatment with oxygen, furosemide, and erythromycin resulted in rapid relief of her dyspnea and, 48 hr later, clearing of the pulmonary infiltrates seen on the chest roentgenogram. She remained in Leadville until cardiac catheterization was performed in Denver 17 days later.

Patient 5 (A. Y.), was a 7-year-old boy of Leadville who had coryza, cough, and fever for 1 week and was admitted to the hospital in Leadville where examination showed a temperature of 39.6° C, cyanosis, and a loud systolic murmur and thrill at the lower left sternal border. Arterial blood oxygen tension was 43 mm Hg. Treatment with oxygen and erythromycin resulted in rapid relief of symptoms and lessening of the murmur. The chest roentgenogram was normal 24 hr after admission. When the symptoms and murmur recurred 12 hr after discharge he was treated with oxygen and transferred to Denver for evaluation by catheterization. On arrival, he was free of symptoms and without a murmur. He returned to Leadville where he remained until cardiac catheterization was performed in Denver 3 weeks later.

Patient 6 (M. A.), a 20-month-old female resident at 3060 m in Colorado, had coryza for several days. She awoke with dyspnea, cyanosis, and cough. Examination in Dillon, CO (2750 m) revealed bilateral rales of the lung fields. She was treated with oxygen, with relief of her dyspnea, cyanosis, and cough in 6 hr. The following day she moved with her family to Denver, where she remained until cardiac catheterization was performed 4 months later.

Patient 7 (M. S.), was a 5-year-old boy of Leadville who underwent cardiac catheterization in Denver after having two previous bouts of pulmonary edema at age 3 and 5 years. At age 7 he twice developed cough and cyanosis after returning home from lower altitudes. On both occasions his symptoms rapidly resolved with oxygen and furosomide therapy. Both his brother and sister have also had episodes of pulmonary edema after returning home from lower altitudes.

Catheterization. Before catheterization all patients underwent standard 12-lead electrocardiographic examinations. Criteria used for diagnosis of right ventricular hypertrophy included a mean QRS axis greater than 100 degrees, an R wave in V_1 greater than 1.8 mV, an R/S ratio in V_1 greater than 1.5, and an upright T wave in V_1.[6] Right and left heart catheterization was performed under meperidine (2 mg/kg im, but no more than 50 mg) and hydroxyzine (1 mg/kg im, but no more than 25 mg) sedation and local anesthesia with 1% lidocaine. Catheter insertion was percutaneous by the modified Seldinger technique via the femoral vessels. Aortic and pulmonary arterial pressures were simultaneously measured through fluid-filled catheters, with the level of the midchest as the zero reference, and recorded on an Electronics for Medicine recorder (White Plains, NY). Blood oxygen saturations were measured on an American Optical (Rochester, NY) oxymeter and arterial blood gas tensions were determined on a Corning 165 blood-gas analyzer (Medford, MA). Cardiac output was calculated by the Fick method with the use of hemoglobin and oxygen saturations to calculate arterial and mixed venous contents. We assumed an oxygen consumption of 150 ml/min/m^2.[7] Measurements were repeated during a 5 to 12 min period while the patients breathed 16% oxygen in nitrogen via a head hood. Then 100% oxygen was administered via the head hood for 5 to 10 min and the measurements were repeated.

Control patients. Three control patients were Leadville residents 8 to 14 months old who underwent catheterization during evaluation for a presumed atrial septal defect or pulmonary hypertension but in whom no abnormalities were found. There were three additional control patients. One was a 3-year-old resident of Leadville in whom cardiac catheterization 6 months after surgical closure of an atrial septal defect showed normal hemodynamics, one was a 4-year-old male resident of Leadville and Vail, CO (2300 m) catheterized for L-transposition of the great arteries and found to have normal hemodynamics, and the third was a 3-year-old female resident of Leadville in whom catheterization at 1½ years after closure of a ventricular septal defect showed normal hemodynamics. None of these control patients had symptoms consistent with high-altitude pulmonary edema.

Results

Clinical findings. The seven patients, four boys and three girls, had nine episodes of high-altitude pulmonary edema, all of which were characterized by cough, radiographic infiltrates (table 1), and response to oxygen therapy. Dyspnea, decreased activity, nausea, emesis, and cyanosis were frequent but not invariable findings (table 1). Five of the nine episodes (two in

TABLE 1
Clinical characteristics of patients during episodes of high-altitude pulmonary edema

	Patient								
	E. H.							M. S.	
	Episode 1	Episode 2	D. F.	A. M.	S. S.	A. Y.	M. A.	Episode 1	Episode 2
Cough	+	+	+	+	+	+	+	+	+
Radiographic infiltrate	+	+	+	+	+	+	+	+	+
Dyspnea	−	+	+	+	+	+	+	−	+
Decreased activity[A]	+	+	+	+	+	+		+	+
Nausea/emesis	+	−	+	+	+	+	−	−	−
Fever[B]	−	−	−	+	+	+		−	−
Rales	+	+	−	−	+	−	+	+	+
Cyanosis	−	−	−	+	+	+	+	+	+
Low-altitude trip	+	+	+	−	+	−	−	+	+
Coryza	−	−	−	+	+	+	+	−	−
O_2 therapy	+	+	+	+	+	+	+	+	+
Diuretic therapy	+	+	+	−	+	−	−	+	+

[A]Defined as lethargy, or exercise intolerance by history from parent.
[B]Temperature >38.5° C.

E. H., one in D. F., and two in M. S.) occurred upon return to high altitude after a 1 day to several week stay at a lower altitude. Three of the nine episodes (one each in A. M., M. Y., and M. A.) occurred at the resident altitude during a respiratory illness marked by coryza. One patient (S. S.) had coryza during a 1 day visit to a lower altitude before developing high-altitude pulmonary edema.

Chest roentgenograms revealed exclusively upper lobe infiltrates in four of the nine episodes. Diffuse infiltrates were seen on radiographs obtained during the other five episodes. In two of these five, upper lobe infiltrates predominated. In addition, the two siblings of M. S. had a total of three episodes of high-altitude pulmonary edema in which infiltrates were observed exclusively in the upper lobes. None of the chest roentgenograms showed exclusively lower lobe infiltrates.

The four electrocardiograms obtained during acute episodes of high-altitude pulmonary edema demonstrated right ventricular hypertrophy (table 2). Recovery electrocardiograms obtained shortly before catheterization demonstrated persistent right ventricular hypertrophy in all seven patients. When electrocardiograms were obtained both during the acute episode and recovery there tended to be slight improvement demonstrated at recovery, but right ventricular hypertrophy persisted. The electrocardiograms of all patients except M. A., who had a counterclockwise frontal plane vector loop, demonstrated at least two criteria for right ventricular hypertrophy. However, even M. A. had evidence of right ventricular hypertrophy, i.e., an R wave without an S wave in V_1 (table 2).

Hemodynamics. At the time of catheterization, the mean hemoglobin concentration in the patients (13.8 ± 0.7 g/100 ml) was not different from that in the control subjects (13.6 ± 0.3 g/100 ml). By analysis of variance mean pulmonary arterial pressure (table 3), mean arterial pressure, cardiac output, and arterial oxygen tension were not different between groups.

The administration of 16% O_2 decreased arterial oxygen tension to comparable levels in the two groups (table 3). The mean pulmonary arterial pressure during hypoxia in the susceptible patients was greater than in room air and greater than that in the control subjects during hypoxia (figure 1). Also, patients S. S. and A. M., who developed the most severe pulmonary hypertension during hypoxia, showed the most rapid

TABLE 2
Electrocardiographic data in seven patients during acute high-altitude pulmonary edema and after recovery

	QRS axis (degrees)		RV_1 (mV × 10^{-1})		R/S in V_1	
Patient	Acute	Recovery	Acute	Recovery	Acute	Recovery
E. H.	—	110°	—	9.5	—	3.8
D. F.	165°	150°	12.5	13.0	12.5	2.2
A. M.	—	165°	—	20.0	—	1.3
S. S.	120°	120°	7.0	9.0	∞	3.6
A. Y.[A]	115°	105°	2.0	8.0	1.0	1.0
M. A.	—	−15°	—	3.0	—	∞
M. S.	235°	235°	20.0	15.0	∞	∞

[A]Abnormal T wave in V_1.

TABLE 3

Hemodynamics in patients who recovered from high-altitude pulmonary edema and in control subjects also residing at high altitudes (>10,000 feet)

Patient or subject	Age	PPA (mm Hg)			PAo (mm Hg)			CI [l/(min m²)]			Pa_{O_2} (mm Hg)		
		RA	16% O_2	100% O_2	RA	16% O_2	100% O_2	RA	16% O_2	100% O_2	RA	16% O_2	100% O_2
Patients													
E. H.	10 yr	22	51	15	82	87	90	4.9	5.2	4.5	70	49	449
D. F.	8 yr	22	35	18	82	85	74	3.7	4.0	3.3	73	48	457
A. M.	4 yr	25	63	23	70	73	75	3.8	—	2.7	65[A]	47	414
S. S.	6 yr	20	100	23	88	100	78	2.9	—	—	80[A]	38	—
A. Y.	7 yr	16	52	12	77	77	81	3.1	3.3	2.6	73	40	451
M. A.	20 mo	25	37	20	67	65	70	5.8	6.8	4.3	63[A]	36[A]	426
M. S.	5 yr	25	—	—	83	—	—	3.8	—	—	60[A]	—	—
Mean		21.7	56.3[B,C]	8.5	77.7	81.2[B]	78	4.0	4.8	3.5	70.7	43[C]	439
±SD		3.4	23.8	4.4	8.0	12.2	7.0	1.1	1.5	0.9	6.2	5.7	18
Control subjects													
1	8 mo	18	18	—	63	60	—	4.3	—	—	74	52	—
2	11 mo	14	15	—	70	66	—	4.0	—	—	72	48	—
3	14 mo	18	20	—	68	65	—	3.6	—	—	70	57	—
4	3 yr	16	18	11	77	72	75	4.9	4.1	4.4	67	53	328
5	4 yr	13	16	14	82	70	80	3.9	3.9	5.2	62	40	414
6	3 yr	21	26	21	72	62	72	2.3	2.4	2.0	62	41	423
Mean		16.7	18.8	15.3	72.0	65.8	75.7	3.8	3.4	3.9	66.8	48.5[C]	380
±SD		2.9	3.9	5.1	6.7	4.6	4.0	0.9	0.9	1.7	5.1	6.8	52

All patients underwent catheterization in Denver. A. M., M. A., and control subject 5 were catheterized 10 days, 5 months, and 4 months, respectively, after their arrival in Denver; the remaining patients and subjects were catheterized within 3 days. Pa_{CO_2} values in room air and during hypoxia, respectively, in the patients in whom it was measured were as follows: 37 and 32 mm Hg for E. H., 33 and 33 mm Hg for D. F., 38 mm Hg (during hypoxia only) for A. M., and 44 and 44 mm Hg for A. Y. The values for the control subjects in whom it was measured were: 37 and 34 mm Hg for subject 4, 41 and 43 mm Hg for subject 5, and 38 and 38 mm Hg for subject 6.

RA = room air.

[A]Calculated from arterial oxygen saturation, assuming pH of 7.4.

[B]Significant at $p < .05$ by analysis of variance when compared with control subjects at similar inspired oxygen levels.

[C]Significant at $p < .05$ by analysis of variance when compared with same group at room air.

rate of pressure increase (figure 2). There was no change in aortic pressure in the susceptible patients, whereas in the controls there was a significant decline (table 3). The cardiac output values in the susceptible patients were not different from the three values in the control patients. In the two patients in whom wedge pressure was determined, no change was noted with hypoxia (E. H. 4 and 4 mm Hg; A. Y. 3 and 3 mm Hg). While the percent change in total pulmonary resistance in room air to that during hypoxia for the three susceptible patients in whom it could be calculated (138 ± 58%) was greater than that for control patients (29 ± 5%), insufficient data was available to accurately analyze changes in pulmonary arteriolar resistance. Instead, the ratio of the pulmonary-to-aortic pressure was calculated. The ratio for the susceptible patients (0.28 ± 0.07) was not different from that for control subjects (0.23 ± 0.05) while breathing room air. With hypoxia the ratio in the susceptible patients (0.68 ± 0.21) was greater than during normoxia and was greater than the ratio in the control subjects during hypoxia (0.29 ± 0.02), despite a lower mean aortic pressure in the latter.

Discussion

The results of this study show that children living at high altitude who have experienced at least one episode of high-altitude pulmonary edema have increased pulmonary arterial vasoreactivity to hypoxia when compared with children who reside at a similar altitude but who have not developed high-altitude pulmonary edema. Thus, hypoxia caused a large but variable increase in pulmonary arterial pressure in the susceptible patients, but only a small change in the control subjects, although the two groups had comparable arterial oxygen tensions. One major drawback of our study was that the control subjects tended to be younger than those with a history of pulmonary edema. This difficulty arises because catheterization and hypoxic challenge of normal children is not a routine or ethical practice. However, previously published data[8, 9] indicate that infants are more reactive to hypoxia than

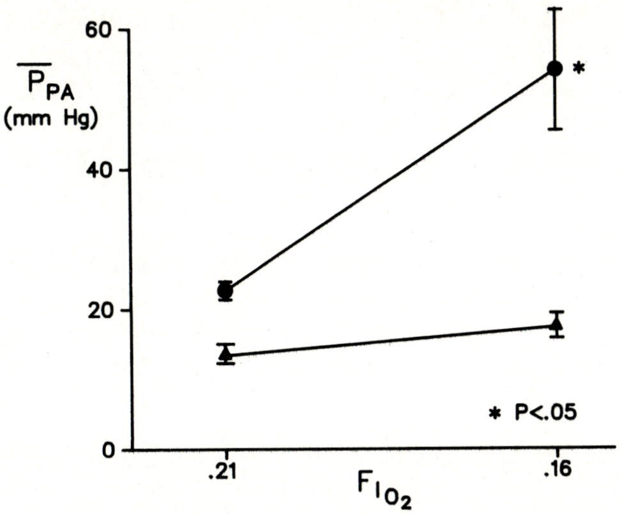

FIGURE 1. Mean and SEM pulmonary arterial pressure at inspired oxygen fractions of 0.21 and 0.16 for high-altitude pulmonary edema (HAPE)–susceptible children and normal children. Closed circles indicate children catheterized in Denver after recovery from high-altitude (> 3000 m) pulmonary edema; open circles indicate healthy children from a similar altitude of residence without a history of edema. The values for the two patient groups were statistically ($p < .05$) different when 16% O_2 was breathed.

adults. Thus, the three infants who served as control subjects would be expected to show greater responses at their age than when they reached the age of the susceptible patients. An additional approach was to use the data of Vogel et al.[10] obtained from normal school-age children who underwent cardiac catheterization in Leadville. In this study population were six adolescents in whom pulmonary arterial pressure and hemoglobin saturation data were recorded in room air and during hypoxia. A comparison of the data of Vogel et al. with that from our susceptible children was made with the arterial oxygen tension as a measure of stimulus and the pulmonary arterial pressure as a measure of response (figure 3). Even though our susceptible patients underwent cardiac catheterization in Denver, they showed a larger increase in pulmonary arterial pressure, beginning at higher oxygen tensions, suggesting an increased pulmonary vasoreactivity to hypoxia. We conclude that an increased vasoreactivity to hypoxia is present after recovery in children who have had high-altitude pulmonary edema. Whether or not increased vasoreactivity has a role in the adult who develops high-altitude pulmonary edema when journeying from low to high altitude cannot be concluded from this investigation.

Although as a group susceptible patients showed an excessive rise in pulmonary arterial pressure during acute hypoxia, one patient in this group did not show such a response when compared with the data of Vogel et al.[10] Indeed, a large range of pressure increases were seen in the susceptible group. This finding is reminiscent of that by Hultgren and Grover,[4] who also showed that some adults with a history of high-altitude pulmonary edema did not show an increased pulmonary pressor response to hypoxia when tested at low altitude,

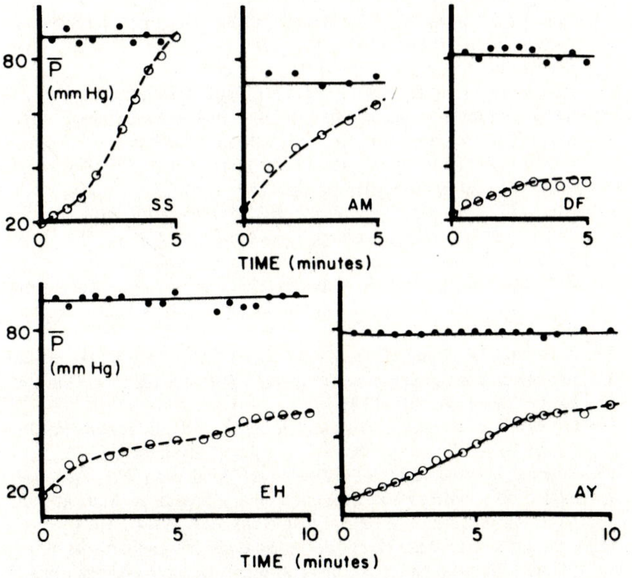

FIGURE 2. Time course of mean pulmonary arterial pressure (open circles) and mean aortic pressure (closed circles) after administration of 16% oxygen to children with a history of high-altitude pulmonary edema. Two patients with very large pulmonary arterial pressor responses also had a rapid rate of pressure rise.

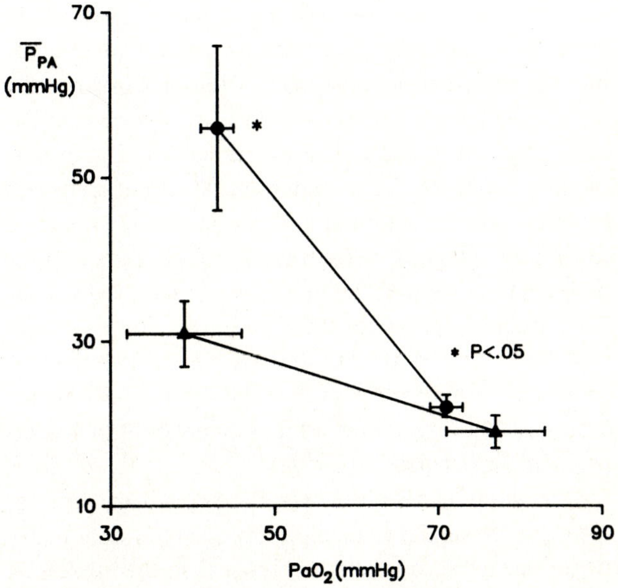

FIGURE 3. Mean and SEM pulmonary arterial pressure vs arterial oxygen tension in children susceptible to high-altitude pulmonary edema as measured in Denver (filled circles). Shown for comparison are values from six normal children undergoing pulmonary arterial catheterization in Leadville, CO as reported by Vogel et al.[10] (filled triangles). Pa_{O_2} for the data of Vogel et al. were calculated from the reported saturations assuming a pH of 7.40.

indicating that pulmonary vascular reactivity may not in itself cause high-altitude pulmonary edema. Furthermore, a report from this institution has previously described infants from areas of high altitude with symptomatic high-altitude pulmonary hypertension.[11] These infants present with failure to thrive and cor pulmonale and have a high mortality rate if not moved to lower elevations. On evaluation they show an exaggerated and rapid pulmonary arterial vasoconstrictive response to hypoxia. Yet, none has been known to have had an episode or illness resembling high-altitude pulmonary edema. Thus, vasoreactivity by itself may not be sufficient to cause pulmonary edema. Although our findings indicate a relationship between susceptibility to high-altitude pulmonary edema and increased pulmonary vasoreactivity to hypoxia, some other factor or factors must be involved.

Clues to other factors may have been that several of the children in the present study developed pulmonary edema during an upper respiratory illness while residing at high altitude, i.e., without a prior trip to lower altitude. We suspect that a propensity of some Leadville children to develop pulmonary edema during a coryza-like illness indicates a susceptibility to high-altitude pulmonary edema. If so, the finding is unique to our study, although others have indicated the presence of upper respiratory illness in their case reports.[3, 12] A possible explanation for the association of upper respiratory illness and pulmonary edema at high altitudes is that nasal obstruction further intensifies the hypoxia of altitude. In particular, nasal obstruction increases the frequency and duration of apneic spells during sleep.[13] Another possibility is that viral respiratory infections could increase permeability in the pulmonary vascular bed or alter the alveolar epithelial barrier.[14] The recent finding of high protein in the fluid from lung lavage of patients with high-altitude pulmonary edema indicates the presence of increased vascular permeability.[15] The combination of increased vascular pressure plus an increase in endothelial or epithelial permeability may result in a much higher extravascular lung water content than would increased pressure or permeability alone.[16]

One would anticipate that the pulmonary arterial pressure during the acute high-altitude pulmonary edema in our patients would be higher than that observed after recovey.[3, 17] Clinical evidence of acute elevation of pressure was observed on the electrocardiograms available for study. That pressures were higher during the acute episode than after recovery was suggested by more rightward QRS vectors and higher right-sided voltages during edema. However, even after recovery, the seven susceptible patients continued to show increased right ventricular forces, suggesting persistent pulmonary hypertension during continued high-altitude residence. If this is the case, the clinical data are consistent with increased pulmonary pressures in the susceptible children during continued residence at high altitude. Perhaps electrocardiographic manifestations of augmented pulmonary hypertension may prove to be a screening technique to uncover those children susceptible to high-altitude pulmonary edema.

We wish to thank the referring physicians Drs. Leonardi, Cullen, Perna, Quakenbush and Vanhardenbrook for their assistance. Also, Dr. John T. Reeves for his invaluable help in the preparation of this manuscript.

References

1. Scoggin CH, Hyers TM, Reeves JT, Grover RF: High altitude pulmonary edema in the children and young adults of Leadville, Colorado. N Engl J Med **297:** 1269, 1977
2. Sophocles A, Bachman J: High altitude pulmonary edema among visitors to Summit County, Colorado. J Fam Pract **17:** 1015, 1983
3. Hultgren HN, Lopez CE, Lundberg E, Miller H: Physiologic studies of pulmonary edema at high altitude. Circulation **29:** 393, 1964
4. Hultgren HN, Grover RF, Hartley LH: Abnormal circulatory responses to high altitude in subjects with a previous history of high altitude pulmonary edema. Circulation **44:** 759, 1971
5. Viswanathan R, Jain SK, Subramanian S, Subramanian TAV, Dua GL, Giri J: Pulmonary edema at high altitude: II. Clinical aerohemodynamic and biochemical studies in a group with history of pulmonary edema of high altitude. Am Rev Respir Dis **100:** 334, 1969
6. Garson A, Gillette PC, McNamara DG: A guide to cardiac dysrhythmias in children. New York, 1980, Grune and Stratton
7. LaFarge CG, Miettinen OS: The estimation of oxygen consumption. Cardiovasc Res **4:** 23, 1970
8. James LS, Rowe RD: The pattern of response of pulmonary and systemic arterial pressures on newborn and older infants to short periods of hypoxia. J Pediatr **51:** 5, 1957
9. Rudolph AM, Auld AM, Golinko RJ, Paul MH: Pulmonary vascular adjustments in the neonatal period. Pediatrics **28:** 28, 1961
10. Vogel JHK, Weaver WF, Rose RL, Blount SG, Grover RF: Pulmonary hypertension on exertion in normal man at 10,150 feet (Leadville, Colorado). Med Thorac **19:** 269, 1962
11. Jones TK, Wiggins JW, Wolfe RR: Symptomatic high altitude pulmonary hypertension of infancy. Circulation **66**(suppl II): II-48, 1982
12. Fred HL, Schmidt AM, Bates T, Hecht HH: Acute pulmonary edema of altitude: clinical and physiologic observations. Circulation **25:** 929, 1962
13. Zwillich CW, Pickett C, Hanson FN, Weil JV: Disturbed sleep and prolonged apnea during nasal obstruction in normal men. Am Rev Respir Dis **124:** 158, 1981
14. Gorin AB, Stewart PA: Differential permeability of endothelial and epithelial barriers to albumin flux. J Appl Physiol **47:** 1315, 1979
15. Schoene RB, Martin TR, Hackett PH, Henderson WR, Sage EH, Roach RC, Miles WJ: Bronchoalveolar lavage in high altitude pulmonary edema. Am Rev Respir Dis **129:** A104, 1984
16. Ohkuda K, Nakahara K, Binder A, Staub NC: Venous air emboli in sheep: reversible increase in lung microvascular permeability. J Appl Physiol **51:** 887, 1981
17. Penaloza D, Sime F: Circulatory dynamics during high altitude pulmonary edema. Am J Cardiol **23:** 369, 1969

Complex ventricular arrhythmias in patients with Q wave versus non–Q wave myocardial infarction

ALAN S. MAISEL, M.D., NEIL SCOTT, M.D., ELIZABETH GILPIN, M.S., STAFFAN AHNVE, M.D., MARTIN LE WINTER, M.D., HARTMUT HENNING, M.D., DANIEL COLLINS, M.D., AND JOHN ROSS JR., M.D.

ABSTRACT We examined whether or not subsets of patients with complex ventricular arrhythmias after myocardial infarction are at high risk with respect to 1 year mortality after hospital discharge. Based on previous studies showing increased risk for those with non–Q wave infarcts, we hypothesized that complex PVCs (premature ventricular complexes) in this group might be associated with a poorer prognosis than complex PVCs in patients with Q wave infarcts. Seven hundred seventy-seven patients entering our study with acute infarction were followed prospectively for 1 year after undergoing a predischarge 24 hr ambulatory electrocardiographic examination. Patients were classified by electrocardiographic criteria into the following groups: Non–Q wave (n = 191), Q wave anterior (n = 261), and Q wave inferior infarction (n = 325). The following arrhythmias were classified as complex: multiform PVCs, couplets, and ventricular tachycardia. Sixty-two percent of patients with non–Q wave infarcts who did not survive 1 year had complex PVCs, compared with 32% of survivors ($p < .01$). No differences were seen in the Q wave subgroup. The survival for patients with Q wave and non–Q wave infarction without complex PVCs were nearly identical at 1 year (93% and 90%), whereas in patients with complex PVCs survival for those with Q wave and non–Q wave infarction was 92% and 76%, respectively ($p < .001$). Of those with non–Q wave infarction, only 4% of nonsurvivors were free of any PVCs, as compared with 28% of nonsurvivors in the Q wave group ($p < .02$). Stepwise linear discrimination analysis revealed that complex PVCs were independent of ejection fraction in those with non–Q wave infarction, but were closely associated with ejection fraction in those with Q wave infarction. Thus, the presence of complex PVCs at the time of hospital discharge is an important predictor of 1 year mortality in the presence of non–Q wave, but not Q wave infarction.
Circulation 72, No. 5, 963–970, 1985.

RISK STRATIFICATION during the course of acute myocardial infarction may identify patients who are subsequently at high risk for recurrent infarction or death afer recovery. Recognition of high-risk patients may permit specific interventions to be directed toward the factors responsible. Although the presence of complex ventricular arrhythmias recorded in the late hospital phase of acute infarction have been a strong predictor of subsequent mortality,[1-12] attempts to improve survival by pharmacologic suppression have resulted in little success.[13-15]

It seems possible that if subsets of patients with complex arrhythmias who are at particularly high risk can be identified, treatment could be selectively aimed at such groups. Although non–Q wave and Q wave infarctions as classified by electrocardiography cannot always be differentiated anatomically, it is clear that they differ clinically and prognostically.[16, 17] Data suggest that patients with non–Q wave infarction, despite an initially favorable prognosis, have a long-term mortality similar to or greater than that of patients with Q wave infarction.[18, 19] Recently we have suggested that a non–Q wave infarction may be an unstable event and that variables such as infarct extension during the course of the acute infarction may be markers for late mortality.[20, 21] Accordingly, the present study was undertaken to test the hypothesis that complex PVCs (premature ventricular complexes) occurring in the late hospital phase of acute infarction signify a poorer

From the Divison of Cardiology, Department of Medicine, University of California, San Diego, Division of Cardiology, Department of Medicine, University of British Columbia, Vancouver, The San Diego Veterans Administration Medical Center, and United States Naval Regional Medical Center, San Diego.

Supported by National Institutes of Health Research grant HL 17682, Ischemic Heart Disease Specialized Center of Research (SCOR) awarded by the National Heart, Lung, and Blood Institute, Bethesda.

Address for correspondence: John Ross, Jr., M.D., Head, Division of Cardiology, Department of Medicine, M-013, University of California, San Diego, School of Medicine, La Jolla, CA 92093.

Received April 1, 1985; revision accepted Aug. 8, 1985.

Presented at the 34th Annual Scientific Session American College of Cardiology, Anaheim, CA, March 1985.

prognosis for patients with non–Q wave infarction compared with the prognosis for those with Q wave infarction.

Methods

Patients. The study group consisted of 1783 patients with acute infarction who were admitted to the hospital within 24 hr after onset of symptoms. Of the 1658 patients eventually discharged from the hospital, 1406 had been followed for 1 year at the time of the study. Of this group, 777 patients underwent predischarge 24 hr ambulatory electrocardiographic (ECG) monitoring, and only this group was analyzed in this study for 1 year outcome. Ambulatory ECG monitoring was not required as part of our protocol and its performance was at the discretion of the attending physician. This could have led to some bias toward ECG monitoring in more gravely ill patients. However, statistical analysis comparing this group with the group of patients who did not undergo predischarge ECG monitoring showed no differences in arrhythmias in the intensive care unit, discharge ejection fraction, or 1 year survival. However, there were higher peak creatine kinase (CK) levels, a longer stay in the intensive care unit, and more evidence of heart failure while in the hospital in the patients electrocardiographically monitored.

Q wave infarction was diagnosed by development of pathologic Q waves (as described below) and at least one of the following: (1) chest pain considered characteristic of myocardial ischemia, and (2) elevation of total creatine kinase. Q waves acceptable for diagnosis were as follows: (1) anterior = Q $\geq$ 0.04 sec in any precordial lead, (2) inferior = Q in leads III and aVF $\geq$0.04 sec or >25% of R wave in depth, and (3) lateral = Q in leads I and aVL $\geq$0.04 sec or >25% of R wave. Posterior infarctions were those resulting in an initial R wave in lead V_1 or V_2 of 0.04 sec with an R/S greater than 1. Infarctions resulting in both anterior and lateral Q waves were classified as anterior, and those resulting in inferior and posterior or inferior and lateral Q waves were classified as inferior. Non–Q wave infarction was diagnosed by (1) the presence of characteristic chest pain, (2) elevation of CK-MB, and (3) the following electrocardiographic criteria: (a) persistent new T wave inversion and/or ST segment changes, and (b) absence of new pathologic Q waves.

Two-channel (leads V_1 and V_5) 24 hr ambulatory electrocardiograms were analyzed by computer with manual overread by a technician, with final review by a physician. Complex PVCs were identified as one or more of the following: multiform PVCs, couplets, and/or ventricular tachycardia (3 or more beats with heart rate >100 beats/min).

Data concerning these patients were available from a data base maintained by the Specialized Center of Research (SCOR) on Ischemic Heart Disease at the University of California San Diego Medical Center. These patients were recruited during the period from 1979 to 1983 from the University of California San Diego Medical Center, the San Diego Veterans Administration Medical Center, the United States Naval Regional Medical Center in San Diego, and the Vancouver General Hospital, Vancouver, British Columbia.

Clinical and laboratory variables. The methods of data acquisition and definitions of variables have been reported in detail previously.[22, 23] Data from the history and physical examination and laboratory findings, chest x-rays, and electrocardiograms were assessed. The data base was examined univariately for variables related to complex PVCs in both the Q wave and the non–Q wave groups. Multivariate analyses were done on variables for which univariate screening showed an association with mortality at a significance level of $p \leq .05$. Historical variables selected included age, sex, previous infarction, congestive heart failure, typical angina pectoris, chronic obstructive pulmonary disease, hypertension, bundle branch block, and new or changing angina within 1 month before hospital admission. The following clinical parameters were assessed throughout the period in the intensive care unit: maximal heart rate, minimum systolic blood pressure, maximal respiratory rate, the presence of S_3 gallop, systolic murmur suggesting mitral regurgitation, apex impulse to the left of the midclavicular line, the presence and extent of rales, peripheral or sacral edema, and mental confusion. From chest radiographs, the maximal degree of pulmonary venous congestion was graded (0 to 4) as previously described.[24]

Laboratory findings included maximal levels of CK, maximum leukocyte count, and maximum creatinine and blood urea nitrogen. From the ECG tracings, the maximal measured QRS duration, infarct location, maximal PR interval, arrhythmias, and conduction disturbances were noted. At discharge, the administration of digitalis, diuretics, procainamide, quinidine, and β-blocking agents was recorded. The cardiothoracic ratio and degree of pulmonary congestion were measured on the discharge chest radiograph. In a subgroup of 496 patients, a discharge left ventricular ejection fraction was measured by radionuclide techniques or cardiac catheterization.

Follow-up. All patients were followed by telephone at 3, 6, and 12 months after hospital discharge. Information regarding death was obtained from death certificates, hospital records, or telephone interviews with the personal physician or family members. Only cardiac deaths were included in the analyses. A committee reviewed all available data to determine cause of death. Sudden death was defined as death presumed to occur within 24 hr after onset of symptoms. Sixty percent of these occurred within the first 1 hr. There was greater than 98% follow-up at 1 year.

Statistical methods. Univariate statistical analyses were performed by the chi-square test for discrete variables or t tests for continuous variables to assess differences in characteristics between patients with and without complex PVCs, as well as to study the influence of these variables on prognosis. To evaluate the independent importance of prognostic variables, the stepwise linear discrimination model (P7M) available in the Biomedical Computer Programs package of statistical programs was used.[25] We have previously shown tht this approach provides similar results to logistic regression analysis.[26] Survival curves for the different populations were compared with the Mantel-Cox statistic as calculated by the survival function program (PIL) provided in the same software package.

Results

The occurrence of noncomplex and complex PVCs in patients with Q wave and non–Q wave infarctions in relation to selected clinical variables is presented in table 1. Among the 791 patients studied (616 men and 175 women, mean age 61 years, range 29 to 89 yr), the location of infarction was classified as Q wave in 75% (inferior 41%, anterior 34%) and as non–Q wave in 25%. Complex PVCs were present on predischarge 24 hr ambulatory monitoring in 41% of patients with non–Q wave infarction and 36% of those with Q wave infarction (p = NS). In patients without complex PVCs, 1 year mortality after hospital discharge was similar in the non–Q wave and Q wave groups (9% vs

7%, p = NS). Among patients with complex PVCs, the 1 year mortality in the non–Q wave group was 27% vs 9% in the Q wave group (p < .01).

Sixty-five variables were examined for association with complex PVCs in the Q wave and non–Q wave categories. Prior history of angina pectoris, myocardial infarction, and heart failure were not associated with complex PVCs in either group. Peak CK levels were higher in patients with Q wave infarctions, but were not significantly higher in those with complex PVCs in either group (table 1). There was no association between early arrhythmias in the coronary care unit and subsequent complex PVCs in either the Q wave or non–Q wave group. In the Q wave group, complex PVCs were associated with a significantly higher incidence of postinfarction left ventricular failure than that in the non–Q wave group, as evidenced by the occurrence of an S_3 gallop (56% vs 45%, p < .01), bibasilar rales (73% vs 54%, p < .001), rales above scapulae (11% vs 2%, p < .05), and increased cardiothoracic ratio (0.49 ± 0.05 vs 0.47 ± 0.05, p < .01). In the non–Q wave group, there was no significant association between complex PVCs and heart failure (table 1).

Complex PVCs were present in 39% of the patients with non–Q wave infarctions who survived 1 year (n = 126) (figure 1), while in those patients who did not survive one year (n = 26), complex PVCs occurred in 69% (p < .01). No such differences between survivors and nonsurvivors with respect to complex PVCs were seen in the anterior or inferior Q wave infarct groups. The cumulative survival curves beginning at discharge for patients with Q wave and non–Q wave infarctions with and without complex PVCs are illustrated in figure 2. In patients without complex PVCs (figure 2, *A*), the survival curves for patients with Q wave infarctions and the curves for those with non–Q wave infarctions were not significantly different, with a 1 year survival of 93% for the Q wave (inferior = 95%, anterior = 92%) and of 91% for the non–Q wave group. However, when survival was compared among patients with complex PVCs, signifi-

TABLE 1
Patient characteristics

Variable	Non–Q wave infarction (n = 191) Noncomplex PVCs	Complex PVCs	p value	Q wave infarction (n = 586) Noncomplex PVCs	Complex PVCs	p value
Total patients	113	78		380	206	
Mean age (years)	62 ± 13	67 ± 10	.002	59 ± 12	63 ± 12	.002
Males (%)	76	80	NS	82	76	NS
Hx heart failure (%)	17	18	NS	5	8	NS
Hx angina (%)	57	64	NS	31	38	NS
Hx infarction (%)	33	36	NS	15	20	NS
Deaths — 1 year (%)	10	27	.01	7	9	NS
Survivors — 1 year (%)	90	73	.01	93	91	NS
Hospitalization						
Mean peak CK	639 ± 725	589 ± 408	NS	1344 ± 999	1431 ± 999	NS
CTR	0.48 ± 0.05	0.49 ± 0.04	NS	0.48 ± 0.05	0.50 ± 0.05	.01
Mean ejection fraction	0.54 ± 13	0.50 ± 15	NS	0.49 ± 13	0.43 ± 14	.003
S_3 (%)	30	37	NS	44	58	.001
Bibasilar rales	59	62	NS	55	74	.001
RAS	12	10	NS	5	10	.05
Arrhythmias — CCU						
PVCs > 6/min	15	19	NS	24	27	NS
V-tachycardia	22	18	NS	30	33	NS
V-fibrillation	3	0	NS	6	4	NS
Discharge medicines						
Digitalis	36	35	NS	35	44	.05
β-Blockers	58	49	NS	44	35	.03
Procainamide	12	16	NS	7	13	NS
Quinidine	17	18	NS	18	18	NS
Diuretic	34	35	NS	26	28	NS

Mean values are ± 1 SD. Probability values based on Chi-square or t test.

CCU = coronary care unit; CTR = cardiothoracic ratio; Hx = history; RAS = rales above scapulae; V-tach = ventricular tachycardia; V-fib = ventricular fibrillation.

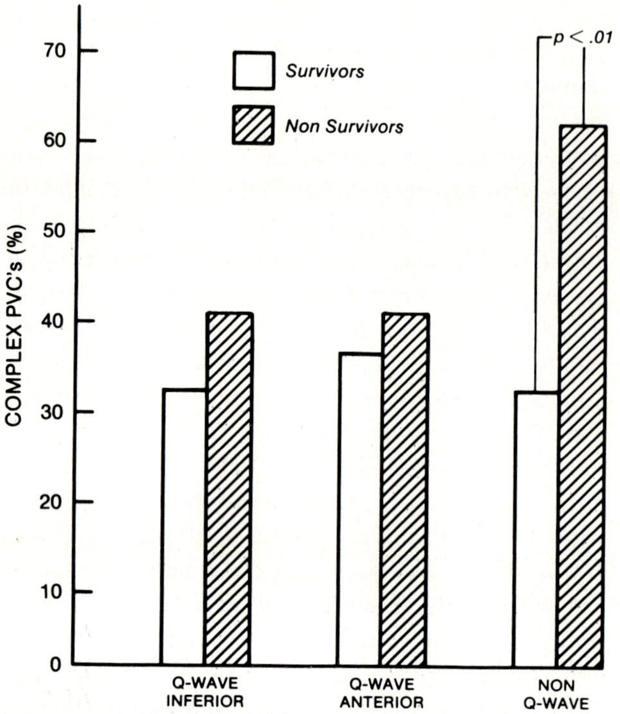

FIGURE 1. Relationship between complex PVCs on discharge Holter recordings and 1 year survival.

wave infarction, 30% had no complex ventricular arrhythmias.

Relationship of left ventricular ejection fraction to complex PVCs. Table 1 reveals an association between the presence of complex PVCs and a decreased ejection fraction in the Q wave (ejection fractions without and with complex PVCs: 49 ± 13% vs 43 ± 14%, respectively, mean ± SD, $p < .01$), but not in the non–Q wave group (54 ± 12% vs 50 ± 14%, p = NS). This lack of association between complex PVCs and ejection fraction in patients with non–Q wave infarction remains when the relationship is examined in terms of mortality. We have recently found that an ejection fraction of 45% best discriminates between survival and death in our population data base and thus used this dichotomized ejection fraction for comparison.[27] The 1 year survival of non–Q wave infarction in all patients with complex PVCs compared with that in patients with complex PVCs and an ejection fraction less than 45% is presented in figure 4. The inclusion of lowered

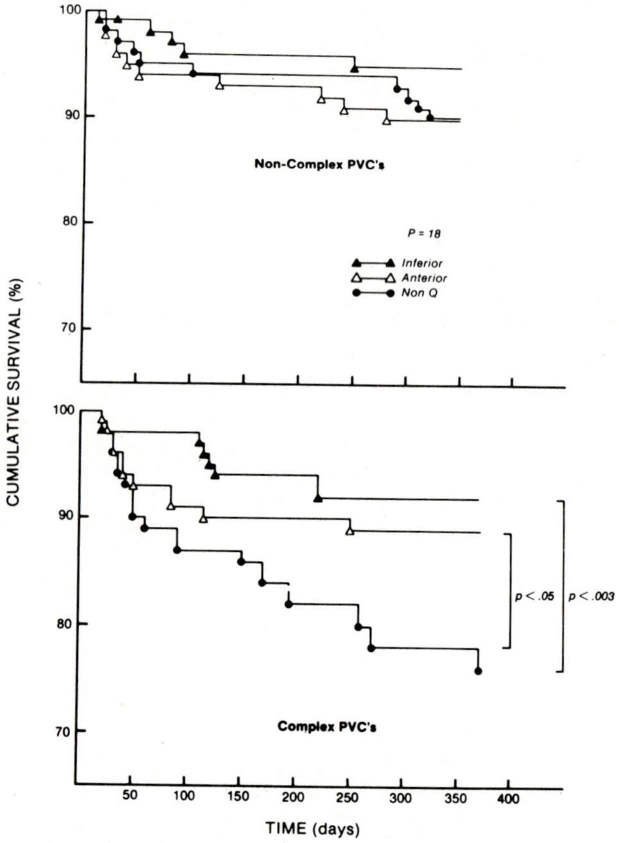

FIGURE 2. Cumulative survival in patients with Q wave vs those with non–Q wave infarction with and without complex PVCs. *A*, In patients without complex PVCs followed for 1 year after discharge there was an 8% mortality in the Q wave (inferior = 5%, anterior = 10%) and a 10% mortality for non–Q wave group. *B*, In patients with complex PVCs, the cumulative survival at 1 year in the non–Q wave group was 76% as compared with 90% in the Q wave anterior ($p<.05$) and 93% in the Q wave inferior group ($p<.001$).

cant differences were seen (figure 2, *B*). The survival at 1 year for the non–Q wave group was 73%, as compared with 90% for the Q wave anterior group ($p < .05$) and 94% for the Q wave inferior group ($p < .001$). Approximately 50% of deaths in each group were classified as "sudden," irrespective of whether or not complex PVCs were present.

Types of ventricular arrhythmias detected on 24 hr monitoring. Figure 3 shows the breakdown of arrhythmias detected by 24 hr ambulatory ECG monitoring as related to survival in Q wave and non–Q wave infarction groups. Of all the types of arrhythmias present, the greatest differences in survivors vs nonsurvivors were in the categories of multiform PVCs and couplets. These were present with greater frequency in nonsurvivors with non–Q wave infarctions than in survivors (33% vs 16% for multiform and 24% vs 7% for couplets, $p < .01$), but their incidence did not differ in survivors and nonsurvivors of Q wave infarctions. In fact, there was no category of arrhythmia alone that was able to discriminate between survivors and nonsurvivors of Q wave infarction, although the small numbers of patients having ventricular tachycardia or R on T PVCs preclude accurate statistical analysis for those groups. Of all nonsurvivors of non–Q wave infarction, only one patient (4%) was totally free of any ventricular arrhythmias, as compared with 31 (25%) of the survivors ($p < .01$). Among nonsurvivors of Q

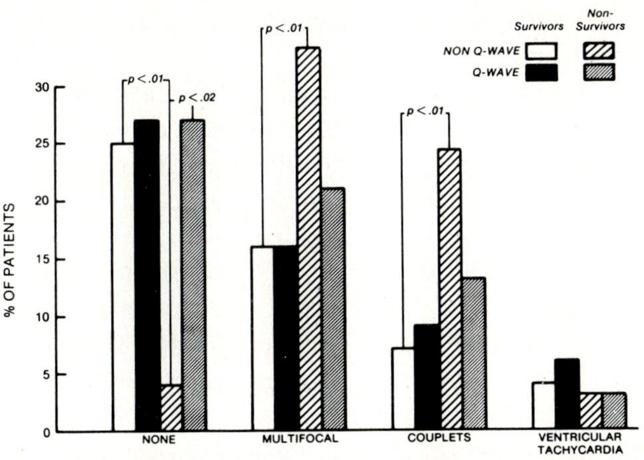

FIGURE 3. Arrhythmias present at discharge (Holter) as related to 1 year survival in Q wave and non–Q wave infarction groups. Multifocal PVCs and couplets were present with greater frequency in nonsurvivors with non–Q wave infarction than in surivors (33% and 24% vs 16% and 7%, respectively, $p<.01$), but did not differ in survivors and nonsurvivors of Q wave infarctions. Only 4% of nonsurvivors of non–Q wave infarction were free of any ventricular arrhythmias as compared with 25% of survivors ($p<.01$).

ejection fraction in the analysis adds only 5% to predicted mortality over 1 year. The *inset* of figure 4 separates patients with and without complex PVCs into groups with normal and low ejection fractions. In the Q wave group, patients with complex PVCs were equally divided into the groups of those with ejection fractions less than and greater than 45%. Among those with non–Q wave infarctions and complex PVCs, twice as many patients had ejection fractions greater than 45%.

Multivariate analysis of predictors of mortality. Stepwise linear discriminant analysis was performed to evaluate independent contributions of ventricular arrhythmias and other variables to postinfarction mortality. No independent contribution to mortality could be attributed to ejection fraction in the non–Q wave group. In this group, the combination of complex PVCs, age, and pulmonary congestion predicted 74% of subsequent deaths. As expected, in contrast to the case in the non–Q wave group, there was no independent influence of complex PVCs on mortality. In the group of patients with Q wave infarction and PVCs the combination of ejection fraction, radiographic pulmonary congestion, and rales above the scapulae predicted 88% of subsequent deaths.

Complex PVCs and antiarrhythmic therapy at discharge. As can be seen in table 1, antiarrhythmic therapy at discharge was not related to type or location of infarction, and such therapy was given to a similar percentage of patients with and without complex PVCs on their discharge 24 hr electrocardiogram. The small numbers of patients in each group discharged on antiarrhythmic medication preclude accurate statistical assessment of the effect of this variable on survival. However, among those discharged on antiarrhythmic therapy, there was a trend toward increased 1 year survival in patients with non–Q wave infarction compared with that in patients with Q wave infarction. Thus, of the 17 patients with non–Q wave infarction discharged on therapy, 11 were dead after 1 year, compared with 21 of 24 patients with Q wave infarction similarly followed and on therapy ($p = .08$).

Discussion

The present study emphasizes the importance of complex PVCs occurring in the late hospital phase of acute myocardial infarction in predicting late cardiac death after non–Q wave myocardial infarction. In patients with Q wave infarction, complex PVCs alone were not associated with increased late mortality. In agreement with Moss[28] and Vismara et al,[11] we found no relationship between PVCs in the coronary care unit and the occurrence of similar arrhythmias on ambulatory recordings 1 to 3 weeks later in either group.

One of the first studies to show an association between ventricular arrhythmias after recovery from myocardial infarction and late cardiac death was the coronary drug project,[12] which reported that the presence of one or more PVCs on a 12-lead electrocardiogram was associated with an increased risk of sudden death over the ensuing 2 to 5 years. More recently,

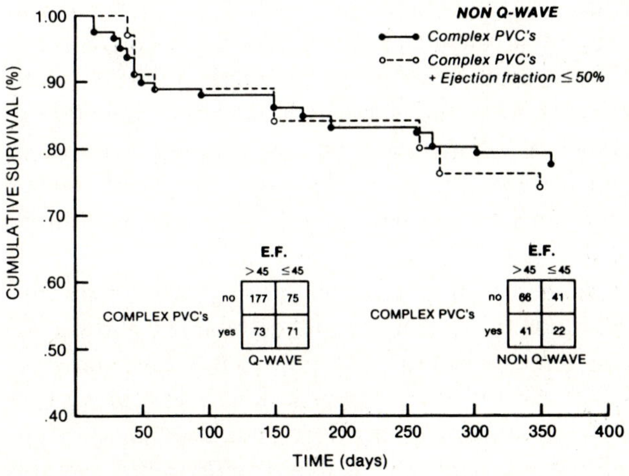

FIGURE 4. Cumulative survival of non–Q wave myocardial infarction: effects of ejection fraction in patients with complex PVCs. The inclusion of lowered ejection fraction in the analysis adds only 5% to predicted mortality over 1 year. The *inset* reveals a strong association between complex PVCs and a low ejection fraction in patients with Q wave infarction. In patients with non–Q wave infarction, complex PVCs were twice as common in those with ejection fractions greater than 45%.

ambulatory ECG monitoring of 1 to 24 hr has been used. Ruberman et al.[7] examined the 1 hr recordings of 1739 men with recent myocardial infarction. Complex PVCs were associated with a threefold increase in risk of cardiac death at 24 months. Moss et al.,[29] in analyzing survivors of acute myocardial infarction, found that arrhythmias of Lown grade 2 or greater identified patients at high risk of cardiac death or new infarction. Subsequent analysis revealed complex PVCs to be an independent contributor to cardiac death.[1]

The criteria proposed by Lown and Wolf[30] for grading the severity of ventricular arrhythmias remain in common use, although objections have been raised to their validity.[31] Our index of complex arrhythmias included repetitive ventricular arrhythmias (couplets and ventricular tachycardia) and multiform beats. The Multicenter Investigation of the Limitation of Infarct Size (MILIS) found that both repetitive PVCs and multiform beats provides strong indexes of sudden cardiac death.[32] In a recent study to determine the relationship of Holter monitoring to programmed electrical stimulation, Gradman et al.[33] found that 100% of patients with induced sustained ventricular tachycardia, and 95% of those with nonsustained induced tachycardia, had multiform PVCs on their preceding 24 hr ambulatory electrocardiograms.

The results of the present study strongly suggest that complex PVCs in the recovery phase of acute infarction indicate high-risk status only in patients with non–Q wave infarction. The 1 year survival for these patients was 73%, compared with 90% for the Q wave group ($p < .01$). Few other studies have examined this relationship. Vismara et al.[11] followed 64 patients who had a 10 hr ambulatory ECG recording before hospital discharge after acute infarction. Of the 12 patients who subsequently died, eight of whom had complex PVCs, there was no difference in the incidence of Q wave and non–Q wave infarctions. However, the small number of patients in that study severely limited the possibility of distinguishing between the two infarct categories. Davis et al.[34] followed 940 patients with myocardial infarction for 12 to 60 months and found that the combination of anterior infarction, left ventricular dysfunction, and PVCs identified a high-risk subset with a 6 month mortality of 15%. Patients with non–Q wave infarctions were not analyzed separately, and the above combination would be expected to yield a high proportion of patients with a poor ejection fraction. Kotler et al.[4] followed 162 patients less than 65 years of age and in New York Heart Association class I or II for 30 to 54 months. Complex PVCs were found to be an independent risk factor, and there were no differences between patients with Q wave and non–Q wave infarctions.

Again the discrepancy from the present study may be explained by the smaller number of patients, a younger age group with possibly less severe coronary heart disease, and a longer follow-up period. Kotler et al.[4] did find that in the patients with non–Q wave infarction and no complex PVCs, no deaths occurred during follow-up. This supports the view that, in patients with non–Q wave infarction, freedom from complex PVCs carries a favorable prognosis, as indicated by our study. Of all nonsurvivors of non–Q wave infarction, only one (4%) was totally free of all ventricular arrhythmias, as compared with 25% of survivors ($p < .01$). In patients with Q wave infarctions, freedom from PVCs was no more common in survivors than nonsurvivors.

Relationship of complex PVCs to left ventricular function. The relationship between ventricular arrhythmias, left ventricular function, and prognosis after myocardial infarction has been controversial. While several studies show an independent effect of ventricular arrhythmias on mortality after adjustments are made for ventricular dysfunction,[1,2] others have concluded that ventricular arrhythmias are so strongly associated with left ventricular dysfunction that this association accounts for the relationship between arrhythmias and subsequent death.[35] Much of the above controversy stems from the variety of methods used in previous studies. Arrhythmias were often detected on resting 12-lead electrocardiograms, 1 to 4 hr ambulatory or resting recordings, or recordings made later than 1 month after discharge; left ventricular dysfunction was often inferred from the clinical findings only. Recently, Bigger et al.[10] examined the relationship between ventricular arrhythmias, left ventricular dysfunction, and mortality after infarction in 760 patients in whom predischarge 24 hr ECG recordings as well as radionuclide ventriculograms were obtained. They concluded that ventricular arrhythmias and ventricular dysfunction were independently related to high risk of death. MILIS presented results in 386 patients followed 2 years, and reported a strong univariate association between repetitive and multiform PVCs and mortality, as well as an independent association with left ventricular dysfunction.[32]

The present study indicates that complex PVCs predict mortality only in the subgroup of patients with non–Q wave infarction, whereas mortality in the Q wave infarction group was closely related to poor ventricular function and did not relate to the presence or absence of complex PVCs. Shultze et al.[3] found that

90% of 81 patients with complex PVCs had ejection fractions of 0.40 or less. In the present study, only one-third of the patients in the non–Q wave infarction group with complex PVCs had ejection fractions of less than 45%, while in the Q wave group complex PVCs were equally distributed among those with fractions of greater or less than 45%.

Implications for treatment. Non–Q wave infarction is generally associated with a relatively small amount of necrosis and a low initial mortality when compared with Q wave infarctions.[21] Despite the initial favorable prognosis, prospective follow-up in our patients has confirmed previous reports[18, 19] that the 1 to 2 year mortality for patients with non–Q wave infarctions is similar to and possibly greater than that for patients with Q wave infarctions.[21] The present study indicates that this late equalization of mortality may largely be due to the death of patients with non–Q wave infarcts who have complex PVCs. Although the mechanisms of late death in patients with non–Q wave infarctions is not known, Rigo et al.,[36] in a long-term study of 49 patients with non–Q wave and 111 patients with Q wave infarcts, suggested the possibility that patients with non–Q wave infarcts may have a higher incidence of fatal arrhythmias after discharge than patients with Q wave infarcts, based on a higher incidence of recurrent ischemia in the non–Q wave group. However, it is possible that the increased incidence of complex ventricular arrhythmias is causally unrelated to the increased late mortality in such patients with non–Q wave infarction, and that an unstable ischemic state[21] with recurrent myocardial infarction is the cause. Nevertheless, it is also possible that death during recurrent ischemia or infarction occurs primarily in those with ongoing arrhythmias, or that primary arrhythmic death without concurrent ischemia occurs in some of these patients.

The best current evidence favors an independent association between ventricular arhythmias after myocardial infarction and subsequent mortality, and therefore it seems reasonable to recommend antiarrhythmic therapy in an effort to reduce this risk. To date, randomized, double-blind studies have not shown antiarrhythmic drugs to be of great benefit, as reviewed elsewhere.[14, 37] However, most of the studies have focused on patients who have recovered from myocardial infarction, without attempts at categorization of arrhythmias or type of infarction. The present study demonstrates that patients with non–Q wave infarcts who have complex PVCs on a predischarge ambulatory recording are at high risk for cardiac death in the subsequent year, irrespective of the ejection fraction. This group may provide one logical choice of patients in whom to test the efficacy of antiarrhythmic therapy in the setting of a randomized clinical trial.

References

1. Moss AJ, Davis HT, DeCamilla J, Bayer LW: Ventricular ectopic beats and their relation to sudden and nonsudden cardiac death after myocardial infarction. Circulation **60:** 998, 1978
2. Ruberman W, Weinblatt E, Goldberg JD, Frank CW, Shapiro S: Ventricular premature beats and mortality after myocardial infarction. N Engl J Med **297:** 750, 1977
3. Schultze RA Jr, Strauss HW, Pitt B: Sudden death in the 1 year following myocardial infarction: relation to ventricular premature contractions in the late hospital phase and left ventricular ejection fraction. Am J Med **62:** 192, 1977
4. Kotler MN, Tabatznik B, Mower MM, Tominaga S: Prognostic significance of ventricular ectopic beats with respect to sudden death in the late post-infarction period. Circulation **47:** 959, 1973
5. Anderson KP, DeCamilla J, Moss AJ: Clinical significance of ventricular tachycardia detected during ambulatory monitoring after myocardial infarction. Circulation **57:** 890, 1978
6. Bigger JT, Weld FM: Analysis of prognostic significance of ventricular arrhythmias after myocardial infarction. Br Heart J **45:** 717, 1981
7. Ruberman W, Weinblatt E, Goldberg JDD, Frank CW, Chaudhary BS, Shapiro S: Ventricular premature complexes and sudden death after myocardial infarction. Circulation **64:** 297, 1981
8. Rehnqvist N, Lundman T, Sjogren A: Prognostic implications of ventricular arrhythmias registered before discharge and one year after acute myocardial infarction. Acta Med Scand **204:** 203, 1978
9. Bigger JT Jr, Weld FM, Rolnitzky LM: The prevalence and significance of ventricular tachycardia detected by ambulatory ECG recording in the late hospital phase of acute myocardial infarction. Am J Cardiol **48:** 815, 1981
10. Bigger JT Jr, Fleiss JL, Kleiger R, Miller PJ, Rolnitzky LM, Multicenter Post-Infarction Research Group: The relationship among ventricular arrhythmias, left ventricular dysfunction, and mortality in the 2 years after myocardial infarction. Circulation **69:** 250, 1984
11. Vismara LA, Amsterdam EA, Mason DT: Relation of ventricular arrhythmias in the late hospital phase of acute myocardial infarction to sudden death after hospital discharge. Am J Med **59:** 6, 1975
12. Tominaga S, Blackburn H: The Coronary Drug Project Research Group: prognostic importance of premature beats following myocardial infarction. JAMA **223:** 1116, 1973
13. May GS, Eberlein KA, Passamani ER, De Mets DL: Secondary prevention after myocardial infarction: a review of long-term trials. Prog Cardiovasc Dis **24:** 3331, 1982
14. Graboys TB, Lown B, Podrid PJ, DeSilva R: Long term survival of patients with ventricular arrhythmia treated with antiarrhythmic drugs. Am J Cardiol **50:** 437, 1982
15. Swerdlow CD, Winkle RA, Mason JW: Determinants of survival in patients with ventricular tachyarrhythmias. N Engl J Med **308:** 1436, 1983
16. Savage RM, Wagne GS, Ideker RE: Correlation of post mortem anatomic findings with electrocardiographic changes in patients with myocardial infarction. Circulation **55:** 729, 1977
17. Spodick DH: Q-wave infarction versus S-T infarction: non specificity of electrocardiographic criteria for differentiating transmural and non transmural lesions. Am J Cardiol **51:** 913, 1983
18. Cannon DS, Levy W, Cohen LS: The short and long term prognosis of patients with transmural and non-transmural myocardial infarction. Am J Med **61:** 452, 1976
19. Hutter AM, DeSanctis RW, Flynn T, Yeatman LA: Non transmural myocardial infarction: a comparison of hospital and late clinical course of patients with that of matched patients with transmural anterior and transmural inferior myocardial infarction. Am J Cardiol **48:** 595, 1981
20. Connolly DC, Fustes V, Danielson M, Frye RL: Effects of collateral circulation following transmural and subendocardial myocardial infarction. Circulation **54**(suppl II): II-77, 1976
21. Maisel AS, Ahnve S, Gilpin EA, Henning H, Goldberger AL,

Collins D, LeWinter M, Ross J Jr: Prognosis after myocardial infarct extension: the role of Q wave and non–Q wave infarction. Circulation (in press)
22. Henning H, Gilpin EA, Covell JW, Swan EA, O'Rourke RA, Ross J Jr: Prognosis after acute myocardial infarction: a multivariate analysis of mortality and survival. Circulation **59:** 1124, 1979
23. Madsen EB, Gilpin EA, Henning H, Ahnve S, Ross J Jr: Prediction of late mortality after myocardial infarction from variables measured at different times during hospitalization. Am J Cardiol **53:** 47, 1984
24. Battler A, Karliner JS, Higgins CB: The initial chest x-ray in acute myocardial infarction. Circulation **61:** 1004, 1980
25. BMDP statistical software. Berkeley, CA, 1981, University of California Press, vol 19, p 519
26. Gilpin E, Olsen R, Henning H, Ross J Jr: Risk prediction after myocardial infarction; comparison of 3 multivariate methodologies. Cardiology **70:** 73, 1983
27. Ahnve S, Gilpin EA, Henning H, Curtis G, Shabetai R, Collins D, Ross J Jr: Prognostic value of left ventricular ejection fraction after myocardial infarction. Clin Res **33:** 2A, 1985 (abst)
28. Moss AJ: Clinical significance of ventricular arrhythmias in patients with and without coronary artery disease. Prog Cardiovasc Dis **23:** 33, 1980
29. Moss AJ, De Camilla J, Davis HP, Bayer L: Clinical significance of ventricular ectopic beats in the early post hospital phase of myocardial infarction. Am J Cardiol **39:** 635, 1977
30. Lown B, Wolf M: Approaches to sudden death from coronary heart disease. Circulation **44:** 130, 1971
31. Bigger JT, Wenger TL, Heissenbuttel RH: Limitations of the Lown grading system for the study of human ventricular arrhythmias. Am Heart J **93:** 27, 1977
32. Mukharji J, Rude RE, Poole WK, Gustafson N, Thomas LJ Jr, Strauss HW, Jaffe AS, Muller JE, Roberts R, Raabe DS, Croft CH, Passamani E, Braunwald E, Willerson JT, MILIS Study Group: Risk factors for sudden death after acute myocardial infarction: two year follow-up. Am J Cardiol **54:** 31, 1984
33. Gradman AH, Batsford WP, Rieur EC, Leon L, Van Zetta AM: Ambulatory electrocardiogrphic correlates of ventricular inducibility during programmed electrical stimulation. Am Coll Cardiol **5:** 1087, 1985
34. Davis HT, DeCamilla J, Bayer LW: Survivorship patterns in the posthospital phase of myocardial infarction. Circulation **60:** 1252, 1979
35. Califf M, Burks JM, Behar VS, Margolis JR, Wagner GS: Relationships among ventricular arrhythmias, coronary artery disease and angiographic and electrocardiographic indicators of myocardial fibrosis. Circulation **57:** 725, 1978
36. Rigo P, Murray M, Taylor DR, Weisfeldt ML, Strauss HW, Pitt B: Hemodynamic and prognostic findings in patients with transmural and non transmural infarction. Circulation **51:** 1064, 1975
37. Bigger JT, Weld FM, Rolnitzky LM: Which post infarction ventricular arrhythmias should be treated? Am Heart J **103:** 660, 1982

The relationship of white cell count, platelet count, and hematocrit to cigarette smoking in adolescents: the Oslo Youth Study

G. S. TELL, D.SC., R. H. GRIMM, JR., M.D., PH.D., O. D. VELLAR, M.D., D.P.H., AND L. THEODORSEN, M.D.

ABSTRACT This article reports on the relationship between cigarette smoking, white blood cell count (WBC), platelet count (PC), and hematocrit in a Norwegian adolescent population. Data were obtained on 439 youths, 14 to 16 years old, as part of the Oslo Youth Study, an investigation of risk factors and behaviors for cardiovascular disease and cancer among adolescents. Analyses of covariance, controlling for height, weight, age, sexual maturation, high-density lipoprotein (HDL) cholesterol, and hematocrit revealed that both male and female regular smokers (those reporting smoking at least once a week) had significantly higher mean WBCs. Male regular smokers also had significantly higher PCs than nonsmokers, and female regular smokers had higher PCs than young women who smoked less often than once a month. Hematocrit, after adjustment for height, weight, age, sexual maturation, and HDL cholesterol, was significantly lower in male regular smokers, while female regular smokers had higher hematocrit values than nonsmokers or occasional smokers. Results of this study show that WBC and PC were increased in adolescents who started smoking relatively recently. This indicates that the increase in white cell count observed in smokers is unlikely to be due to a long-standing smoking-induced chronic disease condition.
Circulation 72, No. 5, 971–974, 1985.

STUDIES have shown that for adults, white blood cell count (WBC) is significantly higher in current cigarette smokers than in nonsmokers or former smokers.[1–3] Furthermore, WBC has been found to be a strong predictor of myocardial infarction[4, 5] and to be independently related to cardiovascular disease (CVD) and cancer mortality.[3] Although these associations do not necessarily indicate causality, one hypothesis that has been put forward is that increased WBC reflects cellular injury of importance in both CVD and cancer. While cardiovascular and cancer mortality end points obviously cannot readily be studied in preadult populations, the relationship between cigarette smoking, WBC, and other related variables can be studied in any age group in which cigarette smoking is prevalent. However, such studies have typically been conducted in adult populations.

Most regular adult smokers have been smoking for a number of years and are likely to have started during adolescence. Therefore, the present analyses were undertaken to investigate whether the relationship between WBC and cigarette smoking could also be demonstrated in a younger population that had been exposed to cigarettes only relatively recently. In addition, we also examined the relationship of cigarette smoking to platelet count (PC), other hematologic parameters, and levels of high-density lipoprotein (HDL) cholesterol.

Methods

The Oslo Youth Study was a mixed cross-sectional and longitudinal school-based study including two surveys, the first in 1979 and the last in 1981.[6, 7] Since smoking frequencies were low in 1979 (students then being 11 to 14 years of age), only data collected in 1981 are used in these analyses. Written parental consent was obtained from all study participants. Between the two surveys, approximately half of the students participated in an intervention program aimed at reducing the onset of cigarette smoking and alcohol consumption and to improve eating and exercise habits. Since the intervention program had no apparent effect on the hematologic variables in the intervention group relative to the comparison group (analyses not presented), data from both groups are combined here. All data reported were analyzed with BMDP Statistical Software.[8]

Blood was drawn from an antecubital vein of each student while he or she was in a standardized seated position. A tourniquet was applied for the shortest time possible and released when the actual blood sampling began. No blood sampling was performed on Mondays or days directly after holidays, and

From the Institute of Preventive Medicine, University of Oslo, the Central Laboratory, the Norwegian Radium Hospital, Oslo, and the Division of Epidemiology, University of Minnesota, Minneapolis.

The Oslo Youth Study was supported by the Norwegian Cancer Society. Preparation of this manuscript was supported by a grant from the National Heart, Lung, and Blood Institute (5–T32–HL–07328) (G. S. T.).

Address for correspondence: Grethe S. Tell, Division of Epidemiology, University of Minnesota, Stadium Gate 27, Minneapolis, MN 55455.

Received May 20, 1985; revision accepted Aug. 8, 1985.

students had been fasting overnight. Plasma was obtained by drawing blood into a Vacutainer tube containing EDTA (K_3) and was analyzed within 2 hr.

Hematologic analyses were done on the Coulter Counter (R) Model S Plus, which is an automated multiparameter hematologic analyzer. Other measurements included those of serum total cholesterol and HDL cholesterol (both measured by the catalase method[9]), HDL cholesterol after precipitation with $MgCl_2$ and dextran sulfate,[10] fasting triglycerides, blood pressure, height, weight, skinfold thickness, assessment of sexual maturity according to the method modified by Tanner,[11] and serum thiocyanate. Self-reports were obtained on smoking behavior and other health behaviors.

Results

Table 1 shows smoking frequencies by gender and age for the examined population, based on the question "How often do you smoke?" We classified students by their smoking frequency status as nonsmokers if they reported no current smoking, as occasional smokers if they reported current smoking of less than once a week, and as regular smokers if they reported smoking at least once a week. None of the three 12-year-olds reported smoking. Because very few 13-year-old students smoke regularly (8.2% of boys and 7.9% of girls smoke one to two times per week or daily), only data from 14-, 15-, and 16-year-olds ($n = 439$) are used in the analyses reported here. Among these, and according to our classification of smokers, 9.0% of male students reported smoking occasionally and 15.0% smoked regularly. Among female students, 12.6% smoked occasionally and 22.3% smoked regularly. Students who reported smoking occasionally or regularly were asked to specify how many cigarettes they had smoked during the week before the survey. Male occasional smokers averaged 5.3 and female smokers 2.9 cigarettes the previous week. Male regular smokers reported an average of 30.1 and female smokers 35.3 cigarettes during the week before the survey. To test the validity of self-reports of cigarette smoking, we measured thiocyanate in serum. No statistically significant relationship was observed between the number of cigarettes reportedly smoked during the prior week and thiocyanate level. However, frequency of cigarette smoking was significantly correlated with serum thiocyanate in both male ($r = .21$, $p < .005$) and female students ($r = .59$, $p < .001$). To determine if inhalation patterns influence levels of thiocyanate, WBC, PC, and hematocrit, we investigated whether students who reported inhaling cigarette smoke had different levels of these parameters than noninhalers. About 95% of smokers of both genders reported inhaling, and no differences were detected between inhalers and noninhalers. Data from both groups are used in analyses presented here.

The smoking variable most frequently used to describe adult populations is the number of cigarettes smoked per day. Among regular smokers in our study, the average number of cigarettes smoked was lower than among most adult regular smokers; male regular smokers averaged 4.3 cigarettes per day and female regular smokers averaged 5.0 cigarettes per day in our population. We therefore used self–reported cigarette smoking *frequency* as the major smoking variable in our analyses, according to the previously described classification.

We compared smokers to nonsmokers with respect to other salient characteristics, including chronologic age, sexual maturity, height, weight, body mass index (weight/height^2), and total cholesterol. None of these characteristics were significantly different between nonsmokers and smokers (occasional and regular).

As can be seen in table 2, smoking frequency (used

TABLE 1
Frequency of cigarette smoking by age and sex

Age (yr)	Never		Less than once a month		One to two times per month		One to two times per week		Almost daily		Total
	n	%	n	%	n	%	n	%	n	%	(n)
Males											
12	1	100.0	—	—	—	—	—	—	—	—	1
13	49	80.3	6	9.8	1	1.6	2	3.3	3	4.9	61
14	80	73.4	9	8.3	3	2.8	1	0.9	16	14.7	109
15	76	82.6	3	3.3	2	2.2	1	1.1	10	10.9	92
16	21	65.6	3	9.4	1	3.1	—	—	7	21.9	32
Females											
12	2	100.0	—	—	—	—	—	—	—	—	2
13	66	86.8	2	2.6	2	2.6	2	2.6	4	5.3	76
14	69	66.3	6	5.8	7	6.7	4	3.8	18	17.3	104
15	51	64.6	8	10.1	2	2.5	3	3.8	15	19.0	79
16	14	60.9	2	8.7	1	4.3	—	—	6	26.1	23

TABLE 2
Simple linear correlations (male students)

	Smoking frequency	WBC	PC	Hematocrit
WBC	.17[A]			
PC	.14[B]	.17[A]		
Hematocrit	−.04	.18[A]	−.08	
HDL cholesterol	−.21[A]	−.14[B]	.17[A]	.21[A]

[A]$p < .005$; [B]$p < .01$.

as a continuous variable with five categories, as shown in table 1) for male students was significantly and positively correlated with total WBC and PC. Smoking frequency was also significantly negatively correlated with levels of HDL cholesterol. Among female students (table 3) there was a significant positive correlation between frequency of cigarette smoking and WBC and hematocrit, but a statistically significant correlation was not observed with PC or HDL cholesterol level.

Analyses of covariance, adjusting for height, weight, age, sexual maturation, HDL cholesterol level, and hematocrit revealed a gradient of total WBC from nonsmokers to occasional smokers to regular smokers (figure 1). This gradient was of borderline significance by the F test with an analyses of variance of the adjusted means ($F = 2.79$, $p = .063$). However, a t test of the adjusted values showed that regular smokers had significantly higher WBCs than nonsmokers (5900/μl vs 5239/μl, respectively; $t = 2.25$, $p = .025$). The same analyses of data from female students revealed a similar overall pattern ($F = 5.45$, $p = .005$); the lower level in occasional smokers was not significantly different from that in nonsmokers.

Mean adjusted PCs in male students showed a relationship with cigarette smoking similar to that for WBC, with regular smokers having significantly higher PCs ($F = 4.05$, $p = .019$). For female students, mean adjusted PC showed a pattern similar to that for WBC. The overall F was of borderline significance ($F = 2.67$, $p = .072$), but a t test on the adjusted means showed that regular smokers had significantly higher PCs than occasional smokers ($t = 2.31$, $p = .022$).

Hematocrit, adjusted for height, weight, age in years, sexual maturation, and HDL cholesterol level, was significantly lower for male regular smokers than occasional smokers ($t = -1.96$, $p = .052$) or nonsmokers ($t = -2.27$, $p = .024$), the overall F was of borderline significance ($F = 2.87$, $p = .059$). For female students there was a trend toward increasing hematocrit with increasing smoking frequency ($F = 2.98$, $p = .053$), with regular smokers having significantly higher levels than nonsmokers ($t = 2.40$, $p = .017$).

For the other variables investigated by analysis of covariance, female smokers had significantly increased hemoglobin ($F = 3.51$, $p = .032$), mean red cell volume ($F = 3.48$, $p = .033$), and mean corpuscular hemoglobin ($F = 3.11$, $p = .047$) than nonsmokers. Male regular smokers had significantly lower levels of HDL cholesterol than nonsmokers ($t = 2.16$, $p = .033$).

TABLE 3
Simple linear correlations (female students)

	Smoking frequency	WBC	PC	Hematocrit
WBC	.19[A]			
PC	.06	.13[C]		
Hematocrit	.16[B]	.14[C]	−.02	
HDL cholesterol	−.05	−.05	−.08	−.01

[A]$p < .005$; [B]$p < .01$; [C]$p < .05$.

Discussion

Results of the present study indicate that there appears to be a relatively rapid effect of cigarette smoking on WBC, PC, hematocrit, and other hematologic variables. For WBC, this is consistent with what

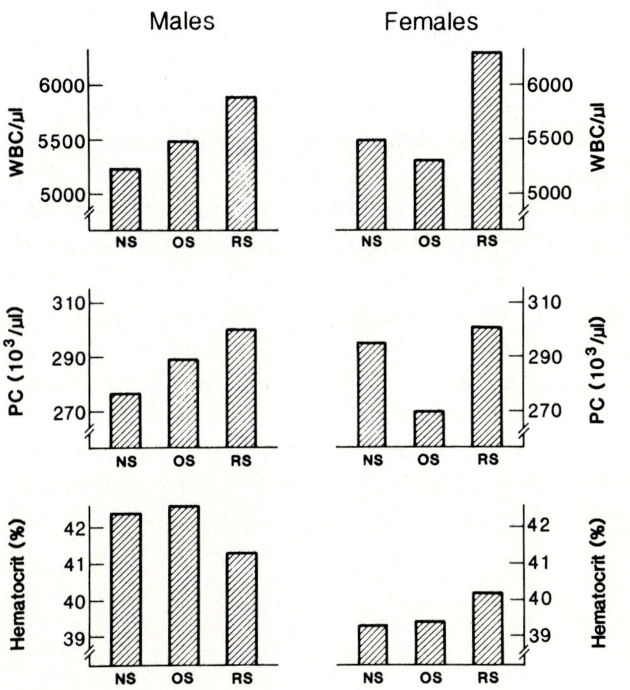

FIGURE 1. WBC, PC, and hematocrit by smoking status, for male and female students. Values are adjusted for chronologic age, sexual maturation, height, weight, HDL cholesterol level, and hematocrit (the latter for WBC and PC only). NS = nonsmokers; OS = occasional smokers; RS = regular smokers.

Scheer[12] found more than 40 years ago, namely an acute transient increase in WBC after smoking one to three cigarettes.

The mechanisms by which smoking increases WBC and PC are unknown. In addition to the possibility that there may be constitutional differences in the individual WBC and PC response to an external stimulus such as cigarette smoking, other mechanisms have been suggested. One of the postulates is that nicotine induces release of catecholamines that can raise WBC. Another proposal is that there is an irritant effect of smoke on the respiratory tree with resultant inflammation. Our findings that adolescents who smoke have elevated WBCs and PCs are consistent with the hypothesis that inhalation of cigarette smoke causes inflammatory reactions. It has been suggested that elevated WBC in smokers is partly due to the presence of chronic bronchitis. The presence of chronic, inflammatory lung disease, however, cannot account for the increase in WBCs in adolescents who started to smoke relatively recently and who smoke on average only four to five cigarettes per day.

As far as we are aware, an increase in PC among cigarette smokers has not been previously reported. A possible explanation for the observed higher PCs in smokers may be that one or more chemical constituents in cigarette smoke stimulate the bone marrow to increase production of certain blood elements, including white cells and platelets. The finding that young men who smoke have elevated WBCs and PCs and lower hematocrit than nonsmokers is consistent with the hypothesis that inhalation of cigarette smoke causes inflammatory reactions, although studies in adults have found that smokers have elevated hematocrit levels.[13] It is not clear why the relationship between smoking and hematocrit is different in male and female subjects. It could be related to the fact that the smoking rates of male regular smokers were lower than were those of female smokers. Since hematologic variables can vary as a function of the menstrual cycle, this should be adjusted for when studying hematologic variables among women. Since in the present study, along with many other hematologic studies in women, we did not control for time of the menstrual cycle, interpretations of the pattern in female smokers is difficult. However, our finding that young women who smoked had higher WBCs, hemoglobin, and mean cell volume is in accordance with previous studies.[14, 15] Elevations in WBC and PC in adolescent smokers indicate that these blood components may have an early role in the pathogenesis of arteriosclerosis.

We suggest that future studies investigate the relationship between cigarette smoking and hemotologic parameters in other adolescent populations, analyze differential WBCs, and also study effects of changes in cigarette smoking habits on these hematologic parameters.

References

1. Yeung MC, Buncio AD: Leukocyte count, smoking, and lung function. Am J Med **76:** 31, 1984
2. Friedman GD, Siegelaub AB, Seltzer CC, Feldman R, Collen MF: Smoking habits and the leukocyte count. Arch Environ Health **26:** 137, 1973
3. Grimm RH Jr, Neaton JD, Ludwig WP: The prognostic importance of total white blood cell count for all cause, cardiovascular and cancer mortality. JAMA (in press)
4. Friedman GD, Klatsky AL, Siegelaub AB: The leukocyte count as a predictor of myocardial infarction. N Engl J Med **290:** 1275, 1974
5. Zalokar JB, Richard JL, Claude JR: Leukocyte count, smoking, and myocardial infarction. N Engl J Med **304:** 465, 1981
6. Tell GS, Vellar OD, Monrad–Hansen HP: Risk factors for chronic diseases in Norwegian schoolchildren: preliminary findings of a baseline survey as part of an intervention study (the Oslo Youth Study). Prev Med **10:** 211, 1981
7. Tell GS, Klepp KI, Vellar OD, McAlister A: Preventing the onset of cigarette smoking in Norwegian adolescents: The Oslo Youth Study. Prev Med **13:** 256, 1984
8. Dixon WJ, editor: BMDP statistical software. Berkeley, CA, 1983, University of California Press
9. Roschlau P, Bernt E, Gruber W: Enzymatische Bestimmung des Gesamt — Cholesterins im Serum. Z Klin Chem Klin Biochem **12:** 226, 1974
10. Finley PR, Schifman RB, Williams RJ: Cholesterol in high density lipoprotein: use of Mg^{2+}/dextran sulfate in its enzymic measurement. Clin Chem **24:** 931, 1978
11. Tanner JM: Growth at adolescence. Oxford, 1962, Blackwell Scientific Publications
12. Scheer P: Uber den Einfluss des Nicotins auf das leukocytare Blutbild des Menschen. Z Gesamte Exp Med **107:** 219, 1940
13. Lowe GDO, Forbes CD, Barbenel JC: The effects of age and cigarette–smoking on blood and plasma viscosity in men. Scott Med J **25:** 13, 1980
14. Eisen ME, Hammond EC: The effect of smoking on packed cell volume, red blood cell counts, haemoglobin and platelet counts. Can Med Assoc J **75:** 520, 1956
15. Helman N, Rubenstein LS: The effects of age, sex and smoking on erythrocytes and leukocytes. Am J Clin Pathol **63:** 35, 1975

Isometric exercise in patients with chronic advanced heart failure: hemodynamic and neurohumoral evaluation

URI ELKAYAM, M.D., ARIE ROTH, M.D., LAURA WEBER, R.N., WILLA HSUEH, M.D., MICHELE NANNA, M.D., LINDALEE FREIDENBERGER, R.N., P. ANTHONY N. CHANDRARATNA, M.D., AND SHAHBUDIN H. RAHIMTOOLA, M.B., F.R.C.P.

ABSTRACT We evaluated the hemodynamic effects of isometric exercise in 53 patients with congestive heart failure (CHF) and compared them with those found in 10 normal subjects. In both groups, isometric exercise increased heart rate and blood pressure. Systemic resistance increased in patients with CHF (1862 ± 520 vs 2126 ± 642 dyne-sec-cm^{-5}; $p < .001$) but not in normal subjects (1359 ± 268 vs 1380 ± 252 dyne-sec-cm^{-5}). Cardiac index and stroke volume index increased mildly but not significantly in the normal subjects (2.8 ± 0.5 vs 3.1 ± 0.7 liters/min/m^2 and 46 ± 8 vs 47 ± 7 ml/m^2) and showed a significant fall in the patients with CHF (2.1 ± 0.6 to 1.9 ± 0.6 liters/min/m^2, $p < .01$ and 23 ± 7 vs 20 ± 7 ml/m^2, $p < .01$). Mean pulmonary arterial wedge pressure increased in patients with CHF from 26 ± 7 to 30 ± 8 mm Hg ($p < .001$). Although no significant change was found in mean value for stroke work index (21 ± 9 vs 20 ± 9 g-m/m^2), the individual changes were variable, with marked decrease (>15%) in 17 of the patients. This hemodynamic deterioration could not be predicted from resting hemodynamics, left ventricular ejection fraction, or functional classification. Isometric exercise resulted in no significant change in circulatory catecholamine levels or plasma renin concentration in our 10 normal subjects. In the patients with CHF renin (measured in 12 patients) and epinephrine (measured in 16 patients) also did not change during isometric exercise, but norepinephrine levels (measured in 16 patients) increased significantly. No correlation was found between changes in hormonal levels and any of the hemodynamic changes during static exercise. We conclude that in patients with chronic CHF, isometric exercise can lead to a significant increase in left ventricular outflow resistance and filling pressure and to a fall in cardiac performance. In the presence of CHF, this form of exercise results in a consistent elevation in norepinephrine levels, but there is no correlation between changes in its plasma level and in hemodynamic values. There is considerable individual variation in the hemodynamic response, with a significant deterioration in cardiac performance in some patients, which cannot be separated by resting hemodynamic values, left ventricular ejection fraction, or clinical status.
Circulation 72, No. 5, 975–981, 1985.

THE EFFECTS of isometric exercise on the cardiovascular system and their neurohumoral mechanisms have been extensively investigated in animals and in normal individuals.[1-4] In contrast, few data are available on the consequences of isometric exercise in patients with chronic congestive heart failure (CHF), in whom both hemodynamic and neurohumoral status is significantly altered. In this study we evaluated the hemodynamic effects of isometric exercise and the response of plasma catecholamines and renin concentration in patients with severe advanced CHF.

From the Department of Medicine, Sections of Cardiology and Endocrinology, LAC/USC Medical Center, University of Southern California School of Medicine, Los Angeles.

Address for correspondence: Uri Elkayam, M.D., USC School of Medicine, Section of Cardiology, 2025 Zonal Ave., Los Angeles, CA 90033.

Received April 22, 1985; revision accepted July 18, 1985.

Methods

Patients with CHF. Hemodynamic effects of isometric exercise were evaluated in 53 patients who were admitted to the University of Southern California/Los Angeles County Medical Center for inadequate control of chronic CHF. There were 39 men and 14 women, ranging in age from 20 to 80 years (mean $\pm$ SD 51 ± 6 years). The cause of CHF was coronary artery disease in 14 patients and congestive cardiomyopathy in 39 patients. Thirty-two of the patients were classified on admission into the NYHA functional class III and 21 were class IV. The diagnosis of left ventricular systolic dysfunction was confirmed by cardiac catheterization in 26 patients, by radionuclide ventriculography in 22 patients, and by echocardiography in five patients. Left ventricular ejection fraction was measured either by contrast or radionuclide ventriculography in 48 patients and ranged from 0.08 to 0.41 (mean 0.20 ± 0.07). None of the patients had evidence of a primary valvular disease, congenital disease, or active myocardial ischemia at the time of the study.

All patients were in a clinically and hemodynamically stable condition at the time of the study. Hemodynamic stability was ensured by repeated measurements 30 min apart to obtain two consecutive measurements with 10% or less variation in heart rate, blood pressure, cardiac output, and mean pulmonary arterial wedge pressure. Digitalis and diuretic therapy were continued in their prestudy doses and given at least 4 hr before the initiation of the study. Further administration of diuretic agents was not allowed until the termination of the hemodynamic study. Orally administered vasodilator agents, including isosorbide dinitrate, hydralazine, and nifedipine, were discontinued at least 16 hr before the initiation of the study.

Hemodynamic measurements and computations. Right-sided cardiac catheterization was performed with a balloon-tipped, triple-lumen Swan-Ganz catheter at least 24 hr before the initiation of the study. Pressure in the right atrium and pulmonary artery and left ventricular filling pressure, determined indirectly from the mean pulmonary arterial wedge pressure, were recorded on Electronics for Medicine VR-12 or AR-6 recorders. Mean pressures were obtained with the use of electronic integration. Heart rate was determined from the electrocardiographic recording, and arterial blood pressure was measured by the standard cuff method. Cardiac output was determined by thermodilution as previously described.[5] Calculations of mean arterial blood pressure, cardiac index, stroke volume index, stroke work index, systemic vascular resistance, and pulmonary vascular resistance were performed by standard formulas.

In 16 patients plasma levels of catecholamines was measured before and during exercise. In 12 of these patients plasma renin concentration was also determined. Blood for hormonal determinations was drawn from the right atrium through the Swan-Ganz catheter.

Control group. Hemodynamic and hormonal studies were also carried out in 10 normal male volunteers (mean age 33 ± 4 years). None of these subjects had a history, symptoms, or signs of heart disease or any other disease. All subjects were studied in the morning after eating a light breakfast without drinking caffeinated beverages or smoking cigarettes. All measurements were done in the same examining room with subjects in the supine position. Cardiac output was measured noninvasively by Doppler technique (Ultracom Lawrence Medical Systems, Inc.) in triplicate. This method for cardiac output determination has been previously validated in our laboratory, demonstrating high correlation ($r = .97$, $p < .001$) with thermodilution cardiac output in patients and excellent interobserver and intraobserver variability in normal subjects ($r = .98$, $p < .001$; $r = .97$, $p < .001$, respectively).[6] In addition, the Doppler technique used in this study has been shown to be reliable in detecting changes in cardiac output and has correlated well ($r = .88$, $p < .001$) with the thermodilution technique.[7] Measurements of blood pressure and heart rate were obtained in methods identical to those used for the CHF patients. Because right atrial pressure was not obtained in the normal subjects, total systemic resistance was calculated as follows: total systemic resistance = 80 (mean blood pressure/cardiac output). Venous blood for hormonal determination was drawn through a heparin-lock needle that was placed in the nonexercising forearm at least 15 min before the beginning of the study.

Plasma hormones. Plasma catecholamines were determined at baseline and 1 to 2 min after the beginning of isometric exercise in 16 patients and in all 10 normal subjects. The determination of both epinephrine and norepineprhine was performed with an isotope radioenzymatic technique.[8] Plasma renin concentration was measured at baseline and during exercise in 12 patients and in all 10 normal subjects by a radioimmunoassay of angiotensin I after addition of excess sheep angiotensinogen.[9]

Isometric exercise. Isometric exercise was performed with a commercially available, calibrated hand dynamometer. After the patients and the normal subjects had been instructed and had practiced the handgrip exercise, they were asked to compress the dynamometer once to maximum extent possible with the dominant arm and then to maintain 30% of their previously determined maximal compression pressures while maintaining normal ventilation and avoiding the Valsalva maneuver. In both the control subjects and patients, hemodynamic measurements were started 1 min after initiation of handgrip and were followed by determination of cadiac output. The duration of handgrip exercise ranged between 5 to 7 min in both groups.

Statistical analysis. The data were anlayzed by paired and nonpaired t tests and by correlation and regression analysis. All group values were expressed as mean ± SD.

Results

CHF patients

Hemodynamic effect of isometric exercise. Figures 1 and 2 demonstrate mean hemodynamic values at rest and during isometric exercise in all 53 patients. Isometric exercise was associated with an increase in heart rate in 36 of the patients. Group values showed a mild but significant increase in heart rate from 94 ± 15 to 99 ± 16 beats/min ($p < .001$). Mean blood pressure increased in most patients ($n = 46$), with a change in mean value from 93 ± 12 to 101 ± 14 mm Hg ($p < .001$). Cardiac index decreased in 36 patients and showed a fall from 2.1 ± 0.6 to 1.9 ± 0.6 liters/min/m^2 ($p < .01$), and stroke volume index fell from 23 ± 7 to 20 ± 7 ml/m^2 ($p < .01$). Mean right atrial pressure increased in the majority of the patients ($n = 41$) during exercise and changed from 11 ± 6 to 14 ± 7 mm Hg ($p < .001$), and mean pulmonary arterial wedge pressure increased from 26 ± 7 to 30 ± 8 mm Hg ($p < .001$). Mean pulmonary arterial wedge pressure increased in 44 patients. Baseline pulmonary arterial wedge pressure was greater than 30 mm Hg in 21 patients and exceeded 40 mm Hg in only one of them. During isometric exercise this parameter measured 30 mm Hg or greater in 33 patients and was 40 mm Hg or greater in 10 of them (figure 3). Isometric exercise also resulted in a rise in systemic vascular resistance in 36 patients (from 1862 ± 520 vs 2126 ± 642 dyne-sec-cm^{-5}; $p < .001$). No change, however, was noted in group values for pulmonary vascular resistance (267 ± 139 vs 281 ± 138 dyne-sec-cm^{-5}) and left ventricular stroke work index (21 ± 9 vs 20 ± 9 g-m/m^2).

Although mean values for stroke work index did not change significantly during exercise, individual analysis has shown variable changes. We divided our patients into groups A and B according to the response of

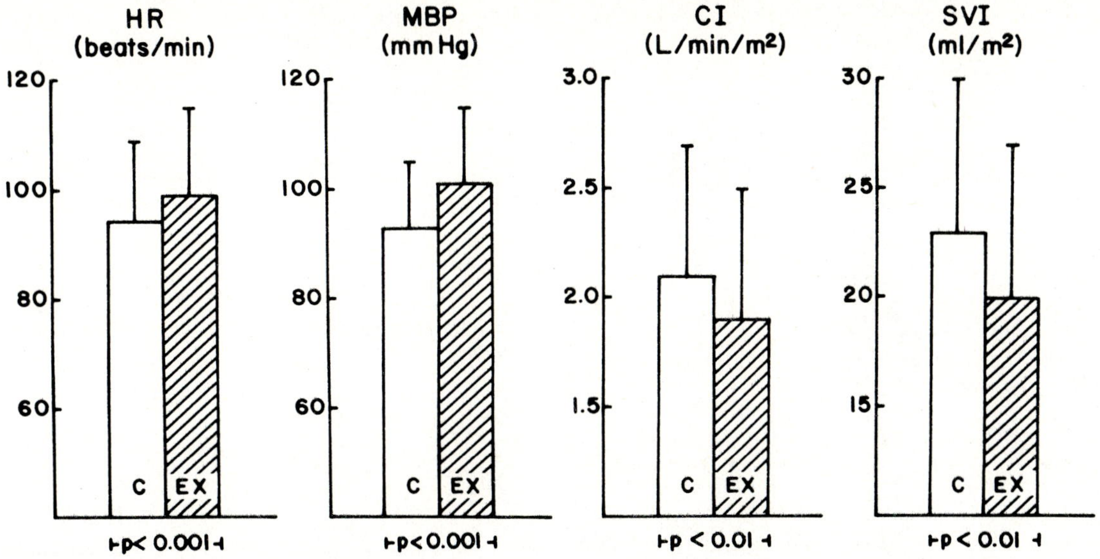

FIGURE 1. Group mean values in heart rate (HR), mean blood pressure (MBP), cardiac index (CI), and stroke volume index (SVI) at baseline (C) and during handgrip isometric exercise (EX) in 53 patients with CHF.

their stroke work index to isometric exercise. To identify clinically important changes, we included in group A 17 patients with a greater than 15% fall in stroke work index (−17% to −56%). Group B included the other 35 patients, who showed either no change, a small decrease (−4% to −11%), or an increase (3% to 50%) in stroke work index. Figures 4 and 5 demonstrate the hemodynamic measurements at baseline and during isometric exercise in these two groups of patients. No significant difference was found in baseline hemodynamic values and ejection fraction (0.21 ± 0.08 vs 0.19 ± 0.07) between the two groups. Nine group A patients were classified in the NYHA class III and eight were in class IV. The incidence of functional class IV in group A did not differ significantly from that found in group B (12 class III patients and 24 class IV patients; $p = .232$). Hemodynamic values as measured during the performance of isometric exercise, however, were significantly different in these two groups. Cardiac index and stroke volume index were lower in group A than in group B (1.7 ± 0.4 vs 2.1 ± 0.7 liters/min/m^2, $p < .005$; 17 ± 4 vs 21 ± 7 ml/m^2, $p < .01$). Mean pulmonary arterial wedge pressure was 34 ± 7 mm Hg in group A and 28 ± 8 mm Hg in

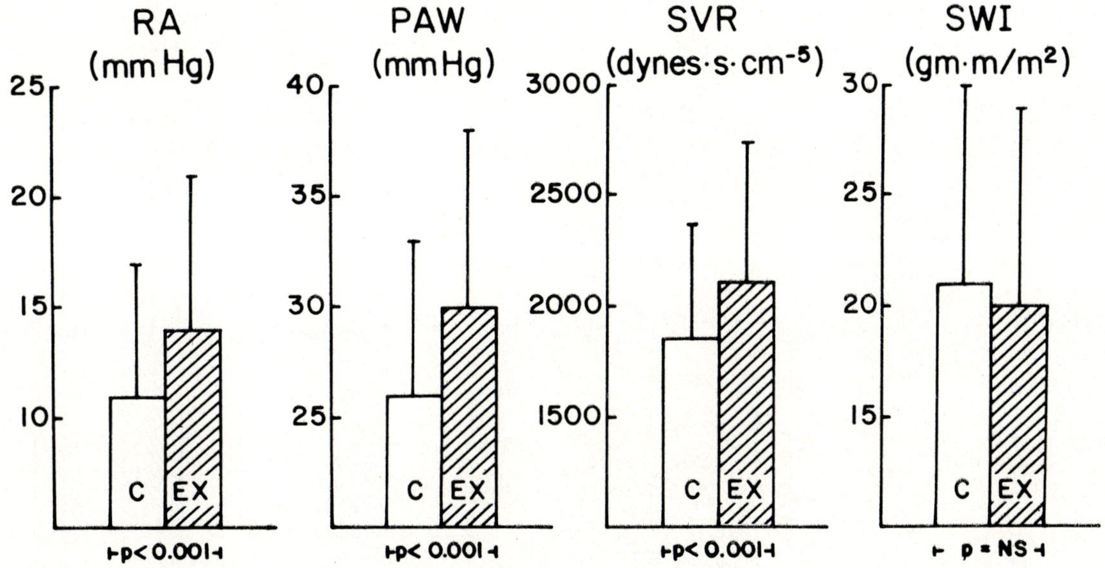

FIGURE 2. Group mean values in mean right atrial pressure (RA), mean pulmonary arterial wedge pressure (PAW), systemic vascular resistance (SVR), and left ventricular stroke work index (SWI) at baseline (C) and during handgrip isometric exercise (EX).

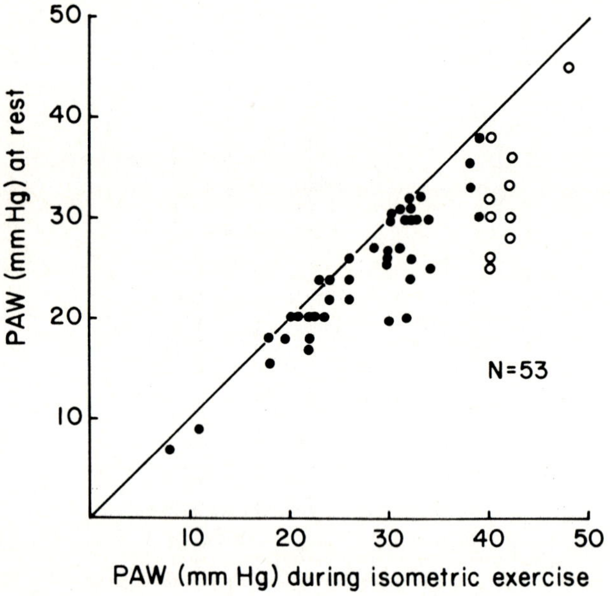

FIGURE 3. Relationships between mean pulmonary arterial wedge pressure (PAW) at rest and during isometric exercise. Baseline PAW was greater than 30 mm Hg in 21 patients and greater than 40 mm Hg in only one of them (pressures ≥40 mm Hg are shown by the open circles); during isometric exercise PAW was 30 mm Hg or greater in 33 patients and 40 mm Hg or greater in 10 of them.

group B ($p < .001$). Exercise stroke work index, as expected by definition of our analysis, was significantly lower in group A. (14 ± 5 vs 23 ± 9 g-m/m^2; $p < .001$). No statistically significant differences were found between exercise values of heart rate (104 ± 14 vs 97 ± 16 beats/min), mean blood pressure (99 ± 16 vs 102 ± 13 mm Hg), mean right atrial pressures (15 $\pm$ 8 vs 13 ± 7 mm Hg), and systemic vascular resistance (2268 ± 535 vs 2059 ± 683 dyne-sec-cm^{-5}).

Neurohumoral effects of isometric exercise. Figure 6 demonstrates the effect of isometric exercise on group values of both catecholamines and renin. A mild increase was seen in the levels of all three measured hormones; however, only the change in norepinephrine level was statistically significant (from 721 ± 520 to 842 ± 634 pg/ml; $p < .02$). Regression analysis between hormonal changes and changes in the various hemodynamic

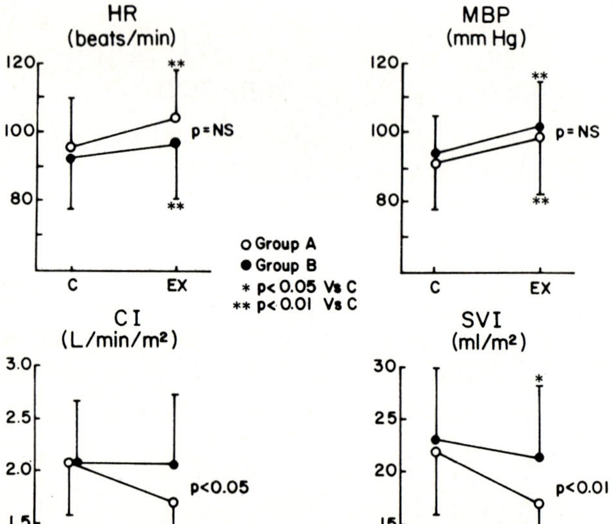

FIGURE 4. Mean hemodynamic values for groups A and B at baseline (C) and during isometric exercise (EX). HR = heart rate; MBP = mean blood pressure; CI = cardiac index; SVI = stroke volume index.

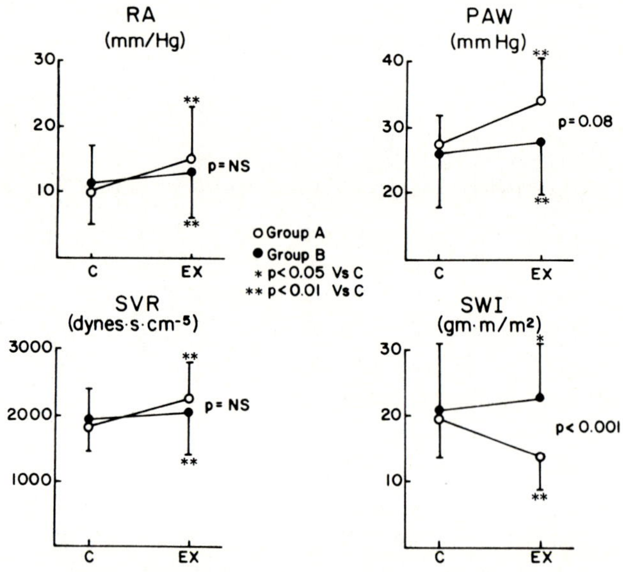

FIGURE 5. Mean hemodynamic values for groups A and B at baseline (C) and during isometric exercise (EX). RA = mean right atrial pressure; PAW = mean pulmonary arterial wedge pressure; SVR = systemic vascular resistance; SWI = left ventricular stroke work index.

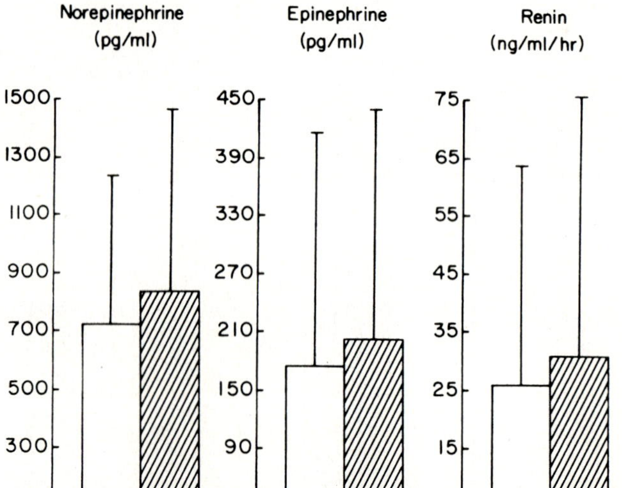

FIGURE 6. Group values of norepinephrine and epinephrine (16 patients) and renin (12 patients) at baseline (C) and during isometric exercise (EX).

parameters revealed no significant correlation. The highest correlation coefficient ($r = .435$) was found between percent change in norepinephrine and systemic vascular resistance. This correlation, however, was not statistically significant ($p = .09$).

Control group

Hemodynamic and neurohumoral response to isometric exercise (table 1). The performance of handgrip isometric exercise in our 10 normal volunteers resulted in a significant increase in heart rate (from 62 ± 11 to 66 ± 9 beats/min; $p < .05$) and mean blood pressure (from 88 ± 7 to 95 ± 11 mm Hg; $p < .05$). Both cardiac index and stroke volume index increased slightly but not significantly (from 2.8 ± 0.5 to 3.1 ± 0.7 liters/min/m^2 and from 46 ± 8 to 47 ± 7 ml/m^2, respectively). Calculated total systemic resistance showed no significant change during exercise (1359 ± 268 vs 1380 ± 252 dyne-sec-cm^{-5}). The measurement of hormonal values before and during isometric exercise also revealed no significant changes (196 ± 61 vs 182 ± 58 pg/ml for norepinephrine, 51 ± 11 vs 52 ± 16 pg/ml for epinephrine, and 5.5 ± 1.8 vs 6.0 ± 2.9 ng/ml/hr for plasma renin concentration).

Discussion

The hemodynamic response of isometric exercise seen in our normal subjects is in accordance with results of previous studies demonstrating an elevation in heart rate and blood pressure and augmentation of cardiac output, presumably caused by an increase in left ventricular contractility.[1-3] The relatively small changes in both stroke volume and cardiac output seen in our study were most probably related to a lower level and shorter duration of exercise.[10, 11] With an identical protocol, the performance of handgrip isometric exercise in our patients with CHF resulted in a similar increase in heart rate and blood pressure. However, whereas the increase in blood pressure in normal subjects was mostly caused by an increase in cardiac output, a significant increase in systemic vascular resistance was responsible for the change in blood pressure in patients with CHF. This rise in systemic vascular resistance in patients with heart failure was accompanied by depression of cardiac performance demonstrated by marked fall in both stroke volume and left ventricular stroke work occurring simultaneously with either no change or a substantial increase in left ventricular filling pressure in many of the patients.

A significant relationship was found in this study between the changes in systemic vascular resistance and the changes in left ventricular stroke volume ($r = .807$, $p < .001$) and cardiac output ($r = -.843$, $p < .001$), emphasizing the dependency and the potentially deleterious effect of further increase in left ventricular afterload in patients with advanced CHF. Ross and Braunwald[12] used angiotensin to increase arterial blood pressure and demonstrated the importance of increasing left ventricular afterload as a test of ventricular reserve. The potential use of sustained handgrip as a test of ventricular performance has been demonstrated in patients with various cardiovascular diseases, including hypertension,[13, 14] coronary artery disease, and valvular abnormalities.[15-23] The reported experience with this technique in patients with chronic severe CHF has been limited to a few patients.[3, 14, 23] Our study demonstrates significant deterioration of stroke work index in a third of our patients during handgrip exercise. This change was accompanied by either no change or an increase in left ventricular filling pressure and suggests a decrease in myocardial inotropic reserve. Although a large number of patients showed marked deterioration in ventricular performance, some demonstrated a normal response to isometric exercise with augmentation of left ventricular performance. Kivowitz et al.[20] reported a correlation between a response to isometric exercise and clinical status as determined by the NYHA functional classification in patients with coronary artery disease and valvular disease. Our results in a large group of patients with CHF in NYHA functional classes III and IV showed that the hemodynamic response to exercise in these patients was not uniform and could not be predicted on the basis of the functional classification. Hemodynamic deterioration as a response to isometric exercise in our patients was also not distinguishable on the basis of their resting hemodynamic measurements or left ven-

TABLE 1

Hemodynamics and hormonal response to isometric exercise in 10 normal men

	HR (beats/min)	MBP (mm Hg)	CI (l/min/m^2)	SVI (ml/m^2)	TSR (dyne-sec-cm^{-5})	Norepinephrine (pg/ml)	Epinephrine (pg/ml)	Renin (ng/ml/hr)
Baseline	62±11	89±7	2.8±0.5	46±8	1359±268	196±61	51±11	5.5±1.8
Isometric exercise	66±9	95±11	3.1±0.7	47±7	1380±252	182±58	52±16	6.0±2.9
p value	<.05	<.05	NS	NS	NS	NS	NS	NS

HR = heart rate; MBP = mean blood pressure; CI = cardiac index; SVI = stroke volume index; SVR = systemic vascular resistance.

tricular ejection fraction. Whether the response to isometric exercise in this patient population is of prognostic and/or therapeutic importance needs to be further investigated.

Left ventricular filling pressure increased during isometric exercise in the majority of our patients (figure 3). Resting mean pulmonary arterial wedge pressure was greater than 30 mm Hg in 21 patients and was greater than 40 mm Hg in only one of them. During exercise this parameter was found to be 30 mm Hg or greater in 33 patients and 40 mm Hg or greater in 10 of them. This rise in left ventricular filling pressure during isometric exercise in patients with CHF can be explained by several mechanisms. Constriction of capacitance vessels caused by increased sympathetic activity has been described during isometric exercise and can result in an increase of both right and left ventricular filling pressures because of increased blood return to the heart.[24, 25] However, no significant correlation was found in the present study between changes in either right or left ventricular filling pressure and changes in catecholamine levels. The significant fall in stroke volume during exercise should also result in an increased left ventricular end-diastolic volume and thus lead to elevation of left ventricular filling pressure. However, analysis of the relationship between changes in stroke volume and mean pulmonary arterial wedge pressure revealed only weak correlation ($r = .3$, $p < .05$). An increase in systemic vascular resistance may also lead to the development of worsening of mitral regurgitation and thus to an elevation in left atrial pressures. An alternative mechanism has been suggested by Ludbrook et al.,[26] who found a change in left ventricular compliance and displacement of its pressure-volume curve during isometric exercise. These investigators postulated an interaction between right ventricular hemodynamics and left ventricular diastolic pressure-volume function due to constraining effect of the pericardium. The significant correlation between changes in mean right atrial and pulmonary arterial wedge pressures found in our study ($r = .55$, $p < .001$) may support this theory. Modification of left ventricular diastolic function during isometric exercise could also be related to myocardial ischemia caused by increased rate-pressure product and thus myocardial oxygen demand or caused by coronary vasoconstriction previously described in experimental animals during static exercise.[27]

Measurements of plasma catecholamines and renin concentration in our normal subjects demonstrated no significant change during isometric exercise in spite of a substantial increase in both heart rate and blood pressure. These findings confirm previous reports showing little change in circulatory catecholamines during short-lasting isometric contractions in normal subjects[28] and reemphasizes the role of vagal withdrawal and the fact that sympathetic nerve stimulation rather than humoral mechanisms are involved in the early circulatory response to isometric exercise.[2, 29, 30] The response of circulatory catecholamines and renin to isometric exercise has not been previously reported in patients with severe CHF. The increase in circulating plasma norepinephrine in our patients with CHF performing an identical exercise protocol to that used for the normal subjects may have been caused by a fall in cardiac output as a result of failure of the myocardium to overcome the rise in peripheral vascular resistance. A previous report has shown an increase with age in the response of norepinephrine to stress in normal subjects.[31] Therefore the difference in norepineprhine response seen between our patients with CHF and our normal subjects could be attributable to the age difference between these two groups. No relationship was found, however, between the age of our patients with CHF and their norepinephrine response to exercise ($r = .234$, $p = .382$). The hemodynamic significance of the increase in circulating norepineprhine level in our patients during exercise is not entirely clear from our data. Although the rise in norepinephrine is expected to increase systemic vascular tone further via stimulation of the α-adrenergic receptors, we found no significant relationship between the magnitude of changes in both systemic vascular resistance and norepinephrine levels. This finding may suggest that the measurement of circulating plasma norepineprhine does not directly reflect stimulation of the sympathetic nerves. In addition, an increase in total vascular resistance may be partially caused by increased intramuscular pressure and compression of the afferent vessels by the exercising muscles.[11, 32] The general relationship between plasma norepinephrine and hemodynamic changes in patients with CHF has been recently challenged by Goldsmith et al.,[33] who showed no significant hemodynamic effects after infusion of exogenous norepinephrine. Whether this observation could be extended to the relationship between changes in endogenous norepinephrine and hemodynamic response needs further evaluation.

Resting plasma renin concentration was elevated in most of our patients. However no change was seen in renin concentration during exercise, suggesting that the renin-angiotensin system does not contribute to the hemodynamic changes mediated by this form and level of muscle activity.

In conclusion, our results demonstrate a variable hemodynamic response to isometric exercise in patients with chronic advanced (class III or IV) CHF. This form of exercise can lead to a significant deterioration in left ventricular performance, which cannot be predicted from resting hemodynamics, left ventricular ejection fraction, and clinical status and may be useful in the evaluation of myocardial inotropic reserve.

We thank the nurses in the Intensive Cardiac Care Unit, LAC/USC Medical Center, for their assistance in the performance of this study. We also thank Dione Fosdick and Linda Meyer for their excellent secretarial work.

References

1. Donald KW, Lind AR, McNicol GW, Humphries PW, Taylor SH, Staunton HR: Cardiovascular response to sustained (static) contraction. Circ Res **20**(suppl I): I-15, 1967
2. Freyschuss U: Elicitation of heart rate and blood pressure increase on muscle contraction. J Appl Physiol **28:** 758, 1970
3. Grossman W, McLaurin LP, Saltz SB, Paraskos JA, Dalen JE, Dexter L: Changes in the inotropic state of the left ventricle during isometric exercise. Br Heart J **35:** 697, 1973
4. Gonyea WJ, Diepstra G, Muntz KH, Mitchell JH: Cardiovascular response to static exercise in the conscious cat. Circ Res **48**(suppl I): I-63, 1981
5. Elkayam U, Berkley R, Azen S, Weber L, Geva B, Henry WL: Cardiac output by thermodilution technique, effect of injectates volume and temperature on accuracy and reproducibility in the critically ill patient. Chest **84:** 418, 1983
6. Chandraratna PAN, Nanna M, McKay C, Nimalasuriya A, Swinney R, Elkayam U, Rahimtoola SH: Determination of cardiac output by transcutaneous continuous-wave ultrasonic Doppler computer. Am J Cardiol **53:** 234, 1984
7. Rose JS, Nanna M, Rahimtoola SH, Elkayam U, McKay C, Chandraratna PAN: Accuracy of determination of changes in cardiac output by transcutaneous continuous-wave Doppler computer. Am J Cardiol **54:** 1099, 1984
8. Peuler JD, Johnson GA: Simultaneous single isotope radioenzymatic assay of plasma norepinephrine, epinephrine and dopamine. Life Sci **21:** 625, 1977
9. Hsueh WA, Carlson EJ, Dzau VJ: Characterization of inactive renin from human kidney and plasma: evidence of renal source of circulating inactive renin. J Clin Invest **71:** 506, 1983
10. Ehsani AA, Heath GW, Hagberg JM, Schechtman K: Noninvasive assessment of changes in left ventricular function induced by graded isometric exercise in healthy subjects. Chest **80:** 51, 1981
11. Asmussen E: Similarities and dissimilarities between static and dynamic exercise. Circ Res **48**(suppl I): I-3, 1981
12. Ross J Jr, Braunwald E: The study of left ventricular function in man by increasing resistance to ventricular ejection with angiotensin. Circulation **29:** 739, 1964
13. Goldstein DS: Arterial baroreflex sensitivity, plasma catecholamines, and pressor responsiveness in essential hypertension. Circulation **68:** 234, 1983
14. Ewing DJ, Irving JB, Kerr F, Kirby BJ: Static exercise in untreated systemic hypertension. Br Heart J **35:** 413, 1973
15. Peter CA, Jones RH: Effects of isometric handgrip and dynamic exercise on left-ventricular function. J Nucl Med **21:** 1131, 1980
16. Krayenbuehl HP, Grimm J, Turina M, Senning A: Assessment of left ventricular function in aortic valve disease by isometric exercise. Circ Res **48**(suppl I): I-149, 1981
17. Huikuri HV, Atteimo MJ, Linnaluoto MM, Takkunen JT: Left ventricular response to isometric exercise and its value in predicting the change in ventricular function after mitral valve replacement for mitral regurgitation. Am J Cardiol **51:** 1110, 1983
18. Elkayam U, McKay CR, Weber L, Eisenberg D, Rahimtoola SH: Favorable effects of hydralazine on the hemodynamic response to isometric exercise in chronic severe aortic regurgitation. Am J Cardiol **54:** 1603, 1984
19. Perez-Gonzales JF, Schiller NB, Parmley WW: Direct and noninvasive evaluation of the cardiovascular response to isometric exercise. Circ Res **48**(suppl I): I-138, 1981
20. Kivowitz C, Parmley WW, Donoso R, Marcus H, Ganz W, Swan HJC: Effects of isometric exercise on cardiac performance: the grip test. Circulation **44:** 994, 1971
21. Huikuri HV, Takkunen JT: Value of isometric exercise testing during cardiac catheterization in mitral stenosis. Am J Cardiol **52:** 540, 1983
22. Bodenheimer MM, Banka VS, Fooshee CM, Gillespie JA, Helfant RH: Detection of coronary heart disease using radionuclide determined regional ejection fraction at rest and during handgrip exercise: correlation with coronary arteriography. Circulation **58:** 640, 1978
23. Helfant RH, Devilla FMA, Meister SG: Effect of sustained isometric handgrip exercise on left ventricular performance. Circulation **44:** 982, 1971
24. Bevejard BS, Shepherd JT: Reaction in man of resistance and capacity vessels in forearm and hand to leg exercise. J Appl Physiol **21:** 123, 1966
25. Shepherd JT, Blomquist CG, Lind AR, Mitchell JH, Altin B: Static (isometric) exercise retrospection and introspection. Circ Res **48**(suppl I): I-179, 1981
26. Ludbrook PA, Byrne JD, Reed FR, McKnight RC: Modification of left ventricular diastolic behavior by isometric handgrip exercise. Circulation **62:** 357, 1980
27. Aung-Din R, Mitchell JH, Loughurst JC: Reflex and adrenergic coronary vasoconstriction during hindlimb static exercise in dogs. Circ Res **48:** 502, 1981
28. Kozlowski SA, Brzezinska SA, Nazar A, Kawalski W, Franczy UM: Plasma catecholamines during sustained isometric exercise. Clin Sci Mol Med **45:** 723, 1973
29. MacDonald HR, Sapru RP, Taylor SH, Donald KW: Effect of intravenous propranolol on the systemic circulatory response to sustained handgrip. Am J Cardiol **18:** 333, 1966
30. Haskel WL, Savin WM, Schroeder JS, Alderman EA, Ingles NB, Daughters GT, Stimson EB: Cardiovascular responses to handgrip isometric exercise in patients following cardiac transplantation. Circ Res **48**(suppl I): I-156, 1981
31. Palmer GJ, Ziegler MG, Lake CR: Response of norepinephrine and blood pressure to stress increases with age. J Gerontol **33:** 482, 1978
32. Lind AR, Taylor SH, Humphreys PW, Kennelly BM, Donald KW: The circulatory effects of sustained voluntary muscle contraction. Clin Sci **27:** 229, 1964
33. Goldsmith SG, Francis GS, Cohn JN: Effects of infused norepinephrine on hemodynamics and renin in patients with congestive heart failure. Circulation **70**(suppl II): II-309, 1984 (abstr)

The nature of opioid involvement in the hemodynamic respiratory and humoral responses to exercise

J. Staessen, M.D., R. Fiocchi, M.D., R. Bouillon, M.D., R. Fagard, M.D., P. Lijnen, Ph.D., E. Moerman, M.D., A. De Schaepdryver, M.D., and A. Amery, M.D.

ABSTRACT After 30 min rest in the lying position, 12 healthy male volunteers (average age 22 years) received, in a randomized double-blind cross-over protocol, either saline or naloxone (10 mg iv followed by a continuous infusion of 10 mg/hr). Thereafter they rested for a further 30 min in the recumbent position and for 15 min sitting on a bicycle ergometer; they then exercised to exhaustion. At rest plasma levels of adrenocorticotropin (ACTH), cortisol, and aldosterone increased during infusion of naloxone, while body temperature decreased. During exercise the difference in plasma ACTH between naloxone and saline periods was abolished, while the differences in plasma cortisol and aldosterone lost statistical significance. Intra-arterial pressure, heart rate, ventilation, O_2 uptake, and CO_2 output were continuously monitored throughout the experiment and were not affected by naloxone. This was also the case for several hormonal and biochemical measurements, including those of plasma renin, angiotensin II, norepinephrine, 13,14-dihydro-15-keto-prostaglandin $F_{2\alpha}$, glucose and lactate, and serum insulin and growth hormone. Exercise performance was not changed by naloxone. In conclusion (1) during exhaustive graded exercise of short duration opioidergic inhibition of the pituitary-adrenocortical axis is probably not sustained, (2) apart from the latter mechanism, the present study does not support the hypothesis that endogenous opioids are involved in various hemodynamic, respiratory, and hormonal responses to this type of exercise.
Circulation 72, No. 5, 982–990, 1985.

THE SENSITIVITY of the human cardiovascular and endocrine systems to exogenous opiates has been recognized for a long time. More recently, the interest in opioid-mediated mechanisms in cardiovascular and neuroendocrine physiology has been revived by the discovery of an endogenous opiate system. Opioid peptides and receptors have been shown to be densely distributed not only in nociceptive anatomic sites, but also in autonomic centers closely involved in cardiorespiratory and hormonal regulation.[1] These localizations include the brainstem, the hypothalamopituitary axis, the sympathetic ganglia, and the adrenal medulla.[1] In addition, since the discovery of immunoreactive β-endorphin in normal human plasma,[2] several investigators have demonstrated that the levels of circulating β-endorphin[3–5] and its precursor β-lipotropin[6] are stimulated by both maximal and submaximal exercise and that this increase is related to the intensity of effort[4] and is augmented by training.[6]

In view of these findings, the present study aimed to investigate in healthy human volunteers the role of opioid mechanisms in various hemodynamic, respiratory, and humoral responses to exercise with the use of naloxone as a pharmacologic probe. Accordingly, throughout this article the term opioid refers to any directly acting endogenous compound, the actions of which are sterospecifically antagonized by naloxone.

From the Hypertension and Cardiovascular Rehabilitation Unit, Department of Pathophysiology, and the Laboratory for Experimental Medicine and Endocrinology, University of Leuven; and Heymans Institute of Pharmacology, University of Ghent, Belgium.

The present study was partially supported by a research grant of the Bekales Foundation, Vaduz, Liechtenstein, and by a grant of the Belgian Research Council "Nationaal Fonds voor Wetenschappelijk Onderzoek."

Address for correspondence: J. Staessen, M.D., Inwendige Geneeskunde-Cardiologie, U. Z. Sint Rafaël-Gasthuisberg, Herestraat 49, B-3000 Leuven, Belgium.

Received March 21, 1985; revision accepted July 25, 1985.

Methods

Subjects. Twelve normal male volunteers from 21.7 ± 0.4 (SE) years old and weighing at initial examination 69.5 ± 1.9 kg gave their informed written consent and participated in the present study. Their mean height was 180 ± 2 cm. They remained on a liberal diet. Their 24 hr urinary sodium and potassium excretion averaged 142 ± 16 and 72 ± 7 mmol, respectively, and remained constant throughout the study.

Experimental protocol. All experiments were performed in an air-conditioned laboratory, where room temperature was stabilized between 18° and 22° C. The protocol, which was approved by the Ethical Committee of the Faculty of Medicine (K. U. Leuven), is summarized in figure 1. The subjects, sitting on a bicycle ergometer, performed graded and uninterrupted exercise tests until exhaustion. A pretest, meant to assess the subjects' maximal exercise capacity, antedated the subsequent experiments on average by 1 month. For this pretest the initial external workload of 10 W was increased by 10 W every minute. Oxygen uptake, carbon dioxide output, and ventilation at the maximal workload were determined and the external workloads, corresponding to incremental steps of 10% of the maximal exercise capacity, were computed.

On the morning of the two subsequent "experimental" tests, which were on average 2 months apart, the subjects had a light breakfast without caffeine-containing beverages. Thereafter they came to the laboratory. First a small catheter (Vygon 115.09) was introduced into the brachial artery for continuous registration of arterial pressure and for sampling of blood. For drug administration a cannula (Abbocath-T, 18G) was inserted in an antecubital vein and kept patent with a 0.9% sodium chloride solution. Throughout the experiments the intravenous infusion rate was kept constant at a speed of 0.33 ml/min with a Harvard pump, model 906.

After the aforementioned manipulations, the subjects were allowed to rest in the recumbent position for 30 min (RR control period). Then, according to a double-blind cross-over design with balanced randomization, either 10 mg naloxone (Endo Laboratories Inc., New York, USA) dissolved in 25 ml 0.9% sodium chloride or a dose of volume-matched saline were injected intravenously over 5 min. Throughout the remaining part of the experiments the intravenous infusion was continued, delivering 10 mg naloxone in a 0.9% sodium chloride solution or volume-matched dose of saline per hour. Apart from the two physicians supervising each experiment neither the subjects nor any of the other investigators who contributed to the acquisition and processing of the data were aware of the nature of the infusion administered.

After the start of the experimental intervention, the subjects remained recumbent for a further 30 min (RR experimental period). The subjects then assumed the sitting position on the bicycle ergometer for 15 min (RS period). Finally, the exercise test was started at an external workload corresponding to 10% of the maximal exercise capacity determined on the occasion of the pretest. Every 3 min the external workload was augmented by a further 10% of the pretest maximum. The volunteers were asked to continue cycling up to 3 min at 100% of their previously determined maximal exercise capacity, but could stop the two exercise tests earlier if they reached complete exhaustion. The subjects were not informed about the maximal exercise level they attained during any of the tests.

Hemodynamic and respiratory measurements and body temperature. Systolic and diastolic intra-arterial pressure were measured directly through the indwelling catheter in the brachial artery with an electronic transducer (Elema Schönander EMT 34) and recorded continuously on a Mingograph 81 ink-jet recorder. The zero reference point for arterial pressure was kept constant at the midchest level independent of the position of the body. Mean arterial pressure was obtained by electrical damping every 5 min during the RR control and experimental periods and every minute during RS and cycling. Heart rate was determined from the electrocardiogram, which was continuously registered throughout each experiment.

Expired gas was collected in a mixing box by an open-circuit method. Oxygen uptake and carbon dioxide output were continuously calculated from the volume of the expired gas and its O_2 and CO_2 concentrations, determined by electronic gas analyzers that were calibrated before each experiment with test gases of known composition (Siregnost FD, Siemens). The

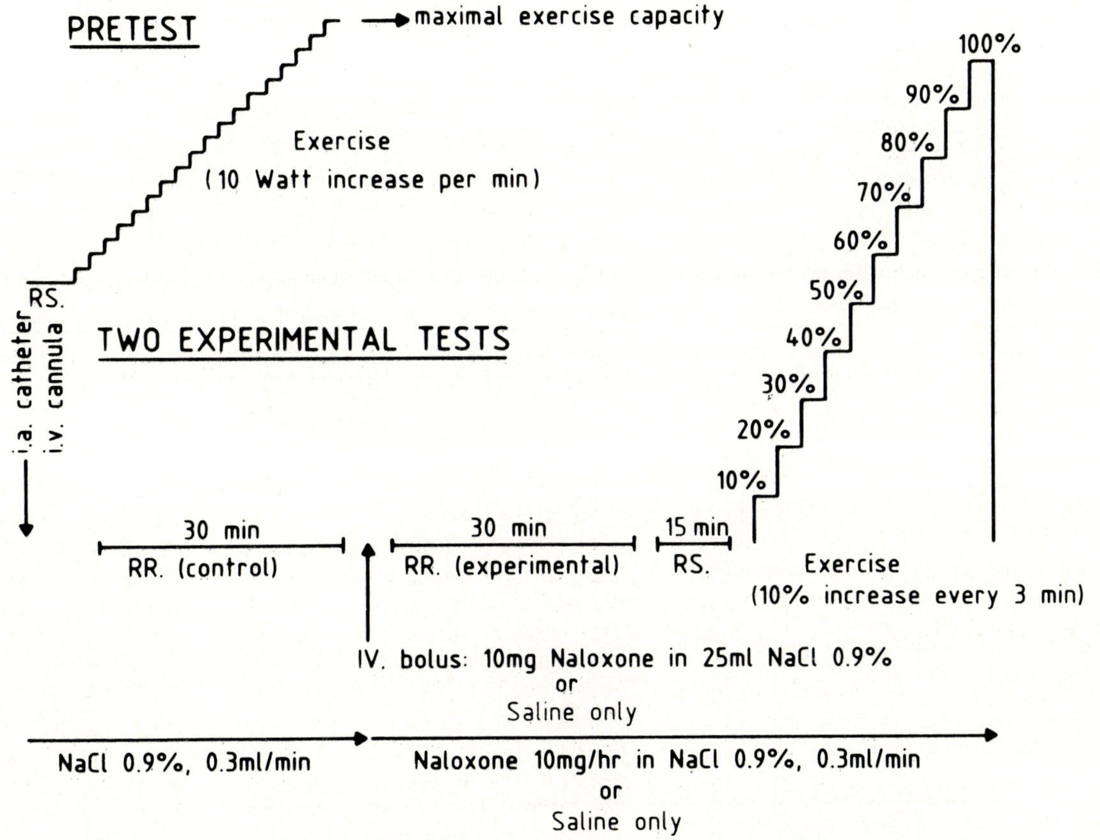

FIGURE 1. Study protocol. See Methods for further explanation.

respiratory gas exchange ratio was calculated as carbon dioxide output divided by oxygen uptake.

Body temperature was measured sublingually at the end of the RR control and RR experimental periods. The same regular mercury thermometer was used for all experiments and read to the nearest 0.05° C after having been applied for exactly 5 min. The subjects were dressed in sportswear, consisting of a sleeveless shirt and shorts, and remained covered by a blanket throughout both the RR control and RR experimental periods.

Biochemical measurements. On both experimental days arterial blood (160 to 180 ml per experiment) was sampled for the following determinations: hemoglobin; plasma renin activity; plasma angiotensin II, aldosterone, norepinephrine, adrenocorticotropin, cortisol, glucose, lactate, and immunoreactive 13, 14-dihydro-15-keto-prostaglandin $F_{2\alpha}$; and serum insulin, growth hormone, electrolytes, bicarbonate, and protein. Arterial blood samples were obtained at the end of the RR control and RR experimental periods, at 10 min of RS, at 30% and 60% of the previously determined maximal exercise capacity, and immediately after the interruption of peak exercise. Arterial blood for hormonal measurements was collected in chilled test tubes and immediately spun at 4° C, the supernatant being instantly frozen and stored at −20° C until assay.

Electrolytes were measured by flame photometry and plasma lactate was determined by an enzymatic method. The plasma concentration of cortisol was determined by a technique based on competitive binding and displacement of radiolabeled cortisol from transcortin. Plasma norepinephrine was assayed by high-performance liquid chromatography with electrochemical detection[7] and the other plasma hormones were assayed by standard radioimmunologic methods, with the use of a double antibody technique for serum insulin and growth hormone.

Statistical analyses. Blood pressure, heart rate, and the respiratory measurements were analyzed by three-way analysis of variance, taking into account as main sources of variation (1) subjects, (2) experimental days or treatments (saline vs naloxone), and (3) time or levels of physical activity. For all other variables comparisons between RR control and RR experimental periods and between experimental days or treatments were performed by Student's two-tailed t test for paired observations.

The distributions of several hormonal measurements were positively skewed. These distributions were linearized by a logarithmic transformation before parametric statistical tests were computed. For these distributions geometric means and ranges are reported, while for other items arithmetic means ± SE are given.

Results

Pretest. At the pretest the volunteers attained a maximal workload of 298 ± 11 W (mean ± SE). At maximal exercise, peak ventilation, oxygen uptake, and carbon dioxide output averaged 114 ± 5, 3.54 ± 0.10, and 3.82 liters/min, respectively.

Measurements obtained before the injection of saline or naloxone. In the comparison of the two experimental days before the injection of saline or naloxone, no differences were found in body weight (69.6 ± 2.1 vs 69.7 ± 1.9 kg, respectively), temperature (36.64 ± 0.08° vs 36.62 ± 0.10° C), blood pressure (figure 2), heart rate (table 1), or any respiratory (table 1), hormonal (figure 3 and table 2), or biochemical measurements (table 3).

Influence of opioid antagonism at recumbent rest (RR experimental). Compared with the administration of saline, opioid antagonism by naloxone did not influence systolic, diastolic, or mean intra-arterial pressure (figure 2), or heart rate (table 1) and the respiratory measurements (table 1). In subjects on saline, body temperature as compared with RR control remained unchanged, averaging 36.64 ± 0.07° C, whereas in those on naloxone a decrease of 0.12 ± 0.04° C (p = .02) to 36.50 ± 0.11° C was observed.

In subjects on saline none of the hormonal (figure 3 and table 2) or biochemical measurements were statistically different between the RR control and RR ex-

TABLE 1

Heart rate and respiratory measurements obtained during the RR and RS periods, at 30% and 60% of the previously determined maximal exercise capacity, and at peak exercise

		RR control	RR experimental	RS	30%	60%	Peak exercise
Workload (W)	S	—	—	—	28 ± 1	170 ± 6	278 ± 12
	N	—	—	—	28 ± 1	170 ± 6	278 ± 10
Heart rate (bpm)	S	69 ± 5	69 ± 4	78 ± 4	102 ± 3	148 ± 4	195 ± 3
	N	68 ± 4	66 ± 4	74 ± 2	102 ± 4	145 ± 4	192 ± 2
Oxygen uptake (ml/min)	S	283 ± 22	271 ± 23	325 ± 21	1239 ± 65	2328 ± 105	3683 ± 155
	N	268 ± 14	271 ± 14	307 ± 20	1179 ± 46	2251 ± 86	3736 ± 158
Carbon dioxide output (ml/min)	S	230 ± 19	222 ± 18	270 ± 22	998 ± 48	2144 ± 86	4035 ± 195
	N	233 ± 14	231 ± 16	258 ± 16	965 ± 33	2120 ± 86	4162 ± 185
Respiratory gas exchange ratio	S	0.81 ± 0.02	0.82 ± 0.02	0.83 ± 0.03	0.81 ± 0.02	0.93 ± 0.02	1.10 ± 0.03
	N	0.87 ± 0.04	0.85 ± 0.02	0.84 ± 0.03	0.82 ± 0.02	0.94 ± 0.01	1.12 ± 0.02
Ventilation (l/min)	S	8.5 ± 1.0	8.2 ± 0.9	10.7 ± 1.1	27.6 ± 1.2	54.4 ± 2.6	108.5 ± 5.4
	N	7.8 ± 0.6	8.0 ± 0.6	9.8 ± 0.8	26.0 ± 1.0	53.8 ± 2.3	112.6 ± 4.8
Respiratory rate (cycles/min)	S	12.7 ± 1.3	12.9 ± 1.4	12.9 ± 1.0	21.5 ± 0.9	26.6 ± 1.8	40.2 ± 2.1
	N	11.1 ± 1.0	12.0 ± 1.2	12.1 ± 0.9	20.0 ± 0.7	24.6 ± 1.0	38.7 ± 1.8

Values are mean ± SE.

S = saline; N = naloxone.

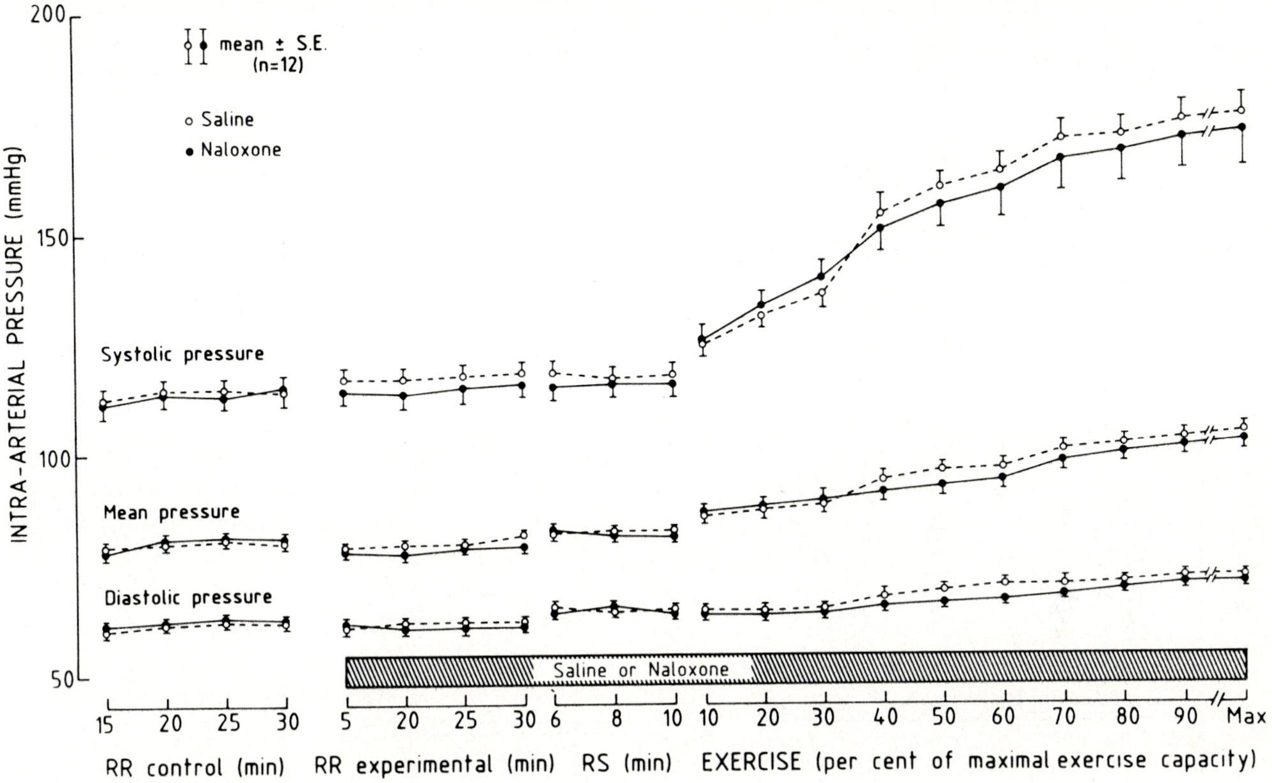

FIGURE 2. Systolic, mean, and diastolic intra-arterial pressure, measured in the RR and RS periods and during exercise, before and during intravenous administration of naloxone (●) or saline (○).

perimental periods. In those on naloxone, however, plasma adrenocorticotropin rose by 450% ($p < .01$), plasma cortisol rose by 80% ($p < .001$), and plasma aldosterone rose by 50% ($p < .001$) (figure 3). Thus, at the end of the RR experimental period higher concentrations were observed during naloxone than during saline administration for plasma adrenocorticotropin (66 vs 21 pg/ml; $p < .01$), plasma cortisol (20.8 vs 13.9 μg/dl; $p < .03$), and plasma aldosterone (10.8 vs 7.2 ng/dl; $p < .01$) (figure 3). None of the remaining hormonal (table 2) or biochemical (table 3) measurements were significantly affected by opioid antagonism and were therefore similar at the end of the RR experimental period on both experimental days.

Influence of opioid antagonism at sitting rest and during exercise. At sitting rest and at each level of exercise, systolic, diastolic, and mean intra-arterial pressure (figure 2), heart rate (table 1), and the respiratory measurements (table 1) were similar on both days.

At sitting rest, plasma concentrations were still higher with naloxone than with saline for adrenocorticotropin (59 vs 32 pg/ml; $p = .08$), cortisol (22.9 vs 17.7 μg/dl; $p = .03$), and aldosterone (12.8 vs 10.2 ng/dl; $p = .02$). Thereafter, during cycling and at the end of exercise, the differences in plasma adrenocorticotropin between tests were abolished, while the differences in plasma cortisol and aldosterone tended to become smaller, and lost statistical significance (figure 3). However, the 95% confidence limits for the changes in plasma cortisol produced by naloxone during and immediately after exercise ranged from an increase in plasma cortisol of 9.6 μg/dl to a decrease of 1.8 μg/dl. The corresponding 95% confidence limits for the naloxone-induced changes in plasma aldosterone embraced +6.3 ng/dl and −1.4 ng/dl, respectively.

Apart from levels of adrenocorticotropin, cortisol, and aldosterone, all other hormonal (table 2) and biochemical (table 3) measurements obtained at sitting rest and during exercise were similar on both experimental days.

Exercise capacity was not different in those on saline and those on naloxone, as evidenced by the maximal attained workload (table 1) and peak oxygen uptake (table 2) and the total duration of exercise (27.8 ± 0.4 vs 27.5 ± 0.2 min, respectively). Two volunteers on saline and two other subjects on naloxone only reached 90% of their previously determined maximal exercise capacity.

Side effects. Subjective complaints were not reported and adverse reactions were not observed, either after the administration of saline or naloxone.

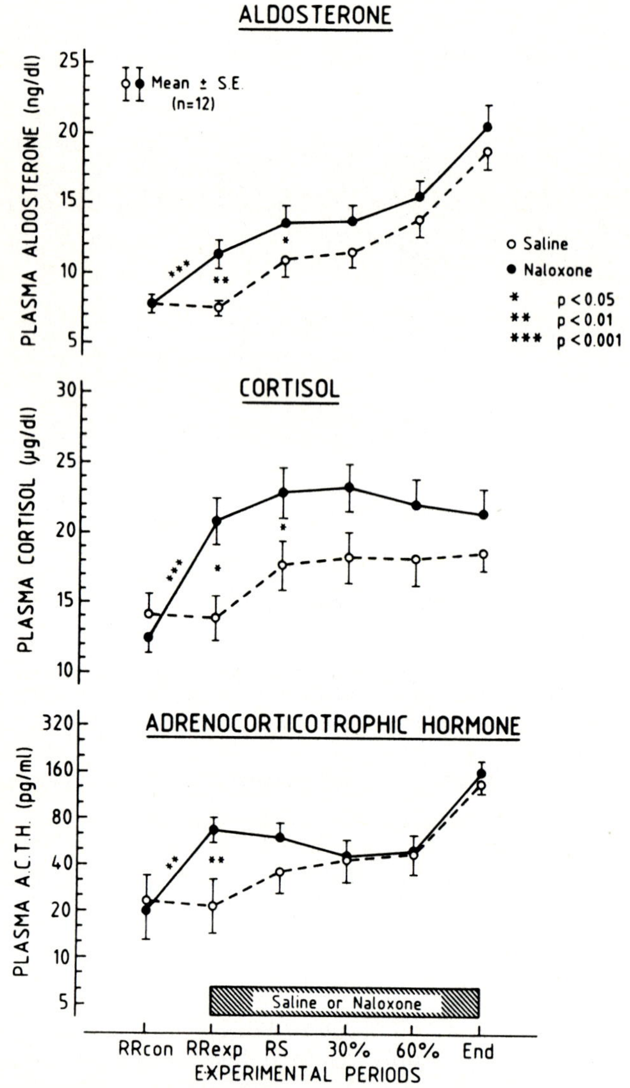

FIGURE 3. Plasma concentrations of aldosterone, cortisol, and adrenocorticotrophic hormone before and during intravenous administration of naloxone (●) or saline (○). Blood samples were obtained in the RR and RS periods, at 30% and 60% of the previously determined maximal exercise capacity, and at the end of peak exercise. Values are mean ± SE. Asterisks refer to the significance of the difference between the experimental sessions (● vs ○) and between control and experimental conditions (RR control vs RR experimental).

Discussion

Antagonism by naloxone has been widely used as a pharmacologic tool to disentangle the involvement of opioid mechanism in human physiology at rest.[1, 9–14] In contrast, only few studies have used this drug in the investigation of the hormonal response to physical effort[15–17] or to study exercise performance.[18] A major concern of the present study was therefore to validate its methodology. This goal was achieved by also recording observations at rest and by testing their reproducibility in comparison with previously reported data from the literature.

Findings in subjects at rest. The present study demonstrated that opioid antagonism in subjects at rest in both the supine and sitting positions did not produce significant changes in intra-arterial pressure. This is in agreement with the work of other investigators,[13, 19] who reported that naloxone, although possibly increasing the sensitivity of baroreflex function,[19] does not alter blood pressure in man, either in the supine position or during 6 hr of 70 degree head-up tilt. The hypothesis that opioid mechanisms do not play a key role in the regulation of systemic arterial pressure in healthy resting but awake subjects is furthermore substantiated by the observation that, similar to naloxone most,[19–22] although not all,[13] studies using opioid agonists such as morphine[20] or met-enkephalin analogues[13, 21, 22] failed to demonstrate a significant effect on blood pressure.

In agreement with earlier findings, the present study confirmed that opioid antagonism by naloxone in normal resting but awake men does not interfere with heart rate[19, 23, 24] or respiration,[23, 25] whereas body temperature is reduced by the drug.[24, 26]

Furthermore, in accordance with previous studies conducted in resting human subjects, opioid antagonism by naloxone did not change the serum levels of growth hormone measured under basal resting conditions,[9–11] but did produce an elevation of the plasma levels of adrenocorticotropin[12, 13] and cortisol.[8–11, 13] Thus, results of the present study also support the concept that inhibitory opiate receptors contribute to the modulation of the pituitary release of adrenocorticotropin in resting human subjects.[12, 13] In addition, we found that opioid antagonism increased the plasma aldosterone concentration at rest, while apart from adrenocorticotropin, several other known determinants of adrenal mineralocorticoid secretion were unaffected throughout the study. These determinants included plasma renin and angiotensin II and serum sodium and potassium. The simultaneously occurring increase in the plasma levels of the two adrenal hormones cortisol and aldosterone on treatment with naloxone is therefore likely to be caused by the enhanced adrenocortical stimulation by adrenocorticotropin, although direct interference with a local opiate–mediated inhibitory mechanism in the adrenal gland itself cannot be ruled out on the basis of the present experiments in vivo.[27, 28]

Opiate agonists have previously been shown to interfere with carbohydrate metabolism at various levels: they stimulate the pancreatic islet secretion of glucagon and insulin,[14, 29, 30] but may also reduce hepatic glucose production.[31] In contrast to these agonist effects the opiate antagonist naloxone, when given under basal conditions to human subjects at rest, has been shown to have no influence on insulin[14, 29, 30] or on plasma glucose.[14, 30] These observations again were confirmed by the present study.

From the results obtained in subjects at rest, one may conclude that the methodology of this study was sufficiently accurate to reproduce most of the effects of opioid antagonism reported by other researchers. In addition, opioid antagonism by naloxone was demonstrated to stimulate plasma aldosterone in healthy human subjects at rest.

Findings during exercise. Several independent groups of investigators have reported that various stimuli, such as metyrapone[2] and physical exercise, produce a concomitant increase in the plasma levels of immunoreactive β-endorphin and adrenocorticotropin.[3–6] Both hormones are derived from the same precursor molecule,[32] are released together from the pituitary gland into the circulation,[32] and share a common circadian rhythm.[13, 33] The present study demonstrated an increase in plasma adrenocorticotropin, from which an enhanced release of β-endorphin can be inferred.[3–6, 13, 32, 33]

Apparently, during exercise opioid receptors accessible via the systemic circulation are exposed to a higher concentration of β-endorphin and possibly other endogenous opiate agonists. The most logical approach to the exploration of the involvement of the endogenous neuroendocrine opiate system in the response to exercise was therefore to inhibit the action of the endogenous ligands at the level of their receptor with the use of naloxone as a pharmacologic probe.

Hemodynamic and respiratory responses to exhaustive graded exercise of short duration. The present study demonstrated that during exercise neither the hemodynamic nor the respiratory measurements were significantly different between the two experimental days. To explain this lack of effect, the possibility should be considered that, as exercise progressed, naloxone no longer reached the endogenous opiate receptors in an amount sufficiently large to sustain their inhibition. Naloxone, however, with its extremely rapid penetration into the brain[34] and its reported serum half-life of 64 min,[34] was infused continuously throughout the experiments. In addition, a further study of similar design in 10 normal volunteers showed that the plasma concentration of naloxone, determined by high-pressure liquid chromatography with electrochemical detection, rose to 43.5 ± 4.0 ng/ml (mean ± SE) in subjects at rest and was subsequently maintained during exercise, averaging 37.2 ± 3.0 and 51.4 ± 4.3 ng/ml at 30% and 60% of peak exercise and 50.9 ± 4.3 ng/ml at the end of cycling.* This is higher than the 5 to 10 ng/ml peak serum concentrations of naloxone obtained within 5 min after a 0.4 mg intravenous bolus,[34] which reportedly sufficed to reverse the effects of exogenously administered morphine for approximately 45 min.[35]

Acidosis may lower the potency of narcotic agonists and antagonists in vivo.[36] It is, however, improbable that exercise-induced changes in pH had a major influence on the outcome of the present study. Indeed, Fagard et al.,[37] using the same exercise protocol in seven normal volunteers, demonstrated that from rest up to 80% of these volunteers' maximal exercise capacity, arterial pH declined only slightly (from 7.40 ± 0.01 to 7.34 ± 0.01, mean ± SE). Moreover, although at higher workloads arterial pH was shown to decrease more sharply, reaching 7.26 ± 0.02 at peak exercise,[37] the lack of effect of naloxone in this study was already apparent at low and moderate exercising levels, when no acidosis was present.

Assuming that the above mechanisms are excluded, our results do not support the view that opioid mechanisms contribute markedly to various hemodynamic and respiratory responses to exhaustive graded exercise of short duration. On the other hand, the present results do not exclude an effect of endogenous opiates on the regional regulation of venous capacitance and arteriolar resistance.[20] Furthermore, under various conditions other than exercise, which was used in the present study, opiates may be involved in cardiorespiratory homeostasis. Indeed, opiates have been reported to interfere with the hypoxic and hypercapnic drive of ventilation in normal human subjects,[38] and with blood pressure regulation during shock,[1] during prolonged head-up tilt,[19, 22] and during acute expansion of intravascular volume.[24] Opiates may also contribute to the fall of systolic blood pressure during sleep[39] and to the blood pressure reduction produced by converting-enzyme inhibition[40] and by central α-adrenergic stimulation,[33] although the latter issue still remains controversial.[41]

Finally, our results confirm earlier findings showing that exercise performance of normal human subjects is not affected by opioid antagonism.[18]

Hormonal responses to exhaustive graded exercise of short duration. At exercise the differences in plasma adrenocorticotropin concentrations, which at rest were apparent between both experimental sessions, were abolished. Concomitantly the differences in the plasma

*Bianchi G: Unpublished data

TABLE 2

Hormonal measurements obtained during RR and RS periods, at 30% and 60% of the previously determined maximal exercise capacity, and at the interruption of peak exercise

		RR control	RR experimental	RS
Serum insulin				
(μU/ml)	S	12.8 (6.0–45.4)	11.9 (3.0–57.1)	14.9 (6.0–43.1)
	N	13.5 (7.0–45.0)	10.9 (5.9–20.0)	14.3 (6.2–24.0)
Plasma 13,14-DH-15K-$PGF_{2\alpha}$				
(pg/ml)	S	43 (19–164)	49 (36–84)	63 (24–132)
	N	43 (28–108)	53 (32–109)	54 (30–110)
Plasma renin activity				
(ng/ml/hr)	S	0.61 (0.01–1.07)	0.41 (0.16–1.05)	0.76 (0.20–2.94)
	N	0.63 (0.28–1.90)	0.63 (0.30–1.40)	0.78 (0.32–1.59)
Plasma angiotensin II				
(pg/ml)	S	19.4 (10.6–35.3)	19.1 (10.3–49.0)	22.9 (11.8–41.8)
	N	20.0 (12.3–31.4)	21.1 (11.6–55.6)	21.1 (12.0–44.3)
Plasma norepinephrine				
(ng/ml)	S	0.26 (0.08–0.50)	0.15 (0.01–0.53)	0.32 (0.19–0.56)
	N	0.23 (0.10–0.65)	0.19 (0.01–0.77)	0.28 (0.01–0.85)
Serum growth hormone				
(ng/ml)	S	2.5 (1.0–21.4)	2.7 (1.0–27.0)	3.1 (1.0–12.2)
	N	1.4 (1.0–5.3)	3.2 (1.0–30.7)	3.5 (1.0–28.0)

Values are geometric means (and ranges).
S = saline; N = naloxone; PG = prostaglandin.

concentrations of the adrenocorticosteroids cortisol and aldosterone tended to be reduced. However, in view of the wide confidence intervals one cannot exclude with certainty that at exercise the plasma concentration of these steroids were persistently higher with naloxone. The observation that the differences in the plasma levels of the adrenal hormones lagged behind those in adrenocorticotropin can be explained by several mechanisms. These include a differential clearance of these hormones from the circulation, a lasting effect of adrenocorticotropin on the adrenal gland,[42] and direct interference of naloxone with the adrenal cortex.[27, 28] With respect to aldosterone the present study also excluded any interaction during exercise of naloxone with other glomerulosa-regulating factors, such as the plasma renin-angiotensin system or serum sodium and potassium. The mechanisms that provoked the exercise-induced rise in plasma adrenocorticotropin have not yet been elucidated. The present data do suggest, however, that the opioid-mediated inhibitory

TABLE 3

Biochemical measurements obtained during RR and RS periods, at 30% and 60% of the previously determined maximal exercise capacity, and at the interruption of peak exercise

		RR control	RR experimental	RS	30%	60%	End of exercise
Hemoglobin (g/dl)	S	14.6±0.2	14.6±0.2	—	—	15.8±0.2	16.2±0.2
	N	14.3±0.2	14.4±0.2	—	—	15.5±0.2	16.0±0.2
Serum protein (meq/l)	S	16.1±0.3	16.1±0.2	—	—	17.9±0.3	18.6±0.3
	N	15.8±0.3	15.9±0.3	—	—	17.7±0.2	18.4±0.2
Serum sodium (meq/l)	S	141.2±0.3	140.5±0.3	—	—	142.2±0.4	142.5±0.5
	N	140.6±0.5	139.8±0.9	—	—	141.6±0.8	142.2±0.9
Serum potassium (meq/l)	S	4.05±0.04	4.06±0.04	—	—	4.84±0.05	4.23±0.11
	N	4.10±0.06	4.12±0.08	—	—	4.92±0.10	4.22±0.13
Serum bicarbonate (meq/l)	S	25.8±0.5	25.9±0.6	—	—	22.3±0.7	14.2±0.9
	N	25.7±0.5	26.0±0.5	—	—	22.0±0.5	12.3±0.9
Plasma lactate (mg/dl)	S	9.1±0.8	7.8±0.6	7.5±0.7	11.4±1.1	31.2±3.5	107.7±9.0
	N	9.2±0.8	7.3±0.8	7.2±0.8	10.8±1.1	32.2±6.6	102.8±8.4
Plasma glucose (mg/dl)	S	89±2	91±3	95±2	95±2	93±2	120±6
	N	89±2	90±1	96±2	94±2	93±2	113±6

Values are arithmetic means ± SE.
S = saline; N = naloxone.

TABLE 2
(Continued)

30%	60%	End of exercise
8.2 (4.0–26.5)	7.4 (4.0–11.2)	19.0 (7.0–62.9)
7.7 (4.0–14.0)	6.9 (4.0–13.1)	18.3 (8.2–56.0)
64 (34–135)	70 (44–133)	117 (65–169)
66 (38–130)	68 (40–131)	119 (74–185)
1.05 (0.45–2.63)	1.40 (0.61–3.03)	2.59 (1.27–4.93)
0.88 (0.33–1.82)	1.29 (0.53–2.34)	2.58 (1.12–4.36)
23.8 (11.4–43.0)	37.2 (13.9–74.4)	176.6 (79.7–823.0)
22.6 (16.0–56.3)	33.5 (20.8–62.9)	131.2 (58.8–429.0)
0.51 (0.25–0.70)	1.10 (0.78–1.70)	2.89 (1.57–6.90)
0.54 (0.27–0.95)	1.09 (0.48–1.59)	2.79 (1.20–4.83)
3.7 (1.0–24.6)	5.5 (1.0–33.5)	20.1 (8.1–43.6)
3.3 (1.0–30.6)	4.7 (1.0–35.6)	20.5 (5.6–42.6)

tone of the pituitary-adrenocortical axis, which prevails at rest[12, 13] and can be unmasked by naloxone, disappeared during exhaustive graded exercise of short duration by subjects in the sitting position. It is not yet known whether this observation also applies to other types of exercise, for instance more prolonged exertion, which would yield a greater increase in plasma cortisol than that induced in the present study.

Since plasma norepinephrine levels followed a similar pattern on both experimental days, the present study suggests that the noradrenergic activation induced by physical effort is not modulated by endogenous opiates. Similarly, the exercise-induced activation of carbohydrate metabolism and of glucose utilization do not seem to be influenced by endogenous opiate-mediated mechanisms, since plasma insulin, glucose, and lactate levels remained similar throughout the two tests. The brisk rise in plasma insulin, which occurred at the end of peak exercise, followed the concurrent overshoot of plasma glucose, when suddenly energy demand decreased. Finally, our findings on growth hormone are in agreement with those of Mayer et al.,[15] but at variance with those of other researchers, who reported that naloxone blunted the maximum incremental response of growth hormone to exercise in normal subjects[16] as well as in athletes.[17]

We gratefully acknowledge the secretarial and technical assistance of L. Cockx, J. Delsupehe, J. Huysecom, M. Laermans, L. Lommelen, V. Mariën, Y. Piccart, J. Romont, M. Stinissen, and Y. Toremans. We are also indebted to R. Grauwels for his help in the computerization of the data. Dr. F. Van Stalle, Continental Pharma, Brussels, Belgium, kindly supplied naloxone.

References

1. Holaday JW: Cardiovascular consequences of endogenous opiate antagonism. Biochem Pharmacol **32:** 573, 1983
2. Nakao K, Nakai Y, Oki S, Horii K, Imura H: Presence of immunoreactive β-endorphin in normal human plasma: a concomitant release of β-endorphin with adrenocorticotropin after metyrapone administration. J Appl Physiol **62:** 1395, 1978
3. Fraioli F, Moretti C, Paolucci D, Alicicco E, Crescenzi F, Fortunio G: Physical exercise stimulates marked concomitant release of β-endorphin and adrenocorticotropic hormone (ACTH) in peripheral blood in man. Experientia **36:** 987, 1980
4. Colt EWD, Wardlaw SL, Frantz AG: The effect of running on plasma β-endorphin. Life Sci **28:** 1637, 1981
5. Gambert SR, Garthwaite TL, Pontzer CH, Cook EE, Tristani FE, Duthie EH, Martinson DR, Hagen TC, McCarty DJ: Running elevates plasma β-endorphin immunoreactivity and ACTH in untrained human subjects. Proc Soc Exp Biol Med **168:** 1, 1981
6. Carr DB, Bullen BA, Skrinar GS, Arnold MA, Rosenblatt M, Beitins IZ, Martin JB, McArthur JW: Physical conditioning facilitates the exercise-induced secretion of beta-endorphin and beta-lipotropin in women. N Engl J Med **305:** 560, 1981
7. Moerman EJ, De Schaepdryver AF: Quantitation of catecholamines in urine and in plasma. Clin Chim Acta **139:** 321, 1984
8. Blankstein J, Reyes FI, Winter JSD, Faiman C: Effects of naloxone upon prolactin and cortisol in normal women. Proc Soc Exp Biol Med **164:** 363, 1980
9. Morley JE, Baranetsky NG, Wingert TD, Carlson HE, Hershman JM, Melmed S, Levin SR, Jamison KR, Weitzman R, Chang RJ, Varner AA: Endocrine effects of naloxone-induced opiate receptor blockade. J Clin Endocrinol Metab **50:** 251, 1980
10. Delitala G, Devilla L, Arata L: Opiate receptors and anterior pituitary hormone secretion in man. Effect of naloxone infusion. Acta Endocrinol **97:** 150, 1981
11. Delitala G, Giusti M, Borsi L, Devilla L, Mazzochi G, Lotti G, Giordano G: Effects of a met-enkephalin analogue and naloxone infusion on anterior pituitary hormone secretion in acromegaly. Hormone Res **15:** 88, 1981
12. Grossman A, Besser GM: Opiates control ACTH through a noradrenergic mechanism. Clin Endocrinol **17:** 287, 1982
13. Grossman A, Gaillard RC, McCartney P, Rees LH, Besser GM: Opiate modulation of the pituitary-adrenal axis: effects of stress and circadian rhythm. Clin Endocrinol **17:** 279, 1982
14. Feldman M, Kiser RS, Unger RH, Li CH: Beta-endorphin and the endocrine pancreas. N Engl J Med **308:** 349, 1983
15. Mayer G, Wessel J, Köbberling J: Failure of naloxone to alter exercise-induced growth hormone and prolactin release in normal men. Clin Endocrinol **13:** 413, 1980
16. Spiler IJ, Molitch ME: Lack of modulation of pituitary hormone stress response by neural pathways involving opiate receptors. J Clin Endocrinol Metab **50:** 516, 1980
17. Moretti C, Fabbri A, Gnessi L, Cappa M, Calzolari A, Fraioli F, Grossman A, Besser GM: Naloxone inhibits exercise-induced release of PRL and GH in athletes. Clin Endocrin **18:** 135, 1983
18. Surbey GD, Andrew GM, Cervenko FW, Hamilton PP: Effects of naloxone on exercise performance. J Appl Physiol **57:** 674, 1984
19. Rubin PC, McLean K, Reid JL: Endogenous opioids modulate central nervous system blood pressure control in man. Clin Sci **63:** 331s, 1982
20. Zelis R, Mansour EJ, Capone RJ, Mason DT: The cardiovasular effects of morphine: the peripheral capacitance and resistance vessels in human subjects. J Clin Invest **54:** 1247, 1974
21. von Graffenried B, del Pozo E, Roubicek J, Krebs E, Pöldinger W, Burgmeister P, Kerp L: Effects of the synthetic enkephalin analogue FK 33-824 in man. Nature **272:** 729, 1978
22. Lightman SL, Forsling ML: The effect of methionin enkephalin analogue DAMME on the vasopressor response to tilt in man. Clin Sci **59:** 501, 1980
23. Willer JC, Boureau F, Dauthier C, Bonora M: Study of naloxone in normal awake man: effects on heart rate and respiration. Neuropharmacology **18:** 469, 1979

24. Zilm DH: Naloxone response in non-dependent man: effect on six physiological variables. Neuropharmacology **19:** 591, 1980
25. Fleetham JA, Clarke H, Dhingra S, Chernick V, Anthonisen NR: Endogenous opiates and chemical control of breathing in humans. Am Rev Respir Dis **121:** 1045, 1980
26. Volavka J, James B, Reker D, Pollock V, Cho D: Electroencephalographic and other effects of naloxone in normal men. Life Sci **25:** 1267, 1979
27. Szalay K Sz, Stark E: Effect of beta-endorphin on the steroid production of isolated zona glomerulosa and zona fasciculata cells. Life Sci **29:** 1355, 1981
28. Rácz K, Varga I, Gláz E, Kiss R, Vida S, Lada G, di Gleria K. Medzihradszky K, Lichtwald K, Vecsei P: Met-enkephalin inhibits mineralocorticoid production in isolated human aldosteronoma cells. J Clin Endocrinol Metab **54:** 656, 1982
29. Ipp E, Dobbs R, Unger RH: Morphine and β-endorphin influence the secretion of the endocrine pancreas. Nature **276:** 190, 1978
30. Reid RL, Yen SSC: β-Endorphin stimulates the secretion of insulin and glucagon in humans. J Clin Endocrinol Metab **52:** 592, 1981
31. Radosevich PM, Williams PE, McRae JR, Lacy WW, Orth DN, Abumrad NN: β-Endorphin inhibits glucose production in the conscious dog. J Clin Invest **73:** 1237, 1984
32. Guillemin R, Vargo T, Rossier J, Minick S, Ling N, Rivier C, Vale W, Bloom F: β-Endorphin and adrenocorticotropin are secreted concomitantly by the pituitary gland. Science **197:** 1367, 1977
33. Farsang C, Vajda L, Kapocsi J, Malisák Z, Alföldi S, Varga K, Juhasz I, Kunos G: Diurnal rhythm of beta-endorphin in normotensive and hypertensive patients: the effect of clonidine. J Clin Endocrinol Metab **56:** 865, 1983
34. Ngai SH, Berkowitz BA, Yang JC, Hempstead J, Spector S: Pharmacokinetics of naloxone in rats and in man: basis for its potency and short duration of action. Anesthesiology **44:** 398, 1976
35. Evans JM, Hogg MIJ, Lunn JM, Rosen M: Degree and duration of reversal by naloxone of effects of morphine in conscious subjects. Br Med J **2:** 589, 1974
36. Kaufman JJ: Acidosis lowers in-vivo potency of narcotics and narcotic antagonists and can even abolish narcotic antagonist activity. Lancet **1:** 559, 1982
37. Fagard R, Lijnen P, Amery A: The pressor effect of exogenous angiotensin II is diminished during dynamic exercise. J Hypertension **1**(suppl 2): 49, 1983
38. Weil JV, McCullough RE, Kline JS, Sodal IE: Diminished ventilatory response to hypoxia and hypercapnia after morphine in normal man. N Engl J Med **292:** 1103, 1975
39. Rubin P, Blaschke TF, Guilleminault C: Effect of naloxone, a specific opioid inhibitor, on blood pressure fall during sleep. Circulation **63:** 117, 1981
40. Millar JA, Sturani A, Rubin PC, Lawrie C, Reid JL: Attenuation of the antihypertensive effect of captopril by the opioid receptor antagonist naloxone. Clin Exp Pharmacol Physiol **10:** 253, 1983
41. Watkins J, FitzGerald G, Zamboulis C, Brown MJ, Dollery CT: Absence of opiate and histamine H_2 receptor–mediated effects of clonidine. Clin Pharmacol Ther **28:** 605, 1980
42. Grower MF, Bransome Jr ED: Adenosine-3′,5′-monophosphate, adrenocorticotropic hormone and adrenocortical cytosol protein synthesis. Science **168:** 483, 1970

Effects of reduced left ventricular mass on chamber architecture, load, and function: a study of anorexia nervosa

MARTIN G. ST. JOHN SUTTON, M.D., TED PLAPPERT, C.V.T., LON CROSBY, PH.D., PAMELA DOUGLAS, M.D., JAMES MULLEN, M.D., AND NATHANIEL REICHEK, M.D.

ABSTRACT We investigated the effects of reduction in left ventricular mass on cavity geometry, afterload, pump function, and exercise performance in 17 patients with anorexia nervosa and in 10 age- and sex-matched normal subjects. Left ventricular mass index determined by two-dimensional echocardiography was significantly lower than that in normal subjects (53 ± 15 vs 79 ± 18 g/m^2; $p < .005$). Left ventricular end-diastolic and end-systolic volume indexes were also reduced in patients with anorexia nervosa compared with normal subjects (49 ± 11 vs 65 ± 17 ml/m^2, $p < .005$; 14 ± 5 vs 19 ± 4 ml/m^2, $p < .025$). In spite of the reductions in left ventricular mass and volume indexes, left ventricular chamber architecture described as h/R ratio, mass to volume ratio, and short/long left ventricular axis ratio were normal. Left ventricular afterload assessed as end-systolic meridional and circumferential wall stress was normal (59 ± 18 vs 79 ± 19 $dyne/cm^2 \times 10^3$ and 170 ± 26 vs 167 ± 23 $dyne/cm^2 \times 10^3$). Ejection fraction, percent fractional shortening, and the relationship between end-systolic wall stress and ejection fraction were all within normal limits. In seven patients restudied after a 15% to 20% weight gain, left ventricular mass and volume indexes increased significantly but end-systolic wall stress and ejection fraction did not change. Ten patients with anorexia nervosa and resting heart rates and systolic blood pressures significantly lower than control values underwent treadmill testing. Exercise duration, peak heart rate, peak systolic blood pressure, and peak oxygen consumption in these patients were all significantly lower than normal. The hypotensive effect of fasting resulted in an initial decrease in afterload, which was the stimulus for reduction in left ventricular mass. The left ventricular remodeling associated with the mass reduction occurred in such a way that (1) orthogonal, meridional, and circumferential wall stresses were normalized, (2) normal chamber shape and architecture were maintained, and (3) chamber function and stress-shortening relationships were preserved. Thus down-regulation of left ventricular mass per se, like up-regulation of left ventricular mass, is not associated with abnormal left ventricular function.
Circulation 72, No. 5, 991–1000, 1985.

THE EFFECTS of left ventricular hypertrophy on cavity geometry and function, and the role of afterload in regulating left ventricular mass and ejection fraction have been clearly demonstrated in pressure and volume overload.[1–6] In addition, the magnitude and time course of regression of left ventricular hypertrophy toward normal following afterload reduction have also been well documented.[7–9] However, the effects of reduction of left ventricular muscle mass to subnormal levels on cardiac mechanics and afterload have not been fully characterized in man. Patients with anorexia nervosa afford an unusual opportunity to examine the biological regulatory mechanisms involved in the left ventricular remodeling associated with reduction in muscle mass and to assess whether the same relationships exist between afterload, pump function, and myocardial mass that operate when left ventricular mass is normal or increased.

From the Section of Cardiology, Department of Medicine, and Section of Nutrition, Department of Surgery, Hospital of the University of Pennsylvania, Philadelphia.

Address for correspondence: Martin G. St. John Sutton, M.D., Division of Cardiology, Brigham and Women's Hospital, Harvard Medical School, 75 Francis St., Boston, MA 02115.

Received March 21, 1985; revision accepted Aug. 1, 1985.

Previous studies of severe caloric deprivation in animals and man have demonstrated decreased heart size, myocardial mass, blood pressure, and heart rate with varying degrees of reversibility after refeeding.[10–17] However, assessment of left ventricular contractile function has produced conflicting results — some have shown it to be supernormal[15] and some normal,[10, 11, 17] whereas others have demonstrated marked left ventricular dysfunction.[16] Postmortem examination of hearts from animals and man dying of starvation has demonstrated marked histologic abnormalities, including vacuolation and fragmentation of myofibrils, replacement fibrosis, and considerable loss of muscle fibers that would provide a substrate for left ventricular dysfunction.[18–20]

We studied patients with anorexia nervosa prospectively to assess the physiologic consequences of marked reduction of left ventricular mass on (1) left ventricular architecture and its remodeling, (2) left ventricular afterload, (3) left ventricular stress-shortening relations, (4) resting pump function, and (5) exercise performance during treadmill testing to assess cardiac reserve.

Methods

Patients with anorexia nervosa. We studied 17 female patients with anorexia nervosa, ages 16 to 37 years (mean 26). The diagnosis of anorexia nervosa was defined by the DSM III criteria, which include (1) loss of more than 25% the original total body weight secondary to self-imposed dietary restriction and (2) absence of any coexistent physical illness that could account for such weight loss.[21] Total body weight in each patient was stable and ranged from 29.7 to 42.1 kg (mean 36.4). Body surface area varied between 1.23 and 1.40 m^2 (mean 1.31).

No patient had any history, symptoms, or signs of heart disease or systemic hypertension. All patients were clinically and biochemically euthyroid, had normal electrolyte balance, and had normal 12-lead electrocardiograms. All patients were participants in a behavior modification program to encourage weight gain. Informed consent was obtained from each patient included in the study.

Normal subjects. We studied 10 normal female volunteers, ages 18 to 35 years (mean 27). Total body weights varied from 42.3 to 69.3 kg (mean 55.2), and body surface areas ranged from 1.47 to 1.71 m^2 (mean 1.60). None had any history, symptoms, or signs of cardiac disease or systemic hypertension. All had normal physical examinations, 12-lead electrocardiograms, and M mode and two-dimensional echocardiograms.

Data acquisition. The following data were recorded from each subject in the resting state: (1) Heart rate was monitored with standard electrocardiographic lead 2. (2) Cuff systolic arterial blood pressure was measured in triplicate in the left arm in each patient after 3 min of recumbency, and mean values were calculated. Cuff arterial pressure was used to represent end-systolic left ventricular pressure, with which it correlates closely as previously demonstrated,[22, 23] to calculate end-systolic circumferential and meridional wall stress. Systolic blood pressure recordings were obtained simultaneously with M mode and two-dimensional echocardiograms. (3) Two-dimensionally directed M mode left ventricular echocardiograms were obtained at the level of chordae tendineae with a Varian 3400R ultrasonoscope at paper speeds of 50 to 100 mm/sec to ensure that the M mode beam sampled the same location on the left ventricular long axis in each subject (figure 1A). (4) Two-dimensional left ventricular echocardiographic images were obtained in (a) the parasternal left ventricular short-axis view at the level of the tips of the papillary muscles (figure 1B) and (b) the apical four-chamber view, so the left ventricular long axis could be measured. Approximately 20 cardiac cycles of the left ventricular short axis were recorded, and the transducer was quickly moved to the left ventricular apex to obtain 20 cardiac cycles of the four-chamber view to minimize the time interval between acquisition of orthogonal left ventricular images.

Treadmill exercise tests. Incremental exercise tests were performed in 10 of the patients with anorexia nervosa and in the 10 normal subjects by means of a modified Naughton protocol. This consisted of a 3 min practice period at 1 mph and 0 degree grade, followed by a constant speed of 2 mph with an increase in grade of 3.5 degrees every 3 min. Heart rate was displayed digitally throughout, blood pressure was measured at 1 min intervals, three simultaneous electrocardiographic leads were monitored continuously, and 12-lead electrocardiograms were printed out every minute.

Expiratory gas flow and partial pressures of oxygen and carbon dioxide were measured breath by breath with the Beckman MMCI metabolic cart. Minute ventilation (V_E, liters/min), oxygen consumption (VO_2, liters/min), and carbon dioxide production (VCO_2, liters/min) were recorded at baseline and after each minute of exercise. Duration of exercise was recorded.

Seven of the 17 patients with anorexia gained weight and had repeat echocardiograms, but only four had repeat treadmill exercise tests.

Data processing and analysis

M mode echocardiograms. M mode left ventricular echocardiograms containing a minimum of three cardiac cycles of similar cycle length were calibrated and digitized on a Hewlett-Packard 9821A microcomputer. End-diastolic and end-systolic left ventricular cavity diameter (LVD) and wall thickness (WT) were measured according to the convention recommended by the American Society of Echocardiography.[24] From these data, end-diastolic relative wall thickness (h/R ratio = WT/LVD/2), fractional left ventricular shortening, and velocity of circumferential fiber shortening (VCF) were computed and used as an index of left ventricular short-axis architecture and pump function, respectively.

End-systolic meridional wall stress was computed with the formula[25]: stress $\sigma = P \times R_i/2h\,(1 + h/2/R_i)$, modified in our

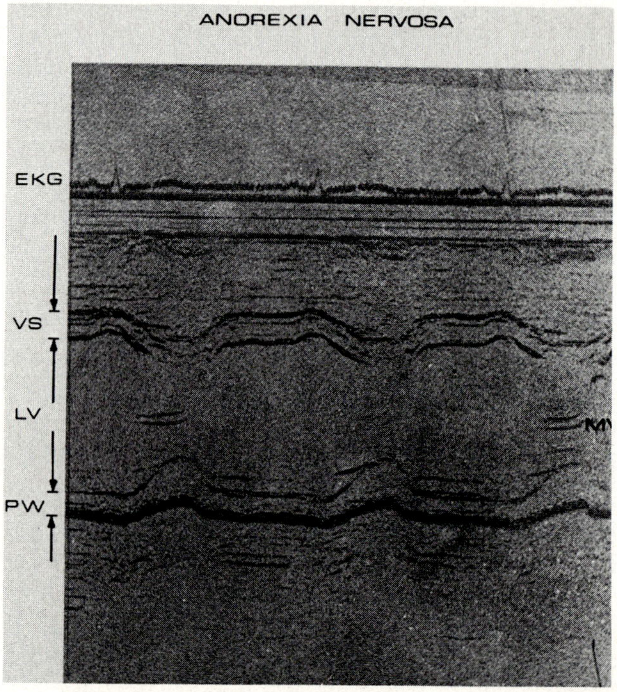

FIGURE 1A. M mode left ventricular echocardiogram from a patient with anorexia nervosa. VS = ventricular septum; LV = left ventricle; PW = posterior wall; MV = mitral valve.

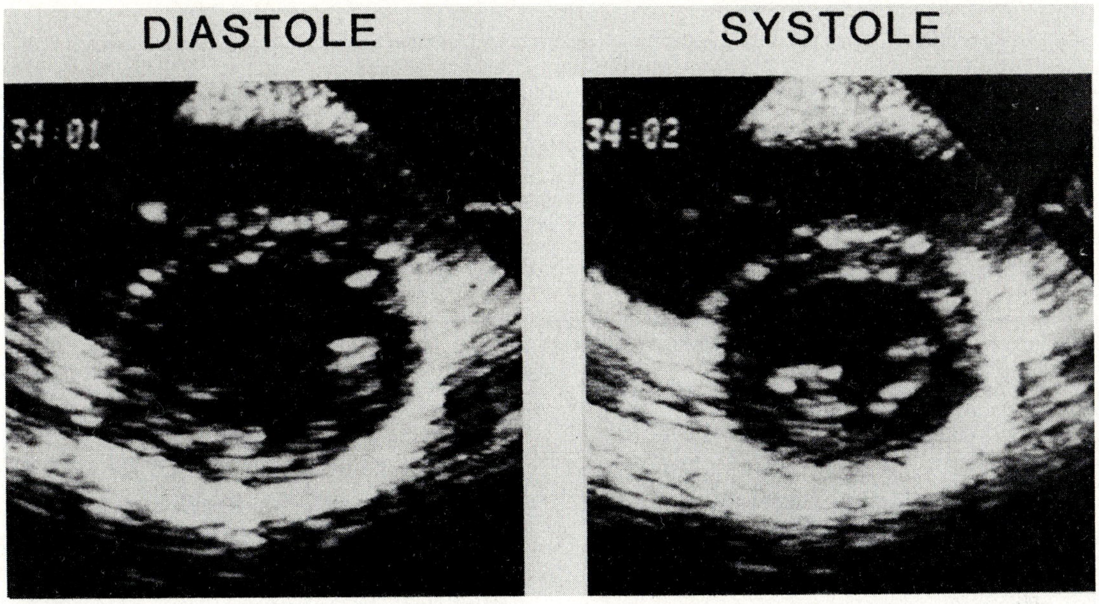

FIGURE 1B. Two-dimensional echocardiographic short-axis view of the left ventricle in a patient with anorexia nervosa at end-diastole and end-systole.

laboratory to $\sigma = 0.25 \times 1.33\,P(LVD)/WT\,(1 + WT/LVD)$ as previously reported,[22, 23] where P is cuff-determined systolic arterial pressure and the constant 1.33 converts mm Hg to dyne/cm$^2 \times 10^3$. (We used cuff systolic pressure to calculate an approximation to "end-systolic" meridional stress, to which it correlated closely.[7])

Two-dimensional left ventricular echocardiograms

Parasternal short-axis view. Short-axis endocardial and epicardial images of the left ventricle from five high-quality, stop-action end-diastolic and end-systolic frames were traced with their calibration factors on clear plastic overlays from a high-contrast scan converter. Tracings of endocardium and epicardium from each subject were digitized on a Hewlett Packard 9825A microcomputer to obtain: (1) total area (A_t) enclosed by the left ventricular epicardium and right side of the septum; (2) cavity area (A_c) by two previously validated methods,[22, 23, 26, 27] in which the papillary muscles were regarded (a) as part of the cavity for stress determinations and (b) as the left ventricular wall for left ventricular volume and mass determinations; and (3) muscle area (A_m) obtained by subtracting A_c (including papillary muscles) from A_t, i.e. ($A_t - A_c$) for wall stress calculations.

Apical four-chamber view. Endocardial and epicardial left ventricular lengths (L) were traced from five end-diastolic and five end-systolic stop-action frames and digitized. Cavity length was defined as the distance between the apical endocardium and the midpoint of the plane of the mitral valve anulus.

The raw values for A_c, A_m, A_t, and L were corrected with regression equations developed in vitro for the two-dimensional echocardiographic instrument used in this study. These corrected values were used to calculate the following: (1) end-diastolic and end-systolic volumes by the short-axis area-length method[26]: $V = 5/6 A_c L$; (2) fractional shortening assessed as the percent change in left ventricular short-axis area; (3) ejection fraction; (4) left ventricular shape expressed as the ratio of short-to-long left ventricular axes $\sqrt{A_c/\pi}/L$; (5) left ventricular muscle mass (LVM) calculated as $LVM = 1.055 \times 5/6\,(A_t L_t - A_c L_c)$ (the constant 1.055 is the density of myocardial muscle); (6) left ventricular end-systolic meridional wall stress (σ_m): $\sigma_m = (1.33 \times P \times A_c)/(A_t - A_c)$; (7) left ventricular end-systolic circumferential wall stress (o_c): $o_c = (1.33 \times P \times \sqrt{A_c})/(\sqrt{A_t}\sqrt{A_c}) \cdot 1 - (A_c^{3/2}/[\pi(0.5L)^2(\sqrt{A_c} + \sqrt{A_t})]$. The formula used to calculate circumferential wall stress was modified from Mirsky.[25] The constant 1.33 is the conversion factor from mm Hg to dyne/cm^2 (we used cuff systolic pressure to calculate an approximation to "end-systolic" meridional and circumferential stresses); and (8) ratio of myocardial area A_m to cavity area A_c: (A_m/A_c).

In addition we compared (1) the end-systolic meridional and circumferential stress-shortening relationships and (2) the relationships among end-systolic meridional and circumferential wall stresses and ejection fraction in patients with anorexia nervosa and in normal subjects. The reproducibility and interobserver variability of left ventricular volume and mass determinations by two-dimensional echocardiography has been previously reported by our laboratory.[22, 26, 27]

Statistical methods. The significance of differences in measured and derived parameters of left ventricular function and exercise performance between patients with anorexia nervosa and normal control subjects was assessed by unpaired Student t tests. Paired t tests were used to compare within-population differences after gain in body weight.

Results are reported as mean $\pm$ 1 SD.

Results

Resting heart rates in patients with anorexia nervosa varied over a similarly wide range as those of the age- and sex-matched normal subjects, whereas resting systolic and diastolic blood pressures were consistently lower than those in normal subjects (table 1).

End-diastolic and end-systolic left ventricular cavity diameters and end-diastolic posterior wall thicknesses measured from two-dimensionally directed M mode echocardiograms were all significantly smaller than normal (table 1). End-diastolic and end-systolic volume indexes determined by two-dimensional echocardiography were also significantly reduced in patients

TABLE 1

Comparison of resting heart rate, blood pressure, and left ventricular size and function between patients with anorexia nervosa and age- and sex-matched normal subjects

	Resting heart rate (beats/min)	Resting blood pressure (mm Hg)		LV diameter (cm)		LV wall thickness–diastole (cm)	h/R ratio	Shape ratio short/long axis	VCE (circumferences/sec)
		Systole	Diastole	Diastole	Systole				
Normals (n = 10)	69±13	110±9	74±9	4.4±0.5	2.9±0.3	0.7±0.1	0.32±0.05	0.62±0.05	0.95±0.32
Anorexia nervosa (n = 17)	63±16	93±8[A]	65±8[A]	3.9±0.3[A]	2.6±0.3[A]	0.6±0.1[B]	0.31±0.04	0.63±0.04	0.98±0.26

LV = left ventricular; VCF = velocity of circumferential fiber shortening.
Statistical comparisons: [A]$p < .01$; [B]$p < .02$.

with anorexia nervosa (49 ± 11 vs 65 ± 17 ml/m^2, $p < .005$; 14 ± 5 vs 19 ± 4 ml/m^2, ($p < .025$) (figure 2). Left ventricular mass indexes were 53 ± 15 g/m^2 compared with 79 ± 18 g/m^2 in normal subjects ($p < .005$) (figure 3), which represented a reduction of between 30% and 50%.

The reduction in left ventricular mass in patients with anorexia nervosa was not accompanied by changes in left ventricular chamber shape; the short/long left ventricular axis ratio at end-diastole was 0.63 ± 0.04, similar to that in the normal control subjects (0.62 ± 0.05) (table 1). End-diastolic relative wall thickness (h/R ratio) determined by M mode echocardiography did not differ significantly from normal (0.31 ± 0.04 vs 0.32 ± 0.05, table 1) and left ventricular mass-to-volume ratio determined by two-dimensional echocardiography in patients with anorexia was indistinguishable from that in normal subjects (1.20 ± 0.20 vs 1.33 ± 0.24, figure 3), indicating that left ventricular architecture in patients with anorexia nervosa was normal.

End-systolic meridional and circumferential wall stresses in patients with anorexia nervosa varied over the same ranges as in normal subjects, and their respective mean values of 59 ± 18 vs 74 ± 19 × 10^3 dyne/cm^2 and 170 ± 26 vs 167 ± 23 × 10^3 dyne/cm^2 were not significantly different (figure 4). Resting left ventricular function was assessed as fractional shortening and ejection fraction, which were both normal (32 ± 4% vs 34 ± 3% and 71 ± 8% vs 71 ± 5%, respectively) (figure 5). The velocity of circumferential fiber shortening in patients with anorexia nervosa was also similar to that in normal subjects (0.98 ±

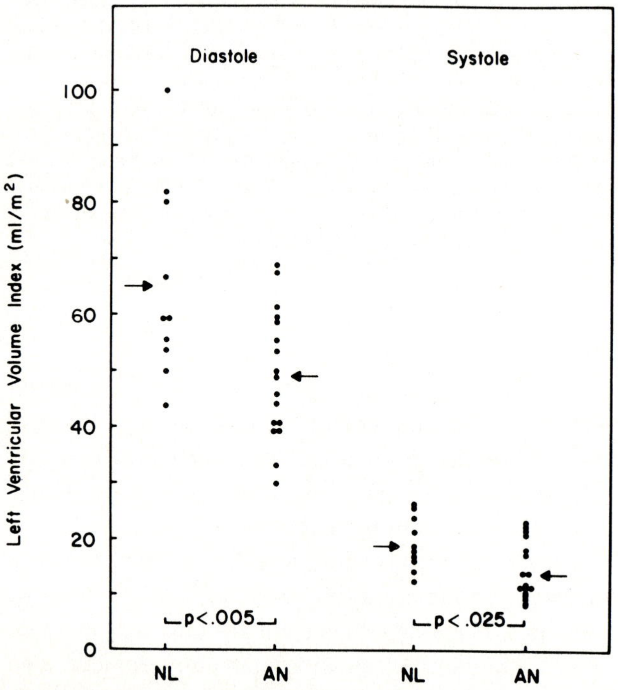

FIGURE 2. Plots comparing left ventricular end-diastolic and end-systolic volume indexes in patients with anorexia nervosa and in age- and sex-matched control subjects.

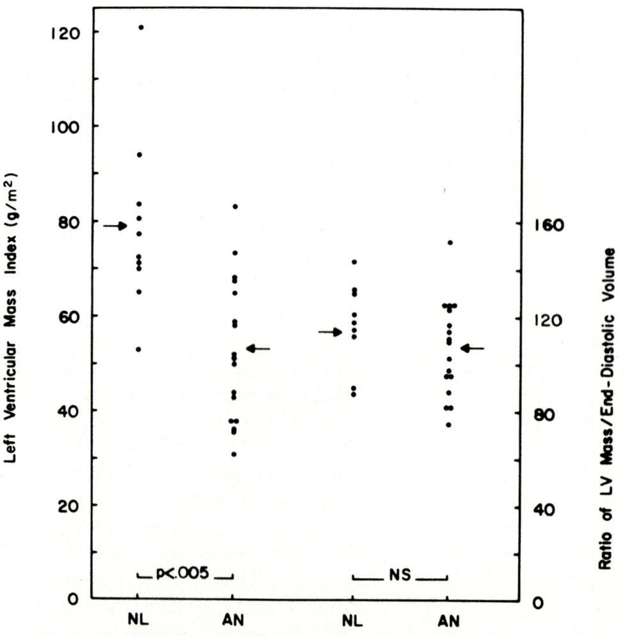

FIGURE 3. Plots of left ventricular mass index and the ratio of left ventricular mass/end-diastolic volume in patients with anorexia nervosa and age- and sex-matched control subjects.

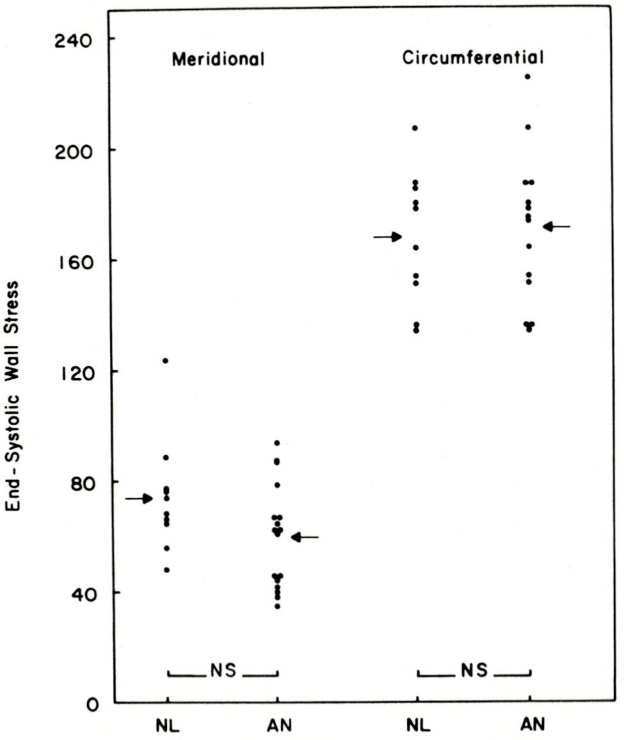

FIGURE 4. Plots of end-systolic meridional and circumferential wall stresses in patients with anorexia nervosa and in normal control subjects.

0.26 vs 0.95 ± 0.32 circumferences/sec) (table 1). The relationships between the percent change in left ventricular diameter and end-systolic wall stress (i.e., the stress-shortening relationships) and between ejection fraction and end-systolic wall stress in patients with anorexia were within normal limits (figure 6). We plotted end-systolic circumferential wall stress against ejection fraction and percent change in left ventricular diameter, since it has been shown to relate more closely to left ventricular emptying than meridional stress because it takes into account chamber length.

Seven patients were restudied with M mode and two-dimensional echocardiography after a mean gain in total body weight of 6.3 kg. Left ventricular mass indexes and end-diastolic volume indexes increased from 61.7 ± 13.3 to 71.2 ± 17.7 g/m^2 ($p < .02$) and from 57.0 ± 7.8 to 63.4 ± 14.6 ml/m^2 ($p < .02$), respectively, but fractional shortening, ejection fraction, and end-systolic wall stresses did not change (table 2).

Exercise testing. In the 10 patients with anorexia nervosa who performed treadmill exercise tests, resting heart rate was significantly lower than that in the normal subjects (table 3), although this difference was not apparent when the population with anorexia nervosa (17 patients) was considered as a whole. Systolic blood pressures at rest were also significantly less than normal (96 ± 7 vs 119 ± 12 mm Hg; $p < .01$), but resting oxygen consumption values were similar (3.20 ± 0.45 vs 3.10 ± 0.60 ml/min/m^2) (table 3, figure 7).

Exercise tests were terminated by fatigue in all subjects. Exercise duration in patients with anorexia nervosa was 22 ± 5 min compared with 37 ± 20 mins ($p < .01$) in normal subjects (table 3). Heart rate and blood pressure responses to exercise were markedly blunted in anorexia nervosa in that both were consistently less at each matched workload throughout treadmill testing. The following mean values were recorded: peak heart rate, 136 ± 19 vs 176 ± 12 beats/min ($p < .01$); peak systolic blood pressure, 122 ± 7 vs 164 ± 9 mm Hg ($p < .01$); peak oxygen consumption, 19.4 ± 4.0 vs 28.9 ± 5.3 ml/min/m^2 ($p < .001$), all significantly lower in patients with anorexia nervosa (table 3, figure 7).

Four patients underwent repeat treadmill exercise testing after a mean gain in body weight of 5.4 kg; left ventricular mass index and end-diastolic volume had increased from 58.0 ± 16.6 to 75.1 ± 23.5 g/m^2 ($p < .05$) and 56.8 ± 6.6 to 74.9 ± 15.9 ml/m^2 ($p < .05$), respectively. Exercise duration increased from a mean of 23 ± 5 to 30 ± 10 min (NS), peak heart rate from 127 ± 12 to 143 ± 5 beats/min ($p < .05$), peak systolic blood pressure from 125 ± 7 to 146 ± 11 mm Hg ($p < .05$), and peak oxygen consumption from 18.9 ± 2.0 to 22.1 ± 1.8 ml/min/m^2 (NS) (figure 8).

Discussion

We assessed the effects of major reduction of left ventricular muscle mass on chamber architecture and

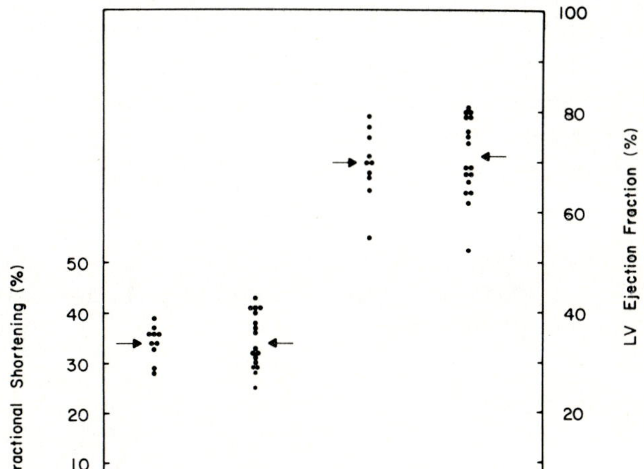

FIGURE 5. Plots of left ventricular fractional shortening and ejection fraction in patients with anorexia nervosa and in normal control subjects.

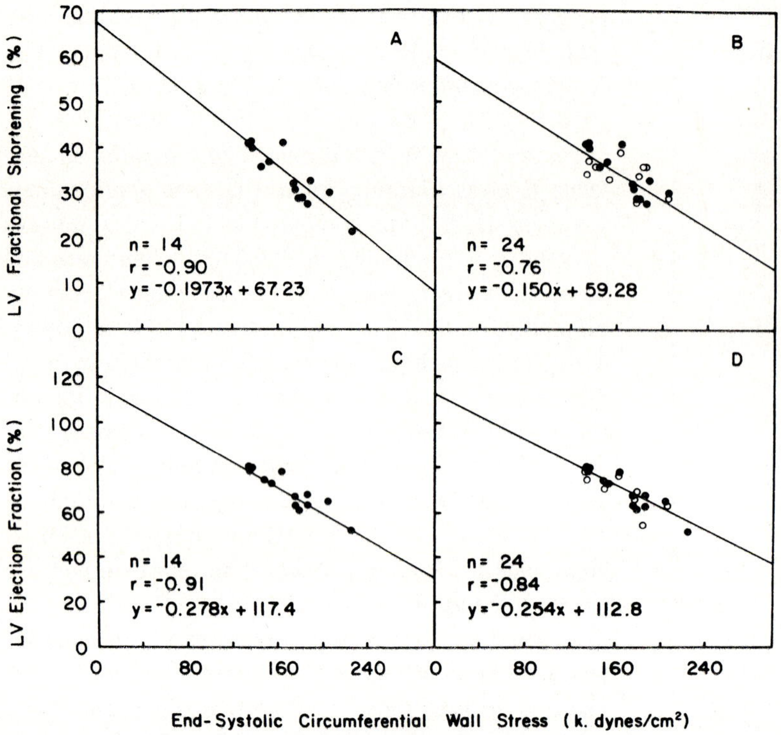

FIGURE 6. Plots demonstrating the relationships between left ventricular fractional shortening and end-systolic circumferential wall stress in patients with anorexia nervosa alone (*A*) and in normal subjects and patients with anorexia nervosa combined (*B*). Plots demonstrating the relationship between ejection fraction and end-systolic circumferential stress in patients with anorexia alone (*C*) and in subjects and patients with anorexia combined (*D*).

mechanics in patients with anorexia nervosa. In addition we examined the interrelationships between left ventricular afterload, chamber function, and muscle mass when left ventricular mass was subnormal. We chose patients with anorexia nervosa as a model for three reasons. First, left ventricular muscle mass was reduced by between 30% and 50%. Second, their age and sex made the presence of coronary artery disease and associated left ventricular dysfunction extremely unlikely. Third, they were normally hydrated, in electrolyte balance, and clinically and biochemically euthyroid.

Left ventricular mass in patients with anorexia nervosa ranged between one-half and two-thirds of that in age- and sex-matched normal control subjects. This reduction in myocardial mass was disproportionately greater than the fall in total body weight; when normalized to unit body weight or unit surface area, these mass indexes remained consistently less than normal. This finding is concordant with a recent report in children with anorexia nervosa[17] but is in sharp contrast to initial beliefs that the heart, like the brain, is spared during starvation.[14]

Major left ventricular remodeling accompanied the reduction in left ventricular mass. Left ventricular end-systolic and end-diastolic cavity diameters and volumes were significantly decreased, whereas cavity shape remained normal. The distribution of left ventricular muscle, expressed as relative wall thickness (h/R ratio) by M mode echocardiography, and the ratio of left ventricular muscle mass to end-diastolic volume determined by two-dimensional echocardiography were also both normal. Although left ventricular muscle mass was down-regulated by between 30% and

TABLE 2

Changes in left ventricular architecture, afterload, and pump function in patients with anorexia nervosa after gain in total body weight

	LV mass index (g/m²)	LV end-diastolic volume index (ml/m²)	% change in LV diameter	Ejection fraction (%)	End-systolic meridional stress (dyne/cm² × 10³)
Before weight gain (n = 7)	61.7±13.3	57.0±7.8	35±5	72±6	58.6±7.3
After weight gain (n = 7)	71.2±17.7[A]	63.4±14.6[A]	36±4	73±5	61.3±12.3

LV = left ventricular.
[A]p < .02.

TABLE 3
Comparison of exercise performance between patients with anorexia nervosa and normal control subjects

	Resting heart rate (beats/min)	Peak heart rate (beats/min)	Resting systolic blood pressure (mm Hg)	Peak systolic blood pressure (mm Hg)	Exercise duration (min)	Resting O_2 uptake (ml/min/m^2)	Peak O_2 uptake (ml/min/m^2)
Normals (n = 10)	88±17	176±12	119±12	164±9	37±20	3.1±0.6	28.9±5.3
Anorexia nervosa (n = 10)	75±18^A	136±19^B	96±7^B	122±7^B	22±5^B	3.2±0.5	19.4±4.0^C

Statistical comparisons: $^A p < .02$; $^B p < .01$; $^C p < .001$.

50%, normal left ventricular architecture was maintained, and this was also true after the increases in muscle mass and volume that accompanied gain in total body weight.

Left ventricular afterload, which we assessed in our patients with anorexia nervosa as end-systolic meridional and circumferential wall stresses, was consistently normal and remained within normal limits even after the increases in left ventricular mass and chamber volume that accompanied gain in total body weight. Thus left ventricular remodeling in patients with anorexia nervosa occurred in such a way that circumferential and meridional wall stresses were maintained within normal limits and normal left ventricular chamber architecture was preserved.

Resting left ventricular function, expressed as percent fractional shortening, velocity of circumferential fiber shortening, and ejection fraction, was normal before and after gain in body weight. In addition, the inverse relationships between left ventricular fractional shortening or ejection fraction and end-systolic wall stress were similar to those in the normal subjects, indicating that stress-shortening relationships, in patients with anorexia nervosa were normal.

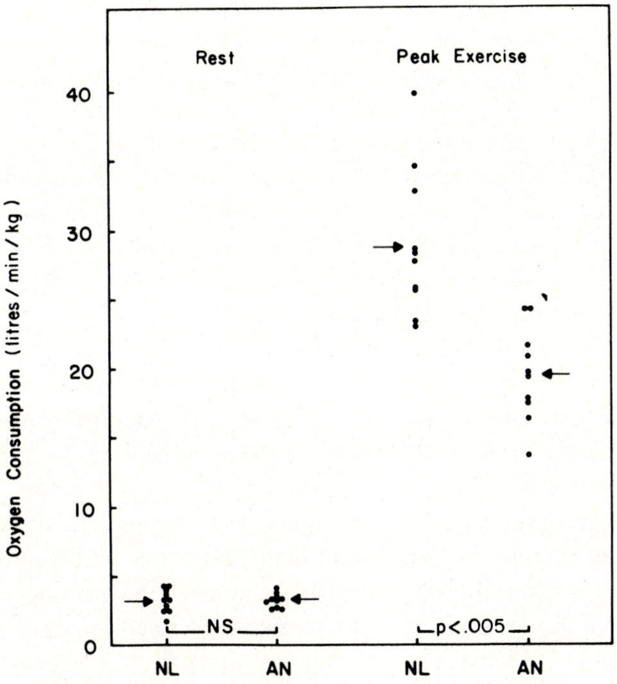

FIGURE 7. Plots demonstrating oxygen consumption in patients with anorexia nervosa and in normal control subjects at rest and at peak exercise.

We were unable to assess myocardial contractility as the slopes of force-length lines or end-systolic stress-dimension lines in individual patients. This would have required perturbations in left ventricular loading conditions with intravenous infusions to increase systolic blood pressure, since it was already below normal at rest. This was not thought to be advisable in our patients on account of their emotional fragility. Thus to determine whether the reduction in left ventricular mass was accompanied by cardiovascular dysfunction not apparent at rest, we assessed cardiac performance during dynamic exercise by breath-by-breath analysis of oxygen uptake.

Exercise tests were terminated by fatigue in the patients with anorexia and in the normal subjects. Exercise duration in patients with anorexia nervosa was shorter than in normal subjects despite a similar degree of fatigue. However, this may have been caused by peripheral factors such as the decreased skeletal muscle mass in these patients. Heart rate and blood pressure were also significantly less than normal at each matched workload throughout the treadmill tests. Although oxygen consumption in patients with anorexia nervosa was normal at rest, it was significantly lower at peak exercise than in the normal subjects. Four patients repeated the exercise test after a 15% gain in total body weight. Peak heart rates and peak systolic blood pressures increased significantly on exercise, although the increases in exercise duration and oxygen consumption were not statistically significant.

The temporal sequence and exact mechanism of left ventricular mass reduction in patients with anorexia

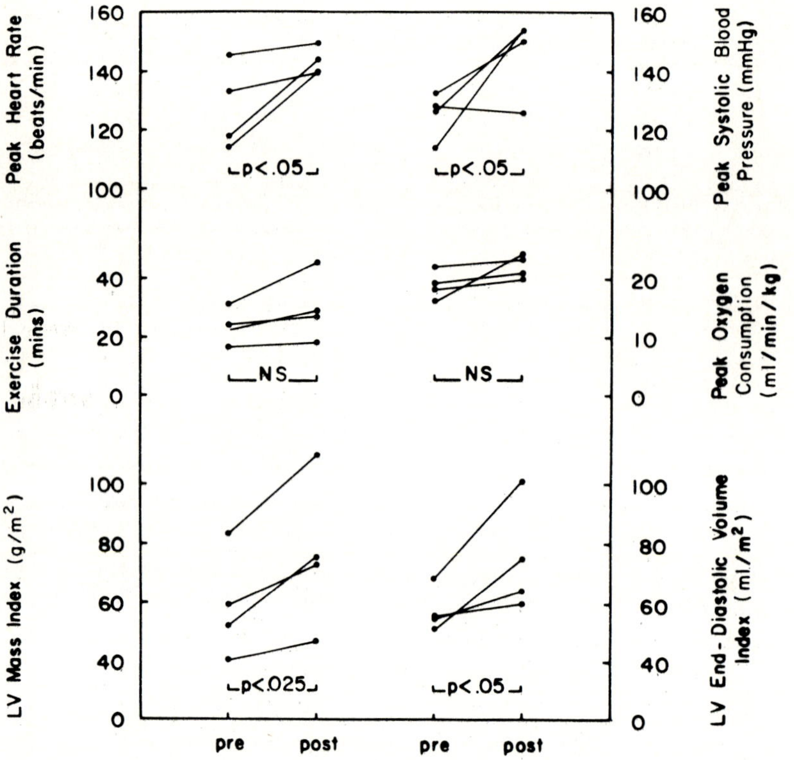

FIGURE 8. Plots showing the changes in peak heart rate, peak systolic blood pressure, exercise duration, peak oxygen consumption, left ventricular mass indexes, and left ventricular end-diastolic volume indexes in four patients with anorexia nervosa after gain in total body weight.

nervosa could not be elucidated from our study because we assessed patients only during the long-term steady state when their body weights were stable. The decrease in left ventricular mass could theoretically have resulted from failure to deliver the metabolic requirements to the myocardium. However, this is inconsistent with the normal left ventricular chamber architecture and normal pump function. The reduction in left ventricular mass more likely resulted from alteration in left ventricular afterload. Systolic arterial pressure decreases early after the onset of fasting in experimental animals, and there is strong evidence that this is caused by decreased norepinephrine biosynthesis and turnover and reduced α-adrenergic receptor activity.[28, 29] This hypotensive effect of fasting also occurs in patients with anorexia nervosa.[10–12, 17] Furthermore, catecholamine metabolism is similarly decreased and the levels of norepinephrine and its active metabolites in plasma, urine, and cerebrospinal fluid in patients with anorexia nervosa are significantly lower than normal.[30–38] The fall in systemic arterial pressure in the early stages of decreased caloric intake would result in a reduction in afterload and act as the stimulus for down-regulation of left ventricular mass to subnormal levels. This is the exact corollary of the increase in afterload in pressure overload that has been demonstrated to up-regulate left ventricular mass in man.

Increased left ventricular afterload results in increased left ventricular muscle mass, which normalizes wall stress and thereby preserves ejection function.[1, 3–5] By contrast, a decrease in afterload, achieved for example by treating systemic hypertension, can result in regression of left ventricular mass and normalization of wall stress.[8] Normalization of systolic wall stress is thought to be the feedback signal that governs the rate and extent of ventricular hypertrophy.[39] In patients with anorexia nervosa, end-systolic meridional and circumferential wall stresses were consistently normal. However, theoretically we could have overlooked physiologically meaningful differences in systolic wall stresses between the two populations because of our relatively small sample sizes. Although we could not establish a direct cause-and-effect relationship between afterload and the reduced left ventricular muscle mass from this study, the disproportionately greater fall in left ventricular mass than in total body weight suggests that it more likely resulted from reduction in afterload, since afterload may vary independently of body weight and surface area.

Our inability to document left ventricular dysfunction in patients with anorexia nervosa either at rest or on exercise, except for a blunted heart rate and blood pressure response, is in sharp contrast to the histologic abnormalities in the myocardium described in starvation.[10–12] One possible reason for this discrepancy might be that histologic abnormalities and associated ventricular dysfunction reported in starvation develop only in the terminal stages, and our patients with anorexia nervosa had not approached this severity of caloric deprivation. An alternative explanation for the development of left ventricular dysfunction might relate to the previously reported high incidence of hypothyroidism.[35] However, several recent studies in patients with anorexia nervosa have demonstrated that thyroxine (T_4) and thyroid-stimulating hormone (TSH) levels are normal and that tri-iodothyronine (T_3) is adaptively down-regulated proportional to the reduction in body weight, which thus spares muscle wasting and does not indicate the presence of hypothyroidism.[36–38] Moreover, all our patients were both clinically and biochemically euthyroid.

We submit that the reduction in left ventricular mass to subnormal levels in patients with anorexia nervosa probably resulted from decreased left ventricular afterload. The decrease in left ventricular afterload and the blunted heart rate and blood pressure responses to exercise may well be mediated by reduced α-adrenergic receptor activity and reduced catecholamine biosynthesis. The fall in left ventricular myocardial mass was associated with major left ventricular remodeling, which occurred in such a way that (1) orthogonal meridional and circumferential wall stresses remained normal, (2) normal chamber shape and architecture were maintained, and (3) normal chamber function and stress-shortening relationships were preserved. Furthermore, these parameters remained normal after the increase in left ventricular mass and volume observed with refeeding. Thus down-regulation of left ventricular mass per se, like adaptive up-regulation of left ventricular mass, was not associated with abnormal left ventricular function.

Hitherto afterload has been shown to increase left ventricular mass only above normal levels. We examined afterload when left ventricular mass was reduced to subnormal levels. Thus these observations extend previous studies of afterload and demonstrate that the same physiologic relationships exist between afterload, left ventricular mass, and chamber function when left ventricular mass is well below normal as exist when left ventricular mass is normal or increased.

We are indebted to Eileen Slattery for the illustrations.

References

1. Grossman W, Jones D, McLaurin LP: Wall stress and patterns of hypertrophy in the human left ventricle. J Clin Invest **56:** 14, 1975
2. Carabello BA, Nolan SP, McGuire LB: Assessment of preoperative left ventricular function in patients with mitral regurgitation: value of the end-systolic wall stress end-systolic volume ratio. Circulation **64:** 1212, 1981
3. Grossman W, Carabello BA, Gunther S, Fifer MA: Ventricular wall stress and the development of cardiac hypertrophy and failure. *In* Alpert NR, editor: Perspectives in cardiovascular research. Vol 7: Myocardial hypertrophy and failure. New York, 1983, Raven Press, p 1
4. Grossman W: Cardiac hypertrophy: useful adaptation or pathologic process? Am J Med **69:** 576, 1980
5. Grossman W, Braunwald E, Mann T, McLaurin LP, Green LH: Contractile state of the left ventricle in man as evaluated from end-systolic pressure-volume relations. Circulation **56:** 845, 1977
6. Gunther S, Grossman W: Determinations of ventricular function in pressure overload hypertrophy in man. Circulation **59:** 679, 1979
7. Reichek N, Wilson J, St. John Sutton M, Plappert TA, Goldberg S, Hirshfeld JW: Non-invasive determination of left ventricular end-systolic stress: validation of the method and initial application. Circulation **65:** 99, 1982
8. Reichek N, Franklin BB, Chandler T, Muhammad A, Plappert T, St. John Sutton MG: Reversal of left ventricular hypertrophy by antihypertensive therapy. Eur Heart J **3**(suppl A): 165, 1982
9. St. John Sutton M, Spiegel A, Reichek R, Douglas P, Edmunds LH: Differing effects of aortic valve replacement in chronic pressure and volume overload. Circulation **70**(suppl II): II-48, 1984 (abst)
10. Gottdiener JS, Gross HA, Henry WL, Borer JS, Ebert MH: Effects of self-induced starvation on cardiac size and function in anorexia nervosa. Circulation **58:** 425, 1978
11. Heymsfield SB, Bethel RA, Ansley JD, Gibbs DM, Feliver JM, Nutter DO: Cardiac abnormalities in cachectic patients before and during nutritional repletion. Am Heart J **95:** 584, 1978
12. Keys A, Henschel A, Taylor HL: The size and function of the human heart at rest in semi-starvation and in subsequent rehabilitation. Am J Physiol **50:** 153, 1947
13. Keys A, Friedell HL, Garland LH, Madrazo MF, Rigler LG: The roentgen evaluation of the size and function of the heart. Am J Roentgenol Radium Ther **44:** 865, 1946
14. Keys A: Cardiovascular effects of undernutrition and starvation. Mod Concepts Cardiovasc Dis **27:** 21, 1948
15. Nutter DO, Murray TG, Heymsfeld SB, Fuller EO: The effect of chronic protein-caloric undernutrition in the rat on myocardial function and cardiac function. Circ Res **45:** 144, 1979
16. Abel RM, Grimes JB, Alonso M: Adverse hemodynamic and ultrastructural changes in dog hearts subjected to protein caloric malnutrition. Am Heart J **97:** 733, 1979
17. Moodie DS, Salcedo E: Cardiac function in adolescents and young adults with anorexia nervosa. J Adolescent Health Care **4:** 9, 1983
18. Wharton BA, Balmer SF, Somers: The myocardium in Kwashiorkor. Q J Med **149:** 107, 1969
19. Smythe PM, Swanepoel A, Campbell JAH: The heart in Kwashiorkor. Br Med J **2:** 67, 1962
20. Chavan S, Nayak NC, Ramalingaswami V: The heart and skeletal muscle in experimental protein malnutrition in rhesus monkeys. J Pathol Bacteriol **90:** 301, 1965
21. Williams JBW: Diagnostic and statistical manual of mental disorders (DSM III), ed. 3. Washington, DC, 1980, American Psychiatric Association, p 69
22. Reichek N, Helak J, Plappert T, St. John Sutton M, Weber KT: Anatomic validation of left ventricular mass estimates from clinical two-dimensional echocardiography: initial results. Circulation **67:** 348, 1983
23. St. John Sutton MG, Plappert TA, Hirshfeld JW, Reichek N: Assessment of left ventricular mechanics in patients with asymptomatic aortic regurgitation: a two-dimensional echocardiographic study. Circulation **69:** 259, 1984
24. Sahn DJ, DeMaria A, Kisslo J, Weyman A: Recommendations regarding quantitation in M-mode echocardiography: results of a survey of echocardiographic measurements. Circultion **58:** 1072, 1978
25. Mirsky I: Review of various theories for evaluation of left ventricular wall stresses. *In* Mirsky I, Chidsey DN, Sandler H, editors: Cardiac mechanics: physiological, chemical and mathematical considerations. New York, 1974, John Wiley and Sons, Inc., Ch 13
26. Helak JW, Reichek N: Quantitation of human left ventricular mass and volume by two dimensional echocardiography; in vitro validation. Circulation **63:** 1398, 1981
27. Helak JW, Plappert T, Muhammad A, Reichek N: Two-dimensional echographic imaging of the left ventricle: comparison of me-

chanical and phased array systems in vitro. Am J Cardiol **48:** 728, 1981
28. Einhorn D, Young JB, Landsberg L: Hypotensive effect of fasting: possible involvement of the sympathetic nervous system and endogenous opiates. Science **217:** 727, 1982
29. Jhanwar-Uniyal M, Fleischer F, Levin BE, Leibowitz SF: Impact of food deprivation on hypothalamic α-adrenergic receptor activity and norepinephrine turnover (NE) in rat brain. Neuroscience **8:** 711, 1982 (abst)
30. Gross HA, Lake CR, Eber MH, Ziegler MG, Kopin IJ: Catecholamine metabolism in primary anorexia nervosa. J Clin Endocrinol Metab **49:** 805, 1979
31. Halmi KA, Dekirmenjian H, Davis JM, Casper R, Goldberg S: Catecholamine metabolism in anorexia nervosa. Arch Gen Psychiatry **35:** 458, 1978
32. Van Loon GR: Abnormal catecholamine mechanisms in hypothalamic-pituitary disorders. Metabolism **29**(suppl I): 1198, 1980
33. Darby PL, Van Loon G, Garfinkel PE, Brown GM: LH, growth hormone, prolactin and catecholamine responses to LHRF and bromo-cryptine in anorexia nervosa. Psychosom Med **41:** 585, 1979
34. Leibowitz SF: Hypothalamic catecholamine systems controlling eating behaviour: a potential model for anorexia nervosa. *In* Anorexia nervosa: Recent developments in research. New York, Alan R. Liss, Inc., pp 221–229
35. Croxson MS, Ibbertson HK: Low serum tri-iodothyroxine (T_3) and hypothyroidism in anorexia nervosa. J Clin Endocinol Metab **44:** 1967, 1977
36. Hurd HP, Palumbo PG, Gharid H: Hypothalamic-endocrine dysfunction in anorexia nervosa. Mayo Clin Proc **52:** 711, 1977
37. Brown GM, Garfinkel PE, Jeuniewic N, Moldofsky H, Stanler HC: Endocrine profile in anorexia nervosa. *In* Vigersky RA, editor: New York, 1977, Raven Press, pp 123–125
38. Boyar RM, Hellman LD, Roffwarg H, Katz J, Zumoff B, O'Connor J, Bradlow L, Fukushima DK: Cortisol secretion and metabolism in anorexia nervosa. N Engl J Med **296:** 190, 1977
39. Alpert NR: Cardiac hypertrophy. New York, 1977, Academic Press

Effects of sublingual nifedipine on hemodynamics and systolic and diastolic function in patients with hypertrophic cardiomyopathy

SANDRO BETOCCHI, M.D., RICHARD O. CANNON III, M.D., RITA M. WATSON, M.D., ROBERT O. BONOW, M.D., HAROLD G. OSTROW, M.S., STEPHEN E. EPSTEIN, M.D., AND DOUGLAS R. ROSING, M.D.

ABSTRACT The hemodynamic effects of sublingual nifedipine were examined in 36 patients with hypertrophic cardiomyopathy. Twenty-one patients were initially given 20 mg and 15 patients were given 10 mg of the drug; 30 min after this first dose 26 patients received 10 mg and one patient 20 mg as a second dose. Hemodynamic findings in patients who received different doses of the drug were similar. Peak effects included an increase in heart rate from 79 ± 12 to 91 ± 14 (mean ± 1 SD) beats/min ($p < .01$), and a decrease in mean blood pressure from 89 ± 12 to 77 ± 10 mm Hg ($p < .01$). Cardiac index increased after nifedipine (2.8 ± 0.6 to 3.3 ± 0.8 liters/min/m^2; $p < .01$); stroke volume index, however, did not change (36 ± 7 to 36 ± 8 ml/beat/m^2; NS). Peripheral vascular resistance index fell significantly from 822 ± 261 to 610 ± 197 dynes·sec·cm^{-5} ($p < .01$). Overall, left ventricular outflow tract gradient (LVOTG) did not change in patients with significant (≥30 mm Hg) basal LVOTG (75 ± 22 to 83 ± 22 mm Hg; NS), but it increased significantly in those six patients in whom peripheral vascular resistance fell by 25% or more (73 ± 28 to 99 ± 22 mm Hg; $p < .05$). Pulmonary arterial wedge pressure increased significantly in patients with normal (≤15 mm Hg) basal values (9 ± 3 to 14 ± 7 mm Hg; $p < .01$) and in patients with significant basal LVOTG (15 ± 8 to 20 ± 10 mm Hg; $p < .01$). In 10 patients, systolic and diastolic function were studied simultaneously by a nonimaging scintillation probe. No changes in systolic or diastolic function were detected when determinations obtained at the time of the peak nifedipine effect were compared with control values recorded at similar heart rates obtained by atrial pacing. The pattern of change in the pressure-counts loops after administration of nifedipine was not consistent; in only three of 10 patients was an improvement in the diastolic pressure-volume relationship observed. These results indicate that in patients with hypertrophic cardiomyopathy sublingual nifedipine induces a marked reduction in afterload without demonstrating any beneficial effects on LVOT obstruction and diastolic function. Moreover, in patients with normal pulmonary arterial wedge pressures and/or significant LVOTGs, nifedipine seems to be detrimental because it increases filling pressures, with these changes being exaggerated in patients with more marked falls in peripheral vascular resistance.
Circulation 72, No. 5, 1001–1007, 1985.

SEVERAL STUDIES have demonstrated that verapamil, the prototype calcium channel–blocking drug, is an effective therapeutic agent for patients with hypertrophic cardiomyopathy.[1–5] The administration of verapamil to these patients reduces left ventricular outflow tract (LVOT) obstruction,[1, 6] enhances diastolic function,[7–11] and increases exercise capacity and reduces symptoms when given either over the short[2] or long term.[3–5, 11]

Approximately one-third of patients who have been started on verapamil treatment, however, do not find this drug beneficial either because of its inability to reduce symptoms[4, 5] or because of adverse drug effects.[4, 5, 12] Therefore, since the calcium channel-blocking drugs differ in their molecular structures, electrophysiologic properties, and hemodynamic effects, it seemed reasonable to examine the effects of another one of this category of drugs in patients with hypertrophic cardiomyopathy.

From the Cardiology Branch, National Heart, Lung, and Blood Institute, and the Computer Systems Laboratory, Division of Computer Research and Technology, National Institutes of Health, Bethesda.

Address for correspondence: Douglas R. Rosing, M.D., Building 10, Room 7B-15, National Institutes of Health, Bethesda, MD 20205.

Received Jan. 14, 1985; revision accepted Aug. 1, 1985.

Dr. Betocchi was a recipient of a NIH-Fogarty International Research Fellowship FO5 TW03350. His present address is: Clinica Medica I, 2a Facolta di Medicina, Via S. Pansini, 5, 80131 Naples, Italy.

Although some reports indicate that administration of nifedipine to patients with hypertrophic cardiomyopathy has beneficial hemodynamic effects,[13] the relatively small number of such patients treated with this drug, as well as some conflicting data,[14, 15] make its clinical usefulness in the treatment of hypertrophic cardiomyopathy still unclear. Nifedipine, however, has the potential advantage over verapamil that it does not produce atrioventricular conduction disturbances or sinus node depression, which are the most frequent side effects encountered during verapamil therapy.[12, 16] In the present study we examined the hemodynamic effects of nifedipine in a large number of patients with hypertrophic cardiomyopathy, with and without LVOT obstruction.

Methods

Patient population. Thirty-six patients, 20 men and 16 women from 14 to 68 years old (mean 46), had echocardiographic evidence of hypertrophic cardiomyopathy (a nondilated hypertrophied left ventricle in the absence of other congenital or acquired heart diseases that produce left ventricular hypertrophy[17]). Twenty-three patients (64%) had no evidence of mitral insufficiency on their left ventriculograms, whereas five patients (14%) had mild and eight (22%) had moderate-to-severe mitral regurgitation. No patient had 50% or more narrowing of the coronary artery luminal diameter. All agreed to participate in the study according to a protocol approved by the Institutional Clinical Research Subpanel of the National Heart, Lung, and Blood Institute. Cardiac catheterizations were performed for diagnostic reasons and/or to guide therapy. No patient underwent an invasive procedure solely for the purpose of determining effects of nifedipine.

At admission, only one patient (3%) was asymptomatic (NYHA functional class I), 15 (42%) patients were functional class II, 18 (50%) were functional class III, and two (6%) were functional class IV. Only three patients (8%) were free of chest pain; 21 (59%) had a history of mild chest pain and 12 (33%) had moderate-to-severe chest pain, compatible with angina. Propranolol had been administered to 33 patients. Cardiac medications were discontinued at least five drug half-lives before catheterization. Each patient received 10 mg of oral diazepam 1 hr before study and had been in a fasting state for a least 8 hr before coming to the catheterization laboratory.

Hemodynamic measurements. Left ventricular pressure was obtained through a pig-tail catheter (end-hole only, no side holes) in 25 patients and through a micromanometer-tipped catheter (Millar Instruments, Inc., Houston) in 11. Catheters were placed at the apex of the left ventricle by the retrograde femoral technique. Catheter entrapment[18] was excluded by the guidelines proposed by Wigle et al.[19] Pulmonary arterial wedge pressure was determined with a Swan–Ganz catheter placed by the antegrade femoral technique. Cardiac output was measured with the right heart catheter by the thermodilution technique with a cardiac output computer (Edwards Laboratories, Inc., Santa Ana, CA) and by averaging at least three replicate determinations. Left ventricular stroke volume was calculated from the cardiac output. Systemic blood pressure was measured by means of a No. 20 4 inch Teflon brachial artery catheter. Left ventricular outflow tract gradient was defined as the difference between the peak left ventricular and peak systemic systolic pressures. In 18 patients, measurements of LVOT gradient (LVOTG) were repeated during a Valsalva maneuver, amyl nitrite inhalation, or isoproterenol infusion. Systemic resistances were measured in units of dynes·sec·cm^{-5}.

In the 11 patients studied with micromanometer catheters, left ventricular relaxation was assessed by digitizing the left ventricular pressure curve and computing the time constant (T) of the fall in left ventricular pressure.[20] In patients in whom a single exponential equation did not adequately fit the actual points of the digitized left ventricular pressure curve, a biexponential fitting was used and two time constants were calculated. The first constant (T1) described the behavior of the left ventricular pressure curve during the first 40 msec after peak negative dP/dt and second one (T2) described that during the following 40 msec.[21]

Radionuclide measurements. In 10 patients studied with micromanometer catheters, left ventricular time-activity curves and pressure-counts loops were obtained by use of a nonimaging scintillation probe, the characteristics of which have been described in detail elsewhere.[10, 22] At the beginning of right heart catheterization, red blood cells were labeled in vivo with 15 to 20 mCi^{99m} TC.[23] After 10 min, systemic antiocoagulation with heparin (5000 units iv) was instituted and left heart catheterization was begun.

The probe was positioned over the patient's chest in a 35 degree left anterior oblique projection with a 15 degree caudad tilt, and adjusted over the precordium to maximize the background-uncorrected ejection fraction. Electrocardiographically gated equilibrium scintillation data and digitized left ventricular pressure values were collected for the first 140 cardiac cycles falling within a preset range of cycle lengths.

The following measurements were made[10]: end-diastolic volume (EDV; normalized by setting the control number of counts = 100); ejection fraction; and peak filling rate (PFR in end-diastolic volumes per second = EDV/sec) and time to PFR (TPFR), defined as the time interval from the nadir of the time-activity curve, i.e., end-systole to PFR.

Instantaneous relationships between left ventricular pressure and volume were analyzed by generating high temporal resolution (25 msec) pressure-counts loops, representing the average of 140 cardiac cycles. Since it was anticipated that nifedipine would increase heart rate, control radionuclide studies were obtained during atrial pacing at heart rates 10 to 30 beats/min faster than those recorded in the initial control study to avoid any effect of heart rate on left ventricular filling.

Administration of nifedipine. Nifedipine was administered buccally with the patients breaking the capsule(s) in their mouths and chewing them until the contained liquid appeared to be absorbed or diluted; the capsule(s) were then swallowed. Hemodynamic measurements were repeated 10, 20, and 30 min after swallowing the remnants of the capsule(s), whereas radionuclide studies were performed only once after each dose: at 20 minutes in five patients and at 30 min in the remaining five patients.

Initial nifedipine dose was 20 or 10 mg, determined by the investigator performing the catheterization, and based on the control blood pressure, outflow tract obstruction, and symptomatic status of the patient. A second dose was administered 30 min after the first if systolic blood pressure remained above 99 mm Hg.

Data analysis. Peak effect of nifedipine was defined for each parameter as the maximal change from the control value. Control values were compared with peak effect values with the two-tailed Student t test for paired samples. The difference between doses was assessed by comparing the percentage changes from the control values by means of the two-tailed Student t test for unpaired samples. The chi-square test was performed to determine whether the occurrence of peak effect after the first or the second dose was affected by the total nifedipine dosage.

Results

Nifedipine dosage. Twenty-one patients received 20 mg as their first dose and the remaining 15 patients were given 10 mg. Nine patients did not recieve the second dose, six because their systolic blood pressures dropped below 99 mm Hg and the remaining three for various clinical reasons. Of these nine, seven had been given a first dose of 20 mg and two a first dose of 10 mg. Twenty-six patients were given 10 mg as their second dose and one patient received 20 mg. A total nifedipine dose of 10 mg was administered to two patients (5%) and 20 patients (56%) received 20 mg; 30 mg was the total dose in 13 patients (36%) and only one patient received 40 mg. For practical purposes, in the analysis of the data this latter patient's hemodynamic responses to the drug will be included with those of patients receiving 20 + 10 mg of nifedipine.

Dose-effect relationship. Table 1 illustrates the maximal changes after nifedipine expressed as a percentage of the control value. No significant differences were observed between patients receiving 10 mg and those receiving 20 mg as their first dose, neither during the 30 min after the first dose nor during the 30 min after the second dose.

Maximal effect on heart rate occurred more frequently after the second dose than after the first (63% vs 37%), whereas peak effect of nifedipine on mean blood pressure, pulmonary arterial wedge pressure, cardiac index, and index of peripheral vascular resistance occurred with comparable frequencies after the first and second doses of nifedipine. No significant differences in the timing of the peak effects of the drug were found when results were analyzed separately according to the first dose. Moreover, no differences in hemodynamic measurements were observed when they were analyzed according to the total dose instead of the first dose.

Hemodynamics. One patient (3%) had a basal heart rate faster than 100 beats/min (105 beats/min) and none had a rate slower than 60 beats/min. In eight patients (22%), cardiac index was less than our established lower limits of normal (2.5 liters/min/m^2). Fourteen patients (39%) had pulmonary wedge pressures higher than the upper limit of normal in our laboratory (15 mm Hg) and 24 (67%) had higher than normal left ventricular end-diastolic pressures (>12 mm Hg). An LVOTG of 30 mm Hg or more in the control study was present in 17 patients (47%) (range 35 to 105 mm Hg, median 85 mm Hg). Of the remaining 19 patients, 11 developed LVOTGs of 30 mm Hg or more during provocative maneuvers (Valsalva in two patients, amyl nitrite inhalation in four, and isoproterenol infusion in five). Thus, 28 of the 36 patients (78%) met our criteria for the diagnosis of obstructive hypertrophic cardiomyopathy.

Since no difference had been observed among patients receiving different doses of nifedipine, all results were analyzed for the group as a whole, independent of the dosage. Table 2 lists the mean hemodynanic values ± 1 SD at control and at peak effect of nifedipine. Nifedipine produced a significant increase in heart rate and a decrease in mean blood pressure. Mean pulmonary arterial wedge pressure significantly increased with nifedipine, but this was confined primarily to those patients who started out with a normal wedge pressure (figure 1). In this group, mean wedge pressure increased from 9 ± 3 to 14 ± 7 mm Hg ($p < .01$) while in those patients who had an elevated control wedge pressure (>15 mm Hg), it did not change significantly (23 ± 6 to 24 ± 7 mm Hg; NS). In the group that started with a normal wedge pressure, pressure became abnormal in nine (41%) after nifedipine, while the drug resulted in normalization of pressure in only two patients (14%) with initially abnormal values. Five patients developed wedge pressures equal to or greater than 30 mm Hg after receiving nifedipine.

TABLE 1
Peak nifedipine effects, expressed as percentage change from control values, during the 30 min after each dose

	First dose		p value	Second dose of 10 mg after first dose of:		p value
	10 mg	20 mg		10 mg	20 mg	
Heart rate	14±12	15±15	NS	15±16	12±16	NS
Mean blood pressure	−12±7	−8±10	NS	−14±11	−9±11	NS
Mean pulmonary artery wedge pressure	8±42	47±78	NS	6±44	25±37	NS
Cardiac index	16±26	15±20	NS	12±22	15±16	NS
Index of peripheral vascular resistance	−23±19	−20±17	NS	−26±16	−23±14	NS

Values are mean ± SD.

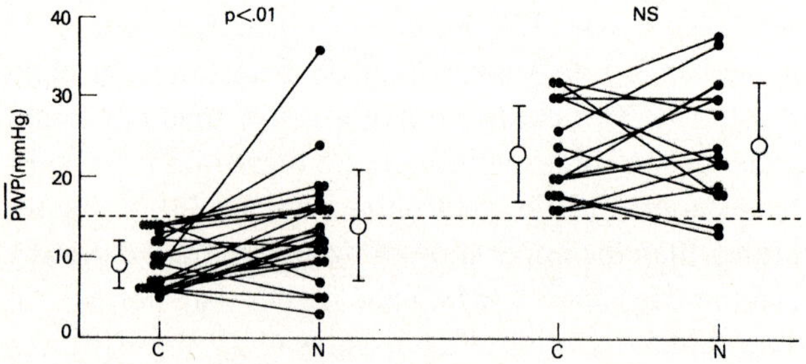

FIGURE 1. Influence of nifedipine on pulmonary arterial wedge pressure (PWP) in patients with normal (*left*) or elevated (*right*) basal PWPs. Dashed line indicates upper limit of normal (15 mm Hg). Open circles with vertical bars represent mean values ± 1 SD. C = control values; N = peak values after administration of nifedipine.

One had started out with normal pressure and one had begun with wedge pressure of 30 mm Hg that increased to 36 mm Hg.

Left ventricular end-diastolic pressure exhibited a similar pattern: it rose significantly after nifedipine for the group as a whole (table 2). In patients who initially had normal values, it rose from 10 ± 1 to 16 ± 4 mm Hg ($p < .01$), but it did not change in patients who had elevated pressures (>12 mm Hg) at control (23 ± 6 to 26 ± 9 mm Hg; NS). In six patients, left ventricular end-diastolic pressure rose above 30 mm Hg after nifedipine administration; none of these patients had normal left ventricular end-diastolic pressures before nifedipine and one had a basal left ventricular end-diastolic pressure of 30 mm Hg that rose to 34 mm Hg.

TABLE 2
Hemodynamic data recorded during the control study and at the peak effect of nifedipine

	Control	Nifedipine	p value
Heart rate (beats/min)	79 ± 12	91 ± 14	<.01
Mean blood pressure (mm Hg)	89 ± 12	77 ± 10	<.01
Pulmonary arterial wedge pressure (mm Hg)	15 ± 8	18 ± 9	<.05
LV end-diastolic pressure (mm Hg)	18 ± 8	22 ± 9	<.01
Cardiac index (l/mm/m^2)	2.8 ± .6	3.3 ± .8	<.01
Stroke volume index (m/beat/m^2)	36 ± 7	36 ± 8	NS
Index of peripheral vascular resistance (dynes·sec·cm^{-5})	822 ± 261	610 ± 197	<.01
LVOTG (mm Hg)[A]	75 ± 22	83 ± 32	NS
Time constant of relaxation (msec)[B]			
T	49.1 ± 9.6	47.1 ± 13.7	NS
T1	47.4 ± 11.1	50.6 ± 18.4	NS
T2	35.5 ± 11.6	45.9 ± 14.7	NS

Values are mean ± SD.

[A]Measured in 17 patients with LVOTGs ≥ 30 mm Hg in the control study.

[B]Measured in 11 patients in whom left ventricular pressure was obtained with micromanometer-tipped catheters.

Cardiac index increased significantly after administration of nifedipine, but stroke volume index remained unchanged (table 2), even when data of patients with moderate-to-severe mitral regurgitation were excluded (36 ± 6 to 37 ± 8 ml/beat/m^2; NS). The index of peripheral vascular resistance fell significantly with nifedipine.

Nifedipine had no effect on the magnitude of the LVOTG (table 2). Among 17 patients with significant basal gradients (≥30 mm Hg) at control, the gradient decreased below 30 mm Hg in one patient, whereas it rose to 30 mm Hg or more in two of 19 patients who started out with a nonsignificant gradient (figure 2). Six patients who initially had LVOTGs of less than 100 mm Hg developed gradients of 100 mm Hg or more after nifedipine, including one patient whose initial gradient was 35 mm Hg. In a subgroup of six patients in whom vascular peripheral resistance decreased by 25% or more after nifedipine, the LVOTG increased from 73 ± 28 to 99 ± 22 mm Hg ($p < .05$; figure 3). In all six patients, both pulmonary arterial wedge pressure (figure 4) and left ventricular end-diastolic pressure increased (11 ± 4 to 20 ± 9 mm Hg [NS], and 15 ± 8 TO 27 ± 12 mm Hg [$p < .05$], respectively). Valsalva maneuver or amyl nitrite inhalation were repeated after nifedipine in those patients in whom (1) a significant LVOTG was not present in the control study, but it developed with interventions, and (2) the drug itself did not induce a significant LVOTG. Gradients obtained with provocation were compared in seven patients before and after administration of nifedipine, and were not significantly different (63 ± 33 to 67 ± 28 mm Hg; NS).

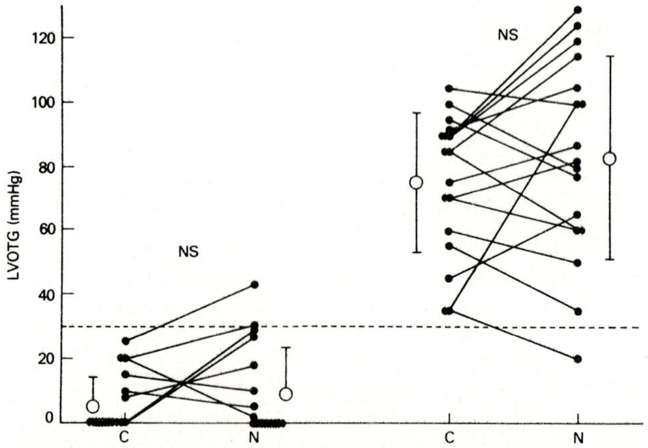

FIGURE 2. Influence of nifedipine on LVOTG in patients without (*left*) or with (*right*) significant (≥ 30 mm Hg; dashed line) basal LVOT obstruction. Open circles with vertical bars represent mean values ± 1 SD. C = control values; N = peak values after nifedipine.

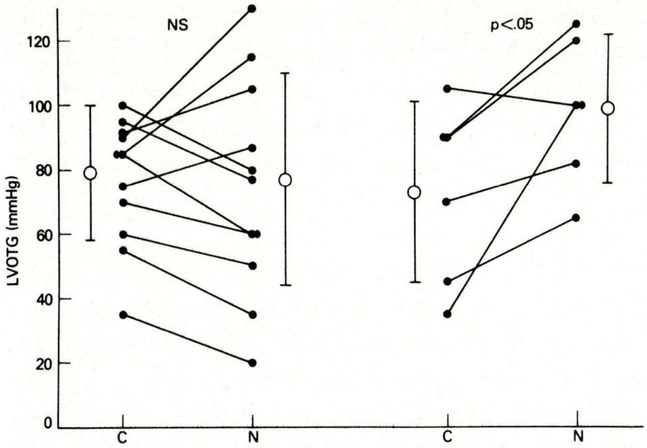

FIGURE 3. Influence of nifedipine on LVOTG in patients in whom administration of nifedipine led to a decrease in peripheral vascular resistance of less than 25% (*left*) or of 25% or greater (*right*). Open circles with vertical bars represent mean values ± 1 SD. C = control values; N = peak values after nifedipine.

Figure 4 illustrates the effects of nifedipine on pulmonary arterial wedge pressure in patients with and without significant basal LVOTGs. Pulmonary arterial wedge pressure increased in all but three patients with significant gradients and for the group rose from 15 ± 8 to 20 ± 10 mm Hg ($p < .01$). This change was not seen in patients without obstruction in the control study (14 ± 9 to 15 ± 7 mm Hg; NS). No further differences between patients with and without obstruction were noted with respect to nifedipine effects on the other hemodynamic parameters.

Left ventricular relaxation, as assessed by the time constants T, T1, and T2, was not affected by nifedipine (table 2).

Radionuclide data. To avoid any effect of heart rate on diastolic function measurements, we compared values obtained at the time of peak effect of nifedipine with those recorded at comparable heart rates obtained by atrial pacing in the control period. The results are

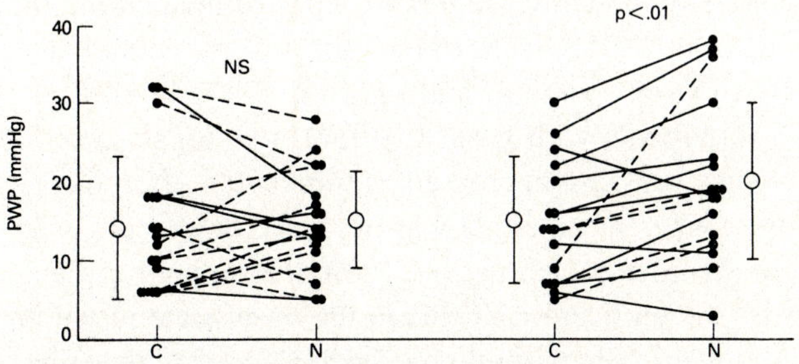

FIGURE 4. Influence of nifedipine on pulmonary arterial wedge pressure (PWP) in patients without *(left)* and with *(right)* significant basal LVOT obstruction. Dashed lines indicate patients in whom peripheral vascular resistance fell by 25% or more after administration of nifedipine. Open circles with vertical bars represent mean values ± 1 SD. C = control values; N = peak values after nifedipine.

TABLE 3
Effects of nifedipine on radionuclide measurements

	Control	Nifedipine	p value
Heart rate (beats/min)	88 ± 14	89 ± 16	NS
End diastolic (% of control)	100	124 ± 39	NS
Ejection fraction (%)	72 ± 14	70 ± 17	NS
PFR (EDV/sec)	4.5 ± 1.7	4.3 ± 2.0	NS
TPFR (msec)	228 ± 72	203 ± 86	NS

presented in table 3. No changes were observed in end-diastolic volume and in ejection fraction. Rapid diastolic filling, as assessed by PFR and TPFR, was also unchanged. The analysis of responses of the diastolic pressure-counts curves showed improvement in three patients (rightward or rightward-downward shift), no modification in three patients (no changes or rightward-upward shift), and deterioration of the diastolic pressure-volume relationship in the remaining four patients (upward or leftward or upward-leftward shift) (figure 5).

Among the 10 patients who underwent radionuclide study, four had significant LVOTGs during the baseline study. Although the small number of such patients does not allow statistically meaningful analysis, no trend was observed suggesting a difference in systolic and diastolic function responses to nifedipine between

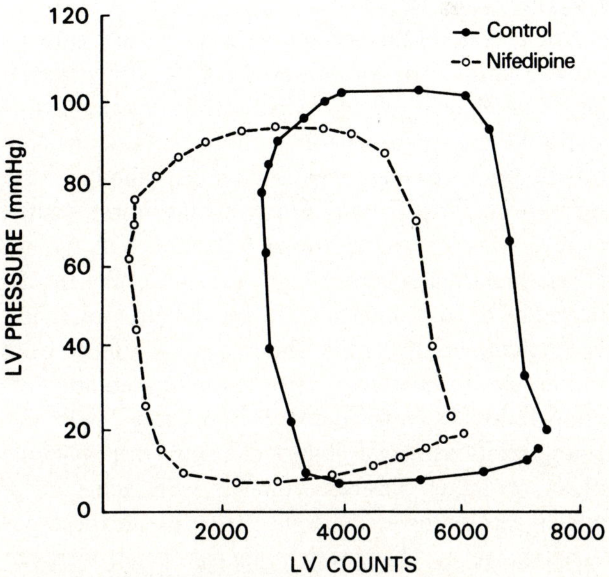

FIGURE 5. Relationship between left ventricular (LV) pressure and counts (proportional to left ventricular volume) before and after administration of nifedipine to one patient. Each point represents the number of counts collected during 25 msec and the corresponding left ventricular pressure, averaged for 140 beats. Nifedipine shifts the diastolic pressure-volume relationship leftward and slightly upward as compared with that during the control study, which was recorded at a comparable heart rate obtained by artrial pacing (104 beats/min for both studies).

patients with and those without LVOT obstruction. When data from three patients with moderate-to-severe mitral regurgitation were excluded from the analysis, a significant increase in relative end-diastolic volume was observed (100 to 136 ± 39; $p < .05$), whereas no changes occurred in any of the other parameters.

Discussion

The hemodynamic effects of nifedipine in patients with hypertrophic cardiomyopathy in this study were unrelated to the dose administered, as has already been shown by others in patients with coronary artery disease.[24] In another aspect of this study, we also demonstrated no difference in nifedipine plasma concentrations over 60 min in two groups of subjects taking different sublingual doses of the drug. The hemodynamic effects of nifedipine, however, were related to plasma concentrations of the drug. Therefore, the failure to show a correlation between dose and effect appears to be the consequence of the lack of relationship between dose and plasma concentration of the drug.

As anticipated, the predominant hemodynamic response of these patients to nifedipine was the fall in blood pressure as a result of diminished peripheral vascular resistance. This finding is similar to that seen when verapamil is administered to these patients,[6] but in contrast to the effects of verapamil, no decrease in LVOTG was observed.

The reason for this lack of beneficial effect seems to be severalfold. The administration of nifedipine had no apparent effect on systolic and diastolic function in this study. Relative end-diastolic volume was not changed by nifedipine for the group as a whole, although it did increase in patients without significant mitral insufficiency. Despite the afterload reduction and the increase in cardiac output, relaxation and filling (as assessed by the time constant of isovolumetric fall in left ventricular pressure, peak filling rate, and time to peak filling rate, respectively) were not improved after administration of nifedipine. The diastolic pressure-counts relationship was improved in only three patients in whom larger diastolic volumes were achieved at unchanged or lower diastolic pressures; in these patients, however, changes in filling parameters were not consistent in that PFR did not increase in any, and TPFR shortened in two.

These results contrast with the data in patients with hypertrophic cardiomyopathy who were studied before and after verapamil. After oral verapamil, an increase in PFR and shortening of TPFR were observed.[8] After intravenous verapamil, the diastolic pressure-counts relationship shifted rightward and/or downward in five of 10 patients and this improvement was associated with an amelioration of filling parameters[10]: improved diastolic function after verapamil occurred in these patients despite significant negative inotropic effects.

Thus, the relative lack of effect of nifedipine, which appears to contrast with the more consistent beneficial effects of verapamil, on LVOT obstruction can be explained by its pronounced vasodilative action, which was unopposed by either a tendency to enhance diastolic function or depress systolic performance.

The fact that we did not observe any improvement in diastolic function with nifedipine contrasts with findings of Lorell et al.[13] They used M mode echocardiography to measure volumes and observed no increase in left ventricular systolic and diastolic dimension after administration of nifedipine. However, left ventricular relaxation and diastolic filling, assessed by the peak rate of changes in left ventricular dimension, were reported to be improved by sublingual administration of the drug. Several factors could account for the discrepancy between their results and ours. First, in Lorell's study, heart rate increased by 10% and diastole shortened by 27%, whereas in our radionuclide study we avoided heart rate–induced effects by using atrial pacing in the control study. Second, the M mode echocardiography used by the authors is suboptimal for the evaluation of volume changes because of the abnormalities of shape and the structural inhomogeneity of the left ventricle in patients with hypertrophic cardiomyopathy. Finally, different degrees of left ventricular hypertrophy and subendocardial ischemia in their patients and ours could be responsible for the different results. Although none of the patients in our study had angiographic evidence of conorary artery disease, most had been experiencing chest pain that was compatible with angina and the presence of myocardial ischemia. It is noteworthy that, among the patients in whom radionuclide studies were performed, nifedipine increased PFR in three of the four patients with moderate to severe angina, and reduced TPFR in all four.

In patients with basal LVOTG, pulmonary arterial wedge pressure increased significantly after nifedipine, whereas no effect was observed in patients without significant obstruction. Moreover, among patients with a significant LVOTG in the basal state in whom administration of nifedipine led to a decrease in peripheral vascular resistance of 25% or more, pulmonary arterial wedge pressure increased in all and was associated with an increase in LVOTGs in five of six patients (figures 3 and 4). Hence, the elevation in filling pressures that occurred in many patients (26/36, 72%) after nifedipine may have been caused by the increase in LVOT obstruction (due to nifedipine-induced decreases in afterload) in addition to the lack of a consistent beneficial effect on diastolic function.

Nifedipine, like verapamil,[6,11] increased pulmonary arterial wedge and end-diastolic pressures in patients with normal baseline values. Verapamil, however, tended to decrease elevated pressures,[6] a trend that was not observed with nifedipine. Moreover, it should be noted that although 39% of the patients started out with abnormal pulmonary wedge pressure, after nifedipine pulmonary wedge pressure was elevated in 58% of the patients, reaching a value of 30 mm Hg or more in 14%.

In conclusion, the predominant effect of short-term administration of nifedipine to patients with hypertrophic cardiomyopathy was a lowering of systemic pressure as a result of peripheral vasodilation; this was unassociated with any consistent effect on systolic or diastolic performance. In some patients with basal outflow obstruction, the drop in blood pressure produced some results that could induce hemodynamic instability, including (1) an increase in left ventricular filling pressures, and (2) an increase in LVOTG. Our data also suggest that left ventricular diastolic filling might improve after nifedipine in those patients with more severe myocardial ischemia. Verapamil exerts a similar, although less pronounced, effect on peripheral vascular resistance; however, such an effect is counterbalanced by a direct action on the systolic and diastolic performance of the myocardium. Although data obtained after sublingual, acute nifedipine administration cannot be extrapolated to the clinical results of long-term therapy, we have demonstrated that oral therapy with nifedipine does not favorably affect short-term symptomatic status and exercise tolerance.[14]

We acknowledge the technical assistance of Frederick Bullock, Rita Mincemoyer, Kathleen Nonnemacher, Marjorie Rimmer, and Gail Tauscher in the acquistion of data for this manuscript.

References

1. Kaltenbach M, Hopf R, Kober G, Bussmann WD, Keller M, Petersen Y: Treatment of hypertrophic obstructive cardiomyopathy with verapamil. Br Heart J **42:** 35, 1979
2. Rosing DR, Kent KM, Maron BJ, Epstein SE: Verapamil therapy: a new approach to the pharmacologic treatment of hypertophic cardiomyopathy. II. Effects on exercise capacity and symptomatic status. Circulation **60:** 1208, 1979
3. Rosing DR, Condit JR, Maron BJ, Kent KM, Leon MB, Bonow RO, Lipson LC, Epstein SE: Verapamil therapy: a new approach to the pharmacologic treatment of hypertrophic cardiomyopathy. III. Effects of long-term administration. Am J Cardiol **48:** 545, 1981
4. Hasin Y, Lewis BS, Lewis N, Weiss AT, Gotsman MS: Long-term effect of verapamil in hypertrophic cardiomyopathy. Int J Cardiol **1:** 243, 1982
5. Rosing DR, Idänpään-Heikkilä U, Maron BJ, Bonow RO, Epstein SE: Use of calcium-channel blocking drugs in hypertrophic cardiomyopathy. Am J Cardiol **55:** 185B, 1985
6. Rosing DR, Kent KM, Borer JS, Seides SF, Maron BJ, Epstein SE: Verapamil therapy: a new approach to the pharmacologic treatment of hypertrophic cardiomyopathy. I. Hemodynamic effects. Circulation **60:** 1202, 1979
7. Hanrath P, Mathey DG, Kremer P, Sonntag F, Bleifeld W: Effect of verapamil on left ventricular isovolumic relaxation time and regional left ventricular filling in hypertrophic cardiomyopathy. Am J Cardiol **45:** 1258, 1980
8. Bonow RO, Rosing DR, Bacharach SL, Green MV, Kent KM, Lipson LC, Maron BJ, Leon MB, Epstein SE: Effects of verapamil on left ventricular systolic function and diastolic filling in patients with hypertrophic cardiomyopathy. Circulation **64:** 787, 1981
9. Hess OM, Grimm J, Krayenbuehl HP: Diastolic function in hypertrophic cardiomyopathy: effects of propranolol and verapamil on diastolic stiffness. Eur Heart J **4**(suppl F): 47, 1983
10. Bonow RO, Ostrow HG, Rosing DR, Cannon RO, Lipson LC, Maron BJ, Kent KM, Bacharach SL, Green MV: Effects of verapamil on left ventricular systolic and diastolic function in patients with hypertrophic cardiomyopathy: pressure-volume analysis with a nonimaging scintillation probe. Circulation **68:** 1062, 1983
11. Anderson DM, Raff GL, Ports TA, Brundage BH, Parmley W, Chatterjee K: Hypertrophic obstructive cardiomyopathy. Effects of acute and chronic verapamil treatment on left ventricular systolic and diastolic function. Br Heart J **51:** 523, 1984
12. Epstein SE, Rosing DR: Verapamil: its potential for causing serious complications in patients with hypertrophic cardiomyopathy. Circulation **64:** 437, 1981
13. Lorell BH, Paulus WJ, Grossman W, Wynne J, Cohn PF: Modification of abnormal left ventricular diastolic properties by nifedipine in patients with hypertrophic cardiomyopathy. Circulation **65:** 499, 1982
14. Rosing DR, Cannon RO, Watson RM, Kent KM, Lakatos E, Epstein SE: Comparison of verapamil and nifedipine effects on symptoms and exercise capacity in patients with hypertrophic cardiomyopathy. Circulation **66**(suppl II): II-24, 1982 (abst)
15. Landmark K, Sire S, Thaulow E, Amlie JP, Nilter-Hauge S: Haemodynamic effects of nifedipine and propranolol in patients with hypertrophic cardiomyopathy. Br Heart J **48:** 19, 1982
16. Rowland E, Evans T, Krikler D: Effect of nifedipine on atrioventricular conduction as compared with verapamil. Br Heart J **42:** 124, 1979
17. Maron BJ, Epstein SE: Hypertrophic cardiomyopathy: recent observations regarding the specificity of three hallmarks of the disease: asymmetric septal hypertrophy, septal disorganization, and systolic anterior motion of the anterior mitral leaflet. Am J Cardiol **45:** 141, 1980
18. White RI Jr, Criley JM, Lewis KB, Ross RS: Experimental production of intracavity pressure differences: possible significance in the interpretation of human hemodynamic studies. Am J Cardiol **19:** 806, 1967
19. Wigle ED, Marquis Y, Auger P: Muscular subaortic stenosis: initial left ventricular inflow tract pressure in the assessment of intraventricular pressure differences in man. Circulation **35:** 1100, 1967
20. Weiss JL, Frederiksen JW, Weisfeldt ML: Hemodynamic determinants of the time-course of fall in canine left ventricular pressure. J Clin Invest **58:** 751, 1976
21. Rousseau MF, Veriter C, Detry JMR, Brasseur L, Pouleur H: Impaired early left ventricular relaxation in coronary artery disease: effects of intracoronary nifedipine. Circulation **62:** 764, 1980
22. Bacharach SL, Green MV, Borer JS, Ostrow HC, Redwood DR, Johnson GS: ECG-gated scintillation probe measurements of left ventricular function. J Nucl Med **18:** 1176, 1977
23. Thrall JH, Freitas JE, Swanson D, Rogers WL, Clare JM, Brown ML, Pitt B: Clinical comparison of cardiac blood pool visualization with technetium 99m human serum albumin. J Nucl Med **19:** 796, 1978
24. Deanfield J, Wright C, Fox K: Treatment of angina pectoris with nifedipine; importance of dose titration. Br Med J **296:** 1467, 1983

Global and regional right ventricular function in normal infants and infants with transposition of the great arteries after Senning operation

ECKARDT TROWITZSCH, M.D., STEVEN D. COLAN, M.D., AND STEPHEN P. SANDERS, M.D.

ABSTRACT Echocardiographic assessment of right ventricular size, global function, and regional wall motion was performed in 29 normal infants and 19 infants with transposition of the great arteries 1 to 41 months after they underwent the Senning procedure. Sixteen of the patients with transposition of the great arteries were in clinically good condition and three had congestive heart failure. The right ventricular endocardial surface was digitized frame by frame for a complete cardiac cycle in both subxiphoid long-axis (coronal plane) and short-axis (parasagittal plane) views, and the cross-sectional area and the area change fraction (AF) were calculated. In each plane the right ventricular wall was subdivided into four anatomic regions (infundibular, free wall, diaphragmatic,and septal). With the use of a floating point center of mass model the direction and average extent of motion of the endocardium was determined for each region. In normal infants the infundibular and free wall portions of the right ventricle exhibited the greatest inward motion and the septal segments the least inward motion. Although the maximal area in both long-axis ($r = .85$) and short-axis ($r = .85$) views was highly correlated with body surface area (BSA), neither global nor regional function was significantly correlated with age or BSA. In clinically well patients after Senning procedure regional right ventricular function followed an entirely different pattern than that seen in normal infants. The endocardium of the septal segments showed the greatest inward motion in systole. In contrast to those in normal infants, maximal and minimal cross-sectional areas did not correlate significantly with BSA. The mean AF was not significantly different from that in normal subjects, although both end-diastolic and end-systolic cross-sectional areas were significantly larger, even when adjusted for body surface area. The three postoperative patients with congestive heart failure had dyskinetic areas in free wall and septal segments. In two of the three patients the cross-sectional area of the right ventricle was enlarged compared with that in the postoperative patients without congestive heart failure. The AF was reduced in all three patients. Analysis of right ventricular regional wall motion and calculation of AF provide new information concerning the manner in which the right ventricle adapts to the systemic workload and may provide clues to the mechanics of right ventricular dysfunction. Documentation of the normal pattern of right ventricular wall motion permits recognition and quantification of regional and global dysfunction.

Circulation 72, No. 5, 1008–1014, 1985.

A SEGMENTAL APPROACH to the analysis of regional wall motion of the left ventricle with the use of quantitative two-dimensional echocardiography to localize areas of ventricular asynergy and infarction was published in 1979 by Heger et al.[1] In the last 5 years, numerous articles have appeared describing the analysis of regional wall motion of the left ventricle and applying this methodology to the detection of abnormally contracting segments under various conditions.[2–9] A computerized segmental analysis of the time relationship of regional events and wall motion velocities for the left ventricle in adults by angiographic techniques demonstrated that even in normal subjects left ventricular contraction cannot be assumed to be symmetrical or uniform.[6]

The evaluation of the right ventricle by noninvasive methods has been complicated by its retrosternal location and irregular shape. Accessibility of the right ventricle to echocardiographic examination can be im-

From the Department of Cardiology, Children's Hospital and the Department of Pediatrics, Harvard Medical School, Boston.

Supported in part by Deutsche Forschungsgemeinschaft grant Tr 201/2-1, Bad Gudesberg Bonn, F.R.G.

Address for correspondence: Stephen P. Sanders, M.D., Department of Cardiology, The Children's Hospital, 300 Longwood Ave., Boston, MA 02115.

Received Feb. 26, 1985; revision accepted Aug. 8, 1985.

*Present address: Department of Pediatric Cardiology, The Children's Hospital, Medical School of Hannover, P.O. Box 6100180, D-3000 Hannover, F.R.G.

proved through the use of a subxiphoid approach. Problems with analysis of global function presented by the irregular shape of the right ventricle can be overcome at least in part by regional analysis of function. For example, right ventricular segmental wall motion abnormalities after infarction can be detected.[10, 11]

Similar analysis of right ventricular wall motion has not been performed either in normal children or in infants with congenital heart defects. This issue assumes particular importance because of the occurrence of lesions in which the right ventricle must serve as the ventricle supporting the systemic circulation. We therefore analyzed right ventricular wall motion in a group of normal infants and children and in a group of patients with transposition of the great arteries who had previously undergone an atrial switch (Senning) operation.

Methods

The study population consisted of 29 patients (age 1 day to 24 months, mean 3.3 months) without structural heart disease and 19 patients with transposition of the great arteries after Senning operation, 16 of whom (age 1 to 37 months, mean = 12 months) were clinically well, and three of whom (age 32 to 82 months) were in congestive heart failure. All normal subjects were referred because of functional heart murmur and two-dimensional echocardiographic examination was performed to exclude structural heart disease. Echocardiographic evaluation was performed 1 to 41 months after surgery in subjects with transposition. All clinically well postoperative patients were investigated at the time of routine late postoperative cardiac catheterization. The three remaining patients were evaluated at the time of presentation with symptoms of congestive heart failure.

Echocardiograms were performed with either a Diasonics CV 100 or an Advanced Technology Laboratories Mark 600 echocardiograph with the use of a 3.0, 3.5, or 5 MHz transducer. The images were recorded on standard 1/2 inch videocassette tape for subsequent computer analysis. Two subxiphoid views of the right ventricle were used for wall motion analysis: a long-axis or coronal plane view just anterior to the tricuspid valve (figure 1A) and a short-axis or parasagittal plane view through the right ventricular outflow tract and the pulmonary valve (figure 1B).

A Franklin Quantic 1200 echocardiographic review center was used for wall motion analysis. The end-diastolic and end-systolic frames were selected as the ones showing the largest and smallest right ventricular cross-sectional areas, respectively. The endocardial borders of these two frames were hand digitized. Minor irregularities in the endocardial border caused by trabeculations were smoothed during digitization. The endocardial border for each intervening frame was then obtained with an automatic edge-detection algorithm (Bruce Franklin, Inc.). The computer-generated borders were reviewed for accuracy and corrected as needed. The center of mass was calculated for each frame (see Appendix), and 64 equally spaced radii were drawn outward from the center of mass for each frame. The centers of mass of the end-diastolic and end-systolic frames were superimposed and the motion of each endocardial segment along its respective radius was determined. The 64 segments were then divided into four anatomic segments in each plane (infundibular, free wall, diaphragmatic, and septal; figures 1A, 1B), and the inward motion of each anatomic segment was calculated as the average inward endocardial motion along the radii contained within that segment.

Cross-sectional long- and short-axis areas were obtained by planimetry for end-diastolic and end-systolic frames. Fractional area change (AF) was calculated as the difference between the end-systolic and end-diastolic areas divided by the end-diastolic area. Areas were adjusted for the square root of body surface area ($\sqrt{BSA}$).

The relation of cross-sectional areas, AF, and segmental wall excursion to body surface area was determined by simple linear regression analysis. Segmental wall excursion values for each of the anatomic segments were compared within and between

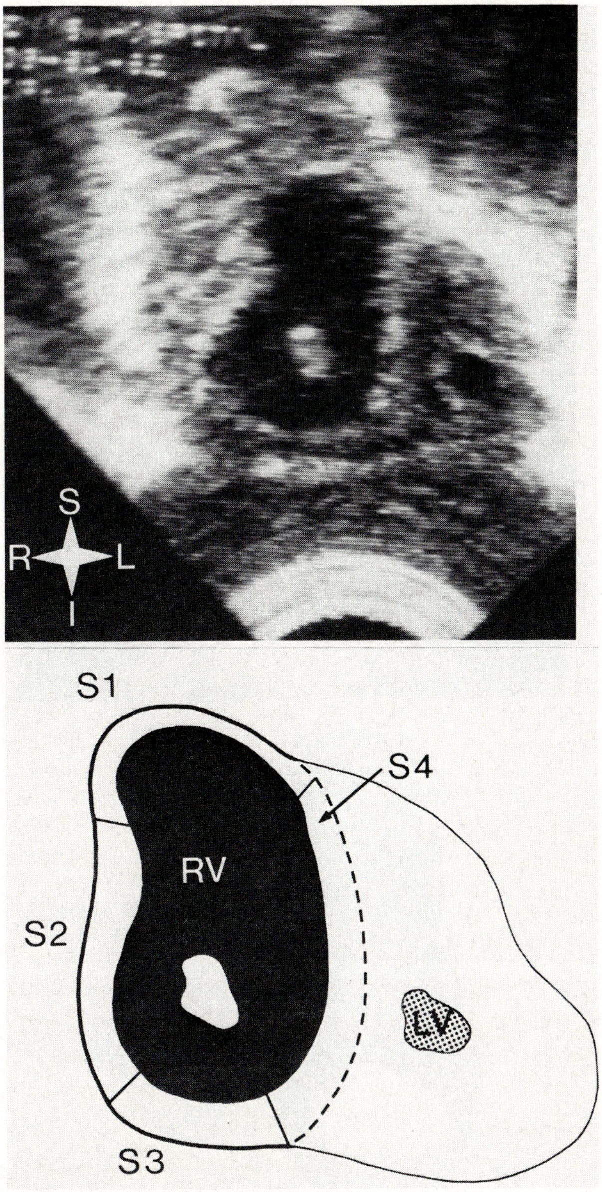

FIGURE 1A. Diagram and subxiphoid echocardiogram used for regional wall motion analysis in the long-axis right ventricular (RV) view. The segmental divisions are illustrated. S1 = infundibulum, S2 = free wall, S3 = diaphragmatic wall, and S4 = septum. LV = left ventricle, LA = left atrium, S = superior, I = inferior, A = anterior, P = posterior, R = right, L = left.

groups by analysis of variance. A p value of .05 or less was considered statistically significant.

Results

Normal subjects. Segmental wall excursion data, cross-sectional areas and AF values for normal infants are listed in table 1. The inward motion of the endocardium for all segments was greater in long-axis views than in corresponding short-axis views ($p < .05$). Inward motion in the long-axis plane was greatest in the infundibular and free wall segments, while the septal segment had the smallest excursion (figure 2, *A*). The extent of inward motion of the infundibular and septal segments was significantly different ($p < .05$) in the

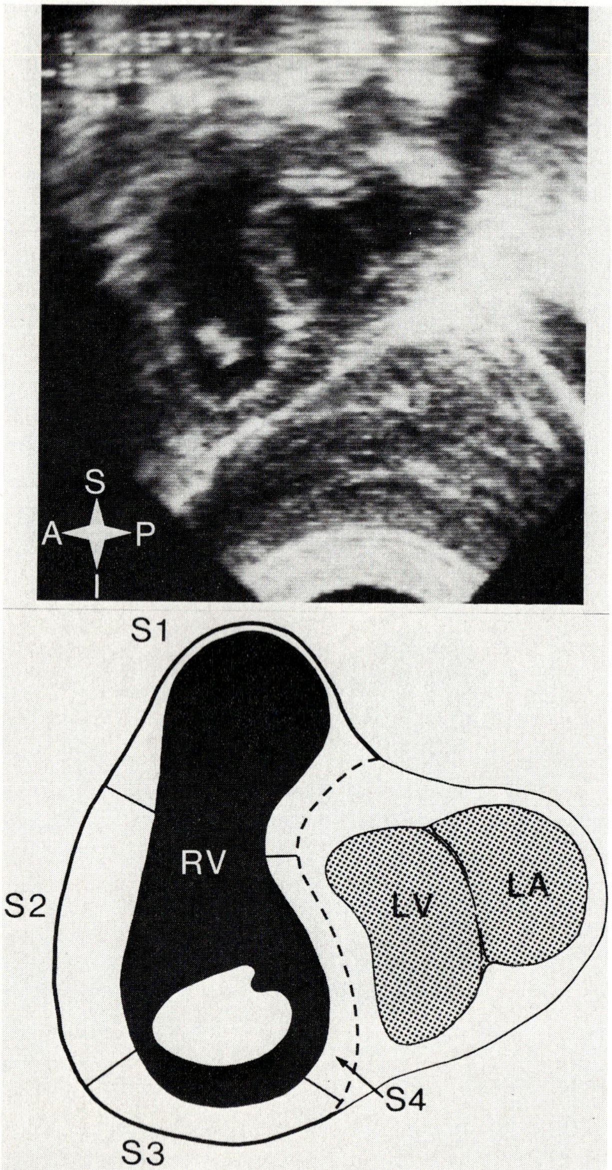

FIGURE 1B. Diagram and subxiphoid echocardiogram used for regional wall motion analysis in the short-axis right ventricular view. Abbreviations are as in figure 1B.

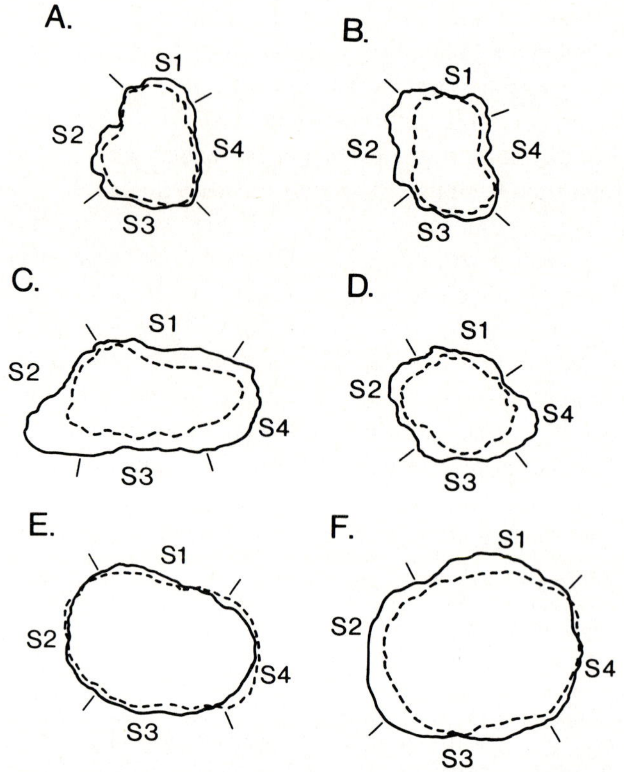

FIGURE 2. Endocardial borders of the right ventricle at end-diastole (solid line) and end-systole (broken line), illustrating various patterns of wall motion. *A* and *B*, Long- and short-axis views in a normal subject. *C* and *D*, Long- and short-axis views in a clinically well patient with transposition. *E* and *F*, Long- and short-axis views in a patient with transposition of the great arteries and congestive heart failure.

long-axis view. In short-axis view, the greatest inward motion was seen in the infundibulum and the least was seen in the septum (figure 2, *B*). The excursion of the infundibular and diaphragmatic segments was significantly greater than the excursion of the septal segment ($p < .005$ and $p < .05$, respectively). The maximal and minimal cross-sectional areas in the long-axis plane were significantly higher than the corresponding area in short-axis view. Long- and short-axis end-diastolic areas were highly correlated with the $\sqrt{BSA}$ ($r = .85$ for both) (table 2). The end-systolic areas were also significantly correlated with $\sqrt{BSA}$ (long-axis $r = .72$ and short-axis $r = .76$; table 2). The AF was not significantly different between the two planes.

Well patients with transposition of the great arteries. The results in patients who had undergone surgery for transposition of the great arteries and did not have congestive heart failure are given in table 3. The inward motion of the endocardium was greatest at the free wall and septal segments and least at the diaphragmatic segment (figure 2, *C*). The excursion of the free wall segment was significantly greater than that of the infundibular or diaphragmatic segment ($p < .005$ and $p < .001$, respectively), but was not significantly dif-

TABLE 1

Clinical and echocardiographic data on normal infants

			Maximal segmental motion (mm)								Area/√BSA)				AF (%)	
			Long axis				Short axis				Long axis		Short axis			
Patient No.	Age	BSA (m^2)	S1	S2	S3	S4	S1	S2	S3	S4	Max	Min	Max	Min	Long axis	Short axis
1	7 days	0.10	2.0	2.7	1.9	1.9	1.3	1.3	0.9	0.5	5.9	2.7	3.5	2.5	55	29
2	2 days	0.20	—	—	—	—	1.8	1.3	1.5	0.3	13.4	8.2	8.4	5.5	39	35
3	4 days	0.25	0.8	1.0	1.0	0.0	1.0	2.8	2.3	2.5	8.5	7.5	5.0	2.7	12	45
4	2 days	0.25	2.0	3.5	2.3	2.5	2.8	3.0	1.8	3.3	9.6	6.0	5.9	3.4	37	41
5	12 days	0.25	2.5	5.0	2.3	4.3	3.0	0.0	6.0	0.8	16.3	9.8	7.2	4.5	39	38
6	6 days	0.20	1.5	2.3	1.8	1.3	1.8	1.0	3.5	0.5	9.8	7.2	8.1	6.0	27	25
7	3 days	0.21	4.0	2.7	3.0	1.5	3.0	2.2	2.5	1.7	14.5	9.0	6.0	3.2	38	47
8	1 day	0.23	2.0	1.5	1.5	0.8	2.5	1.5	2.3	1.0	12.7	9.4	6.5	4.4	26	32
9	1 day	0.21	4.8	3.5	4.5	1.8	0.8	0.7	1.5	0.5	9.6	4.3	5.6	4.5	55	20
10	15 days	0.23	4.8	3.5	4.5	4.8	1.5	2.7	1.5	2.7	11.8	4.9	6.6	4.5	58	31
11	1 day	0.15	1.2	1.3	0.5	1.5	2.0	1.3	1.5	1.5	5.2	3.6	4.8	3.1	30	35
12	3 days	0.21	3.3	2.5	3.3	2.0	2.5	1.3	2.5	0.5	8.2	4.7	7.5	4.5	42	41
13	4 days	0.20	1.0	2.0	0.8	1.3	1.5	1.5	1.0	2.8	10.0	8.4	9.7	6.5	16	13
14	10 days	0.30	0.0	1.5	3.3	2.8	2.5	1.5	3.0	1.5	5.5	2.6	5.2	3.3	53	37
15	2 days	0.24	2.3	2.0	1.5	0.8	0.3	0.0	0.5	0.3	19.5	14.4	8.8	8.3	26	6
16	2 mo	0.24	2.3	3.8	2.3	4.5	2.5	2.5	0.5	2.3	10.7	5.8	9.0	5.9	46	34
17	6 mo	0.34	8.5	8.0	6.3	6.5	5.0	3.2	3.3	2.8	17.3	6.4	9.7	4.9	63	49
18	2 mo	0.34	5.0	5.3	4.0	3.3	3.3	3.0	2.5	1.3	16.4	9.7	13.7	9.4	41	32
19	8 mo	0.33	6.0	5.0	6.0	3.3	5.0	4.8	6.0	3.3	15.4	5.5	12.7	6.6	64	48
20	1 mo	0.24	4.3	5.5	3.5	2.8	4.0	3.5	3.5	1.5	11.3	4.6	7.1	3.6	59	50
21	4 mo	0.35	4.5	9.0	3.3	0.0	2.0	1.3	2.0	1.5	14.1	6.7	6.9	5.1	53	26
22	6 mo	0.30	5.3	4.5	5.3	3.0	3.0	0.5	1.3	1.0	12.0	4.8	9.8	7.3	61	25
23	9 mo	0.32	3.8	4.3	3.0	3.3	3.0	1.7	3.0	1.3	15.0	8.2	11.2	8.4	45	26
24	6 mo	0.30	7.0	4.5	6.5	2.8	4.0	4.0	2.0	3.8	10.9	3.3	9.2	3.9	70	58
25	2 mo	0.25	1.4	1.0	1.8	0.5	1.0	0.8	2.0	0.8	8.2	6.2	6.6	5.3	24	19
26	24 mo	0.53	3.0	5.3	1.8	4.8	5.5	1.3	5.0	2.0	23.1	16.6	12.4	7.5	28	39
27	13 mo	0.40	3.5	0.0	3.5	1.0	1.0	1.7	0.8	0.0	16.1	10.7	13.2	9.9	34	25
28	6 mo	0.35	2.3	4.3	1.5	3.0	2.5	2.5	3.0	2.0	19.3	13.4	11.7	7.8	31	33
29	2 mo	0.26	2.5	3.3	2.0	3.3	2.8	2.1	2.5	1.3	16.7	10.9	11.5	7.9	36	31
Mean	3.3 mo	0.27	3.1	3.4	2.8	2.3	2.5	1.9	2.4	1.5	12.7	7.4	8.4	5.5	41	34
SD	5.2 mo	0.08	2.1	2.2	1.8	1.7	1.3	1.2	1.4	1.0	4.4	3.5	2.8	2.1	15	11

max = maximal; min = minimal; s = segment; S1 = infundibulum; S2 = free wall; S3 = diaphragmatic wall; S4 = septum.

ferent from that of the septal segment. All short-axis segmental wall motion values were very similar; they did not differ significantly from one another (figure 2, *D*). Long-axis maximal and minimal area measurements were significantly larger than the corresponding short-axis measurements. Neither long-axis maximal or minimal areas nor short-axis maximal or minimal areas (table 2) were significantly correlated to $\sqrt{BSA}$. The AF was not significantly different in the two planes.

Comparison of normal infants with the group of well patients after Senning procedure revealed that both end-systolic and end-diastolic areas were significantly larger ($p < .005$) in the patient group, even after adjustment for BSA. AF, however, did not differ between the two groups. Comparison of segmental wall motion between the two groups revealed a significant difference only in septal motion, which was greater in the patient group.

Patients with transposition of the great arteries and congestive heart failure. The findings in patients with congestive heart failure are listed in table 4. Patient 1 showed paradoxic outward motion of parts of the free

TABLE 2

Correlation (r) of ventricular cross-sectional areas with the $\sqrt{BSA}$ in normal infants and patients with transposition of the great arteries

	End-diastole		End-systole	
	Long axis	Short axis	Long axis	Short axis
Normals	.83	.84	.69	.76
Patients	.39	.59	.37	.37

TABLE 3

Personal and echocardiographic data on patients with transposition of the great arteries after Senning operation

Patient No.	Age (mo)	BSA (m^2)	Maximal segmental motion (mm) Long axis S1	S2	S3	S4	Short axis S1	S2	S3	S4	Area/$\sqrt{BSA}$) Long axis Max	Min	Short axis Max	Min	AF (%) Long axis	Short axis
1	15	0.49	3.0	3.8	3.7	3.0	4.0	4.8	6.0	4.0	10.7	4.7	10.4	4.6	56	56
2	5	0.27	1.5	3.5	2.3	2.8	3.0	1.5	2.8	1.0	17.8	12.4	16.5	12.7	30	23
3	14	0.60	4.0	3.0	3.8	3.5	4.3	1.8	4.0	2.7	12.9	8.2	10.5	5.3	36	50
4	1	0.23	2.0	2.8	2.5	3.3	2.3	4.0	2.0	4.0	13.0	8.5	10.3	5.9	34	42
5	37	0.57	1.0	6.5	4.0	6.7	3.0	2.8	3.8	3.0	26.6	15.4	19.5	13.9	42	29
6	7	0.42	4.0	3.5	3.5	4.0	6.0	2.0	5.8	3.7	18.2	11.5	11.3	6.0	37	47
7	2	0.24	4.0	3.8	2.0	1.8	1.7	0.5	1.0	1.0	39.4	29.0	16.2	13.8	26	15
8	24	0.48	5.0	10.0	2.8	9.0	2.5	4.8	2.0	4.5	57.2	32.3	28.4	19.2	43	32
9	25	0.44	2.0	5.0	1.0	3.8	3.0	1.3	2.5	2.0	20.4	14.4	10.2	7.3	29	28
10	5	0.33	2.0	5.8	1.5	5.2	1.5	1.8	1.8	1.8	18.6	11.5	12.8	10.1	38	21
11	12	0.40	4.0	4.5	4.5	4.7	0.0	2.5	3.0	2.8	22.6	13.6	16.6	12.0	40	28
12	1	0.25	4.5	5.0	1.5	3.3	1.5	1.8	1.5	1.8	14.0	7.7	8.1	5.4	45	33
13	5	0.28	2.0	7.0	2.3	5.2	2.0	2.5	2.3	2.7	16.7	9.2	9.6	6.1	45	36
14	4	0.26	3.5	6.0	3.7	4.5	4.0	2.8	3.8	3.2	23.5	14.3	14.0	9.4	39	33
15	32	0.51	3.3	3.3	3.0	1.8	6.3	4.5	6.5	6.2	29.0	23.4	17.5	8.4	19	52
16	3	0.30	4.0	5.0	3.8	2.8	2.8	1.3	2.3	1.8	18.4	9.5	12.6	9.3	48	26
Mean	12	0.38	3.1	4.9	2.9	4.1	3.0	2.5	3.2	2.9	22.4	14.1	14.0	9.3	38	34
SD	12	0.13	1.2	1.9	1.1	1.8	1.6	1.3	1.7	1.4	11.7	7.7	5.1	4.1	9	12
p value			NS	NS	NS	<.01	NS	NS	NS	<.01	<.01	<.01	<.01	<.01	NS	NS

Probability value indicates comparison with normal infants. Abbreviations as in table 1.

wall and septal segments in the long-axis view, whereas all other segments exhibited normal motion (figure 2, *E* and *F*). Similarly, parodoxic outward motion of the free wall and septal segment was seen in the short-axis view in patient 2, with all long-axis segments having an exaggerated inward motion. Outward motion of parts of the free wall segment in both planes and of the septal segment in the long-axis view was noted in patient 3, with the portion of the septal segment adjacent to the diaphragmatic wall being akinetic in the short-axis view. Inward motion of all other segments was decreased.

The end-diastolic cross-sectional area of the right ventricle in patient 1 was within the range of values seen in the well patients after Senning operation, while the end-diastolic cross-sectional areas of the right ventricle in the other two patients were grossly enlarged. In those planes in which dyskinetic areas were seen the AF was significantly lower than that in the other postoperative group.

Discussion

In patients with various congenital heart defects, the right ventricle may be subjected to pressure and/or volume overload and, under some circumstances, may function as the systemic ventricle. The longevity of the right ventricle under these conditions is unknown but clearly of great interest. Evaluation of this issue requires the ability to perform longitudinal studies of right ventricular performance. Nevertheless, few re-

TABLE 4

Personal and echocardiographic data on three patients with transposition of the great arteries after Senning operation in congestive heart failure

Patient no.	Age (mo)	Time since op (mo)	BSA (m^2)	Maximal segmental motion (mm) Long axis S1	S2	S3	S4	Short axis S1	S2	S3	S4	Area/BSA (cm^2/m^2) Max	Min	Max	Min	AF (%) Long axis	Short axis
1	82	41	0.77	2.5	−4	2	−3	3.0	3.5	2.5	4.0	19.3	18.5	12.5	7.9	4.1	36.8
2	32	29	0.60	6.0	5.0	5.5	6.0	2.0	−3	2.0	−4	56.8	40.4	41.2	37.9	28.9	8.0
3	46	35	0.7	1.0	−2	1.0	−3	3.0	−1.5	3.0	0	59.9	48.4	43.1	34.5	19.2	20.0

The negative values represent systolic outward motion. Abbreviations as in table 1.

ports of echocardiographic evaluation of right ventricular function in children have appeared,[12–14] and segmental wall motion analyses and calculation of area and AF in normal children or in infants with congenital heart disease have not been published. The noninvasive technique reported here using echocardiography employs two orthogonal subxiphoid planes in which the right ventricular sinus and infundibular walls are imaged simultaneously (figures 1*A* and 1*B*), enabling analysis of regional wall motion of the entire circumference of the right ventricle.

A floating center of mass method was used to determine the inward motion of the right ventricular wall. In each frame the centroid was calculated, and the wall motion was measured with reference to this point. By this method, all right ventricular segments for all normal subjects and patients without congestive heart failure move toward the center of mass. When this analysis was repeated with use of a fixed reference point method similar results were obtained, except in four older normal subjects in whom the septal segment moved "outward" or toward the left ventricle. D'Arcy and Nanda[15] and Lopez-Sendon et al.[10] independently examined right ventricular wall motion using a fixed reference point system in adult patients after ventricular infarction and considered septal motion to be normal when the septum was displaced toward the left ventricular cavity in systole and dyskinetic or paradoxic when both sides of the septum were displaced toward the right ventricular cavity. In normal infants, however, the septal surface of the right ventricle was found to move toward the ventricle during systole whether a fixed or floating point of reference was used. Only in four older subjects and by the fixed reference point method was "outward" systolic motion of the right ventricular septal surface toward the left ventricle noted. This may be related in part to the normal translational or rotational motion of the heart during contraction.[16] It is our impression that gross motion of the heart is small in newborns and infants but increases with age. The floating center of mass model may compensate for the effect of translational motion on the analysis of regional wall motion.

The patients with transpositon of the great arteries were significantly older than the normal subjects in this study. However, if there is a progression from the pattern of septal motion seen in our controls to the pattern described in adults,[10, 15] inclusion of older normal subjects would have accentuated the difference in wall motion detected in our study.

Regional wall motion. In normal subjects, all segments viewed in the long axis demonstrated a greater net excursion than the corresponding short-axis segments. Anterior-posterior motion of the heart due to contraction might result in a more anterior cross-sectional plane being recorded in systole compared with diastole, artifactually exaggerating right ventricular wall motion in the long-axis plane. However, this would not account for differences between segments or between patients. Additionally, there was no difference between AF values in the two planes, suggesting this difference was due to the greater relative size in the long-axis view.

In normal infants, the septal segment exhibited the least inward motion. In contrast, the free wall and the septal segments exhibited the greatest inward motion in the long axis in patients with transposition of the great arteries. In these patients with the right ventricle as the systemic ventricle, the transseptal pressure difference leads to displacement of the interventricular septum into the left ventricle. The resulting ventricular configuration, with the septal concavity toward the right ventricle, would be expected to facilitate motion of the septal endocardium toward the right ventricular centroid during fiber shortening.

In the three patients with transposition of the great arteries and congestive heart failure clearly different patterns of regional wall motion were observed. In patient 1, dyskinetic areas of free wall and septum, only evident in the long-axis view, were associated with poor overall systolic performance, documented by an AF of 4.4% in the long-axis view. However, in the short-axis view normal inward motion of all segments was observed. In patient 2, on the other hand, dyskinetic segments (free wall and septal) were visible only in the short-axis view, with a resulting AF in the short axis of only 3.4%. In patient 3, the dyskinetic area in the free wall segment could be seen in both planes. Additionally, decreased inward motion of all other segments led to a very low AF in both planes. In patients 1 and 2 the dyskinetic areas alone might account for the observed congestive heart failure, whereas in patient 3, global right ventricular dysfunction was present in addition to regional dyskinesis.

Right ventricular area and area changes. As expected there was a high correlation in normal subjects between the BSA and the end-diastolic area in both planes. The minimal or end-systolic areas correlated less well with $\sqrt{BSA}$, perhaps because of a greater relative error in measuring a smaller end-systolic area[12] and variations in right ventricular systolic performance. In contrast, end-diastolic and end-systolic areas correlated poorly with $\sqrt{BSA}$ in postoperative patients with or without congestive heart failure. The right ventricular enlargement in these patients might have been influenced by several factors. First, the high afterload faced by the right ventricle functioning as the systemic ventricle may result in dilatation, although this is not the typical response of the nonfailing pressure-overloaded ventricle except during acute afterload stress. Second, hypoxia or acidosis before surgery, inadequate myocardial preservation during cardiopulmonary bypass, or complications after the Senning operation (e.g., rhythm disturbances) may have contributed to the wide range of cross-sectional areas measured. Finally, residual dilation from preoperative right ventricular volume overload may be a causative factor in some subjects. However, the AF values, as parameters of systolic performance,[16] in the normal subjects and well infants who had undergone the Senning procedure were not significantly different.

The three patients with congestive heart failure were significantly older as a group than the well patients, although the relationship between this and the presence of right ventricular dysfunction is uncertain. The poor correlation between the maximal and minimal areas and the BSA of patients after the Senning operation makes delineation of the "normal" area for these patients difficult, but at least in patients 2 and 3 the right ventricular cross-sectional areas appeared to be excessively large. Of interest is the fact that all patients with congestive heart failure were found to have abnormalities of regional wall motion, suggesting that this was at least in part the result of a local injury rather than a more globally acting noxious influence such as cyanosis or pressure overload.

This method of regional wall motion analysis combined with AF measurements provides normal values for segmental inward motion and maximal and minimal right ventricular cross-sectional areas and AF in infants. This appears to be a sensitive technique for evaluating regional and global right ventricular function in patients with congenital heart disease. The preliminary data derived from our three patients with congestive heart failure suggest that this method will be of value in detecting the specific mechanism for poor systolic peformance of the right ventricle. Additionally, this method should be applicable to the investigation of the various patterns in which the right ventricle adapts to pressure and volume overload.

Appendix

The center of mass is calculated on a single frame with the following formula:

$$xn = \Sigma(x_i + x_{i+1})/2^* (x_i - x_{i+1}) (y_i + y_{i+1})/2$$
$$yn = \Sigma(y_i + y_{i+1})/2^* (y_i - y_{i+1}) (x_i + x_{i+1})/2$$
$$xd = \Sigma(x_i - x_{i+1}) (y_i + y_{i+1})/2$$
$$yd = \Sigma(y_i - y_{i+1}) (x_i + x_{i+1})/2$$

center of mass = (xn/xd, yn/yd) i = 1,2 ... 64, where x_i and y_i represent the coordinates of the i-th point on an endocardial border.

References

1. Heger JJ, Weymann AE, Wann LS, Dillon JC, Feigenbaum H: Cross-sectional echocardiography in acute myocardial infarction: detection and localization of regional left ventricular asynergy. Circulation **60:** 531, 1979
2. Greenbaum RA, Gibson DG: Regional non-uniformity of left ventricular wall movement in man. Br Heart J **45:** 29, 1981
3. Moynihan PF, Parisi AF, Feldman CL: Quantitative detection of regional left ventricular contraction abnormalities by two-dimensional echocardiography. I. Analysis of methods. Circulation **63:** 752, 1981
4. Parisi AF, Moynihan PF, Folland ED, Feldman CL: Quantitative detection of regional left ventricular contraction abnormalities by two-dimensional echocardiography. II. Accuracy in coronary artery disease. Circulation **63:** 761, 1981
5. Rubenson DS, Tucker CR, London E, Miller DC, Stinson EB, Popp RL: Two-dimensional echocardiographic analysis of segmental left ventricular wall motion before and after coronary artery bypass surgery. Circulation **66:** 1025, 1982
6. Klausner SC, Blair TJ, Bulawa WF, Jeppson GM, Jensen JL, Clayton PD: Quantitative analysis of segmental wall motion throughout systole and diastole in the normal human left ventricle. Circulation **65:** 580, 1982
7. Haendchen RV, Wyatt HL, Maurer G, Zwehl W, Bear M, Meerbaum S, Corday E: Quantitation of regional cardiac function by two-dimensional echocardiogrphy I. Patterns of contraction in the normal left ventricle. Circulation **67:** 1234, 1983
8. Ginzton LE, Conant R, Brizendine M, Lee F, Mena I, Laks MM: Exercise subcostal two-dimensional echocardiography: a new method of segmental wall motion analysis. Am J Cardiol **53:** 805, 1984
9. Greenbaum RA, Evans TR: Investigation of left ventricular function by digital subtraction angiography. Br Heart J **51:** 163, 1984
10. Lopez-Sendon J, Garcia-Fernandez MA, Coma-Canella I, Yanguela MM, Banuelos F: Segmental right ventricular function after acute myocardial infarction: two-dimensional echocardiographic study in 63 patients. Am J Crdiol **51:** 390, 1983
11. Jugdutt BI, Sussex BA, Sivaram CA, Rossall RE: Right ventricular infarction: Two-dimensional echocardiographic evaluation. Am Heart J **107:** 505, 1984
12. Hiraishi S, DiSessa TG, Jarmakani JM, Nakanishi T, Isabel-Jones JB, Friedman WF: Two-dimensional echocardiographic assessment of right ventricular volume in children with congenital heart disease. Am J Cardiol **50:** 1368, 1982
13. Silverman NH, Hudson S: Evaluation of right ventricular volume and ejection fraction in children by two-dimensional echocardiography. Pediatr Cardiol **4:** 197, 1983
14. Lange PE, Seiffert PA, Pries F, Wessel A, Onnasch DGW, Radtke W, Heintzen PH: Improvement of 2D-echo volume determination of the right ventricle by image enhancement and injection of contrast media. Biarritz-Mai, 1984, Premier Colloque Image, Traitement, Synthese, Technologie et Applications
15. D'Arcy B, Nanda NC: Two-dimensional echocardiographic features of right ventricular function. Circulation **65:** 167, 1982
16. Horn HR, Teicholz LE, Cohn PF, Herman MV, Gorlin R: Augmentation of left ventricular contraction pattern in coronary artery disease by inotropic catecholamine. The epinephrine ventriculogram. Circulation **49:** 1963, 1974
17. Kaul S, Tei C, Hopkins JM, Shah PM: Assessment of right ventricular function using two-dimensional echocardiography. Pediatr Cardiol **4:** 197, 1983

Intraoperative detection of myocardial ischemia in high-risk patients: electrocardiography versus two-dimensional transesophageal echocardiography

JOHN S. SMITH, M.D., MICHAEL K. CAHALAN, M.D., DAVID J. BENEFIEL, M.D., BENJAMIN F. BYRD, M.D., FRANCIS W. LURZ, M.A., WILLIAM A. SHAPIRO, M.D., MICHAEL F. ROIZEN, M.D., ALAIN BOUCHARD, M.D., AND NELSON B. SCHILLER, M.D.

ABSTRACT Because acute segmental wall motion abnormalities (SWMAs) of the left ventricle are highly sensitive and specific indicators of myocardial ischemia, this study compared the incidence and significance of ischemia, as detected by two-dimensional transesophageal echocardiography and surface electrocardiography, during anesthesia and surgery in patients at high risk of myocardial ischemia. During surgery, 24 of the 50 patients studied had new SWMAs, whereas only six had ST segment changes. All patients with ST segment changes also had new SWMAs: in three instances, SWMAs occurred before the ST segment change, and in three instances, they occurred simultaneously. All three patients who had intraoperative myocardial infarctions also had persistent intraoperative SWMAs, whereas only one patient had ST segment changes. Ten healthy patients requiring noncardiovascular surgery were monitored similarly; none of these had SWMAs, ST segment changes, or myocardial infarction. This study demonstrates the superiority of two-dimensional transesophageal echocardiography over electrocardiography for the intraoperative detection of myocardial ischemia. Furthermore, when new SWMAs persist to the conclusion of surgery, myocardial infarction is likely to have occurred.
Circulation **72, No. 5, 1015–1021, 1985.**

DESPITE THE AVAILABILITY of aggressive intraoperative cardiac monitoring and therapy, myocardial ischemia and infarction remain common causes of perioperative morbidity and mortality.[1, 2] The standard surface electrocardiogram (ECG) may not reveal subendocardial ischemia.[3] Even severe transmural ischemia may go undetected if only a single electrocardiographic lead is monitored,[4] if excessive filtration is used, or if signal standardization is inappropriate. Furthermore, electrocardiographic monitoring for the detection of ischemia may be impossible if certain conduction disturbances or paced rhythms are present.[5, 6] Nevertheless, the ECG remains the monitor most commonly used to diagnose intraoperative myocardial ischemia.

From the Departments of Anesthesia and Medicine, Division of Cardiology, University of California, San Francisco.

Supported by NIH grants No. 1R23GM-28502-03 and NIA 1 PO 1 AGO3104-02,3 and the Anesthesia Research Foundation.

Address for correspondence: Michael K. Cahalan, M.D., Department of Anesthesia, University of California, Third and Parnassus Avenues, Room S436, San Francisco, CA 94109.

Presented in part at the annual meetings of the Society of Cardiovascular Anesthesiologists and the American Society of Anesthesiologists in 1984.

In 1935 Tennant and Wiggers[7] demonstrated that acute coronary ligation results in paradoxical motion in the ischemic area. Subsequently, wall motion abnormalities have been shown to occur within seconds of the onset of regional ischemia,[8–11] simultaneously with regional lactate production,[12] but before (and even in the absence of) changes on the surface ECG.[13] Because two-dimensional echocardiography reliably detects segmental wall motion abnormalities (SWMAs),[14] this technique may be a more sensitive measure of intraoperative myocardial ischemia than electrocardiography. However, precordial echocardiographic methods are impractical during surgery. In contrast, two-dimensional transesophageal echocardiography can be used during surgery and has been shown to provide safe, reproducible images of the left ventricle.[15, 16]

To compare the incidence of myocardial ischemia, as detected by the occurrence of new SWMAs on echocardiograms, with the incidence as detected by ST segment changes on ECGs, we studied patients at high risk of myocardial ischemia during anesthesia and surgery. Furthermore, we tested whether these changes accurately predicted perioperative myocardial infarction.

Methods

With approval from our committee on human experimentation and informed consent, we prospectively studied 50 patients: 29 undergoing vascular surgery and 21 undergoing coronary artery bypass grafting (CABG). We documented preoperatively any history of angina or myocardial infarction and extent of coronary disease revealed on the angiogram (when available). On the morning of surgery, patients were given their usual medications and appropriate preanesthetic medications. In the operating room, a conventional electrocardiographic system (Marquette MAC-1; Marquette Electronics, Milwaukee, WI), standardized to 10 mm/mV, was attached to the patient. A baseline ECG consisting of leads I, II, III, aVR, aVL, aVF, and V_5 was recorded, and induction of anesthesia was begun. In the last 30 patients, we recorded the ECG every 3 min during induction of anesthesia and endotracheal intubation. Once the endotracheal tube was in place, we introduced into the esophagus a 9 mm (diameter) gastroscope that had a 3.5 MHz phased-array transducer (Diasonics, Inc.; Milpitas, CA) on its tip.

The transducer was connected to an ultrasonograph (Diasonics 3400R or CV-60) focused at 10 cm. We positioned the transducer behind the heart to obtain a short-axis, cross-sectional view of the left ventricle at the level of the papillary muscles (figure 1, *A*). After insertion of the transducer (routinely requiring 15 to 30 sec), we recorded echocardiographic images at predetermined intervals for 60 sec on ½ inch VHS videotape. At the same time, ECGs were recorded. For all patients, one baseline echocardiogram was recorded before skin incision, and a second one within 3 min after skin incision. In those undergoing vascular surgery, recordings were made 3 min before vascular cross-clamping, 3 min after cross-clamping, 30 min after cross-clamping (if the clamp was still in place), and after unclamping. In those undergoing CABG, recordings were made after sternal split, before institution of cardiopulmonary bypass, 5 min after cessation of bypass, 30 min after bypass (if the chest was still open), and after sternal closure. The concluding echocardiogram and ECG were recorded in all patients during skin closure.

The diagnosis of myocardial infarction was based on postoperative ECGs and creatine kinase (CK) isoenzyme levels, which were determined in all patients. Additionally, technetium pyrophosphate scans were obtained in 18 of 21 patients undergoing CABG.

Data analysis. After surgery, ECGs were analyzed with the use of conventional criteria for the diagnosis of ischemia: horizontal or downsloping ST segment depression of at least 1 mm, or ST segment elevation of more than 1 mm (compared with baseline) 80 msec after the J point. The echocardiograms of all intervals were transcribed into a standard format for analysis and were analyzed by modification of the method of Van Reet et al.[17] The cross-sectional image was divided into quadrants with the papillary muscles as guides. This floating-reference system keyed to the papillary muscles compensated for translational and rotational movements of the heart. Only the short-axis view at the level of the papillary muscles was analyzed because this view was maintained throughout the study in each patient. Based on our studies in patients without cardiovascular disease,[18] a segment was considered to contract normally if an imaginary radius to the center of the left ventricle shortened by more than 30% and the wall thickened considerably. Mild hypokinesia was considered to occur if shortening of the radius was less than 30% but more than 10% and the wall thickened. Severe hypokinesia was diagnosed if the wall thickened minimally and radial shortening was less than 10%. An akinetic segment was defined as one in which the wall did not thicken during systole, and a dyskinetic segment as one in which the wall bulged and thinned during systole. This analysis system is qualitative and the estimates of endocardial motion and myocardial thickening are made visually. With the use of the first echocardiogram as a baseline recording, we subsequently judged a segment to be ischemic if it worsened by two or more classifications without the entire image doing likewise. A change was considered transient if it resolved before skin closure (figure 1), and persistent if it did not. Echocardiograms were considered unreadable if the short-axis view was unobtainable, if the orientation changed, or if image definition was insufficient to detect wall thickening. The echocardiograms were analyzed by two independent observers who were unaware of the patient's clinical course or the results of electrocardiographic analysis. All disagreements were arbitrated by a third observer, our senior echocardiographer (N.B.S.).

To describe and compare echocardiographic results with electrocardiographic findings, we used a modification of the method of Heger et al.[19]: the cross section was considered to consist of four regions, each of which could be subdivided for analysis if necessary (figure 2).

Verification of probe position. To ensure the ability to regain consistently the same cross section when the probe or the heart was moved, we performed the following procedure in 10 consecutive patients undergoing CABG. After recording during skin closure, we deliberately unlocked and advanced the probe 2 cm into the esophagus, and then attempted to locate the previous image and record it. Similarly, we pulled the probe back 2 cm toward the mouth and repeated the same procedure. These images were edited and retaped to disguise any association and were submitted for analysis. All images were graded by the same two observers, and the wall motion scores from the two relocated echocardiograms were compared with those from the echocardiograms taken at skin closure. Additionally, using a semiautomatic light-pen system (Diasonics), we compared cross-sectional areas at end-diastole and end-systole.

Incidence of intraoperative SWMAs in non-high-risk patients. To determine the incidence of intraoperative SWMAs in healthy adults, we studied 10 patients (28 to 54 yr of age) who had no evidence of cardiovascular disease and required noncardiovascular surgical procedures. In these patients two-dimensional transesophageal echocardiograms were recorded after induction of anesthesia, 1 to 3 min after skin incision, and 10 to 20 min after skin incision. These images were rerecorded onto the same tapes that contained the images from our high-risk patients, but were disguised to prevent observers from knowing their origins.

Results

High-risk patients. Thirty-four of the 50 patients in this study had at least one prior myocardial infarction. In 28 of these 34 patients SWMAs were detected on the baseline echocardiogram. Of the 16 patients having no history of myocardial infarction, one patient had a baseline area of hypokinesis, and 15 had no SWMAs. Forty-three patients had a history of angina. Of the 21 patients studied with coronary angiography, 16 had triple-vessel disease and five double-vessel disease.

We obtained echocardiograms adequate for analysis of SWMAs in 339 of the 350 measurement intervals attempted. In only one patient were we unable to obtain the appropriate cross section at any time. Four patients had a single interval for which the echocardiogram could not be analyzed. Each of these four instances occurred after cardiopulmonary bypass.

We were able to analyze the ST segment of the ECG for 342 of 400 intervals. Five patients had either left bundle branch block or a ventricularly paced rhythm throughout the surgical procedure. Eleven other patients had at least one interval in which the ST segment could not be analyzed because of a transient conduction disturbance or because heart rhythm was controlled: for one patient (undergoing vascular surgery), this interval occurred after aortic cross-clamping, at which time rhythm was controlled by a demand pacemaker; for 10 patients, this interval occurred after cardiopulmonary bypass.

Five of the 30 patients studied with sequential ECGs during induction of anesthesia had ST segment changes diagnostic of ischemia at this time: the ST segments changed in all leads in two patients; in leads II, III, and aVF in two patients; and in only lead V_5 in

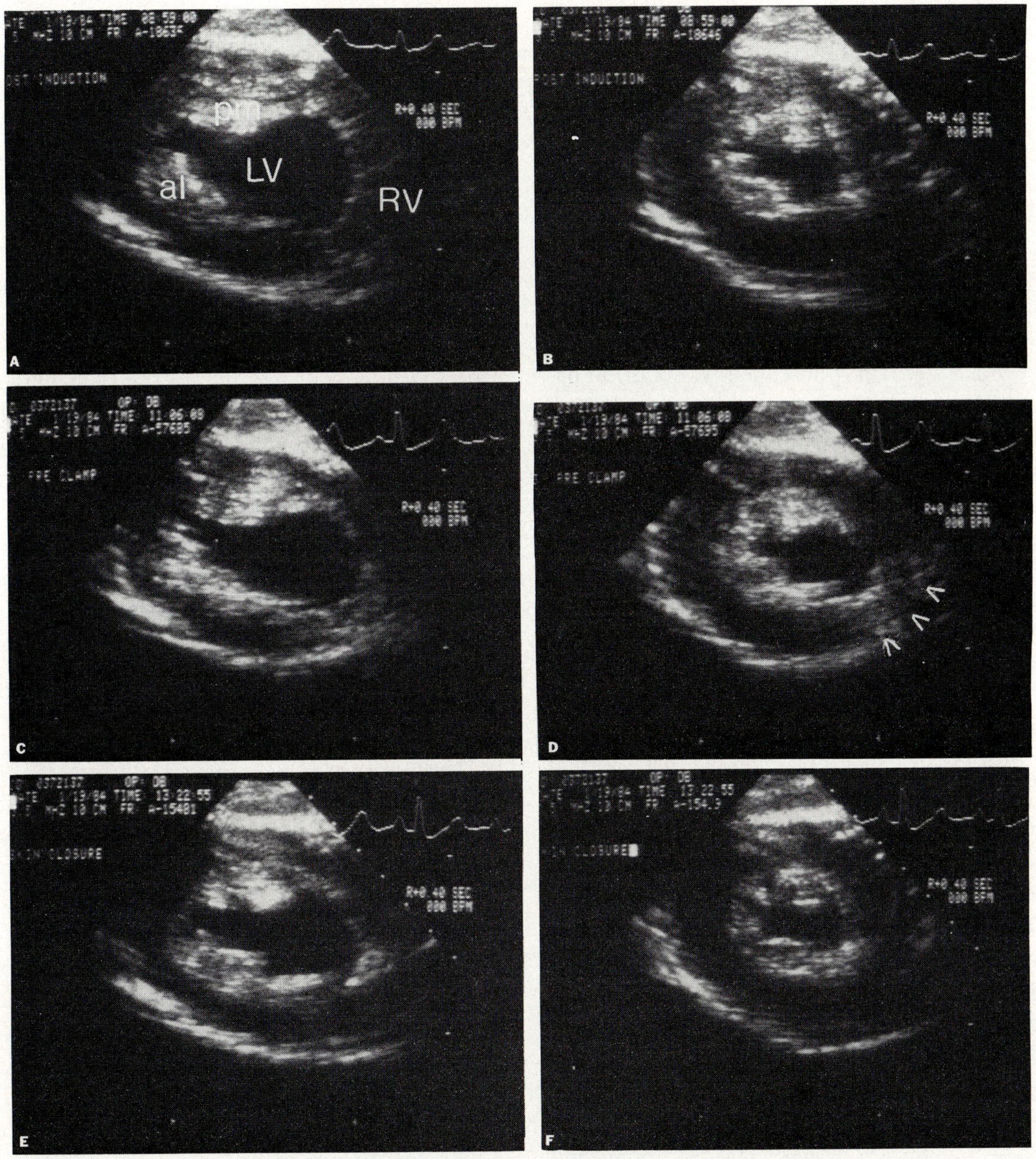

FIGURE 1. Recorded after induction of anesthesia, short-axis echocardiographic images at end-diastole (*A*) and end-systole (*B*) show the left ventricle at the level of the papillary muscles. The inferior wall is nearest to the intraesophageal transducer. The orientation of all other figures is identical. LV = left ventricular cavity; RV = right ventricular cavity; pm = posteromedial papillary muscle; al = anterolateral papillary muscle. Segmental wall motion is normal. Approximately 1 hr later, the end-diastolic image (*C*) has not changed, but the end-systolic image (*D*) reveals a segmental wall motion abnormality (arrows) of the anterior-septal myocardium that resolves before completion of the surgery (*E* and *F*).

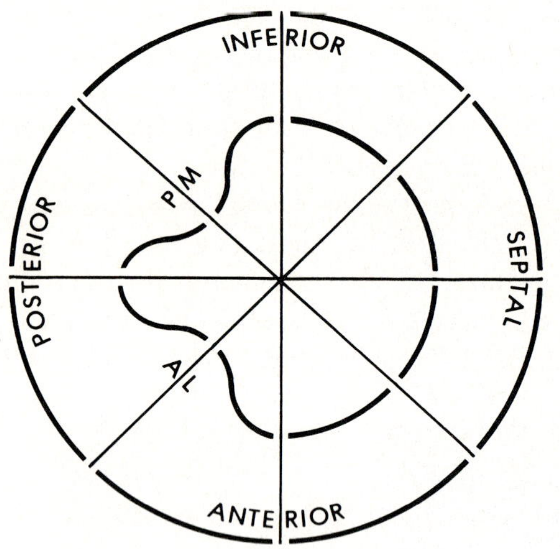

FIGURE 2. Schematic cross-sectional view of the left ventricle at the level of the papillary muscles depicting the octants into which the ventricle is divided and the corresponding walls. PM = posteromedial papillary muscle; AL = anterolateral papillary muscle.

one patient. These changes reverted to normal by the first postinduction recording; thereafter, none of these patients had any episode of ischemia detected on the ECG or echocardiogram. Subsequently, six of 50 patients had ST segment changes during surgery. Three changes were transient, and three were still present at skin closure. The ST segments changed in lead V_5 in one patient; in leads II, III, and aVF in two patients; in leads II, III, aVF, and aVL in two patients; and in lead aVF in one patient.

During the course of surgery, 24 patients had a total of 32 new SWMAs. The locations of the SWMAs were as follows: 10, septal wall; nine, inferior wall; nine, anterior wall; and four, posterior wall. Two patients had baseline hypokinetic segments that subsequently became dyskinetic. The remaining 22 had normal baseline wall motion in the segment that subsequently developed an abnormality. Of these 22, four had segmental dyskinesis; nine, segmental akinesis; and nine, severe segmental hypokinesis. New SWMAs were detected during all intervals without a preponderance of occurrence during any one interval. Changes were transient in 16 patients but persisted through skin closure in eight. Four of five patients with double-vessel disease had new SWMAs, and these changes were in regions of myocardium supplied by the diseased coronary arteries and never in the "risk free" myocardium. Two of these patients had disease in the circumflex and anterior descending arteries and they had both anterior and septal SWMAs. The remaining two patients had circumflex and right coronary disease and had inferior SWMAs.

The six patients who had ST segment changes diagnostic of ischemia during surgery also had new SWMAs (table 1). In three of these patients, the wall motion abnormality appeared at least one interval before the change on the ECG. Four patients had a new SWMA when the ST segment could not be analyzed. One of these patients had left bundle branch block throughout surgery, whereas the other three had conduction disturbances after bypass. No patient had an ST segment change during an interval in which the echocardiogram could not be analyzed.

Four patients had perioperative myocardial infarction, three of which appear to have occurred intraoperatively because isoenzyme levels peaked at 8 hr after surgery. One patient had persistent inferior and posterior wall motion abnormalities; ST segment elevation in leads II, III, and aVF; and ST segment depression in lead aVL. Two patients had persistent wall motion abnormalities but no intraoperative changes on the ECG. One of these patients died, and myocardial infarction was confirmed at autopsy; the other patient had an inferior wall infarction that corresponded with the intraoperative wall motion abnormality. Finally, the fourth patient had only a transient intraoperative wall motion abnormality and no change on the ECG; myocardial infarction occurred 48 hr after surgery, and CK isoenzyme levels peaked on the third postoperative day. As determined by chi-square analysis, the patients with persistent SWMAs had a significantly higher incidence of intraoperative infarction than did patients with transient SWMAs or those without SWMAs ($p < .05$).

No complications related to the use of two-dimensional transesophageal echocardiography occurred in any of our patients.

Verification of probe position. Deliberate repositioning of the probe never caused a change in wall motion rating of greater than one classification or any significant change in the end-systolic or end-diastolic cross-sectional area (table 2).

Intraoperative SWMAs in non-high-risk patients. The 10 normal patients that we examined had normal baseline wall motion, no intraoperative wall motion changes, and no postoperative evidence of myocardial infarction, as assessed by routine clinical surveillance.

Discussion

Studies in animals have demonstrated that wall motion abnormalities progress as coronary artery constriction and myocardial ischemia increase,[9-13, 20, 21] and that subendocardial ischemia alone can cause severe segmental wall dysfunction.[10] Echocardiography has been used to detect SWMAs due to ischemia and

TABLE 1
Patients with intraoperative evidence of ischemia

Patient No.	Ischemic changes detected by: Leads of the ECG	SWMA on echocardiograms	Perioperative myocardial infarction
6	V_5[A]	Anterior[A]	No
9	II, III, aVF[A]	Inferior[A]	No
17	II, III, avF	Anterior/septal	No
26	II, III, aVF, aVL	Anterior/septal	No
34	II, III, aVF, aVL[A]	Inferior/posterior[A]	Yes
46	aVF	Inferior	No
3	None	Septal	No
4	None	Anterior	No
8	None	Septal	No
10	None	Posterior	No
12	None	Anterior[A]	Yes
14	None	Septal/inferior	No
16	None	Septal[A]	No
20	None	Inferior	No
22	None	Posterior	No
24	None	Anterior/posterior	No
29	None	Inferior[A]	No
31	None	Anterior/septal	Yes[B]
35	None	Inferior	No
37	None	Anterior/septal[A]	No
38	None	Anterior	No
40	None	Inferior[A]	Yes
43	None	Septal	No
48	None	Inferior/septal	No

[A]Changes were persistent.
[B]This patient had infarction 2 days postoperatively.

infarction in experimental preparations and in patients.[14, 19, 22–26] For example, echocardiographically detected wall motion changes during exercise testing were shown to be sensitive and specific indicators of the presence and location of coronary artery disease.[27] In another study, adequate two-dimensional precordial echocardiograms were obtained in 65 of 80 consecutive patients with acute chest pain.[28] SWMAs occurred in 31 of the 33 patients with acute myocardial infarction, 18 of whom had nondiagnostic changes on the ECG. Additionally, 27 of 32 who did not have myocardial infarction had normal wall motion. The extent of wall motion abnormalities in patients with acute myocardial infarctions correlated with the incidence of ventricular arrhythimas, congestive heart failure, and death.[29]

Like Horowtiz, Limacher, and others, we used a qualitative analysis of regional wall motion to detect ischemia. Since our interpretations were read by two independent observers who were guided by established criteria and were unaware of the patients' clinical courses, the chance for observer bias was minimized. In our control patients, the two observers did not detect abnormalities, whereas in the high-risk patients, when new SWMAs persisted, the chance of myocardial infarction was high. No patient in whom there were not new intraoperative SWMAs had an immediate postoperative infarction.

Although not all patients with persistent wall motion changes had myocardial infarction, this is not surprising, and may represent either ongoing ischemia or postischemic ventricular dysfunction.[30] Owing to biological differences in normal patients, not all hearts contract uniformly[31]; however, only a pathophysiologic change would cause an acute alteration in segmental wall motion. In patients with coronary artery disease, a likely factor is regional myocardial ischemia. In fact, in our patients with angiographically demonstrated regional disease, SWMAs occurred only in the areas of myocardium at risk. Unmasking of areas of scarring and incoordinate contraction secondary to abnormal conduction are also possible causes of regional wall motion abnormalities. However, 92% of patients with wall motion changes developed abnormalities in previously normal segments.

Although we cannot exclude the possibility that scarring was a factor, the results of analysis of wall thickening as well as inward radial motion throughout the cardiac cycle make scarring an unlikely cause. Additionally, we described new wall motion abnormalities in only 25% of the patients with conduction defects, one of whom had left bundle branch block throughout the entire surgical procedure. Previous investigators have documented a high incidence of septal motion abnormalities after cardiac surgery.[32–34] Opening the sternum and pericardium may alter the motion of the heart within the chest and introduce a factitious decrease in the motion of the septal endocardium if a fixed-reference system is used.[35] However, thickening of the septal wall will not occur if the wall is ischemic.[36] We used a floating-reference system in this

TABLE 2
Changes in cross-sectional area with repositioning of the probe

	Cross-sectional area: Skin closure	+2 cm, then repositioned	−2 cm, then repositioned
End-diastolic area (cm^2)	19.8 ± 6.4	19.8 ± 6.3	20.0 ± 6.0
End-systolic area (cm^2)	11.8 ± 6.3	11.8 ± 6.1	12.1 ± 6.1

As determined by repeated-measures analysis of variance, no significant difference was found in cross-sectional areas after deliberate repositioning of the transducer.

study and evaluated both endocardial motion and wall thickening. Only three of 21 patients developed a SWMA of the septum after sternotomy or pericardiotomy. Therefore, we believe that the wall motion abnormalities we detected were most likely due to myocardial ischemia.

In experimental preparations, electrophysiologic changes rapidly follow the imposition of myocardial ischemia. However, the transthoracic ECG is relatively insensitive to subendocardial ischemia[3] and does not reflect changes until minutes after changes in wall motion and lactate metabolism. Another major limitation of electrocardiography is the difficulty of detecting ischemia in the presence of conduction defects or ventricularly paced rhythms. The new occurrence of such a conduction system defect is relatively common after cardiopulmonary bypass and does not accurately predict perioperative myocardial ischemia.[37, 38] Although monitoring the anterior precordial leads may have provided additional electrocardiographic evidence of ischemia, this area of the chest is inaccessible during cardiac and upper abdominal vascular procedures.

During anesthesia and surgery, we found four presumed episodes of ischemia by analysis of wall motion for every one episode detected by our electrocardiographic system. Three of the four patients with perioperative infarction had no electrocardiographic evidence of intraoperative ischemia, whereas all had SWMAs. Thus, our multilead electrocardiographic system failed to detect 75% of the intraoperative episodes of myocardial ischemia and was no better at predicting perioperative infarction. Moreover, the custom of relying on any single ECG lead would further diminish diagnostic efficacy.

Using one single cross section, we detected baseline wall motion abnormalities in 76% of patients with old myocardial infactions. Although all major coronary vessels supply areas of myocardium at this level, it is conceivable that we may have missed wall motion abnormalities elsewhere. By not moving the probe, we simplified the process of monitoring, minimized the chances of introducing false positives secondary to changes in orientation of the transducer, and diminished the remote possibility of esophageal trauma. Despite this, we did not miss a single episode of intraoperative ischemia detected by electrocardiography.

During induction of anesthesia, we found a 16% incidence of ischemia detected by electrocardiography. This is a period of high risk during which transesophageal echocardiographic monitoring is not feasible. Additionally, ischemia occurring at this time may have caused wall motion abnormalities that we took for baseline defects, thus diminishing the number of new wall motion changes detected.

In summary, we were able to detect intraoperative wall motion changes (presumed to be secondary to myocardial ischemia) by echocardiogram not only four times more frequently than we were able to detect ST segment changes on the ECG, but also when the ECG could not be analyzed because of conduction disturbances or paced rhythms. Patients experiencing persistent wall motion abnormalities were more likely to have myocardial infarction than those having only transient changes. No patient without a new wall motion abnormality had myocardial infarction. Two-dimensional transesophageal echocardiography seems superior to the ECG for the detection of intraoperative myocardial ischemia and should allow earlier identification of patients at higher risk of postoperative cardiovascular complications. Additionally, the ability to detect ischemia earlier may improve treatment of ischemic events and thereby reduce morbidity and mortality.

We thank Diasonics, Inc., and Marquette Electronics for supplying equipment; Pauline Snider and E.I. Eger II, M.D. for editorial advice; and Celeste Mangold for manuscript preparation.

References

1. Marx GF, Mateo CV, Orkin LR: Computer analysis of postanesthetic deaths. Anesthesiology **39:** 54, 1973
2. Lunn JN, Mushin WW: Mortality associated with anaesthesia. London, Nuffield Provincial Hospitals Trust, 1982
3. Barnard RJ, Buckberg GD, Duncan HW: Limitations of the standard transthoracic electrocardiogram in detecting subendocardial ischemia. Am Heart J **99:** 476, 1980
4. Chaitman BR, Bourassa MG, Wagniart P, Corbara F, Ferguson RJ: Improved efficacy of treadmill exercise testing multiple lead ECG system and basic hemodynamic response. Circulation **57:** 71, 1978
5. Whinnery JE, Froelicher VF Jr, Stewart AJ, Longo MR, Triebwasser JH, Lancaster MC: The electrocardiographic response to maximal treadmill exercise of asymptomatic men with left bundle branch block. Am Heart J **94:** 316, 1977
6. Orzan F, Garcia E, Mathur VS, Hall RJ: Is the treadmill exercise test useful for evaluating coronary artery disease in patients with complete left bundle branch block? Am J Cardiol **42:** 36, 1978
7. Tennant R, Wiggers CJ: The effect of coronary occlusion on myocardial contraction. Am J Physiol **112:** 351, 1935
8. Vatner SF: Correlation between acute reductions in myocardial blood flow and function in conscious dogs. Circ Res **47:** 201, 1980
9. Forrester JS, Wyatt HL, Protasio L, Tyberg JV, Diamond GA, Swan HJC: Functional significance of regional ischemic contraction abnormalities. Circulation **54:** 64, 1976
10. Gallagher KP, Kumada T, Koziol JA, McKown MD, Kemper WS, Ross J Jr: Significance of regional wall thickening abnormalities relative to transmural myocardial perfusion in anesthetized dogs. Circulation **62:** 1266, 1980
11. Kerber RE, Marcus ML, Ehrhardt J, Wilson R, Abboud FM: Correlation between echocardiographically demonstrated segmental dyskinesis and regional myocardial perfusion. Circulation **52:** 1097, 1975
12. Waters DD, Luz PD, Wyatt HL, Swan HJC, Forrster JS: Early changes in regional and global left ventricular function induced by graded reductions in regional coronary perfusion. Am J Cardiol **39:** 537, 1977

13. Battler A, Froelicher VF, Gallagher KP, Kemper WS, Ross J Jr: Dissociation between regional myocardial dysfunction and ECG changes during ischemia in the conscious dog. Circulation **62:** 735, 1980
14. Pandian NG, Kerber RE: Two-dimensional echocardiography in experimental coronary stenosis. I. Sensitivity and specificity in detecting transient myocardial dyskinesis: comparison with sonomicrometers. Circulation **66:** 597, 1982
15. Schlüter M, Langenstein BA, Polster J, Kremer P, Souquet J, Engel S, Hanrath P: Transesophageal cross-sectional echocardiography with a phased array transducer system. Technique and initial clinical results. Br Heart J **48:** 67, 1982
16. Schlüter M, Hinrichs A, Thier W, Kremer P, Schröder S, Cahalan MK, Hanrath P: Transesophageal two-dimensional echocardiography: comparison of ultrasonic and anatomic sections. Am J Cardiol **53:** 1173, 1984
17. Van Reet RE, Quinones MA, Poliner LR, Nelson JG, Waggoner AD, Kanon D, Lubetkin SJ, Pratt CM, Winters WL Jr: Comparison of two-dimensional echocardiography with gated radionuclide ventriculography in the evaluation of global and regional left ventricular function in acute myocardial infarction. J Am Coll Cardiol **3:** 243, 1984
18. Cahalan MK, Kremer PF, Beaupre PW, Lurz FW, Roizen MF, Cronnelly R, Robinson S, Hamilton WK, Eger EI, Schiller NB: Consistency and reproducibility of transesophageal two-dimensional echocardiography. Anesth Analg **63:** 194, 1984
19. Heger JJ, Weyman AE, Wann LS, Dillon JC, Feigenbaum H: Cross-sectional echocardiography in acute myocardial infarction: detection and localization of regional left ventricular asynergy. Circulation **60:** 531, 1979
20. Gallagher KP, Osakada G, Hess OM, Koziol JA, Kemper WS, Ross J Jr: Subepicardial segmental function during coronary stenosis and role of myocardial fiber orientation. Circ Res **50:** 352, 1982
21. St. John Sutton MG, Ritman EL: Effects of progressive reduction in coronary blood flow on regional and global left ventricular contraction and relaxation during normal and increased afterload: a roentgen videometric study. Cardiovasc Res **16:** 535, 1982
22. Kisslo JA, Robertson D, Gilbert BW, Von Ramm O, Behar VS: A comparison of real-time, two-dimensional echocardiography and cineangiography in detecting left ventricular asynergy. Circulation **55:** 134, 1977
23. Weiss JL, Bulkley BH, Hutchins GM, Mason SJ: Two-dimensional echocardiographic recognition of myocardial injury in man: comparison with postmortem studies. Circulation **63:** 401, 1981
24. Lieberman AN, Weiss JL, Jugdutt BI, Becker LC, Bulkley BH, Garrison JG, Hutchins GM, Kallman CA, Weisfeldt ML: Two-dimensional echocardiography and infarct size: relationship of regional wall motion and thickening to the extent of myocardial infarction in the dog. Circulation **63:** 739, 1981
25. Wann LS, Faris JV, Childress RH, Dillon JC, Weyman AE, Feigenbaum H: Exercise cross-sectional echocardiography in ischemic heart disease. Circulation **60:** 1300, 1979
26. Gibson RS, Bishop HL, Stamm RB, Crampton RS, Beller GA, Martin RP: Value of early two dimensional echocardiography in patients with acute myocardial infarction. Am J Cardiol **49:** 1110, 1982
27. Limacher MC, Quinones MA, Poliner LR, Nelson JG, Winters WL, Waggoner AD: Detection of coronary artery disease with exercise two-dimensional echocardiography. Description of a clinically applicable method and comparison with radionuclide ventriculography. Circulation **67:** 1211, 1983
28. Horowitz RS, Morganroth J, Parrotto C, Chen CC, Soffer J, Pauletto FJ: Immediate diagnosis of acute myocardial infarction by two-dimensional echocardiography. Circulation **65:** 323, 1982
29. Horowtiz RS, Morganroth J: Immediate detection of early high-risk patients with acute myocardial infarction using two-dimensional echocardiographic evaluation of left ventricular regional wall motion abnormalities. Am Heart J **103:** 814, 1982
30. Braunwald E, Kloner RA: The stunned myocardium: prolonged, postischemic ventricular dysfunction. Circulation **66:** 1146, 1982
31. Pandian NG, Skorton DJ, Collins SM, Falsetti HL, Burke ER, Kerber RE: Heterogeneity of left ventricular segmental wall thickening and excursion in 2-dimensional echocardiograms of normal human subjects. Am J Cardiol **51:** 1667, 1983
32. Burggraf GW, Craige E: Echocardiographic studies of left ventricular wall motion and dimensions after valvular heart surgery. Am J Cardiol **35:** 473, 1975
33. Righetti A, Crawford MH, O'Rourke RA, Schelbert H, Daily PO, Ross J Jr: Interventricular septal motion and left ventricular function after coronary bypass surgery. Am J Cardiol **39:** 372, 1977
34. Vignola PA, Boucher CA, Curfman GD, Walker HJ, Shea WH, Dinsmore RE, Pohost GM: Abnormal interventricular septal motion following cardiac surgery: Clinical, surgical, echocardiographic and radionuclide correlates. Am Heart J **97:** 27, 1979
35. Kerber RE, Litchfield R: Postoperative abnormalities of interventricular septal motion: Two-dimensional and M-mode echocardiographic correlations. Am Heart J **104:** 263, 1982
36. Kerber RE, Marcus ML, Wilson R, Ehrhardt J, Abbound FM: Effects of acute coronary occlusion on the motion and perfusion of the normal and ischemic interventricular septum. An experimental echocardiographic study. Circulation **54:** 928, 1976
37. Zeldis SM, Morganroth J, Horowitz LN, Michelson EL, Josephson ME, Lozner EC, MacVaugh H, Kastor JA: Fascicular conduction disturbances after coronary bypass surgery. Am J Cardiol **41:** 860, 1978
38. O'Connell JB, Wallis D, Johnson SA, Pifarre R, Gunnar RM: Transient bundle branch block following use of hypothermic cardioplegia in coronary artery bypass surgery: high incidence without perioperative myocardial infarction. Am Heart J **103:** 85, 1982

Transcutaneous oxygen recovery and toe pulse reappearance time in the assessment of peripheral vascular disease

HARRY B. KRAM, M.D., RODNEY A. WHITE, M.D., JOSEPH TABRISKY, M.D., PAUL L. APPEL, M.P.A., ARTHUR W. FLEMING, M.D., AND WILLIAM C. SHOEMAKER, M.D.

ABSTRACT The accuracy of measurements of transcutaneous oxygen tension ($Ptco_2$) in the diagnosis of peripheral vascular disease (PVD) may be significantly increased by stressing limb circulation with the use of temporary ischemia. The purpose of this study was to compare the transcutaneous oxygen recovery half-time (TORT) and the toe pulse reappearance time (PRT/2) in a series of patients with symptomatic PVD before and after vascular reconstruction. The TORT was defined as the time required to recover half of the decrease in the limb/chest $Ptco_2$ ratio caused by temporary limb ischemia, and is conceptually comparable to the toe PRT/2, the time required to recover half of the control toe pulse amplitude. Measurement of TORT was found to be more feasible (100% vs 58%) and to have a greater diagnostic yield (100% vs 92%) than that of the toe PRT/2. When measured on the dorsum of the foot, TORT values were found to correlate well with the severity of symptoms of PVD; toe PRT/2 values did not correlate with severity of symptoms. Patients who underwent successful vascular reconstruction had significant improvement in their calf and foot TORT values after surgery ($p < .005$ and .0005, respectively); postoperative values were similar to those obtained in normal subjects. Toe PRT/2 values usually improved postoperatively, but in many patients postoperative values overlapped with values that were considered abnormal. There was no overlap of TORT values in normal subjects with those in patients with symtomatic PVD. The measurement of TORT may be clinically useful for screening patients with suspected PVD and for assessing quantitatively the results of conservative and surgical therapy. Use of the TORT to diagnose and quantitate PVD may lead to development of more refined selection criteria for angiography and to improved limb salvage as a result of the early discovery of potentially reconstructible vascular disease.
Circulation 72, No. 5, 1022–1027, 1985.

LOWER EXTREMITY blood flow in a resting subject is usually fairly stable and it does not differ between healthy subjects and patients with peripheral vascular disease (PVD).[1–4] Stressing limb circulation by temporary ischemia, on the other hand, exaggerates circulatory deficits secondary to stenotic arterial lesions, thereby accentuating differences in blood flow between healthy and diseased limbs. This phenomenon has been quantified by measurement of the toe pulse reappearance time (PRT/2),[5] as well as by determination of segmental pressure changes during postocclusive reactive hyperemia. Although a valuable method for assessing overall blood flow impairment in patients with PVD, the toe PRT/2 is often impossible to measure because of the absence of a toe pulse, the presence of gangrene, or prior amputation. Furthermore, abnormal values do not accurately quantify tissue perfusion, nor do they localize areas of critical arterial narrowing.

Transcutaneous oxygen tension ($Ptco_2$), which reflects both local blood flow and oxygenation,[6–8] has been evaluated extensively in the diagnosis and perioperative management of atherosclerotic and traumatic arterial disease.[9–15] Although prior studies have attempted to assess limb circulation in patients with PVD by measuring resting limb $Ptco_2$, this technique has only limited diagnostic value, since a stenotic inflow system may still permit a normal resting limb $Ptco_2$. This is because measured $Ptco_2$ values reflect the balance between local oxygen supply and demand, and this balance is frequently normal in the resting limbs of patients with PVD. Many symptomatic patients, par-

From the Department of Surgery and Radiology, Los Angeles County Harbor–UCLA Medical Center, Torrance, the Department of Surgery, King-Drew Medical Center, Los Angeles, and the UCLA School of Medicine, Los Angeles, CA.

Address for correspondence: William C. Shoemaker, M.D., Harbor/UCLA Medical Center, Box 15, 1000 West Carson St., Torrance, CA 90509.

Received Feb. 12, 1985; revision accepted Aug. 1, 1985.

ticularly those with intermittent claudication, manifest tissue hypoxia only when limb oxygen demand is increased. Diagnostic methods that increase limb oxygen demand include temporary limb ischemia and treadmill exercise testing. However, the latter may cause muscular contractions that hinder local blood flow,[16] thereby obscuring the $Ptco_2$ response. Moreover, treadmill exercise testing may be unsuited for routine clinical screening, particularly in patients with pain at rest, ischemic ulceration, amputation, or cardiopulmonary disease.

Stressing limb circulation by temporary ischemia, on the other hand, exaggerates reduced limb perfusion secondary to stenotic arterial lesions without the inherent limitations of treadmill exercise testing. The transcutaneous oxygen recovery half-time (TORT), defined as the time required to recover half of the decrease in the limb/chest $Ptco_2$ ratio caused by 4 min of pneumatic cuff occlusion below the knee, was found to be superior to resting $Ptco_2$ measurements in the diagnosis of PVD.[10, 12] This report describes a prospective study designed to compare the utility of postocclusive TORT and toe PRT/2 measurements in the assessment of limb circulation in patients with PVD.

Materials and methods

Patient selection. Paired measurements of calf and foot TORT were performed on 106 occasions in 90 limbs of 47 subjects. Of these, 36 were consecutive readmissions for operative therapy of symptomatic PVD; the remaining subjects were healthy volunteers who were evaluated to establish the normal range of TORT values. All symptomatic patients had angiographic evidence of high-grade large-vessel PVD; the status of each limb was assessed by the admitting surgeon on the basis of the history and physical examination. Patients ranged in age from 21 to 71 years; their mean age was 55 ± 9 (SD) years and 25 were men and 11 were women. Twenty-five of the patients were heavy smokers and 11 had diabetes; four patients had undergone prior vascular reconstruction and presented with failed vascular bypass grafts.

Group 1, the control group, comprised 22 limbs of healthy, normal volunteer subjects. These control subjects had no signs or symptoms of PVD and ranged in age from 20 to 70 years (mean 50 ± 17 [SD]). Group 2 comprised 18 asymptomatic limbs of patients with symptomatic PVD in their contralateral extremities. Group 3a included 32 symptomatic limbs of patients who had a clinical diagnosis of intermittent claudication and group 3b included 18 symptomatic limbs of patients who had a clinical diagnosis of pain at rest. Group 4 comprised 16 limbs of patients in groups 3a and 3b who were restudied 1 to 2 weeks after having undergone successful vascular reconstruction. Nine of these patients had undergone aortofemoral bypass, six had femoropopliteal bypass, and one had an axillofemoral bypass. Successful vascular reconstruction was defined as that resulting in significant relief of symptoms and improvement in conventional vascular hemodynamic measurements.

TORT. Transcutaneous oxygen sensors (Kontron, Roche Inc., Everett, MA) were set at 44° C and calibrated to room air. Areas on the anterior chest, medial midcalf, and dorsum of the foot were cleansed with an alcohol pad and the sensors were affixed to the skin with the double-sided adhesive rings and contact gel supplied by the manufacturer. A standard blood pressure cuff with an inflatable bladder 8 cm wide and of sufficient length to encircle the limb was loosely applied below the knee. The distance from the lower border of the cuff to the calf sensor was approximately 3 to 4 inches to allow adequate sensor contact during cuff inflation. Sensors were allowed to equilibrate with the subject in the supine position for 10 min. The pneumatic cuff was then inflated to 50 mm Hg above the systolic arterial pressure for a period of 4 min and then rapidly deflated. This duration of ischemia is identical to that used for measurement of the toe PRT/2[5] because oxygen stores in skin and muscle become exhausted less than 4 min after circulatory arrest.[17] Simultaneous chest, calf, and foot $Ptco_2$ values were recorded (1) during the control period, (2) after 4 min of cuff inflation, and (3) at 30 sec intervals for 5 min after cuff deflation. Because the $Ptco_2$ after transient limb ischemia returns to baseline levels in an exponential fashion and with a large time constant, extrapolation of the data is unnecessary; TORT values are measured to the nearest 30 sec interval.[12] Calibration of the $Ptco_2$ sensors was rechecked at the end of each study. The $Ptco_2$ response to temporary limb ischemia was determined by the TORT.

Toe PRT/2. Measurement of the toe PRT/2 was performed in all symptomatic patients by a conventional method[18] using a mercury-in-rubber gauge (Life Sciences, Inc, Greenwich, CT). The pulse volume response to temporary limb ischemia was determined by the toe PRT/2, defined as the time required to recover half of the control pulse amplitude.[5] To reduce bias, measurements of TORT and toe PRT/2 were performed and analyzed by two different researchers, neither of which was aware of the other's test results. Instances in which testing was not feasible were also noted.

Data analysis. The significance of the differences in TORT and toe PRT/2 values in the clinical groups was determined by unpaired Student's t test; the significance of the improvement in TORT and toe PRT/2 values after vascular reconstruction was determined by paired Student's t test. The 95% confidence intervals for values of calf and foot TORT in healthy volunteers were determined to establish normal ranges. Results are reported as mean ± SD.

Results

Normal subjects. The resting limb $Ptco_2$ values and limb/chest $Ptco_2$ ratios in subjects in group 1 varied considerably (table 1; figure 1). However, TORT values were remarkably similar in all normal subjects. The coefficient of variation for calf and foot TORT values in normal subjects was less between limbs of the same subject than between limbs of different subjects. Coefficients of variation for calf and foot TORT values in group 1 subjects were 0.37 and 0.27, respectively. The mean calf and foot TORT values were 0.8 ± 0.3 and 1.1 ± 0.3 min, respectively; only one limb had a TORT value greater than two standard deviations above the mean at either calf or foot location. Based on these data, calf TORT values greater than 1.4 and foot TORT values greater than 1.7 min were considered pathologic, since they were outside the 95% confidence level for normal subjects.

Patients with PVD. Group 2 patients frequently had

TABLE 1
TORT: $Ptco_2$ values before and after arterial occlusion

Sensor position	Subject group	Control	Arterial occlusion	Minutes after arterial occlusion									
				0.5	1.0	1.5	2.0	2.5	3.0	3.5	4.0	4.5	5.0
Chest	1	55±9	63±9	62±9	64±10	65±10	65±10	64±11	65±11	64±10	65±11	64±10	66±10
	2	49±13	52±12	52±10	52±12	51±11	52±11	52±10	52±11	51±11	52±11	51±11	53±12
	3a	50±11	55±11	54±11	55±12	55±11	55±11	55±11	56±11	55±11	55±11	55±11	56±12
	3b	51±24	56±21	57±20	57±20	57±20	57±20	57±19	57±20	56±20	56±19	55±19	55±19
	4	47±13	51±14	51±15	51±15	51±15	51±15	51±14	51±14	51±14	51±14	51±14	51±14
Calf	1	53±15	5±2	30±11	47±11	54±10	58±10	61±11	62±11	62±11	62±11	63±11	62±11
	2	43±8	6±6	14±12[A]	26±14	34±13	40±11	43±11	46±11	46±10	47±10	47±10	49±11
	3a	37±13	4±2	6±5[A]	13±10	21±15	27±16	33±16	37±15	40±14	41±13	43±13	43±13
	3b	29±20	4±2	6±5[A]	12±11	19±16	24±18	28±20	31±21	33±21	35±20	36±19	37±18
	4	42±15	7±4	16±12	28±15	36±15	41±15	44±15	46±15	46±15	47±15	47±15	47±14
Foot	1	47±12	7±8	19±10	35±12	45±11	51±11	54±11	60±11	57±10	58±11	58±11	58±11
	2	35±11	5±4	9±7[A]	19±13	25±13	33±13	37±11	41±11	42±10	43±10	43±9	45±11
	3a	33±14	5±3	5±3[A]	9±6	15±11	21±14	27±16	32±16	34±17	37±16	38±17	39±16
	3b	20±16	4±3	5±3[A]	6±5	10±9	13±12	15±15	17±16	20±17	21±18	21±17	22±18
	4	41±16	7±5	14±14	26±16	34±16	36±16	42±16	44±16	45±16	45±16	46±16	46±15

$Ptco_2$ values at rest, after 4 min of limb ischemia, and at 30 sec intervals during recovery. Values were recorded simultaneously at all three levels: chest, calf, and foot. Results are in mm Hg expressed as mean ± 1 SD. See Materials and methods for description of groups. Group 2, 3a, and 3b patients with PVD had lower control $Ptco_2$ values, but in most instances standard deviations overlap with $Ptco_2$ values that would be considered normal.
[A] $p < .001$ by unpaired t test for the differences between group 1 and group 2, 3a, and 3b values.

TORT values that were minimally or moderately prolonged in their asymptomatic limbs, suggesting poor circulatory reserve in these limbs. The mean calf and foot TORT values in patients in group 2 were 1.4 ± 0.4 and 1.6 ± 0.6 min, respectively.

In group 3a patients, both calf and foot TORT values were significantly longer in duration than those in normal subjects ($p < .001$). The mean calf and foot TORT values in patients with claudication (group 3a) were 2.1 ± 0.7 and 2.6 ± 1.0 min, respectively. All symptomatic limbs had a prolonged TORT value in either the calf or foot. An abnormal TORT value in conjunction with a normal TORT value at another site was occasionally found, suggesting variable segmental limb perfusion due to unevenly distributed disease and collateral circulation.

In patients with pain at rest, both calf and foot TORT values were also significantly longer in duration than those in normal subjects ($p < .001$). The mean calf and foot TORT values in patients in group 3b were 2.1 ± 1.1 and 3.4 ± 1.3 min, respectively. Although the diagnosis of symptomatic PVD was frequently obvious in these limbs, measurement of TORT was still a useful way to determine the adequacy of collateral blood flow to the foot. For example, in the three group 3b patients with prolonged calf TORT values but normal foot TORT values, angiograms revealed proximal occlusive disease with good collateral circulation to the foot.

By use of the strict diagnostic criteria of Fronek et al.[5] and Bernstein and Fronek,[18] toe PRT/2 values greater than 6 sec were considered pathologic. In our series, two patients had unequivocally normal toe PRT/2 values and six had minimally prolonged toe PRT/2 values in their symptomatic limbs, despite angiographic evidence of high-grade large-vessel PVD. All eight of these patients had abnormal TORT values in either the calf or foot.

Vascular reconstruction. Patients that underwent vascular reconstruction had significant improvement in their calf and foot TORT values postoperatively ($p < .005$ and $p < .0005$, respectively) (table 2; figure 2). In three of 16 limbs, the foot TORT significantly improved postoperatively, while there was no change in measured calf TORT values; this may be attributed to the topography of the bypassing vessel or prosthesis and to variations in segmental limb perfusion. The postoperative decrease in foot TORT values in these limbs, however, still indicated an improvement in overall limb perfusion after reconstructive surgery. Mean calf and foot TORT values in limbs that underwent vascular reconstruction (group 4) were 1.2 ± 0.4 and 1.2 ± 0.5 min, respectively.

Toe PRT/2 values usually improved postoperatively after vascular reconstruction; however, this improvement was not statistically significant in our series (table 2). Furthermore, toe pulses were unobtainable perioperatively in nine of 16 limbs (figure 2), thereby

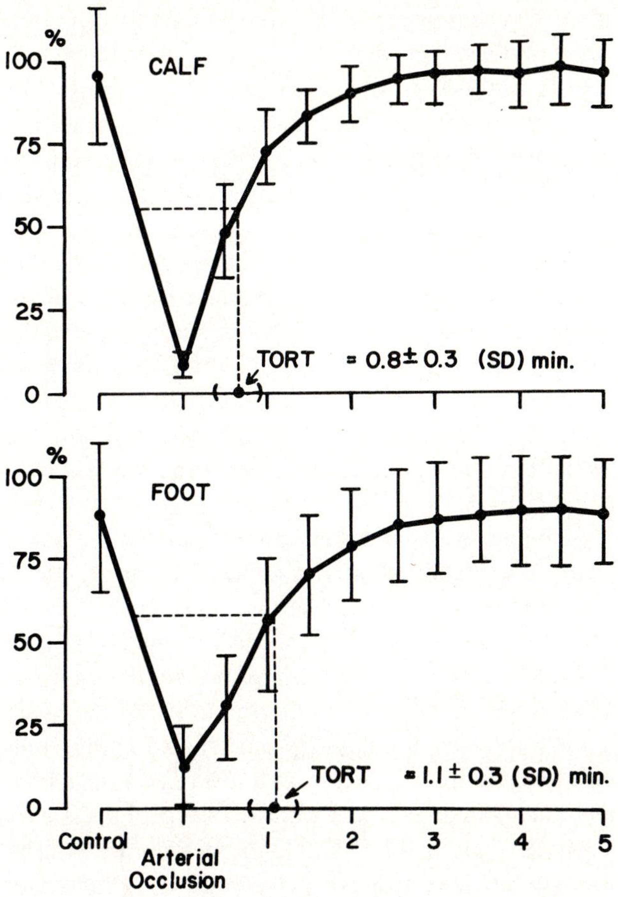

FIGURE 1. Effect of temporary limb ischemia on calf and foot $Ptco_2$ values, expressed as a percentage of the simultaneously recorded chest $Ptco_2$, in limbs of normal subjects ($n = 22$). Values shown represent mean ± 1 SD. Note the small variation in TORT values despite a large variation in resting $Ptco_2$ measurements.

precluding quantitative assessment of the results of surgical therapy in these limbs.

Correlation with symptoms. Foot TORT values correlated well with the severity of symptoms of PVD (figure 3). Patients in group 3b had significantly poorer foot TORT values than those in group 3a, who in turn

TABLE 2
Calf and foot TORT and toe PRT/2 values before and after vascular reconstruction

	Calf TORT (min)	Foot TORT (min)	Toe PRT/2 (sec)
Before vascular reconstruction	2.1±0.8	2.5±1.1	47±27
After vascular reconstruction	1.2±0.4	1.2±0.5	15±20
n	16	16	7[A]
p value	<.005	<.0005	NS

Results are expressed as mean ± 1 SD and compared by paired t test.
[A]Toe pulses were unobtainable perioperatively in nine of 16 limbs.

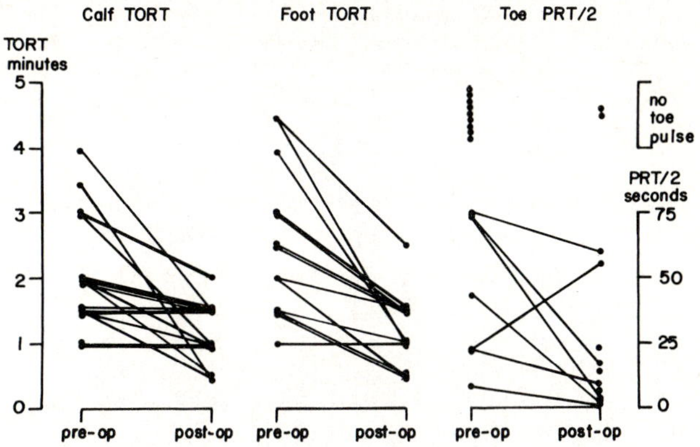

FIGURE 2. Calf and foot TORT values before and after vascular reconstruction in limbs of patients with PVD.

had significantly poorer values than those in asymptomatic limbs of patients in group 2. Foot TORT values in asymptomatic limbs of group 2 patients were significantly poorer than those obtained in normal subjects. There was no significant difference between foot TORT values in limbs of patients that underwent successful vascular reconstruction and values in limbs of normal subjects.

In limbs with measurable toe pulses, toe PRT/2 values did not correlate with the severity of symptoms of PVD since values in patients with intermittent claudication tended to be poorer than those in patients with pain at rest (figure 4). More important, toe pulses were unobtainable overall in 42% of limbs tested. Absent toe pulses did not necessarily indicate symptomatic PVD since the toe pulse was absent in nine asymptomatic limbs, two of which had undergone successful vascular reconstruction. Foot TORT values obtained in limbs with undetectable toe pulses, on the other

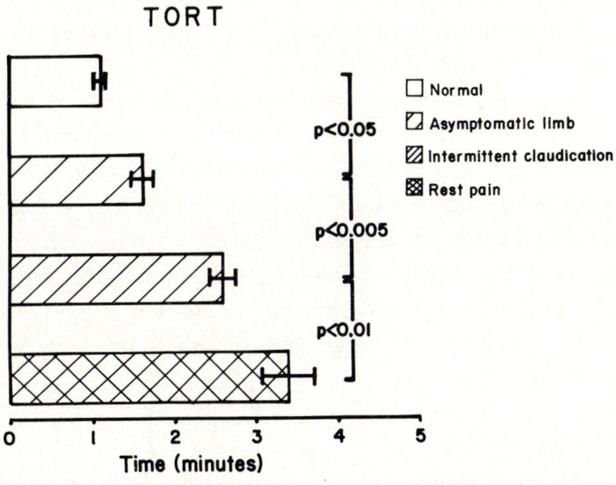

FIGURE 3. Foot TORT values classified according to severity of symptoms. Results are expressed as mean ± SEM and are compared by nonpaired Student's t test.

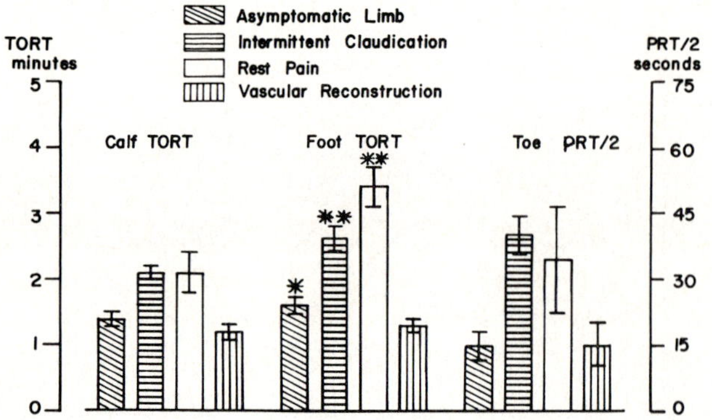

FIGURE 4. Calf and foot TORT and toe PRT/2 values, classified according to clinical status, in patients with PVD. Results are expressed as mean ± SEM. Note that foot TORT values correlated well with clinical status. $^{*}p < .05$, $^{**}p < .01$ by unpaired Student's t test for the differences between clinical groups (asymptomatic limbs vs intermittent claudication, intermittent claudication vs pain at rest, and normal vs asymptomatic limbs).

hand, correlated well with the severity of symptoms of PVD.

Foot ulcers. In our series, 12 patients presented with nonhealing foot ulcers. There was no significant difference in resting Pco_2 values, limb/chest $Ptco_2$ ratios, or TORT values in symptomatic patients with and without foot ulcers. Of these 12 patients, eight had diabetes and two had severe venous disease. Although diabetics represented only 22% of patients with pain at rest, 67% of patients with foot ulcers had diabetes. This is in agreement with the clinically recognized finding that diabetic patients are far more prone to develop nonhealing foot ulcers, perhaps due to neuropathic loss of sensation and decreased resistance to infection.

Of the 12 patients with foot ulcers, toe pulses were measurable in only seven (58%). In the remaining patients, toe PRT/2 values were not significantly different from those in symptomatic patients without foot ulcers.

Angiography. All patients with symptomatic PVD underwent monoplane angiographic examination of their lower extremities via the groin or axillary approach. Patients with intermittent claudication or pain at rest uniformly had angiographically defined high-grade large-vessel PVD in their symptomatic limbs. Asymptomatic limbs showed variable findings, including frequent large-vessel complete arterial obstructions.

Discussion

A simple method for the noninvasive assessment of limb circulation in patients with PVD based on the measurement of the TORT after temporary limb ischemia was compared with conventionally employed measurements of toe PRT/2. The measurement of TORT, defined as the time required to recover half of the decrease in the limb/chest $Ptco_2$ ratio caused by temporary limb ischemia, was found to be more feasible (100% vs 58%) and to have a higher correlation with symptoms and diagnostic yield (100% vs 92%) than the toe PRT/2. In addition, measurements of the PRT/2 and TORT may be obtained simultaneously, reducing the need for additional monitoring personnel or time. Previously, the use of TORT measurements were found to be superior to resting $Ptco_2$ values and limb/chest $Ptco_2$ ratios in the diagnosis of disease and quantification of limb perfusion in patients with PVD.[10, 12]

A major inclusion criteria for patients in the present study was readmission to the hospital for scheduled vascular reconstruction; the necessary baseline measurements from normal limbs was provided by healthy volunteers of similar age who were used in initial standardization studies. This criterion modifies the distribution of vascular pathology represented in this study and excludes most patients with severe end-stage PVD not amenable to surgical therapy, whose PVD is easiest to diagnose with resting $Ptco_2$ measurements. This is indicated by the large percentage of symptomatic limbs of patients with intermittent claudication (64%) vs those with pain at rest (36%).

In the present series, toe pulses were unobtainable in 12 of 32 (37%) of symptomatic limbs in patients with intermittent claudication. Furthermore, toe pulses were absent in 42% of all limbs tested, including nine asymptomatic limbs, two of which had undergone successful vascular reconstruction. This severely limits the application of toe PRT/2 measurements in the diagnosis of PVD. The reduction in local pulse pressure often seen in limbs of patients with PVD may make detection of toe pulses difficult, if not impossible. In addition, toe pulse pressure may give little indication of the circulatory state of the limb, since collateral pathways may permit a normal resting blood flow despite diminished local pulse pressure.[1]

Even if toe pulses are present, it is still desirable to have an objective quantitative measurement that correlates with the patient's degree of disability to evaluate the results of conservative and surgical therapy. The foot TORT was found to correlate well with severity of symptoms (table 3). Moreover, the TORT may have prognostic value, since it has been reported that patients with limb pain at rest usually have a poorer surgical outcome than those with intermittent claudication after vascular reconstruction.[19–22] The toe PRT/2

TABLE 3
Foot TORT values classified according to severity of symptoms

Patient group	Foot TORT (min)	n	p value
1	1.1±0.3	22	
			<.05
2	1.6±0.6	18	
			<.005
3a	2.6±1.0	32	
			<.01
3b	3.4±1.3	18	

Results are expressed as mean ± 1 SD and compared by nonpaired t test. See Materials and methods for description of groups.

has previously been shown to be of value in predicting the outcome of aortofemoral bypass surgery.[23]

Use of the TORT as an index of limb perfusion represents a significant advance in the noninvasive assessment of limb circulation with the use of $Ptco_2$ sensors. The TORT has been shown to be more sensitive and specific than resting $Ptco_2$ values and limb/chest $Ptco_2$ ratios in the diagnosis and quantification of limb circulation in patients with PVD.[12] Data from the present study indicate that TORT measurements also offer certain advantages over conventional noninvasive toe PRT/2 measurements. Use of the TORT in addition to conventional noninvasive vascular diagnostic techniques may lead to refined selection criteria for angiography and improved limb salvage as a result of the early discovery of potentially reconstructable disease.

References

1. Edholm OG, Howarth S, Sharpey-Shafer EP: Resting blood flow and blood pressure in limbs with arterial obstruction. Clin Sci **10:** 361, 1951
2. Lassen NA: Muscle blood flow in normal man and in patients with intermittent claudication evaluated by simultaneous Xe (133) and Na (24) clearance. J Clin Invest **43:** 1805, 1964
3. Strandell T, Wahren J: Circulation in the calf at rest, after arterial occlusion and after exercise in normal subjects and in patients with intermittent claudication. Acta Med Scand **173:** 99, 1963
4. Tonneson KH: The blood flow through the calf muscle during rhythmic contraction and in rest in patients with occlusive vascular disease measured by (133) Xenon. Scand J Clin Lab Invest **17:** 433, 1965
5. Fronek A, Coel M, Bernstein EF: The pulse-reappearance time: An index of over-all blood flow impairment in the ischemic extremity. Surgery **81:** 376, 1977
6. Tremper KK, Waxman K, Shoemaker WC: Effects of hypoxia and shock on transcutaneous PO_2 values in dogs. Crit Care Med **7:** 526, 1979
7. Huch A, Huch R, Menzer K, et al.: Eine Schuelle, behizte proberlachenelektrode zur koninuier lichen uberwache ung des PO_2 beim menschen. Elektrodenautbau und-eigen schaften. Stuttgart, Proc Medizin-Technik, May 16, 1972
8. Eberhard P, Mindt W, Hammacher K: Perkutane messung des sauerstat partaldnuckes. Methodik und Anwendungen. Stuttgart, Proc Medizin-Technik, May 16, 1972
9. Matsen FA, Wyss CR, Pedegana LR, Krugmire RB, Simmons CW, King RV, Burgess EM: Transcutaneous oxygen tension measurement in peripheral vascular disease. Surg Gynecol Obstet **150:** 525, 1980
10. Franzeck VK, Talke P, Bernstein EF, Golbranson FL, Fronek A: Transcutaneous PO_2 measurements in health and peripheral arterial occlusive disease. Surgery **91:** 156, 1982
11. White RA, Nolan L, Harley D, Long J, Klein S, Tremper K, Nelson R, Tabrisky J, Shoemaker W: Noninvasive evaluation of peripheral vascular disease using transcutaneous oxygen tension. Am J Surg **144:** 68, 1982
12. Kram HB, Appel PL, White RA, Shoemaker WC: Assessment of peripheral vascular disease by postocclusive transcutaneous oxygen recovery time. J Vasc Surg **1:** 628, 1984
13. Kram HB, Shoemaker WC: Diagnosis of major peripheral arterial trauma by transcutaneous oxygen monitoring. Am J Surg **147:** 776, 1984
14. Kram HB, Shoemaker WC: Use of transcutaneous O_2 monitoring in the intraoperative management of severe peripheral vascular disease. Crit Care Med **11:** 482, 1983
15. Kram HB, Wright J, Shoemaker WC, Klein S: Perioperative transcutaneous O_2 monitoring in the management of major peripheral arterial trauma. J Trauma **24:** 443, 1984
16. Dornhorst AC: Hyperaemia induced by exercise and ischemia. Br Med Bull **19:** 137, 1963
17. Barcroft H: The mechanism of vasodilation in the limbs during and after arrest of the circulation. Angiology **23:** 595, 1972
18. Bernstein EF, Fronek A: Current status of noninvasive tests in the diagnosis of peripheral arterial disease. Surg Clin North Am **62:** 473, 1982
19. Dean RH, Yao JST, Stanton PE, Bergan JJ: Prognostic indicators in femoropopliteal reconstructions. Arch Surg **110:** 1287, 1978
20. Lee BY, Thoden WF, McCann WJ, Kavner D, Trainor FS, Madden JL: Prognosis of reconstructions for femoropopliteal occlusive disease. Cont Surg **20:** 61, 1982
21. Darling RC, Linton RR: Durability of femoropopliteal reconstructions: Endarterectomy versus vein bypass grafts. Am J Surg **123:** 472, 1972
22. DeWeese JA, Rob CG: Autogenous venous bypass grafts five years later. Am Surg **174:** 346, 1971
23. Bernstein EF, Rhodes GA, Stuart SH, Coel MN, Fronek A: Toe pulse reappearance time in prediction of aortofemoral bypass success. Ann Surg **193:** 201, 1981

Computer detection of atrioventricular dissociation from surface electrocardiograms during wide QRS complex tachycardias

JANET SLOCUM, M.S., ERNEST BYROM, PH.D., LYNN MCCARTHY, R.N., ALAN SAHAKIAN, PH.D., AND STEVEN SWIRYN, M.D.

ABSTRACT Differentiation of wide QRS complex tachycardias on surface electrocardiograms is difficult for physicians and computers due in part to their inability to identify atrial activity, specifically atrioventricular (AV) dissociation. We studied 20 examples of AV associated rhythms and 17 examples of AV dissociated ventricular tachycardia. We applied an algorithm consisting of subtraction of a mean beat from each individual beat in leads II and V_1 to generate remainder electrocardiograms. The remainder electrocardiograms were visually inspected for the presence of P wave candidates and then autocorrelated. AV dissociated P wave candidates were evident on visual inspection of remainder electrocardiograms in none of 20 AV associated and 15 of 17 AV dissociated rhythms. Atrial cycle length and the presence of AV dissociation were automatically detected by applying a peak selection algorithm to the autocorrelation function. AV association was detected in all 20 AV associated rhythms and AV dissociation was detected for 11 of 17 AV dissociated rhythms (sensitivity 65%, specificity 100%, positive and negative predictive accuracy 100%, 77%). The correlation coefficient of detected vs true atrial cycle length for the 11 correctly detected AV dissociated rhythms was r = .98. Visual inspection of the remainder electrocardiograms along with the original electrocardiogram may increase the ease with which human readers can identify the presence of AV dissociation and thus diagnose ventricular tachycardia. Computer diagnosis of wide QRS complex tachycardias should be significantly improved by use of this algorithm.
Circulation 72, No. 5, 1028–1036, 1985.

DETECTION of atrial activity is the most significant limiting factor of the accuracy of current algorithms for diagnosis of arrhythmias by computer.[1] The reason for this is that on the surface electrocardiogram, atrial activity is often represented by small amplitude waves that may be buried in QRS complexes or T waves. Of particular clinical significance is the detection of atrial activity, specifically atrioventricular (AV) dissociation, during a wide QRS complex tachycardia. While occasional instances of supraventricular tachycardias with AV dissociation have been reported, AV dissociation during a wide QRS complex tachycardia is considered virtually diagnostic for ventricular tachycardia.[2] Wellens et al.[3] found that approximately half of ventricular tachycardias are AV dissociated and fewer than one-third had a 1 : 1 ventriculoatrial conduction ratio. The percentage of AV dissociated ventricular tachycardias increases somewhat when the ventricular rate exceeds 200 beats/min.

Historically, arrhythmia algorithms have determined atrial activity by searching the isoelectric region between the end of the T wave and the beginning of the following QRS complex for P wave candidates.[4–19] P waves have been found by a variety of approaches, such as slope measurement,[4–16] difference functions,[17, 18] and matched filters.[19] Some algorithms for interpretation of arrhythmias assume any detected P wave candidate a valid P wave, while in others additional criteria must be fulfilled (e.g., those relating to expected P wave width, slope, and PR interval) to validate a P wave candidate. All of these methods of P wave detection depend on detectable P waves occurring between the end of the T wave and the beginning of the following QRS complex. Such methods are unlikely to be reliable at rapid ventricular rates since little

From the Department of Electrical Engineering and Computer Science, Northwestern University, and the Division of Cardiology, Department of Medicine, Evanston Hospital, Evanston, IL, and Northwestern University Medical School, Chicago.

Supported in part by a grant from Marquette Electronics, Inc.

Address for correspondence: Steven Swiryn, M.D., Director, Cardiac Electrophysiology, Evanston Hospital, 2650 Ridge Ave., Evanston, IL 60201.

Received March 18, 1985; revision accepted Aug. 8, 1985.

or no isoelectric region is present between the end of the T wave and the beginning of the following QRS complex.

Stark et al.[20] reported a method for the detection of AV dissociated P waves that involves taking the average of several consecutive QRST segments to generate a template. The template is then lined up and subtracted from each individual beat. The AV dissociated P waves can then be detected on the remaining signal. Unfortunately, no results with this method have been reported. Additional studies have used similar algorithms involving calculations of a template and subtraction to identify changes in the morphology of the QRS complex.[21]

Recent studies of two widely used computerized electrocardiographic analysis systems have shown poor or no ability to diagnose ventricular tachycardia.[22, 23] In both cases failure was attributed to the inability of the systems to detect P waves, and neither system attempts to identify AV dissociation.

Differentiation of wide QRS complex tachycardias is difficult for the physician as well as for the computer. It has been suggested that based on the surface electrocardiogram, expert electrocardiographers can be certain of the diagnosis in only 50% of cases.[2] Physicians also attribute this to the difficulty with detecting atrial activity. To accurately assess atrial activity, intra-atrial electrodes[24] and esophageal leads[25] have been used.

We present a method that detects AV dissociation by looking for a series of P waves that may appear in any part of the RR interval instead of attempting to detect individual P waves. Our method involves subtracting a mean beat from surface leads to generate a remainder electrocardiogram. The remainder electrocardiogram is visually inspected for P wave candidates and autocorrelated. The output of the autocorrelation function is then used to automatically detect the presence of AV dissociation and the atrial cycle length for AV dissociated rhythms.

Methods

The data base for this study consisted of electrocardiograms from two sources. The first was analog tape recordings from the electrophysiology laboratory and included both surface leads and simultaneous intra-atrial electrograms. The second source was a commercial computerized electrocardiogram system (Marquette Electronics; Milwaukee, WI) that provided standard 12-lead electrocardiograms in digital form. Each data source provided 10 sec rhythm strips. Both leads II and V_1 were analyzed, except in six cases in which lead II was unavailable. In all cases, the diagnosis of ventricular tachycardia was confirmed in the electrophysiology laboratory by standard criteria.[26] Other rhythm diagnoses were determined in the electrophysiology laboratory or with the use of standard electrocardiographic criteria.

For each rhythm, the presence or absence of AV dissociation and true atrial cycle length were determined from simultaneous intra-atrial recordings (when available) or from surface leads. For the purposes of this study we use the term AV dissociation to mean the presence of P waves at a rate slower than the ventricular rate. While not technically correct, we refer in this report to rhythms with intact ventriculoatrial conduction but conduction ratios greater than or equal to 2:1 as AV dissociated rhythms (one of 17 rhythms). This is because the algorithm cannot currently distinguish such rhythms from those that are truly AV dissociated and the implication of both types of atrial activity for the differential diagnosis of wide QRS complex tachycardias is the same. In addition, the detection of AV dissociation by our algorithm requires that P waves be present and therefore rhythms with atrial fibrillation were excluded from the analysis. Unstable rhythms such as polymorphic tachycardias were also excluded. Computer processing was done with a Masscomp MCS-563 system (Massachusetts Computer; Littleton, MA).

Preprocessing. Data from the electrophysiology laboratory were played back from analog tape through an antialiasing filter with a cutoff frequency of 500 Hz and then digitized at 1200 Hz. The waveform was then low-pass filtered at 60 Hz. Data from the commercial electrocardiogram system had been digitized at 250 Hz, filtered, and compressed for the commercial system, and were decompressed and transferred to our computer.

When long strips of data were available (i.e., from the electrophysiology laboratory), 10 sec strips of data without premature ventricular complexes, fusion beats, or amplifier saturation were obtained. No special attempt was made to avoid otherwise noisy electrocardiograms. Each beat in the 10 sec rhythm strip was classified as either a dominant or anomalous beat. Beats that contained QRS complexes of the most common morphology for the rhythm strip were defined as dominant beats. Premature ventricular beats, fusion beats, or beats that saturated the amplifiers were defined as anomalous beats.

Fiducial points were marked for both dominant and anomalous beats and a baseline wander correction was applied. The baseline correction algorithm calculated the mean of successive 2 beat intervals and subtracted the linear trend. Fiducial point marking and beat classification were done by hand for electrophysiology laboratory data. The commercial electrocardiogram system automatically determined fiducial points and classified beats as part of its routine processing. These data were obtained in digital form along with the rhythm strips.

Mean beat and remainder electrocardiogram calculation. The mean ventricular cycle length for each rhythm strip was calculated by averaging the intervals between the fiducial points of consecutive dominant beats. For each beat in the 10 sec rhythm, a beat window was defined as a segment of the rhythm strip equal in length to the mean ventricular cycle length with the fiducial point at its center. A mean beat was generated for leads II and V_1 by averaging every dominant beat window. The mean beat was then lined up against all beat windows in the 10 sec strip and subtracted to generate remainder electrocardiograms.

We reasoned that some anomalous beats may be capture beats with fusion and would therefore be preceded by P waves. It would be desirable in these cases to zero the QRS complex of the anomalous beats to prevent their large remainders from contributing to the autocorrelation function (see below), while attempting to preserve the P waves that occur before them. We therefore zeroed only the part of the beat windows containing anomalous beats beginning at 120 msec before the fiducial points and ending at the end of the window. The earlier part of the window was retained with the appropriate segment of the mean beat subtracted from it.

After subtraction, the data from the electrophysiology laboratory were reduced to 240 Hz for further processing, while the commercial electrocardiogram data were kept at 250 Hz. The remainder electrocardiograms were smoothed by taking the mean of five consecutive data points as the value for the center point. The subtraction process was found to subtract between 71% and 97% of the original signal. Remainder electrocardiograms were examined subjectively and autocorrelated.

Autocorrelation. The autocorrelation function gives a measure of similarity of a signal and the same signal shifted in time. The value of the autocorrelation function at each time shift of interest equals the sum of data points in the product of the original signal and the shifted signal (figure 1). The autocorrelation function of a periodic signal will have a peak at the cycle length of the repetitive waveform. This feature makes the autocorrelation function useful for detecting the periodicity of a signal in noise.[27]

After subtraction of the mean beat, the remainder electrocardiogram will contain signals that are not synchronous with the QRS complexes, such as AV dissociated P waves, muscle artifacts, and noise in addition to the beat to beat fluctuations of QRST morphology. If the atrial activity is periodic and AV dissociated, the autocorrelation of the remainder electrocardiogram will contain a peak at the atrial cycle length and multiples of the cycle length. A suitable peak selection algorithm may then automatically detect the atrial cycle length.

Autocorrelation was performed on two consecutive 1024-point segments of the remainder electrocardiogram giving a resolution of one sample period of from 0 to 2.5 sec.[28] The autocorrelations were then averaged and a peak detection algorithm (see below) was applied.

Computer detection of AV dissociation. Autocorrelation functions for leads II and V_1 were processed separately. Since AV dissociated P waves were expected to have a cycle length longer than the ventricular cycle length and shorter than 1200 msec, only this portion of the autocorrelation function was examined. A peak selection algorithm applied slope and amplitude criteria to the maximum of the examined portion of the autocorrelation function. Values for the slope and amplitude criteria were chosen empirically to avoid falsely identifying AV associated rhythms as AV dissociated rhythms. If the criteria were met, the cycle length at the maximum of the autocorrelation function was identified as the "detected cycle length." If the maximum did not meet the criteria, the rhythm was identified as AV associated and the computer processing was complete.

If a detected cycle length was identified, the computer continued processing to determine whether this cycle length was different from the ventricular cycle length. If the detected cycle length was within an allowable error of the true ventricular cycle length then the computer identified the rhythm as AV associated and the detected cycle length as the ventricular cycle length. Otherwise, the rhythm was identified as AV dissociated and the detected cycle length was identified as the detected atrial cycle length. The allowable error for detected cycle length was chosen

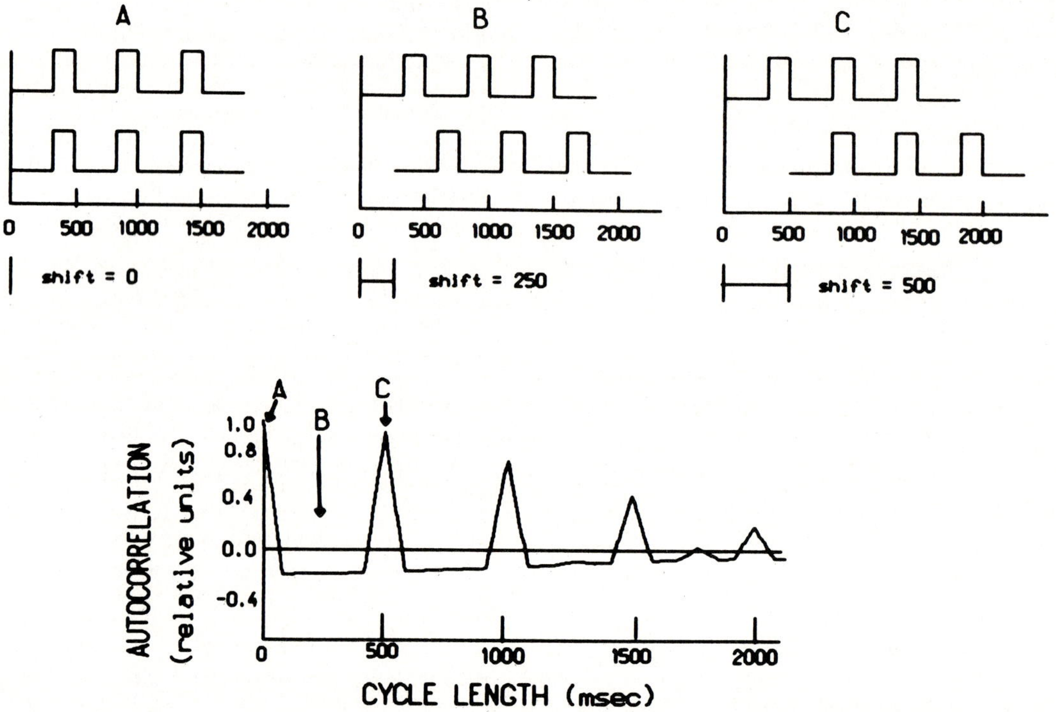

FIGURE 1. The autocorrelation of a rectangular wave with a 500 msec cycle length. The autocorrelation function has three time shifts marked on it that correspond to each of the three panels above it. *A*, The original signal and the signal with a time shift of 0 msec below it. The autocorrelation function is calculated by multiplying the value of the signal by the value of the shifted signal for each data point and summing the results. The autocorrelation of a time shift of 0 always equals the maximum of the autocorrelation function since the signal is identical to itself at that time. (In *A*, large values within the rectangular waves of the original signal are multiplied by large values within the rectangular waves of the shifted signal, while data points with a small value are multiplied by small values in the shifted signal. The result is a large sum.) *B*, The original signal and the signal with a shift of 250 msec. The rectangular waves no longer overlap and the autocorrelation at this time shift will be small, since large values within the rectangular waves are now multiplied by small values within the shifted signal. *C*, The original signal and the signal with a shift of 500 msec. The rectangular waves line up again at this time shift, producing a peak in the autocorrelation function.

as the standard deviation of RR invervals of consecutive dominant beats plus 8 msec. Thus, the greater the variation in RR intervals, the greater the allowable error.

A peak detected at a cycle length different from the ventricular cycle length is likely to represent a meaningful waveform, specifically AV dissociated P waves. By contrast, a peak detected at the ventricular cycle length is most likely to represent artifacts from subtraction of QRS complexes and T waves.

The results of applying the peak selection algorithm to data from the two leads were output by the computer and compared. If AV dissociation was found in either lead, the rhythm was considered AV dissociated with the corresponding detected atrial cycle length. If both leads were detected as AV associated, the rhythm was considered AV associated.

Results

The data base for this study consisted of 37 rhythms. Of these rhythms, 20 were recorded in the electrophysiology laboratory and the remaining 17 were routinely recorded by the commercial computerized electrocardiogram system. The true presence or absence of AV dissociation and the true atrial cycle length were determined from simultaneously recorded intra-atrial electrograms (20 rhythms, 12 associated and eight dissociated) or from surface leads (17 rhythms, nine associated and eight dissociated). Both leads II and V_1 were analyzed (31 rhythms), except when lead II was unavailable (six rhythms). All rhythms obtained from the computerized electrocardiogram system were first analyzed by the Marquette 12SL system. None of the rhythms was called AV dissociated by their algorithm.

Twenty of the 37 rhythms analyzed were AV associated. Eleven of the 20 were wide QRS tachycardias (ventricular tachycardias with intact ventriculoatrial conduction, three; assorted supraventricular tachycardias, eight). The ventricular cycle length of the AV associated tachycardias ranged from 552 to 272 msec (mean $\pm$SD 432 $\pm$ 98 msec). The remaining nine of the 20 AV associated rhythms were narrow QRS rhythms (sinus rhythm, seven; supraventricular tachycardia, two).

Seventeen of the 37 rhythms analyzed were AV dissociated. All 17 were ventricular tachycardias with cycle lengths ranging from 628 to 192 msec (399 $\pm$ 117 msec). The mean cycle lengths of the AV associated and AV dissociated tachycardias were not significantly different ($p = .21$).

Computer detection of AV dissociation. The computer correctly identified all 20 AV associated rhythms and 11 of the 17 AV dissociated rhythms (six of eight from the electrophysiology laboratory and five of nine from the commercial system) and incorrectly identified six of the latter as AV associated. This algorithm for detection of AV dissociation therefore had a sensitivity of 65% and a specificity of 100% for this data set. The algorithm had a positive predictive value of 100% and a negative predictive value of 77%. Of the 11 correctly identified AV dissociated rhythms, the detected atrial cycle length was within 20 msec of the true atrial cycle length in all but one rhythm in which the detected atrial cycle length was 77 msec less than the true cycle length. The correlation coefficient of the true vs detected atrial cycle length was $r = .98$. Of the 11 correctly identified AV dissociated rhythms, atrial cycle length was detected in all analyzed leads (6/11 rhythms) or in one of the two leads (1/11 rhythms in lead V_1, 4/11 rhythms in lead II). For all rhythms in which AV dissociation was found in both analyzed leads, the atrial cycle lengths detected in leads V_1 and II were identical.

Remainder electrocardiograms. Visual inspection of remainder electrocardiograms was performed. Major features of the remainder electrocardiograms from AV associated rhythms usually occurred coincident with the most prominent features of the original electrocardiograms, namely QRS complexes and T waves (figure 2). Thus, prominent features often recurred at regular intervals equal ot the ventricular cycle length. Of the 20 remainder electrocardiograms from AV associated rhythms, visible features recurring at the ventricular cycle length were evident in all analyzed leads (15/20 rhythms), in one of two leads (4/20 rhythms), or in neither lead (1/20 rhythms). There were no prominent features that recurred at an interval other than the ventricular cycle length in any of the 20 remainder electrocardiograms from AV associated rhythms.

Major features of the remainder electrocardiograms of the AV dissociated rhythms often recurred coincident with the most prominent features of the original electrocardiogram, as they did for AV associated rhythms, and thus they also often recurred at regular intervals equal to the ventricular cycle length. Of the 17 AV dissociated rhythms, visible features recurring at the ventricular cycle length were evident in remainder electrocardiograms of all analyzed leads (4/17 rhythms), in one of the two leads (6/17 rhythms), or in neither lead (7/17 rhythms). However, in addition to features recurring at the ventricular cycle length, 15 of the 17 remainder electrocardiograms for AV dissociated rhythms also had prominent features that recurred at a cycle length different than the ventricular cycle length (figure 3). In each case, these features were coincident with atrial activity as assessed by simultaneous intra-atrial electrograms or from surface leads and were therefore labeled P wave candidates. P wave candidates were evident in all analyzed leads (13/17

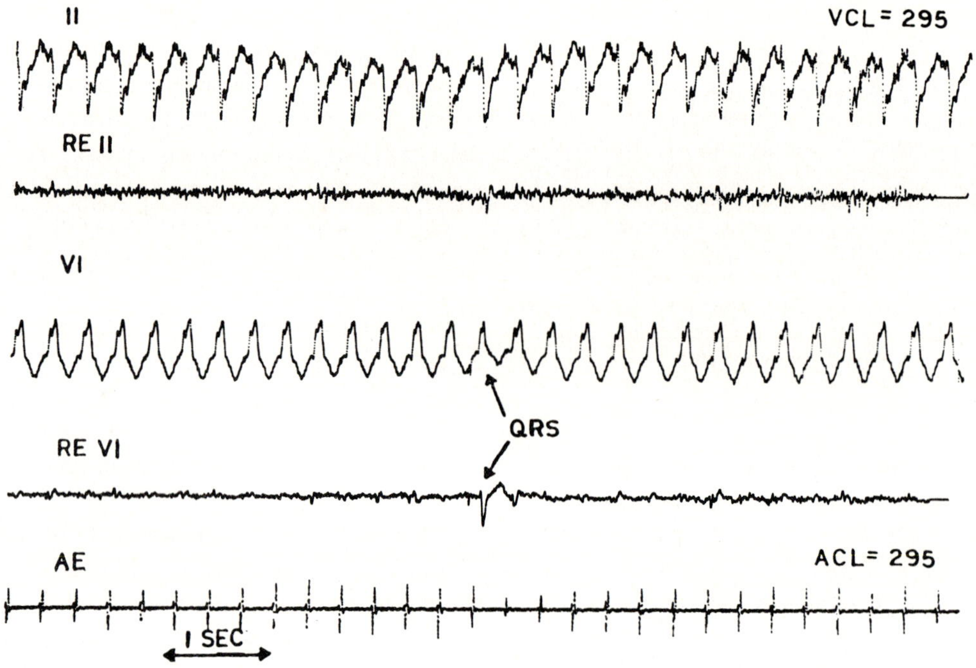

FIGURE 2. Leads II and V_1 and their respective remainder electrocardiograms (RE) from a patient with AV nodal reentrant tachycardia and rate-dependent right bundle branch block with left-axis deviation. Atrial electrograms (AE) show the presence of AV association. The remainder electrocardiograms show repetitive features coincident only with QRS complexes (arrows). The atrial (ACL) and ventricular cycle lengths (VCL) are in msec.

rhythms), in one of the two leads (2/17 rhythms), or in neither lead (2/17 rhythms). When P wave candidates were visible in a given remainder electrocardiogram, most but not all true P waves had a corresponding P wave candidate and some P wave candidates were visible in only one lead (figures 4 and 5).

Autocorrelation function. Plots of the autocorrelation functions of remainder electrocardiograms were varied in shape. Allowable error used to determine how far a peak could be from the mean ventricular cycle length and still be labeled as such ranged from 16 to 104 msec (33 ± 18 msec). Remainder electrocardiograms with major features recurring at the ventricular cycle length usually produced autocorrelation functions with peaks at the ventricular cycle length and multiples of the cycle length. Signals with substantial 60 cycle noise or with very little amplitude in the remainder electrocardiogram produced plots that showed little correlation and no clear peaks (figure 6). Some remainder electrocardiograms that contained wide deflections with no repetitive patterns produced autocorrelation plots with small peaks at many different intervals. Remainder electrocardiograms with P wave candidates usually produced autocorrelation plots with peaks at the cycle length of the P wave candidates and multiples of the cycle length (figures 7 and 8), thus allowing detection of AV dissociation.

Description of errors. The computer incorrectly identified six of the AV dissociated rhythms as AV associated. For two of these rhythms only lead V_1 was available for study. Three additional rhythms, one with frequent anomalous beats, had the true atrial cycle length as the maximum of the autocorrelation function but the peak failed the amplitude criteria.

The final AV dissociated rhythm that was incorrectly identified by the computer had a true atrial cycle length that was only 5 msec different than the true ventricular cycle length, thus making detection of AV dissociation with a cutoff of more than 8 msec in allowable error impossible. The computer correctly identified the atrial cycle length. In addition, P wave candidates were visible in the remainder electrocardiogram.

Discussion

The computer correctly identified all of the 20 AV associated rhythms and 11 of the 17 AV dissociated rhythms. This is comparable to the reported success of human electrocardiographers[2] and superior to currently available computer algorithms.[22, 23] For the 11 correctly identified AV dissociated rhythms, a close correlation was found between detected and true atrial cycle lengths. Of the 17 AV dissociated rhythms, P wave candidates were evident by visual inspection of the remainder electrocardiogram in 15.

For two undetected AV dissociated rhythms and the one that was detected with an incorrect atrial cycle

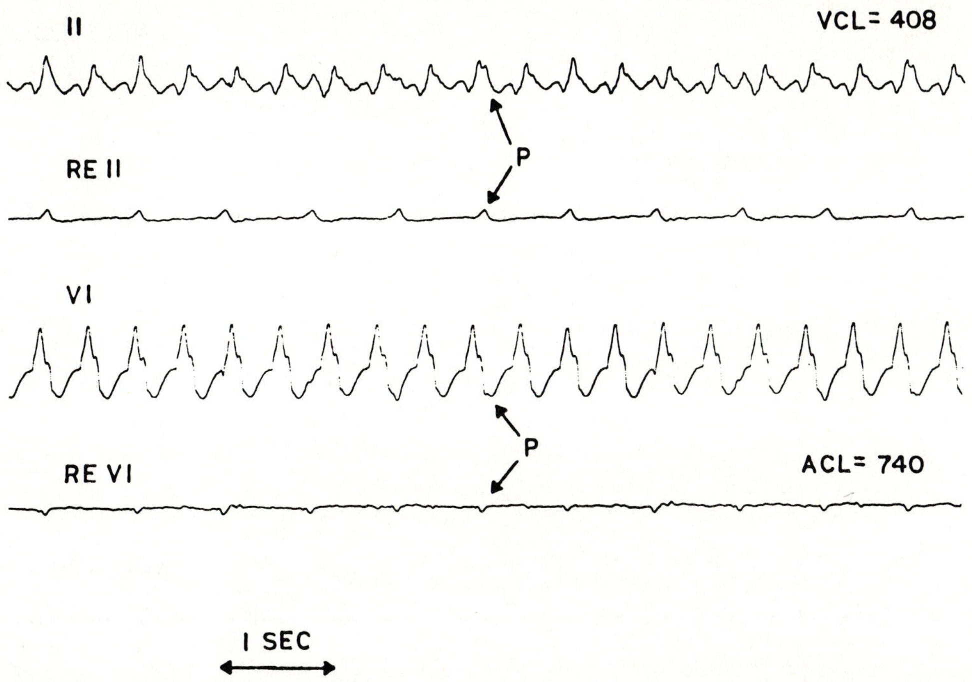

FIGURE 3. Leads II and V_1 and their respective remainder electrocardiograms (RE) from a patient with ventricular tachycardia. True atrial (ACL) and ventricular (VCL) cycle lengths are given in msec. Both remainder electrocardiograms show prominent P wave candidates (P). It is easily verified by the reader of the electrocardiogram that these P wave candidates correspond to P waves in the original signal. While the presence of AV dissociation may be diagnosed in this rhythm with the use of surface leads alone, the display of remainder electrocardiograms along with the original rhythms makes the presence of AV dissociation easily observable.

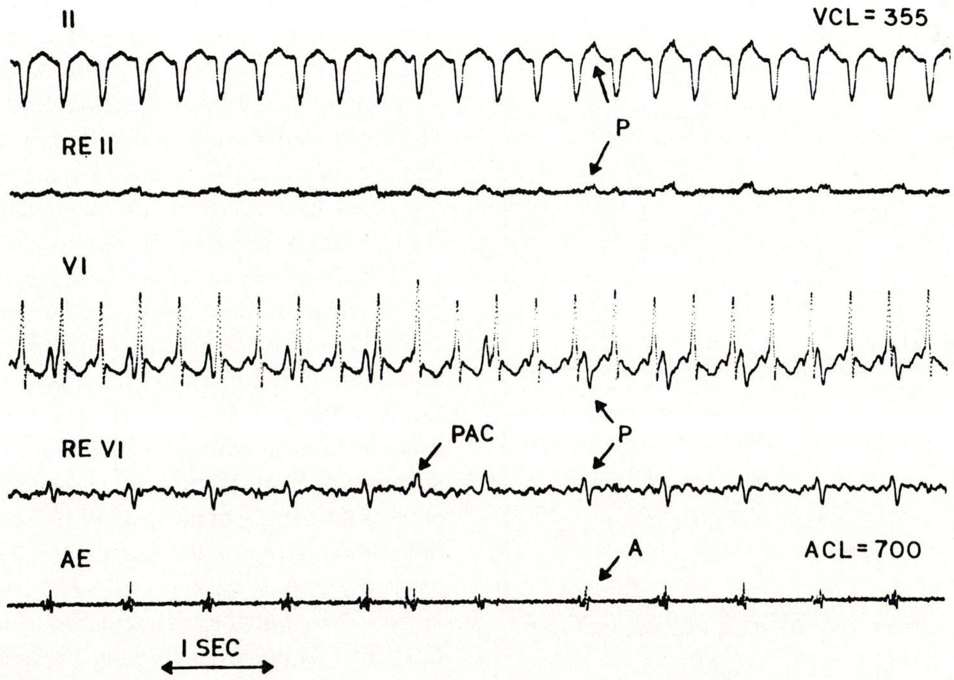

FIGURE 4. Leads II and V_1 and their respective remainder electrocardiograms (RE) from a patient with ventricular tachycardia. Atrial electrograms (AE) show the presence of AV dissociation. True atrial (ACL) and ventricular (VCL) cycle lengths are given in msec. On the remainder electrocardiograms, the repetitive features occurring simultaneously with the atrial electrogram (A) are termed P wave candidates (P). The remainder electrocardiogram from lead V_1 demonstrates two P wave candidate morphologies consistent with sinus P waves and two premature atrial complexes (PAC).

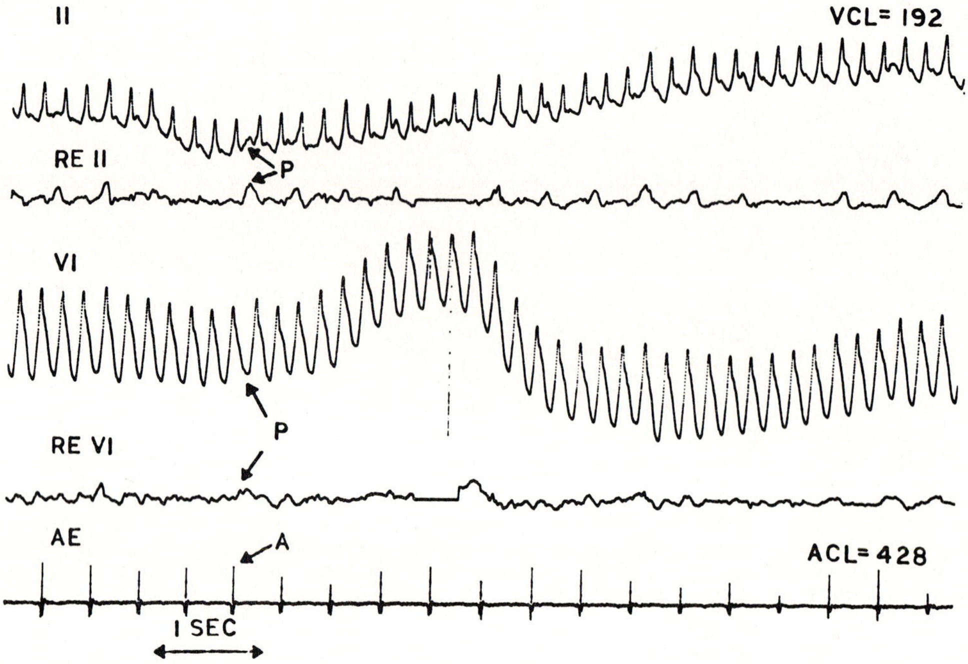

FIGURE 5. Leads II and V_1 and their respective remainder electrocardiograms (RE) from a patient with ventricular tachycardia. Atrial electrograms (AE) show the presence of AV dissociation. True atrial (ACL) and ventricular (VCL) cycle lengths are given in msec. Most, but not all, atrial electrograms (A) have P wave candidates (P) that can be visually detected on the remainder electrocardiograms in lead II despite substantial baseline wander and a short ventricular cycle length.

length only lead V_1 was available for analysis. Lead V_1 is a good choice for visual inspection of the remainder electrocardiogram since P waves tend to be large compared with the QRS complex, but it may not be the best choice for analysis by autocorrelation because the P waves are biphasic. The biphasic P waves cause negative and positive peaks in the autocorrelation function and reduce the amplitude of the peak of the detected atrial cycle length. Of the 11 correctly detected AV dissociated rhythms, seven were detected in lead V_1 and 10 were in lead II. It might be possible to take advantage of the large P waves in lead V_1 by integrating the remainder electrocardiogram to get P waves that are only positive in excursion. Use of a different choice of leads, such as the magnitude of the Frank lead system or lead I or III, might also be considered.

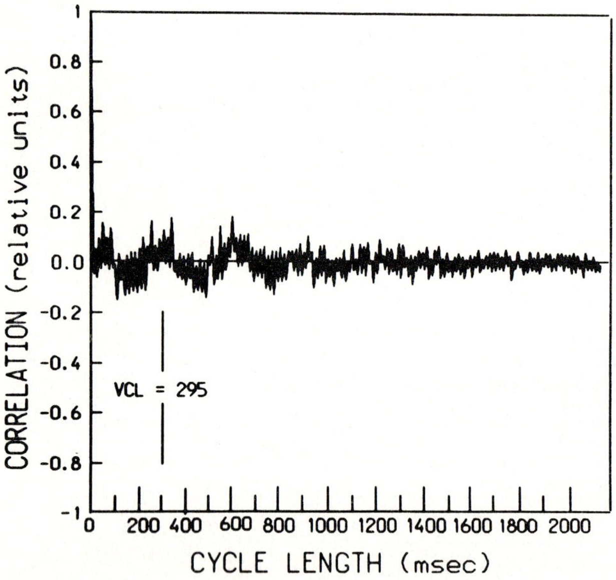

FIGURE 6. Autocorrelation function of the remainder electrocardiogram of lead II of the AV associated rhythm shown in figure 2. The ventricular cycle length (VCL) is marked in msec. The autocorrelation plot shows no peaks meeting slope and amplitude criteria and the rhythm is detected as AV associated.

Three of the six errors occurred when the peak of the autocorrelation function was at the atrial cycle length but did not pass the amplitude criterion. Lowering the amplitude criterion would decrease the specificity of the algorithm. This situation might be improved by implementing some signal conditioning before or after subtraction. Any type of signal conditioning that decreases the energy of noise in the remainder electrocardiogram relative to the energy of the P waves will cause the peak at the detected atrial cycle length to be larger. This might be accomplished by variety of methods, such as use of a different low-pass filter for the original signal, bandpass filtering of the remainder electrocardiogram, or use of different smoothing algorithms for the remainder electrocardiogram.

The final undetected AV dissociated rhythm had a true ventricular cycle length 5 msec less than the true

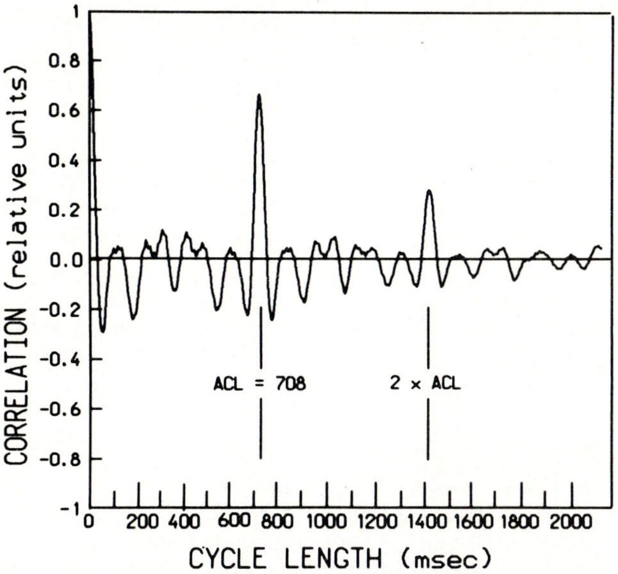

FIGURE 7. Autocorrelation function of the remainder electrocardiogram of lead V_1 of the AV dissociated rhythm shown in figure 4. The large peak was detected by the computer and labeled as the detected atrial cycle length (ACL) equal to 708 msec. True atrial cycle length was 700 msec. A significant peak was also detected at twice the atrial cycle length.

atrial cycle length and 12 msec less than the detected cycle length. The P waves were easily recognizable on the remainder electrocardiogram and the computer-detected cycle length represented the true atrial cycle length. However, the allowable error was larger than 12 msec and the rhythm was called AV associated. The problem of the detection of AV dissociation in those rhythms in which the atrial and ventricular cycle lengths are either close to each other or multiples of each other is an interesting one. We made some assumptions about the rhythms we could diagnose by choosing to use the methods of mean beat calculation and autocorrelation. The rhythms were required to have a relatively constant QRS morphology, PP interval, P wave morphology, and variable PR intervals if the rhythm was to be detected as AV dissociated. In addition, the atrial and ventricular cycle lengths had to be more than an allowable error apart. Rhythms such as those with close atrial and ventricular cycle lengths (e.g., isorhythmic AV dissociation) and rhythms with Wenckebach conduction, multiform atrial tachycardia, and atrial fibrillation are examples of rhythms that do not comply with these assumptions.

The results presented in this report were obtained with a study data set and it remains to be seen whether results from a future test set will be as good. Further investigation must be done with a much larger data set to rigorously test the specificity of this algorithm. If it proves to be capable of accurately detecting AV dissociation, then processing should continue after detection of AV dissociation to detection of individual P waves in the remainder electrocardiograms. The technique of mean beat subtraction might also be applied to detection of single AV dissociated beats during otherwise normal rhythms. Similar computer algorithms might detect second- and third-degree AV block.

The algorithm for detection of AV dissociation presented here is not intended as a stand-alone system but should be used as a software module that may be added to existing arrhythmia interpretation systems. By obtaining half of our data from a commercially available electrocardiogram system, we have shown that it is possible to use the automatic preprocessing from such a system as input to our algorithm with successful results.

Although ventricular tachycardia appears on a very small percentage of the 12-lead electrocardiograms recorded, when it is recorded it is usually in an acutely ill patient requiring immediate therapy. While intravenous verapamil is the current drug of choice for therapy for paroxysmal supraventricular tachycardia with functional or preexisting bundle branch block, administration of this drug to patients with ventricular tachycardia most often results in failure to convert the tachycardia combined with negative inotropy and thus, the risk of hemodynamic collapse. The availability of an algorithm for detection of AV dissociation (both for inspection of the remainder electrocardiogram and the final computer interpretation) in an emergency room or

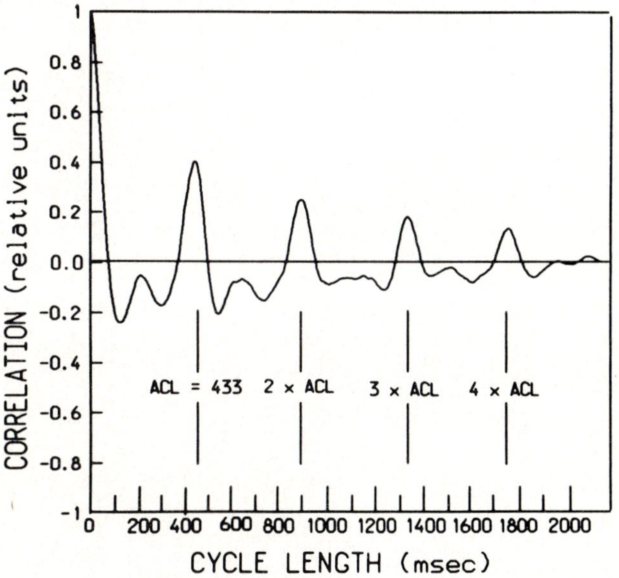

FIGURE 8. Autocorrelation function of the remainder electrogram of lead II of the AV dissociated rhythm in figure 5. The plot shows large peaks at the detected atrial cycle length (ACL) and multiples of the atrial cycle length.

coronary care setting could be of significant benefit, especially when house staff, nurses, or other nonexpert electrocardiographers are called upon to make the diagnosis. Improvements in the algorithm and addition of other diagnostic criteria relating to QRS morphology[3] may improve sensitivity. Extension of the algorithm to coronary care monitors or ambulatory monitors in addition to 12-lead electrocardiograms may be feasible. Whether this algorithm will improve upon the ability of expert electrocardiographers to detect AV dissociation remains to be determined.

We express our appreciation to Marquette Electronics and specifically to Ian Rowlandson, without whose enthusiastic support this study would not have been possible, and to Dr. Jose Gallastegui and Darrel Prechel for assistance in data collection.

References

1. LeBlanc AR, Roberge FA: III. Present state of arrhythmia analysis by computer. Can Med Assoc J **108:** 1239, 1973
2. Kastor JA, Horowitz LN, Harken AH, Josephson ME: Clinical electrophysiology of ventricular tachycardia. N Engl J Med **304:** 1004, 1981
3. Wellens HJJ, Bar FWHM, Lie KL: The value of the electrocardiogram in differential diagnosis of a tachycardia with a widened QRS complex. AM J Med **64:** 27, 1978
4. McFarlane PW, Lorimer AR, Lawrie TDV: ECG reporting by computer. Scot Med J **15:** 363, 1970
5. McFarlane PW: ECG waveform identification by digital computer. Cardiovasc Res **5:** 141, 1971
6. Willems JL, Pipberger HV: Arrhythmia detection by digital computer. Comput Biomed Res **5:** 263, 1972
7. Rey W, Laird JD, Hugenholtz PG: P-wave detection by digital computer. Comput Biomed Res **4:** 509, 1971
8. Pordy LP, Jaffe H, Chesky K, Friedberg CK, Bonner RE, Schwerman HD, Alexander D: Computer analysis of the electrocardiogram. A joint project. J Mount Sanai Hosp **24:** 69, 1967
9. Bonner RE, Crevasse L, Ferrer MI, Greenfield JC: A new computer program for the analysis of scalar electrocardiograms. Comput Biomed Res **5:** 629, 1972
10. Bonner RE, Schwetman HD: Computer diagnosis of electrocardiograms III. A computer program for arrhythmia diagnosis. Comput Biomed Res **1:** 387, 1968
11. Bonner RE, Schwetman HD: Computer diagnosis of electrocardiograms II. A computer program for EKG measurements. Comput Biomed Res **1:** 366, 1968
12. Pordy L, Jaffe H, Chesky K, Friedberg CK, Fallowes L: Computer diagnosis of electrocardiograms IV. A computer program for contour analysis with clinical results of rhythm and contour interpretation. Comput Biomed Res **1:** 408, 1968
13. Stallman FW, Pipberger HV: Automatic recognition of electrocardiographic waves by digital computer. Circ Res **9:** 1138, 1961
14. Brody D, Woolsey MD, Arzbaecher RC: Application of computer techniques to the detection and analysis of spontaneous P-wave variations. Circulation **36:** 359, 1967
15. Hengeveld JJ, van Bemmel JH: Computer detection of P waves. Comput Biomed Res **9:** 125, 1976
16. Cellar BG, Bason PT: Hardware detection of P-waves in the electrocardiogram. Med Biol Eng Comput **14:** 501, 1976
17. Yokoi M, Watanabe Y, Okamoto N, Yasui S, Mizuno Y: On-line computer diagnosis of arrhythmias on ECG using small scale digital computer system. Jpn Circ J **33:** 129, 1969
18. Watanabe Y: Automated diagnosis of arrhythmias by small scale digital computers. Jpn Heart J **11:** 223, 1970
19. Strauss JP: Optimum digital filtering for electrocardiographic waveform detection, thesis. 1973, Northwestern University
20. Stark L, Dickson J, Whipple G, Horibe H: Remote real-time diagnosis of clinical electrograms by a digital computer system. Ann NY Acad Sci **127:** 851, 1966
21. Blumlein SL, Harvey G, Murthy VK and Haywood JJ: New technique for detection of changes in QRS morphology of ECG signals. Am J Physiol **244:** H560, 1983
22. Swiryn S, Jenkins J: Arrhythmia diagnosis by computer. The Marquette 12SL program. *In* Computerized interpretation of the electrocardiogram. Proceedings of the Engineering Foundation Conference, New York, 1983, Engineering Foundation, pp 35–54
23. Floro J, Laks MM: Evaluation of computer interpretation of cardiac arrhythmias. *In* Computerized interpretation of the electrocardiogram. Proceedings of the Engineering Foundation Conference, New York, 1983, Engineering Foundation, pp 11–33
24. Bernard R, Rey W, Vainsel H, Boothroyd M, Demeester M: Computerized dysrhythmia monitoring with an intra-auricular lead. *In* Proceedings of the Computers in Cardiology Conference. Long Beach, 1974, CA, IEEE Press, p 17
25. Jenkins J, Wu D, Arzbaecher R. Computer diagnosis of supraventricular and ventricular arrhythmias. A new esophageal technique. Circulation **60:** 978, 1979
26. Josephson ME, Horowitz LN, Farshidi A, Kastor JA: Recurrent sustained ventricular tachycardia 1. Mechanisms. Circulation **57:** 431, 1978
27. Schwartz M, Shaw L: Signal processing: discrete spectral analysis, detection, and estimation. New York, 1975, McGraw-Hill, Inc., pp 109–125
28. Digital Signal Processing Committee: Programs for digital signal processing. New York, 1979, IEEE Press

Maintenance of exercise stroke volume during ventricular versus atrial synchronous pacing: role of contractility

KALMAN AUSUBEL, M.D., RICHARD M. STEINGART, M.D., MONA SHIMSHI, M.D., PETER KLEMENTOWICZ, M.D., AND SEYMOUR FURMAN, M.D.

ABSTRACT Although atrial synchronous and rate-responsive ventricular pacing have been compared, the importance of maintaining synchronized atrial systole in addition to rate responsiveness has been incompletely defined. That is, the effects of these two pacing modes on cardiac volumes and contractility have not been studied. Accordingly, 16 patients with normal ventricular function were studied while in the upright position and at rest with gated radionuclide ventriculography during both atrial synchronous and ventricular pacing. Twelve of these patients were also studied during low-level upright exercise (300 kilopond-meters). Rest and exercise ventricular pacing heart rates were matched to those recorded with synchronous pacing. Ventricular volumes were determined with a counts-based method. The ejection fraction and peak systolic pressure/end-systolic volume ratio were used as measures of contracility. At rest there were no significant differences in either volumes or contractility between the two pacing modes. However, during exercise to identical heart rates, blood pressures, and workloads, although stroke volume was the same during exercise with atrial synchronous and ventricular pacing (78 ± 13 vs 75 ± 12 ml), end-diastolic and end-systolic volumes were lower with ventricular pacing than with atrial synchronous pacing (end-diastolic volume 101 ± 13 vs 113 ± 16 ml, $p < .001$; end-systolic volume 26 ± 4 vs 35 ± 7 ml, $p < .001$). Stroke volume during ventricular paced exercise was maintained at atrial synchronous pacing levels by means of increased contractility (ejection fraction of 74 ± 4% during ventricular pacing vs 69 ± 5% during atrial synchronous pacing, $p = .002$; peak systolic pressure/end-systolic volume ratio of 6.51 ± 1 during ventricular pacing vs 4.85 ± 1 during atrial synchronous pacing, $p < .001$). Thus, during upright bicycle exercise to workloads corresponding to those of usual daily activities, rate-responsive atrial synchronous pacing results in enhanced ventricular filling and spares contractile reserve when compared with rate-responsive ventricular pacing.
Circulation **72, No. 5, 1037–1043, 1985.**

DUAL-CHAMBER (DDD) pacemakers allow atrioventricular synchronization and a chronotropic response to exercise or stress. By comparison, rate-responsive pacemakers that respond to various physiologic sensors, i.e., evoked QT, respiratory rate, etc., afford an increase in ventricular rate alone. Work done to date has shown similar cardiac outputs and exercise capacities with the two pacing modes.[1] How cardiac output is maintained with rate-responsive ventricular pacing and whether hemodynamic differences exist between the two pacing modes is of importance in assessing the need for maintenance of atrioventricular synchrony in patients with pacemakers.[2] Accordingly, we used previously validated radionuclide ventriculographic techniques in patients with normal ventricular function to examine cardiac volumes and contractility at upright rest and with low-level exercise during both atrial synchronous pacing and rate-adjusted ventricular pacing. In addition to the ejection fraction, the peak systolic pressure/end-systolic volume ratio was used as an index of contractility, since it has been shown to be more sensitive in detecting subtle changes in myocardial function.[3, 4]

Methods

Patient population. Patients with implanted DDD pacemakers and normal ventricular function who were not receiving

From the Division of Cardiology and Department of Surgery, Montefiore Medical Center, New York.

Address for correspondence: Richard M. Steingart, M.D., Montefiore Medical Center, 111 East 210th St., Bronx, NY 10467.

Received April 16, 1985; revision accepted July 18, 1985.

Dr. Ausubel is the 1984–85 Albert S. Hyman Fellow in Cardiac Pacing of the North American Society of Pacing and Electrophysiology.

Presented in part at the Young Investigator Awards Competition of the Sixth Annual Scientific Session of the North American Society of Pacing and Electrophysiology, Toronto, Ontario, May 9–11, 1985.

TABLE 1

Upright rest: comparison of atrial synchronous pacing and rate-matched ventricular pacing

Patient No.	Age (yr)	Sex	Diagnosis	Implant	Ventricular pacing HR	SBP	EDV	ESV	SV	EF	CO	P/V
1	23	M	CHB	12.5 mo	70	130	108	28	80	74	5.60	4.60
2	67	M	IHB	2 days	70	135	90	30	60	67	4.20	4.50
3	58	M	CSS	5 days	70	135	88	30	58	66	4.06	4.50
4	61	M	SND	5 days	70	155	100	31	69	69	4.83	5.00
5	60	F	IHB	7.5 mo	75	105	75	20	55	73	4.13	5.25
6	48	M	CSS	16 mo	80	110	102	33	69	68	5.52	3.33
7	79	M	SND	10 mo	70	120	74	33	41	55	2.87	3.64
8	65	F	SND	6 days	70	130	95	32	63	66	4.41	4.06
9	56	M	SND	4 days	70	110	80	22	58	73	4.06	5.00
10	66	F	CHB	10 days	70	130	90	31	59	66	4.13	4.19
11	86	M	IHB	8 mo	75	150	110	35	75	68	5.63	4.29
12	68	M	SND	1.5 mo	70	120	106	36	70	66	4.90	3.33
13[A]	58	F	IHB	4 mo	75	150	90	35	55	61	4.13	4.29
14[A]	69	M	SND	10 days	70	140	90	29	61	68	4.27	4.83
15[A]	40	M	CHB	5 days	70	110	104	36	68	65	4.76	3.05
16[A]	49	F	SND	14 mo	75	120	87	24	63	72	4.73	5.00
Mean	60				72	128	93	30	63	67	4.51	4.30
SD	±15				±3	±16	±11	±5	±9	±5	±0.7	±0.7

HR = heart rate (beats/min); SBP = systolic blood pressure (mm Hg); EDV = end-diastolic volume (ml); ESV = end-systolic volume (ml); SV = stroke volume (ml); EF = ejection fraction (%); CO = cardiac output (1/min); P/V = peak systolic pressure/end-systolic volume ratio; CHB = complete heart block; CSS = carotid sinus sensitivity; IHB = incomplete heart block; SND = sinus node dysfunction.

[A]Studied at rest only.

cardiac medications were prospectively screened from the Montefiore Medical Center Pacemaker Clinic. Sixteen patients (11 men and five women; mean age 60 ± 15 years) gave informed written consent for the study. All were asymptomatic after pacemaker implantation programmed to the DDD pacing mode, and none had a history of hypertension, diabetes, chest pain, or previous myocardial infarction. Results of physical examinations and chest x-rays were normal. None of the patients had electrocardiographic evidence of a prior myocardial infarction. All patients had normal ventricular function at rest, prospectively defined as an ejection fraction of 55% or greater without any regional wall motion abnormalities. Seven patients had received pacemakers for symptomatic sinus node dysfunction, three for complete heart block, four for incomplete or intermittent heart block, and two for carotid sinus hypersensitivity. The time from implantation was less than 11 days in seven of the patients, and ranged from 1.5 to 16 months in the other nine. None of the subjects were trained athletes and none were receiving cardiac medications.

Four patients studied at rest could not be studied completely during exercise. Two patients developed severe discomfort (shortness of breath, chest pulsations, and weakness) during exercise in the ventricular mode — symptoms consistent with intolerance of ventricular pacing, or the pacemaker syndrome.[5] One was too tired to exercise, and one developed a higher sinus rate with ventricular paced exercise and could not be studied at a rate comparable to that produced by atrial synchronous pacing. These four patients were studied in the two pacing modes at rest only.

Pacing protocol. On the day before the radionuclide study, subjects underwent a 5 min period of bicycling in the DDD pacing mode with electrocardiographic monitoring to determine their heart rate at the end of the exercise period. During the actual exercise study, this heart rate was programmed in the ventricular pacing mode at the onset of exercise. During exercise in the atrial synchronous mode, the ventricular pacing rate was dictated by the patient's atrial rate. This procedure allowed us to randomly alternate the initial pacing mode used in consecutive patients and resulted in similar exercise heart rates with ventricular pacing (VVI) and atrial synchronous pacing (atrial tracking with synchronous ventricular pacing in the DDD mode), with an atrioventricular interval of 150 msec. Continuous electrocardiographic monitoring demonstrated that the patients were paced in the programmed mode at all times. During all parts of the protocol, ventricular contraction was precipitated by a pacemaker stimulus (i.e., atrioventricular conduction through the normal pathway did not occur during synchronous pacing) to eliminate pacemaker-induced vs normal ventricular depolarization and contraction as a potential confounding variable.[6]

Exercise protocol. The patients were studied while in the 90 degree upright position and in the postabsorptive state. Ten minutes after each patient was in the starting position in the first pacing mode, scanning was done while he or she was at rest with a heart rate as close to 70 beats/min as possible. After the resting scans were obtained, the patients exercised in the same pacing mode on a bicycle ergometer–imaging table combination (Nuclear Associates, Carle Place, NY) that allowed the subject to exercise vigorously in the 90 degree upright posture while maintaining a stable position under the gamma camera. Continuous bicycle exercise was done at a constant workload of 300 kilopond-meters (kpm) at a pedal speed of 60 to 70 rpm. After 3 min of exercise, a scan was acquired spanning the subsequent 2.5 min of exercise. Blood pressure measurements were taken at rest and at each minute of exercise and recovery by a single observer who was unaware of the pacing mode. After a 30 min rest period, scanning was repeated in the same pacing mode at upright rest to ensure return to baseline. Pacemakers were then programmed to the alternate pacing mode and, again, to maintain a heart rate as close to 70 beats/min as possible, and the

TABLE 1
(Continued)

Synchronous pacing							
HR	SBP	EDV	ESV	SV	EF	CO	P/V
64	120	105	40	65	62	4.16	3.00
70	120	87	28	59	68	4.13	4.29
70	130	86	28	58	67	4.06	4.60
65	140	105	33	72	69	4.68	4.24
77	105	73	23	50	68	3.85	4.57
75	120	116	44	72	62	5.40	2.72
70	130	79	32	47	60	3.29	4.06
70	130	100	35	65	65	4.55	3.71
70	110	85	26	59	69	4.13	4.23
70	125	86	32	54	63	3.78	3.91
75	150	108	33	75	69	5.63	4.55
70	120	103	38	65	63	4.55	3.16
75	130	89	34	55	62	4.12	3.82
70	130	101	30	71	70	4.97	4.33
70	110	105	37	68	65	4.76	2.97
75	115	94	21	73	78	5.48	5.48
71	124	95	32	63	66	4.47	3.98
±4	±12	±12	±6	±9	±4	±0.7	±0.7

patient was allowed to rest for an additional 10 min. The rest and exercise protocol was then repeated with the patient in the second pacing mode.

Radionuclide methods. Upright gated blood pool cardiac imaging was used to assess changes in global and regional left ventricular function and volume. The details of the acquisition and imaging procedures have been published elsewhere[7] and are briefly summarized here. The subjects red blood cells were incubated in vivo with stannous pyrophosphate and labeled with 25 mCi of ^{99m}Tc pertechnetate.[8] A mobile, standard-field-of-view gamma camera with a high-sensitivity collimator (Picker Corp., North Ford, CT) interfaced with a computer (Digital Equipment Corp., Marlborough, MA) dedicated to the acquisition and processing of nuclear medicine data was used. The camera was positioned in the left anterior oblique projection that best separated the left and right ventricles and the left atrium from the left ventricle. Triplicate resting acquisitions were obtained, and radionuclide data were averaged from these acquisitions. The exercise scan was acquired for 2.5 min as described above. Each acquisition consisted of 28 frames per RR interval in zoomed 64×64 matrixes and a minimum of 4×10^6 counts.

Scans were processed by a single experienced operator with a semiautomated variable-region-of-interest method. Background-corrected end-diastolic and end-systolic count data were calculated from mathematically smoothed time-activity curves, corrected for frame duration, and normalized to 20 msec. Stroke counts were then determined as the difference between end-diastolic and end-systolic counts. All count data were corrected for the 4.5 hr effective half-life of the ^{99m}Tc-labeled red blood cell complex. For multiple determination of end-diastolic, end-systolic, and stroke counts, the percent standard deviations in this laboratory are 6.48, 8.31, and 12.49, respectively.[9] The correlation between changes in stroke counts and in thermodilution stroke volume during intervention is $r = .90$, $p < .001$.[10] Absolute volumes were determined by a modification[11] of the method of Slutsky,[12] in which counts in 5 ml samples of labeled blood, drawn at the time of the rest and exercise scans, are used to convert scintigraphic count data into volume data. In this laboratory, volume (scintigraphic) = volume (angiographic) − 17.3 (n = 25, SEE 5.83, $r = .953$, $p < .001$).

Cardiac output was calculated according to the formula: cardiac output = heart rate × stroke volume, and left ventricular ejection fraction from: stroke volume/end-diastolic volume. Correlation between left ventricular ejection fraction determined by this method and that obtained with contrast cineangiography in this laboratory has been demonstrated to be $r = .90$, $p < .001$.[13] The peak systolic pressure/end-systolic volume ratio was calculated as the sphygmanometrically determined systolic blood pressure divided by end-systolic volume.[3]

Statistical analysis. Left ventricular end-diastolic, end-systolic, and stroke volumes, cardiac output, ejection fraction, and peak systolic pressure/end-systolic volume ratio were measured at rest and during exercise with both ventricular and atrial synchronous pacing at similar heart rates. Results at rest and during exercise as well as with the two pacing modes were compared. All data were mean ± 1 SD. Statistical analysis was performed with the paired t test, and a p value (after Bonferroni adjustment) of <.0125 was considered indicative of statistical significance.[14]

Results

Resting heart rate (71 ± 4 vs 72 ± 3 beats/min, atrial vs ventricular), systolic blood pressure (124 ± 12 vs 128 ± 15 mm Hg), and diastolic blood pressure (77 ± 7 vs 79 ± 9 mm Hg) were similar in the atrial synchronous and ventricular pacing modes. Left ventricular volumes were also comparable in the two pacing modes: end-diastolic volume was 95 ± 12 ml during atrial synchronous pacing vs 93 ± 11 ml during ventricular pacing and end-systolic volume was 32 ± 6 ml during atrial synchronous pacing vs 30 ± 5 ml during ventricular pacing with identical stroke volumes (63 ± 9 ml). The ejection fraction (66 ± 4% atrial synchronous pacing vs 67 ± 5% ventricular pacing) and peak systolic pressure/end-systolic volume ratio (3.98 ± 7 atrial synchronous pacing vs 4.30 ± 8 ventricular pacing) were also not significantly different. Individual results are given in table 1. In the four patients who were studied only at rest, two of whom were symptomatic with ventricular pacing, clinical and hemodynamic findings were similar to those in the other 12. Retrograde ventriculoatrial conduction was not observed on the surface electrocardiogram of any patient at rest or with exercise.

No patient developed chest pain or shortness of breath with exercise. Individual exercise results are in table 2. During exercise at a workload of 300 kpm for 5.5 min in each pacing mode, heart rate (101 ± 9 beats/min during atrial synchronous pacing vs 102 ± 9 beats/min during ventricular pacing), systolic blood pressure (165 ± 18 mm Hg during atrial synchronous pacing vs 168 ± 15 mm Hg during ventricular pacing), and diastolic blood pressure (81 ± 9 mm Hg during atrial synchronous pacing vs 83 ± 10 mm Hg during ventricular pacing) were not different. End-

TABLE 2
Upright exercise: comparison of atrial synchronous pacing and rate-matched ventricular pacing

Patient	Ventricular pacing								Synchronous pacing							
No.	HR	SBP	EDV	ESV	SV	EF	CO	P/V	HR	SBP	EDV	ESV	SV	EF	CO	P/V
1	95	152	119	27	92	77	8.74	5.60	93	155	118	45	73	65	6.79	3.40
2	100	170	104	27	77	74	7.70	6.30	100	150	116	36	80	69	8.00	3.19
3	120	160	86	25	61	71	7.32	6.40	120	180	100	31	69	69	8.30	5.80
4	95	175	108	30	78	72	7.41	5.83	93	160	130	35	95	73	8.84	4.57
5	110	160	91	17	74	81	8.14	9.40	105	150	106	20	86	81	9.03	7.50
6	95	150	118	26	92	78	8.74	5.77	95	150	144	43	101	70	9.60	3.49
7	95	170	76	25	51	67	4.85	6.80	95	165	81	32	49	61	4.66	5.16
8	100	160	100	27	73	73	7.30	5.93	100	150	112	33	79	71	7.90	4.73
9	95	155	90	22	68	76	6.46	7.05	95	150	100	28	72	72	6.84	5.36
10	100	160	100	27	73	73	7.30	5.93	100	150	112	33	79	71	7.90	4.55
11	120	200	115	30	85	74	10.20	6.67	120	200	120	34	86	72	10.32	5.88
12	100	185	108	33	75	69	7.50	5.61	100	190	115	42	73	63	7.30	4.52
Mean	102	168	101^{A}	26^{A}	75	74^{B}	7.65	6.51^{A}	101	165	113^{A}	35^{A}	78	69^{B}	7.97	4.85^{A}
SD	±9	±15	±13	±4	±12	±4	±1	±1	±9	±18	±16	±7	±13	±5	±2	±1

HR = heart rate (beats/min); SBP = systolic blood pressure (mm Hg); EDV = end-diastolic volume (ml); ESV = end-systolic volume (ml); SV = stroke volume (ml); EF = ejection fraction (%); CO = cardiac output (l/min); P/V = peak systolic pressure/end-systolic volume ratio; VP = ventricular pacing; SP = synchronous pacing.

p value, ventricular pacing vs atrial synchronous pacing: $^{A}p < .001$; $^{B}p = .002$.

diastolic volume rose from rest to exercise during both pacing modes, but it increased more with atrial synchronous pacing (increase with ventricular pacing of from 93 ± 11 to 101 ± 13 ml or 9%, p < .001, and increase with atrial synchronous pacing of from 95 ± 12 to 113 ± 16 ml or 19%, p < .001), resulting in a larger end-diastolic volume during exercise with atrial synchronous pacing compared with during ventricular pacing (113 ± 16 vs 101 ± 13 ml, p < .001). End-systolic volume did not change from rest to exercise with atrial synchronous pacing (32 ± 6 vs 35 ± 7 ml), but decreased 13% with ventricular pacing (30 ± 5 to 26 ± 4 ml, p < .001). These differences in end-systolic volume between the two pacing modes during exercise were also highly significant (p < .001).

Stroke volume rose during ventricular paced exercise to a level similar to that during atrial synchronous paced exercise (75 ± 12 vs 78 ± 13 ml, p = NS). Ejection fraction and peak systolic pressure/end-systolic volume ratio, which are measures of ventricular contractility, rose from rest to exercise during both atrial synchronous pacing (ejection fraction 66 ± 4% to 69 ± 5%, p = .004; peak systolic pressure/end-systolic volume ratio 3.98 ± 0.7 to 4.85 ± 1, p = .005) and ventricular pacing (ejection fraction 67 ± 5 to 74 ± 4%, p < .001; peak systolic pressure/end-systolic volume ratio 4.30 ± 0.7 to 6.51 ± 1, p < .001), but increased more with ventricular pacing so that levels during exercise with ventricular pacing were greater (for ejection fraction, ventricular pacing vs atrial synchronous pacing = 74 ± 4% vs 69 ± 5%, p = .002; for peak systolic pressure/end-systolic volume ratio, ventricular pacing vs atrial synchronous pacing = 6.51 ± 1 vs 4.85 ± 1, p < .001) (figure 1).

Discussion

The purpose of this study was to compare ventricular performance at rest and with upright exercise during atrioventricular sequential and ventricular pacing to the same heart rate. Three new findings were that (1) end-diastolic volume at upright rest is similar in both pacing modes, (2) end-diastolic volume during exercise is greater with synchronous than with ventricular pacing, and (3) stroke volume is maintained at atrial synchronous pacing levels during ventricular paced exercise through increased contractility.

Previous studies have examined the contribution of atrial systole to ventricular function, but in patients with abnormal ventricles who were at supine rest. Under these conditions, well-timed atrial systole variably improves cardiac output.[15-23] Fewer data are available on normal subjects, particularly in the upright posture,[24-26] and cardiovascular hemodynamics and volumes differ in supine and upright subjects.[7, 27, 28]

At upright rest, in contrast to findings of previous studies in supine subjects, we found that end-diastolic, end-systolic, and thus stroke volume were similar in the two pacing modes. Furthermore, the volumes and measures of contractile function were equal to those of normal subjects at upright rest in sinus rhythm.[3, 28] A

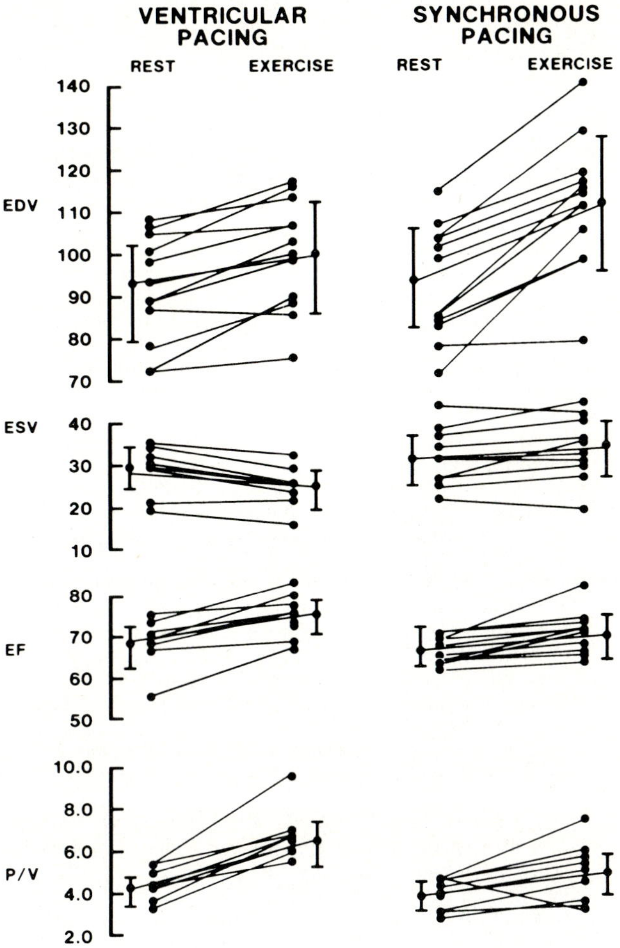

FIGURE 1. Changes in volumes and contractility from rest to exercise with ventricular and atrial synchronous pacing. Thin lines represent individual patient responses and heavy lines represent mean changes ± SD. EDV = end-diastolic volume (ml); ESV = end-systolic volume (ml); EF = ejection fraction (%); P/V = peak systolic pressure/end-systolic volume ratio (arbitrary units).

possible explanation for these observations is that with the assumption of the upright posture, diminished venous return "underfills" the central circulation, making the contribution of atrial systole (which varies with filling) relatively insignificant.[29, 30] Alternatively, changes in ventricular relaxation, which is load-dependent and responsive to metabolic and neurohumoral controls[31] or venous tone,[32] might maintain end-diastolic volume during ventricular pacing at synchronous paced levels in subjects at upright rest. Further work will be needed to clarify which mechanisms underlie our observations.

Many studies have demonstrated superior exercise capacity and cardiac output with rate-responsive than with fixed low-rate ventricular pacing.[33–39] With the development of rate-responsive ventricular pacemakers,[40] the important question is whether cardiac performance differs at matched heart rates. This question has been addressed, in part, previously. In a group of patients with heterogenous cardiac disease, cardiac output was only 8% higher and stroke volume only slightly greater with synchronous than with rate-matched ventricular pacing during supine exercise.[33] These data are similar to our results in upright subjects and suggest that the ventricular rate response to exercise rather than atrioventricular synchrony accounts for most of the observed improvement in cardiac output in patients with synchronous pacing systems.[1]

Cardiac volumes and contractility during exercise with atrial synchronous and rate-matched ventricular pacing have not previously been compared. With upright low-level exercise in unpaced individuals, end-diastolic volume rises and end-systolic volume remains the same, with a resultant increase in stroke volume and hence cardiac output, and no change or a mild increase in contractility.[28] These directional changes in end-diastolic volume were seen with both pacing modes, but with ventricular pacing end-diastolic volume did not increase as much as with atrial synchronous pacing (9% increase as compared with 20%). Thus, atrial synchrony apparently becomes important only during upright exercise, perhaps due to better filling of the central circulation through increased venous return.[32] Responses of end-systolic volume were also different during exercise in the two pacing modes. End-systolic volume did not change with atrial synchronous pacing, while it fell 13% with rate-matched ventricular pacing. Given that systolic blood pressure rose to similar levels in both pacing modes, contractility increased more with ventricular than atrial synchronous pacing. Thus, during ventricular paced exercise, with the loss of consistent atrioventricular synchrony, stroke volume and cardiac output are maintained by means of lowered end-systolic volume, the result of increased ventricular contractility (figure 2). Although a single point of peak systolic pressure/end-systolic volume ratio does not necessarily reflect the slope of the end-systolic pressure/volume relationship as originally described,[41] several clinical studies have empirically demonstrated the utility of this index of contractility.[3, 4] Our conclusions are supported by the directional changes in ejection fraction, which also indicate a greater increase in contractility with ventricular paced than with synchronous paced exercise.[42]

Certain limitations of the study design warrant discussion. Conclusions are limited to a fixed workload of 300 kpm, chosen to allow steady-state measurements that would reflect the physiology of daily activities (i.e., walking).[43] It is possible that biases introduced by the experimental protocol may have influenced the

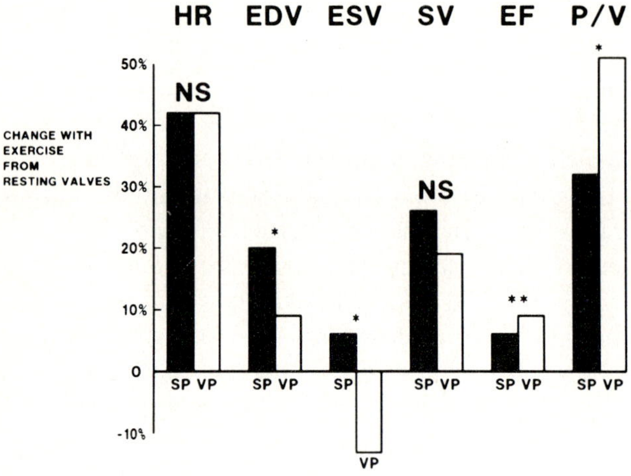

FIGURE 2. Percent changes in heart rate, volumes, and contractility from resting values with ventricular and atrial synchronous pacing during exercise. Level of significance of changes between pacing modes indicated above bars. HR = heart rate (beats/min); EDV = end-diastolic volume (ml); EF = ejection fraction (%); P/V = peak systolic pressure/end-systolic volume ratio (arbitrary units). *$p < .001$; **$p = .002$; NS = not significant.

comparisons between ventricular and atrial synchronous paced exercise. We did avoid the confounding variable of differing ventricular contraction patterns by pacing the ventricle during all parts of the study.[6] However, with synchronous pacing, ventricular rate rose during the first 30 sec of exercise as a function of atrial rate, whereas the exercise rate was programmed immediately at the onset of exercise with ventricular pacing. All measurements, however, were made after the patient had been exercising for 3 min, minimizing the influence of this variable. Also, all measurements in this study were made immediately after changes in pacing mode, but these have been shown to reflect hemodynamic changes that occur with long-term pacing in a given mode.[34, 35] Finally, we have no explanation for the symptomatic intolerance of two patients to ventricular pacing. Our results are therefore applicable only to patients with symptomatic tolerance to ventricular pacing.

In summary, ventricular volumes and contractility are similar with the two pacing modes in subjects at upright rest. During low-level exercise with atrial synchronous and rate-matched ventricular pacing cardiac output was similar, but ventricular volumes and contractility differed in the two pacing modes. During atrial synchronous pacing, as in normal subjects in sinus rhythm, stroke volume increased primarily as a function of the Frank-Starling effect. With ventricular pacing, a situation in which constant atrioventricular synchrony is absent, stroke volume was increased both by an increase in end-diastolic volume and a decrease in end-systolic volume, the latter reflecting a greater increase in myocardial contractility.

References

1. Fananapazir L, Bennett DH, Monks P: Atrial synchronized ventricular pacing: contribution of the chronotropic response to improved exercise performance. PACE **6:** 601, 1983
2. Furman S: AV Synchrony and cardiac rate. PACE **6:** 513, 1983 (editorial)
3. Slutsky R, Karliner J, Gerber K: Peak systolic blood pressure/end-systolic volume ratio: assessment at rest and during exercise in normal subjects and patients with coronary heart disease. Am J Cardiol **46:** 813, 1980
4. Nivatpumin T, Katz S, Scheuer J: Peak left ventricular systolic pressure/end-systolic volume ratio: a sensitive detector of left ventricular disease. Am J Cardiol **43:** 969, 1979
5. Ausubel K, Furman S: The pacemaker syndrome. Ann Intern Med (in press)
6. Askenazi J, Alexander JH, Koenigsberg DI, Belic N, Lesch M: Alteration of left ventricular performance by left bundle branch block simulated with atrioventricular sequential pacing. Am J Cardiol **53:** 99, 1984
7. Steingart RM, Wexler J, Slagle S, Scheuer J: Radionuclide ventriculographic responses to graded supine and upright exercise: critical role of the Frank-Starling mechanism at submaximal exercise. Am J Cardiol **53:** 1671, 1984
8. Pavel DG, Zimmer AM, Patterson BN: In vivo labelling of red blood cells with ^{99m}Tc: a new approach to blood pool visualization. J Nucl Med **18:** 305, 1977
9. Ganz WI, Wexler JP, Brenner AI, Bontemps R, Steingart RM, Blaufox MD: Variability of resting gated ejection fraction. J Nucl Med **21:** 63, 1980
10. Steingart RM, Grose R, Wexler JP, Greenberg M, Weinstein L: Validation of stroke volume determinations by radionuclide ventriculography during intervention. Circulation **64:** 106, 1981 (abst)
11. Konstam MA, Tu'meh S, Wynne J, Beck JR, Kozlowski J, Holman BL: Effect of exercise on erythrocyte count and blood activity concentration after technetium-99m in vivo red blood cell labelling. Circulation **66:** 638, 1982
12. Slutsky R, Karliner J, Ricci D, Kaiser R, Pfisterer M, Gordon D, Peterson K, Ashburn W: Left ventricular volumes by gated equilibrium radionuclide angiography: A new method. Circulation **60:** 556, 1979
13. Ganz WI, Wexler J, Rabinowitz AM, Brenner AI, Steingart RM, Blaufox MD: Methods of improving the precision of left ventricular volume and ejection fraction determination. J Nucl Med **21:** 48, 1980 (abstr)
14. Cupples LA, Heeren T, Schatzkin A, Colton T: Multiple testing of hypotheses in comparing two groups. Ann Intern Med **100:** 122, 1984
15. Braunwald E: Symposium on cardiac arrhythmias with comments on the hemodynamic significance of atrial systole. Am J Med **37:** 655, 1964
16. Samet P, Bernstein WH, Levine S: Significance of the atrial contribution to ventricular filling. Am J Cardiol **16:** 195, 1965
17. Benchimol A, Li YB, Dimond EG: Cardiovascular dynamics in complete heart block at various heart rates: effect of exercise at a fixed heart rate. Circulation **30:** 542, 1964
18. Benchimol A, Duenas A, Liggett MS, Dimond EG: Contribution of atrial systole to the cardiac function at a variable ventricular rate. Am J Cardiol **16:** 11, 1965
19. Samet P, Jacobs W, Bernstein WH, Shane R: Hemodynamic sequelae of idioventricular pacemaking in complete heart block. Am J Cardiol **11:** 594, 1963
20. Morris JJ Jr, Entman M, North WC, Kong Y, McIntosh H: The changes in cardiac output with reversion of atrial fibrillation to sinus rhythm. Circulation **31:** 670, 1965
21. Sowton E: Artificial pacemaking and sinus rhythm. Br Heart J **37:** 311, 1965
22. Samet P, Bernstein WH, Levine S, Lopez A: Hemodynamic effects

of tachycardias produced by atrial and ventricular pacing. Am J Med **39:** 905, 1965
23. Leinbach RC, Chamberlain DA, Kastor JA, Harthorne JW, Sanders CA: A comparison of the hemodynamic effects of ventricular and sequential AV pacing in patients with heart block. Am Heart J **78:** 502, 1969
24. Benchimol A, Ellis JG, Dimond EG: Hemodynamic consequences of atrial and ventricular pacing in patients with normal and abnormal hearts. Am J Med **39:** 911, 1965
25. Samet P, Castillo C, Bernstein WH: Hemodynamic consequences of atrial and ventricular pacing in subjects with normal hearts. Am J Cardiol **18:** 522, 1966
26. Greenberg B, Chatterjee K, Parmley WW: The influence of left ventricular filling pressure on atrial contribution to cardiac output. Am Heart J **98:** 742, 1979
27. Manyari DE, Kostk WJ: Left and right ventricular function at rest and during bicycle exercise in the supine and sitting positions in normal subjects and patients with coronary artery disease. Am J Cardiol **51:** 36, 1983
28. Poliner LR, Dehmer GJ, Lewis SE, Parkey RW, Blomqvist CG, Willerson JT: Left ventricular performance in normal subjects: a comparison of the responses to exercise in the upright and supine positions. Circulation **62:** 528, 1980
29. Braunwald E, Frahm CJ: Studies in Starling's law of the heart, IV: observations on the haemodynamic functions of the left atrium in man. Circulation **24:** 633, 1961
30. Kramer B, Massie B, Topic N: Hemodynamic differences between suine and upright exercise in patients with congestive heart failure. Circulation **66:** 820, 1982
31. Brutsaert DL, Housmans PR, Goethals MA: Dual control of relaxation. Its role in the ventricular function in the mammalian heart. Circ Res **47:** 637, 1980
32. Shepherd JT: Role of the veins in the circulation. Circulation **33:** 484, 1966
33. Karlof I: Haemodynamic effect of atrial triggered versus fixed rate pacing at rest and during exercise in complete heart block. Acta Med Scand **197:** 195, 1975
34. Kruse I, Arnaman K, Conradson TB, Ryden L: A comparison of the acute and long term hemodynamic effects of ventricular inhibited and atrial synchronous ventricular inhibited pacing. Circulation **65:** 846, 1982
35. Kappenberger L, Gloor HO, Babotai I, Steinbrunn W, Turina M: Hemodynamic effects of atrial synchronization in acute and long term ventricular pacing. PACE **5:** 639, 1982
36. Perrins EJ, Morley CA, Chan SL, Sutton R: Randomized controlled trial of physiological and ventricular pacing. Br Heart J **50:** 112, 1983
37. Fananapazir L, Srinivas V, Bennett DH: Comparison of resting hemodynamic indices and exercise performance during atrial synchronized and asynchronous ventricular pacing. PACE **6:** 202, 1983
38. Shapland JE, MacCarter D, Tockman B, Knudson M: Physiologic benefits of rate responsiveness. PACE **6:** 329, 1983
39. Donaldson RM, Rickards AF: Rate responsive pacing using the evoked QT principle. A physiological alternative to atrial synchronous pacemakers. PACE **6:** 1344, 1983
40. Hauser RG: Techniques for improving cardiac performance with implantable devices. PACE **7:** 1234, 1984
41. Sagawa K: The ventricular pressure-volume diagram revisited. Circ Res **43:** 677, 1978
42. Sonnenblick EN, Strobeck JE: Derived indexes of ventricular and myocardial function. N Engl J Med **296:** 978, 1977
43. Passmore R, Durnin JVGA: Human energy expenditure. Physiol Rev **35:** 801, 1955

In-hospital morbidity and mortality in patients undergoing elective coronary angioplasty

CLAYTON E. BREDLAU, M.D., GARY S. ROUBIN, M.B., PH.D., PIERRE P. LEIMGRUBER, M.D., JOHN S. DOUGLAS, JR., M.D., SPENCER B. KING III, M.D., AND ANDREAS R. GRUENTZIG, M.D.

ABSTRACT We prospectively recorded all in-hospital complications of the first 3500 consecutive patients to undergo elective coronary angioplasty (PTCA) at Emory University Hospitals from July 14, 1980, to August 28, 1984, by three operators. PTCA was attempted in a total of 3933 lesions, with a primary success rate of 91%. Multiple-lesion PTCA was performed in 401 patients, and PTCA of saphenous vein grafts was attempted in 172. No complications were recorded in 3116 (89%) cases, isolated minor complications occurred in 241 (6.9%), and major complications (emergency surgery, myocardial infarction, death) were observed in 145 (4.1%). Emergency coronary artery bypass graft surgery (CABG) was performed in 96 patients (2.7%), with a myocardial infarction rate of 49% (47/96), a Q wave infarction rate of 23% (22/96), and an emergency surgery mortality rate of 2% (2/96). Hospital discharge occurred within 2 weeks of attempted PTCA in 91% (87/96) of patients undergoing emergency CABG. The overall myocardial infarction rate was 2.6% (94/3500). There were two nonsurgical deaths, giving a total mortality rate of 0.1% (4/3500). Univariate and multivariate analysis of 3099 patients undergoing single-lesion PTCA identified five preprocedure predictors of a major complication: multivessel coronary disease, lesion eccentricity, presence of calcium in the lesion, female gender, and lesion length. Unstable angina, duration of angina, lesion severity, previous CABG, and vein graft dilatation were not associated with an increased incidence of major complications. The strongest predictor of a major complication was the procedural appearance of an intimal dissection. Intimal dissection was evident in 894/3099 (29%) patients. Of these, 93 (10.4%) patients developed a major complication vs only 35 of 2205 (1.6%) patients without evidence of an intimal dissection ($p < .0001$). Angiographic evidence of intimal dissection resulted in a 6.5-fold increase in the risk of a major complication. In conclusion, these results illustrate what can be expected when elective PTCA is performed with current techniques and good surgical and anesthetic support.
Circulation 72, No. 5, 1044–1052, 1985.

IN PATIENTS with critical stenoses in proximal segments of major arteries, coronary revascularization is now favored over medical management for relief of symptoms.[1] If myocardial ischemia, left ventricular damage, and progressive deterioration in left ventricular function can be avoided, prognosis may also be improved.[2–5] However, comparative trials of medical and surgical therapy have provided clear answers only in left main and severe triple-vessel disease.[6–8]

Percutaneous transluminal coronary angioplasty (PTCA) in selected patients can provide the same degree of effective coronary revascularization as surgery by means of a less invasive approach.[9–11] The widespread use of PTCA has nonetheless been impaired by the incidence of short-term complications associated with the procedure.[12, 13] To date, assessment of complications has been based on reports of limited series[14–16] and data available from the NHLBI PTCA Registry.[17–21] The latter represents the pooled results of many centers performing PTCA on relatively small numbers of patients with what are now considered to be outdated techniques. In the last 4 years, technical advances[22–24] have occurred and physician experience has increased.[25, 26] The Emory University experience comprises a large series of patients, which enables us to analyze the initial results obtained in over 3500 consecutive PTCA attempts to determine (1) the complication rates when PTCA is performed by three experienced operators at a single center using updated techniques and (2) the clinical, arteriographic, and

From the Department of Medicine, Division of Cardiology, Emory University School of Medicine, Atlanta.

Address for correspondence: Andreas R. Gruentzig, M.D., Interventional Cardiovascular Medicine, Emory University Hospital, 1364 Clifton Rd., Atlanta, GA 30322.

Received May 6, 1985; revision accepted July 18, 1985.

Presented in part at the 57th Scientific Sessions of the American Heart Association, Miami Beach, November 1984.

technical factors that predispose to these complications.

Methods

Patients. From July 14, 1980, through August 28, 1984, a total of 3530 PTCA procedures were undertaken at Emory University Hospitals. During this 50 month interval, 30 procedures were done in the setting of an acute myocardial infarction defined as typical ischemic chest pain (≥30 min) with associated electrocardiographic changes. These patients were excluded from the analysis. The remaining 3500 attempts form the basis for this study.

PTCA procedure. All procedures were performed by one of three independent operators. The technique used has been described elsewhere.[27] With Seldinger's entry technique from the groin, arterial and venous sheaths with PTCA guiding and pacemaker catheters were inserted, followed by the administration of heparin (10,000 U iv bolus), nitroglycerin (0.4 mg sublingually), and nifedipine (10 mg sublingually). Heparin boluses (5000 U) were repeated hourly during the procedure. Preliminary angiography of the coronary artery to be dilated was performed in at least two projections with biplane angiographic equipment. The balloon catheter system was inserted and selective intracoronary nitroglycerin (200 μg) was given. The balloon was positioned across the stenosis, a pressure gradient was recorded, and the balloon was inflated as many times as needed to produce the optimal hemodynamic and angiographic result. At the end of the procedure, all catheters were removed and the sheaths were left in place. Sheaths were removed 2 to 3 hr later unless angiographic evidence of intimal dissection or coronary thrombus was seen. These patients were maintained on heparin infusion overnight, with removal of sheaths 2 to 3 hr after discontinuing heparin the next morning.

All patients were taken to a postprocedure monitoring ward or coronary care unit, where they were on telemetry for at least 16 hr after PTCA. A 12-lead electrocardiogram was obtained immediately after PTCA and daily for 2 days. Creatine kinase (CK) levels, including isoenzyme determinations, were performed immediately after PTCA and at 8 and 16 hr. All patients were medicated with cutaneous nitroglycerin (1 inch every 4 hr), isosorbide dinitrate (5 mg sublingually every 4 hr), calcium-blocking agent, and aspirin (325 mg/day orally). If stable, they were discharged 2 days after PTCA.

Data collection and entry. Clinical information, angiographic measurement, and intra- and post-PTCA complication data were recorded during the hospitalization by a physician on standard forms. Specific laboratory data, including electrocardiographic results, creatine kinase levels (including CK-MB fractions), and other post-PTCA complication information, was recorded by a physician at the time of hospital discharge. This information was audited for completeness and entered into a computerized data bank.

Definitions. In accordance with the NHLBI definition,[18] major complications were defined as (1) emergency surgery, (2) nonfatal myocardial infarction, or (3) death before hospital discharge. Emergency surgery[18] was defined as the need for urgent operation because of complications during or after PTCA. A myocardial infarction[18] was defined by the presence of two of the three following criteria: (1) prolonged angina, (2) electrocardiographic evidence of infarction by the Minnesota code,[28] (3) total CK elevation greater than three times the upper limit of normal values with positive MB fraction. Minor complications are detailed in table 3.

Primary success was defined as in the NHLBI Registry as a 20% or greater reduction in percent diameter stenosis.[17] All angiographic measurements were performed in diastole with a computerized electronic caliper system, using the mean diameter stenosis calculated in at least two angiographic views.[29] In patients undergoing multiple-lesion PTCA, primary success was defined as 20% or greater reduction in percent diameter stenosis of at least one lesion. Intimal dissection was defined as in the NHLBI Registry as the presence of angiographically evident intimal damage producing an intraluminal filling defect, extraluminal extravasation of contrast material, linear luminal density, or luminal staining.[19] Multivessel coronary artery disease was defined as at least 50% diameter stenosis in a major branch of at least two of the three main arterial systems: left anterior descending (LAD), left circumflex (LCX), and right (RCA) coronary arteries. Unstable angina was defined as new onset of angina or progressive symptoms during the previous 2 months.

Statistical analysis. Statistical analysis with the chi-square significance test was used to assess differences in categorical variables. Univariate and multivariate analysis was performed to determine clinical and angiographic predictors of a major complication.[30] This analysis was performed on (1) the entire study population of 3500 patients and (2) the more homogeneous subset of 3099 patients who had only single-lesion PTCA. Baseline data analyzed included age, sex, hypertension, diabetes, smoking, previous myocardial infarction, previous coronary artery bypass graft surgery (CABG), unstable angina, anginal functional class, β-blocker therapy, extent of coronary artery disease, PTCA vessel, number of PTCA sites attempted, number of vessel systems in which PTCA was attempted, lesion severity (% diameter stenosis), lesion length, lesion morphology, presence of calcium in the lesion, transstenotic gradient before PTCA, and angiographic appearance of intimal tear or dissection during PTCA.

Results

Patient characteristics. The baseline clinical characteristics of our study population closely approximate those reported in the NHLBI Registry population as shown in table 1. Thirty-six percent of patients gave a history of having undergone medical treatment for hypertension, 30% had a positive family history for coronary artery disease (first-degree relative under 55 years old), 20% were current cigarette smokers, and 9% had diabetes mellitus.

The location of coronary artery lesions undergoing attempted PTCA are listed in table 2. In the subset of 3099 patients undergoing single-lesion PTCA, the location of attempted PTCA was as follows: LAD 1790, RCA 785, LCX 379, left main 10, saphenous vein graft 135. Multiple lesions in one or more coronary arteries were attempted in 401 patients. Six of 11 patients with left main coronary dilatation had patent saphenous bypass grafts to the LAD, LCX, or both and one patient had excellent collateral flow from a native RCA.

Primary success rate. The primary success rate per lesion for the 3933 lesions attempted was 91%; that by lesion location was as follows: LAD 92.5%, RCA 87.5%, LCX 91.3%, saphenous vein graft 91.3%. The primary success rate per lesion was 88.8% in first

PTCA attempts and 93.7% in repeat PTCA attempts performed for restenosis after a previously successful PTCA.

The primary success rate per patient was 90% for the entire study population. The primary success rate per patient in those patients with single-vessel disease was 92%, and that in patients with multivessel disease was 88%. To evaluate trends in the primary success rate over time, we arbitrarily divided the study population into three equal groups that embraced the time periods shown in figure 1. In the first period the primary success rate per patient was 87%. It rose to 92% and remained stable during the last 2334 attempts.

Complications. The distribution of in-hospital complications that occurred during or after attempted PTCA is shown in figure 2. No complication occurred in 3114 (89%) attempts. Major complications occurred in 145 (4.1%) patients and minor complications not associated with a major complication occurred in 241 (6.9%) patients (table 3).

As illustrated in figure 3, a total of 194 major complications occurred in 145 patients (4.1%). More than one major complication occurred in 45 patients who had emergency surgery and myocardial infarction and in two patients who had emergency surgery, myocardial infarction, and death.

The incidence of major complications during each of the three periods outlined previously is summarized in figure 4. The major complication rate was highest

TABLE 1
Baseline patient characteristics

	EUH	NHLBI[36]
Total patients	3500	3079
Age (mean)	55 yr	54 yr
Males (%)	79	77
Previous MI (%)	28	25
Previous CABG (%)	9	9
Unstable angina (%)	50	40
Angina CHC III or IV (%)	42	63
Coronary artery disease (%)		
Single vessel	81	72.5
Multiple vessel	19	27.5
Previous PTCA (%)[A]	12.7	7
Lesion morphology (%)		
Eccentric lesions	37	—
Calcium in lesion	5	—
Lesion length ≥10 mm	17	—
Lesion % diameter stenosis ≥90	13	35

EUH = Emory University Hospital; NHLBI = National Heart, Lung, and Blood Institute PTCA Registry; MI = myocardial infarction; CHC = Canadian Heart Class; CAD = coronary artery disease.

[A]Same lesion site, initial PTCA successful.

TABLE 2
Location of attempted PTCA

Total lesions	3933
Native sites	3761 (95.6%)
LAD	2231 (59.3%)
RCA	1019 (27.1%)
LCX	500 (13.3%)
Left main	11 (0.3%)
Bypass grafts	172 (4.4%)
Multiple lesion attempts	401 (11.5%)

for period 1 (4.8%) but has remained stable over periods 2 (3.7%) and 3 (3.9%).

Major complications

Emergency surgery. Emergency CABG was the most frequent major complication and was performed in 96 patients (2.7%). The mean age of patients undergoing emergency surgery was 56 years, with seven patients over 70 years old. Sixty-nine patients (72%) were men, five had had prior CABG, and five had akinetic myocardial wall segments on ventriculography as a result of prior myocardial infarction. Unstable angina was present in 54 patients (56%). The vessel dilated was the LAD in 60 (62%), the RCA in 29 (30%), the LCX in five (5%), the left main in one, and a saphenous vein graft in two patients, the overall distribution not being significantly different from that of the total study population. The indication for emergency surgery was clinical or angiographic evidence of compromised coronary blood flow in 93 patients and cardiac tamponade in three patients. The latter was caused by

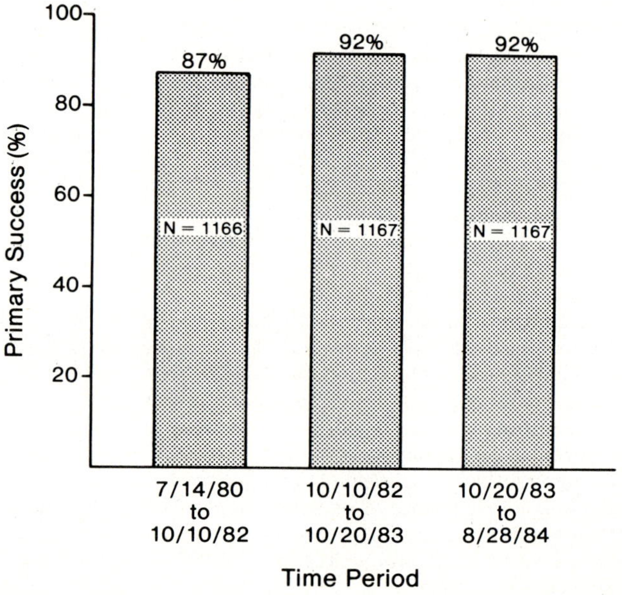

FIGURE 1. Primary success rate of PTCA in 3500 patients. The study population is divided into three periods. N = number of PTCA attempts in each period.

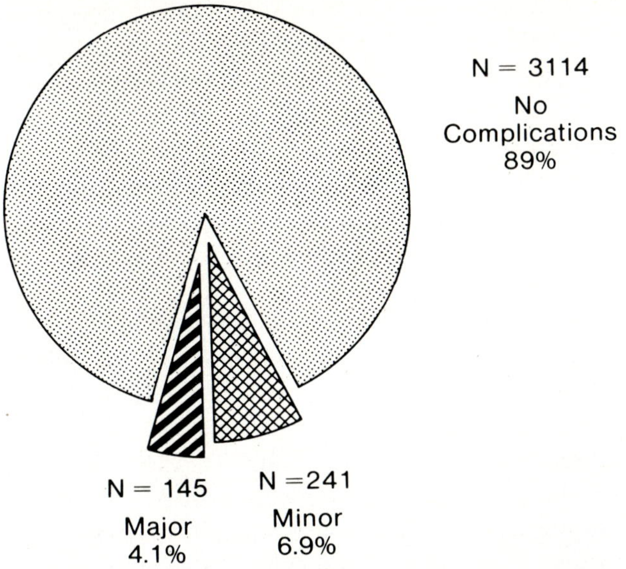

FIGURE 2. Complications in 3500 elective PTCA attempts. N = number of patients with major, minor, or no complications. The major complication group (4.1%) includes all patients who had a myocardial infarction or emergency surgery or who died, whether or not they also had minor complications. The minor complication group (6.9%) includes those patients that had only minor complications.

perforation of the right ventricle by a pacemaker catheter (No. 6F).

All emergency surgery procedures took place within 20 hr of the PTCA. The majority of emergency surgery patients (67/96, 70%) went directly from the catheterization suite to the operating room. There were 29 patients (30%) who initially left the catheterization laboratory in stable condition but subsequently developed evidence of acute coronary ischemia. Twenty-three of these initially stable patients were transported directly to operating room from the ward or the coronary care unit. Emergency repeat PTCA was attempted in the remaining six patients, all of whom then went

TABLE 3
Minor complications of PTCA (n = 3500)

	Episodes	%
Side-branch closure	59	1.7
Ventricular arrhythmia (DC shock)	54	1.5
New conduction defect	31	0.9
Emergency recath.	27	0.8
Repair of femoral artery	22	0.6
Atrial fibrillation/flutter	14	0.4
Excessive blood loss requiring transfusion	9	0.3
Coronary embolus	5	0.1
Tamponade	3	0.1
Stroke	1	0.03
Miscellaneous	19	0.5
Total episodes	244	7.0
Total patients	241	6.9

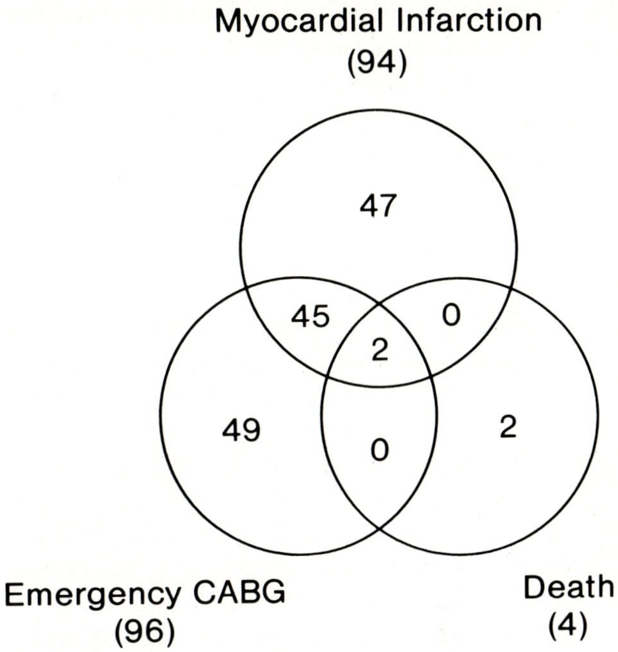

FIGURE 3. Interrelationship of myocardial infarction, emergency surgery, and death in 145 patients with a major complication.

directly from the catheterization laboratory to the operating room. Preoperative insertion of an intra-aortic balloon pump was necessary in 32 of 96 (33%) patients, 21 of whom underwent LAD angioplasty. Ventricular arrhythmias requiring cardioversion occurred in 13 of 96 (14%) patients and preoperative cardiopul-

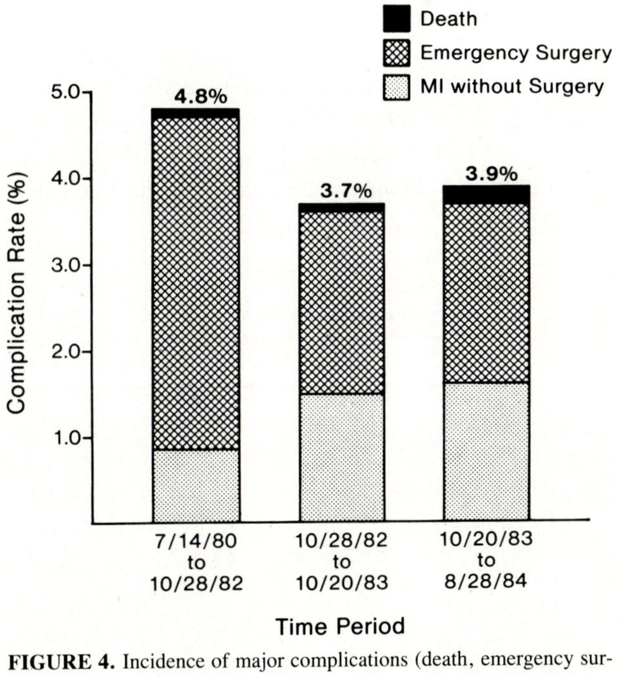

FIGURE 4. Incidence of major complications (death, emergency surgery, and myocardial infarction [MI] not associated with emergency surgery) in 3500 patients undergoing elective PTCA attempts. The total study population is divided into three periods with an equal number of patients in each time period, as in figure 1.

monary resuscitation (sustained closed-chest massage) was necessary in seven of 96 (7%) patients (six of whom had LAD angioplasty).

Initially successful emergency CABG was performed in all 96 patients, with the exception of one patient who underwent a thoracotomy for relief of pericardial tamponade. A total of 165 bypass grafts were placed. Reverse saphenous vein grafts were used in 160 vessels and internal mammary artery grafts to the LAD were used in five. Revascularization was performed to a single coronary arterial system (i.e., LAD or LCX or RCA) in 64 patients (90 grafts), a double arterial system in 30 patients (70 grafts), and all three arterial systems in one patient (five grafts).

The mortality rate for the 96 emergency surgery patients was 2%. Both patients who died had multivessel coronary artery disease, and abnormal left ventricular function caused by previous myocardial infarction, underwent LAD angioplasty attempt, and were hemodynamically unstable in the catheterization laboratory. There were no deaths among patients with single-vessel coronary artery disease or with normal left ventricular function undergoing emergency surgery for failed PTCA. In addition, there were no deaths in the five patients with a history of previous CABG who underwent emergency surgery for a failed PTCA. The duration of hospital stay for the 94 patients who survived surgery was 7 days or less for 53 patients, 8 to 14 days for 33 patients, and over 14 days for eight patients. Fifty-six percent of the emergency surgery patients were discharged within 1 week and 91% were discharged within 2 weeks of attempted PTCA.

An additional 89 patients who had an unsuccessful PTCA went on to elective CABG during the same hospitalization. None of these patients died and only one developed a myocardial infarction.

Myocardial infarction. The overall myocardial infarction rate was 2.6% (94/3500) and the Q-wave infarction rate was 1.1% (38/3500). In the emergency surgery group there was a total of 47 myocardial infarctions (49%), of which 22 (47%) were Q-wave infarctions. In the 3404 patients who did not have emergency surgery there was a total of 47 myocardial infarctions (1.4%), of which 16 (0.5%) were associated with new Q waves.

Fatal complications. The in-hospital mortality rate was 0.1% for the entire study population of 3500 patients. All four deaths occurred in patients undergoing LAD angioplasty (table 4). Two patients had single-vessel disease and initially successful PTCA. In one case, a 51-year-old man with a residual post-PTCA coronary thrombus was treated with 144,000 U of intracoronary streptokinase and a continuous inufusion of heparin. The patient died of an intracerebral hemorrhage 5 hr after PTCA. The second patient was a 69-year-old woman in whom ventricular fibrillation (successfully cardioverted) occurred during the pre-PTCA guiding angiogram. A subsequent left ventricular angiogram showed new anterior/apical akinesis, but this wall motion abnormality improved after successful LAD angioplasty. Sudden refractory electromechanical dissociation occurred 16 hours after PTCA. Total CK, including isoenzyme determination, performed 2 hr before death (14 hr after PTCA) was normal. Autopsy revealed an occlusive LAD thrombus at the PTCA site.

Two other fatal complications occurred in patients with multivessel disease and LAD dissection requiring emergency CABG. Both patients had previous myocardial infarction and impaired left ventricular function. Brief occlusion of the LAD resulted in severe hemodynamic deterioration in spite of intra-aortic balloon pump support and emergency surgery. Both died

TABLE 4
Fatal complications of PTCA

Age	Sex	PTCA site	CAD	Complication	Cause of death
51	M	LAD	SVD	Success/IC thrombus Streptokinase 144,000 U IC Heparin	Cerebral bleeding (5 hr)
69	F	LAD	SVD	Success/acute reocclusion	3° Heart block (16 hr)
63	F	LAD	MVD	Dissection/unstable IABP/EM-CABG	Renal failure Bradyarrhythmia (36 hr)
68	M	LAD	MVD	Dissection/stable EM-RePTCA (3 hr) IABP/EM-CABG	Multiple organ failure (2 wk)

SVD = single-vessel disease; MVD = multivessel disease; IC = intracoronary; IABP = intra-aortic balloon pump; EM-CABG = emergency coronary artery bypass graft surgery; EM-RePTCA = emergency repeat coronary angioplasty.

in the postoperative period from complications related to a low cardiac output state.

Predictors of major complications. To determine the preprocedure predictors of a major complication in patients undergoing single-lesion PTCA, we analyzed the relatively homogeneous subgroup of 3099 patients who had PTCA at only one coronary site in the presence of either single-vessel or multivessel disease (table 5). In this subgroup there was a total of 128 patients who experienced at least one major complication (emergency surgery, 85; myocardial infarction without surgery, 41; death without emergency surgery, two). Patients were at a higher risk of developing a major complication if they had multivessel disease (6.1%) vs single-vessel disease (3.7%), an eccentric lesion (5.2%) vs a concentric lesion (3.5%), or calcification of the lesion (8.0%) vs no calcification (3.9%). There was a trend toward increased complications in women but this did not reach statistical significance.

The strongest independent preprocedure predictor of a major complication by multivariate analysis was multivessel coronary disease ($p = .0099$) followed by lesion eccentricity ($p = .0136$), calcification of the lesion ($p = .0197$), female gender ($p = .0298$), and lesion length ($p = .0706$). However, only 64% of the patients were correctly classified. Unstable angina, duration of angina, lesion severity, previous CABG, and vein graft dilatation were not associated with an increased incidence of major complications. Inclusion of the smaller, heterogeneous subgroup of highly selected patients undergoing multiple-site PTCA in single-vessel or multivessel disease did not change the factors selected in the analysis.

The strongest predictor of a major complication by univariate ($p < .0001$) and multivariate analysis was

TABLE 5
Incidence of major complications in patients with/without a preprocedure risk factor (n = 3099)

Risk factor	No. of patients with risk factor	No. of patients with major complications	p value
Multivessel CAD	523 (17%)	32 (6.1%)	<.025
Single-vessel CAD	2576 (83%)	96 (3.7%)	
Eccentric lesion[A]	1198 (39%)	62 (5.2%)	<.05
Concentric lesion	1853 (61%)	65 (3.5%)	
Calcium in lesion	152 (5%)	12 (8.0%)	<.03
No calcium in lesion	2947 (95%)	116 (3.9%)	
Female	687 (22%)	37 (5.4%)	<.08
Male	2412 (78%)	91 (3.8%)	

[A]Total coronary occlusions in 48 patients could not be classified as eccentric or concentric lesions.

the procedural appearance of an intimal dissection. An intimal dissection was evident in 894 patients (29%). Of these, 93 patients (10.4%) developed a major complication. Of the 2205 patients without an intimal dissection, only 35 (1.6%) developed a major complication. Angiographic evidence of intimal dissection at the time of PTCA resulted in a 6.5-fold increase in the risk of developing a major complication. The other relatively weak procedural predictor of a major complication was a pre-PTCA transstenotic gradient of 50 mm Hg or greater.

Minor complications. A total of 244 isolated minor complications occurred in 241 patients (6.9%) who did not experience a major complication (table 3). Closure of a sidebranch artery at the site of PTCA was recorded only when documented by angiography at the time of the procedure. Ventricular arrhythmia requiring cardioversion was statistically more frequent during RCA angioplasty ($p < .001$) and was successfully treated without sequelae in all patients in whom it occurred. New conduction defects (right bundle branch block, 20; first-degree atrioventricular block, six; left bundle branch block, two; Wenckebach block, one; second-degree atrioventricular block, one; sinus bradycardia requiring temporary pacer, one) resolved before discharge in all but one patient. Emergency repeat catheterization for unstable chest pain with or without electrocardiographic evidence of ischemia revealed a patent PTCA artery site in nine patients, restenosis followed by a successful emergency repeat PTCA in 14, restenosis successfully treated with intracoronary nitroglycerin in three, and restenosis with good collateral perfusion treated with elective surgery in one. Surgical exploration to repair a pseudoaneurysm or persistent hemorrhage at the femoral puncture was required in 17 women and eight men. New-onset atrial fibrillation or flutter requiring medical therapy returned to normal sinus rhythm in all but one patient. Angiographic evidence of coronary embolization occurred in the presence of residual coronary thrombus after myocardial infarction, total occlusion, and saphenous vein graft dilatations. Uncomplicated tamponade caused by perforation of the right ventricle by a No. 6F pacing catheter was treated by pericardiocentesis in only three patients. Since switching to more flexible No. 5F pacing catheters, we have had no further episodes of tamponade. One patient developed a left hemianopsia after PTCA with an occipital lobe infarct documented on computed tomographic scan. Miscellaneous complications included elective repeat angiography and repeat PTCA, use of intra-aortic balloon pump for unstable symptoms, *Staphylococcus aureus* groin infection, transient ischemic attack, LAD closure during RCA angioplasty, and pulmonary edema.

Discussion

The efficacy of any therapeutic procedure depends on its risk-benefit ratio. When this is applied to management of single-vessel coronary disease by PTCA the question of short-term complications assumes particular importance. The natural history of patients with single-vessel disease has been well described.[31–34] In a recent report,[31] the 5 year survival in potential ideal candidates for PTCA with single vessel disease treated medically was 97%. If PTCA is to be offered to improve functional capacity in these patients, the risks of the procedure must be comparable to the most favorable surgical results available in similar groups.

In this consecutive series of 3500 patients undergoing elective PTCA, the mortality rate of 0.1% is better than reported surgical results[7, 35] and the 0.9% mortality recorded from the NHLBI PTCA Registry.[20] The Registry study population is of comparable size (3079 patients) but it differs in that data were collected from 106 institutions during an earlier, although overlapping, time period (1977 to 1982 vs 1980 to 1984). Nevertheless, the baseline patient characteristics and the anatomic location of attempted PTCA are similar to those of our study.[36] The major complication rate for the two series is shown in figure 5.[19, 20]

The lower incidence of major complications in this series can be explained in part by greater experience in case selection, technical expertise, and clinical judgment and by improvements in angioplasty equipment that have evolved since the NHLBI Registry data were collected.[22, 23, 26, 37–39] The routine use of biplane angiographic eqipment and intracoronary hemodynamic measurements may play a role as well as increased familiarity and training of supporting hospital personnel. There has been no significant decrease in the incidence of major complications in our series over the 50 month period, as shown in figure 4, probably because of the increasing difficulty of attempted PTCA procedures.

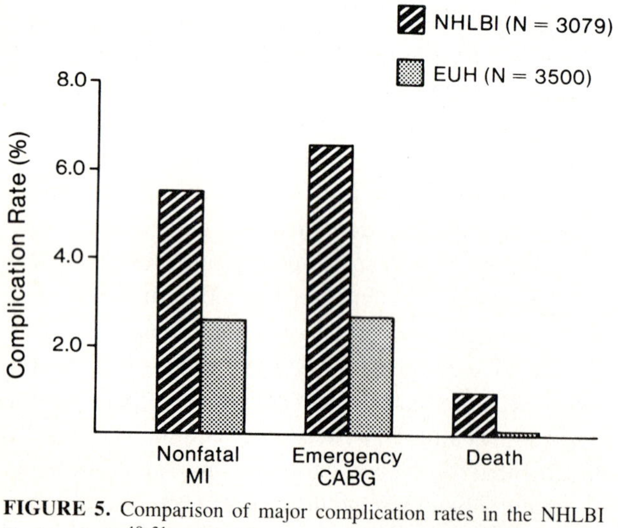

FIGURE 5. Comparison of major complication rates in the NHLBI Registry series[19–21] and the Emory University Hospital (EUH) series. N = total number of patients in each series.

Specifically, the lower mortality in this series may be related to the surgical treatment of failed PTCA at our institution.[15, 40, 41] The emergency surgery mortality was 2% (2/96) in our series vs 6.4% (13/202) in the NHLBI Registry.[20] Emergency surgery initiated during full cardiac arrest appeared to be a life-saving procedure in six patients. In addition, there were no deaths in 89 elective post-PTCA CABG procedures in our series vs 10 deaths during elective post-PTCA surgery in the NHLBI Registry.[20] These data suggest that when elective coronary angioplasty is performed for single-vessel coronary disease with good surgical and anesthetic support, the mortality should approach zero.

It is more difficult to find a surgical series of similar patients suitable for comparison. The overall mortality figures from the five centers with the best surgical results in the Coronary Artery Surgery Study ranged from 0.3% to 1%.[6] For patients with single-vessel disease the overall mortality was 1.4%, and for patients with ejection fractions of 50% or greater the mortality was 1.9%.[6] In our series, 19% of the patients had multivessel disease, 28% had a history of myocardial infarction, and 50% had a recent history of unstable symptoms. This last descriptor may have placed our patients at a higher risk, since patients with class III to IV symptoms were not randomized in the CASS study. These differences not withstanding, the mortality data for PTCA in our series (0.1%) appears to be better than one might have expected for CABG.

In an attempt to improve patient selection for PTCA and to identify high-risk patients, a univariate and multivariate analysis was performed on 20 clinical and angiographic potential predictors of a major complication. Five significant risk factors were identified: multivessel coronary artery disease, eccentric lesions, lesion calcification, female gender, and lesion length.

The only baseline clinical characteristic that was an independent predictor of a major complication was female gender. There were no baseline clinical characteristics identified as predictors of mortality in our series. This is in contrast to the NHLBI Registry data in which five clinical predictors of mortality were identified (female gender, age >60 yr, prior CABG, angina >6 months, and vein graft PTCA).[20] In particular,

Cowley et al.[42] showed that women had a sixfold higher PTCA-related mortality and a fivefold higher mortality with emergency surgery. In our series, the female mortality was increased (0.26% vs 0.073%) but this did not reach statistical significance because of the small number of deaths.

The angiographic predictors of a major complication were related to lesion morphology, and this is in agreement with data from the NHLBI Registry.[19, 21] However, the importance of multivessel disease as an independent risk factor has not previously been reported. The critical link between the morphologic extent of atherosclerosis and development of a major complication appears to be the appearance of angiographically evident intimal dissection.[19] In our series, once this had occurred, 10% of the patients in this subgroup evolved a major complication. In the NHLBI series an intimal dissection was associated with a 30% incidence of major complications.[19] The apparent discrepancy between these results may be related to the coding of patients with intimal dissection, since the recorded incidence of dissection was almost threefold higher in our series than in the NHLBI series (30% vs 12.9%). In addition, intimal dissection in our series was significantly correlated only with female gender and increasing lesion length. In the NHLBI series intimal dissection was associated with female gender, RCA dilatation, multivessel disease, eccentric lesions, and nondiscrete lesions.[19]

In conclusion, the NHLBI Registry provided valuable information about PTCA during its early development. However, such data represent the initial results that were obtained with what are now considered to be outmoded techniques, and must be interpreted from this perspective. They no longer represent the state of the art of coronary angioplasty. The results presented in this article indicate what can now be expected when elective PTCA is performed by current techniques.

We thank Johnny Tate and George Cotsonis for computer programming and statistical assistance. We also thank Linda Greene, Allyson Bakewell, Diana Nelson, Clair Rice, Eileen Ball, Ann Cofer, and Elizabeth Quilter for technical assistance and Diana Williams for typing the manuscript.

References

1. Killip T, Ryan TJ: Randomized trials in coronary bypass surgery. Circulation **71:** 418, 1985
2. Harris PJ, Harrell FE, Lee KL, Behar VS, Rosati RA: Survival in medically treated coronary artery disease. Circulation **60:** 1259, 1979
3. Bruschke AVG, Proudfit WL, Sones FM: Progress study of 590 consecutive nonsurgical cases of coronary disease followed 5–9 years. 1. Arteriographic correlations. Circulation **47:** 1147, 1973
4. Schulze RA, Strauss HW, Pitt B: Sudden death in the year following myocardial infarction: relation to ventricular premature contractions in the late hospital phase and left ventricular ejection fraction. Am J Med 62: 192, 1977
5. Shah PK, Pichler M, Berman DS, Singh BN, Swan HJ: Left ventricular ejection fraction determined by radionuclide ventriculography in early stages of first transluminal myocardial infarction: relation to short-term prognosis. Am J Cardiol **45:** 542, 1980
6. Kennedy JW, Kaiser GC, Fisher LD, Fritz JK, Myers W, Mudd JG, Ryan TJ: Clinical and angiographic predictors of operative mortality from the Collaborative Study in Coronary Artery Surgery (CASS). Circulation **63:** 793, 1981
7. Kennedy JW, Kaiser GC, Fisher LD, Maynard C, Fritz JK, Myers W, Mudd JG, Ryan TJ, Coggin J: Multivariate discriminant analysis of the clinical and angiographic predictors of operative mortality from the Collaborative Study in Coronary Artery Surgery (CASS). J Thorac Cardiovasc Surg **80:** 876, 1980
8. CASS Principal Investigators and their associates: Coronary artery surgery study (CASS): a randomized trial of coronary artery bypass surgery. Survival data. Circulation **68:** 939, 1983
9. Gruentzig A: Transluminal dilatation of coronary artery stenosis. Lancet **1:** 263, 1978
10. Gruentzig A, Senning A, Siegenthaler WE: Nonoperative dilatation of coronary artery stenoses: percutaneous transluminal coronary angioplasty. N Engl J Med **301:** 61, 1979
11. Gruentzig A, Schlumpf M, Siegenthaler W: Long-term results after coronary angioplasty. Circulation **70**(suppl II): II-323, 1984 (abst)
12. Gunnar RM, Loeb HS: An alternative interpretation of the results of the Coronary Artery Surgery Study. Circulation **71:** 193, 1985
13. Health and Public Policy Committee, American College of Physicians: Percutaneous transluminal angioplasty. Ann Intern Med **99:** 864, 1983
14. Reul GJ, Cooley DA, Hallman GL, Duncan JM, Livesay JJ, Frazier OH, Ott DA, Angelini P, Massumi A, Mathur VS: Coronary artery bypass for unsuccessful percutaneous transluminal coronary angioplasty. J Thorac Cardiovasc Surg **88:** 685, 1984
15. Jones EL, Craver JM, Gruentzig AR, King SB, Douglas JS, Bone DK, Guyton RG, Hatcher CR: Percutaneous transluminal coronary angioplasty: role of the surgeon. Ann Thorac Surg **34:** 493, 1982
16. Vlietstra RE, Holmes DR, Reeder GS, Mock MB, Smith HC, Bove AA, Bresnahan JF, Prehler JM: Balloon angioplasty in multivessel coronary artery disease. Mayo Clin Proc **58:** 563, 1983
17. Kent KM, Bentivoglio LG, Block PC, Cowley MJ, Dorros G, Gosselin A, Gruentzig A, Myler RK, Simpson J, Stertzer SH, Williams DO, Fisher L, Gillespie MJ, Mullin JM, Mock MB: Percutaneous transluminal coronary angioplasty: report from the NHLBI Registry. Am J Cardiol **49:** 2011, 1982
18. Dorros G, Cowley MJ, Simpson J, Bentivoglio LG, Block PC, Bourassa M, Detre K, Gosselin AJ, Gruentzig AR, Kelsey SF, Kent KM, Mock MB, Mullin SM, Myler RK, Passamani ER, Stertzer SH, Williams DO: Percutaneous transluminal coronary angioplasty: report of complications from the National Heart, Lung and Blood Institute PTCA Registry. Circulation **67:** 723, 1983
19. Cowley MJ, Dorros G, Kelsey SF, Van Raden M, Detre KM: Acute coronary events associated with percutaneous transluminal coronary angioplasty. Am J Cardiol **53:** 12C, 1984
20. Dorros G, Cowley MJ, Janke L, Kelsey SF, Mullin SM, Van Raden M: In-hospital mortality rate in the National Heart, Lung and Blood Institute PTCA Registry. Am J Cardiol **53:** 17C, 1984
21. Cowley MJ, Dorros G, Kelsey SF, Van Raden M, Detre KM: Emergency coronary bypass surgery after coronary angioplasty: the National Heart, Lung and Blood Institute's PTCA Registry experience. Am J Cardiol **53:** 22C, 1984
22. Anderson HV, Roubin GS, Leimgruber PP, Douglas JS, King SB, Gruentzig AR: Primary angiographic success rates of percutaneous transluminal coronary angioplasty. Am J Cardiol (in press; Oct. 1985)
23. Gruentzig AR, Hollman J: Improved primary success rate in transluminal coronary angioplasty using a steerable guidewire system. Circulation **66**(suppl II): II-330, 1982
24. Simpson JB, Baim DS, Robert EW, Harrison DC: A new catheter system for coronary angioplasty. Am J Cardiol **49:** 1216, 1982
25. Kelsey SF, Mullin SM, Detre KM, Mitchell H, Cowley MJ, Gruentzig AR, Kent KM: Effect of investigator experience on percutaneous transluminal coronary angioplasty. Am J Cardiol **53:** 56C, 1984
26. Meier B, Gruentzig AR: Learning curve for percutaneous translu-

minal coronary angioplasty: skill, technology or patient selection. Am J Cardiol **53:** 65C, 1984
27. Gruentzig AR: Technique of percutaneous transluminal coronary angioplasty. *In* Hurst JW, editor: The Heart. New York, 1982, McGraw-Hill, p 1904
28. Blackburn H, Keys A, Simonson E, Rantalarja P, Pursar S: The electrocardiogram in population studies, a classified system. Circulation **21:** 1160, 1960
29. Meier B, Gruentzig A, Goebel N, Pyle N, von Gossler W, Schlumpf M: Assessment of stenoses in coronary angioplasty. Inter and intraobserver variability. Int J Cardiol **8:** 159, 1983
30. Lochenbruch PA: Discriminant analysis. New York, 1975, Hafner Press
31. Hlatky MA, Califf RM, Kong Yihong, Harrell FE, Rosati RA: Natural history of patients with single vessel disease suitable for percutaneous transluminal coronary angioplasty. Am J Cardiol **52:** 225, 1983
32. Califf RM, Tomabechi Y, Lee KL, Phillips H, Pryor DB, Harrell FE, Harris PJ, Peter RH, Behar VS, Kong Y, Rosati RA: Outcome in one-vessel coronary artery disease. Circulation **67:** 283, 1983
33. Mock M, Ringqvist I, Fisher L, Davis KB, Chairman BR, Konchoukos NT, Kaiser G, Alderman E, Ryan TJ, Russell RO Jr, Mullin S, Fray D, Killip T, and the participants in CASS: Survival of medically treated patients in Coronary Artery Surgery Study (CASS) registry. Circulation **66:** 562, 1982
34. Ringqvist J, Fisher LD, Mock M, Davis KB, Wedel H, Chaitman BR, Passamani E, Russell RO Jr, Alderman EL, Kouchoukas NT, Kaiser GC, Ryan TJ, Killip T, Fray D: Prognostic value of angiographic indices of coronary artery disease from the Coronary Artery Surgery Study (CASS). J Clin Invest **71:** 1854, 1983
35. Council on Scientific Affairs: Percutaneous transluminal angioplasty. JAMA **251:** 764, 1984
36. Detre KM, Myler R, Kelsey SF, Van Roden M, To T, Mitchell H: Baseline characteristics of patients in the National Heart, Lung and Blood Institute PTCA Registry. Am J Cardiol **53:** 7C, 1984
37. Gruentzig AR: PTCA: Technical aspects and indications. *In* Vecht RJ, editor: Angioplasty. London 1984, Pitman Publishing Ltd., pp 83–91
38. McAuley BJ, Oesterle S, Simpson JB: Advances in guidewire technology. Am J Cardiol **53:** 94C, 1984
39. Fogerty TJ, Kinney TB, Finn JC: Current status of dilatation catheters and guiding systems. Am J Cardiol **53:** 97C, 1984
40. Murphy D, Craver J, Jones E, Curling P, Guyton R, King S, Gruentzig A, Hatcher CR: Surgical management of acute myocardial ischemia following percutaneous transluminal coronary angioplasty. J Thorac Cardiovasc Surg **87:** 332, 1984
41. Murphy DA, Craver JM, Jones EL, King SB, Curling PE, Douglas JS: Hemodynamic deterioration after coronary angioplasty in the presence of previous left ventricular infarction. Am J Cardiol **54:** 448, 1984
42. Cowley MJ, Mullin S, Kelsey SF, Kent KM, Gruentzig AR, Detre KM, Passamani ER: Sex differences in early and long-term results of coronary angioplasty in the NHLBI PTCA Registry. Circulation **71:** 91, 1985

The effects of the rate of intravenous infusion of streptokinase and the duration of symptoms on the time interval to reperfusion in patients with acute myocardial infarction

ALLAN S. LEW, M.D., PIERRE LARAMEE, M.D., BOJAN CERCEK, M.D., LOIS RODRIGUEZ, R.N., PREDIMAN K. SHAH, M.D., AND WILLIAM GANZ, M.D., C.SC.

ABSTRACT We studied the influence of the following variables on the time interval from initiation of an intravenous infusion of 750,000 U of streptokinase until reperfusion (reperfusion time) in 140 consecutive patients with an evolving acute myocardial infarction: (1) the rate of infusion of streptokinase, (2) the duration of chest pain before initiation of treatment, (3) patient age, (4) patient sex, (5) location of infarction, (6) history of previous myocardial infarction, and (7) pretreatment pathologic Q waves. The time of reperfusion was recognized by clinical criteria that were completely concordant with the anatomic findings in all 119 patients in whom patency or occlusion of the artery of infarction was established at delayed angiography (n = 116) or at postmortem examination (n = 3). The mean reperfusion time for the 129 patients for whom data were available was 49 ± 36 min. The reperfusion time was inversely related to the rate of infusion of streptokinase (r = .41, p < .001), but this effect of infusion rate appeared to plateau at rates of greater than 500 U/kg/min. In the 64 patients receiving infusions at rates of 500 U/kg/min or less, the mean reperfusion time was 60 ± 40 min, whereas in the 58 patients receiving the drug at rates greater than 500 U/kg/min it was 35 ± 22 min (p < .001). The duration of chest pain before treatment was the only other studied variable found to influence the reperfusion time, but only at infusion rates of less than 250 U/kg/min (r = .6, p < .01). Our findings indicate that in patients with acute myocardial infarction who receive high-dose intravenous streptokinase, the time interval to reperfusion can be minimized by increasing the infusion rate up to at least 500 U/kg/min and by shortening the delay from onset of symptoms to treatment.

Circulation 72, No. 5, 1053–1058, 1985.

EARLY REPERFUSION of the artery of infarction may limit the extent of myocardial necrosis in patients with an evolving acute myocardial infarction[1–3] and improve ventricular function[4–8] and survival.[8, 9] Both experimental[10–12] and clinical[13–15] studies indicate that the critical determinant of the extent of myocardial necrosis and salvage is the duration of myocardial ischemia before reperfusion. In clinical practice, this ischemic period comprises (1) the time interval from the onset of infarction to the commencement of treatment, which is predominantly a logistical problem,[16–20] and (2) the time interval from commencement of treatment until reperfusion, which is predominantly a biological variable.

From the Division of Cardiology, Department of Medicine, Cedars-Sinai Medical Center and the Department of Medicine, UCLA School of Medicine, Los Angeles.

Supported in part by NIH SCOR grant No. 17651.

Address for correspondence: Allan S. Lew, M.D., Room No. 5314, Division of Cardiology, Cedars-Sinai Medical Center, 8700 Beverly Blvd., Los Angeles, CA, 90048.

Received June 13, 1985; revision accepted Aug. 8, 1985.

Presented in part at the 34th Annual Scientific Sessions of the American College of Cardiology in Anaheim, CA, March 12, 1985.

In this study, we investigate the potential effect of the following factors on the time interval from treatment until reperfusion by intravenous streptokinase: (1) the rate of infusion of streptokinase, (2) the duration of chest pain before initiation of treatment, (3) patient age, (4) patient sex, (5) the location of infarction, (6) the presence of eletrocardiographic and/or historical evidence of a previous infarction, and (7) the presence of pretreatment, pathologic Q waves in the region of the current infarction.

Methods

Patient population. The study population consisted of 140 consecutive patients with acute myocardial infarction (107 men, 33 women) who were 62 ± 12 years old (range 32 to 86) and were included in a prospective study of intravenous streptokinase. All fulfilled the following criteria: (1) chest pain of less than 3 hr duration at the time of evaluation by the cardiology team, (2) ST segment elevation indicative of transmural ischemia, (3) persistent chest pain and electrocardiographic changes after sublingual nitroglycerin, (4) absence of contraindications to thrombolytic or anticoagulant therapy, and (5) consent from both the patient's physician and the patient.

Administration of streptokinase. A 750,000 U dose of

streptokinase (Hoechst-Roussel) in 45 to 75 ml of normal saline was administered by infusion into a peripheral vein over a period of 3 to 78 min (mean 26 ± 16). The rate of infusion of streptokinase (U of streptokinase/kg body weight/min) could be determined in 133 of the 140 patients as the total dose of streptokinase divided by the weight of the patient and by the time interval over which the drug was administered.

One hundred and thirty-one of the 140 patients received an intravenous bolus of either 100 mg hydrocortisone or 4 mg dexamethasone before they received streptokinase. All patients were begun on a continuous infusion of heparin immediately after the infusion of streptokinase. Eight patients in whom reperfusion had not occurred by 90 min received a second infusion of 750,000 U of streptokinase at the same rate as the first infusion.

Recognition of reperfusion. To minimize delay in treatment, pretreatment coronary angiography was not performed and reperfusion was recognized by the following nonangiographic criteria.

Abatement of symptoms. Before beginning the infusion of streptokinase, the patient was asked to immediately report any change in chest pain or other symptoms.

Decrease in ST segment elevation. A 12-lead electrocardiogram was recorded before the infusion of streptokinase was begun and a lead with distinct ST segment elevation was continuously monitored and observed by at least one, and usually two, of the authors until either there was evidence of reperfusion or for a period of up to 4 hr in patients with no signs of reperfusion. Short recordings of the monitored lead or a 12-lead electrocardiogram were obtained at 5 to 15 min intervals during the procedure and also whenever there was a change in symptoms, a change in ST segment elevation on the monitor, or a change in cardiac rhythm.

Cardiac enzyme washout. Blood for determination of serum creatine kinase (CK) and CK-MB activity was drawn at 15 to 30 min intervals for the initial 2 to 4 hr and 1 to 4 hourly for the remainder of the first 24 hr after streptokinase. The CK time-activity curves were plotted and the time of an abrupt rise in CK level (CK washout) was determined.

Reperfusion was considered to have occurred when the following three events occurred in a close temporal relationship: (1) an abrupt abatement or progressive reduction of chest pain, (2) a reduction in the magnitude of ST segment elevation with its progressive decrease in sequential electrocardiograms that continued until the ST segments were isoelectric or reached a stable baseline, and (3) an abrupt and rapid rise in serum levels of CK.

In 15 patients, the chest pain had resolved before commencement of the streptokinase infusion, in two patients there was no CK data, and in six patients the onset of the abrupt and rapid rise in CK was delayed. In these 23 patients, reperfusion was considered to have occurred when there was a sustained and progressive resolution of the ST segment elevation temporally related to either an abrupt abatement or reduction in chest pain or an abrupt and rapid rise in serum CK. Because a progressive resolution of the ST segment elevation was always required as a criterion of reperfusion, the time of reperfusion was defined as the time of onset of the resolution of the ST segment elevation. The time interval to reperfusion (reperfusion time) was defined as the interval from commencement of the steptokinase infusion to the time of reperfusion.

Coronary anatomy. In 116 patients, coronary angiography and contrast left ventriculography were performed 4 ± 3 days (range 1 to 15) after admission and were analyzed by two angiographers who were unaware of the results of the other investigations and did not otherwise participate in the study. In three patients who died in-hospital before coronary angiography could be performed, the coronary arteries were examined at a postmortem examination.

Patency or occlusion of the artery of infarction was verified without difficulty in 115 of the 119 patients. In the remaining four patients with both a prior and current inferior infarction in whom either the right or circumflex coronary artery was occluded, determination of the artery of infarction was based on (1) angiographic evidence of an ulcerated atheromatous plaque, i.e., indistinct luminal margins and subintimal defect of the coronary artery following lysis of the clot,[21] and (2) the distribution of regional dysfunction and ^{201}Tl perfusion on sequential radionuclide studies.

Statistical methods. Continuous Gaussian variables are described by their mean and standard deviation. The unpaired Student t test and one-way analysis of variance were used for comparisons between two or more subgroups, respectively. Proportional differences between subgroups were compared with the use of Fisher's exact test. The relationship between continuous variables was analyzed by the unweighted linear least squares method. All analyses were performed with BMDP biostatistical programs and a two-tailed p value of $<.05$ was considered to indicate statistical significance.

Results

One hundred and thirty-four of the 140 patients had nonangiographic evidence of coronary artery reperfusion and the remaining six patients did not. Of the 119 patients with known coronary anatomy, the artery of infarction was found to be patent in all 113 patients with clinical signs of reperfusion and the artery was occluded in the six patients without clinical signs of reperfusion. The reperfusion time could be determined in 129 of the 134 patients with clinical evidence of reperfusion and was 49 ± 35 min (range 5 to 228).

The effect of the rate of infusion of streptokinase on reperfusion time. Figure 1 illustrates that in the 122 patients in whom both the rate of infusion of streptokin-

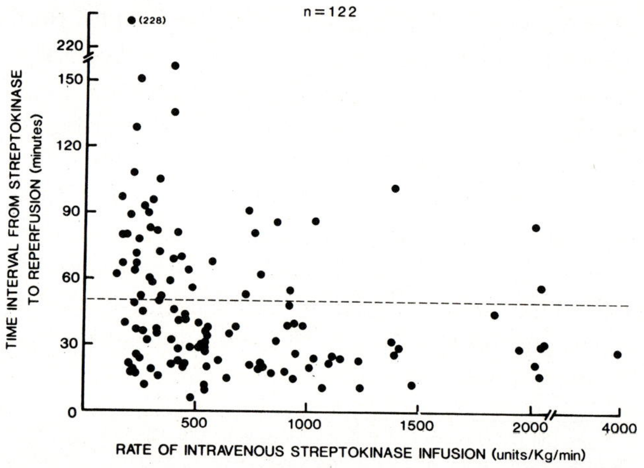

FIGURE 1. Graphic representation of the inverse relationship between the rate of intravenous infusion of streptokinase and the time interval from commencement of streptokinase to reperfusion. The broken line at a reperfusion time of 50 min (mean value) indicates that most patients with a time interval to reperfusion longer than 50 min received an infusion of streptokinase at a rate slower than 500 U/kg/min.

ase and the reperfusion time were available, there was an inverse relationship between the rate of infusion of streptokinase and the time interval to reperfusion ($r = .41$, $p < .001$), which was similar for patients with anterior and those with inferior infarction. This relationship appeared to plateau at infusion rates of about 500 U/kg/min. In the 64 patients receiving infusions at rates of 500 U/kg/min or less, the mean reperfusion time was 60 ± 40 min compared with 35 ± 22 min in the 58 patients who received infusions at rates of greater than 500 U/kg/min ($p < .001$). Figure 1 also indicates that reperfusion time was less than 50 min in only 45% of the 64 patients who received a slower infusion rate compared with 83% of the 58 patients who received a faster infusion rate ($p < .001$).

Further analysis of the influence of the rate of streptokinase infusion on the reperfusion time was performed by dividing the study population into five subgroups according to the rate of intravenous infusion (table 1). In 24 patients the infusion rate was 250 U/kg/min or less (very slow group), in 39 patients it was 260 to 500 U/kg/min (slow group), in 20 patients it was 510 to 750 U/kg/min (intermediate group), in 16 patients it was 760 to 1000 U/kg/min (rapid group), and in 23 patients it was greater than 1000 U/kg/min (very rapid group). The difference in the mean reperfusion times between the very slow and slow infusion rate groups (70 ± 49 and 54 ± 34 min, respectively) was not statistically significant ($p = .07$), but they were both significantly longer ($p < .01$) than the mean reperfusion times in the intermediate (34 ± 19 min), rapid (38 ± 23 min), and very rapid (34 ± 25 min) infusion rate groups. There was no difference in mean reperfusion time among the latter three groups.

The effect of the duration of chest pain on reperfusion time. For the entire study population, there was no correlation between the duration of chest pain before streptokinase and reperfusion time ($r = .13$). To minimize the influence of the infusion rate of streptokinase, the relationship was separately analyzed in five subgroups, each including patients receiving a narrow range of infusion rates defined as the mean value ±15% of each of the subgroups described in table 1. The corresponding infusion rate ranges were 210 ± 30 U/kg/min (17 patients), 370 ± 50 U/kg/min (19 patients), 600 ± 90 U/kg/min (17 patients), 880 ± 130 U/kg/min (16 patients), and greater than 1450 U/kg/min (10 patients). Only in the 17 patients from the slowest infusion rate group (180 to 240 U/kg/min) was there a significant correlation ($r = .6$, $p = .005$) between the duration of chest pain and the reperfusion time (figure 2). There was no correlation, or even a trend, for any of the subgroups receiving faster infusion rates of streptokinase.

Other clinical variables (table 2). The reperfusion time was not influenced by any of the other clinical variables that were studied, including patient age, patient sex, location of infarction, the presence of electrocardiographic and/or historical evidence of a previous infarction, and the presence of pathologic Q waves in the region of the current infarction before initiation of streptokinase therapy.

Discussion

The wide range of infusion rates in this study reflects our progressive experience with intravenous streptokinase. Initially, streptokinase was administered very rapidly (in 5 to 15 min) to achieve a high serum concentration similar to that achieved with intracoronary administration; however, these very rapid infusion rates frequently caused hypotension.[17, 19, 22, 23] Subsequently, a range of slower infusion rate protocols were used in an attempt to prevent the hypotensive effect. Therefore, our total experience provided the data necessary to study the effect of varying infusion rates on reperfusion time.

Our data indicate that in patients with evolving acute myocardial infarction, the reperfusion time is inversely related to the rate of streptokinase infusion and, at slow infusion rates, is also directly related to the duration of chest pain before initiation of treatment.

Since the rate of infusion affects the serum concentration of streptokinase,[24, 25] our results imply that the rate of thrombolysis is a function of the serum concentration of this drug. This finding is consistent with the known direct relationships between the concentration

TABLE 1
Influence of intravenous streptokinase (IV-SK) infusion rate on time interval to reperfusion

	Very slow (n = 24)	Slow (n = 39)	Intermed. (n = 20)	Rapid (n = 16)	Very rapid (n = 19)	p value
Rate IV-SK (U/kg/min)	210±30	370±70	600±80	880±70	1700±710	<.001
Pain to SK (min)	135±53	150±48	137±43	131±55	130±89	NS
SK to reperfusion (min)	70±49	54±34	34±19	38±23	34±25	<.01

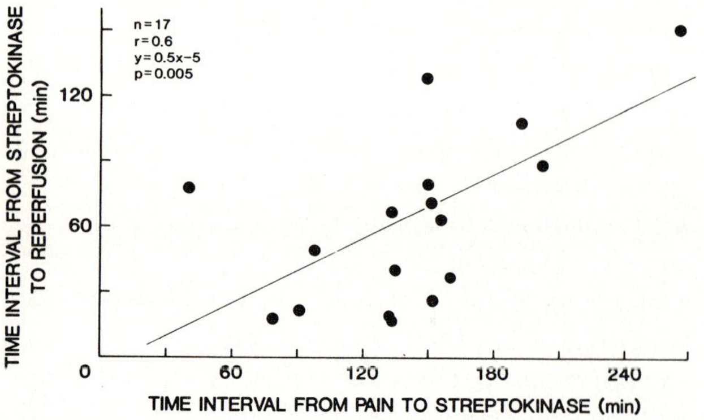

FIGURE 2. Graphic representation of the direct relationship between the duration of chest pain before initiation of streptokinase and the time interval from commencement of streptokinase infusion to reperfusion in patients receiving a slow rate infusion.

of streptokinase, the concentration of plasminogen activator complex,[26, 27] and the rate of thrombolysis.[27, 28] The effect of the streptokinase infusion rate on the reperfusion time appears to plateau at a rate of about 500 U/kg/min and therefore, faster infusion rates, which are more likely to produce significant hypotension, appear to have no advantage with respect to earlier reperfusion.

If one accepts that the chest pain of acute myocardial infarction commences at about the time of thrombotic occlusion of the artery of infarction, then the duration of chest pain in patients with acute infarction is an indirect approximation of age of thrombus, or at least the age of the final occlusive portion of the thrombus. Our finding that at slow infusion rates of streptokinase, the duration of chest pain was a determinant of the reperfusion time, suggests that the age of the thrombus influenced the results of thrombolytic therapy. This is in accordance with clinical studies using streptokinase in which the duration of symptoms before initiation of treatment was shown to be a determinant of both the rate of successful reperfusion[16, 29–31] and the rapidity of thrombolysis,[29, 32] and is also consistent with experimental studies showing that older thrombi are more resistant to lysis.[33, 34] This age-related resistance of the thrombus to lysis may be due to an increased degree of fibrin cross-linking within the thrombus,[35] a decrease in plasminogen content of the thrombus due to its retraction,[27, 36] or thrombus growth with time.[37] The finding that the age of the thrombus was a factor only in patients who received streptokinase at slow infusion rates is consistent with the experimental data reported by McDonagh et al.,[38] who found the presence of fibrin cross-linking to be a determinant of the rate of thrombolysis at low concentrations of urokinase, but not at high concentrations.

The considerable scatter of our data suggests that reperfusion time after intravenous streptokinase is probably affected by other factors,[39] such as the size of the thrombus independent of its age,[40] serum levels of plasminogen, antiplasmins,[41, 42] and neutralizing antistreptokinase antibodies,[42–44] and especially access of streptokinase to the thrombus.[24, 45, 46] The latter depends on the surface area of the thrombus exposed to the lytic agent[24] and the antegrade and collateral blood flow reaching the occlusive thrombus,[46] which may be especially important when the thrombus is situated distal to a tight stenosis.

A potential limitation of this study is that the determination and timing of reperfusion was based on nonangiographic criteria. However, this reperfusion syndrome, consisting of relief of chest pain, resolution of ST segment elevation, and CK washout, has a sound physiologic basis and its validity is supported by (1) experimental studies,[47–49] (2) the complete concordance between the occurrence of this syndrome and the finding of patency of the artery of infarction in our study, and (3) the excellent concordance between these signs and angiographically recognized reperfusion in several intracoronary streptokinase studies.[29, 50–57] In the intracoronary studies of Lee, Rentrop, Mathey, and Ganz and their colleagues,[29, 50–52] the clinical signs of reperfusion usually occurred within minutes of the angiographic demonstration of arterial patency and in some studies, these clinical signs were used to indicate when to check the patency of the artery of infarction by angiography.[50, 58, 59] Furthermore, these clinical signs of reperfusion have also been adopted by several other investigators using intravenous streptokinase.[16, 19, 59, 60]

TABLE 2
Relation of clinical variables to the time interval to reperfusion

Variable	Minutes
Age	
≤60 years (n = 55)	50±34
>60 years (n = 74)	49±37
Sex	
Male (n = 98)	48±40
Female (n = 31)	50±33
Location of infarction	
Anterior (n = 58)	53±36
Inferior (n = 71)	47±35
Previous MI	
Yes (n = 32)	44±27
No (n = 97)	51±38
Pretreatment Q waves	
Yes (n = 53)	55±33
No (n = 68)	46±38

MI = myocardial infarction; SK = streptokinase.

The delay in the abrupt washout of CK relative to the relief of chest pain and resolution of ST segment elevation in six of our patients was similar to that observed in four patients in our intracoronary streptokinase study.[52] In these four patients, the delay in CK washout relative to angiographic patency, as well as relief of chest pain and resolution of ST segment elevation, was associated with initially partial reperfusion and sluggish coronary flow. However, in all four patients, a rapid washout of CK occurred when the flow in the artery of infarction improved and the progression of contrast became similar to that in the other arteries.

Although our definition of reperfusion time has some inherent error, it was based on a sampling frequency of electrocardiographic recordings similar to the usual 15 min interval between coronary angiograms used in intracoronary studies. Since our definition was applied consistently throughout our study, this inaccuracy is not likely to have distorted our conclusions that the reperfusion time is affected by the streptokinase infusion rate and by the duration of chest pain before treatment.

Clinical implications. Our data indicate that in patients with acute myocardial infarction who are treated with high-dose intravenous streptokinase, the reperfusion time can be reduced by starting the infusion of streptokinase as soon as possible after the onset of symptoms and infusing streptokinase at a rate of about 500 U/kg/min, if this dose can be tolerated. Infusion of streptokinase at rates faster than 500 U/kg/min does not appear to be advantageous with respect to reperfusion time.

We are grateful to Rosa Goldsmith for preparation of artwork and to Ann Lew for research assistance.

References

1. Markis JE, Malagold M, Parker A, Silverman KJ, Barry WH, Als AV, Paulin S, Grossman W, Braunwald E: Myocardial salvage after intracoronary thrombolysis with streptokinase in acute myocardial infarction. Assessment by intracoronary thallium-201. N Engl J Med **305:** 777, 1981
2. Maddahi J, Ganz W, Ninomiya K, Hashida J, Fishbein MC, Mondkar A, Buchbinder N, Marcus H, Geft I, Shah PK, Rozanski A, Swan HJC, Berman DS: Myocardial salvage by intracoronary thrombolysis in evolving acute myocardial infarction: evaluation using intracoronary injection of thallium-201. Am Heart J **102:** 664, 1981
3. Sobel BE, Geltman EM, Tiefenbrunn AJ, Jaffe AS, Spadaro JJ, Ter-Pogossian MM, Collen D, Ludbrook PA: Improvement of regional myocardial metabolism after coronary thrombolysis induced with tissue-type plasminogen activator or streptokinase. Circulation **69:** 983, 1984
4. Anderson JL, Marshall HW, Bray BE, Lutz JR, Frederick PR, Yanowitz FG, Datz FL, Klausner SC, Hagan AD: A randomized trial of intracoronary streptokinase in the treatment of acute myocardial infarction. N Engl J Med **308:** 1312, 1983
5. Rogers WJ, Hood WP Jr, Mantle JA, Baxley WA, Kirklin JK, Zorn GL, Nath HP: Return of left ventricular function after reperfusion in patients with myocardial infarction: importance of subtotal stenoses or intact collaterals. Circulation **69:** 338, 1984
6. Sheehan FH, Mathey DG, Schofer J, Krebber HJ, Dodge HT: Effect of interventions in salvaging left ventricular function in acute myocardial infarction: A study of intracoronary streptokinase. Am J Cardiol **52:** 431, 1983
7. Charuzi Y, Beder C, Marshall LA, Sasaki H, Pack NB, Geft I, Ganz W: Improvement in regional and global left ventricular function after intracoronary thrombolysis: assessment with two-dimensional echocardiography. Am J Cardiol **53:** 662, 1984
8. Smalling RW, Fuentes F, Mathews MW, Freund GC, Hicks CH, Reduto LA, Walker WE, Sterling RP, Gould KL: Sustained improvement in left ventricular function and mortality by intracoronary streptokinase adminstration during evolving myocardial infarction. Circulation **68:** 131, 1983
9. Kennedy JW, Ritchie JL, Davis KB, Stadius ML, Maynard C, Fritz JK: The Western Washington randomized trial of intracoronary streptokinase in acute myocardial infarction. A 12 month follow-up report. N Engl J Med **312:** 1073, 1985
10. Jennings RB, Reimer KA: Factors involved in salvaging ischemic myocardium: effect of reperfusion of arterial blood. Circulation **68**(suppl I): I–25, 1983
11. Kloner RA, Ellis SG, Lange R, Braunwald E: Studies of experimental coronary artery reperfusion. Effects on infarct size, myocardial function, biochemistry, ultrastructure and microvascular damage. Circulation **68**(suppl I): I–8, 1983
12. Bergmann SR, Lerch RA, Fox KA, Ludbrook PA, Welch MJ, Ter-Pogossian M, Sobel BE: Temporal dependence of beneficial effects of coronary thrombolysis characterized by positron tomography. Am J Med **73:** 573, 1982
13. Schwarz F, Schuler G, Katus H, Hofmann M, Manthey J, Tillmanns H, Mehmel HC, Kubler W: Intracoronary thrombolysis in acute myocardial infarction: duration of ischemia as a major determinant of late results after recanalization. Am J Cardiol **50:** 933, 1982
14. Mathey DG, Schofer J, Sheehan F, Becher H, Tilsner V, Dodge HT: Intravenous urokinase in acute myocardial infarction. Am J Cardiol **55:** 878, 1985
15. Swan HJC: Thrombolysis in acute evolving myocardial infarction. N Engl J Med **308:** 1354, 1983
16. Schroder R, Biamino G, Leitner ER, Linderer T, Bruggemann T, Heitz J, Vohringer HF, Wegschreider K: Intravenous short-term infusion of streptokinase in acute myocardial infarction. Circulation **67:** 536, 548, 1983
17. Ganz W, Geft I, Shah PK, Lew AS, Rodriguez L, Weiss T, Maddahi J, Berman DS, Charuzi Y, Swan HJC: Intravenous streptokinase in evolving myocardial infarction. Am J Cardiol **53:** 1209, 1984
18. Anderson JL, Marshall HW, Askins JC, Lutz JR, Sorensen SG, Menlove RL, Yanowitz FG, Hagan AD: A randomized trial of intravenous and intracoronary streptokinase in patients with acute myocardial infarction. Circulation **70:** 606, 1984
19. Taylor GJ, Mikell FL, Moses HW, Dove JT, Batchelder JE, Thull A, Hansen S, Wellons HA, Schneider JA: Intravenous versus intracoronary streptokinase therapy for acute myocardial infarction in community hospitals. Am J Cardiol **54:** 256, 1984
20. Valentine RP, Pitts DE, Brooks-Brunn JA, Williams JG, Van Hove E, Schmidt PE: Intravenous versus intracoronary streptokinase in acute myocardial infarction. Am J Cardiol **55:** 309, 1985
21. Ambrose JA, Winters SL, Stern A, Eng A, Teichholz LE, Gorlin R, Fuster V: Angiographic morphology and the pathogenesis of unstable angina. J Am Coll Cardiol **5:** 609, 1985
22. Alderman EL, Jutzy KR, Berte LE, Miller RG, Friedman JP, Creger WP, Eliastam M: Randomized comparison of intravenous versus intracoronary streptokinase for acute myocardial infarction. Am J Cardiol **54:** 14, 1984
23. Lew AS, Laramee P, Shah PK, Rodriguez L, Ganz W: The effect of the rate of intravenous infusion of streptokinase on systolic blood pressure and on the time interval to reperfusion. J Am Coll Cardiol **5:** 421, 1985 (abst)
24. Udall JA: Recent advances using streptokinase for acute coronary thrombosis. Clin Cardiol **7:** 138, 1984
25. Brogden RN, Speight TM, Avery GS: Streptokinase: A review of

its clinical pharmacology, mechanism of action and therapeutic uses. Drugs **5:** 357, 1973
26. Martin M: Studies on activator formation in human plasma with streptokinase. III. Investigation of activator kinetics in undiluted plasma in terms of urokinase equivalents. Thromb Haemost **36:** 566, 1976
27. Alkjaersig N, Fletcher AP, Sherry S: The mechanism of clot dissolution by plasmin. J Clin Invest **38:** 1086, 1959
28. Collen D: On the regulation and control of fibrinolysis. Thromb Haemost **73:** 77, 1980
29. Lee G, Joye JA, Amsterdam EA, Low R, DeMaria AN, Krieg P, Mason DT: Determinants of beneficial coronary streptokinase therapy in acute myocardial infarction: success and rapidity of thrombolysis depends on minimal time from symptom onset to treatment. Am J Cardiol **49:** 973, 1982
30. Weinstein J: Treatment of myocardial infarction with intracoronary streptokinase: Efficacy and safety data from 209 United States cases in the Hoechst-Roussel registry. Am Heart J **104:** 894, 1982
31. Kennedy JW, Gensini GG, Timmis GC, Maynard C: Acute myocardial infarction treated with intracoronary streptokinase: a report of the Society for Cardiac Angiography. Am J Cardiol **55:** 871, 1985
32. Rutsch W, Schartl M, Mathey D, Kuck K, Merx W, Dorr R, Rentrop P, Blanke H: Percutaneous transluminal coronary recanalization: procedure, results, and acute complications. Am Heart J **102:** 1178, 1981
33. Karsch KR, Hofmann M, Rentrop KP, Blanke H, Schaper W: Thrombolysis in acute experimental myocardial infarction. J Am Coll Cardiol **1:** 427, 1983
34. Collen D, Stassen JM, Verstraete M: Thrombolysis with human extrinsic (tissue-type) plasminogen activator in rabbits with experimental jugular vein thrombosis. Effect of molecular form and dose of activator, age of thrombus and route of administration. J Clin Invest **71:** 368, 1983
35. McDonagh J: Structure and function of factor XIII. *In* Colman RW, Hirsh J, Marder VJ, Salzman EW, editors: Hemostasis and thrombosis: basic principles and clinical practice. Philadelphia, 1982, J.B. Lippincott Company, pp 168–169
36. Gottlob R, Blumel G, Piza F, Brucke P, Bohmig HJ: Studies on thrombolysis with streptokinase II. The influence of changes due to age in thrombi and whole blood clots. Thromb Diathes Haemorrh **19:** 156, 1968
37. Erhardt LR, Lundman T, Mellstedt H: Incorporation of ^{125}I-labelled fibrinogen into coronary arterial thrombi in acute myocardial infarction in man Lancet **1:** 387, 1973
38. McDonagh RP, McDonagh J, Duckert F: The influence of fibrin crosslinking on the kinetics of urokinase-induced clot lysis. Br J Haematol **21:** 323, 1971
39. Rothbard RL, Fitzpatrick PG, Francis CW, Caton DM, Hood WB, Marder VJ: Relationship of the lytic state to successful reperfusion with standard-and low-dose intracoronary streptokinase. Circulation **71:** 562, 1985
40. Brosius FC, Roberts WC: Significance of coronary arterial thrombus in transmural acute myocardial infarction. A survey of 54 necropsy patients. Circulation **63:** 810, 1981
41. Spottl F, Holzknecht F: The influence of inhibitors of plasmin and plasminogen activation on the streptokinase-induced fibrinolytic state. Thromb Diathes Haemorrh **24:** 101, 1970
42. Fletcher AP, Alkjaersig N, Sherry S: The clearance of heterologous protein from the circulation of normal and immunized man. J Clin Invest **37:** 1306, 1958
43. Moran DM, Standring R, Lavender EA, Harris GS: Assessment of antistreptokinase antibody levels in human sera using a microradioimmunoassay procedure. Thromb Haemost **52:** 281, 1984
44. Lew AS, Laramee P, Ganz W: Measurement of antistreptokinase antibodies. J Am Coll Cardiol **5:** 1500, 1985 (letter)
45. Tendera MP, Campbell WB, Tennant SN, Ray WA: Factors influencing probability of reperfusion with intracoronary ostial infusion of thrombolytic agent in patients with acute myocardial infarction. Circulation **71:** 124, 1985
46. Cowley MJ: Methodologic aspects of intracoronary thrombolysis. Drugs, dosage and duration. Circulation **68**(suppl I): I–90, 1983
47. Blumenthal MR, Wang HH, Liu LMP: Experimental coronary artery occusion and release. Effect on enzymes, electrocardiograms, myocardial contractility and reactive hyperemia. Am J Cardiol **36:** 225, 1975
48. Muller JE, Maroko PR, Braunwald E: Evaluation of precordial electrocardiographic mapping as a means of assessing changes in myocardial ischemic injury. Circulation **52:** 16, 1975
49. Beller GA, Hood WB Jr, Smith TW: Effects of ischaemia and coronary reperfusion on regional myocardial blood flow and on the epicardial electrogram. Cardiovasc Res **11:** 489, 1977
50. Rentrop P, Blanke H, Karsch KR, Kaiser H, Kostering H, Leitz K: Selective intracoronary thrombolysis in acute myocardial infarction and unstable angina pectoris. Circulation **63:** 307, 1981
51. Mathey DG, Kuck KH, Tilsner V, Krebber HJ, Bleifeld W: Nonsurgical coronary artery recanalization in acute transmural myocardial infarction. Circulation **63:** 489, 1981
52. Ganz W, Geft I, Maddahi J, Berman D, Charuzi Y, Shah PK, Swan HJC: Nonsurgical reperfusion in evolving myocardial infarction. J Am Coll Cardiol **1:** 1247, 1983
53. Goldberg S, Urban P, Greenspon A, Berger B, Walinsky P, Muza B, Kusiak V, Maroko PR: Limitation of infarct size with thrombolytic agents — electrocardiographic indexes. Circulation **68:**(suppl I): I–77, 1983
54. Blanke H, Scherff F, Karsch KR, Levine RA, Smith H, Rentrop P: Electrocardiograpic changes after streptokinase-induced recanalization in patients with acute left anterior descending artery obstruction. Circulation **68:** 406, 1983
55. Tamaki S, Murakami T, Kadota K, Kambara H, Yui Y, Nakajima H, Suzuki Y, Nohara R, Takatsu Y, Kawai C, Tamaki N, Mukai T, Torizuka K: Effects of coronary artery reperfusion on relation between creatine kinase-MB release and infarct size estimated by myocardial emission tomography with thallium-201 in man. J Am Coll Cardiol **2:** 1031, 1983
56. Shell W, Mickle DK, Swan HJC: Effects of nonsurgical myocardial reperfusion of plasma creatine kinase kinetics in man. Am Heart J **106:** 665, 1983
57. Little T, Ellis AK, Masud AZ, Klocke FJ: Non-invasive detection of successful coronary arterial reperfusion in acute myocardial infarction. Clin Res **32:** 205A, 1985 (abst)
58. Ferguson DW, White CW, Schwartz JL, Brayden GP, Kelly KJ, Kioschos JM, Kirchner PT, Marcus ML: Influence of baseline ejection fraction and success of thrombolysis on mortality and ventricular function after acute myocardial infarction. Am J Cardiol **54:** 705, 1984
59. Neuhaus KL, Tebbe U, Sauer G, Kreuzer H, Kostering H: High dose intravenous streptokinase in acute myocardial infarction. Clin Cardiol **6:** 426, 1983
60. Eisenberg PR, Sherman L, Schwartz D, Reich M, Sobel BE, Jaffe AS: Unmasking continued thrombin activity and rethrombosis as a determinant of clinical failure of coronary thrombolysis. J Am Coll Cardiol **5:** 398, 1985 (abst)

Warfarin versus dipyridamole-aspirin and pentoxifylline-aspirin for the prevention of prosthetic heart valve thromboembolism: a prospective randomized clinical trial

C. K. Mok, M.B.,B.S., John Boey, M.D., Rebecca Wang, M.D., T. K. Chan, M.D., K. L. Cheung, M.B.,B.S., P. K. Lee, M.B.,B.S., Joseph Chow, M.B.,B.S., Ronald P. Ng,* M.B.,B.S., and T. F. Tse, M.B.,B.S.

ABSTRACT In a prospective, randomized, parallel study, two regimens of platelet-suppressant therapy (PST) — dipyridamole-aspirin and pentoxifylline-aspirin — were compared with standard oral anticoagulation with warfarin in the prevention of prosthetic heart valve thromboembolism. In the entire group of 254 patients followed for 395.6 patient-years, the thromboembolic rate was significantly less in the warfarin group (warfarin vs dipyridamole-aspirin, $p < .005$; warfarin vs pentoxifylline-aspirin, $p < .05$). Subgroup analysis disclosed that, in patients with isolated mitral valve replacement, warfarin was superior to both of the PSTs with respect to the prevention of thromboembolism (warfarin vs dipyridamole-aspirin, $p = .005$; warfarin vs pentoxifylline-aspirin, $p < .05$). Furthermore, a significant number of our patients could not tolerate the antiplatelet agents. However, in the rare situation in which repeated significant bleeding occurs despite careful adjustment of the dosage of warfarin, PST may be an acceptable alternate method of thromboembolism prophylaxis.
Circulation 72, No. 5, 1059–1063, 1985.

WHEN THE EFFECT of anticoagulant is maintained within a therapeutic range it significantly reduces, but does not eliminate, the risk of thromboembolism in patients with prosthetic heart valves.[1] However, adequate anticoagulation at all times is difficult to achieve,[2] and it carries a definite risk of its own.[3] In clinical practice, whenever the use of oral anticoagulation is complicated, e.g., in children with prosthetic heart valves or when adequate facilities for careful anticoagulation are not available, antiplatelet agents have been used as the alternatives.[4, 5] It would be advantageous to patients with prosthetic heart valves if platelet-suppressant therapy (PST) could be used in place of oral anticoagulation. We undertook a prospective, randomized, parallel study to evaluate the efficacy of PST for the prevention of thromboembolism in patients with mechanical prosthetic heart valves. Anticoagulation with warfarin was used as the control. The regimens of antiplatelet agents used in the present study were derived from our previous study on platelet survival among patients with mechanical prosthetic heart valves.[6] The present report is an analysis of the relevant data from the prospective trial.

From the Departments of Surgery and Medicine, University of Hong Kong, Grantham Hospital, Hong Kong.

Supported by grants from the Hong Kong Heart Foundation Ltd., Hong Kong, and Boehringer Ingelheim and Hoechst, West Germany.

Address for correspondence: C. K. Mok, Grantham Hospital, 125 Wong Chuk Hang Road, Hong Kong.

Received Nov. 26, 1984; revision accepted June 27, 1985.

*Present address: 11A Jalan Ilmu, Singapore 1129.

Methods

From January 1979 to January 1984, patients with mechanical prosthetic heart valves (models 1260 and 6120 Starr-Edwards and standard Björk-Shiley) discharged to our valvular clinic were interviewed. The risks and benefits of anticoagulation, PST, and the proposed drug trial were explained to them in detail. Informed consent was obtained from those who agreed to participate in the prospective study. After 6 months of warfarin therapy, they were assigned to one of the three treatment groups (warfarin, dipyridamole-aspirin, and pentoxifylline-aspirin) by means of random-numbered tables and irrespective of the location and type of the prosthesis they had received. It was thought that 6 months would be required for the sewing ring of the prosthesis to become endothelialized.

Patients in the warfarin group continued to receive the drug in doses that maintained their prothrombin times within the therapeutic range ($1.8 \leq$ prothrombin time/control ≤ 2.5). The dipyridamole-aspirin group received 75 mg dipyridamole twice daily and slow-releasing aspirin, 650 mg once daily; since January 1982, they have received Persantin Plus (dipyridamole 75 mg + aspirin 330 mg), one tablet three times daily. The change was made for the convenience of patients and the dispenser. The pentoxifylline-aspirin group received 400 mg pentoxifylline twice daily and slow-releasing aspirin, 650 mg daily. Dosing with warfarin was discontinued in the two groups of patients who had been assigned to receive PSTs. All participants were instructed not to take any other medications, including herbal medicines, on their own.

Participants were evaluated at monthly intervals or earlier when required. At each visit, compliance with all regimens was assessed by counting of tablets and in those receiving warfarin prothrombin times were also measured. All participants were also checked for significant bleeding complications, i.e., bleeding necessitating hospitalization.

Follow-up end points included the following: (1) Thromboembolism, defined as an embolic episode resulting in transient or permanent neurologic deficit with focal motor weakness or visual deficit or loss of pulses in an extremity and of sudden onset and unexplained by other causes. Cerebral bleeding was excluded at autopsy or by a computerized tomographic scan. Thrombosed prostheses were verified either at autopsy or reoperation. A coronary embolus was diagnosed only when the coronary arteries were known to be normal or when a myocardial infarction occurred in a patient younger than 40 years of age without apparent risk factors other than the presence of the prosthetic valve. (2) Drug intolerance, i.e., appearance of drug-related symptoms that prevented continuation of therapy with the drug.

When a thromboembolic episode occurred in a patient in the warfarin group, he or she was given a larger dose of warfarin if the prothrombin time was below the therapeutic range; when the prothrombin time was within the therapeutic range dipyridamole (400 mg daily) was added. Patients on PST who had an episode of thromboembolism or required discontinuation therapy with antiplatelet drugs were put back on warfarin. Data on the subsequent clinical courses of these patients, both in the warfarin and the PST groups, were not included in the analysis.

Statistical analysis was by the corrected chi-square test, the unpaired Student's t test, and the generalized Wilcoxon comparison of incident-free rates determined by the Kaplan-Meier product-limit actuarial method.[7] Statistical significance was assumed at the 5% level.

TABLE 1
Clinical characteristics of the patients (n)

	Warfarin (n = 97; mean age 42.5 yr)	Dipyridamole-aspirin (n = 81; mean age 40.9 yr)	Pentoxi-fylline-aspirin (n = 76; mean age 42.9 yr; p = .65)
Sex (p = .20)			
Men	41	29	38
Women	56	52	38
Prior thrombo-embolism (p = .61)	9	6	4
Left atrial enlargement^A (p = .14)	80	63	53
LA thrombus at operation (p = .62)	17	10	8
Postoperative atrial fibrillation (p = .36)	57	48	37
Valve type (p = .20)			
Starr-Edwards	24	30	23
Björk-Shiley	73	51	53
Valve position (p = .10)			
Mitral	62	54	41
Aortic	14	15	21
Both mitral and aortic	21	12	12

LA = left atrial.
^ADetermined with M mode echocardiography (>5 mm in size).

Results

Of the 254 patients randomly assigned to drug therapy, 251 received the medications assigned to them. Two patients withdrew consent after randomization and one patient was withdrawn because she became pregnant before PST was to commence. Data from these three patients were included in the final analysis. The comparability in clinical characteristics of the 254 patients in the three randomized treatment groups is shown in table 1.

Follow-up was complete. The mean follow-up periods and overall results are listed in table 2. The manifestations and distribution of the thromboembolic and bleeding episodes are listed in table 3. During the study period, six patients died of causes unrelated to the prosthesis or thromboembolic prophylactic therapy. Death was due to congestive heart failure in two patients, arrhythmia in one patient, infective endocarditis in one patient, ruptured aortic aneurysm in one patient, and carcinoma of the ovary in one patient.

Adequacy of anticoagulation. There were 3132 prothrombin times and corresponding control values tabulated during the follow-up of patients in the warfarin group. The prothrombin times of approximately 50% of the patients were within, those of 30% were above, and those of 20% were below the therapeutic range (1.8 ≤ prothrombin time/control ≤ 2.5).

Incidence of thromboembolism

Warfarin group. There were four thromboembolic events (2.2 per 100 patient-years), and one patient died following coronary embolism.

Dipyridamole-aspirin groups. Eleven patients developed thromboembolism (8.6 per 100 patient-years), and two patients died. Coronary embolism was the cause of death in one, and a thrombosed prothesis was the cause in the other patient.

Pentoxifylline-aspirin group. Eight thromboembolic events occurred (7.9 per 100 patient-years). All eight patients survived the thromboembolic episode.

TABLE 2
Overall results in the three treatment groups

	Warfarin (n = 97; mean FU period 24.4 mo)	Dipyrida-mole-aspirin (n = 81; mean FU period 18.0 mo)	Pentoxi-fylline-aspirin (n = 76; mean FU period 17.3 mo)
Treatment "failure" (n)			
Thromboembolism	4 (4.1%)	11 (13.6%)	8 (10.5%)
(death)	(1)	(2)	(0)
Drug intolerance	0	22 (27.2%)	24 (31.6%)
Bleeding	5 (5.2%)	0	1
Treatment "success" (patients without emboli, on drugs; n)	93 (95.9%)	47 (58.0%)	42 (55.3%)
Death not related to treatment (n)	4	0	2

FU = follow-up.

Episodes of bleeding. There were six episodes of bleeding. All patients survived. Five episodes occurred in the warfarin group and one occurred in the pentoxifylline-aspirin group. Of the five patients who bled in the warfarin group, four had markedly prolonged prothrombin times. One patient in the pentoxifylline-aspirin group developed spontaneous hemoperitoneum that was diagnosed at laparotomy. Both the cause and source of bleeding were obscured.

Drug intolerance. Antiplatelet therapy was discontinued in 46 patients (22 of 81 [27.2%] in the dipyridamole-aspirin group and 24 of 76 [31.6%] in the pentoxifylline-aspirin group). With the exception of one patient who developed a skin rash, intolerable gastrointestinal upset was the reason for cessation of therapy.

Comparison between treatment groups. The actuarial curves depicting the thromboembolic-free intervals in the three groups of patients are shown in figure 1. There was a significant difference between the warfarin and each of the 2 PST groups (warfarin vs dipyridamole-aspirin, $p < .005$; warfarin vs pentoxifylline-aspirin, $p < .05$). Results of subgroup analysis according to the position of the valve are summarized in table 4. Among the patients who had undergone single mitral valve replacement (figure 2), there was a significant difference in the incidence of thromboembolism between those in the warfarin and those in each of the two PST groups (warfarin vs dipyridamole-aspirin, $p = .005$; warfarin vs pentoxifylline-aspirin, $p < .05$). Given the small number of patients in the other two subgroups (aortic and double) no significant difference was found in the thromboembolic-free intervals in the three treatment groups.

When significant bleeding and thromboembolism were considered together as undesirable events, the difference in the event-free intervals between the warfarin and dipyridamole-aspirin groups was significant ($p < .05$), but no such difference was observed between the warfarin and pentoxifylline-aspirin groups

TABLE 3
Manifestations of thromboembolic and bleeding episodes

	Warfarin (n = 97)	Dipyrida-mole-aspirin (n = 81)	Pentoxi-fylline-aspirin (n = 76)
Thromboembolic episodes (n)			
Hemiparesis/hemiplegia with residue	1	2	1
Transient hemiparesis	1	6	5
Thrombosed prosthesis	0	2	1
Acute myocardial infarction	1	1	1
Peripheral arterial embolism	1	0	0
Bleeding episodes (n)			
Gum bleeding	1	0	0
Hematuria	1	0	0
Hemarthrosis	1	0	0
Hemoperitoneum	0	0	1
Intracerebral hematoma	1	0	0
Menorrhagia	1	0	0

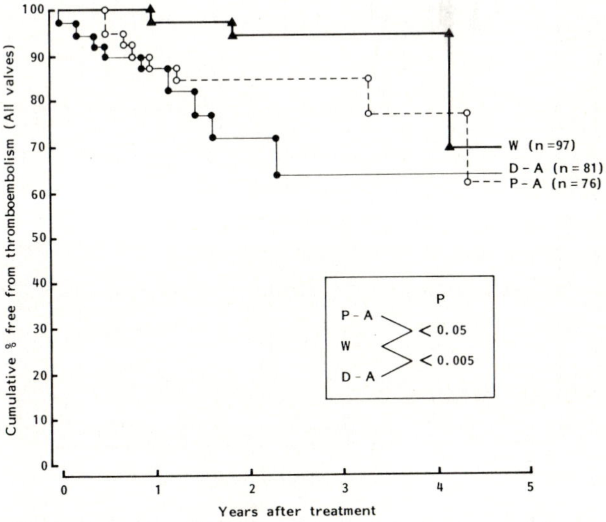

FIGURE 1. Actuarial curves depicting the thromboembolic-free intervals in the three groups of patients. D-A = dipyridamole-aspirin; P-A = pentoxifylline-aspirin; W = warfarin.

TABLE 4
Subgroup analysis according to valve positions

	TE (per 100 patient-years)			p value (comparison of TE-free periods)		p value (comparison of event-free periods)	
	W	D-A	P-A	W vs D-A	W vs P-A	W vs D-A	W vs P-A
All valves	4/97 (2.2)	11/81 (9.8)	8/76 (7.9)	.004	.04	.04	.14
Mitral	2/62 (1.9)	9/54 (12.4)	6/43 (11.5)	.005	.03	.07	.21
Aortic	1/14 (3.6)	1/15 (3.8)	2/21 (5.6)	.86	.79	.44	.35
Double	1/21 (2.1)	1/12 (7.4)	0/12 (0)	.19	.62	.36	.42

TE = thromboembolism; W = warfarin; D-A = dipyridamole-aspirin; P-A = pentoxifylline-aspirin.

nor among the treatment groups when they were further subdivided according to the position of the valves they had received (table 4).

We did not find any significant difference in the thromboembolic or event-free rates nor the percentages of "successful treatment" (table 2) for the two PST groups. Within each treatment group, there was no demonstrable difference in the thromboembolic rate between patients with the two types of prosthesis.

Discussion

Prophylaxis against thromboembolism is unavoidable in the majority of our patients after prosthetic heart valve replacement because they prefer the more durable mechanical valves, and many of them have a large left atrium and are in atrial fibrillation. Because of the lack of resources and the common occurrence of self administration of herbal medicines that may interact with oral anticoagulants in our patients, we have had difficulties with running a conventional anticoagulation clinic. We therefore felt justified in conducting the present trial in a search for an acceptable substitute for conventional anticoagulant therapy.

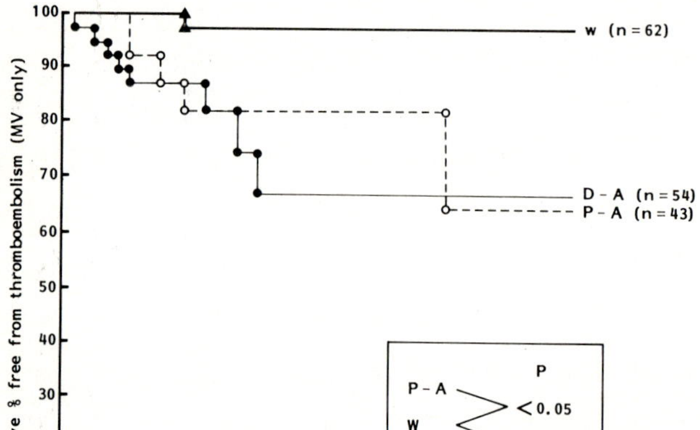

FIGURE 2. Actuarial curves depicting the thromboembolic-free intervals in individuals who underwent single mitral valve replacement. D-A = dipyridamole-aspirin; MV = mitral valve; P-A = pentoxifylline-aspirin; W = warfarin.

As mentioned before, the two regimens of PST were derived from our previous study on platelet survival in patients with mechanical prosthetic heart valves.[6] The study demonstrated that 100 mg dipyridamole plus 1200 mg aspirin daily and 600 mg pentoxifylline plus 1200 mg aspirin daily normalized platelet survival. The minor modifications that were made in dosages for use in the present study were made to attempt to improve patient compliance and allow use of slow-releasing preparations.

The present study conclusively demonstrated that our two regimens of PST were inferior to warfarin therapy in the prevention of thromboembolism among patients with mechanical mitral prostheses. Although there were no significant differences in the incidence of thromboembolism between the treatment groups in patients with aortic or double valve replacement, we hesitate to conclude that our regimens of PST can replace oral anticoagulation in these subsets of patients because the number of patients in each of these subgroups was small. Since analysis of the event-free intervals demonstrated no difference among the subgroups (table 4), PST may be of value in the rare situation in which repeated significant bleeding occurs despite careful adjustment of dosages of warfarin.

Side effects of use of antiplatelet agents that led to discontinuation of therapy were common in previous studies of PST.[8] However, the incidence of drug intolerance we found (dipyridamole-aspirin, 27.2%; pentoxifylline-aspirin, 31.6%) was higher than that observed in other studies[9, 10] in which similar drugs were used (7.5% to 17.6%). The most significant symptom among our patients was intolerable gastrointestinal upset. In that the drugs and dosages used were comparable to those reported in previous studies,[9, 10] these reactions may perhaps be attributable to increased sensitivity in the indigenous population studied.

Our results show that PST by itself, when given arbitrarily, is not as effective as conventional anticoagulation in the prevention of thromboembolism in an unselected group of patients with mechanical prosthetic heart valves. On the other hand, it is generally accepted that the addition of dipyridamole to a regimen of anticoagulant reduces the incidence of prosthetic valve–related thromboembolism.[11, 12] Thus, the exact role of antiplatelet drugs in prophylaxis of prosthetic valve thromboembolism is still largely unknown. This will remain undefined until the effective agents, the optimal dosage to be used, and a laboratory test of platelet reactivity that correlates with thromboembolism are discovered.

We thank W. C. C. Chen, K. K. Hui, and P. H. C. Wong for their assistance in patient follow-up and data entry and Kelly Wong for her assistance with the computer analysis. The dipyridamole and Persantin Plus were kindly supplied by Boehringer Ingelheim, West Germany. The pentoxifylline was kindly provided by Hoechst, West Germany.

References

1. Gadboys HC, Litwak RS, Niemetz J, Wisch N: Role of anticoagulants in preventing embolization from prosthetic heart valves. JAMA **202:** 134, 1967
2. Duvoisin GE, Brandenburg RO, McGoon DC: Factors affecting thromboembolism associated with prosthetic heart valves. Circulation **35** (suppl I): I-70, 1967
3. Forfar JC: A 7-year analysis of haemorrhage in patients on long-term anticoagulant treatment. Br Heart J **42:** 128, 1979
4. Weinstein GS, Mavroudis C, Ebert PA: Preliminary experience with aspirin for anticoagulation in children with prosthetic cardiac valves. Ann Thorac Surg **33:** 549, 1982
5. St. John Sutton MG, Miller GAH, Oldershaw PJ, Paneth M: Anticoagulants and the Bjork Shiley prosthesis. Experience of 390 patients. Br Heart J **40:** 558, 1978
6. Ng RP, Tse TF, Chan TK: Platelet survival in patients with artificial heart valves and the effect of anti-platelet agents. Singapore Med J **20** (suppl I): I-30, 1979
7. Kaplan EL, Meier P: Nonparametric estimation from incomplete observation. J Am Stat Assos **53:** 457, 1958
8. Genton E: A perspective on platelet-suppressant drug treatment in coronary artery and cerebrovascular disease. Circulation **62** (suppl V): V-111, 1980
9. Taguchi K, Matsumura H, Washizu T, Hirao M, Kato K, Kato E, Mochizuki T, Takamura K, Mashimo I, Morifuji K, Nakagaki M, Suma T: Effect of athrombogenic therapy, especially high dose therapy of dipyridamole, after prosthetic valve replacement. J Cardiovasc Surg **16:** 8, 1975
10. Porter JM, Cutler BS, Lee BY, Reich T, Reichle FA, Scogin JT, Strandness DE: Pentoxifylline efficacy in the treatment of intermittent claudication: multicenter controlled double-blind trial with objective assessment of chronic occlusive arterial disease patients. Am Heart J **104:** 66, 1982
11. Sullivan JM, Harken DE, Gorlin R: Pharmacologic control of thromboembolic complications of cardiac-valve replacement. N Engl J Med **284:** 1391, 1971
12. Chesebro JH, Fuster V, Elveback LR, McGoon DC, Pluth JR, Pugo FJ, Wallace RB, Danielson GK, Orszulak TA, Piehler JM, Sehaff HV: Trial of combined warfarin plus dipyridamole or aspirin therapy in prosthetic heart valve replacement. Danger of aspirin compared with dipyridamole. Am J Cardiol **51:** 1537, 1983

Amiodarone and its desethyl metabolite: tissue distribution and morphologic changes during long-term therapy

P. C. ADAMS, B.A., M.R.C.P., D. W. HOLT, B.SC., PH.D., G. C. A. STOREY, B.SC., PH.D., A. R. MORLEY, M.D., J. CALLAGHAN, M.R.C.PATH., AND R. W. F. CAMPBELL, F.R.C.P.

With the technical assistance of P. J. Thompson and Terry Coaker

ABSTRACT The pharmacokinetic characteristics of amiodarone suggest extensive tissue deposition. We confirmed this by measuring tissue concentrations of the drug and of its major metabolite, desethylamiodarone, in human tissues. These were obtained at autopsy (n = 9), surgery (n = 7), or biopsy (n = 2) from 18 patients who had been treated with amiodarone for varying periods of time. High concentrations of amiodarone were found in fat (316 mg/kg wet weight in autopsy specimens, 344 mg/kg wet weight in biopsy specimens). Amiodarone and desethylamiodarone concentrations (mg/kg wet weight, autopsy samples) were also high in liver (391 and 2354), lung (198 and 952), adrenal gland (137 and 437), testis (89 and 470), and lymph node (83 and 316). We also found high concentrations of amiodarone (306 mg/kg wet weight) and desethylamiodarone (943 mg/kg wet weight) in abnormally pigmented ("blue") skin from patients with amiodarone-induced skin pigmentation. These values were 10-fold higher than those in unpigmented skin from the same patients. These high concentrations were associated with lysosomal inclusion bodies in dermal macrophages in the pigmented skin. The inclusion bodies were intrinsically electron dense and were shown to contain iodine by energy dispersive x-ray microanalysis. Lysosomal inclusion bodies shown by electron microscopy to be multilamellar were seen in other tissues. These tissues included terminal nerve fibers in pigmented skin, pulmonary macrophages, blood neutrophils, and hepatocytes and Kupffer cells. These characteristic ultrastructural findings occur in both genetic lipidoses and lipidoses induced by other drugs, e.g., perhexiline. We conclude that during therapy with amiodarone, widespread deposition of amiodarone and desethylamiodarone occurs. This leads to ultrastructural changes typical of a lipidosis. These changes are seen clearly in tissues associated with the unwanted effects of amiodarone, e.g., skin, liver and lung.
Circulation 72, No. 5, 1064–1075, 1985.

AMIODARONE is recognized as an orally effective agent in the treatment of atrial and ventricular arrhythmias refractory to conventional therapy. It is a benzofuran derivative containing two iodine atoms per molecule. In man, only one major metabolite has been identified, desethylamiodarone.[1] During long-term therapy this compound reaches similar plasma concentrations to amiodarone, and both compounds show long terminal elimination half-lives reflecting a comparatively low clearance and an exceptionally large volume of distribution.[2,3] The pharmacologic and toxicologic effects of desethylamiodarone are not well defined.

Unwanted effects occur commonly during therapy with amiodarone.[3,4] Thyroid disturbance is well recognized,[4–6] as is the almost uniform development of corneal microdeposits.[7] Photosensitivity is common (occurring in up to 75% of patients after 2 years' therapy in northwest England),[8] whereas a small number of patients develop slate-blue pigmentation affecting light-exposed skin.[9] A number of recent reports document pulmonary toxicity.[10–12] Peripheral neuropathy has been noted in several patients.[13,14] Abnormalities of plasma concentrations of hepatic enzymes occur in 15% to 50% of patients,[4,15] and more severe hepatic

From the Academic Department of Cardiology, Freeman Hospital, and University Department of Pathology, Royal Victory Infirmary, Newcastle upon Tyne, and Poison's Unit, Guy's Hospital, London.

Supported by a grant from the British Heart Foundation (Dr. Adams) and by Labaz UK.

Address for correspondence: R. W. F. Campbell, M.B., Ch.B., Department of Cardiology, Freeman Hospital, Newcastle upon Tyne, NE7 7DN, England.

Received March 1, 1985; revision accepted July 25, 1985.

disorders have been recognized,[16, 17] including fatal hepatitis.[14]

We have investigated the tissue distribution of amiodarone and desethylamiodarone in man and have noted ultrastructural changes in various organs during therapy with amiodarone. These observations throw light on the association between the drug's unwanted effects and the accumulation of amiodarone and its desethyl metabolite in the body.

Methods

Study population. The clinical details of the 18 patients from whom tissue samples were obtained are shown in table 1. There were 12 men and six women (mean age ± SD 59 ± 16 years, see table 1). The duration of treatment with amiodarone ranged from 11 days to 53 months and the total cumulative dose varied from 9 to 810 g. Daily dose varied both within and between patients, but the range for long-term dosing was 200 to 800 mg/day. Patients 2, 4, 12, and 13 had received no amiodarone for 3 to 41 days before tissue was obtained. The patients had received a median of six (range 0 to 11) other drugs in the 2 years before sampling. Amiodarone was the only drug taken by all patients.

Tissue samples. In nine patients, samples were obtained at autopsy 1 to 4 days after death. In seven patients, biopsy specimens were obtained during surgery (thoracotomy in four and laparotomy in three). All samples were taken during routine surgery or were part of clinically necessary biopsies. In two patients (17 and 18) with amiodarone-induced skin pigmentation, elliptic skin specimens were obtained from affected skin of either the face or the dorsum of the hand.

Unaffected skin was obtained from the trunk or upper arm in the same patients. Similar samples were also obtained from one patient at autopsy (No. 9). In patient 5, pulmonary macrophages were examined after bronchoalveolar lavage and a small lung specimen for histologic examination was also obtained during bronchoscopy.

TABLE 1
Clinical features

Patient	Age (yr)	Sex	Cardiac diagnosis	Duration of therapy	Mean maintenance dose (mg)	Total cum. dose (g)	Time without therapy (days)	Cause of death	Samples obtained at	Body wt. at time of samples (kg)	Unwanted effects
1	34	F	VF, "normal heart"	53 mo	384	610	—	—	Thoracotomy	51	Photosensitivity, goiter (euthyroid), corneal deposits[A]
2	41	F	WPW, RT	22 mo	367	250	14 days	—	Thoracotomy	59	Nausea, bradycardia, corneal deposits[A]
3	60	M	VT, IHD	33 days	600	20	—	—	Thoracotomy	81	—
4	17	M	Ebstein's WPW, RT	12 wk	280	25	3 days	—	Thoracotomy	57	Anorexia
5	64	M	WPW, IHD, RT	28 mo	400	340	—	—	Laparotomy Skin biopsy	55	↑ AST, pulmonary fibrosis, blue pigmentation
6	67	F	AF, Pacer, SSS	4 wk	340	10	—	—	Laparotomy	52	—
7	78	F	WPW, RT	48 mo	540	810	—	—	Laparotomy	47	Hypothyroid ? Hepatitis
8	52	M	SVT, IHD, aneurysm	44 wk	253	79	—	Ischemic CM	Autopsy	67	—
9	70	M	VT, IHD	28 wk	514	100	—	Ischemic CM	Autopsy	72	Photosensitivity, hepatitis
10	59	M	VT, IHD	41 days	644	26	—	VT	Autopsy	72	—
11	76	M	VT, VF, IHD	11 days	800	9		VF	Autopsy	78	—
12	73	F	Recurr. VF, MVD	21 mo	400	240	6 days	Mitral stenosis	Autopsy	58	Hypothyroidism
13	53	M	VT, IHD	20 mo	405	230	41 days	VT	Autopsy	NA	Nausea
14	74	M	VT, IHD	14 days	600	11	—	VF	Autopsy	70	—
15	67	M	Recurr. VF, IHD	29 wk	286	60	—	Sudden death	Autopsy	54	—
16	48	F	AF, complex congenital	9 wk	228	13	—	Congestive failure	Autopsy	41	—
17	63	M	VT, IHD	44 mo	402	530	—	—	Skin biopsy	62	Blue pigmentation
18	65	M	VT, IHD	39 mo	402	476	—	—	Skin biopsy	73	Blue pigmentation, ↑AST, corneal deposits[A]

VF = ventricular fibrillation; WPW = Wolff-Parkinson-White syndrome; RT = reentry tachycardia; VT = ventricular tachycardia; IHD = ischemic heart disease; AF = atrial fibrillation; SSS = sick sinus syndrome; SVT = supraventricular tachycardia; MVD = mitral valve disease; CM = cardiomyopathy; AST = aspartate transaminase; NA = not available.

[A]Examined only in these patients.

Where appropriate, tissue samples for measurement of amiodarone and desethylamiodarone concentrations were dissected free of fat. They were stored at − 20° C in stoppered glass tubes until analysis.

Measurement of drug and metabolite concentrations. The analytical technique is described in full elsewhere.[18] Tissue samples (10 to 100 mg) were digested with a proteolytic enzyme with the exception of fat, which was digested with crude lipase. The analytes were extracted from the homogeneous digest into an organic solvent, and their concentrations were measured by high-performance liquid chromatography. The limit of sensitivity for this method was 0.1 mg/kg wet weight with a 100 mg tissue sample. No endogenous sources of interference in the assay have been identified. The assay is highly specific for amiodarone and for desethylamiodarone; other drugs do not cross-react significantly.

Histologic examination

Light microscopy. Tissue samples were fixed in 10% formalin for a minimum of 12 hr, postfixed in formol sublimate, and embedded in paraffin wax. Five-micrometer sections cut in single batches were stained by standard techniques. Appropriate control sections were included.

Electron microscopy. Samples were received fresh, fixed in 2.5% glutaraldehyde in sucrose-cacodylate buffer (pH 7.3), and postfixed in osmic acid (1% aqueous osmium tetroxide). The samples were embedded in araldite. Sections of 60 to 90 nm thickness were cut on an ultratome (Ultracut, Reichert Jung) with glass knives. Sections were stained with uranyl acetate and lead nitrate. In some cases paraffin–wax embedded tissues were used. The wax was removed, and small blocks were processed for electron microscopy (JEOL JEM-100S, Tokyo). In one patient (No. 5) skin sections were prepared without heavy metal exposure. Buffy coat specimens were prepared by centrifugation of EDTA-treated blood samples for 10 min at 3000 rpm. The plasma was discarded and carefully replaced by buffered glutaraldehyde. After 30 min the buffy coat "plug" was removed, fixed again in buffered glutaraldehyde, and processed for electron microscopy.

Energy-dispersive x-ray analysis. Energy-dispersive x-ray analysis of skin biopsy specimens and bronchoalveolar lavage samples was performed on a modified Corinth 500 transmission electron microscope (A.E.I. Ltd.), with a CORA system (LINK Ltd.); 0.5 μm araldite-embedded sections were mounted on 200 mesh carbon/Formvar–coated copper grids. The probe size was adjusted so that it equaled the size of the granule being analyzed.

Results

Amiodarone and desethylamiodarone tissue concentrations

Autopsy vs biopsy samples. It was necessary to demonstrate comparability of autopsy and biopsy results, but a direct comparison of these results for individual tissues was not possible because patients could not be matched for dose and duration of therapy. However, inspection of the results for tissue concentrations in both groups (tables 2 and 3) showed that they were of the same magnitude, with overlap between the two groups, suggesting that results from the autopsy material can be regarded as an accurate reflection of the tissue concentrations during therapy with amiodarone. Furthermore, in patients 9 and 12, concentrations of amiodarone and desethylamiodarone were compared in liver biopsy specimens taken around the time of death with those in autopsy specimens obtained 3 and 4 days later, respectively. Concentrations of amiodarone (patient 9: premortem 1170 mg/kg wet weight, autopsy 1040 mg/kg wet weight; patient 12: premortem 706 mg/kg wet weight, autopsy 702 mg/kg wet weight) and of desethylamiodarone (patient 9: premortem 5900 mg/kg wet weight, autopsy 6830 mg/kg wet weight; patient 12: premortem 4300 mg/kg wet weight, autopsy 3970 mg/kg wet weight) were similar between the two sets of samples. Over this period, amiodarone and desethylamiodarone concentrations were not affected by the time after death.

Tissue distribution of amiodarone and desethylamiodarone (tables 2 and 3). Blood samples were collected in six patients undergoing biopsy and in eight of the nine patients studied at autopsy. Postmortem blood was collected from the left ventricle in five patients (see table 3) and in most instances was lysed.

TABLE 2

Tissue concentrations of amiodarone (A) and desethylamiodarone (DA) (both mg/kg wet weight) in biopsy samples

	Plasma		Skin		Fat		Skeletal muscle		Heart		Liver		Spleen		Lymph node		Pancreas	
Patient	A	DA	A	DA	A	DA	A	DA	A	DA	A	DA	A	DA	A	DA	A	DA
1	2.1	2.4	8.3	24	470	125	23	46	47	95								
2	0.2	0.3	3.5	14	154	45	5.4	13	12	24								
3	1.4	1.3	4.6	9.3	117	30	8.3	12	12	47								
4			8.9	20	320	42	8.7	15	22	77								
5	3.2	3.7	34	45	856	216	57	71			1640	8150						
6	0.4	0.8	29	10	156	41	11	23			51	370						
7	0.6	0.9			333	65	16	30			286	1486	41	170	57	230	46	123
17			17	72														
18			35	46														
Mean	1.3	1.6	17.5	29.9	344	80.5	18.5	30.0	23.3	60.7	659	3335						
SEM	0.5	0.6	4.7	7.9	97.8	25.6	6.8	8.2	8.2	15.8	495	2429						

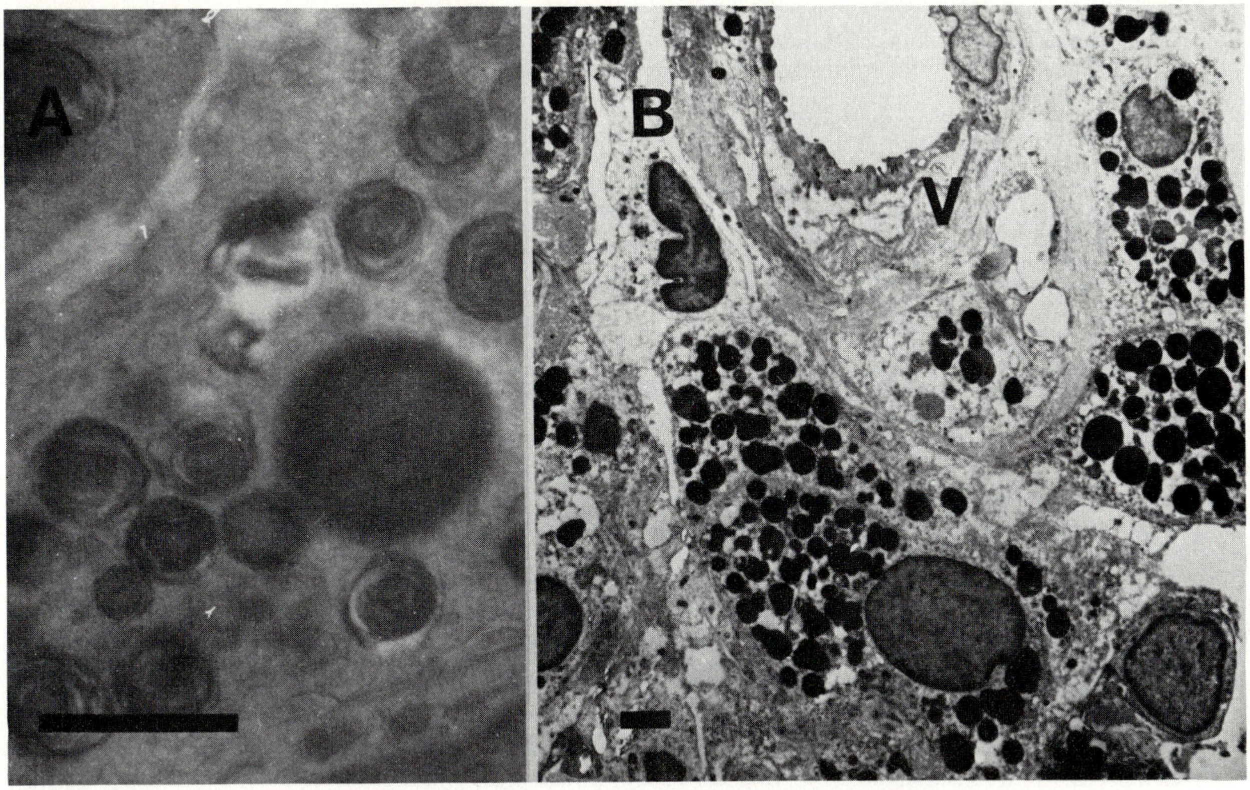

FIGURE 1. Electron micrographs of pigmented skin from a patient with amiodarone-induced skin pigmentation (No. 17). *A*, Structure of multilamellar bodies occasionally seen. The appearance can be contrasted with the electron-dense relatively homogeneous granules seen more commonly (*B*). *B*, Perivascular location of the granules in papillary dermal macrophages (v = vessel). Scale bar = 2 μm.

In biopsy samples the mean (± SEM) concentrations of amiodarone and desethylamiodarone were 1.3 ± 0.5 and 1.6 ± 0.6 mg/liter, respectively. For autopsy samples the results were 1.9 ± 1.0 and 3.0 ± 0.3 mg/liter, respectively. In the autopsy samples the lysing process probably contributed to the lower ratio of amiodarone to desethylamiodarone concentrations because of the higher concentrations of the latter compound in red cells than in plasma.[19] In addition, postmortem changes in blood concentrations depending on the sampling site cannot be ruled out.[20]

High concentrations of amiodarone and desethylamiodarone were found in tissue (tables 2 and 3); the highest concentrations were found in liver, with mean concentrations (amiodarone/desethylamiodarone, mg/kg wet weight) of 659/3335 in biopsy specimens (n = 3) and 391/2354 in autopsy samples (n = 9). The range of concentrations of amiodarone and of desethylamiodarone in a particular tissue was wide, reflecting differences in dose and duration of therapy and the time since therapy had been discontinued (patients 2, 4, 12, and 13). However, the concentrations of both of the compounds were consistently highest in liver, lung, adrenal gland, testis, spleen, and lymph node and were lowest in skeletal muscle, thyroid gland, skin, and brain. This pattern was seen in all of the patients.

The ratio of amiodarone to desethylamiodarone concentrations was lower in tissues than in plasma (table 4), ranging from 0.13 to 0.72. In fat, however, the ratio of amiodarone to desethylamiodarone was 4.67. Mean concentrations in fat were as follows: biopsy specimens, amiodarone 344 mg/kg wet weight, desethylamiodarone 80.5 mg/kg; autopsy specimens, amiodarone 316 mg/kg wet weight, desethylamiodarone 76.5 mg/kg.

Drug and metabolite concentrations in pigmented and unpigmented skin. Concentrations of amiodarone and desethylamiodarone were compared in normal and pigmented skin from the three patients with amiodarone-induced cutaneous pigmentation (Nos. 5, 17, and 18) (table 5). In all three patients the concentrations of both compounds were much higher in pigmented than in unpigmented skin.

Histology

Skin. In skin affected by amiodarone-induced cutaneous pigmentation there was a striking accumulation of dermal macrophages with a perivascular localiza-

TABLE 3
Tissue concentrations of amiodarone (A) and desethylamiodarone (DA) (mg/kg wet weight) in samples obtained at autopsy

	Plasma		Skin		Fat		Skeletal muscle		Heart		Liver		Spleen		Lymph node	
Patient	A	DA	A	DA	A	DA	A	DA	A	DA	A	DA	A	DA	A	DA
8			43	46	479	112	10	30			188	573	94	277	41	133
9	3.9	3.7[A]	60	138	805	240	95	195	147	624	1040	6830	360	2050	272	1070
10	2.3	2.0[B]			210	45	8	19	21	72	430	1520	114	385		
11	2.1	2.5[B]	2.7	7.9	61	14	12	17	25	103	44	202	28	92	22	29
12	1.3	2.6[B]	13	25	359	77			40	199	702	3970	153	893	71	337
13	0.4	3.2[B]	8.3	26	305	53	6.6	31	12	85	69	1180	49	59		
14	1.2	4.6[B]	10	6.5	61	8.7			13	44	24	42	11	50	8.7	8.9
15	2.1	2.5[A]			243	87	7.5	33	35	161	890	6500				
16	2.0	3.1[B]	15	39	321	52	17	29	27	64	131	365	95	342		
Mean	1.9	3.0	21.7	41.2	316	76.5	22	50.6	40.0	169	391	2354	113	519	82.9	316
SEM	0.4	0.3	8.0	17.1	75.6	23.2	12.2	24.2	15.7	67.5	131	905	39	239	48.6	197

[A]Collected before death.
[B]Collected at autopsy from left ventricle or femoral vein (patient 12).

tion in the papillary dermis. Within these macrophages were many golden brown pigment granules, resembling lipofuscin. The staining characteristics of the granules were the same in samples from all patients with pigmentation (Nos. 5, 17, and 18). The pigment was positive in the periodic acid–Schiff test, both before and after diastase extraction, and Perl's technique for ferric iron yielded negative results. Masson-Fontana and long Ziehl-Neelsen techniques were positive. The pigment was resistant to treatment with potassium permanganate and oxalic acid (melanin bleach stable). These findings suggest lipid deposition in secondary lysosomes with little melanin content. Unpigmented skin showed only occasional pigment granules.

Electron microscopy of pigmented skin (figure 1) showed 10 to 40 homogeneous granules per cell profile, 0.5 to 1.5 μm in diameter, in the cytoplasm of papillary dermal histiocytes. Figure 1 shows that many of the bodies appeared electron dense and relatively homogeneous but that some (at higher magnification) were multilamellar with a single limiting membrane. Similar dense bodies and occasional multilamellar inclusions were seen in terminal nerve fibers and infrequently in vascular endothelial cells.

Energy-dispersive x-ray microanalysis was performed on sections from the same blocks. In figure 2 a typical energy spectrum obtained from an electron-dense granule (*top*) in pigmented skin is contrasted with that from background cytoplasm (*bottom*) in the dermal macrophages. There was a high concentration of iodine and phosphorus in the electron-dense granule, the high phosphorus content probably reflecting phospholipid accumulation. The high iodine concentration was consistent with local accumulation of amiodarone or desethylamiodarone or other iodine-containing metabolites. Even without exposure to heavy metal during processing and when unstained, the granules appeared electron dense during routine transmission electron microscopy, further supporting the presence of an element with high atomic number, presumably iodine. The patient from whom the sample for energy-dispersive microanalysis was taken had never received iodine-containing contrast media.

Lung. Light microscopy of lung sections was performed in patients 8, 9, 10, 12, 15, and 16 (autopsy samples) and in patient 5 (transbronchial biopsy, araldite-embedded specimens only). In patient 5, amiodarone pulmonary toxicity was suspected because of a reduced carbon monoxide diffusion capacity, associat-

TABLE 4
Mean ratio of amiodarone to desethylamiodarone concentrations in human tissue

Tissue	Mean ratio (± SD)	No. of cases
Plasma	0.72 (0.30)	14
Skin	0.71 (0.70)	15
Fat	4.67 (1.37)	16
Skeletal muscle	0.50 (0.17)	14
Heart	0.31 (0.13)	12
Liver	0.23 (0.13)	12
Spleen	0.32 (0.20)	9
Lymph node	0.46 (0.32)	6
Pancreas	0.44 (0.20)	7
Lung	0.22 (0.08)	7
Adrenal gland	0.51 (0.37)	7
Testis	0.29 (0.12)	4
Thyroid gland	0.28 (0.14)	8
Kidney	0.26 (0.11)	7
Brain	0.13 (0.05)	9

TABLE 3
(Continued)

Pancreas		Lung		Adrenal gland		Testis		Thyroid gland		Kidney		Brain		Bile		Femoral nerve	
A	DA	A	DA	A	DA	A	DA	A	DA	A	DA	A	DA	A	DA	A	DA
64	114	183	623	103	292	113	357	12	44	37	102	3.0	25				
		600	2540	515	1890					215	960	36	209	150	420		
		180	793					12	40			8.1	44				
28	77			50	177	52	132	13	37	15	62	2.3	20				
38	136	224	1150	81	67			34	159	85	456	12	72			43	116
44	247	81	1140	42	372	167	1320	6.7	102	13	156	1.2	29	10	64	70	69
17	21	26	119	31	38	25	72	10	29	7.7	28	2.3	16			15	15
								15	92			3.7	49				
47	96	96	301	134	223			7.6	14	29	69	4.3	27				
39.8	115	198	952	137	437	89.1	470	13.8	64.5	57.4	262	8.1	54.4	80.1	242	42.7	66.7
6.7	30.8	71.9	302	64.5	246	31.9	290	3.1	17.3	28.1	129	3.7	20.2	70.0	178	15.8	29.1

ed with apical shadowing on the chest radiograph. In patient 12, large numbers and in patients 8 and 9 moderate numbers of intra-alveolar foamy macrophages were present. In patients 10, 15, and 16 similar cells were absent or sparse. In the araldite-embedded specimens from patients 5 toluidine blue staining showed the macrophages to be full of densely staining granules.

Electron microscopy was performed in lung specimens from patient 5 (figure 3). The granules seen by light microscopy in pulmonary macrophages were revealed to be multilamellar inclusions similar to those seen in some dermal macrophages and in terminal nerve fibers in pigmented skin. Macrophages in bronchoalveolar lavage specimens were of identical appearance. Energy-dispersive x-ray microanalysis showed that the multilamellar bodies in macrophages obtained by lavage contained considerable quantities of iodine. The patient had had an intravenous urogram 1 year before biopsy and we cannot exclude a contribution of iodine from the contrast medium used at that time.

Peripheral neutrophils. Electron microscopy of neutrophils was possible in patients 5 and 17. In patient 5, between five and 10 multilamellar bodies with a single limiting membrane were seen in each cell profile (figure 4). These were very similar to those seen in other tissues. In patient 17 somewhat abnormal lysosomal bodies were seen but they did not have similar multilamellar contents.

Liver. In patient 9, liver biopsy was performed because of evidence of hepatitis with a low plasma albumin concentration. Light microscopy revealed preservation of normal lobular architecture with a mild inflammatory infiltrate, predominantly lymphocytic. Many hepatocytes were swollen with large lipid vacuoles. Kupffer cells were prominent with diastase-resistant, periodic acid–Schiff positive granules. Electron microscopy (figure 5) revealed that the vacuoles in hepatocytes and granules in Kupffer cells represented multilamellar bodies, similar in appearance to those seen in skin, neutrophils, and lung. Similar but less marked changes were seen in patient 5, in whom aspartate transaminase concentrations were persistently elevated to twice normal. Similar changes were also seen in patient 7, but interpretation was complicated by the presence of a lymphoma. In patient 12, changes of long-standing cardiac failure were the only abnormalities seen. In this case the aspartate transaminase concentrations were normal.

Energy dispersive x-ray analysis by the same technique as before consistently failed to reveal iodine in

TABLE 5
Concentrations of amiodarone and desethylamiodarone in pigmented and unpigmented skin from the same patients

	Pigmented		Unpigmented	
Patient	Amiodarone (mg/kg wet weight)	Desethylamiodarone (mg/kg wet weight)	Amiodarone (mg/kg wet weight)	Desethylamiodarone (mg/kg wet weight)
9	297	699	60	138
17	119	539	17	72
18	502	1590	35	46

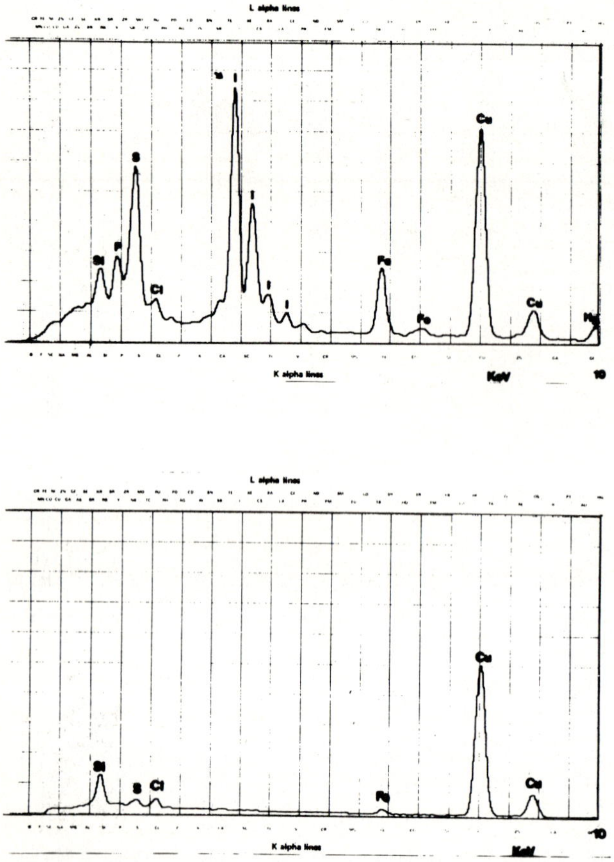

FIGURE 2. Energy-dispersive x-ray analysis spectrum from granule in macrophage from pigmented skin in a patient (No. 17) with amiodarone-induced skin pigmentation (*top*). *Bottom*, Spectrum from cytoplasm of macrophage. There is marked accumulation of iodine (arrow, I) in the granule, not seen in the cytoplasm. There is also more iron and sulphur than in the cytoplasm. The copper (Cu) is derived from the grid and the mercury (Hg) from the staining process.

any part of the hepatic sections. The high tissue concentrations of amiodarone and desethylamiodarone found in these samples are inconsistent with the failure to demonstrate iodine in the samples. If amiodarone was lost during electron microscopy processing, this was most probably caused by loss of lipid. Because iodine was demonstrated in other tissues processed in the same manner, this may indicate a different form of binding.

Discussion

Pharmacokinetic implications. Data concerning the tissue distribution of amiodarone and desethylamiodarone in man are sparse, being restricted to isolated case reports[11, 14, 17, 21, 22] or to cardiac distribution.[23] Yet for a drug with a mean terminal elimination half-life of 53 days and a mean volume of distribution of several thousand liters,[2] tissue drug deposition is likely to be important. Indeed, studies in the rat show extensive tissue deposition of amiodarone, even after brief intravenous therapy.[24] Our results show that high concentrations of amiodarone and of its desethyl metabolite are indeed found in human tissue during long-term therapy. The highest concentrations of both amiodarone and desethylamiodarone were found in liver, lung, adrenal gland, testis, spleen, and lymph node and lowest in skeletal muscle, thyroid gland, skin, and brain. High concentrations of amiodarone were also found in fat. Although the dosage and duration of amiodarone therapy varied widely in the study population, the pattern of distribution was virtually identical in all cases. Relatively large amounts of amiodarone, and particularly of desethylamiodarone, were found in bile. This suggests that biliary excretion may be important and is consistent with the observation that renal elimination of both compounds is negligible.[25] The low concentrations of both compounds in brain suggest an active blood brain barrier. This observation is consistent with the minor central nervous system toxicity associated with the drug, particularly in comparison with other antiarrhythmic agents.

With mean values derived from our autopsy data, the tissue of a 70 kg man with a normal body distribution would contain 3 g of amiodarone and 7 g of desethylamiodarone. The major store for amiodarone is fat, which contains 41% of the total, followed by skeletal muscle with 22% (figure 6). These stores represent therapeutically significant amounts of the drug. Thus, for instance, a tissue content of 3 g of amiodarone would provide therapy for over 30 days on a maintenance dose of 200 mg daily, assuming a bioavailability of 40%. As well as providing an explanation for the persistence of clinical effects after cessation of amiodarone therapy, our results suggest that obesity may well influence the dosage requirements for the drug. The pharmacologic and toxicologic significance of the large amounts of desethylamiodarone are unknown.

Amiodarone and desethylamiodarone distribution. The patterns of distribution of amiodarone and desethylamiodarone were strikingly similar. Does this pattern give any clue about the mechanism responsible for this distribution? The high concentrations of amiodarone in fat are consistent with its lipid solubility, but desethylamiodarone is also highly lipid soluble. The high concentrations of both compounds in liver, lung, adrenal gland, and testis would in themselves be consistent with the lipid solubility of these compounds. However, the disproportionately high concentrations of desethylamiodarone in these tissues (table 4) suggest the possibility of another mechanism. The observation of high amiodarone and desethylamiodarone concentrations in pigmented skin in association with large num-

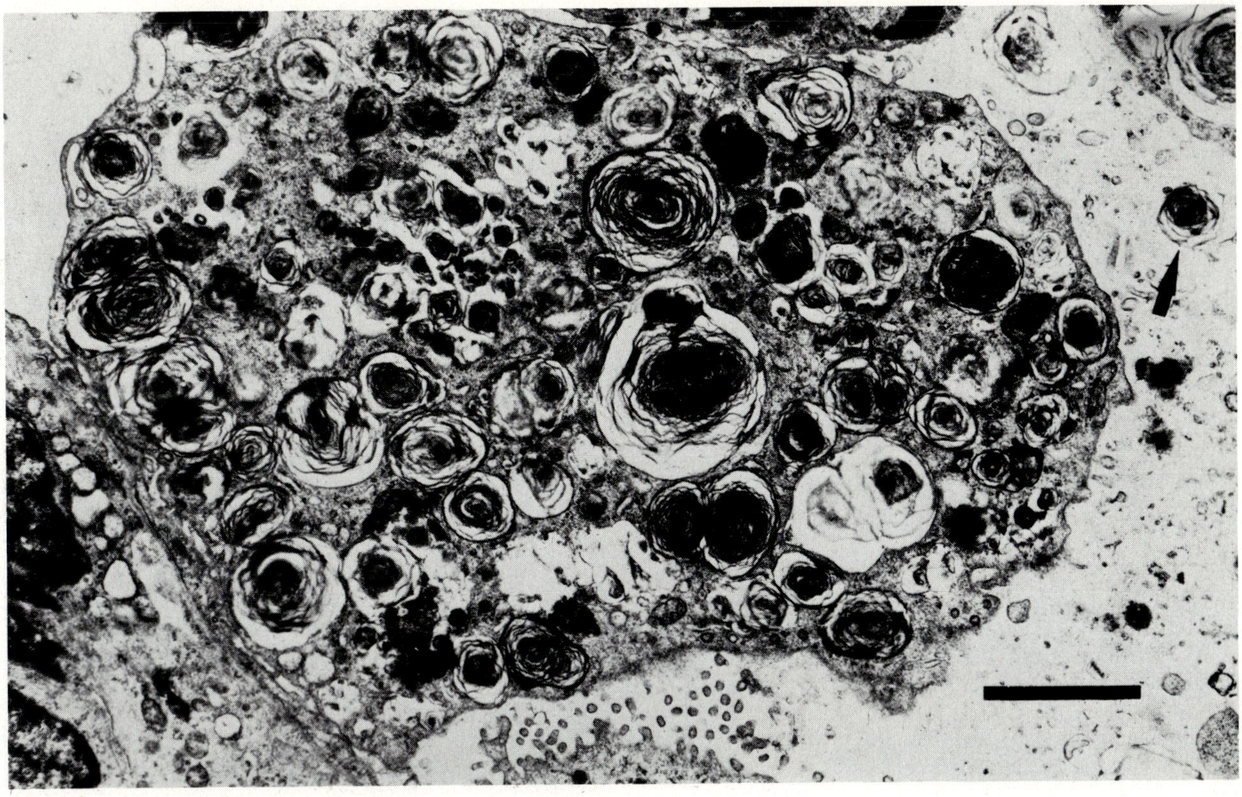

FIGURE 3. Pulmonary macrophage in lung biopsy specimen (patient 5). The cell is stuffed with multilamellar bodies, which in places are coalescent. Note a multilamellar body free in the alveolus (arrow). Scale bar = 2 μm.

bers of macrophages laden with secondary lysosomes suggested that the tissue distribution could be related to varying uptake of drug and metabolite by macrophages. Liver, lung, spleen, adrenal gland, and testis all contain large numbers of macrophages or other cells that actively take up lipid or lipid-rich membrane fragments into lysosomes; we have shown that all these tissues accumulate amiodarone and desethylamiodarone in large amounts.

Ultrastructure and drug and metabolite concentrations. The ultrastructural changes seen in skin, i.e., iodine-containing, lipid-rich inclusions within macrophages, were associated with high concentrations of amiodarone and desethylamiodarone. Similar inclusions were seen in pulmonary macrophages, Kupffer cells, hepatocytes, and peripheral neutrophils. Electron microscopic and histochemical analysis of these bodies suggested they were of lysosomal origin.

Our results are consistent with the inclusion bodies containing amiodarone and desethylamiodarone. Evidence for this comes from the electron density of inclusions in skin sections observed in electron microscopy, even without heavy metal stains; high local concentrations of an electron-dense element, such as iodine, would produce this appearance. Furthermore, the energy-dispersive x-ray microanalysis findings of high local concentrations of iodine in the inclusion bodies, with none in the cytoplasm, strongly support this notion. Computed tomography of the abdomen has demonstrated high hepatic radiodensity in patients receiving amiodarone.[26, 27] These results also suggest high tissue concentrations of an element with large atomic number, presumably iodine.

We suggest, therefore, that during therapy with amiodarone high tissue concentrations of amiodarone and desethylamiodarone accumulate in some sites, associated with characteristic lipid-rich abnormal lysosomal bodies that contain iodine. At least some of this iodine is likely to be within the amiodarone or desethylamiodarone molecule.

Significance of ultrastructural changes. The ultrastructural changes we describe are not seen in normal tissue. This unusual appearance, quite strikingly similar from tissue to tissue, was associated only with amiodarone therapy, this factor being the only factor common to patients 5, 7, 8, 9, 12, 17, and 18, in which the electron microscopic abnormality (or its light microscopic equivalent) was seen. No other drug was common to this group of patients. Although there were slight variations from site to site, with multilamellar

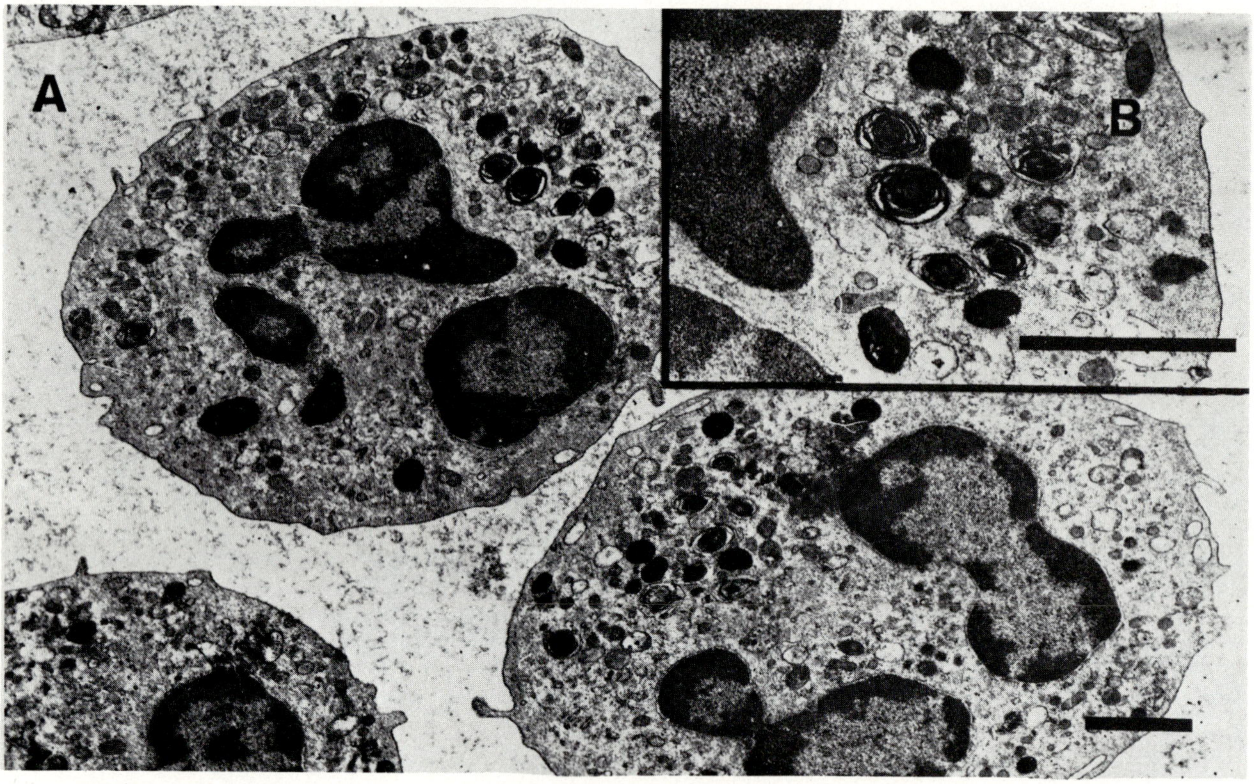

FIGURE 4. *A*, Peripheral neutrophils (electron microscopy) in buffy coat (patient 5). Several abnormal multilamellar bodies with single limiting membranes are seen in each neutrophil. *B*, Higher magnification, showing that the most dense bodies have paler centers and a suggestion of multilamellar contents. Their apparent density may therefore be due to overstaining. Scale bar = 2 μm.

bodies being less prominent in the skin, some were clearly multilamellar (figure 1, *A*). Slight variations in binding may explain these differences.

In our patients ultrastructural changes were associated most strongly with a clinically recognized unwanted effect. Other authors have recognized this association. The corneal deposits that develop in almost all patients receiving long-term amiodarone therapy are caused by multilamellar inclusions in corneal and conjunctival epithelial tissue[28] and are associated with high iodine concentrations.[29] Similar multilamellar bodies have been recognized in pulmonary macrophages, type II pneumocytes, and vascular endothelial cells in patients with pulmonary toxicity ascribed to amiodarone.[10, 12] We have confirmed these findings in patient 5 of this series and in other patients.[30] Multilamellar hepatic inclusions have also been seen by other authors.[14, 16, 17] Similar inclusions have been seen in peripheral nerve in patients with amiodarone-associated neuropathy.[31] Thus inclusions are seen in association with amiodarone-related adverse effects in some patients and probably in the corneal epithelium of most patients taking the drug. These findings, together with our data on tissue concentrations, again indicate that widespread tissue deposition of amiodarone and desethylamiodarone leads to ultrastructural changes in many sites. These changes, some of which are associated with adverse reactions to amiodarone, are of the type seen in lipid storage disorders, both drug induced and genetically determined.

Other drugs produce such ultrastructural changes in animals and in man.[32] The association of drug accumulation in body tissues with lipid-rich lamellar or crystalloid cytoplasmic inclusions in a variety of cell types suggests the development of a drug-induced lipid storage disorder.

Several drugs have been implicated in the production of a lipidosis in man. Chloroquine produces a corneal dystrophy with gross and ultrastructural features similar to those produced by amiodarone,[29] and in a patient with chloroquine-associated myopathy, multilamellar inclusions were found in muscle.[33] Similar changes were seen in hepatocytes in the rat.[34] Perhexiline produces adverse hepatic[35] and neural effects,[36] both of which are associated with the development of multilamellar inclusions in the affected tissue. 4,4′-DH (bis-diethyl-amino-ethoxy-hexestrol, Coralgil, a coronary vasodilator at one time used in the Far East),

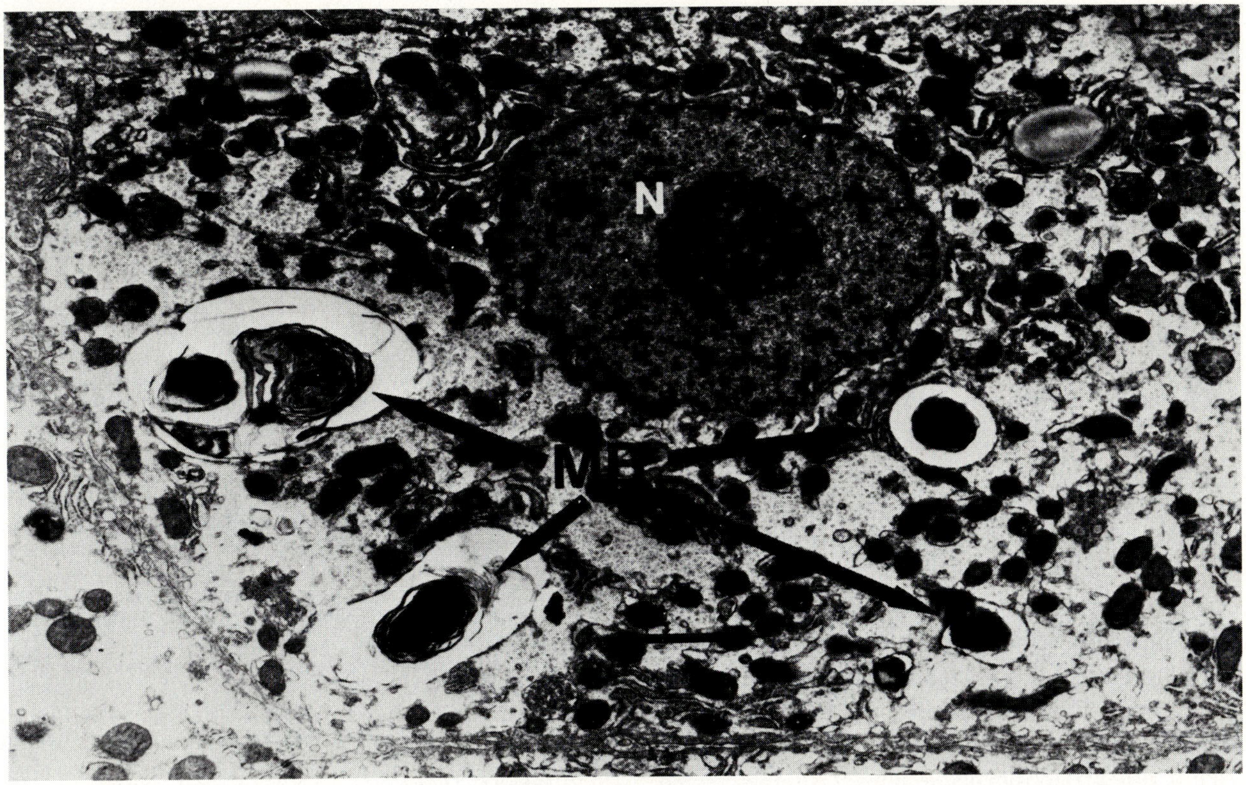

FIGURE 5. Hepatocyte (electron microscopy) from liver biopsy specimen (patient 9). Multilamellar inclusion bodies (MB) are shown in relation to the nucleus (N). The bodies are larger (up to 4 μm) in liver than in neutrophils and skin (0.5 to 1.5 μm). Scale bar = 2 μm.

produced frequent "phospholipid fatty liver"[37] characterized by abnormal lipid metabolism and frequent multilamellar bodies in Kupffer cells and in hepatocytes. These changes were also seen in other tissues.[38] These common morphologic changes are paralleled by a tendency for all these compounds to accumulate in tissues. 4,4′-DH can be found in tissue 18 months after the drug is discontinued, whereas the half-life of perhexiline in patients with neuropathy ranges between 9 and 22 days.[39]

Similar morphologic changes to those described with amiodarone and other drugs occur during the de-

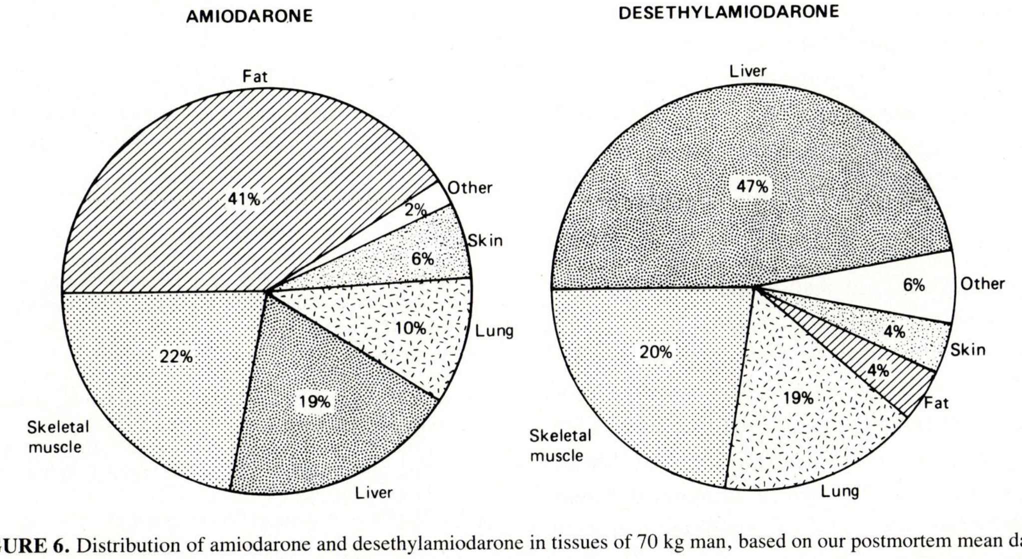

FIGURE 6. Distribution of amiodarone and desethylamiodarone in tissues of 70 kg man, based on our postmortem mean data. The 3.1 g of amiodarone is distributed as shown on the left, with fat, skeletal muscle, and liver being the important stores. Most of the 7.5 g desethylamiodarone is in liver, smaller amounts are in skeletal muscle and lung, and fat is relatively unimportant. This suggests that different factors govern the distribution of the two compounds.

velopment of the genetic lipid storage disorders, e.g., sphingomyelin lipidosis (Niemann-Pick) and glucosyl ceramide lipidosis (Gaucher's disease), in which large quantities of lipid are laid down in tissue, usually of the reticuloendothelial system or the central nervous system. Deposition of lipids in these cases is caused by an inherited deficiency of enzymes essential for lipid metabolism. It has been postulated that drug-induced lipid storage disorders may be caused by similar enzymatic abnormalities in lysosomes, caused by the drug.[32] For example, chloroquine inhibits lysosomal α-galactosidase; however, amiodarone therapy is associated with normal α-galactosidase activity.[40]

These observations suggest that amiodarone produces a generalized lipid storage disorder. They are reinforced by the demonstration that the drug is a potent inhibitor of phospholipase,[41] a lysosomal enzyme; the effects of desethylamiodarone on this enzyme are not documented. Although the ultrastructural changes occur most clearly in association with adverse effects, a lipid storage disorder probably occurs in almost all patients treated with amiodarone for a long enough period. Corneal deposits occur in most patients treated with the drug,[7] and abnormalities in liver function tests, which are frequent in patients taking amiodarone[4] may well reflect early hepatic effects. Furthermore, we have shown that changes in pulmonary gas transfer occur in up to 30% of patients treated with a mean dose of amiodarone of 360 mg/day for 11.6 months[30]; these changes may well represent early pulmonary involvement in the lipid storage disorder. Indeed, some authors,[42] drawing on animal experiments and a single patient, suggest that the pulmonary reaction is a lipid pneumonia.

Conclusions. Our results show that during amiodarone therapy high concentrations of amiodarone and desethylamiodarone accumulate in tissue. The distribution of these compounds may be caused in part by the development of a generalized lipid storage disorder in which drug and metabolite accumulate in the lysosomes of many tissues. The corneal microdeposits seen with amiodarone and also some of the drug's more important adverse effects are related to this property. Similarities with other drugs suggest a mechanism that should be considered in the spectrum of drug-induced disorders. Our observations have also pointed to the value of routine monitoring of morphologic changes in tissues obtained at autopsy or where possible during life, after the introduction of a new drug.

We gratefully acknowledge the help given by staff in many departments, including Freeman Hospital Departments of Histopathology and University Departments of Pathology and Dermatology. We thank Dr. D. M. Adams for practical help and useful discussions. Mrs. M. J. Gray's secretarial skills are gratefully acknowledged.

References

1. Flanagan RJ, Storey GCA, Holt DW, Farmer PB: Identification and measurement of desethylamiodarone in blood plasma specimens from amiodarone-treated patients. J Pharm Pharmacol **34:** 638, 1982
2. Holt DW, Tucker GT, Jackson PR, Storey GCA: Amiodarone pharmacokinetics. Am Heart J **106:** 840, 1983
3. Haffajee CI, Love JC, Canada AT, Lesko LJ, Asdourian G, Alpert JS: Clinical pharmacokinetics and efficacy of amiodarone for refractory tachyarrhythmias. Circulation **67:** 1347, 1983
4. Harris L, McKenna WJ, Rowland E, Holt DW, Storey GCA, Krikler DM: Side effects of long-term amiodarone therapy. Circulation **67:** 45, 1983
5. Burger A, Dinichert D, Nicod P, Jenny M, Lemarchand-Beraud T, Vallotton MB: Effect of amiodarone on serum triiodothyronine, reverse triiodothyronine, thyroxin and thyrotropin. J Clin Invest **58:** 255, 1976
6. Keidar S, Grenadier E, Palant A: Amiodarone-induced thyrotoxicosis: four cases and a review of the literature. Postgrad Med J **56:** 356, 1980
7. Ingram DV: Ocular effects in long-term amiodarone therapy. Am Heart J **106:** 902, 1983
8. Chalmers RJG, Muston HL, Srinivas V, Bennett DH: High incidence of amiodarone-induced photosensitivity in north-west England. Br Med J **285:** 341, 1982
9. Delage C, Lagace R, Huard J: Pseudocyanotic pigmentation of the skin induced by amiodarone: a light and electron microscopic study. Can Med Assoc J **112:** 1205, 1975
10. Marchlinski FE, Gansler TS, Waxman HL, Josephson ME: Amiodarone pulmonary toxicity. Ann Intern Med **97:** 839, 1982
11. Darmanata JI, van Zandwijk N, Duren DR, van Royen EA, Mooi WJ, Plomp TA, Jansen HM, Durrer D: Amiodarone pneumonitis: three further cases with a review of published reports. Thorax **39:** 57, 1984
12. Gefter WB, Epstein DE, Pietra GG, Miller WT: Lung disease caused by amiodarone, a new antiarrhythmic agent. Radiology **147:** 339, 1983
13. Dudognon P, Hauw JJ, de Baecque C, Derrida JP, Escourolle R, Nick J: Neuropathie au chlorohydrate d'amiodarone. Rev Neurol (Paris) **135:** 527, 1979
14. Lim PK, Trewby PN, Storey GCA, Holt DW: Neuropathy and fatal hepatitis in a patient receiving amiodarone. Br Med J **288:** 1638, 1984
15. Heger JJ, Prystowsky EN, Jackman WM, Naccarelli GV, Warfel KA, Rinkenberger RL, Zipes DP: Amiodarone: clinical efficacy and electrophysiology during long-term therapy for recurrent ventricular tachycardia or ventricular fibrillation. N Engl J Med **305:** 539, 1981
16. Poucell S, Ireton J, Valencia-Mayoral P, Downar E, Larratt L, Patterson J, Blendis L, Phillips MJ: Amiodarone-associated phospholipidosis and fibrosis of the liver: light, immunohistochemical and electron microscopic studies. Gastroenterology **86:** 926, 1984
17. Simon JB, Manley PN, Brien JF, Armstrong PW: Amiodarone hepatotoxicity simulating alcoholic liver disease. N Engl J Med **311:** 167, 1984
18. Storey GCA, Adams PC, Campbell RWF, Holt DW: High-performance liquid chromatographic measurement of amiodarone and desethylamiodarone in small tissue samples following enzymatic digestion. J Clin Pathol **36:** 785, 1983
19. Heger JJ, Solow EB, Prystowsky EN, Zipes DP: Plasma and red blood cell concentrations of amiodarone during chronic therapy. Am J Cardiol **53:** 912, 1984
20. Holt DW, Benstead JG: Post mortem assay of digoxin by radioimmunoassay. J Clin Pathol **25:** 483, 1975
21. Maggioni AP, Maggie A, Volpi A, D'Aranno V, Tognoni G, Giani P: Amiodarone distribution in human tissues after sudden death during Holter recording. Am J Cardiol **52:** 217, 1983
22. Zachary CB, Slater DN, Holt DW, Storey GCA, Macdonald DM:

The pathogenesis of amiodarone-induced pigmentation and photosensitivity. Br J Dermatol **110:** 451, 1984

23. Debbas NMG, Cailar C, Bexton RS, Demaille JG, Camm AJ, Puech P: The QT interval: a predictor of the plasma and myocardial concentrations of amiodarone. Br Heart J **51:** 316, 1984
24. Riva E, Gerna M, Neyroz P, Urso R, Bartosek I, Guaitani A: Pharmacokinetics of amiodarone in rats. J Cardiovasc Pharmacol **4:** 270, 1982
25. Harris L, Hing CRK, McKenna WJ, Savage C, Krikler SJ, Storey GCA, Holt DW: Renal elimination of amiodarone and its desethyl metabolite. Postgrad Med J **59:** 440, 1983
26. Patrick D, White FE, Adams PC: Long-term amiodarone therapy: a cause of increased attenuation on CT. Br J Radiol **57:** 573, 1984
27. Shenasa M, Vaisman U, Wojciechowski M, Denker S, Murthy V, Akhtar M: Abnormal abdominal computerized tomography with amiodarone therapy and clinical significance. Am Heart J **107:** 929, 1984
28. D'Amico DJ, Kenyon KR, Ruskin JN: Amiodarone keratopathy: drug-induced lipid storage disorder. Arch Ophthalmol **99:** 257, 1981
29. Francois J: Cornea verticillata. Doc Ophthalmol **27:** 235, 1969
30. Adams PC, Wright AJ, Corris PA, Morley AR, Campbell RWF, Gibson GJ: Amiodarone pulmonary toxicity. Clinical Sci **66:** 7P, 1984
31. Lemaire JF, Autret A, Biziere K, Romet-Lemone JL, Gray F: Amiodaron neuropathy: further arguments for human drug-induced neurolipidosis. Eur Neurol **21:** 65, 1982
32. Lüllmann-Rauch R: Drug-induced lysosomal storage disorders. *In* Dingle JT, Jacques PJ, Shaw IH, editors: Lysosomes in applied biology and therapeutics. Oxford, 1979, North Holland Publishing Co., p 49
33. Mastaglia FL, Papadimitrious JM, Dawkins RL, Beveridge B: Vacuolar myopathy associated with chloroquine, lupus erythematosus and thymoma. J Neurol Sci **34:** 315, 1977
34. Matsuzawa Y, Hostetler KY: Studies on drug-induced lipidosis: subcellular localization of phospholipid and cholesterol in the liver of rats treated with chloroquine or 4,4′-bis(diethylaminoethoxy) - diethyldiphenylethane. J Lipid Res **21:** 202, 1980
35. Beaugrand M, Poupon R, Levy V-G, Callard P, Lageron A, Lecomte D, Darnis F, Ferrier J-P: Lesions hepatiques dues au maleate de perhexiline. Gastroenterol Clin Biol **2:** 579, 1978
36. Mussini JM, Hauw J-J, Escourolle R: Etude en microscopie electronique des lesions, nerveuses musculaires et cutanees determinees par le maleate de perhexiline. Acta Neuropathol (Berlin) **38:** 53, 1977
37. de la Iglesia FA, Feuer G, Takada A, Matsuda Y: Morphologic studies on secondary phospholipidosis in human liver. Lab Invest **30:** 539, 1974
38. Shikata T, Kanetaka T, Endo Y, Nagashima K: Drug-induced generalized phospholipidosis. Acta Pathol (Japan) **22:** 517, 1972
39. Singlas E, Goujet MA, Simon P: Pharmacokinetics of perhexiline maleate in anginal patients with and without peripheral neuropathy. Eur J Clin Pharmacol **14:** 195, 1978
40. Tsai MY, Heger JJ, Prystowski EN, Zipes DP, Frampton BJ, Whitley CB: The amiodarone-induced phenocopy of Fabry keratopathy: normal α-galactosidase A activity in vivo. Am J Hum Genet **32:** 64a, 1982
41. Downar E, Shaikh N, Butany J: Amiodarone — a potent phospholipase inhibitor. J Am Coll Cardiol **3:** 604, 1984
42. Costa-Jussa FR, Corrin B, Jacob JM: Amiodarone lung toxicity: a human and experimental study. J Pathol **143:** 73, 1984

Effects of intravascular volume state on the value of pulsus paradoxus and right ventricular diastolic collapse in predicting cardiac tamponade

TERRENCE L. COGSWELL, M.D., GREGORY A. BERNATH, M.D., L. SAMUEL WANN, M.D., RAYMOND G. HOFFMAN, PH.D., HAROLD L. BROOKS, M.D., AND H. SIDNEY KLOPFENSTEIN, M.D., PH.D.

With the technical assistance of Dennis J. Janzer, M.S.B.E., and R. Keith Tipton, B.S.B.E.

ABSTRACT Both pulsus paradoxus and right ventricular diastolic collapse detected by two-dimensional echocardiography are noninvasive markers of impaired cardiac function in cardiac tamponade, yet the reliability of each may vary with the patient's state of hydration. To examine the relative value of these noninvasive markers at various states of hydration, we studied five chronically prepared, conscious mongrel dogs during 37 episodes of cardiac tamponade at three different intravascular volumes. We continuously measured cardiac output (electromagnetic flowmeter), aortic blood pressure, right atrial blood pressure, intrapericardial pressure, and respirations. Intravascular volume was varied by adjusting the mean right atrial blood pressure to hypovolemic (−2 to −6 mm Hg), euvolemic (0 to 4 mm Hg), or hypervolemic (6 to 10 mm Hg) levels. The sensitivity and specificity of right ventricular diastolic collapse in predicting increases in intrapericardial pressure remained high at all levels of hydration. Pulsus paradoxus showed good sensitivity and specificity at low intravascular volumes, but both sensitivity and specificity declined at higher intravascular volumes. Thus right ventricular diastolic collapse was more sensitive and more specific than pulsus paradoxus in detecting increases in intrapericardial pressure during euvolemia and hypervolemia whereas the two tests were equally valuable in hypovolemic states.
Circulation 72, No. 5, 1076–1080, 1985.

CARDIAC TAMPONADE should be viewed as a continuous spectrum ranging from pericardial effusion with minimal hemodynamic impairment, which may be asymptomatic, to effusion with severe cardiac compression and circulatory collapse.[1-3] The use of a 10 mm Hg inspiratory decline in systemic arterial blood pressure (i.e., pulsus paradoxus) has been suggested to identify hemodynamically significant cardiac tamponade.[4-6] In clinical studies of cardiac tamponade, Guberman et al.[4] have suggested the following criteria for diagnosis: pericardial effusion, an elevated systemic venous pressure, usually a paradoxical arterial pulse (10 mm Hg), and loss of the high venous pressure and paradoxical pulse with the removal of the effusion. The sign of right ventricular diastolic collapse seen on two-dimensional echocardiography provides an additional means of detecting cardiac tamponade.

The most desirable noninvasive test should reliably detect impaired cardiac function during cardiac tamponade early in its hemodynamic progression before arterial blood pressure falls. Right ventricular diastolic collapse has proved to be a very sensitive and specific marker of cardiac tamponade in patients with pericardial effusion.[7-9] We have shown in a euvolemic animal preparation that right ventricular diastolic collapse has a higher sensitivity and specificity than pulsus paradoxus in detecting changes in intrapericardial pressure early in cardiac tamponade.[10] Furthermore, right ventricular diastolic collapse was more strongly related to cardiac output, stroke volume, and heart rate than was pulsus paradoxus.

Changes in intravascular volume may alter our abili-

From the Cardiology Division, Department of Medicine, Medical College of Wisconsin and Wood Veterans Administration Medical Center, Milwaukee.

Supported in part by grants from the NIH-NHLBI, the Veterans Administration, the American Heart Association of Wisconsin, and the Heath Foundation, Milwaukee.

Address for correspondence: H. Sidney Klopfenstein, M.D., Ph.D., Cardiology Division, Medical College of Wisconsin, 8700 West Wisconsin Ave., Milwaukee, WI 53226.

Received March 12, 1985; revision accepted June 27, 1985.

ty to detect these markers in cardiac tamponade. Pulsus paradoxus, for example, may be absent in cardiac tamponade in the circumstance of extreme hypovolemia or hypotension[11, 12] and the time of onset of right ventricular diastolic collapse in cardiac tamponade may be affected by the state of hydration.[13] The purpose of this study was to examine the influence that alterations in intravascular volume have on the relative ability of pulsus paradoxus and right ventricular diastolic collapse to detect changes in intrapericardial pressure early in cardiac tamponade.

Methods

Five adult mongrel dogs weighing from 24 to 29 kg were selected for study, screened for parasites, and brought to the laboratory after an overnight fast. By techniques previously described,[2, 10] a left thoracotomy in the fifth intercostal space was performed and the animals were instrumented to measure cardiac output, aortic blood pressure, right atrial blood pressure, intrapericardial pressure, and heart rate. A chronically instrumented, conscious canine preparation of inducible cardiac tamponade was thus created.

Five days after surgery, the conscious animal was brought to the laboratory and allowed to stand comfortably in a sling. One pericardial, the aortic, and the right atrial catheters were attached directly to pressure transducers as described earlier.[2, 10] Respirations were measured by recording the change in electrical resistance in a small mercury-filled Silastic tube (Whitney gauge) placed around the thorax. Three separate intravascular volume states were investigated with mean right atrial blood pressure used as an index: hypovolemic (−2 to −6 mm Hg), euvolemic (0 to 4 mm Hg), and hypervolemic (6 to 10 mm Hg). Sterile normal saline and dextran 40 (Rheomacrodex 10%, Pharmacia Laboratories) were used to increase intravascular volume, and hemorrhaging was used to lower the mean right atrial blood pressure to the prescribed limits. Animals received 10,000 U of heparin intravenously before hemorrhage and all shed blood was replaced at the conclusion of the experimental period. Baseline data at each intravascular volume state were recorded after the pleural and pericardial cavities had been drained, 5 to 10 ml of normal saline replaced in the pericardial space, and a hemodynamic steady state achieved. Cardiac tamponade was produced by continuous infusion of warmed normal saline into the pericardial space and hemodynamic data were continuously recorded as described previously.[10] Short-axis two-dimensional echocardiograms were obtained with a handheld transducer in the right fourth or fifth intercostal space by means of an Irex HSP-1 phased-array ultrasonoscope (Johnson and Johnson). The echocardiograms were reviewed by two independent observers in real time and right ventricular diastolic collapse was considered to be present if there was indentation or abnormal inward motion of the right ventricular free wall or right ventricular outflow tract during diastole.

The state of intravascular volume was varied so that each animal was randomly exposed to any state only once in a given day. Once a steady-state baseline at any volume level was established, decompensated cardiac tamponade was produced. A maximum of three episodes of cardiac tamponade were produced per day per animal, allowing adequate time for recovery between episodes. Decompensated cardiac tamponade was defined as a drop in mean aortic blood pressure to 70% of the level present when the pericardium was empty (baseline). After achieving decompensated cardiac tamponade, the pericardial fluid was immediately removed and mean right atrial blood pressure was measured to ensure that the intravascular volume remained within the prescribed limits. All hemodynamic data were averaged over a 30 sec period at baseline, at each 2 mm Hg increment of intrapericardial pressure above baseline, at the onset of right ventricular diastolic collapse, and at decompensated cardiac tamponade. Each 30 sec data file included several respiratory cycles. All studies were performed between 5 and 15 days after surgery and each dog underwent between seven and 11 experiments (mean of eight).

All data were stored on analog magnetic tape and subsequently transferred to a digital computer (DEC LSI 11/23). By means of sequential interactive programs, individual beats in the 30 sec file were defined, respiratory phases were established, and mean pressures for intervals were calculated. For the determination of pulsus paradoxus, the largest difference in peak systolic blood pressure that occurred during each respiratory cycle of the 30 sec data file was measured. "Mean" pulsus paradoxus was defined as the average value for all respiratory cycles within the data file. All data files with a respiratory rate of more than 25 respirations/min for the collection were excluded from study because pulsus paradoxus could not be determined accurately. The timing of each interval with respect to the onset of right ventricular diastolic collapse was recorded, and when all the data intervals had been tallied, a final file was created for statistical analysis. All curves generated for analysis from the data file were adjusted for infusion episode before statistical comparison.[10]

A stepwise maximum likelihood logistic analysis was used to estimate the sensitivity and specificity of the onset of right ventricular diastolic collapse, pulsus paradoxus greater than 8 mm Hg, and pulsus paradoxus greater than 10 mm Hg.[14] Comparisons between the hypovolemic, euvolemic, and hypervolemic states were made by testing the differences of the regression coefficients obtained from the logistic analysis.[15] The same statistical method was used to compare the onset of right ventricular diastolic collapse, pulsus paradoxus greater than 8 mm Hg, and pulsus paradoxus greater than 10 mm Hg within each state of hydration.

Results

In chronically prepared, conscious dogs, a total of 37 episodes of cardiac tamponade were analyzed: 11 hypovolemic, 14 euvolemic, and 12 hypervolemic. For our analysis of pulsus paradoxus, an inspiratory decline in mean arterial blood pressure both greater than 8 mm Hg and greater than 10 mm Hg was examined. In our previous study, a degree of pulsus paradoxus greater than 8 mm Hg was associated with a higher sensitivity in detecting increases in intrapericardial pressure than was pulsus paradoxus greater than 10 mm Hg.[10] The values for mean pulsus paradoxus at baseline (empty pericardium), the onset of right ventricular diastolic collapse, and decompensated cardiac tamponade are shown in table 1. Pulsus paradoxus equals or exceeds 10 mm Hg at the time of onset of right ventricular diastolic collapse only for the hypervolemic group. Although present at all intravascular volumes during decompensated cardiac tamponade, this marker clearly occurs later in the progression of

TABLE 1
Mean values for pulsus paradoxus during cardiac tamponade

	Hypovolemia		Euvolemia		Hypervolemia
Baseline	4.44±1.24	p < .01	8.71±0.99	NS	8.45±1.12
Onset of RVDC	5.46±0.97	p < .02	9.76±0.81	p < .01	13.62±0.96
Decompensation	14.80±0.60	NS	12.80±1.40	NS	13.57±1.35
Observations[A]	11		14		12

RVDC = right ventricular diastolic collapse.

Mean values of pulsus paradoxus (mm Hg ± SEM) at baseline (empty pericardium), right ventricular diastolic collapse, and decompensated cardiac tamponade are given for all episodes of cardiac tamponade at each level of intravascular volume.

[A]Observations = the number of episodes of cardiac tamponade analyzed in each volume state. The levels of significance comparing values of mean pulsus paradoxus between volume states at analogous points in time are shown.

cardiac tamponade than does the onset of right ventricular diastolic collapse. When pulsus paradoxus greater than 8 mm Hg is chosen, the specificity of the marker decreases because the euvolemic and hypervolemic populations exhibit this level of paradoxical pulse when the pericardium is empty. When the pericardium is empty, increasing intravascular volume causes an increase in pulsus paradoxus only between the hypovolemic and euvolemic states, whereas early in cardiac tamponade (at the time of onset of right ventricular diastolic collapse) pulsus paradoxus increases continuously as intravascular volume is increased.

In figure 1, *A*, the sensitivity and specificity of pulsus paradoxus greater than 8 mm Hg in detecting a change in intrapericardial pressure from baseline is shown. All three curves differ significantly from each other ($p < .05$ to $p < .001$). The rate of rise in sensitivity for this degree of pulsus paradoxus is low in both the euvolemic and hypervolemic populations. Furthermore, the specificity of pulsus paradoxus greater than 8 mm Hg in detecting changes in intrapericardial pressure declines abruptly as the magnitude of intravascular volume increases.

Figure 1, *B*, illustrates the sensitivity of the more classic 10 mm Hg inspiratory decline in systolic arterial blood pressure in predicting an increase in intrapericardial pressure during cardiac tamponade. All curves differ from one another significantly ($p < .01$). As with pulsus paradoxus of greater than 8 mm Hg, this level of pulsus paradoxus shows a slow rate of rise in sensitivity for the euvolemic and hypervolemic groups and the specificity of the test declines at higher levels of intravascular volume.

By contrast, the ability of right ventricular diastolic collapse to detect an increase in intrapericardial pressure is shown in figure 1, *C*. Hypovolemic and hypervolemic curves differ ($p < .01$), but neither is significantly different from the euvolemic situation. For each level of intravascular volume, the onset of right ventricular diastolic collapse exhibits excellent specificity with a rapid rate of rise in sensitivity over the range of intrapericardial pressures of interest. There is a signifi-

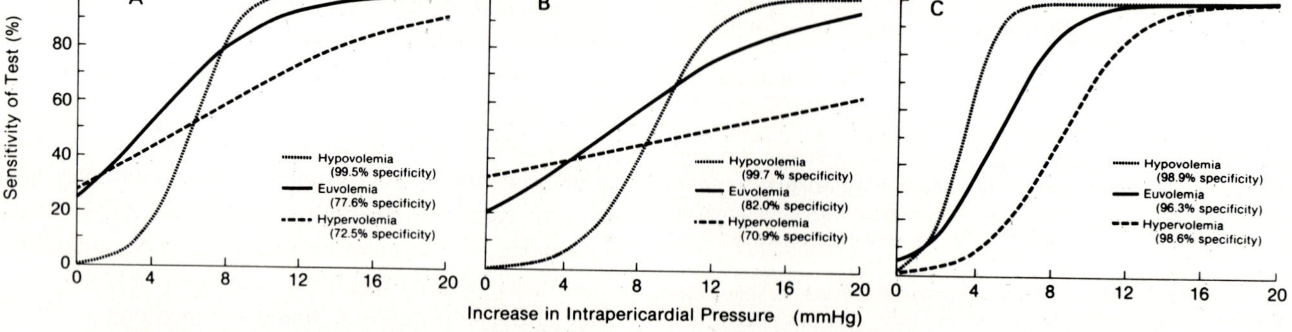

FIGURE 1. *A*, Sensitivity and specificity of pulsus paradoxus greater than 8 mm Hg in detecting an increase in intrapericardial pressure from baseline during cardiac tamponade. The hypovolemic curve differs from the other curves by $p < .001$, and the euvolemic and hypervolemic curves differ from each other by $p < .01$. *B*, Sensitivity and specificity of pulsus paradoxus greater than 10 mm Hg in detecting an increase in intrapericardial pressure from baseline during cardiac tamponade. The hypovolemic curve differs from the other curves by $p < .001$, and the euvolemic and hypervolemic curves are not significantly different. *C*, Sensitivity and specificity of the onset of right ventricular diastolic collapse in detecting an increase in intrapericardial pressure above baseline during cardiac tamponade. All of the curves differ significantly from one another ($p < .05$ for all comparisons).

cant trend toward decreased sensitivity of this test as intravascular volume is increased ($p < .02$).

Figure 2, *A* to *C*, illustrates the relative value of the three indicators of increasing intrapericardial pressure for each intravascular volume studied. The curves for pulsus paradoxus greater than 8 mm Hg and pulsus paradoxus greater than 10 mm Hg do not differ significantly within any volume state. There were no significant differences among any of the curves in the hypovolemic animals (panel *A*). During euvolemia and hypervolemia (panels *B* and *C*), the onset of right ventricular diastolic collapse was more sensitive and specific than either degree of pulsus paradoxus in detecting an increase in intrapericardial pressure from baseline during cardiac tamponade ($p < .001$).

Discussion

We recently examined the relative merits of right ventricular diastolic collapse and pulsus paradoxus in detecting increases in intrapericardial pressure from baseline during cardiac tamponade in a chronically instrumented, euvolemic animal preparation.[10] In that study, we found right ventricular diastolic collapse to be more strongly related to changes in cardiac output, stroke volume, and intrapericardial pressure during cardiac tamponade than pulsus paradoxus of greater than 8 mm Hg or pulsus paradoxus greater than 10 mm Hg. Indeed, pulsus paradoxus provided little additional information concerning hemodynamic parameters to that provided by right ventricular diastolic collapse. Both tests together were better predictors of increased intrapericardial pressure than was either alone.

Although right ventricular diastolic collapse is a better independent marker for hemodynamically significant cardiac tamponade than pulsus paradoxus in a euvolemic animal population, alterations in intravascular volume are known to affect the appearance and reliability of both of these tests.[11-13] Because it is difficult at times to know the status of intravascular volume in a patient with impending cardiac tamponade, a marker of increasing intrapericardial pressure that is reliable, regardless of volume status, would be most advantageous. Hence, in this study we have examined the relative sensitivity and specificity of these two markers in detecting changes in intrapericardial pressure during cardiac tamponade as the intravascular volume was varied.

The ideal marker for significant cardiac tamponade should detect increasing intrapericardial pressure early in the hemodynamic progression of events and long before the point of circulatory collapse. Its usefulness to the clinician would improve if both the sensitivity and specificity of the test remained high regardless of the influence of such factors as the state of hydration of the patient being evaluated.

The results of this study clearly show the limitations of pulsus paradoxus greater than 8 mm Hg or pulsus paradoxus greater than 10 mm Hg as noninvasive markers for an increase in intrapericardial pressure during cardiac tamponade. Both the sensitivity and

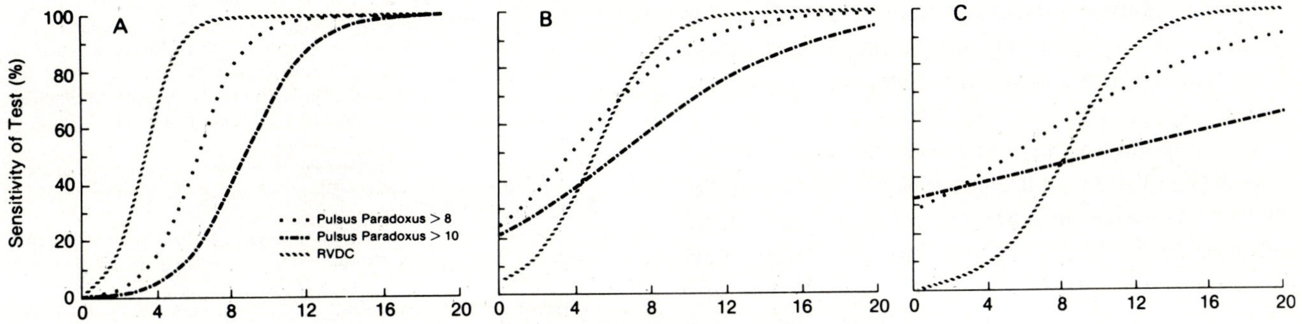

FIGURE 2. *A*, Comparison of the relative sensitivities of the onset of right ventricular diastolic collapse (RVDC), pulsus paradoxus greater than 8 mm Hg, and pulsus paradoxus greater than 10 mm Hg in detecting increases in intrapericardial pressure from baseline during hypovolemic cardiac tamponade. The curve for right ventricular diastolic collapse differs from the other curves by $p < .001$, and the curves for pulsus paradoxus greater than 8 mm Hg and pulsus paradoxus greater than 10 mm Hg are not significantly different. *B*, Relative sensitivities of the onset of right ventricular diastolic collapse, pulsus paradoxus greater than 8 mm Hg, and pulsus paradoxus greater than 10 mm Hg in detecting increases in intrapericardial pressure from baseline during euvolemic cardiac tamponade. The curve for right ventricular diastolic collapse differs from the other curves by $p < .001$, and the curves for pulsus paradoxus greater than 8 mm Hg and pulsus paradoxus greater than 10 mm Hg are not significantly different. *C*, Relative sensitivity of the onset of right ventricular diastolic collapse, pulsus paradoxus greater than 8 mm Hg, and pulsus paradoxus greater than 10 mm Hg in detecting increases in intrapericardial pressure from baseline during hypervolemic cardiac tamponade. The curve for right ventricular diastolic collapse differs from the other curves by $p < .001$, and the curves for pulsus paradoxus greater than 8 mm Hg and pulsus paradoxus greater than 10 mm Hg do not differ.

specificity of each degree of pulsus paradoxus decrease as the intravascular volume increases (figure 1, *A* and *B*). Although the sensitivity of pulsus paradoxus exceeds that of right ventricular diastolic collapse in detecting small changes in intrapericardial pressure at low intrapericardial pressures in euvolemic and hypervolemic populations (figure 2, *B* and *C*), it does so with very low specificity. In these two populations, the onset of right ventricular diastolic collapse is a far better indicator of increasing intrapericardial pressure because it is both sensitive and specific.

Despite the relative positions of the curves in the hypovolemic population (figure 2, *A*), right ventricular diastolic collapse has no clear statistical advantage over pulsus paradoxus in predicting an increase in intrapericardial pressure during cardiac tamponade. All three indicators have excellent specificities for this state of hydration. Although there is a trend toward a higher sensitivity for right ventricular diastolic collapse in detecting small elevations in intrapericardial pressure compared with either degree of pulsus paradoxus in this group, this relationship does not reach statistical significance.

It is interesting that pulsus paradoxus showed a lower percentage of false negatives (better sensitivity) in the hypovolemic group than in the euvolemic or hypervolemic groups (figure 1, *A* and *B*). One might reasonably expect a higher percentage of false negatives in this population.[11, 12] Although we were able to effect a significant reduction in resting cardiac output and aortic blood pressure from the euvolemic situation with the degree of hypovolemia we studied, perhaps further volume contraction in our animal preparation would have resulted in the lower sensitivity others have observed.

It is important to note that both the sensitivity and specificity of right ventricular diastolic collapse in detecting increases in intrapericardial pressure from baseline during cardiac tamponade remain high at low intravascular volumes. It has been suggested that right ventricular diastolic collapse may be too sensitive in volume-contracted states with the potential for false-positive identification of significant cardiac tamponade.[13] The specificity of right ventricular diastolic collapse we observed in our hypovolemic population (98.9%) suggests few false-positive identifications in this animal preparation.

In conclusion, in this chronically instrumented, conscious animal preparation of cardiac tamponade, we have shown that the state of hydration does affect the ability of pulsus paradoxus to detect changes in intrapericardial pressure with worsened sensitivity and specificity at higher intravascular volumes, whereas there appears to be no major affect of the state of hydration on the ability of right ventricular diastolic collapse to detect increases in intrapericardial pressure. Right ventricular diastolic collapse is both more sensitive and more specific than pulsus paradoxus in detecting increases in intrapericardial pressure during cardiac tamponade in euvolemic or hypervolemic states, whereas right ventricular diastolic collapse and pulsus paradoxus are equally valuable in detecting elevations in intrapericardial pressure during hypovolemia.

We thank Dennis J. Janzer, M.S.B.E., and R. Keith Tipton, B.S.B.E., for their technical expertise. We are grateful to Donna Weitzer for her efforts in the preparation of this manuscript.

References

1. Fowler NO: Physiology of cardiac tamponade and pulsus paradoxus. Mod Concepts Cardiovasc Dis **47:** 115, 1978
2. Leimgruber PP, Klopfenstein HS, Wann LS, Brooks HL: The hemodynamic derangement associated with right ventricular diastolic collapse in cardiac tamponade: an experimental echocardiographic study. Circulation **68:** 612, 1983
3. Shabetai R, Mangiard L, Bhargava V, Ross J Jr, Higgins CB: The pericardium and cardiac function. Prog Cardiovasc Dis **22:** 107, 1979
4. Guberman BA, Fowler NO, Engel PJ: Cardiac tamponade in medical patients. Circulation **64:** 633, 1981
5. Spodick DH: Acute cardiac tamponade pathologic physiology, diagnosis, and management. Prog Cardiovasc Dis **10:** 64, 1967
6. Reddy PS, Curtiss EI, O'Toole JD, Shaver JA: Cardiac tamponade: hemodynamic observations in man. Circulation **58:** 265, 1978
7. Armstrong WF, Schilt BF, Helper DJ, Dillon JC, Feigenbaum H: Diastolic collapse of the right ventricle with cardiac tamponade: an echocardiographic study. Circulation **65:** 1491, 1982
8. Shiina A, Yaginuma T, Kondo K, Kawai N, Hosoda S: Echocardiographic evaluation of impending cardiac tamponade. J Cardiogr **9:** 555, 1979
9. Engel PJ, Hon H, Fowler NO, Plummer S: Echocardiographic study of right ventricular wall motion in cardiac tamponade. Am J Cardiol **50:** 1018, 1982
10. Klopfenstein HS, Schuchard GH, Wann LS, Palmer TE, Hartz AJ, Gross CM, Singh S, Brooks HL: The relative merits of pulsus paradoxus and right ventricular diastolic collapse in the early detection of cardiac tamponade: an experimental echocardiographic study. Circulation **71:** 829, 1985
11. Fowler NO: The pericardium in health and disease. Mount Kisco, NY, 1985, Futura Publishing Co, Inc., p 235
12. Antman EM, Cargill V, Grossman W: Low-pressure cardiac tamponade. Ann Intern Med **91:** 403, 1979
13. Gaffney FA, Keller AM, Peshock RM, Lin J-C, Firth BG: Pathophysiologic mechanisms of cardiac tamponade and pulsus alternans shown by echocardiography. Am J Cardiol **53:** 1662, 1984
14. Cox DR: Analysis of binary data. New York, 1970, Halstead Press
15. Kleinbaum DG, Kupper LL: Applied regression analysis and other multivariate methods. North Scituate, 1978, Duxbury Press

Comparison of pathologic and angiographic findings in a porcine preparation of coronary atherosclerosis

BONNIE H. WEINER, M.D., IRA S. OCKENE, M.D., JOHN JARMOLYCH, M.D., KATHERINE E. FRITZ, PH.D., AND ASSAAD S. DAOUD, M.D.

ABSTRACT Coronary atherosclerosis was induced in Yorkshire swine by diet-induced hyperlipidemia and balloon intimal abrasion of a coronary artery. Severe stenoses pathologically similar to the lesions of human atherosclerosis were seen after 8 months of the atherogenic regimen. To examine the relationship between the angiogram and pathology in the assessment of the extent and location of coronary atherosclerosis, antemortem angiographic results were compared with results of pathologic examination. Vernier caliper measurements of the coronary angiogram were compared with results of morphometric evaluation of perfusion-fixed coronary arteries. Isolated focal stenoses were correctly localized and quantified, as were focal lesions within vessels diffusely diseased. Both overestimation and underestimation of lesions occurred at bifurcation sites. Diffuse disease without focal stenoses was not well demonstrated angiographically. Vessels that were angiographically thought to be normal or only minimally diseased demonstrated significantly larger lumens angiographically than pathologically. This is believed to be due to fixation and paraffin-processing artifact, even though fixation was performed by perfusion at physiologic pressure. The demonstration of an excellent correlation between the luminal size as determined angiographically and morphometrically at sites of focal obstruction confirms the value of quantitation of coronary angiograms in vivo as a diagnostic tool in coronary atherosclerosis.
Circulation 72, No. 5, 1081–1086, 1985.

CORONARY ANGIOGRAPHY has become the most widely used tool for determining the status of the coronary arteries in man. Controversy exists, however, over the relationship between the angiographic and the histopathologic assessments of the extent of atherosclerosis.[1-6] Arnett et al.,[1] in studies comparing meticulous pathologic examinations of nonperfusion-fixed hearts to antemortem angiograms obtained at various times relative to death of the patient, has stated that angiography underestimates the severity of coronary atherosclerosis. More recently, Marcus et al.[7] studied a primate model of atherosclerosis and suggested that nondistended pathologic arterial specimens do not accurately reflect the physiologic status of these vessels.

The current study uses a model of coronary atherosclerosis in swine to address the relationship between the degree of atherosclerosis as assessed by antemortem coronary angiographic examination and that seen in pathologic examination of the coronary arteries fixed by perfusion at physiologic pressure.[8-13]

From the Division of Cardiology, Department of Medicine, University of Massachusetts Medical School, Worcester, MA, and Department of Pathology, U.S. Veterans Administration Hospital, Albany, N.Y.

Address for correspondence: Bonnie H. Weiner, M.D., Cardiovascular Medicine, University of Massachusetts Medical Center, 55 Lake Avenue North, Worcester, MA 01605.

Received April 19, 1983; revision accepted Aug. 1, 1985.

Methods

Seven 12 to 15-week-old male Yorkshire pigs from a stable breeding stock were studied. After initial determination of plasma lipid levels, the animals were placed on a high-cholesterol, high-fat diet (table 1), which was continued for the duration of the study. At the end of 2 weeks, to allow for the development of hyperlipidmia, determination of lipid levels, including levels of total cholesterol, low-density lipoprotein (LDL), high-density lipoprotein (HDL), very low-density lipoprotein (VLDL), and triglycerides, was performed with a Beckman airfuge ultracentrifuge and the technique of Bonzert and Brewer.[14]

The animals then underwent cardiac catheterization and balloon abrasion of the proximal left anterior descending coronary artery (LAD) by the following technique: Each animal was sedated with 35 mg/kg ketamine hydrochloride. After intubation, anesthesia was maintained with a Bird respirator (Palm Springs, CA) with 1% halothane, 30% nitrous oxide, and 70%

TABLE 1
Atherogenic diet

	g/day	kcal/day	% total
Peanut oil	15.4	135.5	3.8
Sodium cholate	10.3	91.7	2.6
Cholesterol	15.4	144.8	4.1
Lard	190.4	1711.8	48.5
Milk powder	51.4	283.2	8.0
Vitamin mix (Teklad Mills)	10.3		
Salt mix (U.S. Biochemical Co.)	15.4		
Mash (Agway)	341.8	1162.1	32.9
Total	650	3529.1	

oxygen. The electrocardiogram was monitored with the use of needle electrodes placed in each extremity and displayed on an Electronics for Medicine VR12 oscilloscope and recorder (Pleasantville, NY). A six-lead electrocardiogram was recorded during each procedure.

The neck of each animal was shaved and prepared with betadine. The skin was incised in a longitudinal manner from the mandible caudally. The carotid artery was isolated for a length of 1.0 cm by blunt dissection. The artery was entered under direct vision by the Seldinger technique and a No. 8F Cordis arterial sheath was inserted. Each animal was then anticoagulated with 1500 units of intra arterial heparin.

A No. 8F Teflon-lined polyurethane guiding catheter preformed to a No. 2.0 right Judkins configuration was then inserted (USCI, Billerica, MA). The catheter was positioned at the origin of the left coronary artery and cineangiography was performed in anteroposterior, left anterior oblique, and right anterior oblique projections and filmed on Kodak 35 mm CFR cineangiographic film at 30 frames/sec with a Siemens Corp. cineangiographic system with a resloution of 3.7 line pairs/mm. A No. 3F Fogarty embolectomy catheter was then advanced through the guide catheter and positioned in the proximal left anterior descending coronary artery. The balloon was inflated with 0.3 ml of a 50/50 mixture of saline and meglumine diatrizoate. The embolectomy catheter was then withdrawn to the ascending aorta with the balloon inflated. This procedure was repeated twice.

The balloon catheter was then removed and repeat coronary cineangiography was performed to assess the immediate effect of the abrasion procedure. The catheter and sheath were then removed and the carotid artery was repaired with interrupted 6-0 cardiovascular Tevdek sutures. The skin was closed with interrupted 3-0 nylon sutures.

The animals were kept at our institution for observation for 1 to 2 days after the procedure. Long-term housing was provided at the Tufts University School of Veterinary Medicine farm facility (Grafton, MA). At 4 months intervals, the animals underwent repeat lipid and coronary arteriographic studies. After completion of these studies, the animals were killed (two at 4 months and five at 8 months) by perfusion of 2.5% gluteraldahyde (two animals) or 10% formalin (five animals) into the aortic root at mean arterial pressure for 20 min following anesthetization.[15,16] The aorta was cross-clamped distal to the arch vessels before perfusion was initiated. The hearts were removed intact and were maintained in fixative until processing.

The coronary arteries were dissected free from the myocardium and were sectioned at 3.0 mm intervals. Careful maps of the blocks with definitions of branch points were made for comparison to the angiograms. The sections were then paraffin embedded. For quantitation of the size and components of lesions, a representative hematoxylin and eosin-stained section from each block was projected onto a vertical surface, using a 4× objective in a Leitz Tele-Promar 500 projecting microscope, 3.5 feet from the vertical surface.

Elements of the lesion, including the ideal and the residual lumen, the area occupied by lesions, and areas of necrosis and calcification within the lesion, as projected, were traced and the tracings were subjected to quantitative analysis using a Zeiss MOP-3 digital image analyzer system.

Ideal luminal area was calculated from the perimeter of the internal elastic membrane, assuming that the true vessel shape was circular. The intimal area within this membrane was considered to be the lesion area and was planed directly. The difference between these values was residual luminal area, from which luminal diameter could be calculated. Areas of calcification or necrosis were determined directly by digital planimetry. Comparison with adjacent areas was not performed for the purpose of calculation of percent diameter reduction.

The antemortem angiograms obtained within 24 hr of the animals being killed were independently evaluated both quantitatively and qualitatively by two experienced angiographers (B. H. W., I. S. O.). For each angiogram, the epicardial coronary arteries and their branches were reviewed for the presence or absence of disease and six areas of focal narrowing were indentified. The films were projected on a screen with a Vanguard XR-35 projector, resulting in a total magnification of 5×. The magnification correction factor was calculated with a standard 1 cm × 1 cm grid positioned at the level of the left ventricle. The areas of focal narrowing were measured with a Vernier caliper with 0.1 mm divisions and their locations were identified relative to vessel branch points. Segments proximal or distal to lesions were measured in a similar manner. Sites were chosen that could be easily identified to facilitate comparison between the angiographic and pathologic data. Percent stenosis, based on these values, was not compared. If no areas of focal disease were indentified, locations that could be clearly defined on the basis of proximity to a branch point were measured by the same technique for comparison to the pathologic specimens.

To further evaluate the angiographic-pathologic discrepancy found in the study animals, three normal animals were studied and 12 angiographically identified sites were examined. The animals were sedated, anesthetized, and prepared and catheters were inserted as described above. An initial angiogram was obtained. The chest and pericardium were then opened and a second angiogram was obtained. A segment of the LAD was then dissected free and the external dimension was measured with a Vernier caliper. Coronary angiography was again performed. After perfusion fixation by the same procedure described above, similar measurements and postmortem angiographic examinations were performed. The coronary arteries were then subjected to the same morphometric evaluation described above.

Results

The plasma lipid levels in the study animals are listed in table 2. Their baseline lipids were distributed among the lipoprotein classes in much the same way as in humans. The absolute values, however, were lower. With the antherogenic diet, a marked increase in total cholesterol, LDL, HDL, and VLDL occurred. Although HDL_C was not measured, the elevation in HDL is likely to be in that fraction, as has been shown in other lipid-fed animal preparations.[17,18] These elevations persisted throughout the study. There was no significant change in triglyceride levels.

TABLE 2
Plasma lipoprotein levels (mean ± SD)

	Total cholesterol (mg%)	LDL (mg%)	HDL (mg%)	VLDL (mg%)	Triglyceride (mg%)
Baseline	116±59	68±28	52±14	11±8	139±112
2 weeks	568±287	322±285	118±78	128±125	196±272
4 months	559±256	359±249	116±44	60±55	77±56
8 months	589±261	283±94	186±120	124±80	126±114

Two animals were studied 4 months after the abrasion procedure. Ninety-five coronary arterial sections were examined morphometrically. Forty-five sections had no disease. The other 50 sections (53%) had pathologic evidence of disease, with a mean lesion area of 0.25 + 0.35 mm² (range 0.003 to 1.5 mm²). This represents a mean luminal encroachment of 7.8% in these segments (range 0.3% to 42.1%). Eleven sections (12%) had intimal calcification (mean 7.7% of the lesion area in those segments). No necrosis was seen in any of these lesions.

Five animals were studies 8 months after the abrasion procedure. Two hundred and six sections were examined morphometrically. One hundred and eighty-two (88%) of the sections had lesions. The mean lesion area in these sections was 2.75 ± 2.68 mm² (range 0.004 to 14.8 mm²). The mean luminal encroachment was 48.5 ± 35% (range 0.02% to 100%). Of the 182 segments with disease, 102 had calcification (56%) (9.5 ± 11.5% of the lesion area, range 0.2% to 54.2%). Similarly, 122 (67%) sections had areas of necrosis (mean 43.5 ± 21.3% of the lesion area).

Figure 1 is a representative section from one of the animals studied at 8 months. It demonstrates the major features of complex atherosclerotic disease in man. There is a fibrous cap, intimal necrosis, calcification, and cholesterol clefts. Variable amounts of foam cells are seen in these animals. The two animals studied at 4 months had more focal disease, less overall involvement, and less complex disease, with some calcification but without necrosis.

No evidence of myocardial infarction was found on gross examination of any heart. No electrocardiographic evidence of myocardial infarction was indentified on serial tracings.

Comparison of angiographic and pathologic results

Atherosclerotic animals. Three focal areas of stenosis could be identified in the two animals studied at 4 months and comparable angiograms were available for two of them. The third was in the right coronary artery of an animal in which, for technical reasons, no angiogram of that vessel was obtained. One of the focal lesions was correctly identified both as to significance and location. The other lesion occurred at a bifurcation and was not identified by angiography.

Ten of 12 vessels from the five animals studied at 8 months were described angiographically as having some or multiple areas of irregularity (figure 2). Pathologically, nine of these 10 vessels had severe, diffuse atherosclerosis, defined as greater than 75% of segments being involved with severe atherosclerosis similar to that shown in figure 1. The remaining vessel had

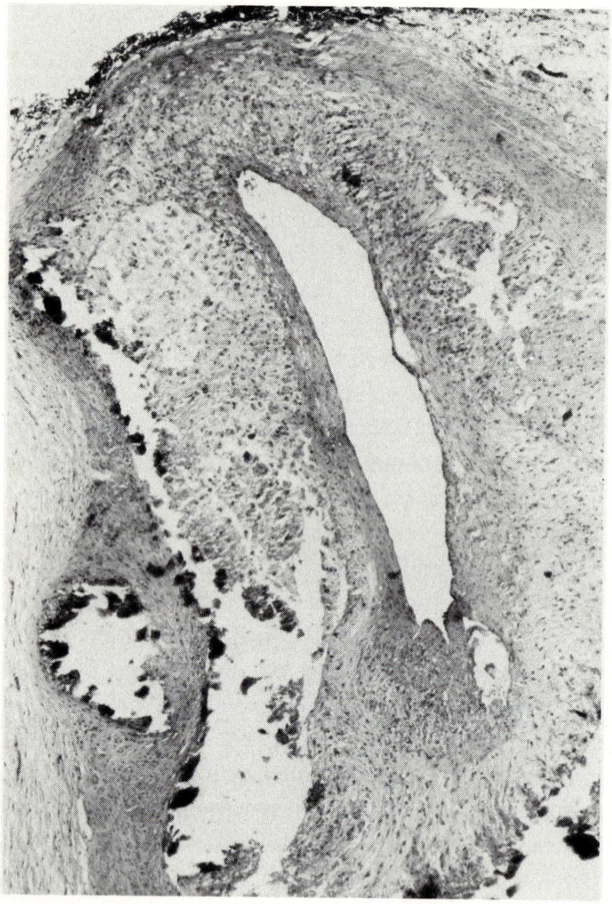

FIGURE 1. Photomicrograph of section of proximal left circumflex coronary artery showing fibrous cap, intimal necrosis, and calcification.

mild disease but was diffusely involved. The other two vessels were pathologically normal. Two focal lesions within diffusely diseased vessels were correctly identified angiographically. An additional lesion, at a bifurcation, was thought to be present angiographically, but was not demonstrated pathologically. In one animal, an area of ostial tapering was comented on as unusual, but the readers could not decide if this represented disease or normal variation. On pathologic evaluation, a significant lesion was found. Two vessels that were interpreted as angiographically normal were "normal" pathologically. No lesion, focal or otherwise, resulting in less than 20% reduction in luminal area as determined pathologically was detected by angiography. Similarly, no area of greater focal stenosis was missed in these animals.

When the luminal areas and diameters of the vessels determined angiographically and morphologically were compared (tables 3 and 4), there was near identity in the values for focal lesions defined angiographically. In areas without focal lesions, however, whether or not the vessel was normal or diffusely diseased, the antemortem angiogram demonstrated significantly greated luminal diameter and area as compared with the pathologic specimens ($p < .001$ for both diameter and area).

Normal animals. There were no significant differences among the angiographically determined luminal sizes at the first three determinations (baseline, open chest/pericardium, and after isolation of a segment of the LAD). There was, however, a mean 35.7 ± 5.2% reduction in luminal diameter after fixation. There was an additional 12.0 ± 4.5% diminution of measured luminal size when the pathologic specimens were compared before and after paraffin imbedding. This would completely account for the 44% difference in angiographic and pathologic assessments of the diffusely diseased and normal segments described in table 4. Although the time sequence of fixation and the use of perfusion for fixation differs from the method routinely used in humans, it seems likely that similar (or greater) fixation artifacts occur in the examination of human pathologic specimens.

Discussion

Arnett et al.[1] studied 10 patients who had undergone coronary angiography and bypass graft surgery within 69 days of their death. Although the hearts were not perfused, the pathologic specimens were quantitated in a manner similar to that used in our study. Only per-

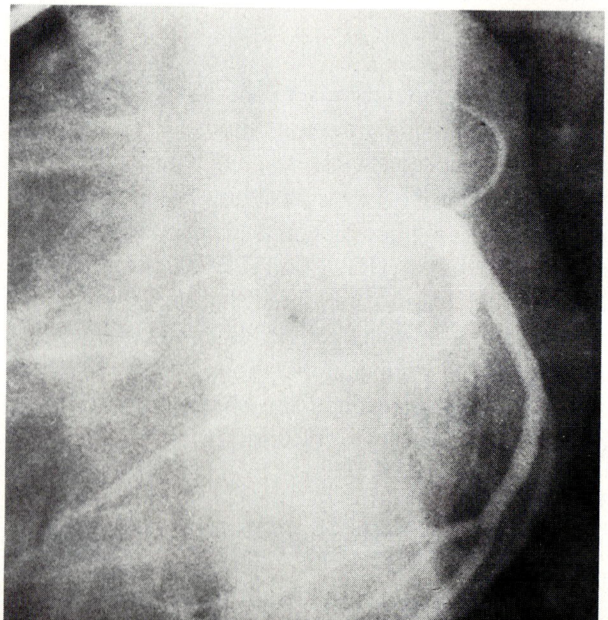

FIGURE 2. Left coronary angiogram in left anterior oblique projection showing multiple irregularities in both the left anterior descending and left circumflex coronary arteries.

TABLE 3
Luminal area and diameter of angiographically defined focal lesions

Angio diameter (mm)	Path diameter (mm)	Angio area (mm^2)	Path area (mm^2)
1.4	1.3	1.5	1.4
1.0	0.9	0.8	0.7
2.3	2.1	4.1	3.6
2.0	2.0	3.2	3.0
1.6	2.0	1.5	1.8
2.0	2.0	3.1	3.0
r = 0.91		r = 0.99	
y = 0.95x + 0.1		y = 0.86x + 0.21	

cent reductions in area or diameter were compared; residual luminal size was not. As seen in our pigs, diffuse disease was present. Arnett et al. conclude that comparing clearly abnormal segments to less but still abnormal adjacent segments does not accurately reflect the status of the artery. On the other hand, since absolute vessel size is not reported, only inaccuracies of the angiograms are discussed, and no comment as to potential errors of pathologic assessment is made.

Vladover et al.[5] reached similar conclusions after study of a comparable group of patients. Although a statement was made that some plaques may be intramural during life, no evidence was supplied to support this concept. This study also used nonperfused specimens, and eccentric luminal contours (slit-like lumen) were the major explanation offered for the observed discrepancies.

Hutchins et al.[3] demonstrated reasonable correlations between antemortem and postmortem coronary angiograms in determining site and percent stenosis of lesions. Luminal diameters or areas were not reported. They also compared postmortem angiograms and pathologic specimens. The hearts were fixed at 20 to 40 cm H_2O; the coronary arteries were not specifically perfused. The major errors in detection of lesions occurred at ostia and branch points. These authors believed that the major sources of error in the antemortem angiograms were radiographic overlap and catheter-induced arterial spasm.

To evaluate the relationship between angiographic and pathologic assessment of atherosclerosis, techniques of similar quantitative ability must be used. Our technique for angiographic evaluation is similar to that described by Gensini et al.[19] This type of evaluation allows for direct comparison of luminal size between angiograms and pathologic specimens while obviating the inaccuracies inherent in discussing percent diameter stenosis, although human pathologic specimens are not routinely perfusion fixed.

In the present study, errors in the evaluation of focal lesions occurred only at sites of bifurcation or at the coronary ostia; no other focal lesions were misinterpreted. This is in accord with the findings of Hutchins et al.[3] that the overlap of vessels makes bifurcation sites particularly difficult to interpret. Furthermore, the normal tapering of the porcine coronary ostium makes evaluation of that segment more difficult. However, pathologically proven diffuse lesions of major severity and extent were missed completely. This presumably results from the visual interpretation of stenosis in the angiogram as the difference between markedly narrowed and adjacent less narrowed sites without taking into account the absolute luminal size. In addition, there is evidence that atherosclerosis is associated with vessel dilatation, and therefore, even in diffusely diseased arteries the lumen may appear angiographically normal.[20]

Our data demonstrate that at sites of focal narrowing, there is excellent agreement between the luminal size determined angiographically and that observed pathologically. This finding validates coronary angiography as a measure of clinical disease in humans, in whom hemodynamically significant disease is often segmental in nature.

In contrast, there was considerable discrepancy between angiographic and pathologic assessment of segments that were read as either normal or mildly diseased angiographically. This discrepancy was uniformly in the direction of smaller luminal size as assesed pathologically. In a study of left main coronary

TABLE 4
Luminal diameter and area of sites defined angiographically as normal or irregular

Angio diameter (mm)	Path diameter (mm)	Angio area (mm^2)	Path area (mm^2)
Diseased vessels			
2.4	1.6	4.5	2.0
2.7	1.6	5.7	2.1
3.0	1.2	7.1	1.1
2.2	0.6	3.8	0.3
2.0	1.1	3.1	0.9
Normal vessels			
4.2	2.3	13.9	4.2
2.1	1.4	3.5	1.5
3.2	2.3	8.3	4.3
4.0	2.3	12.6	4.1
p < .001		p < .001	
y = 0.6x − 0.14		y = 0.33x + 0.005	

artery disease, Isner et al.[21] found a discrepancy between angiographic and morphologic results in 71% of cases. Underestimation by angiography was found chiefly in markedly narrowed segments, whereas overestimation was found in the less narrowed segments.

Zarins et al.[22] demonstrated a 20% to 31% reduction in luminal diameter when antemortem femoral and aortic angiograms were compared with pathologic specimens.[22] The major shrinkage occurred with fixation (22%), with an additional 11% decrease related to paraffin processing. Similarly, Bahr et al.[23] showed 30% to 40% reduction in aortic size related to the preparation of pathologic specimens. The coronary vessels, however, may react differently than the large muscular arteries.

Siegel et al.[24] studied 12 human, nonperfused hearts. In vessels with minimal disease there was a 35% reduction in luminal area, the majority of which was related to paraffin processing, not fixation (25% vs 10%). There was only 7.7% total shrinkage in vessels that were moderately to severely diseased, suggesting that more severely diseased segments of the coronary arteries react less to fixation and processing.

Our data in normal animals demonstrate a 44% reduction in luminal size with perfusion fixation and processing. The major change resulted from the fixation process in these vessels. The difference between our data and Siegel's may be related to use of perfusion fixation rather than immersion as well as to the fact that our initial measurements were made antemortem. In our diseased animals, focal lesions did not show this reduction in measurement as a result of fixation and processing, suggesting that because of extensive fibrosis and calcification these areas could no longer react to the fixation process.

We believe that angiography more accurately reflects luminal caliber in vivo than does pathologic examination and that the decrease in the size of the lumen in the histologic section is due to processing artifact. It is likely that focal lesions are less capable of reacting to the fixation and embedding process.

References

1. Arnett EN, Isner JM, Redwood DR, Kent KM, Baker WP, Ackerstein H, Roberts WC: Coronary artery norrowing in coronary heart disease: comparison of cineangiographic and necropsy findings. Ann Intern Med **91:** 350, 1979
2. Schwartz JN, Kong Y, Hackel DB, Bartel AG: Comparison of angiographic and postmortem findings in patients with coronary artery disease. Am J Cardiol **36:** 174, 1975
3. Hutchins GM, Bulkley BH, Ridolfi RL, Griffith LSC, Lohr FT, Piasio MA: Correlation of coronary arteriograms and left ventriculograms with post mortem studies. Circulation **30:** 654, 1974
4. Kemp HG, Evans H, Elliot WC, Gorlin R: Diagnostic accuracy of selective coronary cineangiography. Circulation **36:** 526, 1967
5. Vlodaver Z, Frech R, Van Tassel RA, Edwards JE: Correlation of the antemortem coronary angiogram and the postmortem specimen. Circulation **47:** 162, 1973
6. Grondin CM, Dyrda I, Pasternac A, Campeau L, Bourassa MC, Lesperance J: Discrepancies between cineangiographic and postmortem findings in patients with coronary artery disease and recent myocardial revascularization. Circulation **49:** 703, 1974
7. Marcus ML, Armstrong ML, Heistad DO, Eastman CL, Mark AL: Comparison of three methods of evaluating coronary obstructive lesions: postmortem arteriography, pathologic examination and measurement of regional myocardial perfusion during maximal vasodilatation. Am J Cardiol **49:** 1699, 1982
8. Wissler RW, Vesselinovitch D: Evaluation of animal models for the study of the pathogenesis of atherosclerosis. *In* Hauss WH, Wissler RW, Lehmann R, editors: International Symposium–State of Prevention and Therapy in Human Arteriosclerosis in Animal Models. Opladen, Germany, 1978, Westdeutscher Verlag, p 13
9. French JE, Jennings MA, Florey HW: Morphologic studies on atherosclerosis in swine. Ann NY Acad Sci **127:** 780, 1963
10. Rowsell HC, Mustard JF, Downie HG: Experimental atherosclerosis in swine. Ann NY Acad Sci **127:** 743, 1965
11. Goldsmith DPJ, Jacob HP: Atherogenesis in swine fed several types of lipid-cholesterol diets. Lipids **13:** 174, 1977
12. Lee KT, Lee WM: Advanced coronary atherosclerosis in swine produced by combination of balloon-catheter injury and cholesterol feeding. Adv Exp Biol Med **82:** 597, 1977
13. Lee KT, Jarmolych J, Kim DM, Grant C, Krasney JA, Thomas WA, Bruno AM: Production of advanced coronary atherosclerosis, myocardial infarction and "sudden death" in swine. Exp Mol Pathol **15:** 170, 1971
14. Bonzert TJ, Brewer HB Jr: New micro method for measuring cholesterol in plasma lipoprotein fractions. Clin Chem **23:** 2089, 1977
15. Clark JM, Glago VS: Luminal surface of distended arteries by scanning electron microscopy: Eliminating configurational and technical artifact. Br J Exp Pathol **57:** 129, 1976
16. Hirsch EZ, Chisolm GM III, Gibbons A: Quantitative assessment of changes in aortic dimensions in response to in situ perfusion fixation at physiologic pressures. Atherosclerosis **38:** 63, 1981
17. Mahley, RW: Cholesterol Feeding: Effects on lipoprotein structure and metabolism. In Gotto AM Jr, Smith LC, Allen B editors: Atherosclerosis V. New York, 1980, Springer-Verlag, p 641
18. Mahley RW, Weisgraber KH, Inmerarity T, Brewer HB Jr. Assman GA: Swine lipoproteins and atherosclerosis. Changes in the plasma lipoproteins and apoproteins induced by cholesterol feeding. Biochemistry **14:** 2817, 1975
19. Gensini GG, Kelly AE, Da Costa BCB, Huntington PP: Quantitative angiography: The measurement of coronary vasomobility in the intact animal and man. Chest **60:** 522, 1971
20. Bond MG, Sawyer JK, Bullock WC, Barnes RW, Ball MR: Animal studies of atherosclerosis progression and regression. *In* Bond MG, Insull W, Glagov S, Chandler AB, Cornhill JF, editors: Clinical diagnosis of atherosclerosis: quantitative methods of evaluation. New York, 1983, Springer-Verlag, pp 435-449
21. Isner JM, Kishel J, Kent KM, Ronan JA, Ross AM, Roberts WC: Accuracy of angiographic determination of left main coronary arterial narrowing. Circulation **63:** 1056, 1981
22. Zarins CK, Zatina MA, Glagov S: Correlation of postmortem angiography with pathologic anatomy: quantitation of atherosclerotic lesions. *In* Bond MG, Insull W, Glagov S, Chandler AB, Cornhill JF, editors: Clinical diagnosis of atherosclerosis: quantitative methods of evaluation. New York, 1983, Springer-Verlag, pp 283-302
23. Bahr GF, Bloom G, Friberg U: Volume changes of tissues in physiological fluids during fixation in osmium tetroxide or formaldehyde and during subsequent treatment. Exp Cell Res **12:** 342, 1957
24. Siegel RJ, Swan K, Edwalds G, Fishbein HC: Limitations of postmortem assessment of human coronary artery size and luminal narrowing: differential effects of tissue fixation and processing on vessels with different degrees of atherosclerosis. J Am Coll Cardiol, 1985

Uptake of hematoporphyrin derivative by valvular vegetations in experimental infective endocarditis

ARTUR M. SPOKOJNY, M.D., I. NIGEL SINCLAIR, M.B., STUART SCHNITT, M.D., SVEN PAULIN, M.D., AND J. RICHARD SPEARS, M.D.

ABSTRACT Drugs that localize in valvular vegetations may be useful in the diagnosis and treatment of infective endocarditis. We therefore tested the hypothesis that parenterally injected hematoporphyrin derivative (HPD), which is concentrated in tumors and atherosclerotic plaques, localizes in the vegetations of experimental infective endocarditis. In 14 rabbits, various bacteria were given intra-arterially immediately after injury to the aortic valve. In 12 additional rabbits, sterile vegetations on the aortic valve were produced by the trauma caused by an indwelling catheter that had been in place over a long period. HPD, 2.5 mg/kg, was injected intravenously 1 to 2 days before the animals were killed in six rabbits with sterile vegetations and in seven rabbits with infected vegetations. In all rabbits, multiple vegetations on the aortic valve leaflets were identified. On exposure to ultraviolet light, strong porphyrin fluorescence of all vegetations, whether sterile or infected, was observed only in rabbits given HPD. In two rabbits given HPD 10 weeks after catheter implantation across the aortic valve, however, only mild fluorescence could be detected in healing endocardial vegetations. In frozen sections of HPD-laden lesions, a patchy distribution of fluorescence was observed that was similar to the pattern of HPD localization in atheromatous plaques. Since vegetations in experimental infective endocarditis selectively concentrate HPD, porphyrins could be useful in the diagnosis and treatment of infective endocarditis.

Circulation **72, No. 5, 1087–1091, 1985.**

THE MORTALITY and morbidity from infective endocarditis are still significant. Classic symptoms and objective signs of infective endocarditis are often lacking, and the initial clinical management of patients with this disease is often empirical, particularly when the results of blood cultures are either pending or negative.[1] Therefore, it is important to investigate new techniques that may improve the diagnosis and treatment of infective endocarditis. Parenterally injected porphyrins have long been known to localize preferentially in certain pathologic lesions, including malignant neoplasms and mechanically injured tissues.[2] The characteristic fluorescence of hematoporphyrin derivative (HPD) on exposure to ultraviolet light has been used to detect occult neoplasms.[3] In addition, photodynamic therapy for tumors, consisting of light-activation of HPD with resultant local release of cytotoxic singlet oxygen,[4,5] has recently been introduced clinically as a new therapeutic modality.[6]

Recent studies have shown that atheromatous plaques in rabbits and humans selectively (as compared with the normal arterial wall) concentrate HPD,[7] and that mechanical injury to the endothelial lining results in uptake of HPD by the arterial wall.[8] Furthermore, the uptake of HPD by several species of bacteria has been demonstrated, and on exposure to light a bactericidal effect of about 99.5% could be achieved.[9]

Valvular vegetations, which characterize infective endocarditis, usually further traumatize valves that have previously suffered a variety of injuries.[10,11] If valvular vegetations selectively concentrate HPD, in addition to the known uptake of HPD by bacteria, improvement in methods of diagnosis by the use of labeled HPD might be achieved and photodynamic therapy of vegetations might be possible. We therefore tested the hypothesis that sterile and infected vegeta-

From the Charles A. Dana Research Institute and the Harvard-Thorndike Laboratory of Beth Israel Hospital, and Department of Medicine, Cardiovascular Division, Department of Pathology, and the Radiology Research Center of the Department of Radiology, Harvard Medical School, Boston.

Supported in part by NHLBI grant R01-HL33252-01.

Address for correspondence: J. Richard Spears, M.D., Cardiovascular Division, Beth Israel Hospital, 330 Brookline Ave., Boston, MA 02215.

Received Feb. 12, 1985; revision accepted Aug. 8, 1985.

Dr. Spokojny was the recipient of a fellowship grant from the Max-Kade Foundation, New York. Dr. Sinclair was a recipient of the Saw Medical Research Fellowship of the University of Western Australia.

Parts of this study were presented at the 57th meeting of the American Heart Association in Miami Beach, November 1984.

tions in a commonly used experimental preparation of infective endocarditis will, compared with the uninjured valve, selectively concentrate HPD after parenteral injection of this material.

Methods

Sterile vegetations. The experimental preparation chosen was similar to that described by Garrison and Freedman,[12] which has been widely used in recent studies for determining the efficacy of various antibiotics in the treatment of endocarditis.[13, 14] Under ketamine and diazepam anesthesia, a longitudinal cutdown in the neck was performed in 14 New Zealand White male rabbits. Polyethylene 90 tubing was advanced under fluoroscopy via the carotid artery across the aortic valve over a guidewire, and the latter was removed. The catheter was filled with contrast medium to visualize and document the position of the tip, and the catheter was then fixed in position. Four to six days later in six rabbits, and 10 weeks later in two rabbits, HPD (Photofrin II, donated by Photofrin Medical, Cheektowoga, NY) was injected in doses of 2.5 mg/kg body weight iv. One day later, all 14 rabbits were killed and their hearts and aortic valves were examined.

Infected vegetations. In 14 other rabbits, a cutdown was performed as described above. Under fluoroscopic control, via the carotid artery, a 0.38 inch flexible guidewire was repeatedly advanced across the aortic valve to mechanically injure the valve. Immediately after injury, 1 ml of a Tryp-Soybroth (Scott, Inc., Fawkesville, RI) suspension containing bacteria in various concentrations was injected intra-arterially. Each type of bacteria was obtained from positive blood cultures of patients with known infective endocarditis. Eight animals were injected with *Staphylococcus aureus* in concentrations of 10^4/ml (n = 3), 10^6/ml (n = 3), or 10^8/ml (n = 2). Six animals were inoculated with *Streptococcus viridans*, 10^7/ml (n = 4) and 10^8/ml (n = 2), and in four animals either 10^7/ml (n = 2) or 10^8/ml (n = 2) of β-hemolytic *Streptococcus* was injected. Since the number of the days of survival correlated well with the concentration of bacteria injected, 2.5 mg/kg iv HPD was injected 1 day before expected death or sacrifice.

The heart and the aortic valves containing infected and sterile vegetations were exposed to ultraviolet light from a Wood's lamp to detect HPD fluorescence. Aortic valves and vegetations from four rabbits with sterile vegetations and four rabbits with infected vegetations were stained with hematoxylin-eosin, formalin fixed, and embedded in paraffin. Tissue from three HPD-injected rabbits with sterile and two with infected (n = 2) vegetations was removed immediately after the animals were killed and fluorescence microscopic examination of frozen sections of the aortic valve and vegetations was performed.

Results

Sterile vegetations up to 4 mm in size appeared whitish and were usually identified on the aortic surface of the aortic valve. Fluorescence was detected upon exposure to ultraviolet light only in rabbits given HPD (figure 1). In the two rabbits in which the catheter had been in place for over 10 weeks, vegetations (1 mm) were detected, but only mild fluorescence was observed. Interestingly, weak fluorescence was also noted in traumatized valvular and myocardial tissues adjacent to the vegetations, although no gross abnormalities were apparent in those tissues under ordinary white light. Furthermore, myocardial injury due to infection (abscess) showed strong porphyrin fluorescence with clear demarcation from normal tissue.

Infected vegetations. In rabbits with infective endocarditis, the size of the vegetations varied with the species and concentration of the bacteria injected. Animals injected with 10^8/ml *S. aureus* died after 2 days with only minimal vegetations, while 10^6/ml *S. aureus* produced large vegetations (1 to 2 mm in size) that fluoresced only after prior injection of HPD. Rabbits injected with *S. viridans* either died or were killed 6 days after injection, and at necropsy were noted to have 2 to 3 cm long, 4 to 5 mm wide vegetations that frequently obstructed the aortic root. Similar findings were noted in rabbits infected with β-hemolytic *Streptococcus;* these animals were also killed or died 6 days after injection of bacteria.

Light microscopy. On hematoxylin-eosin stained sections, the vegetations were composed predominantly of fibrin, with occasional admixed platelets, leukocytes, and erythrocytes. In some areas, the endocardium immediately adjacent to the vegetations showed fibroblastic proliferation and neovascularity that focally extended into the base of the vegetations, consistent with early organization. Vegetations in rabbits with infective endocarditis appeared histologically similar to sterile vegetations, except for the presence of bacteria, as determined by Gram's stain, and a large number of leukocytes. No difference in the histology of vegetations from HPD-injected and control rabbits was found. These findings are identical to those previously described for this preparation of infective endocarditis.[12]

Fluorescence microscopy. The microscopic pattern of fluorescence consisted of small patches within the vegetation and the adjacent injured aortic valve. No difference in fluorescence between injected and sterile vegetations was observed.

Discussion

The effectiveness of antimicrobial therapy in valvular endocarditis has been studied by many investigators in a reproducible preparation of this disease in rabbits.[12] Valvular injury is produced by a polyethylene catheter inserted into either ventricle via a jugular vein or carotid artery. The presence of the catheter in the right or left side of the heart provokes rapid deposition of fibrin-platelet vegetations on traumatized valves and endocardium.[12–14] These sterile vegetations may then be infected by inoculation with microorganisms. Pathologically, the infected vegetations are remarkably similar to those found in man and consist of a

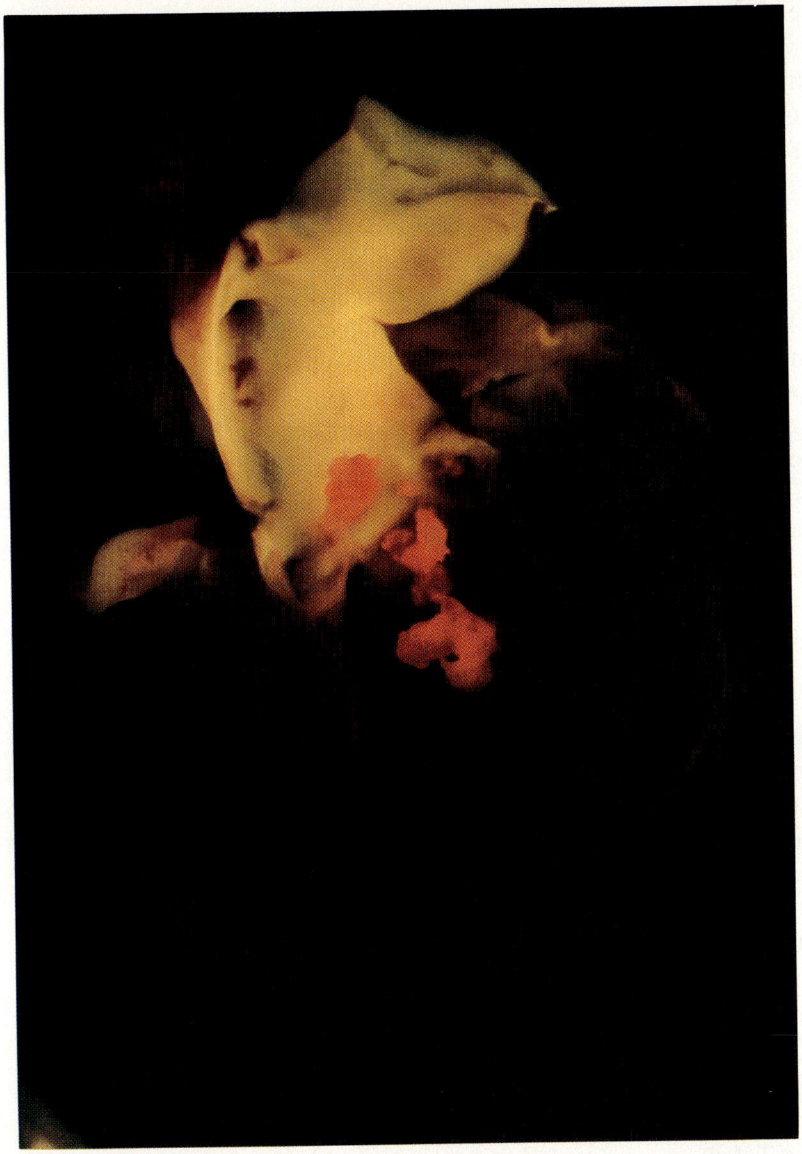

FIGURE 1. Upon exposure to ultraviolet light, only fresh vegetations in rabbits given HPD show intense fluorescence.

relatively amorphous mass of fibrin, platelets, platelet debris, occasional leukocytes, and bacteria.[13, 14] Using a similar rabbit preparation, we found the same histopathology previously described.[12] Furthermore, we were able to produce infective endocarditis without the use of an indwelling catheter. Our findings confirm the hypothesis that HPD is selectively concentrated in sterile and infected vegetations, as compared with uninjured valve tissue, in an experimental preparation of infective endocarditis. To our knowledge, this observation has not been previously reported. The similarity of the pathology of valvular vegetations in the rabbit to the pathology of those in man makes it likely that human vegetations will also selectively concentrate HPD.

Since the exact mechanism and cellular site of HPD uptake by tumors and atheromatous plaques still remains to be elucidated, it is beyond the scope of this study to define the mechanism and site of HPD uptake by endocardial vegetations. It should be noted, however, that fluorescence microscopic examination of frozen sections of neoplastic and atherosclerotic tissues show patterns of HPD uptake similar to those in valvular vegetations, thereby suggesting analogous mechanisms.[8] Recent evidence from our laboratory suggests that increased endothelial permeability of atheromatous plaques[15–20] may be an important factor in the localization of HPD within this tissue,* and endocardial vegetations that consist primarily of a fibrin-platelet mesh lack the endothelial barrier of normal valves. In addition, a variety of porphyrins, including hematoporphyrin, have been shown to have an affinity for fibrinogen and platelets,[21, 22] and fibrin matrixes are known to selectively concentrate HPD.[23]

*Spokojny A, et al: Unpublished observations.

The diagnosis and treatment of infective endocarditis is often difficult, especially in subacute and chronic cases in which symptoms and signs are subtle or lacking.[1] Gallium-64 scintillation scanning results in a high incidence of false-negative results because of poor spatial resolution and is, therefore, unreliable in the diagnosis of infective endocarditis.[24, 25] The usefulness of echocardiography is often limited by the small size of most vegetations and is unreliable in the diagnosis of prosthetic valve endocarditis.[1] Hence, labeled porphyrins might be useful in the diagnosis of endocardial vegetations. However, the use of radiolabeled porphyrins might be limited by the inadequate spatial resolution inherent in radionuclear scintigraphy. Porphyrin labeling with paramagnetic metals such as Mn^{++} could be helpful in the noninvasive diagnosis of endocardial vegetations,[26–28] since nuclear magnetic resonance scanning with electrocardiographic gating may potentially provide sufficient spatial resolution to image vegetations 1 to 2 mm in size.

It should be noted, however, that in patients with atherosclerotic disease of the ascending aorta, identification of vegetations may be difficult, since atherosclerotic lesions probably would also take up HPD. To evaluate the specificity of HPD uptake in acute infective endocarditis vs that in areas of degeneration and fibrotic thickening of the valve, we examined the HPD uptake in rabbits in which an indwelling catheter was in place over a period of 10 weeks. The natural history of these noninfected vegetations is that they regress in size over period of time and endothelialize.[29] Hence, despite previous injury to the valve and presence of a catheter, less fluorescence, when viewed with a Wood's lamp, was observed compared with that in rabbits with fresh lesions. These findings suggest a quantitative difference in HPD uptake by fresh vs older lesions. Further studies are necessary to quantitate HPD uptake. If endothelial permeability or rapid proliferation are substantial for HPD uptake, it is not surprising that freshly grown lesions localize larger amounts of HPD.

Photodynamic therapy with HPD might be of potential use in the treatment of infective endocarditis for several reasons. It has been shown that this substance binds to cellular components of several aerobic and anaerobic microorganisms, including *S. aureus*, several strains of streptococci and *Clostridium perfringens*.[9] Upon light activation, HPD was 99.9% bactericidal for gram-positive strains. Combinations of light-activated HPD and polymorphonuclear leukocytes had a 99.99% bactericidal effect on both intracellular and extracellular *S. aureus*.[9] Hence, photodynamic sterilization of infected valves and myocardium might be possible with HPD by application of light, either with a fiberoptic system during cardiac catheterization or directly during open heart surgery.

In addition, since vegetations concentrate HPD, irrespective of the presence of bacteria, photodynamic treatment might reduce the integrity of the fibrin-platelet matrix barrier of the vegetation, which in turn would amplify the effect of antibiotic treatment, especially in infective endocarditis with gram-negative rods, which are not susceptible to HPD photodynamic therapy. However, potential HPD photoactivation within valvular vegetations might be limited by various factors. Hypoxia, if present within the vegetation, would reduce the photodynamic response, which requires generation of singlet oxygen.[4, 5] In addition, vascular reactions may play an important role in HPD-mediated photodynamic tissue reactions,[6] and avascular portions of vegetations would not be amenable to therapy by this mechanism. Furthermore, even if a photodynamic response could be elicited, sloughing of necrotic debris might occur after treatment and would lead to peripheral embolization.

Although the potential utility of HPD in the clinical management of endocarditis is uncertain, our observation that vegetations in experimental infective endocarditis selectively (compared with normal adjacent tissue) concentrate HPD suggests that the use of HPD in the management of infective endocarditis merits further study.

We thankfully acknowledge the expert and technical assistance of Deborah L. Mattson and the typing of Carol Anne Centauro.

References

1. Weinstein L: Infective endocarditis. *In* Braunwald E, editor: Heart disease. A textbook of cardiovascular medicine. Philadelphia, 1984, WB Saunder, p 1136
2. Figge FHJ, Weiland GS, Morganiello LOJ: Cancer detection and therapy: affinity of neoplastic, embryonic, and traumatized tissues for porphyrins and metalloporphyrins. Proc Soc Exp Biol Med **68:** 640, 1948
3. Lipson RI, Baldes EJ, Olsen AM: The use of a derivative of hematoporphyrin in tumor detection. J Natl Center Inst **26:** 1, 1961
4. Weishaupt KR, Gomer CJ, Dougherty TJ: Identification of singlet oxygen as the cytotoxic agent in photo-inactivation of a murine tumor. Cancer Res **36:** 2326, 1976
5. Fowlks WL: The mechanism of the photodynamic effect. J Clin Invest **32:** 233, 1976
6. Dougherty TJ, Kaufman JE, Goldfarb A, Weishaupt KR, Mittleman A: Photoradiation therapy for the treatment of malignant tumors. Cancer Res **38:** 26, 1978
7. Spears JR, Serur J, Shropshire D, Paulin S: Fluorescence of experimental atheromatous plaques within hematoporphyrin derivative. J Clin Invest **71:** 395, 1983
8. Spokojny AM, Serur J, Paulin S, Spears JR: Selective uptake of hematoporphyrin derivative by human atheromatous plaque in vitro. J Am Coll Cardiol (in press)
9. Venezio FR, DiVincenzo C, Sherman R, Reichman M, Origitano

TC, Thompson K, Reichmann OH: Bactericidal effects of photoradiation therapy with hematoporphyrin derivative. J Infect Dis **151:** 166, 1985
10. Lepeschkin E: On the relation between the site of valvular involvement in endocarditis and the blood pressure resting on the valve. Am J Med Sci **124:** 318, 1952
11. Robard S: Blood velocity and endocarditis. Circulation **22:** 18, 1963
12. Garrison PK, Freedman LR: Experimental Endocarditis: I. Staphylococcal endocarditis in rabbits resulting from placement of a polyethylene catheter in the right side of the heart. Yale J Biol Med **42:** 394, 1970
13. Durack DT, Beeson PB: Experimental bacterial endocarditis. I. Colonization of a sterile vegetation. Br J Exp Pathol **53:** 44, 1972
14. Wright AJ, Wilson WR: Experimental animal endocarditis. Mayo Clin Proc **57:** 10, 1982
15. Friedman M, Byers SO: Endothelial permeability in atherosclerosis. Arch Pathol **76:** 99, 1963
16. Adams CWM, Bayliss OB, Orton CC: Plasma-protein accumulation in arterial degeneration. J Atheroscler Res **7:** 473, 1967
17. Zilversmit DB: Cholesterol Flux in the atherosclerotic plaque. Ann Ny Acad Sci **149:** 710, 1968
18. Veress B, Balint A, Kocze A, Nagy Z, Jellinek H: Increasing aortic permeability by atherogenic diet. Atherosclerosis **11:** 369, 1970
19. Bylock A, Bjorkernd S, Brattsand R, Hansson GK, Hansson H-A, Bondjero G: Endothelial structure in rabbits with moderate hypercholesterolemia. Acta Pathol Microbiol Scand (Sect A) **85:** 67, 1977
20. Ross R, Glomset JA: The pathogenesis of atherosclerosis. N Engl J Med **295:** 369, 1976
21. Zieve PD, Solomon HM: Effect of photodynamic action on human platelets. Fed Proc **24:** 519, 1965
22. Zieve PD, Solomon HM: Effect of hematoporphyrin and light on human fibrinogen. Am J Physiol **210:** 1391, 1966
23. Mussar DA, Sayne JM, Weber FJ, Dalta-Gupta N: The effect of tumor localizing porphyrins on the conversion of fibrinogen to fibrin. Res Commun Chem Pathol Pharmacol **26:** 357, 1979
24. Wiseman J, Rouleau J, Rijo P, Stauss HW, Pitt B: Gallium-67, myocardial imaging for the detection of bacterial endocarditis. Radiology **120:** 135, 1976
25. Miller MH, Casery JI: Infective endocarditis: new diagnostic techniques. Am Heart J **96:** 123, 1978
26. LaMar GN, Viscio DB, Smith VM, Caighey WS, Smith RL: NMR studies of low spin ferric complexes of natural porphyrin derivatives. I. Effect of peripheral substitutes on the electronic asymmetric in Byscyano complexes. J Am Chem Soc **100:** 8085, 1978
27. Chen CW, Cohen JS, Myers CE, Sohn M: Paramagnetic metalloporphyrins as potential contrast agents in NMR imaging. FEBS Lett **168:** 70, 1984
28. Sohn M, Roberts MF, Spokojny AM, Sinclair IN, Muldahy J, Fossel ET, Serur JR, Davis M, Adams DF, Spears JR: Metalloporphyrins: MRI-contrast agents for atherosclerotic vascular disease. Fourth Annual Meeting of the Society for Magnetic Research in Medicine, London, August 1985, Abstract vol II, p 902
29. Carrisoza J, Kaye D, Kobasa W: Experimental streptococcal endocarditis. Arch Pathol Lab Med **102:** 58, 1978

Cesium chloride–induced long QT syndrome: demonstration of afterdepolarizations and triggered activity in vivo

JOSEPH H. LEVINE, M.D., JOSEPH F. SPEAR, PH.D., THOMAS GUARNIERI, M.D., MYRON L. WEISFELDT, M.D., CEES D.J. DE LANGEN, PH.D., LEWIS C. BECKER, M.D., AND E. NEIL MOORE, D.V.M., PH.D.

ABSTRACT The identification of afterdepolarizations and their relationship to arrhythmias in vivo is not available. Experiments were undertaken to determine whether afterdepolarizations could be detected in monophasic action potentials (MAPs) recorded in vivo and whether they were related to arrhythmias in an intact canine preparation of the long QT syndrome. Isolated cardiac tissues from six dogs were studied to validate the technique. In simultaneous MAP and transmembrane recordings, afterdepolarizations induced with barium (early) or acetylstrophanthidin (delayed) were detected in MAPs when present in microelectrode recordings. MAPs were then recorded in situ in eight dogs with cesium chloride–induced long QT syndrome associated with ventricular arrhythmias. Afterdepolarizations were identified in each of the dogs and were similar to early afterdepolarizations identified in vitro; they occurred during phase 3 and were attenuated during overdrive pacing. The afterdepolarizations were closely related to arrhythmias: (1) afterdepolarizations always preceded ventricular arrhythmias, (2) the coupling intervals (CI) of the afterdepolarizations (AD) and the ventricular premature beats (VPB) were nearly identical (VPB CI = 1.06 AD CI − 10.24; r^2 = .87), (3) the take-off potentials of the ventricular premature beats were nearly identical to the amplitude of the afterdepolarizations (take-off potential = 0.98 afterdepolarization amplitude + 0.46, r^2 = .87), and (4) afterdepolarizations and ventricular arrhythmias resolved concurrently during overdrive pacing and with time. Thus, a new catheter technique has been validated and has been used to directly identify afterdepolarizations and triggered activity in vivo.

Circulation 72, No. 5, 1092–1103, 1985.

CURRENT electrophysiologic techniques do not allow for the unequivocal identification of arrhythmia mechanisms in vivo. The characteristic response of an arrhythmia to pacing has been used to differentiate reentrant rhythms from enhanced automaticity; however, direct proof of a reentrant mechanism in vivo is available only in the case of reciprocating tachycardia using an accessory pathway.[1] At present no technique is available to distinguish triggered activity from other arrhythmic mechanisms.[2] Although there have been reports of rhythm disturbances that fulfill the criteria for triggered activity,[3–5] conclusive identification of afterdepolarizations or their relationship to atrial or ventricular arrhythmias in vivo is not available. The mechanisms of the tachyarrhythmias associated with a prolonged QT is one example. That programmed electrical stimulation does not lead to reproducibly inducible tachycardia suggests that the arrhythmias may not be due to reentry.[6] Recent data obtained in vitro indicates that the ventricular ectopic activity that develops in this situation may be a result of triggered activity. Early afterdepolarizations and triggered activity have been identified in isolated canine ventricular muscle and Purkinje fibers after exposure to agents or conditions known to cause ventricular tachyarrhythmias, torsade de pointes, and a long QT interval in animal preparations.[7, 8] However, the conclusive identification of afterdepolarizations and triggered activity in vivo in this or other settings is not available.

Monophasic action potentials (MAPs) can be re-

From the Department of Physiology, The School of Veterinary Medicine, The University of Pennsylvania, Philadelphia, and the Peter Belfer Laboratories for Myocardial Research and The Divison of Cardiology, The Johns Hopkins Medical Institutions, Baltimore.

Supported by grants from the National Institutes of Health (HL–28393, HL–25213, HL–33593, HL–07220–08) and the W. W. Smith Charitable Trust.

Address for correspondence: Joseph H. Levine, M.D., Division of Cardiology, Carnegie 568, The Johns Hopkins Hospital, 600 N. Wolfe St., Baltimore, MD. 21205.

Received April 2, 1985; revision accepted Aug. 8, 1985.

Dr. de Langen is a receipient of a NATO fellowship granted by The Dutch Organization for the Advancement of Pure Scientific Research.

corded in situ from the beating canine left ventricle with a contact or suction electrode.[9–12] The time course of repolarization of MAPs has been shown to correlate closely with that of simultaneous transmembrane action potentials under a variety of conditions.[9, 13] MAPs arise as a result of passive current flow from electrically coupled adjacent normal tissue into a region of injury caused by the contact or suction electrode and vary according to the voltage gradient.[9] Depolarization of the MAP is thought to be due to a change in this gradient during the depolarization of adjacent cells. It follows that any reduction in this gradient would lead to apparent depolarization of the MAP and therefore the MAP should also be able to be used to detect membrane phenomena such as afterdepolarizations.

The present article describes a series of studies designed to document afterdepolarizations and triggered activity in vivo. The detection of afterdepolarizations in MAPs was first validated in vitro and the characteristics of the MAPs and afterdepolarizations that developed after the administration of cesium chloride were then determined in a canine preparation with a prolonged QT interval and torsade de pointes. The behavior of the afterdepolarizations and ventricular ectopic activity was compared during ventricular pacing to provide additional evidence of triggered activity in vivo.

Methods

Experiments in vitro. To validate that afterdepolarizations can be detected in MAPs experiments were performed on tissues removed from six adult mongrel dogs weighing between 8 and 16 kg. The animals were anesthetized with intravenous sodium pentobarbital (30 mg/kg), their chests were opened via a left lateral thoracotomy, and their hearts were removed. Endocardial or epicardial tissue samples 1 to 2 mm thick, 2 cm wide, and 2 to 3 cm long were removed and placed in a 100 ml tissue bath filled with oxygenated Tyrode's solution (standard unless otherwise stated). The methods used have been described previously.[14] The tissues were paced at a basic cyle length of 1000 msec with a bipolar stimulating electrode consisting of two Teflon-coated silver wires positioned at one end of the tissue. Constant-current square-wave pulses of 2 msec duration and twice diastolic threshold intensity were used.

MAP and transmembrane potential recordings. MAPs were recorded with a silver–silver chloride electrode.[12] The distal tip (1 mm in diameter) was used as the recording electrode and a distal bath ground was used as the reference electrode.

In addition, with the use of standard 3M potassium-filled microelectrodes, transmembrane action potentials were recorded from Purkinje fibers or superficial muscle cell layers within 4 mm of the contact electrode. Both MAP and microelectrode recordings were displayed on a memory oscilloscope (Tektronix) and recorded on an electrostatic paper recorder (Gould) at paper speeds of 25 to 250 mm/sec.

Afterdepolarization experiments. In tissues from three animals, early afterdepolarizations were induced with 10^{-7}M barium chloride in standard Tyrode's solution. Epicardial tissue preparations were used to ensure homogeneity of local repolarization in the baseline state. Simultaneous MAP and transmembrane recordings were made. A stable MAP and a continuous, stable microelectrode impalement were required for the data to be accepted.

Delayed afterdepolarizations were induced with acetylstrophanthidin (5 x 10^{-8} g/liter) in endocardial tissues taken from the left ventricles of three different animals. For these experiments, the Tyrode solution was altered: The concentration of K^+ was increased to 4 meq/liter and that of Ca^{++} to 2.5 meq/liter. The contact electrode was placed either over free-running Purkinje fibers or muscle. Transmembrane recordings were also made from Purkinje or muscle cells.

Once afterdepolarizations were induced with acetylstrophanthidin, the tissues were paced at the following cycle lengths: 1000, 800, 600, 500, 400, and 300 msec. The changes induced by pacing in the MAP and transmembrane recordings were compared. Specifically, amplitude changes of the afterdepolarizations and coupling intervals were determined in each case for both recording methods. Afterdepolarization amplitude was defined as the difference in voltage between the peak amplitude and the most negative membrane voltage noted preceding their onset. Afterdepolarization coupling interval was defined as the time from the onset of the action potential to the time of peak amplitude. Amplitude and coupling interval were measured to the nearest millivolt and 5 msec with a Hewlett-Packard 9825A computer and 9864 manual digitizer.

Experiments in vivo. Experiments were performed on eight mongrel dogs of both sexes that ranged in weight from 10 to 24 kg. Animals were anesthetized with pentobarbital (30 mg/kg) and ventilated with room air with the use of a constant-volume ventilator. Catheters were placed in the jugular or femoral vein for infusion of drugs. After a median sternotomy, the pericardium was opened and the heart exposed.

Bipolar pacing leads consisting of two Teflon-coated silver wires exposed at the tip were placed in the right atrial appendage and in the left and right ventricle. Pacing was performed at twice diastolic threshold with a programmed stimulator and a constant-current source (Bloom). MAPs were recorded from the left ventricular epicardium in all eight animals and were simultaneously recorded from the left ventricular endocardium and epicardium in four animals. A bipolar catheter consisting of a silver–silver chloride distal electrode and a reference lead 5 mm away was advanced into the left ventricular cavity via the left carotid artery and positioned against the anterior-apical endocardial surface.[12] Epicardial recordings were obtained from the left anterior ventricular surface by a similar catheter arrangement modified to allow for stable recordings from the beating heart in situ.[15] The MAP signals were amplified and filtered at a frequency of 0.1 to 10 kHz. The surface electrocardiographic lead, amplified MAP signals, and left and right ventricular local bipolar electrograms were simultaneously displayed on an oscilloscope (Tektronix) and recorded on an electrostatic paper recorder (Gould). After this preparation was completed, baseline recordings were obtained sequentially from five to 10 epicardial sites at the sinus heart rate and during pacing at several other more rapid rates. The duration, amplitude, and morphology of the MAPs were noted and the absence of afterdepolarizations was verified. The epicardial probe was then placed in a position that allowed for long-term stable recording from the left ventricular surface.

Cesium chloride (1 mM/kg) was administered as an intravenous bolus over 15 sec via a central venous catheter positioned in the femoral or jugular vein. When either a prolonged QT interval, afterdepolarizations in the MAP, or ventricular ectopic activity developed and reached a steady state, atrial and ventricular pacing was performed at several cycle lengths that were shorter than the sinus cycle length. The behavior of the ventricular ectopic activity and changes in the MAP after 8 to 10 paced beats were analyzed.

Phases 0 to 4 of the MAP were defined in the same way as the phases of a conventional transmembrane action potential.[12, 15] The amplitude of the MAP was defined as the potential difference between phase 2 and phase 4 of the MAP.[15] The duration of the MAP was determined at 90% repolarization. Either delay in repolarization or true depolarizations occurring during phase 2 or phase 3 of the MAP were termed MAP afterdepolarizations. The coupling interval was defined as the interval between phase 0 of the MAP and the peak or shoulder of the afterdepolarization that developed. The amplitude of the MAP afterdepolarizations were defined and determined in a manner analgous to that described for early afterdepolarizations in conventional transmembrane recordings.[8] Only data from recordings considered stable were included in the pooled data. The first criteria for stability was a stable resting potential. In those cases in which ectopic activity arose from the afterdepolarizations, stable resting potentials for each ectopic beat and for the first beat after cessation of the tachycardia, although different from each other, were required. Second, a stable relationship between the amplitudes of phase 2 and phase 0 was required.

The QTU interval was defined as the time between the first deviation from an isolectric PR interval until the last deviation from baseline before the isolectric UP interval.

Controls for changes in MAP induced by motion. To determine whether an increase in contractility and an accentuation of regional wall motion might lead to motion-induced changes in the repolarization phase, epinephrine was infused in six dogs. These animals were anesthetized and prepared in the same manner as the dogs that were to receive cesium chloride. In addition, two pairs of ultrasonic crystals were implanted in the midwall of the left ventricle parallel to the minor axis of the heart.[16] One pair was positioned in the anterior and another in the posterior wall of the left ventricle. Left ventricular pressure and dP/dT were monitored with a catheter-tipped pressure transducer (Millar). In each animal, MAPs were sequentially recorded from 10 to 20 ventricular sites during atrial overdrive pacing at baseline. Epinephrine was then infused at increasing infusion rates intravenously and the dose that led to a maximal hemodynamic response was determined. MAPs were then recorded again from 10 to 20 ventricular sites during atrial overdrive pacing and their characteristics were noted. In each experiment, changes occurred in the MAP, but were limited to a decrease in MAP duration. These changes were not statistically significant. An example is presented in figure 1. Stable recordings were consistently acquired in spite of an increase in heart rate, regional wall motion, blood pressure, and contractility, Furthermore, neither discontinuity in the repolarization phase nor afterdepolarizations were noted at any site in any animal at baseline or after epinephrine.

These results suggest that wall motion, per se, does not lead to abnormalities in repolarization of MAPs. Nevertheless, instability of the MAP recording (as well as of intracellular recordings for that matter) may exist. To avoid artifacts and ensure stable recordings in the present series of experiments, the following were carefully considered when designing the experimental protocol: (1) Control recordings from several sites were made in each animal. (2) A stable baseline recording position was identified in each animal, only after which cesium chloride was administered. (3) The current experimental preparation was used because the genesis of arrhythmias in vivo and afterdepolarizations and triggered activity in vitro have been shown to occur in a matter of minutes. Although prolonged MAP recordings have not been associated with abnormalities in repolarization, this feature of the preparation made it particularly easy to maintain stable, continuous recordings throughout the experimental protocol. (4) Several experiments were performed while monitoring left ventricular pressure and regional wall motion.

Statistical methods. Pooled data are expressed as mean ± SD. Comparison of means was performed with the use of a paired t test. Correlations between variables was determined by linear regression. A p value less than or equal to .05 was considered indicative of a significant difference and an r^2 value greater than or equal to .70 was considered to indicate a significant positive correlation between variables.

Results

Validation in vitro. In tissue samples from six dogs in which simultaneous MAPs and conventional trans-

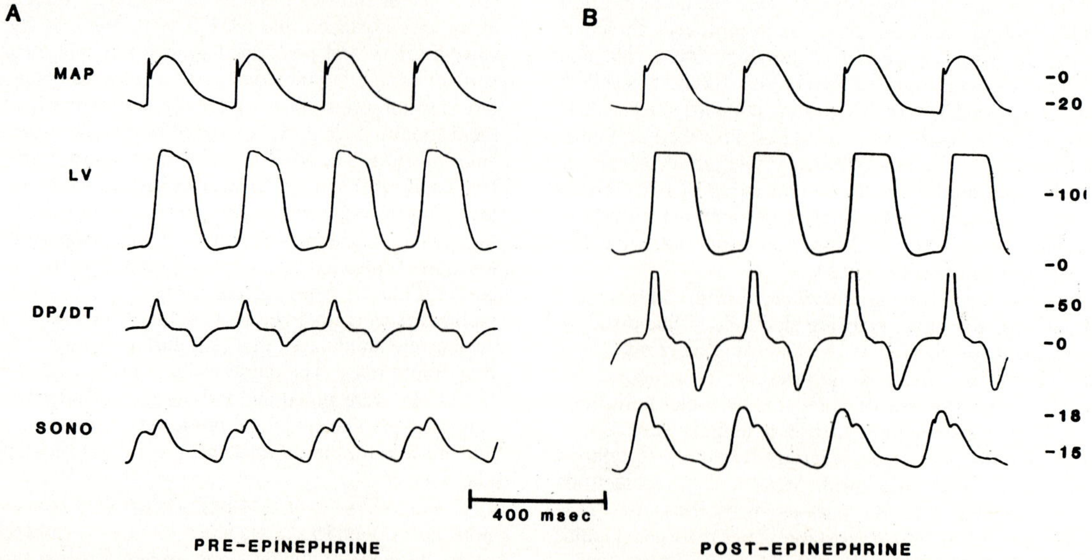

FIGURE 1. Simultaneous recordings of left ventricular pressure (LV), regional wall motion (SONO), dP/dT, and MAPs before (*A*) and after (*B*) the administration of epinephrine. Tracings were obtained during overdrive atrial pacing. Note that although there is a significant increase in blood pressure and regional wall motion, the repolarization phase of the MAP is unchanged. Units are as follows: MAP in mV, LV in mm Hg; dP/dT in mm Hg/msec, SONO in mm.

membrane action potentials were recorded, afterdepolarizations were induced with barium chloride (early) or acetylstrophanthidin (delayed).

Delayed afterdepolarizations and triggered activity were induced in endocardial tissue preparations containing Purkinje fibers taken from the left ventricle. Delayed afterdepolarizations were noted in Purkinje fibers but not in adjacent ventricular muscle under the conditions of the tissue bath. Triggered activity arose from the Purkinje cells and was able to capture neighboring muscle cells in all cases. Shown in figure 2, *A* are analog records from one tissue before and after

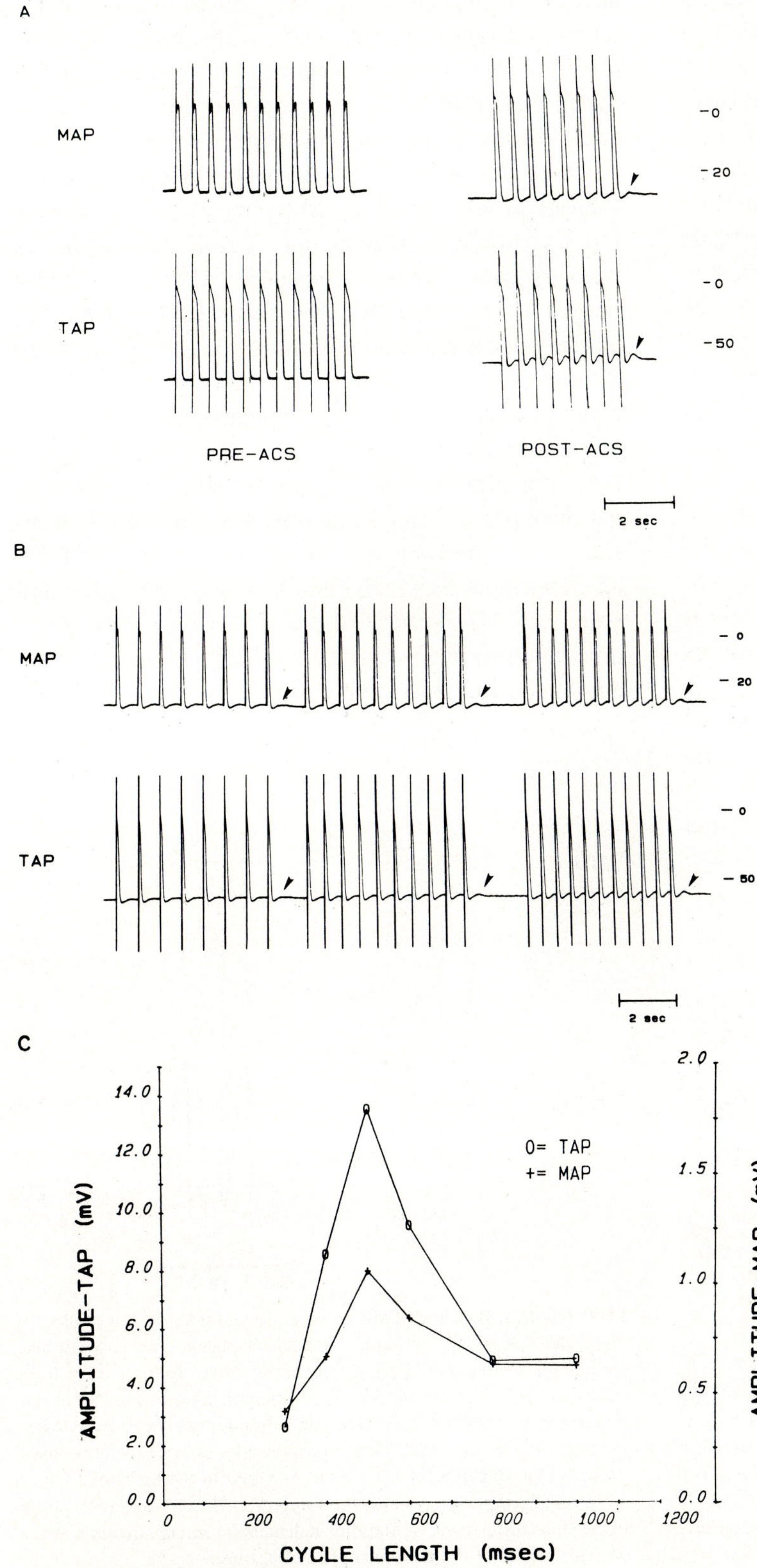

FIGURE 2. Afterdepolarizations that developed in an endocardial preparation exposed to acetylstrophanthidin (5 × 10^{-8} g/liter). *A*, Analog records of simultaneous monophasic and transmembrane action potentials before and after acetylstrophanthidin (ACS). Note that the delayed afterdepolarization present in the transmembrane recording after acetylstrophanthidin is accurately detected by the contact electrode (arrows). *B*, An analog recording from the same tissue sample demonstrating the effect of pacing on the afterdepolarizations of the MAP and transmembrane recordings. An increase in the pacing rate leads to an increase in the prominence of the afterdepolarizations in both the MAP and TAP recordings (arrows). Note also that the characteristic changes in phase 4 during pacing are apparent in the MAP as well. *C*, Results from a different tissue sample in which pacing-induced changes in afterdepolarizations in simultaneous monophasic and transmembrane recordings were compared. Again, although of lower amplitude, delayed afterdepolarizations detected in MAPs behaved the way afterdepolarizations in conventional recordings did during pacing experiments. This tissue was paced for 10 beats at various cycle lengths and afterdepolarization amplitude in transmembrane and monophasic recordings were compared. Afterdepolarization amplitude in both types of recordings increased at decreasing pacing cycle lengths and reached a maximal amplitude at a basic cycle length of 500 msec. At shorter pacing cycle lengths, afterdepolarizations amplitude decreased in both records. The left and right amplitude scales refer to the transmembrane and monophasic recordings, respectively. TAP = transmembrane action potential.

exposure to acetylstrophanthidin; certain features of the MAPs are well shown in the baseline recordings. The time course and configuration of the repolarization phase of the transmembrane action potential were similar to those of the repolarization phase of the MAP. The amplitude of the MAP, on the other hand, was lower than that of the corresponding transmembrane action potential. At baseline, afterdepolarizations were not present in either the transmembrane or monophasic recordings. After exposure to acetylstrophanthidine, afterdepolarizations developed. Afterdepolarizations and changes in phase 4 depolarization were noted in MAPs that were recorded from Purkinje fibers when present in simultaneous microelectrode recordings. In addition, during overdrive pacing at different cycle lengths, changes in the amplitude of the first delayed afterdepolarization in the transmembrane recordings were accurately detected by the MAP. Figure 2, *B* shows a continuous analog recording that demonstrates these effects. As illustrated in this figure, shorter pacing cycle lengths led to more prominent afterdepolarizations in both the monophasic and transmembrane recordings. Figure 2, *C* demonstrates the same findings in a different tissue sample. Although of different absolute amplitude, changes in afterdepolarization amplitude in the transmembrane recordings were accurately detected in the MAPs. In this tissue, peak afterdepolarization amplitude in both transmembrane potentials and MAPs occurred at a pacing cycle length of 500 msec.

Early afterdepolarizations induced in epicardial preparations with barium chloride (10^{-7} M) were also detected in MAPs (figure 3). In this experiment the transmembrane action potential was recorded within 2 mm of the contact electrode. The afterdepolarization present in the transmembrane action potential was accurately recorded in the MAP and the phase 4 depolarization was also detected. As with delayed afterdepolarizations, changes in the amplitude of early afterdepolarizations associated with changes in coupling interval were also accurately reflected in the MAP. Specifically, longer coupling intervals led to early afterdepolarization of greater amplitude.

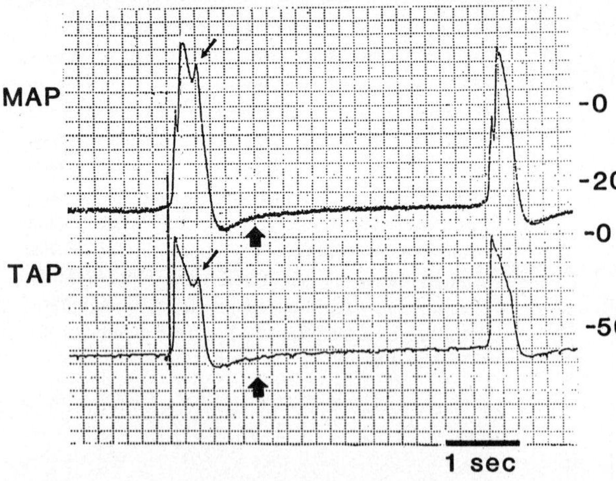

FIGURE 3. Early afterdepolarizations (small arrows) were induced in an epicardial preparation by barium chloride (10^{-7}M). The afterdepolarizations were present, in both the transmembrane action potentials (TAPs) and MAPs for the first beat but not the second beat. Phase 4 depolarization present in the transmembrane potential was also accurately detected by the MAP (large arrows).

Characteristics of the MAP: changes induced by cesium chloride in vivo. Baseline MAP recordings showed a rapid upstroke, a plateau, and a smooth, continuous repolarization phase. Epicardial MAP amplitudes ranged from 12.0 to 49.2 mV (mean 32.4 ± 8.6 mV), while endocardial MAP amplitudes ranged from 6.5 to 21.4 mV (mean ± SD = 12.7 ± 4.4 mV). No delayed repolarization or afterdepolarizations during either phase 2 or 3 were noted in baseline recordings. After the administration of cesium chloride, a prolongation of phase 2 and the development of afterdepolarizations occurred. Figure 4 is an analog recording from an experiment in which simultaneous endocardial and epicardial MAPs were recorded. Baseline recordings are shown in panel *A* and recordings 15 sec after the administration of cesium chloride are shown in panel

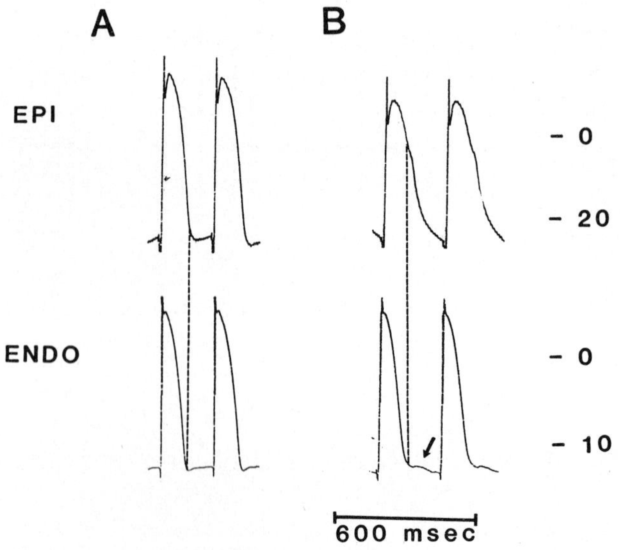

FIGURE 4. *A*, Baseline MAPs recorded simultaneously from endocardium and epicardium. A rapid upstroke, a plateau, and smooth and continuous repolarization phase are noted. Note that relatively little dispersion of onset of activity or of repolarization is present in the baseline state. *B*, MAPs recorded from the same positions approximately 15 sec after the administration of cesium chloride demonstrate several changes. Prolongation of the plateau is noted in the epicardial trace, while an afterdepolarization (arrow) interrupts the repolarization phase of the endocardial trace. A significant dispersion in repolarization arises (dotted line) after the administration of cesium.

B. Very soon after the administration of cesium, a prolongation of phase 2 occurred in the epicardial recording while an afterdepolarization developed in the endocardial recording. These initial changes were seen in all of the experiments. Subsequently, afterdepolarizations were the predominant finding. The amplitude of the afterdepolarizations ranged from 0.7 to 15.6 mV (mean 5.0 ± 4.2 mV) in the epicardial recordings and from 0.5 to 4.6 mV (mean 2.7 ± 1.3 mV) in the endocardial recordings. The afterdepolarizations were seen with equal frequency and relative prominence on both endocardial and epicardial recordings. In addition, prominent TU waves were occasionally noted in the local bipolar electrograms and they correlated in time with the afterdepolarizations. The QTU interval prolonged concurrently with the development of the MAP changes (QTU_c before infusion 360.3 ± 30.5 msec; QTU_c after infusion 453.0 ± 31.2 msec). The QTU interval correlated with the MAP duration before as well as after the cesium-induced changes. These data and their regression are shown in figure 5.

When the cesium effect had reached a steady state the afterdepolarizations that developed responded in a characteristic way to overdrive pacing. Pacing at short cycle length led to the attenuation of afterdepolarizations. Figure 6 is an example of analog recordings from one such experiment. At each shorter pacing cycle length, the amplitude of the afterdepolarizations and the area under the afterdepolarization[8] progressively diminished. At the shortest cycle length (in this case, 300 msec), the afterdepolarizations are nearly abolished. This same behavior was noted in each of the experiments. Figure 7 presents the sumary data for the eight experiments. In each case, pacing at shorter cycle lengths led to attenuation of the afterdepolarizations.

The afterdepolarizations that developed were relatively short-lived. They became less prominent over time and finally disappeared after 10 to 15 min. Of interest is that in all cases the time course of the disappearance of the MAP afterdepolarizations followed that of normalization of the QTU interval.

Relationship of the afterdepolarizations to ventricular ectopy. After the administration of cesium chloride, ventricular ectopy developed in seven of eight experiments. In the animal that did not develop ventricular arrhythmias, sinus arrest, atrioventricular block, and a narrow, junctional tachycardia developed after administration of cesium. Ventricular arrhythmias were spontaneous in all cases. Four animals developed sustained ventricular tachycardia (at least 30 consecutive sec of tachycardia) and three animals developed torsade de pointes (figure 8). Ventricular fibrillation re-

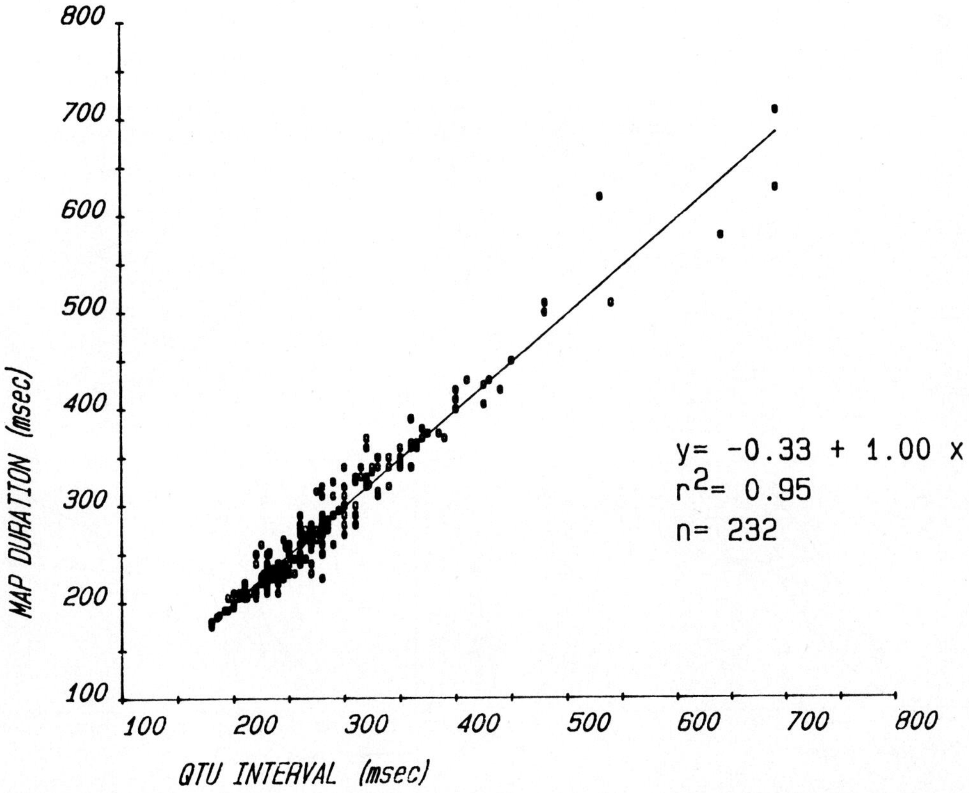

FIGURE 5. MAP duration and QTU interval duration are strongly correlated and nearly identical. The equation of the regression line, its r^2 value, and the number of measurements (n) are shown at the lower right. See text for details.

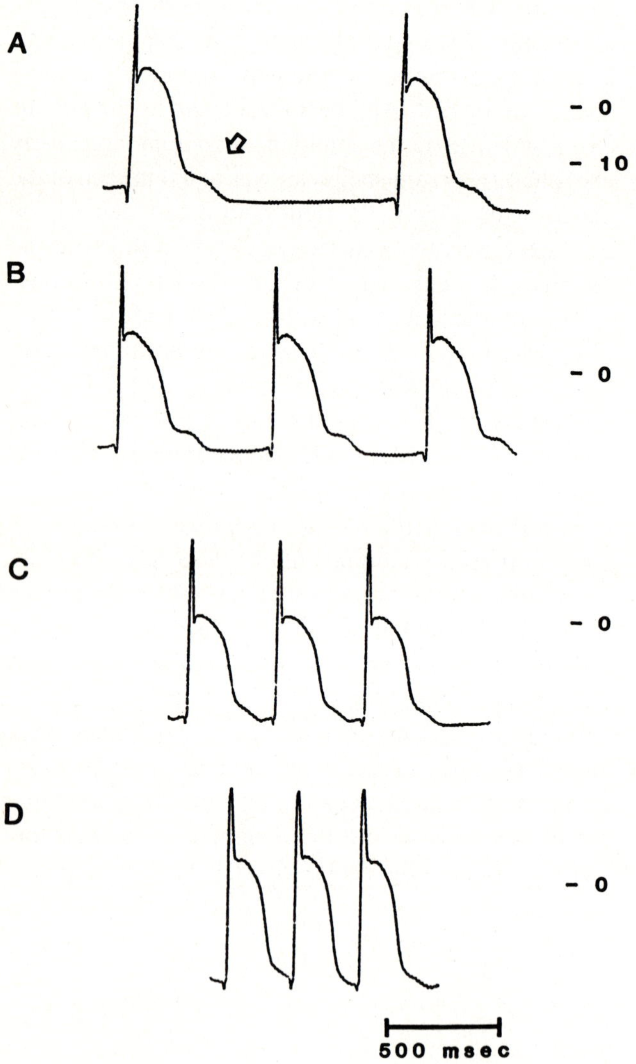

quiring cardioversion occurred in one dog. Bigeminy or short salvos of nonsustained ventricular tachycardia were noted in all but the one experiment.

MAP afterdepolarizations were associated with the development of ventricular ectopy in each case. In all experiments, there was a progressive increase in afterdepolarization amplitude during the first minute after the administration of the cesium chloride. In no case did ventricular ectopy develop without the prior development of the afterdepolarizations. Figure 9 presents typical analog tracings recorded in an animal approximately 1 min after the administration of cesium chloride. An afterdepolarization developed in phase 3 of the MAP, it became progressively larger, and was associated with the development of an ectopic ventricular beat. The coupling interval of the ventricular ectopic beat was very similar to that of the afterdepolarization in this case. This relationship was present in each experiment. Figure 10 presents the summary data relating the coupling intervals of the ectopic beats to the afterdepolarization coupling intervals. These variables are closely related and the coupling intervals of the afterdepolarizations are nearly identical to those of the corresponding ectopic beats.

Moreover, the take-off potential for each ectopic beat was related to the afterdepolarization amplitude in

FIGURE 6. The response of the afterdepolarizations to overdrive pacing. *A* to *D*, Analog epicardial recordings from an experiment in which afterdepolarizations developed after the administration of cesium chloride. Atrial overdrive pacing led to progressive attenuation of the afterdepolarizations (arrow) at shorter cycle lengths.

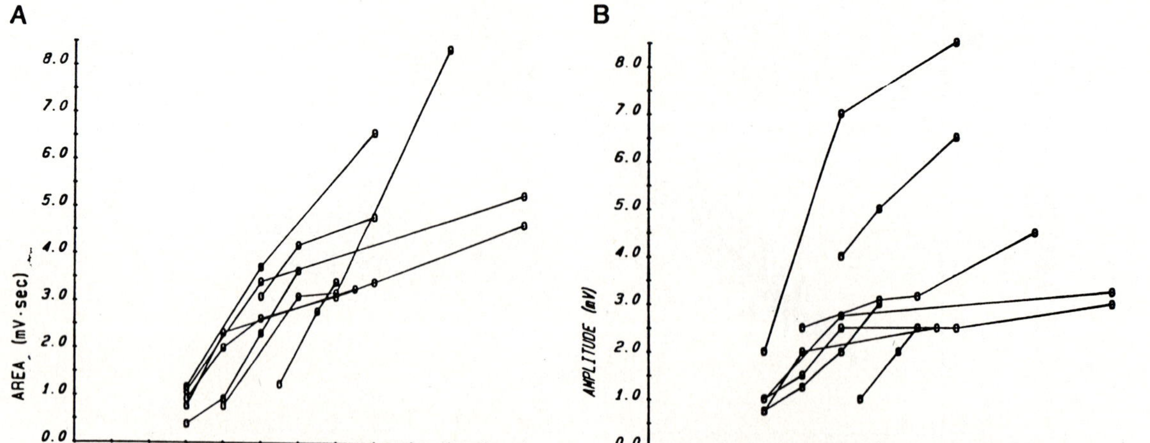

FIGURE 7. The effect of overdrive pacing at various cycle lengths on the amplitude of the afterdepolarization (*A*) as well as the area under the afterdepolarization (*B*) for each experiment. Both of these measured variables decreased at progressively shorter pacing cycle lengths in each experiment. (Each line represents a separate experiment).

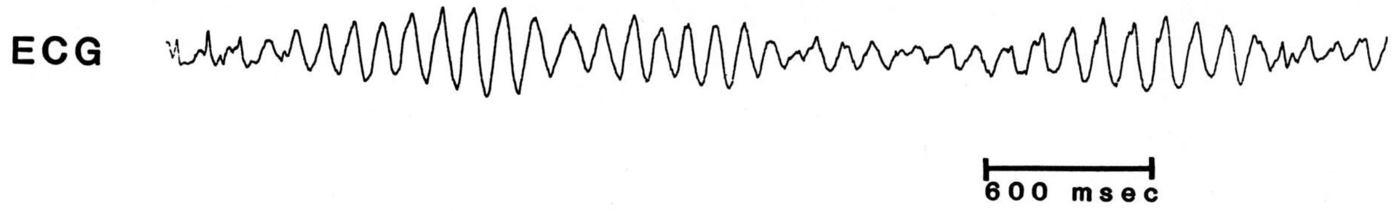

FIGURE 8. An example of the torsade de pointes that developed after the administration of cesium chloride. Note the typical "twisting of points" present in this tracing characteristic of the rhythm identified in patients with the long QT syndrome.

each experiment; that is, the take-off potential in every case approximated the baseline resting potential plus the afterdepolarization amplitude. Figure 11 illustrates analog recordings in which endocardial and epicardial MAPs were recorded simultaneously with right and left ventricular electrograms and a surface electrocardiographic lead. Salvos of nonsustained ventricular tachycardia developed in this animal approximately 45 sec after the administration of cesium. The MAP of the terminal beat in each salvo was associated with an afterdepolarization. The take-off potentials of the last ectopic beat in each salvo were nearly the same and approximate the amplitude of the subthreshold afterdepolarizations. Also, the resting potential from which the first beat after the termination of each salvo arose was relatively constant, demonstrating a stable recording throughout. In addition, the afterdepolarizations present in the epicardial and endocardial tracings, although of different absolute amplitudes, were proportionally the same relative to the MAP amplitude. The close relationship of the take-off potential of the ectopy and the amplitude of the afterdepolarization is summarized in figure 12.

Termination of ventricular ectopy was also related to the properties of the afterdepolarizations. The afterdepolarizations became attenuated during atrial or ventricular overdrive pacing at short cycle lengths (figures 6 and 7) as well as after 10 to 15 min elapsed time following the administration of cesium chloride. Ventricular ectopy was also suppressed during overdrive pacing. In addition, all spontaneous ventricular ectopy ceased as the afterdepolarizations became attenuated with elapsed time (after the initial injection). Thus, the genesis and termination of the ventricular ectopic beats were correlated with the presence or absence of MAP afterdepolarizations.

Discussion

In this study, a new technique for recording MAPs was validated, its sensitivity to record membrane phenomena was determined in vitro, and its application for recording these membrane phenomena was demon-

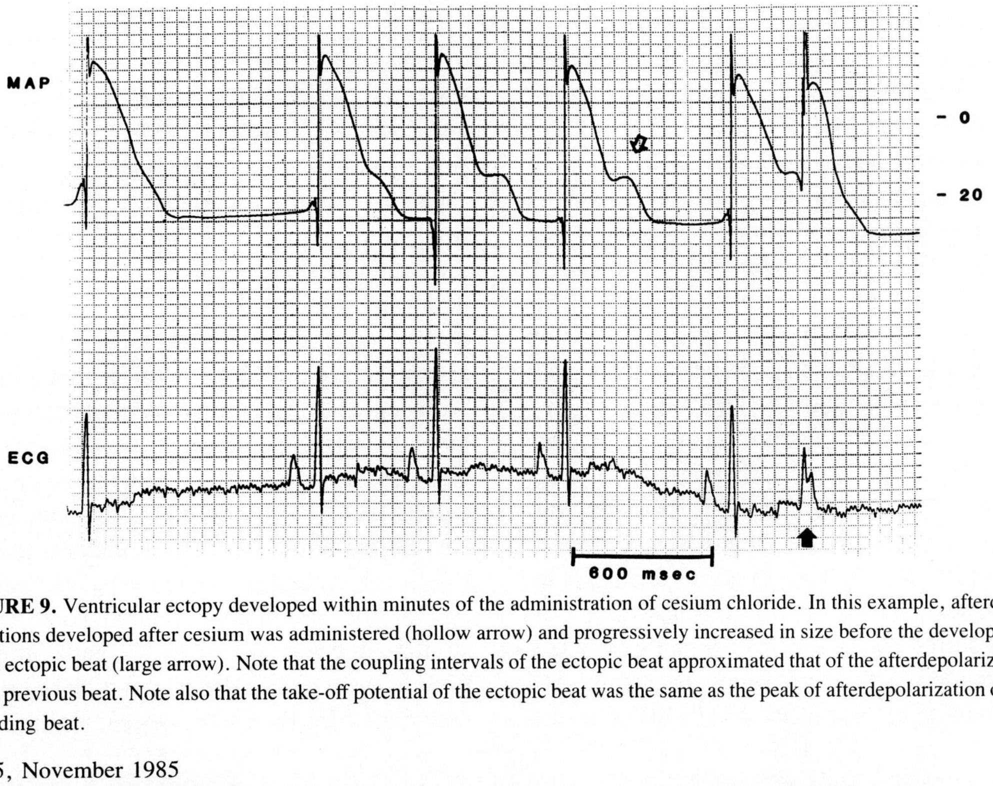

FIGURE 9. Ventricular ectopy developed within minutes of the administration of cesium chloride. In this example, afterdepolarizations developed after cesium was administered (hollow arrow) and progressively increased in size before the development of the ectopic beat (large arrow). Note that the coupling intervals of the ectopic beat approximated that of the afterdepolarization in the previous beat. Note also that the take-off potential of the ectopic beat was the same as the peak of afterdepolarization of the preceding beat.

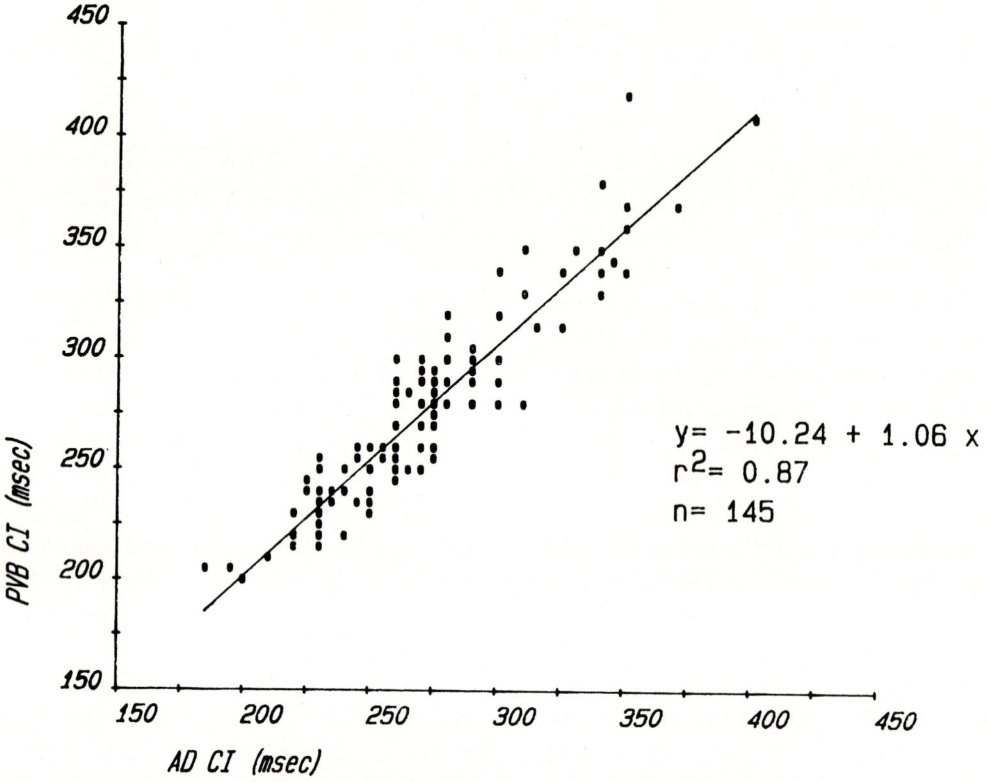

FIGURE 10. The coupling intervals of the afterdepolarizations (AD CI) and the premature ventricular beats (PVB CI) were strongly correlated and nearly identical. The graph is arranged similar to that of figure 5.

strated in vivo. The major finding in this study is that afterdepolarizations and triggered activity occur in vivo and that they underly the genesis of ventricular arrhythmias and torsade de pointes in an animal preparation of the long QT syndrome. In addition, it was shown that the afterdepolarizations and ventricular ectopy that developed behaved in a manner predicted from studies in vitro in isolated tissue preparations exposed to cesium chloride.[7, 8]

MAPs can be recorded from cardiac tissue that has been injured by suction or pressure and are thought to result from current flow from immediately adjacent normal cells that remain electrically coupled to injured tissue beneath the suction or contact electrode.[9–13] The time course of the plateau and repolarization phases of the MAP have been shown to correlate with that of neighboring action potentials.[9, 13] One might predict that other perturbations in the transmembrane voltage either during phase 2 or 3 (early afterdepolarizations) or during phase 4 (delayed afterdepolarizations, enhanced phase 4 depolarization) should also be detectable. This, in fact, was the case in our experiments in vitro. Membrane effects that perturbed phase 2 or 3 or that occurred during phase 4 were accurately detected in MAPs recorded with the contact electrode. Although the absolute voltage of the MAPs differed significantly from that of transmembrane action potentials, enhanced phase 4 depolarization as well as early and delayed afterdepolarizations present in transmembrane action potentials were also recorded in MAPs in vitro (figures 2 and 3).

After the administration of cesium chloride in vivo, afterdepolarizations were also noted during phase 3 of the MAP. We have not proven that these afterdepolarizations recorded in the MAPs in our animal preparation in vivo represent the same phenomenon as that represented by afterdepolarizations noted in conventional transmembrane action potentials recorded in isolated preparations exposed to cesium chloride. Our data, however, do suggest that this may be the case. MAPs and the afterdepolarizations that develop in response to cesium chloride share many characteristics with conventional action potentials recorded from isolated preparations exposed to cesium chloride.[7, 8] Cesium chloride-induced prolongation of the MAP in vivo (figure 4) is similar to the phenomenon described for transmembrane recordings under similar conditions (figure 3). In addition, the time course and morphology of the afterdepolarizations noted in MAPs are similar to those described for early afterdepolarizations of the type that develop at high resting membrane potentials.[8] Furthermore, the pacing-induced changes

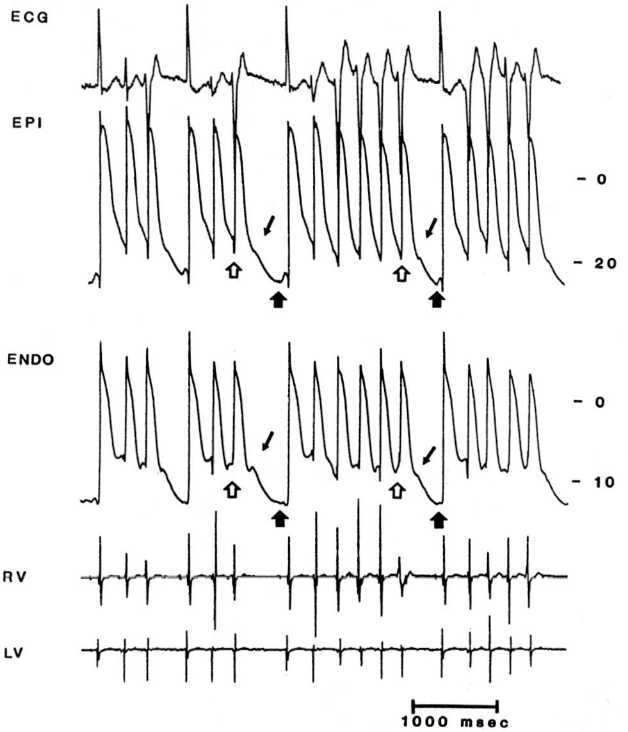

FIGURE 11. An example of an analog recording in which frequent salvos of nonsustained ventricular tachycardia developed after administration of cesium. An electrocardiogram (ECG), an epicardial MAP (EPI), an endocardial MAP (ENDO), and a left (LV) and a right (RV) ventricular bipolar electrogram are shown. Note that afterdepolarizations are present in both the endocardial and epicardial MAPs (small arrows), that their amplitude is related to the take-off potential of the ectopic beats (hollow arrow), that they are of the same polarity and relative magnitude, and that their coupling interval is related to the coupling interval of the ectopic beats present in the tracing. Note also that the baseline resting potential of the supraventricular beats is relatively constant (large arrow), implying a stable recording.

in the afterdepolarizations (figures 6 and 7) that were noted in our experiments are similar to those described for early afterdepolarizations identified in vitro.[8] It thus seems highly probable that the phenomena we have recorded in vivo are the same as those identified in conventional transmembrane recordings in isolated preparations.

The afterdepolarizations seemed to play an important role in the genesis of the ventricular ectopic activity that arose. The development of afterdepolarizations preceded the development of arrhythmias in all cases. In addition, in several dogs, a clear progression in afterdepolarization amplitude before a spontaneous premature beat was noted, thereby suggesting that the premature beat resulted from a threshold respone (figure 9). Furthermore, the coupling intervals of the afterdepolarizations were closely related to and nearly the same as the coupling intervals of the associated ventricular premature beats (figures 9 and 10). In addition, the take-off potential of the premature beats in the MAP recording was related to the afterdepolarization amplitude (figures 11 and 12). Finally, both the ectopy and the afterdepolarizations resolved concurrently during overdrive pacing or with time; the animals returned to a near-baseline electrophysiologic condition 5 to 10 min after the cesium infusion. Thus, a clear relationship between the MAP afterdepolarizations and the ventricular ectopy that developed was present in this in vivo preparation. It should be noted that the arrhythmias that arose in vivo were considerably faster than those described in vitro and that the initial coupling intervals of the ectopic beats were shorter.[7, 8] While the exact reason for this difference is unknown, it is likely related to sympathetic tone that is present in vivo.

The mechanism underlying the development of the afterdepolarizations that occur after the administration of cesium chloride is unknown. Early afterdepolarizations develop in vitro in ventricular muscle or Purkinje fibers exposed to agents or conditions that favor prolonged repolarization.[7, 8] Their genesis is thought to be due in part to cesium-induced depression of potassium currents.[17] However, definite evidence for the presence of an altered ionic current leading to the genesis of early afterdepolarizations is not available. Furthermore, the possibility that some early afterdepolarizations might represent an electrotonic membrane phenomenon has not been ruled out in our experiments nor in most experiments in vitro. In fact, data from our studies suggest that electrotonic phenomena may have been involved in the genesis of some afterdepolarizations. Figure 4 is taken from an experiment in which simultaneous endocardial and epicardial MAPs were recorded. Cesium chloride induced a similar prolongation of the MAP duration within 15 sec in both tracings. However, the prolongation found in the epicardial recording was due to a prolongation of phase 2, while that in the endocardial tracing was due to the development of an afterdepolarization with relatively little change in phase 2. This suggests that the afterdepolarizations found in this case may have been due to electrotonic phenomena resulting from dispersion of repolarization. In addition, the ectopy that developed could have arisen via current flow between cells with prolonged and shortened repolarization phases by a mechanism similar to that described for ischemia.[18]

The possibility that the afterdepolarizations arose as a result of ventricular wall motion or an unstable catheter position seems unlikely. First, control recordings under baseline conditions as well as after an epinephrine-induced increased contractile state (over 100 recording positions) failed to show similar changes dur-

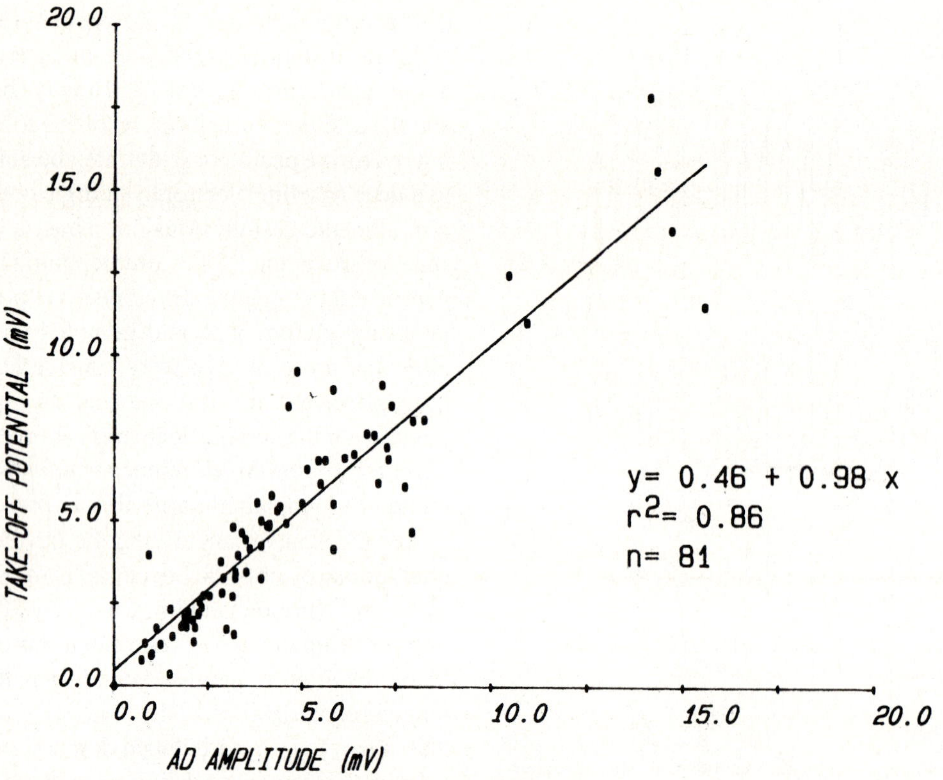

FIGURE 12. The take-off potential and the afterdepolarization (AD) amplitude are closely correlated and very close in magnitude. The graph is arranged similar to that of figure 10. See text for details.

ing phase 2 or 3 (figure 1). If these recordings of afterdepolarizations in vivo were due to motion-induced changes in contact pressure, they should have been accentuated under these conditions. Second, simultaneous endocardial and epicardial tracings were made after administration of cesium chloride and afterdepolarizations of the same relative magnitude and polarity were demonstrated in both MAP recordings (figure 11). If wall motion affecting the electrode-myocardial interface were the cause of the afterdepolarizations (i.e., during contraction or filling) one might predict humps of opposite polarity in the two recordings; i.e., the ventricular wall is always moving toward one of the catheters thereby potentially increasing contact pressure while moving away from the other. Third, if motion underlied their genesis, one would not expect the close correlation between the MAP duration and the QTU interval (figure 5), or the close relationship between the afterdepolarizations and the ventricular ectopic activity documented in our experiments (figures 9 to 12). Fourth, in three experiments in which simultaneous left ventricular pressure was monitored, and in two experiments in which regional wall motion was measured with ultrasonic crystals, no relationship was found between the afterdepolarizations and changes in the hemodynamic parameters. Fifth, the afterdepolarizations became attenuated during rapid overdrive pacing (figures 6 and 7). If they resulted from instability due to ventricular wall motion, one would expect them to be accentuated by pacing at rapid rates. Finally, afterdepolarizations such as these have been noted in vitro during simultaneous MAP and transmembrane recordings under similar conditions, and that the MAP catheter can clearly detect these membrane phenomena has been validated in vitro (figures 2 and 3). Thus, the evidence is in favor of the fact that the afterdepolarizations recorded in our experiments are representative of similar phenomena present in nearby myocardial cell action potentials.

The findings in this study are clinically relevant. The long QT syndrome, acquired or congenital, has been associated with ventricular ectopic activity and torsade de pointes.[19, 20] Although assumed to be due to triggered activity, the mechanism of these arrhythmias in vivo have not been defined.[6–8, 19] The present studies provide direct evidence linking afterdepolarizations, the characteristics of which are similar to early afterdepolarizations defined in vitro, with ventricular ectopy in this animal preparation of the long QT syndrome. We have further defined a mechanism by which conventional management of these patients, such as overdrive pacing, may exert a beneficial effect. That the findings in this study may be relevant to the long QT syndrome in man is further suggested by the demonstration of similar afterdepolarizations in right ventricular MAPs in patients with acquired or congenital long QT syndrome and severe ventricular arrhythmias.[20] Thus, recording MAPs in patients with the long QT syndrome may help to identify those at risk for the development of tachyarrhythmias as well as provide an assay in the electrophysiology laboratory against which drugs, pacemakers, or other therapeutic interventions can be measured.

We thank Ralph Iannuzzi, William Moore and Chuck Prood for their technical assistance and Bejay Moore for typing the manuscript.

References

1. Josephson ME, Seides SF: Clinical cardiac electrophysiology, 1979, Philadelphia, Lea and Febiger, pp 211–280
2. Rosen MR, Reder RF: Does triggered activity have a role in the genesis of cardiac arrhythmias? Ann Intern Med **94:** 794, 1981
3. Levine, JH, Michael JR, Guarnieri TG: The treatment of multifocal atrial tachycardia with verapamil. N Engl Med **312:** 21, 1985
4. Sung RJ, Shapiro WA, Shen EN, Morady F, Davis J: Effects of verapamil on ventricular tachycardia possibly caused by reentry, automaticity, and triggered activity. J Clin Invest **72:** 350, 1983
5. Mason JW: Efficacy of verapamil in recurrent ventricular tachycardia. Am J Cardiol **49:** 105, 1982 (abst)
6. Bhandari AK, Shapiro WA, Morady F, Shen EN, Mason J, Scheinman MM: Electrophysiologic testing in patients with the long QT syndrome. Circulation **71:** 63, 1985
7. Brachmann J, Scherlag BJ, Rosenshtraukh LV, Lazzara R: Bradycardia-dependent triggered activity: relevance to drug-induced multiform ventricular tachycardia. Circulation **68:** 846, 1983
8. Damiano BP, Rosen MR: Effects of pacing on triggered activity induced by early afterdepolarizations. Circualtion **69:** 1013, 1984
9. Hoffman BF, Cranefield PF, Lepeshkin E, Surawicz B, Herrlich HC: Comparison of cardiac monophasic action potentials recorded by intracellular and suction electrodes. Am J Physiol **196:** 1297, 1959
10. Shabetai R, Surawicz B, Hammel W: Monophasic action potentials in man. Circulation **38:** 341, 1968
11. Sjostand U: A method for intracardiac recording of monophasic action potentials in the dog heart in situ. Acta Physiol Scand **68:** 58, 1966
12. Franz MR: Long-term recording of monophasic action potentials from human endocardium. Am J Cardiol **51:** 1629, 1983
13. Franz MR, Burkhoff D, Weisfeldt ML, Lakatta EG: Quantitative comparison of monophasic action potentials recorded simultaneously with an intra- and a new extracellular electrode. J Am Coll Cardiol **32:** 498, 1984 (abst)
14. Spear JF, Michelson EL, Moore EN: Cellular electrophysiologic characteristics of chronically infarcted myocardium in dogs susceptible to sustained ventricular tachyarrhythmias. J Am Coll Cardiol **1:** 1099, 1983
15. Franz MR, Flaherty JT, Platia EV, Bulkley BH, Weisfeldt ML: Localization of regional myocardial ischemia by recording of monophasic action potentials. Circulation **69:** 593, 1984
16. Hermisch W, Hagl S, Gebhardt K, Meisner H, Medler N, Sebening F: Direct measurement of cycle changes in regional wall geometry in the left ventricle of the dog. Innov Tech Biol Med **2:** 487, 1981
17. Gay LA, Stanfield PR: Cs^+ causes a voltage dependent block of inward K^+ current in resting skeletal muscle fibers. Nature **267:** 169, 1977
18. Janse MJ, Kleber AG: Electrophysiological changes and ventricular arrhythmias in the early phase of regional myocardial ischemia. Circ Res **49:** 1069, 1981
19. Moss AJ, Schwartz PJ, Crampton RS, Locati E, Carleen E: The long QT syndrome: a prospective international study. Circulation **71:** 17, 1985
20. Bonatti V, Rolli A, Botti G: Recording of monophasic action potentials of the right ventricle in the long QT syndrome complicated by severe ventricular arrhythmias. Eur Heart J **4:** 168, 1983

Effects of right ventricular ischemia on left ventricular geometry and the end-diastolic pressure-volume relationship in the dog

YOICHI GOTO, JIN YAMAMOTO, MUNEYASU SAITO, KAZUO HAZE, TETSUYA SUMIYOSHI, KENICHI FUKAMI, AND KATSUHIKO HIRAMORI

ABSTRACT We studied the effects of right ventricular ischemia on left ventricular three-dimensional geometry and the end-diastolic pressure-volume relationship in 16 open-chest dogs before and after pericardiectomy. Left ventricular volume was calculated from three internal dimensions measured with ultrasonic crystals. In one group of eight dogs, right coronary artery (RCA) occlusion for 2 min with the pericardium intact reduced aortic flow by 24 ± 9% ($p < .001$) and septal-lateral dimension by 8 ± 5% ($p < .01$), without changing anterior-posterior and apical-basal dimensions. However, parameters of left ventricular systolic function (aortic flow, left ventricular systolic pressure, peak dP/dt, and mean percent systolic shortening) were similar to those observed at a comparable level of left ventricular end-diastolic volume during inferior vena caval occlusion. In the other group of eight dogs, during RCA occlusion before pericardiectomy the left ventricular end-diastolic pressure-volume relationship determined during rapid blood transfusion shifted leftward and upward significantly from the preocclusion relationship. After pericardiectomy, RCA occlusion caused less significant changes in aortic flow and septal-lateral dimension as well as in the left ventricular end-diastolic pressure-volume relationship. We concluded that right ventricular ischemia causes a leftward shift of the interventricular septum in end-diastole and an alteration of the left ventricular end-diastolic pressure-volume relationship without changing left ventricular myocardial performance. These changes are enhanced by the intact pericardium.

Circulation 72, No. 5, 1104–1114, 1985.

AN INCREASE in right ventricular filling[1] and the presence of the pericardium[2] have been shown to cause a leftward and upward shift of left ventricular diastolic pressure-volume curves.[3] Also, there is experimental evidence that the interventricular septum shifts leftward in end-diastole and left ventricular geometry is distorted when right ventricular loading is induced by pulmonary artery constrictions,[4, 5] atrial septal defect,[6] the Mueller maneuver[7] or positive end-expiratory pressure ventilation.[8] However, the effects of right ventricular infarction or ischemia on left ventricular diastolic properties have not yet been reported. Although Goldstein et al.[9] showed that elevated intrapericardial pressure after right ventricular infarction could reduce left ventricular preload and cardiac output, they neither evaluated left ventricular geometry nor measured left ventricular volume.

The goal of the present study was to elucidate the effects of right ventricular ischemia on left ventricular geometry and the end-diastolic pressure-volume relationship in dogs, and to consider the importance of the intact pericardium. To this end, we measured septal-lateral, anterior-posterior, and apical-basal dimensions of the left ventricle with three pairs of ultrasonic dimension gauges, during right coronary artery (RCA) occlusions with the pericardium intact and open.

Methods

Animal preparation and instrumentation. Sixteen mongrel dogs weighing 13 to 24 kg (average 16.9) were anesthetized with ketamine hydrochloride (5 to 7 mg/kg im) followed by intravenous α-chloralose (50 mg/kg) and urethane (500 mg/kg). After endotracheal intubation, ventilation was maintained, by a volume respirator, with room air. A bilateral thoracotomy was performed in each dog in the fifth intercostal space with transection of the sternum. The electrocardiogram was continuously monitored in a limb lead (lead II). Arterial blood was repeatedly sampled for measurements of pH, Po_2, and Pco_2 with a blood gas analyzer (Acid-Base Laboratory, ABL2d), and supplemen-

From the Departments of Cardiovascular Dynamics and Internal Medicine, National Cardiovascular Center, Osaka, Japan.

Address for correspondence: Yoichi Goto, M.D., Department of Cardiovascular Dynamics, National Cardiovascular Center, 5-7-1, Fujishirodai, Suita, Osaka, 565, Japan.

Received Dec. 31, 1984; revision accepted July 5, 1985.

Presented in part at the 56th Scientific Sessions of The American Heart Association, Anaheim, CA, 1983.

tal oxygen and intravenous sodium bicarbonate were given when necessary to maintain values for these parameters within their physiologic ranges.

Instrumentation was performed with the pericardium virtually intact. A micromanometer-tipped catheter with a fluid-filled lumen (Millar Instruments, PC-470) was inserted into the left ventricle through the right common carotid artery to measure left ventricular pressure. A fluid-filled polyvinyl catheter (1 mm internal diameter) was placed in the right ventricle through the right external jugular vein. Both the fluid-filled lumens were connected to Statham P23ID pressure transducers. The electronic micromanometer in the left ventricle, connected to a direct-current amplifier (NEC San-Ei, model 1170) and calibrated and balanced at 37° C with a mercury manometer before each experiment, was rechecked in vivo with the use of the left ventricular systolic and end-diastolic pressure signals obtained simultaneously through the fluid-filled lumen. An occlusive snare (3–0 silk thread) was placed around the RCA near its origin, and a pair of pacing electrodes was sutured to the right atrial appendage. The RCA snare and pacing electrodes were placed through two small incisions (2 to 3 mm in length) in the pericardium. When incisions were made in the pericardium, care was taken to minimize their size.

Placement of ultrasonic crystals. The three types of ultrasonic crystals used in this study are illustrated in figure 1. These crystals were made of 5 MHz piezoelectric crystals (Murata Mfg. Co., 7R-30-20-5000) that were coated with polyester resin in our laboratory. As shown in figure 1, three pairs of ultrasonic crystals (2.5 mm in diameter) were placed through small incisions (3 mm in length) in the pericardium to measure the three internal dimensions of the left ventricle. The septal-lateral dimension was measured with a pair of crystals between the left ventricular endocardial surface of the septum and the subendocardium of the lateral free wall. These crystals were placed by the following method. A small stab incision was made into the lateral wall of the left ventricle, a needle carrying a crystal was thrust through the incision to the right ventricle, and the wires were pulled through the interventricular septum and the right ventricular free wall until the crystal lay flat against the septum. A second crystal was inserted through the same stab incision into the subendocardium of the lateral wall. The anterior-posterior dimension was measured with another pair of crystals implanted in the subendocardium through small stab incisions adjacent to the anterior and posterior descending coronary arteries. These two pairs of crystals were on the equatorial plane of the left ventricle.

A third pair of crystals was implanted to measure the longitudinal (apical-basal) internal dimension of the left ventricle. The apical crystal was placed in the subendocardium near the apical dimple, and the basal crystal was placed in the subendocardium just below the bifurcation of the left main coronary artery. In addition, to measure the right ventricular segment length, a fourth pair of crystals (2 mm in diameter) was placed in the mid portion of the right ventricular free wall in the circumferential direction. When the crystals were implanted, great care was taken not to injure any epicardial coronary arteries or veins.

The ultrasonic signals were continuously monitored with a four-channel ultrasonic dimension system (NEC San-Ei, model 4105). This instrument applied a pinging voltage to a piezoelectric crystal of 1024 times/sec/channel, measured the transit-time of ultrasound bursts across each pair of crystals, and generated a proportional analog voltage. Calibration was made electronically with gain (0.4 to 20 mm/0.5 V) and offset (0 to 100 mm) adjustments. The instantaneous distance between the crystals was calculated electronically according to the velocity of sound in blood (1.57×10^5 cm/sec). The linearity of this system in combination with 5 MHz crystals was $\pm 0.5\%$ over full scale (= 100 mm), and the noise level was below 0.05 mm.

The small incisions in the pericardium were not closed with sutures because suturing of the pericardium might have caused a leftward shift in the left ventricular diastolic pressure-volume relationship.[10] Thee was no blood in the pericardial space at the end of the period of instrumentation.

Experimental protocol. After the instrumentation with the pericardium intact, the dogs were divided into two groups. In group 1 (eight dogs), we assessed the effects of right ventricular ischemia on left ventricular geometry before and after pericardiectomy and compared them with those observed during inferi-

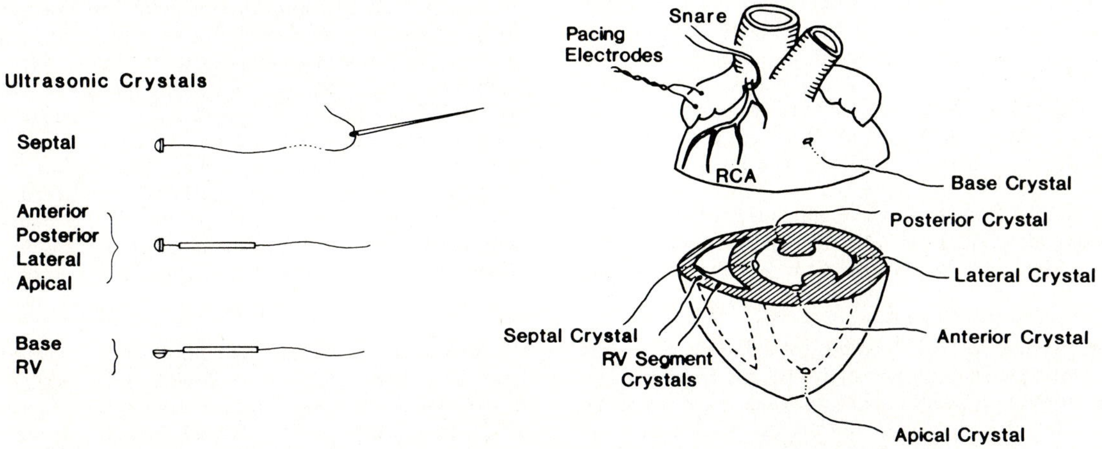

FIGURE 1. Schematic drawing of ultrasonic crystals (*left*) and cardiac instrumentation (*right*). There were three types of ultrasonic crystals used in this study. The septal crystal has a long twisted pair of multistranded flexible wires attached perpendicularly to the disk; it is threaded through the eye of a 9 cm long stainless steel needle for implantation. Anterior, posterior, lateral, and apical crystals also have perpendicularly attached wires that are passed through the lumen of a 3 cm long plastic tubing with a 1.7 mm diameter. Basal and right ventricular (RV) crystals have wires attached to the edge of the disk, and the wires are also passed through the plastic tubing. These were implanted to measure the anterior-posterior, septal-lateral, and longitudinal (apical-basal) dimensions of the left ventricle and the right ventricular segment length in the area to be rendered ischemic when the RCA was occluded by the snare. Pacing electrodes were sutured to the right atrial appendage. The instrumentation was performed through small incisions in the pericardium so that the pericardium was kept virtually intact.

or vena caval (IVC) occlusion. In group 2 (eight dogs), we assessed alterations in the left ventricular end-diastolic pressure-volume relationship during right ventricular ischemia before and after pericardiectomy. All experiments were carried out while the heart rate was held constant by right atrial pacing.

Group 1. In eight dogs, an electromagnetic flow probe was placed on the descending aorta because it was technically difficult to place it on the ascending aorta with the pericardium intact. The probe was connected to an electromagnetic flowmeter (Narco Bio-systems, RT-500). An occlusive snare (1–0 silk thread) was placed around the IVC to induce a transient reduction in left ventricular preload.

A first control recording was made, and then left ventricular preload was reduced for 30 sec by partial IVC occlusion with the IVC snare. The degree of IVC occlusion was adjusted to obtain a 20% to 30% reduction in aortic flow below the control level so that the end-diastolic volume would be similar to that during RCA occlusion. Hemodynamic and dimensional measurements were made, and then the snare was released.

After the hemodynamic and dimensional parameters had returned to the basal level, a second control recording was made. To produce right ventricular ischemia, the RCA was completely occluded with the RCA snare for 2 min. Measurements were made at 2 min of occlusion when hemodynamic and dimensional parameters became steady, and then the RCA snare was completely released.

When hemodynamic and dimensional parameters had completely returned to the control level, the pericardium was widely opened and a pericardial cradle was produced. When the hemodynamic values reached a new steady state, a third control recording was made. A second RCA occlusion was then induced, and the measurements were repeated.

Group 2. In the other eight dogs, a polyvinyl catheter (3 mm internal diameter) for blood transfusion was placed into the IVC through the right femoral vein. To prevent ventricular arrhythmias during transfusion, an intravenous infusion of lidocaine (0.03 mg/kg/min) was maintained throughout the experiments. A control volume loading with heparinized fresh blood withdrawn from donor dogs and kept at 37° C was carried out to obtain a control left ventricular end-diastolic pressure-volume relationship with the pericardium intact. Blood was rapidly transfused with a roller pump (Cole-Parmer Instrument, Masterflex PA-51B) at a constant speed of 400 ml/min through the IVC catheter until left ventricular end-diastolic pressure reached 16 to 18 mm Hg. Usually this level of left ventricular end-diastolic pressure was achieved within 35 to 50 sec of transfusion with the pericardium intact, and within 45 to 60 sec with the pericardium open.

During volume loading, pressure and dimensions were measured continuously. After left ventricular end-diastolic pressure reached 16 to 18 mm Hg, blood was withdrawn at a slower speed until left ventricular pressure returned to the control level. At least 15 min were allowed to elapse for restabilization of overall hemodynamics. A second control volume loading was performed to check the reproducibility of the hemodynamic responses to blood transfusion and to avoid errors due to an anaphylactic response to the first transfusion. Almost the same hemodynamic and dimensional responses were observed in all dogs and therefore we used the second control volume loading values for analysis.

After restabilization of hemodynamics, the RCA was occluded for 3 min, and during the last 1 min, rapid volume loading was performed as described above. After measurements were made, the RCA snare was released and blood was withdrawn. The pericardium was then opened widely to produce a pericardial cradle, and after hemodynamics had stabilized, a second series of control volume loading and volume loading during RCA occlusion was repeated in the same manner as in the first series.

After the completion of each experiment, the proper position of the ultrasonic crystals was verified by autopsy. In two dogs mercury was injected into the RCA through a No. 5F Judkins' catheter under x-ray fluoroscopic monitoring before they were killed, and in four dogs barium sulfate suspension was injected into the RCA after they were killed. Postmortem x-ray films of the hearts were taken to assess the RCA distribution.

Data analysis. All data were recorded on both a multichannel thermal-pen recorder (NEC San-Ei, Polygraph 360) and magnetic tape. In group 1 we measured mean aortic flow, peak systolic and end-diastolic pressures of the right and left ventricles, dP/dt, and end-systolic and end-diastolic values for the dimensional data. These were averaged over 6 to 8 beats under steady-state conditions. Data obtained during the earliest phase of IVC occlusion were not used because decreases in right ventricular pressure in this phase often permit rightward displacement of the interventricular septum.[5] We visually identified end-systole at the time when the left ventricular dimensions reached their nadir near peak negative dP/dt, and end-diastole at the time immediately before left ventricular pressure started its rapid upstroke. Percent systolic shortening of each dimension was calculated as the end-diastolic dimension minus the end-systolic dimension, divided by the end-diastolic dimension, times 100. Mean left ventricular percent systolic shortening was obtained by averaging percent systolic shortening of the three dimensions. In group 2 we measured left ventricular peak systolic and end-diastolic pressures and dimensions during blood transfusions, as well as right ventricular pressures and dimensions. Pleural pressure was not measured, and respiratory variation was neglected because these experiments were performed in an open-chest preparation.

Left ventricular volume was calculated from the three internal dimensions by a nonprolate ellipsoid model with the formula

$$V_{calc} = \frac{\Pi}{6} D_{SL}\, D_{AP}\, D_{L} \times 10^{-3} \qquad (1)$$

where V_{calc} = calculated left ventricular volume (ml); D_{SL} = left ventricular septal-lateral dimension (mm); D_{AP} = anterior-posterior dimension (mm); D_L = longitudinal dimension (mm). This calculation was validated by comparing calculated volume and directly measured volume obtained in five excised hearts after the experiments in the following manner. The heart was suspended in a beaker filled with blood. A known amount of blood (directly measured volume) was injected into a well-fitted left ventricular balloon that was placed through the aortic valve with the mitral valve sutured, and simultaneously the three left ventricular dimensions were measured, for determination of the calculated volume, with the ultrasonic cyrstals. Using a total of 71 data points, we obtained the following regression equation:

$$V_{calc} = 0.93\, V_{meas} + 2.5 \qquad (2)$$

where V_{calc} = calculated volume (ml); V_{meas} = measured volume (ml). The correlation coefficient of the pooled data was .94. Although there was a slight underestimation in the calculated volume, the correlation between the values obtained by the two techniques was highly linear for each of five hearts (correlation coefficients = .994, .996, .996, .998, and .998). These data were comparable to those of Rankin et al.[11] On the basis of these results, we used calculated volume as left ventricular volume for subsequent analysis.

Alterations of the left ventricular end-diastolic pressure-volume relationship during RCA occlusion were evaluated in two ways. First, left ventricular end-diastolic volume during RCA occlusion was compared with the preocclusion value at several matched left ventricular end-diastolic pressures. By this analysis, a leftward shift in the pressure-volume relationship was tested. Second, an upward shift in the left ventricular end-diastolic pressure-volume relationship was evaluated by approximating the pressure-volume data during blood transfusion as a fourth-order polynomial according to the method of Glantz[12]:

$$P = a_4V^4 + a_3V^3 + a_2V^2 + a_1V + a_0 + bS \quad (3)$$

where P = left ventricular end-diastolic pressure (mm Hg); V = left ventricular end-diastolic volume (ml); S = 0 for data obtained during control volume loading and 1 for data obtained during volume loading with RCA occlusion; a_4, a_3, a_2, a_1, a_0, and b = constants. The bS term shifts the entire pressure-volume relationship upward or downward in the presence of RCA occlusion, and thus the b value represents the amount of the shift of the relationship.

Statistics. In group 1, statistical comparison of data obtained during first control period, IVC occlusion, second control period, RCA occlusion before pericardiectomy, third control period, and RCA occlusion after pericardiectomy were performed by the analysis of variance for repeated measurements.[13] In group 2 the same method was also used for comparisons of data obtained during control and RCA occlusion before and after pericardiectomy. When the analysis of variance offered F values for $p < .05$ among the measurements, the paired t test was used to determine the statistical significance of differences between corresponding control and intervention values. Statistical comparisons were also made by the paired t test between parameters of left ventricular systolic function during IVC and RCA occlusions, and between changes in the observed values during RCA occlusion with the pericardium intact and open. Probability values smaller than .05 were considered indicative of statistical significance. Data are presented as mean ± SD unless otherwise indicated.

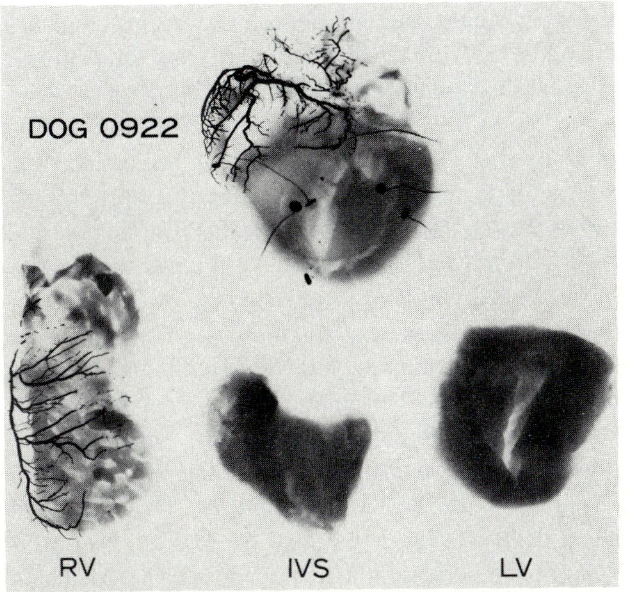

FIGURE 2. Postmortem x-ray of an excised heart that shows the distribution of the right coronary artery filled with mercury. After the picture of the whole heart (*top*) was taken, the heart was dissected into three separate sections (*bottom*): the right ventricular free wall (RV), the interventricular septum (IVS), and the left ventricular free wall (LV). Mercury was distributed only to the right ventricular free wall, not to the interventricular septum or the left ventricle. The pairs of ultrasonic crystals implanted in the heart can be seen.

Results

In all of the six dogs in which postmortem radiographic findings were obtained, the mercury injected into the RCA was distributed only to the right ventricular free wall, not to the left ventricle or the interventricular septum (figure 2).

Group 1. Representative tracings obtained in one dog during RCA occlusion are shown in figure 3, and hemodynamic and dimensional data are summarized in table 1 and figure 4.

During partial IVC occlusion, there were significant decreases in aortic flow (−24.5 ± 5.8%), left ventricular systolic pressure (−15.5 ± 4.0%), left ventricular end-diastolic pressure (−1.3 ± 0.7 mm Hg), right ventricular systolic pressure (−7.9 ± 1.8 mm Hg), and right ventricular end-diastolic pressure (−1.2 ±

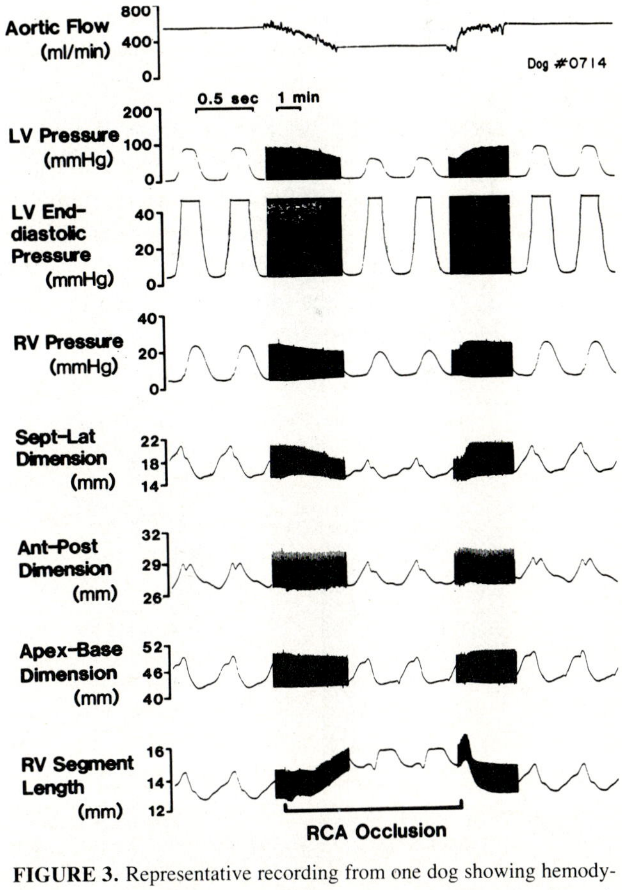

FIGURE 3. Representative recording from one dog showing hemodynamic and dimensional changes during RCA occlusion with the pericardium intact. Decreases in aortic flow, left ventricular (LV), and right ventricular (RV) systolic pressures and an increase in right ventricular end-diastolic pressure occurred during 2 min of RCA occlusion. Interestingly, among the left ventricular dimensions, the septal-lateral dimension showed a striking decrease compared with other two dimensions. The right ventricular semgent length extended markedly and showed systolic bulging, indicating right ventricular ischemia. After the release of RCA occlusion, the hemodynamic and dimensional parameter values returned to the control level within a few minutes.

TABLE 1
Effects of interventions on hemodynamics and dimensions in group 1 dogs

	C_1	IVCO	C_2	$RCAO_{Pi}$	C_3	$RCAO_{Po}$
AoF (ml/min)	526±74	400±51^C	510±92	387±84^C	494±154	429±134^C
LVSP (mm Hg)	103±15	87±14^C	101±17	85±22^B	91±17	83±18^A
LVEDP (mm Hg)	5.2±1.8	3.8±2.0^C	4.7±1.9	4.8±1.7	3.7±1.1	3.4±1.1^A
RVSP (mm Hg)	33±8	25±8^C	34±10	29±5	29±5	27±4^A
RVEDP (mm Hg)	4.7±1.2	3.6±1.0^C	4.7±1.2	6.1±1.0^C	4.6±1.2	5.5±0.7^B
EDD_{SL} (mm)	23.1±3.4	22.1±3.2^B	22.7±3.5	20.9±4.0^B	23.4±3.1	22.6±3.3^B
EDD_{AP} (mm)	31.3±2.8	29.9±2.7^C	30.9±3.2	30.8±3.3	30.7±3.1	30.7±3.0
EDD_L (mm)	46.0±3.4	45.6±3.7^A	45.8±3.5	45.7±3.4	46.3±3.4	46.4±3.5
RVEDL (mm)	15.4±2.4	15.1±2.3^B	15.4±2.7	16.8±3.0^B	16.2±2.5	17.1±2.8^A
RV %SS (%)	12.6±4.0	11.3±3.1^A	11.8±3.8	−2.6±5.8^C	15.1±3.8	0.1±5.9^C

Values are mean ± SD.

AoF = aortic flow; LVSP = left ventricular systolic pressure; LVEDP = left ventricular end-diastolic pressure; RVSP = right ventricular systolic pressure; RVEDP = right ventricular end-diastolic pressure; EDD_{SL} = end-diastolic septal-lateral dimension; EDD_{AP} = end-diastolic anterior-posterior dimension; EDD_L = end-diastolic longitudinal dimension; RVEDL = right ventricular end-diastolic segment length; RV %SS = right ventricular percent systolic shortening; C_1 = the first control; IVCO = inferior vena cava occlusion; C_2 = the second control; $RCAO_{Pi}$ = right coronary artery occlusion with the pericardium intact; C_3 = the third control; $RCAO_{Po}$ = right coronary artery occlusion with the pericardium open.

$^Ap < .05$; $^Bp < .01$; $^Cp < .001$ compared with each control value by paired t test.

0.5 mm Hg), compared with the respective control values. There were concomitant decreases in all three end-diastolic dimensions of the left ventricle, namely, septal-lateral (−4.3 ± 2.1%), anterior-posterior (−4.6 ± 1.4%), and longitudinal (−1.1 ± 1.3%) dimensions. As a result, the ratio of end-diastolic septal-lateral to anterior-posterior dimensions (D_{SL}/D_{AP}), which is considered to be an index of eccentricity of the left ventricular equatorial plane, did not change (0.74 ± 0.07 to 0.74 ± 0.07). Right ventricular end-diastolic segment length (15.4 ± 2.4 to 15.1 ± 2.3 mm) and its percent systolic shortening (12.6 ± 4.0% to 11.3 ± 3.1%) also decreased slightly during IVC occlusion.

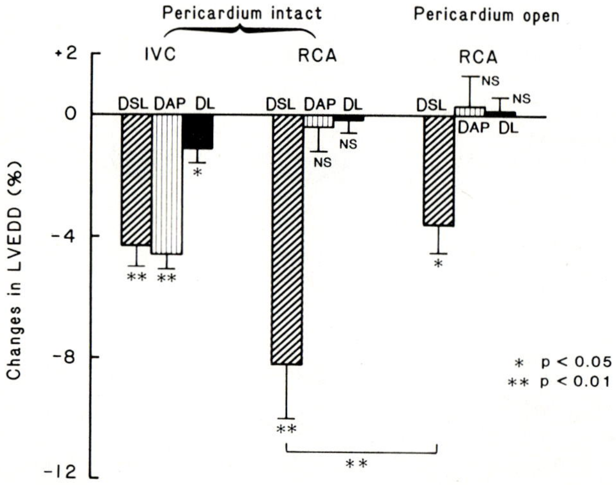

FIGURE 4. Changes in left ventricular end-diastolic dimensions (LVEDD) during IVC or RCA occlusion with the pericardium intact and open (group 1). Data are expressed as the percentage of change from each control value. During IVC occlusion, septal-lateral (D_{SL}), anterior-posterior (D_{AP}), and longitudinal (D_L) dimensions all decreased significantly. However, during RCA occlusion, only the D_{SL} decreased significantly. The decrease in the D_{SL} was significantly less with the pericardium open than with it intact in spite of the fact that the coronary occlusions were of the same duration (2 min). Means ± SE are indicated.

During RCA occlusion with the pericardium intact, the right ventricular end-diastolic segment length increased (15.4 ± 2.7 to 16.8 ± 3.0 mm), its percent systolic shortening decreased markedly (11.8 ± 3.8% to −2.6 ± 5.8%), and right ventricular end-diastolic pressure rose (+1.4 ± 0.6 mm Hg), indicating right ventricular ischemia. Concomitantly, aortic flow (−24.0 ± 9.4%) and left ventricular systolic pressure (−17.2 ± 12.1%) decreased by similar degrees to those seen during IVC occlusion, but left ventricular end-diastolic pressure did not change. In contrast to IVC occlusion, among left ventricular end-diastolic dimensions, only the septal-lateral dimension showed a significant decrease (−8.2 ± 5.0%), while anterior-posterior and longitudinal dimensions remained unchanged (figure 4). As a result, D_{SL}/D_{AP} decreased significantly (0.73 ± 0.06 to 0.68 ± 0.08, $p < .01$).

After the pericardium was opened, RCA occlusion also increased right ventricular end-diastolic segment length (16.2 ± 2.5 to 17.1 ± 2.8 mm), markedly decreased the percent systolic shortening (15.1 ± 3.8 to 0.1 ± 5.9%), and elevated right ventricular end-diastolic pressure (+0.9 ± 0.5 mm Hg). Aortic flow (−12.9 ± 4.9%) and left ventricular systolic pressure (−9.6 ± 10.6%) decreased concomitantly, but these

TABLE 2
Left ventricular end-diastolic volume and systolic function during IVC or RCA occlusion

	IVCO	$RCAO_{Pi}$	p value (paired t test)
LVEDV (ml)	15.7±2.6	15.4±3.6	NS
AoF (ml/min)	400±51	387±84	NS
LVSP (mm Hg)	87±14	85±22	NS
Peak dP/dt (mm Hg/sec)	1980±530	1904±761	NS
LV %SS (%)	12.3±2.6	11.4±3.3	NS

Values are mean ± SD.
LVEDV = left ventricular end-diastolic volume; AoF = aortic flow; LVSP = left ventricular systolic pressure; mean LV %SS = mean left ventricular percent systolic shortening; IVCO = IVC occlusion; $RCAO_{Pi}$ = RCA occlusion with the pericardium intact.

reductions were significantly less ($p < .01$) than those observed with the pericardium intact, despite the same duration (2 min) of occlusion. There were slight decreases in end-diastolic septal-lateral dimension ($-3.6 \pm 2.5\%$) and D_{SL}/D_{AP} (0.76 ± 0.08 to 0.74 ± 0.09, $p < .05$) without changes in anterior-posterior and longitudinal dimensions. The decrease in end-diastolic septal-lateral dimension was significantly less ($p < .01$) with the pericardium open than with it intact, although the procedure was the same (figure 4).

To evaluate the effects of RCA occlusion on left ventricular myocardial performance, left ventricular end-diastolic volume and parameters of left ventricular systolic function during RCA occlusion with the pericardium intact were compared with those observed during IVC occlusion (table 2). Left ventricular end-diastolic volume was not different, and all parameters, i.e., aortic flow, left ventricular systolic pressure, peak dP/dt, and mean left ventricular percent systolic shortening, were similar in the two conditions.

Group 2. Hemodynamic and right ventricular segment length data determined during blood transfusion under control conditions and during RCA occlusion in group 2 dogs are summarized in table 3. When the data obtained during RCA occlusion were compared with the respective control values at matched left ventricular end-diastolic pressures (8 and 16 mm Hg), the changes were similar to those observed in group 1 dogs. Data observed at other end-diastolic pressures (6, 10, 12, and 14 mm Hg) were similar.

The end-diastolic pressure-diameter relationship before and during RCA occlusions with the pericardium intact and open are presented in figure 5. Among the three end-diastolic pressure-diameter relationships of the left ventricle, the most remarkable shift to the left was in the septal-lateral dimension whether the pericardium was intact or open. Furthermore, the leftward shift was greater with the pericardium intact or at high end-diastolic pressure than with the pericardium open or at low end-diastolic pressure. End-diastolic pressure-diameter relationships of anterior-posterior and longitudinal dimensions showed only minimal or no changes.

Left ventricular end-diastolic pressure-volume rela-

TABLE 3
Effects of RCA occlusion on hemodynamics and right ventricular segment length in group 2 dogs

	Pericardium intact		Pericardium open	
	Control	RCAO	Control	RCAO
LVSP (mm Hg)				
LVEDP 8 mm Hg	116.4±19.1	109.0±20.2^B	121.6±14.8	124.4±15.3
LVEDP 16 mm Hg	139.8±22.5	134.9±21.6^A	153.3±17.2	154.4±18.6
RVSP (mm Hg)				
LVEDP 8 mm Hg	33.8±6.3	31.9±5.9^B	33.8±7.5	32.8±7.2
LVEDP 16 mm Hg	41.0±6.7	37.1±5.8^A	42.1±8.8	39.6±7.4^A
RVEDP (mm Hg)				
LVEDP 8 mm Hg	7.8±0.7	8.6±1.2	6.9±1.8	8.4±2.0^B
LVEDP 16 mm Hg	13.0±1.6	15.9±2.1^C	9.8±1.9	12.9±2.5^A
RVEDL (mm)				
LVEDP 8 mm Hg	18.1±4.1	19.0±4.2^B	19.4±3.9	20.6±4.7^A
LVEDP 16 mm Hg	19.6±4.4	20.9±4.2^B	20.8±4.3	21.7±4.7^B
RV %SS (%)				
LVEDP 8 mm Hg	13.7±4.8	0.8±4.7^C	14.6±4.8	3.9±4.7^B
LVEDP 16 mm Hg	17.4±4.5	3.6±5.1^C	12.8±4.6	2.9±2.4^C

Values are means ± SD.
RCAO = RCA occlusion; other abbreviations as in table 1.
^A$p < .05$; ^B$p < .01$; ^C$p < .001$ compared with each control value by paired t test.

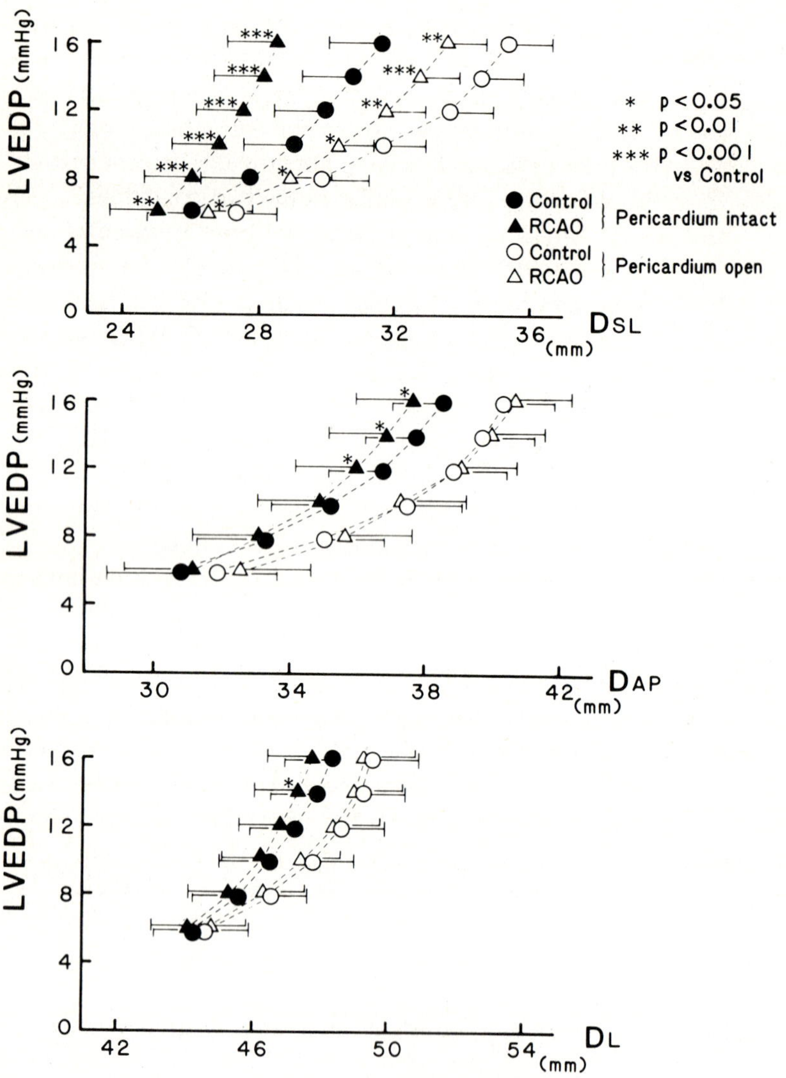

FIGURE 5. Left ventricular end-diastolic pressure-diameter relationship before and during RCA occlusion (RCAO) with the pericardium intact and open (group 2). Comparisons were performed by the paired t test with the respective control values at matched left ventricular end-diastolic pressures (LVEDP). Among the three end-diastolic pressure-diameter relationships, the most remarkable shift to the left was shown in the septal-lateral dimension, whether the pericardium was intact or open. Furthermore, the leftward shift was greater with the pericardium intact or at high end-diastolic pressure than with the pericardium open or at low end-diastolic pressure. D_{SL} = septal-lateral dimension; D_{AP} = anterior-posterior dimension; D_L = longitudinal dimension. Means ± SE are indicated.

tionships before and during RCA occlusion with the pericardium intact and open are shown in figure 6. At matched end-distolic pressures over 8 mm Hg, RCA occlusion with the pericardium intact significantly reduced left ventricular end-diastolic volume. Also, after the pericardium was opened, RCA occlusion reduced end-diastolic volume at matched end-diastolic pressure over 10 mm Hg. The reductions in end-diastolic volume were significantly greater with the pericardium intact than with it open except at end-diastolic pressures of 6 and 10 mm Hg (table 4).

Left ventricular end-diastolic pressure-volume data during control volume loading closely approximated the fourth-order polynomial (equation 3) in all animals, and the correlation coefficient averaged .998 ± .001 with the pericardium intact and .998 ± .002 with it open (table 5). Except in one dog with the pericardium intact (p = .060) and in one other dog with the pericardium open (p = .064), the b values during RCA occlusion were significant in all animals whether the pericardium was intact or open. However, compared with the values with the pericardium intact, the b values with the pericardium open were significantly smaller ($p < .001$), both by paired and pooled data analysis.

Discussion

The major new findings of the present study are (1) right ventricular ischemia shifts the interventricular septum to the left in end-diastole without changing left ventricular myocardial performance, (2) right ventricular ischemia causes a leftward and upward shift of the left ventricular end-diastolic pressure-volume relationship, and (3) the intact pericardium augments these effects.

The hemodynamic and dimensional changes during IVC occlusion in group 1 dogs indicate that the reduction of stroke volume was primarily due to the reduction of left ventricular end-diastolic volume. These findings are consistent with previous findings[5, 14] that

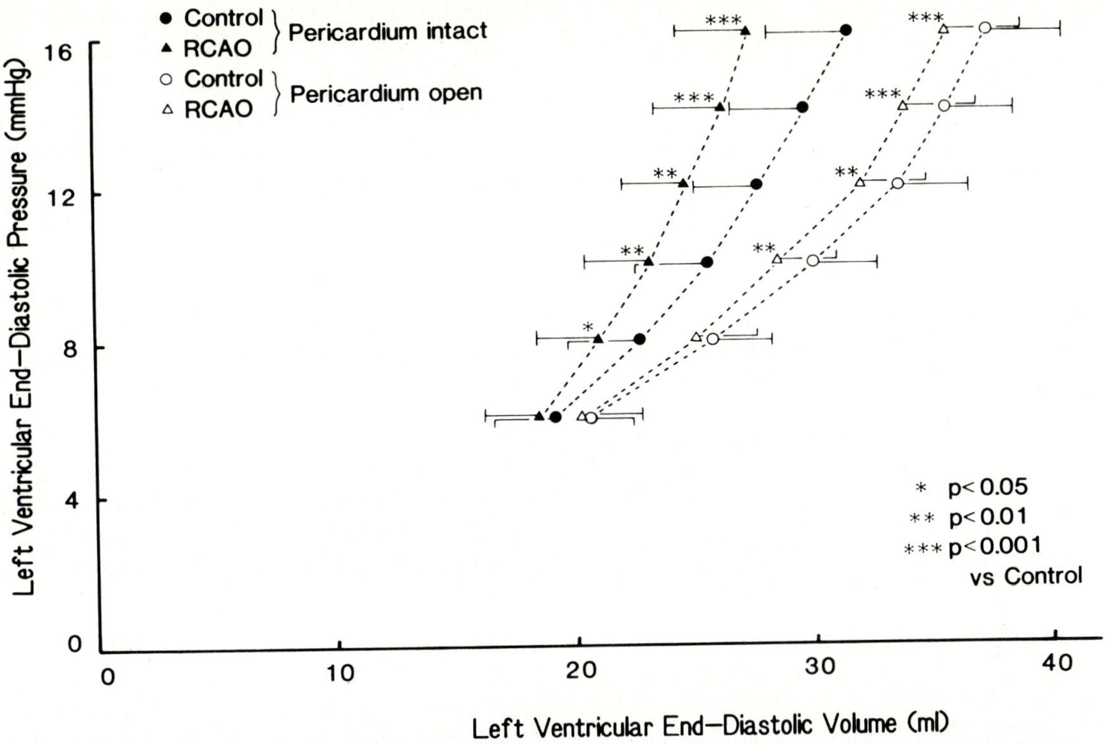

FIGURE 6. Left ventricular end-diastolic pressure-volume relationship obtained by rapid blood transfusion before and during RCA occlusion (RCAO) with the pericardium intact and open in group 2 dogs. Compared with the respective control values, RCAO significantly shifted the relationship to the left at end-diastolic pressures over 8 mm Hg with the pericardium intact and over 10 mm Hg with the pericardium open.

IVC occlusion simply reduces left ventricular preload, with no change in geometry except in the earliest phase when the interventricular septum often shifts rightward.[5] In contrast, the hemodynamic and dimensional changes during RCA occlusion indicate that ischemic right ventricular dysfunction causes a disproportionate decrease in septal-lateral dimension, and hence distorted the left ventricular end-diastolic geometry, despite a reduction similar to that during IVC occlusion in end-diastolic volume, aortic flow, and left ventricular systolic pressure. These geometric changes, as well as the reductions of aortic flow and left ventricular systolic pressure observed during RCA occlusion, were significantly attenuated after the pericardium was opened. Because the degree of right ventricular ischemia probably remained unchanged, these attenuations can be attributed to opening of the intact pericardium.

In group 2 dogs, the left ventricular end-diastolic pressure-volume relationship during RCA occlusion shifted leftward and upward significantly (figure 6; tables 4 and 5). These changes can be attributed to the leftward shift of the end-diastolic pressure-diameter relationship of the septal-lateral dimension during RCA occlusion (figure 5). These findings indicate that an acute dilatation and end-diastolic pressure elevation of the right ventricle causes encroachment on the left ventricle by the interventricular septum, resulting in a leftward and upward shift of the pressure-volume relationship. The intact pericardium augments these effects. We can assume that, in this situation, the right and left ventricles not only are aligned in series, but also interact directly through the interventricular septum.[5]

On the basis of these results, we can at least partly attribute the absent or minimal circulatory derangement in previous studies in which the right ventricular free wall was damaged by cauterization[15–18] or RCA

TABLE 4
Reduction in left ventricular end-diastolic volume (ml) during RCA occlusion in group 2 dogs

	Pericardium intact	Pericardium open
LVEDP 6 mm Hg	0.6±1.0	0.0±1.1
LVEDP 8 mm Hg	1.9±1.7	0.5±1.0[A]
LVEDP 10 mm Hg	2.4±1.6	1.6±1.2
LVEDP 12 mm Hg	2.9±1.6	1.5±0.9[A]
LVEDP 14 mm Hg	3.3±1.4	1.7±0.8[A]
LVEDP 16 mm Hg	4.1±1.7	1.7±0.6[B]

Values are mean ± SD.

LVEDP = left ventricular end-diastolic pressure.

[A]$p < .05$; [B]$p < .01$ compared with the pericardium intact value by paired t test.

TABLE 5
Effects of RCA occlusion on the left ventricular end-diastolic pressure-volume relationship in group 2 dogs

Dog No.	Pericardial condition	Control n	Control r	RCAO n	RCAO b±SD	p value
1	Intact	7	.999	7	2.55±1.64	<.01
	Open	7	.995	8	0.88±0.85	<.05
2	Intact	7	.995	6	3.45±1.57	<.01
	Open	7	.998	7	1.38±1.15	<.05
3	Intact	9	.999	9	1.63±1.73	<.05
	Open	9	.998	8	0.88±0.62	<.01
4	Intact	9	.999	8	2.66±1.81	<.01
	Open	10	.999	8	1.10±1.07	<.05
5	Intact	6	.999	6	0.60±0.60	.060
	Open	6	.996	6	0.51±0.43	<.05
6	Intact	9	.997	9	1.88±2.11	<.05
	Open	8	.998	10	0.78±1.00	<.05
7	Intact	11	.999	11	2.21±2.23	<.01
	Open	10	.997	10	1.00±1.06	<.05
8	Intact	8	.998	8	2.13±2.28	<.05
	Open	8	.999	8	1.00±1.29	.064
Paired data						
Pericardium intact (n = 8)					2.14±0.83	
Pericardium open (n = 8)					0.94±0.25	<.001[A]
Pooled data						
Pericardium intact (n = 64)					2.13±1.91	
Pericardium open (n = 65)					0.94±0.96	<.001[B]

Left ventricular end-diastolic pressure-volume data were approximated as fourth-order polynomials (equation 3). See text for details.

RCAO = RCA occlusion; r = correlation coefficient of fitting to equation 3; b = coefficient in equation 3 that indicates the amount of the upward shift of the end-diastolic pressure-volume relationship during RCAO; p value = significance of b during RCAO compared with each control by unpaired t test.

[A]Significance of difference in b for intact and open pericardium by paired t test.

[B]Significance of difference in b for intact and open pericardium based on analysis of pooled data (unpaired t test).

ligation[19] to the use of a preparation with an open pericardium. Recently, Goldstein et al.[9] produced right ventricular infarction by RCA occlusion with the pericardium intact and observed an elevation of intrapericardial pressure and significant reductions of mean aortic pressure and cardiac output. However, they did not evaluate left ventricular geometry or the diastolic pressure-volume relationship. Our present study is therefore the first one showing that right ventricular ischemia is a pathologic condition that causes a leftward shift of the interventricular septum and a leftward and upward shift of the left ventricular diastolic pressure-volume relationship.

The effects of right ventricular ischemia on left ventricular geometry and hemodynamics have some resemblance to those of pulmonary artery constriction during which the interventricular septum shifts leftward, the diastolic pressure-volume curve also shifts leftward, and left ventricular stroke volume decreases.[5, 14] However, when our data are compared with those from studies of acute pulmonary artery constriction,[5, 14] the increase in right ventricular end-diastolic pressure during our RCA occlusion seems smaller (1.4 vs 3.0 and 3.7 mm Hg), despite a similar decrease in left ventricular stroke volume. This might be attributable to the difference in the degree of right ventricular dilatation between the two conditions. Using two-dimensional echocardiography, Goldstein et al.[9] reported a 110% increase in right ventricular end-diastolic size after RCA occlusion in the dog, while Stool et al.[4] reported only a 46% to 52% increase in right ventricular end-diastolic volume during acute pulmonary artery hypertension that reduced stroke volume by 19% to 39%. In addition, although a significant increase in intrapericardial pressure has been reported during RCA occlusion,[9] Kenner and Wood[20] found no increase in this pressure during acute pulmonary artery obstruction. Thus, during right ventricular ischemia, the acute and marked right ventricular dilatation within the relatively stiff pericardium might affect left ventricular geometry and hemodynamics by increasing intrapericardial pressure even when the increase in right ventricular end-diastolic pressure is relatively small.

One potential limitation in our study is related to the accuracy of the left ventricular volume measurement. Although we validated our crystal method in excised hearts, we could not validate the method in a beating heart. Also, there seems to have been a slight underestimation in our calculated volume, probably because the position of the basal crystal had to be slightly lower than the level of the aortic valve. However, the correlation between calculated and directly measured volume was highly linear in each animal, and changes in left ventricular geometry would not have affected the measurement.[14] Therefore, the present method provides a reliable index of left ventricular volume.

Another potential problem is that the brief periods of right ventricular ischemia have resulted in persistent diastolic abnormalities in the right ventricle. However, right ventricular systolic pressure, end-diastolic pressure, and percent systolic shortening during the third control period were not significantly different ($p > 0.1$) from those during the second control period (table 1). Therefore, the prolonged effects of brief ischemia, if any, were negligible.

The leftward and upward shift of the left ventricular end-diastolic pressure-volume relationship could be caused by changes in viscous properties or by acute ischemia of the left ventricle.[3, 21] In group 2 dogs use of the rapid blood transfusion itself might raise the possibility that the changes in viscous properties of the left ventricle altered the end-diastolic pressure-volume relationship.[22] However, we infused blood at the same rate during both control and RCA occlusion periods. The choice to read end-diastolic values also tends to minimize viscous effects since ventricular filling is relatively slow near end-diastole. Therefore, the observed shift in the relationship during RCA occlusion could not be attributed to changes in viscous properties. Also, we found that the RCA territory was confined to the right ventricular free wall, as Blair[23] reported, and that the indexes of left ventricular systolic function during RCA occlusion were not different from those observed at a comparable level of left ventricular end-diastolic volume during IVC occlusion (table 2), so that left ventricular ischemia would not have occurred during our RCA occlusion.

The results of the present study indicate that the primary mechanism by which aortic flow is decreased during right ventricular ischemia is a reduction of left ventricular end-diastolic volume, because parameters of left ventricular systolic function remain relatively constant when compared with those observed during IVC occlusion (table 2). Olsen et al.[14] reported that the parameters of left ventricular systolic function measured during pulmonary artery and IVC occlusions were similar at a matched left ventricular end-diastolic volume, despite significant interventricular septal shift and alteration of left ventricular shape. Our results suggest that their conclusion that end-diastolic volume or mean myocardial fiber length is the major preload determinant of left ventricular systolic function independent of chamber pressure and shape also holds true under conditions of right ventricular ischemia.

In addition, our results suggest that the reduction of left ventricular end-diastolic volume during right ventricular ischemia can itself be attributed to two mechanisms. One is right ventricular systolic dysfunction,[9] which reduces right ventricular output. This was suggested in our study by the decrease in right ventricular systolic pressure during RCA occlusion. The other mechanism is the leftward and upward shift of the left ventricular end-diastolic pressure-volume relationship. When right ventricular systolic function is constant, i.e., when left ventricular filling pressure is constant, the leftward and upward shift of the pressure-volume relationship itself results in a decrease in left ventricular end-diastolic volume for a given end-diastolic pressure. The presence of the latter mechanism was suggested by our finding that the greater shift in the pressure-volume relationship during RCA occlusion was accompanied by a greater decrease in aortic flow with the pericardium intact than with the pericardium open, because the degree of ischemic right ventricular dysfunction was similar and left ventricular myocardial performance would be the same under the two conditions. Thus, series ventricular interaction, together with substantial direct interaction, seems responsible for the reduction in left ventricular end-diastolic volume during right ventricular ischemia.

The findings shown in the present study cannot be applied directly to the clinical setting, because clinical right ventricular infarction is usually accompanied by left ventricular inferior or posterior infarction.[24, 25] However, there is one case report of a patient with right ventricular infarction who had interventricular septum convexity toward the left ventricle during diastole on the two-dimensional echocardiogram.[26] Therefore, the present results merit further studies of ventricular interaction in clinical right ventricular infarction.

In summary, right ventricular ischemia causes a leftward shift of the interventricular septum in end-diastole, distorts left ventricular geometry, and also causes a leftward and upward displacement of the left ventricular end-diastolic pressure-volume relationship, without changing left ventricular myocardial performance. The presence of the intact pericardium augments these changes. The reduction of aortic flow during right ventricular ischemia seems to be primarily due to the reduction of left ventricular end-diastolic volume, which may be attributable to right ventricular systolic dysfunction and the leftward and upward shift in the left ventricular end-diastolic pressure-volume relationship.

We thank Nobuko Ishitsubo for her technical assistance and Dr. Hiroyuki Suga and Dr. Alice S. Cary for their helpful advice in the preparation and revision of this manuscript.

References

1. Taylor RR, Covell JW, Sonnenblick EH, Ross J Jr: Dependence of ventricular distensibility on filling of the opposite ventricle. Am J Physiol **213:** 711, 1967
2. Glantz SA, Misbach GA, Moores WY, Mathey DG, Lekven J, Stowe DF, Parmley WW, Tyberg JV: The pericardium substantially affects the left ventricular diastolic pressure-volume relationship in the dog. Circ Res **42:** 433, 1978
3. Glantz SA, Parmley WW: Factors which affect the diastolic pressure-volume curve. Circ Res **42:** 171, 1978
4. Stool EW, Mullins CB, Leshin SJ, Mitchell JH: Dimensional changes of the left ventricle during acute pulmonary arterial hypertension in dogs. Am J Cardiol **33:** 868, 1974
5. Visner MS, Arentzen CE, O'Connor MJ, Larson EV, Anderson RW: Alterations in left ventricular three-dimensional dynamic ge-

ometry and systolic function during acute right ventricular hypertension in the conscious dog. Circulation **67:** 353, 1983

6. Weyman AE, Wann S, Feigenbaum H, Dillon JC: Mechanism of abnormal septal motion in patients with right ventricular volume overload. A cross-sectional echocardiographic study. Circulation **54:** 179, 1976
7. Brinker JA, Weiss JL, Lappe DL, Rabson JL, Summer WR, Permutt S, Weisfeldt ML: Leftward septal displacement during right ventricular loading in man. Circulation **61:** 626, 1980
8. Scharf SM, Brown R, Saunders N, Green LH, Ingram RH: Changes in canine left ventricular size and configuration with positive end-expiratory pressure. Circ Res **44:** 672, 1979
9. Goldstein JA, Vlahakes GJ, Verrier ED, Schiller NB, Tyberg JV, Ports TA, Parmley WW, Chatterjee K: The role of right ventricular systolic dysfunction and elevated intrapericardial pressure in the genesis of low output in experimental right ventricular infarction. Circulation **65:** 513, 1982
10. Spadaro J, Bing OHL, Gaasch WH, Weintraub RM: Pericardial modulation of right and left ventricular diastolic interaction. Circ Res **48:** 233, 1981
11. Rankin JS, McHale PA, Arentzen CE, Ling D, Greenfield JC, Anderson RW: The three-dimensional dynamic geometry of the left ventricle in the conscious dog. Circ Res **39:** 304, 1976
12. Glantz S: Computing indices of diastolic stiffness has been counterproductive. Fed Proc **39:** 162, 1980
13. Wallenstein S, Zucker CL, Fleiss J: Some statistical methods useful in circulation research. Circ Res **47:** 1, 1980
14. Olsen CO, Tyberg GS, Maier GW, Spratt JA, Davis JW, Rankin JS: Dynamic ventricular interaction in the conscious dog. Circ Res **52:** 85, 1983
15. Starr I, Jeffers WA, Meade RH: The absence of conspicuous increments of venous pressure after severe damage to the right ventricle of the dog, with a discussion of the relation between clinical congestive failure and heart disease. Am Heart J **26:** 291, 1943
16. Bacos ACP: The question of the function of the right ventricular myocardium: An experimental study. Circulation **1:** 724, 1950
17. Kagan A: Dynamic responses of the right ventricle following extensive damage by cauterization. Circulation **5:** 816, 1952
18. Guiha NH, Constantinos JL, Cohn JN: Predominant right ventricular dysfunction after right ventricular destruction in the dog. Am J Cardiol **33:** 254, 1974
19. Brooks H, Kirk ES, Vokonas PS, Urschel CW, Sonnenblick EH: Performance of the right ventricle under stress: Relation to right coronary flow. J Clin Invest **50:** 2176, 1971
20. Kenner HM, Wood EH: Intrapericardial, intrapleural, and intracardiac pressures during acute heart failure in dogs studied without thoracotomy. Circ Res **19:** 1071, 1966
21. Ross J Jr: Acute displacement of the diastolic pressure-volume curve of the left ventricle: role of the pericardium and the right ventricle. Circulation **59:** 32, 1979
22. LeWinter MM, Engler R, Pavelec RS: Time dependent shifts of the left ventricular diastolic filling relationship in conscious dogs. Circ Res **45:** 641, 1979
23. Blair E: Anatomy of the ventricular coronary arteries in the dog. Circ Res **9:** 333, 1961
24. Isne JM, Roberts WC: Right ventricular infarction complicating left ventricular infarction secondary to coronary heart disease. Am J Cardiol **42:** 885, 1978
25. Ratliff NB, Hackel DB: Combined right and left ventricular infarction: Pathogenesis and clinicopathologic correlations. Am J Cardiol **45:** 217, 1980
26. Coma-Canella I, Lopez-Sendon J, Oliver J: Premature pulmonic valve opening and inverted septal convexity in acute ischemic right ventricular dysfunction. Am Heart J **101:** 684, 1981

Contrast echocardiographic estimation of regional myocardial blood flow after acute coronary occlusion

ANDREW J. KEMPER, M.D., THOMAS FORCE, M.D., ROBERT KLONER, M.D., MICHELE GILFOIL, B.A., LORRI PERKINS, B.A., SHARON HALE, M.S., KEVIN ALKER, B.S., AND ALFRED F. PARISI, M.D.

ABSTRACT Contrast echocardiography can predict pathologic area at risk during acute coronary occlusion. In this study we evaluated (1) whether the intensity and timing of contrast appearance in ischemic regions can provide a quantitative measure of residual myocardial perfusion, and (2) whether changes in these parameters observed after serial injections reflect changes in blood flow to acutely ischemic tissue. Supra-aortic hydrogen peroxide contrast echocardiography was performed in 12 consecutive dogs at 1, 20, and 120 min after acute circumflex coronary occlusion. Contrast enhancement was determined qualitatively with a segmental four-point scoring system based on the appearance time and peak perceived intensity of contrast enhancement and quantitatively with a computer algorithm designed to reflect these parameters. Comparison was made in each segment to concomitant radioactive microsphere blood flow. Qualitative scoring related systematically to normalized segmental blood flow (3+ = 93%; 2+ = 61%; 1+ = 32%; 0 = 18%; $p < .01$ for each vs adjacent value), as did quantitative analysis including all segments ($r = .78$; $p < .01$) and isolated to the ischemic region (flow = 1.13 intensity change + 6.8%; $r = .83$, $p < .001$). Changes in microsphere flow in ischemic regions between sequential observations were correlated with changes in qualitative score ($r = .88$, $p < .001$) and results of quantitative analysis ($r = 0.70$, $p < .01$). The amount of contrast enhancement can provide quantitative information about residual myocardial blood flow in ischemic regions and can also be used to track changing patterns of flow in vivo after acute coronary occlusion.
Circulation **72, No. 5, 1115–1124, 1985.**

THE SUPRA-AORTIC INJECTION of microbubble-containing solutions during echocardiographic imaging of the heart results in an intense increase in myocardial contrast in regions that receive normal blood flow. Regions that are severely malperfused do not enhance and can be seen as a contrast defect. Studies in our laboratory and others indicate that the size of this contrast defect accurately predicts the size in vivo of the region that is at risk of infarction after acute coronary occlusion.[1–5] Contrast analyses have not previously been evaluated for their ability to quantify the amount, rather than the presence or absence, of flow within the ischemic region.

During our previous studies of supra-aortic hydrogen peroxide contrast echocardiography in canine infarction we observed in some animals a pattern of delayed contrast appearance in the initially ischemic region on observation later after an acute occlusion. In others, the pattern and amount of contrast did not change on sequential observations.

The canine preparation of acute coronary ligation and infarction is notable because a substantial proportion of these animals have preformed epicardial collateral vessels that dilate in response to regional ischemia. Animals that have epicardial collaterals may show a spontaneous improvement in blood flow to the ischemic region during the first several hours after occlusion.[6–7] We hypothesized that the changing pattern of the intensity of echocardiographic myocardial contrast enhancement we observed in prior experiments represented changes in regional myocardial blood flow. Therefore, the present study was designed to compare serial observations of the pattern and intensity of myocardial contrast enhancement with concomitant regional blood flow after acute coronary occlusion. Contrast enhancement resulting from supra-aortic injection of hydrogen peroxide was assessed qualitatively, based on the perceived intensity and

From the Department of Medicine, Cardiology Section of the Veterans Administration Medical Center, West Roxbury and Brockton, MA, and the Department of Medicine, Brigham and Women's Hospital and Harvard Medical School, Boston.
Supported by the Research Service of the U.S. Veterans Administration.
Address for correspondence: Andrew J. Kemper, M.D., Department of Medicine, Cardiology Section, Veterans Administration Medical Center, 1400 VFW Parkway, West Roxbury, MA 02132.
Received Jan. 14, 1985; revision accepted Aug. 8, 1985.

temporal course of appearance in the myocardium, and quantitatively, with a computer-based analysis of regional pixel intensity. Comparison was made with regional microsphere blood flow by use of echocardiographic markers and a grid system.

Methods

Experimental animal preparation. After preliminary imaging to ensure adequate two-dimensional echocardiographic epicardial and endocardial target definition, 12 mongrel dogs were selected for study. They were premedicated with 1 mg/kg morphine, anesthetized with 10 mg/kg pentobarbitol, intubated, and placed on a Harvard respirator. The heart was exposed through a standard left thoracotomy and the circumflex artery distal to the origin of the first obtuse marginal was dissected free. To maintain correct anatomic location for sequential studies, a stainless steel clip, 2 mm × 6 mm, was inserted under echocardiographic guidance into the anterior wall of the left ventricle at the level of the mitral chordae. The jugular vein and carotid artery were cannulated. Five minutes after the intravenous injection of 1 mg/kg of lidocaine, the coronary artery was occluded with a Schwartz clamp. The occlusion was maintained for 6 hr.

Echocardiographic techniques. The myocardial contrast echocardiographic technique using supra-aortic hydrogen peroxide injection is described in detail elsewhere.[4-5] Briefly, a modified pigtail catheter was inserted into the left femoral artery and advanced to a level just above the aortic cusps with the use of echocardiographic guidance. The catheter was attached to bulb flush extension tubing and a constant drip was maintained. To prevent clotting of the catheter side holes, 2000 units heparin was added to the drip saline solution.

The left ventricle was imaged with the standard closed-chest right sternal border approach. A short-axis view was obtained at the level of the myocardial marker (mitral chordae) with a two-dimensional ultrasonograph with a 3 MHz/13 mm transducer (ATL/ADR). The ultrasonograph was interfaced with a commercial color videodensitometer (Colorado Video) that displays a color image where all echo image gray scale intensities are translated into a predetermined eight-step color scale ranging from blue to red. The preprocessing settings on the echocardiograph (enh 1, comp b) were maintained constant throughout all studies. Gain, reject, and brightness controls were adjusted before the initial injection by interaction with the color image to obtain a low-level homogeneous video output throughout the myocardium. Subsequent injections were made with the same settings. Echocardiographic images were recorded for future analysis (Panasonic model No. NV8950) on a ½ inch T-60 VHS cassette.

Contrast echocardiograms were recorded for a period of 1 to 2 min after supra-aortic injection of 2 ml of 0.3% H_2O_2 solution and 1 ml heparinized blood at 1, 20, 120 min after occlusion. Before the animals were killed, to assist in accurate localization of pathologic material, a second steel clip was placed circumferentially approximately 3 cm from the first clip within the image plane with the use of echocardiographic guidance. Monastral blue pigment (0.5 ml/kg) was injected via the left atrial line. Twenty seconds after the injection, the animals were killed with KCl solution and their hearts were removed. The left ventricle was dissected free and an 8 mm thick section was made centered on the echocardiographic markers parallel to the atrioventricular groove.

Regional myocardial blood flow (RMBF). Radioactive microspheres (4.0 x 10^6, 9 to 11 μm) labeled with ^{46}Sc, ^{113}Sn or ^{141}Ce were injected into the left atrium immediately before contrast echocardiographic studies at 1, 20, and 120 min of occlusion. A reference blood sample was drawn simultaneously from the carotid artery at a rate of 15.3 ml/min.

After the animals were killed, zones for measurement of regional myocardial blood flow were determined with the use of the monastral blue boundaries as a guide. Transmural tissue samples (approximately 4 mm wide) were cut sequentially from the entire region unperfused by the monastral blue dye and from areas 3 to 4 cm on both sides of the unperfused zone. Normal reference samples were obtained from the anterior wall directly opposite the center of the nonperfused zone. Tissue samples were weighed and counted along with the reference blood samples in a gamma well counter. Regional myocardial blood flow was then calculated as previously described.[9] All individual values in the region of interest were expressed as a percentage of the normal flow for each study. The reference microsphere flow, central ischemic flow, and normalized central flow are presented in Appendix 1.

Data analysis. For qualitative echocardiographic analyses, the echocardiographic studies were replayed in real time by an observer blinded to the microsphere flow data. A 24 segment radial grid was superimposed on the monitor face and centered on the end-diastolic center of mass, with the junction of segments 4 and 5 corresponding to the posterolateral right ventricular/septal junction (figure 1). The course of contrast enhancement in each segment was reviewed in slow motion and selected end-diastolic stop frames were used for reference.

A small region of contrast enhancement was initially seen in the region of the anterior wall. A wave of intense enhancement of both endocardium and epicardium could be seen to progress circumferentially in both directions from this region toward the posterior wall over the next two to three diastoles. Segments receiving intense contrast by the fourth diastole were graded 3+ (immediate).

In some animals, a secondary wave of contrast enhancement could be seen within portions of the previously nonenhanced region. This enhancement appeared to proceed from epicardium

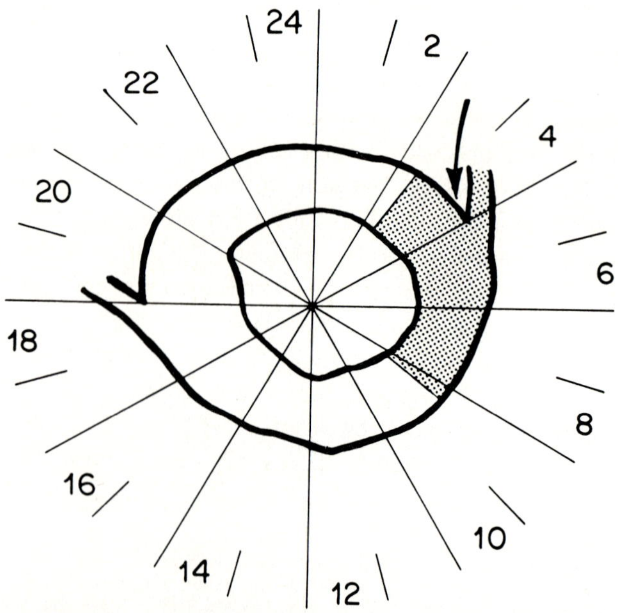

FIGURE 1. Orientation of 24-segment radial grid for echocardiographic contrast analysis and matching of microsphere flow samples. The grid was centered on the epicardial center of mass with the junction of segments 4 and 5 placed at the posterior right ventriculoseptal junction (arrow). The shaded area represents an echocardiographic contrast defect.

toward endocardium. If the intensity level reached was perceived as greater than 50% of surrounding grade 3 segments by the twelfth end-diastole, the segment was graded 2+. If the intensity increase was less striking (<50% of 3+ level), but perceptible by the twentieth diastole after injection, the segment was graded 1+. Regions that received minimal (<10% of 3+ level) or no contrast enhancement were graded 0.

Segmental interobserver and intraobserver variability for the qualitative analysis was determined by review of a summary tape of 20 randomly selected contrast studies. Two observers each reviewed the tape twice at 1 month intervals. Intraobserver correlations were r = .91 and r = .86, respectively. Interobserver correlations ranged from r = .84 to r = .90. A total of 108 of 1548 (6.5%) paired segment ratings varied by more than 1 grade; 78 of 108 occurred at the borders of the ischemic region and represent alignments of the axis system differing by one segment. The raw data for those values are presented in Appendix 2.

Quantitative echocardiographic analyses were performed with a commercial computerized analysis system (Microsonics CAD 888). Single end-diastolic echocardiographic stop frames, as indicated by the initial upslope of the R wave on an accompanying electrocardiogram, were digitized with an arbitrary linear 252-step brightness scale with maximum and minimum brightness set to 252 and 0, respectively. Two end-diastoles immediately before and end-diastoles 2, 4, 10, and 12 immediately after the first appearance of intramyocardial contrast were selected for analysis for each injection. Each echocardiographic cross section was divided into 12 circumferential segments with the use of the posterior right ventriculoseptal junction as a landmark (figure 2). In each segment, a free-form crescent-shaped region was drawn that circumscribed the myocardial region of interest but carefully excluded specular endocardial and epicardial echocardiographic signals. At least six regions were drawn for each study and each included at least two segments on either side of the ensuing contrast defect. To assess the effect of contrast injection on the strength of echocardiographic signals returning from deeper myocardial structures, a background figure, 10 pixels deep and three segments wide and centered on the posterior pericardium, was also drawn. The mean pixel intensity encompassed in each of the above areas was calculated with a computer algorithm. The regions defined for the first preinjection end-diastolic frame were transferred to the second and successive frames and intensity values were similarly calculated.

To determine the change in intensity resulting from contrast injection, the background intensity (mean of frames 1 and 2) for each segment was subtracted from the intensity value of each postinjection frame. Despite our use of the color videodensitometer to normalize preinjection baseline intensity settings, when all 35 studies are considered, the mean background intensity for any individual segment varied widely (from 6 to 210 units). Therefore, to express intensity changes in comparable units between segments with varying backgrounds, all values were expressed as a percentage of the gray-scale steps remaining after background subtraction. The mean of the intensity change seen in the four postinjection frames for each segment was defined as the contrast intensity change for that segment.

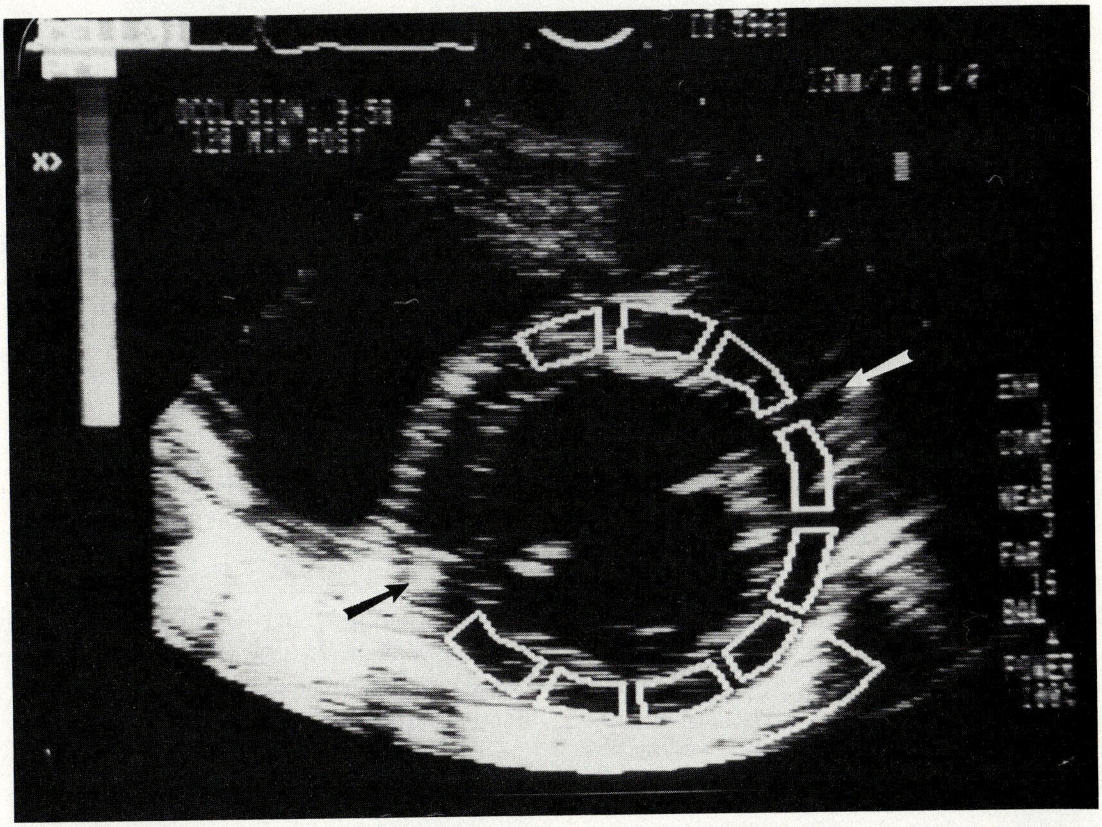

FIGURE 2. Representative frame from the computer screen demonstrating method of region delineation. A digitized short-axis echocardiographic end-diastolic frame is shown with segmental contrast regions drawn in. The regions, which correspond clockwise to segments 0 through 8, are oriented with the border of segments 2 and 3 at the posterior right ventriculoseptal junction (white arrow). The region drawn below the short axis gave a baseline brightness reading. The echocardiographic marker is visible at the anterior right ventriculoseptal junction (dark arrow).

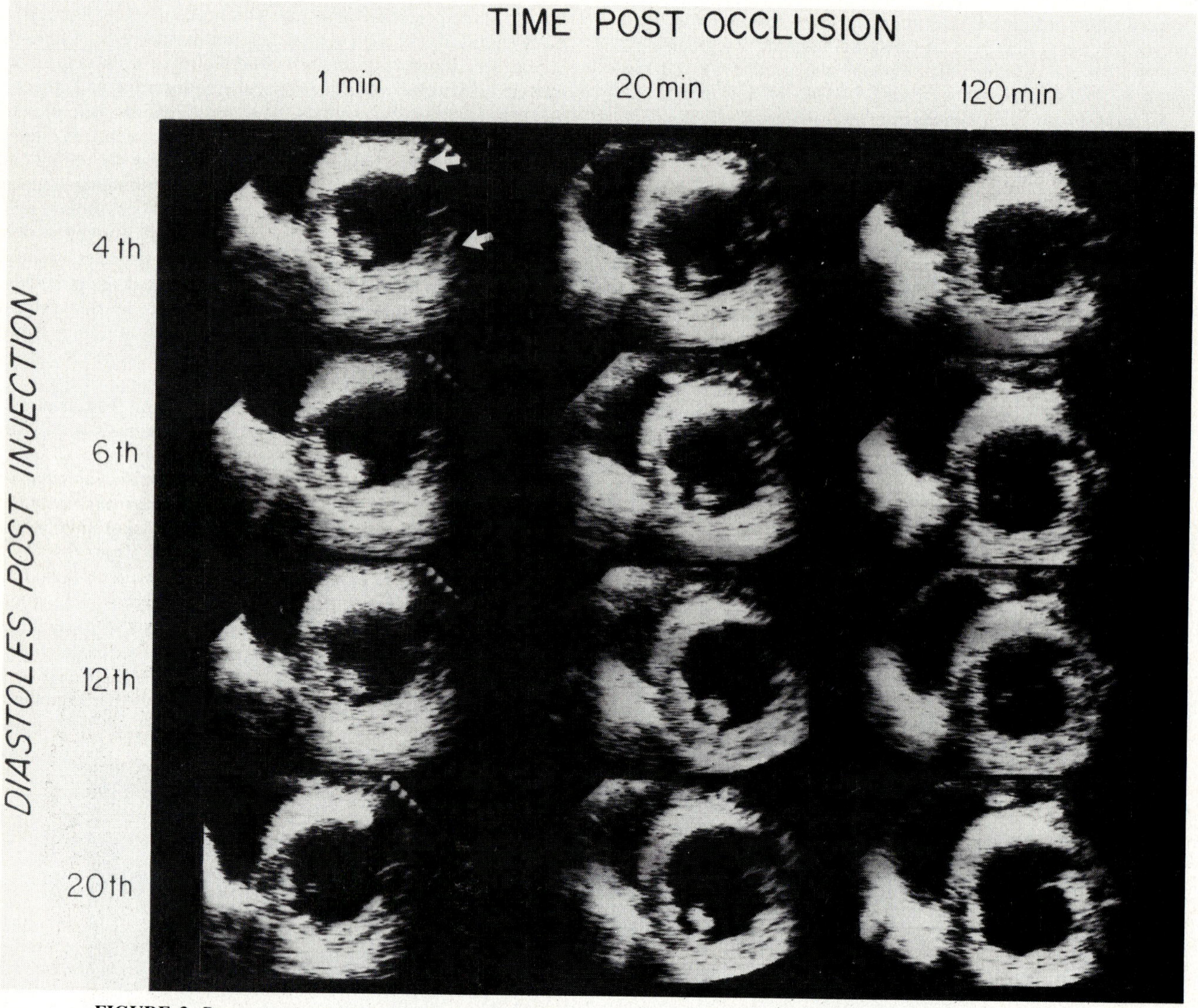

FIGURE 3. Representative still frames during contrast injections at 1, 20, and 120 min after occlusion in an animal that demonstrated increasing contrast enhancement in the ischemic region over time. Still frames for each contrast injection sequence are shown for the fourth, sixth, twelfth, and twentieth end-diastoles after myocardial contrast appearance. The region enhancing by the fourth diastole (arrows) changed little on sequential studies. Progressively more intense and earlier appearing contrast enhancement occurred within the ischemic region during the 20 and 120 min studies.

To determine the intraobserver variability for performance of the quantitative analysis, the analysis was repeated for the 120 min observations after 6 weeks. For 97 segment pairs, the correlation was r = .92, with a SEE of 10.5%. The mean enhancement value within the ischemic area comparing analyses for 12 data pairs had a correlation coefficient of r = .97, with a SEE of 4.8%.

Radial microsphere blood flow maps divided into 24 segments corresponding to the qualitative echocardiographic ratings were made by assigning flow values to each segment by superimposition of the grid system on a map of tissue samples drawn at the time of sectioning. One to two samples were assigned to each echocardiographic segment. Adjacent segments, i.e., 1 and 2, 3 and 4, etc., were combined to yield 12 segments corresponding to the quantitative analysis system.

Statistical analyses were performed with a commercial software system (NWA Statpak). Statistical significance for group data were determined by one-way analysis of variance. If significant differences were found, multiple comparisons were made with the Tukey formula for samples of equal size and Sheffe's formula for samples of unequal size.

Results

All 12 animals survived to complete the protocol. Contrast enhancement was analyzed for 35 periods of observation. One contrast study at 1 min was inadvertently erased and could not be analyzed.

Patterns of contrast enhancement over time. Although the circumferential extent of immediate (3+) contrast enhancement did not change after sequential contrast injections, lesser grades of enhancement within the immediate defect area followed highly individualized patterns. In five animals, virtually the entire region encompassed within the immediate contrast defect

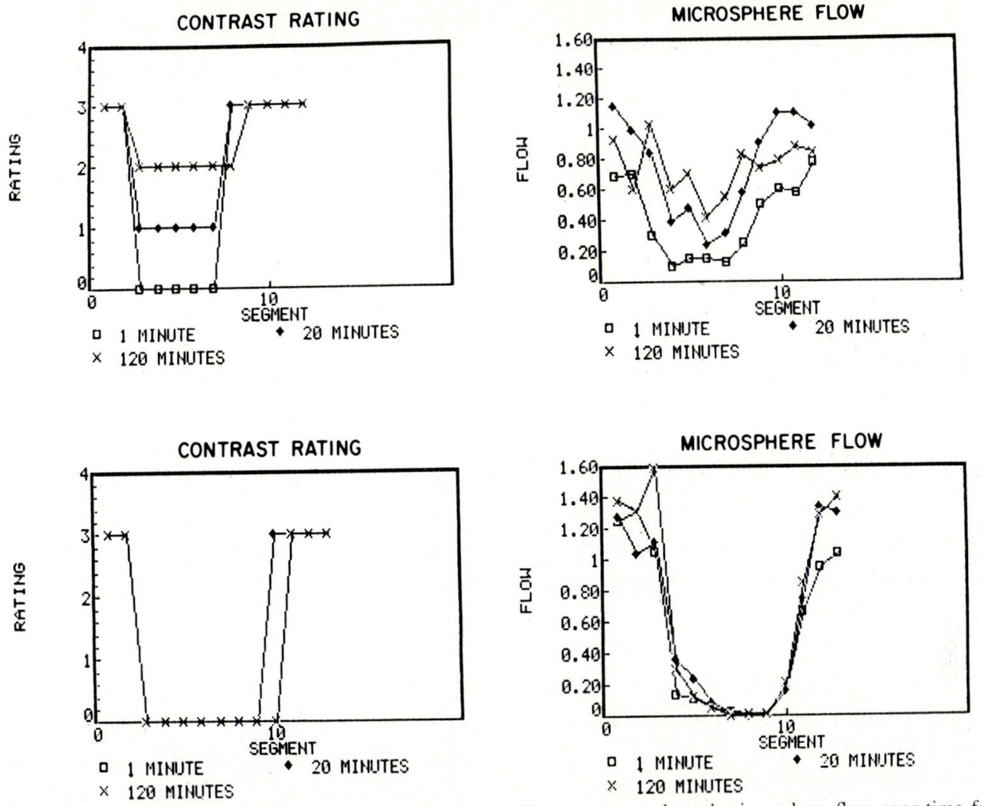

FIGURE 4. Computer-generated radial maps for echocardiographic contrast grade and microsphere flow over time for two representative animals. *Top*, The contrast rating map (*left*) and flow map (*right*) for the animal shown in figure 2, in which there was increasing contrast enhancement within the ischemic region on sequential studies. *Bottom*, Contrast (*left*) and flow (*right*) maps for an animal in which there was no late contrast enhancement within the ischemic region on any study.

showed progressively increasing levels of contrast enhancement after subsequent injections. Figure 3 shows a series of echocardiographic still frames recorded during the fourth, sixth, twelfth, and twentieth postinjection diastoles for the 1, 20, and 120 min observations in one of these animals. At 1 min, no delayed enhancement was seen inside the immediate contrast defect. After the 20 min injection, delayed (+1) enhancement occurred that was maximal by the twentieth postinjection diastole. After the 120 min injection, delayed (2+) enhancement was maximal and was similar in intensity to the immediate level by the twelfth diastolic image. The radial contrast enhancement and radial microsphere flow maps for this animal are presented in figure 4, *top*.

In the other seven animals, delayed contrast enhancement on later studies was seen in one or two segments adjacent to the immediately enhanced myocardium (n = 4) or did not occur inside the immediate contrast defect after any injection (n = 3). No contrast enhancement occurred in the center of the original contrast-negative zone in these animals. The contrast enhancement map and radial flow map for such an animal are presented in figure 4, *bottom*.

Relationship of contrast enhancement to microsphere flow. The mean normalized microsphere flow found in each segment as related to the qualitative echocardiographic contrast enhancement grade is presented in table 1. Microsphere flow increased progressively from 18% of normal in segments graded as zero to 93% of normal in grade 3+ segments ($p < .01$).

The quantitative value of contrast intensity for all segments correlated linearly with the mean normalized microsphere flow (mean flow [percent] = 0.78 intensity + 10%; r = .78, SEE 26%, $p < .01$). To ascertain that the correlation was not unduly dependent on a large number of segments with normal flows, the mean flow and mean intensity within the ischemic region were determined. The ischemic region was defined as that containing all segments with a mean flow less than 50% of normal at the 1 min observation. Contrast intensity also correlated with normalized microsphere flow within the ischemic region (flow [percent] = 1.13 intensity + 6.8%; r = .83, SEE = 14%, $p < .001$; figure 5).

Serial changes in contrast enhancement and microsphere flow. To determine whether changes in the level of contrast enhancement reflect changes in blood flow,

TABLE 1

Concomitant segmental microsphere flow according to echocardiographic contrast rating

Echocardiographic rating	% Nl flow	SD	SEM	Samples
0	18[A]	24	2	134
1	32[A]	27	3	63
2	61[A]	20	3	34
3	93[A]	32	2	278

% Nl flow = percent of segmental microsphere flow in unaffected LAD distribution.

[A]$p < .01$ vs all other values.

changes in the qualitative contrast grade in the central ischemic zone between sequential studies were compared with changes in microsphere blood flow. The mean contrast score in the central three segments, as defined by the immediate contrast defect for the 1 min study, was compared for sequential studies. The change in the contrast rating in the central zone correlated well with the change in microsphere flow ($r = .88$, $p < .001$; figure 6).

The change in sequential value for quantitative contrast intensity also correlated, although less well, with sequential changes in mean normalized microsphere flow within the ischemic region (flow change [percent] = 0.83 intensity change + 9.3%; $r = .70$, SEE = 10.3%, $p < .01$).

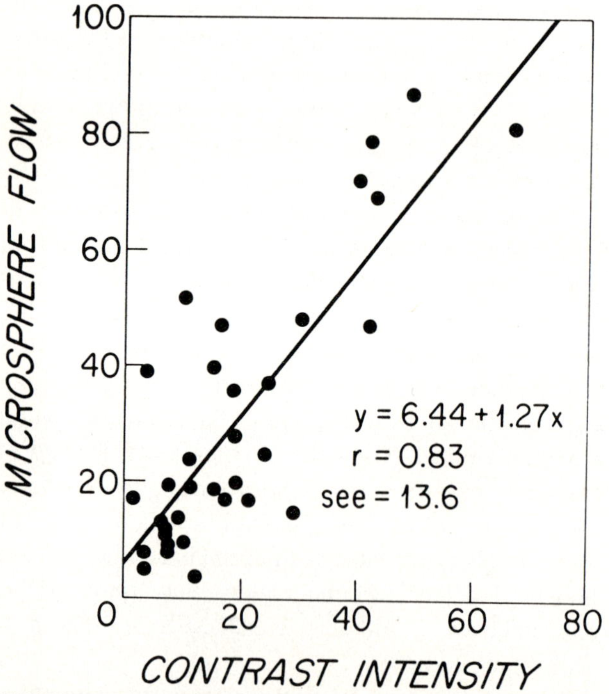

FIGURE 5. Relationship of quantitative intensity change within the ischemic region during contrast injection and concomitant microsphere-derived normalized blood flow. The regression line is shown.

Discussion

Most previous work with myocardial contrast echocardiography during acute coronary occlusion has focussed on a visual determination of the presence or absence of regional contrast enhancement to define the size of a region that is "at risk" of infarction.[2-5] The present study is the first in which serial contrast studies performed during the critical early hours after acute occlusion have been compared directly with regional myocardial blood flow. Contrast enhancement, assessed both qualitatively and quantitatively based on the time of contrast appearance and the peak intensity achieved, bore an important relationship to the amount of residual myocardial blood flow within the ischemic region. Blood flow to this region changed in a highly individualized manner during the 2 hr after occlusion and was reflected by changes in the amount of contrast enhancement observed.

Recent studies suggest that collateral function and residual blood flow may play an important role in determining the time available for successful myocardial salvage. Rogers et al.,[10] who studied 63 patients a mean of 7 hr after the onset of acute ischemia, found that subsequent improvement in regional and global left ventricular function was related primarily to the presence of subtotal stenosis or intact collateral circulation. Nohara et al.[11] also found that the presence of collateral vessels or subtotal occlusion was the most important predictor of subsequent functional improvement in their study of 34 patients undergoing thrombolysis 6 hr after acute infarction. In animal experiments,

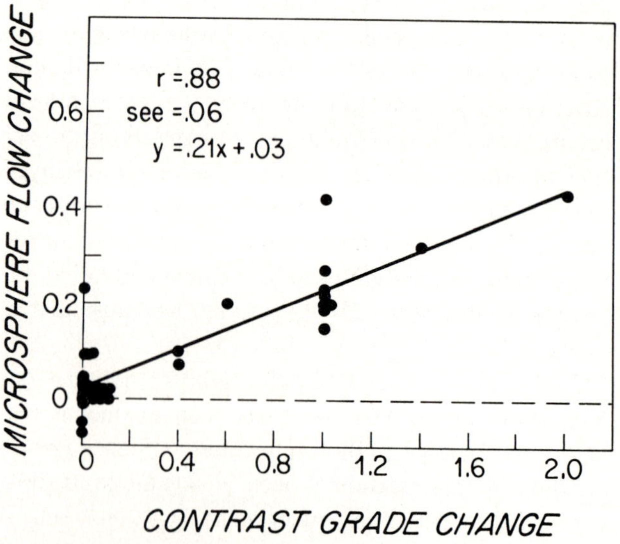

FIGURE 6. Relationship of the change in qualitative contrast grade to the change in normalized microsphere-determined blood flow in the central ischemic region between any two successive observations. The regression line is solid.

Reimer et al.[12] and Koyanagi et al.[13] have shown, using the radioactive microsphere technique, that myocardial survival is prolonged in ischemic regions that receive more than 30% of normal blood flow. Our data indicate that contrast echocardiography can detect flows in this range in the ischemic region and suggest that, if fully developed and proven safe, this method could potentially assist in the selection of patients with large amounts of jeopardized yet viable myocardium who are likely to benefit from aggressive interventional approaches.

At present, myocardial contrast echocardiography requires the supraaortic or intracoronary injection of microbubble-containing contrast agents. Although the exact methods used in the present study are not yet applicable to the clinical situation, there have been several recent encouraging preliminary reports. Left-sided injections of microbubble-containing agitated saline,[14] carbon dioxide solution,[15] and polygellin colloid[16] have been performed safely in small numbers of patients in the catheterization laboratory. Our study was performed with a pigtail catheter that was modified by introducing a 90 degree bend just above the first catheter side holes and therefore was easily advanced to the level of the aortic root solely by the use of echocardiographic guidance. This experience suggests that aortic root injection of echocardiographic contrast may be possible in a monitored situation outside the catheterization laboratory, such as in the coronary care unit.

No agent such as hydrogen peroxide and blood solution that is capable of producing intense myocardial contrast by supra-aortic injection has as yet been proven safe for use in man. Studies have been reported by Gaffney et al.[17] and Wang et al.[18] of the safe use of doses of hydrogen peroxide similar to ours for right-sided injections in over 100 patients. Our experience with an animal preparation[4, 5] shows only occasional transient and relatively minor alterations in hemodynamics, and is similar to that reported by Gaffney,[17] who observed no changes in hemodynamics or alertness and no sign of distress in five conscious dogs receiving 10 ml bolus injections of 0.2% solution into the left atrium. Recent preliminary reports by Levine et al.[19] and Holt et al.[20] indicate that transient decreases in contractility can be observed after the intracoronary injection of contrast agents such as meglumine/saline, Fluosol DA, 50% dextrose, and hydrogen peroxide solution. The degree of the subjectively assessed decrease in contraction seen in Levine's study appeared to be proportional to the amount of contrast enhancement.[19] The amount of regional contractile depression measured by ultrasonic crystals by Holt[20] was too small and transient to affect ventricular dP/dt. The occurrence of these contractile changes does suggest that at least some transient microcirculatory blockage may occur as a result of the contrast bubbles. Further studies will be necessary to determine whether these transient changes result in any long-term deleterious consequences.

The contrast agent used in this study was a mixture of dilute hydrogen peroxide solution and autologous blood, which results in the generation of heterogeneous oxygen microbubbles ranging from 10 to 100 μm in diameter (mean 52 μm).[10] Although a constant volume of this solution was injected by a standardized approach, there was undoubtedly some variability in the number and size of the microbubbles delivered to the coronary circulation. With our agent, the mean increase in intensity reached in normal segments averaged 61 $\pm$ 20% of the available gray scale with 23 of 111 segment pairs varying by more than 20% on two successive injections. No injection sequences were excluded in our study for inadequate or overabundant contrast enhancement because these criteria had not been established; however, close attention to values in normal areas, both in terms of adequacy of enhancement and study-to-study reproducibility, might be expected to improve the predictive value of changes in contrast enhancement for changes in myocardial flow within the ischemic region. The exact relationship between microbubble size, number, and time/gain compensation has not yet been defined, but the relationship between bubble distribution and echo intensity is likely to be closest for homogeneously sized bubbles. Investigations of the relationship between flow and contrast enhancement with agents with more uniformly sized microbubbles such as ultrasonicated meglumine/saline[21] or polysorbate[22] should be pursued to elucidate this point.

The qualitative approach taken has several important pragmatic advantages. It is relatively easy to perform and is relatively independent of the background level of echo intensities. The pattern of contrast appearance and intensity in relatively small areas can be visually integrated into a topographic map by close attention to surrounding myocardial landmarks and repeated playback with the use of selected stop frames as reference. Its major limitations are those inherent to all visually oriented qualitative techniques: a relatively coarse discrimination between different visual intensities and a dependence on subjective, although trained, observations. The technique was quite reproducible for each observer, but was more variable between observers, primarily because of differences in axis orientation.

The quantitative approach taken was based on our qualitative observations and was a primitive attempt to take into account both the temporal course of contrast appearance and the peak intensity of contrast achieved in each segment by calculation of the mean segmental intensity for several postinjection end-diastolic frames and comparing them with a mean preinjection value. The end-diastoles chosen for analysis, (second, fourth, tenth, and twelfth) were arbitrarily selected on the basis of our qualitative experience and the relatively small amount of computer memory available to us. We mathematically normalized for the baseline inhomogeneity of regional echo signal intensities by subtracting background intensity and rescaling the residual available gray scale for each segment to 100 arbitrary units. Our approach is limited in both temporal and spatial resolution. One image-processing approach might allow for regional rescaling of gray-scale assignments before injection of contrast. Presuming that the major image-processing problems of misregistration and misalignment can be overcome, multiple background frames could be spatially smoothed. By an approach similar to that used in radionuclide angiography to calculate ventricular filling and emptying rates, backgrounds could be subtracted from temporally smoothed end-diastoles after injection of contrast. Regional contrast appearance rates and peak intensities could then be directly calculated.

One key variable affecting quantitative analysis that was not completely appreciated at the time the studies were performed is the effect of preinjection region intensity on analyses of the amount of change in that intensity. High regional intensities before injection limit the available dynamic range for display of contrast enhancement. In addition, there is a modest decrease in echo intensity for deeper target levels during the course of contrast injection that occurs as a result of interference induced by the presence of contrast material at levels closer to the transducer. With very high baseline intensities, this attenuation may be quantitatively similar to the increase in echo signal strength that occurs in a region as a result of contrast appearance. In our study, the two points farthest from the regression line for the quantitative analysis (4, 39 and 9, 52; figure 5) occurred in the same animal. Although a color videodensitometer was used interactively before the initial injection in each study in an attempt to achieve a homogeneous low baseline level of regional pixel intensity, the baseline intensity in the ischemic region was 210 units for that animal, or approximately two to three times the baseline intensity for the other animals and 84% of the total available dynamic range. Close attention paid to the absolute baseline level should obviate this problem in the future.

Contrast echocardiography with analysis of the pattern and intensity of contrast appearance allows serial estimation of relative myocardial blood flow within the region subserved by an occluded coronary artery. Changes in the amount of contrast enhancement within this region bear an important relationship to changes in myocardial blood flow. The qualitative analysis system presented can be performed virtually in real time.

APPENDIX 1

Microsphere flow in reference (Ref) and central ischemic (CI) regions

Dog	1 min			20 min			120 min		
No.	Ref	CI	NCI	Ref	CI	NCI	Ref	CI	NCI
5935	1.31	0.18	0.14	1.91	0.28	0.15	2.51	0.24	0.10
5940	1.49	0.03	0.02	0.90	0.02	0.02	0.97	0.02	0.02
5943	2.25	0.05	0.02	1.60	0.04	0.03	1.98	0.07	0.04
5946	1.29	0.01	0.01	1.89	0.01	0.01	1.63	0	0
5949	1.06	0.07	0.07	0.96	0.10	0.10	0.63	0.10	0.16
5954	0.95	0.01	0.01	1.58	0.03	0.02	0.85	0.04	0.05
5956	1.20	0.46	0.38	0.97	0.74	0.76	1.03	0.78	0.76
5962	1.92	0.03	0.02	1.56	0.05	0.03	1.73	0.04	0.02
5968	2.57	0.16	0.06	1.67	0.36	0.22	1.55	0.57	0.37
5970	1.42	0.48	0.34	1.14	0.81	0.71	1.18	0.79	0.67
5989	1.72	0.17	0.10	1.40	0.09	0.06	1.77	0.11	0.06
5994	1.86	0.07	0.04	2.39	0.12	0.05	1.58	0.34	0.22
Mean	1.59	0.14	0.10	1.50	0.22	0.18	1.45	0.26	0.21
SD	0.49	0.16	0.13	0.45	0.28	0.27	0.54	0.30	0.26

NCI = normalized microsphere flow in central ischemic segment.

Presuming that our agent, dilute hydrogen peroxide and blood solution, or another agent can be proved safe for administration to humans, this method is applicable for the detection of patients likely to benefit from aggressive intervention for acute myocardial infarction. The quantitative analysis presented represents a first approximation and indicates directions for future research in developing a means of serially depicting the pattern of regional myocardial flow in vivo during acute myocardial infarction.

References

1. Armstrong WF, Mueller TM, Kinney EL, Tickner EG, Dillon JC, Feigen- baum H: Assessment of myocardial perfusion abnormalities with contrast-enhanced two-dimensional echocardiography. Circulation **66:** 166, 1982
2. Tei C, Sakamaki T, Shah PM, Meerbaum S, Shimoura K, Kondo S, Corday E: Myocardial contrast echocardiography: a reproducible technique of myocardial opacification for identifying regional perfusion defects. Circulation **67:** 585, 1983
3. Armstrong WF, West SR, Mueller TM, Dillion JC, Feigenbaum H: Assessment of location and size of myocardial infarction with contrast enhanced echocardiography. J Am Coll Cardiol **2:** 63, 1983
4. Kemper AJ, O'Boyle JE, Sharma S, Cohen CA, Kloner RA, Khuri SF, Parisi AF: Hydrogen peroxide contrast-enhanced two-dimensional echocardiography: real-time in vivo delineation of regional myocardial perfusion. Circulation **68:** 603, 1983
5. Kemper AJ, O'Boyle JE, Cohen CA, Taylor A, Parisi AF: Hydrogen peroxide contrast echocardiography: quantification in vivo of myocardial risk area during coronary occlusion and of the necrotic area remaining after myocardial reperfusion. Circulation **70:** 309, 1984
6. Jugdutt BI, Hutchins GM, Bulkley BH, Becker LC: Myocardial infarction in the conscious dog: three-dimensional mapping of infarct, collateral flow and region at risk. Circulation **60:** 1141, 1979
7. White FC, Sanders M, Bloor CM: Regional redistribution of myocardial blood flow after coronary occlusion and reperfusion in the conscious dog. Am J Cardiol **42:** 234, 1978
8. Jugdutt BI, Becker LC, Hutchins GM. Early changes in collateral blood flow during myocardial infarction in conscious dogs. Am J Physiol **237:** H371, 1979
9. Domenech RJ, Hoffman JI, Noble MI, Saunders KB, Henson JR, Subijanto S: Total and regional coronary blood flow measured by radioactive microspheres in conscious and anesthetized dogs. Circ Res **25:** 581, 1969
10. Rogers WJ, Hood WP, Mantle JA, Baxley WA, Kirklin JK, Zorn GL, Nath HP: Return of left ventricular function after reperfusion in patients with myocardial infarction: importance of subtotal stenosis or intact collaterals. Circulation **69:** 338, 1984
11. Nohara R, Kambara H, Murakami T, Kadota K, Tamaki S, Kawai C: Collateral function in acute myocardial infarction. Am J Cardiol **52:** 955, 1983
12. Reimer KA, Jennings RB: The "wavefront phenomenon" of myocardial cell death. Transmural progression of necrosis within the framework of ischemic bed size (myocardium at risk) and collateral flow. Lab Invest **40:** 633, 1979
13. Koyanagi S, Eastham CL, Harrison DG, Marcus ML: Transmural variation in the relationship between myocardial infarct size and risk area. Am J Physiol **242:** H867, 1982
14. Bailey BP, Fletcher PJ: Two-dimensional echo-contrast studies of the left heart during cardiac catheterization. Circulation **70**(suppl II): II-5, 1984 (abst)
15. Jiang L, Pu SY, Yang MZ, Lu YZ, Chen HZ: Left heart contrast echocardiography using a carbon dioxide producing agent. Circulation **70**(suppl II): II-5, 1984 (abst)
16. Santoso T, Roelandt J, Masjoer J, Abjurahman N, Meltzer R, Hugenholtz P: Myocardial perfusion imaging in humans by contrast echocardiography using polygellin colloid solution. J Am Coll Cardiol **5:** 474, 1985 (abst)
17. Gaffney FA, Lin J-C, Peshock RM, Bush L, Buja M: Hydrogen peroxide contrast echocardiography. Am J Cardiol **52:** 607, 1983

APPENDIX 2

Intraobserver and interobserver variability: first and second ratings for observers 1 and 2

	Observer 1: second rating			
	0	1	2	3
Observer 1: first rating				
0	87	8	0	4
1	6	17	3	5
2	0	1	12	3
3	3	1	1	107

	Observer 2: second rating			
	0	1	2	3
Observer 2: first rating				
0	92	8	1	4
1	4	11	6	4
2	0	1	3	1
3	9	2	3	109

	Observer 2: second rating			
	0	1	2	3
Observer 1: first rating				
0	87	5	0	4
1	6	14	7	4
2	1	1	6	8
3	10	2	0	103

	Observer 2: second rating			
	0	1	2	3
Observer 1: second rating				
0	86	6	2	2
1	8	11	5	1
2	1	2	5	8
3	10	3	1	107

	Observer 2: first rating			
	0	1	2	3
Observer 1: first rating				
0	94	0	0	3
1	6	21	1	3
2	1	0	3	12
3	4	4	1	105

	Observer 2: first rating			
	0	1	2	3
Observer 1: second rating				
0	90	2	0	4
1	6	17	0	2
2	2	1	4	9
3	7	5	1	108

18. Wang H, Wang J, Chen H, Lu C: Contrast echocardiography with hydrogen peroxide. II. Clinical application. Chinese Med J **92:** 693, 1979
19. Levine RA, Gillam LD, Guerrero JL, Weyman AE: Wall motion abnormalities following myocardial echo contrast injection are caused by microbubbles. J Am Coll Cardiol **5:** 474, 1985
20. Holt G, Reeves W, Rieder M, Daley L, Murthy V, Christensen C: Negative inotropic effects of intracoronary echo-contrast agents. J Am Coll Cardiol **5:** 474, 1985 (abst)
21. Feinstein SB, Ten Cate FJ, Zwehl W, Ong K, Maurer G, Tei C, Shah PM, Meerbaum S, Corday E: Two-dimensional contrast echocardiography. I. In vitro development and quantitative analysis of echo contrast agents. J Am Coll Cardiol **3:** 14, 1984
22. Smith MD, Kwan QL, Reiser J, Demaria AN: Intensity and reproducibility of ultrasonic contrast agents: superiority of a new substance, SHU 454R, to conventional agents. Circulation **68**(suppl III): II-92, 1983 (abst).

Mechanisms of improving regional and global ventricular function by preload alterations during acute ischemia in the canine left ventricle

WILBUR Y. W. LEW, M.D., AND ERNESTO BAN-HAYASHI, M.D.*

ABSTRACT We examined the influence of left ventricular end-diastolic pressure (LVEDP) on the mechanical interaction between ischemic and nonischemic areas during acute myocardial ischemia. Circumferentially oriented ultrasonic segment gauges were implanted in the midwall of the anterior apex and posterior apex of the left ventricle in seven anesthetized dogs. Stroke volume was measured with a flow probe around the ascending aorta in five of these animals. We varied LVEDP with vena caval occlusion and dextran infusions to three matched levels (7, 12, and 19 mm Hg) before and 30 min after complete occlusion of the mid left anterior descending coronary artery. With acute ischemia, the anterior apex or ischemic zone demonstrated marked segmental lengthening during isovolumetric systole (end-diastole to aortic valve opening) and akinesis during the ejection phase (aortic valve opening to closure). In the posterior apex or nonischemic area, isovolumetric shortening increased and ejection phase shortening decreased during acute ischemia when compared with those under control conditions at the same LVEDP. Thus, a portion of the shortening generated by the nonischemic area was expended in stretching the ischemic zone during isovolumetric systole, thereby reducing the amount of ejection phase shortening. As LVEDP was increased, there was a parallel decrease in both the amount of isovolumetric lengthening in the ischemic zone and the isovolumetric shortening in the nonischemic area. As a result, acute ischemia produced less of a reduction in ejection phase shortening in the nonischemic area and in stroke volume at high as compared with low LVEDP. We conclude that the ischemic zone imposes a mechanical disadvantage on the nonischemic area, the magnitude of which is directly proportional to the amount of isovolumetric lengthening or bulge in the ischemic zone. An increase in LVEDP during acute ischemia improves regional and global ventricular function by both the Frank-Starling mechanism in the nonischemic (but not the ischemic) area and by reducing the mechanical disadvantage that the ischemic zone imposes on the nonischemic area.
Circulation 72, No. 5, 1125–1134, 1985.

IN PATIENTS with acute myocardial infarction, therapeutic alteration of the left ventricular filling pressure to an "optimal" level improves stroke volume while minimizing adverse hemodynamic effects.[1-6] Although much of this improvement is due to the Frank-Starling mechanism in nonischemic areas, additional alterations in regional function may be involved. Accordingly, this study was designed to examine the effects of preload manipulation during acute ischemia on regional function in the ischemic zone and on the mechanical interaction between ischemic and nonischemic areas.

Recently, we postulated that a mechanical interaction between ischemic and nonischemic areas occurs during acute myocardial ischemia.[7] After occlusion of a coronary artery, paradoxical lengthening during isovolumetric systole was observed in the ischemic zone. In nonischemic areas, end-diastolic segmental length increased due to the increase in left ventricular end-diastolic pressure (LVEDP), and total segmental shortening (from end-diastole to aortic valve closure) increased due to the Frank-Starling mechanism. However, all of the increase in nonischemic area shortening occurred during isovolumetric systole (from end-diastole to aortic valve opening), and developed coincident with the development of paradoxical isovo-

From the Cardiovascular Division, University of California, San Diego, and the San Diego Veterans Administration Medical Center.

Supported by the National Institutes of Health grant HL-28644 and by the Research Service of the Veterans Administration.

Address for correspondence: Wilbur Y. W. Lew, M.D., Cardiovascular Division 111A, VA Medical Center, 3350 La Jolla Village Dr., San Diego, CA 92161.

Received Feb. 26, 1985; revision accepted Aug. 19, 1985.

*Current address: Instituto Nacional de Cardiologia, Servicio de Medicina Nuclear, Juan Badiano No. 1, Tlalpan D.F. CP 14080, Mexico.

lumetric lengthening in the ischemic zone. Therefore, we suggested that a significant portion of the shortening generated by the nonischemic segments was expended in stretching the ischemic zone during isovolumetric systole. Although there was hyperfunction of nonischemic areas, there was no significant "compensatory" increase in nonischemic area shortening during the ejection phase (aortic valve opening to closure).

The current study was designed to more completely explore the mechanical interaction between ischemic and nonischemic areas and its consequences. First, we hypothesized that during acute ischemia, the ischemic zone imposes a mechanical disadvantage on the nonischemic areas, due to the regional intraventricular unloading effect during isovolumetric systole. However, this mechanical disadvantage may be masked by the increased effect of the Frank-Starling mechanism in nonischemic areas. Thus, we proposed to examine the effects of acute ischemia under conditions in which LVEDP and end-diastolic segmental length of nonischemic areas do not change. Under these conditions, we predicted that the shortening expended by the nonischemic areas to stretch the ischemic zone during isovolumetric systole would result in an actual decrease in ejection phase shortening by nonischemic areas.

Second, we hypothesized that the magnitude of the mechanical disadvantage imposed by the ischemic zone is directly proportional to the amount of its paradoxical isovolumetric lengthening, which in turn is inversely proportional to its stiffness. We postulated that when LVEDP is increased during acute ischemia, the ischemic segment is placed at a steeper (stiffer) position on its passive pressure-length curve, and thus offers greater resistance to passive (paradoxical) isovolumetric lengthening. If less shortening is expended by the nonischemic areas in stretching the ischemic zone during isovolumetric systole, the reduction in nonischemic area ejection phase shortening with acute ischemia would be less severe. This reduction in the mechanical disadvantage imposed by the ischemic zone on nonischemic areas would be an additional mechanism by which an increase in LVEDP to an "optimal" level improves regional and global ventricular function during acute myocardial ischemia.

Methods

Instrumentation. Seven mongrel dogs of both sexes and weighing between 20 and 33 kg were anesthetized with intravenous pentobarbital (25 mg/kg) and intubated. Respiration was supported with a Harvard respirator. A midline sternotomy and bilateral fifth interspace thoracotomy were performed in each and the heart exposed and supported in a pericardial cradle. An inflatable occlusion cuff was placed around the inferior vena cava and a large-bore cannula was placed in a femoral vein for administration of intravenous fluids. A fluid-filled pigtail catheter, attached to a Statham P23 DB transducer, was placed into the left ventricle through a femoral artery. The zero level was established at the level of the right atrium. A Konigsberg P20 high-fidelity micromanometer catheter was placed into the left ventricle through a stab wound in the apex and secured in place with a purse-string suture. After the left ventricular pressure waveform from the micromanometer was matched to that of the fluid-filled catheter, the fluid-filled catheter was withdrawn into the ascending aorta just above the aortic valve for measurement of central aortic pressure. A limb-lead electrocardiogram was recorded throughout.

The mid left anterior descending coronary artery was isolated just distal to the first or second acute diagonal branch and dissected free over a 3 to 5 mm course. Any large visible collateral vessels from the right coronary or left circumflex systems supplying the anterior wall were ligated near the ventricular apex.

Regional ventricular function was measured with ultrasonic segmental length gauges comprised of two 5 MHz piezoelectric crystals (2 mm diameter). The crystals were implanted approximately 1 cm apart through small stab wounds into the midwall of the left ventricle (4 to 6 mm below the epicardial surface) and oriented in the circumferential direction of the midwall hoop axis fibers.[8] One gauge was placed in the anterior apex within the perfusion bed of the mid left anterior descending coronary artery so it would be within the ischemic zone after acute coronary artery occlusion. This gauge was placed at a level approximately one-third of the distance from the apical dimple to the bifurcation of the left coronary artery along an external (epicardial) long axis. The second midwall segmental length gauge was placed in the posterior apex in a region that would remain nonischemic. This gauge was approximately one-third to one-half of the distance from the apex to the inferior pulmonary veins along the posterior wall. The circumferential orientation and midwall depth of the gauges were confirmed on postmortem examination.

In five of the seven animals, a Biotronix electromagnetic flow probe attached to an electromagnetic flowmeter (Biotronix Model BL620) was placed around the ascending aorta. The aortic flow signal was integrated on-line such that the area under the flow curve was proportional to the stroke volume. The aortic flow curve was calibrated over several cardiac cycles by determining the simultaneous stroke volume. Cardiac output was determined with thermodilution techniques (Instrumentation Laboratory Cardiac Output System 601) by the use of a No. 7F balloon-tipped catheter (Instrumentation Laboratory Model 44166) introduced through the right jugular vein, through the right heart, and placed into the pulmonary artery. Cardiac output was divided by heart rate to obtain the average stroke volume, which was compared with the average area from the integrated aortic flow curve over the same cardiac cycles. At least three cardiac output and calibration determinations were made and the results were averaged.

The electrocardiogram, central aortic pressure, left ventricular pressure, ultrasonic segmental length signals from the anterior and posterior apexes, and the central aortic flow signal (in five animals) were recorded on an eight-channel forced-ink polygraph (Brush Clevite) at a paper speed of 200 mm/sec (figure 1) and on FM magnetic tape for subsequent playback. All measurements were obtained under steady-state conditions with respiration suspended at end-expiration; at least 20 consecutive beats were recorded.

Experimental protocol. LVEDP was varied by a combination of inferior vena caval occlusion by inflatable cuff and infusion of 6% dextran dissolved in 0.9% saline. Control measurements were obtained under steady-state conditions at three

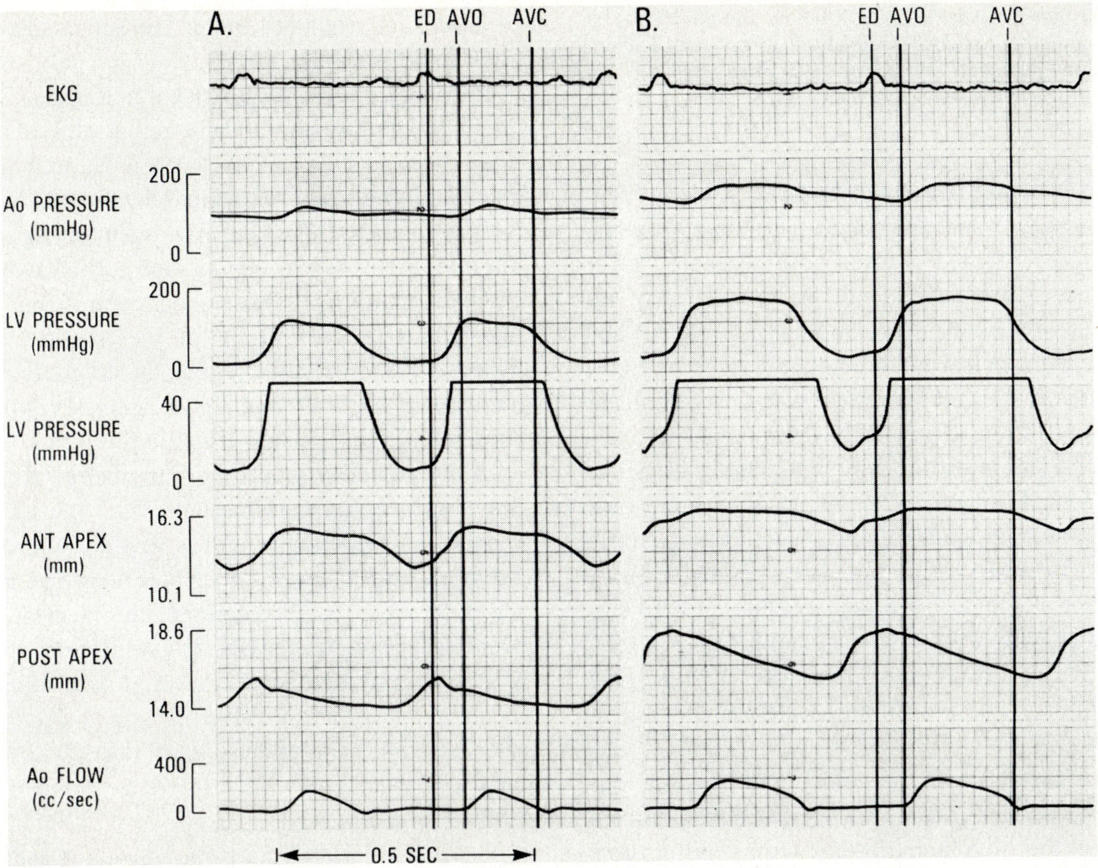

FIGURE 1. A typical tracing obtained after 30 min of ischemia including the electrocardiogram (EKG), central aortic (Ao) pressure, left ventricular (LV) pressure low and high gain, segmental length signals from the anterior (ANT) and posterior (POST) apexes, and the aortic flow signal (Ao FLOW). The time scale is at the bottom. The vertical lines denote the time of end-diastole (ED), aortic valve opening (AVO), and aortic valve closure (AVC). *A*, Low LVEDP; *B*, high LVEDP. Note in *A* that the anterior apex or ischemic zone demonstrates marked segmental lengthening during isovolumetric systole (from ED to AVO) and akinesis during the ejection phase (from AVO to AVC). The posterior apex or nonischemic area demonstrates a significant amount of shortening during early isovolumetric systole. When LVEDP is increased (from *A* to *B*), there is a significant decrease in the amount of isovolumetric lengthening or bulge in the ischemic zone and a parallel decrease in the amount of isovolumetric shortening in the nonischemic area. Although an increase in LVEDP increased ejection phase shortening in the nonischemic area, there is no improvement in the akinesis of the ischemic zone during the ejection phase.

levels of LVEDP (7, 12, and 19 mm Hg). After a recovery period of at least 30 min, acute anterior wall ischemia was induced by occluding the mid left anterior descending coronary artery with a Schwartz clamp. Although the majority of changes in regional function and hemodynamics occurred within the first 5 min, the animals were allowed to stabilize for at least 30 min after occlusion of the coronary artery to ensure that nearly steady-state conditions had been achieved. Repeat measurements then were made during ischemia at the three levels of LVEDP, which were chosen to closely simulate those under control conditions.

Data analysis. The aortic and left ventricular pressures and anterior and posterior apical lengths and aortic flow signals were all played back from FM tape and converted from analog to digital data at 5 msec intervals. Data from 20 consecutive cardiac cycles were averaged. Thus, in each animal, averaged data were obtained at the same three levels of LVEDP (7, 12, and 19 mm Hg) under control conditions and after 30 min of ischemia.

Regional segmental lengths were determined at three times during the cardiac cycle: at end-diastole, at aortic valve opening, and at aortic valve closure (figure 1). End-diastole was determined from the high-gain left ventricular pressure tracing by the trough following atrial contraction. If this was not obvious, the peak of the R wave on the electrocardiogram was used. In the five animals with aortic flow probes, the time of zero crossover of the aortic flow tracing was used to time aortic valve opening and closure (figure 1). In the other two animals, the central aortic pressures at the onset of ejection and at the dicrotic notch were transposed onto the high-fidelity left ventricular pressure tracing to time aortic valve opening and closure, respectively.

Total segmental shortening, defined as the percent change in segmental length from end-diastole to aortic valve closure, was subdivided into isovolumetric shortening (from end-diastole to aortic valve opening) and ejection phase shortening (from aortic valve opening to closure), as in our previous study.[7] The times from end-diastole to aortic valve opening (isovolumetric time) and from aortic valve opening to closure (ejection time) were measured from the original tracings, and the intervals from five cardiac cycles were averaged.

Statistical analysis. Hemodynamic and timing data, segmental lengths, and segmental shortening were compared for the same region at the same LVEDP before and after acute ischemia by a repeated-measure analysis of variance and Tukey's test for comparing mean values. A p value of less than .05 was considered to indicate statistical significance.

Results

Hemodynamic and timing measurements (table 1). Measurements before and after acute ischemia were obtained at three matched levels of LVEDP (table 1). For convenience, these levels will be subsequently referred to as LVEDP 7, 12, and 19 mm Hg. When compared with control conditions at the same LVEDP, acute ischemia was not associated with any significant change in heart rate at any of the three matched levels of LVEDP. The heart rate was significantly higher at LVEDP 7 mm Hg than at 12 or 19 mm Hg during acute ischemia, but not under control conditions. Aortic pressures at the time of aortic valve opening and closure at control and during acute ischemia differed significantly at only one of the matched LVEDP levels: the aortic valve closure pressure at LVEDP 7 mm Hg was significantly lower during acute ischemia than during control.

When compared with that under control conditions at the same LVEDP, there was a slight but significant increase in the isovolumetric time (from end-diastole to aortic valve opening) after acute ischemia at LVEDP 7 and 19 mm Hg, but not at LVEDP 12 mm Hg. Both at control and after acute ischemia, isovolumetric time decreased similarly as LVEDP increased. The left ventricular ejection time (from aortic valve opening to closure) did not differ under control conditions and after acute ischemia at any of the matched LVEDP levels. With increasing LVEDP, ejection time increased similarly both under control conditions and after acute ischemia.

Regional segmental lengths (table 2). Regional segmental lengths before and after ischemia were obtained at three matched LVEDP levels (table 2). In the anterior apical or ischemic zone, acute ischemia was associated with a significant increase in segmental length at end-diastole, aortic valve opening, and aortic valve closure when compared with those under control conditions at the same matched LVEDP. In the anterior apex, the increase in end-diastolic segmental length for the same increase in LVEDP was significantly less after ischemia than under control conditions.

In the posterior apical or nonischemic area, acute ischemia was not associated with any significant change in segmental length at end-diastole or aortic valve closure at any of the three matched levels of LVEDP. As LVEDP increased, the increase in end-diastolic segmental length was similar under control conditions and after acute ischemia. Although the segmental length at aortic valve opening tended to be less after ischemia than under control conditions (particularly at low LVEDP), this difference was not statistically significant.

Regional segmental shortening (figures 2 and 3). Regional isovolumetric and ejection phase shortening measurements obtained at different LVEDPs before and after ischemia are shown in figure 2. Under control conditions, segmental shortening occurred predominantly during the ejection phase, with minimal motion during isovolumetric systole in both the anterior and posterior apexes. In both the anterior and posterior apexes, the ejection phase shortening increased sig-

TABLE 1

Hemodynamic and timing measurements for three levels of LVEDP before (control) and after acute ischemia in seven animals

LVEDP (mm Hg)	HR (beats/min)	AVO P (mm Hg)	AVC P (mm Hg)	ISOVOL T (msec)	EJECT T (msec)
Control					
6.8 ± 0.7	118 ± 17	94 ± 11	108 ± 10	60 ± 11	185 ± 28
12.3 ± 1.1	117 ± 15	98 ± 7	118 ± 12	51 ± 10	207 ± 27
19.1 ± 2.5	115 ± 12	103 ± 11	126 ± 18	52 ± 10	227 ± 25
Ischemia					
7.3 ± 1.2	124 ± 23	83 ± 19	93 ± 22[A]	65 ± 12[A]	186 ± 44
12.3 ± 1.3	112 ± 14	94 ± 19	113 ± 18	55 ± 7	224 ± 40
19.1 ± 2.3	109 ± 14	102 ± 13	122 ± 12	58 ± 11[A]	240 ± 40

Measurements are given as mean ± 1 SD.

HR = heart rate; AVO P = aortic pressure at the time of aortic valve opening; AVC P = aortic pressure at aortic valve closure; ISOVOL T = isovolumetric time interval; EJEC T = ejection phase time.

[A]Significantly different from control measurements at the same LVEDP ($p < .05$). See text for additional statistical analysis and discussion.

TABLE 2
Regional segmental lengths (mm)

LVEDP (mm Hg)	Anterior apex			Posterior apex		
	ED	AVO	AVC	ED	AVO	AVC
Control						
7	12.7±2.6	12.5±2.4	10.5±2.7	15.0±4.5	14.9±4.6	13.3±4.0
12	14.7±2.2	14.8±2.2	11.8±2.6	16.3±5.0	16.4±5.0	14.2±4.4
19	15.7±1.7	15.8±1.6	12.6±2.1	17.0±5.2	17.0±5.1	14.6±4.4
Ischemia						
7	15.0±2.4^A	16.9±2.3^A	16.7±2.3^A	14.9±3.8	14.2±3.7	13.0±3.5
12	16.5±2.5^A	17.6±2.4^A	17.4±2.4^A	16.4±4.6	16.1±4.5	14.2±4.0
19	17.1±2.3^A	17.9±2.3^A	17.6±2.3^A	17.1±5.0	16.9±4.9	14.7±4.2

Segmental lengths (mean ± 1 SD) from the anterior apex and posterior apex are given at three levels of LVEDP before (control) and after acute ischemia in seven animals.

ED = end-diastole; AVO = aortic valve opening; AVC = aortic valve closure.

[A]Segmental lengths during ischemia that are significantly different from control values at the same LVEDP ($p < .01$). The trends also differed in the anterior apex. For the same increase in LVEDP, end-diastolic segmental length in the anterior apex increased significantly less after ischemia than under control conditions ($p < .01$).

nificantly when LVEDP increased from 7 mm Hg to 12 or 19 mm Hg. In neither region was there a significant difference in ejection phase shortening at LVEDP 12 and 19 mm Hg. Isovolumetric shortening in both regions tended to decrease as LVEDP inreased, but this was not a statistically significant change.

After acute ischemia, there was virtual akinesis during the ejection phase in the anterior apex or ischemic zone and most of the changes in segmental length occurred during isovolumetric systole, with marked paradoxical lengthening or bulge (figure 1). With acute ischemia, ejection phase shortening in the anterior apex decreased significantly for all three levels of LVEDP. During ischemia, there was no significant change in ejection phase shortening of the ischemic zone as LVEDP increased. However, there was a significant decrease in the amount of isovolumetric lengthening or bulge in the ischemic zone as LVEDP increased from 7 mm Hg to 12 or 19 mm Hg. The amount of isovolumetric lengthening in the ischemic zone was not significantly different between LVEDP 12 and 19 mm Hg.

In the posterior apex or nonischemic area, acute ischemia was associated with a significant increase in isovolumetric segmental shortening when compared with that under control conditions at the same LVEDP. This was true at all three levels of LVEDP. During ischemia, the amount of isovolumetric shortening in the nonischemic posterior apex decreased significantly as LVEDP increased from 7 mm Hg to 12 or 19 mm Hg. There was no significant difference in isovolumetric shortening at LVEDP 12 and 19 mm Hg.

The amount of isovolumetric shortening in the non-

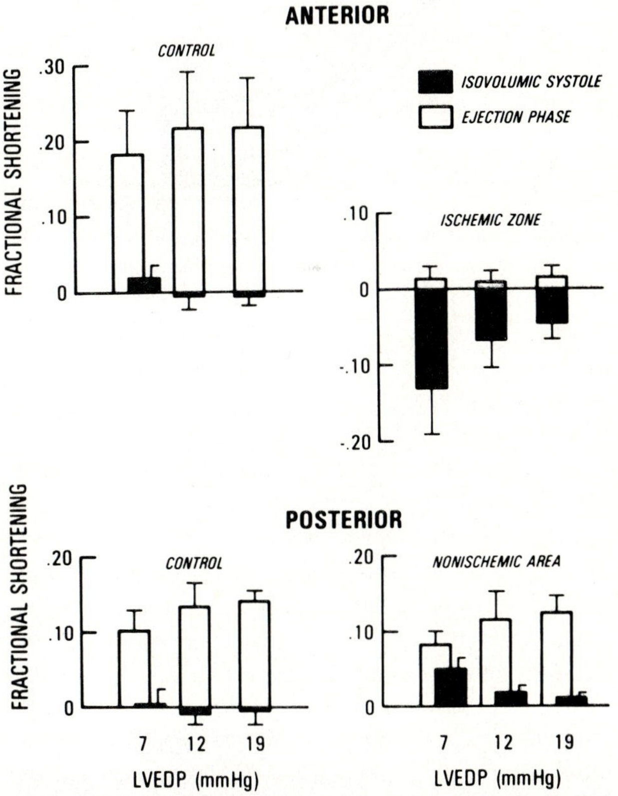

FIGURE 2. Regional segmental shortening in the seven animals. Values are with error bars denoting one standard deviation. The filled bars represent isovolumetric shortening (measured as the fractional change in segmental length from end-diastole to aortic valve opening) and the open bars are ejection phase shortening (from aortic valve opening to closure). Within each panel, three sets of bars are given for the three levels of LVEDP of 7, 12, and 19 mm Hg. The two *top panels* represent shortening in the anterior apex and the two *bottom panels* illustrate shortening in the posterior apex. In each case, the panel on the *left* is during control conditions and the panel on the *right* is after 30 (or more) min of acute ischemia when the anterior apex becomes the ischemic zone (*top right*) and the posterior apex is the nonischemic area (*lower right*). See text for statistical analysis and discussion.

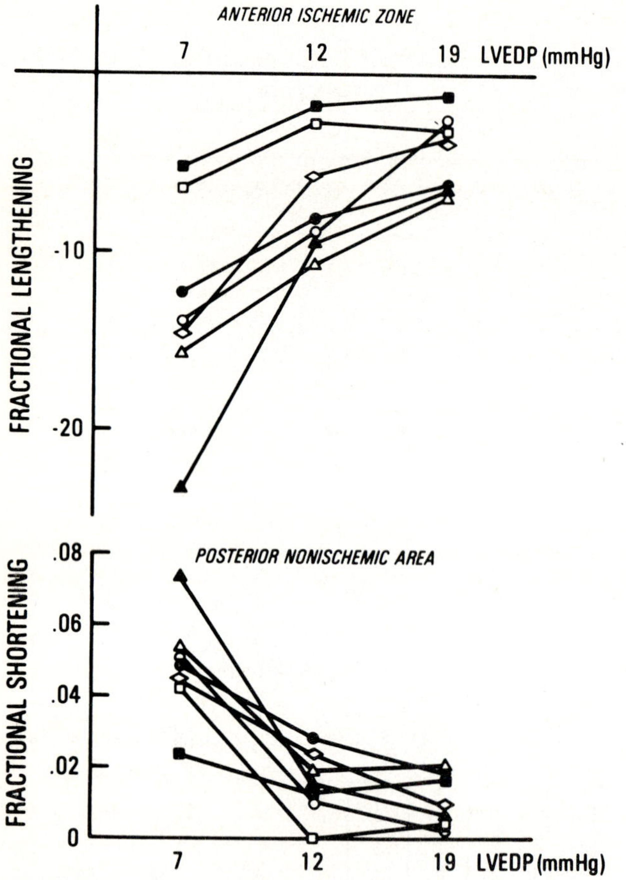

FIGURE 3. The simultaneous isovolumetric lengthening in the ischemic zone and isovolumetric shortening in the nonischemic area during acute ischemia are shown individually for each of the seven animals with the use of seven different symbols. For each animal, the symbols are connected by lines to demonstrate the change in isovolumetric shortening or lengthening as LVEDP is increased from 7 to 12 to 19 mm Hg. See text for discussion.

ischemic area directly paralleled the amount of isovolumetric lengthening in the ischemic zone. Figure 3 illustrates the regional isovolumetric data during acute ischemia for each of the seven animals at three levels of LVEDP. At LVEDP 7 mm Hg, the animals with the greatest amount of isovolumetric lengthening in the ischemic zone also had the greatest amount of isovolumetric shortening in the nonischemic areas (as shown with the filled and open triangles). Conversely, the animals with the least amount of isovolumetric lengthening in the ischemic zone were the same ones with the least amount of isovolumetric shortening in nonischemic areas (as shown with the filled and open boxes). As LVEDP increased, there was a significant decrease in isovolumetric lenthening of the ischemic zone that was directly paralleled by a significant decrease in isovolumetric shortening in nonischemic areas in each of the seven animals. An example of these changes is shown in figure 1.

The relationship between changes in isovolumetric length in the anterior and posterior apexes was examined by linear regression analysis. We defined x as the change in fractional isovolumetric shortening or lengthening in the anterior apex as LVEDP increased from 7 to 12 mm Hg, or from 12 to 19 mm Hg, and y as the change in fractional isovolumetric shortening in the posterior apex, also as LVEDP increased from 7 to 12 mm Hg or from 12 to 19 mm Hg. During the control period, there was no statistically significant correlation between x and y, i.e., between the fractional changes in isovolumetric shortening in the anterior apex and posterior apex. The correlation coefficient was .44. After acute ischemia, there was a significant ($p < .01$) correlation between the change in isovolumetric lengthening or bulge in the ischemic zone and the change in isovolumetric shortening in the nonischemic area. This was defined by the regression equation $y = -0.32x + 0.49$. The correlation coefficient was $-.64$. Thus, during acute ischemia, there was a direct correlation between the decrease in isovolumetric lengthening or bulge in the ischemic zone and the decrease in isovolumetric shortening in the nonischemic area as LVEDP increased.

In the posterior apex or nonischemic area, acute ischemia was associated with a significant decrease in ejection phase shortening when compared with that under control conditions at the same LVEDP. This was true at all three levels of LVEDP. However, the reduction in ejection phase shortening was less at high than at low LVEDP. When compared with that under control conditions at the same LVEDP, the reduction in ejection phase shortening in the nonischemic area with acute ischemia was 10 ± 8% at LVEDP 19 mm Hg, significantly less than the 21 ± 10% reduction at LVEDP 7 mm Hg.

Stroke volume and cardiac output (table 3). Stroke volume and cardiac output were measured in five of the seven animals (table 3). When compared with control conditions at the same LVEDP, acute ischemia was associated with a significant reduction in stroke vol-

TABLE 3
Stroke volume and cardiac output (mean ± 1 SD) at three levels of LVEDP before (Control) and after acute ischemia (Ischemia) in five animals

LVEDP	Stroke volume (ml/beat)		Cardiac output (l/min)	
(mm Hg)	Control	Ischemia	Control	Ischemia
7	24±3	16±4	2.9±0.5	1.9±0.3
12	40±8	30±6	4.9±1.0	3.3±0.7
19	49±11	38±10	5.9±1.5	4.2±1.1

See text for statistical comparisons.

ume and cardiac output. However, the magnitude of this reduction was less at high than at low LVEDP. When compared with that under control conditions at the same LVEDP, there was a reduction in stroke volume of 21 ± 16% during acute ischemia at LVEDP 19 mm Hg, which was significantly less than the 32 ± 15% reduction at LVEDP 7 mm Hg. This milder impairment of stroke volume with acute ischemia at high as compared with low LVEDP occurred in each of the five animals.

Discussion

The characteristic alterations in regional ventricular function that develop with acute ischemia include paradoxical systolic lengthening or bulge in the ischemic zone[9–15] and an increase in segmental shortening,[13, 14, 16–19] wall thickening,[20–22] or endocardial wall motion[23] in nonischemic areas. The concept that the ischemic zone may impose a mechanical disadvantage on the nonischemic area has evolved from theoretical studies of regional ischemia,[24–26] studies placing hypoxic and normal muscle strips in series,[27, 28] and studies of ventricular aneurysms.[29] It has been proposed that the magnitude of the mechanical disadvantage imposed by a "weak" ischemic[24–26] or aneurysmal muscle[29] is directly proportional to its size and inversely proportional to its stiffness.

Recently, we postulated that a mechanical interaction between ischemic and nonischemic areas occurs during acute ischemia in the intact ventricle.[7] We found an increase in segmental shortening in nonischemic areas during acute ischemia due to the increase in LVEDP and the Frank-Starling mechanism. However, all of the increase in nonischemic area shortening occurred during isovolumetric systole (end-diastole to aortic valve opening) and developed with a time course that paralleled the development of paradoxical isovolumetric lengthening or bulge in the ischemic zone. These findings suggested that all of the increase in nonischemic area shortening was expended in stretching the ischemic zone during isovolumetric systole. Although the hyperfunction of nonischemic areas has been thought to "compensate" for the loss of systolic function in the ischemic zone, we did not find any significant "compensatory" increase in ejection phase shortening (aortic valve opening to aortic valve closure) in the nonischemic areas.

The current study was designed to further examine the mechanical interaction between ischemic and nonischemic areas. We used techniques to measure regional ventricular function similar to those used in our previous study.[7] Ultrasonic segmental length gauges were implanted in the midwall and oriented in the circumferential direction. Thus, gauges were in line with the direction of local midwall fibers[8] and could detect the maximal amount of midwall segmental shortening.[30] Measuring regional function in the circumferential direction is important since there are many more circumferential than longitudinal fibers across the ventricular wall[8] and the predominant direction of left ventricular shortening and work is circumferential.[31, 32] This is also a sensitive method for the detection of alterations in regional function, as occurs with ischemia. For example, a circumferentially oriented segmental gauge in the subepicardium will be more sensitive to impairments in subendocardial blood flow and function than a segmental gauge placed in line with the local subepicardial fiber direction.[33] Thus, midwall circumferential segmental length gauges measure maximal midwall segmental shortening under normal conditions, and provide a sensitive measure of functional alterations induced by even mild degrees of myocardial ischemia.

The first hypothesis examined in the current study was that the ischemic zone imposes a mechanical disadvantage on the nonischemic areas. We postulated that this was due to the regional intraventricular unloading effect during isovolumetric systole that was observed in our prior study.[7] However, the increase in LVEDP with acute ischemia increases end-diastolic segmental length in the nonischemic area and may mask any mechanical disadvantage. Thus, to examine the first hypothesis, we compared regional function before and after acute ischemia at the same matched LVEDP. We found a significant increase in isovolumetric shortening and a decrease in ejection phase shortening in the nonischemic area under these conditions of acute ischemia at a matched LVEDP. These findings were present at each of the three matched levels of LVEDP (7, 12, and 19 mm Hg). The reduction in ejection phase shortening in the nonischemic area was primarily due to the significant amount of shortening that had been expended in stretching the ischemic zone during isovolumetric systole. Thus, the regional intraventricular unloading effect during isovolumetric systole resulted in a decrease in ejection phase shortening in the nonischemic area, a manifestation of the mechanical disadvantage imposed by the ischemic zone.

The second hypothesis examined in this study was that the magnitude of the mechanical disadvantage imposed by the ischemic zone is directly proportional to the amount of its paradoxical isovolumetric lengthening, which in turn is inversely related to its stiffness.

We found a direct parallel between the isovolumetric behavior of the ischemic zone and the nonischemic area in this study (figure 3). As LVEDP increased during acute ischemia, the amount of isovolumetric lenthening or bulge in the ischemic zone and the amount of isovolumetric shortening in the nonischemic area decreased in parallel. Since less shortening generated by the nonischemic area was expended in stretching the ischemic zone during isovolumetric systole at a high LVEDP, relatively more shortening was available during the ejection phase. Therefore, the reduction in ejection phase shortening in the nonischemic area during acute ischemia was less severe at high than low LVEDP. This was also reflected by a less severe reduction in stroke volume with acute ischemia at high than at low LVEDP (when compared with that under control conditions at the same matched LVEDP). These findings support the concept that the magnitude of the mechanical disadvantage imposed by the ischemic zone is directly related to the amount of its isovolumetric lengthening or bulge.

The mechanism for the reduction of the mechanical disadvantage imposed by the ischemic zone by an increase in LVEDP may be related to the passive properties of the ischemic zone. At higher LVEDP, the ischemic segment is at a steeper (stiffer) position on its passive pressure-length relationship. Less isovolumetric shortening would be expended by the nonischemic area in stretching an ischemic segment that offers greater resistance to passive (paradoxical) isovolumetric lengthing. Thus, the reduction in nonischemic area ejection phase shortening with acute ischemia would be less severe at high than at low LVEDP. This inverse relationship between the stiffness of the ischemic zone and its mechanical disadvantage supports the conclusions drawn from the theoretical studies examining "weak" and "strong" muscles in series.[24–26, 29]

The ischemic zone may also be particularly sensitive to changes in LVEDP since the end-diastolic pressure-length relationship is steeper after acute ischemia. Our findings are consistent with prior studies that have demonstrated an increase in ischemic zone stiffness with acute regional ischemia[13, 14, 34, 35] and an increase in global left ventricular stiffness with global hypoxia[36] or global ischemia.[37] However, these findings remain controversial because some investigators have found no change[25, 38] or a decrease[39, 40] in left ventricular stiffness with acute ischemia. Furthermore, it is difficult to use measurements of regional segmental length to assess regional myocardial stiffness or its change with ischemia. Elastic stiffness is more precisely defined by the stress-strain relationship than by the pressure-length relationship. Estimates of regional wall stress frequently are derived from mathematic models that require several assumptions that are controversial and difficult to validate.[41, 42] These calculations require a measure of the local radius of curvature, which cannot be accurately assessed from local measurements of segmental length. Furthermore, with myocardial ischemia, there are local shape changes that will significantly alter the local radius of curvature, particularly in the ischemic zone. Thus, segmental length data cannot be used reliably to describe changes in regional shape or wall stress that occur with ischemia, or the resultant change in myocardial wall stiffness.

The ischemic zone may not behave as a strictly passive tissure during isovolumetric systole. Studies with theoretical models[24, 27, 28] and in the intact ventricle[43] suggest that the ischemic zone retains some residual contractile function. If this were the case, then an increase in LVEDP could conceivably improve residual contractile function in the ischemic zone. A Frank-Starling effect has been demonstrated in the ischemic zone in a model of coronary stenosis,[44] but not with complete coronary occlusion.[45] If the ischemic zone is able to generate active tension during early isovolumetric systole, as in the model of Elings et al.,[24] then greater tension may develop with an increased LVEDP. This would be an additional mechanism by which the ischemic zone resists passive stretch during isovolumetric systole at high LVEDP. However, an increased LVEDP did not improve the akinesis of the ischemic zone during the ejection phase. Therefore, it is unlikely that the ischemic zone can utilize the Frank-Starling mechanism sufficiently to make any direct or effective contribution to ventricular ejection.

The results of our study can be related to the clinical setting of acute myocardial infarction. Bedside hemodynamic estimates of left ventricular filling pressure are frequently obtained in patients with acute myocardial infarction to guide therapy and to provide prognostic information.[5, 6, 46, 47] At an "optimal" left ventricular filling pressure, stroke volume is optimized while adverse hemodynamic effects are minimized.[1–6] Ventricular filling pressures above this optimal level are associated with pulmonary venous congestion, exacerbation of myocardial perfusion deficits, a possible decrease in stroke volume, and a poor prognosis.[5, 6, 38, 46, 47, 48] When ventricular filling pressure is below the optimal level, a significant increase in stroke volume can be obtained by therapy designed to increase LVEDP. The current study demonstrates that therapeutic preload manipulations to increase LVEDP to an optimal level during acute ischemia results in increased utilization of the Frank–Starling mechanism in the nonischemic area but not in the ischemic zone. In addition, at an optimal LVEDP, the ischemic zone imposes less of a mechanical disadvantage on the nonischemic area. As a result, acute ischemia is associated with a less severe reduction in nonischemic area ejection phase function and in stroke volume at high as compared with low LVEDP.

We conclude that during acute myocardial ischemia, the ischemic zone imposes a mechanical disadvantage on the nonischemic area due to the regional intraventricular unloading effect during isovolumetric systole. This mechanical disadvantage results in a reduction in ejection phase shortening in the nonischemic area, a finding that may be masked if the increase in LVEDP that normally accompanies acute ischemia occurs. The magnitude of the mechanical disadvantage of the ischemic zone is directly related to the amount of its paradoxical isovolumetric lengthening. Increases in LVEDP to an optimal level during acute ischemia improve regional and global ventricular function as a result of the Frank–Starling mechanism in the nonischemic (but not the ischemic) area, and by reducing the mechanical disadvantage that the ischemic zone imposes on the nonischemic area.

We gratefully acknowledge the assistance of Ms. Elizabeth Gilpin in the statistical analysis and Ms. Janeen McCracken for word processing.

References

1. Russell RO Jr, Rackley CE, Pombo J, Hunt D, Potanin C, Dodge HT: Effects of increasing left ventricular filling pressure in patients with acute myocardial infarction. J Clin Invest **49:** 1539, 1970
2. Broder MI, Cohn JN: Evolution of abnormalities in left ventricular function after acute myocardial infarction. Circulation **46:** 731, 1972
3. Crexells C, Chatterjee K, Forrester JS, Dikshit K, Swan HJC: Optimal level of filling pressure in the left side of the heart in acute myocardial infarction. N Engl J Med **289:** 1263, 1973
4. Chatterjee K, Parmley WW, Ganz W, Forrester J, Walinsky P, Crexells C, Swan HJC: Hemodynamic and metabolic responses to vasodilator therapy in acute myocardial infarction. Circulation **48:** 1183, 1973
5. Forrester JS, Diamond G, Chatterjee K, Swan HJC: Medical therapy of acute myocardial infarction by application of hemodynamic subsets. N Engl J Med **295:** 1356; 1404, 1976
6. Forrester JS, Diamond GA, Swan HJC: Correlative classification of clinical and hemodynamic function after acute myocardial infarction Am J Cardiol **39:** 137, 1977
7. Lew YW, Chen Z, Guth B, Covell J: Mechanisms of augmented segment shortening in nonischemic areas during acute ischemia of the canine left ventricle. Circ Res **56:** 351, 1985
8. Streeter DD Jr, Spotnitz HM, Patel DP, Ross J Jr, Sonnenblick EH: Fiber orientation in the canine left ventricle during diastole and systole. Circ Res **24:** 339, 1969
9. Tennant R, Wiggers CS: The effect of coronary occlusion on myocardial contraction. Am J Physiol **112:** 351, 1935
10. Prinzmetal M, Schwartz LL, Corday E, Spritzler R, Bergman HC, Kruger HE: Studies on the coronary circulation VI: Loss of myocardial contractility after coronary artery occlusion. Ann Intern Med **31:** 429, 1949
11. Tatooles CJ, Randall WC: Local ventricular bulging after acute coronary occlusion. Am J Physiol **201:** 451, 1961
12. Tyberg JV, Forrester JS, Wyatt HL, Goldner SJ, Parmley WW, Swan HJC: An analysis of segmental ischemic dysfunction utilizing the pressure-length loop. Circulation **49:** 748, 1974
13. Theroux P, Franklin D, Ross J Jr, Kemper WS: Regional myocardial function during acute coronary artery occlusion and its modification by pharmacologic agents in the dog. Circ Res **35:** 896, 1974
14. Theroux P, Ross J Jr, Franklin D, Covell JW, Bloor CM, Sasayama S: Regional myocardial function and dimensions early and late after myocardial infarction in the unanesthetized dog. Circ Res **40:** 158, 1977
15. Ringertz HG, Carlsson E, Tyberg JV: A method for the study of regional ischemic dysfunction in the intact dog. Invest Radiol **11:** 556, 1976
16. Nakano J: Effect of changes in coronary arterial blood flow on the myocardial contractile force. Jpn Heart J **7:** 78, 1966
17. Heyndrickx GR, Baig H, Nellens P, Leusen I, Fishbein MC, Vatner SF: Depression of regional blood flow and wall thickening after brief coronary occlusions. Am J Physiol **234:** H653, 1978
18. Pashkow F, Holland R, Brooks H: Early changes in contractility and coronary blood flow in the normal areas of the ischemic porcine heart. Am Heart J **93:** 349, 1977
19. Molaug M, Geiran O, Kiil F: Compensatory cardiac mechanisms evoked by septal ischemia in dogs. Am J Cardiol **51:** 201, 1983
20. Kerber RE, Marcus ML, Wilson R, Ehrhardt J, Abboud FM: Effects of acute coronary occlusion on the motion and perfusion of the normal and ischemic interventricular septum: an experimental echocardiographic study. Circulation **54:** 928, 1976
21. Savage RM, Guth B, White FC, Hagan AD, Bloor CM: Correlation of regional myocardial blood flow and function with myocardial infarct size during acute myocardial ischemia in the conscious pig. Circulation **64:** 699, 1981
22. Nakamura M, Sasayama S, Takahashi M, Ohyagi A, Yamamoto A, Lee JD, Kawai C: Regional dysfunction of the interventricular septum during acute coronary artery occlusion. Cardiovasc Res **16:** 144, 1982
23. Rigaud M, Rocha P, Boschat J, Farcot JC, Bardet J, Bourdarias JP: Regional left ventricular function assessed by contrast angiography in acute myocardial infarction. Circulation **60:** 130, 1979
24. Elings VB, Jahn GE, Vogel JHK: A theoretical model of regionally ischemic myocardium. Circ Res **41:** 722, 1977
25. Laird JD, Vellekoop HP: Time course of passive elasticity of myocardial tissue following experimental infarction in rabbits and its relation to mechanical dysfunction. Circ Res **41:** 715, 1977
26. Bogen DK, Rabinowitz SA, Needleman A, McMahon TA, Abelmann WH: An analysis of the mechanical disadvantage of myocardial infarction in the canine left ventricle. Circ Res **47:** 728, 1980
27. Tyberg JV, Parmley WW, Sonnenblick EH: In-vitro studies of myocardial asynchrony and regional hypoxia. Circ Res **25:** 569, 1969
28. Wiegner AW, Allen GJ, Bing OHL: Weak and strong myocardium in series: implications for segmental dysfunction. Am J Physiol **235:** H776, 1978
29. Parmley WW, Chuck L, Kivowitz C, Matloff JM, Swan HJC: In vitro length-tension relations of human ventricular aneurysms: relation of stiffness to mechanical disadvantage. Am J Cardiol **32:** 889, 1973
30. Freeman GL, LeWinter MM, Engler RL, Covell JW: Relationship between myocardial fiber direction and segment shortening in the midwall of the canine left ventricle. Circ Res **56:** 31, 1985
31. Rankin JS, McHale PA, Arentzen CE, Ling D, Greenfield JC Jr, Anderson RW: The three-dimensional dynamic geometry of the left ventricle in the conscious dog. Circ Res **39:** 304, 1976
32. Phillips CA, Grood ES, Schuster B, Petrofsky JS: Left ventricular work and power: circumferential, radial and longitudinal components. Mathematical derivation and characteristic variation with left ventricular dysfunction. J Biomechanics **15:** 427, 1982
33. Gallagher KP, Osakada G, Hess OM, Koziol JA, Kemper WS, Ross J Jr: Subepicardial segmental function during coronary stenosis and the role of myocardial fiber orientation. Circ Res **50:** 352, 1982
34. Edwards CH II, Rankin JS, McHale PA, Ling D, Anderson RW: Effects of ischemia on left ventricular regional function in the conscious dog. Am J Physiol **240:** H413, 1981

35. Hess OM, Osakada G, Lavelle JF, Gallagher KP, Kemper WS, Ross J Jr: Diastolic myocardial wall stiffness and ventricular relaxation during partial and complete coronary occlusions in the conscious dog. Circ Res **52:** 387, 1983
36. Serizawa T, Vogel WM, Apstein CS, Grossman W: Comparison of acute alterations in left ventricular relaxation and diastolic chamber stiffness induced by hypoxia and ischemia. J Clin Invest **68:** 91, 1981
37. Wong BYS, Toyama M, Reis RL, Goodyer AVN: Sequential changes in left ventricular compliance during acute coronary occlusion in the isovolumic working canine heart. Circ Res **43:** 274, 1978
38. Palacios I, Johnson RA, Newell JB, Powell WJ Jr: Left ventricular end-diastolic pressure-volume relationships with experimental acute global ischemia. Circulation **53:** 428, 1976
39. Forrester JS, Diamond G, Parmley WW, Swan HJC: Early increase in left ventricular compliance after myocardial infarction. J Clin Invest **51:** 598, 1972
40. Pirzada FA, Ekong EA, Vokonas PS, Apstein CS, Hood WB Jr: Experimental myocardial infarction XIII: Sequential Changes in left ventricular pressure-length relationships in the acute phase. Circulation **53:** 970, 1976
41. Huisman RM, Sipkema P, Westerhof N, Elzinga G: Comparison of models used to calculate left ventricular wall force. Med Biol Eng Comput **18:** 133, 1980
42. Yin FCP: Ventricular wall stress. Circ Res **49:** 829, 1981
43. Yoran C, Sonnenblick EH, Kirk ES: Contractile reserve and left ventricular function in regional myocardial ischemia in the dog. Circulation **66:** 121, 1982
44. Wyatt HL, da Luz PL, Waters DD, Swan HJC, Forrester JS: Contrasting influences of alterations in ventricular preload and afterload upon systemic hemodynamics, function, and metabolism of ischemic myocardium. Circulation **55:** 318, 1977
45. Wyatt HL, Forrester JS, da Luz PL, Diamond GA, Chagrasulis R, Swan HJC: Functional abnormalities in nonoccluded regions of myocardium after experimental coronary occlusion. Am J Cardiol **37:** 366, 1976
46. Ratshin RA, Rackley CE, Russell RO Jr: Hemodynamic evaluation of left ventricular function in shock complicating myocardial infarction. Circulation **45:** 127, 1972
47. Weber KT, Janicki JS, Russell RO, Rackley CE: Indentification of high risk subsets of acute myocardial infarction: derived from the Myocardial Infarction Research Units Cooperative Study data bank. Am J Cardiol **41:** 197, 1978
48. Kjekshus JK: Mechanism for flow distribution in normal and ischemic myocardium during increased ventricular preload in the dog. Circ Res **33:** 489, 1973

Circulation

VOL 72 NO 6
DECEMBER 1985

An Official Journal of the American Heart Association, Inc.®

FEATURES

Physicians confront the nuclear peril

BERNARD LOWN, M.D.

Dedicated to Paul D. White, one of the founders of the American Heart Association, who inspired many cardiologists with a global and charitable view of the human condition.

Into the eternal darkness, into fire, into ice.
— Dante, The Inferno

We must behave as though the world was created for man.
— Thomas Mann

We live in an age of unprecedented uncertainty. Life on Earth is perilously poised at the precipice of history. No public health threat ever faced by humankind equals the threat of nuclear war. Never before has man possessed the destructive resources to make his planet uninhabitable. This fact, although widely acknowledged, is not fully comprehended. Our comprehension is defined by the boundaries of our experience and the world has never experienced multimegaton detonations.

Should physicians become mired in what appear to be global, political issues? Does our commitment as physicians involve addressing these issues? Is such involvement consonant with medical values? Does it confuse our medical responsibilities with our responsibilities as citizens? What, if any, are our special areas of expertise or insight that permit us, as physicians, to take a stance on the nuclear arms race without undermining our credibility? Finally, does physician involvement make a difference?

A remarkable aspect of the growing public concern about nuclear war is the prominent role of the medical profession.[1] A group calling itself Physicians for Social Responsibility (PSR), nearly a quarter of a century ago, wrote a landmark study on the medical consequences of nuclear war.[2-6] In recent years, with escalation of the arms race and intensification of the cold war, increasing numbers of leading medical figures as well as traditional professional organizations have voiced concern and are speaking out. Prestigious medical organizations including the American Medical Association, the British Medical Association, the World Health Organization, the Institute of Medicine, the American College of Physicians, the American Public Health Association, the American Academy of Pediatrics, the American Academy of Family Practice, the American College of Emergency Physicians, and many others are addressing the nuclear dilemma.[7-14] To date, however, the great majority of physicians remain uninvolved and deem the nuclear threat remote from their medical concerns. In large measure, this lack of involvement is due to inadequate appreciation of the magnitude of the danger and of the intimate link between the nuclear threat and medicine. It is therefore appropriate to examine the issues concretely and systematically.

What is at stake?

The medical and ecologic consequences. It is now 40 years since physicians first confronted the medical consequences of nuclear war. In Hiroshima a primitive uranium bomb with the explosive power of 13 kilotons (13,000 tons of TNT) killed more than 100,000 people and injured nearly 100,000 others out of a total population of 245,000. Ninety percent of the buildings within the city limits were demolished in a few seconds. Of the nearly 300 doctors in Hiroshima, only 28 were available to attend the thousands of victims. Of the 1780 nurses, 1654 were dead or too badly injured to work. Forty-two out of 45 hospitals were destroyed or rendered useless.[15, 16]

Compared with the Hiroshima bomb, nuclear weapons have grown a thousandfold in destructiveness. Today, we speak of megatons, not kilotons. In terms of destructive magnitude, a megaton is equivalent to 1 million tons of dynamite. Were this amount of dynamite to be transported by rail, the train of boxcars

This *Editorial* is based on the First Annual Edward Massie Lecture in Cardiovascular Disease, Washington University School of Medicine, St. Louis, October 1983.

Dr. Lown is Co-President of the International Physicians for the Prevention of Nuclear War, recipients of the 1985 Nobel Peace Prize.

Address for correspondence: Bernard Lown, M.D., Professor of Cardiology, Lown Cardiovascular Laboratories, Harvard School of Public Health, 221 Longwood Ave., Boston, MA 02115.

would stretch over 400 miles. There are almost 18,000 thermonuclear weapons with plutonium fission triggers, each sufficient to devastate a city of more than 100,000 inhabitants. But worldwide there are fewer than 3000 cities of this size.[17]

Early studies. The first physicians' study, conducted in the early 1960s, examined the medical effect of a modest multimegaton attack against Boston.[2–6] From a population of 2,875,000 then residing in the metropolitan area, it was determined that 1 million would be killed immediately, 1 million would be fatally injured, and 500,000 would be injured but would survive. How many physicians would be available to attend the millions of victims? Out of greater Boston's 6500 physicians only 10 percent would themselves remain alive and uninjured. In the postattack period, one physician would be available for approximately 1700 acutely injured persons. This ratio has staggering implications. If the physician were to spend only 10 minutes on diagnosis and treatment of each injured patient, and if the work day were 20 hours, 8 to 14 days would be required before every injured person would be seen for the first time.[4]

Each 10 minute consultation would have to be performed without x-rays, laboratory equipment, diagnostic aids, medical supplies, drugs, blood, plasma, beds, and other medical equipment. Unlike Hiroshima and Nagasaki, no help could be anticipated from the "outside." No rational medical organization would remain, even to render primitive care. There could be no meaningful medical response.

Those physicians able and willing to serve would confront injuries and illnesses unique to their experience and remote from their area of expertise. Patients would be afflicted with fractures, trauma to internal organs, penetrating wounds of thorax and abdomen, multiple lacerations, hemorrhage, shock, and second- and third-degree burns. Many, if not all, would have received sublethal or lethal doses of radiation. Many would be psychologically shocked and psychiatrically deranged. Indeed, 50 percent or more of the immediate survivors would have combined injuries with synergistic effects. For example, a dose of 100 rads of external body radiation to a standard burn victim increases mortality eightfold. A dose of even 25 rads to such a burn doubles the mortality.[18]

Over one-third of the survivors would perish in epidemics in the 12 months following a nuclear attack due to the combined impact of malnutrition, crowded shelters, poor sanitation, immunologic deficiency, contaminated water supply, proliferation of insect and rodent vectors, inadequate disposal of the dead, lack of antibiotic supplies, and poor medical care.[19] Those afflicted would be ideal candidates for AIDS, which may constitute the ultimate malady for all survivors.[20]

Physicians would be unequipped psychologically or morally for the medical and ethical problems they would confront after a nuclear attack.[4] When faced with thousands of victims, how does the physician select those to be treated first, if at all? How is one to choose between saving the lives of the few and easing the pain of many? When pain-relieving narcotics and analgesics are in scarce supply, what is the physician's responsibility to the fatally injured or those with incurable disease? Which of the duties — prolongation of life or relief of pain — takes precedence? How is the physician to respond to those who are in great pain and demand euthanasia? What then substitutes for the sacred and cherished oaths that have guided medical practice for several millennia? Modern medicine has nothing to offer, not even a token benefit, in the case of thermonuclear war.

Contemporary studies. The ethical questions posed above were pondered nearly a quarter of a century ago.[2–6] They represent oversimplifications when considering the magnitude and sophistication of current nuclear arsenals. New data have provided the scientific underpinning for the apocalyptic predictions of the most demented of Cassandras. The World Health Organization, in a recent authoritative study, concluded that in an all-out nuclear war using only one-half of the world's nuclear stockpiles, over 1 billion people would be killed instantly, mainly in the United States, the Soviet Union, Europe, China, and Japan.[14] More than 1 billion immediate survivors would suffer serious injuries and radiation sickness, for which medical help would be either unavailable or unavailing. It is thus possible that almost half of all the inhabitants on Earth would be killed in the immediate aftermath of a global nuclear war. Organized society and civilized life, at least in the northern hemisphere, would be reduced to a state of prolonged barbarism and brutality. Yet these grim and foreboding conclusions do not depict the full gravity of the consequences. Indeed the real situation is likely to be much worse.

Nuclear winter. Astonishingly, 40 years into the atomic age, scientists first discovered unforeseen catastrophic global consequences of nuclear war. Nuclear explosions, particularly groundbursts, lift enormous quantities of fine soil into the atmosphere — more than 100,000 tons of dust for every megaton detonated at ground level.[21] With explosions of 1 megaton or greater, these particles are likely to be transported into the higher layers of the stratosphere and would spread within weeks over the greater part of the northern hemisphere, where they could remain for years. Airbursts would cause massive fire storms. The urban environment is surfeited with asphalt, plastic, and petroleum products, which, when they burn, generate extraordinary amounts of black soot and smoke. Such particulates would shield sunlight, cooling the Earth's surface. Within a week after a nuclear war, only a small percentage of the sunlight that normally reaches the Earth would penetrate the haze. Subfreezing temperatures would jeopardize the lives of survivors. Land temperatures away from coastlines would plummet to $-15°$ C and possibly to $-25°$ C.[22] The impact of these climatic changes would spare neither the tropics, where subfreezing temperatures would be especially devastating, nor the southern hemisphere.

The raging urban fires resulting from nuclear war would have additional consequences, not fully appreciated before. Large amounts of deadly toxins would be released into the air because cities are storehouses for enormous quantities of combustible synthetic materials. As these materials burned, they would release pyrotoxins, including carbon monoxide, cyanides, dioxins, and furans. Such a release would place additional, unpredictable stresses on the global ecosystem. An estimated 30% of the northern hemisphere's mid-latitude land areas would receive a radiation dose greater than 500 rads.[23] Such radiation exposure, from external gamma-emitting radioactive fission products in fallout, would be more than the median lethal dose (LD-50) for healthy adults. Over the ensuing weeks, fallout would contribute at least another 100 rads of external dose radiation, from radioiodine, radiostronthium, and radiocesium. These substances would concentrate in specific body systems, such as the thyroid, bones, the gastrointestinal tract, and in the milk of lactating mothers.

Survivors would face extremes of cold; water shortages; scarcity or total lack of food and fuel; severe radiation exposure; chemical poisoning of the air, water, and food; raging epidemics; and unprecedented psychologic stresses — all to be endured in a pall of pervading frigid darkness.[22]

When the dust, soot, and poisons ultimately clear, the radioactivity dissipates, and the sun mercifully reappears, an additional plague would afflict the unfortunate survivors. The nitrous oxides generated by the nuclear fireball would have depleted the ozone layer high in the atmosphere, thereby increasing short-wave ultraviolet radiation several fold for many years. Increased ultraviolet exposure is known to suppress the immune system of men and animals[24] and to induce corneal damage and cataracts leading to blindness.[25]

The studies that form the basis for the tragic scenario outlined above assumed an exchange of 5000 megatons.[22] But severe climatic effects would result even from a "small" war with the explosive power of 100 megatons. The implications of these findings are as profound as they are disquieting. A first strike by the United States against Soviet land-based missiles, without any retaliation by them, would make the United States uninhabitable. Extinction of our species cannot be excluded.[23] These findings have been widely confirmed and accepted by scientists in the East and the West.

We know little or nothing of the synergistic effects on our fragile ecosystem of subfreezing temperatures, darkness, high levels of radiation, diverse toxins from combustibles, excessive ultraviolet rays, and other unforeseen consequences of nuclear war. It is sheer hubris to pretend that there would be human survival after such a man-made catastrophe. Talk by politicians of winning or surviving a nuclear war represents a crass abrogation of these stark medical and ecologic facts.

The likelihood of nuclear war. The notion is widespread that nuclear war will never happen. Common sense dictates that these weapons never be used because they are capable of simultaneously inflicting genocide on the victim and suicide on the attacker. But nuclear reality compels a different assessment.[8, 26] Although no national interest could justify nuclear war, sober appraisal suggests that if the present course of multiplying megatonnage continues, it will be short of miraculous if we reach the end of the century, a mere 15 years away, without a nuclear catastrophe. Seven considerations lead to this sobering conclusion.

(1) *Historic precedents.* In 5 thousand years of recorded human history, only 125 years have been free of war. All nations have armed themselves in order to defend themselves. The old Roman adage reigned, *vis pacem para bellum.* History teaches that weapons that have been continuously and massively stockpiled are invariably used.

(2) *Growth in nuclear arsenals.* During the initial decades of the atomic age, the military policy of the two superpowers was one of deterrence. Cities were the primary targets; the populations of the United States and Soviet Union were held hostage. Only a finite and limited arsenal was required to eliminate a dozen or more major urban centers on either side. In the early 1960s, then Secretary of Defense Robert McNamara concluded that if 400 nuclear warheads were dropped on either the United States or the Soviet Union, 30% of the population and 75% of the industri-

al capacity of each country would be destroyed instantly.[27] A military policy based on deterrence provided crisis stability. Since then, the two superpowers have acquired at least 50,000 strategic and tactical nuclear warheads, equivalent in the aggregate to more than four tons of TNT for every man, woman, and child on Earth.

If deterrence is the objective of military policy, what is the purpose of accumulating an overkill capacity equivalent in destructiveness to more than 1 million Hiroshimas? If the aim is to deter the Soviets, a single modern Trident submarine would suffice. A Trident, with its 24 MIRVed missiles, carries 240 nuclear warheads of 100 kilotons each, totalling 24 megatons, eight times the total firepower used in World War II. This is sufficient to destroy not only the Soviet Union but every major city in the northern hemisphere. An identical threat is posed to the United States by Soviet nuclear submarines.

The spiralling accumulation of massive overkill capacity makes the world less secure and invites each side to preempt a strike by the other. If preemption or first strike becomes a nation's nuclear policy, there is no limit to the number of weapons that can be justified under one or more strategic scenarios. The sheer increase in nuclear bombs year by year invites their use. In this race, the runners are no longer in control of their legs.

(3) *Military technologic developments.* An even more compelling provocation for nuclear war is the growing precision of missile delivery systems. Recent advances in microminiaturization of electronic components have significantly improved the accuracy of ballistic missiles, and constitute the technologic basis for a new "counterforce" strategy.[28] This strategy calls for targeting the opponent's land-based missile systems in their hardened silos. The ability to destroy a large fraction of an opponent's intercontinental ballistic missiles in a first strike represents a dramatic shift from deterrence, the prevailing strategy for the past 30 years, to a fantasy about the possibility of "winning" a nuclear war.

The adoption of this counterforce strategy diminishes the time between detection of a presumed attack and a retaliatory response. Delay in firing one's own missiles increases the risk of their loss. To avoid such destruction, each side must plan to launch nuclear weapons early, even on warning of an attack and before such an attack can be verified. It takes about 20 minutes for a missile to traverse the distance between the Soviet Union and the United States. This time has been reduced to less than 10 minutes by the American emplacement of Pershing II missiles in West Germany and the Soviets' response in placing missiles on ships off the U.S. coast. In no previous age were adversaries so totally and continuously mobilized for instant war. It is unlikely that hair-trigger readiness can endure as a permanent condition.

(4) *Technologic malfunctions.* The stability of the nuclear establishment is linked to the reliability of early warning systems. These systems involve sophisticated computers that must cope with many potentially confusing signals. With the increase in nuclear weapons and the multiplication of information networks, there has been an exponential growth in false alarms. In one 18 month period, there were 3703 false alerts.[29] Most of these were routinely assessed and dismissed, but 147 false alarms were deemed serious enough to require further evaluation to determine whether or not they represented actual nuclear attacks.[30] In a period of 8 months there were six major computer failures that placed the United States on nuclear alert.

Detection of increased nuclear readiness on one side leads inevitably to increased readiness on the other side. These preparations could in turn provide "verification" of nuclear-launch preparation by the opponent, thereby activating the feedback loop of responses and leading inexorably to a nuclear exchange.

In this age of ubiquitous high technology, seldom does a day pass when physicians in hospitals do not encounter some malfunctioning hardware. Whereas the failure of a pacemaker, defibrillator, or oxygenator might jeopardize a single life, a malfunctioning military computer threatens the life of a nation if not of life itself.

(5) *Human fallibility.* Military systems involve the complex interactions of man and machine. As these systems become ever more complex, geographically dispersed and technologically sophisticated, there is an increase in system failure rates. Alcoholism, drug addiction, mental illness, and other related problems are pervasive in our society. Military personnel have no special immunity from such afflictions. About 5% to 6% of U.S. military personnel, or around 115,000 people, have critical access to nuclear weapons or their control systems. In a single year, the Department of Defense separates nearly 5000 people from this cadre for behavior that is deemed to render them unreliable.[31] Of these, nearly a third are removed because of the use of hard drugs, including LSD. A major problem in Soviet society is the prevalence of chronic alcoholism. This problem, no doubt, pervades the Soviet military as well.

An additional and no less potent threat is a possible

lapse in rational behavior by the decision makers who hold the nuclear systems in check. In times of political crisis, as history shows, miscalculation, misunderstanding, impetuosity, and operational rigidities shape events. Just as World War I spiralled out of a local conflict, when mounting tensions and misperceptions overwhelmed European leaders, so too, a small crisis anywhere in this tension-ridden world could escalate into a nuclear conflagration.[32] "The balance of terror is now threatened by the balance of error."[33]

(6) *Proliferation of nuclear weapons.* At present, three nations (France, England, and China), in addition to the United States and the Soviet Union, are known to possess nuclear weapons. India has exploded a nuclear device, and Israel and South Africa are suspected to have a dozen or more nuclear bombs. A number of small nations already have the necessary technology and could develop nuclear weapons without much difficulty. It is estimated that 10 to 20 additional nations will obtain nuclear weapons during the 1990s.[34]

As more countries and more people gain access to nuclear materials and nuclear weapons, the likelihood of accident, nuclear terrorism, or deliberately initiated nuclear war increases. The possession by many different nations of the capacity to launch a nuclear strike multiplies the possibility of its occurrence. It is not difficult to imagine fanatical leaders engaging in nuclear blackmail when faced with serious threats to their power. In an age of shifting and intricate alliances, a nuclear exchange, once begun, will be difficult to contain.

In 1970 a substantial step forward was taken to stop the spread of nuclear weapons when the Non-Proliferation Treaty was signed. In exchange for the renunciation of nuclear weapons by the nonnuclear states, the superpowers assumed obligations to pursue negotiations in good faith to achieve an early end to the nuclear arms race.[35] The United States and the Soviet Union can exert little moral leadership in preventing proliferation since they have failed so conspicuously to exercise restraint in weapons production.

(7) *Incentives for preemption.* A prevalent misconception is that newer technologies and greater weapon sophistication provide increasing precision, control, and security. Valid command, control, and communication systems* on which putative deterrence is based must, however, be able to survive a first strike, even a modest one. A single nuclear blast high above the United States or the Soviet Union could shut down the nation's power grid and knock out the entire communication system of either country.[36, 37] When a nuclear explosion occurs at high altitude, it generates an electromagnetic pulse (EMP) of enormous electrical currents; its effect would extend over thousands of miles. A 10 megaton burst at an altitude of 400 km would destroy electrical equipment from coast to coast.

Furthermore, there are a limited number of critical targets that, if hit, would decapitate the military command structures.[38] Neither side will permit itself to be made militarily deaf, blind, and dumb, with individual commanders left isolated, uninformed, and able only to engage in a genocidal götterdammerung. The incentive, therefore, is to strike first. Thus, it becomes imperative to launch one's own missile before detonation of the first attacking weapon, while the military communication network is still intact.

Forces have been set in motion that threaten human survival. These forces are increasingly out of human control. Ultimately the bomb, the robot, and the computer will preempt man's decision-making role and take command.

The price we are already paying

Even if war is prevented, the arms race is exacting enormous economic, psychological, and moral costs. The current global economic crisis is largely the result of the mortgaging of scarce world resources to the military. In dollar equivalent terms, military expenditures exceed the annual income of half the world's population — its poorest two and half billion people.[39, 40] The resources allocated to the military far exceed total world health care expenditures. In 1985 world military spending exceeded $800 billion or $100 million each and every hour. This is occurring at a time when life expectancy at birth in Africa is 30 years less than in Europe, when more than 40,000 children die daily from malnutrition and infection, when 5 million under the age of 5 die annually from disease that could be prevented by inexpensive immunization,[41] and when over 300 million children are chronically hungry.

We are bereft of resources to combat hunger. Yet the solution of world health problems requires but picayune investments, compared to the enormity of military expenditures. The total cost for eradicating smallpox from the Earth, a major public health achievement, is spent during a mere 150 minutes of the arms race. Access to sanitary water (the lack of which accounts for 80 percent of all sickness) could be pro-

*The network of communications by which a country discovers it is under attack, evaluates the nature of the attack, and grades its response.

vided to the entire world for the cost of only 5 months of military spending.[42]

The arms race also diverts the intellectually gifted from health and other human services to military activities. Research funds are increasingly diverted from vital societal needs. In 1980, $30.7 billion was spent by the United States on research and development; of this, $15.1 billion (49 percent) was allocated to the military and $3.7 billion (12 percent) to health. The disparities are even more striking today. Similarly distorted priorities are a global phenomenon. Of the world's research physicists and engineering scientists, more than half are employed by the military.[43]

The United States is not spared the adverse consequences of the arms race. A physicians task force on hunger reported that 20 million Americans suffer a "growing epidemic" of hunger.[44] They found that one in 12 Americans is hungry at least part of every month and countless numbers border on starvation. In some areas, malnutrition is comparable to that found in Third World nations. Rampant protein, calorie, and vitamin deficiencies stunt growth, permanently impair intellectual development, and cause lethargy and disease. No section of the United States is free of "the human face of hunger."[45] Physicians and health workers increasingly confront wrenching ethical choices in allocating scarce economic resources.

The reason for this state of affairs is not obscure. When a team of physicians toured the United States in 1979 searching for hunger, they found almost none.[44] From 1982 to 1985, however, the U.S. government cut $12 billion from federal food stamps for the poor and from child-nutrition programs, while food outreach programs have been eliminated and eligibility for food relief restricted. The situation has worsened. The medical experts of this task force concluded that hunger in America could be eliminated in 6 months if the government allocated $7 billion or the cost of two nuclear-powered aircraft carriers to combat hunger. We are already living in the rubble of World War III.

Moral implications

The arms race has been galloping without moral brakes, like cancer cells that multiply because they have been genetically programmed to do so. Pointing nuclear-tipped missiles at entire nations is a virtually unprecedented act of moral depravity.[46] The world recoiled with horror when the Nazis murdered innocent hostages held accountable for the behavior of their compatriots. There is little outrage now when billions of people are being held hostage, threatened with extinction, accountable for actions of governments they have little control over. More than 30 years ago the British philosopher and mathematician Bertrand Russell called attention to the prevalent distortion of values: "Our world has sprouted a weird concept of security and a warped sense of morality. Weapons are sheltered like treasures while children are exposed to incineration."

This moral abnegation results in part from our failure to dispel a myth in confronting the unthinkable. Nuclear war is seen as war with but magnified consequences. We need to break this intellectual stranglehold — this habitual mode of thinking. Nuclear "war" is a term of deception. Nuclear conflict is not war as we have known war. Everyone resides in the combat zone and every human being on Earth is targeted. No political differences can be adjudicated with nuclear bombs. No victory can be snatched in the global holocaust. Nuclear missiles are not weapons; they are instruments of genocide. Nuclear war between the superpowers will be the most brutal verdict ever rendered against humankind. It will be an incomprehensible act of suicide. It will be Jonestown in Guyana on a grand scale.

The role for physicians

Although many in our profession would agree that the medical, economic, and ecologic consequences of the arms race and nuclear war are as I have described them, they would demur from acting on this issue *in their capacity as physicians.* Almost all would agree with the commitment of various medical societies to educate both the public and political leaders on the medical consequences of a nuclear war or with the stance that "prevention is the only reasonable medical response."[12] But must a physician's activities be limited to descriptions of the medical and environmental consequences of nuclear war? Or should physicians advocate and lobby for policies that will reduce the likelihood of nuclear war?

Historically, the medical profession has not shied away from involvement in diverse social and political issues when these have impacted on the health of their communities. Health hazards have not been excluded from the province of medical concerns because their remedy required political activity.[47] The imperatives of preventive medicine have compelled physicians to engage in a variety of social and political struggles. Physicians have worked to improve nutrition of impoverished families and have supported legislation to remove asbestos from insulation and lead paint from school rooms. Pediatricians have pressed successfully for legislation to require safety caps on household chemical and medication containers to reduce the chances of childhood poisoning. Certainly nuclear war is an issue of no lesser magnitude than lead paint, safety caps, seat belts, smoking, highway safety, gun control, and the like.

Physicians must respond to the moral imperatives of their commitment to life and health rather than worry about crossing the ill-defined boundary of the political realm. Although the nuclear issue is a highly charged political issue, it is also a public health issue of the greatest importance. The highest duty of physicians in the nuclear age is marshalling professional resources to work for preventing the final epidemic. The struggle for human survival requires no apologies. It is consonant with the most hallowed traditions of medicine. Over a century ago, Rudolf Virchow, a principal architect of scientific medicine, maintained that "Medicine was a social science, and politics nothing but medicine on a grand scale."[48] He taught that to improve the health of the public, the physician must not shy away from social action. The principles that Virchow espoused have even greater relevance today when the question concerns not only the health but the very survival of life on Earth.

Achievements of the physicians antinuclear movement

Physicians are pragmatists. Overwhelmed with burdensome responsibilities for which there is rarely enough time, they are not prone to dissipate their energies tilting at windmills. Physicians need to be persuaded that their labors will be productive.

The experience of the physicians antinuclear movement is instructive. Its accomplishments, both in the United States and worldwide, have been significant.[49] Millions of people have been persuaded to confront the reality of the nuclear threat for the first time. Physicians' activities have exposed to public view the litany of horrors resulting from blast, fire, and radiation. A large segment of the public has been convinced that there can be no useful medical response to nuclear war, that most of the fatally injured will never see a health worker even for the relief of pain before they die.

The physicians movement has also exerted an effect on the political process. Because our message has been heard, one no longer hears about the possibility of keeping nuclear war limited, nor talk about nuclear demonstration shots to prove national resolve. Nor is there discourse about winning or prevailing in a nuclear conflict. The subject of civil defense has become a butt for social satire. In many countries concern about the nuclear arms race has gained respectability as a legitimate issue among political parties.[50]

In less than 5 years the International Physicians for the Prevention of Nuclear War (IPPNW) has grown to over 135,000 members in 41 countries. Of interest to the readers of this Journal is that this antinuclear movement was founded by American and Soviet cardiologists. Indeed, the most signal accomplishment of the IPPNW has been the broad-based, free-flowing dialogue between physicians of the two contending power blocs.[51] Its success stems largely from an insistent avoidance of linkage with problems that have embittered relations between the superpowers. The IPPNW has resisted being sidetracked to other issues, even those that are morally compelling. Combatting the nuclear threat has been IPPNW's total and exclusive preoccupation.

The IPPNW has not limited itself to dire prognostication. A year ago, at its fourth annual congress in Helsinki, IPPNW offered a medical prescription for peace. That prescription called for a comprehensive moratorium on all nuclear explosions.[52] Such a moratorium is an achievable first step in slowing and then reversing the arms race. Underground testing is readily verifiable; it does not require trust between the superpowers. A ban on testing would cap the most dangerous aspect of the nuclear arms race, the ongoing qualitative improvement and introduction of ever more sophisticated first strike weapons. A complete testing moratorium is a prescription simple in concept, devoid of complexity, free of risk to either party, verifiable without need for intrusive on-site inspection, and will, if enacted, begin unwinding the potential doomsday process.

The IPPNW has also addressed the causes that propel the arms race. In large measure the cause is the distrust pervading Soviet-American relations. The complex differences between our social systems have been reduced to martial combat between the forces of good and evil. We physicians are well equipped by training and background to counteract such simplistic, dehumanized, and dangerous stereotyping of fellow human beings. IPPNW has sponsored extensive physician exchanges in which Soviet and American physicians have traversed each other's country engaging in a free-flowing dialogue on nuclear issues. As physicians, we can set an example and demonstrate that people can work together in spite of their political and cultural differences.

IPPNW has also stimulated cooperation by others in the health field. At the fifth IPPNW Congress in Budapest, leading virologists and public health workers were brought together to promote immunization of children in the Third World. At a time when disease and hunger are rampant in the world, physicians have many opportunities to contrast the dismal investment made in health care with the profligate spending for war preparations.

These are but some of the accomplishments of the physicians antinuclear movement. Although the nuclear genie may never again be forced back into the bottle, greater involvement by the medical profession will hasten the day when it does not threaten our extinction.

Final thoughts

The world today is in danger. But still greater is the opportunity. Although science and technology have catapulted us to the brink of extinction, the same ingenuity has brought humankind to the frontier of an age of abundance. Never before was it possible to feed all the hungry, to shelter all the homeless, to teach all the illiterates, to assuage much of the affliction. Science and medicine can liberate us from drudgery and pain. Only those who see the invisible can do the impossible. But in order to do the impossible, in the words of Jonathan Schell we ask "not for our personal survival: we ask only that we be survived. We ask for assurance that when we die as individuals, as we know we must, mankind will live on."[53]

References

1. Relman AS: Physicians, nuclear war, and politics. N Engl J Med **307:** 744, 1982
2. Garland J: The medical consequences of nuclear war: Editor's note. N Engl J Med **266:** 1127, 1962
3. Ervin FR, Glazier JB, Aronow S, Nathan S, Coleman R, Avery N, Shohet S, Leeman C: The medical consequences of thermonuclear war. I. Human and ecologic effects in Massachusetts of an assumed thermonuclear attack on the United States. N Engl J Med **266:** 1127, 1962
4. Sidel VW, Geiger HJ, Lown B: The medical consequences of thermonuclear war. II. The physician's role in the postattack period. N Engl J Med **266:** 1137, 1962
5. Aronow S: The medical consequences of thermonuclear war. III. A glossary of radiation terminology. N Engl J Med **266:** 1145, 1962
6. Leiderman PH, Mendelson JH: The medical consequences of thermonuclear war. IV. Some psychiatric and social aspects of the defense-shelter program. N Engl J Med **266:** 1149, 1962
7. Geiger HJ: Addressing apocalypse now: the effects of nuclear warfare as a public health concern. Am J Pub Health **70:** 958, 1980
8. Lown B, Chivian E, Muller J, Abrams H: The nuclear arms race and the physician. N Engl J Med **304:** 726, 1981
9. Hiatt HH: Preventing the last epidemic. JAMA **244:** 2314, 1981
10. Beeson PB: Consequences of nuclear warfare. West J Med **138:** 254, 1983
11. American Medical Association: Physician and public education on the medical consequences of thermonuclear war. *In* Proceedings of the House of Delegates, 35th Interim Meeting. Report of the Board of Trustees. Chicago, 1981, American Medical Association, pp 59–60
12. American College of Physicians: The medical consequences of radiation accidents and nuclear war. Ann Intern Med **97:** 447, 1982
13. The Report of the British Medical Association's Board of Science and Education: The medical effects of nuclear war. Published on behalf of the British Medical Association by John Wiley & Son, Chicester, New York, Brisbane, Toronto, Singapore, 1983
14. Bergstrom S: Effects of nuclear war on health and health services (Report of the International Committee of Experts in Medical Sciences to Implement Resolution WHA 34.38.). World Health Organization Publ. A36.12, 1983
15. Yuzaki M: Disintegration of community by the atomic bombs; working documents (Proceedings of the International Symposium on Damage and After Effects of the Atomic Bombing of Hiroshima and Nagasaki, July 21 to August 9, 1977). Tokyo, Asahi Evening News, 1978, p 105
16. Hersey J: Hiroshima. New York, 1946, Alfred A. Knopf, pp 33–34
17. Sagan C: Nuclear war and climatic catastrophe: some policy implications. Foreign Affairs **62:** 257, 1983–84
18. Constable JD: Burn casualties. *In* Adams R, Cullen S, editors: The final epidemic: physicians and scientists on nuclear war. Chicago, 1981, Public Education Foundation for Nuclear Science, pp 182–191
19. Abrams H, Von Kaenel WE: Medical problems of survivors of nuclear war: infection and the spread of communicable disease. N Engl J Med **305:** 1226, 1981
20. Greer D: The immunological impact of nuclear warfare. Paper presented at Institute of Medicine Symposium on Medical Effects of Nuclear War, Washington, DC, September 1985
21. Crutzen PJ, Birks JW: The atmosphere after a nuclear war: twilight at noon. Ambio **11:** 114, 1982
22. Turco RP, Toon OB, Ackerman TP, Pollack JB, Sagan C: Nuclear winter: global consequences of multiple nuclear explosions. Science **222:** 1283, 1983
23. Ehrlich PR, Harte J, Harwell MA, Raven PH, Sagan C, Woodwell GM, Berry J, Ayensu ES, Ehrlich AH, Eisner T, Gould SJ, Grover HD, Herrera R, May RH, Mayr E, McKay CP, Mooney HA, Myers N, Pimentel D, Teal JM: Long term biological consequences of nuclear war. Science **222:** 1293, 1983
24. DeFabo EC, Kripke ML: Dose-response characteristics of immunologic unresponsiveness to UV-induced tumors produced by UV irradiation of mice. Photochem Photobiol **30:** 385, 1979
25. Pitts DM: *In* Hearing on the Consequences of Nuclear War on the Global Environment, 197th Congress, 2nd Session, Serial No. 171. Washington, DC, 1983, U.S. Government Printing Office, pp 83–101
26. Lown B: Physicians and nuclear war. JAMA **246:** 2331, 1981
27. U.S. Congress Office of Technology Assessment: The Effects of Nuclear War OTA-NS 089 (1979). Washington, DC, 1979, US Government Printing Office
28. Tsipis K: The accuracy of strategic missiles. Sci Am **233:** 14, 1975
29. Halloran R: Senators report: False warning of Soviet strikes. New York Times, October 29, 1980, p 16
30. Cox AM: Russian roulette. New York, 1982, Times Books
31. Dumas L: Human fallibility and weapons. Bull Atom Sci **36:** 15, 1980
32. Alexandrov VV, Britten S, Abrams H: Risks of unintentional nuclear war: an overview. Working Paper Fourth Congress. IPPNW Report **2:** 15, 1984
33. Wieseltier L: The great nuclear debate (special issue). New Republic **188:** 7, 1983
34. Kapur A: International nuclear proliferation: multilateral diplomacy and regional aspects. New York, 1979, Praeger, p 79
35. Tovish A: The Non-Proliferation Treaty and nuclear disarmament. IPPNW Report **3:** 11, 1985
36. Broad WJ: Nuclear pulse. I. Awakening to the chaos factor. Science **212:** 1009, 1981
37. Lerner EJ: Electromagnetic pulses: potential crippler. IEE Spectrum **18:** 41, 1981
38. Ford D: The button: the Pentagon's strategic command and control system. New York, 1985, Simon and Schuster
39. Sidel VW: Buying death with taxes: Impact of arms race on health care. *In* Adams R, Cullen S, editors: The final epidemic. Chicago, 1981, Public Education Foundation for Nuclear Science, pp 35–47
40. Sivard RF: World military and social expenditures. Washington, DC, 1984, Arms Control Association
41. Henderson RH: Vaccine preventable diseases of children. *In* Protecting the World's Children, Bellagio Conference, 1984. New York, 1984, Rockefeller Foundation, pp 1–16
42. Hiatt HH: The final epidemic: prescriptions for prevention. JAMA **252:** 635, 1984
43. Pringle EP, Spigelman J: The nuclear barons. London, 1982, Michael Joseph

44. Physician Task Force on Hunger in America: Hunger in America: the growing epidemic. Boston, 1985, Harvard University School of Public Health
45. Hunger in America (editorial): Boston Sunday Globe, March 3, 1985, p A18
46. Lown B: President's message. IPPNW Report **1:** 2, 1983
47. Cassel C, Jameton A: Medical responsibility and thermonuclear war. Ann Intern Med **97:** 426, 1982
48. Eisenberg L, Ludwig R, Virchow K: Where are you now that we need you? Am J Med **77:** 524, 1984
49. Boyer P: Physicians confront the apocalypse: the American medical profession and the threat of nuclear war. JAMA **254:** 633, 1985
50. Lown B: The burden of the arms race: an international perspective. Co-President's message. IPPNW Report **3:** 2, 1985
51. Lown B, Chazov E: Cooperation not confrontation: the imperative of a nuclear age. The message from Budapest. JAMA **254:** 655, 1985
52. Lown B: Physicians need to devise a prescription. IPPNW Report **2:** 2, 1984
53. Schell J: The fate of the Earth. New York, 1982, Alfred A. Knopf

Percutaneous transluminal coronary angioplasty: a surgeon's view

NICHOLAS T. KOUCHOUKOS, M.D.

AS PHYSICIANS, we are becoming increasingly aware of and increasingly committed to the need for cost containment in the delivery of health care. When new modes of therapy become available, we must evaluate critically not only their effectiveness, but also their cost in relation to that of alternative, potentially equally effective modalities. A case in point is percutaneous transluminal angioplasty (PTCA) of the coronary arteries. Most PTCA procedures are performed in symptomatic patients with proximal, discrete high-grade stenosis of one of the three major coronary arteries, most commonly the anterior descending.[1] Advocates maintain that PTCA is a good alternative to coronary artery bypass grafting (CABG) in patients with single-vessel disease because it is effective, it is associated with less morbidity and lower cost, and it may delay or obviate the need for subsequent CABG. A role for PTCA in patients with multivessel disease has been advocated as well. The number of PTCA procedures performed annually in the United States is unclear. In the 1 year interval ending in March 1983, approximately 27,000 procedures were done.* In 1984, the figure may have approached 85,000.[2]

Individual studies and several multicenter randomized trials[3,4] have shown conclusively that CABG cannot enhance the already excellent survival of patients with single-vessel disease who have stable or unstable angina or who are asymptomatic. Accordingly, CABG for patients with single-vessel disease has been reserved primarily for individuals whose symptoms cannot be controlled with medical therapy. Among the 6564 patients in the Coronary Artery Surgery Study (CASS) who had CABG between August 1975, and December 1978, 18.5% had single-vessel disease.[5] In our experience during the 1974 to 1977 corresponding interval, only 7% of 2467 patients undergoing CABG had single-vessel disease.[6] The fraction of CABG procedures currently performed for single-vessel disease is not likely to exceed that in the CASS study and is probably substantially lower.

Although virtually all patients presently treated with PTCA are suitable candidates for CABG, not all patients undergoing coronary bypass grafting are candidates for PTCA. In the CASS Registry, approximately 20% to 25% of patients with single-vessel disease who had CABG met conventional criteria for PTCA (proximal, discrete, subtotal, noncalcified stenosis in patients with well preserved ventricular function).[5,7] Based on the assumption that 200,000 CABG procedures are performed annually, no more than 37,000 (18.5%) would involve patients with single-vessel disease and only 9250 (25% of 37,000) of the surgically treated patients would be candidates for PTCA. If 50,000 PTCAs are being performed annually (a conservative estimate) and if 75% involve patients with single-vessel disease, a minimum of 37,500 patients with single-vessel disease are undergoing PTCA annually. Thus PTCA is being implemented in many patients (at least 28,000 per year) *not* currently considered candidates for CABG who would otherwise be managed medically. This phenomenon is extant even though PTCA may not be demonstrably more effective than medical management for this group of patients. The trend seems particulary questionable for treatment of patients with stable angina, since many of them experience improvement in functional capacity and maintain their employment status with medical therapy.[7,8]

Results of PTCA. The NHLBI Registry for PTCA has accumulated data from over 3000 patients treated in 105 centers between September 1977 and September 1981. Complete follow-up data are available for 2272 patients from 65 of the centers.[9] Angiographic success was defined as a reduction in diameter narrowing of at least 20%. It was achieved in 1397 patients (61%). Seventy-two percent of these successfully treated patients (or 44% of the original group) were improved

From the Division of Cardiothoracic Surgery, Washington University School of Medicine, St. Louis.

Address for correspondence: Nicholas T. Kouchoukos, M.D., Department of Surgery, Jewish Hospital at Washington University Medical Center, 216 S. Kingshighway Blvd., St. Louis, MO 63110.

*Personal communication, K. M. Detre, Member, Executive Committee of the National Heart, Lung, and Blood Institute Percutaneous Transluminal Coronary Angioplasty Registry.

and required no further procedures 1 year after the procedure, 14% had repeat PTCA, 12% required CABG, 3% sustained a myocardial infarction, and 1.6% died. Among the initially successfully treated patients, 67% were asymptomatic after 1 year. Recently reported higher initial success rates (80% to 85%) may reflect improved techniques and favorable patient selection. Despite improvement in initial success rate, angiographically determined rates of recurrent stenosis 6 to 12 months after PTCA have not been reduced, remaining 30% to 35%. Consequently, increasing numbers of patients are undergoing repeat procedures. Preliminary studies indicate that the restenosis rate after repeat PTCA may be lower than that after initial PTCA.

Approximately 5% to 10% of patients treated with PTCA require urgent or emergent CABG. Hospital mortality, perioperative myocardial infarction, and postoperative complication rates are substantially higher for patients requiring emergent operation after PTCA than for those who undergo elective operation, particularly in the presence of multivessel disease.[10–12]

Relief of symptoms by PTCA has been satisfactory in most patients with single-vessel disease. However, neither the extent of relief nor improvement in functional capacity have been shown to exceed appreciably those in candidates for PTCA treated medically.[7, 8] Symptomatic improvement may be less marked among patients with multivessel disease after PTCA, since all of the occlusive lesions may not be suitable for dilation and "incomplete revascularization" results. Incomplete revascularization among CABG patients results in a higher incidence of persistent or recurrent angina and this is also true for patients who undergo PTCA.[13] Employment status is maintained in a high percentage of patients after successful PTCA. However, it is also maintained in an equally high percentage of patients who have unsuccessful PTCA followed by CABG.[14] Not surprisingly, patients return to work more quickly after PTCA than after CABG. Despite these and other uncertainties regarding the effectiveness of PTCA in comparison with medical therapy and CABG, it has an established role in the treatment of symptomatic patients with coronary artery disease.

Costs. Costs of PTCA have been compared generally with those of CABG rather than with the costs of medical treatment per se. Using data acquired from patients with single-vessel disease in the NHLBI PTCA Registry at 11 centers and assuming an 80% initial success rate and a follow-up interval of 6 to 12 months, Jang et al.[15] reported that PTCA saved an average of $7149 per patient compared with CABG. However, several occult and additional costs associated with PTCA were ignored, such as costs for standby of surgeons, anesthesiologists, and operating room facilities. In a survey of 276 cardiac surgeons and surgical groups in 39 states of whom 175 (63%) responded anonymously to a questionnaire,* I found that 163 are available on a standby basis to respond to complications of PTCA and that 99 (57%) among these submit a charge for *being available* that ranges from $100 to $1000. Forty-six percent charge between $250 and $750. Thirty-nine percent of the standby anesthesiologists submit a charge of $100 to $750. An operating room is made available on a standby basis at 76% of the centers polled with charges levied for *its availability* ranging from $100 to $1000. Assuming that 50% of all centers (a conservative estimate) submit charges ($500 for the surgeon, $300 for the anesthesiologist, and $500 for the operating room), at least $650 should be added to the cost of each PTCA performed in the United States.

The analysis of Jang et al.[15] failed to consider costs of repeat catheterization, repeat angioplasty, or subsequent bypass grafting. In the PTCA Registry, 26% of patients required either repeat PTCA or CABG within 1 year after initial angioplasty.[9] All of these (and probably many others in the Registry as a whole) had at least one repeat catheterization. Jang and co-workers failed to recognize that the patients undergoing CABG to which the PTCA group was compared contained a significantly higher percentage of patients over age 65 (27% vs 9% in the angioplasty group). Costs of CABG in elderly patients exceed those in younger patients because the duration of hospitalization is longer.[16] Thus, the calculated average cost for CABG is too high for comparative purposes.

A recent report from the Mayo Clinic compared expenditures for PTCA and CABG in patients with single-vessel disease during a 3 year interval ending in December 1981.[17] One year after the procedures, the mean monetary outlay was modestly (15%) lower for the PTCA-treated group. Charges for standby of surgeons and anesthesiologists were not included. A major component of the expense of PTCA was associated with the treatment of recurrent stenosis evident in 33% of patients within 1 year. Fifteen of the 55 patients in whom PTCA was sucessful initially required repeat PTCA (n = 6) or CABG (n = 9) during this interval. Only two of the 89 surgically treated patients required reoperation within the first year. The PTCA patients

*A list of geographic locations of the surgeons responding is available on request.

had a greater number of subsequent hospitalizations and hospital days.

It seems clear that unless the initial failure and restenosis rates of PTCA can be reduced substantially, cost savings from the widespread application of PTCA may be more apparent than real. Studies with longer intervals for follow-up are urgently needed to define the durabiity of PTCA.

Unresolved issues. In my view, the data available at present are insufficient to justify the inference that PTCA is more effective than medical management for patients with stable, mild, or moderate angina, or that it is more effective than CABG for patients with severe or unstable angina. The potential benefit of lower morbidity associated with PTCA may be offset by the increased mortality and rates of infarction associated with emergent operation, the need for repeat catheterization and repeat angioplasty, and risks associated with subsequently required CABG. Furthermore, the available analyses of costs suffer from incompleteness and limited follow-up. They do not conclusively document cost-effectiveness of PTCA compared with CABG. Of most importance, the durability of PTCA is questionable. The goal of postponement for 3 to 5 years of the need for CABG or for repeat PTCA may not be realized for most patients.

When CABG was first developing, critics and skeptics argued that it was being applied indiscriminately and that randomized trials were needed to determine whether or not it had a bona fide role in the treatment of coronary artery disease. Modern CABG was performed initially in 1967. The first large-scale randomized trial comparing CABG with medical therapy was initiated by the Veterans Administration in 1972. The NHLBI-sponsored randomized trial comparing medical and surgical treatment of patients with unstable angina was initiated in 1972. The CASS was initiated in 1974. Numerous single-center, randomized trials have been performed as well. Coronary PTCA was first reported in 1977. Remarkably, in the past 8 years not one multicenter prospective randomized trial comparing PTCA with medical therapy or with CABG has been initiated. The techniques for PTCA are now sufficiently standardized to permit valid comparison with current medical therapy and CABG.

Because most patients who undergo CABG are not candidates for PTCA according to current criteria, and because increasing numbers of patients are undergoing PTCA, one cannot escape the conclusion that large numbers of patients are being *added* to the pool of those subjected to aggressive interventions rather than being benefited by assignment to a less expensive procedure as implied by the lay press.[18] The cost of this subtle excursion is not inconsequential.

Under conditions when an invasive procedure is clearly indicated and in our current social and economic climate, the implicit assumption that angioplasty is less expensive than CABG can lead to inappropriate therapeutic decisions. As an example, overt reimbursement for PTCA under the prospective payment system (diagnostic related groups, DRGs) entails payment through an ICD-9 category of 36.0 (direct surgery on the coronary arteries) — in most hospitals placing the procedure in the DRG No. 108 (cardiothoracic surgery with pump except coronary bypass and valves).[19] This categorization may make PTCA seem to be a "bargain" to hospitals. Hospital administrators may therefore exert undue pressure on cardiologists and internists to perform the less expensive procedure, regardless of its therapeutic merit in comparison with CABG.

PTCA is being applied increasingly to patients with multivessel disease and with more extensive single-vessel disease including totally occluded vessels. Data available are insufficient to justify this trend on a large scale. Prospective, randomized trials comparing PTCA with medical therapy and with CABG are needed to define objectively the utility of PTCA. Subgroups of patients suitable for randomization have been recently proposed by Mock et al.[20] Significant differences in survival may not be found even among patients with multivessel disease because of the favorable natural history of the patterns of coronary artery disease in many patients deemed suitable for PTCA. However, other end points such as the extent and duration of relief of symptoms and improvement in functional capacity, subsequent infarction rate, need for secondary procedures, and cumulative costs can and must be characterized.

References

1. Detre KM, Myler RK, Kelsey SF, Van Raden M, To T, Mitchell H: Baseline characteristics of patients in the National Heart, Lung, and Blood Institute Percutaneous Transluminal Coronary Angioplasty Registry. Am J Cardiol **53:** 7C, 1984
2. Block PC: Emergency surgery after percutaneous transluminal coronary angioplasty: he who calls the tune may have to pay the piper. Ann Thorac Surg **40:** 1, 1985
3. Russell RO, Moraski RE, Kouchoukos N, et al: Unstable angina pectoris: national cooperative study group to compare surgical and medical therapy. Am J Cardiol **42:** 839, 1978
4. CASS Principal Investigators and their Associates: Coronary artery surgery study (CASS): a randomized trial of coronary artery bypass surgery; survival data. Circulation **68:** 939, 1983
5. Kennedy JW, Kaiser GC, Fisher LD, Fritz JK, Myers W, Mudd G, Ryan TJ: Clinical and angiographic predictors of operative mortality from the collaborative study in coronary artery surgery (CASS). Circulation **63:** 793, 1981
6. Kouchoukos NT, Oberman A, Kirklin JW, Russell RO, Karp RB, Pacifico AD, Zorn GL: Coronary bypass surgery: analysis of fac-

tors affecting hospital mortality. Circulation **62**(suppl I): I-84, 1980
7. Holmes DR, Vlietstra RE, Fisher LD, Smith HC, Mock MB, Faxon DP, Gosselin AJ, Ryan TJ, Judkins MP, Pettinger M, participants in the Coronary Artery Surgery Study: Follow-up of patients from the Coronary Artery Surgery Study (CASS) potentially suitable for percutaneous transluminal coronary angioplasty. Am Heart J **106:** 981, 1983
8. Hlatky MA, Califf RM, Kong Y, Harrell FE, Rosati RA: Natural history of patients with single-vessel disease suitable for percutaneous transluminal coronary angioplasty. Am J Cardiol **52:** 225, 1983
9. National Heart, Lung, and Blood Institute PTCA Registry: Long-term efficacy of percutaneous transluminal coronary angioplasty (PTCA): report from the National Heart, Lung, and Blood Institute PTCA Registry. Am J Cardiol **53:** 27C, 1984
10. Jones E, Craver JM, Grüntzig AR, King SB III, Douglas JS, Bone DK, Guyton RG, Hatcher CR Jr: Percutaneous transluminal coronary angioplasty: role of the surgeon. Ann Thorac Surg **34:** 493, 1982
11. Reul GJ, Cooley DA, Hallman GL, Duncan JM, Livesay JJ, Frazier OH, Ott DA, Angelini P, Massumi A, Mathur VS: Coronary artery bypass for unsuccessful percutaneous transluminal coronary angioplasty. J Thorac Cardiovasc Surg **88:** 685, 1984
12. Killen DA, Hamaker WR, Reed WA: Coronary artery bypass following percutaneous transluminal coronary angioplasty. Ann Thorac Surg **40:** 133, 1985
13. Mabin TA, Holmes DR Jr, Smith HC, Vlietstra RE, Reeder GS, Bresnahan JF, Bove AA, Hammes LN, Elveback LR, Orszulak TA: Follow-up clinical results in patients undergoing percutaneous transluminal coronary angioplasty. Circulation **71:** 754, 1985
14. Holmes DR Jr, Vlietstra RE, Mock MB, Smith HC, Dorros G, Cowley MJ, Kent KM, Hammes LN, Janke L, Elveback LR, Vetrovec GW: Employment and recreation patterns in patients treated by percutaneous translminal coronary angioplasty: a multicenter study. Am J Cardiol **52:** 710, 1983
15. Jang GC, Block PC, Cowley MJ, Gruentzig AR, Dorros G, Holmes DR Jr, Kent KM, Leatherman LL, Myler RK, Sjolander SME, Stertzer SH, Vetrovec GW, Willis WH Jr, Williams DO: Relative cost of coronary angioplasty and bypass surgery in a one-vessel disease model. Am J Cardiol **53:** 52C, 1984
16. Montague NT, Kouchoukos NT, Wilson TAS, Bennett AL III, Knott HW, Lochridge SK, Erath HG Jr, Clayton OW: Morbidity and mortality of coronary bypass grafting in patients 70 years of age and older. Ann Thorac Surg **39:** 552, 1985
17. Reeder GS, Krishnan I, Nobrega FT, Naessens J, Kelly M, Christianson JB, McAFee MK: Is percutaneous coronary angioplasty less expensive than bypass surgery? N Engl J Med **311:** 1157, 1984
18. Angioplasty for milder CAD may soon bypass the bypass, cardiologists say. Medical World News, October 22, 1984, p 22
19. Thoracic surgery and diagnosis related groups (DRG's). The American Board of Thoracic Surgery Newsletter, vol 2, Fall, 1984
20. Mock MB, Reeder GS, Schaff HV, Holmes DR Jr, Vlietstra RE, Smith HC, Gersh BJ: Percutaneous transluminal coronary angioplasty versus coronary artery bypass: isn't it time for a randomized trial? N Engl J Med **312:** 916, 1985

PERSPECTIVE

Has 'obstruction' hindered our understanding of hypertrophic cardiomyopathy?

JOHN MICHAEL CRILEY, M.D., AND ROBERT J. SIEGEL, M.D.

The ill and unfit choice of words wonderfully obstructs the understanding. — *Sir Francis Bacon*

The presence of an outflow tract pressure gradient in patients with hypertrophic cardiomyopathy (HCM) has been equated with an obstruction deemed primarily responsible for significant morbidity and mortality. Over 40 names containing variations of the words obstruction or stenosis have been applied to this disease. So strong was the belief in the presence and primacy of obstruction in the early 1960s that angiocardiograms and surgical observations were perceived to demonstrate a muscular sphincter or "contraction ring"[1] that later proved to be mythical. We believe that hindered or impeded outflow is rarely, if ever, present in HCM and that the equation gradient = obstruction has wonderfully obstructed the understanding of this disease process for nearly 3 decades. The bases for our questioning the primacy of obstruction and suggesting that impaired diastolic function and life-threatening arrhythmias are of more significance in HCM will be developed in this article. Since it was the outflow tract pressure gradient that initially led to the assumption that an obstruction was present, mechanisms responsible for the development of pressure gradients will first be discussed.

Pressure gradients. At least four different mechanisms capable of producing physiologic or pathologic outflow tract pressure gradients have been characterized. The left ventricular and aortic pressure, aortic flow, and left ventricular volumetric events associated with these gradients will be depicted.

Impulse gradients (figure 1) are instantaneous pressure differences between the left ventricle and aorta that occur in normal hearts and are generated in early systole during the time when peak flow acceleration (dQ/dT) and velocity are achieved.[2] After peak flow there is a deceleration with reversal of the early systolic pressure gradient so that the aortic pressure exceeds left ventricle pressure and the rate of outflow declines. Impulse gradients are related to flow acceleration in early systole as left ventricle pressure rapidly increases and aortic pressure lags behind. They are of greater magnitude in high flow states such as during exercise or after a premature ventricular contraction.[2]

The normal ventricle ejects approximately 60% of its stroke volume in the first half of systole, and the ventricular volumetric curve has achieved an asymptote at the time of aortic valve closure. In the following two figures, these normal contours for aortic flow and left ventricular volume are reproduced in open lines and circles for comparison with the contours in the disease states depicted.

Discrete obstructive pressure gradients (figure 2) across localized regions of stenosis, as in aortic stenosis, are associated with a reduction in the rate of ejection and ventricular emptying. There is a diminished rate of rise (dP/dT) of the pressure pulse distal to the stenosis. The orifice size calculated by hydrodynamic formulation remains constant over a wide range of flow.[1] An inverse relationship has been demonstrated between the magnitude of the pressure gradient in aortic stenosis and the rate of ventricular emptying—the more severe the gradient, the more retarded the rate of emptying.[3] Peak flow and velocity occur later than normal and flow is distributed almost symmetrically (58%/42%) over the entire ejection period, which is longer than normal. Thus, both the systolic ejection period (measured from the onset of aortic pressure rise to the dicrotic notch) and the ejection time (duration of aortic outflow) are prolonged. Aortic valve closure occurs shortly after the onset of retrograde aortic flow, which results from relaxation of the left ventricle and the development of an adequate negative pressure gradient and negative dP/dT. The ventricle both empties and fills more slowly than the normal ventricle (solid dots vs open circles), and augmented atrial transport function (prominent increase in left ventricular volume with the "a" wave) is evident.

Dynamic gradients (figure 3) between the body and outflow tract of the left ventricle are recorded at rest or after provocation in some patients with HCM. Pressure gradients with similar waveform appearance (brisk

From the Divisions of Cardiology, Harbor–UCLA Medical Center, Torrance, and Cedars–Sinai Medical Center, Los Angeles, CA.
Address for correspondence: John Michael Criley, M.D., Harbor–UCLA Medical Center, 1000 West Carson St., Torrance, CA 90509.
Received Aug. 2, 1985; accepted Aug. 8, 1985.

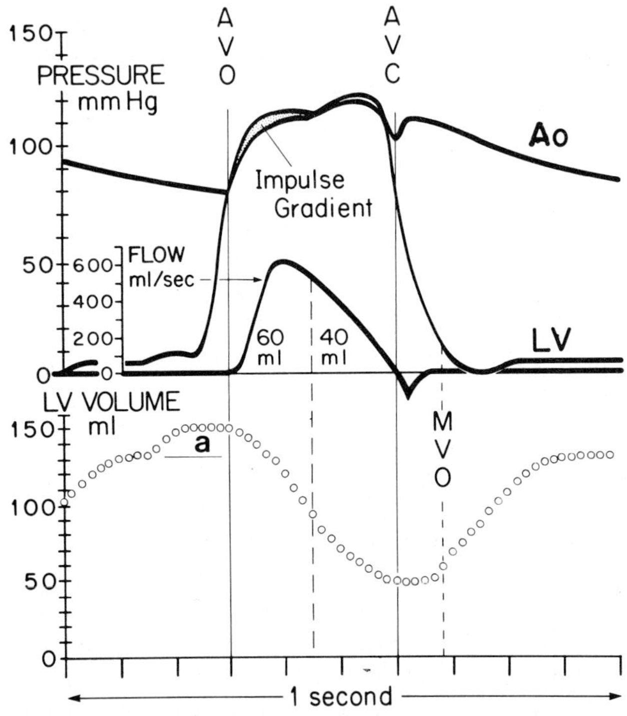

FIGURE 1. Impulse gradient in a normal ventricle. Left ventricular (LV) and aortic (Ao) pressure, aortic flow, and ventricular volumetric relationships are displayed. Vertical solid lines indicate aortic valve opening (AVO) and aortic valve closure (AVC), and encompass the systolic ejection period. Dashed lines indicate the midpoint of systole and mitral valve opening (MVO). a = atrial contribution to ventricular filling.

aortic upstroke, mid and late systolic gradient) can also be induced in normal or hypertrophied ventricles subjected to inotropic, hypovolemic, or vasodilator provocations.[4-6] Calculations of outflow orifice area based on hydrodynamic formulae suggest progressive constriction during systole, and perturbations that increase the magnitude of the gradient result in marked decreases in calculated orifice size.[1] The pressure and flow relationships[1, 7, 8] associated with dynamic gradients in a patient with HCM can be divided into three time periods, which are designated in figure 3 by encircled numbers and are referred to throughout this article as phases 1 to 3.

In phase 1, the body, outflow tract (dashed line), and aortic pressures rise while peak flow acceleration and velocity are enhanced and achieved earlier than in the outflow tract of the normal left ventricle. As a consequence, there is a larger impulse gradient than in a normal ventricle and the emptying slope of the left ventricle volumetric plot is correspondingly steeper (solid dots vs open circles).[1, 8, 9]

Phase 2 is characterized by a divergence of the pressure in the body of the left ventricle from that in the outflow tract and aorta. There is a decline in aortic flow to zero or near zero. The pressure gradient reaches its maximum during this phase, as the ventricular pressure reaches a midsystolic peak and the outflow tract and aortic pressures a midsystolic trough.[1, 7-9] Left ventricular ejection ends as the ventricle achieves a small volume and a supernormal ejection fraction.[8-10]

In phase 3 there is virtually no aortic outflow,[1, 7-11] and the ventricle is essentially isovolumetric.[8-10] There is a persistent but declining pressure gradient as the ventricular pressure falls, while there is a secondary rise in outflow tract and aortic pressures. The pressures in the ventricular body and outflow tract then equalize as they decline below the aortic pressure. Complete aortic valve closure and the aortic dicrotic notch occur after a negative gradient and an adequate negative dP/dT have developed between the outflow tract and aorta to initiate retrograde aortic flow. The systolic ejection period is prolonged, while ejection time measured from the flow signal is short.[1, 7-10] As in aortic stenosis, passive ventricular filling is impeded in HCM, reflecting decreased distensibility, and augmented atrial transport function is required to achieve an adequate end-diastolic volume.

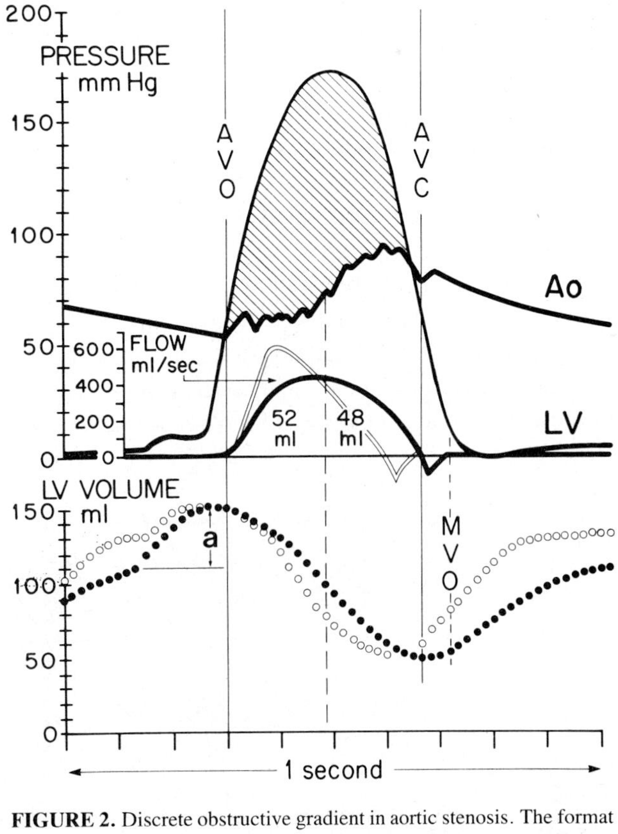

FIGURE 2. Discrete obstructive gradient in aortic stenosis. The format is similar to that of figure 1. Normal contours for aortic flow and instantaneous volume curves are depicted in open lines and circles for comparison. Abbreviations are as in figure 1.

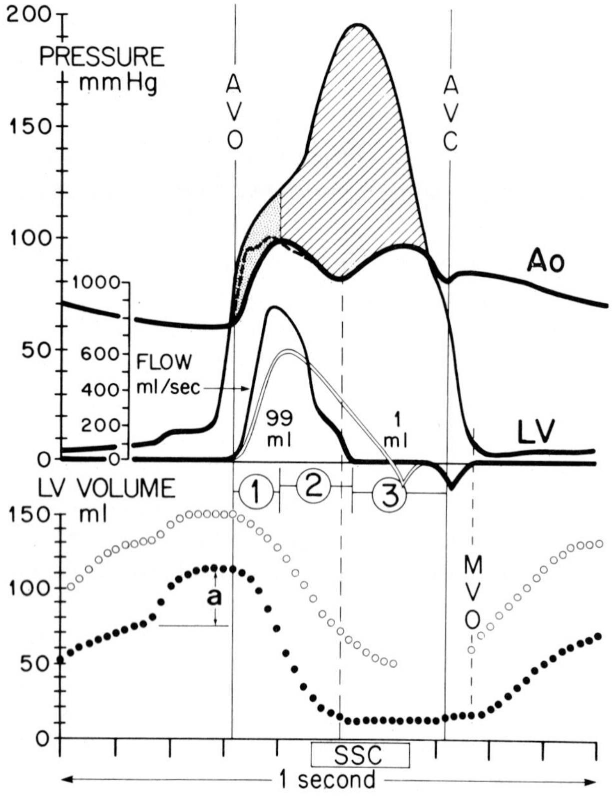

FIGURE 3. Dynamic gradient in HCM. The format is similar to that of figures 1 and 2. The contour depicted by a dashed line following aortic valve opening represents left ventricular outflow tract pressure. See text for explanation of phases (encircled numbers). SSC = onset and duration of SAM-septal contact; other abbreviations are as in figure 1.

Catheter entrapment (figure 4) results in an artifactually high pressure when the catheter is embedded in the ventricular wall during systole and records intramyocardial and not intracavitary pressure.[12] The recording illustrated in figure 4 was made during advancement of a retrograde left ventricular catheter. The pressure waveform demonstrates a mid and late systolic "pressure gradient" with a delay in the decline of pressure, so that the ventricular downstroke follows the central aortic dicrotic notch. The entrapped catheter does not eject blood nor permit blood sampling through its lumen during systole.[12]

Obstructive vs nonobstructive interpretations of dynamic pressure gradients. Two diametrically opposite interpretations of dynamic pressure gradients have been put forth: midsystolic obstruction and excessively rapid and complete elimination of left ventricular cavitary contents. Advocates of the obstruction theory have postulated that the outflow tract is widely patent during phase 1, progressively impedes outflow during phase 2 as ejection occurs in the face of a pressure gradient, and is totally obstructed during phase 3.[1,7] In the first decade after the discovery of HCM this contention was supported by intraoperative central aortic flowmeter recordings demonstrating cessation of flow in midsystole, angiocardiograms that were thought to show "a long area of subvalvular narrowing," and intraoperative findings of a "forceful contraction of the outflow tract on the examining finger."[1] Surgical interruption of the septal aspect of the contraction ring by myotomy/myectomy was devised as an operation analogous to resection of pyloric stenosis. The relief of the gradient and concurrent symptomatic improvement have been considered further confirmation of the obstructive nature of the pressure gradient.[1,7]

When the long area of angiographic subvalvular narrowing was acknowledged to be a result of the diastolic excursion of the anterior mitral leaflet[7,13] and the presence of a contraction ring could not be corroborated by angiography,[13] the site of obstruction was translocated to the systolic apposition of the anterior mitral leaflet and the interventricular septum. This new zone of obstruction appeared as a subtle horizontal lucent line on angiocardiograms[7] and as systolic anterior motion (SAM) on echocardiograms.[14] Despite this translocation of the presumed obstruction, myotomy-myectomy designed to interrupt the "contraction ring" has re-

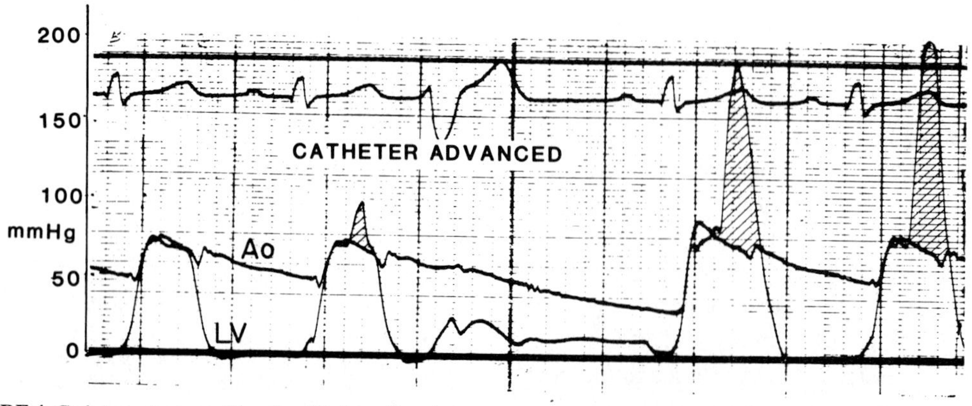

FIGURE 4. Catheter entrapment "gradient" induced by advancement of a retrograde left ventricular catheter while recording left ventricular (LV) and aortic (Ao) root pressure.

mained the most commonly performed surgical procedure for this condition.

It has been postulated that SAM is a result of a Venturi phenomenon, in which the high outflow velocity in the narrowed left ventricle draws the anterior leaflet forward against the septum.[12, 15] The temporal and quantitative relationship between SAM-septal contact (SSC, figure 3) and the interventricular pressure gradient, as well as the presence of flow during the development of the pressure gradient, are used to support the contention that the mitral valve imposes a significant impediment to outflow.[11, 12, 15]

A nonobstructive explanation of the dynamic pressure gradient is that the ventricle rapidly ejects during phase 1, decreases its rate of ejection while achieving its minimal residual volume ("dead space") during phase 2, and is isovolumetric with a sustained isometric contraction during phase 3.[4, 5, 10, 13] This phenomenon has been termed cavity obliteration[13] or cavity elimination.[16] The paradox of a pressure gradient without obstruction was elucidated by Gauer and Henry[4] in studies during hemorrhagic shock and during application of negative gravitational force in animals. They recorded dynamic gradients (as shown in figure 3) and demonstrated that continued isometric contraction after the ventricle had emptied the pathologically small intracavitary contents produced a high pressure in the obliterated cavity. This phenomenon could also account for the sensation of a contraction ring when the surgeon's exploring finger enters the obliterating cavity.[13]

The Gauer phenomenon can be studied in a hydrodynamic model of the left ventricle and aorta that is anatomically incapable of outflow obstruction, as described by White et al.[5] The contractile force, aortic resistance, and ventricular filling can be controlled independently, and dynamic intracavitary gradients can be readily generated by perturbations that match those that provoke gradients in experimental animals and patients with HCM. For example, if the systolic ventricular pressure is held constant and the aortic resistance is reduced, there is a rapid aortic upstroke, a mid-systolic trough, and a mid and late systolic gradient similar to the three phases in figure 3. The ventricle rapidly eliminates its contents as the gradient is developing in phases 1 and 2, and is isovolumetric during phase 3. White et al. noted "as the cavity becomes smaller, the body and the outflow tract of the ventricle become progressively isolated from one another and a pressure difference develops between these two areas. These two regions are not separated by an obstruction, but by the tightly opposed walls of an essentially empty ventricle below."[5] It is important to emphasize that the pressure gradient develops during ejection as the ventricle progressively isolates the obliterating body from the noncontractile outflow tract, which is in free communication with the aorta beyond, and shares its lower pressure.

Hemodynamic and cineangiographic studies of the ventricle in the presence of dynamic pressure gradients in patients with HCM,[3, 9, 10, 13] normal subjects undergoing the Valsalva maneuver and inotropic stimuli,[6] and animals with intraventricular gradients induced with isoproterenol[5] reveal cavitary obliteration compatible with Gauer's phenomenon. These studies have demonstrated the development of the peak pressure gradient during rapid obliteration of the ventricle, phase 2. When the left ventricular ejection fractions of patients with HCM are grouped according to hemodynamic subsets, patients with resting gradients have the highest ejection fractions, those with inducible gradients intermediate ejection fractions, and those without resting or inducible gradients the lowest ejection fractions.[10] In patients with HCM studied with and without an intracavitary gradient, the left ventricle empties more rapidly and the ejection fraction increases when the gradient is induced or augmented.[3, 9, 10] Thus, the imposition of a pressure gradient is associated with enhanced left ventricular emptying (both rate and degree) and belies the concept of impeded or obstructed outflow. If an obstruction were responsible for the gradient, it would be expected to retard emptying when present.

Since some degree of mitral regurgitation, which might represent a low resistance alternate pathway for left ventricular ejection, is usually present in patients with HCM it has been argued that the rapidity of emptying is a result of mitral regurgitation.[12, 15] However, this hyperdynamic emptying pattern is also seen when trivial or no mitral regurgitation is present.[8–10]

Although there are important differences in the genesis of dynamic gradients due to cavity obliteration and the artifactually high pressures recorded from catheters embedded or entrapped in the left ventricular wall, these two phenomena have unfortunately been confused and equated.[12]

Echocardiography in HCM. The relationship between SAM-septal contact and dynamic pressure gradients need not be cause and effect; both may be the result of rapid and complete left ventricular emptying. In support of this alternative, the rate of emptying of the left ventricle is enhanced (and therefore not impeded) during the presence of the gradient and SAM.[10]

Patients with resting pressure gradients in excess of

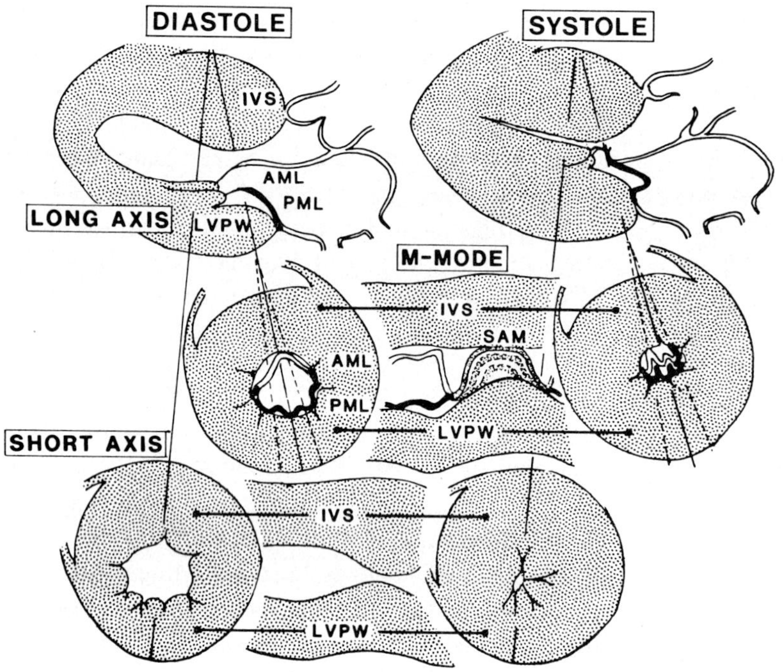

FIGURE 5. Echocardiography in HCM. IVS = interventricular septum; AML = anterior mitral leaflet; PML = posterior mitral leaflet; LVPW = left ventricular posterior wall.

90 mm Hg studied in our laboratory by angiography and two-dimensional echocardiography were found by both techniques to have cavitary obliteration.[17] Figure 5 diagrammatically depicts the typical echocardiographic findings in these patients. Two-dimensional parasternal long-axis (*top*) and short-axis (*middle* and *bottom*) images are related to the M mode images at the level of the mitral valve (center of *middle* row) and body of the ventricle (center of *bottom* row). The posterior mitral leaflet (black area) originates from the mitral anulus and occupies roughly two-thirds of the circumference of the mitral sleeve while the anterior leaflet (white area) has no annular attachment and is in continuity with the posterior wall of the aorta.

In diastole, the mitral sleeve is confined by the walls of the inflow region of the left ventricle, so that the anterior leaflet impacts on the interventricular septum and the posterior leaflet on the left ventricular posterior and lateral walls. During systole vigorous systolic constriction of the anulus and circumferential contraction of the ventricular walls causes the posterior leaflet to engulf the anterior leaflet, and the sleeve is corrugated like a folded umbrella. Because of the lateral divergence of the ultrasound beam (dashed lines) the interdigitated peaks and valleys of the puckered leaflets are superimposed to yeild a laminated multilayer SAM on the one-dimensional M mode image (*center*). The distal mitral apparatus has a hockey-stick configuration (*top right*) or crossed-swords appearance on apical four-chamber views (not shown) because folds of the posterior leaflet often project anterior to the anterior leaflet. In systolic long- and short-axis views (*top* and *bottom right*), obliteration of the submitral cavity is seen.

The onset of SAM-septal contact occurs at the midpoint of phase 2, near the nadir of the radidly declining aortic flow signal and as the ventricle has nearly achieved its dead space (SSC, figure 3).[9, 10] If SAM-septal contact was due to the Venturi phenomenon, the decline to zero velocity in the outflow tract would not be expected to sustain the anterior displacement of the mitral valve throughout the remainder of systole. The relationship of SAM-septal contact to a small left ventricular volume and its appearance with rapid and complete emptying of the ventricle[9, 10] are consistent with the view that the mitral valve becomes distorted as the left ventricle empties convulsively up to the level of the mitral apparatus, as depicted in figure 5.

The aortic valve may partially "preclose" in midsystole when outflow diminishes, but complete closure (and the second heart sound) does not occur until ventricular relaxation permits retrograde aortic root flow.

Is obstruction necessary to explain the clinical picture of HCM? There are many observations that are not in concert with the presence of an important or clinically relevant impediment to left ventricular outflow in HCM. Natural history studies[18, 19] demonstrate the lack of correlation between the presence and magnitude of an outflow tract gradient and symptoms or mortality. In a study of a group of 126 patients in which 10 cardiac deaths were reported, seven deaths occurred in 49 patients with insignificant gradients (0 to 30 mm Hg), and none occurred in 34 patients with gradients over 90 mm Hg.[18] Thus, the presence of a pressure gradient is not predictive of cardiogenic death. More recent studies have demonstrated that the appearance of ventricular tachyarrhythmias on ambulatory electrocardiographic monitoring is predictive of sudden death.[20]

The morphologic hallmark of the disease process is inordinate hypertrophy, which is not dependent on the presence of a pressure gradient. The triad of symptoms (angina, syncope, and dyspnea) can be attributed to the consequences of pathologic hypertrophy, since these symptoms are frequently present in patients with HCM but without pressure gradients. The hypertrophied muscle has the potential for myocardial supply/demand imbalance, which can readily explain the triad on the bases of ischemia, arrhythmias, and diminished ventricular distensibility. Medications (e.g., β-adrenergic receptor– or calcium channel–blocking drugs) that do not consistently alter the pressure gradient but that decrease myocardial oxygen consumption and/or improve ventricular distensibility have been demonstrated to ameliorate symptoms.[21]

While the results of operative intervention suggested a link between relief of symptoms and reduction of the pressure gradient, the aforementioned natural history studies do not support any consistent relationship between symptoms and pressure gradients.[18, 19, 21] This lack of correlation would suggest that the symptomatic benefits imparted by operative intervention may not be directly related to the reduction of the pressure gradient, but to other factors (pericardotomy, decreased contractility, enlargement of cavity size, cardiac denervation, etc.). Despite the reported symptomatic benefits, septal myotomy-myectomy carries a substantial morbidity and mortality and has little if any impact on the occurrence of sudden death.[22]

The cardiovascular physical findings in HCM can be explained by cavity obliteration/elimination. The arterial "spike and dome" represents the rapid ejection of blood in phase 1 followed by a reflected wave from the peripheral reflecting sites. The prolongation of the systolic ejection period results from delayed closure of the aortic valve. This delay in aortic valve closure and the late systolic wave in the apical impulse result from the sustained contraction and delayed rate of relaxation[16] in the body of the left ventricle in phase 3. The aortic valve does not close fully (and cause the dicrotic notch) until relaxation of the left ventricle results in a negative gradient across the valve and initiates retrograde aortic flow.

The Brockenbrough-Braunwald-Morrow phenomenon,[1] the failure of the postextrasystolic arterial pulse pressure to rise, has been attributed to increased obstruction. Since the rapidity and degree of emptying are enhanced rather than retarded in the beat with a gradient,[3, 9, 10] three nonobstructive mechanisms can be invoked for the attenuation of the arterial pulse pressure: (1) reduced diastolic left ventricular compliance preventing increased filling during the postextrasystolic pause, (2) an emptier, more compliant aortic bed as a result of enhanced runoff time, and (3) increased mitral regurgitation due to earlier and more profound distortion of the mitral apparatus in the inotropically stimulated ventricle.

The characteristic mid–late systolic murmur of HCM is considered a cardinal manifestation of an outflow tract stenosis, but is often present in the absence of a gradient. Unlike aortic stenosis, the magnitude of the murmur fails to track consistently with the magnitude of the gradient.[23] The murmur is best heard at the apex and lower sternal border and is rarely transmitted to the base and carotid arteries, unlike murmurs generated in the outflow tract. A mid–late systolic murmur is recorded in the left atrium by intracardiac phonocardiography, while a typical "ejection murmur," peaking in early systole, is recorded during phase 1 in the aortic root.[9] The response of the murmur to postural maneuvers is similar to that of the murmur of mitral prolapse (increased intensity on standing, decreased with squatting) because both HCM and mitral prolapse have a significant ventriculovalvular disproportion in which the ventricle is too small to support the mitral valve in a competent subannular position in mid and late systole. Each of these observations support the contention that the principal murmur is caused by mitral regurgitation through the distorted mitral valve.

Summary and conclusions. HCM is a disorder associated with significant morbidity and mortality and a propensity to cause sudden, often unexpected death. The similarity to the symptom complex of aortic stenosis and the presence of a pressure gradient justified the initial assumption that obstruction was of prime importance in HCM and that relief of obstruction was the focal point of rational therapy. However, it is our belief that the dogma of obstruction has impeded progress in and obscured the understanding of HCM and interpretation of its manifestations. The purpose of this article is to call attention to significant discrepancies in the obstructive concept that have been reinforced as new techniques emerged that have allowed further study of the disease.

Since neither the presence of a gradient nor SAM can be justifiably equated with the presence of an obstruction, it is proposed that the appellation "obstruction" be reserved for those cases in which the rate of outflow or the rate or degree of ventricular emptying are demonstrably impeded, as in aortic stenosis.

Therapy with β-adrenergic–receptor and calcium channel–blocking agents have shown promise for alleviating symptoms and possibly prolonging life without systematically or predictably affecting the pressure gradient, probably because of their beneficial effects on ventricular relaxation and diastolic filling.[21, 22] Antiarrhythmic therapy has been effective in reducing mortality.[20, 22] Ideally, prevention or regression of the pathologic hypertrophy should be the major focus of future therapeutic interventions in hypertrophic cardiomyopathy.

References

1. Braunwald E, Lambrew CT, Morrow AG, Pierce GE, Rockoff SD, Ross J Jr: Idiopathic hypertrophic subaortic stenosis. Circulation **30** (suppl IV): IV-1, 1964
2. Murgo JP, Altobelli SA, Dorethy JF, Logdson JR, McGranahan GM: Normal ventricular ejection dynamics in man during rest and exercise. Am Heart Assoc Mongr **46:** 92, 1975
3. Wilson WS, Criley JM, Ross RS: Dynamics of left ventricular emptying in hypertrophic subaortic stenosis: a cineangiographic and hemodynamic study. Am Heart J **73:** 4, 1967
4. Gauer OH, Henry JP: Negative (-Gz) acceleration in relation to arterial oxygen saturation, subendocardial hemorrhage and venous pressure in the forehead. Aerospace Med **35:** 533, 1964
5. White RI, Criley JM, Lewis KB, Ross RS: Experimental production of intracavity pressure differences: possible significance in the interpretation of human hemodynamic studies. Am J Cardiol **19:** 806, 1967
6. Grose R, Maskin C, Spindola-Franco H, Yipintsoi T: Production of left ventricular cavitary obliteration in normal man. Circulation **64:** 448, 1981
7. Ross J Jr, Braunwald E, Gault JH, Mason DT, Morrow AG: The mechanism of the intraventricular pressure gradient in idiopathic hypertrophic subaortic stenosis. Circulation **34:** 558, 1966
8. Murgo JP, Alter BR, Dorethy JF, Altobelli SA, McGranahan GM Jr: Dynamics of left ventricular ejection in obstructive and nonobstructive hypertrophic cardiomyopathy. J Clin Invest **66:** 1369, 1980
9. Murgo JP, Miller JW: Hemodynamic, angiographic and echocardiographic evidence against impeded ejection in hypertrophic cardiomyopathy. *In* Goodwin JF, editor: Heart muscle disease. Lancaster, England, 1985, MIP Press Limited, p 187
10. Siegel RJ, Criley JM: A comparison of ventricular emptying with and without a pressure gradient in patients with hypertrophic cardiomyopathy. Br Heart J: **53:** 283, 1985
11. Maron BJ, Gottdiener JS, Arce J, Rosing DR, Wesley YE, Epstein SE: Dynamic subaortic obstruction in hypertrophic cardiomyopathy: analysis by pulsed Doppler echocardiography. J Am Coll Cardiol **6:** 1, 1985
12. Wigle ED, Marquis Y, Auger P: Muscular subaortic stenosis: initial left ventricular inflow tract pressure in the assessment of intraventricular pressure differences in man. Circulation **35:** 1100, 1967
13. Criley JM, Lewis KB, White RI, Ross RS: Pressure gradients without obstruction: a new concept of "hypertrophic subaortic stenosis." Circulation **22:** 881, 1965
14. Shah PM, Gramiak R, Kramer DH: Ultrasound localization of left ventricular outflow obstruction in hypertrophic obstructive cardiomyopathy. Circulation **40:** 3, 1969
15. Pollick C, Rakowski, Wigle ED: Muscular subaortic stenosis: the quantitative relationship between systolic anterior motion and the pressure gradient. Circulation **69:** 43, 1984
16. Goodwin JF: The frontiers of cardiomyopathy. Br Heart J **48:** 1, 1982
17. Ginzton LE, Criley JM: "Obstructive" systolic anterior motion of the mitral valve in cavity obliteration. Circulation **64** (suppl IV): IV-30, 1981 (abst)
18. Frank S, Braunwald E: Idiopathic hypertrophic subaortic stenosis: clinical analysis of 126 patients with emphasis on the natural history. Circulation **37:** 759, 1968
19. Powell WJ Jr, Whiting RB, Dinsmore RE, Sanders CA: Symptomatic Prognosis in patients with idiopathic hypertrophic subaortic stenosis (IHSS). Am J Med **55:** 1973
20. McKenna WJ, Oakley CM, Krickler DM, Goodwin JF: Improved survival with amiodarone in patients with hypertrophic cardiomyopathy and ventricular tachycardia. Br Heart J **53:** 412, 1985
21. Bonow RO, Rosing DR, Bacharach SL, Green MV, Kent KM, Lipson LC, Maron BJ, Leon MB, Epstein SE: Effect of verapamil on left ventricular systolic function and diastolic filling in patients with hypertrophic cardiomyopathy. Circulation **64:** 787, 1981
22. Canedo MI, Frank MJ: Therapy of hypertrophic cardiomyopathy: medical or surgical? Clinical and pathophysiologic considerations. Am J Cardiol **48:** 383, 1981
23. Kramer DS, French WJ, Criley JM: The postextrasystolic murmur response in hypertrophic cardiomyopathy and aortic stenosis. J Am Coll Cardiol **5:** 395, 1985 (abst)

The virtual disappearance of rheumatic fever in the United States: lessons in the rise and fall of disease

T. Duckett Jones Memorial Lecture

LEON GORDIS, M.D., DR.P.H.

I AM DEEPLY HONORED to have been invited to give the 1984 T. Duckett Jones Memorial Lecture. This year marks 40 years since Dr. Jones first published his paper entitled "The Diagnosis of Rheumatic Fever."[1] Jones had the foresight to recognize the importance of standardized diagnostic criteria from three points of view. He wrote: "(1) Otherwise, [without standardized criteria] the incidence of rheumatic fever may be interpreted as varying greatly whether the data are collected by surveys, the development of a rheumatic fever register, making the disease reportable, or the study of hospital records. (2) The interpretation of study programs of prevention and care is obviously dependent on such diagnostic criteria." Jones' third point dealt with the importance of standardized diagnostic criteria if valid information regarding ultimate prognosis were to be obtained and provided to patients and their families. It is noteworthy that the primary benefits he described were not so much the improved clinical management of individual patients with rheumatic fever, but rather facilitation of the collection of meaningful incidence data and evaluation of the effectiveness of prevention programs. In this article I would like to discuss the dramatically changing incidence of rheumatic fever and its relation to our preventive efforts. The studies I will present were possible only because of the broad acceptance and utilization of the diagnostic criteria promulgated by Dr. Jones 40 years ago.

Throughout history people have been intrigued by the apparent appearance and disappearance of human disease, believed by many to be actions of the gods in direct response to human behavior. Over the years there have been attempts to develop a scientific rationale for explaining these phenomena. I would like to review the picture of rheumatic fever as it has emerged in studies we have carried out in Baltimore over a period of more than two decades. I shall then try to place the changes that have occurred in the context of other diseases that have either increased or decreased in incidence or mortality in the United States during the 20th century.

The Baltimore studies. The earliest of these studies were carried out in collaboration with Dr. Milton Markowitz. In the ensuing years he has continued to be a stimulus and constructive critic and is, in essence, a spiritual collaborator in all these investigations. Our first study in Baltimore examined the incidence patterns of acute rheumatic fever from 1960 to 1964.[2] The findings were marked by dramatic racial differences. Rates of both initial and recurrent attacks were more than twice as frequent in blacks as in whites. These findings were consistent with the observation that the disease tended to cluster in the predominantly black areas of the inner city of Baltimore. Relatively few of the cases occurred in suburban areas.

In a second study we found that from 1960-64 to 1968-70, the rates in blacks in Baltimore dropped dramatically while the rates in whites remained relatively unchanged. To explain this change we asked the question: Could the decline in incidence in black children be due to the inner city comprehensive care programs for children and youth that had been established in the mid-1960s? A study was therefore carried out to compare the incidence of rheumatic fever in census tracts eligible for comprehensive care compared to census tracts not eligible for comprehensive care.[3] As seen in figure 1, in the census tracts that were eligible for comprehensive care, incidence of rheumatic fever dropped 60% from 1960-64 to 1968-70. In contrast, there was virtually no change in noneligible census tracts.

Because many social and economic changes had taken place during this time, it would be difficult to ascribe the decline in rheumatic fever specifically to

From the Department of Epidemiology, Johns Hopkins School of Hygiene and Public Health, Baltimore.

Supported in part by NHLBI grant T32HL07024.

Address for correspondence: Leon Gordis, M.D., Dr. P.H., Department of Epidemiology, Johns Hopkins School of Hygiene and Public Health, 615 N. Wolfe St., Baltimore, MD 21205.

This *Perspective* summarizes Dr. Gordis' presentation as the T. Duckett Jones Memorial Lecturer at the Annual Meeting of the American Heart Association, Miami Beach, November 1984.

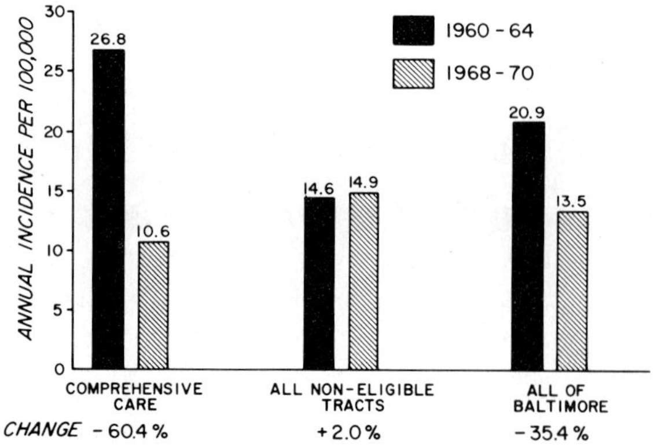

FIGURE 1. Comprehensive care and changes in rheumatic fever incidence, 1960–64 to 1968–70 (Baltimore, black population, ages 5 to 14 years).

comprehensive care solely on the basis of these findings. A further analysis was therefore carried out with the following rationale: If the comprehensive care programs were indeed responsible for the observed decline in rheumatic fever by providing quality ambulatory care to children, they could have had such an impact only in children who had clinically overt pharyngitis. If so, we would expect the decline observed in rheumatic fever to have been limited to those cases that had been preceded by clinical pharyngitis and to see relatively little change in the incidence of cases preceded by subclinical pharyngitis, since such children would have had no reason to seek medical care and consequently the comprehensive care programs would not be expected to have any impact in this group. As seen in figure 2, when analyzed in this fashion the entire decline in rheumatic fever was found in cases that had been preceded by clinically overt acute pharyngitis. Thus the data up to 1970 were highly consistent with the hypothesis that in Baltimore, the decline in rheumatic fever, which was limited to blacks, was primarily a result of the comprehensive care programs in the inner city.

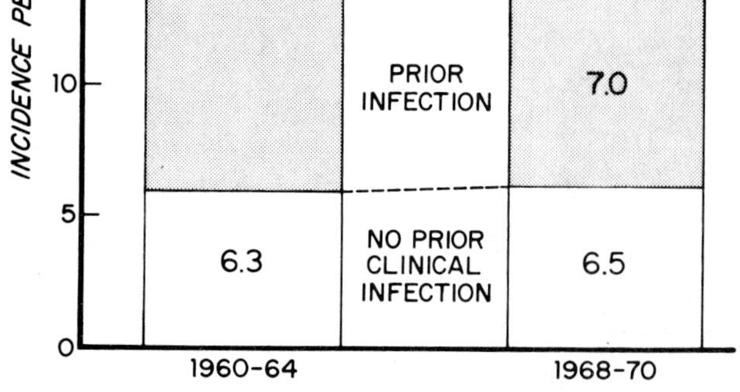

FIGURE 2. Changes in the annual incidence of first attacks of rheumatic fever in relation to preceding clinical respiratory infection.

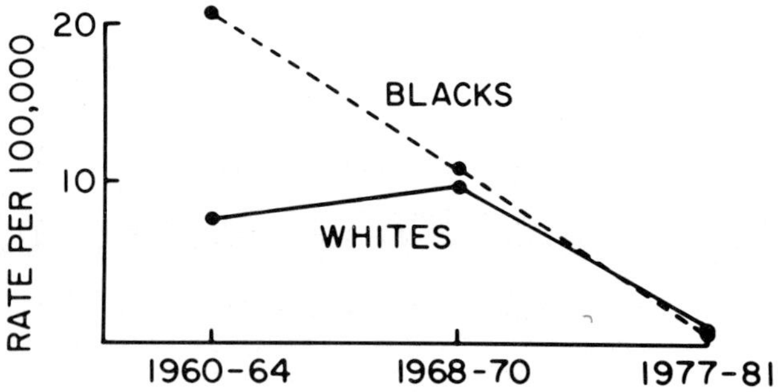

FIGURE 3. Average annual incidence of first attacks of rheumatic fever ages 5 to 19, by race, Baltimore, 1960–81.

More recently, we carried out a third study in Baltimore utilizing the same methods as the two previous investigations. As seen in figure 3, from 1968-70 to 1977-81, incidence rates of rheumatic fever dropped dramatically in both whites and blacks to extremely low rates. Perhaps the most dramatic view of these changes is seen in figure 4, which shows spot maps for rheumatic fever cases for the first and last 5 year periods of this study, 1960-64 on the left and 1977-81 on the right. Only five cases were seen in Baltimore from 1977 to 1981, and all were clinically mild.

National data for the United States. These findings are consistent with data reported from other communities, such as those of Land and Bisno from Memphis, Tennessee.[4] Available evidence suggests that this is also the pattern in other cities in the United States in most populations. National data for hospital discharges with a diagnosis of rheumatic fever from the National Hospital Discharge Survey conducted by the National Center for Health Statistics, and kindly provided by Dr. Edward Bacon of the Center, confirm this decline (table 1). The decline is also seen when the rates are

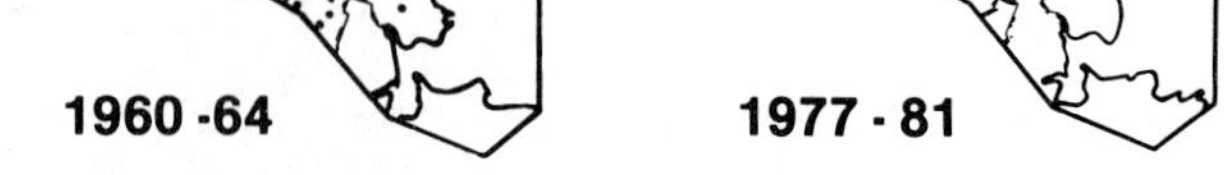

FIGURE 4. Spot maps for rheumatic fever cases in Baltimore 1960–64 and 1977–81.

TABLE 1
Annual rates (per 100,000) of discharges of patients with rheumatic fever from short-stay non-federal hospitals in the United States, 1965–83

Year	Discharge rate	Year	Discharge rate
1965	14.0	1973	5.1
1966	13.3	1974	4.8
1967	10.2	1975	4.1
1968	8.4	1976	3.3
1969	NA[A]	1977	3.5
1970	7.8	1978	3.0
1971	8.1	1979–80	2.0[B]
1972	5.6	1981–83	1.0[B]

Source: National Hospital Discharge Survey, NCHS.
[A]Data not available.
[B]Average annual rate per time period.

examined by age and race (table 2). Thus we have a marked decline in rheumatic fever, indeed a virtual disappearance of the disease in both blacks and whites in Baltimore, and this appears consistent with most available data from elsewhere in the United States.

"New" and "disappearing" diseases. What can account for the extraordinary phenomenon we are observing in acute rheumatic fever in the United States? To address this issue I would like to discuss briefly other diseases that have either appeared or at least increased in incidence or disappeared or declined in incidence in the course of the 20th century. Among the "new" diseases, or those that have at least increased markedly in incidence during the last few decades, are: lung cancer, clear cell carcinoma of the vagina, phocomelia, toxic shock syndrome, legionnaires disease, Kawasaki disease, Reye syndrome, Lyme arthritis, and AIDS. Each has attracted considerable interest, including perhaps most notably the rapid increase in AIDS.

What can account for the relatively rapid appearance

TABLE 2
Annual rates of hospital discharges of patients with rheumatic fever by age and race, United States, 1965–67, 1972–76, and 1979–83[A]

	Rates per 100,000		
	1965–67	1972–76	1979–83
Age			
0–19 yr	19.2	7.0	2.8
20 yr and older	8.0	3.2	0.8
Race			
White	11.8	4.4	1.4
Nonwhite	17.3	5.6	1.4[B]

[A]Short-stay non-federal hospitals (source: National Hospital Discharge Survey, NCHS).
[B]Based on a small sample of records.

of a disease? Certainly better diagnosis and recognition or differences in artifacts of coding can also play a role. Increased physician awareness of infectious agents and changes in the prevalence of the agents or in the biological characteristics of the agents that relate to virulence may also be critical. For diseases having other causes, new agents introduced into the environment or new exposures to them may account for the increase. Finally, removal of certain protective mechanisms may play a role. For example, it has been suggested that Hodgkin's disease has a higher incidence in upper socioeconomic individuals because such individuals are protected from certain early childhood infections such as Epstein-Barr virus, a model similar to that seen in polio.[5]

Below are listed some diseases that seem to have disappeared or at least declined in incidence during the 20th century:

- As a result of planned eradication campaigns:
  - Infectious diseases
    - Smallpox
    - Polio
  - Nutritional rickets
- As a result of changes in medical practice:
  - Retrolental fibroplasia
- Not completely understood:
  - Stomach cancer
  - Uterine cancer
  - Peptic ulcer
  - Celiac disease
  - Stroke
  - Myocardial infarction
  - Endocardial fibroelastosis

Some of these diseases seem to have declined primarily as a result of planned and well-organized eradication campaigns. These include infectious diseases such as smallpox and poliomyelitis and diseases such as nutritional rickets, which have declined in incidence as a result of specific dietary supplementation. Second, we have diseases that have almost disappeared as a result of changes in medical practice. Perhaps the most dramatic example is retrolental fibroplasia.

Other diseases have disappeared without any specific eradication campaign. For example, stomach cancer has declined markedly in the United States, as has uterine cancer, with no explanation immediately at hand to account for these changes. Other diseases such as peptic ulcer and celiac disease have also declined and the causes for the declines remain unknown. Isolated endocardial fibroelastosis, without aortic disease, appears to be much less frequent than in previous years. Finally, and perhaps most noteworthy are the declines in mortality from stroke and coronary heart disease.

What can account for dramatic decreases in incidence and mortality of disease? Changing diagnostic approaches and changes in coding can play a role and produce artifactual changes. For diseases caused by infectious agents, it is at least theoretically possible that the virulence of the agent may diminish or the prevalence of human exposure to the agent may decline. If caused by exposures to other etiologic agents in the environment, such may change over time as existing hazards are recognized and controlled. Finally, changes in lifestyle or changes in the quality and accessibility of medical care may play a role in declines observed in the incidence of disease.

Possible explanations for the virtual disappearance of rheumatic fever. With this background, how can we explain the changes observed in the incidence of rheumatic fever? Reasonably valid population-based incidence data for rheumatic fever did not become available until the 20th century. Hence, although rheumatic fever has been present for centuries and according to some, may have been present in antiquity, it is difficult to state whether at some point in time there was a sudden appearance of the disease or a sudden rise in the incidence of the disease. What is clear, however, is that the 20th century has witnessed a sharp decline in rheumatic fever, at least in the United States and in other economically developed countries.

Could the decline in rheumatic fever be due to changes in the streptococcus itself? Let us examine the possibilities. The first would be that the incidence of streptococcal infections has declined. Although some experts believe that there has, in fact, been a decline in the incidence of streptococcal infections, it is difficult to document such a change. In fact, Hall and Breese have reported from Rochester, New York, that the number of throat cultures positive for group A streptococci did not decline during a time period when a decline in rheumatic fever was observed (unpublished observations). Unfortunately, there is no ongoing systematic data collection system in the United States that could provide the information needed to address this issue.

If the incidence of streptococcal infections has in fact declined, the decline could be part of a cyclical pattern of increases and decreases in incidence of streptococcal infections and that we may just be on the down side of the curve at this point in time. If indeed there is such a cyclic phenomenon, we might anticipate another rise in streptococcal incidence in the future and with it a possible rise in rheumatic fever incidence.

Could there have been a change in the prevalence of rheumatogenic types in our communities or in the incidence of infections produced by rheumatogenic types? Although there is strong evidence that there are nephritogenic types, the case for rheumatogenic types is not clear. Support for this contention comes from several types of evidence: (1) The temporal and geographic variations observed in rheumatic fever incidence are consistent with the existence of rheumatogenic and nonrheumatogenic types. (2) Early data from Kuttner and Krumweide[6] suggested differences in rheumatic fever attack rates depending on the serologic type of streptococcus in the outbreak. (3) Data from Potter et al.[7] suggest that in Trinidad the serologic types of streptococci causing rheumatic fever differ from those causing nephritis even in the same families. (4) Seasonal differences reported in occurrence of rheumatic fever and of glomerulonephritis are also consistent with different rheumatogenic potential of different serotypes.[8] (5) Rheumatic fever and nephritis rarely occur simultaneously.

Could there have been a change in the virulence of the streptococcus over time? This is certainly a possibility, although as McCarty has suggested, given the fact that no single serologic type has been demonstrated to be rheumatogenic, any changes in virulence would have had to occur in several serologic types of streptococci simultaneously.[9] Nevertheless, we do see some evidence consistent with changes in the virulence of the streptococcus. Scarlet fever has become a much milder disease over the last few decades and its incidence has perhaps declined. Data from Baltimore suggest that the incidence of poststreptococcal acute glomerulonephritis may also have declined, although not as markedly as that of rheumatic fever (figure 5). Further evidence consistent with a possible change in virulence of the organism is the changing pattern of antibiotic sensitivity of the streptococcus. High rates of resistance of streptococci to tetracycline, and to a lesser extent to erythromycin and lincomycin, have been reported.[10]

There is some ambiguity associated with the term "virulence." Virulence may refer to the capacity of the streptococcus to adhere to human epithelium, to its ability to evoke an antibody response, to its ability to produce clincial pharyngitis or other infection, or to its rheumatogenic or nephritogenic potential. Streptococcal virulence has been associated with the M protein of the cell surface, which has antiphagocytic properties and may also enhance the adherence of the streptococcus to epithelial cells by forming a complex with lipoteichoic acid.[11] To date, there is no evidence that the

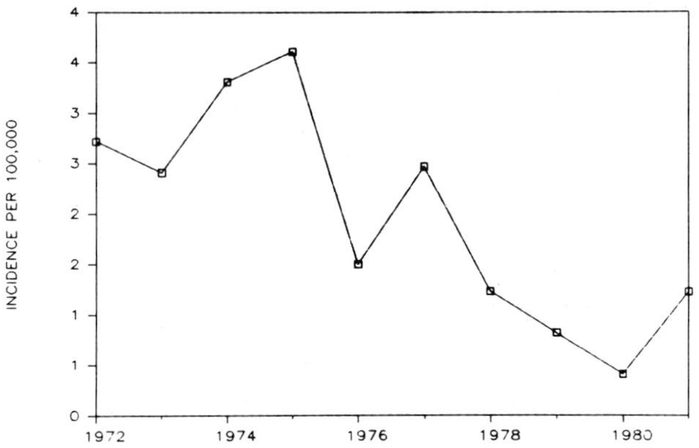

FIGURE 5. Incidence of hospitalized glomerulonephritis, Baltimore residents, ages 0–19 years, 1972–81.

percentage of streptococcal strains isolated that are M-typeable has decreased and, in fact, data from Rochester suggest that the percentage of streptococcal isolates that are M-typeable may have increased in recent years. Data are needed on changes in the adherence ability of streptococcal strains isolated over time.

If a change in the virulence of the streptococcus has indeed taken place, what could have produced it? It has been suggested that the relatively high proportion of people in the population who have serum penicillin levels at any time may serve to interrupt the chain of transmission, which is often also associated with enhanced virulence. If this were the case, one would expect a decrease in the percentage of isolated strains that were M-typeable. It is also possible that nowadays the streptococcus more frequently encounters people with specific antibodies that prevent this transmission. Unfortunately, population-based data on the prevalence rates of anti-M antibodies are not available.

Another possibility for explaining the decline in rheumatic fever is the disappearance of a cofactor that may operate together with the streptococcus to produce rheumatic fever. Viruses have been known to affect host resistance and responses to bacterial infections.[12] It is well recognized that during influenza epidemics there is an increased risk for both systemic and pulmonary infections caused by many organisms, including *Hemophilus influenzae, Staphylococcus aureus, Neisseria Meningitidis, Escherichia coli,* and *Streptococcus* pneumoniae.[13] Newborns with upper respiratory viral infections were reported long ago by Eichenwald to be particularly susceptible to infections by staphylococci, streptococci, and *H. influenzae*.[14] Bacterial adherence had been found to be enhanced by experimentally and naturally acquired viral infections.[15] Antecedent viral infection potentiates the growth of several organisms in the lung, including group B streptococci.[16] Viral infections have also been shown to inhibit normal antibacterial defenses, and all measures of macrophage function seem to be affected.[13] Thus the possibility that viruses may act as a cofactor in promoting the establishment of streptococcal infections or in some other fashion is not unreasonable. Although studies in the past of possible associations of viral and streptococcal infections were not rewarding, the markedly improved technology for viral studies available only in recent years has not yet been adequately applied to exploring this possibility.

It is also possible that some other environmental agent could be serving as a cofactor. Fainstein and Musher[17] found that smokers had increased adherence of pneumococci compared with nonsmokers. Although they did not observe such differences for streptococci, their findings exemplify the possibility that environmental factors may, in principle, affect bacterial adherence and that such a mechanism could be operating with the streptococcus, although the possible agent or agents that may be involved is not known.

To what extent can we attribute the decline in rheumatic fever to medical care and primary prevention efforts? It seems an inescapable conclusion that at least part of the observed decline in rheumatic fever must be due to the prompt and appropriate antistreptococcal treatment given by physicians throughout the country. However, although the data in Baltimore for 1968-70 suggest such an explanation, it is difficult to reconcile the more recent decline in rheumatic fever that has occurred in both blacks and whites in Baltimore, with changes in medical care and in the way health services are delivered. In assessing any decline in disease incidence, however, there are potential hazards in assuming that the changes observed are in fact due to medical advances and to the care provided. Rene Dubos wrote, "When the tide is receding from the beach, it is easy to have the illusion that one can empty the ocean by removing water with a pail."[18] Some years ago, Dr. Edward Kass pointed out that major scientific advances that have enhanced our medical care for diseases such as tuberculosis have not been clearly related to the major declines in incidence and mortality of such diseases[19] (figure 6). When we examine a similar presentation of the data for rheumatic fever as shown in figure 7, we see that the decline in rheumatic fever mortality clearly began before antistreptococcal agents became available.

Could the decline in rheumatic fever be due to some change or changes in the host? Given the relatively short period of time during which the incidence of the disease has declined, the changes cannot be accounted for by genetic alterations in human populations. It is

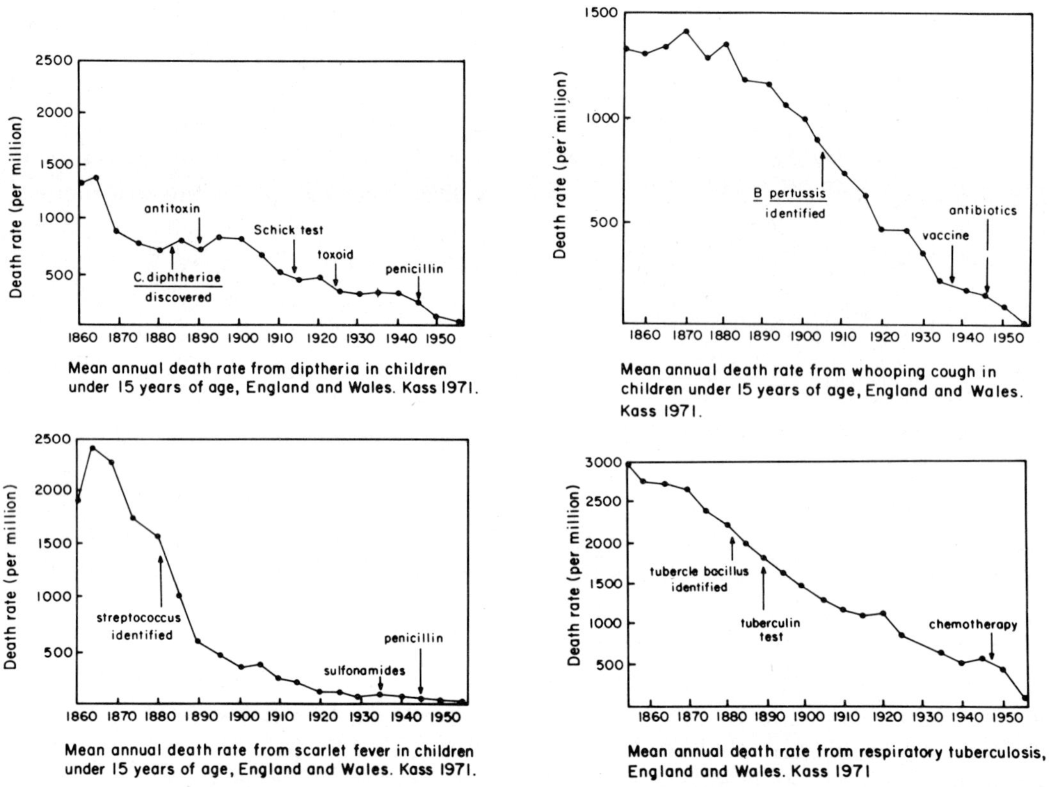

FIGURE 6. Decline in death rates of diphtheria, whooping cough, Scarlet fever, and respiratory tuberculosis in England and Wales. (Reprinted, with permission, from Kass.[19])

conceivable, however, that improved life-style factors such as nutrition may have affected the host and made him more resistant to streptococcal infections.

It is important to note that host factors have long been recognized as playing a role in the risk of rheumatic fever. The higher risk of rheumatic fever in children has generally been attributed to their greater exposure to streptococcal infections. However, it has been reported that streptococci adhere more vigorously to cells from young compared with middle-aged subjects.[17] This suggests the possibility that endocrine factors, for example, may affect infectivity and rheumatogenicity. Examples from other diseases support the notion that such host factors above and beyond any genetically determined susceptibility may play a role. For example, it is well recognized that pregnancy places a woman at increased risk of acquiring poliomyelitis. Particularly in the prevaccine era, it was also recognized that tonsillectomy increased the risk for bulbar poliomyelitis.

It is interesting to reflect on the reasons we have so much difficulty today in explaining the marked decline in the incidence of rheumatic fever. One aspect of this problem specifically merits discussion because it may have implications for our approaches to the etiologies of other diseases in the future. After Lancefield published her landmark work on the streptococcus, investigators interested in rheumatic fever quite appropriately focused their attention on confirming the relationship between the streptococcus and rheumatic fever and on elucidating the pathogenetic pathways involved. As the streptococcus was pursued, the possible etiologic role of factors other than the streptococcus in rheumatic fever received relatively little attention. That such factors — genetic, environmental, or a combination thereof — are in fact probably playing

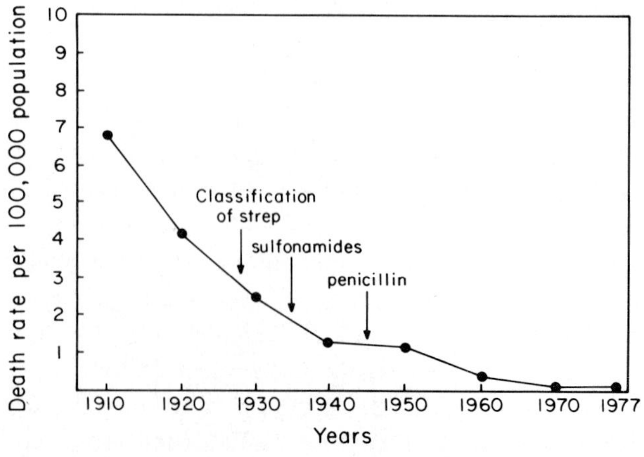

FIGURE 7. Crude death rates from rheumatic fever, United States, 1910–1977.

such a role is suggested by the data from the studies that yielded estimated rheumatic fever attack rates of 3% in the military and of 0.3% in civilian populations of children. Thus 97 of every 100 recruits who acquired a streptococcal infection did *not* develop rheumatic fever and 997 of every 1000 children who acquired streptococcal infections did *not* develop rheumatic fever. Why not? What factors could account for the small percentage of individuals with streptococcal sore throats who subsequently developed rheumatic fever, even in days when rheumatic fever was more common in the United States?

In this context, it is worthwhile to look at the approaches taken by epidemiologists to study the etiology of chronic diseases today, particularly when it is desired to explore the possible role of a number of etiologic agents. The approach often used initially is the case-control study (figure 8). In this design, patients with the disease ("cases") are compared with control subjects without the disease and the proportions of cases and controls with specific characteristics or exposures are compared. In the case of rheumatic fever, in which the streptococcus had been clearly implicated, case-control studies addressing genetic and environmental factors other than the streptococcus would have been very valuable. Thus a study of viral factors in rheumatic fever in association with streptococcal infections could be carried out by comparing cases of rheumatic fever with appropriately selected controls and determining what proportion of cases and of controls had specific prior viral infections of interest. Because the case-control design permits the investigation of a number of possible etiologic factors at the same time, it would be possible to develop a predictive model of which patients with streptococcal infections are at high risk for rheumatic fever. Until now, prediction of development of rheumatic fever has primarily been addressed by focusing on the characteristics of the streptococcus. Although this is a reasonable approach, it should not exclude consideration of host and other environmental characteristics. In his 1982 T. Duckett Jones Lecture, Dr. Elia Ayoub addressed host genetic factors in the genesis of rheumatic fever.[20] I

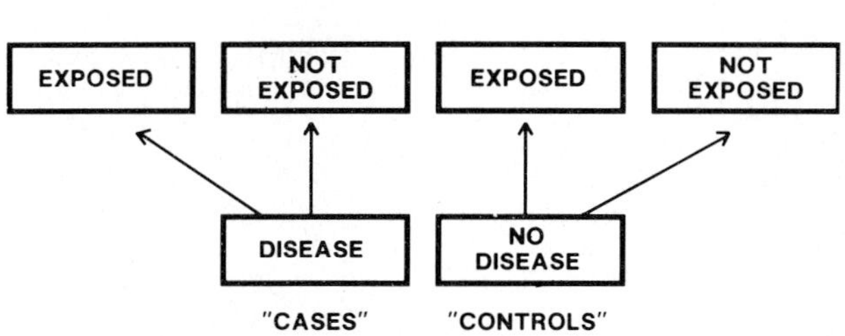

FIGURE 8. Schematic design of a case-control study.

would suggest that other host and environmental characteristics should also be considered.

The relative lack of rigorously designed and conducted case-control studies in the search for a full understanding of the etiology of rheumatic fever is understandable, since much of Lancefield's work was published at a time when the case-control design had not yet received full recognition and acceptability and was ony sporadically used. Not until the 1950s, when the case-control study design played a major role in establishing the relationship between cigarette smoking and lung cancer, was the case-control study fully legitimized. By this time the streptococcus was viewed as the full solution to the etiology of rheumatic fever, and as a result, a diligent search for other variables that might be involved was never carried out. Thus rheumatic fever began its dramatic decline in the United States before adequate attempts had been made to investigate the role of other etiologic agents above and beyond the streptococcus. Consequently, in the absence of a full understanding of the etiology of rheumatic fever today, we are unable to definitively explain its decline.

Rheumatic fever in the third world. Although the risk of rheumatic fever has been sharply declining in the United States, the picture is far different in developing countries. Worldwide, rheumatic heart disease remains the most common form of acquired heart disease in children and young adults and an important cause of all heart disease seen in adults. The status of rheumatic fever and rheumatic heart disease in developing countries has been succinctly summarized by Markowitz[21]: (1) Rheumatic fever is the most frequent cause of heart disease in the 5 to 30 year age group. (2) Acute rheumatic fever and rheumatic heart disease are two of the most common causes of death in young people. (3) Rheumatic heart disease causes 25% to 40% of all cardiovascular disease. Estimated prevalence of rheumatic heart disease in India schoolchildren is six to 11 per 1000.[22] Thirty-three to fifty percent of all hospital admissions for heart disease are for rheumatic heart disease.

Even in the United States, however, there are areas and population groups that have not clearly shared in the decline in incidence of rheumatic fever. For example, in the Navajo from 1962 to 1977, the annual attack rate was 12.4 per 100,000 for all ages, with the highest rate of 23.4 per 100,000 in the 10 to 14 year age group.[23] Rates of 96.5 per 100,000 have been reported in Samoans living in Hawaii, with 50% of the patients having carditis.[24] Recently, the Colorado Department of Health reported 14 confirmed cases of rheumatic fever in the first 6 months of 1984 compared with only two to three cases reported annually in recent years.[25] Two points emerge: First, any hypothesis developed to explain the decline observed in rheumatic fever in most of the United States must also explain its persistence in certain American population subgroups and in the developing world. Second, this persistence both in the United States and abroad should preclude any complacency on our part in regard to rheumatic fever.

Conclusion. In conclusion, although the group A streptococcus is the critical etiologic agent of rheumatic fever, the disease may well be multifactorial in origin. While improved medical care and the use of penicillin and other antibiotics have contributed significantly to the decline of rheumatic fever in the United States, the decline antedated the availability of antibiotics, and in addition the changes in rheumatic fever in the United States cannot be fully accounted for solely by medical care and antibiotic use. The difficulty is that we lack adequate information regarding other possible cofactors. Studies of such factors are not feasible in the United States today in view of the very low incidence of the disease, but such etiologic investigations could be initiated and conducted in developing countries.

From the clinical standpoint, the low risk of rheumatic fever today suggests that perhaps we should reassess present policies regarding our hunt for the streptococcus and our determination to eradicate it. However, any relaxation of our currently recommended approaches to streptococcal infections should be undertaken with great caution, since we do not understand the reasons for the decline and consequently cannot fully anticipate the possible results of any relaxation in policy. In any case, such a relaxation would be highly inappropriate for developing countries in which the risks of rheumatic fever and rheumatic heart disease remain so high.

Finally, there is an urgent need for additional research both on the biology of the streptococcus and the pathogenetic mechanisms involved in the development of rheumatic fever as well as on other factors that may interact with the streptococcus and influence the risk of disease. Such research may not only be valuable in improving the health of populations that are at high risk for rheumatic fever in developing countries, but may also shed light on the pathogenesis of other nonsuppurative sequelae of infectious diseases.

References

1. Jones TD: The diagnosis of rheumatic fever. JAMA **126:** 481, 1944
2. Gordis L, Lilienfeld A, Rodriguez R: Studies in the epidemiology and preventability of rheumatic fever. I. Demographic factors and the incidence of acute attacks. J Chron Dis **21:** 645, 1969
3. Gordis L: Effectiveness of comprehensive-care programs in preventing rheumatic fever. N Engl J Med **289:** 331, 1973
4. Land MA, Bisno AL: Acute rheumatic fever: a vanishing disease in suburbia. JAMA **249:** 895, 1983
5. Gutensohn N, Cole P: Epidemiology of Hodgkin's disease in the young. Int J Cancer **19:** 595, 1977
6. Kuttner AG, Krumwiede E: Observations on the effect of streptococcal upper respiratory infections on rheumatic children: a three-year study. J Clin Invest **20:** 273, 1941
7. Potter EV, Svartman M, Poon-King T, Earle DP: The families of patients with acute rheumatic fever or glomerulonephritis in Trinidad. Am J Epidemiol **106:** 130, 1977
8. Bisno AL, Pearce IA, Wall HP, Moody MD, Stollerman GH: Contrasting epidemiology of acute rheumatic fever and acute glomerulonephritis: nature of the antecedent streptococcal infection. N Engl J Med **283:** 561, 1970
9. McCarty M: The streptococcus and human disease. Am J Med **65:** 717, 1978
10. Maruyama S, Yoshioka H, Fujita K, Takimoto M, Satake Y: Sensitivity of group A streptococci to antibiotics: prevalence of resistance to erythromycin in Japan. Am J Dis Child **133:** 1143, 1979
11. Beachey EH: Bacterial adherence: adhesin-receptor interactions mediating the attachment of bacteria to mucosal surfaces. J Infect Dis **143:** 325, 1981
12. Jakab GJ: Viral-bacterial interactions in pulmonary infection. Adv Vet Sci Comparat Med **26:** 155, 1982
13. Mills EL: Viral infections predisposing to bacterial infections. Annu Rev Med **35:** 469, 1984
14. Eichenwald HF, Kotsevalov D, Fasso LA: Some effect of viral infections on aerial dissemination of staphylococci and on susceptibility to bacterial colonization. Bacteriol Rev **25:** 274, 1961
15. Fainstein V, Musher DM, Cate TR: Bacterial adherence to pharyngeal cells during viral infection. J Infect Dis **141:** 172, 1980
16. Jones WT, Menna JH, Wennerstrom DE: Lethal synergism induced in mice by influenza type A virus and type Ia group B streptococci. Infect Immun **41:** 618, 1983
17. Fainstein V, Musher DM: Bacterial adherence to pharyngeal cells in smokers, nonsmokers, and chronic bronchitics. Infect Immun **26:** 178, 1979
18. Dubos R: Mirage of health. Perennial Library, 1959, New York, p 23, Cited in McKinlay JB, McKinlay SM: The questionable contribution of medical measures to the decline of mortality in the United States in the Twentieth century. Millbank Mem Fund Q Summer 1977, pp 405–428
19. Kass EH: Infectious diseases and social change. J Infect Dis **123:** 110, 1971
20. Ayoub EM: The search for host determinants of susceptibility to rheumatic fever: the missing link. T. Duckett Jones Memorial Lecture. Circulation **69:** 197, 1984
21. Markowitz M: Observations on the epidemiology and preventability of rheumatic fever in developing countries. Clin Ther **4:** 240, 1981
22. Community control of rheumatic heart disease in developing countries. 1. A major public health problem. WHO Chronicle **34:** 336, 1980
23. Coulehan J, Grant S, Reisinger K, Killian P, Rogers KD, Kaltenbach C: Acute rheumatic fever and rheumatic heart disease on the Navajo reservation, 1962-77. Public Health Rep **95:** 62, 1980
24. Chun LT, Reddy V, Rhoads GG: Occurrence and prevention of rheumatic fever among ethnic groups of Hawaii. AJDC **138:** 476, 1984
25. Rheumatic fever, forgotten but not gone. Colorado Dis Bull **12**(16):1, 1984

PLATELETS AND VASCULAR OCCLUSION: PHARMACOLOGY OF PLATELET INHIBITION

Part II

The potential contribution of platelets to atherogenesis, thrombogenesis, and vasospasm has prompted considerable interest in their role in syndromes of vascular occlusion. Recently identified, novel platelet-derived products and pharmacologic problems have helped to illuminate these areas. This continues our series on key advances in cell biology, biochemistry, and pharmacology of platelet–vessel wall interactions based on presentations at a recent symposium entitled "Platelet inhibition and vascular occlusion in man" held in London, England, in August 1984. To provide our readers with an in-depth presentation of the basic science and clinical implications of platelet biology, the material is being published as a featured symposium. Selection of reviewers and editorial decisions for the manuscripts from the symposium were made with the help of Drs. Garret A. FitzGerald, Nashville, Tennessee, and Carlo Patrono, Rome, Italy, chairmen of the meeting.

Part III, "Therapeutic implications of platelet activation," will appear in the February 1986 issue of *Circulation*.

The human pharmacology of platelet inhibition: pharmacokinetics relevant to drug action

ANDERS KIRSTEIN PEDERSEN, M.D., AND GARRET A. FITZGERALD, M.D.

THE RATIONALE for antithrombotic intervention by pharmacologic inhibition of platelet reactivity derives from experimental evidence that platelet aggregation or adhesion to vascular endothelium is a primary event in the development of arterial thrombosis and thromboembolism and possibly, in the development of atherosclerotic lesions.[1]

A large number of drugs and other chemicals inhibit human platelet function in vitro.[2] Very few of them have been used in vivo. This is because the concentrations necessary to achieve platelet inhibitory effects are, with few exceptions, associated with significant toxicity.

Inhibition of platelet function is not a well-characterized biological phenomenon. It is best defined as inhibition of the reactivity-associated aspects of platelet physiology: the shape change, changes in glycoprotein structure on the surface membrane, adhesion, initiation of the granule release reaction, aggregation, and generation of procoagulant activity.[3] The term "antiplatelet drugs" covers a range of compounds with very different mechanisms of action. Many of the drugs under current clinical evaluation were originally developed for other therapeutic purposes. Common to all of them is the characteristic that, in certain preparations in vitro or in vivo, they inhibit platelet-dependent events.

The requirements for rational clinical use of a drug include detailed information about the pharmacokinetics and pharmacodynamics of the compounds, i.e., the relationship between drug dose and drug effect. A model for this relationship can be schematized[4] as depicted in figure 1.

Drug concentrations in different parts of the body are determined by drug absorption, distribution, metabolism, and excretion. The purpose of pharmacokinetic studies is to quantitatively characterize these processes to explain or predict the concentrations of drug at the site(s) of effect. Drug concentration at this site should in theory be related to effect. Pharmacodynamic modeling analyzes this relationship.

The clinical evaluation of antiplatelet drugs, in conditions in which platelets were thought to be of pathophysiologic importance, was initiated at a time when sufficient information on bioavailability, disposition, or dose-effect relationships was not available. Many of the trials had a negative outcome; in retrospect, some of these negative results may have been associated with the selection of less-than-optimal dose regimens because of incomplete understanding of the basic pharmacology of the compounds involved. Such information is now accumulating. The aim of this review is to present and discuss some of the more important antiplatelet drugs under current clinical evaluation.

Pharmacokinetic modeling. Pharmacokinetic models are based primarily on determination of the concentrations of drugs or metabolites in plasma or urine. The validity of the analytical method is crucial for the interpretation of the results. In many cases, insufficient sensitivity or selectivity may have resulted in errors of interpretation. For example, salicylate levels are often used in describing "aspirin" pharmacokinetics[5]; many analytic methods for the determination of sulfinpyrazone do not include selective determination of the active sulfone or sulfide metabolites.[6]

During the past decade, selective and sensitive methods involving gas chromatography (GC) or high-performance liquid chromatography (HPLC) have been used for pharmacokinetic studies. GC-mass spectrometry, combining high sensitivity and high selectivity with the possibility of chemical structural analysis of unknown compounds, has been particularly useful in analysis of the metabolism and kinetics of antiplatelet drugs.[7–9]

Once obtained, the concentration data are usually "fitted" to a mathematical model of the body, combining monoexponential or multiexponential functions to

From the Department of Medicine I, Aarhus Amssygehus, Arhus, Denmark, and the Division of Clinical Pharmacology, Vanderbilt University Medical School, Nashville, Tennessee.

Supported by grants from the National Institutes of Health (HL 30400) and the Danish Medical Research Council. Dr. FitzGerald is an Established Investigator of the American Heart Association.

Address for correspondence: Anders Pedersen, M.D., Department of Medicine I, Aarhus Amssygehus, DK-8000, Aarhus C, Denmark.

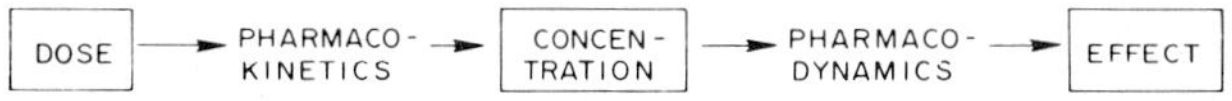

FIGURE 1. The relationship between drug administration and pharmacologic effect.

describe drug absorption, elimination, and distribution in one or more hypothetical body compartments.[10]

The compartments rarely correspond to physiologically defined volumes like the plasma volume or the extracellular volume; on the other hand, drug concentrations in a compartment might change in parallel to the concentrations in a physiologic volume or to the concentrations at the site of effect. Pharmacokinetic modeling gives useful information about bioavailability and clearance of drugs and in many cases has had a high predictive value.[11]

Pharmacokinetic modeling has several important implications for clinical medicine. The rational design of a dosage regimen relies on pharmacokinetic data. Failure to recognize variability in bioavailability, elimination, cumulation, or significant metabolism might result in excessive or insufficient drug concentrations and invalidate clinical trials of the drugs under study. Detection of large intraindividual or interindividual variability in pharmacokinetics or identification of subgroups with special metabolic patterns are important for the interpretation of drug effects or side effects. Convergence or divergence of drug concentrations and effects are often discovered by pharmacokinetic modeling and might, as described below, lead to identification of active metabolites or provide insights into unknown mechanisms of action.

Pharmacodynamic modeling. Inhibition of platelet function may be reversible or irreversible. Reversible inhibition of platelet function is associated with the presence of the parent drug or of a metabolite at the site of effect and is related to the pharmacokinetics of the compounds. In practice, such inhibition of function is caused by reversible inhibitors of cyclooxygenase (sulfinpyrazone and metabolites), thromboxane synthase (dazoxiben and similar drugs), or phosphodiesterase (dipyridamole and theophylline); by antagonists of the thromboxane/endoperoxide receptor[12]; by inhibitors of adenosine binding (dipyridamole); or by stimulators of adenylate cyclase (PGI_2 and other prostaglandins).

Because platelets are cells without a nucleus and have a very limited capacity for protein synthesis,[13] irreversible inhibition of a cellular function usually lasts for the lifespan of the platelet, which in normal situations is approximately 10 days.[14] The recovery from irreversible inhibition after a single drug exposure is therefore not a function of the drug involved, but is rather directly related to the platelet renewal rate. This rate is normally a function of the platelet survival time, i.e., the lifespan of the platelet. Aspirin and ticlopidine inhibit platelet function irreversibly.

The pharmacodynamics of reversible inhibition. Reversible effects of drugs are seen much more commonly than irreversible effects, and several pharmacodynamic dose-effect models have been suggested.[4]

The linear model, in which the effect is linearly proportional to the dose, is often used in very simple plots to investigate whether a certain effect correlates with drug dose or drug concentration:

$$E = k*D \qquad (1)$$

where E = the effect, k = a constant, and D = the drug dose or concentration.

The predictive value of this model is limited because it does not describe a maximum effect, and the linear relationship often overestimates the increase in effect caused by increases in drug doses.

The log-linear model permits a linear increase in drug effect with logarithmic increases in the dose and is usually more suited to biological data:

$$E = k*\log D \qquad (2)$$

It does not, however, provide information on maximum or zero effect and there is no particular theoretical rationale for using this model; data that correlate with this model will, in most cases, fit the Emax model (see below), which has a much greater biological relevance.

Derived from classical binding studies and extensively used in general pharmacology, receptor studies, and enzyme kinetics, the law of mass action equation gives a simple, and in most cases adequate, description of drug effects over a large range of doses[15]:

$$E = Emax*D\gamma/D\gamma + K) \qquad (3)$$

where E = the effect, Emax = the maximum effect, D = the drug concentration, K = the drug concentration necessary to give 50% of the maximum effect, and γ = an arbitrary constant (often set to unity) (figure 2).

In a linear plot, the model describes a hyperbolic function and in a log-linear plot demonstrates a limited sigmoid shape with approximate linearity in the middle 70% of the curve. A particular feature of the model is the variable change in drug effect caused by decreasing or increasing the dose or concentration at different parts of the curve. At the lower part of the curve, the dose-effect relationship is almost linear; at the steep

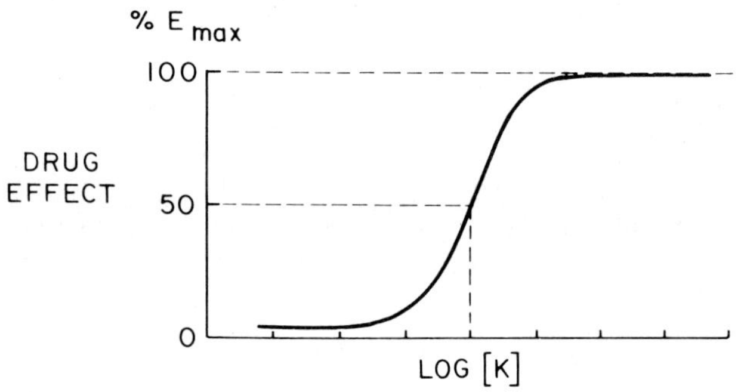

FIGURE 2. The relationship of plasma concentration and effect as predicted by the law of mass action, where E is the drug effect and K is the drug concentration in plasma.

middle part of the curve, the relationship is approximately log-linear, whereas at the upper part, only small increases in drug effect are seen with log-increases in dose or concentration.

The pharmacodynamics of irreversible inhibition. The models for irreversible inhibition of cellular function are more complex than the models for concentration-effect relationships of reversible inhibitors. For reversible inhibitors, a certain concentration of the drug at the effector site is associated with a certain effect. This relationship should, in theory, be valid under all circumstances: during short- or long-term therapy, during absorption, or during elimination. After distribution equilibrium has been achieved, plasma concentration may also be used, assuming active metabolites are not present.

This direct relationship between drug concentration and effect is not valid for irreversible inhibitors. The mechanism of irreversible inhibition is usually a process in which the drug damages a target cellular component. Because the damage is cumulative, the effect of this process is dependent not only on drug concentration but also on the duration of exposure to the compound. The effect is still present when the drug is eliminated from the environment so that a subsequent drug exposure results in a cumulative effect. This phenomenon is usually limited by a renewal of the cellular component, allowing some degree of functional recovery between doses.

Whereas the effect of reversible inhibitions is generally determined by the local drug concentration at any given time, the effect of irreversible inhibitors is influenced by additional factors. In fact, failure of concentration and effect to be correlated should raise the possibility that such a mechanism may be operative. In acute situations, the effect is determined by drug concentration and the exposure time, i.e., the area under the plasma drug concentration-time curve (AUC); the disappearance of effect is determined by the rate of replacement of the defective component. In long-term therapy, the single-dose effect is cumulative. This accumulation is a function of the rate of renewal of the defective component and the dose interval. With a rapid renewal rate and a long dose interval, the defective component is replaced between the doses and accumulation of drug effects is negligible. With a slow rate of renewal and a short dose interval, the accumulation of even a small initial effect is substantial.

Aspirin is the classic example of a drug with this mechanism of action, and the pharmacodynamics of aspirin have been studies most intensively.[16–19] Ticlopidine has a pharmacodynamic profile compatible with irreversible inhibition,[20] but the exact mechanism of its action has not been established.

Concentration-effect relationships: convergence or divergence. When different pharmacokinetic or pharmacodynamic models are compared with the experimental results, convergence of the data according to the specific model indicates that the drug concentration and drug effect are directly related. The alternative finding, a divergence of concentration and effect, requires further analysis. Two common situations are discussed below.

Figure 3 illustrates the situation with rapid drug elimination but prolonged effect after administration of a single dose. Several models could, in theory, explain this finding and should be considered:

(1) An irreversible effect of the drug. The recovery from the effect is not determined by the rate of removal of the drug but by the replacement of a "defective" cellular or enzymatic component.

(2) Formation of active metabolites with similar properties as the parent drug but with a slower rate of elimination. The decay of effect is then related to the half-life of the metabolites, not the drug.

(3) Penetration of the drug or a metabolite into a "deep" effect-related compartment, containing small amounts of drug. The drug concentration at this site is directly related to the effect, but drug clearance from the relevant compartment is much slower than from plasma.

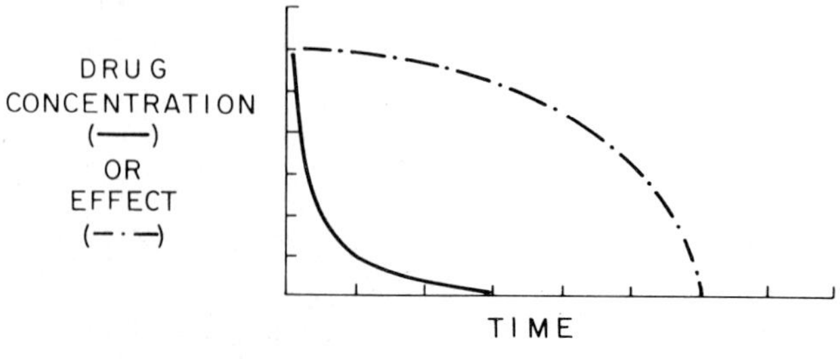

FIGURE 3. Rapid drug elimination but prolonged pharmacodynamic effect.

(4) "Supramaximal" drug dose, i.e., a dose larger than needed for maximal effect. In an Emax model, the dose would be located far to the right of the dose-effect curve. Even dramatic reductions in plasma concentrations of the drug would then be followed by only modest changes in effect until the concentration range close to K was reached.

An alternative situation would be a very short duration of drug effect despite a prolonged presence of the drug in the circulation (figure 4).

At least four explanations should be considered:

(1) Rapid tachyphylaxis. Despite drug concentrations, the effect disappears with the development of tolerance.

(2) Inactive metabolites measured instead of or in addition to (nonspecific assay) the active drug. The active drug is associated with the effect but is cleared much more rapidly than metabolites.

(3) Small changes in concentrations followed by large changes in effect on a very steep concentration-effect curve.

(4) Generation of an antagonistic active metabolite.

A careful analysis of the pharmacokinetic and pharmacodynamic profile of a drug often leads to new insight into the clinical pharmacology of the compound. The recognition of irreversible drug effects, the potential for biologically active metabolites, and the determination of dose-effect relationships have been important advances in our understanding of the clinical pharmacology of drugs with platelet-inhibitory activity.

Dipyridamole. Dipyridamole is a drug with strong fluorescence, a property that has been utilized in the assay of the drug.[21] Early methods with extraction followed by spectrofluorometry did not permit measurement of low plasma concentrations[22]; HPLC-methods were consequently developed with detection limits in the low nanogram per milliliter range.[23, 24] These methods allow determination of the compound as well as its glucuronide metabolite with sensitivity and selectivity sufficient for pharmacokinetic studies.

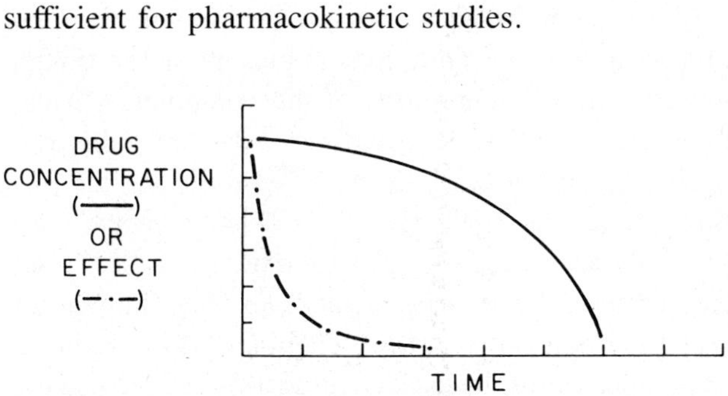

FIGURE 4. Delayed drug elimination but rapid offset of pharmacodynamic effect.

Pharmacokinetics. The elimination of dipyridamole is primarily by biliary excretion as a glucuronide conjugate.[25] After oral and intravenous administration, dipyridamole exhibits biexponential elimination with a terminal half-life of about 100 min.[26] When the sampling time is extended, a longer apparent terminal elimination phase has been described.[27] In this situation, elimination can be described by a triexponential function with a terminal half-life of about 10 hr, confounded to some extent by enterohepatic recirculation, which produces one or several late reabsortion peaks in the concentration curve.[27] An independent estimate of the terminal rate of elimination was obtained in experiments comparing steady-state with single-dose kinetics.[28] An accumulation factor of 2.4 consistent with a prolonged half-life was found.[29] A difficulty with this approach is the low and highly variable nature of absorption resulting in an intersubject variability in peak plasma concentrations of seven- to 15-fold.[26, 29] The intrasubject variability is not known. The drug is highly bound to α-1-acid glycoprotein in plasma.[24, 30]

A pharmacokinetic interaction between salicylate and dipyridamole, perhaps resulting from an alteration in hepatic blood flow, has been suggested, leading to increased concentrations of both drugs.[31] The significance of this putative interaction is unclear. A recent report[32] indicates that coadministration of dipyridamole significantly increases both the peak plasma concentrations and the area under the plasma concentration-time curve (AUC) of aspirin.

The steady-state plasma concentrations of the drug during administration of 75 mg three times daily have generally been in the range of 1 to 2 μg/ml, although higher and lower levels have been reported.[26, 28, 33, 34] This difference is most likely a result of the variable bioavailability of the drug. Some pharmaceutical brands have a documented low bioavailability.[35] Analytical artifacts, probably associated with instability of the drug, might play a role as well.[23]

Pharmacodynamics. Dipyridamole was originally introduced as a vasodilator and this activity has been attributed to inhibition of adenosine uptake and degradation by the vasculature, thus potentiating the effect of endogenous adenosine.[36] With regard to platelet function, dipyridamole is a very weak inhibitor of most platelet agonists in vitro, requiring concentrations of more than 10 to 50 μg/ml.[37–39] It does not affect prostaglandin-dependent pathways, but several other mechanisms of action have been proposed. Dipyridamole inhibits adenosine biding and uptake in the platelet,[31, 40] and this effect is significant at 0.1 μg/ml. On the other hand, no clear relationship between adenosine binding and platelet aggregation has been established. Alternatively, dipyridamole inhibits cyclic AMP phosphodiesterase in platelets in the concentration range of 1 to 10 μg/ml.[41–43] This inhibition may potentiate the effects of PGI_2[44, 41]; however, because PGI_2 is not a circulating hormone,[45, 46] any effect must be exerted at the local level. Other drugs (like theophylline) are more effective enzyme inhibitors in therapeutic concentrations.[41]

Based on experiments in vitro and bioassays in vivo it has been reported that dipyridamole stimulates PGI_2 biosynthesis, but the data have not been supported by specific noninvasive methods.[44–48] The most convincing evidence that the drug has antiplatelet activity in vivo comes from platelet survival studies. In nonhuman primate preparations and in patients with increased platelet consumption and decreased survival, the drug produces a decrease in platelet turnover.[49–51]

Dipyridamole has been investigated extensively as an adjunct to aspirin and is claimed to be effective in the prevention of myocardial infarction, embolic incidents associated with prosthetic heart valves, and occlusion of coronary artery grafts.[52–54] At present, it is not clear whether the drug is necessary for the beneficial effects of the combination.

Sulfinpyrazone. Sulfinpyrazone is a uricosuric drug that has a chemical structure similar to that of phenylbutazone and was developed in the late 1950s. The development of phenylbutazone, the first effective anti-inflammatory drug after aspirin, encouraged the search for new and more effective drugs with related molecular structures. In a series of sulfur-substituted biphenyl-pyrazolidines, CG-25671 showed promising antiinflammatory and uricosuric effects.[55] In urine from subjects treated with this substance, sulfinpyrazone was isolated as the sulfoxide metabolite. This compound had almost selective uricosuric properties and only weak anti-inflammatory effects in animal preparations. It was introduced in clinical medicine in 1960 as an effective therapeutic agent against gout. The discovery of the antiplatelet activity of this compound prompted substantial clinical and basic research aimed at defining the mechanisms of action and possible clinical applications of the drug.

Investigating platelet survival time in patients with gout, Smythe et al.[56] reported that the drug restored an abnormally shortened platelet survival time in some patients. Several clinical and laboratory investigations have since suggested that the drug might be useful as a platelet inhibitory drug in thromboembolic disorders.

Sulfinpyrazone inhibits cyclooxygenase, but some experimental evidence suggests that the drug possesses antiplatelet activity distinct from that of cyclooxygenase inhibition.[57, 58] Although two major clinical trials in the secondary prevention of myocardial infarction reported positive effects in terms of reducing the incidence of sudden death or reinfarction, a consensus on the role of the drug in prevention of these events has not been obtained.[59–61] Beneficial effects in other thrombosis-related diseases have been reported but not sufficiently documented.[62]

Pharmacokinetics. Analysis of sulfinpyrazone levels was performed by spectrophotometry in the early studies of the drug.[63] Since the development of HPLC, alternative analytical methods have been described.[64] Gas chromatography with selective mass-spectrometric detection was used in the characterization of the complex metabolic disposition of the drug,[7, 8] and after the identification of the circulating metabolites, an HPLC method with simultaneous detection of the parent drug and four metabolites in plasma was developed for routine use.[65]

The absorption of sulfinpyrazone is quite complete,[6] although a dose-related difference in metabolism might be related to preabsorptive metabolism (for review see ref. 64). The elimination kinetics conform to a three-compartment open model[6] with a terminal half-life of 6 hr. The β-phase half-life of approximately 2 to 3 hr seems more in accordance with the "terminal" half-life observed in other studies.[66–69] The parent drug is highly bound to plasma albumin[70] and is eliminated by metabolism and urinary excretion.[71, 72, 74]

The first chemical analysis of the metabolic products identified a C-conjugated glucoronide, a sulfone and a p-OH-metabolite.[71] A new metabolic pathway involving reduction of the sulfoxide was identified in the rabbit[73] and later in man.[8, 74] The principal product of this pathway, the sulfide accumulates to high concentrations in plasma, probably because of slower rate of elimination. The sulfone has a similar half-life to that of the parent drug and is detectable early after drug administration. The para-hydroxylated metabolites of sulfinpyrazone and its primary metabolites are only present in low concentrations in plasma. Mean trough steady-state concentrations of the compounds in patients receiving 200 mg four times a day are: sulfinpyrazone 7.1 μg/ml, the sulfone 1.7 μg/ml, and the sulfide 2.8 μg/ml.[74] Whereas the oxidative metabolites probably are formed by hepatic oxidation, the site of formation of the reduced metabolites is not known for certain. Analogous to the formation of other reduced drug metabolites, bacterial degradation[75, 76] may be the source of these compounds. Such a possibility is consistent with the slow formation of the sulfide, suggesting biliary excretion of the parent drug with subsequent reduction.[76] Both metabolites are strongly protein bound.[70] Short-term studies in normal subjects indicate that the steady-state plasma concentrations are reached within a few days of therapy.[66, 69]

Pharmacodynamics. Early studies by Packham et al.[77] demonstrated that sulfinpyrazone inhibited the release of serotonin from platelets stimulated with low concentrations of collagen. The inhibition of thrombin-induced release was less pronounced. These effects were associated with the inhibition of platelet cyclooxygenase. Sulfinpyrazone had, on a molecular basis, an activity similar to that of phenylbutazone but much less than that of aspirin.[77] Since the conversion of ^{14}C-arachidonate to PGD_2 and thromboxane B_2 was suppressed to a similar degree, no indication of selective inhibition of thromboxane synthase was found.[78, 79]

These results have largely been confirmed in more recent studies (for review see ref. 80). The concentrations needed for inhibitory activity have usually been in the range of 100 to 200 μg/ml; greater activity was found in protein-free media.[79] A few investigators report inhibition at much lower plasma concentrations.[78, 81] Since sulfinpyrazone is tightly bound to plasma albumin, the unbound fraction of the drug probably determines the antiplatelet effect in whole blood or platelet-rich plasma.[82]

The platelet-inhibitory effects of sulfinpyrazone are not restricted to the parent drug. Buchanan et al.[83] reported a prolonged antiplatelet activity after intravenous injection of sulfinpyrazone in the rabbit, which was unrelated to the plasma concentration of the drug. The formation of one or several active metabolites was suggested and a sulfide and a p-OH-sulfide metabolite were identified in rabbits and guinea pigs[73, 84] at time points corresponding to the prolonged effect. In vitro, the sulfide was five to 12 times as active as the parent compound in inhibiting collagen- or arachidonate-induced aggregation. In purified cyclooxygenase preparations, the sulfide was nearly 100 times as active.[82] The sulfone was twice as active as sulfinpyrazone itself; the hydroxylated metabolites were approximately equipotent with the parent drug.[73, 74]

A possible differential effect on endothelial cell vs platelet cyclooxygenase has been suggested from investigations of endothelial cell cultures and isolated platelets in vitro.[85] Noninvasive approaches based on determination of urinary prostaglandin metabolites indicate no differences in the degree of inhibition or formation of products by the two cyclooxygenases.[66]

In high doses, sulfinpyrazone inhibits the thrombocytopenia and bronchoconstriction triggered by intravascular platelet sequestration during the Forssman reaction in the guinea pig.[58] Neither aspirin nor indomethacin has any effect in this model. Sulfinpyrazone appears to inhibit some of the phenomena associated with intravenous injection of platelet activating factor.[86] It has been suggested that the drug acts as a specific inhibitor of this pathway of activation. Other experiments, however, found no additional antiplatelet activity of the drug apart from that associated with inhibition of cyclooxygenase.[66]

The prolongation of a shortened platelet survival by sulfinpyrazone has been demonstrated in several patient groups.[56, 87, 88] In baboons, the drug protects the vascular endothelium against damage induced by homocysteine. The mechanism of action in these models seems distinct from that of cyclooxygenase inhibition, since aspirin has no effect. Studies in patients with arteriovenous shunt thrombosis indicated that at least 1 week of treatment with 800 mg/day was required before effective antiplatelet activity was achieved.[90] This finding led to the controversial "7-day rule" in the "Anturane Reinfarction Trial,"[59] which excluded patients in the early treatment period from the statistical analysis. The basis for this strategy is not well documented. Some studies seem to indicate that a cumulative antiplatelet effect is seen during prolonged treatment[91]; other investigations produced inconclusive or no evidence of this phenomenon.[66] Metabolism of sulfinpyrazone to the active sulfide and sulfone metabolites is probably necessary to produce a maximal antiplatelet effect.[82] At present, divergent results on the accumulation of these metabolites have been published.[66, 67, 69] A combined drug activity index determined by multiplying the plasma concentrations of the compounds by their activity seems to correlate with the inhibition of cyclooxygenase during therapy.[66] The lack of correlation with individual drug or metabolite levels underlines the complexity of relating kinetics to pharmacodynamic responses.

The dose most commonly used, 800 mg/day, leaves little room for investigating dose-related effects, since it is at the lower end of the dose-response curve and close to the maximum tolerable level. The equivocal results from clinical trials of sulfinpyrazone in the prevention of thromboembolic events may reflect the limited tissue selectivity with respect to cyclooxygenase as well as the relatively poor pharmacologic potency of the drug and its metabolites.

Thromboxane synthase inhibitors. Thromboxane A_2 is a major metabolite of arachidonic acid in the platelet.[92] The discovery of prostacyclin synthase in the vessel wall,[93] which led to the proposal of the "endoperoxide shunt" hypothesis,[94] made cyclooxygenase inhibition a theoretically less attractive antithrombotic strategy. Cyclooxygenase inhibitors, such as aspirin and sulfinpyrazone, inhibit both thromboxane A_2 and prostacyclin biosynthesis. Selective inhibition of thromboxane synthase would preserve the capacity of the vasculature to produce prostacyclin. Furthermore, accumulation of endoperoxides, which are the substrate for thromboxane synthase, is likely to occur in circulating platelets, especially if stimulated. This might permit shunting of platelet-derived endoperoxides to prostacyclin synthase located in adjacent endothelium.[95] The increased supply of the substrate for the enzyme might then stimulate the biosynthesis of prostacyclin.

On the other hand, the proaggregatory effects of the accumulated endoperoxides might attenuate the inhibitory effect caused by inhibition of thromboxane A_2 formation.[96] Several structurally different thromboxane synthetase inhibitors have now been tested in controlled clinical studies. Although only limited information on the pharmacokinetics of these compounds is available, some important conclusions can be drawn from the data published.

Pharmacokinetics. Several structurally distinct thromboxane synthase inhibitors have been administered to man.[97–100] Only scattered pharmacokinetic data are available; it seems that all compounds are cleared rapidly from the blood with a half-life of around 60 min. The metabolic pattern is not yet elucidated, but no active metabolites are suspected.

Pharmacodynamics. The effect in vivo of thromboxane synthase inhibitors is most conveniently measured using platelets as test cells *ex vivo*. Inhibition of stimulated thromboxane generation as in the assay of thromboxane B_2, the stable hydration product of thromboxane A_2, in serum, provides an attractive and reproducible parameter of drug effect.[101] Platelet aggregation is much less sensitive to thromboxane synthase inhibition. In most studies, only weak effects have been reported, mainly inhibition of aggregation of the release reaction caused by threshold concentrations of collagen or arachidonate.[93, 101] The lack of effect on platelet aggregation in general has been taken as evidence for the agonistic effects of endoperoxides. This explanation is supported by the finding that further addition of endoperoxide-thromboxane receptor antagonists results in a complete inhibition of aggregation.[102] On the other hand, synthase inhibitors seem to inhibit aggregation consistently in some individuals, the so-called responders.[103] Whether this is caused by generation of endoperoxide products[104] with modulating antiplatelet activity (PGE_2, PGD_2) is not known. A contributing factor may be the slow entry of some of the drugs into the platelet.[102, 105]

Whereas inhibition of platelet thromboxane generation is easy to quantitate, the examination of the endoperoxide "shunt" in vivo is a more difficult analytical task. Radioimmunoassay of serum 6-keto-$PGF_{1\alpha}$, the hydration product of prostacyclin, is an unreliable parameter under conditions where other endoperoxide products are produced in large amounts.[106] Initial reports that plasma 6-keto-$PGF_{1\alpha}$ was increased substantially during thromboxane synthase inhibition have not been confirmed.[97, 98, 106] Determination of 2,3-dinor-6-keto-$PGF_{1\alpha}$ in urine during thromboxane synthase inhibition has demonstrated the existence of endoperoxide rediversion in vivo.[99, 101] Whether this is caused by platelet-endothelial endoperoxide transfer or simply caused by rediversion within cells containing both thromboxane and prostacyclin synthase is not known.

One of the major disadvantages of thromboxane synthase inhibitors compared with aspirin is the lack of prolonged inhibition of thromboxane formation. This is difficult to achieve by the drugs under current evaluation because of their rapid elimination. This example clearly illustrates the necessity of a thorough pharmacokinetic evaluation in the investigation of antiplatelet drugs. With further pharmacokinetic and pharmacodynamic information improved dosing strategies may evolve.

In the clinical studies of two inhibitors of thromboxane synthase, a discrepancy between the elimination of the drug from plasma and the disappearance of the effect on serum thromboxane B_2 have been noted.[100, 107] Based on HPLC determinations of the drug concentrations, the half-life in plasma was calculated to be about 1 hr; the effect on serum thromboxane B_2 lasts much longer, with greater than 50% inhibition at eight half-lives after maximum inhibition. Several explanations have been offered for this phenomenon; either slow elimination from a deep compartment (for example, the platelet) or the existence of unknown active metabolites. An additional likely explanation is that the plasma concentration-effect curve follows the law of mass action relationship. The maximum effect of the dose given (figure 3) is about 99%, probably very close to the Emax. At the flat upper part of the log dose-response curve, even a rapid clearance of the drug does not change the effect very much initially. The dose given is "supramaximal" and located to the right of the slope of the curve. Together with slow elimination of the drug from the platelet, such phenomena would explain the disparity between offset of plasma drug levels and inhibition of platelet cyclooxygenase. The slow decrease of effect gives a false image of the real half-life of the drug. If this half-life was as long as indicated from the effect curve, significant accumulation would be expected in long-term therapy, which is not the case.[107]

The potential of thromboxane synthase inhibitors as a therapeutic strategy in thrombotic disease has been reviewed elsewhere.[102, 108]

Aspirin. Aspirin is unstable at alkaline and acidic pH and is susceptible to spontaneous or enzymatic hydrolysis.[109] The rate of hydrolysis in human blood or plasma at room temperature is fast; the half-life is about 1 hr. When plasma is maintained at $-20°$ C, the half-life is 2 to 3 weeks.[11] The rate of degradation is slowed by addition of esterase inhibitors (eserine or fluoride). Because of the hydrolysis of aspirin into salicylic acid in vitro and in vivo, selective determinations of the compounds involves separation by TLC, GC, or HPLC before analysis.[111–115] Spectrophotometric and spectrofluorimetric methods are not specific in that respect. The conventional limit of detection by GC or HPLC is around 50 to 100 ng/ml. GC–mass spectrometric detection allows determination in the low nanogram per millliter range.[9] Selective ion monitoring also permits detection of heavy isotope-labeled analogues. This is useful in the exact pharmacokinetic experiments with simultaneous administration of isotopes by different routes.[9, 116]

Pharmacokinetics. Aspirin is hydrolyzed in the gastrointestinal tract[117] and is absorbed partly as salicylate. Esterases present in the stomach and jejunal wall probably mediate this presystemic metabolism.[115, 118, 119] Absorption from aqueous solutions is rapid,[120] whereas the absorption from tablet preparations is variable; the presystemic metabolism renders systemic bioavailability susceptible to fluid and food ingestion.[121] Low systemic availability has been reported from enteric coated tablets and sustained release microencapsulated preparations.[122]

After absorption, aspirin is hydrolyzed by esterases present in the plasma, the red blood cells, the liver, and the lungs. The half-life of aspirin in plasma in vivo is about 15 to 20 min; the half-life of the hydrolysis product, salicylate, is about 2 to 3 hr.[117, 123] Hydrolysis is intimately associated with transfer of the free acetyl group to a number of proteins that are covalently acetylated. This has been demonstrated for cyclooxygenase,[16] albumin, hemoglobin, some of the plasma esterases, and several proteins present in cell membranes.[113] Acetylation of cyclooxygenase accounts for the irreversible inhibition of this enzyme.

Salicylate is further metabolized into glucuronic acid and glycine conjugates and, to a minor degree, to dihydroxy acids. Several of the enzymatic steps in this biotransformation are saturable,[124] resulting in mixed zero-order/first-order elimination kinetics of salicylate at higher plasma concentrations.

The pharmacokinetics of aspirin has been approximated by an open two-compartment model with first-order absorption and elimination and metabolism from the central compartment.[117] The pharmacokinetics of aspirin seem unaffected by long-term therapy or by a range of doses from 20 to 1300 mg.[116]

Pharmacodynamics. The inhibitory effect of aspirin on prostaglandin biosynthesis results from acetylation of the cyclooxygenases enzyme.[125] The effect is irreversible and persists for the lifetime of the enzyme. This is readily demonstrable in the platelet, which has no capacity for protein synthesis.[126, 127] The discovery of thromboxane A_2 and prostacyclin as the predominent endoperoxide products in the platelet and in the endothelium, respectively, raised the possibility of a differential inhibitory effect of aspirin on cyclooxygenase in the two tissues.[94] According to this hypothesis, low doses of aspirin might preferentially inhibit platelet thromboxane synthesis leaving endothelial prostacyclin synthesis relatively intact. Thus low doses of aspirin would presumably be more effective in the prevention of thrombosis than the doses of 300 to 1000 mg/day used in the early clinical trials of the drug.

In a pharmacologic sense, the requirement for such evidence is a statistically significant separation of the doses-inhibition curves for platelet cyclooxygenase and arterial cyclooxygenase, during short- and long-term therapy.[128–131] Biologically, the hypothesis of a selective dose is more complicated to test. In addition to inhibition of cyclooxygenase, some investigators have reported nonspecific inhibition of platelet function by high doses of aspirin.[132] In man, no additional platelet effects have been reported with high doses.[133] Maximum inhibition of platelet aggregation and the release reaction was associated with $\geq$95% inhibition of cyclooxygenase activity.

Since the function of prostacyclin as an antithrombotic agent in vivo has not been definitively established, the biological significance of a certain degree of inhibition is more unclear. Whether, for instance, 60% rather than 90% inhibition of vascular cyclooxygenase has a differential impact on the biological function of prostacyclin is unknown. Local differences in prostacyclin generation might have different biological effects: "upstream" release, i.e., proximal to a thrombogenic lesion, might be important in the prevention of thrombotic occlusion of the vessel, whereas "downstream" release, i.e., distal to the lesion, might be important for the dissolution of platelet emboli. As discussed in the section on irreversible inhibition, the turnover of cyclooxygenase is the major single determinant of the efficacy of aspirin. The renewal rate of this enzyme under normal conditions is not known. It might differ from atherosclerotic areas to normal areas of the vasculature, resulting in local differences in the degree of inhibition.

The mechanism by which selectivity might be related to dose is not clear. A differential sensitivity of the platelet and endothelial cell cyclooxygenase to aspirin has been reported in some studies but not confirmed in others.[134, 135] The recovery from inhibition and the accumulation of effect by repeated dosing is determined by the synthesis of new enzyme. After exposure to aspirin, recovery of prostacyclin production by endothelial cells in culture is more rapid than that of platelet thromboxane A_2.[19, 135, 136] However, there is more prolonged depression of vascular prostacyclin release ex vivo and reduced excretion of a major urinary prostacyclin metabolite after high-dose aspirin administration.[128, 137]

An alternative explanation for the biochemical selectivity of aspirin relates to its kinetics.[116] Platelets passing through the intestinal capillaries and portal vein during the absorptive phase of aspirin are exposed to higher concentrations of aspirin than in the peripheral circulation. These concentrations of aspirin might be sufficient to inhibit platelet cyclooxygenase in the portal circulation. Since aspirin is extensively cleared by the liver and the lung, the concentrations in the peripheral circulation might not be sufficient to inhibit vascular cyclooxygenase. Experimental evidence supports this hypothesis.[116] Substantial depression of serum thromboxane was found in the early absorption phase after a 20 mg oral dose of aspirin and before any aspirin was detected in the systemic circulation. Furthermore, the effect in vivo of aspirin on platelet cyclooxygenase is larger than predicted from the concentrations measured in peripheral venous blood. Both findings are consistent with presystemic inhibition of platelets.

Due to its affinity for the active site of cyclooxygenase[138] salicylate interferes with the acetylation of that site by aspirin.[139] Accumulation of salicylate during long-term aspirin therapy has been proposed as a mechanism for selectivity; salicylate appears to be more efficient as an inhibitor of vascular cyclooxygenase acetylation than of platelet cyclooxygenase acetylation.[140] The importance of this interaction for the antithrombotic efficacy of aspirin in man is unclear.

Some experimental evidence supports the selective dose hypothesis. In animal preparations, high doses of aspirin appear to be thrombogenic,[141, 142] although the doses used in the experimental preparations were much higher than the doses used in humans. The hemostatic function of platelets as assessed by determination of the bleeding time reportedly showed the same paradoxic pattern: high doses of aspirin did not change the bleeding time whereas lower doses significantly prolonged it.[143] This finding, however, was not reproduced in controlled, double-blind studies.[144] Even though prostacyclin infused intravenously prolongs the bleeding time in man,[145] it is not clear to what extent local production of prostacyclin at the capillary level influences the bleeding time. It has been suggested that the bleeding time might be an index of a putative prostacyclin/thromboxane "balance" and that age, sex, and disease-related changes in the balance are reflected in different bleeding times.[146]

Clinical studies addressing the hypothesis of a selective dose of aspirin have reached varied conclusions, depending on the trial design and analytic method used.[128–131, 137, 147] Most studies have not focused on the cumulative effect of aspirin on cyclooxygenase.[127] The cumulative effect is particularly obvious at low doses and has been demonstrated clearly in the platelet. The threshold dose for a steady-state inhibition of more than 90% to 95% of platelet thromboxane generation is 20 to 40 mg/day, both for normal subjects as well as for patients with coronary heart disease.[18, 133] Determination of systemic prostacyclin biosynthesis by analysis of the excretion of 2,3-dinor-6-keto-$PGF_{1\alpha}$, using a long-term dosing schedule from 20 to 2600 mg/day, showed significant inhibition at doses from 40 mg/day upward and maximum inhibition at 650 mg/day.[137] Although this metabolite may, in part, be derived from extravascular sources of prostacyclin, quantitation of the excretion rate accurately reflects the entry of prostacyclin into the circulation.[45, 148] Alternative estimates of vascular prostacyclin biosynthesis during aspirin therapy have been derived from bioassay or radioimmunoassay of whole blood or plasma,[13] from determination of the production capacity of excised venous or arterial segments in vitro,[129, 131] or from the urinary excretion of 6-keto-$PGF_{1\alpha}$.[17, 149] However, whole blood and plasma do not contain any significant amount of prostacyclin under physiologic conditions.[46, 106]

The use of ex vivo vascular generation of prostacyclin is a capacity-related index,[150] which probably accurately reflects the degree of cyclooxygenase inhibition. A problem with this approach is that the local capacity may differ from venous to arterial tissue, and because of the distribution and metabolism of aspirin, the effect would be expected to differ as well.

In summary, none of the studies published so far has presented conclusive evidence for a selective dose of aspirin. The most convincing studies suggest doses of 20 to 40 mg/day. During long-term therapy, this regimen secures effective inhibition of platelet aggregation and release with inhibition of prostacyclin biosynthesis. Whether such selectivity has any biological relevance would be appropriately examined by a comparative clinical trial of biochemically selective and nonselective dosing regimens.

Conclusion. Pharmacokinetic considerations may be of the utmost importance when considering the effects of antiplatelet therapy in vivo. Variability in absorption, distribution, metabolism, and excretion of these compounds, as well as in their pharmacodynamics, may contribute significantly to determining their efficacy in the prevention of thrombotic disease.

References

1. Harker LA, Ritchie JL: The role of platelets in acute vascular events. Circulation **62** (suppl V): V-13, 1980
2. Packham MA, Mustard JF: Pharmacology of platelet-affecting drugs. Circulation **62** (suppl V): V-26, 1980
3. Vermylen J, Badenhorst PN, Deckmyn H, Arnout J: Normal mechanisms of platelet function. Clin Haematol **12:** 107, 1983
4. Hölford NHG, Scheiner LB: Understanding the dose-effect relationship: clinical applications of pharmacokinetic-pharmacodynamic models. Clin Pharmacokin **6:** 429, 1981
5. Levy G, Anelino NJ: Clinical pharmacokinetics of salicylates: a re-assessment. Br J Clin Pharmacol **10** (suppl 1): 285, 1980
6. Lecaillon JB, Souppart CM, Schoeller JP, Humbert G, Massias P: Sulfinpyrazone kinetics after intravenous and oral administration. Clin Pharmacol Ther **26:** 611, 1979
7. Jakobsen P, Pedersen AK: Determination of sulfinpyrazone and two of its metabolites in human plasma and urine by gas chromatography and selective detection. J Chromatgr **163:** 259, 1979
8. Jakobsen P, Pedersen AK: Two metabolites of sulfinpyrazone and their identification and determination by mass spectrometry. J Pharm Pharmacol **33:** 89, 1981
9. Pedersen AK, FitzGerald GA: Preparation and analysis of deuterium labelled aspirin: application to pharmacokinetic studies. J Pharm Sci **74:** 188, 1984
10. Gibaldi M, Perrier D: Pharmacokinetics. New York, 1975, Marcel Dekker Co., p 329
11. Greenblatt DJ, Koch-Weser J: Clinical pharmacokinetics. N Engl J Med **293:** 702, 1975
12. Gresele P, Deckmyn H, Arnout J, Lemmens J, Janssens W, Vermylen J: BM 13-177, a selective blocker of platelet and vessel wall thromboxane receptors, is active in man. Lancet **1:** 991, 1984
13. White JG: Platelet morphology. *In* Johnson SA, editor: The circulating platelet. New York, 1971, Academic Press, p 41
14. Mustard JF: Platelet survival. Thromb Haemost **40:** 154, 1978
15. Ariens EJ, Simonis AM: A molecular basis for drug action: the interaction of one or more drugs with different receptor. J Pharm Pharmacol **16:** 289, 1964
16. Roth GJ, Majerus PW: The mechanism of the effect of aspirin on human platelets. I. Acetylation of a particulate fraction protein. J Clin Invest **56:** 624, 1975
17. Patrignani P, Filabozzi P, Patrono C: Selective cumulative inhibition of platelet thromboxane production by low-dose aspirin in healthy subjects. J Clin Invest **71:** 676, 1982
18. Catalano PM, Smith JB, Murphy S: Platelet recovery from aspirin inhibition *in vivo*: differing patterns under various assay conditions. Blood **57:** 88, 1981
19. Patrono C, Patrignani P, Davi G, Ciabattoni G, Forni L, Cochavi S: Variables affecting cumulative inhibition of human platelet cyclooxygenase activity by low-dose aspirin. Clin Res **32:** 319A, 1984
20. Ellis DJ, Roe RL, Bruno JJ, Cranston BJ, McSpadden MM: The effects of ticlopidine on bleeding time and platelet function in man. Thromb Haemost **46:** 1976, 1981
21. Zak SB, Tallan HH, Quinn GP, Fratta I, Greengard P: The determination and physiological distribution of dipyridamole and its glucuronides in biological material. J Pharmacol Exp Ther **141:** 382, 1963
22. Mellinger TJ, Bohorfoush JG: Blood levels of dipyridamole in humans. Arch Intern Pharmacodyn **163:** 471, 1966
23. Pedersen AK: Specific determination of dipyridamole in serum by high-performance liquid chromatography. J Chromatogr **162:** 98, 1979
24. Wolfram KM, Bjornsson RD: HPLC analysis of dipyridamole in plasma and whole blood. J Chromat **183:** 57, 1980
25. Beisenhertz G, Koss FW, Schule A, Gebauer I, Baerisch R, Froede R: The metabolism of 2,6-bis(diethanolamine)-4,8-dipiperidino-pyrimido(5,4-d)-pyrimidine. Arzneimittelforsch **10:** 307, 1960
26. Nielsen-Kudsk F, Pedersen AK: Pharmacokinetics of dipyridamole. Acta Pharmacol Toxicol **44:** 381, 1979
27. Mahony C, Wolfram KM, Cochetto D, Bjornsson TD: Dipyridamole kinetics. Clin Pharmacol Ther **31:** 330, 1982
28. Mahony C, Cox JL, Bjornsson TD: Plasma dipyridamole concentrations after two different dosage regimens in patients. J Clin Pharmacol **23:** 123, 1983
29. Bjornsson TD, Shand DG: Estimation of kinetic parameters from two point determination of the drug cumulation factor. Clin Pharmacol Ther **26:** 540, 1979
30. Subbarao K, Rucinski B, Rausch MA, Schmid K, Niewiaroski S: Binding of dipyridamole to human platelets and to alpha-l-acid glycoprotein and its significance for the inhibition of adenosine uptake. J Clin Invest **60:** 936, 1977
31. Buchanan MR, Rosenfeld J, Gent M, Lawrence W, Hirsh J: Increased dipyridamole plasma concentrations associated with salicylate administration: relationship to effects on platelet aggregation in vivo. Thromb Res **15:** 803, 1979
32. Nitelius E, Melander A, Wahlin-Boll E: Pharmacokinetic interaction of acetylsalicylic acid and dipyridamole. Br J Clin Pharmacol **19:** 379, 1985
33. Rajah SM, Crow MJ, Penny AF, Ahmad R, Watson DA: The effect of dipyridamole on platelet function: correlation with blood levels in man. Br J Clin Pharmacol **4:** 129, 1977
34. Tyce GM, Fuster V, Owen CA: Dipyridamole levels in plasma of man and other species. Res Commun Chem Pathol Pharmacol **26:** 495, 1979
35. Mahony C, Wolfram KM, Nash PV, Bjornsson TD: Kinetics and metabolism of sulfinpyrazone. Clin Pharmacol Ther **33:** 491, 1983
36. Crutchley DJ, Ryan US, Ryan JW: Effects of aspirin and dipyridamole on the degradation of ADP by cultured cells derived from bovine pulmonary artery. J Clin Invest **68:** 29, 1980
37. Emmons PR, Harrison MJG, Honour AJ, Mitchell JRA: Effect of dipyridamole on human platelet behavior. Lancet **2:** 803, 1965
38. Niewiarowski S, Lukasienicz H, Nrapendra N, Tai Sha A: Inhibition of human platelet aggregation by dipyridamole and its modification by acid glycoproteins of human plasma. J Lab Clin Med **86:** 64, 1975
39. Cucuianu MP, Nishizawa E, Mustard JF: Effect of pyrimido-pyrimidine compounds on platelet function. J Lab Clin Med **77:** 958, 1971
40. Summers A, Subbarao K, Rucinski B, Niewiarowski S: The effect of dipyridamole on adenosine uptake by platelets *ex vivo*. Thromb Res **11:** 611, 1977
41. Pedersen AK: Dipyridamole and platelet aggregation. Lancet **2:** 270, 1978
42. Vigdahl RL, Mongin J, Marquis NR: Platelet aggregation. IV.

Platelet phosphodiesterase and its inhibiton by vasodilators. Biochem Biophys Res Commun **42:** 1088, 1971
43. Best LC, Mcguire MB, Jones PBB, Holland TK, Martin TJ, Preston FE, Segal DS, Russel RG: Mode of action of dipyridamole on human platelets. Thromb Res **16:** 367, 1979
44. Moncada S, Korbut R: Dipyridamole and other phosphodiesterase inhibitors act as antithrombotic agents by poteniating endogenous prostacyclin. Lancet **1:** 1286, 1978
45. FitzGerald GA, Brash AR, Falardeau P, Oates JA: Estimated rate of prostacyclin secretion into the circulation of normal man. J Clin Invest **68:** 1271, 1981
46. Blair IA, Barrow SE, Wadell KA, Lewis PJ, Dollery CT: Prostacyclin is not a circulating hormone in man. Prostaglandins **23:** 579, 1982
47. Pickles H, Fish A, Hasan S, Burke C, Warrington S, O'Grady J: Effects of intravenous epoprostenol on platelets and the cardiovascular system are not potentiatead by dipyridamole. Clin Pharmacol Ther **33:** 178, 1982
48. Neri Serneri G, Masotti G, Poggesi L, Galanti G, Morettini A: Enhanced prostacyclin production by dipyridamole in man. Eur J Clin Pharmacol **21:** 9, 1981
49. Harker LA, Slichter SJ: Platelet and fibrinogen consumption in man. N Engl J Med **297:** 999, 1972
50. Harker LA, Slichter SJ: Studies in platelet and fibrinogen kinetics in patients with prosthetic heart valves. N Engl J Med **283:** 1302, 1970
51. Harker LA, Hanson SR: Experimental arterial thromboembolism in baboon: mechanism, quantitation and pharmacological prevention. J Clin Invest **64:** 559, 1979
52. The Persantine Aspirin Reinfarction Study Research Group: Persantine and aspirin in coronary heart disease. Circulation **62:** 449, 1980
53. Sullivan JM, Harken DE, Gorlin R: Pharmacological control of thromboembolic complications of cardiac-valve replacement: N Engl J Med **284:** 1391, 1971
54. Chesebro JH, Clements IP, Fuster V, Elveback LR, Smith HC, Bardsley WT, Frye RL, Holmes DR Jr, Vlietstra RE, Pluth JR, Wallace RB, Puga FJ, Orszulak TA, Piehler JM, Schaff HV, Danielson GK: A platelet inhibitor drug trial in coronary-artery bypass operations. N Engl J Med **307:** 73, 1982
55. Burns JJ, Yu TF, Ritterband A, Perel JM, Gutman A, Brodie BB: A new potent uricosuric agent, the sulfoxide metabolite of the phenylbutazone analogue CG 25671. J Pharmacol Exp Ther **119:** 418, 1957
56. Smythe HA, Ogryzlo MA, Murphy EA, Mustard JF: The effect of sulfinpyrazone on platelet economy in man. Can Med Assoc J **92:** 818, 1965
57. Butler KD, Pay GF, Roberts JM, White AM: The effect of sulfinpyrazone and other drugs on the platelet response during the acute phase of the active Arthus reaction in the guinea pig. Thromb Res **15:** 319, 1979
58. Butler KD, Smith JR: Mechanisms of Forssman-induced bronchospasm and their inhibition. Br J Pharmacol **73:** 25, 1981
59. The Anturane Reinfarction Trial Research Group: Sulfinpyrazone in the prevention of sudden death after myocardial infarction. N Engl J Med **302:** 250, 1980
60. The Anturane Reinfarction Trial Policy Committee: The Anturane Reinfarction Trial: reevaluation of the outcome. N Engl J Med **306:** 1005, 1982
61. The Anturane Reinfarction Italian Study Group: Sulpinpyrazone in postmyocardial infarction. Lancet **1:** 237, 1982
62. Kelton JG: Antiplatelet agents: rationale and results. Clin Haematol **12:** 311, 1983
63. Alridge A, Johnson GE: Excretion of sulfinpyrazone in the rat. Can J Physiol Pharmacol **50:** 1061, 1972
64. Pedersen AK, Jakobsen P, Kampmann JP, Hansen JM: Clinical pharmacokinetics and potentially important drug interactions of sulfinpyrazone. Clin Pharmacokin **7:** 42, 1982
65. Jakobsen P, Pedersen AK: Simultaneous determination of sulfinpyrazone and four of its metabolites by high-performance liquid chromatography. J Chromatogr **223:** 460, 1981
66. Pedersen AK, FitzGerald GA: Cyclooxygenase inhibiton, platelet function and drug metabolite formation during chronic administration of sulfinpyrazone in man. Clin Pharmacol Ther **37:** 36, 1985
67. Rosenkranz B, Fischer C, Jakobsen P, Pedersen AK, Frohlich JC: Plasma levels of sulfinpyrazone and two of its metabolites after a single dose and during steady-state. Eur J Clin Pharmacol **24:** 231, 1983
68. Bradbrook ID, John VA, Morrison PJ, Rogers HJ, Spector RG: Pharmacokinetics of single doses of sulfinpyrazone and its major metabolites in plasma and urine. Br J Clin Pharmacol **13:** 177, 1982
69. Schlicht F, Staiger C, Vries J, Gundert-Remy V, Hildebrandt R, Harenberg J, Wang JS, Weber E: Pharmacokinetics of sulfinpyrazone and its major metabolites after a single dose and during chronic treatment. Eur J Clin Pharmacol **28:** 97, 1985
70. Jakobsen P, Pedersen AK, Andreassen FA: Binding of sulfinpyrazone and its metabolites in human serum and in solutions of human serum albumin. Acta Pharmacol Toxicol **51:** 243, 1982
71. Dieterle W, Faigle JW, Mory H, Richter W, Theobald W: Biotransformation and pharmacokinetics of sulfinpyrazone in man. Eur J Clin Pharmacol **9:** 135, 1975
72. Dieterle W, Faigle JW, Moppert J: New metabolites of sulfinpyrazone in man. Arzneimittelforschung **30:** 989, 1980
73. Pedersen AK, Jakobsen P: Two new metabolites of sulfinpyrazone in the rabbit: a possible cause of prolonged *in vivo* effect. Thromb Res **16:** 871, 1979
74. Pedersen AK, Jakobsen P: Sulfinpyrazone metabolism during long term therapy. Br J Clin Pharmacol **11:** 597, 1981
75. Duggan DE, Hare LE, Dizler CA, Lei BW, Kwan KC: The disposition of sulindac. Clin Pharmacol Ther **21:** 326, 1977
76. Renwick AG, Evans SP, Sweatman TW, Cumberland J, George CF: The role of gut flora in the reduction of sulfinpyrazone in the rat. Biochem Pharmacol **31:** 2649, 1982
77. Packham MA, Warrior ES, Glynn MF, Senyi AS, Mustard JF: Alteration of the response of platelets to surface stimuli by pyrazole compounds. J Exp Med **126:** 171, 1967
78. Ali M, McDonald JWD: Effects of sulfinpyrazone on platelet prostaglandin synthesis and platelet release of serotonin. J Lab Clin Med **89:** 868, 1977
79. McDonald JWD, Ali M, Cerskus AL: Effects of sulfinpyrazone on synthesis of prostaglandins and thromboxanes by platelets *in vitro* and *in vivo*. *In* McGregor M, Mustard JF, Oliver MF, Sherry S, editors: Cardiovascular actions of sulfinpyrazone — basic and clinical research. Miami, 1980, Symposia Specialists, Inc., p 37
80. Margulies EH, White AM, Sherry S: Sulfinpyrazone: a review of its pharmacological properties and therapeutic use. Drugs **20:** 179, 1980
81. Wiley JS, Chesterman CN, Morgan F, Castaldi PA: The effects of sulfinpyrazone on the aggregation and release reactions of human platelets. Thromb Res **15:** 181, 1979
82. Wallis RB: Mechanisms of actions of sulfinpyrazone. Thromb Res **S-IV:** 31, 1983
83. Buchanan MR, Rosenfeld J, Hirsh J: The prolonged effect of sulfinpyrazone in collagen-induced platelet aggregation *in vivo*. Thromb Res **13:** 883, 1979
84. Butler KD, Wallis RB, White AM: A study of the relationship between *ex vivo* and *in vivo* effects of sulfinpyrazone in the guinea pig. Haemostasis **8:** 353, 1979
85. Gordon JL, Pearson JD: Effects of sulfinpyrazone and aspirin on PGI_2 synthesis by endothelial cells. Br J Pharmacol **64:** 481, 1978
86. Chignard M, Wal F, Lefort J, Vargaftig BB: Inhibition by sulfinpyrazone of the platelet-dependent bronchoconstriction due to platelet activating factor (PAF-acether) in guinea pigs. Eur J Pharmacol **78:** 71, 1982
87. Steele P, Carrol J, Overfield D, Genton E: Effect of sulfinpyrazone on platelet survival time in patients with transient cerebral ischemic attacks. Stroke **8:** 398, 1977
88. Steele P, Weily HS, Davies H, Genton E: Platelet survival in patients with rheumatic heart disease. N Engl J Med **290:** 537, 1974
89. Harker LA, Wall RI, Harlan JM, Ross R: Sulfinpyrazone prevention of homocysteine-induced endothelial cell injury and atherosclerosis. Clin Res **26:** 554 A, 1978
90. Kaegi A, Pineo GF, Shimuzu A, Trivedi H, Hirsh J, Gent M: Arterio-venous shunt thrombosis: prevention by sulfinpyrazone. N Engl J Med **290:** 304, 1974
91. Walter E, Hodok-Laibach P, Zimmermann R, Weber E: Action

and interaction of sulfinpyrazone in anticoagulated patients. Thromb Haemost **42:** 62, 1979
92. Hamberg M, Svensson J, Samuelsson B: Thromboxanes: a new group of biologically-active compounds derived from prostaglandin endoperoxides: Proc Natl Acad Sci USA **72:** 2994, 1975
93. Moncada S, Gryglewski RJ, Bunting S, Vane JR: An enzyme isolated from arteries transforms prostaglandin endoperoxides to an unstable substance that inhibits platelet aggregation. Nature **263:** 663, 1976
94. Moncada S, Vane JR: Unstable metabolites of arachidonic acid and their role in haemostasis and thrombosis. Br Med Bull **34:** 129, 1979
95. Marcus AJ, Weksler BB, Jaffe EA, Broekman MJ: Synthesis of prostacyclin from platelet-derived endoperoxides by cultured human endothelial cells. J Clin Invest **66:** 979, 1980
96. Hamberg M, Svensson J, Wakabayashi T, Samuelsson B: Isolation and structure of two prostaglandin endoperoxides that cause platelet aggregation. Proc Natl Acad Sci USA **71:** 345, 1974
97. Vermylen J, Defreyn G, Carreas L, Machin S, Van Schaeren J, Verstraete M: Thromboxane synthetase inhibition as an antithrombotic strategy. Lancet **1:** 1073, 1981
98. Tyler HM, Saxton CA, Parry MJ: Administration to man of UK-37248-01, a selective inhibitor of thromboxane synthetase. Lancet **1:** 629, 1981
99. FitzGerald GA, Oates JA: Selective and nonselective inhibition of thromboxane formation. Clin Pharmacol Ther **35:** 633, 1984
100. McNab MW, Foltz EL, Graves BS, Rinehart RK, Tripp SL, Feliciano NR, Sen S: The effects of a new thromboxane synthetase inhibitor, CGS-13080 in man. J Clin Pharmacol **24:** 76, 1984
101. FitzGerald GA, Brash AR, Oates JA, Pedersen AK: Endogenous prostacyclin biosynthesis and platelet function during selective inhibition of thromboxane synthase in man. J Clin Invest **71:** 1336, 1983
102. FitzGerald GA, Reilly IAG, Pedersen AK: The biochemical pharmacology of thromboxane synthase inhibition in man. Circulation **72:** 1194, 1985
103. Bertele V, Cerletti C, Schiepatti A, Di Minno G, de Gaetano G: Inhibition of thromboxane synthetase does not necessarily prevent platelet aggregation. Lancet **1:** 1057, 1981
104. Defreyn G, Deckmyn H, Vermylen J: A thromboxane synthetase inhibitor reorients endoperoxide metabolism in whole blood towards prostacyclin and PGE_2. Thromb Res **26:** 389, 1982
105. Parry MJ: Effects of thromboxane synthetase inhibition on arachidonate metabolism and platelet behavior. Br J Clin Pharmacol **15:** 23-S, 1983
106. Pedersen AK, Watson ML, FitzGerald GA: Inhibition of thromboxane biosynthesis in serum: limitations of the measurement of immunoreactive 6-keto-$PGF_{1\alpha}$.
107. Reilly IAG, Doran J, Smith B, FitzGerald GA: Continued platelet activation in severe atherosclerosis despite chronic administration of a thromboxane synthase inhibitor. Circ Res **33:** 287A, 1985 (abst)
108. Lewis P, Tyler HM: Clinical prospects for a thromboxane synthetase inhibitor. Br J Clin Pharmacol **15:** S-1, 1983
109. Harris PA, Riegelman S: Acetylsalicylic acid hydrolysis in human blood and plasma. I. Methodology and *in vitro* studies. J Pharmacol Sci **59:** 713, 1967
110. Rowland M, Riegelman S: Determination of acetylsalicylic acid and salicylic acid in plasma. J Pharmacol Sci **56:** 717, 1968
111. Walter LJ, Biggs DF, Coutts RT: Simultaneous GLC estimation of salicylic acid and aspirin in plasma. J Pharmacl Sci **63:** 1754, 1974
112. Rainsford KD: Aspirin and the salicylates. London, 1984, Butterworths, p 32
113. Trinder P: Rapid determination of salicylate in biological fluids. Biochem J **57:** 301, 1954
114. Peng GW, Gadella AF, Smith V, Peng A, Chiou WL: Simple and rapid high-pressure liquid chromatographic simultaneous determination of aspirin, salicylic acid and salicyluric acid in plasma. J Pharmacol Sci **67:** 710, 1978
115. Dawson I, Pryse-Davies J: The distribution of certain enzyme systems in the normal gastrointestinal tract. Gastroenteroloy **44:** 745, 1968
116. Pedersen AK, FitzGerald GA: Dose-related kinetics of aspirin: presystemic acetylation of platelet cyclooxygenase. N Engl J Med **311:** 1206, 1984
117. Rowland M, Riegelman S: Pharmacokinetics of acetylsalicylic acid and salicylic acid after intravenous administration in man. J Pharmacol Sci **57:** 1313, 1968
118. Harris PA, Riegelman S: Influence of the route of administration on the area under the plasma concentration-time curve. J Pharmacol Sci **59:** 71, 1969
119. Levy G, Angelino NJ: Hydrolysis of aspirin by rat small intestine. J Pharmacol Sci **57:** 1449, 1968
120. Rowland M, Riegelman S, Harris PA, Sholokoff SD: Absorption kinetics of aspirin in man following oral administration of an aqueous solution. J Pharmacol Sci **61:** 379, 1972
121. Koch PA, Schultz CA, Willis AJ, Hallquist SL, Welling PG: Influence of food and fluid ingestion on aspirin bioavailability. J Pharmacol Sci **67:** 1533, 1978
122. Thiessen JJ: Aspirin: plasma concentration and effects. Thromb Res **S-IV:** 105, 1983
123. Levy G: Clinical pharmacology of salicylates: a reassessment. Br J Clin Pharmacol **10,S-1:** 285, 1980
124. Levy G, Tsuchiya T: Salicylate accumulation kinetics in man. N Engl J Med **297:** 430, 1972
125. Roth GJ, Stanford N, Majerus PW: Acetylation of prostaglandin synthetase by aspirin. Proc Natl Acad Sci USA **72:** 3075, 1975
126. Stuart MJ, Murphy S, Oski FA: A simple non-radioisotopic technique for the determination of platelet lifespan. N Engl J Med **292:** 1310, 1975
127. Burch JW, Stanford N, Majerus PW: Inhibition of platelet prostaglandin synthetase by oral aspirin. J Clin Invest **61:** 314, 1978
128. Preston FE, Whipps S, Jackson C, French A, Wyld P, Stoddard J: Inhibition of prostacyclin and platelet thromboxane A_2 after low-dose aspirin. N Engl J Med **304:** 76, 1981
129. Hanley SP, Bevan J, Cockbill SR, Heptinstall S: Differential inhibition by low-dose aspirin of human venous prostacyclin synthesis and platelet thromboxane synthesis. Lancet **1:** 969, 1981
130. Masotti G, Galanti G, Poggessi L, Abbate R, Neri Serneri G: Differential inhibition of prostacyclin production and platelet aggregation by aspirin. Lancet **2:** 1213, 1979
131. Weksler BB, Pett SB, Alonso D, Richter RC, Stelzer P, SubraManian V, Tack-Goldman K, Gay W: Differential inhibition by aspirin of vascular and platelet protaglandin synthesis in atherosclerotic patients. N Engl J Med **308:** 800, 1983
132. Buchanan MR, Rischke JA, Hirsh J: Aspirin inhibits platelet function independent of the acetylation of cyclooxygenase. Thromb Res **25:** 363, 1982
133. deCaterina R, Patrono C: Selective inhibition of thromboxane-related platelet function by low-dose aspirin in patients after myocardial infarction. Am J Cardiol **55:** 589, 1985
134. Baenziger NL, Dillenden MJ, Majerus PW: Cultured human skin fibroblasts and arterial cells produce a labile platelet inhibitory prostaglandin. Biochem Biophys Res Commun **78:** 294, 1977
135. Jaffe EA, Weksler BB: Recovery of endothelial cell prostacyclin production after low doses of aspirin. J Clin Invest **63:** 532, 1979
136. Czervionke RL, Smith JB, Fry GL, Hoak JC: Inhibition of prostacyclin by treatment of endothelium with aspirin. J Clin Invest **63:** 1089, 1979
137. FitzGerald GA, Oates JA, Hawiger J, Maas RL, Roberts LJ II, Lawson JA, Brash AL: Endogenous biosynthesis of prostacyclin and thromboxane and platelet function during chronic administration of aspirin in man. J Clin Invest **71:** 876, 1983
138. Vargaftig BB: The inhibition of cyclooxygenase of rabbit platelets by aspirin is prevented by salicylic acid and by phenanthrolines. Eur J Pharmacol **50:** 231, 1978
139. Cerletti C, Livio M, de Gaetano G: Non-steroidal anti-inflammatory drugs react with two sites on platelet cyclooxygenase. Biochim Biophys Acta **714:** 122, 1982
140. Dejana E, Cerletti C, De Castellarnau C, Livio M, Galletti F, Latini R, de Gaetano G: Evidence that salicylate accumulating during aspirin administration may protect vascular prostacyclin. J Clin Invest **68:** 1108, 1981
141. Kelton JG, Hirsh J, Carter CJ, Buchanan MR: Thrombogenic effect of high-dose aspirin in rabbits: relationship to inhibition of vessel wall synthesis of PGI_{21}-like activity. J Clin Invest **62:** 892, 1978
142. Buchanan MR, Dejana E, Gent M, Mustard JF, Hirsh J: Enhanced

platelet accumulation onto injured rabbit carotid arteries in rabbits after aspirin treatment. J Clin Invest **67:** 503, 1981
143. O'Grady J, Moncada S: Aspirin: a paradoxical effect on bleeding time. Lancet **2:** 780, 1978
144. Dybdahl JH, Daae LNW, Eika C, Godal HC, Larsen S: Acetylsalicylic-induced prolongation of bleeding time in healthy men. Scand J Haematol **26:** 50, 1981
145. Moncada S, Vane JR: Pharmacology and endogenous roles of prostaglandin endoperoxides, thromboxane A_2 and prostacyclin. Pharmacol Rev **30:** 293, 1979
146. Jorgensen KA: Studies on the biological balance between thromboxanes and prostacyclins in relation to the platelet vessel-wall interaction. Danish Med Bull **29:** 169, 1982
147. Villa S, Livio M, de Gaetano G: The inhibitory effect of aspirin on platelet and vascular prostaglandins in rats cannot be completely dissociated. Br J Haematol **42:** 425, 1979
148. FitzGerald GA, Smith B, Pedersen AK, Brash AR: Increased prostacyclin biosynthesis in patients with severe atherosclerosis and platelet activation. N Engl J Med **310:** 1065, 1984
149. Patrono C, Pugliese F, Ciabattoni G, Patrignani P, Maseri A, Chierchia S, Peskar BA, Cinotti GA, Simonetti BM, Pierucci A: Evidence for a direct stimulatory effect of prostacyclin on renin release in man. J Clin Invest **69:** 231, 1982
150. FitzGerald GA, Pedersen AK, Patrono C: Analysis of prostacyclin and thromboxane A_2 biosynthesis in cardiovascular disease. Circulation **67:** 1174, 1983

Clinical pharmacology of platelet cyclooxygenase inhibition

CARLO PATRONO, M.D., GIOVANNI CIABATTONI, M.D., PAOLA PATRIGNANI, D.SCI., FRANCESCO PUGLIESE, M.D., PAOLA FILABOZZI, M.D., FRANCESCA CATELLA, M.D., GIOVANNI DAVÌ, M.D., AND LAURA FORNI, M.D.

ABSTRACT Nonsteroidal anti-inflammatory drugs and sulfinpyrazone compete dose-dependently with arachidonate for binding to platelet cyclooxygenase. Such a process closely follows systemic plasma drug concentrations and is reversible as a function of drug elimination. Peak inhibition and extent of its reversibility at 24 hr varies consistently with individual pharmacokinetic profile. Inhibition of platelet cyclooxygenase activity by these agents is associated with variable effects on prostaglandin (PG) synthesis in the gastric mucosa and the kidney. Aspirin acetylates platelet cyclooxygenase and permanently inhibits thromboxane (TX) A_2 production in a dose-dependent fashion when single doses of 0.1 to 2.0 mg/kg are given. Acetylation of the enzyme by low-dose aspirin is cumulative on repeated dosing. The fractional dose of aspirin necessary to achieve a given level of acetylation by virtue of cumulative effects approximately equals the fractional daily platelet turnover. Serum TXB_2 measurements obtained during long-term dosing with 0.11, 0.22, and 0.44 mg/kg aspirin in four healthy subjects could be fitted by a theoretical model assuming identical acetylation of platelet (irreversible) and megakaryocyte (reversible) cyclooxygenase. For a given dose within this range, both the rate at which cumulative acetylation occurs and its maximal extent largely depend upon the rate of platelet turnover. Continuous administration of low-dose aspirin (20 to 40 mg/day) has no statistically significant effect on urinary excretion of either 6-keto-$PGF_{1\alpha}$ or 2,3-dinor-6-keto-$PGF_{1\alpha}$, i.e., indexes of renal and extrarenal PGI_2 biosynthesis in vivo. Whether a selective sparing of extraplatelet cyclooxygenase activity by low-dose aspirin will result in increased antithrombotic efficacy, fewer toxic reactions, or both remains to be established in prospective clinical trials.
Circulation 72, No. 6, 1177–1184, 1985.

PLATELET CYCLOOXYGENASE or prostaglandin (PG) H synthase (i.e., the enzyme that converts arachidonate released from membrane phospholipids into PG endoperoxides) is the target of several antiplatelet agents that can reversibly or irreversibly block the activity of the enzyme by competing with the substrate or permanently altering the active site, respectively.[1] Such drugs belong to the class of so-called nonsteroidal anti-inflammatory agents (e.g., indomethacin, aspirin), but also include a uricosuric agent, i.e., sulfinpyrazone. This article will review the available information on platelet cyclooxygenase inhibition, as derived from human studies in health and disease, and present novel findings related to the mechanism of and variables affecting cumulative inhibition of the enzyme by low-dose aspirin.

From the Department of Pharmacology, Catholic University School of Medicine, Rome.

Supported by grants from Consiglio Nazionale delle Ricerche (82.00389.96 and 83.02535.04) and Ministero della Pubblica Istruzione (60/82, 60/83).

Address for correspondence: Dr. Carlo Patrono, Department of Pharmacology, Catholic University School of Medicine, Largo Francesco Vito 1, 00168 Rome, Italy.

Assessment of human platelet cyclooxygenase activity. Platelet PGH synthase levels can be determined with an immunoradiometric assay.[2] However, PGH synthase immunoreactivity is not influenced by inactivation of the enzyme with aspirin.[2] Similarly, a dissociation between platelet PGH synthase concentration and activity has been shown in uremic patients.[3] Also, the enzyme can be measured by its ability to interact selectively with (acetyl-^{3}H) aspirin and undergo a site-specific acetylation reaction, giving rise to (acetyl-^{3}H) PGH synthase.[4] Inactivation of platelet cyclooxygenase by aspirin in vivo can be measured as a reduction in the ability of (acetyl-^{3}H) aspirin to acetylate the enzyme in washed platelets in vitro.[5]

In the vast majority of studies assessing pharmacologic inhibition of platelet cyclooxygenase enzyme activity was measured ex vivo by quantitative analysis of the main product(s). These analyses may include measurement of (1) thromboxane (TX) A_2–like biological activity released by exogenous arachidonate in platelet-rich plasma (PRP),[6] (2) malondialdehyde (MDA) production in PRP stimulated with *N*-ethyl-maleimide,[7] and (3) TXB_2 production in whole blood,[8] agonist-stimulated PRP,[9, 10] or bleeding-time blood.[11] The latter have gained wider acceptance as indicators of platelet inhibition because of the more accurate and specific determination of TXB_2 by radioimmunoassay (RIA) or gas chromatography/mass spectrometry (GC/MS). These methods assess the capacity of platelets to synthesize TXB_2 in response to native or exogenously added stimuli and by no means reflect the actual production rate of TXB_2 in vivo.[12] Such platelet-specific indexes can be used appropriately in pharmacologic studies in which drug-induced changes in cyclooxygenase or TX synthase are being investigated.

In our studies, we have used serum TXB_2 determinations as a reflection of thrombin-induced platelet TXA_2 production during whole blood clotting.[8] Serum levels of this eicosanoid averaged 300 ± 108 ng/ml (mean ± SD) in a group of 177 healthy subjects, with no statistically significant differences between men and women.[13] In this study, no statistically significant correlation was found between serum TXB_2 and any of the continuous variables examined (age, body mass index, blood pressure, cigarette smoking, and serum cholesterol, triglyceride, and glucose) except for the number of platelets. Upon repeated blood sampling on successive days in healthy subjects, the intrasubject variability in serum TXB_2 determinations averaged 14 ± 5%,[14] a value allowing accurate determination of marginal inhibition of enzyme activity. Consistent results have been reported from different laboratories, whether serum TXB_2 was measured by RIA[14–16] or GC/MS.[17]

The dinor metabolite of TXB_2 is the most abundant urinary derivative of systemically administered radioactive TXB_2 in man,[18] and it largely reflects systemic (extrarenal) TXB_2 synthesis in vivo.[12] The relative contribution of platelet and extraplatelet sources to urinary 2,3-dinor-TXB_2 remains to be determined under pathophysiologic conditions. The finding that daily dosing with 20 mg aspirin can reduce urinary 2,3-dinor-TXB_2 excretion by 67% in healthy subjects[9] suggests that it may represent primarily platelet TXB_2 production under physiologic conditions.

Reversible inhibition of platelet cyclooxygenase. Nonsteroidal anti-inflammatory drugs (with the exception of aspirin) and sulfinpyrazone compete dose dependently with arachidonate for binding to cyclooxygenase. Such a process closely follows systemic plasma drug concentrations and is reversible as a function of drug elinination. The extent and duration of inhibition of human platelet cyclooxygenase activity after a single dose of each of several of the currently available nonsteroidal anti-inflammatory drugs is detailed in table 1. Peak inhibition and extent of its reversibility at 24 hr varied consistently with individual pharmacokinetic profile.

TABLE 1

Reversible inhibition of platelet cyclooxygenase activity (as reflected by serum TXB_2 levels) by single oral doses of nonsteroidal anti-inflammatory drugs in humans (n = 5 for each drug)

Drug	Dose (mg)	Percentage of initial enzyme activity		
		At 1 hr	At 3 hr	At 24 hr
Indomethacin	75	2±2	2±1	50±23
Diflunisal	750	46±20	35±17	65±21
Naproxen	250	11±3	12±3	22±12
Diclofenac	50	19±7	34±6	57±3
Sulindac	200	38±16	22±2	62±33
Piroxicam	20	68±22	41±16	27±18
Ibuprofen	300	33±14	12±4	59±39

Values are mean ± SD.

Upon repeated dosing, no evidence of cumulative inhibition of platelet cyclooxygenase activity was found with ibuprofen or sulindac in patients with chronic glomerular disease.[19] Thus, 85% reduction of platelet TXB_2 production was measured after 1 week of treatment with 200 mg bid sulindac.[19]

With the notable exception of indomethacin, it appears that none of these inhibitors with reversible effects can achieve and sustain greater than 95% inhibition of platelet enzyme activity. Inasmuch as virtually complete and long-lasting suppression of TXA_2 production may be required for maximal inhibition of platelet function,[9] it appears likely that these and similar agents have limited antiplatelet efficacy.

Similar considerations might apply to partial reversible inhibition of platelet cyclooxygenase activity by sulfinpyrazone. Inhibition of cyclooxygenase activity is dependent on reduction to an active sulfide metabolite.[20] When added to human whole blood in vitro this metabolite inhibits TXB_2 production with 50% inhibitory concentration of 11 μM as compared with the 247 μM of the parent sulfoxide.* When given to healthy volunteers, sulfinpyrazone (200 mg qid) reduced platelet TXB_2 production by 65%, with no evidence of cumulative inhibition over 7 days.[21] This finding is consistent with similar sulfide levels measured after 1 and 5 days of sulfinpyrazone dosing in healthy subjects.[22] The contribution of such limited suppression of platelet cyclooxygenase activity to the reported clinical efficacy of therapy[22a] remains to be established.

Inhibition of platelet cyclooxygenase activity by

*Patrono C, et al: Unpublished results.

these agents is associated with variable effects on PG synthesis in the gastric mucosa and the kidney.[23] Such a differential pattern of inhibition may account for the diverse incidence of gastric and renal side effects associated with long-term use of cyclooxygenase inhibitors. One clear example of tissue-selective inhibition of cyclooxygenase activity is provided by sulindac and sulfinpyrazone. We have previously shown that sulindac does not inhibit renal PG synthesis in man.[19] This property is probably related to reoxidation of the active sulfide metabolite to its prodrug form within the kidney.[24] Sulindac and sulfinpyrazone share the following pharmacokinetic and pharmacodynamic features: (1) the major biotransformations involve valence changes at the sulfur atom, (2) inhibition of cyclooxygenase activity is dependent on reduction to an active sulfide metabolite, and (3) the sulfide metabolite is not detected in urine after oral dosing of the prodrug. Sulfinpyrazone, similar to sulindac, does not inhibit renal cyclooxygenase activity when given to healthy subjects at a dosage (200 mg qid for 7 days) that significantly reduces platelet TXB_2 production[21] and urinary 2,3-dinor-6-keto-$PGF_{1\alpha}$ excretion,[22] i.e., that reducing cyclooxygenase activity at platelet and vascular sites.[12] The finding of a selective sparing of renal cyclooxygenase activity by sulfinpyrazone is consistent with the absence of short-term effects on glomerular filtration rate both in healthy subjects[25] and patients with myocardial infarction.[26]

Irreversible inactivation of platelet cyclooxygenase. Aspirin selectively acetylates the hydroxyl group of a single serine residue within the polypeptide chain of PGH_2 synthase, thereby inactivating the enzyme.[27, 28] The serine side chain is probably located near the active site of the enzyme. As a consequence of this acetylation, the cyclooxygenase activity (arachidonate $\rightarrow$ PGG_2) of the enzyme is lost, while the peroxidase activity ($PGG_2 \rightarrow PGH_2$) is unaffected. The stoichiometry of this reaction is 1:1, with one acetyl group transferred per enzyme monomer (M_r = 70,000).[27, 28] At low concentrations, aspirin acetylates PGH_2 synthase rapidly (within minutes) and selectively. At high concentrations, over longer time periods, aspirin will also acetylate nonspecifically a variety of proteins and nucleic acids.[4] When given orally to healthy subjects, aspirin acetylates circulating platelet cyclooxygenase[5] and inhibits TXB_2 production[14] in a dose- and time-dependent fashion. A linear inhibition of platelet cyclooxygenase activity was found after a single dose in the range of 0.1 to 2 mg/kg.[14] Moreover, such a dose-response relationship is substantially identical in healthy subjects[14] and in patients with atherosclerosis[15] when assessed by the same technique of determination of TXB_2 production ex vivo in whole blood. No sex-related difference in the effect of aspirin was noted in these studies.

Evidence has been presented that the return of cyclooxygenase activity after a single dose (100 to 400 mg) of aspirin does not occur for approximately 48 hr.[5, 8] The 2 day lag in the return of unacetylated enzyme to the circulation has been interpreted as evidence that aspirin acetylates cyclooxygenase in the megakaryocyte.[5] However, platelet aggregation and secretion have been reported to occur as early as 4 hr after ingestion of aspirin (650 mg) in response to a combination of arachidonate with epinephrine, collagen, or ADP.[10] This finding may suggest the early entry into the circulation of platelets originating from megakaryocytes in which cyclooxygenase has not been completely acetylated.[10] It should be pointed out that the functional significance of a small percentage of aspirin-free platelets may be greatly enhanced by the performance of platelet aggregation studies in vitro, under conditions in which both removal (by flow) and metabolism (by lung and liver enzymes) of TXA_2 are absent.

Because of irreversible enzyme inactivation and lack of enzyme synthesis in platelets de novo, acetylation of platelet cyclooxygenase and consequent inhibition of TXA_2 production by low-dose (20 to 40 mg) aspirin is cumulative on repeated dosing.[5, 14] To investigate the variables affecting the rate and maximal degree of cumulative inhibition, we studied seven healthy subjects (four men and three women 23 to 38 yr old) receiving short- and/or long-term therapy with oral aspirin, 5 to 40 mg. As shown in figure 1, a single oral 20 mg dose of aspirin caused a time-dependent reduction in serum TXB_2 levels. Serum TXB_2 was significantly reduced to 82% of the control value, as early as 5 min after dosing. Inasmuch as no acetylsalicylic acid can be detected in peripheral venous blood at this time, acetylation of cyclooxygenase during the first 5 min may occur by exposure of platelets to the drug in the presystemic circulation.[29]

Serum TXB_2 reached a 52% nadir at between 30 and 60 min and remained stable thereafter up to 24 hr. Upon repeated daily dosing with 20 mg aspirin, each dose caused a time-dependent reduction in serum TXB_2 that reached a nadir at 60 min and persisted after 24 hr (data not shown). This pattern is consistent with acetylation of megakaryocyte cyclooxygenase by low-dose aspirin. Serum TXB_2 was reduced to 46% of the control value after the first dose, to 27% after the second dose, and to 11% after the third dose. Platelet

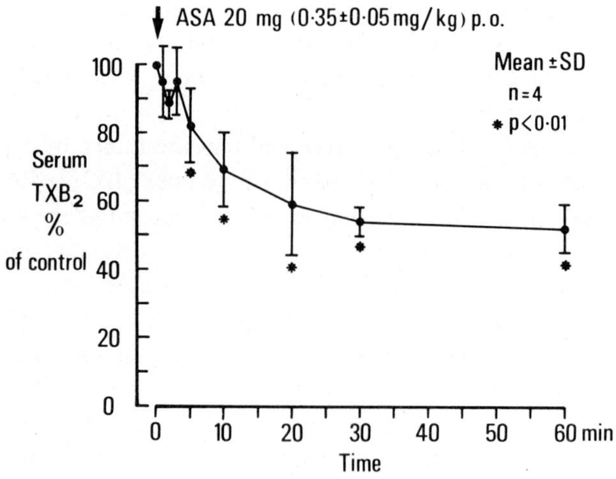

FIGURE 1. Time course of aspirin-induced inhibition of platelet TXB_2 production. Mean ($\pm$ SD) serum TXB_2 level, expressed as percentage of control, is plotted as a function of time after the oral administration of 20 mg aspirin to four healthy volunteers. The asterisk denotes statistically significant ($p < .01$) changes from the predosing level, as assessed by analysis of variance.

cyclooxygenase activity, as reflected by TXB_2 generation in serum measured after daily administration of 20 mg aspirin for 3 days, is illustrated in figure 2 as a percentage of basal activity before drug in the same subject. Serum TXB_2 was reduced to 46% of control 60 min after the first dose, to 53% after the second dose, and to 43% after the third dose, with a similar time course. Given a 14% intrasubject coefficient of variation in serum TXB_2 determinations in our laboratory,[14] the data presented in figure 2 demonstrate induction of a virtually identical acetylation process of platelet cyclooxygenase by successive doses of aspirin, irrespective of the initial level of acetylation of the enzyme.

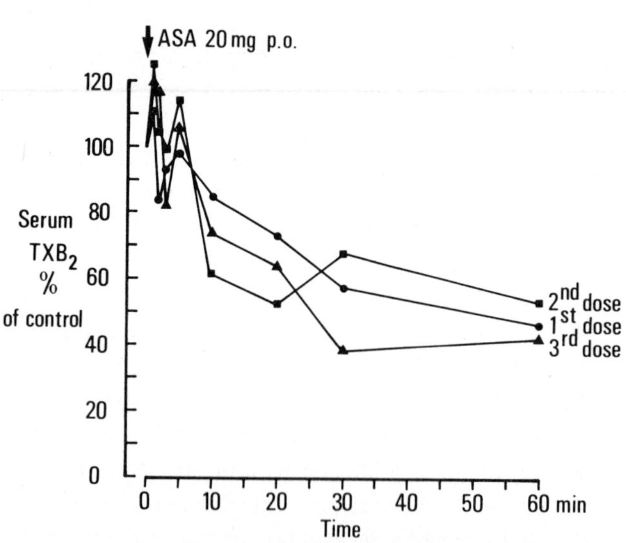

FIGURE 2. Time course of aspirin-induced inhibition of platelet TXB_2 production on repeated dosing. Platelet cyclooxygenase activity, as reflected by TXB_2 generation in serum, was measured before and after daily administration of 20 mg aspirin for 3 days in the same subject. Values are expressed as percentage of basal activity before each dose. The three symbols denote the three consecutive studies.

To study the time and dose dependence of cumulative inhibition, four healthy subjects received aspirin in daily doses of 0.44, 0.22, and 0.11 mg/kg on separate occasions. Each dose was given for 1 month and serum TXB_2 was measured before, during, and for 2 weeks after aspirin was given. Daily dosing with 5 to 10 mg aspirin (0.11 $\pm$ 0.02 mg/kg, mean $\pm$ SD; n = 4) caused a maximal inhibition of cyclooxygenase activity of 56% to 76% within 18 to 30 days. Daily dosing in the same subjects with 10 to 20 mg (0.22 $\pm$ 0.03 mg/kg) caused a maximal inhibition of 68% to 90% within 10 to 20 days. Daily dosing with 20 to 40 mg (0.44 $\pm$ 0.06 mg/kg) caused a maximal inhibition of 92% to 95% within 6 to 12 days. As shown in figure 3, a linear relationship exists between the oral aspirin dose and the percentage inhibition of platelet TXB_2 production, both after single and daily dosing. The 50% inhibitory dose for one-time dosing was 26 mg, while that for repeated dosing (measured at steady-state) was 3.2 mg, or only 12.5% of the former.

This finding suggests that the fractional dose of aspirin necessary for achieving a given level of acetylation by virtue of cumulative effects approximately equals the fractional daily platelet turnover (10% to 15%). Such an interpretation is further supported by an experiment in which virtually complete suppression of platelet TXB_2 production was achieved by a single dose of 4 mg/kg and maintained over 5 weeks by daily dosing with 11% of this dose (0.44 mg/kg; data not shown). The inverse linear relationship (r = −.92, n

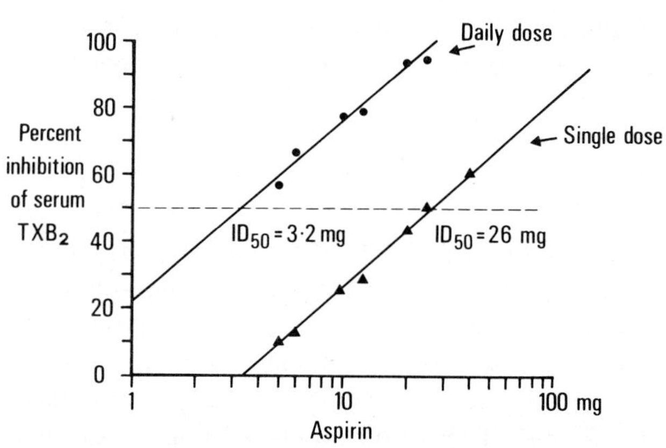

FIGURE 3. Dose dependence of the inhibition of platelet TXB_2 production by aspirin. Serum TXB_2 was measured before and after single (▲) or daily (●) dosing with aspirin in four healthy subjects. Individual data are expressed as percent inhibition, with each subject serving as his or her own control. Daily dosing values represent measurements obtained at steady-state inhibition. ID_{50} = 50% inhibitory dose.

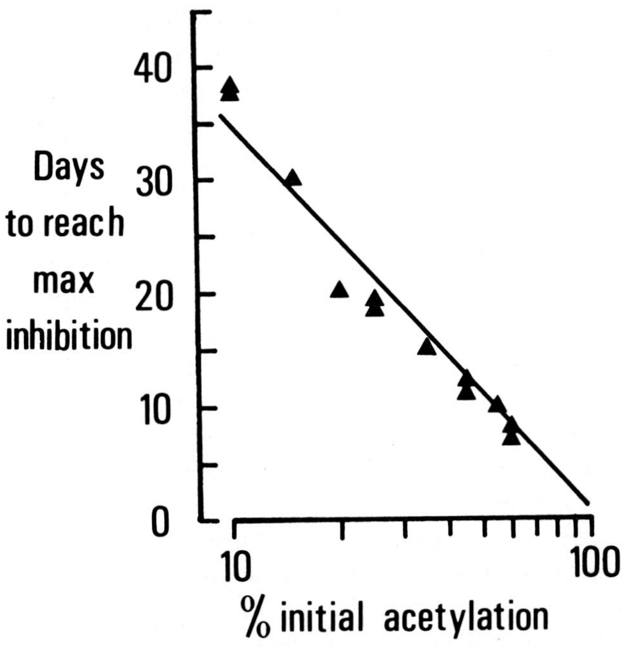

FIGURE 4. Relationship between the time interval necessary to achieve steady-state inhibition with long-term dosing, and percentage inactivation of platelet cyclooxygenase after first dosing with aspirin. Individual data from 12 experiments are plotted. Each of four healthy subjects underwent daily treatment for 1 month with three different doses in the range of 5 to 40 mg. Serum TXB_2 was measured as a reflection of platelet cyclooxygenase activity.

= 12, $p < .001$) between the time interval necessary to achieve steady inhibition with long-term dosing and percentage inactivation of platelet cyclooxygenase after the first dose is shown in figure 4. Each set of experimental data could be fitted by a theoretical model assuming that (1) aspirin acetylates platelet as well as megakaryocyte cyclooxygenase, (2) the two enzymes are equally sensitive to aspirin, (3) synthesis of the enzyme de novo occurs within 24 hr in megakaryocytes but not in platelets, and (4) platelets with acetylated and those with unacetylated cyclooxygenase have a similar life span. As shown in figure 5, which illustrates results of three monthly experiments performed in the same subject, the computer-simulated pattern of inhibition closely matched the experimental data obtained at three dose levels. As an average, the two sets of data (computer-generated vs actual measurements of serum TXB_2) did not differ from each other by a greater interval than the intrasubject coefficient of variation for the method.

In view of the above findings and of recent studies of Pedersen and FitzGerald[29] demonstrating unchanged systemic bioavailability of aspirin in doses of 20 to 1300 mg and presystemic acetylation of platelet cyclooxygenase by low doses (20 to 40 mg) of the drug, it

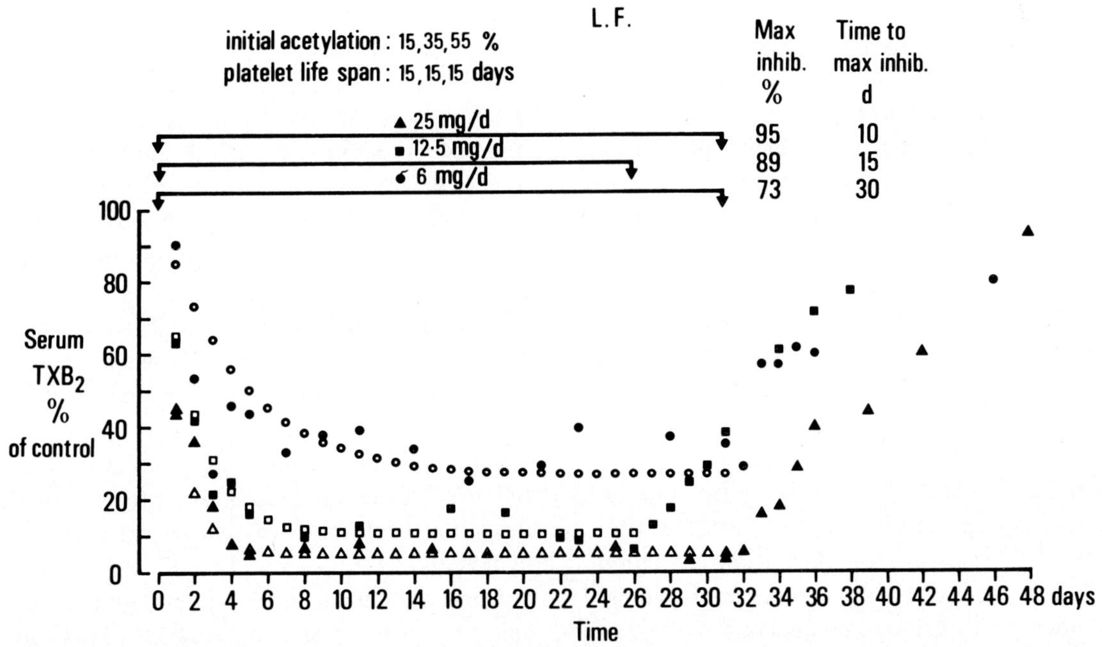

FIGURE 5. Time course of platelet cyclooxygenase inactivation and reappearance as a function of aspirin dosage. Results of three monthly experiments performed in the same healthy subject are depicted. Serum TXB_2 was measured as a reflection of platelet cyclooxygenase activity before, during, and after dosing with 6 (●), 12.5 (■), and 25 (▲) mg/day. The open symbols represent computer-simulated daily levels of enzyme activity. The best fit of experimental data was provided by a combination of 15%, 35%, and 55% initial acetylation (after first dosing) at 6, 12.5, and 25 mg, respectively, and a platelet life span of 15 days. Percentage maximal inactivation and time interval necessary to achieve steady-state inhibition of platelet cyclooxygenase, as obtained by computer simulation, is also indicated.

appears likely that platelet life span represents a major variable affecting cumulative inhibition within this particular dose range. For a given dose, both the rate at which cumulative acetylation occurs and its maximal extent would essentially depend on the rate of platelet turnover and dosing interval.

Although the long-lasting suppression of TXA_2-related platelet function by aspirin has been disputed on the basis of studies using pairs of aggregating agents,[10] the likely occurrence of this phenomenon in vivo is suggested by the positive results (>50% reduction in thrombotic events) of three clinical trials of once-daily dosing: a study of 160 mg in patients on hemodialysis,[30] one of 324 mg in men with unstable angina,[31] and one of 100 mg in patients with aortocoronary bypass.[32] These results are consistent with the hypothesis that the antithrombotic effect of aspirin is largely or entirely related to irreversible inactivation of platelet cyclooxygenase and consequent suppression of TXA_2-related platelet function. Further support for this contention derives from recent studies of Steele et al.[33] demonstrating that low-dose aspirin (1 mg/kg/day) is as effective as high-dose aspirin (20 mg/kg/day) combined with dipyridamole in preventing platelet deposition and mural thrombus formation after arterial balloon angioplasty in pigs. Although mechanisms other than acetylation of platelet cyclooxygenase may be operative after doses of aspirin of 10 to 20 mg/kg, the likelihood of this occurring at doses 10 to 20 times lower is limited by the stoichiometry of the acetylation reaction[4] and its dose dependence in vivo.[5, 14]

Is low-dose aspirin a selective inhibitor of platelet cyclooxygenase? Dissociation of the vascular from the platelet inhibiting effects of aspirin has been attempted on the assumption that intact PGI_2 production might enhance the antithrombotic efficacy of the drug. Although probably not serving the role of a circulating antiplatelet hormone, as originally proposed, PGI_2 may still be important in the local modulation of platelet-endothelial interactions, particularly in patients with severe atherosclerosis and platelet activation.[34] Complete separation of platelet-inhibiting from vascular effects of aspirin can not be demonstrated after single doses.[15, 35] However, continuous administration of aspirin in low doses (20 to 40 mg/day) has no statistically significant effects on urinary excretion of either 6-keto-$PGF_{1\alpha}$[14] or 2,3-dinor-6-keto-$PGF_{1\alpha}$,[9] two indexes of renal and extrarenal PGI_2 biosynthesis in vivo.[12] Inasmuch as the cumulative nature of aspirin-induced inhibition of cyclooxygenase activity is a function of the different rates of daily acetylation and turnover of the enzyme (cell turnover or synthesis de novo), careful consideration should be given to the possibility of variable effects of the drug when pathologic processes affect platelet and/or endothelial behavior. Thus, enhanced platelet turnover and/or endothelial damage might decrease the effectiveness and/or selectivity of low doses of aspirin.

De Caterina et al.[36] have reported that in patients recovering from myocardial infarction, low-dose aspirin (0.4 mg/kg/day) persistently inhibits platelet cyclooxygenase activity and TXA_2-dependent platelet function over 1 month of therapy without significantly reducing urinary 6-keto-$PGF_{1\alpha}$ excretion. In contrast, Weksler et al.[37] have reported evidence for a significant cumulative inhibition of vascular PGI_2 synthesis in atherosclerotic patients given 20 mg aspirin daily for 7 days. This study showed that there was a cumulative inhibition of maximal production of PGI_2 ex vivo in vascular tissue, but that synthesis was 50% preserved.[37] This may indicate that sufficient reserve exists, that urinary 6-keto-$PGF_{1\alpha}$ or 2,3-dinor-6-keto-$PGF_{1\alpha}$ might not be depressed, and that sufficient PGI_2 for local modulation of platelet function might persist. The long-term effects of intermittent aspirin regimens[38] have not been explored, although evidence exists that they may effectively abolish platelet TXA_2 production in healthy subjects.[8] On theoretical grounds, it appears that the alleged benefit of giving a single fully effective dose (2 to 3 mg/kg) every 2 or 3 days might be offset by the profound and long-lasting inhibition of vascular PGI_2 production after each dose.[15, 35] An alternative regimen of 40 mg every 48 hr has been proposed recently.[39] However, it does not appear that this regimen offers any appreciable advantage with respect to sparing venous PGI_2 production when compared with the daily administration of the same dose.

Is selective inhibition of platelet cyclooxygenase activity by low-dose aspirin clinically important? The observation that aspirin can exert an antithrombotic effect when given in a dose that largely suppresses vascular PGI_2 production[40] and a critical appraisal of its role in platelet-vessel wall homeostasis[41] have raised skepticism on the clinical relevance of sparing extraplatelet sites of cyclooxygenase activity. To the extent that PGI_2 biosynthesis is enhanced in patients with severe atherosclerosis, possibly as a consequence of platelet interactions with endothelium or other vascular insults,[34] preservation of the capacity of the vessel wall to produce this natural platelet-inhibitory compound would be desirable in the setting of platelet activation in vivo. Moreover, aspirin-induced reduction of PGI_2 production in the gastric mucosa[42] and in glomeruli[43] has been proposed to contribute importantly to gastric and renal side effects, respectively, that are associated with long-term use of the drug at high dosage.

Whether a selective sparing of extraplatelet cyclooxygenase activity by low-dose aspirin will result in increased antithrombotic efficacy, fewer toxic reactions, or both remains to be established in prospective clinical trials.

We gratefully acknowledge the expert editorial assistance of Ms. Angelamaria Zampini and the generous support of the Upjohn Company, through the courtesy of Dr. J. E. Pike, in providing samples of authentic PGs and TXB_2.

References

1. FitzGerald GA, Sherry S: Pharmacology and pharmacokinetics of platelet-active drugs under current clinical investigation. *In* Oates JA, editor: Prostaglandins and the cardiovascular system. New York, 1982, Raven Press, p 107
2. De Witt DL, Day JS, Gauger JA, Smith WL: Monoclonal antibodies against PGH synthase: an immunoradiometric assay for quantitating the enzyme. Methods Enzymol **86:** 229, 1982
3. Remuzzi G, Benigni A, Dodesini P, Schieppati A, Livio M, De Gaetano G, Day JS, Smith WL, Pinca E, Patrignani P, Patrono C: Reduced platelet thromboxane formation in uremia. Evidence for a functional cyclooxygenase defect. J Clin Invest **71:** 762, 1983
4. Roth GJ: Preparation of (acetyl-^{3}H) aspirin and use in quantitating PGH synthase. *In* Lands WEM, Smith WL, editors: Methods in enzymology. New York, 1982, Academic Press, Inc., vol 86, p 392
5. Burch JW, Stanford N, Majerus PW: Inhibition of platelet prostaglandin synthetase by oral aspirin. J Clin Invest **61:** 314, 1978
6. Szczeklik A, Gryglewski RJ, Grodzinska L, Musial J, Serwonska M, Marcinkiewicz E: Platelet aggregability, thromboxane A_2 and malonaldehyde formation following administration of aspirin to man. Thromb Res **15:** 405, 1979
7. Stuart MJ, Murphy S, Oski FA: A simple nonradioisotope technique for the determination of platelet life-span. N Engl J Med **292:** 1310, 1975
8. Patrono C, Ciabattoni G, Pinca E, Pugliese F, Castrucci G, De Salvo A, Satta MA, Peskar BA: Low dose aspirin and inhibition of thromboxane B_2 production in healthy subjects. Thromb Res **17:** 317, 1980
9. FitzGerald GA, Oates JA, Hawiger J, Maas RL, Roberts LJ II, Lawson JA, Brash AR: Endogenous biosynthesis of prostacyclin and thromboxane and platelet function during chronic administration of aspirin in man. J Clin Invest **71:** 676, 1983
10. Di Minno G, Silver MJ, Murphy S: Monitoring the entry of new platelets into the circulation after ingestion of aspirin. Blood **61:** 1081, 1983
11. Thorngren M, Shafi S, Born GVR: Thromboxane A_2 in skin-bleeding-time blood and in clotted venous blood before and after administration of acetylsalicylic acid. Lancet **1:** 1075, 1983
12. FitzGerald GA, Pedersen AK, Patrono C: Analysis of prostacyclin and thromboxane biosynthesis in cardiovascular disease. Circulation **67:** 1174, 1983
13. Alessandrini P, Avogaro P, Bittolo Bon G, Patrignani P, Patrono C: Physiologic variables affecting thromboxane B_2 production in human whole blood. Thromb Res **37:** 1, 1985
14. Patrignani P, Filabozzi P, Patrono C: Selective cumulative inhibition of platelet thromboxane production by low-dose aspirin in healthy subjects. J Clin Invest **69:** 1366, 1982
15. Weksler BB, Pett SB, Alonso D, Richter RC, Stelzer P, Subramanian V, Tack-Goldman K, Gay WA: Differential inhibition by aspirin of vascular and platelet prostaglandin synthesis in atherosclerotic patients. N Engl J Med **308:** 800, 1983
16. Fischer S, Struppler M, Böhlig B, Bernutz C, Wober W, Weber P: The influence of selective thromboxane synthetase inhibition with a novel imidazole derivative, UK-38,485, on prostanoid formation in man. Circulation **68:** 821, 1983
17. Pedersen AK, Watson ML, FitzGerald GA: Inhibition of thromboxane biosynthesis in serum: limitations of the measurement of immunoreactive 6-keto-$PGF_{1\alpha}$. Thromb Res **33:** 99, 1984
18. Roberts LJ II, Sweetman BJ, Oates JA: Metabolism of thromboxane B_2 in man: identification of twenty metabolites. J Biol Chem **256:** 8384, 1981
19. Ciabattoni G, Cinotti GA, Pierucci A, Simonetti BM, Manzi M, Pugliese F, Barsotti P, Pecci G, Taggi F, Patrono C: Effects of sulindac and ibuprofen in patients with chronic glomerular disease. Evidence for the dependence of renal function on Prostacyclin. N Engl J Med **310:** 279, 1984
20. Kirstein Pedersen A, Jakobsen P: Sulphinpyrazone metabolism during long-term therapy. Br J Clin Pharmacol **11:** 597, 1981
21. Catella F, Pugliese F, Patrignani P, Filabozzi P, Ciabattoni G, Patrono C: Differential platelet and renal effects of sulfinpyrazone in man. Clin Res **32:** 239A, 1984 (abst)
22. Pedersen AK, FitzGerald GA: Cyclooxygenase inhibition, platelet function, and metabolite formation during chronic sulfinpyrazone dosing. Clin Pharmacol Ther **37:** 36, 1985

22a. Pederson AK, FitzGerald GA: The human pharmacology of platelet inhibition: pharmacokinetics relevant to drug action. Circulation **72:** 1164, 1985

23. Ciabattoni G, Bianchi Porro G, Caruso I, Fumagalli M, Pugliese F, Patrono C: Differential inhibition of prostaglandin and thromboxane synthesis in human tissues by non-steroidal antiinflammatory drugs. Clin Res **32:** 462A, 1984 (abst)
24. Miller MJ, Bednar MM, McGiff JC: Renal metabolism of sulindac, a novel nonsteroidal antiinflammatory agent. *In* Samuelsson B, Paoletti R, Ramwell P, editors: Advances in prostaglandin thromboxane and leukotriene research. New York, 1983, Raven Press, vol 11, p 487
25. Rosenkranz B, Frölich JC: Effects of sulfinpyrazone on renal function and prostaglandin synthesis in man. Clin Res **31:** 253A, 1983 (abst)
26. Choudhury SL, Taylor SH, Wieringa G, Swaminathan R, Morgan DB: Sulphinpyrazone and renal function following myocardial infarction. Eur J Clin Pharmacol **24:** 747, 1983
27. Roth GJ, Stanford NS, Majerus PW: Acetylation of prostaglandin synthetase by aspirin. Proc Natl Acad Sci USA **72:** 3073, 1975
28. Van Der Ouderaa FJ, Buytenhek M, Nugteren DH, Van Dorp DA: Acetylation of Prostaglandin endoperoxide synthetase with acetylsalicylic acid. Eur J Biochem **109:** 1, 1980
29. Pedersen AK, FitzGerald GA: Dose related kinetics of aspirin: presystemic acetylation of platelet cyclooxygenase. N Engl J Med **311:** 1206, 1984
30. Harter HR, Burch JW, Majerus PW, Stanford N, Delmez JA, Anderson CB, Weerts CA: Prevention of thrombosis in patients on hemodialysis by low-dose aspirin. N Engl J Med **301:** 577, 1979
31. Lewis HD, Davis JW, Archibald DG, Steinke WE, Smitherman TC, Doherty JE, Schnaper HW, LeWinter MM, Linares E, Pouget JM, Sabharwal SC, Chesler E, DeMots H: Protective effects of aspirin against acute myocardial infarction and death in men with unstable angina. Results of a Veterans Administration Cooperative Study. N Engl J Med **309:** 396, 1983
32. Lorenz RL, Weber M, Kotzur J, Theisen K, Schacky CV, Meister W, Reichardt B, Weber PC: Improved aortocoronary bypass patency by low-dose aspirin (100 mg daily). Effects on platelet aggregation and thromboxane formation. Lancet **1:** 1261, 1984
33. Steele PM, Chesebro JH, Fuster V: The natural history of arterial balloon angioplasty in pigs and intervention with platelet-inhibitor therapy: implications for clinical trials. Clin Res **32:** 209A, 1984 (abst)
34. FitzGerald GA, Smith B, Pedersen AK, Brash AR: Increased prostacyclin biosynthesis in patients with severe atherosclerosis and platelet activation. N Engl J Med **310:** 1065, 1984
35. Preston FE, Whipps S, Jackson CA, French AJ, Wyld PJ, Stoddard CJ: Inhibition of prostacyclin and platelet thromboxane A_2 after low-dose aspirin. N Engl J Med **304:** 76, 1981
36. De Caterina R, Giannessi D, Bernini W, Gazzetti P, Michelassi C, L'Abbate A, Donato L, Patrignani P, Filabozzi P, Patrono C: Selective inhibition of thromboxane-related platelet function by low-dose aspirin in patients after myocardial infarction. Am J Cardiol **55:** 589, 1985
37. Weksler BB, Tack-Goldman K, Subramanian VA, Gay WA Jr: Cumulative inhibitory effect of low-dose aspirin on vascular pros-

tacyclin and platelet thromboxane production in patients with atherosclerosis. Circulation **71:** 332, 1985
38. Masotti G, Galanti G, Poggesi L, Abbate R, Neri Serneri GG: Differential inhibition of prostacyclin production and platelet aggregation by aspirin. Lancet **2:** 1213, 1979
39. Hanley SP, Bevan J, Cockbill SR, Heptinstall S: A regimen for low-dose aspirin? Br Med J **285:** 1299, 1982
40. Marcus AJ: Editorial retrospective. Aspirin as an antithrombotic medication. N Engl J Med **309:** 1515, 1983
41. Majerus PW: Arachidonate metabolism in vascular disorders. J Clin Invest **72:** 1521, 1983
42. Whittle BJR, Higgs GA, Eakins KE, Moncada S, Vane JR: Selective inhibition of prostaglandin production in inflammatory exudates and gastric mucosa. Nature **284:** 271, 1980
43. Sraer J, Ardaillou N, Sraer J-D, Ardaillou R: In vitro prostaglandin synthesis by human glomeruli and papillae. Prostaglandins **23:** 855, 1982

Pharmacology of platelet inhibition in humans: implications of the salicylate-aspirin interaction

Giovanni de Gaetano, M.D., Ph.D., Chiara Cerletti, Ph.D., Elisabetta Dejana, Ph.D., and Roberto Latini, M.D.

ABSTRACT The current dispute over the effects of "low" vs "high"doses of aspirin should take into consideration the pharmacokinetics of this drug. In fact, different pharmaceutical formulations of aspirin may deliver little or no aspirin to the systemic blood. This was the case, for instance, in healthy volunteers taking 320 mg of compressed aspirin or 800 mg of enteric-coated aspirin. In all instances thromboxane B_2 generation in serum was fully inhibited. Platelet cyclooxygenase might therefore be effectively acetylated by exposure to aspirin in the portal circulation, whereas vascular cyclooxygenase could be spared. Thus aspirin formulations ensuring complete first-pass deacetylation should be sought rather than "low" or "high" doses of unspecified aspirin formulations. Regardless of the type and dose of aspirin administered, salicylate is formed and accumulates in the circulation. It may antagonize the effects of aspirin on cyclooxygenase, at least in acute conditions. As an example, after administration of 1 g of salicylate to healthy volunteers, when plasma levels of the drug were about 75 μg/ml, the effect of 40 mg iv aspirin (given 40 min later) on platelet cyclooxygenase and aggregation was significantly diminished. In contrast, in patients undergoing saphenectomy, the same dose of salicylate (1 g) gave plasma drug levels of about 25 μg/ml; salicylate was unable to prevent the inhibitory effect on platelets of 40 mg iv aspirin (given 1 hr later) but did act on vascular prostacyclin. Thus the combination of salicylate with aspirin at an appropriate dose and blood level ratio may result in almost complete dissociation of the drug's effect on platelets and vessels in man. Because the studies outlined in this review address only the short-term outcome of the salicylate-aspirin interaction, the possibility should be tested that inactivation of cyclooxygenase would occur after long-term administration of salicylate-aspirin. A pharmacokinetic approach to the "aspirin dilemma" should also consider the possibility that salicylate and/or its metabolites (e.g., gentisic acid) may interfere with lipoxygenase activity, synthesis of the prothrombin complex coagulation factors, and fibrinolysis.

Circulation 72, No. 6, 1185–1193, 1985.

Aspirin, salicylate, and inhibition of platelet aggregation and cyclooxygenase activity. Aspirin inhibits platelet aggregation and the concomitant release reaction.[1-4] This exciting discovery, made more than 15 years ago, was characterized by three main facts: (1) aspirin was active in man at oral doses as low as 150 mg (about 2 mg/kg), (2) its effects were long lasting (at least 24 to 48 hr), and (3) salicylate, the main metabolite of aspirin, was virtually inactive. The last two observations suggested that the effect of aspirin on platelets was the result of irreversible acetylation. Consequently, the salicylate moiety of aspirin was considered irrelevant for the drug's action on platelets.

From the Laboratory of Cardiovascular Clinical Pharmacology, Istituto di Ricerche Farmacologiche Mario Negri, Milano, Italy.

Supported by the Italian National Research Council, Progetto Finalizzato "Medicina Preventiva," Sottoprogetto "Malattie Degenerative," Contract No. 84.02277.56.

Address for correspondence: Giovanni de Gaetano, M.D., Ph.D.,Laboratory of Cardiovascular Clinical Pharmacology, Istituto di Ricerche Farmacologiche Mario Negri, via Eritrea, 62-20157 Milano, Italy.

In the early seventies, aspirin and other nonsteroidal anti-inflammatory drugs (NSAID) were shown to inhibit prostaglandin formation in human platelets.[5] Again salicylate was inactive. Acetylation of platelet proteins by aspirin was subsequently reported.[6] Because one of these proteins was a subunit of fatty acid cyclooxygenase, the role of this enzyme in the aspirin action was considered to be crucial. Although the nonspecific acetylation of other platelet proteins is currently of unknown biological significance, the inhibition of cyclooxygenase by aspirin does not appear to explain fully the antithrombotic effects of this drug.[7-10]

Aspirin is quickly deacetylated in vivo to salicylate. It has been suggested that in sites readily accessible to aspirin, such as circulating platelet cyclooxygenase, it might be expected to act in its own right as the acetylsalicylate ion and hence to be more potent than salicylate.[7] It would also be expected that the salicylate ion, into which aspirin is converted, would contribute to the overall activity of aspirin, for instance in actions that need persistent presence of an anti-inflammatory drug or that are located at poorly accessible sites; this might apply for example in rheumatic joints.[7] Additionally, salicylate may antagonize some effects of aspirin, such as its gastrointestinal ulcerogenicity.[11]

Our aim in this article is to review the available evidence on (1) the occurrence and the possible clinical relevance of the interaction between salicylate (or other NSAID) and aspirin on platelet and vascular cyclooxygenase and (2) the existence of additional mechanism(s) related to salicylate and possibly involved in the antithrombotic effects of aspirin.

Salicylate may antagonize the effects of aspirin on cyclooxygenase

Salicylate-aspirin or other NSAID-aspirin interactions on animal platelet cyclooxygenase. Studies in vitro have demonstrated that salicylate, which is not inhibitory by itself, protects cyclooxygenase from aspirin inhibition in rat[12] and rabbit[13] platelets (figure 1). A similar pharmacologic interaction was apparent in vivo.[14, 15] In the rat, administration of salicylate resulted in dose-related prevention of aspirin's effect on platelet cyclooxygenase activity. This interaction appeared to be competitive and closely dose related for both drugs.[15]

Other NSAID structurally related or unrelated to salicylate, such as diflunisal and sulphinpyrazone, respectively, are able in the rat in vivo to counter the effect of aspirin on platelets.[15] This effect was apparent for diflunisal or sulphinpyrazone at doses that did not inhibit platelet cyclooxygenase. The prevention by indomethacin of the effect of aspirin on platelets was apparent 24 hr after administration of aspirin. Actually the effect of indomethacin on platelet cyclooxygenase is short lasting, whereas that of aspirin lasts at least 24 hr. When the two drugs were given concurrently, the lasting effect of aspirin was no longer detectable and inhibition of cyclooxygenase lasted as if indomethacin alone had been administered. On the other hand, salicylate and diflunisal competitively blunted the inhibitory effect of indomethacin on platelet cyclooxygenase.

All these results could be explained by postulating a common site of interaction for the different NSAID on cyclooxygenase.[15, 16] The observation that salicylate, a virtually inactive compound or ineffective doses of diflunisal and sulphinpyrazone counteract the effect of aspirin suggests that competition does not occur at the *catalytic site* but rather at a supplementary *binding site.* Interaction with this putative supplementary site is necessary but not sufficient for the efficacy of these drugs as cyclooxygenase inhibitors.[15, 16] Thus salicylate interacts with the binding site of cyclooxygenase but does not modify its enzymatic activity. However, neither aspirin nor indomethacin can exert their inhibitory activity on the enzyme when the binding site is occupied by salicylate.

Further experimental evidence of a supplementary binding site on cyclooxygenase was provided by the failure of salicylate to prevent enzyme inhibition by 5,8,11,14-eicosatetraynoic acid (ETYA), a competitive antagonist of arachidonic acid. Moreover, salicylate did not affect either ETYA or nor-dihydroguaiaretic acid inhibition of platelet lipoxygenase.

On the basis of these and other data presented in detail elsewhere,[17] a functional model of pharmacologic inhibition of cyclooxygenase by aspirin and other NSAID can be proposed (figure 2). This model would explain the selectivity of NSAID for the cyclooxygen-

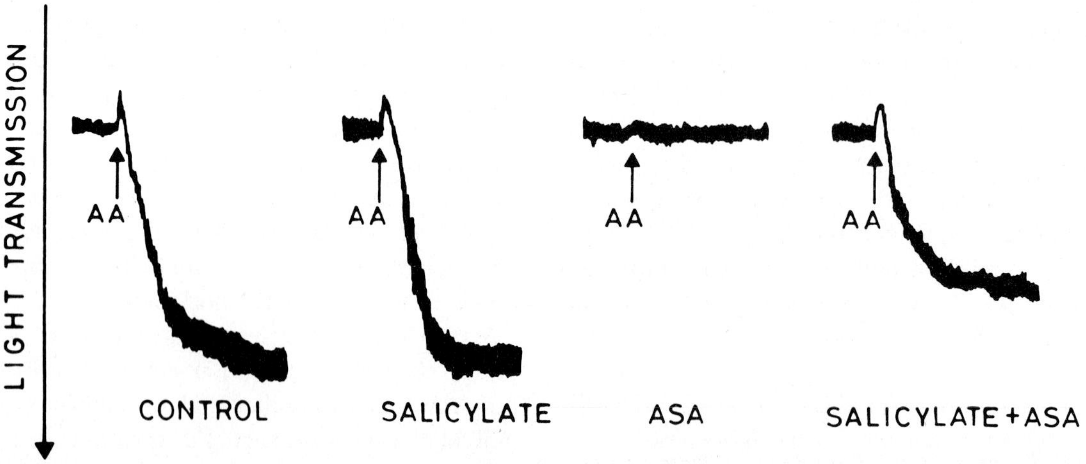

FIGURE 1. Prevention by salicylate of aspirin inhibition of arachidonic acid–induced platelet aggregation. Rat platelet aggregation was induced by threshold concentrations of arachidonic acid (AA 0.5 mM). Aspirin (100 μM) preincubation (1 min) with PRP completely prevented aggregation, whereas sodium salicylate (1 mM) 1 min before was ineffective. The combination of both compounds resulted in an almost normal aggregation. ASA = aspirin; PRP = platelet-rich plasma.

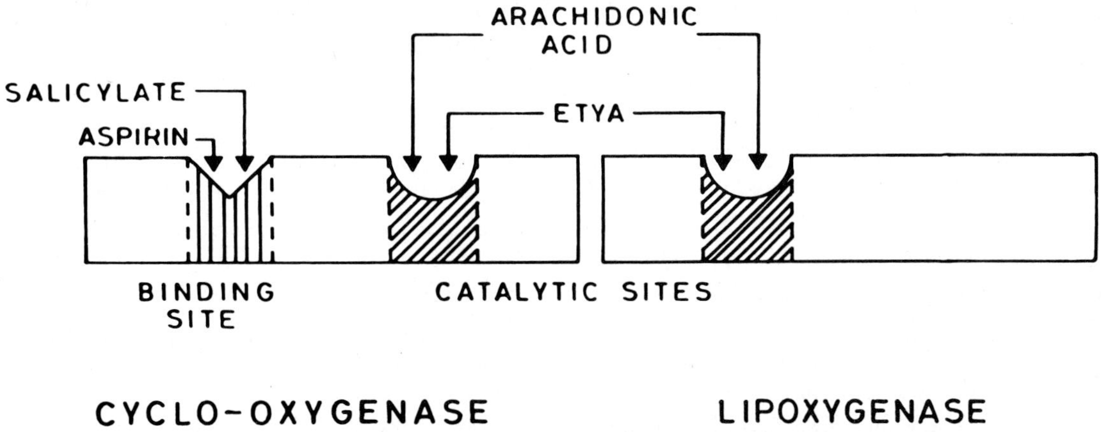

FIGURE 2. Functional model of cyclooxygenase and lipoxygenase inhibition. Salicylate, aspirin, and the other NSAIDs bind to a binding site related to but distinct from the catalytic site of cyclooxygenase. This binding is necessary but not sufficient for enzyme inhibition. 5,8,11,14-Eicosatetraynoic acid (ETYA) competes with arachidonic acid for the catalytic sites of both cyclooxygenase and lipoxygenase. Thus salicylate does not interfere with the effect of ETYA.

ase pathway of arachidonic acid metabolism in relation to lipoxygenase.[16, 17] The intensity of interaction with the supplementary site and the ensuing modifications of the catalytic site would determine these compounds' potency as cyclooxygenase inhibitors. This model might also account for the finding that salicylate, aspirin, and indomethacin equipotently inhibit the lipoxygenase pathway.[18] Recently, additional evidence for two distinct enzymatic sites on rabbit platelet cyclooxygenase has been presented.[19]

Salicylate-aspirin interaction on animal vascular cyclooxygenase. The interaction between salicylate and aspirin is not restricted to platelet cyclooxygenase.[12] In fact, salicylate administered to rats may prevent the inhibitory activity of aspirin on vascular cyclooxygenase.[20] This effect was even more evident than that on platelets. Indeed the doses of salicylate needed to completely counteract the effect of the same dose of aspirin on vascular cyclooxygenase were lower than those on platelets. As a direct consequence of this observation, the administration of salicylate and aspirin at appropriate dose ratios could achieve complete inhibition of platelet cyclooxygenase without affecting the vascular enzyme.

Whether the different efficacy of salicylate in preventing aspirin effect derives from a different sensitivity to or access of the drug at various cellular levels remains to be established.

Salicylate-aspirin interaction at other cellular levels in animals. In the guinea pig, salicylate, inactive by itself, prevents the protective effect of aspirin in arachidonic acid–induced bronchoconstriction in vivo.[21] Because this arachidonate effect was not mediated by platelet aggregation but most likely by endoperoxide and thromboxane A_2 (TxA_2) production by the lung, the salicylate-aspirin interaction could occur in the lungs.

It has been reported that salicylate diminishes the gastric lesions induced by aspirin and other NSAID in rats.[11] This effect seems to be secondary to a depression of prostaglandin synthesis in the stomach, and the counteracting effect of salicylate was correlated to its ability to protect gastric cyclooxygenase from NSAID inhibition.[11, 22]

Salicylate-aspirin interaction on human platelet cyclooxygenase. All the above data have been obtained in vitro or in vivo in animal studies. Interference by salicylate with aspirin inhibition of human platelet cyclooxygenase activity has also been observed.[23–25] The question remains as to whether a similar interaction occurs between salicylate and other NSAID on cyclooxygenase *in vivo* in man and as to its clinical relevance.

In a recent study in human volunteers we observed that orally administered indomethacin (50 mg) prevented the long-lasting effect of a subsequent dose of aspirin (500 mg) on platelet cyclooxygenase activity and on platelet aggregation.[25] Similarly, ingestion of ibuprofen prevented the aspirin effect.[26] More recently we investigated whether salicylate and aspirin interact on platelets in man at doses and plasma levels of clinical relevance.[27] Six volunteers, given oral doses of sodium salicylate (250 or 1000 mg) presented peak plasma salicylate levels averaging 20 and 75 μg/ml, respectively. Neither platelet aggregation nor serum immunoreactive thromboxane B_2 (TxB_2) formation was modified by either salicylate treatment. Forty minutes later, all volunteers received 40 mg iv aspirin, the lowest single dose that suppressed arachidonate-induced platelet aggregation and TxB_2 generation. Aspirin plasma levels were not affected by previous salicylate ingestion. Inhibition by aspirin of both platelet aggregation and TxB_2 generation was significantly prevented by the larger salicylate dose, giving plasma salicylate levels similar to those after an oral dose of 800 mg of enteric-coated aspirin. Pretreatment with 250 mg of salicylate, giving plasma salicylate levels similar to those obtained with an oral dose of 320 mg of compressed aspirin, resulted in proportionally diminished prevention of aspirin's effect on platelet aggregation but did not significantly modify its effect on serum TxB_2 generation.

Salicylate-aspirin interaction in man as a possible pharmacologic solution to the "aspirin dilemma." When it was shown that aspirin, while inhibiting TxA_2 in platelets, equally inhibited antiaggregatory prostacyclin (PGI_2) in vascular cells, the "aspirin dilemma" emerged.[28, 29] Simultaneous inhibition of PGI_2 and TxB_2 synthesis was considered a possible reason for the disappointing results of clinical trials on the drug's antithrombotic effect.[8]

In an effort to solve the "aspirin dilemma," studies were devised to determine the aspirin dose that would inhibit TxA_2 production but would not interfere with PGI_2 synthesis in vascular cells. Platelet cyclooxygenase was believed to be more sensitive than vascular cyclooxygenase to aspirin inhibition. If it had been, the "aspirin dilemma" could have been solved easily by using low doses of the drug. Unfortunately, studies with endothelial cells in culture, laboratory animals, and man have not completely dissociated the inhibitory effect of aspirin on platelets from that on vascular cells (for review see refs. 8 and 30).

We have already mentioned that in the rat, salicylate was more effective in counteracting the inhibitory activity of aspirin on vascular cyclooxygenase than that on platelet cyclooxygenase.[20] We have recently completed a study[31] in patients undergoing saphenectomy, aimed at verifying a similar differential salicylate-aspirin interaction in man. Twenty-one female patients, admitted to the Milan University Institute of Vascular Surgery for removal of varicose veins, entered this study. Seven took no medications, and six were given 40 mg iv aspirin 1 hr before operation. The remaining eight patients took 1000 mg sodium salicylate orally 1 hr before aspirin. During surgery, segments of epigastric vein in close proximity to the saphenous vein were removed for measurements of prostacyclin production. At the same time, venous blood was collected for measurements of serum TxB_2 synthesis.

As reported in table 1, TxB_2 generation was completely inhibited in all patients given aspirin alone, whereas prostacyclin generation was reduced by more than 50%. In the salicylate-aspirin group, TxB_2 generation remained undetectable in three patients and reached about 10% of control values in the other five. In contrast, six patients generated prostacyclin levels within the control range and only two appeared to be partially inhibited. Mean salicylate blood levels at the moment of aspirin administration were 25.9 ± 5 μg/ml.

TABLE 1

Effect of aspirin and salicylate on immunoreactive serum TxB_2 and vascular 6-keto-$PGF_{1\alpha}$ generation in 21 patients undergoing saphenectomy

Treatment	n	Serum TxB_2 (pmol/ml)	Vascular 6-keto-$PGF_{1\alpha}$ (pmol/mg)
Control	7	44.8±4	2.73±0.2
Aspirin (40 mg iv)	6	nd	1.18±0.2[A]
Salicylate (1 g po) + aspirin	8	4.3±1	2.11±0.2

nd = not detectable (<0.075 pmol/ml).

[A]$p < .01$ compared with the other two groups (Duncan's test). 6-Keto-$PGF_{1\alpha}$ was measured by specific radioimmunoassay in the supernatant of epigastric segments of saphenous vein incubated for 5 min with arachidonic acid (50 μM), as described.[31]

This observation confirms in man the results obtained in the rat. In this animal as well as in the present study in man, vascular cells showed lower sensitivity to aspirin than platelets. Salicylate resulted in both instances in an amplification of the difference in response to aspirin of platelets and vascular cells. The mechanism of this property of salicylate (e.g., different access of the drug at various cellular levels) remains to be defined. This observation, however, may constitute an original approach on which to base the clinical use of aspirin in a supposedly beneficial antithrombotic direction.

When analyzed with respect to the study in healthy male volunteers, this study in female patients undergoing saphenectomy merits some comments. As summarized in table 2, the same salicylate-aspirin dose ratio (1000 mg oral vs 40 mg iv) resulted in significant prevention of the aspirin effect on platelet TxB_2 generation in the group of volunteers but not in patients. The most likely explanation is that at the moment of aspirin administration, the plasma levels of salicylate, measured 1 hr after ingestion (abut 25 μg/ml), were markedly lower than those measured 40 min after ingestion in volunteers (about 75 μg/ml). In fact, salicylate levels in patients were similar to those found in volunteers 40 min after 250 mg of salicylate. In the latter condition, as well as in patients, no significant prevention of aspirin's effect on TxB_2 synthesis could be detected. Possibly, gastrointestinal absorption of salicylate was reduced in patients by anesthesia.

TABLE 2
Salicylate-aspirin interaction at platelet and vascular level and plasma salicylate levels in healthy volunteers and in patients undergoing saphenectomy

Subjects	Salicylate (mg, oral)	Interval (min)	Salicylate levels (μg/ml)	SAL/ASA interaction	
				TxB_2	PGI_2
Volunteers	250	40	22.3±1.7	No	—
Volunteers	1000	40	76.3±5.1	Yes	—
Saphenectomy patients	1000	60	25.9±5.0	No	Yes

SAL = salicylate; ASA = aspirin.
Plasma salicylate levels were measured immediately before aspirin (40 mg iv). For other details see table 1.

Independently of the reasons why the same dose of salicylate gave rise to different plasma levels of the drug in the two groups of subjects, it appears that the plasma levels of salicylate rather than the amount of the drug administered are relevant for an optimal interaction with aspirin.

In summary, we have discussed the hypothesis that platelet and/or vascular cyclooxygenase might be spared acetylation by aspirin if the plasma levels of salicylate are carefully balanced with the plasma levels of aspirin. This hypothesis has been tested experimentally both in vitro and ex vivo in short-term animal and human studies. Protection of cyclooxygenase with salicylate acutely prevented irreversible inactivation by aspirin; experimental evidence that salicylate protects cyclooxygenase from inactivation by aspirin after long-term administration of both compounds is still lacking. Cyclooxygenase protection by salicylate might slow the rate of its inactivation by aspirin but not prevent it completely; thus the cyclooxygenase population might be finally inactivated during long-term salicylate-aspirin therapy, despite a careful balance between salicylate and aspirin levels. On the basis of these considerations we addressed our attention to another possible approach to solve the "aspirin dilemma."

Aspirin formulations that deliver only salicylate to the systemic circulation: a pharmacokinetic approach to the "aspirin dilemma." The importance of salicylate plasma levels mentioned in the preceding section suggests that a better knowledge of the pharmacokinetics of aspirin might help solve the "aspirin dilemma." Little attention has been paid to aspirin pharmacokinetics with regard to the different pharmaceutical formulations used in thrombosis prevention trials. This approach seemed of particular interest in view of observations in healthy volunteers[27] that the peak plasma levels of aspirin after either 320 mg of compressed aspirin or 800 mg of enteric-coated aspirin were not statistically different (2.9 ± 0.06 and 3.3 ± 0.3 μg/ml, respectively). Serum TxB_2 generation was almost completely inhibited 1 hr after either aspirin formulation.

Of even greater interest was the observation that similar full TxB_2 inhibition was obtained in five volunteers in whose peripheral circulation aspirin levels were not measurable (figure 3). Three subjects had received a compressed aspirin and two an enteric-coated aspirin. No significant differences in salicylate area under the plasma concentration vs time curve could be found between subjects with detectable or undetectable aspirin plasma levels after either formulation (table 3). On account of the potential for erratic absorption pattern of aspirin, detectable plasma levels of the unchanged drug may depend on fortuitous blood collection times.[32] In our study, however, this was unlikely because as many as eight blood samples were collected within the first hour after compressed aspirin and six

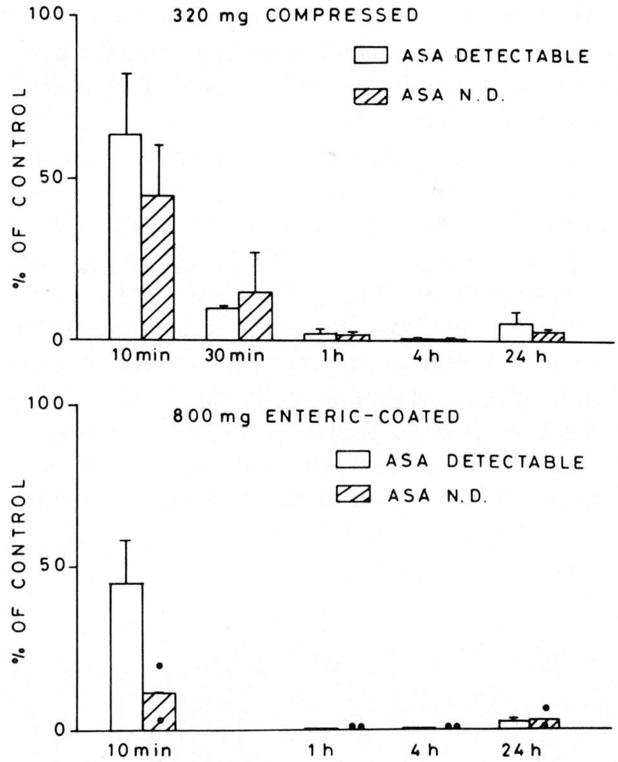

FIGURE 3. Serum TxB_2 measured at different times after ingestion of 320 mg of compressed (*upper panel*) or 800 mg of enteric-coated (*lower panel*) aspirin in subjects with detectable or undetectable aspirin levels. Figures are percent values of predrug serum TxB_2 in each subject and SEM. Three subjects had detectable and three undetectable aspirin plasma levels after 320 mg aspirin, while four had detectable and two undetectable aspirin plasma levels after 800 mg enteric-coated aspirin. In this last group the mean and the two single values are reported, respectively. ASA = aspirin; ND = not detectable.

TABLE 3
Pharmacokinetics of aspirin after ingestion of two different drug formulations in six healthy volunteers

Aspirin preparation (oral dose)	n	AUC (0→∞) (nmol/ml/hr)	
		Aspirin	Salicylate
Compressed	3	17.3±1.4	544±42
(320 mg)	3	undetectable	830±40
Enteric-coated	4	31.9±3.3	2680±153
(800 mg)	2	undetectable	2190–2851

AUC = area under the plasma concentrations between 0 and ∞. Detection limit of aspirin = 0.5 nmol/ml.

during the first 3 hr after enteric-coated aspirin. The time of peak aspirin concentration in subjects in whom it was detectable was 33 min for compressed and 83 min for enteric-coated aspirin.[27]

Experiments in vitro showed that incubation of human whole blood from three different donors with 0.5 μM aspirin (corresponding to the detection limit of the high-performance liquid chromatographic assay method used) for 1 hr at 37° C did not result in any significant reduction of serum TxB_2 generation. As shown in figure 4, concentrations of aspirin at least 50 times this detection limit were required to prevent TxB_2 generation by more than 90%.

It has long been known that aspirin undergoes extensive first-pass deacetylation within the enterohepatic circulation.[33] Whether this first-pass effect is dose-dependent is not yet known. Thus inhibition of serum TxB_2 generation in the absence of measurable aspirin in systemic peripheral blood might result from acetylation of platelet cyclooxygenase by exposure of circulating cells to the drug in the portal circulation. Cyclooxygenase in the peripheral vasculature could thus come into contact only with inactive salicylate, with the possible exception of the mesenteric and portal vessels exposed to aspirin before the first-pass occurs.

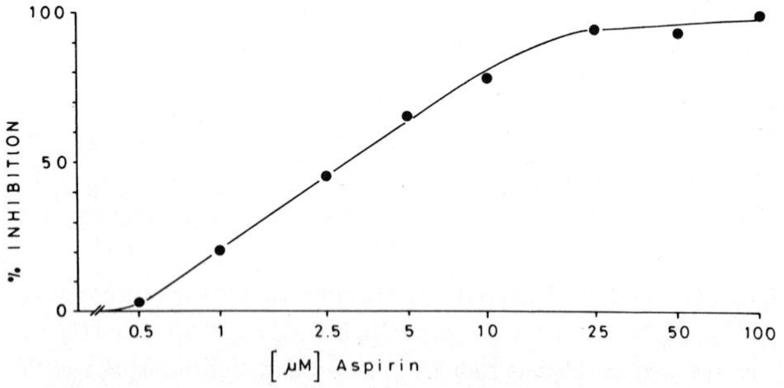

FIGURE 4. Effect of different aspirin concentrations on TxB_2 generation in human serum in vitro. Blood was collected without anticoagulant from the antecubital vein of healthy subjects and incubated in glass tube at 37° C for 1 hr in the presence of aspirin. TxB_2 generation was measured in serum. The values (mean from four experiments) are percent inhibition of control values.

Thus aspirin formulations ensuring extensive first-pass deacetylation rather than merely "low" or "high" doses of unspecified aspirin formulations should be sought as a pharmacologic goal for solving the "aspirin dilemma." The current dispute on the difference in sensitivity to "low" doses of aspirin between platelet and vascular cyclooxygenase may well arise from the wide variability of aspirin pharmacokinetics. Indeed, as in our experiments, the same dose or formulation may or may not deliver measurable amounts of aspirin to the systemic circulation; the inhibitory effect on platelet cyclooxygenase would be achieved in any case, but vascular PGI_2 synthesis would only be spared in the absence of detectable peripheral aspirin levels. Similar conclusions have recently been reached by other investigators.[34, 35]

Salicylate may contribute to the overall activity of aspirin in the prevention of vascular occlusion. Although inhibition of prostanoid synthesis has become an attractive, unifying explanation of the anti-inflammatory activity of aspirin-like drugs, this mechanism does not explain all aspects of the anti-inflammatory action of salicylates, especially in conditions in which aspirin and salicylate are of approximately equal potency.[7] It has therefore been suggested that the anti-inflammatory activity of aspirin-like drugs probably does not arise from a single mechanism but may be mediated through an additional or alternative mechanism, which becomes operative only at doses in excess of those required to suppress cyclooxygenase. The possibility has also been discussed that aspirin has additional components to its mechanism of action not possessed by other NSAIDs, such as flufenamic acid or indomethacin. The major lines of research into alternative mechanisms that might explain the therapeutic action of salicylate have been reviewed extensively.[7]

Because several pathways may be involved in the initiation and growth of thrombi, one would expect aspirin to be inhibitory only in conditions in which prostanoid biosynthesis (cyclic endoperoxides and TxA_2) plays a major role in thrombus formation.

Effects of aspirin and salicylate on blood coagulation and fibrinolysis. A recent study[9] in rabbits with in-dwelling aortic catheters strongly suggests that aspirin at doses that inhibit only platelet cyclooxygenase activity is not a satisfactory inhibitor of arterial thrombosis when there is a significant fibrin component. At very high doses aspirin inhibited thrombosis, but this effect was not mediated through inhibition of platelet function. In fact salicylate was more effective than aspirin. The tendency for high doses of aspirin or salicylate to inhibit thrombus formation appears related to a prolongation of the one-stage prothrombin time and to activation of whole blood fibrinolytic activity; which of these pathways is most important in reducing thrombus formation remains to be established.

This experimental finding is in keeping with some observations in man. There are reports that doses of 2 to 3 g of aspirin per day in man prolong prothrombin time[36, 37] and increase whole blood fibrinolytic activity.[38–40] Moroz[39] reported that aspirin and sodium salicylate (1.8 g) were equipotent in stimulating fibrinolytic activity through the protease action of leukocytes.

The beneficial effect of high doses of aspirin in preventing venous thrombosis and pulmonary embolism after total knee replacement[41] may be due not just to the effect of aspirin on platelets but also to its effect (and/or of the salicylate) on blood coagulation and fibrinolysis. However, in a recent study on healthy human volunteers, aspirin (650 mg given orally both 18 and 2 hr before blood collection) inhibited the rise in vascular plasminogen activity after venous occlusion.[42] Similarly a decrease in fibrinolysis induced by both cellular and plasmatic factors after ingestion of 1 g of aspirin per day for 4 days had been reported.[43]

Recently Roncaglioni et al.[44] have shown in rats that salicylate, like warfarin, with which it may have some common chemical features (figure 5), reduced the plasma concentration of the prothrombin complex clotting factors in vivo. It also caused an accumulation of microsomal substrates for vitamin K–dependent carboxylase in the liver and lung. These effects of salicylate were dose-dependent (between 4 × 50 and 4 × 200 mg/kg) and were counteracted by simultaneous administration of vitamin K (20 mg/kg). The mechanism of salicylate-induced hypoprothrombinemia in the rat and in the rabbit has been extensively investigated by several groups.[45–48] Because the effect of salicylate was additive to that of warfarin,[44] relatively low doses of aspirin or salicylate should interfere with oral anticoagulant therapy. Aspirin-induced fluctuation in clotting factor levels of as little as 5% to 10% of normal might have serious consequences in patients undergoing anticoagulant treatment, although it might not even be measurable in healthy volunteers.

These considerations should be borne in mind when analyzing the results of clinical trials combining aspirin and oral anticoagulants. On the one hand it is not surprising that this drug combination has been reported to be more effective than oral anticoagulants alone in preventing thrombotic complications in patients with aortic ball valves.[49] On the other hand it could explain the high frequency of bleeding complications encountered in other trials.[50] Two recent reports in rabbits[51] and in rats[52] have suggested that high doses of aspirin may prolong bleeding time independently of an effect on platelet cyclooxygenase and also of formation of salicylate.

Effects of aspirin and salicylate on leukocytes. The observation that aspirin and salicylate equipotently inhibit the generation of chemotactic 12-HETE from 12-HPETE in the lipoxygenase pathway of the arachidonic acid metabolism,[18] although controversial, has been considered as diminishing the importance of the cyclooxygenase pathway in the anti-inflammatory activity of salicylate.[7]

A key event in any inflammatory reaction is the migration of leukocytes from the blood into the inflammatory lesion. Leukocytes metabolize arachidonic acid by lipoxygenase[53] and the products of this enzyme are potent chemotactic agents[54] that induce leukocyte aggregation.[55, 56] It has recently been proposed[57] that migrating leukocytes contribute to the tissue injury accompanying myocardial ischemia, possibly by release of proinflammatory mediators and free radicals

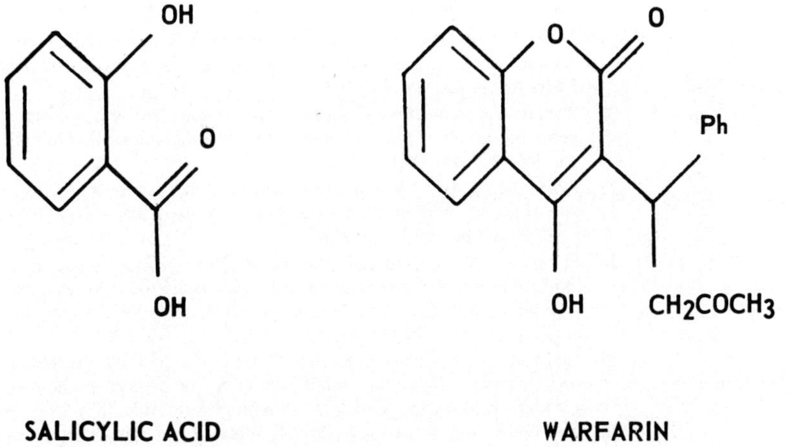

FIGURE 5. Chemical structures of salicylate and warfarin.

(oxygen metabolites). Drugs that reduce the migration and/or activation of leukocytes might be useful in reducing infarct size.

Aspirin and salicylate inhibit the production of superoxide anion by activated leukocytes[7] but do not reduce leukocyte invasion into an inflammatory exudate.[58] Thus, although an interaction with superoxide anion could be considered as a possible additional mechanism of the anti-inflammatory action of salicylates, the biological consequences of this pharmacologic effect are not obvious. A recent observation in our laboratory (A. Lorico and S. Villa, unpublished) may also be of interest in this context: gentisic acid,[59] a hydroxylated metabolite of salicylate, not only prevented superoxide anion production by human leukocytes stimulated with either arachidonic acid or phorbol myristate acetate, but also prevented leukocyte aggregation. The concentrations of gentisic acid active in vitro (0.4 to 1.2 mM) are probably not reached in the human circulation after current therapeutic doses of aspirin.[60] However, this finding merits further investigation.

Conclusions. Aspirin inhibits cyclooxygenase. This effect distinguishes it from salicylate, its major metabolite, with regard to inhibition of the platelet function induced by certain stimuli. Although inactive on cyclooxygenase, salicylate may interfere with the effect of aspirin on this enzyme both in platelets and (even more effectively) in the vasculature. Knowledge of the pharmacokinetics of aspirin and salicylate is essential for optimal use of aspirin as a selective inhibitor of platelet but not of vascular cyclooxygenase activity. The mechanism involving cyclooxygenase does not, however, appear to fully explain the antithrombotic action of aspirin. Therefore, it is best to assume that in preventing thrombosis aspirin acts by at least two mechanisms, one of which is the inhibition of platelet cyclooxygenase.

The best candidate mechanisms, most likely to be linked to the salicylate moiety of aspirin, are the inhibition of vitamin K–dependent clotting factor synthesis, cell-mediated activation of blood fibrinolysis, and interference with the platelet and/or leukocyte lipoxygenase pathway of arachidonic acid metabolism.

Judith Baggott, Antonella Bottazzi, Vincenzo de Ceglie, and Felice de Ceglie helped prepare the manuscript.

References

1. Evans G, Packham MA, Nishizawa EE, Mustard JF, Murphy EA: The effect of acetylsalicylic acid on platelet function. J Exp Med **128:** 877, 1968
2. Weiss HJ, Aledort LM, Kochwa S: The effect of salicylates on the hemostatic properties of platelets in man. J Clin Invest **47:** 2169, 1968
3. O'Brien JR: Effects of salicylates on human platelets. Lancet **1:** 779, 1968
4. Zucker MB, Peterson J: Inhibition of adenosine diphosphate-induced secondary aggregation and other platelet functions by acetylsalicylic acid ingestion. Proc Soc Exp Biol Med **127:** 547, 1968
5. Smith JB, Willis AL: Aspirin selectively inhibits prostaglandin production in human platelets. Nature New Biol **231:** 235, 1971
6. Roth GJ, Stanford N, Majerus PW: Acetylation of prostaglandin synthase by aspirin. Proc Natl Acad Sci USA **72:** 3073, 1975
7. Atkinson DC, Collier HOJ: Salicylates: molecular mechanism of therapeutic action. Adv Pharmacol Chemother **17:** 233, 1980
8. de Gaetano G, Cerletti C, Bertelé V: Pharmacology of antiplatelet drugs and clinical trials on thrombosis prevention: a difficult link. Lancet **2:** 974, 1982
9. Cattaneo M, Chahil A, Somers D, Kinlough-Rathbone RL, Packham MA, Mustard JF: Effect of aspirin and sodium salicylate on thrombosis, fibrinolysis, prothrombin time, and platelet survival in rabbits with indwelling aortic catheters. Blood **61:** 353, 1983
10. Marcus AJ: Aspirin as an antithrombotic medication. N Engl J Med **309:** 1515, 1983
11. Ezer E, Palosi E, Hajos Gy, Szporny L: Antagonism of the gastrointestinal ulcerogenic effect of some non-steroidal anti-inflammatory agents by sodium salicylate. J Pharm Pharmacol **28:** 655, 1976
12. Merino J, Livio M, Rajtar G, de Gaetano G: Salicylate reverses *in vitro* aspirin inhibition of rat platelet and vascular prostaglandin generation. Biochem Pharmacol **29:** 1093, 1980
13. Vargaftig BB: The inhibition of cyclo-oxygenase of rabbit platelets by aspirin is prevented by salicylic acid and by phenanthrolines. Eur J Pharmacol **50:** 231, 1978
14. Vargaftig BB: Salicylic acid fails to inhibit generation of thromboxane A_2 activity in platelets after in vivo administration to the rat. J Pharm Pharmacol **30:** 101, 1978
15. Cerletti C, Livio M, de Gaetano G: Non-steroidal anti-inflammatory drugs react with two sites on platelet cyclo-oxygenase: evidence from *in vivo* drug interaction studies in rats. Biochim Biophys Acta **714:** 122, 1982
16. Humes JL, Winter CA, Sadowski SJ, Kuehl FA Jr: Multiple sites on prostaglandin cyclooxygenase are determinants in the action of nonsteroidal antiinflammatory agents. Proc Natl Acad Sci USA **78:** 2053, 1981
17. Cerletti C, Livio M, Doni MG, de Gaetano G: Salicylate fails to prevent the inhibitory effect of 5,8,11,14-eicosatetraynoic acid on human platelet cyclo-oxygenase and lipoxygenase activities. Biochim Biophys Acta **759:** 125, 1983
18. Siegel MI, McConnell RT, Porter NA, Cuatrecasas P: Arachidonate metabolism via lipoxygenase and 12L-hydroperoxy-5,8,10,14-icosatetraenoic acid peroxidase sensitive to anti-inflammatory drugs. Proc Natl Acad Sci USA **77:** 308, 1980
19. Rotilio D, Joseph D, Hatmi M, Vargaftig BB: Structural requirements for preventing the aspirin- and the arachidonate-induced inactivation of platelet cyclo-oxygense: additional evidence for distinct enzymatic sites. Eur J Pharmacol **97:** 197, 1984
20. Dejana E, Cerletti C, De Castellarnau C, Livio M, Galletti F, Latini R, de Gaetano G: Salicylate-aspirin interaction in the rat: evidence that salicylate accumulating during aspirin administration may protect vascular prostacyclin from aspirin-induced inhibition. J Clin Invest **68:** 1108, 1981
21. Lefort J, Vargaftig BB: Role of platelets in aspirin-sensitive bronchoconstriction in the guinea-pig: interaction with salicylic acid. Br J Pharmacol **63:** 35, 1978
22. Robert A: Antisecretory, antiulcer, cytoprotective and diarrheogenic properties of prostaglandins. Adv Prostaglandins Thromboxane Res **2:** 507, 1976
23. Ali M, McDonald JWD: Interference by sulfinpyrazone and salicylate of aspirin inhibition of platelet cyclooxygenase activity. Prostaglandins Med **3:** 327, 1979
24. Peterson DA, Gerrard JM, Rao GHR, White JG: Salicylic acid inhibition of the irreversible effect of acetylsalicylic acid on prostaglandin synthetase may be due to competition for the enzyme cationic binding site. Prostaglandins Med **6:** 161, 1981
25. Livio M, Del Maschio A, Cerletti C, de Gaetano G: Indomethacin prevents the long-lasting inhibitory effect of aspirin on human platelet cyclooxygenase activity. Prostaglandins **23:** 787, 1982
26. Rao GHR, Johnson GG, Reddy R, White JG: Ibuprofen protects

platelet cyclooxygenase from irreversible inhibition by aspirin. Arteriosclerosis **3:** 383, 1983
27. Cerletti C, Bonati M, Del Maschio A, Galletti F, Dejana E, Tognoni G, de Gaetano G: Plasma levels of salicylate and aspirin in healthy volunteers: relevance to drug interaction on platelet function. J Lab Clin Med **103:** 869, 1984
28. Moncada S, Vane JR: Pharmacology and endogenous roles of prostaglandin endoperoxides, thromboxane A_2, and prostacyclin. Pharmacol Rev **30:** 293, 1979
29. Marcus AJ: Aspirin and thromboembolism: a possible dilemma. N Engl J Med **297:** 1284, 1977
30. Majerus PW: Arachidonate metabolism in vascular disorders. J Clin Invest **72:** 1521, 1983
31. Dejana E, Costantini V, de Amicis G, Cerletti C, Lorenzi G, de Gaetano G: Differential salicylate-aspirin interaction on vascular prostacyclin and platelet thromboxane synthesis in patients undergoing saphenectomy. Proc Soc Exp Biol Med (in press)
32. Ali M, McDonald JWD, Thiessen JJ, Coates PE: Plasma acetylsalicylate and salicylate and platelet cyclo-oxygenase activity following plain and enteric-coated aspirin. Stroke **11:** 9, 1980
33. Rowland M, Riegelman S, Harris PA, Sholkoff SD: Absorption kinetics of aspirin in man following oral administration of an aqueous solution. J Pharm Sci **61:** 379, 1972
34. Siebert DJ, Bochner F, Imhoff DM, Watts S, Lloyd JV, Field J, Gabb BW: Aspirin kinetics and platelet aggregation in man. Clin Pharmacol Ther **33:** 367, 1983
35. FitzGerald GA: Novel aspects of aspirin action. *In* Proceedings of the 4th International Washington Spring Symposium, Washington, May 1984, abst. 52
36. Quick AJ, Clesceri L: Influence of acetylsalicylic acid and salicylamide on the coagulation of blood. J Pharmacol Exp Ther **128:** 95, 1960
37. Loew D, Vinazzer H: Dose-dependent influence of acetylsalicylic acid on platelet functions and plasmatic coagulation factors. Haemostasis **5:** 239, 1976
38. Menon IS: Aspirin and blood fibrinolysis. Lancet **1:** 364, 1970
39. Moroz LA: Increased blood fibrinolytic activity after aspirin ingestion. N Engl J Med **296:** 525, 1977
40. Green D, Davies RO, Holmes GI, Johnson C, Kohl H, Reynolds N, Ts'ao C-h: Fibrinolytic activity after administration of diflunisal and aspirin: a double-blind, randomized, placebo-controlled clinical trial. Haemostasis **13:** 394, 1983
41. McKenna R, Galante J, Bachmann F, Wallace DL, Kaushal SP, Meredith P: Prevention of venous thromboembolism after total knee replacement by high-dose aspirin or intermittent calf and thigh compression. Br Med J **280:** 514, 1980
42. Levin RI, Harpel PC, Weil D, Chang T-S, Rifkin DB: Aspirin inhibits vascular plasminogen activator activity in vivo: studies utilizing a new assay to quantify plasminogen activator activity. J Clin Invest **74:** 571, 1984
43. Ghezzo F, Trinchero P, Pegoraro L: Effects of aspirin treatment upon fibrinolytic activity of peripheral blood granulocytes. Acta Haematol (Basel) **65:** 229, 1981
44. Roncaglioni MC, Ulrich M, Muller AD, Soute BAM, de Boer-van den Berg MAG, Vermeer C: The vitamin K-antagonism of salicylate and warfarin. Thromb Res (in press)
45. Owens MR, Cimino CD: The inhibitory effects of sodium salicylate on synthesis of factor VII by the perfused rat liver. Thromb Res **18:** 839, 1980
46. Park BK, Leck JB: On the mechanism of salicylate-induced hypothrombinaemia. J Pharm Pharmacol **33:** 25, 1981
47. Hildebrand EF, Suttie JW: The effects of salicylate on enzymes of vitamin K metabolism. J Pharm Pharmacol **35:** 421, 1983
48. Owen MR, Cimino CD: The interaction of salicylate and vitamin K in synthesis of factor II (prothrombin). Thromb Res **31:** 135, 1983
49. Dale J, Myhre E, Storstein O, Stormorken H, Efskind L: Prevention of arterial thromboembolism with acetylsalicylic acid: a controlled clinical study in patients with aortic ball valves. Am Heart J **94:** 101, 1977
50. Chesebro JH, Fuster V, Elveback LR, McGoon DC, Pluth JR, Puga FJ, Wallace RB, Danielson GK, Orszulak TA, Piehler JM, Schaff HV: Trial of combined warfarin plus dipyridamole or aspirin therapy in prosthetic heart valve replacement: danger of aspirin compared with dipyridamole. Am J Cardiol **51:** 1537, 1983
51. Buchanan MR, Richke JA, Hirsh J: Aspirin inhibits platelet function independent of the acetylation of cyclo-oxygenase. Thromb Res **25:** 363, 1982
52. Buczko W, de Gaetano G: Effect of high doses of aspirin and salicylate on bleeding time in rats. Thromb Res **32:** 631, 1983
53. Sun FF, McGuire JC: Metabolism of arachidonic acid by human neutrophils: characterization of the enzymatic reactions that lead to the synthesis of leukotriene B_4. Biochim Biophys Acta **772:** 56, 1984
54. Lewis RA, Auster F: The biologically active leukotrienes: biosynthesis, metabolism, receptors, functions, and pharmacology. J Clin Invest **73:** 889, 1984
55. Ford-Hutchinson AW, Bray MA, Doig MV, Shipley ME, Smith MJH: Leukotriene B_4, a potent chemokinetic and aggregating substance released from polymorphonuclear leukocytes. Nature **286:** 264, 1980
56. Villa S, Colotta F, de Gaetano G, Semeraro N: Arachidonic acid and leukotriene B_4 induce aggregation of human peripheral blood mononuclear leukocytes in vitro. Br J Haematol **58:** 137, 1984
57. Mullane KM, Read N, Salmon JA, Moncada S: Role of leukocytes in acute myocardial infarction in anesthetized dogs: relationship to myocardial salvage by anti-inflammatory drugs. J Pharmacol Exp Ther **228:** 510, 1984
58. Higgs GA, Eakins KE, Mugridge KG, Moncada S, Vane JR: The effects of non-steroidal anti-inflammatory drugs on leukocyte migration in carrageenan-induced inflammation. Eur J Pharmacol **66:** 81, 1980
59. Angelico F: Sulla trasformazione dell'acido salicilico nell'organismo animal. Arch Farmacol Sper **31:** 8, 1921
60. Bochner F, Graham GG, Chan E, Imhoff DM, Haavisto TM: Salicylate metabolite kinetics after several salicylates. Clin Pharmacol Ther **30:** 263, 1981

The biochemical pharmacology of thromboxane synthase inhibition in man

GARRET A. FITZGERALD, M.D., IRENE A. G. REILLY, M.B., AND ANDERS K. PEDERSEN, M.D.

ABSTRACT Selective inhibitors of thromboxane synthase have two theoretical advantages over inhibitors of the cyclooxygenase enzyme as potential antithrombotic compounds. First, they do not prevent formation of prostacyclin, a platelet-inhibitory, vasodilator compound, coincident with inhibiting thromboxane biosynthesis. Second, the prostaglandin endoperoxide substrate that accumulates in the platelet in the presence of thromboxane synthase inhibition may be donated to endothelial prostacyclin synthase at the site of platelet-vascular interactions (endoperoxide "steal"). Selective inhibition of thromboxane biosynthesis coincident with enhanced prostacyclin formation in vivo has been observed after administration of these compounds to man. Despite these attractive features and the efficacy of these compounds in diverse short-term animal preparations of thrombosis, investigations of their efficacy in human disease have proven disappointing. This may reflect on the importance of thromboxane A_2 in the diseases that have been investigated. Alternatively, the lack of drug efficacy may have resulted from either incomplete suppression of thromboxane biosynthesis and/or substitution for the biological effects of thromboxane A_2 by prostaglandin endoperoxides during long-term dosing studies. Given that selective inhibition of thromboxane formation can be approached with aspirin, the particular value of these compounds is dependent on enhancing prostacyclin formation. Aspirin inhibits thromboxane-dependent platelet activation, but many platelet agonists are likely to act in concert in vivo and prostacyclin inhibits platelet aggregation induced by both thromboxane-dependent and thromboxane-independent mechanisms. To test the hypothesis that thromboxane synthase inhibitors are efficacious in human disease, compounds of longer duration of action are required. Combination with antagonists of the prostaglandin/thromboxane A_2 receptor may be necessary to reveal their full beneficial action.
Circulation 72, No. 6, 1194–1201, 1985.

ASPIRIN irreversibly acetylates platelet cyclooxygenase and thereby inhibits production of thromboxane A_2 a potent vasoconstrictor and platelet agonist.[1, 2] These observations provided a molecular basis for prospective studies of aspirin in syndromes putatively associated with platelet activation. These trials were initially mounted on the basis of aspirin's effects on platelet aggregation[3] and retrospective data suggesting a reduced cardiovascular mortality in patients with arthritis who consumed aspirin over the long term.[4] In prospective, double-blind, placebo-controlled studies aspirin has since been shown of benefit in the prevention of transient ischemic attack and stroke,[5, 6] the prevention of death and nonfatal myocardial infarction in patients with unstable angina,[7, 8] the prevention of hemodialysis shunt occlusion[9] and, with dipyridamole, the prevention of coronary graft occlusion[10, 11] and renal deterioration in patients with membranoproliferative glomerulonephritis.[12]

The efficacy of aspirin alone in a recent study of coronary graft occlusion[13] and the similar efficacy of aspirin with or without dipyridamole in the prevention of transient ischemic attacks[14] and coronary graft occlusion[15] suggests that dipyridamole may have contributed little benefit in the last three studies cited.[10–12] Residual doubts about the efficacy of aspirin remain, however, particularly fostered by a number of negative studies in the secondary prevention of myocardial infarction.[16–18] Many factors, including delay from the time of presentation to randomization and inadequate sample size may have contributed to these results. However, it has also been suggested that the dosage of aspirin used may have resulted in coincidental depression of formation of prostacyclin, the major cyclooxygenase product of vascular endothelium and a potent inhibitor of platelet aggregation.[19] Consequently, the development of compounds that selectively inhibit thromboxane synthase[20, 21] prompted considerable interest. Unlike cyclooxygenase inhibitors, such agents would prevent formation of thromboxane A_2 with-

From the Division of Clinical Pharmacology, Vanderbilt University, Nashville.

Supported by the National Institute of Health (HL30400). Dr. FitzGerald is an Established Investigator of the American Heart Association.

Address for correspondence: Dr. G. A. FitzGerald, Division of Clinical Pharmacology, Vanderbilt University, Nashville, TN 37232.

out coincident inhibition of prostacyclin biosynthesis. Furthermore, they might actually enhance vascular prostacyclin formation if platelets could "donate" their accumulated prostaglandin endoperoxide substrate to endothelial prostacyclin synthase.[22]

Endoperoxide rediversion. A compound that enhanced vascular prostacyclin formation would be of substantial potential benefit as a platelet inhibitor in vivo. Aspirin-like drugs might be expected to prevent thromboxane-dependent platelet activation. However, many endogenous mediators of platelet activation, such as thrombin and collagen, could stimulate aggregation despite the presence of aspirin. Prostacyclin, by increasing platelet cyclic AMP, prevents platelet aggregation induced by all known agonists and has been shown to disaggregate aggregated platelets in vitro.[23] Multiple agonists are likely to act in concert in vivo, so even in a syndrome of platelet-mediated vascular occlusion, inhibition of thromboxane formation alone would not be expected to be completely effective. Enhanced production of prostacyclin, particularly at the site of platelet-vessel wall interaction, as envisaged by the endoperoxide rediversion or "steal" hypothesis,[24] might represent an important advantage over aspirin.

Initial attempts to demonstrate endoperoxide rediversion were unsuccessful.[25] However, Marcus et al.[26] demonstrated that in a perturbed mixture of endothelial cells and platelets, approximately half of the prostacyclin produced by the endothelial cells originated from platelet endoperoxides. This phenomenon was amplified by thromboxane synthase inhibitors. These observations, which were subsequently confirmed by others,[27] provide important experimental support for the concept of endoperoxide transfer. However, the model lacks important components such as flow, shear stress, and albumin (which avidly binds eicosenoids[28]), which operate in vivo. Early reports that were purported to demonstrate an increase in plasma 6-keto-prostaglandin (PG)$F_{1\alpha}$ after administration of a thromboxane synthase inhibitor to human volunteers[29] were uninterpretable due to methodologic shortcomings.[30] More commonly, inhibitors were screened for evidence of endoperoxide rediversion by measurement of immunoreactive thromboxane B_2 and 6-keto-$PGF_{1\alpha}$ formation in serum in vitro or ex vivo.[31, 32] However, although 6-keto-$PGF_{1\alpha}$ is formed in small amounts in whole blood,[33] immunoreactive 6-keto-$PGF_{1\alpha}$ may greatly overestimate actual 6-keto-$PGF_{1\alpha}$ formation in serum in the presence of a thromboxane synthase inhibitor.[34] PGE_2, $PGF_{2\alpha}$, and PGD_2 are formed in much greater amounts than 6-keto-$PGF_{1\alpha}$ in serum in the presence of a synthase inhibitor.[33] Thus, although cross reactivity of a 6-keto-$PGF_{1\alpha}$ antibody with these compounds may be small in percentage terms, increased PGE_2, $PGF_{2\alpha}$, or PGD_2 production would be likely to introduce a substantial quantitative artifact into estimates of 6-keto-$PGF_{1\alpha}$ production in the presence of a synthase inhibitor. Confirmation of this hypothesis was obtained by measurement of both thromboxane B_2 and 6-keto-$PGF_{1\alpha}$ by radioimmunoassay and gas chromatography–mass spectrometry in serum with and without addition of the thromboxane synthase inhibitor dazoxiben.[34]

An alternative approach to the detection of enhanced prostacyclin formation after the administration of these compounds has been the measurement of 2,3-dinor-6-keto-$PGF_{1\alpha}$ (PGI-M), a major urinary prostacyclin metabolite in man.[35] We have conducted three double-blind, short-term studies with structurally distinct thromboxane synthase inhibitors.[36–38] PGI-M excretion increased approximately two- to threefold after two of these compounds, dazoxiben and CGS 13080, while the increase after dazmagrel was less marked. Assuming that the "basal" level of 6-keto-$PGF_{1\alpha}$ is 2 to 3 pg/ml or less,[39, 40] a threefold increment would result in levels that are still below the limits of sensitivity of most assay systems. This is consistent with the marginal increase in plasma 6-keto-$PGF_{1\alpha}$ reported by Patrignani et al.[41] after administration of dazoxiben to volunteers. Obviously, such an increment would be insufficient to result in circulating concentrations of prostacyclin of biological significance. However, it might reflect production at sites of platelet–vessel wall interaction that could be relevant to local thromboresistance. It is also of interest that in patients with severe peripheral vascular disease, prostacyclin metabolite excretion is increased three- to fourfold.[42] Finally, although these data are consistent with the vascular steal hypothesis, it is important to remember that one cannot definitively attribute a tissue of origin to metabolites measured in urine. It is possible that the increment in PGI-M reflects its production by a tissue other than vascular endothelium.

In summary, information has been provided in constrained circumstances in vitro that demonstrates enhanced transfer of platelet endoperoxides to vascular prostacyclin synthase in the presence of thromboxane synthase inhibitors. Data compatible with this mechanism has been obtained after short-term administration of thromboxane synthase inhibitors in vivo.

"Nonresponse" to thromboxane synthase inhibition. Bertele et al.[43] reported interindividual differences in the platelet-inhibitory response to thromboxane synthase inhibitors in vitro. Despite efficient inhibition of thromboxane formation, some "nonresponders" would fully aggregate in response to collagen or arachidonate.[43] A possible explanation for this phenomenon is substitution for the platelet-aggregatory effects of thromboxane A_2 by prostaglandin endoperoxides at their common receptor site[44] during thromboxane synthase inhibition. An alternative explanation would be differential rates of platelet uptake of the inhibitor between individuals. We performed experiments with the use of the lag time to 50% maximal aggregation induced by arachidonic acid as a sensitive index of inhibition of arachidonate-dependent aggregation.[45, 46] Prolongation of the time platelets were preincubated with a thromboxane synthase inhibitor, dazoxiben, progressively prolonged the lag time and ultimately inhibited aggregation (figure 1). In further experiments, we found that prolongation of the lag time was reflected by increasing inhibition of platelet thromboxane generation and conversion of "nonresponders" into "responders" (figure 2). In some individuals, however, despite prolongation of the preincubation time to 10 min and comparable inhibition of platelet thromboxane production, full aggregation was preserved. In such true nonresponsers, aggregation was completely inhibited by coincubation with both dazoxiben and 5-*endo*-(6′-caboxyhex-2′Z-enyl-6-*exo* *N*-(phenylcarbamoyl) hydrazono methyl-*becyclo* 2,2,1 heptane (EPO45; a gift of Dr. R. L. Jones),[47] an antagonist of the shared thromboxane A_2/prostaglandin endoperoxide receptor (figure 3). Responder status may also be altered by adenylate cyclase inhibitors[48] or influenced by the proaggregatory properties of PGE_2 and the antiaggregatory properties of PGD_2.[49] However, nonresponders and responders do not differ with respect to generation of PGE_2 and PGD_2[49] and complete inhibition of platelet aggregation by thromboxane A_2/endoperoxide antagonists suggests that endoperoxides play the predominant role.

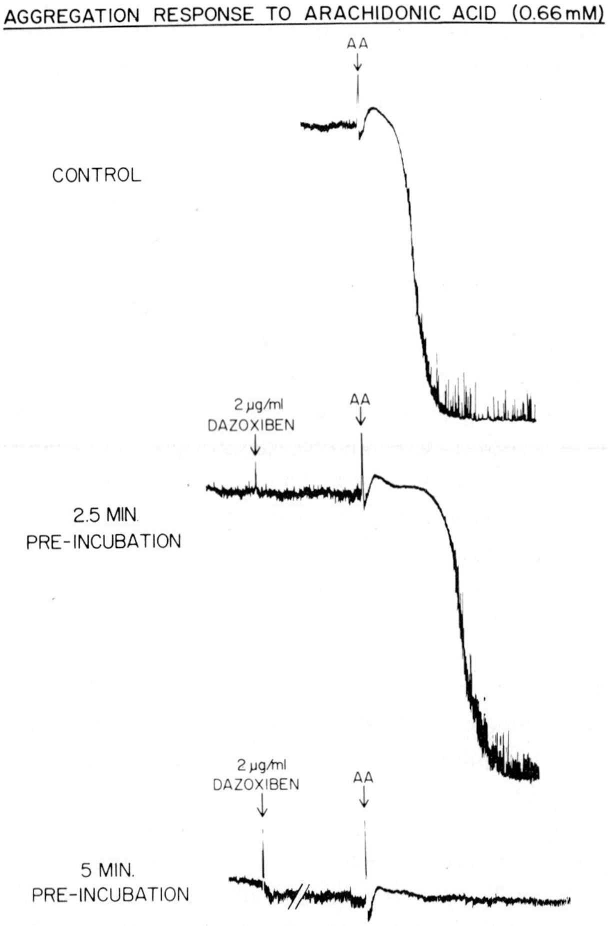

FIGURE 1. Preincubation of platelets for 2.5 min with a thromboxane synthase inhibitor, dazoxiben (2μg/ml), prolonged the lag time to 50% of full aggregation induced by arachidonic acid (1.33 mM). Preincubation of the platelets with dazoxiben for a longer period (5 min) permitted complete inhibition of platelet aggregation.

In summary, experiments in vitro suggest that prostaglandin endoperoxides may substitute for the proaggregatory effects of thromboxane A_2 during efficient synthase inhibition. Even responders demonstrate less marked inhibition of platelet aggregation ex vivo than would be anticipated on the basis of comparable inhibition of thromboxane formation by aspirin.[37]

Clinical trials with thromboxane synthase inhibitors. In contrast to their efficacy in certain short-term models of platelet activation,[50–54] the experience with thromboxane synthase inhibitors in clinical trials has been unencouraging. Although the greatest experience has been gained with dazoxiben, the first of these compounds to be studied in man,[55] the human pharmacology of the subsequently developed inhibitors suggests that their effects would be similar.

Dazoxiben has been studied in human syndromes putatively associated with platelet activation. For example, Belch et al.[56] administered a daily dose of 400 mg for 6 weeks to patients with Raynaud's phenomenon. Subjective clinical improvement occurred in some patients treated with dazoxiben, but there was no improvement in the objective parameters (hand temperature, plasma viscosity, and red cell deformability). Furthermore, two double-blind placebo-controlled studies in patients with Raynaud's phenomenon have failed to detect any benefit from dazoxiben. Luderer et al.[57] found no improvement in total digital blood flow, capillary flow, or forearm blood flow at 28° or 20° C in 21 patients receiving 100 mg dazoxiben four times a day for 2 weeks. Ettinger et al.[58] reported that the subjective evaluation of severity of disease and episode rate were unaltered by dazoxiben. Recently, we have failed to demonstrate efficacy in a double-

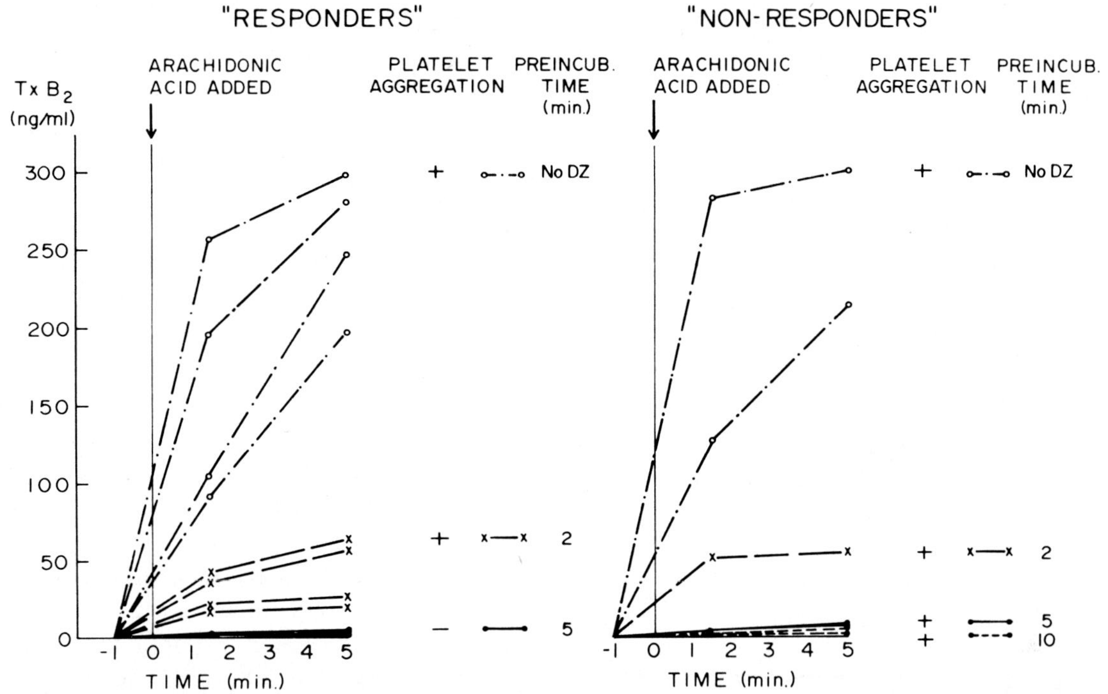

FIGURE 2. In responders platelet aggregation to arachidonic acid (1.33 mM) persisted despite preincubation with dazoxiben (DZ) for 2 min, reducing thromboxane (Tx) B_2 generation in the platelet-rich plasma from 252 ± 19 ng/ml (mean ± SEM) to 47 ± 8 ng/ml. Further prolongation of the DZ preincubation time to 5 min completely prevented thromboxane formation and inhibited arachidonic acid–induced aggregation. In nonresponders, inhibition of thromboxane formation was quantitatively similar to that observed in responders. However, despite prolongation of the DZ preincubation time to 10 min and complete inhibition of thromboxane formation, a full aggregation response to arachidonic acid was observed.

blind placebo-controlled study of another thromboxane synthase inhibitor (CGS 13080 100 mg qid and 200 mg qid) in patients with severe peripheral vascular disease.[59] Zipser et al.[60] have recently reported that the imidazole analog dazmagrel has no effect on renal or hepatic function in patients with the hepatorenal syndrome. A reported benefit of dazoxiben therapy in patients with diabetic nephropathy based on a reduction in microalbuminuria[61] has not been confirmed by a subsequent, larger study.*

Long-term dosing studies with thromboxane synthase inhibitors have not been reported in patients with primary cardiac disease. McGibney et al.[62] have reported that predosing with dazoxiben (100 mg) failed to influence the time to exercise-induced angina despite the inhibition of thromboxane formation in serum ex vivo by 80% or more. Reuben et al.[63] performed a double-blind randomized crossover study of 200 mg dazoxiben four times daily for 7 days in patients with stable angina who had had a positive stress test. Serum thromboxane B_2 was reduced by approximately 80% at the time of exercise testing during dazoxiben therapy. No change was observed in the duration of exercise to angina, the cumulative ST depression, the angina attack rate or in glyceryl trinitrate consumption. Kiff et al.[64] reported that pretreatment with 200 mg dazoxiben had no effect on the hemodynamic response to atrial pacing in patients with chronic stable angina. Lactate extraction and the percentage oxygen uptake were also unaltered. By contrast, Thaulow et al.[65] reported that pretreatment with dazoxiben (200 mg) reduced lactate accumulation and ST depression during pacing-induced angina. Myocardial extraction of free fatty acids and the arteriovenous oxygen difference were unaltered by dazoxiben. However, the changes in lactate accumulation in this study were marginal, and the study did not include a placebo group.

Let us consider several factors that might explain the discrepancy between the efficacy of thromboxane synthase inhibitors in short-term animal preparations of thrombosis and their lack of effect in clinical studies.

The role of thromboxane A_2 in the syndromes studied. Although the clinical conditions that have been studied are putatively associated with platelet activation, evidence of increased thromboxane biosynthesis has generally not been provided. However, despite documentation of increased thromboxane formation in vivo in patients with the hepatorenal syndrome[60] and severe peripheral vascular disease[59] by acceptable methodolo-

*Tyler H: Personal communication.

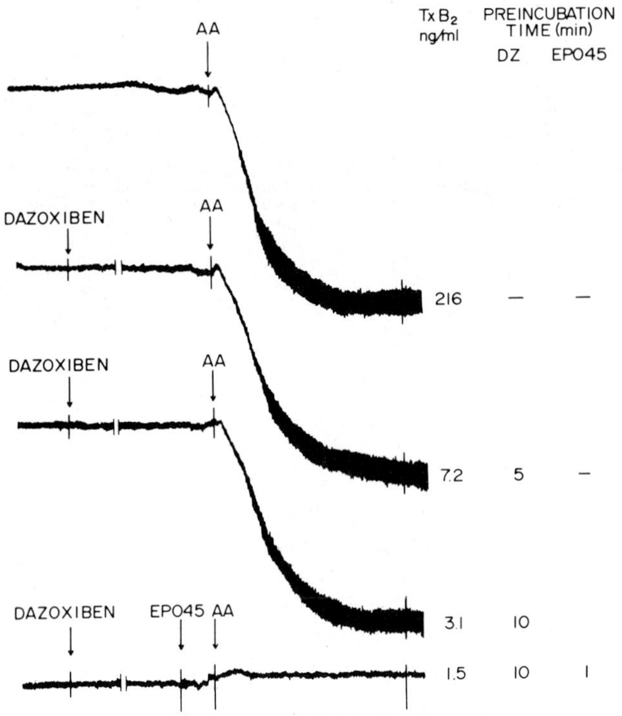

FIGURE 3. Aggregation of platelet-rich plasma to arachidonic acid (1.33 mM) resulted in formation of 216 ng/ml thromboxane (Tx) B_2 6 min after addition of the agonist. Preincubation with the thromboxane synthase inhibitor dazoxiben did not alter the aggregatory response in this nonresponder, despite inhibition of thromboxane formation. Coincubation with dazoxiben and the antagonist of the prostaglandin endoperoxide/thromboxane A_2 receptor EPO45 completely inhibited aggregation.

gy, in controlled studies with synthase inhibitors no effect was observed. Similarly, although increased thromboxane formation was not documented in the studies of patients with Raynaud's phenomenon,[56–58] we have recently found that such patients do indeed excrete excessive quantities of the urinary thromboxane metabolite 2,3-dinor-thromboxane B_2. Thus, in these long-term dosing studies, one assumes that the synthase inhibitors were ineffective either because thromboxane formation was an epiphenomenon of little relevance to the clinical syndrome or that it was of importance but that the compounds studied inadequately blocked its biological action. Although synthase inhibitors fail to alter the response to exercise and pacing in patients with chronic stable angina in short-term dosing studies, the only investigations that have suggested that thromboxane formation is enhanced in these settings have been based on plasma immunoreactive thromboxane B_2. These reports are likely to have been confounded by platelet thromboxane formation ex vivo and/or problems of analytic methodology.[30]

In summary, despite enhanced in vivo thromboxane synthesis in patients with Raynaud's phenomenon, severe peripheral vascular disease, and the hepatorenal syndrome, conventional long-term dosage schedules for thromboxane synthase inhibitors have proven ineffective. The effects of short-term administration of synthase inhibitors in pacing- and exercise-induced angina have also been unconvincing. However, whether thromboxane formation is increased in these settings remains to be determined. Two reports suggest that short-term administration of thromboxane synthase inhibitors may reduce the incidence of ventricular fibrillation after coronary artery occlusion in the dog.[66, 67] Whether thromboxane formation is enhanced in this setting has yet to be established and the antiarrhythmic properties of thromboxane synthase inhibition remain to be explored in man.

Is thromboxane formation adequately suppressed throughout the dosing interval in long-term dosing studies? Studies of platelet function both in vitro and ex vivo indicate that maximal (~100%) inhibition of platelet cyclooxygenase is necessary to inhibit thromboxane-dependent platelet activation. Thus, clinical benefit may be anticipated only when inhibition of thromboxane is complete. All of the compounds that have been developed thus far are reversible inhibitors of thromboxane synthase. Plasma drug half-lives vary from ~45 to ~90 min. However, more attention has been paid to the "biological" half-lives. These are calculated from the recovery of platelet thromboxane formation ex vivo after inhibition by short-term administration of a synthase inhibitor and have varied from ~3 to 6 hr. This discrepancy has not been explained by the identification of active drug metabolites, but can be readily anticipated from well-characterized plasma drug kinetic-dynamic relationships.[68] This factor appears to have been ignored during the design of long-term dosing studies with these inhibitors, since the dosing interval has been based on the biological half-life. When dosing interval is based on plasma drug half-life, the pharmacokinetic assumption of accumulation to a steady-state effect in three to four half-lives is readily verified. However, no such assumptions can be derived from the employment of biological half-life. Thus, in a study of patients with severe peripheral vascular disease,[59] recovery of thromboxane formation ex vivo and in vivo was just as rapid after administration of the twenty-fifth dose as after the first. Recovery of thromboxane formation would also be consistent with the discrepancy between the efficacy of thromboxane synthase inhibition in certain short-term animal preparations — in which observations are usually made during the period of maximal thromboxane inhibition — and the lack of effect during long-term dosing studies in human disease. Although little data are available that permit direct testing of this hypothesis in man, it is noteworthy that despite the failure of long-term dosing with inhibitors to ameliorate Raynaud's phenomenon, a condition associated with enhanced thromboxane biosynthesis, Cowley et al.[69] have demonstrated that short-term administration of dazoxiben suppressed cold-induced vasoconstriction when blood flow was measured at the time of maximal inhibition of thromboxane formation.

In summary, these results suggest that substantial recovery of thromboxane formation is likely to have occurred during the dosing interval in published long-term dosing studies of thromboxane synthase inhibitors. Consequently, even if thromboxane-dependent platelet activation were of relevance to the clinical condition studied, benefit would not be anticipated.

Prostaglandin endoperoxides might substitute for the biological action of thromboxane A_2 during inhibition of the synthase enzyme. Experiments in vitro, as outlined above, combining antagonists of the thromboxane A_2/prostaglandin endoperoxide receptor with synthase inhibitors, suggest that endoperoxides may continue to mediate proaggregatory effects on platelets despite inhibition of thromboxane formation. Data supportive of the concept that this may be of importance in vivo are provided by the observation ex vivo of platelet nonresponders to thromboxane synthase inhibitors. Indeed, even responders demonstrate markedly less inhibition of platelets ex vivo than is obtained after comparable inhibition of thromboxane biosynthesis with aspirin. However, direct evidence in support of this hypothesis is unavailable from human experiments. We have recently addressed this issue by comparing the efficacy of a thromboxane/prostaglandin endoperoxide antagonist, a synthesis inhibitor, and their combination in a canine preparation of coronary vascular occlusion.[70, 71] The parameters of this preparation can be set so that occlusion becomes prostaglandin endoperoxide–dependent in the presence of a synthase inhibitor. Under these circumstances, the antagonist, but not the synthesis inhibitor, prolongs the time to occlusion. This supports the concept of endoperoxide-dependent platelet activation in vivo. Furthermore, combination with the synthase inhibitor improved the efficacy of the antagonist in this preparation, as would be anticipated from increased formation of vasodilator platelet-inhibitory eicosanoids at sites of platelet-vascular interaction.

In conclusion, the future place of thromboxane synthase inhibitors in the treatment of vasoocclusive disease in man is dependent on the importance of thromboxane A_2 and prostacyclin as mediators of platelet and vascular homeostasis in vivo. The development of sensitive methods of measuring enzymatic metabolites of thromboxane in urine[72] and plasma[73] and the availability of receptor antagonists are likely to clarify the role of thromboxane A_2 in the coming years. The efficacy of synthase inhibitors is perhaps especially dependent on a role for prostacyclin in the preservation of endothelial thromboresistance. If prostacyclin is important, inhibition of platelet function without depression of vascular prostacyclin formation would be indeed desirable. However, such "selectivity" can be approached with aspirin.[74–76] More importantly, enhanced formation of prostacyclin at sites of platelet-vascular interaction might be a particular advantage of the use of this class of compounds since prostacyclin inhibits platelet activation by both thromboxane-dependent and thromboxane-independent mechanisms. Finally, even if these assumptions are proven to be facts, modifications of either drug structure or delivery will be necessary to prolong the duration of maximal thromboxane inhibition throughout the dosing interval. Combination of synthesis inhibitors with receptor antagonists may be necessary to realize the full therapeutic potential of these interesting compounds.

References

1. Roth GJ, Majerus PW: The mechanism of the effect of aspirin on human platelets. J Clin Invest **56:** 624, 1975
2. Hamberg M, Svensson J, Samuelsson B: Thromboxanes: a new group of biologically active compounds derived from prostaglandin endoperoxides. Proc Natl Acad Sci USA **72:** 2994, 1975
3. O'Brien JR: Effects of salicylates on human platelets. Lancet **1:** 779, 1968
4. Coronary Drug Project Research Group: Aspirin in coronary heart disease. J Chron Dis **29:** 625, 1978
5. Fields WS, Lemak NA, Frankowski RF, Hardy RJ: Controlled trial of aspirin in cerebral ischemia. Stroke **8:** 301, 1977
6. Aspirin Myocardial Infarction Study Research Group: A randomized controlled trial of aspirin in persons recovering from myocardial infarction. JAMA **243:** 661, 1980
7. Lewis HD, David JW, Archibald DG, Steinke WE, Smitherman TC, Daugherty JE, Schnaper JW, LeWinter MM, Leonaras E, Pouget JM, Sabharwal SC, Chesler C, DeMotte H: Protective effects of aspirin against acute myocardial infarction and death in man with unstable angina. N Engl J Med **309:** 396, 1983
8. Cairns J, Gent M, Singer J, Finnie K, Froggatt G, Holder D, Jablonsky G, Kostuk W, Melendez L, Myers M, Sackett D, Sealey B, Tanzer P: A study of aspirin and/or sulfinpyrazone in unstable angina. Circulation **70**(suppl II): 415, 1984 (abst)
9. Harter HR, Burch JW, Majerus PW, Stanford M, Delmas JA, Anderson CB, Weerts CA: Prevention of thrombosis in patients on hemodialysis by low dose aspirin. N Engl J Med **301:** 577, 1979
10. Chesebro JH, Clements IP, Fuster V, Elveback LR, Smith HC, Bardsley WT, Frye RL, Holmes DR, Vlietstra RE, Pluth JR, Wallace RB, Puga FJ, Orszulak TA, Piehler JM, Schaff HV, Danielson GK: A platelet inhibitor drug trial in coronary artery bypass operations. Benefit of perioperative dipyridamole and aspirin therapy on early postoperative vein graft patency. N Engl J Med **307:** 73, 1982
11. Chesebro JH, Fuster V, Elveback LR, Clements IP, Smith HC, Holmes DR, Bardsley WT, Pluth JR, Wallace RB, Puga FJ, Orszulate TA, Piehler JM, Danielson GK, Schaff HV, Frye RL: Effects

of dipyridamole and aspirin on late vein-graft patency after coronary bypass operations. N Engl J Med **310:** 209, 1984
12. Donadio JV, Anderson CF, Mitchell JC III, Holley KE, Ilstrap DM, Fuster V, Chesebro JH: Membranoproliferative glomerulonephritis: A prospective trial of platelet inhibitor therapy. N Engl J Med **310:** 1421, 1984
13. Lorenz RL, Weber M, Kotzur J, Theisen K, Schacky CV, Meister W, Reichardt B, Weber PC: Improved aortocoronary bypass patency by low-dose aspirin (100 mg daily). Lancet **1:** 1261, 1984
14. Bousser MG, Eschwege E, Hagunau M, Lefaucconnier JM, Thibult N, Touboul D, Touboul PJ: "AICLA" controlled trial of aspirin and dipyridamole in the secondary prevention of athero-thrombotic cerebral ischemia. Stroke **14:** 5, 1983
15. Brown RG, Chukingnan RA, DeRoven T, Geode LV, Fee HJ, Roth JA, Carey JS: Improved graft patency in patients treated with platelet-inhibiting therapy after coronary bypass therapy. Circulation **72:** 138, 1985
16. Elwood PC, Cochran AL, Burr ML, Sweetnam PM, Williams G, Wellsby E, Hughes SJ, Wenton RA: A randomized controlled trial of acetyl salicylic acid in the secondary prevention of mortality from myocardial infarction. Br Med J **1:** 436, 1974
17. Aspirin Myocardial Infarction Study Research Group: A randomized controlled trial of aspirin in persons recovered from myocardial infarction. JAMA **243:** 661, 1980
18. Elwood PC, Sweetnam PM: Aspirin and secondary mortality after myocardial infarction. Lancet **2:** 1313, 1979
19. Bunting SR, Gryglewski R, Moncada SA, Vane JR: Arterial walls generate from prostaglandin endoperoxides a substance (prostaglandin X) which relaxes strips of mesenteric and coeliac arteries and inhibits platelet aggregation. Prostaglandins **12:** 897, 1976
20. Kulkarni P, Eakins KE: N–011064 inhibits generation of thromboxane A_2-like activity from prostaglandin endoperoxides by human platelet microsomes. Prostaglandins **12:** 465, 1976
21. Gorman RR, Bundy GL, Pederson DC, Sun FF, Miller OV, Fitzpatrick FA: Inhibition of human platelet thromboxane synthetase by 9,11-azoprosta-5,13-dienoic acid. Proc Natl Acad Sci USA **74:** 4007, 1977
22. Needleman P: Prostacyclin and blood vessel platelet interactions. Perspectives and questions. Nature **279:** 14, 1979
23. Gryglewski RJ, Bunting S, Moncada S, Flower RJ, Vane JR: Arterial walls are protected against deposition of platelet thrombin by a substance (prostaglandin X) which they make from prostaglandin endoperoxides. Prostaglandins **12:** 685, 1976
24. Fitzpatrick FA, Gorman RR: A comparison on imidazole and 9,11-azoprosta-5,13-dienoic acid: two selective thromboxane synthetase inhibitors. Biochim Biophys Acta **539:** 162, 1978
25. Needleman P, Wyche A, Raz A: Platelet and blood vessel arachidonate metabolism and interactions. J Clin Invest **63:** 345, 1979
26. Marcus AJ, Weksler BB, Jaffe EA, Broekman MJ: Synthesis of prostacyclin from platelet derived endoperoxides by cultured human endothelial cells. J Clin Invest **66:** 979, 1980
27. Schafer AI, Crawford DD, Gimbrone MA: Unidirectional transfer of prostaglandin endoperoxides between platelets and endothelial cells. J Clin Invest **73:** 1105, 1984
28. Wynalda MA, Fitzpatrick FA: Albumins stabilize prostaglandin I_2 Prostaglandins **20:** 853, 1980
29. Vermylen J, Defreyn NG, Carreras AS, Machin SJ, Scaeren JV, Verstraete M: Thromboxane synthetase inhibition as an antithrombotic strategy. Lancet **1:** 1073, 1981
30. FitzGerald GA, Pedersen AK, Patrono C: Analysis of prostacyclin and thromboxane A_2 biosynthesis in cardiovascular disease. Circulation **67:** 1174, 1983
31. Perry MJ, Randall MJ, Tyler HM, Myhre E, Dale J, Thaulow WE: Selective inhibition of thromboxane synthetase by dazoxiben increases prostacyclin production by leukocytes in angina patients and healthy volunteers. Lancet **2:** 164, 1982
32. Maguire ED, Wallis RB: In vivo redirection of prostaglandin endoperoxides into 6-keto-$PGF_{1\alpha}$ formation by thromboxane synthase inhibitors in the rat. Thromb Res **32:** 15, 1983
33. Orchard MA, Blair IA, Dollery CT, Lewis PJ: Blood can synthesize prostacyclin. Lancet **2:** 565, 1983
34. Pedersen AK, Watson M, FitzGerald GA: Inhibition of thromboxane synthase in serum: limitations of the measurement of immunoreactive 6-keto-$PGF_{1\alpha}$. Thromb Res **33:** 99, 1983
35. Brash AR, Jackson EK, Saggese C, Lawson J, Oates JA, FitzGerald GA: The metabolic disposition of prostacyclin in man. J Pharmacol Exp Ther **266:** 78, 1983
36. FitzGerald GA, Brash AR, Oates JA, Pedersen AK: Endogenous prostacyclin biosynthesis and platelet function during selective inhibition of thromboxane synthase in man. J Clin Invest **71:** 1336, 1983
37. FitzGerald GA, Oates JA: Selective and nonselective inhibition of thromboxane formation. Clin Pharmacol Ther **35:** 633, 1984
38. Reilly IAG, FitzGerald GA: Platelet function, prostanoids and combined inhibition of thromboxane synthase and cyclooxygenase. A double blind controlled study. Proceedings of the Ninth International Congress Pharmacology. London, 1985
39. FitzGerald GA, Brash AR, Falardeau P, Oates JA: Estimated rate of prostacyclin secretion into the circulation of normal man. J Clin Invest **68:** 1271, 1981
40. Blair IA, Barrow SE, Waddell KA, Lewis PJ, Dollery CT: Prostacyclin is not a circulating hormone in man. Prostaglandins **23:** 579, 1982
41. Patrignani P, Filabozzi P, Catella F, Pugliese F, Patrono C: Differential effects of dazoxiben, a selective thromboxane synthase inhibitor on platelet and renal prostaglandin endoperoxide metabolism. J Pharmacol Exp Ther **228:** 472, 1984
42. FitzGerald GA, Smith B, Pedersen AK, Brash AR: Prostacyclin biosynthesis is increased in patients with severe atherosclerosis and platelet activation. N Engl J Med **310:** 1065, 1984
43. Bertele V, De Gaetano G: Potentiation by dazoxiben, a thromboxane synthetase inhibitor, of platelet aggregation inhibitory activity of a thromboxane receptor antagonist and of prostacyclin. Eur J Pharmacol **85:** 331, 1982
44. LeBreton GC, Venton DL, Enke SE, Halushka PV: 13-Azoprostanoic acid: a specific antagonist of the human blood thromboxane/endoperoxide receptor. Proc Natl Acad Sci USA **76:** 4097, 1979
45. Pedersen AK, Jacobson P: Sulfinpyrazone metabolism during long-term therapy. Br J Clin Pharmacol **11:** 567, 1981
46. Pedersen AK, FitzGerald GA: Cyclooxygenase inhibition, platelet function and metabolite formation during chronic sulfinpyrazone dosing. Clin Pharmacol Ther **37:** 36, 1985
47. Jones RL, Veesapati V, Wilson NH: Antagonist of the thromboxane sensitive contractile systems of the rabbit aorta, dog saphenous vein and guinea-pig trachea. Br J Pharmacol **76:** 423, 1982
48. Bertele V, Falanga A, Tomasiak M, Cerletti C, deGaetano G: SQ 22536, an adenylate cyclase inhibitor, prevents the antiplatelet effect of dazoxiben, a thromboxane synthetase inhibitor. Thromb Haemost **51:** 125, 1984
49. Bertele V, Falanga A, Tomasiak N, Chiabrando C, Cerletti C, deGaetano G: Pharmacologic inhibition of thromboxane synthetase and platelet aggregation: modulatory role of cyclooxygenase products. Blood **63:** 1460, 1984
50. Aiken JW, Shebuski RJ, Miller OV, Gorman RR: Endogenous prostacyclin contributes to the efficacy of a thromboxane synthetase inhibitor for preventing coronary artery thrombosis. J Pharmacol Exp Ther **219:** 299, 1981
51. Schumacher WA, Lucchesi BR: Effect of the thromboxane synthetase inhibitor UK 37,248 (dazoxiben) upon platelet aggregation, coronary artery thrombosis and vascular reactivity. J Pharmacol Exp Ther **277:** 719, 1983
52. Randall MJ, Wilding RIR: Acute arterial thrombosis in rabbits: Reduced platelet accumulation after treatment with dazoxiben hydrocholoride (UK 37, 248–01). Br J Clin Pharmacol **15:** 495, 1983
53. Lefer AM, Okamatsu S, Smith EF, Smith JB: Beneficial effects of a new thromboxane synthetase inhibitor in arachidonate-induced sudden death. Thromb Res **23:** 265, 1981
54. Fukumori T, Tani E, Mauda Y, Sukenaga A: Effect of a selective inhibitor of thromboxane A_2 synthetase on experimental cerebral vasospasm. Stroke **15:** 306, 1984
55. Tyler HM, Saxton CAPD, Parry MJ: Administration to man of UK 37,248-01, a selective inhibitor of thromboxane synthestase. Lancet **1:** 629, 1981
56. Belch JJF, Cormie J, Newman P, McClaren M, Barbenel LJ, Capell H, Lieberman FP, Forbes C, Prentice CRM: Dazoxiben, a thromboxane synthetase inhibitor, in the treatment of Raynaud's syndrome: a double-blind trial Br J Clin Pharmacol **15:** 113S, 1983
57. Luderer JR, Nicholas GG, Nonamier MM, Riley DL, Vary JE, Garcia G, Schneck DW: Dazoxiben, a thromboxane synthetase

inhibitor, in Raynaud's phenomenon. Clin Pharmacol Ther **36:** 105, 1984
58. Ettinger WH, Wise RR, Schaffhauser D, Wigley FM: Controlled double-blind trial of dazoxiben and nifedipine in the treatment of Raynaud's phenomenon. Am J Med **77:** 451, 1984
59. Reilly IAG, Doran J, Smith B, FitzGerald GA: Continued platelet activation in severe atherosclerosis despite chronic administration of a thromboxane synthase inhibitor. Clin Res **33:** 287A, 1985 (abst)
60. Zipser RD, Kronborg I, Rector W, Reynolds T, Daskalopouls G: Therapeutic trial of thromboxane synthesis inhibition in the hepatorenal syndrome. Gastroenterology **87:** 1228, 1984
61. Barnett AH, Wakelin K, Leatherdale BA, Britton JR, Polak A, Bennett J, Toop M, Rowe D, Dallinger K: Specific thromboxane synthetase inhibition and albumin excretion rate in insulin dependent diabetes. Lancet **1:** 1322, 1984
62. McGibney D, Menys VC, Nelson GIC, Kumar EB, Taylor SH, Davies JA: Effects of UK 37,248, a thromboxane synthetase inhibitor, on platelet behavior in patients with coronary heart disease undergoing exercise to angina. Clin Sci 12p, 1983
63. Reuben SR, Kuan P, Cairns T, Gysle OH: Effects of dazoxiben and exercise performance in chronic stable angina. Br J Clin Pharmacol **15:** 835, 1983
64. Kiff PS, Bergman G, Atkinson L, Jewitt DE, Westwick J, Kakkar VV: Hemodynamic and metabolic effects of dazoxiben at rest and during atrial pacing. Br J Clin Pharmacol **15:** 738, 1983
65. Thaulow E, Dale J, Myhre E: Effects of a selective thromboxane synthetase inhibitor, dazoxiben, and acetyl salicylic acid on myocardial ischemia in patients with coronary heart disease. Am J Cardiol **53:** 1255, 1984
66. Coker SJ, Parrat JR: Effects of dazoxiben on arrhythmias and ventricular fibrillation induced by coronary artery occlusion and reperfusion in anaesthesized greyhounds. Br J Clin Pharmacol **15:** 875, 1983
67. Wehr CJ, Oates JA, Hammond JW: The mechanism of prevention of ventricular fibrillation arrhythmias by thromboxane synthetase inhibitors. Clin Res **33:** 236A, 1985 (abst)
68. Pedersen AK, FitzGerald GA: The human pharmacology of platelet inhibition: pharmacokinetics relevant to drug action. Circulation **72:** 1164, 1985
69. Cowley AJ, Jones EW, Hanley SP: Effects of dazoxiben, an inhibitor of thromboxane synthetase, on forearm vasoconstriction in response to cold stimulation and on human blood vessel prostacyclin production. Br J Clin Pharmacol **15:** 107S, 1983
70. FitzGerald DJ, Doran J, Jackson EK, FitzGerald GA: Coronary vascular occlusion mediated through thromboxane A_2 prostaglandin endoperoxide receptor activation in vivo. J Clin Invest (in press)
71. FitzGerald DJ, Fragetta J, FitzGerald GA: Thromboxane synthase inhibition and thromboxane A_2/endoperoxide receptor antagonism in a canine model of coronary thrombosis. Circulation **72**(suppl III): III-1688, 1985 (abst)
72. FitzGerald GA, Lawson J, Blair IA, Brash AR: Analysis of urinary metabolites of thromboxane and prostacyclin by negative ion chemical ionization gas chromatography mass spectrometry. Adv Prost Thrombox Leukotrienes Res **15:** 87, 1985
73. FitzGerald GA, Lawson J, Catella F, Patrono C: Long lived enzymatic metabolites of thromboxane. Thromb Haemost **54:** 1024, 1985 (abst)
74. Patrignani P, Filabozzi P, Patrono C: Selective cumulative inhibition of platelet thromboxane production by low dose aspirin in healthy subjects. J Clin Invest **69:** 1366, 1982
75. Pedersen AK, FitzGerald GA: Dose related pharmacokinetics of aspirin: Presystemic acetylation of platelet cyclooxygenase in man. N Engl J Med **311:** 1206, 1984
76. Siebert DJ, Bochner F, Imhoff DM, Watts S, Lloyd JV, Fields J, Gable BW: Aspirin kinetics and platelet aggregation in man. Clin Pharmacol Ther **33:** 367, 1983

Thromboxane A_2 and prostaglandin endoperoxide receptors in platelets and vascular smooth muscle

DAVID L. SAUSSY, JR., B.S., DALE E. MAIS, PH.D., DANIEL R. KNAPP, PH.D., AND PERRY V. HALUSHKA, M.D., PH.D.

ABSTRACT 9,11-Dimethylmethano-11,12-methano-16-(3-iodo-4-hydroxyphenyl)-13,14-dihydro-13-aza-15αβ-ω-tetranor-TXA_2 (I-PTA-OH), a recently synthesized thromboxane (TX) A_2/prostaglandin (PG) H_2 receptor antagonist, was shown to be a competitive antagonist of human platelet aggregation induced by the stable endoperoxide analog U46619. This antagonism was due to competitive blockade of the platelet TXA_2/PGH_2 receptor since I-PTA-OH did not antagonize the first phase of ADP-induced aggregation which is TXA_2/PGH_2 independent, nor did it inhibit TXA_2 synthesis. In addition, analysis of dose-response curves to U46619 (0.1 to 40 μM) in the presence of increasing concentrations of I-PTA-OH (0.5 to 10 μM) showed that I-PTA-OH produced a parallel rightward shift of the dose-response curve. Further analysis of the data in the form of a Schild plot yielded a straight line with a slope (m = 1.03) not significantly different from −1. These results are consistent with the notion that I-PTA-OH acts as a competitive antagonist of the TXA_2/PGH_2 receptor.
Circulation 72, No. 6, 1202–1207, 1985.

SINCE THE DISCOVERY of the prostaglandin (PG) endoperoxides PGG_2 and PGH_2[1–3] and thromboxane (TX) A_2,[4] their actions on platelets and vascular smooth muscle have been the subject of numerous investigations. Initial studies were descriptive in nature, characterizing PGG_2, PGH_2, and TXA_2 as potent vasoconstrictors[2–7] and stimulators of platelet aggregation.[3–6, 8, 9] Since the development of TX synthetase inhibitors, the potential roles of the PG endoperoxides and TXA_2 in platelet aggregation[10] and in cardiovascular diseases[11] have been studied. It was anticipated that this group of compounds could provide new therapeutic approaches for the treatment of a variety of cardiovascular diseases.[11]

More recently, the development of stable analogs of the PG endoperoxides and TXA_2, which act as either mimics or antagonists of the actions of the naturally occurring eicosanoids, has provided tools for fundamental investigations into the mechanisms of action of these compounds and the nature of their receptors. Studies with the receptor antagonists have provided some preliminary evidence for more than one class of receptors.[12] Like the TX synthetase inhibitors, the receptor antagonists also provide the promise of potential new therapeutic approaches for the treatment of a variety of cardiovascular diseases.[11]

This report provides information of the effects of 9,11-dimethylmethano-11,12-methano-16-(3-iodo-4-hydroxyphenyl)-13,14-dihydro-13-aza-15αβ-ω-tetranor-TXA_2, (I-PTA-OH), a recently synthesized[13] TXA_2/PGH_2 receptor antagonist, on human platelet aggregation. This compound was originally synthesized for its potential to be radiolabeled with ^{125}I for radioligand binding studies. Current concepts concerning platelet and vascular TXA_2/PGH_2 receptors are also reviewed.

Materials and methods

Platelet aggregation. Blood obtained by venipuncture from four healthy male subjects who had not received any medication for 2 weeks before the study was collected into plastic syringes containing 3.8% trisodium citrate (9:1). Platelet-rich plasma (PRP) was prepared by centrifugation of whole blood at 100 *g* for 30 min at room temperature. The PRP (425 μl) was added to individual silanized glass cuvettes. Platelet aggregation was monitored, by the method of Born,[14] in a Chronolog model 300 aggregometer (Havertown, PA) maintained at 37° C. Platelets were preincubated with 25 μl of indomethacin (10 μM) and 25 μl of the antagonist, I-PTA-OH, 0.5 to 10 μM (figure 1) or vehicle for 1 min before the addition of 25 μl of the aggregating agent, the stable endoperoxide analog U46619 (0.1 to 40 μm). The aggregatory response was followed for 2 min. The percent aggregation was determined 1 min after the addition of U46619. The pA_2 value for I-PTA-OH was determined by constructing

From the Departments of Pharmacology and Medicine, Medical University of South Carolina, and The Drug Science Foundation, Charleston.

Supported in part by NIH grants HL 29566 and HL 07260.

Address for correspondence: Dr. Perry V. Halushka, Department of Pharmacology, Medical University of South Carolina, 171 Ashley Ave., Charleston, SC 29425.

David Saussy is supported by a predoctoral fellowship from the State of South Carolina. Perry V. Halushka is a Burroughs Wellcome Scholar in Clinical Pharmacology.

dose-response curves to U46619 in the presence and absence of varied concentrations of I-PTA-OH, as previously described.[15, 16]

I-PTA-OH was synthesized by a previously described method.[13] A 10 mM stock solution of I-PTA-OH was prepared in ethanol and was diluted appropriately in barbital-buffered saline (final concentration of ethanol in the cuvette was 0.1%). U46619 was a generous gift of Dr. John Pike, Upjohn Company, Kalamazoo, MI.

This study was approved by the Institutional Review Board of the Medical University of South Carolina. Written informed consent was obtained from all subjects.

TX synthetase assay. The effect of I-PTA-OH on platelet TX synthetase was measured in human platelet homogenates. PRP was prepared as described above. Platelet pellets were prepared from PRP by centrifugation at 650 *g* for 20 min and resuspended in 25 mM Tris HC1, pH 7.4. Platelet homogenates were prepared from the resuspended platelet pellets by 20 passes of a tight-fitting Dounce glass homogenizer. Platelet homogenates (1 ml) were preincubated with either vehicle or 10 μM I-PTA-OH for 1 min at 37° C before the addtion of 1 mM arachidonic acid (Nucheck Prep, Elesyian, MN). Samples (100 μl) were removed at 15, 30, and 60 sec intervals, immediately added to 900 μl of 500 μM imidazole to stop synthesis of TXA_2, and quick-frozen in a dry ice–acetone bath. TXA_2 was measured as its stable metabolite, $iTXB_2$ (immunoreactive TXB_2), by a previously described radioimmunoassay.[17] Protein was determined by the method of Lowry et al.[18]

Statistics. $iTXB_2$ levels in control (vehicle) and treated (10 μM I-PTA-OH) platelet homogenates were compared with Student's t test for paired observations.[19]

Results

To determine if I-PTA-OH was an antagonist of the platelet TXA_2/PGH_2 receptor, platelets were aggregated with U46619. The latter is considered to be a TXA_2/PGH_2 receptor agonist. I-PTA-OH produced a dose-dependent inhibition of U46619-induced platelet aggregation (figure 2). As shown in figure 3, increasing concentrations of I-PTA-OH produced successive parallel shifts in the dose-response curves to U46619. The Schild plot[15, 16] of the data (figure 4) revealed a straight line with a slope not significantly different from −1. Thus, I-PTA-OH appears to be a competitive inhibitor of U46619-induced platelet aggregation. The pA_2 value (6.68) yields a K_d of 208 nM for I-PTA-OH. I-PTA-OH had no effect on the first phase of ADP-induced aggregation.[12]

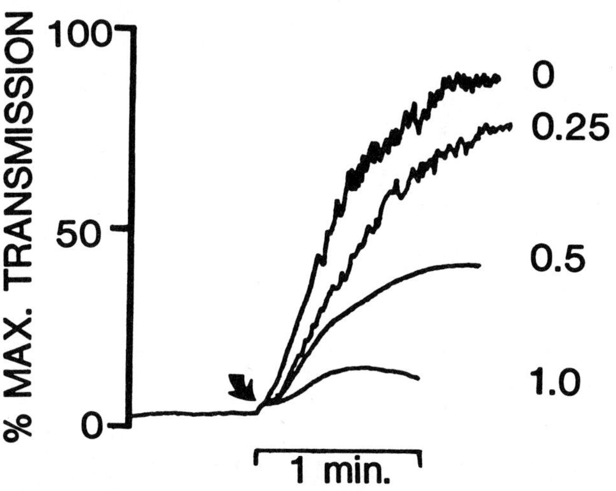

FIGURE 2. Dose-dependent inhibition of U46619-induced human platelet aggregation by I-PTA-OH. U46619 (1 μM) was added to the cuvette containing PRP, 10 μM indomethacin and I-PTA-OH, or vehicle, and the aggregation response was followed for 1 min. Numbers to the right of the trace indicate the concentration (in μM) of I-PTA-OH present. Experiments were performed as described in methods.

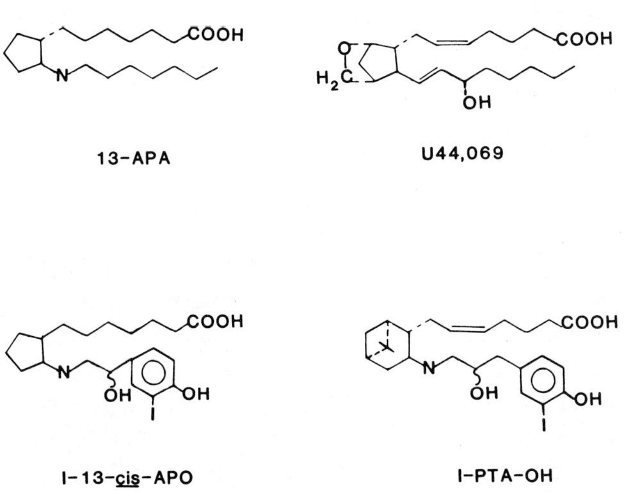

FIGURE 1. Structures of radiolabeled PGH_2/TXA_2 receptor agonists or antagonists used in radioligand binding studies. 13-APA and U44069 are labeled with ^3H, and I-*cis*-13-APO and I-PTA-OH are labeled with ^{125}I.

I-PTA-OH (10 μM) did not have any significant effect on platelet TX synthetase, as assayed in human platelet homogenates. Sixty seconds after the addition of 1 mM arachidonic acid, $iTXB_2$ was 6.5 ± 1.4 ng/mg protein in control samples and 6.4 ± 1.9 ng/mg protein in 10 μM I-PTA-OH–treated samples (n = 3, p > .05).

Discussion

Until recently characterization of TXA_2/PGH_2 receptors has been predominately by pharmacologic approaches. The use of radiolabeled ligands for characterization of the receptors has lagged behind the pharmacologic approach. The major reason for this has been the unavailability of a suitable radiolabeled ligand. In particular, these efforts have been hampered by the lack of molecules with high affinity for the putative receptors and that may be easily radiolabeled to high specific activity and retain biological activity. Figure 1 shows the ligands that have been synthesized and used for radioligand binding studies to date.

The first molecule to be synthesized and used for radioligand binding assays was [^{3}H]-13-azaprostanoic

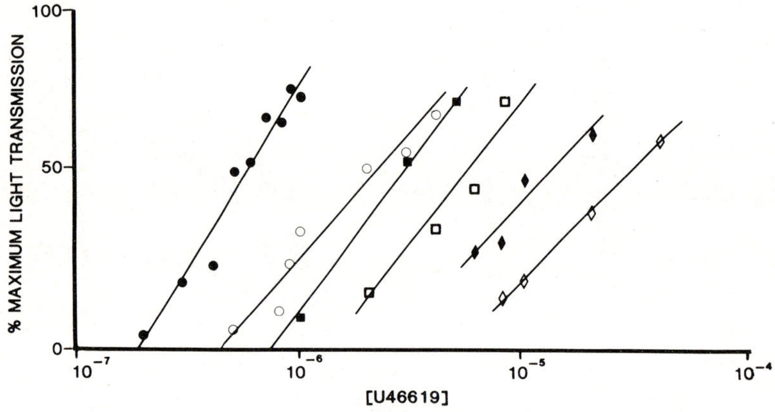

FIGURE 3. Dose-response curves for platelet aggregation induced by U46619 (determined 1 min after U46619) in the presence of vehicle (closed circles), 500 nM I-PTA-OH (open circles), 1 μM I-PTA-OH (closed squares), 2.5 μM I-PTA-OH (open squares), 5 μM I-PTA-OH (closed diamonds), and 10 μM I-PTA-OH (open diamonds). Each point represents the mean of values obtained in PRP of two to four donors. Experiments were performed as indicated in Methods.

acid (13-APA) (figure 1), a TXA_2/PGH_2 antagonist.[20, 21] Experiments with [^{3}H]-13-APA and human platelet membranes demonstrated that the binding of the drug was saturable, stereospecific, and displaceable by a series of compounds thought to interact with TXA_2/PGH_2 receptors in human platelets.[22] However, this compound will probably prove not to be an ideal ligand since its potency is too low to make it suitable for extensive radioligand binding studies. There was also a 100-fold discrepancy between the reported K_d and the concentration at which it inhibited 50% (IC_{50}) of U46619-induced platelet aggregation. In addition, [^{3}H]-13-APA was displaced from its binding site by

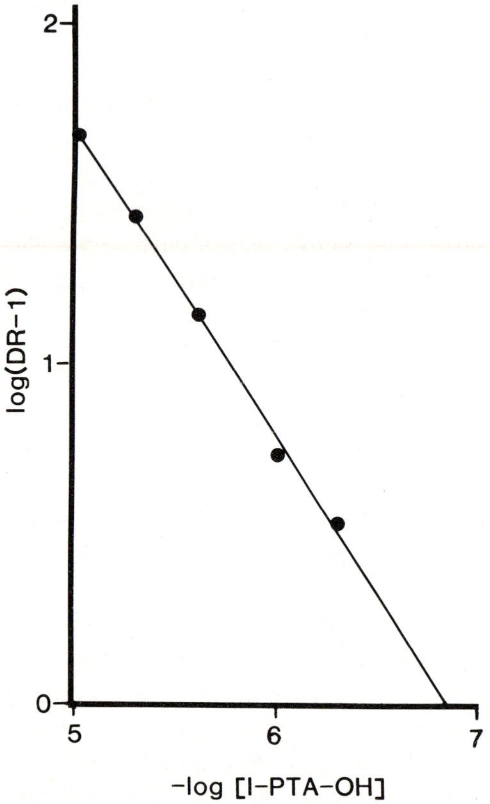

FIGURE 4. Schild plot of data illustrated in figure 3. The equation for the line is y = 1.03x + 6.85.

$PGF_{2\alpha}$, a compound that reportedly does not act at the TXA_2/PGH_2 receptor,[23, 24] although this is somewhat controversial.[25]

Radiolabeled ligand binding studies with [$_3$H]-U44069 (figure 1), a stable PGH_2 analog, have also been conducted with the use of intact washed human platelets.[24] With this ligand, it was shown that binding was sensitive to the stereochemistry of the C-15 OH group. In addition, a series of full and partial agonists and antagonists of TXA_2/PGH_2 displaced the bound ligand with potency ratios similar to those found for their pharmacologic activities in platelets. More recently, with the use of the same ligand,[26] it was found that there was a correlation between receptor occupancy by the ligand, induction of phosphatidate formation, and elevation of cytosolic free calcium levels in human platelets, thus establishing pharmacologic relevance to the binding site.

Work in our laboratory has focused on the synthesis and pharmacologic characterization of a series of TXA_2/PGH_2 antagonists, two of which have been radiolabeled with ^{125}I and used in radioligand binding studies. The first such compound synthesized, *cis*-7-(2-p-hydroxyphenylethanolaminocyclopentyl) heptanoic acid (*cis*-13-APO) (figure 1), a structural analog of 13-APA, was iodinated by a modification of the chloramine T method. It was successfully used in radioligand binding studies, thus demonstrating the utility of ^{125}I-labeled ligands in characterizing platelet TXA_2/ PGH_2 receptors.[27] The iodinated molecule retained the biological activity of the parent compound, although there was some loss of activity. The amount of radioiodinated material that bound to membranes from human platelets was saturable, displaceable, dependent on protein concentration, and was reduced by treatment with trypsin or inactivation of the protein by boiling. In addition, the K_d determined from binding studies agreed well with the IC_{50} obtained from platelet aggregation experiments.

However, I-*cis*-13-APO, like 13-APA, proved to be of insufficient potency to be useful for extensive investigations of platelet TXA_2/PGH_2 receptors. Therefore, a series of compounds were synthesized that are derivatives of 13-azapinane-TXA_2, a series of TXA_2/PGH_2 receptor antagonists that are more potent[12, 13] than 13-APA. One of these compounds was I-PTA-OH (figure 1). Experiments described herein have demonstrated that I-PTA-OH is a competitive antagonist of the human platelet TXA_2/ PGH_2 receptor. In addition, it is considerably more potent than both I-*cis*-13-APO and 13-APA. Thus, it has the characteristics necessary for it to be used as a radioligand in binding assays. Preliminary studies using [^{125}I]-PTA-OH in radioligand binding assays with human platelet membranes have demonstrated that binding is saturable, displaceable, and dependent on protein concentration. The K_d has been estimated to be approximately 30 nM from equilibrium binding studies.* We have recently found that the K_d determined from the pA_2 value for I-PTA-OH in washed human platelets is 7.9 nM.* Thus, these two K_d values agree well with each other. The higher K_d obtained in PRP in this study probably reflects binding of I-PTA-OH to plasma proteins. However, this binding to plasma proteins apparently does not affect the rank orders of potency for agonists or antagonists.* We have found that the rank orders for agonists as stimulators of aggregation in PRP and for antagonists as inhibitors of U46619-induced aggregation in PRP were the same as the rank orders for displacement of [^{125}I]-PTA-OH from its binding sites in washed human platelets.* In addition, binding is displaceable by a number of TXA_2/PGH_2 agonists and antagonists.[28] Thus, [^{125}]I-PTA-OH may prove to be a suitable ligand for use in binding studies of human platelet TXA_2/PGH_2 receptors.

That both the PG endoperoxides and TXA_2 can cause platelet aggregation and contraction of vascular smooth muscle is well documented. In the platelets and blood vessels, TXA_2 seems to be more potent than either of the endoperoxides.[6, 7, 29, 30] It is generally assumed that their effects are mediated at discrete receptors, most commonly termed TXA_2 and/or TXA_2/PGH_2 receptors. However, efforts in which the naturally occurring eicosanoids were used to pharmacologically characterize these receptors were hindered due to their lack of stability under physiologic conditions. In 1975, the first potent stable analogs of PGH_2 were reported,[31, 32] while the corresponding stable TXA_2 analogs were not synthesized until 1979 and 1980.[33, 34] Since that time, a wide variety of synthetic PGH_2 and TXA_2 analogs that act as agonists or antagonists have been described.[35–55] These compounds provided useful tools in the elucidation of the physiologic and pathophysiologic roles of PGH_2 and TXA_2 in the cardiovascular system and platelet function.

As these studies progressed, structure-activity relationships among the various analogs examined became apparent. For example, the most potent derivatives, agonist or antagonist, possess bicyclic ring systems of a variety of types that not only confer biological activity but also lend stability to the molecules.[31–55] Some of these molecules include the pinane,[33, 40] carbocyclic,[34, 41] and sulfur-substituted isosteres[42–45] among the TXA_2 analogs and the azo,[32] ether,[31] and ethano[46] analogs among the PGH_2 derivatives. In general, the retention of electronegative atoms (O,S,N) in the bicyclic nucleus leads to agonist activity, while substitution to an all-carbon system results in both agonist (CTA_2) and antagonist (PTA_2) properties, depending upon the degree of substitution of the bicyclic ring system.[33, 45] However, a notable exception is 11a-carba-TXA_2, which is an antagonist of human platelet aggregation but devoid of any activity in rat aorta.[47]

Certain structural groupings among the side chains of the analogs examined also appear to be important. Among the agonists, both the presence and the orientation of the C-15 hydroxy group in the natural (*S*) configuration is crucial for activity as a mimetic.[41, 44–49] Reversal of the configuration at C-15 often results in lower potency or a loss of mimetic activity, indeed many (*R*)-epimers of agonists are antagonists.[41, 44–49] In contrast, the influence of the orientation of the C-15 hydroxy group upon the activity of antagonists may be unpredictable, and may depend on the tissue that is studied. We have found in platelets, for example, that the 15(*R*)- and 15(*S*)-epimers of PTA-OH, I-PTA-OH, and ONO11120 were equipotent as antagonists of U46619-induced platelet aggregation; in canine saphenous veins the epimers were not equipotent.[50] Other examples exist in which the most potent antagonist is of either the (*R*) or (*S*) configuration,[48] which suggests that other structural features play a more important role in these molecules. In addition, the presence of the Δ^5 and Δ^{13} double bonds are important determinants of potency for compounds with either agonist or antagonist activity.[6, 37, 56] However, the Δ^5 double bond appears to be the most important determinant of activity. For example, pinane TXA_2, an antagonist in platelets and vascular smooth muscle, losses its activity when the Δ^5 double bond is saturated, while carbocyclic TXA_2 loses its agonist effect in smooth muscle.[38] This

*Saussy DL, et al.: Unpublished observations.

loss in activity has also been observed with other molecules both in platelet and vascular smooth muscle.[37]

Previous studies with the "classic" PGs have shown that the lower (ω) side chain could be modified distal to the C-15 position without a loss of agonist activity.[51] Furthermore, 16-*p*-halophenoxy and 16,16-dimethyl derivatives of $PGF_{2\alpha}$, 11-deoxy-$PGF_{2\alpha}$, and PGD_2 and 11-deoxy-16-phenoxy derivatives of PGE exhibit TXA_2/PGH_2-like activity.[24, 39, 52] In addition, 16-*p*-halophenoxy derivatives of stable TXA_2/PGH_2 analogs are more potent agonists than their parents. Indeed, some 16-*p*-halophenoxy derivatives of TXA_2/PGH_2 analogs are agonists, while the parent compound acts as an antagonist.[46] Likewise, many TXA_2/PGH_2 antagonists have undergone significant modifications distal to the C-15 position and retained antagonist activity.[51, 53] Our work with a series of ω-substituted congeners that are analogs of I-PTA-OH and TXA_2/PGH_2 receptor antagonists indicate that the receptors in platelets and vascular smooth muscle are different. It was determined that the potency ratios of the compounds as antagonists of U46619-induced platelet aggregation or contraction of saphenous vein were significantly different in tissues from canine and human sources.[12] Furthermore, while the 15(*R*)- and 15(*S*)-epimers of PTA-OH, I-PTA-OH, and ONO11120 were equipotent as antagonists of U46619-induced platelet aggregation, there were differences in their potencies as inhibitors of U46619-induced canine saphenous vein contraction.[50] This confirms the suggestion put forward by several other investigators[6, 37, 42, 47, 54–56] that the receptors are different in platelets than in blood vessels.

In summary, pharmacologic approaches have begun to characterize the TXA_2/PGH_2 receptor(s) in platelets and vascular smooth muscle. Structure-activity relationships among the variety of analogs synthesized have implicated the existence of different TXA_2/PGH_2 receptors among platelets and vascular smooth muscle. The strongest evidence for this is the presence of agonist activity in vascular smooth muscle and antagonistic activity in platelets[6, 37, 42, 47, 55] within individual molecules and changes in the rank order of potency among a series of 13-azapinane-TXA_2 antagonists.[12, 50] While pharmacologic studies remain a powerful tool for characterizing the TXA_2/PGH_2 receptor(s), studies using radioligand binding assays should provide greater understanding of the nature of the TXA_2/PGH_2 receptor in many tissues, particularly quantitative information on receptor number and regulation.

We acknowledge the secretarial assistance of Ms. Nita Pike and Ms. Virginia Minchoff.

References

1. Nugteren DH, Hazelhof E: Isolation and properties of intermediates in prostaglandin biosynthesis. Biochim Biophys Acta **326:** 448, 1973
2. Hamberg M, Samuelsson B: Detection and isolation of an endoperoxide intermediate in prostaglandin biosynthesis. Proc Natl Acad Sci USA **70:** 899, 1973
3. Hamberg M, Svensson J, Wakabayashi T, Samuelsson B: Isolation and structure of two prostaglandin endoperoxides that cause platelet aggregation. Proc Natl Acad Sci USA **71:** 345, 1974
4. Hamberg M, Svensson J, Sameulsson B: Thromboxanes: a new group of biologically active compounds derived from prostaglandin endoperoxides. Proc Natl Acad Sci USA **72:** 2994, 1975
5. Hamberg M, Hedqvist P, Strandberg K, Svensson J, Samuelsson B: Prostaglandin endoperoxides IV. Effects on smooth muscle. Life Sci **16:** 451, 1975
6. Needleman P, Minkes M, Raz A: Thromboxanes: selective biosynthesis and distinct biological properties. Science **193:** 163, 1976
7. Needleman P, Moncada S, Bunting S, Vane J, Hamberg M, Samuelsson B: Identification of an enzyme in platelet microsome which generates thromboxane A_2 from prostaglandin endoperoxides. Nature **261:** 558, 1976
8. Malmsten C, Hamberg M, Svensson J, Samuelsson B: Physiological role of an endoperoxide in human platelets: hemostatic defect due to platelet cyclooxygenase deficiency. Proc Natl Acad Sci USA **72:** 1446, 1975
9. Hamberg M, Samuelsson B: Prostaglandin endoperoxides. Novel transformations of arachidonic acid in human platelets. Proc Natl Acad Sci USA **71:** 3400, 1974
10. Grimm LJ, Knapp DR, Senator D, Halushka PV: Inhibition of platelet thromboxane synthesis by 7-(1-imidazolyl) heptanoic acid: dissociation from inhibition of aggregation. Thromb Res **24:** 307, 1981
11. Mitchell JRA: Clinical aspects of the arachidonic acid-thromboxane pathway. Br Med Bull **39:** 289, 1983
12. Mais DE, Saussy DL Jr, Chaikhouni A, Kochel PJ, Knapp DR, Hamanaka N, Halushka PV: Pharmacologic characterization of human and canine thromboxane A_2/prostaglandin H_2 receptors in platelets and blood vessels: evidence for different receptors. J Pharmacol Exp Ther **233:** 418, 1985
13. Mais D, Knapp D, Halushka P, Ballard K, Arai Y: Synthesis of thromboxane receptor antagonists with the potential to radiolabel with ^{125}I. Tetrahedron Lett **25:** 4204, 1984
14. Born GVR: Aggregation of blood platelets by adenosine diphosphate and its reversal. Nature **194:** 927, 1962
15. Arunlakshana O, Schild HO: Some quantitative uses of drug antagonists. Br J Pharmacol Chemother **14:** 48, 1959
16. Tallarida RJ, Cowan A, Adler MW: pA_2 and receptor differentiation: a statistical analysis of competitive antagonism. Life Sci **25:** 637, 1979
17. Burch RM, Knapp DR, Halushka PV: Vasopressin stimulates thromboxane synthesis in the toad urinary bladders effects of imidazole. J Pharmacol Exp Ther **210:** 344, 1979
18. Lowry OH, Rosenbrough NJ, Farr AL, Randall RD: Protein measurement with the folin phenol reagent. J Biol Chem **193:** 268, 1951
19. Steel RGD, Torrie JH: Principles and procedures of statistics. New York, 1960, McGraw-Hill, p 78
20. Venton DL, Enke SE: Azaprostanoic acid derivatives. Inhibitors of arachidonic acid induced platelet aggregation. J Med Chem **22:** 824, 1979
21. LeBreton GC, Venton DL, Enke SE, Halushka, PV: 13-Azaprostanoic acid: a specific antagonist of the human blood platelet thromboxane/endoperoxide receptor. Proc Natl Acad Sci USA **76:** 4097, 1979
22. Hung SC, Ghali NI, Venton DL, LeBreton GC: Specific binding of the thromboxane A_2 antagonist 13-azaprostanoic acid to human platelet membranes. Biochim Biophys Acta **728:** 171, 1983
23. Armstrong RA, Jones RL, Wilson NH: $PGF_{2\alpha}$ is not a TXA_2 receptor antagonist on human platelets. Br J Pharmacol **80:** 603P, 1983
24. Armstrong RA, Jones RL, Wilson NH: Ligand binding to throm-

boxane receptors on human platelets: Correlation with biological activity. Br J Pharmacol **79:** 953, 1983
25. Hung SC, Ghali NI, Venton DL, LeBreton GC: Prostaglandin $F_{2\alpha}$ antagonizes thromboxane A_2-induced human platelet aggregation. Prostaglandins **24:** 195, 1982
26. Pollock WK, Armstrong RA, Brydon LJ, Jones RL, MacIntyre DE: Thromboxane-induced phosphatidate formation in human platelets. Relationship to receptor occupancy and to changes in cytosolic free calcium. Biochem J **219:** 833, 1984
27. Halushka PV, MacDermot J, Knapp DR, Eller T, Saussy DL Jr, Mais D, Blair IA, Dollery CT: A novel approach for the study of thromboxane A_2 and prostaglandin H_2 receptors using an ^{125}I-labelled ligand. Biochem Pharmacol **34:** 165, 1985
28. Saussy DL Jr, Mais DE, Knapp DR, Halushka PV: Identification of a putative thromboxane A_2/prostaglandin H_2 receptor in human platelets using a ^{125}I-labeled receptor antagonist. Circulation **70**(suppl II): II-70, 1984 (abst)
29. Svensson J, Hamberg M, Samuelsson B: On the formation and effects of thromboxane A_2 in human platelets. Acta Physiol Scand **98:** 285, 1976
30. Svensson J, Strandberg K, Tuvemo T, Hamberg M: Thromboxane A_2: effects on airway and vascular smooth muscle. Prostaglandins **14:** 425, 1977
31. Bundy GL: The synthesis of prostaglandin endoperoxide analogs. Tetrahedron Lett **24:** 1957, 1975
32. Corey EJ, Nicolaou KC, Machida Y, Malmsten CL, Samuelsson B: Synthesis and biological properties of a 9,11-azo-prostanoid: highly active biochemical mimic of prostaglandin endoperoxides. Proc Natl Acad Sci USA **72:** 3355, 1975
33. Nicolaou KC, Magolda RL, Smith JB, Aharony D, Smith EF, Lefer AM: Synthesis and biological properties of pinane-thromboxane A_2, a selective inhibitor of coronary artery constriction, platelet aggregation, and thromboxane formation. Proc Natl Acad Sci USA **76:** 2566, 1979
34. Nicolaou KC, Magolda RL, Claremon DA: Carbocyclic thromboxane A_2. J Am Chem Soc **102:** 1404, 1980
35. Kálè VN, Clive DLJ: Studies related to thromboxane A_2: a formal synthesis of optically active 9α, 11α-thiathromboxane A_2 methyl ester from levoglucosan. J Org Chem **49:** 1554, 1984
36. Newton RF, Roberts SM, Taylor RJK: Strategies employed in the synthesis of prostacyclins and thromboxanes. Synthesis, p 449, 1984
37. Gorman RR, Shebuski RJ, Aiken JW, Bundy GL: Analysis of the biological activity of azoprostanoids in human platelets. Fed Proc **40:** 1997, 1981
38. Nicolaou KC, Smith JB, Lefer AM: Chemistry and pharmacology of a series of new thromboxane analogs. Drugs Future **7:** 331, 1982
39. Jones RL, Peesapati V, Wilson NH: Antagonism of the thromboxane-sensitive contractile systems of the rabbit aorta, dog saphenous vein, and guinea-pig trachea. Br J Pharmacol **76:** 423, 1982
40. Ansell MF, Caton MPL, Palfreqman MN, Stuttle KAJ: Synthesis of structural analogues of thromboxane A_2. Tetrahedron Lett **46:** 4497, 1983
41. Ohuchida S, Hamanaka N, Hayashi M: Synthesis of thromboxane A_2 analogs -1. ($\pm$)-Dimethanothromboxane A_2. Tetrahedron **39:** 4257, 1983
42. Hamanaka N, Ohuchida S, Hayashi M: Synthesis of thromboxane A_2 analogs: thia- and dithiathromboxane A_2. Adv Prostaglandin Thromboxane Leukotriene Res **11:** 319, 1983
43. Ohuchida S, Hamanaka N, Hayashi M: Synthesis of thromboxane analogs -3. (+)-Thiathromboxane A_2. Tetrahedron **39:** 4269, 1983
44. Ohuchida S, Hamanaka N, Hayashi M: Synthesis of thromboxane A_2 analogs -2. ($\pm$)-Thiathromboxane A_2. Tetrahedron **39:** 4263, 1983
45. Ohuchida S, Hamanaka N, Hayashi M: Synthesis of thromboxane A_2 analogs -4. ($\pm$)-Dithiathromboxane A_2 sodium salt. Tetrahedron **39:** 4273, 1983
46. Wilson NH, Peesapati V, Jones RL, Hamilton K: Synthesis of prostanoids with bicyclo [2,2,1]heptane, bicyclo [3,1,1]heptane and bicyclo [2,2,2]octane ring systems. Activities of 15-hydroxy epimers on human platelets. J Med Chem **25:** 495, 1982
47. Gorman RR, Maxey KM, Bundy GL: Inhibition of human platelet thromboxane synthetase by 11α-carbathromboxane A_2 analogs. Biochem Biophys Res Commun **100:** 184, 1981
48. Sprague PW, Heikes JE, Harris DN, Greenberg R: 7-Oxa-bicyclo [2.2.1]heptane analogs as modulators of the thromboxane A_2 and prostacyclin receptors. Adv Prostaglandin Thromboxane Leukotriene Res **11:** 337, 1983
49. Harris DN, Phillips MB, Michel IM, Goldenberg HJ, Heikes JE, Sprague PW, Antonaccio MJ: 9α-Homo-9,11-epoxy-5,13 prostadienoic acid analogues: Specific stable agonist (SQ 26,538) and antagonist (SQ 26.536) of the human platelet thromboxane receptor. Prostaglandins **22:** 295, 1981
50. Mais DE, Dunlap C, Hamanaka N, Halushka PV: Further studies on the effects of epimers of thromboxane A_2 antagonists on platelets and veins. Eur J Pharmacol **111:** 125, 1985
51. Nelson NA, Kelly RC, Johnson RA: Prostaglandins and the arachidonic acid cascade. Chem Eng News **60:** 30, 1982
52. Banerjee AK, Tuffin DP, Walker JL: Pharmacological effects of ($\pm$)-11-deoxy, 16-phenoxyprostaglandin E_1 derivatives in the cardiovascular system. Br J Pharmacol **84:** 71, 1985
53. Katsura M, Miyamoto T, Hamanaka N, Kondo K, Terada T, Ohgaki Y, Kawasaki A, Tsuboshima M: *In vitro* and *in vivo* effects of new powerful thromboxane antagonists (3-alkylamino pinane derivatives). Adv Prostaglandins Thromboxane Leukotriene Res **11:** 351, 1983
54. Fitzpatrick FA, Bundy GL, Gorman RR, Honohan T: 9,11-Epoxyiminoprosta-5, 13-dienoic acid is a thromboxane A_2 antagonist in human platelets. Nature **275:** 764, 1978
55. Lefer AM, Smith EF III, Araki H, Smith JB, Aharony D, Claremon DA, Magolda RL, Nicolaou KC: Dissociation of vasoconstrictor and platelet aggregatory activities of thromboxane by carbocyclic thromboxane A_2, a stable analog of thromboxane A_2. Proc Natl Acad Sci USA **77:** 1706, 1980
56. LeDuc LE, Wyche AA, Sprecher H, Sankarappe SK, Needleman P: Analogues of arachidonic acid used to evaluate structural determinants of prostaglandin receptor and enzyme specificities. Mol Pharmacol **19:** 242, 1981

AH23848*: a thromboxane receptor–blocking drug that can clarify the pathophysiologic role of thromboxane A_2

R. T. Brittain, D.Sc., L. Boutal, B.Sc., M. C. Carter, B.Sc., R. A. Coleman, Ph.D., E. W. Collington, Ph.D., H. P. Geisow, Ph.D., P. Hallett, Ph.D., E. J. Hornby, B.Sc., P. P. A. Humphrey, Ph.D., D. Jack, Ph.D., I. Kennedy, B.Sc., P. Lumley, Ph.D., P. J. McCabe, Ph.D., I. F. Skidmore, D. Phil, M. Thomas, M.R.C.P.(UK), and C. J. Wallis, Ph.D.

ABSTRACT Despite numerous suggestions in the literature that thromboxane A_2 is involved in a variety of occlusive vascular diseases, no definitive evidence is available. Arguments have been presented to support the view that such evidence can only come from clinical studies with a highly specific thromboxane receptor–blocking drug. We have now identified such a drug, AH23848, in our laboratories. Preliminary experiments with AH23848, ([1α(Z), 2β,5α]-(±)-7-[5-[[(1,1′-biphenyl)-4-yl]methoxy]-2-(4-morpholinyl)-3-oxocyclopentyl]-4-heptenoic acid), show that it is a potent, specific thromboxane receptor–blocking drug that is orally active and has a long duration of action. It should be a valuable tool in elucidating any physiologic or pathologic role of thromboxane A_2.
Circulation **72, No. 6, 1208–1218, 1985.**

THROMBOXANE A_2 (TxA_2), a product of arachidonic acid metabolism in blood platelets, is an exceptionally potent inducer of platelet aggregation and of contraction of vascular and respiratory smooth muscle.[1] Together with prostacyclin, it may play a physiologic role in the maintenance of vascular homeostasis and may also contribute to the pathogenesis of a variety of vascular disorders.[2, 3] As yet, however, there is no rigorous proof that TxA_2 plays a critical role in any disease process. Furthermore, such proof is unlikely to be obtained by observing the consequences of inhibition of the synthesis of TxA_2. If this is achieved by inhibition of fatty acid cyclooxygenase, the formation of other biologically active prostanoids such as prostacyclin and prostaglandin E_2 is also inhibited and, if by inhibition of TxA_2 synthetase, the production of the other products of the cyclooxygenase pathway may be enhanced. Thus, in neither case is it possible to relate the end result solely to a deficiency of TxA_2. Clearly a specific TxA_2 antagonist would, in principle, be a better tool for investigating any putative role of TxA_2 in disease states because it should affect only the actions of TxA_2.

From Glaxo Group Research Limited, Ware Division, Ware, Herts, U.K.

Address for correspondence: Dr. P. P. A. Humphrey, Biology Division, Glaxo Group Research Ltd., Ware, Herts SG12 ODJ, U.K.

*The chemical name for this drug appears in the abstract.

Until recently specific thromboxane receptor–blocking drugs were not available. One of the first available was AH19437 but this, like most subsequently described thromboxane receptor–blockers, such as EP045 and BM 13,177, is relatively weak.[4–7] We now describe the pharmacology of AH23848 (figure 1), which is chemically related to AH19437, but is about 100 times more potent. The high potency and selectivity of action of AH23848 make it a valuable tool for blocking thromboxane receptors. Preliminary studies in both animals and man provide further support for the view that TxA_2 plays a key pathologic role in some types of cardiovascular disorders. However, more detailed and wider ranging clinical studies are needed with drugs like AH23848 before we can be sure about the importance of TxA_2 in various diseases.

Materials and methods

Isolated smooth muscle. Isolated vascular smooth muscle samples from the rat and dog were prepared as spiral strips and set up in a modified Krebs solution gassed with 95% oxygen and 5% carbon dioxide for recording changes in isometric tension, as described previously.[8, 9] The human blood vessels were removed from macroscopically normal lung pieces obtained from surgical resection 12 to 48 hr earlier from patients with carcinoma of the lung. The arteries were cut into spiral strips and set up as described for the rat and dog vessels.

Other isolated smooth muscle preparations examined were the guinea pig ileum, guinea pig fundus, dog fundus, chick ileum, cat iris, and dog iris. These were prepared and set up in

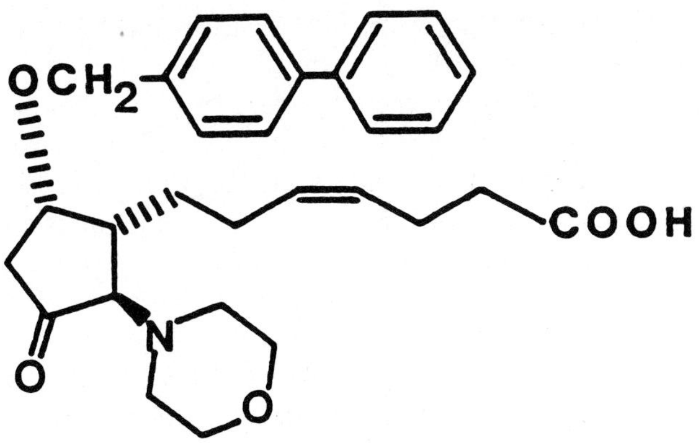

FIGURE 1. Chemical structure of AH23848.

modified Krebs solution to record changes in isometric tension, as described by us elsewhere.[9]

Platelets. Human platelets from healthy male volunteers were examined in platelet-rich plasma with the use of a standard technique of preparation and aggregation was monitored with a photometric aggregometer.[10] Except when examining the effects of collagen and arachidonic acid, aspirin (2.5×10^{-4} mol/liter) was added to the platelet-rich plasma to prevent secondary aggregation resulting from TxA_2 production.

Platelet aggregation was also examined in human whole blood with a novel technique expressly devised for this study.[11] Aliquots of blood (treated with aspirin, 2.0×10^{-3} mol/liter) were equilibrated at 37° C with a 95% air and 5% carbon dioxide mixture to maintain normal blood gas pressures and pH. Aggregation was measured by monitoring the peak percentage fall in the total number of single platelets in each aliquot with an Ultra-Flo 100 whole blood platelet counter. Platelet counts in each aliquot were determined in the absence and presence of different concentrations of aggregating agent so as to construct a concentration-effect curve. The procedure was repeated in the presence of different concentrations of AH23848. The control concentration-aggregation curve was recorded again at the end of the experiment to monitor any spontaneous changes in sensitivity to the aggregating agent.

Isolated enzymes. The effect of AH23848 (1×10^{-5} mol/liter) on the conversion of substrate to product by the following isolated enzymes was examined with methods previously described: fatty acid cyclooxygenase obtained from ram seminal vesicles,[12] thromboxane synthetase obtained from human platelets,[13] prostacyclin synthetase obtained from pig aorta,[14] and cyclic AMP phosphodiesterase obtained from guinea pig lung.[15] In each case the appropriate positive control experiment was run to show the expected activity of known inhibitors, namely indomethacin (1×10^{-4} mol/liter), UK 34787 (1.0×10^{-5} mol/liter)[16] or 1-butyl-imidazole (5.0×10^{-4} mol/liter), tranylcypromine (3×10^{-3} mol/liter),[17] and isobutylmethylxanthine (IBMX; 1×10^{-5} mol/liter), respectively.

Biosynthesis of TxA_2. TxA_2 was biosynthetically generated from prostaglandin endoperoxide, PGH_2, and a suspension of indomethacin-treated human platelet microsomes in 0.1 mol/liter Tris buffer (pH 7.5).[13, 18] The PGH_2 was prepared by incubating arachidonic acid with ram seminal vesicle microsomes as described by Gorman et al.[19] and stored at -70° C in anhydrous diethyl ether until needed.

Platelet deposition. ^{111}In-labeled human platelets were prepared by the method of Hawker et al.[20] and then resuspended in autologous blood, which was circulated over everted deendothelialized segments of rabbit aorta at 160 ml/min for 10 min at 37° C in a Baumgartner chamber.[21] With the use of fresh everted aortic segments the blood was recirculated after addition of different concentrations of AH23848 ($1.0 \times 10^{-9} - 1.0 \times 10^{-5}$ mol/liter). The number of platelets deposited was calculated by measurement of radioactivity in the aortic segments and reference to the platelet count and specific activity of the blood. Comparison of the inhibitory effect of AH23848 was made with the effect of prostacyclin and aspirin at different concentrations.

Anesthetized animals. Guinea pigs were anesthetized with sodium pentobarbital (60 mg/kg ip) and blood pressure and tracheal inflation pressure were monitored. Platelet counts were obtained in arterial blood samples with an Ultra-Flo 100 platelet counter. AH23848, aspirin, or vehicle were administered intravenously as bolus injections to animals before administration of collagen (0.1 mg/kg iv) or ADP (15 μg/kg/min iv). Each animal received only one treatment and one aggregatory challenge. The peak fall in platelet count, change in blood pressure, and tracheal inflation pressure after administration of the aggregating agent were compared with values immediately preceding the challenge.

Beagle dogs were anesthetized with sodium barbital and prepared so that blood pressure, heart rate, tracheal inflation pressure, and mesenteric arterial vascular resistance could be measured as described elsewhere.[22] Dose-response curves for increases in mesenteric arterial vascular resistance were constructed for U-46619 administered intra-arterially close to the bed. When constant, curves were redetermined after administration of increasing intravenous doses of AH23848.

Platelet studies ex vivo. Platelet aggregation induced by collagen and ADP was measured ex vivo in whole blood from conscious dogs before and at intervals after oral administration of AH23848. Similar studies were performed in human volunteers, but the aggregating agents used in these studies were U-46619 and ADP. In both series of experiments platelet aggregation was measured with the Ultra-Flo whole blood platelet counter as described above.

Analysis of data

Estimates of antagonist potency. The interaction of agonists and antagonists on isolated smooth muscle preparations and on isolated platelets in whole blood was examined by the method of Arunlakshana and Schild with the use of established experimental protocols.[8, 9, 23] Agonist concentration ratios were determined by dividing the concentration of agonist required to produce 50% of its maximal effect in the presence of antagonist by the dose or concentration of agonist required to produce the same response in the absence of antagonist. Schild analysis enabled determination of pA_2 values, which are the negative logarithms of the concentration of antagonist required to produce a twofold rightward shift in the agonist concentration-effect curve. More importantly, if (1) the shifts of the agonist concentration-effect curve are parallel over a reasonable antagonist concentration range, (2) there is no reduction in the maximum response to the agonist, and (3) the Schild plot represents a straight line with a slope of unity, then the antagonist can be considered to be acting competitively.[23] If so and there are no complicating factors the pA_2 value can be shown to be equivalent to the negative logarithm of the antagonist dissociation constant for the receptor involved.[24, 25]

Statistical analysis. Where appropriate all data have been presented as the mean ± SEM of n observations.

Drugs used. The drugs used and their suppliers were as follows: aspirin (BDH), AH23848 (Glaxo Group Research), arachidonic acid (Sigma), (-)adrenaline (Sigma), collagen (Hormon Chemie), 5-hydroxytryptamine (5-HT; Koch-Light), indomethacin (Merck, Sharpe & Dohme), IBMX (Aldrich Chemical Co.), prostaglandin D_2 (PGD_2; Glaxo Group Research), prostaglandin E_2 (PGE_2; Ono), prostaglandin $F_{2\alpha}$ ($PGF_{2\alpha}$; tromethamine salt; Upjohn), prostaglandin I_2 (PGI_2; Glaxo Group Research), tranylcypromine (Smith, Kline & French), UK 34787

([2-isopropyl]-3(1-imidazolylmethyl) indole; Pfizer); U-46619 (11,9-expoxymethano-PGH_2; Glaxo Group Research).

All except the following compounds were prepared as stock solutions in distilled water. ADP was dissolved in 5 × 10^{-2} mol/liter Tris HCl, pH 6.5. Aspirin was prepared immediately before use in 1 × 10^{-1} mol/liter Tris HCl, pH 8.5. PGI_2 was dissolved in ice cold 5 × 10^{-2} mol/liter Tris HCl, pH 9.0. Dilutions were prepared in cold 5 × 10^{-2} mol/liter Tris HCl, pH 8.0. PGD_2, U-46619, and indomethacin were each dissolved in 10% weight/volume (wt/vol) sodium bicarbonate. AH23848 was dissolved in ethanol (6% wt/vol) followed by dilution to stock concentrations in saline or 10% wt/vol sodium bicarbonate. Collagen was dissolved in a commercially supplied buffer (pH 2.8) or in 1.5 × 10^{-1} mol/liter sodium chloride. Arachidonic acid was dissolved in 5% wt/vol sodium carbonate followed promptly by dilution with 10% wt/vol sodium bicarbonate. UK 34787 was dissolved in 1 × 10^{-1} mol/liter HCl, followed by dilution to stock concentrations with 1.5 × 10^{-1} mol/liter sodium chloride. Epinephrine was dissolved in 1.5 × 10^{-1} mol/liter sodium chloride or water, both of which contained 5 × 10^{-3} mol/liter ascorbic acid. For all compounds, further dilutions to working concentrations were made with 1.5 × 10^{-1} mol/liter sodium chloride or with physiologic buffers or by direct addition to plasma or blood. In all platelet studies, concentrations refer to those in platelet rich plasma or blood. During experiments all drug solutions were kept on ice.

Results

Isolated smooth muscle. AH23848 (6.0 × 10^{-8} to 6.0 × 10^{-6} mol/liter) was assessed as an antagonist of the contractile actions of the stable TxA_2 mimetic U-46619[18] in isolated vascular smooth muscle. In human pulmonary arteries U-46619 produced sustained concentration-dependent changes in tension to a maximum tension of 0.48 ± 0.02 g at 1.0 × 10^{-6} mol/liter (n = 31). The concentration-effect curve for U-46619 was shifted to the right by AH23848 in a concentration-dependent manner with little or no reduction in the maximum response (figure 2, *A*). The pA_2 value for AH23848 was found to be 7.8 and the slope of the Schild plot was close to unity, indicating competitive antagonism. There was a similar interaction between U-46619 and AH23848 on vascular preparations from rat and dog (table 1). In some experiments in the human pulmonary vessels and dog saphenous vein, but not in the rat aorta, AH23848 by itself produced weak transient contractions (up to about 15% of the maximum response to U-46619), but these waned within minutes.

The antagonistic action of AH23848 was very specific since in isolated preparations of rat aorta it did not antagonize contractions induced by 5-HT or potassium chloride, even at concentrations as high as 10^{-5} mol/liter (table 1). Similarly, AH23848 (1.0 × 10^{-6} mol/liter) did not inhibit contractions induced by PGE_2 or $PGF_{2\alpha}$ in nonvascular smooth muscle preparations such as guinea pig ileum and fundus, dog fundus, chick ileum, and cat and dog iris, which are highly sensitive to PGE_2 or $PGF_{2\alpha}$, but relatively much less so to TxA_2 or U-46619.[9]

Confirmatory evidence that AH23848 is a specific antagonist of TxA_2 per se was obtained with the use of dog saphenous vein preparations suspended for cascade superfusion. AH23848 (1.0 × 10^{-7} mol/liter) almost abolished the contractions produced by TxA_2, but was without effect on contractile responses to 5-HT (figure 3). AH23848 appeared to be about as potent an antagonist of TxA_2 as of U-46619, but the instability of TxA_2 precluded accurate pA_2 determinations.

Platelets. In human platelet-rich plasma AH23848 selectively inhibited aggregation caused by submaximal concentrations of TxA_2, U-46619, PGH_2, arachidonic acid, or collagen (table 2). The antagonistic action of AH23848 at platelet thromboxane receptors was specific since even concentrations as high as 1.0 × 10^{-4} mol/liter did not inhibit the primary phase of aggregation caused by epinephrine, 5-HT, or ADP (table 2). AH23848 (1.0 × 10^{-7} to 1.0 × 10^{-5} mol/liter) did not cause any change in platelet shape or aggregation on its own nor did it affect the antiaggregatory actions of prostacyclin or PGD_2. In addition, AH23848 (1.0 × 10^{-5} mol/liter) had no significant action on the activity of fatty acid cyclooxygenase, thromboxane synthetase, prostacyclin synthetase, or cyclic AMP phosphodiesterase (data not shown).

In human whole blood AH23848 (3.0 × 10^{-8} to 3.0 × 10^{-7} mol/liter) was a specific antagonist of U-46619–induced platelet aggregation, producing a concentration-dependent rightward shift of the U-46619 concentration-effect curve (figure 2, *B*). The pA_2 value obtained for AH23848 of 7.8 was similar to those obtained with the vascular preparations, although unlike in the vascular preparations, the slope of the Schild plot was significantly greater than unity (table 1). AH23848 had no effect on ADP-induced aggregation, even at concentrations as high as 1.0 × 10^{-5} mol/liter (table 1).

With the use of a modified Baumgartner technique, AH23848 was found to inhibit deposition of autologous ^{111}In labeled human platelets from human whole blood onto isolated deendothelialized rabbit aorta. The maximum achievable degree of inhibition was about 70% of the total platelet deposition, which was similar to the maximum inhibition achieved with prostacyclin and aspirin (figure 4). AH23848 produced 50% of its own maximal inhibition at a concentration (IC_{50}) of 5 × 10^{-8} mol/liter being about 17 times weaker than prostacyclin (IC_{50} = 3 × 10^{-9} mol/liter) and 180 times more potent than aspirin (IC_{50} = 3 × 10^{-5} mol/ liter).

Studies in whole animals. In the anesthetized guinea

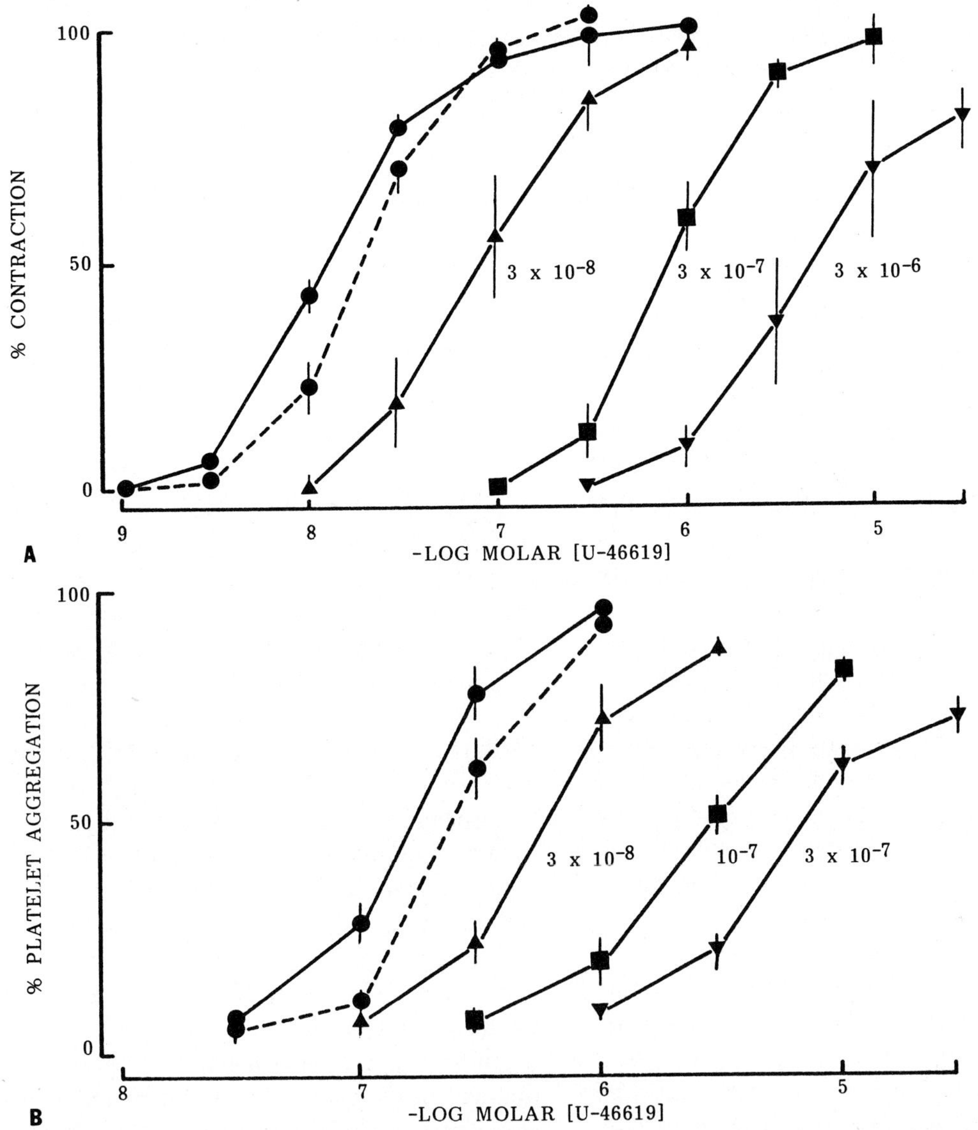

FIGURE 2. *A*, Human isolated pulmonary artery. Antagonism of U-46619–induced contractions by AH23848. Mean time-related agonist concentration-effect curves are shown in untreated preparations (●) and preparations treated with varying concentrations of AH23848, 3×10^{-8} mol/liter (▲), 3×10^{-7} mol/liter (■), and 3×10^{-6} mol/liter (▼) with a contact time of 30 min. Each point is the mean of seven or eight determinations, vertical bars represent ± SEM. *B*, Human platelets in whole blood. Antagonism of U-46619–induced aggregation by AH23848. Agonist concentration-effect curves are shown in the absence (●) and presence of AH23848, 3×10^{-8} mol/liter (▲), 1×10^{-7} ml/liter (■), and 3×10^{-7} mol/liter (▼) with a contact time of 10 min. Each point is the mean from 11 determinations; vertical bars represent ± SEM. Dotted curve represents repeat control data.

pig intravenous injection of collagen (0.1 mg/kg) produced a marked thrombocytopenia (40 ± 4% fall in circulating platelets), a biphasic effect on diastolic blood pressure with a small depressor response (↓ 6 ± 2 mm Hg) followed by a pressor response (↑ 9 ± 4 mm Hg), and bronchoconstriction (114 ± 17% increase in tracheal inflation pressure, n = 8). AH23848, at doses as low as 0.03 mg/kg iv, substantially reduced the thrombocytopenia and almost completely abolished the diastolic pressor response and the bronchoconstriction induced by collagen (figure 5). The thrombocytopenia produced by ADP (15 μg/kg/min iv) was not inhibited by AH23848 at doses as high as 1.0 mg/kg iv.

In the anesthetized dog, AH23848 (0.01 to 0.3 mg/kg iv) had little or no effect on blood pressure or mesenteric arterial blood flow, but specifically antagonized the vasoconstriction produced by close intra-arterial injection of U-46619 into the bed. U-46619 (0.003 to 0.03 μg/kg intra-arterially) produced a dose-dependent decrease in mesenteric blood flow and a mean decrease in vascular conductance of 68% (range 54% to 86%, n = 7) at a dose of 0.03 μg/kg intra-arterially. At a dose of 0.1 mg/kg iv AH23848 caused a

TABLE 1

Potency of AH23848 as an antagonist of the actions of the TxA_2 mimetic, U-46619, and 5-HT, potassium chloride, or ADP in isolated vascular preparations and human platelets

Preparation	Response	U-46619		5-HT	KCl	ADP
		pA_2	Slope	(pA_2)	(pA_2)	(pA_2)
Human platelets[A]	Aggregation	7.79±0.09	1.34±0.10[B]	—	—	<5.0
Human pulmonary artery	Contraction	7.75±0.12	1.02±0.10	—	—	—
Rat aorta	Contraction	7.94±0.17	0.98±0.04	<5.0	<5.0	—
Dog saphenous vein	Contraction	8.25±0.28	0.91±0.07	—	—	—

pA_2 values for AH23848 were determined by the method of Arunlakshana and Schild[25] (see Methods and figure 2). Each value is the mean ± SEM of four to 11 determinations.

[A]Studies in whole blood.

[B]Statistically significantly different from unity, $p < .05$.

mean rightward shift in the U-46619 dose-effect curve of 6.5-fold (range 3- to 13-fold, n = 4), while in separate control experiments the spontaneous shift was less than twofold (n = 3).

In the conscious dog orally administered AH23848 (1 mg/kg) produced a marked inhibition of collagen-induced platelet aggregation in whole blood ex vivo. There was a 23-fold rightward shift (mean peak effect, range 11 to 43, n = 5) of the collagen concentration aggregation curve and a residual effect (twofold shift) was still evident after 11 hr. In the same experiments there was no inhibition of ADP-induced aggregation ex vivo.

Studies in man. The effects of orally administered AH23848 (0.125 to 1.0 mg/kg) in eight healthy volunteers were qualitatively similar to those in the conscious dog. Platelet aggregation induced by U-46619 (but not ADP) ex vivo was inhibited for at least 8 hr after doses of 0.5 mg/kg or greater (figure 6). No cardiovascular or other effects that could be attributed to the drug were observed.

Discussion

The data presented in this study show that AH23848 is a highly specific thromboxane receptor–blocking drug in vitro and in vivo and as such should be a valuable drug tool in defining the physiologic and pathologic roles of TxA_2. In isolated smooth muscle the surmountable nature of the antagonism against the TxA_2 mimetic U-46619 and the linear Schild regression with a slope not significantly different from unity indicate a competitive drug-receptor interaction (see Methods). The anomalously high slope of the Schild regression for human platelets may have resulted from a nonspecific effect of the agonist at the high concentrations required in the presence of AH23848. Thus, high concentrations of U-46619 appear to raise intracellular cyclic AMP levels in platelets,[26] presumably by a mechanism independent of its TxA_2 mimetic action. Such an action by U-46619 would lead to an antiaggregatory effect that would physiologically antagonize its aggregatory action at thromboxane receptors and might explain the apparent reduction in the maximum response in the presence of 3.0×10^{-7} mol/liter AH23848 and the high slope of the Schild plot. The antagonism produced by AH23848 in platelets and smooth muscle was evidently mediated via thromboxane-receptor blockade per se since the actions of agonists acting via other receptors (e.g., 5-HT or ADP) were not inhibited, thus excluding any possible non-

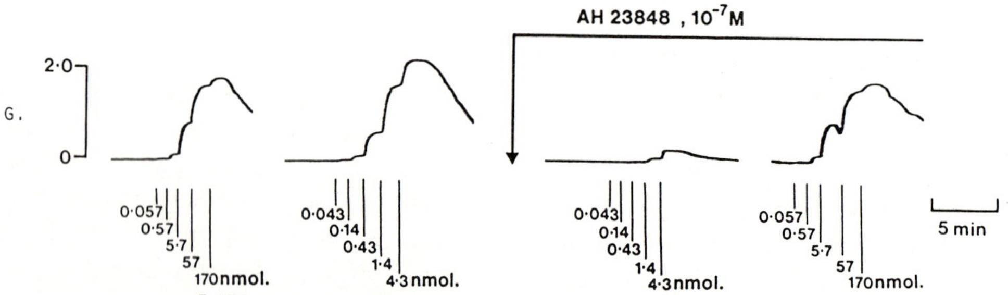

FIGURE 3. Dog isolated superfused saphenous vein. Original tracing showing the specific antagonism by AH23848 (1×10^{-7} ml/liter) of TxA_2 biosynthetically generated and administered to the superfusion medium.[18] Note that the contractile response to TxA_2 was markedly inhibited while that to 5-HT was unaffected.

TABLE 2
Potency of AH23848 as an inhibitor of human platelet aggregation in platelet-rich plasma

Agonist (concentration)	IC_{50} ($\times 10^{-7}$ mol/l) for AH 23848	n
Collagen (1 μg/ml)	6.3 ± 1.2	15
Arachidonic acid (10^{-3} mol/l)	2.95 ± 0.8	4
PGG_2/PGH_2 (10^{-6} mol/l)^A	1.05 ± 0.45	4
TxA_2 (from 10^{-6} mol/l PGH_2)^A	2.62 ± 1.61	3
U-46619 (10^{-6} mol/l)^A	1.62 ± 0.8	4
ADP (10^{-6} mol/l)^A	$>1000^B$	4
5-HT (5×10^{-6} mol/l)^A	$>1000^B$	4
Epinephrine (10^{-6} mol/l)^A	$>1000^B$	4

Platelet aggregation studied in platelet-rich plasma with the use of a Born aggregometer. Each value is the mean ± SEM of n determinations.

IC_{50} = molar concentration of AH23848 causing 50% inhibition of aggregation produced by a submaximal concentration of aggregating agent.

^{A}Platelets pretreated with 2.5×10^{-4}M aspirin.

^{B}No significant effect at 10^{-4} mol/l.

specific effects of AH23848, such as activation of adenylate cyclase or phosphodiesterase inhibition.

The weak contractions produced by AH23848 that were seen occasionally in some isolated vascular preparations (see Results) were transient and did not complicate the measurement of its antagonistic potency since this was always measured in the absence of any agonistic activity 30 min after its administration. The agonistic activity also exhibited marked tachyphylaxis, which was absent if a second dose of AH23848 was administered subsequently.* The mechanism involved is under investigation and will be the subject of a later report. It may result from a degree of partial agonistic activity at thromboxane receptors, but its weak and ephemeral nature makes it unlikely to have any clinical consequence. Indeed, AH23848 had no effect on blood pressure in human volunteers and no proaggregatory effects have ever been observed on platelets.

In human platelet-rich plasma AH23848 potently and specifically antagonized the aggregation induced not only by U-46619 and TxA_2, but also PGH_2, collagen, and arachidonic acid, each of which is known to produce its effects either directly or indirectly via thromboxane-receptor activation.[9, 27] AH23848 also inhibited the deposition of ^{111}In-labeled human platelets onto isolated deendothelialized rabbit aorta and was as effective as prostacyclin in this respect. The deposition of platelets is believed to result from both adherence (platelet monolayer bound to subendothelium) and aggregation (platelets bound to other platelets).[28, 29] The inhibitory effect of AH23848 presumably resulted from inhibition of aggregation per se induced by thromboxane-receptor activation since AH23848 was effective at the same concentrations as those necessary to prevent collagen- or U-46619–induced platelet aggregation in human whole blood. Neither AH23848 nor prostacyclin had any effect on the residual 25% to 30% of platelet deposition, which probably represents platelet adherence, a phenomenon known to be prostacyclin-insensitive.[29]

In the anesthetized guinea pig, AH23848 inhibited the bronchoconstrictor action of collagen, which has been shown to be platelet dependent and like a substantial component of the thrombocytopenic effect to result from the formation of a prostaglandin cyclooxygenase product.[30] The potent inhibition of these responses by AH23848 are consistent with this and indicate that the particular prostanoid involved is TxA_2. The vasopressor effect of collagen was also selectively abolished by AH23848, suggesting that this too results from the endogenous release of TxA_2, which is presumably platelet derived and produces vasoconstriction resulting in an increase in total peripheral resistance. In the anesthetized dog AH23848 was shown to be a potent antagonist against the vasoconstrictor actions of U-46619. Furthermore, the vasoconstrictor responses to endogenously released TxA_2 in the guinea pig were inhibited by doses of AH23848 similar to those necessary to inhibit vasoconstrictor responses to the exogenous synthetic TxA_2 mimetic U-46619 in the dog. These findings are consistent with the view that AH23848 blocks vascular thromboxane receptors in vivo.

Evidence has also been provided that AH23848 will block platelet thromboxane receptors in vivo. Thus, AH23848 not only potently antagonized the collagen-induced thrombocytopenia in the anesthetized guinea pig, but also antagonized collagen-induced platelet aggregation ex vivo. In the dog an oral dose of 1 mg/kg AH23848 produced a sustained inhibition over many hours. The effect was specific for collagen, indicating that the inhibition resulted from thromboxane-receptor blockade. Further evidence for long-lasting platelet thromboxane-receptor blockade in vivo was obtained in man.

Until the development of orally active specific thromboxane receptor–blocking drugs like AH23848 that can be administered to man,[7] it was not possible to obtain good evidence for the involvement of TxA_2 in human disease. Research workers have had to rely, to

*Brittain RT, et al: Unpublished observation.

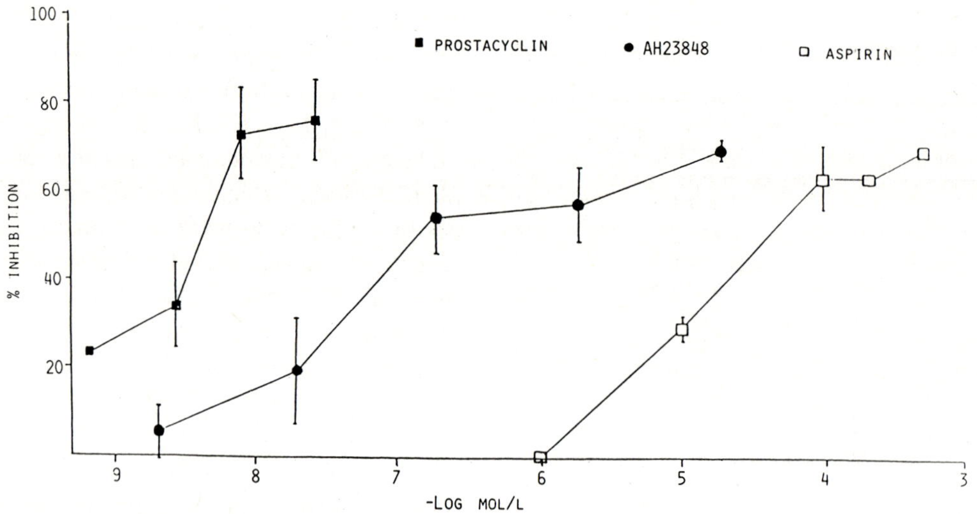

FIGURE 4. Rabbit isolated everted deendothelialized rabbit aorta superfused in a Baumgartner chamber[21] with ^{111}In-labeled platelets in human whole blood. The effects of different concentrations of prostacyclin, AH23848, and aspirin on platelet deposition were compared with those on control (untreated) preparations. Each value is the mean of at least four determinations; vertical bars represent ± SEM.

a large extent, on observing whether or not a cyclo-oxygenase inhibitor, such as aspirin, or a thromboxane-synthestase inhibitor, such as dazoxiben,[31] ameliorated the condition. However, as already discussed (see introduction), none of these tools will provide definitive evidence for or against the involvement of TxA_2. Similarly, measurement of plasma levels of TxB_2 (the stable breakdown product of TxA_2) may be of little value because any increases could be secondary to some other pathologic event, TxA_2 not being the primary mediator, or artifactual as a consequence of blood sampling problems. Alternatively, despite a major involvement, thromboxane levels in peripheral blood might not be raised since there is good reason to believe that TxA_2 (as well as prostacyclin) may be released locally at the site of a pathologic lesion.[32, 33] Thus, for example, after ligation of the left anterior descending coronary artery in the anesthetized greyhound, marked increases in TxB_2 production can be shown in blood from a vein draining the ischemic area

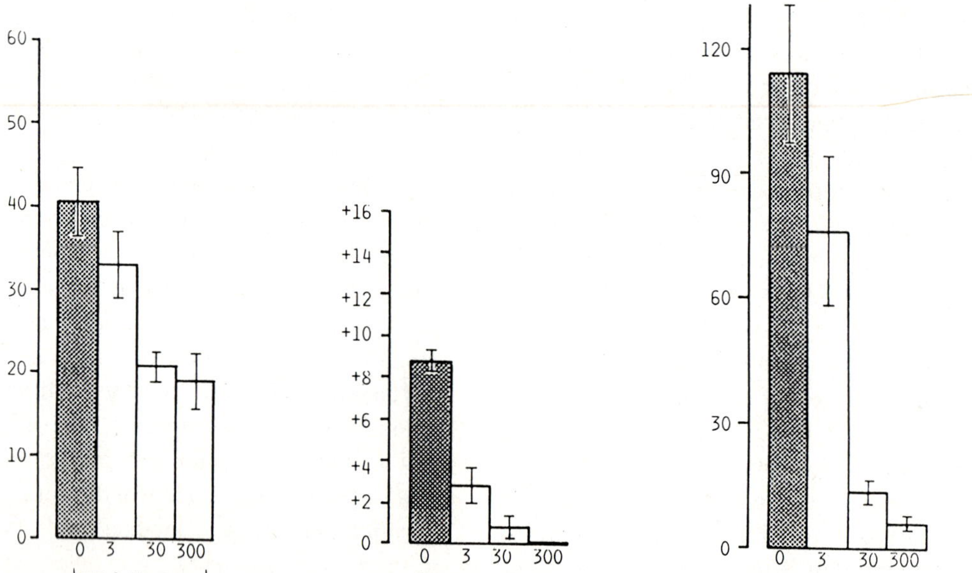

FIGURE 5. Anesthetized guinea pig. The effect of AH23848 (μg/kg) on collagen (0.1 mg/kg iv)-induced thrombocytopenia (*left*), increases in diastolic blood pressure (*center*), and increases in tracheal inflation pressure (*right*). Each value is the mean from four to seven animals in each dosage group; vertical bars represent ± SEM.

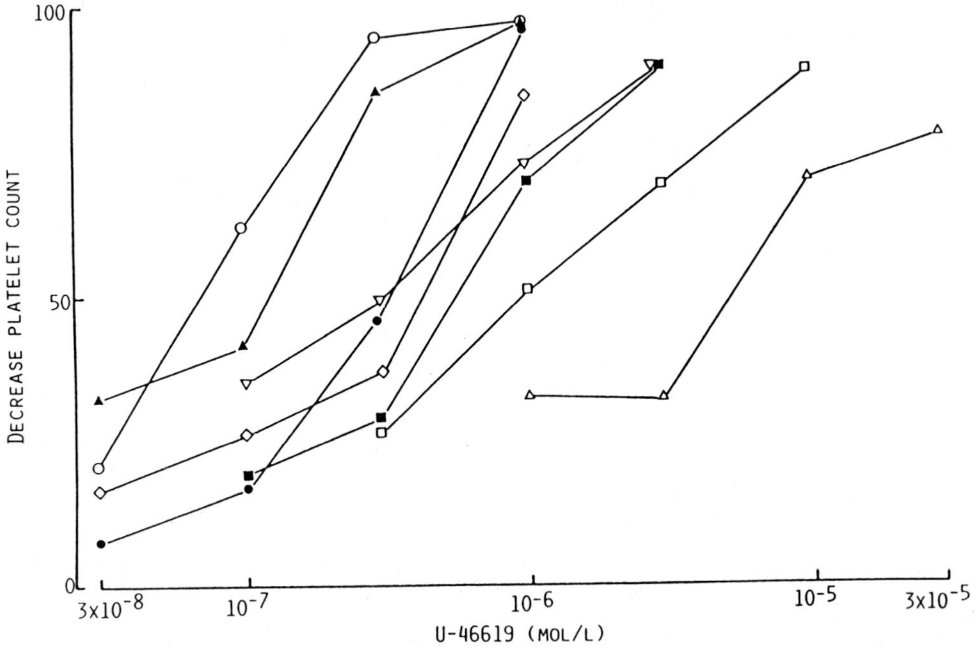

FIGURE 6. Human volunteer. U-46619–induced platelet aggregation was examined ex vivo in whole blood. Concentration-effect curves for U-46619 were constructed before (○) and at intervals (1 hr, △; 3 hr, ■; 4 hr, ▽; 6 hr, ◇; 8 hr, ●; and 24 hr, ▲) after oral administration of 0.5 mg/kg AH23848. The ordinate represents the percentage decrease in platelet count and the abscissa is the log molar concentration of U-46619. The data are from a single study in one of two volunteers given this dose. Similar findings were observed in the other volunteer.

but not in peripheral venous blood or even in blood from the coronary sinus.[32]

If aspirin (or other cyclooxygenase inhibitors) is beneficial in an animal preparation or clinical disease state, this could be considered evidence for the possible involvement of TxA_2. Thus, aspirin would prevent the conversion of arachidonic acid to the endoperoxide intermediate and thereby stop the production of TxA_2. However, it would also prevent the formation of the antithrombotic prostanoids, PGD_2 and prostacyclin, which could be counterproductive and could even be potentially dangerous in the clinical situation. Indeed, aspirin has been shown to have a prothrombotic action in some animal preparations.[34] Nevertheless, "low dose" aspirin has been shown to selectively inhibit thromboxane production in platelets[35–37]; however, whether this can be achieved in the clinical setting in all patients on long-term treatment remains to be seen.[38]

If a thromboxane-synthetase inhibitor were shown to ameliorate a condition clinically or in an animal preparation interpretation of the mechanism involved would be difficult. It could be effective because it reduces the levels of the deleterious primary mediator TxA_2 or alternatively because it increases the levels of circulating antithrombotic prostaglandins (e.g., prostacyclin or PGD_2) by synthesis pathway diversion.[39, 40] If, as has been suggested, thromboxane-synthetase inhibitors rely on conversion of prostaglandin endoperoxides to anti-aggregatory prostaglandins for their efficacy, such conversion may not occur when there is extensive vessel wall disease or a (local) congenital or pathologic enzyme deficiency. Under these conditions excess endoperoxides may accumulate that themselves mimic the biological actions of TxA_2. Indeed, it has been shown that thromboxane-synthetase inhibitors do not have much effect on the platelet aggregation produced by arachidonic acid or PGH_2 in vitro because the endoperoxides cause platelet aggregation (and vasoconstriction) in their own right.[10, 41, 42] Thus, even if a thromboxane-synthetase inhibitor did not work in a given clinical situation, it would not necessarily provide evidence for the lack of involvement of TxA_2.

Definitive evidence for the involvement of TxA_2 can, however, come from clinical studies with a highly specific and potent thromboxane receptor–blocking drug such as AH23848. AH23848 would, if given in a sufficiently high dose, antagonize the effects of TxA_2, even if the levels were as much as a 100 times or more greater than normal. As shown in this study, this could be achieved without inhibiting the normal synthesis of antithrombotic prostaglandins since the compound has no inhibitory effect on the enzymes involved. In addition, AH23848 antagonizes the actions of the endoperoxide PGH_2, which acts directly via thromboxane receptors (table 2).[43, 44] Importantly too, such a compound will not produce potentially undesirable hemodynamic effects such as vasodilation or hypotension that would be expected to compromise further an already ischemic vascular bed by "steal" or a reduction in driving pressure, respectively.

TxA_2 has been suggested to be involved in a variety of pathologic conditions, particularly those embraced by the title of occlusive vascular disease. Thus it has been reported a number of times in the literature that thromboxane levels are markedly raised in pacing-induced angina and that the rise appears to relate specifically to coronary disease since pacing does not induce such changes in healthy volunteers.[45, 46] However, drugs that inhibit the synthesis of TxA_2, such as indomethacin and aspirin, appear to be without effect on the severity or incidence of symptomatic episodes of vasospastic angina.[47, 48] One could argue, as indeed Chierchia et al.[48] have done, that the inhibition of prostacyclin production could explain the negative results in these studies.[48] In keeping with this view it has been shown that prostacyclin levels, as well as thromboxane levels, are markedly elevated in venous blood draining an ischemic myocardial region.[32] The thromboxane-synthetase inhibitor dazoxiben has also been found to have no marked effect on the time to reach pacing- or exercise-induced angina.[49, 50] However, in view of the interpretational problems discussed above, it can be argued that only the investigation of the effects of a thromboxane receptor–blocking drug will provide definitive evidence one way or the other for the involvement of TxA_2.

Importantly, AH23848 has now been examined clinically in pacing- and exercise-induced angina, but has been shown to have no obvious effect.[51] We therefore conclude that TxA_2 is not important in the pathogenesis of pacing- or exercise-induced angina. Nevertheless, it may still be that TxA_2 is important in Prinzmetal's angina or vasospasm and thrombosis, which lead to sudden death or myocardial infarction. In anesthetized greyhounds AH23848 (1 mg/kg iv) protects against death after ventricular fibrillation as a result of reperfusion of an ischemic area of myocardium.[52] Clinically aspirin does appear to have some benefit in myocardial infarction, and it may be that its efficacy is reduced by failure to use the correct dosage.[53, 54] The question of whether elevated thromboxane levels are only secondary to platelet aggregation or whether TxA_2 is the primary etiologic factor in these conditions remains to be determined.[55] Definitive evidence can only come from well-designed clinical trials with a potent effective thromboxane receptor–blocking drug.

Other clinical conditions in which TxA_2 might be important pathologically include postoperative complications resulting from platelet activation, cerebrovascular disease, and septic shock. Evidence has been presented that aspirin and AH23848 will inhibit platelet deposition onto isolated deendothelialized vascular smooth muscle. The inhibitory action might be of value in maintaining the patency of vascular prostheses and in the prophylaxis of organ transplant rejection, particularly the kidney, which synthesizes substantial amounts of TxA_2 under ischemic conditions.[56] Interestingly, it has already been found clinically that AH23848 will inhibit platelet deposition onto aortobifemoral prosthetic grafts and in this respect was perhaps surprisingly superior to a combination of aspirin and dipyridamole.[57] Whether the superior effect of AH23848 will be a consistent finding remains to be determined, but nevertheless a thromboxane receptor–blocking drug has a theoretical advantage over aspirin in that it would spare the production of the protective prostaglandins such as prostacyclin. Thus it may be preferable to use a thromboxane-receptor blocker and avoid the risk of compromising a sick patient's own natural defenses, which may be at least partially functional at the site of the lesion and indeed intact elsewhere in the body.

Patients suffering from transient ischemic attacks commonly have advanced atherosclerosis of the intracranial circulation and this may provide the stimulus for TxA_2 release from aggregating platelets, thus producing a chain reaction for further aggregation and cerebral vasoconstriction.[58, 59] Some evidence that such a pathologic sequence may indeed occur comes from the fact that aspirin is now considered to be an effective prophylactic in the treatment of transient ischemic attacks and cerebral infarction.[60, 61] The rationale for the use of a thromboxane-receptor blocker in patients with cerebrovascular disease is similar to that advanced for the use of such a drug in the prophylaxis of vascular graft occlusion.

There is evidence from animal experiments in preparations of endotoxin shock that plasma levels of thromboxane are raised by up to 10-fold or more.[62, 63] The early hemodynamic effects, which include hypotension, pulmonary vasoconstriction, and splanchnic infarction appear to be due to these high levels of TxA_2.[62] However, there is some doubt about the importance of TxA_2 in the later stages of shock, which are characterized by progressive reductions in blood pressure and cardiac output associated with cellular damage, which leads to death.[64] Certainly studies with prostaglandin cyclooxygenase inhibitors should be interpreted with caution since prostacyclin may have an important protective role in such conditions.[65] Nevertheless, indomethacin has been shown to increase survival rates in dogs and rats.[62] Inhibitors of thromboxane synthetase have also been shown to improve survival rates in rats in endotoxin shock and this seemed not to be dependent on the shunting of arachidonic acid metabolism to prostacyclin.[66] Clinically, thromboxane levels have been shown to be very high in severe cases of septic shock and the condition is characterized by pulmonary complications, hypotension, thrombocytopenia, and hypoxia.[67] Evidence has recently been provided that AH23848 protects against the early cardiopulmonary effects of endotoxin in cats.[68] It may be that a thromboxane receptor–blocking drug like AH23848 would be of clinical value in this potentially fatal condition.

In conclusion, we have provided arguments to support the view that the controversy about the etiologic role of TxA_2 in a variety of cardiovascular diseases can only be definitively resolved by a thorough clinical evaluation of a potent thromboxane receptor–blocking drug such as AH23848. Such studies may also reveal other, as yet unconsidered, pathophysiologic roles of TxA_2.

We gratefully thank Dr. A. Wadsworth (Chemical Research Department, Glaxo Group Research Ltd., Ware) for synthesizing U-46619. We are also very grateful to Pfizer (U.K.), Sandwich, for the supply of UK 34787.

References

1. Moncada S, Vane JR: Unstable metabolites of arachidonic acid and their role in haemostasis and thrombosis. Br Med Bull **34:** 129-135, 1978
2. Hornstra G: Thromboxanes and ischaemic vascular disease. Neth J Med **25:** 6, 1982
3. Moncada S, Vane JR: Prostacyclin and blood coagulation. Drugs **21:** 430, 1981
4. Coleman RA, Collington EW, Geisow HP, Hornby EJ, Humphrey PPA, Kennedy I, Levy GP, Lumley P, McCabe PJ, Wallis CJ: AH19437, a specific thromboxane receptor blocking drug? Br J Pharmacol **72:** 524P, 1981
5. Coleman RA, Humphrey PPA, Kennedy I, Levy GP, Lumley P: Further evidence that AH19437 is a specific thromboxane receptor blocking drug. Br J Pharmacol **73:** 258P, 1981
6. Jones RL, Wilson NH: Thromboxane receptor antagonism shown by a prostanoid with a bicyclo [2,2,1] heptane ring. Br J Pharmacol **73:** 220P, 1981
7. Gresele P, Deckmyn H, Arnout J, Lemmens J, Janssens W, Vermylen, J: BM 13,177, a selective blocker of platelet and vessel wall thromboxane receptors, is active in man. Lancet **1:** 991, 1984
8. Apperley E, Humphrey PPA, Levy GP: Receptors for 5-hydroxytryptamine and noradrenaline in rabbit isolated ear artery and aorta. Br J Pharmacol **58:** 211, 1976
9. Kennedy I, Coleman RA, Humphrey PPA, Levy GP, Lumley P: Studies on the characterisation of prostanoid receptors: a proposed classification. Prostaglandins **24:** 667, 1982
10. Skidmore IF, Hornby EJ: Evidence that prostaglandin endoperoxides can induce platelet aggregation in the absence of thromboxane A_2 production. Biochem Pharmacol **31:** 1158, 1982
11. Lumley P, Humphrey PPA: A method for quantitating platelet aggregation and analysing drug-receptor interactions on platelets in whole blood in vitro. J Pharmacol Meth **6:** 153, 1981
12. Flower RJ, Cheung HS, Cushman DW: Quantitative determination of prostaglandins and malondialdehyde formed by the arachidonic oxygenase (prostaglandin synthetase) system of bovine seminal vesicles. Prostaglandins **4:** 325, 1973
13. Yoshimoto T, Yamamoto S, Hayaishi O: Selective inhibition of prostaglandin endoperoxide thromboxane isomerase by 1-carboxyalkyl imidazole. Prostaglandins **16:** 529, 1978
14. Salmon JA, Smith DR, Flower RJ, Moncada S, Vane JR: Further studies on the enzymatic conversion of prostaglandin endoperoxide into prostacyclin by porcine aorta microsomes. Biochem Biophys Acta **523:** 250, 1978
15. Somerville AR, Rabouhans ML, Smith AA: Adenosine 5′-cyclic monophosphate phosphodiesterase: kinetic and inhibition studies. Biochem J **120:** 11P, 1970
16. Cross PE, Dickinson RP, Parry MJ, Randall MJ: 3-(-1-imidazolymethyl) indoles: potent and selective inhibitors of human blood platelet thromboxane synthetase. Ag Actions **11:** 274, 1981
17. Gryglewski RJ, Bunting S, Moncada S, Flower RJ, Vane JR: Arterial walls are protected against deposition of platelet thrombi by a substance (prostaglandin X) which they make from prostaglandin endoperoxides. Prostaglandins **12:** 685, 1976
18. Coleman RA, Humphrey PPA, Kennedy I, Levy GP, Lumley P: Comparison of the actions of U-46619, a prostaglandin H_2 analogue with those of prostaglandin H_2 and thromboxane A_2 on some isolated smooth muscle preparations. Br J Pharmacol **73:** 773, 1981
19. Gorman R, Sun F, Miller O, Johnson R: Prostaglandin H_1 and H_2. Convenient biochemical synthesis and isolation. Further biological and spectroscopic characterisation. Prostaglandins **13:** 1043, 1977
20. Hawker RJ, Hawker LM, Wilkinson AR: Indium (^{111}In)-labelled human platelets: optimal method. Clin Sci **58:** 243, 1980
21. Baumgartner HR: The role of blood flow in platelet adhesion, fibrin deposition and formation of mural thrombi. Microvas Res **5:** 167, 1973
22. Lumley P, Humphrey PPA, Kennedy I, Coleman RA: Comparision of the potencies of some prostaglandins as vasodilators in three vascular beds of the anaesthetised dog. Eur J Pharmacol **81:** 421, 1982
23. Arunlakshana O, Schild HO: Some quantitative uses of drug antagonists. Br J Pharmacol Chemother **14:** 48, 1959
24. Furchgott RF: The classification of adrenoceptors (adrenergic receptors). An evaluation from the standpoint of receptor theory. *In* Blascho H, Muscholl E, editors: Cathecholamines. Handbook of experimental pharmacology, New Series, Berlin, 1972, Springer Verlag, vol 33, pp 283-335
25. Kenakin TP: The Schild regression in the process of receptor classification. Can J Physiol Pharmacol **60:** 249, 1982
26. Best LC, McGuire MB, Martin TJ, Preston FE, Russell RGG: Effects of epoxymethano analogues of prostaglandin endoperoxides on aggregation, on release of 5-hydroxytryptamine and on the metabolism of 3′,5′- cyclic AMP and cyclic GMP in human platelets. Biochim Biophys Acta **583:** 344, 1979
27. Best LC, Holland TK, Jones PBB, Russell RGG: The inter-relationship between thromboxane biosynthesis, aggregation and 5-hydroxytryptamine secretion in human platelets in vitro. Thromb Haemostas **43:** 38, 1980
28. Tschopp TB, Baumgartner HR: Physiological experiments in haemostasis and thrombosis. Br J Haematol **31:** 221, 1975
29. Higgs EA, Moncada S, Vane JR, Caen JP, Michel H, Tobelem G: Effect of prostacyclin (PGI_2) on platelet adhesion to rabbit arterial sub-endothelium. Prostaglandins **16:** 17, 1978
30. Vargaftig BB, Lefort J, Joseph D, Fonque F: Mechanisms of bronchoconstriction and of thrombocytopenia induced by collagen in the guinea pig. Eur J Pharmacol **58:** 273, 1979
31. Thaulow E, Dale J, Myhre E: Effects of a selective thromboxane synthetase inhibitor, dazoxiben, and of acetylsalicyclic acid on myocardial ischemia in pateints with coronary artery disease. Am J Cardiol **53:** 1255, 1984
32. Coker SJ, Parratt JR, Ledingham I, Zeitlin IJ: Thromboxane and prostacyclin release from ischaemic myocardium in relation to arrhythmias. Nature **291:** 323, 1981
33. Aiken JW, Shebuski J, Miller OV, Gorman RR: Endogenous prostacyclin contributes to the efficacy of a thromboxane synthetase

inhibitor for preventing coronary artery thrombosis. J Pharmacol Exp Ther **219:** 299, 1981
34. Buchanan MR, Dejana E, Gent, M, Fraser Mustard J, Hirsch J: Enhanced platelet accumulation onto injured carotid arteries in rabbits after aspirin treatment. J Clin Invest **67:** 503, 1981
35. Masotti G, Galanti G, Poggesi L, Abbate, R, Neri Serneri GG: Differential inhibition of prostacyclin production and platelet aggregation by aspirin. Lancet **2:** 1213, 1979
36. Patrono C, Ciabattoni G, Pinca E, Pugliese F, Castrucci G, De Salvo A, Satta MA, Peskar BA: Low dose aspirin and inhibition of thromboxane B_2 production in healthy subjects. Thromb Res **17:** 317, 1980
37. Hanley SP, Bevan J, Cockbill SR, Hetinstall S: A regimen for low dose aspirin? Br Med J **285:** 1299, 1982
38. Johnson M, Reece AH, Harrison HE: Abnormal arachidonic acid metabolism in diabetes — effect of drugs. *In* Forster W, editor: Prostaglandins and thromboxanes. Jena, East Germany, VEB Gustar Fischer Verlag, pp 79–83
39. Vermylen J, Defreyn G, Carreras LO, Machin SJ, Schaeren JV, Verstraete M: Thromboxane synthetase inhibition as anti-thrombotic strategy. Lancet **1:** 1073, 1981
40. Randall MJ, Wilding RIR: Acute arterial thrombosis in rabbits: reduced platelet accumulation after treatment with dazoxiben hydrochloride (UK 37,2481-01). Br J Clin Pharmacol **15:** 49S, 1983
41. Bertele V, Cerletti C, Schieppati A, Di Minno G, De Gaetano G: Inhibition of thromboxane synthetase does not necessarily prevent platelet aggregation. Lancet **1:** 1057, 1981
42. Svensson J, Hamberg M: Thromboxane A_2 and prostaglandin H_2: Potent stimulators of the swine coronary artery. Prostaglandins **12:** 943, 1976
43. Armstrong RA, Jones RL, Wilson NH: Ligand binding to thromboxane receptors on human platelets: correlation with biological activity. Br J Pharmacol **79:** 953, 1983
44. Lumley P, Humphrey PPA: AH23848: a novel, potent thromboxane receptor blocking drug on vasculature and platelets. Br J Pharmacol **83:** 378P, 1978
45. Lewy IR, Wiener L, Walinsky P, Lefer AM, Silver MJ, Smith JB: Thromboxane release during pacing-induced angina pectoris: possible vasoconstrictor influence on the coronary vasculature. Circulation **60:** 1165, 1979
46. Tada M, Kuzuy T, Inoue M, Kodama K, Mishima M, Yamada M, Inui M, Hiroshi A: Elevation of thromboxane B_2 levels in patients with classic and variant angina pectoris. Circulation **64:** 1107, 1981
47. Robertson RM, Robertson D, Roberts LJ, Maas RL, Fitzgerald GA, Freisinger GC, Oates JA: Thromboxane A_2 in vasotonic angina pectoris. N Engl J Med **304:** 998, 1981
48. Chierchia S, De Caterina R, Crea F, Patrono C, Maseri A: Failure of thromboxane A_2 blockade to prevent attacks of vasospastic angina. Circulation **66:** 702, 1982
49. Hutton I, Tweddel AC, Rankin AC: Effects of dazoxiben on transcardiac thromboxane levels and haemodynamics in coronary heart disease. Br J Clin Pharmacol **15:** 79S, 1983
50. Reuben SR, Kuan P, Cairns J, Gyde OH: Effects of dazoxiben on exercise performance in chronic stable angina. Br J Clin Pharmacol **15:** 83S, 1983
51. De Bono DP, Lumley P, Been M, Keery R, Ince S, Wooding DF: Clinical trials of a competitive thromboxane A_2 antagonist in pacing and exercise induced angina. Poster presentation at IUPHAR Satellite Symposium on Platelet Inhibition and Vascular Occlusion in Man, London, 1984
52. Coker SJ, Parratt JR: Antiarrhythmic activity of the thromboxane antagonist AH23848 during myocardial ischaemia and reperfusion. Br J Pharmacol **83:** 380P, 1984
53. Elwood PC: Aspirin in the prevention of myocardial infarction current status. Drugs **28:** 1, 1984
54. Lewis HD, Davis JW, Archibald DG, Steinke WE, Smitherman TC, Doherty JE, Schnaper HW, Le Winter MM, Linares E, Pouget JM, Sabharwal SC, Chesler E, DeMots H: Protective effects of aspirin against acute myocardial infarction and death in men with unstable angina. N Engl J Med **309:** 396, 1983
55. Robertson D, Robertson RM: The role of the platelet in vasotonic (Prinzmetal) angina pectoris. *In* Mehta J, Mehta P, editors: Platelets and prostaglandins in cardiovascular disease. New York, 1981, Futura Publishing Co.
56. Scharschmidt LA, Lianos E, Dunn MJ: Arachidonate metabolites and the control of glomerular function. Fed Proc **42:** 3058, 1983
57. Lane IF, Irwin JTC, Poskih KR, Greenhalgh RM, McCollum CN: Thromboxane antagonists: reduction of platelet deposition on human grafts in vivo. Thromb Haemost **54:** 3, 1985
58. Ellis EF, Nies AS, Oates JA: Cerebral arterial smooth muscle contraction by thromboxane A_2. Stroke **8:** 480, 1977
59. Schmidley JW, Caronna JJ: Transient cerebral ischemia: pathophysiology. Prog Cardiovasc Dis **22:** 325, 1980
60. Fields WS, Lemak NA, Frankowski RF, Hardy RJ: Controlled trial of aspirin in cerebral ischemia. Thromb Haemost **40:** 135, 1979
61. Fields WS, Lemak NA, Frankowski RF, Hardy RJ, Bigelow RH: Implications of aspirin trials in transient ischaemic attack and stroke. *In* Aspirin Symposium, Royal Society of Medicine. International Congress and Symposium Series No. 39. London, 1980, Academic Press Inc (London) Ltd & Royal Society of Medicine
62. Wise WC, Cook JA, Halushka PV: Implications for thromboxane A_2 in the pathogenesis of endotoxic shock. Adv Shock Res **6:** 83, 1981
63. Ball HA, Parratt JR, Zeitlin IJ: Effect of dazoxiben, a specific inhibitor of thromboxane synthetase, on acute pulmonary responses to E. coli endotoxin in anesthetized cats. Br J Pharmacol **15:** 127S, 1983
64. Flynn JT: Endotoxic shock in the rabbit: the effects of prostaglandin and arachidonic acid administration. J Pharmacol Exp Ther **206:** 555, 1978
65. Fletcher JR, Ramwell PW: The effects of prostacyclin (PGI_2) on endotoxin shock and endotoxin-induced platelet aggregation in dogs. Circulatory Shock **7:** 299, 1980
66. Halushka PV, Cook JA, Wise WC: Beneficial effects of UK 37248, a thromboxane synthetase inhibitor, in experimental endotoxic shock in the rat. Br J Clin Pharmacol **15:** 133S, 1983
67. Parratt JR, Coker SJ, Hughes B, MacDonald A, Ledingham I, Rodger IW, Zeitlin IJ: The possible role of prostaglandins and thromboxane in the pulmonary consequences of experimental endotoxin shock and clinical sepsis. *In* McConn R, editor: The role of chemical mediators in the pathophysiology of acute illness and injury. New York, 1982, Raven Press, pp 195-218
68. Ball HA, Parratt JR: Effects of a new thromboxane receptor antagonist, AH23848, on the aucte cardiopulmonary responses to E. coli endotoxin in cats. Br J Pharmacol **83:** 379P, 1984

Platelet actions of stable carbocyclic analogues of prostacyclin

BRENDAN J. R. WHITTLE, PH.D., AND SALVADOR MONCADA, M.D., DS.C.

SINCE THE TIME of the discovery of prostacyclin[1] and the elucidation of its chemical structure as prostaglandin (PG) (5Z)-9 deoxy-6, 9 α-epoxy-Δ^5PGF_1,[2] many synthetic prostacyclin analogues have been prepared and reported in the literature. Although prostacyclin (epoprostenol) is now available for clinical use as the freeze-dried sodium salt that, when mixed with the diluent buffer (sodium chloride 0.15% weight per volume [wt/vol] and glycine buffer solution 0.19% wt/vol; pH 10.5), results in a preparation that will remain stable over 24 hr when stored at 2° to 8° C, there is much interest in synthesizing a chemically stable analogue with a biological profile comparable to that of the parent prostacyclin. Furthermore, the definitive separation of the platelet and vascular activities in an orally active synthetic prostacyclin analogue, both for use as a research tool and as a clinically useful agent, is an ultimate objective in the development of prostacyclin mimetics.

Many structural variants of prostacyclin have been synthesized, including 5,6-dihydro analogues, exemplified by 6β-PGI_1,[3–5] thia prostacyclins such as (5Z)-6,9-thia prostacyclin,[6] nitrogen-containing analogues such as 9-deoxy-9α-6-nitrilo-PGF_1,[7] ring-expanded 5,9-epoxy derivatives such as 9-deoxy-5, 9α-epoxy-PGF_1,[7] and interphenylene analogues.[8] However, the synthesis and biological actions of stable carbocyclic analogues of prostacyclin, in which the enol-ether oxygen atom is replaced by a methylene group, has attracted much attention and has been described by several groups.[9–16]

Carbacyclin analogues. Carbacyclin, or (5*E*)-6a carbaprostaglandin I_2 (figure 1, *A*), inhibits human platelet aggregation induced by a variety of agents including ADP, collagen, and arachidonic acid, while also inhibiting aggregation in platelet-rich plasma (PRP) obtained from several species, including the rabbit, rat, and dog.[12–16] In our studies with carbacyclin,[13] this stable analogue was 0.03 times as potent as prostacyclin as an inhibitor of aggregation induced by ADP (table 1), collagen, and arachidonic acid. As with prostacyclin, the antiaggregating activity of carbacyclin was enhanced by preincubation of platelets with theophylline, the phosphodiesterase inhibitor,[13, 15] indicating stimulation of cyclic AMP as its mechanism of inhibitory action. Indeed, other studies have shown an elevation of platelet cyclic AMP after incubation with the analogue.[14]

Carbacyclin has been shown to be a potent inhibitor of platelet aggregation ex vivo when infused intravenously in the dog and rabbit, being 0.1 times as active as the parent, prostacyclin.[13] Likewise, this analogue was effective in vivo in reducing formation of thrombi in canine coronary arteries[16] when infused intravenously. Studies with carbacyclin in anesthetized baboons have likewise shown inhibition of platelet aggregation determined ex vivo after intravenous or intragastric administration.[17]

In our studies in human PRP with analogues synthesized and supplied by the Upjohn Company, (5Z)-carbacyclin was less active than the (5*E*)-analogue, the latter being isosteric[12] with naturally occurring prostacyclin (5Z-PGI_2). As expected, the (15*R*)-epimer had mimimal activity, as did the 2-nor derivative (table 1). Substitution in the 9 position[18] can also alter antiaggregating potency, with (5Z)-9β-ethynyl and 9-cyano groupings enhancing activity and 9β-methyl, 9-pentyl-1-ynyl, and 9-ethyl groupings decreasing activity compared with that induced by carbacyclin itself (table 1).

Studies in human PRP with 9β-methyl-carbacyclin (ciprostene; figure 2, *B*) have shown it to have comparable potency as an antiaggregating agent against several aggregating agents (table 2). This compound is equiactive in vitro in human PRP and whole blood, and elevates platelet cyclic AMP levels.[19]

Studies using further derivatives of carbacyclin have been reported, and the 15-cyclopentyl-ω-pentanor carbacyclin derivative (ONO 41483, figure 1, *B*) has been shown to have 0.1 times the activity of prostacyclin as

From the Department of Mediator Pharmacology, Wellcome Research Laboratories, Beckenham, Kent, U.K.

Address for correspondence: Brendan J. R. Whittle, Ph.D., Department of Mediator Pharmacology, Wellcome Research Laboratories, Langley Court, Beckenham, Kent BR3 3BS, U.K.

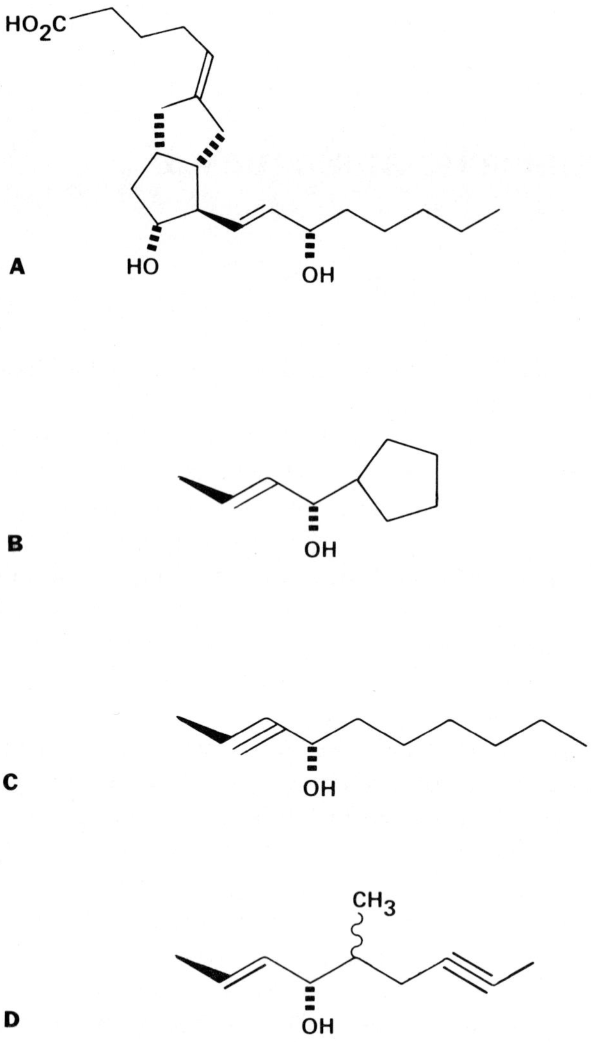

FIGURE 1. Structure of the stable prostacyclin analogue carbacyclin (*A*), its 15-cyclo-pentyl derivative (ONO 41483) (*B*), the 13,14-didehydro-20-methyl derivative (*C*), and iloprost (*D*; the 16-methyl, 18-19-didehydro derivative).

an inhibitor of human platelet aggregation in vitro,[20, 21] as shown in table 3. In addition, this analogue inhibited platelet aggregation, determined ex vivo after intravenous infusion or oral administration in the baboon, and exhibited vasodepressor actions after bolus intravenous administration.[20]

Further chemically stable analogues based on the carbacyclin structure have been reported. The 16-methyl, 18-19-didehydro derivative (figure 1, *D*) has been shown to have potent antiaggregating properties, inhibiting human platelet aggregation in vitro induced by a variety of agents[22] in a concentration range similar to that of prostacyclin (table 3). This analogue (ZK 36374 or iloprost) also induced disaggregation of platelets in vitro in cat whole blood, such platelet aggregates being formed in vivo after surgery.[23] In addition, intravenous infusion reversed the fall in platelet number after coronary artery ligation in the cat.[23] Other studies conducted in the rat have shown this carbocyclic derivative to inhibit platelet aggregation in vitro in PRP, and to have 0.3 times the activity of prostacyclin. This potency ratio is similar to that observed in the rat in vivo with respect to prolonging bleeding time in an extracorporeal circuit after intravenous infusion.[24] Potent relaxation of bovine coronary artery strips in vitro and vasodepressor actions in the cat and rat have also been observed with this carbacyclin derivative.[23]

A series of 13,14-didehydro carbacyclin analogues has also been reported.[25] One such compound (figure 1, *C*), like its 20-carbon homologue, inhibited rabbit platelet aggregation in vitro, while studies in vivo in the guinea pig, in which pulmonary accumulation of indium-labeled platelets was measured after infusion of ADP as an index of aggregation, showed antiaggregating activity after bolus injection.[26]

Metabolic stability. Although the chemical half-life of prostacyclin at physiologic temperatures and pH is short, its antiplatelet activity, and particularly its cardiovascular activity in vivo, is often even more short-lived.[13] This suggests that the pharmacologic effects of prostacyclin in vivo are limited by biological inactivation rather than solely by chemical breakdown. Furthermore, chemically stable prostacyclin analogues such as carbacyclin have only short-lived biological activity in vivo, as determined by cardiovascular actions and inhibition of platelet aggregation ex vivo, suggesting that like prostacyclin, these compounds are rapidly inactivated.[13] The extent and duration of the biological actions of prostacyclin and its analogues

TABLE 1

Inhibition of ADP-induced platelet aggregation by stable 6a-carbocyclic prostacyclin analogues in vitro in human PRP

	IC_{50} ($ng\ ml^{-1}$)	Relative potency
Prostacyclin	0.4±0.1	1
(5*E*)-carbacyclin	11±3	0.036
(5*Z*)-carbacyclin	700±100	0.0006
(5*E*)-carbacyclin-methyl ester	140±40	0.003
5*E*-(15*R*)-carbacyclin	>1600	0.0003
(5*Z*,9β)-ethynyl-carbacyclin	2.2±0.3	0.18
9β-cyano-carbacyclin	7.1±0.3	0.06
9β-methyl-carbacyclin	87±11	0.005
9β-pent-1-ynyl-carbacyclin	475±175	0.0008
9β-ethyl-carbacyclin	1348±439	0.0003

Results given as the IC_{50} value (concentration causing 50% inhibition of platelet aggregation) after 1 min incubation at 37° C in PRP and as potency relative to prostacyclin, are the mean ± SEM from at least four experiments. Carbacyclin and its derivatives were synthesized as described[11, 12, 18] and supplied by the Upjohn Company, Kalamazoo, MI.

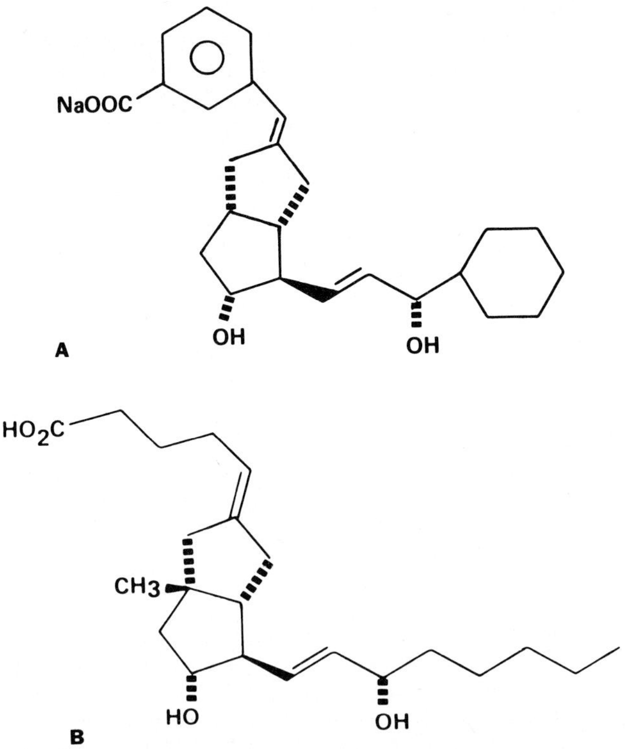

FIGURE 2. Structures of the chemically stable prostacyclin analogues: the β- and ω-modified carbacyclin derivative (*A*; CG 4305) and 9β-methyl carbacyclin (*B*; ciprostene).

in vivo may also be attenuated by the release of endogenous vasoactive substances, including renin and vasopressin.[27–30]

Like prostacyclin, carbacyclin has comparable vasodepressor activity when administered by the intravenous or intra-arterial route, indicating minimal pulmonary inactivation of this analogue.[13] The finding that carbacyclin is a good substrate for the purified 15-hydroxy prostaglandin dehydrogenase derived from monkey lung[31] lends support to the concept that these analogues fail to gain access to the enzyme in the intact lung. Like prostacyclin, these analogues will presumably undergo metabolism elsewhere, including in the liver.

TABLE 2

Comparison of the ID_{50} values[A] of prostacyclin and ciprostene (9β-methyl-carbacyclin) in human PRP aggregated with different aggregating agents, ADP, collagen, U-46619 (epoxy-methano PGH_2), and arachidonic acid

	ID_{50} (ng ml^{-1})		
Aggregating agent	Prostacyclin	Ciprostene	Potency ratio
ADP	0.55±0.1	86.6±11	0.01
Collagen	0.91±0.08	123±32	0.01
Arachidonic acid	1.8±0.7	55.8±17.6	0.03
U-46619	0.15±0.03	15.4±1	0.01

Values are mean ± SEM (n = 4 to 13).
[A]Dose producing 50% inhibition of platelet aggregation.

TABLE 3

Inhibition of platelet aggregation in vitro in PRP from various species by carbocyclic prostacyclin analogues and their potency relative to prostacyclin

Compound	Species	Potency ratio	Reference
Carbacyclin	Human	0.03	13
13,14-didehydro-carbacyclin	Rabbit	0.09	26
20 methyl-didehydro-carbacyclin	Rabbit	0.11	26
15-cyclopentyl-carbacyclin	Human;	0.11	21
	baboon	0.31	20
16-methyl-18,19-didehydro-carbacyclin	Human	1	22
9β-methyl-carbacyclin	Human	0.01	19

The prevention of enzymatic inactivation of prostacyclin analogues in vivo has been attempted by substitution in both β- and ω-chains. Studies of the kinetics of 16-methyl-18,19-didehydro-carbacyclin (figure 1, *D*) after bolus intravenous injection in the rat have indicated a biphasic decline in plasma concentrations, with an initial half-life of 5 min.[32] Although the kinetics of prostacyclin under comparable conditions was not investigated, these results suggest that the analogue does not exhibit a biologically significant longer duration of activity than prostacyclin, despite protection of the 15-hydroxy grouping from enzymatic attack. Studies in the baboon also suggest that this compound did not exhibit enhanced metabolic stability as compared with carbacyclin.[33]

In a further series of carbocyclic analogues, the 15-hydroxy group was protected by modification of the ω-tail, e.g., by insertion of a 15-cyclohexyl grouping, while protection against β-oxidation was afforded by insertion of an *m*-carboxyphenylene residue.[8] Despite such modifications (figure 2, *A*), these prostacyclin analogues still exhibited only a short duration of action, with the hypotensive effects ranging from 0.25 to 1.2 min. Only with supramaximal doses were any differences between the duration of biological action of the analogues detected, and thus such properties have no real clinical or experimental application.

These observations with chemically stable prostacyclin analogues thus suggest that a rapid elimination of the analogues, largely independent of the rate of metabolism of the compound, is of major importance in determining the plasma levels of active drug and hence the duration of cardiovascular and antiaggregating activity in vivo. It would therefore appear that until the pharmacokinetic parameters of these analogues are fully elucidated and some mechanism of controlling the distribution of the analogue from the blood to the various tissue compartments is developed, metabolically stable prostacyclin analogues with long durations of action in vivo will remain to be identified.

Selectivity of action. A preliminary indication of the separation between platelet antiaggregating and cardiovascular actions within a particular prostacyclin analogue series can be gained from consideration of the selectivity ratio. Studies on the potency of such analogues in inhibiting human platelet aggregation in vitro and in lowering blood pressure in the anesthetized rat can be employed as primary screens for biological activity of analogues and thus, the ratio of the relative potency of effects on these parameters can readily be obtained. With the use of this ratio,[13] it has been calculated that carbacyclin has a selectivity ratio close to that of prostacyclin. A favorable ratio of activity for carbacyclin has also been reported by others, whereas the (5*Z*) and (15*R*)-hydroxy derivatives of carbacyclin appeared less selective than carbacyclin itself. This selectivity ratio must be interpreted with caution, since it is derived from studies in two species, and importantly, from a comparison of data obtained in vitro with that obtained in vivo. Thus, for example, modification of a structure to prevent metabolism in the body may reduce its activity in vitro compared with its parent, yet in vivo it may appear more potent as a consequence of reduced metabolism giving a seemingly high ratio and apparent low selectivity. However, platelet studies in vitro of the effects of prostacyclin and carbacyclin in PRP from man, dog, and rabbit have been predictive of the potency as an inhibitor of platelet aggregation ex vivo (table 4).

It is clear that the most valid determination of selectivity between cardiovascular and platelet antiaggregating actions of prostacyclin analogues is obtained from studies in which the compounds are administered in vivo and in which both parameters are measured simultaneously. For this purpose the inhibition of platelet aggregation ex vivo and concurrent cardiovascular changes have been determined in anesthetized rabbits, dogs, and monkeys.[13] To enable a more rapid preparation of samples of PRP so that platelet function could readily and continually be assessed, a rapid-spin method for the centrifugation of blood samples was developed.[13] With this technique, blood samples (3.0 ml) are slowly collected from a cannula inserted into a femoral vein into a plastic syringe containing trisodium citrate (3.18%, 1 volume to 9 volumes of blood), shaken gently, and transferred to two Eppendorf plastic tubes (1.5 ml). Each sample is then spun separately in a modified Eppendorf centrifuge for 2 sec (maximum centrifuge force, 10,000 *g*). The PRP from each tube is collected separately and 0.4 ml aliquots are transferred to the aggregometer and incubated at 37° C for 1 min before addition of sufficient ADP to produce near-maximal aggregation (table 5). The time interval between removal of blood samples and the transference of the PRP to the aggregometer is only 1 min. This technique, which allows continual monitoring of platelet aggregation throughout periods of drug infusion, appears particularly useful in the study of labile or rapidly metabolized substances, the plasma half-

TABLE 4
Inhibition of ADP-induced platelet aggregation in vitro in PRP by prostacyclin and carbacyclin after 1 min incubation, and ex vivo after intravenous infusion in various species

	ID_{50}[A]			
	Prostacyclin		Carbacyclin	
Species	in vitro ($ng\ ml^{-1}$)	ex vivo ($\mu g\ kg^{-1}\ min^{-1}$)	in vitro ($ng\ ml^{-1}$)	ex vivo ($\mu g\ kg^{-1}\ min^{-1}$)
Human	0.3	0.008[B]	11	0.2–0.8[C]
Dog	0.7	0.015	20	0.15
Rabbit	2.0	0.28	25	2.4

[A]Dose producing 50% inhibition of platelet aggregation.

Experimental data taken from Whittle et al.[13] and ex vivo human data from [B]O'Grady et al.[36] or [C]Adaikan et al.[35]

TABLE 5
Actions of prostacyclin and carbacyclin on platelet aggregation and systemic arterial blood pressure (BP) ex vivo in the anesthetized dog and rhesus monkey during intravenous infusion

		Platelet aggregation (% inhibition)[A]		
Compound	Dose	Submax.	Maximum	ΔBP (mm Hg)
Dog				
Prostacyclin	0.01	40 ± 15	37 ± 15	−6 ± 2
	0.02	61 ± 4	54 ± 11	−11 ± 3
Carbacyclin	0.2	67 ± 24	64 ± 22	−4 ± 2
	0.4	86 ± 12	76 ± 21	−10 ± 5
Monkey				
Prostacyclin	0.01	50 ± 10	17 ± 4	−6 ± 5
	0.02	85 ± 8	51 ± 7	−17 ± 6
	0.05	99 ± 1	82 ± 8	−36 ± 10
Carbacyclin	0.4	56 ± 7	22 ± 7	−1 ± 0.5
	0.8	81 ± 7	42 ± 10	−5 ± 3
	2.0	99 ± 1	88 ± 5	−30 ± 14

Results are mean ± SEM from three or four experiments during a 15 min period of intravenous infusion.

[A]Platelet aggregation ex vivo was induced by ADP in doses causing submaximum aggregation (3 and 5 μM in monkey and dog, respectively) and maximum aggregation (10 and 20 μM, respectively).

lives of which may be far shorter than the time taken to prepare PRP by conventional methods (15 to 20 min).

Using this technique, studies of both prostacyclin and carbacyclin in the anesthetized dog[13] have suggested that inhibition of platelet aggregation ex vivo could be achieved after intravenous infusion of doses having minimal action on blood pressure (table 5). While carbacyclin appeared more selective than prostacyclin, producing a greater degree of platelet inhibition for a given vasodepressor response, this selectivity of action cannot be considered of great magnitude. Cardiovascular studies in the anesthetized baboon and determination of platelet inhibition in vitro with carbacyclin and prostacyclin have also suggested that effects of carbacyclin may be more selective than prostacyclin in this species.[17] Studies ex vivo of carbacyclin in the baboon have indicated that near-maximal inhibition of platelet aggregation could be achieved by doses with minimal hypotensive action.[17] However, after oral administration of carbacyclin in the baboon[17] at a dose causing 70% inhibition of platelet aggregation, a rise in the heart rate was observed without a fall in blood pressure. In our studies in the anesthetized monkey, intravenous infusion of carbacyclin in intermediate doses inhibited platelet aggregation with a minimal hypotensive effect, in contrast to the effects of prostacyclin. At higher rates of infusion, however, carbacyclin, like prostacyclin, did lower blood pressure (table 5).

Further studies have been conducted with the stable analogue 9β-methyl-carbacyclin in both anesthetized patas monkeys and greyhounds.[34] After intravenous infusion in the dog, at doses having minimal action on blood pressure, both prostacyclin and 9β-methyl carbacyclin inhibited platelet aggregation, which was determined ex vivo in samples of PRP prepared by the rapid-spin procedure (table 6). Comparison of the potency ratio for either action suggests a minimal difference between the selectivity of 9β-methyl-carbacyclin and that of prostacyclin in this species.[34] Likewise, in the monkey, in which both prostacyclin and 9β-methyl-carbacyclin were less potent with respect to both parameters compared with in the dog, there was no significant difference between the potency ratios and hence selectivity of the compounds (table 6).

Since the potency and intrinsic selectivity of prostacyclin for either parameter can vary between species, it is clear that any claim for selective cardiovascular or antiaggregating actions in a series of analogues must be supported by a direct comparison in which prostacyclin or carbacyclin is tested in the same experimental preparation. Thus, selectivity of action may be more readily demonstrated in certain species and preparations of platelet aggregation.

TABLE 6

Comparison of the hypotensive and platelet antiaggregating effects of prostacyclin and 9β-methyl-carbacyclin (9β-Me) after intravenous infusion in the anesthetized greyhound and the patas monkey

	Blood pressure		Platelets	
	ED_{30} (μg^{-1} min^{-1})	Potency ratio	ID_{50} (μg^{-1} min^{-1})	Potency ratio
Dog				
PGI_2	0.05	1	0.013	1
9β-Me	1.9	0.03	0.31	0.04
Monkey				
PGI_2	0.2	1	0.13	1
9β-Me	14.3	0.014	9.1	0.014

Results, shown as mean from four experiments for each species, are expressed as the ED_{30} (the dose causing a 30 mm Hg fall in diastolic blood pressure) and the ID_{50} (the dose causing a 50% inhibition of ex vivo platelet aggregation induced by ADP) and as the potency ratio to prostacyclin. Data is derived from Allan et al.[34]

Studies with the 16-substituted carbacyclin derivative iloprost (figure 1, *D*) in the anesthetized cat indicate that the decrease in peripheral platelet count after coronary ligation can be abolished by doses having no effect on blood pressure.[22] Results of studies with this derivative in the baboon during intravenous infusion have indicated that platelet aggregation ex vivo could be inhibited with variable effects on blood pressure and heart rate.[33] Investigation of the hypotensive activity after bolus injection in the baboon have suggested selectivity of action of iloprost away from the cardiovascular actions of carbacyclin.[33] Comparative studies with this analogue and with prostacyclin on formation of thrombi in an extracorporeal circuit in the anesthetized rat could not, however, demonstrate any disassociation between the antiaggregatory and vasodepressor actions.[24]

Studies in man. In a preliminary evaluation in human volunteers, intravenous infusion of carbacyclin inhibited platelet aggregation ex vivo yet had no effect on blood pressure or heart rate.[35] Since concurrent studies with prostacyclin in these subjects were not undertaken, the extent of this selectivity of action in man could not be assessed. After oral administration of carbacyclin (25 mg) in two subjects in a dose sufficient to cause approximately 68% inhibition of platelet aggregation ex vivo (determined 30 to 90 min later), a marked rise in heart rate was observed, along with headache and flushing of rapid onset.[35]

In studies in human volunteers, the analogue 15-cyclopentyl carbacyclin (ONO 41483; figure 1, *B*), infused intravenously in the maximum tolerated dose (2.5 ng $kg^{-1}min^{-1}$), caused a 27% inhibition of platelet aggregation ex vivo.[21] Higher doses, both by the intravenous and oral route, produced more substantial inhibition of platelet aggregation, but also induced side effects including flushing of the face and limbs, headache, and phlebitis,[21] effects similar to those observed with high doses of prostacyclin.[36]

In a placebo-controlled study in six patients with peripheral vascular disease, intravenous infusion of the 16-methyl derivative iloprost (figure 1, *A*) in doses of 0.5 to 3 ng $kg^{-1}min^{-1}$ for 2 to 4 hr did not alter systemic arterial blood pressure or heart rate, nor did it increase blood flow in the calf muscle or extremities.[37] At higher doses that inhibited platelet aggregation ex vivo, side effects of facial flushing and headache were observed.[37] In a further study during intravenous infusion of iloprost (4 to 8 $ng^{-1}kg^{-1}min^{-1}$) for 72 hr in nine patients with peripheral vascular disease, marked vasodilation but only a small fall in blood pressure was reported, but a high incidence of side effects (including headache and vomiting) was noted. An increase in urine output, glomerular filtration, and kallikrein excretion was also found, with a decrease in tubular reabsorptions of sodium and water and serum angiotensin-converting activity after infusion of iloprost.[38]

In a double-blind placebo-controlled comparison of the effects of epoprostenol (prostacyclin) and the analogue 9β-methyl-carbacyclin (figure 2, *B*; ciprostene) in healthy volunteers, the two drugs exhibited comparable profiles of pharmacologic activity.[19] During intravenous infusion, 9β-methyl-carbacyclin (150 to 600 ng $kg^{-1}min^{-1}$) significantly displaced the dose-response curve for ADP-induced platelet aggregation ex vivo, being 0.01 times as active as prostacyclin. As with prostacyclin, elevation in heart rate was only observed at the highest rate of infusion, while no change in systolic or diastolic blood pressure or left ventricular ejection time was observed with either compound in the dose range studied. A greater incidence of facial flushing was observed with prostacyclin than with 9β-methyl-carbacyclin in the lower dose range, while headache was only noted at the highest rate of infusion of 9β-methyl-carbacyclin.[19] The pharmacodynamic effects and duration of action of 9β-methyl-carbacyclin and prostacyclin in man are thus comparable, with the analogue being 100 times less active.

The mechanisms underlying peripheral vasodilation, as demonstrated by facial flushing or increased blood flow to the extremities in the absence of a marked fall in blood pressure, as seen with prostacyclin, 9β-methyl-carbacyclin, or other analogues, warrant further investigation and point to potential therapeutic utilities of these compounds, including the treatment of peripheral vascular diseases. Although the carbacyclin analogues described thus far offer the advantage of being more chemically stable than prostacyclin, the development of well-tolerated, orally effective compounds of long duration of activity for use in man is still awaited. Although there is some evidence from experimental studies of a change in selectivity away from the vasodepressor actions of prostacyclin, there is as yet no stable analogue that has a highly selective action on platelets in vivo. Claims for such selectivity in an analogue will require support from rigorous comparisons with prostacyclin in several experimental preparations in different species. The definitive separation of the platelet and cardiovascular properties in further analogues, if demonstrated in man, will have extensive therapeutic possibilities and will also allow a closer analysis of the mechanism of action of prostacyclin in such clinical situations as peripheral vascular disease. The rational design of the pharmacologic profile of such analogues will, however, depend on the clinical experience gained with prostacyclin itself.

We are grateful to Mr. Paul Lidbury and Ms. Sheesh Hamid for technical expertise, and to The Upjohn Company, Kalamazoo, MI, for the supply of the carbacyclin derivatives.

References

1. Moncada S, Gryglewski RJ, Bunting S, Vane JR: An enzyme isolated from arteries transforms prostaglandin endoperoxides to an unstable substance that inhibits platelet aggregation. Nature **263:** 663, 1976
2. Johnson RA, Morton DR, Kinner JH, Gorman RR, McGuire JC, Sun FF, Whittaker N, Bunting S, Salmon JA, Moncada S, Vane JR: The chemical structure of prostaglandin X (prostacyclin). Prostaglandins **12:** 915, 1976
3. Johnson RA, Lincoln FH, Smith HW, Ayer DE, Nidy EG, Thompson JL, Axen U, Aiken JW, Gorman RR, Nishizawa EE, Honohen T: Biological effects of stable prostacyclin analogs. *In* Vane JR, Bergstrom S, editors: Prostacyclin. New York, 1979, Raven Press, p 17
4. Tonga G, Gandolfi C, Andreoni A, Fumagalli A, Passarotti C, Faustini F, Patrono C: Inhibition of human platelet aggregation by stable analogs of prostacyclin. Pharmacol Res Commun **9:** 909, 1977
5. Whittle BJR, Boughton-Smith NK, Moncada S, Vane JR: The relative activity of prostacyclin (PGI_2) and a stable analogue 6β-PGI_1 on the gastrointestinal and cardiovascular systems. J Pharm Pharmacol **30:** 597, 1978
6. Nicolaou KC, Barnette WE, Magolda RL: Synthesis of (5Z)- and (5E)-6,9-thiaprostacyclins. J Am Chem Soc **103:** 3472, 1981
7. Bundy GL, Baldwin JM: The synthesis of nitrogen-containing prostacyclin analogs. Tetrahedron Lett **16:** 1371, 1978
8. Flohé L, Bohlke H, Frankus E, Kim SMA, Lintz W, Loschen G, Michel G, Muller B, Schneider J, Seipp U, Vollenberg W, Wilsmann K: Designing prostacyclin analogues. Arzneimittelforsch **33:** 1240, 1983
9. Nicolaou K, Sipio WJ, Magolda RL, Seitz S, Barnette WE: Total synthesis of carboprostacyclin, a stable and biologically active

analogue of prostacyclin (PGI_2). J Chem Soc Chem Comm 1067, 1978
10. Kojima K, Sakai K: Total synthesis of 9(0)-methanoprostacyclin and its isomers. Tetrahedron Lett **39:** 3743, 1978
11. Morton DR, Brokaw FC: Total synthesis of 6a-carbaprostaglandin I_2 and related isomers. J Organic Chem **44:** 2280, 1979
12. Morton DR, Bundy GL, Nishizawa EE: Five-membered ring-modified prostacyclin analogs. *In* Vane JR, Bergstrom S, editors: Prostacyclin. New York, 1979, Raven Press, p 31
13. Whittle B Jr, Moncada S, Whiting F, Vane JR: Carbacyclin — a potent stable prostacyclin analogue for the inhibition of platelet aggregation. Prostaglandins **19:** 605, 1980
14. Ceserani R, Grossoni M, Longiave D, Mizzotti B, Pozzi O, Dembinska-Kiec A, Bianco S: dl-9a-deoxy-9a-methylene-PGI_2 (a stable prostacyclin derivative): preliminary pharmacological data. Prostaglandins Med **5:** 131, 1980
15. Morita A, Mori M, Hasegawa K, Kojima K, Kobayashi S: Antiplatelet aggregating and disaggregating activities of 6,9-methano PGI_2. Life Sci **27:** 695, 1980
16. Aiken JW, Shebuski RJ: Comparison in anaesthetized dogs of the anti-aggregatory and hemodynamic effects of prostacyclin and a chemically stable prostacyclin analog, 6a-carba-PGI_2 (carbacyclin). Prostaglandins **19:** 629, 1980
17. Adaikan PG, Karim SMM, Lau LC: Platelet and other effects of carboprostacyclin — a stable prostacyclin analogue. Prostaglandins Med **5:** 307, 1980
18. Aristoff PA, Johnson PD, Harrison AW: Synthesis of 9-substituted carbacyclin analogues. J Organic Chem **48:** 5341, 1983
19. O'Grady J, Hedges A, Whittle BJR, Al-Sinawil AH, Mekki QA, Burke C, Moody SG, Moti MJ, Hassan S: A chemically stable analogue, 9β-methyl carbacyclin, with similar effects to epoprostenol (prostacyclin, PGI_2) in man. Br J Clin Pharmacol **18:** 921, 1984
20. Adaikan PG, Kottegada SR, Lau LC, Tai MY, Karim SMM: Inhibition of platelet aggregation and reversal of vasopressin-induced ECG changes by a carboprostacyclin analogue, ONO 41483, in primates. Prostaglandins Leukotrienes Med **9:** 307, 1982
21. Adaikan PG, Lau LC, Tai MY, Karim SMM: Inhibition of platelet aggregation with intravenous and oral administration of a carboprostacyclin analogue, 15-cyclopentyl — pentanor-5(E)-carbacyclin (ONO 41483) in man. Prostaglandins Leukotrienes Med **10:** 53, 1983
22. Schrör K, Darius H, Matzky R, Ohlendorf R: The antiplatelet and cardiovascular actions of a new carbacyclin derivative (ZK 36374) — Equipotent to PGI_2 in vitro. N-S. Arch Pharmacol **316:** 252, 1981
23. Schrör K, Ohlendorf R, Darius H: Beneficial effects of a new carbacyclin derivative, ZK 36 374, in acute myocardial ischemia. J Pharmacol Exp Ther **219:** 243, 1981
24. Casals-Stenzel J, Buse M, Losert W: Comparison of the vasodepressor action of ZK 36 374, a stable prostacyclin derivative, PGI_2 and PGE_2 with their effect on platelet aggregation and bleeding time in rats. Prostaglandins Leukotrienes Med **10:** 197, 1983
25. Gandolfi CA, Ceserani R: Prostacyclin analogs: Structure-activity relationships. *In* Johnson Hegyeli R, editor: Prostaglandins and cardiovascular disease. New York, 1981, Raven Press, p 183
26. Morley J, Page CP, Paul W, Mongelli N, Ceserani R, Gandolfi C: A comparative study of PGI_2 and two analogues (FCE 21292 and FCE 21258) in vitro and in vivo. Prostaglandins Leukotrienes Med **11:** 391, 1983
27. Oates JA, Whorton AR, Gerkens JF, Branch RA, Hollifield JW, Frolich JC: The participation of prostaglandins in the control of renin release. Fed Proc **38:** 72, 1979
28. Patrono C, Pugliese F, Ciabattoni G, Patrignani P, Maseri A, Chierchia S, Peskar BA, Cinotti GA, Simonetti BM, Pierucci A: Evidence for a direct stimulatory effect of prostacyclin on renin release in man. J Clin Invest **69:** 231, 1982
29. Feuerstein G, Zerbe RL, Meyer DK, Kopin IJ: Alterations of cardiovascular, neurogenic and humoral responses to acute hypovolemic hypotension by administered prostacyclin. J Cardiovasc Pharmacol **4:** 246, 1982
30. Muller B, Schneider J, Wilsmann K, Lintz W, Flohé L: Role of renin release in the hemodynamic, renal and dipsogenic actions of the prostacyclin analogue CG 4203 in conscious rats. Prostaglandins Leukotrienes Med **11:** 361, 1983
31. McGuire JC, Morton DR, Brokaw FC, Sun FF: Metabolism of (5E)-6a-carbaprostaglandin I_2 by rhesus monkey lung 15-OH prostaglandin dehydrogenase. Prostaglandins **21:** 609, 1981
32. Krause W, Schubert M, Totzek M: Pharmacokinetics and biotransformation of the prostacyclin analogue ZK 36 374 in the monkey (*Macaca fascicularis*). Prostaglandins Leukotrienes Med **11:** 325, 1983
33. Adaikan PG, Karim SMM, Lau LC, Tai MY, Kottegoda SR: Inhibition of platelet aggregation and antagonism of vasopressin-induced ECG changes in primates by a carboprostacyclin analogue, ZK 36 374. Thromb Res **33:** 333, 1984
34. Allan G, Follenfant MJ, Lidbury P, Oliver PL, Whittle BJR: The cardiovascular and platelet actions of 9β-methyl carbacyclin (ciprostene), a chemically stable analogue of prostacyclin in the dog and monkey. Br J Pharmacol **85:** 547, 1985
35. Karim SMM, Adaikan PG, Lau LC, Tai MY: Inhibition of platelet aggregation with intravenous and oral administration of carboprostacyclin in man. Prostaglandins Med **6:** 521, 1981
36. O'Grady J, Warrington S, Moti MJ, Bunting S, Flower RJ, Fowle ASE, Higgs EA, Moncada S: Effects of intravenous prostacyclin infusions in healthy volunteers. Some preliminary observations. In Vane JR, Bergstrom S, editors: Prostacyclin. New York, 1979, Raven Press, p 409
37. Darius H, Hossmann V, Auel H, Schrör K: Haemodynamic and platelet effects of iloprost (ZK 36 374) in patients with peripheral arterial disease. *In* Proceedings of the Second International Symposium on Prostaglandins and Cardiovascular System. Nurnberg, 1984
38. Vapaatalo H, Ylitalo P, Kaukinen S, Pessi T, Nurimi AK, Krais T: Effects of iloprost, a stable carbaprostacyclin analogue on kidney function, plasma and urine electrolytes and kallikrein-kinin system in man. In Proceedings of the Second International Symposium on Prostaglandins and Cardiovascular System. Nurnberg, 1984

Effect of β-adrenergic blockers on the peripheral circulation in patients with peripheral vascular disease

WILLIAM R. HIATT, M.D., SANDRA STOLL, O.T.R., AND ALAN S. NIES, M.D.

ABSTRACT β-Adrenergic blockers have not been widely used in patients with peripheral vascular disease because these drugs have been reported to worsen the symptoms of intermittent claudication. To test this assumption we studied the effects of a β_1-selective and a nonselective β-adrenergic blocker on postexercise calf blood flow and symptoms of claudication in 19 patients with mild-to-moderate peripheral vascular disease. Subjects received placebo for 3 weeks, and then were randomized to 120 mg/day propranolol or 150 mg/day metoprolol with the use of a crossover design. Blood flow in the calf was measured by strain-gauge plethysmography at rest and immediately after exercise on a bicycle ergometer at a low and a high workload. The symptoms of claudication were monitored during bicycle exercise and by patient diaries maintained between visits. Maximal exercise heart rate was reduced an equivalent amount by metoprolol (19 beats/min) and propranolol (16 beats/min). Mean arterial pressure was reduced by propranolol at rest and by both drugs with exercise. Calf blood flow was not affected by either drug compared with placebo at rest or at either workload. In addition, the symptoms of claudication were not worsened by either drug. We conclude that despite evidence of β_1-adrenergic blockade and a lowering of arterial pressure, neither β-adrenergic blocker adversely affected the peripheral circulation.
Circulation 72, No. 6, 1226–1231, 1985.

β-ADRENERGIC BLOCKING DRUGS are infrequently prescribed in patients with peripheral vascular disease (PVD) because anecdotal reports associate these agents with causing or worsening the symptoms of intermittent claudication.[1–5] As a result, it has been recommended that β-adrenergic blockers should be used cautiously, or not at all, in such patients.[6–8] However, controlled trials have been unable to confirm this adverse effect.[9,10]

β-Adrenergic blockers may interact with the peripheral circulation in serveral ways. A nonselective antagonist could attenuate epinephrine-induced vasodilation during exercise by blocking vascular β_2-adrenergic receptors.[11, 12] Thus, a selective β_1-adrenergic blocker would be preferred because it would maintain epinephrine-mediated vasodilation. In contrast, any drug that reduces systemic blood pressure could decrease blood flow through a stenotic vessel or the collateral circulation and thereby exacerbate the symptoms of claudication. To better define the effects of these drugs on exercise calf blood flow and the symptoms of claudication, we studied patients with PVD during treatment with placebo, propranolol, and metoprolol.

Methods

Patients. Twenty-four patients with chronic stable intermittent claudication were evaluated for the study. The diagnosis of PVD was confirmed by previous noninvasive testing demonstrating that the ratio of ankle to arm systolic blood pressure was less than 0.95 at rest or after exercise.[13, 14] Patients with ischemic pain at rest were excluded because of inability to exercise, as were patients with angina, arrhythmias, or congestive heart failure. Patients with contraindications to the use of β-adrenergic blockers, such as vasospasm, asthma, or insulin-dependent diabetes mellitus were also excluded. Patients on vasoactive medications (vasodilators, sympatholytics, nitrates, etc.) discontinued these drugs before entry into the study. This study was approved by the Human Subjects Committee and informed consent was obtained from all subjects.

During the initial visit, all subjects underwent a symptom-limited, maximal treadmill test. The treadmill protocol began at

From the Department of Medicine, Divisions of General Internal Medicine and Clinical Pharmacology, University of Colorado Health Sciences Center, Denver.

Supported by a grant from Ciba-Geigy Pharmaceuticals Corp., and by a Research and Training Center grant (G008003049) from the National Institute for Handicapped Research, Department of Education, Washington, D.C.

Address for correspondence: William R. Hiatt, M.D., Division of General Internal Medicine, University of Colorado Health Sciences Center, 4200 East 9th Ave., Box B-180, Denver, CO 80262.

Received May 31, 1985; revision accepted Sept. 12, 1985.

Dr. Hiatt is a Henry J. Kaiser Family Foundation Faculty Scholar in General Internal Medicine.

3 mph, 0% grade. Stages were 2 min in duration, with a 2.5% increase in the grade at each successive stage until maximal symptoms of claudication occurred. To be included in the study each subject had to be able to achieve at least the third stage of exertion.

Study design. All subjects participated in a 3 week, single-blind, placebo run-in phase. At the end of each week, measurements of calf blood flow were obtained, and the symptoms of claudication were noted. Patients were excluded if calf blood flow measurements after exercise varied by more than 15% over the three visits. After the placebo phase, subjects were randomly assigned in a double-blind fashion, to receive either propranolol or metoprolol. After 2 weeks on a drug subjects received 2 weeks of placebo and then crossed over to the other drug for the final 2 weeks. Measurements were obtained at the end of each 2 week period.

Drug dosing. Placebo and drugs were administered as identically appearing tablets. The doses were as follows: placebo three times a day, 40 mg propranolol three times a day, and 50 mg metoprolol three times a day. Equivalency of dosing was determined by comparing the reduction in maximal exercise heart rate on drug to the heart rate on placebo.[15]

Vascular testing. Subjects were studied while in the supine position with the calf elevated above the level of the heart. Blood flow to the calf was measured by venous occlusion plethysmography.[16] With this method, a single-stranded, mercury-in-silicone rubber strain gauge was calibrated with a 1 mm stretch, then placed around the maximal calf circumference. The signal from the strain gauge was amplified and recorded on a strip-chart recorder. For the duration of each measurement sequence an ankle cuff was inflated to 250 mm Hg, then a thigh cuff was rapidly inflated to 40 mm Hg for 3 sec. Blood flow (ml/100 ml tissue/min) was calculated from the maximal rate of change of the calf volume. This technique has been validated previously by comparison with direct measurements of flow.[17] The electrocardiogram (lead V_5) was monitored continuously, and blood pressure was measured in the left arm by cuff sphygmomanometry. Mean systemic arterial pressure was calculated as one-third the pulse pressure added to the diastolic pressure. Vascular resistance was calculated by dividing mean blood pressure in the arm by calf blood flow.

At each testing session, initial measurements were taken at rest in the leg with the most severe claudication. Heart rate and blood pressure were recorded once. Calf blood flow was taken as the average of three determinations. Next, both feet were placed on the pedals of a bicycle ergometer, with the fulcrum of the pedal over the distal portion of the foot to facilitate calf exercise. Subjects exercised at a workload of 100 kg·m/min for 2 min, with heart rate and blood pressure recorded during the last 30 sec. Exercise was terminated with an electronically activated catch on the ergometer that allowed the foot to stop in a fixed, reproducible position and the calf to relax rapidly. Beginning 3 sec after the termination of exercise, calf blood flow was measured multiple times to monitor postexercise hyperemia. Subjects were then allowed to rest until heart rate, blood pressure, and calf blood flow had returned to baseline levels. This measurement sequence was repeated three times. The single peak flow after each exercise test was used for analysis. The three determinations of blood pressure, heart rate, and calf blood flow were averaged, and the mean values were used for subsequent analysis.

After exercise at the low workload, subjects performed a final test to maximal exertion. The workload was increased by 100 kg·m/min every 2 min to exhaustion of the subject, and the times of onset of and maximal claudication were noted. Heart rate, blood pressure, and calf blood flow were recorded at the end of exercise, as in the preceding exercise tests.

Between study visits, subjects were instructed to keep a diary recording the frequency of their symptoms of intermittent claudication in the most severely affected leg.

Statistical analysis. Subjects were initially analyzed according to the order in which they received the drugs. Those in sequence I received metoprolol before propranolol and those in sequence II received propranolol before metoprolol. Demographic data on entry were compared with Student's t test for unpaired data or Fisher's exact test.

For a given response variable, the baseline for the first treatment period was determined by averaging responses obtained during the first three visits while the subject was on placebo. The baseline for the second period was determined from the single placebo visit before the final 2 weeks of treatment.

The crossover design was evaluated by the statistical methods of Grizzle[18] and Patel[19] with the use of an analysis of variance with covariate adjustment for the baseline measurements. Once the crossover design was validated, the differences between each drug and placebo were determined by averaging all data from both sequences and comparing the means with a one-way analysis of variance for repeated measures. Multiple comparisons were performed with a modification of the Scheffe test.[20]

A 95% confidence interval was used to describe the potential change in flow caused by each drug at each workload. This was done by subtracting the flow values on drug from those on placebo for each subject.

Results

Baseline data and tests of crossover design. Twenty-four subjects were screened for enrollment into the study. Four were excluded: two were unable to walk 6 min on the treadmill, one had angina, and one did not develop symptoms of claudication during treadmill testing. Twenty subjects were enrolled, but one was disqualified because of a greater than 15% variation in calf blood flow measurements during the placebo period. Of the remaining subjets, 10 had aortoiliac disease, seven had femoropopliteal disease, and two had both. Nine were hypertensive, two had diabetes, seven had coronary artery disease, and three had carotid artery disease. The mean ankle/arm ratio of systolic blood pressure of the most diseased leg was 0.70, with a range of 0.22 to 0.89. The subjects were randomized into comparable groups with respect to age, sex, and treadmill walking time on entry into the study. Demographic data are summarized in table 1.

Subjects in each treatment sequence were found to have equivalent responses during the two placebo periods for heart rate, blood pressure, and calf blood flow at rest and with exercise. The symptoms of claudication during these testing sessions were also equivalent between groups. There were no carryover drug effects and the order in which the drugs were given did not influence the results. Thus, the criteria for validity of the crossover design were satisfied and the results in the two sequences were pooled.

Maximal exercise heart rate. Heart rate during maximal exercise was reduced an equivalent amount by

TABLE 1
Demographics

	n	Sex (male: female)	Age (years)	Treadmill (min:sec)
Sequence I	10	9:1	57±3	8:23±0:54
Sequence II	9	7:2	58±3	7:23±1:00

Values are reported as mean ± SEM. Treadmill refers to the maximal duration of walking exercise at entry. There were no significant differences between the sequences for any of the above variables.

Sequence I = metoprolol before propranolol; sequence II = propranolol before metoprolol.

each drug. The reduction on metoprolol was 19 beats/min and on propranolol is was 16 beats/min ($p<.01$ for both compared with placebo). The maximal workload did not change in either sequence when subjects went from placebo to drug. The effects of each drug at maximal exercise heart rate and workload are summarized in table 2.

Mean blood pressure. Mean blood pressure was lowered by propranolol at rest, and by both drugs at 100 kg·m/min and maximal exercise (figure 1).

Calf blood flow. Flow at rest averaged 3.0 ± 0.3 ml/100 ml/min on placebo and increased progressively at each workload (figure 1). Neither drug caused a significant reduction in calf blood flow compared with placebo at rest or with exercise, nor were there differences in flow in subjects on the two drugs. The 95% confidence limits (in ml/100 ml/min) for the change in blood flow on metoprolol were −0.5 to 0.8 at rest, −0.8 to 1.6 at 100 kg·m/min of exertion, and −0.02 to 2.2 at maximal exercise. For propranolol, the 95% confidence limits were −0.2 to 0.9 at rest, −0.1 to 2.4 at 100 kg·m/min of exertion, and −0.5 to 2.8 at maximal exercise.

Vascular resistance. Calculated vascular resistance in the leg was not changed by either drug compared with placebo. Resistance values are presented in table 3.

Symptoms of claudication. During maximal bicycle exercise the symptoms of claudication initially appeared in all subjects within 2 to 3 min and became maximal at 4 to 5 min. Subjects recorded an average of three to five episodes of claudication per week. Neither the occurrence of these symptoms during bicycle exercise nor the frequency of claudication as recorded in patient diaries was affected by either drug (table 2).

Discussion

Peripheral vascular disease is a common disorder. When an elderly population was surveyed, 11% had definite arterial occlusive disease diagnosed by noninvasive testing.[21] In the Framingham study, PVD occurred at one-fourth the incidence of coronary artery disease.[22]

Among the large population of patients with PVD, coronary artery disease and hypertension are prevalent conditions that often require treatment with β-adrenergic blockers. However, several case reports indicated that patients prescribed these drugs for angina or hypertension were at risk of developing claudication. In some cases,[4] symptoms did not occur until several months after drug therapy was begun, indicating that patients with coronary artery disease are at a four- to five-fold increased risk of developing PVD.[22] In addition, β-adrenergic blockers may improve exercise tolerance in patients with angina and thus unmask intermittent claudication. Symptoms of vasospasm are also reported frequently in these patients,[2, 3] and vasospasm is a well-described potential side effect of β-adrenergic blockers.[23] However, in some patients the drugs were more temporally associated with the development of claudication.[1, 5] These observations have led to the general recommendation that β-adrenergic blockers should be used cautiously, if at all, in patients with PVD.[6–8]

Ingram et al.[24] studied 15 patients with PVD who were being treated with β-adrenergic blockers. In an uncontrolled manner he observed an improvement in exercise calf blood flow on withdrawal of the medication. Smith and Warren[25] randomly assigned eight patients with PVD to placebo or one of three different β-

TABLE 2
Maximal exercise heart rate, workload, and symptoms of claudication

	Placebo	Metoprolol	Placebo	Propranolol
Maximal heart rate (beats/min)	110±4	91±2[A]	110±3	94±3[A]
Maximal workload (kg·m/min)	285±24	268±20	275±26	274±25
Onset of claudication (min)	2.5±0.4	2.4±0.4	2.8±0.6	2.7±0.5
Maximal claudication (min)	4.9±0.5	4.6±0.5	5.1±0.6	5.0±0.6

Subjects exercised once to maximal exertion on a bicycle ergometer for determination of heart rate, workload, and symptoms of claudication. Data are reported as mean ± SEM.

[A]$p < .01$ compared with placebo.

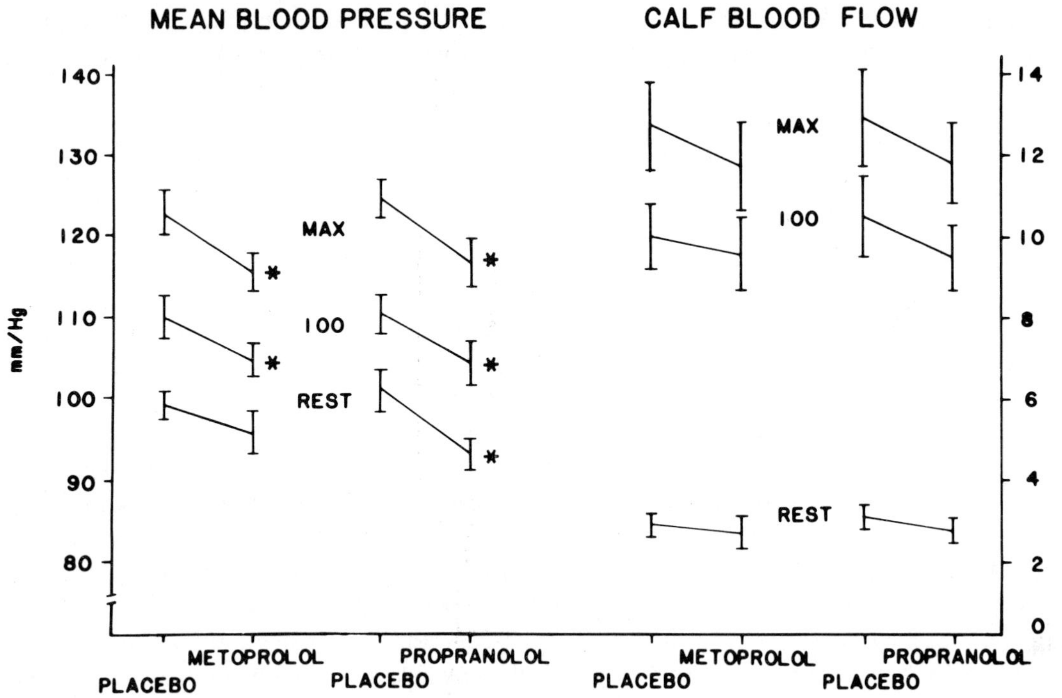

FIGURE 1. Mean blood pressure and calf blood flow at rest and with exercise. Rest = before exercise; 100 = 100 kg·m/min of exertion; Max = maximal exercise. * Analysis of variance significant ($p<.05$) for blood pressure lowered by drug compared with placebo. Data are reported as mean ± SEM.

adrenergic blockers. Those on drug had a 30% to 40% reduction in exercise calf blood flow. In these two studies the exercise involved flexion and extension movements of the foot, an activity that does not stimulate the circulation to the extent of walking or bicycling. In both studies, flow was measured by xenon clearance, a technique that may not accurately measure the true muscle blood flow.[26] Also, in the latter study there were only two subjects per group, making the conclusions difficult to generalize to a larger population.

Lepantalo,[9] in a placebo-controlled, double-blind trial studied seven patients with PVD. Subjects received three different β-adrenergic blockers in a trial of crossover design. Calf blood flow during reactive hyperemia was modestly reduced by some of the drugs, but calf vascular resistance was not affected by any drug compared with placebo. Finally, Clement,[10] using a crossover design, evaluated 10 patients with PVD. Subjects were initially studied on placebo and then randomly assigned to receive high doses of metoprolol or propranolol. Neither drug was found to affect the symptoms of claudication or the walking distance achieved during treadmill exercise. Thus, no conclusive, well-controlled study documents an adverse effect of β-adrenergic–blocking drugs on exercise blood flow and the symptoms of claudication in patients with PVD.

There are several hypotheses to explain the potential interaction of β-adrenergic blockers with the peripheral circulation. First, a decrease in systemic arterial pressure will decrease perfusion pressure to the extremity. This decrease in pressure could reduce flow both in the collateral circulation and in the stenotic vessel.[27, 28] Also, in patients with PVD, calf blood flow had been observed to cease with each muscle contrac-

TABLE 3
Calf vascular resistance

	Placebo	Metoprolol	Placebo	Propranolol
Rest	40.6±4.4	51.2±8.1	40.8±5.6	43.1±5.4
100 kg·m/min exercise	12.3±1.0	13.1±1.5	12.2±1.1	12.4±1.0
Maximal exercise	11.0±1.0	11.5±1.1	11.2±1.0	11.3±1.1

Calf vascular resistance was calculated from mean arm arterial pressurse divided by calf blood flow and is expressed in units. Neither drug caused an increase in calf resistance compared with placebo.

tion during walking exercise. The cessation of flow occurs because the external pressure generated by the muscle exceeds that in the vessels distal to the stenosis, resulting in the collapse of arterioles.[29] By both mechanisms, drugs that lower arterial pressure may worsen skeletal muscle perfusion during walking and exacerbate the symptoms of claudication.

Second, β-adrenergic blockers may alter vascular tone by preventing vasodilation mediated by vascular β-adrenergic receptors. When normal subjects are infused with the adrenergic agonist epinephrine, muscle blood flow increases and vascular resistance falls.[11, 12] This vasodilation can be prevented by use of a nonselective β-adrenergic blocker, but is only partially attenuated by a β_1-selective adrenergic blocker. A drug that blocks vascular β_2-adrenergic receptors could prevent that component of muscle vasodilation mediated by the high levels of circulating epinephrine during exercise. However, findings that argue against this hypothesis are (1) skeletal muscle blood flow during exercise is controlled largely by the release of local metabolic factors,[30] and (2) patients with PVD are generally vasodilated distal to the large vessel stenosis or occlusion.[27] In addition, normal subjects given β-adrenergic blockers do not have diminished calf blood flow during exercise.[31, 32] However, collateral vessels may be under partial sympathetic control and the tone in these vessels could be increased by a β-adrenergic blocker.[28, 33]

Finally, β-adrenergic blockers could impair exercise performance by altering skeletal muscle metabolism. Free fatty acids are an important substrate for skeletal muscle during submaximal exercise.[34] β-Adrenergic blockers have been shown to lower blood levels and availability of this substrate.[35, 36] When propranolol is administered to normal subjects, the ability to sustain prolonged submaximal exercise is decreased, an effect that is correlated with the reduction in free fatty acids.[37] Similar effects are possible in "claudicators," but typically in these patients exercise is of short duration and is limited by the impaired blood flow.

In this study, subjects received equivalent doses of drug as indicated by the equal reduction in maximal exercise heart rate.[15] Mean blood pressure was reduced by both drugs compared with placebo, thus providing evidence that a substantial degree of β-adrenergic blockade was achieved in all subjects.

Calf blood flow was not significantly reduced by either β-adrenergic blocker, although there was a trend for exercise blood flow to be lowered by both drugs in proportion to the fall in mean blood pressure. If a larger sample size had been studied the changes in flow might have become significant, but given the size of the confidence intervals, the potential reduction in flow could not be great. In addition, there is no evidence that either drug induced an increase in calculated vascular resistance.

Importantly, the flow data were corroborated by the observation that the symptoms of claudication, as recorded during bicycle exercise and in patient diaries, were not affected by propranolol or metoprolol. Had the drugs reduced peripheral blood flow or altered skeletal muscle metabolism and availability of substrate, then these symptoms would have worsened. Thus, patient perceptions of claudication are in concordance with the hemodynamic findings.

We conclude that β-adrenergic blockers may be used safely in most patients with mild-to-moderate PVD. However, physicians should not disregard the case reports discussed above. None of our patients had Raynaud's phenomenon or other vasospastic tendencies that, in association with vascular disease, may indeed contraindicate the use of β-adrenergic blockers. Also, in patients with severe PVD small changes in perfusion pressure or vascular tone caused by β-adrenergic blockers could prove to be deleterious. Finally, all patients with PVD should be monitored carefully for changes in their symptoms during the initiation of β-adrenergic–blocker therapy.

We thank the staff of the Cardiac Rehabilitation Center and Drs. H.L. Brammell and Demerick Fradl for assistance with the study. Drs. Harji Patel and Gary Zerbe assisted with the statistical analysis, and Eleanor Swanson, Ph.D. helped edit the manuscript.

References

1. Fogoros R: Exacerbation of intermittent claudication by propranolol. N Engl J Med **302:** 1089, 1980
2. Frohlich E, Tarazi R, Dustan H: Peripheral arterial insufficiency. A complication of beta-adrenergic blocking therapy. JAMA **208:** 2471, 1969
3. Gokal R, Dornam T, Ledingham J: Peripheral skin necrosis complicating beta-blockage. Br Med J **1:** 721, 1979
4. Rodger J, Sheldon C, Lerski R, Livingstone W: Intermittent claudication complicating beta-blockade. Br Med J **1:** 1125, 1976
5. Vale J, Jefferys D: Peripheral gangrene complicating beta-blockade. Lancet **1:** 1216, 1978
6. Frishman W: β-Adrenoceptor antagonists: new drugs and new indications. N Engl J Med **305:** 500, 1981
7. Frishman W, Silverman R, Strom J, Elkayam U, Sonnenblick E: Clinical pharmacology of the new beta-adrenergic blocking drugs. Part 4. Adverse effects. Choosing a beta adrenergic blocker. Am Heart J **98:** 256, 1979
8. Breckenridge A: Which beta blocker? Br Med J **286:** 1085, 1983
9. Lepantalo M: Chronic effects of labetalol, pindolol, and propranolol on calf blood flow in intermittent claudication. Clin Pharmacol Ther **37:** 7, 1985
10. Clement D: Studies on the effect of alpha- and beta-adrenergic blocking agents on the circulation in human limbs. Verh K Acad Geneeskd Belg **42:** 164, 1980
11. Houben H, Thien T, van't Laar A: Effect of low-dose epinephrine

infusion on hemodynamics after selective and nonselective β-blockade in hypertension. Clin Pharmacol Ther **31:** 685, 1982
12. Hiatt W, Wolfel E, Stoll S, Nies A, Zerbe G, Brammell H, Horwitz L: $Beta_2$-adrenergic blockade evaluated with epinephrine after placebo, atenolol or nadolol. Clin Pharmacol Ther **37:** 2, 1985
13. Rutherford R, Lowenstein D, Klein M: Combining segmental systolic pressures and plethysmography to diagnose arterial occlusive disease of the legs. Am J Surg **138:** 211, 1979
14. Carter S: Response of ankle systolic pressure to leg exercise in mild or questionable arterial disease. N Engl J Med **287:** 578, 1972
15. Carruthers S, Shanks R, McDevitt D: Intrinsic heart rate on exercise and the measurement of β-adrenoceptor blockade. Br J Clin Pharmacol **3:** 991, 1976
16. Whitney R: The measurement of volume changes in human limbs. J Physiol **121:** 1, 1953
17. Longhurst J, Capone R, Mason D, Zelis R: Comparison of blood flow measured by plethysmograph and flowmeter during steady state forearm exercise. Circulation **49:** 535, 1974
18. Grizzle J: The two-period change-over design and its use in clinical trials. Biometrics **21:** 467, 1965
19. Patel H: Use of baseline measurements in the two-period crossover design. Commun Statist Theor Meth **12:** 2693, 1983
20. Einot I, Gabriel K: A study of the powers of several methods of multiple comparisons. J Am Stat Assoc **70:** 574, 1975
21. Criqui M, Fronek A, Barrett-Connor E, Klauber M, Gabriel S, Goodman D: The prevalence of peripheral arterial disease in a defined population. Circulation **71:** 510, 1985
22. Kannel W, Skinner J, Schwartz M, Shurtleff D: Intermittent claudication: incidence in the Framingham study. Circulation **41:** 875, 1970
23. Feleke E, Lyngstam O, Rastam L, Ryden L: Complaints of cold extremities among patients on antihypertensive treatment. Acta Med Scand **213:** 381, 1983
24. Ingram D, House A, Thompson G, Stacey M, Castleden W, Lovegrove F: Beta-adrenergic blockade and peripheral vascular disease. Med J Aust **1:** 509, 1982
25. Smith R, Warren D: Effect of β-blocking drugs on peripheral blood flow in intermittent claudication. J Cardiovasc Pharmacol **4:** 2, 1982
26. Rowell L: Cardiovascular adjustments to thermal stress. *In* Shepherd J, Abboud F, Geiger S, editors: Handbook of physiology. Bethesda, 1983, American Physiological Society, p 967
27. Dahn I, Ekman C, Lassen N, Nilsen R, Westling H: On the conservative treatment of severe ischemia of the leg. Scan J Clin Lab Invest **19**(suppl 99): 160, 1967
28. Coffman J: Peripheral collateral blood flow and vascular reactivity in the dog. J Clin Invest **45:** 923, 1966
29. Coffman J, Mannick J: A simple, objective test for arteriosclerosis obliterans. N Engl J Med **273:** 1297, 1965
30. Shepherd J: Circulation to skeletal muscle. *In* Shepherd J, Abboud F, Geiger S, editors: Handbook of physiology. Bethesda, 1983, American Physiological Society, p 319
31. Hiatt W, Fradl D, Zerbe G, Byyny R, Nies A: Selective and nonselective β-blockade of the peripheral circulation. Clin Pharmacol Ther **35:** 12, 1984
32. Juhlin-Dannfelt A, Astrom H: Influence of β-adrenoceptor blockade on leg blood flow and lactate release in man. Scand J Clin Lab Invest **39:** 179, 1979
33. Agerskov K, Henriksen O, Tonnesen K, Lassen N: Constriction of collateral arteries induced by "head-up tilt" in patients with occlusive arterial disease of the legs. Cardiovasc Res **15:** 675, 1981
34. Havel R, Pernow B, Jones N: Uptake and release of free fatty acids and other metabolites in the legs of exercising men. J Appl Physiol **23:** 90, 1967
35. Stankiewicz-Choroszucha B, Gorski J: Effect of beta-adrenergic blockade on intramuscular triglyceride mobilization during exercise. Experientia **34:** 357, 1978
36. Frisk-Holmberg M, Jorfeldt L, Juhlin-Dannfeldt A: Influence of alprenolol on hemodynamic and metabolic responses to prolonged exercise in subjects with hypertension. Clin Pharmacol Ther **21:** 675, 1977
37. Lundborg P, Astrom H, Bengtsson C, Fellenius E, Von Schenck H, Svensson L, Smith U: Effect of β-adrenoceptor blockade on exercise performance and metabolism. Clin Sci **61:** 299, 1981

Significance of cardiac defects in the developing fetus: a study of spontaneous abortuses

PHILIP C. URSELL, M.D., JULIANNE M. BYRNE, PH.D.,* AND BARBARA A. STROBINO, PH.D.

ABSTRACT We investigated the impact of heart defects on the developing human fetus by examining 412 hearts from consecutive spontaneous abortuses. In each case, the cardiac morphology was correlated with the autopsy findings and the karyotype (unavailable in 115 hearts not successfully cultured). Of the 412 hearts, 10 (2.4%) contained structural defects (six ventricular septal defects, one atrial septal defect with ventricular septal defect, and one each coarctation, atrioventricular septal defect, and tetralogy of Fallot). Only one of 10 had major extracardiac malformations. Of the 277 fetuses with normal karyotype, three (1.1%) had heart defects. Of the 20 fetuses with abnormal karyotype, four (20%) had heart defects. In the remaining three fetuses with heart defects, the karyotype was not obtained. Thus (1) 57% of spontaneous abortuses with congenital heart defects contained major chromosomal abnormalities, (2) the spectrum of heart defects among spontaneous abortuses was similar to that among liveborns, and (3) since the prevalence of heart defects among fetuses without other major abnormalities was similar to that among liveborns, heart defects alone may not jeopardize the survival of a developing fetus.
Circulation 72, No. 6, 1232–1236, 1985.

THE SIGNIFICANCE of heart defects in the developing fetus is uncertain. Major structural malformations of the heart that cause shunting and/or obstruction could be detrimental to the fetus. Studies have documented a higher prevalence of heart defects among stillborn infants than among liveborns.[1-3] However, it has never been clear from such studies whether the heart defect per se was responsible for death. In this regard, physiologic studies performed in animal preparations suggest that cardiac defects have little effect in utero.[4] Thus, cardiac defects may be a part of some other abnormal developmental process that results in death of the fetus.

We investigated the impact of heart defects on the developing human fetus by examining hearts from consecutive spontaneous abortuses. Analysis of the products of conception from spontaneous abortions provides an efficient means of evaluating the importance of morphologic and chromosomal anomalies to the survival of the fetus.[5] We correlated the cardiac pathology in each case with the karyotype and pathology manifest in the remainder of the fetus. Our objectives in this study were (1) to determine the prevalence and nature of cardiac defects among spontaneously aborted fetuses, and (2) to develop insight into the significance of these defects in the developing fetus.

From the Department of Pathology, the Gertrude H. Sergievsky Center, Columbia University, and the New York State Psychiatric Institute, New York.

Supported in part by the New York State Department of Mental Hygiene and by NIH grants 5R01HD08838, 5T32HD07040, 5R01HD12207, 5R01DA02090, and 5R01HD15909.

Address for correspondence: Philip C. Ursell, M.D., Department of Pathology, College of Physicians and Surgeons, Columbia University, 630 West 168th St., New York, NY 10032.

Received May 6, 1985; revision accepted Sept. 12, 1985.

Presented in part at the 1984 meeting of the American Heart Association, Miami Beach.

*Present address: Clinical Epidemiology Branch National Cancer Institute, N.I.H.

Materials and methods

Hearts examined in this study were obtained from a large epidemiology-cytogenetic-pathology study of consecutive spontaneous abortions identified at three New York City hospitals between 1976 and 1983. Approximately 4000 specimens were examined as a part of the larger study. However, because most products of conception from spontaneous abortions do not contain an organized fetus[6] and some hearts are not large enough to study, only 412 hearts could be eviscerated and subsequently examined. In each of the 412 cases, a complete autopsy of the fetus and placenta was performed.[7] Developmental age was determined by crown-rump length.[8] Histologic sections of the major organs, placenta, and umbilical cord were examined. The hearts were from relatively nonmacerated fetuses from 8 to 28 weeks of gestation. They were preserved in formaldehyde for subsequent study.

Dissection of the hearts was performed according to standard autopsy techniques. Each heart was opened along the path of blood flow. All observations and measurements were made under 10-fold magnification with a dissecting microscope. Measurements of the circumference of valve anuli and the aorta at the isthmus were made with a small flexible ruler or with a piece of thread and the ruler. The morphologic characteristics of these fetal hearts were described according to the scheme of Tynan et al.[9] A heart defect was defined as any developmental malformation of cardiac structure (and proximal great vessels) that is known to be attended by significant morbidity after birth. In addition to clear-cut abnormalities such as septal defects, more subtle changes due to relative stenoses or dilatations were judged to be true defects if measurements were more than two standard deviations from the mean of those of the normal hearts in the corresponding developmental age range. A secundum atrial septal defect was diagnosed if the untorn primum membrane covered less than one-half of the fossa ovalis. Although all ductus arteriosus vessels were patent, histologic inspection of ductal tissue was not performed.

Karyotypes were determined by tissue culture of fetal tissue and subsequent staining by the G-banding method as described previously.[10] A fetal karyotype was determined from 297 (72%) of the 412 specimens. In the remaining 115 hearts either no fetal tissue was set up in culture, or the specimen was set up but failed to grow.

A chi-square test was used to determine the significance of associations.

Results

The distribution of developmental ages of the 412 fetuses included in this study is shown in figure 1. Of the 412 hearts, 10 (2.4%) contained structural defects. The developmental age, type of defect, karyotype, and other accompanying major malformations are listed for each abortus with a heart defect in table 1. The developmental age of the youngest of the fetuses was 11 weeks, well beyond the period when cardiac morphogenesis is complete.

Ventricular septal defect was the most common cardiac anomaly among the 10 fetuses with heart defects. In each of the six cases of isolated ventricular septal defect, the defect was perimembranous and the diameters of the defects ranged from 50% to 100% of the diameter of the corresponding aortic valve anulus (figure 2). In one other case of ventricular septal defect there was a wide defect of the midportion of the interatrial septum with virtually no membrane covering it. Coarctation of the aorta was diagnosed in one heart in which the circumference of the aorta at the isthmus fell two standard deviations below the mean for fetuses of similar developmental age. There was no discrete "shelf" present in the aorta at the level of the ductus, but the distal portion of the aortic segment between the left subclavian artery and the ductus contained several irregular ridges of tissue that compromised the lumen. The coarctation was present in association with a bicuspid aortic valve. This association is seen in liveborns.[11] Only two of the 10 hearts showed complicated lesions: atrioventricular septal defect and tetralogy of Fallot (figure 3). There were no cases of more complex heart defects. Other major malformations were present in only one of the 10 fetuses with heart defects. This fetus had hydrocephalus and lung hypoplasia.

Karyotypes were documented in 297 fetuses; 277 were normal and 20 were abnormal. Of the 277 fetuses with normal karyotype, three (1.1%; 95% confidence limits 0.0% to 2.3%) had heart defects. Of the 20 fetuses with abnormal karyotype, four (20%; 95% confidence limits 2.5% to 37.5%) had heart defects. Thus, although the numbers are small, heart defects were more common in chromosomally abnormal than in chromosomally normal fetuses ($\chi^2 = 21.4$, $p < .001$). As shown in table 1, the chromosomal anomalies included trisomy 21, trisomy 3 with a normal cell line, and two cases of triploidy.

TABLE 1
Fetal characteristics

Fetus No.	Developmental age (weeks)	Cardiac defect	Karyotype	Other major malformations
1	11	AVSD	unknown	–
2	14	VSD	69XXY	–
3	15	VSD	69XXX	+
4	15	Tetralogy of Fallot	46XX	–
5	16	VSD, ASD-2°	46XX	–
6	18	VSD	47XX+3/46XX	–
7	19	VSD	unknown	–
8	20	VSD	46XY	–
9	21	Coarctation, BAV	unknown	–
10	26	VSD	47XX+21	–

VSD = ventricular septal defect; AVSD = atrioventricular septal defect; ASD-2° = ostium secundum–type atrial septal defect; BAV = bicuspid aortic valve; + = hydrocephalus and hypoplastic lungs present.

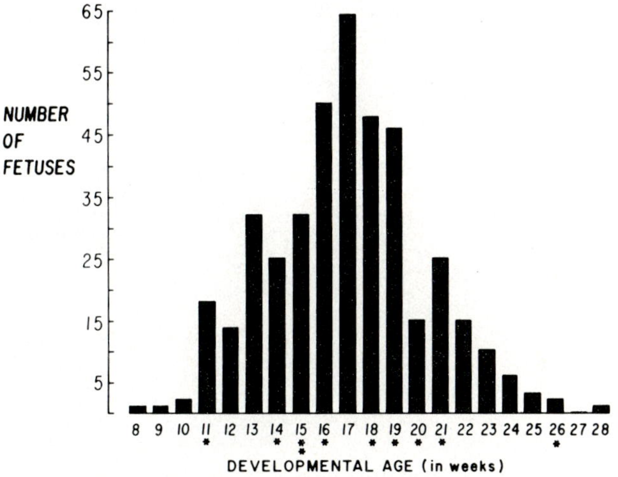

FIGURE 1. Histogram showing the distribution of developmental ages of fetuses from which hearts were obtained for this study. An asterisk denotes a fetus with a cardiac defect.

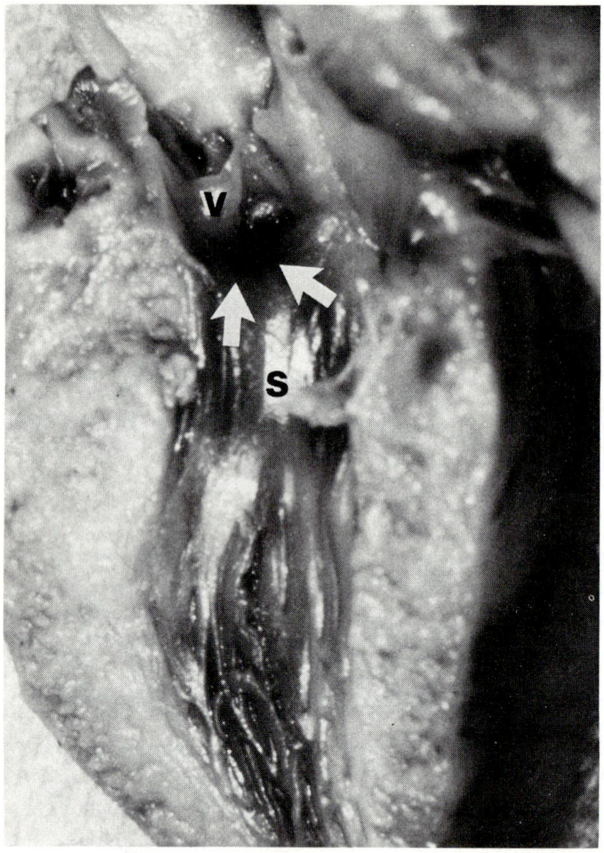

FIGURE 2. Under the dissecting microscopic, a perimembranous ventricular septal defect (arrows) is easily appreciated directly inferior to the aortic valve (V). The defect occupies roughly 10% of the septal surface (S), and the diameter of the defect is 50% of the diameter of the aortic valve anulus.

Discussion

Several studies of stillborn infants have determined the prevalence of cardiovascular defects to be in the range of 1.2% to 5.4%.[1] Our finding of heart defects in 2.4% of spontaneous abortuses of developmental ages 8 to 28 weeks is in accord with these other studies. It is important to recognize, however, that these prevalence figures include fetuses with heart defects and possibly other major malformations or chromosomal abnormalities. Thus, conclusions as to the effect of heart defects alone on the developing fetus should not be made from these data.

Recently, a series of cardiac malformations in spontaneous abortions has been published by Gerlis.[12] Using standard autopsy dissection techniques on larger hearts as well as histologic examination of small hearts, he found the prevalence of cardiac defects to be 15.4% within the gestational age range examined (less than 24 weeks). While this prevalence is considerably higher than what we found, a direct comparison of the two series may be impossible for several reasons. First, although "unselected," the British series of hearts may not have been derived from *consecutive* spontaneous abortions, as ours was. In any epidemiologic study, careful control over inclusion of specimens (preferably at one institution) is critical to ensure an unbiased sample. Second, although cardiac malformation is not specifically defined, the British series included hearts with several minor malformations, such as bilateral superior caval veins and pericardial defects, which were excluded in our series. On the other hand, there is a preponderance of relatively complex cardiac defects — such as valve atresias, transpositions and double-outlet ventricles — in the British series. It is unlikely that histologic analysis (a difference between the two studies) would have yielded many more cardiac malformations in our series, since these structural defects are readily identifiable grossly under the dissecting microscope. By not examining tissue histologically, we may have missed abnormal ductus tissue, a precursor for patent ductus arteriosus. However, from the report it appears that ductus tissue

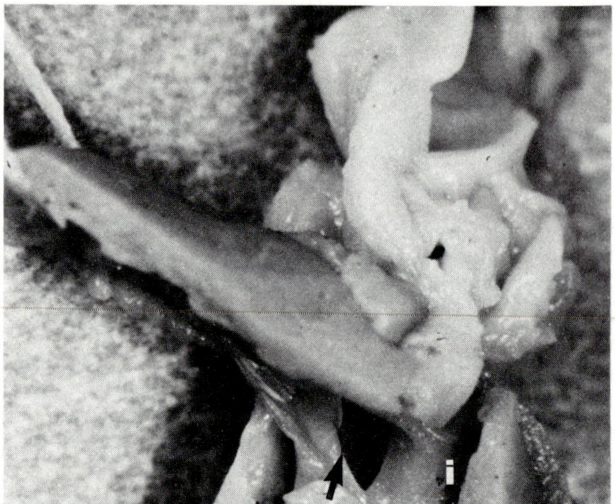

FIGURE 3. The anatomy of tetralogy of Fallot is clearly evident in this view from the opened right ventricle (V). The ventricular septal defect (arrow) is present directly anterior to the tricuspid valve (T) and is separated from the stenotic infundibulum (i) by the conal septum.

was not examined in the British study either, and so this cannot explain the discrepancy in prevalence rates found in the two studies. Instead, we suspect that the British series does not reflect the entire population of spontaneous abortuses — that the heart specimens were unwittingly selected by the referring hospitals for examination by the cardiac pathologist. That cardiac malformations are not so common among spontaneous abortuses in Great Britain is supported by another study in which the prevalence was found to be 0.4%.[13] Problems such as inadvertant introduction of a bias, different observers, and varying definitions of terms commonly plague epidemiologic studies and often make direct comparison difficult.

We have attempted to focus on the significance of cardiac disease in the fetus by separating out fetuses with other conditions that may jeopardize survival. It is generally accepted that certain anatomic malformations are detrimental to the developing fetus, although there are scant data in support of this. For example, an increased frequency of malformation of the central nervous system among spontaneous abortuses has been reported,[14] suggesting that these defects are detrimental in utero. Certain other major malformations may also be harmful to the fetus. In our study, only one fetus with cardiac defects had other major malformations, but it also had an abnormal karyotype.

In contrast to gross structural malformations, chromosomal anomalies were more common in fetuses with heart defects (57.1%), in excess of their frequency among fetuses without heart defects (5.5%) ($p < .001$). The association of heart defects with specific chromosomal anomalies is well known.[2, 15] Trisomy 21 is associated with a 53% frequency of congenital heart disease, while trisomy 13 and trisomy 18 are associated with even higher frequencies of 83% and 95%, respectively. In addition to one case of trisomy 21 with ventricular septal defect, within our group of fetuses with heart defects there were two examples of triploidy with ventricular septal defect. A variety of heart defects, including ventricular septal defects, has been reported in stillbirths and infants with triploid karyotype.[16, 17] The precise manner by which extra chromosomes lead to heart defects has never been determined. Nevertheless, clinically it is important to recognize that a high percentage of patients with heart defects (liveborn infants as well as fetuses) has chromosomal abnormalities, a factor that may influence the prognosis.

In the present study of spontaneous abortuses, three of 277 (1.1%) fetuses with normal karyotypes had heart defects. As best we can determine by our methods (complete autopsy and documentation of karyotype), these three demonstrate no other significant disease processes. In studies of stillborn infants and neonates, the autopsy, including gross and histologic examination, and the determination of karyotype appear sufficient to detect the great majority of abnormalities.[18] We believe that the same should be true for fetuses. However, it is possible that in our study subtle abnormalities were not discovered. For example, cardiac arrhythmias contributing to fetal demise would not have been detected. In this regard, histology of the conduction system may provide clues as to functional abnormality (such as complete heart block), but other more sophisticated techniques would be required to document the dysfunction.

Many investigations have addressed the question of the prevalence of congenital heart defects among liveborn infants.[3, 19–25] Although the results vary widely (in part due to the variety of investigative techniques), most intensive studies show the true prevalence of congenital heart defects, excluding bicuspid aortic valve, to approach 1%.[3] We have used this figure from the literature as a basis for comparison in the present study. That this prevalence among liveborns is similar to what we found among our population of chromosomally normal spontaneous abortions suggests that heart defects per se may not jeopardize the survival of the developing fetus within the developmental age range studied.

In autopsy series such as ours, associations may be established but conclusions as to cause and effect may not follow. For example, the association between cardiac defects and abnormal karyotype emphasizes that other abnormal developmental processes may be present in fetuses with defects. Even in those fetuses with cardiac defects and normal karyotype, an unknown process (for which heart defects may or may not be a marker) may be operant. In those with a normal karyotype, minor chromosomal alterations beyond the resolution of current techniques may be present and affect cardiac development.[15] Similar alterations can be expected to adversely affect the entire developing fetus. Clearly, genetics is a critical influence in cardiac and general fetal development, but environment may be equally, if not more, important.[26] Unfortunately, specific environmental teratogens are difficult to identify. Environmental risk factors associated with spontaneous abortion include cigarette smoking, fever, and alcohol consumption by the mother during pregnancy.[27–30] The latter is associated with a syndrome that may include heart defects. Ultimately, the interaction between genetics and environment may be most important not only in cardiac morphogenesis but also general fetal development. In light of the above, the British study[12] appears incomplete: neither a complete autopsy nor karyotyping was done on the spontaneous abortuses. Without more complete data it is difficult to evaluate the significance of the cardiac defects in developing fetuses. Thus, the statement made in the accompanying editorial[31] that in some cases the heart defect itself leads to fetal loss appears to be a hasty conclusion. Our data suggest that this is not true.

The conclusion that the impact of heart defects on the fetus may be minimal has been deduced from physiologic studies performed in a sheep preparation during the last one-half of gestation.[4] Because of the nature of the circulation in the fetus, pressures and oxygenation in the four chambers of the fetal heart are relatively homogeneous. Thus, most lesions resulting in abnormal shunting and/or obstruction may be expected to have minimal effect. One abnormality, constriction of the ductus arteriosus in utero, may affect the developing fetus by diminishing blood return to the placenta.[4] We did not find this lesion among any of our specimens.

It is possible, although unlikely, that more complex heart malformations adversely affect the survival of the fetus. Since we did not identify any such lesions among the spontaneous abortuses, our data neither support nor refute this thesis. In light of the rarity of complex cardiac defects, an epidemiologic analysis would require much larger numbers than those provided by our study.

We gratefully acknowledge the encouragement and helpful criticism of Drs. Welton M. Gersony, William A. Blanc, Zena Stein, Jennie Kline, and Dorothy Warburton.

References

1. Hoffman JIE: Natural history of congenital heart disease. Problems in its assessment with special reference to ventricular septal defects. Circulation **37:** 97, 1968
2. Polani PE: Chromosomal abnormalities and congenital heart disease. Guys Hosp Report **117:** 323, 1968
3. Hoffman JIE, Christianson R: Congenital heart disease in a cohort of 19,502 births with long-term follow-up. Am J Cardiol **42:** 641, 1978
4. Rudolph AM: Congenital diseases of the heart. Chicago, 1974, Yearbook Medical Publishers Inc.
5. Kline J, Stein Z, Strobino B, Susser M, Warburton D: Surveillance of spontaneous abortions. Power in environmental monitoring. Am J Epidemiol **106:** 345, 1977
6. Byrne J, Warburton D, Kline J, Blanc W, Stein Z: Morphology of early fetal deaths and their chromosomal characteristics. Teratology **32:** 297, 1985
7. Byrne J: Fetal pathology laboratory manual. Birth Defects **19:** 10, 1983
8. Potter EL, Craig JM: Rate of antenatal growth. *In* Pathology of the fetus and the infant, ed 3. Chicago, 1975, Yearbook Medical Publishers Inc., p 19
9. Tynan MJ, Becker AE, Macartney FJ, Jimenez MQ, Shinebourne EA, Anderson RH: Nomenclature and classification of congenital heart disease. Br Heart J **41:** 544, 1979
10. Warburton D, Stein Z, Kline J, Susser M: Chromosome abnormalities in spontaneous abortion: data from the New York City study. *In* Porter IH, Hook EB, editors: Human embryonic and fetal death. New York, 1980, Academic Press, pp 261–288
11. Keith JD: Bicuspid aortic valve. *In* Keith JD, Rowe RD, Vald P, editors: Heart disease in infancy and childhood, ed 3. New York, 1978, MacMillan Publishing Co, Inc., p 732
12. Gerlis LM: Cardiac malformations in sponaneous abortions. Int J Cardiol **7:** 29, 1985
13. Creasy MR, Crolla JA, Alberman ED: A cytogenetic study of human spontaneous abortions using banding techniques. Hum Genet **31:** 177, 1976
14. Creasy MR, Alberman ED: Congenital malformations of the central nervous system in spontaneous abortions. J Med Genetics **13:** 9, 1976
15. German J, Ehlers KH, Crippa LP, Engle MA: The chromosomes in congenital heart disease. Birth Defects **8:** 96, 1972
16. Leisti JT, Raivo KO, Rapola MHJ, Saksela EJ, Aula PP: The phenotype of human triploidy. Birth Defects **10:** 248, 1974
17. Wertelecki W, Graham JM, Sergovich FR: The clinical syndrome of triploidy. Obstet Gynecol **47:** 69, 1976
18. Mueller RF, Sybert VP, Johnson J, Brown ZA, Chen W-J: Evaluation of a protocol for post-mortem examination of stillbirths. N Engl J Med **309:** 586, 1983
19. Richards MR, Meritt KK, Samuels MH, Langmann AG: Congenital malformations of the cardiovascular system in a series of 6053 infants. Pediatrics **15:** 12, 1955
20. Carlgren L-E: The incidence of congenital heart disease in children born in Gothenburg 1941–1950. Br Heart J **21:** 40, 1959
21. Mitchell SC, Korones SB, Berendes HW: Congenital heart disease in 56,109 births. Incidence and natural history. Circulation **43:** 323, 1971
22. Feldt RH, Avasthey P, Yoshimasu F, Kurland LT, Titus JL: Incidence of congenital heart disease in children born to residents of Olmstead County, Minnesota 1950–1969. Mayo Clin Proc **46:** 794, 1971
23. Bound JP, Logan WFWE: Incidence of congenital heart disease in Blackpool 1957–1971. Br Heart J **39:** 445, 1977
24. Heinonen OP, Slone D, Shapiro S: The women, their offspring, and the malformations. *In* Birth defects and drugs in pregnancy. Littleton, MA, 1977, Publishing Sciences Group Inc., p 31
25. Ferencz C, Rubin JD, McCarter RJ, Brenner JI, Neill CA, Perry LW, Hepner SI, Downing JW: Congenital heart disease: prevalence at livebirth. The Baltimore-Washington infant study. Am J Epidemiol **121:** 31, 1985
26. Nora JJ: Update on the etiology of congenital heart disease and genetic counseling. *In* Van Praagh R, Takao A, editors: Etiology and morphogenesis of congenital heart disease. Mount Kisco, NY, 1980, Futura Publishing Company, pp 21–39
27. Kline J, Stein Z, Susser M, Warburton D: Smoking: a risk factor for spontaneous abortion. N Engl J Med **297:** 793, 1977
28. Harlap S, Shiono PH: Alcohol, smoking and incidence of spontaneous abortions in the first and second trimester. Lancet **2:** 173, 1980
29. Kline J, Stein Z, Shrout P, Susser M, Warburton D: Drinking during pregnancy and spontaneous abortion. Lancet **2:** 176, 1980
30. Kline J, Stein Z, Susser M, Warburton D: Fever during pregnancy and spontaneous abortion. Am J Epidemiol **121:** 832, 1985
31. Allan LD: Evidence of congenital cardiac malformations in spontaneous abortions. Int J Cardiol **7:** 45, 1985

Effect of isotonic exercise training on left ventricular volume during upright exercise

MICHAEL H. CRAWFORD, M.D., MICHAEL A. PETRU, M.D., AND CHARLES RABINOWITZ, M.D.
With the technical assistance of K. Wray Amon, B.S.

ABSTRACT To determine the changes in left ventricular volume and their time course during exercise we studied 30 runners. Left ventricular end-diastolic and end-systolic volumes were measured from biapical two-dimensional echocardiograms recorded during graded upright bicycle exercise. The validity of this echocardiographic technique was assessed by comparing measurements at rest and exercise with results obtained by gated equilibrium radionuclide angiography in 10 patients with coronary artery disease. Although the absolute volume measurements were lower by echocardiography, ejection fraction was not significantly different and the directional changes in volume during exercise were comparable. In the runners, resting left ventricular end-diastolic volume measurements by echocardiography correlated with their maximum bicycle exercise endurance times (r = .80). Left ventricular end-diastolic volume, stroke volume, and ejection fraction increased during exercise with the most marked changes occurring in the first half of exercise. Systolic blood pressure/end-systolic volume (SBP/ESV) also increased during exercise, but the largest change occurred during the second half of exercise. Left ventricular volumes were larger in the 12 competitive marathon runners (maximum exercise duration ≥ 27 min) as compared with the 18 noncompetitive runners (exercise duration ≤ 23 min): resting end-diastolic volume 130 ± 29 (SD) ml vs 87 ± 20 ml ($p < .001$), respectively. During exercise the competitive runners exhibited a larger increase in end-diastolic volume and the noncompetitive athletes showed a greater increase in SBP/ESV. Therefore, highly trained competitive marathon runners make greater use of the less energy-consuming Frank-Starling mechanism to accomplish high levels of isotonic exercise performance as compared with less well-trained runners.
Circulation 72, No. 6, 1237–1243, 1985.

LONG-TERM isotonic exercise training results in a reduction in resting heart rate and an increase in left ventricular end-diastolic volume.[1-4] Also, isotonically trained individuals are able to achieve higher values for stroke volume, cardiac output, and exercise workload as compared with untrained individuals, despite similar values for peak exercise heart rate, blood pressure, and ejection phase indexes of left ventricular performance.[5, 6] However, it is unclear whether the increased left ventricular output during exercise in athletes is related simply to the larger resting end-diastolic volume that persists during exercise, or whether further increases in left ventricular volume occur. If the latter is the case, what is the time course of volume changes during exercise? The relative contribution of increases in contractile state as estimated by the systolic pressure-volume relationship and the time course of these changes are poorly understood. Therefore we sought to determine whether the large ventricular end-diastolic volume of the trained individual can be increased further to take advantage of the less energy-consuming Frank-Starling effect and if so, to determine when it occurs during exercise. We also wished to evaluate changes in the systolic pressure-volume relationship during exercise and compare these with the changes in end-diastolic volume. Finally, the response of the left ventricle during exercise in highly trained competitive athletes was compared with that in less well-trained individuals to ascertain any differences during exercise that would explain the greater performance of the former. For this study, two-dimensional echocardiography was used during exercise to measure left ven-

From the Division of Cardiology, Department of Medicine, University of Texas Health Science Center, and The Veterans Administration Hospital, San Antonio.

Supported in part by The Veterans Administration and NIH training grant 5T32 HL07350-05.

Address for correspondence: Michael H. Crawford, M.D., Department of Medicine, Division of Cardiology, University of Texas Health Science Center, 7703 Floyd Curl Dr., San Antonio, TX 78284.

Received Jan. 30, 1985; revision accepted Sept. 5, 1985.

tricular volumes after validation of the technique in comparison with gated equilibrium radionuclide angiography in a group of patients with coronary artery disease.

Methods

Subject selection. Two groups of subjects were selected for this study. The first group consisted of 10 patients with angina pectoris caused by fixed coronary artery disease who agreed to participate in a study of the validation of two-dimensional echocardiographically derived volumes during exercise, with gated radionuclide angiography used as the standard of reference. This validation could not be done in the second group (normal subjects) because of a reluctance by many of them to receive radioactive tracers and questions raised by our Institutional Review Board concerning the advisability of giving radionuclides to young normal individuals. The second group was chosen to evaluate the effect of isotonic conditioning on left ventricular performance during exercise and consisted of 30 members of a YMCA-sponsored running club.

Thirteen men with chronic stable angina pectoris were evaluated for the validation part of the experiment; of these, 10 (77%) had suitable upright biapical two-dimensional echocardiograms for participation in the study. All 10 patients had previously demonstrated exercise-induced ischemia on a Bruce protocol exercise treadmill test as manifested by 0.1 mV of electrocardiographic ST segment depression in an anterolateral precordial lead and typical angina pectoris. Nine of the 10 patients had previous well-documented myocardial infarctions and eight had prior selective coronary cineangiographic results demonstrating at least one vessel with greater than 70% diameter narrowing. All 10 patients had been off antianginal medications for 1 week before the study.

Thirty-four normal individuals were screened and 30 (88%) had suitable upright two-dimensional echocardiograms for inclusion in the study. All 30 were active and asymptomatic and had normal physical examinations and two-dimensional echocardiograms at rest. They varied greatly in their degree of training, from those who were highly trained and regularly competed in marathons to those that had just joined the running club and were practically sedentary. Objective testing readily separated them into two groups: 12 completed 27 min or longer of graded bicycle exercise (range 27 to 33 min), claimed to run more than 50 miles/week, and were regularly competing in marathons. There were three women and nine men. The other 18 had an exercise time of 23 min or less (range 12 to 23), ran less than 30 miles/week, and were considered noncompetitive in the marathon. There were four women and 16 men.

Exercise protocol. All subjects were exercised on an upright mechanically braked bicycle ergometer. Exercise was begun at 150 kpm/min and was increased by the same amount every 3 min. The electrocardiogram was monitored continually and heart rate and cuff blood pressure were recorded at rest and after each minute of exercise. All 10 patients with ischemc heart disease exercised until the onset of both angina pectoris and ischemic ST segment depression in the lateral precordial leads. All the normal subjects exercised to the point of fatigue that they considered near maximal from their experience. The patients exercised twice, 4 to 24 hr apart, with the order of radionuclide angiography and two-dimensional echocardiography being randomized.

Despite the marked differences in exercise duration between the two groups of subjects as noted above, maximum exercise heart rates were not significantly different (177 ± 15 beats/min competitive vs 162 ± 25 beats/min noncompetitive). To compare values of left ventricular size and performance during exercise between the two groups, heart rate was used to identify four points during exercise for each group. Therefore, comparison between groups were made at rest, at 60%, 70%, and 85% of maximum heart rate, and at maximum heart rate. Also, there is a well-known relationship between heart rate and oxygen consumption during exercise.[7]

Exercise two-dimensional echocardiography. Exercise biapical two-dimensional echocardiograms were recorded with a phased-array echocardiograph and an 84 degree wide-angle 2.25 mHz transducer. Two- and four-chamber views were recorded on video tape at rest and after each minute of exercise with the patient upright on the bicycle and leaning slightly forward as we have previously described.[8] The length of time for data acquisition at each exercise point was 10 to 15 sec. Echocardiograms were analyzed from the video tape recordings with a light pen–equipped microprocessor programmed for Simpson's rule. End-diastolic and end-systolic volumes as well as ejection fractions were calculated at rest and at peak exercise from beats at end-expiration. Analysis of the two-dimensional echocardiograms at peak exercise were done at the time corresponding to the midpoint of data acquisition for the radionuclide angiogram. This allowed comparison of the instantaneous single-beat data acquisition for two-dimensional echocardiography with the 2-min data acquisition period for gated equilibrium radionuclide angiography as we have described previously.[9] For the purpose of this study, we did not apply normalizing regression equations to correct for the echocardiographic underestimation of left ventricular end-diastolic volume and end-systolic volume that we have previously demonstrated at rest in comparison with biplane left ventricular cineangiography.[10] There were two reasons for this decision. First, this underestimation was shown to be consistent in the previous study, since ejection fraction was not significantly different by the two techniques. Second, the previous study involved patients, many of whom had wall motion abnormalities. Thus regression equations based on their data may not be applicable to normal individuals.

The ratio of systolic blood pressure (cuff) to end-systolic volume (SBP/ESV) was calculated in the normal subjects at rest and during exercise as an index of contractility. This index has been shown to be reliable even when peak systolic pressure is substituted for end-systolic pressure and has been used to differentiate changes in contractile state vs those induced by the Frank-Starling mechanism.[11–13]

Exercise radionuclide angiography. The patients were taken to the exercise laboratory after injection of 1.7 mg of stannous chloride as pyrophosphate. Twenty minutes later, 20 mCi of 99m-technetium pertechnetate were injected intravenously. The patient was positioned on the exercise ergometer and connected to the leads for an electrocardiographic physiologic gate. A portable 37-photo multiplier tube gamma camera (Ohio Nuclear VIP) was positioned to obtain 45 degree left anterior oblique views centered on the left ventricle. The gamma camera was equipped with a parallel-hole medium-sensitivity collimator. Gated equilibrium radionuclide angiography was performed over a 2 min data acquisition period, with the patient at rest seated on the bicycle. The patient's heart rate and blood pressure and the duration (min) of data acquisition were recorded. During exercise, gated equilibrium radionuclide angiograms were recorded during the last 2 min of each exercise stage and at peak exercise. All data acquisition was performed with 40 msec time frames and a maximum of 16 frames per cardiac cycle.

Rest and peak exercise radionuclide angiograms were analyzed with a semiautomated computer program. After nine-point spatial smoothing, an operator-identified periventricular region of interest was used for background subtraction. An automated left ventricular edge-detection algorithm was used providing for variable regions of interest and definition of the left ventricular time-activity curve. Care was taken to ensure that the left ventricular silhouette excluded left atrial activity and did not overlap the right ventricle. From the left ventricular time-activity curve, left ventricular end-diastolic and end-systolic counts were recorded and ejection fraction was determined by the ratio of stroke counts to end-diastolic counts. Left ventricular end-diastolic and end-systolic counts were converted to left ventricular end-diastolic and end-systolic volumes by a photon attenuation correction method based on a geometric method of attenuation distance quantitation that we have previously described.[14] This method accurately estimates cardiac output determined by the Fick tecnique ($r = .91$). It overestimates left ventricular volumes by approximately 20% as compared with contast cineangiography, but the values are correlated at $r = .80$. Left ventricular volume estimates were not corrected by regression equations because the error has been shown to be systematic and the echocardiographic volumes were not corrected.

Data analysis. The two-dimensional echocardiographic and radionuclide angiographic measurements made at rest and peak exercise in the patients were compared by linear regression analysis and paired Student's t tests. The serial two-dimensional echocardiographic data recorded at rest and during exercise in the two groups of normal subjects were analyzed by a one-way analysis of variance for repeated measures to ascertain differences across time in each group and by a two-way analysis of variance for repeated measures to compare the values across time between the two groups. Individual mean differences were determined by the Newman-Kuels mean comparison test based on the range and a significant difference was defined as $p < .05$.

Results

Validation experiment (table 1). End-diastolic and end-systolic volumes were smaller by two-dimensional echocardiography as compared with radionuclide angiography both at rest and during exercise, but there was a correlation between the values by each technique considering that the former was measured from 1 beat in the midpoint of the 2 min collection for the latter. Ejection fraction values were not significantly different between the two techniques, which supports the concept that the differences in volumes were consistent. Also, the average directional change in volumes during exercise was the same by both techniques, although the change was somewhat greater by radionuclide angiography. End-diastolic volume increased by an average of 8% by echocardiography and 22% by radionuclide angiography; end-systolic volume increased 22% by echocardiography and 38% by radionuclide angiography. The average change in ejection fraction with exercise was almost identical by the two techniques (14% two-dimensional echocardiography vs 15% radionuclide angiography). Thus, in these patients left ventricular volume and ejection fraction measurements by both techniques correlated and their directional changes during exercise were the same.

Effects of conditioning on resting left ventricular performance. Resting left ventricular end-diastolic volume estimates varied considerably between subjects (range 60 to 190 ml). They were related to maximum exercise duration ($r = .80$) (figure 1) but not to resting heart rate ($r = .23$) or body surface area ($r = .38$). Also, the relationship of end-diastolic volume to maximum exercise duration persisted when the former was corrected for body surface area ($r = .70$). Therefore, the major determinant of resting left ventricular size seemed to be the isotonic exercise capability of the individual, which is a reflection of the degree of training.

Maximum isotonic exercise duration readily separated the normal subjects into two groups as described above; a highly trained competitive group and a less well-trained noncompetitive group. The resting left ventricular end-diastolic volume estimate of 130 ± 29 (SD) ml in the 12 competitive marathon runners was significantly larger than the estimate of 87 ± 20 in the 18 noncompetitive subjects ($p < .001$), despite no significant difference in resting heart rate (70 ± 15 vs 68 ± 12 beats/min). The difference persisted when end-diastolic volume was divided by body surface area ($p < .001$). Resting left ventricular ejection fraction was similar in the two groups (55 ± 9% vs 54 ± 11%), but because of the marked difference in end-diastolic volume, resting left ventricular stroke volume

TABLE 1
Comparison of rest and peak exercise left ventricular volume and performance measured by two-dimensional echocardiography and radionuclide angiography in the patients with coronary artery disease

	EDV (ml)		ESV (ml)		EF (%)	
	Rest	Ex.	Rest	Ex.	Rest	Ex.
2DE	92 ± 24 (SD)	99 ± 21	51 ± 18	62 ± 27	46 ± 9	40 ± 13
RNA	177 ± 61	219 ± 91	92 ± 51	127 ± 74	51 ± 12	44 ± 12
p value	<.001	<.001	<.001	<.001	NS	NS
r	.66	.74	.69	.78	—	—

EDV = end-diastolic volume; ESV = end-systolic volume; EF = ejection fraction; Ex. = exercise; 2DE = two-dimensional echocardiography; RNA = radionuclide angiography.

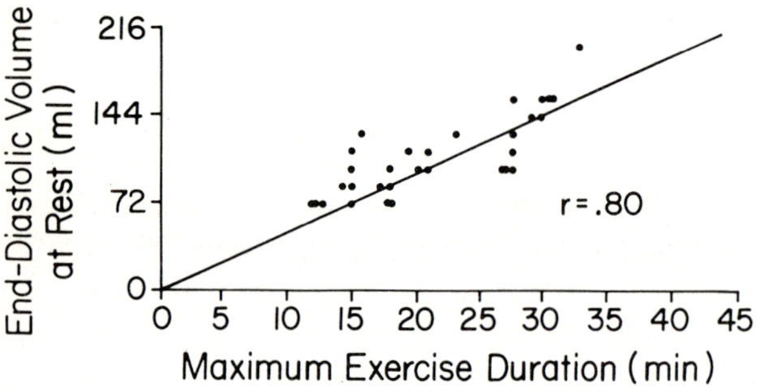

FIGURE 1. Relationship between resting left ventricular end-diastolic volume and maximum exercise duration in all the subjects.

was much greater in the competitive athletes at 72 ± 22 ml vs 48 ± 16 ml in the noncompetitive subjects (p < .001). SBP/ESV was significantly greater in the noncompetitive group as compared with the competitive group (3.3 ± 1.0 vs 2.0 ± 0.5 mm Hg/ml; p < .001), largely because end-systolic volume was larger in the competitive group.

Exercise left ventricular performance. The difference in end-diastolic volume between the competitive and noncompetitive athletes persisted during exercise (figure 2). However, the changes during exercise were not parallel because the difference between the two groups was significantly greater as exercise progressed (p < .01). Also, in each group end-diastolic volume at each point during exercise was significantly different from the resting values (p < .001), but the change from time to time during exercise was not significant after 70% of maximum heart rate was achieved. Thus end-diastolic volume in both groups increased significantly only during the first half of exercise.

The difference in stroke volume between the two groups also persisted during exercise (figure 3). Again, the changes during exercise were not parallel, because the difference between the two groups was significantly greater at higher exercise levels (p < .01). In both groups each value during exercise was significantly different from the resting value (p < .001). However, the change as exercise progressed was no longer significant after 70% of maximum heart rate was achieved. Therefore, as with end-diastolic volume, stroke volume in both groups did not increase significantly after the first half of exercise.

The difference in SBP/ESV between the two groups observed at rest was not consistent during exercise, because SBP/ESV increased more during exercise in the noncompetitive group (p < .03). However, in both groups the changes were most marked during the latter part of exercise (figure 4). Significant increases as compared with the resting value and over time during exercise were observed after 70% of maximum heart rate in the competitive group and after 85% in the noncompetitive group. Therefore, SBP/ESV in both groups increased significantly only during the second half of maximal bicycle exercise.

Throughout exercise there was no significant difference between the ejection fraction values of the two groups and the values paralleled each other (figure 5). In each group ejection fraction was significantly different from control at each point during exercise (p < .001); however, after 70% of maximum heart rate there was no signficant change in ejection fraction as exercise progressed. Therefore, in each group significant changes in ejection fraction only occurred during the first half of exercise.

Discussion

A potential concern regarding our study is the reliability of two-dimensional echocardiographic left ventricular volume and performance measures during exercise. It has been shown that two-dimensional

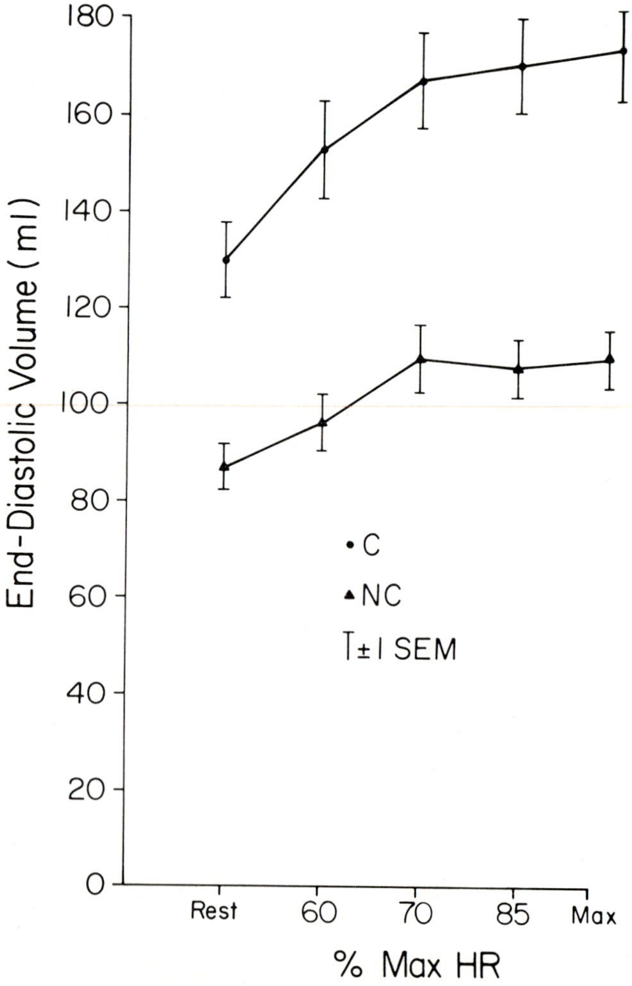

FIGURE 2. End-diastolic volume at rest and at progressive levels of heart rate (HR) during exercise in competitive (C) and noncompetitive (NC) runners.

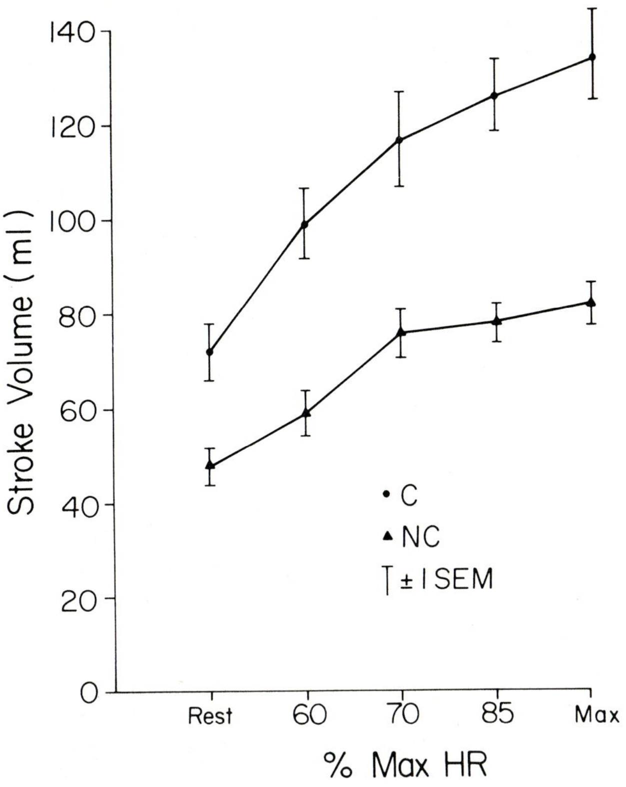

FIGURE 3. Left ventricular stroke volume at rest and during exercise. Abbreviations as in figure 2.

echocardiographically derived resting left ventricular volumes correlate well with those derived by cineangiography but are underestimations.[10, 15] Ejection fraction calculations, on the other hand, are nearly equivalent by two-dimensional echocardiography, cineangiography, and radionuclide angiography at rest.[10, 16] Recent studies have shown the feasibility of recording high-quality two-dimensional echocardiograms during exercise.[8, 17] We recently demonstrated that ejection fraction determinations during upright bicycle exercise by two-dimensional echocardiography are equivalent to those by gated equilibrium radionuclide angiography if the former are measured during the midpoint of data collection for the latter.[9]

Although these data would suggest that the volume estimates from which the ejection fractions were derived were accurate, we decided to further establish their validity as compared with a new radionuclide technique for estimating volume with correction for photon attenuation. We have shown that the latter technique accurately measures cardiac output as compared with the Fick technique but consistently overestimates left ventricular volumes measured by cineangiography with a good correlation.[14] As expected, the two-dimensional echocardiography values measured at rest and during exercise were lower than the radionuclide measures. However, the differences were consistent, since ejection fraction values by the two techniques were similar and the directional changes in volume during exercise were the same by both techniques. Because normal individuals are easier to image by echocardiography than patients, we would anticipate that the results in our athletic subjects would be more accurate than those in previous studies with patients. Also, we have previously demonstrated that the reproducibility of exercise two-dimensional echocardiographic estimates of left ventricular size and performance is not adversely affected by exercise.[8] Similar results have been reported by others.[17]

The results of our study demonstrate that the increase in resting end-diastolic volume observed in isotonically trained athletes was related to their ability to perform exercise. These data are consistent with the results of Zeldis et al.,[18] who found that the resting left ventricular internal dimension by M mode echocardiography was correlated with maximum oxygen consumption during exercise in athletes. It is also consistent with the findings of Cohen et al.,[19] who found that left ventricular end-diastolic volume index estimated by M mode echocardiography was related to the number of hours of dancing per year in ballet dancers. Thus

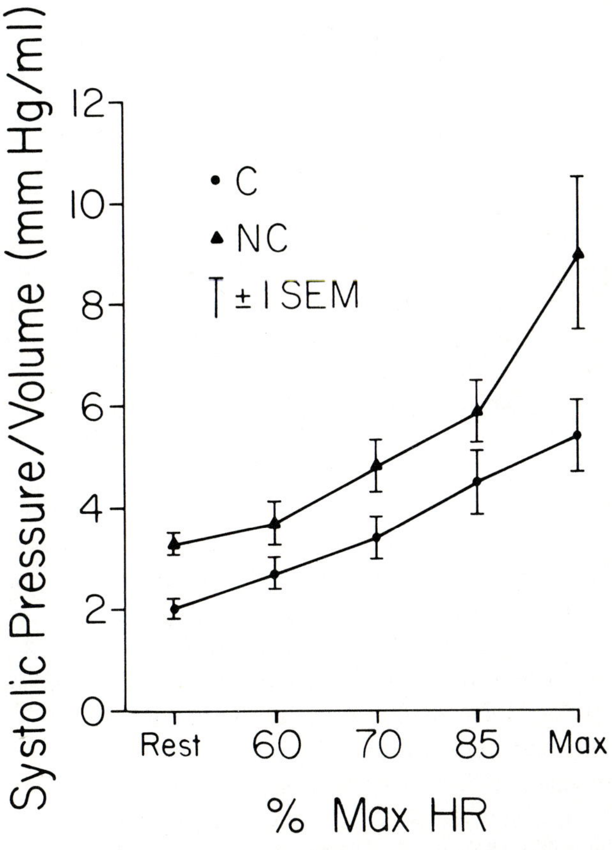

FIGURE 4. SBP/ESV at rest and during exercise. Abbreviations as in figure 2.

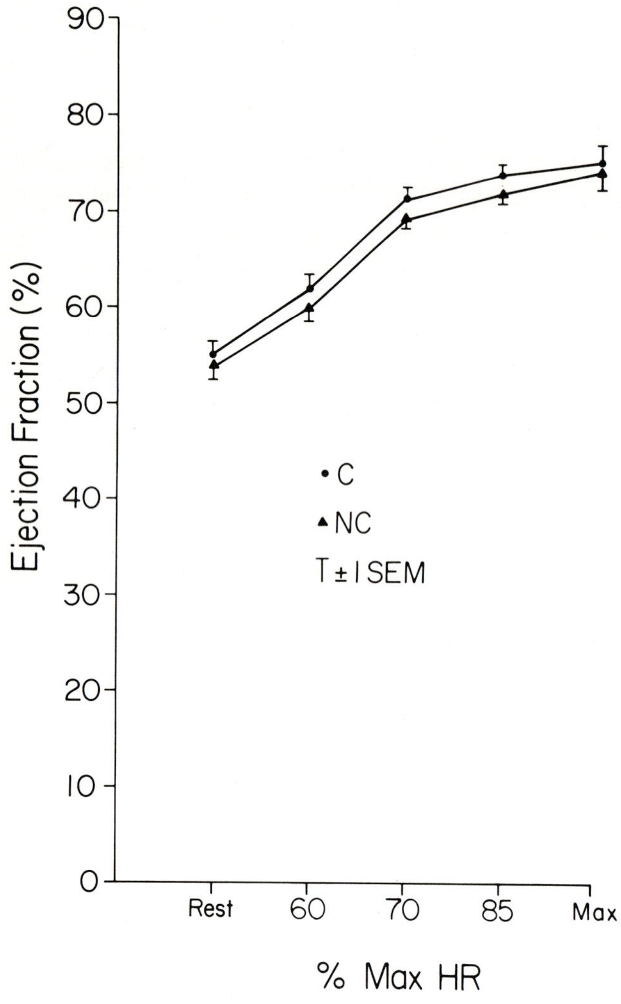

FIGURE 5. Left ventricular ejection fraction at rest and during exercise. Abbreviations as in figure 2.

it appears that the well-recognized phenomenon of increased left ventricular end-diastolic volume in endurance-trained athletes is proportional to their level of training and represents a major adaptive mechanism to isotonic exercise training.

Our data also demonstrated that during upright exercise, left ventricular end-diastolic volume increases in the competitive and noncompetitive athletes and the patients with coronary artery disease. Previous studies have not consistently demonstrated increases in left ventricular size during exercise. The conflicting data concerning whether or not left ventricular end-diastolic volume increases during exercise seems to be explainable if the exercise position and amount of exercise are considered. Almost all studies employing maximum upright isotonic exercise have shown an increase in left ventricular size at peak exercise as compared with rest.[20-24] However, studies using supine exercise often have failed to show an increase in left ventricular size, especially during submaximal exercise.[3, 25] Of interest is that studies employing previously instrumented conscious dogs subjected to severe exercise by swimming or running also showed increases in left ventricular end-diastolic dimensions during maximal exercise.[26, 27]

In our athletes the increase in end-diastolic volume was greatest during the first half of exercise and plateaued during the second half of exercise. These findings are consistent with those of Steingart et al.,[24] who used gated equilibrium radionuclide angiographic changes in end-diastolic counts to estimate left ventricular volume in 17 normal subjects undergoing maximum upright bicycle exercise. However, they are at variance with the results of Weiss et al.,[28] who studied normal subjects during maximal semisupine exercise by M mode echocardiography. They found increases in end-diastolic left ventricular size only at higher levels of exercise. Perhaps this difference is due to the semisupine position, which may augment venous return.

The increases in ejection fraction and stroke volume during exercise in both groups paralleled the changes in end-diastolic volume and thus were significant only during the first half of exercise. By contrast, increases in SBP/ESV were significant only during the second half of exercise. The latter results are consistent with those in the normal subjects studied by Steingart et al.[24] They examined SBP/ESV derived from radionuclide angiography at 150, 300, and 600 kpm of supine bicycle exercise and found significant differences from the resting values only at 600 kpm. Thus it appears that the increase in cardiac performance during upright exercise is more dependent on the Frank-Starling mechanism in early exercise and on increases in contractile state toward the end of exercise. However, the Frank-Starling mechanism is probably still operant at peak exercise, since Sonnenblick et al.[29] have shown that end-diastolic dimensions are larger during exercise than would be anticipated if the heart rate attained was duplicated by atrial pacing at rest.

Another concern regarding our study is the finding that the noncompetitive athletes had higher values for SBP/ESV than the competitive marathon runners. Does this mean that the former group has a higher contractile state than the latter? This index of contractility must be interpreted with caution, since it is an estimate of the slope of the end-systolic pressure-volume relationship based on a single point.[30] To compare such slope estimates, a volume intercept of zero must be assumed. However, we know this is probably not the case, since the competitive athletes have larger hearts. Thus comparing the two groups may be inaccurate, but the measure probably can be used to assess changes during exercise in the same group.

In comparing the response of the left ventricle to exercise in the highly trained competitive athletes vs the less well-trained noncompetitive runners, it is apparent that there are significant differences in the end-diastolic volume, stroke volume, and SBP/ESV at rest and during exercise, despite similar ejection fractions. Also, the differences in these variables between the two groups are always greatest at the end of exercise. More specifically, the left ventricle of the highly trained athlete is not only enlarged but also can increase in size during exercise proportionately more as compared with the left ventricle of less well-trained individuals. In addition, the SBP/ESV of the competitively trained athlete steadily increases during exercise, whereas in noncompetitive runners this measure increases markedly near maximum exercise. Thus it appears that the highly trained competitive athlete makes greater use of the less energy-consuming Frank-Starling mechanism to accomplish high levels of isotonic exercise performance as compared with the less well-trained noncompetitive runner.

The advice of Robert A. O'Rourke, M.D., and William C. Little, M.D., is greatly appreciated. Also, we are grateful for the cooperation of the Northwest Branch of the YMCA of San Antonio.

References

1. DeMaria AN, Neumann A, Lee G, Fowler W, Mason DT: Alterations in ventricular mass and performance induced by exercise training in man evaluated by echocardiography. Circulation **57:** 237, 1978
2. Ehsani AA, Hagberg JM, Hickson RC: Rapid changes in left ventricular dimensions and mass in response to physical conditioning and deconditioning. Am J Cardiol **42:** 52, 1978
3. Stein RA, Michielli D, Diamond J, Horwitz B, Krasnow N: The cardiac response to exercise training: echocardiographic analysis at rest and during exercise. Am J Cardiol **46:** 219, 1980
4. Fagard R, Aubert A, Lysens R, Staessen J, Vanhees L, Amery A: Noninvasive assessment of seasonal variations in cardiac structure and function in cyclists. Circulation **67:** 896, 1983
5. Rerych SK, Scholz PM, Sabiston DC, Jones RH: Effects of exercise training on left ventricular function in normal subjects: a longitudinal study by radionuclide angiography. Am J Cardiol **45:** 244, 1980
6. Anholm JD, Foster C, Carpenter J, Pollock ML, Hellman CK, Schmidt DH: Effect of habitual exercise on left ventricular response to exercise. Am Physiol Soc **52:** 1648, 1982
7. Mitchell JH, Blomqvist G: Maximal oxygen uptake. N Engl J Med **284:** 1018, 1971
8. Crawford MH, Amon KW, Vance WS: Exercise 2-dimensional echocardiography: quantitation of left ventricular performance in patients with severe angina pectoris. Am J Cardiol **51:** 1, 1983
9. Crawford MH, Petru MA, Amon KW, Sorensen SG, Vance WS: Comparative value of 2-dimensional echocardiography and radionuclide angiography for quantitating changes in left ventricular performance during exercise limited by angina pectoris. Am J Cardiol **53:** 42, 1984
10. Starling MR, Crawford MH, Sorensesn SG, Levi B, Richards KL, O'Rourke RA: Comparative accuracy of apical biplane cross-sectional echocardiography and gated equilibrium radionuclide angiography for estimating left ventricular size and performance. Circulation **63:** 1075, 1981
11. Grossman W, Braunwald E, Mann T, McLaurin LP, Green LH: Contractile state of the left ventricle in man as evaluated from end-systolic pressure-volume relations. Circulation **56:** 845, 1977
12. Mehmel HC, Stockins B, Ruffmann K, Olshausen KV, Schuler G, Kubler W: The linearity of the end-systolic pressure-volume relationship in man and its sensitivity for assessment of left ventricular function. Circulation **63:** 1216, 1981
13. Iskandrian AS, Hakki A, Bemis CE, Kane SA, Boston B, Amenta A: Left ventricular end-systolic pressure-volume relation: a combined radionuclide and hemodynamic study. Am J Cardiol **51:** 1057, 1983
14. Petru MA, Sorensen SG, Chaudhuri TL, Rosen P, O'Rourke RA: Attenuation correction of equilibrium radionuclide angiography for noninvasive quantitation of cardiac output and ventricular volumes. Am Heart J **107:** 1221, 1984
15. Erbel R, Schweizer P, Lambertz H, Henn G, Meyer J, Krebs W, Effert S: Echoventriculography — a simultaneous analysis of two-dimensonal echocardiography and cineventriculography. Circulation **67:** 205, 1983
16. Folland ED, Parisi AF, Moynihan PF, Jones DR, Feldman CL, Tow DE: Assessment of left ventricular ejection fraction and volumes by real-time, two-dimensional echocardiography: a comparison of cineangiographic and radionuclide techniques. Circulation **60:** 760, 1979
17. Zwehl W, Gueret P, Meerbaum S, Holt D, Corday E: Quantitative two dimensional echocardiography during bicycle exercise in normal subjects. Am J Cardiol **47:** 866, 1981
18. Zeldis SM, Morganroth J, Rubler S: Cardiac hypertrophy in response to dynamic conditioning in female athletes. J Appl Physiol **44:** 849, 1978
19. Cohen JL, Gupta PK, Lichstein E, Chadda KD: The heart of a dancer: noninvasive cardiac evaluation of professional ballet dancers. Am J Cardiol **45:** 959, 1980
20. Rerych SK, Scholz PM, Newman GE, Sabiston DC, Jones RH: Cardiac function at rest and during exercise in normals and in patients with coronary heart disease: evaluation by radionuclide angiography. Ann Surg **187:** 449, 1978
21. Thadani U, Parker JO: Hemodynamics at rest and during supine and sitting bicycle exercise in normal subjects. Am J Cardiol **41:** 52, 1978
22. Poliner LR, Dehmer GJ, Lewis SE, Parkey RW, Blomqvist CG, Willerson JT: Left ventricular performance in normal subjects: a comparison of the responses to exercise in the upright and supine positions. Circulation **62:** 528, 1980
23. Freeman MR, Berman DS, Staniloff H, Elkayam U, Maddahi J, Swan HJC, Forrester J: Comparison of upright and supine bicycle exercise in the detection and evaluation of extent of coronary artery disease by equilibrium radionuclide ventriculography. Am Heart J **102:** 182, 1981
24. Steingart RM, Wexler J, Slagle S, Scheuer J: Radionuclide ventriculographic responses to graded supine and upright exercise: critical role of the Frank-Starling mechanism at submaximal exercise. Am J Cardiol **53:** 1671, 1984
25. Bar-Shlomo B, Druck MN, Morch JE, Jablonsky G, Hilton JD, Feiglin DH, McLaughlin PR: Left ventricular function in trained and untrained healthy subjects. Circulation **65:** 484, 1982
26. Erickson HH, Bishop VS, Kardon MB, Horwitz LD: Left ventricular internal diameter and cardiac function during exercise. J Appl Physiol **30:** 473, 1971
27. Horwitz LD, Atkins JM, Leshin SJ: Role of the Frank-Starling mechanism in exercise. Circ Res **31:** 868, 1972
28. Weiss JL, Weisfeldt ML, Mason SJ, Garrison JB, Livengood SV, Fortuin NJ: Evidence of Frank-Starling effect in man during severe semisupine exercise. Circulation **59:** 655, 1979
29. Sonnenblick EH, Braunwald E, Williams JF, Glick G: Effects of exercise on myocardial force-velocity relations in intact unanesthetized man: relative roles of changes in heart rate, sympathetic activity, and ventricular dimensions. J Clin Invest **44:** 2051, 1965
30. Sagawa K: The end-systolic pressure-volume relation of the ventricle: definition, modifications and clinical use. Circulation **63:** 1223, 1981

Survival and functional results after valve replacement for aortic regurgitation from 1976 to 1983: impact of preoperative left ventricular function

ROBERT O. BONOW, M.D., ANTHONY L. PICONE, M.D., CHARLES L. MCINTOSH, M.D., PH.D., MICHAEL JONES, M.D., DOUGLAS R. ROSING, M.D., BARRY J. MARON, M.D., EDWARD LAKATOS, PH.D., RICHARD E. CLARK, M.D., AND STEPHEN E. EPSTEIN, M.D.

ABSTRACT Recent studies suggest that preoperative left ventricular function may no longer be an important determinant of survival or functional results after operation for aortic regurgitation because of improved operative techniques. To assess the effect of left ventricular function on prognosis in the current surgical era, we performed echocardiographic and radionuclide angiographic studies in 80 consecutive patients undergoing valve replacement from 1976 to 1983. No patient had associated coronary artery disease. For all patients, 5 year survival was 83 ± 5%, significantly better than the 62 ± 9% 5 year survival in our patients operated on from 1972 to 1976. Preoperative resting left ventricular ejection fraction ($p < .001$), fractional shortening ($p < .001$), and end-systolic dimension ($p < .01$) were the most significant predictors of survival (univariate life-table analysis). Five year survival was 63 ± 12% in patients with subnormal ejection fraction ($n = 50$) compared with 96 ± 3% in those with normal ejection fraction ($n = 30$). Patients with subnormal left ventricular ejection fraction and poor exercise tolerance or prolonged duration of left ventricular dysfunction (>18 months) comprised the high-risk subgroup (5 year survival 52 ± 11%). Patients in this subgroup also had persistent left ventricular dysfunction after operation, with greater left ventricular end-diastolic dimensions and reduced ejection fraction (both $p < .001$) compared with patients with normal preoperative left ventricular ejection fraction or a brief duration of left ventricular dysfunction (<14 months). Cold hyperkalemic cardioplegia was used for myocardial preservation in 46 patients. Survival was not influenced by cardioplegia, nor did cardioplegia alter the influence of left ventricular function on postoperative prognosis. Hence, despite improved operative techniques and better long-term survival compared with earlier results, preoperative resting left ventricular dysfunction continues to identify patients with aortic regurgitation at risk of death or persistent left ventricular dysfunction after aortic valve replacement. Early operation in such patients may result in further improvement in survival and functional results.
Circulation 72, No. 6, 1244–1256, 1985.

LEFT VENTRICULAR systolic function is an important determinant of prognosis in patients with chronic aortic regurgitation. Numerous hemodynamic, angiographic, and echocardiographic studies indicate that indexes of preoperative left ventricular function identify patients at low risk and at high risk of death or persistent left ventricular dysfunction after aortic valve replacement.[1-8] However, a few recent reports suggest that survival after valve replacement for aortic regurgitation is no longer influenced by preoperative left ventricular function.[9-11] These studies suggest that improved operative techniques in the current surgical era have negated the influence of preoperative left ventricular function on postoperative prognosis.

To address this issue and to assess the continued importance of preoperative left ventricular function in aortic regurgitation, we evaluated the results of aortic valve replacement over a 7 year period (from 1976 to 1983) at the National Heart, Lung, and Blood Institute. Our results indicate that preoperative left ventricular systolic function continues to influence postoperative prognosis and suggest that the discordant conclusions of previous studies probably resulted from interpretive differences and differences in patient selection.

From the Cardiology Branch and Cardiac Surgery Branch, National Heart, Lung, and Blood Institute, National Institutes of Health, Bethesda, MD.

Address for correspondence: Robert O. Bonow, M.D., Bldg. 10, Room 7B15, National Institutes of Health, Bethesda, MD 20892.
Received May 17, 1985; revision accepted Aug. 29, 1985.

Methods

Patient selection. We evaluated the results of aortic valve replacement in 96 consecutive patients with chronic aortic regurgitation undergoing operation between August 1976 and September 1983. Sixteen patients had associated coronary artery disease (>50% reduction in luminal diameter of at least one major coronary artery) and were excluded from the current analysis because of the potential impact of coexistent coronary artery stenosis on both survival and left ventricular function after operation. Thus the 80 consecutive patients with chronic aortic regurgitation and no coronary artery disease form the basis of the current study. There were 65 men and 15 women, ranging in age from 15 to 74 years (mean 44). Data analysis was performed in March 1984, resulting in potential follow-up periods ranging from 6 to 90 months (mean 45).

During the course of this study, our indications for valve replacement were the development of moderate to severe cardiac symptoms. Since 1979 we added as an indication for surgery in the absence of symptoms the documentation of consistent and reproducible evidence of depressed left ventricular contractile function at rest by echocardiography and radionuclide angiography. The current operative series represents a consecutive series of patients who fulfilled these criteria for operation, except for one patient with symptoms of congestive heart failure who refused operation, and one asymptomatic patient with a subnormal ejection fraction who had severe kyphoscoliosis. Specifically, no patient was excluded from operation because of extreme symptoms, severely depressed ejection fraction, severely dilated left ventricular chamber, or a combination of these disorders.

Sixty-eight patients underwent aortic valve replacement because of moderate to severe cardiac symptoms (New York Heart Association functional class III to IV). The other 12 patients were either asymptomatic or mildly symptomatic (functional class I to II), and valve replacement was recommended because of consistent evidence of left ventricular dysfunction, based on serial echocardiographic and radionuclide angiographic studies. Nine of these patients were completely asymptomatic. All patients were evaluated preoperatively by echocardiography, radionuclide angiography, graded treadmill exercise testing, and cardiac catheterization, except for one patient in whom echocardiographic studies were of suboptimal quality and one patient who did not undergo radionuclide angiography. All preoperative studies were performed while patients were taking no cardiac medications.

Cardiac catheterization was performed in all patients; coronary arteriography was performed in all patients over 35 years of age as well as all patients under 35 with angina pectoris. Catheterization data confirmed the diagnosis of isolated aortic regurgitation in 76 patients. Four patients had associated small ventricular septal defects with left-to-right shunt ratios less than 1.5:1, which were closed at the time of aortic valve replacement. No patient had associated mitral valve disease or disease of the ascending aorta requiring repair at the time of aortic valve replacement.

Patient stratification. The patients were divided into two subgroups on the basis of preoperative left ventricular ejection fraction at rest as measured by radionuclide angiography. Twenty-nine patients with left ventricular ejection fraction greater than 45% (the lower limit of normal by our technique[12]) were included in the subgroup with normal ejection fraction, while those with ejection fraction of 45% or less were placed in the subgroup with left ventricular dysfunction. In all patients in the left ventricular dysfunction subgroup, impaired contractile function was confirmed by subnormal fractional shortening by echocardiography (<29%). The one patient in whom preoperative radionuclide angiography was not performed was included in the normal left ventricular function subgroup on the basis of echocardiographic demonstration of only moderate left ventricular dilatation (end-diastolic dimension 68 mm, end-systolic dimension 44 mm) with normal fractional shortening (35%).

The 50 patients with left ventricular dysfunction were subdivided further on the basis of exercise tolerance[13]; 17 patients had impaired exercise tolerance, defined as inability to complete the 22.5 min of the first stage of the NIH exercise protocol because of limiting symptoms, while 33 patients manifested preserved exercise tolerance, completing the first stage of exercise without symptoms. These latter 33 patients were stratified again on the basis of duration of preoperative left ventricular dysfunction.[14] In six patients, the duration of left ventricular dysfunction was prolonged, documented by subnormal fractional shortening on previous echocardiographic studies (when all were asymptomatic) performed 18 to 57 months (mean 33 ± 14) before operation and confirmed in four of these six patients by serial radionuclide angiographic studies demonstrating subnormal ejection fraction at rest. In 10 patients the duration of preoperative left ventricular dysfunction was brief, with previous echocardiographic studies performed 1.5 to 14 months before operation (when all were asymptomatic), demonstrating normal fractional shortening and confirmed by serial ejection fraction by radionuclide angiography in seven of these patients; the onset of left ventricular dysfunction occurred within this short time period. In the remaining 17 patients with left ventricular dysfunction and preserved exercise tolerance, the duration of depressed left ventricular systolic function was unknown, since impaired left ventricular systolic function was evident at the time of the initial preoperative evaluation and serial data were not available. In this fashion, the 80 patients were subdivided into five groups on the basis of preoperative left ventricular function, exercise tolerance, and duration of left ventricular dysfunction.

Echocardiography. M mode echocardiograms were obtained with a 2.25 MHz, 1.25 cm diameter unfocused Aerotech transducer and an Ekoline 20A or Hoffrel 201 ultrasound receiver interfaced with a Honeywell 1856 strip-chart recorder, or an Irex System II ultrasound unit with a 2.25 MHz, 1.3 cm diameter transducer. Echocardiographic measurements of left ventricular transverse dimensions were obtained with the ultrasound beam directed through the left ventricle just caudal to the tips of the mitral leaflets.[5, 15] The end-diastolic left ventricular dimension was measured at the R wave of the electrocardiogram. The end-systolic dimension was measured at the peak of systolic posterior wall motion. Left ventricular fractional shortening was calculated as the ratio of the difference between the left ventricular diastolic dimension and systolic dimension to the left ventricular diastolic dimension.[16] Interventricular septal thickness was measured just below the tips of the mitral leaflets, and left ventricular posterior wall thickness was measured at the level of the mitral leaflets. The left ventricular radius-to-wall thickness ratio (an index of the volume-to-mass ratio and a measure of the degree to which left ventricular muscle mass is appropriate for a given chamber volume[8, 17–19]) was computed as one-half the left ventricular end-diastolic dimension divided by the posterior wall thickness. The muscle cross-sectional area, an index of left ventricular myocardial mass,[8, 20, 21] was also computed: cross-sectional area $= \pi[(\text{diastolic dimension}/2) + \text{wall thickness}]^2 - \pi[\text{diastolic dimension}/2]^2$.

Gated blood pool cardiac scintigraphy. Radionuclide cineangiography was performed with patients in the supine position at rest and during maximum symptom-limited exercise. Left ventricular ejection fraction was computed from the scintigraphic data as previously described.[12]

Exercise studies were performed with a bicycle ergometer and a restraining harness to minimize patient motion under the camera. Exercise loads were increased by 25 W increments every 2 min until the development of angina or limiting fatigue or dyspnea. Heart rate and blood pressure (by cuff sphygmomanometry) were monitored during exercise. Imaging was begun shortly after the onset of exercise, but only that portion of the data series that occurred during maximal exercise, encompassing approximately the last 2 to 2.5 min of exercise, was selected for analysis. Exercise data were not obtained in four patients because they were severely symptomatic. Two other patients did not speak English and could not cooperate satisfactorily to obtain adequate exercise images. Hence, exercise radionuclide angiographic data were obtained in 74 of the 80 patients.

Graded treadmill exercise testing. Preoperative exercise capacity was evaluated using the NIH treadmill protocol.[13, 14] In the first stage of the protocol, the treadmill is driven at a constant speed of 2.2 mph at inclination of 0%. Every 2.5 min the inclination is increased by 2.5% until a maximum of 22.5 min elapse. The maximum workload at this final stage is 2.5 mph at 20% incline or approximately 8 mets. Fifty-four of the 80 patients (68%) were able to complete this workload without limiting symptoms, including 33 of 50 patients (66%) in whom the ejection fraction at rest was subnormal. Two patients with severe symptoms at rest (New York Heart Association functional class IV) were not exercised and are included in the subgroup with poor exercise tolerance.

Aortic valve replacement. At operation, 37 patients received Starr-Edwards prostheses (1260 series in 24, 2320 series in four, and 2400 series in nine), 38 received Hancock porcine bioprosthesis model 242, three received Bjork-Shiley prostheses, and two received Ionescu-Shiley prostheses. Cardiopulmonary bypass was performed with disc or bubble oxygenator with a flow rate of 2.2 liters/min/m^2. Cardiopulmonary bypass times ranged from 55 to 158 min (mean 86 $\pm$ 21), and aortic cross-clamp times ranged from 33 to 97 min (mean 55 $\pm$ 15). In addition to systemic hypothermia to 25° to 30° C in all patients, myocardial preservation techniques included topical 4° iced saline with coronary perfusion in 34 patients and hyperkalemic cold cardioplegia and topical hypothermia in 46. Myocardial preservation techniques, cardiopulmonary bypass and aortic cross-clamp times, and the type of prosthetic valve implanted were not different among the five subgroups of patients.

Postoperative studies. Seventy-three of the 75 patients who survived 6 months returned within 4 to 8 months after operation for repeat echocardiographic and radionuclide angiographic studies. Repeat cardiac catheterization was performed in 69 of the 73 patients. These studies were performed after patients were withdrawn from all cardiac medications, except for antiarrhythmic drugs in 11 patients (procainamide in six, quinidine in three, and disopyramide in two patients). Left heart catheterization was performed with either the transseptal or the left ventricular puncture technique. Echocardiographic left ventricular end-systolic dimension and fractional shortening were not analyzed for the group because of the frequent occurrence of abnormal septal motion after operation.[5, 22]

Postoperative hemodynamic data demonstrated peak systolic gradients across the prosthetic valve of less than 10 mm Hg in 50 patients, between 10 and 20 mm Hg in 13 patients, and 20 mm Hg or greater in six patients. No patient had a prosthetic valve gradient greater than 40 mm Hg. One patient with left ventricular dysfunction of unknown duration had persistent severe (4+ out of 4+) aortic regurgitation 7 months after operation because of a perivalvular leak. He underwent a second operation 8 months after the initial valve replacement and was asymptomatic 32 months after repair of the perivalvular leak. For comparison with other patients, the 6 month data in this patient were derived from the studies obtained 6 months after the second operation.

Statistical methods. Comparison of preoperative or postoperative data among the five subgroups was performed by analysis of variance. Changes in echocardiographic and radionuclide angiographic data from before to after operation within subgroups were analyzed by the paired t test. The association between preoperative echocardiographic, radionuclide angiographic, and hemodynamic variables and subsequent postoperative survival was tested by the Cox method of life-table analysis.[23] Life-table curves were plotted by modification of the method of Kaplan and Meier,[24] and differences between subgroups were analyzed by the method of Mantel and Haenszel.[25]

Results

Preoperative data. Preoperative hemodynamic, echocardiographic, and radionuclide angiographic data are presented in table 1 for the five subgroups of patients. Patients with normal preoperative left ventricular ejection fraction by radionuclide angiography had significantly higher fractional shortening and smaller end-systolic dimensions by echocardiography compared with patients with subnormal ejection fraction ($p <$ .001). However, hemodynamic measurements of left ventricular function and echocardiographic indexes of left ventricular diastolic size and myocardial mass were not different between patients with normal or subnormal ejection fraction. Among the four patient subgroups with depressed preoperative ejection fractions, patients with impaired exercise tolerance were older, had greater systolic dysfunction, and had higher pulmonary wedge pressures than patients with good exercise tolerance, but there were no differences in degree of left ventricular dilatation or hypertrophy.

Postoperative survival. The postoperative survival curve for the 80 patients derived by life-table analysis is shown in figure 1. There were no intraoperative deaths, but three patients died within 35 days, yielding an early postoperative mortality rate of 4%. In two of these patients, in whom death occurred in hospital, there was evidence of heart failure and reduced cardiac output; the third patient died suddenly shortly before hospital discharge. A total of 11 patients died after operation. The preoperative data obtained in these 11 patients are presented in table 2. Two of the postoperative deaths were related to the prosthetic valve: prosthetic valve endocarditis and severe regurgitation of a porcine bioprosthesis. The other nine deaths were cardiac in origin and not apparently related to the prosthetic valve: three patients died suddenly and six patients died from congestive heart failure. These latter six patients all had postoperative symptoms of pulmonary congestion and low cardiac output as well as objective evidence of left ventricular dysfunction after operation. The 5 year postoperative survival rate was 83 $\pm$ 5% ($\pm$SE), yielding an annual postoperative

TABLE 1
Preoperative data

	Patients with normal LV EF at rest (n = 30)	p value[A]	Patients with subnormal LV EF at rest: All patients (n = 50)	Good exercise tolerance: Brief duration (n = 10)	Good exercise tolerance: Unknown duration (n = 17)	Good exercise tolerance: Prolonged duration (n = 6)	Patients with poor exercise tolerance (n = 17)
Age (yr)	41±15	NS	46±14	44±14	42±15	35±5	55±10[D,E]
Echocardiographic data							
LV diastolic dimension (mm)	74±6	NS	75±7	75±4	76±6	75±10	76±7
LV systolic dimension (mm)	51±6	<.001	58±7	55±3	58±6[E]	56±8	59±8[E]
LV fractional shortening (%)	31±4	<.001	24±4	26±2[E]	24±3[E]	25±3[E]	21±5[D,E]
R/Th ratio	2.9±0.5	NS	3.0±0.4	3.1±0.5	3.3±0.4	3.1±0.4	2.9±0.7
Cross-sectional area (cm^2)	35±6	NS	35±7	34±5	36±5	35±13	36±7
Radionuclide angiographic data							
LV EF at rest (%)	52±7	C	37±7	40±6	38±5	40±6	33±9[D]
LV EF during exercise (%)	45±8	C	30±7	30±9	31±6	30±6	27±7
LV EF exercise response (%)[B]	−7±7	NS	−8±5	−10±7	−7±4	−9±5	−7±5
Hemodynamic data							
Pulmonary wedge pressure (mm Hg)	13±8	NS	15±7	11±4	16±6	13±4	20±9[D,E]
LV end-diastolic pressure (mm Hg)	14±8	NS	17±9	16±8	16±7	13±8	21±10[E]
Cardiac index ($l/min/m^2$)	2.8±0.5	NS	2.6±0.7	2.7±0.7	2.9±0.7	3.0±0.6	2.2±0.6[E]

Data are mean ± SD; statistical significance by analysis of variance.
EF = ejection fraction; LV = left ventricular; R/Th = radius–to–wall thickness ratio.
[A]Comparison between patients with normal ejection fraction and all patients with subnormal ejection fraction.
[B]Exercise LV ejection fraction minus resting ejection fraction.
[C]Comparison not made since patient subgroups defined on basis of ejection fraction.
[D]$p < .05$ compared with all other subgroups with subnormal ejection fraction at rest.
[E]$p < .05$ compared with patients with normal ejection fraction.

mortality rate (including the three in-hospital deaths) of less than 4% per year.

By the Cox univariate life-table analysis, several preoperative echocardiographic and radionuclide angiographic indexes of left ventricular systolic size and systolic function were associated with subsequent postoperative cardiac mortality (table 3). Significant echocardiographic indexes were the left ventricular fractional shortening and end-systolic dimension. The left ventricular end-diastolic dimension, the diastolic radius–to–wall thickness ratio, and the myocardial cross-sectional area were not significantly related to postoperative death. Among the radionuclide angiographic indexes, the association between left ventricular ejection fraction at rest and postoperative death was highly significant. Although the value of the ejection fraction during supine exercise was also significantly related to mortality, the ejection fraction response to exercise (i.e., the magnitude of the change from rest to exercise) was not. Preoperative echocardiographic and radionuclide angiographic variables are shown in figure 2 for patients who died after operation compared with survivors. Although age at operation was marginally associated with subsequent cardiac mortality (table 3), four of nine patients with cardiac death (and four of six who died from left ventricular dysfunction) were age 42 or less (table 2). No preoperative hemody-

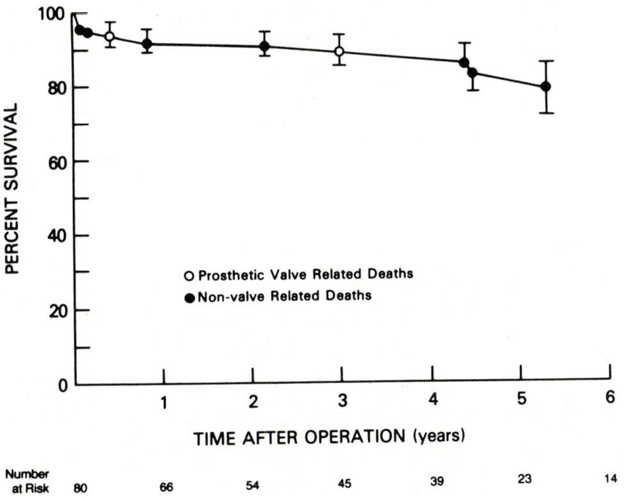

FIGURE 1. Life table depicting postoperative survival in the 80 patients undergoing operation from 1976 to 1983. Brackets indicate standard error. Two patients with death related to the aortic valve prosthesis are indicated by open symbols.

TABLE 2

Preoperative data in 11 patients who died after aortic valve replacement

Patient	Age (yr)	Sex	Postoperative survival (mo)	Cause of death	Echocardiographic data LVDD (mm)	LVSD (mm)	LVFS (%)	CSA (cm^2)	Radionuclide angiographic data Rest EF (%)	Exercise EF (%)	Exercise response (%)
1	66	M	1	LV dysfunction	76	64	16	30	30	—	—
2	37	M	1	LV dysfunction	75	60	20	36	26	20	−6
3	62	M	1	Sudden	90	75	17	38	23	—	—
4	69	M	2	Sudden	84	72	14	40	13	—	—
5	26	M	5	Valve[A]	65	48	26	35	45	41	−4
6	36	M	10	LV dysfunction	75	58	23	36	29	22	−7
7	62	F	26	Sudden	62	41	34	25	50	46	−4
8	30	M	36	Valve[B]	85	70	18	40	36	24	−12
9	42	M	53	LV dysfunction	74	58	22	32	29	22	−7
10	58	M	54	LV dysfunction	72	54	25	41	38	32	−6
11	34	M	64	LV dysfunction	94	70	26	59	40	27	−13

CI = cardiac index; CSA = cross-sectional area; DD = diastolic dimension; EDP = end-diastolic pressure; EF = ejection fraction; FS = fractional shortening; LV = left ventricular; PAW = pulmonary arterial wedge pressure; SD = systolic dimension.

[A]Prosthetic valve endocarditis.

[B]Severe regurgitation of aortic porcine bioprosthesis; died after second valve replacement operation.

namic variable was significantly associated with subsequent mortality (table 3). The method of myocardial preservation used at operation also did not influence outcome. At 5.5 years after operation, the survival rate in patients treated with hyperkalemic cardioplegia was 81 ± 8%, compared with 82 ± 8% in patients who did not receive hyperkalemic cardioplegia (preoperative hemodynamic, echocardiographic, and radionuclide angiographic data were similar between these two groups). No relationship was evident between the type of prosthetic valve used and postoperative survival.

TABLE 3

Association between preoperative variables and subsequent postoperative mortality

Variable	p value: All deaths (n = 11)	Deaths not related to prosthetic valve (n = 9)
Echocardiographic data		
LV fractional shortening	<.001[A]	<.005[A]
LV systolic dimension	<.01[A]	<.01[A]
LV diastolic dimension	.25	.21
LV R/Th ratio	.42	.38
LV myocardial cross-sectional area	.47	.52
Radionuclide angiographic data		
LV EF at rest	<.001[A]	<.001[A]
LV EF during exercise	<.02[A]	<.02[A]
LV EF response to exercise[B]	.81	.76
Hemodynamic data		
Pulmonary wedge pressure	.20	.07
LV end-diastolic pressure	.18	.052
Cardiac index	.88	.80
Age	.26	.047[A]
Sex	.29	.43
Hyperkalemic cardioplegia	.29	.74

EF = ejection fraction; LV = left ventricular; R/Th = diastolic radius-to-wall thickness ratio.

[A]Significant value by Cox univariate analysis.

[B]LV EF response to exercise = exercise EF minus rest EF.

Subgroup analysis. The influence of preoperative left ventricular function, assessed by resting radionuclide angiographic ejection fraction, on postoperative survival is demonstrated in figure 3. Among the 30 patients with normal preoperative ejection fraction, there was only one late death, a 64-year-old woman who died suddenly after 26 months. In contrast, the other 10 deaths, including all in-hospital deaths, occurred in patients with subnormal preoperative ejection fraction. The survival rate at 5.5 years was 96 ± 3% in patients with normal preoperative ejection fraction compared with 63 ± 12% in patients with subnormal ejection fraction ($p < .01$). Among subgroups of patients with subnormal preoperative ejection fraction (figure 4), postoperative survival was excellent in the subgroup with preserved exercise tolerance and only a brief duration of left ventricular dysfunction (no deaths). In contrast, postoperative survival rates were very similar in the other three subgroups with subnormal preoperative ejection fraction: patients with poor exercise tolerance, or those with good exercise tolerance but prolonged or unknown duration of preoperative left ventricular dysfunction. In these latter three subgroups, the survival rate was reduced below 60% at 5 years.

These survival trends in the patient subgroups were

TABLE 2
(Continued)

Hemodynamic data			Postoperative prosthetic valve gradient (mm Hg)
PAW (mm Hg)	LVEDP (mm Hg)	CI (l/min/m²)	
20	18	1.9	—
14	23	3.4	—
34	32	2.7	—
22	20	2.5	—
10	13	3.4	—
19	20	3.9	15
28	32	1.7	3
8	6	2.7	20
8	7	2.2	12
18	25	2.6	0
14	23	2.4	5

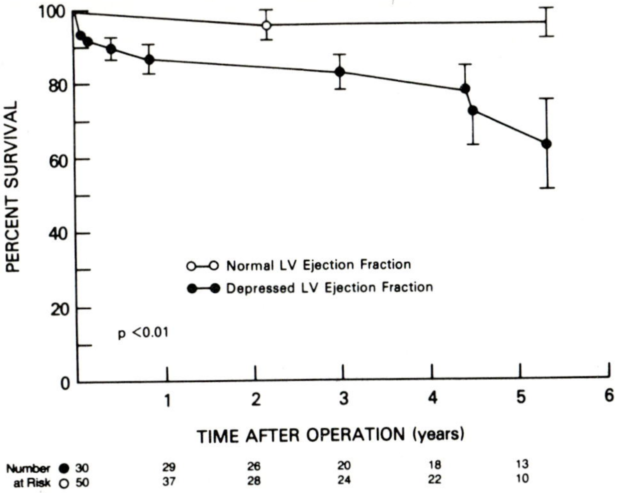

FIGURE 3. Survival after aortic valve replacement. Patients are subgrouped on the basis of preoperative left ventricular (LV) ejection fraction at rest.

paralleled by changes in left ventricular function after operation. In patients with preoperative left ventricular dysfunction, the ejection fraction at rest did not change significantly 6 months after operation in either the subgroup with poor exercise tolerance or the subgroup with good exercise tolerance but prolonged duration of dysfunction (table 4, figure 5). In contrast, patients with good exercise tolerance and only a brief duration of left ventricular dysfunction manifested a significantly greater increase in ejection fraction after operation, and the postoperative ejection fraction in this group was identical to that observed in patients in whom the preoperative ejection fraction was normal. Nearly identical results were obtained when the postoperative changes in the ejection fraction during exer-

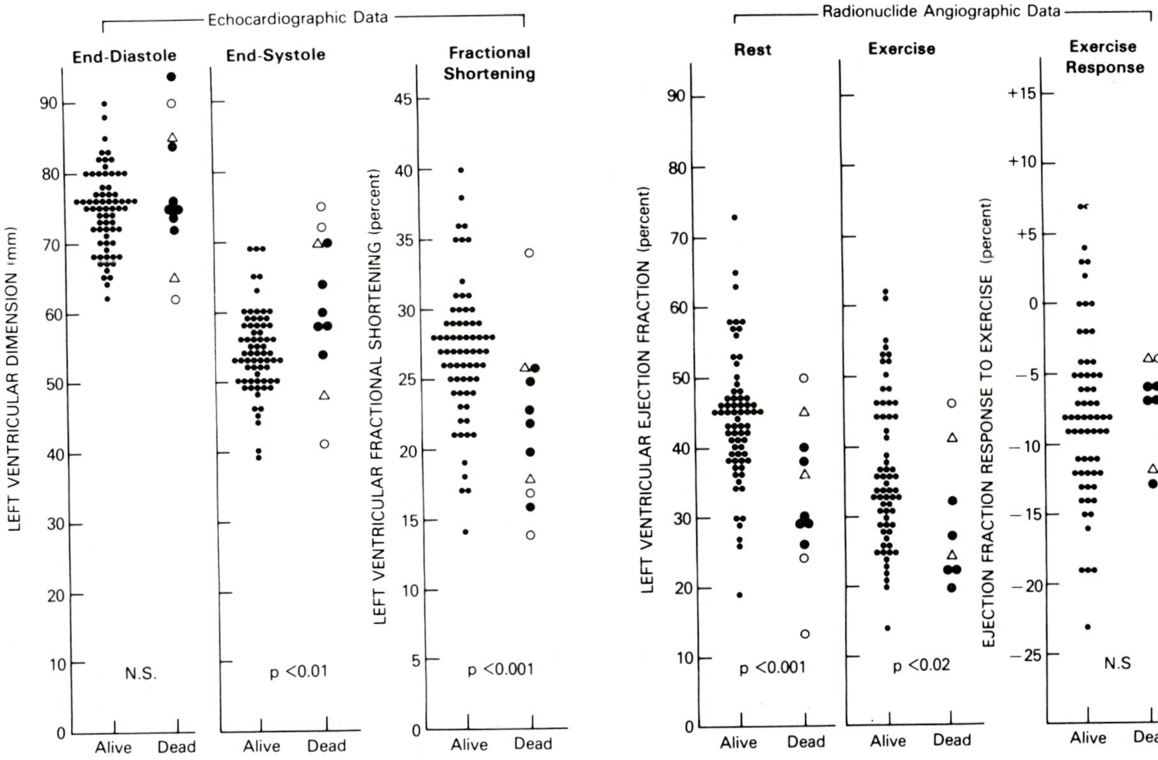

FIGURE 2. Preoperative echocardiographic and radionuclide angiographic data for 69 patients surviving after aortic valve replacement and the 11 patients who died after operation. Significance values indicate the ability of each variable to predict subsequent mortality by life-table analysis rather than direct differences between the two groups. Cause of death is indicated by different symbols: left ventricular dysfunction (closed circles), sudden death (open circles), valve-related deaths (open triangles).

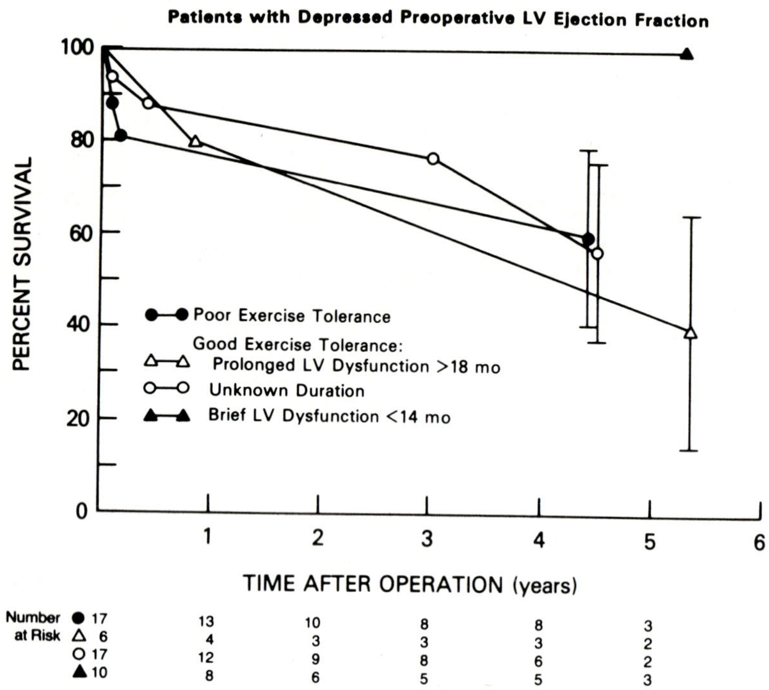

FIGURE 4. Survival after aortic valve replacement in subgroups of patients with subnormal preoperative left ventricular (LV) ejection fraction at rest.

cise were analyzed (table 4, figure 6). Patients with a brief duration of preoperative left ventricular dysfunction manifested a significant increase in exercise ejection fraction after operation to a value comparable to that observed in patients in whom the preoperative ejection fraction at rest was normal. However, the exercise ejection fraction did not change significantly after operation in those patients with preoperative left ventricular dysfunction at rest who either manifested poor preoperative exercise tolerance or a prolonged

TABLE 4
Postoperative data

	Patients with normal preoperative EF at rest	p value[A]	Patients with subnormal preoperative EF at rest				
				Good preoperative exercise tolerance			Patients with poor preoperative exercise tolerance
			All patients	Brief duration	Unknown duration	Prolonged duration	
Echocardiographic data							
LV diastolic dimension (mm)	53±7	<.01	58±9	49±3[C]	58±8[D]	60±10[D]	64±8[E]
Change in LV diastolic dimension (mm)[B]	−21±8	NS	−18±9	−26±5[C]	−19±10	−16±7	−11±7[E]
Radionuclide angiographic data							
LV EF at rest (%)	57±16	<.001	45±15	63±7[C]	47±10[E]	37±12[E]	34±15[E]
Change in LV EF at rest (%)[B]	9±10	NS	7±14	23±9[C]	8±11	−2±9[D]	−2±11[E]
LV EF during exercise (%)	61±14	<.001	45±16	62±9[C]	46±12[E]	36±13[E]	33±11[E]
Change in LV EF during exercise (%)[B]	15±10	NS	15±15	32±13[C]	15±12	6±10	4±9[E]
Hemodynamic data							
Prosthetic valve gradient	9±9	NS	7±9	11±13	8±8	5±6	5±5
LV end-diastolic pressure (mm Hg)	9±4	NS	10±4	7±3	11±4	8±1	12±5[D]
Cardiac index (l/min/m²)	3.1±0.8	NS	3.0±0.9	3.0±0.6	2.8±0.7	2.9±0.8	3.3±0.4

See table 1 for abbreviations.
[A]Comparison between patients with normal preoperative ejection fraction and all patients with subnormal ejection fraction.
[B]Compared with preoperative value.
[C]$p < .01$ compared with all other subgroups with subnormal preoperative ejection fraction at rest.
[D]$p < .05$ compared with patients with normal preoperative ejection fraction at rest.
[E]$p < .01$ compared with patients with normal preoperative ejection fraction at rest.

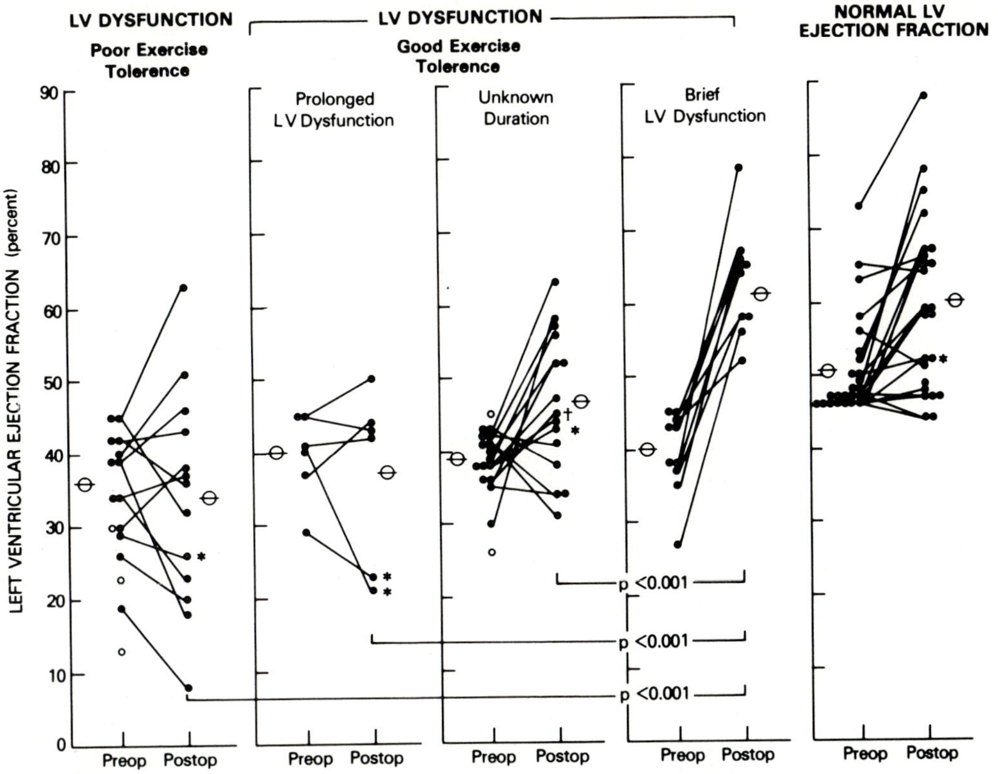

FIGURE 5. Change in radionuclide angiographic ejection fraction at rest from before (Preop) to 6 months after (Postop) operation in patients with normal preoperative left ventricular (LV) ejection fraction at rest and the four subgroups with subnormal preoperative ejection fraction. Open symbols, patients who died before the 6 month repeat evaluation; asterisks, cardiac deaths after 6 month study; cross, valve-related death after 6 month study. Significance values by analysis by variance.

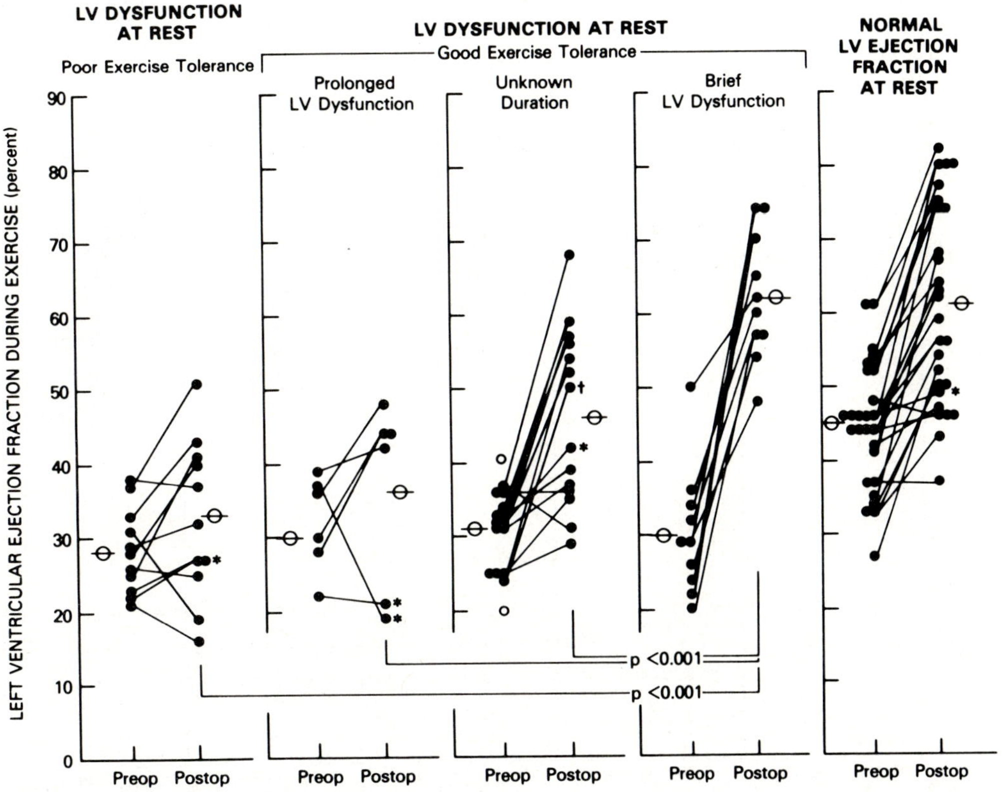

FIGURE 6. Change in ejection fraction during exercise from before to 6 months after operation in the five patient subgroups. Symbols are defined in legend to figure 5.

duration of left ventricular dysfunction. In any individual patient, the value of the preoperative ejection fraction during exercise per se did not indicate whether or not a patient was likely to manifest a substantial improvement in left ventricular ejection fraction after operation, either at rest or during exercise (figure 6).

The changes in left ventricular ejection fraction after operation were paralleled closely by the magnitude of reduction in left ventricular diastolic dimension after operation (table 4, figure 7). Preoperative left ventricular diastolic dimension was not different among the five subgroups of patients but was reduced to a greater extent after operation in those patients with normal preoperative ejection fraction or preoperative left ventricular dysfunction of only brief duration, compared with that in patients with preoperative left ventricular dysfunction and poor exercise tolerance or a prolonged duration of left ventricular dysfunction.

Eleven patients were receiving antiarrhythmic drugs at the time of the postoperative studies. Although seven of these patients had depressed preoperative ejection fractions, none was in the subgroup with poor exercise tolerance or prolonged duration of preoperative left ventricular dysfunction. Similarly, although six patients had prosthetic valve gradients of 20 mm Hg or greater at the postoperative study, none of these patients was in the subgroup with preoperative left ventricular dysfunction and either poor exercise tolerance or prolonged duration of dysfunction. Hence, postoperative data in subgroups at highest risk of persistent left ventricular dysfunction were not influenced by potential drug effects or prosthetic valve gradients.

On the basis of these functional changes after operation, the survival analysis was repeated to assess postoperative prognoses in subgroups with a high likelihood of normal postoperative left ventricular function compared with subgroups with a likelihood of persistent dysfunction (figure 8). Patients with either normal preoperative ejection fraction or a brief duration of left ventricular dysfunction with good exercise tolerance had an excellent postoperative survival rate (97 ± 3% at 5.5 years). In contrast, postoperative survival was significantly reduced in those patients with left ventricular dysfunction and poor exercise tolerance or prolonged duration of left ventricular dysfunction. The survival rate at 5.5 years was 52 ± 17% in this combined subgroup of patients. Hence, patients with left ventricular dysfunction and impaired exercise tolerance, and those with a prolonged duration of preoperative dysfunction, define the high-risk group.

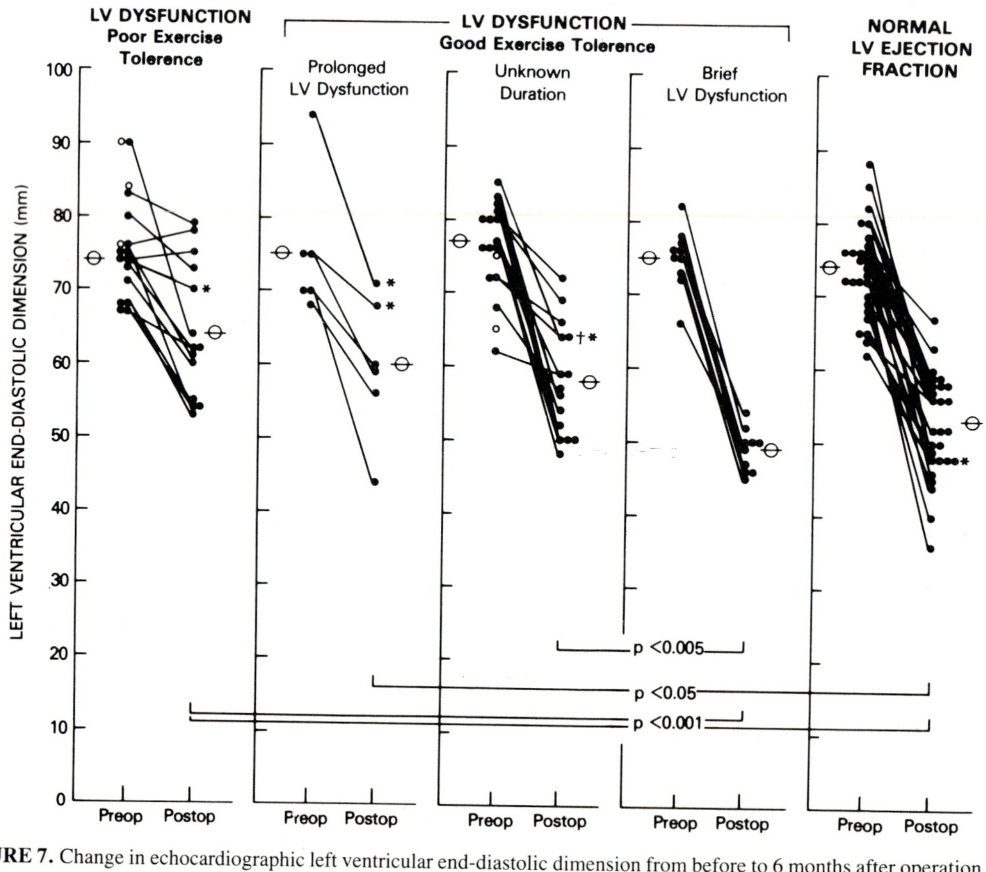

FIGURE 7. Change in echocardiographic left ventricular end-diastolic dimension from before to 6 months after operation in the five patient subgroups. Symbols are defined in legend to figure 5.

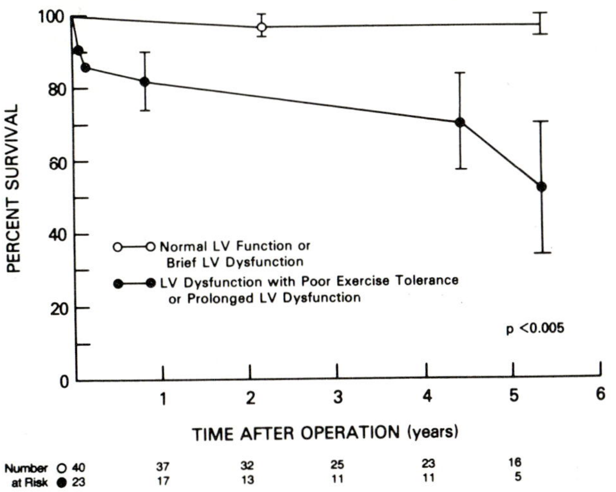

FIGURE 8. Survival after aortic valve replacement in high-risk and low-risk subgroups of patients.

Discussion

The impact of preoperative left ventricular dysfunction on postoperative survival in patients with aortic regurgitation remains a subject of controversy. Numerous studies demonstrate that patients who exhibit impaired preoperative left ventricular systolic function are at risk of manifesting irreversible myocardial dysfunction and of dying postoperatively from congestive heart failure despite technically successful valve replacement.[1–8] Other reports emphasize, however, that impaired preoperative left ventricular function may improve dramatically, and even normalize, in many patients after operation.[9–11, 13, 14, 17, 20, 21, 26–28] Some investigators have interpreted this potential for improvement as an indication that survival and functional results after valve replacement for aortic regurgitation may no longer be influenced by preoperative left ventricular function.[9–11]

We believe the principal reason for the disparate conclusions of recent studies regarding survival and functional results of aortic valve replacement relate to patient selection factors and to interpretive differences. The influence of patient selection on the results is evident from the following analysis. In the current study, our in-hospital mortality rate was 4% and the annual postoperative mortality rate (including perioperative deaths) was less than 4% per year, yielding a 5 year survival rate of 83%. This represents a significant improvement in postoperative survival compared with our previous experience from 1972 to 1976 (figure 9), in which survival at 4 years was only 62%. Similar improvement in postoperative survival in the late 1970s compared with the early 1970s has been reported by Turina et al.[29] These improved survival results in the recent era probably represent, in part, differences in selection of patients for operation. During the course of the current study, our strategy for patient management in aortic regurgitation was changed because of data implicating left ventricular function and severity of symptoms as important determinants of postoperative prognosis.[1–8, 13, 17, 20, 30–35] Hence, many patients with left ventricular dysfunction in the current study underwent operation before the development of severe symptoms or impaired exercise capacity. Fifty-four of the 80 patients (68%) were able to complete stage I of our treadmill protocol, including 33 of 50 (67%) with subnormal ejection fractions. In contrast, from 1971 to 1976, our only indication for aortic valve replacement was moderate to severe cardiac symptoms (New York Heart Association functional class III to IV), and only 12% of patients were able to complete stage I. Turina et al.[29] also suggested that improved late survival in their recent operative experience was the result of earlier operation before the onset of severe clinical and hemodynamic impairment.

The improved survival may also reflect advances in operative techniques. Our study was not designed to study the effects of different myocardial preservation techniques, and the two procedures used in this study were historically controlled rather than concurrently performed. Nonetheless, we could not demonstrate a beneficial effect of hyperkalemic cardioplegia in enhancing postoperative survival in our study. It is possible, however, that other subtle operative factors developed over the course of a decade may have important effects that would not be apparent simply by description of myocardial preservation techniques.

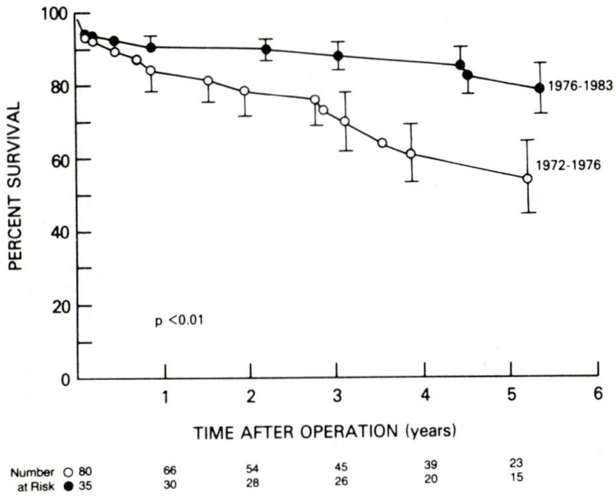

FIGURE 9. Survival after aortic valve replacement for the 80 patients in the current study (1976 to 1983) compared with 35 patients undergoing isolated aortic valve replacement for aortic regurgitation at our institution from 1972 to 1976.

Despite the recent improvement in postoperative survival, our current results demonstrate that ejection phase indexes of left ventricular function remain significantly associated with subsequent postoperative cardiac mortality (table 3). In addition to the significant association between postoperative mortality and reduced preoperative left ventricular fractional shortening and increased systolic dimension by echocardiography, as in our previous experience,[5] mortality in the current study was also highly associated with low values of resting left ventricular ejection fraction by an independent noninvasive technique, radionuclide angiography, which does not have the potential limitations of echocardiography in assessing left ventricular systolic performance in the volume-loaded left ventricle.[36-39] Because of the ongoing controversy surrounding the use of echocardiography in the diagnosis of aortic regurgitation, we used resting ejection fraction by radionuclide angiography as the standard with which to subgroup patients in this study into those with normal vs subnormal systolic function. Patients with normal ejection fraction before operation had a significantly higher postoperative survival rate than patients with preoperative left ventricular dysfunction (figure 3).

Importantly, within the group with depressed ejection fraction, we also identified patients who constituted subgroups at low and high risk (figures 4 and 8). Patients with subnormal ejection fraction but preserved exercise tolerance and only a brief duration left ventricular dysfunction had excellent postoperative survival (no patient died), whereas patients with either impaired exercise tolerance or good exercise tolerance but prolonged left ventricular dysfunction had survival rates less than 60% at 5 years. These survival results were paralleled by changes in left ventricular function after operation (table 4, figures 5 to 7). These data suggest that differences in patient selection might explain discordant results in previous studies regarding the frequency and magnitude of reversal of left ventricular dysfunction after valve replacement. These data also indicate that delaying operation in an asymptomatic or mildly symptomatic patient with impaired left ventricular function until the development of more severe symptoms places the patient at greater risk of death or irreversible ventricular dysfunction.

These findings relate to three recent studies in which discrepancies between preoperative left ventricular function and postoperative results were apparently identified, insofar as the authors concluded that echocardiographic evidence of preoperative left ventricular systolic dysfunction did not identify subgroups of patients at risk of death or persistent left ventricular dysfunction after operation.[9-11] These investigators suggested that improved operative techniques and valve design have in effect negated the impact of left ventricular function on postoperative survival, so that indexes of left ventricular dilatation and function cannot be used in the timing of operation. We believe that the results of these studies and our current results are quite similar and that the disparate conclusions arise from interpretive differences.

The reason echocardiography was of no predictive value regarding survival in the studies by Fioretti et al.[9, 11] is readily apparent: there was only one postoperative death. Despite improved postoperative results, however, all other centers continue to report a more finite risk to life of aortic valve replacement,[29, 40-44] as was our experience in the current study. Fioretti and associates excluded from study all patients who had "complicated" postoperative courses, an action that may have influenced their results importantly. Moreover, although Fioretti's group did not demonstrate a relationship between left ventricular function and postoperative survival, 50% of their patients with preoperative left ventricular dysfunction by echocardiography had persistent left ventricular dilatation after operation.

Although Daniel et al.[10] were also critical of the predictive value of echocardiographic indexes of left ventricular function in assessing postoperative prognosis, their data actually demonstrate poor postoperative survival in patients with preoperative left ventricular dysfunction. Survival curves were not presented in that study; however, only 79% of patients with left ventricular dysfunction (assessed echocardiographically) were alive at a mean follow-up of 29.5 months. This translates into an average mortality rate in such patients of 8.6% per year. In contrast, 91% of patients without left ventricular dysfunction were alive during the same postoperative period, representing an annual mortality rate of 3.7%. All but four of the deaths in that series were related to the prosthetic valve. Such complications must be considered chance events and would not be predicted by preoperative left ventricular function. In the four patients with cardiac deaths, however, all four had subnormal preoperative left ventricular fractional shortening (less than 29%); three of the four had end-systolic dimensions greater than 60 mm, and the fourth had an end-systolic dimension of 53 mm. Patients with preoperative left ventricular dysfunction also had a greater prevalence of persistent severe postoperative left ventricular dilatation.

The prognostic value of the resting ejection fraction

in our study was not enhanced further by analysis of the ejection fraction response to exercise (table 3). The majority of patients with normal ejection fraction at rest manifested an abnormal exercise response (that is, a decrease in ejection fraction compared to the value at rest). However, since survival in these patients was excellent, the abnormal ejection fraction response did not identify patients with normal ejection fractions in whom survival after operation was reduced. In addition, neither the value of the exercise ejection fraction nor the magnitude of the ejection fraction response to exercise predicted which patients with subnormal ejection fraction at rest were at risk of death or persistent left ventricular dysfunction after operation (tables 1 and 3, figure 7). Thus, despite the good correlation between the decrease in ejection fraction during exercise and increased left ventricular dimensions,[28, 45] increased left ventricular wall stress,[45–47] and perhaps abnormal exercise hemodynamic data,[48, 49] the ejection fraction response to exercise does not appear to provide meaningful information regarding postoperative prognosis over the initial 5 to 7 years after aortic valve replacement.

Our data demonstrate improved long-term postoperative survival in the current operative series compared with our earlier results. Despite this improvement, preoperative left ventricular systolic dysfunction continues to identify patients with aortic regurgitation at risk of death or persistent left ventricular dysfunction after aortic valve replacement. Indexes of left ventricular systolic size and systolic function are the most important determinants of prognosis. Patients with left ventricular dysfunction and impaired exercise tolerance, or those with a prolonged duration of preoperative left ventricular dysfunction, define the high-risk subgroup. We emphasize, however, that operation is not contraindicated in such patients; many will do well after operation, although the probability of survival and normalization of left ventricular function is considerably less than in patients in the low-risk group. Our data indicate that early operation in such patients should result in further improvement in long-term survival.

We appreciate the important assistance of Gale G. White in acquisition of data and of Elizabeth Todd and June Moon in preparation of the manuscript.

References

1. Cohn PF, Gorlin R, Cohn LH, Collins JJ Jr: Left ventricular ejection fraction as a prognostic guide in surgical treatment of coronary and valvular heart disease. Am J Cardiol **34:** 136, 1974
2. Fischl SJ, Gorlin R, Herman MV: Cardiac shape and function in aortic valve disease: physiologic and clinical implications. Am J Cardiol **39:** 170, 1977
3. Copeland JG, Griepp RB, Stinson EB, Shumway NE: Long-term follow-up after isolated aortic valve replacement. J Thorac Cardiovasc Surg **74:** 875, 1977
4. Forman R, Firth BF, Barnard MS: Prognostic significance of preoperative left ventricular ejection fraction and valve lesion in patients with aortic valve replacement. Am J Cardiol **45:** 1120, 1980
5. Henry WL, Bonow RO, Borer JS, Ware JH, Kent KM, Redwood DR, McIntosh CL, Morrow AG, Epstein SE: Observations on the optimum time for operative intervention for aortic regurgitation. I. Evaluation of the results of aortic valve replacement in symptomatic patients. Circulation **61:** 471, 1980
6. Cunha CLP, Giuliani ER, Fuster V, Seward JB, Brandenburg RO, McGoon DC: Preoperative M-mode echocardiography as a predictor of surgical results in chronic aortic insufficiency. J Thorac Cardiovasc Surg **79:** 256, 1980
7. Greves J, Rahimtoola SH, McAnulty JH, DeMots H, Clark DG, Greenberg B, Starr A: Preoperative criteria predictive of late survival following valve replacement for severe aortic regurgitation. Am Heart J **101:** 300, 1981
8. Gaasch WH, Carroll JD, Levine HJ, Criscitiello MG: Chronic aortic regurgitation: prognostic value of left ventricular end-systolic dimension and end-diastolic radius/thickness ratio. J Am Coll Cardiol **1:** 775, 1983
9. Fioretti P, Roelandt J, Bos RJ, Meltzer RS, van Hoogenhuijze D, Serruys PW, Nauta A, Hugenholtz PG: Echocardiography in chronic aortic insufficiency: is valve replacement too late when left ventricular systolic dimension reaches 55 mm? Circulation **67:** 216, 1983
10. Daniel WG, Hood WP, Siart A, Hausmann D, Nellesen V, Oelert H, Lichtlen PR: Chronic aortic regurgitation: reassessment of the prognostic value of preoperative left ventricular end-systolic dimension and fractional shortening. Circulation **71:** 669, 1985
11. Fioretti P, Roelandt J, Sclavo M, Domenicucci S, Haalebos M, Bos E, Hugenholtz PG: Postoperative regression of left ventricular dimensions in aortic insufficiency: a long-term echocardiographic study. J Am Coll Cardiol **5:** 856, 1985
12. Borer JS, Bacharach SL, Green MV, Kent KM, Henry WL, Rosing DR, Seides SF, Johnston GS, Epstein SE: Exercise-induced left ventricular dysfunction in symptomatic and asymptomatic patients with aortic regurgitation. Am J Cardiol **42:** 351, 1978
13. Bonow RO, Borer JS, Rosing DR, Henry WL, Pearlman AS, McIntosh CL, Morrow AG, Epstein SE: Preoperative exercise capacity in symptomatic patients with aortic regurgitation as a predictor of post-operative left ventricular function and long-term prognosis. Circulation **62:** 1280, 1980
14. Bonow RO, Rosing DR, Maron BJ, McIntosh CL, Jones M, Bacharach SL, Green MV, Clark RE, Epstein SE: Reversal of left ventricular dysfunction after aortic valve replacement for chronic aortic regurgitation: influence of duration of preoperative left ventricular dysfunction. Circulation **70:** 570, 1984
15. Feigenbaum H: Echocardiography, ed 2. Philadelphia, 1976, Lea and Febiger, p 464
16. Fortuin NJ, Hood WP, Sherman ME, Craige E: Determination of left ventricular volumes by ultrasound. Circulation **44:** 575, 1971
17. Gaasch WH, Andrias CW, Levine HJ: Chronic aortic regurgitation: the effect of aortic valve replacement on left ventricular volume, mass, and function. Circulation **58:** 825, 1978
18. Grossman W, Jones D, McLaurin LP: Wall stress and patterns of hypertrophy in the human left ventricle. J Clin Invest **56:** 56, 1975
19. Gaasch WH: Left ventricular radius to wall thickness ratio. Am J Cardiol **43:** 1189, 1979
20. Schuler G, Peterson KL, Johnson AD, Francis G, Ashburn W, Dennish G, Daily PO, Ross J: Serial noninvasive assessment of left ventricular hypertrophy and function after surgical correction of aortic regurgitation. Am J Cardiol **44:** 585, 1979
21. Carroll JD, Gaasch WH, Zile MR, Levine HJ: Serial changes in left ventricular function after correction of chronic aortic regurgitation: dependence on early changes in preload and subsequent regression of hypertrophy. Am J Cardiol **51:** 476, 1983
22. Burggraf GW, Craig E: Echocardiographic studies of left ventricular wall motion and dimension after valvular heart surgery. Am J Cardiol **35:** 473, 1975
23. Cox DR: Regression models and life tables (with discussion). J R Stat Soc **34:** 187, 1972
24. Kaplan EL, Meier P: Non-parametric estimation from incomplete observations. J Am Stat Soc **53:** 457, 1958

25. Mantel N: Chi square test with one degree of freedom: extension of the Mantel-Haenszel procedure. J Am Stat Soc **58:** 690, 1963
26. Schwarz F, Flameng W, Langebartels F, Sesto M, Walter P, Schlepper M: Impaired left ventricular function in chronic aortic valve disease: survival and function after replacement by Bjork-Shiley prosthesis. Circulation **60:** 48, 1979
27. Clark DG, McAnulty JH, Rahimtoola SH: Valve replacement in aortic insufficiency with left ventricular dysfunction. Circulation **61:** 411, 1980
28. Bonow RO, Rosing DR, McIntosh CL, Jones M, Maron BJ, Lan KKG, Lakatos E, Bacharach SL, Green MV, Epstein SE: The natural history of asymptomatic patients with aortic regurgitation and normal left ventricular function. Circulation **68:** 509, 1983
29. Turina J, Turina M, Rothlin M, Krayenbuehl HP: Improved late survival in patients with chronic aortic regurgitation by earlier operation. Circulation **70**(suppl I): I-147, 1984
30. Rahimtoola SH: Valve replacement should not be performed in all asymptomatic patients with severe aortic incompetence. J Thorac Cardiovasc Surg **79:** 163, 1980
31. Kennedy JW, Doces J, Stewart DK: Left ventricular function before and following aortic valve replacement. Circulation **56:** 944, 1977
32. Herreman F, Ameur A, deVernejoul F, Bourgin JH, Gueret P, Guerin F, Degorges M: Pre- and post-operative hemodynamic and cineangiographic assessment of left ventricular function in patients with aortic regurgitation. Am Heart J **98:** 63, 1979
33. Ross J Jr: Left ventricular function and the timing of surgical treatment in valvular heart disease. Ann Intern Med **94:** 498, 1981
34. Toussaint C, Cribier A, Cazor JL, Sayer R, Letac B: Hemodynamic and angiographic evaluation of aortic regurgitation 7 and 27 months after aortic valve replacement. Circulation **64:** 456, 1981
35. Bonow RO, Rosing DR, Kent KM, Epstein SE: Timing of operation for chronic aortic regurgitation. Am J Cardiol **50:** 325, 1982
36. Johnson AD, Alpert JS, Francis GS, Vieweg VR, Ockene I, Hagan AD: Assessment of left ventricular function in severe aortic regurgitation. Circulation **54:** 975, 1976
37. Bhatt DR, Isabel-Jones JB, Villoria GJ, Nakazawa M, Yabek SM, Marks RA, Jarmakani JM: Accuracy of echocardiography in assessing left ventricular dimensions and volume. Circulation **57:** 699, 1978
38. Abdulla AM, Frank MJ, Canedo MI, Stefadouros MA: Limitations of echocardiography in the assessment of left ventricular size and function in aortic regurgitation. Circulation **61:** 148, 1980
39. O'Rourke RA, Crawford MH: Timing of valve replacement in patients with chronic aortic regurgitation. Circulation **61:** 493, 1980
40. Acar J, Luxereau P, Ducimetiere P, Cadilhac M, Jallut H, Vahanian A: Prognosis of surgically treated chronic aortic valve disease. J Thorac Cardiovasc Surg **82:** 114, 1981
41. Schwarz F, Bauman P, Manthey J, Hoffmann M, Schuler G, Mehmel HC, Schmitz W, Kubler W: The effect of aortic valve replacement on survival. Circulation **66:** 1105, 1982
42. Nunley DL, Grunkemeier GL, Starr A: Aortic valve replacement with coronary bypass grafting: significant determinants of ten year survival. J Thorac Cardiovasc Surg **85:** 705, 1983
43. Cohn LH, Allred EN, DiSesa VJ, Sawtelle K, Shemin RJ, Collins JJ Jr: Early and late risk of aortic valve replacement: a 12 year concomitant comparison of the porcine bioprosthetic and tilting disc prosthetic aortic valves. J Thorac Cardiovasc Surg **88:** 695, 1984
44. Scott WC, Miller DC, Haverich A, Dawkins K, Mitchell RC, Jamieson SW, Oyer PE, Stinson EB, Baldwin JC, Shumway NE: Determinants of operative mortality for patients undergoing aortic valve replacement: discriminant analysis of 1,479 operations. J Thorac Cardiovasc Surg **89:** 400, 1985
45. Goldman M, Packer M, Horowitz SF, Meller J, Patterson RE, Kukin M, Teichholz LE, Gorlin R: Relation between exercise-induced changes in ejection fraction and systolic loading conditions at rest in aortic regurgitation. J Am Coll Cardiol **3:** 924, 1984
46. Shen WF, Roubin GS, Choong CYP, Hutton BF, Harris PJ, Fletcher PJ, Kelly DT: Evaluation of relationship between myocardial contractile state and left ventricular function in patients with aortic regurgitation. Circulation **71:** 31, 1985
47. Greenberg B, Massie B, Thomas D, Bristow JD, Cheitlin M, Broudy D, Szlachcic J, Krishnamurthy G: Association between the exercise ejection response and systolic wall stress in patients with chronic aortic insufficiency. Circulation **71:** 458, 1985
48. Boucher CA, Wilson RA, Kanarek DJ, Hutter AM, Okada RD, Liberthson RR, Strauss HW, Pohost GM: Exercise testing in asymptomatic or minimally symptomatic aortic regurgitation: relationship of left ventricular ejection fraction to left ventricular filling pressure during exercise. Circulation **67:** 1091, 1983
49. Massie BM, Kramer BL, Loge D, Topic N, Greenberg BH, Cheitlin MD, Bristow JD, Byrd RC: Ejection fraction response to supine exercise in asymptomatic aortic regurgitation: relation to simultaneous hemodynamic measurements. J Am Coll Cardiol **5:** 847, 1985

Regional wave travel and reflections along the human aorta: a study with six simultaneous micromanometric pressures

RICKY D. LATHAM, M.D., MAJ., M.C., NICO WESTERHOF, PH.D., PIETER SIPKEMA, PH.D., BERNARD J. RUBAL, PH.D., PETER REUDERINK, B.S., AND JOSEPH P. MURGO, M.D., COL., M.C.

ABSTRACT The human aorta and its terminal branches were investigated in normal subjects during elective cardiac catheterization to evaluate regional wave travel and arterial wave reflections. A specially designed catheter with six micromanometers equally spaced at 10 cm intervals was positioned with the tip sensor in the distal external iliac artery and the proximal sensor in the aortic arch. Simultaneous pressures were obtained and analyzed for foot-to-foot wave velocity, and Fourier analysis was used to derive apparent phase velocity. These quantities were assessed during control (n = 9), during Valsalva (n = 8) and Müller (n = 4) maneuvers, and during femoral artery occlusion by bilateral manual compression (n = 8). During control, regional cross-sectional areas, determined from aortography, and regional foot-to-foot pulse wave velocities were used to calculate the local reflection coefficient in the proximal descending aorta ($\Gamma = 0.05$), at the junction of the renal arteries ($\Gamma = 0.43$), and at the terminal aortic bifurcation ($\Gamma = 0.13$). To test the hypothesis that significant reflections originate in the aorta, at the level of the renal arteries, aortograms were used to design a latex tube model with geometric properties similar to the descending aorta. Velocities and reflection characteristics in the model and in vivo were compared. Inspection of thoracic aortic pressures under control conditions revealed a reflected wave originating from the region of the aorta at the level of the renal arterial branches while abdominal pressures exhibited reflection from a site peripheral to the terminal aortic bifurcation. In the low frequency range, apparent phase velocity was found to be higher proximal to the renal arteries as compared with at the distal sites. In addition, the minimum value occurred at a higher frequency in the lower thoracic aorta than at more distal sites. The effects of reflection on apparent wave velocity in the tube model were consistent with data obtained in vivo. The Valsalva maneuver diminished the reflection from the aortic region of the renal arteries, thus allowing the distal reflected wave to become more evident on the thoracic pressure waveforms. Bilateral femoral artery occlusion usually enhanced the distal reflection and the Müller maneuver usually resulted in small increases in reflections. In conclusion, the geometric and elastic nonuniformity of the aorta results in two major sites of arterial wave reflection that influence the aortic pressure waveforms in man. The first major reflection site is located at the aortic level of the renal arterial branches and the second reflection site is located distal to the terminal aortic bifurcation.
Circulation 72, No. 6, 1257–1269, 1985.

ALTERATIONS in the contour of the pressure wave along the aorta have been noted since the turn of the century,[1–5] but the mechanisms responsible for these changes have not been fully explained.[4] There have been few detailed investigations of the transmission characteristics of pressure along the human aorta.[2, 3, 6–9] Studies by Luchsinger et al.[2] and O'Rourke[3] described and analyzed pressure waveforms in the human aorta, but pressures were not obtained simultaneously and a fluid-filled manometer system was used. Most of the previous laboratory investigations on this subject have been in animal preparations[10–15]; however, it has been shown that the proximal aortic pulse contour in man differs from that of most laboratory animals,[1, 9, 16] making it difficult to extrapolate all results in animals to man. Furthermore, quantitative assessment of changes in the arterial pressure waveform in man has been attempted in few laboratories because of the complex-

From the Cardiology Service, Department of Medicine, Brooke Army Medical Center, Fort Sam Houston, TX, and Laboratory for Physiology, Free University, Amsterdam.

Address for correspondence: Ricky D. Latham, MAJ, MC, Cardiology Service, Department of Medicine, Brooke Army Medical Center, Fort Sam Houston, TX 78234.

Received Dec. 27, 1984; revision accepted Sept. 19, 1985.

The opinions or assertions contained herein are the private views of the authors and are not to be construed as reflecting the views of the Department of the Army or the Department of Defense.

ity in recording and analyzing multiple simultaneous high-fidelity arterial pressure signals.

Investigations performed in adult humans have shown that the proximal aortic pressure waveform commonly exhibits a secondary systolic wave (figure 1). This secondary systolic wave was generally considered to be associated with arterial wave reflections,[1, 7, 8] the significance of which remains controversial.[1, 7, 8, 11, 13, 17] Although there is strong theoretical and experimental support for the existence of arterial wave reflections,[18] the site(s) of origin of these reflected waves is debated. Most often, arterial reflection sites have been ascribed to the region of the terminal aorta[7, 9, 19] and/or the peripheral arteriolar bed.[1, 5, 20]

Arterial wave reflections are affected by local characteristic impedances that are directly proportional to pulse wave velocity and have been scrutinized frequently.[21–24] Various methods have been used to obtain wave velocity,[4, 20, 25–29] but due to the nonuniformities of the human aorta and technical limitations in its measurement, it is presently unclear which method best approximates true pulse wave velocity.

It is generally known that clinical maneuvers influence systemic arterial pressure, pulse wave velocity, and wave reflections.[6, 8, 30] Previous studies have shown that the Valsalva maneuver reduces the secondary systolic wave in proximal aortic pressure waveforms (Figure 1) and makes the systemic input impedance spectrum less oscillatory, suggesting a diminution of reflections measured in the ascending aorta.[8] An alternative explanation may be based on the observation by Kroeker and Wood,[30] who reported a significant decrease in the duration of systole and a decrease in wave velocity during the Valsalva maneuver.[3, 30] This may lead to a delay of reflected waves so that they arrive in diastole. Previous studies performed

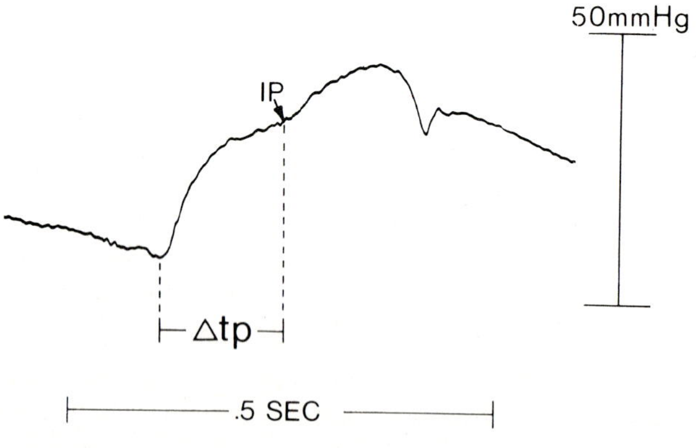

FIGURE 1. Example of a pressure waveform from the ascending aorta of patient D. N. demonstrating a secondary systolic wave resulting from reflections. IP is the inflection point; Δtp is the transmission time of the reflected wave.

in our laboratory were confined to the ascending aorta so that the exact mechanisms of reduction of the secondary systolic wave were difficult to ascertain. Accordingly, this study was designed to investigate the entire human aorta and its terminal branches with simultaneous, equidistant (10 cm), micromanometric pressure measurements in order to determine regional pulse wave velocities, identify the major arterial reflection site(s), and assess the influence of clinical maneuvers on reflected waves. To aid in the interpretation of the results in vivo, a branching latex tube model was constructed based on the dimensions obtained from aortography.

Methods

Data acquisition. The patient population consisted of nine patients studied at Brooke Army Medical Center by elective cardiac catheterization for various chest pain syndromes. Patients included in this study were found to have normal coronary arteries and ventriculograms, as well as normal hemodynamic variables and ejection phase index values (table 1). Patients with hypertensive or clinical evidence of peripheral vascular disease were excluded.

This project was approved by the Clinical Investigation Committee and the Institutional Review Board at Brooke Army Medical Center. Informed consent was obtained for each study. All patients were studied by the right brachial artery approach. Cardiac outputs were obtained with a flow-directed thermodilution catheter positioned in the pulmonary artery. Pressures were initially obtained with a three-sensor catheter with transducers located at the tip, 4 cm proximal to the tip, and a third sensor 5 cm proximal to the middle one (Millar VPC-684H). This catheter was positioned with the tip in the cavity of the left ventricle, the middle sensor located just above the aortic valve, and the proximal sensor positioned in the aortic root. After a steady state was obtained and pressure waveforms were recorded in the control condition, the patient was asked to perform a standardized Valsalva maneuver[8, 30] by exhaling into a mouthpiece connected to a one-way Rudolph valve. The effort expended was measured with a pressure gauge distal to the valve. A 40 mm Hg expiratory effort was maintained for about 20 sec. The Müller maneuver was performed by reversing the valve and having the patient inhale with maximal inspiratory effort. Simultaneous femoral artery occlusions were then performed by bilateral manual compression at the level of the inguinal ligament. The patients rested until there was a return to control conditions between maneuvers.

The triple-sensor catheter was then withdrawn and replaced with a custom-designed catheter with six micromanometers mounted at 10 cm intervals [Millar PC-786(K)]. The catheter was advanced under fluoroscopic guidance until the tip sensor (No. 1) was in the distal external iliac artery and the most proximal sensor (No. 6) was positioned in the arch of the aorta (figure 2). All transducers were simultaneously calibrated with a precision laboratory mercury manometer before insertion.

Pressures from the six micromanometers were recorded under control conditions, during Valsalva and Müller maneuvers, and during bilateral femoral artery occlusion in the manner described above. The catheter position was documented by cinefluoroscopy and the distance between sensors was used to calibrate the measurements of aortic dimensions derived from the subsequent aortograms. Without altering the relationship between x-ray tube, patient, and image intensifier, the six-sensor catheter was withdrawn and then replaced with a No. 8F

TABLE 1
Patient data

Patient[A]	Age (yr)	BSA (m^2)	CO (l/min)	LVEDP (mm Hg)	LVEF (%)	HR (bpm)	MAP (mm Hg)	SVR dynes-sec-cm^{-5}
G. W.	49	2.12	7.1	10	77	68	88	1241
C. H.	35	1.88	5.8	7	57	76	90	945
P. S.	51	2.00	5.6	10	74	75	92	1271
A. B.	41	1.94	6.6	8	74	78	100	1333
J. I.	40	1.91	6.9	10	66	66	90	949
C. W.	37	2.20	6.4	9	79	71	95	1075
D. N.	42	1.92	8.1	12	74	58	105	1171
J. O.	39	2.00	5.4	10	68	63	87	1206
K. K.	40	1.78	6.3	7	84	69	75	899
Mean ± SD	42±5	1.97±0.12	6.5±0.8	9±1.6	73±8	69±6	91±8	1121±160

BSA = body surface area; CO = cardiac output; LVEDP = left ventricular end-diastolic pressure; LVEF = left ventricular ejection fraction; HR = heart rate; MAP = mean aortic root pressure; SVR = systemic vascular resistance.

[A]K. K. is the only female patient.

NIH angiographic catheter. This catheter was advanced to the aortic root, which was examined by single-plane aortography while approximately 100 ml of meglumine diatrizoate was injected at 20 ml/sec. Full-length cineangiograms were obtained by panning from the aortic arch to the femoral arteries.

Data recording and analysis. Data were recorded on FM analog tape (Honeywell 5600C) and converted offline to digital format at a sampling rate of 200 Hz after passing the signals through a low-pass filter (corner frequency 80 Hz, roll-off 12 dB/octave) to avoid aliasing. The foot of the pressure wave was determined by the intersection of slopes of the terminal diastolic and initial upstroke of the pressure wave at a paper speed of 200 mm/sec. Foot-to-foot wave velocity was measured as the time interval between intersection points of adjacent sensors. The time Δtp was determined similarly. Fourier analysis was performed on individual beats to derive apparent phase velocity (see equation 4 below) and amplitudes of harmonics as a function of frequency.[27, 31] Mean apparent phase velocity was calculated by averaging values greater than 3 Hz.[32] When the amplitude of pressure harmonics was less than 0.5 mm Hg, harmonics were considered to be too contaminated by noise to give useful information and discarded. Data from five to 10 cardiac cycles were averaged for each patient during control periods and interventions, where only plateau phases were analyzed. Harmonic amplitude changes along the aorta were calculated by taking the ratio of the pressure modulus at the specified location to the modulus of the same frequency of the most proximal pressure sensor (No. 6).

Tube model. With dimensions obtained from averaged radii of the aortograms, a latex model of the human descending aorta was constructed to compare the results of measurement of wave travel in vivo with results in the model. Dimensions were ob-

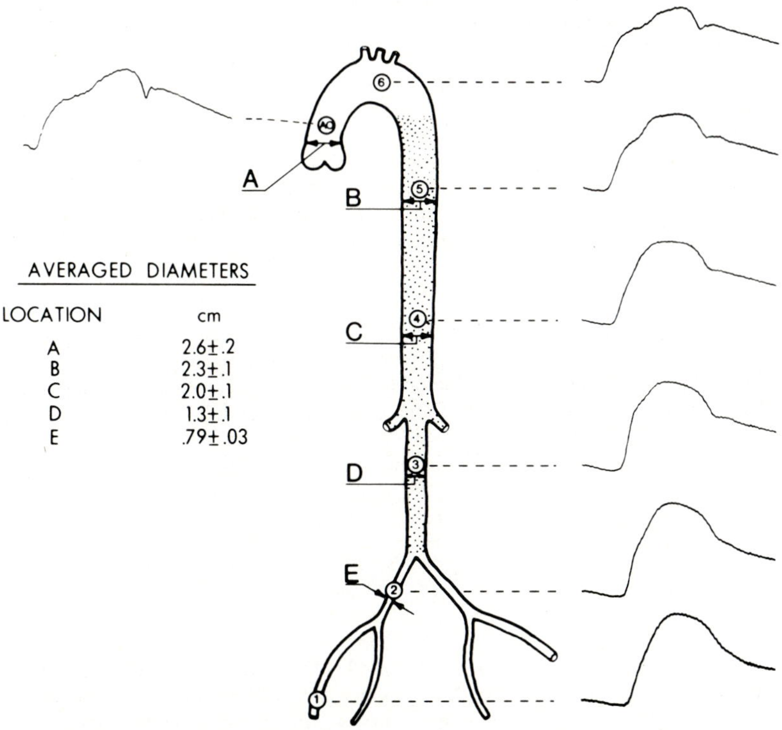

FIGURE 2. Schema of the descending aorta identifying catheter sensor positions, indicated by numerals, and examples of pressure waveforms from patient C. H. Only one of the two ascending aortic pressure waveforms is depicted. The shaded area depicts the region of the aorta modeled by the elastic tube. The length of the tube model was constructed to accommodate the entire length of the six-sensor catheter. Diameter values ± SD are given.

TABLE 2
Model parameters

	Internal diameter (cm)	Wall thickness (cm)	Length (cm)	c_{ff} ($msec^{-1}$)	Z_c (dynes-sec-cm^{-5})
Thoracic aorta	2.32	0.029	28.0	6.8	171
Abdominal aorta	1.40	0.039	25.0	8.8	606
Renal artery	0.96	0.026	8.8	11.1	1630

Dimensions of a latex tube constructed based on averaged values from aortograms of the patient population. All segments of the model are nontapering, and the elastic modulus of the material used was 15×10^6 dynes/cm^2.

c_{ff} = foot-to-foot wave velocity measured from impulse stimuli; Z_c = characteristic impedance.

tained from averaged radii of the aortograms from the studies in vivo. The model consisted of a proximal uniform tube ("descending thoracic aorta") connected to a uniform distal tube ("abdominal aorta") and two branches ("renal arteries"). Dimensions for the model when mounted under 10% longitudinal stretch are given in table 2. The modulus of the elasticity for the material used was 15×10^6 dynes/cm^2 and the Moens-Korteweg equation (see equation 5 below) was used to adjust wall thickness to achieve pulse wave velocities resembling those measured in vivo. The resistances loading the "renal arteries" and the "abdominal aorta" were adjustable. Flow velocity was measured by a cannulated flow probe positioned at the proximal end of the model. Bench testing was performed with the use of sine waves and impulse stimuli. Pressure measurements were obtained with the same catheter [Millar PC-786(K)] used for in vivo measurements and sensors were placed in the same relative positions as in man (figure 2). The model differed from anatomy in vivo in that all three distal sensors were in a uniform tube referred to as the "abdominal aorta." No attempt was made to duplicate the terminal bifurcation or pelvic vessels, rather the resistor located at the terminus of the "abdominal" segment was used to represent total peripheral reflection. The tube system was filled with a 40% glycerin/60% NaCl mixture (0.9%) that had approximately the same viscosity (3.3 cP at 22° C) as blood at body temperature. Impulse stimuli were measured to obtain foot-to-foot wave velocity. Analog-to-digital conversion was performed on-line (sample rates of 500 Hz) with a PDP-11 Digital computer. The sine wave excitation was used to calculate apparent phase velocity (see equation 4). Wave velocities could be obtained for various settings of terminal resistances.

Statistical methods. A two-way analysis of variance (ANOVA) was used to test for significant differences between control and interventions. ANOVA also was used to test regional variances. We compared wave velocities of adjacent regions and control vs interventions. A paired t test was used to test for significant differences between foot-to-foot wave velocity and mean apparent wave velocity as well as differences in amplification of the first four harmonics between control and interventions. A value of $p < .05$ was accepted as indicative of statistic significance.

Theory. The time of the inflection point is the sum of the travel time of the forward wave and transmission time of the reflected wave, and may be determined from the foot of the pressure pulse to the inflection point, IP (figure 1).[7] If the true pulse wave velocity (c_{ph}) is known, then one may use the transmission time to calculate the distance (L) to the reflection site as follows:

$$L = c_{ph} \times \Delta tp/2 \quad (1)$$

With the first minimum of the modulus of systemic input impedance (f_{min}) and the quarter-wave length formula, a second estimate of the distance to the reflection site or "effective length" (L) may be derived[46]:

$$L = c_{ph}/4f_{min} \quad (2)$$

Regional foot-to-foot wave velocity (c_{ff}) was found by the measurement of the time interval (Δt) of the initial upstroke between two pressures a known distance (Δz) apart:

$$c_{ff} = \Delta z/\Delta t \quad (3)$$

Limitations to the technique arise from the difficulty in exactly determining the "foot" of the wave. Various methods have been proposed for measuring the foot of the wave and have been elucidated elsewhere.[4, 20, 22] On the basis of experiments with uniform rubber tubes, it may be assumed that the foot of the wave is not affected by reflections and the foot-to-foot wave velocity therefore should approximate the c_{ph}.[4, 20]

Regional apparent phase velocity (c_{app}) was calculated over each interval (Δz = 10 cm) by subtracting the phase angles of corresponding harmonics ($\Delta\phi$) at the two locations[2]:

$$c_{app} = 2\pi nf\Delta z/\Delta\phi_n \quad (4)$$

where f is heart rate, i.e., fundamental frequency and n is harmonic number.

Phase velocity may be estimated from the Moens Korteweg equation[4, 20]:

$$c_{ph} = \sqrt{\frac{Eh}{2\rho R}} \quad (5)$$

where E is the elastic (Young) modulus, h is the wall thickness, ρ is blood density, and R is the radius of the vessel. In a reflectionless system, the three velocities, c_{ff}, mean c_{app}, and c_{ph} should approach each other.[33]

Reflections at arterial junctions are due to the mismatch in characteristic impedance on either side.[4, 23, 24] The local reflection coefficient is calculated as:

$$\Gamma = \frac{1 - Z_p/Z_d}{1 + Z_p/Z_d} \quad (6)$$

where Z_p is the characteristic impedance of the proximal tube and Z_d is the characteristic impedance of the distal tube. The relationship between characteristic impedance (Z_c) and c_{ph} is:

$$Z_c = \rho c_{ph}/A \quad (7)$$

where A is cross-sectional area. For parallel tubes (distal to bifurcations or trifurcations),[1] impedances should be summed as parallel resistances. In equations 6 and 7 impedances used are real numbers, which is permitted for large arteries so that phases are zero and equations remain simple. Thus, one may calculate the reflection coefficient at an arterial junction when pulse wave velocities and areas are known, i.e., inserting equation 7 in equation 6.[23] For a symmetrical bifurcation, the reflection coefficient is found to be:

$$\Gamma = \frac{1 - (2A_dc_p/A_pc_d)}{1 + (2A_dc_p/A_pc_d)} \quad (8)$$

where the proximal area and velocity are A_p and c_p and the distal parameters are A_d, c_d. For a trifurcation with two equal distal vessels, and a third vessel with different properties (A_1, c_1):

$$\Gamma = \frac{1 - \frac{c_p}{A_p} \div \left(\frac{A_l}{c_l} + \frac{2A_d}{c_d}\right)}{1 + \frac{c_p}{A_p} \div \left(\frac{A_l}{c_l} + \frac{2A_d}{c_d}\right)} \qquad (9)$$

Results

Patient data are summarized in table 1. The population consisted of eight men and one woman with a mean age of 42 years. All patients were found to have normal coronary arteries and hemodynamic characteristics.

Aortic diameters were averaged at the aortic valve and sensor positions 5, 4, 3 and 2 (figure 2). Averaged diameters ($\pm$SD) were 2.6 $\pm$ 0.2, 2.3 $\pm$ 0.1, 2.0 $\pm$ 0.1, 1.3 $\pm$ 0.1, and 0.79 $\pm$ 0.03 cm, respectively. The diameter of the renal arteries was 0.78 $\pm$ 0.17 cm. These data revealed a significant taper ($p < .0005$) of the aorta, with the greatest change in diameter from proximal to distal of the origin of the renal arteries in the renal segment (34%).

During control, the proximal aortic pressure contour revealed an initial rise in pressure followed by an inflection point and a secondary systolic wave (figure 2). This inflection point occurred earlier (relative to the foot) in more distal waveforms until it was almost masked in the initial upstroke at location 4 (5 to 7 cm proximal to the renal arterial branches). The next sensor, No. 3, demonstrated another inflection point early in the waveshape, which again was obscured in the upstroke of the most distal sensor (No. 1). Measurements of the transmission time Δtp (figure 1) at the aortic valve, the ascending aorta (i.e., 5 cm distal, both from the triple tip sensor), and sensors 6, 5, and 4 from the six-sensor catheter were 140 $\pm$ 7, 120 $\pm$ 11, 107 $\pm$ 12, 71 $\pm$ 10, and 35 $\pm$ 9 msec, respectively. With the use of the average foot-to-foot velocity of the thoracic aorta (5.2 m/sec, see below), the distances calculated (equation 1) to the site of reflection were 36, 31, 28, 18, and 9 cm, respectively. The site of reflection determined by these distances was in the aortic segment at the level of the renal arterial branches. Furthermore, the total transmission time of the foot of the wave from the aortic valve to the renal artery branches was 68 $\pm$ 3 msec, which is almost exactly one-half Δtp of the waveform measured at the aortic valve (figure 1). Another inflection point at more distal sites was evident, with Δtp at sensor 2 being 27 $\pm$ 2 msec.

During the Müller maneuver, the foot of the reflected wave in the aortic root pressure occurred earlier than at control. The amplitude of the secondary wave was slightly increased (figure 3, *A* and *B*) in most cases. Bilateral femoral artery occlusion usually changed the character of the secondary systolic wave, which was increased in amplitude and more sharply peaked than at control in some patients (figure 3, *A* and *C*). During the plateau phase of the Valsalva maneuver, the most proximal aortic waveforms showed a loss of the secondary systolic wave (figure 3, *A* and *D*). At location 5 (10 cm distal to the arch), however, a small late systolic peak became manifest that increased in amplitude and occurred earlier in more distal waveforms.

The foot-to-foot wave velocity for each sensor pair is given in table 3. Each sensor pair defines a pulse wave velocity over a 10 cm segment of the aorta (5 cm in aortic root), with sensor pair 6–5 representing the most proximal portion of the descending aorta and sensor pair 2–1 located in the iliac artery segment. During control, there was regional variance in foot-to-foot wave velocity, with a significant increase ($p < .01$) at the region measured by sensor pair 3–2 from that at the adjacent proximal segment (sensor pair 4–3). During control, the Valsalva maneuver, and bilateral femoral artery occlusion, the velocities in the abdominal aorta were greater ($p < .05$) than the velocities in the thoracic aorta (not shown in table 3). During the Müller maneuver, proximal velocities were increased from control values ($p < .05$), resulting in a more uniform distribution of velocities throughout the aorta. Regional foot-to-foot velocities during the interventions were compared with their corresponding control values and significant differences are indicated in table 3.

The degree of amplification or attenuation of the individual harmonics with respect to location, averaged for all patients, is depicted in figure 4 for control and the three interventions. During control, amplitude of the fundamental harmonic tended to increase slightly from proximal to distal sites. The third and fourth harmonics increased significantly and plateaued by location 3. The rate of increase, however, was greatest between locations 5 and 4. During the Müller maneuver, little difference from control was noted in percent amplification of the first four harmonics, except at location 2 ($p > .05$). During the Valsalva maneuver, the first two harmonics continuously increased from proximal to distal sites; the relative increase being greater than during control ($p < .005$). The third and fourth harmonics, in contrast to control, exhibited an initial attenuation with an increase noted only in more distal sensors. Bilateral femoral artery occlusion produced an exaggerated degree of amplification in all

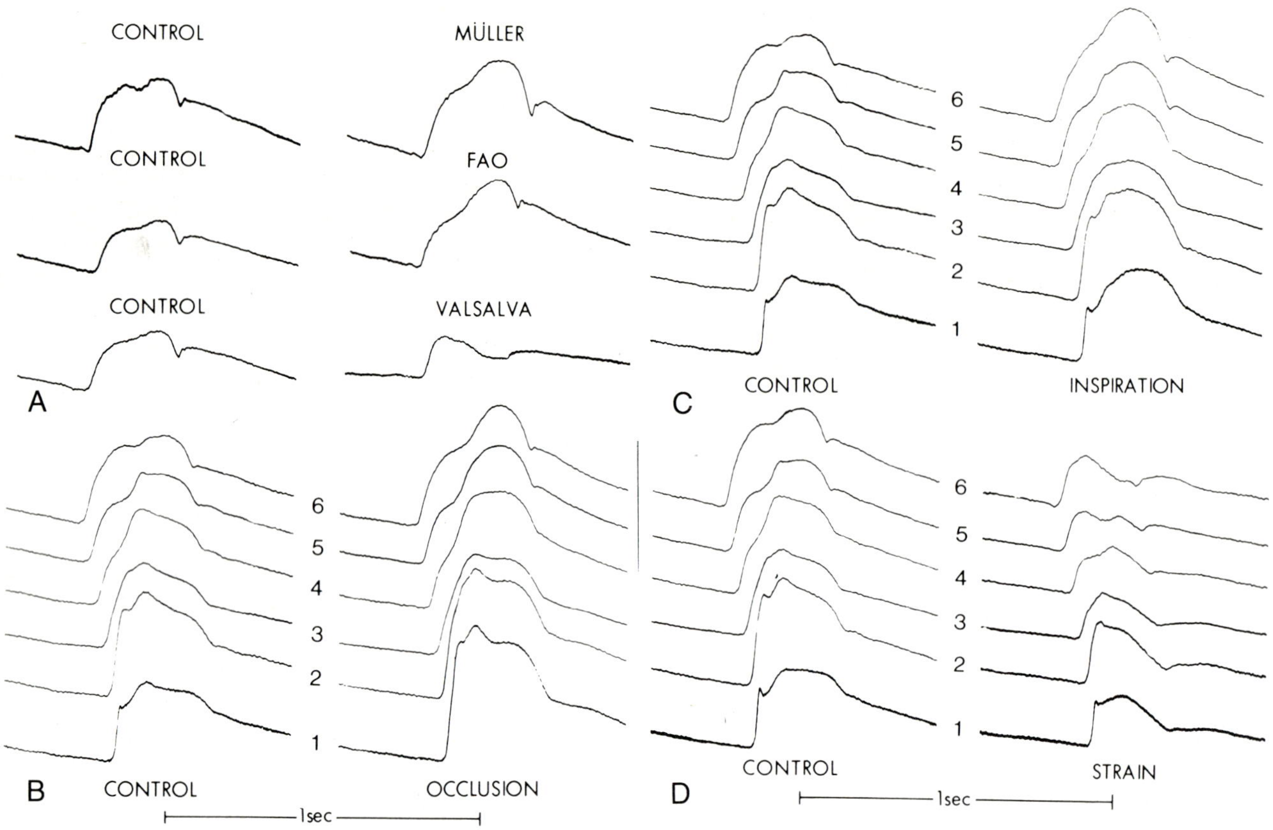

FIGURE 3. Simultaneously obtained pressures throughout the aorta and terminal branches during control, Müller and Valsalva maneuvers, and bilateral femoral artery occlusion. The aortic root pressures are from patient J. O. and are presented in *A*. *B*, *C*, and *D*, Representative waveforms recorded from patient K. K. during the Müller maneuver, femoral artery occlusion, and the Valsalva maneuver, respectively. For anatomic location of sensors, see figure 2.

harmonics except the first, which was not significantly different from control (p > .05).

Regional apparent phase velocity was derived by applying equation 4. Mean apparent wave velocity as a function of location is shown in table 4 and is compared with foot-to-foot velocity in figure 5. It was found that during control the two wave velocities differed significantly (p < .01) at the region given by sensor pair 4–3. It is this region of the aorta in which the renal arteries have their origin and in which the aortic diameter significantly decreases (figure 2). The differences between the wave speeds were maintained during the Müller maneuver and femoral artery occlusion (p < .05 and p < .01, respectively), but disappeared during the Valsalva maneuver.

Apparent phase velocities as a function of frequency are presented in figure 6, together with the mean apparent phase velocities. Under control conditions apparent phase velocity in the low frequency range was found to be higher proximal to the renal arteries (sen-

TABLE 3
Regional foot-to-foot velocities (m/sec)

	Sensor pair					
Condition	Aortic root	6–5	5–4	4–3	3–2	2–1
Control	4.4±0.4	5.3±0.2	5.2±0.1	5.7±0.4	9.2±0.5^{B}	8.8±0.4
Valsalva	3.6±0.2^{A}	5.1±0.3	4.5±0.3^{B}	4.5±0.4^{A}	7.0±0.7^{B}	7.5±0.6^{A}
Müller	7.2±0.1^{A}	6.6±0.5^{A}	7.0±1.2^{A}	5.5±0.5	7.2±1.2	7.3±0.7
FAO	4.2±0.8	5.5±0.3	5.2±0.2	5.3±0.3^{A}	8.9±0.7	9.5±1.3

Values are means ± SEM. The aortic root velocity was measured with the triple-tip catheter with sensors 5 cm apart. The multiple-sensor catheter was used to determine velocity over 10 cm intervals. For locations, see figure 2.

FAO = femoral artery occlusion.

Comparison for each region is with its control value; comparison of control values is with adjacent regions: ^{A}p < .05; ^{B}p < .01.

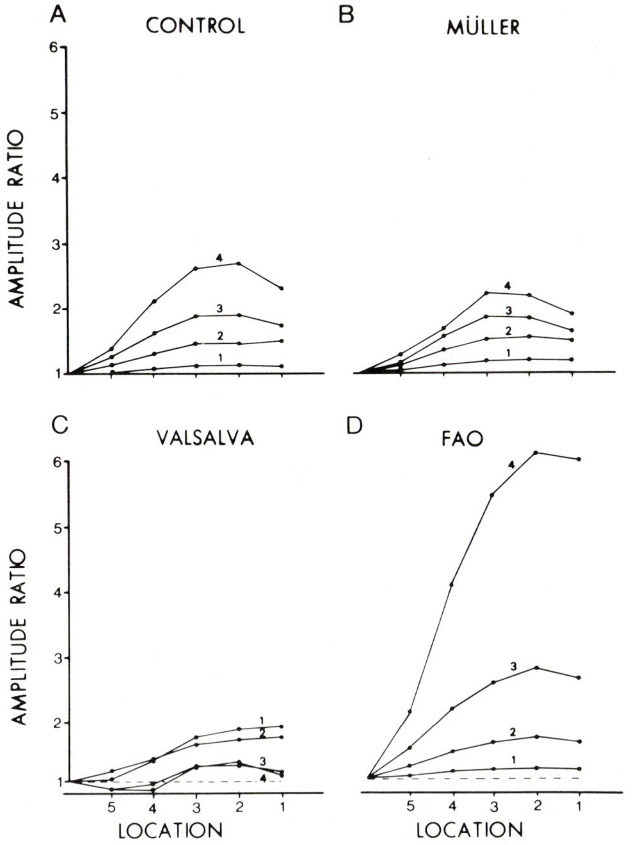

FIGURE 4. Amplification of the first four harmonics as a function of location during control, Valsalva and Müller maneuvers, and bilateral femoral artery occlusion averaged for all patients.

sors 5, 4) than in the distal segment (sensors 3, 2). A minimum was reached at higher frequencies in the more proximal segments. The Valsalva maneuver attenuated the differences between proximal and distal segments. During bilateral femoral artery occlusion, the velocities at low frequencies in the proximal and distal aortic segments both deviated from the mean apparent wave velocity.

Reflection coefficients were calculated for the proximal descending aorta, the level of the renal arteries, and the region of the terminal bifurcation of the aorta with equations 6 to 9. Averaged aortic cross-sectional areas are given above and the foot-to-foot velocities are taken from table 3 (control). Pulse wave velocity in the renal arteries was assumed to be 1 m/sec greater than that in the abdominal segment. The local reflection coefficients were found to be small in the proximal descending aorta (from foot-to-foot velocities 6–5 and 5–4; cross-sectional area at locations A and B of figure 2, $\Gamma = 0.05$) and at the terminal aortic bifurcation (from foot-to-foot velocities 3–2 and 2–1; cross-sectional areas of locations D and E of figure 2, $\Gamma = 0.13$). The estimated characteristic impedances of the lower thoracic aorta, abdominal aorta, and renal arteries were 175, 730, and 2250 dynes-sec-cm^{-5}, respectively. The reflection coefficient in the aorta at the level of the renal arterial branches was calculated to be 0.43.

Model. A tube model was constructed so that the effects of peripheral resistance and the mismatch around the renal arteries on reflections could be separated. The variability of apparent phase velocities, with frequency measured at sensor pair 3–2 (distal to "renal arteries"), demonstrated small oscillations around mean apparent phase velocity when peripheral reflections were small (figure 7). On the other hand, when the terminal resistor was completely closed, reflections were increased and the plot of apparent phase velocity was significantly altered (figure 7). Thus, with increased peripheral reflections, apparent phase velocity varies more with frequency, as demonstrated by previous investigators.[30, 34] More deviation of apparent phase velocity from its mean value was found in the model at sensor pair 5–4 (immediately proximal to the "renal arteries") than in sensor pair 3–2 (distal to the "renal" branches), implying more reflections proximal to these branches (figure 8). In a similar fashion, the frequency variation of apparent phase velocity from sensor pair 5–4 in man indicated there was a stronger reflection there than in the abdominal aorta (figure 6). These data imply that the geometric config-

TABLE 4
Regional mean apparent phase velocity (m/sec)

	Sensor pair					
Condition	Aortic root	6–5	5–4	4–3	3–2	2–1
Control	4.3±0.2	5.4±0.5	5.3±0.3	10.4±0.9	8.8±0.7	6.4±0.4
Valsalva	4.0±0.3	4.8±0.3	4.0±0.2[A]	4.9±0.6[B]	7.7±0.6[B]	6.3±0.3
Müller	7.2±0.5[A]	6.4±1.2[A]	4.9±0.4	9.0±1.6	9.8±1.9	6.6±0.7
FAO	4.5±0.4	6.4±1.0	5.3±0.5	10.9±0.8	10.3±1.0	11.8±3.1

Values are ± SEM.

FAO = femoral artery occlusion.

Comparison for each region with control value: [A]$p < .05$; [B]$p < .01$.

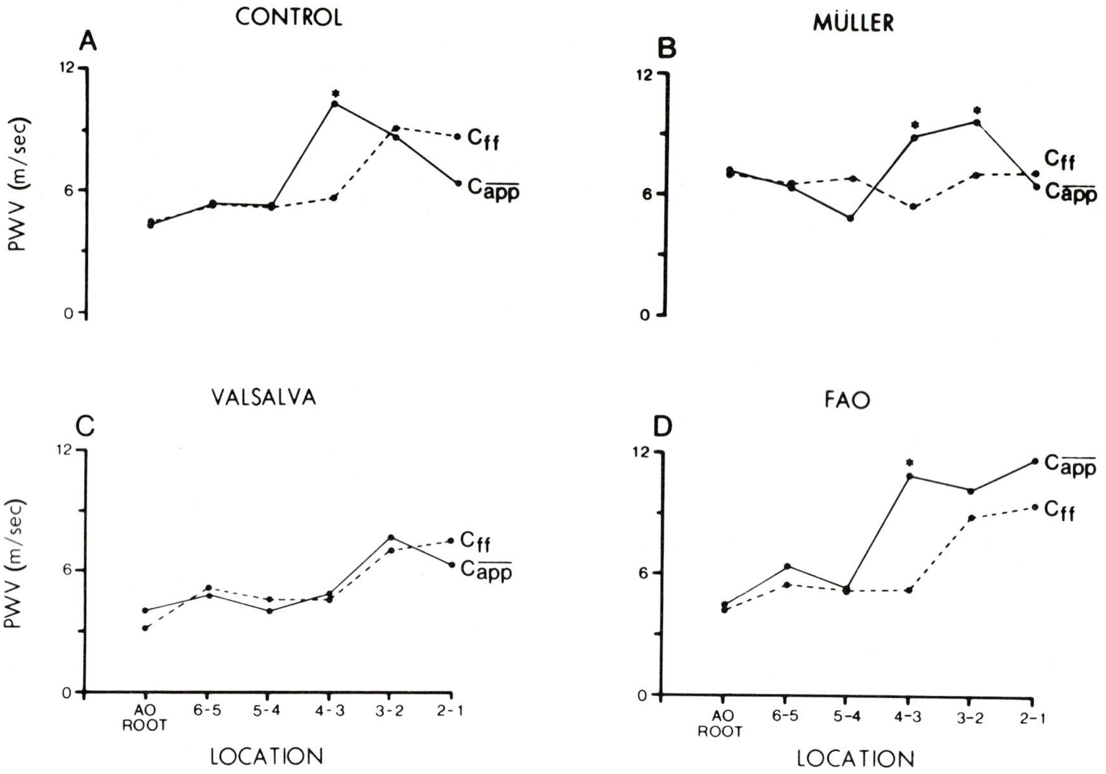

FIGURE 5. Foot-to-foot wave velocity (c_{ff}; dashed line) and mean apparent phase velocity ($c_{\overline{app}}$; fully drawn) as functions of location during control, Valsalva and Müller maneuvers, and bilateral femoral artery occlusion averaged for all patients. *$p < .01$, comparison between c_{ff} and $c_{\overline{app}}$.

uration of the descending aorta at the level of the renal arterial branches is a very likely site for the production of a major local reflection. Finally, the reflection coefficient could be precisely calculated in the model since foot-to-foot wave velocity in the "renal" segments was measured and tube diameters were determined by a micrometer. The renal reflection coefficient was found to be 0.34, which closely corresponded to our estimate in vivo of 0.43. The value of this model lies in its simplicity in testing the possibility of wave reflection from a particular geometric configuration analogous to the taper of the human aorta at the level of the renal arteries.

Discussion

This study is the first to employ simultaneous pressure measurements at multiple sites along the human aorta and to compare pressure wave transmission in a geometrically similar tube model to describe the effects of regional architecture on wave travel and wave reflection. The initial goal of our investigation was to identify the major site(s) of wave reflection in the aorta. To help identify these site(s), several characteristics of pulse wave propagation were analyzed: (1) inspection of regional waveform contours, (2) regional differences in wave velocity and pressure amplification, and (3) regional differences in the apparent phase velocity. Finally, a tube model of the human descending aorta was used to test the hypothesis that geometric nonuniformities in the aorta are capable of producing a reflected wave that is manifested in more proximal waveforms.

Luchsinger,[2] O'Rourke,[3] and Mills[9] and their colleagues have reported pressure waveforms measured at different sites along the human aorta. Several mechanisms responsible for the differences in proximal and distal waveforms have been proposed,[16, 35–37] but the most widely accepted one is that of wave reflections. Reflection characteristics of the systemic circulation have been studied in a number of ways. McDonald[38] and O'Rourke[11, 39] have proposed an "eccentric" or asymmetric T-tube model of the human circulation, implying that reflections are "effectively" summated at peripheral locations on opposite ends of the circulation. On the other hand, Murgo et al.[7] concluded that, in addition to diffuse reflections from the periphery, the region of the terminal aortic bifurcation was a major reflection site. This conclusion is similar to those reached by other investigators.[9] Both the inflection point on the aortic root waveform and the impedance spectrum were previously used to calculate the distance to a single dominant reflection site.[7] With equa-

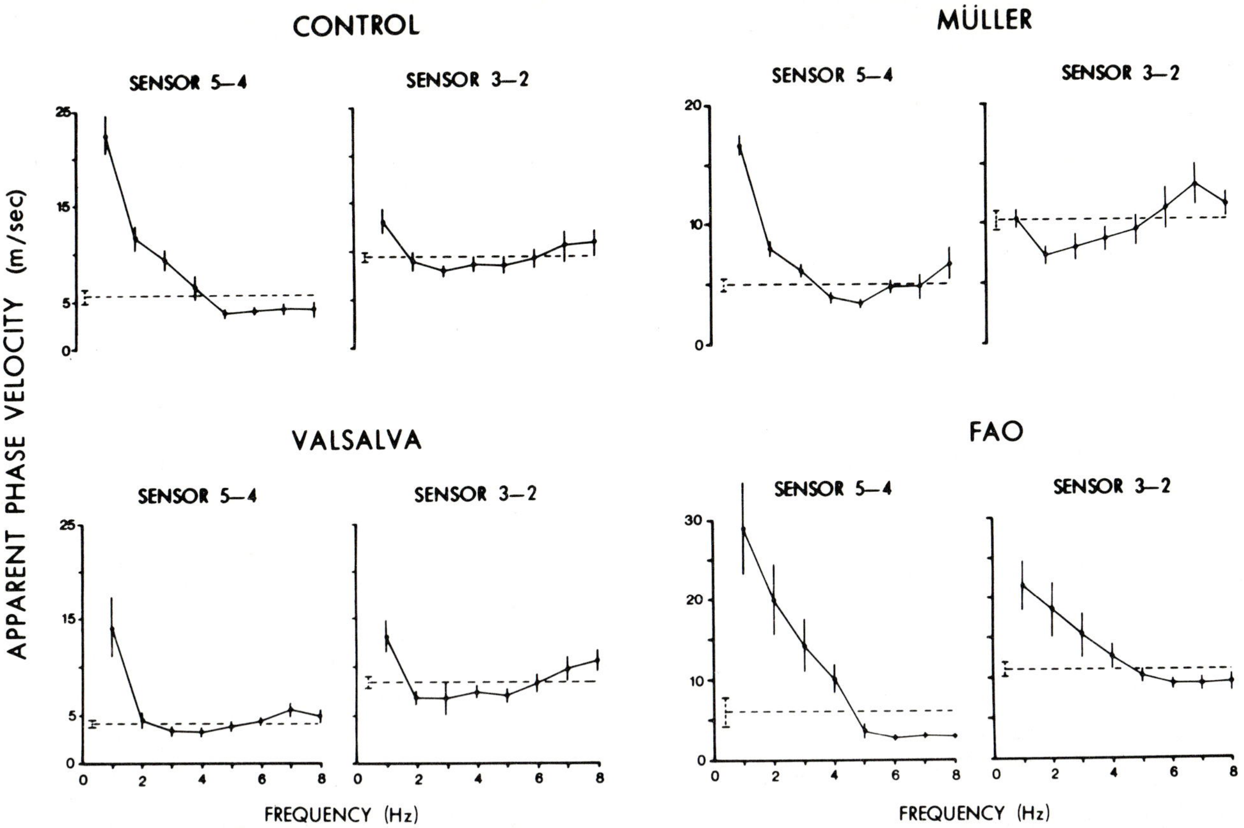

FIGURE 6. Apparent phase velocity as a function of frequency at locations immediately proximal and distal to the renal branches during control, Valsalva and Müller maneuvers, and femoral artery occlusion. Data averaged (± SE) for all patients. Horizontal dashed lines represent mean apparent phase velocity.

tions 1 and 2 and the pulse wave velocity measured in the aortic root, an average distance of 44 cm was calculated. One recognized limitation of this earlier study was the use of an aortic root wave velocity to estimate average wave velocity of the entire aorta. The use of the regional variation in pulse wave velocity

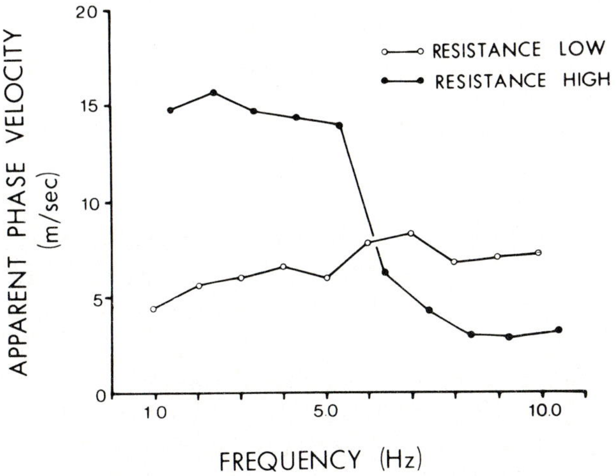

FIGURE 7. Effect of reflections on apparent phase velocity as a function of frequency in the "abdominal" segment (sensor pair 3–2) of the model. Open circles refer to low resistance, i.e., little reflection, and closed circles represent high resistance, i.e., increased reflection.

could result in a length different from the distance to the reflection site derived earlier. The present study was undertaken to overcome these limitations and to analyze the mechanisms by which reflections are generated and transmitted in more detail.

The aortic root wave velocity in the present study is significantly different from that in the previous report.[7] In that study a different catheter was used for the ascending aorta. The previously used catheter had only two sensors and when it was withdrawn from the left ventricle into the aortic root the native curve in the distal segment of the catheter resulted in a shorter axial distance between the two sensors. A special catheter, mounted with three micromanometers on which the two proximal transducers (5 cm apart) were mounted on a straight portion of the catheter, was used for the ascending aorta in our current study. This eliminated the possible error inherent in the previous study and resulted in pulse wave velocities we believe are more accurate and similar to previously reported values by King (1950),[40] Barnett et al. (1961),[41] and Merillon et al. (1978).[42]

The waveforms recorded also were similar in contour to those previously reported.[2,7] The inflection

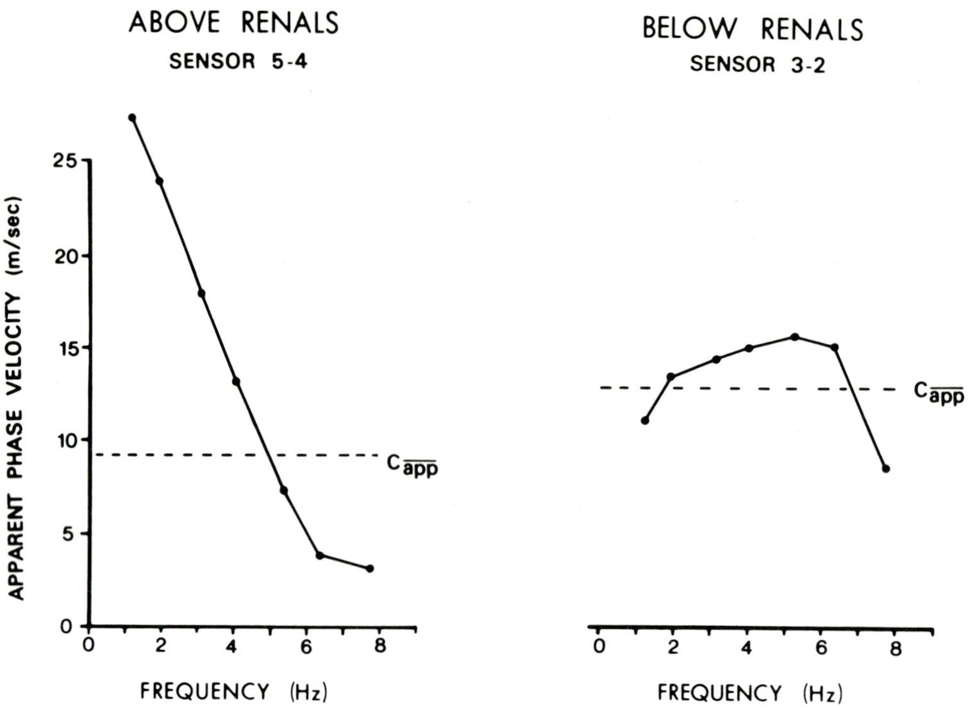

FIGURE 8. Apparent phase velocity as a function of frequency immediately proximal and distal to the "renal" branches in the tube model. Dashed line is mean apparent phase velocity.

point occurred earlier on the pressure waveform, proceeding from proximal to distal locations until it was manifest early on the initial upstroke at sensor 4, just above the renal arteries. A second inflection point, although less prominent, often was seen in more distal pressures and lost in the most distal waveform. Under control conditions, the time to the first inflection point and the foot-to-foot wave velocity from aortic root to renal arteries were used to calculate the site of reflection. This calculation showed the region of the aorta at about the level of the renal arterial branches to be a major reflection site. In support of this theory, the finding of a secondary systolic wave, as seen in aortic waveforms in man, was exactly reproduced by others by occluding the aorta of the dog at the level of the diaphragm.[36, 43] The second, more distal site was calculated to a distance slightly beyond the inguinal ligament. Wave speeds are high in the most distal segments and, although the reflected wave appears functionally discrete, it probably represents the summation of effects from the pelvic and lower extremity arteriolar beds, as previously described by O'Rourke.[1] Therefore, we would suggest that the major local reflections in the human aorta can be described by two tubes of different properties in series, as proposed by Wetterer and Kenner.[44] It is also possible there are other contributing regions to the total reflection, as proposed by Remington and O'Brien,[45] which could not be evaluated in our study.

Although regional pulse wave velocity has been measured in animal preparations,[21] there have been few analyses in man. It is very important when comparing results between laboratories that the criteria used to define the mean apparent phase velocity be specified. For the present study, mean apparent phase velocity represents the mean of values greater than 3 Hz.[32] Both foot-to-foot and apparent wave velocity showed significant regional variation, although neither changed with location in a simple linear fashion. It is generally accepted that the wavefront used to measure foot-to-foot velocity is not affected by arterial reflections.[4, 20] When the two velocities are compared for each region, a significant difference is found in the aortic region at the level of the renal arteries, which can be interpreted to be the result of strong local reflections influencing the calculation of mean apparent phase velocity (figure 5).[22] Thus, our data confirm that mean apparent phase velocity in arterial segments with strong local reflections should not be taken to be equivalent to foot-to-foot wave velocity or true phase velocity.

Furthermore, we found that the apparent phase velocity deviates more from its mean value with increased reflection, as shown by previous investigators.[32, 34] Under control conditions in vivo, the apparent phase velocity in the low frequency range was found to be higher in the aortic segment just proximal to the renal arteries than in that distal to the renal arteries.

The apparent phase velocity also reached a minimum at higher frequencies in the more proximal segment than in the distal segment. We conclude these findings to be consistent with a prominent local reflection in this region of the aorta.

The frequency of the first minimum of apparent phase velocity was not used to calculate the distance to the site of reflection ("effective length") by the quarter-wavelength formula (equation 2). The effective length calculated in this way is correct only for a uniform tube with frequency-independent load where the frequency of the first minimum of modulus of impedance (f_{min}) equals the frequency of the first crossover of the phase angle ($f\phi$).[46] This concept is questionable in a nonuniform tapering tube like the aorta. It has been shown in latex tubes[46] and recently in vivo in our laboratory,[47] that when f_{min} is not equal to $f\phi$, the calculated effective length significantly overestimates the actual distance to the site of reflection. Therefore, the frequency of the first minimum of the apparent phase velocity should only be used with caution to verify the distance to the site of reflection.

By means of Fourier analysis, pressure amplification was computed as well. Under control conditions, the greatest degree of amplification is in the region just proximal to the renal arterial branches, which also supports the conclusion of a prominent local reflection in the aortic segment incorporating the renal artery branches (figure 4). The maximal amplification of the third and fourth harmonic during the Valsalva maneuver and femoral occlusion differs considerably from control. This may be interpreted to mean that the aortic reflection from the renal artery level plays a lesser role during these interventions.

In addition to the above analyses, regional anatomic tapering of the aorta and its terminal branches was documented angiographically. The 10 cm segment of aorta measured by sensor pair 4–3 includes the region of transition of the thoracic aorta to the abdominal segment. It is also the section that passes through the diaphragm and incorporates the origin of the renal arteries. Inspection of aortograms from all patients revealed significant reduction in diameter of arteries distal to the renal arterial branches. This section contains the branching into the superior mesenteric artery, the coeliac artery, and two renal arteries and the continuing moderately sized abdominal aorta.

The importance of the discontinuity due to geometric and/or elastic factors at this segment is also supported by the calculated reflection coefficient that can be expressed in terms of the ratio of wave velocities and cross-sectional areas of proximal and distal sections of branching segments. We did not measure renal wave velocities in vivo, but if the region of the aorta at the level of the renal arteries were reflectionless, one would have to assume an unphysiologically low renal artery pulse wave velocity of about 1.5 m/sec. Assuming a renal artery pulse wave velocity approximately 1 m/sec greater than that of the abdominal aorta results in an estimated reflection coefficient of 0.43. A more detailed study of this aortic segment, including the effect of mesenteric and coeliac arteries, is necessary to fully understand reflections in this aortic segment.

Reported data on reflection coefficients in the aorta of man[25, 33] were obtained by determination of cross-sectional area in cadaver specimens and estimation of elastic wall properties. These studies arrived at a value of $\Gamma = 0.16$ for the terminal aortic bifurcation, and $\Gamma = 0.25$ at the level of the renal arteries. Our calculation of the reflection coefficients at the terminal aortic bifurcation and at the level of the renal arteries resulted in values of 0.13 and 0.43, respectively. The older data also indicate a relatively matched terminal aortic bifurcation compared with a rather large impedance mismatch of the aorta at the region of the renal artery branches.

The hydraulic model was chosen since other approaches (e.g., electrical[25, 33, 48] and mathematic[49, 50]) are not able to incorporate all the detailed effects of bifurcations on pressure-flow relationships. The geometrically similar tube model was studied with the same multisensor catheter as was used for the determinations in vivo. From the tube model, we confirmed that apparent phase velocity was increased in the lower frequency range when the larger peripheral resistance was present (figure 7). The apparent phase velocity in the segment proximal to the "renal arteries" deviated more from its mean value than did the velocity in the distal segment (figure 8), consistent with a significant local reflection in the aortic region of the "renal" branches. If mean apparent phase velocity is calculated by averaging values larger than 3 Hz in the presence of strong local reflections, a value significantly different from the foot-to-foot velocity will be derived (figure 8 and table 2). Transmission times measured from impulse stimuli in the tube model also demonstrated a reflection from the geometric taper of the aorta at the region of the "renal" branches, which is consistent with findings in vivo.

Previous investigations have shown that clinical interventions in man may influence wave reflections.[6, 8, 30] We have studied simultaneous pressures along the aorta during the physiologic stress induced by Valsalva and Müller maneuvers and bilateral femoral artery occlusion. During the Valsalva maneuver, the increased intrathoracic pressure reduces the transmural pressure across the thoracic aortic wall significantly and decreases proximal aortic diameter by an average of 17%.[6] The result is a thoracic aorta that is more compliant than during control. During the maneuver, foot-to-foot pulse wave velocity was significantly reduced throughout the aorta, with a relatively greater reduction of velocities in the abdominal segment. If the aortic diameters change with the same percentage, and the reduction in wave velocity is greater in the abdominal aorta than in the descending thoracic aorta (table 3), the renal junction becomes more matched (see equations 7, 8, and 9). Since this proximal reflection was reduced during Valsalva, reflection from a distal location, already seen in the control pressures, became more apparent.

During the Müller maneuver, there was a significant increase in pulse wave velocity in the proximal aorta to the extent that it approximated velocities of the distal segments (tables 3 and 4). The pressure waveforms during the Müller maneuver showed only slight increases in pulse pressure that mainly resulted from the increase in the amplitude of the secondary wave. Amplification (figure 4) was of a similar pattern compared with that under control conditions, indicating that reflection from the region of the renal artery branches was not further increased. The increase in uniformity of wave velocities throughout the aorta further implies that reflections are not necessarily increased. It may be speculated that the forward wave[8] is larger during the Müller maneuver and returns earlier, leading to the observed pressure waveform. The normalized data in figure 4 do not account for different inputs.

In contrast, femoral artery occlusion by bilateral manual compression usually enhanced the reflected wave from the point of occlusion (figure 4). This was also manifested in proximal aortic pressure waveforms as an increase in the amplitude of the secondary systolic wave. The wave speeds in the proximal aorta were unchanged, and the time of the inflection point remained the same. Only the amplitude of the secondary wave was larger, thus indicating that this peak was the summation of reflection from both proximal (renal) and distal sites. The distal effective load is strongly frequency dependent,[38, 39] and the reflection coefficient may contain a significant phase angle, but it was not appropriate to calculate the location of this distal reflection site from the data presented here.

The present results do not reconcile all theories on arterial wave reflection in man, but provide a basis from which other studies may be performed to gain further insight into the hydrodynamic principles of the human circulation. A knowledge of wave propagation characteristics and vascular architecture gives the physician greater insight into the physiologic interpretation of wave shapes routinely measured in the proximal aorta. Reflection may be of importance for the cardiac workload (tension time index) and in future design of artificial grafts involving extensive segments of the human aorta.

We conclude that the physiologic stresses on the arterial system induced by clinical maneuvers produce alterations in regional wave reflections. The Valsalva maneuver diminishes reflection from the proximal site. The Müller maneuver affects reflection little, but equalizes wave speeds in the aorta, and femoral artery occlusion increases reflection from a distal site. We further conclude that there are two major sites of wave reflection from the lower part of the body that, along with the diffuse reflections from the periphery, affect aortic pressure waveforms in man. The first major reflection site appears to be at the aortic level of the renal artery branches and the second is distal to the terminal aortic bifurcation.

Our appreciation to Mr. R. J. Th. Braak of the Physiology Department, Free University, The Netherlands, for making the tube model. We also appreciate SP6 Michael R. Cornett and the cardiac catheterization technicians of the Cardiovascular Laboratories at Brooke Army Medical Center for their expert assistance with collection of the data in vivo, and Sgt. Noel Diaz for his assistance with the graphics. We are grateful to Mrs. Bettye Jo Hairston for her assistance in the preparation of this manuscript.

References

1. O'Rourke MF: Arterial function in health and disease. Edinburgh, 1982, Churchill Livingstone
2. Luchsinger PC, Snell RE, Patel DJ, Fry DL: Instantaneous pressure distribution along the human aorta. Circ Res **15:** 510, 1964
3. O'Rourke MF, Blazek JV, Morrcels CO Jr, Krovetz LJ: Pressure wave transmission along the human aorta. Circ Res **23:** 567, 1968
4. McDonald DA: Blood flow in arteries, ed 2. Baltimore, 1974, Williams and Wilkins Company, pp 254, 309, 351, 392
5. Hamilton WF: The patterns of the arterial pressure pulse. Am J Physiol **41:** 235, 1944
6. Greenfield JC Jr, Cox RL, Hernandez RL, Thomas C, Schoonmaker FW: Pressure-flow studies in man during the Valsalva maneuver with observations on the mechanical properties of the ascending aorta. Circulation **35:** 653, 1967
7. Murgo JP, Westerhof N, Giolma JP, Altobelli SA: Aortic input impedance in normal man: relationship to pressure waveforms. Circulation **62:** 105, 1980
8. Murgo JP, Westerhof N, Giolma JP, Altobelli SA: Manipulation of ascending aortic pressure and flow wave reflections with the Valsalva maneuver: relationship to input impedance. Circulation **63:** 122, 1981
9. Mills CJ, Gabe IT, Gault JH, Mason DT, Ross J Jr, Braunwald E, Shillingford JP: Pressure-flow relationships and vascular impedance in man. Cardiovasc Res **4:** 405, 1970
10. Busse R, Bauer RD, Schabert A, Summa Y, Wetterer E: An improved method for the determination of the pulse transmission characteristics of arteries in vivo. Circ Res **44:** 630, 1979

11. O'Rourke MF: Pressure and flow waves in systemic arteries and the anatomical design of the arterial system. J Appl Physiol **23:** 139, 1967
12. Van den Bos GC, Westerhof N, Elzinga G, Sipkema P: Reflection in the systemic arterial system: effects of aortic and carotid occlusion. Cardiovasc Res **10:** 565, 1976
13. Peterson LH, Gerst PH: Significance of reflected waves within the arterial system. Fed Proc **15:** 469, 1956
14. Greenwald SE, Newman DL, Bowden NLR: Comparison between theoretical and directly measured pulse propagation velocities in the aorta of the unaesthetised dog. Cardiovasc Res **12:** 407, 1978
15. Newman D, King D, Gosling R, Willie S: Reflections of aortic-iliac functions. *In* Roberts C, editor: Blood flow measurement. Baltimore, 1972, Williams and Wilkins Co., p 44
16. Alexander RS: Factors determining the contour of pressure pulses recorded from the aorta. Fed Proc **11:** 738, 1952
17. O'Rourke MF: Vascular impedance in studies of arterial and cardiac function. Phys Rev **62:** 570, 1982
18. Womersley JR: Oscillatory flow in arteries: reflection of the pulse wave at junctions and rigid inserts in the arterial system. Phys Med Biol **2:** 313, 1958
19. Gosling RG, Newman DL, Bowden NLR, Twinn KW: The area ratio of normal aortic junctions: aortic configuration and pulse wave reflection. Br J Radiol **44:** 850, 1971
20. Milnor W: Hemodynamics. Baltimore, 1982, Williams and Wilkins, pp 93, 192, 218, 325
21. McDonald DA: Regional pulse wave velocity in the arterial tree. J Appl Physiol **24:** 73, 1968
22. Nichols WW, McDonald DA: Wave velocity in the proximal aorta. Med Biol Eng Comput **10:** 327, 1972
23. Greenwald SE, Newman DL: Impulse propagation through junctions. Med Biol Eng Comput **20:** 343, 1982
24. Skalak R: Wave propagation in blood flow. *In* Fung YC, editor: Biomechanics. New York, 1969, American Society of Mechanical Engineers. p 20
25. Westerhof N, Bosman F, DeVries CJ, Noordergraaf A: Analog studies of the human systemic arterial tree. J Biomech **2:** 121, 1969
26. Taylor MG: Wave travel in a nonuniform transmission line in relation to pulses in arteries. Phys Med Biol **10:** 539, 1965
27. Cox RH: Determination of the true phase velocity of arterial pressure waves in vivo. Circ Res **29:** 407, 1971
28. Milnor WR, Bertram CD: The relation between arterial viscoelasticity and wave propagation in the canine femoral artery in vivo. Circ Res **43:** 870, 1978
29. Li JK-J, Melbin J, Riffle RA, Noordergraaf A: Pulse wave propagation. Circ Res **49:** 442, 1981
30. Kroeker EJ, Wood EH: Beat-to-beat alterations in relationship of simultaneously recorded central and peripheral arterial pressure pulses during Valsalva maneuver and prolonged expiration in man. J Appl Physiol **8:** 483, 1956
31. Westerhof N, Sipkema P, Elzinga G, Murgo JP, Giolma JP: Arterial impedance. *In* Hwang NHB, Gross DR, Patel DJ, editors: Quantitative cardiovascular studies. Baltimore, 1979, University Park Press, p 111
32. Gabe IT, Karnell J, Porjé IG, Rudewald B: The measurement of input impedance and apparent phase velocity in the human aorta. Acta Physiol Scand **61:** 73, 1964
33. Westerhof N: Analog studies of human arterial hemodynamics, doctoral thesis. University of Pennsylvania, Philadelphia, 1968
34. Porjé JG: Studies of the arterial pulse wave, particularly in the aorta. Acta Physiol Scand **13**(suppl): 42, 1946
35. Remington JW: Volume quantification of the aortic pressure pulse. Fed Proc **11:** 750, 1952
36. Alexander RS: The genesis of the aortic standing wave. Circ Res **1:** 145, 1953
37. Hamilton WF, Dow P: An experimental study of the standing waves in the pulse propagated through the aorta. Am J Physiol **125:** 48, 1939
38. McDonald DA: Hemodynamics. Ann Rev Physiol **9:** 525, 1968
39. O'Rourke MF: The arterial pulse in health and disease. Am Heart J **82:** 687, 1971
40. King AL: Circulatory system: arterial pulse wave velocity. *In* Glasser O, editor: Medical physiology. Chicago, 1950, The Year Book Publishers, Inc., vol II, pp 188–191
41. Barnett GO, Greenfield JC Jr, Cox SM: The technique of estimating the instantaneous aortic blood velocity in man from the pressure gradient. Am Heart J **62:** 349, 1961
42. Merillon JP, Motte G, Fruchaud J, Masquet C, Gourgon R: Evaluation of the elasticity and characteristic impedance of the ascending aorta in man. Cardiovasc Res **12:** 401, 1978
43. Westerhof N, Elzinga G, Van den Bos GC: Influence of central and peripheral changes on the hydraulic input impedance of the systemic arterial tree. Med Biol Eng **11:** 710, 1973
44. Wetterer E, Kenner TH: Grundlagen der Dynamik des Arterien pulses. Berlin, 1968, Springer-Verlag
45. Remington JW, O'Brien LJ: Construction of aortic flow pulse from the pressure pulse. Am J Physiol **218:** 437, 1970
46. Sipkema P, Westerhof N: Effective length of the arterial system. Ann Biomed Eng **3:** 296, 1975
47. Latham RD, Westerhof N, Sipkema P, Rubal BJ, Murgo JP: Effective length of the arterial circulation in man: limitations on use of systemic input impedance. Fed Proc **44:** 1889, 1985 (abst)
48. Jager GN, Westerhof N, Noordergraaf A: Oscillatory flow impedance in an electrical analog of the arterial system. Circ Res **16:** 121, 1965
49. Taylor MG: Wave transmission through an assembly of randomly branching elastic tubes. Biophys J **6:** 29, 1966
50. Avolio AP: Multi-branched model of the human arterial system. Med Biol Eng Comput **18:** 709, 1980

The pressure-flow response of the pulmonary circulation in patients with heart failure and pulmonary vascular disease

JOSEPH S. JANICKI, PH.D.,* KARL T. WEBER, M.D.,* MARIELL J. LIKOFF, M.D.,** AND ALFRED P. FISHMAN, M.D.

ABSTRACT Although it is well known that the pulmonary circulation is altered in patients with pulmonary arterial or venous hypertension, the resultant hemodynamic behavior has not been systematically studied. We undertook to do so in a group of patients with pulmonary hypertension of diverse etiology. We measured pulmonary arterial (PAP) and occlusive wedge pressures and cardiac output at rest (i.e., standing) and during progressive upright treadmill exercise in 51 patients. Forty-two had chronic, stable, cardiac failure secondary to ischemic, myopathic or valvular heart disease and were grouped according to whether their mean PAP was less than (normotensive) or greater than (hypertensive) 19 mm Hg, and nine had pulmonary vascular disease of diverse etiology and were considered separately. In the majority of patients, we found that irrespective of whether the hypertension was arterial or venous in origin or etiology: (1) the mean PAP-flow relationship was linear; (2) pulmonary capillary wedge pressure was greater than or equal to the average closure pressure of the pulmonary vascular bed and could therefore be used as the downstream pressure in calculating pulmonary vascular resistance; and (3) pulmonary vascular resistance declined with exercise. Notable exceptions to the third observation were patients with valvular heart disease or a resting pulmonary vascular resistance greater than 800 dyne-sec-cm^{-5}.
Circulation 72, No. 6, 1270–1278, 1985.

THE HEMODYNAMIC behavior of a vascular bed can be characterized by the relationship between blood flow and the pressure gradient. In the absence of external forces, the pressure gradient is simply the difference between the upstream or arterial and the downstream or venous pressure. However, because most of the pulmonary vasculature is contained within the parenchyma of the lung, it is subjected to extravascular pressures that result in a critical closure pressure.[1, 2] It is not certain whether this pressure normally exceeds the venous pressure and therefore the calculation of the true pressure gradient of the pulmonary circulation remains uncertain. In the isolated lung preparation, in which a curvilinear relationship exists between arterial pressure and flow, the nonlinear portion is most evident at either low levels of blood flow[1,2] or high lung volumes.[2] In intact ventilated animals, in which it is possible to control pulmonary venous and alveolar pressure and to keep both constant, the pressure drop or gradient to flow relationship is linear over a wide range of flows in the physiologic range.[3]

The nature of the pressure-flow relationship in the pulmonary circulation of man has previously been explored by various techniques to alter pulmonary blood flow such as exercise, balloon occlusion, or crystalloid infusion.[4] However, few observations are available on this relationship for abnormal pulmonary circulation in which disease has created pulmonary arterial or venous hypertension. For example, in patients with left heart failure, mitral valve disease, or pulmonary vascular disease, the critical closure pressure and the hemodynamic behavior of the pulmonary circulation may be seriously altered.[5, 6] Therefore, the purpose of this study was to estimate the average closure pressure and to characterize the relationship between pressure drop and flow in the pulmonary circulation of patients with

From the Department of Medicine, University of Pennsylvania, Philadelphia.

Supported in part by program project grant HL08805, NHLBI, NIH, and by NIH grant MO1 RR00040 to the Clinical Research Center of the Hospital of the University of Pennsylvania.

Address for correspondence: Alfred P. Fishman, M.D., Cardiovascular Pulmonary Division, University of Pennsylvania, Philadelphia, PA 19104.

Received March 8, 1984; revision accepted Aug. 22, 1985.

*Current address: Cardiovascular Institute, Michael Reese Hospital and Medical Center, Chicago, IL 60616.

**Current address: Cardiovascular Institute, Hahnemann University, Philadelphia, PA 19102.

and without pulmonary arterial or venous hypertension of different degrees of severity and etiology. To obtain multiple pressure and flow data points, hemodynamic monitoring was performed in these patients during progressive upright treadmill exercise.[7, 8]

Methods

Fifty-one patients form the basis of this report. They were selected from a larger group of 68 patients, which represented the total number of patients referred to the Cardio-Pulmonary Evaluation Laboratory for a cardiopulmonary exercise evaluation with hemodynamics over a 4 year period. Patients were rejected because of an inability to complete more than one stage of exercise or because pertinent hemodynamic data were not obtained. Of those selected, 42 had chronic stable left ventricular heart failure of varying severity secondary to either idiopathic dilated cardiomyopathy (24 patients), valvular heart disease (nine patients), or ischemic heart disease (nine patients). Of the nine patients with valvular heart disease, three had mitral valve incompetence, four aortic valve incompetence, and two combined mitral and tricuspid valve incompetence. Nine other patients had biopsy-proven pulmonary vascular disease; in five the vascular disease was attributable to pulmonary emboli, scleroderma, hypersensitivity pneumonitis, sarcoidosis, or berylliosis, and in four the etiology was unknown.

At the time of study, all patients had been clinically stable for at least 6 months. All but two of the patients with cardiac disease were receiving diuretics and digitalis, whereas only one patient with pulmonary vascular disease was receiving medication (warfarin). Six patients had chronic atrial fibrillation while the others were in sinus rhythm. Three of the patients with pulmonary vascular disease had severe gas transfer abnormalities (i.e., the diffusing capacity, as measured by the single-breath CO uptake method was less than 30% of predicted). Two of these patients had either mild or moderate obstructive lung disease, with the ratio of forced expired volume in 1 sec to forced vital capacity being 65% and 45%, respectively. The third patient had restrictive lung disease as demonstrated by a reduced vital capacity (i.e., 48% of predicted) and normal airflow. In the remainder of the patients the presence of significant intrinsic pulmonary disease was excluded either by history or routine pulmonary function tests.

Protocol and measurements. The protocol and consent form were approved by the institutional review board of this hospital. After obtaining informed consent, all patients underwent right heart catheterization using a flotation catheter that was advanced into the pulmonary artery through an antecubital vein. Each patient was then exercised in the upright position to exhaustion according to a treadmill program (table 1) that consisted of 2 min stages of progressive work.[7] Increments in work were obtained by varying either treadmill speed, treadmill grade, or both.

The electrocardiogram (modified V_5) and pulsatile pulmonary artery pressure, together with measurements of breath-by-breath expired oxygen and carbon dioxide partial pressures and air flow, were monitored continuously during exercise as described in detail elsewhere.[8] Briefly, the breathing apparatus consisted of a mouthpiece, a nose clamp, and a low-resistance two-port, unidirectional valve with a pneumotachygraph connected to the expiratory port of the valve. Air was removed from the valve chamber at a constant rate and sampled by rapidly responding oxygen and carbon dioxide analyzers. The pressure transducer (Statham P23ID) was positioned approximately at the midheart level (i.e., midway between the sternal angle and the xiphoid process), and this level served as the zero reference throughout the protocol for measurements of pulmonary capillary wedge pressure and pulsatile and mean pulmonary arterial pressure (PAP). Pulsatile pulmonary arterial and pulmonary capillary wedge pressure data reported herein were obtained at the end of expiration. At this point in the respiratory cycle, intrathoracic pressure is close to atmospheric pressure and therefore the intravascular pressures measured with respect to atmosphere come close to approximating transmural pressures. Cuff blood pressure and mixed venous blood oxygen content and lactate concentration were measured at rest and during the last minute of each stage. Timed expired gas collections were also obtained at rest and each stage. Finally, arterial oxygen saturation was continuously monitored by an ear oximeter in all patients with pulmonary vascular disease and in all but seven of the patients with heart failure. These seven were deeply pigmented blacks and reliable ear oximetry data could not be obtained. However, because patients with chronic heart failure typically do not experience a fall in oxygen saturation during exercise[9, 10] and because the presence of pulmonary disease was excluded, it is unlikely that they would have desaturated during exercise. Ear oximetry has been found to closely approximate arterial oxygen saturation over a wide range of saturations (standard error of estimate <3% of arterial oxygen saturation).[11]

Derivations. From the above measurements, the following quantities were derived: heart rate, oxygen uptake ($\dot{V}O_2$, ml/min) from both the breath-by-breath and timed gas collection measurements, and mixed venous oxygen content from the percent oxygen saturation, hemoglobin, and oxygen combining capacity. Systemic arterial oxygen saturation was assumed to be 98% for those patients who were not monitored by ear oximetry. Maximum $\dot{V}O_2$ ($\dot{V}O_2$max) was considered to have been achieved when $\dot{V}O_2$ increased by less than 1 ml/min/kg after an increment in work. The degree of aerobic impairment, which reflects the severity of circulatory or cardiac failure, was determined by $\dot{V}O_2$max and criteria previously reported from this laboratory[8]: minimum to no impairment (class A) when $\dot{V}O_2$max exceeded 20 ml/min/kg; mild to moderate impairment (class B) when $\dot{V}O_2$max was between 16 and 20 ml/min/kg; moderate to marked impairment (class C) when $\dot{V}O_2$max was between 10 and 16 ml/min/kg; and severe impairment (class D) when $\dot{V}O_2$max was less than 10 ml/min/kg. Cardiac output (CO, liters/min) was calculated by the Fick principle, and pulmonary vascular resistance (PVR, dyne-sec-cm^{-5}) was obtained by dividing the mean pulmonary vascular pressure drop (see below) by cardiac

TABLE 1
Treadmill program

	Stage									
	1	2	3	4	5	6	7	8	9	10
Speed	1	1.5	2	2	2	3	3	3	3	3.4
Grade	0	0	3.5	7	10.5	7.5	10	12.5	15	14

The treadmill program is identified by stage, speed (mph), and percent grade.

TABLE 2
Group I: Etiology and rest-exercise hemodynamics

Patient	Etiology	Class[A]	Mean PAP (mm Hg)		PVR (dyne-sec-cm^{-5})		Mean PAP-CO relation		
			Rest	Peak Ex.	Rest	Peak Ex.	Slope	Intercept	r
1	AR	A	10	35	55	120	2.64	1.0	.99
2	CM	A	10	38	130	115	2.56	−3.9	.92
3	MR	B	18	43	70	60	4.22	3.8	.95
4	MR	B	13	26	85	115	2.73	−6.2	.98
5	CM	B	18	60	260	200	8.93	−6.5	.98
6	AR	C	17	37	50	70	4.00	−8.7	.91
7	CM	C	16	34	65	55	3.55	2.4	.94
8	AR	C	8	23	100	110	3.20	−1.8	.92
9	CM	C	17	49	240	160	3.87	0.7	.99
10	CM	C	12	26	165	150	3.51	−2.6	.84
11	CM	C	14	44	215	105	6.20	−4.6	.98
12[B]	MR/TR	D	15	32	325	155	3.82	5.4	.91
Mean			14	37	145	120			
±SD			3	11	95	45			

Ex. = exercise; AR, MR, and TR = aortic, mitral, and tricuspid regurgitation; CM = dilated cardiomyopathy.
[A]Class is based on maximum O_2 uptake being >20 ml/min/kg (A), >16 and <20 ml/min/kg (B), >10 and <16 ml/min/kg (C), and <10 ml/min/kg (D).
[B]Atrial fibrillation.

output and multiplying the result by the unit conversion factor, 80. The average closure pressure for the entire pulmonary vascular bed was estimated as follows: CO and mean PAP data at rest and for each level of exercise were plotted and the best fit line determined by linear regression. The extrapolated, zero-flow pressure intercept of this relation, which has been shown to represent the average closure pressure for the pulmonary circulation,[1] was then used as an estimate of closure pressure. It should be noted that because the CO–mean PAP relation becomes nonlinear as CO approaches zero, the closure pressure is greater than the actual zero-flow pressure intercept. In fact, Graham et al.[2] have shown the average closure pressure to be approximately equal to the true zero-flow pressure plus the alveolar pressure. Finally, this intercept pressure was compared with the resting pulmonary wedge pressure to determine which pressure was greater and should be used as the downstream pressure when calculating the pressure gradient.

Statistical analysis. All combined results are presented as mean ± 1 SD. Linearity of a relationship was assessed on the basis of the correlation coefficient being greater than .9. Comparison of regression line slopes and intercepts were made according to the method described by Brownlee.[12] Intergroup comparisons of resting data were made by the one-factor analysis of variance and the modified t test.[13] Intragroup comparisons were performed with the t test for paired data. Statistical significance for all comparisons was taken to be, according to the Bonferroni method, at a level of $p < .05/m$, where m is the number of comparisons.[13]

Results

Response in pressure and flow to exercise. Patients with cardiac disease were divided into two groups (see tables 2 and 3) according to whether their resting mean PAP was less than or greater than the upper normal value of 19 mm Hg (groups I and II, respectively). Patients with pulmonary vascular disease were considered separately as group III (see table 4). Oxygen saturation in the patients with heart failure (groups I and II) never fell below 90%. There were, however, four patients from group III (Nos. 46, 49, 50, and 51) who were found to have significant desaturation (i.e., oxygen saturation <80%) during exercise; three-fourths had severe gas transfer abnormalities (see Methods) with either restrictive (patient 50) or obstructive (mild, patient 46; moderate, patient 49) lung disease. Nevertheless, all patients, regardless of their disease, were able to exercise beyond their anaerobic threshold and most attained their maximum oxygen uptake. The resting hemodynamics of the upright patients in each group are summarized below.

Group I consisted of 12 patients with normal resting PAP and wedge pressure of 21 ± 4/10 ± 3 mm Hg (mean 14 ± 3) and 8 ± 4 mm Hg, respectively. The 30 group II patients had significantly higher PAPs (42 ± 9/24 ± 8 mm Hg, mean 32 ± 8) in association with significantly higher pulmonary wedge pressures (21 ± 3 mm Hg). Group III patients, on the average, had a significantly greater PAP (63 ± 25/35 ± 12 mm Hg, mean 43 ± 16) than did groups I and II. However, the average pulmonary capillary wedge pressure (8 ± 5 mm Hg) did not differ statistically from that of group I. The resting CO did not differ among the three groups, with average values of 3.8 ± 1.4, 3.5 ± 1.2, and 3.4 ± 0.7 liters/min for groups I, II, and III, respectively.

The average group responses to exercise in terms of systolic, diastolic, and mean PAP, pulmonary capil-

TABLE 3
Group II: Etiology and rest-exercise hemodynamics

			Mean PAP (mm Hg)		PVR (dyne-sec-cm^{-5})		Mean PAP-CO relation		
Patient	Etiology	Class	Rest	Peak Ex.	Rest	Peak Ex.	Slope	Intercept	r
13	CM	C	37	67	345	320	8.72	12.9	.99
14	CM	C	30	48	165	85	3.46	10.5	.89
15	CM	C	25	54	480	180	4.59	15.9	.98
16	IHD	C	30	54	155	110	4.69	18.6	.87
17	CM	C	38	47	410	185	2.40	31.0	.99
18	CM	C	26	46	140	345	10.25	−38.8	.82
19	CM	C	26	42	370	240	5.51	9.4	.96
20	CM	C	25	40	325	215	9.75	−3.6	.89
21	CM	C	23	38	255	160	2.99	15.6	.99
22	CM	C	25	48	150	175	6.32	1.3	.60
23	IHD	C	21	42	155	175	3.72	8.2	.97
24[A]	MR/TR	C	22	47	—	105	4.46	13.8	.96
25	IHD	D	36	83	175	120	7.10	18.6	.98
26	CM	D	38	65	265	165	2.69	35.4	.91
27	CM	D	43	59	295	250	11.57	23.8	.91
28	IHD	D	41	48	455	345	4.39	29.9	.92
29	CM	D	52	66	495	535	6.29	37.3	.91
30	IHD	D	35	57	365	240	7.39	20.0	.83
31	CM	D	30	52	145	300	18.08	−5.4	.99
32[A]	MR	D	33	60	220	115	12.15	−3.1	.86
33	CM	D	39	50	325	185	4.38	30.9	.92
34	CM	D	42	56	—	155	12.07	12.3	.99
35	IHD	D	28	58	255	240	10.15	3.0	.73
36	CM	D	34	42	125	120	0.67	31.4	.11
37	IHD	D	34	46	280	275	4.30	21.1	.80
38	CM	D	28	40	185	165	3.19	17.0	.67
39	IHD	D	43	62	370	240	11.24	6.4	.99
40[A]	AR	D	24	29	130	115	3.55	7.1	.85
41[A]	CM	D	24	57	185	210	11.67	−17.0	.94
42	IHD	D	22	60	170	250	44.08	−164.0	.88
Mean			32	52	265	210			
±SD			8	11	115	95			

IHD = ischemic heart disease. Other abbreviations and notes as in table 2.
[A]Atrial fibrillation.

lary wedge pressure, and cardiac index are shown in figure 1. All values increased as the level of work was incremented. Mean PAP significantly increased in group I from an average resting value of 14 ± 3 to 37 ± 11 mm Hg, in group II from 32 ± 8 to 52 ± 11 mm Hg, and in group III from 43 ± 16 to 81 ± 16 mm Hg. Pulmonary capillary wedge pressure rose from 8 ± 4 to 21 ± 12 mm Hg in group I, from 21 ± 3 to 37 ± 11 mm Hg in Group II, and from 8 ± 5 to 18 ± 7 mm Hg in group III. Cardiac index (liters/min/m^2) increased in group I from 2.2 ± 0.6 to 6.8 ± 1.4, in group II from 1.9 ± 0.6 to 3.6 ± 1.4, and in group III from 1.9 ± 0.3 to 5.0 ± 1.5. However, at each level of work, cardiac index did not differ among the three groups.

As can be seen from the pressure responses for groups I and II in figure 1, the increases in PAP closely follow that of pulmonary capillary wedge pressure. Regression line analysis revealed a close correlation (range of r, .85 to .92) between PAP (i.e., diastolic, mean, and systolic) and pulmonary capillary wedge pressure for these two groups, while for group III the correlation coefficients were all less than .60. If, instead of grouping the patients with heart failure by mean PAP they are grouped by etiology, similar results are obtained (range of r, .70 to .92). The three lowest correlation coefficients of .70, .78, and .83 were obtained for the patients with valvular heart disease when systolic, mean, and diastolic PAPs were correlated, respectively with pulmonary capillary wedge pressure. All other correlation coefficients were greater than .86.

Pressure-flow relationship during exercise. The number

TABLE 4
Group III: Etiology and rest-exercise hemodynamics

			PAP (mm Hg)		PVR (dyne-sec-cm^{-5})		PAP-CO relation		
Patient	Etiology	Class[A]	Rest	Peak Ex.	Rest	Peak Ex.	Slope	Intercept	r
43	PPH	D	61	81	1740	1740	31.45	−22.7	.90
44	PSS	D	40	100	860	900	12.52	−1.4	.98
45	PPH	D	69	102	1290	—	25.32	−18.9	.77
46[A]	HP	D	44	80	980	920	17.42	−4.8	.95
47	PE	C	26	65	600	—	7.03	6.2	.98
48	PPH	B	36	90	500	450	6.86	7.4	.98
49[A]	BE	B	26	80	460	440	8.67	−7.8	.98
50[A]	SA	C	28	52	420	300	3.12	14.5	.96
51[A]	PPH	D	58	76	990	700	8.23	32.0	.95
Mean			43	81	850	780			
±SD			16	16	460	490			

PPH = primary pulmonary hypertension; PSS = scleroderma; HP = hypersensitivity pneumonitis; PE = pulmonary emboli; BE = berylliois; SA = sarcoidosis. Other notes as in table 2.

[A]Hypoxemia during exercise.

of data points per patient ranged from three to 11, averaging six. The relationship between mean PAP and CO during exercise was linear (i.e., $r > .9$) in most (69%) of the patients. As can be seen in tables 2, 3, and 4, the individual correlation coefficients were greater than .9 in 11 (92%) group I, 17 (57%) group II, and eight (89%) group III patients, whereas only four (13%) patients from group II and one (11%) patient from group III had values less than .8.

The average pressure-flow relationships (mean PAP–cardiac index) for each group are given in figure 2 along with the slope (±95% confidence limit) and correlation coefficient for each relationship; each slope differed significantly ($p < .01$) from the others. The pressure-flow relationship of the pulmonary circulation tended to be shifted upward and became steeper as the level of resting PAP increased. The correlation between slope and resting mean PAP was .66 for all patients, .74 for group I, and .79 for group III; no significant correlation was found in group II.

As discussed in Methods, the zero-flow pressure intercept of the mean PAP–cardiac index relation was used to approximate the average closure pressure for the pulmonary circulation. To investigate whether

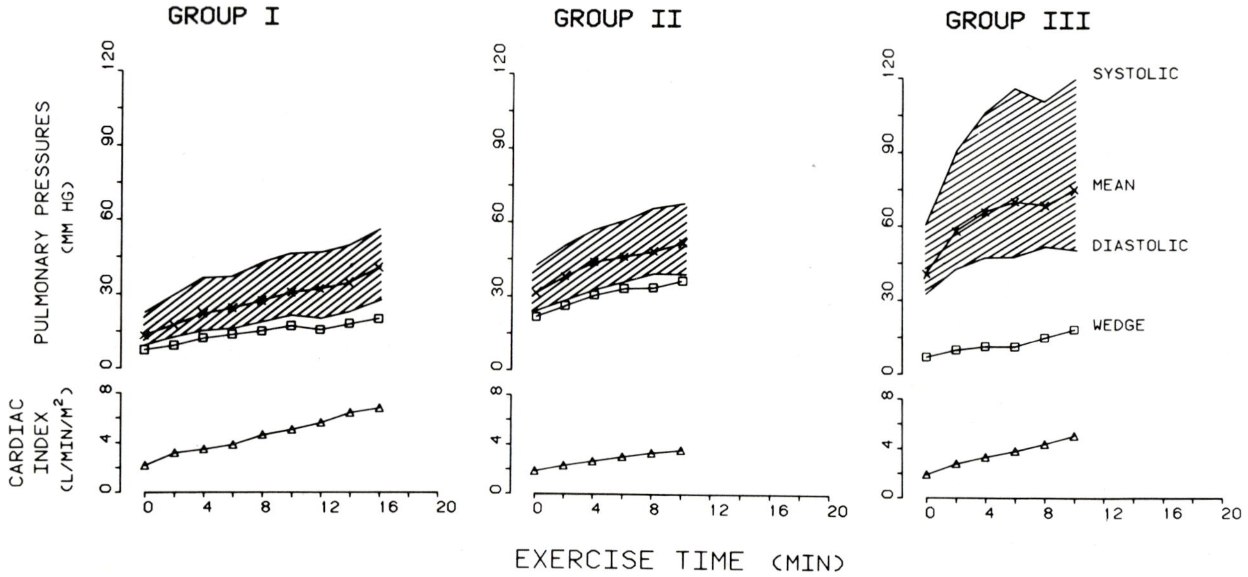

FIGURE 1. Average responses in systolic, mean, and diastolic PAP, wedge pressures, and cardiac index to progressive upright treadmill exercise. Data at zero time are resting data and at each 2 min interval the level of muscular work was increased. Groups I and II represent patients with chronic, stable heart failure with resting mean PAP < and > 19 mm Hg, respectively. Group III consists of patients with pulmonary vascular disease.

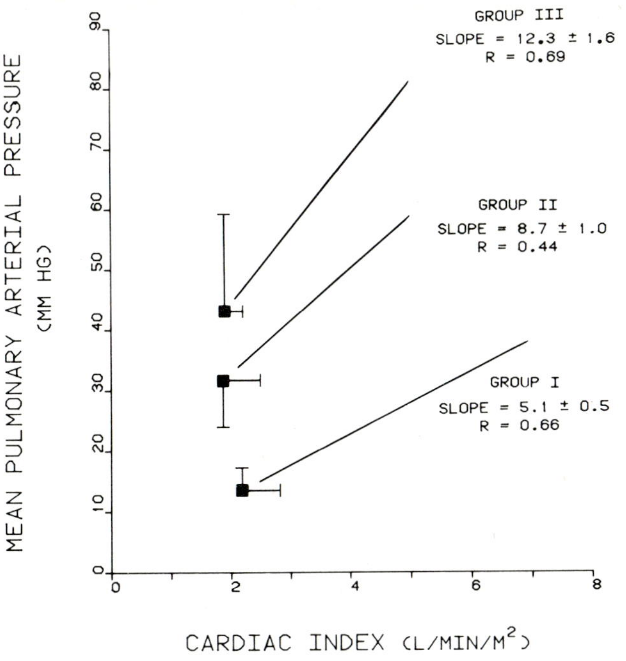

FIGURE 2. Average relationships between mean PAP and cardiac index during exercise for patients with heart failure (groups I and II) and patients with pulmonary vascular disease (group III). Solid squares and bars represent resting data and SD and solid lines are regression lines. Listed for each regression line is slope ±95% confidence limits and correlation coefficient (R).

average closure pressure exceeded the resting pulmonary capillary wedge pressure in these patients, the resting pulmonary capillary wedge pressure was compared with the extrapolated y-intercept pressure for each patient. The results are shown in figure 3. Eighty-two percent of the points lie on, or to the left of, the line of identity, indicating that the resting pulmonary capillary wedge pressure was equal to or exceeded the average closure pressure. Accordingly, pulmonary capillary wedge pressure was used as the downstream pressure in calculating the pressure drop and vascular resistance of the pulmonary circulation.

Of the nine patients whose data fell to the right of the line of identity, none were from group I, seven were from group II, and two were from group III. Two of the group II patients (Nos. 15 and 17) were functional class C, whereas the other five (Nos. 26, 28, 29, 33, and 36) were class D. As can be seen from table 3, the etiology of all but one (i.e., patient 28, ischemic heart disease) was a cardiomyopathy. The two patients from group III (Nos. 50 and 51) belonged to the subset of four patients who developed hypoxemia during exercise (see table 4).

PVR during exercise. In tables 2, 3, and 4, PVR values at rest and during peak exercise are listed for each of the patients in groups I, II, and III, respectively. As can be seen from the average values, there was a trend for PVR to decrease modestly (17%, 21%, and 8% in groups 1, II, and III) during exercise. The amount of decrease ranged from 10 to 170 (avg. 60), 5 to 300 (avg. 90), and 20 to 290 (avg. 75) dyne-sec-cm^{-5}, respectively, for the three groups. However, only the decrease in group II reached the level of statistical significance ($p < .025$).

Within group I, it was only the patients with valvular heart disease (Nos. 1, 4, 6, and 8) who did not exhibit a decrease in PVR with exercise. Thus, when the six cardiomyopathic patients are considered separately they are found to have a significant ($p < .04$) decrease (28%) from 180 ± 75 to 130 ± 50 dyne-sec-cm^{-5}. The average PVR for the patients with valvular heart disease remained essentially constant from rest (114 ± 105 dyne-sec-cm^{-5}) to peak exercise (105 ± 35 dyne-sec-cm^{-5}).

In group II there were three patients with valvular heart disease (Nos. 24, 32, and 40), and in the two with complete data (Nos. 32 and 40) PVR decreased with exercise. However, when the results of these two are averaged with those of the six patients with valvular disease in group I, the PVR at peak exercise (105 ± 30 dyne-sec-cm^{-5}) was not significantly different from the resting value of 130 ± 95 dyne-sec-cm^{-5} (see table 5).

A significant fall in resistance was observed in 75% or 21 of the patients included in group II (see table 3). Of the seven patients in whom a decrease was not observed, two had ischemic heart disease (Nos. 23 and 42) and five had a cardiomyopathy (Nos. 18, 22, 29, 31, and 41). If instead of being grouped according to mean PAP, the patients with heart failure are grouped on the basis of their etiology, significant decreases in PVR are observed in 78% of the patients with cardiomyopathy (see table 5); the decrease in PVR observed

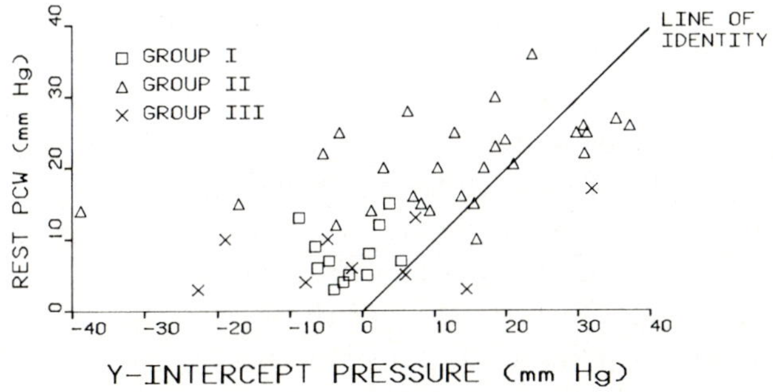

FIGURE 3. Resting pulmonary capillary wedge pressure (PCW) vs the y-intercept pressure, which was obtained by fitting a regression line to each patient's mean PAP and the values for CO at rest and exercise. In most of the patients, the PCW at rest was greater than the y-intercept pressure.

TABLE 5
Hemodynamics of patients with heart failure grouped according to etiology

	Mean PAP (mm Hg)		PVR (dyne-sec-cm^{-5})	
Etiology	Rest	Peak ex.	Rest	Peak ex.
Valve disease	18±8	37±12	130±95	105±30
Cardiomyopathy	28±11	49±10	250±115	200±100^{A}
Ischemia	32±8	57±12	265±110	220±75

$^{A}p < .05$.

in 78% of the patients with ischemic heart disease did not reach the level of significance.

Group III patients who had an invariant or increasing PVR during exercise (Nos. 43 and 44) had resting PVR in excess of 850 dyne-sec-cm^{-5} and were functional class D. As can be seen, a decrease in PVR from rest to peak exercise was obtained in the four patients who developed hypoxemia during exercise.

Discussion

Pulmonary hypertension is said to exist when the resting mean PAP exceeds 19 mm Hg or when the resting peak systolic pressure is greater than 30 mm Hg.[4] The most common causes of pulmonary hypertension are left ventricular failure with its accompanying increase in pulmonary venous pressure, and pulmonary vascular disease with its increase in resistance to flow. The patients and the grouping criteria used in this report created three groups: group I, heart failure with normal pulmonary arterial and venous pressures; group II, heart failure with abnormally high pulmonary venous pressure; and group III, pulmonary vascular disease without left heart failure. Thus, the two most common causes of a hypertensive pulmonary circulation were represented in this study.

To characterize the hemodynamic behavior of the pulmonary circulation, upright progressive treadmill exercise to exhaustion was used as the test. The respiratory impairment present in several of the group III patients did not prevent them from exercising to levels associated with anaerobic metabolism and lactate production. In our laboratory, a lactate level in mixed venous blood that is greater than 12 mg/dl is assumed to indicate lactate production. The onset of lactate production and the appearance of the anaerobic threshold by respiratory gas exchange criteria are closely related and, in a given patient, occur during the same stage of exercise.[8] Accordingly, all patients were able to exercise beyond the anaerobic threshold and most attained their $\dot{V}O_2$max. For groups I, II, and III, these maximal levels of work were associated, on the average, with increases in cardiac index of 3.1, 1.9, and 2.6 times the average resting value, which was essentially the same for the three groups. The fact that group II patients had the smallest increase in CO reflects their greater degree of circulatory dysfunction. Thus the group II patient typically could complete only 4.7 stages of exercise, whereas the group I and group III patient averaged 7.4 and 5.1 stages, respectively.

It should be emphasized that pulmonary vascular disease indirectly impairs the heart's ability to meet the oxygen demands of the body and therefore can be considered to represent a form of circulatory failure. For example, our patients with severe pulmonary vascular disease (i.e., PVR >850 dyne-sec-cm^{-5}) were found to be functional class D on the basis of their $\dot{V}O_2$max being less than 10 ml/min/kg. Functionally, they performed at a level similar to the patient with severe cardiac failure. Therefore, since the functional status of patients in group III ranged from class B to class D, it is not surprising to find their average CO response to be somewhere between those of groups I and II.

In all patients, PAP increased with each increment in work. However, the amount by which it increased and the maximal levels were group dependent, being lowest in group I and greatest in group III. In fact, the systolic and mean PAPs attained by group III patients during maximal exercise typically reached or exceeded systemic levels.

With the exception of very low pressures and flow, the relationship between mean PAP and flow (cardiac index) has been shown to be linear over a wide range of flows in dog[2] and pig[1] isolated lung preparations and in left lung segments of the intact dog.[3] Whether the exercise mean PAP–cardiac index relationship in normal man is also linear is less certain. Fowler[4] found, after averaging group values for pulmonary flow and pressure, the pressure response to changes in flow to be linear. However, there was considerable individual variation; in one of the studies reviewed,[14] all of the individual pressure-flow plots were nonlinear.

To the best of our knowledge, the exercise mean PAP–cardiac index relationship for patients with circulatory dysfunction has not been systematically analyzed from rest to maximum exercise capacity. Moreover, in studies where mean PAP–flow data were reported for patients with heart disease,[5, 6] rest and only one to two data points with increased flow are presented per patient, thus making the assessment of linearity difficult. In the present study an average of six data points (i.e., rest and exercise) per patient were obtained. The results indicated that the mean PAP–cardiac index relationship tended to be linear; in only five patients was the correlation coefficient less than .8.

At maximal exercise the resting pulmonary capillary wedge pressure had increased by an average total amount of 14, 16, and 10 mm Hg in groups I, II, and III, respectively. Although similar increases have been reported in patients with chronic cardiac failure of diverse etiology,[8] little is known regarding the wedge pressure response of the normal left ventricle during upright exercise. Thus it is not clear to what extent the group III response was abnormal.

In healthy young men and women performing supine exercise, Ekelund and Holmgren[15] found mean wedge pressure to increase from 8 to 13 mm Hg as CO rose from 5 to 20 liters/min. In elderly normal men (i.e., >61 years), they frequently observed a 10 to 15 mm Hg increment to levels in excess of 20 mm Hg. Based on observations regarding stroke volume and body position,[15] one would predict some differences in the wedge pressure response obtained during supine and upright exercise. When the position is changed from supine to standing, there is a decrease in the end-diastolic size of the heart and in stroke volume. Then, with progressive muscular work, stroke volume increases to the level observed in the recumbent position. Accordingly, wedge pressure in the upright position would be lower at rest and during mild exercise than that in the supine position; at higher levels of work, the difference, if any, would be much smaller. Therefore the normal increase in wedge pressure from rest to peak upright exercise would be expected to exceed the 5 mm Hg increment obtained during supine exercise.

In the upright position, the increases in stroke volume contribute to the exercise-induced elevation in CO only at the onset of exercise. Then, as workload increases further, changes in heart rate account for most of the subsequent increases in CO. Thus the Frank-Starling mechanism is minimally used during exercise. This appears to be at odds with the observations concerning the wedge pressure response during supine or upright exercise unless the increases in pulmonary capillary wedge pressure were in part the result of the pericardium imposing a mechanical constraint to short-term enlargement of the heart and enhancing the mechanical interplay or interaction between the left and right heart.[16, 17] If this were so, the wedge pressure measurement would include the increase in intrapericardial pressure. The degree to which the wedge pressure response of group III was abnormal is explainable by this mechanism. That is, right ventricular distension, which accompanies large, exercise-induced increases in right ventricular pressure, causes a shift in the left ventricular diastolic pressure-volume relation via ventricular interaction and the pericardium so that a given volume is associated with a higher wedge pressure.

As discussed above, the mean PAP–flow relationship of the pulmonary vasculature has been found to be linear except at very low flows. In this nonlinear region, the slope was much steeper than that of the linear region. As a result, the y-intercept pressure obtained by extrapolating the linear curve to the y-axis was always greater than the actual zero flow pressure.[2, 3] Recently Graham et al.[2] reported the zero-flow PAP for normal lungs to be approximately 7 mm Hg and invariant with respect to the level of alveolar pressure; the latter varied from 3 to 11 mm Hg in their isolated lung preparation. Because the transmural pressure was positive for most of the alveolar pressures, they concluded that 7 mm Hg represented the critical closure pressure as defined by Burton.[18] In contrast, Hyman[3] reported the PAP at zero flow to be only 3.5 mm Hg, and West and Dollery[19] concluded the critical closure pressure of the canine pulmonary vasculature was negligibly small.

Although controversy exists regarding the magnitude of the critical closure pressure, there is little doubt that the linear portion of the mean PAP–flow relationship and the extrapolated pressure are shifted upward with hypoxia[1] and as alveolar pressure is increased.[2, 20] Mitzner and Sylvester[1] on the basis of a parallel-channel Starling resistor model of the pulmonary circulation, have reasoned that the extrapolated y-intercept pressure is equivalent to the average closure pressure of the vascular bed. In our study, the resting wedge pressure was found to equal or exceed the extrapolated y-intercept pressure in most of the patients. There were, however, nine patients in whom this was not the case. Because the extrapolated pressure is shifted upward with hypoxia, this was expected for the two patients from group III who developed hypoxemia during exercise. For the seven patients from group II, and in particular the five who were classified as functional class D, an elevated interstitial pressure may be present, which would result in an abnormally high average closure pressure. Accordingly, in these nine patients it may not have been appropriate to use the wedge pressure as the downstream pressure when calculating the PAP gradient and vascular resistance. However, this still remains an unsettled issue. Harris et al.,[20] for example, observed pulmonary venous pressure to increase by the same amount as alveolar pressure. Moreover, because the wedge pressure increases during exercise, the difference between wedge and extravascular pressure would be continually increasing. Therefore the wedge pressure was used as the downstream pressure in this study.

The PVR in the majority of the patients decreased during exercise. This was particularly true for the patients with heart failure caused by a cardiomyopathy (19/23) or by ischemic heart disease (7/9) and for the patients with pulmonary vascular disease whose resting PVR was less than 850 dyne-sec-cm^{-5}. In contrast, a decline in PVR was observed in only half of the patients with valvular heart disease. Harris et al.[20] also noted a similar, although not statistically significant, tendency for PVR to decrease in the supine patient and predicted that more substantial changes might occur with the patient upright. An explanation as to why an increase in PVR occurred with exercise in some of the patients is not apparent from the data. That is, they could not be distinguished on the basis of their etiology, functional class, or hemodynamics.

If one assumes PVR to be proportional to 1/(effective pulmonary vascular area), then the exercise-induced reductions in PVR were associated with increases in effective area of 5%, 6%, and 2% for groups I, II, and III, respectively. Although these do not indicate, per se, whether the increases in pulmonary vascular area were the result of passive and/or active processes, the magnitude of increase and the fact that both pulmonary arterial and venous pressures increase during exercise suggest that the increase in pulmonary vascular area is predominantly a passive process secondary to recruitment and distension. The findings of Borst et al.[21] in the isolated, in vivo lung preparation and those of Hopkins et al.[22] in the conscious dog support this view. Both groups reported that PVR decreased after short-term increments in left atrial pressure. An analysis of the impedance spectra revealed capillary recruitment had occurred as a result of acute pulmonary venous hypertension.[22] Borst and co-workers also found a reduction in resistance as PAP was elevated and left atrial pressure held constant. This effect on resistance, however, was not as great as that seen with increments in left atrial pressure. Thus, if the exercise induced reductions in PVR are assumed to be the result of a passive increase in the effective vascular area, then the pulmonary circulation of those patients with an invariant PVR behaved as a rigid system.

In summary, hemodynamic data obtained during upright, progressive treadmill exercise were used to estimate the average closure pressure of the pulmonary vascular bed and to characterize the pressure-flow and pressure drop–flow relationships in the pulmonary circulation of patients with and without pulmonary arterial or venous hypertension of different degrees of severity and etiology. In the majority of patients the results indicated that: (1) the mean PAP–flow relationship was linear; (2) pulmonary capillary wedge pressure was greater than or equal to the average closure pressure and could therefore be used as the downstream pressure in calculating PVR; and (3) PVR declined with exercise.

We are grateful for the dedicated technical assistance of Thomas Nusbickel, David Ward, and Virginia Andrews.

References

1. Mitzner W, Sylvester JT: Hypoxic vasoconstriction and fluid filtration in pig lungs. J Appl Physiol **51:** 1065, 1981
2. Graham R, Skoog C, Oppenheimer L, Rabson J, Goldberg HS: Critical closure in the canine pulmonary vasculature. Circ Res **50:** 566, 1982
3. Hyman AL: Effects of large increases in pulmonary blood flow on pulmonary venous pressure. J Appl Physiol **27:** 179, 1969
4. Fowler NO: The normal pulmonary arterial pressure-flow relationships during exercise (editorial). Am J Med **47:** 1, 1969
5. Harris P, Segel N, Bishop JM: The relation between pressure and flow in the pulmonary circulation in normal subjects and in patients with chronic bronchitis and mitral stenosis. Cardiovasc Res **2:** 73, 1968
6. Epstein SE, Beiser GD, Stampfer M, Robinson BF, Braunwald E: Characterization of the circulatory response to maximal upright exercise in normal subjects and patients with heart disease. Circulation **35:** 1049, 1967
7. Weber KT, Kinasewitz GT, West JS, Janicki JS, Reichek N, Fishman AP: Long term vasodilator therapy with trimazosin in chronic cardiac failure. N Engl J Med **303:** 242, 1980
8. Weber KT, Kinasewitz GT, Janicki JS, Fishman AP: Oxygen utilization and ventilation during exercise in patients with chronic cardiac failure. Circulation **65:** 1213, 1982
9. Rubin SA, Brown HV, Swan HJC: Arterial oxygenation and arterial oxygen transport in chronic myocardial failure at rest, during exercise and after hydralazine treatment. Circulation **66:** 143, 1982
10. Wilson JR, Ferraro N: Exercise intolerance in patients with chronic left heart failure: relation to oxygen transport and ventilatory abnormalities. Am J Cardiol **51:** 1358, 1983
11. Sanders NA, Powles ACP, Rebuck AS: Ear oximetry: accuracy and practicability in the assessment of arterial oxygenation. Am Rev Respir Dis **113:** 745, 1976
12. Brownlee KA: Statistical theory and methodology in science and engineering. New York, 1965, John Wiley & Sons, pp 349–351
13. Wallenstein S, Zucker CL, Fleiss JL: Some statistical methods useful in circulation research. Circ Res **47:** 1, 1980
14. DeMato AN, Galante JG, Smith WM: Hemodynamic response to treadmill exercise in normal subjects. J Appl Physiol **21:** 959, 1966
15. Ekelund LG, Holmgren A: Central hemodynamics during exercise. Circ Res **20/21**(suppl I): I-33, 1967
16. Janicki JS, Weber KT: Factors influencing the diastolic pressure-volume relation of the cardiac ventricles. Fed Proc **39:** 133, 1980
17. Janicki JS, Weber KT: The pericardium and ventricular interaction, distensibility and function. Am J Physiol **238:** H494, 1980
18. Burton AC: On the physical equilibrium of small blood vessels. Am J Physiol **164:** 319, 1951
19. West JB, Dollery CT: Distribution of blood flow and the pressure-flow relations of the whole lung. J Appl Physiol **20:** 175, 1965
20. Harris P, Segal N, Green I, Housley E: The influence of the airways resistance and alveolar pressure on the pulmonary vascular resistance in chronic bronchitis. Cardiovasc Res **2:** 84, 1968
21. Borst HG, McGregor M, Whittenberger JL, Berglund E: Influence of pulmonary arterial and left atrial pressures on pulmonary vascular resistance. Circ Res **4:** 393, 1956
22. Hopkins RA, Hammon Jr JW, McHale PA, Smith PK, Anderson RW: An analysis of the pulsatile hemodynamic responses of the pulmonary circulation to acute and chronic pulmonary venous hypertension in the awake dog. Circ Res **47:** 902, 1980

Right ventricular function in an operating room model of mechanical left ventricular assistance and its effects in patients with depressed left ventricular function

DAVID J. FARRAR, PH.D., PETER G. COMPTON, M.S., JAMES J. HERSHON, M.D., AND J. DONALD HILL, M.D.

ABSTRACT Approximately 20% of patients who receive left ventricular assist devices (LVADs) for refractory cardiac failure after open heart surgery have had complications of right ventricular failure. To evaluate this problem in the diseased heart we simulated an LVAD in the operating room by bypassing and unloading the left ventricle with the heart-lung machine before routine open heart surgery. Right ventricular function was assessed in 12 patients with preoperative left ventricular ejection fractions of less than 0.55 (poor left ventricular function) (mean ± SEM 0.40 ± 0.03) and 10 patients with ejection fractions greater than 0.55 (normal left ventricular function) (0.63 ± 0.02). Measurements before and during left ventricular bypass in the normal left ventricular function group revealed no change in cardiac output (from 5.7 ± 0.6 to 5.8 ± 0.4 liters/min), with a decrease in right ventricular end-diastolic pressure (from 8 ± 2 to 6 ± 1 mm Hg). However, in the poor left ventricular function group, cardiac output was increased significantly during left ventricular bypass from 4.5 ± 0.2 to 5.3 ± 0.4 liters/min and right ventricular end-diastolic pressure was decreased significantly from 13 ± 2 to 8 ± 2 mm Hg. During bypass there were significant reductions in mean pulmonary arterial pressure from 17 ± 3 to 10 ± 2 mm Hg in the normal left ventricular function group and from 27 ± 3 to 12 ± 2 mm Hg in the poor left ventricular function group. These measurements reflect passive changes in pulmonary pressures due to reductions in left ventricular filling pressure during left ventricular bypass. The findings show that acute left ventricular unloading results in unchanged to slightly improved right ventricular function in the normal left ventricular function group and in significantly improved right ventricular function in the poor left ventricular function group, principally due to right ventricular afterload reduction. This demonstrates a potential beneficial effect to the right ventricle in patients with pulmonary venous hypertension secondary to poor left ventricular function. The data suggest that acute unloading of the left ventricle is not the cause of right ventricular failure in patients with LVADs, and the pathophysiology of other causes must be investigated.
Circulation 72, No. 6, 1279–1285, 1985.

PREVIOUS CLINICAL EXPERIENCE with left ventricular assist devices (LVADs) used for refractory cardiac failure after open heart surgery has demonstrated right heart failure in a significant fraction of patients.[1] Of 213 patients who received LVADs at 12 different centers, 49 patients either died of right ventricular failure or required biventricular mechanical support.[1] Reports from many of these centers discussed right ventricular failure as a potential limitation to LVAD therapy,[2-11] but others reported adequate management of right ventricular function with isoproterenol[12] or did not mention right ventricular failure as a major problem during left ventricular assistance.[13-15]

In addition, our experimental studies of left ventricular bypass and unloading in the normal dog heart[16, 17] and findings of a preliminary clinical study[18] have provided no evidence of right ventricular failure. Although patient survival during mechanical support of only one ventricle is obviously dependent on the severity of biventricular dysfunction,[8] the problem is not clearly understood in terms of anatomic and hemody-

From the Department of Cardiovascular Surgery, Pacific Presbyterian Medical Center, San Francisco.
Supported in part by grant HL27275 from the National Heart, Lung, and Blood Institute.
Address for correspondence: David J. Farrar, Ph.D., Department of Cardiovascular Surgery, Pacific Presbyterian Medical Center, PO Box 7999, Room P3378, San Francisco, CA 94120.
Received Jan. 28, 1985; revision accepted Sept. 5, 1985.

namic ventricular interaction or in terms of patient selection and patient management. The purpose of the present study is to extend the experimental evaluation of the effects of left ventricular bypass on right ventricular function to the diseased human heart by studying patients during routine open heart surgery.

Methods

Patients for study during left ventricular bypass were selected from the pool of patients referred to the Department of Cardiovascular Surgery at Pacific Presbyterian Medical Center for aortocoronary bypass grafting, aneurysmectomy, and valve replacement surgery. Studies were performed with the signed informed consent of each patient according to a protocol approved by the hospital's Institutional Review Board. Patients (table 1) were divided into the two following groups based on preoperative cineangiographic left ventricular ejection fractions (LVEFs) determined during cardiac catheterization: the normal left ventricular function group (LVEF ≥0.55, 10 patients) and the poor left ventricular function group (LVEF < 0.55, 12 patients). None of the patients had severe pulmonary hypertension preoperatively. All studies were carried out in the operating room immediately before placing the patient on full cardiopulmonary bypass during open heart surgery. The study added 15 to 20 min to the operation and about 10 min to pump time.

TABLE 1
Patient characteristics

Patient	Sex	Age (yr)	Operation	Weight (kg)	BSA (m^2)	LVEF (%)
Normal LV function group (LVEF ≥ 55%)						
R. H.	M	46	ACB (3)	89	2.14	60
D. P.	M	73	ACB (2)	77	1.98	70
W. A.	M	55	ACB (4)	84	2.06	59
D. A.	M	53	ACB (1)	81	2.03	67
J. H.	M	38	ACB (3)	102	2.18	58
I. C.	M	73	ACB (3)	80	2.00	80
T. R.	M	46	ACB (3)	68	1.76	60
P. N.	M	53	ACB (4)	66	1.67	59
A. P.	M	61	ACB (1)	89	2.16	58
O. M.	M	63	ACB (5)	59	1.66	56
Mean ± SEM		56±4		80±4	1.96±0.06	63±2
Poor LV function group (LVEF < 55%)						
W. B.	M	63	AVR	74	1.87	51
D. S.	M	58	AVR	62	1.70	41
E. C.	M	81	LVA	82	1.95	23
C. W.	M	60	ACB (3)	74	1.94	38
J. D.	M	61	ACB (2)	78	1.89	46
E. T.	M	58	ACB (2)	89	2.10	51
S. D.	M	54	ACB (3)	71	1.76	25
J. F.	M	74	ACB (5)	65	1.76	36
W. K.	M	67	ACB (2)	72	1.89	46
R. S.	M	59	ACB (4)	64	1.70	34
A. M.	M	63	ACB (2)	78	1.87	51
D. M.	F	78	ACB (3)	45	1.44	32
Mean ± SEM		65±3		71±3	1.82±0.05	40±3

LV = left ventricular; BSA = body surface area; LVEF = preoperative cineangiographic ejection fraction; ACB = aortocoronary bypass (plus number of vessels bypassed); AVR = aortic valve replacement; LVA = left ventricular aneurysmectomy.

A median sternotomy was performed and the pericardium was opened. Venous blood was returned to the heart-lung machine by No. 40F wire-reinforced Bardic cannulas placed in the vena cavae. Arterial blood was returned to the systemic circulation with a No. 28F wire–reinforced cannula introduced into the ascending aorta. The left side of the heart was unloaded via a No. 32F curved wire–reinforced Bardic cannula introduced into the right superior pulmonary vein, through the left atrium, and across the mitral valve into the left ventricle. To obtain better flow the left ventricular vent cannula that was used was larger than the usual No. 24F to 28F size routinely used at this center. Arterial pressure was measured from the radial or femoral artery. A special triple-lumen Swan-Ganz catheter with a proximal port at 13 cm (Edwards Labs) was used to measure pulmonary arterial and right ventricular pressures and thermodilution cardiac output. Left ventricular pressure was measured through a catheter inserted into the left ventricular chamber via the left ventricular vent cannula. This measurement also confirmed adequate placement of the cannula in the ventricle.

Stroke volume was calculated as cardiac output divided by heart rate. Stroke work index was calculated as stroke volume times right ventricular developed pressure divided by body surface area. Systemic vascular resistance index was calculated as mean aortic pressure minus right ventricular end-diastolic pressure (in mm Hg) times 80 (to convert to dynes · sec · m^2/cm^5) divided by cardiac index. Pulmonary arterial input resistance index was calculated as mean pulmonary arterial pressure times 80 divided by cardiac index. Pulmonary vascular resistance was not calculated because left ventricular filling pressures during the suction effect of left ventricular bypass are not representative of changes in the pulmonary vasculature. All data were recorded on a Gould 2800 eight-channel recorder and analyzed on a PDP 11/23 computer.

At the beginning of the operative procedure, all electronic recording equipment was allowed to warm up; pressure transducers were zeroed and balanced to atmosphere and calibrated with a mercury manometer. During the experimental procedures the right ventricle was not manipulated, and measurements of right ventricular function were made before (control) and during left ventricular bypass. Control measurements were made during three to five thermodilution injections of iced 5% dextrose solution, and each value for each subject was calculated from the average of these findings.

To simulate the unloading effects of an LVAD, left ventricular bypass was initiated by opening the left ventricular vent to the heart-lung machine without opening the venous drainage system from the right atrium. The goal was to use this bypass circuit to pump blood from the left ventricle to the aorta to reduce left ventricular pressure as much as possible. No complications occurred as a result of this procedure. If any patient had become unstable, full bypass would have been initiated immediately. Once pressures had stabilized, measurements of ventricular function were again made during three to five thermodilution injections. Data were averaged by patient group, and statistical tests comparing control with left ventricular bypass for each value were performed with a paired t test. Comparisons between patient groups under control or left ventricular bypass conditions were performed by the Student t test.

Results

Under control conditions, stroke volume and cardiac output were significantly lower in the poor left ventricular function group than in the normal left ventricular function group, and right ventricular end-diastolic pressure, mean pulmonary arterial pressure, and pul-

TABLE 2
Summary of average values (± SEM) for each parameter before (control) and after left ventricular (LV) bypass

	Normal LV function group			Poor LV function group		
	Control	LV bypass	% Change	Control	LV bypass	% Change
SV	77±6	71±5	−3±10	58±3[D]	64±6	12±10
(ml)	(10)	(10)		(12)	(12)	
CO (l/min)	5.7±0.6	5.8±0.4	9±11	4.5±0.2[C]	5.3±0.4[A]	19±8
	(10)	(10)		(12)	(12)	
CI	2.9±0.2	3.0±0.2	9±10	2.5±0.1	2.9±0.2	18±8
(l·m^2/min)	(10)	(10)		(12)	(12)	
SWI	0.128±0.013	0.110±0.016	−13±9	0.129±0.021	0.097±0.020[A]	−22±10
(J/m^2)	(10)	(10)		(12)	(12)	
HR	74±4	84±3[A]	16±5	78±3	86±5	10±6
(beats/min)	(10)	(10)		(12)	(12)	
RVEDP	8±2	6±1[A]	−18±7	13±2[C]	8±2[A]	−37±10
(mm Hg)	(10)	(10)		(12)	(12)	
RVPSP	32±3	27±2	−15±10	42±4	27±3[B]	−34±5
(mm Hg)	(10)	(10)		(12)	(12)	
PAP	17±3	10±2[A]	−36±8	27±3[C]	12±2[B]	−53±5
(mm Hg)	(9)	(9)		(12)	(12)	
LVEDP	15±3	4±3[A]	−59±22	20±3	0±3[B]	−107±29
(mm Hg)	(10)	(9)		(11)	(12)	
LVPSP	108±6	56±11[B]	−45±11	101±6	27±9[B,C]	−79±8
(mm Hg)	(10)	(10)		(12)	(12)	
AOP	81±4	68±3[B]	−15±2	80±2	76±4	−4±4
(mm Hg)	(9)	(9)		(12)	(12)	
RinI	532±97	281±39[A]	−33±15	885±105[C]	354±50[B]	−57±6
(dynes·sec·m^2/cm^5)	(9)	(9)		(12)	(12)	
SVRI	2160±260	1804±206	−11±11	2287±124	2033±160	−10±8
(dynes·sec·m^2/cm^5)	(9)	(9)		(12)	(12)	

The number of patients used to calculate each mean is shown in parentheses.

SV = stroke volume; CO = cardiac output; CI = cardiac index; SWI = stroke work index; HR = heart rate; RVEDP and RVPSP = right ventricular end-diastolic and peak systolic pressures; PAP = mean pulmonary arterial pressure; LVEDP and LVPSP = left ventricular end-diastolic and peak systolic pressures; RinI = pulmonary vascular input resistance index; SVRI = systemic vascular resistance index.

[A]$p < .05$; [B]$p < .01$ compared with control, [C] $< .05$; [D]$p < .01$ compared with normal group.

monary arterial input resistance were higher (table 2). Left ventricular bypass produced significant reductions in left ventricular peak systolic and end-diastolic pressures for both groups, and left ventricular peak systolic pressure was reduced to a lower level in the poor left ventricular function group than in the normal group (figure 1, table 2). There was no change in cardiac output during left ventricular bypass in those patients with normal left ventricular function, but output was increased, with a drop in right ventricular end-diastolic pressure, in those with poor left ventricular function (figure 2, table 2). The relationship between cardiac output and right ventricular end-diastolic pressure (figure 3) shows a slight shift to the left during left ventricular bypass in the normal left ventricular function group but a significant shift upward and to the left in poor function group.

Right ventricular end-diastolic pressure, mean pulmonary arterial pressure (figure 4), and pulmonary arterial input resistance index were all significantly reduced in both groups during left ventricular bypass (table 2). There was a significant increase in heart rate and a decrease in mean aortic pressure during bypass only in the normal left ventricular function group, and there was no change in systemic vascular resistance index.

Discussion

This study indicates that left ventricular assistance in patients with normal left ventricular function produces no change in right ventricular function in terms of cardiac output, but does result in a beneficial reduction in right ventricular filling pressure. In patients with poor left ventricular function, left ventricular assistance results in improved right ventricular function, as demonstrated by an increase in cardiac output and a

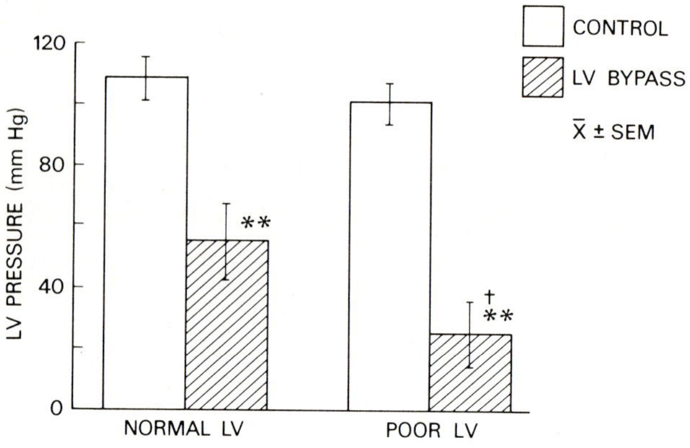

FIGURE 1. Left ventricular (LV) peak systolic pressure was significantly (** $p < .01$) reduced from control during LV bypass in patients with normal (normal LV) and in those with poor (poor LV) preoperative LVEFs. During LV bypass LV peak systolic pressure was significantly (†$p < .05$) lower in the poor LV group than in the normal LV group.

lower filling pressure. Left ventricular assistance in this acute operating room model produces no evidence of right ventricular failure in typical surgical patients with heart disease, and the data suggest that in patients with elevated pulmonary pressures secondary to poor left ventricular function it may offer a beneficial effect to the right heart.

The beneficial effect to the right ventricle during left ventricular bypass is primarily in the form of reduced pulmonary arterial pressure resulting from a reduction in left ventricular filling pressure. In those patients with poor left ventricular function, right ventricular peak systolic pressure and mean pulmonary arterial pressure were reduced 15 mm Hg during bypass, which paralleled the 20 mm Hg drop in left ventricular end-diastolic pressure. In the normal left ventricular function group, mean pulmonary arterial pressures fell 7 mm Hg during an 11 mm Hg drop in left ventricular

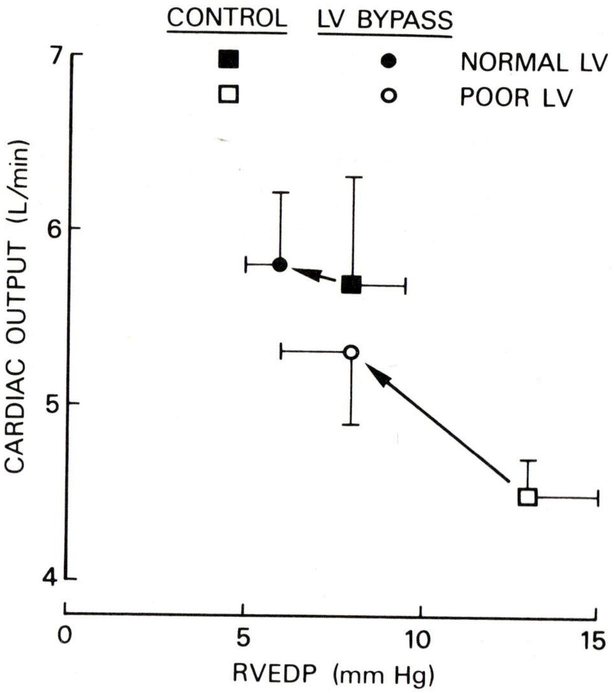

FIGURE 3. The relationship between cardiac output and right ventricular end-diastolic pressure (RVEDP) revealed a slight shift to the left from control to during left ventricular (LV) bypass in the normal LV group, and demonstrated a significant shift upward and to the left in the poor LV group.

end-diastolic pressure. These findings in human subjects compare with a 3 to 7 mm Hg decrease in mean pulmonary arterial pressure in normal dog hearts during a 5 to 16 mm Hg reduction in left ventricular end-diastolic pressure.[16] The decrease in right ventricular afterload produced by left ventricular bypass is more accurately described by a change in pulmonary arterial input resistance index, which is a measure of the resistive portion of the hydraulic afterload of the right ventricle. In the poor left ventricular function group input

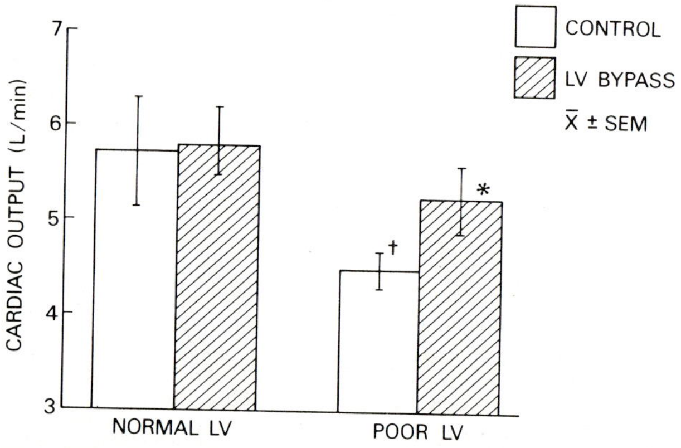

FIGURE 2. There was no change in cardiac output from control to during left ventricular (LV) bypass in the normal LV group, but it was significantly (*$p < .05$) increased in the poor LV group. Under control conditions cardiac output was signifiantly (†$p < .05$) lower in the poor LV group than in the normal group.

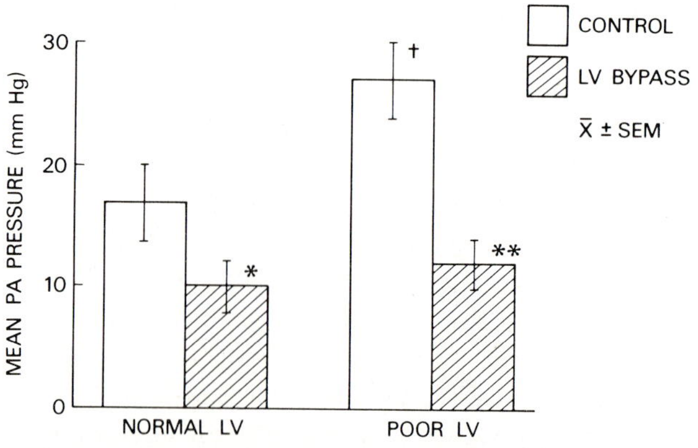

FIGURE 4. Mean pulmonary arterial (PA) pressure was significantly reduced from control to during left ventricular (LV) bypass in the normal LV group (*$p < .05$) and the poor LV group (**$p < .01$). Under control conditions mean PA pressure was significantly (†$p < .05$) greater in the poor LV group than in the normal LV group.

resistance index fell 57%, while in the normal left ventricular function group it decreased 33%; in studies on normal dog hearts input resistance decreased approximately 18%.

The comparison between the two patient groups plus the results from previous animal studies illustrate that the greater the depression of left ventricular function and the associated increase in pulmonary venous and arterial pressures, the greater the effect left ventricular bypass can have on reducing right ventricular afterload. Because of the linear relationship between pulmonary arterial and left atrial pressures in patients without pulmonary vascular obstructive disease,[19] an LVAD should be capable of reducing elevated pulmonary venous and arterial pressures back toward normal levels. However, in the presence of pulmonary vascular obstruction, right heart pressures are in excess of this relationship,[19, 20] and left ventricular assistance may have an opposite and detrimental effect on right ventricular outflow pressure due to augmented flow through the elevated pulmonary vascular resistance.[1] This is apparently what happened in a number of patients with LVADs reported by Pennington et al.,[8] in whom pulmonary vascular resistance increased in the first 12 postoperative hours, probably because of microemboli from multiple blood transfusions.

The most common cause of right ventricular failure is the increase in right ventricular afterload resulting from left ventricular failure.[20] Although at least one study has shown normal right ventricular performance in patients with mitral stenosis and moderate pulmonary hypertension,[21] most studies show the right ventricle to be markedly afterload dependent, with right ventricular ejection fraction being lower in patients with elevated pulmonary arterial pressure than in normal subjects.[22–24] In a preliminary transesophageal echocardiographic study in humans, we have shown right ventricular cross-sectional area to decrease by 29% in diastole and by 54% in systole, and fractional area change to increase from 42% to 63%, in response to a 19 mm Hg decrease in pulmonary arterial pressure during left heart bypass.[18] Similar results were also found in a patient supported with an LVAD for 10 days.[18] These decreases in right ventricular dimensions during left ventricular bypass are consistent with right ventricular afterload dependence, but appear to conflict with results of studies using ultrasonic crystals in dogs indicating an increase in right ventricular free wall-to-septum dimension with no change in fractional shortening during left ventricular unloading.[17] However, the differences can be explained by the fact that the large reduction in pulmonary arterial pressure was the dominant factor in the clinical studies and that the leftward septal shift was the dominant factor in the animal study, in which a much smaller change in pulmonary arterial pressure was noted.

Hypotheses based on studies of ventricular interdependence can explain at least three changes during left ventricular bypass that can affect the preload, afterload, and contractility of the right ventricle.[1] First, a translocation of blood volume from the pulmonary venous circulation to the systemic circulation by the LVAD can result in increased venous return to the right ventricle, thereby modifying right ventricular preload. Second, pulmonary arterial and right ventricular systolic pressures and wall stress (afterload) in patients with normal pulmonary vascular resistance may be reduced indirectly due to a reduction in left ventricular filling pressure produced by the translocation in blood volume away from the pulmonary circulation. Third, the septal contribution to right ventricular contraction may be reduced in some patients due to left ventricular pressure and volume unloading, effectively reducing right ventricular contractility.

The results of the present study support the second hypothesis, especially in the patients with poor preoperative left ventricular ejection fractions. The data from the poor left ventricular function group also show venous return and cardiac output to increase during left heart bypass, as predicted by the first hypothesis. In fact, increased venous return appeared to be handled easily by the right ventricle since the pulmonary arterial and right ventricular end-diastolic pressures decreased during left ventricular bypass. The third hypothesis cannot be tested by the data presented here, but it is supported by studies in normal dog hearts,[16, 25] as well as by studies from isolated hearts that show reduced right ventricular performance and reduced coupling between the ventricles when the left ventricle is pressure unloaded.[26–28]

Because it is easier to pressure unload a left ventricle with poor function (79% decrease in left ventricular peak systolic pressure) than with normal function (45% decrease in left ventricular peak systolic pressure), the effects on interventricular septal wall stress and its contribution to right ventricular function may differ in each group. Further unloading, as in some of the animal preparations, may produce even greater reductions in this contribution. Right ventricular function during left heart assistance is determined, therefore, by the resultant balance among these factors, a balance that most likely varies under different conditions of cardiac pathology.

An illustration of the interaction between these hy-

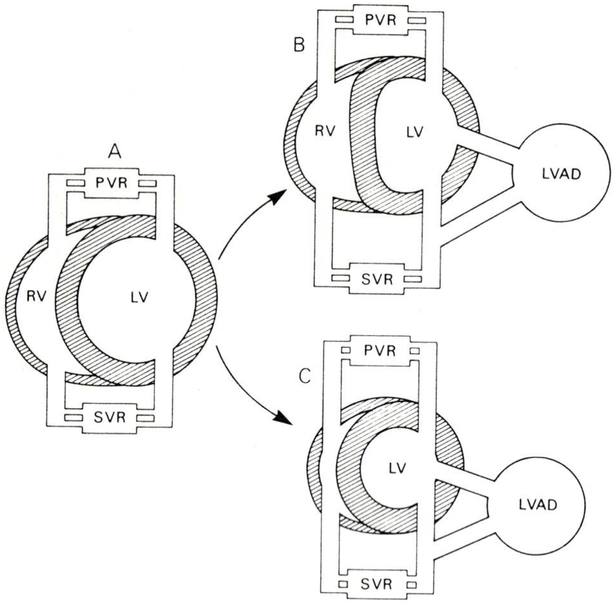

FIGURE 5. Hemodynamic interactions between the right ventricle (RV) and the left ventricle (LV) are due to the two hearts being in series, connected by the systemic (SVR) and pulmonary (PVR) vascular resistances; mechanical interactions are due to the anatomic coupling provided by the shared interventricular septum (*A*). An LVAD in parallel with the left ventricle (*B* and *C*) can alter right ventricular preload and afterload by shifting blood volume from the pulmonary to the systemic vascular systems. An LVAD that unloads the left ventricle can result in a leftward septal shift by reducing the transseptal pressure gradient (*B*). If the pulmonary arterial and right ventricular pressures are also reduced during left ventricular bypass then both ventricles can become dimensionally unloaded (*C*).

potheses is shown in figure 5. Left ventricular unloading with an LVAD may result in a leftward shift of the interventricular septum (figure 5, *B*) as blood is pumped by the LVAD in parallel with the left heart and in series with the right heart.[1, 17] However, if the pulmonary arterial pressure also falls during left ventricular bypass, then the right ventricle as well as the left ventricle may be dimensionally unloaded, as demonstrated by echocardiographic studies[18] and illustrated in figure 5, *C*. The relative septal displacement in each condition is determined by the transseptal pressure gradient,[29] or more accurately by the transseptal force gradient, which includes the effects of chamber configuration.[17]

Caution should be exercised in extending the results of this study of short-term left ventricular assistance to patients with LVADs over the long term or to those who receive LVADs after open heart surgery. Our results demonstrate that acute left ventricular unloading during left ventricular bypass does not result in right ventricular failure in patients undergoing routine open heart surgery. In fact, the resultant reduction in right ventricular afterload in patients with depressed preoperative left ventricular function produced an improvement in right ventricular function. The high incidence of right ventricular failure in the clinical experience with temporary LVADs is probably due to the fact that patients who require LVAD support have much more severely depressed biventricular function, possibly with perioperative infarction,[8] than any of the groups of patients or dogs from the model studies. Mechanical support of only one ventricle in a patient with biventricular failure may unmask the preexisting dysfunction of the other. In addition, patients with LVADs and elevated pulmonary vascular resistance due to obstructive disease or to other factors, such as those reported by Pennington et al.,[8] may not benefit from the right ventricular afterload reduction seen in the present study. In these cases the pumping ability of the right ventricle may not be able to match that of the LVAD. Future research should concentrate on the effect of left ventricular bypass on the three determinants of right ventricular function in patients with biventricular dysfunction or elevated pulmonary vascular resistance. The pathophysiology of other causes of right ventricular failure should also be investigated.

References

1. Farrar DJ, Compton PG, Hershon JJ, Fonger JD, Hill JD: Right heart interaction with the mechanically assisted left heart. World J Surg **9:** 89, 1985
2. Olsen EK, Pierce WS, Donachy JH, Landis DL, Rosenberg G, Phillips WM, Prophet GA, O'Neill MJ, Waldhausen JA: A two and one half year clinical experience with a mechanical left ventricular assist pump in the treatment of profound postoperative heart failure. Int J Artif Organs **2:** 197, 1979
3. Pae WE Jr, Rosenberg G, Donachy JH, Landis DL, Phillips WM, Parr GVS, Prophet GA, Pierce WS: Mechanical circulatory assistance for postoperative cardiogenic shock: a three year experience. Trans Am Soc Artif Intern Organs **26:** 256, 1980
4. Pierce WS, Parr GVS, Myers JL, Pae WE Jr, Bull AP, Waldhausen JA: Ventricular assist pumping in patients with cardiogenic shock after cardiac operations. N Engl J Med **305:** 1606, 1981
5. Parr GVS, Pierce WS, Williams DR, Wisman CB, O'Neill MJ, Waldhausen JA: Ventricular assist devices for shock after cardiac operations. Proc Am Acad Cardiovasc Perfusion **3:** 82, 1982
6. Golding LR, Jacobs G, Groves LK, Gill CC, Nosé Y, Loop FD: Clinical results of mechanical support of the failing left ventricle. J Thorac Cardiovasc Surg **83:** 597, 1982
7. Pennington DG, Merjavy JP, Swartz MT, Willman VL: Clinical experience with a centrifugal pump ventricular assist device. Trans Am Soc Artif Intern Organs **28:** 93, 1982
8. Pennington DG, Merjavy JP, Swartz MT, Codd JE, Barner HB, Lagunoff D, Bashiti H, Kaiser GC, Willman VL: The importance of biventricular failure in patients with postoperative cardiogenic shock. Ann Thorac Surg **39:** 16, 1985
9. Turina MT, Bosio R, Senning A: Paracorporeal artificial heart in postoperative heart failure. Artif Organs **2:** 273, 1978
10. Holub DA, Hibbs CW, Sturm JT, Fuqua JM, Edmonds CH, McGee MG, Fuhrman TM, Trono R, Igo SR, Norman JC: Clinical trials of the abdominal left ventricular assist device (ALVAD): progress report. Trans Am Soc Artif Intern Organs **25:** 197, 1979
11. Norman JC, Duncan JM, Frazier OH, Hallman G, Ott DA, Reul GL, Cooley DA: Intracorporeal (abdominal) left ventricular assist devices or partial artificial hearts. A five-year clinical experience. Arch Surg **116:** 1441, 1981

12. Bernhard WF, Berger RL, Stetz JP, Carr JG, Colo NA, McCormick JR, Fishbein MC: Temporary left ventricular bypass: factors affecting patient survival. Circulation **60** (suppl I): I-131, 1979
13. Koffsky RM, Litwak RS, Mitchell BL, Jurado RA: A simple left heart assist device for use after intracardiac surgery: development, deployment and clinical experience. Artif Organs **2:** 257, 1978
14. Litwak RS, Koffsky RM, Jurado RA, Mindich BP, Fischer AP, Silvay G, Gomez E: Concepts and clinical experience with a left ventricular assist device after intracardiac operation. *In* Unger F, editor: Assisted circulation. Berlin, 1979, Springer Verlag, 199–208
15. Rose DM, Colvin SB, Culliford AT, Isom OW, Cunningham JN Jr, Glassman E, Spencer FC: Late functional and hemodynamic status of surviving patients following insertion of the left heart assist device. J Thorac Cardiovasc Surg **86:** 639, 1983
16. Farrar DJ, Compton PG, Dajee H, Fonger JD, Hill JD: Right heart function during left heart assist and the effects of volume loading in a canine preparation. Circulation **70:** 708, 1984
17. Farrar DJ, Compton PG, Hershon JJ, Fonger JD, Hill JD. Right ventricular pressure dimension relationship during left ventricular assistance in dogs. Trans Am Soc Artif Int Organs **30:** 121, 1984
18. Hershon JJ, Farrar DJ, Compton PG, Hill JD: Right ventricular dimensions with transesophageal echocardiography during an operating room model of left heart assist. Trans Am Soc Artif Int Organs **30:** 129, 1984
19. Walston A, Peter RH, Morris JJ, Kong Y, Behar VS: Clinical implications of pulmonary hypertension in mitral stenosis. Am J Cardiol **32:** 650, 1973
20. Weber KT, Janicki JS, Shroff SG, Likoff MJ, St. John Sutton MG: The right ventricle: physiologic and pathophysiologic considerations. Crit Care Med **11:** 323, 1983
21. Wroblewski E, James F, Spann JF, Bove AA: Right ventricular performance in mitral stenosis. Am J Cardiol **47:** 51, 1981
22. Korr KS, Gandsman EJ, Winkler ML, Shulman RS, Bough EW: Hemodynamic correlates of right ventricular ejection fraction measured with gated radionuclide angiography. Am J Cardiol **49:** 71, 1982
23. Brent BN, Berger HJ, Matthay RA, Mahler D, Pytlik L, Zaret BL: Physiologic correlates of right ventricular ejection fraction in chronic obstructive pulmonary disease: a combined radionuclide and hemodynamic study. Am J Cardiol **50:** 255, 1982
24. Morrison D, Goldman S, Wright AL, Henry R, Sorenson S, Caldwell J, Ritchie J: The effect of pulmonary hypertension on systolic function of the right ventricle. Chest **84:** 250, 1983
25. Miyamoto AT, Tanaka S, Matloff JM: Right ventricular function during left heart bypass. J Thorac Cardiovasc Surg **85:** 49, 1983
26. Santamore WP, Lynch PR, Heckman JL, Bove AA, Meier GD: Left ventricular effects on right ventricular developed pressure. J Appl Physiol **41:**925, 1976
27. Janicki JS, Weber KT: The pericardium and ventricular interaction, distensibility, and function. Am J Physiol **238:** H494, 1980
28. Elzinga G, Piene H, deJong JP: Left and right ventricular pump function and consequences of having two pumps in one heart. Circ Res **46:** 564, 1980
29. Kingma I, Tyberg JV, Smith ER: Effects of diastolic transseptal pressure gradient on ventricular septal position and motion. Circulation **68:** 1304, 1983

Intermittent failure of local conduction during ventricular tachycardia

JOHN M. MILLER, M.D., JOSEPH A. VASSALLO, M.D., W. CLARK HARGROVE, M.D., AND MARK E. JOSEPHSON, M.D.

ABSTRACT Forty-three patients with sustained ventricular tachycardia (VT) caused by prior myocardial infarction underwent intraoperative endocardial activation mapping during a total of 122 episodes of VT. Electrograms obtained during mapping were analyzed to determine the prevalence of local conduction failure during VT (defined as a portion of the local electrogram that did not repeat with every tachycardia cycle). Local conduction failure during VT was observed in 37 (86%) patients and 73 (65%) tachycardias. VT in which local conduction failure was observed were faster than VTs without local conduction failure (cycle length 315 vs 345 msec; $p < .05$). Local conduction failure occurred most frequently at or near sites having the earliest recorded electrical activity during VT ("site of origin"). Twenty-three patients also had sinus rhythm endocardial mapping at the time of surgery. Areas with abnormal or fractionated electrograms in sinus rhythm were more likely to demonstrate local conduction failure in VT than areas with normal electrograms in sinus rhythm (16% vs 8%; $p < .01$). Although the mechanism responsible for local conduction failure in VT is unclear, it is a common occurrence and is significant in that it can occasionally mimic "early" sites of endocardial activation, unless enough VT cycles are observed at a given site.
Circulation **72, No. 6, 1286–1292, 1985.**

INTRAOPERATIVE activation mapping during ventricular tachycardia (VT) has been used for several years to guide surgical therapy of malignant ventricular arrhythmias.[1, 2] With this technique, the local electrical activity from numerous endocardial or epicardial sites is sampled during induced VT with the aim of finding the earliest recorded site of electrical activity, which has been termed the "site of origin" of VT. Occasionally, part of the local electrogram obtained during mapping does not repeat with every tachycardia beat. We have termed this phenomenon intermittent local conduction failure (LCF). This study was undertaken to determine (1) the incidence of intermittent LCF during intraoperative activation mapping in VT, (2) factors associated with the development of LCF during VT, and (3) possible underlying mechanisms for this phenomenon.

From the Clinical Electrophysiology Laboratory, Hospital of the University of Pennsylvania, Cardiology Section, Department of Medicine, University of Pennsylvania School of Medicine, Philadelphia.

Supported in part by grants from the American Heart Association, Southeastern Pennsylvania Chapter, Philadelphia, and grants HL00361 and HL24278 from the NHLBI.

Address for correspondence: Mark E. Josephson, M.D., Cardiovascular Section, Hospital of the University of Pennsylvania, 3400 Spruce St., Room 658, Ravdin Bldg., Philadelphia, PA 19104.

Received May 20, 1985; revision accepted Sept. 5, 1985.

Dr. Josephson is the Robinette Foundation Professor of Medicine (Cardiovascular Diseases).

Methods

The study population consisted of 43 patients who underwent intraoperative mapping-guided subendocardial resection for drug refractory sustained VT. There were 35 men and eight women, with ages ranging from 39 to 72 years (mean 57). All patients had suffered prior transmural myocardial infarctions (37 anterior, six inferior), from 1 month to 10 years before surgery. All patients had failed a mean 4.7 drug trials before the consideration of surgical therapy.

The operative procedure consisted of a median sternotomy and initiation of normothermic cardiopulmonary bypass. The left ventricle was opened at the site of an aneurysm or previous infarction, and sustained VT was induced by programmed electrical stimulation. Endocardial activation mapping during VT was carried out with a single roving bipolar probe electrode (interelectrode distance 1 to 2 mm) according to a predetermined sequence of data acquisition (clockface format).[3] A mean of 36 sites were sampled during each distinct VT morphology. Different VT morphologies in each patient were distinguished by comparison of three to four surface electrocardiographic leads as well as bipolar reference electrograms (using Teflon-coated stainless wires embedded in the endocardium) from each ventricle. Signals from the probe electrogram were amplified, filtered at 50 to 400 Hz, and recorded along with the surface and reference electrograms on paper (Siemens-Elema 16 Channel Ink Jet Recorder, 200 mm/sec paper speed) and on analog tape (Honeywell Model 5600). At least eight VT cycles from each endocardial site were recorded with the probe electrogram and analyzed postoperatively. Procainamide (500 to 1500 mg) was administered to 19 patients during intraoperative mapping to facilitate induction or mapping of VT (by slowing the cycle length). Twenty-three of the patients also underwent extensive sinus rhythm endocardial activation mapping of at least 20 endocardial sites according to a clockface grid as described previously.[3] Endocardial mapping time during normothermic cardiopulmonary bypass was 1 hr or less in all cases.

Definitions. LCF was said to occur when a repetitive portion of an endocardial electrogram did not repeat with every tachycardia beat.

Site of origin of VT was defined as the endocardial site from which the earliest electrogram in the latter half of diastole was recorded in that tachycardia.

Intraoperative sinus rhythm endocardial electrograms were arbitrarily classified as follows:

A normal electrogram was an electrogram with a discrete spike having an amplitude of greater than 1 mV and a duration less than 70 msec. All other electrograms were classified as abnormal.

A fractionated electrogram was an abnormal electrogram with multiple high-frequency components having an amplitude less than 0.3 mV and a duration greater than 90 msec.

Examples of these definitions are seen in figure 1.

Additional electrogram types were as follows:

A split electrogram was an abnormal electrogram with at least two discrete spikes, separated by at least 30 msec.

A late electrogram was one in which electrical activity extended beyond the end of the surface QRS complex.

An individual electrogram could be classified in more than one way, i.e., both fractionated and late.

Statistical analyses. Continuous variables were compared by Students' unpaired t test and categorical variables were compared by the chi-square test with Yates' correction for continuity. All tests were subject to a $p < .05$ level of significance.

Results

Patients. Thirty-seven of the 43 patients (86%) in this series demonstrated intermittent LCF at at least one endocardial site during VT. LCF was observed in all patients with inferior myocardial infarction and 31 out of 37 (84%) patients with previous anterior infarctions ($p =$ NS). The administration of procainamide during mapping did not significantly influence the prevalence of LCF; 18 out of 19 patients who received procainamide demonstrated LCF, and 19 out of 24 who did not receive procainamide demonstrated LCF ($p =$ NS).

VT. Seventy-three out of 112 (65%) tachycardias in this series demonstrated intermittent LCF. The overall incidence of LCF was approximately one out of eight sites recorded. The predominant pattern of conduction failure was 2:1; less common was Wenckebach periodicity (5% to 10% of instances) (figure 2) or variable conduction patterns. The mean cycle length of tachycardias during which LCF was observed was shorter than the cycle length of tachycardias not demonstrating intermittent LCF (315 ± 74 vs 345 ± 77 msec [mean ± SD]; $p < .05$).

Intermittent LCF occurred more frequently at or near sites of origin of the same or another VT. We have shown in a prior study of postinfarction patients with multiple morphologically distinct VT[4] that different VTs are mapped to the same or adjacent areas (<3 cm distant) in 85% to 90% of patients. Twenty-two percent of instances of intermittent LCF were recorded at a site of origin of the same or another VT; 51% were observed within a 1 cm radius of the site from which the earliest electrogram during VT was recorded, and 75% of examples of LCF were recorded from within 2 cm of the site of origin of VT. Twenty-five percent of instances of LCF were recorded from sites more than 2 cm distant from a site of origin of VT. Although the distribution of endocardial sampling was more dense near sites of origin, the prevalences noted above are significantly different from those of all sites recorded during VT ($p < .001$).

The administration of procainamide during mapping again had no statistically significant effect on the prev-

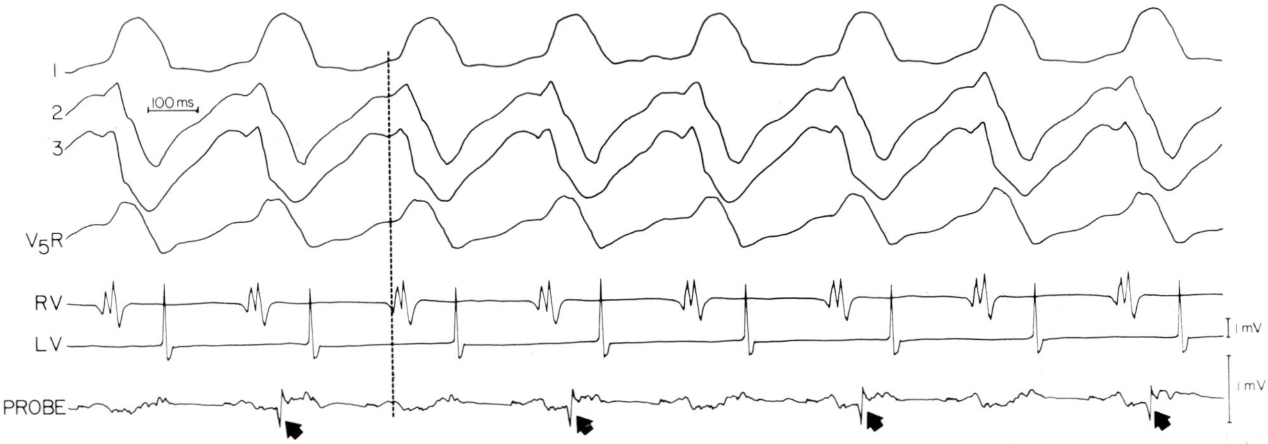

FIGURE 1. LCF recorded during VT. Surface ECG leads I, II, III, and V_5R are displayed with endocardial reference electrograms from the right (RV) and left (LV) ventricles, as well as a roving electrode (PROBE). Time and amplitude scales are also displayed. The vertical dashed line denotes the onset of the surface QRS complex. Part of the PROBE electrogram repeats with every tachycardia beat, but part (arrows) repeats every other beat. This is an example of LCF during VT. The PROBE electrogram is fractionated (see definitions) and was recorded from the "site of origin" of this tachycardia. The LV electrogram is an example of a normal electrogram (see definitions). Analog signals in this and subsequent figures traced from original.

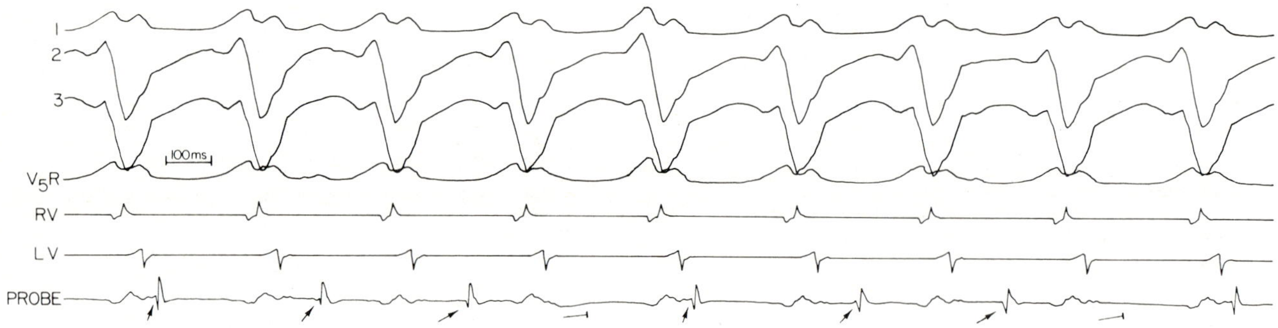

FIGURE 2. LCF demonstrating Wenckebach periodicity. Format and abbreviations as in figure 1. Part of the PROBE electrogram (arrows) occurs at progressively longer intervals from the constant portion of the electrogram, until it finally fails to appear (—|), after which the cycle repeats in a 4:3 conduction ratio.

alence of LCF in individual VTs. Twenty-six out of 39 (67%) of VTs mapped after administration of procainamide demonstrated LCF, and 47 out of 73 (64%) of VTs without drug administration demonstrated LCF (p = NS).

Procainamide was administered after mapping of one VT morphology but before mapping other VT morphologies in 5 patients. LCF was observed in all VTs in two of these patients; LCF was not observed in VTs mapped after procainamide in one patient; and LCF was observed only in VTs mapped after procainamide was given in the other two patients. Of note, in these latter two patients, procainamide facilitated the induction of a more rapid VT (cycle lengths 85 and 90 msec less than previous VT), which may have accounted for the occurrence of LCF in these VTs.

Intermittent LCF was recorded with approximately equal frequency from all regions of the endocardium; among patients in whom LCF was recorded, the percent of septal, anterior wall, and inferior wall sites demonstrating LCF was 15%, 13%, and 10%, respectively (p = NS). The surface electrocardiographic QRS morphology of VT had no influence on the prevalence of LCF during mapping (right vs left bundle branch block pattern, inferior vs superior axis, right or left axis).

Sinus rhythm mapping (table 1). Twenty-three patients had extensive sinus rhythm endocardial activation mapping. A mean 53 ± 15 sites were sampled during sinus rhythm. Eight percent of sites with normal electrograms in sinus rhythm demonstrated intermittent LCF during VT, whereas 16% of sites with abnormal electrograms in sinus rhythm demonstrated LCF in VT ($p < .001$). Among the subclassifications of abnormal electrograms, intermittent LCF was also more likely to occur at sites with fractionated (16%), split (24%), and late (19%) electrograms in sinus rhythm than at normal sites (all $p \leq .01$).

Discussion

Comparison with prior studies. Intermittent LCF has been observed in a canine preparation of infarction-associated VT as reported by Boineau and Cox[5] and El-Sherif et al.[6] These investigators demonstrated 2:1 conduction of late potentials recorded from the infarct zone using intramural and epicardial mapping. Bailey et al.[7] reported a case of intermittent LCF recorded in man with an endocardial catheter. These investigators administered procainamide to the patient and observed a late potential change from 1:1 conduction to 3:2 and finally 2:1 conduction, and believed that procainamide was responsible for this effect. In the current study, administration of procainamide did not influence the incidence of intermittent LCF during the recording of large numbers of endocardial electrograms. LCF was first observed after administration of procainamide in two of our patients but not during the same VT. Procainamide might be expected to facilitate LCF by causing prolonged refractoriness, but this effect may be counterbalanced by the drug's effect on conduction velocity and VT rate (making LCF less frequent).

Gilmour et al.[8] studied cellular electrophysiologic

TABLE 1
Prevalence of local conduction failure in VT according to type of sinus rhythm electrogram

Sinus rhythm electrogram	LCF Present	LCF Absent	p value (vs normal sites)
Normal	45 (8%)	517 (92%)	—
Abnormal	109 (16%)	553 (84%)	.001
Fractionated	28 (16%)	149 (84%)	.001
Split	7 (24%)	22 (76%)	.01
Late	18 (19%)	83 (81%)	.001

characteristics of endocardial resection specimens and observed intermittent LCF during pacing in several instances. Regions from which LCF was recorded had a decrease in resting membrane potential as well as a decrease in upstroke velocity of the action potential (dv/dt). Cellular electrophysiologic studies were not performed on endocardial resection specimens in the present series for comparison with the above studies. Additionally, these studies in vitro must be interpreted with caution because the abnormalities recorded may have resulted from tissue damage during removal or handling and have little relationship to events in vivo.

Cause of LCF. The exact electrophysiologic abnormalities responsible for the phenomenon of intermittent LCF are not clear, but several possibilities exist. Microanatomic factors may be responsible for failure of impulse transmission from one group of cells to another. Cardiac histopathologic findings in a population of patients with prior infarction and VT[9] have shown isolated bundles of ventricular myocardium, five to 10 cells thick, separated by dense fibrous bands. Presumably, these thin bands of muscle are connected to more normal myocardium at the borders of the infarction. These thin bundles of ventricular muscle may be analagous to thin strips of atrial muscle forming a bridge between large muscle segments, as studyed by de La Fuentes et al.[10] These investigations observed 2:1 conduction of impulses across these thin bridges of atrial muscle and ascribed this to "impedance mismatch." Likewise, the direction of impulse propagation relative to microanatomic fiber orientation, and resultant changes in intercellular resistance (anisotropy), may play a critical role in producing abnormal conduction.[11] Spach et al.[12] observed that, even in normal canine atrial muscle, anisotropic influences on impulse propagation could produce conduction delay, unidirectional block, Wenckebach periodicity, or 2:1 conduction failure. The abnormal microanatomy[9] in patients with extensive endocardial scar (nonuniform anisotropy) could also yield abnormal patterns of conduction.

Abnormalities of cellular and tissue electrophysiology, independent of anatomic factors, may also be responsible for intermittent LCF. These would include increased refractoriness (local refractory period greater than VT cycle length), as has been observed in experimental infarctions.[13] Calcium channel–dependent action potential prolongation has been invoked by El Sherif et al.[6] as a cause of LCF in a canine preparation of VT. These investigators abolished LCF in these preparations by administering D-600, a methoxy derivative of verapamil. Altered time dependence of recovery of excitability has been observed to be responsible for the creation of block in certain circumstances.[14, 15] Saltatory conduction via passive electrotonic influences can result in asynchronous and markedly abnormal conduction.[16] Finally, the decreasing efficacy of a wavefront to elicit a downstream action potential, such as occurs normally in the atrioventricular node,[17, 18] may also be responsible for LCF. Regardless of what abnormalities account for LCF on the cellular or tissue level, both the cycle length dependence of intermittent LCF and its occurrence in areas with abnormal sinus rhythm electrograms (as shown in this study) suggest that significantly diseased tissue is involved. The anatomic correlate of abnormal and fractionated sinus rhythm electrograms is not clear, although preliminary studies[19] suggest that fractionated electrograms can be caused by myocardial cells with normal action potentials and upstroke velocity of the action potential, but poor cell-to-cell coupling. Thus, further studies are needed to evaluate the cellular and anatomic features associated with, and perhaps responsible for, intermittent LCF.

It is conceivable that LCF is actually recording atrial electrical activity during VT, which often is observed in a 2:1 or Wenckebach conduction ratio. Atrial electrograms were not routinely recorded during intraoperative studies in this series, but we believe atrial activity is unlikely to be the cause of LCF because (1) LCF was observed frequently in sites near the left ventricular apex, several centimeters removed from atrial tissue; (2) five of the patients who demonstrated LCF were in chronic atrial fibrillation during intraoperative mapping; and (3) LCF was occasionally recorded from extremely localized areas (figure 3). It is also possible that intermittent recording of subendocardial Purkinje fibers could account for examples of LCF. Histopathologic study of endocardial resection specimens[9] has revealed Purkinje fibers in septal and papillary muscle endocardial specimens but not in free-wall endocardium. LCF was observed in equal frequency throughout the left ventricular endocardium in the present study, however, which is at variance with the distribution of endocardial Purkinje fibers in this patient population. Although we cannot exclude Purkinje tissue as the site and source of intermittent LCF, ventricular myocardial cells may be a more plausible source of intermittent LCF. Cellular electrophysiologic abnormalities recorded from surviving ventricular myocardial cells in regions of previous infarction[8] are similar to findings in animal preparations[6, 13] in which intermittent LCF was also observed. Regardless of the cells responsible for intermittent LCF, it is clear that they

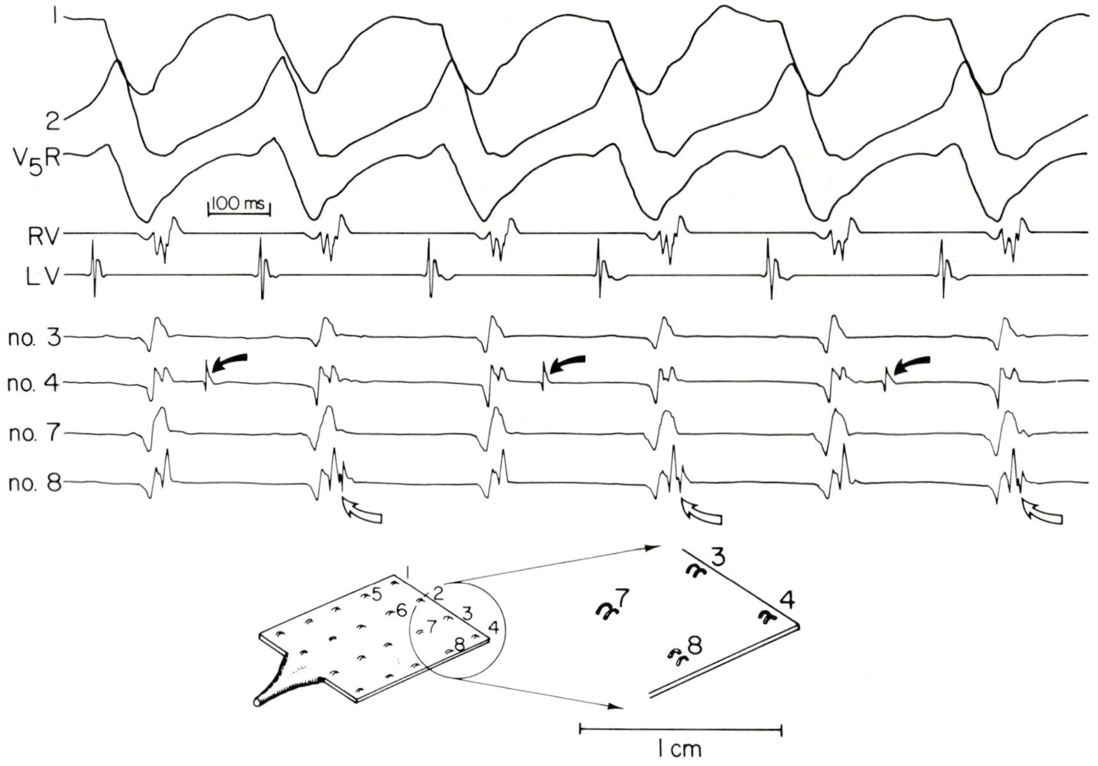

FIGURE 3. Localized nature of LCF in VT. Format and abbreviations as in figure 1. The four lines beneath the LV tracing are recordings from four bipoles on a multipolar electrode matrix, illustrated below. One corner of this matrix containing electrodes 3, 4, 7, and 8 is enlarged at right, with a distance scale beneath. Bipoles are 4 mm apart. In the recordings from these bipoles, local conduction failure is observed in Nos. 4 and 8 (arrows) but not Nos. 3 and 7 (only 4 mm away). Additionally, local conduction failure occurs on opposite beats in bipole Nos. 4 and 8 (open and filled arrows).

are not necessary for the perpetuation of VT, since they are activated only every other beat or less frequently.

Finally, it is also possible that the phenomenon we observed is not really "failure" of local conduction but rather a beat-by-beat change in the direction of part of the excitation wavefront as it passed beneath the recording bipole (perpendicularly) so that no signal was recorded on every other beat, although the tissue was still being activated. This would most likely result in an alteration in configuration or amplitude of part of the electrogram rather than complete absence. Additionally, figure 3 suggests that at least in some instances, LCF is not caused by such changes in wavefront direction relative to the recording bipole, since several closely spaced bipoles still failed to record some of the intermittent potentials. Thus, although changes in wavefront direction could conceivably account for the appearance of LCF in some cases, we believe it is not a frequent cause of the phenomenon.

Significance. Since 75% of sites demonstrating intermittent LCF are found within 2 cm of a VT site of origin, it may be argued that subendocardial resection or other surgical procedures could be directed at areas demonstrating LCF. This would not seem to hold much promise, in that it is still necessary to extensively map VT to find sites with intermittent LCF, and 25% of instances of LCF occur at sites greater than 2 cm distant from any VT site of origin. Thus more extensive resections would be undertaken than would be necessary to eradicate VT, and little would be gained by directing surgery in this way.

Occasionally, intermittent LCF can mimic a site of origin, as shown in figure 4. In this example, the timing of the portion of the local electrogram that undergoes LCF is such that it appears to be significantly presystolic, but if observed for enough cycles, it eventually demonstrates 2:1 or Wenckebach block. The portion of the local electrogram that is repetitive from cycle to cycle (1:1) is clearly not "early." This "pseudo–early site" is fortunately an uncommon phenomenon, occurring in only five of the tachycardias in the present series. Nonetheless, caution must be exercised in interpreting "early" sites that occur in isolation, with sites immediately surrounding it having a substantially later electrogram timing. In each of the five cases in which LCF mimicked an early site in this series, it was recognized as being spurious because of the large dis-

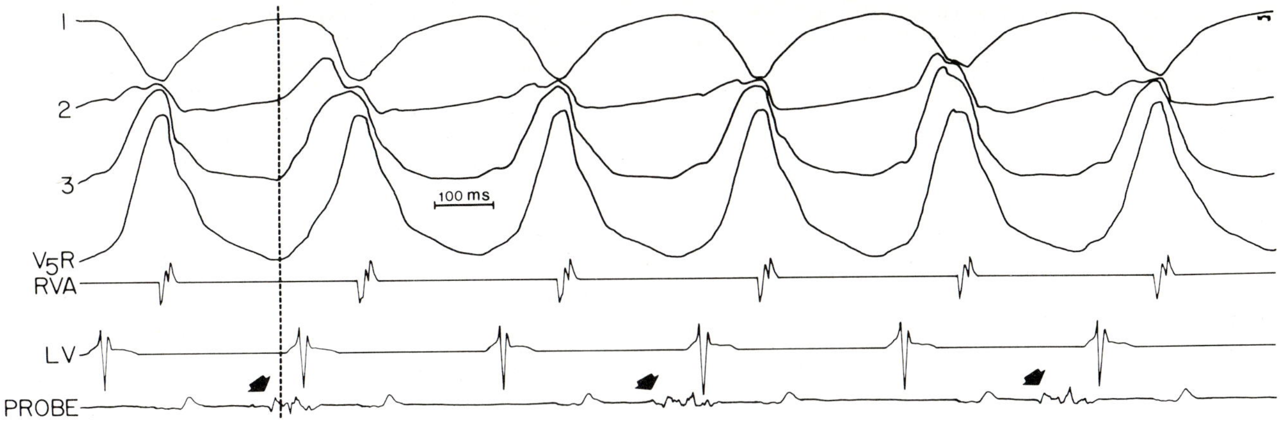

FIGURE 4. LCF simulating a tachycardia site of origin. Format and abbreviations as in figure 1. RVA = RV apex. The vertical dotted line denotes the onset of the surface QRS complex. Where this line crosses the PROBE tracing, a portion of the electrogram (arrow) appears to be some 40 msec presystolic and might be considered a site of origin of this VT; however, this portion of the PROBE electrogram fails to appear on each of the subsequent tachycardia beats and thus demonstrates LCF. The constant portion of the PROBE electrogram occurs some 150 msec *after* the surface QRS complex begins. This illustrates the need to carefully evaluate multiple tachycardia cycles.

parity in timing of electrograms from adjacent sites. The use of sophisticated and expensive computer systems that simultaneously analyze multiple endocardial sites during only a few VT beats could obviously yield misleading information as a result of LCF. Analysis of a large number of VT complexes may thus be required to exclude LCF as a cause of "early" electrograms.

Limitations. The administration of antiarrhythmic drug during intraoperative mapping, which could conceivably produce or eliminate intermittent LCF by altering conduction and/or refractoriness, was not controlled in this series. However, there was no statistical difference in the prevalence of intermittent LCF in patients who received drug vs those not receiving drug during mapping, nor among individual tachycardias that were mapped with or without the influence of antiarrhythmic drug; however, the numbers of patients in each subgroup were small. Additionally, the possibility that intermittent LCF may be caused by the recording of a distant atrial electrogram has not been definitely excluded in this study by systematic recording of atrial activity; this limitation has been discussed above.

A major limitation is the reproducibility of location of endocardial sites in comparing sinus rhythm electrograms and those during VT. This may account for at least some of the instances of intermittent LCF recorded at sites that had normal electrograms in sinus rhythm, although anisotropy or other anatomic or physiologic factors may have been responsible as well. Electrograms of a given variety (normal, abnormal, fractionated) tend to occur in clusters on the endocardium,[3] and thus a small (1 cm) error in location is unlikely to have a profound influence on the type of electrogram obtained. Nonetheless, this is a significant limitation in the current study.

Conclusions. This study demonstrates that intermittent failure of local endocardial conduction during intraoperative endocardial mapping of VT is a frequent finding. LCF is more commonly observed in tachycardias with a shorter cycle length and more frequently occurs at sites having abnormal or fractionated electrical activity than at sites with normal electrograms in sinus rhythm. Intermittent LCF is frequently observed at or near sites of origin of VT and can on occasion mimic a site of origin because of fortuitous timing of the intermittent electrogram relative to the onset of the surface QRS. The exact cause of this phenomenon, as well as the tissues responsible, are unknown at present. Further work is needed to resolve these issues.

We thank Nancy L. Walker for excellent secretarial assistance in the preparation of the manuscript.

References

1. Horowitz LN, Josephson ME, Harken AH: Epicardial and endocardial activation mapping during sustained ventricular tachycardia in man. Circulation **61:** 1227, 1980
2. Waldo AL, Archiniegas JG, Klein H: Surgical treatment of life-threatening arrhythmias: the role of intraoperative mapping and consideration of the presently available surgical techniques. Prog Cardiovasc Dis **23:** 247, 1981
3. Kienzle MG, Miller JM, Falcone RA, Harken AH, Josephson ME: Intraoperative endocardial mapping during sinus rhythm: relation to site of origin of ventricular tachycardia. Circulation **70:** 957, 1984
4. Miller JM, Kienzle MG, Harken AH, Josephson ME: Morphologically distinct sustained ventricular tachycardias in coronary artery disease: significance and surgical results. J Am Coll Cardiol **4:** 1073, 1984

5. Boineau JP, Cox JL: Slow ventricular activation in acute myocardial infarction: a source of reentrant premature ventricular contractions. Circulation **48:** 702, 1973
6. El-Sherif N, Lazzara R: Reentrant ventricular arrhythmias in the late myocardial infarction period. 7. Effect of verapamil and D-600 and the role of the "slow-channel." Circulation **60:** 605, 1979
7. Bailey B, Tan A: The effect of procainamide on delayed action potentials in a patient with ventricular tachycardia. PACE **3:** 695, 1980
8. Gilmour RF, Heger JJ, Prystowsky EN, Zipes DP: Cellular electrophysiologic abnormalities of diseased human ventricular myocardium. Am J Cardiol **51:** 137, 1983
9. Fenoglio JJ, Pham TD, Harken AH, Horowitz LN, Josephson ME, Wit AL: Recurrent sustained ventricular tachycardia: structure and ultrastructure of subendocardial regions in which tachycardia originates. Circulation **68:** 518, 1983
10. de la Fuentes D, Sasyniuk B, Moe GK: Conduction through a narrow isthmus in isolated canine atrial tissue: a model of the Wolff-Parkinson-White syndrome. Circulation **44:** 803, 1971
11. Spach MS, Miller WT, Geselowitz DB, Barr RC, Kootsey JM, Johnson EA: The discontinuous nature of propagation in normal canine cardiac muscle: evidence for recurrent discontinuities of intracellular resistance that affect the membrane currents. Circ Res **48:** 39, 1981
12. Spach MS, Miller WT, Dolber PJ, Kootsey JM, Sommer JR, Mosher CE: The functional role of structural complexities in the propagation of depolarization in the atrium of the dog: cardiac conduction disturbances due to discontinuities of effective axial resistivity. Circ Res **50:** 175, 1982
13. Wong SS, Bassell AL, Cameron JA, Epstein K, Kozlovskis P, Myerburg RJ: Dissimilarities in the electrophysiological abnormalities of lateral border and central infarct zone cells after healing of myocardial infarction in cats. Circ Res **51:** 486, 1982
14. Allessie MA, Bonke FJM, Shopman FJG: Circus movement tachycardia in rabbit atrial muscle as a mechanism of tachycardia. II. The role of nonuniform recovery of excitability in the occurrence of unidirectional block, as studied with multiple microelectrodes. Circ Res **39:** 168, 1976
15. Han J, Moe GK: Nonuniform recovery of excitability in ventricular muscle. Circ Res **14:** 44, 1964
16. Schaffer A, DePasquale NP: Mechanisms of Wenckebach AV block and the obligatory ventricular echo. Cardiovasc Res **7:** 696, 1973
17. Paes de Carvallho A, de Almeida DF: Spread of activity through the atrioventricular node. Circ Res **8:** 801, 1960
18. Wennemark JR, Bandura JP: Microelectrode study of periodicity in canine Purkinje fibers. Am J Cardiol **33:** 390, 1974
19. Gardner PI, Ursell PC, Pham TD, Fenoglio JJ, Wit AL: Experimental chronic ventricular tachycardia: anatomic and electrophysiologic substrates. *In* Josephson ME, Wellens HJJ, editors: Tachycardias: mechanisms, diagnosis, treatment. Philadelphia, 1983, Lea and Febiger, pp 29–60

Further observations on transient entrainment: importance of pacing site and properties of the components of the reentry circuit

KEN OKUMURA, M.D., RICHARD W. HENTHORN, M.D., ANDREW E. EPSTEIN, M.D., VANCE J. PLUMB, M.D., AND ALBERT L. WALDO, M.D.

ABSTRACT Transient entrainment of circus-movement tachycardia utilizing an atrioventricular (AV) bypass pathway was studied in 13 patients (nine with the orthodromic form, two with the antidromic form, and two with both the orthodromic and antidromic forms). All patients had a left-sided AV bypass pathway. Pacing at selected rates faster than the spontaneous rate was performed during the tachycardia at a site proximal or distal to the AV node, an area of slow conduction within the reentry loop. Rapid pacing from a site proximal to the AV node (from the right atrium during the orthodromic form of the arrhythmia or the right ventricle during the antidromic form of the arrhythmia) always demonstrated at least one of the three entrainment criteria: constant fusion beats except for the last captured beat, which was entrained but not fused (first criterion); progressive fusion (second criterion); localized conduction block to a site(s) for 1 paced beat associated with interruption of the tachycardia followed by activation of that site(s) by the next paced beat from a different direction and with a shorter conduction time (third criterion). In contrast, rapid pacing from a site distal to the AV node (from the right ventricle during the orthodromic form of the arrhythmia, or the right atrium during the antidromic form of the arrhythmia) transiently entrained the tachycardia, but never demonstrated any entrainment criteria because the antidromic wave front from the pacing impulse always blocked in the AV node (concealed entrainment). We conclude that the location of the pacing site relative to the components of a reentry loop is critical to the demonstration of the criteria of transient entrainment; i.e., if it is proximal to an area of slow conduction and/or unidirectional block within a reentry loop, transient entrainment should be demonstrable, but if it is distal, it will not be demonstrable.
Circulation 72, No. 6, 1293–1307, 1985.

TRANSIENT ENTRAINMENT of a tachycardia during rapid pacing is an increase in rate of the tachycardia to the faster pacing rate, with resumption of the intrinsic rate of the tachycardia on either termination of pacing or slowing of the pacing rate below the intrinsic rate of the tachycardia.[1–10] We, and subsequently other investigators, have presented evidence that this is best explained by continuous early entrance of the wave front from the pacing impulse into the excitable gap of a tachycardia's reentry loop.[3–8, 10] Furthermore, we[3–5] have suggested three criteria, any one of which, if present, establishes transient entrainment of a tachycardia. These criteria are as follows: (1) The demonstration of constant fusion beats in the electrocardiogram during pacing at a constant rate faster than the rate of the tachycardia, except for the last captured beat, which is entrained but not fused. (2) The demonstration of progressive fusion, i.e., constant fusion beats in the electrocardiogram during rapid pacing at any constant rate faster than the rate of the tachycardia, but different degrees of constant fusion beats at different rapid pacing rates. (3) The interruption of a tachycardia during pacing at a rate faster than the rate of the tachycardia associated with localized conduction block to a site or sites for 1 beat followed by activation of that site or sites from a different direction and with a shorter conduction time by the next pacing impulse. We have, however, emphasized that transient entrainment may be present despite the inability to demonstrate any of these criteria,[3, 4] and recently two studies[10, 11] have suggested the importance of the pacing site for the demonstration of the entrainment criteria.

In this article, using the model of circus-movement tachycardia utilizing an atrioventricular (AV) bypass pathway, a rhythm well accepted to be due to reentry,

From the Department of Medicine and the Cardiovascular Research and Training Center, University of Alabama at Birmingham.

Supported in part by U.S. Public Health Service NHLBI SCOR in Ischemic Heart Disease grant 1P17HL17667 and NHLBI grant 1RO1HL29381-01A2.

Address for correspondence: Albert L. Waldo, M.D., UAB Medical Center, Room 336LHR, University Station, Birmingham, AL 35294.

Received Feb. 7, 1985; revision accepted Aug. 22, 1985.

we further explore transient entrainment and interruption phenomena and demonstrate the importance of the pacing site relative to the components of the reentry loop for the demonstration of transient entrainment.

Methods

Thirteen patients with circus-movement tachycardia utilizing an AV bypass pathway were studied with the use of standard cardiac electrophysiologic techniques. The diagnosis of this tachycardia was made by use of standard criteria.[12–15] All patients had a left-sided AV bypass pathway established by standard electrophysiologic criteria.[12–15] At the time of the study, 12 patients were not receiving any cardioactive drugs, and one was receiving oral amiodarone. All patients gave informed consent before the study.

Studies were divided into two groups based on the type of tachycardia present. Group 1 (table 1) consisted of 11 patients with circus-movement tachycardia of the orthodromic type (five with manifest Wolff-Parkinson-White syndrome and six with a so-called concealed AV bypass pathway). Group 2 (table 1) consisted of four patients with circus-movement tachycardia of the antidromic type (all with manifest Wolff-Parkinson-White syndrome) using a left-sided AV bypass pathway as the antegrade limb of the reentry loop during the tachycardia and the specialized AV conduction system as the retrograde limb. Two patients were included in each group, since they manifested each form of the arrhythmia.

Recording and pacing techniques. By standard techniques,[13–15] quadripolar catheter electrodes (USCI 6F Josephson catheters) were routinely placed in the high right atrium, His bundle position, right ventricular apex, and coronary sinus, and were used selectively to record bipolar electrograms and to pace the heart. In all patients, standard electrocardiographic leads (I, II, III, and V_1 in seven patients; I, II, and V_1 in four patients; I and V_1 in two patients; and II in one patient) were recorded simultaneously along with electrograms from all recording sites. All electrograms were filtered with use of a standard bandpass (30 or 40 to 500 Hz for the His bundle; 10 or 12 to 500 Hz for all others). The electrograms and electrocardiographic

TABLE 1

Patient population, characteristics of the tachycardia, and results of rapid pacing

Patient No.	Age (yr)	Sex	Site of AV-BP	Rate of tachycardia (beats/min)	Rate for interruption (beats/min)	Difference in rates (beats/min)	Site of pacing	Transient entrainment	Criterion for entrainment 1	2	3
Group 1: Orthodromic CMT											
1	22	F	left lateral	143	167	24	RV	+	−	−	−
				141	162	21	HRA	+	+	+	−
2	62	M	left lateral	151	185	34	RV	+	−	−	−
3	3	F	left paraseptal	179	205	26	RV	+	−	−	−
				179	205	26	HRA	+	+	−	−
4	34	M	left lateral	218	252	34	RV	+	−	−	−
5	22	F	left paraseptal	120	143	23	RV	+	−	−	−
6	24	M	left lateral	214	—	—	RV	+	−	−	−
				210	286	76	HRA	+	+	−	+
7	24	M	left lateral	141	170	29	RV	+	−	−	−
8	50	M	left lateral	128	148	20	RV	+	−	−	−
9	52	M	left lateral	147	200	53	RV	+	−	−	−
				147	171	24	HRA	+	+	−	+
10	55	M	left lateral	169	201	32	RV	+	−	−	−
11	15	M	left lateral	222	250	28	RV	+	−	−	−
Group 2: Antidromic CMT											
6	24	M	left lateral	201	216	15	RV	+	+	−[A]	+
11	15	M	left lateral	222	287	65	RV	+	+	+	+
12	55	M	left lateral	190	220	30	RV	+	+	+	+
				188	230	42	LRA	+	−	−	−
13	51	M	left lateral	200	276	76	HRA	+	−	−	−

AV-BP = AV bypass pathway; CMT = circus-movement tachycardia utilizing an AV-BP; HRA = high right atrium; LRA = low right atrium; RV = right ventricle; + = present; − = not present.

[A]Not present because the second pacing rate used interrupted the tachycardia.

leads were recorded simultaneously on photographic paper with either an Electronics-for-Medicine DR-12 or VR-16 switched-beam oscilloscopic recorder. The data were also recorded simultaneously on a Honeywell 5600C FM tape recorder for subsequent playback and analysis. All pacing was performed at twice diastolic threshold with a Medtronic 1349A programmable, battery-powered pacemaker. The pacing procedures in both group 1 and group 2 varied somewhat from patient to patient, depending on the clinical status and requirements of the patient during each study.

Study protocols. In group 1 patients, after the orthodromic form of circus-movement tachycardia utilizing an AV bypass pathway was initiated with standard cardiac pacing techniques,[15] rapid ventricular pacing was performed from the right ventricular apex during the tachycardia. Ventricular pacing was initiated at a rate of 5 to 10 beats/min faster than the spontaneous rate, continued for up to 10 sec, and terminated abruptly. If the tachycardia was not interrupted, rapid ventricular pacing was again initiated, but with an increment in rate of 5 to 10 beats/min. This procedure was repeated until the tachycardia was interrupted. In four of these patients, the same rapid pacing protocol was also performed from the high right atrium during circus-movement tachycardia.

In group 2 patients, the antidromic form of circus-movement tachycardia utilizing an AV bypass pathway was induced with standard techniques.[15] In one patient, both rapid atrial pacing from the low right atrium close to the AV nodal region and rapid ventricular pacing from the right ventricular apex were performed during the tachycardia. In another patient rapid atrial pacing from the high right atrium was performed, and in two others, rapid ventricular pacing from the right ventricular apex was performed during the tachycardia. Consequently, rapid atrial pacing was performed in two patients and rapid ventricular pacing was performed in three patients during antidromic circus-movement tachycardia. For both rapid atrial pacing and rapid ventricular pacing, the pacing protocol was the same as that used in group 1 patients.

Results

Transient entrainment and interruption of the orthodromic form of circus-movement tachycardia utilizing an AV bypass pathway — studies in group 1 patients

Ventricular pacing. Ventricular pacing at a critically rapid rate interrupted the tachycardia in 10 of the group 1 patients, the pacing rate required ranging from 20 to 53 beats/min (mean 30) faster than the spontaneous rate of the tachycardia (table 1). The mean pacing rate required to interrupt the tachycardia was 119% of the spontaneous rate, the range being 113% to 136%. In all instances, rapid ventricular pacing at rates slower than the critically rapid rate only transiently entrained the tachycardia. During ventricular pacing at all rates, the morphology of the QRS complex in all recorded electrocardiographic leads was always the same and was indistinguishable from that during ventricular pacing from the same site during sinus rhythm. Furthermore, the sequence of retrograde atrial activation and morphology of recorded atrial electrograms during the spontaneous tachycardia and during rapid ventricular pacing initiated during the tachycardia were identical. The following is a representative example.

Transient entrainment during ventricular pacing. Figure 1, *A* shows a recording of the tachycardia in a patient (No. 8) with manifest Wolff-Parkinson-White syndrome. This patient was receiving oral amiodarone at the time of the study. The spontaneous rate of the tachycardia was 128 beats/min (cycle length 470 msec) and the earliest recorded activation in the atria was at the distal coronary sinus site. Initially, rapid ventricular pacing at a rate of 138 beats/min (cycle length 434 msec) was performed for 5 sec, completely capturing the ventricles with 1:1 retrograde activation of the atria (figure 1, *B*). Both the morphology of all recorded atrial electrograms (the high right atrial site, coronary sinus site, and low right atrium recorded from the His bundle recording site) and the atrial activation sequence during the spontaneous tachycardia (figure 1, *A*) and during rapid ventricular pacing (figure 1, *B*) were the same. When rapid ventricular pacing was terminated (figure 2, *A*), the spontaneous tachycardia resumed promptly after the last captured atrial beat (indicated by asterisks). The first spontaneous cycle length of the tachycardia was longer than that before pacing, primarily because of a very long AV nodal conduction time.

When the ventricular pacing rate was increased to 143 beats/min (cycle length 419 msec), the ventricles were again captured, the atrial rate again increased to the pacing rate, and the morphology of the atrial electrograms and the atrial activation sequence again remained identical to those during the tachycardia at its spontaneous rate (figure 2, *B*). Once again, with termination of ventricular pacing, the spontaneous tachycardia resumed after the last captured atrial beat (indicated by asterisks). Note that during ventricular pacing at each of these rates (143 and 138 beats/min), although complete capture of the atria and ventricles was evident, and after termination of pacing at each rate, the tachycardia resumed promptly, none of the criteria for the demonstration of transient entrainment was present.

Figure 3 diagrammatically illustrates the cardiac activation sequences consistent with the data obtained during the spontaneous tachycardia, during rapid ventricular pacing, and just after the cessation of the pacing, which resulted in a resumption of the spontaneous tachycardia. During the tachycardia (*left* panel), the excitation wave front enters the ventricles through the normal AV conduction pathway and returns retrogradely to the atria through the left-sided AV bypass pathway. During rapid ventricular pacing (*center* panel), each pacing impulse enters into the excitable gap of the reentry loop and preexcites it antidromically and

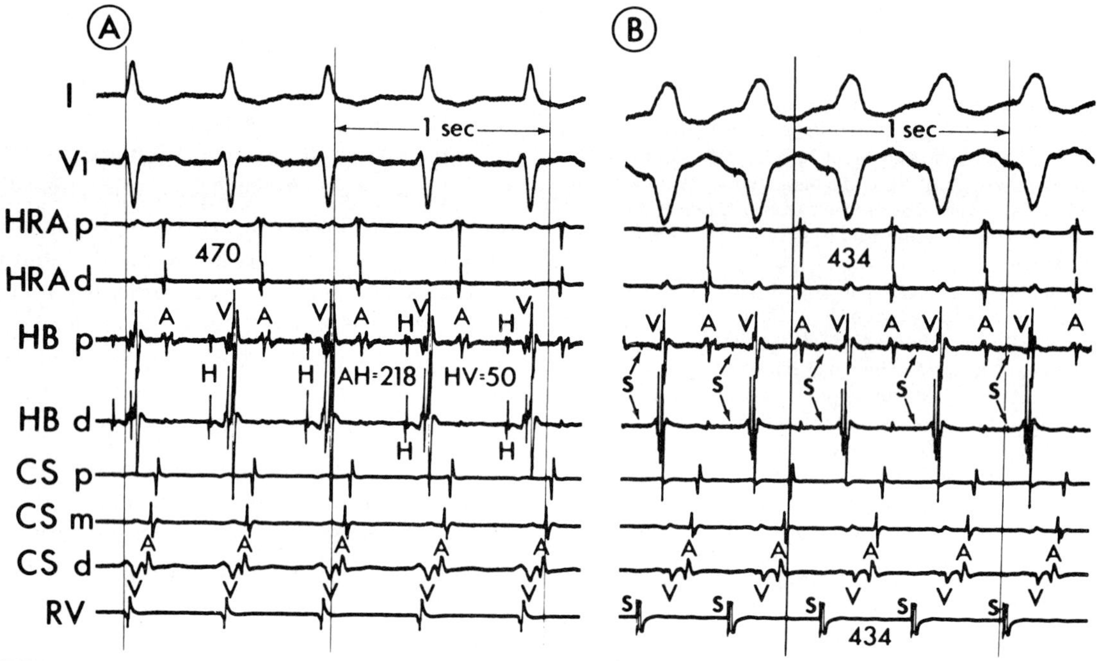

FIGURE 1. Electrocardiographic leads I and V_1 recorded simultaneously with bipolar electrograms from the proximal and distal pairs of electrodes placed in the high right atrium (HRAp and HRAd, respectively), in the His bundle position (HBp and HBd, respectively), from the proximal, middle, and distal pairs of electrodes placed in the coronary sinus (CSp, CSm, and CSd, respectively), and from the electrodes placed in the right ventricular apex (RV) in a patient with the orthodromic form of circus-movement tachycardia utilizing an AV bypass pathway. *A,* The spontaneous tachycardia at a rate of 128 beats/min (cycle length 470 msec). *B,* Rapid ventricular pacing at a rate of 138 beats/min (cycle length 434 msec) initiated during the tachycardia resets the tachycardia rate to the pacing rate. See text for discussion. In this and subsequent figures A = atrial potential; H = His bundle potential; V = ventricular potential; AH = AH interval; S = stimulus artifact; time lines are at 1 sec intervals; and all other numbers are in msec.

orthodromically. Each antidromic wave front from the pacing impulse is blocked retrogradely, either because it collides with the orthodromic wave front from each preceding beat (presumably in the specialized AV conduction system) or because it is simply blocked in the AV node due to AV nodal refractoriness. The early entrance of each orthodromic wave front from the pacing impulse results in repeated resetting of the tachycardia, thereby increasing the tachycardia rate to the pacing rate. The atria are activated only orthodromically. Thus, the atrial activation sequence during rapid ventricular pacing is exactly the same as that during the spontaneous tachycardia. Therefore, the tachycardia is transiently entrained by rapid ventricular pacing without the demonstration of any constant fusion beats. With cessation of rapid ventricular pacing (*right* panel), the orthodromic wave front from the last pacing impulse travels in the atria and reenters the ventricles through the AV node because there is no opposing wave front. This reentering orthodromic wave front then continues the tachycardia. The same was seen in all group 1 patients. Thus, during rapid ventricular pacing, none of the criteria for transient entrainment could be demonstrated, although the tachycardia was, in fact, entrained (concealed entrainment).

Interruption during ventricular pacing. In all patients in group 1, interruption of the tachycardia during ventricular pacing resulted when the antidromic and orthodromic wave fronts of the same pacing impulse blocked during the same beat. Two modes of interruption were observed. One mode is illustrated in figure 4 in the same patient whose recordings are shown in figures 1 and 2. When the ventricular pacing rate was increased to 148 beats/min (cycle length 406 msec), the tachycardia was interrupted due to block of both the antidromic and the orthodromic wave fronts of the same pacing impulse in the specialized AV conduction system, presumably in the AV node.

The second mode of interruption is illustrated in figure 5, *A,* recorded from another patient (No. 1), with a tachycardia at a rate of 143 beats/min. Rapid ventricular pacing at rates slower than 167 beats/min had failed to interrupt the tachycardia, but pacing at a rate of 167 beats/min did interrupt it. During rapid ventricular pacing at this rate, the ventricles were completely captured but, after prolongation of conduction time from the ventricular pacing site to the atria, 2:1 retrograde conduction block to the atria developed. Termination of pacing immediately after a blocked retrograde beat resulted in interruption of the tachycar-

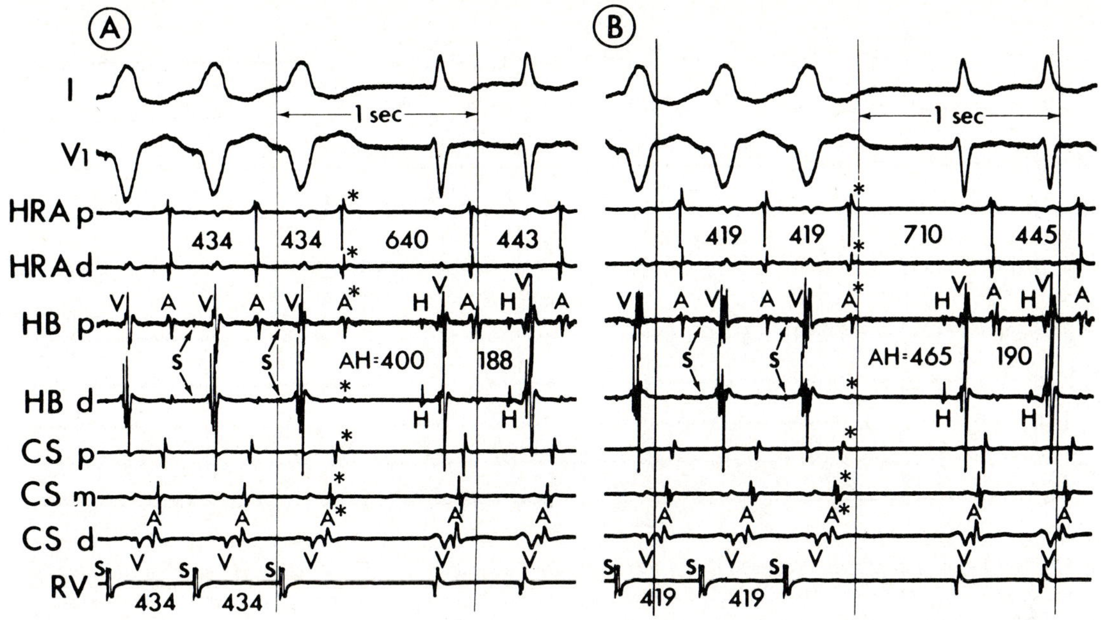

FIGURE 2. Electrocardiographic leads I and V_1 recorded simultaneously with electrograms from the same recording sites in the same patient as in figure 1. Abrupt termination of rapid ventricular pacing at a rate of 138 beats/min (cycle length 434 msec, *A*) and 143 beats/min (cycle length 419 msec, *B*) is shown. Asterisk = last captured atrial beat. See text for discussion. Abbreviations as in figure 1.

dia. When the pacing was not terminated in association with retrograde ventriculoatrial block (figure 5, *B*), resumption of the spontaneous tachycardia occurred (termination with reinitiation),[6, 16, 17] and the sequence of subsequent atrial activation after retrograde conduction block was the same as that before retrograde conduction block developed.

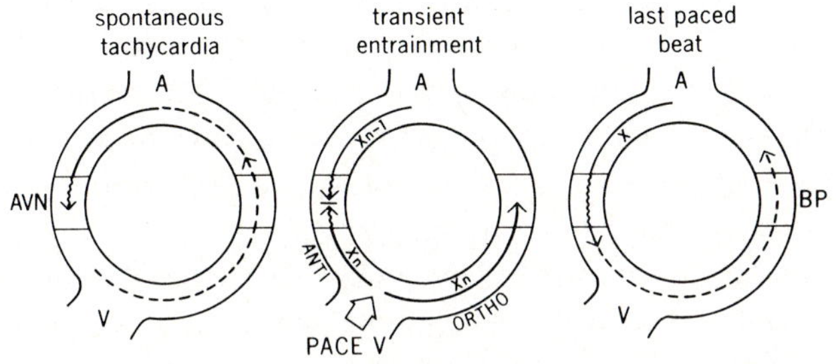

FIGURE 3. Diagrammatic illustrations of cardiac activation sequences consistent with the recordings shown in figures 1 and 2. *Left,* Circus-movement tachycardia utilizing an AV bypass pathway of the orthodromic type. *Center,* Rapid ventricular pacing initiated during the tachycardia. The large arrow indicates the pacing impulse from the right ventricular apex entering the reentry loop both orthodromically (ORTHO) and antidromically (ANTI). The antidromic wave front from the pacing impulse (X_n) collides with the orthodromic wave front of the previous beat (X_n − 1) in the specialized AV conduction system, presumably in the AV node, while the orthodromic wave front from the pacing impulse (X_n) continues the tachycardia, resetting it to the pacing rate. *Right,* Just after the cessation of rapid ventricular pacing. The orthodromic wave front from the last pacing impulse (X) is unopposed by an antidromic wave front, so that it conducts to the ventricles through the normal AV conduction system and restarts the same tachycardia (dashed line). In this and subsequent diagrammatic figures: A = atria; V = ventricles; AVN = atrioventricular node; BP = atrioventricular bypass pathway.

A diagrammatic illustration consistent with the data during each of the two modes of interruption of the orthodromic form of circus-movement tachycardia caused by rapid ventricular pacing is shown in figure 6. During the period of transient entrainment, the antidromic wave front of each pacing impulse was always blocked in the specialized AV conduction system. With interruption of the tachycardia, the orthodromic wave front from the last pacing impulse now also was blocked in the AV node in seven patients (*left* panel) or in the AV bypass pathway in three patients (*center* panel). All patients in the latter group had a so-called concealed AV bypass pathway and, moreover, showed a long ventriculoatrial conduction time during the tachycardia (241, 205, and 214 msec) compared with those in the former group (range 75 to 154 msec, mean 113). The mean pacing rate required for interruption of the tachycardia was 197 beats/min in the former group and 181 beats/min in the latter. In the remaining group 1 patient, rapid ventricular pacing at rates up to 273 beats/min did not interrupt the tachycardia. It was then elected to perform rapid atrial pacing, which interrupted the tachycardia at a rate of 286 beats/min.

The retrograde conduction time through the AV bypass pathway during the critical pacing rate for interruption of the tachycardia was constant in all patients in whom the orthodromic wave front from the pacing impulse blocked in the AV node, while it showed clear

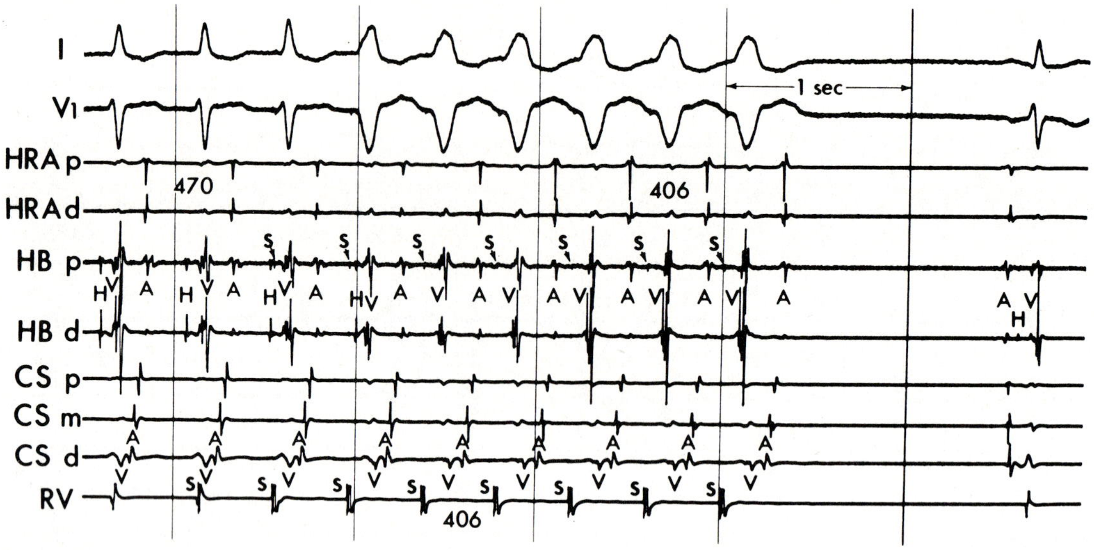

FIGURE 4. Electrocardiographic leads I and V_1 recorded simultaneously with electrograms from the same recording sites in the same patient as in figures 1 and 2. Rapid ventricular pacing at a rate of 148 beats/min (cycle length 406 msec) is initiated during the tachycardia and results in its interruption due to antegrade conduction block in the AV node. Abbreviations as in figure 1.

Wenckebach periodicity and/or 2:1 conduction to the atria in all patients in whom this same wave front blocked in the AV bypass pathway. In the former group, during the critically rapid pacing rate required for interruption of the tachycardia, localized conduction block was not demonstrated. In fact, in this group, only by terminating pacing could one know that interruption of tachycardia had occurred. Therefore, in these patients, the third criterion for transient entrainment also could not be demonstrated. In the latter group, although interruption of the tachycardia was associated with localized conduction block for 1 paced beat in the AV bypass pathway and activation of the site distal to this block by the next paced beat was of shorter conduction time (because of Wenckebach periodicity of retrograde conduction in the AV bypass pathway), it was from the same direction as previously (figure 6, *right*). The third criterion for the demonstration of transient entrainment was therefore not fulfilled. Nevertheless, because of this localized block for 1 beat, one could anticipate interruption of the tachycardia if pacing was terminated with this blocked beat.[3]

Atrial pacing. In four group 1 patients, transient entrainment was also studied with rapid atrial pacing during the orthodromic form of circus-movement tachycardia. Rapid atrial pacing at rates 21 to 76 beats/min (mean 37) faster than the spontaneous rate of the tachycardia was required to interrupt the tachycardia. The mean pacing rate required to interrupt the tachycardia was 120% of the spontaneous rate (range 115% to 136%). Atrial pacing at rates faster than the spontaneous rate of the tachycardia, but slower than the rate required for interruption, always transiently entrained the tachycardia. As described previously,[3] during transient entrainment, the wave front from each pacing impulse entered the reentry circuit via its excitable gap and then traveled both orthodromically and antidromically. Each orthodromic wave front from the atrial pacing impulse repeatedly reset the tachycardia to the pacing rate, while each antidromic wave front from the atrial pacing impulse collided with the orthodromic wave front of the preceding beat. Consequently, during transient entrainment, constant atrial fusion beats, except for the last captured beat (first criterion), were demonstrated in all four patients (table 1). Furthermore, in one of them, progressive atrial fusion (second criterion) was shown in the surface electrocardiogram at different rapid atrial pacing rates.

Interruption of the tachycardia also occurred, as previously described,[3] when both the antidromic and orthodromic wave fronts of the same pacing impulse were blocked during the same beat. In two patients who had Wolff-Parkinson-White syndrome, the orthodromic wave front of the pacing impulse was blocked in the AV node (localized conduction block to the ventricles) for 1 beat, with activation of the ventricles by the next pacing impulse from a different direction (through the AV bypass pathway) and with a shorter conduction time (third criterion). In the other two, who had a concealed AV bypass pathway, the antidromic wave front from the pacing impulse was blocked in the AV bypass pathway due to unidirectional block, and the orthodromic wave front was blocked retrogradely in the AV bypass pathway, so that no localized conduction block was present. Therefore, during rapid atrial pacing performed during orthodromic circus-movement tachycardia, the first criterion of transient entrainment was present in all four patients, the second criterion in one patient, and the third criterion in two of four patients.

Transient entrainment and interruption of the antidromic form of circus-movement tachycardia utilizing an AV bypass pathway — studies in group 2 patients

Ventricular pacing. Rapid ventricular pacing was performed during the antidromic form of circus-movement tachycardia utilizing an AV bypass pathway in

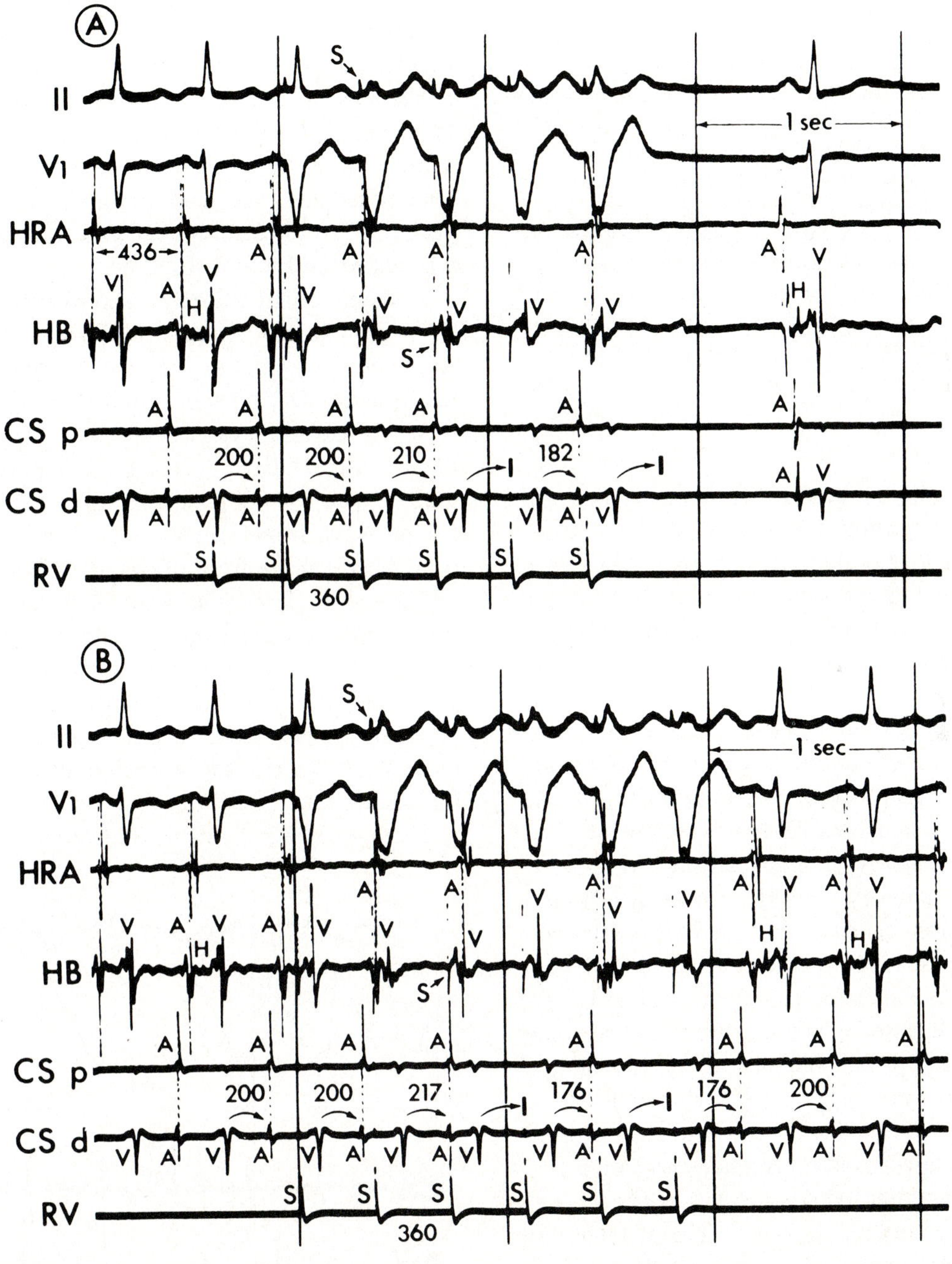

FIGURE 5. Electrocardiographic leads II and V_1 recorded simultaneously with bipolar electrograms from electrodes placed in the high right atrium (HRA), His bundle position (HB), right ventricular apex (RV), and from the proximal and distal pairs of electrodes placed in the coronary sinus (CSp and CSd, respectively) in a group 1 patient. The spontaneous tachycardia rate just before the initiation of rapid ventricular pacing was 138 beats/min (cycle length 436 msec). *A*, Rapid ventricular pacing at a rate of 167 beats/min (cycle length 360 msec) initiated during the tachycardia results in 2:1 ventriculoatrial conduction. The tachycardia is interrupted with the cessation of rapid pacing immediately after retrograde conduction block to the atria. *B*, Rapid ventricular pacing at the same rate initiated during the same tachycardia as in *A*, demonstrating termination with reinitiation of the tachycardia when the pacing is abruptly stopped after retrograde activation of the atria via the AV bypass pathway. See text for discussion. Other abbreviations as in figure 1.

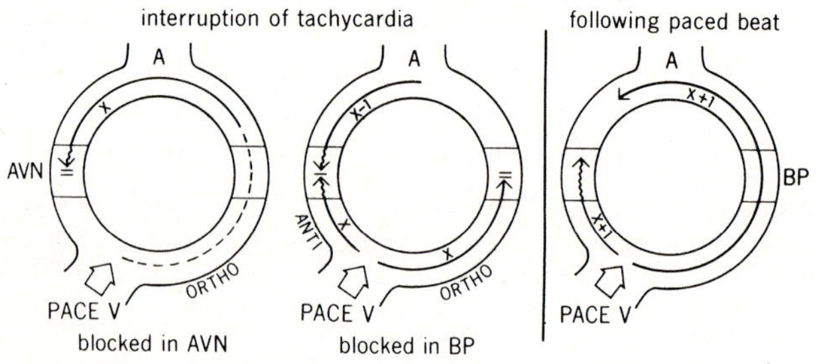

FIGURE 6. Diagrammatic illustrations showing two modes of the interruption of the orthodromic form of circus-movement tachycardia utilizing an AV bypass pathway by rapid ventricular pacing. The orthodromic (ORTHO) wave front from the pacing impulse (X) is blocked in the AV node (*left*) or in the AV bypass pathway (*center*), resulting in interruption of the tachycardia in each example. The antidromic (ANTI) wave front from the pacing impulse (X) is always blocked in the AV node due to collision with the orthodromic wave front of the previous beat (X − 1) in both examples. After retrograde conduction block in the AV bypass pathway shown in the *center* panel, the orthodromic wave front from the pacing impulse (X + 1) enters the atria through the AV bypass pathway and activates them in the same way as before interruption of the tachycardia (*right*). See text for discussion. Other abbreviations as in figure 3.

three patients (table 1). At a critically rapid rate, ventricular pacing interrupted the tachycardia in all three patients. Rapid ventricular pacing at rates faster than the spontaneous rate but slower than this critical rate always transiently entrained the tachycardia, fulfilling the proposed criteria. The following are representative examples.

Transient entrainment during ventricular pacing. Figure 7 was recorded during an antidromic form of circus-movement tachycardia (rate of 190 beats/min; cycle length 316 msec) in patient 12. In this patient who had a left-sided free wall AV bypass pathway, ventricular pacing performed during sinus rhythm always showed an atrial activation sequence starting from the low right atrium, and premature ventricular stimulation produced both a His bundle potential before an atrial potential and an increase in the time interval between the His potential and atrial potential in the His bundle electrogram recording. Therefore, in this patient, the left-sided AV bypass pathway demonstrated unidirectional block, allowing only antegrade conduction.

Initially, rapid ventricular pacing at a rate of 200 beats/min (cycle length 300 msec) was performed for 10 sec. Figure 8, *A* shows the recording at the termination of pacing at this ventricular pacing rate. During rapid ventricular pacing, ventriculoatrial conduction time from the right ventricular recording site to the coronary sinus recording site was 210 msec. In contrast to ventricular pacing during the orthodromic form of circus-movement tachycardia, the QRS complexes during rapid ventricular pacing now clearly demonstrated constant fusion beats. Furthermore, after cessation of ventricular pacing, the spontaneous tachycardia resumed promptly after the last captured ventricular beat, which was entrained but not fused (i.e., it occurred at the pacing cycle length of 300 msec but had the QRS morphology of the spontaneous antidromic tachycardia). A different degree of fusion (progressive fusion) of the QRS complexes occurred when the ventricular pacing rate was increased to 210 beats/min (cycle length 286 msec) (figure 8, *B*). When ventricular pacing at this rate was terminated, the spontaneous antidromic tachycardia resumed in exactly the same manner as observed after termination of ventricular pacing at 200 beats/min; i.e., the last captured beat was entrained but not fused.

A diagrammatic illustration consistent with the data shown in figure 8, *A* and *B* is shown in figure 9. The *left* panel in figure 9, *A* illustrates the spontaneous tachycardia. During the period of transient entrainment during rapid ventricular pacing (*center* panel), the wave front from each pacing impulse enters the reentry loop via the excitable gap. Each antidromic pacing wave front collides in the ventricles with the orthodromic wave front of the preceding beat, resulting in ventricular fusion beats. However, each orthodromic pacing wave front resets the tachycardia to the pacing rate. The orthodromic wave front from the last pacing impulse travels around the reentry circuit unopposed by a subsequent pacing impulse (as pacing has ceased), so that the last ventricular beat is entrained at the pacing rate, but is not fused (*right* panel).

The *left* panel in figure 9, *B* illustrates the spontane-

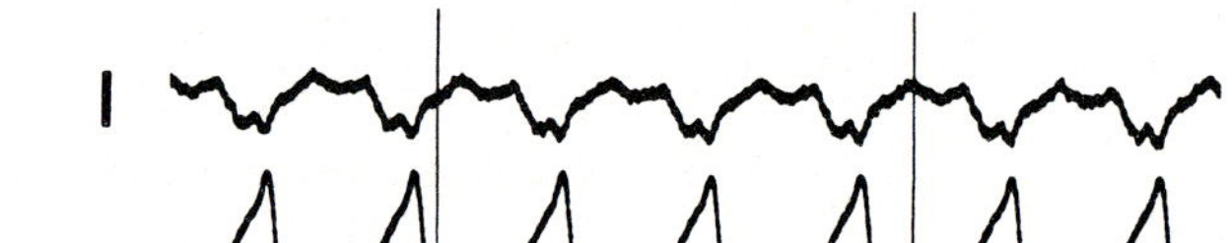

FIGURE 7. Electrocardiographic leads I and V_1 recorded simultaneously with bipolar electrograms from the electrodes placed in the high right atrium (HRA), coronary sinus (CS), and right ventricular apex (RV) during the antidromic form of circus-movement tachycardia utilizing an AV bypass pathway at a rate of 190 beats/min (cycle length 316 msec). Other abbreviations as in figure 1.

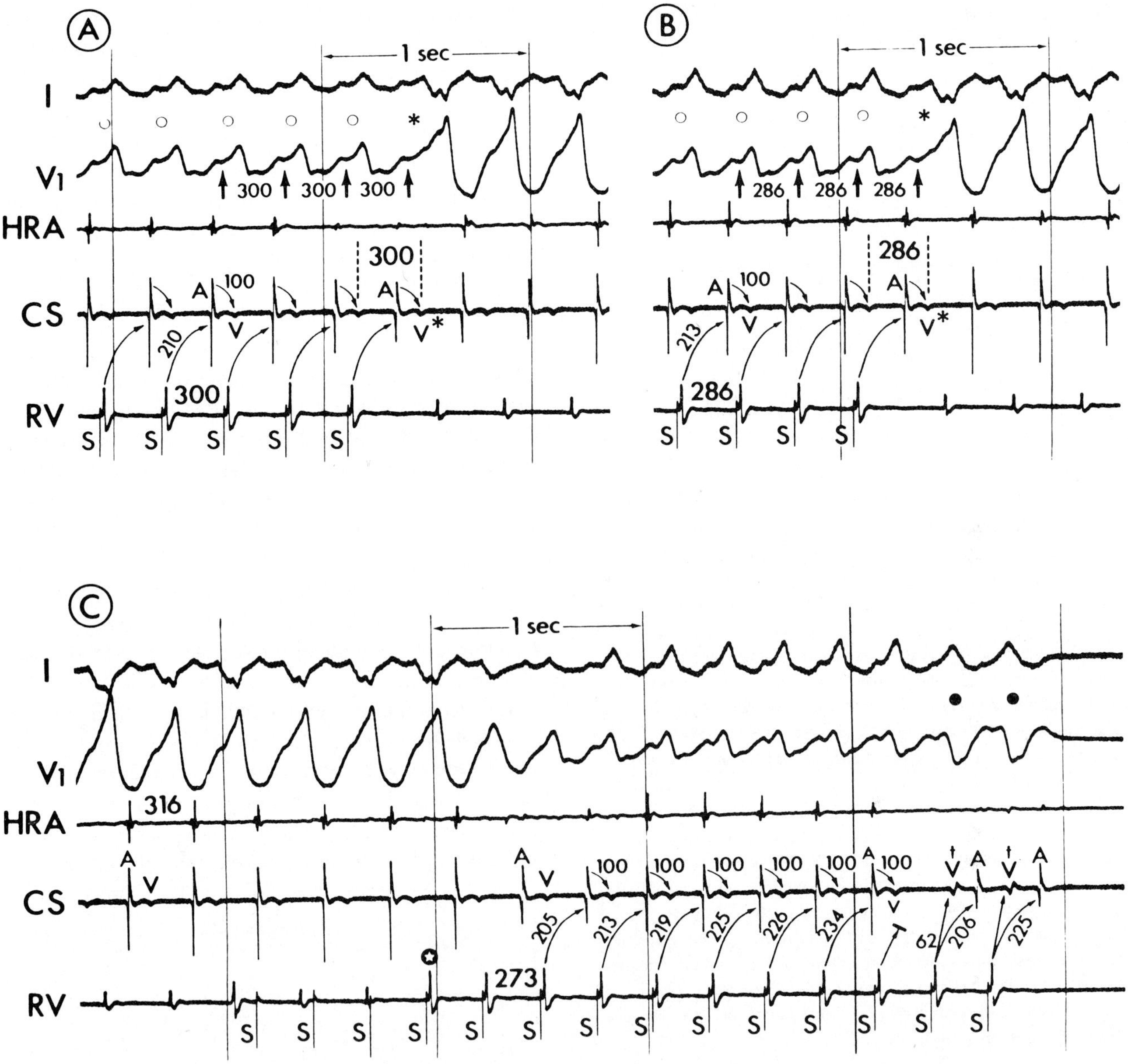

FIGURE 8. Electrocardiographic leads I and V_1 recorded simultaneously with electrogram from the same recording sites in the same patient as in figure 7. The arrows in the V_1 recording indicate the onset of the QRS complexes. *A,* Termination of rapid ventricular pacing initiated during the antidromic form of circus-movement tachycardia utilizing an AV bypass pathway at a rate of 200 beats/min (cycle length 300 msec). During rapid pacing, the ventricular potential recorded in the coronary sinus electrogram results from antegrade activation through the AV bypass pathway. Note the presence of constant ventricular fusion beats, shown in the surface electrocardiogram (indicated by open circles), except for the last captured beat (asterisk), which is entrained (it occurs at the pacing cycle length) but is not fused. The spontaneous tachycardia resumes promptly after the last entrained beat. *B,* Termination of rapid ventricular pacing initiated during the tachycardia at a rate of 210 beats/min (cycle length 286 msec). Note the constant ventricular fusion beats (indicated by open circles), with a different degree of fusion from that shown in *A*. The last captured beat again is entrained at the pacing cycle length, but is not fused (asterisk). The spontaneous tachycardia again resumes after termination of the pacing. *C,* Rapid ventricular pacing initiated during the tachycardia at a rate of 220 beats/min (cycle length 273 msec). After the stimulus captures the ventricles (indicated by the star), ventricular fusion beats occur and ventriculoatrial conduction time (measured from the right ventricular electrogram to the atrial potential in the coronary sinus electrogram) gradually prolongs until finally, retrograde conduction block in the AV node develops (blocked curved arrow). This results in interruption of the tachycardia. The two subsequent ventricular paced beats (indicated by black dots) no longer are ventricular fusion beats (note the sudden change in the morphology of the last two QRS complexes). During these 2 beats, note that the ventricular potential in the coronary sinus electrogram (indicated by the cross), which previously had resulted from antegrade activation through the AV bypass pathway, is now activated from a different direction and with a shorter conduction time. Abbreviations as in figures 1 and 7.

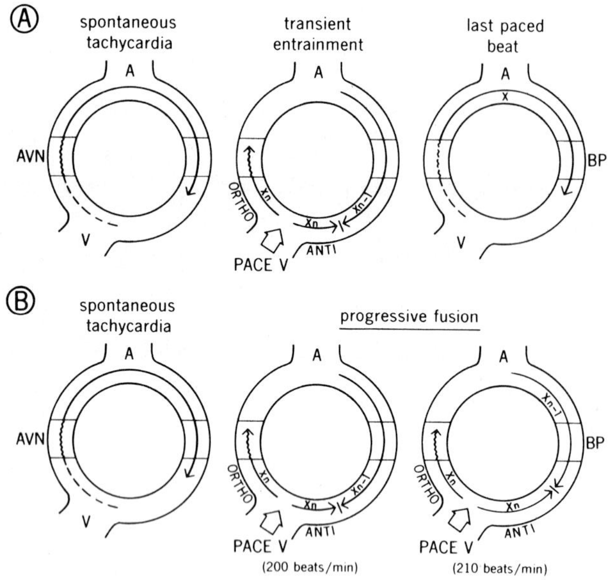

FIGURE 9. Diagrammatic illustrations of cardiac activation sequences consistent with the data shown in figure 8, *A* and *B*. *A*, Activation sequence during the antidromic form of circus-movement tachycardia utilizing an AV bypass pathway is shown (*left*). During rapid ventricular pacing initiated during the tachycardia (*center*), the pacing impulse enters the reentry loop via the excitable gap and the antidromic (ANTI) wave front from the pacing impulse (X_n) collides in the ventricles with the orthodromic (ORTHO) wave front of the preceding beat ($X_n - 1$), thus producing ventricular fusion beats. The orthodromic wave front from the pacing impulse (X_n) continues the tachycardia, resetting it to the pacing rate. The orthodromic wave front from the last paced beat (*right*) travels around the reentry circuit unopposed by a subsequent pacing impulse, so that the last captured ventricular beat is entrained at the pacing cycle length but is not fused. *B*, The mechanism of progressive fusion is shown. During transient entrainment at two different ventricular pacing rates, the antidromic wave front from the pacing impulse at a faster rate (*right*) penetrates the reentry circuit to a greater degree before it collides with the orthodromic wave front of the previous beat than does the antidromic wave front at a slower rate (*center*) and thus, different degrees of fusion at different pacing rates are produced. Other abbreviations as in figure 3.

ous tachycardia. During transient entrainment at two different ventricular pacing rates, the antidromic wave front of the faster pacing rate (210 beats/min, *right* panel) penetrates the reentry circuit to a greater degree before it collides with the orthodromic wave front of the preceding beat than does the antidromic wave front of the slower pacing rate (200 beats/min, *center* panel). Thus, the region of collision of these wave fronts in the ventricle is different for each of the pacing rates. This explains the presence of progressive fusion beats, i.e., constant fusion of QRS complexes at each pacing rate, but different degrees of fusion at different pacing rates. Therefore, rapid ventricular pacing in this patient established the presence of transient entrainment by the demonstration of two of the entrainment criteria.

Interruption during ventricular pacing. Increasing the pacing rate for this same patient to 220 beats/min (cycle length 273 msec) interrupted the tachycardia (figure 8, *C*). Three beats after initiation of ventricular pacing, ventricular capture occurred. This was associated with both ventricular fusion beats and a gradual prolongation of ventriculoatrial conduction time. The latter finally resulted in retrograde block in the specialized AV conduction system, presumably in the AV node, so that for one ventricular paced beat, neither the antidromic nor the orthodromic wave front of that ventricular pacing impulse was conducted to the atria. This was associated with interruption of the tachycardia. The two subsequent ventricular paced beats (black dots) that followed the localized conduction block to the atria captured the ventricles, but did not produce any fusion of the associated QRS complex (note the sudden change in the morphology of the last two QRS complexes). Also, these last two ventricular paced beats were conducted retrograde to the atria over the normal specialized AV conduction system, because retrograde AV conduction over the AV bypass pathway was never demonstrated in this patient.

A diagrammatic illustration consistent with the data recorded in figure 8, *C*, is shown in figure 10. The antidromic wave front from the ventricular pacing impulse is always blocked due to collision with the orthodromic wave front from the preceding beat (*left* panel), while the orthodromic wave front from the pacing im-

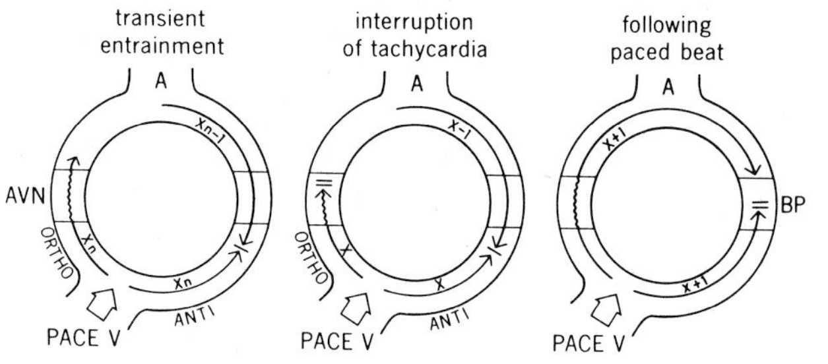

FIGURE 10. Diagrammatic illustrations of cardiac activation sequences consistent with the data shown in figure 8, *C*. During transient entrainment of the antidromic form of circus-movement tachycardia utilizing an AV bypass pathway by rapid ventricular pacing (*left*), the antidromic (ANTI) wave front from the pacing impulse (X_n) is always blocked due to collision with the orthodromic wave front from the previous beat ($X_n - 1$). At a critically rapid ventricular pacing rate, the orthodromic (ORTHO) wave front from the pacing impulse (X_n) is blocked in the AV node (*center*), resulting in interruption of the tachycardia. The following ventricular paced beat totally captures the ventricles, since there is no orthodromic wave front with which to collide (*right*). Note that although the atria are activated in the same manner as before interruption of the tachycardia, a part of the ventricles previously activated by the orthodromic wave front from the pacing impulse is now activated from a different direction and with a shorter conduction time. Other abbreviations as in figure 3.

pulse shows decremental conduction in the AV node, finally resulting in conduction block (*center* panel). The latter resulted in interruption of the tachycardia. The next ventricular paced beat totally captures the ventricles, since there is no orthodromic wave front from a preceding beat with which to collide (*right* panel). Also, this paced beat enters the atria via the normal specialized AV conduction system (because no retrograde conduction via the AV bypass pathway is present), so that the atria are activated in the same manner as before interruption of the tachycardia. However, note that the part of the ventricles previously activated by the orthodromic wave front from the pacing impulse is now activated from a different direction and with a shorter conduction time (thus fulfilling the third criterion for the demonstration of transient entrainment).

In the other two patients (Nos. 6 and 11) in whom rapid ventricular pacing was performed during antidromic circus-movement tachycardia, retrograde conduction via the AV bypass pathway was present. In these patients, localized conduction block in the specialized AV conduction system (presumably in the AV node) occurred during rapid pacing as described above and was associated with interruption of the tachycardia (figure 11). However, during the next pacing impulse, ventricular and atrial activation in the region from which the coronary sinus electrogram was recorded occurred from a different direction (note the change in morphology of the respective complexes in the coronary sinus electrogram recording in figure 11) and with a shorter conduction time, as this pacing impulse, now unopposed by a preceding orthodromic wave front, spread "antidromically" to these sites. Therefore, in these patients, the third criterion was demonstrated more clearly.

Atrial pacing. In contradistinction to rapid ventricular pacing, rapid atrial pacing during the same antidromic form of circus-movement tachycardia utilizing an AV bypass pathway failed to fulfill any transient entrainment criteria. Figure 12 was recorded from the same patient whose recordings are shown in figures 7 and 8. Rapid atrial pacing was performed from the low right atrium close to the region of the AV node. Rapid atrial pacing at a rate of 220 beats/min (cycle length 273 msec) was performed for about 6 sec during the tachycardia. Each atrial pacing impulse captured the atria and consequently the ventricles. When pacing was terminated, the spontaneous tachycardia resumed promptly after the last captured ventricular beat (figure

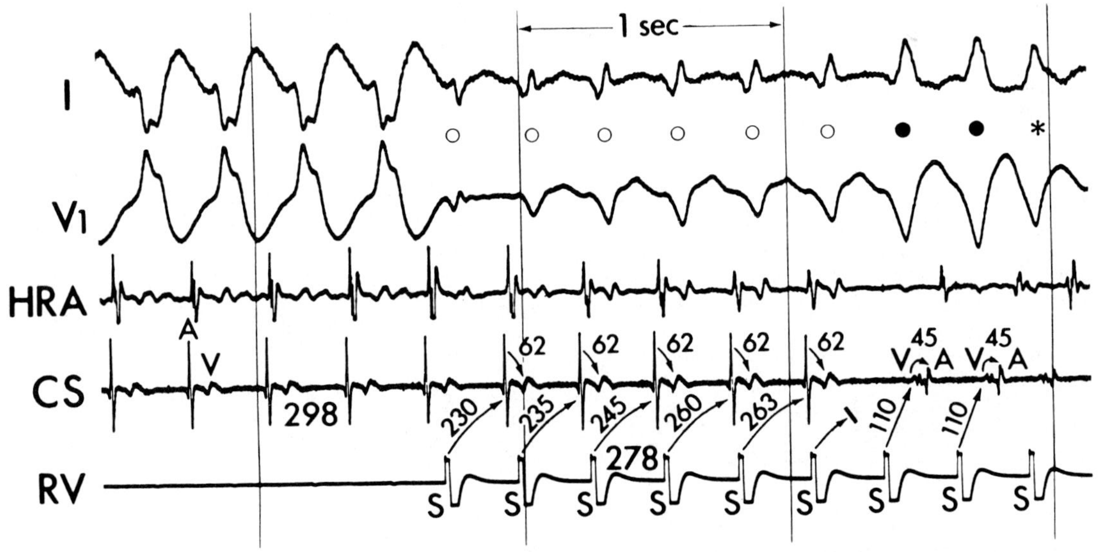

FIGURE 11. Another example of interruption of the antidromic form of circus-movement tachycardia utilizing an AV bypass pathway by rapid ventricular pacing. Electrocardiographic leads I and V_1 are shown simultaneously with bipolar electrograms from electrodes placed in the high right atrium (HRA), coronary sinus (CS), and right ventricular apex (RV). The long and short curved arrows represent ventriculoatrial and AV conduction, respectively. The rate of the spontaneous tachycardia is 201 beats/min (cycle length 298 msec). Rapid ventricular pacing at a rate of 216 beats/min (cycle length 278 msec) initiated during the tachycardia produces ventricular fusion beats (indicated by open circles). Ventriculoatrial conduction time measured from the right ventricular stimulus artifact to the atrial potential in the coronary sinus electrogram gradually prolongs during rapid pacing. Finally, retrograde conduction block develops in the AV node (blocked long curved arrow), resulting in interruption of the tachycardia. The subsequent ventricular paced beats totally capture the ventricles (note the sudden change in the morphology of the QRS complexes indicated by black dots) and, moreover, activate the atria through the AV bypass pathway (i.e., from a different direction and with a shorter conduction time). The last ventricular complex (indicated by an asterisk) is a premature beat. Other abbreviations as in figure 1.

12, *A*). No constant fusion beats were manifest during the pacing. This is because each antidromic wave front of each atrial pacing impulse was either blocked in the AV node or collided in the normal specialized AV conduction system with the orthodromic wave front of the previous beat, while the orthodromic wave front of each atrial pacing impulse activated the ventricles via the AV bypass pathway just as during the spontaneous tachycardia (figure 13, *left*).

Rapid atrial pacing at a rate of 230 beats/min (cycle length 261 msec) caused antegrade conduction block at the AV bypass pathway and terminated the tachycardia (figure 12, *B*). This occurred because both the antidromic and orthodromic wave fronts of the same pacing impulse were blocked during the same beat, the former in the AV conduction system and the latter in the AV bypass pathway (figure 13, *center*). It was critical that the pacing be terminated with this blocked beat, because if the pacing was terminated after conduction of an orthodromic wave front (note the presence of 2:1 AV conduction via the AV bypass pathway in figure 12, *B* and *C*), the tachycardia continued (termination with reinitiation) (figure 12, *C*).[6, 16, 17] Note that although interruption of the tachycardia was associated with localized conduction block in the AV bypass pathway, the next paced beat activated the ventricles via the AV bypass pathway, i.e., from the same direction as before the localized block (figure 13, *right*). Therefore, none of the transient entrainment criteria were demonstrated despite the fact that rapid atrial pacing did in fact transiently entrain the antidromic form of circus-movement tachycardia (concealed entrainment). The same observations were made in the other patient in whom rapid atrial pacing was performed from the high right atrium during the antidromic form of circus-movement tachycardia.

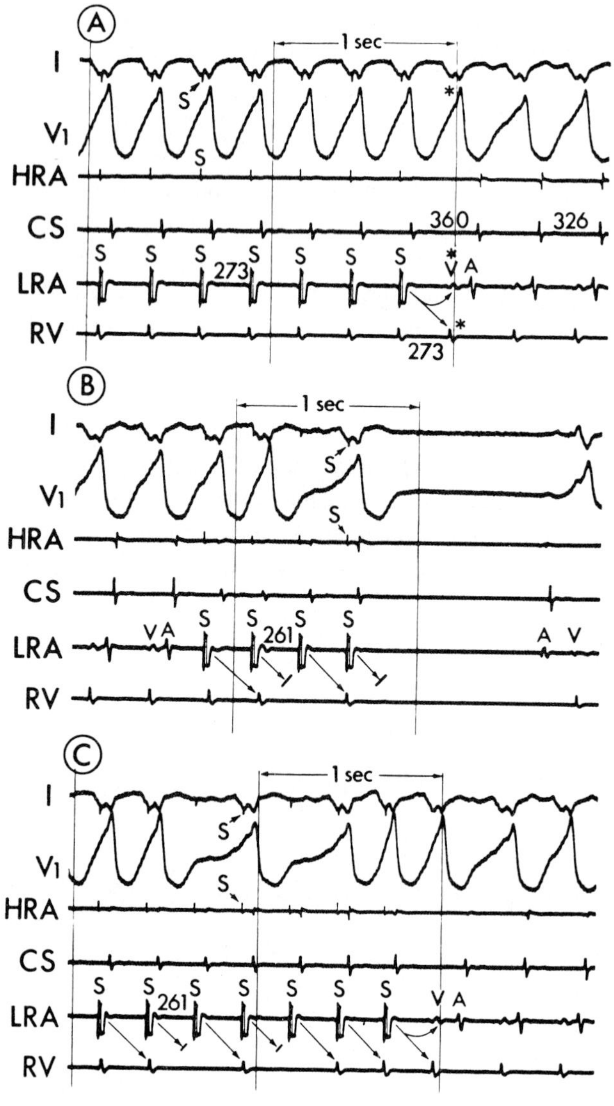

FIGURE 12. Electrocardiographic leads I and V_1 recorded simultaneously with electrograms from the low right atrium (LRA) close to the AV nodal region and at the same recording sites in the same patient as in figures 7 and 8. *A*, Rapid atrial pacing at a rate of 220 beats/min (cycle length 273 msec) is performed from the low right atrial site during the antidromic form of circus-movement tachycardia utilizing an AV bypass pathway. No constant fusion beats are manifest. With termination of rapid atrial pacing, the spontaneous tachycardia resumes after the last entrained beat (indicated by asterisks). *B*, Rapid atrial pacing at a rate of 230 beats/min (cycle length 261 msec) causes 2:1 antegrade conduction block at the AV bypass pathway (blocked arrows) and interrupts the tachycardia. *C*, Rapid atrial pacing at the same rate as shown in *B* demonstrating termination with reinitiation. See text for discussion. Other abbreviations as in figure 1.

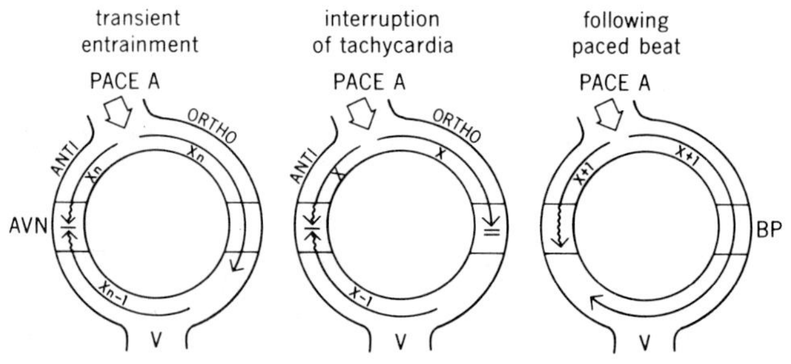

FIGURE 13. Diagrammatic illustrations of cardiac activation sequences consistent with the data shown in figure 12. *Left,* During rapid atrial pacing initiated during the antidromic form of circus-movement tachycardia utilizing an AV bypass pathway, the pacing impulse enters the reentry loop via the excitable gap. The antidromic (ANTI) wave front from the pacing impulse (X_n) collides with the orthodromic wave front of the previous beat ($X_n - 1$), presumably in the AV node, while the orthodromic (ORTHO) wave front from the pacing impulse (X_n) resets the tachycardia to the pacing rate. *Center,* At a critically rapid rate, the orthodromic wave front from the pacing impulse (X) is blocked in the AV bypass pathway. The termination of pacing immediately after the conduction block results in interruption of the tachycardia. *Right,* The following atrial paced beat enters the ventricles through the AV bypass pathway and activates them in the same manner as before interruption of the tachycardia. Other abbreviations as in figure 3.

Discussion

These data both confirm and expand our previous observations of transient entrainment and interruption of tachyarrhythmias.[1–6, 11, 18] They confirm the reliability of the three proposed criteria for its identification, demonstrate and explain that both transient entrainment and interruption of a tachyarrhythmia may occur without fulfilling any of the three criteria (concealed entrainment), permit localization of an area of slow conduction within the reentry loop relative to the pacing site, and force a reexamination of the third criterion concerning localized conduction block associated with interruption of the tachycardia.

Reliability of three criteria proposed for identification of transient entrainment. Through our series of studies of transient entrainment and interruption of tachyarrhythmias during rapid pacing, we have explained its mechanism and have proposed three criteria for its identification,[3–5] any one of which establishes its presence and, we propose, indicates that the underlying mechanism of the arrhythmia can be best explained by reentry. In the present study, we again observed transient entrainment and interruption of the orthodromic form of circus-movement tachycardia utilizing an AV bypass pathway during rapid atrial pacing, and obtained the same results concerning the three criteria as noted in our previous study when pacing was performed proximal to an area of slow conduction.[3] Furthermore, rapid ventricular pacing was performed during the antidromic form of this well-accepted reentrant tachycardia, and the data not only were consistent with our previous explanation of the mechanism of transient entrainment and interruption of tachyarrhythmias, but also demonstrated the three criteria clearly.

During rapid ventricular pacing of the antidromic form of circus-movement tachycardia, transient entrainment was again found to be consistent with the continuous early entrance of the wave front from the pacing impulse into the excitable gap of the tachycardia's reentry loop. Constant ventricular fusion beats, except for the last captured beat, were clearly demonstrated in the electrocardiogram during rapid ventricular pacing (the first criterion). This can best be explained by collision of the antidromic wave front from each pacing impulse with the orthodromic wave front of each previous beat except for the last captured beat, which was entrained but not fused. The latter occurred because the orthodromic wave front of the last paced beat had no antidromic wave front from a subsequent pacing impulse with which to collide. As the pacing rate was increased, the antidromic wave front from each pacing impulse penetrated the reentry loop to a greater degree, thus producing a different degree of constant ventricular fusion beats in the electrocardiogram (progressive fusion, the second criterion). Finally, when the pacing rate was increased to a rate critically faster than the rate of the spontaneous tachycardia, it was interrupted, being associated with localized conduction block (at the AV node) of the orthodromic wave front from the pacing impulse followed by subsequent activation of sites distal to the localized block from a different direction (manifest by a different electrogram morphology) and with a shorter conduction time (the third criterion). This change in the sequence of activation after localized conduction block was well shown in the electrocardiogram by the change in the morphology of QRS complex. Therefore, the present study supports the previous observations about transient entrainment and interruption of tachyarrhythmias and, moreover, confirms the reliability of the three criteria proposed for its demonstration.

Concealed entrainment: the importance of pacing site in the inability to demonstrate transient entrainment despite its being operative. As shown by this study, none of the proposed three criteria necessary to establish transient entrainment of a tachycardia and, ergo, reentry as its mechanism, may be demonstrable despite the fact that transient entrainment during rapid pacing is certainly occurring (concealed entrainment). That is, transient entrainment occurred without fulfilling any of the criteria when rapid pacing was performed at sites orthodromically distal to the AV node, an area of slow conduction within the reentry loop. This was manifest during rapid ventricular pacing of the orthodromic form of circus movement tachycardia utilizing an AV bypass pathway and during rapid atrial pacing of the antidromic form. In each case, the antidromic wave front of each pacing impulse blocked in the specialized AV conduction system, presumably in the AV node, so that the demonstration of fusion beats in the electrocardiogram was not possible. Therefore, fulfillment of either the first or second criterion was impossible.

Recently, the importance of the pacing site in demonstrating the criteria for entrainment has been shown in two studies[10, 11] during rapid ventricular pacing from different sites during ventricular tachycardia. In both studies, rapid ventricular pacing from one site fulfilled all three entrainment criteria, while that from another site did not fulfill any of the criteria. Extrapolating from the data in our present study, the results of these two studies are likely explained by the relationship of the pacing site to an area of slow conduction in the reentry loop of the tachycardia.

In the present study, since the pacing site that failed

to demonstrate the entrainment criteria (the right ventricle in the orthodromic form and the right atrium in the antidromic form of circus-movement tachycardia) was not precisely but rather was relatively distal to the AV node (in terms of the reentry loop), some degree of constant fusion might have been expected during transient entrainment. In fact, no constant fusion beats were demonstrated. This may have been because conduction time of the antidromic wave front from the pacing impulse to the area of slow conduction was not long enough to permit the orthodromic wave front of the previous beat to have conducted through and exited the area of slow conduction and thus permit fusion to occur. In addition, the prolongation of the already slow conduction of the orthodromic wave front in the area of slow conduction in the reentry loop (i.e., in the AV node) caused by the rapid rate of pacing[19] made it even more likely that the antidromic wave front from each pacing impulse would reach and block in the AV node.

The inability to fulfill the third criterion in these same examples can be explained in one of two ways. During rapid pacing at a critical rate, either the antidromic and orthodromic wave fronts from the same pacing impulse both blocked at the same time (the AV node), resulting in the interruption of the tachycardia without producing localized conduction block, or the antidromic wave front from the pacing impulse blocked in the AV node and the orthodromic wave front from the same pacing impulse blocked at the AV bypass pathway, resulting in the interruption of the tachycardia. Actually, in the latter form of interruption, localized conduction block to the atria during rapid ventricular pacing or to the ventricles during rapid atrial pacing did occur (in the AV bypass pathway) and activation of sites distal to the AV bypass pathway by the next pacing impulse occurred with a shorter conduction time than immediately before the appearance of localized conduction block. However, this activation occurred from the same direction as before the appearance of the localized conduction block. The third criterion requires activation of the blocked sites by the next paced beat from a different direction.

The occurrence of these two types of interruption depends on the electrophysiologic properties of the AV bypass pathway. Localized conduction block to the atria during rapid ventricular pacing of the orthodromic form of circus-movement tachycardia occurred at the AV bypass pathway in patients who manifested long ventriculoatrial conduction time during the tachycardia. Furthermore, this block was preceded by decremental conduction in the AV bypass pathway. The prolongation of retrograde conduction time in the AV bypass pathway of these patients was different from that in other patients in this study in whom retrograde conduction time in the AV bypass pathway was constant at each pacing rate. In the latter patients, it was not until the cessation of rapid ventricular pacing that termination of the tachycardia could be appreciated. In the former patients, i.e., those with prolonged retrograde conduction time, if rapid pacing was terminated immediately after localized conduction block, it resulted in the interruption of the tachycardia, but if it was terminated even 1 beat beyond that, the tachycardia would resume because the orthodromic wave front from that pacing impulse would continue around the reentry loop unopposed (termination with reinitiation).[6, 16, 17]

Localization of an area of slow conduction and/or unidirectional block — relationship to the pacing site. This study shows that the location of the pacing site is critical for the demonstration of transient entrainment and interruption of a tachyarrhythmia. When it is relatively proximal to an area of slow conduction within a reentry loop, transient entrainment during rapid pacing usually will be demonstrated by the fulfillment of at least one of the three proposed criteria. If the pacing site is relatively distal to an area of slow conduction, transient entrainment will not be demonstrable, since none of the criteria can be fulfilled.

With the use of the observations obtained in this and previous studies of circus-movement tachycardia utilizing an AV bypass pathway,[3] identification of an area of slow conduction relative to the pacing site may be possible. Thus, if one can demonstrate transient entrainment during rapid pacing initiated during the tachycardia, the pacing site must be located relatively proximal to an area of slow conduction. After transient entrainment is established, and if one paces from another site but cannot demonstrate any of the three criteria (concealed entrainment), the latter pacing site is most likely distal to an area of slow conduction. An exception to the latter might occur when an area of slow conduction and an area of unidirectional block are at separate sites and rapid pacing is performed just distal to an area of unidirectional block but proximal to an area of slow conduction. This will occur during pacing from the coronary sinus just distal to a left-sided AV bypass pathway during the orthodromic form of circus-movement tachycardia utilizing such a pathway when the pathway either doesn't conduct antegradely at all (a so-called concealed AV bypass pathway) or has a very long antegrade effective refractory period. Although such a pacing site is relatively proximal to an area of slow conduction, its being just distal to an area of unidirectional block with the aforementioned properties will not permit any of the proposed criteria for the demonstration of entrainment to occur. Nevertheless, if any of the criteria are demonstrable, the conclusion that a pacing site is proximal to an area of slow conduction can be drawn. Thus, observing for transient entrainment from multiple pacing sites during a tachycardia may permit the localization of an area of slow conduction critical for establishing and/or maintaining a reentrant tachycardia, as, for example, in ventricular tachycardia.

Reexamination of the third criterion for the demonstration of transient entrainment. We have proposed that if interruption of a tachycardia is associated with localized conduction block to a site(s) for 1 beat followed by subsequent activation of that site(s) from a different direction and with a shorter conduction time, transient entrainment has been demonstrated. In this and a previous study[3] we have observed that localized conduction block for 1 beat (second-degree block) may occur either in the AV node or AV bypass pathway, followed by activation of the previously blocked site(s) by the next pacing impulse with a shorter conduction time. However, different from the originally proposed third criterion, this subsequent activation may be from the same direction as before, and rather than maintain interruption of the tachycardia, it may result in its reinitiation (termination with reinitiation phenomenon). Thus, if pacing is stopped 1 beat after the pacing beat that produced the localized conduction block, the tachycardia may resume.

We have wondered whether these events should be considered as evidence of transient entrainment, i.e., whether the originally proposed third criterion should be expanded or otherwise amended. As shown in this study, this form of interruption of a tachyarrhythmia can occur without demonstration of either of the other two proposed criteria. However, rapid pacing of a tachycardia due to any mechanism can possibly produce a second-degree block of the type described above so that this form of block may be "an innocent bystander" to the underlying mechanism of the tachycardia. Therefore, we suggest that because of our currently limited understanding of mechanisms of arrhythmias and the importance of the demonstration of transient entrainment as a tool to establish a reentry mechanism, the third criterion should remain as is.

References

1. Waldo AL, MacLean WAH, Karp RB, Kouchoukos NT, James TN: Entrainment and interruption of atrial flutter with atrial pacing. Studies in man following open heart surgery. Circulation **56:** 737, 1977
2. MacLean WAH, Plumb VJ, Waldo AL: Transient entrainment and interruption of ventricular tachycardia. PACE **4:** 358, 1981
3. Waldo AL, Plumb VJ, Arciniegas JG, MacLean WAH, Cooper TB, Priest MF, James TN: Transient entrainment and interruption of the atrioventricular bypass pathway type of paroxysmal atrial tachycardia. A model for understanding and identifying reentrant arrhythmias. Circulation **67:** 73, 1983
4. Waldo AL, Plumb VJ, Henthorn RW: Observations on the mechanism of atrial flutter. *In* Surawicz B, Reddy CP, Prystowsky EN, editors: Tachycardias. Boston, 1984, Martinus Nijhoff Publishing, p 213
5. Waldo AL, Henthorn RW, Plumb VJ, MacLean WAH: Demonstration of the mechanism of transient entrainment and interruption of ventricular tachycardia with rapid atrial pacing. J Am Coll Cardiol **3:** 422, 1984
6. Waldo AL, Henthorn RW, Plumb VJ: Relevance of electrograms and transient entrainment for antitachycardia devices. PACE **7:** 588, 1984
7. Anderson KP, Swerdlow CD, Mason JW: Entrainment of ventricular tachycardia. Am J Cardiol **53:** 335, 1984
8. Portillo B, Mejias J, Leon-Portillo N, Zaman L, Myerburg RJ, Castellanos A: Entrainment of atrioventricular nodal reentrant tachycardias during overdrive pacing from high right atrium and coronary sinus: with special reference to atrioventricular dissociation and 2:1 retrograde block during tachycardias. Am J Cardiol **53:** 1570, 1984
9. Brugada P, Waldo A, Wellens HJJ: Transient entrainment and interruption of paroxysmal AV nodal tachycardia. J Am Coll Cardiol **3:** 537, 1984 (abst)
10. Mann DE, Lawrie GM, Luck JC, Griffin JC, Magro SA, Wyndham CRC: Importance of pacing site in entrainment of ventricular tachycardia. J Am Coll Cardiol **5:** 781, 1985
11. Plumb VJ, Henthorn RW, Waldo AL: Characteristics of the transient entrainment of ventricular tachycardia by ventricular pacing. PACE **7:** 463, 1984 (abst)
12. Barold SS, Coumel P: Mechanisms of atrioventricular junctional tachycardia. Role of reentry and concealed accessory bypass tracts. Am J Cardiol **39:** 97, 1977
13. Wu D, Denes P, Amat-Y-Leon F, Dhingra R, Wyndham CRC, Bauernfeind R, Latif P, Rosen KM: Clinical, electrocardiographic and electrophysiologic observations in patients with paroxysmal supraventricular tachycardia. Am J Cardiol **41:** 1045, 1978
14. Farshidi A, Josephson ME, Horowitz LN: Electrophysiologic characteristics of concealed bypass tracts: clinical and electrocardiographic correlates. Am J Cardiol **41:** 1052, 1978
15. Wellens HJJ, Farre J, Bar FW: Wolff-Parkinson-White syndrome: Value and limitations of programmed electrical stimulation. *In* Narula OS, editor: Cardiac arrhythmias: electrophysiology, diagnosis and management. Baltimore, 1979, Williams and Wilkins, p 589
16. Josephson ME, Seides SF: Clinical cardiac electrophysiology. Techniques and interpretations. Philadelphia, 1979, Lea and Febiger, p 307
17. Brugada P, Wellens HJJ: Entrainment as an electrophysiologic phenomenon. J Am Coll Cardiol **3:** 451, 1984
18. Henthorn RW, Plumb VJ, Arciniegas JG, Waldo AL: Entrainment of "ectopic atrial tachycardia": Evidence for re-entry. Am J Cardiol **49:** 920, 1982 (abst)
19. Lister JW, Stein E, Kosowsky BD, Lau SH, Damato AN: Atrioventricular conduction in man: Effect of rate, exercise, isoproterenol and atropine on the P-R interval. Am J Cardiol **16:** 516, 1965

Abnormal signal-averaged electrocardiograms in patients with nonischemic congestive cardiomyopathy: relationship to sustained ventricular tachyarrhythmias

DAVID S. POLL, M.D., FRANCIS E. MARCHLINSKI, M.D., RITA A. FALCONE, M.S., MARK E. JOSEPHSON, M.D., AND MICHAEL B. SIMSON, M.D.

ABSTRACT We assessed whether signal-averaged electrocardiography could identify patients with sustained ventricular arrhythmias in 41 patients with non-ischemic cardiomyopathy. Twelve of these patients presented with sustained ventricular arrhythmia and 29 patients had no history of sustained ventricular arrhythmias. The mean ejection fractions in the groups were 30 ± 9% and 24 ± 9%, respectively. Results were compared with signal-averaged electrocardiograms in 55 normal individuals. The filtered QRS duration was longest in patients with sustained ventricular arrhythmias (130.2 ± 19.5 vs 105.0 ± 13.1 msec in the group without sustained ventricular arrhythmia, $p < .001$ and 95.9 ± 9.1 in the normal group, $p < .001$). The voltage in the last 40 msec of the filtered QRS was lower in the sustained ventricular arrhythmia group (11.3 ± 9.3 μV) than the group without sustained ventricular arrhythmia (53.5 ± 28.3 μV; $p < .001$) or the normal group (53.7 ± 25.2 μV; $p < .001$). Eighty-three percent of patients in the sustained ventricular arrhythmia group had an abnormal signal-averaged electrocardiogram characterized by both a long filtered QRS duration and a late potential of low voltage level; only 2% of normal subjects and 14% of patients without sustained ventricular arrhythmias had an abnormal signal-averaged electrocardiogram. The signal-averaged electrocardiogram can identify patients with nonischemic congestive cardiomyopathy and sustained ventricular arrhythmias.

Circulation 72, No. 6, 1308–1313, 1985.

PATIENTS with congestive cardiomyopathy have a high incidence of life-threatening ventricular arrhythmias and sudden cardiac death. To date, however, no clinical predictors of sudden cardiac death have been identified.[1] In recent years, signal-averaged electrocardiography has developed as a technique for the noninvasive evaluation of intracardiac conduction. In patients with coronary artery disease, the presence of abnormalities of the signal-averaged electrocardiogram such as low voltage, high-frequency potentials late in the QRS complex and prolonged QRS duration has successfully identified patients with sustained ventricular tachycardia.[2–8] Thus, this technique may be useful in the noninvasive identification of patients with nonischemic disease who are prone to ventricular arrhythmias.

In this study, we characterize the signal-averaged electrocardiogram in 41 patients with nonischemic congestive cardiomyopathy with and without sustained ventricular arrhythmias and compare them with the signal averaged electrocardiograms of 55 normal individuals.

From the Cardiovascular Section, Hospital of the University of Pennsylvania, Philadelphia.

Supported in part by grant HL27925 from the National Heart, Lung and Blood Institute.

Address for correspondence: Michael B. Simson, M.D., Cardiovascular Section, 945 W. Gates Bldg., Hospital of the University of Pennsylvania, 3400 Spruce St., Philadelphia, PA 19104

Received March 19, 1985; revision accepted Sept. 5, 1985.

Dr. Poll is supported by the AHA Southeastern Chapter and by National Institutional Training grant HL07346 from the NHLBI. His current address is: Cardiovascular Section, Pennsylvania Hospital, 8th and Spruce Streets, Philadelphia, PA 19107. Dr. Marchlinski is supported by the University of Pennsylvania Department of Medicine Measey Foundation. Dr. Josephson is the Robinette Foundation Professor of Cardiology and Medicine of the University of Pennsylvania. Dr. Simson is the Samuel Bellet Associate Professor of Medicine of the Hospital of the University of Pennsylvania.

Methods

Patients. The study population consisted of 26 men and 15 women with nonischemic congestive cardiomyopathy. The mean age was 50 ± 14 years (mean ± SD). All patients met the following criteria for nonischemic congestive cardiomyopathy: (1) left ventricular ejection fraction of 45% or less by angiographic left ventriculography (14 patients), radionuclide angiography (25 patients), or two-dimensional echocardiography (two patients),[9] (2) exclusion of coronary artery disease by (a) absence of significant coronary stenosis by angiography (25 patients) or (b) absence of history of angina or myocardial infarction (16 patients). In addition, no patient had left ventricular dyskinesis. The cause of congestive cardiomyopathy was idiopathic in 35 patients, related to alcohol abuse in five patients, and doxorubicin toxicity in 1 patient. Patients with bundle branch block were not included because of possible masking of low voltages late in the filtered QRS complex.[10]

The study group was divided according to clinical arrhythmia presentation. Twelve patients presented with sustained, uniform ventricular tachycardia (eight patients), defined as a tachycardia lasting longer than 30 sec, or cardiac arrest and ventricular fibrillation (four patients). These patients made up the sustained VT/VF group. Twenty-nine patients had no history of sustained ventricular arrhythmis and made up the no sustained VT/VF group.

The normal group consisted of 55 individuals without clinical evidence of organic heart disease by history, physical examination, and routine electrocardiography. The mean age for the control group was 36 ± 11 years.

Signal averaging. Bipolar X, Y, and Z leads were each recorded for 133 sec and amplified by a high-gain, low-noise amplifier. Each signal was then converted to digital information at 1000 samples/sec with a resolution of 1 to 2.5 μV. A bandpass filtered Z lead served as a reference signal to set a reference time for signal averaging. Signal averaging was performed after each new beat was tested with a template-recognition program to reject ectopic and grossy noisy beats. Acceptable beats were signal averaged over a 512 msec segment beginning 100 msec before the QRS complex. Each averaged lead was then filtered (>25 Hz) in a bidirectional fashion to eliminate impulse ringing of the filter at the end of the QRS complex.[6] The three filtered signals were then combined into a vector magnitude, $\sqrt{(X^2 + Y^2 + Z^2)}$, which allowed the detection of high-frequency voltage in any lead. This filtered vector magnitude is referred to as the "filtered QRS complex." The QRS onset and end were determined by a computer algorithm that found the points at which the mean filtered voltage, measured over a 5 msec interval, exceeded the mean plus 3 SDs of the noise sample.[6] The noise sample (20 to 80 msec) was located in the PR segment for the filtered QRS onset and in the ST segment for the end of the QRS. All voltages reported were measured by the root-mean-square method. Total filtered QRS voltage refers to the amplitude measured over the entire filtered QRS duration. The voltage for the last 40 msec of the filtered QRS complex was calculated separately. These techniques were derived from a study of patients with coronary artery disease.[6]

A late potential is defined as a waveform with voltage not exceeding 25 μV in the last 40 msec of the filtered QRS complex. An abnormal signal-averaged electrocardiogram is defined as that having both a filtered QRS duration of 110 msec or more and a late potential.[6]

Five patients in the sustained VT/VF group and two patients in the no sustained VT/VF group were studied while taking antiarrhythmic drugs. Antiarrhythmic agents have been shown to prolong the filtered QRS complex by 5 to 15 msec, but have no influence on the incidence of late potentials.[11]

Data analysis. Results were analyzed with the unpaired t test, Fischer's exact test, chi square with or without Yate's correction, and R by C contingency analysis. Continuous data are expressed as mean ± SD.

Results

Patient characteristics. The ejection fraction in the study group was 26 ± 10%. The ejection fraction in the sustained VT/VF group was 30 ± 9%, and that in the no sustained VT/VF group was 24 ± 9% (p=NS).

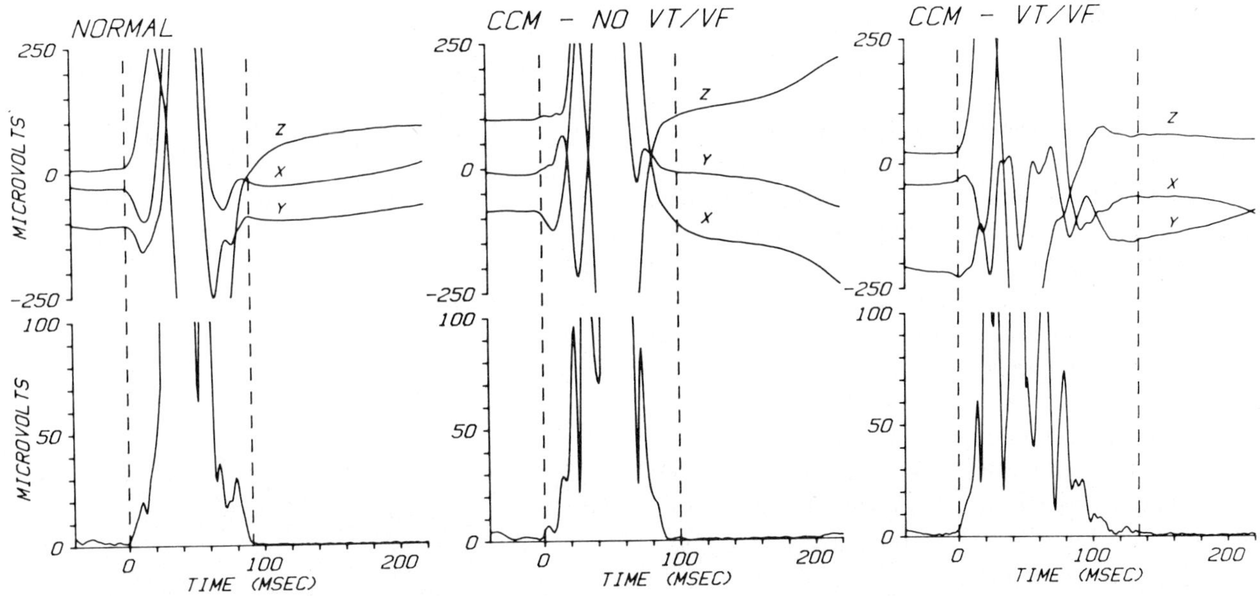

FIGURE 1. Examples of signal-averaged electrocardiograms obtained from each of the three patient groups. On *top* are the signal-averaged bipolar x, y, and z leads shown at high gain. The filtered QRS complex appears on the *bottom*. The dashed lines indicate the end points of the filtered QRS complex as determined by a computer algorithm. The example from a normal individual shows a symmetric filtered QRS complex lasting less than 100 msec and containing no persistent low-amplitude activity in the last 40 msec. The example from a patient with congestive cardiomyopathy and no sustained ventricular arrhythmia shows a normal filtered QRS complex and no late potential. The example from a patient with congestive cardiomyopathy and sustained ventricular arrhythmia shows a prolonged filtered QRS duration with low-level late potential at the end of the filtered QRS complex.

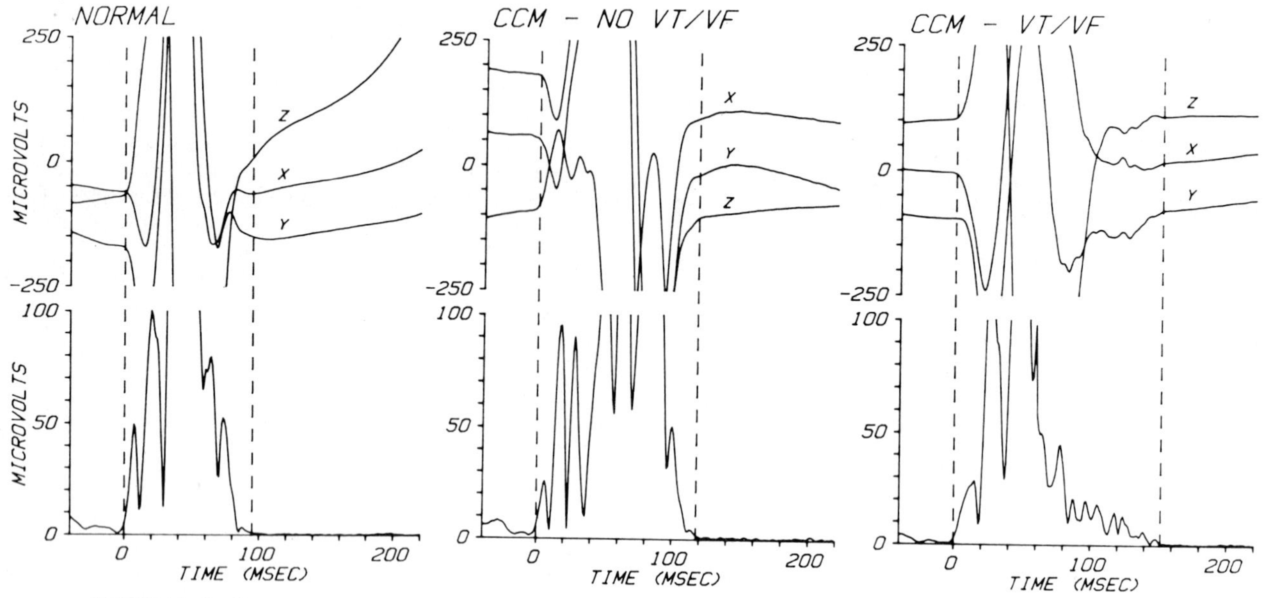

FIGURE 2. Further examples of signal-averaged electrocardiograms from the three patient groups. The example from a patient with cardiomyopathy and no sustained ventricular arrhythmia shows a prolonged filtered QRS complex and no late potential.

Eleven of 16 patients (69%) in the no sustained VT/VF group who underwent 24 hr ambulatory electrocardiographic monitoring had nonsustained ventricular tachycardia lasting up to 10 beats.

Signal averaging. Examples of signal processing from individuals in the normal, cardiomyopathy and no sustained VT/VF, and cardiomyopathy and sustained VT/VF groups are illustrated in figure 1. Patients with cardiomyopathy and no sustained arrhythmias usually had a filtered QRS duration similar to that of normal subjects and no late potentials. Patients with sustained arrhythmias usually had a prolonged filtered QRS duration with a late potential. Ten of 29 (34%) patients with no sustained VT/VF had mildly prolonged filtered QRS duration (figure 2).

The filtered QRS duration was longest in patients in the sustained VT/VF group (130.2 ± 19.5 vs 105.0 ± 13.1 msec in the no sustained arrhythmia group, $p < .001$) and vs 95.9 ± 9.1 in the normal group, $p < .001$) (figure 3). Of note, 11 patients (92%) in the sustained VT/VF group had a QRS duration of 110 msec or more, in contrast to 10 patients (34%) in the no sustained VT/VF group ($p < .001$) and three patients (5%) in the normal group.

The voltage in the last 40 msec of the filtered QRS (figure 4) was 53.7 ± 25.2 μV in the normal and 53.5 ± 28.3 μV in the no sustained VT/VF group. The mean voltage in the sustained VT/VF group was significantly lower at 11.3 ± 9.3 μV ($p < .001$). Eighty-three percent of patients in the sustained VT/VF group had a late potential compared with 17% of those in the no sustained VT/VF group ($p < .001$) and 7% of those in the normal group.

The total QRS voltage was similar in the normal and the cardiomyopathy no VT/VF groups (figure 5), with values of 109.0 ± 29.1 and 102.7 ± 35.1 μV, respectively. The sustained arrhythmia group had lower total voltage (71.4 ± 17.0 μV, $p < .005$), but there was considerable overlap between groups.

Eighty-three percent of patients with sustained

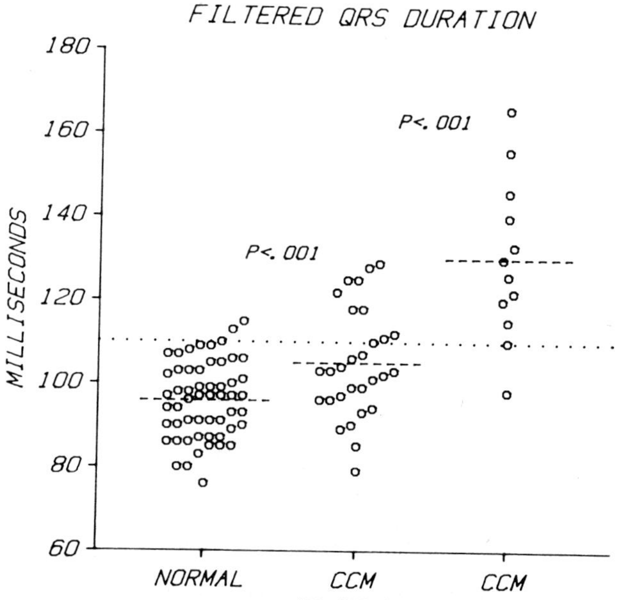

FIGURE 3. Values for filtered QRS duration in the three study groups. The dashed lines represent the mean value for all patients in each group. The dotted line represents a threshold of 110 msec.

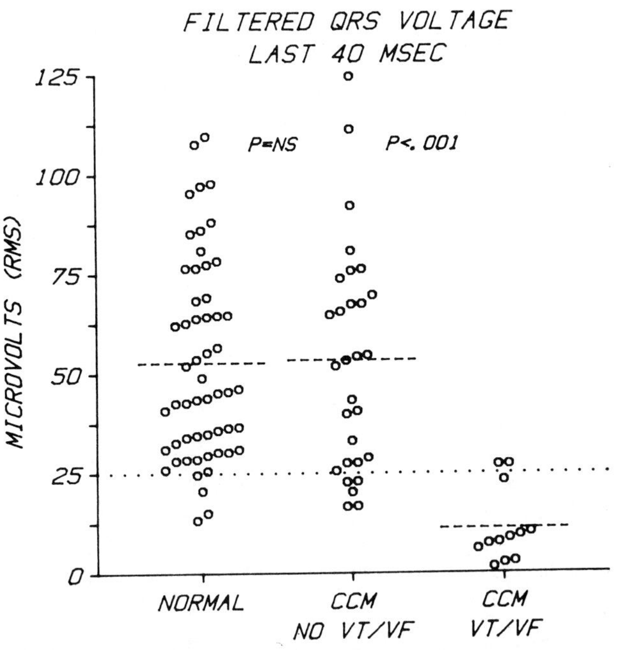

FIGURE 4. Values for filtered QRS voltage in the last 40 msec. The dashed lines represent mean values for patients in each group. The dotted line represents a voltage threshold of 25 μV demonstrating low-level late potentials below it.

VT/VF had abnormal signal-averaged electrocardiograms, i.e., both long filtered QRS duration and a late potential. Only 2% of normal subjects and 14% of patients with no sustained VT/VF had abnormal signal-averaged electrocardiograms. This difference between the cardiomyopathy groups was highly significant ($\chi^2 = 15.3; p < .001$). The combined criteria of a QRS duration of 110 msec or more and presence of a late potential identified patients with cardiomyopathy and sustained ventricular arrhythmias with a sensitivity of 83% and a specificity of 86% in this study.

Exclusion of the seven patients who were taking antiarrhythmic medications did not alter the results. Five of six patients (83%) with sustained VT/VF had an abnormal signal-averaged electrocardiogram in contrast to four of 27 (15%) patients without sustained VT/VF ($p < .003$).

Of the 11 patients with nonsustained ventricular tachycardia, two patients had abnormal signal-averaged electrocardiograms (18%). Additionally, one patient had a late potential only and two patients had a QRS duration of 110 msec or more.

The QRS duration determined by the routine surface electrocardiogram did not distinguish between the cardiomyopathy groups. Fifty-five percent of patients in the no sustained VT/VF group had a routine surface QRS duration of 100 msec or more compared with 67% of patients in the sustained VT/VF group (p=NS). Patients with low-level late potentials on the signal-averaged electrocardiogram had ejection fractions similar to those of patients without late potentials (27.7 ± 9.4% vs 24.5 ± 9.6%, p=NS).

Discussion

Signal-averaged electrocardiography appears to be a useful test for identifying patients with coronary artery disease and ventricular tachycardia.[2–8] This study extends the application of this technique to patients with nonischemic cardiomyopathy and demonstrates that abnormalities of the signal-averaged electrocardiogram can identify patients with sustained ventricular arrhythmias. Patients with cardiomyopathy have longer filtered QRS durations than normal individuals, and the presence of a long filtered QRS duration together with a late potenial differentiated the cardiomyopathy population with sustained ventricular arrhythmias from that with no sustained ventricular arrhythmias. This distinction is not discernible on the routine electrocardiogram and most likely relates to the ability to detect microvolt-level high-frequency potentials by the signal-averaging technique.

Signal-averaged electrocardiography has developed as a noninvasive measure of late and slow activation, which has been associated with reentrant arrhythmias.[12–15] Low-level late potentials detected by signal-averaging techniques have been correlated with localized areas of delayed ventricular activation in animal and human preparations.[10, 16, 17] Additionally, fractionated electrograms have been recorded by endocardial and epicardial mapping techniques in patients with

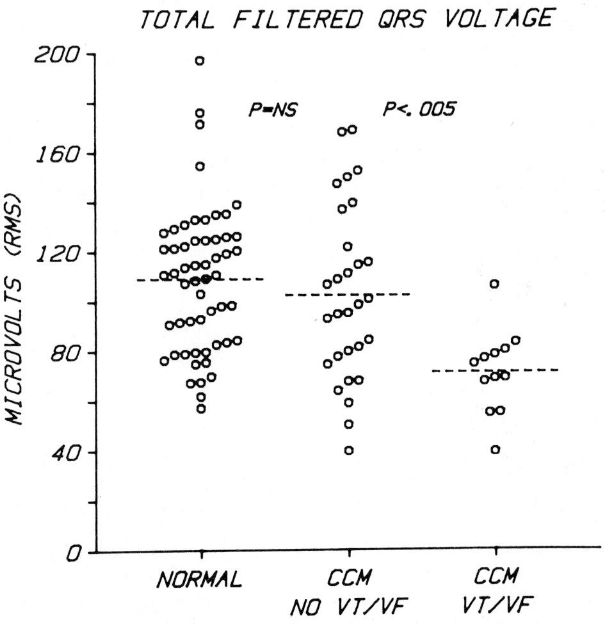

FIGURE 5. Values for total filtered QRS voltage. The dashed lines represent mean values from each group.

ventricular tachycardia and coronary artery disease[18, 19] as well as in those with right ventricular dysplasia, a diffuse myocardial process.[10, 20–22] These fractionated electrograms have been correlated with the surface late potential and the duration of these fragmented electrograms has correlated with the surface filtered QRS duration.[10, 16] The precise role of these abnormal areas of myocardium in arrhythmogenesis has not been established, but it appears that among patients with coronary disease and prior myocardial infarction, the extent and severity of fragmentation is greatest in patients with recurrent sustained ventricular tachycardia.[23, 24]

The substrate for ventricular arrhythmias in patients with nonischemic congestive cardiomyopathy has not been characterized. We recently reported data that supported reentry as a mechanism for uniform ventricular tachycardia in patients with idiopathic cardimyopathy based on initiation and termination of tachycardias and the resetting phenomenon in response to programmed stimulation.[25] Fontaine et al.[20] have reported delayed and abnormal electrograms both endocardially and epicardially in patients with right ventricular dysplasia, suggesting that slow conduction is an element of arrhythmogenesis in that patient population. We present evidence here that patients with nonischemic congestive cardiomyopathy and sustained ventricular arrhythmias have a detectable electrophysiologic substrate. Detection of low-level late potentials and a prolonged filtered QRS duration implies that these patients have delayed ventricular activation. Whether this slow conduction participates in arrhythmogenesis or merely reflects the severity and extent of diseased myocardium remains to be determined. Describing the anatomic and electrophysiologic characteristics of this slow conduction requires further investigation.

The abnormalities of the signal-averaged electrocardiogram we describe appear to be markers of electrical instability in patients with non-ischemic congestive cardiomyopathy. The utility of this test as a noninvasive predictor of risk in this patient population awaits prospective evaluation.

We are grateful to Miss Anita Armellini for her secretarial assistance.

References

1. Wilson JR, Schwartz JS, St. John Sutton M, Ferraro N, Horowitz LN, Reichek N, Josephson ME: Prognosis in severe heart failure: relation to hemodynamic measurements and ventricular ectopic activity. J Am Coll Cardiol **2:** 403, 1983
2. Uther JB, Dennett CJ, Tan A: The detection of delayed activation signals of low amplitude in the vectorcardiogram of patients with recurrent ventricular tachycardia by signal averaging. *In* Sandoe E, Julian DG, Bell JW, editors: Management of ventricular tachycardia — role of mexiletine. Amsterdam, 1978, Excerpta Medica, pp 80–82
3. Hombach V, Hopp HW, Braun V, Behrenbeck DW, Tauchert M, Hilger HH: Die Bedeutung von Nachpotentialen innerhalb des ST-Segmentes im Oberflachen — EKG bei Patienten mit koronarer Herzkrankheit. Dtsch Med Wochenschr **105:** 1457, 1980
4. Breithardt G, Becker G, Seipel L, Abendroth RR, Ostermeyer J: Noninvasive detection of late potentials in man — a new marker for ventricular tachycardia. Eur Heart J **2:** 1, 1981
5. Rozanski JJ, Mortara D, Myerburg RJ, Castellanos A: Body surface detection of delayed depolarizations in patients with recurrent ventricular tachycardia and left ventricular aneurysm. Circulation **63:** 1172, 1981
6. Simson MB: Identification of patients with ventricular tachycardia after myocardial infarction from signals in the terminal QRS complex. Circulation **64:** 235, 1981
7. Denes P, Santarelli P, Hauser RG, Uretz EF: Quantitative analysis of the high-frequency components of the terminal portion of the body surface QRS in normal subjects and in patients with ventricular tachycardia. Circulation **67:** 1129, 1983
8. Cain ME, Ambos HD, Witkowski FX, Sobel BE: Fast-Fourier transform analysis of signal averaged electrocardiograms for identification of patients prone to sustained ventricular tachycardia. Circulation **69:** 711, 1984
9. Stamm RB, Carabello BA, Mayer DL, Martin FP: Two-dimensional echocardiographic measurement of left ventricular ejection fraction: prospective analysis of what constitutes an adequate determination. Am Heart J **104:** 136, 1982
10. Simson MB, Untereker WJ, Spielman SR, Horowitz LN, Marcus NH, Falcone RA, Harken AH, Josephson ME: Relation between late potentials on the body surface and directly recorded fragmented electrograms in patients with ventricular tachycardia. Am J Cardiol **51:** 105, 1983
11. Simson MB, Waxman HL, Falcone RA, Marcus NH, Josephson ME: Effects of antiarrhythmic drugs on noninvasively recorded late potentials. *In* Breithardt G, Loogen F, editors: New aspects in the medical teatment of tachyarrhythmias: role of amiodarone. Munich, 1983, Urban and Schwarzenberg, p 80
12. Boineau JP, Cox JL: Slow ventricular activation in acute myocardial infarction: a source of reentrant premature ventricular contraction. Circulation **48:** 702, 1973
13. Waldo AL, Kaiser GA: A study of ventricular arrhythmias associated with acute myocardial infarction in the canine heart. Circulation **47:** 1222, 1973
14. Wit AL, Cranefield PF, Hoffman BF: Slow conduction and reentry in the ventricular conducting system. Circ Res **30:** 11, 1972
15. El-Sherif N, Scherlag BJ, Lazzara R, Hope RR: Reentrant ventricular arrhythmias in the late myocardial infarction period. 1. Conduction characteristics in the infarction zone. Circulation **55:** 686, 1977
16. Simson MB, Euler D, Michelson EL, Flcone RA, Spear JF, Moore EN: Detection of delayed ventricular activation on the body surface in dogs. Am J Physiol **241:** H363, 1981
17. Berbari EJ, Scherlag BJ, Hope RR, Lazzara R: Recording from the body surface of arrhythmogenic ventricular activity during the ST-segment. Am J Cardiol **41:** 697, 1978
18. Josephson ME, Horowitz LN, Farshidi A: Continuous local electrical activity: a mechanism of recurrent venticular tachycardia. Circulation **57:** 659, 1978
19. Waldo AL, Arciniegas JG, Klein H: Surgical treatment of life-threatening ventricular arrhythmias. The role of intraoperative mapping and consideration of the presently available surgical techniques. Prog Cardiovasc Dis **23:** 247, 1981
20. Fontaine G, Guiraudon G, Frank R, Vedel J, Grosgogeat Y, Cabrol C, Facquet J: Stimulation studies and epicardial mapping in ventricular tachycardia. Study of mechanisms and selections for surgery. *In* Kulbertus HE, editor: Reentrant arrhythmias. Baltimore, 1976, University Park Press, pp 334–350
21. Belhassen B, Caspi A, Miller H, Shapira I, Laniado S: Extensive endocardial mapping during sinus rhythm and ventricular tachycardia in a patient with arrhythmogenic right ventricular dysplasia. J Am Coll Cardiol **4:** 1302, 1984
22. Rosenfeld LE, Batsford WP: Intraventricular Wenckebach conduction and localized reentry in a case of right ventricular dysplasia with recurrent ventricular tachycardia. J Am Coll Cardiol **2:** 585, 1983

23. Wiener I, Mindich B, Pitchon R. Determinants of ventricular tachycardia in patients with ventricular aneurysms: results of intraoperative epicardial and endocardial mapping. Circulation **65:** 856, 1982
24. Klein H, Karp RB, Kouchoukos NT, Zorn GL Jr, James TN, Waldo AL: Intraoperative electrophysiologic mapping of the ventricles during sinus rhythm in patients with a previous myocardial infarction. Identification of the electrophysiologic substrate of ventricular arrhythmias. Circulation **66:** 847, 1982
25. Poll DS, Marchlinski FE, Buxton AE, Doherty JU, Waxman HL, Josephson ME: Sustained ventricular tachycardia in patients with idiopathic dilated cardiomyopathy: electrophysiologic testing and lack of response to antiarrhythmic drug therapy. Circulation **70:** 451, 1984

Coronary angioplasty of multiple vessels: short-term outcome and long-term results

MICHAEL J. COWLEY, M.D., GEORGE W. VETROVEC, M.D., GERMANO DISCIASCIO, M.D., STEPHEN A. LEWIS, M.D., PAUL D. HIRSH, M.D., AND TIMOTHY C. WOLFGANG, M.D.

ABSTRACT Experience with percutaneous transluminal coronary angioplasty (PTCA) of multiple vessels was reviewed to assess short-term outcome and long-term results. PTCA of multiple vessels was performed in 100 of the initial 500 patients (20%) who underwent PTCA at the Medical College of Virginia between July 1979 and August 1984. Eighty-nine percent had class 3 or 4 angina, and 66% had unstable angina. Two-thirds had severe stenosis of two vessels or major branches and one-third had three-vessel disease. One or more significant lesions were dilated in two vessels in 84 patients, in three vessels in 14 patients, and in four vessels in two patients. PTCA of 273 lesions (2.7/patient) was attempted (range two to eight per patient) with angiographic success in 250 lesions (91.6%). Primary success (angiographic and clinical improvement) was achieved in 95 of 100 patients (95%); 84% had success in multiple vessels, and 79% had success in all attempted lesions. Complications occurred in 11 patients (11%); four patients (4%) underwent urgent bypass surgery and four additional patients (4%) had myocardial infarction. Long-term results were assessed in 44 patients with primary success who had follow-up of more than 1 year (mean 26 months) after multiple-vessel PTCA. Twenty-eight patients (64%) remain event-free and improved and 48% are event-free and asymptomatic. Clinical recurrence developed in 15 patients (34%); four had sustained improvement with repeat PTCA, three remain improved with medical therapy, and eight (18%) have undergone bypass surgery during follow-up. One patient (2.3%) developed late myocardial infarction, and no deaths have occurred in the follow-up cohort. Including repeat PTCA, 75% have maintained clinical success during follow-up and 82% remain improved without bypass surgery. These short- and long-term follow-up results suggest that PTCA of multiple vessels is a safe and effective therapy in selected patients with multivessel coronary artery disease.
Circulation 72, No. 6, 1314–1320, 1985.

PERCUTANEOUS transluminal coronary angioplasty (PTCA) is a safe and effective method of myocardial revascularization in selected patients with symptomatic coronary artery disease[1–6] and has been used predominantly in patients with single-vessel disease or selected patients with multivessel disease in whom a single vessel is dilated. Application of PTCA in patients with more extensive coronary artery disease or in multiple vessels has been limited,[7–9] and the safety and short- and long-term efficacy are less clear. This report reviews our experience with PTCA of multiple vessels.

From the Division of Cardiology, Medical College of Virginia, Richmond.

Address for correspondence: Michael J. Cowley, M.D., Division of Cardiology, Medical College of Virginia, Box 59, MCV Station, Richmond, VA 23298.

Presented in part at the American Heart Association 57th Annual Meeting, Anaheim, CA, November 1984.

Received March 12, 1985; revision accepted Aug. 22, 1985.

Methods

PTCA of multiple vessels was performed in selected patients at the Medical College of Virginia after October 1979 under a protocol approved by the institutional Committee for Conduct of Human Research. All patients were considered candidates for coronary bypass surgery based on the presence and severity of angina pectoris, evidence of myocardial ischemia by noninvasive studies (unless contraindicated), and the presence of significant coronary artery disease of more than one major vessel or branch that appeared suitable for revascularization with angioplasty and/or bypass surgery. Multivessel disease was defined by the presence of 50% or greater stenosis in two or more major vessels. However, angioplasty was generally not performed in vessels with less than 70% stenosis. Primary exclusion criteria for multiple-vessel PTCA were left main disease, multiple total occlusions, and severe, diffuse disease with extensive involvement of all major vessels and branches. Patients with distal lesions or total occlusions were not excluded if the lesions appeared accessible for dilatation. In some patients, additional disease was present in vessels not considered suitable for PTCA or for bypass grafting because of small size or diffuse or distal involvement, so that PTCA was considered to offer a reasonable probability of revascularizing the major ischemic segments. In several patients, vessels were dilated that were not considered appropriate for bypass grafting. All procedures were performed with a cardiac surgery team on stand-by. Patients received aspirin (600 mg/day), dipyridamole (150 mg/day), and a calcium antagonist for 1 to 2 days before PTCA and for 6 months after PTCA. All patients received heparin intravenously (5000 to 10,000 IU), nitroglycerin ointment, and intracoronary nitroglycerin during the procedure.

Angioplasty of the vessel considered to be the most important (based on vessel size and lesion severity) was initially performed, and if successful, additional vessels were attempted. When sequential lesions were present in one or more vessels, it was frequently necessary to dilate the more proximal lesion first, regardless of whether it was the more severe lesion. When a vessel with high-grade disease supplied collaterals to another vessel, the collateralized vessel was dilated first to protect its source of collateral flow. A second or third vessel was generally not attempted if dilatation of the preceding vessel was not successful. Angioplasty of additional vessels was also not performed at the same session when angiographic success was equivocal or if major intimal split was evident that might progress to occlusive dissection. Angiographic success was defined as 20% or greater improvement in luminal diameter. A procedure was considered successful when all vessels/lesions were successfully dilated or the most important vessel was successfully dilated and clinical improvement occurred. Definitions of complications have been previously reported.[6] Lesion severity was determined by visual assessment as the average diameter reduction in multiple views before and after PTCA. Angioplasty was performed by standard techniques, with fixed-tip catheters in the early experience and moveable wire (steerable) catheter systems when they became available.

Clinical recurrence was defined as recurrence of symptoms after initial improvement associated with angiographic evidence of restenosis of one or more lesions. Follow-up status was determined at periodic follow-up visits or by telephone interview. Vital status, presence of angina, medication use, occurrence of myocardial infarction, and need for further revascularization with PTCA or bypass surgery were assessed. Long-term follow-up status was analyzed for patients who had a minimum of 12 months follow-up after multiple-vessel PTCA.

Statistical analysis was performed with the chi-square test for discrete variables and t test for continuous variables.

Results

PTCA of multiple vessels was performed in 100 of the first 500 patients (20%) who underwent PTCA at the Medical College of Virginia between July 1979 and August 1984. The baseline clinical and angiographic profiles of the patients are shown in table 1. There were 71 men and 29 women with a mean age of 55 ± 10 years (range 23 to 85). Eighty-six patients (86%) had multivessel disease: 53 patients with two-vessel disease and 33 with three-vessel disease. Fourteen patients (14%) had single-vessel disease by conventional classification; each also had significant stenosis of one or more major branches of the parent vessel. Fifteen patients (15%) had prior coronary bypass surgery, 36% had prior myocardial infarction, and 66 had (66%) unstable angina. Forty-six patients had class 4 angina (Canadian Heart Classification), 41 had class 3, 12 had class 2, and one had postcardiac transplant ischemia.

The proportion of patients having PTCA of multiple vessels increased with increasing experience: first 100 cases, nine; second 100 cases, 12; third 100 cases, 10; fourth 100 cases, 26; fifth 100 cases, 43. The distribution of multiple-vessel PTCA also increased by calendar year: 1979, two patients; 1980, one patient; 1981, five patients; 1982, 11 patients; 1983, 26 patients; 1984, 55 patients.

Angioplasty of two vessels was performed in 84 patients (84%), of three vessels in 14 patients (14%), and of four vessels in two patients (2%). PTCA of multiple vessels was performed in 91 patients at their first PTCA procedure and in nine (who had undergone prior single-vessel PTCA) at a second or third PTCA procedure. In 98 patients, multiple vessels were dilated at the same session and two patients had "staged" PTCA, with the second vessel dilated 1 day later. Two lesions were attempted in 57 patients (57%), three in 25 patients (25%), four in 11 patients (11%), five in four patients (4%), six in two patients (2%), and eight in one patient (1%).

PTCA result by vessels/lesions. Overall, PTCA was attempted in 273 lesions (2.7 lesions/patient) and angiographic success was achieved in 250 lesions (91.6%). Success rate by individual vessel attempted ranged from 96% for right coronary lesions to 79% for circumflex lesions (table 2) and was significantly lower for the circumflex artery than for other vessels ($p < .05$). The combinations of vessels attempted and pa-

TABLE 1
Clinical profiles of 100 patients undergoing multiple-vessel PTCA

	n	%
Age (mean)	55 ± 10 yr (23–85 yr)	
Sex		
Male	71	71
Female	29	29
Unstable angina	66	66
Prior MI	36	36
Prior CABG	15	15
Angina class (CHC)		
Class 2	12	12
Class 3	41	41
Class 4	46	46
Other	1	1
Extent CAD		
1 vessel	14	14
2 vessel	53	53
3 vessel	33	33
1st PTCA	91	91
2nd or 3rd PTCA	9	9

CABG = coronary artery bypass surgery; CAD = coronary artery disease; CHC = Canadian Heart Class; MI = myocardial infarction.

TABLE 2
Success rate by individual vessels in patients undergoing multiple-vessel PTCA

Vessel	n	Success	%
LAD	104	99	95
RCA	72	69	96
LCX	48	38	79[A]
Diagonal	33	29	88
Graft	14	13	93
Left main	1	1	100
Septal	1	1	100
Total	273	250	92

LAD = left anterior descending; LCX = left circumflex; RCA = right coronary artery.

[A]$p < .05$.

tient and lesion success rates are shown in table 3.

The mean severity of the multiple lesions before and after PTCA are shown in table 4. The initial severity of first lesions was greater than that of subsequent lesions ($p < .01$), although the relative severity of first through sixth lesions dilated was similar (range 90% to 82%).

PTCA was not successful in 23 lesions (8%); in 19 the lesion could not be traversed with the balloon catheter (stenosis too tight in 14, tortuosity or unfavorable angulation in five). In four unsuccessful attempts, the lesion was dilated but occlusive dissection developed at the dilated site (one patient) or distally (three patients). Six unsuccessful attempts were of total occlusions.

TABLE 3
Combinations of vessels dilated and patient and lesion success rates with multiple-vessel PTCA

Vessels	Patients[A]	Lesions[A]
LAD/RCA	28/28 (100)	82/80 (98)
LAD/Diag.	20/19 (95)	50/47 (94)
LAD/LCX	18/17 (94)	40/35 (88)
Graft/other	8/ 7 (88)	19/17 (89)
RCA/LCX	7/ 7 (100)	19/16 (84)
LAD/RCA/LCX	5/ 5 (100)	21/19 (90)
RCA/Diag.	5/ 5 (100)	12/11 (92)
LCX/Diag.	3/ 3 (100)	8/ 7 (88)
LAD/RCA/Diag.	2/ 2 (100)	7/ 7 (100)
LCX/marginal	2/ 2 (100)	7/ 7 (100)
LAD/septal	1/ 0 (0)	3/ 2 (67)
LAD/LCX/Diag.	1/ 1 (100)	4/ 2 (50)
Total	100/95 (95)	273/250 (92)

Diag. = diagonal artery; LAD = left anterior descending; LCX = left circumflex; RCA = right coronary artery.

[A]Expressed as total number of patients or lesions/number successful, with the percentage in parentheses.

PTCA of total occlusions was attempted in 11 patients (11%) and was successful in five of 11 occlusions (45%). The occlusion was the primary vessel in four patients, the second vessel in five, and the third vessel in two; PTCA was successful in three of four occlusions in the primary vessel, two of five in the second vessel, and none of two in the third vessel. Success rate for total occlusions was significantly lower than that for patent vessels (45% vs 94%; $p < .001$).

PTCA result by patients. PTCA was clinically successful in 95 of 100 patients (95%). Eighty-seven patients (87%) had successful PTCA of multiple lesions and 84 patients (84%) had successful PTCA of more than one vessel and associated clinical success. In 15 patients, PTCA of only one vessel was successful (11 with clinical success and four with clinical failure). Seventy-nine patients (79%) had successful dilatation of all attempted lesions (range two to eight lesions). Thirty-six patients (36%) also had sequential (tandem) lesions dilated in one or more vessels (31 in one vessel, five in two or three vessels).

In eight additional patients, PTCA of multiple vessels was planned but was not performed because of failure to dilate the primary vessel. Overall clinical success rate of multiple vessel PTCA, including these patients, was 95 of 108 patients (88%). In seven other patients, multiple-vessel PTCA was considered but was not performed despite success of the first vesssel because of the length of the procedure or the small size of the second vessel or because the second vessel lesion was not severe.

PTCA was not successful in five patients (5%) in whom multiple vessels were attempted. In four the first vessel was successfully dilated but PTCA of a second major vessel was not successful or produced deterioration of flow and early bypass surgery was performed. In the other patient with unsuccessful PTCA, although the primary vessel (left anterior descending [LAD]) was unsuccessful, a secondary (large septal) vessel

TABLE 4
Coronary stenosis severity before and after PTCA for multiple lesions

Lesion	n	% Stenosis before	% Stenosis after
1st	100	90 ± 7[A]	43 ± 17
2nd	100	85 ± 11	48 ± 20
3rd	43	84 ± 9	45 ± 24
4th	18	84 ± 11	44 ± 23
5th	7	82 ± 7	32 ± 15
6th	3	83 ± 10	40 ± 10

[A]$p < .01$ for first lesion severity vs other lesions before PTCA.

was dilated despite the need for bypass surgery because the septal artery was considered to be of clinical importance and would not otherwise be revascularized.

Complications. Complications during or after PTCA of multiple vessels occurred in 11 patients (11%). Urgent bypass surgery was performed in four patients (4%): one who had occlusive dissection beyond the dilated site in the left circumflex artery (LCX) after PTCA of an LAD graft, one who developed deterioration of flow in the primary vessel during PTCA of the second vessel, one who developed subtotal occlusion with delayed flow in the LAD whose septal branch was then dilated before surgery, and one patient with unstable angina whose LAD could not be dilated after PTCA of the LCX.

Evidence of myocardial infarction developed in five patients (5%), with Q waves in two patients (2%) and without Q waves in three patients. Both Q wave infarctions occurred after successful PTCA caused by acute occlusion of one of the successfully dilated vessels 4 and 6 hr later. One had early reperfusion with repeat PTCA and had evidence of residual function in the infarct zone despite Q waves. Both had continued patency of major dilated vessels and were clinically improved despite myocardial infarction involving one of the vessels. Both later developed return of angina after restenosis of a primary vessel, indicating that the initial improvement was caused by revascularization with angioplasty. Of the three non–Q wave infarctions, one occurred in a patient who had urgent bypass surgery for occlusion of a major secondary vessel, and two occurred in patients who had dissection of a second or third dilated vessel that was managed without surgery. Three other patients developed asymptomatic occlusion of secondary vessels that were collateralized. The patients with non–Q wave infarction and with asymptomatic occlusion were each improved after PTCA.

TABLE 5
Follow-up outcome after successful multiple-vessel PTCA

	>12 mo follow-up
No. of patients	44
Mean follow-up	26 mo
Follow-up events	16 (36%)
Clinical recurrence	15 (34%)
Repeat PTCA	9
Success	6
2nd/3rd recurrence	1
Sustained improvement	4
CABG	8 (18%)
For initial recurrence	6
After 2nd/3rd recurrence	1
For new disease	1
Medical therapy, improved	3 (7%)
Myocardial infarction	1 (2%)
Death	0
Event-free, improved	28 (64%)
Asymptomatic	21 (48%)
Continued success[A]	33 (75%)
Improved, no CABG[B]	36 (82%)

[A]Includes patients with sustained improvement after repeat PTCA and patient with myocardial infarction.

[B]Includes patients with recurrence managed with medication and improved.

Follow-up. Clinical status was assessed in the 45 patients who had completed at least 1 year of follow-up after multiple-vessel PTCA through January 1985; 44 had successful PTCA and represent the follow-up cohort (table 5). Follow-up ranged from 12 to 62 months (mean 26). The clinical profiles of the follow-up cohort did not differ from those of the total study population.

Twenty-eight of these 44 patients (64%) had sustained clinical improvement and were event-free (no clinical recurrence, myocardial infarction, or death), and 21 patients (48%) were asymptomatic and event-free during follow-up. In the 16 patients who had events, 15 had clinical recurrence, one had myocardial infarction, and none died.

Clinical recurrence (return of angina and angiographic evidence of restenosis) occurred in 15 of 44 patients (34%). Mean time for clinical recurrence was 8.3 $\pm$ 11 months (median 6), with a range of 1.5 to 47 months. Clinical recurrence developed during the first year in 13 patients and occurred in two patients beyond 1 year (at 13 and 47 months). Repeat catheterization was performed in 29 of the 44 follow-up patients (66%), including all 15 with return of symptoms. In the 15 patients with clinical recurrence, repeat PTCA was attempted in nine and was successful in six; five of these six have not had a second recurrence at a mean follow-up of 12 months after the second PTCA. Bypass surgery was performed during follow-up in eight patients (18%): for clinical recurrence in seven patients (three without a second PTCA, three after unsuccessful repeat PTCA, one after a third recurrence) and in one patient at 18 months for progression of disease unsuitable for PTCA. In three patients clinical recurrence was partial associated with minimal return of symptoms; these patients remain improved on a medical regimen without additional revascularization. One patient (2.3%) developed myocardial infarction during follow-up (at 6 months) because of new occlusion of a vessel that had not had significant stenosis; both dilated vessels remained improved at restudy and clinical improvement has been maintained. Myocardial infarction rate during follow-up was 1.25%/year. No deaths have occurred in the follow-up cohort.

Overall 33 of 44 patients (75%) have had continued success of angioplasty: 28 who were event-free and improved, four after repeat PTCA, and one with infarction involving an undilated vessel. Including the three additional patients with partial recurrence managed with medical therapy, 36 of 44 patients (82%) have remained improved or asymptomatic without requiring surgery during the mean follow-up period of 26 months.

Of the 15 patients with clinical recurrence, 12 (80%) developed restenosis of only one dilated vessel or lesion and three patients (20%) had recurrence of multiple vessels or lesions. Overall, 18 of 34 lesions (53%) and 18 of 29 vessels (62%) recurred in these patients.

The overall incidence of clinical recurrence at our institution during this period was 83 of 294 patients (28.2%) with follow-up of more than 12 months after successful PTCA: 68 of 250 patients (27.2%) after PTCA of a single vessel and 15 of 44 (34.1%) in patients after PTCA of multiple vessels (p = NS).

Of the remaining 55 patients who have not reached 1 year after PTCA of multiple vessels, all have reached at least 6 months after multiple vessel angioplasty. For the total population (follow-up range of 6 to 62 months, mean 15), clinical recurrence has developed in 31 of 95 patients (33%), infarction in two patients (2.1%), and repeat PTCA in 25 patients with success in 22 (88%). Bypass surgery was performed in 10 patients (10.4%). One death has occurred during follow-up in a 78-year-old patient who had clinical recurrence involving one of three vessels. Repeat PTCA was successful but the patient died suddenly (presumably of an arrhythmia) 48 hr later. Overall mortality rate during follow-up after multiple-vessel PTCA was 0.8%/year.

Discussion

The initial guidelines for use of PTCA were restricted to patients with single-vessel coronary artery disease and selected patients with multivessel disease in whom a single vessel was attempted and the safety and efficacy of PTCA in these situations has been established.[1-5] With improvements in technology and increased experience, application of PTCA in multiple vessels and more complex anatomic situations has become feasible. However, experience with PTCA in multiple vessels has been limited and the safety and long-term efficacy in this setting are not as well characterized. These results with PTCA of multiple vessels in 100 patients over a 5 year period demonstrate that satisfactory early and longer-term results can be achieved with PTCA of multiple vessels in selected patients. The majority of patients in this experience had two-vessel disease, and only one-third had three-vessel disease. Therefore the study population does not represent a general population of patients with multivessel disease who may require revascularization. However, the study population was severely symptomatic, with nearly 90% having functional class 3 or 4 angina and 66% having unstable angina.

In addition to angioplasty of multiple vessels, 36% also had PTCA of sequential lesions in one or more vessels, 43% had PTCA of three or more lesions, and nearly 20% had dilatation of four or more lesions. An average of 2.7 lesions/patient were dilated with an angiographic success rate of 92%, and clinical improvement was achieved in 95% of patients. In a multicenter experience with complex angioplasty, Dorros et al.[7] have reported success rates in excess of 90% for patients having multiple dilatations in a single vessel or in more than one vessel. Hartzler et al.,[8] in a preliminary report, have reported similar success rates in patients with complex anatomy and with multiple dilatations. Our results with PTCA of multiple vessels confirm high initial angiographic and clinical success rates in selected patients undergoing multiple-vessel angioplasty. The clinical success rate in our multiple-vessel dilatation group is higher than the overall success rate of 81% for our total PTCA population during the same period. This in part reflects careful patient selection for multiple-vessel PTCA and the higher proportion of patients undergoing multiple-vessel angioplasty in our more recent experience, when we had more experience and better technology was available. The proportion of patients undergoing multiple-vessel PTCA progressively increased from 9% of the first 100 cases to 43% of the fifth 100 cases at our institution. The high success rate is also to some extent artifactual, since multiple vessels were not usually attempted if the first was unsuccessful. However, inclusion of patients in whom PTCA of multiple vessels was planned but not performed would have resulted in an overall primary success rate of 88%. All patients with clinical success had improvement and most were asymptomatic. The high frequency of symptomatic improvement likely reflects the high prevalence of successful revascularization of multiple zones, since most patients had high-grade stenoses of multiple vessels and 88% of the 95 patients with primary success had successful PTCA of multiple vessels.

Case selection guidelines were based on the estimated technical feasibility of suitable revascularization of the multiple vessels/lesions with PTCA and reflect evolving experience with the technique. Patients were generally selected as candidates for multiple-vessel angioplasty when they were judged as having a high likelihood of successful revascularization of the major ischemic segments, weighing the individual probabilities of successful dilatation of each lesion. The success rate for circumflex lesions was significantly lower than that for other vessels; a similar relationship was seen in the NHLBI PTCA Registry.[3] Success rate was also lower for total occlusions than for patent vessels ($p < .001$), but nearly 50% of total occlusions were successfully dilated. The mean severity of second or subsequent vessels or lesions dilated was less than the primary lesion but still represented high-grade stenoses (mean 82% to 85%) in the additional vessels.

The incidence of significant complications (myocardial infarction or urgent bypass surgery) of 8% in this experience is comparable to results reported for patients in the NHLBI PTCA Registry,[5, 6] who had less extensive coronary artery disease, and to other reports of complex coronary angioplasty and multiple dilatations.[7, 8] Urgent bypass surgery was performed in 4% and evidence of infarction developed in four additional patients. Each of the four patients with infarction managed nonoperatively was improved despite infarction, probably because of effective revascularization of other major ischemic segments, and two of these four had clinically small (non–Q wave) infarctions. No in-hospital deaths occurred with multiple-vessel angioplasty.

Although angioplasty of multiple vessels may carry a higher potential risk than PTCA of a single vessel, the incidence of important complications in this experience was not appreciably different from published reports predominantly involving patients with single-vessel disease. This may be due in part to improvements in technology and increased experience with PTCA, which appear to have reduced the risk, as well as to have increased success rates.[6, 10–12] The major risks of multiple-vessel PTCA are acute occlusion of multiple vessels or acute extensive ischemia caused by occlusion of a major vessel that supplies collateral flow to other vessels. Certain factors involving patient selection and technical considerations would appear important to minimize these risks. Most patients in our study did not have three-vessel disease and patients with left main stenosis, who are at increased risk with PTCA,[4] were generally not considered candidates for PTCA in our study. Use of a staged or sequenced approach to multiple vessels, with PTCA of the most important or safest vessels initially and additional vessels only if the preceding vessel has an excellent angiographic result, should minimize the risk of multiple occlusions. When the angiographic result was equivocal in one of the vessels, additional vessels were dilated later in a separate session when it was clear that the primary vessel had maintained stable patency. In addition, when severe stenosis was present in a vessel supplying collaterals to other vessels, the collateralized vessel was dilated first to avoid jeopardizing the source of collateral flow.

Long-term follow-up. The long-term results, analyzed in the subset of patients who had a minimum follow-up period of at least 1 year, indicate that sustained improvement was achieved in the majority of patients after multiple-vessel PTCA; 64% are event-free and remain improved and nearly 50% are asymptomatic during the mean follow-up period of more than 2 years. Clinical recurrence, the most common event, has developed in 34% during follow-up. Although clinical recurrence was frequently evident during the first 6 months, the mean time for clinical recurrence was 8.3 months (median 6), suggesting that follow-up of at least 1 year may better characterize the recurrence rate with multiple-vessel PTCA than a shorter follow-up period. Although the recurrence rate after PTCA of multiple vessels was higher (34%) than that with single-vessel PTCA at our institution (28%), the difference was not significant, and our clinical recurrence rate with multiple-vessel PTCA is similar to other reports for recurrence after PTCA.[13, 14] These results suggest that the recurrence rate after multiple-vessel PTCA may not be substantially higher than that with single-vessel PTCA and that recurrence may be patient-related rather than related to the number of vessels or lesions dilated. Of interest, 80% of patients who developed recurrence after PTCA of multiple vessels had restenosis of only one vessel. Repeat PTCA is feasible in most patients with recurrence and often achieves sustained improvement.[15]

Bypass surgery after successful PTCA was performed in 18% of the follow-up cohort, usually for recurrence in multiple vessels or recurrence plus progression of disease in other vessels, and in several patients after unsuccessful repeat PTCA. The incidence of myocardial infarction during follow-up was low (1%/year) and no deaths occurred in the follow-up cohort. Overall, including repeat PTCA, 75% have had continued success of angioplasty and 82% have remained improved or asymptomatic without requiring surgery during the mean follow-up of 26 months. These long-term results with PTCA of multiple vessels are comparable to the follow-up results reported from the NHLBI PTCA Registry in a population composed predominantly of patients with single-vessel disease who were followed for a mean of 18 months.[4] Although the number of patients with follow-up of at least 12 months in our study is relatively small and represents only approximately 50% of the multiple-vessel PTCA group, the incidence of continued improvement, clinical recurrence, and event-free outcome appears similar in the additional patients who have not yet reached 1 year after PTCA of multiple vessels. One death has occurred in the total study group, representing an annual mortality rate of 0.8%/year.

In summary, these short-term outcome and long-term follow-up results after PTCA of multiple vessels indicate that multiple-vessel PTCA can be performed with high success rates and acceptable complication rates in selected patients, that continued success can be achieved in approximately 75% of patients during long-term follow-up, and that PTCA of multiple vessels is a safe and effective therapy in selected patients with multivessel coronary artery disease. However, comparative studies of PTCA with alternative therapies will be necessary to clarify the role of coronary angioplasty in the various subsets of patients with multivessel coronary artery disease.

References

1. Gruentzig AR, Senning A, Siegenthaler WE: Nonoperative dilatation of coronary artery stenosis: percutaneous transluminal coronary angioplasty. N Engl J Med **301:** 61, 1979
2. Cowley MJ, Vetrovec GW, Wolfgang TC: Efficacy of percutaneous transluminal coronary angioplasty: technique, patient selection, salutary results, limitations and complications. Am Heart J **101:** 272, 1981
3. Kent KM, Bentivoglio LG, Block PC, Cowley MJ, Dorros G, Gosselin AJ, Gruentzig A, Myler RK, Simpson J, Stertzer SH, Williams DO, Fisher L, Gillespie MJ, Mullin SM, Mock MB: Percutaneous transluminal coronary angioplasty: report from the NHLBI Registry. Am J Cardiol **49:** 2011, 1983
4. Kent KM, Bentivoglio LG, Block PC, Bourassa MG, Cowley MJ, Dorros G, Detre K, Gosselin AJ, Gruentzig A, Kelsey SF, Mock M, Mullin SM, Passamani E, Myler RK, Simpson J, Stertzer SH, VanRaden M, Williams DO: Long-term efficacy of percutaneous transluminal coronary angioplasty (PTCA): report from NHLBI-PTCA Registry. Am J Cardiol **53:** 27C, 1984
5. Dorros G, Cowley MJ, Simpson J, Bentivoglio LG, Block PC, Bourassa M, Detre K, Gosselin AJ, Gruentzig A, Kelsey SF, Kent KM, Mock MB, Mullin SM, Myler RK, Passamani ER, Stertzer SH, Williams DO: Percutaneous transluminal coronary angioplasty: report of complications from the NHLBI PTCA Registry. Circulation **67:** 723, 1983
6. Cowley MJ, Dorros G, Kelsey SK, VanRaden MJ, Detre KM: Acute coronary events associated with percutaneous transluminal coronary angioplasty: NHLBI PTCA Registry experience. Am J Cardiol **53:** 12C, 1984
7. Dorros G, Stertzer SH, Cowley MJ, Myler RK: Complex coronary angioplasty: multiple coronary dilatations. Am J Cardiol **53:** 126C, 1984
8. Hartzler GO, Rutherford BD, McConahay DR, McCallister BD: Simultaneous multiple lesion coronary angioplasty: a preferred therapy for patients with multiple vessel disease. Circulation **66**(suppl II): II-5, 1982 (abst)
9. Dorros G, Stertzer SH, Cowley MJ, Kent K, Williams DO: Complex transluminal coronary angioplasty: multivessel disease and multiple dilatations. Circulation **66**(suppl II): II-329, 1982 (abst)
10. Cowley MJ, Dorros G, Kelsey SF, Van Raden M, Detre KM: Emergency coronary bypass surgery after coronary angioplasty: The National Heart, Lung, and Blood Institute's percutaneous transluminal coronary angioplasty registry experience. Am J Cardiol **53:** 22C, 1984
11. Meier B, Gruentzig AR: Learning curve for percutaneous transluminal coronary angioplasty: skill, technology or patient selection. Am J Cardiol **53:** 65C, 1984
12. Kelsey SF, Mullin SM, Detre KM, Mitchell H, Cowley MJ, Gruentzig AR, Kent KM: Effect of investigator experience on percutaneous transluminal coronary angioplasty. Am J Cardiol **53:** 56C, 1984
13. Holmes DR Jr, Vlietstra RE, Smith HC, Vetrovec GW, Kent KM, Cowley MJ, Faxon DP, Gruentzig AR, Kelsey SF, Detre KM, Van Raden MJ, Mock MB: Restenosis after percutaneous transluminal coronary angioplasty (PTCA): a report from the PTCA Registry of the National Heart, Lung, and Blood Institute. Am J Cardiol **53:** 77C, 1984
14. Thornton MA, Gruentzig AR, Hollman J, King SB III, Douglas JS: Coumadin and aspirin in prevention of recurrence after transluminal coronary angioplasty: a randomized study. Circulation **69:** 721, 1984
15. Williams DO, Gruentzig AR, Kent KM, Detre KM, Kelsey SF, To T: Efficacy of repeat percutaneous transluminal coronary angioplasty for coronary restenosis. Am J Cardiol **53:** 32C, 1984

The hypotensive effect of intravenous streptokinase in patients with acute myocardial infarction

ALLAN S. LEW, M.D., F.R.A.C.P., PIERRE LARAMEE, M.D., BOJAN CERCEK, M.D., PREDIMAN K. SHAH, M.D., AND WILLIAM GANZ, M.D., C.SC.

ABSTRACT We studied the hypotensive effect of a rapid intravenous infusion of high-dose streptokinase in 98 patients with an acute myocardial infarction. The systolic blood pressure fell from 132 ± 20 (range 90 to 174) to 97 ± 21 mm Hg (range 58 to 152) at 15 ± 8 min (range 4 to 40) after the commencement of the streptokinase infusion ($p < .001$). A fall in diastolic blood pressure from 80 ± 16 (range 51 to 105) to 61 ± 15 mm Hg (range 32 to 92) accompanied the fall in systolic pressure ($p < .001$). The fall in blood pressure was associated with an increase in heart rate (73 ± 14 to 78 ± 17 beats/min, $p < .001$), preceded the appearance of clinical signs of reperfusion by 37 ± 38 min and was similar in magnitude and timing in patients with anterior and inferior infarction. There were direct relationships between the rate of infusion of streptokinase and both the magnitude ($r = .49$, $p < .001$) and the rate of fall of systolic blood pressure ($r = .67$, $p < .001$) as well as both the magnitude and rate of fall of diastolic blood pressure. In most patients, the fall in blood pressure was transient (9 ± 6 min, range = 2 to 30) and easily managed by slowing or stopping the infusion, placing the patient in the Trendelenburg position, or by administering an infusion of low-dose norepinephrine or dopamine. However, in four patients with severe left ventricular dysfunction, severe hypotension persisted for more than 60 min. Our data indicate that in patients with either anterior or inferior myocardial infarction, a rapid infusion of high-dose intravenous streptokinase may frequently cause transient and sometimes severe hypotension, the magnitude of which is directly related to the rate of infusion of streptokinase.
Circulation 72, No. 6, 1321–1326, 1985.

SHORT-TERM INTRAVENOUS INFUSION of high-dose streptokinase is an effective method of coronary thrombolysis and coronary artery reperfusion during an acute myocardial infarction.[1–9] In most recent studies, intravenous streptokinase has been administered rapidly so as to achieve a high concentration of streptokinase in proximity to the coronary thrombus and thereby accelerate thrombolysis.[10–13]

One limitation of the administration of a rapid intravenous infusion of streptokinase is that it can cause a significant fall in systemic blood pressure.[4, 5, 9] This study investigates the frequency and severity of the hypotensive effect of intravenous infusion of streptokinase in patients with acute myocardial infarction and its relationship to the rate of the infusion.

From the Division of Cardiology, Department of Medicine, Cedars-Sinai Medical Center and the Department of Medicine, UCLA School of Medicine, Los Angeles.
Supported in part by NIH SCOR grant No. 17651.
Address for correspondence: Allan S. Lew, M.D., Room No. 5314, Division of Cardiology, Cedars-Sinai Medical Center, 8700 Beverly Blvd, Los Angeles, CA 90048.
Received June 4, 1985; revision accepted Sept. 19, 1985.

Methods

Patient population. The patient population consisted of 101 consecutive patients who were entered into a prospective study of intravenous streptokinase in acute myocardial infarction and in whom ıe systemic blood pressure was continuously monitored duri ̧ the infusion of streptokinase. The study inclusion criteria were (1) chest pain of 3 hr or less duration, (2) ST segment elevation indicative of transmural ischemia, (3) unresponsiveness of both the chest pain and the electrocardiographic changes to sublingual nitroglycerin, (4) no contraindication to thrombolytic or anticoagulant therapy, and (5) consent of both the patient and his or her physician. The diagnosis of acute myocardial infarction was subsequently confirmed by a rise in serum levels of the creatine kinase MB isoenzyme in all patients.

Three patients were excluded from analysis. Two patients were receiving intravenous nitrates to control hypertension and their baseline blood pressures had already been reduced by more than 30 mm Hg before streptokinase and in one patient the fall in blood pressure coincided with the onset of ventricular tachycardia. The remaining 98 patients (76 men and 22 women, 63 ± 11 years old, range 40 to 86) constitute the study population.

Study protocol. An intravenous infusion of 750,000 U of streptokinase (Hoechst-Roussel) in 45 to 75 ml normal saline was administered into a peripheral vein over 30 ± 16 min (range 7 to 78). The rate of infusion of streptokinase (U streptokinase/kg body weight/min) was determined in 92 of the 98 patients by dividing the total dose of streptokinase by the weight of the patient and by the time interval over which the infusion was administered. Eighty-eight patients were given 100 mg iv hydrocortisone before streptokinase.

The brachial arterial blood pressure and the heart rate were monitored at 1 min intervals for at least 5 min before and during the entire streptokinase infusion with a Dinamap automatic oscillometric cuff blood pressure recorder.[14] The blood pressure varied by less than 10% during the interval preceding the commencement of the streptokinase infusion and the lowest value recorded during this interval was accepted as the baseline blood pressure. The fall in blood pressure was defined as the difference between the baseline blood pressure and the minimum blood pressure recorded during the infusion of streptokinase. The rate of fall of blood pressure was defined as the fall in blood pressure (mm Hg) divided by the time interval from the commencement of streptokinase to the time of the minimum value (min). These variables were calculated separately for systolic and diastolic blood pressures.

Statistical methods. Continuous variables are described by their mean and standard deviation. The unpaired Student t test was used for comparisons between two groups and the paired Student t test was used to assess the significance of serial changes in blood pressure and heart rate. Proportional differences between groups were compared with the use of Fisher's exact test. Correlations between the rate of infusion of intravenous streptokinase and the magnitude and rate of fall in systolic and diastolic blood pressures were calculated by the unweighted linear least squares method. All statistical analyses were performed with BMPD biostatistical programs and a p value of $<.05$ was considered to represent statistical significance.

Results

Fall in blood pressure. The mean systolic blood pressure before streptokinase for the entire study population was 132 ± 20 mm Hg (range 90 to 174). During the intravenous infusion of streptokinase, there was a mean fall of 35 ± 19 mm Hg (range 0 to 82) to a minimum value of 97 ± 21 mm Hg (range 58 to 152), which was recorded at 15 ± 8 min (range 4 to 40) after the commencement of the infusion ($p < .001$ for fall in systolic blood pressure). In most patients the duration of the fall was brief, lasting 9 ± 6 min (range 2 to 30). The mean diastolic blood pressure before streptokinase was 80 ± 16 mm Hg (range 51 to 105). A fall of 20 ± 14 mm Hg in diastolic pressure to a minimum value of 61 ± 15 mm Hg (range 32 to 92) accompanied the fall in systolic pressure ($p < .001$ for fall in diastolic blood pressure).

In 85 of the 98 patients (87%), there was a fall in systolic blood pressure of more than 10% of the baseline value (BP fall). In the remaining 13 patients, there was a lesser fall or no fall in blood pressure (no BP fall). In 18 patients the systolic blood pressure fell to a minimum value of 90 to 99 mm Hg, in 17 patients it fell to 80 to 89 mm Hg, in 10 patients it fell to 70 to 79 mm Hg, and in 10 patients the minimum systolic blood pressure was less than 70 mm Hg. Therefore, a fall to a systolic blood pressure of 90 mm Hg or less occurred in 37 of the 98 patients (38%).

Influence of rate of streptokinase infusion on blood pressure. Figure 1 illustrates that both (1) the magnitude and (2) the rate of fall in systolic blood pressure were each directly related to the rate of infusion of streptokinase in patients with either anterior or inferior infarction. There were also similar direct relationships between the rate of infusion of streptokinase and the magnitude of the fall of diastolic blood pressure ($r = .38$, $p < .001$) and the rate of fall of diastolic blood pressure ($r = .53$, $p < .001$) respectively.

Figure 1, *A* shows that a BP fall (points above broken line) was frequent at all rates of streptokinase infusion, but 12 of the 13 patients with no BP fall received an infusion of streptokinase at a rate slower

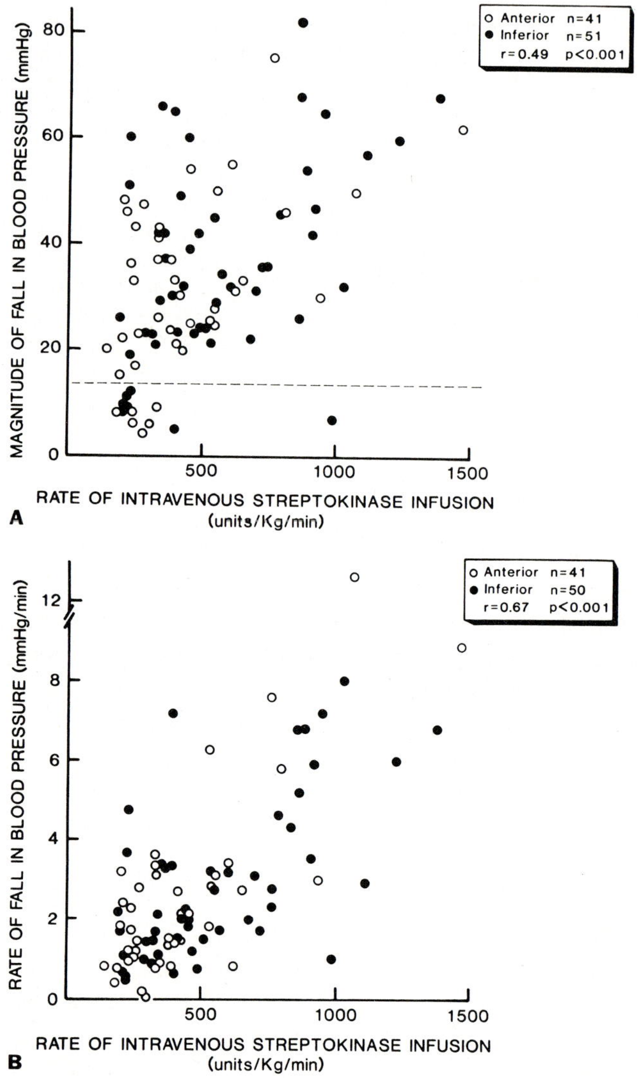

FIGURE 1. Graphic representation of the relationship between the rate of intravenous infusion of streptokinase and *A*, The magnitude of the fall in systolic blood pressurse and *B*, the rate of fall of systolic blood pressure, in patients with anterior and inferior infarction. The broken line on *A* indicates that most patients without a significant fall in systolic blood pressure (below line) received an infusion of streptokinase at a rate slower than 500 U/kg/min.

than 500 U/kg/min (p < .001 for rates <500 vs ≥500 U/kg/min). The exception was a patient in whom streptokinase was completely inactivated by a high titer of neutralizing antibodies.[15]

Relationship between heart rate and fall in blood pressure. The mean heart rate increased from 73 ± 14 beats/min before streptokinase to 78 ± 17 beats/min at the time of maximum fall in blood pressure (p < .001). In only eight patients (five with inferior and three with anterior infarction) did the heart rate fall by 10 beats/min or more (or ≥10%) from the baseline value. The increase in heart rate was similar in patients with and without a significant fall in blood pressure. Two patients with inferior infarction who had a fall in systolic blood pressure that was initially associated with an increase in heart rate developed transient third-degree atrioventricular block when the systolic blood pressure fell below 85 mm Hg. In one of these two patients, the onset of atrioventricular block occurred 22 min before the appearance of any of the clinical signs of reperfusion and in the other patient, reperfusion was not achieved.

Relationship between site of infarction and fall in blood pressure (table 1). There were 45 patients with anterior infarction and 53 patients with inferior infarction. There were no significant differences in blood pressure before streptokinase, the magnitude of the fall in blood pressure, or the rate of fall of blood pressure between patients with anterior or inferior infarction. Both groups of patients also had a similar increase in mean heart rate during the streptokinase infusion.

Relationship between time of reperfusion and time of fall in blood pressure. The onset of the fall in blood pressure always preceded the appearance of any of the clinical signs of reperfusion. The time of maximum blood pressure fall preceded the appearance of clinical signs of reperfusion in 74 of the 78 patients in whom the timing of both events could be determined (mean 37 ± 38 min, range 5 to 216). In the remaining four patients, all with anterior infarction, the minimum blood pressure was recorded up to 10 min after the appearance of clinical signs of reperfusion.

TABLE 1
Relationship of infarct location to blood pressure and heart rate

	Anterior MI (n = 45)	Inferior MI (n = 53)	p value
Pre-SK systolic BP (mm Hg)	132±20	132±20	NS
Minimum systolic BP (mm Hg)	98±22	96±21	NS
Fall in systolic BP (mm Hg)	34±20	36±19	NS
Pre-SK diastolic BP (mm Hg)	82±13	80±13	NS
Minimum diastolic BP (mm Hg)	64±14	60±17	NS
Fall in diastolic BP (mm Hg)	18±14	20±15	NS
Time to minimum BP (min)	15±8	16±8	NS
Rate of fall in systolic BP (mm Hg/min)	4±4	3±2	NS
Pre-SK heart rate (bpm)	76±15	70±14	.06
Heart rate at minimum BP (bpm)	82±16	74±18	<.05

BP = blood pressure; MI = myocardial infarction; SK = streptokinase.

Clinical characteristics of patients with a fall in blood pressure. The most important determinant of the fall in blood pressure was the rate of infusion of streptokinase. Therefore, the clinical characteristics of the BP fall group and the no BP fall group were compared after controlling for infusion rate by restricting the analysis to the 33 patients in the former group and the 12 patients in the latter group receiving infusions at a rate of 400 or less U/kg/min (the fastest effective rate in the no BP fall group). Patients in the BP fall group had evidence of more extensive myocardial damage, as suggested by a higher incidence of prior myocardial infarction (30% vs 8%) and a higher peak serum level of creatine kinase MB (161 ± 82 vs 121 ± 98 IU/liter). There was no difference in (1) age (62 ± 12 vs 57 ± 11 years), (2) sex distribution (85% vs 92% males), (3) location of infarction (58% vs 50% anterior), or (4) baseline blood pressure (130 ± 20 vs 124 ± 16 mm Hg). There was also no difference between these two groups with respect to the frequency of patency of the artery of infarction at delayed angiography or the incidence of hemorrhagic complications.

Recovery of blood pressure. The fall in blood pressure was generally, but not always, transient and easily managed. In 81 of the 85 patients with a fall in systolic blood pressure, recovery to baseline values occurred within 9 ± 6 min (range = 2 to 30). In 28 of these 81 patients (33%) with a mean fall in systolic pressure of 31 ± 12 mm Hg to a minimum blood pressure of 111 ± 19 mm Hg, recovery of blood pressure occurred spontaneously, without any intervention, within 7 ± 4 min (range = 2 to 21). In 35 patients (41%) with a mean fall of 38 ± 16 mm Hg to a minimum systolic pressure of 91 ± 15 mm Hg, the blood pressure recovered in 9 ± 6 min (range = 2 to 30) after the infusion was slowed or stopped, with or without placing the patient in the Trendelenburg position. In the remaining 18 patients, with a mean fall of 51 ± 17 mm Hg to a minimum systolic pressure of 75 ± 11 mm Hg, an infusion of low-dose norepinephrine or dopamine was administered in addition to the other measures and the blood pressure recovered within 11 ± 7 min (range = 2 to 29).

In four patients with severe left ventricular failure

before administration of streptokinase, systolic hypotension of less than 85 mm Hg persisted for more than 60 min despite intravenous infusion of catecholamines.

Discussion

In this study, a transient fall in blood pressure was frequent during intravenous infusion of high-dose streptokinase in patients with acute myocardial infarction and both the magnitude and the rate of the fall in blood pressure were directly related to the rate of infusion of intravenous streptokinase. This hypotensive effect was similar in patients with anterior and inferior infarction and not infrequently resulted in significant hypotension. The fall in blood pressure was usually associated with an increase in heart rate and was not temporally related to clinical signs of reperfusion, suggesting that it was distinct from the Bezold-Jarisch vagal reflex, which has been reported to occur at the time of reperfusion in some patients with inferior infarction.[16, 17]

Although the fall in blood pressure was generally of short duration and easily managed by slowing or interrupting the infusion of streptokinase, in some patients it was severe and prolonged and in about 20% of patients administration of vasopressors was required. Our data suggest that the risk of hypotension was related to the extent of damage to the myocardium; the most severe falls in blood pressure occurred in hemodynamically compromised patients. In such patients, the hemodynamic combination of hypotension and an increase in heart rate can further reduce perfusion to the acutely ischemic myocardium[18–20] and thereby accelerate the rate of progression of myocardial necrosis and reduce the potential for myocardial salvage by reperfusion.[21] Hypotension may also lead to hypoperfusion in the nonischemic myocardium, especially if it is supplied by stenotic coronary arteries or via collaterals.[22]

Because of the frequent prompt recovery of blood pressure after placement of the patients in the Trendelenburg position, patients are now treated in the supine position when possible, with one pillow under the head and another under the legs. Our data suggests that severe falls in blood pressure may be avoided by limiting the rate of infusion of intravenous streptokinase. Therefore, in hemodynamically compromised patients and in those with a baseline systolic blood pressure of less than 100 mm Hg, we now commence the infusion at a slow rate of about 200 to 250 U/kg/min or less and have an infusion of norepinephrine available "on standby." Our findings underscore the importance of continuous monitoring of blood pressure during intravenous infusion of high-dose streptokinase and have important implications for the use of streptokinase in an out-of-hospital setting.

Despite the frequency of its occurrence, the pathophysiology of this hypotensive effect is not known. The symptomatic and visible cutaneous flushing that frequently heralds or accompanies the fall in blood pressure and the associated increase in heart rate are suggestive of a vasomotor effect, but this has not yet been documented. Invasive hemodynamic monitoring that would delay the initiation of treatment is not used in our clinical studies and in our experimental studies in anesthetized dogs, sheep, and monkeys, blood pressure has not been observed to fall during an intravenous bolus injection of high-dose streptokinase. In contrast, a marked fall in blood pressure occurred in dogs given rapid intravenous infusions of streptokinase-activated human plasminogen,[23] streptokinase-plasmin activator complex,[24] and trypsin,[25] an enzyme with a broad spectrum of activity similar to plasmin. This hypotensive effect of the streptokinase-plasmin(ogen) complex has been attributed to a rapid increase in serum plasmin concentration[24] and differs from the effect of streptokinase alone, probably because streptokinase is a weak activator of canine circulating plasminogen.[26] In the study by Green et al.,[24] the hypotensive effect in conscious dogs (mean fall of 56 mm Hg) had a time course and recovery similar to our clinical observations and was related to plasmin activation of kallikrein and production of bradykinin. Their conclusions regarding the role of bradykinin appear to be consistent with the clinical features of marked flushing and the known ability of plasmin to activate Hageman factor and generate bradykinin.[27] Unfortunately, the systemic vascular resistance was not measured during that study.

In addition to the effect of bradykinin, there are several other mechanisms that could reduce systemic vascular resistance during the infusion of streptokinase. Vasodilation may be due to plasmin activation of the complement pathway[28] or to endothelial prostacyclin secretion, which in experimental studies is stimulated by short chain, human fibrinogen degradation products.[29] A direct vasodilative effect of streptokinase is reminiscent of vasoactive properties of many peptides. However, our observations that the effect is short-lived and that a closely timed second infusion of streptokinase may either have no effect or an attenuated effect on blood pressure and the observation in European studies that hypotensive reactions also occur after high-dose intravenous infusions of both urokinase[30] and tissue-type plasminogen activator[31] suggest that the fall in blood pressure is not due to a specific effect of streptokinase.

Allergy has also been postulated as the cause of the fall in blood pressure. Although low titers of antistreptokinase antibodies are almost ubiquitous in man,[32] allergy seems unlikely because allergic reactions to streptokinase are very rare and do not accompany the fall in blood pressure. On the contrary, in our experience, in patients with high titers of neutralizing anti-streptokinase antibodies the fibrinolytic system is not activated and there is no fall in blood pressure during intravenous infusion of streptokinase.[15] Furthermore, allergy could not explain the fall in blood pressure observed with intravenous urokinase or tissue-type plasminogen activator.

Since a depletion of serum fibrinogen lowers serum viscosity[33] and therefore systemic vascular resistance, theoretically this could cause a fall in blood pressure. This mechanism is unlikely, however, because in our experience, hypotension can occur early in the development of plasminemia (a lytic state inducing elevated levels of fibrinogen degradation products) before serum fibrinogen has significantly decreased.

Finally, it was not possible to implicate the administration of opiates, nitroglycerin, antiarrhythmic agents, or any other medication as the cause for the fall in blood pressure.

Clinical implications. In patients with either anterior or inferior myocardial infarction, rapid infusion of high-dose intravenous streptokinase frequently causes a transient and sometimes severe fall in blood pressure, the magnitude of which is directly related to the rate of infusion of streptokinase. To avoid severe hypotensive reactions, the rate of infusion of streptokinase should probably not exceed about 500 U/kg/min in normotensive patients. In hemodynamically unstable patients with reduced myocardial reserve who are more likely to develop significant and sometimes resistant hypotension and in patients with low initial blood pressure, the rate of infusion should be much slower (200 to 250 U/kg/min or less) and a vasopressor infusion should be available "on standby."

We are grateful to Lois Rodriguez and Ann Lew for research assistance and to Rosa Goldsmith for preparation of artwork.

References

1. Schroder R, Biamino G, Leitner ER, Linderer T, Bruggemann T, Heitz J, Vohringer HF, Wegschreider K: Intravenous short-term infusion of streptokinase in acute myocardial infarction. Circulation **67:** 536, 1983
2. Neuhaus KL, Tebbe U, Sauer G, Kreuzer H, Kostering H: High dose intravenous streptokinase in acute myocardial infarction. Clin Cardiol **6:** 426, 1983
3. Spann JF, Sherry S, Carabello BA, Denenberg BS, Mann RH, McCann WD, Gault JH, Gentzler RDE, Belber AD, Maurer AH, Cooper EM: Coronary thrombolysis by intravenous streptokinase in acute myocardial infarction: acute and follow-up studies. Am J Cardiol **53:** 655, 1984
4. Ganz W, Geft I, Shah PK, Lew AS, Rodriguez L, Weiss T, Maddahi J, Berman DS, Charuzi Y, Swan HJC: Intravenous streptokinase in evolving myocardial infarction. Am J Cardiol **53:** 1209, 1984
5. Alderman EL, Jutzy KR, Berte LE, Miller RG, Friedman JP, Creger WP, Eliastam M: Randomized comparison of intravenous versus intracoronary streptokinase for acute myocardial infarction. Am J Cardiol **54:** 14, 1984
6. Taylor GJ, Mikell FL, Moses HW, Dove JT, Batchelder JE, Thull A, Hansen S, Wellons HA, Schneider JA: Intravenous versus intracoronary streptokinase therapy for acute myocardial infarction in community hospitals. Am J Cardiol **54:** 256, 1984
7. Rogers WJ, Hood WP Jr, Reeves RC, Whitlow PL: Randomized trial of intracoronary versus intravenous streptokinase in acute myocardial infarction. J Am Coll Cardiol **3:** 525, 1984 (abst)
8. Anderson JL, Marshall HW, Askins JC, Lutz JR, Sorensen SG, Menlove RL, Yanowitz FG, Hagan AD: A randomized trial of intravenous and intracoronary streptokinase in patients with acute myocardial infarction. Circulation **70:** 606, 1984
9. Valentine RP, Pitts DE, Brooks-Brunn JA, Williams JG, Van Hove E, Schmidt PE: Intravenous versus intracoronary streptokinase in acute myocardial infarction. Am J Cardiol **55:** 309, 1985
10. Alkjaersig N, Fletcher AP, Sherry S: The mechanism of clot dissolution by plasmin. J Clin Invest **38:** 1086, 1959
11. Brogden RN, Speight TM, Avery GS: Streptokinase: a review of its clinical pharmacology, mechanism of action and therapeutic uses. Drugs **5:** 357, 1973
12. Martin M: Studies on activator formation in human plasma with streptokinase. III. Investigation of activator kinetics in undiluted plasma in terms of urokinase equivalents. Thromb Haemost **36:** 566, 1976
13. Collen D: On the regulation and control of fibrinolysis. Thromb Haemost **73:** 77, 1980
14. Borow KM, Newburger JW: Noninvasive estimation of central aortic pressure using the oscillometric method for analyzing systemic artery pulsatile blood flow: comparative study of indirect systolic, diastolic, and mean brachial artery pressure with simultaneous direct ascending aortic pressure measurements. Am Heart J **103:** 879, 1982
15. Lew AS, Neer T, Rodriguez L, Geft IL, Ganz W: Clinical failure of streptokinase due to an unsuspected high titer of antistreptokinase antibody. J Am Coll Cardiol **4:** 183, 1984
16. Wei JY, Markis JE, Malagold M, Braunwald E: Cardiovascular reflexes stimulated by reperfusion of ischemic myocardium in acute myocardial infarction. Circulation **67:** 796, 1983
17. Esente P, Giambartolomei A, Gensini GG, Dator C: Coronary reperfusion and Bezold-Jarisch reflex (bradycardia and hypotension). Am J Cardiol **52:** 221, 1983
18. Hoffman JIE: Maximal coronary flow and the concept of coronary vascular reserve. Circulation **70:** 153, 1984
19. Schaper W, Pasyk S: Influence of collateral flow on the ischemic tolerance of the heart following acute and subacute coronary occlusion. Circulation **53**(suppl I): I-57, 1976
20. Goldberg HL, Goldstein J, Borer JS, Moses JW, Collins MB: Functional importance of coronary collateral vessels. Am J Cardiol **53:** 694, 1984
21. Jennings RB, Reimer KA: Factors involved in salvaging ischemic myocardium: effect of reperfusion of arterial blood. Circulation **68**(suppl I): I-25, 1983
22. Naccarella FF, Weintraub WS, Agarwal JB, Helfant RH: Evaluation of "ischemia at a distance": effects of coronary occlusion on a remote area of left ventricle. Am J Cardiol **54:** 869, 1984
23. Ambrus JL, Ambrus CM, Back N, Sukal JE, Collins GL: Clinical and experimental studies on fibrinolytic enzymes. Ann NY Acad Sci **68:** 97, 1957
24. Green J, Dupe RJ, Smith RAG, Harris GS, English PD: Comparison of the hypotensive effects of streptokinase-(human) plasmin activator complex and BRL 26921 (p-anisoylated streptokinase-plasminogen activator complex) in the dog after high dose, bolus administration. Thromb Res **36:** 29, 1984
25. Agress CM, Jacobs HI, Binder MJ, Clark WG, Kaplan L, Lederer

M, Glassner HF: Intravenous trypsin in experimental myocardial infarction. Circ Res **2:** 397, 1954
26. Summaria L, Arzadon L, Bernabe P, Robbins KC: The interaction of streptokinase with human, cat, dog, and rabbit plasminogens. J Biol Chem **249:** 4760, 1974
27. Kaplan AP, Meier HL, Mandle R: The Hageman factor dependent pathways of coagulation, fibrinolysis and kinin-generation. Sem Thromb Hemost **3:** 1, 1976
28. Ratnoff OD, Naff GB: The conversion of C′1 to C′1 esterase by plasmin and trypsin. J Exp Med **125:** 337, 1967
29. Andersson RGG, Saldeen K, Saldeen T: A fibrin(ogen) derived pentapeptide induces vasodilation, prostacyclin release and an increase in cyclic AMP. Thromb Res **30:** 213, 1983
30. A European Collaborative Study: Controlled trial of urokinase in myocardial infarction. Lancet **2:** 624, 1975
31. Verstraete M, Bory M, Collen D, Erbel R, Lennane RJ, Mathey D, Michels HR, Schartl M, Uebis R, Bernard R, Brower RW, De Bono DP, Huhmann W, Lubsen J, Meyer J, Rutsch W, Schmidt W, Von Essen R: Randomized trial of intravenous recombinant tissue-type plasminogen activator versus intravenous streptokinase in acute myocardial infarction. Report from the European Cooperative Study Group for recombinant tissue-type plasminogen activator. Lancet **1:** 842, 1985
32. Moran DM, Standring R, Lavender EA, Harris GS: Assessment of antistreptokinase antibody levels in human sera using a microradioimmunoassay procedure. Thromb Haemost **52:** 281, 1984
33. Schmid-Schonbein H, Rieger H, Hess H: Quantification of the streptokinase effects on blood microrheology. *In* Martin M, Schoop W, Hirsh J, editors: New concepts in streptokinase dosimetry. Bern, 1978, Hans Huber Publishers, pp 39–48

Comparative effects of volume loading, dobutamine, and nitroprusside in patients with predominant right ventricular infarction

LOUIS J. DELL'ITALIA, M.D., MARK R. STARLING, M.D., RALPH BLUMHARDT, M.D., JOHN C. LASHER, M.D., AND ROBERT A. O'ROURKE, M.D.

ABSTRACT To assess the value of volume loading and to determine the relative efficacy of dobutamine compared with nitroprusside therapy in acute right ventricular infarction (RVMI), 13 patients with clinical, hemodynamic, and radionuclide angiographic evidence of RVMI were evaluated. In 10 patients who had an initial pulmonary arterial wedge pressure less than 18 mm Hg, volume loading did not improve cardiac index (1.9 ± 0.5 [SD] to 2.1 ± 0.4 liters/min/m^2), despite significant increases in mean right atrial pressure (11 ± 2 to 15 ± 2 mm Hg, $p < .001$) and pulmonary arterial wedge pressure (10 ± 4 to 15 ± 2 mm Hg, $p < .001$). Nine patients received dobutamine or nitroprusside in random order, while hemodynamic measurements and radionuclide angiograms were obtained simultaneously. Compared with nitroprusside, dobutamine produced a statistically significant increase in cardiac index (2.0 ± 0.4 to 2.7 ± 0.5 vs 2.1 ± 0.4 to 2.3 ± 0.5 liters/min/m^2, $p < .001$), stroke volume index (29 ± 6 to 36 ± 8 vs 29 ± 6 to 30 ± 6 ml/m^2, $p = .02$), and right ventricular ejection fraction (30 ± 8% to 42 ± 7% vs 34 ± 8% to 37 ± 4%, $p < .01$) by two-way analysis of variance. We conclude that volume loading does not improve cardiac index in patients with acute RVMI despite a rise in cardiac filling pressures and that infusion of dobutamine, after appropriate volume loading, produces a significant improvement in cardiac index and right ventricular ejection fraction over those after infusion of nitroprusside.
Circulation 72, No. 6, 1327–1335, 1985.

INFARCTION of the right ventricle commonly occurs with acute inferior transmural myocardial infarction.[1,2] Because of the variable extent of right ventricular damage, patients may present with a spectrum of hemodynamic characteristics.[3] When right ventricular myocardial infarction (RVMI) is associated with decreased cardiac index and systolic arterial blood pressure, volume loading has been advocated based on work in animals by Guiha and Cohn[4] and Goldstein et al.[5,6] Conversely, in a substantial number of patients with hemodynamically important RVMI, we[7] and others[8] have found that volume loading alone did not improve cardiac index. However, in patients whose conditions are refractory to volume loading alone, other investigators have reported an improvement in cardiac index with the infusion of dobutamine[9,10] or nitroprusside.[11,12] This information concerning the beneficial effects of dobutamine and nitroprusside is derived from case reports involving a total of three patients. Because no study has systematically evaluated these potential therapies in an adequate number of patients with acute RVMI, no rational approach to the treatment of this complex hemodynamic syndrome has evolved. Accordingly, the purpose of this study was to evaluate the potential salutary effects of volume loading and to determine the relative efficacy of dobutamine and nitroprusside therapy, in addition to volume loading, in patients with hemodynamically important RVMI.

From the University of Texas Health Science Center at San Antonio.
Supported in part by AHA-Tex 83-7 from the American Heart Association, Texas Affiliate, Dallas, and NIH New Investigator Research Award No. R23-HL27508 from the National Heart, Lung, and Blood Institute, Bethesda.
Address for correspondence: Louis J Dell'Italia, M.D., Department of Medicine/Cardiology, The University of Texas Health Science Center at San Antonio, 7703 Floyd Curl Dr., San Antonio, TX 78284.
Received July 31, 1985; accepted Aug. 29, 1985.

Methods

Patients. The study group (n = 13) was made up of consecutive patients who presented with (1) a history of prolonged chest pain consistent with myocardial ischemia, (2) pathologic Q waves of at least 0.04 sec in duration with a Q:R ratio of at least 1:4 in leads II, III, and aVF and associated ST-T wave changes, and (3) the elevation of serum levels of total creatine kinase and its MB isoenzyme fraction.[13] Potential study patients with right ventricular infarction were identified within 48 hr of the onset of

TABLE 1

Mean hemodynamic data in the 13 study patients before and after therapy with normal saline (n = 10), dobutamine (n = 12), and nitroprusside (n = 10)

	RAP (mm Hg)	PAWP (mm Hg)	RA:PAWP ratio	$\overline{PA}$ (mm Hg)	CI (l/min/m²)	SVI (ml/m²)	RVSWI (g·m/m²)	LVSWI (g·m/m²)	HR (bpm)
Control	11±2	10±4	1.3±0.9	18±4	1.9±0.5	27±5	2.5±1.4	30±6	73±11
Normal saline	15±2^C	15±2^C	1.0±0.2	22±4^C	2.1±0.4	29±5	2.8±1.5	32±8	72±11
Control	15±2	15±3	1.0±0.2	21±3	2.1±0.4	30±6	2.6±1.6	33±11	71±11
Dobutamine	13±3^A	16±4	0.8±0.2^B	24±3^B	2.8±0.6^C	36±7^C	5.4±2.1^C	41±11^B	79±13^B
Control	14±4	14±5	1.1±0.3	21±4	2.0±0.3	29±6	2.6±1.1	30±4	72±12
Nitroprusside	12±4^A	12±5	1.1±0.3	18±4^A	2.2±0.5^A	30±6	2.5±1.6	28±6	75±12^A

RAP = right atrial pressure; PAWP = pulmonary arterial wedge pressure; $\overline{PA}$ = mean pulmonary arterial pressure; CI = cardiac index; SVI = stroke volume index; RVSWI = right ventricular stroke work index; LVSWI = left ventricular stroke work index; HR = heart rate; $\overline{BP}$ = mean arterial pressure; SVR = systemic vascular resistance; TPR = total pulmonary resistance; PVR = pulmonary vascular resistance.

$^A p < .05$; $^B p < .01$; $^C p < .001$ for control vs intervention.

symptoms by the following combined criteria: (1) elevated jugular venous pressure (≥ 8 cm H_2O) or Kussmaul's sign[14]; and (2) evidence of both reduced equilibrium radionuclide angiographic right ventricular ejection fraction (<40%) and regional right ventricular wall motion abnormalities of akinesia or dyskinesia.[7, 15] After written informed consent was obtained on a form approved by our Institutional Review Board, right heart catheterization was performed in all patients who met the physical examination and radionuclide angiographic criteria for RVMI. The final study group of 13 patients was subsequently defined by the presence of hemodynamic criteria for RVMI either before or after volume infusion.[7, 15] Thus, all study patients fulfilled the clinical, hemodynamic, and radionuclide angiographic criteria for RVMI.

The 13 study patients consisted of nine men and four women with ages ranging from 40 to 75 years (mean 55). Two patients had a history of a prior nontransmural myocardial infarction. Also, eight of the 13 study patients had a well-documented history of hypertension. Patients with a history of severe chronic obstructive lung disease, left-to-right shunts, renal failure, pulmonary embolus, pericardial disease, and biventricular congestive heart failure were excluded from this study.

Hemodynamics. A No. 7 balloon-tip, flow-directed Edward's catheter (American Edwards Laboratories, Santa Anna, CA) was inserted into the right heart within 48 hr of the onset of symptoms in each patient. With Statham P23 Db transducers (Gould Inc., Oxnard, CA) leveled at the mid-axillary line, calibrated pressures were recorded from the right atrium, right ventricle, pulmonary artery, and pulmonary arterial wedge positions. Cardiac output (CO) was determined in triplicate by the thermodilution technique with an Edwards 9520A cardiac output computer (American Edwards Laboratories, Santa Ana, CA); heart rate (HR) and systemic arterial pressure (cuff sphygmomanometer) were recorded. From these data, the cardiac index (CI), stroke volume index (SVI), right ventricular stroke work index (RVSWI), left ventricular stroke work index (LVSWI), systemic vascular resistance (SVR), total pulmonary resistance (TPR), and pulmonary vascular resistance (PVR) were calculated as: CI = CO/BSA (liters/min/m²); SVI = CI/HR × 1000 ml/m²; RVSWI = SVI × (MPA-RAP) × 0.0136 g·m/m²; LVSWI = SVI × (MAP-PAWP) × 0.0136 g·m/m²; SVR = MAP-RAP/CO × 80 dynes·sec/cm⁵; TPR = MPA/CO × 80 dynes·sec/cm⁵; PVR = MPA-PAWP/CO × 80 dynes·sec/cm⁵; where BSA = body surface area (m²); MPA = mean pulmonary arterial pressure; MAP = mean arterial pressure; RAP = right atrial pressure; PAWP = pulmonary arterial wedge pressure.

Radionuclide angiography. Equilibrium radionuclide angiography was performed with a 37 photomultiplier tube single crystal gamma scintillation camera equipped with an all-purpose parallel-hole collimator. Labeling of red blood cells in vivo was accomplished by intravenous administration of stannous pyrophosphate followed in 15 min by 25 mCi of ^{99m}Tc pertechnetate. Images were acquired in the anterior and left anterior oblique projections, which best separated the right and left ventricles in the plane of the interventricular septum. Electrocardiographically gated radionuclide angiographic images were obtained in 64 × 64 byte mode matrix at 30 msec intervals throughout the cardiac cycle to 250,000 counts per frame. A dedicated computer cart was used for data acquisition and processing. The radionuclide angiographic images were initially reviewed in movie format to assess overall qualitative right ventricular wall motion. The apex, inferior and lateral walls, and outflow tract of the right ventricle were evaluated. Right ventricular ejection fraction was calculated by the technique described by Maddahi et al.[16] The radionuclide criteria for RVMI included both a right ventricular ejection fraction of less than 40% and the presence of regional right ventricular wall motion abnormalities of akinesia or dyskinesia.[7] During each phase of the protocol, radionuclide images were obtained and attenuation-corrected right and left ventricular volumes were calculated by a technique that has been previously validated in our laboratory.[17–19]

Protocol. The protocol consisted of the simultaneous acquisition of radionuclide angiograms and hemodynamic measurements at baseline, after volume loading with normal saline if indicated, during the peak drug effect of dobutamine and nitroprusside, and during a control period between the infusion of each drug. Nine of the 13 study patients received both a dobutamine and nitroprusside infusion in the following random sequence of administration: (1) control 1, (2) drug A, (3) control 2 (20 to 30 min after end of infusion of drug A), and (4) drug B. Seven of the nine patients had pulmonary arterial wedge pressures of less than 15 mm Hg at baseline, and these patients received volume infusions as indicated below.

Ten of the 13 study patients received normal saline in 200 ml increments over 5 min for a total infusion ranging from 200 to 800 ml. The volume infusion was continued until the pulmonary arterial wedge pressure was greater than 15 mm Hg. Three patients did not undergo volume loading because their pulmo-

TABLE 1
(Continued)

$\overline{BP}$ (mm Hg)	SVR (dynes·sec·cm^{-5})	TPR (dynes·sec·cm^{-5})	PVR (dynes·sec·cm^{-5})
93±17	1877±584	388±99	169±71
96±16	1714±484	466±115	147±71
96±17	1699±508	445±116	135±59
101±14	1363±352^B	379±93^B	132±57
93±18	1706±556	435±125	140±67
82±16^B	1398±498^B	344±116^B	114±58

nary arterial wedge pressures were greater than 18 mm Hg at baseline. There were no complications of volume loading.

Dobutamine was infused in 12 of the 13 study patients starting at an infusion rate of 2.5 μg/kg/min and increasing to a maximum of 20 μg/kg/min, or until the mean arterial pressure or heart rate increased 10% or more above the baseline value. The infusion rate ranged from 5 to 20 μg/kg/min (mean 13). Three patients had complications related to the dobutamine infusion, including (1) supraventricular tachyarrhythmia requiring cessation of the drug therapy, (2) atrial fibrillation occurring after the discontinuation of the drug, and (3) chest pain, which occurred after the radionuclide and hemodynamic acquisitions, requiring termination of the drug infusion.

Nitroprusside was infused in 10 of the 13 patients. The infusion rate ranged from 0.4 to 2.1 μg/kg/min (mean = 1.2) and was aimed at achieving a 10% decrease in mean arterial pressure with a less than 10% increase in the heart rate. There were no complications associated with nitroprusside infusion. Two patients did not receive a nitroprusside infusion due to the complications that occurred during the prior dobutamine infusion, and one patient, whose mean arterial pressure was elevated at baseline, developed unexplained sinus tachycardia without a 10% decrease in mean arterial pressure.

Statistical analysis. Radionuclide right and left ventricular volumes and ejection fractions were calculated by a technician who was blinded to the hemodynamic results. Continuous data are presented as the mean ± SD. Paired Student's t test was performed to identify differences in hemodynamic and radionuclide angiographic values obtained before and after volume loading (10 patients), dobutamine infusion (12 patients), and nitroprusside infusion (10 patients). In the nine patients who received both dobutamine and nitroprusside infusions, one-way and two-way analyses of variance were performed to determine whether differences existed between the hemodynamic and radionuclide angiographic values obtained during the two control periods and during the nitroprusside and dobutamine infusions. When a difference was found, Bonferroni-corrected multiple t tests were performed to identify intergroup differences. A value of .05 or less was considered to indicate a significant difference.

Results

Volume loading (n = 10)

Hemodynamics (table 1). The mean control cardiac and stroke volume indexes were depressed in the 10 patients who received a normal saline infusion (1.9 ± 0.5 liters/min/m^2 and 27 ± 5 ml/m^2, respectively). Volume infusion increased the right atrial pressure (11 ± 2 to 15 ± 2 mm Hg, $p < .001$) and pulmonary arterial wedge pressure (10 ± 4 to 15 ± 2 mm Hg, $p < .001$). Despite increases in these fillings pressures, cardiac index and stroke volume index did not change significantly. Right and left ventricular stroke work indexes were also initially reduced (2.5 ± 1.4 and 30 ± 6 g·m/m^2, respectively), and they did not change significantly with the volume infusion. Also, heart rate, mean arterial pressure, systemic vascular resistance, total pulmonary resistance, and pulmonary vascular resistance did not change significantly with volume infusion.

Radionuclide angiography (table 2). Baseline right ventricular end-diastolic and end-systolic volumes in the 10 patients who received a volume infusion were elevated, and right ventricular ejection fraction was depressed (34 ± 5%). However, left ventricular end-diastolic and end-systolic volumes were within the normal range, and left ventricular ejection fraction was 60 ± 12%. After an infusion of normal saline, right and left ventricular volumes and ejection fractions did not change significantly.

TABLE 2
Mean radionuclide angiographic volumes and ejection fractions before and after therapy with normal saline (n = 10), dobutamine (n = 12), and nitroprusside (n = 10)

	RVEDV (ml)	RVESV (ml)	RVEF (%)	LVEDV (ml)	LVESV (ml)	LVEF (%)
Control	161±47	107±29	34±5	113±57	49±35	60±12
Normal saline	168±57	115±39	32±8	112±53	48±32	60±11
Control	159±54	110±37	31±7	124±55	53±32	60±12
Dobutamine	154±58	89±30^C	42±7^C	131±59	46±27^B	67±12^C
Control	165±95	117±86	32±10	110±38	43±22	61±12
Nitroprusside	153±92	107±86	34±9	106±33	36±21	68±13^A

RVEDV = right ventricular end-diastolic volume; RVESV = right ventricular end-systolic volume; RVEF = right ventricular ejection fraction; LVEDV = left ventricular end-diastolic volume; LVESV = left ventricular end-systolic volume; LVEF = left ventricular ejection fraction.

$^A p < .05$; $^B p < .01$; $^C p < .001$ for control vs intervention.

Dobutamine infusion (n = 12)

Hemodynamics (table 1). Because 10 of the 12 patients who received a dobutamine infusion also had received normal saline, the control right atrial and pulmonary arterial wedge pressures were 15 ± 2 and 15 ± 3 mm Hg, respectively. During infusion of dobutamine, right atrial pressure decreased to 13 ± 3 mm Hg ($p < .05$), while pulmonary arterial wedge pressure did not change significantly. During infusion of dobutamine, there were significant increases, compared with the control values, in cardiac index (2.1 ± 0.4 to 2.8 ± 0.6 liters/min/m^2, $p < .001$) and stroke volume index (30 ± 6 to 36 ± 7 ml/m^2, $p < .001$). Because of this improvement, there was a decrease in systemic vascular resistance from 1699 ± 508 to 1363 ± 352 dynes·sec/cm^5 ($p < .01$), while mean arterial pressure did not change significantly. In addition, right and left ventricular stroke work indexes increased from 2.6 ± 1.6 to 5.4 ± 2.1 ($p < .001$) and from 33 ± 11 to 41 ± 11 g·m/m^2 ($p < .01$), respectively. The pulmonary vascular resistance did not change significantly.

Radionuclide angiography (table 2). During the infusion of dobutamine right ventricular ejection fraction improved from 31 ± 7 to 42 ± 7% ($p < .001$) as a result of a decrease in right ventricular end-systolic volume (110 ± 37 to 89 ± 30 ml, $p < .001$) and the lack of a significant change in end-diastolic volume. Also, left ventricular ejection fraction increased from 60 ± 12% to 67 ± 12% ($p < .001$) owing to a decrease in left ventricular end-systolic volume from 53 ± 32 to 46 ± 27 ml ($p < .01$) and the lack of a significant change in end-diastolic volume.

Nitroprusside infusion (n = 10)

Hemodynamics (table 1). Eight of the 10 patients received a volume infusion before receiving nitroprusside; consequently, the control right atrial and pulmonary arterial wedge pressures were 14 ± 4 and 14 ± 5 mm Hg, respectively. The right atrial and pulmonary arterial wedge pressures decreased during the infusion of nitroprusside to 12 ± 4 mm Hg ($p < .05$) and 12 ± 5 mm Hg, respectively. As required by the protocol, the mean arterial pressure decreased from 93 ± 18 to 82 ± 16 mm Hg ($p < .01$). There was an increase in cardiac index from 2.0 ± 0.3 to 2.2 ± 0.5 liters/min/m^2 ($p < .05$), which was due to an increase in heart rate (72 ± 12 to 75 ± 12 beats/min, $p < .05$). The stroke volume index did not change significantly. The observed decrease in systemic vascular resistance from 1706 ± 556 to 1398 ± 498 dynes·sec/cm^5 ($p < .01$) was due primarily to the decrease in mean arterial pressure.

Radionuclide angiography (table 2). During the infusion of nitroprusside, the right and left ventricular volumes all decreased, but these changes were not significant. The right ventricular ejection fraction also did not change significantly; however, the left ventricular ejection fraction increased from 61 ± 12% to 68 ± 13% ($p < .05$). This was due to a greater decrease in left ventricular end-systolic volume compared with that in end-diastolic volume.

Comparison of dobutamine and nitroprusside therapy. On data from the nine patients who completed the protocol, a one-way analysis of variance was performed to determine whether differences existed in the loading conditions on the right and left ventricles during the two control periods. The mean right atrial, pulmonary arterial, pulmonary arterial wedge, and systemic arterial pressures and pulmonary and systemic vascular resistances did not differ during the control periods. In addition, the mean right and left ventricular end-diastolic volumes were similar during the two control periods. Therefore, the loading conditions in both ventricles were comparable before initiating the random infusion of each drug.

A two-way analysis of variance was performed to determine whether a significant difference existed between values obtained during the infusion of the two drugs (figure 1). The cardiac and stroke volume indexes increased more during the infusion of dobutamine than during the infusion of nitroprusside (2.0 ± 0.4 to 2.7 ± 0.5 vs 2.1 ± 0.4 to 2.3 ± 0.5 liters/min/m^2, $p < .001$; and 29 ± 6 to 36 ± 8 vs 29 ± 6 to 30 ± 6 ml/m^2, $p = .02$, respectively). The increase in right ventricular ejection fraction during the infusion of dobutamine was greater than that during the infusion of

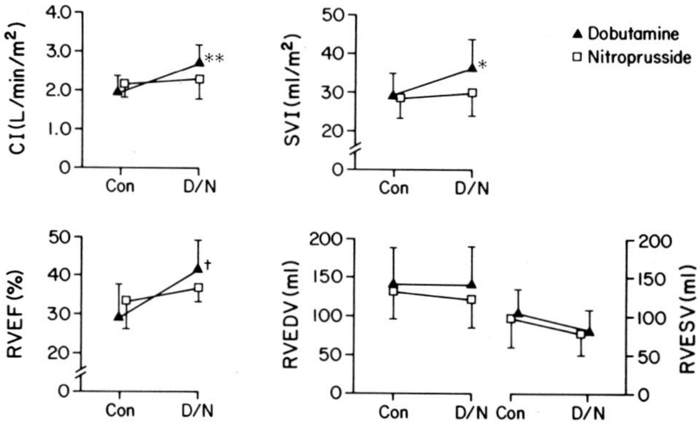

FIGURE 1. Results of two-way analysis of variance comparing the effects of dobutamine (D) and nitroprusside (N) therapy on cardiac index (CI), stroke volume index (SVI), right ventricular ejection fraction (RVEF), right ventricular end-diastolic volume (RVEDV), and right ventricular end-systolic volume (RVESV) in the nine patients receiving both drugs as outlined in the protocol. Significant differences are noted as follows: **$p < .001$; *$p = .02$; †$p < .01$.

nitroprusside (30 ± 8% to 42 ± 7% vs 34 ± 8% to 37 ± 4%, $p < .01$, respectively). This difference reflected a greater increase in stroke volume during the dobutamine infusion, since end-systolic volume decreased significantly ($p < .01$) and end-diastolic volume remained unchanged. In contrast, during the infusion of nitroprusside, there was a commensurate decrease in both end-diastolic and end-systolic volumes, producing no change in stroke volume. These changes paralleled the hemodynamic changes described above.

Discussion

Since the original reports by Cohn and Guiha and their colleagues[4, 11] in 1974, volume loading has been the mainstay of therapy for treatment of the low cardiac output state in acute RVMI. Subsequently, we[7] and others[8] have found that volume therapy did not improve cardiac output in a group of patients with hemodynamically important RVMI. Lopez-Sendon et al.[8] rapidly infused dextran into the right atrium of 36 patients with acute RVMI until either the right atrial or pulmonary arterial wedge pressure increased more than 5 mm Hg, or until cardiac output decreased. They found that volume loading increased filling pressures but did not significantly improve cardiac output for the group, and in many instances, it produced a decrease in cardiac output. They concluded that the pulmonary arterial wedge pressure may not reflect the true preload or end-diastolic volume of the left ventricle. Thus, therapy should aim for an optimal cardiac index rather than a specific pulmonary arterial wedge pressure, since copious volume infusions may produce a decrease in cardiac output.

This concept was nicely demonstrated by Goldstein et al.[5, 6] in their closed pericardial dog preparation of acute RVMI. After acute right coronary arterial occlusion, volume loading increased the left ventricular end-diastolic pressure from 7 to 12 mm Hg, and there was a small but significant increase in cardiac output. However, after the pericardium was removed, the left ventricular end-diastolic pressure decreased to 11 mm Hg and the left ventricular volumes and cardiac output increased significantly over the post-volume load values when the pericardium was intact. Thus, despite a significant increase in the left ventricular end-diastolic pressure after volume loading, the true distending pressure or transmural pressure of the left ventricle was diminished owing to an increased intrapericardial pressure. This finding corroborates other studies in animals and man that suggest that acute distension of the right ventricle encroaches upon the left ventricle, with a subsequent decrease in the septal-to-free wall left ventricular diameter, despite a rise in left ventricular end-diastolic pressure.[20–22]

Volume loading. The basic pathophysiology of acute RVMI as demonstrated in the animal preparation of Goldstein et al. is exemplified in our patient population by the following: an increased right atrial pressure, low cardiac index, increased right ventricular volumes with a markedly depressed right ventricular ejection fraction, and normal left ventricular volumes and ejection fraction. After a volume infusion, the following occurred: (1) both the right atrial and pulmonary arterial wedge pressures increased significantly, but cardiac index did not improve, (2) left ventricular end-diastolic volume and left ventricular ejection fraction did not change, and (3) right ventricular end-diastolic volume increased and right ventricular ejection fraction decreased slightly but not significantly. Thus, by further increasing right ventricular cavity size, volume loading may limit left ventricular filling through a mechanism of ventricular interaction due partly to the effects of the intact pericardium. Furthermore, increases in intracavitary pressure and radius may increase wall stress of the thin-walled right ventricle. This, in turn, may decrease right ventricular ejection fraction and right ventricular stroke volume, thereby further depressing forward cardiac output and systemic arterial pressure as demonstrated in a subset of patients studied by Lopez-Sendon et al.[8]

Dobutamine infusion. Dobutamine significantly increased cardiac and stroke volume indexes in our patients with acute RVMI by a direct augmentation in right ventricular systolic performance, as evidenced by a significant increase in right ventricular ejection fraction. This was accomplished through improved wall motion of hypokinetic wall segments, while akinetic and dyskinetic wall segments remained largely unchanged. In most cases, right ventricular lateral wall and outflow tract demonstrated normal to hypokinetic wall motion during the control study, and these segments became hyperkinetic during the infusion of dobutamine (figure 2). In addition, left ventricular systolic performance improved significantly over generally normal systolic function owing to improvement in normal and hypokinetic wall segments. The increases in hemodynamically determined cardiac and stroke volume indexes were paralleled by increases in radionuclide angiographic stroke volumes of the right and left ventricles.

In the hypotensive patient, there are theoretical contraindications to the use of dobutamine because of its weak systemic vasoconstrictor effect. However, six patients had systolic blood pressures ranging between

TABLE 3

Mean hemodynamic and radionuclide angiographic data before and after dobutamine in six patients with an initial systolic pressure less than 110 mm Hg

	RAP (mm Hg)	PAWP (mm Hg)	PA (mm Hg)	CI (l/min/m^2)	SVI (ml/m^2)	HR (bpm)	MAP (mm Hg)	SVR (dynes·sec·cm^2)	RVEDV (ml)
Control	15±3	15±3	22±3	2.1±0.4	31±6	68±11	83±6	1372±431	185±61
Dobutamine	13±3	17±4	25±4	2.8±0.5^C	39±7^B	71±12	95±13^A	1241±376	183±63

Abbreviations are as in tables 1 and 2.
$^A p < .05$; $^B p < .01$; $^C p < .005$.

90 and 110 mm Hg, and three of these patients had well-documented histories of hypertension. Mean cardiac index, stroke volume index, and systemic arterial pressure increased significantly, and no patient experienced hypotension during the infusion of dobutamine (table 3). Since vascular decompensation resulted from depressed myocardial contractility and not from loss of vascular tone, dobutamine was particularly beneficial in the present study population. However, when a patient presents in profound shock, when loss

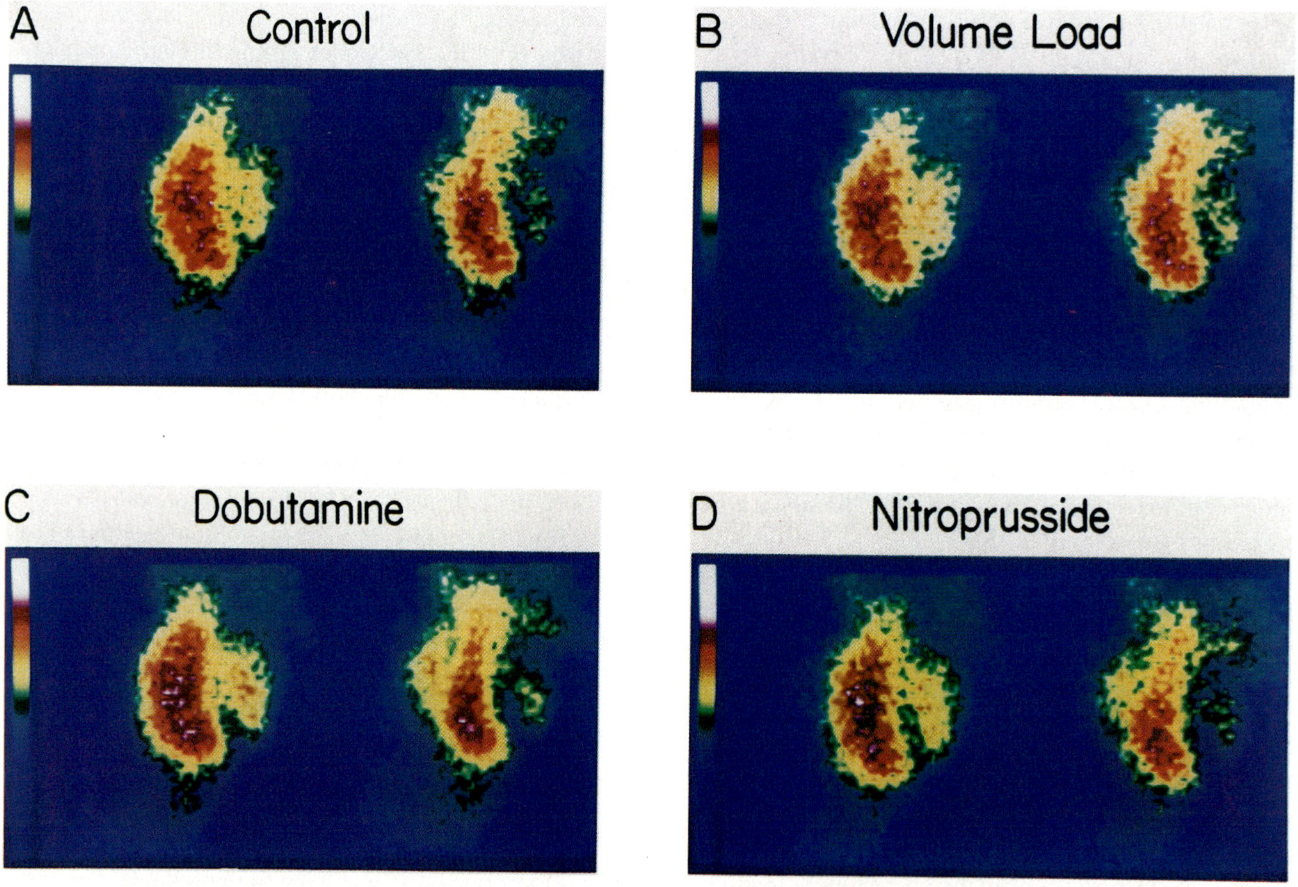

FIGURE 2. End-diastolic (*left*) and end-systolic (*right*) equilibrium radionuclide angiographic images in the left anterior oblique projection during control, volume loading, and administration of dobutamine and nitroprusside in a representative patient with acute RVMI are shown. *A*, The right ventricle is markedly enlarged with akinesis of the apex and inferior walls and hypokinesis of the lateral wall. Right ventricular ejection fraction = 31%. The left ventricle is small and the left ventricular ejection fraction = 58%. *B*, There is no change in right ventricular size and wall motion after a volume load. Right ventricular ejection fraction = 34%; left ventricular ejection fraction = 55%. *C*, During infusion of dobutamine right ventricular lateral and inferior wall motion markedly improve, producing a smaller end-systolic volume. Right ventricular ejection fraction = 43%. The overlying right atrium (yellow) becomes more prominent owing to enhancement of lateral wall motion. Left ventricular contractility increases, and left ventricular ejection fraction = 69%. *D*, A second control study was obtained before infusion of nitroprusside and findings were similar to those in *B*. Nitroprusside did not improve lateral or inferior wall motion. Right ventricular ejection fraction = 33%. Left ventricular contractility is augmented, with a left ventricular ejection fraction = 67%.

TABLE 3
(Continued)

RVESV (ml)	RVEF (%)	LVEDV (ml)	LVESV (ml)	LVEF (%)
129±39	29±8	153±57	68±30	55±11
105±28[B]	42±8[C]	167±55	59±23	63±12[C]

of vascular tone and marked hypotension may play a major role in the decompensated state, a positive inotropic agent with some α -adrenergic vasoconstrictive properties may be preferrable.

Nitroprusside infusion. Despite a significant decrease in mean pulmonary arterial pressure and total pulmonary resistance during the infusion of nitroprusside, there was no improvement in right ventricular systolic performance or stroke volume index in our study population. In contrast, afterload reduction improves right ventricular systolic performance and cardiac index in patients with pulmonary hypertension secondary to chronic obstructive lung disease or chronic left heart failure.[23–25] Because patients with significant right ventricular infarction have primary right ventricular pump failure, they usually present with normal to only mildly elevated pulmonary arterial systolic pressures, low pulmonary arterial pulse pressure, and mildly elevated total pulmonary resistance owing to a low cardiac output. Thus, right ventricular afterload does not present a significant obstacle to right ventricular ejection, either by passive elevation of left heart filling pressures or by increased pulmonary vascular resistance, as long as significant left ventricular dysfunction is not present.

Although both right ventricular end-diastolic volume and right atrial pressure demonstrated a tendency to decrease during the infusion of nitroprusside, these changes did not reach statistical significance. Therefore, the lack of improvement in right ventricular ejection fraction and stroke volume index cannot be totally attributed to an excessive decrease in preload during the infusion of nitroprusside, although this is the most likely explanation. In summary, therapy with nitroprusside in addition to volume loading did not improve the overall hemodynamic status of our patients with predominant RVMI.

Limitations. The results of this study suggest that volume loading does not improve cardiac index in patients with acute ischemic right ventricular dysfunction. However, one may argue that insufficient volume was given to produce a beneficial effect of the Frank-Starling mechanism, since right and left ventricular end-diastolic volume calculations did not increase significantly after this therapeutic intervention. Nonetheless, after a volume load, each patient had at least a 5 mm Hg increase in the pulmonary arterial wedge pressure, or a final pressure of greater than 15 mm Hg (range 15 to 20 mm Hg); the final right atrial pressure ranged between 14 and 19 mm Hg in each patient. According to the Frank-Starling mechanism, this initial rise in right- and left-sided filling pressures should have increased cardiac index, since the early portion of the cardiac function curve demonstrates the steepest slope in the relationship of stroke volume to filling pressure. After the achievement of an initial rise in filling pressures and an adequate sinal pulmonary arterial wedge pressure, a failure to increase cardiac index suggests that function in these patients was on the flat portion of the ventricular function curve and therefore, further volume loading could not improve forward cardiac output.

Although dobutamine significantly improved cardiac and stroke volume indexes, there was a significant increase in heart rate and mean arterial pressure, and the pulmonary arterial wedge pressure rose slightly. These effects in our patients are in direct contrast to the findings in patients with acute myocardial infarction and significant left ventricular dysfunction, in whom the infusion of dobutamine does not change heart rate or mean arterial pressure, while it does cause a decrease in the pulmonary arterial wedge pressure.[26, 27] Recently, Pacold et al.[28] demonstrated a significant increase in heart rate and blood pressure during low dose dobutamine infusion in 13 patients with chronic coronary artery disease and normal to minimally depressed left ventricular function. In these patients, myocardial ischemia was documented by a significant decrease in myocardial lactate extraction and a significant increase in mean ST segment depression. In our patient population with nearly normal left ventricular function, it is unlikely that the increased myocardial oxygen demands of dobutamine were offset by a decrease in left ventricular size and wall tension, as usually occurs in patients with severe congestive heart failure. Therefore, use of dobutamine in patients with predominant right ventricular dysfunction may induce ischemia, as it did in one of our patients. Nonetheless, systemic arterial hypotension and decreased cardiac index are the main indications for treatment of patients with acute RVMI; the subsequent improvement in pressure and cardiac index should augment myocardial blood flow and offset any increase in myocardial oxygen demand by an increase in systemic arterial and coronary perfusion pressures during the infusion of dobutamine.

Although each patient in the protocol had unequivocal clinical, hemodynamic, and radionuclide angiographic evidence of RVMI, no patient was severely hypotensive at the start of the protocol. However, eight of the 13 study patients had a well-documented history of hypertenson, and the mean arterial pressure for the group reflected relative hypotension when compared with preinfarction level. One patient (table 3) presented with a systolic blood pressure of 70 mm Hg, and concomittant volume loading (300 ml normal saline) and dobutamine subsequently raised his systolic arterial pressure to 100 mm Hg. After a stable hemodynamic condition was attained, dobutamine was discontinued and the complete protocol was performed. The protocol excluded patients with chronic left heart failure. In addition, none of our patients with right ventricular infarction had concomitant extensive infarction of the left ventricle. Thus, there were no patients in the study group who had significant right and left ventricular dysfunction. These patients are the most difficult to treat, and we and others have found that this subgroup of patients has the highest acute mortality, irrespective of the mode of therapy employed.[7, 29–30] In addition, Legrand et al.[31] reported that the 6 month mortality in 46 patients with RVMI was related to severe left ventricular disease in five of the six cases.

Conclusions. Right ventricular infarction is a unique clinical syndrome that differs from infarction that is predominantly of the left ventricle with respect to its acute presentation, therapy, and, most importantly its long-term prognosis. Our data[7] and the data from other investigators[32] demonstrate improvement in right ventricular systolic performance over the 6 week to 3 month recovery period. Thus, it appears that if these patients can be supported through the first 2 to 5 days after infarction, the chances of full recovery are excellent if there is predominant right ventricular dysfunction and no extensive impairment of performance of the left ventricle. This underscores the importance of early detection and prompt administration of appropriate therapy to improve acute mortality. In general, an initial volume infusion should be used to achieve an increase of greater than 5 mm Hg, not to exceed a final value of 20 mm Hg, in the pulmonary arterial wedge or right atrial pressure. This initial volume infusion should be carefully administered, and if cardiac output does not improve, then dobutamine should be administered to augment right ventricular systolic performance and improve forward cardiac output.

We appreciate the technical assistance of Ms. Betty Heyl, Suzanne Patrick-Fischer, and Sandra Carr, R.N., and the preparation of this manuscript by Ms. Patricia Krueger.

References

1. Isner JM, Robert WC: Right ventricular infarction complicating left ventricular infarction secondary to coronary heart disease. Am J Cardiol **42:** 885, 1978
2. Ratliff NB, Hackel DB: Combined right and left ventricular infarction: pathogenesis and clinicopathologic correlations. Am J Cardiol **45:** 217, 1980
3. Dell'Italia LJ, Starling MR: Right ventricular infarction: an important clinical entity. Curr Probl Cardiol **9:** 1, 1984
4. Guiha NJ, Limas CJ, Cohn JN: Predominant right ventricular dysfunction after right ventricular destruction in the dog. Am J Cardiol **33:** 254, 1974
5. Goldstein JA, Vlahakes GJ, Verrier ED, Schiller NB, Botvinick E, Tyberg JV, Parmley WW, Chatterjee K: Volume loading improves low cardiac output in experimental right ventricular infarction. J Am Coll Cardiol **2:** 270, 1983
6. Goldstein JA, Vlahakes GJ, Verrier ED, Schiller NB, Tyberg JV, Ports TA, Parmley WW, Chatterjee K: The role of right ventricular systolic dysfunction and elevated intrapericardial pressure in the genesis of low output in experimental right ventricular infarction. Circulation **65:** 513, 1982
7. Dell'Italia LJ, Starling MR, Crawford MH, Boros BL, Chaudhuri TK, O'Rourke RA: Right ventricular infarction: identification by hemodynamic measurements before and after volume loading and correlation with noninvasive techniques. J Am Coll Cardiol **4:** 931, 1984
8. Lopez-Sendon J, Coma-Canella I, Adanez JV: Volume loading in patients with ischemic right ventricular dysfunction. Eur Heart J **2:** 329, 1981
9. Roberts R, Marmor AT: Right ventricular infarction. Annu Rev Med **34:** 377, 1983
10. Clark G, Strauss HD, Roberts R: Dobutamine vs furosemide in the treatment of cardiac failure due to right ventricular infarction. Chest **77:** 220, 1980
11. Cohn JN, Guiha NH, Broder MI, Limas CJ. Right ventricular infarction: Clinical and hemodynamic features. Am J Cardiol **33:** 209, 1974
12. Raabe DS, Chester AC: Right ventricular infarction. Chest **73:** 96, 1978
13. The Criteria Committee of the New York Heart Association: Nomenclature and criteria for diagnosis of disease of the heart and heart vessels, ed. 8. Boston, 1979, Little, Brown and Company, pp 91–95
14. Dell'Italia LJ, Starling MR, O'Rourke RA: Physical examination for exclusion of hemodynamically important right ventricular infarction. Ann Intern Med **99:** 608, 1983
15. Starling MR, Dell'Italia LJ, Chaudhuri TK, Boros BL, O'Rourke RA: First transit and equilibrium radionuclide angiography in patients with inferior transmural myocardial infarction: criteria for the diagnosis of associated hemodynamically significant right ventricular infarction. J Am Coll Cardiol **4:** 923, 1984
16. Maddahi J, Berman DS, Matsuoka DT, Waxman AD, Stankus KE, Forrester JS, Swan HJC: A new technique for assessing right ventricular ejection fraction using rapid multiple-gated equilibrium cardiac blood pool scintigraphy: description, validation and findings in chronic coronary artery disease. Circulation **60:** 581, 1979
17. Dell'Italia LJ, Starling MR, Walsh RA, Badke FR, Lasher JC, Blumhardt R: Validation of attenuation-corrected equilibrium radionuclide angiographic right ventricular volume determinations: comparison with cast-validated biplane cineventriculography. Circulation **72:** 317, 1985
18. Starling MR, Dell'Italia LJ, Nusynowitz ML, Walsh RA, Little WC, Benedetto AR: Estimates of left-ventricular volumes by equilibrium radionuclide angiography: importance of attenuation correction. J Nucl Med **25:** 14, 1984
19. Starling MR, Dell'Italia LJ, Walsh RA, Little WC, Benedetto AR, Nusynowitz ML: Accurate estimates of absolute left ventricular volumes from equilibrium radionuclide angiographic count data using a simple geometric attenuation correction. J Am Coll Cardiol **3:** 789, 1984
20. Lorell BH, Palacios I, Daggett WM, Jacobs ML, Fowler BN, Newell JB: Right ventricular distension and left ventricular compliance. Am J Physiol **240:** H87, 1981

21. Bove AA, Santamore WP: Ventricular interdependence. Prog Cardiovasc Dis **23:** 365, 1981
22. Brinker JA, Weiss JL, Lappe DL, Rabson JL, Summer WR, Permutt S, Weisfeldt ML: Leftward septal displacement during right ventricular loading in man. Circulation **61:** 626, 1980
23. Yin FCP, Guzman PA, Brin KP, Maughan WL, Brinker JA, Traill TA, Weiss JL, Weisfeldt ML: Effect of nitroprusside on hydraulic vascular loads on the right and left ventricle of patients with heart failure. Circulation **67:** 1330, 1983
24. Brent BN, Berger HJ, Matthay RA, Mahler D, Pytlik L, Zaret BL: Contrasting acute effects of vasodilators (nitroglycerin, nitroprusside, and hydralazine) on right ventricular performance in patients with chronic obstructive pulmonary disease and pulmonary hypertension: a combined radionuclide-hemodynamic study. Am J Cardiol **51:** 1682, 1983
25. Colucci WS, Holman BL, Wynne J, Carabello B, Malacoff R, Grossman W, Braunwald E: Improved right ventricular function and reduced pulmonary vascular resistance during prazosin therapy of congestive heart failure. Am J Med **71:** 75, 1981
26. Gillespie TA, Ambos HD, Sobel BE, Roberts R: Effects of dobutamine in patients with acute myocardial infarction. Am J Cardiol **39:** 588, 1977
27. Goldstein RA, Passamani ER, Roberts R: A comparison of digoxin and dobutamine in patients with acute infarction and cardiac failure. N Engl J Med **303:** 846, 1980
28. Pacold I, Kleinman B, Gunnar R, Loeb HS: Effects of low-dose dobutamine on coronary hemodynamics, myocardial metabolism and anginal threshold in patients with coronary artery disease. Circulation **68:** 1044, 1983
29. Jugdutt BI, Sussex BA, Sivaram CA, Rossall RE: Right ventricular infarction: two-dimensional echocardiographic evaluation. Am Heart J **107:** 505, 1984
30. Lopez-Sendon J, Coma-Canella I, Gamallo C: Sensitivity and specificity of hemodynamic criteria in the diagnosis of acute right ventricular infarction. Circulation **64:** 515, 1981
31. Legrand V, Rigo P, Demoulin JC, Collignon P, Kulbertus HE: Right ventricular myocardial infarction diagnosed by 99^{m} pyrophosphate scintigraphy: clinical course and follow-up. Eur Heart J **4:** 9, 1983
32. Klein HO, Tordjman T, Ninio R, Sareli P, Oren V, Lang R, Gefen J, Pauzner C, Di Segni E, David D, Kaplinsky E: The early recognition of right ventricular infarction: diagnostic accuracy of the electrocardiographic V4R Lead. Circulation **67:** 558, 1983

Systemic and transcardiac platelet activity in acute myocardial infarction in man: resistance to prostacyclin

HILTRUD S. MUELLER, M.D., PARINAM S. RAO, PH.D., MARK A. GREENBERG, M.D., PETER M. BUTTRICK, M.D., IRA I. SUSSMAN, M.D., HOWARD A. LEVITE, M.D., RICHARD M. GROSE, M.D., VICENTE PEREZ-DAVILA, M.D., JANET E. STRAIN, M.D., AND THEODORE H. SPAET, M.D.

ABSTRACT There is increasing evidence that platelets play an important role in the pathogenesis of acute ischemic heart disease. Therefore an understanding of factors that influence platelet performance is important. This study was undertaken (1) to characterize during evolving myocardial infarction platelet activity in the peripheral circulation and across the ischemic/infarcting myocardial compartment, the locus of presumed platelet hyperactivity, and (2) to evaluate the effects of prostacyclin (PGI_2), a most potent antiplatelet agent and vasodilator. A total of 59 patients with evolving myocardial infarction were studied. Twenty-two patients were instrumented with arterial and coronary sinus catheters and received intravenous infusion of PGI_2, 13 ± 4.5 ng/kg/min (mean ± SD), for 90 min. In 15 patients with anterior myocardial infarction, transcardiac platelet function and response to PGI_2 were studied. Plasma levels of β-thromboglobulin (β-TG) and of thromboxane B_2 (TxB_2), in vivo measures of platelet activity, were elevated three- and 10-fold. 6-Keto-prostaglandin $F_{1\alpha}$, the stable end product of PGI_2, was less than 10 pg/ml, reflecting a leftward shift of the TxB_2/PGI_2 ratio. Platelets circulating during evolving myocardial infarction ("ischemic platelets") were hyperaggregable in response to ADP and relatively resistant to PGI_2, both in vivo and in vitro. Concentrations of platelet cyclic AMP and the cyclic AMP response to PGI_2 were diminished. The platelet hyperreactivity, expressed by plasma β-TG, platelet aggregation, and PGI_2-induced inhibition of aggregation, was most intense early during infarct evolution and decreased with time. The increased platelet performance resulted in "platelet fatigue," indicated by decreased contents of β-TG of the ischemic platelet and decreased TxA_2 production in response to collagen. However, the ischemic platelet produced twice normal TxA_2 in response to arachidonic acid (stimulus and substrate), demonstrating a heightened metabolic capacity. TxA_2 was produced across the ischemic/infarcting compartment in 10 of 15 patients with anterior myocardial infarction. The antiplatelet effect of PGI_2 was greatly diminished. In summary, the data define an abnormal pattern of platelet behavior during evolving myocardial infarction, characterized by a proaggregatory environment, heightened platelet reactivity in both the peripheral and coronary circulation, and relative resistance to PGI_2. The clinical consequences of the data are that the patient in the acute phase of myocardial infarction may benefit from suppression of platelet function and requires significantly greater doses of PGI_2 than normal subjects. The data also suggest future directions for therapeutic manipulation of platelet hyperreactivity in the setting of acute myocardial ischemia.

Circulation 72, No. 6, 1336–1345, 1985.

INCREASING EVIDENCE is accumulating that platelets play an important role in the pathogenesis of ischemic heart disease.[1, 2] Previous studies have demonstrated increased circulating platelet release products[3–5] and platelet aggregates[6] as well as enhanced platelet aggregability in patients with acute myocardial infarction.[7] Clinical and autopsy studies have shown obstructive thrombi and platelet aggre-

From the Department of Medicine, Montefiore Medical Center, Albert Einstein College of Medicine of Yeshiva University, Bronx, NY.

Supported by NHLBI grant R01HL2944902 and by the Upjohn Co., Kalamazoo, MI. Drs. Buttrick and Levite were supported by USPHS Institutional Training Grant HL07071. Dr. Buttrick is the recipient of an ACC/Merck Fellowship Award. Dr. Strain is the recipient of NHLBI Clinical Investigator Award HL01179.

Address for correspondence: Hiltrud S. Mueller, M.D., Division of Cardiology–Central I, Montefiore Medical Center, 111 E. 210th St., Bronx, NY 10467.

Received June 5, 1985; revision accepted Sept. 12, 1985.

gates in acutely occluded coronary vessels.[8, 9] In animal experiments, cyclical flow reduction by platelet aggregates proximal to the obstructive coronary lesion[10–12] and thromboxane formation distal to the obstruction have been observed.[11, 12] These results have led to the suggestion that increased platelet activity and its consequences contribute to the development of unstable angina, acute myocardial infarction, and sudden cardiac death.[13] Therefore an understanding of platelet function and factors that influence platelet performance is important.

This study was undertaken to characterize both the platelets circulating during acute myocardial infarction and also local and systemic factors that might influence platelet behavior in this setting. Descriptors of platelet function in vivo, such as circulating release products, and platelet responsiveness in vitro to various stimuli were investigated and, whenever feasible, correlated in the attempt to characterize platelet behavior as completely as possible. Transcardiac alterations in platelet function across the ischemic/infarcting myocardial compartment were investigated, since this tissue bed is the locus of presumed platelet hyperactivity.

In addition to these empiric studies, the effect of a potent antiplatelet agent, prostacyclin (PGI_2), on platelet behavior during acute myocardial infarction was evaluated. This prostaglandin is of interest for several reasons: first, it is considered the most potent antiaggregating agent yet described; second, it is synthesized by vascular endothelium and is postulated to provide endogenous biological protection against platelet microthrombi;[14] and third, it has a short serum half-life, making it an attractive agent for the treatment of patients with unstable coronary disease. From this study it was hoped that an approach to the manipulation of platelet function in acute myocardial infarction would emerge.

Methods

Patients. Two groups of patients with acute transmural myocardial infarction were studied: group I patients received only a peripheral venous line, and group II patients were instrumented with two intravascular catheters. Characteristics of the two groups are shown in table 1.

Criteria for acute myocardial infarction were (1) typical anginal pain for more than 30 min and (2) ST segment elevation greater than 1 mm in at least two leads in the extremity and/or precordial electrocardiogram. Myocardial infarction was confirmed retrospectively by serial creatine kinase–MB elevations. In a third group of 20 normal volunteers, platelet activity was studied for comparison; 12 were men, and the average age was 43 ± 10 years.

None of the patients or normal volunteers had taken aspirin or related drugs that might have interferred with the cyclooxygenase pathway during the previous 2 weeks. All patients had received sublingual or topical nitroglycerin, and most also had been given morphine in the emergency room. All patients received lidocaine as bolus and continuous intravenous infusion (2 mg/min). Two patients in group I and one patient in group II had taken propranolol (not exceeding 10 mg tid), which was discontinued before the study. None of the patients had received calcium-channel blockers. None of the patients showed evidence of cardiac failure based on clinical findings and chest roentgenogram.

Procedure. The protocol was approved by the Institutional Review Board for Clinical Research, Montefiore Medical Center. All patients gave written informed consent.

In group I, blood was obtained by a single 19 gauge needle stick, with the first few milliliters discarded. Patients in group II were instrumented with an intra-arterial and a coronary sinus catheter: (1) a No. 6F catheter (USCI, Billerica, MA) was inserted via a femoral artery into the descending aorta in 14 patients, and a No. 20 gauge Angiocath (Deseret Medical Inc., Sandy, UT) was inserted via a radial artery in eight patients; (2) a No. 7F Baim catheter[15] (Electro-Catheter Co., Rahway, NJ) was inserted via the right internal jugular vein into the coronary sinus and advanced into the great cardiac vein. In seven of 15 patients in whom transcardiac platelet studies were performed, the catheters were coated with heparin (provided by supplier). The catheters were positioned in the coronary care unit by means of radiolucent beds and portable fluoroscopic equipment. They were flushed by a constant infusion pump with isotonic saline without heparin. A multichannel oscilliscope VR 6 (Electronics for Medicine) was used for recording. Measurements of arterial blood pressure, heart rate, and coronary blood flow and blood samples were obtained at baseline, during the end of a 90 min infusion of PGI_2, and 30 min after discontinuation of the infusion.

Plasma thromboxane B_2 (TxB_2) and β-thromboglobulin (β-TG) were determined from blood samples obtained under the following conditions: before instrumentation by venipuncture and shortly after through the catheter (n = 5), after approximately 40 (n = 5) and 90 min (n = 5), and simultaneously by venipuncture and through the catheter (n = 4).

Specific methods. Thromboxane A_2 (TxA_2) and PGI_2 in plasma were assayed by measuring the stable end products, TxB_2 and 6-keto-prostaglandin $F_{1\alpha}$ (6-keto-$PGF_{1\alpha}$), with a radioimmunoassay kit (New England Nuclear RIA-NEK007/008). The method was modified by us[16] as follows: To avoid falsely elevated TxB_2 levels caused by the buffer matrix and nonspecific impurities introduced during the extraction procedure, we measured TxB_2 directly in plasma without ethyl acetate extraction, and we used human plasma control, 0 ng/ml TxB_2 (New England Nuclear) instead of 50 mM phosphate buffer. To increase the sensitivity, 20 pg of TxB_2 or 6-keto-$PGF_{1\alpha}$ in human plasma control was added to duplicate specimens. Normal values were 7.3 ± 6.9 (SD) pg/ml TxB_2 and less than 10 pg/ml 6-keto-$PGF_{1\alpha}$ (n = 20). The reproducibility of

TABLE 1
Patient characteristics

	Group I	Group II
n	37	22
Age (yr)	62 ± 10	62 ± 11
Sex (No. of men)	30	17
Infarct site		
Anterior/lateral	25	15
Inferior/posterior	12	7
Infarct size (CK_{MB} g-Eq/m^2)	—	44 ± 18
Infarct onset to study (hr)	7.0 ± 3.4	8.5 ± 2.8

the assay for duplicate determinations was 5.6%. Our normal values for TxB_2 and 6-keto-$PGF_1\alpha$ are comparable to those reported in the literature using direct assays[17–19] or extraction followed by purification with reverse-phase high-pressure liquid chromotography.[20]

β-TG was assayed in plasma with a commercially available radioimmunoassay kit according to the manufacturer's instruction (Code IM 88; Amersham Corp., Arlington Heights, IL). Normal values averaged 34 ± 10 ng/ml (n = 20).

Norepinephrine and epinephrine in plasma were determined by high-pressure liquid chromatography (HPLC, Waters 6000A) with an LC-4 electrochemical detector.[21] Standards containing 200 pg/ml of norepinephrine and epinephrine were run in parallel. Plasma contents in normal volunteers, obtained after 20 min rest in a supine position, were 168 ± 41 pg/ml for norepinephrine and 47 ± 14 pg/ml for epinephrine (n = 13). The coefficient of variation of 30 duplicate determinations was 2.1 ± 1.2% (norepinephrine) and 4.5 ± 4.2% (epinephrine).

Platelet aggregation in response to ADP (Sigma Chemical Co.) and collagen (Bio Data Corp.) was measured by methods standard in our laboratory.[22] In brief, blood was carefully drawn and transferred into polypropylene tubes containing 3.2% sodium citrate. This was then centrifuged at room temperature for 2 min 45 sec at 1000 *g* to obtain platelet-rich plasma (PRP). Platelet-poor plasma (PPP) was obtained by centrifuging the remaining pellet at 2200 *g* for 10 min at +4° C. Platelet cell counts were determined in an ultraflow blood counter (Clay Adams), and final PRP concentration was adjusted to 250 to 400 × 10^6 platelets/ml with autologous PPP.

Aggregometry was performed in a Payton dual-chamber aggregometer at 37° C with constant stirring (1000 rpm). Serial studies using various concentrations of ADP (0.5 to 8 μM) and of collagen (0.5 to 8 μg/ml) were done to generate dose-response curves. Results are expressed as aggregation to 50% (AG_{50}; μM ADP or μg/ml collagen), indicating the amount of ADP or collagen required to achieve 50% change in optical density. Normal values averaged 1.46 ± 0.35 μM ADP (n = 20) and 1.26 ± 0.53 μg/ml collagen (n = 11). Total time from initial phlebotomy to aggregation was greater than 30 min, and all studies were performed within 120 min. Duplicate studies were done at the beginning and end of this study interval to verify internal consistency.

Inhibiton of platelet aggregation (INH_{50}): Maximal aggregation in response to ADP was determined as described above. PRP was exposed in the aggregometer to varying concentrations of PGI_2 (0.5 to 4 ng/ml) for 3 min, followed by addition of 4 μM ADP, and aggregation was determined. Results are expressed as inhibition to 50% (INH_{50}; ng/ml PGI_2), indicating the amount of PGI_2 required to inhibit the maximal change in optical density by 50%.

β-TG release was measured after 5 min exposure to ADP (0.5 to 8 μM) or collagen (0.5 to 8 μg/ml) in the aggregometer under the conditions described above. Release of β-TG was stopped by the addition of 10 μ M PGE_1 and 8 μM indomethacin. The specimen was subsequently centrifuged at 9000 *g* for 2 min and the supernatant diluted in saline buffer containing 10 μM PGE_1 and 8 μM indomethacin. β-TG was assayed with an Amersham radioimmunoassay kit (see above). Normal values averaged 34 ± 8.7 μg/10^9 platelets after ADP exposure (n = 15) and 37 ± 10 μg/10^9 platelets after collagen exposure (n = 10).

Platelet β-TG content: PRP was frozen at −20° C for 15 min and thawed (room temperature) six times.[23] The lysate was diluted (100×) with saline containing 10 μM indomethacin and 10 μM PGE_1. A 50 μl volume of the solution was assayed for β-TG with an Amersham radioimmunoassay kit (see above). Normal values were 44 ± 9.3 μg/10^9 platelets (n = 15).

Platelet thromboxane production was determined according to the method of Ludlam et al.[24] Briefly, samples of PRP were stimulated in the aggregometer as described above with 50 to 500 μg/ml arachidonic acid (AA), (Bio Data Corp) for 8 min or with 0.5 to 8 μg/ml collagen for 5 min and then centrifuged at 900 *g* for 2 min. A 50 μl aliquot of supernatant was then transferred into phosphate buffer containing 10 μg/ml diclofenac sodium. TxB_2 contents were measured as indicated above with the exception that phosphate buffer was used as a matrix system. Results are expressed as maximum TxA_2 production; normal values were 2.5 ± 0.9 ng/10^7 platelets after arachidonic acid exposure to AA (n = 20) and 1.0 ± 0.35 ng/10^7 platelets after collagen (n = 10).

Cyclic AMP (cAMP) contents in PRP alone and in PRP exposed to 1 ng/ml PGI_2 at 37° C for 3 min in the aggregometer were measured by a standard radioimmunoassay kit (DuPont, NEK-0033) modified by us as follows: PRP after stimulation was precipitated with equal volumes of 10% trichloroacetic acid, centrifuged at 9000 *g* for 2 min, and the supernatant washed four times with fivefold excess volume of ether. The aqueous phase was dried under nitrogen and the residue was resuspended in 1 ml of sodium acetate (0.5 M). cAMP determinations were made with a nonacetylated technique. Normal values in unstimulated platelets were 8.8 ± 3.7 pmol/10^8 platelets (n = 20).

Infarct size was measured by serial determinations of plasma creatine kinase–MB (CK-MB) sampling every 2 hr for 12 hr, every 6 hr for 48 hr, and every 12 hr thereafter, until baseline values were reached. Analysis of plasma CK-MB was performed with the ESKACHEM Kit for CK-MB (No. 86239; Smith Kline Co., Sunnyvale, CA), with an immunoinhibition assay at 30 °C. Infarct size was calculated according to the formula of Sobel et al.,[25] applying a constant rate of disappearance (K_d). The following values were used for calculation: plasma volume, 4.4% of body weight; K_d, 0.0017/min; CK-MB content of normal myocardium at 30° C, 170 U/g wet weight, of infarcted myocardium, 46 U/g.

Coronary blood flow was measured by thermodilution technique and a Baim double-lumen catheter.[15] The design of the catheter allows measurement of both coronary blood flow and blood substances.

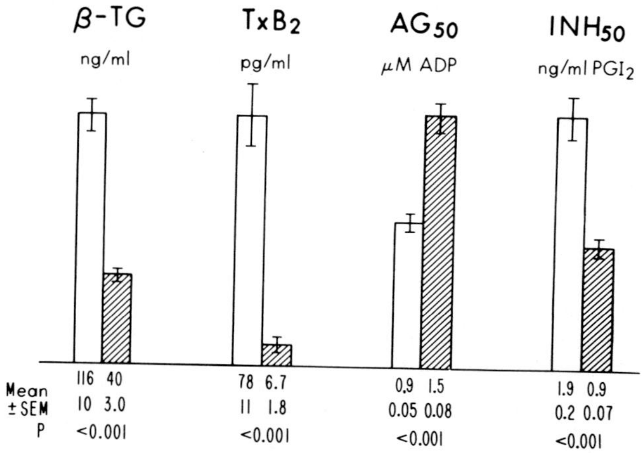

FIGURE 1. Platelet function profile in 37 patients with acute myocardial infarction (open bar) and in 20 normal volunteers (hatched bar), mean ± SEM. Plasma concentrations of β-TG and TxB_2 are strikingly increased in patients with infarction. Platelet aggregation is enhanced, indicated by the smaller amount of ADP (μM) required for 50% aggregation (AG_{50}). Inhibition of aggregation by PGI_2 is diminished, indicated by twice the amount of PGI_2 required to inhibit the maximal change in optical density by 50% (INH_{50}).

PGI_2 was kindly provided by Upjohn Co., Kalamazoo, MI. Intravenous infusion of PGI_2 was begun at 2 ng/kg/min and increased at 3 min intervals at increments of 2 ng/kg/min. Limiting end points for the infusion were: (1) increase in heart rate of 20% of baseline and/or absolute heart rate greater than 115 beats/min, (2) decrease in mean arterial pressure of 20% below baseline and/or absolute mean blood pressure less than 65 mm Hg, (3) side effects such as nausea, vomiting, headache, or excess anxiety. The maximum dose tolerated by patients with myocardial infarction for 90 min was 13 ± 4.5 ng/kg/min.

Data analysis. Statistical analysis was performed with Student's t test for paired and unpaired data. Data with three study points on the same patient were compared by analysis of variance.[26] A p value <.05 was considered significant. Data were expressed as mean ± 1 SD. To reduce the impact of the skewness of the original thromboxane levels in the artery and great cardiac vein on test statistics, which assumes some degree of normality, and to adjust for the exaggeration of the impact of small negative great cardiac vein–arterial differences with large arterial levels (see below), we used percent change and log transformation of the data. Statistical significance of the log of the ratios was calculated by t test. The use of the log and reciprocal functions for calculating relationships between time and the measurements for AG_{50}, INH_{50}, and plasma β-TG concentration was based on analyzing several different types of data transformation and displaying those that provided the best linear fit.

Results

Platelet function in peripheral blood

Group I (not instrumented). Data of 37 patients with myocardial infarction and of 20 normal volunteers are shown in figures 1 and 2. In the patients with infarction, plasma contents of β-TG and TxB_2 were significantly elevated compared with normal. Plasma contents of 6-keto-$PGF_{1\alpha}$ (not shown) averaged less than 10 pg/ml in both groups. Thus the TxB_2/PGI_2 ratio was shifted toward thromboxane. The platelets circulating in the acute phase of infarction ("ischemic platelets") were highly aggregable: significantly less ADP was required for 50% aggregation compared with normal. Furthermore, the ischemic platelets were relatively resistant to PGI_2; twice the amount of PGI_2 was required for inhibition of aggregation by 50%. Concentrations of cAMP, a biochemical mediator for the inhibitory effect of PGI_2 on aggregation, were decreased in the PRP of patients with infarction compared with normals. PGI_2 (1 ng/ml) increased the cAMP concentrations to 10 ($p < .001$) and 14 ($p = .001$) pmol/10^8 platelets, respectively. The PGI_2-induced changes were similar in both groups, although the maximal cAMP levels in the infarct group remained lower than in normal subjects. The maximal thromboxane production by the ischemic platelet in response to AA was twice that of normal. Plasma contents of norepinephrine and epinephrine (not shown) were approximately fourfold elevated in the infarct group (725 ± 282 vs 176 ± 49 pg/ml, $p < .001$; 140 ± 112 vs 41 ± 14 pg/ml, $p < .001$). Platelet counts were similar in both groups (351 ± 109 [infarct] and 384 ± 121 × $10^3/\mu l$ [normals]).

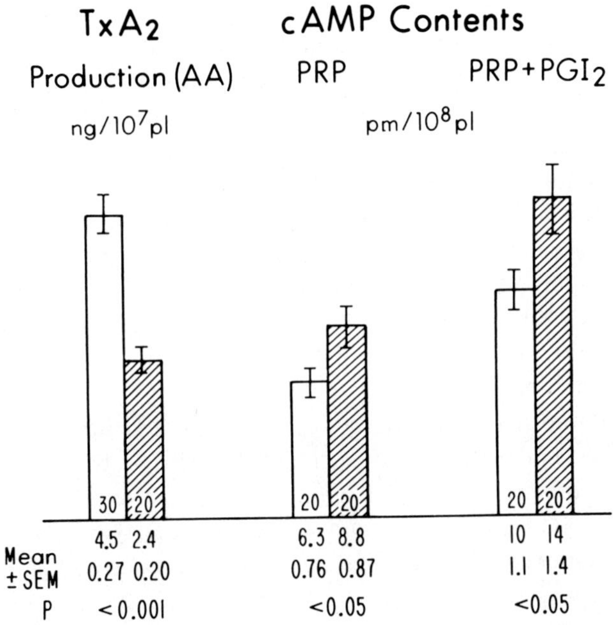

FIGURE 2. Platelet function profile. Arrangement as in figure 1. Maximal TxA_2 production in response to AA is twice as high in the infarct group compared with normal. cAMP concentrations in PRP are lower in patients with infarction vs normals and remain lower in response to 1 ng/ml PGI_2.

Separation of the platelet function data described above according to anterior/lateral (AMI, n = 25) and inferior/posterior infarction (IMI, n = 12) showed no statistically significant differences between the two subgroups: plasma contents averaged for β-TG, 121 ± 56 (AMI) and 107 ± 74 (IMI) ng/ml; for TxB_2, 73 ± 62 and 82 ± 59 pg/ml; for AG_{50}, 0.88 ± 0.28 and 0.93 ± 0.37 μM ADP; for INH_{50}, 1.79 ± 0.93 and 1.98 ± 1.69 ng/ml PGI_2; for maximal TxA_2 production, 4.38 ± 1.64 (n = 19) and 4.70 ± 1.24 (n = 11) μg/ml AA.

In order to evaluate the impact of the increased release of β-TG and production of thromboxane in vivo on the functional capacity of the ischemic platelet, we studied the platelet response to maximal stimulation in vitro (table 2). In response to collagen, the production of thromboxane was reduced by 46% compared with normal. However, if AA was used as stimulus (*and* substrate) (figure 2), the ischemic platelet produced twice as much thromboxane as the normal. Platelet β-TG contents of the ischemic platelet were half of normal. Maximal β-TG release in response to collagen approximated 80% in both groups. The amounts released averaged 17 and 37 μg/10^9 platelets.

Group II (instrumented with two catheters). Baseline

TABLE 2
Maximal platelet responses to graded stimulation in vitro (mean ± SD)

Measurement	Infarct	Normal	p value
Maximal TxA_2 production ($ng/10^7$ platelets)			
Collagen	0.55±0.20 (10)	1.02±0.35 (10)	<.01
Maximal β-TG release ($\mu g/10^9$ platelets)			
Collagen	17±11 (12)	37±10 (10)	<.001
ADP	10±8.5 (12)	34±8.7 (15)	<.001
Platelet β-TG content ($\mu g/10^9$ platelets)	22±7.9 (12)	44±9.3 (15)	<.001

Data in parentheses are number of subjects.

data demonstrate that mean values did not significantly differ between groups I and II: plasma contents averaged for β-TG, 110 ± 51 (group II) and 116 ± 60 (Group I) ng/ml; for TxB_2, 89 ± 62 and 78 ± 69 pg/ml; for AG_{50}, 1.0 ± 0.42 and 0.89 ± 0.31 μM ADP; for norepinephrine, 683 ± 307 and 725 ± 282 pg/ml; and for epinephrine 166 ± 126 and 140 ± 112 pg/ml.

Figure 3 compares plasma contents of TxB_2 and β-TG from blood samples obtained before placement of catheters and shortly after through the catheter, after approximately 40 and 90 min, and simultaneously by venipuncture and through the catheter. The distribution of the data points is similar above and below the line of identity. The mean values for TxB_2 are 69 ± 37 (venipuncture) and 65 ± 38 pg/ml (catheter) and those for β-TG are 100 ± 42 and 102 ± 50 ng/ml.

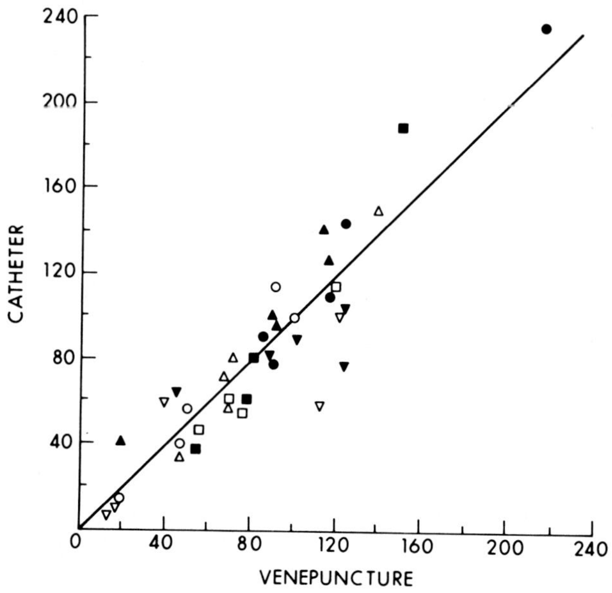

FIGURE 3. Comparison of plasma contents of TxB_2 (open symbols) and β-TG (solid symbols). Samples were obtained by venipuncture before catheter placement and shortly afterwards through the catheter (○●), after 40 min (△▲), after 90 min (▽▼), and simultaneously by venipuncture and through the catheter (□■). Results do not significantly differ over a period of up to 90 min or when sampled simultaneously. In particular, there is no consistent increase in plasma concentrations attributable to catheter exposure. The distribution of data points is similar above and below the line of identity.

Platelet function in relation to infarct duration. Platelet aggregability was highest during the early phase of infarction and decreased with time (figure 6, *A*): $AG_{50} = 0.54 \times \log_e (hr)$, $r = .71$, $p < .0001$, $n = 37$. Inhibition of aggregation by PGI_2 was least effective in the early infarct phase and improved with infarct duration (figure 6, *B*): $INH_{50} = 9.61/hr$, $r = .67$, $p < .0001$, $n = 26$. Plasma contents of β-TG were highest early after infarct onset: $246 - 54 \times \log_e (hr)$, $r = -.44$, $p < .005$, $n = 41$. There was no relationship between plasma TxB_2 and infarct duration. When the data obtained within 4 hr ($n = 7$) and within 10 to 15 hr ($n = 9$) after clinical onset of infarction were separated, the differences became accentuated. The average data for AG_{50} were 0.54 ± 0.35 (early) and 1.0 ± 0.13 (late) μM ADP ($p < .01$) and the data for β-TG were 194 ± 31 and 106 ± 35 ng/ml ($p < .01$). Thromboxane contents of the two subgroups did not significantly differ.

Platelet function across the infarcting myocardial compartment. We obtained transcardiac measurements in 15 patients with transmural anterior wall infarction, sampling from the aorta and great cardiac vein. We did not include patients with inferior wall infarction because of the inability to sample selectively from the infarcting compartment. Platelet counts were similar in the arterial and great cardiac vein blood: 311 ± 70 and 309 ± 85 × $10^3/\mu l$. Ten of the 15 patients produced thromboxane across the infarcting compartment (figure 4); the TxB_2 contents averaged 76 ± 101 pg/ml in the artery and 211 ± 273 pg/ml in the great cardiac vein. In the remaining five patients, no changes in transcardiac thromboxane contents were seen. For the entire group, the arterial–great cardiac vein differences did not reach statistical significance ($p = .068$). The geometric mean value of the great cardiac vein–arterial ratio of the entire group was 1.85 ($p < .005$). β-TG contents did not change across the infarcting compartment.

Effect of PGI_2 on platelet function. PGI_2 was infused for 90 min at the maximal tolerated dose, 13 ± 4.5 ng/kg/min. Data are reported for baseline, after 90 min of infusion, and 30 min after termination of infusion (table 3). PGI_2 caused a sharp rise in the plasma con-

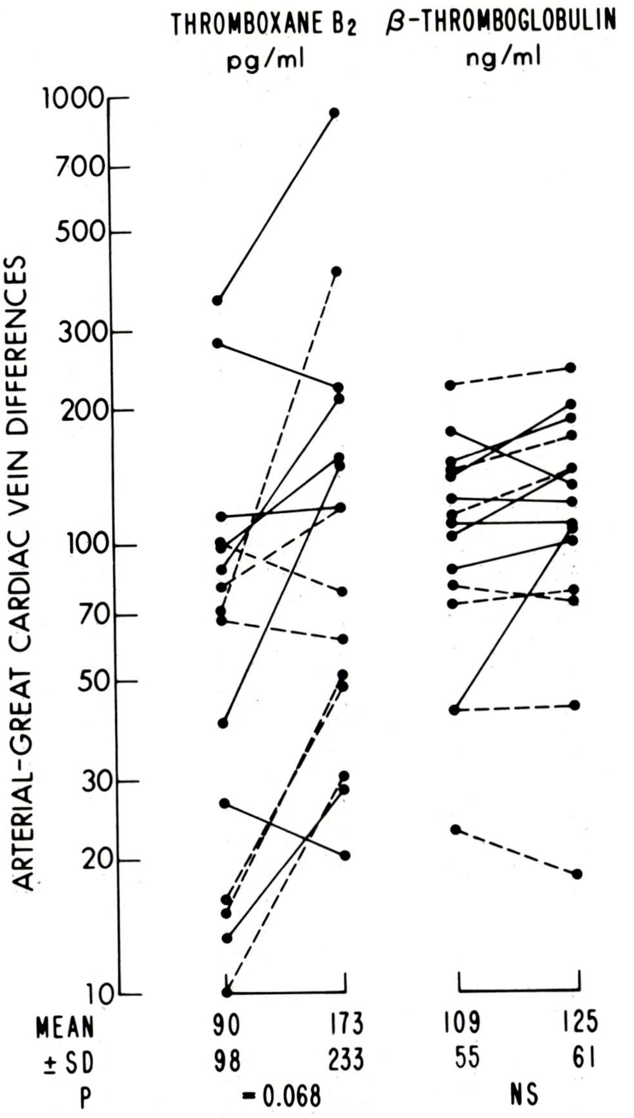

FIGURE 4. Arterial–great cardiac vein differences in plasma levels of TxB_2 and β-TG. Dotted lines represent data obtained with heparin-coated catheters. In two-thirds of the patients, TxB_2 levels in the great cardiac vein are twofold to threefold higher. There is no difference in the transcardiac β-TG levels, except in one patient.

tents of 6-keto-$PGF_{1\alpha}$, the stable metabolite of PGI_2. The agent decreased plasma β-TG and reduced platelet aggregation; the amount of ADP required for 50% aggregation doubled. These PGI_2-induced changes were reversible after termination of the infusion. PGI_2 tended to decrease plasma TxB_2 levels; however, the responses varied widely. Plasma levels of norepinephrine and epinephrine remained unchanged during the infusion.

We evaluated the effect of prostacyclin on platelet reactivity across the infarcting compartment. Data are reported as ratios of great cardiac vein/arterial contents (figure 5). During infusion of PGI_2, the TxB_2 ratios decreased in six of the eight "thromboxane producers" receiving the agent; the ratios remained essentially unchanged in four patients and increased in two. The mean values of the ratios of the entire group were 2.2 and 1.5 (NS); the geometric mean values were 1.85 and 1.38 (NS), respectively. The great cardiac vein/arterial ratios for β-TG (figure 5) were distributed essentially around unity at control measurements and during infusion of PGI_2. The mean values were 1.1 and 1.2. Blood flow in the great cardiac vein remained essentially unchanged during administration of PGI_2: 62 ± 23 ml/min before and 66 ± 26 ml/min during the infusion, excluding a dilutional effect on the transcardiac PGI_2 and β-TG values.

Discussion

Our data clearly demonstrate enhanced platelet reactivity during the early hours of myocardial infarction. In vivo, release of β-TG and formation of thromboxane are increased, and the relationship between thromboxane and PGI_2 is strikingly shifted in favor of thromboxane. In vitro, platelet aggregation in response to exogenous stimuli is enhanced. The ADP dose-response curve of the ischemic platelets is left shifted when contrasted with normal. The alteration in platelet behavior in patients with acute myocardial infarction is also marked by a reduced response to exogenous (and probably to endogenous) PGI_2. In vivo, infusion of 10 to 20 ng/kg/min PGI_2 increases the required amount of ADP for 50% aggregation from 1.1 to only 2.1 μM, in contrast to normal volunteers[27] in whom infusion of 10 to 12 ng/kg/min increased the required ADP from 1.8 to 4.5 μM. In vitro, twice the amount of PGI_2 is required to inhibit platelet aggregation by 50%. Similarly, concentrations of cAMP, a biochemical mediator for the antiaggregatory effects of PGI_2, are lower in the ischemic platelet compared with normal and remain lower after exposure to PGI_2 in vitro.

These results in patients with acute myocardial infarction and endogenously elevated catecholamines support previous observations by us[28] and others[29, 30] that catecholamines change the platelet response to PGI_2, presumably by altering the bioavailability of platelet membrane receptors.[31–33] Using platelets from normal volunteers, we have shown[28] that subaggregatory doses of epinephrine and norepinephrine abolish the inhibitory effect of PGI_2 on aggregation and also the cAMP increase in response to PGI_2. α-Adrenergic blockade reestablishes both PGI_2 effects.

The platelet hyperreactivity in vivo is reflected by alterations of the metabolic capacity of the ischemic platelet as studied in vitro. We realize that in vitro tests may not accurately represent actual physiologic condi-

TABLE 3
Effect of PGI_{α} on platelet function and plasma catecholamines (mean ± SD)

Measurement (n = 19)	Baseline		PGI_{α} 90 min on		PGI_{α} 30 min off	
6-keto-$PGF_{1\alpha}$ (pg/ml)	<10	(<.001)	454±332	(<.001)	39±64	(NS)[A]
β-TG (ng/ml)	117±51	(<.05)	83±42	(<.025)	133±62	(NS)
AG_{50} (μM ADP)	1.09±0.44	(<.001)	2.08±1.09	(<.005)	1.22±0.51	(NS)
TxB_2 (pg/ml)	109±87	(NS)	87±71	(NS)	103±94	(NS)
Norepinephrine (pg/ml)	674±278	(NS)	713±375	(NS)	103±94	(NS)
Epinephrine (pg/ml) (n = 15)	139±59	(NS)	126±57	(NS)	114±36	(NS)

Data in parentheses are p values.
[A]Compared with baseline values.

tions. Given this limitation, the various measures obtained, however, appear to be consistent with each other. β-TG contents in ischemic platelets are 50% lower than normal. However, the maximal percentage of β-TG released by the two platelet groups is the same, implying that the ischemic platelet has a functioning release pathway but has undergone partial α-degranulation. Furthermore, maximal thromboxane formation by the ischemic platelet in response to collagen is decreased by 46%, whereas AA, providing both stimulus and substrate, elicits twice as much thromboxane formation as control. These data emphasize that the ischemic platelet has a heightened metabolic capacity that may, at least in vitro, be dampened by limited substrate availability. Consistent with these results are studies in experimental myocardial infarction demonstrating an accumulation of malondialdehyde,[34] a breakdown product of AA, and decreased concentrations of phospholipids in the infarcting myocardium.[35] The clinical relevance of these data is unclear, since the potential substrate limitation does not seem to interfere with enhanced platelet performance. That ischemic platelets remain hyperaggregable in the face of reduced thromboxane formation may imply that additional pathways of platelet aggregation are activated during myocardial ischemia[36–38] and that antiplatelet therapy aimed only at the cyclooxygenase pathway (such as aspirin) may be less effective than combination therapy in suppressing platelet hyperactivity. Furthermore, it is conceivable that compounds such as TxA_2, serotonin,[12, 39] and catecholamines[12, 40–42] remain bound to their respective receptors after removal of platelets from the circulation, contributing to the hyperaggregability of the ischemic platelets.

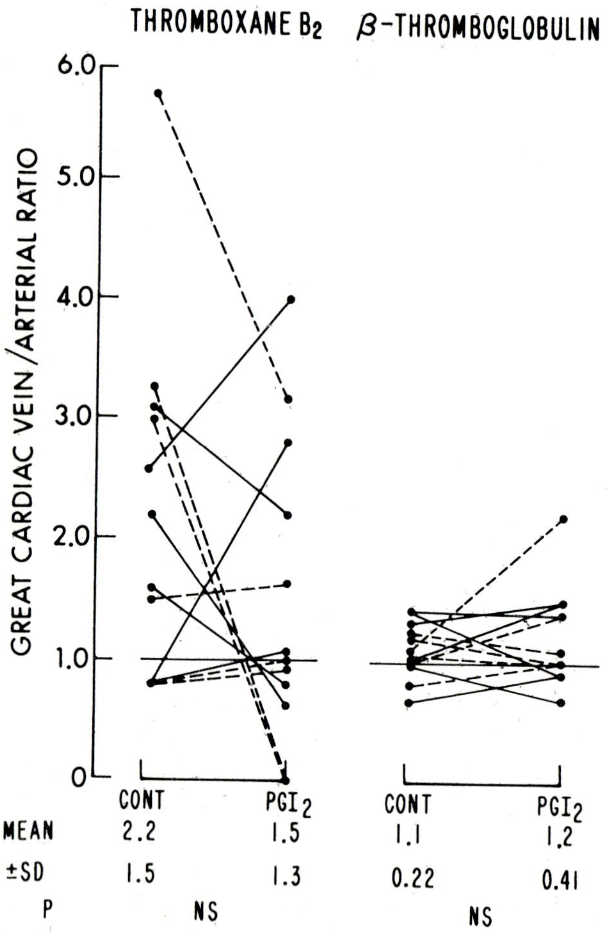

FIGURE 5. Great cardiac vein/arterial ratios of plasma levels of TxB_2 *(left)* and β-TG *(right)*. At control measurements (Cont) the thromboxane ratios are increased in eight of the 12 patients. PGI_2 decreases or abolishes the ratio in six instances. β-TG ratios are distributed around unity at control and during infusion of PGI_2.

When platelet activity is related to infarct duration, it is evident that the most striking alterations are seen early after onset of infarction. Aggregation (figure 6, *A*) is most abnormal in the hyperacute phase and tends to normalize as time from clinical onset increases although aggregation remains abnormal. Inhibition of aggregation (figure 6, *B*) is least effective in the hyperacute infarct phase and improves with time. Plasma contents of β-TG, an in vivo indicator of platelet activity, are highest early after onset of infarction and decline with increasing infarct duration. Whether or not

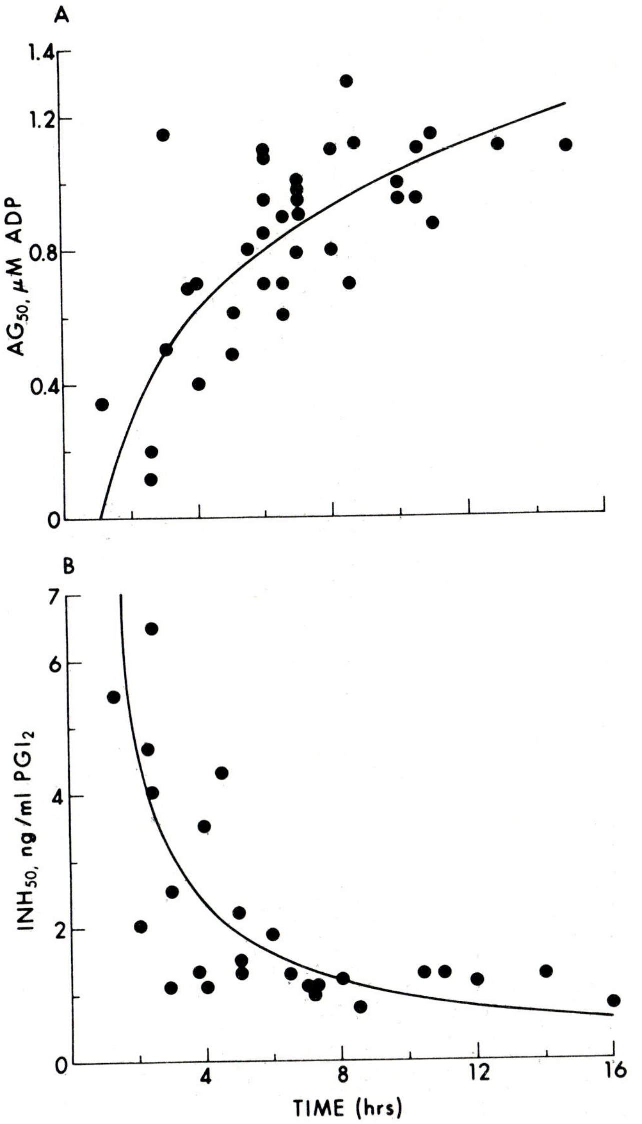

FIGURE 6. *A*, Relationship between clinical onset of infarction (hr) and platelet aggregation (AG_{50}). Aggregation is greatest in the hypera cute phase of infarction and decreases with time. $AG_{50} = 0.45 \times \log_e(hr)$; $r = .71$, $p < .0001$, $n = 37$. *B*, Relationship between clinical onset of infarction (hr) and PGI_2-induced inhibition of aggregation (INH_{50}). Inhibition is least effective in the hyperacute infarct phase and improves with time. $INH_{50} = 0.61/hr$; $r = .67$, $p < .0001$, $n = 26$.

these early changes in platelet activity have biological significance in triggering or contributing to infarction cannot be answered by our results. An important caveat is that our patients were studied relatively late after onset of infarction, making it impossible to distinguish primary events from those secondary to infarction and tissue damage. However, if tissue damage were responsible for platelet hyperactivity, one might predict an increase rather than a decrease in platelet activity with time.

Our data suggest that platelet reactivity is enhanced across the infarcting myocardial compartment. Thromboxane is produced across the coronary circulation in two-thirds of patients with evolving anterior wall infarction. The reason that this response is not universal is unclear, and no factor can be identified that predicts thromboxane production. Plasma catecholamine contents are elevated in both groups, there is no consistent transcardiac catecholamine increase in the thromboxane producers, and time from onset of infarction to study and size of infarct are not different among groups. We cannot demonstrate transcardiac release of β-TG, in contrast to thromboxane, perhaps because the amount released at the infarct site is insufficient to influence the high serum concentrations given the long half-life of the compound. It is also possible that α-granule function is exhausted in the ischemic compartment, since release is independent of thromboxane production[43] and responds to less potent stimulation.[43, 44]

Transcardiac formation of thromboxane in patients with acute myocardial infarction has been reported previously, although results have varied.[11, 45–48] Hirsh et al.[45, 46] have shown that thromboxane is produced in patients with unstable angina or recent myocardial infarction but not in patients with stable angina, suggesting that the dynamic character of the coronary lesion may be important. Autopsy studies in patients with sudden cardiac death have identified layers of thrombus of different ages and platelet thrombi in occluded coronary vessels.[9]

There is concern that platelets might be activated by catheter placement, exposure over time, and blood sampling.[49] Our data indicate that catheter-induced platelet activation is unimportant in patients with increased platelet activity before instrumentation. As demonstrated in figure 3, plasma contents of TxB_2 and β-TG do not significantly differ when obtained before and after catheter placement over a period of up to 90 min, or simultaneously by venipuncture and through the catheter. In particular, there is no consistent increase over time. The distribution of the data points is similar above and below the line of identity. Other investigators[50] have failed to show consistent alterations in platelet activity attributable to catheter exposure. Furthermore, we have established the platelet function profile in a matched group of patients with acute myocardial infarction without instrumentation, and the data of the instrumented infarct group are similar to the data of this group.

Intravenous infusion of PGI_2 to patients with evolving myocardial infarction produces an attenuated antiplatelet effect. Patients with infarction tolerate higher doses of PGI_2 (10 to 20 ng/kg/min) over a longer period of time than either normal volunteers[51–53] or cardiac patients without acute myocardial ischemia (8 to 12 ng/kg/min).[27, 54] The few studies using higher doses report infusions of only 10 to 15 min.[55, 56] In spite of the higher doses of PGI_2, the inhibitory effect on platelet aggregation is small. At an equivalent infusion rate of 10 to 12 ng/kg/min, the rightward shift of the ADP dose-response curve of the patients with infarction is only 20% of the shift observed in normal volunteers.[51] These data obtained during intravenous infusion of PGI_2 support the results in vitro discussed above in which PGI_2 added to PRP of patients with evolving myocardial infarction has an attenuated inhibitory effect on aggregation of ischemic platelets in vitro. The PGI_2-induced decrease in plasma β-TG (table 3) is moderate, and there is no effect on coronary sinus β-TG levels. PGI_2 does not consistently affect peripheral or transcardiac TxB_2 concentrations.

In summary, we have defined a pattern of abnormal platelet behavior in the acute phase of myocardial infarction. This is characterized by a proaggregatory environment (elevated thromboxane-to-PGI_2 ratio in both systemic and coronary circulation), evidence of heightened platelet activity in vivo (increased circulating β-TG) and increased platelet aggregability in vitro. Platelets from patients with myocardial infarction are relatively resistant to the antiaggregatory effects of exogenous PGI_2. These data and the finding that the platelet abnormalities are most striking in the hyperacute phase of infarction support the contention that platelet aggregation and thrombus formation are important participants in the events of acute myocardial ischemia/infarction.

On the basis of the characterization of the platelet abnormalities, acknowledging the limitations that our patients were studied relatively late after onset of infarction and not allowing a separation of primary from secondary events, future directions for the manipulation of platelet hyperactivity in acute myocardial infarction can be suggested. Conventional antiplatelet agents and PGI_2 are probably insufficient by themselves to influence the proaggregatory environment. Alternative approaches would include agents that decrease the release of catecholamines and thus ameliorate their synergistic effects on endogenous inducers of platelet activity,[12, 40–42] agents that block the platelet α_2-adrenergic receptors so as to make platelets more responsive to the antiaggregatory effects of PGI_2,[28–30] agents that potentiate the effect of PGI_2 such as phosphodiesterase inhibitors,[57] and agents that reduce the effect of thromboxane such as thromboxane synthetase inhibitors or thromboxane receptor antagonists.[12, 39] The recognition that the event of myocardial infarction likely involves dynamic thrombus formation, in which both platelets and plasma proteins participate, and that the ischemic platelet has a heightened sensitivity to these plasma constituents might suggest use of both antiplatelet and anticoagulant modalities.

We appreciate the assistance of the nurse specialists, Miss Anne Dyer, Miss Eileen Ferrick, and Mr. Michael Behrens. We thank Miss Joyce Milinowicz for performance of the laboratory tests and Mrs. Virginia Wengerter for preparation of the manuscript.

References

1. Mehta J, Mehta P: Role of blood platelets and prostaglandins in coronary artery disease. Am J Cardiol **48:** 366, 1981
2. Pitt B, Shea MJ, Romson JL, Lucchesi BR: Prostaglandins and prostaglandin inhibitors in ischemic heart disease. Ann Intern Med **99:** 83, 1983
3. Smitherman TC, Halam M, Woo J, Willerson JT, Frenkel EP: Elevated β-thromboglobulin in peripheral venous blood of patients with acute myocardial ischemia: direct evidence of enhanced platelet reactivity in vivo. Am J Cardiol **48:** 375, 1981
4. DeBoer AC, Turpie AGG, Butt RW, Johnston RV, Genton E: Platelet release and thromboxane synthesis in symptomatic coronary artery disease. Circulation **66:** 327, 1982
5. Handin RI, McDonough M, Lesch M: Elevation of platelet factor four in acute myocardial infarction: measurement by radioimmunoassay. J Lab Clin Med **91:** 340, 1978
6. Sobel M, Salzman EW, Davies GC, Handin RI, Sweeney J, Ploetz J, Kurland G: Circulating platelet products in unstable angina pectoris. Circulation **63:** 300, 1981
7. Szczeklik A, Gryglewski RJ, Musial J, Grodzinska L, Serwonska M, Marcinkiewicz E: Thromboxane generation and platelet activation in survivors of myocardial infarction. Thromb Haemost **40:** 66, 1978
8. DeWood MA, Spores J, Notske R, Mouser LT, Burroughs R, Golden MS, Lang HT: Prevalence of total coronary occlusion during early hours of transmural myocardial infarction. N Engl J Med **303:** 897, 1980
9. Falk E: Unstable angina with fatal outcome: dynamic coronary thrombosis leading to infarction and/or sudden death. Circulation **71:** 699, 1985
10. Folts JD, Crowell EB Jr, Rowe CG: Platelet aggregation in partially obstructed vessels and its elimination by aspirin. Circulation **54:** 365, 1976
11. Bush LR, Campbell WB, Tilton GD, Buja LM, Willerson JT: Effects of the selective thromboxane synthetase inhibitor, dazoxiben, on variations in cyclic blood flow in stenosed canine coronary arteries. Circulation **69:** 1161, 1984
12. Bush LR, Campbell WB, Buja LM, Tilton GD, Willerson JT: Effects of α_2-adrenergic and serotoninergic antagonists on cyclic flow reductions in stenosed canine coronary arteries. Circ Res **55:** 642, 1984
13. Willerson JT, Campbell WB, Winniford MD, Schmitz J, Aprill P, Firth BG, Ashton J, Smitherman T, Bush L, Buja LM: Conversion from chronic to acute coronary artery disease: speculation regarding mechanisms. Am J Cardiol **54:** 1349, 1984
14. Dusting GJ, Moncada S, Vane JR: Prostacyclin is the endogenous metabolite response for relaxation of coronary arteries induced by arachidonic acid. Prostaglandins **13:** 3, 1977
15. Baim DS, Rothman MT, Harrison DC: Improved catheter for regional coronary sinus flow and metabolic studies. Am J Cardiol **46:** 997, 1980
16. Rao PS, Mueller HS: Direct radioimmunoassay of plasma thromboxane B_2 and 6-keto-$PGF_{1\alpha}$. Clin Chem **29:** 1252A, 1983
17. Morris HG, Sherman NA, Shepperdson FT, Selner JC: Radioimmunoassay of TxB_2 in plasma of normal and asthmatic subjects. *In* Samuelsson B, Ramwell PW, Paoletti R, editors: Advances in prostaglandin and thromboxane research. New York, 1980, Raven Press, p 1759

18. Steele PP, Sklar J: Relationship between the release of thromboxane and the occurrence and extent of myocardial ischemia during exercise. Am J Cardiol **49:** 902, 1982 (abst)
19. Walinsky P, Smith JB, Lefer AM, Lebenthal M, Urban P, Goldberg S, Greenspon A: Thromboxane A_2 in acute myocardial infarction. Am J Cardiol 49: 901, 1982 (abst)
20. Siess W, Dray F: Very low levels of 6-keto-prostaglandin $F_{1\alpha}$ in human plasma. J Lab Clin Med **99:** 388, 1981
21. Hallman H, Farnebo LO, Hamberger B, Johnson G: Selective method for the determination of plasma catecholamines using liquid chromatography with electrochemical detection. Life Sci **23:** 1049, 1978
22. Shevde N, Sussman II, Rosner F, Pacholuk K: Oral contraceptives and platelet aggregation. Am J Obstet Gynecol **132:** 303, 1978
23. Verheugt FW, Serruys PW, vanVliet H, Spijkers A, Hugenholtz PG: Intracoronary platelet release in patients with and without coronary artery disease. Thromb Haemost **49:** 28, 1983
24. Ludlam CA, Moore S, Bolton AE, Pepper DS, Cash JD: The release of a human platelet-specific protein measured by a radioimmunoassay. Thromb Res **6:** 543, 1975
25. Sobel BE, Roberts R, Larson KB: Estimation of infarct size from serum MB creatine phosphokinase activity: applications and limitations. Am J Cardiol **37:** 474, 1976
26. Zar JH: Biostatistical analysis. Englewood Cliffs, NJ, 1974, Prentice-Hall, p 29
27. Bergman G, Atkinson L, Richardson PJ, Daly K, Rothman M, Jackson G: Prostacyclin: haemodynamic and metabolic effects in patients with coronary artery disease. Lancet **1:** 569, 1981
28. Buttrick PM, Forscher CA, Sussman II, Mueller HS: Sub-aggregatory doses of catecholamines prevent prostacyclin induced inhibition of platelet aggregation. Am Heart J **109:** 1258, 1985
29. Mehta P, Mehta J: Platelet function studies in coronary heart disease. VIII. Decreased platelet sensitivity to prostacyclin in patients with myocardial ischemia. Thromb Res **18:** 273, 1980
30. Sinzinger H, Silberbauer K, Horsch AK, Gall A: Decreased sensitivity of human platelets to PGI_2 during long-term intraarterial prostacyclin infusion in patients with peripheral vascular disease — a rebound phenomenon? Prostaglandins **21:** 49, 1981
31. Haslam RJ, Davidson MML, Davies T, Lynham JA, McClenaghan MD: Regulation of blood platelet function by cyclic nucleotides. *In* George WJ, Ignarro LJ, editors: Advances in cyclic nucleotide research. New York, 1978, Raven Press, p 533
32. Peerschke EJ: Induction of human fibrinogen receptors by epinephrine in the absence of released ADP. Blood **60:** 71, 1982
33. Neri Serneri GG, Modesti PA, Fortini A, Abbate R, Lombardi A, Gensini GF: Reduction in prostacyclin platelet receptors in active spontaneous angina. Lancet **2:** 838, 1984
34. Rao PS, Cohen MV, Mueller HS: Production of free radicals and lipid peroxides in early experimental myocardial ischemia. J Mol Cell Cardiol **15:** 713, 1983
35. Rao PS, Mueller HS: Lipid peroxidation and acute myocardial ischemia. *In* Spitzer JJ, editor: Advances in experimental medicine and biology. New York, 1982, Plenum Publishing Co., p 347
36. Rao GHR, Gerrard JM, Witkop CJ, White JG: Platelet aggregation independent of ADP release of prostaglandin synthesis in patients with Hermansky-Pudlak syndrome. Prostaglandins Med **6:** 459, 1981
37. Packham MA, Mustard JF: Normal and abnormal platelet activity. *In* Lasslo A, editor: Blood platelet function and medicinal chemistry. New York, 1984, Elsevier Biomedical, p 72
38. Kaplan KL, Broekman MJ, Chernoff A, Lesznik GR, Drillings M: Platelet α-granule proteins: studies on release and subcellular localization. Blood **53:** 604, 1979
39. Baumgartner HR, Born GVR: The effects of 5-hydroxytryptamine on platelet aggregation. Nature (Lond) **218:** 137, 1968
40. O'Brien JR: Some effects of adrenaline and antiadrenaline compounds on platelets in vitro and in vivo. Nature (Lond) **200:** 763, 1963
41. Mills DCB, Roberts GCK: Effects of adrenaline on human platelets. J Physiol (Lond) **193:** 443, 1967
42. Grant JA, Scrutton MC: Positive interaction between agonists in the aggregation of human blood platelets: interaction between ADP, adrenaline and vasopressin. Br J Haematol **44:** 109, 1980
43. Levy-Toledano S, Caen JP, Breton-Gorius J, Rendu F, Cywiner-Golenzer C, Dupuy E, Legrand Y, Maclouf J: Gray platelet syndrome: α-granule deficiency: its influence on platelet function. J Lab Clin Med **98:** 831, 1981
44. Witte LD, Kaplan KL, Nossel HL, Lages BA, Weiss HJ, Goodman DS: Studies of the release from human platelets of the growth factor for cultured human arterial smooth muscle cells. Circ Res **42:** 402, 1978
45. Hirsh PD, Hillis LD, Campbell WB, Firth BG, Willerson JT: Release of prostaglandins and thromboxane into the coronary circulation in patients with ischemic heart disease. N Engl J Med **304:** 685, 1981
46. Hirsh PD, Firth BG, Campbell WB, Dehmer GJ, Willerson JT, Hillis LD: Effects of provocation on transcardiac thromboxane in patients with coronary artery disease. Am J Cardiol **51:** 727, 1983
47. Lewy RI, Wiener L, Walinsky P, Lefer AM, Silver MJ, Smith JB: Thromboxane release during pacing-induced angina pectoris: possible vasoconstrictor influence on the coronary vasculature. Circulation **61:** 1165, 1980
48. Robertson RM, Robertson D, Roberts LJ, Maas RL, FitzGerald GA, Friesinger GC, Oates JA: Thromboxane A_2 in vasotonic angina pectoris: evidence from direct measurement and inhibitor trials. N Engl J Med **304:** 998, 1981
49. Nichols AB, Owen J, Grossman BA, Marcella JJ, Fleisher LN, Lee MML: Effect of heparin bonding on catheter-induced fibrin formation and platelet activation. Circulation **70:** 843, 1984
50. Hirsh PD, Firth BG, Campbell WB, Willerson JT, Hillis LD: Influence of blood sampling site and technique on thromboxane concentrations in patients with ischemic heart disease. Am Heart J **104:** 234, 1982
51. Data JL, Molony BA, Meinzinger MM, Gorman RR: Intravenous infusion of prostacyclin sodium in man: clinical effects and influence on platelet adenosine diphosphate sensitivity and adenosine 3′:5′-cyclic monophosphate levels. Circulation **64:** 4, 1981
52. Eklund B, Joreteg T, Kaijser L: Dissimilar effects of prostacyclin on cardiac output and forearm blood flow in healthy men. Clin Physiol **1:** 123, 1981
53. Fitzgerald GA, Friedman LA, Miyamori I, O'Grady J, Lewis PJ: A double-blind placebo controlled crossover study of prostacyclin in man. Life Sci **24:** 665, 1979
54. Szczeklik J, Szczeklik A, Nizankowski R: Hemodynamic changes induced by prostacyclin in man. Br Heart J **44:** 254, 1980
55. Chelly J, Fabiani J-N, Chahine R, Tricot A-M, Carpentier A, Passelecq J, Dubost C: Hemodynamic and metabolic effects of prostacyclin after coronary bypass surgery. Circulation **66** (suppl I): I-45, 1982
56. O'Grady J, Warrington S, Moti MJ, Bunting S, Flower R, Fowle ASE, Higgs EA, Moncada S: Effects of intravenous prostacyclin infusions in healthy volunteers — some preliminary observations. Prostaglandins **19:** 319, 1980
57. Lam SC-T, Guccione MA, Packham MA, Mustard JF: Effect of cAMP phosphodiesterase shape change, cAMP and nucleoside diphosphokinase activity of rabbit platelets. Thromb Haemost **47:** 90, 1982

Prevention of coronary thrombosis with subthrombolytic doses of tissue-type plasminogen activator*

KEITH A. A. FOX, M.B., CH.B., ALICE K. ROBISON, PH.D., ROBERT M. KNABB, PH.D., THOMAS L. ROSAMOND, M.D., BURTON E. SOBEL, M.D., AND STEVEN R. BERGMANN, M.D., PH.D.

ABSTRACT To determine whether tissue-type plasminogen activator (t-PA) may prevent coronary thrombosis or accelerate the lysis of clot formed under conditions in which increased concentration of the activator is present before thrombosis, clot lysis studies were undertaken in vitro and in vivo. In vitro, exogenous t-PA (6 to 100,000 ng/ml) accelerated the lysis of clot in a dose-dependent fashion when the clot was formed either from whole plasma or from euglobulin fractions (n = 316 determinations). Adding t-PA before clot formation shortened the time to lysis by at least threefold with euglobulin fractions and by at least 10-fold with whole plasma clots, which is consistent with the presence of inhibitors of fibrinolysis in whole plasma and with the binding of t-PA to nascent fibrin. In an intact dog preparation of coronary thrombosis (n = 25), occlusive thrombus formation was prevented when t-PA was present in subthrombolytic concentrations (430 to 1200 ng/ml, n = 5). Occlusive thrombus formation occurred after only discontinuation of the t-PA infusion and clearance of t-PA. Lower concentrations of t-PA (147 to 427 ng/ml, n = 6) significantly delayed occlusion (26 ± 6.5 vs 7.8 ± 2.8 min for controls). In animals with t-PA concentrations of less than 140 ng/ml (n = 4), the time to occlusion was unaltered (7.7 ± 4.5 min). The present study demonstrates that t-PA present before clot formation inhibits thrombosis or accelerates thrombolysis depending on concentration, and that subthrombolytic doses of t-PA can prevent thrombus formation in vivo. The findings of this study provide a rationale for clinical strategies aimed at augmenting t-PA concentrations in patients at high risk for coronary thrombosis or at risk for reocclusion after thrombolysis.
Circulation 72, No. 6, 1346–1354, 1985.

WE HAVE RECENTLY demonstrated that tissue-type plasminogen activator (t-PA) is an effective agent for the induction of coronary thrombolysis in experimental animals and in patients.[1-4] Either intravenous[1-4] or intramuscular[5] administration of t-PA can lyse established thrombi. However, despite successful lysis of macrovascular clot, salutary effects on the ischemic heart depend on minimization of the delay before reperfusion.[6-8] Thus, attention has focused on early implementation of thrombolysis so that myocardial perfusion can be restored before irreversible injury in jeopardized tissue is complete.

Minimization of the duration of coronary occlusion is facilitated by the use of agents that are effective after systemic rather than intracoronary administration. Recently, we have shown that effective blood levels of t-PA can be achieved promptly when t-PA is administered intramuscularly in association with an absorption-enhancing agent.[5] Although the levels of t-PA attainable are lower than those achieved with intravenous administration, they are of the same order of magnitude that has been demonstrated to be effective in inducing thrombolysis in experimental studies.

An additional strategy could involve the identification of patients at high risk for occlusion or reocclusion and pretreatment of incipient thrombosis. Patients presenting with unstable angina and high-grade critical lesions are at increased risk for coronary occlusion,

From the Cardiovascular Division, Washington University School of Medicine, St. Louis.
Supported in part by National Institute of Health grants HL17646, SCOR in Ischemic Heart Disease.
Address for correspondence: Keith A. A. Fox, M.B., Ch.B., Cardiovascular Division, Washington University School of Medicine, 660 South Euclid Ave., Box 8086, St. Louis, MO 63110.
Received July 25, 1985; revision accepted Sept. 5, 1985.
*All editorial decisions for this article, including selection of reviewers and the final disposition, were made by a guest editor. This procedure applies to all manuscripts with authors from the Washington University School of Medicine.

and in patients in whom successful thrombolysis has been achieved, residual high-grade coronary lesions predispose to reocclusion despite administration of anticoagulants or antiplatelet agents.[4, 9–11]

In view of these considerations, the present study was performed to determine whether t-PA can prevent coronary thrombosis or can accelerate thrombolysis of clots that form under conditions in which an increased concentration of the activator is already present. Its rationale depends in part on the kinetic properties of t-PA, including its high affinity for fibrin and its facilitated activation of plasminogen within clot as opposed to in the circulation.[12–15]

The key properties of t-PA that distinguish it from conventionally available pharmacologic activators of the fibrinolytic system include its high fibrinolytic activity,[12, 14] despite a short half-life in the circulation,[2, 16] coupled with only modest induction of proteolytic activity in the circulating blood when t-PA is administered in therapeutically effective doses.[3, 4, 11, 17] t-PA has a high affinity for fibrin. The fibrin–t-PA complex in turn has a high affinity for plasminogen. The Michaelis constant (Km) of t-PA for circulating free plasminogen in plasma is much higher (approximately 65 μM) than the Km of fibrin-bound t-PA for plasminogen (0.16 μM).[12, 13] Accordingly, little or no conversion of circulating plasminogen (generally 2 μM) to plasmin occurs despite activation of plasminogen at the fibrin surface.[15, 18] Thus, plasmin is formed locally without marked fibrinogenolysis or proteolysis in the systemic circulation.

To characterize dose-response relationships for lysis of clot by t-PA when the agent was present before clot formation in comparison with those when the activator added after clot formation, we measured clot dissolution in euglobulin and plasma fractions in vitro with exogenous t-PA over a wide range of concentrations. In contrast to clots formed in plasma, those formed in euglobulin fractions contain diminished levels of fibrinolytic inhibitors and, primarily, α_2-antiplasmin. Previous investigations have not characterized this relationship in plasma clots over concentration ranges that may be applicable in vivo for rapid coronary thrombolysis. An additional aim of this study was to determine whether pretreatment in vivo with subthrombolytic doses of t-PA, before induction of coronary thrombi, could prevent or retard coronary thrombosis. Accordingly, infusions of t-PA were administered to dogs before induction of occlusive thrombus with a copper coil introduced under fluoroscopic guidance into the coronary artery. This experimental animal preparation has been characterized extensively in studies of more than 300 animals in our laboratory.

Methods

Studies in vitro. Venous blood was obtained without the use of a tourniquet from 10 healthy male volunteers on two different occasions. It was collected into citrated Vacutainer tubes at 0° to 4° C, with a final concentration of citrate-10 mM. Plasma was harvested at 4° C by centrifugation for 10 min at 2000 *g* and stored at −70° C until assay.

For studies in vitro, clot was formed by the addition of thrombin and clot lysis time was measured as the interval required for total dissolution of a clot. Clot lysis in vitro was assessed under the four following sets of conditions, in samples with a concentration range of t-PA of 6 to 100,000 ng/ml: (1) "prethrombosis" conditions with whole plasma in which exogenous t-PA was added before formation of clot and lysis time was compared with that occurring spontaneously in samples in which no exogenous t-PA had been added, (2) "postthrombosis" conditions with whole plasma in which exogenous t-PA was added 5 min after coagulation had been induced, (3) "prethrombosis" conditions with euglobulin fractions of plasma samples in which t-PA was added before formation of clot, and (4) "postthrombosis" conditions with euglobulin fractions in which exogenous t-PA was added 5 min after clot had been formed. Prethrombosis conditions were used to permit maximal incorporation of t-PA into interstices of the clot while it was being formed. Postthrombosis conditions were used to mimic conditions in vivo in which only endogenous t-PA would have maximal access to the interstices of a fibrin clot being formed, with exogenous t-PA available to penetrate the clot after it was established.

The t-PA used (Genentech, Inc., lot BH001DAX) was produced by recombinant DNA technology in a mammalian cell culture system.

The euglobulin fraction of plasma contains fibrinogen, plasminogen, and endogenous plasminogen activator. However, it contains reduced levels of most of the plasma inhibitors of fibrinolysis such as α_2-antiplasmin. Euglobulin fractions were prepared from thawed plasma samples by diluting 0.5 ml aliquots with 9.5 ml of distilled water at 4° C, adjustment of pH to 5.9 with acetic acid, centrifugation for 10 min at 3000 *g* at 4° C, removal of the supernatant fraction, and solubilization of the precipitate in 0.5 ml of imidazole-buffered saline (0.025M imidazole HCl, 0.113M NaCl, pH 7.4), containing 0.8 mg/ml bovine serum albumin.

Clots were induced in vitro by addition of 50 μl of a solution containing 0.5 IU of freshly prepared thrombin in imidazole-buffered saline to 0.2 ml aliquots of either whole plasma or euglobulin fractions in 10 mm × 75 mm clear-glass test tubes at melting ice-bath temperature. After immediate mixing and formation of clot, tubes were incubated at 37° C. The interval required for clot lysis was assessed visually and recorded as the time required for complete dissolution of clot. Lysis time was expressed in units defined by Marsh,[19] i.e., $10^6/(\text{lysis time in min})^2$. Either t-PA or buffered saline vehicle was added in 20 μl aliquots either before or 5 min after addition of thrombin to yield a final concentration of 6 to 100,000 ng/ml, approximately equivalent to the range of 10 to 200,000 IU/ml for the International Reference Preparation of t-PA (IRP-t-PA, used for calibration). Fibrinogen content was assayed in pooled plasma by the method of Clauss.[20] For each set of conditions, assays at each concentration were performed in quadruplicate and each set of conditions was reassessed with a second batch of pooled plasma from the same subjects.

Studies in vivo

Animal preparations. Twenty-five mongrel dogs weighing

23 to 35 kg were anesthetized with 12.5 mg/kg of intravenously administered thiopental and 60 mg/kg α-chloralose after premedication with 1 mg/kg morphine sulfate given subcutaneously. After a cuffed endotracheal tube had been inserted, ventilation was maintained with room air and a Harvard respirator. Catheters were placed in the abdominal aorta and vena cava via the left femoral artery and vein and flushed with normal saline without heparin. A cannula was placed in a peripheral vein of the right leg of each animal for administration of 50 μg/kg/min lidocaine in saline. The left common carotid artery was isolated for introduction of coronary artery catheters and insertion of a copper coil was used to induce coronary thrombosis. Coronary arteriography was performed with meglumine diatrizoate with the use of a Siemens radiographic unit.

For the induction of coronary thrombi, a copper coil, 5 mm in length, was inserted into the left anterior descending coronary artery. The coil was formed by wrapping a copper wire (0.5 mm diameter) in a spiral around a 19-gauge needle, as previously described.[8] With the animal in the right anterior oblique position, a modified USCI No. 1 Amplatz coronary catheter was inserted selectively into the left anterior descending coronary artery under fluoroscopic guidance. A Teflon-coated guidewire, 0.021 inch in diameter, was inserted, and the angiographic catheter was removed. The copper coil was advanced into the artery over the guidewire with the use of a narrow gauge (0.025 inch internal diameter, 0.038 inch external diameter) Formacath catheter, the guide wire was removed, and the coil was lodged in the midportion of the left anterior descending coronary artery. The Formacath catheter was withdrawn slightly to a position 1 cm proximal to the coil.

Experimental protocol. Thirty minutes after baseline coronary angiography had been performed, control blood samples were obtained. These and subsequent samples were drawn into ice-cold 5 ml Vacutainer tubes containing sodium citrate for assay of fibrinolytic activity and immunoradiometrically detectable human t-PA.[21] After collection at 0° to 4° C, samples were centrifuged at the same temperature. Plasma was frozen promptly and stored at −70° C before assay within 2 weeks.

To rapidly attain constant plasma concentrations of exogenous t-PA, infusions were initiated with a bolus injection of t-PA providing 7.7 times the amount subsequently infused per minute. This dosage was based on considerations of blood levels anticipated, the known rates of clearance from plasma in dogs defined in preliminary studies, and the calculations outlined in the Appendix. An initial sample was obtained at zero time, before administration of t-PA. The next sample was obtained 10 min after onset of administration of t-PA. The thrombogenic copper coil was placed in the left anterior descending coronary artery immediately after acquisition of the second sample. Subsequent samples were obtained at frequent intervals throughout the infusion of t-PA.

t-PA was infused at one of the following rates: 1 to 1.75 μg/kg/min, n = 4; 2.5 μg/kg/min, n = 6; 3.75 μg/kg/min, n = 4; 5.0 μg/kg/min, n = 2; and 10.0 μg/kg/min, n = 1. Control dogs (n = 8) underwent angiography and coil insertion, but did not receive exogenous t-PA. The time to coronary occlusion was recorded in each case, and the electrocardiogram was monitored throughout for detection of ischemia and reperfusion arrhythmia. For continuing evaluation of coronary patency, low-dose injections of coronary contrast were given and fluoroscopy was performed at 5 min intervals. When electrocardiographic criteria of ischemia or fluoroscopic criteria of occlusion appeared, thrombotic occlusion was confirmed by repeat cineangiography.

Infusion of t-PA was discontinued 70 min after its initiation. Subsequent blood samples were obtained at 5 min intervals for an additional 40 min for determination of the rate of clearance of t-PA from the circulation. In those animals in which coronary occlusion occurred before the end of the infusion, the infusion was stopped, and sampling for determination of clearance of t-PA was initiated immediately after acquisition of the confirmatory angiogram. In those animals in which coronary patency was maintained throughout the entire infusion of t-PA, repeat fluoroscopy was performed during the interval in which clearance of t-PA from the circulation was being assessed. During the interval in which plasma concentrations of t-PA were declining, the time of occurrence of coronary occlusion induced by the indwelling coronary thrombogenic coil was identified.

Assay of plasma samples. t-PA antigen was assayed with a two-site immunoradiometric assay, as previously described.[21] The procedure involves binding of t-PA to anti-t-PA adsorbed to wells in a microtiter plate and subsequent binding of radiolabeled ^{125}I-anti-t-PA to bound t-PA. After removal of excess ^{125}I-anti-t-PA, the amount of bound ^{125}I-t-PA is determined with a gamma counter. Canine t-PA does not cross react in the immunoradiometric assay system used. Anti-t-PA antiserum and purified human melanoma t-PA for the reference standards were provided by Professor Désiré Collen.

t-PA functional activity was assayed conventionally with fibrin plates[19] as follows: Circular zones of fibrinolysis were measured by planimetry on fibrin plates exposed to serial dilutions of euglobulin fractions of samples. These were prepared by dilution of citrated plasma (1:20) with distilled water, adjustment to pH 5.6 with acetic acid, centrifugation, and solubilization of precipitates in imidazole-buffered saline (pH 7.4) containing 0.8% bovine serum albumin. Fibrin plates were prepared with fibrinogen (Kabi Diagnostica), thrombin (Sigma), and $CaCl_2$ (0.05M), and were incubated at 37° C for 16 hr. Zones of lysis were quantified by comparison with those induced with IRP-t-PA.

Results

Studies in vitro. Pooled plasma was found to contain 1.9 mg/ml fibrinogen and 7.5 ng/ml of endogenous t-PA, equivalent to approximately 14 U/ml of IRP-t-PA cocalibrated with the fibrin-plate assay. Lysis of clot in euglobulin fractions and in whole plasma was assessed in 316 samples with exogenous t-PA in the sample in concentrations ranging from 0 to 100,000 ng/ml.

As shown in figure 1, clot lysis was accelerated in a concentration-dependent fashion in response to t-PA in whole plasma. For each concentration, when t-PA was present before clot formation, more rapid lysis of clot occurred than was the case when the same concentration of t-PA was present only after clot formation.

As shown in figure 2, clots formed from euglobulin fractions of plasma exhibited more prompt lysis at a given concentration of t-PA than those formed in whole plasma because of the diminished quantities of inhibitors of components of the fibrinolytic system in euglobulin fractions compared with those in plasma.

With addition of t-PA after thrombin-coagulation in euglobulin fractions and in whole plasma samples, the response to a given concentration of exogenous t-PA was diminished (figure 2) compared with that which

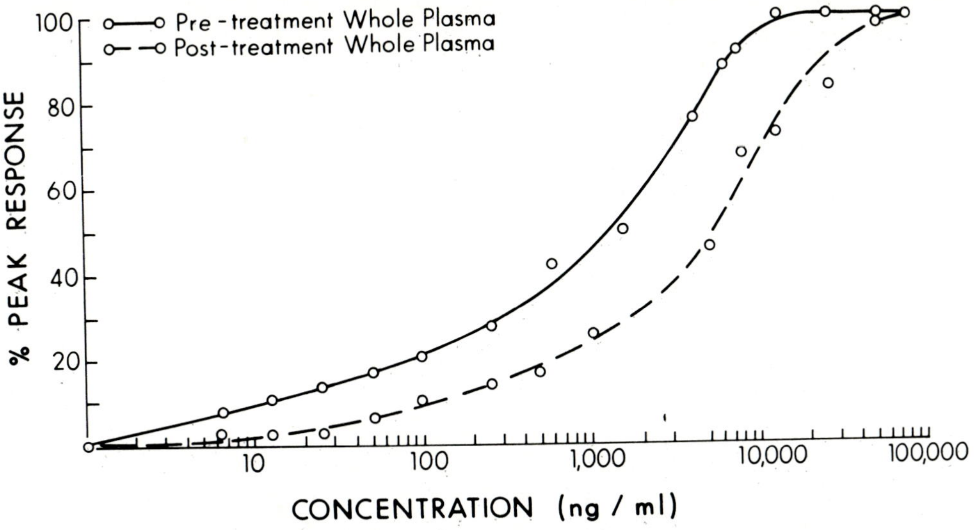

FIGURE 1. Studies in vitro. Relationship between the rate of lysis and concentration of t-PA. Results are expressed as a percentage of the maximal rate of lysis. The results shown are for whole plasma samples in which exogenous t-PA was present at the time of clot formation (pretreatment) or after clot formation (posttreatment). Administration of t-PA before, in comparison with after, clot formation resulted in a shift of the dose-response curve to the left such that lower concentrations of t-PA were required to achieve similar rates of lysis. The concentration of t-PA that achieved the maximal rate of lysis as a result of pretreatment achieved only 70% of the maximal rate of lysis under posttreatment conditions. The results are consistent with the influence of plasma inhibitors in the posttreatment group and with different access of t-PA to established compared with nascent clot.

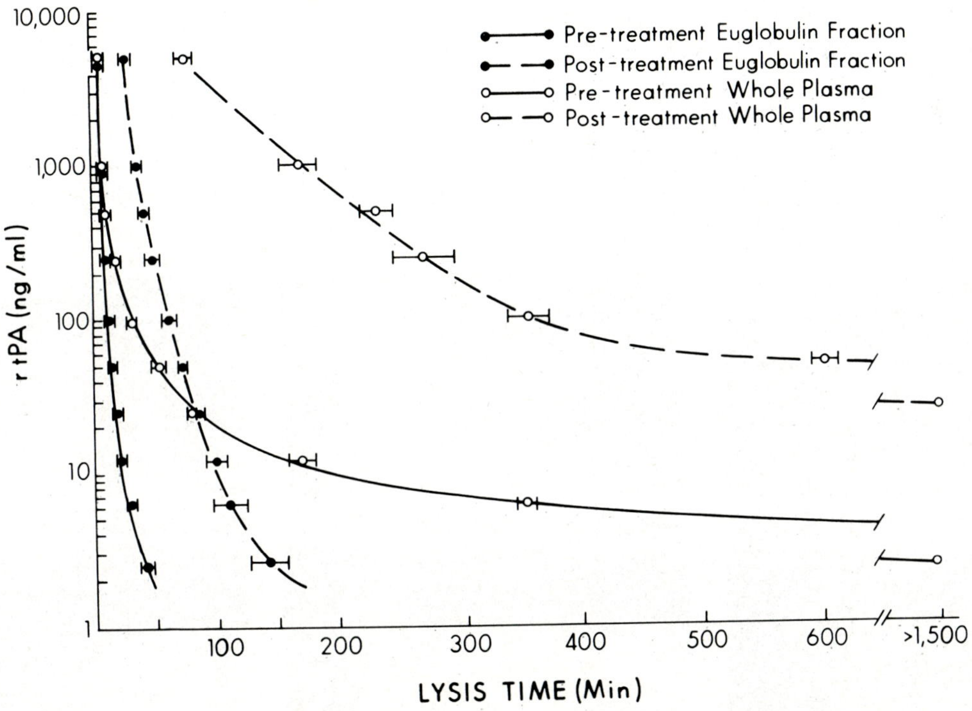

FIGURE 2. Studies in vitro. Data for the four groups of conditions are shown. Values are means ± SD. Pretreatment and posttreatment refer to the groups in which exogenous t-PA was present at the time of clot formation or added after formation. The euglobulin fractions exclude the majority of circulating inhibitors. The results demonstrate that for either whole plasma or euglobulin fractions, the presence of t-PA at the time of clot formation results in substantially shorter times to lysis in comparison with those when the same concentrations of t-PA are added after clot formation. At the lowest concentrations of administered t-PA, lysis did not occur for up to 1500 min in the pretreatment whole plasma (t-PA concentrations less than or equal to 3.75 ng/ml) or posttreatment whole plasma groups (t-PA concentrations less than or equal to 12.5 ng/ml).

TABLE 1
Concentrations (ng/ml) of t-PA required to achieve 50% of the maximal rate of lysis in vitro

Time of addition of t-PA to whole plasma		Time of addition of t-PA to euglobulin fraction	
Before clot	Subsequent to clot	Before clot	Subsequent to clot
2670	6800	260	650

Results are for t-PA antigen activity (n = 316 analyses).

occurred when t-PA was present during clot formation. The displacement to the right of the dose-response curve for t-PA was consistent with decreased penetration of t-PA into established as opposed to nascent thrombi and the probable influence of inhibitors of t-PA and plasmin in the sample when t-PA was added after clot formation. In contrast, when t-PA is bound to fibrin, activation of plasminogen occurs at the fibrin surface and in the absence of the majority of plasmin inhibitors.

Table 1 summarizes the concentrations of t-PA required for acceleration of clot lysis to 50% maximum. To elicit lysis at comparable rates, only 40% as much t-PA was needed before clot formation in comparison with that needed after clot formation. The findings pertained to both euglobulin fractions and whole plasma studies.

Studies in vivo. Twenty-five dogs were studied. Eight were controls and 17 were given infusions of t-PA. Two animals given t-PA sustained ventricular fibrillation almost immediately after insertion of the coronary coil but before thrombotic coronary occlusion. They were excluded. Angiographically documented occlusive thrombus formed in control dogs in an average of 7.8 ± 2.5 (SD) min. Coronary angiograms documented induction, localization, and dissolution of coronary thrombi in each case. An example is shown in figure 3. The distribution of persistent clot was confirmed by dissection of each of the coronary arteries at autopsy.

Because the immunoradiometric assay used is specific for human t-PA, endogenous canine t-PA was not detected. Hence, values in all baseline samples and all samples from control dogs were zero. The fibrin-plate assay detects functional fibrinolytic activity whether it is attributable to endogenous canine or exogenous human t-PA or other activators. Thus, baseline samples exhibited fibrinolytic activity equivalent to 16.8 ± 8.8 IU/ml (range 7 to 35 IU/ml). Sequential samples in control dogs exhibited values indistinguishable from baseline values.

Bolus administration followed by constant infusion of t-PA elicited plateaus of concentrations of t-PA within 10 min (figure 4). Close concordance was observed between determinations of t-PA antigen and determinations of functional, fibrin plate–assayable activity at both higher and lower doses (figure 4). Clearance of either t-PA antigen or functional activity after cessation of infusion of t-PA conformed to a biexponential function with fast and slow components. The apparent disappearance rates exhibited considerable variability for both early and late components.

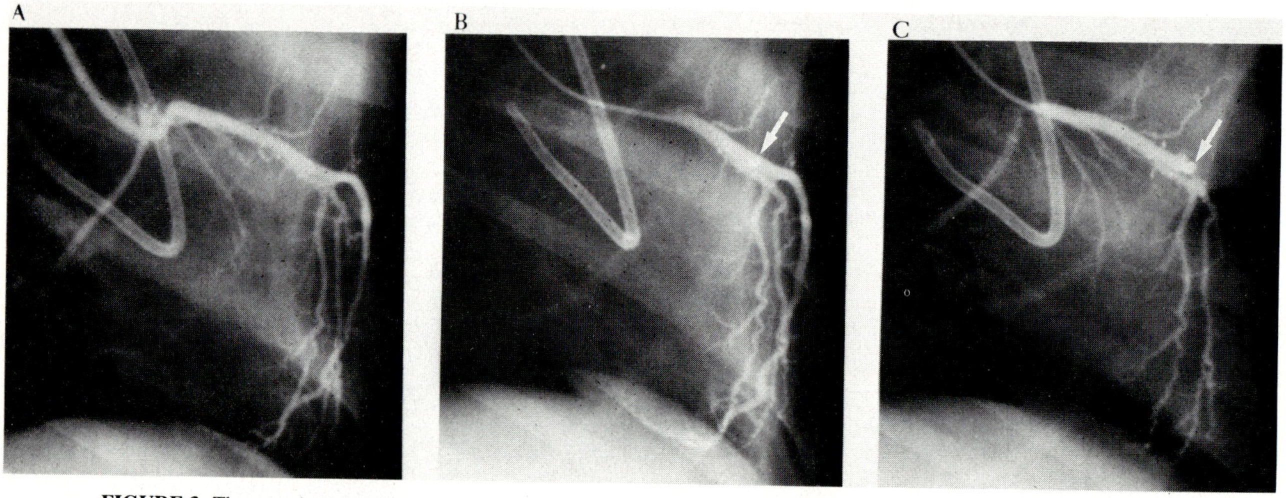

FIGURE 3. Three angiograms obtained in the right anterior oblique projection from a dog in which t-PA was administered by constant infusion before insertion of the thrombogenic copper coil. *A*, Control angiogram obtained before initiation of t-PA infusion. Distal left anterior descending artery (LAD) is patent. *B*, Angiogram obtained 60 min after copper coil insertion (arrow) during t-PA infusion at a rate of 5 μg/kg/min (t-PA concentration 761 ± 23 ng/ml). Patency of the distal LAD is demonstrated. *C*, Repeat angiogram from the same animal taken 40 min after discontinuation of infusion (plasma t-PA concentration 90.5 ng/ml). Total occlusion of the vessel is demonstrated at the site of the coil. Occlusive thrombus was confirmed by dissection of the vessel after the animal was killed.

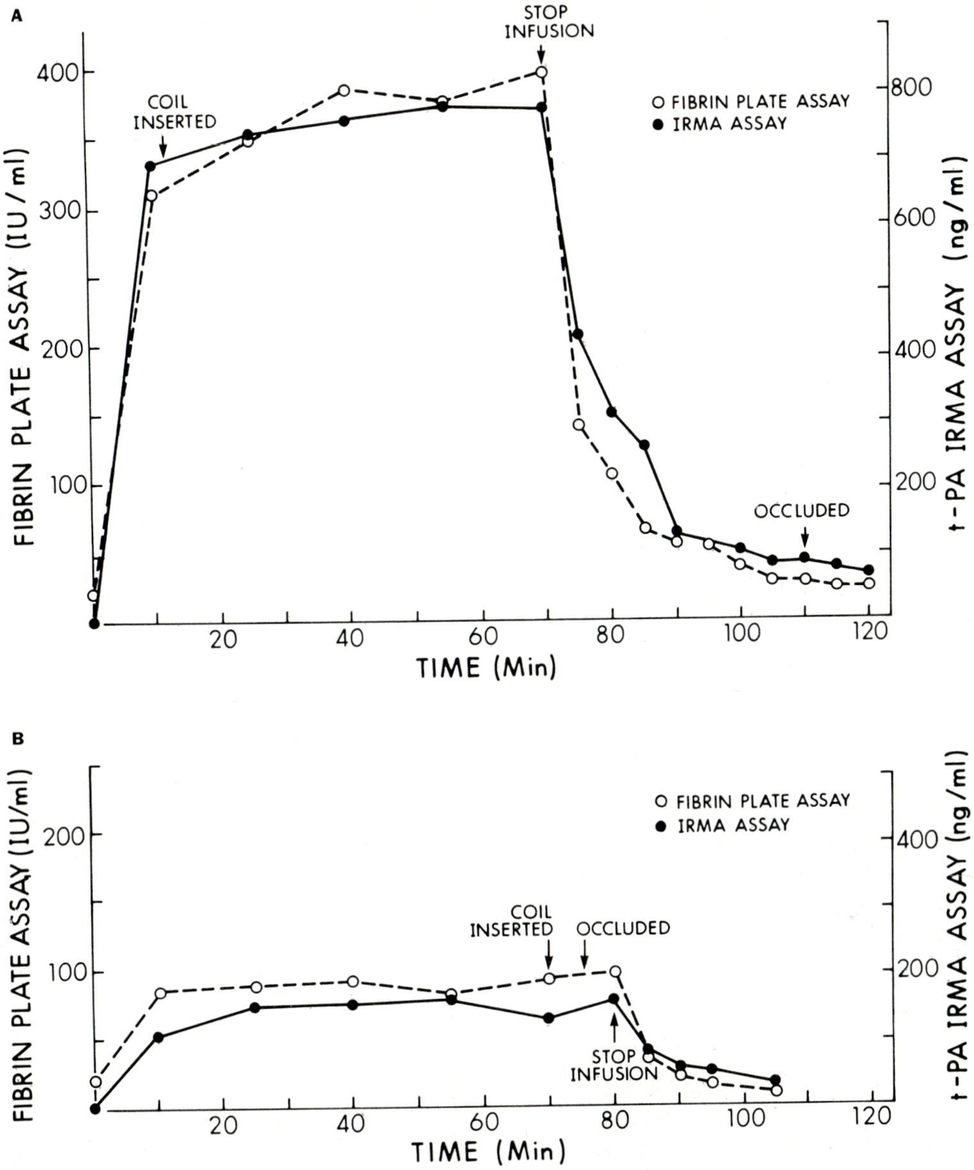

FIGURE 4. t-PA antigen and fibrinolytic activity in animals that received a constant infusion of 5 μg/kg/min (*A*) or 1 μm/kg/min t-PA (*B*). The concordance of fibrinolytic and t-PA antigen activity is apparent. Whereas the artery of the animal in *A* did not occlude until 40 min after discontinuation of the infusion, that of the animal in *B* occluded 5.3 min after insertion of the coil. Clearance of t-PA antigen and fibrinolytic activity was determined by assessing samples after discontinuation of the infusion.

Thus, the half-time of disappearance (t½) ranged from 6.6 to 16.6 min for the fast component and from 26.8 to 56 min for the slow (late) component.

Steady-state infusions of t-PA precluded apparent clot formation when prevailing concentrations of t-PA in plasma exceeded 430 ng/ml. This was achieved with doses of 3.75 to 10 μg/kg/min (n = 5). When prevailing plasma levels of t-PA ranged from 147 to 427 ng/ml, the onset of coronary occlusion was significantly delayed (n = 6). Under these conditions, occlusion occurred 26 ± 6.5 min after insertion of the thrombogenic coil in four dogs, but was precluded throughout the duration of infusion in two. For animals given the lowest dose of t-PA, less than 1.75 μg/kg/min (n = 4), the onset of coronary occlusion was not delayed compared with that in control dogs (7.7 ± 4.5 min). Prevailing concentrations of t-PA antigen in plasma and corresponding functional activity results are shown in table 2.

In each of four animals in which coronary patency was maintained throughout the infusion, the time of onset of occlusion after cessation of infusion was compared with the simultaneous plasma concentration of t-PA while plasma t-PA was declining. Occlusion oc-

TABLE 2
t-PA antigen and functional activity and time to coronary occlusion

Infusion rate of t-PA (μg/kg/min)	t-PA antigen (ng/ml)	Fibrinolytic activity (IU)	Time to occlusion (min)
5–10			
(n = 3)	610–1198	78–152	>60
3.75			
(n = 2)	467–609	81–122	>60
2.5			
(n = 2)	165–387	65–108	>60
(n = 4)	147–427	33–128	18–33
1–1.7			
(n = 4)	129–150	29–123	5–13
Zero (control)			
(n = 8)	0	7–35	5–12

Results are expressed as the range of values for each set of conditions.

curred when the plasma concentration of t-PA had declined to a value within the range of 85.1 to 91.0 ng/ml.

Discussion

Results of studies in vitro demonstrate that for clots in which t-PA is incorporated at the time of clot formation, lysis is more rapid than for similar clots exposed to equivalent concentrations of t-PA only after clot is formed. Results with euglobulin fractions indicate that reduction of concentrations of inhibitors of the fibrinolytic system shifts the dose-response curve for t-PA such that less activator is necessary to elicit lysis at a comparable rate. These results are consistent with those of earlier studies suggesting that inhibitors of fibrinolysis are not concentrated in clots.[22] Brommer[23] has incubated plasminogen activator with clot before or after induction of coagulation in vitro. However, in contrast to his findings, we observed a close correlation between lysis time and the concentration of t-PA when activator was added after as well as before clot formation. Concentrations of t-PA necessary to elicit lysis were higher than those employed by Brommer, who used washed clots, possibly with limiting amounts of native plasminogen.

Zammaron et al.[22] showed that elevations in concentration of exogenous t-PA accelerate thrombolysis. However, the dose range was limited and the endpoint used was clot dissolution over a 5 hr interval. In our study conditions were consistent with the rapidity of lysis required and temporal constraints associated with coronary thrombolysis.

A major inhibitor of plasmin present in plasma but not present in euglobulin fractions, α_2-antiplasmin, rapidly inactivates circulating plasmin (t½ = approximately 100 msec).[24] In addition, plasma, but not euglobulin fractions, has been found to contain rapidly acting ("fast inhibitors") inhibitors of t-PA. Our findings, which indicate that the fibrinolytic activity of t-PA is diminished in whole plasma as compared with euglobulin fractions, are consistent with these observations.

A concentration of t-PA of 3560 ng/ml was required to induce a half-maximal rate of lysis of clots formed from whole plasma samples. Acceleration of thrombolysis resulted from pretreatment of the samples even when exogenous t-PA was present in concentrations as low as 6.25 ng/ml (figures 1 and 2). Although results in vitro cannot be extrapolated directly to conditions in vivo, they indicate the likelihood of substantial augmentation of the rate of fibrinolysis in vivo over a wide range of concentrations of t-PA by exposure of nascent as opposed to established clots to exogenous t-PA. Furthermore, they confirm that augmentation of clot lysis is readily accomplished in whole plasma samples containing inhibitors.

The results of our studies in vivo indicate that concentrations of t-PA in plasma that are too low to induce lysis of established clots are nevertheless capable of preventing or retarding coronary thrombosis. In clinical studies, coronary thrombolysis has been accomplished with elevation of plasma t-PA to concentrations of 1000 to 5000 ng/ml.[3, 4, 10, 17] In previous studies from our laboratory with the same experimental preparation as was used here, thrombolysis was elicited in dogs with elevation of plasma t-PA to concentrations in excess of 1000 ng/ml.[2] In the present study, coronary thrombosis was prevented when concentrations of t-PA in plasma were in the range of 430 to 1200 ng/ml. Significant delay of the onset of coronary occlusion was demonstrated with even lower concentrations (147 to 427 ng/ml). Nevertheless, it should be appreciated that achievement of blood levels of this magnitude requires pharmacologic administration of exogenous t-PA and is not yet possible by utilization of any known stimulus to release or inhibition of catabolism of endogenous t-PA.

The efficacy of subthrombolytic concentrations of t-PA for prevention of coronary thrombosis may reflect the high affinity of t-PA for fibrin, the increased affinity of fibrin-bound t-PA for plasminogen, and the relative protection of t-PA and plasmin bound to fibrin from inhibitors. In addition, previous studies indicate that nascent fibrin with incomplete cross-linkage is likely to be more susceptible to lysis.[25, 26] The resistance to lysis of cross-linked α-chains of fibrin may represent a rate-limiting factor of fibrinolysis of mature clot.[25]

In contrast to t-PA, neither streptokinase nor urokinase binds selectively to fibrin.[27, 28] In clinical studies in which reduced doses of these agents have been administered, systemic proteolysis nevertheless occurred.[29–31] Thus, with either streptokinase or urokinase it appears unlikely that inhibition of clot formation will occur in vivo without induction of systemic proteolysis.

Several clinical speculations may be warranted. Clinically effective coronary thrombolysis must be implemented as soon as possible after the onset of myocardial ischemia if appreciable functional and metabolic recovery of myocardium is to be elicited. If incipient thrombosis can be recognized promptly and if a relatively clot-selective activator can be administered with dispatch, benefit may be maximized. Patients with unstable angina with high-grade coronary lesions and a high risk of coronary thrombosis may be shown ultimately to benefit from prevention of coronary occlusion with low doses of t-PA before angioplasty or coronary surgery. An obvious advantage of use of low-dose regimens in these settings is the avoidance of activation of the fibrinolytic system in circulating blood, which might otherwise compromise patients requiring immediate invasive or surgical intervention. Patients with high-grade residual stenoses that predispose to early reocclusion[9] after initially successful thrombolysis and for whom antiplatelet agents and systemic anticoagulation may not provide suitable protection[9–11, 17] may be particularly benefitted during the interval before bypass surgery or angioplasty. Despite the relatively fibrin-specific properties of t-PA and the lower doses required for prevention compared with dissolution of established coronary thrombi, prolonged administration of t-PA in inappropriately high doses can result in depletion of circulating α_2-antiplasmin and fibrinogenolysis. Nevertheless, our results suggest that approaches designed to modestly augment concentrations of t-PA in plasma before or concomitantly with the onset of coronary thrombosis may be useful. Although the experimental animal preparation used in our study does not necessarily simulate thrombosis in an atherosclerotic human coronary artery, the results obtained provide a framework for hypotheses readily testable in clinical investigations.

The potential for application of alternative methods for activation of fibrinolysis may merit reappraisal. Several agents, such as the oral anabolic steroid stanozolol, and the vasopressin analog 1-desamino-8-D-arginine vasopressin (DDAVP), have been shown to raise fibrinolytic activity and increase endogenous t-PA activity.[32, 33] Stanozolol appears also to diminish the concentration of the fast inhibitor of t-PA, thereby increasing t-PA activity.[34] In the context of pretreatment of incipient thrombosis, this potential may be considerable. Concentrations of t-PA insufficient to induce lysis of established clot may nevertheless inhibit or prevent clot formation.

We thank Joanne Markham for assistance with the mathematic derivations used in the appendix, Amelia Grace and Denise Nachowiak for technical assistance with assays of fibrinolysis, Richard Rodriquez for assistance with the studies in animals, and Barbara Donnelly and Lori Dales for preparation of the typescript.

References

1. Bergmann SR, Fox KAA, Ter-Pogossian MM, Sobel BE, Collen D: Clot-selective coronary thrombolysis with tissue-type plasminogen activator. Science **220:** 1181, 1983
2. Van de Werf F, Bergmann SR, Fox KAA, deGeest H, Hoyng CF, Sobel BE, Collen D: Coronary thrombolysis with intravenously administered human tissue-type plasminogen activator produced by recombinant DNA technology. Circulation **69:** 605, 1984
3. Van de Werf F, Ludbrook PA, Bergmann SR, Tiefenbrunn AJ, Fox KAA, deGeest H, Verstraete M, Collen D, Sobel BE: Coronary thrombolysis with tissue-type plasminogen activator in patients with evolving myocardial infarction. N Engl J Med **310:** 609, 1984
4. Collen D, Topol EJ, Tiefenbrunn AJ, Gold HK, Weisfeldt ML, Sobel BE, Leinbach RC, Brinker JA, Ludbrook PA, Yasuda I, Bulkley BE, Robison AK, Hutter AM Jr, Bell WR, Sparado JJ Jr, Khaw BA, Grossbard EB: Coronary thrombolysis with recombinant human tissue-type plasminogen activator: a prospective, randomized, placebo-controlled trial. Circulation **70:** 1012, 1984
5. Sobel BE, Fields LE, Robison AK, Fox KAA, Sarnoff SJ: Coronary thrombolysis with facilitated absorption of intramuscularly injected tissue-type plasminogen activator. Proc Natl Acad Sci USA **82:** 4258, 1985
6. Reimer KA, Lowe JE, Rasmussen MM, Jennings RB: The wavefront phenomenon of ischemic cell death. I. Myocardial infarct size vs duration of coronary occlusion in dogs. Circulation **56:** 786, 1977
7. Kloner RA, Ellis SG, Lange R, Braunwald E: Studies of experimental coronary artery reperfusion. Effects on infarct size, myocardial function, biochemistry, ultrastructure and microvascular damage. Circulation **68** (suppl I): I-8, 1983
8. Bergmann SR, Lerch RA, Fox KAA, Ludbrook PA, Welch MJ, Ter-Pogossian MM, Sobel BE: Temporal dependence of beneficial effects of coronary thrombolysis characterized by positron tomography. Am J Med **73:** 573, 1982
9. Harrison DG, Ferguson DW, Collins SM, Skorton DJ, Ericksen EE, Kioschos JM, Marcus ML, White CW: Rethrombosis after reperfusion with streptokinase: importance of geometry of residual lesions. Circulation **69:** 991, 1984
10. The TIMI study group: The thrombolysis in myocardial infarction (TIMI) trial. Phase I findings. N Engl J Med **312:** 932, 1985
11. Gash AK, Spann JF, Sherry S, Belber AR, Carabello BA, McDonough M, Mann R, McCann R, Gault J, Gentzler R: Factors influencing reocclusion after coronary thrombolysis. Circulation **70** (suppl II): II-256, 1984
12. Rijken DC, Hoylaerts M, Collen D: Fibrinolytic properties of one-chain and two-chain human extrinsic (tissue-type) plasminogen activator. J Biol Chem **257:** 2920, 1982
13. Hoylaerts M, Rijken DC, Lijnen HR, Collen D: Kinetics of the activation of plasminogen by human tissue plasminogen activator. Role of fibrin. J Biol Chem **257:** 2912, 1982
14. Matsuo O, Rijken DC, Collen D: Comparison of the relative fibrinogenolytic, fibrinolytic and thrombolytic properties of tissue plasminogen activator and urokinase in vitro. Thromb Haemost **45:** 225, 1981

15. Fox KAA, Bergmann SR, Sobel BE: Coronary thrombolysis: Pharmacological considerations with emphasis on tissue-type plasminogen activator (t-PA). Biochem Pharmacol **33:** 1831, 1984
16. Korninger C, Stassen JM, Collen D: Turnover of human extrinsic (tissue-type) plasminogen activator in rabbits. Thromb Haemost **46:** 658, 1981
17. Verstraete M, Bory M, Collen D, Erbel R, Lennane RJ, Mathey D, Michels HR, Schartl M, Uebis R, Bernard R, Brower RW, De-Bono DP, Huhmann W, Lubsen J, Meyer J, Rutsch W, Schmidt W, von Essen R: Randomised trial of intravenous recombinant tissue-type plasminogen activator versus intravenous streptokinase in acute myocardial infarction. Lancet **1:** 842, 1985
18. Wiman B, Collen D: Molecular mechanism of physiological fibrinolysis. Nature **272:** 549, 1978
19. Marsh N: Fibrinolysis. Chichester, England, 1981, John Wiley & Sons, pp 206–241
20. Clauss VA: Gerinnungsphysiologische Schnellmethode zur Bestimmung des Fibrinogens. Acta Haematol **17:** 237, 1957
21. Rijken DC, Juhan-Vague I, De Cock F, Collen D: Measurement of human tissue-type plasminogen activator by a two-site immunoradiometric assay. J Lab Clin Med **101:** 274, 1983
22. Zamarron C, Lijnen HR, Collen D: Influence of exogenous and endogenous tissue-type plasminogen activator on the lysability of clots in a plasma milieu in vitro. Thromb Res **35:** 335, 1984
23. Brommer EJP: The level of extrinsic plasminogen activator (t-PA) during clotting as a determinant of the rate of fibrinolysis: inefficiency of activators added afterwards. Thromb Res **34:** 109, 1984
24. Collen D: On the regulation and control of fibrinolysis. Thromb Haemost **43:** 77, 1980
25. Gaffney PJ, Brasher M: Subunit structure of the plasmin-induced degradation products of crosslinked fibrin. Biochim Biophys Acta **295:** 308, 1973
26. Schwartz ML, Pizzo SV, Hill RL, McKee PA: Human factor XIII from plasma and platelets. Molecular weights, subunit structures, proteolytic activation, and cross-linking of fibrinogen and fibrin. J Biol Chem **248:** 1395, 1973
27. Castellino FJ, Sodetz JM, Brockway WJ, Siefring GE: Streptokinase. Methods Enzymol **45:** 244, 1976
28. Thorsen S, Glas-Greenwalt P, Astrup T: Differences in the binding to fibrin of urokinase and tissue plasminogen activator. Thromb Diathes Haemorrh **28:** 65, 1972
29. Timmis GC, Gangadharan V, Ramos RG, Hauser AM, Westveer DC, Stewart J, Goodfliesh R, Gordon S. Hemorrhage and the products of fibrinogen digestion after intracoronary administration of streptokinase. Circulation **69:** 1146, 1984
30. Hayashi S, Yamada K: Role of α_2-plasmin inhibitor in the appearance of fibrinolytic activity during urokinase administration, and an evaluation of the optimal urokinase dosage. Thromb Res **16:** 393, 1979
31. Juhan I, Calas MF, Buonocore M, Mathieu P, Isnard G, Cazenave B, Serradimigni A: Modifications of coagulation parameters induced by treatment associating urokinase (2000μ CTA/kg/h) with heparin. Thromb Haemost **42:** 945, 1979
32. Walker ID, Davidson JF, Young P, Conkie JA: Plasma fibrinolytic activity following oral anabolic steroid therapy. Thromb Diathes Haemorrh **34:** 236, 1975
33. Mannucci PM, Rota L: Plasminogen activator response after DDAVP: a clinico-pharmacological study. Thromb Res **20:** 69, 1980
34. Verheijen JH, Rijken DC, Chang GTG, Preston FE, Kluft C: Modulation of rapid plasminogen activator inhibitor in plasma by Stanozolol. Thromb Haemost **51:** 396, 1984

Appendix: Derivation of formula for determination of appropriate t-PA bolus

Judging from results in studies of dogs, in which we found that the t½ for the first phase of t-PA from plasma was on the order of 5.5 min, a peak concentration of t-PA in plasma was achieved within 30 min with a constant input:

$$a = \frac{\text{Ln } 2}{t_{1/2}} = 0.126/\text{min and } V\frac{dC(t)}{dt} = I - aVC(t) \qquad (1)$$

where a = elimination rate constant ng/min^{-1}; t½ = half-time in plasma of t-PA (min); V = volume of distribution of t-PA (ml); I = constant infusion rate (t-PA ng/min); C(t) = concentration in plasma of t-PA at any time (t-PA ng/min).

Solving equation 1:

$$C(t) = \frac{I}{Va}(1 - e^{-at}) \qquad (2)$$

assuming that the peak concentration is reached in 30 min,

$$C_p = \frac{I}{Va}(1 - e^{-30a}) = 7.754\frac{I}{V}\text{ min} \qquad (3)$$

where C_p = desired peak concentration of t-PA in plasma (ng/ml).

For a bolus injection of B units of t-PA at time zero, the concentration in plasma at any time t is given by $C_b(5)$:

$$C_b(t) = B/V^{e^{-at}} \qquad (4)$$

where B = bolus injection of t-PA at time zero (ng of t-PA). When the initial concentration at time 0 is equal to C_p:

$$C_b(0) = C_p = \frac{B}{V} = 7.754\frac{I}{V}\text{ min},$$

$$B = 7.754 \text{ I min} \qquad (5)$$

Therefore, an amount of t-PA equivalent to 7.754 times the amount given by infusion per minute is required for the bolus to rapidly attain a plateau concentration that can be maintained by constant infusion at a rate of I_m. In this formulation, I_m is insignificantly altered from the original infusion rate I (I_m = 0.981 by derivation).

Determination of left ventricular mass in dogs with rapid-acquisition cardiac computed tomographic scanning

ANDREW J. FEIRING, M.D., JOHN A. RUMBERGER, M.D., PH.D., STEVEN J. REITER, M.D., DAVID J. SKORTON, M.D., STEVE M. COLLINS, PH.D., MARTIN J. LIPTON, M.D.*, CHARLES B. HIGGINS, M.D.*, STEPHEN ELL, PH.D., M.D., AND MELVIN L. MARCUS, M.D.

ABSTRACT The development of left ventricular hypertrophy in patients with heart disease often has far-reaching clinical implications with respect to overall morbidity and mortality. Approaches used to assess left ventricular mass include electrocardiography, echocardiography, contrast ventriculography, single photon–emission tomography, and conventional computed tomography. However, all of these modalities suffer from some major draw back that precludes widespread application to all patients. In this study we assessed the accuracy of determinations of left ventricular mass in 22 dogs by rapid-acquisition (50 msec) computed axial tomography (RACAT), an ultrafast computed tomographic (CT) instrument. Electrocardiographically triggered, end-diastolic, short-axis cardiac scans were obtained from apex to base during administration of intravenous iodinated contrast. Myocardial edges were determined for each tomographic scan by two methods: the regional half-contour method (the CT density half way between that of the left ventricular myocardium and adjacent ventricular cavities or lung) and "interactive plateau thresholding" of the cardiac borders. Left ventricular mass by RACAT was calculated as the sum of the mass of each individual scan from apex to base (modified Simpson's rule). Postmortem left ventricular mass ranged from 58 to 160 g. The correlation between true left ventricular mass and tomographically determined mass was excellent (r = .99), with the slope and y intercept not statistically different from 1 and 0, respectively. The standard error of the estimate was 4.1 g. Interobserver and intraobserver variability for determining left ventricular mass demonstrated excellent agreement (r = .99 and r = .99, respectively). We conclude that quantitative assessment of left ventricular mass can be accurately and reproducibly performed in dogs by rapid acquisition CT scanning. It is likely that this technique will be readily transferable to the clinical settings and prove to be an important method for quantifying left ventricular mass in patients.
Circulation 72, No. 6, 1355–1364, 1985.

DEVELOPMENT of left ventricular hypertrophy is often a harbinger of adverse clinical consequences. It is known that the incidence of sudden death associated with acute myocardial infarction is increased threefold among patients with concomitant left ventricular hypertrophy and hypertension.[1] Regardless of the cause, left ventricular hypertrophy has recently been implicated as a cause for diminished coronary artery reserve.[2, 3] Furthermore, in patients with left ventricular hypertrophy the functional integrity of the ventricle tends to deteriorate over time and may eventually result in overt heart failure.

Determination of left ventricular mass in vivo has been attempted by various techniques, including electrocardiography,[4] biplane left ventricular angiography,[5, 6] M mode and two-dimensional echocardiography[7–12] and ^{201}Tl imaging in conjunction with single photon–emission tomography[13] and gated and dynamic computed tomography,[14, 15] however, none are ideal.

A rapid-acquisition computed axial tomographic (RACAT) system is now available that is capable of obtaining real-time, stop-action tomographic images of the left ventricle in conjunction with excellent spa-

From the Cardiovascular Center, Departments of Internal Medicine, Electrical and Computer Engineering and Radiology, University of Iowa, Iowa City VA Medical Center, and Department of Radiology University of California at San Francisco.

Supported by grants NIH — HL20827, Ischemic SCOR — HL32295, PPG — HL14388-145, and by Imatron, Inc.

Address for correspondence: Andrew J. Feiring, M.D., Department of Internal Medicine, Cardiovascular Division, University of Iowa Hospitals and Clinics, Iowa City, IA 52242.

Received Jan. 3, 1985; revision accepted Aug. 22, 1985.

Dr. Feiring is a recipient of the Veterans Administration Associate Investigator Award.

Dr. Rumberger is a recipient of the American Heart Association Clinician Scientist Award.

Dr. Skorton is a recipient of a Research Career Development Award from the National Heart, Lung and Blood Institute.

tial resolution.[16] The intent of this study was twofold: (1) to determine whether the theoretical advantages of RACAT scanning could be used to accurately determine left ventricular mass in dogs under conditions that would be potentially clinically applicable, and (2) to evaluate a myocardial identification algorithm that would facilitate determination of left ventricular mass.

Methods

RACAT scanner. The computed tomographic (CT) scanner used in this study was the Imatron C-100 (Cine CT). A prototype scanner was used for the first nine dog studies. The remaining 13 dogs were scanned on a production model. The scanner uses four semicircular x-ray–generating tungsten target rings that may be sequentially activated by focusing and sweeping an electrocardiographically triggered election beam along each target ring. Each target ring may be activated in 50 msec, producing two contiguous, 8 mm thick tomographic slices. Each of the four targets is separated from its neighbor by 4 mm (figure 1). An individual target may be activated up to 17 times per second, thus effectively producing a tomographic cine composed of 50 msec tomographic frame images.

Animal preparation. Twenty-two dogs (weight 15 to 30 kg) were used in this study. Each was anesthetized with a combination of droperidol and fentanyl (Innovar-Vet, 1.0 ml/10 kg iv) and sodium pentobarbital (10 mg/kg iv). The dogs were mechanically ventilated via a cuffed endotracheal tube (tidal volume 12 ml/kg, rate 10/minute. Anesthesia was maintained by supplemental doses of sodium pentobarbital as needed. Electrocardiographic electrodes were attached to each dog to provide continuous monitoring of the heart rate as well as providing a trigger signal to the scanner. An angiographic catheter (No. 6F) was placed in the inferior or superior vena cava via a jugular or femoral vein. This catheter was to be used for contrast media injection. An 18-gauge catheter was placed in the femoral artery for continuous monitoring of arterial pressure.

Data acquisition

Experimental animal studies. Each dog was oriented in the scanner such that short-axis tomographic scans could be obtained from cardiac apex to base. This was accomplished by placing the dog right-side down with a shallow degree (15 to 25 degrees) of caudocranial slew (the dog's head pointing approximately to 11:15–11:30 with respect to the scanner gantry in the y plane) of the imaging table with respect to the body's long axis

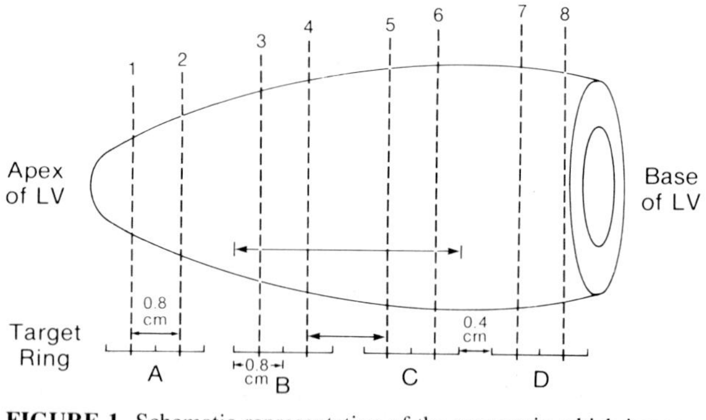

FIGURE 1. Schematic representation of the manner in which images for a myocardial mass study were acquired. Four Tungsten target rings (A, B, C, and D) lie beneath the scanning table. Activation of each target produces a pair of 8 mm thick tomographic slices separated from their neighbors by a 4 mm interscan gap. The interrupted line denotes the centers of the tomographic slices.

and scanner gantry. One or two localization scans were obtained without contrast to determine the scan level immediately below the cardiac apex. Once this level was identified, an intravenous injection of iodinated contrast (meglumine sodium diatrizoate) was administered over 15 sec. The dogs' respirations were suspended at end inspiration and maintained for approximately 3 sec while scanning was performed. Electrocardiographically triggered scanning was begun 2 sec before the completion of the injection of the contrast media, thus assuring that adequate contrast enhancement would be present on both sides of the interventricular septum during data acquisition. The electrocardiogram triggered scans were initiated at 80% of the RR interval, thus allowing for acquisition of data during mid- to end-diastole. Sequential activation of the lowest and next highest target rings produced two pairs of scans (four contiguous slices) within 108 msec in a single cardiac cycle.

Two scanning methods of determining left ventricular mass were evaluated in this study. In the first method 15 dogs were evaluated by use of contrast injection 0.75 ml/kg of meglumine sodium diatrizoate for every four tomographic slices obtained. In this group only the central two target rings (figure 1, *B* and *C*) were sequentially activated during a 108 msec interval of a single cardiac diastole. With this method the completion of an apex-to-base mass study necessitated two injections. In the second method seven dogs were studied after a single contrast injection of 0.6 ml/kg was used to radiographically interrogate 8 cm of myocardium (four pairs of slices). This was accomplished by sequentially activating target rings D and C during the first cardiac diastole and then rings B and A on the second diastole. The rate administration of contrast was similar to that in the first set, although myocardial scanning was performed 3 to 4 sec before the completion of the bolus injection.

Postmortem measurement of myocardial mass. After the completion of the study, the animals were killed with an intravenous injection of potassium chloride. Their hearts were removed, the left ventricle was dissected free from the adjacent right ventricular free wall, and the atrium and right ventricular free wall were dissected from the anatomic left ventricle. Free-hanging right ventricular trabeculae were trimmed to the septal wall. Valvular tissue, atrioventricular groove fat, and epicardial fat surrounding the coronary arteries were carefully excised. The unfixed left ventricle was blotted dry and immediately weighed to the nearest 0.1 g.

Analysis of data. During the acquisition of each scan the projection data are supplied continuously to the scanner acquisition system and subsequently to the computer. Image reconstruction was performed by the filtered back projection technique.[17] The data were processed to provide images composed of 256 × 256 picture elements (pixels). For the animal studies a reconstruction circle of 25 cm was used, so that each pixel represented a cross-sectional area of 1.02 × 1.02 mm^2. Each scan "thickness" was 8 mm. The resulting tomographic image were displayed on a monochrome video monitor with the brightness of each pixel linearly proportional to the x-ray attenuation coefficient of the tissues examined. The data are expressed in a quantitative manner in terms of Houndsfield numbers (Hn) derived from the equation

$$Hn = 1000 (A - A_w)/A_w$$

where A is the calculated x-ray attenuation coefficient of the tissue and A_w is the attenuation coefficient of water. Thus water is assigned a Houndsfield number of 0. All tissue attenuation coefficients with and without contrast were compressed into a scale that ranged from −1000 (air) to +1000 (bone). Computer programs allowed selection for regularly or irregularly shaped regions of interest within a displayed image. The absolute Houndsfield numbers of these regions could be determined regardless of the window level and width chosen for image display.

Border identification. There were four myocardial borders in a tomographic image of the left ventricle that required separate identification before the left ventricular mass could be accurately determined. These four regions were the interface between the lung and epicardium, left ventricular cavity and adjacent endocardium, right ventricular cavity and right endocardial edge of the septum, and anterior chest wall and myocardium (figure 2). Individual determination of these four interfaces were necessary because the Houndsfield numbers of tissues adjacent to the left ventricular myocardial edges are highly variable between individual scan levels in the same animal as well as between individual dogs. Consequently, specific criteria were developed for identifying each of these edges.

Two algorithms for myocardial border identification were evaluated. The first method was a regional half-height contour algorithm that has previously been described.[14, 18] The second method of border detection we term interactive plateau thresholding. With this technique the border in question was defined by evaluating the rate of change in distance vs CT density across a border. With each of these computer-assisted border identification methods the endocardial and epicardial borders of the left ventricle were traced superimposed on the displayed image with a trackball controlled cursor. The areas enclosed by the traced

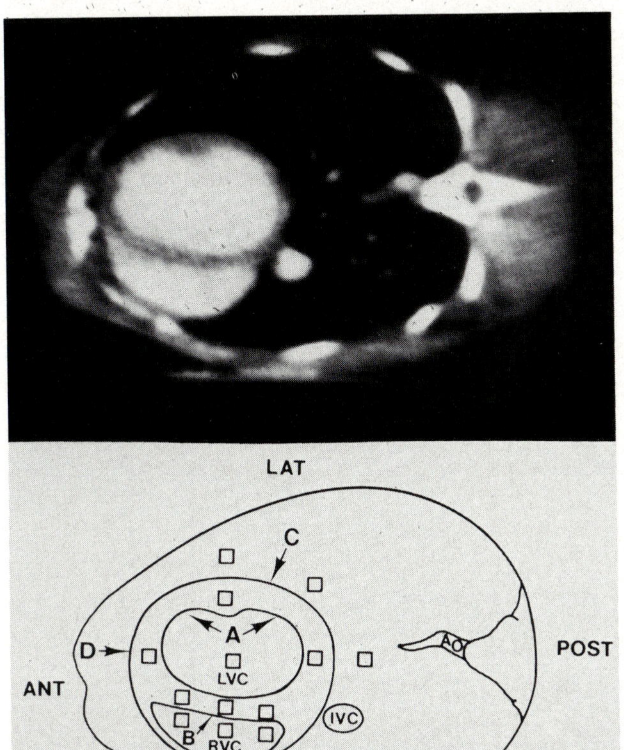

FIGURE 2. *Top,* A short-axis RACAT scan obtained at the mid papillary muscle level. On the *bottom* is a schematic representation of the four distinct myocardial boundaries (A, B, C, and D) that were identified as well as the 13 separate regions of interest used to determine edge-detection parameters. LVC = left ventricular cavity; RVC = right ventricular cavity; IVC = inferior vena cava; Ao = descending aorta; A = left ventricular cavity/endocardial edge; B = right ventricular cavity/septal (myocardial) edge; C = lung/epicardial edge; D = anterior chest wall/myocardial edge.

borders were automatically planimetered. The border of the papillary muscles were included in calculation in vivo of the left ventricular mass.

Image analysis

Regional half-contour border detection. At each corresponding tomographic scan level from cardiac apex to base 13 distinct regions of interest were defined: three in the right ventricular cavity, three in the left ventricular septum, one in the left ventricular cavity, three myocardial areas corresponding to the anterior lateral and posterior aspects of the heart, and three areas in the lung (figure 2). From these regions of interest average Houndsfield numbers were calculated for the lung, myocardium, septum, and right ventricular cavity, and appropriate window and level settings were determined.

Left ventricular cavity/endocardial edge. Without the aid of contrast administration it is virtually impossible to identify the interface between the ventricular cavity and endocardium because the CT tissue densities of myocardium and blood are nearly identical. However, with intravenous injection of iodinated contrast the ventricular cavities are clearly delineated. Six regions of interest, each approximately 5 mm/^{2}, were positioned midway between the epicardial and endocardial borders along the anterior, free wall, and posterior myocardium and left ventricular septum. In addition, a region of interest (7×7 mm^2) was placed in the center of the left ventricular cavity (figure 2). Definition of the endocardial cavity edge was determined by setting the Houndsfield window level display setting half way between the average Houndsfield numbers of the four myocardial regions and that of the opacified left ventricular cavity. These window level settings varied for each image and between individual dogs, but ranged from approximately $+50$ to $+150$ Houndsfield units. After setting the window level the window width was set at 1, thus converting the image to a black and white binary image. With the aid of a track ball the black-white interface was traced. The outline of the papillary muscles was traced from the same binary image. The heterogeneity of CT numbers within the left ventricular cavity was less than 10% or ± 20 units in a given image at the center of the left ventricular cavity.

Right ventricular cavity/myocardial edge. In contradistinction to the left ventricular cavity, which demonstrated a fairly homogeneous Houndsfield number distribution after contrast injection, the right ventricular cavity was less uniform. This difference may be related to the irregular shape of the right ventricle, heavy trabeculations in the right ventricle, and inhomogeneous admixture of contrast agent and blood following a right-sided contrast injection. Three separate regions of interest were placed in the interventricular septum. The average of these three was obtained. An additional three regions of interest were then placed in the right ventricular cavity close to the interventricular septum and the average Houndsfield number of these three was determined. Analogous to the determination of the left ventricular cavity endocardial border the septal border of the right ventricle was defined as the half-counter Houndsfield number between the average Houndsfield number of the right ventricular cavity and the average number for the interventricular septum. In a short-axis scan this edge defines approximately 33% of the left ventricular myocardium outer circumference.

Lung/epicardial edge. The placement of the lung/epicardial edge was facilitated by the large differences between the Houndsfield numbers of the myocardium (usually between $+50$ to $+150$) and the adjacent lung (less than -400). Unlike the ventricular cavity/endocardial edge the visual placement of the lung/epicardial edge is highly dependent on the Houndsfield window level chosen for display. The left ventricular–lung edge was defined with the use of the half-contour edge detection algorithm by analogy to the edge-detection method described above. The resulting values of the Houndsfield numbers ranged from −250 to −400, within the "plateau" range of Houndsfield numbers as described above. This edge defines approximately 56% of the left ventricular epicardial surface in the short axis.

Anterior chest wall/myocardial edge. The identification of the anterior chest wall/myocardial edge was facilitated by the observation that in the closed-chest dog there is a distinct visual plane separating these areas. A simple mathematic approach to defining this interface could not be developed because the Houndsfield numbers of the anterior mediastinum and adjacent myocardium are roughly the same. Consequently, the placement of the anterior chest wall/myocardial edge was made directly from the image display. This interface usually involved less than 10% of the total circumference and thus minor errors in this edge placement would not result in significant errors in estimation of left ventricular mass.

Interactive "plateau" thresholding method of edge detection. The computer software permits the operator to highlight, by means of the "blink" or "identify" mode, all those pixels within a range of CT densities. This highlighting is accomplished by alternation of the displayed intensity (grey level) of the pixel between bright white and the original grey-level values. For example, a window level of 100 and a window width of 1 will identify only those pixels with a CT density of 100. At a window level of 100 and a window width of 10 the identify mode will highlight all those pixels from 95 to 105 CT units. When the window width is set equivalent to the inherent background noise level of this instrument (approximately 15 CT units), as the window level blink is progressively increased from negative to positive numbers (lung to myocardium), the myocardial borders can be determined by observing that at various times the CT numbers in the blink mode align themselves in a uniform curvilinear pattern identifying first the epicardial and then the endocardial edges. The CT numbers at which this alignment occurred represented the values of the border of interest and corresponded closely to the CT density defined by the half-contour method previously described. Initially, with the use of the blink mode with a window level set at the mean lung density (−600 to −900), a random distribution of highlighted CT pixels was produced within the thorax. As the window level was progressively increased, the ragged and disorderly appearance of the highlighted pixels was suddenly outlined by a smooth curvilinear pattern in the epicardial edge. This pattern circumscribing the perimeter of the epicardium persisted without significant alteration as the threshold was increased over a range of CT numbers of approximately −250 to −350 CT units (the plateau) (figure 3). With further reduction in the window level, the highlighted pixels of the edge rapidly dispersed into the left ventricular myocardium and remained in a disorganized pattern for the next 150 to 300 CT units.

Further increases of the window level eventually produced a clear and well-organized curvilinear outline of the left ventricular endocardial border. Once again the position of the highlighted endocardial border remained constant and uniform for a plateau range of approximately 50 to 75 CT units. Further increase in the window level resulted in an abrupt and chaotic disorganization of the highlighted pixels that rapidly dispersed into the ventricular cavity. The right ventricular cavity and endocardial edge were determined in a similar manner. The limits of the threshold plateau for the endocardial, epicardial, and right ventricular endocardial interfaces were determined. After determining the CT limits of each border "plateau," the window blink level was set at one-half this number. With a track ball the pixels highlighted by the blink CT numbers outlining each myocardial interface was traced.

Calculation of in vivo left ventricular mass. The mass of each short-axis left ventricular slice was then calculated as a product of the planimetered myocardial area, scan slice thickness (0.8), and specific gravity of the myocardium (1.05 g/cm^3). The data for the 4 mm gap of unscanned myocardium was estimated by linear interpolation between the slice above and below the gap. The cardiac apex was defined as occurring at the lowest chest level scan that contained definable myocardium. The cardiac base was identified as occurring at the scan level immediately below the scan level at which the aorta appeared as a distinct structure (i.e., a circle). The left ventricular myocardial mass was calculated as a sum of the masses of the individual scanned sections (modified Simpson's rule).

Statistical analysis. Statistical analysis of the 22 data points comparing the left ventricular mass derived by RACAT scan-

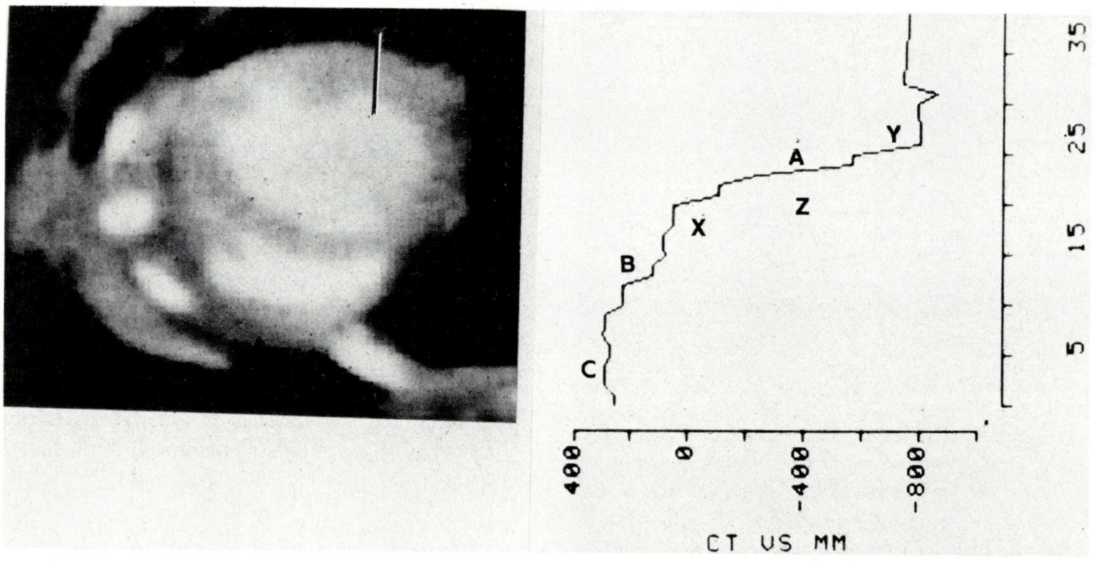

FIGURE 3. Relationship between CT number and distance along a line traversing from lung through myocardium and left ventricular cavity. Lung-epicardial and endocardial left ventricular cavity plateaus are denoted respectively by letters "A" and "B." Points X and Y represent mean myocardial and lung CT densities. Point Z corresponds to calculated half-contour CT value for the lung-myocardium interface. Point C represents mean CT number in the left ventricular cavity.

ning in vivo and the postmortem left ventricular mass were analyzed by linear regression. The first seven dogs comprised a training set in which the two edge-detection algorithms were validated. The remaining 15 dogs comprised the test set of experimental animals. The linear correlation coefficient, slope, and y intercept were calculated. Standard error of the estimate was determined in the usual fashion. Interobserver and intraobserver variability were calculated for representative animals in which left ventricular masses spanned the full range of those in all animals studied. The reproducibility of determinations of left ventricular mass was examined in six animals scanned for left ventricular mass between two and five times each.

Results

Data on left ventricular mass are presented for 22 dogs. In these dogs, heart rate varied from 60 to 90 beats/min and mean aortic blood pressure varied from 70 to 110 mm Hg.

A representative series of short-axis scans from cardiac apex to base in one experimental animal is shown in figure 4. The right ventricular tree wall is not readily apparent because of technical limitations in photo-

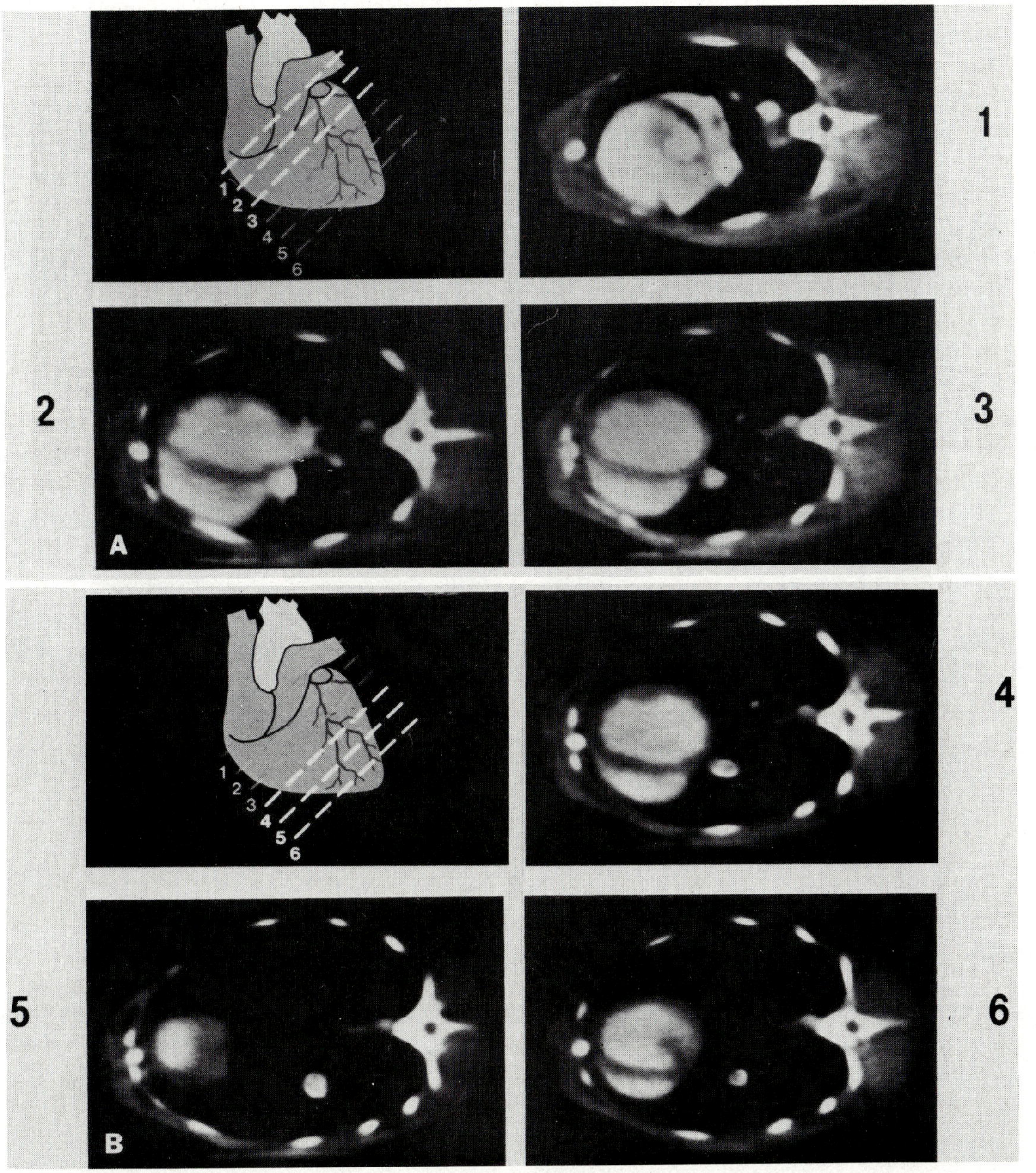

FIGURE 4. Typical short-axis scans in one dog from cardiac base to apex (right to left, top to bottom). The graphic at the *upper left* of each panel demonstrates the relative cardiac level at which each tomographic scan was obtained. *A*, The three most basal slices; *B* the midventricular through apical slices. All scans were obtained near end-diastole. Note the excellent spatial resolution of the left ventricular cavity, anterior and posterior papillary muscles, right ventricular cavity, and anterior, lateral, posterior, and septal myocardial surfaces. (The right ventricular free wall is not well visualized as a consequence of limitations in photographic reproduction.)

graphic reproduction. The data acquisition time for two pairs of 8 mm thick contiguous scans was 108 msec (4 cm of myocardium). All scans were obtained at mid- to end-diastole by electrocardiographic triggering at 80% of the RR interval. This method of scan acquisition provides excellent delineation of the left and right ventricular cavities and structure and clearly demonstrates the anterior, lateral, and posterior myocardial walls and interventricular septum.

Between six and 10 tomographic slices were required to scan the entire left ventricle from apex to base. In four animals in which the entire ventricle could not be scanned with the initial eight tomographic sections the table was incremented by 8 cm and the remainder of the ventricle scanned. Figure 5 shows the results of RACAT determination of left ventricular mass as compared with left ventricular mass at autopsy in all 22 dogs. Left ventricular mass ranged from 58 to 160 g, with a mean of 98.7 ± 33 g. The correlation coefficient and linear regression equation for the entire animal population (n = 22) by the interactive plateau thresholding technique were r = .99, y = 0.97x + 1.98, SEE = 4.1 g (figure 5). The slope and y intercept were not statistically different than 1 and 0, respectively. By the interactive plateau thresholding edge-detection method, the respective correlation coefficient, linear regression equation, and standard error of the estimate for the initial training set (n = 7) and testing set (n = 15) were r = .97, y = 1.02x − 1.09, SEE = 3.5 g and r = .99 y = 0.97x + 1.88, SEE = 4.3 g. There was no statistical difference between the slope and intercept for either the testing or training data set.

Observer variability for left ventricular mass determined by RACAT scanning. With the interactive plateau thresholding technique the intraobserver and interobserver variability for analysis of 42 ventricular scans from six dogs with myocardial masses of between 58 and 150 g was excellent (intraobserver variability r = .99, y = 0.96x + 3.5 [figure 6, *A*]; interobserver variability r = .99, y = 0.96x + 4.8 [figure 6, *B*]).

Variability between edge-detection algorithms. Fifteen random animals were evaluated with both the half-contour and interactive plateau thresholding edge-detection algorithms. The correlation coefficients, linear regression equations, and standard errors of the estimate for the two edge-detection methods were virtually identical. The autocorrelation between left ventricular mass determined by the half-contour and interactive plateau thresholding techniques was r = .99, y = 1.02x − 1.83, SEE = 3.25. The range of error for determination of the left ventricular mass with the half-contour method was from 0 to 7 g with an average of 3.3 g vs a range of 0 to 8 g with an average of 3.7 g for the plateau threshold technique.

Reproducibility of determinations of left ventricular mass. Studies of the reproducibility of scanning and determination of left ventricular mass was performed in six animals. Figure 7 demonstrates that determination of left ventricular mass in the same animal after repositioning and rescanning was highly reproducible with a small range of error (0 to 5 g).

Effect of positioning on determination of left ventricular mass. The relationship between position of the animal and accuracy of mass determination was evaluated in five dogs (range of mass 85 to 133 g). The dogs were

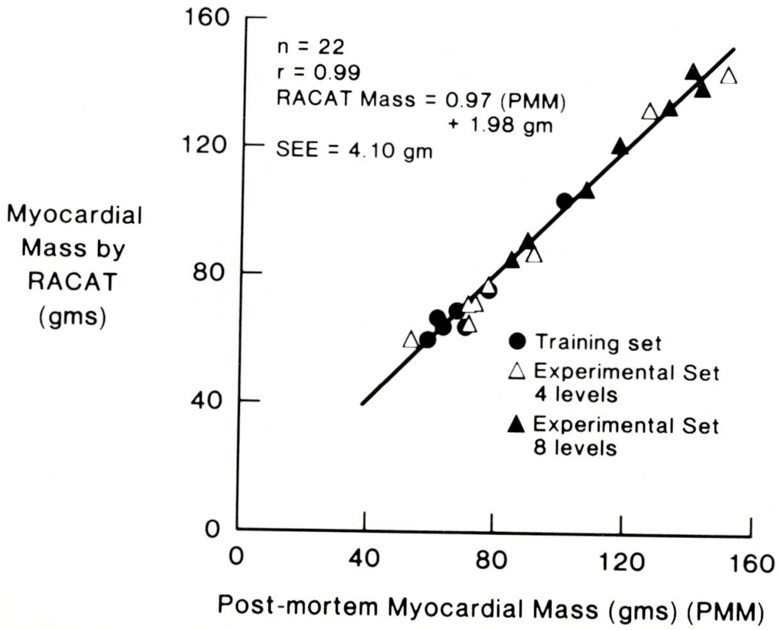

FIGURE 5. Relationship between RACAT and postmortem left ventricular mass. Regression equation slope (0.97) and y intercept (1.98) are not significantly different from 1.0 and 0.0, respectively. Standard error of the estimate is 4.1 g.

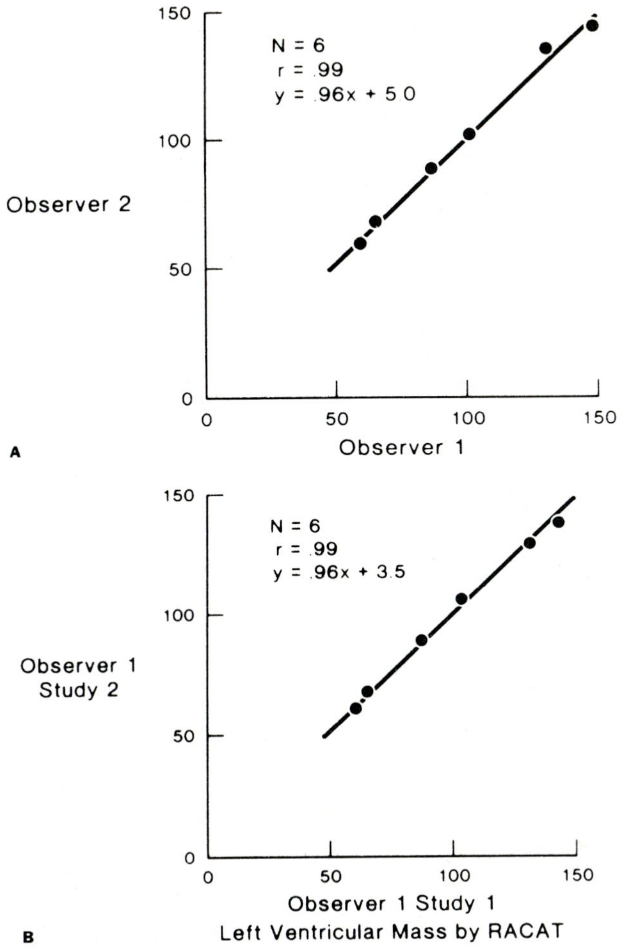

FIGURE 6. Intraobserver (*A*) and interobserver variability (*B*) in determinations of left ventricular mass from six representative dogs with masses ranging from 50 to 150 g. These data represent the result of analysis of 42 separate ventricular tomographic scans.

positioned in the scanner right-side down, with the table slewed clockwise 20 degrees with respect to the center of the gantry (figure 7, second data point in lines A thru E). The range of error for determination of left ventricular mass for the half-contour edge-detection method was 0 to 5 g and the range of error for plateau thresholding was 0 to 4 g.

Discussion

This study represents the first attempt to determine left ventricular mass in vivo with a commercially available RACAT instrument. The data demonstrate that by use of the RACAT technique and the method of cardiac edge definition described, left ventricular mass in the dog can consistently and accurately be determined.

The discussion section will be divided into three components: (1) comparison of RACAT determination of left ventricular mass with other methods, (2) myocardial edge detection and partial volume effect, and (3) potential problems, risks, and benefits when this technique is applied to patients.

Comparison of methods of determination of left ventricular mass in vivo. There are four clinical methods, in addition to computerized tomography, that have been used to determine left ventricular mass in vivo. These are (1) electrocardiography, (2) contrast ventriculography, (3) single photo–emission computed tomography, and (4) echocardiography. Determination of left ventricular mass from the surface electrogram is unreliable.[4, 5] Biplane angiographic estimates of left ventricular mass have been shown to correlate reasonably well with postmortem left ventricular mass despite its inherent dependency on fixed geometric assumptions of left ventricular shape.[6, 7] Unfortunately, the invasive nature of this procedure limits its practical application, especially for serial determination of left ventricular mass. The experimental accuracy of single photon–emission tomography with ^{201}Tl is comparable to that of biplane angiography.[13] However, since the distribution of ^{201}Tl parallels myocardial perfusion, determination of left ventricular mass in patients would be severely limited by prior myocardial infarction or severe coronary artery disease. Compared with the earlier estimates of left ventricular mass with M mode echocardiography,[8] two-dimensional echocardiographic imaging has substantially improved the accuracy of determination of left ventricular mass.[9–11] Unfortunately, high-quality two-dimensional echocardiograms from standard transducer positions may not be obtained in a substantial number of adult patients. This limitation has hindered the widespread ap-

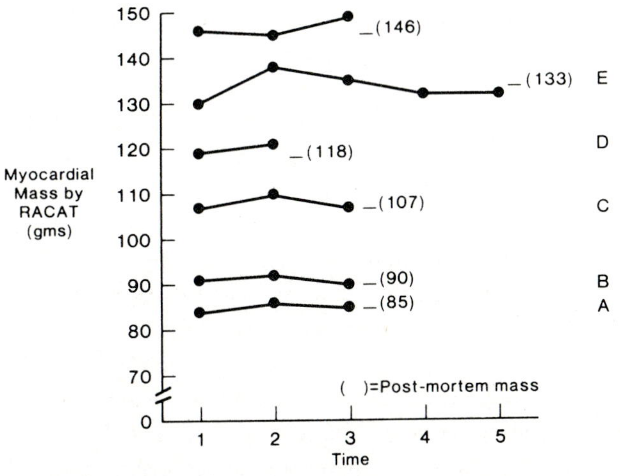

FIGURE 7. Reproducibility of scans and determinations of left ventricular mass in each of six animals. Each was rescanned between two to six times. The second point on each line A to E represents animals that were scanned at a 40 degree angle clockwise to the usual short-axis orientation.

plication of echocardiographic estimation of left ventricular mass to the majority of patients with cardiac disease.

Studies by Skioldebrand et al.[14] and Peck et al.[15] have demonstrated the feasibility of the use of computerized tomography to determine left ventricular mass in dogs. The results of these studies demonstrated that CT estimates of left ventricular mass were highly correlated with postmortem mass (r = .94, .95; SEE 8.4, 8.1 g, respectively). However, because of the excessively long scanning time (2 to 4 sec per tomographic image), these studies were performed under less than ideal physiologic conditions that included prolonged breath holding or respiratory paralysis. In addition, because only one scan could be acquired at a time the study necessitated multiple couch incrementations as well as continuous infusion of contrast medium. Despite these shortcomings, the potential applicability of computed tomography to the determination of myocardial mass was established.

Iwasaki et al.,[19] using the dynamic spatial reconstructor (DSR) (an ultrafast CT research scanner capable of obtaining millimeter-thin multiple-level tomographic scans in under 20 msec), have recently reported highly accurate estimates of left ventricular mass (r = .99, SEE = 4.1 g) in eight dogs. In that study left ventricular mass was determined after three-dimensional reconstruction of a left ventricle from 1.8 mm slices and reformatting the section to obtain 3.6 mm short-axis scans from apex to base. This is in contrast to our method whereby short-axis scans were directly obtained through the majority of the left ventricle. The tomographic thickness in the study by Iwasaki et al. was approximately one-half that of the present study (3.6 vs 8 mm). Theoretically, thinner tomographic slices should result in more accurate estimates of ventricular mass.[20] However, despite significant differences in slice thickness, the results of the present study are virtually identical to those of Iwasaki's. These findings demonstrate that subsecond tomographic techniques such as the DSR and RACAT methods provide the most accurate experimental estimates of left ventricular mass in vivo.

Accuracy of border identification. In this study we have used two algorithms for border detection. Interactive plateau thresholding in the blink mode allows for a rapid and accurate method of edge detection. Regional edge detection by the half-contour algorithm is time-consuming, but is equally as accurate. Figure 3 demonstrates a plot of CT numbers vs pixel location in a profile traversing the lung, myocardium, left ventricular cavity, septum, and right ventricular cavity in the right ventricular free wall. A clearly defined plateau (or steepest descent) corresponding to the myocardial border is observed. Plateau A defines the edge between the lung and the partial volume corona of the epicardial surface. Note that this plateau defines the area of least rate of change whereas change in CT numbers from −650 to −200 is accompanied by only a minimal (less than 1.5 mm) change in distance. Likewise, the endocardial edge is found along plateau B, whereas the change in CT numbers from +100 to +230 is accompanied by a minimal change in distance. In a sense the half-contour method and interactive plateau thresholding techniques are quite similar. If the mean CT numbers of the myocardium (x = 100) and the lung (y = −700) are used to compute the half-contour CT number (−400), then it is observed that this number will always fall along the lung-epicardial plateau.[2] Consequently, it is likely that the regional half-contour algorithm for border detection works because it fortuitously falls within this plateau.

Myocardial edge detection and the partial volume effect. In this experiment each display pixel represented a voxel of 1.02 mm × 1.02 mm × 8 mm. The attenuation number (Houndsfield units) computed for each voxel is dependent on the relative proportion of the various tissue constituents that it contains. The partial volume effect results from inclusion of two dissimilar tissues (i.e., lung/myocardial or contrast-enhanced cavity/myocardial interface) in a voxel that is to be investigated. For example, in a voxel that contains 3 mm of myocardium and 5 mm of lung tissue (i.e., an apical slice) the Houndsfield number for the myocardium will be a negative number, although it is known that tissue density structures are all above zero. Consequently, if the myocardial borders were drawn with the use of set display parameters for all scans, centering only about positive Houndsfield numbers, a serious underestimation of myocardial mass would occur. Moreover, partial volume problems are more pronounced at the apex and base of the heart. The presently used algorithms for border detection are validated by the highly correlative relationships demonstrated in this study.

Potential problems, risks, and benefits of determination of left ventricular mass in patients by RACAT. Determination of left ventricular mass in patients would be facilitated by serial short-axis tomographic acquisition from apex to base. Although previous reports of patient studies employing cardiac computed tomography have not used short-axis projections, evaluation of the left ventricle in the short axis-view is important for a number of reasons. Theoretically, myocardial edge detection is facilitated and the compounding influences of partial volume effect are minimized in this view. Second, Simpson's approximation for determining left ventricular mass and volumes should be facilitated by use of scans perpendicular to the left ventricular long axis. Finally, the short-axis view is one of the most clinically desirable projections since it allows the inspection of the entire circumference of the heart at any level, with the exception of the apex. This is in contrast to the usual transaxial view obtained with conventional computed tomography, which obscures the posterior and inferior walls. Preliminary studies in our laboratory have demonstrated that by the use of a combination of cranial tilt and clockwise slew of the imaging table multiple short-axis views can be acquired in patients. One potential problem with this mode of acquisition is that a portion of the ventricular circumference of the lowest apical tomograms lies adjacent to the liver and thus edge detection in this area may be imprecise. However, the absolute error of border identification would be small compared with the total left ventricular mass.

The presence of irregular cardiac rhythms of frequent premature beats may cause inaccuracies in determination of left ventricular mass since this method involves nonsimultaneous acquisition of tomographic changes. Consequently, for the present time it would seem prudent to avoid determination of ventricular mass in subjects with grossly irregular rhythms.

The risks of RACAT determination of left ventricular mass in man relate to the cumulative exposure to radiation as well as the known risk of intravenous injection of iodinated contrast material. The dose of radiation to the heart is approximately 250 mrads.[21] If only left ventricular mass is to be determined each section of the heart is scanned only once. Since the x-ray beam is well collimated, the cumulative dose to the whole organ per mass study is 250 mrads. In comparative terms the total dose of radiation for a RACAT mass study is about 2 to 2½ times greater than that for a routine posterior-anterior and lateral chest x-ray (100 mrads) or equivalent to 2 to 3 sec of fluoroscopy (exposure 80 to 160 mrads/sec).[22]

Intravenous administration of iodinated contrast agents has been associated with a wide variety of minor side effects, although significant adverse reactions rarely occur.[23, 24] With the emergence of the newer isosmotic, nonionic contrast agents,[25] the potential hazards associated with intravenous contrast agents should be substantially reduced.

In conclusion, we have measured left ventricular mass in 22 dogs with a high degree of accuracy using a RACAT scanner. This report presents a highly accurate method of estimation of left ventricular mass in vivo. The extremely favorable interobserver and intraobserver concordance for analysis of ventricular slices lend support to the algorithms for myocardial border identification used. Rapid-acquisition computed tomography represents a precise and minimally invasive approach for determination of left ventricular mass that should readily translate to the clinical arena.

We gratefully acknowledge the assistance of Dr. Douglas Boyd and Dr. Robert Gould and Imatron Corp. for their technical assistance. We wish to express our thanks and gratitude to Lauranne Cox, Cindy Haughland, Reginald Pike, and Peter Martins for their help and guidance. Finally we thank Mary McDermott and Marlene Blakley for their assistance in preparing the manuscript.

References

1. Kannel WB, Gordon T, Offuth D: Left ventricular hypertrophy by electrocardiograms. Prevelance, incidence and mortality in the Framingham Study. Ann Intern Med **71:** 89, 1969
2. Marcus ML, Doty DB, Hiratzka LF, Wright CB, Eastham CL: Decreased coronary reserve: a mechanism for angina pectoris in patients with aortic stenosis and normal coronary arteries. N Engl J Med **307:** 1662, 1982
3. Marcus ML: *In* The coronary circulation in health and disease. New York, 1983, McGraw-Hill Book Company, p 303
4. Romhilt DW, Bove KE, Norris RJ, Conyers E, Comadi S, Rowlands DT, Scott RC: A critical appraisal of the electrocardiographic criteria for the diagnosis of left ventricular hypertrophy. Circulation **40:** 185, 1969
5. Baxely WA, Dodge HT, Sandler H: A quantitative angiocardiographic study of left ventricular hypertrophy and the electrocardiogram. Circulation **37:** 509, 1968
6. Rackley CE, Dodge HT, Coble YD, Hay RE: A method for determining left ventricular mass in man. Circulation **29:** 666, 1964
7. Kennedy JW, Reichenbach DD, Baxley WA, Dodge HT: Left ventricular mass. A comparison of angiographic measurements with autopsy weight. Am J Cardiol **19:** 221, 1967
8. Devereux RB, Reicheck N: Echocardiographic determination of left ventricular mass in man. Circulation **55:** 613, 1976
9. Wyatt HL, Heng MK, Neirbaum S, Hestines JD, Cobo JM, Davidson RM, Corday E: Cross-sectional echocardiography. I. Analysis of mathematical models for quantifying mass of the left ventricle in dogs. Circulation **60:** 1104, 1979
10. Schiller NB, Skioldebrand CG, Schiller EJ, Mavrodius CC, Silverman NH, Rahimtodla SH, Lipton MJ: Canine left ventricular mass estimation by two-dimensional echocardiography. Circulation **68:** 210, 1983
11. Reicheck N, Helak J, Plappert T, Sutton MSJ, Weber KT: Anatomic validation of left ventricular mass estimates from clinical two-dimensional echocardiography: Initial results. Circulation **67:** 348, 1983
12. Teichholz LE, Krenlin T, Herman MV, Gorlin R: Problems in echocardiographic volume determinations: echocardiographic-angiographic correlations in the presence or absence of asynergy. Am J Cardiol **37:** 7, 1976
13. Wolfe CL, Corbett JR, Lewis SE, Buja LM, Willerson JT: Determination of left ventricular mass by single-photon emission computed tomography with thallium-201. Am J Cardiol **53:** 1365, 1984
14. Skioldebrand CG, Lipton MJ, Mavroudis C, Hayaski TT: Determination of left ventricular mass by computed tomography. Am J Cardiol **49:** 63, 1982
15. Peck WW, Maurini GBJ, Slutsky RA, Mathey RF, Higgins CB: In vivo assessment by computed tomography of the natural progression of infarct size, left ventricular muscle mass and function after acute myocardial infarction in the dog. Am J Cardiol **53:** 929, 1984
16. Boyd DP, Lipton MJ: IEEE Proc **71:** 298, 1983

17. Brooks RA, DiChiro G: Theory of image reconstruction in computed tomography. Radiology **117:** 561, 1975
18. Skioldebrand CG, Ovenfors CO, Mavroudis C, Lipton MJ: Assessment of ventricular wall thickness in vivo by computed transmission tomography. Circulation **61:** 960, 1980
19. Iwasaki T, Sinak LJ, Hoffman EA, Robb RA, Harris LD, Bahn RC, Ritman EL: Mass of left ventricular myocardium estimated with dynamic spatial reconstructor. Am J Physiol **?:** H138, 1984
20. Janicki JS, Weber KT, Gochman RF, Shroff S, Geheb FT: Three-dimensional myocardial and ventricular shape: a surface representation. Am J Physiol **241:** H1, 1981
21. Gould RG, Couch JL, Napel S, Peschmann KR, Rand RE, Boyd DP: Performance characteristics of an ultrafast scanning electron beam CT scanner. Med Phys **10:** 526, 1983
22. John HE, editor: The physics of radiology, ed 4. Springfield, IL, 1984, Charles C Thomas Publisher, p 648
23. Toniolo G, Biua L: Fatal reactions following injection of iodinated contrast media. Radiol Med **52:** 625, 1966
24. Hessel SJ, Adams DF, Abrams HL: Complications of angiography. Radiology **138:** 273, 1981
25. Higgins CB: Overview of cardiovascular effects of contrast media. Invest Radiol **19** (suppl 5): 187, 1984

Treatment of canine permeability pulmonary edema: short-term effects of dobutamine, furosemide, and hydralazine

WILLIAM D. MOLLOY, M.B., K. Y. LEE, M.B., LINDA GIRLING, B.SC.,
AND RICHARD M. PREWITT, M.D.

ABSTRACT The effects of treatment of oleic acid pulmonary edema with dobutamine, furosemide, and hydralazine on cardiopulmonary function in 24 dogs were investigated. Pulmonary capillary wedge pressure (PCWP) was adjusted to approximately 7 mm Hg; 45 min after oleic acid (0.08 ml/kg), dogs were randomly divided into a control group, in which PCWP was maintained at approximately 7 mm Hg, and into treatment groups as described above. Mean time-averaged PCWP was 2.3 mm Hg in dogs treated with dobutamine, 4.1 mm Hg with furosemide, and 4.4 mm Hg with hydralazine. Four hours of treatment with dobutamine and furosemide significantly ($p < .01$) reduced accumulation of lung water compared with the control and hydralazine groups. Qs/Qt was lower ($p < .05$) with dobutamine and furosemide compared with the other groups. In dogs given hydralazine, cardiac output (CO) and systemic vascular resistance (SVR) remained constant over the 4 hr treatment interval. In contrast, in all other groups, SVR increased and CO decreased (both $p < .05$). The short-term pulmonary effects of the above drugs are probably explained by differences in PCWP and/or by regional pulmonary vascular effects.

Circulation 72, No. 6, 1365–1371, 1985.

IN CONTRAST to cardiogenic pulmonary edema, in the adult respiratory distress syndrome severe edema develops in spite of normal or low left ventricular filling pressure. Acute respiratory failure occurs because alveolar and/or pulmonary endothelial damage results in excess accumulation of extravascular lung water, leading to alveolar edema and collapse, which causes a large right-to-left intrapulmonary shunt (Qs/Qt).[1-3] Although therapy designed to reduce pulmonary capillary wedge pressure (PCWP) effectively treats cardiogenic pulmonary edema, this approach has only recently been tested in low-pressure pulmonary edema.[4, 5] In a canine study, phlebotomy and infusion of nitroprusside reduced PCWP from 11 to 6 mm Hg over a 4 hr period, and compared with a control group in which the 4 hr time-averaged PCWP was 11 mm Hg, pulmonary edema was significantly reduced.[5] Although phlebotomy reduced edema, it resulted in a large fall in cardiac output (CO), an effect clearly to be avoided in critically ill patients. Although nitroprusside maintained CO despite reduced PCWP, it had adverse effects on blood pressure and gas exchange. These adverse effects were confirmed in two short-term experiments in which infusion of nitroprusside increased CO, increased Qs/Qt, and reduced Pa_{O_2}.[6, 7] Similar results with nitroprusside are reported in patients with acute respiratory failure.[8]

This study was designed to determine the short-term cardiopulmonary effects of several drugs in canine low-pressure pulmonary edema induced by intravenous injection of oleic acid.

Current inotropic agents used to increase CO include dobutamine and dopamine. In patients with congestive heart failure, dopamine increased PCWP when it increased CO.[9, 10] On the other hand, in the same patients, for an equal change in CO, PCWP fell with dobutamine. Because the subacute cardiopulmonary effects of dobutamine have not been investigated in a model of low pressure pulmonary edema, we chose to study this drug and test the hypothesis that PCWP and lung water will decrease with dobutamine.

From the Department of Medicine, University of Manitoba Health Sciences Centre, Winnipeg.

Address for correspondence: Richard M. Prewitt, M.D., Department of Medicine, Section of Cardiology, F-2 Health Sciences Centre, 700 Williams Ave., Winnipeg, Manitoba R3E 0Z3 Canada.

Received March 4, 1985; revision accepted Aug. 15, 1985.

Dr. Molloy is a fellow of the Canadian Heart Foundation. Dr. Prewitt is the Manitoba Heart Foundation Research Professor.

Previous work in canine oleic acid edema demonstrated that over a two 2 hr interval, intravenous furosemide (1 mg/kg) improved gas exchange but did not affect formation of pulmonary edema.[11] Most likely, edema was not reduced with furosemide because PCWP remained constant. Accordingly, in the current study, furosemide was given to reduce PCWP.

In patients with congestive heart failure, primary pulmonary hypertension and chronic obstructive pulmonary disease, hydralazine decreases resistance and increases CO.[12-14] Two recent studies investigated the short-term cardiopulmonary effects of hydralazine in canine oleic acid pulmonary edema.[6, 15] In both, there was a small decrease in PCWP with hydralazine and an increase in CO. Lung water was not measured in these studies. Accordingly, the current study was designed to determine the subacute cardiopulmonary effects of hydralazine in low-pressure pulmonary edema.

We emphasize that the value of observations in this study is not dependent on how closely oleic acid pulmonary edema mimics clinical adult respiratory distress syndrome; rather, our objective was to investigate several commonly used drugs in a model of permeability pulmonary edema.

Methods

Twenty-four dogs of mixed breed were anesthetized with pentobarbital (30 mg/kg) and given small maintenance doses as required. They were artificially ventilated (20 ml/kg) in the supine position via an endotracheal tube with 100% O_2. End expiratory pressure was zero. Respiratory rate was adjusted to maintain Pco_2 between 35 and 40 mm Hg. Sodium bicarbonate was given as required to correct metabolic acidosis and maintain pH above 7.3. A catheter was placed in the aorta to record blood pressure and to sample arterial blood. A Swan-Ganz catheter was flow directed into the right ventricle via the external jugular vein. A thermistor-tipped Swan-Ganz catheter that was flow directed to the pulmonary artery through the external jugular vein was used to sample mixed venous blood and to measure pulmonary arterial pressure and PCWP. These catheters were connected to Statham P23 ID transducers and leveled to the center of the chest, and their outputs were displayed and recorded on an Electronics for Medicine oscillograph. The pressures were recorded at a sensitivity at which 1 mm Hg corresponds to a 1 mm deflection. Another catheter was placed in the right atrium for injection of boluses of saline, and a thermal dilution curve was recorded and analyzed by a cardiac output computer (Columbus Instruments). A large-bore polyethylene catheter was inserted into the superior vena cava through the external jugular vein for volume infusion and drug administration.

When the surgical preparation was completed, the PCWP was adjusted to approximately 7 mm Hg by intravenous infusion of approximately 250 ml of 6% dextran; after the preparation was stable for approximately 10 min, baseline measurements were taken. Simultaneous samples of arterial and venous blood were taken before hemodynamic measurements were obtained. They were analyzed for blood gas tension with a Corning 165/2 (Corning Scientific Instruments, Medfield, MA) and O_2 contents were measured by a carbon monoxide scrubbing technique.[16] Qs/Qt was calculated in a standard manner[5] as $Qs/Qt = (Cc'O_2 - CaO_2)/(Cc'O_2 - CvO_2)$.

With the animals' breath held at end expiration, heart rate, blood pressure, pulmonary arterial pressure, mean PCWP, right ventricular pressure, and CO were measured. Measurements of oncotic pressure (π IV) were obtained from samples of arterial blood.

After baseline measurements, during a 20 sec breath hold, oleic acid (0.08 ml/kg) was infused into the right atrium. The PCWP was maintained at 7 to 8 mm Hg for 45 min by intravenous infusion of approximately 250 ml of 6% dextran.

Forty-five minutes after injection of oleic acid, dogs were randomized into the following groups:

(1) Untreated group. In this group, PCWP was maintained at approximately 8 mm Hg for the 4 hr treatment interval. This was achieved with infusion of 6% dextran, as required. Dogs received 250 to 400 ml of dextran over the treatment period. In all groups, measurements of PCWP, pulmonary arterial pressure, and blood pressure were obtained at 10 min intervals throughout the study. The reported values represent the mean of all measurements during the treatment period in this and the three treated groups. Furthermore, in all groups transducers were frequently balanced and the zero position confirmed during each experiment.

(2) Furosemide-treated group. Intravenous furosemide was given as required to reduce and maintain PCWP at approximately 3 mm Hg. It took approximately 20 min to reduce PCWP to the desired level, and over the 4 hr treatment interval the PCWP was stable and varied less than 2 mm Hg. Dogs received aliquots of 20 to 40 mg and the total dose received varied between 5 and 20 mg/kg. Blood pressure fell less than 10% with furosemide and it remained relatively constant over the treatment interval.

(3) Hydralazine-treated group. Intravenous hydralazine was initially given in 2 mg aliquots until mean blood pressure had fallen approximately 15%. This was usually achieved in less than 20 min at an average dose of 12 mg. Subsequently, the drug was given by continuous infusion at a rate of 2 to 4 mg/hr. At this rate of infusion the mean blood pressure and PCWP remained relatively stable.

(4) Dobutamine-treated group. Dobutamine was infused at an increasing rate until mean blood pressure decreased by 15%, until mean heart rate increased by approximately 15 beats/min, or until PCWP fell to approximately 3 mm Hg. PCWP always fell with dobutamine and the desired reduction in left ventricular filling pressure was always achieved within 20 min. The rate of infusion varied among dogs between 8 to 15 μg/kg/min.

After dogs had been treated for 4 hr and just before they were killed, 100 ml of blood was taken and weighed. Twenty-five microcuries of chromium-51 tagged to autologous red blood cells was then injected into the right atrium. After adequate mixing, 9 ml of blood was withdrawn and divided into 3 × 3 ml aliquots. The dogs were then killed by an intravenous bolus of concentrated KCl, and almost immediately the chests were opened, the hila clamped, and the lungs removed. The lungs were then homogenated and blood was taken and counted in a gamma camera.

The lungs and 100 ml of blood were placed in a vacuum-sealed oven at 60° C and dried over the next few days. Lungs and blood were weighed each day until weights changed less than 1 g in 2 consecutive days. The following formulas were used to calculate lung composition: (1) lung blood weight = (count in homogenate sample)/(count in blood sample) × (volume blood)/(volume homogenate) × density of homogenate; (2) lung wet weight blood free (LWWBF) = lung wet weight − lung blood weight; (3) extravascular lung water (EVLW) = LWWBF − lung dry weight blood free.

TABLE 1
Short-term cardiopulmonary effects of oleic acid

	CO (l/min)	BP (mm Hg)	Ppa (mm Hg)	πIV (mm Hg)	RVEDP (mm Hg)	SVR (mm Hg/ l/min)	PVR (mm Hg/ l/min)	PO_2 (mm Hg)	Qs/Qt (%)	PCWP (mm Hg)
Baseline	6.0	140	17.2	18.6	4.3	25.3	2.0	502	17	7.9
	±1.2	±4.9	±2.3	±1.9	±0.9	±4.4	±0.2	±16.7	±3.1	±0.1
45 min	5.3	133	15.9	18.5	4.1	28.0	1.9	239[A]	37.4[A]	7.4
After OA	±0.9	±7.8	±2.2	±2.4	±0.8	±3.2	±0.1	±41.3	±5.2	±0.2

Values are mean ±SD for all 24 dogs.
OA = oleic acid; BP = blood pressure; Ppa = pulmonary arterial pressure; PO_2 = partial pressure of oxygen in arterial blood.
[A]$p < .05$ compared with preceding value.

Results

Table 1 depicts measured values before and 45 min after oleic acid. Analysis of variance showed no significant differences among the five groups for any of the measured variables in either baseline or 45 min measurements. Oleic acid caused a marked deterioration in gas exchange, i.e. mean Qs/Qt more than doubled ($p < .05$, paired t test). There was no significant change in the values of CO, πIV, PCWP, pulmonary arterial pressure, and systemic (SVR) or pulmonary vascular resistance (PVR) with oleic acid.

Table 2 summarizes the mean (±SD) values for PCWP, right ventricular end-diastolic pressure (RVEDP), and πIV for each group over the 4 hr treatment intervals. Analysis of variance demonstrated a highly significant F ratio for PCWP. Duncan's multiple comparison test confirmed that PCWP was significantly lower in the treated groups compared with the untreated group. Also note that, compared with hydralazine, dobutamine produced lower PCWP values. Values for πIV were similar in all groups and RVEDP was reduced in two groups.

Table 3 illustrates the effects of treatment on formation of pulmonary edema.

Lung weights are normalized for body weight. Analysis of variance of lung wet weight (WW)/body weight (BW) ratios resulted in a significant F statistic. Dogs treated with furosemide and dobutamine had a significantly smaller WW/BW ratio compared with the hydralazine and control groups by analysis of variance and Duncan's test ($p < .01$). In the same groups there was also a significant reduction ($p < .01$) in the ratio of LWWBF to BW.

When groups were compared by EVLW/BW ratios, the F statistic was again significant. Compared with the control and hydralazine groups, treatment with furosemide and dobutamine significantly ($p < .05$) reduced this ratio. Compared with controls, all treatments except hydralazine significantly ($p < .05$) reduced the EVLW/BF dry lung ratio. The compara-

TABLE 2
Effects of treatment on ventricular filling pressures and oncotic pressure

	Control	H	F	D
PCWP (mm Hg)				
45 min after OA	7.4±0.8	7.3±0.4	7.7±0.5	7.1±0.4
4 hr	7.4±0.7	4.4±0.3[A,C]	4.1±0.2[A,D]	2.3±1.1[A,B,D]
RVEDP (mm Hg)				
45 min after OA	5.0±1.4	4.8±2.4	3.5±1.0	4.0±1.7
4 hr	5.2±2.3	4.0±2.8	1.8±1.7[A,D]	0.5±1.2[A,C]
πIV (mm Hg)				
45 min after OA	18.3±3.2	22.5±1.5	17.0±6.4	17.3±2.8
4 hr	18.3±4.7	16.0±2.8	14.3±3.3	14.4±1.2

Values are mean ±SD.
H = hydralazine; F = furosemide; D = dobutamine; OA = oleic acid.
[A]Significant difference ($p < .05$) compared with controls.
[B]Significant difference ($p < .05$) compared with hydralazine.
[C]Significant difference ($p < .05$) compared with 45 min values.
[D]Significant difference ($p < .01$) compared with 45 min values.

TABLE 3
Effects of treatment on lung water

	WW/BW (g/kg)	WWBF/BW (g/kg)	EVLW/BW (ml/kg)	EVLW/BFDL (ml/g)
Control	47.3 ± 12.2	41.0 ± 6.2	38 ± 5	11.4 ± 1.2
Furosemide	32.6 ± 6.8[B,D]	25.0 ± 3.6[B,D]	22 ± 5.7[A,C]	8.1 ± 1.3[A]
Dobutamine	32.0 ± 4.0[B,D]	27.2 ± 3.9[B,D]	26 ± 4.9[A,C]	9.7 ± 1.7[A]
Hydralazine	43.8 ± 8.6	36.0 ± 6.6	32 ± 6.2	9.7 ± 3.0

Values are mean ± SD.
BW = body weight; WW = wet weight; WWBF = wet weight blood free; EVLW = extravascular lung water; BFDL = blood free dry lung.
[A]Difference from control group ($p < .05$).
[B]Difference from control group ($p < .01$).
[C]Difference from H group ($p < .05$).
[D]Difference from H group ($p < .01$).

tively low ratio obtained with hydralazine is explained by the high value for lung dry weight in two dogs that had marked edema as assessed by the other indexes.

The nonsignificant F statistic from analysis of variance of lung dry weight to BW suggested no difference among groups. However, mean values were highest in controls and in dogs given hydralazine.

Table 4 illustrates effects of oleic acid and treatment on gas exchange. Compared with the 45 min values, there was a large ($p < .05$, paired t test) increase in Qs/Qt over the treatment interval in the control group and in dogs treated with hydralazine. In contrast, mean Qs/Qt remained constant in dogs treated with furosemide and dobutamine. Analysis of variance of measurements obtained after 4 hr of treatment resulted in a significant F ratio. Compared with the other groups, Duncan's test confirmed that Qs/Qt was lower ($p < .05$) in groups treated with furosemide and dobutamine. Edema and Qs/Qt at 4 hr were similar in the latter two groups. In the control group and in dogs given hydralazine, the deterioration in gas exchange paralleled the increase in lung water. Changes in PaO^2 followed the trend for Qs/Qt but no significant differences were detected by analysis of variance.

As illustrated in figure 1, mean CO expressed as a percent of the 45 min (control) value fell over the treatment interval in all groups except that given hydralazine. Comparing values obtained at 4 hr with those obtained at 45 min, CO decreased in all dogs ($p < .05$, paired t test) except those treated with hydralazine.

Over the treatment interval, mean arterial blood pressure remained constant with dobutamine and in controls but tended to decrease in other groups (table 5). Over the 4 hr interval, SVR increased in all groups ($p < .05$, paired t test) except those dogs treated with hydralazine. The initial high value for SVR in the hydralazine groups is explained by the observation that two dogs in this group had low CO and thus high SVR 45 min after oleic acid. Values for blood pressure, pulmonary arterial pressure, and PVR were similar between groups after 4 hr of treatment and there were no differences by analysis of variance.

Discussion

This study confirms previous work describing the pathophysiology of oleic acid pulmonary edema.[5, 6] Despite normal PCWP, 45 min after oleic acid, mean

TABLE 4
Effects of treatment on gas exchange

	Control	H	F	D
Qs/Qt (%)				
45 min after OA	37 ± 15	37 ± 18	31 ± 13	34 ± 8
4 hr	58 ± 12[B]	50 ± 7[B]	30 ± 16[A]	33 ± 12.7[A]
Pao_2 (mm Hg)				
45 min after OA	239 ± 135	278 ± 140	284 ± 126	236 ± 84
4 hr	76 ± 66[B]	97 ± 49[B]	159 ± 143[B]	147 ± 92[B]

Values are mean ± SD. Abbreviations as in table 2.
[A]$p < .05$ compared with controls and hydralazine.
[B]$p < .05$ compared with 45 min value.

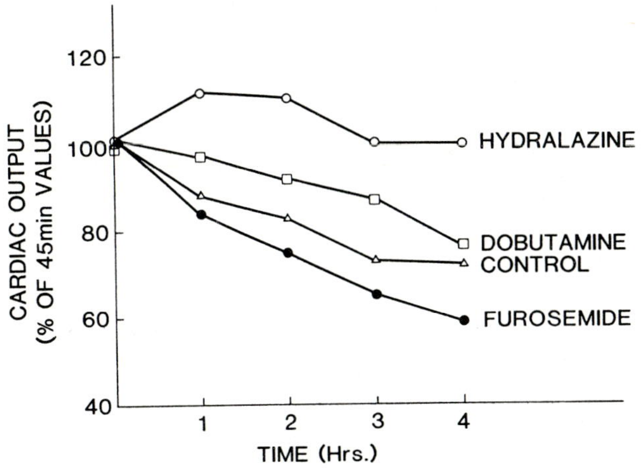

FIGURE 1. Effects of treatment on CO. CO increased at 1 and 2 hr after treatment in dogs given hydralazine. Although CO decreased progressively in controls and in dogs given furosemide, in those treated with dobutamine and combination therapy, CO remained constant over the first 2 hr. For further discussion, see text.

Qs/Qt had more than doubled. The deterioration in gas exchange most likely resulted from accumulation of excess lung water, which occurred because oleic acid disrupted pulmonary vascular integrity. Two of our interventions caused a small but significant decrease in a normal left ventricular filling pressure and substantially decreased accumulation of lung water. In an earlier study of canine oleic acid edema, phlebotomy and a 4 hr infusion of nitroprusside decreased PCWP from 11 to 6 mm Hg and significantly reduced pulmonary edema.[5] Other canine studies have also demonstrated that relatively small changes in PCWP can affect accumulation of lung water when vascular permeability is increased.[4]

We emphasize that because the pathophysiology of oleic acid pulmonary edema is different from clinical acute respiratory failure, direct clinical extension of the current results is limited. However, the adult respiratory distress syndrome is also characterized by increased pulmonary vascular permeability,[17] and in this condition relatively small changes in PCWP may influence accumulation of pulmonary edema.

A previous study demonstrated that despite no effect on edema, furosemide improved gas exchange in canine oleic acid pulmonary edema.[11] The improvement in gas exchange was attributed to pulmonary vasoactive effects of the drug. In that study, the dose of furosemide was relatively low (0.1 mg/kg) and had no effect on PCWP. Most likely, edema was not reduced because PCWP remained constant. In the current study, furosemide decreased PCWP from 7 to 4 mm Hg and significantly reduced pulmonary edema.

Compared with the control group and dogs treated with hydralazine, gas exchange did not deteriorate over 4 hr in dogs given furosemide. As reflected in figure 1, corresponding to the decrease in PCWP, there was a large fall in CO over the treatment interval. The decrease in CO with furosemide is explained by a decrease in ventricular preload and by an increase in SVR. Note that despite constant ventricular filling pressures and unchanged PVR, CO fell over the 4 hr interval in controls. The decrease in flow in this group may be explained by the increase in systemic resistance. Since SVR increased a similar amount in controls and in dogs given furosemide, the greater decrease in mean flow in the treated group (29% vs 19%)

TABLE 5
Hemodynamic effects of oleic acid and treatment

	Control	H	F	D
CO (l/min)				
45 min	5.6±1.2	4.2±1.1	5.1±0.5	4.5±0.6
4 hr	4.7±0.4[A]	4.4±0.2	3.6±0.4[A]	3.8±0.6[A]
BP (mm Hg)				
45 min	140±30	132±26	141±19	133±11
4 hr	140±32	103±20	131±14	133±23
Ppa (mm Hg)				
45 min	18±2.8	16±4.0	17±3.0	16±1.7
4 hr	20±3.8	16±4.1	14±3.5	15±4.1
PVR (mm Hg/l/min)				
45 min	2.1±0.5	1.8±1.4	1.7±0.44	1.9±0.8
4 hr	3.0±0.3	2.8±0.4	2.9±0.4	3.4±0.8
SVR (mm Hg/l/min)				
45 min	24±5	32±4	26±5	29±6
4 hr	31±3[A]	24±4	38±5[A]	35±3[A]

BP = blood pressure; Ppa = pulmonary artery pressure; other abbreviations as in table 2.
[A]$p < .05$ compared with 45 min value.

may be explained by the fall in preload with furosemide. Other studies have described similar changes in CO after oleic acid and attributed the decrease in flow to increased systemic resistance.[6,7]

A 4 hr continuous infusion of dobutamine maintained mean time-averaged PCWP at 2.3 mm Hg, and compared with controls and dogs given hydralazine, dobutamine substantially reduced formation of pulmonary edema. Corresponding to the reduction in edema, gas exchange did not deteriorate over the treatment interval. Note that lung water and values for Qs/Qt and Pao_2 were similar in dogs given dobutamine and in those treated with furosemide. Despite a significant fall in PCWP, after 2 and 3 hr of treatment, mean CO remained constant with dobutamine. In contrast over the same interval, despite constant PCWP in the controls, CO decreased. In patients with established left ventricular failure, CO increases when PCWP decreases with dobutamine.[10] The different effects of dobutamine are probably explained by the marked differences in subjects, i.e. patients with left ventricular failure vs dogs with oleic acid pulmonary edema and low PCWP. The improvement in left ventricular pump performance with dobutamine is most likely explained by its positive inotropic effects. That is, with respect to the current study, the increased contractile state allowed increased ventricular shortening to a smaller end-systolic volume so that stroke volume and CO remained constant despite a decrease in ventricular preload. Note that compared with controls, RVEDP also decreased with dobutamine, signaling an improvement in right ventricular pump performance. After 4 hr of treatment CO decreased. The fall may in part be explained by an increase in systemic resistance. SVR increased ($p < .05$) from 29 mm Hg/liter/min at baseline to 38 mm Hg/liter/min after 4 hr of treatment. Compared with other groups by analysis of variance, dobutamine did not affect other cardiopulmonary parameters. Although cardiovascular effects of dobutamine have been carefully investigated in patients with left ventricular failure,[9,10] the current study is one of first to systematically investigate subacute effects of this agent on cardiopulmonary function in a model of low-pressure pulmonary edema.

Hydralazine is commonly used to decrease afterload and improved left ventricular function in patients with long-term left ventricular failure.[12] One study of patients with congestive heart failure demonstrated that the increase in CO with hydralazine was greater when ventricular end-diastolic dimensions were larger.[18] Furthermore, oral hydralazine has also been shown to be effective in decreasing resistance and increasing CO in patients with primary pulmonary hypertension and in patients with raised pulmonary artery pressure secondary to chronic pulmonary disease.[13,14]

In two recent canine studies, we demonstrated that in the presence of oleic acid edema, hydralazine acutely decreased SVR and increased CO.[6,15] In both studies, there was a small decrease in PCWP with hydralazine. In this study, despite a decrease in left ventricular filling pressure and in contrast to controls and treatment with furosemide and dobutamine, CO did not decrease with hydralazine. Compared to other groups, the most likely explanation for the improvement in left ventricular function with hydralazine is that the drug prevented the increases in systemic resistance. However, an increased inotropic state with hydralazine cannot be ruled out.

Although all indexes of lung water (table 3) were consistently lower in dogs treated with hydralazine than in controls because of the variability within groups, those changes were not significant. Since PCWP decreased a similar amount with all interventions, the failure of edema to decrease with hydralazine indicates that in addition to changes in PCWP, other factors influence formation of pulmonary edema in this model. For example, CO was highest in those dogs given hydralazine and the increased flow in concert with regional vascular effects of the drug could have resulted in higher intravascular pressures in damaged areas. Such changes could increase local lung water accumulation and offset effects of a lower mean PCWP. In this regard, the decrease in lung water seen with furosemide and dobutamine may also be partially explained by local pulmonary vascular effects of the drugs.

Current results indicate that in permeability pulmonary edema, relatively small changes in PCWP and/or regional pulmonary vascular effects of certain drugs may affect accumulation of lung water.

References

1. Murray JF: Mechanisms of acute respiratory failure: conference report. Am Rev Respir Dis **115:** 1071, 1977
2. Pontoppidin H, Wilson RS, Rie MA, Schneider RC: Respiratory intensive care. Anesthesiology **47:** 96, 1977
3. Robin ED, Carey LC, Grenvib A, Glauser F, Gaudio R: Capillary leak syndrome with pulmonary edema. Arch Intern Med **130:** 66, 1972
4. Gottlieb SS, Hansen DH, Wood LDH, Long GR: The effect of nitroprusside on edema and O_2 delivery (QO_2) in canine hydrochloric acid (HCl) aspiration. Am Rev Respir Dis **129:** A94, 1984
5. Prewitt RM, McCarthy J, Wood LDH: Treatment of acute low pressure edema in dogs: relative effects of hydrostatic and oncotic pressure, nitroprusside and PEEP. J Clin Invest **67:** 409, 1981
6. Harrison WD, Raizen M, Ghignone M, Girling L, Slykerman LJ, Prewitt RM: Treatment of canine low pressure pulmonary edema. Am Rev Respir Dis **128:** 857, 1983
7. Prewitt RM, Wood LDH: Effect of sodium nitroprusside on cardio-

vascular function and pulmonary shunt in canine oleic acid pulmonary edema. Anesthesiology **55:** 537, 1981
8. Wood LDH, Prewitt RM: Cardiovascular management in acute hypoxemic respiratory failure. Am J Cardiol **47:** 963, 1981
9. Leier CV, Heban PT, Huss P, Bush CA, Lewis RP: Comparative systemic and regional hemodynamic effects of dopamine and dobutamine in patients with cardiomyopathic heart failure. Circulation **58:** 466, 1978
10. Loeb HS, Bredakis J, Gunner RM: Superiority of dobutamine over dopamine for augmentation of cardiac output in patients with chronic low output cardiac failure. Circulation **55:** 375, 1977
11. Ali J, Chernicki W, Wood LDH: The effect of furosemide in canine low pressure pulmonary edema. J Clin Invest **64:** 1494, 1979
12. Franciosa JA, Cohn JN: Hemodynamic responsiveness of short and long-acting vasodilators in left ventricular failure. Am J Med **65:** 126, 1975
13. Rubin LJ, Peter RH: Oral hydralazine therapy for primary pulmonary hypertension. N Engl J Med **302:** 69, 1980
14. Rubin LJ, Peter RH: Hemodynamics at rest and during exercise alter oral hydralazine in patients with cor pulmonale. Am J Cardiol **47:** 116, 1981
15. Ghignone M, Girling L, Prewitt RM: Effects of hydralazine on cardiopulmonary function in canine low pressure pulmonary edema. Anesthesiology **59:** 15, 1983
16. Kirk BW, Raber MB: A practical apparatus for rapid determinations of blood oxygen content. J Appl Physiol **34:** 724, 1973
17. Gelb AF, Klein E: Hemodynamic and alveolar protein studies in noncardiac pulmonary edema. Am Rev Respir Dis **114:** 831, 1976
18. Packer M, Meller J, Medina N, Gorlin R, Herman MV: Importance of left ventricular chamber size in determining the response to hydralazine in severe chronic heart failure. N Engl J Med **303:** 250, 1980

Correlation between refractory periods and activation-recovery intervals from electrograms: effects of rate and adrenergic interventions

C. KAY MILLAR, M.D., FANY A. KRALIOS, M.D., AND ROBERT L. LUX, PH.D.

ABSTRACT Unipolar electrograms from ventricular epicardium in dogs were analyzed for the timing of local excitation and repolarization with computer assistance. The most rapid decrease in voltage in the QRS (dV/dt min) was used to determine local excitation time, and the maximum rate of voltage increase (dV/dt max) near the peak of the T wave was used to time local repolarization. The difference between dV/dt min and dV/dt max, the activation-recovery interval, is theoretically related to the net effect of the durations of the action potentials at that site. Paired data for refractory periods and activation-recovery intervals obtained from the same electrodes during fixed activation orders were obtained before and during repolarization changes induced by changes in cycle length, infusion of norepinephrine, and cardiac sympathetic nerve stimulation. Correlation coefficients were close to 1.00 and standard errors were 2.0 to 4.3 msec for changes at individual sites. Pooling of data from multiple sites increased standard errors and reduced correlation coefficients. Results provide quantification of errors in the use of unipolar electrograms to time local repolarization changes induced by variations in rate and adrenergic tone. They should increase the practical usefulness of the unipolar electrogram as a tool for assessing the time course and spatial distribution of repolarization changes.
Circulation 72, No. 6, 1372–1379, 1985.

IMPROVED METHODS for assessing spatial distributions and rapid temporal changes in cardiac repolarization properties would enhance studies of repolarization effects on arrhythmiogenesis. The measurement of refractory period has been widely used to assess repolarization, since it is known to approximate the duration of the transmembrane action potential in certain circumstances,[1] and individual measurements can be obtained easily and reproducibly. However, there are limitations to using refractory periods for assessing spatial distributions and rapid changes, since only one site can be sampled at a time and each determination of refractory period requires several seconds for completion.

Information regarding the timing of regional repolarization is present in electrograms recorded from the heart, and such recordings have the advantage that multiple sites may be sampled simultaneously and beat-to-beat measures of repolarization changes thus are possible. In spite of this important advantage, because the relationship between the T waveform in electrograms and regional electrophysiologic properties is a complex one,[2] direct recording methods for assessing local repolarization times have not been optimally investigated and validated.

A method has been reported from our laboratory by Wyatt et al,[3, 4] in which the timing of the maximum rate of rise in voltage (dV/dt max) in the T wave of direct unipolar electrograms is related to the timing of the downstroke of the intracellular action potential. An activation-recovery interval is obtained between the time of local activation and repolarization, which is comparable to the duration of the local action potential and refractory period. Although correlations between transmembrane action potential durations and the electrogram-derived values were sufficiently high in those studies to support the theoretical validity of the method, the data were not adequate to optimally evaluate its practical utility, particularly for repolarization changes caused by adrenergic interventions.

The purposes of this study are (1) to provide further

From the Nora Eccles Harrison Cardiovascular Research and Training Institute and the Department of Internal Medicine, University of Utah School of Medicine, Salt Lake City.

Supported by Program Project grant HL13480 and grant HL17367 from the NHLBI, and by awards from the Nora Eccles Treadwell Foundation and the Richard A. and Nora Eccles Harrison Fund for Cardiovascular Research.

Address for correspondence: C. Kay Millar, M.D., Nora Eccles Harrison Cardiovascular Research and Training Institute, University of Utah School of Medicine, Salt Lake City, UT 84112.

Received Oct. 30, 1984; revision accepted August 22, 1985.

evaluation of activation-recovery intervals from unipolar electrograms in relation to the durations of regional refractoriness, (2) to estimate the errors in using unipolar electrograms to measure changes in repolarization time at individual sites and between sites during changes in cycle length and adrenergic influences, and (3) to improve the practical utility of the method as a laboratory and clinical tool.

Methods

Experimental protocol. Experiments were done in 11 dogs anesthetized with sodium pentobarbital (30 mg/kg) and additional smaller doses as needed. The heart was exposed by a midsternal incision and cradled in the opened pericardium. The sinus node was crushed to permit pacing at slow heart rates. A bipolar electrode on the right atrial appendage was used for S_1 pacing. The central connections of the vagi and stellate ganglia were cut to diminish spontaneous fluctuations in autonomic neural effects on ventricular repolarization. In some dogs the ventral lateral cardiac nerve and/or left ventral ansa were isolated for later stimulation. An array of 75 fine silver wire unipolar electrodes, mounted on a nylon sock to produce uniform electrode spacing over the entire heart, was stretched over the heart and anchored near the pericardial reflexion. This array was alternately connected by a switch to the output of the stimulator for measuring refractory periods and to the system for recording electrograms.

In each experiment, refractory periods and activation-recovery intervals were measured as described below at six to eight sites. Sites varied among experiments and were selected from the 75 available leads in the sock array from the anterior, lateral, and posterior left ventricle and variable locations on the right ventricle. Immediately after completion of refractory period measurements, electrograms were recorded from those sites during three activation orders induced by bipolar pacing of the atrium, the left ventricle and atrium simultaneously, and the right ventricle and atrium simultaneously, at the same rate. Electrograms were analyzed later, as described below, to determine activation-recovery intervals. The relationship between paired refractory periods and activation-recovery intervals was studied during repolarization changes induced by variable pacing rate in one experiment, by variable pacing rate and graded norepinephrine (8 μg/ml iv) in six other experiments, and by variable pacing rate and cardiac sympathetic neural stimulation in four others. Stimulus parameters for cardiac sympathetic neural stimulations were 5 Hz, 4 msec pulse duration, and current adequate to induce T wave changes in lead II of the body surface electrocardiogram. All data considered stable and acceptable at the time of collection were included in the final analysis. A total of 76 sites was sampled, and there were 2312 paired observations.

Refractory period measurements. Heart rate was controlled by simultaneous fixed rate bipolar pacing (S_1) of the atrium and unipolar pacing (S_1) of the ventricular site being tested. S_1 ventricular stimuli and S_2 ventricular premature test stimuli were 2 msec cathodal unipolar square pulses at two times diastolic threshold voltage. The S_2 stimulus was delivered to the ventricular test site after every eighth S_1, starting with a short S_1-S_2 and incrementing S_2 in 1 msec steps. The refractory period was the shortest S_1-S_2 at which a propagated response to S_2 occurred. Rate was controlled by atrial pacing between observations and for at least 5 min at a new rate before refractory period determinations. Refractory periods at six to eight sites on the sock array were obtained in sequence and the bank was repeated until each site was reproducible to 2 msec or less. Thresholds were determined before each set of refractory periods in the baseline state and during adrenergic interventions. Data collection was discontinued from sites at which thresholds or refractory periods were unstable. Most such deletions occurred at the beginning of experiments, and an alternative site was studied.

Activation-recovery interval. The amplification-multiplexing system for unipolar mapping of the body surface or cardiac surface has been described previously.[5] All 75 epicardial sites from the sock array were recorded against a Wilson central terminal, although only the six to eight test sites were finally analyzed. In two additional experiments, the results of which are presented separately, comparisons of activation-recovery intervals were made during recording of electrograms against a Wilson central terminal an a left hind leg electrode.

Electrograms were displayed on an oscilloscope for monitoring the quality of records and initial selection of test sites. Electrograms were recorded at a band width of 0.03 to 500 Hz, gain of 50 or 82, and sampling rate of 1000 samples/sec/channel. Input impedence was 10^{12} ohms and noise referred to input was 2 μV P-P. An analog-to-digital converter with input range of ± 5 V was used to transfer the multiplexed signals at 10 bits resolution to digital magnetic tape.

Data were analyzed later with a semiautomated computer program for recognizing the maximum negative slope in the QRS (dV/dt min) and the maximum positive slope in the T wave (dV/dt max) of individual complexes, without signal averaging. A smoothing procedure using parabolic least-squares fit was done to minimize effects of noise. The first-pass used broad time windows for finding dV/dt min and dV/dt max to make the program accept a wide range of heart rates and waveforms. Each electrogram, its first derivative, and first-pass computer-calculated timing indicators for dV/dt min and dV/dt were displayed on a graphics terminal. When timing indicators were obviously incorrect, a second-pass calculation was done with a manually operated cursor after narrower time windows were set on the electrogram. For negative T waves dV/dt max occurred after the nadir of the T, while for positive T waves dV/dt max was before the peak of the T. Notched positive T waves were frequently encountered, and dV/dt max was taken on the upslope of the second peak. When T waves were diphasic, the positive phase occurred after the negative phase, and dV/dt max was taken on the upslope of the positive peak. Hard copies were made of accepted waveforms, timing indicators, and calculations of activation-recovery intervals derived from the difference between the times of dV/dt min and dV/dt max. The computer operator had no knowledge of determinations of refractory period when processing electrogram data.

Data analysis. Paired data comparing refractory periods to activation-recovery intervals during each of the three activation orders and classified according to T waveform were analyzed by linear regression analysis. Correlations were examined for individual sites and for data pooled from all sites in the same experiment.

Results

Sample data from three experiments are shown in figures 1 to 3. These computer printouts show waveforms of simultaneously recorded electrograms and graphic and numeric time indicators for dV/dt min and dV/dt max. Comparison of the activation-recovery interval with the refractory period for that site is tabulated to the right of each electrogram.

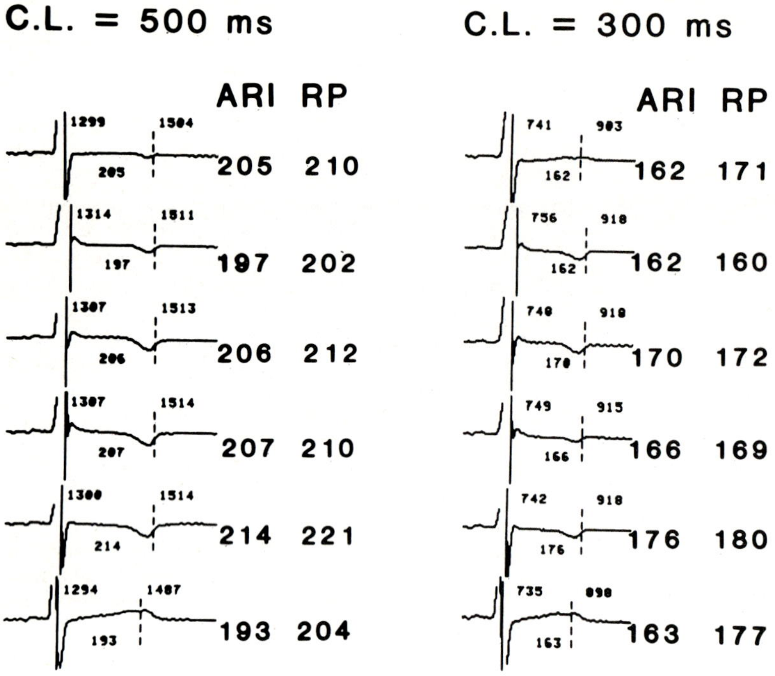

FIGURE 1. Comparison of refractory periods with activation-recovery intervals at six simultaneously recorded sites at two paced cycle lengths during atrial drive. RP = refractory period; ARI = activation-recovery interval; C.L. = cycle length. Vertical solid line in each QRS complex and number above each QRS represents the computer calculation of activation time (dV/dt min) at that site. Dotted vertical line in each T wave and number above each T wave represents the computer calculation of recovery time (dV/dt max) at that site. Calculated ARIs are computer printed below each waveform. Errors in timing dV/dt min and dV/dt max, due to noise, are reflected in the lower two complexes.

Figure 1 illustrates unipolar electrogram–derived activation-recovery interval and changes in refractory period induced by changing cycle length during atrial pacing. Repolarization changes were of the order of 30 to 40 msec. For these data, differences between the two measurements for individual comparisons ranged from 2 to 11 msec, with a mean ± SD of 4 ± 4.2 msec. For rate changes, the repolarization changes at individual sites assessed by the two methods differed by 3.5 ± 2.3 msec, with a range of 0 to 7 msec. This illustrates a finding supported by analysis of all experiments, summarized below, that the unipolar electrogram method is better for estimating changes in refractory period at individual sites than for estimating the absolute value of individual refractory period measurements. In the case illustrated in figure 1, the mean differences are similar but there is less variability in the estimates of changes in refractory period than of the absolute values.

In figure 2, refractory periods and activation-recov-

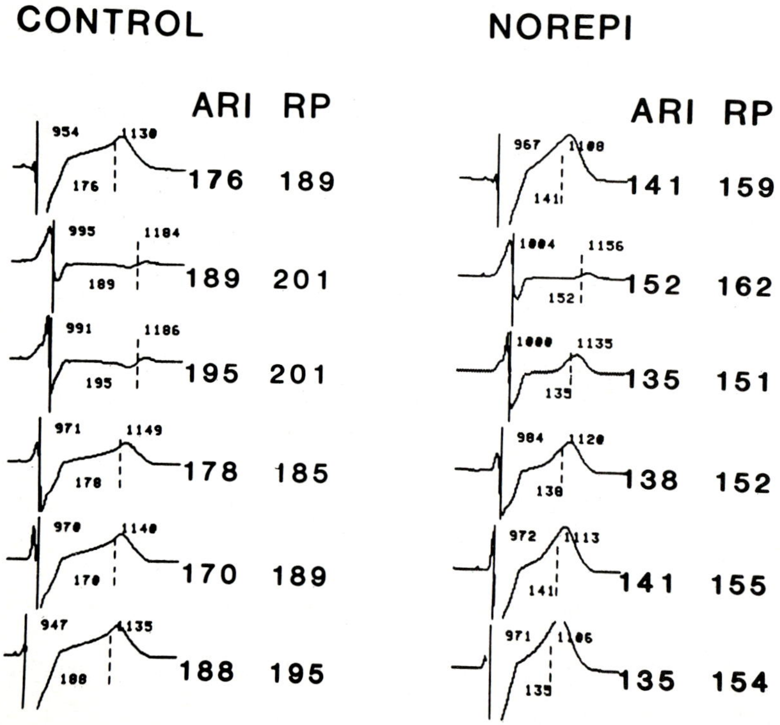

FIGURE 2. Comparison of refractory periods with activation-recovery intervals at six simultaneously recorded sites before and during infusion of norepinephrine. The right ventricle was paced at a fixed cycle length of 400 msec. Norepi = norepinephrine. Other abbreviations and format are the same as for figure 1.

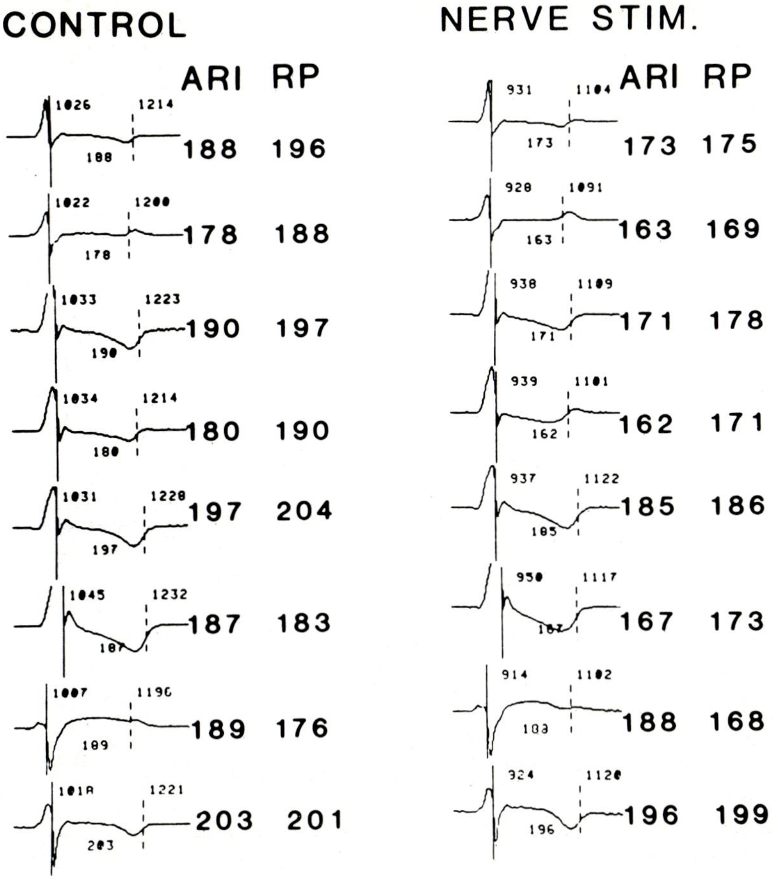

FIGURE 3. Comparison of refractory periods with activation-recovery intervals at eight simultaneously recorded sites before and during stimulation of the ventral lateral cardiac nerve. The left ventricle was paced at a fixed cycle length of 400 msec. The upper six electrograms are from sites on the posterior heart surface, and the lower two are from the anterior surface. Format and abbreviations are as in figure 1.

ery intervals are compared during changes induced by graded infusion of norepinephrine in another experiment. There were major changes in repolarization times and T waveforms, and in one lead there was reversal of T wave polarity.

Figure 3 shows repolarization changes at eight simultaneously recorded sites in another experiment during fixed rate pacing of the left ventricle, before and during stimulation of the ventral lateral cardiac nerve. The upper six traces are from sites on the posterior surface of the heart in the known functional distribution of the nerve,[6] showing refractory period and activation-recovery interval shortening of 10 to 21 msec during nerve stimulation. The lower two traces are from sites on the anterior heart surface, where stimulation of the ventral lateral nerve is expected to have less effect on repolarization. Repolarization changes were not as great as those illustrated for rate changes and infusion of norepinephrine in figures 1 and 2. End points were taken when refractory period measurements had stabilized, after the peak of refractory period and T wave changes.

Plots of data points and regression coefficients from one experiment are shown in figure 4. Refractory period vs activation-recovery interval from electrograms during left ventricular pacing for six sites are shown, with paired observations at variable cycle lengths (*A*) and during infusion of norepinephrine at fixed rate (*B*). For variable rate, correlation coefficients (r) ranged from .98 to 1.00 for individual sites. For pooled data from all sites, r was slightly less at .97. Standard errors were 0.2 to 2.6 msec for individual sites and 4.3 msec for pooled sites. For individual sites there was considerable variation in slopes of the regression lines, while the slope for pooled sites was 1.05, very close to the theoretical prediction of 1.00. For changes caused by norepinephrine, slopes of regression lines are less steep than those for rate interventions. Standard errors are comparable to those for rate interventions. The paired data from figure 4, *A* and *B*, are combined in panel *C*, showing a slight increase in standard errors with the combined intervention, but which are still less than 5 msec.

Regression analysis of data from each of the experiments is summarized in table 1. For repolarization changes at individual sites caused by rate changes, norepinephrine, and sympathetic nerve stimulation, correlation coefficients averaged .97 to .99 for fixed activation sequences. Standard errors for these correlations were small, with those induced by nerve stimula-

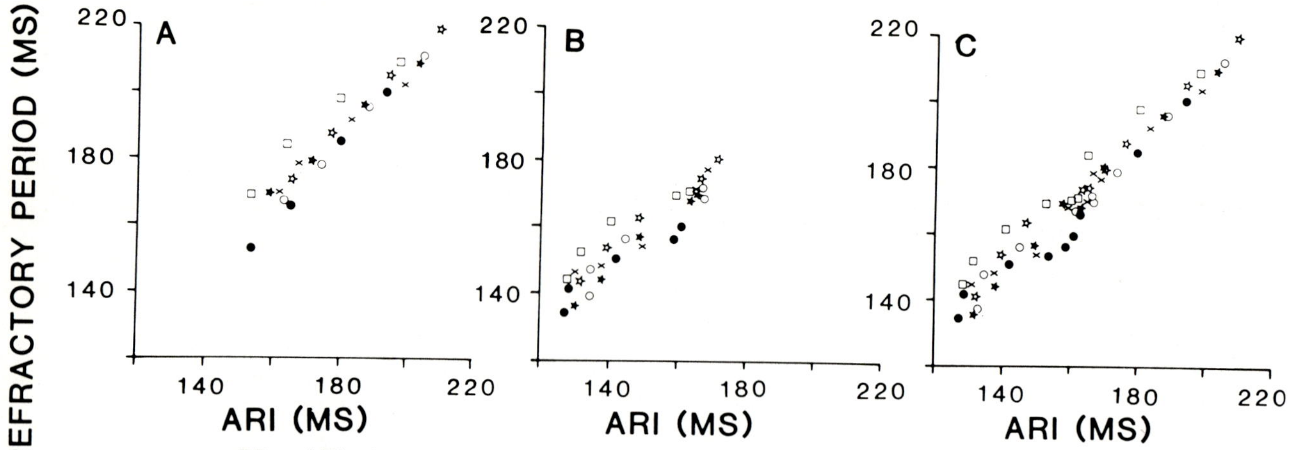

A — RP = aARI + b

Site	a	b	r	SEE
□	0.92	30	0.98	2.6
●	1.20	−30	1.00	0.5
○	1.08	−8	1.00	0.9
✶	0.96	16	1.00	0.2
☆	1.06	−1	1.00	0.6
×	0.90	28	1.00	1.1
×☆✶○□●	1.05	−5	0.97	4.3

B — RP = aARI + b

Site	a	b	r	SEE
□	0.70	58	0.96	2.9
●	0.61	61	0.96	2.4
○	0.83	32	0.97	2.9
✶	0.99	8	1.00	0.9
☆	0.89	27	0.99	2.0
×	0.87	28	0.98	2.4
×☆✶○□●	0.82	35	0.94	4.3

C — RP = aARI + b

Site	a	b	r	SEE
□	0.93	26	0.98	4.2
●	0.92	17	0.97	4.7
○	0.98	11	0.99	3.0
✶	1.00	3	1.00	1.3
☆	0.99	13	1.00	2.1
×	0.94	18	0.99	2.4
×☆✶○□●	0.97	14	0.98	4.7

FIGURE 4. Refractory period vs activation-recovery interval during repolarization changes. RP = aARI + b is the regression equation with a = slope, b = RP intercept, r = correlation coefficient, and SEE = standard error of the estimate. ARIs were obtained during left ventricular pacing. *A*, RP vs ARI at variable cycle lengths from 300 to 500 msec (n = 4 for each individual site). *B*, RP vs ARI during graded infusion of norepinephrine in the same animal, at a fixed cycle length of 300 msec (n = 5 for each individual site). *C*, RP vs ARI for rate and iv norepinephrine interventions combined (n = 9 for each site).

tions slightly higher than those for other interventions. Pooling data from multiple sites reduced r values and increased standard errors. Correlations appear closer, on average, for ventricular pacing sites when compared with results during atrial pacing. However, there were experiments in which atrial pacing gave better correlations than did ventricular drive. The ranges shown in parentheses at the bottom of the table indicate the range of slopes for individual sites for all experiments. For rate interventions, slopes averaged close to 1.00 when data were pooled for each experiment. Slopes for individual sites during infusion of norepinephrine also showed variation and on average were less than 1.00.

Most, but not all, of the values for activation-recovery intervals were smaller than their paired refractory periods. Table 2, which summarizes data pooled from all experiments, shows the average differences between the values for activation-recovery intervals and refractory periods when calculated algebraically with sign preserved and when calculated for the absolute difference between the two. For all three activation orders, activation-recovery intervals were less than RPs. Average absolute differences were only slightly greater than average algebraic differences because of the few pairs in which refractory periods were shorter than activation-recovery intervals. Table 2 also summarizes average slopes of regression lines for all interventions, with pooled data from all experiments.

The relationship between basic cycle length and the slope (a) of the regression line in response to infusion of norepinephrine was examined for those six experiments. For pooled data from experiments in which the basic pacing cycle length was 300 (n = 3), 325 (n = 2), and 400 msec (n = 1), the respective slopes were .78, .85, and .92. In the one experiment with a basic cycle length of 400 msec, the noradrenalin induced repolarization changes were as marked as in the other five experiments and were of the order of 60 to 70 msec.

Refractory period vs activation-recovery interval for rate and norepinephrine interventions was examined in relation to T wave polarity, rather than pacing site, using the same data as in tables 1 and 2. Results are summarized in table 3. Negative T waves gave activation-recovery intervals that were closest, on average, to corresponding refractory periods. Correlation coefficients (r) and standard errors (SEE) were approximately the same for all T waveforms during rate changes, but change in T polarity during norepineph-

TABLE 1
Summary for changes at individual sites and pooled data for individual experiments

	Variable rate	Variable IV norepi.	Var. rate & var. norepi.	Var. rate & symp. nerve stm.
No. of experiments	11	6	6	4
No. of sites	76	36	36	32
Average r for RP vs ARI for individual sites				
AT DR	.98	.97	.98	.98
RV DR	.99	.98	.99	.99
LV DR	.98	.98	.99	.99
Average SEE (msec) for RP vs ARI for individual sites				
AT DR	2.7	2.8	3.6	4.3
RV DR	2.7	2.2	3.3	3.9
LV DR	2.5	2.0	2.9	3.5
Average r for pooled data (6–8 sites) in each dog				
AT DR	.95	.91	.96	.94
RV DR	.96	.96	.98	.96
LV DR	.96	.94	.98	.96
Average SEE (msec) for pooled data				
AT DR	6.1	6.0	6.1	8.6
RV DR	4.9	4.0	4.4	7.0
LV DR	5.5	4.7	4.9	7.8
For RP = aARI + b: avg. & range of a (slope)				
AT DR	.99 (.50–1.46)	.84 (.45–1.56)	.89 (.62–1.13)	1.01 (.78–1.15)
RV DR	1.04 (.54–1.47)	.80 (.52–1.11)	.89 (.59–1.07)	1.02 (.88–1.15)
LV DR	.98 (.48–1.43)	.86 (.45–1.33)	.87 (.56–1.09)	1.02 (.78–1.20)

AT = atrial; RV = right ventricular; LV = left ventricular; DR = drive. See legend to figure 4 for additional abbreviations.

TABLE 2
Summary for pooled data from all experiments

	Variable rate	Variable IV norepi.	Variable symp. nerve stm.	All interventions
No. of experiments	11	6	4	11
No. of sites	76	36	32	76
ARI minus RP; avg. ± SD (msec)				
AT DR	−8.9±8.1	−10.5±8.7	−11.5±10.5	−9.5±8.7
RV DR	−12.5±6.3	−14.6±6.1	−14.9±8.8	−13.6±6.8
LV DR	−9.3±7.4	−10.9±6.2	−12.5±9.5	−10.2±7.5
Absolute value of ARI minus RP; avg. ± SD (msec)				
AT DR	9.7±7.1	10.8±8.2	12.3±9.6	10.2±7.9
RV DR	12.6±6.2	14.6±6.0	14.9±8.8	13.6±6.7
LV DR	9.9±6.6	11.0±6.0	12.9±9.0	10.7±6.8
For RP = aARI + b; avg. slope (a)				
AT DR	.96	.82	.81	.93
RV DR	1.00	.89	.86	.96
LV DR	.98	.90	.85	.95
No. of paired observations				
AT DR	502	234	128	784
RV DR	502	234	128	776
LV DR	478	234	120	752

See table 1 and legend to figure 4 for abbreviations.

TABLE 3
Summary of data from all experiments with rate and norepinephrine interventions, according to T wave polarity

	Variable rate	Variable IV norepi.
ARI minus RP; average (msec)		
pooled data		
T (−)	−5.7	−8.2
T (+)	−11.7	−14.1
T (− +)	−5.4	−7.2
TΔ	A	−8.7
For RP = aARI + b; r		
T (−)	.99 (.97)	.99 (.97)
T (+)	.99 (.97)	.97 (.95)
T (− +)	.99 (.97)	.96 (.92)
TΔ	A	.98 (.96)
For RP = aARI + b; SEE (msec)		
T (−)	1.6 (6.3)	1.8 (4.4)
T (+)	1.0 (5.4)	2.4 (5.0)
T (− +)	1.5 (5.4)	2.7 (5.0)
TΔ	A	2.6 (5.9)
For RP = aARI + b; average slope (a); pooled data		
T (−)	.95	.87
T (+)	.97	.79
T (− +)	.89	.69
TΔ	A	.80

T (−) = negative T waves; T (+) = positive T waves; T (− +) = biphasic T waves; TΔ = T wave polarity change with intervention. See table 1 and legend to figure 4 for other abbreviations. Correlation coefficients (r) and SEE are averages of r and SEE for individual sites, with average r and SEE for pooled data from all experiments in parentheses.

[A]Too few data for analysis.

rine had a small adverse effect on r and SEE. T polarity change during rate interventions was a rare event and was not statistically evaluated.

For 37 electrograms in two additional dogs, activation-recovery intervals were compared for Wilson central terminal and left hind limb indifferent electrodes. The absolute difference in the intervals was 0 to 0.3 msec, with an average of 1.3 msec. There was no systematic relationship of the magnitude or sign of the difference to T wave polarity or pacing site.

Discussion

This study was undertaken to provide further evaluation of a method for measurement of the timing of regional myocardial repolarization directly from unipolar electrograms. Unlike another method for assessing repolarization changes from electrograms, which uses changes in QRST areas,[7,8] the present method results in a number that approximates the refractory period.

The results document a close correlation between the unipolar electrogram measure of activation-recovery interval and refractory periods during the interventions of altered rate and adrenergic influences. The correlations obtained were considerably higher than those reported for the same method in previous studies from this laboratory, in which intervals derived from unipolar and bipolar electrograms were also compared with the durations of transmembrane action potentials.[3,4] The major reasons for this are, we believe, the much greater ease of determining refractory periods than of maintaining stable transmembrane action potentials, the larger number of paired data in the present experiments, and because measurements at identical sites rather than adjacent sites were compared in the present experiments.

The findings of the present study indicate a close correlation between the electrogram method and refractory periods during changes in rate and infusion of norepinephrine and somewhat lower correlations during repolarization changes induced by neural stimulation. In our opinion the reason for this is more likely the difficulty of obtaining stable and comparable refractory periods during the changing state associated with nerve stimulation than diminished applicability of the method to neurally induced repolarization changes. In these and previous experiments we have observed that refractory period shortening induced by cardiac sympathetic neural stimulation subsides during continued nerve stimulation in the absence of threshold changes and that the accompanying electrocardiographic changes do not defervesce as rapidly as do the refractory period changes.[6]

Although recovery time should correlate with the timing of action potential downstroke, the activation-recovery interval is not expected to be precisely equal in duration to refractory period. Because timing of the effective refractory period is expected to occur a little later than the most rapid portion of the action potential downstroke,[1] the activation-recovery interval should be systematically a little shorter than the corresponding refractory period. The finding in this study that activation-recovery intervals averaged on the order of 10 msec shorter than refractory periods while maintaining high correlations during changes is consistent with the theoretic basis of the method.

The activation-recovery interval provides a more precise estimate of repolarization changes at a particular site than of repolarization differences between sites. As shown in table 1, the standard error of the estimate for changes at individual sites averaged 2 to 4 msec and between sites (pooled data) averaged 4 to 9 msec. This degree of precison makes the method useful for many experimental purposes, and the ability to evaluate changes at many sites simultaneously can be exploited statistically to further minimize the effect of errors in individual estimates.

Although the activation-recovery interval should be largely independent of activation order, the three activation orders did not generally result in near identical activation-recovery intervals for individual observations. Pooling of data from all three activation orders, not shown in the tables, increased standard errors. This finding and the deviation of regression slopes for paired data from the predicted value of 1.00 may be due at least in part to distant electrocardiographic effects that vary from site to site and with activation order. This explanation is supported by the findings that use of pooled data from multiple sites during cycle length changes resulted in regression slopes close to 1.00 (table 1) and average activation-recovery intervals that were within 3 msec for the three activation orders (table 2). Because of the variable distant electrocardiographic effects in unipolar electrograms, measurements from fixed activation orders are recommended for assessing local repolarization changes.

An additional source of error for regression slopes calculated for individual sites may be sample size, since for many of the regression calculations n was as small as four for single interventions at individual sites. Sample size, however, cannot entirely explain the variations in regression slopes for individual sites, since the associated r values were high.

For repolarization changes caused by infusion of norepinephrine, average slopes were less than 1.0, and the reason for this is not certain. Norepinephrine resulted in marked repolarization shortening, probably exceeding changes that occur clinically or physiologically. T wave morphology changed substantially, displacing ST segments and possibly inducing errors in determining the dV/dt max end point. The finding that regression slopes were closer to 1.00 for norepinephrine-induced changes when the basic pacing rate was slower, supports this explanation. Other sources of error with marked norepinephrine effect are change in action potential waveform and in the relationship between action potential downstroke and refractoriness.

Of the three T waveform classes (negative, positive, and biphasic) negative T waves gave activation-recovery intervals that were closer to refractory period values, gave higher correlation coefficients and lower standard errors more often than other waveforms, and gave regression slopes closer to 1.0 during infusion of norepinephrine. It was our impression that positive T waves were more likely than negative T waves to have ambiguous end points due to increased ST elevation and T wave rounding during infusion of norepinephrine and during very fast rates. These data were not excluded and may be at least a partial explanation for the apparent statistical advantage of negative as compared with positive T waves. The theoretical and practical reasons for T polarity influence on the method deserve further investigation.

The experiments presented here do not address the issue of the relative merits of unipolar vs bipolar recordings for timing ventricular repolarization. For bipolar electrograms, the peak of the T wave should represent the time of most rapid action potential downstrokes at sampled sites, in the same way that the dV/dt max does so in unipolar recordings, and a limited validation of the bipolar method in comparison to refractory periods has been reported by Martins et al.[9] In that report, correlations were statistically significant, but r values were considerably less than those obtained in the present report, standard errors were not presented, and data scatter appeared greater. The two studies are not comparable, however, because of the limited scope of the validation portion of that study and the different interventions used in these two studies.

References

1. Hoffman BF, Kao CY, Suckling EE: Refractoriness in cardiac muscle. Am J Physiol **190:** 473, 1957
2. Spach MS, Barr RC, Serwer GA, Kootsey JM, Johnson EA: Extracellular potentials related to intracellular action potentials in the dog Purkinje system. Circ Res **30:** 505, 1972
3. Wyatt RF: Comparison of estimates of activation and recovery times from bipolar and unipolar electrograms to *in vivo* transmembrane action potential durations. Proc. IEEE/Engineering in Medicine and Biology Society 2nd Annual Conference, Washington, DC, pp 22–25, Sept. 1980
4. Wyatt RF, Burgess MJ, Evans AK, Lux RL, Abildskov JA, Tsutsumi T: Estimation of ventricular transmembrane action potential durations and repolarization times from unipolar electrograms. Am J Cardiol **47:** 488, 1981
5. Wyatt RF: Instrumentation for mapping electrocardiographic potential distributions. IEEE Engineering in Medicine and Biology Society First Annual Conference, Oct. 1979, p 141
6. Kralios FA, Martin L, Burgess MJ, Millar CK: Local ventricular repolarization changes due to sympathetic nerve branch stimulation. Am J Physiol **228:** 1621, 1975
7. Abildskov JA, Evans AK, Lux RL, Burgess MJ: Ventricular recovery properties and the QRST deflection area in cardiac electrograms. Am J Physiol **239:** H227, 1980
8. Lux RL, Abildskov JA, Wyatt RF, Evans AK, Burgess MJ: Estimation of ventricular repolarization duration and disparity from distributions of QRST area. Am J Cardiol **47:** 489, 1981
9. Martins JB, Zipes DP, Lund DD: Distribution of local repolarization changes produced by efferent vagal stimulation in the canine ventricles. J Am Coll Cardiol **2:** 1191, 1983

Kinetics of electrophysiologic changes during oral loading of amiodarone and after withdrawal of amiodarone in the unsedated dog*

ISHIK C. TUNA, M.D., ANCHEN QI, M.D., CHARLES GORNICK, M.D.,
R. MORTON BOLMAN III, M.D.,** AND DAVID G. BENDITT, M.D.

ABSTRACT We examined the temporal kinetics of onset and offset of the cardiac electrophysiologic effects of orally administered amiodarone in chronically instrumented, unsedated adult dogs (n = 8). Right atrial (RA), atrioventricular nodal (AVN), and right ventricular (RV) effective refractory period (ERP), and AVN functional refractory period (FRP), were determined daily for 21 days during amiodarone loading (24 mg/kg/day) and for 21 days after cessation of amiodarone. Left ventricular (LV) ERP was assessed in four of eight animals. Group mean RA-ERP peaked and plateaued early during amiodarone loading (time to reach one-half observed peak change [$t_{1/2}$ onset] = 1.2 ± 0.5 days) and rapidly returned toward baseline after cessation of drug (decay time to one-half peak value [$t_{1/2}$ offset] = 2.0 ± 1.7 days). Group mean RV-ERP rose in a linear manner throughout the loading period ($t_{1/2}$ onset = 9.3 ± 2.1 days) and remained elevated after cessation of drug ($t_{1/2}$ offset > 21.0 days). Group mean AVN-ERP and FRP exhibited temporal kinetics intermediate between those of the RA-ERP and RV-ERP, both during amiodarone loading and after cessation of the drug. Group mean LV-ERP onset kinetics (assessed in a limited number of animals, n = 4) appeared to differ from RV-ERP onset kinetics ($t_{1/2}$ onset = 2.5 ± 2.5 days), whereas LV-ERP and RV-ERP offset kinetics appeared similar ($t_{1/2}$ offset > 21 days). In summary, our findings demonstrate that during oral loading, the temporal sequence of onset of amiodarone-induced electrophysiologic effects is site dependent. Similarly, after cessation of amiodarone, the persistence of drug-induced electrophysiologic effects is both variable and site dependent.
Circulation 72, No. 6, 1380–1385, 1985.

AMIODARONE is an investigational antiarrhythmic drug, undergoing evaluation for treatment of both ventricular and supraventricular tachyarrhythmias.[1–7] Clinical studies have revealed that amiodarone possesses many novel properties, the foremost being a delayed onset of antiarrhythmic activity and a variable but prolonged half-life of antiarrhythmic activity after oral loading; the latter is estimated to be from 10 to 40 days.[1, 4, 5, 8, 9] To understand the onset and offset characteristics of amiodarone's cardiac electrophysiologic effects more fully, we sought to quantify the time course and magnitude of changes in atrial, atrioventricular nodal and ventricular refractory periods, His-ventricular conduction intervals, and pacing thresholds, during oral loading of amiodarone in an unsedated, chronically instrumented canine preparation. We further sought to determine the time course and magnitude of cardiac electrophysiologic changes after cessation of amiodarone loading. Finally, we wished to determine whether the onset and offset characteristics (i.e., temporal kinetics) of amiodarone-induced cardiac electrophysiologic changes differed among the cardiac tissues evaluated.

From the Departments of Medicine and Surgery, University of Minnesota Medical School, Minneapolis.

Supported in part by Grant-in-Aid funds (HL-29460) from the NIH (Dr. Benditt) and by Grant-in-Aid and Fellowship funds from the American Heart Association, Minnesota Affiliate (Dr. Tuna). These studies were completed during Dr. Benditt's tenure as an Established Investigator of the American Heart Association.

Address for correspondence: Ishik C. Tuna, M.D., Department of Surgery, Box 347 Mayo Memorial Bldg., University of Minnesota Hospitals, Minneapolis, MN 55455.

Received April 29, 1985; revision accepted Aug. 29, 1985.

Presented at the 57th Annual Scientific Sessions of the American Heart Association.

*All editorial decisions for this article, including selection of reviewers and the final disposition, were made by a guest editor. This procedure applies to all manuscripts with authors from the Washington University School of Medicine.

**Present address: Department of Surgery, Washington University School of Medicine, St. Louis.

Methods

Experimental preparation. Adult mongrel dogs under inhalational anesthesia (n = 8) and weighing 21 to 26 kg (mean 24) were instrumented with pairs of bipolar epicardial electrodes for pacing/sensing the right atrium, right ventricle, and in four of eight animals, the left ventricle. A custom-manufactured bipolar epicardial His bundle electrode was additionally implanted in all animals, adjacent to the noncoronary sinus of Valsalva (figure 1).[10] Animals were allowed 3 weeks to recuperate from surgery and conditioned to lie quietly in an unsedated state for subsequent electrophysiologic studies. This preparation yielded stable atrial, ventricular, and His bundle electrograms in all animals throughout the duration of the study.

Experimental protocol. Baseline determinations of atrial, atrioventricular (AV) nodal, and ventricular refractory periods, His-ventricular (HV) conduction intervals, and pacing thresholds were obtained in all animals before administration of amiodarone (Cordarone, LABAZ). Amiodarone (24 mg/kg/day) was administered in a single daily oral dose for 21 days. Electrophysiologic measurements were obtained before each oral dose during the 21 day loading period. Daily electrophysiologic studies were continued for 21 days after cessation of amiodarone. The duration of the loading period (arbitrarily selected) was based on a desire to encompass the conventional 2 to 3 week loading periods typically used clinically.

Electrophysiologic studies. Electrophysiologic studies were carried out in awake unsedated animals conditioned to lie quietly. Right atrial effective refractory period (RA-ERP), AV nodal effective refractory period (AVN-ERP), AV nodal functional refractory period (AVN-FRP), and right and left ventricular effective refractory periods (RV-ERP and LV-ERP) were determined during bipolar pacing at cycle lengths of 450, 400, and 350 msec by means of an 8 beat drive train followed by a single extrastimulus.[11] HV conduction intervals were measured during right atrial pacing at a cycle length of 450 msec.

Pacing and extrastimulus studies were performed at twice diastolic pacing threshold of the tissue being studied (Medtronic 5325 Programmable Stimulator). Electrograms were bandpass filtered (50 to 500 Hz) and amplified (Hewlett-Packard bioelectric amplifier, model 8811A) before being recorded on a multichannel recorder (Hewlett-Packard model 7404A) at a paper

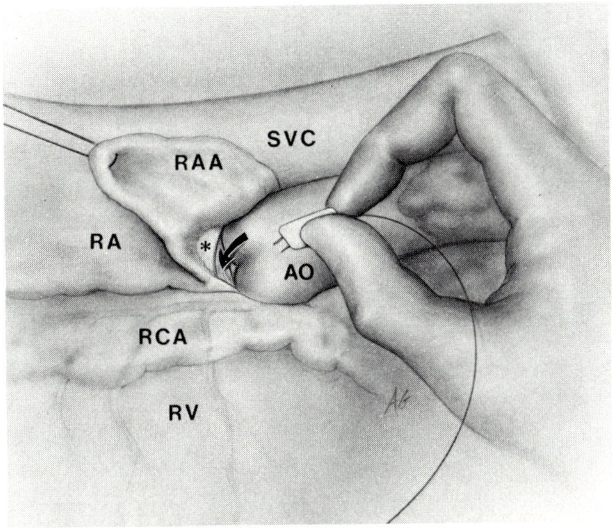

FIGURE 1. Representation of epicardial His bundle electrode implantation. The right atrial appendage (RAA) is retracted to show the aortoatrial groove, developed through dissection of the base of the right atrial appendage (asterisk) off the aorta (AO). The site of electrode implantation (arrow), typically at the junction of the right and noncoronary sinuses of Valsalva, in the aortoatrial groove, is determined via intraoperative His bundle mapping. SVC = superior vena cava; RA = right atrium; RCA = right coronary artery; RV = right ventricle.

speed of 100 mm/sec. A digitizing tablet and interactive computer system (Complot Series 7000 digitizer, DEC, PDP 11/34 digital computer) were used to measure interstimulus and interelectrogram intervals.

Data analysis. Measurements of refractory period were normalized with respect to predrug baseline values and expressed as percent of baseline value. Normalized group mean values (with 95% confidence intervals) were plotted as a function of the day of drug administration (day 0 to day 21) or discontinuance (day 0 to day 21), with day 21 of drug administration corresponding to day 0 of drug discontinuance. Times to reach one-half peak observed change in refractory period during amiodarone loading ($t_{1/2}$ onset) and time to decay to one-half peak observed change in refractory period after cessation of amiodarone ($t_{1/2}$ offset) were determined for each animal at each site evaluated. Student's t test was used to compare group mean $t_{1/2}$ onset values and $t_{1/2}$ offset data. Group mean HV intervals and right atrial, right ventricular, and left ventricular pacing thresholds during amiodarone administration (day 0 vs day 21) and after cessation of amiodarone (day 0 vs day 21) were similarly evaluated.

Results

Changes in measured variables from comparable sites were qualitatively and quantitatively similar among all animals. Group mean values at each site evaluated are therefore presented.

Right atrial refractory periods. Group mean RA-ERP (cycle length [CL] = 450 msec) peaked by approximately day 3 after initiation of oral amiodarone loading and appeared to remain relatively constant for the duration of the 21 day loading period (figure 2, *A*). Mean RA-ERP (CL = 450 msec) plateaued at 18 ± 5% above baseline, with a $t_{1/2}$ onset of 1.2 ± 0.5 days.

After cessation of amiodarone loading, group mean RA-ERP (CL = 450 msec) returned toward baseline with a $t_{1/2}$ offset of 2.0 ± 1.7 days (figure 2, *B*). Findings were comparable at other cycle lengths tested (table 1).

AV nodal refractory periods. Group mean AVN-ERP (CL = 450 msec) increased more slowly and variably than did RA-ERP, reaching an apparent plateau approximately 12 days after initiation of amiodarone loading (figure 3, *A*). Mean AVN-ERP (CL = 450 msec) plateaued at 54 ± 31% above baseline, with a $t_{1/2}$ onset of 5.8 ± 5.2 days. With cessation of amiodarone, group mean AVN-ERP (CL = 450 msec) varied in a complex, biphasic manner (figure 3, *B*), precluding calculation of $t_{1/2}$ offset. AVN-ERP demonstrated a primary return toward baseline occurring within 2 days after cessation of amiodarone, followed by rebound elevation and a secondary decay at 16 days after withdrawal of drug. Group mean AVN-FRP changes paralleled AVN-ERP changes both during and after cessation of oral amiodarone loading. Mean AVN-FRP (CL = 450 msec) plateaued at 36 ± 15% above baseline,

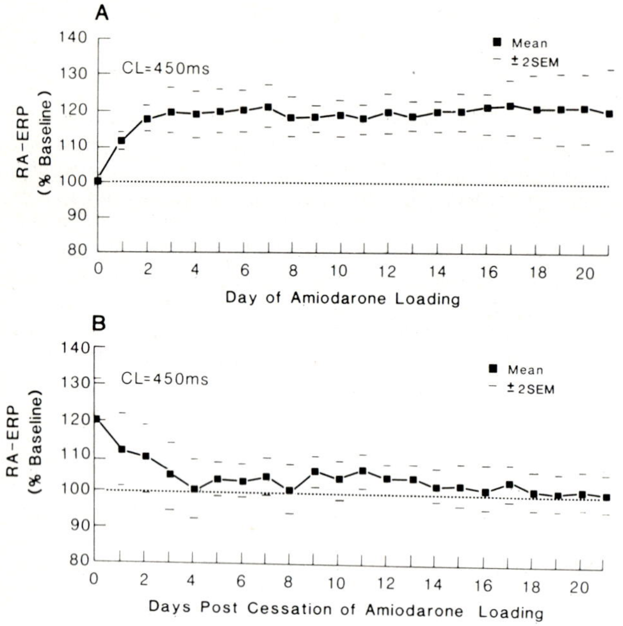

FIGURE 2. Graph depicting the temporal effect of orally administered amiodarone (*A*), or cessation of amiodarone (*B*) on group mean RA-ERP (CL = 450 msec) measured in dogs (n = 8). The ordinate indicates RA-ERP expressed as a percentage of predrug baseline value. The abscissa indicates day of amiodarone administration or withdrawal. Panels *A* and *B* depict measurements of RA-ERP over 42 consecutive days, with day 21 in panel *A* corresponding to day 0 in panel *B*. 95% confidence intervals are indicated for each data point (±2 SEM).

with a $t_{1/2}$ onset of 4.3 ± 3.7 days. AVN-FRP (CL = 450 msec) values, like those of AVN-ERP, decayed in a complex manner after cessation of amiodarone loading. Findings at shorter cycle lengths (400 or 350 msec) could not be evaluated because drug-induced increases in AVN-ERP and AVN-FRP precluded assessment at these cycle lengths.

Right ventricular refractory periods. Group mean RV-ERP (CL = 450 msec) increased in a linear manner throughout the entire 21 day loading period (figure 4, *A*). RV-ERP (CL = 450 msec) rose 21 ± 5% above baseline, with a $t_{1/2}$ onset of 9.3 ± 2.1 days. After cessation of amiodarone, group mean RV-ERP (CL = 450 msec) remained elevated above baseline for the duration of the study, with a $t_{1/2}$ offset of greater than 21 days (figure 4, *B*). Findings at other cycle lengths were similar (table 1).

Left ventricular refractory periods. Group mean LV-ERP (CL = 450 msec) (based on observations in four animals) appeared to peak early, then plateaued at 15 ± 5% above baseline, with a $t_{1/2}$ onset of 2.5 ± 2.5 days (figure 5, *A*). After cessation of amiodarone, group mean LV-ERP (CL = 450 msec) remained elevated above baseline (figure 5, *B*), with a $t_{1/2}$ offset of greater than 21 days. Findings at other cycle lengths were comparable (table 1).

TABLE 1
Kinetics of electrophysiologic change

Refractory period (CL, msec)	$t_{1/2}$ onset (mean ± SD, days)	$t_{1/2}$ offset (mean ± SD, days)	Maximum value (% increase from baseline)
RA-ERP			
450	1.2±0.5[A]	2.0±1.7[A]	18±5
400	1.3±0.5[A]	2.1±1.5[A]	20±8
350	1.2±0.3[A]	2.1±1.2[A]	19±3
AVN-ERP			
450	5.8±5.2	B	56±31
AVN-FRP			
450	4.3±3.7	B	36±15
RV-ERP			
450	9.3±2.1[A]	>21[A]	21±5
400	9.4±3.0[A]	>21[A]	20±5
350	9.3±2.7[A]	>21[A]	20±5
LV-ERP			
450	2.5±2.5	>21	15±5
400	2.5±2.6	>21	15±5
350	2.4±2.5	>21	14±3

[A]$p < .05$, RA vs RV.
[B]Not measured.

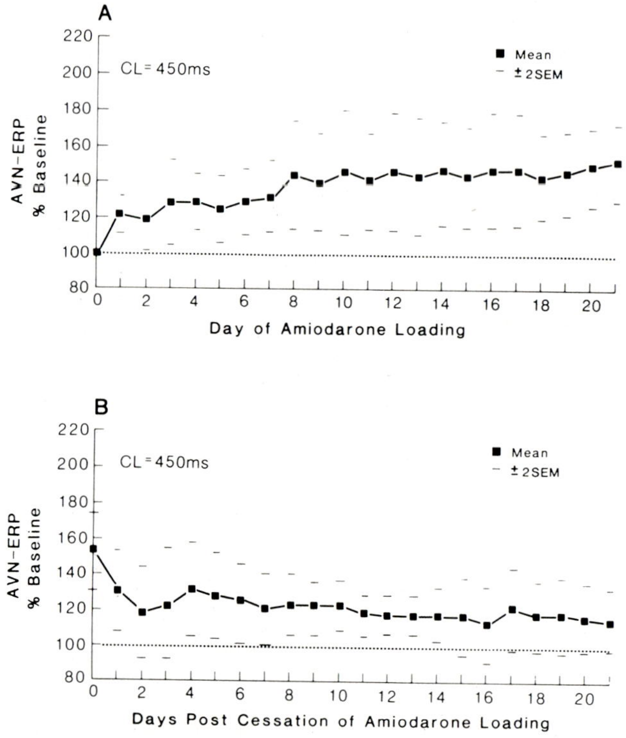

FIGURE 3. Graph depicting the temporal effect of orally administered amiodarone (*A*) or cessation of amiodarone (*B*) on group mean AVN-ERP (CL = 450 msec) measured in dogs (n = 8). The ordinate indicates AVN-ERP expressed as a percentage of predrug baseline value. The abscissa indicates day of amiodarone administration or withdrawal. The format of the figure is otherwise the same as figure 2. 95% confidence intervals are indicated for each data point (±2 SEM).

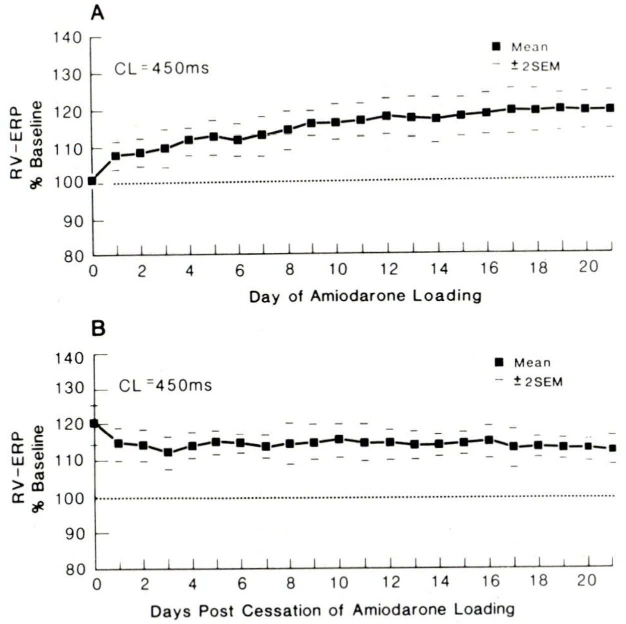

FIGURE 4. Graph depicting the temporal effect of orally administered amiodarone (*A*) or cessation of amiodarone (*B*) on group mean RV-ERP (CL = 450 msec) measured in dogs (n = 8). The ordinate indicates RV-ERP expressed as a percentage of predrug baseline value. The abscissa indicates day of amiodarone administration or withdrawal. The format of the figure is otherwise the same as figure 2. 95% confidence intervals are indicated for each data point (±2 SEM).

HV intervals. Group mean HV intervals (CL = 450 msec) were not significantly altered by amiodarone loading (day 0, 29.1 ± 2.7 msec; day 21, 30.0 ± 2.5 msec, p = NS) or by cessation of amiodarone (day 0, 30.0 ± 2.5 msec; day 21, 29.5 ± 2.9 msec, p = NS).

Pacing thresholds. Although group mean right atrial pacing threshold appeared to rise minimally during oral amiodarone loading, the difference was not statistically significant (day 0, 1.6 ± 0.5 mA; day 21, 1.8 ± 0.8 mA, p = NS), and reversal did not occur after cessation of amiodarone (day 0, 1.8 ± 0.8 mA; day 21, 1.9 ± 0.7 mA, p = NS). Group mean right ventricular pacing threshold behaved similarly during amiodarone loading (day 0, 1.7 ± 0.9 mA; day 21, 1.9 ± 0.9 mA, p = NS) and after cessation of amiodarone (day 0, 1.9 ± 0.9 mA; day 21, 2.0 ± 0.9 mA, p = NS), as did group mean left ventricular pacing threshold (amiodarone loading: day 0, 0.8 ± 0.4 mA, day 21, 3.0 ± 2.7 mA, p = NS; cessation of amiodarone administration: day 0, 3.0 ± 2.7 mA, day 21, 3.2 ± 2.6 mA, p = NS).

Discussion

Four principal observations regarding the temporal sequence of electrophysiologic effects of orally administered amiodarone were made in this study: (1) The temporal onset of amiodarone's electrophysiologic actions progressed at variable, site-dependent rates. Specifically, the maximal effect of amiodarone on right atrial refractoriness occurred before its maximal effect on AV nodal refractoriness, which in turn occurred before its maximal effect on right ventricular refractoriness. (2) Offset kinetics of electrophysiologic effects after cessation of amiodarone demonstrated similar site-dependent characteristics, with right atrial effects regressing before AV nodal effects, while regression of right and left ventricular effects were minimal during this time. (3) Amiodarone-induced changes in the electrophysiologic properties of the right atrium, AV node, right ventricle and left ventricle regressed in a complex, biphasic manner after withdrawal of drug. (4) Amiodarone had no effect on conduction through the His-Purkinje system, as assessed by HV interval measurements.

Changes in refractory period during administration of amiodarone. Clinical studies have attempted to assess the electrophysiologic effects of amiodarone serially during oral loading. Wellens et al.[3] assessed RA-ERP, AVN-ERP, and RV-ERP in 15 patients before and after 14 days of oral amiodarone loading (6.3 g total loading dose); RA-ERP and AVN-ERP rose 20% and 39% above predrug levels, respectively, whereas RV-

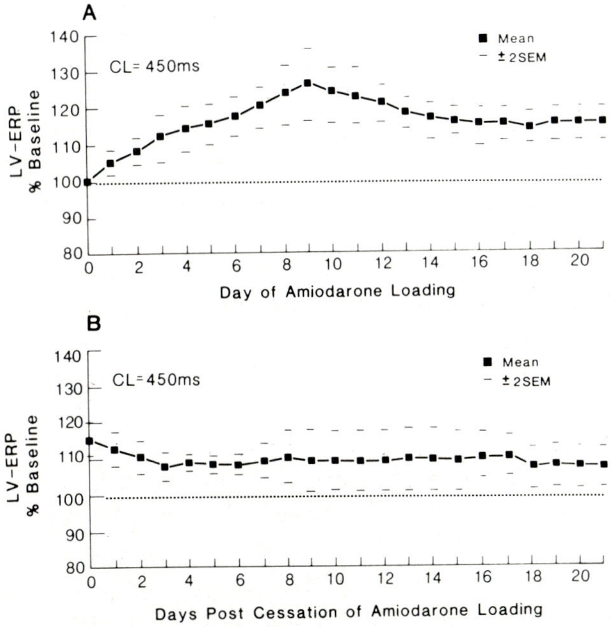

FIGURE 5. Graph depicting the temporal effect of orally administered amiodarone (*A*) or cessation of amiodarone (*B*) on group mean LV-ERP (CL = 450 msec) measured in dogs (n = 4). The ordinate indicates LV-ERP expressed as a percentage of predrug baseline value. The abscissa indicates day of amiodarone administration or withdrawal. The format of the figure is otherwise the same as figure 2. 95% confidence intervals are indicated for each data point (±2 SEM).

ERP rose only 10%. The magnitude of RA-ERP and AVN-ERP changes are comparable to our findings, while smaller RV-ERP changes may be interpreted as indicating that maximal effect had not yet occurred. This interpretation is supported by the results of clinical studies, which indicate that RV-ERP may be expected to rise 15% to 20% above baseline after 2 to 4 months of amiodarone administration.[12-19] Mitchell et al.[13] evaluated seven patients at 2, 6, and 10 weeks after onset of amiodarone loading (22.4 g total loading dose over 21 days, 400 mg/day maintenance dose) and noted that Wenckebach cycle lengths maximized within 2 weeks of therapy, whereas RV-ERP required 6 weeks to maximize at 18% above control. In a similar study, Kennedy et al.[14] evaluated 25 patients with electrophysiologic studies at 8 and 69 days after onset of oral amiodarone loading (9.6 g total loading dose over 8 days, 660 mg/day maintenance dose). RA-ERP and Wenckebach cycle length changes (20% and 38% above baseline, respectively) plateaued by day 8, while RV-ERP rose 15% above baseline by day 69. In summary, the temporal sequence of onset of amiodarone's cardiac electrophysiologic actions in these clinical studies appears consistent with site-specific differences in the temporal onset of amiodarone's electrophysiologic actions identified in this study.

Changes in refractory period after withdrawal of amiodarone. Studies serially evaluating the regression of amiodarone-induced electrophysiologic changes after drug withdrawal have not been performed in humans. In the present study, electrophysiologic changes regressed in a complex, site-dependent manner after the cessation of amiodarone. A primary decay in refractory periods occurring 2 to 4 days after cessation of amiodarone, followed by rebound elevation and a secondary decay at 15 to 18 days after withdrawal of drug, is qualitatively present in measurements from all sites (figure 2, *B*, and 5, *B*), but is most apparent in AVN-ERP measurements (figure 5, *B*). These electrophysiologic findings mimic the biphasic plasma amiodarone elimination profile reported by Holt et al.[9] in humans after withdrawal of long-term amiodarone therapy (200 to 600 mg/day, administered for longer than 30 days). In the latter study, plasma amiodarone levels fell to half steady-state levels by day 2.5, demonstrated rebound elevation, and fell again at 12 to 21 days after cessation of therapy.

Effect of amiodarone on intraventricular conduction. The reported effects of oral amiodarone on conduction through the His-Purkinje system have been variable. Zipes et al.[20] noted a 10% to 20% prolongation in HV intervals in patients treated with a variety of oral amiodarone regimens (dosages typically lower than those in the present study). Reports on the effects of amiodarone on HV conduction intervals have ranged from infra-Hisian block to lack of a measurable effect.[1, 4, 15, 18, 19, 21-23] In the present study, mean HV conduction intervals varied less than 2% throughout the loading and withdrawal periods and demonstrated no significant deviation from control values.

Clinical implications. Our findings are consistent with the observations of Rosenbaum et al.[24] on latency and duration of amiodarone's antiarrhythmic effects. Among 2000 patients undergoing treatment for a variety of arrhythmias, supraventricular tachyarrhythmias (including atrial fibrillation/flutter) were reported to respond maximally to amiodarone within 5 to 20 days of initiation of therapy, whereas ventricular arrhythmias (in the setting of ischemic heart disease) required 20 to 30 days of therapy before maximal response was achieved. Similarly, atrial arrhythmias were reported to recur as soon as 15 days after drug withdrawal, whereas ventricular arrhythmias typically recurred after drug had been withheld for 30 to 40 days. Our observations suggest that underlying these site-specific differences in latency and duration of amiodarone's antiarrhythmic effects may be site-specific differences in drug-induced electrophysiologic effects on the atria, AV node, and ventricles.

The basis for site-dependence in the electrophysiologic effects of amiodarone is not clearly understood. Whether differential binding and storage of amiodarone and its metabolites (already demonstrated among various noncardiac tissues[25]) exists between atrial, AV nodal, and ventricular tissues, contributing to site-specific differences in local tissue amiodarone levels, remains to be determined but may be a potential mechanism underlying these observations. Indeed, our findings of qualitatively similar biphasic changes in refractory period measurements at all cardiac sites after amiodarone withdrawal (mimicking regression of plasma amiodarone levels after cessation of amiodarone in humans[9]) in the presence of significant quantitative electrophysiologic differences between cardiac sites suggests that factors in addition to plasma drug concentration may be involved in local tissue response to amiodarone.

In summary, our findings indicate that the time course of amiodarone's electrophysiologic effects differs among various cardiac tissues, both during amiodarone loading and after withdrawal of drug. Although the basis for this site dependence is not clearly understood, these observations provide insight into previously reported temporal differences in onset and duration of maximal antiarrhythmic effect during oral amiodarone therapy for supraventricular and ventricular arrhythmias.

Wc acknowledge the technical contributions of Leslie McGregor, Barry Detloff, Thomas Gohman, Gil Lewandowski, and Michael Walker, the assistance of Thomas S. Rector, Ph.D., with statistical analysis, and the aid of D. Woodrow Benson, M.D., Ph.D., in preparation of the manuscript.

References

1. Marcus F, Fontaine G, Frank R, Grosgogeat Y: Clinical pharmacology and therapeutic applications of the antiarrhythmic agent amiodarone. Am Heart J **101:** 480, 1981
2. Alboni D, Shantha N, Pirani R, Baggioni F, Scarpo S, Tomasi A, Masoni A: Effects of amiodarone on supraventricular tachycardia involving bypass tracts. Am J Cardiol **53:** 93, 1984
3. Wellens H, Lie K, Bar F, Wesdorp J, Dohman H, Duren D, Durrer D: Effect of amiodarone in the Wolff-Parkinson-White syndrome. Am J Cardiol **38:** 189, 1976
4. Rosenbaum M, Chiale P, Halpern M, Nau G, Przybylski J, Levi R, Lazzari J, Elizari M: Clinical efficacy of amiodarone as an antiarrhythmic agent. Am J Cardiol **38:** 934, 1976
5. Kaski J, Girotti L, Messuti H, Rutitzky B, Rosenbaum M: Long-term management of sustained, recurrent symptomatic ventricular tachycardia with amiodarone. Circulation **64:** 273, 1981
6. Rowland E, Krikler D: Electrophysiologic assessment of amiodarone in treatment of resistant supraventricular arrhythmias. Br Heart J **44:** 82, 1980
7. Heger J, Prystowky E, Zipes D: Clinical efficacy of amiodarone in treatment of recurrent ventricular tachycardia and ventricular fibrillation. Am Heart J **106:** 887, 1983
8. Latini R, Connolly S, Kates R: Myocardial disposition of amiodarone in the dog. J Pharmacol Exp Ther **224:** 603, 1983
9. Holt D, Tucker G, Jackson P, Storey G: Amiodarone pharmacokinetics. Am Heart J **106:** 840, 1983
10. Karpawich P, Gillette P, Lewis R, Zinner A, McNamara D: Chronic epicardial His bundle recordings in awake nonsedated dogs: a new method. Am Heart J **150:** 16, 1983
11. Josephson M, Seides S: Definitions of electrophysiologic terms. *In* Clinical cardiac electrophysiology. Philadelphia, 1979, Lea & Febiger, p 41
12. Hamer A, Finerman W, Peter T, Mandel W: Disparity between the clinical and electrophysiologic effects of amiodarone in the treatment of recurrent ventricular tachyarrhythmias. Am Heart J **102:** 992, 1981
13. Mitchell L, Wyse D, Hinton M, Duff H: Amiodarone loading: disparate time courses of electrophysiologic changes assessed by serial studies. Circulation **70**(suppl II): II-3, 1984 (abst)
14. Kennedy E, Rosenfeld L, McPherson C, Batsford W: Time course of amiodarone electrophysiologic effects: evaluation of an oral loading and maintenance regimen. Circulation **70**(suppl II): II-4, 1984 (abst)
15. Senasa M, Denker S, Mahmud R, Lehmann M, Estrada A, Akhtar M: Effect of amiodarone on conduction and refractoriness of the His-Purkinje system in the human heart. J Am Coll Cardiol **4:** 105, 1984
16. Hariman R, Gomes J, Kang P, El-Sherif N: Effects of intravenous amiodarone in patients with inducible repetitive ventricular responses and ventricular tachycardia. Am Heart J **107:** 1109, 1984
17. Saksena S, Rothbart S, Cappello G: Chronic effects of amiodarone in patients with refractory ventricular tachycardia. Int J Cardiol **3:** 339, 1983
18. Waxman H, Groh W, Marchlinski F, Buxton A, Sadowski L, Horowitz L, Josephson M, Kastor J: Amiodarone for control of sustained ventricular tachyarrhythmia: clinical and electrophysiologic effects in 51 patients. Am J Cardiol **50:** 1066, 1982
19. Finerman W, Hamer A, Peter T, Weiss D, Mandel W: Electrophysiologic effects of chronic amiodarone therapy in patients with ventricular arrhythmias. Am Heart J **104:** 987, 1982
20. Zipes D, Prystowsky E, Heger J: Amiodarone: electrophysiologic actions, pharmacokinetics and clinical effects. J Am Coll Cardiol **3:** 1059, 1984
21. Reddy C, Kuo C: Effect of amiodarone on retrograde conduction and refractoriness of the His-Purkinje system in man. Br Heart J **51:**648, 1984
22. Santinelli V, Chiariello M, Ambrosio G, Stanislao M: Further observations on the electrophysiologic effects of oral amiodarone therapy. Chest **82:** 117, 1982
23. Feld G, Nademanee K, Weiss J, Stevenson W, Singh B: Electrophysiologic basis for the suppression by amiodarone of orthodromic supraventricular tachycardias complicating pre-excitation syndromes. J Am Coll Cardiol **3:** 1298, 1984
24. Rosenbaum M, Chiale P, Kaski J, Elizari M: Is amiodarone an ideal antiarrhythmic drug. PACE **7:** 272, 1984
25. Nitsch J, Luderitz B: Serum and tissue concentrations of amiodarone in man and animals. *In* Breithardt G, Loogen F, editors: New aspects in the medical treatment of tachyarrhythmias: role of amiodarone. Dusseldorf, 1982, Urban and Schwarzenberg, p 74

IN APPRECIATION

The Editors gratefully acknowledge the valuable assistance of the following reviewers[1] and the Editorial Office staff.[2]

Abdul Abbasi
Shimon Abboud
George Abela
Walter Abelmann
Dana Abendschein
J. Abildskov
Jonathan Abrams
J. Joseph Ackerman
Harry Acquatella
A. A. Jennifer Adgey
Gail Ahumada
Masood Akhtar
John Albers
Edwin Alderman
J. Alger
Hugh Allen
A. Allessie
Bruce Alpert
Joseph Alpert
Martin Alpert
Ezra Amsterdam
Jeffrey Anderson
Gary Anderson
Page Anderson
Robert Anderson
Elliott Antman
Michael Antonaccio
Charles Antzelevitch
William Armstrong
Morton Arnsdorf
Stephen Ayres
Charles Babbs
Robert Bache
F. Bachmann
Nancy Baenziger
Donald Baim
Harold Baltaxe
Vidya Banka
Clyde Barlow
Robert Barnes
Roger Barr
Elizabeth Barrett-Connor
William Barry
Benico Barzilai
Ludwik Bass
Arthur Bassett
James Bassingthwaighte
John Batty
Lewis Becker
Luiz Belardinelli
William Bell
George Beller
David Benditt
Bruno Benfey
Joseph Benotti
D. Woodrow Benson, Jr.
Jonathan Benumof
Edward Berbari
Harvey Berger
Martin Berger
Steven Bergmann
Robert Berliner
Daniel Berman
Robert Berne
Jesus Bianco
Daniel Biello
J. Thomas Bigger, Jr.
Joseph Billadello
Oscar H. Bing
Richard Bing
Vermon Bishop
Joe Bissette
Henry Blackburn
David Blankenhorn
Terrence Blaschke
Walter Bleifeld
Peter Block
C. Gunnar Blomqvist
Colin Bloor
Sidney Blumenthal
Monty Bodenheimer
David Bohr
John Boineau
Ralph Bolman
Hooshang Bolooki
I. M. Felix Bonke
Robert Bonow
Fred Bonte
Kenneth Borow
Elias Botvinick
Charles Boucher
Martial Bourassa
Patrick D. Bourdillon
Alfred Bove
A. Brash
Eugene Braunwald
Gunter Breithardt
J. David Bristow
Michael Bristow
Harold Brooks
B. Greg Brown
Truman Brown
Robert Bruce
Pedro Brugada
Bruce Brundage
Dirk Brutsaert
Mortimer Buckley
Thomas Budinger
Fritz Buhler
L. Maximilian Buja
Ivan Bunnell
George Burch
Mary Jo Burgess
Gary Burggraf
Larry Bush
Alfred Buxton
David Bylund
Henry Cabin
Paul Calabresi
James Caldwell Jr.
Paul Cannon
Richard Cannon III
Balse Carabello
Joseph Carey
Robert Carney
John Caronna
Dan Carr
David Case
Joan Casey
Aldo Castaneda
Agustin Castellanos
William Castelli
Bernard Chaitman
Britton Chance
Kanu Chatterjee
Melvin Cheitlin
James Chesebro
Kenneth Chien
Francis Chinard
Frederick Cobb
Leonard Cobb
Jay Coffman
Jerome Cohen
Marc Cohen
Michael Cohen
Peter Cohn
R. Edward Coleman
Desire Collen
Steve Collins
Wilson Colucci
Patricia Come
C. Richard Conti
Theodore Cooper
James Coramilas
James Corbette
Eliot Corday
Betty Corya
James Covell
Marie Cowan
Michael Cowley
James Cox
Jerome Cox Jr.
Edward Coyle
Ernest Craige
Michael Crawford
J. Michael Criley
Michael Criqui
Karl Crossen
Richard Crow
Philip Cryer
Lawrence Czer
James Dalen
Kenneth Dangman
Dolores Danilowicz
Harold Dash
Allan Daugherty
George Daughters
M. Davies
Andrew Davis
Adolfo de Bold
Jan Willem de Jong
Robert DeBusk
Raffaele DeCaterina
Anthony DeMaria
Henry DeMots
Marcus DeWood
Gregory Dehmer
John Demakis
Quentin Deming
Pablo Denes
Katherine Detre
Jean-Marie Detry
Richard Devereux
Michael Devous
Stephen Devries
Mrinal Dewanjee
James Deweese
N. Dhalla
Ramesh Dhingra
Robert Di Bianco
John DiMarco
George Diamond
James Dillon
Emily Diltz
Roy Ditchey
William Dixon
Harold Dodge
Donald Doty
Eugene Downar
S. Evans Downing
Leonard Dreifus
David Driscoll
Dirk Durrer
Harriet Dustan
Duncan Dymond
Paul Ebert
Debra Echt
Dwain Eckberg
David Effeney
Richard Egdahl
Ali Ehsani
Stanley Einzig
Joel Eisenberg
Mickey Eisenberg
Paul Eisenberg
Nabil El-Sherif
Victor Elharrar
Uri Elkayam
Myrvin Ellestad
Larry Elliott
Avery Ellis
Robert Ellis
Mary Allen Engel
Peter Engel
Toby Engel
Mark Entman
Stephen Epstein
David Euler
Ronald Evans
Alex Evers
John Fallon
David Faxon
Harvey Feigenbaum
Eric Feigl

[1]These reviewers served from September 1, 1984 through August 31, 1985.

[2]Melanie Miller, Managing Editor; Kevin Brennan, Assistant Managing Editor; Beth Engeszer, Editorial Copyeditor; Mary Henderson and Judy Pyne, Editorial Assistants.

Manning Feinleib
Alvan Feinstein
Andrew Feiring
Frederick Feit
Robert Felder
Robert Feldman
Ross Feldman
John Fenoglio Jr.
Jack Ferlinz
Victor Ferrans
Gregory Ferrier
Larry Fields
Charles Fisch
Edwin Fisher Jr.
John Fisher
Garret FitzGerald
Stephen Flaim
Gerald Fletcher
Nancy Flowers
John Folts
James Forrester
Nicholas Fortuin
James Foster
Michael Fowler
Nobel Fowler
Arthur Fox
Keith A. A. Fox
Lawrence Frame
Joseph Franciosa
Charles Francis
Gary Francis
Robert Francis
Dean Franklin
Roger Freedman
Edward Freis
Gary Friedman
Gottlieb Friesinger
William Frishman
Victor Froelicher
Edward Frohlich
Arnest Fronek
Curt Furberg
Seymour Furman
William Gaasch
Thomas Gaffney
Pierre Galetti
Kim Gallagher
Peter Gallerstein
Peter Ganz
William Ganz
Julius Gardin
Timothy Gardner
Tim Garson
James Gault
Leslie Geddes
Jacques Genest
Edward Genton
Lawrence German
Ross Gerrity
Lawrence Gessman
Leonard Gettes
Henry Gewirtz
Elsa-Grace Giardina
Paul Gillette
Richard Gillis
Richard Gillum
Robert Gilmour, Jr.
Robert Ginsburg
Albert Gjedda
Stanton Glantz
Ephrain Glassman
Gerald Glick
Charles Glueck
Robert Glueck
John Gohagan
Herman Gold
Emanuel Goldberg
Sheldon Goldberg
Stanley Goldberg
Mark Goldman
Merv Goldman
Nora Goldschlager
Joseph Goldstein
Richard Goldstein
Robert Goldstein
Tavia Gordon
Carl Goresky
Antonio Gotto Jr.
K. Lance Gould
Thomas Graboys
Michael Graham
Raymond Gramiak
Augustus Grant
Michael Green
H. Leon Greene
Joseph Greenfield Jr.
Allan Greenspan
Jerry Griffin
Lawrence Griffith
Richard Gross
William Grossman
Maleah Grover-McKay
Andreas Gruentzig
Scott Grundy
Rolf Gunnar
Warren Guntheroth
Victor Gurewich
Howard Gutgesell
Fernando Gutierrez
Edgar Haber
Jacob Haft
James Hagberg
Donald Hagler
K. Hammermeister
E. William Hancock
Lawrence Harker
Thomas Harris
David Harrison
W. Proctor Harvey
William Haskell
Liv Hatle
Richard Havlik
L. Julian Haywood
Jame Hazelrig
William Hazzard
David Hearse
James Heger
Donald Heistad
Richard Helfant
Philip Henry
Eberhard Henze
R. Herfkins
Michael Herman
Antonio Hernandez, Jr.
Michael Hess
Otto Hess
Guy Heyndrickx
Alan Higgins
Charles Higgins
L. David Hillis
Ake Hjalmarson
David Hoelzer
Brian Hoffman
Eric Hoffman
Julien I. Hoffman
Jay Hollman
John Holloszy
David Holmans
David Holmes, Jr.
Luc Hondeghem
William Hood, Jr.
Philip Hopewell
Richard Hopkins
Leo Horan
Leonard Horowitz
Lawrence Horwitz
Kenneth Hossack
Paul Hugenholtz
Bernadette Hughes
James Huhta
Russell Hull
Lee Huntsman
J. Willis Hurst
Grover Hutchins
Peter Hutt
Adolph Hutter, Jr.
Raymond Ideker
Roger Illingworth
Joanne Ingwall
Paul Insel
William Insull, Jr.
Lloyd Iseri
Abhulmassih Iskandrian
William Jacobus
Allan Jaffe
Jose Jalife
Joseph Janicki
Michiel Janse
Jay Jarmakani
Robert Jennings
Robert Jeresaty
Robert Jones
Terry Jones
Mark Josephson
William Joyner
Bodh Jugdutt
D. Julian
Jack Juni
Stanley Kalsner
Jean Kan
John Kane
William Kannel
Norman Kaplan
Karen Kaplan
Joel Karliner
Ronald Karlsberg
Robert Karp
Karl Karsch
John Kastor
Arnold Katz
Bert Katzung
Leon Kaufman
Chuichi Kawai
Harry Keiser
Harvey Kemp, Jr.
Andrew Kemper
Harold Kennedy
J. Ward Kennedy
Joseph Kenzora
Richard Kerber
Ban An Khaw
Iris Kingma
David Kipnis
Joseph Kisslo, Jr.
John Kjekshus
Andre Kleber
Robert Kleiger
George Klein
Lloyd Klein
Peter Klementowicz
Paul Kligfield
Francis Klocke
Robert Kloner
Maureen Knabb
Robert Knabb
Suzanne Knoebel
Marvin Konstam
Donald Kornfeld
William Kostuk
Morris Kotler
Nicholas Kouchoukos
Sandor Kovacs
Jeffrey Kramer
Dieter Kramsch
Hans Krayenbuehl
Dennis Krikler
Kenneth Krone
Ronald Krone
Marvin Kronenberg
Itzhak Kronzon
Wolfgang Kubler
Lewis Kuller
Peter Kurnik
Martin Kushmerick
Peter Kwiterovich
Kathryn LaNoue
M. J. Lab
Edward Lakatta
Charles Lambert
Louis Lange
John Laragh
Pierre Larochelle
Kenneth Larson
Claire Lathers
Ronald Lauer
Gerald Lawrie
Ralph Lazzara
Thierry LeJemtel
Carwile LeRoy
Martin LeWinter
Aubrey Leatham
Benjamin Lee
Kerry Lee
Allan Lefer
Robert Lefkowitz
Marianne Legato
Roy Leiboff
Robert Leinbach

Martin Leon
Rene Lerch
Michael Lesch
Charles Leven
David Levin
Harold Levine
Herbert Levine
Theodore Levine
Sidney Levitsky
Robert Levitt
Matthew Levy
Robert Levy
Samuel Lewis
Chang-seng Liang
Richard Liberthson
Paul Lichtlen
Bruce Lindsay
Martin Lipton
William Little
William Littler
James Lock
Floyd Loop
Beverly Lorell
David Loskutoff
Benedict Lucchesi
John Luce
Kenneth Ludmerer
Robert Lux
Rex MacAlpin
R. MacFarlane
Jamshid Maddahi
David Mailman
Philip Majerus
Alberto Malliani
James Malm
Francis Marchlinski
Frank Marcus
Melvin Marcus
Victor Marder
Allyn Mark
John Markis
Barry Maron
Henry J. Marriott
Barry Marterson
Gregorio Martin
Randolph Martin
Richard Martin
Thomas Martin
Wade Martin
J. Danie Marx
Dean Mason
Jay Mason
Barry Massie
Shaul Massry
Jack Morton Matloff
Jeffrey Matos
Michael Matthey
W. Lowell Maughan
Morton Maxwell
John McAnulty
David McCarthy
Walter McDonald
Mary Ann McDonnell
Edward McFadden, Jr.
J. Denis McGarry
John McGiff
Henry McGill, Jr.
Robert McGilvery
Philip McHale
Paul McHenry
Malcolm McIlroy
Raymond McKay
William McKenzie
Robert McKnight
Alan McLaughlin
Jeanie McMillin-Wood
Dan McNamara
M. T. McNamara
Irma Mebane
Gerald Medoff
Samuel Meerbaum
Jawahar Mehta
Richard Melker
G. Leland Melson
Franz Messerli
Richard Meyer
Eric Michelson
Joseph Miletich
C. Kay Millar
D. Craig Miller
Fletcher Miller, Jr.
James Miller
Thomas Miller
William Miller
Noel Lang Mills
Stephen Mills
William Milnor
Mark Mintun
Gary Mintz
Mieczyslaw Mirowski
Israel Mirsky
David Mirvis
Jere Mitchell
Michael Mock
Gordon Moe
Terrence Montague
E. Neil Moore
Fred Morady
Jon Moran
Howard Morelli
Joel Morganroth
Eugene Morkin
Aubrey Morrison
John Morrison
Mark Morton
Arthur Moss
Albert Most
John Mowbray
Morton Mower
H. Mudd
Hiltrud Mueller
Amal Mukherjee
James Muller
Rebecca Mullis
Eldred Mundth
Daniel Murphy, Jr.
Marvin Murphy
Robert Myerburg
Alexander Nadas
Koonlawee Nademanee
Navin Nanda
Winifred Nayler
Philip Needleman
James Neely
William Neill
Stephen Nellis
Jeffrey Newhouse
Allen Nichols
Wilmer Nichols
Alan Nies
J. Nixon
Jacqueline Noonan
Carl Norden
William Norwood, Jr.
Ray Nunnally
John O'Connell
Matthew O'Donnell
Michael O'Rourke
Robert O'Rourke
Allen Oboler
Seiji Ogawa
Robert Okada
Philip Oliva
Michael Oliver
Eckhardt G. Olsen
Joseph Ornato
Leon Ostrander, Jr.
Catherine Otto
Albert Pacifico
Milton Packer
Ralph Paffenbarger, Jr.
Natesa Pandian
J. Frank Pantridge
Alfred Parisi
Brent Parker
Robert Parkey
Loren Parmley
William Parmley
J. Parratt
Victor Parsonnet
Eugene Passamani
Randolph Patterson
Sven Paulin
Dan Pavel
Alan Pearlman
Thomas Pearson
Amir Pelleg
Patricia Penkoske
Glenn Pennington
Carl Pepine
Julio Perez
Joseph Perloff
H. Mitchell Perry, Jr.
Ronald Peshock
Robert Petersdorf
Janice Pfeffer
Marc Pfeffer
David Phillips
Nancy Phillips
John Pierce
Daniel Pieroni
Hubert Pipberger
Farouk Pirzada
Bertram Pitt
Edward Platia
Philip Podrid
Steven Pogwizd
Gerald Pohost
Michael Pollock
P. Poole-Wilson
Richard Popp
Herbert Pouleur
William Powell
Eric Powers
William Powers
Stephen Prescott
Edward L. Pritchett
Jeffrey Probstfield
William Proudfit
Eric Prystowsky
Miguel Quinones
Simon Rabkin
Charles Rackley
Edward Raftery
Shahbudin Rahimtoola
Marcus Raichle
Walter Randall
A. Koneti Rao
Dabeeru Rao
Elliot Rapaport
Adam Ratner
Timothy Regan
Johan Reiber
Nathaniel Reichek
Philip Reid
James Reiffel
Keith Reimer
Peter Rentrop
Leon Resnekov
Stuart Rich
Kent Richards
David Richardson
Basil Rifkind
Pierre Rigo
Jorge Rios
James Ritchie
Erik Ritman
Robert Roberts
Francis Robicsek
Thomas Robinson
Dan Roden
Benson Roe
Joseph Roelandt
William Roeske
J. Carlos Romero
Thomas Rosamond
Robert Rosati
Ray Roseman
Michael Rosen
Allan Ross
John Ross, Jr.
Richard Ross
Michel Rousseau
George Rowe
Stanley Rubin
Rafael Rubio
Robert Rude
Abraham Rudolph
Rodolphe Ruffy
John Rumberger
Robert Rushmer
Jeremy Ruskin
Thomas Ryan
David Sabiston, Jr.
Frank Sacks
Peter Safar
Jeffrey Saffitz
Kiichi Sagawa

Circulation

An Official Journal of the American Heart Association

AUTHOR/SUBJECT INDEX TO

VOLUME 72

JULY-DECEMBER 1985

*

Cardiovascular Medicine:
Opportunities for Enhanced University-Industry Collaboration
Part II, Volume 72, Number 2, August 1985
Supplement I

*

Cardiovascular Surgery 1984
Part II, Volume 72, Number 3, September 1985
Supplement II

*

Cardiovascular Metabolic Imaging:
Physiologic and Biochemical Dynamics In Vivo
Part II, Volume 72, Number 5, November 1985
Supplement IV

*

Surgery in the Treatment of Coronary Artery Disease
Part II, Volume 72, Number 6, December 1985
Supplement V

AMERICAN HEART ASSOCIATION, INC.

David Sahn
Timothy Sanborn
Merle Sande
Steve Sanders
Harold Sandler
William Santamore
Julio Santiago
Arthur Sasahara
Betty Sasyniuk
Lowell Satler
Wolfgang Schaper
Kenneth Schechtman
Melvin Scheinman
Heinrich Schelbert
Benjamin Scherlag
James Scheuer
Barbara Schick
Nelson Schiller
Robert Schlant
Phillip Schmid
Donald Schmidt
Ingela Schnittger
John Schroeder
R. Schuessler
Daniel Schuster
Marcus Schwaiger
Benjamin Schwartz
Peter Schwartz
Kate Scott
Steve Sedlis
Ronald Selvester
Andrew Selwyn
Patrick Serruys
Gerald Serwer
James Seward
Ralph Shabetai
Kenneth Shafer
David Shand
Jeffrey Shanes
Arjun Sharma
Florence Sheehan
L. Thomas Sheffield
Richard Shekelle
William Shell
Albert Shepherd, Jr.
John Shepherd
Desmond Sheridan
Laurence Sherman
Earl Shrago
Barry Siegel
Mark Siegler
Norman Silverman
A. Simon
Martin Simoons
John Simpson
Michael Simson
Bramah Singh
David Skorton
Brian Slinker
Robert Slutsky
Eldon Smith
W. McFate Smith
Thomas Smitherman
Peter Snell
Allan Sniderman
Louis Sokoloff
Michael Sole
Madison Spach
James Spadaro, Jr.
Joseph Spear
Scott Spielman
John Spittell, Jr.
David Spodick
Thomas Spray
Martin St. John Sutton
Howard Staniloff
Mark Starling
Albert Starr
Charles Steenbergen
Paul Stein
Richard Steingart
Michael Stern
Ester Sternberg
Edward Brad Stinson
Joseph Stokes III
Neil Stone
Janet Strain
H. William Strauss
Hans Strauss
C. M. Harold Strauss
Bala Subramanian
Timothy Sullivan
Ruey Sung
Henry Sung-Cheng
Borys Surawicz
Judith Swain
Karl Swedberg
Harley Sybers
W. Tacker
Michihiko Tada
Heinrich Taegtmeyer
Timothy Takaro
Robert Tarazi
Morton Tavel
Anne Taylor
Michel Ter-Pogossian
Pierre Theroux
Peter Thoren
Alan Tiefenbrunn
Gregory Tilton
Gerald Timmis
Thomas Traill
Elbert Trulock III
Zoltan Turi
Peter Tuteur
John Tyberg
Daniel Ullyot
Patrick Umeda
Donald Unverferth
Ferdinand Urthaler
Anthony Vagnucci
Lilliam Valdes-Cruz
Cornelis van Breeman
Richard Van Praagh
Michel Vandormael
Paul Vanhoutte
Michael Vannier
Stephen Vatner
John Vavra
Richard Verrier
Victoria Vetter
Ronald Victor
J. Vinten-Hohansen
Marc Visner
Ronald Vlietstra
John H. Vogel
Robert Vogel
Frans Wackers
Galen Wagner
Henry Wagner, Jr.
J. Deane Waldman
Albert Waldo
Andrew Wallace
Robert Wallace
L. Samuel Wann
James Ware
Lawrence Waspe
David Waters
R. D. Watson
Rita Watson
Harvey Waxman
Menashe Waxman
Karl Weber
William Weglicki
Max Weil
Donald Weiner
Milton Weinstein
Myron Weisfeldt
James Weiss
Babette Weksler
Francis Weld
Clarence Weldon
Hein J. Wellens
Nanette Wenger
Milton Wessel
G. Alexander West
Arthur Weyman
Carl White
Michael Whyte
Samuel Wickline
James Willerson
David Williams
George Williams
R. Sanders Williams
Robert Gay Williams
John Wilson
Roger Winkle
Judith Wisneski
Andrew Wit
Francis Witkowski
Joseph Witztum
Ernst Wolner
Peter Wood
Charles Wooley
Raymond Woosley
Gregory Wright
Christopher Wyndham
Joshua Wynne
Kathryn Yamada
James S. Yao
Lawrence Yeatman, Jr.
Edward Yellin
Frank Yin
Mitsuhiro Yokoyama
Barry Zaret
Arno Zaritsky
Kenneth Zierler
Douglas Zipes
Lenore Zohman
Irving Zucker

AUTHOR INDEX*

NOTE

Committee and Special Reports are published in rear forms as part of AHA News. The reports follow text and are continued into rear ad pages.

Indexes to ABSTRACTS, AHA 58th Scientific Sessions, Supplement III, October 1985, are included in that issue.

A

Abbott JA, 170
Abe H, 280
Ackell PH, 82
Adams PC, 1064
Agnelli G, 178
Ahnve S, 963
Akaishi M, 632
Alam M, II-129
Alderman EL, II-207
Alferness C, 612
Ali S, II-35
Alker K, 1115
Amery A, 982
Anderson HV, 530
Anoal M, 272
Antman EM, 873
Appel PL, 1022
Appleton S, II-45
Apprill P, 397, 413
Arky R, 1135A
Armstrong ML, 82
Arom KV, II-153
Ascah KJ, 377
Ash JM, 471
Ashihara T, 747
Ashton J, 397, 413
Asseman P, 205
Atarashi H, 370
Aueron FM, 833
Ausubel K, 1037
Ayelsworth CA, II-231

B

Baan J, 440
Bacharach SL, 853
Badke FR, 317
Baird RJ, II-120
Bakhos M, II-185
Baldwin JC, II-108
Balschi JA, IV-89
Ban-Hayashi E, 1125
Barber MJ, 623
Bardy GH, 612
Barnhart GR, II-227
Barreca P, 105
Barrett-Connor E, 53
Bass L, IV-47
Bassingthwaighte JB, IV-39
Bates ER, 833
Baumann FG, II-13
Baur HR, 27
Bear G, II-13
Becker LC, 1092
Becker RE, I-53
Beller GA, V-9
Bellotti P, 310, 774
Bender HW, II-45
Benditt DG, 147, 1380
Benefiel DJ, 1015
Benjamin D, II-13
Bensasson D, II-140
Benson DW Jr, 147
Benveniste J, 713
Berger RL, II-216
Bergmann SR, 1346
Berman MA, II-35
Bernath GA, 1076
Bernhard WF, II-216
Berns MW, II-200
Bernstein JS, II-191
Berry TE, II-101
Bessou JP, II-140
Betocchi S, 1001
Bieber LL, IV-9
Billingham ME, 193, 302
Blackstone EH, 753, II-175
Blake GJ, 214
Bleifeld W, 112
Block PC, V-161
Blondeau P, II-140
Bloomfield P, 781
Blumhardt R, 317, 1327
Boccadamo R, 153
Bode H, IV-103
Boey J, 1059
Boineau JP, 249
Bolli R, 915
Bolman RM III, 1380
Boneu B, 178
Bonow RO, 853, 1001, 1244, V-23
Born GVR, 741
Borow KM, 495, 515
Botvinick EH, 334
Boucek RJ Jr, II-45
Bouchard A, 1015
Bouillon R, 982
Bourassa MG, 487, V-71
Boutal L, 1208
Bouvagnet P, 272
Bove AA, 389
Bowen-Pope DF, 735
Brachmann J, 200
Brady TJ, II-231
Brash AR, 702
Braunwald E, 873, V-1
Bray GA, 1135A
Brazzamano S, 225
Breazeale DG, 612
Bredlau CE, 530, 1044
Brenner JI, II-35
Breyer RH, II-259
Brittain RT, 1208
Broekman MJ, 698
Brooks HL, 1076
Brown BG, 138, V-39
Brown TR, IV-18
Brown WV, 1135A
Brugada P, 1
Buchanan MR, 178
Buckley MJ, 31, II-231
Budinger TF, IV-53
Buja LM, 327, 397, 413
Bull C, II-52
Bundy GL, 708
Burger J, II-45
Burkhoff D, 440, 654
Burnett JC Jr, 892
Burns J, II-35
Bush LR, 413
Buttrick PM, 1336
Byrd BF, 1015
Byrne JM, 1232
Byrom E, 1028

C

Cahalan MK, 1015
Calderwood SB, 31
Califf RM, V-136
Callaghan J, 1064
Campbell RWF, 1064
Campbell WB, 397
Campeau L, V-71
Cannon RO III, 1001
Carey JS, 138
Carpentier A, II-140
Carroll JD, 119
Carter MC, 1208
Castaneda AR, II-77
Catella F, 1177
Cercek B, 1053, 1321
Cerletti C, 1185
Chachques JC, II-140
Chadwick B, 364, 846
Chaitman BR, V-31
Chan TK, 1059
Chance B, IV-103
Chandran P, 153
Chandraratna PAN, 865, 975
Chauvaud S, II-140
Chesebro JH, V-65
Cheung KL, 1059
Chiarella F, 310, 774
Chignard M, 713
Childers RW, 495
Chilian WM, 82
Chin A, II-61
Chow J, 1059
Chræmmer-Jørgensen B, 502
Christakis GT, II-120
Chu A, 632
Chu SC, IV-89
Ciabattoni G, 1177
Clark BJ, IV-103
Clark RE, 1244
Clarke RH, II-191
Cloutier A, 471
Cobb FR, 632
Cobbe SM, 200
Coffman JD, 466
Cogswell TL, 1076
Cohen LS, I-1
Cohen MV, 881
Colan SD, 515, 1008
Colavita PG, 344

*Roman numbers indicate articles published in supplements.

Coleman RA, 1208
Collen D, 18, 178, 384
Collington EW, 1208
Collins D, 963
Collins SM, 1355
Coltorti F, 612
Compton PC, 1279
Condorelli M, 38
Cooper GR, 93
Copel JA, 825
Copeland J, II-7
Copeland JG, II-7
Copenhaver GL, 353
Corbett JR, 327
Cordell RA, 431
Coronary Artery Surgery Study Principal Investigators and their Associates, V-102, V-117
Cosgrove DM, II-146, II-170
Coughlin SS, 768
Coulibaly AO, II-274
Cousineau D, IV-81
Cowley MJ, 1314
Crawford MH, 1237
Criley JM, 1148
Criqui MH, 768
Crosby L, 991
Cukingnan RA, 138
Cuocolo A, 38

D

Dae M, 334
Daggett WM, II-241
d'Allaines C, II-140
D'Ambra MN, II-231
Danielson GK, 130, II-70, II-84, II-88, II-93
Daoud AS, 1081
Dash H, 353
Daughters GT, II-207
Davi G, 1177
David TE, II-18
Davies BG, 623
Davis JC, 170
Davis JW, 668
Davis K, 292, V-102, V-110
Davis KB, V-31, V-117
Davis SC, II-97
de Gaetano G, 1185
De Geest H, II-179
de Langen CDJ, 1092
de Leval M, II-52
De Luca N, 38
De Roo M, II-179
De Schaepdryver A, 982
De Simone A, 38
de Zuttere D, 819
Deanfield J, II-52
DeBoer LWV, II-241
Dechesne CA, 272
Deckelbaum LI, II-191
Dejana E, 1185
DeLeon SY, II-101
Dell'Italia LJ, 317, 1327
Deloche A, II-140
Den Hollander W, 565
Derby GC, II-207
DeRouen T, 138
Detre KM, V-79, V-84
DiCarlo LA Jr, 170
Dilsizian V, 853
Director BA, 193
DiSciascio G, 1314
Distante A, 572
Ditchey RV, 660
Dodge HT, V-39
Dollery CT, I-51
Domenicucci S, 774
Donaldson RF, II-191
Douglas JS Jr, 530, 1044
Douglas PS, 991, II-135, II-159
Downing TP, II-84
Dresdale AR, II-237
Driscoll DJ, II-70, II-84
Drop LJ, II-241
Drusin RE, II-237
Duffy CE, II-101
Dunnigan A, 147
Dureau G, 272
Durrer D, 585
Duwel CMB, 565

E

Edgerton TA, 431
Edie RN, II-135
Edmunds LH Jr, II-135, II-159
Edwards WD, II-84
El-Sherif N, 105
Eldar M, 170
Elkayam U, 865, 975
Elkins RC, 840
Ell S, 1355
Ellenbogen KA, 344
Ellis AK, 639
Ellis SG, 193
Emanuelsson H, 287
Emery RW, II-7
Enderlein MA, 825
Engelman RM, II-259
Engelmeier RS, 536
Ensminger S, 353
Epstein AE, 1293
Epstein SE, 1001, 1244, V-23
Ernst ND, 1135A
Eugene J, II-200
European Coronary Surgery Study Group, V-90
Evanochko WT, IV-111
Evans J, 648

F

Fabiani JN, II-140
Fabri BM, II-231
Fagard R, 982
Falcone RA, 1308
Fallon JT, II-231, II-241
Farrar DJ, 1279
Fasules JW, 957
Fedor JM, 225
Fee HJ, 138
Feiring AJ, 1355
Feld G, 555
Feld H, 364
Feldman RD, 547
Feldman T, 495
Fenoglio JJ Jr, 596
Fenyvesi T, 480
Fernandez F, 178
Ferraro N, 72
Fiebig R, 112
Filabozzi P, 1177
Filipchuk N, 327
Finn P, 406
Fiocchi R, 982
Fiol CJ, IV-9
Fisher LD, V-31, V-71, V-110, V-117
Fishman AP, 1270
FitzGerald GA, 1164, 1194
Flameng W, II-179
Fleet WF, 922
Fodor GJ, 692
Force T, 781, 1115
Forni L, 1177
Foster ED, V-59
Fox KAA, 1346
Frazier JC, IV-89
Freed MD, II-77
Freidenberger L, 975
Fremes SE, II-120
Fritz JK, 292
Fritz KE, 1081
Fronek A, 768
Fujii K, 523
Fukami K, 1104
Funai JT, II-191
Furman S, 1037
Fuster V, V-65
Fye WB, 21, 262

G

Gabliani G, 327
Gadsbøll N, 502
Gallino A, 27
Galva MD, 38
Ganz W, 1053, 1321
Gardner PI, 596
Gayheart PA, 431
Geffin GA, II-241
Geisow HP, 1208
George B, II-61
German LD, 344
Gersh BJ, 130
Gersony W, II-52
Gettes LS, 922
Gibson RS, V-9
Gilbert MR, 344
Gilfoil M, 1115
Gill CC, II-170
Gill RM, 623
Gillam LD, 377
Gillespie MJ, V-71
Gilpin E, 963
Ginsburg ME, II-254
Girling L, 1365
Girod DA, II-93
Goede LV, 138
Golbus M, 825
Goldberg LI, 245
Golding LR, II-170, II-216
Goldman BS, II-120
Goldman MH, II-227
Gomes JA, 105
Goor DA, II-164
Goormastic M, II-170
Gordis L, 1155
Goresky CA, IV-81
Gorman RR, 698, 708
Gornick C, 1380
Goto A, 280
Goto Y, 1104
Gotto AM Jr, 8
Gourgon R, 819

Graebner CA, 922
Graham MM, IV-63
Graham TP Jr, II-45
Graves WL Jr, 654
Green MS, 93
Green MV, 853
Green TP, 147
Greenberg MA, 1336
Greene HL, 612
Greenfield JC Jr, 225
Griffin JC, 170
Grimm RH Jr, 971
Grogan EW, 660
Grose RM, 1336
Gruentzig AR, 530, 1044
Grundy SM, 1135A
Guarnieri T, 1092
Guerrero JL, 377
Guiraudon GM, 161
Gunnar RM, 536
Guth B, 233
Guyton RA, II-97

H

Haeberli A, 27
Hagler DJ, II-88
Hale S, 1115
Halushka PV, 1202
Hamano Y, 280
Hammer-Wilson M, II-200
Hammon JW, II-45
Hanrahan J, II-227
Hargrove WC, 1286
Hariman R, 105
Harken AH, II-135
Hartley CJ, 82, 915
Hastillo A, II-227
Hatcher CR Jr, II-97
Hatle L, 810
Hattner RS, 334
Haverich A, II-22, II-108
Haze K, 1104
Hegrenaes L, 810
Heidendal GAK, 565
Heiserman JE, 193
Heiss G, 93
Heitmiller RF, II-241
Hellenbrand W, II-61
Hendrickson JA, 555
Henning H, 963
Henry PD, 456
Henthorn RW, 1293
Herrell FE Jr, V-136
Hershon JJ, 1279
Herst JA, II-120
Hess ML, II-227
Hess OM, 119
Heyden S, 692
Hiatt WR, 1226
Hicks GL, II-254
Higgins CB, 1355
Hill JD, 1279
Hiramori K, 1104
Hirsh J, 178
Hirsh PD, 1314
Hirshfeld JW Jr, 61, II-135, II-159
Hirzel HO, 119
Hlatky MA, V-136
Hodgson JM, 833
Hoffman RG, 1076
Hoffmann E, 200
Høilund-Carlsen PF, 502
Holden JE, IV-72
Holida MD, 82
Hollingsworth C, V-1
Holmberg S, 287
Holt DW, 1064
Holtzman R, 105
Holvoet G, II-179
Hopkins NK, 708
Hopkins R, II-52
Hori M, 523
Hornby EJ, 1208
Houston DS, 728
Howard G, 431
Howe HR, 431
Hsueh W, 975
Huang S, IV-77
Huberty J, 334
Huesman RH, IV-53
Hultgren HN, V-79, V-84
Humphrey PPA, 1208
Hunter WC, 654

I

Idriss FS, II-101
Igarashi A, 801
Ikeda K, 801
Ilbawi MN, II-101
Imaizumi T, 747
Imparato AM, II-13
Ingels NB Jr, II-207
Ingwall JS, IV-89
Inoue M, 523
Ishihara K, 523
Islam N, 698
Isner JM, II-191
Ito H, 523
Ivey TD, 612

J

Jack D, 1208
Jaffe AS, 327
Jamieson SW, II-108
Jang IK, 384
Janicki JS, 1270
Janse MJ, 585
Jansen DE, 327
Jarmolych J, 1081
Jefferis JE, I-21
Jiang L, 377
Johnson SA, II-185
Johnson TA, 922
Jonas RA, II-77
Jones M, 1244
Josa M, 781
Josephson ME, 1286, 1308
Jugdutt BI, 907
Julsrud PR, II-93

K

Kaiser GC, V-46
Kamada T, 280, 523
Kaplan NM, I-31
Karchmer AW, 31
Karp RB, II-175
Kass D, 440
Katz MR, II-227
Kawanishi DT, 865
Kemper AJ, 781, 1115
Kemper WS, 233
Kennedy I, 1208
Kennedy JW, 292, V-39
Kent KM, V-166
Keren A, 302
Kernoff RS, 193
Kersten TE, II-153
Khaw KT, 53
Khuri SF, 781, II-216
Killip T, V-102
King SB III, 530, 1044
Kirklin JK, II-175
Kirklin JW, 753, II-175
Kirshenbaum JM, 873
Kitabatake A, 523
Kleaveland JP, 61
Klein GJ, 161
Kleinman CS, 825
Klementowicz P, 1037
Klocke RJ, 639
Kloner RA, 873, 1115
Klopfenstein HS, 1076
Knabb RM, 1346
Knapp DR, 1202
Konstam MA, II-191
Kormos RL, II-120
Kouchoukos NT, 1144
Kralios FA, 1372
Kram HB, 1022
Kramer E, II-13
Krayenbuehl HP, 119
Kremer P, 112
Krivosic I, 205
Kübler W, 200
Kubota I, 801
Kuo CS, 370
Kussmaul WG, 61
Kwiterovich PO Jr, 1135A

L

L'Abbate A, 572
Lai CYC, 547
Lakatos E, 1244
Laks H, II-61
Lamb J, II-237
Lamparello PJ, II-13
Landini L, 572
Lane GE, 389
Lane MM, 840
Lang RM, 495
LaRaia PJ, II-231
Laramee P, 1053, 1321
Lasher JC, 317, 1327
Laskey WK, 61
Latham RD, 1257
Latini R, 1185
Lattanzi F, 572
Laughlin DE, 82
Le Winter M, 963
Lee KL, V-136
Lee KY, 1365
Lee PK, 1059
LeFree MT, 833
Léger J, 272
Léger JJ, 272

Legrand V, 833
Leimgruber PP, 530, 1044
LeJemtel TH, 364, 846
Lekich RF, 915
Lemeshow S, II-259
Lenfant C, I-44
Lesperance J, V-71
Levine HD, 790
Levine JH, 1092
Levine RJ, I-48
Levinson MM, II-7
Levite HA, 1336
Levy RI, 686
Lew AS, 1053, 1321
Lew WYW, 1125
Lewis HD Jr, V-155
Lewis SA, 1314
Lewis SE, 327
Lijnen HR, 384
Lijnen P, 982
Likoff MJ, 1270
Lindenfeld JA, 660
Lindsay WG, II-153
Lipton MJ, 1355
Little T, 639
Littmann L, 480
Loop FD, II-1, II-170
Lower RR, II-227
Lown B, 1135
Lumley P, 1208
Lurz FW, 1015
Lux RL, 1372
Lytle BW, II-146, II-170

M

Macartney FJ, II-52
Magilligan DJ Jr, II-129
Mahley RW, 943
Maier GW, 668
Mair DD, II-70, II-88, II-93
Mais DE, 1202
Maisel AS, 963
Mancini D, 364
Mancini GBJ, 833
Marchand E, 487
Marchese AC, 344
Marchlinski FE, 1308
Marcus AJ, 698
Marcus ML, 82, 1355
Maris JM, IV-103
Mark DB, V-136
Maron BJ, 310, 853, 1244
Martin JL, 61
Martins JB, 933
Marving J, 502
Masini M, 572
Maskin CS, 364, 846
Masud ARZ, 639
Masuyama T, 523
Matherne GP, 840
Mathey D, 112
Mathey DG, V-39
Matsumoto M, 280
Matsuzaki M, 233
Mattson F, 1135A
Maughan WL, 440, 654
Mayer JE Jr, II-77
Maynard C, 292
McAleer MJ, II-7
McCabe CA, V-31
McCabe PJ, 1208
McCarthy L, 1028
McColgan SJ, II-200
McConney M, V-71
McGoon DC, 130, II-88
McIntosh CL, 1244
McIntyre TM, 718
McKay CR, 865
McKeever LS, II-185
McMillin-Wood JB, IV-145
Meeran MK, II-259
Mehra R, 105
Meijer AEFH, 205
Metras D, II-274
Michalik RE, II-97
Mickleborough LL, II-120
Millar CK, 1372
Miller DC, II-22, II-108, II-207, II-264
Miller JG, 183
Miller JM, 1286
Miller PS, I-41
Milliken JC, II-61
Mills SA, 431
Milstein S, 161
Minamino T, 280
Mitchell RS, II-22, II-108, II-207
Moerman E, 982
Mohanakumar T, II-227
Mohr R, II-164
Mok CK, 1059
Molloy WD, 1365
Moncada S, 1219
Montoya A, II-185
Moore EN, 214, 1092
Moore-Jeffries EW, II-200
Morady F, 170
Morita T, 523
Morley AR, 1064
Morris KG, 632
Moulton AL, II-35
Mueller HS, 1336
Mueller TM, 623
Mullen J, 991
Müller FB, 47
Mullins CB, I-8
Murgo JP, 1257
Murray CK, 840
Myers ML, 915

N

Nademanee K, 555
Nakamura M, 747
Nanna M, 865, 975
Nattel S, 898
Neumann A, 495, 515
Newell JB, 377, II-231
Ng RP, 1059
Nicoloff DM, II-153
Nies AS, 1226
Nightingale SL, I-25
Nioka S, IV-103
Nitenberg A, 819
Nobuhara M, 384
Nordenberg A, II-35
Northrup WF III, II-153

O

O'Callaghan WG, 344
Ocken S, 846
Ockene IS, 1081
O'Connell JB, 536
O'Connell JW, 334
Oesterle SN, II-264
Oglesby TD, 698, 708
O'Keefe DD, II-241
Okumura K, 1293
Olsen CO, 668
O'Rourke RA, 258, 1327
Orszulak TA, 130
Ostrow HG, 1001
Ouattara K, II-274
Ouriel K, II-254
Oyama C, II-129
Oyer PE, II-22, II-108, II-264

P

Pacifico AD, II-175
Packer M, 681
Pandian NG, II-191
Pantopoulos D, 153
Parisi AF, 781, 1115
Park GD, 547
Parkey RW, 327
Passamani E, V-1, V-102
Pasternack PF, II-13
Patrignani P, 1177
Patrono C, 1177
Patti CS, II-254
Paul MH, II-101
Paulin S, 1087
Pearce FJ, II-254
Pedersen AK, 1164, 1194
Peduzzi P, V-79, V-84
Pelletier GB, 487
Pennington DG, II-216
Pérez JE, 183
Perez-Davila V, 1336
Perier P, II-140
Perkins L, 1115
Peters RJG, 585
Petru MA, 1237
Pfeffer JM, 406
Pfeffer MA, 406
Phelps ME, IV-77
Picano E, 572
Picone AL, 1244
Picotti GB, 38
Piehler JM, 130
Pifarre R, II-185
Pike MM, IV-89
Plappert T, 991
Plumb VJ, 1293
Pluth JR, 130
Pohoryles L, II-164
Pohost GM, IV-111
Poll DS, 1308
Pollock ME, II-200
Popp RL, 193, 302, 577
Ports TA, 334
Pozzoli M, 310
Prasquier R, 819
Prescott SM, 718
Prewitt RM, 1365
Price FD, I-13
Pryor DB, V-136
Puga FJ, 130, II-84, II-88, II-93
Pugliese F, 1177

R

Rabinovitch M, 471
Rabinowitz C, 1237

Rad N, 536
Raheja S, 397
Rahimtoola SH, 449, 865, 975, V-123
Rajfer SI, 245
Rankin JS, 668
Rao PS, 1336
Rasmussen HM, 466
Razook JD, 840
Reddy CP, 370
Redish G, 327
Reemtsma K, II-237
Rees P, II-52
Reeves RC, IV-111
Reichek N, 991
Reichenbach D, 612
Reilly IAG, 1194
Reiter SJ, 1355
Rembert JC, 225
Reuderink P, 1257
Ricciardelli B, 38
Rice MJ, II-88, II-93
Richards DA, 214
Rider S, II-227
Rifkind BM, 93
Riles TS, II-13
Riley JE, II-7
Ringel R, II-35
Ritchie JL, 292
Ritzenhoff A, 200
Roberts R, 915, V-145
Robison AK, 1346
Rodriguez L, 1053
Rogers WJ, II-175
Rohla M, 480
Roizen MF, 1015
Roos JP, 565
Rosamond TL, 1346
Rosati RA, V-136
Rose CP, IV-81
Rose EA, II-237
Rosing DR, 853, 1001, 1244
Ross J Jr, 233, 963
Ross R, 735
Roth A, 975
Roth JA, 138
Rothbart ST, 153
Roubin GS, 530, 1044
Rousou JA, II-259
Rovetto MJ, IV-134
Rowe RD, 471
Roy D, 487
Rubal BJ, 1257
Rude R, 327
Ruder M, 170
Rudolph AM, 825
Rumberger JA, 1355
Ruvolo G, II-164
Ruy R, II-179
Ryan TJ, V-31

S

Safier LB, 698
Sagawa K, 440, 654
Sahakian A, 1028
St. John Sutton MG, 991
Saito M, 1104
Saksena S, 153
Salem DN, II-191
Salvadori M, 572
Sanders SP, 1008
Sanger J, II-13
Sasaguri S, II-231
Saussy DL Jr, 1202
Scanlon PJ, 536, II-185
Schaff HV, 130, II-84
Schechtmann N, 334
Scheinman MM, 170
Schelbert HR, IV-122
Scheuer J, IV-139
Schiller NB, 1015
Schlant RC, I-18
Schmitz JJ, 397
Schneider K, 692
Schneider RM, 632
Schneider SP, 147
Schnitt S, 1087
Schnittger I, 193
Schonfeld G, 1135A
Schwartz L, II-120
Schwartz PJ, 585
Scott N, 963
Scott WC, II-22, II-108
Scriven TA, 892
Scully HE, II-120
Seifert FC, II-264
Seifert RA, 735
Selin K, 287
Selwyn AP, IV-31
Sementa A, 774
Senges J, 200
Sergeant P, II-179
Seward JB, II-70
Shah PK, 1053, 1321
Shah Y, 153
Shapiro WA, 1015
Sharma AD, 161
Sheehan F, 292
Sheehan FH, V-39
Sheffield LT, V-31
Shimski M, 1037
Shoemaker WC, 1022
Shroff S, 61
Shumway NE, II-22, II-108, II-264
Siegel RJ, 1148
Silverman NH, 825
Simson MB, 214, 1308
Sinclair N, 1087
Singh BN, 555
Singh PN, 555
Sinoway L, 364
Sipkema P, 1257
Skidmore IF, 1208
Skjaerpe T, 810
Skorton DJ, 1355
Slocum J, 1028
Smallhorn JF, 471
Smith CR, II-237
Smith JS, 1015
Smith TW, IV-31, IV-89
Smolinsky A, II-164
Sobel BE, 183, 327, 1346, I-36, IV-22
Spaet TH, 1336
Spear JF, 214, 1092
Spears JR, 1087
Spirito P, 310, 774
Spokojny AM, 1087
Springer CS Jr, IV-89
Stadius ML, 292
Staessen J, 982
Stark J, II-52
Starling MR, 317, 1327
Steinberg C, 406
Steingart RM, 881, 1037
Stephenson LW, II-135
Stevenson WG, 1
Stewart RW, II-170
Stewart WJ, 377
Stinson EB, 302, II-22, II-108, II-207, II-264
Stoll S, 1226
Storey GCA, 1064
Strain JE, 1336
Straub PW, 27
Strauss MC, 344
Strobino BA, 1232
Strong JP, 1135A
Stump D, 384
Subramanian H, IV-103
Sullivan HJ, II-185
Sumiyoshi T, 1104
Sunagawa K, 654
Surawicz B, 370
Sussmann II, 1336
Swanson JS, II-140
Swinski LA, 31
Swiryn S, 1028
Szentpetery S, II-227

T

Tabrisky J, 1022
Taegtmeyer H, IV-1
Tajimi T, 233
Takamoto T, 193
Takaro T, V-79, V-84
Takeshita A, 747
Tanouchi J, 523
Taylor JFN, II-52
Teirstein PS, 577
Tell GS, 971
Tenczer J, 480
Teplick RS, II-241
Theodorsen L, 971
Théroux P, 487
Théry C, 205
Thomas LJ III, 183
Thomas M, 1208
Thomas R, 612
Thompson WM Jr, 840
Tilsner V, 112
Tilton G, 397, 413
Toal KW, II-241
Tong CP, II-120
Touche T, 819
Tow DE, 781
Tramarin R, 310
Trimarco B, 38, 47
Tristani FE, V-31
Trowitzsch E, 1008
Trusler GA, 471
Tse TF, 1059
Tsuiki K, 801
Tuna IC, 1380
Turina M, 119
Turley K, 334
Tyroler HA, 93
Tyson GS, 668

U

Uğurbil K, IV-94
Ullman HL, 698
Ursell PC, 596, 1232

V

Van de Werf F, 384
van der Velde E, 440
van der Wall EE, 565
van Eenige MJ, 565
Van Ryn J, 178
Vanhaecke J, II-179
Vanhoutte PM, 728
Varnauskas E, V-90
Vassallo JA, 1286
Vatterott PJ, 130
Vecchio C, 310, 774
Vellar OD, 971
Veterans Administration Cooperative Study Group, V-155
Vetrovec GW, 1314
Vieli A, 193
Vinten-Johansen J, 431
Visser FC, 565
Vogel RA, 460, 833
Volpe M, 47

W

Wahr DW, 334
Waldo AL, 1293
Wallin J, 287
Wallis CJ, 1208
Walsh R, 536
Walsh RA, 317
Wang R, 1059
Wann LS, 1076
Ward JW, 698
Watanabe F, 280
Waternaux CM, 31
Waters DD, 487
Wathen M, 413
Watson DD, V-9
Watson JT, II-216
Watson RM, 1001
Weber KT, 1270
Weber L, 975
Wehrli FW, IV-97
Weidman WH, 1135A
Weinberger M, 1135A
Weiner BH, 1081
Weiner DA, V-31
Weinstein EM, 825
Weintraub D, 302
Weintraub WS, 632
Weisel RD, II-120
Weisfeldt ML, 1092
Weiss JN, 865
Wellens HJJ, 1
Westera G, 565
Westerhof N, 1257
Weyman AE, 377
White CW, 82
White RA, 1022
Whittle BJR, 1219
Whitworth HB, 530
Wickline SA, 183
Wiener DH, 72
Wiggins JW, 957
Willerson JT, 327, 397, 413, V-3
Williams GW, II-146
Williams OD, 93
Williams RG, II-61
Williams WG, 471
Williams WH, II-97
Wilms-Schopman F, 585
Wilson JR, 72
Wilson RF, 82
Winston SA, 170
Wisenbaugh T, 648
Wit AL, 596
Wolfe CL, 327
Wolfe RR, 957
Wolfgang TC, 1314, II-227
Wong M, 138
Wroblewski R, I-1, I-3

Y

Yamaki M, 801
Yamamoto J, 1104
Yasui K, 280
Yasui S, 801
Yock PG, 577
Yoshida Y, 523
Yoshima H, 523
Yu G, 648

Z

Zak R, IV-13
Zerbe GO, 660
Zierler K, IV-69
Zimmerman GA, 718
Zipes DP, 623, 949
Ziskind Z, II-164
Zorn GL Jr, II-175

SUBJECT INDEX*

A

Abdominal aortic surgery
Combined cardiac and abdominal aortic surgery, II-18
Adolescents
The relationship of white cell count, platelet count, and hematocrit to cigarette smoking in adolescents: the Oslo Youth Study, 971
Afterdepolarizations
Cesium chloride–induced long QT syndrome: demonstration of afterdepolarizations and triggered activity in vivo, 1092
Allograft rejection
Early detection of cardiac allograft rejection with proton nuclear magnetic resonance, II-231
α-Adrenergic receptors
Cyclic blood flow variations induced by platelet-activating factor in stenosed canine coronary arteries despite inhibition of thromboxane synthetase, serotonin receptors, and α-adrenergic receptors, 397
Amiodarone
Amiodarone and its desethyl metabolite: tissue distribution and morphologic changes during long-term therapy, 1064
Kinetics of electrophysiologic changes during oral loading of amiodarone and after withdrawal of amiodarone in the unsedated dog, 1380
Amitriptyline
Frequency-dependent effects of amitriptyline on ventricular conduction and cardiac rhythm in dogs, 898
Aneurysm
Left ventricular aneurysm and the prediction of left ventricular enlargement studied by two-dimensional echocardiography: quantitative assessment of aneurysm size in relation to clinical course, 280
Angina
The 5 year effect of bypass surgery on relief of angina and exercise performance, V-79
Indications for coronary artery bypass surgery in patients with chronic angina pectoris: implications of the multicenter randomized trials, V-23
Stable angina as a manifestation of ischemic heart disease: medical management, V-145
Unstable angina: status of aspirin and other forms of therapy, V-155
Angioplasty
Comparative long-term effects of coronary artery bypass graft surgery and percutaneous transluminal coronary angioplasty on regional coronary flow reserve, 833
Coronary angioplasty of multiple vessels: short-term outcome and long-term results, 1314
The effects of coronary angioplasty and reperfusion on distribution of myocardial flow, 334
Factors contributing to perforations from laser coronary angioplasty: observations in an intact human postmortem preparation of intraoperative laser coronary angioplasty, II-191
In-hospital morbidity and mortality in patients undergoing elective coronary angioplasty, 1044
Indications for transluminal coronary angioplasty, V-166
Influence of intimal dissection on restenosis after successful coronary angioplasty, 530
Percutaneous transluminal coronary angioplasty: a surgeon's view, 1144
Percutaneous transluminal coronary angioplasty: role in the treatment of coronary artery disease, V-161
Usefulness of coronary artery bypass graft surgery or percutaneous transluminal angioplasty after thrombolytic therapy, V-39
Animal preparations
Animal preparations relevant for study with positron-emission tomography or nuclear magnetic resonance, IV-139
Requirements for animal preparations for metabolic imaging, IV-134
Anorexia nervosa
Effects of reduced left ventricular mass on chamber architecture, load, and function: a study of anorexia nervosa, 991
Aortic disease
Altered left ventricular mechanics in patients with valvular aortic stenosis and coarctation of the aorta: effects on systolic performance and late outcome, 515
Aortic dissection
Acute and chronic aortic dissections—determinants of long-term outcome for operative survivors, II-22
Aortic elasticity
Regional wave travel and reflections along the human aorta: a study with six simultaneous micromanometric pressures, 1257
Aortic regurgitation
Assessment and follow-up of patients with aortic regurgitation by an updated Doppler echocardiographic measurement of the regurgitant fraction in the aortic arch, 819
Importance of internal controls, statistical methods, and side effects in short-term trials of vasodilators: a study of hydralazine kinetics in patients with aortic regurgitation, 865
A new approach to noninvasive evaluation of aortic regurgitant fraction by two-dimensional Doppler echocardiography, 523
Survival and functional results after valve replacement for aortic regurgitation from 1976 to 1983: impact of preoperative left ventricular function, 1244
Aortic stenosis
Noninvasive estimation of valve area in patients with aortic stenosis by Doppler ultrasound and two-dimensional echocardiography, 810
Arrhythmia
Abnormal signal-averaged electrocardiograms in patients with nonischemic congestive cardiomyopathy: relationship to sustained ventricular tachyarrhythmias, 1308
Amiodarone and its desethyl metabolite: tissue distribution and morphologic changes during long-term therapy, 1064
Atrial fibrillation in patients with Wolff-Parkinson-White syndrome: incidence after surgical ablation of the accessory pathway, 161
Atrial flutter: a synthesis of concepts, 249
Autonomic control of ventricular tachycardia: sympathetic neural influence on spontaneous tachycardia 24 hours after coronary occlusion, 933
Catheter-mediated electrical ablation of the posterior septum via the coronary sinus: electrophysiologic and histologic observations in dogs, 612
Clinical correlates of atrial tachyarrhythmias after valve replacement for aortic stenosis, II-159
Comparative efficacy of transvenous cardioversion and pacing in patients with sustained ventricular tachycardia: a prospective, randomized, crossover study, 153
Complex ventricular arrhythmias in Q wave and non–Q wave myocardial infarction, 963
Computer detection of atrioventricular dissociation from surface electrocardiograms during wide QRS complex tachycardias, 1028
A consideration of antiarrhythmic therapy, 949
Day-to-day variations in inducibility of ventricular tachyarrhythmias during the late postmyocardial infarction phase in conscious dogs, 200
Dispersion of ventricular repolarization and arrhythmia: study of two consecutive ventricular premature complexes, 370
Does the type of venous drainage or cardioplegia affect postoperative conduction and atrial arrhythmias? II-259
The effects of premature stimulation of the His bundle on epicardial activation and body surface late potentials in dogs susceptible to sustained ventricular tachyarrhythmias, 214
Electrophysiologic and antiarrhythmic effects of sotalol in patients with life-threatening ventricular tachyarrhythmias, 555
Frequency-dependent effects of amitriptyline on ventricular conduction and cardiac rhythm in dogs, 898
Programmed electrical stimulation of the heart in patients with life-threatening ventricular arrhythmias: What is the significance of induced arrhythmias and what is the correct stimulation protocol? 1
Arteriosclerosis
Experimental arteriosclerosis treated by argon ion and neodymium-YAG laser endarterectomy, II-200
Some reflections on arteriosclerosis: past, present, and future. Presidential Address, 8
Aspirin
Unstable angina: status of aspirin and other forms of therapy, V-155

*Roman numbers indicate articles published in supplements.

Warfarin versus dipyridamole-aspirin and pentoxifylline-aspirin for the prevention of prosthetic heart valve thromboembolism: a prospective randomized clinical trial, 1059
Atenolol
Effect of the combination of diltiazem and atenolol on exercise-induced regional myocardial ischemia in conscious dogs, 233
Atherosclerosis
Angle dependence of ultrasonic backscatter in arterial tissues: a study in vitro, 572
Atherogenic lipoproteins and coronary artery disease: concepts derived from recent advances in cellular and molecular biology, 943
Atherosclerosis, calcium, and calcium antagonists, 456
Cholesterol and cardiovascular disease: no longer whether, but rather when, in whom, and how? 686
Comparison of pathologic and angiographic findings in a porcine preparation of coronary atherosclerosis, 1081
Noninvasively diagnosed peripheral arterial disease as a predictor of mortality: results from a prospective study, 768
ATPase
Magnetization transfer measurements of creatine kinase and ATPase rates in intact hearts, IV-94
Atrial fibrillation
Atrial fibrillation in patients with Wolff-Parkinson-White syndrome: incidence after surgical ablation of the accessory pathway, 161
Atrial flutter
Atrial flutter: a synthesis of concepts, 249
Atrial natriuretic peptide
Effects of synthetic atrial natriuretic peptide on renal function and renin release in acute experimental heart failure, 892
Atrioventricular node conduction
Frequency-dependent effects of verapamil on atrioventricular nodal conduction in man, 344

B

β-Adrenergic receptors
The interaction of verapamil and norverapamil with β-adrenergic receptors, 547
β-Blockers
Effect of β-adrenergic blockers on the peripheral circulation in patients with peripheral vascular disease, 1226
Effect of the combination of diltiazem and atenolol on exercise-induced regional myocardial ischemia in conscious dogs, 233
Effects of β-adrenoreceptor–blocking drugs in patients with Raynaud's phenomenon, 466
Use of an ultra short–acting β-blocker in patients with acute myocardial ischemia, 873
Blalock-Taussig shunt
Classic versus modified Blalock-Taussig shunts in neonates and infants, II-35
Blood flow
The accuracy of Doppler ultrasound measurement of pressure gradients across irregular, dual, and tunnellike obstructions to blood flow, 577
Contrast echocardiographic estimation of regional myocardial blood flow after acute coronary occlusion, 1115
Cyclic blood flow variations induced by platelet-activating factor in stenosed canine coronary arteries despite inhibition of thromboxane synthetase, serotonin receptors, and α-adrenergic receptors, 397
Effect of the sympathetic nervous system on limb circulation and metabolism during exercise in patients with heart failure, 72
Effects of blood flow on the positron-emission tomographic determination of substrate transport rates, IV-72
The effects of coronary angioplasty and reperfusion on distribution of myocardial flow, 334
Error in parameter estimates with variations in flow: measurement of oxygen utilization with positron-emission tomography, IV-77
Exercise thallium-201 scintigraphy in dogs: effects of long-term coronary occlusion and collateral development on early and late scintigraphic images, 881
Factors that modify the flow response to intracoronary injections, 287
The radiographic assessment of coronary blood flow parameters, 460
Transluminal, subselective measurement of coronary artery blood flow velocity and vasodilator reserve in man, 82
Blood pressure
The nature of opioid involvement in the hemodynamic, respiratory, and humoral responses to exercise, 982
Body surface mapping
Detection of local abnormalities in ventricular activation sequence by body surface isochrone mapping in patients with previous myocardial infarction, 801

C

Calcium antagonists
Atherosclerosis, calcium, and calcium antagonists, 456
Frequency-dependent effects of verapamil on atrioventricular nodal conduction in man, 344
Captopril
Survival after an experimental myocardial infarction: beneficial effects of long-term therapy with captopril, 406
Systemic and regional hemodynamic effects of captopril and milrinone administered alone and concomitantly in patients with heart failure, 364
Carbohydrates
Carbohydrate interconversions and energy production, IV-1
Cardiac catheterization
Accuracy of volume measurement by conductance catheter in isolated, ejecting canine hearts, 440
Cardiac metabolism
Overview of the process of delivery: flow, transmembrane transport, reaction, and retention, IV-39
Cardiac surgery
Combined cardiac and abdominal aortic surgery, II-18
Hemodynamic effects of intravenous nitroglycerin in pediatric patients after heart surgery, II-101
Cardiac tamponade
Effects of intravascular volume state on the value of pulsus paradoxus and right ventricular diastolic collapse in predicting cardiac tamponade, 1076
Cardiac transplantation
Early detection of cardiac allograft rejection with proton nuclear magnetic resonance, II-231
A prospective randomized trial of pretransfusion/azathioprine-/prednisone versus cyclosporine/prednisone immunosuppression in cardiac transplant recipients: preliminary results, II-227
Reduced infection in cardiac transplant recipients, II-237
The role of mechanical support and transplantation in treatment of patients with end-stage cardiomyopathy, II-7
Cardiogenic shock
Long-term follow-up of postcardiotomy patients with profound cardiogenic shock treated with ventricular assist devices, II-216
Cardiomyopathy
Abnormal signal-averaged electrocardiograms in patients with nonischemic congestive cardiomyopathy: relationship to sustained ventricular tachyarrhythmias, 1308
Diastolic abnormalities in patients with hypertrophic cardiomyopathy: relation to magnitude of left ventricular hypertrophy, 310
Effects of sublingual nifedipine on hemodynamics and systolic and diastolic function in patients with hypertrophic cardiomyopathy, 1001
Has 'obstruction' hindered our understanding of hypertrophic cardiomyopathy? 1148
Improvement in symptoms and exercise tolerance by metoprolol in patients with dilated cardiomyopathy: a double-blind, randomized, placebo-controlled trial, 536
Mildly dilated congestive cardiomyopathy, 302
The role of mechanical support and transplantation in treatment of patients with end-stage cardiomyopathy, II-7
Cardioplegia
Does the type of venous drainage or cardioplegia affect postoperative conduction and atrial arrhythmias? II-259
Myocardial recovery after hypothermic arrest: a comparison of oxy-

genated crystalloid to blood cardioplegia. The role of calcium, II-241
Cardioversion
Comparative efficacy of transvenous cardioversion and pacing in patients with sustained ventricular tachycardia: a prospective, randomized, crossover study, 153
Catecholamines
Participation of endogenous catecholamines in the regulation of left ventricular mass in progeny of hypertensive parents, 38
Catheter ablation
Catheter-mediated electrical ablation of the posterior septum via the coronary sinus: electrophysiologic and histologic observations in dogs, 612
Cesium chloride
Cesium chloride–induced long QT syndrome: demonstration of afterdepolarizations and triggered activity in vivo, 1092
Cholesterol
Atherogenic lipoproteins and coronary artery disease: concepts derived from recent advances in cellular and molecular biology, 943
Cholesterol and cardiovascular disease: no longer whether, but rather when, in whom, and how? 686
The ratio of plasma high-density lipoprotein cholesterol to total and low-density lipoprotein cholesterol: age-related changes and race and sex differences in selected North American populations. The Lipid Research Clinics Program Prevalence Study, 93
Cineventriculography
Validation of attenuation-corrected equilibrium radionuclide angiographic determinations of right ventricular volume: comparison with cast-validated biplane cineventriculography, 317
Clinical trials
Some unexpected lessons from large multicenter randomized clinical trials, 449
Coarctation
Altered left ventricular mechanics in patients with valvular aortic stenosis and coarctation of the aorta: effects on systolic performance and late outcome, 515
Collateral vessels
Collateral conductance changes during a brief coronary occlusion in awake dogs, 225
Computed tomography
Determination of left ventricular mass in dogs with rapid-acquisition cardiac computed tomographic scanning, 1355
Conductance
Collateral conductance changes during a brief coronary occlusion in awake dogs, 225
Congenital heart disease
Abnormal distribution of pulmonary blood flow after the Glenn shunt or Fontan procedure: risk of development of arteriovenous fistulae, 471
Fetal atrioventricular valve insufficiency associated with nonimmune hydrops: a two-dimensional echocardiographic and pulsed Doppler ultrasound study, 825
Hemodynamic effects of intravenous nitroglycerin in pediatric patients after heart surgery, II-101
Right heart assist by intermittent abdominal compression after surgery for congenital heart disease, II-97
Significance of cardiac defects in the developing fetus: a study of spontaneous abortuses, 1232
Congestive heart failure
Characteristics of vascular hydraulic load in patients with heart failure, 61
Comparative systemic and renal effects of dopamine and angiotensin-converting enzyme inhibition with enalaprilat in patients with heart failure, 846
Effect of the sympathetic nervous system on limb circulation and metabolism during exercise in patients with heart failure, 72
The effects of sublingually administered nitroglycerin on forearm vascular resistance in patients with heart failure and in normal subjects, 747
Isometric exercise in patients with chronic advanced heart failure: hemodynamic and neurohumoral evaluation, 975
Mildly dilated congestive cardiomyopathy, 302
The pressure-flow response of the pulmonary circulation in patients with heart failure and pulmonary vascular disease, 1270
Sudden unexpected death in patients with congestive heart failure: a second frontier, 681
Systemic and regional hemodynamic effects of captopril and milrinone administered alone and concomitantly in patients with heart failure, 364
Contractility
The dependence of myocardial ultrasonic integrated backscatter on contractile performance, 183
Coronary angiography
Comparison of pathologic and angiographic findings in a porcine preparation of coronary atherosclerosis, 1081
Coronary arteriography
The radiographic assessment of coronary blood flow parameters, 460
Selection of patients for coronary arteriography, V-3
Coronary artery disease
Fibrin formation and platelet aggregation in patients with severe coronary artery disease: relationship with the degree of myocardial ischemia, 27
Improvement in regional wall motion and left ventricular relaxation after administration of diltiazem in patients with coronary artery disease, 353
Left ventricular systolic and diastolic function in coronary artery disease: effects of revascularization on exercise-induced ischemia, 119
Percutaneous transluminal coronary angioplasty: role in the treatment of coronary artery disease, V-161
Reoperation for coronary artery disease, V-59
Surgery in the treatment of coronary artery disease: introduction, V-1
Coronary artery surgery
CABG 1984: technical aspects of bypass surgery, V-46
Comparative long-term effects of coronary artery bypass graft surgery and percutaneous transluminal coronary angioplasty on regional coronary flow reserve, 833
Coronary Artery Surgery Study (CASS): a randomized trial of coronary bypass surgery. Eight years follow-up and survival in patients with reduced ejection fraction, V-102
Design and study similarities and contrasts: the Veterans Administration, European, and CASS randomized trials of coronary artery bypass graft surgery, V-110
Does mammary artery grafting increase surgical risk? II-170
The effect of clinical characteristics on the comparison of medical and surgical therapy in the Coronary Artery Surgery Study (CASS) and the Veterans Administration Cooperative Trial, V-117
Emergency bypass surgery: late effects on size of infarction and ventricular function, II-179
The 5 year effect of bypass surgery on relief of angina and exercise performance, V-79
Improved graft patency in patients treated with platelet-inhibiting therapy after coronary bypass surgery, 138
Indications for coronary artery bypass surgery in patients with chronic angina pectoris: implications of the multicenter randomized trials, V-23
Intermediate-term results of coronary artery bypass grafting for acute myocardial infarction, II-175
Long-term fate of bypass grafts: the Coronary Artery Surgery Study (CASS) and Montreal Heart Institute experiences, V-71
Long-term mortality and morbidity results of the Veterans Administration randomized trial of coronary artery bypass surgery, V-84
A perspective on the three large multicenter randomized clinical trials of coronary bypass surgery for chronic stable angina, V-123
Radionuclide methods of identifying patients who may require coronary artery bypass surgery, V-9
Randomized trials of coronary artery bypass surgery: impact on clinical practice at Duke University Medical Center, V-136
Survival, myocardial infarction, and employment status in a prospective randomized study of coronary bypass surgery, V-90
Usefulness of coronary artery bypass graft surgery or percutaneous transluminal angioplasty after thrombolytic therapy, V-39
Coronary Artery Surgery Study (CASS)
CASS continued, II-1
Coronary Artery Surgery Study (CASS): a randomized trial of coronary bypass surgery. Eight years follow-up and survival in patients with reduced ejection fraction, V-102
The effect of clinical characteristics on the comparison of medical and surgical therapy in the Coronary Artery Surgery Study (CASS)

and the Veterans Administration Cooperative Trial, V-117
Exercise testing in the Coronary Artery Surgery Study randomized population, V-31
Long-term fate of bypass grafts: the Coronary Artery Surgery Study (CASS) and Montreal Heart Institute experiences, V-71

Coronary occlusion
Collateral conductance changes during a brief coronary occlusion in awake dogs, 225

Coronary sinus
An enzyme histochemical study of human sinus node, coronary sinus, and mitral valve muscle, 205

Creatine kinase
Magnetization transfer measurements of creatine kinase and ATPase rates in intact hearts, IV-94

Cyclooxygenase
The effect of cyclooxygenase inhibition on vasomotion of proximal coronary arteries with endothelial damage, 389

Cyclosporine
A prospective randomized trial of pretransfusion/azathioprine-/prednisone versus cyclosporine/prednisone immunosuppression in cardiac transplant recipients: preliminary results, II-227

D

Data analysis
Ten precepts for quantitative data acquisition and analysis, IV-53

Digital radiography
The radiographic assessment of coronary blood flow parameters, 460

Diltiazem
Effect of the combination of diltiazem and atenolol on exercise-induced regional myocardial ischemia in conscious dogs, 233
Effects of propranolol and diltiazem alone and in combination on the recovery of left ventricular segmental function after temporary coronary occlusion and long-term reperfusion in conscious dogs, 413
Improvement in regional wall motion and left ventricular relaxation after administration of diltiazem in patients with coronary artery disease, 353

Dobutamine
Comparative effects of volume loading, dobutamine, and nitroprusside in patients with predominant right ventricular infarction, 1327
Treatment of canine permeability pulmonary edema: short-term effects of dobutamine, furosemide, and hydralazine, 1365

Dopamine
Comparative systemic and renal effects of dopamine and angiotensin-converting enzyme inhibition with enalaprilat in patients with heart failure, 846

Dopamine receptors
Dopamine receptors: applications in clinical cardiology, 245

E

Ebstein's anomaly
Surgical repair of Ebstein's anomaly: selection of patients and early and late operative results, II-70

Echocardiography
The accuracy of Doppler ultrasound measurement of pressure gradients across irregular, dual, and tunnellike obstructions to blood flow, 577
Assessment and follow-up of patients with aortic regurgitation by an updated Doppler echocardiographic measurement of the regurgitant fraction in the aortic arch, 819
Contrast echocardiographic estimation of regional myocardial blood flow after acute coronary occlusion, 1115
Diastolic abnormalities in patients with hypertrophic cardiomyopathy: relation to magnitude of left ventricular hypertrophy, 310
A Doppler–two-dimensional echocardiographic method for quantitation of mitral regurgitation, 377
Fetal atrioventricular valve insufficiency associated with nonimmune hydrops: a two-dimensional echocardiographic and pulsed Doppler ultrasound study, 825
Intraoperative detection of myocardial ischemia in high-risk patients: electrocardiography vs two-dimensional transesophageal echocardiography, 1015
Left ventricular aneurysm and the prediction of left ventricular enlargement studied by two-dimensional echocardiography: quantitative assessment of aneurysm size in relation to clinical course, 280
A new approach to noninvasive evaluation of aortic regurgitant fraction by two-dimensional Doppler echocardiography, 523
Non–Q wave perioperative myocardial infarction: assessment of the incidence and severity of regional dysfunction with quantitative two-dimensional echocardiography, 781
Noninvasive estimation of valve area in patients with aortic stenosis by Doppler ultrasound and two-dimensional echocardiography, 810
Prognostic significance and natural history of left ventricular thrombi in patients with acute anterior myocardial infarction: a two-dimensional echocardiographic study, 774
Transluminal, subselective measurement of coronary artery blood flow velocity and vasodilator reserve in man, 82

Editorials
Cardiology at a precipice, 258
Comprehensive health care and noncardiovascular mortality: an unlikely explanation of the findings from the Hypertension Detection and Follow-up Program, 692
Human tissue-type plasminogen activator: from the laboratory to the bedside, 18
Percutaneous transluminal coronary angioplasty: a surgeon's view, 1144
Physicians confront the nuclear peril, 1135
Some unexpected lessons from large multicenter randomized clinical trials, 449

Ejection fraction
Are right and left ventricular ejection fractions equal? Ejection fractions in normal subjects and in patients with first acute myocardial infarction, 502
Effect of early postoperative volume loading on left ventricular systolic function (including left ventricular ejection fraction determined by myocardial marker) after myocardial revascularization, II-207
Left ventricular ejection fraction after acute coronary occlusion in conscious dogs: relation to the extent and site of myocardial infarction, 632

Electrocardiography
Change in ventricular cavity size: differential effects on QRS and T wave amplitude, 495
Computer detection of atrioventricular dissociation from surface electrocardiograms during wide QRS complex tachycardias, 1028
Intraoperative detection of myocardial ischemia in high-risk patients: electrocardiography vs two-dimensional transesophageal echocardiography, 1015

Electrophysiology
Catheter-mediated electrical ablation of the posterior septum via the coronary sinus: electrophysiologic and histologic observations in dogs, 612
Correlation between refractory periods and activation-recovery intervals from electrograms: effects of rate and adrenergic interventions, 1372
Day-to-day variations in inducibility of ventricular tachyarrhythmias during the late postmyocardial infarction phase in conscious dogs, 200
Detection of local abnormalities in ventricular activation sequence by body surface isochrone mapping in patients with previous myocardial infarction, 801
Dispersion of ventricular repolarization and arrhythmia: study of two consecutive ventricular premature complexes, 370
Effect of serial brief ischemic episodes on extracellular K^+, pH, and activation in the pig, 922
The effects of overdrive pacing and lidocaine on atrioventricular junctional rhythm in man: the role of abnormal automaticity, 480
Effects of unilateral stellate ganglion stimulation and ablation on electrophysiologic changes induced by acute myocardial ischemia in dogs, 585

Efficacy and safety of transcatheter ablation of posteroseptal accessory pathways, 170
Electrophysiologic and anatomic basis for fractionated electrograms recorded from healed myocardial infarcts, 596
Electrophysiologic and antiarrhythmic effects of sotalol in patients with life-threatening ventricular tachyarrhythmias, 555
Frequency-dependent effects of amitriptyline on ventricular conduction and cardiac rhythm in dogs, 898
Further observations on transient entrainment: importance of pacing site and properties of the components of the reentry circuit, 1293
Intermittent failure of local conduction during ventricular tachycardia, 1286
Kinetics of electrophysiologic changes during oral loading of amiodarone and after withdrawal of amiodarone in the unsedated dog, 1380
Periodic procainamide for paroxysmal tachycardia, 147
Programmed ventricular stimulation in survivors of an acute myocardial infarction, 487
Quantitative analysis of the high-frequency components of the signal-averaged QRS complex in patients with acute myocardial infarction: a prospective study, 105

Enalaprilat
Comparative systemic and renal effects of dopamine and angiotensin-converting enzyme inhibition with enalaprilat in patients with heart failure, 846

Endocarditis
Risk factors for the development of prosthetic valve endocarditis, 31
Uptake of hematoporphyrin by valvular vegetations in experimental infective endocarditis, 1087

Endomyocardial fibrosis
The surgical treatment of endomyocardial fibrosis: results in 55 patients, II-274

Energy metabolism
Cardiac energy metabolism: contributions from nuclear magnetic resonance, IV-18

Energy production
Carbohydrate interconversions and energy production, IV-1

Epicardial activation
The effects of premature stimulation of the His bundle on epicardial activation and body surface late potentials in dogs susceptible to sustained ventricular tachyarrhythmias, 214

Esmolol
Use of an ultra short–acting β-blocker in patients with acute myocardial ischemia, 873

Exercise
Effect of isotonic exercise training on left ventricular volume during upright exercise, 1237
Effect of the sympathetic nervous system on limb circulation and metabolism during exercise in patients with heart failure, 72
The 5 year effect of bypass surgery on relief of angina and exercise performance, V-79
Isometric exercise in patients with chronic advanced heart failure: hemodynamic and neurohumoral evaluation, 975
Left ventricular systolic and diastolic function in coronary artery disease: effects of revascularization on exercise-induced ischemia, 119
Maintenance of exercise stroke volume during ventricular versus atrial synchronous pacing: rate of contractility, 1037
The nature of opioid involvement in the hemodynamic, respiratory, and humoral responses to exercise, 982

Exercise testing
Exercise testing in the Coronary Artery Surgery Study randomized population, V-31

F

Fatty acids
Fatty acid and ketone metabolism, IV-9

Fibrin
Fibrin formation and platelet aggregation in patients with severe coronary artery disease: relationship with the degree of myocardial ischemia, 27

Fontan procedure
Abnormal distribution of pulmonary blood flow after the Glenn shunt or Fontan procedure: risk of development of arteriovenous fistulae, 471
Outcome of the Fontan procedure in patients with tricuspid atresia, II-88
Relationship of pulmonary artery size to mortality in patients undergoing the Fontan operation, II-93

Fractionated electrograms
Electrophysiologic and anatomic basis for fractionated electrograms recorded from healed myocardial infarcts, 596

Furosemide
Treatment of canine permeability pulmonary edema: short-term effects of dobutamine, furosemide, and hydralazine, 1365

G

Glenn shunt
Abnormal distribution of pulmonary blood flow after the Glenn shunt or Fontan procedure: risk of development of arteriovenous fistulae, 471

Graft patency
Improved graft patency in patients treated with platelet-inhibiting therapy after coronary bypass surgery, 138

H

Heart failure
Effects of synthetic atrial natriuretic peptide on renal function and renin release in acute experimental heart failure, 892

Heart rate
Effect of heart rate on the canine end-systolic pressure-volume relationship, 654

Hematology
The relationship of white cell count, platelet count, and hematocrit to cigarette smoking in adolescents: the Oslo Youth Study, 971

Hematoporphyrin
Uptake of hematoporphyrin by valvular vegetations in experimental infective endocarditis, 1087

Hemodynamics
Effects of sublingual nifedipine on hemodynamics and systolic and diastolic function in patients with hypertrophic cardiomyopathy, 1001
Isometric exercise in patients with chronic advanced heart failure: hemodynamic and neurohumoral evaluation, 975
Maintenance of exercise stroke volume during ventricular versus atrial synchronous pacing: rate of contractility, 1037

Heterogeneity
Heterogeneity within observed regions: physiologic basis and effects on estimation of rates of biodynamic processes, IV-47

Histochemistry
An enzyme histochemical study of human sinus node, coronary sinus, and mitral valve muscle, 205

Hydralazine
Importance of internal controls, statistical methods, and side effects in short-term trials of vasodilators: a study of hydralazine kinetics in patients with aortic regurgitation, 865
Treatment of canine permeability pulmonary edema: short-term effects of dobutamine, furosemide, and hydralazine, 1365

Hydraulic load
Characteristics of vascular hydraulic load in patients with heart failure, 61

Hyperlipoproteinemia
Atherogenic lipoproteins and coronary artery disease: concepts derived from recent advances in cellular and molecular biology, 943

Hypertension
Comprehensive health care and noncardiovascular mortality: an unlikely explanation of the findings from the Hypertension Detection and Follow-up Program, 692

Is hypertension more benign when associated with obesity? 53
Participation of endogenous catecholamines in the regulation of left ventricular mass in progeny of hypertensive parents, 38
Transient enhancement of sympathetic nervous system activity by long-term restriction of sodium intake, 47
Hypertrophic cardiomyopathy
Verapamil-induced improvement in left ventricular diastolic filling and increased exercise tolerance in patients with hypertropic cardiomyopathy: short- and long-term effects, 853

I

Immunofluorescence
Local changes in myosin types in diseased human atrial myocardium: a quantitative immunofluorescence study, 272
Immunosuppression
A prospective randomized trial of pretransfusion/azathioprine-/prednisone versus cyclosporine/prednisone immunosuppression in cardiac transplant recipients: preliminary results, II-227
Internal mammary artery
Does mammary artery grafting increase surgical risk? II-170
Intracoronary injection
Factors that modify the flow response to intracoronary injections, 287
Ischemia
The dependence of myocardial ultrasonic integrated backscatter on contractile performance, 183
Effect of the combination of diltiazem and atenolol on exercise-induced regional myocardial ischemia in conscious dogs, 233
Effect of serial brief ischemic episodes on extracellular K^+, pH, and activation in the pig, 922
Effects of right ventricular ischemia on left ventricular geometry and the end-diastolic pressure-volume relationship in the dog, 1104
Effects of unilateral stellate ganglion stimulation and ablation on electrophysiologic changes induced by acute myocardial ischemia in dogs, 585
Enhancement of recovery of myocardial function by oxygen free-radical scavengers after reversible regional ischemia, 915
Fibrin formation and platelet aggregation in patients with severe coronary artery disease: relationship with the degree of myocardial ischemia, 27
Immediate functional recovery and avoidance of reperfusion injury with surgical revascularization of short-term coronary occlusion, 431
Intraoperative detection of myocardial ischemia in high-risk patients: electrocardiography vs two-dimensional transesophageal echocardiography, 1015
Left ventricular systolic and diastolic function in coronary artery disease: effects of revascularization on exercise-induced ischemia, 119
Mechanisms of improving regional and global ventricular function by preload alterations during acute ischemia in the canine left ventricle, 1125
Stable angina as a manifestation of ischemic heart disease: medical management, V-145
Ultrasonic tissue characterization: detection of acute myocardial ischemia in dogs, 193
Use of an ultra short–acting β-blocker in patients with acute myocardial ischemia, 873

J

Jones, T. Duckett, Memorial Lecture
The virtual disappearance of rheumatic fever in the United States: lessons in the rise and fall of disease. T. Duckett Jones Memorial Lecture, 1155
Junctional rhythms
The effects of overdrive pacing and lidocaine on atrioventricular junctional rhythm in man: the role of abnormal automaticity, 480

K

Ketone
Fatty acid and ketone metabolism, IV-9

L

Laser coronary angioplasty
Factors contributing to perforations from laser coronary angioplasty: observations in an intact human postmortem preparation of intraoperative laser coronary angioplasty, II-191
Laser endarterectomy
Experimental arteriosclerosis treated by argon ion and neodymium-YAG laser endarterectomy, II-200
Late potentials
The effects of premature stimulation of the His bundle on epicardial activation and body surface late potentials in dogs susceptible to sustained ventricular tachyarrhythmias, 214
Left ventricular assistance
Right ventricular function in an operating room model of mechanical left ventricular assistance and its effects in patients with depressed left ventricular function, 1279
Left ventricular function
Left ventricular systolic and diastolic function in coronary artery disease: effects of revascularization on exercise-induced ischemia, 119
Lipids
Atherogenic lipoproteins and coronary artery disease: concepts derived from recent advances in cellular and molecular biology, 943
Cholesterol and cardiovascular disease: no longer whether, but rather when, in whom, and how? 686
The ratio of plasma high-density lipoprotein cholesterol to total and low-density lipoprotein cholesterol: age-related changes and race and sex differences in selected North American populations. The Lipid Research Clinics Program Prevalence Study, 93
Lipoproteins
The ratio of plasma high-density lipoprotein cholesterol to total and low-density lipoprotein cholesterol: age-related changes and race and sex differences in selected North American populations. The Lipid Research Clinics Program Prevalence Study, 93
Long QT syndrome
Cesium chloride–induced long QT syndrome: demonstration of afterdepolarizations and triggered activity in vivo, 1092

M

Mannitol
Preservation of myocardial function with mannitol reperfusate, II-254
Mechanical support
The role of mechanical support and transplantation in treatment of patients with end-stage cardiomyopathy, II-7
Metabolic imaging
Requirements for animal preparations for metabolic imaging, IV-134
Workshop on Cardiovascular Metabolic Imaging: kinetics of substrate transport and reaction. Critique of the session, IV-69
Metabolism
Heterogeneity within observed regions: physiologic basis and effects on estimation of rates of biodynamic processes, IV-47
Metoprolol
Improvement in symptoms and exercise tolerance by metoprolol in patients with dilated cardiomyopathy: a double-blind, randomized, placebo-controlled trial, 536
Milrinone
Systemic and regional hemodynamic effects of captopril and milrinone administered alone and concomitantly in patients with heart failure, 364

Mitral regurgitation
A Doppler–two-dimensional echocardiographic method for quantitation of mitral regurgitation, 377
Mitral valve
An enzyme histochemical study of human sinus node, coronary sinus, and mitral valve muscle, 205
Model simplification
Model simplification: complexity versus reduction, IV-63
Mortality
Comprehensive health care and noncardiovascular mortality: an unlikely explanation of the findings from the Hypertension Detection and Follow-up Program, 692
In-hospital morbidity and mortality in patients undergoing elective coronary angioplasty, 1044
Noninvasively diagnosed peripheral arterial disease as a predictor of mortality: results from a prospective study, 768
Results of triple valve replacement in 91 patients: perioperative mortality and long-term follow-up, 130
Myocardial function
Preservation of myocardial function with mannitol reperfusate, II-254
Myocardial infarction
Are right and left ventricular ejection fractions equal? Ejection fractions in normal subjects and in patients with first acute myocardial infarction, 502
Comparative effects of volume loading, dobutamine, and nitroprusside in patients with predominant right ventricular infarction, 1327
Complex ventricular arrhythmias in Q wave and non–Q wave myocardial infarction, 963
Coronary anatomy and left ventricular function in the first 12 hours of acute myocardial infarction: the Western Washington Randomized Intracoronary Streptokinase Trial, 292
Day-to-day variations in inducibility of ventricular tachyarrhythmias during the late postmyocardial infarction phase in conscious dogs, 200
The delayed diagnosis of myocardial infarction: it took half a century! 262
Delayed effects of early infarct-limiting therapies on healing after myocardial infarction, 907
Detection of local abnormalities in ventricular activation sequence by body surface isochrone mapping in patients with previous myocardial infarction, 801
The effects of the rate of intravenous infusion of streptokinase and the duration of symptoms on the time interval to reperfusion in patients with acute myocardial infarction, 1053
Electrophysiologic and anatomic basis for fractionated electrograms recorded from healed myocardial infarcts, 596
Emergency bypass surgery: late effects on size of infarction and ventricular function, II-179
Human tissue-type plasminogen activator: from the laboratory to the bedside, 18
The hypotensive effect of intravenous streptokinase in patients with acute myocardial infarction, 1321
Intermediate-term results of coronary artery bypass grafting for acute myocardial infarction, II-175
Interruption of sympathetic and vagal-mediated afferent responses by transmural myocardial infarction, 623
Intraoperative detection of myocardial ischemia in high-risk patients: electrocardiography vs two-dimensional transesophageal echocardiography, 1015
Left ventricular aneurysm and the prediction of left ventricular enlargement studied by two-dimensional echocardiography: quantitative assessment of aneurysm size in relation to clinical course, 280
Left ventricular ejection fraction after acute coronary occlusion in conscious dogs: relation to the extent and site of myocardial infarction, 632
Mechanisms of improving regional and global ventricular function by preload alterations during acute ischemia in the canine left ventricle, 1125
Non–Q wave perioperative myocardial infarction: assessment of the incidence and severity of regional dysfunction with quantitative two-dimensional echocardiography, 781
Patterns of myoglobin release after reperfusion of injured myocardium, 639
Prognostic significance and natural history of left ventricular thrombi in patients with acute anterior myocardial infarction: a two-dimensional echocardiographic study, 774
Programmed ventricular stimulation in survivors of an acute myocardial infarction, 487
Quantification of myocardial infarction: a comparison of single photon–emission computed tomography with pyrophosphate to serial plasma MB–creatine kinase measurements, 327
Quantitative analysis of the high-frequency components of the signal-averaged QRS complex in patients with acute myocardial infarction: a prospective study, 105
Subendocardial infarction in retrospect: pathologic, cardiographic, and ancillary features, 790
Survival after an experimental myocardial infarction: beneficial effects of long-term therapy with captopril, 406
Survival, myocardial infarction, and employment status in a prospective randomized study of coronary bypass surgery, V-90
Systemic and transcardiac platelet activity in acute myocardial infarction in man: resistance to prostacyclin, 1336
Urgent surgery for ventricular septal rupture complicating acute myocardial infarction, II-185
The value of the radionuclide angiogram in the prediction of perioperative myocardial infarction in patients undergoing lower extremity revascularization procedures, II-13
Myocardial metabolism
Metabolic fate of radioiodinated heptadecanoic acid in the normal canine heart, 565
Positron tomography and myocardial metabolism: an overview, IV-22
Myocardial protection
Enhancement of recovery of myocardial function by oxygen free–radical scavengers after reversible regional ischemia, 915
Myoglobin
Patterns of myoglobin release after reperfusion of injured myocardium, 639
Myosin
Local changes in myosin types in diseased human atrial myocardium: a quantitative immunofluorescence study, 272

N

Naloxone
The nature of opioid involvement in the hemodynamic, respiratory, and humoral responses to exercise, 982
Nifedipine
Effects of sublingual nifedipine on hemodynamics and systolic and diastolic function in patients with hypertrophic cardiomyopathy, 1001
Nitrogen
Nitrogen metabolism and mechanisms of protein synthesis and degradation, IV-13
Nitroglycerin
The effect of low-dose intravenous nitroglycerin on pulmonary hypertension immediately after replacement of a stenotic mitral valve, II-164
The effects of sublingually administered nitroglycerin on forearm vascular resistance in patients with heart failure and in normal subjects, 747
Hemodynamic effects of intravenous nitroglycerin in pediatric patients after heart surgery, II-101
Nitroprusside
Comparative effects of volume loading, dobutamine, and nitroprusside in patients with predominant right ventricular infarction, 1327
Nonimmune hydrops
Fetal atrioventricular valve insufficiency associated with nonimmune hydrops: a two-dimensional echocardiographic and pulsed Doppler ultrasound study, 825
Norverapamil
The interaction of verapamil and norverapamil with β-adrenergic receptors, 547
Nuclear cardiology
Validation of attenuation-corrected equilibrium radionuclide angio-

graphic determinations of right ventricular volume: comparison with cast-validated biplane cineventriculography, 317
Nuclear magnetic resonance
Cardiac energy metabolism: contributions from nuclear magnetic resonance, IV-18
Early detection of cardiac allograft rejection with proton nuclear magnetic resonance, II-231
Localization methods for nuclear magnetic resonance spectroscopy in vivo, IV-97
Nuclear magnetic resonance: potential clinical relevance to the cardiovascular system, IV-111
Phosphorus nuclear magnetic resonance spectroscopy in vivo, IV-103
Use of shift reagents for nuclear magnetic resonance studies of the kinetics of ion transfer in cells and perfused hearts, IV-89

O

Obesity
Is hypertension more benign when associated with obesity? 53
Occlusion
Autonomic control of ventricular tachycardia: sympathetic neural influence on spontaneous tachycardia 24 hours after coronary occlusion, 933
Contrast echocardiographic estimation of regional myocardial blood flow after acute coronary occlusion, 1115
Exercise thallium-201 scintigraphy in dogs: effects of long-term coronary occlusion and collateral development on early and late scintigraphic images, 881
Oxygen free radicals
Enhancement of recovery of myocardial function by oxygen free-radical scavengers after reversible regional ischemia, 915

P

Pacing
Comparative efficacy of transvenous cardioversion and pacing in patients with sustained ventricular tachycardia: a prospective, randomized, crossover study, 153
The effects of overdrive pacing and lidocaine on atrioventricular junctional rhythm in man: the role of abnormal automaticity, 480
Further observations on transient entrainment: importance of pacing site and properties of the components of the reentry circuit, 1293
Maintenance of exercise stroke volume during ventricular versus atrial synchronous pacing: rate of contractility, 1037
Pediatrics
Significance of cardiac defects in the developing fetus: a study of spontaneous abortuses, 1232
Pericardial valve
Hemodynamic performance of the Carpentier-Edwards pericardial valve in the aortic position in vivo, II-146
Pericarditis
Surgical treatment of constrictive pericarditis: analysis of outcome and diagnostic error, II-264
Peripheral vascular disease
Effect of β-adrenergic blockers on the peripheral circulation in patients with peripheral vascular disease, 1226
Noninvasively diagnosed peripheral arterial disease as a predictor of mortality: results from a prospective study, 768
Transcutaneous oxygen recovery and toe pulse reappearance time in the assessment of peripheral vascular disease, 1022
Perspectives
Atherosclerosis, calcium, and calcium antagonists, 456
Atrial flutter: a synthesis of concepts, 249
Cholesterol and cardiovascular disease: no longer whether, but rather when, in whom, and how? 686
A consideration of antiarrhythmic therapy, 949
Has 'obstruction' hindered our understanding of hypertrophic cardiomyopathy? 1148
Programmed electrical stimulation of the heart in patients with life-threatening ventricular arrhythmias: What is the significance of induced arrhythmias and what is the correct stimulation protocol? 1
The radiographic assessment of coronary blood flow parameters, 460
Some reflections on arteriosclerosis: past, present, and future. Presidential Address, 8
Sudden unexpected death in patients with congestive heart failure: a second frontier, 681
Pharmacology
Dopamine receptors: applications in clinical cardiology, 245
Systemic and regional hemodynamic effects of captopril and milrinone administered alone and concomitantly in patients with heart failure, 364
Photon-emission tomography
Quantification of myocardial infarction: a comparison of single photon-emission computed tomography with pyrophosphate to serial plasma MB-creatine kinase measurements, 327
Platelets
Aortocoronary artery vein-graft disease: experimental and clinical approach for the understanding of the role of platelets and platelet inhibitors, V-65
Cyclic blood flow variations induced by platelet-activating factor in stenosed canine coronary arteries despite inhibition of thromboxane synthetase, serotonin receptors, and α-adrenergic receptors, 397
Fibrin formation and platelet aggregation in patients with severe coronary artery disease: relationship with the degree of myocardial ischemia, 27
Improved graft patency in patients treated with platelet-inhibiting therapy after coronary bypass surgery, 138
Systemic and transcardiac platelet activity in acute myocardial infarction in man: resistance to prostacyclin, 1336
Platelets and vascular occlusion
Adenosine diphosphate as a mediator of platelet aggregation in vivo: an editorial view, 741
AH23848: a thromboxane receptor-blocking drug that can clarify the pathophysiologic role of thromboxane A_2, 1208
The biochemical pharmacology of thromboxane synthase inhibition in man, 1194
Clinical pharmacology of platelet cyclooxygenase inhibition, 1177
Evidence for 15-HETE synthesis by human umbilical vein endothelial cells, 708
The human pharmacology of platelet inhibition: pharmacokinetics relevant to drug action, 1164
Inhibition of platelet function in thrombosis, 698
Locally acting growth factors for vascular smooth muscle cells: endogenous synthesis and release from platelets, 735
Pharmacology of platelet inhibition in humans: implications of the salicylate-aspirin interaction, 1185
Platelet actions of stable carbocyclic analogues of prostacyclin, 1219
Platelets, endothelium, and vasospasm, 728
Production of platelet-activating factor by human vascular endothelial cells: evidence for a requirement for specific agonists and modulation by prostacyclin, 718
A review of possible roles of the platelet 12-lipoxygenase, 702
A role for PAF-acether (platelet-activating factor) in platelet-dependent vascular diseases? 713
Thromboxane A_2 and prostaglandin endoperoxide receptors in platelets and vascular smooth muscle, 1202
Positive end-expiratory airway pressure
A potential method of correcting intracavitary left ventricular filling pressures for the effects of positive end-expiratory airway pressure, 660
Positron-emission tomography
Animal preparations relevant for study with positron-emission tomography or nuclear magnetic resonance, IV-139
Biochemical approaches to metabolism: application to positron-emission tomography, IV-145
Current and future directions for clinical investigation of the heart with positron-emission tomography, IV-31
Effects of blood flow on the positron-emission tomographic determination of substrate transport rates, IV-72
Error in parameter estimates with variations in flow: measurement of oxygen utilization with positron-emission tomography, IV-77

Positron-emission tomography: assessment of myocardial blood flow and metabolism, IV-122
Positron tomography and myocardial metabolism: an overview, IV-22
Preludes and Progress
Cardiology in 1885, 21
The delayed diagnosis of myocardial infarction: it took half a century! 262
Presidential Address
Some reflections on arteriosclerosis: past, present, and future. Presidential Address, 8
Pressure-volume relationship
Effect of heart rate on the canine end-systolic pressure-volume relationship, 654
Effects of right ventricular ischemia on left ventricular geometry and the end-diastolic pressure-volume relationship in the dog, 1104
Procainamide
Periodic procainamide for paroxysmal tachycardia, 147
Programmed electrical stimulation
The effects of premature stimulation of the His bundle on epicardial activation and body surface late potentials in dogs susceptible to sustained ventricular tachyarrhythmias, 214
Programmed electrical stimulation of the heart in patients with life-threatening ventricular arrhythmias: What is the significance of induced arrhythmias and what is the correct stimulation protocol? 1
Propranolol
Effects of propranolol and diltiazem alone and in combination on the recovery of left ventricular segmental function after temporary coronary occlusion and long-term reperfusion in conscious dogs, 413
Prostacyclin
Systemic and transcardiac platelet activity in acute myocardial infarction in man: resistance to prostacyclin, 1336
Prosthetic valve thrombosis
Warfarin versus dipyridamole-aspirin and pentoxifylline-aspirin for the prevention of prosthetic heart valve thromboembolism: a prospective randomized clinical trial, 1059
Prosthetic valves
Clinical comparison of St. Jude and porcine aortic valve prostheses, II-135
Comparative evaluation of aortic valve replacement with Starr, Björk, and porcine valve prostheses, II-140
Comparison of dysfunction with mechanical and porcine mitral valve prostheses, II-129
Hemodynamic performance of the Carpentier-Edwards pericardial valve in the aortic position in vivo, II-146
Risk factors for the development of prosthetic valve endocarditis, 31
Six years of experience with the St. Jude Medical valvular prosthesis, II-153
Protein
Local changes in myosin types in diseased human atrial myocardium: a quantitative immunofluorescence study, 272
Nitrogen metabolism and mechanisms of protein synthesis and degradation, IV-13
Pro-urokinase
Coronary thrombolysis in dogs with intravenously administered human pro-urokinase, 384
Pulmonary artery
Relationship of pulmonary artery size to mortality in patients undergoing the Fontan operation, II-93
Pulmonary atresia
Early and late results in the treatment of patients with pulmonary atresia and intact ventricular septum, II-61
Pulmonary edema
Increased lung vasoreactivity in children from Leadville, Colorado, after recovery from high-altitude pulmonary edema, 957
Treatment of canine permeability pulmonary edema: short-term effects of dobutamine, furosemide, and hydralazine, 1365
Pulmonary hypertension
The effect of low-dose intravenous nitroglycerin on pulmonary hypertension immediately after replacement of a stenotic mitral valve, II-164
Pulmonary vascular disease
The pressure-flow response of the pulmonary circulation in patients with heart failure and pulmonary vascular disease, 1270
Pulsus paradoxus
Effects of intravascular volume state on the value of pulsus paradoxus and right ventricular diastolic collapse in predicting cardiac tamponade, 1076

Q

QRS complex
Quantitative analysis of the high-frequency components of the signal-averaged QRS complex in patients with acute myocardial infarction: a prospective study, 105

R

Race differences
The ratio of plasma high-density lipoprotein cholesterol to total and low-density lipoprotein cholesterol: age-related changes and race and sex differences in selected North American populations. The Lipid Research Clinics Program Prevalence Study, 93
Radionuclide angiography
Validation of attenuation-corrected equilibrium radionuclide angiographic determinations of right ventricular volume: comparison with cast-validated biplane cineventriculography, 317
The value of the radionuclide angiogram in the prediction of perioperative myocardial infarction in patients undergoing lower extremity revascularization procedures, II-13
Radionuclide studies
Radionuclide methods of identifying patients who may require coronary artery bypass surgery, V-9
Randomized trials
Design and study similarities and contrasts: the Veterans Administration, European, and CASS randomized trials of coronary artery bypass graft surgery, V-110
A perspective on the three large multicenter randomized clinical trials of coronary bypass surgery for chronic stable angina, V-123
Raynaud's phenomenon
Effects of β-adrenoreceptor–blocking drugs in patients with Raynaud's phenomenon, 466
Reperfusion
The effects of coronary angioplasty and reperfusion on distribution of myocardial flow, 334
Effects of propranolol and diltiazem alone and in combination on the recovery of left ventricular segmental function after temporary coronary occlusion and long-term reperfusion in conscious dogs, 413
Immediate functional recovery and avoidance of reperfusion injury with surgical revascularization of short-term coronary occlusion, 431
Patterns of myoglobin release after reperfusion of injured myocardium, 639
Repolarization
Change in ventricular cavity size: differential effects on QRS and T wave amplitude, 495
Dispersion of ventricular repolarization and arrhythmia: study of two consecutive ventricular premature complexes, 370
Restenosis
Influence of intimal dissection on restenosis after successful coronary angioplasty, 530
Revascularization
Effect of early postoperative volume loading on left ventricular systolic function (including left ventricular ejection fraction determined by myocardial marker) after myocardial revascularization, II-207
Left ventricular systolic and diastolic function in coronary artery disease: effects of revascularization on exercise-induced ischemia, 119
The value of the radionuclide angiogram in the prediction of perioperative myocardial infarction in patients undergoing lower extremity revascularization procedures, II-13

Rheumatic fever
The virtual disappearance of rheumatic fever in the United States: lessons in the rise and fall of disease. T. Duckett Jones Memorial Lecture, 1155
Right heart assist
Right heart assist by intermittent abdominal compression after surgery for congenital heart disease, II-97
Right heart conduits
Long-term follow-up of patients with synthetic right heart conduits, II-77
Right ventricle
Decision making in the definitive repair of the heart with a small right ventricle, II-52
Risk factors
Coronary risk factor statement for the American public, 1135A
Risk factors for the development of prosthetic valve endocarditis, 31

S

Scintigraphy
Exercise thallium-201 scintigraphy in dogs: effects of long-term coronary occlusion and collateral development on early and late scintigraphic images, 881
Senning operation
Global and regional right ventricular function in normal infants and infants with transposition of the great arteries after Senning operation, 1008
Senning repair for transposition of the great arteries in the first week of life, 840
Serotonin
Cyclic blood flow variations induced by platelet-activating factor in stenosed canine coronary arteries despite inhibition of thromboxane synthetase, serotonin receptors, and α-adrenergic receptors, 397
Sex differences
The ratio of plasma high-density lipoprotein cholesterol to total and low-density lipoprotein cholesterol: age-related changes and race and sex differences in selected North American populations. The Lipid Research Clinics Program Prevalence Study, 93
Signal averaging
Abnormal signal-averaged electrocardiograms in patients with nonischemic congestive cardiomyopathy: relationship to sustained ventricular tachyarrhythmias, 1308
Quantitative analysis of the high-frequency components of the signal-averaged QRS complex in patients with acute myocardial infarction: a prospective study, 105
Sinus node
An enzyme histochemical study of human sinus node, coronary sinus, and mitral valve muscle, 205
Smoking
The relationship of white cell count, platelet count, and hematocrit to cigarette smoking in adolescents: the Oslo Youth Study, 971
Sodium
Transient enhancement of sympathetic nervous system activity by long-term restriction of sodium intake, 47
Sotalol
Electrophysiologic and antiarrhythmic effects of sotalol in patients with life-threatening ventricular tachyarrhythmias, 555
Special Report
Coronary risk factor statement for the American public, 1135A
Streptokinase
A comparison of the thrombolytic and hemorrhagic effects of tissue-type plasminogen activator and streptokinase in rabbits, 178
Coronary anatomy and left ventricular function in the first 12 hours of acute myocardial infarction: the Western Washington Randomized Intracoronary Streptokinase Trial, 292
The effects of the rate of intravenous infusion of streptokinase and the duration of symptoms on the time interval to reperfusion in patients with acute myocardial infarction, 1053
The hypotensive effect of intravenous streptokinase in patients with acute myocardial infarction, 1321
Patterns of myoglobin release after reperfusion of injured myocardium, 639
Stroke volume
Diminished stroke volume during inspiration: a reverse thoracic pump, 668
Substrate transport
A clinically applicable method for the estimation of substrate transport in the coronary circulation in vivo, IV-81
Sudden death
Programmed ventricular stimulation in survivors of an acute myocardial infarction, 487
Sudden unexpected death in patients with congestive heart failure: a second frontier, 681
Surgery
Abnormal distribution of pulmonary blood flow after the Glenn shunt or Fontan procedure: risk of development of arteriovenous fistulae, 471
Comparative long-term effects of coronary artery bypass graft surgery and percutaneous transluminal coronary angioplasty on regional coronary flow reserve, 833
Death and other time-related events after valve replacement, 753
Global and regional right ventricular function in normal infants and infants with transposition of the great arteries after Senning operation, 1008
In-hospital morbidity and mortality in patients undergoing elective coronary angioplasty, 1044
Reoperation for coronary artery disease, V-59
Senning repair for transposition of the great arteries in the first week of life, 840
Surgery in the treatment of coronary artery disease: introduction, V-1
Sympathetic afferents
Interruption of sympathetic and vagal-mediated afferent responses by transmural myocardial infarction, 623
Sympathetic nervous system
Effect of the sympathetic nervous system on limb circulation and metabolism during exercise in patients with heart failure, 72
Transient enhancement of sympathetic nervous system activity by long-term restriction of sodium intake, 47

T

Tachycardia
Autonomic control of ventricular tachycardia: sympathetic neural influence on spontaneous tachycardia 24 hours after coronary occlusion, 933
Comparative efficacy of transvenous cardioversion and pacing in patients with sustained ventricular tachycardia: a prospective, randomized, crossover study, 153
Computer detection of atrioventricular dissociation from surface electrocardiograms during wide QRS complex tachycardias, 1028
Intermittent failure of local conduction during ventricular tachycardia, 1286
Periodic procainamide for paroxysmal tachycardia, 147
Thallium
Exercise thallium-201 scintigraphy in dogs: effects of long-term coronary occlusion and collateral development on early and late scintigraphic images, 881
Thoracic pump
Diminished stroke volume during inspiration: a reverse thoracic pump, 668
Thrombolysis
A comparison of the thrombolytic and hemorrhagic effects of tissue-type plasminogen activator and streptokinase in rabbits, 178
Coronary thrombolysis in dogs with intravenously administered human pro-urokinase, 384
The effects of the rate of intravenous infusion of streptokinase and the duration of symptoms on the time interval to reperfusion in patients with acute myocardial infarction, 1053
Human tissue-type plasminogen activator: from the laboratory to the bedside, 18
The hypotensive effect of intravenous streptokinase in patients with acute myocardial infarction, 1321

Lysis of left ventricular thrombi with urokinase, 112
Prevention of coronary thrombosis with subthrombolytic doses of tissue-type plasminogen activator, 1346
Usefulness of coronary artery bypass graft surgery or percutaneous transluminal angioplasty after thrombolytic therapy, V-39
Thromboxane
Cyclic blood flow variations induced by platelet-activating factor in stenosed canine coronary arteries despite inhibition of thromboxane synthetase, serotonin receptors, and α-adrenergic receptors, 397
Thrombus
Lysis of left ventricular thrombi with urokinase, 112
Tissue characterization
Angle dependence of ultrasonic backscatter in arterial tissues: a study in vitro, 572
Ultrasonic tissue characterization: detection of acute myocardial ischemia in dogs, 193
Tissue-type plasminogen activator
A comparison of the thrombolytic and hemorrhagic effects of tissue-type plasminogen activator and streptokinase in rabbits, 178
Human tissue-type plasminogen activator: from the laboratory to the bedside, 18
Prevention of coronary thrombosis with subthrombolytic doses of tissue-type plasminogen activator, 1346
Transcatheter ablation
Efficacy and safety of transcatheter ablation of posteroseptal accessory pathways, 170
Transposition of the great arteries
Global and regional right ventricular function in normal infants and infants with transposition of the great arteries after Senning operation, 1008
Improved right ventricular function after intra-atrial repair of transposition of the great arteries, II-45
Senning repair for transposition of the great arteries in the first week of life, 840
Tricuspid atresia
Abnormal distribution of pulmonary blood flow after the Glenn shunt or Fontan procedure: risk of development of arteriovenous fistulae, 471
Outcome of the Fontan procedure in patients with tricuspid atresia, II-88
Triggered activity
Cesium chloride–induced long QT syndrome: demonstration of afterdepolarizations and triggered activity in vivo, 1092

U

Ultrasonic backscatter
Angle dependence of ultrasonic backscatter in arterial tissues: a study in vitro, 572
The dependence of myocardial ultrasonic integrated backscatter on contractile performance, 183
Ultrasound
The accuracy of Doppler ultrasound measurement of pressure gradients across irregular, dual, and tunnellike obstructions to blood flow, 577
Ultrasonic tissue characterization: detection of acute myocardial ischemia in dogs, 193
University-industry collaboration
Academia-industry collaborative research programs—a legal perspective, I-41
Academia-industry dialogue: a step toward mutual understanding, I-53
Academic-industrial relations in the United Kingdom, I-51
Cardiovascular medicine: opportunities for enhanced university-industry collaboration. Introduction, I-1
The changing climate for cardiovascular research: stresses and opportunities, I-36
Educating physicians in the use of pharmaceuticals, I-31
Industry and academia in collaboration: the Pfizer experience, I-13
Institutional review boards and collaborations between academia and industry: some counterproductive policies and practices, I-48
The pharmaceutical industry and academic medicine in collaboration, I-3
The pharmaceutical industry and academic medicine: opportunities for physician collaboration, I-21
Policy directions for the National Heart, Lung, and Blood Institute: implications for academia and industry, I-44
Principles of partnership in research, I-18
Shared responsibility in clinical research, I-25
A university administrator's view of academia-industry collaboration, I-8
Urokinase
Lysis of left ventricular thrombi with urokinase, 112

V

Vagal afferents
Interruption of sympathetic and vagal-mediated afferent responses by transmural myocardial infarction, 623
Valve replacement
Clinical correlates of atrial tachyarrhythmias after valve replacement for aortic stenosis, II-159
Comparative evaluation of aortic valve replacement with Starr, Björk, and porcine valve prostheses, II-140
Death and other time-related events after valve replacement, 753
The effect of low-dose intravenous nitroglycerin on pulmonary hypertension immediately after replacement of a stenotic mitral valve, II-164
Hemodynamic performance of the Carpentier-Edwards pericardial valve in the aortic position in vivo, II-146
Morbidity and mortality in mitral valve surgery, II-120
Operative risk of mitral valve replacement: discriminant analysis of 1329 procedures, II-108
Results of triple valve replacement in 91 patients: perioperative mortality and long-term follow-up, 130
Survival and functional results after valve replacement for aortic regurgitation from 1976 to 1983: impact of preoperative left ventricular function, 1244
Valved conduits
Replacement of obstructed right ventricular–pulmonary arterial valved conduits with nonvalved conduits in children, II-84
Valvular heart disease
Assessment and follow-up of patients with aortic regurgitation by an updated Doppler echocardiographic measurement of the regurgitant fraction in the aortic arch, 819
A Doppler–two-dimensional echocardiographic method for quantitation of mitral regurgitation, 377
Morbidity and mortality in mitral valve surgery, II-120
A new approach to noninvasive evaluation of aortic regurgitant fraction by two-dimensional Doppler echocardiography, 523
Noninvasive estimation of valve area in patients with aortic stenosis by Doppler ultrasound and two-dimensional echocardiography, 810
Operative risk of mitral valve replacement: discriminant analysis of 1329 procedures, II-108
Results of triple valve replacement in 91 patients: perioperative mortality and long-term follow-up, 130
Vasodilator reserve
Transluminal, subselective measurement of coronary artery blood flow velocity and vasodilator reserve in man, 82
Vasodilators
Importance of internal controls, statistical methods, and side effects in short-term trials of vasodilators: a study of hydralazine kinetics in patients with aortic regurgitation, 865
Vasoreactivity
Increased lung vasoreactivity in children from Leadville, Colorado, after recovery from high-altitude pulmonary edema, 957
Vasospasm
The effect of cyclooxygenase inhibition on vasomotion of proximal coronary arteries with endothelial damage, 389

Vein graft disease
Aortocoronary artery vein-graft disease: experimental and clinical approach for the understanding of the role of platelets and platelet inhibitors, V-65
Ventricular assist devices
Long-term follow-up of postcardiotomy patients with profound cardiogenic shock treated with ventricular assist devices, II-216
Ventricular fibrillation
Effect of serial brief ischemic episodes on extracellular K^+, pH, and activation in the pig, 922
Ventricular function
Altered left ventricular mechanics in patients with valvular aortic stenosis and coarctation of the aorta: effects on systolic performance and late outcome, 515
Are right and left ventricular ejection fractions equal? Ejection fractions in normal subjects and in patients with first acute myocardial infarction, 502
Coronary anatomy and left ventricular function in the first 12 hours of acute myocardial infarction: the Western Washington Randomized Intracoronary Streptokinase Trial, 292
Effect of early postoperative volume loading on left ventricular systolic function (including left ventricular ejection fraction determined by myocardial marker) after myocardial revascularization, II-207
Effects of propranolol and diltiazem alone and in combination on the recovery of left ventricular segmental function after temporary coronary occlusion and long-term reperfusion in conscious dogs, 413
Effects of reduced left ventricular mass on chamber architecture, load, and function: a study of anorexia nervosa, 991
Effects of right ventricular ischemia on left ventricular geometry and the end-diastolic pressure-volume relationship in the dog, 1104
Emergency bypass surgery: late effects on size of infarction and ventricular function, II-179
Global and regional right ventricular function in normal infants and infants with transposition of the great arteries after Senning operation, 1008
Immediate functional recovery and avoidance of reperfusion injury with surgical revascularization of short-term coronary occlusion, 431
Improved right ventricular function after intra-atrial repair of transposition of the great arteries, II-45
Improvement in regional wall motion and left ventricular relaxation after administration of diltiazem in patients with coronary artery disease, 353
Left ventricular ejection fraction after acute coronary occlusion in conscious dogs: relation to the extent and site of myocardial infarction, 632
Maintenance of exercise stroke volume during ventricular versus atrial synchronous pacing: rate of contractility, 1037
Mechanisms of improving regional and global ventricular function by preload alterations during acute ischemia in the canine left ventricle, 1125
A potential method of correcting intracavitary left ventricular filling pressures for the effects of positive end-expiratory airway pressure, 660
Right ventricular function in an operating room model of mechanical left ventricular assistance and its effects in patients with depressed left ventricular function, 1279
The superiority of maximum fiber elastance over maximum stress-volume ratio as an index of contractile state, 648
Survival and functional results after valve replacement for aortic regurgitation from 1976 to 1983: impact of preoperative left ventricular function, 1244
Ventricular hypertrophy
Diastolic abnormalities in patients with hypertrophic cardiomyopathy: relation to magnitude of left ventricular hypertrophy, 310
Participation of endogenous catecholamines in the regulation of left ventricular mass in progeny of hypertensive parents, 38
Ventricular septal rupture
Urgent surgery for ventricular septal rupture complicating acute myocardial infarction, II-185
Ventricular size
Change in ventricular cavity size: differential effects on QRS and T wave amplitude, 495
Ventricular thrombi
Prognostic significance and natural history of left ventricular thrombi in patients with acute anterior myocardial infarction: a two-dimensional echocardiographic study, 774
Ventricular volume
Accuracy of volume measurement by conductance catheter in isolated, ejecting canine hearts, 440
Validation of attenuation-corrected equilibrium radionuclide angiographic determinations of right ventricular volume: comparison with cast-validated biplane cineventriculography, 317
Verapamil
Frequency-dependent effects of verapamil on atrioventricular nodal conduction in man, 344
The interaction of verapamil and norverapamil with β-adrenergic receptors, 547
Verapamil-induced improvement in left ventricular diastolic filling and increased exercise tolerance in patients with hypertropic cardiomyopathy: short- and long-term effects, 853
Volume loading
Effect of early postoperative volume loading on left ventricular systolic function (including left ventricular ejection fraction determined by myocardial marker) after myocardial revascularization, II-207

W

Warfarin
Warfarin versus dipyridamole-aspirin and pentoxifylline-aspirin for the prevention of prosthetic heart valve thromboembolism: a prospective randomized clinical trial, 1059
Wolff-Parkinson-White syndrome
Atrial fibrillation in patients with Wolff-Parkinson-White syndrome: incidence after surgical ablation of the accessory pathway, 161
Efficacy and safety of transcatheter ablation of posteroseptal accessory pathways, 170

News from the American Heart Association

7320 Greenville Ave., Dallas, Texas 75231
Telephone: 214 750-5300

Program Being Prepared For 58th Scientific Sessions To Be In Washington, DC

The program for the 58th Annual Scientific Sessions of the American Heart Association will be developed this month (July) at a meeting of the Committee on Scientific Sessions Program in Dallas. The Scientific Sessions will be held at the Washington Convention Center, Washington, D.C., November 11–14.

A two-day session of the Program Committee, chaired for the third year by Dr. Bernadine Healy Bulkley, will consider the abstracts submitted for the Sessions. Approximately 100 volunteer abstract readers, most of whom are members of program committees of the scientific councils, select about 35 percent of the best submissions. The top 20 percent are easily identified; the next 15 percent are selected because they are unusually creative or even controversial. The final 65% report important investigations. Each abstract is considered by at least five graders. Abstracts will be published in a supplement to October CIRCULATION.

In 1954, for the Miami Beach Sessions, 5,750 abstracts were submitted and 1,852 presented.

Poster Sessions

Abstracts will also be selected for the poster sessions. In these, space is assigned where research workers can present on poster boards material pertaining to their abstracts.

Special lectures and their presenters (six to eight) will be selected and the program structured for symposia, lectures, and awards announcements. Scientific Council functions and programs will be set.

Other Functions

Arrangements will be made for clinical sessions, Cardiovascular Conferences, and "How To" sessions. Postgraduate Symposia, arranged by the Scientific Councils, will be programmed. More than 300 industry exhibits are expected.

Among the lecturers to be selected by various groups in AHA are those who will deliver the Lewis A. Conner Memorial, Dickinson W. Richards Memorial, George Lyman Duff Memorial, International, George E. Brown Memorial, Helen B. Taussig Lecture, and the Excellence in Nursing Lecture.

Awards

Awards to be selected by groups in the Heart Association are Research Achievement, Louis N. Katz, Irvine H. Page for Young Investigators, James B. Herrick Award, Richard and Hinda Rosenthal Foundation, Scientific Council Distinguished Achievement and 2nd annual Excellence in Nursing.

Meeting with the Sessions will be the Scientific Sessions for Nurses.

Advance Arrangements

Advance registration, including hotel reservations, may now be arranged on forms available from affiliates and the National Center in Dallas. Forms are also published in MODERN CONCEPTS OF CARDIOVASCULAR DISEASE and CARDIOVASCULAR NURSING. Information may be obtained from the Coordinator, Scientific Sessions, AHA, 7320 Greenville Ave., Dallas, TX 75231. Tel. for housing and reservations, 1-214-750-5425.

Symposia Selected For World Congress

Twenty-eight symposia have been selected for the World Congress of Cardiology to be held in Washington, D.C. Sept. 14 to 19, **1986.** The American Heart Association is host for the Congress which will be dediated to the memory of Dr. Paul Dudley White, one of the founders of AHA and of the International Society and Federation of Cardiology, on the 100th anniversary of his birth.

Dr. Thomas N. James, president of the Congress, said the planning committee, headed by Dr. Elliot Rapaport, former Editor of CIRCULATION, had selected the following symposia:

Hyperlipidemia, outcome after congenital heart disease surgery, pacemakers update, pulmonary hypertension, cardiovascular adaptation during space flight, electrolytes in hypertension, mitral valve prolapse, stroke, angioplasty and related techniques.

Other Symposia Topics

Additional symposia topics include sodium channels and arrhythmias, myocarditis and cardiomyopathies, ventricular function, rheumatic fever and rheumatic heart disease, worldwide trends of coronary heart disease and mortality/possible explanations, biology of the vascular wall, basic mechanisms and clinical applications of reperfusion of ischemic myocardium.

Also, management of early phase of acute MI, exercise tolerance testing, echo/Doppler, newer imaging techniques, anti-arrhythmic drugs in prevention and causation of sudden cardiac death, coronary artery bypass surgery, treatment of recurrent cardiac arrhythmias, Chagas disease, primary prevention of coronary heart disease, emergence of CV disease within developing countries, toxic oil syndrome, worldwide problem of rheumatic fever, diagnosis and management of infective endocarditis, adrenergic receptors in CV disease, Kawasaki disease, genetic control of lipoprotein receptors in atherosclerosis.

Program for Nurses

The program for nurses will include symposia on:

CV nursing/international perspectives, an approach to nursing the patient with CV problems, rheumatic fever and rheumatic heart disease, myocardial revascularization, pharmacological interventions for CV problems, hypertension, stroke and aging, heart replacement, management of pump failure, computers in CV nursing practice.

cont'd on ad page 25

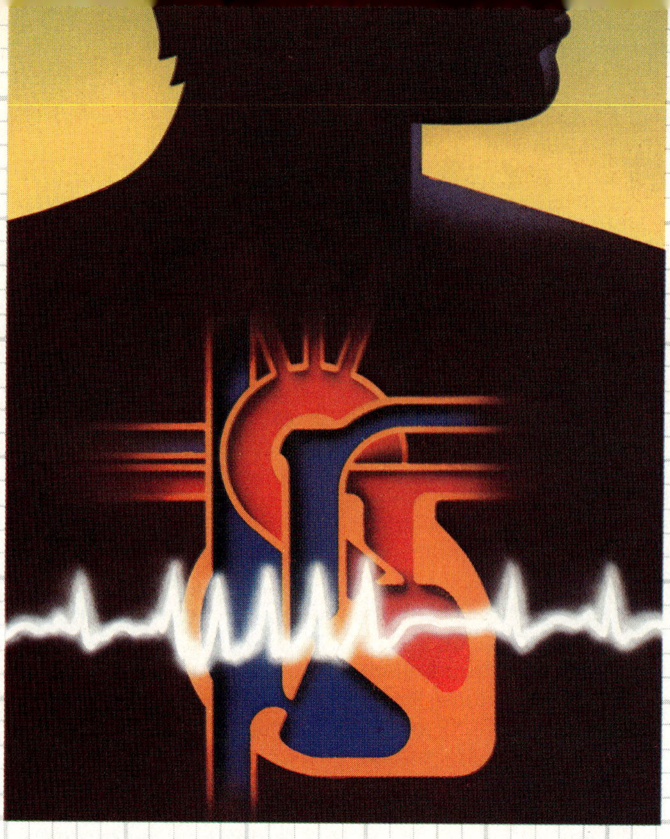

From the Astra/Merck Research Programs

New, for symptomatic ventricular arrhythmias

TONOCARD®

(TOCAINIDE HCl | MSD)

Like lidocaine.

But it's oral.

For a Brief Summary of Prescribing Information, please see last page of this advertisement.

cont'd from ad page 13

Papers and Posters

The program will offer more than 500 free communications and poster presentations. There will be a public education program spaced over four days for lay members of Heart Foundations.

Opening and Closing

The Congress will open the evening of Sept. 14, **1986** with a concert by the Washington National Symphony Orchestra. The closing general session on Friday, Sept. 19, will present the International Society and Federation of Cardiology Lecture and the Xth World Congress Young Investigator's Award.

AHA Hosts Conference On CPR, ECC in July

The National Conference on Standards and Guidelines for Cardiopulmonary Resuscitation (CPR) and Emergency Cardiac Care (ECC) will be held July 11–13 at the Dallas-Fort Worth Hilton Hotel in Dallas. It will mark the 25th anniversary of modern techniques in this field and explore new findings for possible incorporation in basic life support, advanced cardiac life support, pediatric resuscitation, medicolegal aspects and emergency cardiac care systems.

The meeting, following conferences held in 1966, 1973, and 1979, is cosponsored by the American Heart Association, the American College of Cardiology, the American Red Cross, the National Academy of Sciences, and the National Heart, Lung, and Blood Institute.

Program Outlined

The program includes talks on standards and guidelines for cardiopulmonary resuscitation and emergency cardiac care, review of changes in science and clinical data since 1980, and the status of CPR training in 1985. Each afternoon will be devoted to 10 to 12 panel discussions and the Conference will conclude with panel reports and an evaluation of the state of the algorithms after decisions of the meeting.

Subscription Renewels Entered as Requested

Subscriptions to American Heart Association Scientific Journals are now entered as the subscribers request in order to spread expiration times over the year.

Subscriptions to CIRCULATION, CIRCULATION RESEARCH, STROKE, HYPERTENSION and ARTERIOSCLEROSIS can be entered at any time of the year instead of only for fiscal and calendar years as in the past. Subscribers may still request fiscal and calendar year subscriptions but an attempt is now being made to lighten the load of expirations at those periods.

Readers of the fiscal year subscriptions should now renew to preserve continuity. Renewal notices should be returned with payment. All checks should be payable to AHA in U.S. dollars.

Subscribers in **Japan** should renew through Nankodo Co. Ltd., 42-5 Hongo 3-Chome, Bunkyo-Ku, Tokyo, Japan. Orders from **Europe** should be directed to Bailliere Tindall, 1 St. Anne's Rd., Eastbourne, East Sussex BN21 3UN, England.

Other orders should go to the AHA Scientific Journals Subscription Department, 7320 Greenville Ave., Dallas, TX 75231. Tel. 214-750-5466.

Special rates for *research fellows, residents, interns* and *medical students* are available for subscribers in the United States, Canada, and Mexico. A letter from the department chairperson stating the post held is required with payment. (U.S.: CIRCULATION $28, Canada and Mexico $36; U.S.; CIRCULATION RESEARCH, $43, Canada and Mexico $52.50; U.S.; STROKE $25, Canada and Mexico $32.50; HYPERTENSION $27.50, Canada and Mexico $35; U.S.; ARTERIOSCLEROSIS $30, Canada and Mexico $37.50).

Airmail is available upon request for all subscriptions.

All subscription rates include postage, indexes at the end of volumes and supplements. CIRCULATION subscribers receive the Abstracts of the Annual AHA Scientific Sessions.

Three periodicals — MODERN CONCEPTS OF CARDIOVASCULAR DISEASE, CURRENT CONCEPTS OF CEREBROVASCULAR DISEASE/STROKE, and CARDIOVASCULAR NURSING — are distributed in the United States by Heart Association affiliates only. (MODERN CONCEPTS is available on subscription outside the U.S. at $10 (U.S.) annually).

Rates for 1985

	U.S.	Outside U.S.
CIRCULATION	$56	$ 72
CIRCULATION RESEARCH	86	105
HYPERTENSION	55	70
STROKE	50	65
ARTERIOSCLEROSIS	60	75

Attack on Smoking Moves to New Goals

On the heels of success in strengthening advertising cautions against smoking, the American Heart Association and its more than 30 allies in the Coalition on Smoking OR Health, have set new goals to pursue in the 99th Congress:

- Increase in the federal cigarette excise tax to 32¢ per pack.
- Creation of a smoking-free society by the year 2000.
- Elimination of deceptive advertising aimed at young people.
- Providing assistance to state and local agencies for drug education programs.
- Prohibiting advertising of all tobacco products on any electronic medium.
- Clamping down on import of foreign tobacco using domestically unapproved pesticides.
- Enhancing anti-smoking initiatives in the military.

cont'd on ad page 28

Reference
1. McAreavey D, Ramsey LE, Latham L, et al: "Third drug" trial: comparative study of antihypertensive agents added to treatment when blood pressure remains uncontrolled by a beta blocker plus thiazide diuretic. *Br Med J* 1984(Jan 14); 288:106-111.

Apresoline® hydrochloride

hydralazine hydrochloride USP

TABLETS

INDICATIONS

Essential hypertension, alone or as an adjunct.

CONTRAINDICATIONS

Hypersensitivity to hydralazine; coronary artery disease; and mitral valvular rheumatic heart disease.

WARNINGS

Hydralazine may produce in a few patients a clinical picture simulating systemic lupus erythematosus. In such patients hydralazine should be discontinued unless the benefit-to-risk determination requires continued antihypertensive therapy with this drug. Symptoms and signs usually regress when the drug is discontinued but residua have been detected many years later. Long-term treatment with steroids may be necessary.

Complete blood counts, L.E. cell preparations, and antinuclear antibody titer determinations are indicated before and periodically during prolonged therapy with hydralazine even though the patient is asymptomatic. These studies are also indicated if the patient develops arthralgia, fever, chest pain, continued malaise or other unexplained signs or symptoms.

A positive antinuclear antibody titer and/or positive L.E. cell reaction requires that the physician carefully weigh the implications of the test results against the benefits to be derived from antihypertensive therapy with hydralazine.

Use MAO inhibitors with caution in patients receiving hydralazine.

When other potent parenteral antihypertensive drugs, such as diazoxide, are used in combination with hydralazine, patients should be continuously observed for several hours for any excessive fall in blood pressure. Profound hypotensive episodes may occur when diazoxide injection and Apresoline (hydralazine hydrochloride) are used concomitantly.

Usage in Pregnancy

Animal studies indicate that hydralazine is teratogenic in mice, possibly in rabbits, and not in rats. Teratogenic effects observed were cleft palate and malformations of facial and cranial bones. Although clinical experience does not include any positive evidence of adverse effects on the human fetus, hydralazine should not be used during pregnancy unless the expected benefit clearly justifies the potential risk to the fetus.

PRECAUTIONS

Myocardial stimulation produced by Apresoline can cause anginal attacks and ECG changes of myocardial ischemia. The drug has been implicated in the production of myocardial infarction. It must, therefore, be used with caution in patients with suspected coronary artery disease.

The "hyperdynamic" circulation caused by Apresoline may accentuate specific cardiovascular inadequacies. An example is that Apresoline may increase pulmonary artery pressure in patients with mitral valvular disease. The drug may reduce the pressor responses to epinephrine. Postural hypotension may result from Apresoline, but is less common than with ganglionic blocking agents. Use with caution in patients with cerebral vascular accidents.

In hypertensive patients with normal kidneys who are treated with Apresoline, there is evidence of increased renal blood flow and a maintenance of glomerular filtration rate. In some instances improv

cont'd from ad page 25

AHA Food Festival To Enter Groceries

The American Heart Food Festival, a national program event, will be conducted Sept. 8–14 in supermarkets and groceries to focus attention on the benefits of low-fat eating patterns and heart health.

Several national supermarket chains have accepted AHA's invitation to join in the event and affiliates are expected to recruit smaller stores.

As part of the program, stores will provide a "help your heart" nutrition message on grocery bags, display window posters promoting the Festival, have employees wear stickers to promote the event, print ads displaying a "help your heart" message, and use literature with a nutrition message as bag stuffers. Collateral projects, such as food preparation demonstrations, store tours, and literature distribution will also be encouraged.

It is planned in coming years to extend the program to restaurant dining, cooking classes and other outlets where the eating patterns which can help reduce the risk of heart disease can be explained.

Heart To Join Program On Living with HBP

The American Heart Association is joining with the American Health Care Association (AHCA) to implement a program on living with high blood pressure as the patient grows older.

The program is aimed at active and alert people over 50 and will attempt to inform them about hypertension and especially to motivate them to continue prescribed treatment. The program is supported by a grant from Merck Sharp and Dohme.

Included in the plans is a color film in 16 mm and a ½ inch video cassette which includes medical advice from Ray Gifford, M.D. A selection of materials to aid the program coordinator, including a discussion guide, posters, and medical record calendars are part of the program.

The program will be continued to May 1, 1986, when its effectiveness and popularity will be assessed.

Heart-At-Work

A slide/tape presentation for the Heart-At-Work program, as well as a flip chart, have been developed for an AHA program for businesses. The program, tested in seven affiliates, is designed to bring AHA educational programs to executives and workers. Albuquerque and Los Angeles have been used for extended field tests of materials.

Obesity/Lipid/CVD Pattern Unusual in Pima Indians

A study of 3,000 Pima Indians of Arizona appears to show a high prevalence of obesity but a significantly lower rate of heart disease than in Caucasians. Total amounts of cholesterol were lower than Caucasian levels and in Pima males total levels of cholesterol remained unchanged after age 20.

The study is being conducted by Dr. Barbara V. Howard and colleagues of the National Institute of Arthritis, Diabetes, and Digestive and Kidney Diseases in Phoenix. The aim is to explain the role of lipoproteins in maintaining plasma cholesterol levels. Pima indians without diabetes, who have a high level of obesity, were compared with a similar group of Caucasians.

Among findings in the Pimas reported by the investigators were:

- There was a lower level of LDL cholesterol and lower prevalence of cardiovascular disease in the Pimas despite a high incidence of obesity.
- Pima catabolism of LDL, the major carrier of plasma cholesterol, was high suggesting LDL is metabolized more rapidly.
- Almost half the precursor VLDL metabolized by the Pimas was not converted to LDL as was found in the Caucasians.
- Investigators speculated that an alternate VLDL metabolic pathway might exist in the Pimas to prevent buildup of cholesterol normally seen in the obese and resulting in less Pima heart disease.
- HDL cholesterol levels measured lower in the Pimas than in Caucasians supporting the theory that an inverse relationship existed between obesity and HDL levels in the Pimas.
- Both sexes of Pimas had relatively equal amounts of HDL cholesterol. But Pima females had a lower rate of heart disease than Pima males.

AHA Briefs . . .

- **Modern Concepts of Cardiovascular Disease** for July is "Acute Myocardial Infarction. Thoughts About Pathogenesis and Treatment," by C. Richard Conti, M.D., and Robert L. Feldman, M.D., of the University of Florida College of Medicine.
- **Current Concepts of Cerebrovascular Disease/Stroke** for July/August is "Intracerebral Hemorrhage: Common Nonhypertensive Causes," by Carlos S. Kase, M.D., Boston University.
- **High Blood Pressure Measurement Training Programs** in five affiliates of the Heart Association have been recommended by the National Office to other affiliates seeking such programs. The programs were reviewed and recommended for use by the Subcommittee on Hypertension for Teaching Accurate BP Measurement to Lay and Professional Persons. The affiliates with manuals are Connecticut, Maryland, Texas, Wisconsin, and Chicago.

Meetings Calendar

1985

July 15–18: **Clinical Cardiology.** Hilton Head Inn, Hilton Head Island, SC. Sponsored by the School of Medicine, Medical College of Georgia. Inquiries: Medical College of Georgia, Augusta, GA 30912. Tel. 1-404-828-3967.

July 15–19: **Cardiac Rehabilitation Workshop.** (Also Nov. 18–22). La Crosse Exercise Program, University of Wisconsin. Inquiries: Philip K. Wilson, Univ. of Wisconsin-LaCrosse, WI 54601. Tel 1-608-785-8686.

July 18–21: **Pulmonary Diseases.** Kiawah Island Inn, Kiawah Island,

cont'd on ad page 37

cont'd from ad page 28

SC. Sponsored by School of Medicine, Medical College of Georgia. Inquiries: See Medical College of Georgia, July 15–18.

July 21–24: **Nutrition in Cardiovascular Disease and Diabetes Mellitus. 26th Annual Meeting of American College of Nutrition.** Donaldson Brown Center for Continuing Education of Virginia Polytechnic Institute and State University, Blacksburg, VA. Inquiries: Mildred S. Seelig, M.D., M.P.H., F.A.C.N., American College of Nutrition, POB 831, White Plains, NY 10602. Tel. 1-914-948-4848.

July 21–26: **37th Annual Meeting American Association of Clinical Chemistry.** Georgia World Congress Center, Atlanta. Inquiries: AACC, 1725 K St., NW, Washington, DC 20006. Tel. 1-202-857-0717.

July 22–26: **Interdisciplinary Symposium on Plant Flavonoids in Biology and Medicine.** Biochemical, Pharmacological, and Structure-Activity Relationships. Buffalo, NY. Inquiries: Dr. Elliott Middleton, Jr., Dept. Med., Buffalo General Hospital, 100 High St., Buffalo, NY 14203. Tel. 1-716-845-2985.

July 22–26: **Topics in Clinical Nuclear Medicine.** Colby College, Waterville, ME. Henry N. Wagner, Jr., M.D., course director. Inquiries: R. Kany, Colby College, Waterville, ME 04901. Tel. 1-207-873-3386.

July 22–26: **Fitness and Weight Control Workshop.** La Crosse Exercise Program, University of Wisconsin-La Crosse. Inquiries: See July 15–19.

July 24–28: **Critical Care Medicine.** Kiawah Island Inn, Kiawah Island, SC. Sponsored by School of Medicine, Medical College of Georgia. Inquiries: See Medical College of Georgia, July 15–18.

July 24–28: **4th International Symposium on Magnesium.** Magnesium in Cardiovascular Diseases, Open Heart and Other Surgery, Stress, Epidemiology, and Diagnosis. Donaldson Brown Center for Continuing Education, Virginia Polytechnic Institute and State University, Blacksburg, VA. Inquiries: See July 21–24.

July 31–Aug. 2: **Interventional Radiology: An Update for Radiologic Technologists and Nurses.** Hyatt Regency Hotel, San Francisco. Ernest J. Ring, M.D., Robert Marco, Kathleen Marr, R.T., program directors. Sponsored by Dept. of Radiology, University of California San Francisco. Inquiries: Dept. Radiology, UCSF, San Francisco CA 94143.

Aug. 18–24: **Health Care Expo '85:** Washington, DC, Convention Center. Sponsored by Health Care Expositions. Inquiries: S. K. Herlitz, Health Care Expo, 404 Park Ave. S., New York, NY 10016. Tel. 1-212-532-9400.

Aug. 27–30: **Research Conference on Regulation of Bile Acid Synthesis.** Given Institute of Pathobiology, Aspen, CO. Sponsored by American Gastroenterological Association. Inquiries: Bile Acid Research, 740 Krameria St., Denver, CO 80220.

Sept. 9–14: **4th Annual Symposium in Doppler and 2-D Echocardiography.** Washington, D.C. Sponsored by the Johns Hopkins University School of Medicine and the Institute for Medical Studies. James Weiss, M.D., program director. Inquiries: K. Stroich, Inst. for Med. Studies, 30131 Town Center Dr., Suite 215, Laguna Niguel, CA 92677. Tel. 1-714-495-4499.

Sept. 11–14: **15th Annual Peripheral Vascular Disease Symposium: Critical Issues and Controversies in Vascular Surgery.** The Hyatt on Capitol Square, Columbus, OH. William E. Evans, M.D., and Blair D. Vermillion, M.D., co-chairmen. Sponsored by St. Anthony Medical Center. Inquiries: S. Hershberger, St. Anthony Medical Center, 1492 E. Broad St., Suite 1100, Columbus, OH 43205. Tel. 1-614-251-3680.

Sept. 12–14: **International Symposium on Cardiovascular Surgery — 1985. 15th Annual Symposium of Texas Heart Institute.** Houston. Inquiries: Medical Director, Texas Heart Institute, POB 20269, Houston, TX 77225. Tel. 1-713-791-2157.

Sept. 30–Oct. 1: **2nd Annual Graduate Hospital Symposium: Acute Myocardial Infarction — Emerging Concepts of Pathogenesis and Treatment.** Philadelphia. Inquiries: M. Blob, Bockus Research Institute, The Graduate Hospital, Philadelphia, PA 19146. Tel. 1-215-893-2375.

Oct. 3–5: **3rd Biannual Symposium in Cardiac Imaging.** Hotel Meridian, San Francisco. Sponsored by University of California, San Francisco School of Medicine and Institute for Medical Studies. Drs. Nelson Schiller, Martin Lipton, Charles Higgins and Elias Botvinick, program directors. Inquiries: K. Stroich — See Sept. 9–14.

Oct. 3–5: **Clinical Doppler Echocardiography. Practical Educational Approach.** Costa Mesa, CA. Stanley J. Goldberg, M.D., course director. Inquiries: Clinical Doppler Echocardiography, 5650 E. 9th St., Tucson, AZ 85711. Tel. 1-602-626-7303.

Oct. 10–13: **4th Annual Chicago Critical Care Symposium.** Chicago Marriott (Downtown). Inquiries: E. C. Rackow, M.D., Dept. Med., University of Health Sciences/Chicago Medical School, 3333 Green Bay Rd., North Chicago, IL 60064. Tel. 1-312-578-3291.

Oct. 11–12: **4th Southern Biomedical Engineering Conference.** Jackson, MS. Inquiries: Dr. Barry W. Sauer, SBEC, Div. Cont. Health Profess. Ed., University of Mississippi Medical Center, 2500 N. State St., Jackson, MS 39216-4505.

Oct. 13–18: **Clinical Congress, American College of Surgeons.** Chicago. Inquiries: ACS, 55 East Erie St., Chicago, IL 60611.

Oct. 14–16: **4th Annual Cardiac Rehabilitation Symposium.** Hotel Meridien, New Orleans. Sponsored by East Jefferson General Hospital. Inquiries: S. Weigel, East Jefferson General Hospital, 4200 Houma Blvd., POB 8213, Metairie LA 70011. Tel. 1-504-454-4147.

Oct. 19–20: **Head and Neck Radiology: Advanced Techniques in Diagnostic Imaging.** Hyatt Regency Hotel, San Francisco. William P. Dillon, M.D., and Gretchen A.W. Gooding, M.D., course directors. Sponsored by Radiology Research and Education Foundation, UCSF. Inquiries: Dept. Radiology, UCSF, San Francisco, CA 94143. Tel. 1-415-666-5731.

Oct. 21–25: **Clinical Magnetic Resonance Imaging.** Hyatt Regency Hotel, San Francisco. Charles B. Higgins, M.D., Hedvig Hricak, Ph.D., program directors. Sponsored by UCSF Dept. of Radiology. Inquiries: Dept. of Radiology, UCSF School of Medicine, San Francisco, CA 94143. Tel. 1-415-666-5731.

Oct. 25: **Annual Meeting, Society of Neurological Anesthesia and Neurological Supportive Care.** San Francisco. Inquiries: Society of Neurological Anesthesia, POB 238, Univ. of Virginia Medical Center, Charlottesville, VA 22908.

Nov. 4–8: **Diagnostic Radiology Seminars.** Maui Marriott Hotel, Maui, Hawaii. Neil Chafetz, M.D. course director. Sponsored by UCSF Dept. of Radiology. Inquiries: Radiology PG Education, UCSF Room C-324, Third & Parnassus Ave., San Francisco, CA 94143. Tel. 1-415-666-5731 (between 7:30 am-4:30 pm Pacific Time).

Nov. 11–14: **58th Annual Scientific Sessions, American Heart Association, Washington, DC. Inquiries: Coordinator Scientific Sessions, AHA, 7320 Greenville Ave., Dallas, TX 75231. Tel. for abstracts: 1-214-750-5439, for housing and reservations 1-214-750-5425.**

Nov. 19–20: **Subspecialty Boards in Cardiovascular Disease.** Philadelphia. Inquiries: American Board of Internal Medicine, 3624 Market St., Philadelphia, PA 19104. Tel. 1-215-243-1500. (New date.)

Dec. 2–6: **Chest Radiology — Update and Review.** Hotel Del Coronado, San Diego. Sponsored by Chest Division of Dept. of Radiology, UCSD. David S. Feigin, M.D., and Paul J. Friedman, M.D., program directors. Inquiries: D. Ryals. Ryals Associates, POB 610203, Dallas-Fort Worth, TX 75261-0203. Tel. 1-214-659-9590.

1986

Jan. 24–25: **Current Controversies and Techniques in Congenital Heart Surgery.** Baltimore, MD. (Immediately prior to Annual Meeting, Society of Thoracic Surgeons, Washington, DC). Sponsored by Div. of Thoracic and Cardiovascular Surgery, University of Maryland School of Medicine. Inquiries: Program Cont. Ed., University of Maryland School of Medicine, 10 South Pine St., Suite 300, Baltimore, MD 21201. Tel. 1-301-528-3956.

Feb. 19–22: **11th International Joint Conference on Stroke and Cerebral Circulation.** Vacation Village, San Diego. Inquiries: Admin. Assist., Scientific Sessions, AHA, Dallas, TX 75231. Tel. 1-214-750-5441.

cont'd on ad page 43

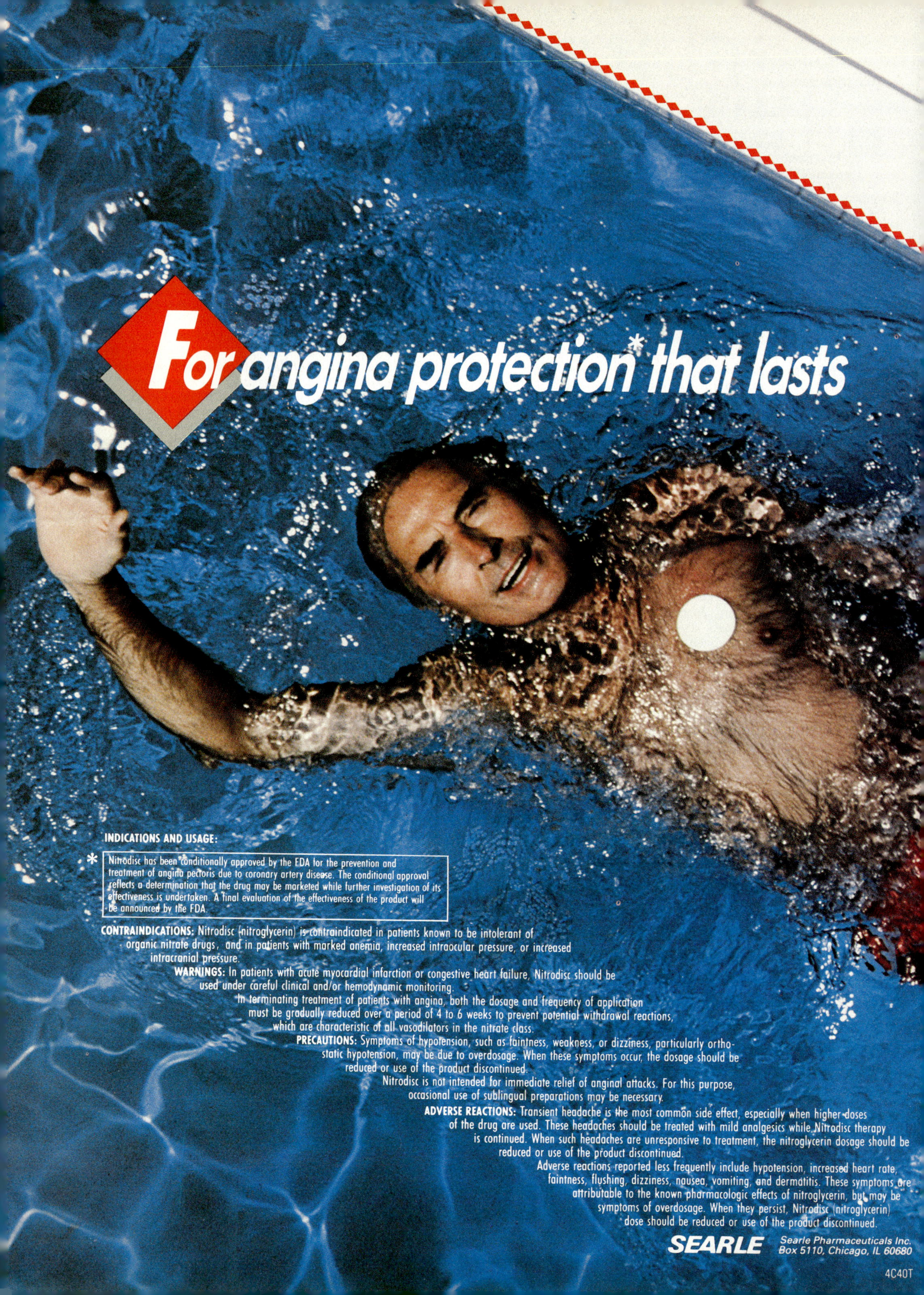
For angina protection* that lasts
INDICATIONS AND USAGE:
* Nitrodisc has been conditionally approved by the FDA for the prevention and treatment of angina pectoris due to coronary artery disease. The conditional approval reflects a determination that the drug may be marketed while further investigation of its effectiveness is undertaken. A final evaluation of the effectiveness of the product will be announced by the FDA.
CONTRAINDICATIONS: Nitrodisc (nitroglycerin) is contraindicated in patients known to be intolerant of organic nitrate drugs, and in patients with marked anemia, increased intraocular pressure, or increased intracranial pressure.
WARNINGS: In patients with acute myocardial infarction or congestive heart failure, Nitrodisc should be used under careful clinical and/or hemodynamic monitoring.
In terminating treatment of patients with angina, both the dosage and frequency of application must be gradually reduced over a period of 4 to 6 weeks to prevent potential withdrawal reactions, which are characteristic of all vasodilators in the nitrate class.
PRECAUTIONS: Symptoms of hypotension, such as faintness, weakness, or dizziness, particularly orthostatic hypotension, may be due to overdosage. When these symptoms occur, the dosage should be reduced or use of the product discontinued.
Nitrodisc is not intended for immediate relief of anginal attacks. For this purpose, occasional use of sublingual preparations may be necessary.
ADVERSE REACTIONS: Transient headache is the most common side effect, especially when higher doses of the drug are used. These headaches should be treated with mild analgesics while Nitrodisc therapy is continued. When such headaches are unresponsive to treatment, the nitroglycerin dosage should be reduced or use of the product discontinued.
Adverse reactions reported less frequently include hypotension, increased heart rate, faintness, flushing, dizziness, nausea, vomiting, and dermatitis. These symptoms are attributable to the known pharmacologic effects of nitroglycerin, but may be symptoms of overdosage. When they persist, Nitrodisc (nitroglycerin) dose should be reduced or use of the product discontinued.
SEARLE
Searle Pharmaceuticals Inc.
Box 5110, Chicago, IL 60680
4C40T

cont'd from ad page 37

July 10–12: **4th International Symposium on Mechanisms of Vasodilatation.** Rochester, MN. Satellite of International Congress of Physiological Sciences. Cerebral, coronary, and limb circulation. Paul M. Vanhoutte, M.D., chairman organizing committee. Abstracts by Oct. 30, 1985. Inquiries: J. Beckman, 942C Guggenheim Bldg., Mayo Clinic, Rochester, MN 55905.

Sept. 14–19: **Xth World Congress of Cardiology,** Washington, DC. Inquiries: Secretariat, 7320 Greenville Ave., Dallas, TX 75231. Tel. 1-214-750-5429. Cable: Tencard, Dallas, TX.

Abroad

1985

July 15–19: **4th Meeting, World Federation on Ultrasound in Medicine and Biology.** Sydney, Australia. Inquiries: WFUMB, POB 1441 GPO, Sydney, NSW, Australia 2001.

Aug. 3–17: **5th Annual Roentgen Revisited.** Postgraduate Radiology Course with NMR Symposium. Switzerland, Austria, Germany. Sponsored by University of California San Francisco Medical Center and University of Munich. Charles B. Higgins, M.D., course director. Inquiries: Travel Planners, POB 32366, San Antonio, TX 78216 Tel. 1-512-341-8131.

Aug. 23–25: **Vascular Update. 3rd Annual Seminar on Peripheral Vascular Disease and Hypertension.** Four Seasons Hotel, Toronto, Ont., Canada. Mill Creek Community Hospital and Cleveland Clinic Foundation, sponsors. J.A.M. Smith, D.O., program director. Inquiries: Dept. Med. Ed., Millcreek Community Hospital, 5515 Peach St., Erie, PA 16509. Tel. 1-814-864-4031 Ext. 448.

Aug. 31–Sept. 7: **Diagnosis of Diseases of the Chest.** Italy. (Also in Greece, Sept. 8–14). 2nd Great Teachers Foundation International Postgraduate Medical Education Program. Eric N.C. Milne, M.D., program director. Inquiries: Ryals, POB 610203, Dallas/Fort Worth Airport TX 75261 USA. Tel 1-214-659-0590.

Sept. 1–6: **13th World Federation of Neurology International Conference on Cerebrovascular Disease.** Salzburg, Austria. Inquiries: Prof. Helmut Lechner, Chief, Clinic of Neurology and Psychiatry, University of Graz, Graz, Austria.

Sept. 1–6: **13th World Congress of Neurology.** Hamburg FRG. Inquiries T. Sober, M.D., Dept. Neurology, Faculty of Medicine, University of Saarland D-6650, Hamburg-Saar, Federal Republic of Germany.

Sept. 1–7: **3rd Postgraduate International Course on Pain Therapy.** Vicenza, Italy. Inquiries: Ruggiero Rizzi, M.D., Ospedale Generale Regionale, 36100 Vicenza, Italy.

Sept. 1–15: **Interpreting the Chest X-Ray — Problems and Advances.** Italy — Greece/Greek Isles. Drs. Eric Milne, Norah Milne, Anthony Proto and E.G. Theros, faculty. Inquiries: D. Ryals, POB 610203, DFW Airport, TX 75261-0203. Tel. 1-214-659-9590.

Sept. 3–6: **European Nuclear Medicine Congress.** Barbican Centre, London, England. Incorporates 23rd Meeting Society of Nuclear Medicine Europe, 8th Meeting European Nuclear Medicine Society, 13th Meeting British Nuclear Medicine Society. Inquiries: Congress, Institute of Nuclear Medicine, Middlesex Hospital Medical School, Mortimer St., London, WIN 8AA, United Kingdom. Tel. OI 631 1066.

Sept. 4–6: **Symposium on Factors Affecting Platelet Adhesion and Aggregation.** Buenos Aires, Argentina. Organized by the Latin American Cooperative Group on Hemostasis and Thrombosis and sponsored by the Boehringer Ingelheim Program for Thrombosis Research in Latin America. Dr. Raúl Altman, chairman scientific committee. Inquiries: Dr. Altman, Viamonte 2008, 1056 Buenos Aires, Argentina.

Sept. 4–7: **Sclerosis in Plaques. Annual World Meeting of the International Federation of National Societies (FISEP).** Hamburg, FRG. Inquiries: German Society of Sclerosis in Plaques, Rosental 5, Aufgang D-8, Munich 2, Federal Republic of Germany.

Sept. 5–7: **1st Asian-Pacific Conference on Doppler and Echocardiography.** Tokyo. Inquiries: Pravin M. Shah, M.D., Coordinator for North America, Cardiology Section (691/111E), Wadsworth VA Medical Center, Wilshire & Sawtelle Blvds, Los Angeles, CA. Tel. 1-213-824-3126.

Sept. 7–9: **3rd International Brain Heart Conference.** Trier, Germany. Inquiries: Dr. T. Stober, Dept. Neurology, Faculty of Med. University of Saarland, D-6650, Homburg/Saar, Federal Republic of Germany.

Sept. 8–11: **6th Meeting of the European Section of the International Society on Research in Cardiology.** Stockholm, Sweden. Inquiries: Dr. L. Kaijser, Dept. Clinical Physiology, Karolinska Hospital, SU-1041, Stockholm, Sweden.

Sept. 8–12: **1st International Congress on Hospital Laws, Procedures, and Ethics.** Tel Aviv, Israel. Judge Amnon Carmi, organizing chairman. Inquiries: Hospitalaw, 28 Ahad Ha'am St., POB 394, Tel Aviv 61003, Israel. Tel. 03-650862. Telex: 33803 TLV. Cable: PELTOURS TELAVIV.

Sept. 9: **Workshop on Cardioembolic Stroke (During 3rd International Brain/Heart Conference,** Sept. 7–9). Trier, Germany, Inquiries: David G. Sherman, M.D., and Robert G. Hart, M.D., co-chairmen, Dept. of Medicine, University of Texas Health Science Center, 7703 Floyd Curl Dr., San Antonio, TX 78284. Tel. 1-512-691-6521.

Sept. 9–12: **8th Annual European Conference on Lipoproteins.** Evangelische Akademie, Tutzing (near Munich), West Germany. Apolipoprotein mutants and dyslipoproteinemias; cellular processing of lipoproteins. Sponsored by European Lipoprotein Club. Inquiries: Dr. J. Shepherd, Secretary European Lipoprotein Club, Dept. Pathological Biochemistry, Royal Infirmary, Glasgow, Scotland, GF OSF.

Sept. 11–14: **4th European Conference on Mechanocardiography.** Budapest, Hungary. Organized by the European-African Div. of the International Society of Mechanocardiography and the Hungarian Society of Cardiology. Prof. J. Simonyi, chairman scientific committee. Inquiries: Mechanocardiography Organizing Committee, Budapest, Pf 88, H-1450, Hungary.

Sept. 11–14: **Acute Brain Ischemia 1985: Medical and Surgical Therapy.** University of Siena, Italy. Satellite of 13th World Congress of Neurology, Sept. 7–9, Hamburg, Germany. Prof. Noè Battistini, organizer. Inquiries: GIBI s.a.s., M. P. Gerini, Via Orlona, 7, 00198 Rome, Italy.

Sept. 16–19: **12th European Congress for Artificial Organs. Pre-Congress Meeting of the International Diabetes Federation.** Athens, Greece. (Artificial endocrine pancreas, insulin delivery devices, pancreas and islet transplantation). Inquiries Prof. S. Raptis, M.D., POB 14127, 11510, Athens, Greece.

Sept. 16–20: **International Symposium on Cardiogenic Reflexes.** University of Leeds, England. Organized by Dept. of CV Studies, Univ. Leeds, and Commission on CV Physiology of International Union of Physiological Sciences. Inquiries: Dr. R. Hainsworth, Dept. CV Studies, University of Leeds, Leeds LS2 93T, England.

Oct. 3–4: **Hemodynamics and Atherosclerosis.** Wellington, New Zealand. Inquiries: Dr. W.E. Stehbens, Dept. Pathology, Wellington Clinical School of Med., Wellington, 2, New Zealand.

Oct. 3–18: **Frontiers in Imaging and Cardiopulmonary Diagnosis.** In USSR. Drs. Benjamin Felson, Eric Milne and Jack Westcott, faculty. Inquiries: See Ryals Sept. 1–15.

Oct. 6–10: **7th International Symposium on Atherosclerosis.** Melbourne, Australia. Inquiries: Dr. P.J. Nestel, Baker Medical Research Inst., Commercial Rd., Prahran, Vic., Australia 3181.

Oct. 8–10: **1st Latin American Congress of Cardiac Pacing.** Buenos Aires, Argentina. Organized by Latin American Society of Cardiac Pacing and Argentine Chamber of Cardiac Pacing. Dr. Alejandro Dussaut, president organizing committee. Inquiries: Congresos Internacionales S.A., Moreno 854 — 9° piso, 1091 Buenos Aires, Argentina. Tel. 14-3216/3408/3283. Telex 22036 JECON AR.

Oct. 11–12: **2nd International Symposium on Hypertension in Children and Adolescents.** Heidelberg, FRG. Organized by Dept. of Pediatrics, Univ. of Heidelberg, and German Institute for High Blood Pressure Research. Inquiries: German Institute HBP Research, University of Heidelberg, Im Neuenheimer Feld 366, D-6900 Heidelberg, FRG.

Oct. 11–18: **Cell Biology of the Artery Wall.** Hayman Island, Great Barrier Reef, Australia. Satellite of 7th International Symposium on Arteriosclerosis, Oct. 6–10, Melbourne. Inquiries: Dr. Gordon H. Campbell, Dept. Anatomy, University of Melbourne, Parkville, 3052, Australia.

Oct. 14–18: **International Congress on Cardiac Doppler.** Pisa, Italy.

cont'd on ad page 47

cont'd from ad page 43

(Tutorial sessions Oct. 14–15; Scientific Sessions Oct. 16–18). Prof. Luigi Donato and Dr. Merrill Spencer, presidents. Inquiries: Istituto di Fisiologia Clinica, C.N.R., University of Pisa, Via Savi 8, 1-567100 Pisa, Italy. Tel. 050-47231/502109. Telex: 590549 IFCI.

Oct. 17–19: **18th Danube Symposium for Neurological Sciences.** University Clinic for Neurology. Innsbruck, Austria. Inquiries: Danube Symposium for Neurological Sciences, c/o Vienna Academy of Medicine, Alser Str. 4,A-1090 Vienna, Austria. Tel. (0222) 42 71 65. Cable MEDACAD, Wien. Telex 134743 MEDAK A.

Oct. 20–22: **5th International Symposium on Rats with Spontaneous Hypertension and Related Studies.** Kyoto, Japan. Yukio Yamori, M.D., program director. Inquiries: 5th SHR Symposium, Shimane Medical University, Izumo 693, Japan. Tel. 0853-23-2111 Ext. 2375. Cable: WHOCOLLAB IZUMO.

Oct. 20–23: **3rd World Congress of Cardiac Rehabilitation.** Caracas, Venezuela. Sponsored by the International Society and Federation of Cardiology: Scientific Council on Rehabilitation of Cardiac Patients and AHA Council on Clinical Cardiology. Inquiries Dr. Deyanira Almeida, Congresa C.A., POB 17422, Caracas 1015A, Venezuela.

Oct. 23–24: **International Symposium on Mechanisms and Treatment in Essential Hypertension: Calcium and Calcium Antagonists.** Hotel Nagoya Castle, Nagoya, Japan. (Satellite of 5th International Symposium on Rats with Spontaneous Hypertension, Oct. 20–22, Kyoto, Japan). Inquiries: Kyuzo Aoki, M.D., 2nd Dept. Internal Med., Nagoya City University Medical School, Mizuho-ku, Nagoya 467, Japan. Tel. 052-851-5511, Ext. 2204.

Oct. 25–27: **International Symposium on Brain and Blood Pressure Control.** Kikai-Shinkoh Hall, Shiba Park, Tokyo, Japan. Dr. Keiji Nakamura organizing chairman. Inquiries: Brain and Blood Pressure, Dept. of Pharmacology, Nippon Roche Research Center, Kamakura 247, Japan. Tel. 0467-45-3191-Ext. 380 or 381. Telex 2222861 PANROCHE J.

Oct. 27–30: **3rd Asian Pacific Symposium on Cardiac Pacing and Electrophysiology.** Hilton Hotel, Melbourne, Australia. Sponsored by Cardiac Society of Australia and New Zealand under auspices of International Cardiac Pacing Society. Inquiries: 3rd Asian Pacific Symposium on Cardiac Pacing and Electrophysiology, Dept. of Cardiology, Suite 3.5, Epworth Medical Centre, 62 Erin St., Richmond, Vic. 3121, Australia.

Oct. 28–31: **1st International Congress on Food and Health.** Salsomaggiore Terme, Italy. Sponsored by International Association for Advancement of Biomedical Research, by Society of Medical Gastronomy, and Institute of Pharmacology of University of Pisa. Inquiries: ALM s.r.l., Via Lattuada, 26, 20135 Milan, Italy. Telex: 313063 HOTALM I.

Nov. 2–4: **3rd International Symposium on Ischemic Heart Disease, Exercise, and Related Topics.** Royal York Hotel, Toronto, Canada. Sponsored by Toronto Rehabilitation Center. Inquiries: J. Kennedy or A. Ceci, Toronto Rehab. Center, 345 Rumsey Rd., Toronto, Ont. Canada M4G 1RT. Tel. 1-416-425-1117 Ext. 236.

Nov. 28–30: **7th Biennial Congress of Cardiology.** Rawalpindi/Islamabad, Pakistan. Inquiries: Pakistan Cardiac Society, Brig. Muhammad Zulfiqar Ali Khan, AFIC/NIHD, Rawalpindi, Pakistan. Tel. 64946, 61-31113, 61-33911.

Dec. 1–4: **International Symposium on Left Ventricular Dysfunction.** Jerusalem Hilton Hotel, Israel. Jan J. Kellermann, M.D. of Israel and David Spodick, M.D. of Worcester, MA, co-chairmen. Under the auspices of the Universities of Tel Aviv and Massachusetts. Inquiries: POB 50006, Tel Aviv 61500, Israel. Tel. 03-654571. Telex 341171 KENS IL.

1986

Jan. 8–11: **7th Annual European Conference on Vascular Biology.** Bad Buchau, FR Germany. Growth and Differentiation of Vascular Cells. Organized by European Artery Club. Inquiries: Dr. G. Bondjers, Dept. Med. 1, Salgren's Hospital, 5-413 45 Göteborg, Sweden.

Feb. 9–13: **12th World Congress of the International Society for Heart Research,** Melbourne, Australia. Inquiries: Dr. N.S. Dhalla, Dept. Physiology, Faculty of Medicine, University of Manitoba, Winnipeg, Canada R3E OW3.

March 23–25: **2nd International Symposium on Holter Monitoring.** Jerusalem, Israel. V. Hombach, Cologne, and S. Stern, Jerusalem, co-chairmen. Inquiries: Prof. Shlomo Stern, c/o Stier Group, Ltd., 203 Dizengoff St., Tel Aviv 63115 Israel. Tel. (03) 224-153/4/5. Telex 35570 STI COIN IL.

April 23–25: **1st International Symposium on Cardiology.** Hospital de Clinicas, University of Buenos Aires, Argentina. Inquiries: Dr. Luis D. Suárez, Dean Funes 1075-(1231), Buenos Aires, Argentina. Tel. 821-6041.

July 8–11: **8th Annual Meeting American Section of the International Society For Heart Research and Satellite Symposium on Heart Metabolism for the 30th International Congress of Physiological Sciences.** Winnipeg, Canada. Inquiries: Dr. R. E. Beamish, Experimental Cardiology Section, Dept. of Physiology, Faculty of Medicine, University of Manitoba, Winnipeg, Canada R3E OW3.

July 13–18: **30th International Congress of Physiological Sciences.** The University of British Columbia, Vancouver, Canada. Dr. H. McLennan, chairman program committee. Inquiries: IUPS, Suite 801, 750 Jervis St., Vancouver, B.C., Canada V6E 2A9. Tel. 604-681-5226. Telex 04-352848 VCR.

Aug. 31–Sept. 7: **11th Congress of International Society of Hypertension.** Heidelberg, Federal Republic of Germany. Organized by German Institute of High Blood Pressure Research and German Hypertension League. Dr. Detlev Ganten, Congress chairman. Inquiries: GKV, Frankfurter Str. 57, D-6050 Offenbach 1, Heidelberg, FR Germany.

Sept. 14–17: **8th International Symposium on Microsurgical Anastomoses for Cerebral Ischemia.** Florence, Italy. Inquiries: Rolando Gagliardi, M.D., Dept. of Neurosurgery, USL 10/D, Careggi Hospital, 50100 Florence, Italy.

Sept. 14–18: **2nd International Conference on Diet and Nutrition and 5th International Congress on Obesity.** Jerusalem, Israel. Inquiries: C. Horwitz, Ph.D., and S. H. Blondheim, M.D., POB 983, Jerusalem 91009, Israel.

1987

Sept. 2–4: **International Conference on Management of Cardiac Arrhythmias.** London, England. Sponsored by the British Heart Foundation. Professor A. J. Camm and Dr. A. W. Nathan, members organizing committee. Inquiries: British Heart Foundation, 102 Gloucester Pl., London W1H 4DH England. Tel. 01-935-0185.

AHA Scientific Sessions Future Meeting Dates

1985	Washington, DC	Nov. 11–14
1986	Dallas, TX	Nov. 17–20
1987	Anaheim, CA	Nov. 16–19
1988	Locale Not Set	Nov. 14–17
1989	New Orleans	Nov. 13–16
1990	Dallas	Nov. 12–15

Xth World Congress of Cardiology, 1986

The Xth World Congress of Cardiology will be held in Washington, DC, Sept. 14–19, 1986. Official languages English, Spanish, and French. Inquiries: Secretariat, Xth World Congress Cardiology, 7320 Greenville Ave., Dallas, TX 75231. Tel. 1-214-750-5429. Cable: TenCard, Dallas.

settings insure COSMOS senses only cardiac activity.

On the pacing side, this new COSMOS sends the pacing impulse from the lead tip to the pacemaker can, giving you a strong, easily identified and interpreted pacing spike on your DDD ECG tracing. Eliminating any need for special equipment for analysis.

For you, the result is a reliable COSMOS with superior interference signal rejection as well as far-field QRS rejection by the atrial channel. And a bipolar sensing DDD pacemaker that is much easier to follow-up on standard ECG equipment.

Best of all, it's a COSMOS.

Our new model 284-02 offers you pacing sophistication that is more clinically useful because its wide-range programmability is simple, fast, effective and safe to use.

The Rx2000 programmer puts everything you need to know about your COSMOS patient's condition at your fingertips. Its built-in printer even makes copies for your files.

Diagnostic capabilities in a class by themselves.

A complete history of your patients' COSMOS/cardiac activity begins at the moment of implant. A simple press of the light pen displays it. Another press of the light pen and your patient's original pacing regime is displayed. Press one key, and COSMOS telemetry measures exactly how the pacer is functioning at any given moment. So you have a complete picture of cause, and effect and result in your follow-up care program.

Patient safety is a matter of superior design and painstaking quality control.

In developing a pacemaker as advanced as the COSMOS 284-02, our first concern was producing a system with no unexpected clinical results. Which is why COSMOS was the first DDD to effectively deal with problems such as pacemaker mediated tachycardia. Why every COSMOS features multiple backup systems for critical circuitry. And why our new COSMOS is the very first to combine the advantages of bipolar sensing with the ECG clarity of unipolar pacing.

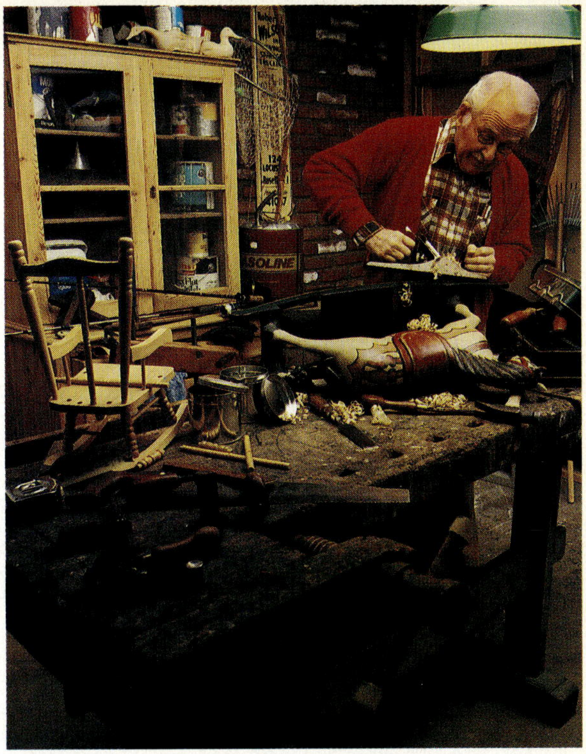

Bipolar sensing of the COSMOS 284-02 *allows normal patient activity virtually free from myopotentials and* EMI.

Getting to know COSMOS is very simple.

Intermedics has a complete range of educational video tapes that cover everything from implant techniques to advanced DDD pacing concepts. Just ask your Intermedics Representative to show you COSMOS, the DDD pacing system that's as unique as the heart it serves.

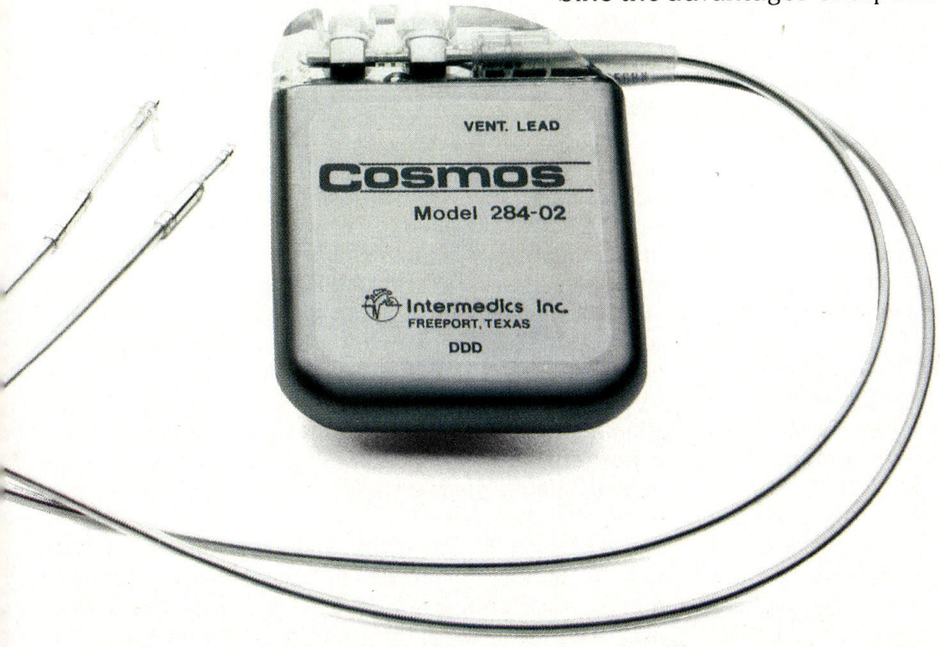

Intended Uses: All Intermedics implantable pulse generators are intended for use in long-term cardiac pacing therapy. The applications for long-term cardiac pacing are many and varied and are discussed as they apply to the particular pulse generator in the Physician's Manual accompanying the device along with Contraindications, Possible Complications and Precautions.

The choice of pacing modes and/or programmable features that best meet the therapeutic requirements of the individual patient is at the discretion of the prescribing physician.

For further information, see the Physician's Manual packaged with the pulse generator, or contact your Intermedics Sales Representative or Intermedics directly.

Intermedics Inc.®
Quality comes to life.™

P.O. Box 617, Freeport, Texas 77541-0617
Toll Free: 1-800-231-2330 In Texas: 1-800-392-3726
Telex: 4620584 INTL UI

News from the American Heart Association

7320 Greenville Ave., Dallas, Texas 75231
Telephone: 214 750-5300

Stroke Council Provides 10 Scholarships in CBVD Aiding Medical Students

The AHA Stroke Council has awarded ten scholarships in Cerebrovascular Disease (CBVD) in order to stimulate medical students' interest, knowledge, and investigative work.

The winners, including institution and sponsor, are: *Max Robert Steuer,* Baylor College of Medicine, sponsored by David S. Baskin, M.D.; *Douglas Ziedonis* (one other to be named), M. S. Hershey Medical Center, sponsored by Richard S. K. Young, M.D., and Robert B. Duckrow, M.D.; *Jeffrey Frank, B.S.,* Southern Illinois University, sponsored by David Good, M.D.; *Jessie E. Taber, B.S.,* University of Illinois, sponsored by Philip B. Gorelick, M.D.; *Bruce Ballon,* Virginia Commonwealth University, sponsored by Hermes A. Kontos, M.D., Ph.D.

Also, To be named, Massachusetts General Hospital, sponsored by Michael A. Moskowitz, M.D.; *Mark Hospodar,* University of Pittsburgh, sponsored by Oscar M. Reinmuth, M.D.; *Charles Semba, B.A.,* University of Minnesota, sponsored by James G. White, M.D.; To be named, University of Cincinnati, sponsored by Hwa-Shain Yeh, M.D.; To be named, Duke University, sponsored by James W. Davis, M.D.

1984 HBP Proceedings Printed as Supplement

The "Proceedings of the AHA Council for High Blood Pressure (1984)" has been published as a supplement to HYPERTENSION, May/June, 1985. The volume is also available as AHA Monograph No. 111.

The volume, guest edited by Michael J. Dunn, M.D., of Cleveland, contained 26 papers, selected from the meetings on Oct. 10–12, 1984.

Announced in the publication was the CIBA Award for Hypertension Research to David F. Bohr, M.D., "for elaborating the interactions of ions, nerves, and hormones affecting behavior of vascular smooth muscle. The studies, spanning three decades, demonstrated the overriding importance of the chemical environment to the reactivity of blood vessels in hypertension."

Also announced was the first award of the Marion Hypertension Research Clinical Fellowship to Christine Seidman, M.D. of Harvard Medical School. Dr. Seidman presented the winning paper in a competition among physicians in training prior to the HBP Council meeting in Cleveland. Her paper concerned the genetic structure regulating the atrial natriuretic factor and established that the regulation for the production of this new natriuretic polypeptide occurs exclusively in atrial tissue.

The award is funded by a grant from Marion Laboratories.

Mortality Rates Decline In Provisional 1983 Data

Provisional data released by the National Center for Health Statistics show a continuing declinc in thc crudc and age adjusted U.S. mortality rates through 1983.

Cardiovascular diseases as a group also continued to show a decline in both the crude and age adjusted rates.

U.S. life expectancy reached a new high of 78.8 years for white females, 71.6 years for white males, 73.8 years for black females, and 65.2 years for black males.

CVD continued as the leading cause of death, accounting for an estimated 989,364 deaths in 1983, 49.2% of the deaths from all causes.

CVD declines from 1972 to 1983 were: Total CVD −30.7%, Coronary Heart Disease −31.2%, Stroke −47.1%, Hypertensive Disease −40.7%, and Rheumatic Fever/Rheumatic Heart Disease −47.4%.

NIH Panel Agrees With AHA On Lowering Cholesterol

Dietary recommendations, similar to those of the American Heart Association and the Inter-Society Commission for Heart Disease Resources, have been issued by a National Institutes of Health Consensus Panel.

The recommendations came after a conference earlier in 1985 under the auspices of the NHLBI and the Office of Medical Applications of Research in Bethesda, MD. A panel of experts, which considered scientific evidence, issued the report on lowering blood cholesterol to prevent heart disease.

In addition to five recommendations similar to those of the AHA, the panel called for establishment of a National Cholesterol Education Program, greater efforts by the food industry to market and label food adhering to diet recommendations, encouraging physicians to include blood cholesterol levels in examining patients, and further research on diets and their assessment.

Free single copies of the NIH consensus statement may be obtained from the Office of Medical Applications of Research, NIH, Bldg. 1, Rm. 216, Bethesda, MD 20205.

cont'd on ad page 18

cont'd from ad page 8

81 U.S. Medical Schools Report Courses on ACLS

Eighty-one of 101 U.S. medical schools responding, reported to the American Heart Association that they offered courses in Advanced Cardiac Life Support (ACLS). The replies were in response to a survey of 200 medical schools by the AHA Emergency Cardiac Care Subcommittee.

The Subcommittee has distributed the results and has recommended that ACLS National Faculty Members encourage medical schools which did not respond to develop Life Support programs for medical students.

2 Groups Grant Credits

The Heart Association has been advised by the American College of Emergency Physicians (ACEP) that Life Support courses approved for American Medical Association Category 1 accreditation will also be eligible for ACEP accreditation.

The American Academy of Family Physicians has given national approval for prescribed credit for Life Support programs — 16 hours for ACLS Provider and 20 hours for instructor.

"Heart Research" Funds Asked by Unknown Group

The American Heart Association has been unable to obtain information on a group identified as the "American Heart Research Foundation," which has conducted a mass mailing survey on stress and cardiovascular disease and is soliciting funds.

AHA has written to this organization at Washington, D.C., and Toms River, NJ, addresses advising them that the "American Heart Research Foundation" name is confusingly similar to the American Heart Association name. It demanded that the new group immediately change its name to prevent confusion or the false perception that it is related to the American Heart Association.

Inquiries are also being made by AHA to government offices in New Jersey and the District of Columbia.

"On the basis of our inquiries so far," an AHA statement said, "we cannot now confirm that 'American Heart Research Foundation' is a reputable charitable organization conducting bona fide research, education, or programs in the cardiovascular health area."

Phone Solicitation Scheme

AHA affiliates have also reported a phone solicitation scheme to sell office supplies. The caller identifies himself as the son of a recently deceased parent who was a friend of a key AHA volunteer. The volunteer, he adds, recommended that the affiliate buy stationery from the caller.

"This is fraud," an AHA representative stated, "we are trying to stop this."

Atherosclerosis Meeting In Australia, Oct. 6–10

The 7th International Symposium on Atherosclerosis will be held in the Regent Melbourne Hotel in Melbourne, Australia, Oct. 6–10. The session is supported by 12 international societies including the American Heart Association.

Inquiries may go to the 7th International Symposium, Baker Medical Research Institute, Commercial Road, Prahan, Melbourne, Vic., 3181 Australia.

Satellite Session

A satellite symposium, "Cell Biology of the Artery Wall," will be held at Hayman Island, Great Barrier Reef, Oct. 11–15. Inquiries may go to Dr. Gordon H. Campbell, Dept. of Anatomy, University of Melbourne, Parkville, 3052 Australia.

A meeting on Hemodynamics and Atherosclerosis will be held Oct. 3–4 in Wellington, New Zealand, under the direction of Dr. W. E. Stehbens, Dept. of Pathology, Wellington Clinical School of Medicine, Wellington 2, New Zealand.

Cardiology Tutorial "In the Wilderness"

The University of California San Diego School of Medicine has announced plans for a continuing medical education conference: "Cardiology Tutorial in the Wilderness."

Dates and locations are:

1985

Sept. 7–14 — Exploring the Colorado Plateau.

Sept. 15–22 — Hiking Inn to Inn in Vermont.

1986

Jan. 18–25 — Canoe trip in the Everglades.

March 8–15 — Royal Gorge Cross Country Ski Resort.

May 10–17 — Scuba diving.

Aug. 8–16 — San Juan River Canyon rafting.

A brochure, giving credit hours and fees, may be obtained from the Office of Continuing Medical Education, UC San Diego School of Medicine, M-017, La Jolla CA 92093. Tel. 1-619-452-3940.

Kyoto Symposium on SHR To Note Rat Model Value

"Contribution of Spontaneously Hypertensive and Stroke-Prone Rat Models to Medicine, Past, Present and Future," will be the theme of the 5th International Symposium on SHR and Related Studies to be held in Kyoto, Japan, Oct. 20–22. The meeting will honor the 77th birthday of Dr. Koso Okamoto who first bred the animals in Kyoto.

Among papers scheduled at the meeting will be "Cardiovascular complications in SHR," "Identification of possible pathogenic components of essential hypertension in rat models," "Cardiovascular factors," "Electrolytes and humoral factors," and "Pharmacological intervention in SHR."

cont'd on ad page 27

cont'd from ad page 18

Honorary president of the Symposium is Dr. Okamoto and president is Dr. Yumiko Yamori. The working language is English. Inquiries may go to: Secretariat, 5th SHR Symposium, Shimane Medical University, Izumo 693, Japan. Tel. 0853-23-2111, Ext. 2375. Cable WHOCOLLAB IZUMO.

Satellite Meeting

A satellite symposium in Nagoya, Japan, Oct. 23–4, will be the "International Symposium on Mechanisms and Treatment in Essential Hypertension — Calcium and Calcium Antagonists." Attendance is limited to 100. Twenty invited speakers will present their work in English. (Dr. Kyuzo Aoki, Hinokuchi-cho, Nishi-ku, Nagoya 467, Japan. Tel. 052-521-2121).

Heart Position Papers Offered on Smoking, RF

Two important AHA position papers on cigarette smoking and on rheumatic fever have been reprinted from CIRCULATION (**70**, No. 6, December, 1984) and may be obtained from affiliates or the National Center (ask for 71-001-C and 71-006-C).

The reprint of "Cigarette Smoking and Cardiovascular Disease," is a statement for health professionals prepared by a task force appointed by the Steering Committee. It give details of the case against cigarette smoking and makes recommendations for patient management.

Rheumatic Fever

"Prevention of Rheumatic Fever" was prepared by the Committee on Rheumatic Fever and Infective Endocarditis of the Council of Cardiovascular Disease in the Young. It points out that acute RF and rheumatic heart disease remain important preventable disorders throughout the world. The revised statement gives recommendations on the prevention of initial attacks ("primary" prevention) and recurrent attacks ("secondary" prevention).

Manual for Basic Life Support

A revised "Instructors Manual for Basic Life Support" (70-029-C) is now available from affiliates. Prepared by the AHA Subcommittee on Emergency Cardiac Care, the manual is a loose-leaf, three-hole punched source book for new instructors as well as the experienced instructor.

Plan to Increase Community Groups

A Three-Year Community Organization Plan to increase AHA community organizations from 1,040 to 2,030 by June 30, 1988, and to raise more dollars for research, has been adopted by the Board of Directors.

The plan charts a course for the National Center and is expected to serve as a guideline for affiliates to expand community organizations. The importance of broad-based volunteer support has been a National priority since 1983.

Three Year Goal

Community organizations in each affiliate are expected to aid in programs, increasing public awareness of cardiovascular disease, and help raise more money for research.

The Three-Year Plan said that by 1988 it is hoped to have 2030 communities with a group of volunteers "who are addressing the cardiovascular health needs of their communities through public education and service programs, as well as raising funds to support cardiovascular research. This represents approximately two-thirds of the counties in the U.S."

One County, One Group

Beyond the Three-Year Plan, it is expected to have one Community Organization or Division in every county and multiple Divisions or Branches in counties or towns with major populations.

A task force based in the affiliates will be formed to serve as advisers, a pool of National staff members will be formed to assist with commnity organization upon affiliate request, a slide/tape will help volunteer awareness and a revised Self-Instruction Kit will be available.

Organ Procurement Group Handled 170 Phone Calls

The North American Transplant Coordinators Organization (NATCO), established in 1983, has reported that as of July, 1984, over 170 inquiries on organ procurement had been processed.

The majority of calls, NATCO said, were inquiries from physicians and other medical professionals seeking the nearest organ procurement agency. There were also 71 calls reporting a potential organ donor, 14 of which led to retrieval.

The organization, which maintains a 24-hour hot line — 800/24-DONOR — is staffed by organ procurement professionals for the referral of potential organ donors by physicians and other health professionals. All donor referrals and information requests are directed to local programs. It also assists hospitals not affiliated with a local program.

Risk Factors in Stroke Now Available as Reprint

"Risk Factors in Stroke," originally printed as a Special Report in the November/December issue of STROKE has been issued by AHA as a reprint.

The report, subtitled "A Statement for Physicians by the Subcommittee on Risk Factors and Stroke of the Stroke Council," is available from AHA affiliates or the National Center. (Ask for 71-022-A)

"Risk Factors" states that in the past twelve years impressive declines in mortality due to stroke and heart disease have occurred. Circumstantial evidence suggests that this change was related chiefly to more effective treatment of hypertension. However, other factors may also have contributed to the decline, and the

cont'd on ad page 36

cont'd from ad page 27

Stroke Council deemed it appropriate to issue an updated review of risk factors."

HBP Structural Changes

Also available as a Monograph (No. 110; 73-096 A) is "Pathophysiology and Clinical Implications of Early Structural Changes in Hypertension," published as a supplement to November/December HYPERTENSION. Editors of the Monograph — Björn Folkow, M.D., Margareta I.L. Nordlander, Ph.D., Bodo-Eckehard Strauer, F.A.C.C., and John Wikstrand, M.D., Ph.D. — said the symposium was arranged in collaboration with the Universities of Göteborg and Munich as a "Midnight Sun Symposium." They said no previous meeting had broadly considered the issues of structural adaptation to primary hypertension which had wide consequences in all areas of CV research.

BE Wallet Cards

A revised Bacterial Endocarditis (BE) wallet card, suitable for patients with rheumatic fever or congenital heart disease who need protection from BE during medical or dental treatment, is now available from Heart Association affiliates (ask for 70-004-D). The card carries the regimens adapted from "Prevention of Bacterial Endocarditis — A Statement for Health Professionals" by the Committee on Rheumatic Fever and Infective Endocarditis of the Council on Cardiovascular Disease in the Young. (CIRCULATION, 1984, **70:** 1123A–1127A — also excerpted in J Am Dent Assoc, 1985, **110:**96–100)

AHA Briefs . . .

• **Modern Concepts of Cardiovascular Disease** for August is "Clinical Applications of Cardiac CT Imaging," by Bruce H. Brundage, M.D., and Eva Chomka, M.D., of the University of Illinois at Chicago.

• The **Society of Magnetic Resonance in Medicine** will hold its 4th Annual Meeting August 19–23 at the Barbican Center, London, United Kingdom. A one-day teaching symposium will be held Aug. 19. Inquiries may go to SMRM, 15 Shattuck Square, Suite 204, Berkeley, CA 94704. Tel. 1-415-841-1899. Also to POB 26 Hitchin, Hertfordshire, SG5 ISA, United Kingdom. Tel. 01-240 1871 Ext. 222. Telex: 261176 IEE LDN G.

• The AHA **Instructor's Manual for Basic Life Support** (70-029C) has been revised in a two-year study by the Basic Life Support Working Group. The revision does not change existing standards but is an expansion and reorganization of previous material.

• A new **Cardiology Training Program** beginning July 1, **1986** has been announced by St. Vincent Hospital, Worcester, MA, affiliated with the University of Massachusetts Medical School. Candidates must have completed internal medicine training. Two and three year training periods will be available. Inquiries may go to David H. Spodick, M.D., D.Sc., Professor of Medicine, University of Massachusetts, Cardiology Divison, St. Vincent Hospital, 25 Winthrop St., Worcester, MA 01604.

• **Dr. Sharon Seltzer** has joined the National Institute of Neurological and Communicative Disorders and Stroke (NINCDS) as grants officer in the extramural Communicative Disorders Program. Her specialty will be otolaryngology and the communicative sciences, as well as magnetic resonance spectroscopy and theoretical chemistry.

• **Dr. John Barranger** of NINCDS has received the Arthur S. Flemming Award as one of the year's 10 outstanding federal employees under age 40. His specialty is studies of inherited metabolic disease.

• **Dr. John J. Pisano,** head of the Section on Physiological Chemistry of the Laboratory of Chemistry, National Heart, Lung, and Blood Institute, has died of a heart attack. He was 56 years old.

Meetings Calendar

1985

Aug. 18–24: **Health Care Expo '85:** Washington, DC, Convention Center. Sponsored by Health Care Expositions. Inquiries: S. K. Herlitz, Health Care Expo, 404 Park Ave. S., New York, NY 10016. Tel. 1-212-532-9400.

Aug. 27–30: **Research Conference on Regulation of Bile Acid Synthesis.** Given Institute of Pathobiology, Aspen, CO. Sponsored by American Gastroenterological Association. Inquiries: Bile Acid Research, 740 Krameria St., Denver, CO 80220.

Sept. 7: **Heart and Mind: Neurocardiology Update.** Hyatt Regency Hotel, Kansas City, MO. Sponsored by University of Kansas Medical Center. Inquiries: J. Johnston, OCE, Univ. of Kansas Medical Center, 39th and Rainbow Blvd., Kansas City, KS 66103. Tel. 1-913-588-4480.

Sept. 9–14: **4th Annual Symposium in Doppler and 2-D Echocardiography.** Washington, D.C. Sponsored by the Johns Hopkins University School of Medicine and the Institute for Medical Studies. James Weiss, M.D., program director. Inquiries: K. Stroich, Inst. for Med. Studies, 30131 Town Center Dr., Suite 215, Laguna Niguel, CA 92677. Tel. 1-714-495-4499.

Sept. 11–14: **15th Annual Peripheral Vascular Disease Symposium: Critical Issues and Controversies in Vascular Surgery.** The Hyatt on Capitol Square, Columbus, OH. William E. Evans, M.D., and Blair D. Vermillion, M.D., co-chairmen. Sponsored by St. Anthony Medical Center. Inquiries: S. Hershberger, St. Anthony Medical Center, 1492 E. Broad St., Suite 1100, Columbus, OH 43205. Tel. 1-614-251-3680.

Sept. 12–14: **International Symposium on Cardiovascular Surgery — 1985. 15th Annual Symposium of Texas Heart Institute.** Houston. Inquiries: Medical Director, Texas Heart Institute, POB 20269, Houston, TX 77225. Tel. 1-713-791-2157.

Sept. 18–20: **10th Annual Nuclear Cardiology Symposium.** Red Carpet Hotel, Madison, WI. Sponsored by CVD Program, Milwaukee Clinical Campus, School of Medicine; Univ. of Wisconsin CME, and American Heart Association, Wisconsin Affiliate. Inquiries: S. Aslakson, CME, 4658 WARF Bldg., 610 Walnut St., Madison, WI 53705. Tel. 1-608-263-2856.

Sept. 20–21: **Coronary Care Update '85.** Wisconsin Center, Madison. Sponsored by CME Univ. of Wisconsin Extension and Dept. Med., School of Med., Univ. of Wis. — Madison. Inquiries: See Sept. 18–20, Aslakson.

Sept. 25–26: **Advanced Cardiac Life Support Provider Course.** University of Kansas, KS, Medical Center. (Also Nov. 6–8). Inquiries: See Sept. 7, J. Johnston.

Sept. 27–29: **2nd Midwest Regional Conference on Women in Medicine.** Alameda Plaza Hotel, Kansas City, MO. Sponsored by University of Kansas Medical Center. Ellen L. Shulman, M.D., guest speaker. Inquiries: See Sept. 7, J. Johnston.

Sept. 30–Oct. 1: **2nd Annual Graduate Hospital Symposium: Acute Myocardial Infarction — Emerging Concepts of Pathogene-**

cont'd on ad page 48

cont'd from ad page 36

sis and Treatment. Philadelphia. Inquiries: M. Blob, Bockus Research Institute, The Graduate Hospital, Philadelphia, PA 19146. Tel. 1-215-893-2375.

Oct. 3–5: **3rd Biannual Symposium in Cardiac Imaging.** Hotel Meridian, San Francisco. Sponsored by University of California, San Francisco School of Medicine and Institute for Medical Studies. Drs. Nelson Schiller, Martin Lipton, Charles Higgins and Elias Botvinick, program directors. Inquiries: K. Stroich — See Sept. 9–14.

Oct. 3–5: **Clinical Doppler Echocardiography. Practical Educational Approach.** Costa Mesa, CA. Stanley J. Goldberg, M.D., course director. Inquiries: Clinical Doppler Echocardiography, 5650 E. 9th St., Tucson, AZ 85711. Tel. 1-602-626-7303.

Oct. 9–11: **Physiology and Techniques of Dual Chamber Pacing.** Waldorf Astoria Hotel, New York City. Doris J. W. Escher, M.D., and Seymour Furman, M.D., co-chairmen. Inquiries: North American Society of Pacing and Electrophysiology, 13 Easton Court, Wellesley Hills, MA 02181. Tel. 1-617-237-1866.

Oct. 10–13: **4th Annual Chicago Critical Care Symposium.** Chicago Marriott (Downtown). Inquiries: E. C. Rackow, M.D., Dept. Med., University of Health Sciences/Chicago Medical School, 3333 Green Bay Rd., North Chicago, IL 60064. Tel. 1-312-578-3291.

Oct. 10–Nov. 1: **New Issues in Stroke: Diagnosis, Treatment and Rehabilitation Among the Elderly.** Hollenden House Hotel, Cleveland. Inquiries: R. Dunkle, Center on Aging, 2009 Adelbert Rd., Rm. 101, Cleveland, OH 44106.

Oct. 11–12: **4th Southern Biomedical Engineering Conference.** Jackson, MS. Inquiries: Dr. Barry W. Sauer, SBEC, Div. Cont. Health Profess. Ed., University of Mississippi Medical Center, 2500 N. State St., Jackson, MS 39216-4505.

Oct. 13–18: **Clinical Congress, American College of Surgeons.** Chicago. Inquiries: ACS, 55 East Erie St., Chicago, IL 60611.

Oct. 14–16: **4th Annual Cardiac Rehabilitation Symposium.** Hotel Meridien, New Orleans. Sponsored by East Jefferson General Hospital. Inquiries: S. Weigel, East Jefferson General Hospital, 4200 Houma Blvd., POB 8213, Metairie LA 70011. Tel. 1-504-454-4147.

Oct. 15–18: **Angiography and Interventional Radiology: 1985.** 15th Annual Postgraduate Course. Marriott-Copley Place, Boston. Drs. L.M. Boxt, M.A. Bettmann, and D.C. Levin, program directors. Inquiries: Dept. Cont. Ed., Harvard Medical School, 25 Shattuck St., Boston, MA 02115. Tel. 1-617-732-6265.

Oct. 19: **Common Problems with Coronary Artery Disease.** Somerset Inn, Troy, MI. Inquiries: E.D. Peterson, R.N., AHA of Michigan, 16310 W. 12 Mile Road, POB 160, Lathrup Village, MI 48076. Tel. 1-313-557-9500.

Oct. 19–20: **Head and Neck Radiology: Advanced Techniques in Diagnostic Imaging.** Hyatt Regency Hotel, San Francisco. William P. Dillon, M.D., and Gretchen A.W. Gooding, M.D., course directors. Sponsored by Radiology Research and Education Foundation, UCSF. Inquiries: Dept. Radiology, UCSF, San Francisco, CA 94143. Tel. 1-415-666-5731.

Oct. 19–20: **Magnetic Resonance Imaging for Technologists.** Hyatt Regency Hotel, San Francisco. A.R. Margulis, M.D., program chairman. Inquiries: See Oct. 21–25, UCSF Dept. Radiology.

Oct. 21–22: **Myocardial Revascularization During Acute MI.** Towsley Center, Ann Arbor, MI. Sponsored by CME, Univ. of Michigan Medical School. Inquiries: B. Phillips, CME, Towsley Center Box 057, Univ. of Mich. Med. School, Ann Arbor, MI 48109-0010. Tel. 1-313-763-1400.

Oct. 21–25: **Clinical Magnetic Resonance Imaging.** Hyatt Regency Hotel, San Francisco. Charles B. Higgins, M.D., Hedvig Hricak, Ph.D., program directors. Sponsored by UCSF Dept. of Radiology. Inquiries: Dept. of Radiology, UCSF School of Medicine, San Francisco, CA 94143. Tel. 1-415-666-5731.

Oct. 25: **Annual Meeting, Society of Neurological Anesthesia and Neurological Supportive Care.** San Francisco. Inquiries: Society of Neurological Anesthesia, POB 238, Univ. of Virginia Medical Center, Charlottesville, VA 22908.

Oct. 30–Nov. 1: **La Crosse Health and Sports Science Symposium.** La Crosse, WI. Inquiries: La Crosse Exercise, 221 Mitchell Hall, UWI, La Crosse, WI 54601. Tel. 1-608-785-8686.

Nov. 4–8: **Diagnostic Radiology Seminars.** Maui Marriott Hotel, Maui, Hawaii. Neil Chafetz, M.D. course director. Sponsored by UCSF Dept. of Radiology. Inquiries: Radiology PG Education, UCSF Room C-324, Third & Parnassus Ave., San Francisco, CA 94143. Tel. 1-415-666-5731 (between 7:30 am-4:30 pm Pacific Time).

Nov. 11–14: **58th Annual Scientific Sessions, American Heart Association, Washington, DC. Inquiries: Coordinator Scientific Sessions, AHA, 7320 Greenville Ave., Dallas, TX 75231. Tel. for abstracts: 1-214-750-5439, for housing and reservations 1-214-750-5425.**

Nov. 19–20: **Subspecialty Boards in Cardiovascular Disease.** Philadelphia. Inquiries: American Board of Internal Medicine, 3624 Market St., Philadelphia, PA 19104. Tel. 1-215-243-1500. (New date.)

Nov. 22–24: **3rd Annual Emergency Cardiac Care Symposium.** Chicago O'Hare Marriott. Inquiries: M.H. Weil, M.D., chairman, Dept. Med., University of Health Sciences/Chicago Medical School, 3333 Green Bay Rd., North Chicago, IL 60064. Tel. 1-312-578-3291.

Dec. 2–6: **Chest Radiology — Update and Review.** Hotel Del Coronado, San Diego. Sponsored by Chest Division of Dept. of Radiology, UCSD. David S. Feigin, M.D., and Paul J. Friedman, M.D., program directors. Inquiries: D. Ryals. Ryals Associates, POB 610203, Dallas-Fort Worth, TX 75261-0203. Tel. 1-214-659-9590.

1986

Jan. 24–25: **Current Controversies and Techniques in Congenital Heart Surgery.** Baltimore, MD. (Immediately prior to Annual Meeting, Society of Thoracic Surgeons, Washington, DC). Sponsored by Div. of Thoracic and Cardiovascular Surgery, University of Maryland School of Medicine. Inquiries: Program Cont. Ed., University of Maryland School of Medicine, 10 South Pine St., Suite 300, Baltimore, MD 21201. Tel. 1-301-528-3956.

Feb. 17–20: **Annual Postgraduate Course on Thoracic Imaging.** Newporter Beach Hotel, Newport Beach, CA. (Feb. 15–16: Scientific Sessions, Society of Thoracic Radiology). H. Baltaxe, M.D., program director. Inquiries: Ryals, POB 610203, DFW Airport, TX 75261-0203. Tel. 1-214-659-9590.

Feb. 19–22: **11th International Joint Conference on Stroke and Cerebral Circulation.** Vacation Village, San Diego. Inquiries: Admin. Assist., Scientific Sessions, AHA, Dallas, TX 75231. Tel. 1-214-750-5441.

April 3–5: **Electrocardiography of Pacemaker Rhythms.** Parker House Hotel, Boston. P.A. Levine, M.D., chairman. Sponsored by North American Society of Pacing and Electrophysiology. Inquiries: NASPE, 13 Eaton Court, Wellesley Hills, MA 02181. Tel. 1-617-237-1866.

May 15–17: **7th Annual Scientific Session, North American Society of Pacing and Electrophysiology.** Marriott Hotel, New Orleans. P.C. Gillette, M.D., program chairman. Inquiries: See April 3–5, 1986, NASPE.

July 10–12: **4th International Symposium on Mechanisms of Vasodilatation.** Rochester, MN. Satellite of International Congress of Physiological Sciences. Cerebral, coronary, and limb circulation. Paul M. Vanhoutte, M.D., chairman organizing committee. Abstracts by Oct. 30, 1985. Inquiries: J. Beckman, 942C Guggenheim Bldg., Mayo Clinic, Rochester, MN 55905.

Sept. 14–19: **Xth World Congress of Cardiology,** Washington, DC. Inquiries: Secretariat, 7320 Greenville Ave., Dallas, TX 75231. Tel. 1-214-750-5429. Cable: Tencard, Dallas, TX.

Abroad

1985

Aug. 23–25: **Vascular Update. 3rd Annual Seminar on Peripheral Vascular Disease and Hypertension.** Four Seasons Hotel, Toronto, Ont., Canada. Mill Creek Community Hospital and Cleveland Clinic Foundation, sponsors. J.A.M. Smith, D.O., program director. Inquiries: Dept. Med. Ed., Millcreek Com-

cont'd on ad page 65

cont'd from ad page 48

munity Hospital, 5515 Peach St., Erie, PA 16509. Tel. 1-814-864-4031 Ext. 448.

Aug. 29–Sept. 1: **15th Annual Meeting European Association for Behavior Therapy — 15 Years of Progress: Research Outcome and Practical Application.** Munich (FRG). Inquiries: EABT '85, S. Winner, Max-Planck-Institute of Psychiatry, Psychological Dept., Kraepelin Str. 2, D-8000 München 40, Federal Republic of Germany. Tel. 089/30622-544.

Aug. 31–Sept. 7: **Diagnosis of Diseases of the Chest.** Italy. (Also in Greece, Sept. 8–14). 2nd Great Teachers Foundation International Postgraduate Medical Education Program. Eric N.C. Milne, M.D., program director. Inquiries: Ryals, POB 610203, Dallas/Fort Worth Airport TX 75261 USA. Tel 1-214-659-0590.

Sept. 1–6: **13th World Federation of Neurology International Conference on Cerebrovascular Disease.** Salzburg, Austria. Inquiries: Prof. Helmut Lechner, Chief, Clinic of Neurology and Psychiatry, University of Graz, Graz, Austria.

Sept. 1–6: **13th World Congress of Neurology.** Hamburg FRG. Inquiries T. Sober, M.D., Dept. Neurology, Faculty of Medicine, University of Saarland D-6650, Hamburg-Saar, Federal Republic of Germany.

Sept. 1–7: **3rd Postgraduate International Course on Pain Therapy.** Vicenza, Italy. Inquiries: Ruggiero Rizzi, M.D., Ospedale Generale Regionale, 36100 Vicenza, Italy.

Sept. 1–15: **Interpreting the Chest X-Ray — Problems and Advances.** Italy — Greece/Greek Isles. Drs. Eric Milne, Norah Milne, Anthony Proto and E.G. Theros, faculty. Inquiries: D. Ryals, POB 610203, DFW Airport, TX 75261-0203. Tel. 1-214-659-9590.

Sept. 3–6: **European Nuclear Medicine Congress.** Barbican Centre, London, England. Incorporates 23rd Meeting Society of Nuclear Medicine Europe, 8th Meeting European Nuclear Medicine Society, 13th Meeting British Nuclear Medicine Society. Inquiries: Congress, Institute of Nuclear Medicine, Middlesex Hospital Medical School, Mortimer St., London, WIN 8AA, United Kingdom. Tel. OI 631 1066.

Sept. 4–6: **Symposium on Factors Affecting Platelet Adhesion and Aggregation.** Buenos Aires, Argentina. Organized by the Latin American Cooperative Group on Hemostasis and Thrombosis and sponsored by the Boehringer Ingelheim Program for Thrombosis Research in Latin America. Dr. Raúl Altman, chairman scientific committee. Inquiries: Dr. Altman, Viamonte 2008, 1056 Buenos Aires, Argentina.

Sept. 4–7: **Sclerosis in Plaques. Annual World Meeting of the International Federation of National Societies (FISEP).** Hamburg, FRG. Inquiries: German Society of Sclerosis in Plaques, Rosental 5, Aufgang D-8, Munich 2, Federal Republic of Germany.

Sept. 5–7: **1st Asian-Pacific Conference on Doppler and Echocardiography.** Tokyo. Inquiries: Pravin M. Shah, M.D., Coordinator for North America, Cardiology Section (691/111E), Wadsworth VA Medical Center, Wilshire & Sawtelle Blvds, Los Angeles, CA. Tel. 1-213-824-3126.

Sept. 7–9: **3rd International Brain Heart Conference.** Trier, Germany. Inquiries: Dr. T. Stober, Dept. Neurology, Faculty of Med. University of Saarland, D-6650, Homburg/Saar, Federal Republic of Germany.

Sept. 8–11: **6th Meeting of the European Section of the International Society on Research in Cardiology.** Stockholm, Sweden. Inquiries: Dr. L. Kaijser, Dept. Clinical Physiology, Karolinska Hospital, SU-1041, Stockholm, Sweden.

Sept. 8–12: **1st International Congress on Hospital Laws, Procedures, and Ethics.** Tel Aviv, Israel. Judge Amnon Carmi, organizing chairman. Inquiries: Hospitalaw, 28 Ahad Ha'am St., POB 394, Tel Aviv 61003, Israel. Tel. 03-650862. Telex: 33803 TLV. Cable: PELTOURS TELAVIV.

Sept. 9: **Workshop on Cardioembolic Stroke (During 3rd International Brain/Heart Conference,** Sept. 7–9). Trier, Germany, Inquiries: David G. Sherman, M.D., and Robert G. Hart, M.D., co-chairmen, Dept. of Medicine, University of Texas Health Science Center, 7703 Floyd Curl Dr., San Antonio, TX 78284. Tel. 1-512-691-6521.

Sept. 9–12: **8th Annual European Conference on Lipoproteins.** Evangelische Akademie, Tutzing (near Munich), West Germany. Apolipoprotein mutants and dyslipoproteinemias; cellular processing of lipoproteins. Sponsored by European Lipoprotein Club. Inquiries: Dr. J. Shepherd, Secretary European Lipoprotein Club, Dept. Pathological Biochemistry, Royal Infirmary, Glasgow, Scotland, GF OSF.

Sept. 11–14: **4th European Conference on Mechanocardiography.** Budapest, Hungary. Organized by the European-African Div. of the International Society of Mechanocardiography and the Hungarian Society of Cardiology. Prof. J. Simonyi, chairman scientific committee. Inquiries: Mechanocardiography Organizing Committee, Budapest, Pf 88, H-1450, Hungary.

Sept. 11–14: **Acute Brain Ischemia 1985: Medical and Surgical Therapy.** University of Siena, Italy. Satellite of 13th World Congress of Neurology, Sept. 7–9, Hamburg, Germany. Prof. Noè Battistini, organizer. Inquiries: GIBI s.a.s., M. P. Gerini, Via Orlona, 7, 00198 Rome, Italy.

Sept. 16–19: **12th European Congress for Artificial Organs. Pre-Congress Meeting of the International Diabetes Federation.** Athens, Greece. (Artificial endocrine pancreas, insulin delivery devices, pancreas and islet transplantation). Inquiries Prof. S. Raptis, M.D., POB 14127, 11510, Athens, Greece.

Sept. 16–20: **International Symposium on Cardiogenic Reflexes.** University of Leeds, England. Organized by Dept. of CV Studies, Univ. Leeds, and Commission on CV Physiology of International Union of Physiological Sciences. Inquiries: Dr. R. Hainsworth, Dept. CV Studies, University of Leeds, Leeds LS2 93T, England.

Oct. 3–4: **Hemodynamics and Atherosclerosis.** Wellington, New Zealand. Inquiries: Dr. W.E. Stehbens, Dept. Pathology, Wellington Clinical School of Med., Wellington, 2, New Zealand.

Oct. 3–18: **Frontiers in Imaging and Cardiopulmonary Diagnosis.** In USSR. Drs. Benjamin Felson, Eric Milne and Jack Westcott, faculty. Inquiries: See Ryals Sept. 1–15.

Oct. 6–10: **7th International Symposium on Atherosclerosis.** Melbourne, Australia. Inquiries: Dr. P.J. Nestel, Baker Medical Research Inst., Commercial Rd., Prahran, Vic., Australia 3181.

Oct. 8–10: **1st Latin American Congress of Cardiac Pacing.** Buenos Aires, Argentina. Organized by Latin American Society of Cardiac Pacing and Argentine Chamber of Cardiac Pacing. Dr. Alejandro Dussaut, president organizing committee. Inquiries: Congresos Internacionales S.A., Moreno 854 — 9° piso, 1091 Buenos Aires, Argentina. Tel. 14-3216/3408/3283. Telex 22036 JECON AR.

Oct. 11–12: **2nd International Symposium on Hypertension in Children and Adolescents.** Heidelberg, FRG. Organized by Dept. of Pediatrics, Univ. of Heidelberg, and German Institute for High Blood Pressure Research. Inquiries: German Institute HBP Research, University of Heidelberg, Im Neuenheimer Feld 366, D-6900 Heidelberg, FRG.

Oct. 11–18: **Cell Biology of the Artery Wall.** Hayman Island, Great Barrier Reef, Australia. Satellite of 7th International Symposium on Arteriosclerosis, Oct. 6–10, Melbourne. Inquiries: Dr. Gordon H. Campbell, Dept. Anatomy, University of Melbourne, Parkville, 3052, Australia.

Oct. 13–15: **6th International Congress, International Society for Laser Surgery and Medicine.** Jerusalem, Israel. Inquiries: POB 50006, Tel Aviv 61500, Israel.

Oct. 14–18: **International Congress on Cardiac Doppler.** Pisa, Italy. (Tutorial sessions Oct. 14–15; Scientific Sessions Oct. 16–18). Prof. Luigi Donato and Dr. Merrill Spencer, presidents. Inquiries: Istituto di Fisiologia Clinica, C.N.R., University of Pisa, Via Savi 8, 1-567100 Pisa, Italy. Tel. 050-47231/502109. Telex: 590549 IFCI.

Oct. 17–19: **18th Danube Symposium for Neurological Sciences.** University Clinic for Neurology. Innsbruck, Austria. Inquiries: Danube Symposium for Neurological Sciences, c/o Vienna Academy of Medicine, Alser Str. 4,A-1090 Vienna, Austria. Tel. (0222) 42 71 65. Cable MEDACAD, Wien. Telex 134743, MEDAK A.

Oct. 20–22: **5th International Symposium on Rats with Spontaneous Hypertension and Related Studies.** Kyoto, Japan. Yukio Yamori, M.D., program director. Inquiries: 5th SHR Symposium, Shimane Medical University, Izumo 693, Japan. Tel. 0853-23-2111 Ext. 2375. Cable: WHOCOLLAB IZUMO.

Oct. 20–23: **3rd World Congress of Cardiac Rehabilitation.** Caracas, Venezuela. Sponsored by the International Society and

cont'd on ad page 71

cont'd from ad page 65

Federation of Cardiology: Scientific Council on Rehabilitation of Cardiac Patients and AHA Council on Clinical Cardiology. Inquiries Dr. Deyanira Almeida, Congresa C.A., POB 17422, Caracas 1015A, Venezuela.

Oct. 23–24: **International Symposium on Mechanisms and Treatment in Essential Hypertension: Calcium and Calcium Antagonists.** Hotel Nagoya Castle, Nagoya, Japan. (Satellite of 5th International Symposium on Rats with Spontaneous Hypertension, Oct. 20–22, Kyoto, Japan). Inquiries: Kyuzo Aoki, M.D., 2nd Dept. Internal Med., Nagoya City University Medical School, Mizuho-ku, Nagoya 467, Japan. Tel. 052-851-5511, Ext. 2204.

Oct. 25–27: **International Symposium on Brain and Blood Pressure Control.** Kikai-Shinkoh Hall, Shiba Park, Tokyo, Japan. Dr. Keiji Nakamura organizing chairman. Inquiries: Brain and Blood Pressure, Dept. of Pharmacology, Nippon Roche Research Center, Kamakura 247, Japan. Tel. 0467-45-3191-Ext. 380 or 381. Telex 2222861 PANROCHE J.

Oct. 27–30: **3rd Asian Pacific Symposium on Cardiac Pacing and Electrophysiology.** Hilton Hotel, Melbourne, Australia. Sponsored by Cardiac Society of Australia and New Zealand under auspices of International Cardiac Pacing Society. Inquiries: 3rd Asian Pacific Symposium on Cardiac Pacing and Electrophysiology, Dept. of Cardiology, Suite 3.5, Epworth Medical Centre, 62 Erin St., Richmond, Vic. 3121, Australia.

Oct. 28–31: **1st International Congress on Food and Health.** Salsomaggiore Terme, Italy. Sponsored by International Association for Advancement of Biomedical Research, by Society of Medical Gastronomy, and Institute of Pharmacology of University of Pisa. Inquiries: ALM s.r.l., Via Lattuada, 26, 20135 Milan, Italy. Telex: 313063 HOTALM I.

Nov. 2–4: **3rd International Symposium on Ischemic Heart Disease, Exercise, and Related Topics.** Royal York Hotel, Toronto, Canada. Sponsored by Toronto Rehabilitation Center. Inquiries: J. Kennedy or A. Ceci, Toronto Rehab. Center, 345 Rumsey Rd., Toronto, Ont. Canada M4G 1RT. Tel. 1-416-425-1117 Ext. 236.

Nov. 28–30: **7th Biennial Congress of Cardiology.** Rawalpindi/Islamabad, Pakistan. Inquiries: Pakistan Cardiac Society, Brig. Muhammad Zulfiqar Ali Khan, AFIC/NIHD, Rawalpindi, Pakistan. Tel. 64946, 61-31113, 61-33911.

Dec. 1–4: **International Symposium on Left Ventricular Dysfunction.** Jerusalem Hilton Hotel, Israel. Jan J. Kellermann, M.D. of Israel and David Spodick, M.D. of Worcester, MA, co-chairmen. Under the auspices of the Universities of Tel Aviv and Massachusetts. Inquiries: POB 50006, Tel Aviv 61500, Israel. Tel. 03-654571. Telex 341171 KENS IL.

Dec. 8–12: **2nd International Symposium on Hypertension in the Community.** Jerusalem, Israel. Prof. Talma Rosenthal, POB 50006, Tel Aviv, 61500, Israel. Tel. 03-654571. Telex 341171 KENS IL.

1986

Jan. 8–11: **7th Annual European Conference on Vascular Biology.** Bad Buchau, FR Germany. Growth and Differentiation of Vascular Cells. Organized by European Artery Club. Inquiries: Dr. G. Bondjers, Dept. Med. 1, Salgren's Hospital, 5-413 45 Göteborg, Sweden.

Feb. 9–13: **12th World Congress of the International Society for Heart Research,** Melbourne, Australia. Inquiries: Dr. N.S. Dhalla, Dept. Physiology, Faculty of Medicine, University of Manitoba, Winnipeg, Canada R3E OW3.

Feb. 16–21: **1st International Congress on Stress, Behavior and Coronary Disease.** Southern Cross Hotel, Melbourne, Australia. Prof. G.D. Burrows, president, Dr. M. Jelinek, scientific program chairman. Inquiries: Mental Health Foundation, Suite 23, 20 Commercial Rd., Melbourne 3004, Vic., Australia.

March 23–25: **2nd International Symposium on Holter Monitoring.** Jerusalem, Israel. V. Hombach, Cologne, and S. Stern, Jerusalem, co-chairmen. Inquiries: Prof. Shlomo Stern, c/o Stier Group, Ltd., 203 Dizengoff St., Tel Aviv 63115 Israel. Tel. (03) 224-153/4/5. Telex 35570 STI COIN IL.

April 23–25: **1st International Symposium on Cardiology.** Hospital de Clinicas, University of Buenos Aires, Argentina. Inquiries: Dr. Luis D. Suárez, Dean Funes 1075-(1231), Buenos Aires, Argentina. Tel. 821-6041.

June 5–7: **International Congress for Clinical Neuroimaging.** Palais Auersperg, Vienna, Austria. Inquiries: International Congress for Clinical Neuroimaging, c/o Vienna Academy of Medicine, Alser Str. 4, A-1090, Vienna, Austria. Tel. 0222 42 71 65. Cable MEDACAD Wien, Telex: 134743 medak a.

June 23–27: **6th Asean Congress of Cardiology.** Jakarta, Indonesia. Working language, English. Organized by Indonesian Heart Association. L.I. Rilantono, M.D., chairman. Inquiries: Asean Congress Cardiology, Dept. Cardiology, Cipto Mangunkusumo Hospital, Jalan Diponegoro 69, Jakarta 10453, Indonesia.

July 2–5: **35th International Conference European Society for CV Surgery.** Metropole Hotel, Brighton, England. Prof. H.H. Bentall, chairman. Inquiries: European Society for CV Surgery, Concorde Services Ltd., 10 Wendell Rd., London W12 9RT, United Kingdom.

July 8–11: **8th Annual Meeting American Section of the International Society For Heart Research and Satellite Symposium on Heart Metabolism for the 30th International Congress of Physiological Sciences.** Winnipeg, Canada. Inquiries: Dr. R. E. Beamish, Experimental Cardiology Section, Dept. of Physiology, Faculty of Medicine, University of Manitoba, Winnipeg, Canada R3E OW3.

July 13–18: **30th International Congress of Physiological Sciences.** The University of British Columbia, Vancouver, Canada. Dr. H. McLennan, chairman program committee. Inquiries: IUPS, Suite 801, 750 Jervis St., Vancouver, B.C., Canada V6E 2A9. Tel. 604-681-5226. Telex 04-352848 VCR.

Aug. 31–Sept. 7: **11th Congress of International Society of Hypertension.** Heidelberg, Federal Republic of Germany. Organized by German Institute of High Blood Pressure Research and German Hypertension League. Dr. Detlev Ganten, Congress chairman. Inquiries: GKV, Frankfurter Str. 57, D-6050 Offenbach 1, Heidelberg, FR Germany.

Sept. 14–17: **8th International Symposium on Microsurgical Anastomoses for Cerebral Ischemia.** Florence, Italy. Inquiries: Rolando Gagliardi, M.D., Dept. of Neurosurgery, USL 10/D, Careggi Hospital, 50100 Florence, Italy.

Sept. 14–18: **2nd International Conference on Diet and Nutrition and 5th International Congress on Obesity.** Jerusalem, Israel. Inquiries: C. Horwitz, Ph.D., and S. H. Blondheim, M.D., POB 983, Jerusalem 91009, Israel.

1987

Sept. 2–4: **International Conference on Management of Cardiac Arrhythmias.** London, England. Sponsored by the British Heart Foundation. Professor A. J. Camm and Dr. A. W. Nathan, members organizing committee. Inquiries: British Heart Foundation, 102 Gloucester Pl., London W1H 4DH England. Tel. 01-935-0185.

AHA Scientific Sessions Future Meeting Dates

1985	Washington, DC	Nov. 11–14
1986	Dallas, TX	Nov. 17–20
1987	Anaheim, CA	Nov. 16–19
1988	Locale Not Set	Nov. 14–17
1989	New Orleans	Nov. 13–16
1990	Dallas	Nov. 12–15

Xth World Congress of Cardiology, 1986

The Xth World Congress of Cardiology will be held in Washington, DC, Sept. 14–19, 1986. Official languages English, Spanish, and French. Inquiries: Secretariat, Xth World Congress Cardiology, 7320 Greenville Ave., Dallas, TX 75231. Tel. 1-214-750-5429. Cable: TenCard, Dallas.

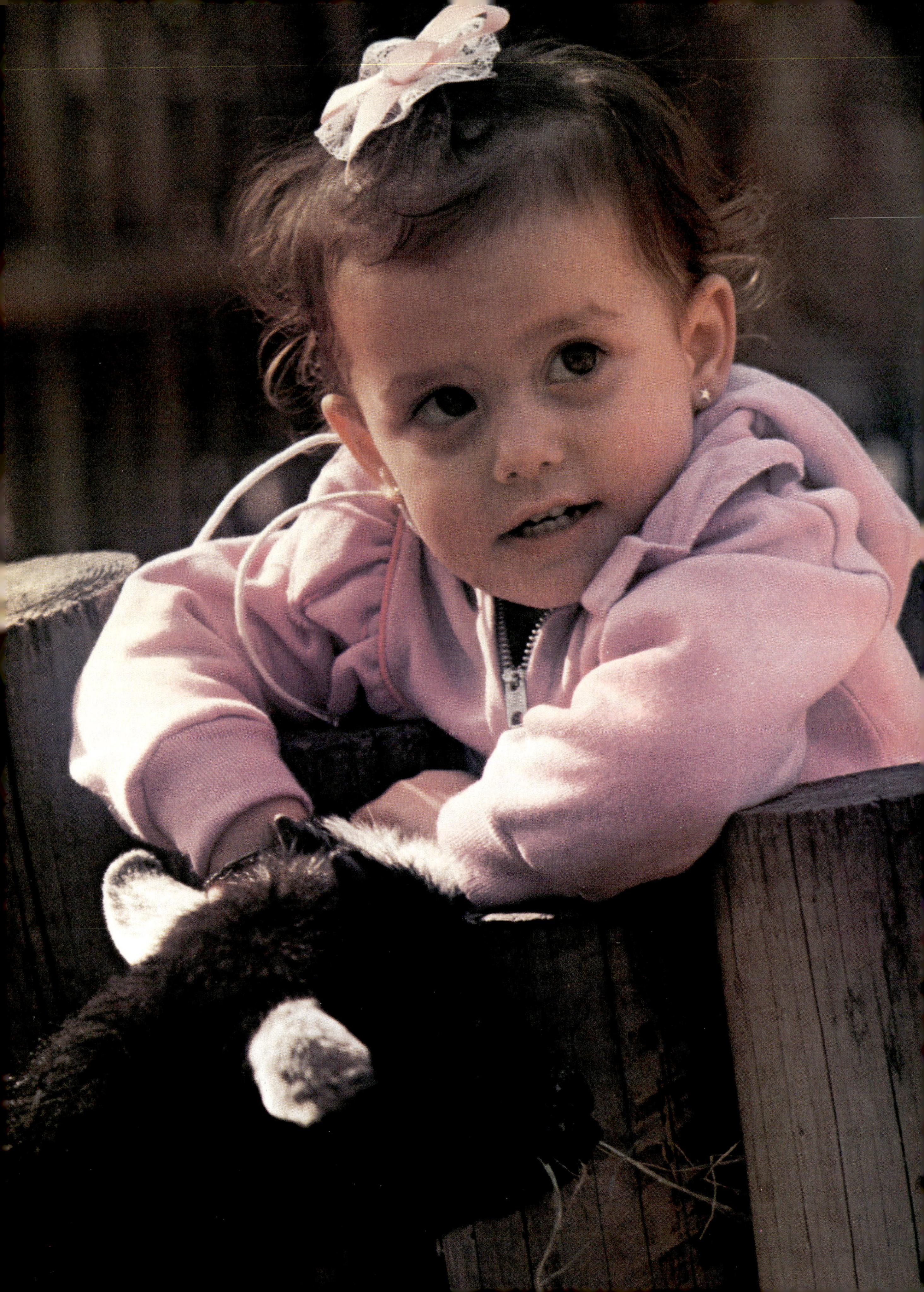

News from the American Heart Association

7320 Greenville Ave., Dallas, Texas 75231
Telephone: 214 750-5300

AHA Statement of Mission Amended

At the recent Delegate Assembly/Futures Conference held in Chicago, members voted to amend AHA's mission statement to emphasize the Association's involvement in stroke. The mission statement now reads:

> It is the mission of the American Heart Association to reduce premature death and disability from cardiovascular diseases and stroke.

In another action, the Assembly adopted goals and expected outcomes which had been drafted by the Futures Conference. Additionally, the 1985–86 Board of Directors was elected. The officers include: Thomas J. Ryan, M.D., President; Richard A. Boehning, Esq., Chairman of the Board; William B. Dulany, Esq., Secretary; and W.W. Aston, Treasurer.

Scientific Meeting of the Councils on Circulation and Basic Science

A combined scientific meeting of the Councils on Circulation and Basic Science of the American Heart Association will be held February 25–March 2, 1986, in Keystone, Colorado.

The theme of this meeting, which will be chaired by Dr. Stephen Vatner (Council on Circulation) and Dr. Harold Strauss (Council on Basic Science), will be **Autonomic Cardiovascular Control,** with invited lectures on *Ca^{++} Channels, Adrenergic Receptors, Neural Recordings in Man and Conscious Animals, Neural-Hormonal Mechanisms in Control of Cerebral Circulation and Microcirculation.* Additional topics may be added, including *Measurement of Myocardial Perfusion in Man and Experimental Animals* and *Autonomic Alterations in Heart Failure.*

Investigators are encouraged to submit abstracts on related topics for presentation as posters.

A proposed new feature of this meeting is the support of the young investigator, i.e., one below the rank of associate professor. However, support is still tentative pending availability of funds. No support will be available for the more senior investigators.

Support of the young investigator will enable both presentation of research in poster format and discussion of results with faculty members. The young investigator is encourged to submit an abstract and enclose a curriculum vitae. A statement in a covering letter should indicate whether attendance is dependent upon funding.

Abstract forms can be obtained from the Administrative Assistant for Scientific Sessions at the American Heart Association, 7320 Greenville Avenue, Dallas, Texas 75231, and must be postmarked no later than October 28, 1985, and received at the same address by November 1, 1985.

Student Scholarships in Cerebrovascular Disease

The Stroke Council of the American Heart Association has awarded ten student scholarships in stroke. The scholarships' intent is to stimulate the interest, knowledge, and investigative work of medical students.

The 1985 awardees, institutions, and sponsors are: *Max Robert Steuer,* Baylor College of Medicine, sponsored by David S. Baskin, M.D.; *Douglas Ziedonis* and one other to be named, M.S. Hershey Medical Center, sponsored by Richard S.K. Young, M.D., and Robert B. Duckrow, M.D.; *Jeffrey Frank, B.S.,* Southern Illinois University, sponsored by David Good, M.D.; *Jessie E. Taber, B.S.,* University of Illinois, sponsored by Philip B. Gorelick, M.D.; *Bruce Ballon,* Virginia Commonwealth University, sponsored by Hermes A. Kontos, M.D., Ph.D.

Also, a student to be named, Massachusetts General Hospital, sponsored by Michael A. Moskowitz, M.D.; *Mark Hospodar,* University of Pittsburgh, sponsored by Oscar M. Reinmuth, M.D.; *Charles Semba, B.A.,* University of Minnesota, sponsored by James G. White, M.D.; To be named, University of Cincinnati, sponsored by Hwa-Shain Yeh, M.D.; To be named, Duke University, sponsored by James W. Davis, M.D.

NIH Consensus Panel Issues Report: Health Implications of Obesity

A National Institutes of Health (NIH) consensus development statement on health implications of obesity may now be obtained from the NIH Office of Medical Applications of Research.

A panel of experts prepared the report, which considered scientific evidence presented at a consensus development conference at the NIH. It contains recommendations and conclusions concerning health implications of obesity.

At NIH, consensus conferences bring together researchers, practicing physicians, representatives of public interest groups, consumers, and others to carry out scientific assessments of drugs, devices, and procedures in an effort to evaluate their safety and effectiveness.

Free single copies of the consensus statement on health implications of obesity are available from Michael J. Bernstein, Office of Medical Applications of Research, National Institutes of Health, Bldg. 1, Room 216, Bethesda, MD, 20205.

cont'd on ad page 11

cont'd from page 8

NHLBI Investigates Clot-Dissolving Drugs

The preliminary conclusion of the first phase of the Thrombolysis in Myocardial Infarction (TIMI) study indicates that intravenously injected tissue-type plasminogen activator (tPA) was nearly two times as effective as streptokinase in reopening the blocked coronary arteries of patients suffering acute heart attack.

Investigators from the National Heart, Lung, and Blood Institute studied a group of 316 patients who had experienced at least 30 minutes of chest pain and shown ST-segment elevation in two leads of the electrocardiogram. Participants underwent heart catheterization, during which coronary blood flow was graded from 0 (no flow) to 3 (normal). Patients with less than 50 percent narrowing were not treated with either drug.

At 90 minutes, 36 percent of the 122 patients with closed arteries who received streptokinase had restored blood supply (grade 2 or 3). Sixty-six percent of 118 patients who received tPA had reopened arteries at 90 minutes.

It has not yet been established if reopening of the coronary arteries will affect morbidity or mortality, a question which will be addressed in the second phase of the TIMI study. Phase II will be a larger placebo-controlled, double-blind trial with a longer follow-up period.

NINCDS Notes

- **Dr. Henry deForest Webster,** chief of the Laboratory of Experimental Neuropathology, National Institute of Neurological and Communicative Disorders and Stroke (NINCDS), is the recipient of a Senior U.S. Scientist Award from the Alexander von Humboldt Foundation of the Federal Republic of Germany. The award honors American scientists with an international reputation and promotes the exchange of ideas between German and American investigators and research institutions.
- **Stroke** is the subject of one of four reports now available from the Office of Scientific and Health Reports. The report was prepared in conjunction with Congressional appropriations hearings. It describes research on the causes, diagnosis, treatment, and prevention of stroke, as well as progress made during 1984 and future areas of investigation. To receive a copy, contact the Office of Scientific and Health Reports, NINCDS, Bldg. 31, Room 8A06, Bethesda, MD, 20205.

AHA Briefs

- **Modern Concepts of Cardiovascular Disease** for September is "The Long QT Syndrome," by Anil K. Bhandari, M.D., and Melvin Scheinman, M.D., of the University of Southern California, Los Angeles and University of California San Francisco School of Medicine.
- On Nov. 8 and 9, 1985, the American Heart Association, New York City Affiliate, will present **"Cardiology in Psychosocial, Economic, Political and Ethical Perspectives."** The meeting takes place at the Halloran House Hotel, New York City, and is presented in cooperation with the International Society for Humanism in Cardiology. For a preliminary program, contact the Humanism Conference, American Heart Association, New York City Affiliate, 205 East 42 Street, New York, NY 10017. Telephone 212-661-5335.
- The National Heart, Lung, and Blood Institute has announced the availability of **competitive renewals** of Clinical Investigator Awards and Physician Scientist Awards to assist awardees in achieving the status of independent investigator. Application receipt date for 1985 was August 1; the 1986 deadline is June 1. For further information, contact the program staff shown on the Notice of Grant Award: Fann Harding, Ph.D., Division of Blood Diseases and Resources, NHLBI, Federal Building, Room 5A08, Bethesda, MD 20205; Max A. Heinrich, Jr., Ph.D., Division of Heart and Vascular Diseases, NHLBI, Federal Building, Room 3A12, Bethesda, MD 20205.
- The **Association of Teachers of Preventive Medicine** has announced an agreement with the Centers for Disease Control. The two organizations are joining together in a series of activities designed to enhance the professional education of physicians in the areas of disease prevention and health promotion. For more information, contact Katherine Lacy, Project Director, ATPM/CDC Cooperative Agreement, Association of Teachers of Preventive Medicine, 1015 15th Street, N.W., Suite 403, Washington, D.C. 20005. Telephone (202) 682-1698.
- The National Center for Health Statistics is planning a third **National Health and Nutrition Examination Survey** to occur in 1988. Its purpose is to measure and monitor the health and nutritional status of the American population. The Center is now soliciting suggestions for research topics to be included in the survey. Specific suggestions, which briefly describe the public health importance and available data collection methodologies, should be submitted to: Kurt R. Maurer, Chief, Survey Planning and Development Branch, Division of Health Examination Statistics, National Center for Health Statistics, 3700 East-West Highway, Room 2-58, Hyattsville, MD 20783.
- **Dr. Martha Vaughan,** chief of the Laboratory of Cellular Metabolism, National Heart, Lung, and Blood Institute, has been elected to the National Academy of Sciences. She is one of 60 newly elected members chosen for their achievements in original research.
- **Leonore Wagner** of the National Institutes of Health has died. At NIH, Ms. Wagner developed a database of information on U.S. support of health-related research which is an important resource for decisionmakers in health policy.

Meetings Calendar

1985

Sept. 18–20: **10th Annual Nuclear Cardiology Symposium.** Red Carpet Hotel, Madison, WI. Sponsored by CVD Program, Milwaukee Clinical Campus, School of Medicine; Univ. of Wis-

cont'd on ad page 14

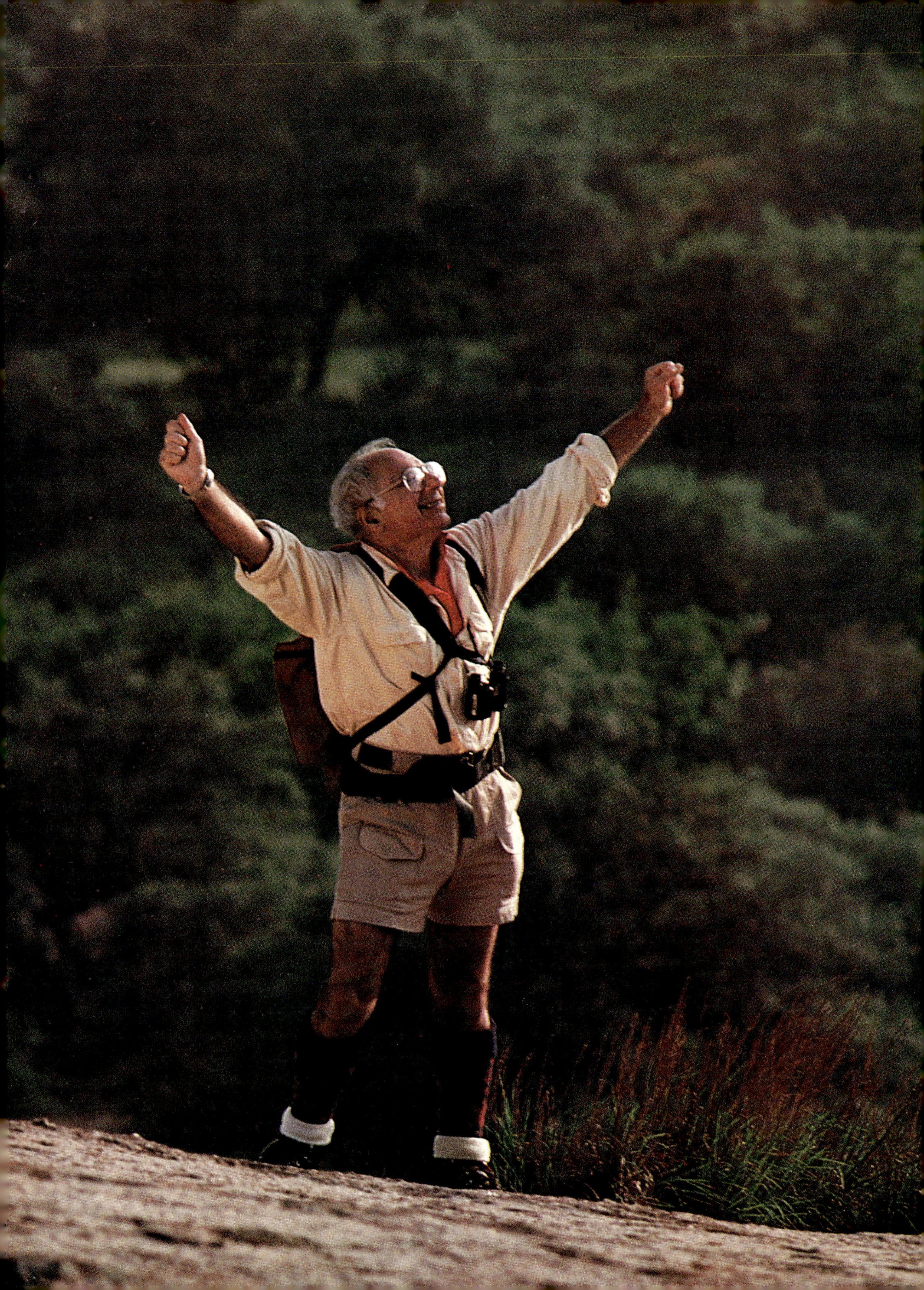

A life like Marcel Malden's is worth every extra step we take.

Safety backup systems. It's a simple concept, but it represents one of the extra steps we take to bring you and your patients the most reliable pacemakers available today.

At Intermedics, we design critical function redundancy into every pacemaker we develop. Such as the primary timing control in the Quantum®–a crystal oscillator. It's backed up by a resistor-capacitor oscillator that takes over and continues pacing. Or the programmed bypass parameters that back up the magnetic reed switch in our COSMOS pulse generators. Or the multiple elective replacement indicators in both the Quantum and COSMOS. And the Rx2000 programmer that gives a clear indication if any of these safety systems activate.

Multiple backup systems like these assure that pacing continues even in the unlikely event of a critical component failure. It is this attention to detail that has earned Intermedics the highest reliability rating (and the lowest recall statistics) of any major pacemaker manufacturer.

When the fullness of life depends on the flawless performance of a sophisticated implant, there is no such thing as excessive quality control. Because there's more at stake than our reputation.

We believe these extra steps have helped make us the world's second largest pacemaker company in just eleven years. We know they are the reason Intermedics has consistently produced the most dependable line of pacemakers ever offered.

For documentation of our product reliability, just ask your Intermedics Representative. Or call us toll-free at 1-800-231-2330. (In Texas, 1-800-392-3726.) You'll see a record worth every extra step.

Intermedics Inc.®

Quality comes to life.™

cont'd from ad page 11

consin CME, and American Heart Association, Wisconsin Affiliate. Inquiries: S. Aslakson, CME, 4658 WARF Bldg., 610 Walnut St., Madison, WI 53705. Tel. 1-608-263-2856.

Sept. 18–29: **39th Annual Fall Conference and Scientific Sessions of the Council for High Blood Pressure Research.** Sponsored by AHA Council for High Blood Pressure Research.

Sept. 20–21: **Coronary Care Update '85.** Wisconsin Center, Madison. Sponsored by CME Univ. of Wisconsin Extension and Dept. Med., School of Med., Univ. of Wis. — Madison. Inquiries: See Sept. 18–20, Aslakson.

Sept. 25–26: **Advanced Cardiac Life Support Provider Course.** University of Kansas, KS, Medical Center. (Also Nov. 6–8). Inquiries: See Sept. 7, J. Johnston.

Sept. 27–29: **Second Midwest Regional Conference on Women in Medicine.** Alameda Plaza Hotel, Kansas City, MO. Sponsored by University of Kansas Medical Center. Ellen L. Shulman, M.D., guest speaker. Inquiries: See Sept. 7, J. Johnston.

Sept. 30–Oct. 1: **Second Annual Graduate Hospital Symposium: Acute Myocardial Infarction — Emerging Concepts of Pathogenesis and Treatment.** Philadelphia. Inquiries: M. Blob, Bockus Research Institute, The Graduate Hospital, Philadelphia, PA 19146. Tel. 1-215-893-2375.

Oct. 1–3: **Neurological/Neurosurgical ICU Course.** Massachusetts General Hospital — Harvard Medical School. Inquiries: Allan H. Ropper, M.D., Massachusetts General Hospital, Boston, MA 02114. Tel. 1-617-726-2921.

Oct. 3–5: **Third Biannual Symposium in Cardiac Imaging.** Hotel Meridian, San Francisco. Sponsored by University of California, San Francisco School of Medicine and Institute for Medical Studies. Drs. Nelson Schiller, Martin Lipton, Charles Higgins and Elias Botvinick, program directors. Inquiries: K. Stroich, The Institute for Medical Studies, 30131 Town Center Drive, Suite 215, Laguna Niguel, CA 92677. Tel. 1-714-495-4499.

Oct. 3–5: **Clinical Doppler Echocardiography. Practical Educational Approach.** Costa Mesa, CA. Stanley J. Goldberg, M.D., course director. Inquiries: Clinical Doppler Echocardiography, 5650 E. 9th St., Tucson, AZ 85711. Tel. 1-602-626-7303.

Oct. 9–11: **Physiology and Techniques of Dual Chamber Pacing.** Waldorf Astoria Hotel, New York City. Doris J. W. Escher, M.D., and Seymour Furman, M.D., co-chairmen. Inquiries: North American Society of Pacing and Electrophysiology, 13 Easton Court, Wellesley Hills, MA 02181. Tel. 1-617-237-1866.

Oct. 9–12: **The Assessment of Extracranial Arterial Disease by Duplex Scanning.** Chicago. Anthony Comerota, M.D., and Barton Bean, R.V.T., program directors. Sponsored by Temple University School of Medicine and the Institute for Medical Studies. Inquiries: See Oct. 3–5 — K. Stroich.

Oct. 10–13: **Fourth Annual Chicago Critical Care Symposium.** Chicago Marriott (Downtown). Inquiries: E. C. Rackow, M.D., Dept. Med., University of Health Sciences/Chicago Medical School, 3333 Green Bay Rd., North Chicago, IL 60064. Tel. 1-312-578-3291.

Oct. 10–Nov. 1: **New Issues in Stroke: Diagnosis, Treatment and Rehabilitation Among the Elderly.** Hollenden House Hotel, Cleveland. Inquiries: R. Dunkle, Center on Aging, 2009 Adelbert Rd., Rm. 101, Cleveland, OH 44106.

Oct. 11–12: **Fourth Southern Biomedical Engineering Conference.** Jackson, MS. Inquiries: Dr. Barry W. Sauer, SBEC, Div. Cont. Health Profess. Ed., University of Mississippi Medical Center, 2500 N. State St., Jackson, MS 39216-4505.

Oct. 11–12: **Exercise Stress Testing in the 80s** New Clinical Techniques and Applications (Lecture and Workshop Sessions). Radisson South Plaza, Minneapolis, Minnesota. Jay N. Cohn, chairman. Sponsored by University of Minnesota Continuing Medical Education Department through a grant from Medical Graphics Corporation. Inquiries: Medical Graphics Corporation, 501 West Country Road E, St. Paul, MN 55126. Tel. 1-612-484-4874 or 1-800-328-4138.

Oct. 13–18: **Clinical Congress, American College of Surgeons.** Chicago. Inquiries: ACS, 55 East Erie St., Chicago, IL 60611.

Oct. 14–16: **Fourth Annual Cardiac Rehabilitation Symposium.** Hotel Meridien, New Orleans. Sponsored by East Jefferson General Hospital. Inquiries: S. Weigel, East Jefferson General Hospital, 4200 Houma Blvd., P.O. Box 8213, Metairie LA 70011. Tel. 1-504-454-4147.

Oct. 15–18: **Angiography and Interventional Radiology: 1985.** 15th Annual Postgraduate Course. Marriott-Copley Place, Boston. Drs. L.M. Boxt, M.A. Bettmann, and D.C. Levin, program directors. Inquiries: Dept. Cont. Ed., Harvard Medical School, 25 Shattuck St., Boston, MA 02115. Tel. 1-617-732-6265.

Oct. 18–20: **Interventional Cardiology.** Las Vegas, Nevada. Drs. James Forrester and Robert Kraus, program directors. Sponsored by the Institute for Medical Studies. Inquiries: See Oct. 3–5 — K. Stroich.

Oct. 19: **Common Problems with Coronary Artery Disease.** Somerset Inn, Troy, MI. Inquiries: E.D. Peterson, R.N., AHA of Michigan, 16310 W. 12 Mile Road, P.O. Box 160, Lathrup Village, MI 48076. Tel. 1-313-557-9500.

Oct. 19–20: **Head and Neck Radiology: Advanced Techniques in Diagnostic Imaging.** Hyatt Regency Hotel, San Francisco. William P. Dillon, M.D., and Gretchen A.W. Gooding, M.D., course directors. Sponsored by Radiology Research and Education Foundation, UCSF. Inquiries: Dept. Radiology, UCSF, San Francisco, CA 94143. Tel. 1-415-666-5731.

Oct. 19–20: **Magnetic Resonance Imaging for Technologists.** Hyatt Regency Hotel, San Francisco. A.R. Margulis, M.D., program chairman. Inquiries: See Oct. 21–25, UCSF Dept. Radiology.

Oct. 21–22: **Myocardial Revascularization During Acute MI.** Towsley Center, Ann Arbor, MI. Sponsored by CME, Univ. of Michigan Medical School. Inquiries: B. Phillips, CME, Towsley Center Box 057, Univ. of Mich. Med. School, Ann Arbor, MI 48109-0010. Tel. 1-313-763-1400.

Oct. 21–25: **Clinical Magnetic Resonance Imaging.** Hyatt Regency Hotel, San Francisco. Charles B. Higgins, M.D., Hedvig Hricak, Ph.D., program directors. Sponsored by UCSF Dept. of Radiology. Inquiries: Dept. of Radiology, UCSF School of Medicine, San Francisco, CA 94143. Tel. 1-415-666-5731.

Oct. 25: **Annual Meeting, Society of Neurological Anesthesia and Neurological Supportive Care.** San Francisco. Inquiries: Society of Neurological Anesthesia, P.O. Box 238, Univ. of Virginia Medical Center, Charlottesville, VA 22908.

Oct. 25–27: **Diagnostic Radiology Update.** Mandalay Four Seasons Hotel, Dallas. Sponsored by University of Texas Health Science Center at Dallas. Inquiries: Dolly Christensen, Director of Radiology Postgraduate Education, UT Health Science Center, 5323 Harry Hines Blvd., Dallas, TX 75235. Tel. 1-214-688-2502 or 688-2166.

Oct. 28–Nov. 2: **Doppler and 2-D Echocardiography.** Tulsa, Oklahoma. Dr. Arthur Hagan, program director. Sponsored by Hillcrest Medical Center, University of Oklahoma, Tulsa Medical College, and the Institute for Medical Studies. Inquiries: See Oct. 3–5 — K. Stroich.

Oct. 30–Nov. 1: **La Crosse Health and Sports Science Symposium.** La Crosse, WI. Inquiries: La Crosse Exercise, 221 Mitchell Hall, UWI, La Crosse, WI 54601. Tel. 1-608-785-8686.

Nov. 4–8: **Diagnostic Radiology Seminars.** Maui Marriott Hotel, Maui, Hawaii. Neil Chafetz, M.D. course director. Sponsored by UCSF Dept. of Radiology. Inquiries: Radiology PG Education, UCSF Room C-324, Third and Parnassus Ave., San Francisco, CA 94143. Tel. 1-415-666-5731 (between 7:30 am-4:30 pm Pacific Time).

Nov. 8–9: **Cardiology in Psychosocial, Economic, Political and Ethical Perspectives.** The Halloran House Hotel, New York City. Sponsored by AHA New York City Affiliate in cooperation with the International Society for Humanism in Cardiology. Inquiries: Humanism Conference, AHA, New York City Affiliate, 205 East 42 Street, New York, NY 10017. Tel. 1-212-661-5335.

Nov. 10: **Current Events in Clinical Cardiology.** (Special Sunday Afternoon Program). Sponsored by the AHA Council on Clinical Cardiology, European Society of Cardiology.

Nov. 10: **Cardiovascular Risk Factors in the Young.** Sponsored by the AHA Councils on Cardiovascular Nursing, Cardiovascular Disease in the Young, Epidemiology.

Nov. 10: **Central Neural Cardiovascular Control.** Sponsored by the AHA Councils on Basic Science, Circulation, High Blood Pressure Research.

Nov. 10: **The Changing Role of Echocardiography in Coronary**

cont'd on ad page 24

cont'd from ad page 14

Artery Disease. Washington, D.C. Harvey Feigenbaum, M.D., program director. Sponsored by Indiana University Department of Medicine and the Institute for Medical Studies. Inquiries: See Oct. 3–5 — K. Stroich.

Nov. 11–14: **58th Annual Scientific Sessions, American Heart Association, Washington, DC. Inquiries: Coordinator Scientific Sessions, AHA, 7320 Greenville Ave., Dallas, TX 75231. Tel. for abstracts: 1-214-750-5439, for housing and reservations 1-214-750-5425.**

Nov. 19–20: **Subspecialty Boards in Cardiovascular Disease.** Philadelphia. Inquiries: American Board of Internal Medicine, 3624 Market St., Philadelphia, PA 19104. Tel. 1-215-243-1500. (New date.)

Nov. 22–24: **Third Annual Emergency Cardiac Care Symposium.** Chicago O'Hare Marriott. Inquiries: M.H. Weil, M.D., chairman, Dept. Med., University of Health Sciences/Chicago Medical School, 3333 Green Bay Rd., North Chicago, IL 60064. Tel. 1-312-578-3291.

Dec. 2–6: **Chest Radiology — Update and Review.** Hotel Del Coronado, San Diego. Sponsored by Chest Division of Dept. of Radiology, UCSD. David S. Feigin, M.D., and Paul J. Friedman, M.D., program directors. Inquiries: Dawne Ryals, Ryals and Associates, P.O. Box 610203, DFW Airport, TX 75261-0203. Tel. 1-214-659-9590.

Dec. 4–7: **Second Annual Seminar and Workshop in Doppler Echocardiography.** Hotel Meridien, San Francisco. Julius Gardin, M.D., program director. Sponsored by the University of California, Irvine, California College of Medicine and the Institute for Medical Studies. Inquiries: See Oct. 3–5 — K. Stroich.

Dec. 9–10: **Second Antwerp/La Jolla Research Conference on Cardiac Function.** Inotropic Mechanisms and Heart Failure. Hotel Inter-Continental, San Diego. John Ross, Jr., M.D., chairman. Sponsored by La Jolla/San Diego Heart Institute and University of California, San Diego School of Medicine. Inquiries: Antwerp/La Jolla Conference, P.O. Box 33185, San Diego, CA 92103. Tel. 1-619-692-9115.

Dec. 9–12: **Chest Imaging — (PRE) 1986.** Hotel Del Coronado, San Diego. David S. Feigin, M.D., program director. Sponsored by the Chest Division of the Department of Radiology, University of California, San Diego. Inquiries: See Dec. 2–6 — D. Ryals.

1986

Jan. 13–17: **Interventional, MRI and Neuroradiology.** Fairmont Hotel, San Francisco. Sponsored by University of California, San Francisco.

Jan. 24–25: **Current Controversies and Techniques in Congenital Heart Surgery.** Baltimore, MD. (Immediately prior to Annual Meeting, Society of Thoracic Surgeons, Washington, DC). Sponsored by Div. of Thoracic and Cardiovascular Surgery, University of Maryland School of Medicine. Inquiries: Program Cont. Ed., University of Maryland School of Medicine, 10 South Pine St., Suite 300, Baltimore, MD 21201. Tel. 1-301-528-3956.

Feb. 17–20: **Annual Postgraduate Course on Thoracic Imaging.** Newporter Beach Hotel, Newport Beach, CA. (Feb. 15–16: Scientific Sessions, Society of Thoracic Radiology). H. Baltaxe, M.D., program director. Inquiries: D. Ryals, P.O. Box 610203, DFW Airport, TX 75261-0203. Tel. 1-214-659-9590.

Feb. 19–22: **11th International Joint Conference on Stroke and Cerebral Circulation.** Vacation Village, San Diego. Inquiries: Admin. Assist., Scientific Sessions, AHA, Dallas, TX 75231. Tel. 1-214-750-5441.

Feb. 24–27: **Fourth Annual Cardiology Update.** Honolulu, Hawaii. Roger White, M.D., program director. Sponsored by Straub Clinic and Hospital and the Institute for Medical Studies. Inquiries: See Oct. 3–5, 1985 — K. Stroich.

Feb. 24–28: **Diagnostic Radiology Seminars.** Park City, Utah. Sponsored by University of California, San Francisco.

Mar. 5–8: **Seventh Annual Scientific Sessions, the Society of Behavioral Medicine.** Sheraton Palace Hotel, San Francisco. Abstracts by September 20, 1985. Inquiries: Society of Behavioral Medicine, P.O. Box 8530, University Station, Knoxville, TN 37996. Tel. 1-615-974-5164 or 974-5248.

Mar. 5: **Combined Meeting of the Society of Behavioral Medicine and the Epidemiology Council of the AHA.** Seventh Annual Scientific Sessions, Society of Behavioral Medicine, Sheraton Palace Hotel, San Francisco. Inquiries: Society of Behavioral Medicine, P.O. Box 8530, University Station, Knoxville, TN 37996. Tel. 1-615-974-5164 or 974-5248.

Mar. 9–13: **35th Annual Scientific Sessions, American College of Cardiology.** Atlanta. Inquiries: ACC, Meeting Services Department, 9111 Old Georgetown Road, Bethesda, MD 20814. Tel. 1-301-897-5400.

Mar. 9–14: **Diagnostic Imaging: 1986.** Waiohai Hotel, Kauai, Hawaii. Sponsored by University of California, San Francisco.

Mar. 20–22: **87th Annual Meeting of the American Society for Clinical Pharmacology and Therapeutics.** Sheraton Washington Hotel, Washington, D.C. Inquiries: ACSPT, 1718 Gallagher Road, Norristown, Pennsylvania 19401-2810. Tel. 1-215-825-3838.

Mar. 22–23: **Advances in Uroradiology.** Fairmont Hotel, San Francisco. Sponsored by University of California, San Francisco.

April 3–5: **Electrocardiography of Pacemaker Rhythms.** Parker House Hotel, Boston. P.A. Levine, M.D., chairman. Sponsored by North American Society of Pacing and Electrophysiology. Inquiries: NASPE, 13 Eaton Court, Wellesley Hills, MA 02181. Tel. 1-617-237-1866.

April 12–16: **1986 AAMI 21st Annual Meeting and Exhibit Program.** Hyatt Regency, Chicago. Abstracts by September 20, 1985. Inquiries: Marguerite Leishman, AAMI, 1901 North Fort Myer Drive, Suite 602, Arlington, VA 22209-1699. Tel. 1-703-525-4890.

April 17–19: **Thoracic Imaging Update, 1986.** Hyatt Regency Hotel, Monterey, CA. Sponsored by University of California, San Francisco.

April 23–25: **National Student Research Forum.** The University of Texas Medical Branch, Galveston, TX. Abstracts by Dec. 1, 1985. Supported by American Medical Association — Education and Research Foundation, Mead Johnson Nutritional Division, Roche Laboratories, and American Academy of Family Physicians. Inquiries: National Student Research Forum, P.O. Box 54, Station 1, UT Medical Branch, Galveston, TX 77550. Tel. 1-409-761-3762.

May 15–17: **Seventh Annual Scientific Session, North American Society of Pacing and Electrophysiology.** Marriott Hotel, New Orleans. P.C. Gillette, M.D., program chairman. Inquiries: See April 3–5, 1986, NASPE.

May 20–23: **Cardiovascular Disease '86: Molecular and Cellular Mechanisms, Prevention, Treatment.** Sixth International Washington Spring Symposium. Washington, D.C. Linda L. Gallo, Ph.D., G.V. Vahouny, Ph.D., co-chairs. Inquiries: Symposium '86. Department of Biochemistry, The George Washington University, School of Medicine and Health Sciences, 2300 Eye Street, N.W., Washington, DC 20037. U.S.A.

July 10–12: **Fourth International Symposium on Mechanisms of Vasodilatation.** Rochester, MN. Satellite of International Congress of Physiological Sciences. Cerebral, coronary, and limb circulation. Paul M. Vanhoutte, M.D., chairman organizing committee. Abstracts by Oct. 30, 1985. Inquiries: J. Beckman, 942C Guggenheim Bldg., Mayo Clinic, Rochester, MN 55905.

Sept. 1–5: **Biology and Physics of Radiology.** Department of Radiology, the University of California, San Diego School of Medicine. Inquiries: See Dec. 2–6, 1985 — D. Ryals.

Sept. 12–14: **Sonographers Update and Review.** Hanalei Hotel, San Diego. Sponsored by the Department of Radiology of the University of California, San Diego School of Medicine. Inquiries: See Dec. 2–6, 1985 — D. Ryals.

Sept. 14–19: **Xth World Congress of Cardiology,** Washington, DC. Inquiries: Secretariat, 7320 Greenville Ave., Dallas, TX 75231. Tel. 1-214-750-5429. Cable: Tencard, Dallas, TX.

Oct. 18: **Imaging of the Lumbar Spine and Pelvis.** Department of Radiology of the University of California, San Diego School of Medicine. Inquiries: See Dec. 2–6, 1985 — D. Ryals.

cont'd on ad page 40

cont'd from ad page 24

Abroad

1985

Aug. 23–25: **Vascular Update. Third Annual Seminar on Peripheral Vascular Disease and Hypertension.** Four Seasons Hotel, Toronto, Ont., Canada. Mill Creek Community Hospital and Cleveland Clinic Foundation, sponsors. J.A.M. Smith, D.O., program director. Inquiries: Dept. Med. Ed., Millcreek Community Hospital, 5515 Peach St., Erie, PA 16509. Tel. 1-814-864-4031 Ext. 448.

Aug. 29–Sept. 1: **15th Annual Meeting European Association for Behavior Therapy — 15 Years of Progress: Research Outcome and Practical Application.** Munich (FRG). Inquiries: EABT '85, S. Winner, Max-Planck-Institute of Psychiatry, Psychological Dept., Kraepelin Str. 2, D-8000 München 40, Federal Republic of Germany. Tel. 089/30622-544.

Aug. 31–Sept. 7: **Diagnosis of Diseases of the Chest.** Italy. (Also in Greece, Sept. 8–14). Second Great Teachers Foundation International Postgraduate Medical Education Program. Eric N.C. Milne, M.D., program director. Inquiries: D. Ryals, P.O. Box 610203, DFW Airport TX 75261. Tel. 1-214-659-0590.

Sept. 1–6: **13th World Federation of Neurology International Conference on Cerebrovascular Disease.** Salzburg, Austria. Inquiries: Prof. Helmut Lechner, Chief, Clinic of Neurology and Psychiatry, University of Graz, Graz, Austria.

Sept. 1–6: **13th World Congress of Neurology.** Hamburg FRG. Inquiries T. Sober, M.D., Dept. Neurology, Faculty of Medicine, University of Saarland D-6650, Hamburg-Saar, Federal Republic of Germany.

Sept. 1–7: **Third Postgraduate International Course on Pain Therapy.** Vicenza, Italy. Inquiries: Ruggiero Rizzi, M.D., Ospedale Generale Regionale, 36100 Vicenza, Italy.

Sept. 1–15: **Interpreting the Chest X-Ray — Problems and Advances.** Italy — Greece/Greek Isles. Drs. Eric Milne, Norah Milne, Anthony Proto and E.G. Theros, faculty. Inquiries: See Aug. 31–Sept. 7. — D. Ryals.

Sept. 3–6: **European Nuclear Medicine Congress.** Barbican Centre, London, England. Incorporates 23rd Meeting Society of Nuclear Medicine Europe, 8th Meeting European Nuclear Medicine Society, 13th Meeting British Nuclear Medicine Society. Inquiries: Congress, Institute of Nuclear Medicine, Middlesex Hospital Medical School, Mortimer St., London, WIN 8AA, United Kingdom. Tel. OI 631 1066.

Sept. 4–6: **Symposium on Factors Affecting Platelet Adhesion and Aggregation.** Buenos Aires, Argentina. Organized by the Latin American Cooperative Group on Hemostasis and Thrombosis and sponsored by the Boehringer Ingelheim Program for Thrombosis Research in Latin America. Dr. Raúl Altman, chairman scientific committee. Inquiries: Dr. Altman, Viamonte 2008, 1056 Buenos Aires, Argentina.

Sept. 4–7: **Sclerosis in Plaques. Annual World Meeting of the International Federation of National Societies (FISEP).** Hamburg, FRG. Inquiries: German Society of Sclerosis in Plaques, Rosental 5, Aufgang D-8, Munich 2, Federal Republic of Germany.

Sept. 5–7: **First Asian-Pacific Conference on Doppler and Echocardiography.** Tokyo. Inquiries: Pravin M. Shah, M.D., Coordinator for North America, Cardiology Section (691/111E), Wadsworth VA Medical Center, Wilshire and Sawtelle Blvds, Los Angeles, CA. Tel. 1-213-824-3126.

Sept. 7–9: **Third International Brain Heart Conference.** Trier, Germany. Inquiries: Dr. T. Stober, Dept. Neurology, Faculty of Med. University of Saarland, D-6650, Homburg/Saar, Federal Republic of Germany.

Sept. 8–11: **Sixth Meeting of the European Section of the International Society on Research in Cardiology.** Stockholm, Sweden. Inquiries: Dr. L. Kaijser, Dept. Clinical Physiology, Karolinska Hospital, SU-1041, Stockholm, Sweden.

Sept. 8–12: **First International Congress on Hospital Laws, Procedures, and Ethics.** Tel Aviv, Israel. Judge Amnon Carmi, organizing chairman. Inquiries: Hospitalaw, 28 Ahad Ha'am St., P.O. Box 394, Tel Aviv 61003, Israel. Tel. 03-650862. Telex: 33803 TLV. Cable: PELTOURS TELAVIV.

Sept. 9: **Workshop on Cardioembolic Stroke (During Third International Brain/Heart Conference,** Sept. 7–9). Trier, Germany, Inquiries: David G. Sherman, M.D., and Robert G. Hart, M.D., co-chairmen, Dept. of Medicine, University of Texas Health Science Center, 7703 Floyd Curl Dr., San Antonio, TX 78284. Tel. 1-512-691-6521.

Sept. 9–12: **Eighth Annual European Conference on Lipoproteins.** Evangelische Akademie, Tutzing (near Munich), West Germany. Apolipoprotein mutants and dyslipoproteinemias; cellular processing of lipoproteins. Sponsored by European Lipoprotein Club. Inquiries: Dr. J. Shepherd, Secretary European Lipoprotein Club, Dept. Pathological Biochemistry, Royal Infirmary, Glasgow, Scotland, GF OSF.

Sept. 11–14: **Fourth European Conference on Mechanocardiography.** Budapest, Hungary. Organized by the European-African Div. of the International Society of Mechanocardiography and the Hungarian Society of Cardiology. Prof. J. Simonyi, chairman scientific committee. Inquiries: Mechanocardiography Organizing Committee, Budapest, Pf 88, H-1450, Hungary.

Sept. 11–14: **Acute Brain Ischemia 1985: Medical and Surgical Therapy.** University of Siena, Italy. Satellite of 13th World Congress of Neurology, Sept. 7–9, Hamburg, Germany. Prof. Noè Battistini, organizer. Inquiries: GIBI s.a.s., M. P. Gerini, Via Orlona, 7, 00198 Rome, Italy.

Sept. 16–19: **12th European Congress for Artificial Organs. Pre-Congress Meeting of the International Diabetes Federation.** Athens, Greece. (Artificial endocrine pancreas, insulin delivery devices, pancreas and islet transplantation). Inquiries Prof. S. Raptis, M.D., P.O. Box 14127, 11510, Athens, Greece.

Sept. 16–20: **International Symposium on Cardiogenic Reflexes.** University of Leeds, England. Organized by Dept. of CV Studies, Univ. Leeds, and Commission on CV Physiology of International Union of Physiological Sciences. Inquiries: Dr. R. Hainsworth, Dept. CV Studies, University of Leeds, Leeds LS2 93T, England.

Oct. 3–4: **Hemodynamics and Atherosclerosis.** Wellington, New Zealand. Inquiries: Dr. W.E. Stehbens, Dept. Pathology, Wellington Clinical School of Med., Wellington, 2, New Zealand.

Oct. 3–18: **Frontiers in Imaging and Cardiopulmonary Diagnosis.** In USSR. Drs. Benjamin Felson, Eric Milne and Jack Westcott, faculty. Inquiries: See Aug. 31–Sept. 7. — D. Ryals.

Oct. 6–10: **Seventh International Symposium on Atherosclerosis.** Melbourne, Australia. Inquiries: Dr. P.J. Nestel, Baker Medical Research Inst., Commercial Rd., Prahran, Vic., Australia 3181.

Oct. 8–10: **First Latin American Congress of Cardiac Pacing.** Buenos Aires, Argentina. Organized by Latin American Society of Cardiac Pacing and Argentine Chamber of Cardiac Pacing. Dr. Alejandro Dussaut, president organizing committee. Inquiries: Congresos Internacionales S.A., Moreno 854 — 9° piso, 1091 Buenos Aires, Argentina. Tel. 14-3216/3408/3283. Telex 22036 JECON AR.

Oct. 11–12: **Second International Symposium on Hypertension in Children and Adolescents.** Heidelberg, FRG. Organized by Dept. of Pediatrics, Univ. of Heidelberg, and German Institute for High Blood Pressure Research. Inquiries: German Institute HBP Research, University of Heidelberg, Im Neuenheimer Feld 366, D-6900 Heidelberg, FRG.

Oct. 11–18: **Cell Biology of the Artery Wall.** Hayman Island, Great Barrier Reef, Australia. Satellite of Seventh International Symposium on Arteriosclerosis, Oct. 6–10, Melbourne. Inquiries: Dr. Gordon H. Campbell, Dept. Anatomy, University of Melbourne, Parkville, 3052, Australia.

Oct. 12–19: **Cardiopulmonary Emergencies.** Grand Cayman Island, B.W.I. Sponsored by the University of California, San Diego School of Medicine, the American Institute of Postgraduate Education, Scripps Memorial Hospital — Encinitas, Encinitas, California. Inquiries: Edith Bookstein/AIPE, P.O. Box 2586, La Jolla, CA 92038. Tel. 1-619-454-3212.

Oct. 13–15: **Sixth International Congress, International Society for Laser Surgery and Medicine.** Jerusalem, Israel. Inquiries: P.O. Box 50006, Tel Aviv 61500, Israel.

Oct. 14–18: **International Congress on Cardiac Doppler.** Pisa, Italy. (Tutorial sessions Oct. 14–15; Scientific Sessions Oct. 16–18). Prof. Luigi Donato and Dr. Merrill Spencer, presidents. Inquiries: Istituto di Fisiologia Clinica, C.N.R., University of Pisa, Via Savi 8, 1-567100 Pisa, Italy. Tel. 050-47231/502109. Telex: 590549 IFCI.

cont'd on ad page 54

cont'd from ad page 40

Oct. 17–19: **18th Danube Symposium for Neurological Sciences.** University Clinic for Neurology. Innsbruck, Austria. Inquiries: Danube Symposium for Neurological Sciences, c/o Vienna Academy of Medicine, Alser Str. 4,A-1090 Vienna, Austria. Tel. (0222) 42 71 65. Cable MEDACAD, Wien. Telex 134743 MEDAK A.

Oct. 20–22: **Fifth International Symposium on Rats with Spontaneous Hypertension and Related Studies.** Kyoto, Japan. Yukio Yamori, M.D., program director. Inquiries: Fifth SHR Symposium, Shimane Medical University, Izumo 693, Japan. Tel. 0853-23-2111 Ext. 2375. Cable: WHOCOLLAB IZUMO.

Oct. 20–23: **Third World Congress of Cardiac Rehabilitation.** Caracas, Venezuela. Sponsored by the International Society and Federation of Cardiology: Scientific Council on Rehabilitation of Cardiac Patients and AHA Council on Clinical Cardiology. Inquiries Dr. Deyanira Almeida, Congresa C.A., P.O. Box 17422, Caracas 1015A, Venezuela.

Oct. 23–24: **International Symposium on Mechanisms and Treatment in Essential Hypertension: Calcium and Calcium Antagonists.** Hotel Nagoya Castle, Nagoya, Japan. (Satellite of 5th International Symposium on Rats with Spontaneous Hypertension, Oct. 20–22, Kyoto, Japan). Inquiries: Kyuzo Aoki, M.D., 2nd Dept. Internal Med., Nagoya City University Medical School, Mizuho-ku, Nagoya 467, Japan. Tel. 052-851-5511, Ext. 2204.

Oct. 24–25: **Animals and the Scientist: Institutional Responsibilities.** The Hart House, University of Toronto, Toronto, Canada. Sponsored by the Scientists Center for Animal Welfare and the University of Toronto. Inquiries: Dr. F. Barbara Orlans, Director, Scientists Center for Animal Welfare, 4805 St. Elmo Avenue, Bethesda, MD 20814. Tel. 1-301-654-6390.

Oct. 25–27: **International Symposium on Brain and Blood Pressure Control.** Kikai-Shinkoh Hall, Shiba Park, Tokyo, Japan. Dr. Keiji Nakamura organizing chairman. Inquiries: Brain and Blood Pressure, Dept. of Pharmacology, Nippon Roche Research Center, Kamakura 247, Japan. Tel. 0467-45-3191-Ext. 380 or 381. Telex 2222861 PANROCHE J.

Oct. 27–30: **Third Asian Pacific Symposium on Cardiac Pacing and Electrophysiology.** Hilton Hotel, Melbourne, Australia. Sponsored by Cardiac Society of Australia and New Zealand under auspices of International Cardiac Pacing Society. Inquiries: Third Asian Pacific Symposium on Cardiac Pacing and Electrophysiology, Dept. of Cardiology, Suite 3.5, Epworth Medical Centre, 62 Erin St., Richmond, Vic. 3121, Australia.

Oct. 28–31: **First International Congress on Food and Health.** Salsomaggiore Terme, Italy. Sponsored by International Association for Advancement of Biomedical Research, by Society of Medical Gastronomy, and Institute of Pharmacology of University of Pisa. Inquiries: ALM s.r.l., Via Lattuada, 26, 20135 Milan, Italy. Telex: 313063 HOTALM I.

Nov. 2–4: **Third International Symposium on Ischemic Heart Disease, Exercise, and Related Topics.** Royal York Hotel, Toronto, Canada. Sponsored by Toronto Rehabilitation Center. Inquiries: J. Kennedy or A. Ceci, Toronto Rehab. Center, 345 Rumsey Rd., Toronto, Ont. Canada M4G 1RT. Tel. 1-416-425-1117 Ext. 236.

Nov. 28–30: **Seventh Biennial Congress of Cardiology.** Rawalpindi/Islamabad, Pakistan. Inquiries: Pakistan Cardiac Society, Brig. Muhammad Zulfiqar Ali Khan, AFIC/NIHD, Rawalpindi, Pakistan. Tel. 64946, 61-31113, 61-33911.

Dec. 1–4: **International Symposium on Left Ventricular Dysfunction.** Jerusalem Hilton Hotel, Israel. Jan J. Kellermann, M.D. of Israel and David Spodick, M.D. of Worcester, MA, cochairmen. Under the auspices of the Universities of Tel Aviv and Massachusetts. Inquiries: P.O. Box 50006, Tel Aviv 61500, Israel. Tel. 03-654571. Telex 341171 KENS IL.

Dec. 8–12: **Second International Symposium on Hypertension in the Community.** Jerusalem, Israel. Prof. Talma Rosenthal, P.O. Box 50006, Tel Aviv, 61500, Israel. Tel. 03-654571. Telex 341171 KENS IL.

1986

To be announced: **The 35th National Meeting of the Italian Neurosurgical Society.** Pavia, Italy. Inquiries: Prof. Pietro Paoletti, Department of Surgery, Neurosurgical Clinic, University of Pavia, San Matteo Hospital, 27100 Pavia, Italy. Tel 0382/422231.

Jan. 8–11: **Seventh Annual European Conference on Vascular Biology.** Bad Buchau, FR Germany. Growth and Differentiation of Vascular Cells. Organized by European Artery Club. Inquiries: Dr. G. Bondjers, Dept. Med. 1, Salgren's Hospital, 5-413 45 Göteborg, Sweden.

Jan. 16–21: **Basic Principles of Pacing and Electrophysiology — Dual Chamber and Antitachycardia Pacing.** Frenchman's Reef, St. Thomas, Virgin Islands. Sponsored by Cardiostim America. Seymour Furman, course director. Inquiries: Cardiostim America, P.O. Box 428, Mount Kisco, NY 10549, U.S.A. Tel. 1-914-241-3295.

Jan. 20–21: **Diagnostic Radiology Seminars.** Camino Real, Ixtapa, Mexico. University of California, San Francisco.

Jan. 31–Feb. 8: **Fifth Annual Winter Congress in Medical Diagnostic Imaging.** Zermatt, Switzerland. Inquiries: Winter Congress, West Park Hospital, Department of Radiology, 22141 Roscoe Blvd., Canoga Park, CA 91304. Tel. 1-818-340-9580, Ext. 280.

Feb. 8–12: **The Fourth Annual London Winter Seminar in Medical Diagnostic Imaging.** Inquiries: Winter Seminar, West Park Hospital Department of Radiology, 22141 Roscoe Blvd., Canoga Park, CA 91304. Tel. 1-818-340-0580, Ext. 280.

Feb. 9–13: **12th World Congress of the International Society for Heart Research,** Melbourne, Australia. Inquiries: Dr. N.S. Dhalla, Dept. Physiology, Faculty of Medicine, University of Manitoba, Winnipeg, Canada R3E OW3.

Feb. 16–21: **First International Congress on Stress, Behavior and Coronary Disease.** Southern Cross Hotel, Melbourne, Australia. Prof. G.D. Burrows, president, Dr. M. Jelinek, scientific program chairman. Inquiries: Mental Health Foundation, Suite 23, 20 Commercial Rd., Melbourne 3004, Vic., Australia.

March 23–25: **Second International Symposium on Holter Monitoring.** Jerusalem, Israel. V. Hombach, Cologne, and S. Stern, Jerusalem, co-chairmen. Inquiries: Prof. Shlomo Stern, c/o Stier Group, Ltd., 203 Dizengoff St., Tel Aviv 63115 Israel. Tel. (03) 224-153/4/5. Telex 35570 STI COIN IL.

April 17–19: **Exercise Testing in the Diagnosis and Evaluation of Treatment of Arrhythmias.** Athens, Greece. Inquiries: Prof. D. Cokkinos, 5 Dorylaiou, 115 21 Athens, Greece.

April 23–25: **First International Symposium on Cardiology.** Hospital de Clinicas, University of Buenos Aires, Argentina. Inquiries: Dr. Luis D. Suárez, Dean Funes 1075-(1231), Buenos Aires, Argentina. Tel. 821-6041.

May 1–3: **First Verona Seminar on Nephrology: Hypertension and Renal Disease.** Camera di Commercio, corso Porta Nuova 96, 37100 Verona-Italy. Inquiries: Lamberto Oldrizzi, M.D., Divisione Nefrologia, Istituti Ospitalieri, 37126 Verona-Italy, Tel. 045-932528-932694.

May 1–3: **First Vienna Shock Forum.** Hotel Hilton, Vienna, Austria. Held by the Ludwig Boltzmann Institute for Experimental Traumatology. Abstracts by December 31, 1985. Inquiries: Wiener Schockgespräche, Ludwig Boltzmann Institut für experimentelle, Traumatologie, Donaueschingenstraße 13, A-1200 Wien, A-1200 Vienna-Austria. Tel. 222-33-55-33/464.

May 11–14: **The Seventh Annual Meeting of the Society for Clinical Trials.** Montreal, Quebec, Canada. Abstracts by January 2, 1986. Inquiries: Mary A. Finch, Meeting Coordinator, Society for Clinical Trials, Inc., 600 Wyndhurst Avenue, Baltimore, MD 21210, U.S.A.

May 29–30: **35 Years of Electrocardiology in Amsterdam.** Sponsored by the Interuniversity Cardiology Institute in The Netherlands. Inquiries: F.L. Meijler, M.D., F.A.C.C., Professor of Cardiology, Interuniversity Cardiology Institute, P.O. Box 19258, 3501 DG Utrecht, The Netherlands.

June 5–7: **International Congress for Clinical Neuroimaging.** Palais Auersperg, Vienna, Austria. Inquiries: International Congress for Clinical Neuroimaging, c/o Vienna Academy of Medicine, Alser Str. 4, A-1090, Vienna, Austria. Tel. 0222 42 71 65. Cable MEDACAD Wien, Telex: 134743 medak a.

June 17–20: **Second World Meeting on Impotence.** Fifth Conference on Vasculogenic Impotence and Corpus Cavernosum Revascularization. Prague, Czechoslovakia. Sponsored by the International Society for Impotence Research. Inquiries: Czechoslovak

cont'd on ad page 63

cont'd from ad page 54

Medical Society, J.E. Purkyně, P.O. Box 88, Vítězného února 31, 120 26 Praha, Czechoslovakia. Tel. 29-41-41-4.

June 22–25: **Seventh Congress of the European Section, International Society for Heart Research.** Reykjavík, Iceland. Inquiries: Guomundur Thorgeirsson, M.D., Ph.D., Department of Medicine, Landspítalinn, 101 Reykjavík, Iceland.

June 23–27: **Sixth Asian Congress of Cardiology.** Jakarta, Indonesia. Working language, English. Organized by Indonesian Heart Association. L.I. Rilantono, M.D., chairman. Inquiries: Asean Congress Cardiology, Dept. Cardiology, Cipto Mangunkusumo Hospital, Jalan Diponegoro 69, Jakarta 10453, Indonesia.

June 26–28: **Annual Scientific Meeting of the International Medical Society of Paraplegia.** Oslo, Norway. Abstracts by Dec. 1, 1985. Inquiries: IMSP Annual Scientific Meeting in Scandinavia 1986, Dept. of Neurology, Rikshospitalet, University Hospital, Oslo, 1 Norway.

July 2–5: **35th International Conference European Society for CV Surgery.** Metropole Hotel, Brighton, England. Prof. H.H. Bentall, chairman. Inquiries: European Society for CV Surgery, Concorde Services Ltd., 10 Wendell Rd., London W12 9RT, United Kingdom.

July 8–11: **Eighth Annual Meeting American Section of the International Society for Heart Research and Satellite Symposium on Heart Metabolism for the 30th International Congress of Physiological Sciences.** Winnipeg, Canada. Inquiries: Dr. R. E. Beamish, Experimental Cardiology Section, Dept. of Physiology, Faculty of Medicine, University of Manitoba, Winnipeg, Canada R3E OW3.

July 13–18: **30th International Congress of Physiological Sciences.** The University of British Columbia, Vancouver, Canada. Dr. H. McLennan, chairman program committee. Inquiries: IUPS, Suite 801, 750 Jervis St., Vancouver, B.C., Canada V6E 2A9. Tel. 604-681-5226. Telex 04-352848 VCR.

Aug. 21–23: **International Symposium.** Recent Aspects on Diagnosis and Treatment of Lipoprotein Disorders: Impact on Prevention of Atherosclerotic Diseases. Palais Auersperg, Vienna, Austria. Inquiries: Dr. K. Widhalm, Dept. Pediatrics, University of Vienna, Währinger Gürtel 18, A-1090 Vienna, Austria.

Aug. 31–Sept. 7: **11th Congress of International Society of Hypertension.** Heidelberg, Federal Republic of Germany. Organized by German Institute of High Blood Pressure Research and German Hypertension League. Dr. Detlev Ganten, Congress chairman. Inquiries: GKV, Frankfurter Str. 57, D-6050 Offenbach 1, Heidelberg, FR Germany.

Sept. 14–17: **Eighth International Symposium on Microsurgical Anastomoses for Cerebral Ischemia.** Florence, Italy. Inquiries: Rolando Gagliardi, M.D., Dept. of Neurosurgery, USL 10/D, Careggi Hospital, 50100 Florence, Italy.

Sept. 14–18: **Second International Conference on Diet and Nutrition and Fifth International Congress on Obesity.** Jerusalem, Israel. Inquiries: C. Horwitz, Ph.D., and S. H. Blondheim, M.D., P.O. Box 983, Jerusalem 91009, Israel.

Sept. 22–23: **International Symposium on Lipid Metabolism in the Normoxic and Ischemic Heart.** Erasmus University, Rotterdam, The Netherlands. Inquiries: Dr. H. Stam, Dept. Biochemistry I, Med. Fac., Erasmus University Rotterdam, P.O. Box 1738, 3000 DR Rotterdam, The Netherlands.

Oct. 22–25: **Ninth International Symposium on Drugs Affecting Lipid Metabolism.** Florence, Italy. Dr. Kritchevsky, R. Paoletti, chairmen. Inquiries: Fondazione Giovanni Lorenzini, Via Monte Napoleone, 23-20121 Milan, Italy. Tel. 02-702.267-783.868.

1987

Sept. 2–4: **International Conference on Management of Cardiac Arrhythmias.** London, England. Sponsored by the British Heart Foundation. Professor A. J. Camm and Dr. A. W. Nathan, members organizing committee. Inquiries: British Heart Foundation, 102 Gloucester Pl., London W1H 4DH England. Tel. 01-935-0185.

AHA Scientific Sessions Future Meeting Dates

1985	Washington, DC	Nov. 11–14
1986	Dallas, TX	Nov. 17–20
1987	Anaheim, CA	Nov. 16–19
1988	Locale Not Set	Nov. 14–17
1989	New Orleans	Nov. 13–16
1990	Dallas	Nov. 12–15

Xth World Congress of Cardiology, 1986

The Xth World Congress of Cardiology will be held in Washington, DC, Sept. 14–19, 1986. Official languages English, Spanish, and French. Inquiries: Secretariat, Xth World Congress Cardiology, 7320 Greenville Ave., Dallas, TX 75231. Tel. 1-214-750-5429. Cable: TenCard, Dallas.

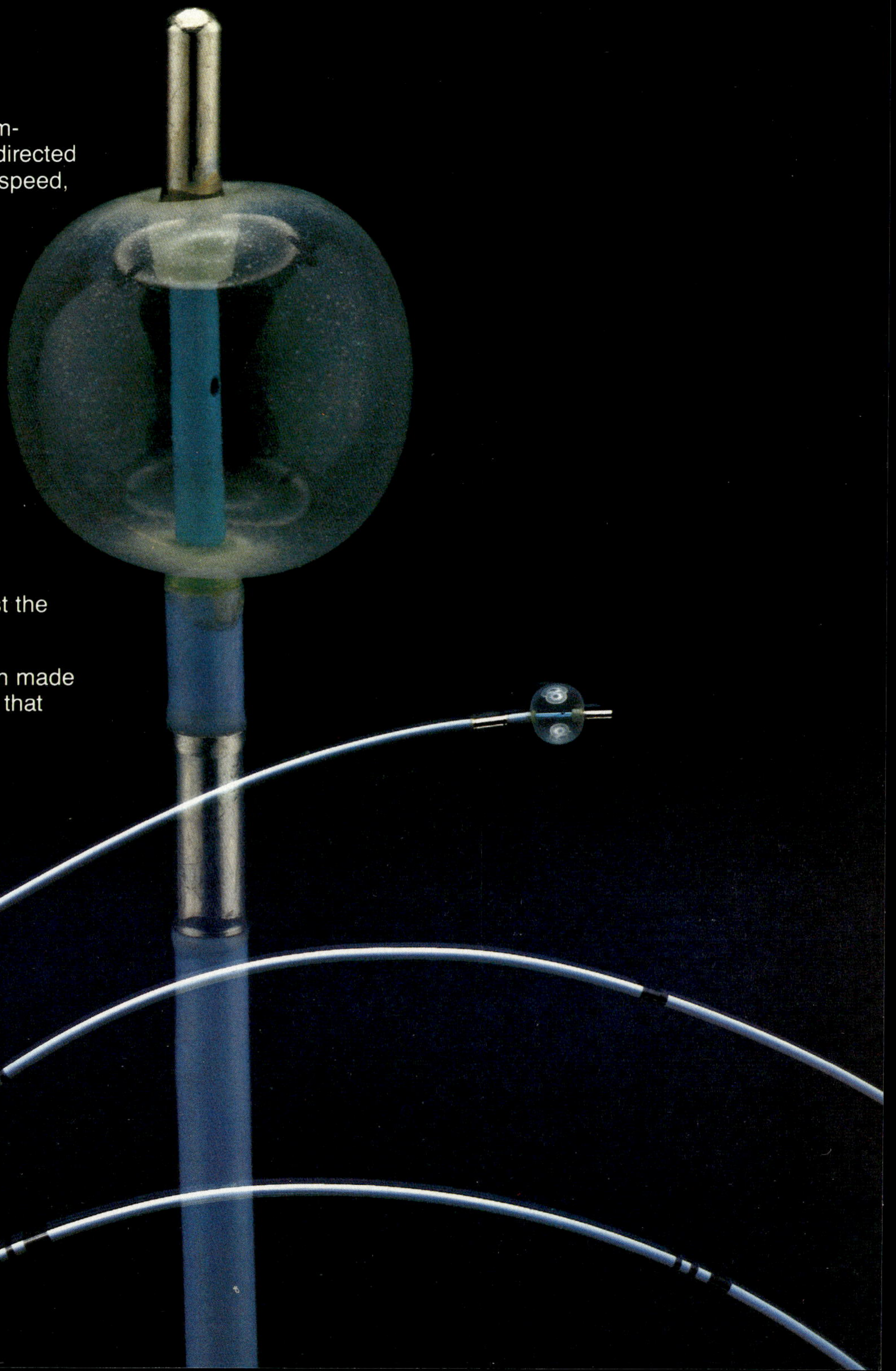

News from the American Heart Association

7320 Greenville Ave., Dallas, Texas 75231
Telephone: 214 750-5300

State of the Art: The 58th Scientific Sessions of the American Heart Association

Four days of comprehensive medical education are planned for the American Heart Association's 58th Scientific Sessions, which open November 11 in Washington, D.C. This event is sponsored annually by the AHA in an effort to improve the care of the cardiovascular patient. It provides medical professionals with an opportunity to acquire new insight into the pathophysiology, diagnosis, treatment, and prevention of heart disease.

New developments in clinical and basic research will be presented in simultaneous sessions on adult and pediatric cardiology, surgery, radiology and nursing, with focus on cardiopulmonary medicine, hypertension, stroke, renal disease, thrombosis and preventive medicine. State-of-the-art lectures by experts in the field will present information important to both practicing physicians and researchers. Teaching exhibits will provide an opportunity for self-assessment.

This year's program will include: 1941 oral and poster presentations; 11 plenary sessions designed to provide physicians with new theories in cardiovascular medicine; 15 postgraduate seminars on state-of-the-art topics; 28 cardiovascular conferences and 26 how-to sessions, both of which offer informal discussion with noted authorities; 12 teaching and public service exhibits which provide an opportunity for self-assessment in clinically relevant topics; and 300 industrial exhibits of the latest products and services.

Three special programs will be offered on the Sunday afternoon preceding the opening of the Sessions. "Current Events in Clinical Cardiology" will present European and American viewpoints on several topics of interest in cardiology, including thrombolytic therapy in acute infarction, the role of coronary artery bypass surgery, and electrophysiology testing for ventricular arrhythmias. The second program, "Central Neural Cardiovascular Control," will include presentation and discussions on such topics as brain stem control of blood pressure, hypothalamic control of the cardiovascular system and cardiovascular control during exercise. The third program, "Cardiovascular Risk Factors in the Young," will include presentations on epidemiological background, risk reduction in children and families at high risk, and role of the multidisciplinary approach in outpatient clinics for the high-risk children and families.

Request for Application AHA/Bugher Foundation Centers for Molecular Biology in the Cardiovascular System

The American Heart Association, in response to a grant from the Bugher Foundation, has announced a competition for a five-year award for three institutions to establish Centers for Molecular Biology in the Cardiovascular System. The purpose of the award is to stimulate and enhance the application of the science of molecular biology to the study of components of the cardiovascular system. Molecular biology relates to those studies of cell biology which address the molecular bases of the structure and functions of genes, proteins, and cells.

The deadline for receipt of application is December 1, 1985. First review of applications will be complete by February 7, 1986, followed by a finalist reverse-site visit by April 7. Awards will be announced on April 15, 1986.

Forms and specific guidelines for preparation may be obtained from the AHA Division of Research Awards. Inquiries may be directed to the program administrator, Wallace G. Frasher, M.D., Vice President for Research, American Heart Association, 7320 Greenville Avenue, Dallas, TX 75231. Telephone 214-750-5445.

Council on Clinical Cardiology Announces 1985 Teaching Awards

The AHA Council on Clinical Cardiology has announced the recipients of its 1985 Medical School Teaching Awards. The awards are presented annually to full- or part-time faculty members of U.S. medical schools engaged in teaching cardiovascular diseases. Their purpose is to recognize and encourage excellence in teaching.

Award recipients are: *Harry R. Gibbs, M.D.*, assistant professor, University of Missouri–Kansas City School of Medicine; *William P. Follansbee, M.D.*, assistant professor of medicine (cardiology), University of Pittsburgh School of Medicine; *Eugene E. Nattie Jr., M.D.*, associate professor of physiology medicine, Dartmouth Medical School; *Joseph Francis Majdan, M.D.*, instructor in medicine, Jefferson Medical College, Thomas Jefferson University; *Joseph Carver, M.D.*, Hahnemann University School of Medicine;

cont'd on ad page 21

cont'd from ad page 14

Arthur J. Moss, M.D., clinical professor of medicine, University of Rochester Medical Center.

Also, *Eric Schenk, M.D.*, professor of pathology and laboratory medicine, University of Rochester Medical Center; *Modestino G. Criscitiello, M.D.*, professor of medicine and physiology, Tufts University School of Medicine; *Richard A. Gillis, Ph.D.*, professor of pharmacology, Georgetown University School of Medicine; *George T. Kondos, M.D.*, University of Illinois College of Medicine; *Philip R. Liebson, M.D.*, Rush Medical College; and *Joseph D. Lynch, M.D.*, Creighton University School of Medicine.

NHLBI Issues Appeal to Physicians

The Cardiology Branch of the National Heart, Lung, and Blood Institute is initiating a new protocol on hypertrophic cardiomyopathy (HCM) and has issued an appeal to physicians to refer patients into the study.

Patients with HCM have an increased risk for sudden death, and sudden death may be the first clinical presentation of HCM. It is likely that ventricular fibrillation is the most frequent event immediately preceding sudden death in these patients. Holter monitor studies have shown that about 20 percent of patients with HCM not previously known to have arrhythmias exhibited ventricular tachycardia.

Follow-up of these individuals found that 24 percent of those with ventricular tachycardia died within three years; only 3 percent of those without this arrhythmia died. Having identified this subgroup at high risk of death, two tasks remain: distinguish those patients with ventricular tachycardia who will die from those who will not; and develop a therapeutic regimen that will best prevent sudden death.

Patient referrals are sought; specifically, patients with one or more of the following factors: an episode of cardiac arrest; a "malignant" family history characterized by two or more first-order relatives who died from the disease before the age of 55; ventricular tachycardia documented on ambulatory monitoring or telemetry; a septal thickness greater than 30 mm and no left ventricular outflow tract obstruction; or syncope that is believed secondary to the disease.

Additional details are available from Cynthia M. Tracy, M.D., Cardiology Branch, or Stephen E. Epstein, M.D., Chief, Cardiology Branch, NHLBI, National Institutes of Health, Bethesda, MD 20205. Telephone 1-301-496-4236.

Hypothermia Thermometers: A National Education Campaign

The Center for Environmental Physiology, with assistance from the Administration on Aging, U.S. Department of Health and Human Services, is conducting a national public awareness campaign on the subject of hypothermia thermometers.

The purpose of the campaign is to educate the public concerning the role of these special thermometers in the early recognition and management of hypothermia. Hypothermia is a life-threatening medical condition that afflicts older Americans. Data from the National Center for Health Statistics reveals that nearly 35,000 deaths a year are caused by cold stress; 81 percent of those deaths were in persons over 65 years of age.

Temperatures do not have to fall below freezing to cause hypothermia. Experts consider indoor cold exposure the most common cause of hypothermia in the U.S. Most elderly victims become ill at temperatures between 50 and 65° F.

The only real means of determining if a person has hypothermia is to take his or her body temperature. However, standard clinical glass "fever" thermometers have a maximal lower limit of 94° F — they cannot detect hypothermia. As a result, special purpose low-reading thermometers have been designed to allow early diagnosis and treatment of the illness.

The Center for Environmental Physiology is a nonprofit organization located in Washington, D.C. It works in partnership with government agencies, national associations, and industry to promote public awareness of heat and cold stress.

1986 Competition for The Lita Annenberg Hazen Awards

Nomination material is now available for The 1986 Lita Annenberg Hazen Awards for Excellence in Clinical Research. The purpose of the awards is to encourage increased participation in clinical research by physicians. Prizes total $100,000. Nominations will be accepted until February 28, 1986.

For further information, contact the chairman of the awards program, James F. Glenn, M.D., One Gustave L. Levy Place, New York, NY 10029. Telephone 1-212-650-8832

NASPE Fellowships to be Awarded

The North American Society of Pacing and Electrophysiology is planning to award full-year fellowships in cardiac pacing and cardiac electrophysiology for the academic year beginning July 1, 1986 and ending June 30, 1987. The fellowships are open to applicants who have a degree of doctor of medicine, philosophy, osteopathy, science, or equivalent training or experience in biomedical engineering. Applicants must be citizens or permanent residents of a country in North America. Award recipients must include cardiac pacing or cardiac electrophysiology in their long-range career plans. Traveling fellowships are also available. The deadline for applications is December 1, 1985. For additional information, write or call the NASPE office at 13 Eaton Court, Wellesley Hills, MA 02181. Telephone 1-617-237-1866.

AHA Briefs

- **Modern Concepts of Cardiovascular Disease** for October is "Acute Dissection of the Aorta — Continuing Need for Earlier Diagnosis and Treatment" by D. Craig Miller, M.D., of Stanford, California.
- **"Common Problems with Coronary Artery Disease"** is a program scheduled for October 19 at the

cont'd on ad page 24

cont'd from ad page 21

Somerset Inn, 2601 W. Big Beaver Road, Troy, MI 48084. For more information, contact Eleanor D. Peterson, R.N., American Heart Association of Michigan, 16310 W. 12 Mile Road, P.O. Box 160, Lathrup Village, MI 48076. Telephone 1-313-557-9500.

- **"Rehabilitation of the Coronary Patient"** is the title of a program scheduled to take place October 17–20 in Pine Mountain, Georgia. The program is sponsored by the American College of Cardiology, Emory University School of Medicine, and the AHA Georgia Affiliate. For further information, contact the Registration Secretary, Extramural Programs Department, American College of Cardiology, 9111 Old Georgetown Road, Bethesda, MD 20814.
- A comprehensive food and nutrition course designed for use in hospitals, schools, and community groups is now available through AHA affiliates. The **Culinary Hearts Kitchen** was developed by the New York City Affiliate. Each package includes an instructor's manual, slides, recipes, and more.
- The National Institute of Neurological and Communicative Disorders and Stroke (NINCDS) recently announced its **Clinical Investigator Development Awards** (CIDA). The new award is designed to prepare physicians or persons with doctorates in clinical areas for a career in research in an academic setting. It replaces the Teacher Investigator Development Award. CIDA application deadlines are October 1, February 1, and June 1 of each year. For more information, contact Dr. Donald H. Luecke, Deputy Director, Extramural Activities Program, NINCDS, NIH, Bethesda, MD 20205. Telephone 1-301-496-4188.

Meetings Calendar

1985

To be arranged individually: **Preceptorships in Cardiology.** Pacific Medical Center, San Francisco. Arthur Selzer, M.D., F.A.C.C., director. Sponsored by American College of Cardiology and Pacific Medical Center, San Francisco. Inquiries: Registration Secretary, Extramural Programs Department, American College of Cardiology, 9111 Old Georgetown Road, Bethesda, MD 20814.

To be arranged individually: **Preceptorships in Cardiology.** Buffalo General Hospital, Buffalo, NY. Jules Constant, M.D., F.A.C.C., director. Sponsored by American College of Cardiology and State University of New York at Buffalo, School of Medicine. Inquiries: Registration Secretary, Extramural Programs Dept., ACC, 9111 Old Georgetown Rd., Bethesda, MD 20814.

Oct. 15–18: **Angiography and Interventional Radiology: 1985.** 15th Annual Postgraduate Course. Marriott-Copley Place, Boston. Drs. L.M. Boxt, M.A. Bettmann, and D.C. Levin, program directors. Inquiries: Dept. Cont. Ed., Harvard Medical School, 25 Shattuck St., Boston, MA 02115. Tel. 1-617-732-6265.

Oct. 17–20: **Rehabilitation of the Coronary Patient.** Callaway Gardens, Pine Mountain, GA. Gerald F. Fletcher, M.D., F.A.C.C., Nanette K. Wenger, M.D., F.A.C.C., directors. Sponsored by American College of Cardiology; Emory University School of Medicine; and the American Heart Association, Georgia Affiliate. Inquiries: Registration Secy., Extramural Programs Dept., American College of Cardiology, 9111 Old Georgetown Rd., Bethesda, MD 20814.

Oct. 18–20: **Interventional Cardiology.** Las Vegas, Nevada. Drs. James Forrester and Robert Kraus, program directors. Sponsored by the Institute for Medical Studies. Inquiries: K. Stroich, The Institute for Medical Studies, 30131 Town Center Drive, Suite 215, Laguna Niguel, CA 92677. Tel. 1-714-495-4499.

Oct. 19: **Common Problems with Coronary Artery Disease.** Somerset Inn, Troy, MI. Inquiries: E.D. Peterson, R.N., AHA of Michigan, 16310 W. 12 Mile Road, P.O. Box 160, Lathrup Village, MI 48076. Tel. 1-313-557-9500.

Oct. 19–20: **Head and Neck Radiology: Advanced Techniques in Diagnostic Imaging.** Hyatt Regency Hotel, San Francisco. William P. Dillon, M.D., and Gretchen A.W. Gooding, M.D., course directors. Sponsored by Radiology Research and Education Foundation, UCSF. Inquiries: Dept. Radiology, UCSF, San Francisco, CA 94143. Tel. 1-415-666-5731.

Oct. 19–20: **Magnetic Resonance Imaging for Technologists.** Hyatt Regency Hotel, San Francisco. A.R. Margulis, M.D., program chairman. Inquiries: See Oct. 21–25, UCSF Dept. Radiology.

Oct. 19–20: **Stanford Weekend Workshop in Coronary Angioplasty.** Fairchild Auditorium, Stanford University Medical Center, Stanford, CA. Stephen N. Oesterle, M.D., course director. Inquiries: PTCA Workshop, Division of Cardiology, CVRB 287, Stanford University Medical Center, Stanford, CA 94305. Tel. 1-415-497-6895.

Oct. 21–22: **Myocardial Revascularization During Acute MI.** Towsley Center, Ann Arbor, MI. Sponsored by CME, Univ. of Michigan Medical School. Inquiries: B. Phillips, CME, Towsley Center Box 057, Univ. of Mich. Med. School, Ann Arbor, MI 48109-0010. Tel. 1-313-763-1400.

Oct. 21–25: **Clinical Magnetic Resonance Imaging.** Hyatt Regency Hotel, San Francisco. Charles B. Higgins, M.D., Hedvig Hricak, Ph.D., program directors. Sponsored by UCSF Dept. of Radiology. Inquiries: Dept. of Radiology, UCSF School of Medicine, San Francisco, CA 94143. Tel. 1-415-666-5731.

Oct. 24–26: **New Techniques and Concepts in Cardiology.** Hyatt Regency Hotel, Washington, DC. Stephen E. Epstein, M.D., F.A.C.C., director. Sponsored by American College of Cardiology. Inquiries: See Oct. 17–20 — Registration Secy., ACC.

Oct. 25: **Annual Meeting, Society of Neurological Anesthesia and Neurological Supportive Care.** San Francisco. Inquiries: Society of Neurological Anesthesia, P.O. Box 238, Univ. of Virginia Medical Center, Charlottesville, VA 22908.

Oct. 25–27: **Diagnostic Radiology Update.** Mandalay Four Seasons Hotel, Dallas. Sponsored by University of Texas Health Science Center at Dallas. Inquiries: Dolly Christensen, Director of Radiology Postgraduate Education, UT Health Science Center, 5323 Harry Hines Blvd., Dallas, TX 75235. Tel. 1-214-688-2502 or 688-2166.

Oct. 28–Nov. 2: **Doppler and 2-D Echocardiography.** Tulsa, Oklahoma. Dr. Arthur Hagan, program director. Sponsored by Hillcrest Medical Center, University of Oklahoma, Tulsa Medical College, and the Institute for Medical Studies. Inquiries: See Oct. 18–20 — K. Stroich.

Oct. 30–Nov. 1: **La Crosse Health and Sports Science Symposium.** La Crosse, WI. Inquiries: La Crosse Exercise, 221 Mitchell Hall, UWI, La Crosse, WI 54601. Tel. 1-608-785-8686.

Nov. 2–3: **Hemodynamic Monitoring/Patient Care and Pulmonary Artery Catheterization.** The Preclinical Teaching Bldg., The Johns Hopkins Medical Institutions, Baltimore, MD. James F. Schauble, M.D., course director. Sponsored by the Department of Anesthesiology and Critical Care Medicine, The Johns Hopkins Medical Institutions. Inquiries: Jeanne Ryan, Program Coordinator, Office of Continuing Education, The Johns Hopkins University School of Medicine, 720 Rutland Avenue, Turner 22, Baltimore, MD 21205. Tel. 1-301-955-6046.

Nov. 4–8: **Diagnostic Radiology Seminars.** Maui Marriott Hotel, Maui, Hawaii. Neil Chafetz, M.D. course director. Sponsored by UCSF Dept. of Radiology. Inquiries: Radiology PG Education, UCSF Room C-324, Third and Parnassus Ave., San Francisco, CA 94143. Tel. 1-415-666-5731 (between 7:30 am-4:30 pm Pacific Time).

Nov. 8–9: **Cardiology in Psychosocial, Economic, Political and Ethical Perspectives.** The Halloran House Hotel, New York City. Sponsored by AHA New York City Affiliate in cooperation with the International Society for Humanism in Cardiology. Inquiries: Humanism Conference, AHA, New York City Affiliate, 205 East 42 Street, New York, NY 10017. Tel. 1-212-661-5335.

cont'd on ad page 27

cont'd from ad page 24

Nov. 10: **Current Events in Clinical Cardiology.** (Special Sunday Afternoon Program). Sponsored by the AHA Council on Clinical Cardiology, European Society of Cardiology.

Nov. 10: **Cardiovascular Risk Factors in the Young.** Sponsored by the AHA Councils on Cardiovascular Nursing, Cardiovascular Disease in the Young, Epidemiology.

Nov. 10: **Central Neural Cardiovascular Control.** Sponsored by the AHA Councils on Basic Science, Circulation, High Blood Pressure Research.

Nov. 10: **The Changing Role of Echocardiography in Coronary Artery Disease.** Washington, D.C. Harvey Feigenbaum, M.D., program director. Sponsored by Indiana University Department of Medicine and the Institute for Medical Studies. Inquiries: See Oct. 18–20 — K. Stroich.

Nov. 10: **Thrombolytic and Interventional Therapy in Acute Myocardial Infarction.** An international workshop. Sponsored by the George Washington University Medical Center. Inquiries: The Office of Continuing Medical Education, Tel. 1-202-676-4285.

Nov. 11–14: **58th Annual Scientific Sessions, American Heart Association, Washington, DC. Inquiries: Coordinator Scientific Sessions, AHA, 7320 Greenville Ave., Dallas, TX 75231. Tel. for abstracts: 1-214-750-5439, for housing and reservations 1-214-750-5425.**

Nov. 15: **Hypertension Symposium.** Hyatt Regency, Baltimore, MD. Sponsored by The Johns Hopkins Medical Institutions, Baltimore. Inquiries: Catherine Sentman, Program Coordinator, Turner 22, 720 Rutland Avenue, Baltimore, MD 21205. Tel. 1-301-955-6046.

Nov. 19–20: **Subspecialty Boards in Cardiovascular Disease.** Philadelphia. Inquiries: American Board of Internal Medicine, 3624 Market St., Philadelphia, PA 19104. Tel. 1-215-243-1500. (New date.)

Nov. 22–24: **Third Annual Emergency Cardiac Care Symposium.** Chicago O'Hare Marriott. Inquiries: M.H. Weil, M.D., chairman, Dept. Med., University of Health Sciences/Chicago Medical School, 3333 Green Bay Rd., North Chicago, IL 60064. Tel. 1-312-578-3291.

Dec. 1–4: **Coronary, Hypertensive, Valvular, and Myocardial Heart Diseases: The Multidisciplinary Approach.** Williamsburg Lodge, Williamsburg, VA. William C. Roberts, M.D., F.A.C.C., director. Sponsored by American College of Cardiology. Inquiries: See Oct. 17–20 — Registration Secy., ACC.

Dec. 2–6: **Chest Radiology — Update and Review.** Hotel Del Coronado, San Diego. Sponsored by Chest Division of Dept. of Radiology, UCSD. David S. Feigin, M.D., and Paul J. Friedman, M.D., program directors. Inquiries: Dawne Ryals, Ryals and Associates, P.O. Box 610203, DFW Airport, TX 75261-0203. Tel. 1-214-659-9590.

Dec. 4–7: **Second Annual Seminar and Workshop in Doppler Echocardiography.** Hotel Meridien, San Francisco. Julius Gardin, M.D., program director. Sponsored by the University of California, Irvine, California College of Medicine and the Institute for Medical Studies. Inquiries: See Oct. 18–20 — K. Stroich.

Dec. 5–7: **Mechanisms and Treatment of Cardiac Arrhythmias.** Hershey Philadelphia Hotel, Philadelphia. Leonard S. Dreifus, M.D., F.A.C.C., Eric L. Michelson, M.D., F.A.C.C., and Yoshio Watanabe, M.D., F.A.C.C., directors. Sponsored by American College of Cardiology and Lankenau Hospital, Philadelphia. Inquiries: See Oct. 17–20 — Registration Secy., ACC.

Dec. 9–10: **Second Antwerp/La Jolla Research Conference on Cardiac Function.** Inotropic Mechanisms and Heart Failure. Hotel Inter-Continental, San Diego. John Ross, Jr., M.D., chairman. Sponsored by La Jolla/San Diego Heart Institute and University of California, San Diego School of Medicine. Inquiries: Antwerp/La Jolla Conference, P.O. Box 33185, San Diego, CA 92103. Tel. 1-619-692-9115.

Dec. 9–12: **Chest Imaging — (PRE) 1986.** Hotel Del Coronado, San Diego. David S. Feigin, M.D., program director. Sponsored by the Chest Division of the Department of Radiology, University of California, San Diego. Inquiries: See Dec. 2–6 — D. Ryals.

Dec. 13–15: **Advances in Heart Disease.** Hyatt Regency Hotel, San Francisco. Elliot Rapaport, M.D., F.A.C.C., director. Sponsored by American College of Cardiology. Inquiries: See Oct. 17–20 — Registration Secy., ACC.

Dec. 13–15: **Cardiovascular Disease 1986 — Changes, Choices, Challenges.** Grand Hyatt Hotel, New York City. Henry I. Russek, M.D., F.A.C.C., director. Sponsored by American College of Cardiology and Hahnemann University, Philadelphia. Inquiries: See Oct. 17–20 — Registration Secy., ACC.

Dec. 27–30: **The Third International Symposium on Electrophysiologic Basis for Diagnosis and Management of Cardiac Arrhythmias.** Wyndham Hotel, Orlando, FL. Sponsored by the University of Wisconsin Continuing Medical Education; Mt. Sinai Medical Center, Milwaukee, WI: American Heart Association, Central Florida and Wisconsin Affiliates; Florida Heart Institute in Orlando; and the Continuing Education and Research Foundation, Elm Grove, WI. Inquiries: Sarah Aslakson, University of Wisconsin Medical School, Continuing Medical Education, Room 465B, 610 Walnut Street, Madison, WI 53705. Tel 1-608-263-2856.

1986

Jan. 13–17: **Interventional, MRI and Neuroradiology.** Fairmont Hotel, San Francisco. Sponsored by University of California, San Francisco.

Jan. 13–17: **17th Annual Cardiovascular Conference at Snowmass.** New Snowmass Conference Center, Snowmass Resort, Snowmass, CO. John H.K. Vogel, M.D., F.A.C.C., and Bruce C. Paton, M.D., F.A.C.C., directors. Sponsored by American College of Cardiology and Santa Barbara Heart and Lung Institute, Santa Barbara, CA. Inquiries: Registration Secy., Extramural Programs Dept., ACC, 9111 Old Georgetown Rd., Bethesda, MD 20814.

Jan. 24–25: **Current Controversies and Techniques in Congenital Heart Surgery.** Baltimore, MD. (Immediately prior to Annual Meeting, Society of Thoracic Surgeons, Washington, DC). Sponsored by Div. of Thoracic and Cardiovascular Surgery, University of Maryland School of Medicine. Inquiries: Program Cont. Ed., University of Maryland School of Medicine, 10 South Pine St., Suite 300, Baltimore, MD 21201. Tel. 1-301-528-3956.

Jan. 30–Feb. 1: **Fifth Annual Perspectives on New Diagnostic and Therapeutic Techniques in Clinical Cardiology.** Buena Vista Palace, Walt Disney World, FL. C. Richard Conti, M.D., F.A.C.C., director. Sponsored by American College of Cardiology and the University of Florida College of Medicine, Gainesville. Inquiries: See Jan. 13–17 — Registration Secy., ACC.

Feb. 1–4: **Evolution of the Human Atherosclerotic Plaque.** Reston, VA. Sponsored by the Council on Arteriosclerosis of the AHA. Inquiries: Administrative Assistant, Scientific Sessions, AHA, 7320 Greenville Ave., Dallas, TX 75231. Tel. 1-214-750-5441.

Feb. 2–7: **13th Annual New Clinical Applications in Doppler Echocardiography, Coronary Angioplasty, Thrombolytic Therapy, Electrophysiologic Testing, Arrhythmia Management, Heart Failure and Cardiac Drugs.** Prospector Square Resort Hotel, Park City, UT. Arthur D. Hagan, M.D., F.A.C.C., Anthony N. DeMaria, M.D., F.A.C.C., Jay W. Mason, M.D., F.A.C.C., Jeffrey L. Anderson, M.D., F.A.C.C., directors. Sponsored by American College of Cardiology; Tulsa Heart Center and University of Oklahoma Tulsa Medical College; LDS Hospital and University of Utah School of Medicine, Salt Lake City. Inquiries: See Jan. 13–17 — Registration Secy., ACC.

Feb. 6–8: **11th International Joint Conference on Stroke and Cerebral Circulation.** San Francisco. Sponsored by the Council on Stroke of the AHA. Inquiries: Administrative Assistant, Scientific Sessions, AHA, 7320 Greenville Ave., Dallas, TX 75231. Tel. 1-214-750-5441.

Feb. 10–14: **First Annual Cardiovascular Conference at Hawaii.** Sheraton Waikoloa, Kona Coast, HI. John H.K. Vogel, M.D., F.A.C.C., director. Sponsored by American College of Cardiology and Santa Barbara Heart and Lung Institute. Inquiries: See Jan. 13–17 — Registration Secy., ACC.

Feb. 14–16: **Pathophysiology and Techniques of Cardiopulmonary Bypass: VI.** Sheraton Harbor Island East, San Diego, CA. Joe

cont'd on ad page 37

cont'd from ad page 27

R. Utley, M.D., program director. Sponsored by the Cardiothoracic Research and Education Foundation. Inquiries: CREF, P.O. Box 33185, San Diego, CA 92103. Tel. 1-619-692-9115.

Feb. 17–20: **Annual Postgraduate Course on Thoracic Imaging.** Newporter Beach Hotel, Newport Beach, CA. (Feb. 15–16: Scientific Sessions, Society of Thoracic Radiology). H. Baltaxe, M.D., program director. Inquiries: D. Ryals, P.O. Box 610203, DFW Airport, TX 75261-0203. Tel. 1-214-659-9590.

Feb. 19–22: **11th International Joint Conference on Stroke and Cerebral Circulation.** Vacation Village, San Diego. Inquiries: Admin. Assist., Scientific Sessions, AHA, Dallas, TX 75231. Tel. 1-214-750-5441.

Feb. 24–27: **Fourth Annual Cardiology Update.** Honolulu, Hawaii. Roger White, M.D., program director. Sponsored by Straub Clinic and Hospital and the Institute for Medical Studies. Inquiries: See Oct. 18–20, 1985 — K. Stroich.

Feb. 24–28: **Diagnostic Radiology Seminars.** Park City, Utah. Sponsored by University of California, San Francisco.

Feb. 25–Mar. 2: **Joint Scientific Sessions of the Councils on Circulation and Basic Science.** Keystone, CO. Sponsored by the Councils on Circulation and Basic Science. Dr. Stephen Vatner and Dr. Harold Strauss, chairpersons. Abstracts by Nov. 1, 1985. Inquiries: Administrative Assistant for the Scientific Sessions of the AHA, 7320 Greenville Ave., Dallas, TX 75231. Tel. 1-214-750-5441.

March 3–5: **26th Annual Conference on Cardiovascular Disease Epidemiology.** San Francisco. Sponsored by the Council on Epidemiology of the AHA. Inquiries: Coordinator, Scientific Sessions, AHA, 7320 Greenville Ave., Dallas, TX 75231. Tel. 1-214-750-5439.

March 5: **Combined Meeting of the Society of Behavioral Medicine and the Epidemiology Council of the AHA.** Seventh Annual Scientific Sessions, Society of Behavioral Medicine, Sheraton Palace Hotel, San Francisco. Inquiries: Society of Behavioral Medicine, P.O. Box 8530, University Station, Knoxville, TN 37996. Tel. 1-615-974-5164 or 974-5248.

March 5–8: **Seventh Annual Scientific Sessions, the Society of Behavioral Medicine.** Sheraton Palace Hotel, San Francisco. Abstracts by September 20, 1985. Inquiries: Society of Behavioral Medicine, P.O. Box 8530, University Station, Knoxville, TN 37996. Tel. 1-615-974-5164 or 974-5248.

March 6–8: **FOCUS '86.** A national, bi-annual conference on chest diseases. Doubletree Inn. Scottsdale, AZ. Sponsored by the Heart Lung Center at St. Luke's Medical Center, Phoenix. Inquiries: Christine Campbell, Director, Department of Medical Meetings, St. Luke's Medical Center, 1800 E. Van Buren, Phoenix, AZ 85006. Tel. 1-602-251-8402.

March 9–13: **35th Annual Scientific Sessions, American College of Cardiology.** Atlanta. Inquiries: ACC, Meeting Services Department, 9111 Old Georgetown Road, Bethesda, MD 20814. Tel. 1-301-897-5400.

March 9–14: **Diagnostic Imaging: 1986.** Waiohai Hotel, Kauai, Hawaii. Sponsored by University of California, San Francisco.

March 14–16: **15th Princeton Conference on Cerebrovascular Diseases.** St. Louis, MO. Abstracts by Dec. 1, 1985. Invitations to participants will be issued by Jan. 16, 1986. Inquiries: Dr. Marcus E. Raichle, Division of Radiation Sciences, Washington University School of Medicine, 510 South Kingshighway, St. Louis, MO 63110.

March 20–22: **87th Annual Meeting of the American Society for Clinical Pharmacology and Therapeutics.** Sheraton Washington Hotel, Washington, D.C. Inquiries: ACSPT, 1718 Gallagher Road, Norristown, Pennsylvania 19401-2810. Tel. 1-215-825-3838.

March 22–23: **Advances in Uroradiology.** Fairmont Hotel, San Francisco. Sponsored by University of California, San Francisco.

March 24–26: **New Directions in Cardiac Rehabilitation.** Stanford University School of Medicine, Stanford, CA. Robert DeBusk, M.D., F.A.C.C., director. Sponsored by American College of Cardiology and Stanford University School of Medicine. Inquiries: See Jan. 13–17 — Registration Secy., ACC.

March 24–26: **Cardiovascular Conference at Lake Louise.** Chateau Lake Louise, Lake Louise, Alberta, BC. W. Peter Klinke, M.D., F.A.C.C., Israel Belenkie, M.D., F.A.C.C., and James Wayne Warnica, M.D., F.A.C.C., directors. Sponsored by American College of Cardiology and the Alberta Cardiovascular Society and Continuing Medical Education, University of Alberta. Inquiries: See Jan. 13–17 — Registration Secy., ACC.

March 24–26: **Practical Cardiology for the Family Physician — 1986.** Red Lion's La Posada Resort Hotel, Scottsdale, AZ. Robert S. Eliot, M.D., F.A.C.C., director. Sponsored by American College of Cardiology; Heart Lung Center, St. Luke's Medical Center; and Arizona Academy of Family Physicians, Phoenix. Inquiries: See Jan. 13–17 — Registration Secy., ACC.

March 24–28: **Electrocardiographic Interpretation of Complex Arrhythmias: A Physiological Approach.** Krannert Institute of Cardiology, Indianapolis. Charles Fisch, M.D., F.A.C.C., and Douglas P. Zipes, M.D., F.A.C.C., directors. Sponsored by American College of Cardiology; Indiana University School of Medicine; and Krannert Institute of Cardiology. Inquiries: See Jan. 13–17 — Registration Secy., ACC.

April 3–5: **Electrocardiography of Pacemaker Rhythms.** Parker House Hotel, Boston. P.A. Levine, M.D., chairman. Sponsored by North American Society of Pacing and Electrophysiology. Inquiries: NASPE, 13 Eaton Court, Wellesley Hills, MA 02181. Tel. 1-617-237-1866.

April 9–11: **Cardiology Update 1986.** The Houstonian Hotel and Club, Houston. Robert Roberts, M.D., F.A.C.C., Antonio M. Gotto, M.D., D. Phil., F.A.C.C., and Michael E. DeBakey, M.D., F.A.C.C., directors. Sponsored by American College of Cardiology, Baylor College of Medicine, and the Methodist Hospital, Houston. Inquiries: See Jan. 13–17 — Registration Secy., ACC.

April 10–12: **The Fourth Charleston Symposium on Congenital Heart Disease.** Mills House Hotel, Charleston, SC. Robert Sade, M.D., F.A.C.C., Paul C. Gillette, M.D., F.A.C.C., Fred Crawford, M.D., F.A.C.C., and Arno Hohn, M.D., F.A.C.C., directors. Sponsored by American College of Cardiology. Inquiries: See Jan. 13–17 — Registration Secy., ACC.

April 12–16: **1986 AAMI 21st Annual Meeting and Exhibit Program.** Hyatt Regency, Chicago. Abstracts by September 20, 1985. Inquiries: Marguerite Leishman, AAMI, 1901 North Fort Myer Drive, Suite 602, Arlington, VA 22209-1699. Tel. 1-703-525-4890.

April 17–19: **Thoracic Imaging Update, 1986.** Hyatt Regency Hotel, Monterey, CA. Sponsored by University of California, San Francisco.

April 17–19: **The Pathology of the Heart.** Palmer House Hotel, Chicago. Saroja Bharati, M.D., F.A.C.C., Jesse E. Edwards, M.D., F.A.C.C., and Maurice Lev, M.D., F.A.C.C., directors. Sponsored by American College of Cardiology; United Hospital of St. Paul, St. Paul, MN; and Deborah Heart and Lung Center, Browns Mills, NJ. Inquiries: See Jan. 13–17 — Registration Secy., ACC.

April 17–19: **New Strategies in Cardiology.** Boca Raton Hotel and Beach Club, Boca Raton, FL. David O. Williams, M.D., F.A.C.C., director. Sponsored by American College of Cardiology, Brown University, and Rhode Island Hospital, Providence. Inquiries: See Jan. 13–17 — Registration Secy., ACC.

April 23–25: **National Student Research Forum.** The University of Texas Medical Branch, Galveston, TX. Abstracts by Dec. 1, 1985. Supported by American Medical Association — Education and Research Foundation, Mead Johnson Nutritional Division, Roche Laboratories, and American Academy of Family Physicians. Inquiries: National Student Research Forum, P.O. Box 54, Station 1, UT Medical Branch, Galveston, TX 77550. Tel. 1-409-761-3762.

May 7–9: **Clinical Auscultation of the Heart.** Georgetown University Medical Center, Washington, DC. W. Proctor Harvey, M.D., F.A.C.C., John F. Stapleton, M.D., F.A.C.C., and James A. Ronan, M.D., F.A.C.C., directors. Sponsored by American College of Cardiology and Georgetown University School of Medicine, Division of Cardiology. Inquiries: See Jan. 13–17 — Registration Secy., ACC.

May 12–16: **Consultant's Course in Cardiology.** The Mount Sinai Medical Center, New York City. Valentin Fuster, M.D., F.A.C.C., Richard Gorlin, M.D., F.A.C.C., Louis E. Teichholz, M.D., F.A.C.C., Simon Dack, M.D., F.A.C.C., and Ephraim Donoso, M.D., F.A.C.C., directors. Sponsored by American College of Cardiology and the Page and William

cont'd on ad page 52

BEHIND THE FACE OF HYPERTENSION

Continuing evidence for central control

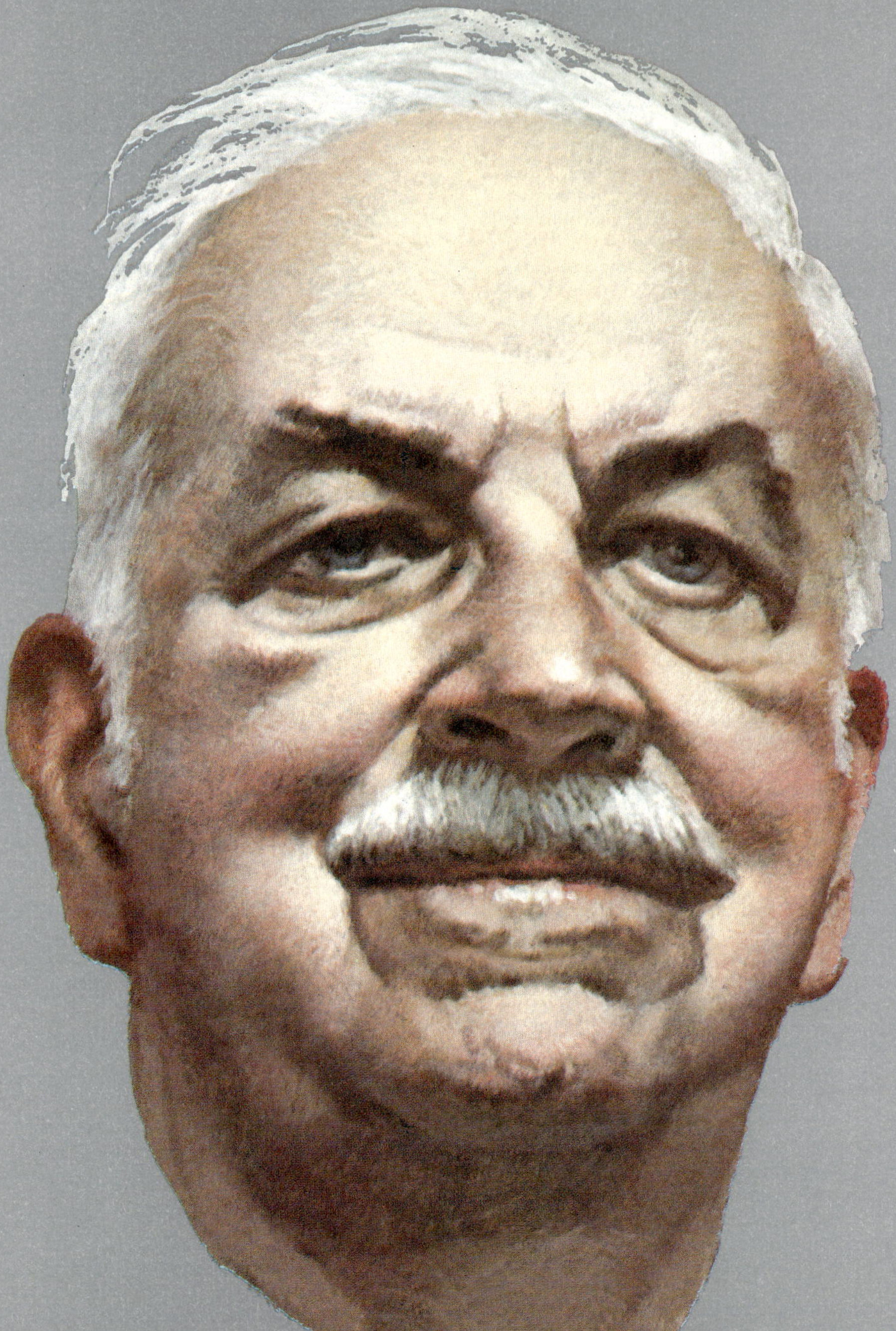

cont'd from ad page 37

AHA NEWS

Black Postgraduate School of Medicine of the Mount Sinai School of Medicine, New York City. Inquiries: See Jan. 13–17 — Registration Secy., ACC.

May 15–17: **Seventh Annual Scientific Session, North American Society of Pacing and Electrophysiology.** Marriott Hotel, New Orleans. Abstracts and Young Investigator Awards by Dec. 1, 1985. P.C. Gillette, M.D., program chairman. Inquiries: See April 3–5, 1986, NASPE.

May 16–18: **Update in Cardiac Catheterization and Invasive Cardiology: 1986 — A Weekend Review.** Hyatt Regency Cambridge Overlooking Boston, Cambridge, MA. William Grossman, M.D., F.A.C.C., and Donald S. Baim, M.D., F.A.C.C., directors. Sponsored by American College of Cardiology and the Harvard Medical School Dept. of Medicine at the Beth Israel Hospital, Boston. Inquiries: See Jan. 13–17 — Registration Secy., ACC.

May 20–23: **Cardiovascular Disease '86: Molecular and Cellular Mechanisms, Prevention, Treatment.** Sixth International Washington Spring Symposium. Washington, D.C. Linda L. Gallo, Ph.D., G.V. Vahouny, Ph.D., co-chairs. Inquiries: Symposium '86. Department of Biochemistry, The George Washington University, School of Medicine and Health Sciences, 2300 Eye Street, N.W., Washington, DC 20037.

May 27–31: **15th Annual Educational and Scientific Symposium, Society of Critical Care Medicine.** Washington, DC. Sponsored by SCCM. Inquiries: Tracy Schultz, Program Coordinator, SCCM, 223 E. Imperial Highway, Suite 110, Fullerton, CA 92635. Tel. 1-714-870-5243.

June 5–7: **10th Annual Update Cardiology for the Primary Physician During Spoleto Festival USA 1986.** Mills House Hotel, Charleston, SC. Peter C. Gazes, M.D., F.A.C.C., Michael E. Assey, M.D., F.A.C.C., William H. Barnwell, M.D., F.A.C.C., Grady H. Hendrix, M.D., F.A.C.C., Robert B. Leman, M.D., F.A.C.C., Charles P. Summerall III, M.D., F.A.C.C., and Bruce W. Usher, M.D., F.A.C.C., directors. Sponsored by American College of Cardiology; Cardiovascular Division, Department of Medicine and Division of Continuing Education, Medical University of South Carolina, Charleston. Inquiries: See Jan. 13–17 — Registration Secy., ACC.

June 8–11: **Advanced Echocardiography and Doppler Ultrasound 1986.** Sheraton Harbor Island, San Diego, CA. Pravin M. Shah, M.D., F.A.C.C., John S. Child, M.D., F.A.C.C., Joseph K. Perloff, M.D., F.A.C.C., and Maylene Wong, M.D., F.A.C.C., directors. Sponsored by American College of Cardiology. Inquiries: See Jan. 13–17 — Registration Secy., ACC.

June 23–27: **Two-Dimensional Echocardiography and Cardiac Doppler: Second Annual Core Curriculum and Self-Assessment.** Buena Vista Palace, Lake Buena Vista, FL. Arthur D. Hagan, M.D., F.A.C.C., and Anthony N. DeMaria, M.D., F.A.C.C., directors. Sponsored by American College of Cardiology; Tulsa Heart Center and University of Oklahoma Tulsa Medical College, Tulsa; and the University of Kentucky School of Medicine, Lexington. Inquiries: See Jan. 13–17 — Registration Secy., ACC.

July 10–12: **Fourth International Symposium on Mechanisms of Vasodilatation.** Rochester, MN. Satellite of International Congress of Physiological Sciences. Cerebral, coronary, and limb circulation. Paul M. Vanhoutte, M.D., chairman organizing committee. Abstracts by Oct. 30, 1985. Inquiries: J. Beckman, 942C Guggenheim Bldg., Mayo Clinic, Rochester, MN 55905.

July 27–Aug. 9: **12th Ten-Day Seminar on Epidemiology and Prevention of Cardiovascular Disease.** Lake Tahoe, CA. Sponsored by the Council on Epidemiology of the AHA. Inquiries: Executive Secretary, Scientific Sessions, AHA, 7320 Greenville Ave., Dallas, TX 75231. Tel. 1-214-750-5438.

Sept. 1–5: **Biology and Physics of Radiology.** Department of Radiology, the University of California, San Diego School of Medicine. Inquiries: See Dec. 2–6, 1985 — D. Ryals.

Sept. 12–14: **Sonographers Update and Review.** Hanalei Hotel, San Diego. Sponsored by the Department of Radiology of the University of California, San Diego School of Medicine. Inquiries: See Dec. 2–6, 1985 — D. Ryals.

Sept. 14–19: **Xth World Congress of Cardiology,** Washington, DC. Inquiries: Secretariat, 7320 Greenville Ave., Dallas, TX 75231. Tel. 1-214-750-5429. Cable: Tencard, Dallas, TX.

Oct. 8–10: **40th Annual Fall Conference and Scientific Sessions of the Council for High Blood Pressure.** Cleveland. Sponsored by the Council on High Blood Pressure Research of the AHA. Inquiries: Administrative Assistant, Scientific Sessions, AHA, 7320 Greenville Ave., Dallax, TX 75231. Tel. 1-214-750-5441.

Oct. 18: **Imaging of the Lumbar Spine and Pelvis.** Department of Radiology of the University of California, San Diego School of Medicine. Inquiries: See Dec. 2–6, 1985 — D. Ryals.

1987

July 1–3: **Stress and the Heart.** Jackson Lake Lodge, Grand Teton National Park, Moran, WY. Robert S. Eliot, M.D., F.A.C.C., director. Sponsored by American College of Cardiology and St. Luke's Heart Lung Center, Phoenix. Inquiries: Registration Secy., Extramural Programs Dept., American College of Cardiology, 9111 Old Georgetown Road, Bethesda, MD 20814.

Aug. 25–27: **Tutorials in the Tetons: Clinical Cardiology — Diagnostic and Therapeutic Advances.** Jackson Lake Lodge, Grand Teton National Park, Moran, WY. Robert S. Eliot, M.D., F.A.C.C., James C. Buell, M.D., F.A.C.C., and Timothy Fleming, M.D., F.A.C.C., directors. Sponsored by American College of Cardiology and St. Luke's Heart Lung Center, Phoenix. Inquiries: See July 1–3 — Registration Secy., ACC.

Abroad

1985

Oct. 14–18: **International Congress on Cardiac Doppler.** Pisa, Italy. (Tutorial sessions Oct. 14–15; Scientific Sessions Oct. 16–18). Prof. Luigi Donato and Dr. Merrill Spencer, presidents. Inquiries: Istituto di Fisiologia Clinica, C.N.R., University of Pisa, Via Savi 8, 1-567100 Pisa, Italy. Tel. 050-47231/502109. Telex: 590549 IFCI.

Oct. 17–19: **18th Danube Symposium for Neurological Sciences.** University Clinic for Neurology. Innsbruck, Austria. Inquiries: Danube Symposium for Neurological Sciences, c/o Vienna Academy of Medicine, Alser Str. 4,A-1090 Vienna, Austria. Tel. (0222) 42 71 65. Cable MEDACAD, Wien. Telex 134743 MEDAK A.

Oct. 20–22: **Fifth International Symposium on Rats with Spontaneous Hypertension and Related Studies.** Kyoto, Japan. Yukio Yamori, M.D., program director. Inquiries: Fifth SHR Symposium, Shimane Medical University, Izumo 693, Japan. Tel. 0853-23-2111 Ext. 2375. Cable: WHOCOLLAB IZUMO.

Oct. 20–23: **Third World Congress of Cardiac Rehabilitation.** Caracas, Venezuela. Sponsored by the International Society and Federation of Cardiology: Scientific Council on Rehabilitation of Cardiac Patients and AHA Council on Clinical Cardiology. Inquiries Dr. Deyanira Almeida, Congresa C.A., P.O. Box 17422, Caracas 1015A, Venezuela.

Oct. 20–25: **Conference on Leukotrienes and Prostanoids in Health and Disease.** Jerusalem and Rehovot, Israel. Inquiries: Prof. Uriel Zor, Weizmann Institute of Science, Rehovot, Israel 76100. Tel. 1081 483557. Telex 361900. Cable: WEIZINST.

Oct. 23–24: **International Symposium on Mechanisms and Treatment in Essential Hypertension: Calcium and Calcium Antagonists.** Hotel Nagoya Castle, Nagoya, Japan. (Satellite of Fifth International Symposium on Rats with Spontaneous Hypertension, Oct. 20–22, Kyoto, Japan). Inquiries: Kyuzo Aoki, M.D., 2nd Dept. Internal Med., Nagoya City University Medical School, Mizuho-ku, Nagoya 467, Japan. Tel. 052-851-5511, Ext. 2204.

Oct. 24–25: **Animals and the Scientist: Institutional Responsibilities.** The Hart House, University of Toronto, Toronto, Canada. Sponsored by the Scientists Center for Animal Welfare and the University of Toronto. Inquiries: Dr. F. Barbara Orlans, Director, Scientists Center for Animal Welfare, 4805 St. Elmo Avenue, Bethesda, MD 20814. Tel. 1-301-654-6390.

Oct. 25–27: **International Symposium on Brain and Blood Pressure Control.** Kikai-Shinkoh Hall, Shiba Park, Tokyo, Japan. Dr.

cont'd on ad page 62

cont'd from ad page 52

AHA NEWS

Keiji Nakamura organizing chairman. Inquiries: Brain and Blood Pressure, Dept. of Pharmacology, Nippon Roche Research Center, Kamakura 247, Japan. Tel. 0467-45-3191-Ext. 380 or 381. Telex 2222861 PANROCHE J.

Oct. 27–30: **Third Asian Pacific Symposium on Cardiac Pacing and Electrophysiology.** Hilton Hotel, Melbourne, Australia. Sponsored by Cardiac Society of Australia and New Zealand under auspices of International Cardiac Pacing Society. Inquiries: Third Asian Pacific Symposium on Cardiac Pacing and Electrophysiology, Dept. of Cardiology, Suite 3.5, Epworth Medical Centre, 62 Erin St., Richmond, Vic. 3121, Australia.

Oct. 28–31: **First International Congress on Food and Health.** Salsomaggiore Terme, Italy. Sponsored by International Association for Advancement of Biomedical Research, by Society of Medical Gastronomy, and Institute of Pharmacology of University of Pisa. Inquiries: ALM s.r.l., Via Lattuada, 26, 20135 Milan, Italy. Telex: 313063 HOTALM I.

Nov. 2–4: **Third International Symposium on Ischemic Heart Disease, Exercise, and Related Topics.** Royal York Hotel, Toronto, Canada. Sponsored by Toronto Rehabilitation Center. Inquiries: J. Kennedy or A. Ceci, Toronto Rehab. Center, 345 Rumsey Rd., Toronto, Ont. Canada M4G 1RT. Tel. 1-416-425-1117 Ext. 236.

Nov. 28–30: **Seventh Biennial Congress of Cardiology.** Rawalpindi/Islamabad, Pakistan. Inquiries: Pakistan Cardiac Society, Brig. Muhammad Zulfiqar Ali Khan, AFIC/NIHD, Rawalpindi, Pakistan. Tel. 64946, 61-31113, 61-33911.

Dec. 1–4: **International Symposium on Left Ventricular Dysfunction.** Jerusalem Hilton Hotel, Israel. Jan J. Kellermann, M.D. of Israel and David Spodick, M.D. of Worcester, MA, co-chairmen. Under the auspices of the Universities of Tel Aviv and Massachusetts. Inquiries: P.O. Box 50006, Tel Aviv 61500, Israel. Tel. 03-654571. Telex 341171 KENS IL.

Dec. 8–12: **Second International Symposium on Hypertension in the Community.** Jerusalem, Israel. Prof. Talma Rosenthal, P.O. Box 50006, Tel Aviv, 61500, Israel. Tel. 03-654571. Telex 341171 KENS IL.

1986

To be announced: **The 35th National Meeting of the Italian Neurosurgical Society.** Pavia, Italy. Inquiries: Prof. Pietro Paoletti, Department of Surgery, Neurosurgical Clinic, University of Pavia, San Matteo Hospital, 27100 Pavia, Italy. Tel 0382/422231.

Jan. 8–11: **Seventh Annual European Conference on Vascular Biology.** Bad Buchau, FR Germany. Growth and Differentiation of Vascular Cells. Organized by European Artery Club. Inquiries: Dr. G. Bondjers, Dept. Med. 1, Salgren's Hospital, 5-413 45 Göteborg, Sweden.

Jan. 16–21: **Basic Principles of Pacing and Electrophysiology — Dual Chamber and Antitachycardia Pacing.** Frenchman's Reef, St. Thomas, Virgin Islands. Sponsored by Cardiostim America. Seymour Furman, course director. Inquiries: Cardiostim America, P.O. Box 428, Mount Kisco, NY 10549, U.S.A. Tel. 1-914-241-3295.

Jan. 20–21: **Diagnostic Radiology Seminars.** Camino Real, Ixtapa, Mexico. University of California, San Francisco.

Jan. 31–Feb. 8: **Fifth Annual Winter Congress in Medical Diagnostic Imaging.** Zermatt, Switzerland. Inquiries: Winter Congress, West Park Hospital, Department of Radiology, 22141 Roscoe Blvd., Canoga Park, CA 91304. Tel. 1-818-340-9580, Ext. 280.

Feb. 8–12: **The Fourth Annual London Winter Seminar in Medical Diagnostic Imaging.** Inquiries: Winter Seminar, West Park Hospital Department of Radiology, 22141 Roscoe Blvd., Canoga Park, CA 91304. Tel. 1-818-340-0580, Ext. 280.

Feb. 9–13: **12th World Congress of the International Society for Heart Research,** Melbourne, Australia. Inquiries: Dr. N.S. Dhalla, Dept. Physiology, Faculty of Medicine, University of Manitoba, Winnipeg, Canada R3E OW3.

Feb. 16–21: **First International Congress on Stress, Behavior and Coronary Disease.** Southern Cross Hotel, Melbourne, Australia. Prof. G.D. Burrows, president, Dr. M. Jelinek, scientific program chairman. Inquiries: Mental Health Foundation, Suite 23, 20 Commercial Rd., Melbourne 3004, Vic., Australia.

March 23–25: **Second International Symposium on Holter Monitoring.** Jerusalem, Israel. V. Hombach, Cologne, and S. Stern, Jerusalem, co-chairmen. Inquiries: Prof. Shlomo Stern, c/o Stier Group, Ltd., 203 Dizengoff St., Tel Aviv 63115 Israel. Tel. (03) 224-153/4/5. Telex 35570 STI COIN IL.

April 1–3: **International Symposium on Noninvasive Cardiac Imaging. 1986.** Tel Aviv, Israel. Abstracts by Nov. 15, 1985. Sponsored by the Page and William Black Postgraduate School of Medicine, Mt. Sinai School of Medicine, New York City, and the Heart Institute, Chaim Sheba Medical Center and Sackler School of Medicine, Tel Aviv. Inquiries: Richard Meltzer, M.D., Cardiology Division, Mt. Sinai Medical Center, One Gustave Levy Place, New York, NY 10029.

April 17–19: **Exercise Testing in the Diagnosis and Evaluation of Treatment of Arrhythmias.** Athens, Greece. Inquiries: Prof. D. Cokkinos, 5 Dorylaiou, 115 21 Athens, Greece.

April 21–23: **The First Portuguese Congress.** Lisbon, Portugal. Inquiries: Prof. Martins Prata, Chairman, Dept. of Nephrology, Hospital Univ. Santa Maria, Av. Prof. Egas Moniz, 1600 Lisboa/Portugal.

April 23–25: **First International Symposium on Cardiology.** Hospital de Clinicas, University of Buenos Aires, Argentina. Inquiries: Dr. Luis D. Suárez, Dean Funes 1075-(1231), Buenos Aires, Argentina. Tel. 821-6041.

May 1–3: **First Verona Seminar on Nephrology: Hypertension and Renal Disease.** Camera di Commercio, corso Porta Nuova 96, 37100 Verona-Italy. Inquiries: Lamberto Oldrizzi, M.D., Divisione Nefrologia, Istituti Ospitalieri, 37126 Verona-Italy, Tel. 045-932528-932694.

May 1–3: **First Vienna Shock Forum.** Hotel Hilton, Vienna, Austria. Held by the Ludwig Boltzmann Institute for Experimental Traumatology. Abstracts by December 31, 1985. Inquiries: Wiener Schockgespräche, Ludwig Boltzmann Institut für experimentelle, Traumatologie, Donaueschingenstraße 13, A-1200 Wien, A-1200 Vienna-Austria. Tel. 222-33-55-33/464.

May 11–14: **The Seventh Annual Meeting of the Society for Clinical Trials.** Montreal, Quebec, Canada. Abstracts by January 2, 1986. Inquiries: Mary A. Finch, Meeting Coordinator, Society for Clinical Trials, Inc., 600 Wyndhurst Avenue, Baltimore, MD 21210, U.S.A.

May 29–30: **35 Years of Electrocardiology in Amsterdam.** Sponsored by the Interuniversity Cardiology Institute in The Netherlands. Inquiries: F.L. Meijler, M.D., F.A.C.C., Professor of Cardiology, Interuniversity Cardiology Institute, P.O. Box 19258, 3501 DG Utrecht, The Netherlands.

June 5–7: **International Congress for Clinical Neuroimaging.** Palais Auersperg, Vienna, Austria. Inquiries: International Congress for Clinical Neuroimaging, c/o Vienna Academy of Medicine, Alser Str. 4, A-1090, Vienna, Austria. Tel. 0222 42 71 65. Cable MEDACAD Wien, Telex: 134743 medak a.

June 15–20: **The First International Congress on Complementary Medicine.** Jerusalem, Israel. Open to physicians and researchers of basic sciences. Abstracts by Oct. 15, 1985. Inquiries: Dr. Z. Singer, Secretary of the Scientific Committee, The International Congress on Complementary Medicine, c/o OMEGA Tours, P.O. Box 482, Jerusalem, 91004, Israel.

June 17–20: **Second World Meeting on Impotence.** Fifth Conference on Vasculogenic Impotence and Corpus Cavernosum Revascularization. Prague, Czechoslovakia. Sponsored by the International Society for Impotence Research. Inquiries: Czechoslovak Medical Society, J.E. Purkyně, P.O. Box 88, Vítězného února 31, 120 26 Praha, Czechoslovakia. Tel. 29-41-41-4.

June 19–21: **CARDIOIMAGE 86.** International Congress on Recent Advances in Cardiac Imaging. Congress Center, Monaco. Inquiries: Dr. J.P. Letouzey, Centre d'Echographie et d'Explorations médicales, 6, avenue de Messine, 75008 PARIS. Tel. 1 45639807. Telex 211897 F TECEXPO.

June 22–25: **Seventh Congress of the European Section, International Society for Heart Research.** Reykjavík, Iceland. Inquiries: Guðmundur Thorgeirsson, M.D., Ph.D., Department of Medicine, Landspítalinn, 101 Reykjavík, Iceland.

June 23–27: **Sixth Asian Congress of Cardiology.** Jakarta, Indonesia. Working language, English. Organized by Indonesian Heart

cont'd on ad page 68

cont'd from ad page 62

Association. L.I. Rilantono, M.D., chairman. Inquiries: Asean Congress Cardiology, Dept. Cardiology, Cipto Mangunkusumo Hospital, Jalan Diponegoro 69, Jakarta 10453, Indonesia.

June 26–28: **Annual Scientific Meeting of the International Medical Society of Paraplegia.** Oslo, Norway. Abstracts by Dec. 1, 1985. Inquiries: IMSP Annual Scientific Meeting in Scandinavia 1986, Dept. of Neurology, Rikshospitalet, University Hospital, Oslo, 1 Norway.

July 2–5: **35th International Conference European Society for CV Surgery.** Metropole Hotel, Brighton, England. Prof. H.H. Bentall, chairman. Inquiries: European Society for CV Surgery, Concorde Services Ltd., 10 Wendell Rd., London W12 9RT, United Kingdom.

July 8–11: **Eighth Annual Meeting American Section of the International Society for Heart Research and Satellite Symposium on Heart Metabolism for the 30th International Congress of Physiological Sciences.** Winnipeg, Canada. Inquiries: Dr. R. E. Beamish, Experimental Cardiology Section, Dept. of Physiology, Faculty of Medicine, University of Manitoba, Winnipeg, Canada R3E OW3.

July 13–18: **30th International Congress of Physiological Sciences.** The University of British Columbia, Vancouver, Canada. Dr. H. McLennan, chairman program committee. Inquiries: IUPS, Suite 801, 750 Jervis St., Vancouver, B.C., Canada V6E 2A9. Tel. 604-681-5226. Telex 04-352848 VCR.

Aug. 21–23: **International Symposium.** Recent Aspects on Diagnosis and Treatment of Lipoprotein Disorders: Impact on Prevention of Atherosclerotic Diseases. Palais Auersperg, Vienna, Austria. Inquiries: Dr. K. Widhalm, Dept. Pediatrics, University of Vienna, Währinger Gürtel 18, A-1090 Vienna, Austria.

Aug. 31–Sept. 7: **11th Congress of International Society of Hypertension.** Heidelberg, Federal Republic of Germany. Organized by German Institute of High Blood Pressure Research and German Hypertension League. Dr. Detlev Ganten, Congress chairman. Inquiries: GKV, Frankfurter Str. 57, D-6050 Offenbach 1, Heidelberg, FR Germany.

Sept. 14–17: **Eighth International Symposium on Microsurgical Anastomoses for Cerebral Ischemia.** Florence, Italy. Inquiries: Rolando Gagliardi, M.D., Dept. of Neurosurgery, USL 10/D, Careggi Hospital, 50100 Florence, Italy.

Sept. 14–18: **Second International Conference on Diet and Nutrition and Fifth International Congress on Obesity.** Jerusalem, Israel. Inquiries: C. Horwitz, Ph.D., and S. H. Blondheim, M.D., P.O. Box 983, Jerusalem 91009, Israel.

Sept. 22–23: **International Symposium on Lipid Metabolism in the Normoxic and Ischemic Heart.** Erasmus University, Rotterdam, The Netherlands. Inquiries: Dr. H. Stam, Dept. Biochemistry I, Med. Fac., Erasmus University Rotterdam, P.O. Box 1738, 3000 DR Rotterdam, The Netherlands.

Oct. 22–25: **Ninth International Symposium on Drugs Affecting Lipid Metabolism.** Florence, Italy. Dr. Kritchevsky, R. Paoletti, chairmen. Inquiries: Fondazione Giovanni Lorenzini, Via Monte Napoleone, 23-20121 Milan, Italy. Tel. 02-702.267-783.868.

1987

Sept. 2–4: **International Conference on Management of Cardiac Arrhythmias.** London, England. Sponsored by the British Heart Foundation. Professor A. J. Camm and Dr. A. W. Nathan, members organizing committee. Inquiries: British Heart Foundation, 102 Gloucester Pl., London W1H 4DH England. Tel. 01-935-0185.

AHA Scientific Sessions Future Meeting Dates

1985	Washington, DC	Nov. 11–14
1986	Dallas, TX	Nov. 17–20
1987	Anaheim, CA	Nov. 16–19
1988	Locale Not Set	Nov. 14–17
1989	New Orleans	Nov. 13–16
1990	Dallas	Nov. 12–15

Xth World Congress of Cardiology, 1986

The Xth World Congress of Cardiology will be held in Washington, DC, Sept. 14–19, 1986. Official languages English, Spanish, and French. Inquiries: Secretariat, Xth World Congress Cardiology, 7320 Greenville Ave., Dallas, TX 75231. Tel. 1-214-750-5429. Cable: TenCard, Dallas.

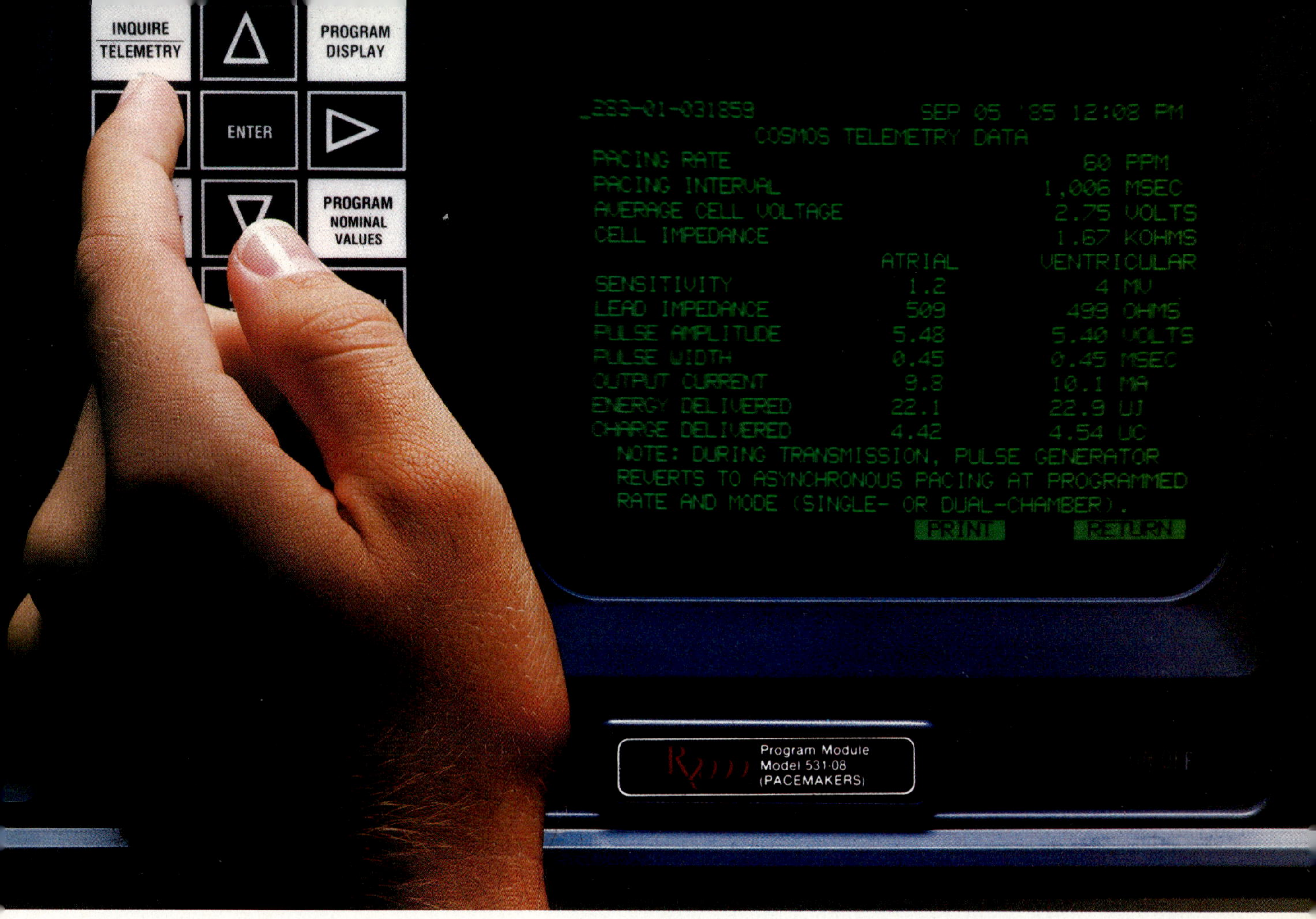
INQUIRE
TELEMETRY
PROGRAM
DISPLAY
ENTER
PROGRAM
NOMINAL
VALUES
_233-01-031859 SEP 05 '85 12:08 PM
COSMOS TELEMETRY DATA
PACING RATE 60 PPM
PACING INTERVAL 1,006 MSEC
AVERAGE CELL VOLTAGE 2.75 VOLTS
CELL IMPEDANCE 1.67 KOHMS
ATRIAL VENTRICULAR
SENSITIVITY 1.2 4 MV
LEAD IMPEDANCE 509 499 OHMS
PULSE AMPLITUDE 5.48 5.40 VOLTS
PULSE WIDTH 0.45 0.45 MSEC
OUTPUT CURRENT 9.8 10.1 MA
ENERGY DELIVERED 22.1 22.9 UJ
CHARGE DELIVERED 4.42 4.54 UC
NOTE: DURING TRANSMISSION, PULSE GENERATOR
REVERTS TO ASYNCHRONOUS PACING AT PROGRAMMED
RATE AND MODE (SINGLE- OR DUAL-CHAMBER).
PRINT
RETURN
Program Module
Model 531-08
(PACEMAKERS)

cont'd from ad page 19

International Society for Humanism in Cardiology. Contact the AHA New York City Affiliate for further information. Telephone 212-661-5335.

• **The Third International Symposium on Electrophysiologic Basis for Diagnosis and Management of Cardiac Arrhythmias** is planned for December 27–30 at the Wyndham Hotel in Orlando, Florida. The event is sponsored by the University of Wisconsin Continuing Medical Education; the Mount Sinai Medical Center, Milwaukee; the AHA Central Florida and Wisconsin Affiliates; the Florida Heart Institute in Orlando; and the Continuing Education and Research Foundation, Elm Grove, Wisconsin. For more information, contact Sarah Aslakson, University of Wisconsin Medical School, Continuing Medical Education, Room 465B, 610 Walnut Street, Madison, WI 53705. Telephone 608-263-2856.

• **"Seafood and Health '85: Issues, Questions, and Answers"** is a national conference planned for November 15–16 in Seattle. The program is designed for medical researchers, nutritionists, health and science journalists, and others interested in health and food. Keynote speakers for the event include Dr. William P. Castelli, director of the Framingham Heart Study; and Jane Brody, *New York Times* reporter and best-selling author. Edwin L. Bierman, editor of *Arteriosclerosis*, is among others scheduled to speak.

• The deadline for receipt of applications for **AHA/Bugher Foundation Centers for Molecular Biology in the Cardiovascular System** award is December 1, 1985. First review of applications will be completed by February 7, 1986, followed by a finalist reverse-site visit by April 7. Awards will be announced April 15. Forms and guidelines for preparation are available from the AHA Division of Research Awards, 7320 Greenville Avenue, Dallas, TX 75231. Inquiries go to the program administrator, Wallace G. Frasher, M.D., Vice-President for Research. Telephone 214-750-5445.

• Researchers at the **University of Rochester Medical Center** have begun a study to determine whether death and disability from congestive heart failure can be substantially reduced by early treatment with drugs. The study is funded by a six-year grant from the National Heart, Lung, and Blood Institute. It will include 255 patients over a three-year period from Rochester-area hospitals.

• **F. Mason Sones, M.D.,** a senior physician in The Cleveland Clinic Foundation's department of cardiology, has been awarded the Galen Medal. The Worshipful Society of Apothecaries of London presented the award for "pioneer research leading to cardiac bypass surgery." Dr. Sones is renowned for his work in coronary angiography. His method involves the insertion of a catheter he designed, now called the "Sones Catheter," into the coronary arteries.

• **Dr. John Hopps** is recovering at home following the insertion of a cardiac pacemaker at the National Defense Medical Centre in Ottawa. Dr. Hopps developed the pacemaker while working with Dr. Wilfred Bigelow at the Banting Institute, University of Toronto. He was also involved in the development of the cardiac defibrillator. The North American Society for Pacing and Electrophysiology recently presented Dr. Hopps with its Distinguished Scientist Award.

Meetings Calendar

1985

To be arranged individually: **Preceptorships in Cardiology.** Pacific Medical Center, San Francisco. Arthur Selzer, M.D., F.A.C.C., director. Sponsored by American College of Cardiology and Pacific Medical Center, San Francisco. Inquiries: Registration Secretary, Extramural Programs Department, American College of Cardiology, 9111 Old Georgetown Road, Bethesda, MD 20814.

To be arranged individually: **Preceptorships in Cardiology.** Buffalo General Hospital, Buffalo, NY. Jules Constant, M.D., F.A.C.C., director. Sponsored by American College of Cardiology and State University of New York at Buffalo, School of Medicine. Inquiries: Registration Secretary, Extramural Programs Dept., ACC, 9111 Old Georgetown Rd., Bethesda, MD 20814.

Nov. 2–3: **Hemodynamic Monitoring/Patient Care and Pulmonary Artery Catheterization.** The Preclinical Teaching Bldg., The Johns Hopkins Medical Institutions, Baltimore, MD. James F. Schauble, M.D., course director. Sponsored by the Department of Anesthesiology and Critical Care Medicine, The Johns Hopkins Medical Institutions. Inquiries: Jeanne Ryan, Program Coordinator, Office of Continuing Education, The Johns Hopkins University School of Medicine, 720 Rutland Avenue, Turner 22, Baltimore, MD 21205. Tel. 1-301-955-6046.

Nov. 4–8: **Diagnostic Radiology Seminars.** Maui Marriott Hotel, Maui, Hawaii. Neil Chafetz, M.D., course director. Sponsored by UCSF Dept. of Radiology. Inquiries: Radiology PG Education, UCSF Room C-324, Third and Parnassus Ave., San Francisco, CA 94143. Tel. 1-415-666-5731 (between 7:30 am-4:30 pm Pacific Time).

Nov. 8–9: **Cardiology in Psychosocial, Economic, Political and Ethical Perspectives.** The Halloran House Hotel, New York City. Sponsored by AHA New York City Affiliate in cooperation with the International Society for Humanism in Cardiology. Inquiries: Humanism Conference, AHA, New York City Affiliate, 205 East 42 Street, New York, NY 10017. Tel. 1-212-661-5335.

Nov. 10: **The Changing Role of Echocardiography in Coronary Artery Disease.** Washington, DC. Harvey Feigenbaum, M.D., program director. Sponsored by Indiana University Department of Medicine and the Institute for Medical Studies. Inquiries: K. Stroich, The Institute for Medical Studies, 30131 Town Center Drive, Suite 215, Laguna Niguel, CA 92677. Tel. 1-714-495-4499.

Nov. 10: **Thrombolytic and Interventional Therapy in Acute Myocardial Infarction.** An international workshop. Sponsored by the George Washington University Medical Center. Inquiries: The Office of Continuing Medical Education, Tel. 1-202-676-4285.

Nov. 10: **Digital Cardiac Imaging '85.** J.W. Marriott Hotel, Washington, DC. Anthony N. DeMaria, M.D.; Jonathan L. Elion, M.D.; and Steven E. Nissen, M.D., symposium co-directors. Sponsored by the University of Kentucky. Inquiries: Digital Cardiac Imaging, P.O. Box 25610, Lexington, KY 40524-5610. Tel. 606-233-5479.

Nov. 10: **Current Events in Clinical Cardiology.** (Special Sunday afternoon program of the AHA Scientific Sessions). Washington, DC. Sponsored by the AHA Council on Clinical Cardiology, European Society of Cardiology. Inquiries: Executive Secretary for the Scientific Sessions of the AHA, 7320 Greenville Ave., Dallas, TX 75231. Tel. 214-750-5438.

Nov. 10: **Cardiovascular Risk Factors in the Young.** (Special Sunday afternoon program of the AHA Scientific Sessions). Washington, DC. Sponsored by the AHA Councils on Cardiovascular Nursing, Cardiovascular Disease in the Young, Epidemiology. Inquiries: Executive Secretary for the Scientific Sessions of the

cont'd on ad page 36

WE ADDED ONE THING TO THE MOST RESPONSIVE BALLOON PUMP

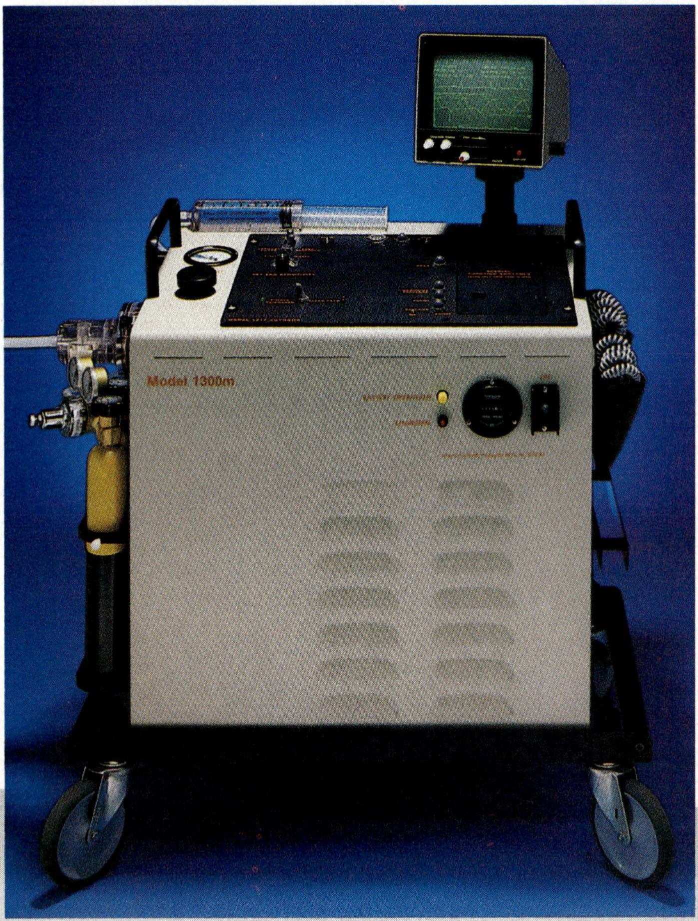

HOUSE CALLS.

This is the intra-aortic balloon pump hat tracks the heart more responsively han any other—with real-time trigger-ng and the fastest inflate/deflate time.

This is the pump with a Video nformation Center that responds to perator's needs by instructing, inform-ng, and alerting.

And this is the pump that travels most easily with the patient. It's the lightest and smallest, yet has the largest battery capacity.

What we've added is Mansfield's national organization of over 200 professionals in 66 cities, ready to respond to all customer needs: Education, sales, service, and technical support. We call it 15/4 technical support: 15 minutes or less for answers by telephone, 4 hours or less for on-site service. No one else has it.

Remember the new name: Mansfield 1300m. It describes the most responsive balloon pump and the company that is committed to keeping it that way. Mansfield, 135 Forbes Boulevard, Mansfield, MA 02048. Call 800 225-2732 (in Mass. 617 339-4112). Telex 951959.

Mansfield

cont'd from ad page 24

AHA, 7320 Greenville Ave., Dallas, TX 75231. Tel. 214-750-5438.

Nov. 10: **Central Neural Cardiovascular Control.** (Special Sunday afternoon program of the AHA Scientific Sessions). Washington, DC. Sponsored by the AHA Councils on Basic Science, Circulation, High Blood Pressure Research. Inquiries: Executive Secretary for the Scientific Sessions of the AHA, 7320 Greenville Ave., Dallas, TX 75231. Tel. 214-750-5438.

Nov. 11–14: **58th Annual Scientific Sessions, American Heart Association, Washington, DC. Inquiries: Coordinator, Scientific Sessions, AHA, 7320 Greenville Ave., Dallas, TX 75231. Tel. for abstracts: 1-214-750-5439, for housing and registration 1-214-750-5425.**

Nov. 13–15: **Biomedical High Technology.** Columbus, OH. Inquiries: Ohio State University Conferences and Institutes, 2400 Olentangy River Road, Columbus, OH 43210. Tel. 614-422-8571.

Nov. 15: **Hypertension Symposium.** Hyatt Regency, Baltimore, MD. Sponsored by The Johns Hopkins Medical Institutions, Baltimore. Inquiries: Catherine Sentman, Program Coordinator, Turner 22, 720 Rutland Avenue, Baltimore, MD 21205. Tel. 1-301-955-6046.

Nov. 15–16: **Seafood and Health '85: Issues, Questions and Answers.** Seattle Sheraton, Seattle. Sponsored by the West Coast Fisheries Development Foundation. Inquiries: Seafood and Health '85, 1932 First Avenue, No. 815, Seattle, WA 98101. Tel. 206-441-0260.

Nov. 19–20: **Subspecialty Boards in Cardiovascular Disease.** Philadelphia. Inquiries: American Board of Internal Medicine, 3624 Market St., Philadelphia, PA 19104. Tel. 1-215-243-1500. (New date.)

Nov. 22–24: **Third Annual Emergency Cardiac Care Symposium.** Chicago O'Hare Marriott. Inquiries: M.H. Weil, M.D., chairman, Dept. Med., University of Health Sciences/Chicago Medical School, 3333 Green Bay Rd., North Chicago, IL 60064. Tel. 1-312-578-3291.

Dec. 1–4: **Coronary, Hypertensive, Valvular, and Myocardial Heart Diseases: The Multidisciplinary Approach.** Williamsburg Lodge, Williamsburg, VA. William C. Roberts, M.D., F.A.C.C., director. Sponsored by American College of Cardiology. Inquiries: Registration Secy., ACC, Extramural Programs Dept., 9111 Old Georgetown Rd., Bethesda, MD 20814.

Dec. 2–6: **Chest Radiology — Update and Review.** Hotel Del Coronado, San Diego. Sponsored by Chest Division of Dept. of Radiology, UCSD. David S. Feigin, M.D., and Paul J. Friedman, M.D., program directors. Inquiries: Dawne Ryals, Ryals and Associates, P.O. Box 610203, DFW Airport, TX 75261-0203. Tel. 1-214-659-9590.

Dec. 4–7: **Second Annual Seminar and Workshop in Doppler Echocardiography.** Hotel Meridien, San Francisco. Julius Gardin, M.D., program director. Sponsored by the University of California, Irvine, California College of Medicine and the Institute for Medical Studies. Inquiries: K. Stroich, The Institute for Medical Studies, 30131 Town Center Drive, Suite 215, Laguna Niguel, CA 92677. Tel. 1-714-495-4499.

Dec. 5–7: **Mechanisms and Treatment of Cardiac Arrhythmias.** Hershey Philadelphia Hotel, Philadelphia. Leonard S. Dreifus, M.D., F.A.C.C., Eric L. Michelson, M.D., F.A.C.C., and Yoshio Watanabe, M.D., F.A.C.C., directors. Sponsored by American College of Cardiology and Lankenau Hospital, Philadelphia. Inquiries: Registration Secy., ACC, Extramural Programs Dept., 9111 Old Georgetown Rd., Bethesda, MD 20814.

Dec. 6: **Hypertension Update.** Baltimore, MD. Sponsored by the University of Maryland Hypertension Center and the University of Maryland School of Medicine. Inquiries: Program of Continuing Education, University of Maryland School of Medicine, 10 South Pine St., Suite 300, Baltimore, MD 21201. Tel. 301-528-3956.

Dec. 6–7: **Intervention in Acute Myocardial Infarction and Contemporary Topics in Cardiology.** Thunderbird Inn, Portland, OR. Inquiries: Continuing Medical Education, c/o Educational Services, St. Vincent Hospital and Medical Center, 9205 SW Barnes Rd., Portland, OR 97225. Tel. 503-299-2010.

Dec. 6–7: **Fifth Annual Conference on Heart Diseases: Imaging Comes to Cardiology.** Wisconsin Center, University of Wisconsin, Madison. Sponsored by the University of Wisconsin Medical School and the University of Wisconsin Hospital and Clinics. Inquiries: Sarah Z. Aslakson, Continuing Medical Education, 465B WARF Bldg., 610 Walnut St., Madison, WI 53705. Tel. 608-263-2856.

Dec. 9–10: **Second Antwerp/La Jolla Research Conference on Cardiac Function.** Inotropic Mechanisms and Heart Failure. Hotel Inter-Continental, San Diego. John Ross, Jr., M.D., chairman. Sponsored by La Jolla/San Diego Heart Institute and University of California, San Diego School of Medicine. Inquiries: Antwerp/La Jolla Conference, P.O. Box 33185, San Diego, CA 92103. Tel. 1-619-692-9115.

Dec. 9–12: **Chest Imaging — (PRE) 1986.** Hotel Del Coronado, San Diego. David S. Feigin, M.D., program director. Sponsored by the Chest Division of the Department of Radiology, University of California, San Diego. Inquiries: D. Ryals, Ryals and Assoc., P.O. Box 610203, DFW Airport, TX 75261-0203. Tel. 214-659-9590.

Dec. 13–15: **Advances in Heart Disease.** Hyatt Regency Hotel, San Francisco. Elliot Rapaport, M.D., F.A.C.C., director. Sponsored by American College of Cardiology. Inquiries: Registration Secy., ACC, Extramural Programs Dept., 9111 Old Georgetown Rd., Bethesda, MD 20814.

Dec. 13–15: **Cardiovascular Disease 1986 — Changes, Choices, Challenges.** Grand Hyatt Hotel, New York City. Henry I. Russek, M.D., F.A.C.C., director. Sponsored by American College of Cardiology and Hahnemann University, Philadelphia. Inquiries: Registration Secy., ACC, Extramural Programs Dept., 9111 Old Georgetown Rd., Bethesda, MD 20814

Dec. 27–30: **The Third International Symposium on Electrophysiologic Basis for Diagnosis and Management of Cardiac Arrhythmias.** Wyndham Hotel, Orlando, FL. Sponsored by the University of Wisconsin Continuing Medical Education; Mt. Sinai Medical Center, Milwaukee, WI; American Heart Association, Central Florida and Wisconsin Affiliates; Florida Heart Institute in Orlando; and the Continuing Education and Research Foundation, Elm Grove, WI. Inquiries: Sarah Aslakson, University of Wisconsin Medical School, Continuing Medical Education, Room 465B, 610 Walnut Street, Madison, WI 53705. Tel 1-608-263-2856.

1986

Jan. 13–17: **Interventional, MRI and Neuroradiology.** Fairmont Hotel, San Francisco. Sponsored by University of California, San Francisco.

Jan. 13–17: **17th Annual Cardiovascular Conference at Snowmass.** New Snowmass Conference Center, Snowmass Resort, Snowmass, CO. John H.K. Vogel, M.D., F.A.C.C., and Bruce C. Paton, M.D., F.A.C.C., directors. Sponsored by American College of Cardiology and Santa Barbara Heart and Lung Institute, Santa Barbara, CA. Inquiries: Registration Secy., Extramural Programs Dept., ACC, 9111 Old Georgetown Rd., Bethesda, MD 20814.

Jan. 19–23: **Advanced Coronary Angioplasty Principles and Techniques.** Stouffer's Wailea Beach Resort, Maui, HI. David O. Williams, director. Sponsored by Brown University Program in Medicine and Rhode Island Hospital, Providence. Inquiries: Course Coordinator, Division of Cardiology, Rhode Island Hospital, Providence, RI 02903.

Jan. 24–25: **Current Controversies and Techniques in Congenital Heart Surgery.** Baltimore, MD. (Immediately prior to Annual Meeting, Society of Thoracic Surgeons, Washington, DC.) Sponsored by Div. of Thoracic and Cardiovascular Surgery, University of Maryland School of Medicine. Inquiries: Program Cont. Ed., University of Maryland School of Medicine, 10 South Pine St., Suite 300, Baltimore, MD 21201. Tel. 1-301-528-3956.

Jan. 30–Feb. 1: **Fifth Annual Perspectives on New Diagnostic and Therapeutic Techniques in Clinical Cardiology.** Buena Vista Palace, Walt Disney World, FL. C. Richard Conti, M.D., F.A.C.C., director. Sponsored by American College of Cardiology and the University of Florida College of Medicine, Gainesville. Inquiries: Registration Secy., ACC, Extramural Programs Dept., 9111 Old Georgetown Rd., Bethesda, MD 20814.

cont'd on ad page 42

cont'd from ad page 36

Feb. 1–4: **Evolution of the Human Atherosclerotic Plaque.** Reston, VA. Sponsored by the Council on Arteriosclerosis of the AHA. Inquiries: Administrative Assistant, Scientific Sessions, AHA, 7320 Greenville Ave., Dallas, TX 75231. Tel. 1-214-750-5441.

Feb. 2–7: **13th Annual New Clinical Applications in Doppler Echocardiography, Coronary Angioplasty, Thrombolytic Therapy, Electrophysiologic Testing, Arrhythmia Management, Heart Failure and Cardiac Drugs.** Prospector Square Resort Hotel, Park City, UT. Arthur D. Hagan, M.D., F.A.C.C., Anthony N. DeMaria, M.D., F.A.C.C., Jay W. Mason, M.D., F.A.C.C., Jeffrey L. Anderson, M.D., F.A.C.C., directors. Sponsored by American College of Cardiology; Tulsa Heart Center and University of Oklahoma Tulsa Medical College; LDS Hospital and University of Utah School of Medicine, Salt Lake City. Inquiries: Registration Secy., ACC, Extramural Programs Dept., 9111 Old Georgetown Rd., Bethesda, MD 20814.

Feb. 6–8: **11th International Joint Conference on Stroke and Cerebral Circulation.** San Francisco. Sponsored by the Stroke Council of the AHA. Inquiries: Administrative Assistant, Scientific Sessions of the AHA, 7320 Greenville Ave., Dallas, TX 75231. Tel. 1-214-750-5441.

Feb. 10–14: **First Annual Cardiovascular Conference at Hawaii.** Sheraton Waikoloa, Kona Coast, HI. John H.K. Vogel, M.D., F.A.C.C., director. Sponsored by American College of Cardiology and Santa Barbara Heart and Lung Institute. Inquiries: Registration Secy., ACC, Extramural Programs Dept., 9111 Old Georgetown Rd., Bethesda, MD 20814.

Feb. 14–16: **Pathophysiology and Techniques of Cardiopulmonary Bypass: VI.** Sheraton Harbor Island East, San Diego, CA. Joe R. Utley, M.D., program director. Sponsored by the Cardiothoracic Research and Education Foundation. Inquiries: CREF, P.O. Box 33185, San Diego, CA 92103. Tel. 1-619-692-9115.

Feb. 17–20: **Annual Postgraduate Course on Thoracic Imaging.** Newporter Beach Hotel, Newport Beach, CA. (Feb. 15–16: Scientific Sessions, Society of Thoracic Radiology). H. Baltaxe, M.D., program director. Inquiries: D. Ryals, P.O. Box 610203, DFW Airport, TX 75261-0203. Tel. 1-214-659-9590.

Feb. 23–28: **General Internal Medicine and Cardiology: A Practical Approach.** Hyatt Lake Tahoe, Incline Village, NV. Sponsored by the University of California, San Francisco. Inquiries: Postgraduate Programs, Dept. of Medicine, 505 Parnassus, M979, University of California, San Francisco, CA 94143. Tel. 415-666-5208.

Feb. 24–27: **Fourth Annual Cardiology Update.** Honolulu, Hawaii. Roger White, M.D., program director. Sponsored by Straub Clinic and Hospital and the Institute for Medical Studies. Inquiries: K. Stroich, The Institute for Medical Studies, 30131 Town Center Drive. Suite 215, Laguna Niguel, CA 92677. Tel. 1-714-495-4499.

Feb. 24–28: **Diagnostic Radiology Seminars.** Park City, Utah. Sponsored by University of California, San Francisco.

Feb. 25–March 2: **Joint Scientific Sessions of the Councils on Circulation and Basic Science.** Keystone, CO. Sponsored by the Councils on Circulation and Basic Science of the AHA. Dr. Stephen Vatner and Dr. Harold Strauss, chairpersons. Abstracts by Dec. 6, 1985. Inquiries: Administrative Assistant for the Scientific Sessions of the AHA, 7320 Greenville Ave., Dallas, TX 75231. Tel. 1-214-750-5441.

Feb. 27–March 1: **13th Annual Symposium. Barrow Neurological Institute of St. Joseph's Hospital and Medical Center.** La Posada Resort Hotel, Phoenix. Inquiries: Richard A. Thompson, M.D., Barrow Neurological Institute, 222 West Thomas Rd., Suite 415, Phoenix, AZ 85013.

Feb. 27–March 2: **24th Annual Symposium on Critical Care Medicine.** MGM Grand Hotel, Las Vegas. Sponsored by the University of Southern California School of Medicine, Postgraduate Division. Inquiries: Associate Dean, USC School of Medicine, Postgraduate Division, 2025 Zonal Avenue, KAM 307, Los Angeles, CA 90033. Tel. 213-224-7051 or 800-421-6729 (outside California) or 800-321-1929 (inside California).

March 3–5: **26th Annual Conference on Cardiovascular Disease Epidemiology.** San Francisco. Sponsored by the Council on Epidemiology of the AHA. Inquiries: Coordinator, Scientific Sessions of the AHA, 7320 Greenville Ave., Dallas, TX 75231. Tel. 1-214-750-5439.

March 5: **Combined Meeting of the Society of Behavioral Medicine and the Epidemiology Council of the AHA.** Seventh Annual Scientific Sessions, Society of Behavioral Medicine, Sheraton Palace Hotel, San Francisco. Inquiries: Society of Behavioral Medicine, P.O. Box 8530, University Station, Knoxville, TN 37996. Tel. 1-615-974-5164 or 974-5248.

March 5–8: **Seventh Annual Scientific Sessions of the Society of Behavioral Medicine.** Sheraton Palace Hotel, San Francisco. Inquiries: Society of Behavioral Medicine, P.O. Box 8530, University Station, Knoxville, TN 37996. Tel. 1-615-974-5164 or 974-5248.

March 6–8: **FOCUS '86.** A national, bi-annual conference on chest diseases. Doubletree Inn. Scottsdale, AZ. Sponsored by the Heart Lung Center at St. Luke's Medical Center, Phoenix. Inquiries: Christine Campbell, Director, Dept. of Medical Meetings, St. Luke's Medical Center, 1800 E. Van Buren, Phoenix, AZ 85006. Tel. 1-602-251-8402.

March 9–13: **35th Annual Scientific Sessions, American College of Cardiology.** Atlanta. Inquiries: ACC, Meeting Services Department, 9111 Old Georgetown Rd., Bethesda, MD 20814. Tel. 1-301-897-5400.

March 9–14: **Diagnostic Imaging: 1986.** Waiohai Hotel, Kauai, Hawaii. Sponsored by University of California, San Francisco.

March 14–16: **15th Princeton Conference on Cerebrovascular Diseases.** St. Louis, MO. Abstracts by Dec. 1, 1985. Invitations to participants will be issued by Jan. 16, 1986. Inquiries: Dr. Marcus E. Raichle, Division of Radiation Sciences, Washington University School of Medicine, 510 South Kingshighway, St. Louis, MO 63110.

March 20–22: **87th Annual Meeting of the American Society for Clinical Pharmacology and Therapeutics.** Sheraton Washington Hotel, Washington, DC. Inquiries: ACSPT, 1718 Gallagher Road, Norristown, PA 19401-2810. Tel. 1-215-825-3838.

March 22–23: **Advances in Uroradiology.** Fairmont Hotel, San Francisco. Sponsored by University of California, San Francisco.

March 24–26: **New Directions in Cardiac Rehabilitation.** Stanford University School of Medicine, Stanford, CA. Robert DeBusk, M.D., F.A.C.C., director. Sponsored by American College of Cardiology and Stanford University School of Medicine. Inquiries: Registration Secy., ACC, Extramural Programs Dept., 9111 Old Georgetown Rd., Bethesda, MD 20814.

March 24–26: **Cardiovascular Conference at Lake Louise.** Chateau Lake Louise, Lake Louise, Alberta, BC. W. Peter Klinke, M.D., F.A.C.C., Israel Belenkie, M.D., F.A.C.C., and James Wayne Warnica, M.D., F.A.C.C., directors. Sponsored by American College of Cardiology and the Alberta Cardiovascular Society and Continuing Medical Education, University of Alberta. Inquiries: Registration Secy., ACC, Extramural Programs Dept., 9111 Old Georgetown Rd., Bethesda, MD 20814.

March 24–26: **Practical Cardiology for the Family Physician — 1986.** Red Lion's La Posada Resort Hotel, Scottsdale, AZ. Robert S. Eliot, M.D., F.A.C.C., director. Sponsored by American College of Cardiology; Heart Lung Center, St. Luke's Medical Center; and Arizona Academy of Family Physicians, Phoenix. Inquiries: Registration Secy., ACC, Extramural Programs Dept., 9111 Old Georgetown Rd., Bethesda, MD 20814.

March 24–28: **Electrocardiographic Interpretation of Complex Arrhythmias: A Physiological Approach.** Krannert Institute of Cardiology, Indianapolis. Charles Fisch, M.D., F.A.C.C., and Douglas P. Zipes, M.D., F.A.C.C., directors. Sponsored by American College of Cardiology; Indiana University School of Medicine; and Krannert Institute of Cardiology. Inquiries: Registration Secy., ACC, Extramural Programs Dept., 9111 Old Georgetown Rd., Bethesda, MD 20814.

April 3–5: **Electrocardiography of Pacemaker Rhythms.** Parker House Hotel, Boston. P.A. Levine, M.D., chairman. Sponsored by North American Society of Pacing and Electrophysiology. Inquiries: NASPE, 13 Eaton Court, Wellesley Hills, MA 02181. Tel. 1-617-237-1866.

April 9–11: **Cardiology Update 1986.** The Houstonian Hotel and Club, Houston. Robert Roberts, M.D., F.A.C.C., Antonio M. Gotto, M.D., D. Phil., F.A.C.C., and Michael E. DeBakey, M.D., F.A.C.C., directors. Sponsored by American College of Cardiology, Baylor College of Medicine, and the Methodist Hospital, Houston. Inquiries: Registration Secy., ACC, Extra-

cont'd on ad page 56

The new PASS II system gives you instant access to 2-D, M-mode and three Doppler modes through a single transducer

You're in the middle of an echocardiographic procedure and you want to switch to Doppler. You stop what you're doing and hook up another transducer. Or, if you're using a system that has Doppler through a "single" probe (actually two probes in one housing), you realign the device until the fixed Doppler beam is in the correct orientation.

The PASS™ II system changes all that. It provides 2-D, M-mode and three Doppler modes through a single electronic phased array transducer.

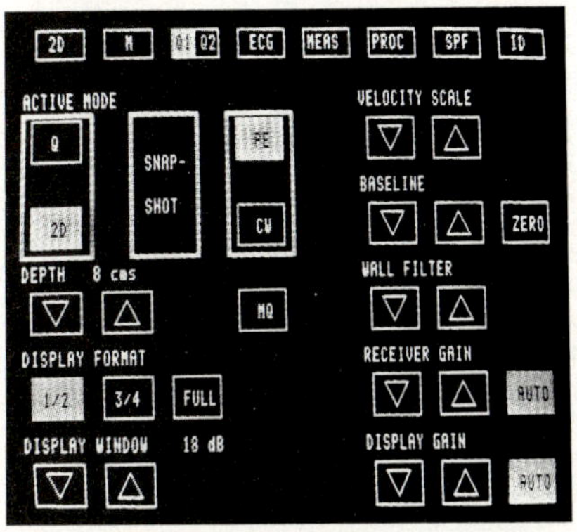

Press the appropriate entry on the PASS II system's easy to use touch screen menu, and you're presented with two Doppler choices. Press pulsed echo and you're able to assess blood flow deep in the body. Should the sample volume be very near the transducer, you can switch to high pulse repetition frequency for accurate near field assessments. Press continuous wave and you can steer the Doppler beam electronically. That means when you're doing difficult studies such as aortic flow assessments via the suprasternal notch, you don't have to move the probe to get better beam orientation... helping make studies faster, easier and more accurate.

Fast, comprehensive calculations

Often, echocardiographic scan data must be quantified, a difficult and time-consuming task. The PASS II system is available with an on-line calculations package option that automatically calculates from operator-initiated measurements for virtually any region and function you'll ever have to quantify. Simply press the CALC software key for access to all calculation functions. Use the preprogrammed equations as they exist, or change them to meet your specific needs. The system will even generate a standard report based on measurements and calculations made.

Image resolution only phased array can provide

The PASS II system's 100% electronic phased array engineering permits construction of smaller probes for better acoustic access. Our

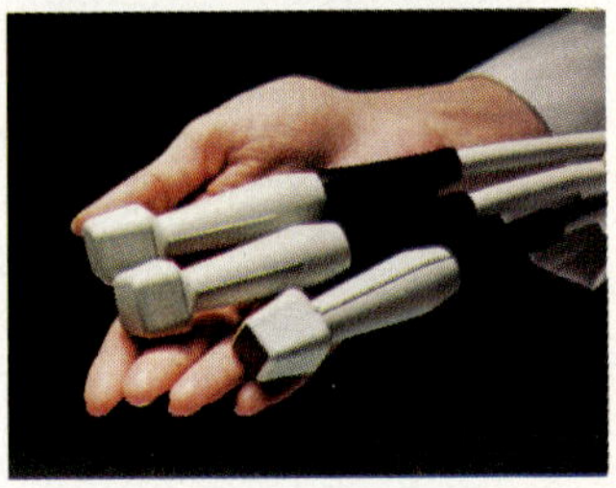

phased array probes have no moving parts, no water path to de-bubble—and all electronic components are solidly encased for resistance to damage. Most important, electronic phased array provides enhanced image resolution, free of many artifacts found with other technologies.

Call 1-800-433-5566 to arrange a demonstration. See how the PASS II ultrasound system can change your practice.

GENERAL ELECTRIC

cont'd from ad page 42

mural Programs Dept., 9111 Old Georgetown Rd., Bethesda, MD 20814.

April 10–12: **The Fourth Charleston Symposium on Congenital Heart Disease.** Mills House Hotel, Charleston, SC. Robert Sade, M.D., F.A.C.C., Paul C. Gillette, M.D., F.A.C.C., Fred Crawford, M.D., F.A.C.C., and Arno Hohn, M.D., F.A.C.C., directors. Sponsored by American College of Cardiology. Inquiries: Registration Secy., ACC, Extramural Programs Dept., 9111 Old Georgetown Rd., Bethesda, MD 20814.

April 12–16: **1986 AAMI 21st Annual Meeting and Exhibit Program.** Hyatt Regency, Chicago. Inquiries: Marguerite Leishman, AAMI, 1901 North Fort Myer Drive, Suite 602, Arlington, VA 22209-1699. Tel. 1-703-525-4890.

April 17–19: **Thoracic Imaging Update, 1986.** Hyatt Regency Hotel, Monterey, CA. Sponsored by University of California, San Francisco.

April 17–19: **The Pathology of the Heart.** Palmer House Hotel, Chicago. Saroja Bharati, M.D., F.A.C.C., Jesse E. Edwards, M.D., F.A.C.C., and Maurice Lev, M.D., F.A.C.C., directors. Sponsored by American College of Cardiology; United Hospital of St. Paul, St. Paul, MN; and Deborah Heart and Lung Center, Browns Mills, NJ. Inquiries: Registration Secy., ACC, Extramural Programs Dept., 9111 Old Georgetown Rd., Bethesda, MD 20814.

April 17–19: **New Strategies in Cardiology.** Boca Raton Hotel and Beach Club, Boca Raton, FL. David O. Williams, M.D., F.A.C.C., director. Sponsored by American College of Cardiology, Brown University, and Rhode Island Hospital, Providence. Inquiries: Registration Secy., ACC, Extramural Programs Dept., 9111 Old Georgetown Rd., Bethesda, MD 20814.

April 23–25: **National Student Research Forum.** The University of Texas Medical Branch, Galveston, TX. Abstracts by Dec. 1, 1985. Supported by American Medical Association — Education and Research Foundation, Mead Johnson Nutritional Division, Roche Laboratories, and American Academy of Family Physicians. Inquiries: National Student Research Forum, P.O. Box 54, Station 1, UT Medical Branch, Galveston, TX 77550. Tel. 1-409-761-3762.

May 1–3: **Second Annual Echocardiography Symposium: Update in Doppler and Two-Dimensional Echocardiography.** Sheraton-Boston Hotel, Boston. Natesa G. Pandian, M.D., course director. Inquiries: Tufts University School of Medicine, Office of Continuing Education, 136 Harrison Ave., Box 36, Boston, MA 02111. Tel. 617-956-6579.

May 7–9: **Clinical Auscultation of the Heart.** Georgetown University Medical Center, Washington, DC. W. Proctor Harvey, M.D., F.A.C.C., John F. Stapleton, M.D., F.A.C.C., and James A. Ronan, M.D., F.A.C.C., directors. Sponsored by American College of Cardiology and Georgetown University School of Medicine, Division of Cardiology. Inquiries: Registration Secy., ACC, Extramural Programs Dept., 9111 Old Georgetown Rd., Bethesda, MD 20814.

May 11–14: **Annual Meeting of the American Thoracic Society.** Kansas City, MO. (In conjunction with the annual meeting of the American Lung Association.) Abstracts by Dec. 2, 1985. Inquiries: American Thoracic Society, 1740 Broadway, New York, NY 10019. Tel. 212-315-8779.

May 12–16: **Consultant's Course in Cardiology.** The Mount Sinai Medical Center, New York City. Valentin Fuster, M.D., F.A.C.C., Richard Gorlin, M.D., F.A.C.C., Louis E. Teichholz, M.D., F.A.C.C., Simon Dack, M.D., F.A.C.C., and Ephraim Donoso, M.D., F.A.C.C., directors. Sponsored by American College of Cardiology and the Page and William Black Postgraduate School of Medicine of the Mount Sinai School of Medicine, New York City. Inquiries: Registration Secy., ACC, Extramural Programs Dept., 9111 Old Georgetown Rd., Bethesda, MD 20814.

May 15–17: **Seventh Annual Scientific Session of the North American Society of Pacing and Electrophysiology.** Marriott Hotel, New Orleans. Abstracts and Young Investigator Awards by Dec. 1, 1985. P.C. Gillette, M.D., program chairman. Inquiries: NASPE, 13 Eaton Court, Wellesley Hills, MA 02181. Tel. 617-237-1866.

May 16–18: **Update in Cardiac Catheterization and Invasive Cardiology: 1986 — A Weekend Review.** Hyatt Regency Cambridge Overlooking Boston, Cambridge, MA. William Grossman, M.D., F.A.C.C., and Donald S. Baim, M.D., F.A.C.C., directors. Sponsored by American College of Cardiology and the Harvard Medical School Dept. of Medicine at the Beth Israel Hospital, Boston. Inquiries: Registration Secy., ACC, Extramural Programs Dept., 9111 Old Georgetown Rd., Bethesda, MD 20814

May 20–23: **Cardiovascular Disease '86: Molecular and Cellular Mechanisms, Prevention, Treatment.** Sixth International Washington Spring Symposium. Washington, DC. Linda L. Gallo, Ph.D., G.V. Vahouny, Ph.D., co-chairs. Inquiries: Symposium '86. Department of Biochemistry, The George Washington University, School of Medicine and Health Sciences, 2300 Eye Street, N.W., Washington, DC 20037.

May 27–31: **15th Annual Educational and Scientific Symposium, Society of Critical Care Medicine.** Washington, DC. Sponsored by SCCM. Inquiries: Tracy Schultz, Program Coordinator, SCCM, 223 E. Imperial Highway, Suite 110, Fullerton, CA 92635. Tel. 1-714-870-5243.

June 5–7: **10th Annual Update Cardiology for the Primary Physician During Spoleto Festival USA 1986.** Mills House Hotel, Charleston, SC. Peter C. Gazes, M.D., F.A.C.C., Michael E. Assey, M.D., F.A.C.C., William H. Barnwell, M.D., F.A.C.C., Grady H. Hendrix, M.D., F.A.C.C., Robert B. Leman, M.D., F.A.C.C., Charles P. Summerall III, M.D., F.A.C.C., and Bruce W. Usher, M.D., F.A.C.C., directors. Sponsored by American College of Cardiology; Cardiovascular Division, Department of Medicine and Division of Continuing Education, Medical University of South Carolina, Charleston. Inquiries: Registration Secy., ACC, Extramural Programs Dept., 9111 Old Georgetown Rd., Bethesda, MD 20814.

June 8–11: **Advanced Echocardiography and Doppler Ultrasound 1986.** Sheraton Harbor Island, San Diego, CA. Pravin M. Shah, M.D., F.A.C.C., John S. Child, M.D., F.A.C.C., Joseph K. Perloff, M.D., F.A.C.C., and Maylene Wong, M.D., F.A.C.C., directors. Sponsored by American College of Cardiology. Inquiries: Registration Secy., ACC, Extramural Programs Dept., 9111 Old Georgetown Rd., Bethesda, MD 20814.

June 23–27: **Two-Dimensional Echocardiography and Cardiac Doppler: Second Annual Core Curriculum and Self-Assessment.** Buena Vista Palace, Lake Buena Vista, FL. Arthur D. Hagan, M.D., F.A.C.C., and Anthony N. DeMaria, M.D., F.A.C.C., directors. Sponsored by American College of Cardiology; Tulsa Heart Center and University of Oklahoma Tulsa Medical College, Tulsa; and the University of Kentucky School of Medicine, Lexington. Inquiries: Registration Secy., ACC, Extramural Programs Dept., 9111 Old Georgetown Rd., Bethesda, MD 20814.

July 10–12: **Fourth International Symposium on Mechanisms of Vasodilatation.** Rochester, MN. Satellite of International Congress of Physiological Sciences. Cerebral, coronary, and limb circulation. Paul M. Vanhoutte, M.D., organizing committee chairman. Inquiries: J. Beckman, 942C Guggenheim Bldg., Mayo Clinic, Rochester, MN 55905.

July 20–25: **FASEB Summer Research Conference, "Physiology and Pathophysiology of the Splanchnic Circulations."** Vail, CO. D. Neil Granger, chairman. Inquiries: Federation of American Societies for Experimental Biology, Splanchnic Circulation Conference, 9650 Rockville Pike, Bethesda, MD 20814.

July 27–Aug. 9: **12th Ten-Day Seminar on Epidemiology and Prevention of Cardiovascular Disease.** Lake Tahoe, CA. Sponsored by the Council on Epidemiology of the AHA. Inquiries: Executive Secretary of the Scientific Sessions of the AHA, 7320 Greenville Ave., Dallas, TX 75231. Tel. 1-214-750-5438.

Sept. 1–5: **Biology and Physics of Radiology.** Department of Radiology, the University of California, San Diego School of Medicine. Inquiries: D. Ryals, Ryals and Assoc., P.O. Box 610203, DFW Airport, TX 75261-0203. Tel. 214-659-9590.

Sept. 10–12: **13th International Congress on Electrocardiology and the 27th International Symposium on Vectorcardiography.** Washington, DC. Official language of the Congress will be English. Inquiries: Jorge C. Rios, M.D., Professor and Chairman, Dept. of Medicine, The George Washington University

cont'd on ad page 58

cont'd from ad page 56

Medical Center, 2150 Pennsylvania Ave. NW, Room 407, Washington, DC 20037. Tel. 202-676-8007.

Sept. 12–14: **Sonographers Update and Review.** Hanalei Hotel, San Diego. Sponsored by the Department of Radiology of the University of California, San Diego School of Medicine. Inquiries: D. Ryals, Ryals and Assoc., P.O. Box 610203, DFW Airport, TX 75261-0203. Tel. 214-659-9590.

Sept. 14–19: **Xth World Congress of Cardiology,** Washington, DC. Inquiries: Secretariat, Xth World Congress of Cardiology, 7320 Greenville Ave., Dallas, TX 75231. Tel. 1-214-750-5429. Cable: Tencard, Dallas, TX.

Sept. 28–Oct. 1: **Sixth Conference on Neural Trauma: Brain Injury and Ischemia.** Charlottesville, VA. Inquiries: J. Jane, M.D., Ph.D., Brain Injury Research Program, Box 180, School of Medicine, University of Virginia, Charlottesville, VA 22908.

Oct. 8–10: **40th Annual Fall Conference and Scientific Sessions of the Council for High Blood Pressure.** Cleveland, OH. Sponsored by the Council on High Blood Pressure Research of the AHA. Inquiries: Administrative Assistant, Scientific Sessions of the AHA, 7320 Greenville Ave., Dallas, TX 75231. Tel. 1-214-750-5441.

Oct. 18: **Imaging of the Lumbar Spine and Pelvis.** Department of Radiology of the University of California, San Diego School of Medicine. Inquiries: D. Ryals, Ryals and Assoc., P.O. Box 610203, DFW Airport, TX 75261-0203. Tel. 214-659-9590.

1987

July 1–3: **Stress and the Heart.** Jackson Lake Lodge, Grand Teton National Park, Moran, WY. Robert S. Eliot, M.D., F.A.C.C., director. Sponsored by American College of Cardiology and St. Luke's Heart Lung Center, Phoenix. Inquiries: Registration Secy., Extramural Programs Dept., ACC, 9111 Old Georgetown Road, Bethesda, MD 20814.

Aug. 25–27: **Tutorials in the Tetons: Clinical Cardiology — Diagnostic and Therapeutic Advances.** Jackson Lake Lodge, Grand Teton National Park, Moran, WY. Robert S. Eliot, M.D., F.A.C.C., James C. Buell, M.D., F.A.C.C., and Timothy Fleming, M.D., F.A.C.C., directors. Sponsored by American College of Cardiology and St. Luke's Heart Lung Center, Phoenix. Inquiries: Registration Secy., ACC, Extramural Programs Dept., 9111 Old Georgetown Rd., Bethesda, MD 20814.

Abroad

1985

Nov. 2–4: **Third International Symposium on Ischemic Heart Disease, Exercise, and Related Topics.** Royal York Hotel, Toronto, Canada. Sponsored by Toronto Rehabilitation Center. Inquiries: J. Kennedy or A. Ceci, Toronto Rehab. Center, 345 Rumsey Rd., Toronto, Ont. Canada M4G 1RT. Tel. 1-416-425-1117 Ext. 236.

Nov. 28–30: **Seventh Biennial Congress of Cardiology.** Rawalpindi/Islamabad, Pakistan. Inquiries: Pakistan Cardiac Society, Brig. Muhammad Zulfiqar Ali Khan, AFIC/NIHD, Rawalpindi, Pakistan. Tel. 64946, 61-31113, 61-33911.

Dec. 1–4: **International Symposium on Left Ventricular Dysfunction.** Jerusalem Hilton Hotel, Israel. Jan J. Kellermann, M.D. of Israel and David Spodick, M.D. of Worcester, MA, co-chairmen. Under the auspices of the Universities of Tel Aviv and Massachusetts. Inquiries: P.O. Box 50006, Tel Aviv 61500, Israel. Tel. 03-654571. Telex 341171 KENS IL.

Dec. 8–12: **Second International Symposium on Hypertension in the Community.** Jerusalem, Israel. Prof. Talma Rosenthal, P.O. Box 50006, Tel Aviv, 61500, Israel. Tel. 03-654571. Telex 341171 KENS IL.

1986

To be announced: **The 35th National Meeting of the Italian Neurosurgical Society.** Pavia, Italy. Inquiries: Prof. Pietro Paoletti, Department of Surgery, Neurosurgical Clinic, University of Pavia, San Matteo Hospital, 27100 Pavia, Italy. Tel 0382/422231.

Jan. 8–11: **Seventh Annual European Conference on Vascular Biology.** Bad Buchau, FR Germany. Growth and Differentiation of Vascular Cells. Organized by European Artery Club. Inquiries: Dr. G. Bondjers, Dept. Med. 1, Salgren's Hospital, 5-413 45 Göteborg, Sweden.

Jan. 16–21: **Basic Principles of Pacing and Electrophysiology — Dual Chamber and Antitachycardia Pacing.** Frenchman's Reef, St. Thomas, Virgin Islands. Sponsored by Cardiostim America. Seymour Furman, course director. Inquiries: Cardiostim America, P.O. Box 428, Mount Kisco, NY 10549, U.S.A. Tel. 1-914-241-3295.

Jan. 20–21: **Diagnostic Radiology Seminars.** Camino Real, Ixtapa, Mexico. University of California, San Francisco.

Jan. 31–Feb. 8: **Fifth Annual Winter Congress in Medical Diagnostic Imaging.** Zermatt, Switzerland. Inquiries: Winter Congress, West Park Hospital, Department of Radiology, 22141 Roscoe Blvd., Canoga Park, CA 91304. Tel. 1-818-340-9580, Ext. 280.

Feb. 3–4: **International Symposium on Cardiovascular Therapy.** Calouste Gulbenkian Foundation, Lisbon, Portugal. The official language is English. Sponsored by the Clinical Council of the International Society and Federation of Cardiology, the European Society of Cardiology and its Working Group on Cardiovascular Drug Therapy. Inquiries: Prof. Salomão S. Amram, Portuguese Society of Cardiology, Campo Grande, 28-4C, 1700 Lisbon, Portugal.

Feb. 4–5: **Second Bangladesh–Japan Joint Conference on Cardiovascular Diseases.** Dhaka, Bangladesh. Sponsored by the Government of Bangladesh and Japan International Cooperation Agency. Abstracts by Dec. 15, 1985. Inquiries: Secretary General, Second Bangladesh–Japan Joint Conference, Institute of Cardiovascular Diseases, Shaheed Suhrawardy Hospital Complex, Sher-e-Bangla Nagar, Dhaka, Bangladesh. Tel. 325150-54.

Feb. 8–12: **The Fourth Annual London Winter Seminar in Medical Diagnostic Imaging.** Inquiries: Winter Seminar, West Park Hospital Dept. of Radiology, 22141 Roscoe Blvd., Canoga Park, CA 91304. Tel. 1-818-340-0580, Ext. 280.

Feb. 9–13: **12th World Congress of the International Society for Heart Research,** Melbourne, Australia. Inquiries: Dr. N.S. Dhalla, Dept. Physiology, Faculty of Medicine, University of Manitoba, Winnipeg, Canada R3E OW3.

Feb. 16–21: **First International Congress on Stress, Behavior and Coronary Disease.** Southern Cross Hotel, Melbourne, Australia. Prof. G.D. Burrows, president, Dr. M. Jelinek, scientific program chairman. Inquiries: Mental Health Foundation, Suite 23, 20 Commercial Rd., Melbourne 3004, Vic., Australia.

March 23–26: **Second International Symposium on Holter Monitoring.** Jerusalem, Israel. Inquiries: Dr. S. Stern, c/o Stier Group, Secretariet-Holter Monitoring, 203 Dizengoff St., 63115 Tel Aviv, Israel.

April 1–3: **International Symposium on Noninvasive Cardiac Imaging. 1986.** Tel Aviv, Israel. Abstracts by Nov. 15, 1985. Sponsored by the Page and William Black Postgraduate School of Medicine, Mt. Sinai School of Medicine, New York City, and the Heart Institute, Chaim Sheba Medical Center and Sackler School of Medicine, Tel Aviv. Inquiries: Richard Meltzer, M.D., Cardiology Division, Mt. Sinai Medical Center, One Gustave Levy Place, New York, NY 10029.

April 8–9: **Obstetric and Neonatal Blood Flow.** Kings College Hospital, London. Inquiries: Biological Engineering Society, Royal College of Surgeons, 35/43 Lincoln's Inn Fields, London WC2A 3PN, United Kingdom. Tel. 01 242 7750.

April 17–19: **Exercise Testing in the Diagnosis and Evaluation of Treatment of Arrhythmias.** Athens, Greece. Inquiries: Prof. D. Cokkinos, 5 Dorylaiou, 115 21 Athens, Greece.

April 21–23: **The First Portuguese Congress.** Lisbon, Portugal. Inquiries: Prof. Martins Prata, Chairman, Dept. of Nephrology, Hospital Univ. Santa Maria, Av. Prof. Egas Moniz, 1600 Lisboa/Portugal.

April 23–25: **First International Symposium on Cardiology.** Hospital de Clinicas, University of Buenos Aires, Argentina. Inquiries: Dr. Luis D. Suárez, Dean Funes 1075-(1231), Buenos Aires, Argentina. Tel. 821-6041.

cont'd on ad page 84

cont'd from ad page 58

AHA NEWS

May 1–3: **First Verona Seminar on Nephrology: Hypertension and Renal Disease.** Camera di Commercio, corso Porta Nuova 96, 37100 Verona-Italy. Inquiries: Lamberto Oldrizzi, M.D., Divisione Nefrologia, Istituti Ospitalieri, 37126 Verona-Italy, Tel. 045-932528-932694.

May 1–3: **First Vienna Shock Forum.** Hotel Hilton, Vienna, Austria. Held by the Ludwig Boltzmann Institute for Experimental Traumatology. Abstracts by Dec. 31, 1985. Inquiries: Wiener Schockgespräche, Ludwig Boltzmann Institut für experimentelle, Traumatologie, Donaueschingenstraße 13, A-1200 Wien, A-1200 Vienna-Austria. Tel. 222-33-55-33/464.

May 4–7: **International Symposium. Ventricular Tachycardias. "From Mechanism to Therapy."** Vittel, France. The official languages will be French and English. Inquiries: Service de Cardiologie, Hôpital Central, Case officielle n⁰ 34, 54037 Nancy Cedex-France" Tél. 83.32.37.86.

May 11–14: **The Seventh Annual Meeting of the Society for Clinical Trials.** Montreal, Quebec, Canada. Abstracts by Jan. 2, 1986. Inquiries: Mary A. Finch, Meeting Coordinator, Society for Clinical Trials, Inc., 600 Wyndhurst Avenue, Baltimore, MD 21210, U.S.A.

May 29–30: **35 Years of Electrocardiology in Amsterdam.** Sponsored by the Interuniversity Cardiology Institute in The Netherlands. Inquiries: F.L. Meijler, M.D., F.A.C.C., Professor of Cardiology, Interuniversity Cardiology Institute, P.O. Box 19258, 3501 DG Utrecht, The Netherlands.

June 5–7: **International Congress for Clinical Neuroimaging.** Palais Auersperg, Vienna, Austria. Inquiries: International Congress for Clinical Neuroimaging, c/o Vienna Academy of Medicine, Alser Str. 4, A-1090, Vienna, Austria. Tel. 0222 42 71 65. Cable MEDACAD Wien, Telex: 134743 medak a.

June 15–20: **The First International Congress on Complementary Medicine.** Jerusalem, Israel. Open to physicians and researchers of basic sciences. Inquiries: Dr. Z. Singer, Secretary of the Scientific Committee, The International Congress on Complementary Medicine, c/o OMEGA Tours, P.O. Box 482, Jerusalem, 91004, Israel.

June 17–20: **Second World Meeting on Impotence.** Fifth Conference on Vasculogenic Impotence and Corpus Cavernosum Revascularization. Prague, Czechoslovakia. Sponsored by the International Society for Impotence Research. Inquiries: Czechoslovak Medical Society, J.E. Purkyně, P.O. Box 88, Vítězného února 31, 120 26 Praha, Czechoslovakia. Tel. 29-41-41-4.

June 19–21: **CARDIOIMAGE 86.** International Congress on Recent Advances in Cardiac Imaging. Congress Center, Monaco. Inquiries: Dr. J.P. Letouzey, Centre d'Echographie et d'Explorations médicales, 6, avenue de Messine, 75008 PARIS. Tel. 1 45639807. Telex 211897 F TECEXPO.

June 22–25: **Seventh Congress of the European Section, International Society for Heart Research.** Reykjavík, Iceland. Inquiries: Guðmundur Thorgeirsson, M.D., Ph.D., Department of Medicine, Landspítalinn, 101 Reykjavík, Iceland.

June 23–27: **Sixth Asean Congress of Cardiology.** Jakarta, Indonesia. Working language, English. Organized by Indonesian Heart Association. L.I. Rilantono, M.D., chairman. Inquiries: Asean Congress Cardiology, Dept. Cardiology, Cipto Mangunkusumo Hospital, Jalan Diponegoro 69, Jakarta 10453, Indonesia.

June 26–28: **Annual Scientific Meeting of the International Medical Society of Paraplegia.** Oslo, Norway. Abstracts by Dec. 1, 1985. Inquiries: IMSP Annual Scientific Meeting in Scandinavia 1986, Dept. of Neurology, Rikshospitalet, University Hospital, Oslo, 1 Norway.

July 2–5: **35th International Conference European Society for CV Surgery.** Metropole Hotel, Brighton, England. Prof. H.H. Bentall, chairman. Inquiries: European Society for CV Surgery, Concorde Services Ltd., 10 Wendell Rd., London W12 9RT, United Kingdom.

July 8–11: **Eighth Annual Meeting American Section of the International Society for Heart Research and Satellite Symposium on Heart Metabolism for the 30th International Congress of Physiological Sciences.** Winnipeg, Canada. Inquiries: Dr. R. E. Beamish, Experimental Cardiology Section, Dept. of Physiology, Faculty of Medicine, University of Manitoba, Winnipeg, Canada R3E OW3.

July 13–18: **30th International Congress of Physiological Sciences.** The University of British Columbia, Vancouver, Canada. Dr. H. McLennan, chairman program committee. Inquiries: IUPS, Suite 801, 750 Jervis St., Vancouver, B.C., Canada V6E 2A9. Tel. 604-681-5226. Telex 04-352848 VCR.

Aug. 21–23: **International Symposium.** Recent Aspects on Diagnosis and Treatment of Lipoprotein Disorders: Impact on Prevention of Atherosclerotic Diseases. Palais Auersperg, Vienna, Austria. Inquiries: Dr. K. Widhalm, Dept. Pediatrics, University of Vienna, Währinger Gürtel 18, A-1090 Vienna, Austria.

Aug. 31–Sept. 7: **11th Congress of International Society of Hypertension.** Heidelberg, Federal Republic of Germany. Organized by German Institute of High Blood Pressure Research and German Hypertension League. Dr. Detlev Ganten, Congress chairman. Inquiries: GKV, Frankfurter Str. 57, D-6050 Offenbach 1, Heidelberg, FR Germany.

Sept. 7–8: **Satellite Symposium to the 11th Congress of the International Society of Hypertension.** Applied Psychophysiology in Hypertension. August Wilhelm von Eiff, chairman. Inquiries: Dr. H. Rüddel, Dept. of Internal Medicine, University of Bonn, Sigmund-Freud-Straße 25, D-5300 Bonn 1, West Germany. Tel 02 28-2 80 32 99. Telex: 8 869 546 KLBO D.

Sept. 14–17: **Eighth International Symposium on Microsurgical Anastomoses for Cerebral Ischemia.** Florence, Italy. Inquiries: Rolando Gagliardi, M.D., Dept. of Neurosurgery, USL 10/D, Careggi Hospital, 50100 Florence, Italy.

Sept. 14–18: **Second International Conference on Diet and Nutrition and Fifth International Congress on Obesity.** Jerusalem, Israel. Inquiries: C. Horwitz, Ph.D., and S.H. Blondheim, M.D., P.O. Box 983, Jerusalem 91009, Israel.

Sept. 22–23: **International Symposium on Lipid Metabolism in the Normoxic and Ischemic Heart.** Erasmus University, Rotterdam, The Netherlands. Inquiries: Dr. H. Stam, Dept. Biochemistry I, Med. Fac., Erasmus University Rotterdam, P.O. Box 1738, 3000 DR Rotterdam, The Netherlands.

Oct. 22–25: **Ninth International Symposium on Drugs Affecting Lipid Metabolism.** Florence, Italy. Dr. Kritchevsky, R. Paoletti, chairmen. Inquiries: Fondazione Giovanni Lorenzini, Via Monte Napoleone, 23-20121 Milan, Italy. Tel. 02-702.267-783.868.

1987

Sept. 2–4: **International Conference on Management of Cardiac Arrhythmias.** London, England. Sponsored by the British Heart Foundation. Professor A.J. Camm and Dr. A.W. Nathan, organizing committee members. Inquiries: British Heart Foundation, 102 Gloucester Pl., London W1H 4DH England. Tel. 01-935-0185.

1988

Aug. 29–Sept. 2: **XIX International Congress of Internal Medicine.** Palais de Congrès, Belgium. Inquiries: Scientific Secretariat, Dr. A. Dupont, Dept. of Pharmacology, University Hospital VUB, Laarbeeklaan 103, B-1090 Brussels; Administrative Secretariat, Mrs. D. Shanni, SDR Associated, Rue Vilain XIIII 17a, B-1050 Brussels.

AHA Scientific Sessions Future Meeting Dates

1985	Washington, DC	Nov. 11–14
1986	Dallas, TX	Nov. 17–20
1987	Anaheim, CA	Nov. 16–19
1988	Locale Not Set	Nov. 14–17
1989	New Orleans	Nov. 13–16
1990	Dallas	Nov. 12–15

Xth World Congress of Cardiology, 1986

The Xth World Congress of Cardiology will be held in Washington, DC, Sept. 14–19, 1986. Official languages English, Spanish, and French. Inquiries: Secretariat, Xth World Congress Cardiology, 7320 Greenville Ave., Dallas, TX 75231. Tel. 1-214-750-5429. Cable: TenCard, Dallas.

News from the American Heart Association

7320 Greenville Ave., Dallas, Texas 75231
Telephone: 214 750-5300

58th Scientific Sessions to Open November 11 in Washington, D.C.

Researchers, cardiologists, surgeons, internists, nurses, nutritionists, medical students — these and other medical professionals from around the world will be on hand for the American Heart Association's annual Scientific Sessions. This year's meeting will be held November 11–14 in the nation's capital at the Washington Convention Center.

The latest findings in clinical and basic research related to cardiovascular diseases will be presented in simultaneous sessions. The program includes 1,941 oral and poster presentations, as well as plenary sessions, postgraduate seminars, cardiovascular conferences, how-to sessions, teaching and public service exhibits, and industrial exhibits.

This year's named lecture series features several distinguished speakers. *Richard Gorlin,* Murray M. Rosenberg Professor of Medicine and chairman of the department of medicine at Mount Sinai Medical Center in New York, will deliver the Lewis Conner Memorial Lecture. *Sir John Vane* of Great Britain's Wellcome Research Laboratories will present the International Lecture. The George E. Brown Memorial Lecture will be given by *Barry M. Brenner,* Samuel A. Levine Professor of Medicine at Harvard Medical School and director of the renal division at Brigham and Women's Hospital, Boston. The G. Lyman Duff Memorial Lecture will feature *Thomas B. Clarkson,* professor of comparative medicine and director of the Arteriosclerosis Research Center, Bowman Gray School of Medicine at Wake Forest University. The Dickinson W. Richards Lecture will be given by *Solbert Permutt,* director of the Pulmonary Research Division of Pulmonary Medicine, Francis Scott Key Medical Center, and professor of medicine, The Johns Hopkins Medical Institutions, Baltimore. The Helen B. Taussig Lecture will be presented by *Dan G. McNamara,* professor of pediatrics, Baylor College of Medicine and Texas Children's Hospital, Houston.

Six AHA Scientific Council Distinguished Achievement Awards will be presented at the meeting. Recipients of the awards are: *Howard A. Eder,* Bronx, New York (Council on Arteriosclerosis); *M. Jeanne Pontious,* Indianapolis, Indiana (Council on Cardiovascular Nursing); *Jacques Genest,* Montreal, Quebec (Council on High Blood Pressure Research); *Donald C. Harrison,* Stanford, California (Council on Clinical Cardiology); *William H. Weidman,* Rochester, Minnesota (Council on Cardiovascular Disease in the Young); and *Brian F. Hoffman,* New York, New York (Council on Basic Science).

Two awards are presented annually to young investigators. *Kenneth Lee Luskey,* Dallas, Texas, is the winner of the Irvine H. Page Award for 1985. He was chosen by the AHA Council on Arteriosclerosis.

Five finalists for the Louis N. Katz Award were selected from a field of 57 entrants. They are: *Makoto Inui,* Nashville, Tennessee; *Ralph A. Kelly,* Boston, Massachusetts; *Dale E. Mais,* Charleston, South Carolina; *Alan Stewart Maisel,* La Jolla, California; and *David W. Russell,* Dallas, Texas. Finalists' abstracts are published in the Abstracts supplement to October *Circulation*.

Other awards to be presented during the sessions include the Research Achievement Award, given to *Harold T. Dodge,* Seattle, Washington; the James B. Herrick Award, given to *H.J.C. Swan,* Los Angeles, California; and the Richard and Hinda Rosenthal Foundation Award, which goes to *Gerald M. Pohost* of Birmingham, Alabama.

Task Force Issues Three Statements

The following three statements were approved by the Steering Committee on September 5, 1985. These statements were written by the Task Force on New and Unestablished Therapies.

I. Percutaneous Transluminal Coronary Angioplasty

Percutaneous transluminal coronary angioplasty (PTCA), also known as coronary artery balloon dilatation, is an established and effective therapy for patients with symptomatic ischemic heart disease. PTCA, as currently practiced, is useful therapy for a minority of patients with coronary artery disease. Complications requiring emergency coronary bypass surgery occur in 3 percent to 5 percent of patients. The dilated segment of coronary artery renarrows in 25 percent to 30 percent, requiring either repeat PTCA or coronary artery bypass surgery. PTCA procedures should only be performed by experienced operators in hospitals where emergency coronary artery surgery is available.

II. Cardiac Transplantation

Cardiac transplantation is now recognized to be a proven procedure in appropriately screened patients. It should be carried out only in medical centers skilled in cardiac surgery.

cont'd on ad page 19

cont'd from ad page 11

III. Chelation Therapy

The American Heart Association's Task Force on New and Unestablished Therapies has reviewed the available literature on the use of chelation (EDTA) in the treatment of arteriosclerotic heart disease and finds no scientific evidence to demonstrate any benefit of this form of therapy. The Task Force recognizes that there have been no adequate trials utilizing currently approved scientific methodology to support this therapy. Furthermore, employment of this form of unproven treatment may deprive patients of the well-established benefits attendant to the many other valuable methods of treating these diseases.

For answers to questions concerning these statements, please write the Office of Medical Programs, American Heart Association, 7320 Greenville Avenue, Dallas, TX 75231.

11th International Joint Conference on Stroke and Cerebral Circulation to Be Held February 6–8, 1986

The 11th International Joint Conference on Stroke and Cerebral Circulation will be held February 6, 7, and 8 at the Hyatt Regency Hotel in San Francisco. The meeting is sponsored by the Council on Stroke of the American Heart Association.

The program provides a two and one-half day educational experience for neurologists, surgeons and general physicians in major facets of cerebrovascular disease — its pathophysiology, diagnosis, treatment, and management. New developments in clinical and basic research will be presented. Abstracts will be published in the January/February 1986 issue of *Stroke*.

For more information, contact the Administrative Assistant for the Scientific Sessions of the AHA, 7320 Greenville Avenue, Dallas, TX 75231. Telephone 214-750-5441.

Council on Stroke Invites Applications for Student Scholarships

The American Heart Association's Council on Stroke invites applications for student scholarships in cerebrovascular disease. The purpose of the scholarships is to stimulate the interest, knowledge, and investigative work of medical students in the area of stroke.

Awards of $1,500 each are available to institutions in the United States where clinical and research training in stroke is available to medical students.

The deadline for receipt of applications is December 13, 1985. Applications and inquiries should be addressed to Edna M. Wilson, Administrative Assistant, American Heart Association, 7320 Greenville Avenue, Dallas, TX 75231.

Erratum

A recently published book, *Perioperative Cardiac Dysrhythmias,* by John L. Attlee III, M.D., contains an error involving a dangerously wrong dosage of the drug bretylium. On page 404, table 9-2, the dosage for bretylium is presently stated as 1–2 mg/kg/minute. It should read 1–2 mg/minute. Errata sheets are available from Year Book Medical Publishers, Inc., 35 E. Wacker Drive, Chicago, IL 60601. Telephone 1-800-621-9262.

Smokeless Tobacco: How Safe Is It?

The increasing popularity of snuff and chewing tobacco has caused growing concern over the safety of smokeless tobacco. What are the current trends in the use of smokeless tobacco in the U.S.? What are the behavioral consequences of smokeless tobacco use? What issues regarding the health consequences of smokeless tobacco use require further research?

The National Institutes of Health (NIH), along with the National Cancer Institute and the National Institute of Dental Research, will join in a Consensus Development Conference on the Health Implications of Smokeless Tobacco Use. The conference, to be held at the NIH on January 13–15, 1986, will consider the health and behavioral effects resulting from the use of smokeless tobacco. Following discussion by a panel of scientists, medical professionals, clinical investigators and public representatives, a consensus statement will be issued.

To register for the conference, or for further information, contact Barbara McChesney, Prospect Associates, Suite 401, 2115 East Jefferson Street, Rockville, MD 20852. Telephone 301-468-6555.

American Federation for Aging Research Grants

The American Federation for Aging Research has announced its 1986 General Grants Program for Biomedical Research in Gerontology and Geriatrics. The one-year grants, up to $25,000 each, support clinical and basic research on all biomedical aspects of aging. Applications must be postmarked no later than January 15, 1986; funding will begin July 1, 1986. To apply, write or call Harold Epstein, Executive Vice-President, American Federation for Aging Research, 335 Madison Avenue, Fourth Floor, New York, NY 10017. Telephone 212-503-7600.

News Briefs

- **Modern Concepts of Cardiovascular Disease** for November and December is "Congestive Heart Failure" by David McCall, M.D., Ph.D., and Robert A. O'Rourke, M.D., San Antonio. Part I, which appears in the November issue, is "Biochemistry, Pathophysiology and Neurohumoral Mechanisms." Part II, to be published in December, is "Therapeutic Options, Old and New."
- **"Cardiology in Psychosocial, Economic, Political and Ethical Perspectives"** is the title of an event scheduled for November 8–9 at the Halloran House Hotel in New York City. It is sponsored by the AHA New York City Affiliate in cooperation with the

cont'd on ad page 24

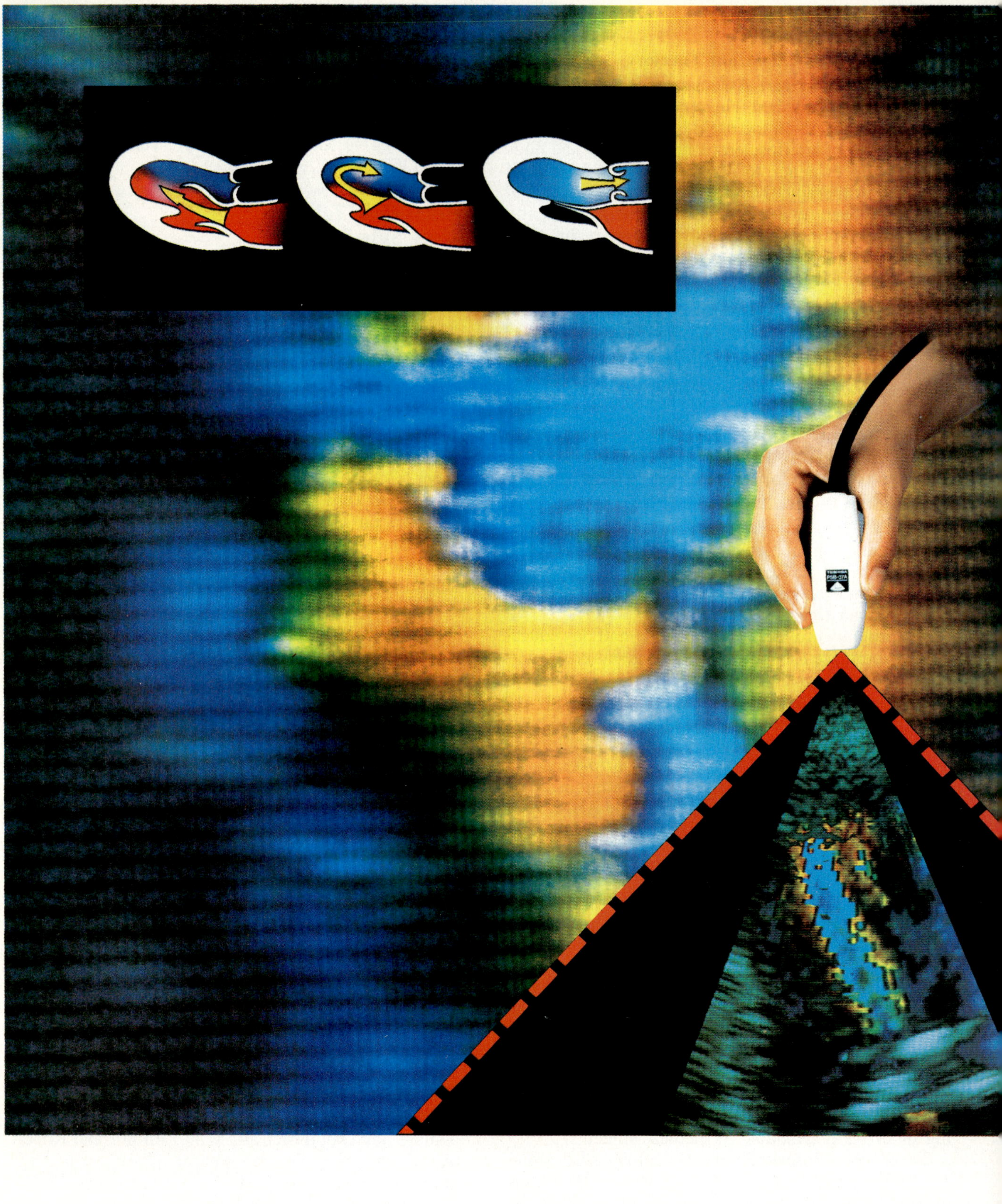

News from the American Heart Association

7320 Greenyille Ave., Dallas, Texas 75231
Telephone: 214 750-5300

Brown and Goldstein Named 1985 Nobel Prize Winners

The co-recipients of the 1984 AHA Research Achievement Award have won the 1985 Nobel Prize for Medicine.

Michael Brown and Joseph Goldstein, researchers at the University of Texas Health Science Center in Dallas, received the prize, medicine's highest honor, for their discoveries involving cholesterol and cholesterol-related diseases. Specifically, the award was given for their discovery in 1974 of the LDL receptor and its relationship to blood cholesterol levels. In presenting the award, the Nobel Institute stated that Brown and Goldstein's research could lead to new treatment of cholesterol-related coronary artery disease.

Dr. David Bilheimer, professor of internal medicine at the UT Health Science Center, and a former AHA established investigator, has already applied the Nobel winners' research in the treatment of patients with high cholesterol levels. Bilheimer's most famous patient is Stormie Jones, the six-year-old recipient of the world's first heart and liver transplant in 1984. Surgery alone lowered Stormie's blood cholesterol reading from its 1,000–1,200 level to 280–300. Medication has dropped it still further to the 180–200 level, enabling Stormie to lead a nearly normal life.

Brown and Goldstein's association dates back to the 1960s, when both completed internships and residencies at Massachusetts General Hospital in Boston. Joseph Goldstein is a graduate of the University of Texas Southwestern Medical School, where he received the school's Ho Din Award naming him outstanding medical school graduate in 1966. Brown also received his medical degree in 1966. His work at the University of Pennsylvania School of Medicine led to his receiving the 1966 Frederick L. Packard Prize in Internal Medicine. Upon leaving Massachusetts General, they pursued parallel careers in research until they were reunited at Southwestern Medical School in the early 1970s.

In their 13 years of research together since then, they have shared numerous honors, which include the 1974 Heinrich Wieland Prize, the 1977 Albion O. Bernstein Award, and the 1978 Passano Award. They were the 1982 recipients of The Lita Annenberg Hazen Award for excellence in clinical research and in 1984 won awards from Columbia University and the Roche Institute of Molecular Biology.

Brown and Goldstein were honored at the 57th annual Scientific Sessions of the American Heart Association with its 1984 Research Achievement Award. The award, presented annually since 1953, recognizes distinguished scientific work in cardiovascular research. It is the highest honor given by the AHA.

AHA Warns Donors "Look, Before You Give"

The American Heart Association is urging donors not to confuse the AHA with other organizations soliciting funds to support cardiovascular research.

"We are particularly concerned that the public may be confused about the relationship between the American Heart Association and the American Heart Research Foundation," said Richard A. Boehning, AHA's chairman of the board.

He said that AHA offices across the nation have received numerous requests for information about AHRF. "We believe prospective donors might think that when they contribute to the American Heart Research Foundation they are giving to the American Heart Association."

The AHRF recently sent out a nationwide request for donations accompanied by a survey on stress and heart disease. A similar plea for funds and a survey on stress were mailed about the same time by the American Cancer Research Fund, which listed the same New Jersey address as AHRF.

Both the AHRF and ACRF are under investigation in several states, Boehning pointed out. "In New Hampshire and New Jersey for example, federal authorities have been probing the two organizations. And New York's Department of State also has been investigating the Heart Foundation.

"The American Heart Association has no desire to harm any legitimate nonprofit agency," Boehning said. "However, we have been unsuccessful in obtaining information concerning AHRF's operations."

Boehning offered these suggestions for donors who are not certain about the legitimacy of organizations asking for contributions: (1) Determine if it has tax-exempt status by asking to see a letter from the Internal Revenue Service. (2) Contact the local office of the Better Business Bureau for information about the organization or write to the Council of Better Business Bureaus, 1515 Wilson Blvd., Arlington, VA 22209. (3) The National Charities Information Bureau issues a free "Wise Giving Guide" every two months. It may be obtained by writing 19 Union Square West, New York, NY 10003.

Blue Cross/Blue Shield of Michigan to Underwrite Health and Nutrition Program

Blue Cross/Blue Shield of Michigan has agreed to underwrite a $262,000 physical education and nutrition program which will benefit an estimated 8,000 children in three Michigan school districts.

Guy Reiff of the University of Michigan Fitness

cont'd on ad page 18

Lidocaine in the hospital

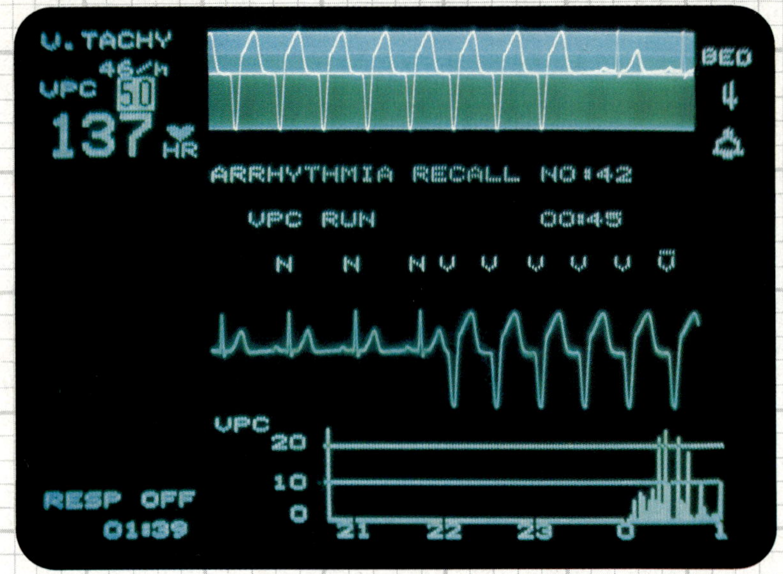

Like other antiarrhythmics, tocainide has not been shown to prevent sudden death, and also, like other antiarrhythmics, it has potentially serious adverse effects including the ability to worsen arrhythmias. Clinical and electrocardiographic evaluation should be used to periodically assess the need for therapy.

TONOCARD® (Tocainide HCl, MSD) is contraindicated in patients who are hypersensitive to this product or to local anesthetics of the amide type and in patients with second- or third-degree atrioventricular block in the absence of an artificial ventricular pacemaker.

Agranulocytosis, bone marrow depression, leukopenia, hypoplastic anemia, and thrombocytopenia have been reported in patients receiving TONOCARD; fatalities have occurred. Blood counts are recommended within the first two to three weeks of therapy and periodically thereafter. See Prescribing Information for details.

For a Brief Summary of Prescribing Information, please see last page of this advertisement.

The Original

...the only clinically-tested dipyridamole

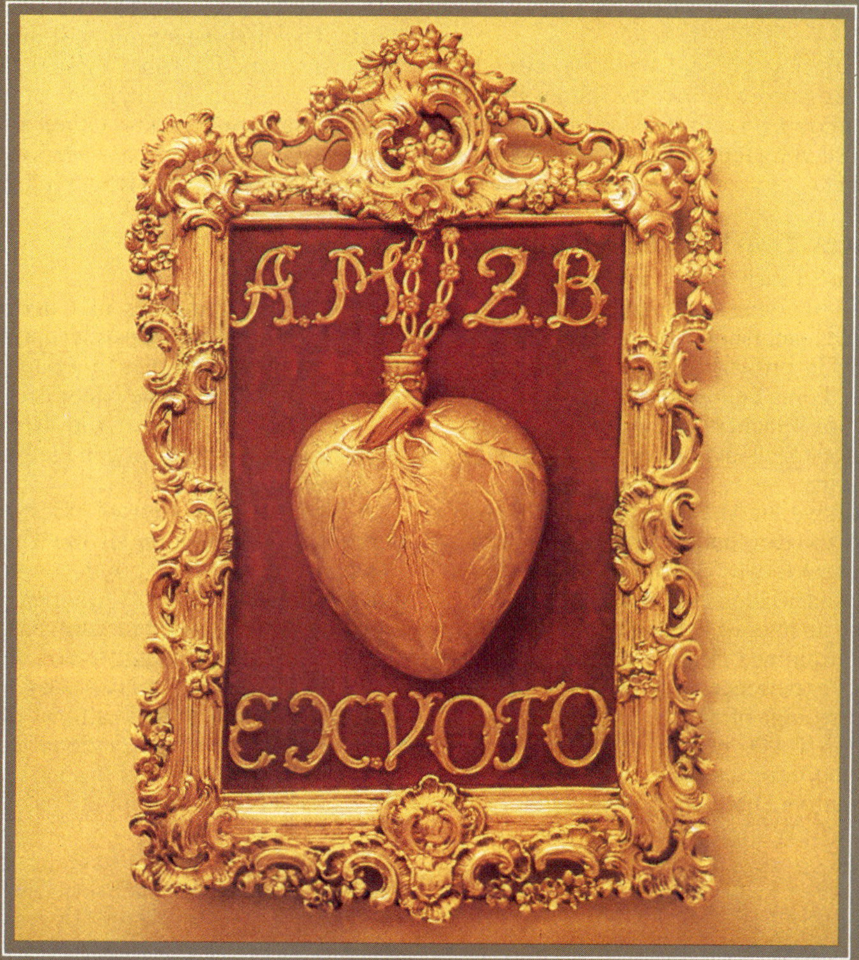

Votive Heart
c. 1770
Thought to be the work of the craftsman Georg Ignaz Bauer. The heart and lettering are made of gold; the frame is gilded silver. Originally placed in the chapel at Bickesheim in southwestern Germany, the heart was later acquired by the monastery at Lichtental.

dipyridamole

Tablets of 25, 50 and 75 mg

Persantine®

The experienced dipyridamole

BRIEF SUMMARY

INDICATIONS—Based on a review of this drug by the National Academy of Sciences-National Research Council and/or other information, FDA has classified the indication as follows:
"Possibly" effective: For long-term therapy of chronic angina pectoris. Prolonged therapy may reduce the frequency of, or eliminate, anginal episodes, improve exercise tolerance, and reduce nitroglycerin requirements. The drug is not intended to abort the acute anginal attack. Final classification of the less-than-effective indications requires further investigation.

CONTRAINDICATIONS—No specific contraindications are known.
PRECAUTIONS—Since excessive doses can produce peripheral vasodilation, the drug should be used cautiously in patients with hypotension.
ADVERSE REACTIONS—Adverse reactions are minimal and transient at recommended dosages. Instances of headache, dizziness, nausea, flushing, weakness or syncope, mild gastrointestinal distress and skin rash have been noted during therapy. Rare cases of what appeared to be an aggravation of angina pectoris have been reported, usually at the initiation of therapy. On those uncommon occasions when adverse reactions have been persistent or intolerable, withdrawal of medication has been followed promptly by cessation of undesirable symptoms.
DOSAGE AND ADMINISTRATION—The recommended dosage is 50 mg three times a day, taken at least one hour before meals. In some cases higher doses may be necessary but a significantly increased incidence of side effects is associated with increased dosage. Clinical response may not be evident before the second or third month of continuous therapy. Tablets of 25, 50 and 75 mg. For complete details, please see the full prescribing information.

Boehringer Ingelheim®

Boehringer Ingelheim Ltd.
Ridgefield, CT 06877

PE 3026 7/84 – 1

cont'd from ad page 13

Research Center will initiate the program, called "Fitness for Youth." According to Reiff, the program is designed "to help youngsters understand how exercise and nutrition can benefit them and to provide the information they need to monitor their own physical well-being."

In addition to offering aerobic exercise periods twice weekly, the program will modify school lunch programs by cutting down on fats and sugars in lunchroom menus while retaining federally subsidized foods to stay within budget.

ATPM Announces Two-Year Fellowship

The Association of Teachers of Preventive Medicine has announced a two-year senior level position for a physician to provide leadership in the development of preventive medicine in primary care. The Luther L. Terry Preventive Medicine Fellowship is sponsored by ATPM, the Society of Teachers of Family Medicine, and the Society for Research and Education in Primary Care Internal Medicine.

Applicants must have an M.D. degree with board certification in primary care and/or preventive medicine disciplines; current faculty appointment or equivalent position; oral and written communication skills; leadership skills; and an interest in health policy. Additional postgraduate training, clinical experience, research, and training experience is desired.

The deadline for receipt of applications is January 15, 1986. Salary is $70,000 per year plus travel expenses. For additional information, contact Dennis J. Barbour, J.D., Executive Director, ATPM, 1030 15th Street NW, Suite 1020, Washington, DC 20005. Telephone 202-682-1698.

Notes

- **Simeon Margolis** is one of nine new members appointed to the National Diabetes Advisory Board. Dr. Margolis is the associate dean for academic affairs at Johns Hopkins University in Baltimore. He is renowned for his work in biomedical research related to the cardiovascular complications of diabetes mellitus.
- **Richard E. Clark,** chief of the NHLBI's surgery branch, has been voted president-elect by the Association for the Advancement of Medical Instrumentation (AAMI). Clark has done research in such areas as pathophysiologic studies of cardiopulmonary bypass, development of a synthetic trileaflet heart valve, and studies of biomaterials for small-diameter vascular prostheses. He assumed the position of surgery branch chief in September 1983.
- Ground-breaking ceremonies were held in September for two **new heart research facilities.** The Minneapolis Heart Clinic and the Minneapolis Heart Institute will be housed in the new five-level Heart Building being constructed in Minneapolis. The building will contain research, education and cardiac rehabilitation programs in addition to patient service facilities. And in Danville, Pennsylvania, the Geisinger Clinic has broken ground for a 65,000 square foot research center that will be completed late in 1987. The center's first investigative emphasis will be cardiovascular research.
- **The University of Texas Southwestern Medical School** has received an $825,000 grant for basic medical research from the Lucille P. Markey Charitable Trust. The three-year grant will support the work of the Texas institution's Nobel winners, Michael Brown and Joseph Goldstein, in the fields of cholesterol metabolism and atherosclerosis. Other grants from the Markey Trust went to Carnegie-Mellon University in Pittsburgh and the Eleanor Roosevelt Institute for Cancer Research, Denver.

AHA Briefs

- **Modern Concepts of Cardiovascular Disease** for December is "Therapeutic Options, Old and New," which is the second part of a paper entitled "Congestive Heart Failure." The paper is coauthored by David McCall, M.D., Ph.D., and Robert A. O'Rourke, M.D. Part I was published in the November 1985 issue of *Modern Concepts*.
- The AHA has revised its estimates of the **prevalence of hypertension in the United States.** *Heart Facts* and other AHA publications now state that approximately 57,700,000 Americans six years old and older have high blood pressure, based on a threshold of 140/90 mm Hg. This figure was determined by a subcommittee of the Joint National Committee on Detection, Evaluation, and Treatment of High Blood Pressure. Projections of the National Health and Nutrition Examination Survey and the Systolic Hypertension in the Elderly Program were the basis of the subcommittee's data.
- **Three task forces** have been commissioned by AHA president Thomas Ryan. They are charged with confronting scientific issues of great importance to the AHA. The Task Force on Health Care Issues is investigating and evaluating the impact of economic constraints on health care and on the quality of medical care. The Task Force on Evaluation and Treatment of Hyperlipidemia is charged with reviewing the results of the Coronary Primary Prevention Trial (CPPT) and the Consensus Document on CPPT. The Task Force on New and Unestablished Therapies has issued statements on percutaneous transluminal coronary angioplasty, cardiac transplantation, and chelation therapy. The statements appeared in the AHA News section of all five scientific journals during the month of November.
- The **AHA ventricular arrhythmia data base** was designed for use in validating ambulatory EKG monitoring systems. The data base is now available on tapes developed by the Committee on Electrocardiography and Cardiac Electrophysiology of the Council on Clinical Cardiology. The tapes can be ordered through ECRI, 5200 Butler Pike, Plymouth, PA 19462.
- The second annual **American Heart Food Festival** has been scheduled for September 1986. This year's event brought AHA's nutrition message to 92 million Americans through the efforts of 8,000 supermarkets and thousands of volunteers. President Rea-

cont'd on ad page 20

cont'd from ad page 18

gan lent his assistance by issuing a statement urging Americans to participate in the event.

- On December 27–30, the AHA Central Florida Chapter and the Wisconsin Affiliate will cosponsor the **Third International Symposium on Electrophysiologic Basis for Diagnosis and Management of Cardiac Arrhythmias.** The conference will be held in Orlando, Florida at the Wyndham Hotel. For further details, contact Sarah Aslakson at the University of Wisconsin Medical School, Continuing Medical Education, 610 Walnut Street, Room 465B, Madison, WI 53705. Telephone 608-263-2856.

Meetings Calendar

1985

To be arranged individually: **Preceptorships in Cardiology.** Pacific Medical Center, San Francisco. Arthur Selzer, M.D., F.A.C.C., director. Sponsored by American College of Cardiology and Pacific Medical Center, San Francisco. Inquiries: Registration Secretary, Extramural Programs Department, American College of Cardiology, 9111 Old Georgetown Road, Bethesda, MD 20814.

To be arranged individually: **Preceptorships in Cardiology.** Buffalo General Hospital, Buffalo, NY. Jules Constant, M.D., F.A.C.C., director. Sponsored by American College of Cardiology and State University of New York at Buffalo, School of Medicine. Inquiries: Registration Secretary, Extramural Programs Dept., ACC, 9111 Old Georgetown Rd., Bethesda, MD 20814.

Dec. 1–4: **Coronary, Hypertensive, Valvular, and Myocardial Heart Diseases: The Multidisciplinary Approach.** Williamsburg Lodge, Williamsburg, VA. William C. Roberts, M.D., F.A.C.C., director. Sponsored by American College of Cardiology. Inquiries: Registration Secy., ACC, Extramural Programs Dept., 9111 Old Georgetown Rd., Bethesda, MD 20814.

Dec. 2–6: **Chest Radiology — Update and Review.** Hotel Del Coronado, San Diego. Sponsored by Chest Division of Dept. of Radiology, UCSD. David S. Feigin, M.D., and Paul J. Friedman, M.D., program directors. Inquiries: Dawne Ryals, Ryals and Associates, P.O. Box 610203, DFW Airport, TX 75261-0203. Tel. 1-214-659-9590.

Dec. 4–7: **Second Annual Seminar and Workshop in Doppler Echocardiography.** Hotel Meridien, San Francisco. Julius Gardin, M.D., program director. Sponsored by the University of California, Irvine, California College of Medicine and the Institute for Medical Studies. Inquiries: K. Stroich, The Institute for Medical Studies, 30131 Town Center Drive, Suite 215, Laguna Niguel, CA 92677. Tel. 1-714-495-4499.

Dec. 5–7: **Mechanisms and Treatment of Cardiac Arrhythmias.** Hershey Philadelphia Hotel, Philadelphia. Leonard S. Dreifus, M.D., F.A.C.C., Eric L. Michelson, M.D., F.A.C.C., and Yoshio Watanabe, M.D., F.A.C.C., directors. Sponsored by American College of Cardiology and Lankenau Hospital, Philadelphia. Inquiries: Registration Secy., ACC, Extramural Programs Dept., 9111 Old Georgetown Rd., Bethesda, MD 20814.

Dec. 6: **Hypertension Update.** Baltimore, MD. Sponsored by the University of Maryland Hypertension Center and the University of Maryland School of Medicine. Inquiries: Program of Continuing Education, University of Maryland School of Medicine, 10 South Pine St., Suite 300, Baltimore, MD 21201. Tel. 301-528-3956.

Dec. 6–7: **Intervention in Acute Myocardial Infarction and Contemporary Topics in Cardiology.** Thunderbird Inn, Portland, OR. Inquiries: Continuing Medical Education, c/o Educational Services, St. Vincent Hospital and Medical Center, 9205 SW Barnes Rd., Portland, OR 97225. Tel. 503-299-2010.

Dec. 6–7: **Fifth Annual Conference on Heart Diseases: Imaging Comes to Cardiology.** Wisconsin Center, University of Wisconsin, Madison. Sponsored by the University of Wisconsin Medical School and the University of Wisconsin Hospital and Clinics. Inquiries: Sarah Z. Aslakson, Continuing Medical Education, 465B WARF Bldg., 610 Walnut St., Madison, WI 53705. Tel. 608-263-2856.

Dec. 9–10: **Second Antwerp/La Jolla Research Conference on Cardiac Function.** Inotropic Mechanisms and Heart Failure. Hotel Inter-Continental, San Diego. John Ross, Jr., M.D., chairman. Sponsored by La Jolla/San Diego Heart Institute and University of California, San Diego School of Medicine. Inquiries: Antwerp/La Jolla Conference, P.O. Box 33185, San Diego, CA 92103. Tel. 1-619-692-9115.

Dec. 9–12: **Chest Imaging — (PRE) 1986.** Hotel Del Coronado, San Diego. David S. Feigin, M.D., program director. Sponsored by the Chest Division of the Department of Radiology, University of California, San Diego. Inquiries: D. Ryals, Ryals and Assoc., P.O. Box 610203, DFW Airport, TX 75261-0203. Tel. 214-659-9590.

Dec. 13–15: **Advances in Heart Disease.** Hyatt Regency Hotel, San Francisco. Elliot Rapaport, M.D., F.A.C.C., director. Sponsored by American College of Cardiology. Inquiries: Registration Secy., ACC, Extramural Programs Dept., 9111 Old Georgetown Rd., Bethesda, MD 20814.

Dec. 13–15: **Cardiovascular Disease 1986 — Changes, Choices, Challenges.** Grand Hyatt Hotel, New York City. Henry I. Russek, M.D., F.A.C.C., director. Sponsored by American College of Cardiology and Hahnemann University, Philadelphia. Inquiries: Registration Secy., ACC, Extramural Programs Dept., 9111 Old Georgetown Rd., Bethesda, MD 20814

Dec. 27–30: **The Third International Symposium on Electrophysiologic Basis for Diagnosis and Management of Cardiac Arrhythmias.** Wyndham Hotel, Orlando, FL. Sponsored by the University of Wisconsin Continuing Medical Education; Mt. Sinai Medical Center, Milwaukee, WI; American Heart Association, Central Florida Chapter and Wisconsin Affiliate; Florida Heart Institute in Orlando; and the Continuing Education and Research Foundation, Elm Grove, WI. Inquiries: Sarah Aslakson, University of Wisconsin Medical School, Continuing Medical Education, Room 465B, 610 Walnut Street, Madison, WI 53705. Tel 1-608-263-2856.

1986

Jan. 13–17: **Interventional, MRI and Neuroradiology.** Fairmont Hotel, San Francisco. Sponsored by University of California, San Francisco.

Jan. 13–17: **17th Annual Cardiovascular Conference at Snowmass.** New Snowmass Conference Center, Snowmass Resort, Snowmass, CO. John H.K. Vogel, M.D., F.A.C.C., and Bruce C. Paton, M.D., F.A.C.C., directors. Sponsored by American College of Cardiology and Santa Barbara Heart and Lung Institute, Santa Barbara, CA. Inquiries: Registration Secy., Extramural Programs Dept., ACC, 9111 Old Georgetown Rd., Bethesda, MD 20814.

Jan. 19–23: **Advanced Coronary Angioplasty Principles and Techniques.** Stouffer's Wailea Beach Resort, Maui, HI. David O. Williams, director. Sponsored by Brown University Program in Medicine and Rhode Island Hospital, Providence. Inquiries: Course Coordinator, Division of Cardiology, Rhode Island Hospital, Providence, RI 02903.

Jan. 24–25: **Current Controversies and Techniques in Congenital Heart Surgery.** Baltimore, MD. (Immediately prior to Annual Meeting, Society of Thoracic Surgeons, Washington, DC.) Sponsored by Div. of Thoracic and Cardiovascular Surgery, University of Maryland School of Medicine. Inquiries: Program Cont. Ed., University of Maryland School of Medicine, 10 South Pine St., Suite 300, Baltimore, MD 21201. Tel. 1-301-528-3956.

Jan. 30–Feb. 1: **Fifth Annual Perspectives on New Diagnostic and Therapeutic Techniques in Clinical Cardiology.** Buena Vista Palace, Walt Disney World, FL. C. Richard Conti, M.D., F.A.C.C., director. Sponsored by American College of Cardiology and the University of Florida College of Medicine, Gainesville. Inquiries: Registration Secy., ACC, Extramural Programs Dept., 9111 Old Georgetown Rd., Bethesda, MD 20814.

cont'd on ad page 26

cont'd from ad page 20

AHA NEWS

Feb. 1–4: **Evolution of the Human Atherosclerotic Plaque.** Reston, VA. Seymour Glagov, M.D. and William P. Newman III, M.D., co-chairpersons. Sponsored by the Council on Arteriosclerosis of the AHA. Inquiries: Administrative Assistant, Scientific Sessions, AHA, 7320 Greenville Ave., Dallas, TX 75231. Tel. 1-214-750-5441.

Feb. 2–7: **13th Annual New Clinical Applications in Doppler Echocardiography, Coronary Angioplasty, Thrombolytic Therapy, Electrophysiologic Testing, Arrhythmia Management, Heart Failure and Cardiac Drugs.** Prospector Square Resort Hotel, Park City, UT. Arthur D. Hagan, M.D., F.A.C.C., Anthony N. DeMaria, M.D., F.A.C.C., Jay W. Mason, M.D., F.A.C.C., Jeffrey L. Anderson, M.D., F.A.C.C., directors. Sponsored by American College of Cardiology; Tulsa Heart Center and University of Oklahoma Tulsa Medical College; LDS Hospital and University of Utah School of Medicine, Salt Lake City. Inquiries: Registration Secy., ACC, Extramural Programs Dept., 9111 Old Georgetown Rd., Bethesda, MD 20814.

Feb. 2–7: **Diagnostic Radiology Seminars.** The Gant, Aspen, CO. Gorden Gamsu, M.D., course director. Sponsored by University of California, San Francisco, School of Medicine. Inquiries: Radiology Postgraduate Education, University of California, Room C324, Third and Parnassus Ave., San Francisco, CA 94143. Tel. 415-666-5731.

Feb. 6–8: **11th International Joint Conference on Stroke and Cerebral Circulation.** San Francisco. Dr. J. Donald Easton and Dr. Vladimir C. Hachinski, co-chairpersons. Sponsored by the Stroke Council of the AHA. Inquiries: Administrative Assistant, Scientific Sessions of the AHA, 7320 Greenville Ave., Dallas, TX 75231. Tel. 1-214-750-5441.

Feb. 10–14: **First Annual Cardiovascular Conference at Hawaii.** Sheraton Waikoloa, Kona Coast, HI. John H.K. Vogel, M.D., F.A.C.C., director. Sponsored by American College of Cardiology and Santa Barbara Heart and Lung Institute. Inquiries: Registration Secy., ACC, Extramural Programs Dept., 9111 Old Georgetown Rd., Bethesda, MD 20814.

Feb. 14–16: **Pathophysiology and Techniques of Cardiopulmonary Bypass: VI.** Sheraton Harbor Island East, San Diego, CA. Joe R. Utley, M.D., program director. Sponsored by the Cardiothoracic Research and Education Foundation. Inquiries: CREF, P.O. Box 33185, San Diego, CA 92103. Tel. 1-619-692-9115.

Feb. 17–20: **Annual Postgraduate Course on Thoracic Imaging.** Newporter Beach Hotel, Newport Beach, CA. (Feb. 15–16: Scientific Sessions, Society of Thoracic Radiology). H. Baltaxe, M.D., program director. Inquiries: D. Ryals, P.O. Box 610203, DFW Airport, TX 75261-0203. Tel. 1-214-659-9590.

Feb. 23–28: **General Internal Medicine and Cardiology: A Practical Approach.** Hyatt Lake Tahoe, Incline Village, NV. Sponsored by the University of California, San Francisco. Inquiries: Postgraduate Programs, Dept. of Medicine, 505 Parnassus, M979, University of California, San Francisco, CA 94143. Tel. 415-666-5208.

Feb. 23–28: **Diagnostic Imaging: Update 1986.** Shadow Ridge, Park City, UT. Faye C. Laing, M.D., course director. Sponsored by the University of California, San Francisco, School of Medicine. Inquiries: Radiology Postgraduate Education, University of California, Room C324, Third and Parnassus Ave., San Francisco, CA 94143. Tel. 415-666-5731.

Feb. 23–March 1: **Steamboat Springs Cardiology Symposium: Update in Management 1986.** Sheraton Hotel at Steamboat Springs, CO. Harold H. Kennedy, M.D.; Richard I. Blum, M.D.; and Bernard R. Chaitman, M.D., program directors. Sponsored by St. Louis University School of Medicine, Division of Cardiology. Inquiries: Anita Herbst, CME Coordinator, St. Louis University School of Medicine, 1402 South Grand Blvd., St. Louis, MO 63104. Tel. 314-577-8167.

Feb. 24–27: **Fourth Annual Cardiology Update.** Honolulu, Hawaii. Roger White, M.D., program director. Sponsored by Straub Clinic and Hospital and the Institute for Medical Studies. Inquiries: K. Stroich, The Institute for Medical Studies, 30131 Town Center Drive, Suite 215, Laguna Niguel, CA 92677. Tel. 1-714-495-4499.

Feb. 25–March 2: **Joint Scientific Sessions of the Councils on Circulation and Basic Science.** Keystone, CO. Sponsored by the Councils on Circulation and Basic Science of the AHA. Dr. Stephen Vatner and Dr. Harold Strauss, chairpersons. Abstracts by Dec. 6, 1985. Inquiries: Administrative Assistant for the Scientific Sessions of the AHA, 7320 Greenville Ave., Dallas, TX 75231. Tel. 1-214-750-5441.

Feb. 27–March 1: **13th Annual Symposium. Barrow Neurological Institute of St. Joseph's Hospital and Medical Center.** La Posada Resort Hotel, Phoenix. Inquiries: Richard A. Thompson, M.D., Barrow Neurological Institute, 222 West Thomas Rd., Suite 415, Phoenix, AZ 85013.

Feb. 27–March 2: **24th Annual Symposium on Critical Care Medicine.** MGM Grand Hotel, Las Vegas. Sponsored by the University of Southern California School of Medicine, Postgraduate Division. Inquiries: Associate Dean, USC School of Medicine, Postgraduate Division, 2025 Zonal Ave., KAM 307, Los Angeles, CA 90033. Tel. 213-224-7051 or 800-421-6729 (outside California) or 800-321-1929 (inside California).

March 1–8: **Primary Care: Current Diagnosis and Treatment.** Park City, UT. Gilbert S. Gordan, M.D., program chairman. Sponsored by the University of California, San Francisco, School of Medicine; Veterans Administration Medical Center, Martinez, CA; and the Merrit Peralta Health Education Center, Oakland, CA. Inquiries: University of California, San Francisco, Division of Infectious Diseases, San Francisco General Hospital, 1001 Potrero Ave., San Francisco, CA 94110.

March 3–5: **26th Annual Conference on Cardiovascular Disease Epidemiology.** San Francisco. Dr. Albert Oberman, chairperson. Sponsored by the Council on Epidemiology of the AHA. Inquiries: Coordinator, Scientific Sessions of the AHA, 7320 Greenville Ave., Dallas, TX 75231. Tel. 1-214-750-5439.

March 5: **Combined Meeting of the Society of Behavioral Medicine and the Epidemiology Council of the AHA.** Seventh Annual Scientific Sessions, Society of Behavioral Medicine, Sheraton Palace Hotel, San Francisco. Inquiries: Society of Behavioral Medicine, P.O. Box 8530, University Station, Knoxville, TN 37996. Tel. 1-615-974-5164 or 974-5248.

March 5–8: **Seventh Annual Scientific Sessions of the Society of Behavioral Medicine.** Sheraton Palace Hotel, San Francisco. Inquiries: Society of Behavioral Medicine, P.O. Box 8530, University Station, Knoxville, TN 37996. Tel. 1-615-974-5164 or 974-5248.

March 6–8: **FOCUS '86.** A national, bi-annual conference on chest diseases. Doubletree Inn. Scottsdale, AZ. Sponsored by the Heart Lung Center at St. Luke's Medical Center, Phoenix. Inquiries: Christine Campbell, Director, Dept. of Medical Meetings, St. Luke's Medical Center, 1800 E. Van Buren, Phoenix, AZ 85006. Tel. 1-602-251-8402.

March 9–13: **35th Annual Scientific Sessions, American College of Cardiology.** Atlanta. Inquiries: ACC, Meeting Services Department, 9111 Old Georgetown Rd., Bethesda, MD 20814. Tel. 1-301-897-5400.

March 9–14: **Seventh Annual Mammoth Mountain Emergency Medicine Ski Conference.** Mammoth Lakes, CA. Daniel L. Abbott, M.D., program director. Co-sponsored by the University of California, Irvine, and the Orange County Emergency Department Nurses Association. Inquiries: Medical Conferences, Inc., P.O. Box 52-B, Newport Beach, CA 92662. Tel. 714-650-4156.

March 10–14: **Diagnostic Imaging 1986.** CT, Ultrasound, MRI and Interventional Radiology. Waiohai Hotel, Poipu Beach, Kauai, HI. Vivian W. Wing, M.D., course director. Sponsored by the University of California, San Francisco, School of Medicine. Inquiries: Radiology Postgraduate Education, University of California, Room C324, Third and Parnassus Ave., San Francisco, CA 94143. Tel. 415-666-5731.

March 14–16: **15th Princeton Conference on Cerebrovascular Diseases.** St. Louis, MO. Abstracts by Dec. 1, 1985. Invitations to participants will be issued by Jan. 16, 1986. Inquiries: Dr. Marcus E. Raichle, Division of Radiation Sciences, Washington University School of Medicine, 510 South Kingshighway, St. Louis, MO 63110.

March 20–22: **87th Annual Meeting of the American Society for Clinical Pharmacology and Therapeutics.** Sheraton Washington Hotel, Washington, DC. Inquiries: ACSPT, 1718 Gallagher Rd., Norristown, PA 19401-2810. Tel. 1-215-825-3838.

March 20–22: **Spring Auscultation Session of the Texas Heart Insti-**

cont'd on ad page 31

cont'd from ad page 26

AHA NEWS

tute. Inquiries: Medical Director, Texas Heart Institute, P.O. Box 20269, Houston, TX 77225. Tel. 713-791-2157.

March 24–26: **New Directions in Cardiac Rehabilitation.** Stanford University School of Medicine, Stanford, CA. Robert DeBusk, M.D., F.A.C.C., director. Sponsored by American College of Cardiology and Stanford University School of Medicine. Inquiries: Registration Secy., ACC, Extramural Programs Dept., 9111 Old Georgetown Rd., Bethesda, MD 20814.

March 24–26: **Cardiovascular Conference at Lake Louise.** Chateau Lake Louise, Lake Louise, Alberta, BC. W. Peter Klinke, M.D., F.A.C.C., Israel Belenkie, M.D., F.A.C.C., and James Wayne Warnica, M.D., F.A.C.C., directors. Sponsored by American College of Cardiology and the Alberta Cardiovascular Society and Continuing Medical Education, University of Alberta. Inquiries: Registration Secy., ACC, Extramural Programs Dept., 9111 Old Georgetown Rd., Bethesda, MD 20814.

March 24–26: **Practical Cardiology for the Family Physician — 1986.** Red Lion's La Posada Resort Hotel, Scottsdale, AZ. Robert S. Eliot, M.D., F.A.C.C., director. Sponsored by American College of Cardiology; Heart Lung Center, St. Luke's Medical Center; and Arizona Academy of Family Physicians, Phoenix. Inquiries: Registration Secy., ACC, Extramural Programs Dept., 9111 Old Georgetown Rd., Bethesda, MD 20814.

March 24–28: **Electrocardiographic Interpretation of Complex Arrhythmias: A Physiological Approach.** Krannert Institute of Cardiology, Indianapolis. Charles Fisch, M.D., F.A.C.C., and Douglas P. Zipes, M.D., F.A.C.C., directors. Sponsored by American College of Cardiology, Indiana University School of Medicine, and Krannert Institute of Cardiology. Inquiries: Registration Secy., ACC, Extramural Programs Dept., 9111 Old Georgetown Rd., Bethesda, MD 20814.

March 24–28: **Diagnostic Radiology.** Fairmont Hotel, San Francisco. Alexander R. Margulis, M.D., program chairman; Charles A. Gooding, M.D., program director. Sponsored by the University of California, San Francisco, School of Medicine; and the Radiology Research and Education Foundation. Inquiries: Radiology Postgraduate Education, University of California, Room C324, Third and Parnassus Ave., San Francisco, CA 94143. Tel. 415-666-5731.

April 3–5: **Electrocardiography of Pacemaker Rhythms.** Parker House Hotel, Boston. P.A. Levine, M.D., chairman. Sponsored by North American Society of Pacing and Electrophysiology. Inquiries: NASPE, 13 Eaton Court, Wellesley Hills, MA 02181. Tel. 1-617-237-1866.

April 9–11: **Cardiology Update 1986.** The Houstonian Hotel and Club, Houston. Robert Roberts, M.D., F.A.C.C., Antonio M. Gotto, M.D., D. Phil., F.A.C.C., and Michael E. DeBakey, M.D., F.A.C.C., directors. Sponsored by American College of Cardiology, Baylor College of Medicine, and the Methodist Hospital, Houston. Inquiries: Registration Secy., ACC, Extramural Programs Dept., 9111 Old Georgetown Rd., Bethesda, MD 20814.

April 10–12: **The Fourth Charleston Symposium on Congenital Heart Disease.** Mills House Hotel, Charleston, SC. Robert Sade, M.D., F.A.C.C., Paul C. Gillette, M.D., F.A.C.C., Fred Crawford, M.D., F.A.C.C., and Arno Hohn, M.D., F.A.C.C., directors. Sponsored by American College of Cardiology. Inquiries: Registration Secy., ACC, Extramural Programs Dept., 9111 Old Georgetown Rd., Bethesda, MD 20814.

April 12–16: **1986 AAMI 21st Annual Meeting and Exhibit Program.** Hyatt Regency, Chicago. Inquiries: Marguerite Leishman, AAMI, 1901 North Fort Myer Drive, Suite 602, Arlington, VA 22209-1699. Tel. 1-703-525-4890.

April 17–19: **Thoracic Imaging Update, 1986.** Hyatt Regency Hotel, Monterey, CA. Sponsored by University of California, San Francisco.

April 17–19: **The Pathology of the Heart.** Palmer House Hotel, Chicago. Saroja Bharati, M.D., F.A.C.C., Jesse E. Edwards, M.D., F.A.C.C., and Maurice Lev, M.D., F.A.C.C., directors. Sponsored by American College of Cardiology; United Hospital of St. Paul, St. Paul, MN; and Deborah Heart and Lung Center, Browns Mills, NJ. Inquiries: Registration Secy., ACC, Extramural Programs Dept., 9111 Old Georgetown Rd., Bethesda, MD 20814.

April 17–19: **New Strategies in Cardiology.** Boca Raton Hotel and Beach Club, Boca Raton, FL. David O. Williams, M.D., F.A.C.C., director. Sponsored by American College of Cardiology, Brown University, and Rhode Island Hospital, Providence. Inquiries: Registration Secy., ACC, Extramural Programs Dept., 9111 Old Georgetown Rd., Bethesda, MD 20814.

April 17–19: **Third Annual Meeting of the Neurovascular Society of North America and Society for Neurovascular Surgery.** Hyatt Downtown Hotel, Chicago. Abstracts by Jan. 31, 1986. Inquiries: NVSNA/SNVS, Box 679, Oak Park, IL 60302. Tel. 312-482-3950.

April 23–25: **National Student Research Forum.** The University of Texas Medical Branch, Galveston, TX. Abstracts by Dec. 1, 1985. Supported by American Medical Association — Education and Research Foundation, Mead Johnson Nutritional Division, Roche Laboratories, and American Academy of Family Physicians. Inquiries: National Student Research Forum, P.O. Box 54, Station 1, UT Medical Branch, Galveston, TX 77550. Tel. 1-409-761-3762.

May 1–3: **Second Annual Echocardiography Symposium: Update in Doppler and Two-Dimensional Echocardiography.** Sheraton-Boston Hotel, Boston. Natesa G. Pandian, M.D., course director. Inquiries: Tufts University School of Medicine, Office of Continuing Education, 136 Harrison Ave., Box 36, Boston, MA 02111. Tel. 617-956-6579.

May 7–9: **Clinical Auscultation of the Heart.** Georgetown University Medical Center, Washington, DC. W. Proctor Harvey, M.D., F.A.C.C., John F. Stapleton, M.D., F.A.C.C., and James A. Ronan, M.D., F.A.C.C., directors. Sponsored by American College of Cardiology and Georgetown University School of Medicine, Division of Cardiology. Inquiries: Registration Secy., ACC, Extramural Programs Dept., 9111 Old Georgetown Rd., Bethesda, MD 20814.

May 11–14: **Annual Meeting of the American Thoracic Society.** Kansas City, MO. (In conjunction with the annual meeting of the American Lung Association.) Abstracts by Dec. 2, 1985. Inquiries: American Thoracic Society, 1740 Broadway, New York, NY 10019. Tel. 212-315-8779.

May 12–16: **Consultant's Course in Cardiology.** The Mount Sinai Medical Center, New York City. Valentin Fuster, M.D., F.A.C.C., Richard Gorlin, M.D., F.A.C.C., Louis E. Teichholz, M.D., F.A.C.C., Simon Dack, M.D., F.A.C.C., and Ephraim Donoso, M.D., F.A.C.C., directors. Sponsored by American College of Cardiology and the Page and William Black Postgraduate School of Medicine of the Mount Sinai School of Medicine, New York City. Inquiries: Registration Secy., ACC, Extramural Programs Dept., 9111 Old Georgetown Rd., Bethesda, MD 20814.

May 15–17: **Seventh Annual Scientific Session of the North American Society of Pacing and Electrophysiology.** Marriott Hotel, New Orleans. Abstracts and Young Investigator Awards by Dec. 1, 1985. P.C. Gillette, M.D., program chairman. Inquiries: NASPE, 13 Eaton Court, Wellesley Hills, MA 02181. Tel. 617-237-1866.

May 16–18: **Update in Cardiac Catheterization and Invasive Cardiology: 1986 — A Weekend Review.** Hyatt Regency Cambridge Overlooking Boston, Cambridge, MA. William Grossman, M.D., F.A.C.C., and Donald S. Baim, M.D., F.A.C.C., directors. Sponsored by American College of Cardiology and the Harvard Medical School Dept. of Medicine at the Beth Israel Hospital, Boston. Inquiries: Registration Secy., ACC, Extramural Programs Dept., 9111 Old Georgetown Rd., Bethesda, MD 20814

May 20–23: **Cardiovascular Disease '86: Molecular and Cellular Mechanisms, Prevention, Treatment.** Sixth International Washington Spring Symposium. Washington, DC. Linda L. Gallo, Ph.D., G.V. Vahouny, Ph.D., co-chairs. Inquiries: Symposium '86. Department of Biochemistry, The George Washington University, School of Medicine and Health Sciences, 2300 Eye Street, N.W., Washington, DC 20037.

May 27–31: **15th Annual Educational and Scientific Symposium, Society of Critical Care Medicine.** Washington, DC. Sponsored by SCCM. Inquiries: Tracy Schultz, Program Coordinator, SCCM, 223 E. Imperial Highway, Suite 110, Fullerton, CA 92635. Tel. 1-714-870-5243.

June 5–7: **10th Annual Update Cardiology for the Primary Physi-**

cont'd on ad page 42

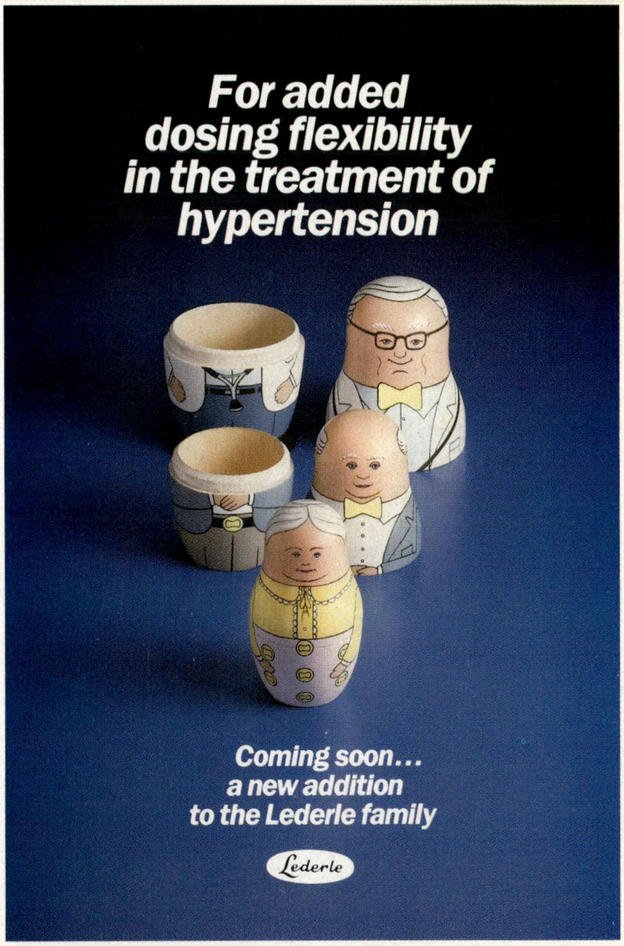

For added dosing flexibility in the treatment of hypertension
Coming soon...
a new addition
to the Lederle family
Lederle

cont'd from ad page 31

cian During Spoleto Festival USA 1986. Mills House Hotel, Charleston, SC. Peter C. Gazes, M.D., F.A.C.C., Michael E. Assey, M.D., F.A.C.C., William H. Barnwell, M.D., F.A.C.C., Grady H. Hendrix, M.D., F.A.C.C., Robert B. Leman, M.D., F.A.C.C., Charles P. Summerall III, M.D., F.A.C.C., and Bruce W. Usher, M.D., F.A.C.C., directors. Sponsored by American College of Cardiology; Cardiovascular Division, Department of Medicine and Division of Continuing Education, Medical University of South Carolina, Charleston. Inquiries: Registration Secy., ACC, Extramural Programs Dept., 9111 Old Georgetown Rd., Bethesda, MD 20814.

June 8–11: **Advanced Echocardiography and Doppler Ultrasound 1986.** Sheraton Harbor Island, San Diego, CA. Pravin M. Shah, M.D., F.A.C.C., John S. Child, M.D., F.A.C.C., Joseph K. Perloff, M.D., F.A.C.C., and Maylene Wong, M.D., F.A.C.C., directors. Sponsored by American College of Cardiology. Inquiries: Registration Secy., ACC, Extramural Programs Dept., 9111 Old Georgetown Rd., Bethesda, MD 20814.

June 9–12: **17th Annual Internal Medicine Symposium.** East Beach Conference Center, Kiawah Island, SC. Sponsored by School of Medicine, Medical College of Georgia. Inquiries: Division of Continuing Education, Medical College of Georgia, Augusta, GA 30912. Tel. 404-828-3967.

June 23–27: **Two-Dimensional Echocardiography and Cardiac Doppler: Second Annual Core Curriculum and Self-Assessment.** Buena Vista Palace, Lake Buena Vista, FL. Arthur D. Hagan, M.D., F.A.C.C., and Anthony N. DeMaria, M.D., F.A.C.C., directors. Sponsored by American College of Cardiology; Tulsa Heart Center and University of Oklahoma Tulsa Medical College, Tulsa; and the University of Kentucky School of Medicine, Lexington. Inquiries: Registration Secy., ACC, Extramural Programs Dept., 9111 Old Georgetown Rd., Bethesda, MD 20814.

July 10–12: **Fourth International Symposium on Mechanisms of Vasodilatation.** Rochester, MN. Satellite of International Congress of Physiological Sciences. Cerebral, coronary, and limb circulation. Paul M. Vanhoutte, M.D., organizing committee chairman. Inquiries: J. Beckman, 942C Guggenheim Bldg., Mayo Clinic, Rochester, MN 55905.

July 20–25: **FASEB Summer Research Conference, "Physiology and Pathophysiology of the Splanchnic Circulations."** Vail, CO. D. Neil Granger, chairman. Inquiries: Federation of American Societies for Experimental Biology, Splanchnic Circulation Conference, 9650 Rockville Pike, Bethesda, MD 20814.

July 23–27: **Critical Care Symposium.** East Beach Conference Center, Kiawah Island, SC. Sponsored by School of Medicine, Medical College of Georgia. Inquiries: Division of Continuing Education, Medical College of Georgia, Augusta, GA 30912. Tel. 404-828-3967.

July 27–Aug. 9: **12th Ten-Day Seminar on Epidemiology and Prevention of Cardiovascular Disease.** Lake Tahoe, CA. Sponsored by the Council on Epidemiology of the AHA. Inquiries: Executive Secretary of the Scientific Sessions of the AHA, 7320 Greenville Ave., Dallas, TX 75231. Tel. 1-214-750-5438.

Sept. 1–5: **Biology and Physics of Radiology.** Department of Radiology, the University of California, San Diego School of Medicine. Inquiries: D. Ryals, Ryals and Assoc., P.O. Box 610203, DFW Airport, TX 75261-0203. Tel. 214-659-9590.

Sept. 10–12: **13th International Congress on Electrocardiology and the 27th International Symposium on Vectorcardiography.** Washington, DC. Official language of the Congress will be English. Inquiries: Jorge C. Rios, M.D., Professor and Chairman, Dept. of Medicine, The George Washington University Medical Center, 2150 Pennsylvania Ave. NW, Room 407, Washington, DC 20037. Tel. 202-676-8007.

Sept. 12–14: **Sonographers Update and Review.** Hanalei Hotel, San Diego. Sponsored by the Department of Radiology of the University of California, San Diego School of Medicine. Inquiries: D. Ryals, Ryals and Assoc., P.O. Box 610203, DFW Airport, TX 75261-0203. Tel. 214-659-9590.

Sept. 14–19: **Xth World Congress of Cardiology,** Washington, DC. Inquiries: Secretariat, Xth World Congress of Cardiology, 7320 Greenville Ave., Dallas, TX 75231. Tel. 1-214-750-5429. Cable: Tencard, Dallas, TX.

Sept. 28–Oct. 1: **Sixth Conference on Neural Trauma: Brain Injury and Ischemia.** Charlottesville, VA. Inquiries: J. Jane, M.D., Ph.D., Brain Injury Research Program, Box 180, School of Medicine, University of Virginia, Charlottesville, VA 22908.

Oct. 7–10: **40th Annual Fall Conference and Scientific Sessions of the Council for High Blood Pressure.** Cleveland, OH. Michael J. Brody, Ph.D., chairperson. Sponsored by the Council on High Blood Pressure Research of the AHA. Inquiries: Administrative Assistant, Scientific Sessions of the AHA, 7320 Greenville Ave., Dallas, TX 75231. Tel. 1-214-750-5441.

Oct. 18: **Imaging of the Lumbar Spine and Pelvis.** Department of Radiology of the University of California, San Diego School of Medicine. Inquiries: D. Ryals, Ryals and Assoc., P.O. Box 610203, DFW Airport, TX 75261-0203. Tel. 214-659-9590.

1987

April 30–May 2: **Eighth Annual Scientific Session of the North American Society of Pacing and Electrophysiology.** Marriott Hotel, Copley Place, Boston. Victor Parsonnet, M.D., chairman. Inquiries: NASPE, 13 Eaton Court, Wellesley Hills, MA 02181.

July 1–3: **Stress and the Heart.** Jackson Lake Lodge, Grand Teton National Park, Moran, WY. Robert S. Eliot, M.D., F.A.C.C., director. Sponsored by American College of Cardiology and St. Luke's Heart Lung Center, Phoenix. Inquiries: Registration Secy., Extramural Programs Dept., ACC, 9111 Old Georgetown Road, Bethesda, MD 20814.

Aug. 25–27: **Tutorials in the Tetons: Clinical Cardiology — Diagnostic and Therapeutic Advances.** Jackson Lake Lodge, Grand Teton National Park, Moran, WY. Robert S. Eliot, M.D., F.A.C.C., James C. Buell, M.D., F.A.C.C., and Timothy Fleming, M.D., F.A.C.C., directors. Sponsored by American College of Cardiology and St. Luke's Heart Lung Center, Phoenix. Inquiries: Registration Secy., ACC, Extramural Programs Dept., 9111 Old Georgetown Rd., Bethesda, MD 20814.

Abroad

1985

Dec. 1–4: **International Symposium on Left Ventricular Dysfunction.** Jerusalem Hilton Hotel, Israel. Jan J. Kellermann, M.D. of Israel and David Spodick, M.D. of Worcester, MA, cochairmen. Under the auspices of the Universities of Tel Aviv and Massachusetts. Inquiries: P.O. Box 50006, Tel Aviv 61500, Israel. Tel. 03-654571. Telex 341171 KENS IL.

Dec. 8–12: **Second International Symposium on Hypertension in the Community.** Jerusalem, Israel. Prof. Talma Rosenthal, P.O. Box 50006, Tel Aviv, 61500, Israel. Tel. 03-654571. Telex 341171 KENS IL.

1986

To be announced: **The 35th National Meeting of the Italian Neurosurgical Society.** Pavia, Italy. Inquiries: Prof. Pietro Paoletti, Department of Surgery, Neurosurgical Clinic, University of Pavia, San Matteo Hospital, 27100 Pavia, Italy. Tel 0382/422231.

Jan. 8–11: **Seventh Annual European Conference on Vascular Biology.** Bad Buchau, FR Germany. Growth and Differentiation of Vascular Cells. Organized by European Artery Club. Inquiries: Dr. G. Bondjers, Dept. Med. 1, Salgren's Hospital, 5-413 45 Göteborg, Sweden.

Jan. 16–21: **Basic Principles of Pacing and Electrophysiology — Dual Chamber and Antitachycardia Pacing.** Frenchmen's Reef, St. Thomas, Virgin Islands. Sponsored by Cardiostim America and North American Society of Pacing and Electrophysiology. Seymour Furman, course director. Inquiries: Cardiostim America, P.O. Box 428, Mount Kisco, NY 10549, U.S.A. Tel. 1-914-241-3295.

Jan. 20–21: **Diagnostic Radiology Seminars.** Camino Real, Ixtapa, Mexico. University of California, San Francisco.

Jan. 31–Feb. 8: **Fifth Annual Winter Congress in Medical Diagnostic Imaging.** Zermatt, Switzerland. Inquiries: Winter Congress,

cont'd on ad page 44

cont'd from ad page 42

AHA NEWS

West Park Hospital, Department of Radiology, 22141 Roscoe Blvd., Canoga Park, CA 91304. Tel. 1-818-340-9580, ext. 280.

Feb. 3–4: **International Symposium on Cardiovascular Therapy.** Calouste Gulbenkian Foundation, Lisbon, Portugal. Official language: English. Sponsored by the Clinical Council of the International Society and Federation of Cardiology, the European Society of Cardiology and its Working Group on Cardiovascular Drug Therapy. Inquiries: Prof. Salomão S. Amram, Portuguese Society of Cardiology, Campo Grande, 28-4C, 1700 Lisbon, Portugal.

Feb. 4–5: **Second Bangladesh–Japan Joint Conference on Cardiovascular Diseases.** Dhaka, Bangladesh. Sponsored by the Government of Bangladesh and Japan International Cooperation Agency. Abstracts by Dec. 15, 1985. Inquiries: Secretary General, Second Bangladesh–Japan Joint Conference, Institute of Cardiovascular Diseases, Shaheed Suhrawardy Hospital Complex, Sher-e-Bangla Nagar, Dhaka, Bangladesh. Tel. 325150-54.

Feb. 8–12: **The Fourth Annual London Winter Seminar in Medical Diagnostic Imaging.** Inquiries: Winter Seminar, West Park Hospital Dept. of Radiology, 22141 Roscoe Blvd., Canoga Park, CA 91304. Tel. 1-818-340-0580, Ext. 280.

Feb. 9–13: **12th World Congress of the International Society for Heart Research,** Melbourne, Australia. Inquiries: Dr. N.S. Dhalla, Dept. Physiology, Faculty of Medicine, University of Manitoba, Winnipeg, Canada R3E OW3.

Feb. 16–21: **First International Congress on Stress, Behavior and Coronary Disease.** Southern Cross Hotel, Melbourne, Australia. Prof. G.D. Burrows, president, Dr. M. Jelinek, scientific program chairman. Inquiries: Mental Health Foundation, Suite 23, 20 Commercial Rd., Melbourne 3004, Vic., Australia.

Feb. 25–28: **Interamerican Cardiac Pacing Symposium.** Rio de Janeiro, Brazil. Robert G. Hauser, M.D., and Decio Kormann, M.D., co-chairs. Co-sponsored by North American Society of Pacing and Electrophysiology and the Brazilian Society of Cardiology. Inquiries: R.G. Hauser, M.D., 1753 W. Congress Parkway, Chicago, IL 60612.

March 23–26: **Second International Symposium on Holter Monitoring.** Jerusalem, Israel. Inquiries: Dr. S. Stern, c/o Stier Group, Secretariet-Holter Monitoring, 203 Dizengoff St., 63115 Tel Aviv, Israel.

April 1–3: **International Symposium on Noninvasive Cardiac Imaging. 1986.** Tel Aviv, Israel. Sponsored by the Page and William Black Postgraduate School of Medicine, Mt. Sinai School of Medicine, New York City, and the Heart Institute, Chaim Sheba Medical Center and Sackler School of Medicine, Tel Aviv. Inquiries: Richard Meltzer, M.D., Cardiology Division, Mt. Sinai Medical Center, One Gustave Levy Place, New York, NY 10029.

April 8–9: **Obstetric and Neonatal Blood Flow.** Kings College Hospital, London. Inquiries: Biological Engineering Society, Royal College of Surgeons, 35/43 Lincoln's Inn Fields, London WC2A 3PN, United Kingdom. Tel. 01 242 7750.

April 17–19: **Exercise Testing in the Diagnosis and Evaluation of Treatment of Arrhythmias.** Athens, Greece. Inquiries: Prof. D. Cokkinos, 5 Dorylaiou, 115 21 Athens, Greece.

April 21–23: **The First Portuguese Congress.** Lisbon, Portugal. Inquiries: Prof. Martins Prata, Chairman, Dept. of Nephrology, Hospital Univ. Santa Maria, Av. Prof. Egas Moniz, 1600 Lisboa/Portugal.

April 23–25: **First International Symposium on Cardiology.** Hospital de Clinicas, University of Buenos Aires, Argentina. Inquiries: Dr. Luis D. Suárez, Dean Funes 1075-(1231), Buenos Aires, Argentina. Tel. 821-6041.

April 25–26: **Current Status and Future Developments in Fetal Cardiovascular Echography.** Erasmus University Rotterdam. Inquiries: Office for Postgraduate Medical Education, Erasmus University Rotterdam, POB 1738, 3000 DR ROTTERDAM, The Netherlands. Tel. 010-63 50 48.

May 1–3: **First Verona Seminar on Nephrology: Hypertension and Renal Disease.** Camera di Commercio, corso Porta Nuova 96, 37100 Verona-Italy. Inquiries: Lamberto Oldrizzi, M.D., Divisione Nefrologia, Istituti Ospitalieri, 37126 Verona-Italy, Tel. 045-932528-932694.

May 1–3: **First Vienna Shock Forum.** Hotel Hilton, Vienna, Austria. Held by the Ludwig Boltzmann Institute for Experimental Traumatology. Abstracts by Dec. 31, 1985. Inquiries: Wiener Schockgespräche, Ludwig Boltzmann Institut für experimentelle, Traumatologie, Donaueschingenstraße 13, A-1200 Wien, A-1200 Vienna-Austria. Tel. 222-33-55-33/464.

May 4–7: **International Symposium. Ventricular Tachycardias. "From Mechanism to Therapy."** Vittel, France. Official languages: French and English. Inquiries: Service de Cardiologie, Hôpital Central, Case officielle n° 34, 54037 Nancy Cedex-France" Tél. 83.32.37.86.

May 10–14: **Fourth Annual London Spring Seminar in Diagnostic Imaging.** London. (Precedes Annual Spring Seminar in Rome, May 14–18.) Inquiries: Medical Seminars International — Spring Seminar, 21915 Roscoe Blvd., Suite 222, Canoga Park, CA 91304. Tel. 818-340-0580, ext. 280; or 818-701-1624; or 800-MED-TOUR.

May 11–14: **The Seventh Annual Meeting of the Society for Clinical Trials.** Montreal, Quebec, Canada. Abstracts by Jan. 2, 1986. Inquiries: Mary A. Finch, Meeting Coordinator, Society for Clinical Trials, Inc., 600 Wyndhurst Avenue, Baltimore, MD 21210, U.S.A.

May 14–18: **Annual Europe Spring Seminar in Diagnostic Imaging.** Rome. (Follows Fourth Annual London Spring Seminar in London, England, May 9–14.) Inquiries: Medical Seminars International — Spring Seminar, 21915 Roscoe Blvd., Suite 222, Canoga Park, CA 91304. Tel. 818-340-0580, ext. 280; or 818-701-1624; or 800-MED-TOUR.

May 29–30: **35 Years of Electrocardiology in Amsterdam.** Sponsored by the Interuniversity Cardiology Institute in The Netherlands. Inquiries: F.L. Meijler, M.D., F.A.C.C., Professor of Cardiology, Interuniversity Cardiology Institute, P.O. Box 19258, 3501 DG Utrecht, The Netherlands.

June 5–7: **International Congress for Clinical Neuroimaging.** Palais Auersperg, Vienna, Austria. Inquiries: International Congress for Clinical Neuroimaging, c/o Vienna Academy of Medicine, Alser Str. 4, A-1090, Vienna, Austria. Tel. 0222 42 71 65. Cable MEDACAD Wien, Telex: 134743 medak a.

June 11–13: **First International Congress of Internal Medicine.** Hospital de Clínicas. University of Buenos Aires, Argentina. Inquiries: Prof. Dr. Albino M. Perosio, Dean Funes 1075 (1231), Buenos Aires, Argentina. Tel. 83-8544.

June 15–20: **The First International Congress on Complementary Medicine.** Jerusalem, Israel. Open to physicians and researchers of basic sciences. Inquiries: Dr. Z. Singer, Secretary of the Scientific Committee, The International Congress on Complementary Medicine, c/o OMEGA Tours, P.O. Box 482, Jerusalem, 91004, Israel.

June 17–20: **Second World Meeting on Impotence.** Fifth Conference on Vasculogenic Impotence and Corpus Cavernosum Revascularization. Prague, Czechoslovakia. Sponsored by the International Society for Impotence Research. Inquiries: Czechoslovak Medical Society, J.E. Purkyně, P.O. Box 88, Vítězného února 31, 120 26 Praha, Czechoslovakia. Tel. 29-41-41-4.

June 19–21: **CARDIOIMAGE 86.** International Congress on Recent Advances in Cardiac Imaging. Congress Center, Monaco. Inquiries: Dr. J.P. Letouzey, Centre d'Echographie et d'Explorations médicales, 6, avenue de Messine, 75008 PARIS. Tel. 1 45639807. Telex 211897 F TECEXPO.

June 19–21: **Cardiostim '86 — An International Congress of Implantable Therapeutic Devices.** Monaco. Jacques Mugica, M.D. and Seymour Furman, M.D., co-chairs. Co-sponsored by North American Society of Pacing and Electrophysiology. Inquiries: Cardiostim America, P.O. Box 428, Mount Kisco, NY 10549.

June 20–29: **Israel 86 — Ultrasound Symposia.** Jerusalem. Presented in coordination with the Israeli Ultrasound Society's Fourth International Ultrasound Meeting in Jerusalem and the Fourth Annual Barry B. Goldberg Lecture. Inquiries: Medical Seminars International — Israel 86, 21915 Roscoe Blvd., Suite 222, Canoga Park, CA 91304. Tel. 818-340-0580, ext. 280; or 818-701-1624; or 800-MED-TOUR.

June 22–25: **Seventh Congress of the European Section, International Society for Heart Research.** Reykjavík, Iceland. Inquiries: Guðmundur Thorgeirsson, M.D., Ph.D., Department of Medicine, Landspítalinn, 101 Reykjavík, Iceland.

cont'd on ad page 48

cont'd from ad page 44

AHA NEWS

June 23–27: **Sixth Asean Congress of Cardiology.** Jakarta, Indonesia. Working language, English. Organized by Indonesian Heart Association. L.I. Rilantono, M.D., chairman. Inquiries: Asean Congress Cardiology, Dept. Cardiology, Cipto Mangunkusumo Hospital, Jalan Diponegoro 69, Jakarta 10453, Indonesia.

June 26–28: **Annual Scientific Meeting of the International Medical Society of Paraplegia.** Oslo, Norway. Abstracts by Dec. 1, 1985. Inquiries: IMSP Annual Scientific Meeting in Scandinavia 1986, Dept. of Neurology, Rikshospitalet, University Hospital, Oslo, 1 Norway.

July 2–5: **35th International Conference European Society for CV Surgery.** Metropole Hotel, Brighton, England. Prof. H.H. Bentall, chairman. Inquiries: European Society for CV Surgery, Concorde Services Ltd., 10 Wendell Rd., London W12 9RT, United Kingdom.

July 7–10: **Fifth International Congress, International Society for the Study of Hypertension in Pregnancy, 1986 Congress.** Nottingham, England. Inquiries: ISSHP, Concorde Services, Ltd., 10 Wendell Rd., London W12 9RT, United Kingdom.

July 8–11: **Eighth Annual Meeting American Section of the International Society for Heart Research and Satellite Symposium on Heart Metabolism for the 30th International Congress of Physiological Sciences.** Winnipeg, Canada. Inquiries: Dr. R. E. Beamish, Experimental Cardiology Section, Dept. of Physiology, Faculty of Medicine, University of Manitoba, Winnipeg, Canada R3E OW3.

July 13–18: **30th International Congress of Physiological Sciences.** The University of British Columbia, Vancouver, Canada. Dr. H. McLennan, chairman program committee. Inquiries: IUPS, Suite 801, 750 Jervis St., Vancouver, B.C., Canada V6E 2A9. Tel. 604-681-5226. Telex 04-352848 VCR.

Aug. 21–23: **International Symposium.** Recent Aspects on Diagnosis and Treatment of Lipoprotein Disorders: Impact on Prevention of Atherosclerotic Diseases. Palais Auersperg, Vienna, Austria. Inquiries: Dr. K. Widhalm, Dept. Pediatrics, University of Vienna, Währinger Gürtel 18, A-1090 Vienna, Austria.

Aug. 31–Sept. 7: **11th Congress of International Society of Hypertension.** Heidelberg, Federal Republic of Germany. Organized by German Institute of High Blood Pressure Research and German Hypertension League. Dr. Detlev Ganten, Congress chairman. Inquiries: GKV, Frankfurter Str. 57, D-6050 Offenbach 1, Heidelberg, FR Germany.

Sept. 7–8: **Satellite Symposium to the 11th Congress of the International Society of Hypertension.** Applied Psychophysiology in Hypertension. Bonn, West Germany. August Wilhelm von Eiff, chairman. Inquiries: Dr. H. Rüddel, Dept. of Internal Medicine, University of Bonn, Sigmund-Freud-Straße 25, D-5300 Bonn 1, West Germany. Tel 02 28-2 80 32 99. Telex: 8 869 546 KLBO D.

Sept. 14–17: **Eighth International Symposium on Microsurgical Anastomoses for Cerebral Ischemia.** Florence, Italy. Inquiries: Rolando Gagliardi, M.D., Dept. of Neurosurgery, USL 10/D, Careggi Hospital, 50100 Florence, Italy.

Sept. 14–18: **Second International Conference on Diet and Nutrition and Fifth International Congress on Obesity.** Jerusalem, Israel. Inquiries: C. Horwitz, Ph.D., and S.H. Blondheim, M.D., P.O. Box 983, Jerusalem 91009, Israel.

Sept. 22–23: **International Symposium on Lipid Metabolism in the Normoxic and Ischemic Heart.** Erasmus University, Rotterdam, The Netherlands. Inquiries: Dr. H. Stam, Dept. Biochemistry I, Med. Fac., Erasmus University Rotterdam, P.O. Box 1738, 3000 DR Rotterdam, The Netherlands.

Sept. 23–25: **Blood Flow in the Brain in Parallel With Blood Flow in Artificial Organs and Cardiovascular Prostheses.** Strathclyde University, Glasgow. In conjunction with the 26th Annual General Meeting of the Biological Engineering Society. Inquiries: Biological Engineering Society, Royal College of Surgeons, 35/43 Lincoln's Inn Fields, LONDON WC2A 3PN, United Kingdom. Tel. 01 242 7750.

Oct. 22–25: **Ninth International Symposium on Drugs Affecting Lipid Metabolism.** Florence, Italy. Dr. Kritchevsky, R. Paoletti, chairmen. Inquiries: Fondazione Giovanni Lorenzini, Via Monte Napoleone, 23-20121 Milan, Italy. Tel. 02-702.267-783.868.

1987

June 7–11: **VIIIth World Symposium on Cardiac Pacing.** Jerusalem. Shlomo Feldman, M.D., secretary general. Co-sponsored by North American Society of Pacing and Electrophysiology. Inquiries: S. Feldman, M.D., Heart Institute, Sheba Medical Center, Tel Hashomer, Tel Aviv University, Sackler Faculty of Medicine, P.O. Box 985, Kiron, ISRAEL.

Sept. 2–4: **International Conference on Management of Cardiac Arrhythmias.** London, England. Sponsored by the British Heart Foundation. Professor A.J. Camm and Dr. A.W. Nathan, organizing committee members. Inquiries: British Heart Foundation, 102 Gloucester Pl., London W1H 4DH England. Tel. 01-935-0185.

1988

Aug. 29–Sept. 2: **XIX International Congress of Internal Medicine.** Palais de Congrès, Belgium. Inquiries: Scientific Secretariat, Dr. A. Dupont, Dept. of Pharmacology, University Hospital VUB, Laarbeeklaan 103, B-1090 Brussels; Administrative Secretariat, Mrs. D. Shanni, SDR Associated, Rue Vilain XIIII 17a, B-1050 Brussels.

AHA Scientific Sessions Future Meeting Dates

1986	Dallas, TX	Nov. 17–20
1987	Anaheim, CA	Nov. 16–19
1988	Locale Not Set	Nov. 14–17
1989	New Orleans	Nov. 13–16
1990	Dallas	Nov. 12–15
1991	Anaheim	Nov. 18–21

Xth World Congress of Cardiology, 1986

The Xth World Congress of Cardiology will be held in Washington, DC, Sept. 14–19, 1986. Official languages English, Spanish, and French. Inquiries: Secretariat, Xth World Congress Cardiology, 7320 Greenville Ave., Dallas, TX 75231. Tel. 1-214-750-5429. Cable: TenCard, Dallas.